Pathologic Basis *of* Veterinary Disease

Fifth Edition

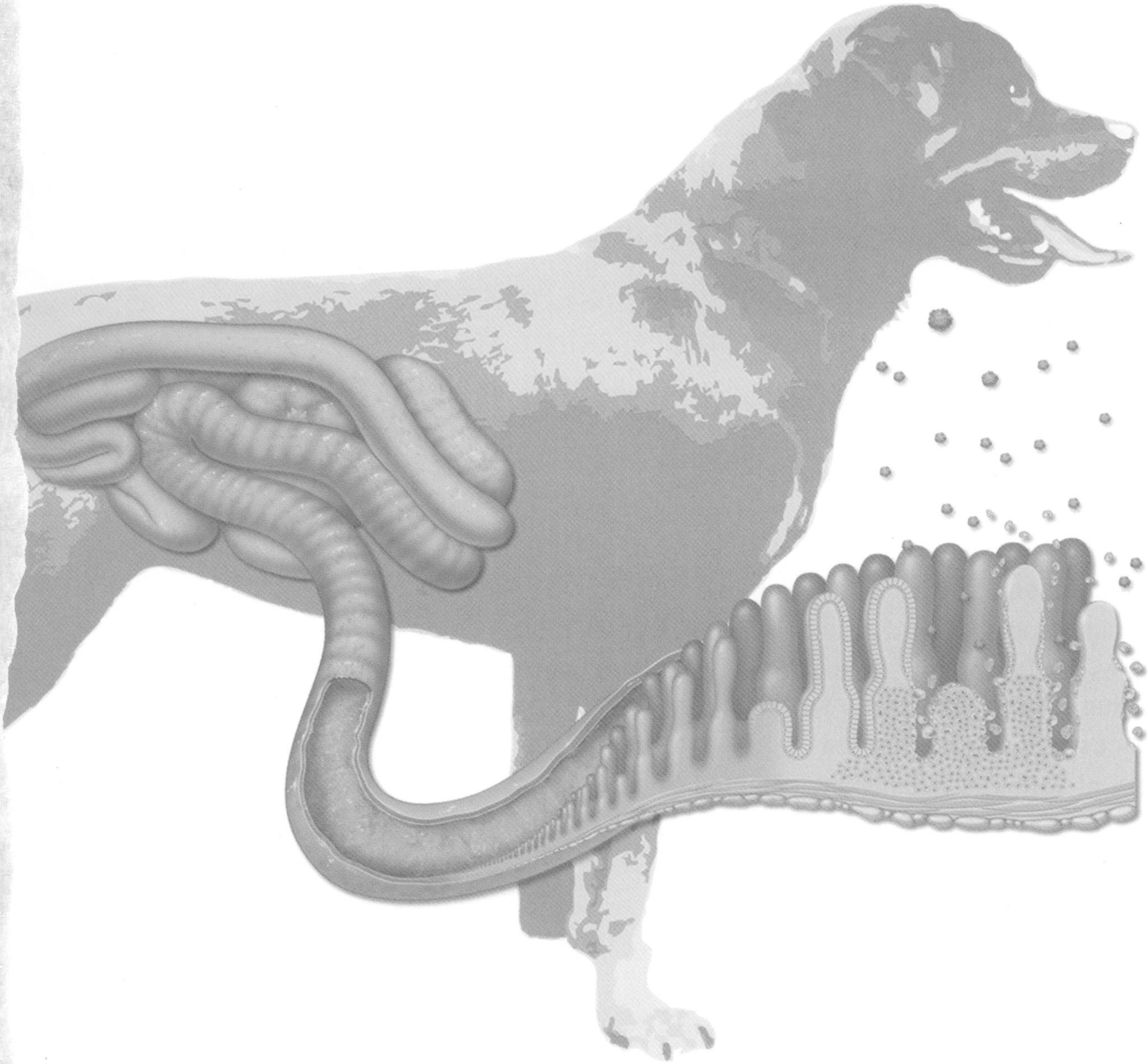

evolve
learning system

ELSEVIER

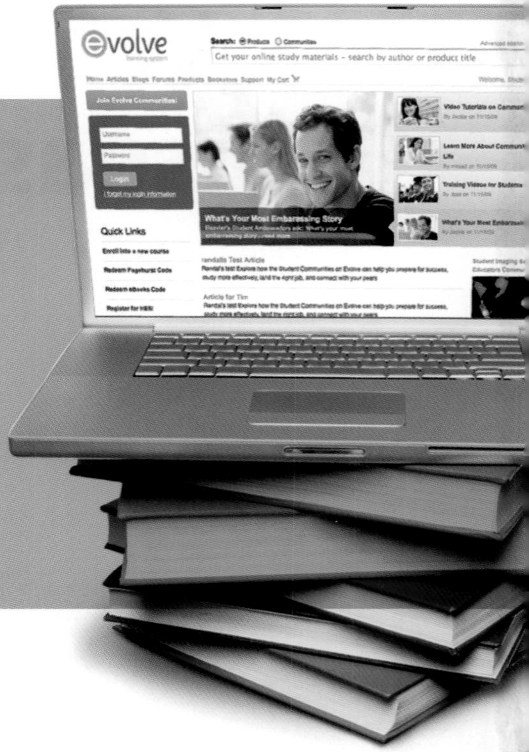

YOU'VE JUST PURCHASED MORE THAN A TEXTBOOK

ACTIVATE THE COMPLETE LEARNING EXPERIENCE THAT COMES WITH YOUR BOOK BY REGISTERING AT

http://evolve.elsevier.com/Zachary/McGavin/

Once you register, you will have access to your
FREE STUDY TOOLS:

- **Image Collection**
  - All images from the book, plus additional images of less common diseases
- **Guidelines for Performing a complete, systematic necropsy and appropriate sample acquisition for selected organ systems**
- **References that link to PubMed**
- **Glossary of Terms to accompany selected organ systems**

REGISTER TODAY!

Pathologic Basis of Veterinary Disease

Fifth Edition

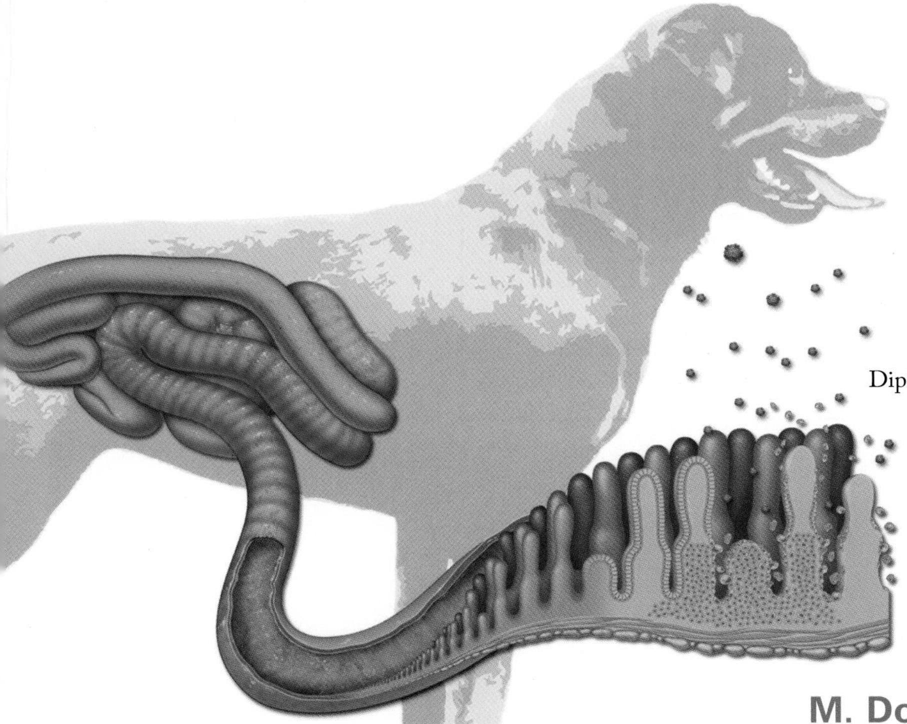

James F. Zachary, DVM, PhD
Diplomate, American College of Veterinary Pathologists
Professor of Veterinary Pathology
Department of Pathobiology
College of Veterinary Medicine
University of Illinois
Urbana, Illinois

M. Donald McGavin, MVSc, PhD, FACVSc
Diplomate, American College of Veterinary Pathologists
Professor Emeritus of Veterinary Pathology
Department of Pathobiology
College of Veterinary Medicine
University of Tennessee
Knoxville, Tennessee

ELSEVIER

ELSEVIER
MOSBY

3251 Riverport Lane
St. Louis, Missouri 63043

PATHOLOGIC BASIS OF VETERINARY DISEASE ISBN: 978-0-323-07533-6

Notices

Knowledge and best practice in this field are constantly changing. As new research and experience broaden our understanding, changes in research methods, professional practices, or medical treatment may become necessary.

Practitioners and researchers must always rely on their own experience and knowledge in evaluating and using any information, methods, compounds, or experiments described herein. In using such information or methods they should be mindful of their own safety and the safety of others, including parties for whom they have a professional responsibility.

With respect to any drug or pharmaceutical products identified, readers are advised to check the most current information provided (i) on procedures featured or (ii) by the manufacturer of each product to be administered, to verify the recommended dose or formula, the method and duration of administration, and contraindications. It is the responsibility of practitioners, relying on their own experience and knowledge of their patients, to make diagnoses, to determine dosages and the best treatment for each individual patient, and to take all appropriate safety precautions.

To the fullest extent of the law, neither the Publisher nor the authors, contributors, or editors, assume any liability for any injury and/or damage to persons or property as a matter of products liability, negligence or otherwise, or from any use or operation of any methods, products, instructions, or ideas contained in the material herein.

ISBN: 978-0-323-07533-6

Publisher: Penny Rudolph
Managing Editor: Shelly Stringer
Publishing Services Manager: Catherine Jackson
Senior Project Manager: David Stein
Design Direction: Paula Catalano
Medical Artist: Theodore G. Huff

Printed in China

Last digit is the print number: 9 8 7 6 5 4 3 2

CONTRIBUTORS

Mark R. Ackermann, DVM, PhD, DACVP
Professor
Department of Veterinary Pathology
College of Veterinary Medicine
Iowa State University
Ames, Iowa
Inflammation and Healing

Danielle L. Brown, DVM, DACVP
Staff Pathologist
WIL-Biotechnics
Hillsborough, North Carolina
Hepatobiliary System and Exocrine Pancreas

Cathy S. Carlson, DVM, PhD, DACVP
Professor
Department of Veterinary Population Medicine
College of Veterinary Medicine
University of Minnesota
St. Paul, Minnesota
Bones, Joints, Tendons, and Ligaments

John M. Cullen, VMD, PhD, DACVP
Professor
Department of Population Health and Pathobiology
College of Veterinary Medicine
North Carolina State University
Raleigh, North Carolina
Hepatobiliary System and Exocrine Pancreas

Robert A. Foster, BVSc, PhD, MACVSc, DACVP
Professor
Department of Pathobiology
Ontario Veterinary College
University of Guelph
Guelph, Ontario, Canada
Female Reproductive System and Mammary Gland
Male Reproductive System

Michael M. Fry, DVM, MS, DACVP
Associate Professor
Department of Pathobiology
College of Veterinary Medicine
University of Tennessee
Knoxville, Tennessee
Bone Marrow, Blood Cells, and the Lymphatic System

Arnon Gal, DVM, MS, DACVIM (SAIM)
Anatomic Pathology Resident
Department of Pathobiology
College of Veterinary Medicine
University of Illinois
Urbana, Illinois
Cardiovascular System and Lymphatic Vessels

Howard B. Gelberg, DVM, PhD, DACVP
Professor of Pathology
Department of Biomedical Sciences
College of Veterinary Medicine
Oregon State University
Corvallis, Oregon
Alimentary System and the Peritoneum, Omentum, Mesentery, and Peritoneal Cavity

Pamela Eve Ginn, DVM, DACVP
Visiting Associate Professor
Department of Infectious Diseases and Pathology
College of Veterinary Medicine
University of Florida
Gainesville, Florida
The Integument

Ann M. Hargis, DVM, MS, DACVP
Owner
DermatoDiagnostics
Edmonds, Washington
Affiliate Associate Professor
Department of Comparative Medicine
University of Washington
School of Medicine
Seattle, Washington
The Integument

Donna F. Kusewitt, DVM, PhD, DACVP
Professor
Department of Molecular Carcinogenesis, Science Park Research Division
University of Texas M.D. Anderson Cancer Center
Smithville, Texas
Neoplasia and Tumor Biology

Krista M.D. La Perle, DVM, PhD, DACVP
Associate Professor
Director of Comparative Pathology & Mouse Phenotyping Shared Resource
Department of Veterinary Biosciences
College of Veterinary Medicine
The Ohio State University
Columbus, Ohio
Endocrine System

Alfonso López, MVZ, MSc, PhD
Professor of Pathology
Department of Pathology and Microbiology
Atlantic Veterinary College
University of Prince Edward Island
Charlottetown, Prince Edward Island, Canada
Respiratory System, Mediastinum, and Pleurae

M. Donald McGavin, MVSc, PhD, FACVSc, DACVP
Professor Emeritus of Veterinary Pathology
Department of Pathobiology
College of Veterinary Medicine
University of Tennessee
Knoxville, Tennessee
Cellular Adaptations, Injury, and Death: Morphologic, Biochemical, and Genetic Bases
Bone Marrow, Blood Cells, and the Lymphatic System
Skeletal Muscle
Photographic Techniques in Veterinary Pathology

Lisa M. Miller, DVM, PhD, DACVP, Med
Professor
Department of Pathology and Microbiology
Atlantic Veterinary College
University of Prince Edward Island
Charlottetown, Prince Edward Island, Canada
Cardiovascular System and Lymphatic Vessels

Derek A. Mosier, DVM, PhD, DACVP
Professor
Department of Diagnostic Medicine/Pathobiology
College of Veterinary Medicine
Kansas State University
Manhattan, Kansas
Vascular Disorders and Thrombosis

Ronald K. Myers, DVM, PhD, DACVP
Professor
Department of Veterinary Pathology
College of Veterinary Medicine
Iowa State University
Ames, Iowa
Cellular Adaptations, Injury, and Death: Morphologic, Biochemical, and Genetic Bases

Shelley J. Newman, DVM, DVSc, DACVP
Associate Professor
Department of Pathobiology
College of Veterinary Medicine
University of Tennessee
Knoxville, Tennessee
The Urinary System

Bradley L. Njaa, DVM, MVSc, DACVP
Associate Professor
Department of Veterinary Pathobiology
Center for Veterinary Health Sciences
Oklahoma State University
Stillwater, Oklahoma
The Ear and Eye

Paul W. Snyder, DVM, PhD, DACVP
Professor of Veterinary Pathology
Comparative Pathobiology
School of Veterinary Medicine
Purdue University
West Lafayette, Indiana
Diseases of Immunity

Beth A. Valentine, DVM, PhD, DACVP
Professor
Department of Biomedical Sciences
College of Veterinary Medicine
Oregon State University
Corvallis, Oregon
Skeletal Muscle

John F. Van Vleet, DVM, PhD, DACVP
Professor Emeritus of Veterinary Pathology
Comparative Pathobiology
School of Veterinary Medicine
Purdue University
West Lafayette, Indiana
Cardiovascular System and Lymphatic Vessels

Steven E. Weisbrode, VMD, PhD, DACVP
Professor Emeritus
Department of Veterinary Biosciences
College of Veterinary Medicine
The Ohio State University
Columbus, Ohio
Bones, Joints, Tendons, and Ligaments

Brian P. Wilcock, DVM, PhD
Senior Pathologist
Histovet Surgical Pathology
Guelph, Ontario, Canada
Professor Emeritus
Department of Pathobiology
Ontario Veterinary College
University of Guelph
Guelph, Ontario, Canada
The Ear and Eye

James F. Zachary, DVM, PhD, DACVP
Professor of Veterinary Pathology
Department of Pathobiology
College of Veterinary Medicine
University of Illinois
Urbana, Illinois
Cellular Adaptations, Injury, and Death: Morphologic, Biochemical, and Genetic Bases
Mechanisms of Microbial Infections
Nervous System

PREFACE

Following the enthusiastic reception of the fourth edition of *Pathologic Basis of Veterinary Disease* both nationally and internationally, the fifth edition continues with the same philosophical approach—explaining pathology and its lesions in the context of understanding disease in a chronological sequence of events from both the morphologic and mechanistic perspectives, and with an emphasis on responses of cells, tissues, and organs to injury.

Veterinary pathology is a dynamic discipline and since the fourth edition was published in 2006, there have been many new insights into the pathogeneses of existing diseases and new or reemerging diseases, many of which have serious economic and health consequences for animals and humans. As a result, to meet the growing scope of the veterinary curriculum we have added to the fifth edition new and revised materials on pets, livestock, and production animal health, including diseases the USDA/APHIS and the World Organization for Animal Health (OIE) consider as "Foreign Animal Diseases" or "OIE Reportable Diseases," respectively.

The book is not meant to be encyclopedic; specific diseases have been selected either because they are of primary importance in the practice of veterinary medicine or because they illustrate a basic mechanism. We also hope this edition will continue to provide a bridge between students' understanding of material learned in the basic sciences and the interpretation of results of physical examinations, differential disease diagnoses, imaging modalities, biochemical and molecular diagnostic methods, and therapeutic strategies presented in the students' clinical years.

NEW TO THIS EDITION

The fifth edition of *Pathologic Basis of Veterinary Disease* has been updated and reorganized such that specific diseases are described under the major domestic animal affected—horses, ruminants (cattle, sheep, and goats), pigs, dogs, and cats. Those disorders and diseases not unique to a single species are grouped under a heading titled "Disorders of Domestic Animals." We continue to describe disease pathogenesis based on sections covering structure, function, portals of entry, defense mechanisms, and responses to injury, augmented by schematic color diagrams and full color illustrations of lesions. Our hope is that this approach will be helpful to the student (and to their instructors) in their understanding of both pathology and the related disciplines of microbiology, immunology, and infectious diseases. Other additions to the fifth edition include new sections on the genetic basis of disease, diseases of the ear, and diseases of ligaments and tendons and a new chapter on mechanisms of microbial infections.

EVOLVE SITE

An enhanced Evolve site accompanies this edition. The Evolve site includes all of the images from the book, plus additional images and schematic illustrations that supplement some common diseases and disease processes discussed in the book. These additional materials may be useful adjuncts for instructors in classroom and/or laboratory presentations.

To avoid adding length and weight to the book, information of historical value and basic clinical information have been removed from the printed book and can be found on the Evolve site. Also included on the Evolve site are guidelines for performing a systematic necropsy and appropriate sample acquisition for selected organ systems; a glossary of terms to accompany selected organ systems; and methods for gross specimen photography and photomicrography. Additionally, all of the selected readings are available on the Evolve site and are linked to original abstracts on PubMed.

The printed book will direct you to the website when there is additional information available.

ABOUT THE COVER

Canine parvovirus enteritis, an important and often fatal disease of dogs, is caused by a cytolytic virus that infects and kills mitotically active cells including crypt enterocytes of the small intestine. Virus in fecal matter is inhaled or ingested and then deposited on and trapped in the mucus layer of oral, nasal, and pharyngeal mucosae, where it infects mucosal macrophages or dendritic cells. These cells spread parvovirus to lymphocytes of the lamina propria of the mucosa, especially that of the tonsil where it infects and replicates in lymphocytes. Many of these cells subsequently lyse, allowing virus to escape free into the lymph, where it and infected macrophages drain to regional lymph nodes and then, via the blood vascular system, systemically to the spleen, thymus, lymph nodes, bone marrow, and mucosa-associated lymphoid nodules (MALT) such as Peyer's patches of the small intestine. In Peyer's patches, chiefly the mitotically active cells of the lymphoid follicle are infected and lysed (lymphocytolysis). From Peyer's patches, parvovirus spreads to adjacent crypts causing enterocyte necrosis, with the result that enterocytes required to replace those lost in normal turnover of absorptive enterocytes sloughed from the tip of a villus, or from destruction by the virus, are not produced. Consequently, villi in a short time are denuded of epithelium, and the primary gross lesion that results is fibrinonecrotic enteritis with hemorrhage and an accompanying serositis. Necrotic crypt enterocytes slough and release virus into the intestinal lumen and then, through diarrheic feces, pass it into the environment.

If no crypt enterocytes are viable, the villi will remain naked, collapse, and fuse together; however, if some crypt enterocytes are still viable, they will become hyperplastic and divide rapidly to re-epithelialize the denuded villi. To facilitate this process, the villi collapse to reduce the volume of their surface area and the crypt enterocytes replicate to produce a less specialized low cuboidal enterocyte that spreads out to cover the exposed basement membrane of the surface area. With time, these less specialized enterocytes will be replaced by fully functioning columnar enterocytes. Thus villus atrophy can be either a transitory stage in regeneration with return to normal structure and function of affected villi or a permanent alteration if there is complete destruction of "regenerative" crypt enterocytes in that segment of the small intestine.

ACKNOWLEDGMENTS

We wish to extend our deepest appreciation and thanks to our colleagues throughout the world (truly an international effort), who have so generously provided their illustrative materials for use in the fifth edition. Although space limitations preclude listing them here, their names are cited in the figure legend credit for each illustration. We also extend our deepest appreciation to Dr. Elizabeth W. Howerth, Director of Noah's Arkive, College of Veterinary Medicine, The University of Georgia for allowing us to use illustrations from the Arkive. We have made every attempt to properly credit each illustration to its original source; however, we recognize that inadvertent errors will be made in the process of assembling a textbook. Please address any concerns about credits to <zacharyj@illinois.edu> or <mmcgavin@utk.edu>. We will make every effort to confirm the origin of the photograph and correct the acknowledgment before the book goes into the next printing.

Although we have used materials from many Elsevier books, we wish to specifically acknowledge the editors of the following books for granting use of some of their illustrative materials:

- Vinay Kumar, Abul K. Abbas, Nelson Fausto, and Jon Aster: *Robbins and Cotran Pathologic Basis of Disease*
- Abraham L. Kierszenbaum: *Histology and Cell Biology: an Introduction to Pathology*
- Lee-Ellen C. Copstead and Jacquelyn L. Banasik: *Pathophysiology: Biological and Behavioral Perspectives*
- Kathryn L. McCance and Sue E. Huether: *Pathophysiology: the Biologic Basis for Disease in Adults and Children*
- Sue E. Huether and Kathryn L. McCance: *Understanding Pathophysiology*

We also wish to acknowledge the contributions of the Elsevier staff: Shelly Stringer (managing editor), David Stein (senior production editor), and Theodore G. Huff (medical artist). We also appreciate the input of Penny Rudolph, publisher at Elsevier. Finally, we wish to thank our families—James Zachary to his daughters, Amanda and Briana, and Donald McGavin to his late wife, Beverley—for their support and encouragement during this process.

No greater impact can be made on students in their veterinary education than by teachers, including veterinary pathologists, who are willing to share their expertise and knowledge with them. We hope that *Pathologic Basis of Veterinary Disease* will aid in this process, foster the student's understanding of mechanistic concepts, and perhaps also alter the way that veterinary pathologists think about teaching pathology.

JAMES F. ZACHARY
M. DONALD McGAVIN

CONTENTS

SECTION 1

General Pathology

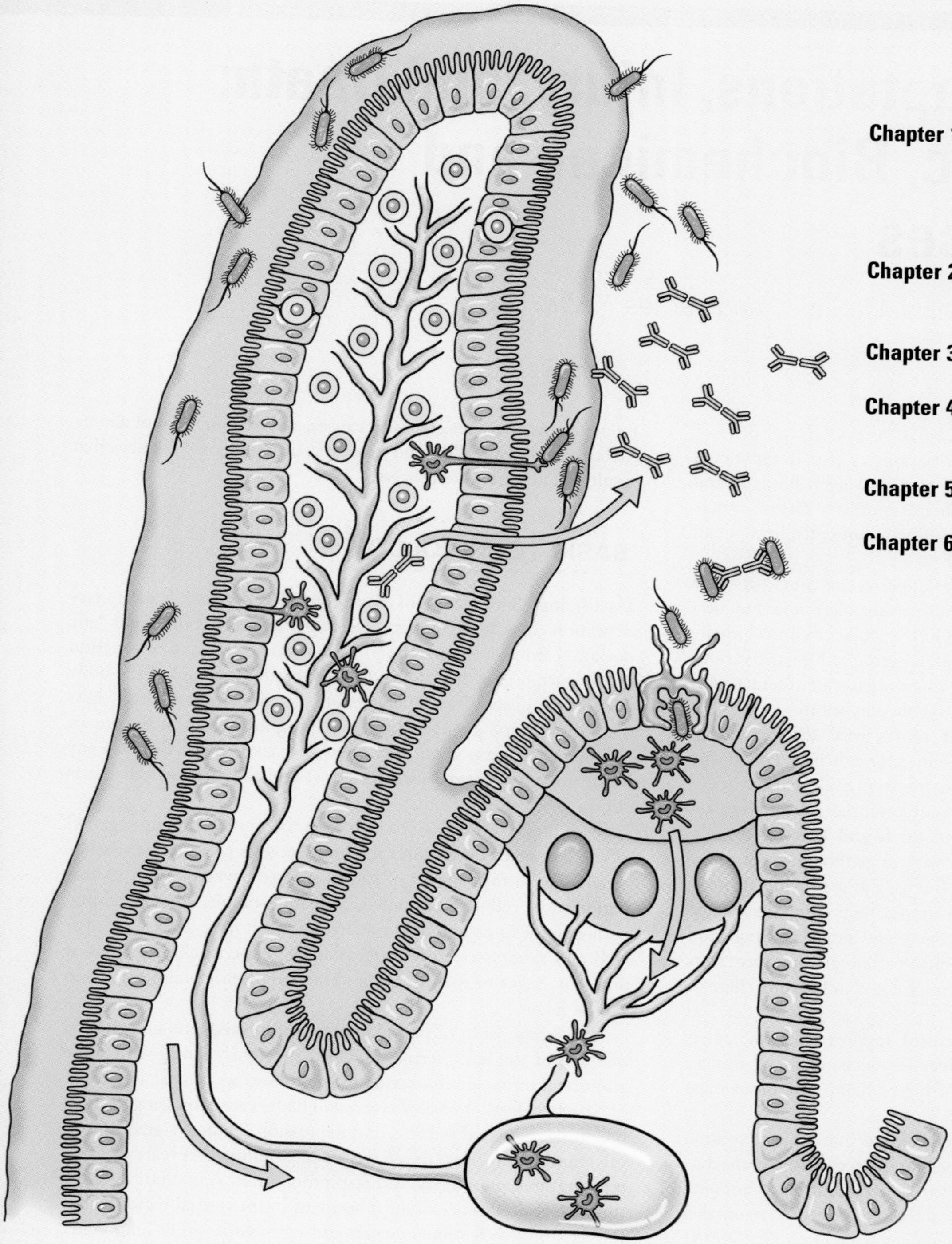

CHAPTER 1

Cellular Adaptations, Injury, and Death: Morphologic, Biochemical, and Genetic Bases

Ronald K. Myers, M. Donald McGavin, and James F. Zachary

The simple definition that pathology is "the study of disease" understates the wide range of contributions of this discipline to modern medicine. An understanding of pathology is fundamental to developing a mechanistic comprehension of how disease occurs in a chronologic sequence of events and consequently, how it can be diagnosed, treated, and prevented.

To students of medical science, pathology is the course of study that finally connects the study of normal structure and function (histology, anatomy, and physiology) to the study of clinical medicine. Pathology is fundamental to making sense of how the various causes of disease such as infectious microorganisms interact with animals and result in clinically identifiable conditions.

Pathology is also an important professional discipline that directly supports the practice of clinical medicine. Diagnostic pathologists, for example, perform postmortem examinations (necropsies), which provide clinicians with essential information on how to manage disease outbreaks in herds and how to improve management of individual cases. Surgical pathologists examine tissue removed from live animals (biopsy) and provide diagnoses that help clinicians treat animals under their care. Toxicologic pathologists test and evaluate the effects and safety of drugs and chemicals in laboratory animals. Clinical pathologists perform tests on blood and other body fluids (hematology and serum chemistry, for example) and examine cells (cytology) to provide detailed and essential information for clinicians. Experimental pathologists study the tissue, cellular, and molecular mechanisms of human and animal diseases in the fields of biomedicine and biomedical engineering.

Pathology is also an experimental science that makes essential contributions to advance our understanding of disease mechanisms through the use of a diverse variety of scientific techniques. Advanced methods of cell and molecular biology are used to unravel the complexities of how cells and animals respond to injury, so that a deeper understanding of disease processes can help improve treatment and prevention.

In summary, pathology is according to one dictionary definition *(Stedman's Medical Dictionary)* "the medical science, and specialty practice, concerned with all aspects of disease, but with special reference to the essential nature, causes, and development of abnormal conditions, as well as the structural and functional changes that result from the disease processes."

BASIC TERMINOLOGY

If pathology is the study of disease, what is disease? A dictionary definition *(Dorland's Medical Dictionary)* states that disease is "any deviation from or interruption of the normal structure or function of any part, organ, or system (or combination thereof) of the body that is manifested by a characteristic set of symptoms and signs and whose etiology, pathology, and prognosis may be known or unknown." Disease is not just illness or sickness but includes any departure from normal form (lesions) and function, whether it is clinically apparent or not.

Pathologists study lesions, as well as the causes (etiologic agents) of the lesions to understand the pathogenesis of a disease. Pathogenesis is the mechanism of how a disease develops from its initiation to its cellular and molecular manifestations. Understanding pathogenesis is essential to understanding how a disease is initiated and progresses, how these changes relate to clinical signs at different stages of the disease, and how appropriate clinical action can be taken.

The relationship of pathology to clinical medicine and the use of some of the basic terms discussed previously along with some additional terms are illustrated in the following clinical scenario.

In a beef feedlot, several steers and heifers are exhibiting difficult breathing, hunched posture, and depression (clinical signs). Physical examination of some of the infected animals reveals elevated temperatures, pulse rates, and respiration rates. Auscultation of the thorax reveals absence of air movement in the cranial region of the thorax along with some crackles and wheezes in other lung fields. A clinical diagnosis of bronchopneumonia is made. Some of the animals die, and a necropsy (postmortem examination) is done. The cranioventral lobes of the lungs are dark red and firm, with fibrin covering the surface (gross lesions). A gross morphologic diagnosis of severe acute fibrinopurulent cranioventral bronchopneumonia is made. Formalin fixed samples are taken for microscopic examination (histopathology), neutrophilic inflammation of airways and alveoli with fibrin are noted (microscopic lesions), and a histologic morphologic diagnosis of severe acute fibrinopurulent bronchopneumonia is made. Fresh samples of lung are taken for bacterial and viral examination, and *Mannheimia haemolytica* and a bovine herpes virus (etiologic agents or causes) are identified. An etiologic diagnosis of *Mannheimia* bronchopneumonia and a disease diagnosis of "shipping fever pneumonia" are made.

The pathogenesis of this disease might be stated in an abbreviated form like the following:

> Various viruses, such as infectious rhinotracheitis virus, and environmental agents, such as dust and noxious gases, disrupt the clearance mechanisms of the airway epithelium allowing opportunistic organisms, such as the bacterium *Mannheimia haemolytica,* to colonize and invade the alveoli. Virulence factors of the bacteria, such as endotoxin and various exotoxins, cause necrosis and inflammation, which result in the filling of alveoli and airways with fibrin and neutrophils.

Although a diagnostic pathologist did the histologic diagnosis of the disease, the details of this pathogenesis were discovered over time by researchers in many fields, including experimental pathologists.

TYPES OF DIAGNOSIS

Note that various levels of diagnosis were made in the previous scenario. Diagnosis is a concise statement or conclusion concerning the nature, cause, or name of a disease. The accuracy of a diagnosis is limited by the evidence (lesions) available for study. A clinical diagnosis is based on the data obtained from the case history, clinical signs, and physical examination. It often suggests only the system involved, or it provides a list of differential diagnoses. The differential diagnosis (often termed *rule outs* in clinical medicine) is a list of diseases that could account for the evidence or lesions of the case. A clinical pathologic diagnosis is based on changes observed in the chemistry of fluids and the hematology, structure, and function of cells collected from the living patient. A morphologic diagnosis or lesion diagnosis is based on the predominant lesion(s) in the tissue(s) (see Chapter 3 and Fig. 3-23). It may be macroscopic (gross) or microscopic (histologic) and describes the severity, duration, distribution, location (organ or tissue), and nature (degenerative, inflammatory, neoplastic) of the lesion. An etiologic diagnosis is even more definitive and names the specific cause of the disease. A disease diagnosis is equally specific and states the common name of the disease.

One of the goals in making a diagnosis in a case is to enable a clinician to predict how the disease will progress or resolve. Prognosis is a statement of what the expected outcome of a condition is likely to be. If the lesion is expected to resolve (return to normal) with no expected lasting harm, the prognosis is good or excellent. If the outcome is uncertain—the lesion could resolve or become worse as a result of unforeseen factors—the prognosis is guarded. If the animal is not expected to recover from the lesion or disease, the prognosis is grave. Accurate determination of the prognosis demands a thorough understanding of the disease, especially pathogenesis.

As in this book, the study of pathology is often divided into two basic parts: general pathology and pathology of organ systems. General pathology is the study of basic responses of cells and tissues to insults and injuries, irrespective of the organs, systems, or species of animal involved. This area of pathology is one of the most complex and rapidly growing fields in the natural sciences, largely as the result of the availability and power of new research techniques. General pathology is studied first, so students will have a thorough understanding of the general principles of disease processes that they will encounter repeatedly in the study of diseases of body systems. Pathology of organ systems (sometimes called systemic or special pathology) involves the study of how each organ system reacts to injury associated with specific diseases.

MORPHOLOGIC CHANGES AND HOW THEY ARE DETECTED AND EVALUATED

The study and practice of pathology historically have been based on the macroscopic and microscopic changes that take place in diseased cells, tissues, and organs, that is to say, the morphology of lesions. Consequently, most pathology texts tend to emphasize anatomic pathology. Morphologic techniques remain the cornerstones of pathology, but progress in our deeper understanding of the mechanisms and in the diagnosis of disease rely more and more on techniques derived from cellular and molecular biology.

The basic tools for the study and practice of pathology begin with an open and inquiring mind, skills in observation, and careful and consistent postmortem techniques. The diagnosis of many diseases can be accurately accomplished with no more than gross examination of a body. Confirmation of gross lesions and discovery and interpretation of microscopic changes typically involves observation of tissue placed on glass microscope slides. Tissues are first fixed (i.e., preserved) usually in 10% formalin, embedded in blocks of paraffin wax, microtome sectioned to about 5 μm thickness, and routinely stained with hematoxylin and eosin (H&E). H&E stained sections are the mainstay of histopathology in both postmortem and surgical pathology, and interpretation of lesions in these specimens can often lead to a final diagnosis. A simplistic explanation of the labeling characteristics of the H&E stain as applied to tissue sections is as follows: Hematoxylin stains nucleic acids (nucleus, ribosomes, mitochondria) blue, whereas eosin stains proteins, such as those found intracellularly (e.g., enzymes, actin, and myosin) or those proteins found extracellularly (e.g., collagen and extracellular matrix [ECM]), red or pink.

A variety of ancillary techniques are also used in histopathology. Histochemistry applies a variety of chemical reactions carried out on tissue sections. Glycogen, for example, can be identified in hepatocytes using periodic acid–Schiff (PAS) reaction. Suspected mast cell tumors are routinely stained to demonstrate the metachromatic mast cell granules using toluidine blue or Giemsa stains.

Increasing use in diagnostic laboratories is being made of immunohistochemistry, in which specific antigens are identified in tissue by antibodies linked to a chromogen. Detection of specific intermediate fibers by immunohistochemistry, in tumors, for example, can separate malignant striated muscle tumors from other sarcomas. Specific infectious agents, such as the coronavirus causing feline infectious peritonitis, can also be identified using immunohistochemistry.

A variety of techniques for identification of molecules or genetic sequences are now in use, with more expected. In situ hybridization, in which labeled nucleic acid probes can identify complementary strands of host or microbe deoxyribonucleic acid (DNA) or ribonucleic acid (RNA) in intact cells and tissues, is particularly useful in the diagnosis and study of viral disease. These techniques are not as sensitive as polymerase chain reaction (PCR), in which small amounts of target DNA in biologic material are amplified and identified. Small amounts of target DNA of microbes (for example) can be identified in tissues, and RNA sequences can be identified after conversion to DNA and subsequent amplification.

The typical light microscope can magnify to about 1000× and is adequate for routine histopathology. Specialized microscopes, such as dark field, phase contrast, and fluorescence microscopes, are also used, often for identification of microbes. In both diagnostic and experimental settings, electron microscopy is used to visualize the subcellular structure of cells and microbes. Transmission electron microscopy of ultrathin sections allows resolution of ultrafine structures of less than a nanometer. Scanning electron microscopy allows the ultrafine observation of surfaces. Specialized analytical electron microscopes are also in use. Finally, laser capture microdissection allows pathologists to isolate and capture groups of similar cells from tumors or a diseased tissue. Using DNA microarrays and other genomic techniques, the genes expressed by these cells can be identified and characterized, thus providing a "genetic fingerprint" of the disease process that clinically can be used to develop therapeutic strategies and assess the outcome. Proteomics, which are molecular techniques used to reveal the protein profiles from genes in tissues and fluids, are also being increasingly used.

THE NORMAL CELL

COMPONENTS OF NORMAL CELLS AND THEIR VULNERABILITIES

The early pathologists Morgagni and Bichat emphasized the importance of organs and tissues as the seat of disease. Virchow later focused on individual cells as the primary cause of abnormal function and structure associated with diseases. Before we can interpret lesions of sick cells, it is essential that we understand normal cell structure and function. The cell can be visualized simplistically as a membrane-enclosed compartment, subdivided into numerous smaller compartments (organelles) by membranes (Fig. 1-1). This vast interconnecting system of membrane-bound spaces is termed the *cytocavitary network*. The function of these organelles is largely determined by the type and quantity of specific enzymes associated with each membrane and in the cytoplasmic matrix.

It is essential to have a clear understanding of the structure and function of the components of normal cells and how they are interrelated in a normally functioning cell. Cell membranes and organelles serve as targets for injury by microbes, harmful environmental agents, and a variety of genetic, metabolic, and toxicologic diseases discussed in greater detail in the Pathology of Organ Systems chapters of this book.

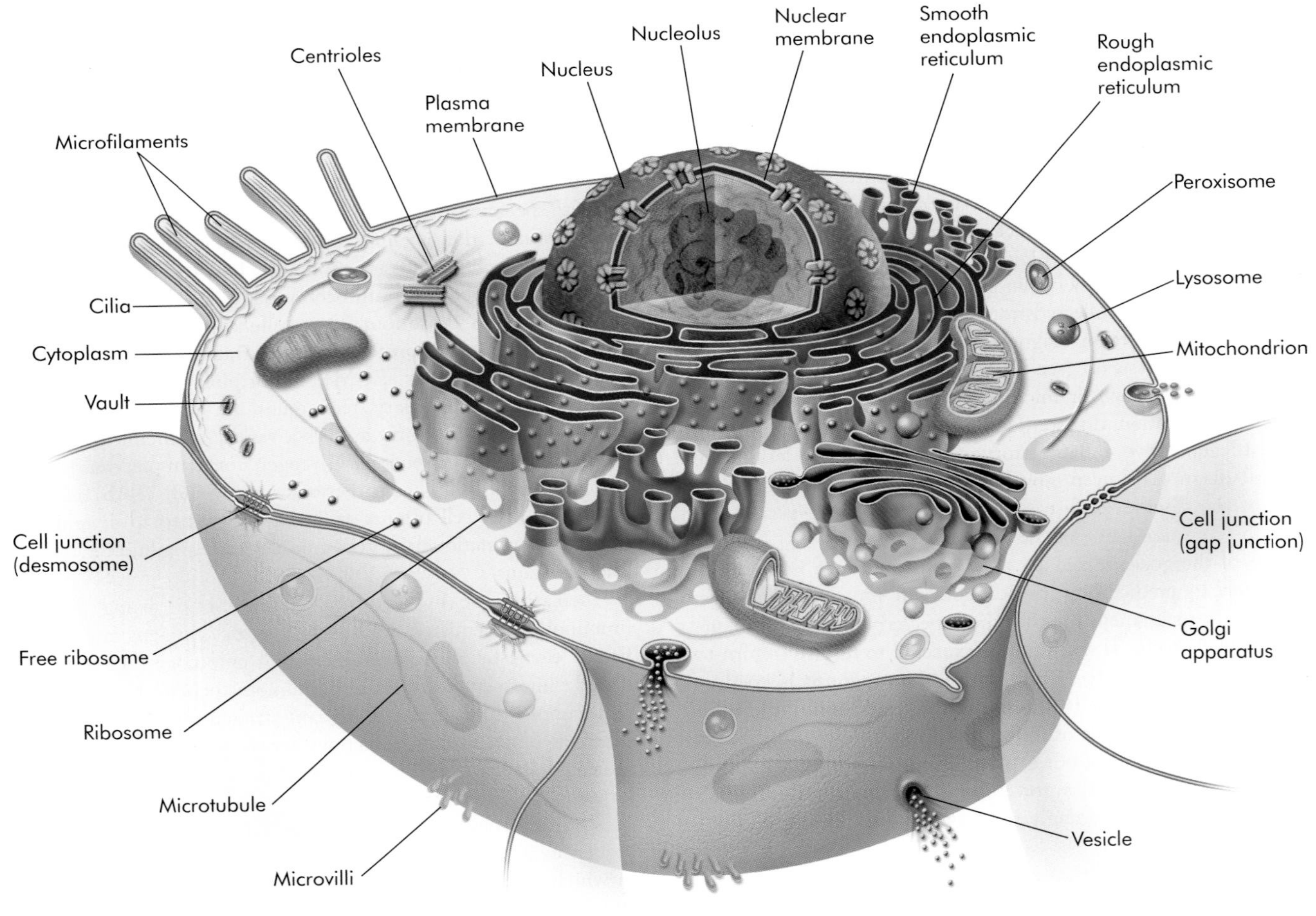

Fig. 1-1 Cell structure and the organization of organelles, cytoskeleton, and membrane enhancements. (From McCance K, Huether S: *Pathophysiology: the biologic basis for disease in adults and children,* ed 5, St Louis, 2006, Mosby.)

Cell Membranes

Cell membranes are a fluid phospholipid bilayer penetrated by numerous specific proteins (Fig. 1-2). The two main biologic functions of these membranes are (1) to serve as selective barriers and (2) to form a structural base for the enzymes and receptors that determine cell function. Cell membranes form the boundaries of many organelles and separate them from the cytosol.

The plasma membrane is the cell's first contact with injurious agents. Microvilli and cilia are specialized areas of the plasma membrane and are often specifically altered in disease (see Fig. 1-1). Plasma membranes separate the interior of the cell from external surfaces, neighboring cells, or surrounding matrix. Surface proteins, such as fibronectin, play a role in cell-to-cell and cell-to-ECM interactions. Transmembrane proteins embedded in the phospholipid bilayer serve in a variety of structural, transport, and enzymatic functions essential to cell viability (Fig. 1-3). It is these transmembrane proteins that are often used by infectious microbes to enter or use cell systems during their life cycles, thus initiating a process that often results in injury to the host cell.

Cytosol

The cytosol is the watery gel in which the cell's organelles and inclusions are dispersed. Many chemical reactions occur in the cytosol mediated by "free" enzymes or macromolecular complexes such as proteasomes. The cytosol is a highly organized microtrabecular network.

Mitochondria

Mitochondria (singular = mitochondrion) are the "powerhouses" of highly specialized eukaryotic cells. They are the site of fatty acid oxidation, the citric acid cycle, and oxidative phosphorylation. Transfer of electrons from reduced cytochrome oxidase to molecular oxygen is the final and critical step culminating in these catabolic pathways. Important structural components of a mitochondrion are the outer membrane, outer compartment, inner

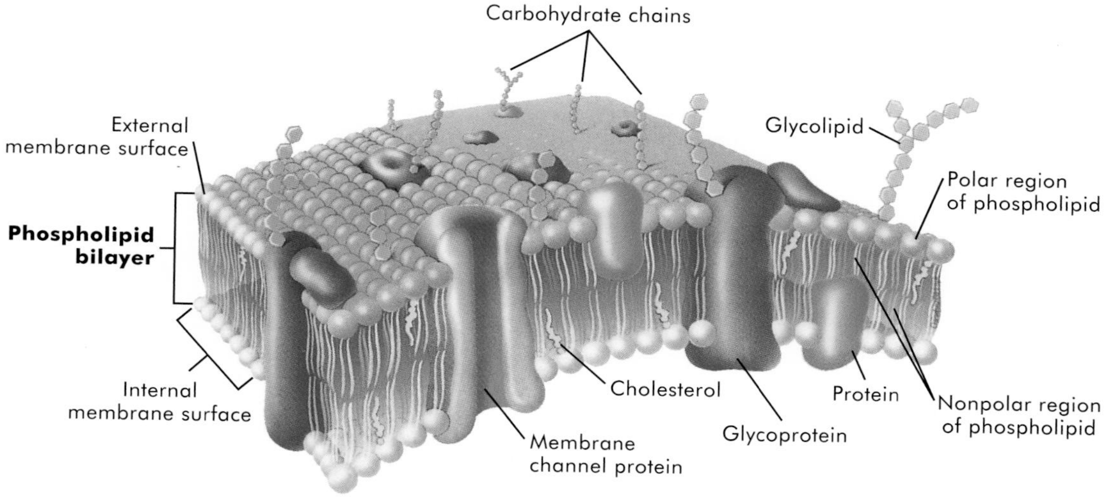

Fig. 1-2 Fluid mosaic model of cell membrane structure.
The lipid bilayer provides the basic structure and serves as a relatively impermeable barrier to most water-soluble molecules. (From McCance K, Huether S: *Pathophysiology: the biologic basis for disease in adults and children,* ed 4, St Louis, 2002, Mosby.)

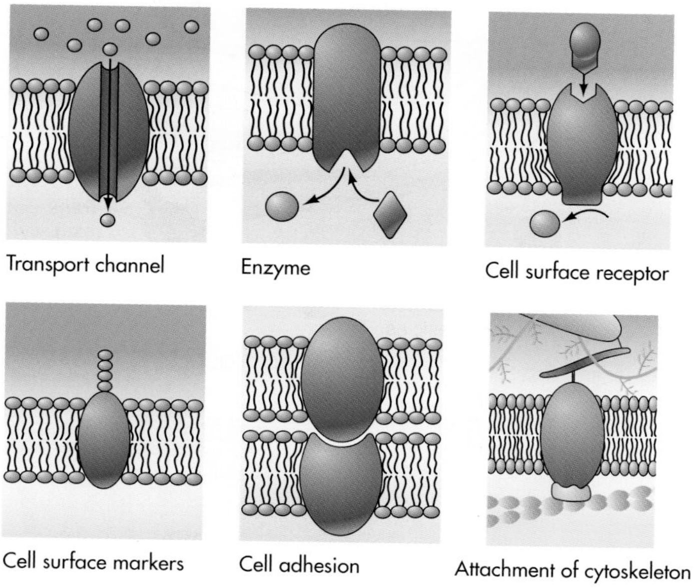

Fig. 1-3 Functions of transmembrane proteins.
A variety of functions are performed by different types of cell membranes as shown. (From McCance K, Huether S: *Pathophysiology: the biologic basis for disease in adults and children,* ed 5, St Louis, 2006, Mosby.)

membrane, inner compartment (matrix), cristae, and mitochondrial DNA. Damage to mitochondria results in diminished adenosine triphosphate (ATP) production and if damage is unchecked, cell death (see Fig. 1-6).

Nucleus

The nucleus is that portion of the cell responsible for storage and transmission of genetic information (see Fig. 1-1). Chains of DNA, complexed to protein, are chromatin. Areas of uncoiled chromatin (euchromatin) are active in the generation of messenger RNA (mRNA) for protein synthesis. Highly coiled chromatin (heterochromatin) is inactive in transcription. The outer nuclear membrane is continuous with that of the rough endoplasmic reticulum (RER).

Nucleolus

The nucleolus is a basic organelle of the nucleus and is composed of RNA, nucleolus-associated chromatin, and protein (see Fig. 1-1). It functions in the synthesis of ribosomal RNA (rRNA), essential in protein synthesis. The nucleolus can be basophilic or eosinophilic, and its prominence is a subjective measure of the cell's synthetic activity.

Rough Endoplasmic Reticulum

The RER is a network of intracellular membranes studded with ribosomes (Fig. 1-4). RER is prominent in cells producing large amounts of extracellular protein (e.g., reactive fibroblasts, hepatocytes, plasma cells, and pancreatic acinar cells). The RER is responsible for the basophilia of the cytoplasm because of the numerous ribosomes, which contain acid (i.e., RNA).

Smooth Endoplasmic Reticulum

Smooth endoplasmic reticulum (SER) is a tubular or vesicular form of cell membrane that lacks ribosomes (see Fig. 1-1). SER is the locus of enzymes that metabolize steroids, drugs, lipids, and glycogen. It gives the cytoplasm a pale, finely vacuolated appearance as viewed in the light microscope.

Golgi Complex

The Golgi complex consists of several lamellar stacks or flattened sacs of membranes, vesicles, and vacuoles (see Fig. 1-4). It functions in the synthesis of complex proteins by the addition of carbohydrate molecules and in the production of secretory vesicles and lysosomes.

Lysosomes

Lysosomes are small membrane-bound vesicles laden with hydrolytic enzymes essential for intracellular digestion (see Fig. 1-1). They are discussed more completely as components of phagocytic cells. Peroxisomes are similar to lysosomes but also play a role in energy metabolism.

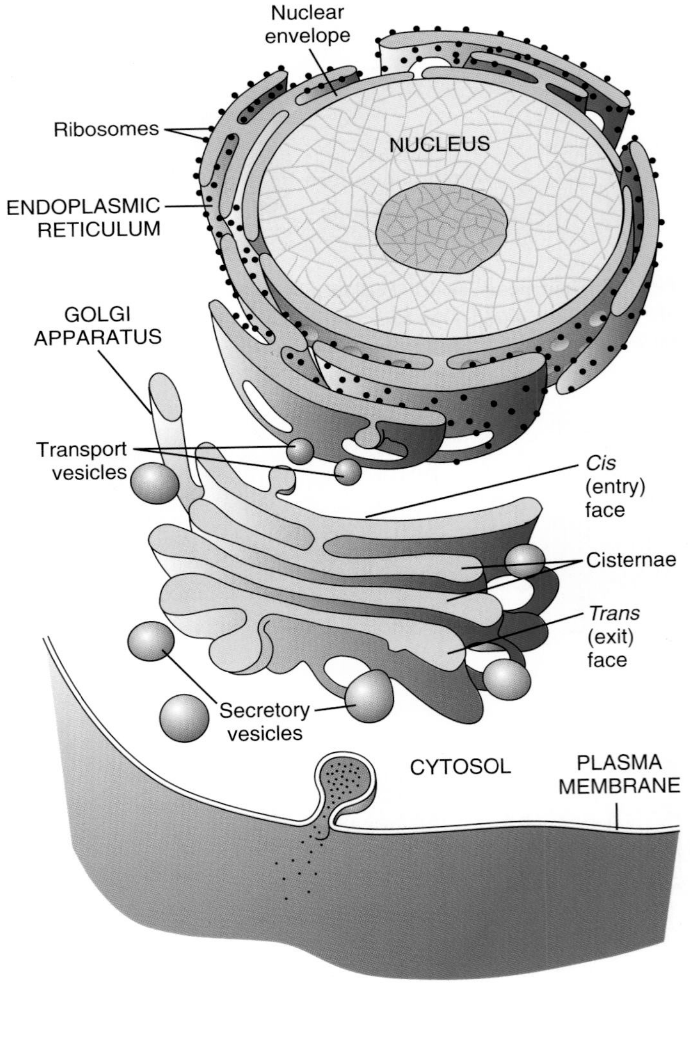

Fig. 1-4 Membrane systems.
The rough endoplasmic reticulum and Golgi apparatus are important organelles in cellular biosynthesis of proteins and glycoproteins inserted into cell membranes and used in and secreted from cells. Transcription, translation, assembly, modification, and packaging of these molecules occur in an orderly sequence from the nucleus to the cell membrane as shown. Alterations in one or more of these steps can result in cell injury and serve as the underlying pathogenesis of a disease process. (From Copstead L, Banasik J: *Pathophysiology,* ed 4, St Louis, 2010, Mosby.)

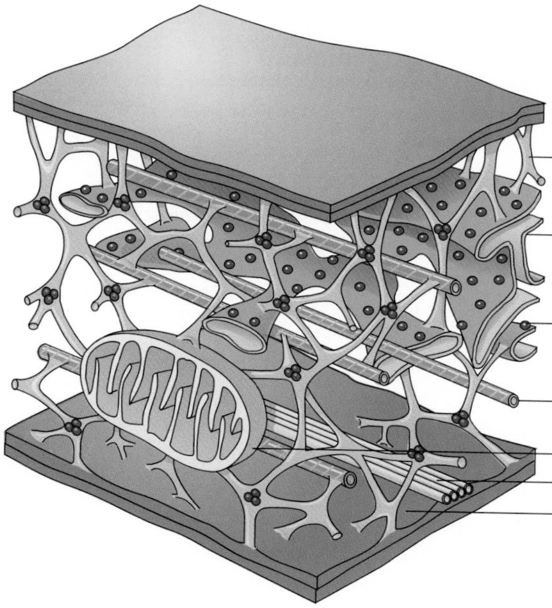

Fig. 1-5 Cytoskeleton. The complexity of and interrelations between intermediate filaments, microtubules, endoplasmic reticulum, and other cytoplasmic organelles that can be involved in the pathogenesis of diseases are shown. (From McCance KL, Huether SE: *Pathophysiology: the biologic basis for disease in adults and children,* ed 5, St Louis, 2006, Mosby.)

Microfilaments, Intermediate Filaments, and Microtubules

These structures are composed of protein subunits and function in the cytoskeleton and in cell movement (Fig. 1-5). They have a prominent role in the mitotic spindle, cilia, microvilli, neurons, myocytes, and phagocytic cells. Many cell types besides muscles, for example, contain actin microfilaments.

Intermediate filaments are about 10 nm in diameter and are important in cell shape and movement. Different cell types have different intermediate filaments; for example, cytokeratins are found in epithelial cells, desmin in muscle cells, and vimentin in cells of mesenchymal origin such as fibroblasts. Intermediate filaments can be useful markers for classifying undifferentiated neoplasms.

Cellular Inclusions

Inclusions include glycogen granules, proteinaceous vacuoles, lipid debris, hemosiderin, viral particles, and calcium granules (discussed in greater detail later in this chapter). Some of these are normal, whereas others are the result of cell injury and are discussed later in this chapter in the section dealing with intracellular and extracellular accumulations.

Extracellular Matrix

Although not part of the cell itself, the ECM and its integrity influences cell health and function (see Chapter 3 and Web Figs. 3-23 and 3-24). ECM includes basement membranes and interstitial matrices composed of various collagens, proteoglycans, and adhesive glycoproteins among a variety of other molecules that interact with cells by means of various integrin molecules. Basement membrane integrity, for example, is essential for the proper structure and functioning of epithelial cells. Other components of the ECM influence how cells grow and differentiate.

CAUSES OF CELL INJURY

Causes of cell injury are numerous and can be classified in a variety of ways. Some causes, such as physical trauma, viruses, and toxins, are clearly extrinsic, whereas others, such as spontaneous genetic mutations, are clearly intrinsic. Others, such as workload imbalance, nutritional abnormalities, and immunologic dysfunctions, can have components of both extrinsic and intrinsic mechanisms. General mechanisms of injury include ATP depletion (often caused by hypoxia), membrane damage (a result of a myriad of causes, including oxygen-derived free radicals), disturbances of cellular metabolism, and genetic damage (Fig. 1-6).

Understanding disease starts with understanding the cell. Until the nineteenth century, the dominant theory of disease in western societies was humoral pathology, wherein disease was attributed to a maldistribution of body fluids or "humors." In the mid-1800s, Rudolph Virchow, a German pathologist now considered to be the founder of modern pathology, redefined pathology and medical science with his idea of the body as an organization of cells, each suited for specific functions. He taught that disease resulted from injury to, or dysfunction of, specific populations of cells. The recent rapid advancement in medical science is owed to a great extent to Virchow's original emphasis on cellular pathology and more recently on molecular pathology.

Cells can be injured through a large number of causes (etiologic agents). Fortunately, the types of responses of the cell to injury are not as large. The responses to injury depend on many factors, including the type of agent, the extent of injury, the duration of injury, and the cell type affected. Renal tubular cells deprived of adequate blood supply, for example, may exhibit only cell swelling, if oxygen is soon restored. Prolonged lack of adequate blood supply (ischemia) can lead to cell death. Diminished but sublethal reduction in blood supply may result in cells adapting by decreasing their metabolic rates, which could lead to recovery or if adaptation is inadequate, eventually death.

Cells respond to stimuli and stressors in a variety of ways to maintain homeostasis. Cell injury takes place when a cell can no longer maintain a steady state. Some types of cell injury, such as cell swelling, can be reversible if the extent and duration of injury are not excessive. But if the injury exceeds certain limits, cell death and irreversible change occur. Not all cell injury results in cell death. Cell injury may be sublethal and result in a variety of types of cell degenerations or accumulations and/or adaptations by the

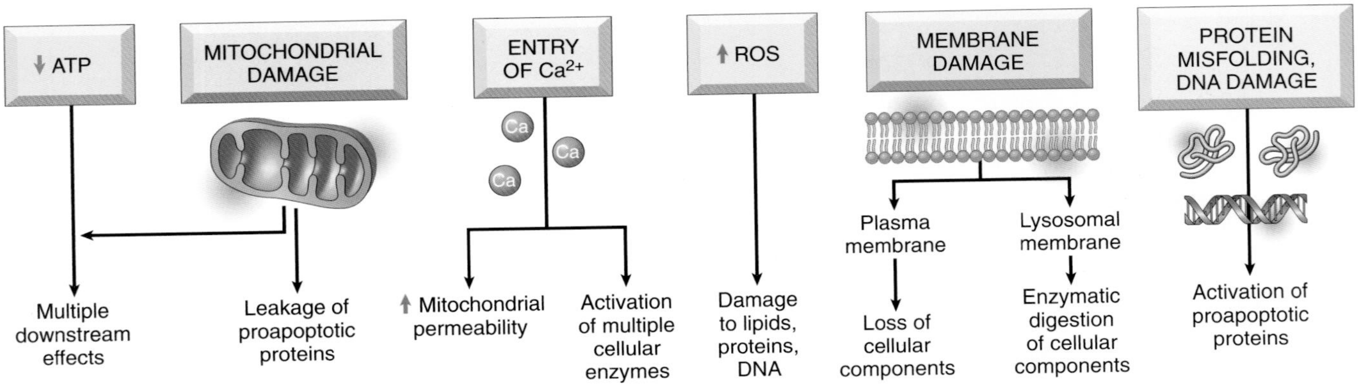

Fig. 1-6 Cellular and biochemical sites of damage in cell injury. *ATP,* Adenosine triphosphate; *ROS,* reactive oxygen species. (From Kumar V, Abbas A, Fausto N, et al: *Robbins & Cotran pathologic basis of disease,* ed 8, Philadelphia, 2009, Saunders.)

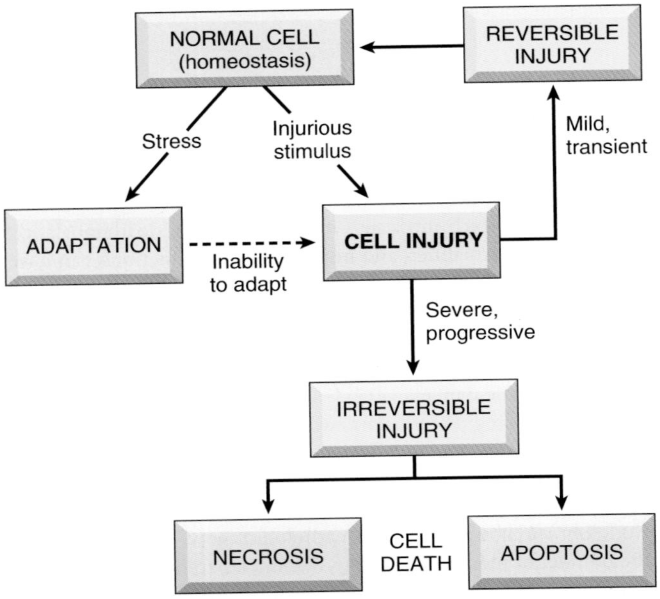

Fig. 1-7 Stages in the cellular response to stress and injurious stimuli. (From Kumar V, Abbas A, Fausto N, et al: *Robbins & Cotran pathologic basis of disease,* ed 8, Philadelphia, 2009, Saunders.)

cell to the injury. In essence, cells or tissues respond to injury (or stress) in three important ways: (1) adaptation, (2) degeneration or intracellular or extracellular accumulations, and (3) death (Fig. 1-7).

Pathologically, reversible cell injury is injury from which the cell can adapt or recover and thus return to normal or nearly normal function. Irreversible cell injury results in a dead cell. This distinction seems clear-cut, but the point at which a cell transitions from reversible cell injury to irreversible cell injury (i.e., "the point of no return") has been a major research challenge for the past few decades and remains so today (Fig. 1-8). The lesions of reversible and irreversible cell injury are discussed in greater detail in subsequent sections; however, in summary, the cytomorphologic changes characteristic of irreversible cell injury include the following:

- Plasma membrane damage
- Calcium entry into the cell
- Mitochondrial swelling and vacuolization
- Amorphous densities (likely calcium) in the mitochondria
- Lysosomal swelling

The causes of reversible and irreversible cell injury resulting in cell death, cell adaptation and degeneration, and finally cellular accumulations are now discussed.

OXYGEN DEFICIENCY

Hypoxia is one of the most common and important causes of cell injury and death (see Fig. 1-8). Hypoxia is a partial reduction in the O_2 concentration supplied to cells or tissue; a complete reduction is referred to as anoxia. Oxygen is critically important for oxidative phosphorylation, especially in highly specialized cells such as neurons, hepatocytes, cardiac myocytes, and renal tubule cells. Hypoxia can result from inadequate oxygenation of blood as a result of heart failure or respiratory failure, loss or reduction of blood supply (ischemia), reduced transport of O_2 in blood (e.g., anemia or carbon monoxide toxicity), and blockage of cell respiratory enzymes (cyanide toxicosis).

PHYSICAL AGENTS

Trauma, extremes of heat and cold, radiation, and electrical energy may seriously injure cells. Trauma may cause direct rupture and death of large numbers of cells, or it may damage the blood supply to cells. Extreme cold impairs the blood flow, and intracellular ice crystals rupture cell membranes. Extreme heat denatures essential cell enzymes and other proteins. Excessive heat can increase the rate of metabolic reactions so that substrates, water, and pH changes reach lethal levels. Electricity generates great heat as it passes through tissue. It also alters conduction of nerves and muscle. Ionizing radiation causes ionization of cellular water with production of highly reactive "free radicals" that injure cell components. Many forms of radiation may damage genetic material, resulting in reproductive death of cells by apoptosis, genetic defects from mutations, and neoplasia.

INFECTIOUS AGENTS

Viruses are obligate intracellular parasites that redirect host cell enzyme systems toward synthesis of viral proteins and genetic materials to the detriment of host cells. Cell changes induced by viral agents vary from little effect to cell death or neoplastic transformation.

Injury caused by bacterial infection varies and can result from the action of potent toxins on specific host cells (clostridial infections, enterotoxigenic *Escherichia coli* infection) or from an overwhelming or ineffective inflammatory response to uncontrolled bacterial replication in tissue. Some bacteria, such as *Lawsonia intracellularis,* can result in excessive intestinal epithelial cell replication.

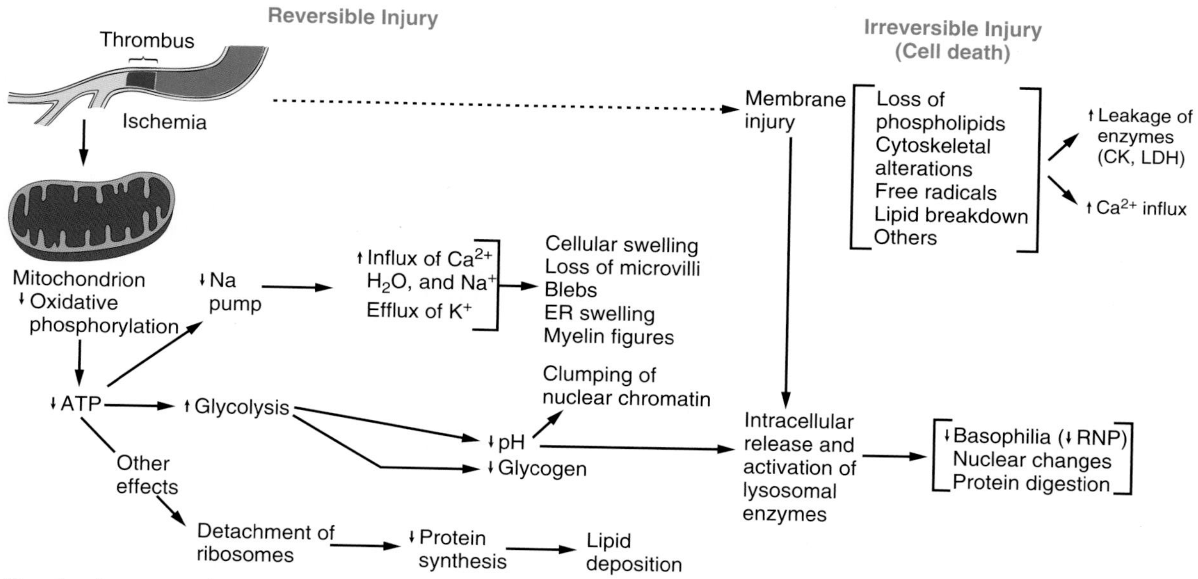

Fig. 1-8 **Postulated sequence of events in reversible and irreversible ischemic cell injury.** Note that although reduced oxidative phosphorylation and adenosine triphosphate (ATP) levels have a central role, ischemia can cause direct membrane damage. *ER,* Endoplasmic reticulum; *CK,* creatine kinase; *LDH,* lactate dehydrogenase; *RNP,* ribonucleoprotein. (From Kumar V, Abbas A, Fausto N: *Robbins & Cotran pathologic basis of disease,* ed 7, Philadelphia, 2005, Saunders.)

Mycotic agents resist destruction by the body that can lead to progressive, chronic inflammatory disease with loss of normal host tissues. Protozoal agents replicate in specific host cells, often resulting in destruction of infected cells. Metazoan parasites cause inflammation, distort tissue, and use host nutrients.

NUTRITIONAL DEFICIENCIES AND IMBALANCES

Dietary protein-calorie deficiencies are seen sporadically in animals and humans (known as kwashiorkor). These deficiencies require metabolic adaptation by large populations of cells. Lipolysis, catabolism of muscle protein, and glycogenolysis enable short-term survival. Calorie excess, as seen in many pets and people of affluent societies, is implicated in cardiovascular disease and several other diseases. Vitamin and mineral imbalances are common due to errors in formulating rations and hypersupplementation by well-meaning animal owners.

GENETIC DERANGEMENT

A normal genetic apparatus is essential for cell homeostasis. Mutations, whatever their origin, may cause no disease, may deprive a cell of a protein (enzyme) critical for normal function, may result in neoplasia, or may be incompatible with cell survival. A few examples of genetic diseases are defects of clotting factors (hemophilia), lysosomal storage disease (mannosidosis), combined immunodeficiency of Arabian foals, and defects of collagen synthesis (dermatosparaxis). Besides causing overt disease, some genotypes cause the host to be more prone to certain types of extrinsic or intrinsic disease, a condition often termed *genetic predisposition.*

WORKLOAD IMBALANCE

Cells that are overworked may adapt to the demand or eventually become exhausted and die. Conversely, cells that are no longer stimulated to work may shrink in size and waste away. An example is the way endocrine tissues react to the presence or absence of specific trophic hormones. Muscle fibers, deprived of work or their nerve supply, will atrophy and ultimately disappear, leaving a fibrous stroma.

CHEMICALS, DRUGS, AND TOXINS

Chemicals, drugs, and toxins influence cells by a multitude of mechanisms. Drugs produce their therapeutic effects by modifying the function (and morphology) of specific populations of cells. Most drugs cause these cells to adapt within a tolerable range of homeostasis. Chemicals, including drugs and toxins, can block or stimulate cell membrane receptors, alter specific enzyme systems, produce toxic free radicals, alter cell permeability, damage chromosomes, modify metabolic pathways, and damage structural components of cells.

IMMUNOLOGIC DYSFUNCTION

The immune system may fail to respond to infectious agents and other antigens as a result of congenital or acquired defects of lymphoid tissue or their products (see Chapter 5). Examples of congenital defects are thymic aplasia of nude mice and combined immunodeficiency of Arabian foals. Affected animals may die at an early age from infection by opportunistic microorganisms. Acquired immunodeficiency disease may be transient and results from damage to lymphoid tissue by viral infection, chemicals, and drugs.

The immune response directed toward foreign antigens (pathogenic organisms) is usually beneficial to the host, but sometimes the response is misdirected against antigens of host cells. This large group of diseases is referred to as *autoimmune disease.* An inappropriate or exaggerated response to certain antigens results in immunologic disease referred to as *hypersensitivity (allergy).* Some examples are anaphylaxis, feline asthma, and flea allergy dermatitis. The activity of the immune system is greatly amplified by its effect on serum complement and inflammation. These reactions often lead to serious injury to the kidney, skin, and joints.

AGING

The diminished capacity of aged cells and tissue to carry out their normal functions can hardly be disputed. One can argue that aging is simply the culmination of life's injuries inflicted by chemicals, infectious agents, work imbalances, or poor nutrition. We use the

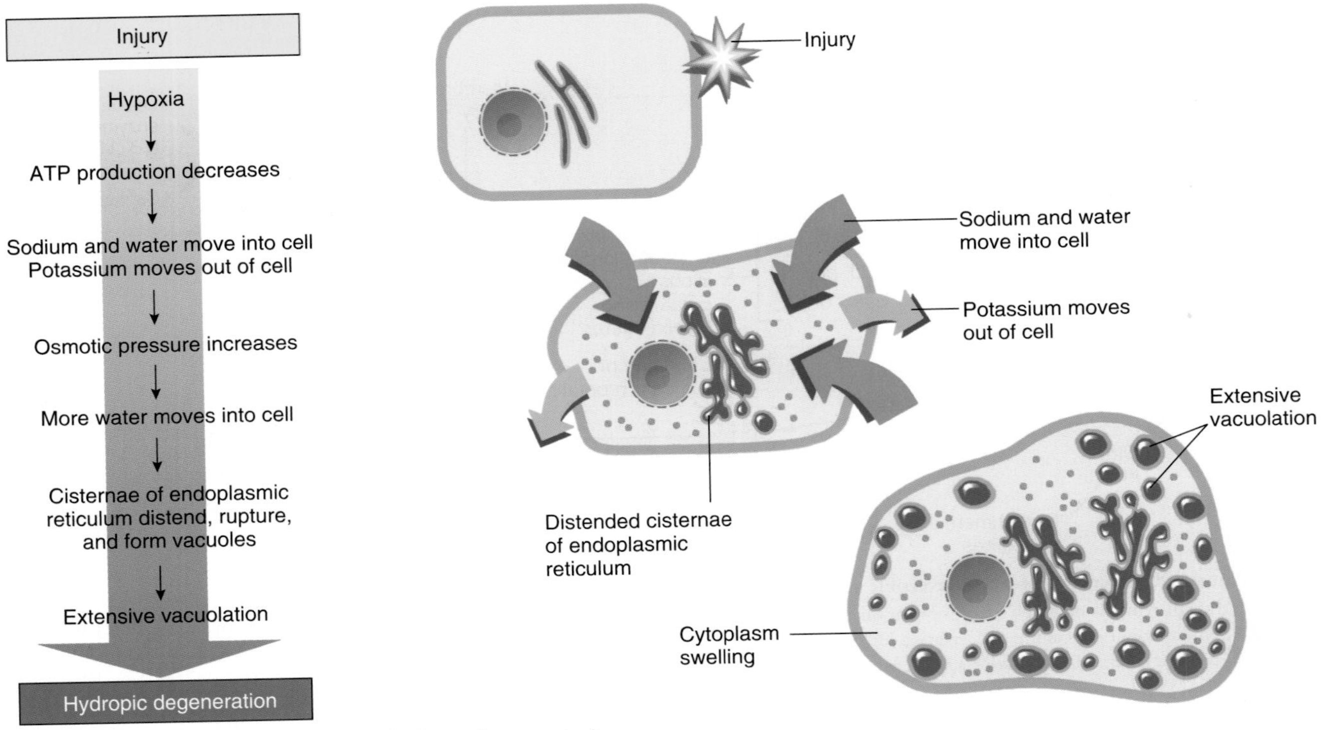

Fig. 1-9 The process of acute cell swelling (hydropic degeneration). *ATP,* Adenosine triphosphate. (From Huether S, McCance K: *Understanding pathophysiology,* ed 3, St Louis, 2004, Mosby.)

aging category for those lesions commonly found in aged animals; lesions for which we have no other defensible mechanistic explanation. Some of the lesions commonly found in older animals include nodular hyperplasia of parenchymal cells in the liver, pancreas, adrenal, spleen, and thyroid. There appear to be defects in growth control of these cell populations, but the cause is unclear. Aged cells may suffer a lifetime of damage to their DNA, or there may be accumulation of cellular debris that interferes with normal cell functions. One could argue that many cancers are caused by old age, rather than by exposure to specific chemicals, foods, viruses, or other insults.

REVERSIBLE CELL INJURY

ACUTE CELL SWELLING

Cell swelling, also called *hydropic degeneration* and by other names in different organ systems (e.g., *cytotoxic edema* in the central nervous system and *ballooning degeneration* in the epidermis), is the most common and fundamental expression of cell injury (Fig. 1-9). It is manifested as increased cell size and volume resulting from an overload of water caused by a failure of the cell to maintain normal homeostasis and regulate the ingress and excretion of water. It is accompanied by modification and degeneration of organelles. Mechanisms responsible for acute cell swelling usually involve damage to cellular membranes, failure of cellular energy production, or injury to enzymes regulating ion channels of membranes. Cell swelling occurs in response to loss of the cell's homeostasis secondary to mechanical, hypoxic, toxic, free radical, viral, bacterial, and immune-mediated injuries.

The functional and morphologic changes begin with increased uptake of water and then to diffuse disintegration of organelles and cytoplasmic proteins. Cell swelling must be distinguished from cell enlargement *(hypertrophy)* that is caused by an increase of normal organelles. Organs composed of swollen cells are themselves swollen. Affected organs are larger and heavier than normal and pale in color. The parenchyma of swollen organs, such as kidney and liver, may bulge a little from beneath their capsule when incised. Because of the increase of intracellular water, the specific gravity of affected tissues is slightly less than those of normal tissues.

Normal Cell Volume Control and Mechanisms of Acute Cell Swelling

In the normal cell, energy derived from ATP drives the Na^+-K^+ ion pumps within cell membranes to continuously drive Na^+ out of the cell in exchange for K^+ moving into the cell. For each molecule of ATP used, the pump moves three Na^+ out of the cell and two K^+ into the cell. By this means, the ion pumps maintain the transmembrane ionic gradients required for normal nerve and muscle function. Because water moves passively across cell membranes in response to the osmotic pressure gradient generated by Na^+ and proteins, the Na^+-K^+ pump is the key to regulation of intracellular water. The best-studied laboratory models of cell swelling are (1) hypoxia-induced failure of ATP synthesis and (2) carbon tetrachloride (CCl_4)–induced membrane damage.

Hypoxic Injury Resulting in Acute Cell Swelling

Hypoxia is probably the most important fundamental cause of acute cell swelling. Hypoxia-induced cell injury results from any defect in the transport of O_2, from inspired air to its role as the final acceptor of electrons from cytochrome oxidase in oxidative phosphorylation. Ischemia is reduced blood flow to a region of the body, usually because of obstruction of the blood supply. Blockage of coronary arteries by atherosclerotic plaque leads to ischemia and hypoxic injury to heart muscle, a common cause of "heart attacks" in humans. Therefore cellular hypoxia occurs with suffocation, anemia, pneumonia, shock or other damage to the circulation, and interference with mitochondrial enzymes.

In acute hypoxic injury, cell O_2 is depleted in moments, aerobic oxidative phosphorylation stops, and ATP levels fall. The drop in cellular ATP stimulates phosphofructokinase, the initial regulator step of anaerobic glycolysis. The metabolic switch to anaerobic metabolism of glucose rapidly depletes the cell's glycogen stores and leads to the accumulation of intracellular lactate and inorganic phosphates. Although the anaerobic generation of ATP is inefficient, it provides for some short-term survival. Some highly specialized cell types, such as neurons, cannot generate ATP anaerobically and thus are especially prone to hypoxic injury. Ultimately, this deficiency of ATP leads to a failure of Na^+-K^+ pumps and loss of cell volume control.

The cardiac glycosides of plant origin, digitalis and ouabain, specifically inhibit the action of the Na^+-K^+ pump. This inhibition modifies the contractility of cardiac myocytes, but it may also cause them to swell.

Cell Membrane Injury in Acute Cell Swelling

Damage to the cell membranes, both plasma membranes and organelle membranes, destroys the selective permeability barrier that retains proteins and electrolytes within the cytosol and that restricts the entry of Na^+, Ca^{2+}, and water from the extracellular space. Failure of the barrier results from chemical modification of phospholipids by free radicals, covalent binding of toxic chemicals to macromolecules, interference with ion channels, and insertion of transmembrane protein complexes (e.g., complement activation).

The hepatotoxicities of CCl_4 and chloroform ($CHCl_3$) provide classic examples of cell membrane injury (Fig. 1-10). Toxic effects of CCl_4 occur when the chemical is converted to the trichloromethyl radical, $CCl_3^•$, by the mixed-function oxidase system of the SER in hepatocytes. The toxic metabolite, $CCl_3^•$, next causes progressive lipid peroxidation of unsaturated fatty acids of cellular membranes, progressing from the SER to mitochondria and other cell membranes. Chloroform is toxic to hepatocytes when it is metabolized to the electrophilic metabolite, phosgene ($COCl_2^•$). The hepatic lesions associated with these two toxins are indistinguishable, and both may result in fatty liver.

Besides toxins, other processes may cause cell membrane injury leading to acute cell swelling. The membrane-attack complex of serum complement (see Chapter 3) and the hemolysin of streptococci (streptolysin-O) penetrate cell membranes to form a channel for free passage of water, proteins, and electrolytes between intracellular and extracellular compartments. Affected cells are quickly lysed by water overload (hypotonic lysis). Cytotoxic effects of natural killer (NK) cells are mediated in part by the implantation of similar hollow protein-complexes into target cell membranes.

The sequence of events in acute cell swelling caused by hypoxia or ischemia (see Fig. 1-8) is as follows:

1. Hypoxia—deficiency of O_2
2. Decrease of oxidative phosphorylation and ATP
3. Increased glycolysis, increased intracellular lactate, and depletion of glycogen stores
4. Failure of Na^+-K^+ pump as the result of ATP deficiency
5. Net influx of Na^+, Ca^{2+}, and H_2O with loss of intracellular K^+ and Mg^{2+}
6. Swelling of mitochondria and the cytocavitary network (RER, SER, Golgi, and outer nuclear membrane)
7. Detachment of ribosomes, clumping of nuclear chromatin, loss of microvilli, vesiculation of endoplasmic reticulum (ER), formation of membrane whorls ("myelin figures")

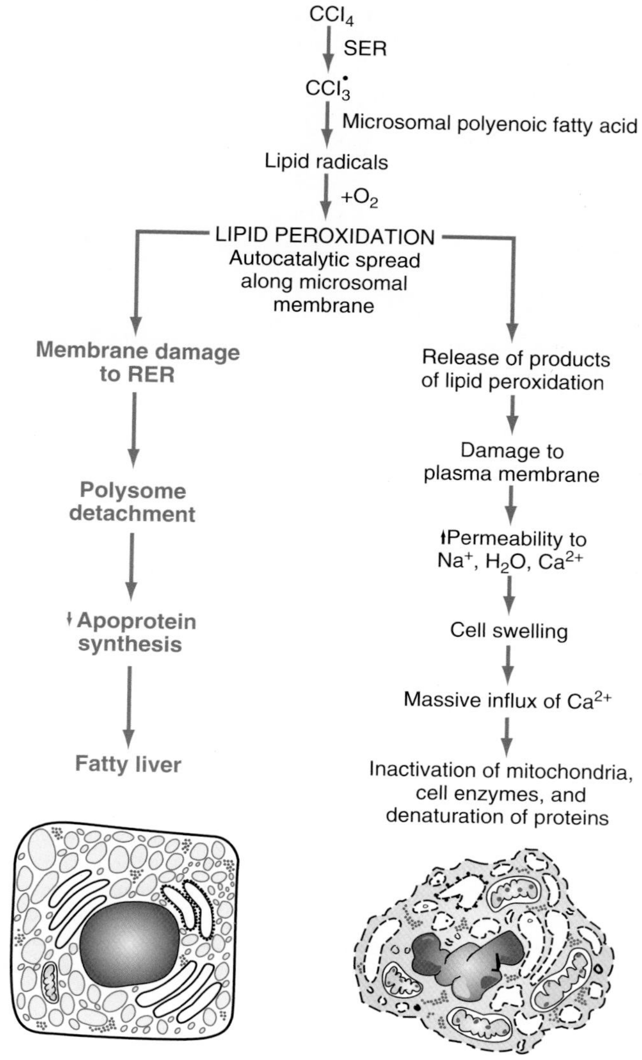

Fig. 1-10 Sequence of events leading to fatty change and cell necrosis in carbon tetrachloride (CCl_4) toxicity.
RER, Rough endoplasmic reticulum; *SER,* smooth endoplasmic reticulum. (From Kumar V, Abbas A, Fausto N: *Robbins & Cotran pathologic basis of disease,* ed 7, Philadelphia, 2005, Saunders.)

8. Severe disruption of cell membranes, influx of Ca^{2+} into mitochondria and cytosol, overall cell enlargement, and clearing of the cytosol
9. Irreversible cell injury, cell death (necrosis)

When acute cell swelling results from membrane injury, the sequence of events is similar to those listed previously, except that changes start at about step 5 or 6.

Morphology of Acute Cell Swelling

Gross Appearance

Acute cell swelling is recognized as pallor, organ swelling, and decreased specific gravity. For example, the liver will be pale and somewhat turgid (Fig. 1-11, *A*). The parenchyma of organs with capsules may bulge when incised.

Microscopic Appearance

The influx of water dilutes the cytoplasmic matrix and dilates organelles to give cells a pale, finely vacuolated appearance (cloudy swelling). Renal tubule epithelial cells bulge and impinge on the

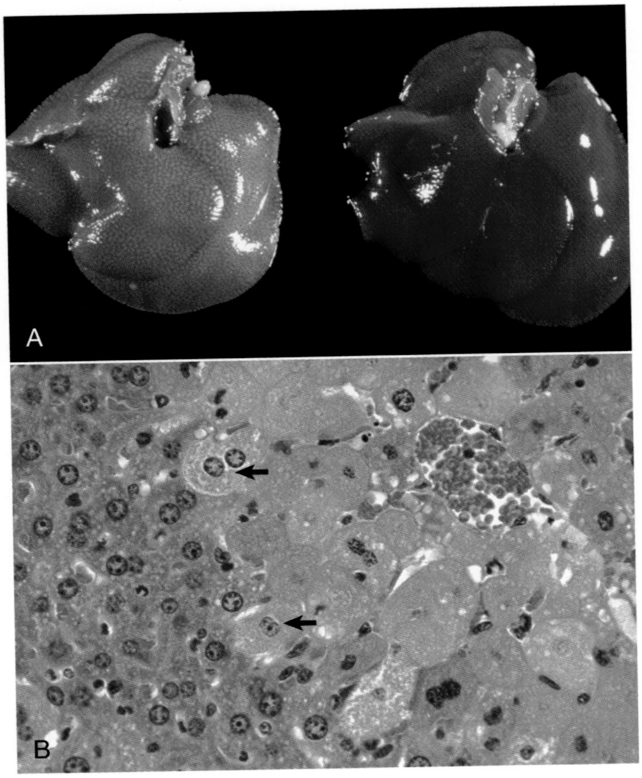

Fig. 1-11 Acute cell swelling, liver, mouse.
A, Hepatic swelling in a mouse exposed to chloroform 24 hours previously. The accentuated lobular pattern and slight pallor in the liver on the left are the result of acute cell swelling (hydropic degeneration) and necrosis of centrilobular hepatocytes. The right liver is normal. **B,** Liver from a mouse with chloroform toxicosis. While many hepatocytes in the centrilobular areas *(at right)* are necrotic, several cells at the interface of normal and necrotic *(arrows)* are still undergoing acute cell swelling (hydropic degeneration). H&E stain. (Courtesy Dr. L.H. Arp.)

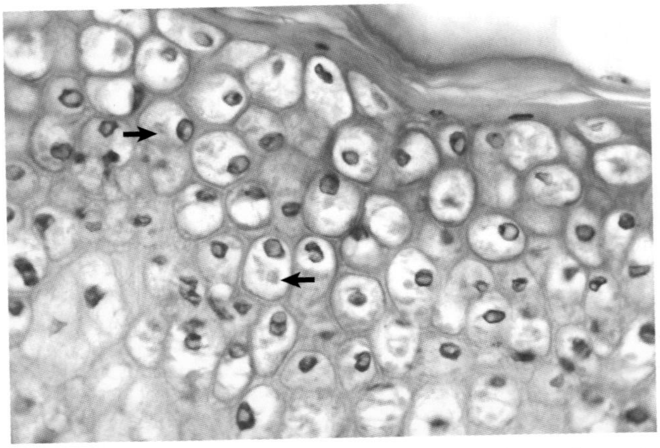

Fig. 1-12 Ballooning degeneration, papular stomatitis, oral mucosa, cow.
Cells infected by some types of virus, such as papular stomatitis virus, are unable to regulate their volume and swell at certain stages of the infection. These cells may become very large (ballooning degeneration) and eventually rupture. Some of the cells have viral inclusion bodies *(arrows)*. H&E stain. (Courtesy Dr. M.D. McGavin, College of Veterinary Medicine, University of Tennessee.)

tubular lumen. Swollen hepatocytes and endothelial cells intrude upon and diminish vascular lumens. Although mechanisms of cell swelling are limited, variations in appearance may occur because of differences in cell type and cause of injury.

Hydropic degeneration is a common term used for the microscopic appearance of acute cell swelling (Fig. 1-11, *B*). It occurs in endothelium, epithelium, alveolar pneumocytes, hepatocytes, renal tubular epithelial cells, and neurons and glial cells of the brain. Cytoplasm of affected cells contains translucent vacuoles that fail to stain for fat or glycogen (two other causes of vacuolar degeneration). These vacuoles represent swollen mitochondria and dilated cisternae of the Golgi and ER. Ballooning degeneration is an extreme variant of hydropic degeneration in which cells are greatly enlarged and the cytoplasm is basically a clear space (Fig. 1-12). Ballooning degeneration is typically seen in epidermal cells infected by epitheliotropic viruses (e.g., poxvirus). This lesion frequently progresses to the formation of vesicles or bullae (blisters) from lysis of the epidermal cells. These viral infections cause both degradation of cytoplasmic proteins (cytoplasmic proteolysis) and net flux of water into the cytoplasm.

Ultrastructural Appearance

As visualized with the electron microscope, swollen epithelial cells have lost and distorted cilia, microvilli, and attachment sites, as well as "blebbing" of cytoplasm at the cell surfaces. The cytoplasm is rarefied, and the cisternae of the ER, Golgi, and mitochondria are dilated. The cytocavitary network becomes fragmented into numerous vesicles. Proteins and Ca^{2+} precipitate in the cytoplasm and in organelles. Acute cell swelling in the central nervous system has other distinctive features (see section on Cerebral Edema in Chapter 14).

Significance and Fate of Acute Cell Swelling

Injured cells that can no longer regulate water and electrolytes are no better equipped to maintain other cell functions. Significance to the patient depends on the number of cells affected and the immediate importance of the lost cell function. Cells highly vulnerable to hypoxia and cell swelling include cardiac myocytes, proximal renal tubule epithelium, hepatocytes, and endothelium. In the central nervous system (CNS), besides endothelium, neurons, oligodendrocytes, and astrocytes also are swollen, and the process in the CNS is called *cytotoxic edema* (see Chapter 14). Swollen neurons fail to conduct nervous impulses, resulting in stupor or coma. Swollen myocardial cells contract with less force or with an abnormal rhythm. Swollen renal epithelium may not only fail to absorb and secrete but also may compress delicate interstitial blood vessels, resulting in further injury. Capillaries lined by swollen endothelium are prone to obstruction, exacerbating the lesions by worsening cellular hypoxia. Injured cells with abnormal membrane permeability may be detected by finding their specific cytoplasmic enzymes in serum.

If adequate oxygen is restored to the cells and membrane injury is repaired before a certain point is reached, the "point of no return," most cells can be restored to normal or nearly normal function. Some cells may retain evidence of previous injury in the form of lipofuscin accumulation after autophagocytosis of damaged organelles. What happens when the stage of reversibility is passed is the topic of the next sections, beginning with cell death.

In summary, cell swelling is a manifestation of reversible, sublethal cell injury. However, unless the cause of injury to critically important cell types is removed quickly, progressive injury to these dependent cells and tissues may culminate in the death of the animal.

IRREVERSIBLE CELL INJURY AND CELL DEATH

As we have just seen, major mechanisms of acute cell swelling are hypoxia, including ischemia, and membrane injury, often by toxins. Cell swelling can be reversible if the extent and duration of injury is not excessive. But if the injury exceeds certain limits (discussed shortly), cell death occurs (Fig. 1-13). Not all cell injury results in cell death. Cell injury may be sublethal and result in a variety of types of cell degenerations and/or adaptations by the cell to the injury. In essence, cells or tissues respond to injury (or stress) in three important ways: (1) adaptation (with or without accumulations or degenerative changes), (2) reversible injury (again with or without subcellular changes), and (3) death. In this section, we deal with cell death. Various types of cell adaptations, degenerations, and accumulations are addressed in subsequent sections.

CELL DEATH

Cell death can occur in many ways. For example, extremes of temperature or direct trauma may result in nearly instantaneous destruction or death of cells. On the other hand, death of an animal (somatic death) results in eventual death of all cells that make up the animal (postmortem autolysis). During most of the last century, cell death and necrosis were thought of as being more or less the same and in most pathologic situations; necrosis was usually thought to be preceded by cell swelling as discussed earlier. It is clear that cells die before macroscopic or histologic evidence can be detected. Although necrosis can be defined as the death of cells in a living animal, it should be understood to mean the specific morphologic changes (either macroscopic or microscopic) indicative of cell death in a living animal.

In the last few decades of the twentieth century, it became clear that cells die also by shrinkage, both under physiologic and

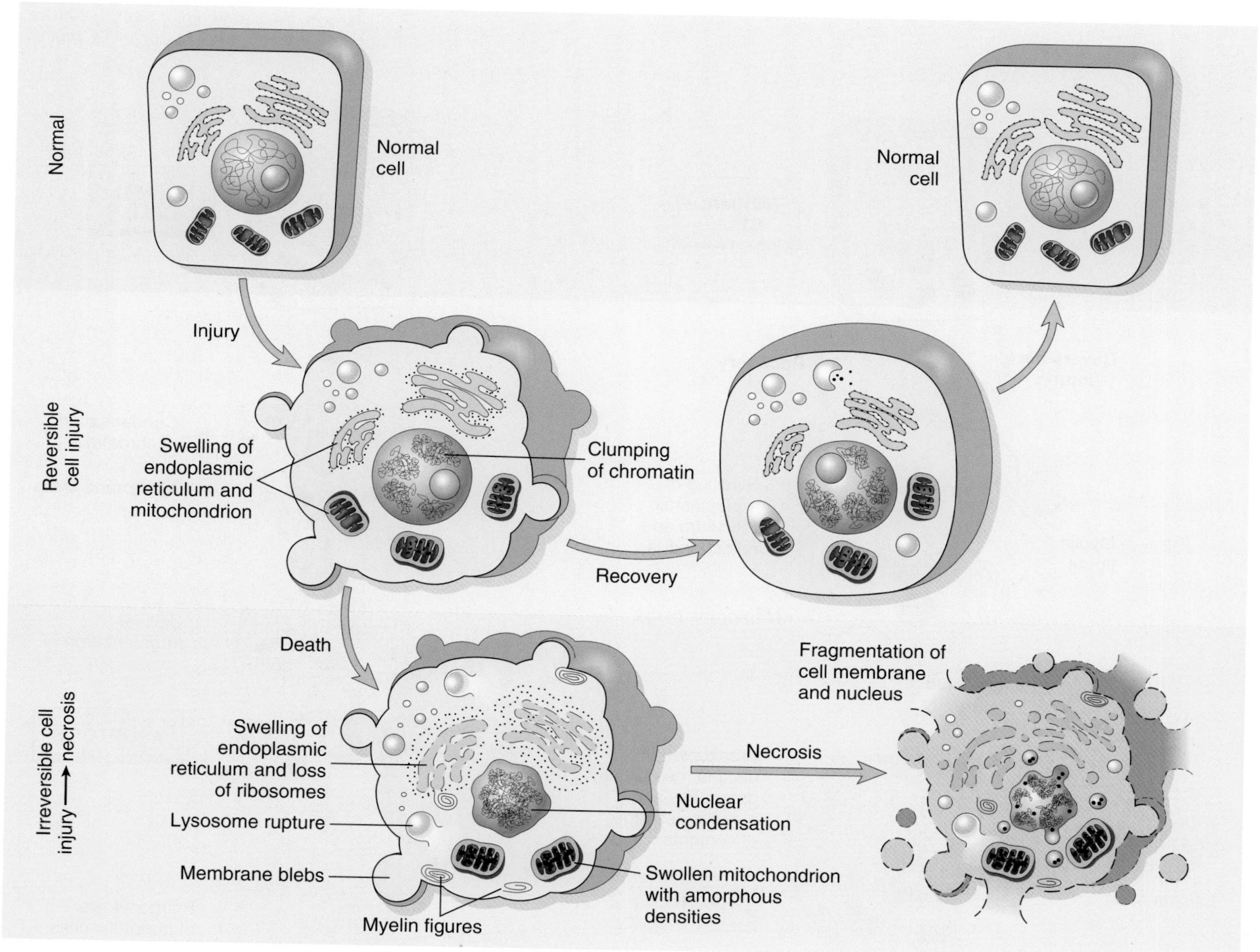

Fig. 1-13 Normal cell and the changes in reversible and irreversible cell injury. Reversible injury is characterized by generalized swelling of the cell and its organelles, blebbing of the plasma membrane, detachment of ribosomes from the endoplasmic reticulum, and clumping of nuclear chromatin. Transition to irreversible injury is characterized by increasing swelling of the cell, swelling and disruption of lysosomes, presence of large amorphous densities in swollen mitochondria, disruption of cellular membranes, and profound nuclear changes. The latter include nuclear condensation (pyknosis), followed by fragmentation (karyorrhexis) and dissolution of the nucleus (karyolysis). Laminated structures (myelin figures) derived from damaged membranes of organelles and the plasma membrane first appear during the reversible stage and become more pronounced in irreversibly damaged cells. (From Kumar V, Abbas A, Fausto N: *Robbins & Cotran pathologic basis of disease,* ed 7, Philadelphia, 2005, Saunders.)

pathologic circumstances, and this complex and now well-studied process has become known as *apoptosis,* a type of programmed cell death. Cell death then began to be classified in two major types: necrosis or apoptosis. Because of the long history of use of necrosis and because apoptosis, cell death with shrinkage, is distinctly different from death following swelling, the term *oncosis* (onco-, meaning swelling) has been proposed for what was previously termed *necrosis.* As in most biologic processes, it is not always possible to make the distinction between these two types of cell death based on histologic examination, and often both swelling and shrinkage are present.

How then are we to use the term *necrosis?* Attempts are being made by toxicologic pathologists to use the term *necrosis* for the histologic changes that occur after cell death by either mechanism, using the terms *oncotic* cell death or *apoptotic* cell death when a distinction needs to be made. We attempt to adhere to this distinction here, but long-used terminology does not easily change. The next sections first discuss cell death after irreversible cell injury by hypoxia and cell membrane damage (oncotic necrosis), and then apoptosis or apoptotic necrosis (Fig. 1-14).

Cell Death by Oncosis (Oncotic Necrosis)

Oncosis is cell death after irreversible cell injury by hypoxia, ischemia, and direct cell membrane injury. Hypoxic injury, as discussed earlier in the section on Acute Cell Swelling, is a common cause of cell death and oncotic necrosis. Cell membrane damage caused by toxins and other substances and mechanisms can also lead to necrosis, but the resulting morphologic changes are similar. Hypoxia is often due to blockage of or markedly diminished blood supply to an area (ischemia). Ischemic injury is typically more severe than hypoxia alone because not only is the amount of oxygen lowered in the tissue, but also the inflow of metabolic substrates and nutrients is decreased and cell waste and by-products accumulate, some of which are injurious in their own right.

Acute cell swelling can result in necrosis or can be reversible. Despite much interest and research about where the exact point of no return is between injury that is reversible and where it is irreversible, resulting in necrosis, is still not clear. There is convincing evidence for the role of Ca^{2+} in the eventual demise of severely injured cells. Earlier work consistently identified two features of

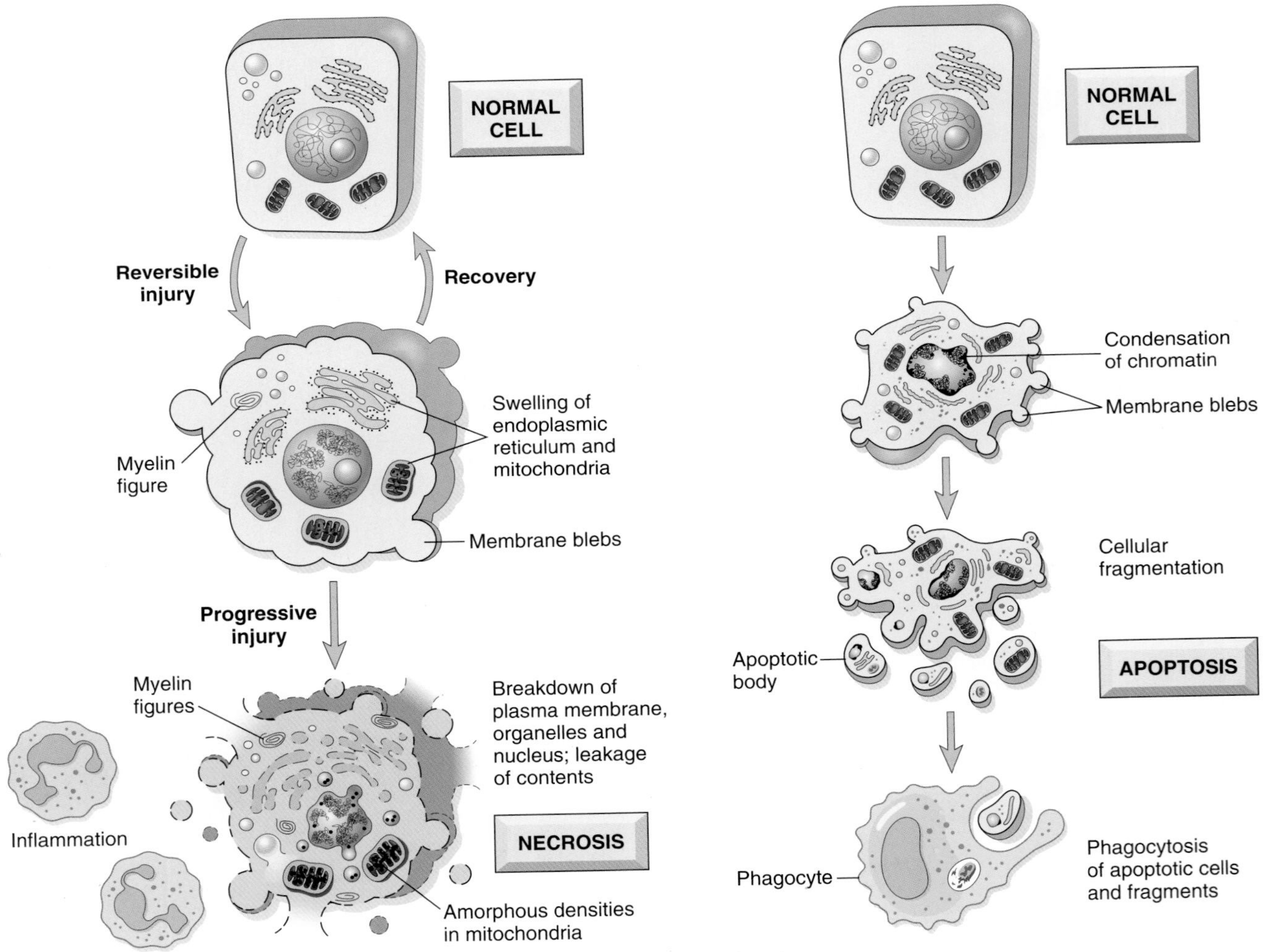

Fig. 1-14 The sequential ultrastructural changes seen in necrosis *(left)* and apoptosis *(right)*. In apoptosis, the initial changes consist of nuclear chromatin condensation and fragmentation, followed by cytoplasmic budding and phagocytosis of the extruded apoptotic bodies. Signs of cytoplasmic blebs, accumulation of myelin figures representing damaged phospholipid membranes, and digestion and leakage of cellular components characterize necrosis. (From Kumar V, Abbas A, Fausto N, et al: *Robbins & Cotran pathologic basis of disease,* ed 8, Philadelphia, 2009, Saunders.)

irreversible cell injury: (1) an inability to restore mitochondrial function and (2) evidence of cellular membrane damage.

Research directed at understanding coronary heart disease has led to improved understanding of the role of Ca^{2+}. Heart muscle deprived of its blood supply (ischemia) suffers from hypoxia and substantial loss of cell volume regulation and the influx of Ca^{2+} because of inadequate ATP to run the ion pumps. If the blood supply is resupplied to the ischemic area, often reversal of the injury is not attained, but instead, injury is accelerated. It has been shown that restored blood flow to areas with potentially viable cells results in added membrane damage shortly after blood supply is reestablished. This phenomenon is termed *ischemia-reperfusion injury.*

Prevention of Ca^{2+} influx can reduce irreversible injury. The reactivity of free Ca^{2+} ion and its role as an intracellular messenger and enzyme activator are known, and these actions are thought to contribute much to the final demise of the cell in necrosis. What does Ca^{2+} do to cause the ultimate demise of many severely injured cells as it influxes from the extracellular space (Fig. 1-15)? At least one endogenous, membrane-bound phospholipase (phospholipase A) is activated by free Ca^{2+}. Activated phospholipases then break down the normal phospholipids of the inner mitochondrial membrane and other cell membranes. These events then preclude any possibility for cell survival. Activation of phospholipases also generates arachidonic acid, the substrate for many lipid mediators of inflammation (to be discussed later). Therefore it is usual to see some degree of inflammation around foci of necrosis. In addition to phospholipases, Ca^{2+} also activates proteases that result in cytoskeleton and membrane damage, adenosine triphosphatases (ATPases) that accelerate depletion of ATP, and endonucleases that result in chromatin degradation. Irreversible injury to mitochondrial membranes appears to be the deathblow to the cell. As if this were not enough, cells injured by ischemia can also die by apoptosis because of the leakage of proapoptotic molecules from injured mitochondria.

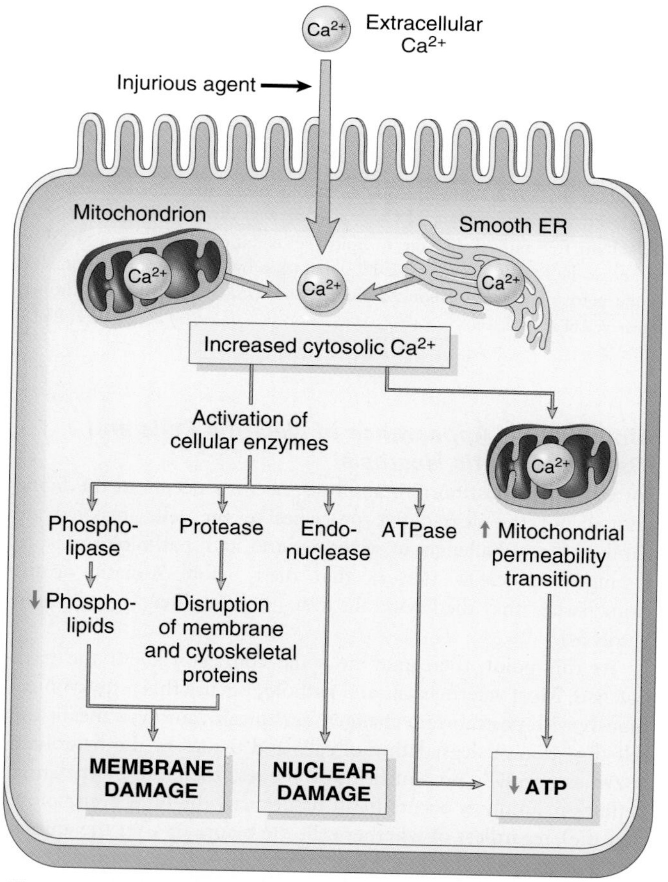

Fig. 1-15 Sources and consequences of increased cytosolic calcium in cell injury.

ER, Endoplasmic reticulum; *ATP,* Adenosine triphosphate. (From Kumar V, Abbas A, Fausto N, et al: *Robbins & Cotran pathologic basis of disease,* ed 8, Philadelphia, 2009, Saunders.)

Ischemia-reperfusion injury, for example, after restoration of blood supply caused by coronary artery blockage and myocardial ischemia (heart attack), has many components that contribute to irreversible injury. Besides the effects of Ca^{2+} influx, generation of free radicals in hypoxic cells combined with restored oxygen results in a variety of reactive oxygen and nitrogen species. These include production of peroxynitrite from nitric oxide (NO), a molecule of endothelial and parenchymal cells that is normally involved in vasodilation, inhibition of platelet aggregation, and prevention of leukocyte adhesion. Free radicals derived from inflammatory cells are also increased as the result of accumulation of neutrophils in reperfused areas after release of cytokines such as tumor necrosis factor-alpha (TNF-α). Reduction of reperfusion injury should theoretically be improved by agents blocking Ca^{2+} influx, by antioxidants such as vitamin E that decrease membrane damage because of the oxygen metabolites (free radicals), and by antiinflammatory agents that decrease the influx of inflammatory cells and impact of inflammatory mediators.

Cell Membrane Injury Leading to Cell Death

Chemical injury to cells in many cases may occur because of organelle and plasma cell membrane damage. Classically studied and referred to in the section on acute cell injury is the toxicity for hepatocytes of CCl_4 (see Fig. 1-10). After ingestion and absorption by the gastrointestinal (GI) tract, CCl_4 is transported via the portal vein to the liver where it enters hepatocytes. CCl_4 itself is fairly innocuous, but metabolism by the cytochrome p450 system in the SER in hepatocytes results in the formation of a toxic metabolite, $CCl_3^{\bullet}$. This free radical causes lipid peroxidation of organelle membranes starting from the SER and spreading to other organelles and eventually to the plasma membrane. This outcome has a variety of consequences. Injury to mitochondria results in decreased oxidative metabolism, decreased ATP production, and consequently an influx of calcium into mitochondria. This outcome results in decreased activity of the Na^+-K^+ pump and dysregulation of cell volume and massive intracellular increase in calcium with its lethal consequences. Direct damage to the plasma membrane itself by lipid peroxidation can have the same consequences to cell volume control and influx of calcium.

Lysosomal swelling and release of hydrolytic enzymes can result in autodigestion of cell components. Injury to RER of the hepatocyte can result in decreased protein synthesis, and this deficiency then causes insufficient production of lipoproteins required to export lipids and then results in increased fatty acid content in the cell and hepatic lipidosis (see discussion later), if the changes are not lethal.

Free Radical Injury

Injury to cell and organelle membranes can occur in many ways. One of the most common and important is free radical injury due especially to reactive oxygen species (Fig. 1-16). A free radical is any molecule that has an unpaired electron. These molecules are highly reactive, transient chemical species, generated as by-products of normal oxidative metabolism or by exposure to radiation, toxic gases, chemicals, and drugs. Most, but not all, are reactive oxygen

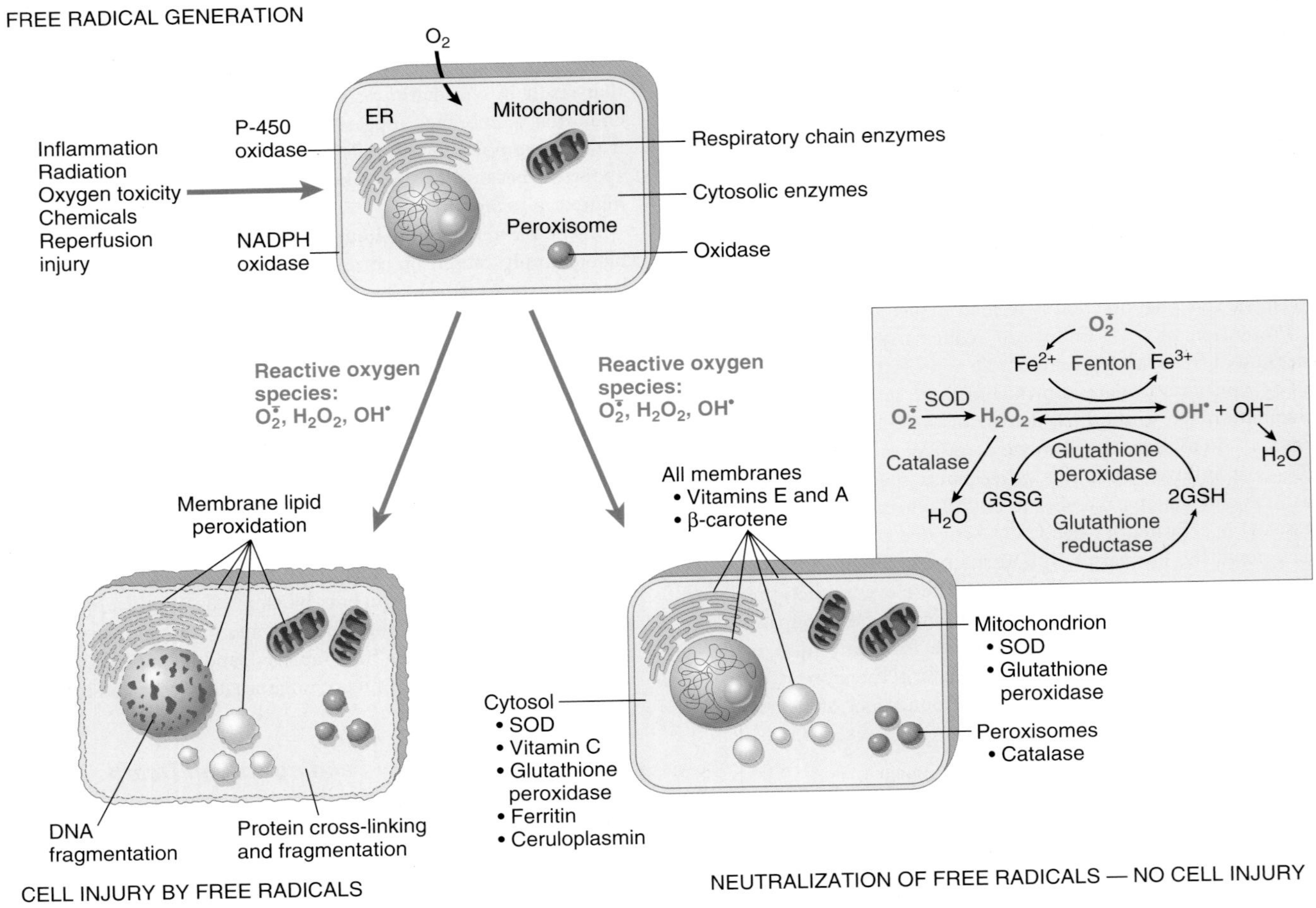

Fig. 1-16 The role of reactive oxygen species in cell injury. Oxygen is converted to superoxide ($O_2^{\bullet}$) by oxidative enzymes in the endoplasmic reticulum (ER), mitochondria, plasma membrane, peroxisomes, and cytosol. $O_2^{\bullet}$ is converted to H_2O_2 by dismutation and thence to $OH^{\bullet}$ by the Cu^{2+}/Fe^{2+}-catalyzed Fenton reaction. H_2O_2 is also derived directly from oxidases in peroxisomes. Not shown is another potentially injurious radical, singlet oxygen. Resultant free radical damage to lipid (peroxidation), proteins, and DNA leads to various forms of cell injury. Note that superoxide catalyzes the reduction of Fe^{3+} to Fe^{2+}, thus enhancing $OH^{\bullet}$ generation by the Fenton reaction. The major antioxidant enzymes are superoxide dismutase (SOD), catalase, and glutathione peroxidase. *GSH,* Reduced glutathione; *GSSG,* oxidized glutathione; *NADPH,* reduced form of nicotinamide adenine dinucleotide phosphate. (From Kumar V, Abbas A, Fausto N: *Robbins & Cotran pathologic basis of disease,* ed 7, Philadelphia, 2005, Saunders.)

radicals. Oxygen radicals are also produced by phagocytic cells in inflammatory lesions and account for significant damage to surrounding tissue. Antineoplastic drugs, such as doxorubicin, generate oxygen radicals that cause significant injury to cardiac myocytes. Cellular components at risk of free radical injury include proteins, membrane lipids, and nucleic acids. Lipid peroxidation of plasma membranes and organelle membranes by free radicals can have similar consequences to those described earlier from CCl_4.

Free radical injury is usually controlled by intracellular antioxidants such as superoxide dismutase (SOD), glutathione peroxidase, and vitamins E and C; however, injury can be catastrophic when these antioxidative systems are defective. In many species of domestic animals, severe cellular damage occurs to heart muscle when there is a deficiency of selenium or vitamin E in the tissues. Vitamin E is one of several cytoprotective molecules that acts as an antioxidant and inhibits production of or quenches free radicals, even in normal cell metabolism. Insufficient antioxidant activity can result in severe cell injury and necrosis as a consequence of the free radicals generated. Selenium is an essential component for some glutathione peroxidases, which also inactivate some free radicals generated within cells.

Morphologic Appearance of Necrotic Cells and Tissues (Oncotic Necrosis)

In contrast to postmortem autolysis, necrosis occurs in the living animal, but the degradative processes of the cells involved are similar. One challenge to veterinarians and pathologists is to distinguish necrosis (tissues that died before somatic death) from tissues that died with the rest of the animal (postmortem autolysis).

At this point, there may be some confusion about the term *autolysis.* Most veterinarians and pathologists use this term synonymously with postmortem changes. Technically, autolysis means the self-digestion or degradation of cells and tissues by the hydrolytic enzymes normally present in those tissues. Therefore by the strict definition, autolysis occurs in all tissues that die (and even before they die), regardless of whether cells die before or after the animal dies. Postmortem change includes both autolysis and putrefaction, which is the process by which bacteria break down tissues.

The appearance of necrotic cells varies with the tissue involved, the cause of cell death, and the duration of time. For our immediate purposes, necrosis here will for the most part be used to mean oncotic necrosis. Apoptotic necrosis will be discussed later.

Ultrastructure of Necrotic Cells (Oncotic Necrosis)

Cells dying after acute cell swelling are first swollen. There is tremendous swelling of all mitochondria, ER is dilated and fragmented, chromatin is clumped, the nuclear membrane is folded, the cytoplasm is pale and structureless, and organelles are poorly visualized. As the intracellular and extracellular compartments reach equilibrium across the altered cell membrane, the cell collapses and shrinks like a hot air balloon that has lost its air. The formerly swollen cell is shrunken; cytoplasm and organelles are homogeneous, electron dense, and hard to identify. Specialized areas of the plasma membrane, such as desmosomes, microvilli, and cilia, are distorted or absent.

Histologic Changes in Necrosis (Oncotic Necrosis)

Nuclear changes of dead cells are strong histologic evidence of cell death. These changes are variable and are described by the terms *pyknosis, karyorrhexis,* and *karyolysis* (Fig. 1-17). All of the following nuclear changes may be visible in necrotic cells in the same necrotic lesion. Basophilic fragments of nuclear debris can be confused with bacteria, protozoa, and calcium deposits. Histomorphology of the nucleus of a necrotic cell includes one or more of the following:

- Pyknosis: The nucleus is shrunken, dark, homogeneous, and round, unlike the dark and dense fragmented nucleus of apoptotic cells. Pyknosis may be a sequel to chromatin clumping of early degeneration.
- Karyorrhexis: The nuclear envelope is ruptured, and dark nuclear fragments are released into the cell cytoplasm.
- Karyolysis: The nucleus is extremely pale due to dissolution of chromatin presumably by action of RNAases and DNAases.
- Absence of nucleus: This is a later stage of karyolysis in which the nucleus has been completely dissolved or lysed.

Some cell lines have a preference for a type of nuclear change in necrosis. Necrotic lymphocytes often become pyknotic, sometimes karyorrhectic, followed by release of nuclear debris. Necrotic renal proximal tubular epithelial cells often have karyolytic nuclei, but the distal tubules may have predominantly pyknotic nuclei.

Cytoplasmic changes in dead cells

Early in cell necrosis, the cytoplasm becomes homogeneous pink in H&E-stained sections (Fig. 1-18). Increased eosinophilia may reflect a loss of rRNA, which is responsible for cytoplasmic basophilia, or a consolidation of cytoplasmic components as the cell collapses. Degradation of cytoplasmic proteins eventually gives the necrotic cell a pale, ghostlike appearance. Necrotic cells usually lose their adherence to basement membranes and neighboring cells become "individualized" so they are found free in tubules, alveoli, follicles, and other lumens or on surfaces. Rupture of cells with loss of cell integrity is the most obvious evidence of cell death.

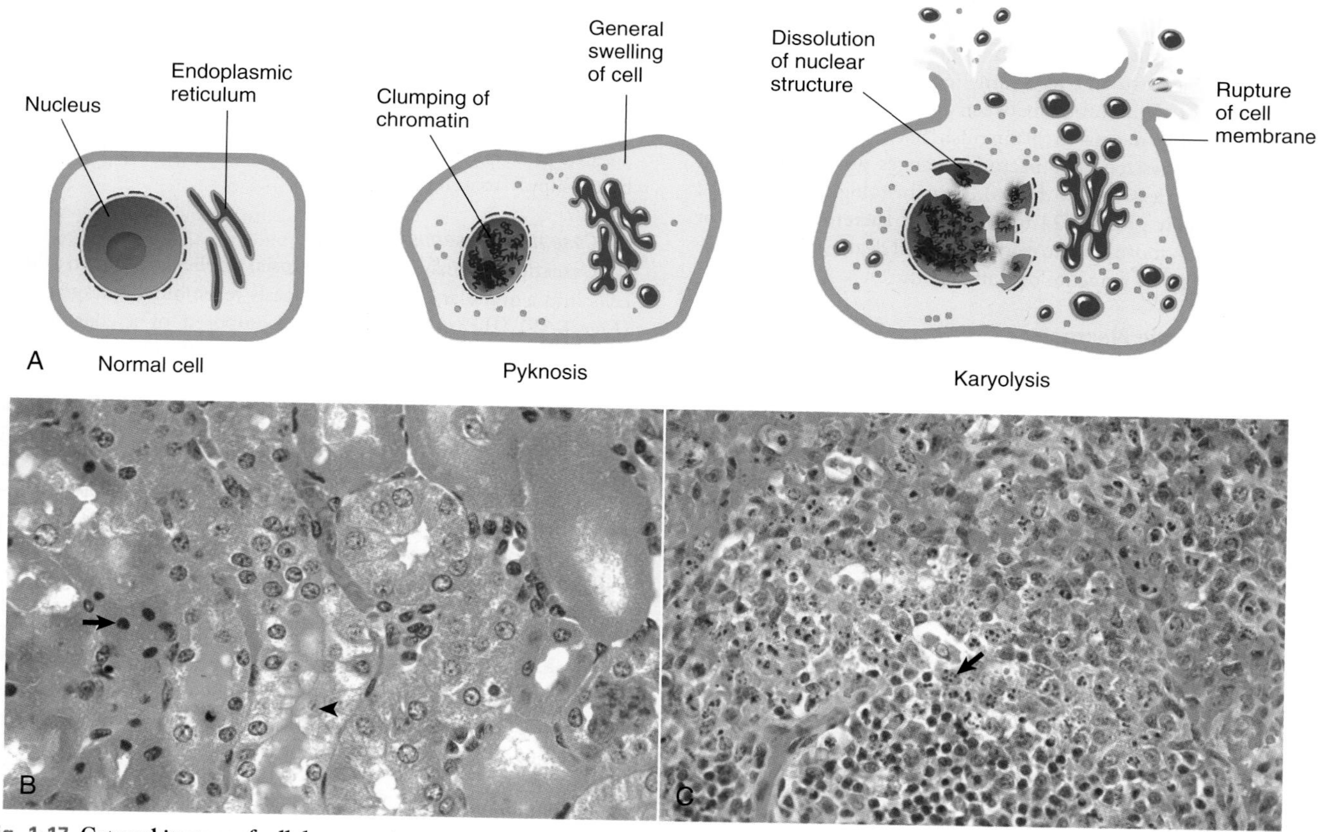

Fig. 1-17 Cytoarchitecture of cellular necrosis.
A, Schematic representation of nuclear and cytoplasmic changes in the stages of necrosis. **B,** Pyknosis and karyolysis, renal cortex, chloroform toxicosis, mouse. Some epithelial cells exhibit hydropic degeneration, whereas others are necrotic. Some necrotic cells exhibit pyknosis *(arrow),* whereas others have lost the nucleus or have a very pale nucleus (karyolysis) *(arrowhead).* H&E stain. **C,** Karyorrhexis, lymphocytes, spleen, dog. Spleen of a dog with parvovirus infection. Lymphocyte nuclei have fragmented because of the infection *(arrow).* H&E stain. (**A** from Huether S, McCance K: *Understanding pathophysiology,* ed 3, St Louis, 2004, Mosby; **B** and **C** courtesy Dr. L.H. Arp.)

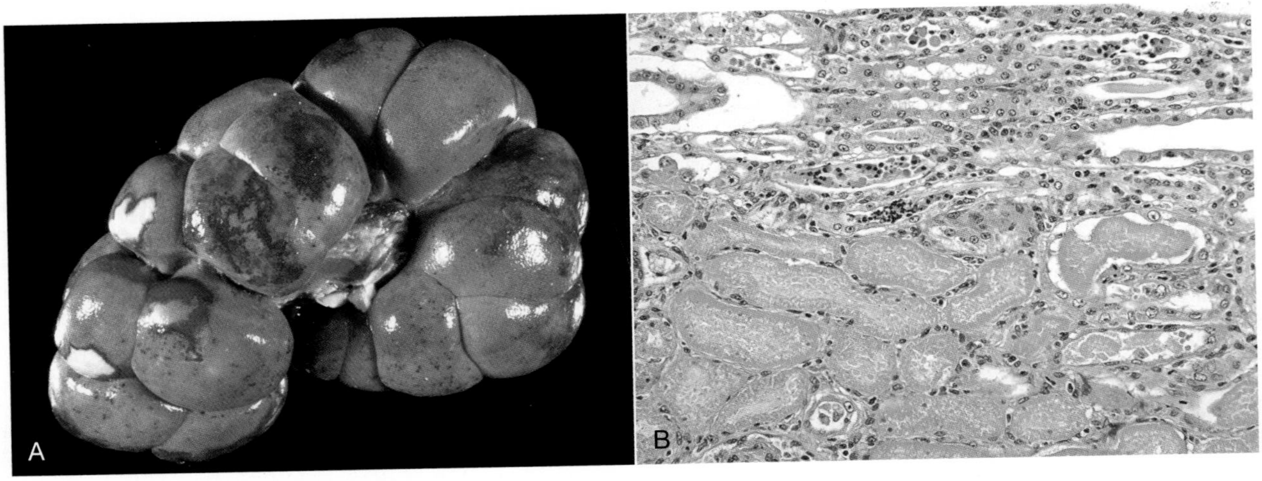

Fig. 1-18 Coagulation necrosis, infarcts, kidney, cow.
A, Note the white-yellow areas of acute coagulation necrosis surrounded by a red rim of active hyperemia and inflammation *(far left).* **B,** Acute coagulation necrosis of renal tubular epithelial cells. Necrotic cells have homogeneous eosinophilic cytoplasm and more or less retained cell outlines *(lower half of figure)* and nuclear changes such as pyknosis and nuclear absence *(upper half of figure).* H&E stain. (**A** courtesy Dr. D.E. Tyler, College of Veterinary Medicine, The University of Georgia; and Noah's Arkive, College of Veterinary Medicine, The University of Georgia. **B** courtesy Dr. J.F. Zachary, College of Veterinary Medicine, University of Illinois.)

Gross Appearance of Necrotic Tissue

Depending on the duration of injury and the type of organ (e.g., liver and kidney), necrotic tissue is usually pale, soft and friable, and sharply demarcated from viable tissue by a zone of inflammation (see Fig. 1-18, *A*). An exception to the pale color occurs when blood oozes into the necrotic tissue from damaged blood vessels in adjacent viable tissue as happens in renal infarcts, which are often surrounded by a narrow (1 to 3 mm) red rim (active hyperemia). A sharp line of demarcation between necrotic and viable tissue is often a reliable means to distinguish necrosis from autolysis. It must be emphasized that necrotic changes are first apparent ultrastructurally (less than 6 hours), then histologically (6 to 12 hours), and finally grossly (24 to 48 hours). Therefore, except for vascular changes, morphologic evidence of cell death is often sparse or absent in cases of peracute or acute death.

Types of Oncotic Necrosis

Foci of necrosis in tissue have a limited number of morphologic appearances, depending on the tissue involved, the cause of cell injury, and somewhat on the time since injury has occurred. Classification of necrotic lesions enables the pathologist to describe the lesion with a minimum of repetitious detail, but more than one pattern or type of necrosis may be seen in an organ or tissue. The recognized types of necrosis in most tissues are the following:

- Coagulation necrosis
- Caseation necrosis
- Liquefactive necrosis
- Gangrenous necrosis

These are classically or historically derived, and although commonly used, do not always accurately describe the complexity of what has happened to the involved cells and tissues.

Coagulation necrosis

Coagulation necrosis (coagulative necrosis) is characterized by preservation of the basic cell outlines of necrotic cells (see Fig. 1-18, *B*). Cytoplasm is homogeneous and eosinophilic due to coagulation of cell proteins, similar to what happens to heat coagulation of proteins of a cooked egg white. Presumably the injury or subsequent cellular acidosis denatures not only structural proteins but also enzymes. This delays proteolysis of the cell. Nuclei are pyknotic, karyorrhectic, karyolytic, or absent. This form of necrosis may occur in any tissue except brain parenchyma, although it does occur initially in individual neurons. It is classically seen in kidney, liver, and muscle, and the necrotic tissue will eventually lyse within several days and be phagocytosed. The presence of coagulation necrosis suggests hypoxic cell injury as seen in local loss of blood supply or in shock. Bacterial exotoxins and chemical toxins also cause the lesion. Infarction is necrosis caused by ischemia. An infarct, for example, occurring in the human heart as a result of the blockage of a coronary artery by an atherosclerotic plaque is an area of coagulation necrosis that results from a sudden loss of blood supply to an area.

Caseation (caseous) necrosis

Caseation necrosis (caseous necrosis) implies conversion of dead cells into a granular friable mass grossly resembling cottage cheese (Fig. 1-19). The necrotic focus is composed of a coagulum of nuclear and cytoplasmic debris. Compared with coagulation necrosis, this is an older (chronic) lesion often associated with poorly degradable lipids of bacterial origin. Any tissue may be affected, and much of the necrotic debris is dead leukocytes. Dystrophic calcification commonly occurs later within the central parts of the lesion. The classic cause of this lesion is tuberculosis. Related bacteria, such as *Corynebacterium,* also cause this lesion in sheep. Delayed degradation of the bacterial cell wall is thought to play a role in the development of a lesion caused by these bacteria and results in a focus of caseous necrosis surrounded by granulomatous inflammatory cells and an outer fibrous connective tissue capsule. In birds and reptiles, necrotic areas are slow to liquefy and often undergo caseation necrosis, likely caused by insignificant amounts of myeloperoxidase in their heterophils, the equivalent inflammatory cell of the neutrophil in mammals.

Liquefactive necrosis

Liquefactive necrosis is the usual type of necrosis in the CNS, although the neuron cell bodies themselves initially show coagulation necrosis, followed by liquefaction (Fig. 1-20). Hypoxic death of cells in the CNS results in rapid enzymatic dissolution of the neuropil (liquefaction), likely the result of the large amount of cell membranes present. With loss of astrocytes and because there

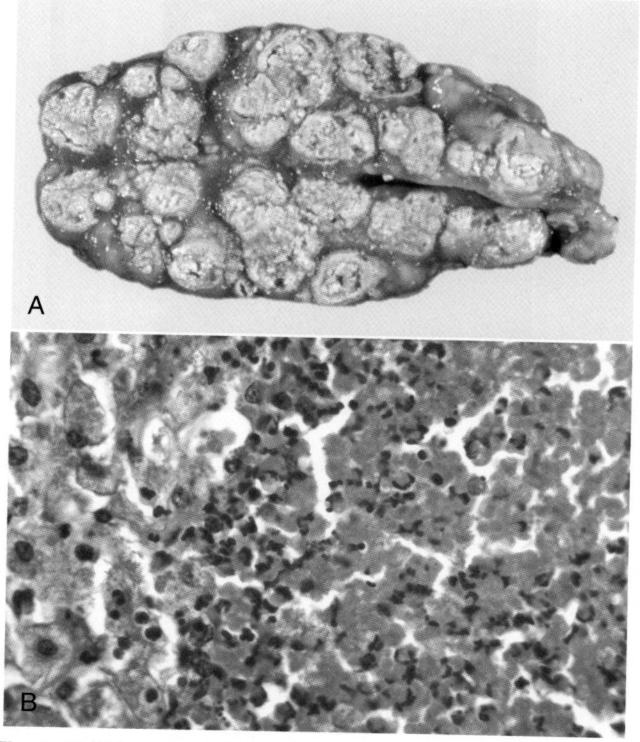

Fig. 1-19 Tuberculosis, lymph node, transverse section, ox. **A,** The lymph has been replaced by a caseating granuloma. Note the caseous necrosis characterized by a pale yellow, crumbly exudate. **B,** Granulomatous inflammation in caseous necrosis. Cell walls are disrupted and tissue architecture is lost. Mineralization (not seen here) is common in this type of necrosis. H&E stain. (**A** courtesy Dr. M. Domingo, Autonomous University of Barcelona; and Noah's Arkive, College of Veterinary Medicine, The University of Georgia. **B** courtesy Dr. M.D. McGavin, College of Veterinary Medicine, University of Tennessee.)

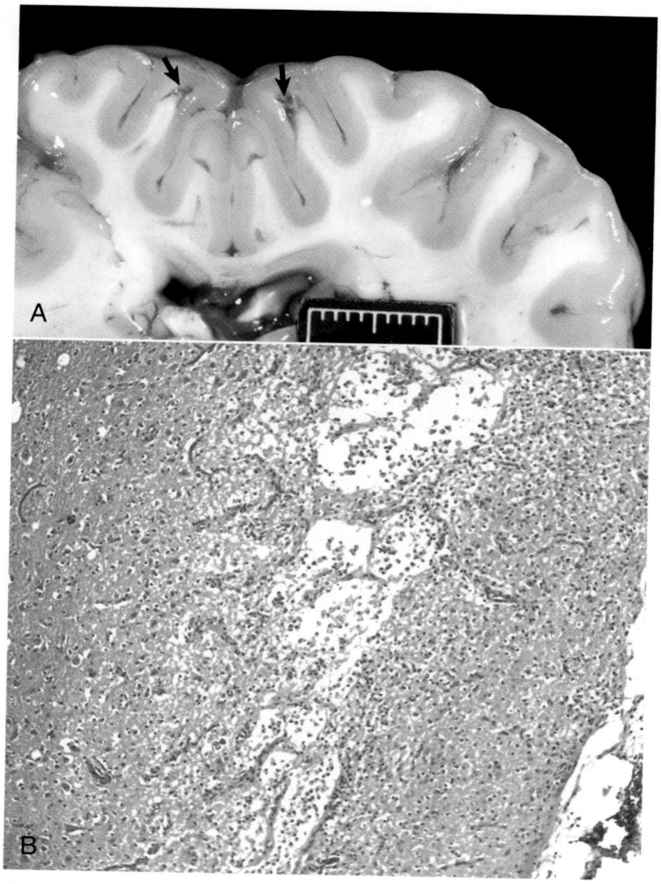

Fig. 1-20 Liquefactive necrosis. **A,** Acute polioencephalomalacia, brain, goat. A thiamine deficiency has resulted in cerebrocortical malacia, which microscopically is liquefactive necrosis and varying degrees of tissue separation *(arrows)*. Scale bar = 2 cm. **B,** Cortical necrosis, cerebrum, dog. The pale horizontal band in the cerebral cortex contains areas of near total loss of cells and tissue loss termed *liquefactive necrosis.* The cells in the spaces are gitter cells. Grossly, this band would have a fluid consistency. H&E stain. (**A** courtesy Dr. R. Storts, College of Veterinary Medicine, Texas A&M University. **B** courtesy Dr. L.H. Arp.)

is normally very little fibrous connective tissue in the CNS, little remains to support the tissue or fill in dead space. The result is a cavity filled with lipid debris and fluid. These cystic areas are cleared of debris by macrophages that become gitter cells (described further in Chapter 14).

In other tissues, focal infection by pyogenic bacteria leads to release of enzymes from accumulating leukocytes. Early in this process, heterolysis leads to a focal liquid collection of necrotic neutrophils and tissue debris (pus), and the lesion is an abscess that is also a type of liquefactive necrosis. If the abscess persists, loss of fluid or inspissation of the pus results in it becoming more caseous.

Gangrenous necrosis

The three types of gangrene are dry gangrene, moist gangrene, and gas gangrene. They are included here because the initial lesion is coagulation necrosis.

- *Moist gangrene* is defined as an area of necrotic tissue (usually coagulation necrosis), which is further degraded by the liquefactive action of saprophytic bacteria (defined as organisms living in dead organic matter) that usually cause putrefaction (defined as the decomposition of organic matter by microorganisms [i.e., rotten]). The initial coagulation necrosis can be caused by infarction of an extremity (too tight a bandage on a limb, penetrating damage to an artery supplying the leg by a bullet or shrapnel) or of a segment of intestine, or as in the case of the lung, by direct action of aspirated irritants such as medicaments or even ruminal fluid. The saprophytic bacteria contaminate the dead tissue from the local environment (air, skin contaminants, and soil) in the case of a limb, from inhaled air in the lung, and from the adjacent ingesta in an intestinal infarct. Grossly, tissues become soft, moist, and reddish-brown to black, and if the saprophytic bacteria produce gas, as they usually do, then gas bubbles and a putrid odor from the hydrogen sulfide, ammonia, and mercaptans may occur (Fig. 1-21, *A*). With time, if death does not supervene from toxemia, gangrenous tissue of the leg and udder are separated from the normal tissue by inflammation and may slough. Microscopically, initially areas of coagulation necrosis contain a few proliferating bacteria. These quickly proliferate and produce liquefaction and depending on the bacteria, gas bubbles. As the lesion progresses, most of the necrotic tissue is liquefied by saprophytic bacteria and infiltrating neutrophils.
- *Dry gangrene* is really coagulation necrosis secondary to infarction, which is followed by mummification. It involves the lower portion of an extremity (leg), tail, ears, and udder and can be caused by ingested toxins (ergot and fescue poisoning) or cold (frostbite). Ergot produces a marked

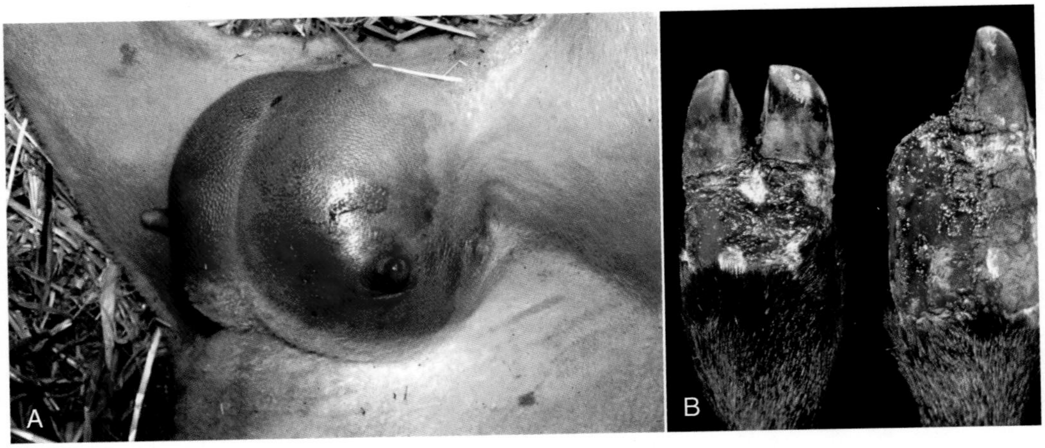

Fig. 1-21 Gangrenous necrosis.
A, Moist gangrene, udder, sheep. The surrounding tissue is well vascularized, which contributes to the wet and bloody nature of the lesion. Often saprophytic bacteria and clostridia contaminate areas of necrosis. **B,** Dry gangrene, fescue toxicity, digits, cow. Fescue toxicity is a disease in which the blood supply to the distal extremities is lost because of vasoconstriction from the toxic effect on vessels. The dry leathery appearance adjacent to the hooves is termed *dry gangrene.* There is still some blood in the skin, indicating that at least a partial blood supply has been retained or restored. Note that one of the claws *(right)* has been lost due to the process. (**A** courtesy Dr. C. Wallace, College of Veterinary Medicine, University of Georgia; and Noah's Arkive, College of Veterinary Medicine, The University of Georgia. **B** courtesy Dr. R.K. Myers, College of Veterinary Medicine, Iowa State University.)

peripheral arteriolar vasoconstriction and damage to capillaries, which leads to thrombosis and infarction. Fescue poisoning in cattle has a similar pathogenesis and lesions. Exposure to very cold temperatures also causes dry gangrene (frostbite). The pathogenesis involves both direct freezing and disruptions of cells by intracellular and extracellular ice crystal formation and vascular damage leading to ischemia and infarction characterized by coagulation necrosis (see Chapter 17). In dry gangrene, after necrosis, the tissues are depleted of water, for example, by low humidity, and this dehydration results in mummification. There is no proliferation of bacteria, as dry tissues do not provide an environment favorable for their proliferation and spread. Grossly, the tissue is shriveled, dry, and brown to black (Fig. 1-21, *B*) and affected parts may slough
- *Gas gangrene* is also an example of bacteria proliferating and producing toxins in necrotic tissue, but in this case the bacteria are anaerobes, usually microbes such as *Clostridium perfringens* and *Clostridium septicum.* Penetrating wounds into muscle or subcutis introduce these bacteria. The necrotic tissue then provides an anaerobic medium for growth of the clostridia. Another example, with similar lesions, is caused by *Clostridium chauvoei* (blackleg), which, unlike the bacteria of gas gangrene, is not introduced by a penetrating wound but from spores spread hematogenously from the intestine and lodged in muscle. Here they stay until by some mechanism, such as trauma, necrosis occurs and thus produces anaerobic conditions in which the spores can germinate and the bacteria proliferate. Grossly, affected tissues are dark red to black with gas bubbles and a fluid exudate that may contain blood. Microscopically, the lesions are characterized by coagulation necrosis of muscle, a serohemorrhagic exudate, and gas bubble formation (see Chapter 15). Some authors do not classify the lesions of blackleg as gas gangrene because it is a result of hematogenously disseminated bacterial spores and not from bacterial contamination of a wound.

Necrosis of Fat (Fat Necrosis)

The three types of fat necrosis, enzymatic necrosis of fat, traumatic necrosis of fat, and necrosis of abdominal fat of cattle, are as follows:

- *Enzymatic necrosis of fat,* also called *pancreatic necrosis of fat,* refers to the destruction of fat in the abdominal cavity and usually adjacent to the pancreas by the action of activated pancreatic lipases in pancreatic fluid that has escaped from the duct system of the pancreas (Fig. 1-22).
- *Traumatic necrosis of fat* is seen when adipose tissue is crushed. It occurs in fat adjacent to the pelvic canal of heifers after dystocia and in subcutaneous tissue that has been injured, for example, in the subcutaneous and intramuscular fat over the sternum of recumbent cattle.
- *Fat necrosis of abdominal fat* of cattle is characterized by large masses of necrotic fat in the mesentery, omentum, and retroperitoneally. The cause is unknown and may not be detected until necropsy. In extreme cases, mesenteric fat may surround the intestine and cause stenosis.

Grossly affected fat is white, firm, and chalky. Histologically, the fat solvents used in the preparation of the paraffin-embedded sections do not remove necrotic fat. Necrotic adipocytes are eosinophilic but become basophilic if free fatty acids react with Ca^{2+} to form soap (saponification of fat).

Sequelae to Oncotic Necrosis

In contrast to apoptosis and obviously postmortem autolysis, necrosis incites a notable inflammatory reaction in most tissues except the CNS in the surrounding viable tissue. Therefore the necrotic foci are often surrounded by a well-demarcated band of white blood cells and the hyperemia of inflammation. The purpose is to digest (by heterolytic enzymes of leukocytes) and liquefy the necrotic tissue so that it can be removed by macrophages and diffusion into blood and lymph vessels and replaced by normal tissue (regeneration) or fibrous connective tissue (healing). Healing of an abscess occurs after the sequestered pus is phagocytosed and/or carried off by the lymphatics. The process is greatly hastened by drainage, either by rupture to the outside or by surgical drainage of the abscess. Material not liquified is phagocytosed by macrophages and removed via lymphatics or veins. A fragment of necrotic material, especially bone, may resist degradation and form a sequestrum. This may cause chronic irritation and delay repair.

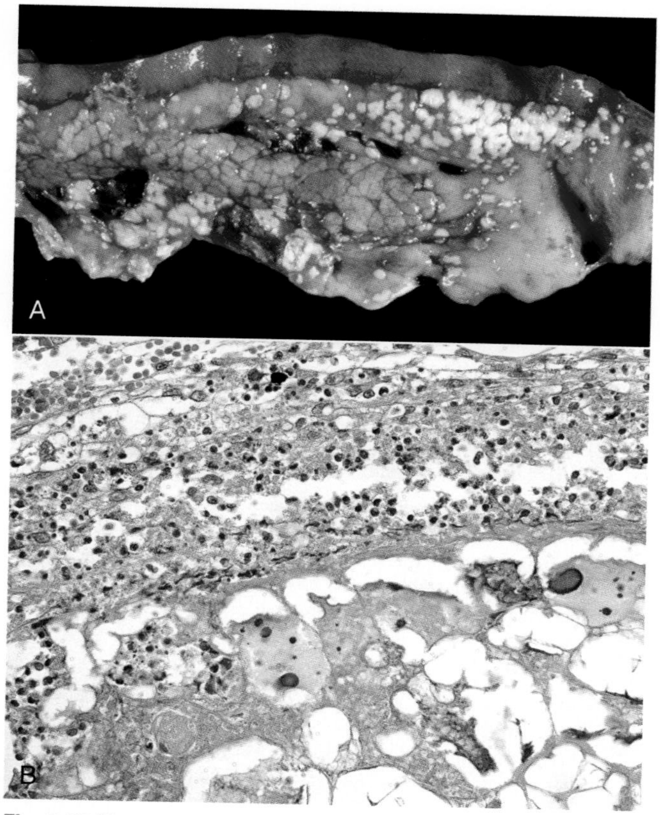

Fig. 1-22 Fat necrosis.
A, Enzymatic necrosis of fat (fat necrosis), dog with previous bouts of pancreatitis. Necrotic fat often becomes saponified and so grossly the lesion is chalky to gritty and pale white. **B,** Pancreas, dog. Note the large area of fat necrosis with acute inflammation and saponification (basophilic areas). H&E stain. (**A** courtesy Dr. J. Wright, College of Veterinary Medicine, North Carolina State University; and Noah's Arkive, College of Veterinary Medicine, The University of Georgia. **B** courtesy Dr. J.F. Zachary, College of Veterinary Medicine, University of Illinois.)

Morphologic Appearance of Postmortem Changes

Postmortem autolysis refers to the autolysis of cells occurring after somatic death. These changes are amplified and accelerated by bacterial decomposition from bacteria that have entered the tissue shortly before death or after death (usually by either direct migration from the lumen of the gut of the dead or dying animal, or from the gut into the blood and then disseminated throughout the body by the final beats of the heart). Postmortem bacterial metabolism and dissolution of host tissues (postmortem decomposition) result in the production of color and texture changes, gas production, and odors collectively termed *putrefaction.*

Somatic death refers to death of the entire body; however, cell types vary greatly in time of viability after cessation of heartbeat, respiration, and brain wave activity. In somatic death, many neurons and cardiac myocytes suffer irreversible injury within minutes; kidney and liver cells may survive for an hour; and fibroblasts and bone survive much longer. Interpretation of lesions is usually clouded by changes that occur between the time of death and the time of necropsy (or fixation of tissue). Postmortem autolysis results from total diffuse hypoxia, and cells degenerate as described for hypoxic cell injury. A long death-to-fixation interval can lead to problems in histopathologic diagnosis of necrosis and other lesions; thus keeping postmortem changes to a minimum is important for accurate gross and histopathologic interpretation.

Postmortem changes vary greatly in onset and rate depending on the cause of death, environmental and body temperature, and microbial flora. Cool environmental temperatures and refrigeration (without freezing if possible because freezing induces artefacts such as intracellular and extracellular ice crystals, which disrupt cells and tissues, respectively) inhibit autolysis and delay putrefaction. Animals examined 24 hours after death, after being maintained at 5° C, have relatively few postmortem changes and artefacts to interpret versus an animal that has been maintained at room temperature for a similar time. An exception is herbivores. In the ruminant forestomach and equine cecum and ascending colon, ingesta will continue to undergo bacterial fermentation after death, with formation of heat and gas. Consequently, these animals, even if refrigerated immediately after death, show considerable intraabdominal postmortem decomposition 24 hours later. High environmental temperatures accelerate autolysis, as does elevated antemortem body temperature caused by fever, high metabolic rate, heat stroke, and exercise. Delay in cooling is especially common in fat animals and those with a heavy coat, especially wool. Young and small animals, such as neonates, cool more rapidly than large obese ones. Determining the time since death has occurred can be difficult because of the many factors just listed that influence the rate of cooling.

In summary, postmortem changes can interfere with accurate interpretation of both gross and histologic changes in tissue. Postmortem changes can be minimized by rapid cooling of the carcass and decreasing the death to tissue fixation time to a minimum. The following are examples of common postmortem changes, with some reference to their sequence of occurrence:

- Rigor mortis is the contraction of muscles occurring after death. It commences 1 to 6 hours after death and persists for 1 to 2 days. When ATP and glycogen (required to relax muscle contraction) are depleted, the contraction is irreversible except by autolysis. Muscular animals often have stronger rigor than those with less muscle mass. High heat and activity before death accelerate the onset of rigor. In animals with cachexia or extreme malnutrition, the energy stores (ATP, glycogen) in the muscles may be so depleted that no contraction of myofibers is possible, and thus these animals do not develop rigor mortis.
- Algor mortis is gradual cooling of the cadaver. Cooling of the carcass depends on temperature of the body at death (e.g., fever, environmental temperature, insulation of the carcass [fat, wool, coverings], body mass, air movement, and other factors) and is difficult to interpret precisely for establishing time of death.
- Livor mortis (hypostatic congestion) (Fig. 1-23) is the gravitational pooling of blood to the down side of the animal. In large vessels, there is clotting followed by separation of blood cells and plasma. This process begins within an hour after death, and the clotted blood can become "fixed" in place (whereby movement of the animal will not influence the distribution of the change) within 12 to 24 hours. It is often not appreciated in animals because of pigmented skin or a thick hair coat and thus is most likely to be evident in white-skinned animals with little hair (e.g., white pigs).
- Postmortem clotting (Fig. 1-24) in the heart and vessels usually occurs within several hours and can be influenced by antemortem changes in blood. Warfarin poisoning and hereditary coagulopathies, for example, will delay or cause failure of blood to clot. Before the blood clots, erythrocytes may settle to the bottom of a large vessel. This results in the clot having two portions: a bottom red mass made up chiefly

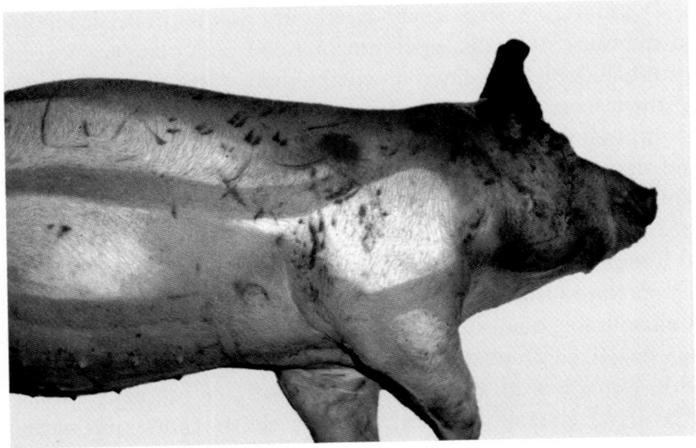

Fig. 1-23 Livor mortis, pig.
Note red to purple staining of the skin on the right side, the side on which the pig was lying when it died. This color change is termed *livor mortis* or *hypostatic congestion*. The pale white areas are pressure points on the down side into which blood could not flow after death. (Courtesy Dr. M.D. McGavin, College of Veterinary Medicine, University of Tennessee.)

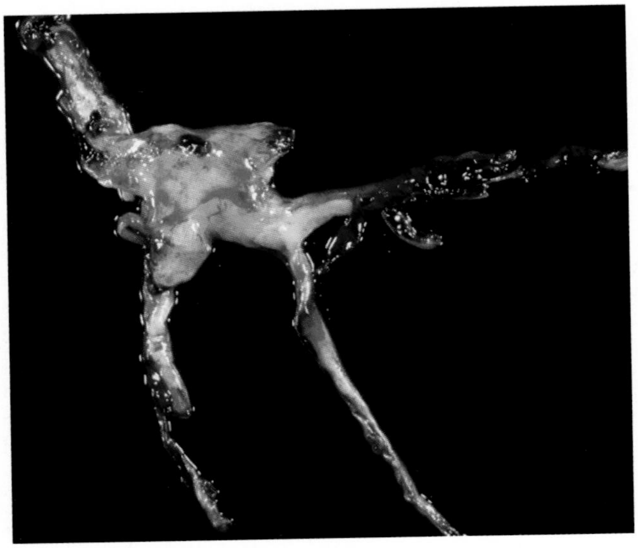

Fig. 1-24 Postmortem clot, dog.
The postmortem clot is pale white to yellow (chicken fat clot) in some areas and shiny red (currant jelly clot) in others. Note how it conforms to the shape of the lumen of the vessels from which it was removed. (Courtesy Dr. R.K. Myers, College of Veterinary Medicine, Iowa State University.)

of erythrocytes and an upper pale yellow mass of clotted serum. The latter type of clot is called a chicken fat clot. This separation depends upon the erythrocyte sedimentation rate (ESR) of the blood. It is high in normal horses and increased in all animals as a systemic inflammatory response. Inflammation results in increased plasma fibrinogen, which causes erythrocytes to form stacks (rouleau formation) that sediment more rapidly. Postmortem clots must be distinguished from antemortem mural thrombi and thromboemboli. Postmortem clots are unattached to vessel walls and tend to be shiny and wet and form a perfect cast of vessel lumens. Antemortem mural arterial thrombi are attached to arterial walls, tend to be dry and duller in color, and are laminated with a tail extending downstream from the point of attachment. Antemortem venous thrombi are also attached, but loosely

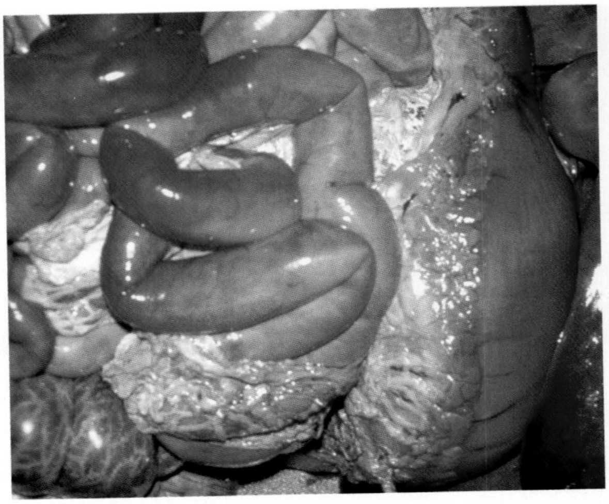

Fig. 1-25 Imbibition of hemoglobin, viscera, pig that has been dead for several hours before being necropsied.
Note the pink color on the serosal surfaces of the stomach and small intestine. This is termed *imbibition of hemoglobin* and is due to staining by hemoglobin that has seeped out of autolyzed red blood cells. (Courtesy Dr. R.K. Myers, College of Veterinary Medicine, Iowa State University.)

so, and in many cases may closely resemble postmortem clots.

- Hemoglobin imbibition (Fig. 1-25) is a term applied to the red staining of tissue, especially evident in the endocardium and tunica intima of arteries (particularly evident in the aorta) and veins beginning some hours after death. Once the integrity of the intima is lost, hemoglobin released by lysed erythrocytes penetrates the vessel wall and extends into the adjacent tissue. Hemoglobin staining of the intima can also occur in acute intravascular hemolysis. It is usually very obvious in aborted fetuses that are retained for hours or days after their in utero deaths.
- Bile imbibition (Fig. 1-26) occurs within hours of death. Bile in the gallbladder starts to penetrate its wall and stain adjacent tissue yellowish, and later this may become greenish brown. Tissues involved include the adjacent liver and any intestine in contact with the gallbladder. Sometimes, similar changes may be seen near the bile ducts.
- Pseudomelanosis is the term used for the blue-green discoloration of the tissue by iron sulfide (FeS) formed by the reaction of hydrogen sulfide (H_2S) generated by putrefactive bacteria and the iron from hemoglobin released from lysed erythrocytes. Because it depends on bacterial action, it usually takes a day or more to develop.
- Bloating (Fig. 1-27) is the result of postmortem bacterial gas formation in the lumen of the GI tract. Herbivores tend to bloat more rapidly and severely than carnivores. Rumen gases are produced normally in the forestomachs of live animals, but the gas is removed by eructation. In ruminants the rumen can become markedly distended by gas within hours of death, and this can be so severe as to rupture the diaphragm. The rate of gas formation depends on the diet, the substrate for the bacteria, and the temperature. Postmortem bloat can sometimes be difficult to distinguish from antemortem bloat (ruminal tympany) in ruminants that have not developed a "bloat line" (see Chapter 7). Bacteria disseminated hematogenously from the GI tract shortly before death can lodge in a variety of tissues and produce gas (postmortem emphysema).

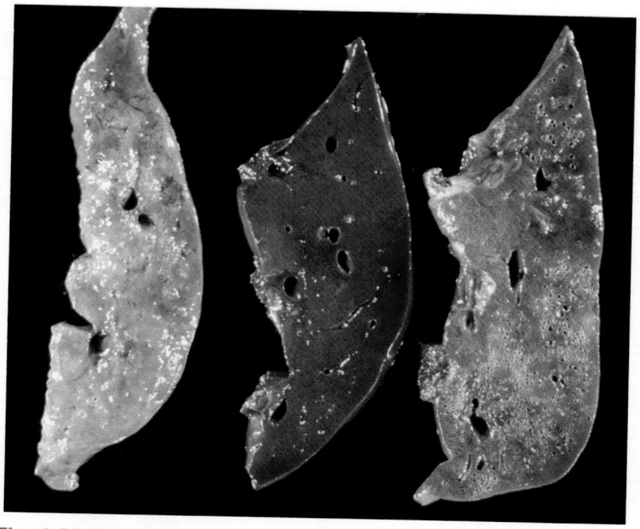

Fig. 1-26 Postmortem autolysis.
Cross-sections of livers from three different pigs at different stages of postmortem autolysis. The section on the right has green staining around the bile ducts caused by leakage of bile into the surrounding parenchyma after death (bile imbibition). All of these livers are softer than normal, but the one on the left is notably softer, another characteristic of autolytic tissue. (Courtesy Dr. R.K. Myers, College of Veterinary Medicine, Iowa State University.)

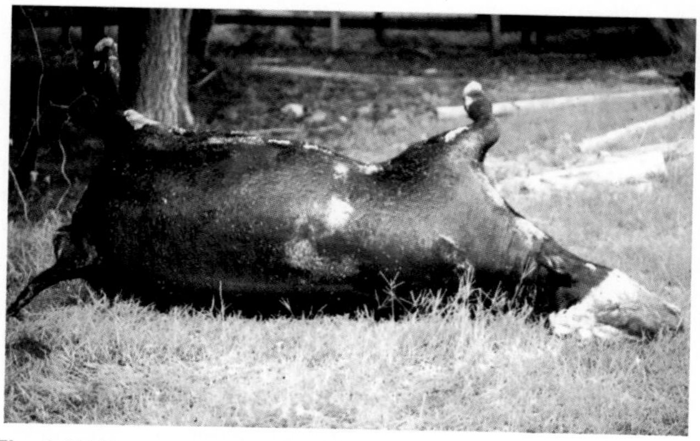

Fig. 1-27 Postmortem bloat or emphysema.
Cow killed by lightning several hours earlier. When animals die, especially ruminants, the bacteria in the gastrointestinal tract continue to grow and produce gas. Rumen microbes may produce very large amounts of gas causing the carcass to swell tremendously. (Courtesy Dr. W. Crowell, College of Veterinary Medicine, The University of Georgia; and Noah's Arkive, College of Veterinary Medicine, The University of Georgia.)

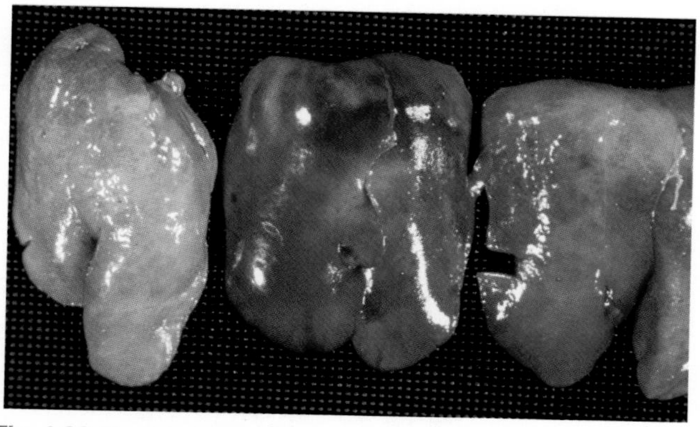

Fig. 1-28 Postmortem autolysis.
Pig livers at various intervals after death. Pale foci on the middle liver are due to blood being forced out of the parenchyma by intestinal swelling (intestinal imprints) and from pressure from the overlying ribs (rib imprints). Multiple small pale foci can sometimes be caused by colonies of postmortem bacteria and can be confused with antemortem necrosis. (Courtesy Dr. R.K. Myers, College of Veterinary Medicine, Iowa State University.)

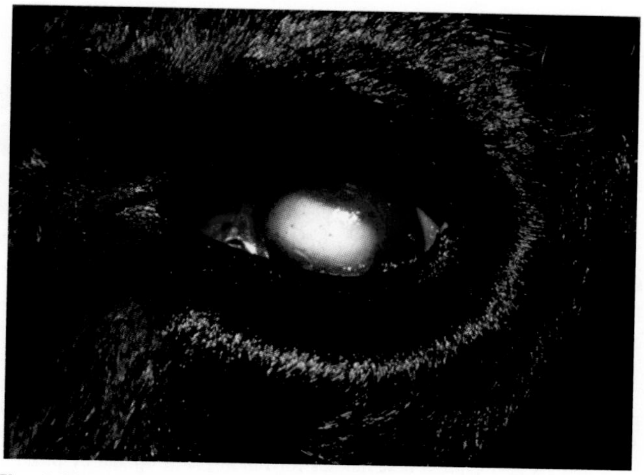

Fig. 1-29 Postmortem autolysis, eye, lens, calf.
Note that the cornea is clear. The cloudiness of the lens is due to cooling or freezing and is reversible as the carcass warms up. It should not be confused with cataracts. (Courtesy Dr. P.N. Nation, University of Alberta; and Noah's Arkive, College of Veterinary Medicine, The University of Georgia.)

- Organ displacement occurs after distention of the viscera; for example, distention of the rumen by gas from fermentation can cause increased intraabdominal pressure, which can result in displacement of abdominal viscera, rectal prolapse, and compression of the diaphragm, which then compresses the thoracic viscera. The latter can result in the expulsion of frothy fluid, originally in the lungs, from the mouth and nose.
- Pale foci subserosally on the liver (Fig. 1-28) can result from two causes: increased intraabdominal pressure, which squeezes blood from these areas (e.g., pressure from the overlying ribs can leave their imprints on the liver), and bacterial action. Under very hot conditions, pale areas can appear on the surface of the bovine liver within hours of death. Histologically, these areas resemble coagulation necrosis in which there are extremely numerous bacteria. Presumably these bacteria have been disseminated agonally from the gut into the portal vein.
- Softening (see Figs. 1-26 and 1-28) of tissue results from autolysis of cells and connective tissue often aided by putrefactive bacteria.
- Mucosal sloughing occurs rapidly in the rumen, often within a few hours as a result of the enzymes within the ingesta and the low rate of cooling.
- Lens opacity (Fig. 1-29, also see Chapter 20) occurs when the carcass is very cold or frozen. The change will reverse to normal transparency on warming, but it can be confused with cataracts in cold carcasses.

Cell Death By Apoptosis

The terms *apoptosis* and *programmed cell death* have been used virtually synonymously to refer to individual cell death in which there is initiation of a self-induced cell death process some refer to as

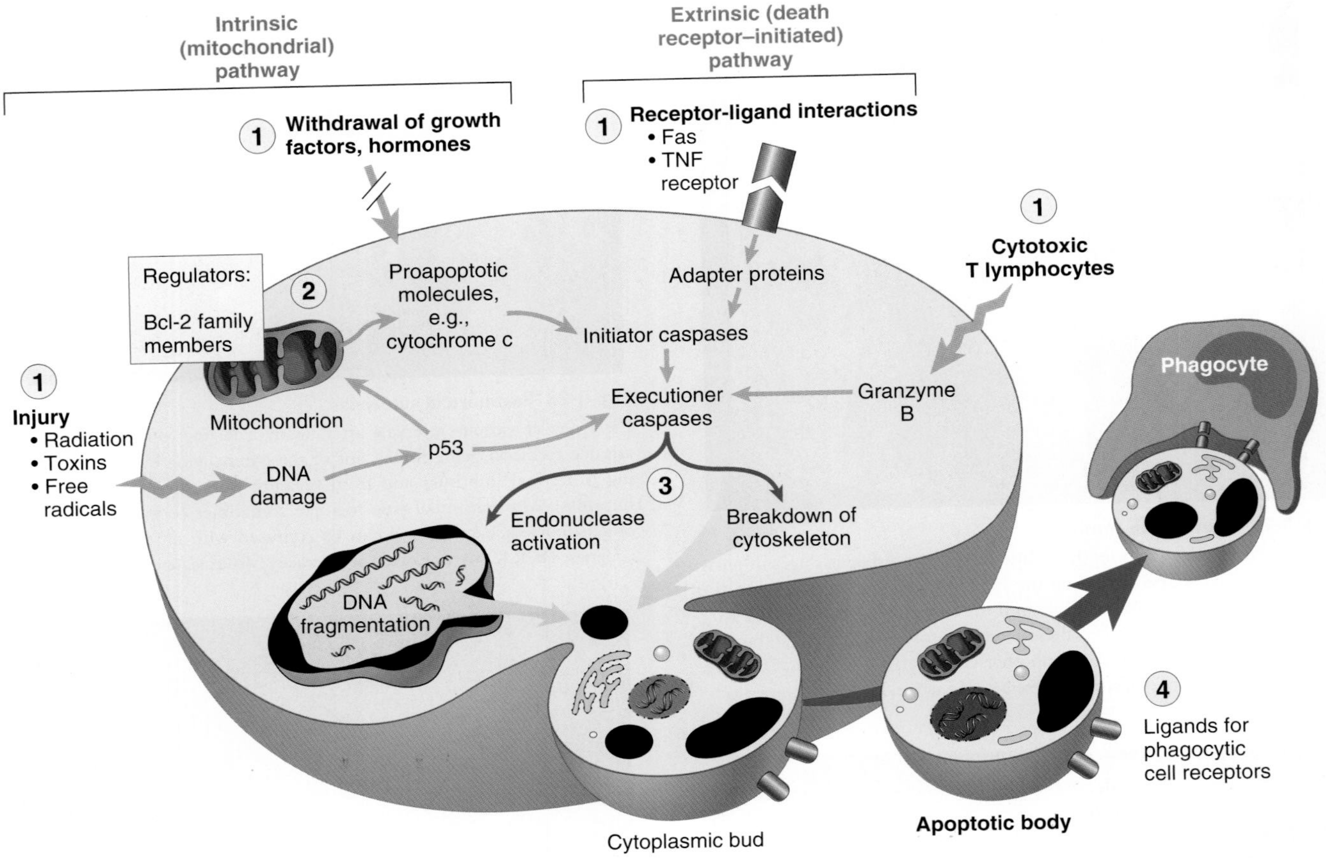

Fig. 1-30 Mechanisms of apoptosis.
Labeled *(1)* are some of the major inducers of apoptosis. These include specific death ligands (tumor necrosis factor [TNF] and Fas ligand), withdrawal of growth factors or hormones, and injurious agents (e.g., radiation). Some stimuli (such as cytotoxic cells) directly activate execution caspases *(right)*. Others act by way of adapter proteins and initiator caspases, or by mitochondrial events involving cytochrome c. *(2)* Control and regulation are influenced by members of the Bcl-2 family of proteins, which can either inhibit or promote the cell's death. *(3)* Executioner caspases activate latent cytoplasmic endonucleases and proteases that degrade nuclear and cytoskeletal proteins. This results in a cascade of intracellular degradation, including fragmentation of nuclear chromatin and breakdown of the cytoskeleton. *(4)* The end result is formation of apoptotic bodies containing intracellular organelles and other cytosolic components; these bodies also express new ligands for binding and uptake by phagocytic cells. (From Kumar V, Abbas A, Fausto N: *Robbins & Cotran pathologic basis of disease,* ed 7, Philadelphia, 2005, Saunders.)

cellular suicide. Apoptosis can be pathologic or physiologic and is only one of types of programmed cell death (others include cell death with autophagy and keratinocyte cornification). Programmed cell death is better reserved for physiologic cell death (which often involves apoptosis) that occurs, for example, in developing animals (embryogenesis and normal growth) and deletion of immune cells. For those circumstances in which pathologic cell death occurs with shrinkage first as a feature, apoptosis or apoptotic necrosis is more appropriately used. Apoptosis occurs in a variety of pathologic circumstances, including viral diseases such as yellow fever in humans, gland involution after duct blockage, immunologic damage by T lymphocytes, and as a component of injury caused by hypoxia and some chemicals and drugs.

*Mechanisms of Apoptosis**

Mechanisms of programmed cell death and apoptosis have been extensively researched within the last decades. A variety of stimuli result in a self-programmed, genetically determined, energy-dependent sequence of molecular events involving initiation by cell signaling, control and integration by regulatory molecules, a common execution phase by caspase family genes, and dead cell removal. Some of these mechanisms are initiated by inflammatory mediators such as TNF and the Fas ligand (FasL). Others involve deprivation of growth factors, mitochondrial damage, DNA damage, accumulation of misfolded proteins, or immune stimulation (Fig. 1-30).

The process of apoptosis may be divided into an initiation phase, during which caspases become catalytically active, and an execution phase, during which these enzymes act to cause cell death. Initiation of apoptosis occurs principally by signals from two distinct but convergent pathways: the extrinsic, or receptor-initiated, pathway and the intrinsic, or mitochondrial, pathway. Both pathways converge to activate caspases. These two pathways are described separately because they involve largely distinct molecular interactions, but it is important to remember that they may be interconnected at numerous steps.

The Extrinsic (Death Receptor–Initiated) Pathway

The extrinsic pathway is initiated by engagement of cell surface death receptors on a variety of cells (see Fig. 1-30). Death receptors are members of the TNF receptor family that contain a cytoplasmic

*Portions of this section are from Kumar V, Abbas A, Fausto N, et al: *Robbins & Cotran pathologic basis of disease,* ed 8, Philadelphia, 2009, Saunders.

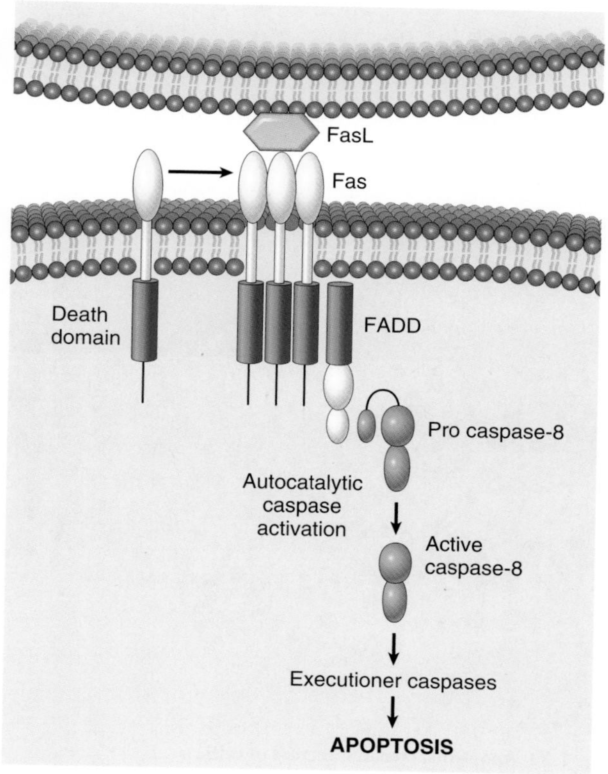

Fig. 1-31 The extrinsic (death receptor–initiated) pathway of apoptosis, illustrated by the events after Fas engagement.
FADD, Fas-associated death domain; *FasL,* Fas ligand. (From Kumar V, Abbas A, Fausto N, et al: *Robbins & Cotran pathologic basis of disease,* ed 8, Philadelphia, 2009, Saunders.)

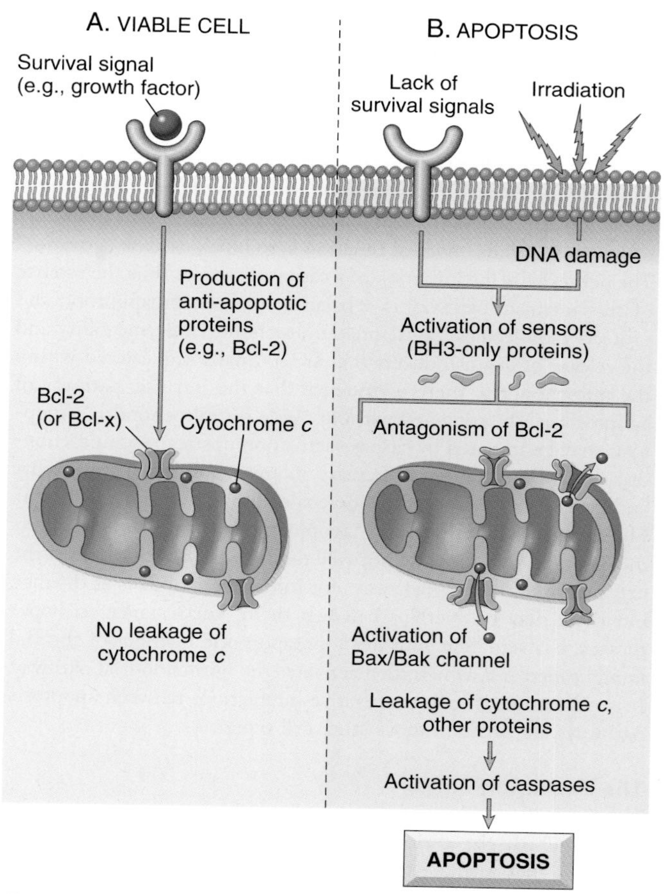

Fig. 1-32 The intrinsic (mitochondrial) pathway of apoptosis.
A, Cell viability is maintained by the induction of antiapoptotic proteins such as Bcl-2 by survival signals. These proteins maintain the integrity of mitochondrial membranes and prevent leakage of mitochondrial proteins. **B,** Loss of survival signals, DNA damage, and other insults activate sensors that antagonize the antiapoptotic proteins and activate the proapoptotic proteins Bax and Bak, which form channels in the mitochondrial membrane. The subsequent leakage of cytochrome c (and other proteins, not shown) leads to caspase activation and apoptosis. (From Kumar V, Abbas A, Fausto N, et al: *Robbins & Cotran pathologic basis of disease,* ed 8, Philadelphia, 2009, Saunders.)

domain involved in protein-protein interactions that is called the *death domain* because it is essential for delivering apoptotic signals. (Some TNF receptor family members do not contain cytoplasmic death domains; their role in triggering apoptosis is much less established.) The best-known death receptors are the type 1 TNF receptor (TNFR1) and a related protein called Fas (CD95), but several others have been described. The mechanism of apoptosis induced by these death receptors is well illustrated by Fas (Fig. 1-31). When Fas is cross-linked by its ligand, membrane-bound FasL, three or more molecules of Fas come together, and their cytoplasmic death domains form a binding site for an adapter protein that also contains a death domain and is called *Fas-associated death domain* (FADD). FADD is attached to the death receptors, which in turn bind an inactive form of caspase-8 (and in humans, caspase-10), again via a death domain. Multiple procaspase-8 molecules are thus brought into proximity, and they cleave one another to generate active caspase-8. The enzyme then triggers a cascade of caspase activation by cleaving and thereby activating other procaspases, and the active enzymes mediate the execution phase of apoptosis (discussed later). This pathway of apoptosis can be inhibited by a protein called *FLIP,* which binds to procaspase-8 but cannot cleave and activate the enzyme because it lacks enzymatic activity. Some viruses and normal cells produce FLIP and use this inhibitor to protect infected and normal cells from Fas-mediated apoptosis. The sphingolipid ceramide has been implicated as an intermediate between death receptors and caspase activation, but the role of this pathway is unclear and remains controversial.

The Intrinsic (Mitochondrial) Pathway

The intrinsic pathway of apoptosis is the result of increased mitochondrial permeability and release of proapoptotic molecules into the cytoplasm, without a role for death receptors (see Fig. 1-30). Growth factors and other survival signals stimulate the production of antiapoptotic members of the Bcl-2 family of proteins. This family is named after Bcl-2, which was identified as an oncogene in a B lymphocyte lymphoma and is homologous to the *Caenorhabditis elegans* protein, Ced-9. There are more than 20 proteins in this family, all of which function to regulate apoptosis; the two main antiapoptotic ones are Bcl-2 and Bcl-x. These antiapoptotic proteins normally reside in mitochondrial membranes and the cytoplasm. When cells are deprived of survival signals or subjected to stress, including misfolded proteins and ER stress, or when DNA is damaged, Bcl-2 and/or Bcl-x are lost from the mitochondrial membrane and are replaced by proapoptotic members of the family such as Bak, Bax, and Bim. When Bcl-2/Bcl-x levels decrease, the permeability of the mitochondrial membrane increases, and several proteins that can activate the caspase cascade leak out (Fig. 1-32).

One of these proteins is cytochrome c, well known for its role in mitochondrial respiration. In the cytosol, cytochrome c binds to a protein called apoptosis activating factor-1 (Apaf-1, homologous to Ced-4 in *Caenorhabditis elegans*), and the complex activates caspase-9. (Bcl-2 and Bcl-x may also directly inhibit Apaf-1 activation, and their loss from cells may permit activation of Apaf-1.) Other mitochondrial proteins, such as apoptosis-inducing factor (AIF), enter the cytoplasm, where they bind to and neutralize various inhibitors of apoptosis, whose normal function is to block caspase activation. The net result is the initiation of a caspase cascade. Thus the essence of this intrinsic pathway is a balance between proapoptotic and protective molecules that regulate mitochondrial permeability and the release of death inducers that are normally sequestered within the mitochondria. There is evidence that the intrinsic pathway of apoptosis can be triggered without a role for mitochondria. Apoptosis may be initiated by caspase activation upstream of mitochondria, and the subsequent increase in mitochondrial permeability and release of proapoptotic molecules amplify the death signal. However, these pathways of apoptosis involving mitochondria-independent initiation are not well defined. We have described the extrinsic and intrinsic pathways for initiating apoptosis as distinct, but there may be overlaps between them. For instance, in hepatocytes, Fas signaling activates a proapoptotic member of the Bcl family called *Bid,* which then activates the mitochondrial pathway. It is not known if such cooperative interactions between apoptosis pathways are active in most other cell types.

The Execution Phase

This final phase of apoptosis is mediated by a proteolytic cascade, toward which the various initiating mechanisms converge. The proteases that mediate the execution phase are highly conserved across species and belong to the caspase family, as previously mentioned. They are mammalian homologues of the Ced-3 gene in *Caenorhabditis elegans.* The term *caspase* is based on two properties of this family of enzymes: The "c" refers to a cysteine protease (i.e., an enzyme with cysteine in its active site), and "aspase" refers to the unique ability of these enzymes to cleave aspartic acid residues. The caspase family, now including more than 10 members, can be divided functionally into two basic groups: initiator and executioner, depending on the order in which they are activated during apoptosis. Initiator caspases, as we have seen, include caspase-8 and caspase-9. Several caspases, including caspase-3 and caspase-6, serve as executioners. Like many proteases, caspases exist as inactive proenzymes, or zymogens, and must undergo an activating cleavage for apoptosis to be initiated. Caspases have their own cleavage sites that can be hydrolyzed not only by other caspases but also autocatalytically. After an initiator caspase is cleaved to generate its active form, the enzymatic death program is set in motion by rapid and sequential activation of other caspases. Execution caspases act on many cellular components. They cleave cytoskeletal and nuclear matrix proteins and thus disrupt the cytoskeleton and lead to breakdown of the nucleus. In the nucleus, the targets of caspase activation include proteins involved in transcription, DNA replication, and DNA repair. In particular, caspase-3 activation converts a cytoplasmic DNAase into an active form by cleaving an inhibitor of the enzyme; this DNAase induces the characteristic internucleosomal cleavage of DNA.

Morphologic Appearance of Apoptosis

Morphologically, apoptotic cells have condensed chromatin and cytoplasm, and fragments of them are often found in adjacent or phagocytic cells as apoptotic bodies (Fig. 1-33). Because single cells are dead, gross changes (and even microscopic changes) are usually not obvious. In addition, because the cell fragments into membrane-bound particles, phagocytosis occurs without the inflammation that is so often seen in necrosis.

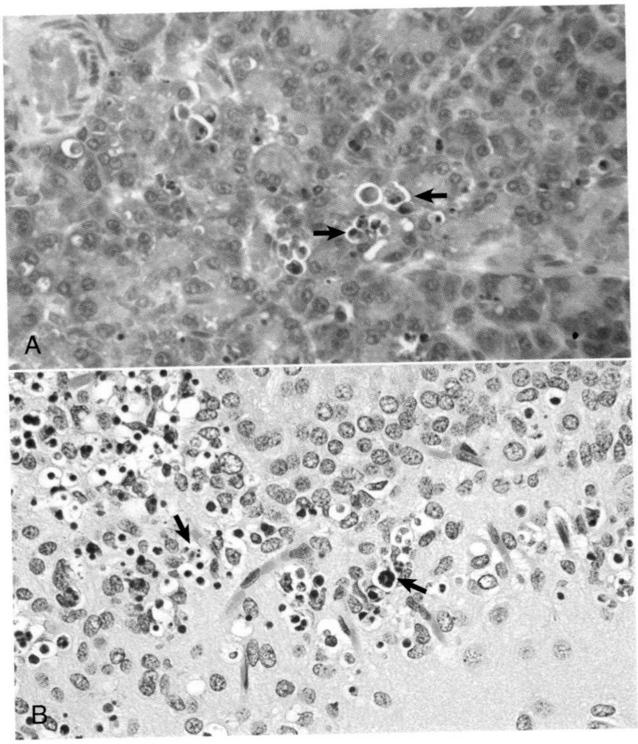

Fig. 1-33 Apoptosis, cytoarchitecture of cells. **A,** Pancreas, rat. Individual acinar cells are shrunken and their chromatin condensed and fragmented *(arrows).* Cytoplasmic buds are found as apoptotic bodies in adjacent cells. Inflammation is absent. H&E stain. **B,** Hippocampal formation, mouse. Individual neurons are shrunken and their chromatin condensed and fragmented *(arrows).* (**A** courtesy Dr. M.A. Wallig, College of Veterinary Medicine, University of Illinois. **B** courtesy Drs. V.E. Valli and J.F. Zachary, College of Veterinary Medicine, University of Illinois.)

Although typically discussed separately, necrosis by oncosis and apoptosis can be seen within the same tissue as the result of the same agent (Fig. 1-34). Cell injury by a chemical, for example, that injures mitochondria may release cytochrome c and initiate the apoptosis program. Cells with more severely affected mitochondria may die from swelling or oncosis.

The histopathologic characteristics of apoptosis are as follows:

- Individual cells are shrunken.
- Chromatin is condensed.
- Cytoplasm is fragmented.
- Cytoplasmic buds often containing a fragment of nucleus form on the surface, separate, and are phagocytosed by adjacent cells as apoptotic bodies, small intracellular eosinophilic inclusions sometimes with dense nuclear fragments.
- Inflammation is absent.

CHRONIC CELL INJURY AND CELL ADAPTATION

As mentioned previously in the discussion of cell swelling and necrosis, cells respond to injury (or stress) in three possible major

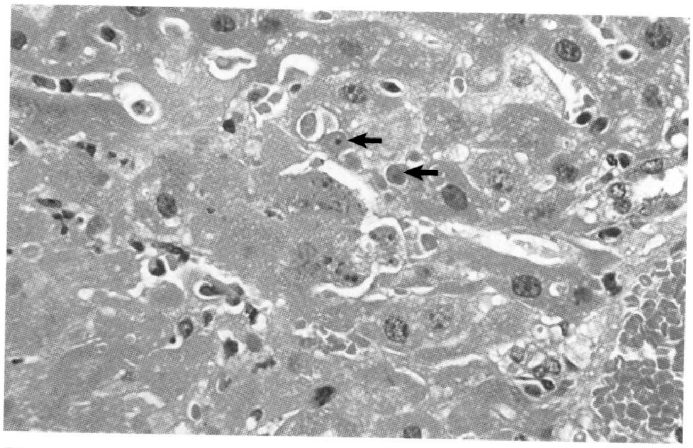

Fig. 1-34 Necrosis and apoptosis, mouse hepatitis virus infection, liver, mouse.
This disease causes hepatocyte death, typically by oncotic necrosis but sometimes by apoptosis. Note areas of coagulation necrosis in the lower left and apoptotic bodies in the center, some of which have been taken up by adjacent hepatocytes *(arrows)*. H&E stain. (Courtesy Dr. R.K. Myers, College of Veterinary Medicine, Iowa State University.)

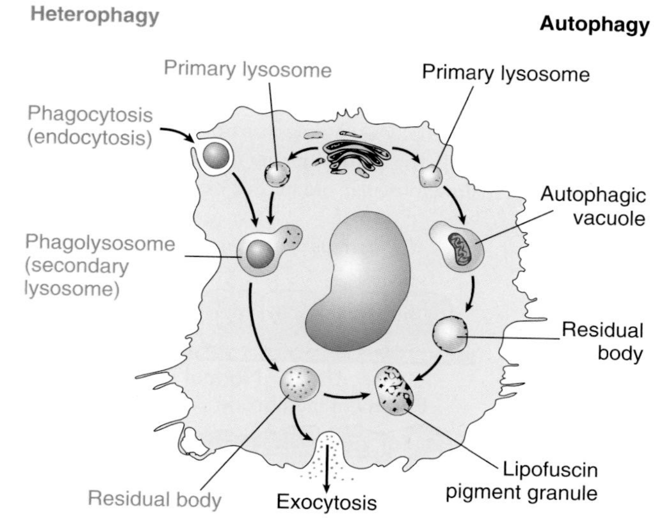

Fig. 1-35 Autophagy and heterophagy.
Schematic representation of heterophagy *(left)* and autophagy *(right)*. The mechanisms are similar for processing cell debris, both from intrinsic sources and extrinsic sources (heterophagy). (From Kumar V, Abbas A, Fausto N: *Robbins & Cotran pathologic basis of disease,* ed 7, Philadelphia, 2005, Saunders.)

ways: (1) adaptation, (2) reversible injury with or without degeneration, and (3) death. Sublethal injury to a cell over time can lead to a variety of cell alterations. Cells may adapt by producing more cells *(hyperplasia)* or by producing more organelles, leading to an increase in size *(hypertrophy)*; in some cases, adaptation results in fewer organelles and a decrease in cell and tissue size *(atrophy)*. Cells may degenerate in a variety of ways, some of which involve the accumulation of excess normal or abnormal substances. Impaired function may result, and morphologic changes in the cell and tissue may give a clue as to the cause of the cell injury.

SEQUELAE TO SUBLETHAL INJURY AND SUBCELLULAR CHANGES

Autophagocytosis

Autophagocytosis is the process by which cells with sublethal injury remove damaged and effete organelles. Cells with sublethal injury often have various amounts of damaged organelles. As in organized societies, the cell has a system to clean up after a "storm." In autophagy, portions of the cytoplasmic matrix and its damaged organelles are enveloped by cell membranes to form autophagosomes, which subsequently fuse with lysosomes (Fig. 1-35). When phagocytic white cells ingest dead or dying cells, the process is very similar and termed *heterophagy*. Autophagy is a common reaction of sublethally injured cells, epithelial cells such as endometrium undergoing cyclic physiologic regression, and in atrophy as the result of many causes. Recent evidence suggests that autophagocytosis pathways may result in a distinct type of cell death termed *autophagic cell death*.

By light microscopy, autophagic vacuoles may appear as eosinophilic inclusions (see section on Intracellular Hyaline Proteins) and are common in the liver and kidney. As digestion progresses, electron-dense and lamellar debris is formed. Some vacuoles are evicted from the cell by exocytosis; others remain as residual bodies, and the contents form lipofuscin, the so-called wear-and-tear pigment.

Misfolded proteins or those otherwise altered occur in a variety of circumstances within the cell, both normally and in disease states. These proteins may be repaired by chaperones, or they may be degraded by the ubiquitin-proteasome pathway. The targeted proteins are conjugated to ubiquitin (one of several heat shock proteins) that through a cascade results in polyubiquitination and direction of the protein into a proteasome, a multisubunit complex with a catalytic core that degrades the protein for removal (see Fig. 1-48). Removal of all sorts of proteins, including cell-signaling molecules, allows proper control of cell function, growth, and replication. This pathway also plays a role in both activation and inhibition of apoptosis as well as in sublethal injury.

ADAPTIVE CHANGES LEADING TO CHANGE IN CELL SIZE, NUMBER, OR APPEARANCE

Adaptive changes to cell stress or injury can lead to an increase in the size of a tissue or organ (by *hyperplasia* and/or *hypertrophy*), a decrease in tissue and cell size *(atrophy)*, or a change to a different cell type *(metaplasia)* (Fig. 1-36). Hypertrophy is an increase in the size of cells or organs. Hyperplasia is an increase in the number of cells in a tissue or organ. The two often occur together as an adaptive change and are considered positive responses to injury or stress.

Hypertrophy

In simple cellular hypertrophy, the number of cells in an organ or tissue does not increase. Cells synthesize more organelles, and cell enlargement occurs. The histologic architecture of the organ is normal, but cells are bigger. Hypertrophy can occur in most organs and tissues but tends to occur in cells that undergo little replication (i.e., stable or permanent cells). It is most common in striated muscle. In response to increased workload, smooth muscle may undergo hypertrophy and hyperplasia. Causes of hypertrophy usually involve demands for increased function (e.g., the increased workload on a muscle and resultant hypertrophy of that muscle in weight lifters).

The size and configuration of organelles reflect the work requirements of the cell. Chronic exposure to drugs, such as phenobarbital, Dilantin, and alcohol, leads to enlargement of the SER in hepatocytes. SER contains the mixed oxidase enzyme systems that function to catabolize these substances. The increased size of the Golgi complex and RER are a reflection of a need for synthesis of extracellular proteins (e.g., immunoglobulin, collagen, and secretions). These organelles increase in size by duplication of membranes. The number of mitochondria adjusts to the ATP requirements of the cell. The size of nucleoli and proportion of euchromatin also reflect the synthetic activity of the cell.

Physiologic hypertrophy is common and expected after work. Compensatory hypertrophy is a response to the loss of a part of an organ or one of the paired organs or from obstruction of the lumen of a hollow muscular organ. For example, hypertrophy occurs in one kidney after the loss of the opposite kidney. The kidney enlarges because of the increased length of nephrons and not the increased numbers of nephrons. Functional capacity increases with the increased size. Hypertrophy of the right ventricle of the heart caused by stenosis of the pulmonary outflow tract is another example of compensatory hypertrophy (Fig. 1-37).

Hypertrophy is common, protective, limited, and reversible and may rarely cause harm to adjacent structures. Hypertrophy may not always be useful. In myocardial hypertrophy, enlargement of myofibers may occur with a corresponding increase in intercellular stroma, making the myocardium stiff. In addition, the blood supply may not increase adequately to serve the needs of the increased mass of myocytes, and this results in hypoxic injury. The term hypertrophy is used in gross pathology to describe lesions that involve gross enlargement of an organ regardless of cause.

Cellular mechanisms leading to hypertrophy vary by tissue and cause, and details are lacking for most entities. Growth factors likely play a role in altering gene expression in many circumstances, whereas in myofiber hypertrophy, the type of mechanical stress can influence the way the muscle enlarges, for example with increased mitochondria, required for oxidative metabolism in endurance training. Muscular hypertrophy of the uterus results from binding of estrogen to cytosolic estrogen-receptors that in turn activate genes leading to muscle protein production. These specific changes and others all are likely due to activation of specific genes.

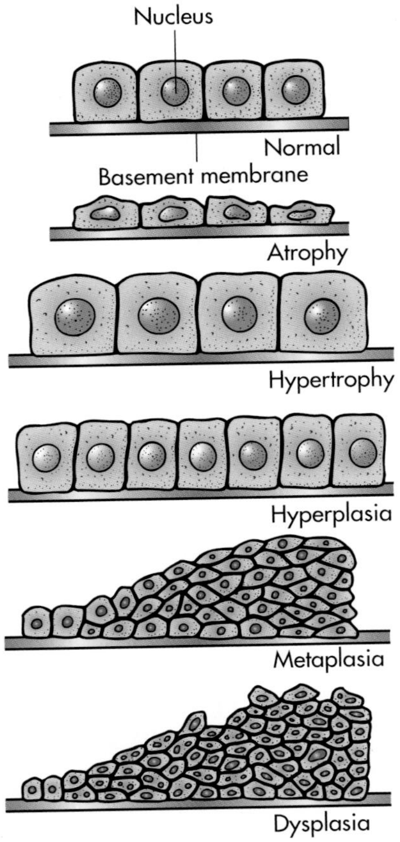

Fig. 1-36 Adaptive changes in epithelium.
(From McCance KL, Huether SE, Brashers VL, et al: *Pathophysiology: the biologic basis for disease in adults and children,* ed 6, St. Louis, 2010, Mosby.)

Hyperplasia

Because hyperplasia is an increase in the number of cells, increased mitotic division is implied. Hyperplasia increases the size of a tissue, an organ, or part of an organ and may appear grossly as hypertrophy. It is a common change. Microscopically, cells resemble normal cells but are increased in numbers. Hyperplastic cells may also be increased in size (i.e., cellular hypertrophy).

The ability of different adult cell types to undergo hyperplasia varies. Labile cells—those that routinely proliferate in normal circumstances, such as those of the epidermis, intestinal epithelium, and bone marrow cells—readily become hyperplastic. Permanent cells, such as neurons and cardiac and skeletal muscle myocytes, have very little capacity to regenerate or become hyperplastic in most situations. Stable cells, such as bone, cartilage, and smooth muscle, are intermediate in their ability to become hyperplastic.

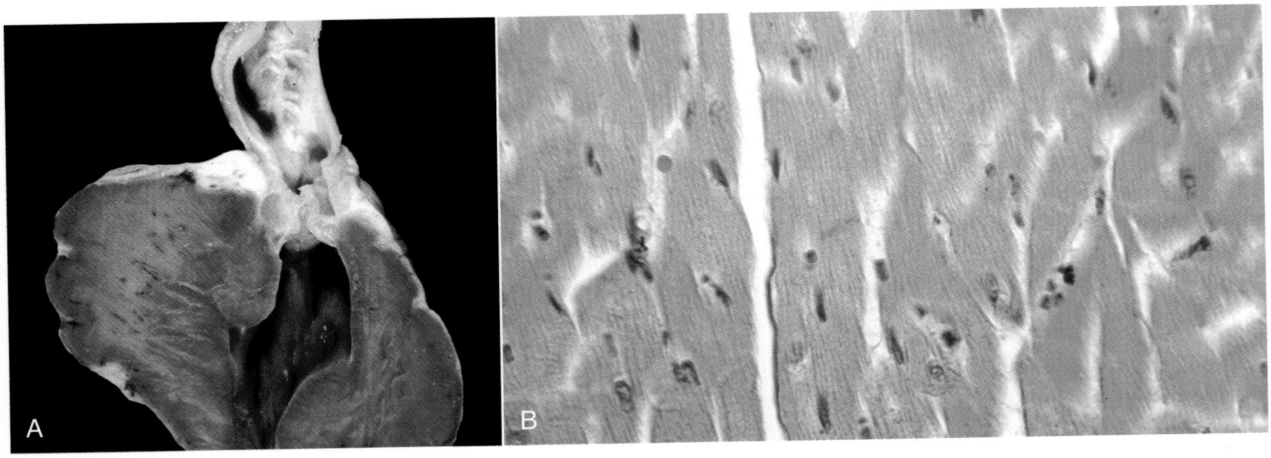

Fig. 1-37 Hypertrophy, heart, dog.
A, Narrowing of the pulmonary outflow tract caused by pulmonic valve stenosis has forced the right ventricle to contract with much more pressure. This increased workload has caused hypertrophy of the wall of the right ventricle, which is much thicker here than it would normally be. **B,** Note the increased size (hypertrophy) of myocytes in the overworked heart muscle. (Courtesy Dr. L. Miller, Atlantic Veterinary College, University of Prince Edward Island; and Noah's Arkive, College of Veterinary Medicine, The University of Georgia.)

Hyperplasia is traditionally divided into physiologic hyperplasia and pathologic hyperplasia, as follows:

- *Physiologic hyperplasia* is usually either hormonal or compensatory. Hormonal hyperplasia includes conditions such as increased mammary gland epithelial proliferation before lactation and enlargement of the pregnant uterus. Compensatory hyperplasia, or regeneration, occurs after a portion of an organ is lost. For example, if the skin is abraded, the basal layer of the epidermis undergoes mitosis to regenerate superficial layers. Removal of part of the liver can cause mitosis in the remaining hepatocytes resulting in the restoration of the liver to its normal size but not necessarily its normal shape. This regenerative process takes as little as 2 weeks in rats after partial hepatectomy.
- *Pathologic hyperplasia* is often caused by excessive hormonal stimulation of target cells or chronic irritation. Cystic endometrial hyperplasia of the canine uterus as a result of prolonged progesterone influence is common. Microscopically, there is folding of increased numbers of epithelial cells into glands and onto the lumen surface. The mucosa thickens and may trap or impair secretions, causing dilation of glands and cyst formation within the mucosa. The process is reversible if the stimulus is removed.

Pathologic hyperplasia may cause diffuse enlargement of an organ, such as in benign prostatic hyperplasia in dogs and in goiter (hyperplasia of the thyroid gland) (Fig. 1-38), or be localized as nodular hyperplasia. Nodular hyperplasia may occur without known cause and occurs in the spleen, liver, and pancreas of old dogs. One must differentiate hyperplasia, particularly nodular hyperplasia, from neoplasia.

The significance of hyperplasia usually lies in determining its cause. If it is hormonal in origin, the disturbance in the source organ should be determined. If chronic irritation is the cause, determining the agent is often important. Hyperplasia is usually induced by known stimuli. It is a controlled process that stops when the stimulus ceases, can serve a useful purpose (e.g., repair defects, compensate for tissue loss, prepare for increased function, and aid in protection), and is subject to regular growth controls. These features are not part of neoplastic processes, which otherwise may be similar to hyperplastic changes in appearance and behavior.

Cellular mechanisms of hyperplasia vary in details, depending on the cell affected and the cause. There are multiple controls as to whether or not a cell enters the replication cycle. In some circumstances hormones trigger cell replication, whereas in others growth factors, increased receptors for growth factors, and activation of cell signaling pathways may all have a role. In some circumstances, cytokines are important. Ultimately, transcription factors may influence the expression of a new cadre of genes leading to cell proliferation. In regeneration for restitution of parenchyma to normal amounts (see later discussion), stem cells turn on and lead to appropriate cell replication.

Metaplasia

Metaplasia is a potentially reversible change in which one adult cell type is replaced by another adult cell type of the same germ line (Fig. 1-39). Usually, specialized epithelium is replaced by less-specialized epithelium. One adult cell type does not transform into another type of adult cell. It is the less-differentiated reserve or stem cells that differentiate along a different line. For example, in cigarette smokers, chronic irritation of the normal columnar ciliated epithelium of the trachea and bronchial tree causes it to be replaced by focal or diffuse areas of stratified squamous epithelium. The squamous cells are more resistant to injury but are less protective to the lung, and, as they lack cilia, there is decreased clearance of mucus.

Metaplasia is often but not always an adaptive change to withstand adverse environmental conditions and is reversible if the cause is removed. Epithelial metaplasia is commonly a change to squamous epithelium and is usually a result of chronic irritation, but it can have other causes (e.g., avitaminosis A). Metaplasia in mesenchymal tissue is less clearly adaptive and is usually a response to change of microenvironment of cells, such as oxygen tension. One type of mesenchymal tissue changes to another, for example, fibrous tissue changes to cartilage or bone.

The following are some examples and causes of metaplasia:

- Chronic irritation from particles and chemicals in the lungs of smokers may cause the normal cuboidal and columnar epithelium of airways to become stratified squamous.
- Vitamin A deficiency causes squamous metaplasia of the transitional epithelium of the urinary tract, cuboidal and

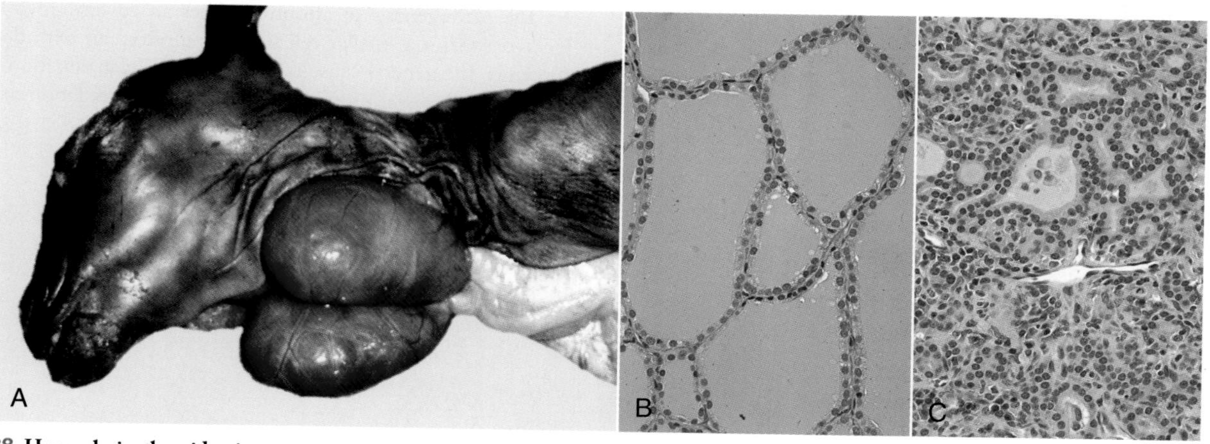

Fig. 1-38 Hyperplasia, thyroid goiter, goat.
A, Deficiency of maternal dietary iodine during pregnancy has resulted in hyperplasia (and hypertrophy) of thyroid follicular epithelial cells in this neonatal goat and thus results in a symmetric enlargement of the glands (goiter). **B,** Thyroid follicular epithelial cells from a normal thyroid gland. H&E stain. **C,** Thyroid follicular epithelial cells from a case of thyroid goiter. Note the increased number (and size) of the follicular epithelial cells. H&E stain. (**A** courtesy Dr. O. Hedstrom, College of Veterinary Medicine, Oregon State University; and Noah's Arkive, College of Veterinary Medicine, The University of Georgia. **B** and **C** courtesy Dr. B. Harmon, College of Veterinary Medicine, The University of Georgia; and Noah's Arkive, College of Veterinary Medicine, The University of Georgia.)

columnar epithelial cells lining the ducts within the salivary glands, and the epithelium of the mucous glands of esophageal mucosa in birds (Fig. 1-40).
- Estrogen toxicity, among other things, causes squamous metaplasia of the urinary tract and prostate.
- Healing of glandular epithelium after mastitis may at first be squamous.
- Squamous metaplasia of salivary, biliary, and pancreatic ducts can occur if they are blocked by stones in the lumen.
- Osseous metaplasia (metaplastic bone) occasionally occurs in injured soft tissue.
- Myeloid metaplasia (extramedullary hematopoiesis) in adult spleens and livers occurs commonly after bone marrow injury or insufficiency.
- Metaplasia occurs in some tumors such as mixed mammary gland tumors of dogs.

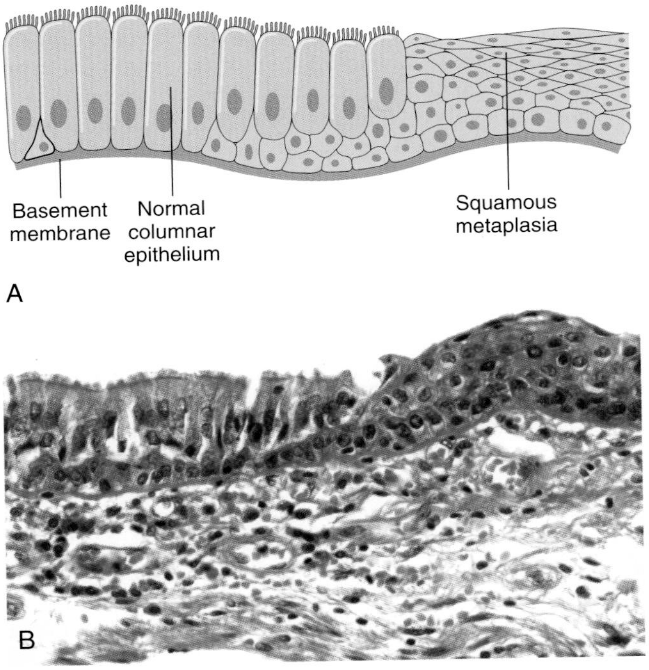

Fig. 1-39 Metaplasia to squamous epithelium.
A, Schematic diagram of columnar to squamous metaplasia. **B,** Metaplasia of columnar epithelium *(left)* to squamous epithelium *(right)* in a bronchus. (From Kumar V, Abbas A, Fausto N, et al: *Robbins & Cotran pathologic basis of disease,* ed 8, Philadelphia, 2009, Saunders.)

Metaplasia is reversible (usually) if the cause is withdrawn. It may, however, be preneoplastic—for example, in the lungs of smokers where it appears before transformation to squamous cell carcinoma.

Cellular mechanisms leading to metaplasia vary. Vitamin A is important in normal differentiation of mucus-secreting epithelium by yet unspecified mechanisms. When vitamin A is deficient, these cells differentiate along squamous lines. Estrogen causes differentiation along squamous lines in specific sex-hormone responsive epithelia. Growth factors and other trophic substances presumably can influence differentiation along certain pathways from stem cells, and ECM can play an important role. How these metaplastic changes take place in response to injury is less clear.

Atrophy

Atrophy is the decrease in size or amount of a cell, tissue, or organ after normal growth has been reached (Fig. 1-41). It is caused by the decreased number and/or size of cells. It may affect virtually any organ or part of an organ. It is a regressive change usually caused by gradual and continuous injury. Some causes and examples of atrophy are as follows:

- Deficient nutritive supply. Starvation and especially a decreased blood supply. For example, liver atrophy results from decreased blood flow through the portal vein (Fig. 1-42).
- Decreased workload. For example, muscle fibers atrophy in sedentary people.
- Disuse. Muscles in a limb in a cast atrophy.
- Denervation. Muscle fibers decrease in size rapidly if their motor neuron is severed.
- Pressure. Atrophy, degeneration, and necrosis occur adjacent to tumors because of pressure and compromised blood supply.
- Loss of endocrine stimulation. Atrophy of the zona fasciculata of the adrenal follows prolonged steroid therapy.
- Senility.

Involution is the decrease in size of a tissue caused by reduction in the number of cells (usually by apoptosis) and is usually used to refer to *physiologic processes.* For example, the thymus involutes with age, and many tissues become smaller because of senile involution. The uterus involutes after parturition, and its smooth muscle cells decrease notably in size and number.

The pathogenesis of atrophy implies an adverse environment. Cells regress to a smaller cell size and survive, but with decreased function. The general cause is inadequate cellular nutrition for any reason. Synthesis of proteins is exceeded by degradation or loss.

Fig. 1-40 Squamous metaplasia, esophagus, parrot.
A, The esophageal mucosa has multiple white raised nodules from squamous metaplasia of mucosal glands. Metaplasia arose from the lack of dietary vitamin A (avitaminosis A). **B,** Note the squamous metaplasia of the esophageal glands. Vitamin A is necessary for maintenance of the normal epithelium. Avitaminosis A results in the replacement of normal mucosal epithelium and goblet cells in the glands by keratinized stratified squamous epithelium. H&E stain. (Courtesy Dr. M.D. McGavin, College of Veterinary Medicine, University of Tennessee.)

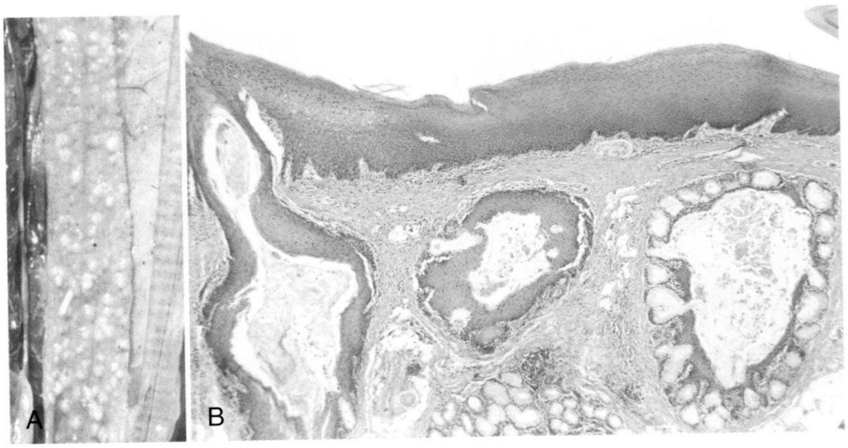

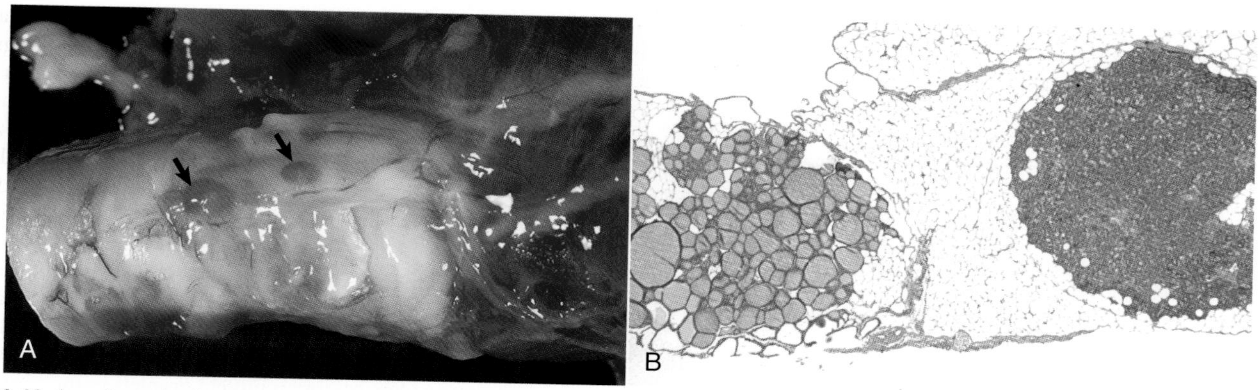

Fig. 1-41 Atrophy, right thyroid gland on trachea, dog.
A, The right thyroid gland is extremely small and difficult to discern. Only small pieces of thyroid tissue remain *(arrows)*. **B,** The thyroid gland is extremely small, follicles are atrophic and of varied sizes, and colloid has a low concentration of thyroglobulin protein (pale pink color). Note that supporting stroma has been replaced by fat cells. The parathyroid gland *(right)* is of normal size. H&E stain. (**A** courtesy Dr. W. Crowell, College of Veterinary Medicine, The University of Georgia; and Noah's Arkive, College of Veterinary Medicine, The University of Georgia. **B** courtesy College of Veterinary Medicine, University of Illinois.)

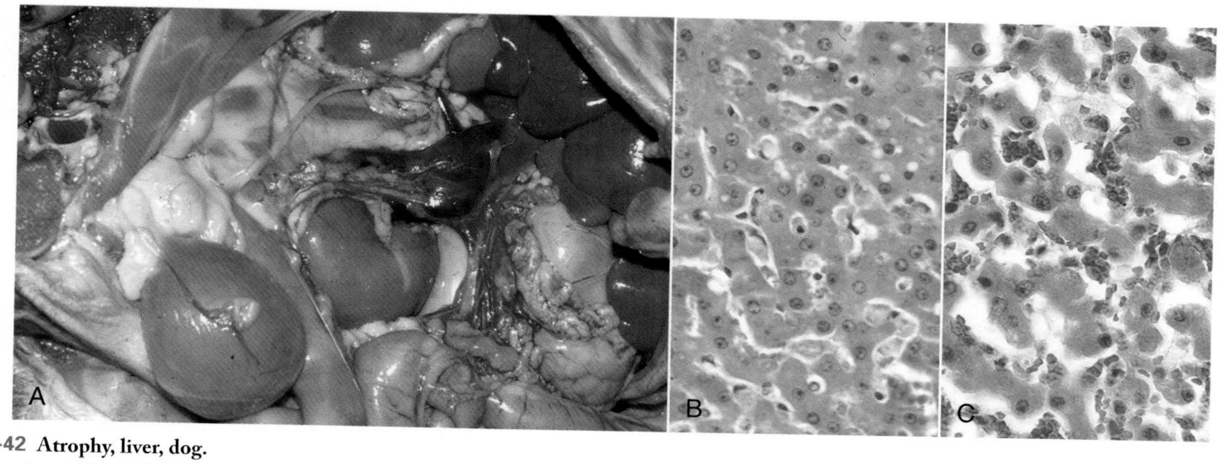

Fig. 1-42 Atrophy, liver, dog.
A, Note the small size (up under the rib cage) but normal color of the liver in this dog and the anomalous size of the caudal vena cava in the mesentery (i.e., shunt between the portal vein and the systemic circulation). This shunt caused bypassing of blood from the liver. The reduction in blood flow to the liver causes decreased nutrients (hepatocyte trophic factors) to the hepatocytes and therefore decreased size of hepatocytes. **B,** Normal liver. H&E stain. **C,** Liver, atrophy. Hepatocytes are smaller and narrower than those in the normal liver **(B).** As a consequence, the sinusoids are correspondingly wider. H&E stain. (**A** courtesy Dr. J. Sagartz, College of Veterinary Medicine, The Ohio State University; and Noah's Arkive, College of Veterinary Medicine, The University of Georgia. **B** courtesy Dr. M.D. McGavin, College of Veterinary Medicine, University of Tennessee. **C** courtesy Dr. R.K. Myers, College of Veterinary Medicine, Iowa State University.)

Autophagocytosis, lysosomes, and the ubiquitin proteasome pathway (see the section on Sublethal Injury and Subcellular Changes) may all play a role in decreasing the organelle and protein content of a cell. The actual triggers and cellular mechanisms are unclear for many circumstances. Atrophy may resolve if the cause is removed. It may persist as is, with or without harm to the organism, or it may progress.

Atrophied organs grossly have a decreased weight and volume, may have a loose covering membrane (e.g., wrinkled skin), have tortuous blood vessels too large for the volume of tissue, and often are firmer because of fibrosis or condensation of remaining collagen. Microscopically, cells are smaller and/or reduced in number. Ultrastructurally, there are fewer mitochondria, ER, and myofilaments (muscle) and often an increase in autophagic vacuoles and maybe lipofuscin.

Serous atrophy of fat is a very important necropsy finding because it may indicate starvation. Grossly, fat deposits are completely or partially depleted, and a clear or yellowish gelatinous material remains. Histologically, adipocytes are smaller, and interstitial hyaluronic acid mucopolysaccharides are increased. It is most evident in the epicardial and perirenal fat but may affect any fat depot, including bone marrow. The cause of starvation may be virtually anything: malnutrition, malabsorption, chronic infection, parasitism, neoplasia, and so forth. It is common in neonates, often the result of mismothering.

INTRACELLULAR ACCUMULATIONS*

One of the manifestations of metabolic derangements in cells is the intracellular accumulation of abnormal amounts of various substances (Fig. 1-43). The stockpiled substances fall into three categories: (1) a normal cellular constituent accumulated in excess, such as water, lipids, proteins, and carbohydrates; (2) an abnormal substance, either exogenous, such as a mineral or products of infectious agents, or endogenous, such as a product of abnormal synthesis or metabolism; or (3) a pigment. These substances may accumulate either transiently or permanently, and they may be harmless to the

*Portions of this section are from Kumar V, Abbas A, Fausto N, et al: *Robbins & Cotran pathologic basis of disease,* ed 8, Philadelphia, 2009, Saunders.

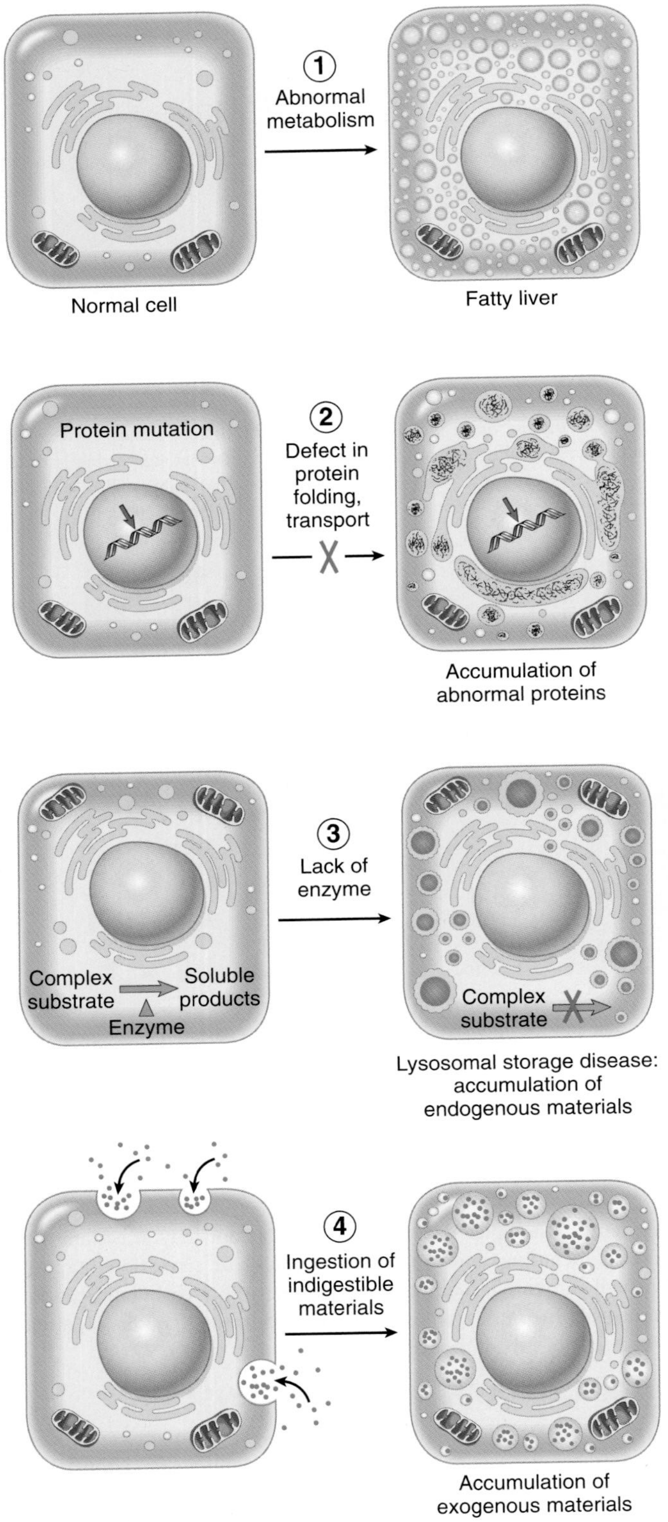

Fig. 1-43 Mechanisms of intracellular accumulations.

A, Abnormal metabolism, as in fatty change in the liver. **B,** Mutations causing alterations in protein folding and transport, as in α_1-antitrypsin deficiency. **C,** Deficiency of critical enzymes that prevent breakdown of substrates that accumulate in lysosomes, as in lysosomal storage diseases;. **D,** Inability to degrade phagocytosed particles, as in hemosiderosis and carbon pigment accumulation. (From Kumar V, Abbas A, Fausto N, et al: *Robbins & Cotran pathologic basis of disease,* ed 8, Philadelphia, 2009, Saunders.)

cells, but on occasion they are severely toxic. The substance may be located in either the cytoplasm (frequently within phagolysosomes) or the nucleus. In some instances, the cell may be producing the abnormal substance, whereas other cells may be merely storing products of pathologic processes occurring elsewhere in the body.

Many processes result in abnormal intracellular accumulations, but most accumulations are attributable to the following three types of abnormalities.

1. A normal endogenous substance is produced at a normal or increased rate, but the rate of metabolism is inadequate to remove it. An example of this type of process is fatty change in the liver because of intracellular accumulation of triglycerides (described in a later section). Another example is the appearance of reabsorption protein droplets in the epithelial cells of renal proximal tubules because of increased leakage of protein from the glomerulus.
2. A normal or abnormal endogenous substance accumulates because of genetic or acquired defects in the metabolism, packaging, transport, or secretion of these substances. One example is the group of conditions caused by genetic defects of specific enzymes involved in the metabolism of lipid and carbohydrates resulting in intracellular deposition of these substances, largely in lysosomes in so-called storage diseases. Another is α_1-antitrypsin deficiency, in which a single amino acid substitution in the enzyme results in defects in protein folding and accumulation of the enzyme in the ER of the liver in the form of globular eosinophilic inclusions.
3. An abnormal exogenous substance is deposited and accumulates because the cell has neither the enzymatic machinery to degrade the substance nor the ability to transport it to other sites. Accumulations of carbon particles and nonmetabolizable chemicals, such as silica particles, are examples of this type of alteration.

Whatever the nature and origin of the intracellular accumulation, it implies the storage of some product by individual cells. If the overload is due to a systemic derangement and can be brought under control, the accumulation is reversible. In genetic storage diseases, accumulation is progressive, and the cells may become so overloaded as to cause secondary injury, leading in some instances to death of the tissue and the patient.

Lipids

Hepatic Lipidosis (Fatty Liver, Fatty Change, Hepatic Steatosis)

All major classes of lipids can accumulate in cells: triglycerides, cholesterol/cholesterol esters, and phospholipids. Phospholipids are components of the myelin figures found in necrotic cells. In addition, abnormal complexes of lipids and carbohydrates accumulate in the lysosomal storage diseases.

Lipidosis is the accumulation of triglycerides and other lipid metabolites (neutral fats and cholesterol) within parenchymal cells. Although it occurs in heart muscle, skeletal muscle, and the kidney, clinical manifestations are most commonly detected as alterations in liver function (elevated liver enzymes, icterus) because the liver is the organ most central to lipid metabolism.

Hepatic lipidosis, the prototype example of this type of cellular degeneration, can occur as the result of one of the following five mechanisms:

1. Excessive delivery of free fatty acids either from the gut or from adipose tissue
2. Decreased β-oxidation of fatty acids to ketones and other substances because of mitochondrial injury (toxins, hypoxia)
3. Impaired synthesis of apoprotein (CCl_4 toxicity, aflatoxicosis)

4. Impaired combination of triglycerides and protein to form lipoprotein (uncommon)
5. Impaired release (secretion) of lipoproteins from the hepatocyte (uncommon)

The underlying pathogenesis of hepatic lipidosis centers on the biochemical pathways of free fatty acid formation and metabolism. Free fatty acids, derived from triglycerides, provide a large component of the basal energy needs for parenchymal cells. They are obtained directly from the diet through digestive processes, from chylomicrons in the blood, or from adipose cells in body fat stores (adipose tissue). Chylomicrons transport dietary lipids consisting predominately of triglycerides from the alimentary system to the liver, muscle, and adipose tissue. Lipoprotein lipase and other proteins act synergistically within the chylomicron to free fatty acids from triglycerides for their use as an energy source. In the liver, free fatty acids are esterified to triglycerides, converted into cholesterol or phospholipids, or oxidized to ketones. Triglycerides can only be transported out of hepatocytes if apolipoprotein converts them to lipoproteins (Fig. 1-44). Alterations in one or more of these biochemical processes can result in the accumulation of triglycerides and other lipid metabolites, resulting in hepatic lipidosis.

In domestic animals, hepatic lipidosis most commonly arises from conditions that cause increased mobilization of body fat stores. Such conditions usually occur when there is increased demand for energy over a short duration, as in late pregnancy and early lactation in dairy cows (pregnancy toxemia and ketosis, respectively). Hepatic lipidosis is also observed with nutritional disorders, including obesity (increased transport of dietary lipids or mobilization from adipose tissue), protein-calorie malnutrition (impaired apolipoprotein synthesis), and starvation (increased mobilization of triglycerides), but it also can occur secondarily in inherited storage diseases, such as Wilson's disease, and in endocrine disease, such as diabetes mellitus (increased mobilization of triglycerides). Poisoning by chemicals, such as CCl_4 (used in industrial applications) and yellow phosphorus (used in manufacturing of incendiary munitions and once in the manufacture of matches), can also induce hepatic lipidosis via decreased oxidation of free fatty acids. These chemicals are strictly regulated and diseases caused by them are rarely seen in clinical medical practice today. In some disorders, such as feline hepatic lipidosis (feline fatty liver syndrome) and fat cow syndrome, the cause of hepatic lipidosis is unclear.

Grossly, mild fatty change may not be detectable, but livers with notable lipidosis are enlarged, yellow, soft and friable, and the edges of the lobes are rounded and broad instead of sharp and flat (Fig. 1-45, *A*). When incised, the cut surface of severely affected livers can bulge and the hepatic parenchyma is soft and friable and has a greasy texture attributable to lipid within hepatocytes. In addition, a 1-cm-thick transverse section from a liver lobe may float in formalin, again indicative of lipid within hepatocytes.

It is important to distinguish these gross lesions from the lesions present in glucocorticoid (steroid) hepatopathy in dogs. The liver in glucocorticoid hepatopathy is also enlarged and has rounded edges, but it is pale beige to tan-white, firm, and nongreasy

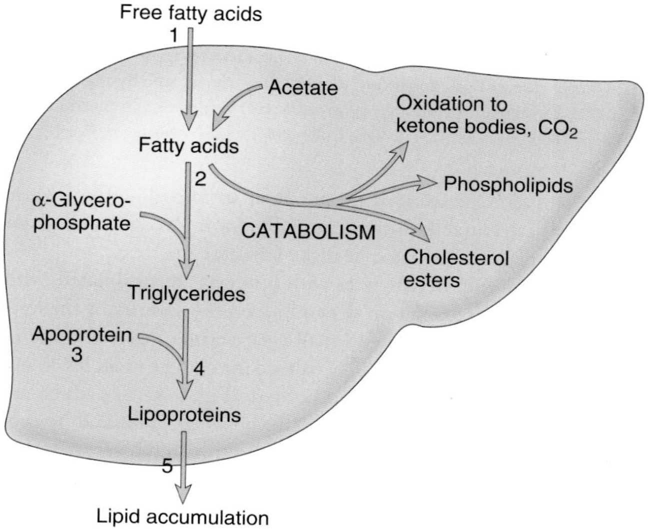

Fig. 1-44 Fatty liver.
Schematic of typical hepatic lipid metabolism (uptake, catabolism, and secretion) and possible mechanisms resulting in lipid accumulation. *1,* Excessive delivery of free fatty acids (FFA) from fat stores or diet. *2,* Decreased oxidation or use of FFAs. *3,* Impaired synthesis of apoprotein. *4,* Impaired combination of protein and triglycerides to form lipoproteins. *5,* Impaired release of lipoproteins from hepatocytes. (Modified from Kumar V, Abbas A, Fausto N, et al: *Robbins & Cotran pathologic basis of disease,* ed 8, Philadelphia, 2009, Saunders.)

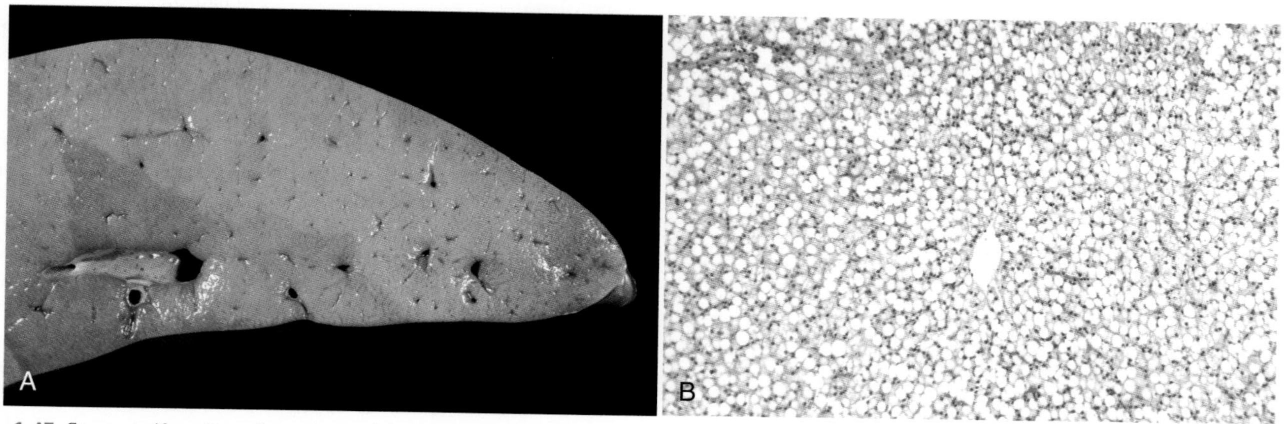

Fig. 1-45 Steatosis (fatty liver, fatty change, hepatic lipidosis), liver, ox.
A, Note the uniformly pale yellow surface. The liver is usually enlarged and the edges rounded. The cut surface bulges on incision and may feel greasy. **B,** In this severely affected liver, all hepatocytes are vacuolated and their nuclei have been displaced to the side. H&E stain. (Courtesy Dr. M.D. McGavin, College of Veterinary Medicine, University of Tennessee.)

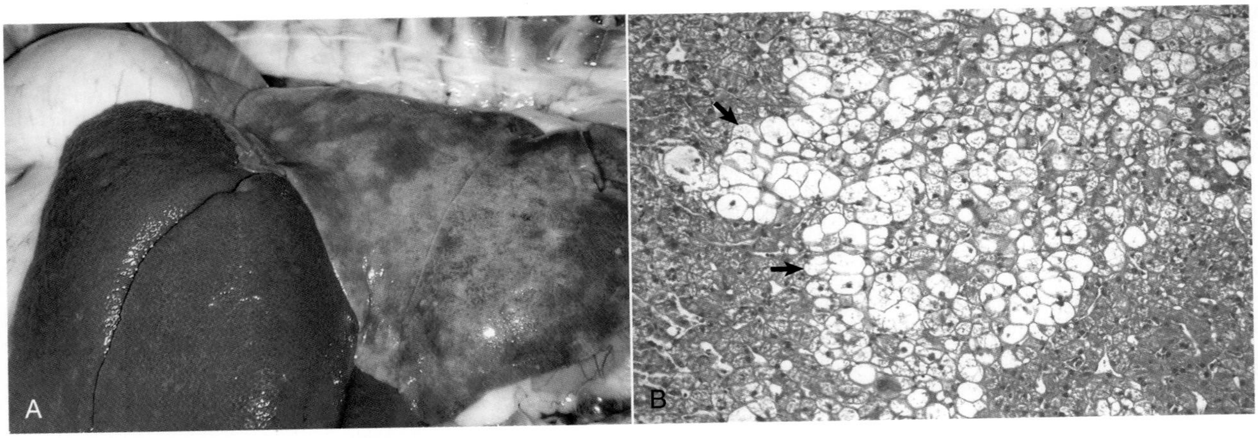

Fig. 1-46 Glucocorticoid hepatopathy, liver, dog.
A, Extensive accumulation of glycogen in hepatocytes leads to an enlarged and pale brown to beige liver in dogs with glucocorticoid excess from endogenous (Cushing's disease) or exogenous sources. The liver is usually enlarged and the edges rounded. This cut surface would bulge on incision and not be greasy. **B,** Note the swollen hepatocytes *(arrows)* with extensive cytoplasmic vacuolation. H&E stain. (**A** courtesy Dr. K. Bailey, College of Veterinary Medicine, University of Illinois. **B** courtesy Dr. J. M. Cullen, College of Veterinary Medicine, North Carolina State University.)

(Fig. 1-46, *A*). Cut sections do not float in formalin. These gross lesions are attributable to the accumulation of glycogen and water in the cytoplasm of hepatocytes (see Chapter 8).

Microscopically, hepatocytes with lipidosis are vacuolated, with the extent of the vacuolation depending on the severity of the lipidosis. Initially, there are a few small clear vacuoles that increase in size and number and eventually coalesce into larger vacuoles. These vacuoles have sharply delineated borders (Fig. 1-45, *B*), which are attributed to the hydrophobic interface between water and lipid in the cell's cytoplasm and should be compared with the vacuoles that result from glycogen accumulation (Fig. 1-46, *B*). In hepatocytes with large amounts of fat, the nucleus can be displaced to the periphery, and the cell can resemble an adipocyte. In extremely affected livers in which all of the hepatocytes are filled with lipid, the liver can resemble fat and can be identifiable only by the presence of portal areas.

Vacuoles in hepatocytes may be due to fat accumulation but can also occur as the result of intracellular accumulation of glycogen or water. Fat is confirmed by special stains, but as alcohol and clearing agents used during the processing of paraffin-embedded sections dissolve fat, formalin-fixed frozen sections—properly stained for fat—must be used to confirm its presence in hepatocytes. Fat stains, which are alcoholic solutions of fat-soluble dyes, include Sudan III, Scharlach R, and Oil-Red-O. Glycogen is confirmed by the PAS and PAS-diastase reactions described later (see section on Glycogen). Vacuoles that do not stain with either fat or PAS are presumed to be a result of the accumulation of water (hydropic degeneration).

Fatty Infiltration

Fatty infiltration should not be confused with fatty change or steatosis, in which the lipid is intracellular (see previous discussion). Adipocytes are normally present in connective tissue and depending on the nutritional state of the animal in limited numbers between fasciculi of skeletal muscle and subepicardially between cardiac myocytes. When increased lipid is to be stored, adipocytes increase in number, and the process is called fatty infiltration. It occurs in old age and in obesity in which there is hyperplasia of adipocytes by means of proliferation of preadipocytes. When myocytes of skeletal muscle atrophy and disappear, the lost myocytes may be replaced by adipocytes (see Chapter 15 and Fig. 15-9).

Glycogen

Variable amounts of glycogen are normally stored in hepatocytes and myocytes (the amount in the liver depends on the interval between sampling and the last meal). Hepatocytes of starved animals are usually devoid of glycogen. Excessive amounts of glycogen are present in animals in which glucose or glycogen metabolism is abnormal, such as in diabetes mellitus, in genetic disorders such as glycogen storage diseases (type Ia and type III), and in animals that have received excess amounts of corticosteroids. Large amounts of glycogen can be found in the livers of young growing animals and in animals that are well nourished and on diets of commercially produced feeds.

In diabetes, glycogen is found not only in hepatocytes but also in the epithelial cells of renal proximal tubules and in B cells of the islets of Langerhans. Hepatocytes are highly permeable to glucose, and hyperglycemia leads to increased glycogen concentration in these cells. Also in diabetes, large amounts of glucose are passed out in the glomerular filtrate and exceed the resorptive capacity of the renal tubule epithelial cells. These cells, when overloaded with glucose, convert it into glycogen, which accumulates intracellularly.

Grossly, physiologic deposits of glycogen cannot be detected, but in steroid-induced hepatopathy, in which massive amounts of glycogen are stored, the liver may be enlarged and pale (see Fig. 1-46).

Microscopically, the amount of glycogen demonstrated in hepatocytes is chiefly a function of the original concentration in the cell, the delay between death and fixation during which time the glycogen is metabolized, and the type of fixation. Despite frequent statements that glycogen is best preserved by fixing tissue in an alcoholic fixative (e.g., absolute alcohol or 10% formalin in absolute alcohol), glycogen can be well preserved by fixation in an ordinary 10% buffered neutral formalin solution at 4° C in a refrigerator during the period of fixation (Fig. 1-47, *A*). This procedure retains most of the glycogen but avoids the excessive shrinkage and distortion of tissues fixed in alcoholic fixatives and also avoids "polarization," the phenomenon whereby the glycogen is displaced to the side of the cell away from the surface. Polarization is seen in fixation at room temperature but is worst with alcoholic fixatives (Fig. 1-47, *B*).

Histologically, glycogen is demonstrated specifically by the PAS reaction using two serial tissue sections mounted on glass slides. The tissue section on the first slide is pretreated with diastase, which digests the glycogen in the tissue, and the tissue section on

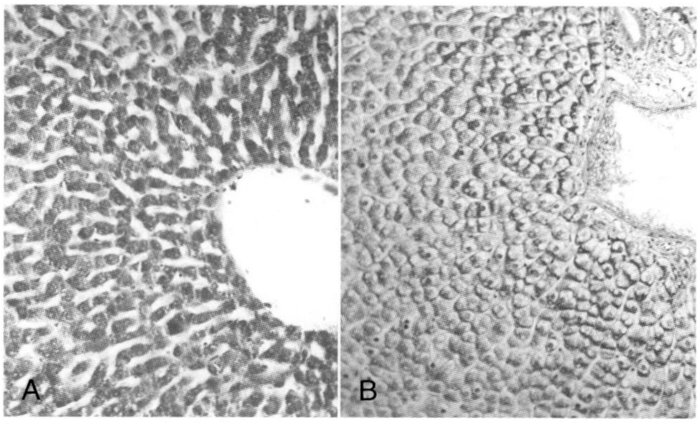

Fig. 1-47 Glycogen, liver, dog.
A, Ten-percent buffered neutral formalin fixation at 4° C. Glycogen (purplish-red) is uniformly dispersed throughout the cytoplasm of all hepatocytes. Periodic acid-Schiff technique. **B,** Absolute alcohol (ethanol) fixation at room temperature. The glycogen in each hepatocyte has been pushed to the side of the cell, so-called polarization of glycogen. Periodic acid-Schiff technique. (Courtesy Dr. M.D. McGavin, College of Veterinary Medicine, University of Tennessee.)

the second glass slide is untreated. Thus the deposits digested by diastase are glycogen. The PAS reaction breaks 1,2-glycol linkages to form aldehydes, which are revealed by Schiff's reagent. These linkages occur in substances other than glycogen, hence the use of two slides, including one pretreated with diastase, to specifically identify glycogen. Microscopically, glycogen appears as clear vacuoles in the cytoplasm of the cell. In contrast to intracellular fat whose vacuoles are rounded and sharply delineated, glycogen forms irregular clear spaces with indistinct outlines. Usually the nucleus remains centrally located in the hepatocyte. However, if very large amounts of glycogen are stored in hepatocytes, as in steroid-induced hepatopathy, hepatocyte nuclei may be displaced peripherally.

In glycogen storage diseases (glycogenoses), glycogen accumulates, sometimes in massive amounts in cells as a result of a defective enzyme. Exactly which cells store glycogen depends on the defective enzyme, but skeletal muscle is frequently involved (see Chapters 14 and 15 for more detail).

Proteins

In histologic sections, intracellular protein accumulations are of several types and include rounded eosinophilic droplets, vacuoles, and aggregates in cells. The causes of these accumulations vary widely.

Hyaline Change

The adjective "hyaline" is defined by *Dorland's Medical Dictionary* as "glassy and transparent or nearly so," and the noun "hyalin" as a "translucent albuminoid substance." However, histologically the term has come to mean having a homogeneous, eosinophilic, and glassy (translucent) appearance. Some pathologists also add "amorphous," and the lesion has been termed both a change and a degeneration, but the term *hyaline* is purely descriptive and rather loosely applied to a variety of changes, none of which is a true cellular degeneration. Hyaline substances may be intracellular or extracellular.

Intracellular Hyaline Proteins

Intracellular hyaline proteins include resorption droplets in the proximal tubule epithelial cells, Russell bodies in plasma cells, and those aggregates caused by defects in protein folding.

Resorption droplets in the epithelial cells of renal proximal tubules

There is normally very little protein in the filtrate from the glomerulus, and the proximal tubule epithelial cells resorb what is present. When the protein concentration of the filtrate is high, as for example in a proteinuria from glomerular damage, this protein is taken up by the proximal tubule epithelial cells into vesicles where, in H&E stained sections, they appear as hyaline droplets in the cytoplasm (Fig. 1-48, *A*). The vesicles fuse with the lysosomes to form phagolysosomes, where the protein is metabolized. If the proteinuria ceases, the formation of hyaline droplets also ceases. This condition was once called *hyaline droplet degeneration.* It is not a degeneration but an exaggeration of a normal process. Also, similar droplets are seen in the intestinal epithelium of neonatal pigs and calves that have recently ingested colostrum.

Excessive production of normal protein

Hyaline bodies called Russell bodies are seen in the cytoplasm of some plasma cells (Mott cells). These bodies are large, eosinophilic, homogeneous, and amorphous and consist of immunoglobulin (γ-globulin). Russell bodies have been described as "manifestations of cellular indigestion" in the ER.

Defects in protein folding

During protein synthesis on ribosomes, proper folding of the protein is essential for its transport in the cell's organelles. Normally, if there is a defect in folding, the protein is eliminated by the proteasome complex (Fig. 1-49). On occasion, these folded proteins accumulate in cells as is seen in some of the human neurodegenerative diseases, including Alzheimer's disease. Sometimes folded proteins may accumulate in tissue, and some types of amyloidosis are examples of this process.

Other Intracellular Inclusions

Autophagic Vacuoles

Autophagic vacuoles are large eosinophilic intracytoplasmic inclusions, which ultrastructurally are autophagosomes (see Fig. 1-35). They are a common response to injury in cells with sublethal damage, particularly hepatocytes, and are a mechanism by which the cell rids itself of damaged or senescent organelles. A portion of the cell membrane invaginates and envelops the affected organelles to form an autophagosome, which then fuses with a lysosome to cause degradation of the contents. Digestion of the material in autophagic vacuoles may leave some lamellar debris, and this debris may either be exocytosed from the cell or remain intracellularly to form lipofuscin (see later discussion of pigments).

Crystalline Protein Inclusion Bodies

Crystalline protein inclusion bodies, sometimes known as *crystalloids,* occur in normal hepatocytes and renal tubular epithelial cells, particularly in old dogs. They are large, eosinophilic, and rhomboidal and may be so large as to distort the nucleus or the cell (Fig. 1-48, *B*). Except for being age related, their significance is unknown. In fact, an increased incidence of these inclusions is the most consistent age-related change in canine hepatocytes.

Viral Inclusion Bodies

Infection of host cells by some types of viruses results in the formation of characteristic inclusion bodies, which may be intranuclear, intracytoplasmic, or both. They contain viral proteins usually mixed with other proteins and are useful diagnostically to confirm a specific viral disease.

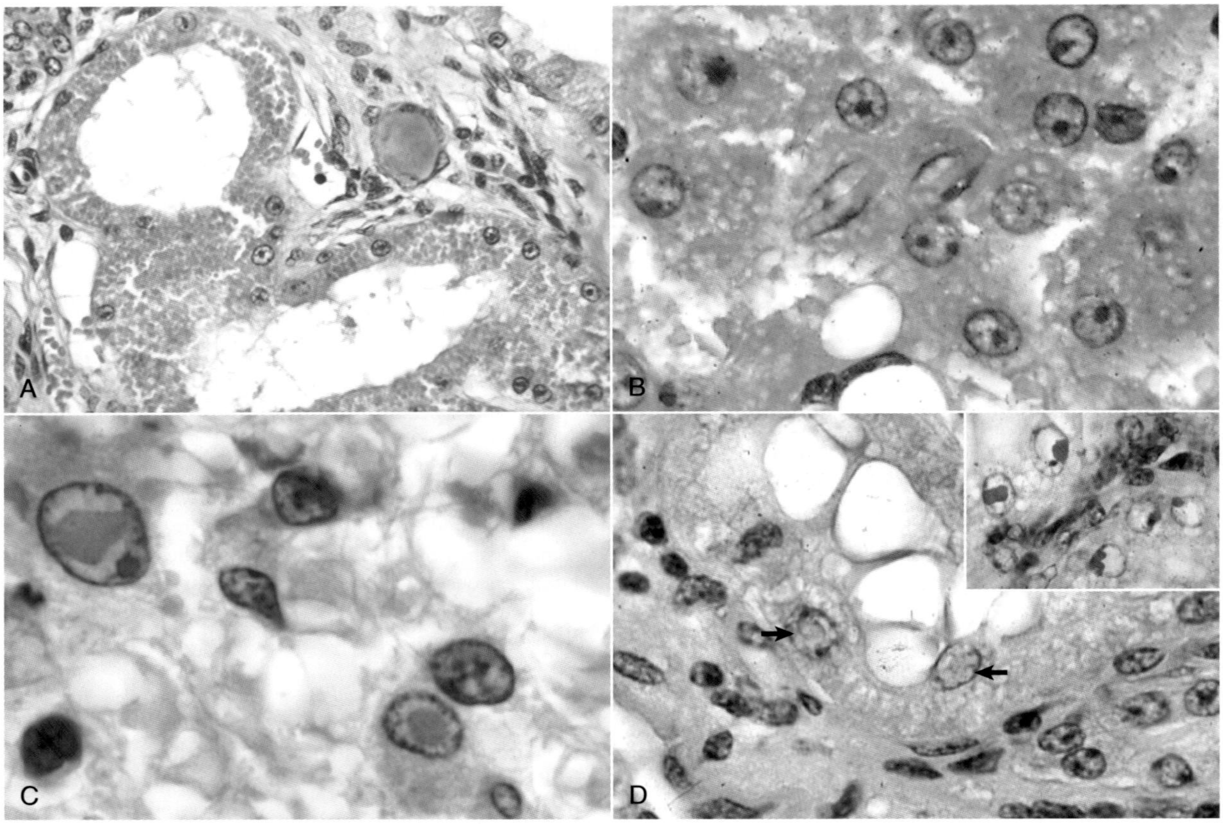

Fig. 1-48 Cell droplets and inclusion bodies.
A, Resorption droplets, proteinuria, kidney, dog. The cytoplasm of the proximal tubule epithelial cells is filled with eosinophilic homogeneous droplets—protein that has been resorbed by the cells from the glomerular filtrate. H&E stain. **B,** Crystalloids, hepatocytes, dog. Note the elongated crystals in the nuclei of the hepatocytes. **C,** Viral inclusion bodies, canine distemper, brain, dog. Note the intranuclear eosinophilic inclusion bodies in glial cells. H&E stain. **D,** Lead inclusion bodies, kidney, dog. The inclusions in the nuclei of these renal tubular epithelial cells are difficult to see with an H&E stain *(arrows). Inset,* An acid-fast stain is useful in identifying lead inclusions, which stain red. Ziehl-Neelsen stain. (**A** and **C** courtesy Dr. M.D. McGavin, College of Veterinary Medicine, University of Tennessee. **B** courtesy Dr. D.D. Harrington, College of Veterinary Medicine, Purdue University; and Noah's Arkive, College of Veterinary Medicine, The University of Georgia. **D** courtesy Dr. W. Crowell, College of Veterinary Medicine, The University of Georgia; and Noah's Arkive, College of Veterinary Medicine, The University of Georgia. **Inset** courtesy Dr. W. Crowell, College of Veterinary Medicine, The University of Georgia; and Noah's Arkive, College of Veterinary Medicine, The University of Georgia.)

DNA viruses, such as herpesviruses, adenoviruses, and parvoviruses, tend to produce only intranuclear inclusions. These inclusions are round to oval and can be eosinophilic (herpesviruses), basophilic, or amphophilic (adenoviruses). Poxviruses are also DNA viruses, but they produce large distinct eosinophilic intracytoplasmic inclusion bodies in infected cells.

A few RNA viruses produce intracytoplasmic inclusions. Examples are the distinctive cytoplasmic neuronal inclusions of rabies (Negri bodies) and the epithelial inclusions of canine distemper. Distemper causes both intranuclear and intracytoplasmic inclusions in nervous tissue (Fig. 1-48, *C*). Viral inclusions are usually surrounded by a clear halo, particularly in the nucleus. Cells with inclusion bodies and adjacent cells usually have signs of degeneration or cell death. Many of these viral inclusion bodies are discussed in the systemic pathology chapters of this book.

Lead Inclusion Bodies

In lead poisoning, irregularly shaped intranuclear inclusion bodies that are acid-fast may be present in renal tubular epithelial cells (Fig. 1-48, *D*). They contain both lead and protein. When they are present, they are helpful in the diagnosis of lead poisoning, but are not present in all cases. In dogs, they must be distinguished from the protein crystalline protein inclusions described previously.

EXTRACELLULAR ACCUMULATIONS

Hyaline Substances

Extracellular hyaline substances include the following:

1. Hyaline casts in the lumens of renal tubules in a proteinuria.
2. Serum or plasma in blood vessels.
3. Plasma proteins in vessel walls (e.g., in porcine edema disease). These substances are subendothelial hyaline deposits, primarily seen in arterioles of the brainstem in pigs with porcine edema disease (see Fig. 1-52).
4. Old scars. With age, the number of nuclei in collagen deposits decreases as the result of cell senescence, and the collagen fibers condense and become hyalinized.
5. Thickened basement membranes (e.g., in glomerulonephritis and in the capillaries of the choroid plexus with old age).
6. Hyaline membranes of the alveolar walls (see Chapter 9).
7. Hyaline microthrombi (e.g., platelet microthrombi) in disseminated intravascular coagulation (DIC); often visible in glomerular capillaries and pulmonary alveolar capillaries.
8. Amyloid (as described next).

Amyloid

The name *amyloid* is given to a chemically diverse group of chiefly extracellular proteinaceous substances that appear histologically

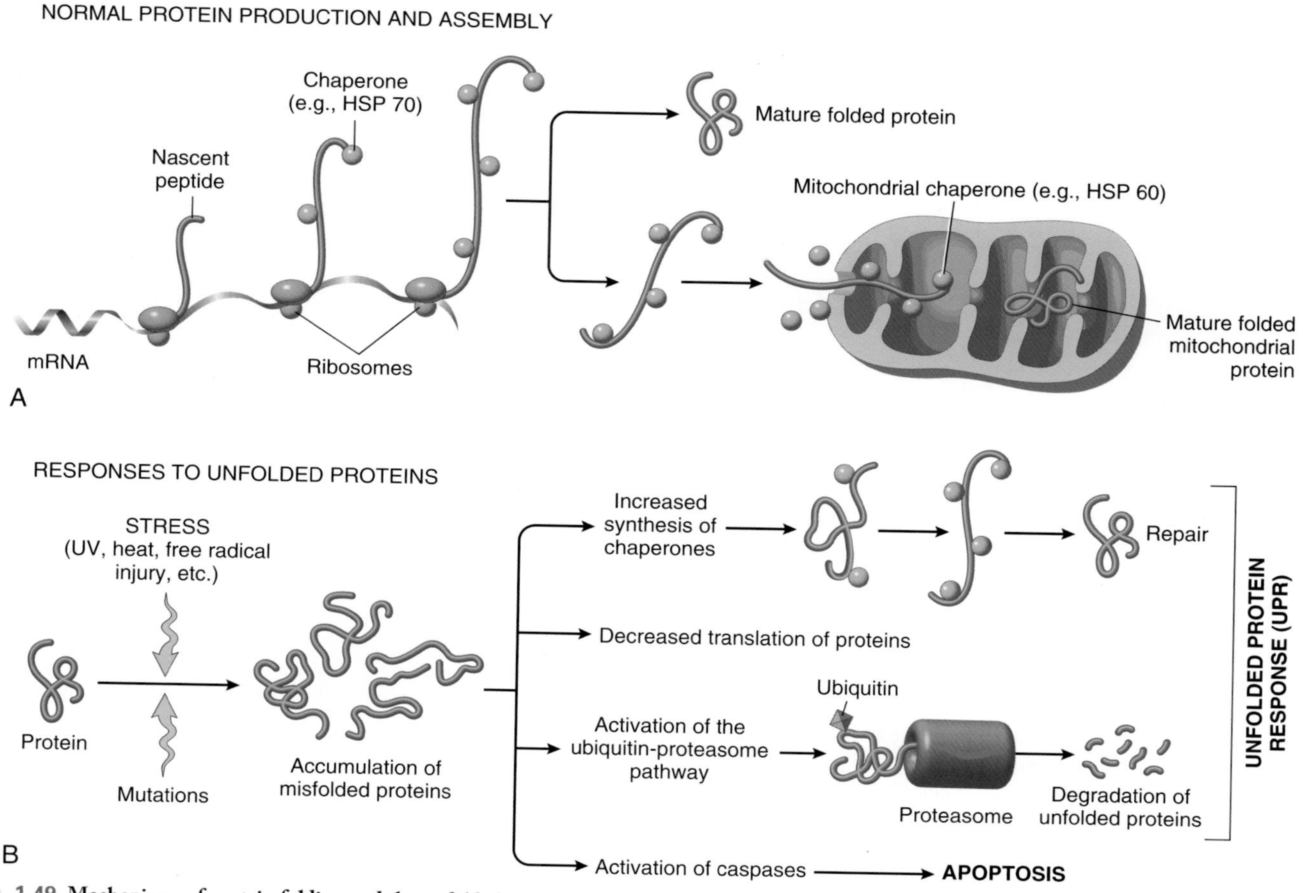

Fig. 1-49 Mechanisms of protein folding and the unfolded protein response.
A, Chaperones, such as heat shock proteins (HSP), protect unfolded proteins from degradation and guide proteins into organelles. **B,** Misfolded proteins trigger a protective unfolded protein response (UPR). If this response is inadequate to cope with the level of misfolded proteins, it induces apoptosis. (From Kumar V, Abbas A, Fausto N, et al: *Robbins & Cotran pathologic basis of disease,* ed 8, Philadelphia, 2009, Saunders.)

and ultrastructurally similar. The name means "starchlike" and was applied to these proteins because when the surface of an affected organ was treated with an iodine solution and then with dilute sulfuric acid, it turned blue, a positive test for starch (Fig. 1-50).

Histologically, amyloid is an eosinophilic amorphous hyaline substance (Fig. 1-51, *A*) and needs to be differentiated from other hyaline substances on histologic examination. It is extracellular and compresses adjacent parenchymal cells, causing atrophy or death from compression and/or ischemia. This outcome is most evident in hepatic amyloidosis, in which the protein is deposited in the space of Disse. Here it compresses the adjacent hepatocytes and interferes with the hepatocytes' access to blood and nutrients in the sinusoids.

The most frequently used special stain for amyloid is Congo red. It stains amyloid orange to orange red (Fig. 1-51, *B*) and under polarized light imparts a light green, the so-called apple green fluorescence (see Chapter 11). Congo red staining is not absolutely specific, and immunohistochemistry or transmission electron microscopy to identify 7.5- to 10-nm filaments may be necessary.

Chemically, amyloid is not one substance. It is a diverse group of glycoproteins whose protein component is configured in a β-pleated sheet pattern, which is responsible for the characteristic staining with Congo red. In humans, there are three major and several minor forms. In animals, there are two major and two minor forms, which are chemically distinct but appear similar histologically.

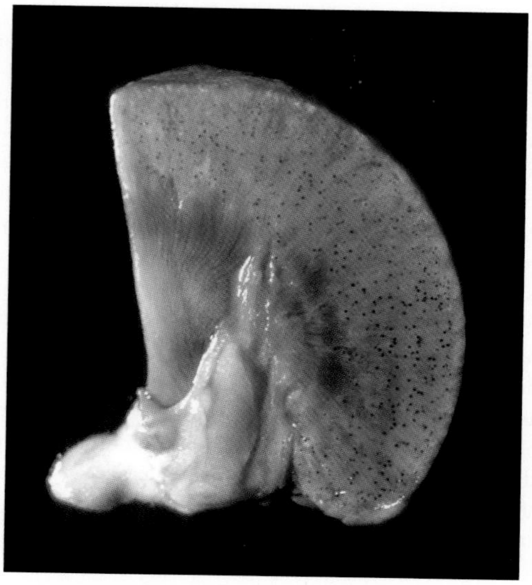

Fig. 1-50 Amyloidosis, kidney, cross section, dog.
Note the blue-black foci, which are glomeruli-containing amyloid stained by Lugol's iodine. (Courtesy Dr. M.D. McGavin, College of Veterinary Medicine, University of Tennessee.)

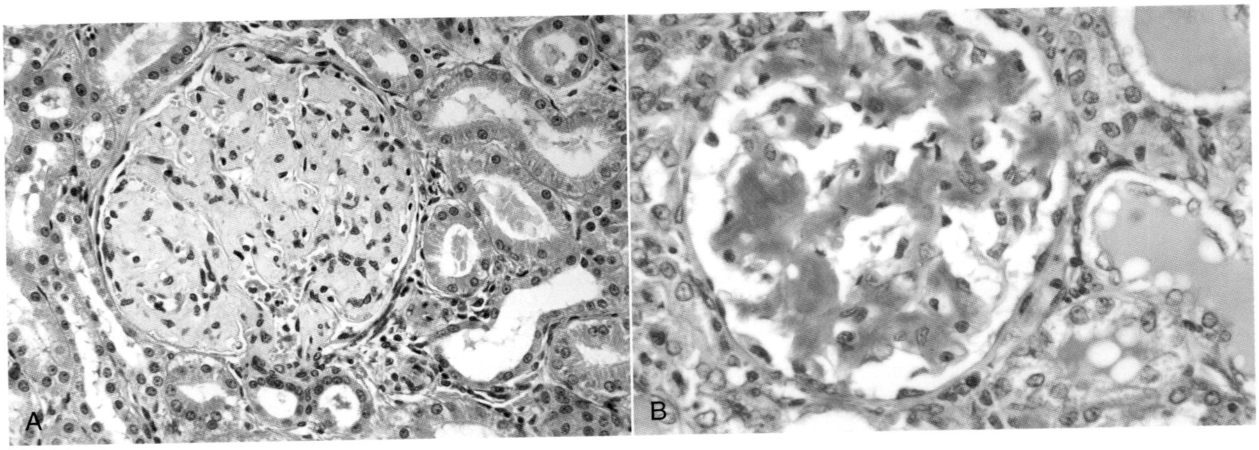

Fig. 1-51 Amyloidosis, kidney, dog.
A, The renal glomerulus contains large amounts of pale homogeneous eosinophilic material, which is amyloid. H&E stain. **B,** The amyloid in the glomeruli stains orange. Congo red stain. (**A** and **B** courtesy Dr. M.D. McGavin, College of Veterinary Medicine, University of Tennessee.)

AL amyloid consists of immunoglobulin light chains, is monoclonal, and is secreted by plasma cells in immunocyte dyscrasias (B lymphocyte proliferative disorders). AA amyloid is not an immunoglobulin but is synthesized from a precursor protein, serum amyloid A (SAA), secreted by the liver. SAA concentration is increased in inflammatory states in response to IL-1 and IL-6, but this increase does not necessarily lead to amyloid deposition in all cases. A minor form of amyloidosis is hereditary amyloidosis found in Shar-Pei dogs and in Abyssinian cats.

β-Amyloid found in Alzheimer's disease in humans has been detected in the brains of aged dogs.

Classification of Amyloidosis

Amyloidosis is discussed in detail in Chapter 5.

Amyloidosis has been classified in several ways (i.e., primary versus secondary, systemic [generalized] versus localized, and a combination of these categories). Systemic amyloidosis (generalized) is also divided into primary amyloidosis (immunocyte dyscrasia) and secondary amyloidosis (reactive systemic amyloidosis).

- *Immunocyte dyscrasia* is the most common form of amyloidosis in humans but not in animals. The amyloid consists of amyloid light chains and is indicative of a plasma cell dyscrasia. These cells also secrete large amounts of γ- and κ-light chains into blood and urine (Bence Jones proteins), which are diagnostically important.
- *Reactive systemic amyloidosis* was initially called *secondary amyloidosis* because it was secondary to chronic inflammatory conditions, particularly those causing a chronic antigenic stimulation with protracted breakdown of cells. It is the most common form of amyloidosis in animals, and the amyloid is deposited in kidney, liver, spleen, and lymph nodes. Functionally, and most often in old dogs, amyloid deposits in the kidney are the most important because they are located in the mesangium and basement membranes of renal glomeruli and cause a proteinuria. The spleen is the most frequent site in reactive systemic amyloidosis, and amyloid is deposited in the periarteriolar lymphoid sheaths and red pulp. The space of Disse of the liver is the usual site for amyloidosis in birds.
- Localized amyloidosis involves a single organ or tissue. Such localized lesions are in the nasal vestibule or rostral portion of the nasal septum and turbinates in horses and in the pancreatic islets in cats.
- β-Amyloidosis. Extracellular accumulation of amyloid-β (Aβ) protein is characteristic of Alzheimer's disease in humans. This type of amyloid has also been identified in the brains of aged dogs, the highest concentration being in the frontal cortex. Dogs older than 13 years had Aβ plaques.

Location of Amyloid Deposits in Animals

The kidney (glomeruli in most animals and medullae in cats), liver (space of Disse in cattle, horses, dogs, and cats), and spleen (germinal centers) are common sites. Other organs affected include the stomach, intestine (lamina propria), thyroid (C-cell tumor), skin (dermis and subcutis of horses), lymph node (germinal centers), adrenal cortex, pancreas (islets of Langerhans in cats), nasal septum and turbinates (walls of submucosal vessels and basement membranes of mucosal glands of horses), and meningeal and cerebral vessels of older dogs. See the appropriate organ chapters for more detail.

Other Extracellular Accumulations

Fibrinoid Change

Fibrinoid change, also known as fibrinoid necrosis and fibrinoid degeneration, is a term applied to a pattern of lesions most often observed in the vascular system. The terms *fibrinoid degeneration* and *fibrinoid necrosis* are inappropriate because the process is not a true regressive alteration of cells. Rather, fibrinoid change is the result of the deposition of immunoglobulin, complement, and/or plasma proteins, including fibrin in the wall of a vessel. This lesion is caused by injury to the intima and media such as occurs in the immune-mediated vasculitides.

Grossly, fibrinoid change cannot be observed; however, it is often accompanied by thrombosis and hemorrhage, and when these two lesions are present in a vascular pattern of distribution, fibrinoid change of the vasculature should be considered. Microscopically, direct injury to endothelial cells, basement membrane, or myocytes, such as caused by viruses or toxins, or indirect injury such as caused by activation of complement proteins, can lead to activation of the acute inflammatory cascade and the deposition of plasma proteins in the vessel walls. These proteins, especially fibrin, stain intensely red (eosinophilic) with H&E stains and involve the vessel wall circumferentially to varying depths of the tunica intima and tunica media (Fig. 1-52). This lesion is also often accompanied by cellular and nuclear debris from injured vascular cells and inflammatory cells. These proteins contribute to the vascular "eosinophilia," which

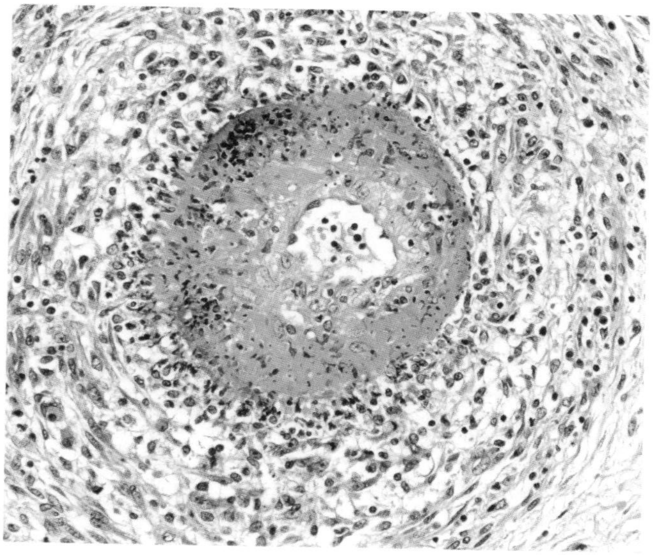

Fig. 1-52 Fibrinoid change, artery.
Note the deeply eosinophilic circumferential band in the tunica media of this artery. It is accompanied by acute inflammation and necrosis. H&E stain. (Courtesy Dr. J.F. Zachary, College of Veterinary Medicine, University of Illinois.)

has been described somewhat differently by different pathologists. There is general agreement that the material is eosinophilic, which is sometimes described as "smudgy" or "deeply eosinophilic." Some pathologists add "homogeneous" and others "amorphous" to the descriptive terminology of fibrinoid change.

Gout

Gout has not been reported in domestic mammals, but does occur in birds and reptiles. Information on this topic is available at evolve.elsevier.com/Zachary/McGavin/.

Pseudogout

Pseudogout has been reported in the dog but is rare. Information on this topic is available at evolve.elsevier.com/Zachary/McGavin/.

Cholesterol

Information on this topic is available at evolve.elsevier.com/Zachary/McGavin/.

PATHOLOGIC CALCIFICATION*

Calcium salts, usually in the form of phosphates or carbonates, may be deposited in dead, dying, or normal tissue. This process is known as *pathologic calcification* and occurs in two forms: dystrophic and metastatic. When the deposition occurs locally in dying tissue, it is known as dystrophic calcification; it occurs despite normal serum concentrations of calcium and in the absence of derangements in calcium metabolism. In contrast, the deposition of calcium salts in otherwise normal tissue is known as *metastatic calcification,* and it almost always results from hypercalcemia secondary to some disturbance in calcium metabolism. Less common forms of calcification are idiopathic (occurs in the absence of tissue injury or abnormalities in calcium or phosphorus metabolism) and iatrogenic (e.g., via ingestation of calcium salts from calcium chloride de-icing solutions).

*Portions of this section are from Kumar V, Abbas A, Fausto N, et al: *Robbins & Cotran pathologic basis of disease,* ed 8, Philadelphia, 2009, Saunders.

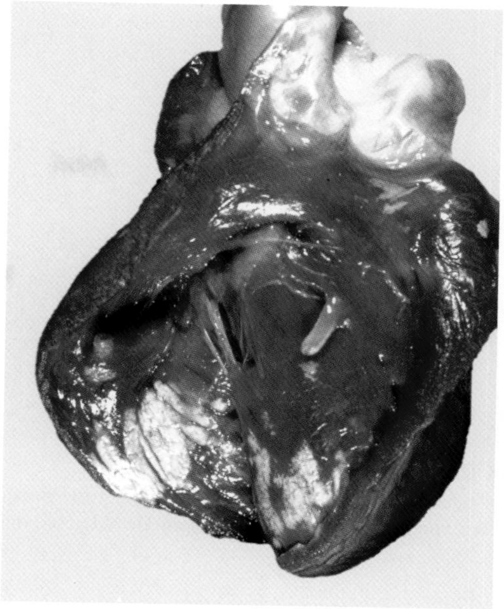

Fig. 1-53 Calcification, vitamin E/selenium deficiency, myodegeneration, heart, lamb.
The multiple white lesions are areas of necrosis of cardiac myocytes that have been calcified. (Courtesy Dr. M.D. McGavin, College of Veterinary Medicine, University of Tennessee.)

Dystrophic Calcification

Dystrophic calcification occurs in areas of necrosis, no matter the type of necrosis-coagulative, caseous, liquefactive, or fat necrosis, but is minimal in liquefactive necrosis. Dead and dying cells can no longer regulate the influx of calcium into their cytosol, and calcium accumulates in the mitochondria.

Common sites include necrotic myocardium (Fig. 1-53), necrotic skeletal muscle, granulomas such as tuberculoid granulomas in cattle, and dead parasites, such as hydatid cysts in cattle and trichinae in pigs. Calcium deposits are relatively permanent but harmless unless they interfere mechanically (e.g., the movement of a calcified heart valve). Their significance is that they are an indicator of previous injury to a tissue.

Calcification in or under the skin has been designated calcinosis. The two main forms are (1) calcinosis cutis and (2) calcinosis circumscripta (see Chapter 17). Calcinosis cutis occurs in dogs with hyperadrenocorticism from either endogenous or exogenous glucocorticoids and has been regarded as idiopathic calcification by some pathologists and dystrophic calcification by others. There is mineralization of the dermal collagen and epidermal and follicular basement membranes. Calcinosis circumscripta is considered to be dystrophic. It has a preference for German shepherds and Great Danes, in which it is familial. Also, it has been associated with repetitive trauma and at the site of buried sutures of polydioxanone.

Grossly, the affected areas of tissue are white and when incised have a gritty feel to them (see Fig. 1-53). Microscopically, calcium salts stain blue with hematoxylin and appear as fine amorphous

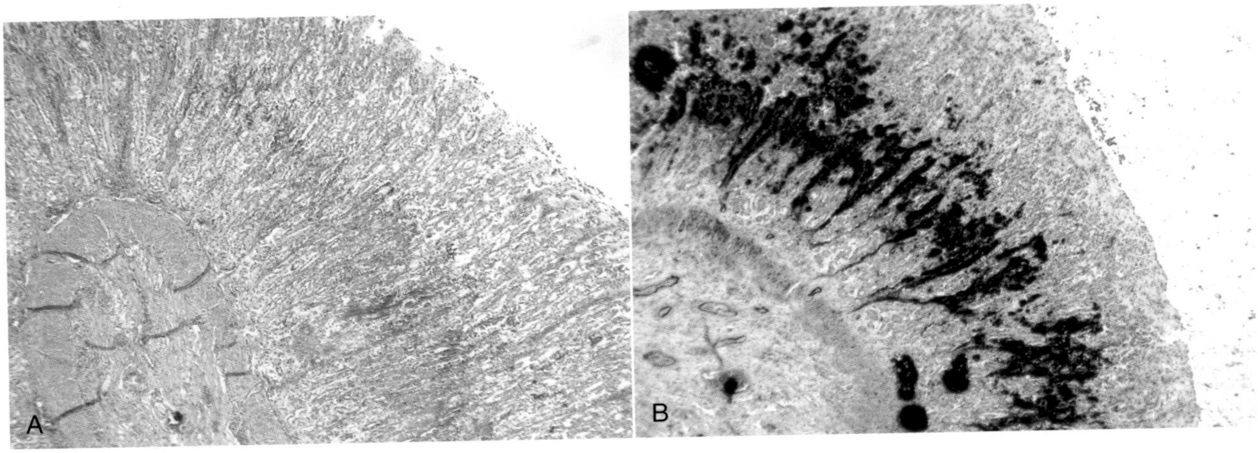

Fig. 1-54 Uremia, stomach, dog.
A band of calcium has been laid down the middle of the gastric mucosa. **A,** The calcium is stained blue with hematoxylin. H&E stain. **B,** The calcium is stained black. von Kossa stain. (**A** and **B** courtesy Dr. M.D. McGavin, College of Veterinary Medicine, University of Tennessee.)

granules or clumps, which can be either intracellular or extracellular. However, the full extent of the calcification may not be evident in H&E-stained sections (Fig. 1-54, *A*) but is revealed more dramatically by special stains, such as von Kossa and Alizarin red S (Fig. 1-54, *B*). The von Kossa method is not specific for calcium but stains phosphates and carbonates. These substances are almost always complexed with calcium.

Metastatic Calcification

Metastatic calcification occurs in normal tissue and is secondary to hypercalcemia. The basic abnormality is the entry of large amounts of calcium ions into cells. These ions precipitate on organelles, particularly mitochondria.

The four causes of metastatic calcification in order of their importance in veterinary medicine are as follows:

1. Renal failure. Renal failure results in retention of phosphates, which induce a secondary renal hyperparathyroidism and hypercalcemia. Calcium is deposited in the gastric mucosa, kidney, and alveolar septa.
2. Vitamin D toxicosis. The ingestion of calcinogenic plants, such as *Cestrum diurnum* by herbivores, results in severe soft tissue mineralization, chiefly involving the aorta, heart, and lungs. In the heart, the endocardium of the right and left atria and left ventricle is often strikingly mineralized. Acute vitamin D toxicosis in dogs and cats is commonly caused by ingestion of rodenticides containing cholecalciferol. Intestinal mucosa, vessel walls, lung, and kidneys are mineralized.
3. Parathormone (PTH) and PTH-related protein. Primary hyperparathyroidism is rare. Hypercalcemia and elevated concentrations of PTH-related protein can be associated with canine malignant lymphomas and canine adenocarcinoma of the apocrine glands of the anal sac. Intestinal mucosa, vessel walls, lung, and kidneys are mineralized.
4. Destruction of bone from primary or metastatic neoplasms.

HETEROTOPIC BONE (ECTOPIC BONE)

Some lesions of dystrophic and metastatic calcification may be confused on gross examination with ectopic ossification, the name given to the process of production of bone at an abnormal site. Ectopic bone is of two types: heterotopic or osseous metaplasia. "Heterotopia" refers to foci of cells or tissues, which are microscopically normal but present at an abnormal location. They are

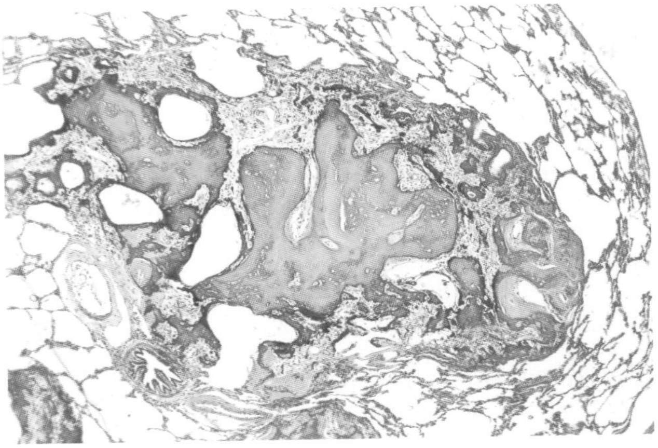

Fig. 1-55 Ectopic bone, lung, dog.
A nodule of mature bone in the connective tissue of the lung. H&E stain. (Courtesy Dr. M.D. McGavin, College of Veterinary Medicine, University of Tennessee.)

considered to arise from embryonic cell rests. The other type of bone is formed by osseous metaplasia, usually from another type of connective tissue. Fibroblasts differentiate into osteoblasts that form osteoid, which is calcified as in normal bone (Fig. 1-55). This is the more common type.

Heterotopic bone is found at many sites, commonly as spicules or nodules of bone in connective tissue of lungs of dogs and cattle, and in the canine dura mater (dural ossification or ossifying pachymeningitis) and at sites of dystrophic and metastatic calcification.

PIGMENTS

It is customary in pathology textbooks to group substances that impart an unusual color to the body (systemic) or its tissues (localized), under the category of pigments. Many of these pigments are unrelated in their origin, but their importance lies in the fact that the clinician and the pathologist need to be able to recognize them grossly, and the pathologist also needs to be able to identify them histologically. Recognition may provide valuable clues in understanding the disease process at hand and its underlying pathogenesis. Because of their diversity, pigments are usually classified broadly into two groups: exogenous (formed outside the body) and endogenous (formed inside the body).

Exogenous Pigments

These pigments include carbon, tattoos, dusts, carotenoids, and tetracycline.

Carbon

Carbon is the most common exogenous pigment. The usual route of entry into the body is via inhalation, and its accumulation in the lung results in a condition called *anthracosis* (also known as *black lung*).

Carbon is ubiquitous in the air and all animals are exposed, but those most likely to show gross lesions live in an environment with substantial air pollution, such as adjacent to busy highways (e.g., animals in a zoo near a highway or animals living in a house with a smoker). In the alveoli, the carbon is phagocytosed by macrophages, which transport it via the lymphatics to the regional tracheobronchial lymph nodes. Because elemental carbon is inert and not metabolized by the body, it remains in the tissue for the life of the animal.

Grossly, the lungs are usually speckled with fine 1- to 2-mm-diameter subpleural black foci, which are most visible if the lungs have been exsanguinated (Fig. 1-56, *A*). In severely affected cases, the medulla of the tracheobronchial lymph nodes may be black. The heavy deposits are in this location because of the concentration of sinus histiocytes (macrophages) in the medulla.

Microscopically, carbon presents as fine black granules and may be extracellular or intracellular (within macrophages). Carbon pigment may be within the alveolar walls or be frequently present as black peribronchiolar or peribronchial foci (Fig. 1-56, *B*). Because of the nonreactiveness of carbon, there are no histochemical tests for it. Unlike many other pigments, it is resistant to solvents and bleaching agents.

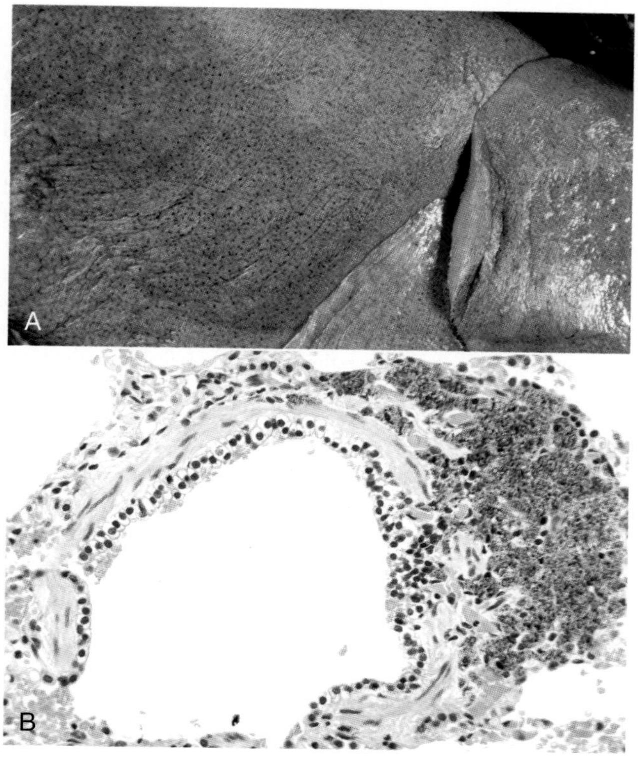

Fig. 1-56 Anthracosis, lung, aged dog.
A, The fine black foci are peribronchiolar deposits of carbon. The animal was exsanguinated at euthanasia to remove the blood from the lung to render the carbon deposits more visible. **B,** Carbon *(black)* inhaled into the alveoli has been phagocytosed by macrophages and transported to the peribronchial region. H&E stain. (**A** and **B** courtesy Dr. M.D. McGavin, College of Veterinary Medicine, University of Tennessee.)

Tattoos

Animals are frequently tattooed as a method of identification. These pigments, which include carbon, are introduced into the dermis. Some of the pigments are phagocytosed by macrophages, whereas the remainder remains free in the dermis where it can remain indefinitely and does not evoke any inflammatory reaction.

Dusts

Pneumoconiosis is the general term used for any dust inhaled into and retained in the lung. Anthracosis, from the inhalation of carbon, is a subtype of pneumoconiosis. Inhalation of silicon (e.g., from quarries) is called *silicosis.* These minute particles enter the lungs by escaping the mucociliary defense mechanisms of the nasal and upper respiratory systems (see Chapter 9) and are deposited in pulmonary alveoli where they may be phagocytosed and carried to the peribronchial regions. Some types of silica evoke a fibrous reaction, which may ultimately form nodules. Microscopically the mineral is visible as birefringent crystals under polarized light.

Carotenoid Pigments

Carotenoid pigments are also called *lipochrome pigments,* although this term is sometimes confused with lipofuscin (see later discussion). They are fat-soluble pigments of plant origin and include the precursor of vitamin A, namely β-carotene.

Grossly, these pigments normally occur in a wide variety of tissue, such as adrenal cortical cells, corpus luteum-lutein cells, Kupffer cells, and testicular cells, and in the plasma/serum and fat of horses and Jersey and Guernsey cattle and sometimes dogs (Fig. 1-57). Carotenoids discolor fat yellow to orange-yellow. The concentration of carotenoids retained in tissue depends on the species of animal. Some animals store little or no carotenoids and have white fat and clear serum. These animals include Holstein cattle, sheep, goats, and cats. As fat stores are depleted (e.g., in starvation or cachexia), carotenoids become concentrated in the adipocytes, giving them a dark yellowish-brown color.

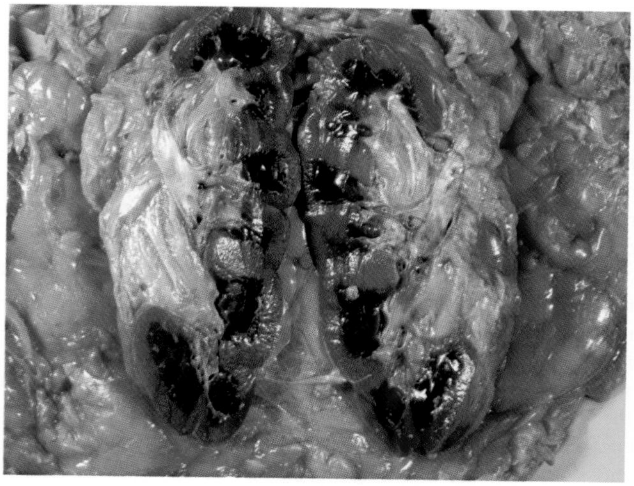

Fig. 1-57 Carotenosis, kidney and the perirenal fat, Jersey ox.
Accumulation of carotenoids in the adipocytes has colored the fat yellow to dark yellow. (Courtesy Dr. M.D. McGavin, College of Veterinary Medicine, University of Tennessee.)

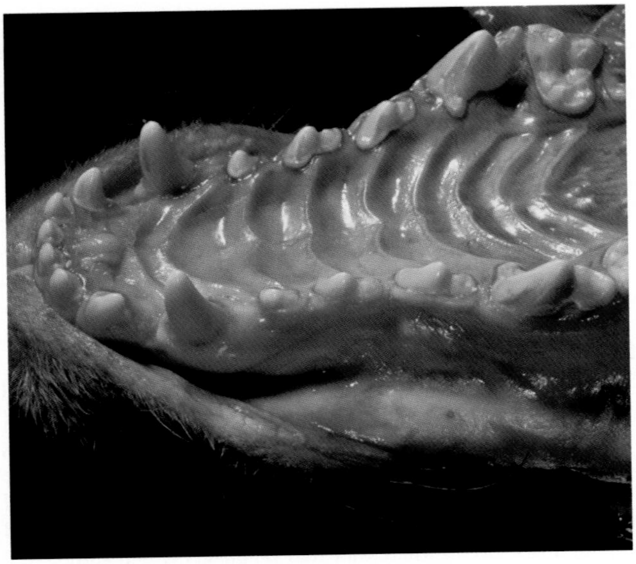

Fig. 1-58 Tetracycline staining, teeth, young dog.
The teeth of this dog have been stained yellow by the tetracycline ingested during their development. (Courtesy Dr. M.D. McGavin, College of Veterinary Medicine, University of Tennessee.)

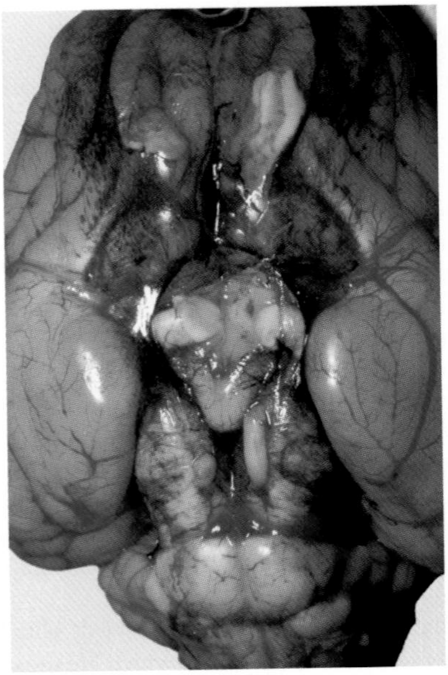

Fig. 1-59 Congenital melanosis, leptomeninges, Suffolk sheep.
The leptomeninges have scattered black areas of melanin. This is normal in black-faced sheep. (Courtesy Dr. M.D. McGavin, College of Veterinary Medicine, University of Tennessee.)

Microscopically, carotenoids are not seen in routine formalin-fixed paraffin-embedded sections because the alcohols and clearing agents remove the fat-soluble pigments.

The significance of carotenoids is that they may obscure or confuse the detection of icterus. In those animals whose fat and serum are devoid of carotenoids, a yellow discoloration is easily detected and is most likely to be caused by bilirubin (i.e., icterus).

Tetracycline

Tetracycline-based antibiotics administered during the development of teeth are deposited in mineralizing dentin, enamel, and cementum, staining the teeth or portions of them yellow or brown (Fig. 1-58). Thus tetracycline administered to a pregnant animal stains the deciduous teeth of the offspring. Tetracycline also stains bone that is being laid down and has been used experimentally as a marker for that bone.

Endogenous Pigments

Melanin

Melanin is the pigment normally present in the epidermis and is responsible for the color of the skin and hair. It is also normally present in the retina, iris, and in small amounts in the pia-arachnoid of black animals (e.g., Suffolk sheep [Fig. 1-59]) and in the oral mucous membrane of some breeds (e.g., Jersey cows and Chow dogs).

Cells called *melanocytes* secrete melanin. In the skin of animals, these cells are in the basal layer and transfer their pigment by means of dendritic processes to adjacent keratinocytes, where the melanin is often arranged as a cap over the nucleus to provide some protection from ultraviolet radiation. Melanin is formed by the oxidation of tyrosine, which requires the copper-containing enzyme tyrosinase. Thus, in copper deficiency, particularly in cattle and sheep, there is a fading of the coat color, and this is most obvious in black wool. A general lack of melanin can be the result of a metabolic defect: a lack of tyrosinase. This condition is called *albinism*, and the affected animal is called an *albino*. Histologically, the melanocytes appear normal.

Pathologically, melanin is present in hyperpigmentation of the skin associated with many types of chronic injury and endocrinopathies, such as hyperadrenalism, and in primary neoplasms of melanocytes (melanocytomas and malignant melanomas), although highly malignant tumors may have little or no pigment.

Microscopically, melanin is stored in melanosomes in the cytoplasm of melanocytes. However, if there is irreversible injury to the cells containing melanin (e.g., necrosis of melanocytes and basal cells of the skin), melanin is released from the dead cells and is phagocytosed by macrophages, which are termed *melanophages*.

Extensive deposits of congenital melanin in tissues are termed *congenital melanosis*. It occurs in the lungs and aorta (intima) of cattle, sheep, and pigs as brown-to-black spots up to a couple of centimeters in diameter (Fig. 1-60). Melanosis of the lung is visible both subpleurally and in cross-sections of the parenchyma. These deposits of melanin have no adverse effects, but organs with extensive melanosis may be aesthetically unacceptable as food and thus will be condemned at the packing plant.

Lipofuscin-Ceroid

Lipofuscin, known as "wear-and-tear" pigment, has in the past been described as accumulating with age and in certain pathologic conditions. However, in recent years, lipofuscin, now referred to as "age" pigment, has been differentiated from a pathologically accumulating similar pigment called *ceroid*, which is described later.

Lipofuscin accumulates in a time-dependent manner in postmitotic cells (neurons, cardiac myocytes [Fig. 1-61], and skeletal muscle myocytes) and in slowly dividing cells, such as hepatocytes and glial cells, and this process is present at a few months of age. Lipofuscin is also found in other cells, but as these replicate, the lipofuscin is divided between the daughter cells and thus does not accumulate to the same extent as it does in postmitotic cells. Lipofuscin is the end result of autophagocytosis of cell constituents, such as organelles, and is the final undegradable remnant of that process. As the pigment cannot be removed by further lysosomal degradation or exocytosis, it accumulates in lysosomes, a form of biologic garbage.

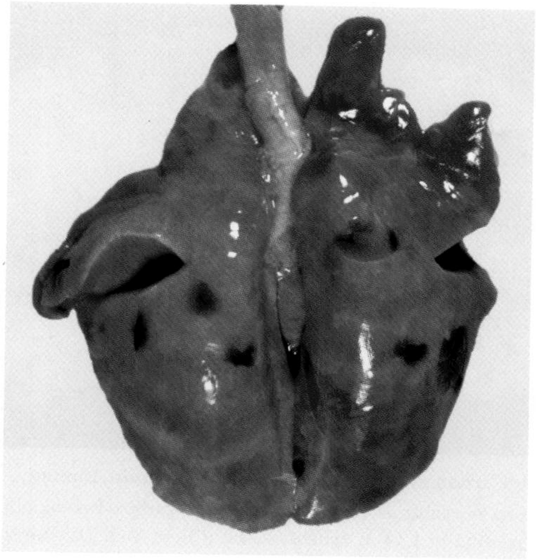

Fig. 1-60 Congenital melanosis, lung, pig.
Melanin deposits are subpleural and extend into the substance of a lung. The lesion has no pathological significance. (Courtesy Dr. M.D. McGavin, College of Veterinary Medicine, University of Tennessee.)

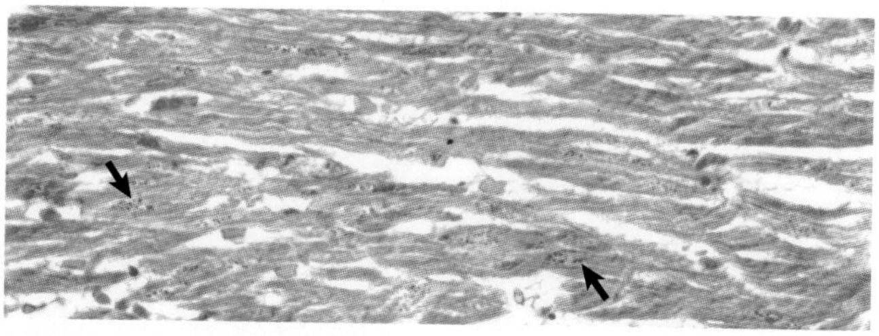

Fig. 1-61 Lipofuscinosis, heart, dog.
Note the brown lipofuscin granules *(arrows)* at the poles of the myocyte nuclei. H&E stain. (Courtesy Dr. J.F. Zachary, College of Veterinary Medicine, University of Illinois.)

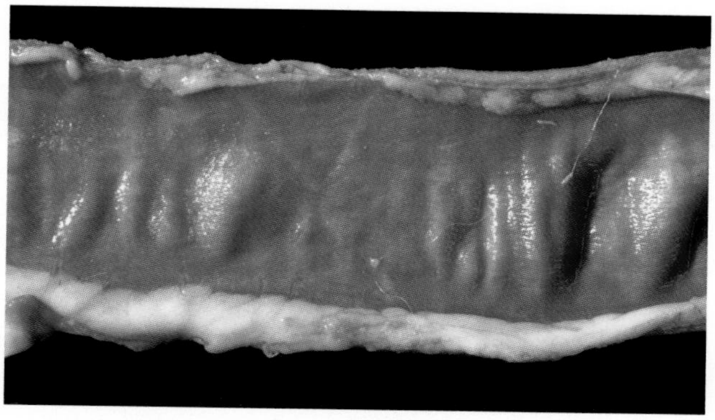

Fig. 1-62 Ceroid, intestine, serosal surface, dog.
Note the brown discoloration of the muscular layer. The condition has been called intestinal lipofuscinosis but is not age related. (Courtesy Dr. M.D. McGavin, College of Veterinary Medicine, University of Tennessee.)

Ceroid has many of the same histochemical features as lipofuscin (see later discussion) but is found in response to severe malnutrition, including vitamin E deficiency, cachexia from cancer, irradiation, and in the inherited disease neuronal ceroid-lipofuscinosis. It accumulates in Kupffer cells and to a lesser extent in hepatocytes, skeletal and smooth muscle myocytes, and in inherited neuronal ceroid-lipofuscinosis, where it accumulates in neurons. It can be either intracellular or extracellular. Unlike lipofuscin, it is considered to have a deleterious effect on the cell.

Both lipofuscin and ceroid have many common histologic and histochemical features, such as autofluorescence (golden yellow) and staining with stains for fat such as Sudan black (sudanophilia), although oil-red-O is more sensitive, PAS positive, and acid-fast (long Ziehl-Neelsen technique). All of these characteristics increase in intensity with age for lipofuscin but not for ceroid. Lipofuscin consists chiefly of proteins and lipids with very little carbohydrate, but lectin-binding histochemistry in humans and rats has revealed differences in the saccharides of lipofuscin and ceroid.

Grossly, large amounts of lipofuscin in the heart and skeletal muscles impart a brown tinge. It is commonly seen in aged dairy cows sent to slaughter. Ceroid is grossly evident in the small intestine of dogs with so-called intestinal lipofuscinosis (Fig. 1-62) (also see Chapter 7) and in nutritional panniculitis in cats, mink, foals, and pigs. Both of these conditions are associated with a vitamin E deficiency and the ingestion of unsaturated fatty acids. In the dog, the tunica muscularis, usually of the caudal small intestine, is discolored brown because of accumulations of ceroid in myocytes. In the cat with nutritional panniculitis, the subcutaneous fat is discolored lemon yellow to orange. This disease is considered to be the result of the ingestion of fish products with a high concentration of unsaturated fatty acids and a vitamin E deficiency, frequently brought about by the fats becoming rancid and destroying the vitamin E.

Microscopically, in routine H&E-stained sections or in unstained sections, lipofuscin varies from a light golden brown to dark brown with advancing age. Because it is intralysosomal, it is perinuclear in neurons and in cardiac, skeletal, and smooth muscle myocytes. In feline nutritional panniculitis, globules of ceroid are extracellular in the interstitial tissue or have been ingested by macrophages and giant cells.

The significance of these two pigments is that lipofuscin is a clear indicator of the age of the cell and ceroid is a pathologic pigment, often associated with vitamin E deficiency. Lectin-binding histochemistry, which has shown differences between lipofuscin and ceroid from rats and humans, may be applicable to differentiating these pigments in domestic animals, but it is a very laborious research tool and only provides semiquantitative data. Isolation and physicochemical analysis is more precise but even more laborious. Thus, until some other specific test becomes available, differentiation between the two pigments for diagnostic purposes will be based on the features listed in Table 1-1.

Hematogenous Pigments

The hematogenous pigment category includes hemoglobin, oxyhemoglobin, unoxygenated hemoglobin, methemoglobin, carboxyhemoglobin, hemosiderin, bilirubin, and hematin. Some are produced normally but can accumulate excessively (unoxygenated hemoglobin, hemosiderin, and bilirubin). Other pigments, such as methemoglobin, carboxyhemoglobin, and hematin, are pathologic.

Hemoglobin

The normal pigment of erythrocytes, hemoglobin, can be responsible for gross changes in the color of the body. Oxygenated hemoglobin is red and imparts the pink appearance to unpigmented skin and tissues. Normally, arterial blood (oxygenated hemoglobin) is red, and venous blood with more unoxygenated blood is bluish. However, if the blood is not sufficiently oxygenated (unoxygenated hemoglobin), the tissues appear blue, exhibiting so-called cyanosis (Fig. 1-63).

TABLE 1-1 Differences between Lipofuscin and Most Ceroid Pigments In Vivo

	Lipofuscin	Ceroid
Universality (invariably present in humans and all domestic animals)	Yes	No
Intrinsically (intracellularly in lysosomes of postmitotic and stable cells)	Yes	No
Time dependence	Yes	No
Initial occurrence	Infancy	Anytime
Deleteriousness	Never demonstrated	Frequent
Accumulation rate	Very slow	Usually rapid
Tissue distribution	Only intracellular	Intracellular and extracellular
Mode of formation	Mainly autophagy	Mainly heterophagy
Origin of precursors	Mainly intracellular	Mainly extracellular

From Porta EA: *Ann N Y Acad Sci* 959:57-65, 2002.

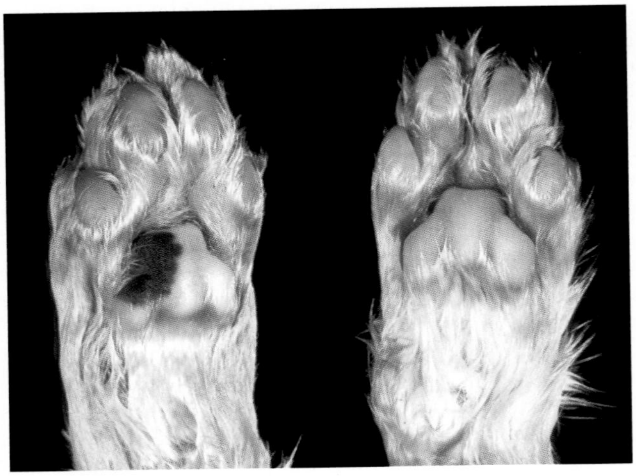

Fig. 1-63 Cyanosis, feet, cat.
The footpads of the paw on the left are bluish due to unoxygenated hemoglobin, the result of a partial obstruction of the iliac artery at the aortic bifurcation by a saddle thrombus. Normal control paw is on the right. (Courtesy Dr. M.D. McGavin, College of Veterinary Medicine, University of Tennessee.)

In acute cyanide poisoning, cyanide binds to cytochrome oxidase, the enzyme in the cell responsible for oxidative phosphorylation, and this results in paralysis of cellular respiration. Tissues cannot use the oxygen delivered by the blood. Consequently, in acute cyanide toxicity the oxygen content and color of venous blood may be similar to those of arterial blood, and the venous blood will be bright red.

In carbon monoxide (CO) poisoning, as from exhaust gases from automobiles, the blood is a bright cherry red from the formation of carboxyhemoglobin (Fig. 1-64). Methemoglobin is an oxide of hemoglobin, in which the ferrous ion of hemoglobin is converted to the ferric ion, resulting in a reddish-brown (chocolate brown) color to the blood and tissue (Fig. 1-65). Methemoglobin is seen most often in poisoning by nitrites, especially after ingestion of nitrate-accumulating plants, but has been reported as a result of ingestion of acetaminophen, naphthalene, and chlorates and of treatment with local anesthetic agents (e.g., lidocaine, benzocaine, and tetracaine).

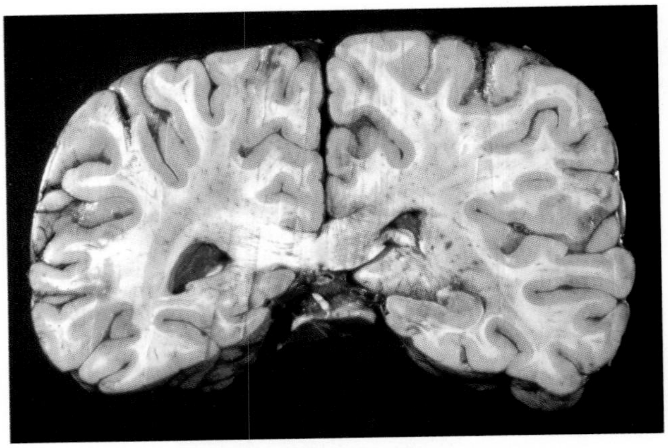

Fig. 1-64 Carbon monoxide (CO) poisoning, brain, human.
The blood in the brain is cherry red from the carboxyhemoglobin formed by the inhalation of CO in exhaust gases. (Courtesy Dr. J.C. Parker, School of Medicine, University of Louisville.)

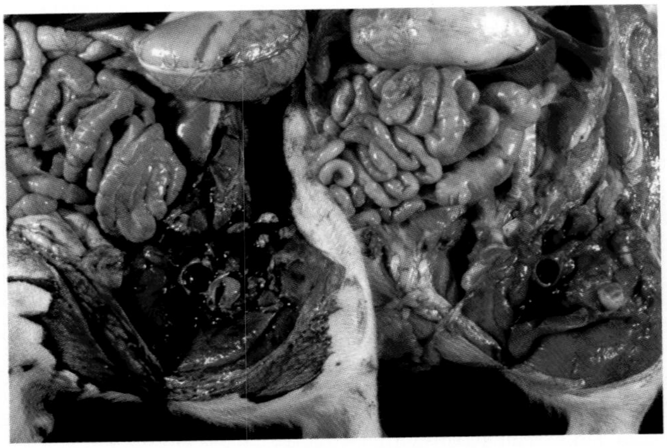

Fig. 1-65 Methemoglobinemia, experimental nitrite poisoning, hindleg, pig.
Left, The methemoglobin in the blood has discolored the blood and muscle chocolate brown. *Right,* Normal control. (Courtesy Dr. L. Nelson, College of Veterinary Medicine, Michigan State University.)

In intravascular hemolysis, hemoglobin is released from the lysed erythrocytes and stains the plasma pink. This hemoglobin may be excreted by the kidney, staining it dark red to reddish-black and the urine red (Fig. 1-66). Similar changes can result from myoglobinuria after the destruction of large numbers of myofibers (see Chapter 15).

Hematins

The hematin category of pigments includes "formalin pigment" and the excreta of parasites such as *Fascioloides magna* (liver fluke) and *Pneumonyssus simicola* (lung mite).

Formalin Pigment

Formalin pigment, also called *acid formalin hematin,* is an annoying microscopic artefact that occurs when tissue rich in blood comes in contact with acid solutions of formalin, particularly if there has been a delay between death and fixation, allowing time for the erythrocytes to lyse and release their hemoglobin.

Grossly, formalin pigment is not visible because this change occurs only after fixation. Microscopically the pigment is brown to almost black, fine, and granular (Fig. 1-67), and can have birefringent spicules. It occurs mainly in blood vessels but also in other

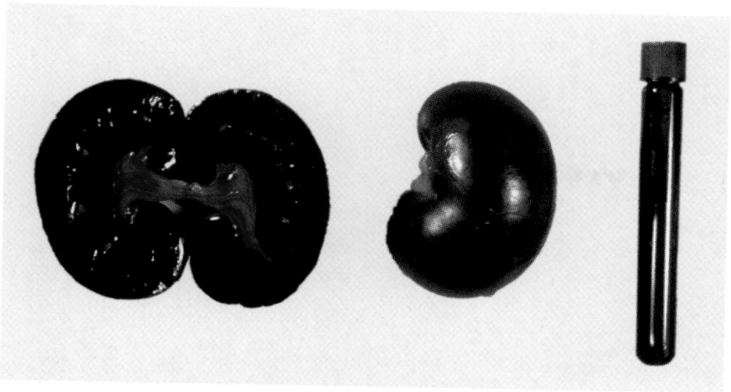

Fig. 1-66 Acute hemolysis from chronic copper poisoning, kidney and urine, sheep.
The dark bluish color of the kidney and the dark red of the urine are caused by hemoglobin excreted via the kidney. (Courtesy Dr. M.D. McGavin, College of Veterinary Medicine, University of Tennessee.)

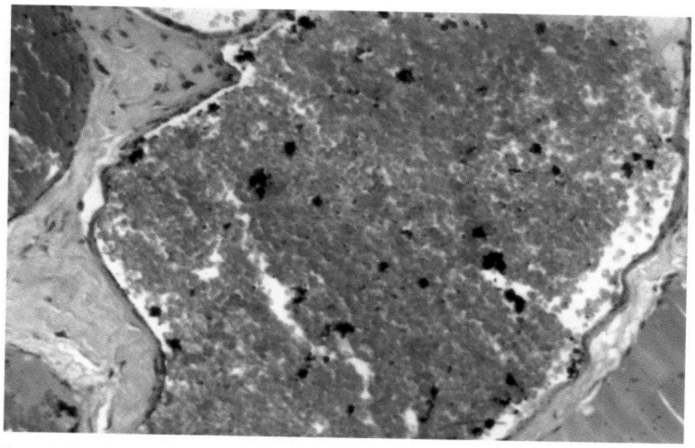

Fig. 1-67 Formalin pigment, blood.
Note the black spicules of hematin that lie between and on the erythrocytes, the result of fixation in unbuffered (acid) 10% formalin. H&E stain. (Courtesy Dr. M.D. McGavin, College of Veterinary Medicine, University of Tennessee.)

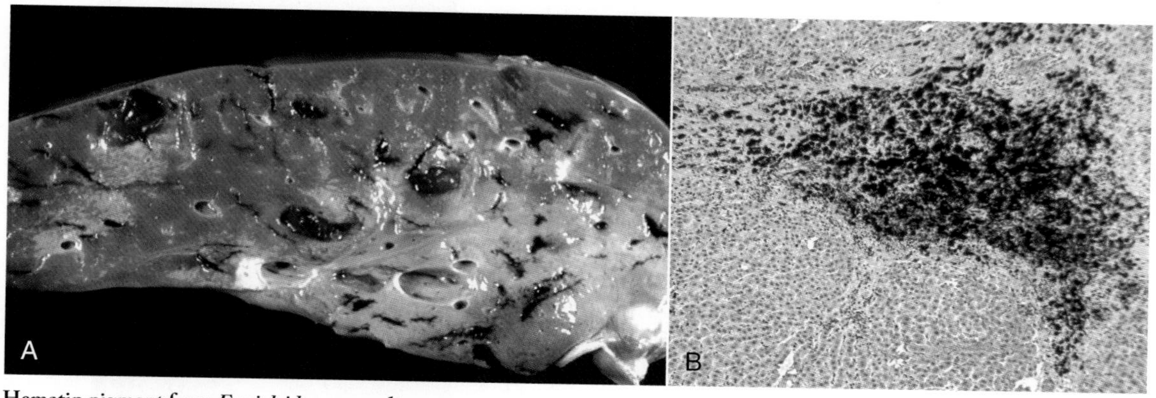

Fig. 1-68 Hematin pigment from *Fascioloides magna*, liver, ox.
A, Large areas of the liver are black from the pigment excreted by the fluke as it migrated through the liver. **B,** Hematin *(black)* pigment deposited in a fluke migration tract in the liver. H&E stain. (**A** courtesy Dr. J. Wright, College of Veterinary Medicine, North Carolina State University; and Noah's Arkive, College of Veterinary Medicine, The University of Georgia. **B** courtesy Dr. M.D. McGavin, College of Veterinary Medicine, University of Tennessee.)

tissues in which there are large accumulations of red blood cells. Pigment can lie between or on top of red blood cells and is negative for iron when stained by the Prussian blue reaction.

Because formalin pigment is formed only during fixation, it has no pathologic significance. Its significance is that it can interfere with the interpretation of histologic sections. Fortunately, it is easy to prevent its formation. Formalin pigment does not form if the pH of the fixative is above 6. Aqueous solutions of unbuffered formalin are highly acid. A common fixative is 10% buffered neutral formalin (really buffered neutral 10% formalin), which is buffered with a Sorensen phosphate buffer, and despite the name "neutral" has a pH of 6.8. It does not cause the formation of formalin pigment. Another commonly used and commercially available formalin fixative is Carson's fixative (also called *modified Millonig's formalin fixative*), with a pH of 7.3 and can be used as a dual-purpose fixative for both routine histopathologic and electron microscopic examinations. If formalin pigment is present in a tissue section, it can be removed by a variety of techniques including soaking the dewaxed tissue section before H&E staining in a saturated alcoholic solution of picric acid.

Parasite Hematin

The two most common causes of parasite hematin in veterinary medicine are *Fascioloides magna* (liver fluke) in ruminants and *Pneumonyssus simicola* in the lungs of macaques.

Parasite hematin from *Fascioloides magna* causes black tracts throughout the liver and is colloquially known as *fluke exhaust* (Fig. 1-68, *A*). This lesion can be so severe that it affects the whole liver. Microscopically, the black pigment accumulates adjacent to the migration tracts of the parasite and is phagocytosed by macrophages (Fig. 1-68, *B*). *Pneumonyssus simicola* produces a similar brown-to-black anisotropic pulmonary pigment presumed to be from the metabolism of hemoglobin by the parasite.

Hemosiderin

Iron is stored in the body in two forms, ferritin and hemosiderin, both of which are protein-iron complexes. Ferritin is in all tissues, but the heaviest concentrations are found in the liver, spleen, bone marrow, and skeletal muscle. Hemosiderin is formed from intracellular aggregates of ferritin (Fig. 1-69). It appears as golden-yellow to golden-brown globules and is the most visible form of storage iron. Normally, most storage iron is found in the spleen.

Excess iron from the breakdown of senescent erythrocytes, or the result of a hemolytic crisis (e.g., because of autoimmune diseases or hemotropic parasites) or reduced erythropoiesis (e.g., from malnutrition), is stored mainly in the spleen. Rarely in veterinary medicine, excess iron can be present in the body because of excessive absorption from the gut, multiple injections of iron, or from multiple blood transfusions.

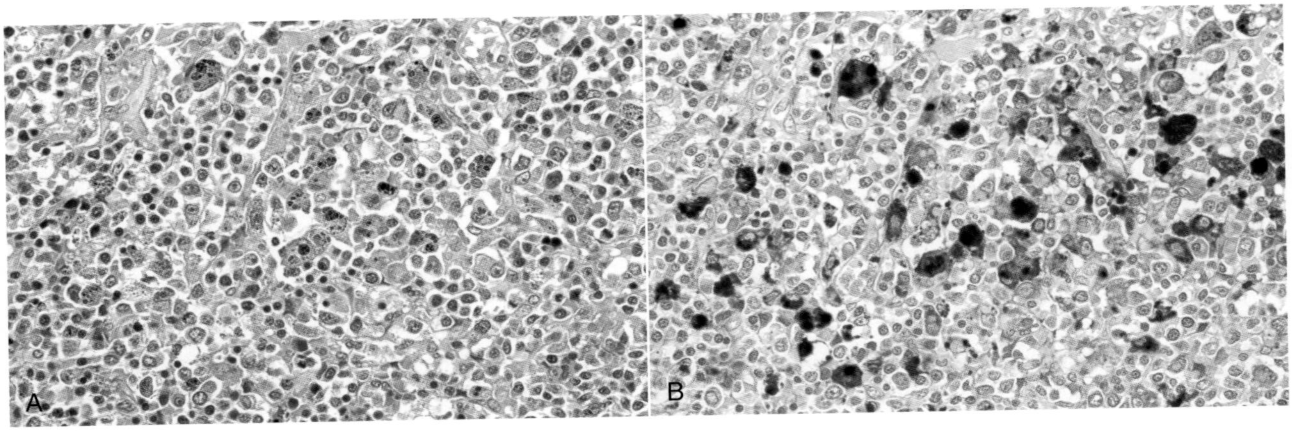

Fig. 1-69 **Hemosiderosis, spleen, dog.**
A, Hemosiderin is present as fine golden brown granules in macrophages. H&E stain. **B,** Granules of hemosiderin are stained dark blue by the Prussian blue reaction, which is specific for iron. Prussian blue reaction. (**A** and **B** courtesy Dr. J.F. Zachary, College of Veterinary Medicine, University of Illinois.)

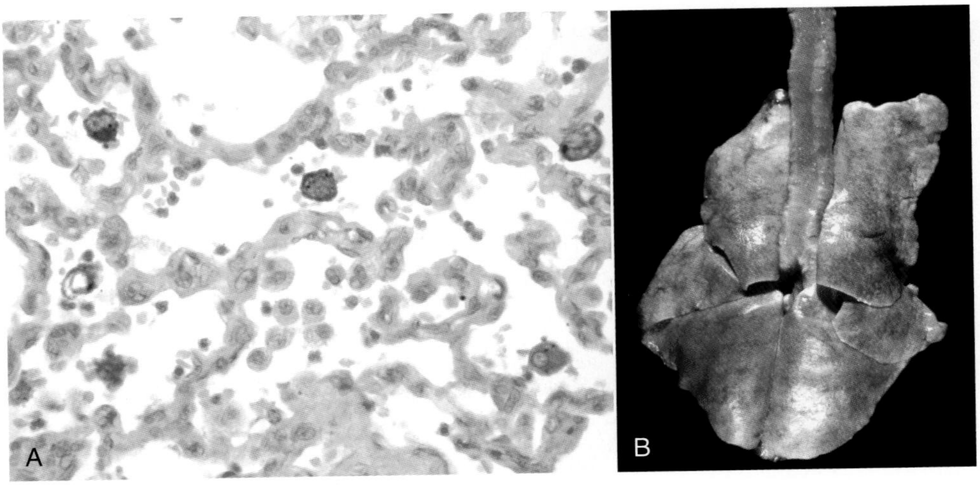

Fig. 1-70 **Chronic passive congestion, lung, dog.**
A, Alveolar macrophages containing hemosiderin *(blue)* are present in the alveoli. Prussian blue reaction. **B,** The lungs have chronic passive congestion attributed to chronic left-sided heart failure. They are moderately firm and yellow-brown caused by alveolar macrophages containing hemosiderin. Inflammatory mediators produced by these macrophages have induced fibroplasia, thus in the long term, there has been extensive formation of interstitial collagen. This collagen is the reason the lungs have failed to collapse after incision of the diaphragm, which releases the negative pressure in the pleural cavity (note the rib impressions in the lung). (**A** courtesy Dr. M.D. McGavin, College of Veterinary Medicine, University of Tennessee. **B** courtesy College of Veterinary Medicine, University of Illinois.)

Besides splenic storage, there may be local iron storage at sites of erythrocyte breakdown, such as in hemorrhages, and in areas of poor blood flow, as in chronic passive congestion of the lungs. In the latter case, because of the poor blood flow through the lungs, erythrocytes may come to the end of their natural life and be lysed or enter the alveoli by diapedesis, where they are phagocytosed by alveolar macrophages. These cells are termed *heart failure cells* (Fig. 1-70). Localized deposits of iron may also be present from the intramuscular injection of iron dextran, and this iron may drain to the regional lymph node.

Grossly, no change is seen in an organ or tissue if there are only small amounts of hemosiderin, but very large amounts cause a yellow-to-brown discoloration (Fig. 1-71). This color change can also be seen at sites of old bruises and other hemorrhages or hematomas. The spleen and the liver in hemolytic disease and the lungs in chronic passive congestion also appear brown. Microscopically, hemosiderin deposits are golden-yellow to golden-brown globules, which may be intracellular or extracellular (see Fig. 1-69, *A*). It can be confirmed by the Prussian blue reaction (see Fig. 1-69, *B*), which is sometimes incorrectly called a stain but is a chemical reaction, of which the end-product is Prussian blue. In the acid solution that liberates ferric iron from the hemosiderin, the ferric iron is reacted with potassium ferrocyanide (colorless) to form ferric ferrocyanide, which is Prussian blue.

The significance of hemosiderin deposits depends on their location and the amount. Normally, the spleen contains some hemosiderin, but excess hemosiderin is seen in the spleen and liver (Kupffer cells and hepatocytes) from hemolytic diseases, such as in autoimmune hemolytic anemia, and hemotropic diseases, such as babesiosis, anaplasmosis, or equine infectious anemia. Local tissue aggregations of hemosiderin are usually the result of the breakdown of erythrocytes in an old hemorrhage.

Excess hemosiderin is called *hemosiderosis* and must be differentiated from hemochromatosis, in which there are extreme accumulations of hemosiderin.

Hematoidin

Grossly, hematoidin is yellow-brown to orange-red pigment derived from hemoglobin but free of iron. Hematoidin closely resembles bilirubin (see next section) but is formed by cells of the

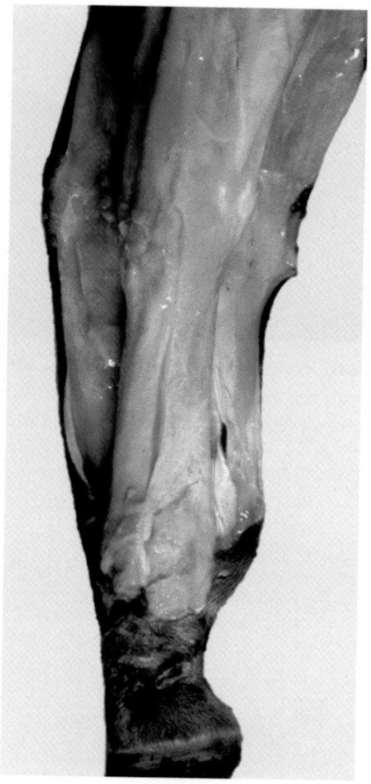

Fig. 1-71 Subcutis, old bruise, leg, horse.
The display of colors—red, yellow, and brown—is due to hemoglobin, bilirubin, and hemosiderin, respectively, from the breakdown of the erythrocytes. (Courtesy Dr. M.D. McGavin, College of Veterinary Medicine, University of Tennessee.)

macrophage-monocyte system when they phagocytose and digest red blood cells and hemoglobin in areas of hemorrhage. Microscopically, hematoidin is crystalline and polarizes light.

Bilirubin

Low concentrations of bilirubin are normally present in the plasma from the breakdown of senescent erythrocytes (see Chapter 13). Briefly, when erythrocytes have come to the end of their natural lifespan (average 70 days for a cat; average 150 days for cattle and horses), they are phagocytosed by the macrophage-monocyte system, chiefly by macrophages of the spleen and to a lesser extent by those of the bone marrow and liver (Kupffer cells). Within these cells, the iron is removed and stored, and the remainder of the porphyrin ring is broken down to bilirubin, which is released into the blood where it attaches to albumin. This bilirubin-albumin complex is too large to be excreted by the kidney. It is carried to the liver, where it enters the space of Disse, is taken up by the microvilli of the hepatocytes, is conjugated to form bilirubin glucuronide or diglucuronide, and is then excreted into the bile canaliculus.

Icterus (jaundice), the yellow staining of the tissue by bilirubin, is the result of an imbalance between production and clearance of bilirubin because there is either excess production or reduced clearance of bilirubin such that it accumulates in the plasma. The mutant Corriedale sheep model is an animal model for Dubin-Johnson syndrome in humans (Fig. 1-72).

Mechanisms leading to icterus can involve one or more of the following:

1. Excess production of bilirubin—as in hemolytic diseases such as babesiosis, anaplasmosis, and equine infectious anemia—or the breakdown of erythrocytes in a large hemorrhage such as a hematoma.
2. Reduced uptake of bilirubin from the plasma by hepatocytes.

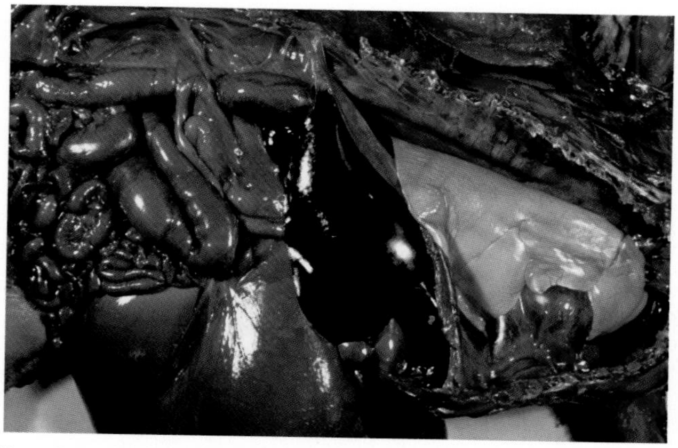

Fig. 1-72 Defective bilirubin excretion, mutant Corriedale sheep, animal model for Dubin-Johnson syndrome.
Note the faint yellow discoloration of the lung from bilirubin. The other tissues are discolored dark green from phylloerythrin, which also has a similar defect in excretion in the liver. (Courtesy Dr. M.D. McGavin, College of Veterinary Medicine, University of Tennessee.)

3. Impaired or absent conjugation in hepatocytes, often a congenital or inherited abnormality, as in the Gunn rat.
4. Hepatic necrosis. Because the cell membranes of several adjacent hepatocytes form the bile canaliculus, any necrosis of these cells will disrupt the wall of the canaliculus and allow leakage of bilirubin into the circulation. Extensive hepatic necrosis can cause icterus.
5. Decreased excretion of conjugated bilirubin by the hepatocytes into the bile canaliculus.
6. Reduced flow of bile from the liver to the intestine caused by either intrahepatic or extrahepatic blockage of the biliary system.

Icterus is classified several different ways. A convenient approach uses the classification of prehepatic, hepatic, and posthepatic. The most common cause of prehepatic icterus is a hemolytic crisis, which produces high plasma concentrations of unconjugated bilirubin that exceed the uptake capacity of the hepatocytes. Hepatic icterus is caused by hepatocellular damage, which results in release of bilirubin, both conjugated and unconjugated into the blood and can be the result of one or more of factors 2 to 4. Posthepatic icterus is secondary to obstruction of the biliary system, either intrahepatic or extrahepatic (hepatic bile ducts and the common bile duct), with reflux of the conjugated bilirubin into the blood. In contrast to unconjugated bilirubin, which is carried in the blood attached to albumin and cannot be excreted by the kidney, conjugated bilirubin is not bound to a plasma protein such as albumin and can be excreted.

Grossly, icteric tissues are discolored yellow, and the color change is distributed systemically. Clinically, icterus is most easily recognized in lightly pigmented animals. In living animals, icterus is detected in mucous membranes of the oral cavity, urogenital systems, and alimentary system and in normally white areas such as the sclera of the eyes. At necropsy, in addition to the sites listed previously, icterus can be identified in the omentum, mesentery, and adipose tissue (Fig. 1-73), except in Jersey and Guernsey cattle, horses, and nonhuman primates, whose sera and fat are normally discolored yellow by carotenoids. The intima of the large vessels is also a good site to detect icterus, and unless the plasma concentration is extremely high, the brain is usually unaffected.

Microscopically, icterus is not detected, but excessive quantities of bilirubin can be seen in the bile ducts and bile canaliculi in obstructive jaundice (Fig. 1-74).

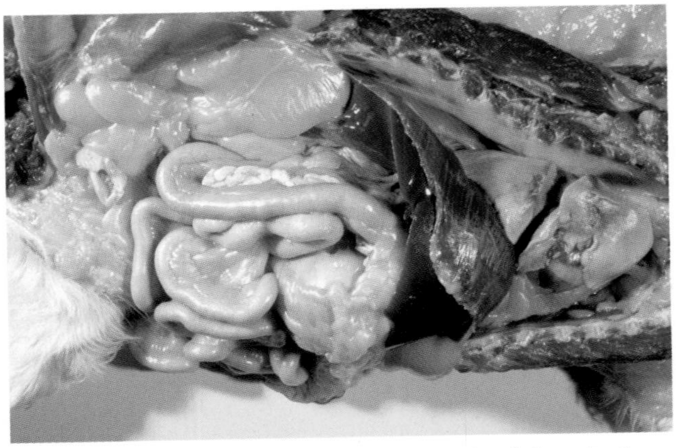

Fig. 1-73 Icterus, hemolytic anemia, abdominal and thoracic viscera, dog.
The yellow discoloration from the bilirubin is particularly evident in fat and mesentery. (Courtesy Dr. M.D. McGavin, College of Veterinary Medicine, University of Tennessee.)

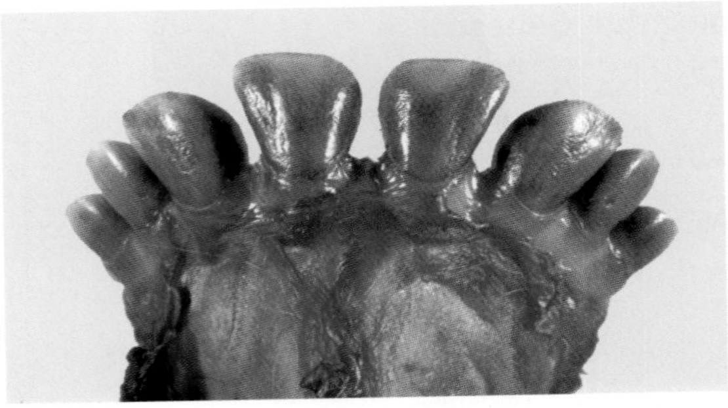

Fig. 1-75 Pink tooth, congenital porphyria teeth, adult ox. The teeth are discolored brown from the accumulation of porphyrins in the dentin. (Courtesy Dr. M.D. McGavin, College of Veterinary Medicine, University of Tennessee.)

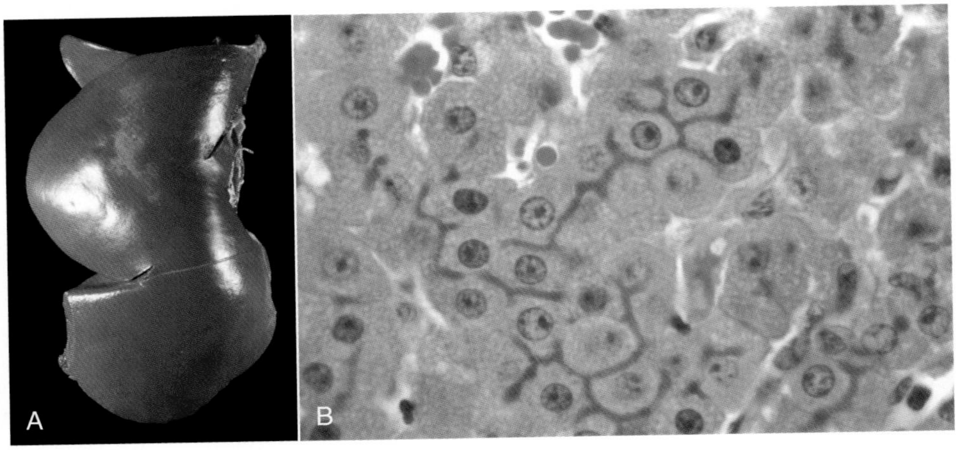

Fig. 1-74 Icterus.
A, Icterus, liver, cat. Note the enlarged liver with rounded edges and yellow-orange color caused by retained bilirubin. **B,** Bile casts in bile canaliculi. Acute hemolytic anemia, babesiosis, liver, cow. The bile casts are the result of a high rate of bilirubin excretion by the liver secondary to intravascular hemolysis. H&E stain. (**A** courtesy College of Veterinary Medicine, University of Illinois. **B** courtesy Dr. M.D. McGavin, College of Veterinary Medicine, University of Tennessee.)

Icterus is a very important clinical sign and may be detected by examination of the sclera, and in cases of anemia, in which the mucous membranes are pale; it may be visible there. Laboratory tests to determine the exact plasma or serum concentrations of bilirubin, and preferably whether it is or is not conjugated, are essential. It is critical to realize that hyperbilirubinemia is not the same as icterus. Most domestic animals normally have very low serum concentrations of bilirubin, usually less than 1 mg/dL, except for the horse, in which it may range from 1 to 3 mg/dL. Icterus is not detected until the serum concentration exceeds 1.5 to 2.0 mg/100 mL. Thus hyperbilirubinemia can be present without causing icterus.

Porphyria

Congenital erythropoietic porphyria of calves, cats, and pigs is an inherited metabolic defect in heme synthesis caused by a deficiency of uroporphyrinogen III cosynthetase. The disease is sometimes incorrectly called *osteohemachromatosis.* It is also known colloquially as *pink tooth* because of the discoloration by the porphyrins accumulating in dentin and bone (Fig. 1-75, also see Chapter 7). The teeth and bones of young animals are reddish (pink tooth) and those of adults are dark brown. In these cases, both bones and teeth fluoresce red under ultraviolet radiation.

CELLULAR AGING*

Information on this topic is available at evolve.elsevier.com/Zachary/McGavin/.

STRUCTURAL AND BIOCHEMICAL CHANGES WITH CELLULAR AGING

Information on this topic is available at evolve.elsevier.com/Zachary/McGavin/.

Replicative Senescence

Information on this topic is available at evolve.elsevier.com/Zachary/McGavin/.

GENETIC BASIS OF AGING

Information on this topic is available at evolve.elsevier.com/Zachary/McGavin/.

Accumulation of Metabolic and Genetic Damage

Information on this topic is available at evolve.elsevier.com/Zachary/McGavin/.

CALORIC RESTRICTION

Information on this topic is available at evolve.elsevier.com/Zachary/McGavin/.

GENETIC BASIS OF DISEASE*

This section provides an overview of (1) the structure and function of chromosomes and genes, (2) the mechanisms of genetic disorders, and (3) the outcomes of specific genetic diseases. The roles of genes have consequences for and are affected by cellular adaptations, cell injury, and cell death. Their roles in controlling immune responses and neoplastic transformation are discussed in Chapters 5 and 6, respectively. The function of microbial genes and their interplay with animal genes in determining host resistance to infectious diseases are discussed in Chapter 4.

CHROMOSOME STRUCTURE AND FUNCTION

Nuclear Chromosomes

Each animal species has a unique chromosomal complement called a *karyotype* (i.e., the number and morphology of the chromosomes that make up its genome). With the exception of cells that develop into ova and spermatozoa (i.e., germline cells), all cells in the body are called *somatic cells* (e.g., soma: body). The genome contained in the nucleus of somatic cells consists of chromosomes arranged in pairs. All except one pair are similar in both males and females and are called *autosomes,* and the remaining pair is the sex chromosomes: two X chromosomes in females and an X and a Y chromosome in males. Although each chromosome has different genes, members of a pair of chromosomes, also called *homologous chromosomes* or *homologues,* carry matching genetic information, that is, they have the same genes in the same sequence. Any specific locus (i.e., the specific location of a gene) on a chromosome may have either identical or slightly different forms of the same gene, called *alleles.* One member of each pair of chromosomes is inherited from the sire, the other from the dam.

Mitochondrial Chromosomes

Mitochondria are the site of aerobic energy production in all cells of the body. In highly active cells, such as type I myofibers of equine athletes, up to 10,000 mitochondria may be present in the cytoplasm of a myofiber. Each mitochondrion contains a single chromosome formed by circular double-stranded DNA, called *mitochondrial DNA* (mtDNA). The genome of a mitochondrial chromosome encodes for 37 genes, including those for messenger RNAs (mRNAs), ribosomal RNAs (rRNAs), transfer RNAs (tRNAs), and 13 protein subunits for enzymes, such as cytochrome b and cytochrome oxidase, which are involved in the production of energy by oxidative phosphorylation. The mitochondrial genome also has distinct transcription and protein-synthesis (i.e., translation) systems. A specialized RNA polymerase, encoded in the nuclear genome, is used to transcribe the mitochondrial genome and then the mitochondrial transcripts are processed to generate the various individual mitochondrial mRNAs, tRNAs, and rRNAs.

GENE STRUCTURE AND FUNCTION

On average, there are approximately 20,000 genes in the nucleus of an individual cell of the different domestic animal species. Genes, the heredity units of the genetic code, determine the structural and functional biologic traits (i.e., expression of genes) necessary to create and maintain cells, tissues, and organs and to pass the genetic code on to offspring. Additionally, genes, especially those of the major histocompatibility complex (see Chapter 5), play important roles in establishing the resistance (or susceptibility) of an animal to infectious diseases. Most biologic traits expressed by genes have a Mendelian pattern of inheritance. They also have varied patterns of expression based on cell structure and function and the responses of cells to injury. Some genes are expressed continually and are called *constitutively expressed genes* and include genes for tRNAs, rRNAs, cell membranes, and enzymes. A different group of genes may be expressed only in a particular tissue such as the gene for galactocerebrosidase in myelinating cells of the nervous system (see the section on Globoid Cell Leukodystrophy in Chapter 14). These tissue-specific genes may be either differentially (i.e., in response to or as a result of cellular perturbations such as neoplastic transformation [see Chapter 6]) or constitutively expressed.

Certain genes may only be active (i.e., turned on and then off) in utero during specific times of fetal development as specific proteins are required for development, differentiation, and growth. Other genes are active continuously or transiently postpartum and are involved in growth, physiologic homeostasis, or reproduction. Thus an important consideration in the occurrence of a genetic disease is the period during which a normal gene is active. If the normal gene is mutated and the mutated gene is expressed during the active period for the normal gene, the outcome may have detrimental effects on structural and functional processes. Mutated genes of those that are normally important for early embryogenesis or organogenesis have earlier and generally more severe consequences than genes not expressed until sexual maturation or after. When the normal functions of genes are lost, disrupted, or altered, the outcome, many of which are heritable, can be harmful and result in congenital development anomalies such as palatoschisis/cheiloschisis (see Chapter 7). Metabolic dysfunction of cells can also occur and result in cell death in diseases such as multisystem neuronal degeneration (see Chapter 14). Examples of known or suspected genetic disorders in domestic animals are listed in

---

*Portions adapted and modified from Nussbaum RL, McInnes RR, Willard HF: *Thompson & Thompson's genetics in medicine,* ed 7, Philadelphia, 2007, Saunders; Jorde LB, Carey JC, Bamshad MJ: *Medical genetics,* ed 4, St Louis, 2010, Mosby; Turnpenny P, Ellard S: *Emery's elements of medical genetics,* ed 13, Edinburgh, 2008, Churchill Livingstone; Adkison L, Brown MS: *Elsevier's integrated genetics,* St. Louis, 2007, Mosby; Kumar V, Abbas AK, Fausto N, et al: *Robbins & Cotran pathologic basis of disease,* ed 8, St Louis, 2010, Elsevier Saunders.

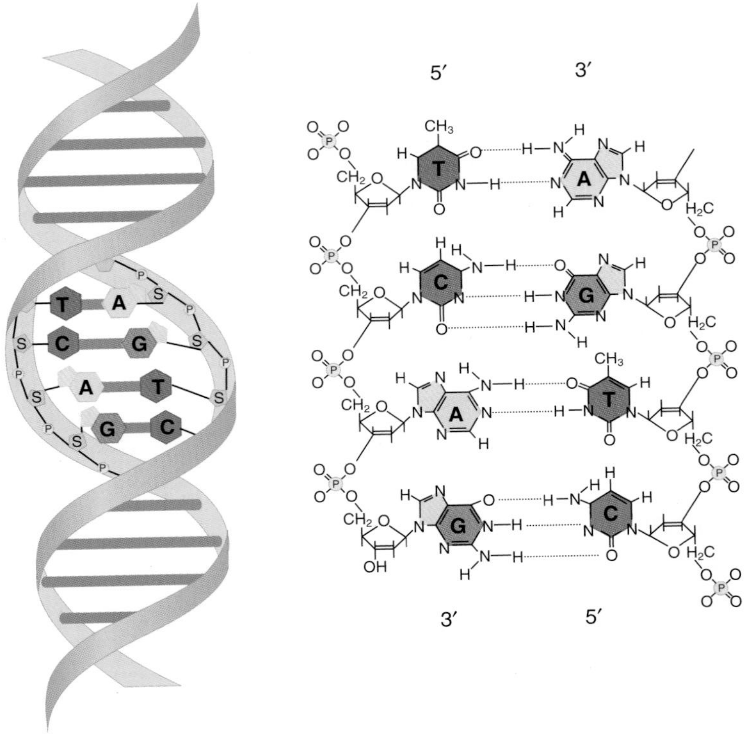

Fig. 1-76 Organization of DNA.
DNA is organized in an antiparallel configuration: one strand is 5′ to 3′ in one direction and the other strand is 5′ to 3′ in the opposite direction. A purine is bound to a pyrimidine by hydrogen bonds: A:T and G:C. The helix occurs naturally because of the bonds in the phosphate backbone. (From Adkison L, Brown MS: *Elsevier's integrated genetics,* St. Louis, 2007, Mosby.)

Web Box 1-1 and are discussed in the chapters covering pathology of organ systems.

In its simplest form, a gene is a segment of a DNA molecule in a chromosome, which contains the nucleotide code for the amino acid sequence of a protein (Fig. 1-76). Genes are arranged in a linear order along each chromosome, each gene having a precise position (e.g., locus). The composition of genes in an animal's genome is determined by the DNA of the chromosomes in the nucleus. In nuclear DNA, each chromosome consists of a single, continuous DNA double helix; in other words, each chromosome is a long, linear double-stranded DNA molecule, and the genome consists therefore of DNA molecules totaling billions of nucleotides (pyrimidines: cytosine [C], thymine [T], uracil [U, found in RNA in place of T in DNA]; purines: adenine [A] and guanine [G]. Chromosomes are not naked DNA double helices within the nucleus. The genome is packaged as chromatin, in which DNA is complexed with one or more of five types of chromosomal proteins called *histones.* Histones have large quantities of arginine and lysine, which are amino acids that carry a positive charge. This charge allows histones to bind tightly to negatively charged DNA, forming complexes called *nucleosomes* that are further condensed into chromosomes. This type of arrangement allows long strands of DNA to be condensed into physically smaller (i.e., less volume) molecules that easily fit into the nucleus (Fig. 1-77). However, for a gene to be active, the condensed DNA must revert to long strands of DNA to allow it to be transcribed.

Genes contain nucleotide sequences that determine what the gene does, and other nucleotide sequences that determine when the gene is to be expressed. When a gene is active, RNA is synthesized from the DNA template through a process known as *transcription* (Fig. 1-78). The RNA carrying the coded information is in a form called *mRNA,* which is then transported from the nucleus to the cytoplasm where the RNA sequence is decoded, or translated, to determine the sequence of amino acids of the protein to be synthesized (e.g., triplet codon in sequence codes for a specific amino acid in sequence). The key to translation is a code along the mRNA that relates specific amino acids to a combination of three adjacent nucleotide bases. Each set of three bases forms a codon that is the "code" for a particular amino acid that is inserted into the protein during translation of the mRNA. In theory, an almost infinite variation in the arrangement of the bases along a polynucleotide chain is possible.

DNA is a macromolecule composed of nucleotides arranged in long chains. For each nucleotide in the chain that forms the chromosome, there are four possible base choices (A, T, C, or G). Thus, with a codon of three nucleotides, there are 64 possible triplet combinations and these 64 codon combinations constitute the genetic code. The process of translation occurs on ribosomes (free in cytoplasm and in RER), which are cytoplasmic organelles with binding sites for all of the interacting molecules, including the mRNA. Ribosomes themselves are made up of many different structural proteins in association with specialized types of RNA known as *rRNA.* Translation also involves a third type of RNA, tRNA, which during synthesis of a protein transfers the appropriate amino acid to the code contained in the base sequence of each mRNA.

Proteins resulting from the expression of genes are responsible for the development (e.g., formation of structural proteins) and function (e.g., formation of enzymes) of cells, tissues, and organs. Many genes belong to gene families, which share closely related DNA sequences and encode polypeptides with closely related amino acid sequences. However, if there is a simple one-to-one correspondence between genes and proteins, then the approximately 20,000 genes in an animal should give rise to about 20,000 different proteins. This number seems insufficient to account for all of the structural needs and functions requiring proteins that occur in animal cells. The answer to this conundrum is found in two features of gene structure and function. Genes are capable of generating multiple different proteins, not just one, and translated proteins can be modified through a process called posttranslational

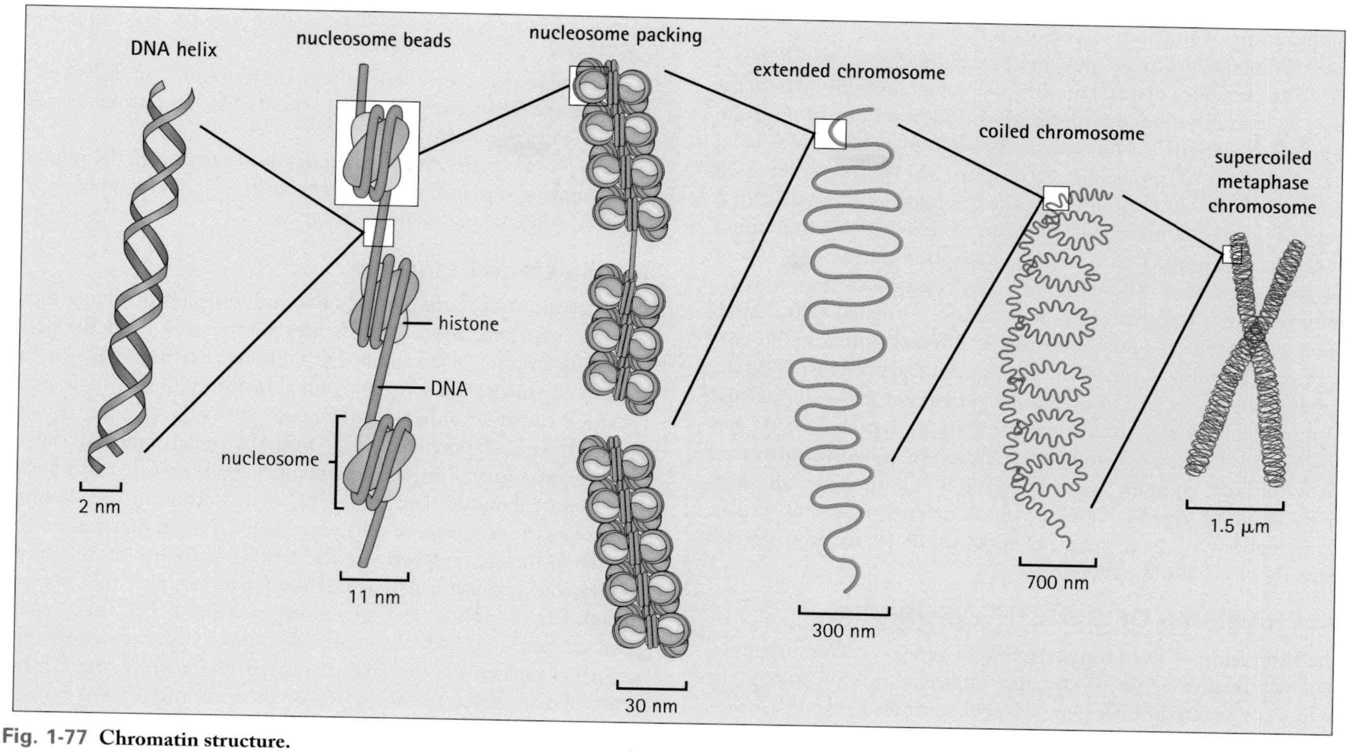

Fig. 1-77 Chromatin structure.

DNA is organized around histones into nucleosomes. The nucleosomes are wound into a helix to form chromatin. In chromosomes, this is then wound again into a supercoiled structure. (From Stevens A, Lowe JS: *Human histology,* ed 3, St. Louis, 2005, Mosby.)

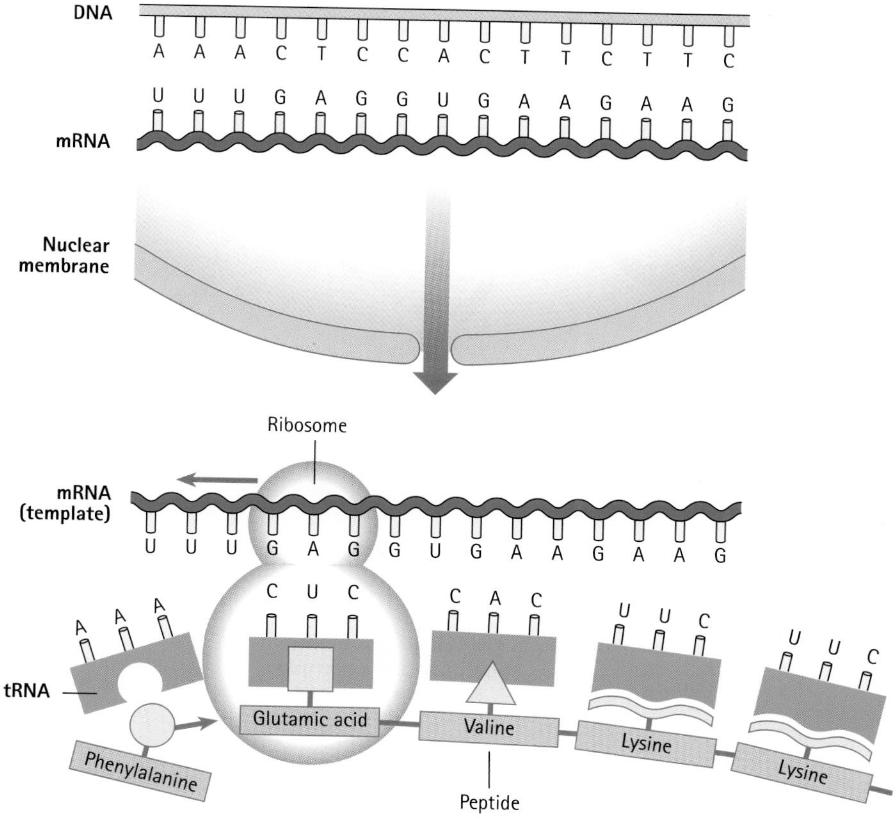

Fig. 1-78 Protein synthesis: transcription and translation.

Schematic representation of the way in which genetic information is transcribed in the nucleus *(upper portion)* and translated into protein in the cytoplasm *(lower portion).* (From Turnpenny P, Ellard S: *Emery's elements of medical genetics,* ed 13, Philadelphia, 2007, Churchill Livingstone.)

modification. Many proteins, before they attain their normal structure or functional activity, undergo posttranslational modification, which can include chemical modification of amino acid side-chains (e.g., by hydroxylation, methylation), the addition of carbohydrate (e.g., glycosylation), or proteolytic cleavage of polypeptides (e.g., the conversion of proinsulin to insulin). The polypeptide chain that is the primary translation product is folded and bonded into a specific three-dimensional structure determined by the amino acid sequence itself. Two or more polypeptide chains, products of the same gene or of different genes, may combine to form a single mature protein complex. Thus it has been estimated that 20,000 genes can encode as many as a million different proteins. This collection of proteins is called the *proteome* and represents all of the proteins expressed by a cell (cellular proteome), tissue, or animal (complete proteome). Individual proteins in a proteome do not function by themselves. They form elaborate networks, involving many different proteins and respond in a coordinated fashion to many different genetic, developmental, or environmental signals. Combinations of such gene networks result in an even greater diversity of cellular functions.

MECHANISMS OF GENETIC DISORDERS

The expression of the estimated 20,000 genes encoded in animal genomes involves a set of complex interrelationships among the factors controlling proper gene dosage (controlled by mechanisms of chromosome replication and segregation), gene structure, and finally, transcription, RNA splicing, mRNA stability, translation, protein processing, and protein degradation. For the normal function of some genes, fluctuations in the level of a functional gene product, resulting from either inherited variation in the structure of a particular gene or changes induced by nongenetic factors such as diet or the environment, are of relatively little importance in genetic disorders. However, for other genes, changes in the level of expression can have dire clinical consequences, reflecting the importance of those gene products in specific biologic pathways. The nature of inherited variation in the structure and function of chromosomes and genes and the influence of this variation on the expression of specific biological traits underlie the mechanisms of genetic disorders.

Genetic disorders can involve germline (i.e., cells that give rise to gametes) or somatic (i.e., cells forming the structure of an animal) cells and can be broadly classified into the following three categories:

1. Single-gene disorders caused by mutations in DNA of a single gene such as point, frameshift, and trinucleotide-repeat mutations
2. Chromosomal disorders caused by alterations in the number and/or structure of chromosomes (i.e., its karyotype)
3. Complex multigenic disorders

Single-Gene Disorders

Most germline cells are meiotic cells, and disorders involving them can be inherited. Somatic cells are mitotic cells, and disorders involving mitotic cells are not heritable but are important in the genesis of cancers and some congenital malformations. Single-gene disorders can affect either germline cells or somatic cells and usually result from mutations in DNA from (1) environmental causes such as exposure to excessive ultraviolet light, excessive radiation, or certain chemicals (i.e., mutagens) or (2) errors in cell division when somatic or germline cells copy their DNA in preparation for mitosis or meiosis, respectively. The actual occurrence of mutations is very low because cells have DNA repair proteins that correct mistakes in the DNA caused by mutagens (Fig. 1-79). These repair proteins determine which nucleotide bases are paired incorrectly, and then replace the incorrect base with the correct one. Mutations of the genes for these repair proteins often have serious outcomes, especially in neoplastic transformation of somatic cells. Single-gene disorders must be differentiated from single nucleotide polymorphisms (SNPs). SNPs represent differences in a single DNA nucleotide between animals of the same species (i.e., different breeds) and are the most common type of genetic variation among animals. They are usually found in regions between genes whose functions are known, thus they have no effect on health or development. However, if they occur within a gene or in a regulatory region near a gene, they may play a more direct role in disease. SNPs most commonly serve as biologic markers to locate genes that are associated with disease or hereditable traits such as muscling, weight gain, and milk production.

Because single-gene disorders arise from a mutation in a single gene, they result in a permanent change of the cell's nuclear DNA (Figs. 1-80 and 1-81). Such mutations can affect the synthesis of proteins by disrupting one or more steps in the

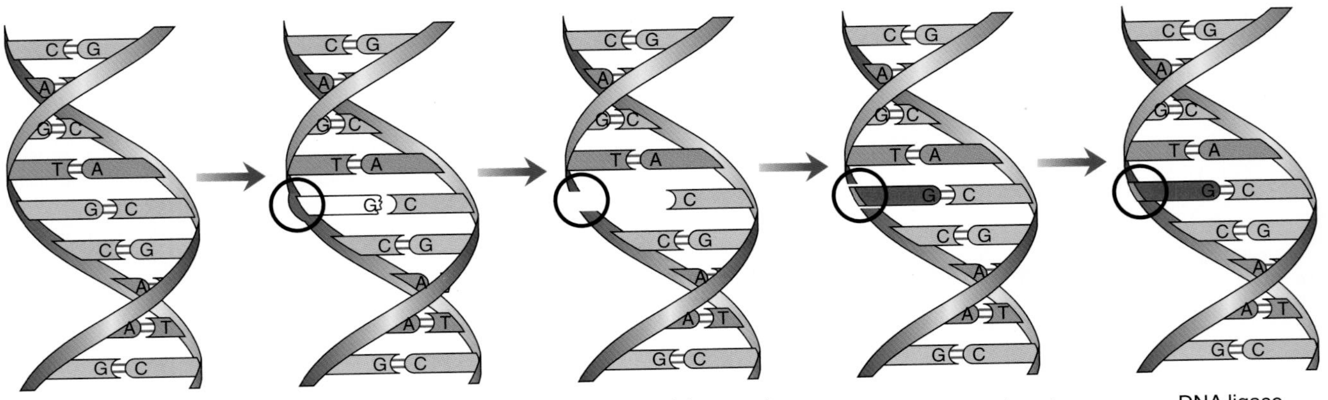

Fig. 1-79 Repair of damaged DNA.
The steps of DNA repair. In step 1, the damaged section is removed; in steps 2 and 3, the original DNA sequence is restored. (From Copstead L, Banasik J: *Pathophysiology*, ed 4, St Louis, 2010, Mosby.)

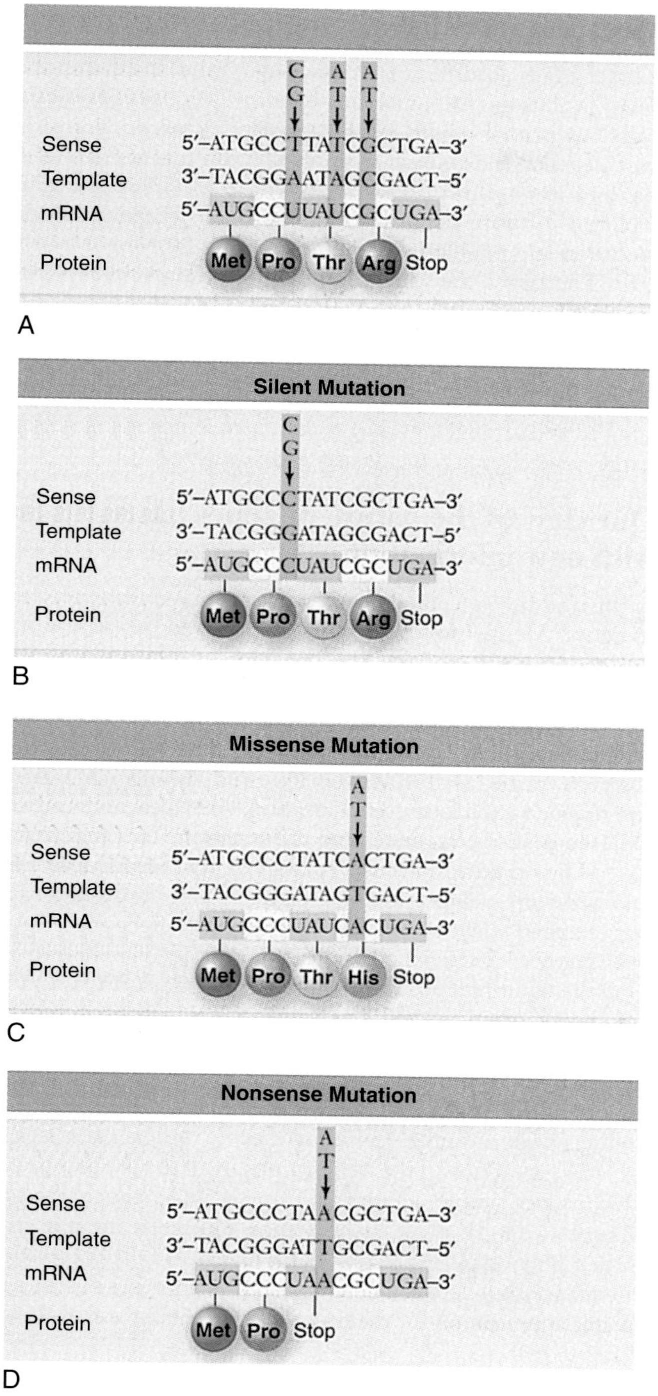

Fig. 1-80 Types of base pair substitutions in gene mutations.
A, Normal process of transcription and translation. **B,** If a base-pair substitution does not result in a change in the amino acid, the mutation is termed a *silent mutation.* **C,** Missense mutation produces a change in a single amino acid. **D,** Nonsense mutation produces a stop codon in the mRNA, which terminates translation of the polypeptide. (From McCance KL, Huether SE, Brashers VL, et al: *Pathophysiology: the biologic basis for disease in adults and children,* ed 6, St. Louis, 2010, Mosby.)

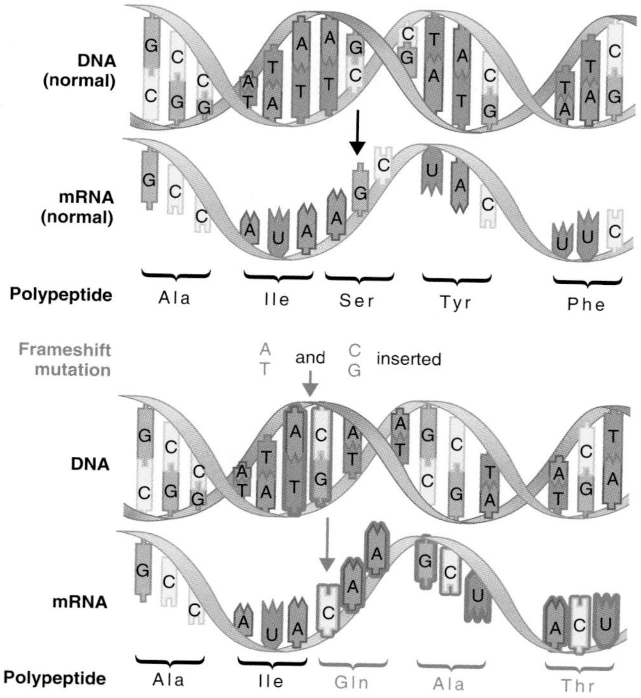

Fig. 1-81 Types of base pair substitutions in gene mutations, frameshift mutations.
Frameshift mutations result from the addition or deletion of a number of bases that is not a multiple of three. This alters all of the codons downstream from the site of insertion or deletion. Thus a frameshift mutation can greatly alter the resulting amino acid sequence. (From Jorde LB, Carey JC, Bamshad MJ: *Medical genetics,* ed 4, St. Louis, 2010, Mosby.)

normal transcriptional and translational processes and lead to the following:

1. The formation of an abnormal protein
2. A reduction in the synthesis of a protein
3. The formation of abnormal proteins without impairing any step in protein synthesis
4. Modification in the rate of synthesis, posttranslational mechanisms, or transporting of proteins out of the cell

Virtually any type of protein may be affected in single-gene disorders, and the mechanisms involved can be classified into the following four categories:

1. Enzyme defects and their consequences
2. Defects in membrane receptors and transport systems
3. Alterations in the structure, function, or quantity of nonenzyme proteins
4. Mutations resulting in unusual reactions to drugs

In enzyme defects, mutations may result in the synthesis of a defective enzyme with reduced activity or in a reduced amount of a normal enzyme. An enzyme defect may lead to three major consequences as follows:

1. Accumulation of a substrate that, depending on the site of the blockage, may be accompanied by accumulation of one or more intermediate substrates. Under these conditions, tissue injury may result if the precursor, the intermediate substrates, or the products of alternative pathways are toxic in high concentrations. For example, excessive accumulation of complex substrates within lysosomes as a result of defect in the degradative enzymes is responsible for a group of diseases generally referred to as storage diseases (see Chapter 14).

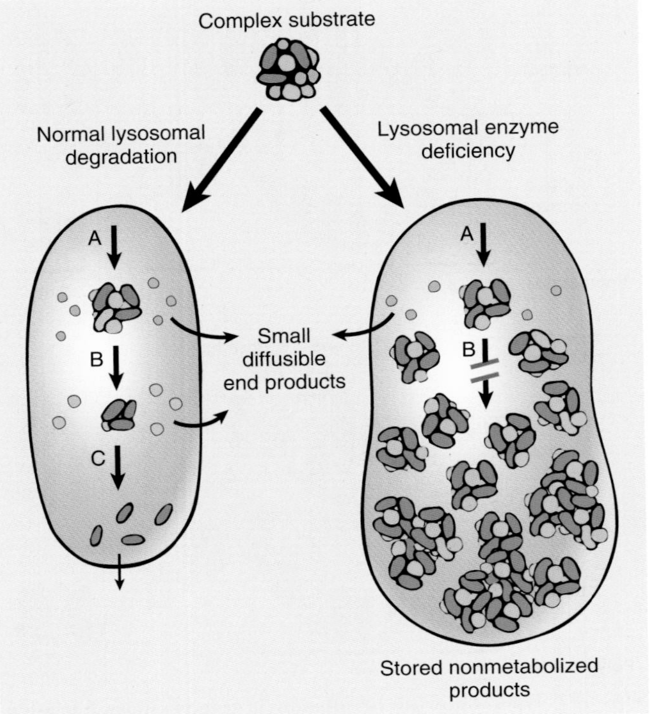

Fig. 1-82 Pathogenesis of lysosomal storage diseases. In the example shown, a complex substrate is normally degraded by a series of lysosomal enzymes (**A** to **C**) into soluble end products. If there is a deficiency or malfunction of one of the enzymes (e.g., **B**), catabolism is incomplete and insoluble intermediates accumulate in the lysosomes. (From Kumar V, Abbas A, Fausto N, et al: *Robbins & Cotran pathologic basis of disease,* ed 8, Philadelphia, 2009, Saunders.)

2. A metabolic block resulting in a decreased amount of end-product that may be necessary for normal function.
3. Failure to inactivate tissue-damaging substrates.

Mutations resulting in the accumulation of substrates or the blockage of normal metabolic pathways are best illustrated by a group of diseases called *storage diseases,* in which defective processing of a metabolic substrate leads to the accumulation of the substrate in cell cytoplasm or within lysosomes in the cell. Such diseases are discussed in the organ system chapters of this book. Storage diseases are commonly grouped as lysosomal storage diseases and glycogen storage diseases. Lysosomal storage diseases are characterized by a deficiency of lysosomal acid hydrolases, in which breakdown of their substrates remain incomplete, leading to the accumulation of the partially degraded insoluble metabolite within the lysosomes (Fig. 1-82). Lysosomal acid hydrolases break down a variety of complex macromolecules derived from the metabolic turnover of intracellular organelles or acquired from outside the cells by phagocytosis. Stuffed with incompletely digested macromolecules, these organelles become large and numerous enough to interfere with normal cell functions. Lysosomal storage diseases are exemplified by globoid cell leukodystrophy in which a deficiency in the function of a lysosomal enzyme called *lysosomal galactocerebroside β-galactosidase* (galactosylceramidase) results in the accumulation of a substrate, galactocerebroside, in lysosomes of macrophages recruited as monocytes from the vascular system (see Fig. 14-64).

Glycogen storage diseases (glycogenoses) are caused by a deficiency of one of the enzymes involved in the synthesis or sequential degradation of glycogen (Figs. 1-83 and 14-63). Glycogen storage diseases are exemplified by glycogenosis type III (Cori's disease), in which a deficiency in the function of an amylo-1, 6-glucosidase (debranching enzyme) results in the accumulation of a structurally abnormal glycogen within hepatocytes.

A failure to inactivate tissue-damaging substrates is illustrated by α_1-antitrypsin deficiency. Animals that have an inherited deficiency of serum α_1-antitrypsin are unable to inactivate neutrophil elastase in their lungs. Unchecked activity of this protease leads to destruction of elastin in the walls of lung alveoli, eventually leading to pulmonary emphysema. The consequences of defects in membrane receptors and transport systems; alterations in the structure, function, or quantity of nonenzyme proteins such as collagen, spectrin, and dystrophin in osteogenesis imperfecta; or mutations resulting in unusual reactions to drugs have not been adequately documented in animals.

Single-Gene Disorders of Germ Cells

Mutations that affect germ cells are transmitted to the progeny and can give rise to inherited diseases that usually follow the classic Mendelian pattern of inheritance. Inherited mutations involving single genes, typically follow one of three patterns: autosomal dominant, autosomal recessive, and X-linked.

Autosomal Dominant Disorders

In autosomal dominant disorders, only one allele of a mutated gene at a given locus is necessary for an animal to be affected by the disorder. This gene may come from the sire or from the dam, thus there is a 50% chance that each offspring will inherit the mutated gene. Examples of autosomal dominant disorders in animals include polycystic kidney disease of the urinary system (see Fig. 11-32, *F*) and osteogenesis imperfecta (see Chapter 16) and chondrodysplasia (see Fig. 16-42) of the skeletal system. In autosomal dominant disorders, most mutations lead to reduced production of a protein or give rise to an inactive protein. The clinical effect of these loss-of-function mutations depends on the biologic activity of the protein affected. If such mutations involve an enzyme in heterozygotic animals, only one allele of the gene is affected. Therefore they are usually clinically normal because up to 50% loss of an enzyme's activity can be compensated for by the normal gene allele for that enzyme. In contrast, nonenzyme structural proteins, such as collagen and cytoskeletal elements of the red cell membrane (e.g., spectrin), are significantly affected in autosomal dominant disorders. As an example, a 50% reduction in the amount of such proteins results in abnormal structure and assembly of collagen and cytoskeletal elements in red blood cells, resulting in a hereditary spectrin deficiency in golden retriever dogs.

Less common than loss-of-function mutations are gain-of-function mutations. In this type of mutation, the protein product acquires new biologic activities not usually associated with the normal-type protein.

Autosomal Recessive Disorders

In autosomal recessive disorders, both alleles at a given gene locus must be mutated for an animal to be affected by the disorder. One mutated allele is provided by the sire and the other by the dam. Thus there is a 25% chance that each offspring from heterozygous parents will inherit both mutated gene alleles. Both parents are clinically normal and serve as carrier animals. Animals with autosomal recessive mutations usually have clinical disease, and the onset is usually early in life. Many of the mutated genes encode enzymes. Examples of autosomal recessive disorders in animals include lysosomal storage diseases (see Figs. 1-82 and 14-63 and 14-64), glycogen storage diseases (see Fig. 14-63) and mucopolysaccharidoses,

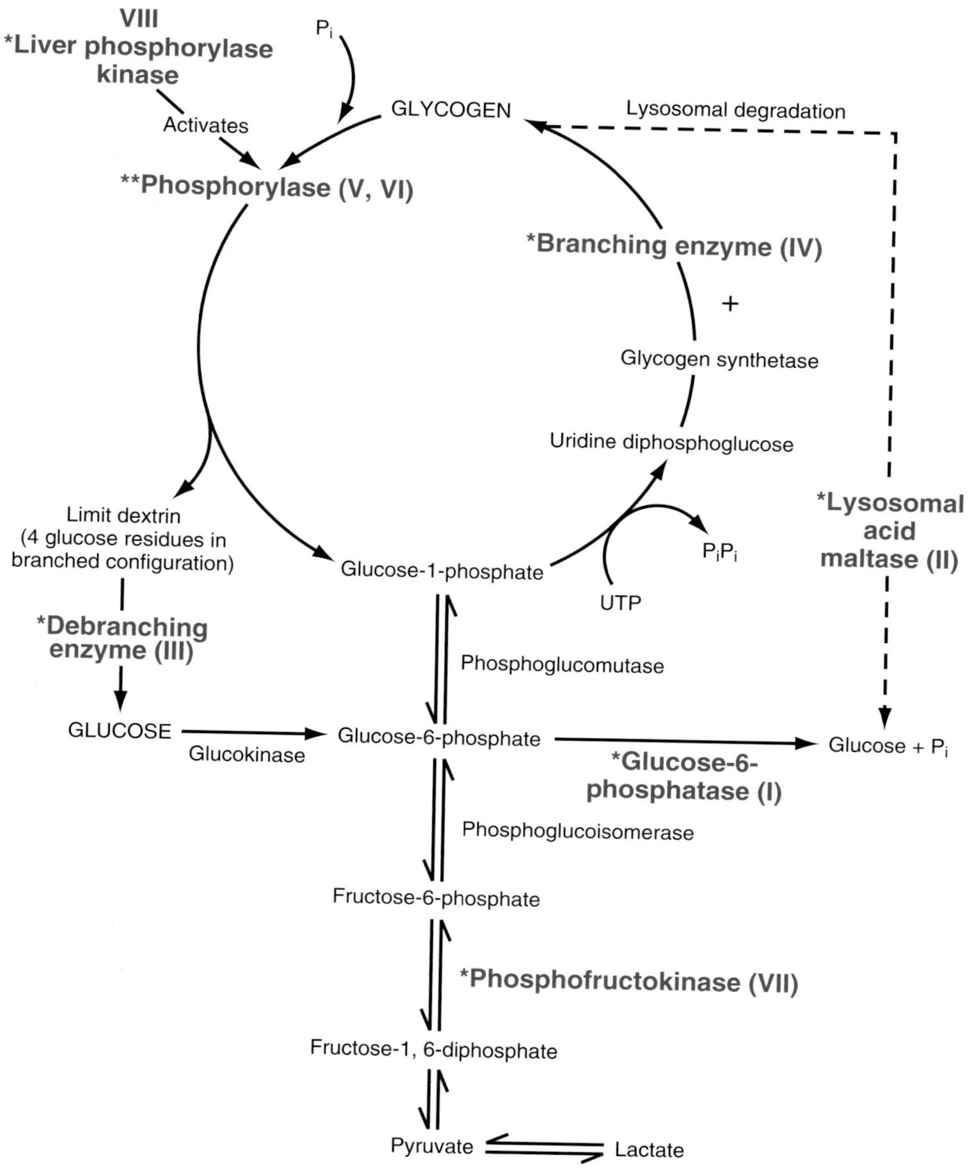

Fig. 1-83 Pathways of glycogen metabolism.
Asterisks mark the enzyme deficiencies associated with glycogen storage diseases. Roman numerals indicate the type of glycogen storage disease associated with the given enzyme deficiency. Types V and VI result from deficiencies of muscle and liver phosphorylases, respectively. (From Kumar V, Abbas A, Fausto N, et al: *Robbins & Cotran pathologic basis of disease*, ed 8, Philadelphia, 2009, Saunders.)

and aminoacidopathies that affect organs such as the brain, spinal cord, skeletal muscle, liver, and kidney.

X-Linked Disorders

All sex-linked disorders are X-linked, and almost all are recessive and caused by mutations in genes on the X chromosome. Examples of autosomal recessive X-linked disorders in animals include Duchenne muscular dystrophy and agammaglobulinemia of the immune system.

Single-Gene Disorders of Somatic Cells

Mutations that arise in somatic cells do not cause hereditary diseases but are important in the genesis of cancers (Fig. 1-84) (see also Chapter 6) and some congenital malformations. Tumor-specific acquired single-gene mutations are expressed in some types of tumors. During the clinical management of cancer, such mutations can serve as a means to detect the growth of a tumor and monitor its response to therapy.

Single-Gene Disorders of Mitochondria

Some single-gene disorders have a non-Mendelian pattern of inheritance and include disorders arising from mutations in mtDNA and those in which the transmission is influenced by trinucleotide-repeat mutations, genomic imprinting, or gonadal mosaicism. In such cases, mitochondrial mutations occur in mtDNA rather than in the nuclear genome and cause mitochondrial encephalopathies in the nervous system.

Diseases resulting from mitochondrial inheritance are rare and many affect the neuromuscular system. There are only 37 mitochondrial genes, and a feature unique to mtDNA is maternal inheritance. Dams and only dams transmit mtDNA to their offspring, both male and female. Sires make no contribution of mtDNA to

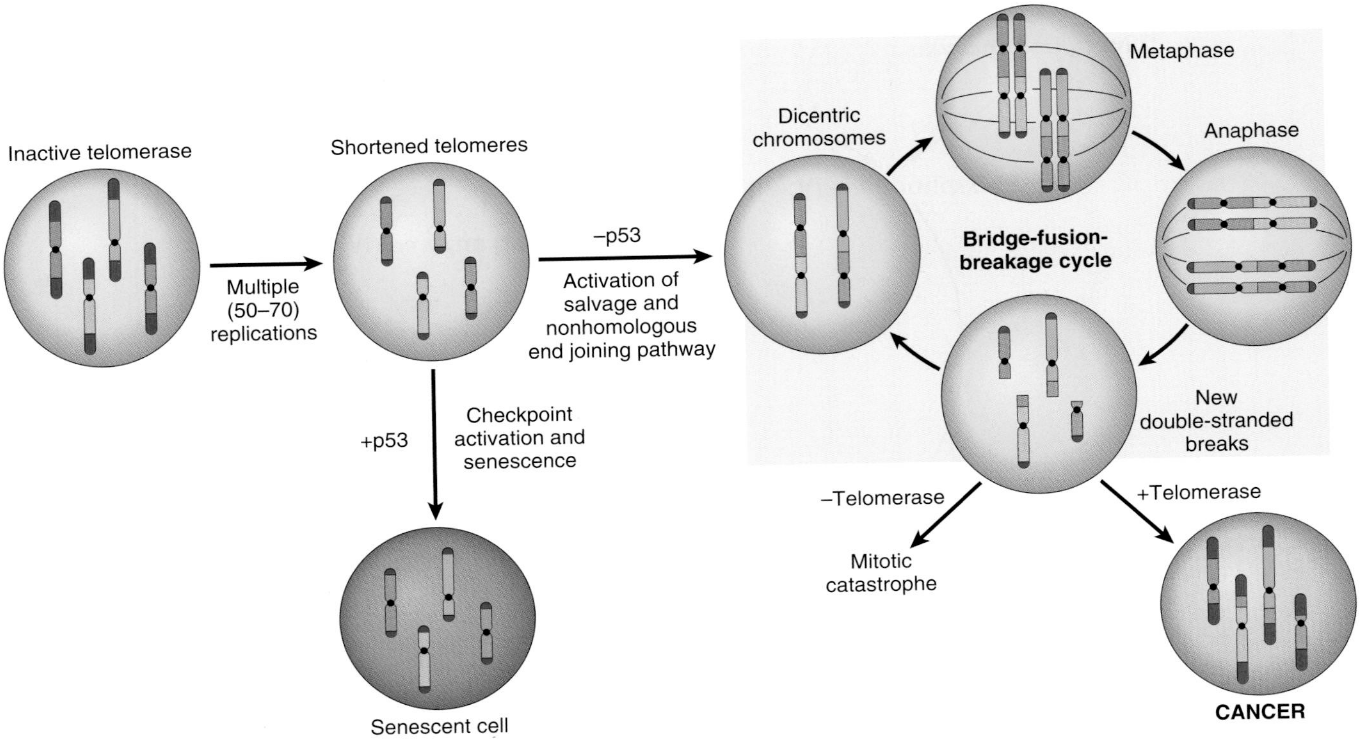

Fig. 1-84 Sequence of events in tumorigenesis.
Replication of somatic cells, which do not express telomerase, leads to shortened telomeres. In the presence of competent checkpoints, cells undergo arrest and enter nonreplicative senescence. In the absence of checkpoints, DNA-repair pathways are inappropriately activated, leading to the formation of dicentric chromosomes. At mitosis the dicentric chromosomes are pulled apart, generating random double-stranded breaks, which then activate DNA-repair pathways, leading to the random association of double-stranded ends and the formation, again, of dicentric chromosomes. Cells undergo numerous rounds of this bridge-fusion-breakage cycle, which generates massive chromosomal instability and numerous mutations. If cells fail to re-express telomerase, they eventually undergo mitotic catastrophe and death. Re-expression of telomerase allows the cells to escape the bridge-fusion-breakage cycle, thus promoting their survival and tumorigenesis. (From Kumar V, Abbas A, Fausto N, et al: *Robbins & Cotran pathologic basis of disease,* ed 8, Philadelphia, 2009, Saunders.)

offspring. This peculiarity exists because ova contain numerous mitochondria within their cytoplasm, whereas spermatozoa contain few, if any. Thus the mtDNA complement of the fertilized ovum is derived entirely from the ovum.

Each type of tissue requires a certain amount of ATP for normal function. Although some variation in ATP levels may be tolerated, there is typically a threshold level below which cells begin to degenerate and die. Organ systems with large ATP requirements and high thresholds tend to be the ones most seriously affected by mitochondrial diseases. Because mtDNA encodes enzymes involved in oxidative phosphorylation, mutations affecting these genes exert their deleterious effects primarily on the organs most dependent on oxidative phosphorylation such as the CNS, skeletal muscle (type 2 myofibers), cardiac muscle, liver, and kidneys. For example, the CNS produces about 20% of the body's ATP production and therefore is often affected by mtDNA mutations. The mutation rate of mtDNA is about 10 times higher than that of nuclear DNA. This difference is caused by a relative lack of DNA repair mechanisms in the mtDNA and also by damage from free oxygen radicals released during the oxidative phosphorylation process.

Chromosomal Disorders

Errors in Cell Division

Abnormalities of chromosome number and/or structure can arise in autosomes (somatic cells) or sex chromosomes (germline cells), by errors in cell division. Cell division transfers genetic disorders within somatic and/or germline cells. Under normal conditions there are two kinds of cell division, mitosis and meiosis (Web Fig. 1-3). Mitosis is somatic cell division by which the body grows and differentiates and tissues regenerate. Mitotic division results in two daughter cells, each with chromosomes and genes identical to those of the parent cell. There may be dozens or even hundreds of successive mitoses of a somatic cell during its lifetime. In contrast, meiosis occurs only in cells of the germline and results in the formation of ova or spermatozoa, with, under normal conditions, each cell type having half of the normal karyotype (one of each kind of autosome and either an X or a Y chromosome).

Most chromosomal disorders are caused by errors in cell division. An animal begins life as a fertilized ovum (e.g., zygote) after fusion of an ovum and spermatogonium, which originate through cell division during meiosis. This single cell zygote gives rise to all cells of the body (estimated at about 100 trillion [1×10^{14} cells]) that are derived from dozens or even hundreds of mitoses crucial for growth and differentiation. The biologic significance of meiosis and mitosis lies in ensuring the constancy of chromosome number and thus the integrity of the genome from one cell to its progeny and from one generation to the next. The medical significance of these processes involves errors of cell division, which lead to the formation of an individual cell or of a cell lineage with an abnormal number of chromosomes and thus an inappropriate amount of genomic material. Such errors are called *nondisjunctions* and represent a failure of chromosome pairs to disjoin (separate) during cell division, and the result is that both chromosomes go to one cell and none to the other. Meiotic nondisjunction, particularly in oogenesis, is a common mutational mechanism, responsible for chromosomally abnormal fetuses. In those fetuses that survive

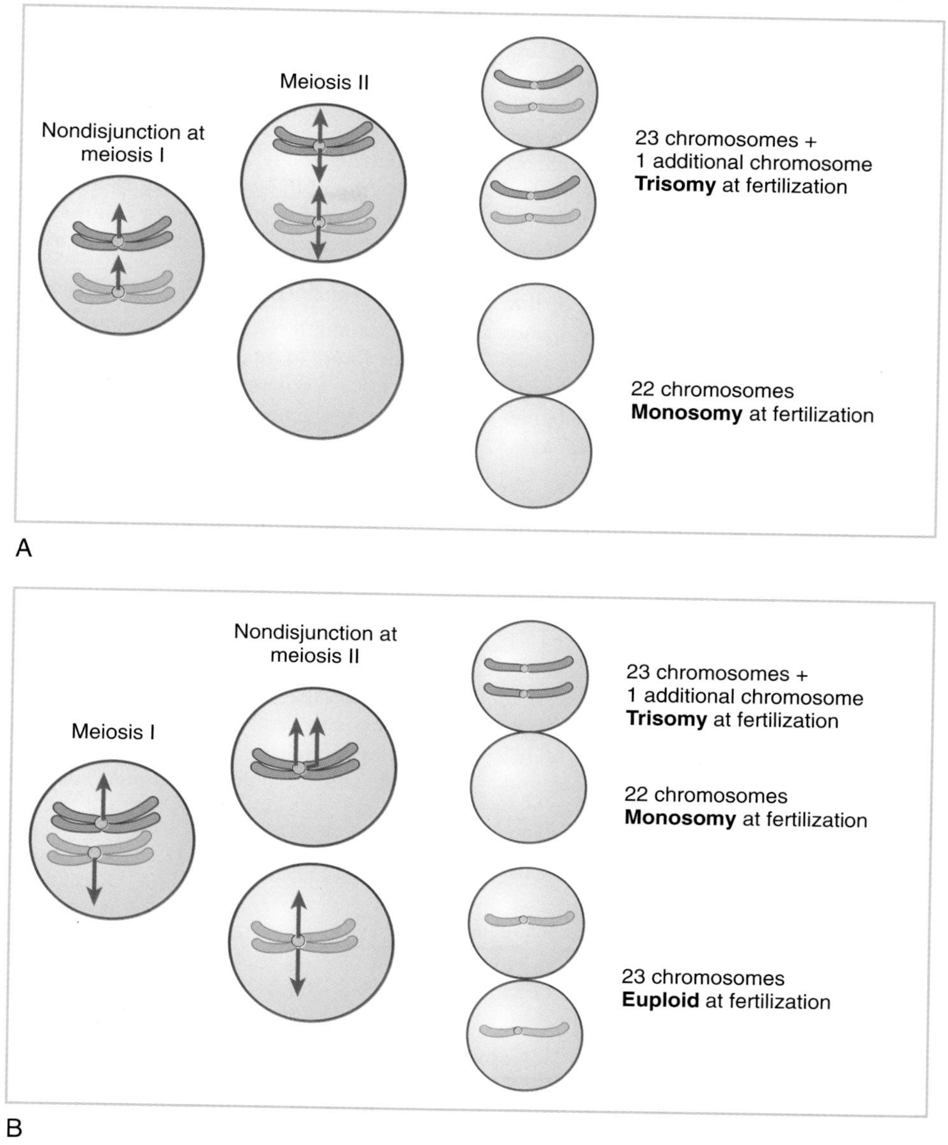

Fig. 1-85 Nondisjunction.
A, Nondisjunction occurs in meiosis I when homologous chromosome pairs segregate to the same daughter cell. **B,** Nondisjunction occurs in meiosis II when sister chromatids segregate to the same daughter cell. When nondisjunction occurs in meiosis I, all gametes are abnormal, whereas when it occurs in meiosis II, there is a 50% chance that a normal gamete will be fertilized. (From Adkison L, Brown MS: *Elsevier's integrated genetics,* St. Louis, 2007, Mosby.)

to term, chromosome abnormalities cause developmental defects, failure to thrive, and reduced mental function. Mitotic nondisjunctions can also be inherited. Nondisjunction soon after fertilization, either in the developing embryo or in extraembryonic tissues like the placenta, leads to chromosomal mosaicism that can be the basis for some genetic disorders. Additionally, abnormal chromosome segregation in rapidly dividing tissues can be a step in the development of tumors.

Numeric Alterations

Cells with normal chromosome numbers have euploid karyotypes (i.e., normal number of chromosomes for a species). If an error occurs in meiosis or mitosis during cell division and a cell acquires a lesser or greater number of chromosomes and thus does not have its normal karyotype, it is referred to as *aneuploidy.* A cause of aneuploidy is nondisjunction during meiosis to form ova or spermatogonia. This outcome result is either extra chromosomes (i.e., trisomy, tetrasomy, and so on) or one less chromosome (i.e., monosomy) (Fig. 1-85). Fertilization of such ova by normal spermatogonia results in two types of zygotes, trisomic (or tetrasomic) or monosomic. Trisomic or tetrasomic offspring are extremely rare in domestic animals, but an autosomal trisomy has been reported in a malformed Italian Friesian calf that had malformed limbs, congenital opisthotonus, brachygnathia, blindness, and absence of external genitalia. Monosomic offspring are more common in domestic animals, in which an X chromosome monosomy (Turner-like syndrome) affecting primarily fillies (mares) has been reported. Affected mares have smaller than normal vulvas, uteri, and ovaries, and most fail to cycle and show estrous behavior.

Occasionally, mitotic errors in early development give rise to two or more populations of cells with different chromosomal karyotypes in the same animal, a condition referred to as *mosaicism.*

Mosaicism can result from mitotic errors during the division of the fertilized ovum or in somatic cells. Mosaicism affecting the sex chromosomes is relatively common. In the division of the fertilized ovum, an error may lead to one of the daughter cells receiving three sex chromosomes, whereas the other receives only one, yielding, for example, an n-1,X/n+1,XXX mosaic. All cells derived from each of these cells will have the same abnormal karyotype. An example of X (sex) chromosome mosaicism occurs in Tortoiseshell and Calico cats. In all female mammalian cells, the function of one X chromosome is inactivated through a random process called *X chromosome inactivation.* In the cells of these cats, approximately 50% of the cells have paternal X chromosomes that have been inactivated and a different 50% of the cells have maternal X chromosomes that have been inactivated. Thus normal female cats have roughly equal populations of two genetically different cell types and are therefore a type of mosaic that is expressed in the patterns of hair coloration (orange, black, and white).

Autosomal mosaicism seems to be much less common than that involving the sex chromosomes. An error in an early mitotic division affecting the autosomes usually leads to a nonviable mosaic fetus.

Structural Alterations

Changes in the structure of chromosomes are caused by deletion, inversion, isochromosome formation, or translocation of a portion of a sex or autosomal chromosome and occur during cell division (Fig. 1-86). During embryogenesis, structural alterations of sex chromosomes are more common than those of autosomes and can result in some cells having XX sex chromosomes and others having XY sex chromosomes. During embryogenesis, these cells coexist and both male and female reproductive structures develop to varying degrees dependent on the expression of the sex chromosomes. As a result, these diseases are characterized by sexual ambiguity of the fetus and include hermaphroditism and pseudohermaphroditism (see Chapters 18 and 19). Structural alterations also likely involve autosomes in animals, but their occurrence and significance have not been adequately characterized.

Complex Multigenic Disorders

Complex multigenic disorders are caused by interactions between variant forms of genes (e.g., polymorphisms) and environmental factors. Each variant gene confers a small increase in disease risk, but no single gene is necessary or able alone to produce disease. It is only when several polymorphisms are present in an animal that disease occurs, hence the terms *multigenic* or *polygenic.* Thus, unlike the single-mutant gene disorders (discussed previously) that commonly cause disease and give rise to Mendelian-inherited disorders, each individual polymorphism has a small effect and rarely causes disease by itself. Because environmental interactions are important in the pathogenesis of these diseases and the complex traits do not follow a Mendelian pattern of inheritance, the genes and polymorphisms that contribute to these diseases have been very difficult to determine. Assigning a disease to this mode of inheritance must be done with caution. Diagnosis of diseases that are considered complex multigenic disorders such as type I diabetes (a known human complex multigenic disorder) depends on many factors and

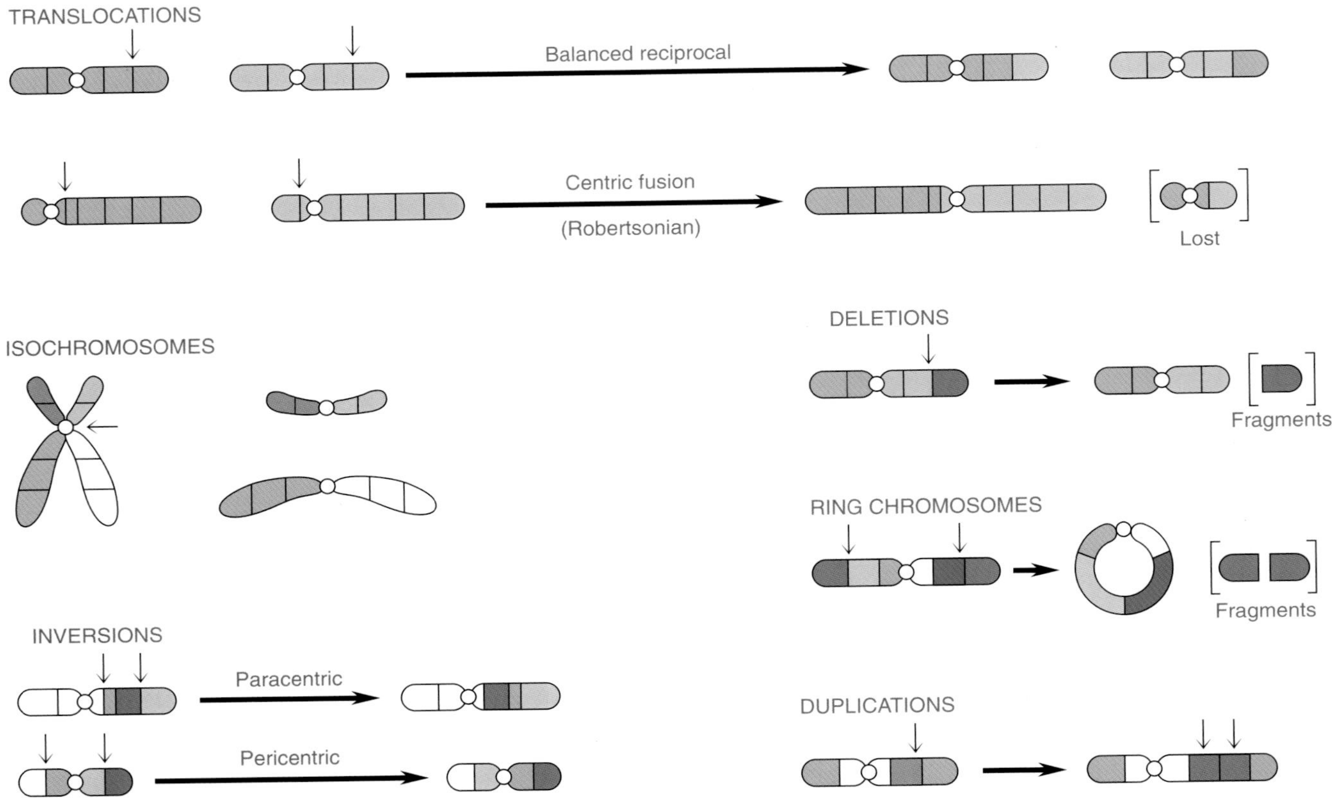

Fig. 1-86 Types of chromosomal rearrangements.
Chromosome rearrangements are structural changes in chromosomes such as deletions, duplications, inversions, and translocations. They are caused by breakage of DNA double helices from errors in DNA replication and from damage caused by mutagens. (From Copstead L, Banasik J: *Pathophysiology,* ed 4, St Louis, 2010, Mosby.)

the exclusion of Mendelian (single-gene) and chromosomal modes of transmission. The occurrence of complex multigenic disorders in animals has not been demonstrated except in laboratory animal models of human disease, but their existence in domestic animal species is highly likely.

SUGGESTED READINGS

Suggested Readings are available at evolve.elsevier.com/Zachary/McGavin/.

CHAPTER 2

Vascular Disorders and Thrombosis

Derek A. Mosier

Free-living unicellular organisms obtain nutrients and eliminate metabolic waste products directly into the external environment. Multicellular organisms require a circulatory system to deliver nutrients to and remove waste products from cells. The movement of fluid and cells through the circulatory system maintains homeostasis and integrates functions of cells and tissues in complex, multicellular organisms. In this chapter, the basic abnormalities that affect fluid circulation and balance within an animal are described.

CIRCULATORY SYSTEM

The circulatory system consists of blood, a central pump (heart), blood distribution (arterial) and collection (venous) networks, and a system for exchange of nutrients and waste products between blood and extravascular tissue (microcirculation) (Fig. 2-1). A network of lymphatic vessels that parallel the veins also contributes to circulation by draining fluid from extravascular spaces into the blood vascular system.

The heart provides the driving force for blood distribution. Equal volumes of blood are normally distributed to the pulmonary circulation by the right side of the heart and the systemic circulation by the left side of the heart. The volume of blood pumped by each half of the heart per minute (cardiac output) is determined by the beats per minute (heart rate) and the volume of blood pumped per beat by the ventricle (stroke volume). Typically, each half of the heart pumps the equivalent of the entire blood volume of the animal per minute.

Arteries have relatively large diameter lumens to facilitate rapid blood flow with minimal resistance. Artery walls are thick and consist predominantly of smooth muscle fibers for tensile strength and elastic fibers for elasticity (Web Fig. 2-1). Elastic fibers allow arteries to act as pressure reservoirs, expanding to hold blood ejected from the heart during contraction and passively recoiling to provide continuous flow and pressure to arterioles between heart contractions.

Arterioles are the major resistance vessels within the circulatory system; intravascular pressure can fall by nearly half after blood passes through an arteriole. Arterioles have relatively narrow lumens, the diameter of which is controlled by the smooth muscle cells that are the major component of their walls. Extrinsic sympathetic innervation and local intrinsic stimuli regulate the degree of arteriolar smooth muscle contraction, causing arterioles to dilate or constrict to selectively distribute blood to the areas of greatest need.

Capillaries are the site of nutrient and waste product exchange between the blood and tissue. Capillaries are the most numerous vessel in the circulatory system, with a total cross-sectional area nearly 1300 times that of the aorta. However, they normally contain only about 5% of the total blood volume. The velocity of blood flow through the capillaries is very slow, and red blood cells generally move through a capillary in single file to further facilitate the diffusion of nutrients and wastes. Capillaries have narrow lumens (approximately 8 μm) and thin walls (approximately 1 μm) consisting of a single epithelial cell layer (endothelium). At the junctions between capillary endothelia are interendothelial pores, which make the capillary semipermeable to facilitate diffusion of nutrients and waste products between the blood and tissues. There are three types of capillaries: continuous, fenestrated, and discontinuous. The basic functions and tissue locations of these types of capillaries are illustrated in Fig. 2-2. They are discussed in greater detail in the chapters covering the diseases of organ systems.

The return trip of blood to the heart begins in the postcapillary venules. Venules have a composition similar to capillaries but may have thin layers of muscle as they become more distant from the capillary bed. Veins are composed mainly of collagen with smaller amounts of elastin and smooth muscle (Web Fig. 2-2). Venules and veins provide a low resistance pathway for the return of blood to the heart. Because of their distensibility, they can store large amounts of blood; nearly 65% of total blood volume is normally present within the systemic veins. Pressure and velocity of flow are low within venules and veins. Therefore other factors are necessary to help move venous blood toward the heart such as venous valves to prevent backflow of blood, skeletal muscle contraction, venous vasoconstriction, an increased pressure gradient due to decreased pressure in the heart during filling (cardiac-suction effect), and

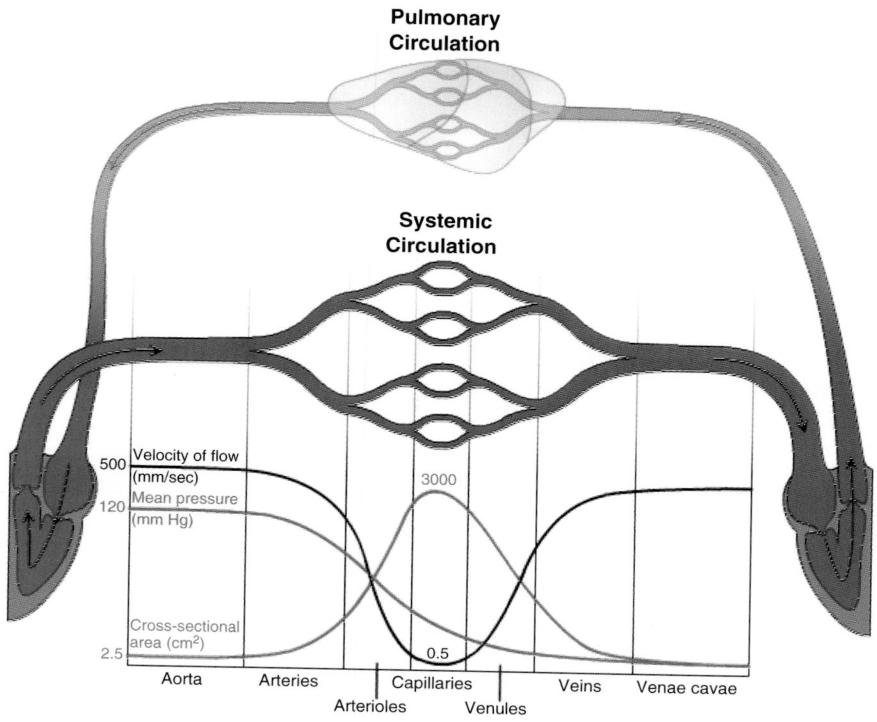

Fig. 2-1 The vascular system. Blood travels from the left to the right side of the heart via the systemic circulation, and from the right to the left side via the pulmonary circulation. Blood flow rate and pressure in the systemic arterial circulation decrease in conjunction with increased arterial cross-sectional area. In the venous systemic circulation, blood flow rate, but not pressure, increases in conjunction with decreased venous cross-sectional area. The flow, pressure, and cross-sectional area relationships are similar but reversed (i.e., veins deliver blood and arteries collect blood) in the pulmonary circulation. (Courtesy Dr. D.A. Mosier and L. Schooley, College of Veterinary Medicine, Kansas State University.)

decreased pressure in the thoracic veins due to negative pressure within the thoracic cavity (respiratory pump).

The lymphatic system originates as blind-ended lymphatic capillaries, which permeate the tissue surrounding the microcirculation (arterioles, metarterioles, capillaries, and postcapillary venules [Fig. 2-3]).Lymphatic capillaries have overlapping endothelial cells and large interendothelial gaps so that external pressure allows movement of fluid and molecules into the vessel. However, intravascular lymphatic pressure forces these overlapping edges together to prevent the flow of lymph out of the vessel. Lymphatic capillary gaps are much larger than those between blood capillary endothelium, so they can accommodate movement of larger particles and substances. Lymphatic capillaries converge into progressively larger lymph vessels that drain into lymph nodes and then ultimately empty into the venous system. Similar to venous vessels, lymphatics are distensible, low-pressure vessels that require lymphatic valves and contraction of surrounding muscles to facilitate return of fluid to the blood.

All components of the circulatory system are lined by a single layer of endothelium. Endothelium forms a dynamic interface between blood and tissue and is a critical participant in fluid distribution, inflammation, immunity, angiogenesis, and hemostasis (Fig. 2-4). Normal endothelium is antithrombotic and profibrinolytic and helps maintain blood in a fluid state, but when injured, endothelium becomes prothrombotic and antifibrinolytic. Endothelial activation by oxidative stress, hypoxia, inflammation, infectious agents, tissue injury, or similar events results in the production and release of numerous substances with wide-ranging roles in physiology and pathology (Fig. 2-5 and Box 2-1). Endothelial activation is typically localized to restrict a host response to a specific area, while not affecting the normal function of endothelium and flow of blood in other parts of the body.

MICROCIRCULATION, INTERSTITIUM, AND CELLS

The exchange of fluid, nutrients, and waste products between blood and cells takes place through the interstitium, the space between cells, and the microcirculation. The interstitium is composed of structural, adhesive, and absorptive components collectively referred to as the *extracellular matrix* (ECM). Type I collagen is the major structural component of the ECM and forms the framework in which cells reside. This is intimately associated with type IV collagen of cell basement membranes. Adhesive glycoproteins provide sites of attachment for structural components and also serve as receptors for cells, such as phagocytes and lymphocytes, which move through the interstitium. Absorptive disaccharide complexes (glycosaminoglycans) and protein-disaccharide polymer complexes (proteoglycans) are hydrophilic and can bind large amounts of water and other soluble molecules. In most cases, no more than 1.0 mm of interstitial space separates a cell from a capillary.

FLUID DISTRIBUTION AND HOMEOSTASIS

Water comprises approximately 60% of body weight, of which about ⅔ is intracellular and ⅓ is extracellular (80% of which is in the interstitium and 20% is in the plasma). The distribution of fluid-nutrients, and waste products between the blood, interstitium, and cells is controlled by physical barriers, as well as pressure and concentration gradients between each compartment. The cell's plasma membrane is a selective barrier that separates interstitial and intracellular compartments. Nonpolar (uncharged) lipid-soluble substances, such as O_2, CO_2, and fatty acids, move relatively freely across the plasma membrane based on concentration

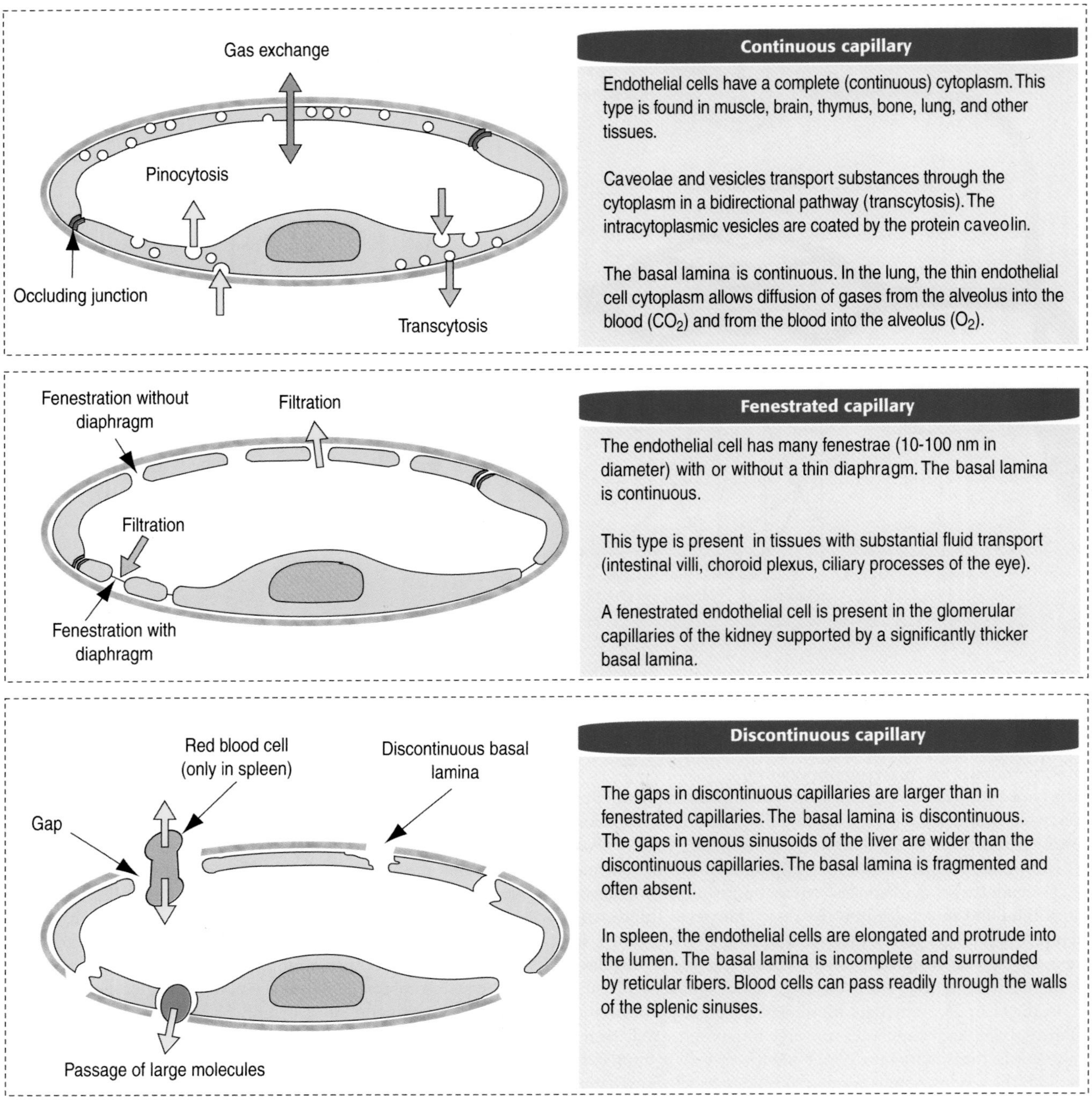

Fig. 2-2 Types of endothelium lining capillaries.
(From Kierszenbaum AL: *Histology and cell biology: an introduction to pathology,* St Louis, 2002, Mosby.)

gradients. Polar (charged) lipid-insoluble particles and molecules, such as electrolytes, calcium, glucose, and amino acids, enter the cell by carrier-mediated transport. Water readily moves across the plasma membrane down its concentration gradient. Although approximately 100 times the volume of water in a cell crosses the plasma membrane in 1 second, cell fluid content remains relatively stable because of the activity of energy-dependent membrane pumps (e.g., Na^+/K^+-adenosine triphosphatase [ATPase] pump) and the balance between osmotic pressures exerted by interstitial and intracellular solutes.

The capillary wall is a semipermeable barrier that influences the movement of fluid, nutrients, and waste products between the blood and interstitium. Lipid-soluble substances can pass through capillary endothelium by dissolving in the membrane lipid bilayer, and large proteins can move through the cell by transport within vesicles. Most importantly, water and polar molecules move through interendothelial pores. Normally, these pores are large enough to allow the passage of water, small nutrients (ions, glucose, amino acids), and waste products, yet small enough to prevent the movement of cells and large proteins (albumin and other plasma proteins such as complement, kinin, and coagulation proteins). Local stimuli, such as inflammation, can cause endothelial cells to contract to widen interendothelial pores and allow the passage of larger molecules. Under normal conditions, the composition of plasma and interstitial fluid is very similar, with the exception of the large plasma proteins.

BOX 2-1 Endothelial Properties in Health and Disease: Endothelial Products

FLUID DISTRIBUTION AND BLOOD FLOW

Semipermeable membrane for fluid distribution
- Interendothelial junctions

Vasodilation
- Nitric oxide
- Prostacyclin (PGI_2)

Vasoconstriction
- Endothelin

HEMOSTASIS

Antihemostatic substances
- PGI_2
- Endothelial cell protein C receptor
- Tissue factor pathway inhibitor (TFPI)
- Tissue plasminogen activator (tPA)
- Heparan sulfate
- Adenosine diphosphatase (ADPase) and adenosine triphosphatase (ATPase)
- Protein S

Prohemostatic substances
- von Willebrand's factor
- Tissue factor (TF) (factor III)
- Plasminogen activator inhibitor-1 (PAI-1)

INFLAMMATORY MEDIATORS

Cytokines
- Interleukin (IL) -1, IL-6, IL-8

Enhanced expression of TF

Expression of leukocyte adhesion molecules:
- Cell adhesion molecule family
  - Mucosal addressin cell adhesion molecule 1 (MAdCAM-1)
  - Intercellular adhesion molecule 1 (ICAM-1),
  - Vascular cell adhesion molecule 1 (VCAM-1)
  - Platelet/endothelial cell adhesion molecule 1 (PECAM-1)
- Selectin family
  - P-selectin
  - E-selectin

GROWTH FACTORS

Platelet-derived growth factor (PDGF)
Colony-stimulating factor (CSF)
Fibroblast growth factor (FGF)
Transforming growth factor-β (TGF-β)
Heparin

FIBRINOLYSIS

Synthesis and secretion of fibrinolytic components under certain circumstances
Regulation of formation of plasmin
tPA
Urokinase plasminogen activator receptor
PAI-1
Annexin II

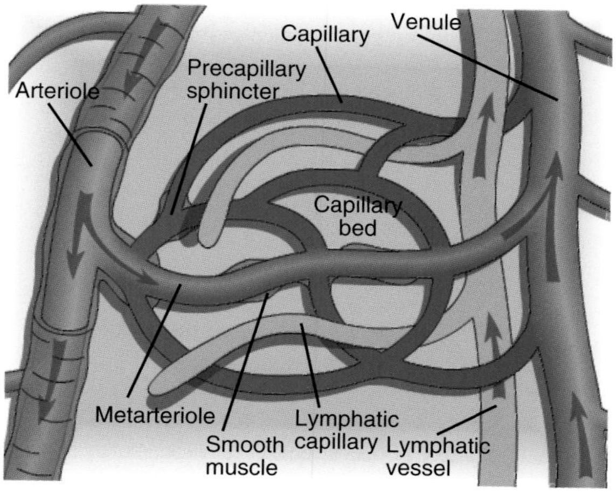

Fig. 2-3 The microcirculation.
The microcirculation consists of arterioles (small arteries proximal to a capillary bed), metarterioles (arterial capillaries), capillaries (thin, semipermeable vessels that connect arterioles and venules), and postcapillary venules (small vessels that merge to form veins after collecting blood from a capillary network). Smooth muscle of the arterioles and metarterioles regulates flow of blood into the capillary bed. There is a dramatic drop in pressure and flow rate from the arterial to the venous side of the microcirculation, facilitating interactions between capillary blood and interstitial fluid. Blind-ended lymphatic vessels that originate near capillary beds interact intimately with the microcirculation. (Courtesy Dr. D.A. Mosier and L. Schooley, College of Veterinary Medicine, Kansas State University.)

Movement of substances through interendothelial pores and cell membranes is generally passive in response to concentration and pressure gradients. Nutrient-rich arterial blood contains O_2, glucose, and amino acids that move down their concentration gradients into the interstitium, where they are available for use by cells. CO_2 and waste products generated by cells accumulate in the interstitium and move down their gradient into the venous blood. These gradients become larger in areas where cells are metabolically active.

Water distribution between the plasma and interstitium is determined mainly by osmotic and hydrostatic pressure differentials between the compartments and is described by the following formula (Fig. 2-6):

$$\text{Net filtration across the endothelium} = K\left[\left(P_{cap} - P_{int}\right) - \sigma\left(\pi_{cap} - \pi_{int}\right)\right]$$

K = Capillary endothelial permeability constant
P = Hydrostatic pressure
σ = Reflection coefficient
π = Colloid osmotic pressure
cap = capillary
int = interstitium

Although sodium and chloride account for approximately 84% of the total osmolality of plasma, free movement of these electrolytes through interendothelial pores balances their concentrations in the plasma and interstitium, so their contribution to differences in osmotic pressure between these compartments is minimal. In contrast, nonpermeable, suspended plasma proteins make up less

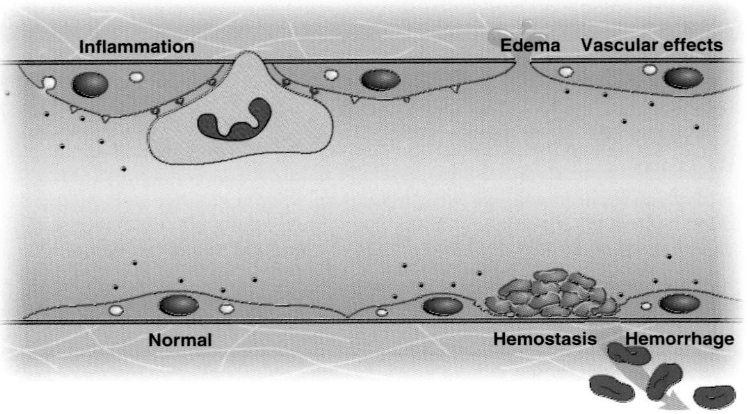

Fig. 2-4 Structure and function of the endothelium.
Endothelium is a physical barrier between intravascular and extravascular spaces, and it is an important mediator of fluid distribution, hemostasis, inflammation, and healing. (Courtesy Dr. D.A. Mosier and L. Schooley, College of Veterinary Medicine, Kansas State University.)

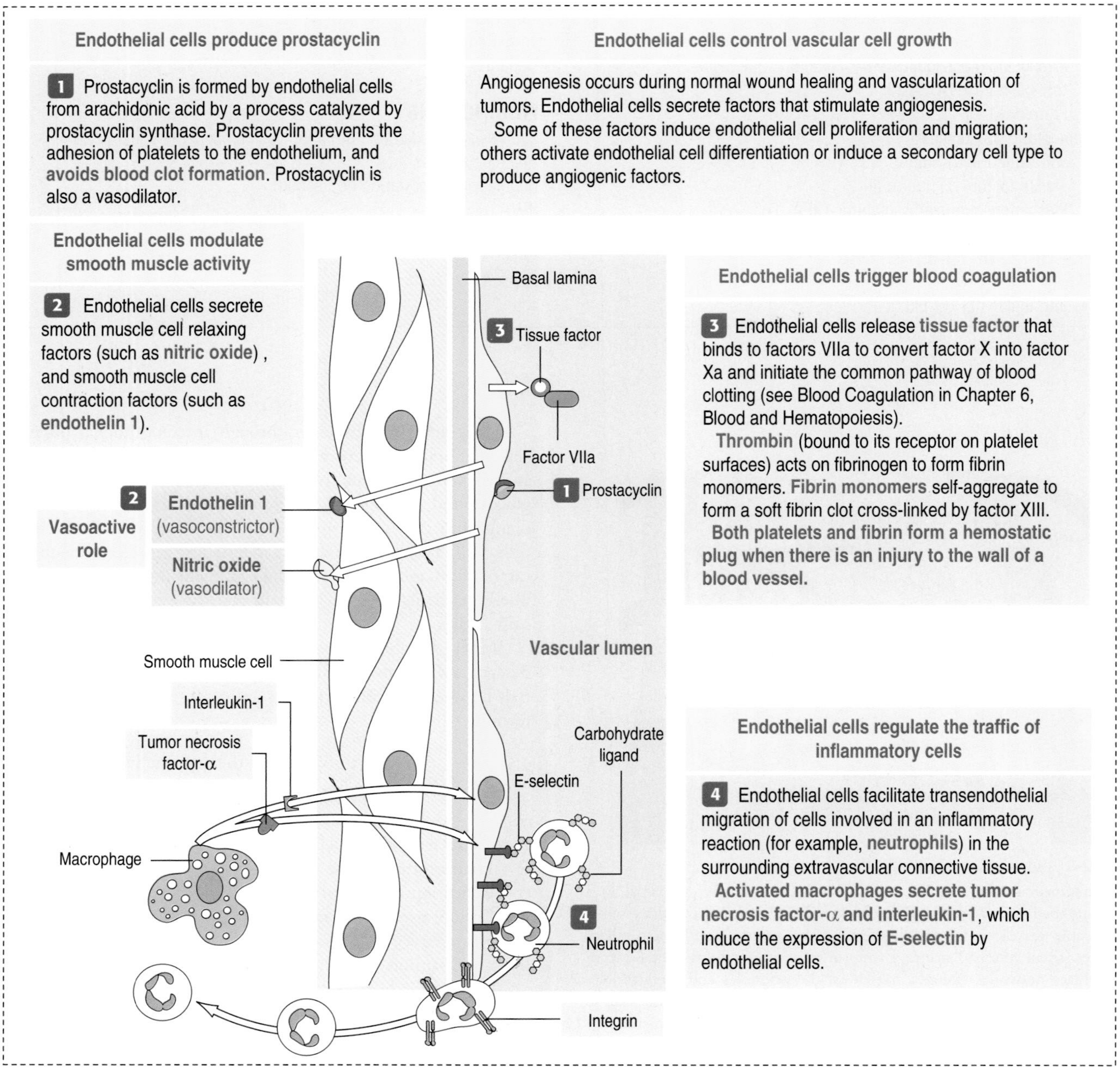

Fig. 2-5 Bioactive mediators from endothelial cells.
(From Kierszenbaum AL: *Histology and cell biology: an introduction to pathology,* St Louis, 2002, Mosby.)

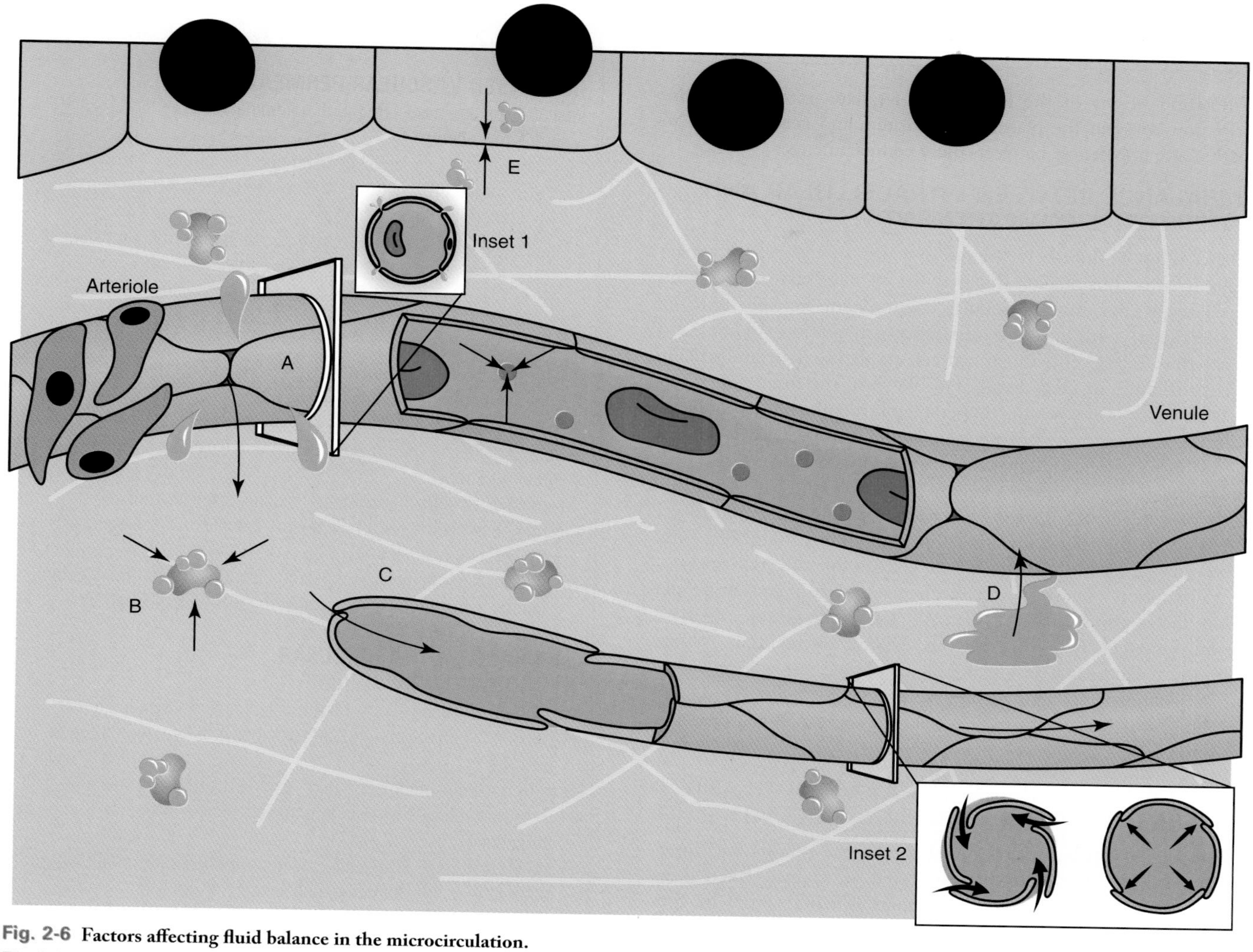

Fig. 2-6 Factors affecting fluid balance in the microcirculation.
Fluid distribution is determined by physical characteristics of the microcirculation and lymphatics and osmotic and hydrostatic forces within the blood and interstitial fluid. Intercellular gaps between endothelium allow movement of fluid and small molecules between the blood and interstitial fluid *(insets 1 and 2)*. **A,** High arteriolar hydrostatic pressure forces fluid into the interstitium. **B,** Plasma proteins (e.g., albumin) and molecules within the ECM exert an osmotic effect to attract and retain water. **C,** Interstitial hydrostatic pressure forces interstitial fluid into lower pressure venules. **D,** The slight excess of interstitial fluid not returned to the venules enters the lymphatics to be drained from the area. **E,** Exchange of intracellular and interstitial fluid is balanced by osmotic forces and concentration gradients of electrolytes and other molecules across the cell plasma membrane. *Inset 1,* Cross-section of a blood vessel capillary showing interendothelial junctions. Endothelium forms end-to-end junctions for movement of fluid and small molecules. *Inset 2,* Cross-section of a lymphatic capillary showing the interendothelial junctions. Endothelium overlaps to allow movement of larger particles and closure when intravascular pressure forces overlapping endothelium together. (Courtesy Dr. D.A. Mosier and L. Schooley, College of Veterinary Medicine, Kansas State University.)

than 1% of the total osmolality of plasma. However, because these proteins (particularly albumin) do not readily move through interendothelial pores, they exert a colloidal osmotic pressure that is responsible for the majority of the difference in osmotic pressure between the plasma and interstitium.

In the microcirculation, intravascular and interstitial osmotic pressures and interstitial hydrostatic forces remain relatively constant and favor intravascular retention of fluid. However, high hydrostatic pressures within the arteriolar end of the capillary bed result in a net filtration of fluid into the interstitium. Lower hydrostatic pressures in the venular end of the capillary bed result in a net absorption pressure and reentry of fluid into the microvasculature. Alternatively, filtration and absorption may not occur because of a drop in hydrostatic pressure across individual capillary beds. Instead, filtration may occur across the entire length of capillary beds with open precapillary sphincters and high rates of blood flow, whereas absorption may occur across the entire length of capillary beds with closed precapillary sphincters and low blood flow rates. The slight excess of fluid that is retained in the interstitium and any plasma proteins that have escaped the vasculature enter lymphatic capillaries to be drained from the area.

The constant flow of fluid between the microcirculation and interstitium allows exchange of nutrients and waste products between these two fluid compartments to support cell functions. Additionally, the interstitium provides a fluid buffer to either increase or decrease the plasma volume to assure effective circulatory function. Excessive fluid intake will expand plasma volume and increase hydrostatic pressure, resulting in greater filtration into the interstitium to maintain a relatively constant plasma volume. Reduced fluid intake will decrease plasma volume, shifting the movement of water from the interstitium into the plasma to increase circulating fluid volume.

ABNORMAL FLUID DISTRIBUTION

Alteration in any of the factors that regulate normal fluid distribution between the plasma, interstitium, and cells can lead to pathologic imbalances between these compartments.

IMBALANCE BETWEEN INTRACELLULAR AND INTERSTITIAL COMPARTMENTS

Distribution of fluid between the interstitium and cells is generally dynamic but stable. This stability is necessary to maintain a relatively constant intracellular environment for cell function. Generalized conditions (e.g., alterations in plasma volume) and local stimuli (e.g., inflammation) can result in slight and usually transient shifts in fluid distribution between the interstitium and cells. Excess plasma volume (hypervolemia) results in movement of additional water into the interstitium and ultimately into the cell along both osmotic and hydrostatic gradients, causing cell swelling. In contrast, reduced plasma volume (hypovolemia) can result in a flow of water in the opposite direction resulting in cell shrinkage and decreased interstitial volume. Increased interstitial volume will also cause a slight flow of fluid into cells in the affected region.

Disruption of any of the mechanisms that maintain proper fluid distribution between the cell and interstitium can have serious consequences for the cell. Failure to maintain proper osmotic balance as a result of cell membrane damage or failure of the energy-dependent plasma membrane pumps results in cell swelling, which if not quickly corrected can lead to cell death by osmotic lysis.

IMBALANCE BETWEEN INTRAVASCULAR AND INTERSTITIAL COMPARTMENTS (EDEMA)

Changes in distribution of fluid between the plasma and interstitium are most commonly manifested as edema, which is an accumulation of excess interstitial fluid. Edema occurs by four major mechanisms: (1) increased microvascular permeability, (2) increased intravascular hydrostatic pressure, (3) decreased intravascular osmotic pressure, and (4) decreased lymphatic drainage (Box 2-2).

MECHANISMS OF EDEMA FORMATION

Increased Microvascular Permeability

Increased microvascular permeability is most commonly associated with the initial microvascular reaction to inflammatory or immunologic stimuli. These stimuli induce localized release of mediators that cause vasodilation and increased microvascular permeability. Immediate increases in permeability are induced by mediators such as histamine, bradykinin, leukotrienes, and substance P, which cause endothelial cell contraction and widening of interendothelial gaps. Subsequent release of cytokines such as interleukin-1 (IL-1), tumor necrosis factor (TNF), and γ-interferon induces cytoskeletal rearrangements within endothelial cells that result in endothelial cell retraction and more persistent widening of interendothelial gaps. Movement of intravascular fluid through these gaps into the interstitium results in localized edema that can dilute an inflammatory agent. The reaction terminates as localized edema and regresses when the stimulus is mild. However, most cases progress to the leakage of plasma proteins and emigration of leukocytes as early events in the formation of an acute inflammatory exudate.

Increased Intravascular Hydrostatic Pressure

Increased intravascular hydrostatic pressure is most often due to increased blood volume in the microvasculature. This can be the result of an active increased flow of blood into the microvasculature (hyperemia), such as occurs with acute inflammation. But more commonly, it results from passive accumulation of blood (congestion), often caused by heart failure or localized venous compression or obstruction. Increased microvascular volume and pressure cause increased filtration and reduced or even reversed fluid absorption back into the vessel. When increased hydrostatic pressure affects a localized portion of microvasculature, the edema is localized. In the

BOX 2-2 Causes of Edema

INCREASED VASCULAR PERMEABILITY

Vascular leakage associated with inflammation
- Infectious agents
  - Viruses (e.g., influenza and other respiratory viruses, canine adenovirus 1, equine and porcine Arterivirus, Morbillivirus)
  - Bacteria (e.g., *Clostridium* sp., Shiga-like toxin–producing *Escherichia coli, Erysipelothrix rhusiopathiae*)
  - Rickettsia (e.g., *Cowdria ruminantium, Ehrlichia risticii, Ehrlichia equi, Rickettsia rickettsii*)
- Immune-mediated
  - Type III hypersensitivity (e.g., feline infectious peritonitis, purpura hemorrhagica)

Neovascularization

Anaphylaxis (e.g., type I hypersensitivity to vaccines, venoms, and other allergens)

Toxins (e.g., endotoxin, paraquat, noxious gases, zootoxins)

Clotting abnormalities (e.g., pulmonary embolism, disseminated intravascular coagulation)

Metabolic abnormalities (e.g., microangiopathy caused by diabetes mellitus, encephalomalacia caused by thiamine deficiency)

INCREASED INTRAVASCULAR HYDROSTATIC PRESSURE

Portal hypertension (e.g., right-side heart failure, hepatic fibrosis)

Pulmonary hypertension (e.g., left-side heart failure, high altitude disease)

Localized venous obstruction (e.g., gastric dilation and volvulus, intestinal volvulus and torsion, uterine torsion or prolapse, venous thrombosis)

Fluid overload (e.g., iatrogenic, sodium retention with renal disease)

Hyperemia (e.g., inflammation, physiologic)

DECREASED INTRAVASCULAR OSMOTIC PRESSURE

Decreased albumin production (e.g., malnutrition/starvation, debilitating diseases, severe hepatic disease)

Excessive albumin loss (e.g., gastrointestinal disease [protein-losing enteropathies] or parasitism [haemonchosis or trichostrongylosis in sheep], renal disease [protein-losing nephropathies], severe burns)

Water intoxication (e.g., hemodilution caused by sodium retention, salt toxicity)

DECREASED LYMPHATIC DRAINAGE

Lymphatic obstruction or compression (e.g., inflammatory or neoplastic masses, fibrosis)

Congenital lymphatic aplasia or hypoplasia

Intestinal lymphangiectasia

Lymphangitis (e.g., paratuberculosis, sporotrichosis, epizootic lymphangitis of horses)

case of heart failure, congestion and increased hydrostatic pressure can occur in the portal venous system (right heart failure) causing ascites; in the pulmonary venous system (left heart failure) causing pulmonary edema; or in both venous systems (generalized heart failure) causing generalized edema. Generalized edema can result in a reduction of circulating plasma volume and renal hypoperfusion, which activate a variety of volume-regulating compensatory responses. Plasma volume is increased through sodium retention induced by activation of the renin-angiotensin-aldosterone pathways, and water retention mediated by antidiuretic hormone (ADH) release following activation of intravascular volume and pressure receptors. The resulting intravascular volume overload further complicates the dynamics of fluid distribution that accompany heart failure.

Decreased Intravascular Osmotic Pressure

Decreased intravascular osmotic pressure most commonly results from decreased concentrations of plasma proteins, particularly albumin. Hypoalbuminemia reduces the intravascular colloidal osmotic pressure, resulting in increased fluid filtration and decreased absorption and culminating in edema. Hypoalbuminemia is caused by either decreased production of albumin by the liver or excessive loss from the plasma. Decreased hepatic production most commonly occurs because of a lack of adequate protein for the synthetic pathway as a result of malnutrition or intestinal malabsorption of protein. Less often, severe liver disease with decreased hepatocyte mass or impaired hepatocyte function can result in inadequate albumin production. Loss of albumin from the plasma can occur in gastrointestinal diseases characterized by severe blood loss, such as that caused by parasitism. Renal disease, in which glomerular and/or tubular function is impaired, can result in loss of albumin into the urine and dilution of remaining albumin caused by sodium retention and expanded intravascular fluid volume (e.g., nephrotic syndrome). Plasma exudation accompanying severe burns is a less frequent cause of albumin loss. Because of the systemic nature of hypoalbuminemia, edema caused by decreased intravascular osmotic pressure tends to be generalized.

Decreased Lymphatic Drainage

Decreased lymphatic drainage reduces the ability of the lymphatic system to remove the slight excess of fluid that normally accumulates in the interstitium during fluid exchange between the plasma and interstitium. This can occur because of lymph vessel compression by a neoplastic or inflammatory swelling, lymph vessel constriction caused by fibrosis, or internal blockage of a lymph vessel by a thrombus. Edema occurs once the capacity of the damaged lymphatics is exceeded and is localized to the area served by the affected lymphatic vessels.

MORPHOLOGIC CHARACTERISTICS OF EDEMA

Edema is morphologically characterized by clear to slightly yellow fluid that generally contains a small amount of protein (transudate), which thickens and expands affected interstitium (Fig. 2-7). When edema occurs in tissues adjacent to body cavities or open spaces, such as alveolar lumens, the increased interstitial pressure often forces fluid into these cavities and spaces. The result can be fluid within alveolar lumens (pulmonary edema; Fig. 2-8), the thoracic cavity (hydrothorax), the pericardial sac (hydropericardium), or the abdominal cavity (ascites or hydroperitoneum; Fig. 2-9). Histologically, edema is an amorphous, pale eosinophilic fluid (hematoxylin and eosin [H&E] stain) because of its protein content (Fig. 2-10). The clinical significance of edema is variable, depending mainly on its location. Subcutaneous edema results in doughy to fluctuant

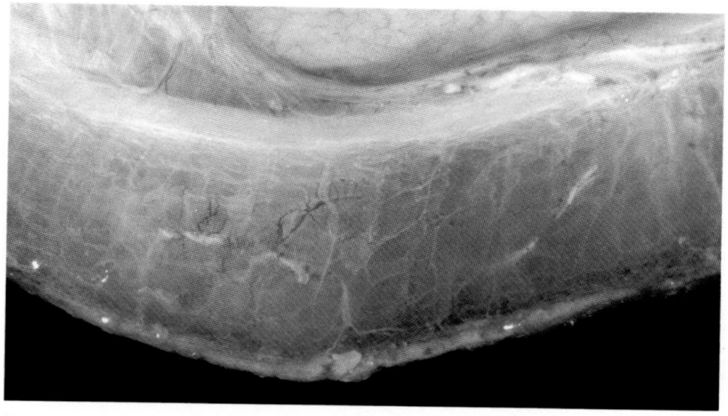

Fig. 2-7 Edema, intestine, submucosa, horse.
Note the clear to slightly yellow fluid (that generally contains a small amount of protein [transudate]), which thickens and expands the affected submucosa. (Courtesy Department of Veterinary Biosciences, The Ohio State University; and Noah's Arkive, College of Veterinary Medicine, The University of Georgia.)

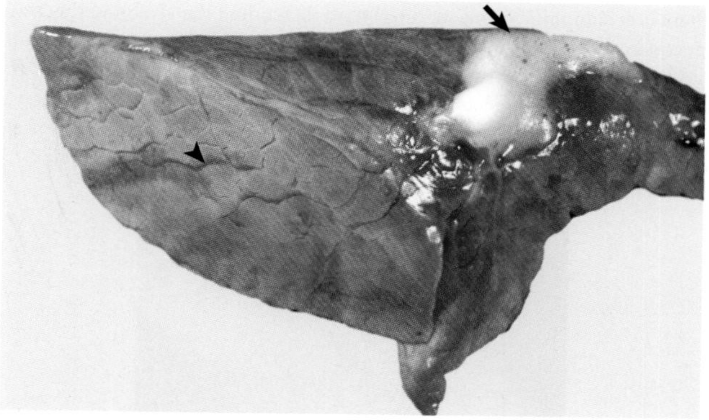

Fig. 2-8 Pulmonary edema, lung, pig.
The lung failed to collapse and is heavy and firm due to edema fluid in alveoli and the interstitium. Note the prominent interlobular septa caused by edema *(arrowhead)* and the frothy edema fluid exuding from the bronchus *(arrow)*. (Courtesy Dr. M.D. McGavin, College of Veterinary Medicine, University of Tennessee.)

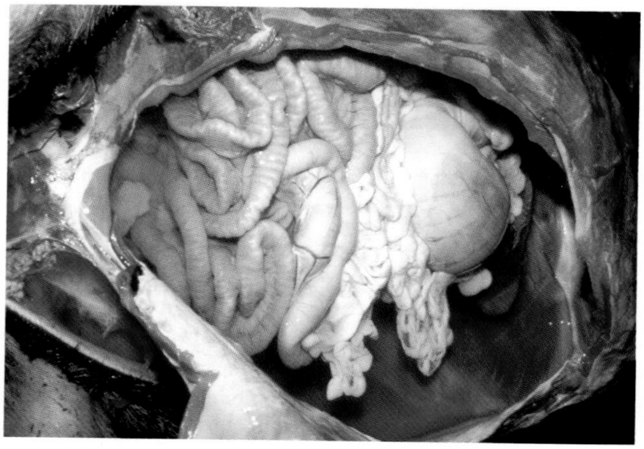

Fig. 2-9 Ascites (hydroperitoneum), peritoneal cavity, dog.
Slightly yellow fluid is present in the peritoneal cavity. When edema occurs in tissue adjacent to body cavities, the increased interstitial pressure forces the edema fluid, which is usually clear to slightly yellow (transudate), into these cavities. (Courtesy Dr. D.A. Mosier, College of Veterinary Medicine, Kansas State University.)

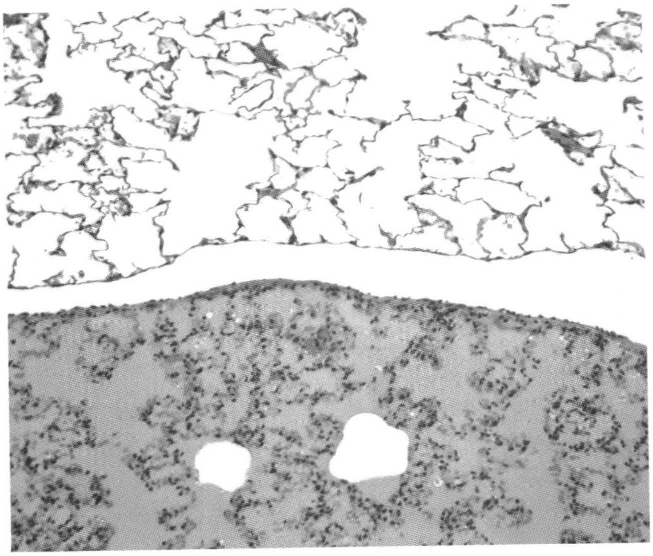

Fig. 2-10 Pulmonary edema, lung, rat.
There is eosinophilic (pink staining) fluid distending the alveoli in the lower specimen. Histologically, edema is an amorphous, pale eosinophilic fluid, and the depth of the eosinophilia is proportional to its protein content. The fluid in this specimen has a high protein content. The upper specimen is normal rat lung. H&E stain. (Courtesy Dr. A. López, Atlantic Veterinary College; and Noah's Arkive, College of Veterinary Medicine, The University of Georgia.)

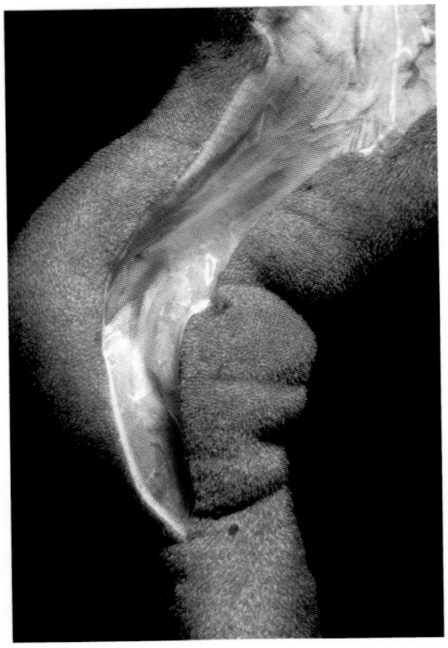

Fig. 2-11 Subcutaneous edema, congenital lymphedema, skin, dog.
This form of edema results in doughy to fluctuant skin and subcutis. Edematous skin is often cooler than adjacent unaffected skin. In congenital lymphedema, the lymph vessels are hypoplastic or aplastic. (Courtesy Dr. H. Liepold, College of Veterinary Medicine, Kansas State University.)

skin and subcutis that is often cooler than adjacent unaffected tissue, but alone has minimal clinical impact (Fig. 2-11). Likewise, ascites does not generally have an impact on the function of abdominal organs. In contrast, edema of a tissue within a confined space, such as the brain in the cranial vault, can result in pressure within the organ that results in serious organ dysfunction. Similarly, filling a confined space with fluid, such as in hydrothorax or hydropericardium, can have a substantial impact on the function of the lungs and heart, respectively. In these situations, edema can have immediate and life-threatening implications.

HEMOSTASIS

Hemostasis is the arrest of bleeding. It is a physiologic response to vascular damage and provides a mechanism to seal an injured vessel to prevent blood loss (*hemo* = blood, *stasis* = halt, slow). Hemostasis is a finely regulated process that predominantly involves interactions between endothelium, platelets, and coagulation factors. It normally occurs only at the site of vascular injury, without affecting fluidity and flow of blood in normal undamaged vasculature. Disruption of the delicate balance of hemostasis can result in the pathologic states of blood loss (hemorrhage) or inappropriate thrombus formation (thrombosis).

Normal endothelium provides a surface that promotes the smooth, nonturbulent flow of blood. It produces and responds to mediators that enhance vasodilation, and inhibit platelet activation and coagulation. In contrast, after injury or activation, endothelium produces or responds to mediators that induce vasoconstriction, enhance platelet adhesion and aggregation, and stimulate coagulation (Box 2-3).

Platelets are anucleate cell fragments derived from megakaryocytes. Their major role in hemostasis is to form the initial plug that covers and seals a small area of vascular damage. After vascular damage, platelets adhere to subendothelial collagen and other ECM components (e.g., fibronectin, adhesive glycoproteins, and proteoglycans). Adhered platelets express receptors that promote aggregation of additional platelets and become activated to release the products of their cytoplasmic granules and produce other mediators of coagulation (e.g., thromboxane; Box 2-4). The phospholipid surfaces of aggregated platelet membranes also provide a surface to concentrate activated coagulation factors to promote coagulation.

Coagulation factors are plasma proteins produced mainly by the liver. Their purpose in hemostasis is to form fibrin. Coagulation factors are divided into (1) a structurally related and functionally interdependent contact group (prekallikrein, high molecular weight kininogen [HMWK], and factors XII and XI); (2) a vitamin K–dependent group (factors II, VII, IX, and X); and (3) a highly labile fibrinogen group (factors I, V, VIII, and XIII). Circulating coagulation factors are activated in a cascade fashion by hydrolysis of arginine- or lysine-containing peptides to convert them to enzymatically active serine proteases (except for factor XIII, which has cysteine-rich active sites). The contact group factors are activated by contact with collagen or subendothelial components to initiate coagulation by the intrinsic pathway. The extrinsic pathway of coagulation is activated by release of tissue factor (TF, factor III) from damaged cells. The vitamin K–dependent coagulation factors play an important role in localizing coagulation by γ-carboxylating glutamic acid residues of N-terminal ends of precursor factors, so they can bind calcium to form calcium bridges with platelet phospholipids.

HEMOSTATIC PROCESS

The sequence of events that contribute to hemostasis are (1) transient vasoconstriction and platelet aggregation to form a platelet plug at the site of damage (primary hemostasis), (2) coagulation to form a meshwork of fibrin (secondary hemostasis), (3) fibrinolysis to remove the platelet/fibrin plug (thrombus retraction), and (4) tissue repair at the damaged site (Fig. 2-12).

Primary Hemostasis

Primary hemostasis includes the initial vascular and platelet response to injury. Neurogenic stimuli and mediators released

BOX 2-3 Endothelial Mediators of Hemostasis

ANTICOAGULANT

Prostacyclin (PGI_2)
Maintains vascular relaxation and inhibits platelet adhesion and activation.

Nitric Oxide (NO)
Maintains vascular relaxation and inhibits platelet aggregation. Acts synergistically with the protein C pathway and antithrombin III (ATIII) to suppress thrombin production.

Thrombomodulin
Membrane protein that binds thrombin to initiate activation of protein C.

Protein S
Cofactor in protein C pathway; independently inhibits activation of factors VIII and X.

Heparin-Like Molecules
Heparan sulfate proteoglycans bind and concentrate ATIII on the endothelial surface.

Tissue Plasminogen Activator (tPA)
Activates fibrinolysis by stimulating plasminogen conversion to plasmin.

Adenosine Diphosphatase (ADP)
Degradation of ADP to inhibit its procoagulant effects.

Annexin V
Binds negatively charged phospholipids and calcium to displace phospholipid-dependent coagulation factors on the endothelial surface to inhibit formation of thrombin and factor Xa.

Tissue Factor Pathway Inhibitor-1 (TFPI-1)
A cell-surface protein that directly inhibits the factor TF:VIIa complex and factor Xa.

PROCOAGULANT

Tissue Factor
Produced after endothelial activation by substances such as cytokines, endotoxin, thrombin, immune complexes, and mitogens.

von Willebrand's Factor
Released after endothelial exposure to substances such as thrombin, histamine, and fibrin.

Plasminogen Activator Inhibitor-1 (PAI-1)
Reduces fibrinolysis by inhibiting tPA and urokinase-like plasminogen activator (uPA).

VASCULAR REPAIR

Platelet-Derived Growth Factor (PDGF)
Stimulates mitogenesis of smooth muscle and fibroblasts.

Fibroblast Growth Factor (FGF)
Stimulates fibroblast proliferation.

Transforming Growth Factor-β (TGF-β)
Modulates vascular repair by inhibition of proliferation of various cell types, including endothelium.

locally by endothelium and platelets cause vasoconstriction immediately after damage (Fig. 2-12, *A*). The nature and effectiveness of vasoconstriction is partially determined by the size of the affected vessel, the amount of smooth muscle it contains, and endothelial integrity. Narrowing of the vessel lumen allows opposing endothelial surfaces to come into contact with and sometimes adhere to each other to reduce the volume of blood flowing through the damaged area. Platelets can directly adhere to the exposed subendothelial matrix of collagen, fibronectin, and other glycoproteins and proteoglycans (Fig. 2-12, *B*). However, more efficient adhesion occurs when von Willebrand's factor released by local activated endothelium coats subendothelial collagen to form a specific bridge between collagen and the glycoprotein platelet receptor GPIb. At this stage and without further stimulation, adhered and aggregated platelets may disaggregate. Otherwise, platelets within the aggregate secrete the contents of their dense bodies and α-granules and produce substances such as thromboxane to accelerate hemostasis. Adenosine diphosphate (ADP) released from dense granules triggers the binding of fibrinogen to platelet receptor GPIIb-IIIa, resulting in the formation of fibrinogen bridges that link platelets into a loose aggregate. Platelet contraction consolidates this loose aggregate into a dense plug, which covers the damaged area. When vascular injury is minimal, platelet plugs alone may resolve the damage. If not, the exposed collagen and aggregated platelet phospholipids promote secondary hemostasis at the site.

Secondary Hemostasis

In most cases of vascular damage, the formation of fibrin is important for the prevention of blood loss. Fibrin is the end-product of a series of enzymatic reactions involving coagulation factors, nonenzymatic cofactors, calcium, and phospholipid membranes derived mainly from platelets (Fig. 2-12, *C*). Three coagulation pathways have been classically used to describe the coagulation process and formation of fibrin in vitro. These pathways provide a useful starting point for understanding coagulation (Figs. 2-13 and 2-14). However, integrated models of coagulation more adequately emphasize the interrelatedness of these pathways, the multiple positive and negative control loops within the system, and amplification of the process on affected cell surfaces.

Intrinsic Pathway

Intrinsic coagulation is a complex and highly interrelated process that is initiated by the contact group of coagulation factors (see Figs. 2-13 and 2-14). Prekallikrein and factor XI normally circulate bound to HMWK, which acts as a catalytic factor for their activation. After vascular injury, circulating prekallikrein-HMWK and factor XII form a complex on negatively charged endothelial or subendothelial surfaces, which results in activation of factor XII (factor XIIa). Factor XIIa initiates a series of reactions that affect coagulation, as well as kinin formation, complement activation, and fibrinolysis. Factor XIIa activates factor XI (XIa), interacts

BOX 2-4 Platelet Mediators in Hemostasis

PROCOAGULANT

Thromboxane A_2 (TXA_2)
Induces vasoconstriction and enhances platelet aggregation.

Phospholipids (i.e., phosphatidyl serine)
Provides sites for coagulation reactions.

Adenosine Diphosphate (ADP)
Mediates platelet aggregation and activation.

Calcium
Cofactor in many coagulation reactions and promotes platelet aggregation.

Platelet Factor 4
Promotes platelet aggregation and inhibits heparin action.

Thrombospondin
Promotes platelet aggregation and inhibits heparin action.

Fibrinogen
Fibrin precursor, concentrated by binding to platelet receptor GpIIb-IIIa.

Factors V, XI, and XIII
Factors involved in coagulation reactions.

von Willebrand's Factor
Promotes platelet adhesion to subendothelial collagen via platelet receptor GpIb.

α_2-Antiplasmin and α_2-Macroglobulin
Inhibition of plasmin.

Plasminogen Activator Inhibitor-1 (PAI-1)
Inhibits tissue plasminogen activator (tPA) and activated protein C to promote clot stabilization.

Serotonin
Promotes vasoconstriction.

ANTICOAGULANT

Adenosine Triphosphate (ATP)
Inhibits platelet aggregation.

Protease Nexin II
Inhibits factor XIa.

Tissue Factor Pathway Inhibitor (TFPI)
Inhibits TF:factor VIIa of the extrinsic pathway.

Protein S
Cofactor in the protein C pathway for inhibition of factors Va and VIIIa.

VASCULAR REPAIR

Platelet-derived Growth Factor (PDGF)
Stimulates mitogenesis of smooth muscle and fibroblasts for vessel repair.

β-Thromboglobulin
Promotes fibroblast chemotaxis for vessel repair.

Vascular Endothelial Growth Factor (VEGF)
Stimulates endothelial cell proliferation.

Transforming Growth Factor-β (TGF-β)
Modulates vascular repair by inhibition of proliferation of various cell types, including endothelium.

Epidermal Growth Factor (EGF)
Promotes fibroblast proliferation.

with prekallikrein to form kallikrein, and interacts with HMWK to form kinins. Cleavage of factor XIIa by kallikrein, plasmin, and other proteolytic enzymes forms fragments (factor XIIf), which have activity that is similar to but much weaker than factor XIIa. Both kallikrein and factor XIa in the presence of Ca^{2+} can activate factor IX (factor IXa). Factor IXa then binds to platelet phospholipids in a complex with Ca^{2+} and factor VIII. After modification of factor VIII by thrombin into factor VIIIa, the complex of factor VIIIa-factor IXa/Ca^{2+}-phospholipid (tenase) activates factor X to initiate the common coagulation pathway.

Extrinsic Pathway

Release of factor III (TF) from cells underlying damaged endothelium, or from activated endothelium, initiates the extrinsic pathway (see Figs. 2-13 and 2-14). TF is a high molecular weight phospholipid-containing glycoprotein found in the plasma membrane of many cells, including activated, but not resting, endothelium. Endothelial cell production of TF is stimulated by substances such as endotoxin, TNF, IL-1, transforming growth factor-β (TGF-β), and thrombin. When circulating factor VII comes into contact with TF, it forms a Ca^{2+}-dependent TF:VII complex on the TF-expressing surface. Although this complex may have some enzymatic activity, activation of factor VII by substances such as factors XIIa, XIIf, IXa, Xa, IIa, and kallikrein results in the much more active TF:VIIa complex. This complex along with Ca^{2+} activates factor X to initiate the common pathway.

Common Pathway

The intrinsic and extrinsic pathways merge with the activation of factor X (see Figs. 2-13 and 2-14). Factor Xa is bound to endothelial or platelet membrane phospholipids where it can directly convert factor II into factor IIa (thrombin). However, when factor Xa is combined with factor Va and Ca^{2+} (prothrombinase complex), this reaction occurs much more rapidly. Thrombin is a multifunctional mediator whose major function is to cleave fibrinopeptides A and B from factor I (fibrinogen) to form fibrin monomers (Fig. 2-15). Removal of these fibrinopeptides reduces intermolecular repulsive forces so that fibrin monomers spontaneously form weak H^+ bonds and self-polymerize into soluble fibrin polymers. Factor XIIIa, formed by the action of factors Xa and IIa on factor XIII in the presence of Ca^{2+}, catalyzes the formation of covalent bonds that cross-link adjacent fibrin molecules to make the polymer insoluble. Cross-linking of the fibrin network, along with concurrent platelet contraction and the presence of abundant calcium, thrombin,

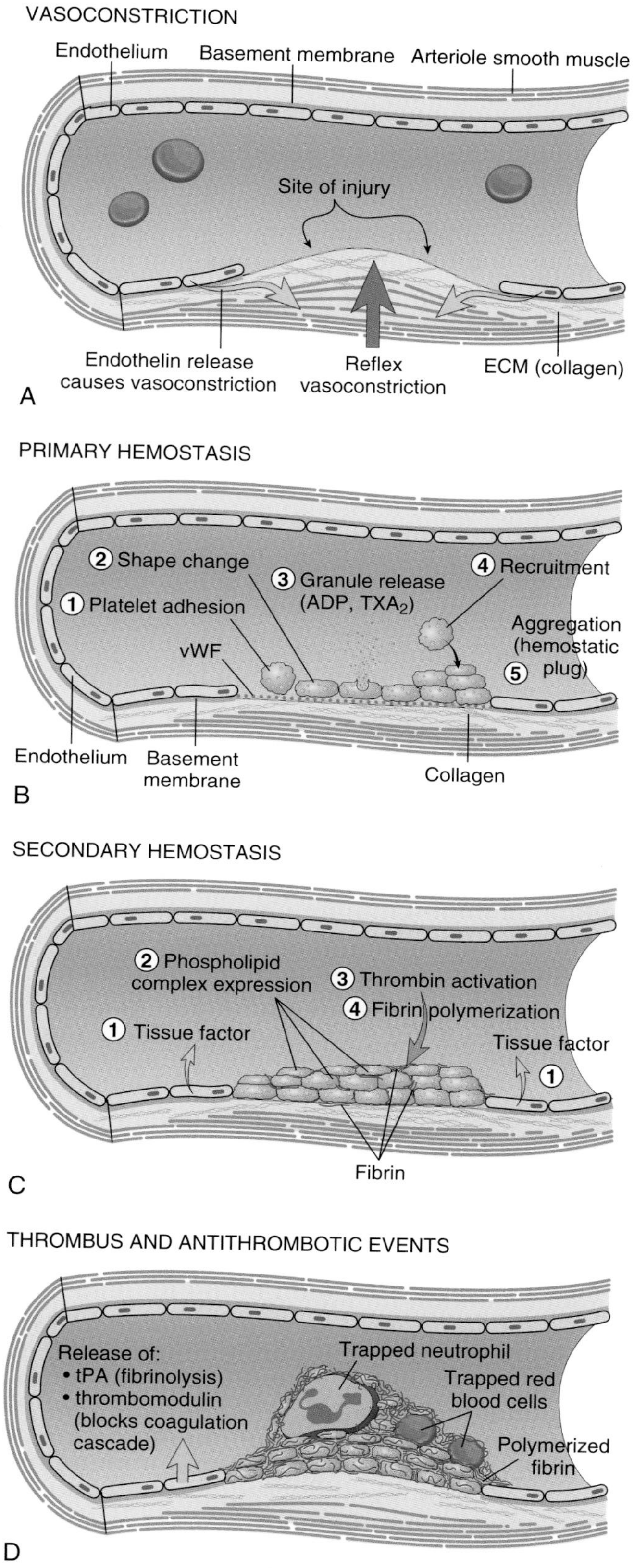

Fig. 2-12 **Diagrammatic representation of the normal hemostatic process.** **A,** After vascular injury, local neurohumoral factors induce a transient vasoconstriction. **B,** After endothelial injury and disruption that exposes the subendothelial extracellular matrix (ECM), platelets adhere to the ECM via von Willebrand's factor (vWF) and are activated, undergoing a shape change and granule release; released adenosine diphosphate (ADP) and thromboxane A_2 (TXA_2) lead to further platelet aggregation to form the primary hemostatic plug. **C,** Local activation of the coagulation cascade (involving tissue factor and platelet phospholipids) results in fibrin polymerization, "cementing" the platelets into a definitive secondary hemostatic plug. **D,** Counter-regulatory mechanisms, such as release of tissue plasminogen activator (tPA) (fibrinolytic) and thrombomodulin (interfering with the coagulation cascade), limit the hemostatic process to the site of injury. (From Kumar V, Abbas AK, Fausto N: *Robbins & Cotran pathologic basis of disease,* ed 8, Philadelphia, 2009, Saunders.)

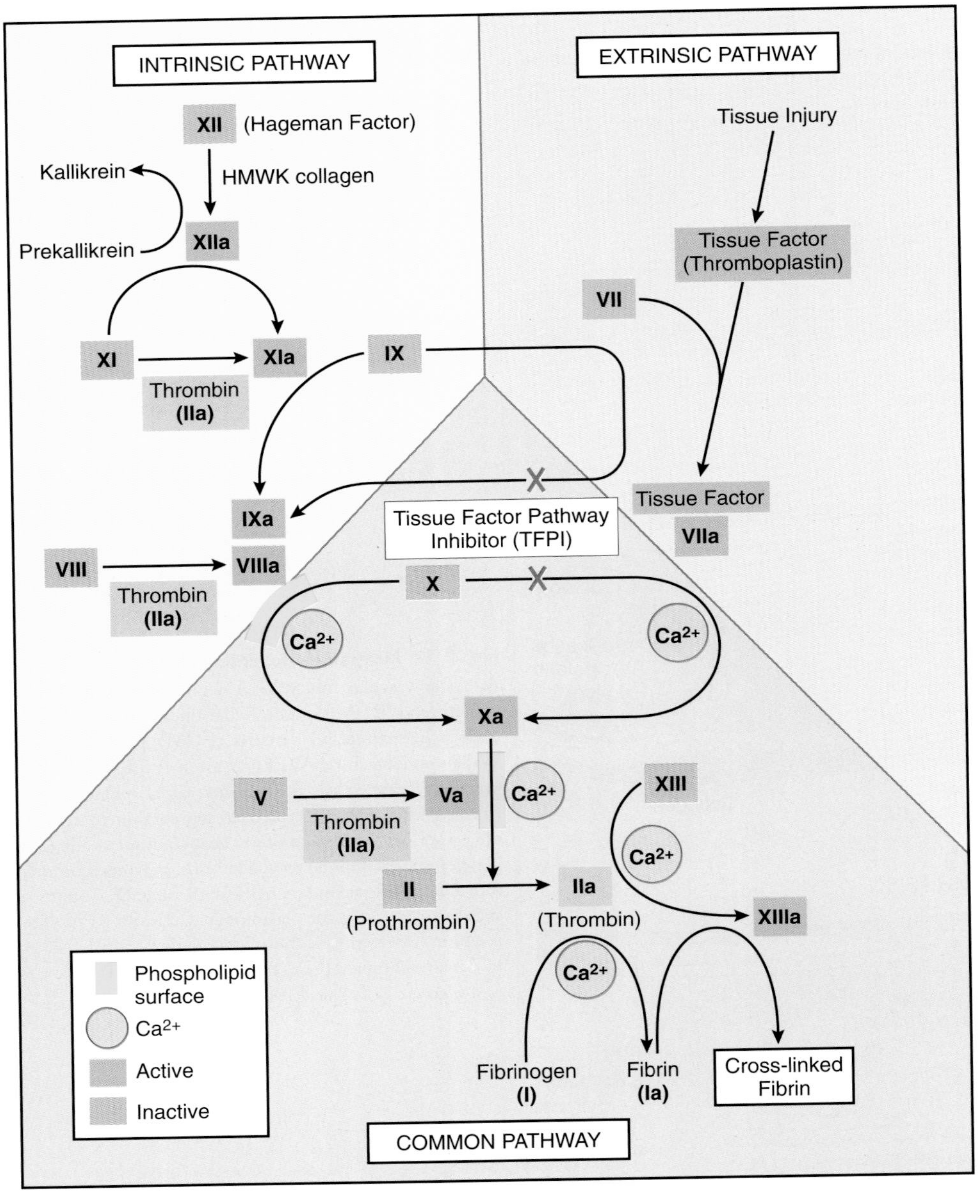

Fig. 2-13 The coagulation cascade.
Note the common link between the intrinsic and extrinsic pathways at the level of factor IX activation. Factors in red boxes represent inactive molecules; activated factors are indicated with a lower case "a" and a green box. *HMWK,* High molecular weight kininogen. Not shown are the anticoagulant inhibitory pathways. (From Kumar V, Abbas AK, Fausto N: *Robbins & Cotran pathologic basis of disease*, ed 8, Philadelphia, 2009, Saunders.)

and adenosine triphosphate (ATP), causes retraction of the fibrin-platelet thrombus. Retraction reduces the size of the thrombus to allow blood flow to continue and to pull damaged vessel edges closer together for efficient healing.

Integrated Model of Coagulation

In vivo coagulation is more like an integrated web rather than a series of independent cascades. The major stimulus for coagulation in vivo is exposure of plasma to TF and subsequent extrinsic coagulation. Two important events occur after the formation of the TF/factor VIIa complex on damaged, TF-expressing surfaces. Factor X is activated as described for the common pathway, and factor IX is activated to allow a bypass of the contact phase of classical intrinsic coagulation. Factor Xa remains localized on the damaged cell surface to initiate the formation of a small amount of thrombin. Although the amount of thrombin generated is insufficient to convert significant amounts of fibrinogen into fibrin, it does activate platelets and factors V, VIII, XI, and XIII on TF-expressing surfaces. Factor IXa can bind to the surface of activated platelets in the area to initiate the formation of tenase complexes, which activates additional factor X of the common pathway. Thrombin-activated or intrinsically activated factor XIa can also participate by activating additional factor XI on platelet surfaces. The thrombin-initiated activation of these different factors provides an amplification of the critical reactions necessary to generate large amounts of thrombin for the subsequent conversion of fibrinogen into fibrin. Other, probably less important links between the pathways also exist. For example, intrinsic factors XIIa, XIIf, and IXa and kallikrein can activate extrinsic factor VII to provide additional amplification of this pathway.

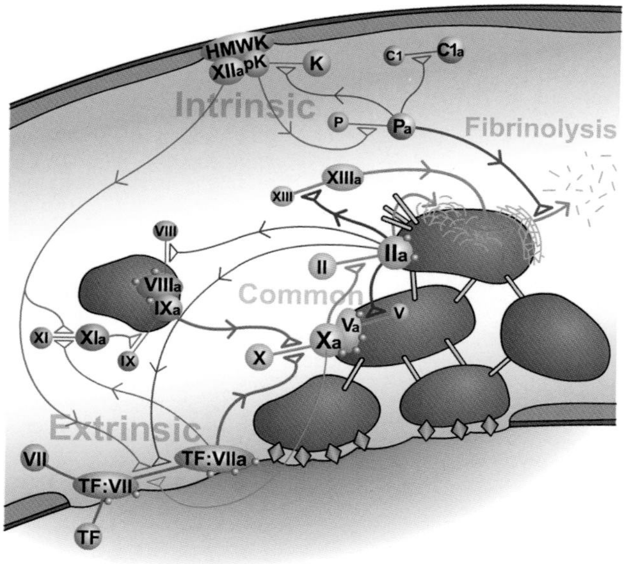

Fig. 2-14 Coagulation, fibrinolysis, and other pathways are highly integrated to balance the host response to injury.
Intrinsic coagulation is initiated by binding of high molecular weight kininogen *(HMWK)*, factor XII, and prekallikrein *(pK)* to altered endothelial surfaces. Activated products of this reaction (factor XIIa and kallikrein *[K]*) directly or indirectly result in the formation of factor XIa (intrinsic coagulation pathway), factor VIIa (extrinsic coagulation pathway), plasmin *(Pa)* (fibrinolysis), and complement fragments C3a, C3b, C5a (complement cascade). Extrinsic coagulation is initiated by release of tissue factor *(TF)* from areas of damaged endothelium, with subsequent binding of TF to factor VII. The TF:VII complex can be activated by a wide variety of agents. Activation of factor X initiates the common cascade to ultimately result in cleavage of fibrinogen into fibrin. In addition to its role in the common pathway, factor IIa (thrombin) also influences both the intrinsic (factors XI and VIII) and extrinsic *(TF:VII)* coagulation pathways. Additional interactions between these factors, which are not shown in the figure, are described in the text. Specific effects of kallikrein include cleavage and activation of factors XII, IX, and VII, plasminogen, HMWK, and complement fragment C5. (Courtesy Dr. D.A. Mosier and L. Schooley, College of Veterinary Medicine, Kansas State University.)

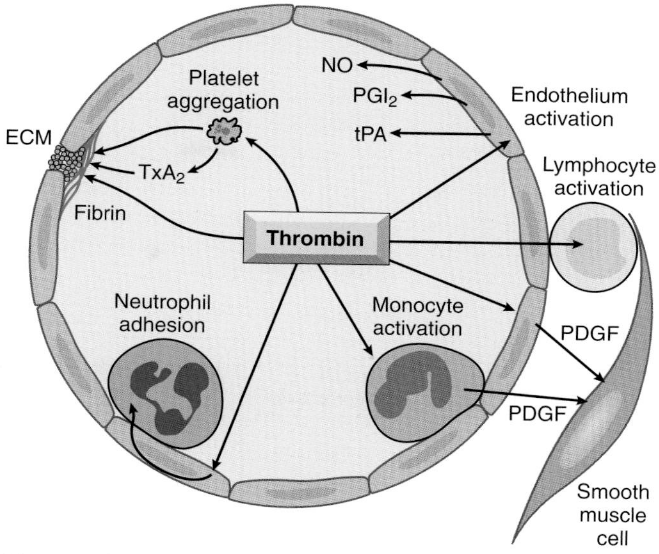

Fig. 2-15 The central roles of thrombin in hemostasis and cellular activation.
In addition to a critical function in generating cross-linked fibrin (via cleavage of fibrinogen to fibrin and activation of factor XIII), thrombin also directly induces platelet aggregation and secretion (e.g., TXA_2). Thrombin also activates endothelium to generate leukocyte adhesion molecules and a variety of fibrinolytic (tPA), vasoactive (NO, PGI_2), or cytokine (PDGF) mediators. Likewise, mononuclear inflammatory cells may be activated by the direct actions of thrombin. *ECM,* Extracellular matrix; *NO,* nitric oxide; *PDGF,* platelet-derived growth factor; *PGI_2,* prostacyclin; *TXA_2,* thromboxane A_2; *tPA,* tissue plasminogen activator. (From Kumar V, Abbas AK, Fausto N: *Robbins & Cotran pathologic basis of disease,* ed 8, Philadelphia, 2009, Saunders.)

The interrelatedness of coagulation pathways also extends to anticoagulant reactions. When excessive levels of thrombin are generated, thrombin destroys rather than activates factors V and VIII. When thrombin binds to thrombomodulin on endothelial surfaces, it activates protein C, a potent anticoagulant (see section on Coagulation Inhibitors). Intrinsic pathway factors XIIa, XIIf, and XIa and kallikrein not only participate in fibrin formation but also initiate fibrinolysis by cleaving plasminogen into plasmin (see section on Thrombus Dissolution).

THROMBUS DISSOLUTION

The purpose of a fibrin-platelet thrombus is to form a temporary patch that is dissolved after healing of the vessel (thrombolysis). The rate of dissolution must be balanced so that it does not occur so quickly that bleeding returns but is not prolonged so that vessel occlusion may occur (Fig. 2-16). Fibrin dissolution (fibrinolysis) is initiated immediately on vessel injury by the cleavage of the plasma protein plasminogen into plasmin (Fig. 2-17). Plasminogen is activated by a wide variety of proteases, including activated contact group coagulation factors, plasminogen activators present within endothelium and other tissues (tissue plasminogen activator [tPA]), and activators present in secretions and fluids. Plasminogen adsorbs to fibrin within a thrombus, so that on activation the plasmin is localized to the site of the thrombus. The presence of fibrin increases the efficiency of tPA-dependent plasmin generation by nearly twofold. Additionally, by binding to fibrin, plasmin is protected from its major inhibitor (α_2-antiplasmin). The bound plasmin restricts thrombus size by degrading both cross-linked (insoluble) fibrin within the thrombus and fibrinogen, so that additional fibrin formation is inhibited. Dissolution of insoluble, but not soluble, fibrin by plasmin results in the formation of fibrin degradation products (FDPs). FDPs are various-sized fragments of fibrin and fibrinogen that can impair hemostasis. Collectively, FDPs inhibit thrombin, interfere with fibrin polymerization, and can coat platelet membranes to inhibit platelet aggregation.

REGULATION OF HEMOSTASIS

The potent biologic effects of hemostatic products must be finely regulated to achieve appropriate hemostasis, without creating detrimental effects associated with too little or too much activity. Coagulation factors are continuously activated at a low, basal level to keep the system primed for a rapid response to an injurious stimulus. Proteins that inhibit or degrade activated hemostatic products are present in the plasma or are locally produced at the site of hemostasis (see Fig. 2-17). These products help confine hemostasis to a site of vascular damage and inhibit hemostatic reactions in normal vasculature. Regulation is also achieved by simple dilution of activated agents as blood removes them from the area, and the factors are removed from the circulation by the liver and spleen.

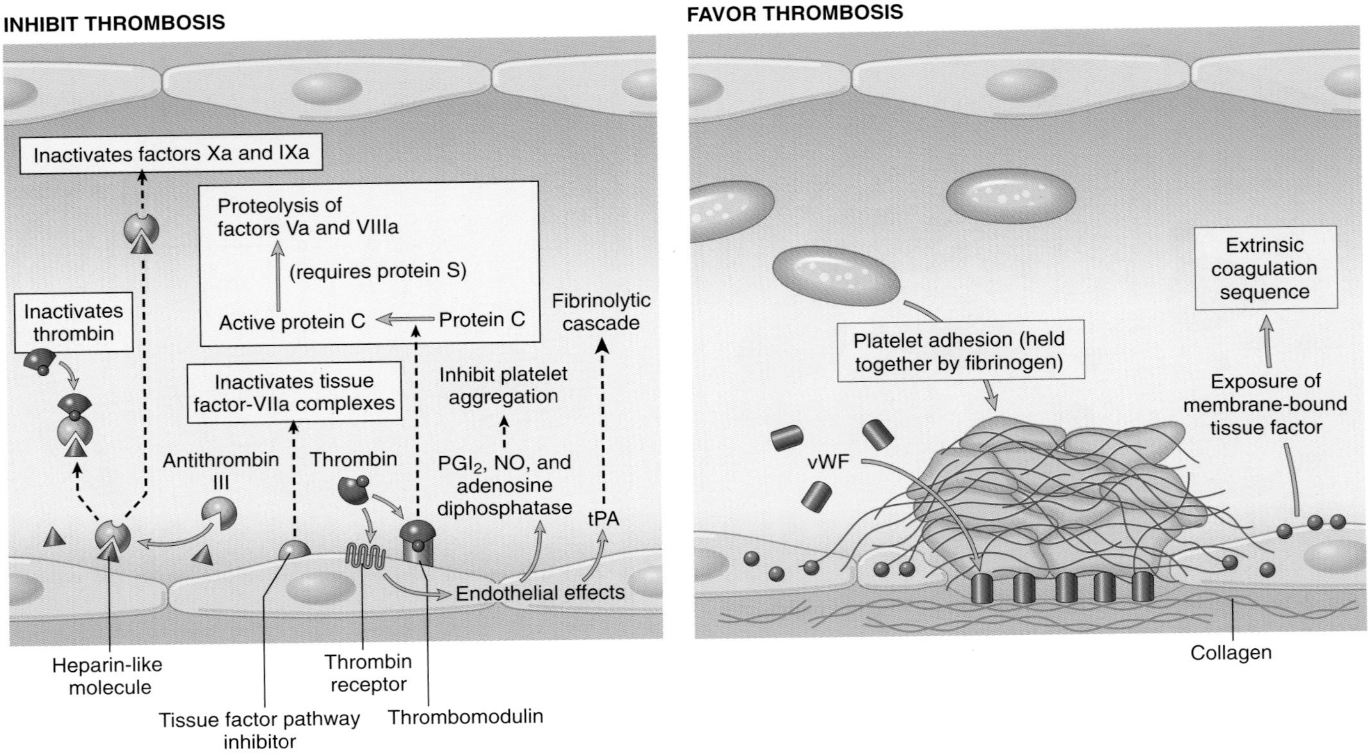

Fig. 2-16 Schematic illustration of some of the procoagulant and anticoagulant activities of endothelial cells. Not shown are the profibrinolytic and antifibrinolytic properties. *vWF,* von Willebrand's factor; *PGI_2,* prostacyclin; *NO,* nitric oxide; *tPA,* tissue plasminogen activator. Thrombin receptor is referred to as protease-activated receptor (PAR). (From Kumar V, Abbas AK, Fausto N: *Robbins & Cotran pathologic basis of disease,* ed 8, Philadelphia, 2009, Saunders.)

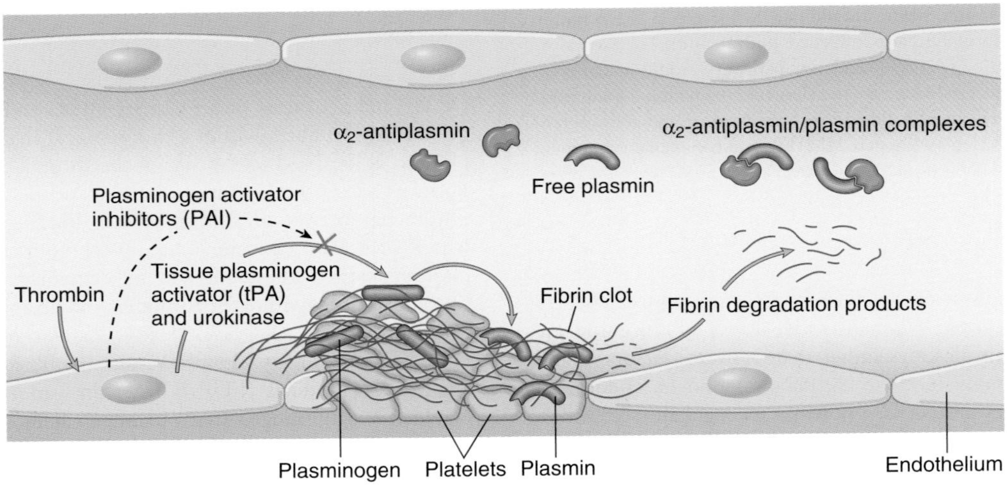

Fig. 2-17 The fibrinolytic system, illustrating the plasminogen activators and inhibitors. (From Kumar V, Abbas AK, Fausto N: *Robbins & Cotran pathologic basis of disease,* ed 8, Philadelphia, 2009, Saunders.)

Coagulation Inhibitors

The major anticoagulant-antithrombotic systems on endothelial cells are the protein C-protein S-thrombomodulin system and endothelial heparan sulfate to which antithrombin III (ATIII) and tissue factor pathway inhibitor (TFPI) are bound. ATIII is the most potent and clinically significant of the coagulation inhibitors, accounting for nearly 80% of the thrombin-inhibitory activity of plasma. ATIII is a circulating serine protease produced by endothelium and hepatocytes that will degrade all activated coagulation factors except for factor VIIa. However, its most important action is the neutralization of thrombin and factor Xa. ATIII can bind heparan sulfate present on the surface of normal endothelium and platelets to localize it to the site where it is most needed to inactivate thrombin and factor Xa. Through this binding, heparin accelerates the rate of ATIII-induced serine protease inactivation by 2000- to 10,000-fold. ATIII also inhibits fibrinolysis (by inhibiting plasmin and kallikrein), kinin formation, and complement activation. Although the major role of heparin is to bind and enhance the activity of ATIII, it also inhibits coagulation by enhancing the release of TFPI from endothelial cells and interfering with binding of platelet receptors to von Willebrand's factor.

The protein C pathway also plays a critical role in preventing thrombosis. Proteins C and S are vitamin K–dependent glycoproteins that, when complexed together on phospholipid surfaces, potently inhibit coagulation by destroying factors Va and VIIIa. An important step in this process is the activation of protein C by thrombin, a reaction that normally occurs at low levels but that increases nearly 20,000-fold after the binding of thrombin to the endothelial receptor thrombomodulin. This reaction is further enhanced by the presence of a protein C receptor on the surface of endothelial cells. Protein S, in addition to serving as a nonenzymatic cofactor with protein C, can independently inhibit factors VIIIa, Xa, and Va. Binding of thrombin to thrombomodulin also results in the loss of the procoagulant functions of thrombin. The protein C-S complex may also enhance fibrinolysis by neutralizing plasminogen activator inhibitors.

TFPI is a significant inhibitor of extrinsic coagulation, which functions synergistically with protein C and ATIII to suppress thrombin formation. TFPI is a plasma protein derived mainly from endothelium and smooth muscle cells that forms a complex with factor Xa on the endothelial-bound TF:VIIa molecule to inhibit subsequent factor X activation. TFPI can interact with VIIa without Xa but at a slow rate. Therefore TFPI does not substantially inhibit extrinsic coagulation until factor Xa levels increase, after which TFPI provides negative feedback for further generation of Xa by the TF:VIIa complex.

Fibrinolytic Inhibitors

Major inhibitors of fibrinolytic agents include plasminogen activator inhibitor-1 (PAI-1) and antiplasmins, which include α_2-antiplasmin, α_2-macroglobulin, α_1-antitrypsin, antithrombin III, and C-1 inactivator. PAI-1 inhibits tPA and urokinase, therefore inhibiting fibrinolysis and promoting fibrin stabilization. PAI-1 also inactivates activated protein C, plasmin, and thrombin. The antiplasmins function in a cooperative fashion to prevent excessive plasmin activity so that a thrombus can dissolve at a slow and appropriate rate. α_2-Antiplasmin is the first to bind and neutralize plasmin. When its binding capacity is saturated, excess plasmin is taken up by α_2-macroglobulin. α_2-Macroglobulin also binds to certain activated factors, such as thrombin, and physically entraps but does not degrade their active sites. When α_2-macroglobulin is saturated, plasmin binds to α_1-antitrypsin. α_1-Antitrypsin is a weak inhibitor of fibrinolysis, but a potent inhibitor of factor XIa. In addition to their fibrinolytic roles, α_1-antitrypsin and α_2-macroglobulin are the major plasma inhibitors of activated protein C.

HEMOSTASIS AND OTHER HOST RESPONSES

Hemostatic pathways are highly integrated, and many factors within the pathways have multiple roles. Thrombin has a major procoagulant role to cleave factor I to yield fibrin monomers. Thrombin also activates factors V, VIII, XI, and XIII and is a potent activator of platelets. In contrast, high concentrations of thrombin destroy, rather than activate, factors V and VIII. When thrombin binds to thrombomodulin on endothelial surfaces, it activates protein C, a potent anticoagulant.

An important link between intrinsic and extrinsic pathways is the TF/factor VIIa complex. This complex is the major component of extrinsic coagulation, but it can also activate factor IX to allow a bypass of the contact phase of intrinsic coagulation. In turn, intrinsic factors XIIa, XIIf, and IXa and kallikrein can activate factor VII, which greatly increases the efficiency of extrinsic coagulation. These features give the TF/factor VIIa complex a central role in efficient hemostasis. Extrinsic coagulation and the TF/factor VIIa complex are probably the most important mechanisms for in vivo hemostasis because bleeding tendencies are not usually associated with factor XII, prekallikrein, and HMWK deficiencies and some factor XI deficiencies in humans and animals. Although the intrinsic pathway does not appear to be essential for in vivo hemostasis, it does appear to play an essential role in the formation of pathologic thrombi in response to major vascular damage.

Hemostasis is closely tied to inflammation and other host responses. A prothrombotic environment is also proinflammatory. Inflammatory stimuli, such as IL-1 and TNF, activate endothelium to produce TF and to increase their expression of leukocyte adhesion molecules. Thrombin and histamine released by degranulating mast cells also stimulate the expression of the adhesin P-selectin. In early stages of inflammation, leukocytes can loosely attach and roll along endothelium or adhered platelets by interacting with endothelial or platelet P-selectin. During this interaction, the neutrophil $\alpha_M\beta_2$ integrin may localize neutrophils to fibrinogen on the surface of activated platelets to promote the conversion of fibrinogen into fibrin. An enhanced prothrombotic environment during inflammation also occurs because of decreased thrombomodulin function in response to inflammatory products such as endotoxin, IL-1, TNF, and TGF-β. Additionally, adhered or migrating neutrophils and platelets can release lysosomal proteases (e.g., elastase, collagenase, and acid hydrolases), which cleave many products on endothelial or platelet surfaces. The conversion of prekallikrein to kallikrein during the contact phase of intrinsic coagulation is another source of integration between hemostatic, fibrinolytic, and inflammatory pathways. Kallikrein is chemotactic, can directly cleave C5 to C5a and C5b, can cleave HMWK to form bradykinin, and can convert plasminogen into plasmin. Plasmin also influences other host responses by cleaving C3 to generate C3a and C3b. Mitogenic factors produced by activated endothelium and platelets (e.g., platelet-derived growth factor [PDGF], TGF-β, and vascular endothelial growth factor [VEGF]) contribute to healing of damaged tissue. Some hemostatic reactions initiate pathways that have multiple and sometimes opposite outcomes. Intrinsic pathway factors XIIa, XIIf, and XIa and kallikrein not only initiate the formation of fibrin but also initiate fibrinolysis by cleaving plasminogen into plasmin. Factor XIIa not only participates directly in intrinsic coagulation and fibrinolysis but also indirectly initiates kinin formation and complement activation by converting prekallikrein to kallikrein. Additionally, both kallikrein and plasmin can directly activate factor XII to result in autoamplification of all factor XIIa pathways. Not all stimuli that activate factor XII lead to fibrin formation. Certain stimuli (e.g., misfolded proteins such as amyloid) activate inflammatory factor XII pathways (kallikrein-kinin) without concurrent activation of coagulation (via subsequent activation of factor XI). Other hemostatic products that influence other host systems include factor Xa, thrombin, and fibrinopeptides, all of which have inflammatory and coagulation functions. These interactions indicate the fine balance within the hemostatic system and the interrelatedness of hemostasis, inflammation, and other host responses.

DISORDERS OF HEMOSTASIS: HEMORRHAGE AND THROMBOSIS

The purpose of hemostasis is to prevent blood loss after vascular damage, while at the same time maintaining blood in a fluid state so that it flows freely through a normal vasculature. Failure of hemostasis can result in the extravascular loss of blood

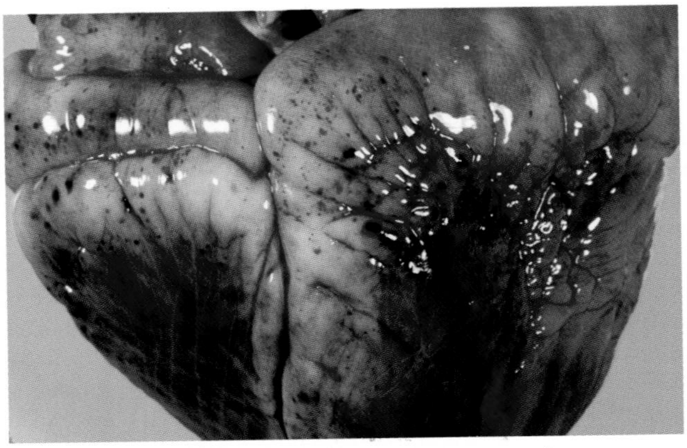

Fig. 2-18 Hemorrhage, endotoxemia, heart, cow. Note the epicardial and subepicardial hemorrhages in the fat of the coronary groove (a common site), from injury to the endothelium from endotoxin (component of the cell wall of Gram-negative bacteria). The smaller, pinpoint hemorrhages (1 to 2 mm) are petechiae. The larger, blotchy hemorrhages (3 to 5 mm) are ecchymoses. (Courtesy Dr. M.D. McGavin, College of Veterinary Medicine, University of Tennessee.)

(hemorrhage) or the inappropriate formation of intravascular clots (thrombosis).

HEMORRHAGE

Hemorrhage occurs because of abnormal function or integrity of one or more of the major factors that influence hemostasis—the endothelium and blood vessels, platelets, or coagulation factors.

Abnormalities in blood vessels can result from various inherited or acquired problems. Trauma can physically disrupt a vessel and cause hemorrhage by rhexis (*rhexis* = breaking forth, bursting). Hemorrhage by rhexis can also occur following vascular erosion by inflammatory reactions or invasive neoplasms. Certain fungi commonly invade and damage blood vessels to cause extensive local hemorrhage (e.g., internal carotid artery erosion secondary to guttural pouch mycosis in horses). More commonly, minor defects in otherwise intact blood vessels allow small numbers of erythrocytes to escape by diapedesis (*dia* = through, *pedian* = leap). Endotoxemia is a common cause of endothelial injury that results in small widespread hemorrhages (Fig. 2-18). Infectious agents, such as canine adenovirus-1, or chemicals, such as uremic toxins, can also damage endothelium. Similarly, immune complexes can become entrapped between endothelial cells and activate complement and neutrophil influx to result in damage to the endothelium and vessel wall (type III hypersensitivity reaction). Developmental collagen disorders, such as the Ehlers-Danlos syndrome, are sometimes accompanied by hemorrhage. Affected blood vessels contain abnormal collagen in their basement membranes and surrounding supportive tissue, resulting in vascular fragility and predisposition to leakage or damage. Similar hemorrhages occur due to collagen defects in guinea pigs or primates with vitamin C deficiency.

Decreased platelet numbers (thrombocytopenia) or abnormal platelet function (thrombocytopathy) can cause hemorrhage. Thrombocytopenia can result from decreased production, increased destruction, or increased use of platelets. Decreased production generally occurs following megakaryocyte damage or destruction as a result of causes such as radiation injury, estrogen toxicity, cytotoxic drugs, and viral or other infectious diseases (e.g., feline and canine parvoviruses). Increased platelet destruction is often immune-mediated. Autoimmune destruction due to antibody production against platelet membrane components, such as GPIIb and GPIIIa, can occur after immune dysregulation (e.g., systemic lupus erythematosus). Alteration of platelet membranes by drugs or infectious agents may also stimulate immune-mediated destruction or removal of platelets from the circulation. Isoimmune destruction of platelets in neonatal pigs has occurred after ingestion of colostrum-containing antiplatelet antibodies. Viral diseases (e.g., equine infectious anemia and feline immunodeficiency syndrome) and arthropod-borne agents are often associated with platelet destruction and their removal by the spleen. The most common cause of increased platelet use is diffuse endothelial damage or generalized platelet activation, which initiates disseminated intravascular coagulation (DIC). With DIC there is widespread intravascular coagulation and platelet activation, which rapidly results in consumption of platelets and coagulation factors (see section on Thrombosis). This results in progressive thrombocytopenia and hemorrhage as the syndrome escalates. Another platelet consumption disease that is not accompanied by coagulation is thrombotic thrombocytopenic purpura. In this condition, platelet aggregates form in the microvasculature, possibly the result of increased release of proagglutinating substances by normal or damaged endothelium.

Decreased platelet function is usually associated with an inability to adhere or aggregate at a site of vascular injury. Inherited problems of platelet function in humans include deficiency of GPIb on the platelet surface (Bernard-Soulier syndrome), deficient or defective GPIIb and GPIIIa on the platelet surface (Glanzmann's thrombasthenia), and deficient release of platelet granule content ("storage pool disease"). Glanzmann's thrombasthenia is a rare disease that has been reported in Otterhound and Great Pyrenees dogs. In these dogs, there is prolonged bleeding and hematoma formation from minor injury and spontaneous epistaxis because of a mutation affecting a Ca^{2+}-binding domain of the extracellular portion of GPIIb. Abnormal synthesis or release of platelet granule content has been reported in Simmental cattle, dogs (Spitz, Basset hound, and American foxhounds), cats, and fawn-hooded rats. Defective platelet storage of ADP occurs in the Chédiak-Higashi syndrome (Aleutian mink, cattle, Persian cats, and killer whales). Acquired platelet inhibition and dysfunction is most often associated with administration of nonsteroidal antiinflammatory drugs such as aspirin. Aspirin inhibits the cyclooxygenase pathway of arachidonic acid metabolism, thus decreasing thromboxane production to result in reduced platelet aggregation. Platelet function is also inhibited by uremia because of renal failure. Secondary platelet dysfunction can also occur because of deficiencies of factors necessary for normal platelet function. In von Willebrand's disease, or in autoimmune or myeloproliferative disorders in which autoantibodies against von Willebrand's factor are produced, the amount of functional von Willebrand's factor is decreased. This results in decreased platelet adhesion following vascular damage with either subclinical or severe hemorrhage.

Decreased concentrations or function of coagulation factors can also result in hemorrhage. Inherited deficiencies in coagulation factors have been recognized in many different breeds of dogs and less often other species (Box 2-5). These conditions are characterized by hemorrhage that can range from subclinical to severe. In many cases, the coagulation factor deficiency is recognized because of prolonged bleeding after venipuncture or surgery, but otherwise has minimal significance to the animal. Other inherited deficiencies are characterized by severe episodes of hemorrhage that begin soon after birth.

Acquired defects in coagulation can be caused by decreased production or increased use of coagulation factors. Severe liver disease results in decreased synthesis of most coagulation factors. Production of coagulation factors II, VII, IX, X and proteins C and S is

BOX 2-5 Examples of Inherited Coagulation Deficiency Disorders

FACTOR I
Rare, goats and dogs (Bernese mountain dogs, borzoi, Lhasa apso, vizsla, collie). Mild bleeding tendencies in dogs, more severe in goats.

FACTOR II
Rare, dogs (boxer, Otterhound, English cocker spaniel). Mild bleeding in adults; epistaxis and umbilical cord bleeding in puppies.

FACTOR VII
Rare, dogs (beagles, also Alaskan malamutes, boxer, bulldog, miniature schnauzer, mix breeds). Mild, more easily bruised.

FACTOR X
Rare, dogs (cocker spaniels, mix breeds, Jack Russell terrier). Fatal in severely affected dogs, mild to moderate hemorrhage in less severe cases.

FACTOR XII
Cats and rarely dogs (miniature poodle, standard poodle, German shorthair pointer, Shar-Pei). No bleeding.

FACTOR XI
Cattle (Holstein and Japanese black) and dogs (Great Pyrenees, English springer spaniel, Kerry blue terrier). Spontaneous hemorrhage is insignificant but can be severe after surgery. Most common hereditary coagulation problem in cattle.

FACTOR IX (HEMOPHILIA B)
Dogs and cats. Variable bleeding depending on the molecular damage; generally mild in cats and small dogs, more severe in large dogs.

FACTOR VIII (HEMOPHILIA A)
Dogs, horses, cattle, sheep, and cats. Bleeding can be severe in large dogs and horses; mildly affected animals do not spontaneously bleed.

VON WILLEBRAND'S DISEASE
Dogs, cats, horses, and pigs. Mild-to-severe hemorrhage depending on form of molecular damage; epistaxis, mucosal hemorrhage, postsurgical bleeding. Most common inherited canine bleeding disorder.

VITAMIN K–DEPENDENT FACTORS (II, VII, IX, X)
Rare, Devon Rex cats. Severe, sometimes fatal hemorrhages.

PREKALLIKREIN
Some dogs and Belgian horses and miniature horses. Mucosal or postsurgical bleeding.

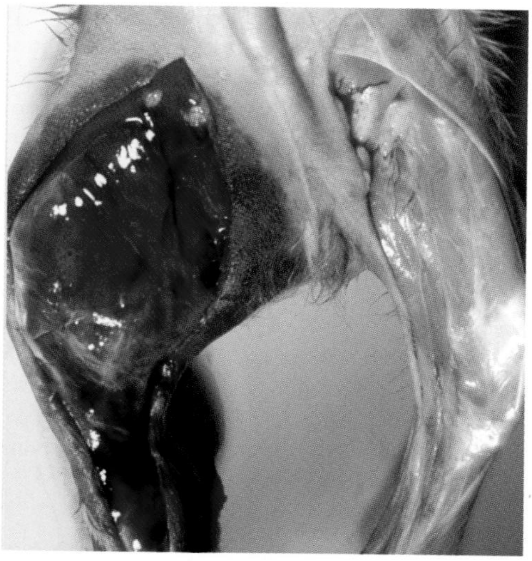

Fig. 2-19 **Hemorrhage, anticoagulant (warfarin-containing) rodenticide toxicosis, skin and subcutis, medial aspect of the right hindleg, dog.** There is a large area of extensive hemorrhage in the subcutis. This lesion was attributed to decreased production of coagulation factors II, VII, IX, and X and proteins C and S resulting from a deficiency of vitamin K induced by warfarin. (Courtesy Dr. D.A. Mosier, College of Veterinary Medicine, Kansas State University.)

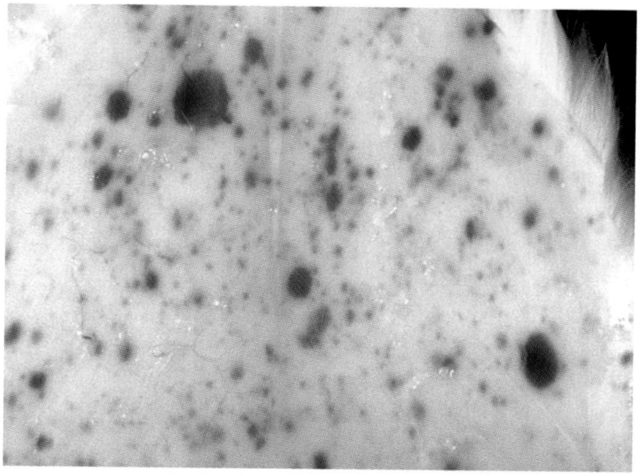

Fig. 2-20 **Ecchymotic hemorrhages (ecchymoses), subcutis, rabbit.** Ecchymoses result from moderate injury to endothelial cells in the capillary beds. (Courtesy Dr. D.A. Mosier, College of Veterinary Medicine, Kansas State University.)

reduced by vitamin K deficiency. Decreased vitamin K production, absorption, or function will reduce conversion of glutamic acid residues into γ-carboxyglutamic acid on these factors. Common substances that competitively inhibit this conversion include dicumarol in moldy sweet clover *(Melilotus alba),* warfarin-containing rodenticides, and sulfaquinoxaline (Fig. 2-19). An inherited deficiency of binding of γ-glutamyl-carboxylase with vitamin K has been reported in British Devon Rex cats. The most common acquired cause of decreased coagulation factors is increased consumption associated with DIC.

The appearance of hemorrhage depends on its cause, location, and severity. Hemorrhage within tissue is often characterized based on size. A petechia (pl. petechiae) is a pinpoint (1 to 2 mm) hemorrhage that occurs mainly because of diapedesis associated with minor vascular damage (see Fig. 2-18). An ecchymosis (pl. ecchymoses) is a larger (up to 2 to 3 cm in diameter) hemorrhage that occurs with more extensive vascular damage (Fig. 2-20), whereas suffusive hemorrhage affects larger contiguous areas of tissue than the other two types (Fig. 2-21). Hemorrhage that occurs in a focal, confined space forms a hematoma. Hematomas are most common

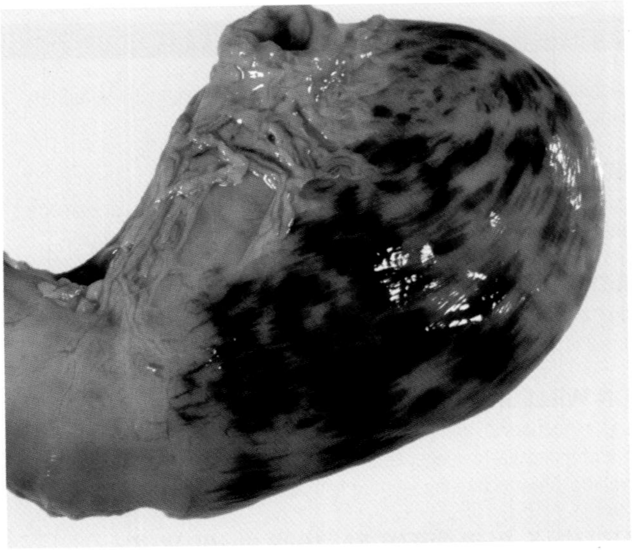

Fig. 2-21 Suffusive hemorrhage, serosa, stomach, dog.
Suffusive hemorrhage results from severe injury to endothelial cells in the capillary beds. (Courtesy Dr. D.A. Mosier, College of Veterinary Medicine, Kansas State University.)

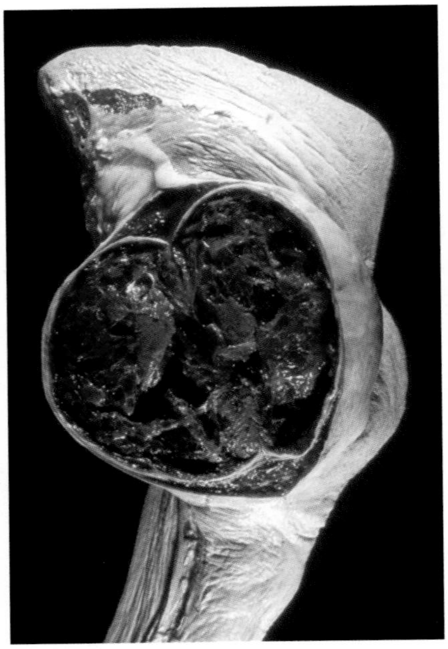

Fig. 2-22 Organizing hematoma, spleen, horse.
Trauma to the spleen has caused damage to the splenic red pulp and its vessels, resulting in bleeding into the splenic parenchyma, forming a hematoma. Note that this hematoma is not acute but is several days old because the blood clot is being degraded. The hematoma is contained by the splenic capsule. (Courtesy Dr. H.B. Gelberg, College of Veterinary Medicine, Oregon State University.)

in the ears of long-eared dogs or pigs and in the spleen after trauma to the vasculature (Fig. 2-22). The hematoma grows in size until the pressure exerted by the extravascular blood matches that within the injured vessel or the vessel seals internally by hemostasis. Hemorrhage into body cavities results in pooling of coagulated or noncoagulated blood within the cavity and is classified by terms such as *hemoperitoneum* (blood in the peritoneal cavity), *hemothorax*

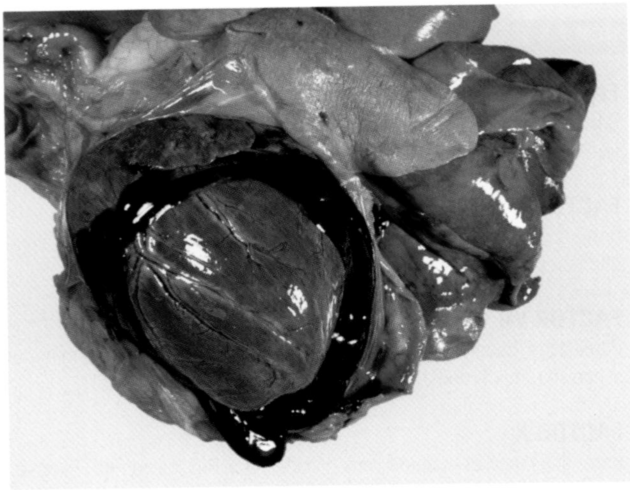

Fig. 2-23 Hemopericardium, pericardial sac, dog.
Hemorrhage into the pericardial sac has caused its distention. Extensive hemopericardium can interfere with the dilatation and contraction of the ventricles, causing cardiac tamponade. Both coagulated and noncoagulated blood are present in the pericardial sac. (Courtesy Dr. D.A. Mosier, College of Veterinary Medicine, Kansas State University.)

(blood in the thoracic cavity), and *hemopericardium* (blood in the pericardial sac) (Fig. 2-23).

The significance of hemorrhage depends mainly on the amount, rate, and location of the blood loss. In most cases, blood loss occurs locally and is quickly stopped by hemostatic processes that seal the damaged vessel. In more severe cases, blood loss continues until local tissue pressure matches intravascular pressure and ends the hemorrhage (such as occurs with hematoma formation). When these mechanisms fail to stop blood loss, significant hemorrhage can occur externally or internally into body cavities. Rapid loss of substantial amounts of blood, such as occurs because of traumatic injury of a large vessel, can lead to hypovolemia, decreased tissue perfusion, and hypovolemic shock (see later discussion in this chapter). In contrast, slow rates of blood loss can be totally or partially compensated for by increased hematopoiesis. Many cases of gastric ulceration and hemorrhage are characterized by persistent but slow rates of blood loss. Some hemorrhages can create pressure that interferes with tissue function. This is most significant in vital organs or in tissue with little room to expand in response to the pressure, such as the brain and heart.

THROMBOSIS

Thrombosis is characterized by the formation of an inappropriate clot of fibrin and/or platelets along with other blood elements (thrombus; pl. thrombi) on the wall of a blood or lymphatic vessel or heart (mural thrombus), or free in their lumens (thromboembolus). Major determinants of thrombosis are historically referred to as Virchow's triad and include the endothelium and blood vessels (vascular injury), coagulation factor and platelet activity (coagulability), and the dynamics of blood flow (stasis or turbulence) (Fig. 2-24 and Box 2-6).

Alterations in the endothelium are the most important factor in thrombosis and can result in increased production of procoagulant substances and decreased production of anticoagulant substances. Endothelial injury and exposure of TF and subendothelial components, such as collagen and fibronectin, are potent stimuli for platelet aggregation and coagulation. Causes of injury are widely varied in their severity and cause and include trauma, vasculitis caused

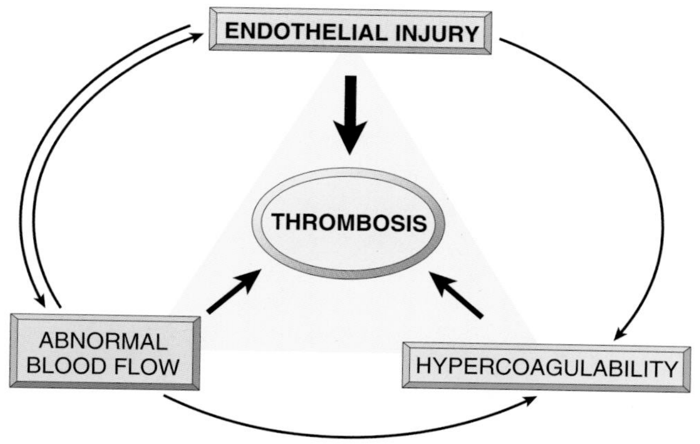

Fig. 2-24 Virchow triad in thrombosis.
Endothelial integrity is the single most important factor. Note that injury to endothelial cells can affect local blood flow and/or coagulability; abnormal blood flow (stasis or turbulence) can, in turn, cause endothelial injury. The elements of the triad may act independently or may combine to cause thrombus formation. (From Kumar V, Abbas AK, Fausto N: *Robbins & Cotran pathologic basis of disease*, ed 8, Philadelphia, 2009, Saunders.)

BOX 2-6 Causes of Thrombosis

ENDOTHELIAL INJURY

Viruses (e.g., canine adenovirus 1, equine Morbillivirus, herpesvirus and Arterivirus, ovine orbivirus, bovine and porcine pestivirus)
Bacteria (e.g., *Salmonella typhimurium, Mannheimia haemolytica, Erysipelothrix rhusiopathiae, Haemophilus somnus*)
Fungi (e.g., *Aspergillus, Mucor, Absidia, Rhizopus*)
Nematode parasites (e.g., *Strongylus vulgaris* larvae, *Dirofilaria, Spirocerca, Aelurostrongylus,* angiostrongylosis)
Immune-mediated vasculitis (e.g., purpura hemorrhagica, feline infectious peritonitis)
Toxins (e.g., endotoxin, *Claviceps*)
Vitamin E/selenium deficiency (microangiopathy)
Local extension of infection (e.g., hepatic abscesses, metritis)
Disseminated intravascular coagulation (DIC)
Faulty intravenous injections
Renal glomerular and cutaneous vasculopathy of greyhounds

ALTERATIONS IN BLOOD FLOW

Local stasis or reduced flow (e.g., gastric dilation and volvulus, intestinal torsion and volvulus, varicocele, external compression of vessel)
Cardiac disease (e.g., cardiomyopathy, cardiac hypertrophy)
Aneurysm (e.g., copper deficiency in pigs, *Strongylus vulgaris, Spirocerca lupi*)
Hypovolemia (e.g., shock, diarrhea, and burns)

HYPERCOAGULABILITY

Inflammation
Enhanced platelet activity (e.g., diabetes mellitus, nephrotic syndrome, malignant neoplasia, heartworm disease, uremia)
Increased clotting factor activation (e.g., nephrotic syndrome, DIC, neoplasia)
Antithrombin III deficiency (e.g., DIC, hepatic disease, glomerular amyloidosis)
Metabolic abnormalities (e.g., hyperadrenocorticism, hypothyroidism)
Glomerulopathies

by infection or immunologic reactions, metabolic disorders, neoplasia, and toxins. Additionally, loss of anticoagulant properties of normal endothelium combined with local release of procoagulant substances can result in fibrin formation. Platelets may also adhere to intact endothelium by interacting with altered proteoglycans in the endothelial glycocalyx. Reduced prostacyclin synthesis may also increase platelet adhesion to endothelium.

Abnormal blood flow increases the risk of thrombosis. Reduced blood flow may occur systemically with heart failure or in a local region of congestion caused by vascular obstruction or vascular dilation. Reduced blood flow is most important in veins, in which the slow flow rate favors accumulation of activated coagulation factors and contact of platelets with the endothelium. Venous thrombosis is common in horses with occlusion of intestinal veins secondary to intestinal torsion. Inactivity can also lead to venous stasis and thrombosis in the limbs, a common problem in humans but not in animals. Dilated heart chambers (e.g., dilatative cardiomyopathy) or dilated vessels (e.g., aneurysms) are also areas in which reduced blood flow predisposes to thrombosis.

Turbulent blood flow also enhances the potential for thrombosis. Turbulence disrupts laminar blood flow so the thin layer of plasma that normally separates the endothelium from cellular elements, particularly platelets, is disrupted, and platelets interact more readily with the endothelium. Similarly, turbulence results in mixing of the blood, which provides greater opportunity for interactions between coagulation factors. Turbulence can also physically damage endothelium, creating a strong stimulus for platelet adhesion and coagulation. Turbulence, along with increased risk of thrombosis, is usually greatest in areas in which vessels branch, there is narrowing of the vessel lumen, or at sites of venous or lymphatic valves.

Increased coagulability of blood (hypercoagulability) is another factor that predisposes to thrombosis. Hypercoagulability usually reflects an increase or decrease in the concentration of activated hemostatic proteins (e.g., coagulation factors and coagulation or fibrinolytic inhibitors) caused by enhanced activation or decreased degradation of these proteins. Less often, an alteration in hemostatic protein function may influence coagulability. Activity of coagulation and fibrinolytic proteins can increase in certain conditions such as inflammation, stress, surgery, neoplasia, pregnancy, and renal disease (e.g., the nephrotic syndrome). Inflammation is the most common cause of hypercoagulability, resulting in a variety of changes such as increased TF, increased platelet reactivity, increased fibrinogen, increased levels of phosphatidylserine, increased PAI-1, and decreased thrombomodulin. Transient increases in fibrinogen can also occur with stress and tissue necrosis. Factor I and factor VIII are elevated by trauma, acute illness, surgery, and increased metabolism that accompanies hyperthyroidism. Deficiency of ATIII, a major inhibitor of thrombin, occurs relatively often in dogs with the nephrotic syndrome. In this syndrome, ATIII is depleted because of loss through damaged glomeruli. In affected dogs, there is an increased incidence of venous thrombosis and pulmonary embolism. Increased platelet activation (e.g., heartworm disease, nephrotic syndrome, and neoplasia) can also contribute to hypercoagulability of blood.

The appearance of a thrombus depends on its underlying cause, location, and composition (relative proportions of platelets, fibrin, and erythrocytes). Thrombi composed predominantly of platelets and fibrin tend to be pale, whereas those containing many erythrocytes are red. Cardiac and arterial thrombi are usually initiated by endothelial damage. This damage provides a site for firm platelet attachment and subsequent incorporation of fibrin. Rapid blood flow in these arteries and arterioles inhibits passive incorporation

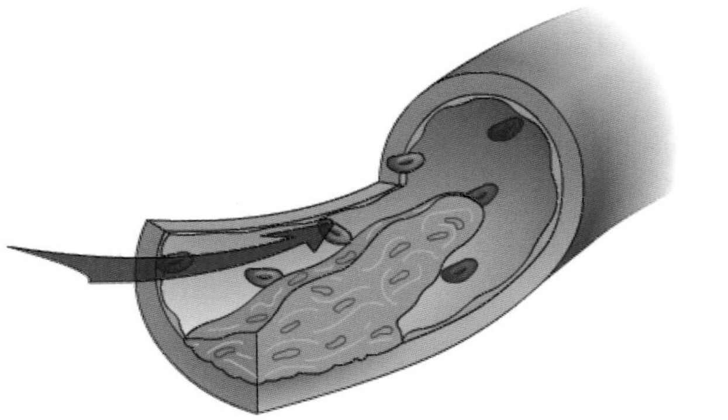

Fig. 2-25 Thrombus (mural), artery.
Thrombus formation is usually initiated by endothelial damage, forming a site of attachment for the thrombus. Growth of the thrombus is downstream, resulting in a tail that is not attached to the vessel wall. Portions of the tail can break off to form thromboemboli. (Courtesy Dr. D.A. Mosier and L. Schooley, College of Veterinary Medicine, Kansas State University.)

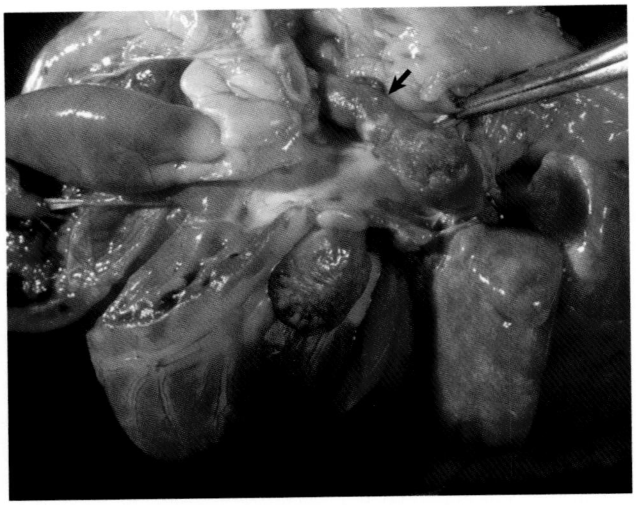

Fig. 2-26 Arterial thrombus, pulmonary artery, dog.
Arterial thrombi are composed primarily of platelets and fibrin because of the rapid flow of blood, which tends to exclude erythrocytes from the thrombus; thus they are usually tan to gray *(arrow)*. (Courtesy Dr. D.A. Mosier, College of Veterinary Medicine, Kansas State University.)

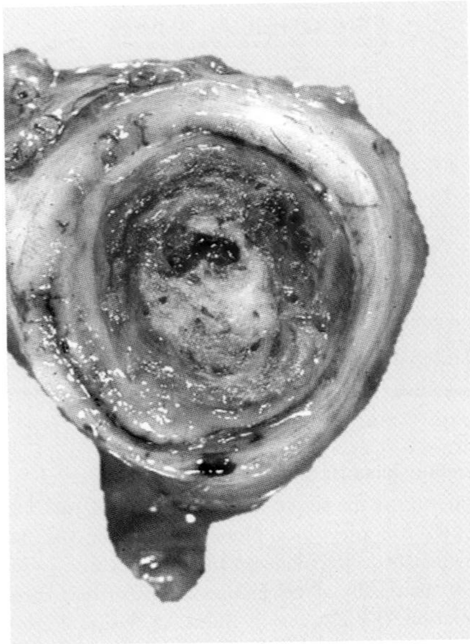

Fig. 2-27 Arterial thrombus, lines of Zahn, cranial mesenteric artery, horse.
Cardiac and larger arterial thrombi often have a laminated appearance characterized by alternating layers of platelets *(white-gray)* and fibrin *(white)* intermixed with erythrocytes and leukocytes (lines of Zahn). These lines are the result of rapid blood flow in the heart and arteries/arterioles that favors the deposition of fibrin and platelets and the exclusion of erythrocytes from the thrombus. This horse had verminous arteritis (*Strongylus vulgaris* fourth stage larvae) in the affected artery. (Courtesy Dr. P.N. Nation, University of Alberta; and Noah's Arkive, College of Veterinary Medicine, The University of Georgia.)

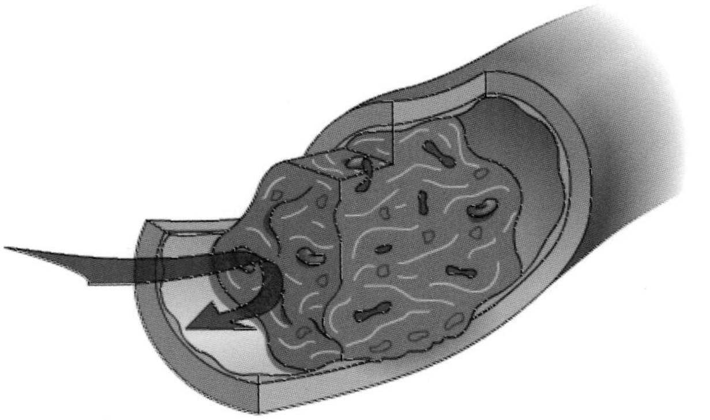

Fig. 2-28 Venous thrombus.
Thrombus formation often occurs in areas of slow blood flow or stasis. Venous thrombi are dark red and gelatinous as a result of large numbers of erythrocytes that are loosely incorporated into the thrombus because of the slow flow. Most venous thrombi are occlusive. (Courtesy Dr. D.A. Mosier and L. Schooley, College of Veterinary Medicine, Kansas State University.)

of erythrocytes into the thrombus (Fig. 2-25). Cardiac and arterial thrombi are dull, usually firmly attached to the vessel wall, and red-gray (pale thrombi) (Fig. 2-26). The thrombus may or may not occlude the vessel lumen, and large thrombi tend to have tails that extend downstream from the point of endothelial attachment. Cardiac and larger arterial thrombi often have a laminated appearance created by rapid blood flow and characterized by alternating layers of platelets, interspersed by fibrin intermixed with erythrocytes and leukocytes (lines of Zahn) (Fig. 2-27).

Venous thrombi often occur in areas of stasis. Because of the slow blood flow and reduced clearance rate of activated clotting factors in these areas, erythrocytes are commonly incorporated into a loose meshwork of fibrin and platelets (Fig. 2-28). Venous thrombi are typically gelatinous, soft, glistening, and dark red (red thrombi) (Fig. 2-29). They are almost always occlusive and molded to the vessel lumen and often extend for a considerable distance upstream from their point of origin. They commonly have points of attachment to the vessel wall, but these are often very loose and difficult to discern. Venous thrombi are morphologically similar to postmortem clots (see Fig. 1-24). Compared with venous thrombi, postmortem clots are softer and do not have a point of vascular attachment. In larger vessels or in the heart, erythrocytes may settle to the bottom of the clot, leaving a yellow upper layer (chicken fat clot) indicative of postmortem formation. The presence or absence of associated lesions is often a major factor in distinguishing between an antemortem venous thrombus and a postmortem clot.

The significance of a thrombus is determined by its location and its ability to disrupt perfusion in a dependent tissue. Disruption of tissue perfusion is influenced mainly by the size of the thrombus, its

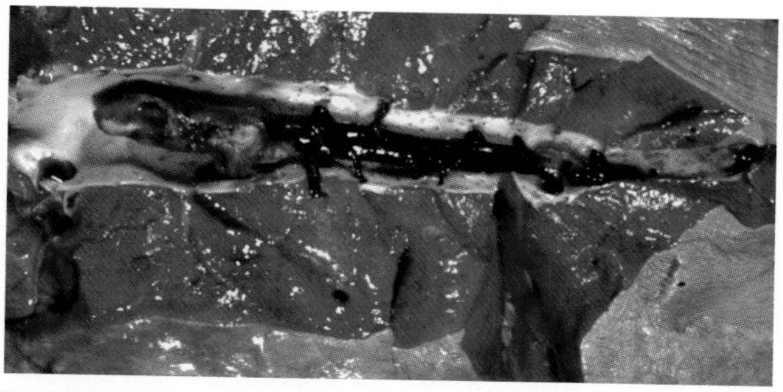

Fig. 2-29 Venous thrombi, pulmonary vein, lung, horse.
Venous thrombi become molded to the shape of the lumen of the vein and grow upstream from the site of initiation. (Courtesy Dr. J. King, College of Veterinary Medicine, Cornell University; and Noah's Arkive, College of Veterinary Medicine, The University of Georgia.)

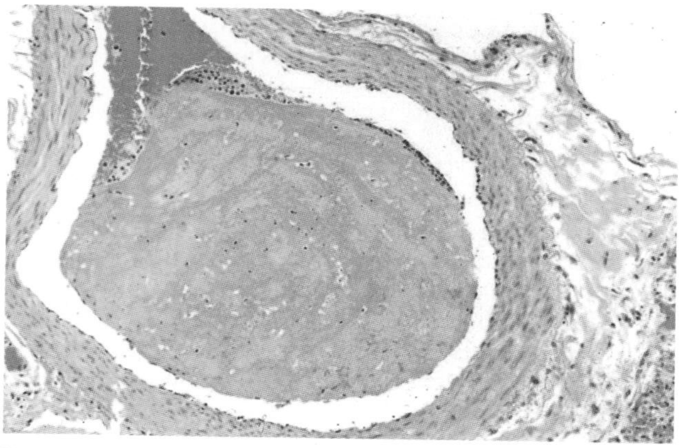

Fig. 2-30 Large thrombus, pulmonary artery, cow.
Large thrombi are less readily dissolved by thrombolysis and therefore heal by other methods. This thrombus consists of a large coagulum of fibrin that has undergone little to no resolution. H&E stain. (Courtesy Dr. M.A. Miller, College of Veterinary Medicine, University of Missouri; and Noah's Arkive, College of Veterinary Medicine, The University of Georgia.)

rate of formation, and its method of resolution or repair. In general, thrombi that rapidly develop are more detrimental than those that slowly develop. A slowly developing thrombus creates progressive narrowing of the vessel lumen, but the slow rate of development provides opportunity for collateral blood flow to increase into the affected area. Small thrombi are usually less damaging than large thrombi. Small thrombi are more easily removed by thrombolysis with little residual vessel damage or tissue compromise. In contrast, large thrombi substantially narrow the vessel lumen to restrict blood flow, are often occlusive, and are less readily dissolved by thrombolysis (Fig. 2-30). Occlusive thrombi block blood flow either into (occlusive arterial thrombus) or out of (occlusive venous thrombus) an area and often result in ischemia (decreased oxygenation of tissue) or infarction (necrosis of tissue caused by lack of oxygen).

Under most circumstances and after removal of the injurious stimulus, the well-regulated cascade of events in thrombosis results in the return to normal function of the endothelium and subendothelial collagen (Fig. 2-31, *A*). However, blood flow through a vessel containing a chronic large or occlusive thrombus can change over time. The thrombus provides an ongoing stimulus for platelet adhesion and coagulation, so thrombus propagation can result in progressive narrowing and possible occlusion of the vessel lumen. A thrombus can also be incorporated into the wall of the vessel by

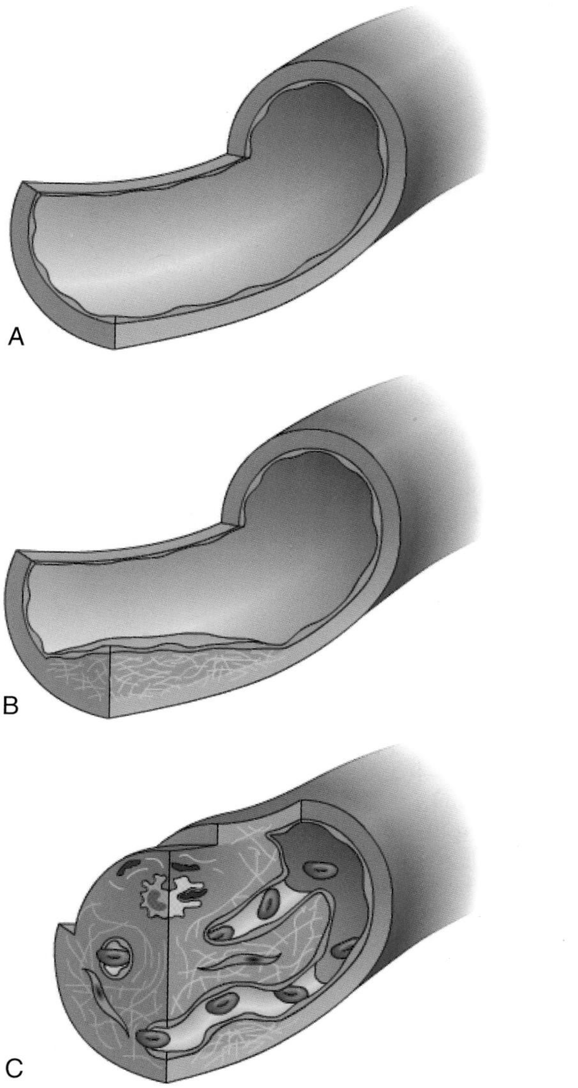

Fig. 2-31 Thrombus resolution.
A, Small thrombi are removed by thrombolysis, and the blood vessel returns to normal structure and function. **B,** Larger, more persistent thrombi are resolved by removal of thrombotic debris by phagocytes with subsequent granulation tissue formation and fibrosis with regrowth of endothelium over the surface to incorporate the affected area into the vessel wall. **C,** In large mural or occlusive thrombi that are not removed by thrombolysis or phagocytosis of the thrombotic debris, the thrombus is organized by the invasion of fibroblasts and later by the formation of new vascular channels (recanalization), which provides alternate routes for blood flow through and around the site of the original thrombus. (**A, B,** and **C** courtesy Dr. D.A. Mosier and L. Schooley, College of Veterinary Medicine, Kansas State University.)

a process similar to that used to replace irreversibly damaged tissue. Products of the aggregated platelets stimulate permanent healing of the damaged area by recruiting fibroblasts to the damaged area. Thrombotic debris is removed by macrophages, and granulation tissue and subsequent fibrosis (organization) occur at the site of the thrombus. Concurrently, there is regrowth of endothelium over the surface of the scar. Although there is a permanent narrowing of the vessel lumen, the regrowth of endothelium over the healed thrombus decreases the stimulus for continued thrombosis (Fig. 2-31, *B*). In occlusive and some large thrombi, this healing process may be accompanied by invasion and growth of endothelial-lined

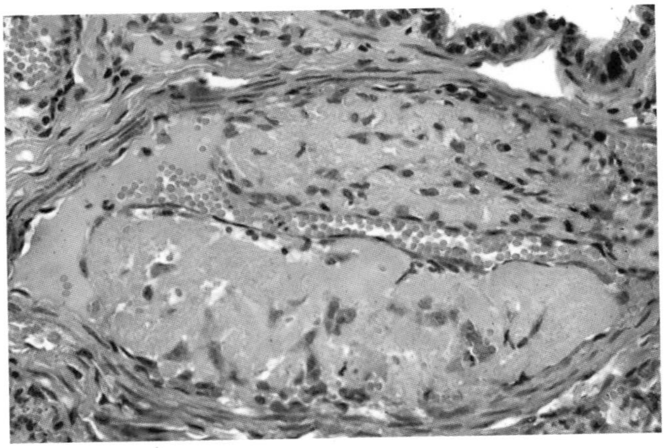

Fig. 2-32 Occlusive mural thrombus, recanalization, cat. In occlusive and large thrombi, the healing process may occur by fibrosis and the invasion and growth of endothelial-lined vascular channels through the fibrosed area (recanalization). Note the vascular channel, horizontally in the middle of the thrombus. This provides alternate routes for blood flow to reestablish through or around the original thrombus. The permanent vascular narrowing and altered, more turbulent blood flow at the site of a healed thrombus result in an increased risk for subsequent thrombosis at the site. H&E stain. (Courtesy Dr. B.C. Ward, College of Veterinary Medicine, University of Mississippi; and Noah's Arkive, College of Veterinary Medicine, The University of Georgia.)

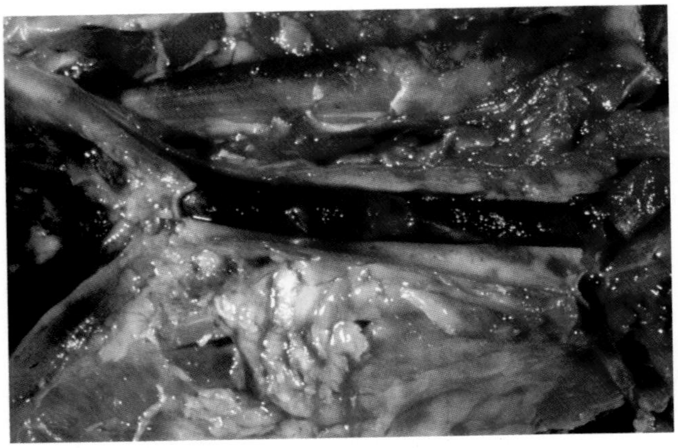

Fig. 2-33 Saddle thrombus, iliac-aortic bifurcation, cat. Cardiac thromboemboli usually lodge at the bifurcation of the aorta into the external iliac arteries with a portion of the thromboembolus entering each iliac vessel to form a saddle thrombus. A saddle thrombus is not attached to the wall of the aorta or iliac arteries and is easily removed at necropsy. The thromboembolus is composed of layers of platelets and fibrin in which there are enmeshed erythrocytes. (Courtesy Dr. M.D. McGavin, College of Veterinary Medicine, University of Tennessee.)

blood channels through the fibrosed area (recanalization) (Fig. 2-31, *C,* and Fig. 2-32). This provides alternate routes for blood flow to reestablish through or around the original thrombus. Although reestablishment of blood flow increases tissue perfusion, the permanent vascular narrowing and altered, more turbulent blood flow at the site of a healed thrombus result in an increased risk for subsequent thrombosis at the site.

In some cases, a thrombus or portions of a thrombus can break loose and enter the circulation as an embolus (pl. emboli), a piece of free-floating foreign material within the blood. Thromboemboli (emboli derived from fragments of a thrombus) eventually become lodged in a smaller-sized vessel as the vessel diameter reaches a size that prevents the passage of the embolus, a process called *embolization.* Venous thromboemboli typically lodge in the pulmonary circulation where they can cause pulmonary infarcts or right-sided heart failure. Arterial thromboemboli typically lodge within a smaller artery downstream from the site of the thrombus, often near sites of vascular bifurcation. Arterial emboli frequently result in infarction of dependent tissue, depending on the tissue and nature of its vascular supply. Cardiac thromboemboli usually lodge at the bifurcation of the external iliac arteries with a portion of the thromboembolus entering each iliac vessel to form a saddle thrombus (Fig. 2-33).

Emboli can also originate from substances other than thrombi. Fat from the bone marrow can be released into the circulation after a fracture of a long bone. Most fat emboli lodge in the pulmonary circulation. Fibrocartilaginous emboli consist of portions of an intervertebral disk, which are released after rupture of a degenerative disk. These can result in occlusion of local vessels and sometimes cause localized spinal cord infarction. Bacteria from inflammatory lesions, such as vegetative valvular endocarditis, or abscesses can enter the blood to form bacterial emboli. When these lodge within vessels, they may cause infarction and secondary sites of infection. Intravascular parasites, such as heartworms (e.g., *Dirofilaria*), or flukes (e.g., schistosomes) can form parasitic emboli. Malignant neoplasms that invade a vessel result in the formation of neoplastic emboli composed of neoplastic cells. Less common sources of emboli include hematopoietic cells from the bone marrow, amniotic fluid, agglutinated erythrocytes, or clumps of other cells, such as hepatocytes, released after tissue trauma. In any case, the significance of these emboli is their potential to occlude a vessel and inhibit blood flow to dependent tissue.

A serious manifestation of abnormal coagulation is DIC. This is a severe dyshomeostasis caused by the generation of excess thrombin. There are many causes, including diffuse vascular damage (e.g., trauma, vasculitis, and burns), which results in exposure of blood to TF. Intravascular generation of TF by endothelial cells and monocytes can also occur in response to bacteremia, other systemic infections, or any other stimuli that activate the release of inflammatory mediators. The result is TF-induced activation of extrinsic coagulation to produce thrombin. Thrombin causes platelet aggregation and activation of coagulation factors V, VIII, and I to form fibrin, resulting in widespread microvascular clots. Concurrently, the high levels of thrombin stimulate clot dissolution by binding to thrombomodulin to activate protein C, by converting plasminogen into plasmin, and by binding to ATIII to become inactivated. The widespread nature of the coagulation response results in the consumption of these and other factors, resulting in widespread hemorrhages. This combination of microthrombosis with concurrent or rapidly sequential hemorrhage represents one of the most profound and dramatic examples of dyshomeostasis in animals.

NORMAL BLOOD FLOW, DISTRIBUTION, AND PERFUSION

The heart provides the driving pressure for blood distribution. Baroreceptors in the carotid sinus and aortic arch signal the cardiovascular control center in the medulla to balance sympathetic and parasympathetic output to maintain appropriate blood pressure. Left atrial volume receptors and hypothalamic osmoreceptors also help regulate pressure by altering water volume and sodium balance. Sodium concentration is an important contributor to blood volume, osmolality, and pressure and is controlled by the renin-angiotensin-aldosterone system. Secretion of ADH by the hypothalamus in response to a water deficit increases renal tubular reabsorption of water to help maintain blood volume.

Distribution of blood within the circulatory system is highly variable. Organs that alter or recondition blood (e.g., lungs, gastrointestinal tract, kidney, and liver) receive substantially greater blood flow than is required for their metabolic needs. O_2 and CO_2 are exchanged in the lungs, nutrients are obtained from the gastrointestinal tract and processed by the liver, wastes are removed and electrolytes are balanced by the kidneys, heat is dissipated in the skin, and regulatory hormones enter from endocrine tissues. Systemic neural and hormonal influences can cause general changes in blood distribution. Blood vessel β_2 receptors, most abundant in cardiac and skeletal muscle, cause vasodilation and increased flow when stimulated by epinephrine. In contrast, vessel α-receptors, notably absent in the brain, induce vasoconstriction and reduced flow in most organs on stimulation with norepinephrine. Local intrinsic controls alter arteriolar diameter to adjust the blood flow to a tissue based on that tissue's metabolic needs. These local controls generally override any central controls to maintain adequate blood flow to support normal cell function. At rest, more than 60% of the circulating blood volume is in the veins, providing a storage pool that can be quickly returned to the heart during periods of increased tissue need. In contrast, most capillary beds are closed at any given time; blood flows through only about 10% of the total capillaries of resting skeletal muscle. The orchestration of central pressure, blood composition, and blood distribution is critical to meet the varying perfusion needs of all the cells in the body despite constantly changing conditions.

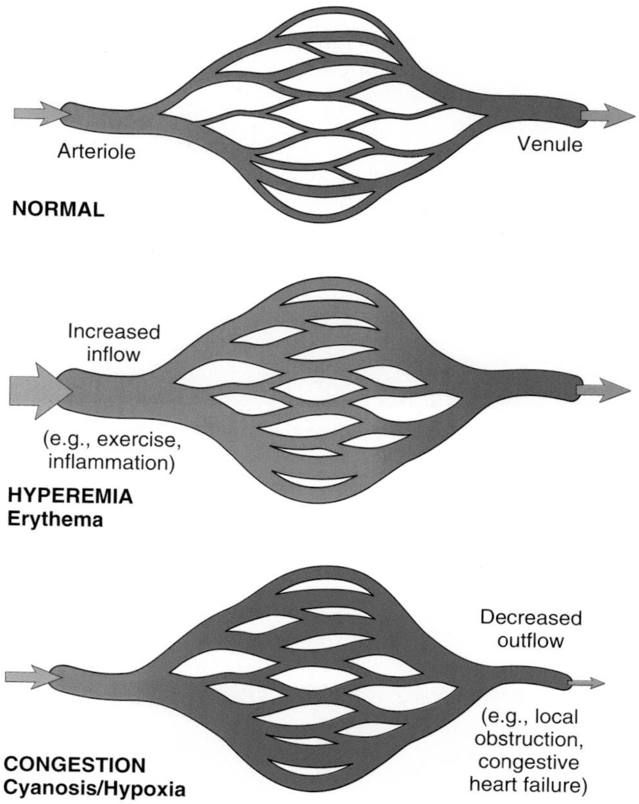

Fig. 2-34 Hyperemia versus congestion.
In both cases, there is an increased volume and pressure of blood in a given tissue with associated capillary dilation and a potential for fluid extravasation. In hyperemia, there is increased inflow leading to engorgement with oxygenated blood. In congestion, diminished outflow leads to a capillary bed swollen with deoxygenated venous blood resulting in cyanosis. (From Kumar V, Abbas AK, Fausto N: *Robbins & Cotran pathologic basis of disease,* ed 7, Philadelphia, 2005, Saunders.)

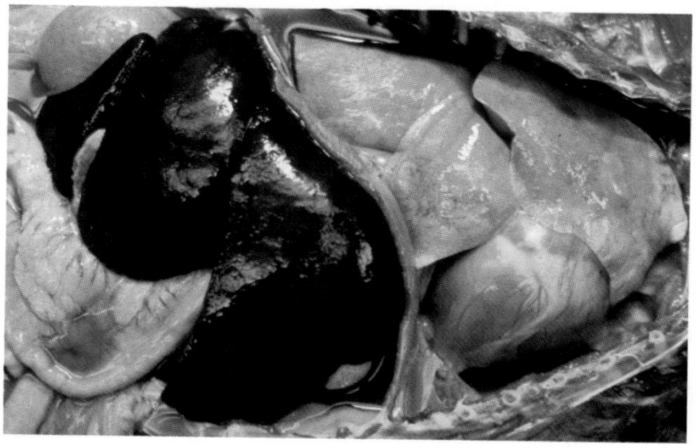

Fig. 2-35 Acute passive congestion, liver, dog.
The liver is enlarged and dark red. Acute passive congestion occurs in the vascular system and dependent organs (heart, lungs, portal system) when there is a sudden interruption of the return of blood to the heart, as occurs in heart failure resulting from arrhythmias and after euthanasia. (Courtesy Dr. D.A. Mosier, College of Veterinary Medicine, Kansas State University.)

ALTERATIONS IN BLOOD FLOW AND PERFUSION

INCREASED BLOOD FLOW

Hyperemia is an active engorgement of vascular beds with a normal or decreased outflow of blood. It occurs because of increased metabolic activity of tissue that results in localized increased concentrations of CO_2, acid, and other metabolites. These cause a local stimulus for vasodilation and increased flow (hyperemia). Hyperemia can occur as a physiologic mechanism within the skin to dissipate heat. It also occurs because of increased need such as increased blood flow to the gastrointestinal tract after a meal. Hyperemia is also one of the first vascular changes that occur in response to an inflammatory stimulus (Fig. 2-34). Neurogenic reflexes and release of vasoactive substances, such as histamine and prostaglandins, mediate the change to promote delivery of inflammatory mediators to the site. Tissues with hyperemic vessels are bright red and warm, and there is engorgement of the arterioles and capillaries.

DECREASED BLOOD FLOW

Congestion is the passive engorgement of a vascular bed generally caused by a decreased outflow with a normal or increased inflow of blood (see Fig. 2-34). Passive congestion can occur acutely (acute passive congestion) or chronically (chronic passive congestion). Acute passive congestion can occur in the liver and lungs in response to acute heart failure (Fig. 2-35), after euthanasia, or in organs in which relaxation of smooth muscle from barbiturate anesthesia/euthanasia results in dilation of the vasculature and vascular sinusoids such as in the spleen. Most passive congestion is recognized clinically as chronic passive congestion. It can occur locally because of the obstruction of venous outflow caused by a neoplastic or inflammatory mass, displacement of an organ, or fibrosis resulting from healed injury. Generalized passive congestion occurs because of decreased passage of blood either through the heart or the lungs. This is most often caused by heart failure or conditions (e.g., pulmonary fibrosis) that inhibit the flow of blood through the lungs. Right-sided heart failure causes portal vein and hepatic congestion (Fig. 2-36). Left-sided heart failure results in pulmonary

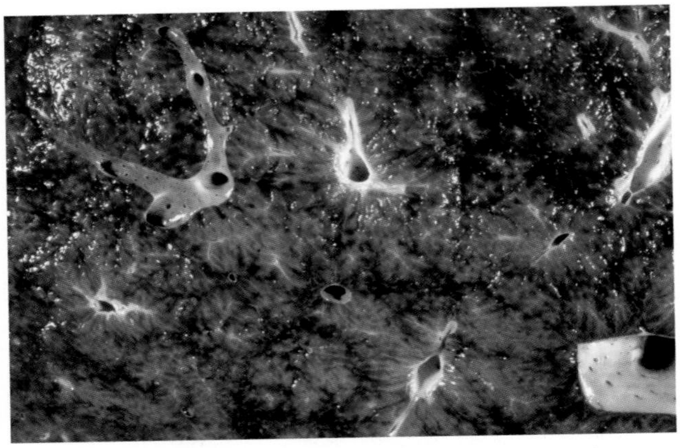

Fig. 2-36 Chronic passive congestion (nutmeg liver), liver, cut surface, dog.
The cut surface has a repeating pattern of red and tan mottling (an accentuated lobular pattern). Chronic passive congestion leads to persistent hypoxia in centrilobular areas and atrophy, degeneration, and/or eventually necrosis of centrilobular hepatocytes. The red areas are dilated central veins and adjacent areas of sinusoidal dilation and congestion caused by centrilobular hepatic necrosis. The tan areas are normal, uncongested parenchyma. (Courtesy Dr. D.A. Mosier, College of Veterinary Medicine, Kansas State University.)

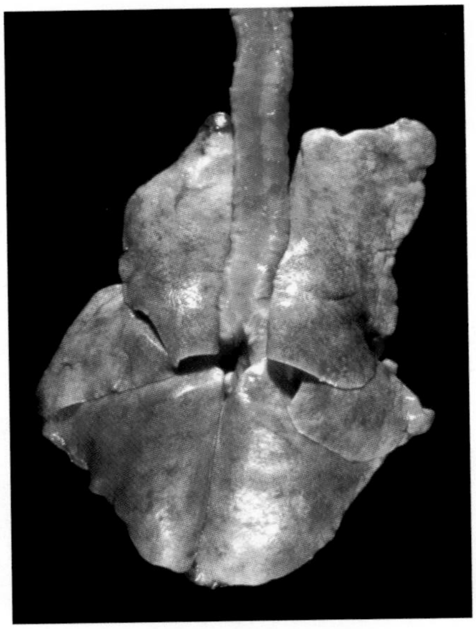

Fig. 2-37 Chronic passive congestion, lung, dog.
The lungs are moderately firm and yellow-brown because of alveolar macrophages containing hemosiderin. Inflammatory mediators produced by these macrophages also induce fibroplasia, thus there is extensive formation of interstitial collagen in the long term. This collagen is the reason the lungs fail to collapse after loss of negative pressure in the pleural cavity when the diaphragm is incised at necropsy. (Courtesy College of Veterinary Medicine, University of Illinois.)

congestion (Fig. 2-37). Chronically, there may be fibrosis caused by the hypoxia and cell injury that accompanies congestion (e.g., chronic hepatic congestion). Congested tissues are dark red, swollen (edema), and cooler than normal. The microvasculature is engorged with blood, and there is often surrounding edema and sometimes hemorrhage caused by diapedesis.

DECREASED TISSUE PERFUSION

Reduced blood flow to an area is usually caused by a local obstruction of a vessel, local congestion, or decreased cardiac output. Local obstruction results in either reduced blood flow into an area or inadequate blood flow out of an area. Ischemia occurs when the perfusion of tissue in the affected area becomes inadequate to meet the metabolic needs of the tissue. Ischemia caused by arterial disease is most commonly the result of incomplete luminal blockage by a thrombus or embolus. The result is a decreased flow of oxygenated blood into the area. Arteriolar vasoconstriction, if prolonged, can also result in ischemia. Ischemia resulting from venous lesions can be caused by intraluminal obstruction such as a venous thrombus. However, external pressure that occludes the vein, such as inflammatory or neoplastic masses, is a common cause. Venous obstruction leads to congestion characterized by slowing and stagnation of blood flow, with loss of tissue oxygenation, local increased hydrostatic pressure, and leakage of fluid into the interstitium (edema). Increased interstitial pressure may partially inhibit arterial inflow into the area to compound the problem. Capillaries can also become occluded by thrombi or external pressure. The severity of ischemia is determined by the local vascular anatomy and degree of anastomoses and collateral circulation, the number of microcirculatory vessels and degree of resistance of the arteriole supplying the capillaries, the extent of the decreased perfusion, the rate at which the occlusion occurred, and the metabolic needs of the tissue. Ischemia can be tolerated to different levels by different tissues. The brain and heart are most susceptible because of a high need for O_2 and nutrients, combined with poor collateral circulation. In contrast, organs that recondition blood (e.g., lungs, gastrointestinal tract, kidneys, and skin) can tolerate substantial reductions in flow because they already receive more blood than necessary for their metabolic needs. Other tissues receive blood based on their immediate needs (e.g., skeletal muscle during physical activity). Rapid and complete occlusion that affects large areas of tissue is generally more severe because collateral circulation may not be able to reestablish flow to certain areas quickly enough to prevent tissue injury.

In tissue in which there has been a return of blood flow after brief ischemia, the tissue often returns to normal. The ATP of ischemic tissue is degraded to adenosine, a potent vasodilator, which relieves the ischemia and allows ATP production to resume. However, after prolonged ischemia, the return of blood flow can result in a variety of detrimental effects. Reflow results in fluid loss to the interstitium, resulting in high tissue pressure, which compresses veins and inhibits local venous return. The congested capillaries hemorrhage, TF is released, and vessels are occluded by thrombi. In ischemic cells, a breakdown product of ATP is hypoxanthine. In the absence of oxygen, this is nonreactive. However, on the return of oxygen, xanthine oxidase converts hypoxanthine into urates, hydrogen peroxide, and superoxide anions. Subsequent reaction of superoxide results in the formation of additional reactive oxygen species such as hydroxyl radicals. Collectively, these oxygen-free radicals formed during reperfusion can induce damage, in addition to that caused by ischemia and energy depletion of the cell.

An infarct is a local area of peracute ischemia that undergoes coagulative necrosis. Infarction is caused by the same events that result in ischemia and is most common secondary to thrombosis or thromboembolism. The characteristics of an infarct are variable based on the type and size of vessel that was occluded (artery or vein), the duration of the occlusion, the tissue in which it occurs, and the prior perfusion and vitality of the tissue. Complete arterial blockage usually results in immediate infarction (Fig. 2-38). In contrast, when venous obstruction occurs, such as from torsions or displacements of the bowel, there is extensive congestion and edema of the affected bowel that precedes and promotes infarction. Concurrent disease, decreased cardiovascular function, anemia, or

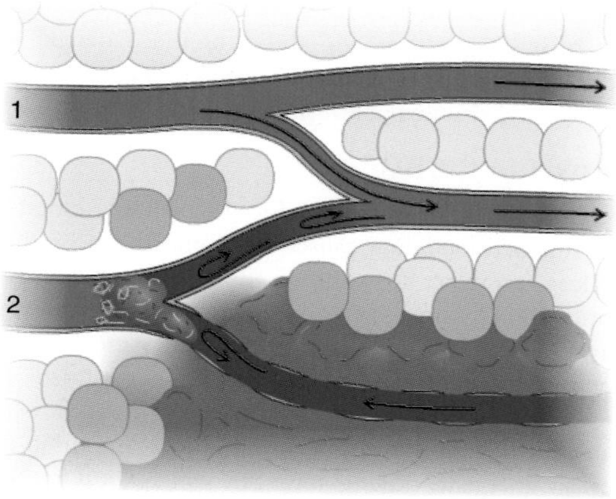

Fig. 2-38 Infarction due to arterial obstruction.
Arterial obstruction results in loss of blood flow to downstream tissue, resulting in abrupt coagulative necrosis. The amount of necrosis depends on factors such as the type and prior health of the tissue affected, its metabolic rate (neurons versus myocytes and fibroblasts), and amount of collateral circulation or alternative blood supply. *1,* Normal arterial flow; *2,* arterial flow obstructed by an arterial thrombus. (Courtesy Dr. D.A. Mosier and L. Schooley, College of Veterinary Medicine, Kansas State University.)

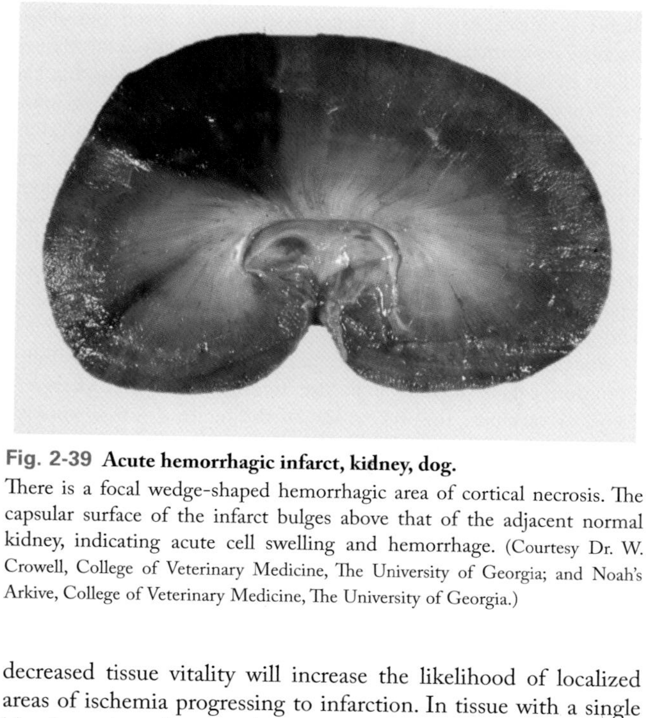

Fig. 2-39 Acute hemorrhagic infarct, kidney, dog.
There is a focal wedge-shaped hemorrhagic area of cortical necrosis. The capsular surface of the infarct bulges above that of the adjacent normal kidney, indicating acute cell swelling and hemorrhage. (Courtesy Dr. W. Crowell, College of Veterinary Medicine, The University of Georgia; and Noah's Arkive, College of Veterinary Medicine, The University of Georgia.)

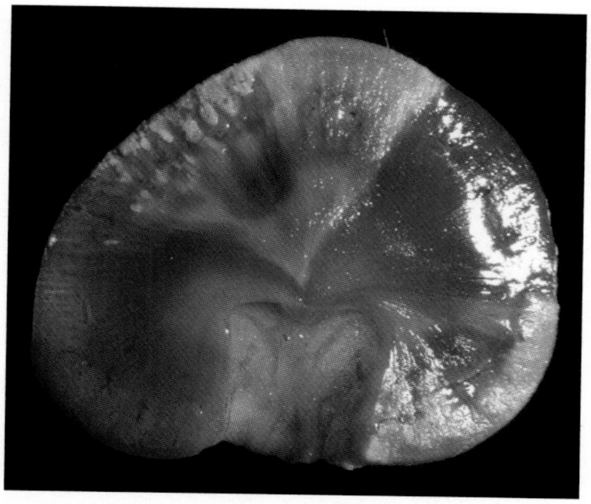

Fig. 2-40 Acute pale infarcts, kidney, rabbit.
Multiple, pale white to tan pyramidal-shaped infarcts extend from the renal cortex to the medulla. The infarcts bulge above the capsular surface *(center top),* indicative of acute cell swelling. The glistening areas on the right are highlights from the photographic lamps. (Courtesy Dr. M.D. McGavin, College of Veterinary Medicine, University of Tennessee.)

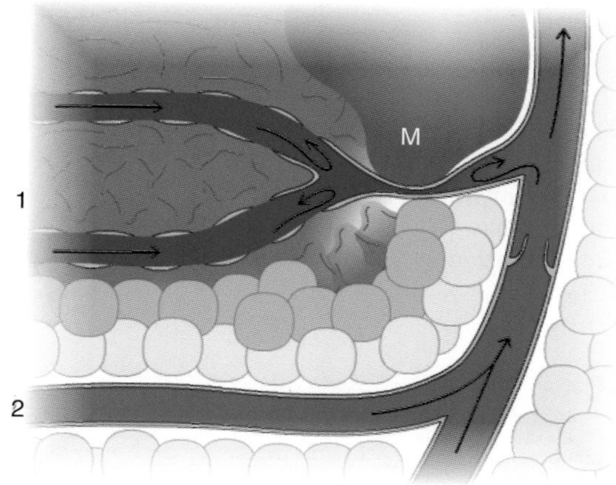

Fig. 2-41 Infarction due to venous obstruction.
Venous obstruction results in stagnation of blood flow and reduction or loss of venous return. There is progressive ischemia and ultimately coagulative necrosis of the tissue upstream of the site of vessel obstruction. The amount of necrosis depends on factors such as the type and prior health of the tissue affected, metabolic rate, and amount of collateral circulation or alternative blood supply. *1,* Venous return to a larger vein (note the valve) obstructed by a mass (M); *2,* normal venous return to a larger vein. (Courtesy Dr. D.A. Mosier and L. Schooley, College of Veterinary Medicine, Kansas State University.)

decreased tissue vitality will increase the likelihood of localized areas of ischemia progressing to infarction. In tissue with a single blood supply and minimal anastomoses (e.g., brain, heart, kidney, and spleen), occlusion of nearly any sized vessel typically results in infarction of the dependent tissue (Fig. 2-39). In tissue with parallel blood supplies that have numerous anastomoses (e.g., skeletal muscle and gastrointestinal tract), occlusion is less serious unless it occurs in a large vessel. Tissues with dual blood supplies (e.g., liver and lung) are not commonly susceptible to infarction unless concurrent underlying disease compromises the overall blood supply.

Most infarcts are dark red soon after their occurrence because of hemorrhage from damaged vessels in the infarcted area and backflow of blood into the area from surrounding vessels (see Fig. 2-39). As cells undergo necrosis, there is swelling of the affected area, which can force blood out of the infarcted region, giving it a pale appearance (Fig. 2-40). Additionally, hemolysis of erythrocytes and degradation and diffusion of hemoglobin give the infarct a progressively paler appearance. This change in color can occur within 1 to 5 days depending on the tissue and extent of the infarction. Certain types of tissue that have a loose (spongy) consistency, such as the lungs and storage-type spleens (e.g., dogs and pigs), usually remain red because the interstitial areas are expandable and necrosis-induced pressure does not build up to force blood out of the infarcted region (Figs. 2-41 and 2-42). Parenchymal tissues with a less expansible interstitium (e.g., kidney) generally become pale over time because of the pressure that forces blood from the necrotic area. Inflammation occurs at the periphery of the dead tissue so that leukocytes, then macrophages, enter the area to clear the necrotic debris, and subsequently neovascularization and granulation occur to replace the necrotic region with fibrous

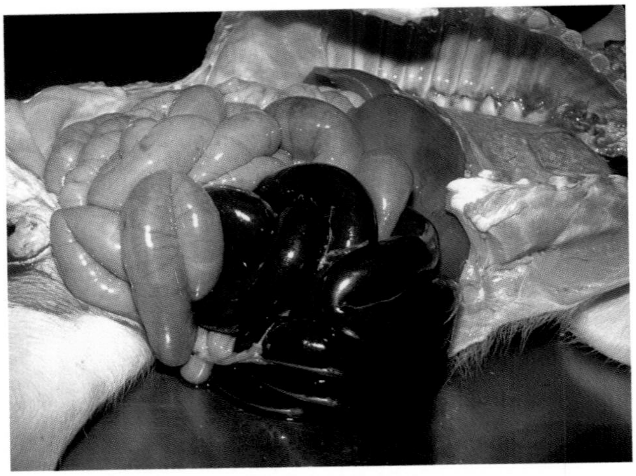

Fig. 2-42 Venous infarction, small intestinal volvulus, pig. Note the intensely congested loops of small intestine undergoing early venous infarction. The veins have been compressed by a volvulus that has compressed the veins but not the arteries, thus preventing the venous return. If the volvulus had rotated further, it would also have compressed the arteries. (Courtesy Dr. D.A. Mosier, College of Veterinary Medicine, Kansas State University.)

tissue. This process can occur over a period of weeks or months depending on the extent of the damage. In contrast to the coagulative necrosis caused by infarction in most tissue, infarction in the brain and nervous tissue is characterized by liquefactive necrosis. Subsequently, there is glial cell removal of damaged tissue and astrocytic production of glial fibers (astrogliosis) to replace the affected area.

SHOCK

Shock (cardiovascular collapse) is a circulatory dyshomeostasis associated with loss of circulating blood volume, reduced cardiac output, and/or inappropriate peripheral vascular resistance. Although causes can be diverse (e.g., severe hemorrhage or diarrhea, burns, tissue trauma, endotoxemia), the underlying events of shock are similar. Hypotension results in impaired tissue perfusion, cellular hypoxia and a shift to anaerobic metabolism, cellular degeneration, and cell death (Fig. 2-43). Although the cellular effects of hypoperfusion are initially reversible, persistence of shock results in irreversible cell and tissue injury. Shock is rapidly progressive and life threatening when compensatory responses are inadequate. Shock can be classified into three different types based on the fundamental underlying problem: (1) cardiogenic, (2) hypovolemic, and (3) blood maldistribution. Shock attributed to blood maldistribution can be further divided into septic shock, anaphylactic shock, and neurogenic shock.

CARDIOGENIC SHOCK

Cardiogenic shock results from failure of the heart to adequately pump blood. Cardiac failure can occur due to myocardial infarction, ventricular tachycardia, fibrillation or other arrhythmias, dilatative or hypertrophic cardiomyopathy, obstruction of blood flow from the heart (e.g., pulmonary embolism and pulmonary or aortic stenosis), or other cardiac dysfunctions. In all cases, there is a decrease in both stroke volume and cardiac output. Major compensatory mechanisms (e.g., sympathetic stimulation of the heart), which increase heart contractility, stroke volume, total cardiac output, and heart rate, are only variably successful depending on the nature of the cardiac damage and the ability of the damaged heart to respond. Unsuccessful compensation leads to stagnation of blood and progressive tissue hypoperfusion.

HYPOVOLEMIC SHOCK

Hypovolemic shock arises from reduced circulating blood volume as the result of blood loss caused by hemorrhage or the result of fluid loss secondary to vomiting, diarrhea, or burns. Reduced circulating blood volume leads to decreased vascular pressure and tissue hypoperfusion. Immediate compensatory mechanisms (e.g., peripheral vasoconstriction and fluid movement into the plasma) act to increase vascular pressure and maintain blood flow to critical tissues such as the heart, brain, and kidney. Increased pressure provides an adequate driving force on which local mechanisms can draw on to increase blood flow based on their needs. When the insult is mild, compensation is generally successful and the animal returns to homeostasis. Loss of about 10% of blood volume can occur without a decrease in blood pressure or cardiac output. However, if greater volumes are lost, adequate pressure and perfusion cannot be maintained and there is insufficient blood flow to meet the needs of the tissues. When blood loss approaches 35% to 45%, blood pressure and cardiac output can fall dramatically.

BLOOD MALDISTRIBUTION

Blood maldistribution is characterized by decreased peripheral vascular resistance and pooling of blood in peripheral tissues. This is caused by neural or cytokine-induced vasodilation that can result from situations such as trauma, emotional stress, systemic hypersensitivity to allergens, or endotoxemia. Systemic vasodilation results in a dramatically increased microvascular area, and although the blood volume is normal, the effective circulating blood volume is decreased. Unless compensatory mechanisms can override the stimulus for vasodilation, there is pooling and stagnation of blood with subsequent tissue hypoperfusion. The three major types of shock caused by blood maldistribution are anaphylactic, neurogenic, and septic shock.

Anaphylactic shock is a generalized type I hypersensitivity. Common causes include exposure to insect or plant allergens, drugs, or vaccines. The interaction of the inciting substance with immunoglobulin E bound to mast cells results in widespread mast cell degranulation and the release of histamine and other vasoactive mediators. Subsequently, there is systemic vasodilation and increased vascular permeability, causing hypotension and tissue hypoperfusion.

Neurogenic shock may be induced by trauma, particularly trauma to the nervous system; electrocution, such as by lightning strike; fear; or emotional stress. In contrast to anaphylactic and endotoxic shock, cytokine release is not a major factor in the initial peripheral vasodilation. Instead, there are autonomic discharges that result in peripheral vasodilation, followed by venous pooling of blood and tissue hypoperfusion.

Septic shock is the most common type of shock associated with blood maldistribution. In septic shock, peripheral vasodilation is caused by components of bacteria or fungi that induce the release of excessive amounts of vascular and inflammatory mediators. The most common cause of septic shock is endotoxin, a lipopolysaccharide (LPS) complex within the cell wall of Gram-negative bacteria. Less often, peptidoglycans and lipoteichoic acids of Gram-positive organisms initiate shock. Local release of LPS from degenerating bacteria is a potent stimulus for many of the host responses induced by the infectious agent. LPS often gains entry from microflora of the bowel, entering the circulation into

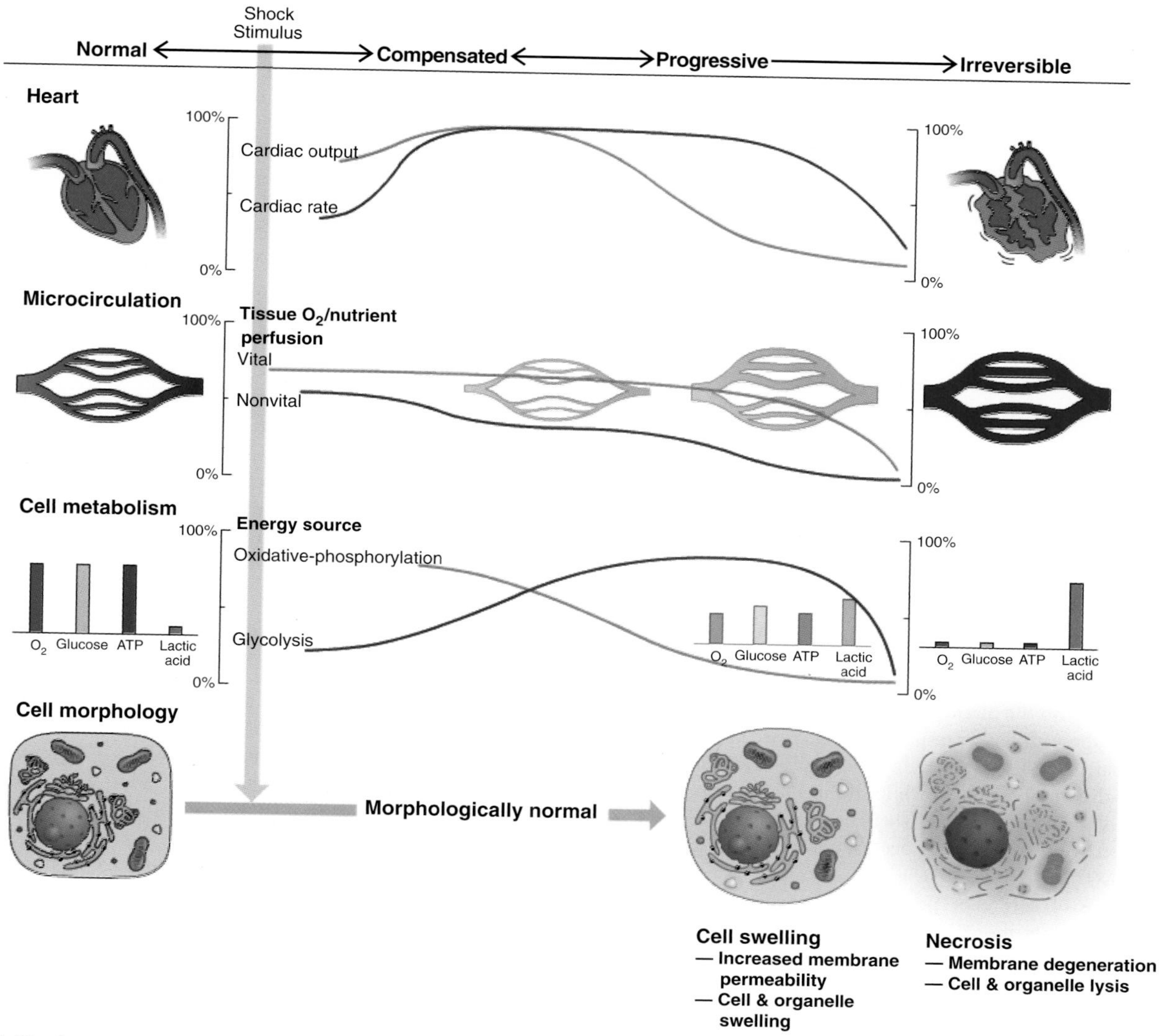

Fig. 2-43 Shock.
In hypovolemic shock, there is initially compensation characterized by increased cardiac rate and output, vasoconstriction of nonessential vascular beds, and predominantly oxidative metabolism by morphologically normal cells. With progression, cardiac output falls as peripheral vasodilation occurs, and cell metabolism shifts to glycolysis with progressive morphologic deterioration of cells. (Courtesy Dr. D.A. Mosier and L. Schooley, College of Veterinary Medicine, Kansas State University.)

the reticuloendothelial system, then accumulating in the liver, spleen, alveoli, and leukocytes. LPS activates cells (mainly endothelium and leukocytes) through a series of reactions involving LPS-binding protein (an acute phase protein), CD14 (a cell membrane protein and soluble plasma protein) and Toll-like receptor 4 (TLR4, a signal-transducing protein). Endothelial activation by LPS inhibits production of anticoagulant substances (e.g., TFPI and thrombomodulin). Activation of monocytes and macrophages by LPS induces the direct or indirect release of TNF and IL-1 and other cytokines (e.g., IL-6, IL-8, chemokines). LPS directly activates factor XII to initiate intrinsic coagulation and other factor XIIa–related pathways (kinins, fibrinolysis, complement). LPS can also directly activate the complement cascade to generate the anaphylatoxins C3a and C5a. Although these events are important for enhancing the inflammatory response to control localized infections associated with relatively low concentrations of LPS, they can be detrimental if the response becomes more pronounced. This may occur with overwhelming infections by bacteria (generating large concentrations of LPS), or when prolonged intestinal ischemia as the result of other types of shock results in breakdown of the mucosal integrity and leakage of bacteria and toxins into the blood. These higher concentrations of LPS induce even more production of TNF, IL-1, and other cytokines, and the secondary effects of these cytokines become more prominent. TNF and IL-1 induce TF expression and endothelial activation of extrinsic coagulation and enhance the expression of endothelial leukocyte adhesion molecules. IL-1 also stimulates the release of platelet-activating factor (PAF) and PAI to enhance platelet aggregation and coagulation. PAF released from leukocytes, platelets, and endothelium can cause platelet aggregation and thrombosis, increased vascular permeability, and similar to TNF and IL-1, stimulation of arachidonic acid metabolite production (particularly prostacyclin [PGI_2] and thromboxane). TNF and IL-1 induce nitric oxide production, which also contributes to vasodilation and hypotension. Neutrophils become activated by TNF and IL-1 to enhance their adhesion to endothelium, which further interferes with blood flow through the microvasculature. The end result of the activation of these myriad vascular, proinflammatory, and procoagulant alterations is the profound systemic vasodilation, hypotension, and tissue hypoperfusion characteristic of septic shock.

STAGES AND PROGRESSION OF SHOCK

Regardless of the underlying cause, shock generally progresses through three different stages: (1) a nonprogressive stage, (2) a progressive stage, and (3) an irreversible stage.

Nonprogressive shock is characterized by compensatory mechanisms that counteract reduced functional circulating blood volume and decreased vascular pressure. Baroreceptors respond to decreased pressure by increasing medullary sympathetic nervous output and epinephrine/norepinephrine release, which increases cardiac output and causes arteriolar vasoconstriction (increased peripheral resistance) in most tissues in an attempt to raise vascular pressure. Notable exceptions are critical tissues, such as the heart, brain, and kidney, to which the blood flow is preserved. Left atrial volume receptors and hypothalamic osmoreceptors help regulate pressure by altering water and sodium balance. Reduced plasma volume stimulates ADH release and water retention and activates angiotensin II production by the renin-angiotensin system to result in aldosterone release and sodium retention. ADH and angiotensin II are also vasoconstrictors and help contribute to increased peripheral resistance. Vasoconstriction also results from endothelial release of endothelin, cold, increased O_2, or decreased CO_2. Decreased microvascular pressure results in a shift in fluid movement from the interstitium into the plasma to also help increase blood volume. The results of these and other responses are increased heart rate and cardiac output, as well as increased vascular pressure. This provides an adequate driving force on which local mechanisms can draw on to increase blood flow based on their needs. When the insult is mild, compensation is generally successful and the animal returns to homeostasis.

In the case of severe or prolonged hypovolemia or cardiac damage that inhibits the ability of the heart to increase output, compensatory mechanisms are inadequate and shock enters the progressive stage. In this stage, there is blood pooling, tissue hypoperfusion, and progressive cell injury. Cellular metabolism becomes less efficient and shifts from aerobic to anaerobic with pyruvate converted to lactate without entering the Krebs cycle. The deficient production of ATP and overproduction of lactic acid inhibits normal cell functions and results in cellular and systemic acidosis. Metabolic products (e.g., adenosine and potassium), increased local osmolarity, local hypoxia, and increased CO_2 eventually result in arteriolar relaxation and dilation. In the case of septic shock, these events exacerbate preexisting cytokine- and mediator-induced vasodilation of the microvasculature. In hypovolemic and cardiogenic shock, the decreased vascular resistance initiates pooling and stagnation of blood within previously closed vascular beds. Widespread arteriolar dilation caused by local influences overrides systemic controls and dramatically contributes to further decreases in vascular plasma volume and pressure. When oxygen and energy stores of the cell are depleted, membrane transport mechanisms are impaired, lysosomal enzymes are released, structural integrity is lost, and cell necrosis occurs. In addition to the detrimental metabolic effects of deficient oxygenation, cell and tissue injury occur in response to the dramatic accumulation of mediators that is characteristic of progressive shock, regardless of its underlying cause. These include histamine, kinins, PAF, complement fragments, and a wide variety of cytokines (e.g., TNF, IL-1, IL-8). These mediators are associated with inappropriate systemic inflammation and systemic activation of complement, coagulation, fibrinolysis, and kinin pathways.

The exact point in which shock enters the irreversible stage is not clear. At the cellular level, metabolic acidosis that results from anaerobic metabolism inhibits enzyme systems needed for energy production. Decreased metabolic efficiency allows vasodilatory substances to accumulate in the ischemic cells and tissues. Once these local products and reflexes override centrally mediated vasoconstriction to produce vasodilation, it is unlikely that shock will be reversed. The fall in peripheral resistance as the result of widespread peripheral vasodilation decreases vascular pressure even more. Irreversibility is generally assured when shock progresses into the syndrome of multiple organ dysfunction. As each organ system fails, particularly the lung, liver, intestine, kidney, and heart, there is a reduction in the metabolic support each system provides to the others. Vicious cycles occur in which the failing function of one organ or tissue contributes to the failure of another (e.g., decreased cardiac output causes renal and pancreatic ischemia; electrolyte imbalances caused by renal ischemia then result in cardiac arrhythmias and myocardial depressant factor released by the ischemic pancreas contribute to even greater reductions in cardiac output). The endpoint of irreversible shock is often manifested as DIC, which is the profound and paradoxic dysfunction of hemostasis.

CLINICAL AND MORPHOLOGIC FEATURES OF SHOCK

Clinical features of shock are rapidly progressive and include hypotension, weak pulse, tachycardia, hyperventilation with pulmonary rales, reduced urine output, and hypothermia. Organ and system failure occurs in later stages, each manifesting with signs specific to that organ or tissue.

The lesions of shock are variable and depend on the nature and severity of the initiating stimulus and the stage of progression of shock. Characteristically, there are vascular changes accompanied by cell degeneration and necrosis. Generalized congestion and pooling of blood are present in most cases, unless there has been substantial blood loss. Edema, hemorrhage (petechial and ecchymotic), and thrombosis may be present as reflections of the vascular deterioration that accompanies shock. Thrombosis and platelet plugging of capillaries can be prominent in septic shock. Vascular abnormalities are most obvious in those cases that progress to DIC. Cell degeneration and necrosis are most prominent in those cells that are most susceptible to hypoxia, such as neurons and cardiac myocytes, and cells that do not obtain adequate preferential blood flow during shock. Hepatocytes, renal tubular epithelium, adrenal cortical epithelium, and gastrointestinal epithelium are often affected. With the exception of loss of neurons and myocytes, virtually all of these tissue changes can revert to normal if the animal survives. Specific changes may include severe pulmonary congestion, edema, and hemorrhage with alveolar epithelial necrosis, fibrin exudation, and hyaline membrane formation. Passive congestion and centrilobular hepatic necrosis, as well as renal tubular necrosis, are often present in these metabolically important organs. Intestinal congestion, edema, and hemorrhage with mucosal necrosis may occur. In the heart, myofibril coagulation is caused by hypercontraction of sarcomeres and is most likely a response to high sarcoplasmic calcium levels as the result of lack of energy and membrane damage. Cerebral edema and in some cases cerebrocortical laminar necrosis as a result of cerebral ischemia may be present.

SUGGESTED READINGS

Suggested Readings are available at evolve.elsevier.com/Zachary/McGavin/.

CHAPTER 3

Inflammation and Healing

Mark R. Ackermann

Injury or death of cells caused by infectious microbes, mechanical trauma, heat, cold, radiation, or cancerous cells can initiate a well-organized cascade of fluidic and cellular changes within living vascularized tissue called *acute inflammation* (Fig. 3-1). These changes result in the accumulation of fluid, electrolytes, and plasma proteins, as well as leukocytes, in extravascular tissue and are recognized clinically by redness, heat, swelling, pain, and loss of function of the affected tissue. Inflammation is often a protective mechanism whose biologic purpose is to dilute, isolate, and eliminate the cause of injury and to repair tissue damage resulting from the injury. Without inflammation, animals would not survive their daily interactions with environmental microbes, foreign materials, and trauma and with degenerate, senescent, and neoplastic cells.

Acute inflammation, a provoked response, is the progressive reaction of vascularized living tissue to injury over time. This process is usually a well-ordered cascade mediated by chemoattractants, vasoactive molecules, proinflammatory and antiinflammatory cytokines and their receptors, and antimicrobial or cytotoxic molecules. Acute inflammation has a short duration, ranging from a few hours to a few days, and its main characteristics are exudation of electrolytes, fluid, and plasma proteins and leukocytic emigration, principally neutrophils from the microvasculature, followed by rapid repair and healing. For convenience, acute inflammation is divided into three sequential phases: fluidic, cellular, and reparative.

Chronic inflammation is considered to be inflammation of prolonged duration, usually weeks to months and even years, in which the response is characterized predominately by lymphocytes and macrophages, tissue necrosis, and accompanied by tissue repair, such as healing, fibrosis, and granulation tissue formation, all of which may occur simultaneously. Chronic inflammation can be a sequela to acute inflammation if there is failure to eliminate the agent or substance that incites the process. With such persistent substances, the inflammatory reaction and exudates gradually transition from seroproteinaceous fluids and neutrophils to macrophages, lymphocytes, and fibroblasts with the potential for formation of granulomas. Alternatively, some inciting substances can invoke chronic inflammation directly and almost immediately. Examples include infections by *Mycobacterium* spp.; exposure to foreign materials, such as silicates and grass awns; and immune-mediated diseases, such as arthritis.

EVOLUTION OF THE CURRENT UNDERSTANDING OF INFLAMMATION

Information on this topic, including Web Table 3-1, is available at evolve.elsevier.com/Zachary/McGavin/. Web Appendix 3-1 on the accompanying website is a list of acronyms and their definitions as used throughout this chapter.

BENEFICIAL AND HARMFUL ASPECTS OF INFLAMMATION

As a general rule, inflammatory responses are beneficial in the following ways:

- Diluting and/or inactivating biologic and chemical toxins
- Killing or sequestering microbes, foreign material, necrotic tissue (e.g., bone sequestrum), and neoplastic cells
- Degrading foreign materials
- Providing wound healing factors to ulcerated surfaces and traumatized tissue
- Restricting movement of appendages and joints to allow time for healing and repair
- Increasing temperature in the body or locally to induce vasodilation and inhibiting replication of some microbial agents

However, in some instances, an excessive and/or prolonged inflammatory response can be detrimental and even more harmful than that of the inciting agent/substance. In several disorders of humans, such as myocardial infarction, cerebral thrombosis and infarction, and atherosclerosis, excessive and prolonged inflammatory responses can exacerbate the severity of the disease process. In veterinary medicine, exuberant or uncontrolled inflammatory responses occurring in the diseases listed in Box 3-1 can also result in increased severity of disease.

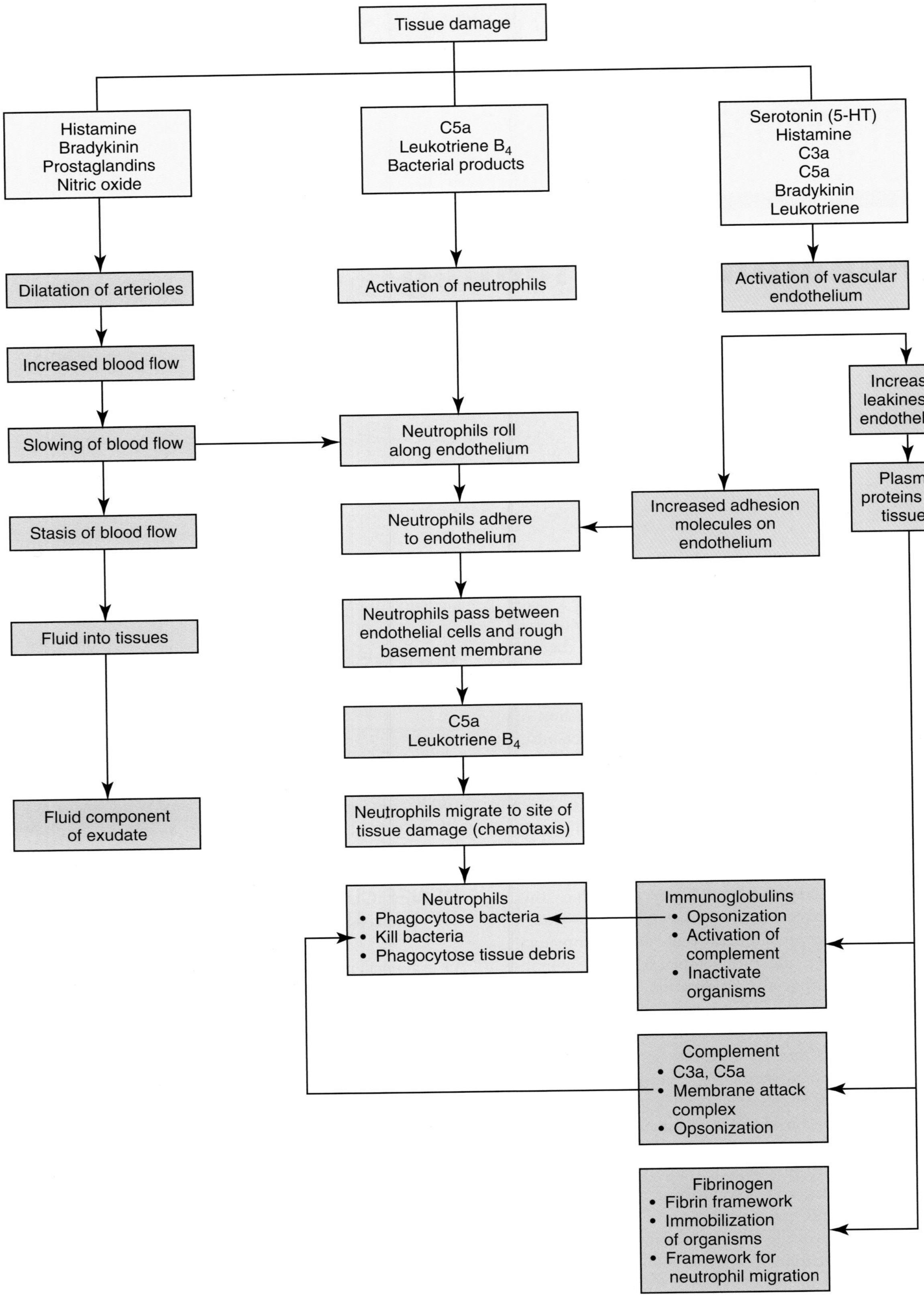

Fig. 3-1 The major steps of the acute inflammatory process.

(Modified from Young B, O'Dowd G, Stewart W: *Wheater's basic pathology: a text, atlas and review of histopathology*, ed 5, New York, 2010, Churchill Livingstone.)

BOX 3-1 Selected Disorders that Are Induced or Exacerbated by Inflammatory Responses

DISORDERS IN WHICH THE MECHANISM OF INJURY IS INFLAMMATION

Humans: Alzheimer's disease, atherosclerosis, atopic dermatitis, chronic obstructive pulmonary disease (COPD), Crohn's disease, gout, graft rejection, Hashimoto's thyroiditis, multiple sclerosis, pemphigus, psoriasis, rheumatoid arthritis, sarcoidosis, systemic lupus erythematosus (SLE), type I diabetes mellitus, ulcerative colitis, vasculitis (Wegener's granulomatosis, polyarteritis nodosa, Goodpasture's disease)

Cats: Eosinophilic stomatitis, lymphoplasmacytic syndrome, pemphigus

Dogs: Granulomatous meningoencephalitis, pemphigus, systemic and discoid lupus erythematosus

Common to many species: Anaphylaxis, spondylitis, asthma, reperfusion injury, osteoarthritis, glomerulonephritis

INFECTIOUS DISEASE EXACERBATED BY INFLAMMATION

Humans: dysentery, Chagas' disease, cystic fibrosis pneumonia, filariasis, *Helicobacter pylori* gastritis, hepatitis C, influenza virus pneumonia, leprosy, *Neisseria*/pneumococcal meningitis, poststreptococcal glomerulonephritis, schistosomiasis, sepsis, tuberculosis

Dogs: *H. pylori* gastritis

Cattle: *Mannheimia haemolytica* pneumonia, mastitis, *Mycobacterium bovis, Mycobacterium avium-intracellularis-paratuberculosis*

Pigs: Circovirus

Ferrets/mink: Aleutian mink disease

Common to many species: Vegetative valvular endocarditis

CONDITIONS IN WHICH POSTINFLAMMATORY FIBROSIS OCCURS

Humans: Bleomycin pulmonary fibrosis, allograft rejection, idiopathic pulmonary fibrosis, hepatic cirrhosis (postviral, alcohol, or toxin), radiation-induced pulmonary fibrosis

Dogs: Idiopathic pulmonary fibrosis (West Highland white dogs)

Cattle/sheep/horses: Plant toxins (hepatic fibrosis)

Modified from Nathan C: *Nature* 420:846-851, 2002.

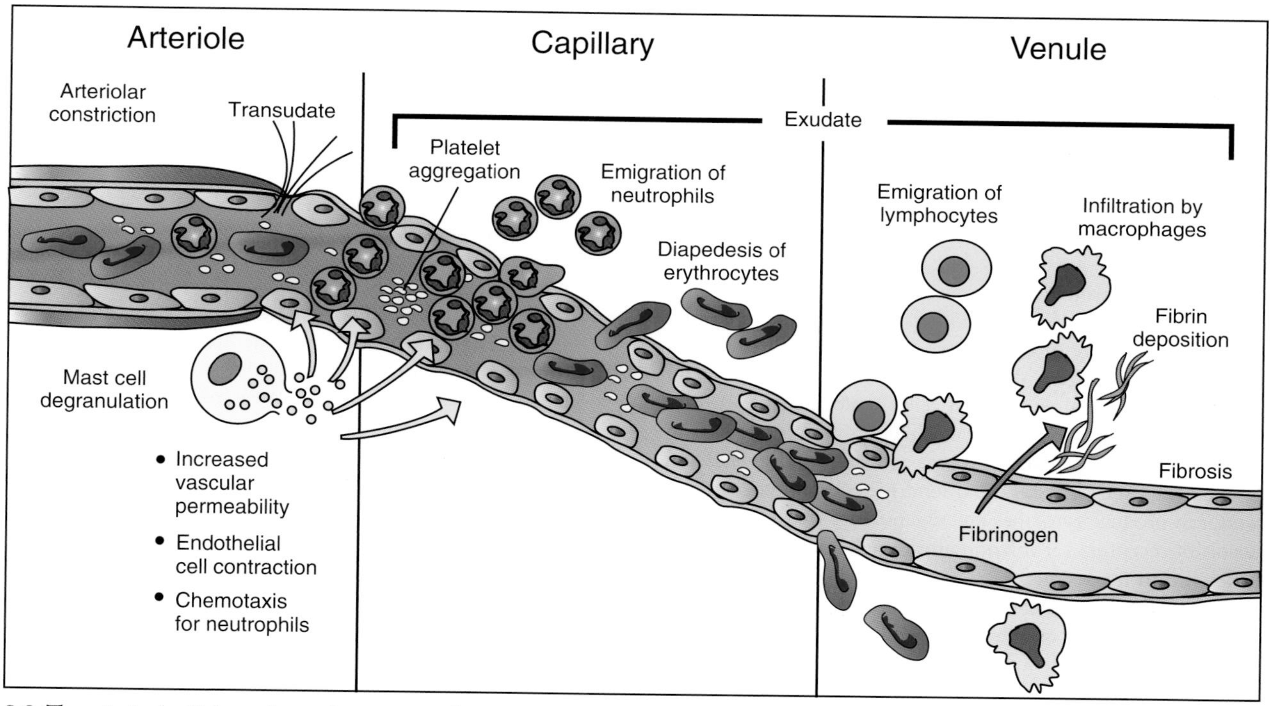

Fig. 3-2 The principal cellular and vascular responses during the inflammatory response.
The majority of leukocyte transmigration and hemorrhage occurs in the capillaries and postcapillary venules. (Modified from McCance KL, Huether SE: *Pathophysiology: the biologic basis for diseases in adults and children*, ed 3, St Louis, 1998, Mosby.)

ACUTE INFLAMMATION

The acute inflammatory response (Fig. 3-2) can be initiated by a variety of exogenous and endogenous substances that injure vascularized tissue. The response to injury begins as active hyperemia, characterized by an increased flow of blood to injured tissue secondary to dilation of arterioles and capillaries (vasodilation), and it is this response that is responsible for redness and heat. It is facilitated by chemical mediators such as prostaglandins, endothelin, and nitric oxide (Box 3-2). With vasodilation, vascular flow is slowed (vascular congestion), allowing time for fluid leakage that occurs as a result of changes in junctional complexes of endothelial cells induced by vasoactive amines, complement components C3a and C5a, bradykinin, leukotrienes, prostaglandins, and platelet-activating factor (PAF), resulting in leakage of plasma and plasma proteins into the extracellular space (swelling and pain [stretching

BOX 3-2 Key Responses of Acute Inflammation and the Principal Inflammatory Mediators that Mediate These Processes

VASODILATION
Nitric oxide
Bradykinin
Prostaglandins: PGD_2
Leukotrienes: LTB_4

INCREASED VASCULAR PERMEABILITY
Vasoactive amines: histamine, substance P, bradykinin
Complement factors: C5a, C3a
Fibrinopeptides and fibrin breakdown products
Prostaglandins: PGE_2
Leukotrienes: LTB_4, LTC_4, LTD_4, LTE_4
PAF, substance P
Cytokines: IL-1, TNF

SMOOTH MUSCLE CONTRACTION
Histamine
Serotonin
C3a
Bradykinin
PAF
Leukotriene D_4

CHEMOTAXIS, LEUKOCYTE ACTIVATION
Complement factors: C5a
Leukotrienes: LTB_4
Chemokines: IL-8
Defensins: α- and β-Defensins
Bacterial products: LPS, peptidoglycan, teichoic acid
Collagenous lectins: Ficolins, surfactant proteins A and D, mannan-binding lectin
Cytokines: IL-1, TNF
Surfactant proteins A and D

FEVER
Cytokines: IL-1, TNF, IL-6
Prostaglandins: PGE_2

NAUSEA
Cytokines: IL-1, TNF, high mobility group factors

PAIN
Bradykinin
Prostaglandins: PGE_2

TISSUE DAMAGE
Neutrophil and macrophage lysosomal/granule contents: Matrix metalloproteinases
Reactive oxygen species: Superoxide anion, hydroxyl radical, nitric oxide

C3a, Complement factor C3a; *C5a,* complement factor C5a; *IL-1,* interleukin-1; *IL-6,* interleukin-6; *IL-8,* interleukin-8; *LTB_4,* leukotriene B_4; *LTC_4,* leukotriene C_4; *LTD_4,* leukotriene D_4; *LTE_4,* leukotriene E_4; *PGD_2,* prostaglandin D_2; *PGE_2,* prostaglandin E_2; *TNF,* tumor necrosis factor.

of pain receptors]) mainly from interendothelial cell gaps in the postcapillary venules.

The volume and protein concentration of leaked fluid is a function of the size of gaps between endothelial cells and the molecular weight, size, and charge of electrolytes and plasma proteins, such as albumin and fibrinogen. With more severe injury resulting in destruction of individual endothelial cells, hemorrhage, as well as plasma and plasma proteins, can leak directly through a breach in the wall of the capillary or venule. Once activated, endothelial and perivascular cells, such as mast cells, dendritic cells, fibroblasts, and pericytes, can produce cytokines and chemokines that regulate the expression of receptors for inflammatory mediators and adhesion molecules within the lesions.

The plasma proteins and fluid that initially accumulate in the extracellular space in response to injury is classified as a transudate (Fig. 3-3). A transudate is a fluid with minimal protein (specific gravity <1.012 [<3 g of protein/dL]) and cellular elements (<1500 leukocytes/mL) and is essentially an electrolyte solution similar to that of plasma. Most commonly, the formation of a transudate occurs with hypertension, hypoproteinemia, and/or early in the acute inflammatory response. With these conditions, there is increased permeability because of small physiologic gaps between endothelial cells. Hypertension in veins and capillaries can be secondary to arterial hypertension or venous/lymphatic obstruction. Hypoproteinemia is often due to loss of albumin, the major intravascular colloidal protein, and an inability of the liver to rapidly synthesize replacement albumin. The loss of albumin allows intravascular fluid to move toward the extravascular colloids (extravascular proteins). Loss of albumin and other intracellular proteins can occur secondary to renal disease (urinary loss), severe burns, and severe hepatic disease (decreased albumin production). During the early stages of the acute inflammatory response, intercellular gaps form between endothelial cells caused by endothelial cell contraction. The gaps are very small and only allow water and electrolytes to pass through them. With persistent and widening endothelial gap formation or with endothelial cell injury, neutrophils and additional protein can enter injured areas resulting in the formation of an exudate (see Fig. 3-3). An exudate is an opaque and often viscous fluid (specific gravity >1.020) that contains more than 3 g of protein/dL and more than 1500 leukocytes/mL. As discussed in a later section, the morphologic classification of inflammatory responses into categories, such as serous, fibrinous, and/or suppurative, is based on the character of the fluid that leaks from the vessel and of the leukocytes that migrate from the vascular lumen into the extracellular space.

Fibrinogen is an important plasma protein in exudates that polymerizes in extravascular tissues to form fibrin (Fig. 3-4). Plasma dilutes the effects of the inciting stimulus, whereas polymerized fibrin confines the stimulus to an isolated area, thus preventing its movement into adjacent tissue. This confinement provides leukocytes with a well-defined target for migration during the cellular phase of the acute inflammatory response. Neutrophils are the first leukocytes to enter the exudate, and their accumulation in the exudate after they liquefy is termed *pus.* Neutrophils have a variety of cytoplasmic granules, such as lysosomes, that contain antimicrobial peptides and proteins, as well as matrix metalloproteinases, elastases, and myeloperoxidases. They kill pathogens and degrade foreign material by two mechanisms: (1) phagocytosis and fusion with primary and secondary lysosomes and (2) secretion of the contents of granules into the exudate. Because of the enzymes

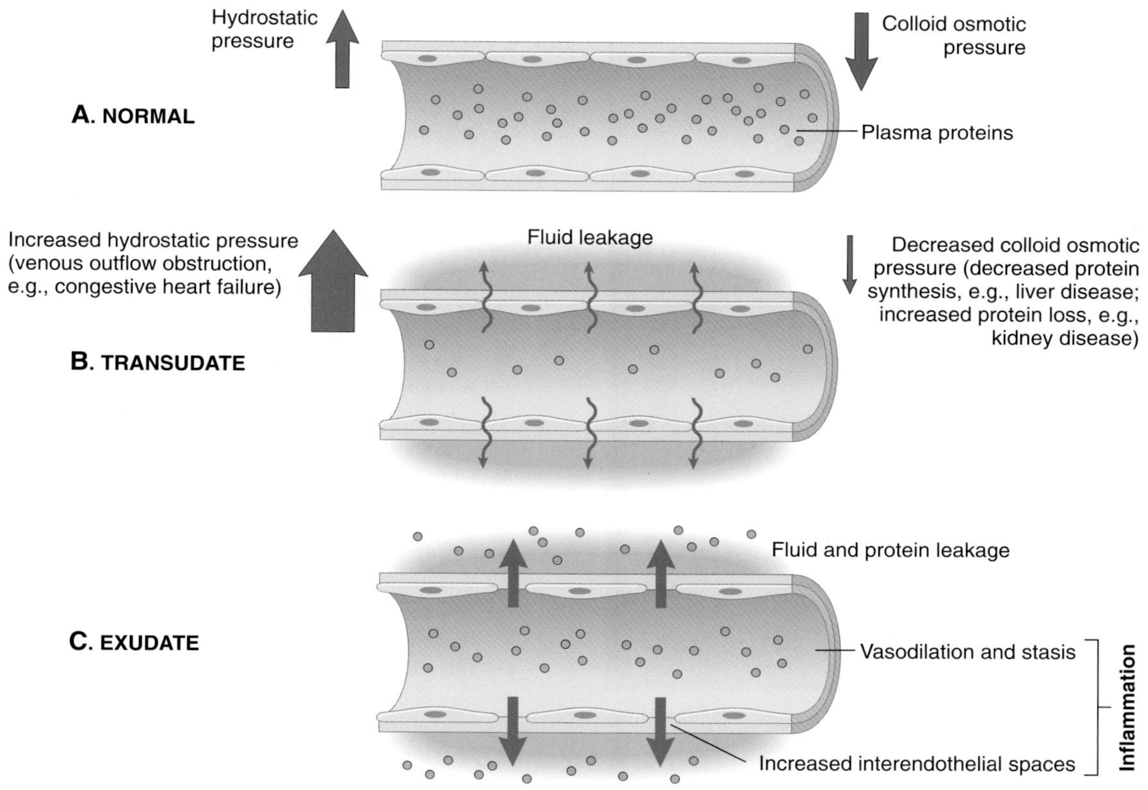

Fig. 3-3 Formation of transudates and exudates.
A, Normal hydrostatic pressure *(blue arrows)* is about 32 mm Hg at the arterial end of a capillary bed and 12 mm Hg at the venous end; the mean colloid osmotic pressure of tissues is approximately 25 mm Hg *(green arrows)*, which is equal to the mean capillary pressure. Therefore the net flow of fluid across the vascular bed is minimal. **B,** A transudate forms when fluid leaks out because of increased hydrostatic pressure or decreased osmotic pressure. **C,** An exudate forms in inflammation because vascular permeability increases as a result of increased interendothelial spaces. (From Kumar V, Abbas A, Fausto N, et al: *Robbins & Cotran pathologic basis of disease*, ed 8, Philadelphia, 2009, Saunders.)

released, these cells can contribute to tissue injury. Fibrin and its products have additional activities, including chemotactic properties and blood clot formation. Fibrin also forms a framework/scaffold for fibroblast and endothelial cell migration during the initial stages of wound healing.

Neutrophils and other leukocytes leave capillaries and venules and migrate into tissue exudates in response to chemoattractant molecules released from host cells, microbes, foreign substances, and some neoplastic cells. As would be expected, the greatest concentration of chemoattractant exists nearest the microbes or foreign substance, and the concentration decreases in a gradient-like manner with increasing distances from the source. This forms a "chemotactic gradient" that essentially creates a pathway for leukocytes to follow to reach the site of tissue injury. Chemoattractants activate receptors and molecules on neutrophils that result in neutrophil (1) movement and attachment to the luminal surface of capillaries and venules, (2) migration through the intercellular junctions formed by gaps between endothelial cells, and (3) migration within the exudate up the concentration gradient to the source of injury. This transmigration process, called the *leukocyte adhesion cascade,* has a well-characterized sequence of events occurring on the luminal surface of endothelial cells. These events, discussed in detail in a later section, lead to the transmigration of leukocytes into the exudate.

The reparative phase of the acute inflammatory response begins early and is only completed after the process or substance causing injury is removed. In the reparative phase, necrotic cells and tissue are replaced by differentiation and regeneration of parenchymal and mesenchymal stem cells, coupled by filling the defect with connective tissue and covering denuded surfaces with a basement membrane and reepithelialization. When the acute inflammatory response has been completed in the proper sequence and the stimulus of injury removed, the inflammatory process is terminated. Failure to remove the stimulus can result in a persistent, unresolved lesion that becomes chronic and can form into granulation tissue or fibrosis.

SUBSTANCES INDUCING THE ACUTE INFLAMMATORY RESPONSE

There are two classes of substances, endogenous and exogenous, capable of injuring cells and tissue and inducing the acute inflammatory response. Endogenous substances include those that primarily cause autoreactive inflammatory responses, such as those induced by newly developed antigens and intracellular molecules released from degenerate, dysplastic, or neoplastic cells, and hypersensitivity reactions. Exogenous substances include microbes, such as viruses, bacteria, protozoa, and metazoan parasites; foreign bodies, such as plant fibers and suture material; mechanical actions, such as traumatic injury; physical actions, such as thermal or freezing injury, ionizing radiation, and microwaves; chemical substances, such as caustic agents, poisons, and venoms; and nutritive actions, such as ischemia and vitamin deficiencies. These substances or actions

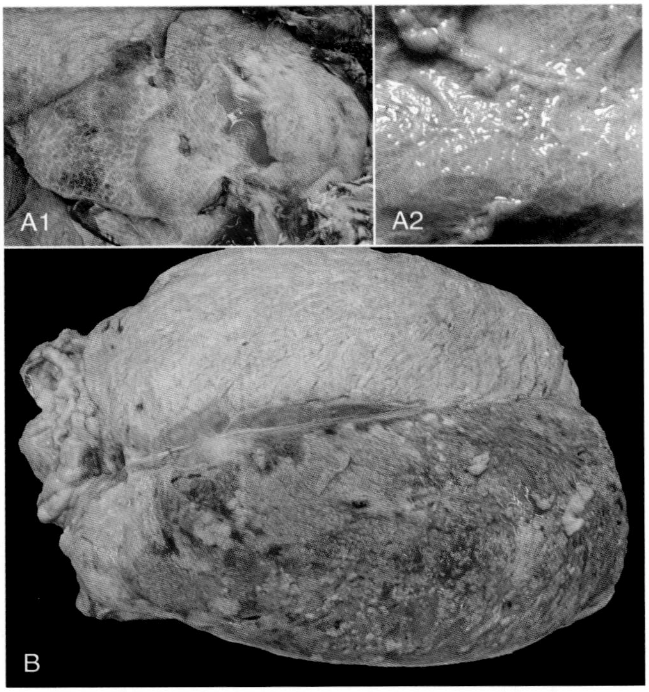

Fig. 3-4 Examples of the appearance of fibrin in acute inflammation in the lung and mammary gland.
A1, Lungs (in situ) from an ox with acute pleuritis. The lungs have a thick mat of fibrin covering the cranioventral region. A small area of fibrin is torn away revealing the subjacent clear, yellow fluid subjacent. The fibrin coating the lung surface was released as fibrinogen from inflamed pleural vessels and polymerized on the serosal surface. The remaining lung surface is less affected. **A2,** Higher magnification of fibrin on the surface of the lung. **B,** Acute fibrinonecrotic mastitis, mammary gland, horizontal section, cow. The left quarters of the mammary gland (lower half of the image) are swollen as a result of edema and fibrin exudation and are reddened because of hyperemia, vascular congestion, and hemorrhage. The right quarters (upper half of the image) are unaffected. (**A1** and **B** courtesy Dr. J.S. Haynes, College of Veterinary Medicine, Iowa State University; **A2** courtesy Dr. M.D. McGavin, College of Veterinary Medicine, University of Tennessee.)

trigger cells to release mediators that lead to an acute inflammatory reaction and include preformed (in cytoplasmic granules) and synthesized (released from cell immediately after synthesis) chemical mediators from effector cells such as mast cells (histamine and tumor necrosis factor-α [TNF-α), leukocytes (cytokines, degradative enzymes), macrophages (cytokines), endothelial and epithelial cells (chemokines, interferons). These cells also produce inflammatory mediators such as prostaglandins, leukotrienes, and PAF from products released from plasma membranes.

The acute inflammatory response to either endogenous or exogenous substances occurs simultaneously with activation of the innate immune system (see Chapter 5). Innate immunity is a nonspecific defense against potentially harmful environmental substances and consists of the following:

- Physical barriers and microenvironments provided by epithelia of the skin (low pH, lactic and fatty acids) and mucosae such as in the respiratory mucociliary escalator, reproductive tracts (secretions), and alimentary system (gastric and duodenal secretions, peristalsis, saliva)
- Molecular products released by mucosae including lactoferrin, antimicrobial peptides (α- and β-defensins, cathelicidins), and collectins. These products have immune activity but also contribute to proinflammatory and antiinflammatory reactions, leukocyte activation, and wound healing.
- Effector molecules in the blood, such as plasma proteases (complement, kinin, and clotting systems), and inflammatory mediators released from nerve fibers (sensory fibers, C-reactive fibers), such as substance P.

The physical and biologic processes that activate the acute inflammatory and innate immune responses can exert their actions directly on the following:

- Effector cells in mucosae and vascularized connective tissue
- Effector molecules in the blood, on endothelial cells
- A combination of these components

The location, severity, and clinical signs of the acute inflammatory response depend on the route of exposure, such as dermal, alimentary, respiratory, urinary, or hematogenous, and the physical or biologic characteristics of the stimulus. More specifically, causes of the acute inflammatory response include but are not limited to the following:

- Visible and ultraviolet light spectra (sunburn and photosensitization)
- Radiation, blunt force trauma (abrasion, bruising, incision, and laceration)
- Thermal injury (hot and cold)
- Chemotherapeutics
- Environmental chemicals
- Microbial molecules (lipids and proteins)
- Venom (insect, snake, and reptile)
- Responses of the adaptive immune system (type I to IV hypersensitivities) to microbial and environmental antigens

These must either penetrate (light spectra) or break/penetrate (microbes and foreign bodies) epithelial barriers of the skin and alimentary, urinary, and respiratory systems to irritate the tissue and incite an acute inflammatory response. Microbes have a few highly conserved ligands called *pathogen-associated molecular patterns* (PAMPs), and when in contact with mucosae, they immediately encounter cells that express membrane *pattern-recognition receptors* (PRRs), which include Toll-like receptors (TLRs), expressed on the cell surface or in its cytoplasm. These patterns include the lipopolysaccharide (LPS; Gram-negative bacterial cell wall), lipoteichoic acids (Gram-positive bacterial cell wall), mannose, peptidoglycan, bacterial DNA, *N*-formylmethionine (in bacterial proteins), double-stranded RNA (dsRNA; viruses), and glucans (fungal cell walls). When these molecular patterns are recognized by receptors, such as TLRs, on macrophages, leukocytes, and mucosal epithelia, they trigger the release of chemokines and cytokines and cellular activation, all of which initiate and/or participate in the acute inflammatory response and the innate immune response.

In contrast to the innate immune system, adaptive immunity results in an antigen-specific immune response characterized by the production of protective antibodies and effector leukocytes that attempt to eliminate the inciting cause of injury and the generation of memory cells that make subsequent adaptive immune responses against a specific microbial antigen more efficient and effective (see Chapter 5). Because acute inflammation is a vasocentric response, it would be reasonable to assume that just about any exogenous or endogenous cause could induce inflammation. This is true, but because the inflammatory response has numerous redundant checks and balances that regulate the occurrence and severity of expression of the response, harmful effects of inflammation are minimized.

The effects of inflammation are mediated through chemical mediators of inflammation, which include the following:

- Vasoactive amines such as histamine and serotonin
- Plasma proteases such as complement, kinin, and clotting system proteins
- Lipid mediators such as arachidonic acid metabolites and platelet-activating factor (PAF)
- Cytokines
- Chemokines
- Chemerin
- Nitric oxide (NO)

Mast cells are rich in histamine and many of the chemical mediators listed previously and are widely distributed in connective tissue adjacent to blood vessels. Changes in the permeability of these vessels in the fluidic phase of the acute inflammatory response often occur as the result of mast cell activation. Histamine, preformed in mast cell granules, is released through a process called *degranulation.* Bradykinin, another vasoactive amine, is produced where there is vascular and/or endothelial cell injury. Both histamine and bradykinin cause changes in the caliber of arterioles, capillaries, and postcapillary venules and permeability in capillaries and postcapillary venules. These occur early in the fluidic phase of the acute inflammatory response and are quickly followed by the cellular phase.

FLUIDIC (EXUDATIVE) PHASE OF THE ACUTE INFLAMMATORY RESPONSE

The principal function of the fluidic phase of the acute inflammatory response is to dilute and localize the inciting agent/substance. In this phase, there is an immediate vasocentric reaction (arterioles, capillaries, and postcapillary venules) to the inciting agent/substance. The sequence of vascular events in the acute inflammatory response includes the following:

- Increased blood flow (active hyperemia) to the site of injury
- Increased permeability of capillaries and postcapillary venules to plasma proteins and leukocytes through release of inflammatory mediators
- Emigration of leukocytes (via the leukocyte adhesion cascade) into the perivascular area

Initially, arterioles dilate and capillary beds in the affected area expand in volume to accommodate an increased blood flow (heat and redness) in response to the stimulus. Second, as a result of permeability changes induced by inflammatory mediators, blood flow through the capillary beds is slowed as a result of increased viscosity and hemoconcentration after leakage of water from capillary beds into extracellular space. Because of the reduced blood flow and pressure, microscopically, capillaries are often packed with erythrocytes and the microenvironment facilitates leukocytic margination along the luminal surface of endothelial cells. This stage precedes leukocyte emigration through intercellular junctions of endothelial cells into the extravascular space. Inflammatory mediators induce endothelial cell contraction, resulting in the formation of interendothelial cell gaps, which further allow fluid leakage and leukocyte migration. In general, the endothelium of the normal vascular capillaries limits exchange of molecules to those less than 69,000 MW, the size of albumin. The exchange of small molecules and water between the vessel lumen and the interstitial space is extremely rapid. For example, the water of plasma is exchanged with the water of the interstitial space 80 times before the plasma can move the entire length of the capillary. Physiologically, increased amounts of fluid can pass across the vascular wall when there is (1) excessive hydrostatic pressure caused by hypertension and/or sodium retention, (2) decreased plasma proteins (colloid), or (3) lymphatic and/or venous obstruction. If fluid leakage is excessive, edema (transudate) develops (see Fig. 3-3). If the leakage is not excessive and postcapillary venules and lymphatic vessels are functioning normally, all of the fluid released from arterioles and small capillaries is returned to the circulation via paracellular gaps of postcapillary venular and lymphatic vessels. During acute inflammatory responses, there is a net outflow of fluid from arterioles, capillaries, and venules into extracellular tissue, which overwhelms the capacity for resorption by postcapillary venules and lymphatic vessels).

ENDOTHELIAL CELL DYNAMICS DURING THE ACUTE INFLAMMATORY RESPONSE

Endothelial cells are the interface between plasma in the lumen and the perivascular connective tissue. They are polarized cells that have specific luminal versus abluminal surfaces, which serve the physiologic needs of the vascular bed of each organ. Transport across the endothelial cell layer occurs by (1) transcytosis (transcellular passage) via small vesicles and caveolae or (2) paracellular passage. Transcytosis, the process of transporting substances across the endothelium by uptake into and release from coated vesicles, facilitates the transport of albumin, low-density lipoproteins (LDLs), metalloproteinases, and insulin. Paracellular passage allows transport of water and ions between cells (cell junctions). Paracellular passage is especially active in postcapillary venules. Roughly 30% of endothelial cell junctions in postcapillary venules can open to a width of 6 mm, roughly the width of a red blood cell. Leakage of fluid from the vasculature can occur within seconds after the acute inflammatory response is induced.

The mechanisms of leakage (Fig. 3-5) depend on the biologic and physical characteristics of the inciting agent or substance and include the following:

- Opening of junctional complexes (endothelial gaps) between endothelial cells responding to inflammatory mediators
- Direct injury that results in necrosis and detachment of endothelial cells, as occurs with certain viral, protozoal infections, toxins, and radiation
- Leukocyte-dependent injury that results in necrosis and detachment of endothelial cells and is induced by enzymes and mediators released from leukocytes during the transmigration phase of the acute inflammatory response
- Increased endothelial cell transcytosis mediated by vascular endothelial growth factor (VEGF)

FORMATION OF ENDOTHELIAL CELL GAPS

Endothelial gaps, resulting in vascular leakage, can occur by (1) contraction (actin/myosin) of adjacent endothelial cells and through (2) the reorganization of the cytoskeletal microtubule and microfilament proteins within the endothelial cells. With both of these changes, gaps result from the opening of junctional complexes between endothelial cells. Gaps by cell contraction in postcapillary venules where there is a high density of receptors for histamine, serotonin, bradykinin, and angiotensin II. Gaps formed by cytoskeletal reorganization occur most commonly in postcapillary venules and to a lesser extent, in capillaries in response to cytokines, such as interleukin-1 (IL-1) and TNF and hypoxia. Gap formation is transient and lasts 15 to 30 minutes after the stimulus occurs.

Vascular leakage resulting from direct injury to endothelial cells can cause detachment of the cell from the underlying basement membrane. Such damage establishes conditions favorable for the activation and attachment of platelets, clotting, and complement cascades. This type of extravasation usually occurs immediately

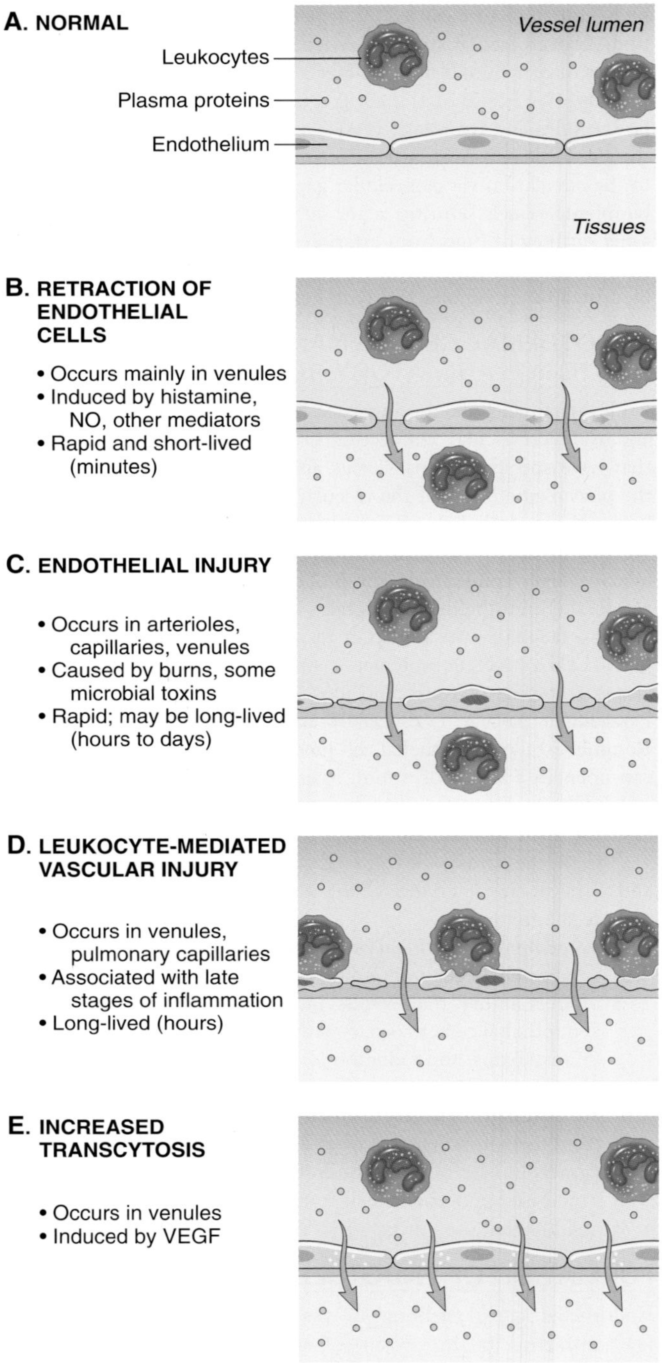

Fig. 3-5 Principal mechanisms of increased vascular permeability in inflammation and their features and underlying causes.
NO, Nitric oxide; *VEGF,* vascular endothelial growth factor. (From Kumar V, Abbas A, Fausto N, et al: *Robbins & Cotran pathologic basis of disease,* ed 8, Philadelphia, 2009, Saunders.)

after necrotizing injury induced by, for example, thermal injury, chemotherapeutic drugs, radiation, bacterial cytotoxins, and inhaled gases such as hydrogen sulfide. It affects arterioles, capillaries, and postcapillary venules. Vascular leakage resulting from leukocyte-induced damage occurs secondary to neutrophils and other leukocytes interacting with endothelial cells during the leukocyte adhesion cascade. Activated leukocytes release reactive oxygen species, such as singlet oxygen and oxygen free radicals, and proteolytic enzymes, such as matrix metalloproteinases and elastase from lysosomes during degranulation of the cells, which then result in endothelial cell necrosis and detachment and thus an increase in vascular permeability. This type of extravasation usually affects capillaries and postcapillary venules.

CELLULAR PHASE OF THE ACUTE INFLAMMATORY RESPONSE

The principal function of the cellular phase of the acute inflammatory response is to deliver leukocytes into the exudate at the site of injury so they can internalize agents/substances through phagocytosis and as required, for killing and/or degradation. Neutrophils, eosinophils, basophils, monocytes, mast cells, lymphocytes, natural killer T (NK-T) cells, and dendritic cells play an integral role in protecting mucosa, skin, and other surfaces of the body, as well as the pleura, pericardium, and peritoneum, from infection by microbes through phagocytosis or release of proteolytic degradative enzymes, chemical mediators, and reactive oxygen species. Neutrophils also have an important role in responding to foreign materials and toxins and in responding to neoplastic cells.

LEUKOCYTE ADHESION CASCADE

The movement of leukocytes from the lumina of capillaries and postcapillary venules into the interstitial connective tissue occurs through a process called the *leukocyte adhesion cascade* (Fig. 3-6). Chemokines, cytokines, and other inflammatory mediators influence this process by modulating the surface expression and/or avidity of adhesion molecules on both endothelial cells and leukocytes. It has a well-characterized sequence of events, including margination, rolling, activation and stable adherence (adhesion), and transmigration of leukocytes toward a chemotactic stimulus.

- *Margination.* As vessels vasodilate and have reduced hydrostatic pressure and blood flow, leukocytes exit the central region of the vascular lumen and move to the periphery of the vascular lumen near the endothelial cell surface (marginization).
- *Rolling.* The initial contact between leukocytes and endothelial cells occurs by transient, weak binding interactions between the selectin family of adhesion molecules and their receptors. During rolling, leukocytes temporarily bind to endothelium and then release, which brings the leukocyte close to endothelial cell surface and reduced velocity of the traveling leukocyte. This process is mediated by selectins, including L-selectin expressed by neutrophils and P-selectin, a carbohydrate binding molecule stored in Weibel-Palade bodies of endothelial cells and α-granules of platelets, as well as E-selectin expressed by endothelial cells. L-selectin is expressed on all leukocytes, but at low concentrations in normal human neutrophils and binds sialyl Lewis X receptor (and other receptors) on endothelial cells. P-selectin molecules expressed on endothelial cell surfaces bind to P selectin glycoprotein ligand 1 (sialyl Lewis X–modified proteins) present on neutrophils, eosinophils, monocytes, and lymphocytes. E-selectin also mediates leukocyte-endothelial cell adherence and is expressed on endothelial cell surfaces for binding glycoprotein receptors expressed on leukocytes. Selectin-mediated attachments are formed at the leading edge of the rolling leukocyte and broken at the trailing edge. Even slight disturbances, such as surgical manipulation, heat, temporary ischemia, and mast cell products, induce rolling of

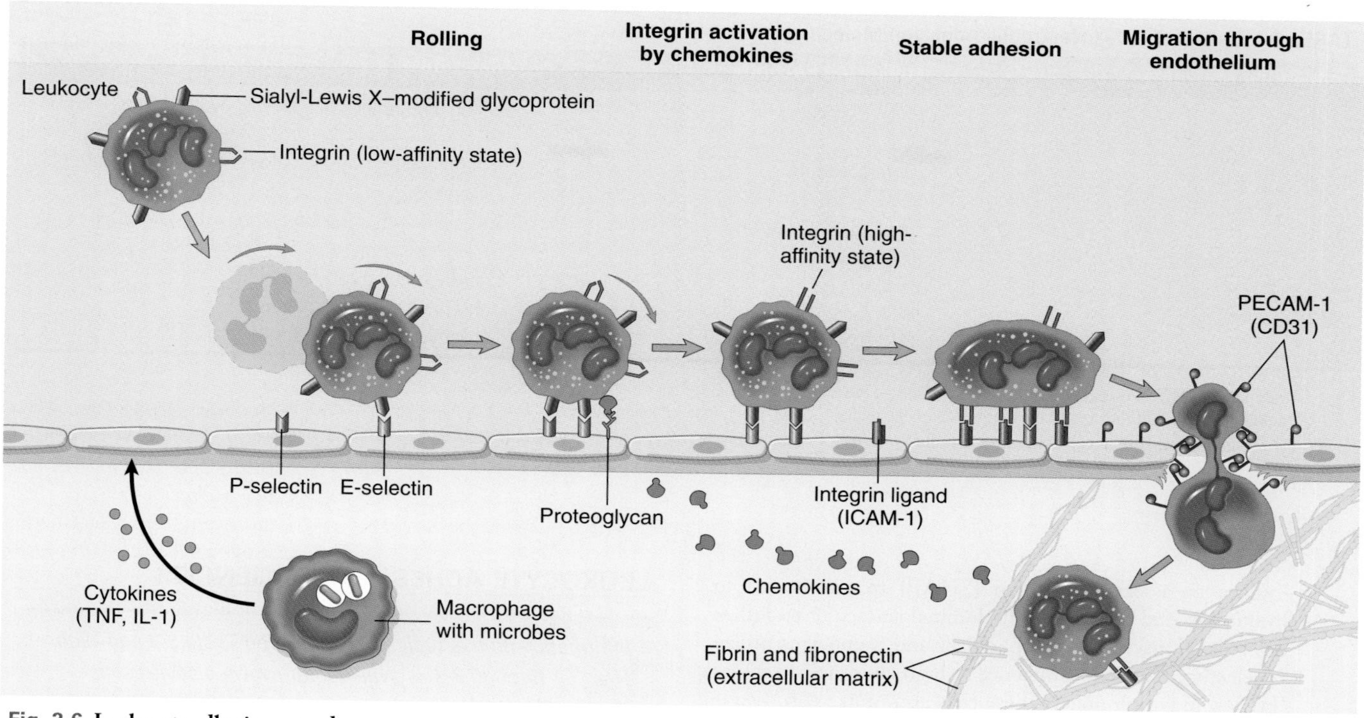

Fig. 3-6 Leukocyte adhesion cascade.
Steps involved with neutrophil migration across the vascular wall include rolling, activation, stable adhesion, and migration across the endothelial layer and vascular wall. Neutrophils express receptors for E- and P-selectin, which bind to ligands expressed on endothelial cells. L-selectin is also expressed by bovine neutrophils and to a varying degree in other species. The rolling process slows neutrophil movement within the vessel and brings the neutrophil closer to the vascular endothelial cell surface. Activation is induced by inflammatory mediators, including chemokines, such as interleukin-8 (IL-8), and cytokines, such as interleukin-1β (IL-1β) and tumor necrosis factor-α (TNF-α), which are released by nearby leukocytes and endothelial cells. These activate both neutrophils and endothelial cells which then changes the conformation of integrins allowing for enhanced binding avidity to integrin receptors and increased expression of additional adhesion molecules. Binding of β_2 integrins (Mac-1; CD11a/CD18) expressed by leukocytes to intercellular adhesion molecule-1 (ICAM-1) expressed by endothelial cells leads to stable adherence of the cell to the endothelial cell surface. Once leukocytes are attached to the vascular endothelium, they adhere to platelet-endothelial cell adhesion (PECAM-1) and other junctional adhesion molecules present at the endothelial cell junction and transmigrate through the junction into the perivascular tissue, where they express β_1 integrins that adhere to extracellular matrix proteins such as laminin, fibronectin, vitronectin, and collagen. The process is mediated by chemokines (CXCL8; IL-8), complement fragments, vasoactive amines, cytokines, and membrane-derived mediators such as platelet-activating factor (PAF) and leukotrienes. (From Kumar V, Abbas A, Fausto N, et al: *Robbins & Cotran pathologic basis of disease*, ed 8, Philadelphia, 2009, Saunders.)

neutrophils along the surface of endothelial cells. By slowing leukocyte transit time through capillaries and postcapillary venules, combined with the continual close proximity of slow rolling leukocytes to the endothelium, and the continued release of chemokines and proinflammatory cytokines, the proper microenvironment for progression to the "stable adhesion" stage occurs.

- *Stable adhesion.* For stable adhesion to occur, neutrophils and endothelial cells become activated by a variety of cytokines (such as IL-1, interleukin-6 [IL-6], TNF), complement factors (C5a), PAF, platelet-derived growth factor (PDGF), chemokines, and other inflammatory mediators. Once neutrophils are activated, L-selectin molecules are proteolytically cleaved from the neutrophil surface by ADAM17, and the neutrophils express a new set of membrane proteins (integrins) by rapid exocytosis of cytoplasmic vesicles. Firm adhesion of neutrophils to endothelial cells is mediated by binding of β_2 integrin molecules, such as Mac-1 (CD11a/CD18), that are expressed on stimulated neutrophils in an active conformation, to intercellular adhesion molecule-1 (ICAM-1) and other ICAM molecules on endothelial cells. P- and E-selectin adherence also contributes to the process of firm adhesion. There are four β_2 integrins (lymphocyte function antigen-1 [LFA-1], Mac-1, p150,95, and $\alpha d\beta_2$), each of which are heterodimers that differ only in their subunit CD11 a, b, c, and d for LFA-1, Mac-1, p150,95, and $\alpha d\beta_2$, respectively. CD18 (the β-subunit) is identical in all four β_2 integrins. Three β_2 integrins (LFA-1, Mac-1, and p150,95) are involved with leukocyte adherence; however, the β_2 integrin $\alpha d\beta_2$, which was first identified in dogs and subsequently in humans, is apparently not meaningfully involved with the adherence of neutrophils or other leukocytes to endothelium. Once stable adherence is achieved, neutrophils move to endothelial cell junctions for transendothelial cell migration.
- *Transendothelial cell migration.* In postcapillary venules, neutrophil movement decreases from 10 μm/sec to a complete stop after margination. Firmly adhered leukocytes emigrate (transmigrate) across the endothelial layer by passing between endothelial cells. A number of leukocyte adhesion molecules are involved in this process (Table 3-1). Adhesion molecule activity and expression differ slightly for different tissues and cell types. In noninflamed skin, for example, there is a higher level of E- and P-selectin expression on endothelial cells, which facilitates rolling of leukocytes. In inflamed liver, CD44 of neutrophils binds serum-derived

TABLE 3-1 Endothelial Cell/Neutrophil Adhesion Molecules

Endothelial Molecule	Leukocyte Receptor	Major Role
P-selectin	Sialyl-Lewis X PSGL-1	Rolling (neutrophils, monocytes, lymphocytes)
E-selectin	Sialyl-Lewis X ESL-1, PSGL-1	Rolling, adhesion to activated endothelium (neutrophils, monocytes, T-lymphocytes)
ICAM-1	CD11/CD18 (integrins) (LFA-1, Mac-1)	Adhesion, arrest, transmigration (all leukocytes)
PECAM-1	PECAM-1	Transendothelial cell migration
JAM A	JAM A, LFA-1	Transendothelial cell migration
JAM C	JAM B, Mac-1	Transendothelial cell migration

From Cotran RS, Kumar V, Collins T, et al: *Robbins pathologic basis of disease*, ed 7, Philadelphia, 2005, Saunders.
ESL-1, E-selectin ligand-1; *ICAM-1*, intercellular adhesion molecule-1; *JAM*, junctional adhesion molecule; *LFA-1*, lymphocyte function antigen-1; *Mac-1*, macrophage antigen-1; *PECAM-1*, platelet endothelial cell adhesion molecule-1; *PSGL-1*, P-selectin glycoprotein ligand-1; *VCAM-1*, vascular cell adhesion molecule-1; *VLA*, very late antigen.

hyaluronan-associated protein (SHAP) that is bound to hyaluronic acid present on the luminal surface of endothelial cells. Nonactivated lymphocytes and monocytes utilize L-selectin to mediate adherence to high endothelial venules (HEVs) in lymph nodes. These cells also utilize $\alpha_4\beta_1$ (very-late antigen-4 [VLA-4]) to mediate stable adherence to the endothelial ligand, vascular cell-adhesion molecule-1 (VCAM-1). Neutrophils and other leukocytes transmigrate between endothelial cells at the intercellular junctions. Platelet-endothelial cell adhesion molecule-1 (PECAM-1), a molecule that is present on endothelial cell membranes, and junctional adhesion molecules (JAM) A, B, and C mediate adherence activities and the adherence process. Contributions to this process also include β_2 integrin binding of ICAM-1 and E-selectin binding. Pseudopodia of neutrophils and other leukocytes extend between endothelial cells and come into contact with and bind to the basement membrane (composed of laminin and collagens) and subjacent extracellular matrix (ECM) proteins (proteoglycans, fibronectin, and vitronectin). This binding interaction is mediated, at least in part, by the β_1 integrins. Neutrophils that pass across the vascular wall accumulate in the perivascular connective tissue stroma within the inflammatory exudate. Once within the perivascular stroma, neutrophils migrate along a pathway established by the chemotactic gradients and inflammatory mediators.

This process is actually initiated during the fluidic phase of the acute inflammatory response and is driven by chemokines, cytokines, and chemoattractant substances such as complement. Temporally, margination, rolling, activation and firm adhesion, and transmigration all occur concurrently, involving different leukocytes in the same capillaries and postcapillary venules. This process is largely mediated by the interaction of ligands expressed on the surface of neutrophils, lymphocytes, and macrophages and their receptors expressed on luminal surfaces of activated endothelial cells (see Table 3-1). Adhesion molecules are divided into (1) selectins (E-, L-, and P-selectin), (2) integrins (VLA family of β_1 integrins; β_2 integrins [Mac-1, LFA-1, p150,95, $\alpha d\beta_2$]), (3) cytoadhesin family (vitronectin, β_3 integrins, and β_7 integrins used predominately by lymphocytes), (4) the immunoglobulin superfamily (ICAM-1 to ICAM-3, VCAM-1, PECAM-1) and mucosal addressin adhesion molecule-1 (MAdCAM-1), and (5) other molecules such as CD44 (Web Table 3-2).

LEUKOCYTE ADHESION DEFICIENCIES

Information on this topic, including Web Table 3-3 and Web Figs. 3-1 through 3-3, is available at evolve.elsevier.com/Zachary/McGavin/.

THERAPEUTIC STRATEGIES TO MODULATE LEUKOCYTE INFILTRATION

Information on this topic is available at evolve.elsevier.com/Zachary/McGavin/.

ADDITIONAL REGULATION OF INFLAMMATION

There are many regulatory mechanisms that closely control the onset, intensity, duration, and resolution of inflammation. In addition to those discussed, additional factors influence the type of inflammatory response by specific individuals. These include mechanisms that affect the expression level and activity of individual inflammatory genes and gene products. First, single nucleotide polymorphisms (SNPs) within the pyrin domain of the inflammasome receptor allow enhanced IL-1β production in patients with familial Mediterranean fever. SNPs in TLR are associated with altered responses to ligands and thus altered inflammatory responses. Similarly, SNP alterations in expression or regulation cytokines, chemokines, and their receptors can change the type and magnitude of inflammatory reactions. Second, premature truncation codons (PTC) are genes with stop codons within a critical location resulting in truncation of the mRNA and protein product. Thus the protein product, whether a cytokine or other inflammatory molecule, has an altered function or may even lack function. Third, gene copy number (the number of copies of a gene in a chromosome) directly affects the amount of protein produced. Some antimicrobial peptides have low gene copy numbers, therefore there is a very limited amount of peptide produced even in the presence of inflammatory stimuli. Fourth, there are latent forms of some molecules such as transforming growth factor-β (TGF-β). The latent forms are present within the tissue stroma and become functional on activation by matrix metalloproteinases. Fifth, there are isoforms of some genes that inhibit activity. VEGF-A, for example, has an isoform that when bound to the VEGF receptor-2 (VEGFR-2) reduces rather than enhances signaling. Sixth, there are soluble receptors such as soluble ICAM-1, which bind ligands but do not transmit signals because the receptor is detached from a cell.

EFFECTOR CELLS OF THE ACUTE INFLAMMATORY RESPONSE

VASCULAR ENDOTHELIAL CELLS

Central to the integrity of the vasculature and any type of acute inflammation is the endothelial cell. Once considered a cell that, in the most simplistic view, forms separation between the blood and the surrounding tissue, endothelial cells are now known to have an extremely sophisticated role in regulating (1) hemostasis/coagulation, (2) vascular pressure, (3) angiogenesis during wound healing, (4) carcinogenesis, (5) leukocyte homing, and (6) inflammation. Under physiologic conditions, transcytosis (transcellular passage) of albumin, LDLs, metalloproteinases, and insulin occur via small vesicles and caveolae in the cytoplasm of the endothelial cell. Paracellular passage (between cell junctions) of water and ions occurs with endothelial cell contraction secondary to physiologic stimuli and/or inflammatory mediators. Secondary to inflammatory mediators, endothelial cells are activated and contract, allowing fluid to lead into the extravascular tissue. Vascular tone is held in check in part by endothelin, a vasoconstrictive molecule and angiotensin II, both of which are produced by endothelial cells, along with vasodilatory substances such as NO and prostacyclin (PGI_2). Activated endothelial cells release these chemical mediators and express adhesion molecules and receptors, including E-selectin, P-selectin, L-selectin ligand, PECAM-1, JAM A, JAM B, and JAM C, and the immunoglobulin superfamily such as ICAM-1. These adhesion molecules serve as ligands for leukocyte adherence. With the onset of inflammation, endothelial cells tend to increase procoagulative properties through release of tissue factor and other procoagulative substances.

MAST CELLS AND BASOPHILS

The origin and relationship between mast cells and basophils has been a traditional point of debate and confusion. Current research clearly indicates that mast cells and basophils represent distinct cell types even though they share several morphologic and functional characteristics. Mast cells and basophils, along with other granulocytes and monocytes, originate and differentiate in bone marrow from a common CD34+ precursor cell. Differentiation of CD34+ precursor cells into mast cells or basophils depends on stem cell factor, a glycoprotein that acts with other cytokines and is produced in the bone marrow by fibroblasts and vascular endothelial cells. There is no evidence to suggest that basophils differentiate into tissue mast cells.

Mammalian mast cells are normally distributed throughout connective tissue adjacent to small blood and lymphatic vessels of skin and mucous membranes. In this location, they respond rapidly to foreign proteins, microbes, and other substances and contribute significantly to the initiation of acute inflammation. This location also allows mast cells to interact with resident dendritic cells and release inflammatory mediators that activate endothelial cells. Experimental studies suggest that cutaneous mast cells in tissue have a lifespan of 4 to 12 weeks, depending on their location. Mast cells represent an extremely heterogeneous population of cells. In the 1960s, Enerback identified two separate types of mast cells: mucosal and connective tissue. The mucosal mast cells are typically located in the respiratory and intestinal mucosa and can increase in numbers during some types of T helper 2 (T_H2) lymphocyte–dependent immune responses. In contrast, the connective tissue mast cells show little or no T lymphocyte dependence. Mast cells express high affinity receptors for immunoglobulin E (IgE; Fc ε-RI) on their surface, and the release of mast cell granules is stimulated by the cross-linking of IgE receptors by antigens such as pollens, allergens, and parasites. Substance P released from sensory (C-reactive) nerve fibers and macrophages also causes degranulation of mast cells. Degranulation results in the release of preformed TNF-α histamine, neutral proteases, proteoglycans (chondroitin sulfates and heparin), serotonin (in rodent species but not humans), tryptase, chymase, and stem cell factor into tissue. Histamine and substance P activity appears interrelated because histamine released by mast cells can downregulate the release of substance P by nerve fibers, thereby reducing excessive amounts of the two proinflammatory molecules. The mast cell–substance P fiber interrelationship is an often-cited example of the neuroinflammatory-neuroimmune pathway.

Mast cells also synthesize leukotriene (LT) C_4 (LTC_4), PAF, prostaglandin (PG) D_2 (PGD_2), numerous cytokines, serotonin (in some species), heparin, and C-C chemokines (macrophage inflammatory protein [MIP]-1-α and macrophage chemotactic protein [MCP]-1). The release of these mediators contributes significantly to the initiation of the acute inflammatory response. In addition, at physiologic concentrations these products likely counteract the effects of dense populations of mast cells in tissue and thus assist in regulating vascular permeability. Mast cells also release proteolytic enzymes, such as tryptase and chymase, which are involved with remodeling of the ECM. Tryptase is mitogenic to epithelial cells and likely contributes to proliferation of epithelial cells during wound repair.

Basophils are similar to neutrophils and eosinophils in that they mature in the bone marrow, circulate in the peripheral blood, are recruited into the tissue, and have a lifespan of several days in tissue. Basophils express high affinity IgE receptors, similar to mast cells, and release granules and inflammatory mediators. Basophils appear to lack heparin, have a more limited cytokine repertoire than mast cells, and release mainly IL-4 and IL-13. Basophils express CD40L and CCR3 (eotaxin receptor). The presence of these suggests that they have a role as a cell that can enter sites of inflammation, release regulatory cytokines where they upregulate VCAM-1 expression by endothelial cells, and switch B lymphocytes to produce IgE, further contributing to the IgE type of response. Basophils can be prominent in IgE-mediated leukocyte infiltration into the mucosa of the nose, sinuses, respiratory tract, and skin, and all of these sites are particularly predisposed to allergic conditions.

The role of mast cells and basophils in IgE-mediated hypersensitivity reactions has been known for decades. These cells are critical effector cells in disorders of IgE-dependent immediate type I hypersensitivities (see Chapter 5). The release of their granules and mediators at inflammatory concentrations in the lung, for example, results in mucus secretion, accumulation of seroproteinaceous fluid in airways, bronchoconstriction, and vasodilation. The excessive release of tryptase and chymase by mast cells may enhance degradation of the ECM, which contributes to fibrosis and tissue remodeling. Chemokines and cytokines from mast cells and basophils contribute to innate immune defenses through chemotaxis and release of antimicrobial peptides. The mediators also enhance adhesion molecule expression on endothelial cells of nearby blood vessels and leukocytes that enter the area.

NEUTROPHILS

Neutrophils are often the first type of leukocyte recruited into the inflammatory exudate. Their purpose is to (1) kill microbes, such as bacteria, fungi, protozoa, and viruses; (2) kill tumor cells; or (3) eliminate foreign materials. The biologic activities of neutrophils are primarily designed to kill microbes through lysosomal degradation, but if killing does not occur, neutrophils can limit the growth of microbes, allowing time for adaptive immunologic responses to develop.

Neutrophils perform two important functions to accomplish their effects: (1) phagocytosis of microbes or foreign material and then fusion of the phagosome with primary lysosomes to form a phagolysosome in which the microbes or foreign material are killed or degraded, respectively (Web Fig. 3-4), and (2) secretion and/or release of the contents of their granules into the inflammatory exudate to enhance the acute inflammatory response. They also infiltrate areas of acute tissue necrosis, such as those that occur in infarcts and necrotic areas of tumors.

Neutrophils are produced in the bone marrow, circulate in the bloodstream, and if not recruited into tissue by an acute inflammatory response, can enter tissue where they eventually are destroyed by macrophages via apoptosis and phagocytosis or are lost from the body by migration across mucosae such as the alimentary and respiratory tracts. The average transit time in the blood is 10 hours, and the half-life in the blood varies between species but ranges from 5 to 10 hours; neutrophils within tissue survive from 1 to 4 days. Cytokines, such as IL-1 and TNF, and growth factors, such as granulocyte-macrophage colony-stimulating factor (GM-CSF), granulocyte colony-stimulating factor (G-CSF), and IL-3 can increase release of neutrophils from the bone marrow and induce granulopoiesis in 2 to 4 days. GM-CSF and G-CSF are also present in tissue during acute inflammatory response and prevent apoptosis of tissue neutrophils. Within areas of intense inflammation, neutrophils and other leukocytes must function under hypoxic conditions and do so through the stabilization of hypoxia-inducible factor-1α (HIF-1α). HIF-1α induces transcription of genes that promote phagocytosis, inhibition of apoptosis, release of antimicrobial peptides, granule proteases, VEGF, cytokine release, and inducible NO synthetase (iNOS). Growth factor withdrawal, which occurs during resolution of acute inflammation, induces apoptosis, and this outcome can be accelerated by TNF. During apoptosis, neutrophils lose the capacity to degranulate and become activated, which prevents release of their lysosomal enzymes and thus excessive tissue damage and allows for their phagocytosis by macrophages.

Neutrophils entering tissue become activated, which enhances migration, phagocytosis, and microbial killing, through stimulation by inflammatory mediators and by adherence to ligands by surface adhesion molecules. Inflammatory mediators bind receptors on neutrophils, such as receptors for PAF, C5a, IL-8 and substance P (the neurokinin-1 receptor), leukotrienes, kallikrein, GM-CSF, and cytokines such as TNF. Many of these mediators induce chemotaxis; when leukocyte adhesion molecules, such as the selectins and integrins, bind to their respective ligands, they induce mitogen-activated protein kinase (MAPK) and G proteins, resulting in migration of neutrophils, usually toward a chemotactic gradient and activation.

Neutrophils can internalize large particles up to 0.5 μm in diameter by phagocytosis, including microbes, foreign bodies, senescent cells, and debris. Although neutrophils can internalize nonopsonized particles, opsonization greatly facilitates phagocytosis. The principal opsonin receptors present on neutrophil membranes are complement (CR1 and CR3) and Fc receptors (Fc γ-receptor I, IIA, IIIB), which bind complement fragments (C3b and C3bi) and the Fc portion of immunoglobulins such as IgG1 and IgG3. Such binding initiates activity of the guanosine triphosphatase (GTPase) Rac1 and the β2 integrin Mac-1 (CD11b/CD18), which also binds complement fragment C3bi and initiates GTPase-ρ. Such binding-inducing proteins and lipid kinases (e.g., protein kinase C and phosphatidylinositol 3-kinase) mediate actin assembly for formation of filopodia or lamellipodia, which surround and then internalize particles via phagocytosis by activated neutrophils. The activation process also leads to the release of calcium stored in the endoplasmic reticulum, which induces a respiratory (oxidative) burst (Table 3-2). Oxidative burst is the process by which nicotinamide adenine dinucleotide phosphate (NADPH) oxidase composed of five phox protein subunits in the membrane of phagosomes is formed. It catalyzes the formation of superoxide free radical that is used to kill microbes or degrade internalized material. Superoxide can react to form hydrogen peroxide, and additional free radicals such as hydroxyl radical, and hypochlorous acid. Neutrophils also express iNOS, which generates NO, and myeloperoxidase, which also produces hypochlorous acid. Superoxide anion and NO can form peroxynitrite, which is highly reactive.

Once a particle is internalized, phagosomes can "mature" by fusing with lysosomes and endosomes or remove parts of internalized particles. The fusion process is likely mediated by calmodulin, a calcium-binding protein, and soluble *N*-ethylmaleimide-sensitive factor (NSF) attachment protein receptors (SNARE; a fusion protein) that bind ligands on another vesicle to bring the membranes together for fusion. The maturation process results in lowering of the pH within the phagosome and the activation of microbicidal enzymes, including NADPH oxidase and myeloperoxidase complexes. Smaller particles are internalized by receptor-mediator endocytosis.

The ability of neutrophils to kill microbes or to degrade foreign material depends largely on the contents of the neutrophil granules, which store degradative enzymes, peroxidative enzymes, adhesion molecules, and antimicrobial peptides and/or proteins (Web Box 3-1). Myeloperoxidase is an enzyme used to convert hydrogen peroxide to hypochlorous acid. Hypochlorous acid, hydrogen peroxide, and a halide cofactor (chloride) form the myeloperoxidase system, which is an effective microbicidal mechanism used by neutrophils to kill internalized microbes and degrade internalized substances. Defensins, cathelicidins, and antimicrobial proteins contribute to the degradation of microbes by forming pores in microbial membranes. They also affect chemotaxis and activation of the adaptive immune response. Lactoferrin inhibits the growth of phagocytosed bacteria by sequestering free iron, and elastase hydrolyzes bacterial cell wall proteins and tissue elastin. The enzymatic contents of granules, such as gelatinase (matrix metalloproteinase-9 [MMP-9]) and myeloperoxidase, and nonenzymatic substances, such as antimicrobial peptides and lactoferrin, are also commonly released by the cell into the extracellular space and contribute to killing of extracellular microbial pathogens and with degradation of the ECM. The effects of extracellular neutrophil proteases, if not inactivated, can cause serious injury to tissue; therefore protease inhibitors are present in plasma and are present in inflammatory lesions after vascular leakage.

Neutrophil granule formation begins during myeloid cell differentiation in the bone marrow (see Web Box 3-1). Granules are observed initially in myeloblasts and promyelocytes when immature transport vesicles bud from Golgi and fuse to form primary granules. Primary granules are also called *azurophilic granules* because of their affinity for the dye azure A. These granules

TABLE 3-2 Antimicrobial Mechanisms in Phagocytic Vacuoles

Oxygen-independent antimicrobial mechanisms			
Cathepsin G and elastase			Damage to microbial membranes
Low molecular weight ***defensins***			
High molecular weight ***cationic proteins***			
Bactericidal ***permeability-increasing protein***			
Lactoferrin			Complex with iron
Lysozyme			Splits proteoglycan
Acid hydrolases			Degrade dead microbes
Oxygen-dependent antimicrobial mechanisms			
Reaction Sequence Generated by NADPH Oxidase:			
Glucose + $NADP^+$	Hexose monophosphate shunt →	pentose phosphate + NADPH	O_2 burst plus generation of superoxide anion
NADPH + O_2	NADPH oxidase →	$NADP^+$ + $\mathbf{O_2^-}$	
$2O_2^-$ + $2H^+$	Spontaneous dismutation →	$\mathbf{H_2O_2}$ + $\mathbf{^1O_2}$	Spontaneous formation of further microbial agents
O_2^- + H_2O_2	→	**•OH** + OH^- + $\mathbf{^1O_2}$	
H_2O_2 + Cl^-	Myeloperoxidase →	$\mathbf{OCl^-}$ + H_2O	Myeloperoxidase generation of microbicidal molecules
OCl^- + H_2O_2	→	$\mathbf{^1O_2}$ + Cl^- + H_2O	
$2{\bullet}O_2O_2^-$ + $2H^+$	Superoxide dismutase →	O_2 + H_2O_2	Protective mechanisms used by host and many microbes
$2H_2O_2$	Catalase →	$2H_2O$ + O_2	
Nitric Oxide Reaction Sequence			
O_2 + L-arginine	NO synthase →	$\mathbf{NO^-}$	Reactive species
NO + O^-_2	→	$\mathbf{{\bullet}ONOO^-}$	
NO + Fe/RSH	→	$Fe(RS)_2$ $(NO)_2$	Complexes iron

Microbicidal species in bold letters. Fe/RSH, a complex of iron with a general sulfhydryl molecule; $Fe(RS)_2$, oxidized Fe/RSH; O_2^-, superoxide anion; $^1O_2$, singlet (activated) oxygen; •OH, hydroxyl free radical; NADPH, reduced nicotinamide adenine dinucleotide phosphate; $NADP^+$, oxidized NADPH; H_2O_2, hydrogen peroxide; OCl^-, hypochlorite anion; NO; nitric oxide; $•ONOO^-$, peroxynitrite radical.

From Goering R, Dockrell H, Roitt I, et al: *Mims' medical microbiology*, ed 4, St Louis, 2008, Mosby.

contain myeloperoxidase, elastase, defensins, and small amounts of lysozyme. Myelocytes and metamyelocytes form secondary (specific) granules that contain defensins, lactoferrin, lysozyme, and lesser amounts of myeloperoxidase, CD11b/CD18, and elastase. Band cells, the penultimate stage of neutrophil development, form tertiary (gelatinase) granules that contain lysozyme, gelatinase (MMP-9), cysteine-rich secretory protein-3 (CRISP-3), and adhesion molecules CD11b/CD18 (Mac-1) but have smaller amounts of myeloperoxidase, lactoferrin, proteinase 3, elastase, and defensins. Band and mature neutrophils also have secretory vesicles that contain plasma proteins, alkaline phosphatase, and numerous CD antigens, including CD11b/CD18 adhesion molecules. The secretory vesicles are mobilized quickly after neutrophil activation resulting in rapid expression of adhesion molecules, which mediate leukocyte infiltration.

Neutrophil granules have evolved phylogenetically and are specially adapted for each species. In most mammals, enzymes released into an exudate from neutrophil granules cause liquefaction of the exudate and the process results in the formation of pus. Reptiles and birds either lack or have reduced concentrations of these enzymes, particularly myeloperoxidase, and cannot liquefy the exudate. Thus a caseous material forms to be degraded by the next available line of inflammatory cells, macrophages. Granules in chicken heterophils (the avian, rabbit, and guinea pig neutrophil equivalent is termed heterophils) have little myeloperoxidase, but concentrations are also reduced in neutrophils of cattle and pigs. Cattle and sheep neutrophils have limited lysozyme levels. α-Defensins are present in rabbits, guinea pigs, hamsters, rats, and cattle neutrophils but have not been identified in those of dogs, cats, mice, pigs, and horses. The effect of these granule differences in various animal species on host defense and neutrophil function is not fully understood.

On cell death, neutrophils can release neutrophil extracellular traps (NETs) composed of a DNA backbone embedded with antimicrobial peptides and proteins and peptides that include histones, primary granule contents, lactoferrin, gelatinase, cathelicidins, and α-defensins. NETs entrap bacteria and can be microbicidal. Actin is also released from dead neutrophils, and in the lung, it can increase the viscosity of respiratory mucus. This outcome may occlude airways in dehydrated animals.

EOSINOPHILS

Eosinophils are recruited from the bloodstream into vascularized connective tissue of most organs in response to eosinophil chemoattractants present in allergic and parasitic diseases. Eosinophils frequently enter lesions during the transition from acute to chronic inflammation. Eosinophils have prominent granules that release basic proteins and when activated produce cytokines, chemokines, proteases, and oxidative radicals. This array of mediators is often released in response to helminthic infections, and eosinophilic infiltration has been more recently implicated in resistance to the development of some cancers. On the other hand, eosinophil products contribute to tissue damage in several organs, including the lungs (asthma), heart, skin, and gastrointestinal tract.

Eosinophils were first recognized as blood cells (leukocytes) having numerous cytoplasmic granules with affinity for acidic dyes such as eosin. Therefore the name *eosinophil* ("eosin-loving") was proposed by Ehrlich in the late 1800s for these unique cells. By 1939, eosinophils were postulated to have a role in the immune response to helminths, and by the 1970s, eosinophils were well known to increase in the blood (eosinophilia) in parasitic and allergic diseases. Eosinophils are slightly larger than neutrophils. The nucleus is lobulated (bilobed) and composed primarily of heterochromatin (condensed). Eosinophil granules are known for their large size, especially in horses, and are rich in arginine with reddish brown tinctorial properties.

Eosinophils have several types of granules listed in Web Table 3-4, including large specific granules, small granules, primary granules, and secondary granules. Large specific granules contain four distinct basic proteins: (1) major basic protein, (2) eosinophil cationic protein, (3) eosinophil-derived neurotoxin, and (4) eosinophil peroxidase. These proteins exert biologic effects on microbes and on the tissue in which the microbes replicate by damaging lipid membranes. In addition, histaminase and a variety of hydrolytic lysosomal enzymes, such as collagenase and gelatinase, are also present in the large specific granules. Small granules contain enzymes such as arylsulphatases, acid phosphatases, MMPs, and gelatinases. Eosinophils also elaborate cytokines such as IL-1 to IL-6, IL-8, IL-10, IL-12, IL-16, GM-CSF, TGF-α and TGF-β, and chemokines. The content of eosinophil granules are released in response to inflammatory stimuli in a manner similar to those used to activate neutrophils. However, products of eosinophil granules can result in extensive tissue degradation, including the degradation of collagen, which is commonly seen in eosinophilic granulomas of cats, horses, and dogs. Nearly all mast cell tumors in dogs and some mast cell tumors in cats contain eosinophils.

Major chemoattractants for eosinophils include histamine and eosinophilic chemotactic factor A (from mast cells), C5a, cytokines (IL-4, IL-5, and IL-13), and chemokines (CCL-5, known as *regulated on activation, normal T lymphocytes expressed and secreted* [RANTES], and CCL-11 [known as *eotaxin]*) released from epithelial cells, eosinophils, mast cells, and helminths. 5-Oxo-6, 8, 11, 14-eicosatetraenoic acid (5-oxo-ETE) is a strong activator of human eosinophils with a chemotactic potency comparable with those of eotaxin and RANTES, both of which enhance 5-oxo-ETE–induced chemotaxis. 5-Oxo-ETE and these chemokines contribute to the accumulation of eosinophils in the respiratory system in diseases such as asthma.

NATURAL KILLER CELLS AND NATURAL KILLER T LYMPHOCYTES

Natural killer (NK) cells are sentinels of the immune system named for lysis of tumor cells and virus-infected cells without previous encounter. These cells enter regions of acute inflammation hours and even days after initiation of the lesion. NK cells kill target cells through release of perforin from cytoplasmic granules. NK cells express CD161, a C-type lectin, but do not express CD3, the T lymphocyte antigen. Roughly 95% of NK cells expression CD56 and produce interferon-γ (IFN-γ); these are type I NK cells. Type II NK cells lack CD56 expression and produce IL-4, IL-5, and IL-13, thus supporting a T_H2 response.

IL-21 regulates differentiation and apoptotic death induced by NK cells. Inactive NK cells can be stimulated by Flt-3 ligand, a hematopoietic cytokine that stimulates proliferation of dendritic cells and antitumor immune responses, and also by IL-4, IL-12, IL-15, and IL-21. Once activated, IL-21 induces NK cell differentiation and upregulation of CD16, the low affinity IgG receptor necessary for antibody-dependent cellular cytotoxicity (ADCC), and also NK release of IFN-γ required for macrophage and dendritic cell activation. Finally, IL-21 initiates a delayed apoptotic program for death of the differentiated NK cell and prevents recruitment of uninvolved NK cells. NK-T lymphocytes are T lymphocytes (express CD3 antigen) that have T and NK cell properties. NK-T lymphocytes recognize CD1d molecule, which is an antigen-presenting molecule that binds self and foreign lipids and glycolipids, and on activation of the NK-T lymphocyte, induce release of IFN-γ, IL-4, and GM-CSF. Because of this close discretion of self and nonself, NK-T lymphocytes can have important roles in the development of autoimmune disease.

MONOCYTES AND MACROPHAGES

Macrophages arise from bone marrow–derived monocytes, which circulate hematogenously with some monocytes localizing in tissues physiologically. They enter acute inflammatory lesions roughly 12 to 48 hours after the initiation of a lesion, depending on the inciting agent/substance. Differentiation of monocyte stem cells into blood monocytes proceeds rapidly in the bone marrow (i.e., 1.5 to 3 days) and is regulated by growth and differentiating factors, cytokines, and adhesion molecules such as IL-3, CSFs, and TNF. Under physiologic conditions, monocytes in the blood localize throughout the body and differentiate into tissue macrophages. Recently, nonclassical monocytes have been identified; they migrate slowly along the luminal side of endothelium and monitor healthy tissue. When these monocytes sense damage or infection, they migrate rapidly into the tissue.

There are two types of tissue macrophages: macrophages that reside within specific organs/tissue (free macrophages and fixed macrophages) and macrophages derived from monocytes in response to inflammatory stimuli. Macrophages residing in organs/connective tissue first enter these sites as blood monocytes under physiologic (rather than inflammatory) conditions. These macrophages form the monocyte-macrophage system and include macrophages in connective tissue (histiocytes [free macrophages]), liver (Kupffer cells [fixed macrophages]), lung (alveolar macrophages [free macrophages], and intravascular macrophages [fixed macrophages]), lymph nodes (free and fixed macrophages), spleen (free and fixed macrophages), bone marrow (fixed macrophages), serous fluids (pleural and peritoneal macrophages [free macrophages]), brain (microglial cells), and skin (histiocytes [fixed macrophages]). The number of macrophages in tissue is maintained by (1) influx of monocytes from the blood, (2) proliferation of recruited monocytes locally in tissue, and (3) biologic turnover of macrophages via apoptotic cell death (lifespan in tissue of less than 3 weeks).

During inflammatory responses, monocytes express receptors (IgG Fc-domains, C3b) for chemical mediators of inflammation that exert migratory, chemotactic, pinocytic, and phagocytic activities in response to inflammatory stimuli. Once within inflammatory lesions, monocyte receptors are bound by cytokines, antigens, and other stimuli, which rapidly activate the maturation of monocytes into macrophages. This process can occur virtually anywhere in the body and often sets the stage for the development of chronic inflammation. In chronic inflammatory lesions, macrophages are the cell of last resort and accumulate in sites of persistent antigen, persistent microbes, foreign material, or repeated injury. Functionally, macrophages are a component of the innate immune system in terms of their role in phagocytosis and cytokine release during the acute inflammatory response. However, macrophages are one of the main triggers of the adaptive immune response because of their ability to process and present antigen and regulate T lymphocyte activity.

CHEMICAL MEDIATORS OF THE ACUTE INFLAMMATORY RESPONSE

Chemical mediators of the acute inflammatory response include molecules such as histamine, serotonin, bradykinin, and tachykinins (Web Fig. 3-5; Web Appendix 3-2). Many are produced as preformed or synthesized molecules in the liver and in neutrophils, basophils, macrophages/monocytes, platelets, mast cells, endothelial cells, smooth muscle cells, fibroblasts, and most epithelial cells. Preformed molecules, such as histamine, are transcribed, translated, processed, and stored, often in granules or vacuoles within inflammatory cells. They can be released immediately on cellular activation and are therefore active in seconds. Other molecules, such as most cytokines, adhesion molecules, and prostaglandins, are largely synthesized after an inflammatory cell becomes activated or injured. Endothelial cells, for example, often express low, basal levels of the adhesion molecule ICAM-1, but after the cells become activated (by cytokines such as IL-1), they rapidly transcribe the ICAM-1 gene to generate ICAM-1 messenger RNA (mRNA), which is translated into ICAM-1 protein, that is, processed, transported, and expressed on the cell surface. This is a quick process, resulting in ICAM-1 expression within hours; however, it is not nearly as rapid as the release of histamine, which occurs in seconds. Inflammatory mediators originating from plasma proteins, such as kinin, and the coagulation and complement system proteins are constantly secreted by the liver in precursor forms that must be activated via proteolytic cleavage in the circulatory system to their active forms; however, once the proteolytic cleavage is initiated, kinin and complement activity is immediate, similar to histamine.

Inflammatory mediators, whether preformed, synthesized, or derived from plasma, generally bind to receptors on target cells and often activate target cells or cause the target cell to secrete additional inflammatory mediators. In the latter case, the mediators may amplify or suppress secretion by target cells of additional mediators. Once activated and released or secreted, most inflammatory mediators:

- Have short half-lives and decay rapidly
- Are destroyed enzymatically
- Are scavenged by protective mechanisms such as antioxidants
- Are blocked by endogenous inhibitors such as complement inhibitors and decoy receptors

This arrangement provides a check and balance system on the severity of the acute inflammatory response and also can be exploited in the development of drugs to inhibit excessive inflammatory responses. Inflammatory mediators, if excessively unregulated, have the potential to cause severe injury to tissue in and surrounding the acute inflammatory response.

In addition to histamine, other preformed inflammatory proteins include serotonin, bradykinin, and tachykinins (substance P and neurokinins). Mast cells and basophils are the principal sources of histamine and serotonin. Bradykinin is released by leukocytes and vascular endothelial cells, and substance P is released by mast cells, basophils, and C-reactive (sensory) nerve fibers. As indicated, the mediators are rapidly active (in seconds to minutes) and contribute to increased vascular permeability that lasts from minutes to hours.

Histamine rapidly enhances vascular permeability and is one of the earliest recognized mediators of inflammation. Experiments by Sir Thomas Lewis in 1927 and Dale and Laidlaw in 1911 indicated the potential role of histamine and other local mediators in acute inflammation. Histamine is derived from the amino acid histidine through the action of histidine decarboxylase. This enzyme catalyzes the decarboxylation of histidine to histamine and carbon dioxide. Histamine is stored in granules of mast cells, basophils, and platelets.

As a mediator of inflammation, major effects of histamine are (1) vasodilation (active hyperemia), (2) increased microvascular, (3) neural reflexes, vagal reflexes, bronchial constriction, (4) release of $PGF_{2\alpha}$, (5) pain and itching, (6) tachycardia, and (7) eosinophil chemotaxis (Web Table 3-5). The acute vascular effects of histamine are immediate (within minutes) and transient (last about 30 to 90 minutes). Whether histamine has a role in chronic inflammation is speculative, but it may act to modulate the inflammatory response and the reactivity of various leukocytes, including lymphocytes. There are four G protein–coupled receptors (GPCR) for histamine. Two of these, H_1 and H_4, are present on leukocytes, whereas H_2 and H_3 are present on gastric mucosa and nerve terminals, respectively.

The release of histamine from mast cells is in response to a variety of stimuli including IgE, C3a, C5a, heat, cold, substance P, adenosine triphosphate (ATP), and products from leukocytes, endothelial cells, and platelets. Free histamine reacts within minutes with H_1 receptors on venular endothelium to cause contraction and gap formation (cytoskeletal reorganization [actinomycin filaments]), resulting in increased vascular permeability. Histamine H_1-receptor activation may lead to the production of cytokines and antibodies by T lymphocytes and B lymphocytes, respectively. In addition, H_1 receptors are also found on a variety of blood leukocytes, such as T lymphocytes, B lymphocytes, and monocytes.

There is substantial overlap of activities by these receptors on many types of cells. Many of the actions of histamine can be mimicked by H_1- and H_2-receptor agonists (a molecule or drug that binds to a receptor and triggers a response by the cell), whereas these actions can be blocked by H_1 and H_2 antagonists, molecules or drugs that block a receptor and prevent a response by the cell. This latter effect is the basis for therapies used in veterinary medicine today. Histamine receptors, for example, are involved in the pathogenesis of allergies, and H_1-receptor antagonists (antihistamines) reduce symptoms associated with allergic rhinitis such as sneezing, pruritus, and rhinorrhea (runny nose). In allergic bronchiolitis of cats and horses, H_1-receptor activation results in increased vascular permeability leading to serous inflammation in the bronchi and bronchioles. If this response can be blocked, the effects of allergens can be minimized in affected patients. Eosinophils produce histaminases that degrade histamine.

Serotonin (5-hydroxytryptamine) is an important preformed vasoactive amine with actions similar to those described previously for histamine. Serotonin is also an important neurotransmitter. Serotonin is found in mast cell granules of rodents and platelets of mammals. Serotonin and histamine are released from platelets after they are activated by the following:

- Aggregation and after contact with collagen in an exposed basement membrane from areas of endothelial necrosis and detached cells
- Thrombin from activation of the coagulation cascade
- Adenosine diphosphate (ADP) released from injured endothelial cells
- Immune complex activation of the complement cascade (C3a, C5a)

Kinins, such as the tachykinins and bradykinin, are chemical mediators of the acute inflammatory response and also act by modulating the responses of the clotting and complement cascades. Kinin system activation leads ultimately to the formation of bradykinin. Bradykinin, a prototype kinin and a vasoactive peptide, has proinflammatory (makes the disease worse) properties that result in the following:

- Increased vascular permeability
- Vasodilation (venules)
- Increased sensitivity to pain
- Smooth muscle contraction
- Increased arachidonic acid metabolism (stimulation of phospholipase A_2)
- Hypotension
- Bronchoconstriction

Kinins are formed by two distinct pathways: the plasma kinin pathway and the tissue kinin pathway. The plasma kinin pathway is activated by contact of a protein complex formed by high molecular weight kininogen (HMWK), factor XI, and prekallikrein with negatively charged surfaces, such as exposed basement membrane. When factor XII (Hageman factor [HF]) binds to this surface and interacts with the bound protein complex, there is reciprocal activation/generation of activated HF (HFa) and kallikrein (contact activation system). Kallikrein then acts on HMWK to yield bradykinin, an oligopeptide containing nine amino acid residues.

The tissue kinin pathway is generated by the action of tissue kallikrein on a low molecular weight kininogen (LMWK) to produce lysyl bradykinin and finally bradykinin. Tissue kallikrein is chemically and antigenically distinct from plasma kallikrein, although it is capable of acting on either HMWK or LMWK to generate bradykinin. Bradykinin binds to two GPCRs, B1R in inflamed tissue and B2R in normal tissues. Control of the proinflammatory effects of kinins is through rapid inactivation of bradykinin and kallikrein. Bradykinin is broken down by aminopeptidase M, neutral endopeptidase, carboxypeptidase (kininase I) and angiotensin-converting enzyme (kininase II). Plasma kallikrein is inhibited by C1-INH esterase (serum $\alpha 2$-macroglobulin), a member of the serpin family of proteases. This family of proteases forms approximately 20% of the proteins in blood plasma and includes α_1-antichymotrypsin, α_1-antitrypsin, and antithrombin III. They act to block proteolytic activity in the clotting and complement systems and thus serve as a regulatory check on these systems.

Tachykinins are a family of vasoactive neuropeptides that includes substance P, neurokinin A and B, neuropeptide Y, and hemokinin-1. Substance P and NK A and B synthesized by sensory afferent nerve fibers of the lungs and alimentary system. These substances are involved in allergic reactions and asthma. Substance P can induce vasoconstriction, vasodilation, increased permeability changes leading to edema, leukocyte activation, and chemotaxis. Substance P also induces activation and degranulation of mast cells, basophils, and eosinophils and their release of histamine and other inflammatory mediators. The released histamine, in a feedback mechanism, binds the H_3 receptors of nerve fibers and partially inhibits the production of substance P, thus regulating the level of activity. One of the main receptors for substance P, neurokinin-1 receptor (NK-1R), is expressed on a variety of cells including mast cells, epithelial cells, endothelial cells, and macrophages. NK-1R is regulated by substance P expression. Frequently, increased levels of substance P result in decreased NK-1R expression. Neurokinin 2 and 3 receptors have a lower affinity for substance P than NK-1R.

The release of substance P from afferent sensory nerve fibers in skin and mucous membranes can also be induced by capsaicinoids such as capsaicin and dihydrocapsaicin. Capsaicinoids are natural compounds present in chile peppers of the genus *Capsicum,* which cause the burning sensation in commercial pepper sprays (less-than-lethal, self-defense weapons). Capsaicin binds the vanilloid receptor-1 of afferent sensory fibers, leading to release of substance P from these fibers. Thus the tachykinins induce inflammatory responses when released by activated and degranulated mast cells, basophils, and eosinophils and also from stimulated nerve fibers.

COMPLEMENT CASCADE

The complement cascade is a unique sequence of molecular events occurring within the vascular system in which inactive complement plasma proteins synthesized by the liver are activated after tissue injury (Fig. 3-7; Web Fig. 3-6), inflammation, clotting, or immune responses. This cascade results in the generation of numerous biologically active molecules, which have effects that are proinflammatory, chemotactic, opsonizing, antigen solubilizing, antibody inducing, permeability enhancing, and microbicidal (cell lysis) and usually beneficial to the animal (Table 3-3). A large number of plasma proteins make up the complement system, and nearly 10% of serum proteins are complement factors. Divided by the "classical," "alternative," and lectin pathways, activation or "fixation" of complement proteins eventually results in formation of a membrane attack complex (MAC) that perforates the cell membranes of foreign invaders and naïve host cells alike. In the generation of MAC, a variety of complement components are elaborated that have important inflammatory and immune effects.

Complement proteins C1 through C9 are inactive components of plasma that are activated by substances, including microbial molecules such as endotoxins, aggregated immunoglobulin, complex polysaccharides, and venoms. The critical step in unleashing the biologic functions of the complement cascade in the classical pathway is activation of C3 through either the classical or alternative complement activation pathways. The classical pathway of the complement cascade can be activated by antibody complexes. Activation occurs when IgG and/or IgM are cross-linked with C1. C1 has three components: C1q, r, and s. C1q binds the Fc regions of IgG and/or IgM and brings C1r, which is proteolytic, into proximity to C1s, which is cleaved, through interactions with C4 and C2. This leads to the formation of classical pathway C3 convertase (C4b2a) and the eventual formation of classical pathway C5 convertase (C4b2a3b). Classical pathway C3 convertase converts C3 to C3a, and classical pathway C5 convertase converts C5 to C5a.

The alternative pathway is initiated by products from microorganisms, including LPS from Gram-negative bacteria and polysaccharides from fungal cell walls (see Web Fig. 3-6). In addition, other activated plasma proteins, including kallikrein, plasmin, and activated factor XII, can cleave C3, resulting in its activation to C3b. C3b combines with factor B and coupled with factor D activity, forms the alternative pathway C3 convertase (C3bBb). Alternative pathway C3 convertase converts C3 to C3b. C3b combines with alternative pathway C3 convertase to form alternative pathway C5 convertase (C3bBb3b), which converts C5 to C5a. Because the alternative pathway can be activated by clotting and kinin factors, once the clotting or the kinin systems are activated, complement activity follows and vice versa. Therefore the clotting, kinin, and

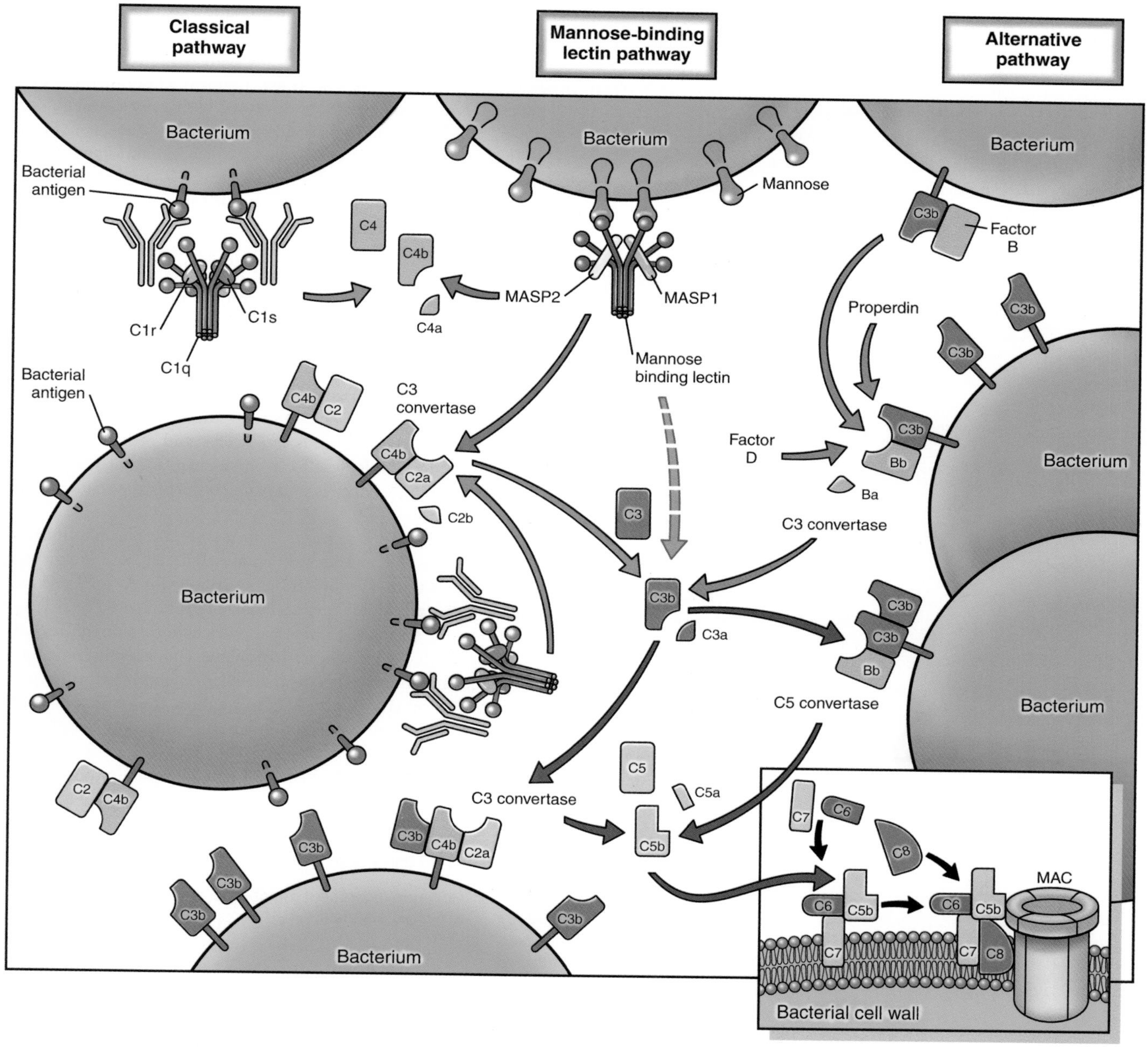

Fig. 3-7 Activation of complement cascade.
Complement is activated by classic, mannose-binding lectin and alternative pathways. The classical pathway is triggered by antibody opsonization, the mannose-binding pathway is induced by binding of the mannose-binding lectin to mannose residue on the surface of microbes, while the alternative pathway is first initiated by binding of C3b to hydroxyl group residues of carbohydrates and proteins and subsequent Factor D cleavage of C3b in plasma. After initiation by these three pathways, the complement cascade continues with formation of C5a and C3a which induce inflammation through attraction of leukocytes, C3b which opsonizes pathogens and induces phagocytosis, and formation of the membrane attack complex (MAC) that creates a pore in the microbial surface. (Redrawn from MJ Walport: Complement, *N Engl J Med* 344:1058-1066, 2001.)

complement systems are closely interactive, and often activation of one system leads to activation of others (Fig. 3-8). When bound to a microbial product, mannose-binding lectins (MBLs) and ficolins can also activate complement through MBL-associated serine proteases (MASPs). MASP-2 cleaves C4 and C2 to activate steps of the classical pathway.

C3a increases vascular permeability by inducing histamine release from mast cells. C5a, once formed, is released into the inflammatory exudate and behaves as an anaphylatoxin (a molecule that causes the release of histamine and other chemical mediators from mast cells or basophils), a chemoattractant for leukocytes, and an inducer of adhesion molecule expression by endothelial cells. C3b and C3bi are important opsonins and enhance neutrophil phagocytosis through CR1 and CR3 receptors. The plasma enzyme carboxypeptidase can degrade both C3a and C5b.

The MAC results from the cleavage of C5 by C5 convertase, leading to the formation of C5a and C5b. C5b serves as the anchor for the assembly of a single molecule composed of C6, C7, and C8. This MAC (C5b with C6, C7, C8) facilitates polymerization of C9 (up to 18 molecules of C9) into a tube that is inserted into the lipid bilayer of the plasma membrane of, for example, a bacterium. A channel is formed through the cell membrane allowing the passage of ions, small molecules, and water into the bacterium by osmosis. Bacterial lysis ensues. This process can also injure naïve host cells such as occurs in hemolytic anemia.

ARACHIDONIC ACID METABOLITES

When inflammation or inflammatory mediators injure cells, the cell membrane lipids are rapidly rearranged to create a variety of biologically active lipid mediators derived from arachidonic acid. Arachidonic acid metabolites are lipid-derived autocoid (acting as a local hormone) mediators of inflammation that serve as intracellular and extracellular signals influencing the coagulation cascade and mediating nearly every step of the acute inflammatory response (Fig. 3-9; Web Fig. 3-7). Effects are short-lived because these lipid metabolites decay rapidly or are destroyed by enzymes. Arachidonic acid metabolites include prostaglandins, leukotrienes, and lipoxins that are produced by cyclooxygenase (COX) and lipoxygenase enzyme pathways.

Arachidonic acid (eicosapentaenoic acid) is an essential 20-carbon, polyunsaturated fatty acid derived from linoleic acid, which is present in plasma membranes of dietary red meats. Arachidonic acid is an integral component of esterified membrane phospholipids that, when cleaved from the plasma membrane by phospholipase, serves as the major precursor for eicosanoids. Eicosanoids are synthesized by two main classes of enzymes: (1) COXs and (2) lipoxygenases and also (3) cytochrome P450 enzymes. Their respective products (eicosanoids) are (1) prostaglandins and thromboxanes and (2) leukotrienes and lipoxins. These molecules are synthesized in endothelial cells, leukocytes, and platelets and principally exert their biologic effects on vascular and airway smooth muscle cells, endothelial cells, and platelets during the acute inflammatory response.

Arachidonic acid is released from membrane phospholipids of many cell types, but particularly endothelial cells and leukocytes, through the action of cytoplasmic phospholipase A_2 ($cPLA_2$) and to a lesser degree, soluble (extracellular) phospholipase A_2 ($sPLA_2$). This occurs in response to physical and chemical stimuli, including C5a. $cPLA_2$ is translocated from the endoplasmic reticulum to plasma membrane when intracellular calcium concentrations increase. The activity of $sPLA_2$ also requires the participation of calcium; however, its contribution to the formation of intracellular arachidonic acid varies among the different cell types when compared with that of $cPLA_2$. Membrane phospholipids contain a

TABLE 3-3 The Main Functions of Complement

Activity	Associated Complement Protein
HOST DEFENSE	
Opsonization	C3 and C4 fragments
Chemotaxis and leukocyte activation	C5a, C3a, C4a, and leukocyte receptors
Lysis of microbial cell walls	Membrane attack complex (C5b-C9)
BRIDGING INNATE AND ADAPTIVE IMMUNITY	
Augmentation of antibody response	C3b, C4b immune complexes and antigen; C3 receptors on B lymphocytes and antigen-presenting cells.
Enhancement of immunologic memory	C3b, C4b immune complexes and antigen; C3 receptors on follicular dendritic cells
DISPOSAL OF WASTE	
Clearance of immune complexes	C1q; C3 and C4 fragments
Clearance of apoptotic cells	C1q; C3 and C4 fragments

Adapted from Mackay IR, Rosen FS: *N Engl J Med* 344:1058, 2001.

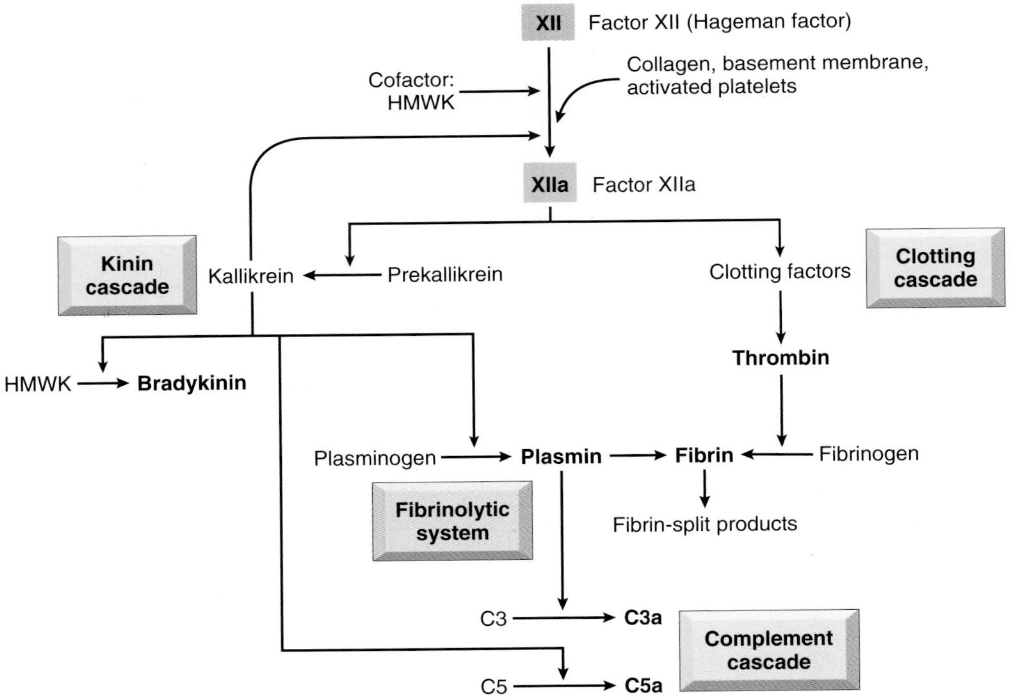

Fig. 3-8 Interrelationships between the four plasma mediator systems triggered by activation of factor XII (Hageman factor). Note that thrombin induces inflammation by binding to protease-activated receptors (PARs) (principally PAR-1) on platelets, endothelium, smooth muscle cells, and other cells. (From Kumar V, Abbas A, Fausto N, et al: *Robbins & Cotran pathologic basis of disease*, ed 8, Philadelphia, 2009, Saunders.)

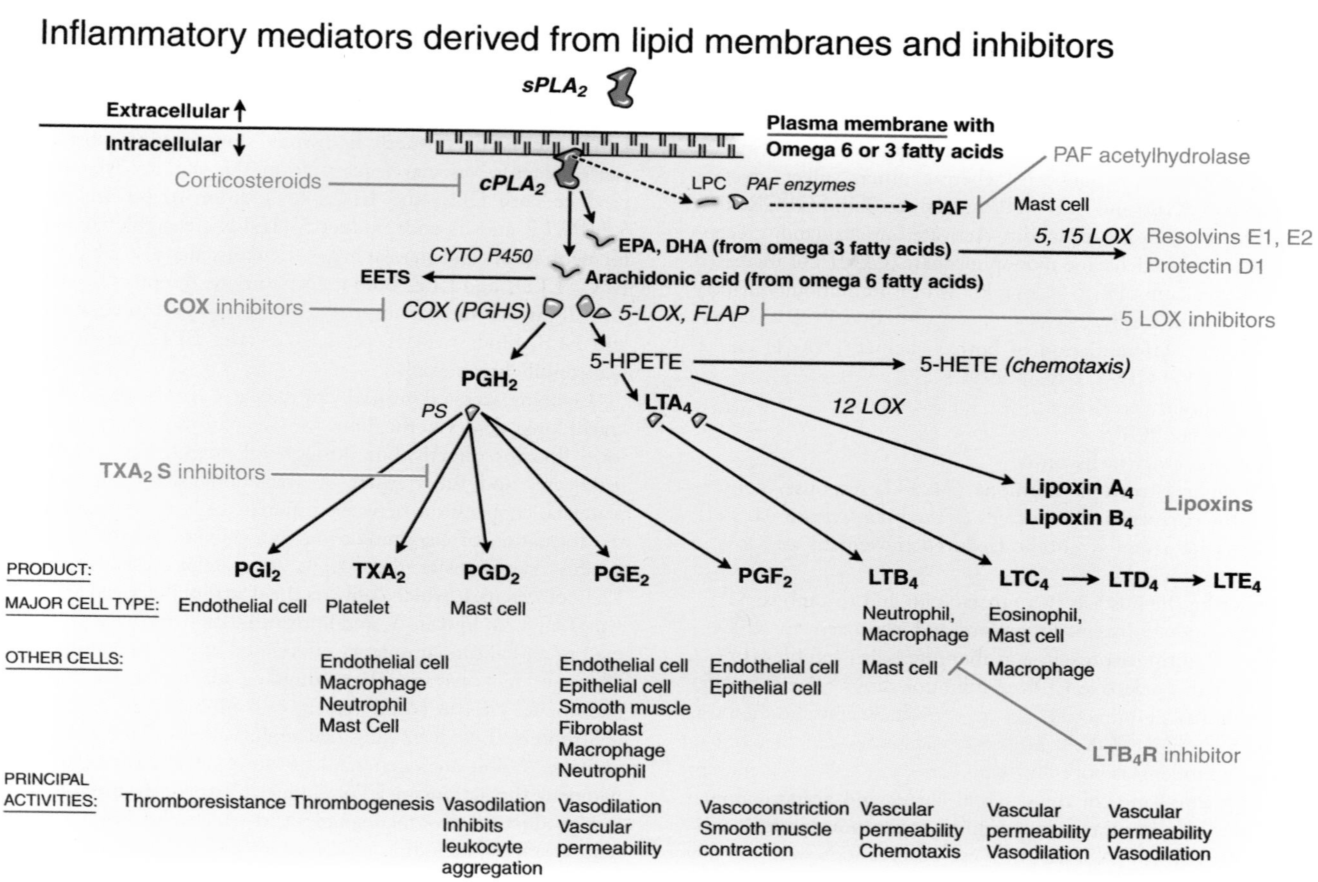

Enzymes are *italicized* and represented by shapes ( ). **Products** are written in bold letters. Abbreviations: sPLA2, soluble phospholipase A2; cPLA2 cytoplasmic phospholipase A2; LPC, lysophosphatidylcholine; PAF, platelet activating factor; AA, arachidonic acid; COX, cyclooxygenase; LOX, Lipoxygenase; FLAP, 5 LO activating protein; PG, prostaglandin; TX, thromboxane; LT, leukotriene; PS, prostanoid synthase; LTA4H, LTA4 hydrolase; LTC4S, LTC4 synthtase, EPA, eicosapentaenoic acid; DHA, docosapentaenoic acid. Inhibitors are listed in red and red lines with cross bars lead to sites of inhibition.

Fig. 3-9 Key inflammatory mediators derived from the plasma membrane.
Cytoplasmic phospholipase A2 *(cPLA2)* activity on the plasma membrane leads to free arachidonic acid *(AA)* and lysophosphatidylcholine *(LPC)*. Arachidonic acid metabolites include prostaglandins and leukotrienes, and LPC is a substrate for platelet-activating factor *(PAF)*. The type of prostaglandin formed by a cell is dependent on the cell type. Platelets, for example, form thromboxane, whereas endothelial cells form prostacyclin. Leukotrienes are formed by leukocytes. Inhibitors specific to the various enzymes or products are indicated in red text and lines. *COX*, Cyclooxygenase; *EETS*, epoxyeicosatrienoics; *FLAP*, 5-lipoxygenase-activating protein; *HETE*, hydroxyeicosatetraenoic acid; *LOX*, lipoxygenase; *LTA_4*, leukotriene A_4; *LTB_4*, leukotriene B_4; *LTC_4*, leukotriene C4; *LTD_4*, leukotriene D_4; *LTE_4*, leukotriene E4; *LTA_4H*, leukotriene A4 hydrolase; *LTC_4S*, leukotriene C_4 synthase; *PGD_2*, prostaglandins D_2; *PGE_2*, prostaglandins E_2; *PGF_2*, prostaglandins F_2; *PGH_2*, prostaglandins H_2; *PGI_2*, prostaglandins I_2; *PGHS*, prostaglandin H synthase; *PS*, polysaccharides; *$sPLA_2$*, soluble phospholipase A_2; *TXA_2*, thromboxane A_2. (Modified from Dr. M.R. Ackermann, College of Veterinary Medicine, Iowa State University.)

glycerol backbone attached to which is often a saturated fatty acid at the sn-1 position, an unsaturated fatty acid at the sn-2 position, and a base at the sn-3 position. Arachidonic acid is often in the sn-2 position and released by $cPLA_2$ or $sPLA_2$ to become free arachidonic acid.

Free arachidonic acid is metabolized in one of three pathways: (1) the COX pathway for the formation of prostaglandins and thromboxanes, (2) the lipoxygenase pathway for the formation of leukotrienes and lipoxins, and (3) the cytochrome p450 pathway for the formation of epoxyeicosatrienoic acids (hydroperoxyeicosatetraenoic acid [HPETE] and hydroxyeicosatetraenoic acid [HETE]). There are three COX isoenzymes—COX-1, COX-2, and COX-3—that are actually components of prostaglandin H synthase and work in concert with a peroxidase heme group. The COX-1 isoenzyme is constitutively expressed, is present in almost all tissues, and is considered a housekeeping enzyme with physiologic roles in hemostasis and gastric mucosa protection. COX-2 isoenzyme expression is induced by exogenous and endogenous stimuli and occurs locally in sites of inflammation. It is present in leukocytes, endothelial cells of blood vessels, and synovial fibroblasts. COX-3 isoenzyme is a splice variant of COX-1 (and also termed *COX-1b* or *COX-1v*). It is present in greatest abundance in the cerebral cortex of dogs and humans and is also detected in human aortas and rodent cerebral endothelia, heart, kidney, and neuronal tissues.

PROSTAGLANDIN FORMATION AND INHIBITION

Arachidonic acid metabolites from COX isoenzymes induce an intermediate prostaglandin, PGH_2, that is converted into at least five metabolites (PGD_2, PGF_2, PGE_2, PGI_2, and thromboxane A_2 [TXA_2]) by prostanoid synthase enzymes unique for each of these five metabolites (see Web Fig. 3-7). The relative concentration of each of these five types of prostaglandins synthesized after stimulation depends on the cell type stimulated. For example, PGI_2—a thromboresistant prostaglandin termed *prostacyclin*—is produced by endothelial cells via PGI_2 (prostacyclin) synthase, whereas

TXA_2—a thrombogenic prostaglandin termed *thromboxane*—is produced by platelets via TXA_2 (thromboxane) synthase. PGD_2 is the major prostanoid produced by mast cells; PGE_2 is the major prostanoid produced by epithelial cells, fibroblasts, and smooth muscle cells. Specific prostaglandins inhibit (PGI_2) or induce (TXA_2) coagulation/thrombosis, whereas others affect vascular permeability (PGD_2 and PGE_2). Prostaglandins bind GPCRs that are specific for each prostaglandin. Activated prostaglandin receptors trigger cyclic adenosine monophosphate (cAMP) or increased cytoplasmic calcium. PGE_2 is long known for immunomodulatory activity; mechanistically, recent work suggests that PGE_2 receptor EP4 promotes differentiation of both T helper 1 (T_H1) and T helper 17 (T_H17) CD4+ T lymphocytes.

Prostaglandins contribute to the following:

- Fever (via PGE_2)
- Inflammatory tachycardia
- Adrenocorticotropic hormone (ACTH) response (neurons of the paraventricular nucleus of the brain release ACTH)
- Behavior stress syndrome (reduced movement and loss of social contact)
- Clotting/hemostasis (via prostacyclin and thromboxane)

Aspirin, indomethacin, ibuprofen, and naproxen are COX-1 inhibitors. Aspirin, naproxen, and ibuprofen also inhibit COX-2, as do the highly selective COX-2 inhibitor drugs celecoxib, rofecoxib, valdecoxib, lumiracoxib, and etoricoxib. Acetaminophen was thought to inhibit COX-3; however, acetaminophen's activity in humans and rodents is not fully defined. Because COX-3 is present in greatest abundance in the cerebral cortex and acetaminophen crosses the blood-brain barrier (unlike other nonsteroidal antiinflammatory drugs [NSAIDs]), these observations were initially thought to explain why acetaminophen was sometimes more effective for treating headaches and pain relief and less effective in inhibiting inflammation in the body. Although this may be the case in dogs, the mechanistic basis of acetaminophen's activity in humans is not fully understood at this time. Acetaminophen may inhibit COX-2 to a minor degree and also slightly inhibit COX-3 (COX-1b), and yet have other activity/activities. Much of the antiinflammatory effect of corticosteroids is due to their inhibition of phospholipase A_2, the enzyme that releases arachidonic acid from membrane phospholipids. Corticosteroids signal the cell to synthesize a polypeptide known as lipocortin (lipomodulin), which then acts to inhibit phospholipase A_2. Therefore the antiinflammatory effect of corticosteroids is delayed. A variety of other natural and synthetic compounds can inhibit phospholipase A_2.

LEUKOTRIENE FORMATION AND INHIBITION

In leukocytes, arachidonic acid can be metabolized through the 5-lipoxygenase pathway to form leukotrienes and lipoxins (see Web Fig. 3-7), which have profound effects on inflammation. 5-Lipoxygenase works in concert with 5-lipoxygenase-activating protein as an arachidonic acid binding protein, which optimizes the proximity of 5-lipoxygenase to interact with arachidonic acid. The complex formed by 5-lipoxygenase and 5-lipoxygenase-activating protein (HPETE) is converted to an intermediate complex, LTA_4, which is subsequently converted to either LTB_4 or LTC_4, via LTA_4 hydrolase or LTC_4 synthetase, respectively. LTC_4 synthetase is a glutathione transferase, and once LTC_4 is secreted from a cell, it is metabolized to LTD_4 and LTE_4 by sequential removal of the glutathione, glutamic acid, and glycine moieties.

The major effects of the leukotrienes include (1) increased vascular permeability, (2) chemotaxis for leukocytes, and (3) vasoconstriction, all of which exacerbate the acute inflammatory response. Neutrophils produce primarily LTB_4, which is one of the most potent chemotactic factors for neutrophils and macrophages. LTB_4 also stimulates leukocytes to release their lysosomal contents further contributing to inflammation. Mast cells and eosinophils produce primarily leukotriene C_4, and the group of leukotrienes—LTC_4, LTD_4, and LTE_4, formerly known as "slow-reacting substance"—causes intense vascular leakage from the venules. Macrophages produce both LTB_4 and LTC_4. In addition to the leukotrienes, 5-HPETE and its end-product 5-HETE are highly chemotactic for neutrophils and macrophages. Leukotrienes also bind GPCR. LTC_4, LTD_4, and LTE_4 bind the leukotriene receptors $CysLT_1$ and $CysLT_2$, which mediate bronchoconstriction and vasoconstriction, and LTB_4 binds two receptors, BLT_1 and BLT_2, which mediate neutrophil chemotaxis.

Lipoxins, secreted primarily by platelets, are also produced from arachidonic acid via the lipoxygenase pathway. Platelets cannot form lipoxins directly, but through cell-to-cell interactions with leukocytes and the transfer of arachidonic acid metabolites to platelets, cooperation between different cells types can result in the formation of eicosanoids via transcellular biosynthesis. Neutrophils can transfer their LTA_4 to platelets. Platelets contain 12-lipooxygenase, which converts the neutrophil derived and transferred LTA_4 to lipoxin A_4 and lipoxin B_4. Lipoxins have proinflammatory and antiinflammatory effects and appear to counteract the effects of leukotrienes. They stimulate macrophage adhesion to endothelial cells in blood vessels, but inhibit LTB_4 activation of neutrophils, thus decreasing neutrophil adhesion and chemotaxis, and also inhibit angiogenesis. Lipoxin A_4 causes vasodilation and dampens the actions of LTC_4–induced vasoconstriction. Resolvin is a product of eicosapentaenoic acid which also has antiinflammatory effects, including inhibition of BLT_1 (LTB_4 receptor) and dendritic cell migration.

The 5-lipoxygenase pathway can be inhibited by a variety of new chemical agents (5-lipoxygenase inhibitors and leukotriene receptor antagonists) (see Fig. 3-9). In addition, eosinophils release arylsulfatase from granules, which inactivates leukotrienes.

OMEGA-3 FATTY ACIDS (FISH OILS) AND INHIBITION OF EICOSANOID ACTIVITY

Information on this topic is available at evolve.elsevier.com/Zachary/McGavin/.

PLATELET-ACTIVATING FACTOR

PAF is another potent molecule of phospholipid origin derived from cell membranes of platelets, basophils, mast cells, neutrophils, macrophages, and endothelial cells. PAF has potent pathophysiologic effects and contributes to inflammation, endotoxic shock, and allergic reactions (asthma) through vasoconstriction, bronchoconstriction, platelet aggregation, and leukocyte adhesion, chemotaxis, and degranulation. However, at low concentrations (experimentally induced), PAF can cause vasodilation and increased vascular permeability. PAF also contributes to the inflammatory response by increasing the oxidative burst in neutrophils following phagocytosis of bacteria and enhances the synthesis of eicosanoids by leukocytes. During IgE-mediated hypersensitivity reaction in the lung, PAF induces mast cell release of serotonin and histamine as well as platelet aggregation. Thus platelet aggregation can increase vascular permeability in acquired immunologic responses and result in inflammation.

Two enzymes, lysoPAF acetyltransferase (lysoPAF-AT) and PAF-synthesizing phosphocholinetransferase (PAF-PCT), control the final synthesis of PAF from lipid membranes and thus promote

PAF production. PAF mediates its effects on target cells through a single GPCR. These receptors have been identified on endothelium, neutrophils, eosinophils, macrophages, smooth muscle, and glial cells in the brain. PAF activity is reduced/regulated by PAF acetylhydrolase, which is expressed by cells expressing PAF receptor. PAF acetylhydrolase degrades PAF through hydrolysis of its acetate moiety in the sn-2 position of glycerol, which inhibits the proinflammatory activity of PAF. PAF acetylhydrolase is thus potentially an enzyme that could be used for the development of drugs to reduce inflammatory responses.

CYTOKINE FAMILY

Overview in Inflammation and Induction of CD4 T_H Subsets

Cytokines are a group of proteins produced by many cell types including lymphocytes, macrophages, endothelial cells, neutrophils, basophils, mast cells, eosinophils, epithelial cells, and connective tissue cells (see Web Appendix 3-2). The primary purpose of cytokines is to modulate, via enhancement or suppression, the functional expression of other cell types during the inflammatory response. Chemokines are produced from almost all cell types and are cytokines that promote leukocyte chemotaxis and migration across capillaries and postcapillary venules. Cytokines also play major roles in (1) hematopoiesis, including granulopoiesis by cytokines such as IL-3, G-CSF, and GM-CSF; and (2) adaptive immunity, such as the proliferation of lymphocytes by cytokines, including IL-2, and activation of T_H1 or T_H2 responses. The CD4 T_H cell response consists of subsets of T-lymphocytes characterized by the secretion of different cytokines, including IFN-γ–producing T_H1 cells and IL-4–producing T_H2 cells, which are involved in cellular or humoral immunity, respectively. The cytokines have been organized into the following categories according to their principal functional activities:

- Hematopoietic growth factors, including IL-3, G-CSF, GM-CSF, possibly IL-9, IL-11, and stem cell factor
- Inflammatory mediators, which induce acute phase reactants and natural immunity (IL-1, IL-6, TNF-α, and TNF-β)
- Chemotactic cytokines (IL-8)
- T lymphocyte proliferation, activation, and differentiation cytokines (IL-2, IL-4, IL-5, IL-7, IL-9, IL-10, IL-12, and IL-17 on up to IL-29)

Stimuli that invoke expression of these families of cytokines are varied and secondary to activation of a wide variety of receptors, including soluble receptors, receptors on the cell surface, endosomal receptors, and cytoplasmic receptors, which activate nuclear factor (NF) kappa B, extracellular signal-related kinase (ERK), Jun, p38, and other signaling pathways.

Concerning T-lymphocyte activity, there are cytokines and proteins that exert T-lymphocyte regulatory activity (IFN-γ, TGF-β). Of particular importance is the presentation of antigen by dendritic cells to T-lymphocyte cells that release cytokines, which mediate formation of lineages of T-lymphocyte helper cells (T_H1, T_H2, T_H17, and T regulatory [T reg] cells). Dendritic cells are present in tissues that are in contact with the environment such as Langerhans' cells of the skin and dendritic cells of the mucosal surfaces of the respiratory and alimentary systems. These dendritic cells are sentinels constantly monitoring for and phagocytosing microbes and foreign materials. In cooperation with lymphocytes and macrophages in lymphoid tissue, they act as antigen-presenting cells to activate T helper lymphocytes and cytotoxic T lymphocytes and B lymphocytes. The T_H1 lineage of CD4 T lymphocytes, normally driven by IL-12, expresses the transcription factor T-bet, releases IFN-γ, and induces cell-mediated immune responses within specific diseases such as the granulomatous inflammatory response to mycobacterial infections. Whereas T_H2 CD4 cells form in response to IL-4, IL-6, and thymic stromal lymphopoietin (TSLP); express transcription factor GATA-3; produce IL-4, IL-5, IL-10, and IL-13; and induce humoral responses and humoral-related diseases, such as asthma and atopy, T_H17 CD4 T lymphocytes form in response to TGF-β, IL-6, and IL-23, express transcription factor Rorγt, and release IL-17. These cells bridge innate and adaptive immune responses through the production of IL-17 cytokines, which promote inflammatory responses such as neutrophil recruitment and development of autoimmune responses. T reg cells develop in the thymus and also in response to antigenic stimulation in the presence of TGF-β, which induces transient or stabile expression of transcription factor forkhead box P3 (FOXP3). T reg cells modulate adaptive responses through the release of IL-10. Follicular CD4 T lymphocytes (T_{FH}) develop in the presence of IL-6 and IL-21, express transcription factor Bcl6 and cMaf (BLIMP-1 is inhibitory), and release IL-21. Through secretion of IL-21, T_{FH} cells support B lymphocyte development and antibody production. Follicular dendritic cells are present in the follicles of lymph nodes and present antigen to B lymphocytes.

Biochemically, cytokines can be divided into type I and type II cytokines. Type I cytokines have four α-helix units. Type II cytokines have six α-helix units and are likely derived from a single ancestral gene. Type I and II cytokines bind receptors specific for the I and II ligand structures. Despite the similarities within type I and type II cytokines and their receptors, there is still much diversity in structure and function of cytokines within each type.

Cytokine Receptors and Signaling

Information on this topic and Web Fig. 3-8 are available at evolve.elsevier.com/Zachary/McGavin/.

Inflammatory Proteins

Interferons

Interferons are glycoprotein cytokines produced by lymphocytes and many other cell types in response to viruses and virus-infected cells, parasites, and neoplastic cells. They inhibit viral replication within host cells, activate NK cells and macrophages, increase antigen presentation to T lymphocytes, and increase the resistance of host cells to viral infection. Type 1 interferons (IFN-α and IFN-β) bind IFN-α receptors (IFNAR) 1 and 2 to signal through JAK1 and STAT1 and STAT2 and mediate antiviral responses; type II interferons (IFN-γ) bind IFN-γ receptors (IFNGR) 1 and 2, signal through JAK1, JAK2, and STAT1, to induce T_H1 and T_H17 responses. Type III interferons bind IL-10 receptors and have been described, but their function is not fully clarified. The antiviral activity of type I interferons involves expression activation of the ISGlyation pathway, MxA protein, 2′,5′-oligoadenylate synthetase 1 (OAS1) activation of ribonuclease L (RNaseL), and protein kinase R (PKR). ISGlyation is a process in which interferon-stimulated gene 15 (ISG15) protein binds key interferon antiviral proteins (e.g., JAK1, STAT1, MxA, PKR, and RNaseL) and prevents their degradation, thus enhancing the antiviral response. MxA protein binds and traps viruses. The OAS1/RNaseL process cleaves viral RNA and PKR protein dimerizes on itself and in the presence of viral RNA phosphorylates, thus inhibiting host cell translation initiation factor-2α (EIF-2α), which blocks viral replication.

High Mobility Group Box Protein-1

High mobility group box protein 1 (HMGB-1) is a proinflammatory cytokine released by monocytes and macrophages. It is a nonhistone nuclear protein that binds DNA to regulate gene expression and the chromosomal architecture. HMGB-1 is released by nearly all cells during necrosis, and once outside the cell, it is an alarmin, which is an endogenous molecule that triggers host inflammatory responses. HMGB-1 binds macrophage receptor for advanced glycosylation end-products (RAGE) and TLRs 2 and 4, activating the innate immune system and pathologic responses that include release of IL-1, TNF-α, and IFN-γ. HMGB-1 and cytokines, such as IL-1, TNF, and IL-6, and prostaglandins, such as PGE_2, are involved with hypothalamic function in food aversion, hypophagia, anorexia, weight loss, and sickness behavior (see section on Febrile Response) and serve to amplify the inflammatory response.

Chemokines

Chemokines, released in response to inflammatory stimuli, are secreted proteins that induce leukocyte chemotaxis into inflammatory exudates (Fig. 3-10). They also activate inflammatory cells, induce antiviral activity, regulate immune responses, and induce hematopoiesis, angiogenesis, and cell growth. Chemokines are produced by all nucleated cells in the body, including epithelial cells, fibroblasts, macrophages, mast cells, keratinocytes, dendritic cells, and endothelial cells. Leukocytes secrete all types of chemokines, except for fractalkine (used for monocyte chemotaxis), which is produced by nonhematopoietic cells such as vascular endothelial cells.

Classification of Chemokines

Information on this topic and Web Table 3-6 are available at evolve.elsevier.com/Zachary/McGavin/.

Chemokine Receptors and Signaling

Information on this topic and Web Tables 3-7 and 3-8 are available at evolve.elsevier.com/Zachary/McGavin/.

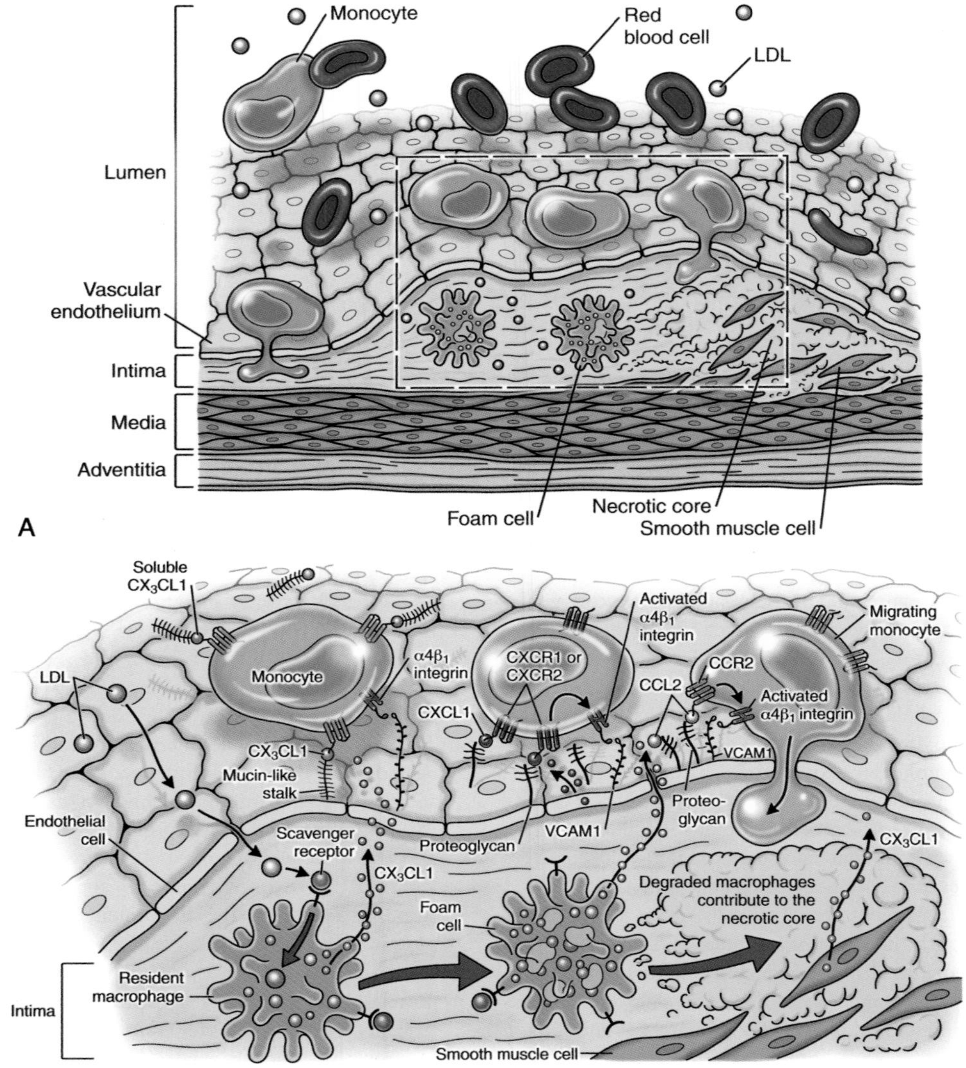

Fig. 3-10 Chemokine responses to vascular injury.
A, The atherosclerotic plaque illustrates the interactions of chemokine ligands with their receptors during an inflammatory reaction. While neutrophils respond to IL-8 (a C-C chemokine), monocytes respond to CX_3CL1, CXCL1, CCL2 and their respective receptors to attract cells along the vascular wall for adhesion molecule adherence and leukocyte infiltration. **B,** Higher magnification of the area defined by the box in **A**. (Redrawn from Charo IF, Ransohoff RM: The many roles of chemokines and chemokine receptors in inflammation, *N Engl J Med* 354(6):610-621, 2006.)

OXYGEN-DERIVED FREE RADICALS AND NITRIC OXIDE

Free radicals, such as superoxide anion, hydroxy radical, and NO derivatives, can (1) injure vascular endothelial cells, leading to increased vascular permeability; (2) inactivate antiproteases, such as α_1-antitrypsin, resulting in damage to ECM proteins; (3) enhance cytokine and chemokine expression secondary to signaling changes and cell damage; (4) activate endothelial cells and increase adhesion molecule expression; and (5) increase the formation of chemotactic factors (LTB_4). They can also inactivate neurotransmitters (adrenaline and noradrenaline), leading to hypotension.

Oxygen-derived free radicals are released from neutrophils and macrophages after exposure to chemokines and immune complexes and after phagocytosis by the leukocyte (see Table 3-2). They damage cells through peroxidation of cell membrane lipids, cross-linking of proteins and oxidizing thiol groups on methionine and cysteine, cleaving glycoconjugates, directly damaging DNA phosphate backbone and bases, and inducing the formation of DNA adducts. Because of damage to proteins, the activity of key enzymes and transcription factors needed by the cell can be impaired. Fortunately, the body has antioxidants that are (1) enzymatic, such as superoxide dismutase (SOD) isoforms 1, 2, and 3, catalase, thioredoxin, peroxiredoxins, and glutathione reductase; (2) nonenzymatic endogenous substances, such as ceruloplasmin, transferrin, metallothionein, uric acid, and melatonin; and (3) nonenzymatic dietary substances, such as vitamins A, C, and E and lycopenes, flavonoids, resveratrol genistein, anthocyanins, naringenin, and reserpines. All of these minimize the damage to tissue caused by free radicals.

NO is a chemical mediator of inflammation that causes vasodilation by relaxing vascular smooth muscle cells. In response to injury and inflammatory stimuli, NO derivatives are synthesized by endothelial cells, macrophages, and specific populations of neurons in the brain from L-arginine, molecular oxygen, NADPH, other cofactors, and the enzyme NO synthetase (NOS). There are three forms of NOS that mediate NO formation: neuronal (nNOS), iNOS, and endothelial (eNOS). In addition to its vasodilatory activities, NO inhibits platelet aggregation and adhesion, inhibits mast cell-induced inflammation, oxidizes lipids and other molecules, and regulates leukocyte chemotaxis.

RECEPTORS FOR EXOGENOUS AND ENDOGENOUS INFLAMMATORY STIMULI AND TOLL-LIKE RECEPTORS

Inflammatory responses occur in response to endogenous and exogenous substances. The body's inflammatory reaction to exogenous pathogens has been understood and studied for many years. Increasingly, it is clear that the body also produces inflammatory reactions to host endogenous molecules released under sterile conditions. Thus both endogenous and exogenous stimuli produce "danger" signals, termed *danger-associated molecular patterns* (DAMPs).

Exogenous microbial products, often with redundant molecular structure, are PAMPs and include substances such as LPS, peptidoglycan, and lipoteichoic acid. PAMPs can bind several types of PRRs (Fig. 3-11; Table 3-4; Web Fig. 3-9). These receptors include secreted receptors that circulate in the blood (LPS binding protein), surface receptors (macrophage mannose receptors; and TLRs), nucleotide-binding oligomerization domain (NOD) -like receptors (NLRs), and endosomal receptors (TLR and endosomal viral receptors). These receptors have different mechanisms by which they activate the cell and some work together. LPS, for example, is bound by LPS-binding protein (LBP), which in turn binds CD14 and TLR4. The formation of a PRR-PAMP complex initiates transmembrane signaling that often involves a MyD88 protein event leading to NF kappa B activation and MAPK (p38) signaling. The NF kappa B family of transcription factors initiates gene transcription and translation, resulting in the expression of proteins involved in many cellular processes such as cell proliferation, differentiation, apoptosis, and cell responses to injury, stress, and external pathogens. NF kappa B and p38 then can induce phagocytosis by leukocytes, dendritic cell activation, release of inflammatory cytokines and chemokines, and the activation of the innate (defensin and antimicrobial peptide release) and adaptive (T_H1, T_H2, T_H17, T_{FH} activity) immune systems. Alternatively, TLR4 signaling does not engage MyD88 (MyD88-independent signaling) and results in the formation of IFN-β and IFN-inducible gene products.

In addition to LBP, other secreted PRRs that can trigger inflammatory reactions through complement activation or receptor binding include collagenous lectins such as mannan-binding lectins A and C, ficolins, surfactant proteins A (SP-A) and D (SP-D), and conglutinin (cattle), which bind glycans of chitin, bacterial capsules, viruses, C-reactive protein, and serum amyloid–binding protein. SP-A, for example, can bind, aggregate, and inhibit respiratory syncytial virus. SP-A can also activate macrophages.

Leukocytes, epithelia, mucosal-lining cells, and other cells can also express PRR on the plasma membrane, including TLR1, TLR2, TLR4, TLR5, TLR6, and TLR11. TLRs are a family of PRRs in mammals that can distinguish between chemically diverse classes of genetically conserved microbial products (see Table 3-4). For example, bacterial lipoprotein binds TLR1 and TLR2/6, flagellin binds TLR5, and LPS binds TLR4. These receptors have a central role in the release of inflammatory cytokines from the innate immune system in response to microbial structures, such as exogenous microbial substances and endogenous products (Web Fig. 3-10). Also, TLRs likely play a role in the adaptive immune response, which develops during the acute inflammatory response.

C-type lectin receptors are also present on the surface of monocytes, macrophages, neutrophils, and dendritic cells and include dectin 1 that binds beta 1,3 glucan, as well as dectin 2, MBL, and dendritic cell-specific intercellular adhesion molecule-grabbing nonintegrins (DC-SIGNs) that bind high mannose and fructose; both glucans and mannose/fructose residues are produced and released by mycobacterial and fungal organisms. Once bound, both TLR and C-type lectins regulate a wide range of innate and adaptive immune responses through NF kappa B, transcription factor activators protein-1 (TFAP-1), and interferon regulatory factors (IRFs).

Intracellular receptors, such as the NLRs, have a leucine-rich repeat domain that binds PAMPs and xenocompounds to induce and/or regulate inflammation. NOD1 binds to peptidoglycan-derived tripeptide structures, whereas NOD2 binds peptidoglycan-derived muramyl dipeptides. Bound NOD1 and NOD2 activate the receptor-interacting protein (RIP) family of serine/threonine protein kinase (RIPK2), which then induces NF kappa B activity and eventual secretion of antimicrobial peptides and inflammatory cytokines such as IL-1β and IL-18 and IL-33, invoking inflammation. Muramyl dipeptides and a variety of xenocompounds and endogenous stimuli can activate another family of NLRs that contain a pyrin domain NLRP3 (also termed *NALP3*), which triggers caspase 1 activation and activation of IL-1β, IL-18, and IL-33.

PRRs for certain viral infections include retinoic acid-inducible gene I (RIG-I) (e.g., paramyxoviridae, influenza viruses) and melanoma differentiation-associated gene 5 (MDA-5) (picornaviridae). These molecules sense viral RNA, alter mitochondrial activity through IPS-1, and invoke IRF3 for IFN-α and -β release and

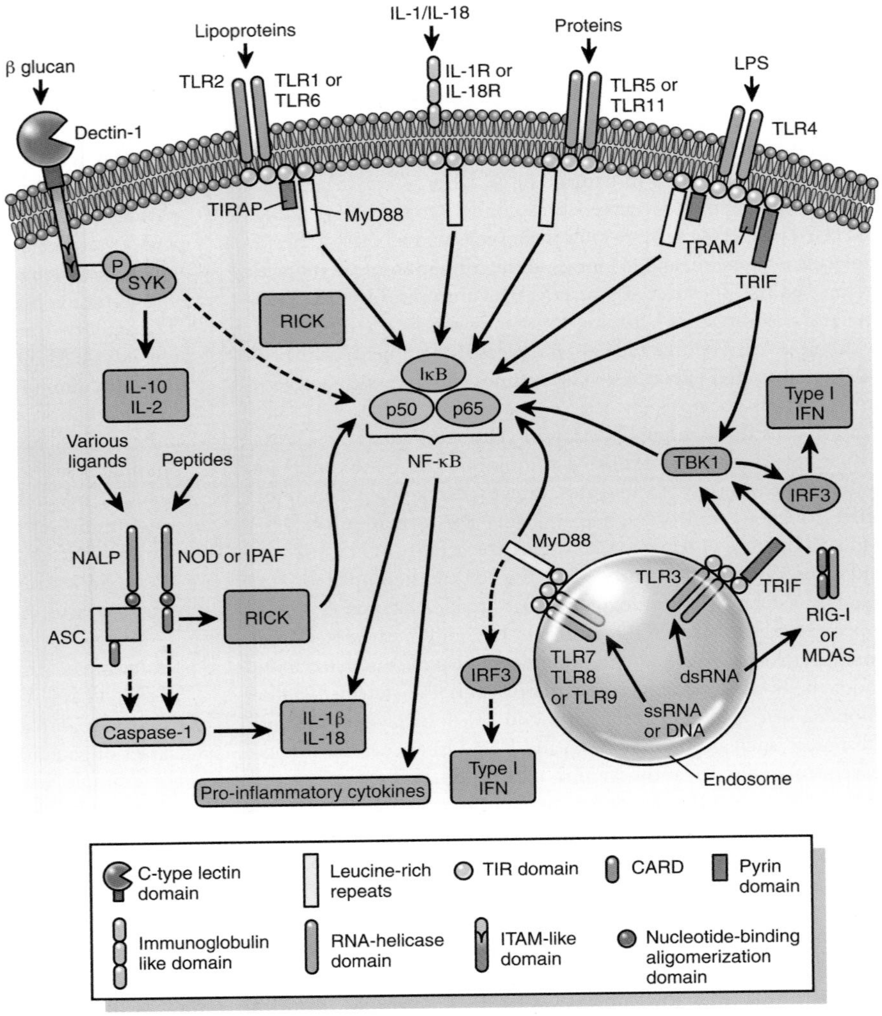

Fig. 3-11 Pathogen-associated molecular patterns (PAMPs), pattern recognition receptors (PRR), and cellular signaling. PAMPs such as lipopolysaccharide (LPS), teichoic acid, beta-glucans, as well as microbial peptides, proteins, RNA, DNA, and CpG, bind specific receptors and trigger activation of the subjacent signaling cascade leading to transcription of proinflammatory genes (cytokines, interferons, chemokines). Receptors are present on the membrane surface (Dectin-1, TLR1, 2, 4, 5, 6, 11, IL-1) in endosomes (TLR3, 7, 8, 9), and in the cytoplasm (NOD, NALP, RIG-1). TLR utilize MyD88 protein for signaling, except for TLR 3 and 4 which can be MyD88-independent. All pictured trigger NF kappa B (NFκB) and some also induce interferon responses. (Redrawn from Dale DC, Boxer L, Liles WC: The phagocytes: neutrophils and monocytes, *Blood* 112(4):935-945, 2008.)

NF kappa B for inflammatory cytokine production along with antimicrobial peptides.

Endosomes express PRRs that also have important roles in sensing viral infection and triggering a cellular response that often results in inflammatory and immune activity. TLR3, TLR7, TLR8, and TLR9 are present along the inner endosomal membrane and bind double-stranded RNA (dsRNA) (TLR3) or single-stranded RNA/DNA (ssRNA/DNA) (TLR7, TLR8, TLR9) and activate IRF7 and NF kappa B.

Endogenous molecules (not produced by microbes) are released in response to noninfectious injury (trauma, toxins, neoplasia, necrosis, or irritation). Because endogenous molecules can trigger an inflammatory reaction, they have been termed *alarmins*. Alarmins include sulfate, hyaluronan, HSP 60 (mitochondria), HSP 70 (cytoplasm), Gp 96 (endoplasmic reticulum), fibronectin, fibrinogen, and SP-A, all of which can bind PRRs or other receptors and initiate cell signaling, inflammation, and activation of the innate immune system (see Table 3-4). These molecules are often overlooked when considering acute inflammation in the context of microbial infections because microbial products, such as teichoic acid and LPS, are very potent activators of acute inflammation. However, endogenous molecules likely have a significant role in inflammation generated against neoplastic cells, toxins, and mechanical injury. For example, a wide variety of xenocompounds, including apoptotic cells, toxins (maitotoxin, valinomycin, nigericin, aerolysin), stress molecules (ultraviolet [UV] radiation, monosodium urate, calcium pyrophosphate, beta amyloid fibrils), xenogeneic compounds (silicates, asbestos, aluminum hydroxide), as well as microbial products (lipoteichoic acid, LPS), can affect lysosomal function which in turn induces NLRP3 (NALP3) activation (Fig. 3-12). Furthermore, adenosine, a by-product of cell injury CD39 hydroxylation of ATP, can bind adenosine receptors present on the surface membrane of leukocytes and modulate inflammatory and immune responses. Endogenous molecules mitigate the intensity of the inflammatory response by regulating signaling intensity.

ANTIMICROBIAL PEPTIDES AND COLLECTINS

Antimicrobial peptides, such as the α- and β-defensins, cathelicidins, and others—such as anionic peptides, histatin, and dermacidins—are small peptides with microbicidal activity against Gram-negative and -positive bacteria, fungi, mycobacteria, and some enveloped viruses such as human immunodeficiency virus (HIV) (Web Table 3-9). They are encoded by genes of the cells involved in the inflammatory response, especially neutrophils, and by epithelial cells forming the skin and the mucosal barriers of the respiratory and alimentary systems. The microbicidal activity likely occurs through the formation of pores within bacterial membranes and viral envelopes. In addition to the microbicidal activity, antimicrobial peptides are increasingly appreciated for their role in other nonmicrobial activities related to inflammation and

TABLE 3-4 Types of Pathogen-Associated Molecular Pattern (PAMP) Exogenous Ligands, Their Pattern Recognition Receptors (PRRs), and the Subsequent Action Related to Acute Inflammation

Exogenous PAMP Ligands	Secreted PRRs	Action
Mannose	MBL	Complement activation
Microbial membranes	CRP and SAP	Opsin, complement activation
LPS	LBP	LPS-binding
	C1q	Complement activation
	Ficollins	Complement activation
Cell-Surface PRRs		
LPS, peptidoglycan	CD14	Co-receptor for TLR4
Mannose	Macrophage mannose receptor	Phagocytosis
Bacterial cell walls	MARCO	Phagocytosis
β-glucan	Dectin-1	IL-10 and NF kappa B
Lipopeptides	TLR1	NF kappa B, MAPK
Lipoteichoic acid, lipoarabinomannan, zymosan	TLR2	NF kappa B, MAPK
LPS	TLR4	NF kappa B, MAPK
Flagellin	TLR5	NF kappa B, MAPK
Diacyl lipopeptides	TLR6	NF kappa B, MAPK
	TLR10	
	TLR11	
	TLR12	
	TLR13	
Intracellular PRRs		
DNA	TLR9	Type 1 IFN, NF kappa B
dsRNA	TLR3	Type 1 IFN, NF kappa B
ssRNA	TLR7/8, RIG-1, MDA5,	Type 1 IFN, NF kappa B
Muramyl tripeptide peptidoglycan (Gram-negative bacteria)	NOD1	IL-1β
Peptidoglycan-muramyl dipeptide (Gram-positive and Gram-negative bacteria)	NOD1	IL-1β
Low K^+ concentration, uric acid, silica, amyloid β, microbial products, dsRNA	NALP3	IL-1β, IL-18, IL-33
Heparin sulfate, hyaluronic acid, heat shock protein 60 and 70, endoplasmic reticulum glycoprotein 96, fibronectin, fibrinogen, surfactant protein A, apoptotic cells, K^+ fluxes via P2X and pannexin 1, adenosine	Growth factor receptors, CD44, TLRs, TGF-βR, gp IIb/IIIa, surfactant protein receptor 210 (myosin XVIIIA), NALP3, adenosine receptor	Numerous cellular responses, including cellular activation, proliferation, and/or apoptosis, IL-1β, IL-18, IL-33 production, T_H2 responses

Data from Medzhitov R: *Nat Rev Immunol* 1:135-142, 2001.
Endogenous inflammatory stimuli are those produced by host cells.
CRP, C-reactive protein; *dsRNA,* double-stranded RNA; *gp,* Glycoprotein; *IFN,* interferon; *IL,* interleukin; *LBP,* LPS-binding protein; *LPS,* lipopolysaccharide; *MAPK,* mitogen-activated protein kinase; *MARCO,* class A scavenger receptor macrophage receptor with collagenous structure; *MDA5,* melanoma differentiation-associated gene 5; *MBL,* Mannan-binding lectin; *NALP3,* ; *NF,* nuclear factor; *NOD1,* nucleotide-binding and oligomerization domain; *RIG-1,* retinoic acid-inducible gene-I; *SAP,* serum amyloid protein; *ssRNA,* single-stranded RNA; *TGF-βR,* transforming growth factor-β receptor; *TLR4,* Toll-like receptor 4.

wound repair. These activities include chemotaxis of leukocytes and dendritic cells, cell proliferation, wound repair, cytokine release, and the protease-antiprotease balance. There is also much evidence that antimicrobial peptides link the innate and adaptive immune responses.

There are a wide variety of antimicrobial peptides; however, the defensins have received the most attention for activities other than microbial killing. There are three types of defensins: the α-, β- and θ-defensins. α-Defensins are produced by neutrophils and Paneth cells. β-Defensins are produced by neutrophils and epithelial cells. θ-Defensins are produced in neutrophils of primates. The defensins are cationic proteins with three pairs of intramolecular disulfide bonds. α-Defensins and β-defensins can stimulate mast cell degranulation, induce IL-8 synthesis, induce T-lymphocyte chemotaxis, and activate T lymphocytes, macrophages, and dendritic cells, thus interconnecting innate and adaptive immunity. The importance of defensins in immunity is underscored by the fact that HIV-1 infected individuals that are healthy and in "remission" have high concentrations of α-defensins, which are thought to enhance T-lymphocyte activity and may also have direct anti–HIV-1 activity.

ACUTE PHASE PROTEINS

Acute phase proteins are plasma proteins synthesized in the liver whose concentrations increase (or decrease) by 25% or more during inflammation. These proteins serve as inhibitors or mediators of the inflammatory processes and include C-reactive protein, α_1-acid glycoprotein, haptoglobin, mannose-binding protein, fibrinogen, α_1-antitrypsin, and complement components C3 and C4. The concentration of these acute phase proteins usually increases during inflammation, whereas the concentration of prealbumin and albumin (also acute phase proteins) decreases in inflammation. Acute inflammatory conditions that are severe enough to raise blood plasma concentrations of cytokines, such as IL-1 and TNF, increase the blood concentrations of acute phase proteins and elevation of fibrinogen in the blood of cattle is used clinically

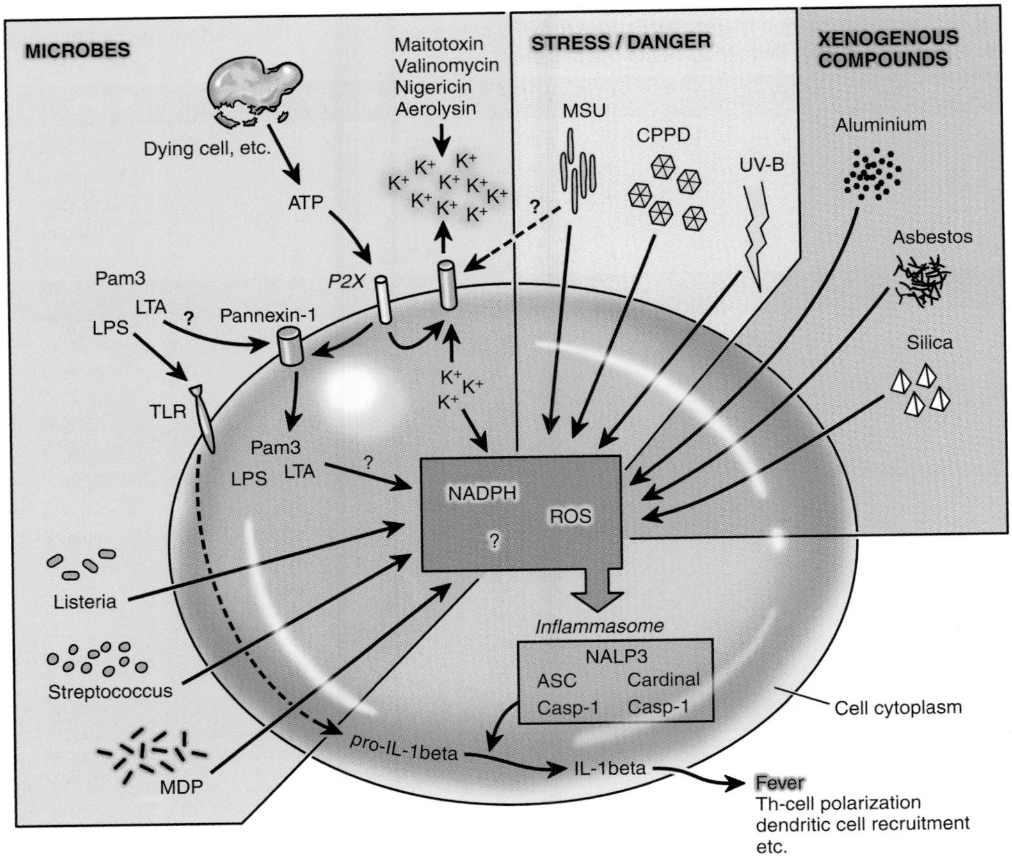

Fig. 3-12 Inflammasome activation by exogenous and endogenous stimuli. Numerous stimuli can result in activation of the NALP3 inflammasome. Exogenous stimuli include lipopolysaccharide (LPS), lipoteichoic acid (LTA), toxins, monosodium urate crystals (MSU), calcium pyrophosphate dehydrate (CPPD) crystals, ultraviolet (UV)-B waves, aluminum, asbestos, and silica. Endogenous stimuli include ATP, potassium, NADPH and reactive oxygen species (ROS). Once engaged, NALP3 activates caspase 1 which cleaves pro-IL-beta into IL-1 beta and also activates IL-18 (not shown). (Redrawn from Benko S, Philpott DJ, Girardin SE: The microbial and danger signals that activate Nod-like receptors, *Cytokine* 43(3):368-373, 2008. Epub 2008 Aug 19.)

as an indicator of systemic inflammation. C-reactive protein has recently received attention as a marker of inflammatory conditions, especially atherosclerosis in humans. In addition to its role diagnostically, C-reactive protein binds to bacteria and fungi and also activates complement. Once acute phase proteins and systemic levels of inflammatory cytokines are elevated, they affect the heart rate, blood pressure, and the hypothalamic regulation of temperature by directly or indirectly stimulating neurons within specific hypothalamic nuclei. The previously described changes also affect respiratory rates and gaseous exchange.

SUMMARY OF THE CHEMICAL MEDIATORS OF ACUTE INFLAMMATION

Various exogenous and endogenous stimuli can activate soluble, surface, or cytoplasmic and endosomal receptors or simply cause mechanical or other damage to invoke an acute inflammatory response. This response can occur very rapidly as the result of the release of preformed or rapidly activated inflammatory mediators such as histamine, kinins, complement factors like C3a and C5a, and tachykinins (substance P). These molecules generally affect vascular caliber and permeability and activate leukocytes and endothelial cells. Concurrently, lipid-based products, such as prostaglandins, leukotrienes, and PAF, contribute to chemotaxis, vascular tone, and leukocyte activity, all of which work in concert with chemokines and cytokines to activate endothelial cells and leukocytes and enhance neutrophil infiltration. NO released by macrophages and endothelia induce vasodilation and also can contribute to tissue damage caused by other reactive oxygen species. Inflammatory mediators bind receptors that subsequently induce cytoplasmic signaling and cellular activation, resulting in the production of additional cytokines, chemokines, adhesion molecules, antimicrobial peptides, and other inflammatory mediators that may either exacerbate or inhibit the inflammatory process. Activated neutrophils expressing leukocyte adhesion molecules, such as the integrins, enter inflamed tissue and can release hydrolytic enzymes and other granule contents that further damage tissue. Systemically, increases in acute phase proteins, cytokines, chemokines, complement, and inflammatory proteins can affect body temperature, cardiovascular function, locomotion, sleep, appetite, and other activities (Table 3-5).

REPARATIVE PHASE OF THE ACUTE INFLAMMATORY RESPONSE

OUTCOMES OF THE ACUTE INFLAMMATORY RESPONSE

The four main outcomes of acute inflammation are as follows:

- Resolution (the return to normal structure and function)
- Healing by fibrosis

TABLE 3-5 Examples of Differing Types of Inflammatory and Clinical Responses to Substances

	TYPE OF INFLAMMATORY SUBSTANCES		
	Skin Allergen	**Gram-Negative Bacterial Infection in Dermis**	**Gram-Negative Septicemia**
Substance	Allergen	LPS, toxins	LPS, toxins
Site	Epidermis/dermis	Dermis	Blood
Molecular trigger	Immunoglobulin E–cross-linking, dendritic cell binding	TLR4, CD14, NOD1	Hageman factor, complement, TLR4
Major response	Histamine, leukotrienes	IL-1, IL-18, TNF, prostaglandins, PAF, neutrophil products	Kinins, bradykinin, PAF, prostaglandins, IL-1, TNF
Extent of response	Local	Local	Systemic
Clinical finding	Swelling, pruritus (bronchoconstriction)	Swelling, exudate (pus)	Fever, nausea, malaise
Desired resolution	Limited, resolves in hours/days	Limited, resolves in days	Transient, resolves
Possible sequelae	Severe wheal and flare, anaphylaxis	Cellulitis leading to ulceration, eventual fibrosis/granuloma	Septic shock

CD14 = receptor for LPS-binding protein.
Hageman factor = clotting factor.
IL-1, Interleukin-1; *IL-18,* interleukin 18; *LPS,* lipopolysaccharide (endotoxin); *PAF,* platelet-activating factor; *NOD1,* nucleotide-binding and oligomerization domain; *TLR4,* Toll-like receptor 4; *TNF,* tumor necrosis factor.

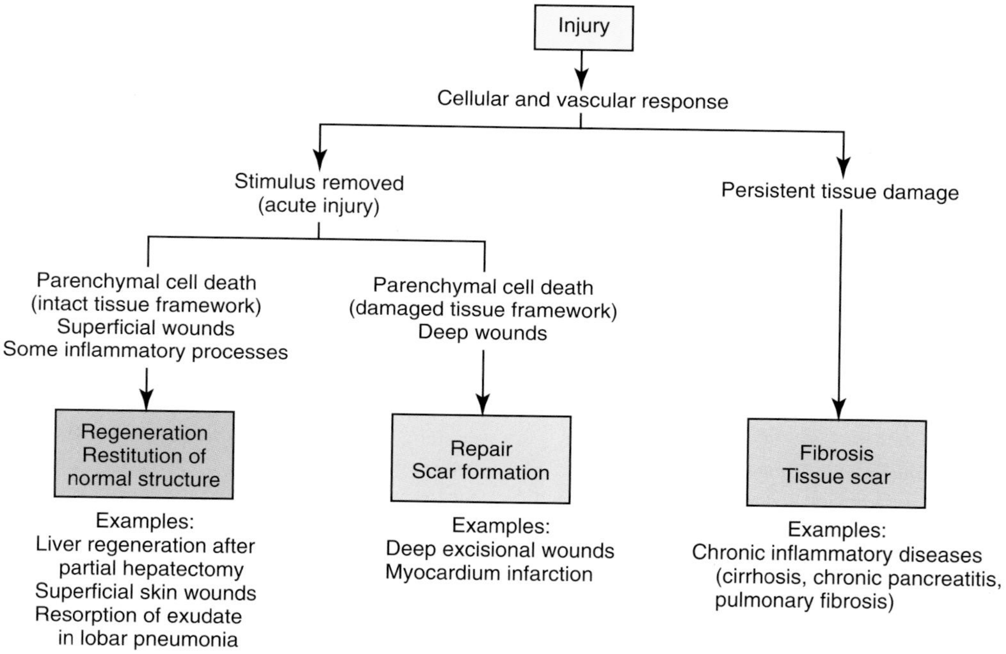

Fig. 3-13 Repair, regeneration, and fibrosis after injury and inflammation.
(From Kumar V, Abbas A, Fausto N, et al: *Robbins & Cotran pathologic basis of disease,* ed 8, Philadelphia, 2009, Saunders.)

- Abscess formation
- Progression to chronic inflammation

The severity of tissue damage, the ability of cells to regenerate, and the physical or biologic characteristics of the cause of the injury determine these outcomes. In the acute inflammatory response (Fig. 3-13), the desired outcome is resolution, that is, the complete return of normal structure and function. Resolution occurs if the following occur:

- The acute inflammatory response is completed in the correct sequence.
- Macrophages and lymphatic vessels remove the exudate.
- The inciting agent or substance is eliminated.
- The stroma (connective tissue) of the affected tissue is intact and can provide support for regeneration of epithelial cells.
- Ulcerated or necrotic epithelial cells are replaced by regeneration of adjacent epithelial cells on an intact basement membrane.

Mechanistically, the critical first stage of resolution involves the killing and/or removal of the inciting cause, removal of chemical mediators by neutralization or decay, return to normal vascular flow and capillary permeability, cessation of leukocyte emigration, apoptotic cell death of remaining neutrophils in the exudate, the removal of the exudate by monocyte-macrophage phagocytosis, and drainage to regional lymph nodes (Fig. 3-14).

Inflammatory responses of neutrophils, monocytes, and macrophages are further inhibited by chemokine inactivation and release of products such as lipoxin A4, resolvins, annexin A, lactoferrin, and lysophosphatidylcholine.

Regeneration is the second stage of resolution and depends on the availability of progenitor epithelial cells and the presence of a supportive stroma and intact basement membrane for orderly cellular migration. As an example, acute renal tubular necrosis can be caused by aminoglycoside antibiotics and results in detachment and necrosis of tubular epithelial cells from the tubular basement membrane. If the supporting stroma and basement membrane remain intact, progenitor epithelial cells can divide and migrate to replace lost cells and thus return the tubule to normal function. If the basement membrane is not intact to guide the proliferating cells, functional tubules will not form. Instead, regenerative tubular epithelial cells will atrophy or form into small aggregates with syncytial giant cells. Simultaneously, the microvascular supply to the region must be restored, which occurs mechanistically by the proliferation of endothelial cells in response to molecules such as VEGF.

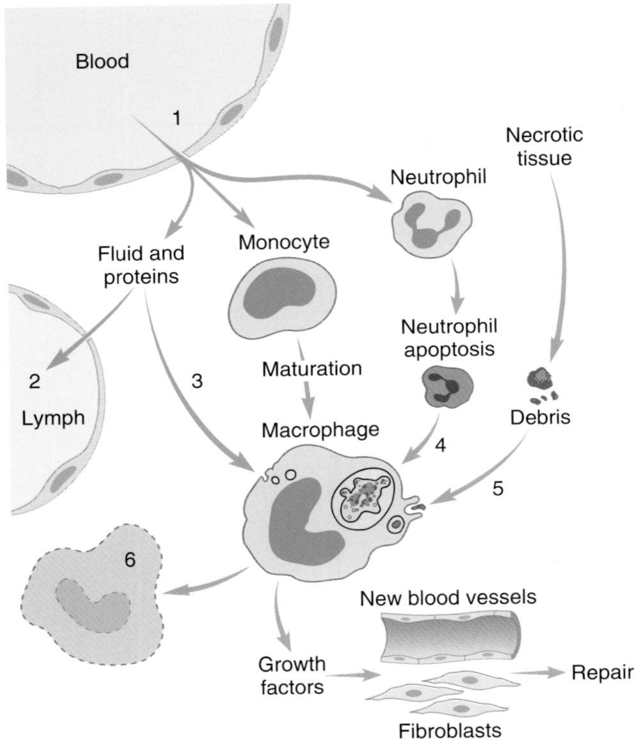

Fig. 3-14 Events in the resolution of inflammation.
1, Return to normal vascular permeability; *2,* drainage of edema fluid and proteins into lymphatics or *3,* by pinocytosis into macrophages; *4,* phagocytosis of apoptotic neutrophils and *5,* phagocytosis of necrotic debris; and *6,* disposal of macrophages. Macrophages also produce growth factors that initiate the subsequent process of repair. Note the central role of macrophages in resolution. (Modified from Haslett C, Henson PM: Resolution of inflammation. In Clark R, Henson PM, editors: *The molecular and cellular biology of wound repair,* New York, 1996, Plenum Press.)

NOMENCLATURE OF THE INFLAMMATORY RESPONSE (MORPHOLOGIC DIAGNOSES)

Nomenclature, a system of names assigned to structures and processes in a scientific discipline, used in veterinary pathology provides clinicians with a morphologic diagnosis, a precise description of the process, type of inflammation, and disease. A morphologic diagnosis has six components listed in the following sequence: degree of severity, duration, distribution, exudate, modifier, and tissue (Table 3-6). Based on the results of a postmortem examination and/or histologic evaluation of tissue specimens, a pathologist will construct a morphologic diagnosis by including in sequential order the components of the nomenclature that best describe the specimens. For example, using the kidney as the injured tissue, the central component of a morphologic diagnosis is the name of the tissue derived from its Latin term, "nephro-." If the kidney is inflamed, the prefix "nephro-" is combined with the suffix "itis" (inflammation or disease of) to form the word "nephritis," meaning inflammation of the kidney. The other components of the morphologic diagnosis, such as degree, duration, distribution, exudate, and modifier, precede nephritis and are used to describe the characteristics of the inflammatory process. The pattern of distribution of the inflammatory lesion not only provides location but also in many instances implies a mechanism of injury. These patterns of distribution as shown in Fig. 3-15 include focal, multifocal, locally extensive, and diffuse. They are covered in greater detail in each organ system. The subtleties of this process are learned through advanced training in the discipline of pathology, and terms describing the degree and duration evolve from years of professional experience and are not likely to be mastered by veterinary students during their professional training.

Morphologic diagnoses can also use the suffixes "osis" (diseased or abnormal condition) or "opathy" (disease). In this context, such diseases or conditions refer to those caused by degenerative or aging processes without inflammation. Therefore the same nomenclature can be used to diagnose a degenerative condition in the kidney by

TABLE 3-6 The Nomenclature of a Morphologic Diagnosis

Degree	Duration	Distribution	Exudate	Modifier	Tissue
Minimal	Acute	Focal	Serous	Necrotizing	Nephritis
Mild	Subacute	Multifocal	Catarrhal	Bronchointerstitial	Cystitis
Moderate	Chronic	Locally extensive	Fibrinous	Hemorrhagic	Enteritis
Marked (severe)	Chronic-active	Diffuse (interstitial)	Suppurative	Embolic	Pneumonia*
		Cranioventral†	Granulomatous		Hepatitis

This table provides an example of how nomenclature can be used to construct a morphologic diagnosis. It is not intended to be all-inclusive and may vary from schemes used in other veterinary colleges.
*In the lung, it is customary to use the term pneumonia to indicate inflammation of the lung.
†Used only for diseases of the lungs.

using the term *nephrosis* or the term *nephropathy*. The other components are then added to nephrosis or nephropathy to describe the characteristics of the degenerative process. Finally, some metabolic and neoplastic diseases do not fit into this nomenclature, but equally valid morphologic diagnoses can be constructed. An enlarged, soft and friable, yellow, and greasy liver can be morphologically diagnosed as "fatty liver" (hepatic lipidosis), whereas a solid, firm, white expansile mass in the liver could be morphologically diagnosed as "hepatic malignant lymphoma."

MORPHOLOGIC CLASSIFICATION OF EXUDATES IN ACUTE INFLAMMATORY LESIONS

The gross and microscopic appearance of different types of acute inflammatory reactions in tissue can often be classified according to the vascular and cellular components of the response, thus providing a mechanistic basis for understanding the pathogenesis. Histopathologic lesions of acute inflammation are most commonly grouped into five categories: serous, catarrhal, fibrinous, suppurative or purulent, and hemorrhagic, or a combination of these lesions such as fibrinosuppurative. Similar histopathologic patterns of lesions also occur in chronic inflammation (lymphohistiocytic or granulomatous [macrophages, multinucleate giant cells, lymphocytes, plasma cells, fibrosis]).

It should be recognized that the histopathologic lesions of acute inflammation often represent (1) a continuum of progressive changes of the same type of inflammation occurring over time or (2) different types of inflammatory responses occurring concurrently in the same or different areas of an affected tissue. Therefore rhinitis, for example, could progress in a sequence from serous to catarrhal to mucopurulent to purulent. If the inciting stimulus is severe, changes could progress rapidly from serous to fibrinous to hemorrhagic.

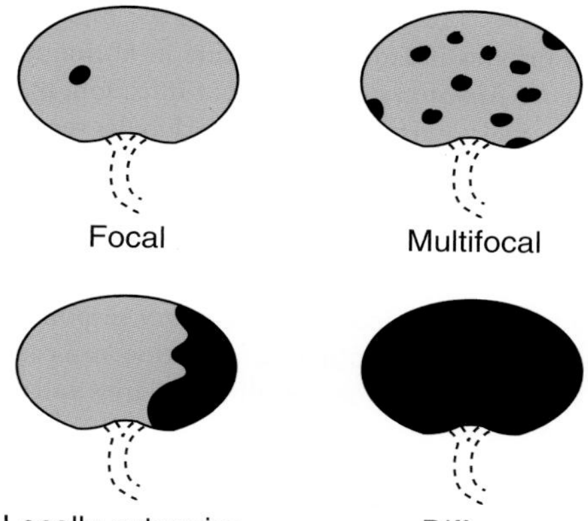

Fig. 3-15 Patterns of lesion distribution used to construct morphologic diagnoses, as an example, in the kidney.

(From Slauson DO, Cooper BJ: *Mechanisms of disease: a textbook of comparative general pathology*, ed 3, St Louis, 2002, Mosby.)

SEROUS INFLAMMATION

Serous inflammation is the term used to describe a pattern of acute inflammation in which the tissue response consists of the leakage or accumulation of fluid with a low concentration of plasma protein and no to low numbers of leukocytes. This watery material is released from small gaps between endothelial cells and from hypersecretion of inflamed serous glands. This response is essentially a transudate (specific gravity <1.012) and is seen with (1) thermal injury to skin, such as burns and photosensitization, in which the lesion can appear as a fluid-filled blisters, or (2) acute allergic responses characterized by watery eyes and a runny nose with a clear, colorless transudate.

Grossly, lesions, for example, with serous inflammation consist of tissue that (1) contains excessive clear to slightly yellow, watery fluid that leaks from the tissue on cut section or (2) forms raised fluid-filled vesicles protruding above the surface of the mucous membrane of the nasal cavity (serous rhinitis) or of the skin (Fig. 3-16). Microscopically, connective tissue fibers are separated, often widely, and capillaries and postcapillary venules are dilated with erythrocytes (active hyperemia). Endothelial cells lining these vessels can vary from flattened to hypertrophied.

CATARRHAL INFLAMMATION

Catarrhal inflammation, or mucoid inflammation, is the term used to describe a pattern of acute inflammation in which the tissue

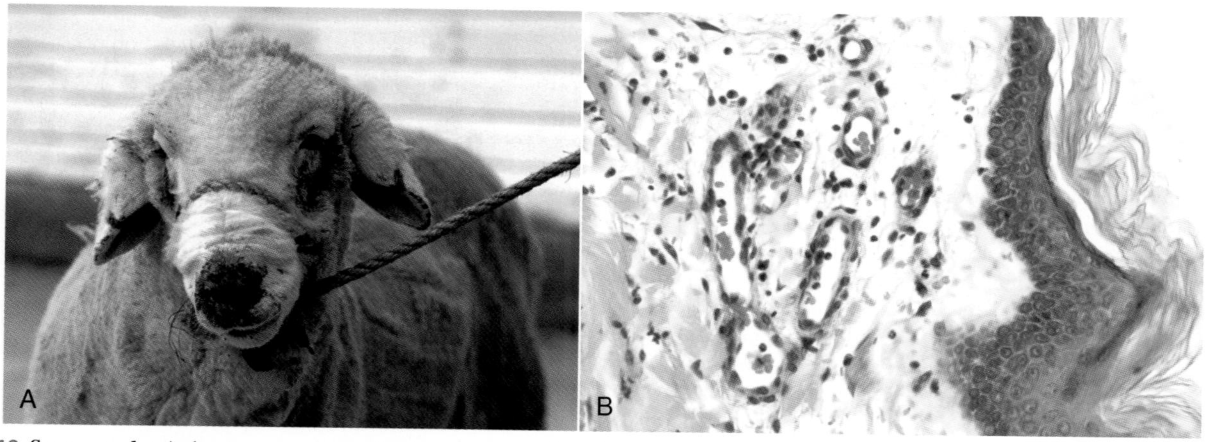

Fig. 3-16 Serous exudate/subcutaneous edema, photosensitization, skin of the nose and ears, ewe.
A, The nonhaired skin of the nose is covered by a crust resulting from dehydration of the serous exudate released from injured blood vessels following a short exposure to the sun. The ears are edematous and droopy. **B,** Microscopically, there is moderate expansion of the superficial dermis with edema secondary to vascular leakage (serous inflammation). The postcapillary venules are dilated (active hyperemia), and leukocytes have marginated on endothelial cells. H&E stain. (Courtesy Dr. M.D. McGavin, College of Veterinary Medicine, University of Tennessee.)

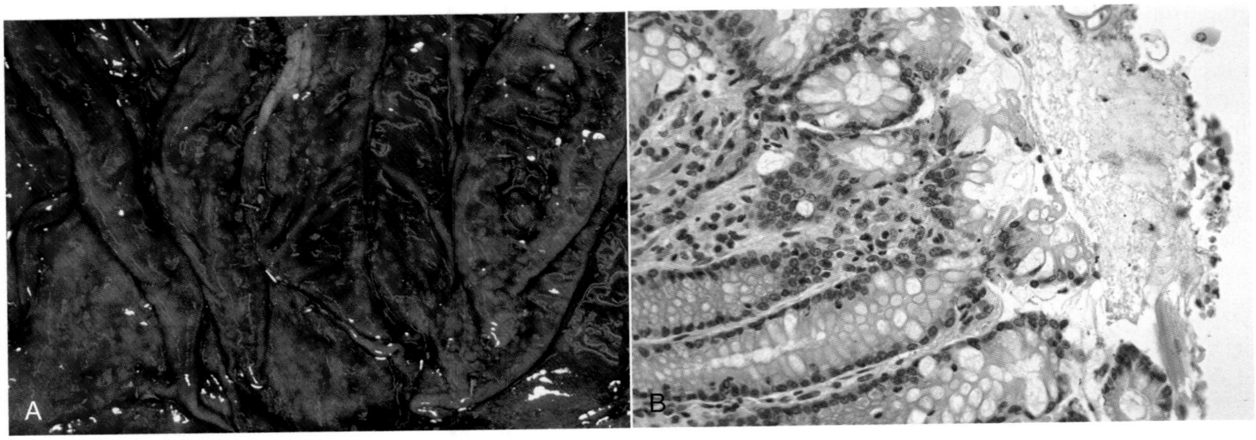

Fig. 3-17 Catarrhal inflammation.
A, Abomasum, cow. The mucosal epithelium is moderately thickened, covered by a glistening layer of clear mucus, and has a subtle nodular appearance caused by accumulation of mucinous secretory products (catarrhal exudate) in the gastric pits. **B,** Colon, cow. Microscopically, there is a catarrhal colitis with hyperplasia of mucosal epithelial cells and increased accumulation of mucus on the mucosal surface. H&E stain. (Courtesy Dr. M.D. McGavin, College of Veterinary Medicine, University of Tennessee.)

response consists of the secretion or accumulation of a thick gelatinous fluid containing abundant mucus and mucins from a mucous membrane. This response occurs most commonly in tissue with abundant goblet cells and mucus glands, such as in certain types of chronic allergic and autoimmune gastrointestinal diseases and with chronic inflammation of the airways of the respiratory system (chronic asthma). Grossly, the surface or cut surface of affected tissue may be covered with or contain a clear to slightly opaque, thick fluid (Fig. 3-17). Microscopically the lesion can include hyperplastic epithelial cells of mucus glands and goblet cells, as well as connective tissue fibers separated by mucins.

FIBRINOUS INFLAMMATION

Fibrinous inflammation is the term used to describe a pattern of acute inflammation in which the tissue response consists of the accumulation of fluid with a high concentration of plasma protein (specific gravity >1.02) and no to low numbers of leukocytes. This response is an exudate. Fibrinous inflammation occurs with more severe endothelial cell injury that allows leakage of large molecular weight proteins such as fibrinogen. Fibrinogen leaks from capillaries and postcapillary venules during the fluidic phase of the acute inflammatory response and polymerizes outside of the vessels to fibrin, a homogeneous and vividly pink (eosinophilic) protein when stained with hematoxylin and eosin (H&E). This lesion is most commonly caused by infectious microbes and is seen in the serous membranes of the body cavities, such as those lined by pleura (fibrinous pleuritis), pericardium (fibrinous pericarditis), peritoneum (fibrinous peritonitis), and in the synovial membranes of joints (fibrinous synovitis) and the meninges (fibrinous leptomeningitis). Common examples include the lesions in pulmonary alveoli in fibrinous pneumonia *(Mannheimia haemolytica),* atypical interstitial pneumonia (3-methyl indol), and respiratory viral infections (bovine herpesvirus-1 in cattle). When fibrin forms a distinct layer covering an ulcer, it is referred to as a *fibrinous pseudomembrane,* whereas when it lines the pneumonocyte surface of lung alveoli in a curvilinear fashion and is mixed with necrotic cell debris, such as occurs with bovine respiratory syncytial virus (BRSV) infection, it is called a *hyaline membrane.*

Grossly, the surfaces of affected tissue are red (active hyperemia) and covered with a thick, stringy, elastic, white-gray to yellow exudate that can be removed from the surface of the tissue (in contrast to a fibrous response) (Fig. 3-18; see Fig. 3-4). A classic example of fibrinous inflammation occurs in fibrinous pneumonia caused by acute *Mannheimia haemolytica* infection, in which both alveoli and stromal connective tissue (interlobular septa and pleura) contain notable fibrinous exudate that rapidly becomes infiltrated by neutrophils, resulting in a fibrinosuppurative exudate. Another example of fibrinous inflammation occurs in bovine herpesvirus-1 infection. This virus injures epithelial cells of the respiratory tract, resulting in an acute fibrinous inflammatory response. Noninfectious causes, such as heat and smoke inhalation, can cause fibrinous exudate in the trachea. Microscopically, capillaries and postcapillary venules are dilated with erythrocytes (active hyperemia), and endothelial cells are reactive (hypertrophied). The stromal connective tissue or the mesothelial surfaces of the affected organ contains or is covered by red to vividly red layers of coagulated and/or polymerized fibrin, albumin, and other plasma proteins. The fibrinous exudate is often rapidly infiltrated by neutrophils, resulting in fibrinosuppurative inflammation.

SUPPURATIVE INFLAMMATION

Suppurative inflammation is the term used to describe a pattern of acute inflammation in which the tissue response consists of the accumulation of fluid with a high concentration of plasma protein (specific gravity >1.02) and high numbers of leukocytes, predominately neutrophils. This material is an exudate commonly known as *pus.* Pus can be a creamy liquid, but if dehydrated, it can be more caseous and firm in consistency and occasionally laminated in diseases such as ovine caseous lymphadenitis. A collection of pus circumscribed by a fibrous capsule that is visible grossly is called an *abscess,* whereas, if visible only microscopically, it is called a *microabscess.*

Dense neutrophil accumulation (pus) can also be distributed in tissue layers such as fascial planes and subcutaneous connective tissue and is referred to as *cellulitis* or *phlegmonous inflammation.* Instead of producing a focal abscess, the neutrophils evoke a watery suppurative exudate distributed along fascial planes and tissue spaces, as in some cases of blackleg or extensive Gram-positive (staphylococcal) infection. Suppurative inflammation, microabscesses, abscesses, and exudates are most commonly caused by bacteria, including *Staphylococcus* spp., *Streptococcus* spp., and *Escherichia coli,* and can occur in many organs. These genera can also

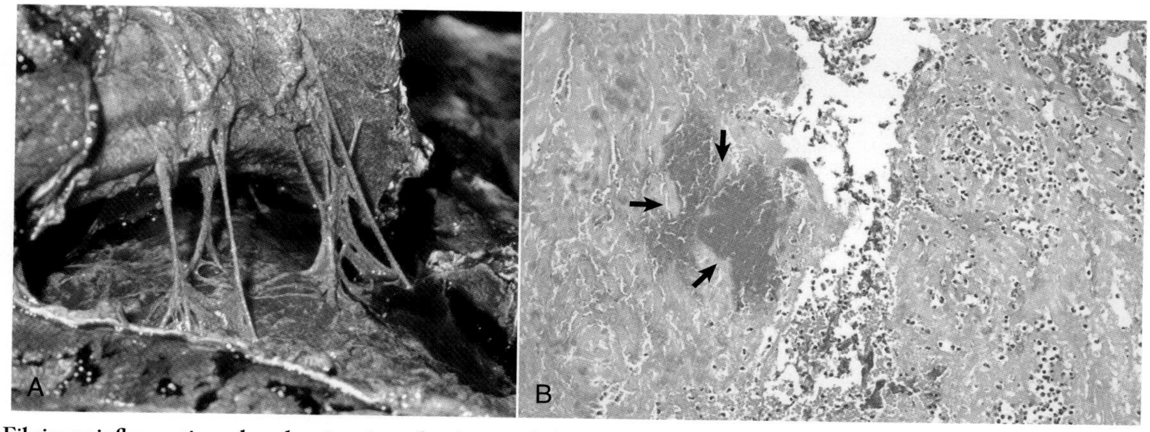

Fig. 3-18 Fibrinous inflammation, pleural cavity, visceral and parietal pleurae, horse.
A, The pleural surfaces are covered by a yellow-gray, thick, friable exudate consisting of fibrin mixed with other plasma proteins. This exudate can be easily pulled apart and should not be confused with fibrous adhesions. The latter response occurs over time and consists of a similar appearing material that contains collagen fibers, which provide tensile strength to the material and form adhesions between opposing surfaces that can only be broken with some difficulty. **B,** Microscopically, there are layers of homogeneous red material (fibrin-fibrinous exudate) that contain occasional neutrophils and a focus of bacteria *(arrows)*. H&E stain. (Courtesy Dr. J.F. Zachary, College of Veterinary Medicine, University of Illinois.)

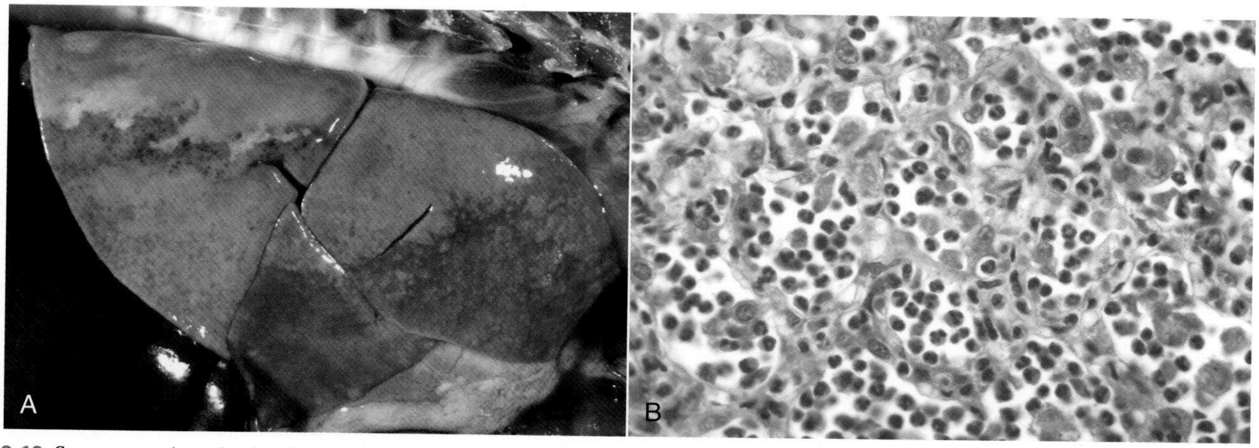

Fig. 3-19 Suppurative (purulent) inflammation, secondary bacterial bronchopneumonia, infectious canine distemper, puppy.
A, The cranioventral areas of the lung are firm and beige to brown. This lesion is caused by neutrophils transmigrating into alveoli in an acute inflammatory response secondary to bacterial infection of the lung. **B,** Microscopically, alveoli contain numerous neutrophils (suppurative exudate) and sloughed pneumocytes. H&E stain. (Courtesy Dr. M.D. McGavin, College of Veterinary Medicine, University of Tennessee.)

cause suppurative bacterial meningitis in the central nervous system (CNS). Abscesses in the brains of horses caused by *Streptococcus equi* and microabscesses in the brains of cows caused by *Listeria monocytogenes* are good examples of suppurative inflammation. Bacteria-induced suppurative inflammation also occurs commonly in (1) the pelvis and tubules (pyelonephritis) of the kidney, (2) the bronchi of the lungs (bronchopneumonia), (3) the nasal and sinus cavities (rhinitis and sinusitis), (4) the glandular epithelium of the prostate (prostatitis), (5) the lumina of the gall bladder (cholecystis) and urinary bladder (urocystitis), and (6) the acini and ducts of the mammary gland (mastitis). Unresolved suppurative inflammation can progress to chronic inflammation.

Grossly the surfaces and/or connective tissues of affected organs are hyperemic and covered by or contain, respectively, a thick white-gray to yellow pus (Fig. 3-19). In some cases, pus will be mixed with fibrin, forming a fibrinosuppurative exudate. Microscopically, affected tissues have large numbers of neutrophils; many degenerate and often are mixed with necrotic cellular debris, bacteria, plasma proteins, and fibrin.

CHRONIC INFLAMMATION

Chronic inflammation is inflammation of prolonged duration (weeks to months to years) that occurs (1) when the acute inflammatory response fails to eliminate the inciting stimulus, (2) after repeated episodes of acute inflammation, or (3) in response to unique biochemical characteristics and/or virulence factors in the inciting stimulus or microbe. Table 3-7 lists some of the most common causes of chronic inflammation in domestic animals. The underlying biologic mechanisms that result in chronic inflammation include persistence/resistance, isolation in tissue, unresponsiveness, autoimmunity, and unidentified mechanisms.

- Persistence/resistance: Persistent infections, such as those caused by *Mycobacterium* spp.; *Nocardia* spp.; deep-seated mycoses, such as *Blastomyces dermatitidis* (Web Fig. 3-11) and *Histoplasma capsulatum*; and parasites, such as *Toxocara canis* larvae, can avoid and/or resist phagocytosis by neutrophils and macrophages—or once internalized by these cells, can prevent fusion of primary and secondary lysosomes or

TABLE 3-7 Selected Examples of Conditions That Can Cause or Lead to Chronic Inflammation in Domestic Animals

Microbial Agents	Toxins	Autoimmune Diseases	Foreign Bodies	Other
Bacteria: *Brucella* spp. *Mycobacteria* spp.: canine/feline leprosy *M. avium-intracellulare* *M. bovis tuberculosis atypical (e.g., M. marinum)* *Rhodococcus equi* Virus: Porcine circovirus Fungi: *Trichophyton* spp. *Microsporum* spp. *Aspergillus* spp. Protozoa/parasites: *Leishmania* spp. *Trypanosoma* spp. *Draschia* spp. *Habronema* spp.	*Vicia villosa* (hairy vetch)	Lupus erythematosus Allergic contact dermatitis Irritant contact dermatitis Rheumatoid arthritis Polyarteritis nodosa	Retained suture Plant fibers Silica Asbestos Beryllium Inhaled smoke Inhaled dust	Canine granulomatous meningoencephalitis Lick granuloma Sterile nodular granuloma Sperm granuloma Chalazion Eosinophilic granulomas of dogs, cats, horses (see Table 3-8)

killing by lysosomes. Such microbes also usually do not produce biologic molecules that cause severe tissue injury, but their presence continually incites chronic inflammatory and immune responses. Some microbial agents can induce macrophages to undergo apoptosis and subsequent internalization by adjacent macrophages. Tissue destruction, granulomatous inflammation, and fibrosis are common sequelae of persistent/resistant infectious agents.

- Isolation: Some microbes, such as *Streptococcus* and *Staphylococcus* spp., are not naturally resistant to phagocytosis and/or destruction but are able to isolate themselves from effective innate and adaptive immune responses and from antimicrobial drugs by "hiding" themselves in pus.
- Unresponsiveness: Certain foreign materials are virtually indestructible and therefore are unresponsive to phagocytosis and/or enzymic breakdown. These include plant material, grass awns, silica dust, asbestos fibers, some suture materials, and surgical prostheses.
- Autoimmunity and leukocyte defects: Alterations in the regulation of adaptive immune responses to self-antigens result in autoimmune diseases, such as polyarteritis nodosa, with a chronic inflammatory response. Defects in leukocyte function can also result in chronic inflammation. For example, loss of NADPH oxidative function in human patients with chronic granulomatous disease, impair leukocyte free radical formation and oxidative killing, thus allowing persistence of microbial agents or internalized material.
- Unidentified mechanisms: In some diseases, such as canine granulomatous meningoencephalitis, the cause of chronic inflammation remains unknown.

The chronic inflammatory response is maintained by cytokines, chemokines, and other inflammatory mediators that are released and incite (1) ongoing inflammation mediated by infiltration and activation of lymphocytes, macrophages, plasma cells, and multinucleated giant cells (MGCs); (2) tissue destruction (necrosis); (3) proliferation of fibroblasts and deposition of collagen (desmoplasia and/or fibroplasia); (4) angiogenesis and neovascularization (granulation tissue formation); and (5) initiation of wound healing (reepithelialization and tissue repair).

BENEFICIAL AND HARMFUL ASPECTS OF CHRONIC INFLAMMATION

The body initially responds to injury through acute inflammation. Once the acute inflammatory response fails to overcome the inciting agent or persistent substance, chronic inflammation ensues as the body attempts to overcome the inciting agent/substance via a variety of cells such as NK cells, lymphocytes, macrophages and the adaptive immune response. If these responses fail, the inciting agent/substance is then "walled-off" with collagen produced by fibroblasts, encapsulating the agent/substance and functionally placing it "outside" of the body. Some types of responses, such as lepromatous (diffuse) granulomatous reactions, do not form defined fibrous capsules or walls and instead separate the agent/substance by dense accumulations of macrophages and fibroblasts that are arranged irregularly. Often, this response can be beneficial and in time can lead to a return to normal activity. Small granulomas or abscesses in the lung, liver, or even in some areas of the skin, with time, eventually go unnoticed by the innate and adaptive immune systems and do not stimulate pain or mechanical interference to movement or function.

On the other hand, chronic inflammation can be detrimental. The mononuclear leukocyte infiltrates (macrophages, lymphocytes, and NK cells) within areas of chronic inflammation take up space and often displace, replace, and sometimes obliterate the original tissue. At the same time, new blood vessels form, fibroblasts proliferate and deposit collagen, and if the lesion expands, the inflammatory response can affect function of adjacent tissues and/or cells and ultimately the function of the entire organ. For example, chronic inflammatory lesions in the intestine of dogs and cats with inflammatory bowel disease (IBD) can induce progressive weight loss and debilitation. Also, chronic inflammation in the brains of dogs with granulomatous meningoencephalitis, can destroy neurons and glia, impinge and obstruct flow of cerebrospinal fluid (CSF) in the ventricular system, and elevate the intracranial pressure, all of which can impair cognition and movement.

The extent of debilitation in animals with chronic inflammatory lesions depends on the location of the lesion and extent of tissue involvement. Even very small chronic lesions in the brain can rapidly incite clinical signs through either the destruction of neuroparenchyma or, perhaps, by impairing flow or resorption of CSF. In contrast, some widespread chronic inflammatory lesions, such as those in inflammatory bowel disease of dogs and cats and Johne's disease of cattle, can involve extensive areas of the intestine and often precede clinical signs (diarrhea) by months or even years. Yet other diseases, such as embolic hepatic or lung abscesses or disseminated tuberculoid granulomas, can be debilitating over time through the loss of parenchymal function and the continual release of inflammatory mediators, such as TNF and IL-1, both of which affect temperature and appetite.

In chronic inflammation, the first clinical intervention is to remove the inciting factor, if possible. Thus antibiotics and antifungal drugs are used against bacterial and mycotic infections. Some foreign bodies can be removed surgically, and it may be possible to identify, opsonize, chelate, or sequester immunologic allergens, antigens, and nondegradable substances. Unfortunately, few medical therapies completely resolve certain types of chronic inflammation, especially if granulomas and/or extensive scar tissue have developed. In the future, perhaps surgical debulking of large lesions may be followed by gene or stem cell therapy to effectively eliminate specific types of granulomas, such as those caused by mycobacterial infection or inducing apoptosis of fibroblasts, myofibroblasts, and macrophages.

PROGRESSION OF THE ACUTE INFLAMMATORY RESPONSE TO CHRONIC INFLAMMATION, FIBROSIS, AND ABSCESS FORMATION

Acute inflammatory responses can either fully resolve with return of the tissue to normal structure and function or repair by healing (Fig. 3-20). If conditions do not allow for complete resolution of the acute inflammatory response, four outcomes can result: (1) progression to chronic/granulomatous inflammation, (2) healing by fibrosis, (3) healing with increased cellularity (cerebral gliosis, Kupffer cell hyperplasia, or glomerular mesangial cell hyperplasia), or (4) abscess formation. These outcomes are determined by the severity of tissue damage, the ability of cells to regenerate, and the biologic characteristics of the agent/substance (e.g., mycobacterial waxes, poorly degradable plant fibers) that caused the injury.

PROGRESSION TO CHRONIC/GRANULOMATOUS INFLAMMATION

Progression to chronic/granulomatous inflammation occurs when the acute inflammatory response fails. Failure is characterized by the following:

- The inciting stimulus persisting for a long period of time (weeks to months)
- Extensive tissue injury and necrosis (third-degree burn)
- A shift of the cellular elements of the inflammatory response from neutrophils to lymphocytes, macrophages, and sometimes multinucleate giant cells
- Extensive connective tissue reorganization followed by fibrosis (fibroplasia)

Examples of agents and substances that often result in chronic inflammatory responses include systemic mycoses, such as *Blastomyces dermatitidis* and *Histoplasma capsulatum*; intracellular bacterial pathogens, such as *Nocardia, Brucella, Mycobacterium, or Salmonella* spp.; protozoa, such as *Leishmania* or *Trypanosoma* spp.; parasites, such as *Toxocara larva* or *Habronema;* autoantigens, such as those occurring in sperm granulomas or in autoimmune diseases like lupus erythematosus; and foreign bodies (plant awns, sticks, metals, asbestos, or suture material). Such agents continually induce the release of inflammatory mediators from indigenous parenchymal cells and leukocytes, leading to macrophage infiltration and activation; T-lymphocyte, NK cell, and perhaps mast cell or eosinophil infiltration; and fibroblast and endothelial cell proliferation. Some of the inflammatory cytokines, such as TGF-β, may interfere with regeneration of epithelial and parenchymal cells (see section on Wound Healing and Angiogenesis).

HEALING BY FIBROSIS

Healing by fibrosis occurs after tissue injury in which there is necrosis of the tissue framework provided by stromal elements

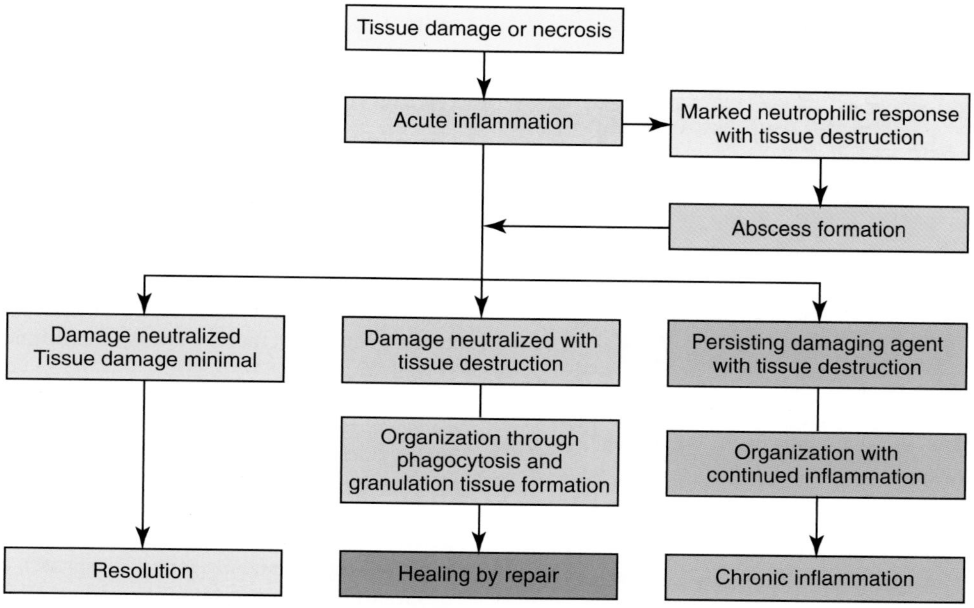

Fig. 3-20 The outcomes of tissue injury and unresolved acute inflammation.
(Modified from Young B, O'Dowd G, Stewart W: *Wheater's basic pathology: a text, atlas and review of histopathology*, ed 5, New York, 2010, Churchill Livingstone.)

(connective tissue) and of the epithelial cells required to regenerate and successfully reconstitute the parenchymatous elements of the tissue. After necrosis, dead tissue and the acute inflammatory exudate are removed by macrophages (phagocytosis by cells of the monocyte-macrophage system), and the space is filled with fibrovascular tissue (granulation tissue) commonly seen in the healing process. Granulation tissue is eventually replaced by immature fibrous connective tissue that is poorly collagenized and then by mature connective tissue that is well collagenized, healing the wound and forming a scar (cicatrix). Structural integrity may be reestablished, but functional integrity depends on the extent of the loss of parenchymal cells. For example, with severe skin burns or extensive lacerations, dermal scarring eventually replaces lost dermal structures and to a limited extent restores structural integrity; however, the skin's functional integrity is extremely limited because of the loss of adnexal glands, hair follicles, and scar tissue that reduces the range of motion in joints of the limbs and digits. The degree and extent of fibroblast and myofibroblast proliferation in such wounds largely depends on mediators such as TGF-β and IL-13 (see the section on Wound Healing and Angiogenesis).

ABSCESS FORMATION

Abscess formation (Fig. 3-21) occurs when the acute inflammatory response fails to rapidly eliminate the inciting stimulus and the enzymes and inflammatory mediators from neutrophils in the exudate liquefy the affected tissue and neutrophils to form pus. Myeloperoxidase enzyme in neutrophils contributes to neutrophil necrosis and liquefaction. The presence of myeloperoxidase is an evolutionary phenomena and reptiles and birds lack this enzyme and are therefore unable to liquefy neutrophils into pus. Abscesses can have a septic or sterile origin. Septic abscesses most commonly originate from bacterial infection, whereas sterile abscesses arise from incompletely degraded foreign bodies or from the failure of injected medications to be completely absorbed. Pyogenic bacteria, such as *Staphylococcus* and *Streptococcus* spp., commonly cause septic abscesses. They enter tissue hematogenously or by direct extension from the skin following trauma. The pus within an abscess can range in consistency from serous to purulent to caseous and in color from white, to yellow, to green, depending on the inciting agent/substance. The color of the exudate often depends on the pigment produced by the inciting bacterium and the species; for example, yellow exudates are caused by abscesses formed by *Staphylococcus, Streptococcus* spp., and *Corynebacterium ovis;* green exudate is caused by abscesses formed by *Pseudomonas aeruginosa;* and red exudate is caused by abscesses formed by *Serratia marcescens.*

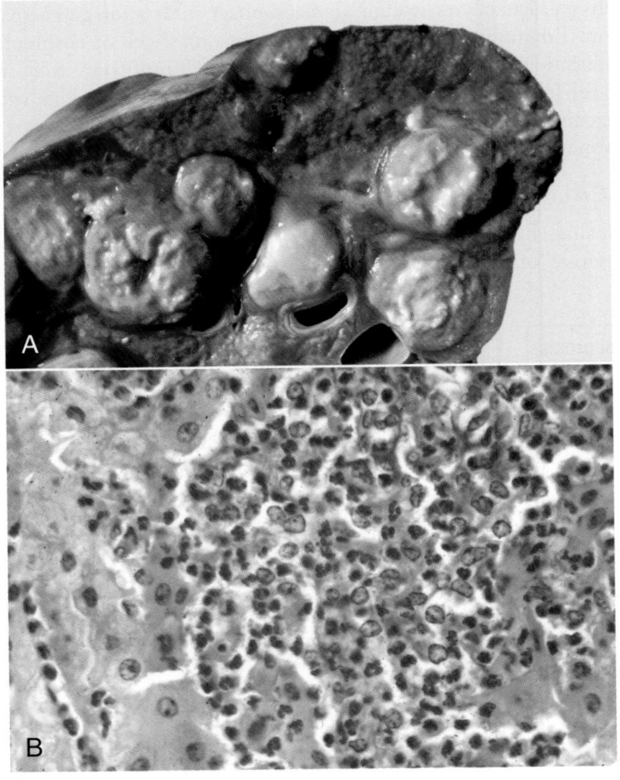

Fig. 3-21 Abscess formation.
A, Abscess, lung, cow. A cut section of lung has numerous abscesses. Note the white-to-gray exudate and how it bulges from the cut surface. **B,** The exudate in **A** consists of cell debris and a large number of neutrophils admixed with lesser numbers of degenerating macrophages and lymphocytes, and bacteria (the latter not visible with H&E stain). H&E stain. (Courtesy Dr. M.D. McGavin, College of Veterinary Medicine, University of Tennessee.)

After an acute inflammatory response has been established, the development of an abscess in this site consists of a collection of neutrophils admixed with cell debris, macrophages, and fibroblasts with variable infiltrates of lymphocytes. Experimentally, such a site can form in 2 to 3 days, depending on the agent/substance. Fibroblasts in this site begin to produce collagen and ECM proteins that can form into a "thin" vascularized connective tissue area. At this point, antibiotics can penetrate this area and enter the exudate. If the septic abscess persists, the initial "thin" connective tissue area surrounding the exudates can mature into a fibrous capsule, which is thick and largely impermeable, in an attempt to "wall-off" the exudates from normal tissue. A capsular wall takes weeks to form. Abscesses with this response can present serious problems in systemic (hematogenous) or local (topical diffusion) antibiotic treatments. In large abscesses with abundant pus, the pus itself may dilute the antibiotic and further prevent the drug from reaching the optimal concentration required to kill the bacteria. It is for these reasons that larger abscesses are often lanced to drain the pus. Sterile abscesses do not require antibiotics or other drugs to kill an inciting agent/substance, but they do require breakdown of the capsule by lancing or some other means.

GRANULOMATOUS INFLAMMATION AND GRANULOMA FORMATION

Granulomatous inflammation is a distinct type of chronic inflammation in which cells of the monocyte-macrophage system are predominant and take the form of macrophages, epithelioid macrophages (activated macrophages), and MGC. In granulomatous inflammation, the cells are dispersed as sheets of cells distributed at random (diffuse or lepromatous) within parenchymal and connective tissue planes (Fig. 3-22, *A*), whereas in a granuloma (tuberculoid granuloma), they are arranged in distinct masses or nodules (Fig. 3-22, *B*).

Granulomatous inflammation occurs secondarily in response to endogenous or exogenous antigens or idiopathically as in granulomatous meningoencephalitis of dogs. Development and regulation of granulomatous inflammation requires multiple factors: (1) the inciting agent, usually with indigestible, poorly degradable, and persistent antigens (e.g., *Mycobacteria* spp.); (2) the host immune response (e.g., T_H and macrophage response); and (3) the interplay of various cytokines, chemokines, and other proinflammatory and antiinflammatory mediators produced by cells within the chronic inflammatory lesion.

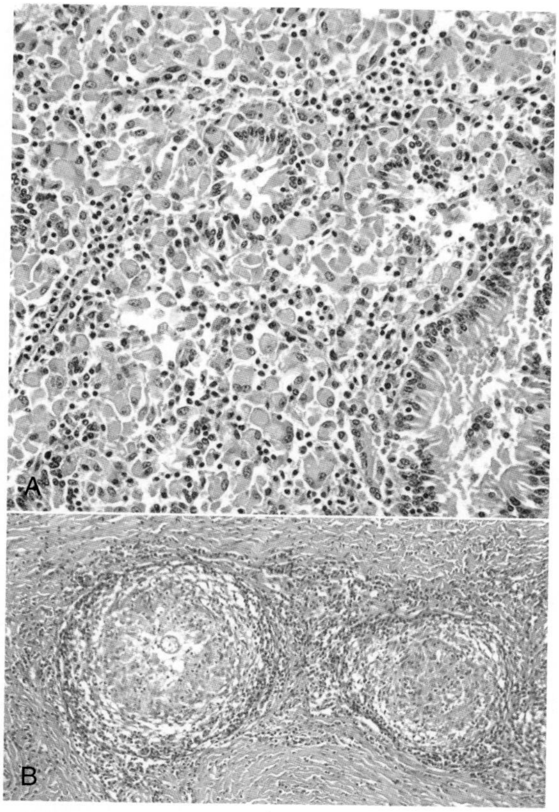

Fig. 3-22 Granulomatous inflammation and granulomas. **A,** Granulomatous inflammation in Johne's disease, ileum. The lamina propria contains a solid sheet of granulomatous inflammatory cells, which is characteristic of lepromatous (diffuse) granulomatous inflammation, H&E stain. **B,** Nodular (tuberculoid) granuloma in coccidioidomycosis. Granulomas are round to oval with a central core of granulomatous inflammatory cells and a peripheral zone of fibroblasts, which may produce a fibrous capsule. The granuloma on the left contains a single central fungal element. H&E stain. (**A** courtesy Dr. J.F. Zachary, College of Veterinary Medicine, University of Illinois. **B** courtesy Dr. M.D. McGavin, College of Veterinary Medicine, University of Tennessee.)

Classification of granulomatous inflammation by pathologists has evolved over the years because of the increased understanding of disease pathogenesis and advances in molecular biology. For simplicity, this chapter discusses two morphologic forms of granulomatous inflammation: diffuse (lepromatous) granulomas, which are currently thought to be consistent with a T_H2-biased immunologic response, and nodular (tuberculoid) granulomas, which are currently thought to be consistent with a T_H1-biased immunologic response. Both of these terms are derived from granulomatous lesions in humans and are increasingly becoming defined and seen as distinct, both immunologically and molecularly.

Nodular (Tuberculoid) Granulomas (T_H1-Biased Granulomas)

Examples of nodular (tuberculoid) granulomas are those that have been classically caused by *Mycobacterium bovis* or *Mycobacterium tuberculosis* (Fig. 3-23) and by some deep fungal infections, such as coccidioidomycosis (Web Fig. 3-12). Grossly, nodular granulomas are often gray to white, round to oval, and firm to hard, whereas diffuse granulomatous inflammation is often gray to white; expansile but poorly demarcated from adjacent tissue; and firm. Tuberculoid (nodular) granulomas develop with a T_H1-type lymphocytic response and occur in many species but have been described extensively from lesions of infected humans, cattle, and rhesus monkeys. Because the portal of entry is often the respiratory tract, these lesions involve the lung with secondary involvement of other parenchymal organs and induce the formation of granuloma. Microscopically, nodular (tuberculoid) granulomas may or may not have a central core of necrotic cell debris (caseating and noncaseating granulomas) (see Fig. 3-23). Granulomas of either type are often oval to round and can be irregular as well as multinodular, vary in size from microscopic to macroscopic, and very large.

Noncaseating granulomas are often round to oval and microscopically composed of numerous macrophages with variable numbers of epithelioid macrophages, perhaps multinucleate giant cells, with a peripheral zone of fibroblasts, lymphocytes, and plasma cells. Caseating granulomas have the same morphologic features as noncaseating granulomas; however, the center is formed by a core of gray-white-yellow pasty (thick-dehydrated) necrotic debris resembling cheese (Latin caseus = cheese). Caseating granulomas most commonly occur in tuberculosis. Microscopically, caseating granulomas have a central core of cell debris, surrounded by a dense zone of macrophages that may contain epithelioid macrophages that are admixed increasingly in the outer layers of granuloma with lymphocytes, plasma cells, and fibroblasts.

The outermost zones of either a noncaseating or caseating granuloma are frequently similar and composed of fibroblasts that deposit collagen and ECM proteins that create a dense fibrous region that can form into a capsule. Thus a well-formed granuloma has three distinctive morphologic areas. The innermost area is often but not always a centrally located region of macrophages and multinucleate giant cells in a noncaseating granuloma and cellular necrosis in a caseating granuloma, which is surrounded by a middle area containing macrophages, epithelioid macrophages, and multinucleate giant cells. The outermost area surrounding the entire lesion consists of T and B lymphocytes, plasma cells, macrophages, and a fibrous capsule (Fig. 3-24).

Mycobacterial organisms and their antigens are very sparse in these granulomas and not commonly detected with acid-fast stains and immunohistochemical stains for mycobacterial antigens. Mineralization can occur in tuberculoid granulomas, but this outcome depends on the species of animal affected. It is common in cattle, present to a lesser degree in pigs, and uncommon in sheep. "Atypical" mycobacteria, such as *Mycobacterium marinum,* can also cause nodular (tuberculoid) granulomas in the subcutaneous tissues of dogs, cats, and other species, and very few organisms are detected with stains. Certain persistent, poorly degradable antigens, such as those in foreign bodies and in microbes, such as *Nocardia* spp., can have eosinophilic proteinaceous aggregates of immunoglobulin on their outer surfaces, which can be seen histologically and are termed *Splendore-Hoeppli proteins.*

Steps in formation of a tuberculoid (nodular) granuloma (see Fig. 3-23) are as follows:

1. Stage I granuloma. Days after infection, the lesion site is infiltrated by neutrophils, monocytes, macrophages, γ/δ T lymphocytes, and NK cells. Epithelioid macrophages also form.
2. Stage II granuloma. From roughly 48 hours to multiple days and weeks, lesions contain macrophages, epithelioid macrophages, thin rims of fibrous connective tissue, variable numbers of NK cells, and γ/δ T lymphocytes, as well as α/β T lymphocytes and B lymphocytes. MGCs can also form.
3. Stage III granuloma. From weeks to 1 month, the central area can caseate or become dense with macrophages and mineralize. Lymphocytes, plasma cells, a zone of fibroblasts, and a fibrous connective tissue capsule surround this core.

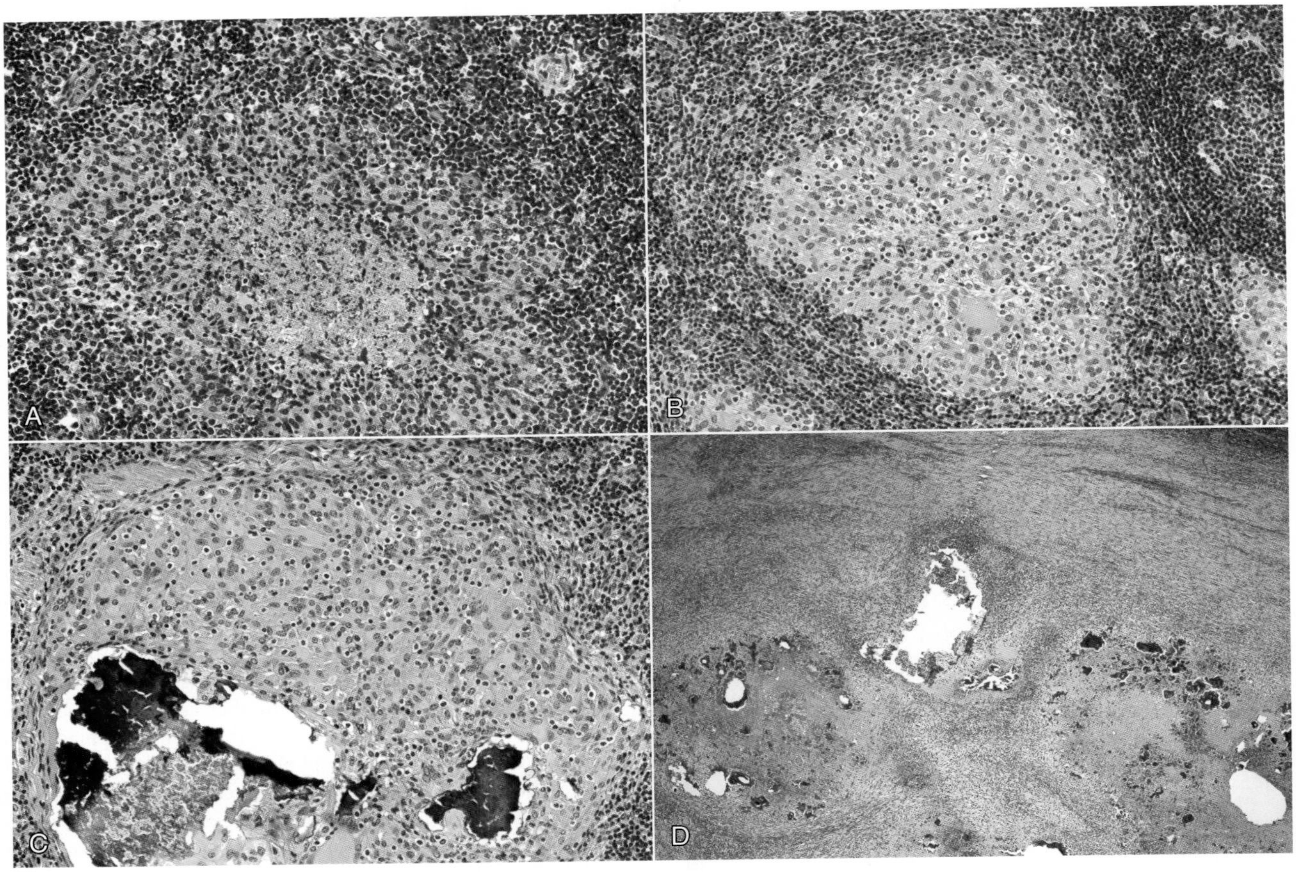

Fig. 3-23 Nodular (tuberculoid, T_H1) type of granulomatous inflammation.
A series of micrographs from lymph nodes of cattle experimentally infected with *Mycobacterium bovis* illustrate stages of T_H1 granuloma formation. **A,** Stage I granuloma. Initial lesions have a central region of cell debris with occasional neutrophils and macrophages that are surrounded by a zone of macrophages that are irregularly arranged and further surrounded by densely associated lymphocytes. **B,** Stage II granuloma. Days later, granulomas are composed of numerous macrophages aggregated in an oval region with occasional epithelioid macrophages and small multinucleate giant cells. This core is surrounded by dense infiltrates of lymphocytes. **C,** Stage III granuloma. The mature granuloma has a central area of mineralization along with numerous macrophages, multinucleate giant cells and epithelioid macrophages. **D,** Stage IV granuloma. With long-term persistence of antigen, the granulomatous reactions with areas of mineralization coalesce and overtake additional surrounding tissue and are bordered by dense infiltrates of lymphocytes. H&E stain. (Courtesy Dr. M. Palmer, USDA/ARS-National Animal Disease Center, Ames, Iowa.)

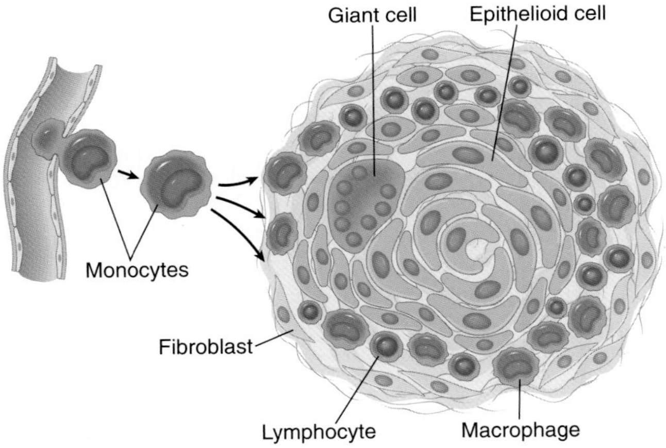

Fig. 3-24 Schematic illustration of the formation of a granuloma.
(Modified from Kumar V, Abbas A, Fausto N, et al: *Robbins & Cotran pathologic basis of disease*, ed 8, Philadelphia, 2009, Saunders.)

4. Stage IV granuloma. From several weeks to months, the lesion can be walled off by a dense capsule and regions within the lesion can become mineralized and overtake the surrounding tissue. The capsule wall can sometimes become degraded when microorganisms are released from the inner regions of the lesion.

Diffuse (Lepromatous) Granulomas (T_H2-Biased Granulomas)

Mycobacterium leprae, the cause of human leprosy, produces noncaseating aggregates of macrophages and chronic inflammatory cells often around nerve fibres in the distal extremities and upper respiratory tract mucosa (sites in the body with temperatures lower than core body temperature) of infected humans. This type of granulomatous inflammation appears to form with a predominantly T_H2-type of adaptive immune response that is seen in veterinary medicine during the clinical stages of Johne's disease in cattle and sheep.

These lesions can be poorly delineated (e.g., poorly defined borders) and have a widespread distribution, a heavy intracellular bacterial burden, relatively few lymphocytes, numerous macrophages that extend into surrounding tissue often without a distinct

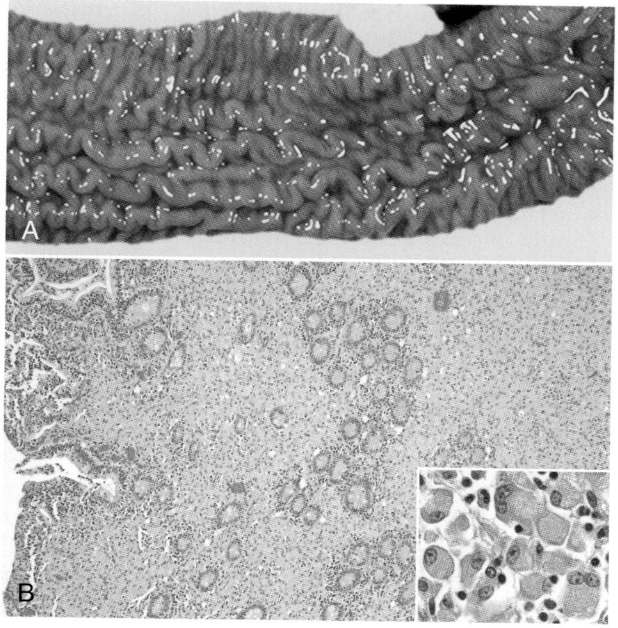

Fig. 3-25 **Diffuse (lepromatous) type of granulomatous inflammation, Johne's disease (*Mycobacterium avium* ssp. *paratuberculosis*), ileum, cow.** **A,** The mucosa is thickened because of a dense infiltrate of granulomatous inflammatory cells in the lamina propria. The lumen of the intestine is to the left. **B,** The lamina propria contains numerous macrophages arranged in sheets. The ileal lumen is to the left; scattered crypts still remain in the central area of the specimen. H&E stain. **Inset,** Higher magnification of macrophages present in the granulomatous inflammatory exudate. H&E stain. (**A** courtesy Dr. M.D. McCracken, College of Veterinary Medicine, University of Tennessee; and Noah's Arkive, College of Veterinary Medicine, The University of Georgia. **B** courtesy Dr. J. Hostetter, College of Veterinary Medicine, Iowa State University. **Inset** courtesy Dr. M.D. McGavin, College of Veterinary Medicine, University of Tennessee.)

capsule, variable degrees of fibrosis, and lack caseation. Similar granulomatous lesions are seen in animals. Feline leprosy and canine lepromatous-like granulomas are somewhat similar to human leprosy in lesion formation. *Mycobacterium avium-intracellulare* paratuberculosis—the cause of Johne's disease in cattle, sheep, and goats—also induces a diffuse (lepromatous) type of granulomatous inflammation consisting of diffuse sheets of macrophages with few lymphocytes and plasma cells. This lesion most commonly occurs in the lamina propria of the ileum and colon (Fig. 3-25) and in mesenteric lymph nodes. Special stains, such as acid-fast and immunohistochemical stains specific to bacterial antigens, can be used to identify these bacteria within the cytoplasm of macrophages and those that are extracellular (Web Fig. 3-13). Because bacteria are present in large numbers in these diseases, they are commonly identified by these techniques. Nodular (tuberculoid) granulomas, defined later, are not seen in Johne's disease lesions. Finally, *Mycobacterium avium* ssp. *paratuberculosis* infection also occurs in the lung and other organs of birds often induces lesions with similar sheets of macrophages containing abundant bacteria detectable with special stains.

SARCOIDS OF HORSES

Sarcoids of human patients are granulomatous-like lesions. In contrast, sarcoids of horses are not a correlate to sarcoids in humans. Sarcoids that occur in the skin of horses are not granulomas as occur in humans but are locally aggressive skin tumors, and the most common dermatologic neoplasm reported in horses. They are composed of proliferating fibroblasts and do not contain the numerous macrophages, lymphocytes, and plasma cells seen in human sarcoids. Bovine papillomavirus (BPV) types 1 and 2 and the major transforming protein, E5, are associated with equine sarcoids but appear not to produce infectious virions. E5 may contribute to the persistence of the virus and development of the lesion by downregulating major histocompatibility complex (MHC) class I expression and thereby reducing immunosurveillance. The mode of transmission of BPV infection has not been determined.

TABLE 3-8 Eosinophilic Granulomas of Domestic Animals

Species	Type of Eosinophilic Granuloma
Feline	Eosinophilic plaque, granuloma, and dermatitis
Canine	Eosinophilic granuloma of the oral cavity of huskies and other dogs
Equine	Equine collagenolytic granuloma, axillary nodular necrosis, and unilateral papular dermatosis
All species	Eosinophilic (T_H2) granulomas secondary to parasitic infections

T_H2, T helper lymphocyte type 2.

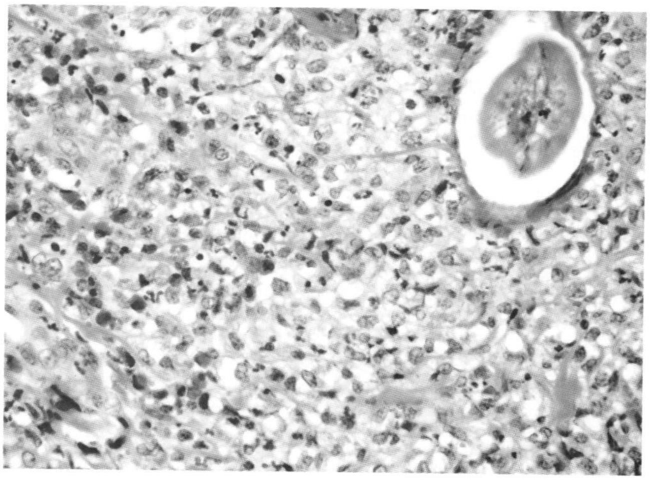

Fig. 3-26 **Granuloma with eosinophils.**
A region of skin from a horse in which there is a parasitic organism (Habronema sp) that has invoked a marked granulomatous reaction of closely associated macrophages admixed with eosinophils. H&E stain. (Courtesy Dr. M.R. Ackermann, College of Veterinary Medicine, Iowa State University.)

EOSINOPHILIC GRANULOMAS

Certain types of chronic inflammation have dense infiltrates of eosinophils with macrophages, and varying numbers of lymphocytes and plasma cells (Web Fig. 3-14). Because of the presence of eosinophils, they are termed *eosinophilic granulomas* (Table 3-8). Some granulomas with numerous eosinophils develop in response to migrating parasites, such as *Toxocara canis* (larval migrans). In eosinophilic granuloma of cats, eosinophilic stomatitis of dogs, and equine eosinophilic dermatitis of horses, it is suspected these conditions form in response to antigen in a T_H2-directed manner; however, no specific antigen has been identified.

Grossly, eosinophilic granulomas in cats appear as papules, nodules, plaques (sometimes linear), and ulcers in the skin. They also occur as nodular or ulcerated lesions in the oral mucosae and footpads. Microscopically, the inflammatory response consists of eosinophils, macrophages, and areas of dense eosinophilia around collagen (Fig. 3-26). For many years, the densely eosinophilic, collagen-rich areas were considered regions of collagen degradation; however, the eosinophilic material is composed largely of major basic protein (MBP), a protein present in large amounts in the granules of eosinophils. Apparently eosinophils degranulate in these regions, releasing MBP, which accumulates over time. Some eosinophilic granulomas do not form distinct nodular granulomas and the cellular content of the lesions (e.g., the numbers of macrophages and eosinophils) can vary widely. But the lesions are chronic in nature and contain enough macrophages and other chronic inflammatory cells to be classified as granulomas by most pathologists.

OTHER CHRONIC INFLAMMATORY/GRANULOMATOUS CONDITIONS

Information on this topic, including visceral leishmaniasis and Web Figs. 3-15 and 3-16, are available at evolve.elsevier.com/Zachary/McGavin/.

GROSS AND MICROSCOPIC LESIONS AND NOMENCLATURE OF THE CHRONIC INFLAMMATORY RESPONSE

The term *chronic inflammation* implies two underlying and often concurrently occurring processes: fibroplasia and cellular infiltration. Often, one of these types of responses predominates. Fibroplasia, the formation of fibrous connective tissue, includes any stage of the process from the formation of fibrous connective tissue that includes newly formed "immature" connective tissue with newly formed blood vessels to "mature" connective tissue that contains well-collagenized and remodeled granulation tissue. Cellular infiltrates are composed of predominantly macrophages, lymphocytes, and plasma cells, depending on the inciting agent/substance and the duration of the inflammatory process. It is important to understand the mechanism of these processes to apply gross and histopathologic diagnoses. To clinicians, these terms imply duration of illness, whereas to pathologists, they imply the characteristics of the tissue's response to injury.

Grossly, chronic inflammatory lesions are often gray-to-white and firm and have either a nodular surface in the case of granulomas or an indented or pitted surface in the case of fibrosis. The gray-to-white color is largely a result of the infiltrates of macrophages and lymphocytes, proliferation of fibroblasts, and deposition of fibrous connective tissue. The firm texture is attributable to fibrous connective tissue (fibroblasts and endothelial cells) and the consolidation (i.e., solidification) of the leukocytes in the exudate. The irregular shape occurs because of the haphazard accumulation of leukocytes and the fibrosis/scarring and contraction of the lesion by myofibroblasts within the fibrous connective tissue (see section on Wound Healing and Angiogenesis).

The lungs of dogs with *Blastomyces dermatitidis* infection often have a nodular appearance because of the formation of numerous granulomas and/or pyogranulomas. The use of and distinction between terms such as *granuloma* and *pyogranuloma* depend on the number of neutrophils in the overall inflammatory exudate or in the center of the granuloma and often reflect the interpretation of the examining pathologist.

The pitted surface of kidneys of dogs, cats, or other species can be seen, for example, with chronic interstitial nephritis or chronic pyelonephritis. Frequently, the pitted surfaces correspond to areas where fibrous tissue formed within renal parenchyma during the chronic inflammatory response that pulls the renal capsule into the parenchyma as part of the healing process. In chronic pyelonephritis, the inflammatory bands often radiate from the renal medulla into the cortex and to the renal capsule and obliterate or surround and separate cortical tubules and glomeruli. Fibrous adhesions between the renal cortex and the capsule can occur. This fibrous connective tissue may also contain lymphocytes, plasma cells, and macrophages.

Grossly, abscesses, granulomas, and areas of fibrosis that occur with the persistence of chronic inflammation are often easily seen. Severe fibrosis results in an area that is generally gray to white with extensive contraction, whereas abscesses are often round with a fibrous capsule and a central area of pus. Grossly, the three main differential diagnoses for a white, firm, oval-to-irregular nodular mass are abscess, granuloma, and neoplasm. Most commonly, histopathology is required to differentiate the three because they can appear very similar grossly.

Microscopically, chronic inflammatory responses are classified into categories based on the types and distribution of the inflammatory cells in the exudate. These categories include (1) chronic lymphocytic/lymphohistiocytic inflammation, (2) fibrosing chronic inflammation, (3) chronic-active (purulent) inflammation, (4) granulomatous (noncaseating) inflammation, (5) pyogranulomatous inflammation, (6) granulomas, and (7) pyogranulomas.

- Chronic inflammation composed of lymphocytes and plasma cells admixed with macrophages occurs commonly in the body (Fig. 3-27). Sometimes, lymphocytes and macrophages predominate over plasma cells, and such lesions can be called lymphohistiocytic. *Histiocytic* is a term used for macrophage infiltration; however, some pathologists use the term *macrophagic*. This type of inflammatory response is characteristically seen in the early stages of the chronic inflammatory response and in response to specific microbes, such as viruses, and in mucosal surfaces in response to antigenic stimulation.

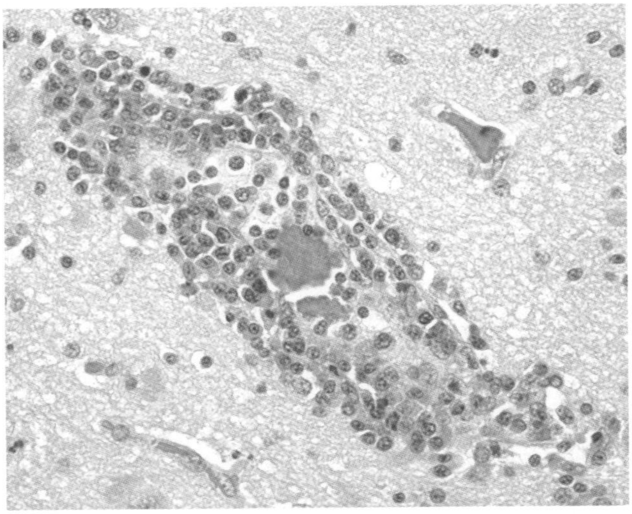

Fig. 3-27 Chronic inflammation, distemper, brain, raccoon. In its simplest form, chronic inflammation, as seen with some viral infections, consists of an exudate of lymphocytes with occasional macrophages and plasma cells. In many tissues, especially in the central nervous system, these cells can have a perivascular pattern of distribution. In certain animal species (exotic wildlife species, horses) and specific disease categories (parasitic, protozoal, viral), perivascular chronic inflammatory exudates may also contain variable numbers of eosinophils. H&E stain. (Courtesy Dr. J.F. Zachary, College of Veterinary Medicine, University of Illinois.)

- Fibrosing chronic inflammation is a region of chronic inflammation that is predominantly composed of fibrous connective tissue. This can occur in chronic traumatic pericarditis (hardware disease) of cattle where there are areas of pericardial fibrosis covered by fibrin and in the chronic fibrosis that surround necrotic regions of lung and form along the pleura of cattle with contagious bovine pleuropneumonia and chronic *Mannheimia haemolytica* pneumonia.
- Chronic-active inflammation has the same cellular components as chronic inflammation but also contains neutrophils, fibrin, and plasma proteins that are constituents of the acute inflammatory response. Chronic-active inflammation occurs when the inciting stimulus has not been removed from the exudate in the chronic inflammatory response, and it continues to elicit an acute inflammatory response. One should be careful not to confuse the morphologic diagnosis of chronic-active inflammation with the hepatic disease entity of dogs termed *chronic-active hepatitis.*
- Granulomatous inflammation has a basic cellular exudate consisting predominantly of activated macrophages and in some cases also epithelioid macrophages, multinucleate giant cells, and lesser numbers of lymphocytes and plasma cells. Granulomatous inflammation can be arranged in a diffuse or haphazard manner as seen in the thickened intestinal mucosa (i.e., lamina propria) of cattle with Johne's disease (see Fig. 3-25). While the presence of a few macrophages in a lesion is indicative of chronic inflammation, these are considered to be granulomatous inflammation when the macrophages aggregate and begin to replace portions of the normal stroma.
- Pyogranulomatous inflammation has the same cellular exudate as granulomatous inflammation but also contains multifocal/random infiltrates of neutrophils, fibrin, and plasma proteins, which are constituents of the acute inflammatory response. Pyogranulomatous inflammation occurs when the inciting stimulus has not been removed from the exudate in the granulomatous inflammatory response, and it continues to elicit an acute inflammatory response. A nodular-like granulomatous area with neutrophils is termed a *pyogranuloma* (see later). Pyogranulomatous inflammation is often seen with infections caused by *Blastomyces dermatitidis* and is frequently multinodular. Pyogranulomatous is sometimes used loosely, with little discretion. For example, it can be used in lesions that are in transition from acute inflammation to chronic inflammation or during the "clean-up" phase of healing.
- Granulomas are a distinct type of granulomatous inflammatory response that occurs when macrophage infiltration is present in a well-defined area and thus form a distinct mass on gross observation. Granulomas can occur as noncaseating and caseating types, as described.
- A pyogranuloma is a nodular granuloma with a central area of neutrophils.

CELLULAR MECHANISMS OF CHRONIC INFLAMMATORY RESPONSES

LYMPHOCYTES

Lymphocytes play a key role in most chronic inflammatory lesions, especially in autoimmune diseases and in diseases with persistent antigen. As with macrophages, lymphocytes enter unresolved areas of acute inflammation within 24 to 48 hours, being attracted by chemokines, cytokines, and other stimuli. Histologically, they are often aggregated around blood vessels and surround granulomas or are distributed haphazardly within injured tissue (see Fig. 3-27). In viral encephalitides, lymphocytes are commonly distributed in a perivascular pattern, primarily in the gray matter. In other types of conditions, such as lymphoplasmacytic stomatitis and pododermatitis of cats, lymphocytes and plasma cells are the predominant cell types in the lesions.

γ/δ–T LYMPHOCYTES

γ/δ–T lymphocytes are often the first type of T lymphocyte to arrive in the lesion of chronic inflammation and can contribute to the development of granulomas. This mechanism is supported by the fact that mice lacking γ/δ–T lymphocytes have defects in granuloma formation. However, the role of γ/δ–T lymphocytes in the establishment and persistence of granulomas has not been fully determined. Cattle have high numbers of circulating γ/δ–T lymphocytes, relative to other T lymphocytes, and are a useful model for assessing the role of γ/δ–T lymphocytes, in the formation of classic granulomas in *Mycobacterium tuberculosis* and *Mycobacterium bovis* infections and in the formation of diffuse granulomatous lesions in *Mycobacterium avium-paratuberculosis* infections.

α/β–T LYMPHOCYTES (CD4/CD8)

α/β–T lymphocytes (CD4 and CD8 lymphocytes) enter areas of chronic inflammation and are key to the regulation of the type of adaptive immune response that ensues, albeit a T_H1, T_H2, or T_H0 response of chronic inflammation and/or granuloma formation. Under the influence of cytokines, these lymphocytes can further differentiate into (1) effector memory lymphocytes, which enter extralymphoid sites of inflammation; and (2) central memory lymphocytes, which settle into the blood and lymphoid organs. Memory lymphocytes contribute to the persistence of the chronic inflammatory response and granuloma formation.

T_H1, T_H2, T_H17, AND T REG IMMUNOLOGIC RESPONSES

The mechanistic basis for chronic inflammation to develop and persist is slightly to profoundly different, depending on the inciting agent or condition. While the cell types (e.g., monocytes, macrophages, T and B lymphocytes, and NK cells) are consistent features of chronic inflammation, their relative numbers and function can vary widely. T lymphocytes expressing CD4+ (T helper lymphocytes) and CD8+ T lymphocytes (cytotoxic cells) play important roles in the adaptive immune response that shapes chronic inflammation. When CD4+ T lymphocytes bind foreign antigens presented by macrophages, dendritic cells, or B lymphocytes, they release lymphokines that attract leukocytes into the lesion site; some of these cells are directed toward T_H1 (cell mediated), T_H2 (humoral), T_H17, T_{FH}, and T reg responses (Web Fig. 3-17). Dendritic cells generally present antigen to naïve CD4 T lymphocytes, whereas macrophages present antigen to committed T lymphocytes. Thus antigen presentation by macrophages is especially active in long-standing regions of chronic inflammation. In the presence of poorly degradable exogenous or endogenous antigens, the biologic characteristics of antigens, including the amount and structure of protein, polysaccharide, and lipid, contribute to the extent to which the T lymphocyte response will be between a T_H1, T_H2, T_H17, T_{FH}, or T reg. However, in most chronic inflammatory conditions, there is a mixed T_H1, T_H2, and T_H17 type cellular response. T reg lymphocytes, regulatory dendritic cells, and other cells (NK type 1 cells, mast cells, eosinophils, or basophils) can affect the strength and the balance of T_H1, T_H2, and T_H17 responses through inhibition of the responses. T_H1 immunologic responses often occur in response to (1) foreign bodies; (2) endogenous antigens, such as those in MBP (which can occur in murine experimental allergic encephalomyelitis [EAE] and is an experimental model of multiple sclerosis); and (3) endogenous antigens, such as those in intracellular microbes like *Mycobacteria* spp., *Listeria monocytogenes, Histoplasma capsulatum, and Leishmania* spp. T_H1 chronic inflammatory responses are composed, histologically, of macrophages with variable numbers of T and B lymphocytes, dendritic cells, and occasionally fibroblasts. The T_H1 response is induced by IL-12, IFN-γ, IL-18, IL-23, and IL-27. Briefly, antigen-presenting cells release IL-12 (also IL-18, IL-23, and IL-27) that induces pre-T_H/CD4+ cells to commit to the T_H1 pathway. The T_H1-committed CD4+ cells then release IL-2 for proliferation of T lymphocytes that produce IFN-γ and TNF-β, which activates macrophages. In addition, IFN-γ can inhibit the commitment of pre-Th_H/CD4+ cells to the T_H2 pathway.

In contrast, theT_H2-predominant responses are often seen in chronic inflammatory conditions with an allergic basis, such as asthma, chronic allergic inhalant, or food allergic dermatitis, or inflammatory bowel disease. The mucosa and skin dermis of these conditions contain T and B lymphocytes, macrophages, dendritic cells, and fibroblasts in the T_H2 inflammatory milieu that leads to increased numbers of mast cells, basophils, and eosinophils associated with IgE and other humoral responses. T_H2 responses are induced by high concentrations of IL-4 and IL-10, as well as IL-5, IL-9, IL-13, IL-17, and to some degree, perhaps IL-19, IL-20, IL-22, IL-24, IL-26, IL-28, and IL-29. Briefly, T_H2 dendritic cells present antigen to pre-T helper/CD4+ lymphocytes committing them to the T_H2 pathway. T_H2-committed CD4+ lymphocytes release IL-4 and IL-5, IL-10, IL-13, IL-17, and IL-19 (also IL-19, IL-20, IL-22, IL-24, IL-26, IL-28, and IL-29) to act on B lymphocytes, thus resulting in antibody production and in some cases, increased activity of eosinophils, mast cells, and basophils that release mediators of acute inflammation and T_H2 cytokines such as IL-4. In addition, IL-4, IL-5, IL-10, and IL-13 can also inhibit pre-T helper/CD4+ lymphocytes from committing to the T_H1 pathway.

T_H17 immunologic responses form in the presence of IL-23 and induce secretion of IL-17A, IL-17F, IL-21, IL-22, IL-26, and CCL20, which are associated with development of autoimmune responses in conditions such as allergic airway inflammation, psoriasis, inflammatory bowel disease, arthritis, and multiple sclerosis (humans). T_H17 lymphocytes function predominantly at mucosal surfaces and trigger neutrophil activation and release of antimicrobial factors to bridge innate and adaptive immune responses. Other cell types, such as γδ T lymphocytes, NK cells, NK-T lymphocytes, and lymphoid tissue inducer (LTi) cells, produce a range of cytokines similar to T_H17 lymphocytes.

MONOCYTES/MACROPHAGES

Monocytes/macrophages are the signature cell types of chronic inflammation. They produce a wide variety of inflammatory mediators, including chemokines, cytokines, and NO, and are often situated at strategic locations within tissues of the body to (1) quickly sense the initial activity of acute inflammation, (2) migrate in response to chemotaxins, (3) remove and kill microbial agents by phagocytosis, (4) remove and degrade particulate matter by phagocytosis, (5) process antigens for presentation to effector cells of the adaptive immune response, and (6) facilitate angiogenesis and remodel the ECM (Fig. 3-28).

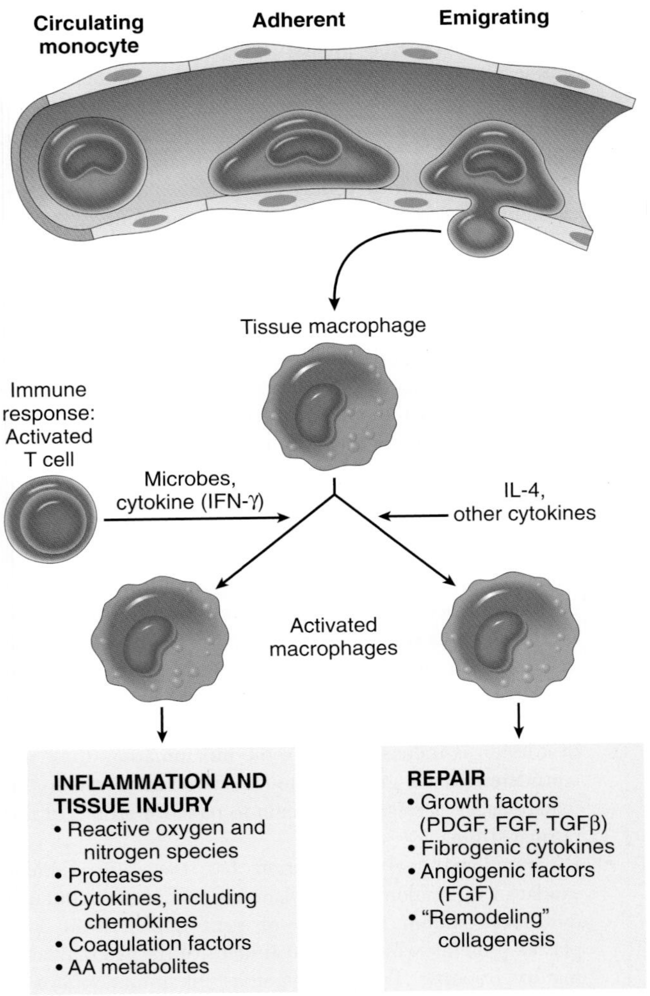

Fig. 3-28 The roles of activated macrophages in chronic inflammation. Macrophages are activated by nonimmunologic stimuli such as endotoxin or by cytokines from immune-activated T lymphocytes (particularly interferon-γ [IFN-γ]). The products made by activated macrophages that cause tissue injury and fibrosis are indicated. *AA,* Arachidonic acid; *PDGF,* platelet-derived growth factor; *FGF,* fibroblast growth factor; *TGF-β,* transforming growth factor-β. (From Kumar V, Abbas A, Fausto N, et al: *Robbins & Cotran pathologic basis of disease*, ed 8, Philadelphia, 2009, Saunders.)

EPITHELIUM

Epithelial cells can contribute to chronic inflammatory responses in a variety of manners. For example, experimental models of granuloma formation have shown that Mycobacteria release an early secretory antigen-6 (ESAT-6), which induces release of MMP-9 from epithelia that is vital for recruitment of macrophage infiltration. Epithelia can also release type I interferons, cytokines, antimicrobial peptides, and chemokines and express adhesion molecules.

MONONUCLEAR CELL MATURATION AND TRAFFICKING IN THE CHRONIC INFLAMMATORY RESPONSE

The macrophage is key to the development and persistence of chronic inflammation. Monocytes, derived from the bone marrow, form the monocyte/macrophage system by entering tissues and

TABLE 3-9 Stimuli That Affect the Activation Status of Macrophages

Type of Activation	Activating Factor	Macrophage Response	Macrophage Activity
Innate activation to microbes	Toll-like receptor CD14 (LPS binding) β-Glucan receptor TREM	Co-stimulatory expression ROS, NO expression Cytokine release	Inflammation, antigen presentation to memory T lymphocytes
Humoral activation	Fc receptor Complement receptors	Ig/Fc internalization Cytolytic activity Cytokine release	Inflammation, antigen presentation to memory T lymphocytes
Classical activation T_H1	IFN-γ	MHC II expression Cytokine release (IL-1, IL-6, TNF) Respiratory burst NO release	Cell-mediated immunity Microbial killing DTH
Alternative activation T_H2	IL-4 IL-13	MHC II expression Mannose receptor expression	Humoral immunity Allergic response Response to parasites Arginase repair
Deactivation by innate/adaptive stimuli	IL-10 TGF-β IFN-α, IFN-β GM-CSF CD47 CD200R CD36 (scavenger receptor) $\alpha_5\beta_3$-Integrin Glucocorticoid receptor Internalized ox LDL	MPH II down-regulation PGE_2 release IL-10 release TGF-β release PPAR inhibition of NF kappa B	Immunosuppress

GM-CSF, Granulocyte-macrophage colony-stimulating factor; *DTH,* delayed type hypersensitivity; *IFN,* interferon; *Ig,* immunoglobulin; *IL,* interleukin; *MHC,* major histocompatibility complex; *NF,* nuclear factor, *NO,* nitric oxide; *ox LDL,* oxidized low-density lipoprotein; *PGE_2,* prostaglandin type E_2; *PPAR,* peroxisome proliferator-activated receptor; *ROS,* reactive oxygen species; *TGF,* transforming growth factor; *T_H1,* T helper cell type 1 lymphocyte response; *T_H2,* T helper cell type 2 lymphocyte response; *TREM,* triggering receptor expressed on myeloid cells.

differentiating into macrophages (e.g., Kupffer cells, alveolar macrophages, and microglial cells) and are central to innate and adaptive immune systems. Recent work also shows that the spleen is a significant reservoir of monocytes, which can exit en masse on tissue injury. Monocytes are then recruited from the bloodstream to enter tissue and differentiate into macrophages that can also respond to tissue injury. Under noninflammatory conditions, the replenishment of tissue macrophages occurs through local proliferation and not via monocyte influx. However, with inflammatory stimuli, monocytes are recruited from the blood into tissue in response to inciting agents/substances.

In noninflamed tissue, monocytes expressing CX3CR1 and CCR5 chemokine receptors are attracted to tissues expressing their respective ligands (i.e., fractalkine (CX3CL) and MIP-1-a [CCL3]). In areas of inflammation, monocytes expressing CCR2 chemokine receptors are attracted by MCP-1 (CCL2). Attracted monocytes enter these areas in a manner similar to that described for the leukocyte adhesion cascade outlined for neutrophils. Slow rolling is mediated by E and P selectins and firm adherence by monocytes to endothelial cells is largely mediated by LFA-1 (CD11a/CD18), VLA-4 ($\alpha_4\beta_1$-integrin), and also Mac-1 (CD11b/CD18) molecules that adhere to the respective endothelial cell ligands: ICAM-1/2, VCAM-1, and ICAM-1/2. Transmigration of monocytes between endothelial cells is mediated by leukocyte adhesion molecules expressed on the monocyte such as LFA-1, VLA-4, Mac-1, PECAM-1, and JAM A, JAM B, and JAM C. These molecules bind to adhesion molecules, such as PECAM-1, and the JAM molecules expressed by endothelial cells at the intracellular junction. As monocytes and other leukocytes pass between endothelial cells, they separate the tight junctions and vascular-endothelial (VE)-cadherins to allow the passage of the leukocyte.

T_H1, T_H2, T_H17, and T reg lymphocytes, along with inflammatory mediators released by somatic cells and macrophages during injury and/or infection, affect the differentiation of monocytes and noncommitted macrophages to macrophages with specific function (see Web Fig. 3-21). In conditions favorable to T_H1 influence, macrophages respond to IFN-γ released by T_H1, NK lymphocytes, and TNF from antigen-presenting cells to form classically-activated macrophages (Table 3-9). Under T_H2 conditions, macrophages respond to IL-4 released by T_H2 lymphocytes and granulocytes (e.g., mast cells, basophils) by forming wound-healing (tissue repair) type macrophages. Under T-reg secretion of IL-10 and other substances, such as immune complexes, prostaglandins, glucocorticoids, and apoptotic cells, macrophages differentiate into regulatory macrophages (antiinflammatory cells), which secrete IL-10 to suppress inflammation. Macrophages committed to the classical-activation, wound-healing/tissue repair, or regulatory pathways greatly influence the anatomic (histopathologic) structure and function of the chronic inflammatory response and granuloma formation (Fig. 3-29; Web Fig. 3-18).

Macrophages activated within lesions enter lymphatic vessels that drain into nearby lymph nodes via the afferent lymphatic vessels. In addition, some macrophages from lesions within the caudal body can enter the thoracic duct, which drains into the cranial vena cava or one of its branches. Macrophages within

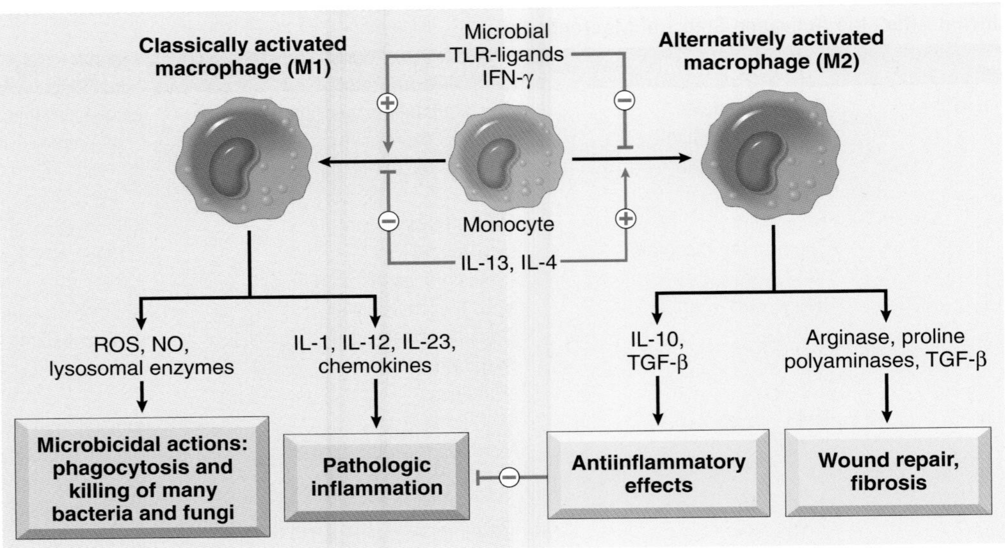

Fig. 3-29 Subsets of activated macrophages.
Different stimuli activate monocytes/macrophages to develop into functionally distinct populations. Classically activated macrophages are induced by microbial products and cytokines, particularly interferon-γ [IFN-γ], and are microbicidal and involved in potentially harmful inflammation. Alternatively activated macrophages are induced by other cytokines and in response to helminths (not shown), and are important in tissue repair and the resolution of inflammation (and may play a role in defense against helminthic parasites, also not shown). (From Kumar V, Abbas A, Fausto N, et al: *Robbins & Cotran pathologic basis of disease*, ed 8, Philadelphia, 2009, Saunders.)

the head and neck can enter right or left tracheal lymphatic ducts. The right tracheal lymphatic duct empties into the cranial vena cava, whereas the left tracheal duct empties into the thoracic duct. Once in the blood, the macrophages are disseminated throughout the body.

The outcome of these different types of macrophage activation leads to the following specific responses (see Fig. 3-29):

- Innate activation can lead to release of reactive oxygen species (ROS), NO, and IFN-α and IFN-β.
- Classic activation with IFN-γ leads to expression of MHC II antigen, respiratory burst, release of IL-1 and TNF for microbial killing, cellular immunity, and delayed type hypersensitivity.
- Alternative activation enhances MHC class II expression and mannose receptor expression for humoral immunity and allergic responses.
- Innate deactivation and reduced inflammatory responses can occur with the uptake of apoptotic cells or storage of oxidized LDLs in lysosomes and release of IL-10.

In addition to T reg lymphocytes and regulatory macrophages, recent work has shown that sialylated IgG molecules can regulate macrophage function. This stems from the observation that certain types of chronic inflammation, particularly autoimmune conditions of humans, have responded favorably to polyclonal IgG given intravenously. The mechanism by which this therapy works is poorly understood. Recently, evidence suggests that the polyclonal IgG activity may be due to a subset of IgG molecules that are sialylated on the Fc chain of the IgG. The sialylated IgGs are thought to interact with sialic acid–specific receptors on regulatory macrophages and upregulate expression of Fc receptor IIB, which is inhibitory, on effector macrophages.

FORMATION OF EPITHELIOID MACROPHAGES AND MULTINUCLEATE GIANT CELLS

Activated macrophages within tissues are relatively large cells histologically (20 to 25 mm in diameter) with abundant, often clear cytoplasm and a single, oval-to-polygonal, often slightly eccentric, reniform nucleus (Fig. 3-30). With time, activated macrophages can sometimes further differentiate into epithelioid macrophages and MGC (Fig. 3-31).

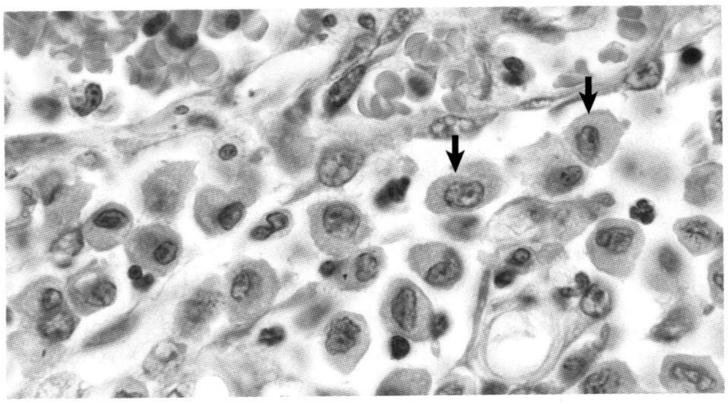

Fig. 3-30 Macrophages, lung, dog.
Macrophages have abundant cytoplasm and slightly eccentric, often reniform nuclei *(arrows)*. Note the small vacuoles in the cytoplasm, probably phagocytosed material. H&E stain. (Courtesy Dr. N. Cheville, College of Veterinary Medicine, Iowa State University.)

Both epithelioid macrophages and multinucleate giant cells often form in response to foreign bodies or persistent intracellular pathogens. The molecular mechanisms by which epithelioid macrophages and multinucleate giant cells form are poorly understood. It is a fascinating biologic phenomenon that requires membrane fusion and integration of the cytoplasm and nuclei of multiple cells. Studies in human patients with sarcoidosis, a special type of granulomatous inflammation in humans (see section on Sarcoidosis) have elucidated some of the important factors and conditions that contribute to MGC formation. Epithelioid macrophages are larger than activated macrophages. They have abundant cytoplasm, and the cell membrane occasionally assumes a polygonal to elongated shape, forming sheets, and thus can resemble to a limited

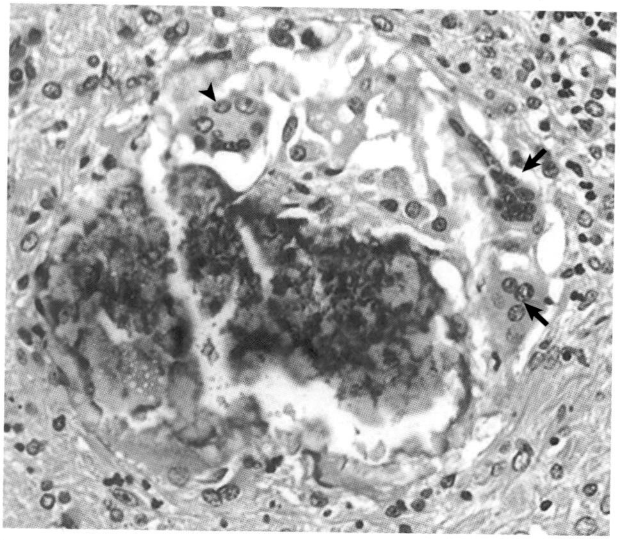

Fig. 3-31 Multinucleate giant cells, chronic granulomatous inflammation, central nervous system, rabbit.
This focus contains both foreign body-type *(arrows)* and Langhans'-type *(arrowhead)* multinucleate giant cells. H&E stain. (Courtesy Dr. A. Loretti, Ontario Veterinary College, University of Guelph.)

degree squamous epithelium. These cells have diminished phagocytic capacity, but they contain large amounts of rough endoplasmic reticulum (RER), Golgi, vesicles, and vacuoles. These latter structures suggest that the main function of epithelioid macrophages involves extracellular secretion; however, the physiologic activity of epithelioid macrophages is poorly understood and requires additional investigation.

MGC are seen frequently in granulomatous inflammation. MGC are syncytial cells formed by the fusion of two or more activated macrophages into one large cell with two or more nuclei (see Fig. 3-31). These nuclei can be distributed in the cell in a haphazard manner or aggregated in the center of the cytoplasm. This form is called a *foreign body type* of MGC. The nuclei can also be arranged in a horseshoe-like semicircle at the periphery of the cell. This form is called a *Langhans'-type cell.* The Langhans'-type giant cell should not be confused with Langerhans' cells, which are dendritic cells (see next discussion) of the skin. Although epithelioid macrophages, foreign body MGC, and Langhans' MGC have distinct cellular morphology, their physiologic activity is poorly understood.

The process of MGC formation (macrophage fusion) is not fully understood. It requires that macrophages be present within a chronic inflammatory milieu and thus likely bathed in cytokines, such as IFN-γ, IL-3, IL-4, IL-13, and GM-CSF; pathogen factors, such as muramyl dipeptide, a peptidoglycan portion of bacterial cells walls; and other inflammatory mediators. In this close proximity, the membranes of adjacent macrophages express fusionogenic molecules such as DC-STAMP (a seven transmembrane receptor), β_1 and β_2 integrins, CD44 (hyaluronic acid receptor), CD47 (integrin-associated protein), macrophage fusion receptor (MFR), fusion regulatory protein (FRP-1; CD98), and P2X7 (a ligand-gated ion channel activated by ATP that forms a pore). The fusion process has similarities to osteoclast formation.

Dendritic Cells

Dendritic cells are central to antigen processing, presentation, and the stimulation of adaptive immunity (Fig. 3-32). Functionally, they serve as sentinel cells of the adaptive immune response. Nearly all tissues and organs contain dendritic cells; however, they are most plentiful in tissues that cover the body, such as the skin and the mucous membranes that line the respiratory and alimentary tracts. Although dendritic cells have some resemblance to macrophages, they have numerous distinct filopodia, which extend from their surface (Web Fig. 3-19). Increasingly, several subtypes of dendritic cells are being identified (Table 3-10). In general, immature dendritic cells (CD34+) migrate to sites of antigen exposure, take up antigen, and migrate to and mature in a lymphoid organ in which they present antigen to T and B lymphocytes (Web Fig. 3-20). This migration process is mediated by chemokines and adhesion molecules, and most dendritic cells enter lymph nodes via the afferent lymphatic vessels in lymph fluid under the influence of chemokines, particularly CCL21. Once in the lymph node, dendritic cells often localize in the parafollicular (T lymphocytes) area in the vicinity of HEVs, a site in which naïve T lymphocytes enter the node. In this location, dendritic cells activate naïve T lymphocytes. Follicular dendritic cells, localized in lymph node follicles, take up antigen from the lymphatic fluid for presentation to follicular B lymphocytes. In addition to their activity as antigen-presenting cells, dendritic cells also contribute to adaptive immune responses through release of chemokines and cytokines. Outside of lymph nodes, dendritic cells, cytokines, and chemokines also contribute to inflammatory and immune responses; however, their contribution to these responses are dwarfed by macrophages, since there are many more macrophages within inflammatory lesions than dendritic cells.

Although macrophages also present antigen to naïve T lymphocytes, macrophage antigen presentation is more efficient for memory T lymphocytes than for naïve T lymphocytes, the forte of dendritic cells. Through recruitment of naïve T lymphocytes within and outside of the lymph node and presentation of antigen, dendritic cells contribute to the ongoing persistence of a stimulus in chronic inflammatory lesions. In contrast, tolerogenic dendritic cells can suppress immune responses. They accomplish this activity through the sampling of small amounts of self-antigens, harmless environmental antigens, and inciting the deletion of self-reactive T lymphocytes.

Dendritic Cell Trafficking

Trafficking immature monocytic dendritic cells released from the bone marrow express chemokine receptors CCR1 and CCR5 and are recruited by chemokine ligands CCL3 and CCL4 released from lymphocytes and macrophages in tissue (see Fig. 3-32). There are several subtypes of dendritic cells, and those dendritic cells that express CD11c antigen express CCR2, which responds to CCL2, CCL7, CCL8, CCL12, and CCL13. After dendritic cells take up antigen and become exposed to an endogenous (e.g., TNF-α) or exogenous (a ligand for a TLR) mediator, the dendritic cell matures and expresses CCR7 (see Web Fig. 3-20). Mature dendritic cells expressing CCR7 migrate from the site of the inflammatory lesion into the vasculature and then spread hematogenously throughout the body until they are recruited by HEVs in the paracortical areas of lymph nodes in which lymphocytes express CCL19 and CCL20. In this location, dendritic cells present antigen and thus contribute to the amplification of the adaptive immune response. Mature dendritic cells from lesion sites that enter the lymphatic vessels travel to the subtrabecular sinus of the lymph node, draining the lesion site and presenting antigen within paracortical regions. Some dendritic cells also drain via the lymphatic vessels to the thoracic duct and enter the blood. Follicular dendritic cells reside in the lymph node follicle and take up antigen present in the lymphatic fluid for presentation to B lymphocytes.

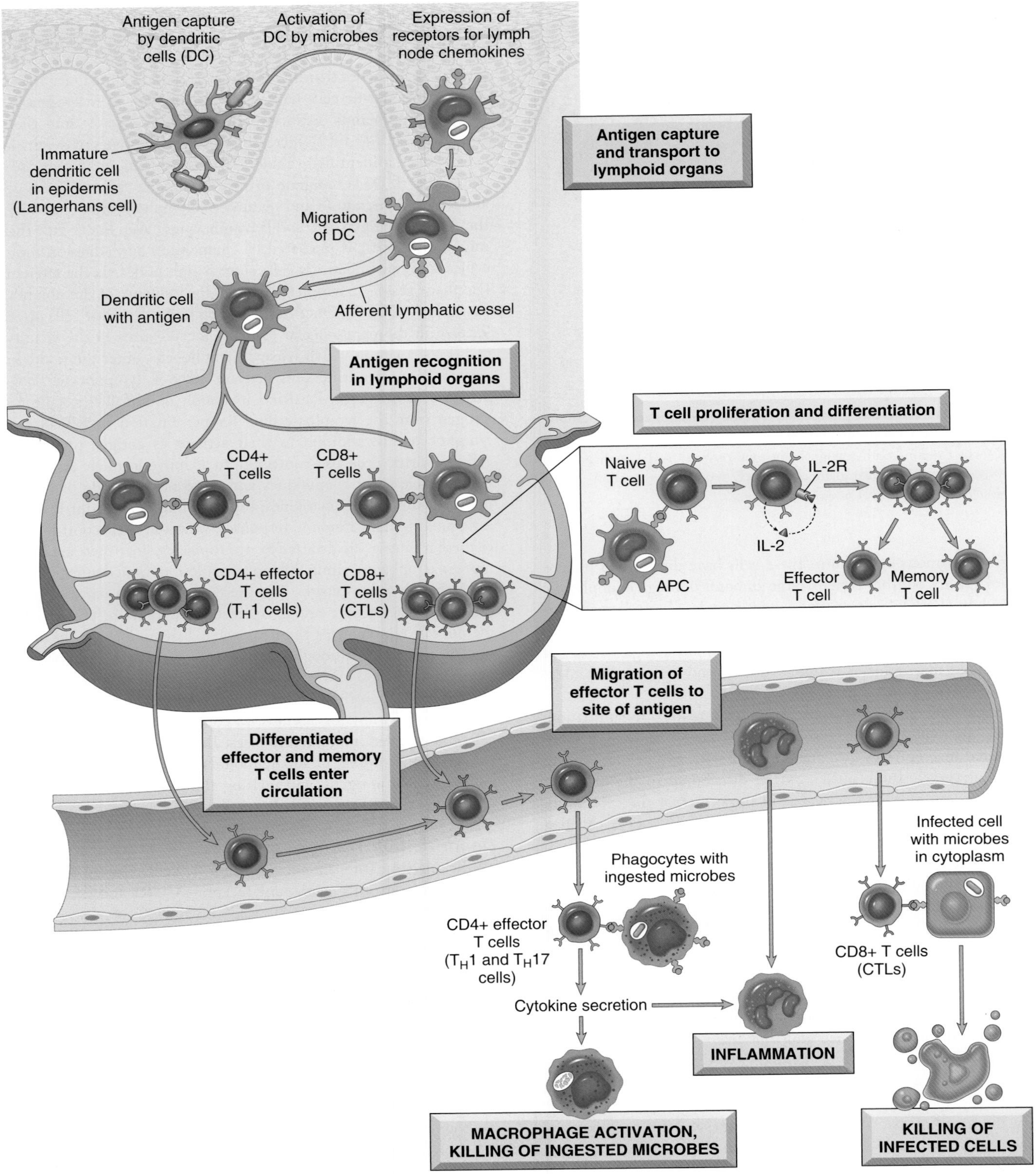

Fig. 3-32 Dendritic cells (DCs).

They capture microbial antigens from epithelia and tissues and transport the antigens to lymph nodes. During this process, the DCs mature, and express high levels of MHC molecules and costimulators. Naïve T lymphocytes recognize MHC-associated peptide antigens displayed on DCs. The T lymphocytes are activated to proliferate and to differentiate into effector and memory cells, which migrate to sites of infection and serve various functions in cell-mediated immunity. CD4+ effector T lymphocytes of the T_H1 subset recognize the antigens of microbes ingested by phagocytes, and activate the phagocytes to kill the microbes. CD4+ T lymphocytes also induce inflammation. CD8+ cytotoxic T lymphocytes (CTLs) kill infected cells harboring microbes in the cytoplasm. Not shown are T_H2 lymphocytes, which are especially important in defense against helminthic infections. Some activated T lymphocytes differentiate into long-lived memory cells. *APC,* Antigen-presenting cell. (From Kumar V, Abbas A, Fausto N, et al: *Robbins & Cotran pathologic basis of disease,* ed 8, Philadelphia, 2009, Saunders.)

TABLE 3-10 Subpopulations of Dendritic Cells (DCs) and Activities

DC Subpopulation	Location	Activity	Other
$CD8^+$ DCs	T, S, LN, PP, L	↓T_H1, ↑T_H2, ↓IL-12	Present antigen
$CD8^+$ DCs	T, S, LN, PP, L	↑T_H1, ↓T_H2, ↑IL-12	Present antigen
$CD8^{int}$ DCs	LN	Enter LN via lymphatics	
Langerhans' cells	Skin epidermis	Antigen capture	Migrate to LN
Dermal DCs	Skin dermis	Antigen capture	Migrate to LN
Plasmacytoid DCs	T, S, LN, PP	Viruses induce type I IFN	Antiviral activity

IFN, Interferon; *IL-12*, interleukin-12; *L*, liver; *LN*, lymph node; *PP*, Peyer's patch; *S*, spleen; *T*, thymus; *T_H1*, T helper cell type 1 lymphocyte response; *T_H2*, T helper cell type 2 lymphocyte response.

B LYMPHOCYTES

B lymphocytes contribute to chronic inflammation in at least two major ways. B lymphocytes can (1) take up and present antigen and (2) differentiate into immunoglobulin-producing cells (plasma cells or immunocytes), which secrete immunoglobulins that bind to and opsonize antigens facilitating phagocytosis. B lymphocytes are present within chronic inflammatory lesions and granulomas. They also populate the medullary sinus of lymph nodes in which they produce immunoglobulin locally or leave the medullary sinus through efferent lymphatic flow.

PLASMA CELLS

Under appropriate stimuli, such as intense antigenic stimulation and B lymphocyte presentation of antigens, B lymphocytes differentiate into plasma cells, which can secrete immunoglobulins that bind to and opsonize antigens and facilitate phagocytosis. Plasma cells form within lymph nodes, mucosal surfaces, and wound sites. The bone marrow also contains a resident population of plasma cells, which can increase in certain disease conditions. Clusters of these cells must be differentiated from neoplastic accumulations as can occur with multiple myelomas. Bone marrow plasma cells can easily migrate into venular walls in the bone marrow to enter the vasculature. Similarly, plasma cells within the medullary sinus of lymph nodes can enter efferent lymphatic vessels and eventually drain into the blood; however, peripheral blood often contains few plasma cells. In the chronic inflammatory exudate, plasma cells are usually found mixed with lymphocytes and macrophages, although in lesser numbers. Plasma cells predominate in certain chronic inflammatory conditions such as inflammatory bowel disease of dogs and cats, lymphoplasmacytic stomatitis and pododermatitis of cats, chronic dermatitis of any domestic animal species, and interstitial nephritis of dogs and cats.

EOSINOPHILS

Different types of chronic inflammatory conditions and granulomas contain a low to high number of eosinophils. Eosinophils are recruited into and stimulated to proliferate within chronic inflammatory exudates by several mediators, most notably IL-5 and eotaxin. In some chronic inflammatory conditions that contain eosinophils, such as asthma in humans, there is a T_H2 shift, resulting in increased concentrations of chemokines, such as eotaxin, in the tissue that contribute to the recruitment of additional eosinophils and exacerbates the T_H2 response. The same result is likely true for other as yet poorly characterized conditions such as the eosinophilic complex of cats, eosinophilic infiltrates in the base of the tongue of Siberian huskies and other dogs, eosinophilic enteritis in boxer dogs, and eosinophilic inflammatory lesions in the skin of horses. For these conditions, it may be that some type of persistent yet unidentified T_H2-inducing antigen is present locally.

MAST CELLS

Mast cells have a central role in triggering acute inflammatory reactions. In chronic inflammation, mast cells tend to look similar to macrophages in H&E-stained tissue sections and therefore are often not considered to be a part of the chronic inflammatory lesion. However, special stains, such as a Giemsa stain, of chronic or granulomatous inflammation frequently reveal a surprisingly large number of mast cells identified by their characteristic metachromatic granules. For example, chronic lung lesions (e.g., fibrosis and alveolar epithelial hyperplasia) that develop following severe *Mannheimia haemolytica* pneumonia often contain increased numbers of mast cells and reduced levels of substance P fibers resulting in persistently altered immune responses.

The reason for the presence of mast cells in chronic inflammatory conditions likely relates to their production of proteolytic enzymes such as chymase and tryptase. Such enzymes likely help physiologically in remodeling and fine tuning components of the ECM. With persistent inflammation and fibrosis, there can be increased proliferation of mast cells. Increased mast cell numbers in such lesions occur by increased infiltration and also by increased proliferation of mast cells in situ. With severe inflammation, there can be loss of substance P fibers, and mast cells can respond to this loss by increasing their expression of c-kit, an important regulator of mast cell proliferation.

NATURAL KILLER CELLS

NK cells are present in chronic inflammatory lesions, but their role varies based on the characteristics of the inflammatory stimulus. NK cells can kill cells recognized as foreign without prior exposure to antigen and thereby lacking antigen specificity as required by T lymphocytes. NK cells are activated by type I interferons and IL-12 and can activate macrophages and dendritic cells, thus contributing to chronic inflammation. NK-T lymphocyte activation can be triggered by lipid antigens in the presence of CD1d and can contribute to autoimmune responses.

Fibroblasts

Fibroblasts are multipurpose cells whose function is often overlooked in tissue responses to injury. Fibroblasts are elongated cells that contribute to the structural integrity of tissue and have abundant RER, which is used for the synthesis of collagen and ECM proteins. In addition, they also produce cytokines, MMPs, and chemokines that regulate the composition of the extracellular microenvironment in physiologic and pathologic conditions.

With tissue injury or certain hypoxic conditions, fibroblasts undergo proliferation in response to the release of fibroblast growth factors (FGFs), TGF-β, IL-13, PDGF, VEGF, and other mediators/molecules. Continued release of these substances in response to chronic inflammatory stimuli leads to the extensive fibrosis characteristic of chronic inflammation (Fig. 3-33; Web Fig. 3-21).

ENDOTHELIAL CELLS

Endothelial cells are essential for neovascularization of chronic inflammatory lesions. The process of angiogenesis (neovascularization) in chronic lesions is similar to that which occurs during wound healing (see section on Wound Healing and Angiogenesis)

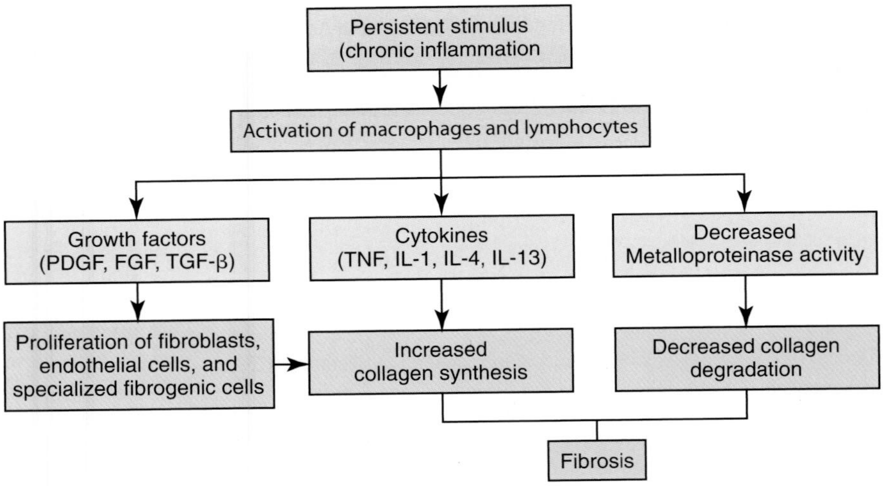

Fig. 3-33 Development of fibrosis in chronic inflammation. The persistent stimulus of chronic inflammation activates macrophages and lymphocytes, leading to the production of growth factors and cytokines, which increase the synthesis of collagen. Deposition of collagen is enhanced by decreased activity of metalloproteinases. (Modified from Kumar V, Abbas A, Fausto N, et al: *Robbins & Cotran pathologic basis of disease*, ed 8, Philadelphia, 2009, Saunders.)

and is induced by hypoxia and release of endothelial cell growth factors, such as FGF, VEGF, and PDGF.

Endothelial cells are interconnected by tight junctions composed of occludins, claudin, and JAMs, as well as adherens junctions composed of VE-cadherins. As leukocytes migrate between endothelial cells, leukocyte adhesion molecules bind some of these intercellular molecules. For example, LFA-1 molecule (CD11-α/CD18) binds JAM A, VLA-4 molecule (α-4/β-1) binds VCAM-1 and JAM B, and Mac-1 (CD11b/CD18) binds JAM C to mediate leukocyte passage between endothelial cells. These molecules are especially important for the transmigration of monocytes and lymphocytes through endothelial cell junctions into sites of chronic inflammation, by providing a stable yet temporary site of attachment of leukocyte filopodia and lamellipodia.

Trafficking of Naïve and Activated T and B Lymphocytes

Homing of Naïve Lymphocytes Via High Endothelial Venules

After naïve T lymphocytes are formed in the thymus and B lymphocytes are formed in the bone marrow, they traffic (home) to various secondary lymphoid organs, including lymph nodes, lymphoid nodules in the mucosal surfaces of the colon and cecum, Peyer's patches in the mucosal surfaces of the small intestine, and organs such as the spleen. These cells express L-selectin and migrate in the blood and often enter these areas through specialized vessels termed *high endothelial venules* (HEVs), which are postcapillary venules that have a thick basal lamina, and plump endothelial cells with abundant cytoplasm. HEVs produce certain chemokines constitutively (CCL19, CCL21, CXCL12, and CXCL13) to attract naïve T and B lymphocytes expressing the corresponding chemokine receptors CCR7 (receptor for CCL19, CCL21) and/or CXCR4 (receptor for CXCL12) and/or CXCR5 (receptor for CXCL12) (Web Table 3-10). HEVs are located principally in T-lymphocyte zones (paracortical areas of lymph nodes, interfollicular areas of Peyer's patches), but some are located in the B-lymphocyte zones, especially the periphery of B-lymphocyte follicles. Both peripheral lymph nodes and Peyer's patch HEVs express the adhesion molecules that mediate T and B lymphocyte adherence, including peripheral node addressin ligand for L-selectin, ICAM 1, ICAM-2, VE-cadherins; however, only Peyer's patch HEVs express MAdCAM-1, a receptor for the α-4/β-7 adhesion molecule expressed by T and B lymphocytes destined for Peyer's patches and mesenteric lymph nodes.

In addition to chemokines, sphingosine-1-phosphate (S1P) is produced by endothelial cells and by local mast cells and platelets and accumulates in the fluid of lymphatic vessels at high levels. S1P receptors are present on T and B lymphocytes, NK-T lymphocytes, and dendritic cells, as well as eosinophils, mast cells, NK cells, and macrophages. S1P mediates homing and also egress of naïve T and B lymphocytes and dendritic cells from the lymph node into the lymphatic fluid.

Adherence and Transendothelial Migration of Activated T Lymphocytes

Lesions developing into sites of chronic inflammation release chemokines, S1P, and other chemoattractant substances that attract and activate T lymphocytes. Although naïve T lymphocytes express high concentrations of L-selectin and the antigen CD45RB, in recently activated T lymphocytes, in effector/memory T lymphocytes, and T-lymphocyte clones, L-selectin expression decreases along with expression of the CD45RB antigen. Instead of L-selectin, acutely activated T_H1 and T_H2 cells, effector and central memory lymphocytes, and T-lymphocyte clones begin to express high to low levels of E- and P-selectin ligands, which bind to E- and P-selectin receptors, which are expressed by endothelial cells, activated in sites of chronic inflammation. Lymphocytes adhere to these areas of endothelium by eventually binding firmly to the vascular wall via adhesions between the LFA-1 adhesion molecule expressed on lymphocytes, which binds to ICAM-1 and ICAM-2 expressed on endothelial cells. Lymphocytes transmigrate across the vascular wall by adherence between LFA-1 integrins and the ICAM-1 molecules, JAM molecules, and also contributions from PECAM-1.

INFLAMMATION AND THE SENSATION OF PAIN

Information on this topic is available at evolve.elsevier.com/Zachary/McGavin/.

THE EFFECT OF INFLAMMATION ON THE FEBRILE RESPONSE AND OTHER ACTIVITIES

Information on this topic is available at evolve.elsevier.com/Zachary/McGavin/.

UNIQUE TYPES OF INFLAMMATION

Septicemia and Endotoxic Shock

Septicemia

Septicemia is a clinically significant form of bacteremia complicated by toxemia, fever, malaise, and often shock (see Table 3-5). Septicemia is characterized by the multiplication of microorganisms within the bloodstream and "seeding" into blood from fixed microcolonies present in one or more tissues. In septicemia, inflammation is not a localized reaction to injury, but instead mediators of inflammation are generated systemically leading to diffuse "leakage" of plasma into the interstitium and sequestration of leukocytes in the microvasculature. Generation of cytokines, kinins, vasoactive amines, and lipid mediators of inflammation, combined with widespread endothelial damage, leads to profound circulatory disturbances. Because of the systemic nature of this host-microbial interaction, quantities of phagocytic cells, antibody, complement components, coagulation proteins, and platelets may become depleted unless septicemia is controlled in the early stages. Septic shock and disseminated intravascular coagulation (DIC) are the usual sequelae of advanced bacterial septicemia.

Septicemia should be differentiated from a bacterial embolism. For example, some strains of *Streptococcus* spp. may break free from vegetative lesions (valvular endocarditis), as large colonies are protected by cell debris and fibrin. The bacterial emboli may then mechanically lodge in the lung, liver, kidney, or brain to produce a secondary focus of infection (abscess), but the whole process remains subclinical. In such a case, the blood sample taken for culture often lacks viable bacteria.

Septic (Endotoxic) Shock

The systemic interaction of microorganisms and their products (toxins) with a spectrum of host cells and chemical mediators results in a clinical syndrome recognized as sepsis or septic shock (see Table 3-5). The host mediators and amplification systems initiating the syndrome vary with the type of organism and the nature of the infectious process (local or systemic). Regardless of the specific cause, the major elements of septic shock form a continuum, including (1) hemodynamic derangements (reduced blood pressure and increased heart rate), (2) abnormal body temperature, (3) progressive hypoperfusion of the microvasculature, (4) hypoxic injury to susceptible cells, (5) quantitative adjustments in blood leukocytes and platelets, (6) DIC, (7) multiple organ failure, and (8) death.

Bacterial endotoxin, the LPS from the outer membrane of Gram-negative bacteria, has been studied extensively as an initiator of septic shock. The peptidoglycan layer of Gram-positive bacteria and bacterial exotoxins can initiate many of the same host responses. Other important initiators are products of the interaction of neutrophils, macrophages, and platelets with microorganisms in the tissue. Endotoxin is bound in the serum by LBP that binds CD14. Endotoxin has numerous ways to induce systemic activation of inflammatory mediators. Three direct effects of endotoxin are the activation of Hageman factor (a clotting factor), the complement cascade, and induction of the TLR4 pathway. These pathways can ultimately activate bradykinin, PAF, arachidonic acid metabolites, and cytokines (IL-1 and TNF), all of which have a role in many of the coagulation, hemodynamic, thermoregulatory, and leukocyte derangements observed in septic shock. TNF is capable of producing most clinical and pathologic features of septic shock, including hypotension, metabolic acidosis, hemoconcentration, intestinal hemorrhage, fever, neutrophil and endothelial activation, and predisposition to thrombosis. IL-1 shares many of the biologic activities of TNF in the mediation of septic shock. Secretion of TNF by activated macrophages can be partially inhibited by pretreatment with glucocorticoids, such as dexamethasone, which have been used therapeutically, often with limited success. In addition, lethal shock is prevented with anti-TNF antibody or TNF-receptor inhibitors. Chelators of endotoxin and other bacterial products are also under development for use in therapeutic intervention.

In severe septicemia, a *systemic inflammatory response syndrome* (SIRS) can develop in which there is extensive accumulation of cytokines, activated neutrophils, and platelets in the circulatory system. This result leads to multiple organ failure (MOF) and shock. Most patients survive initial SIRS insults, but these individuals are at increased risk of secondary or opportunistic infections termed *compensatory antiinflammatory response syndrome* (CARS). The initial activation of innate immunity can lead to decreased macrophage activity, T lymphocyte anergy, and apoptosis of lymphocytes contributing to CARS.

Multiple organ dysfunction syndrome (MODS) represents a late stage in septic shock and accounts for much of the irreversibility of organ failure. Systemic tissue ischemia and hypoxia, associated with progressive cardiovascular derangements, increased vascular leakage, and DIC, lead to generalized organ failure. Organs that are particularly sensitive to these effects include heart, brain, kidney, lung, liver, and intestinal mucosa. Cells injured by ischemia revert to anaerobic energy production (glycolysis), resulting in rapid depletion of substrates (glycogen, glucose), accumulation of lactate, and a deficiency of ATP. Without sufficient ATP, cell membrane ion pumps fail to maintain electrolyte balances, membrane integrity, and protein synthesis. The influx of sodium into cells with water causes cells to swell with further loss of function. Influx of calcium ions activates many intracellular enzymes, including phospholipase, which breaks down cellular membranes and generates arachidonic acid products. Loss of the proton gradient of the inner mitochondrial membrane makes oxidative phosphorylation impossible. Irreversible cell injury is believed to be closely related to generalized failure of mitochondria and loss of selective permeability of cell membranes. In dogs, sepsis of abdominal origin can induce MODS, and dysfunction of any organ system is associated with increased risk of death and mortality rates increase as the number of affected organs increase.

Animals dying of septic shock typically have evidence of fluid in the body cavities, pulmonary edema, petechial hemorrhages, congestion of the liver and intestines, and dehydration. Common microscopic lesions include acute necrosis of renal tubules, centrolobular hepatocytes, cardiac myocytes, adrenals, and tips of intestinal villi.

WOUND HEALING AND ANGIOGENESIS

Almost immediately after a wound develops, the process of healing begins. Injured tissue goes through four temporal phases to repair the wound: hemostasis, acute inflammation, proliferation (granulation), and remodeling (maturation, contraction) (Fig. 3-34). These phases occur in this sequence but may progress at different rates. Even in one lesion site, different areas may be in different phases of repair.

Hemostasis occurs immediately after injury unless there is a clotting disorder. Initially after injury, hemostasis is controlled via vasospasm, a process in which blood vessels constrict in response to injury. But this spasm subsides rapidly, and the injured (transected) blood vessels will subsequently relax, allowing additional bleeding if platelets do not become involved. During the initial period of vasoconstriction, platelets aggregate and adhere to exposed collagen,

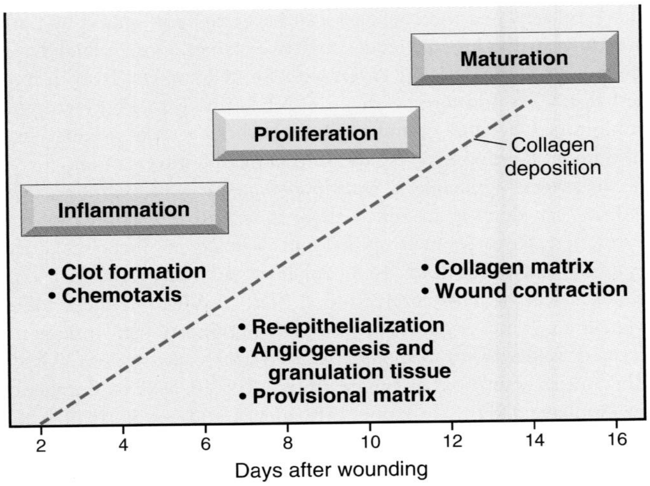

Fig. 3-34 Phases of cutaneous wound healing. Inflammation, proliferation, and maturation (see text for details). (From Kumar V, Abbas A, Fausto N, et al: *Robbins & Cotran pathologic basis of disease*, ed 8, Philadelphia, 2009, Saunders.)

especially collagen in the basement membrane underlying injured endothelial cells. Once adhered, platelets secrete vasoconstrictive substances to (1) maintain constriction of the transected vessels, (2) initiate the process of thrombogenesis to "plug" the leak in the vessel and prevent additional bleeding, and (3) initiate blood vessel healing (angiogenesis). This process also occurs with large blood vessels, but additional physiologic factors, such as blood shunting and decreased blood pressure. are involved.

By 24 hours after vascular injury, the inflammation phase (acute inflammation) of wound healing is fully established and can last up to 96 hours or longer if the healing process is disrupted by infection, trauma, or some other perturbation. It is in this phase that the "cardinal signs" of inflammation—redness, swelling, heart pain, and loss of function are observed. Neutrophils and macrophages, through phagocytosis and their degradative enzymes, breakdown and remove ("clean-up") the cell debris resulting from tissue injury. Macrophages secrete a variety of chemotactic and growth factors that establish the microenvironment for the proliferation (granulation) phase. The "clean-up" activity of neutrophils and macrophages within wounds is necessary, although excessive inflammatory cell infiltration reduces healing.

Some ECM molecules, such as some proteoglycans, have a negative charge thus attracting and binding to more positive-charged growth factors, chemokines, cytokines, MMPs, and other molecules. In addition, fragments of collagen, fibrin, and other molecules in wounds can induce chemotaxis, cell proliferation, and angiogenesis. Thus, with degradation of the ECM in wounds, there is release of these molecules, which contribute to matrix degradation, chemotaxis, and cell proliferation.

In tissues lined by epithelium, migration of basal cells from the overlying epithelium begins early in the healing process and does not require an underlying collagenous matrix. These cells arise from the transected edges of epithelium that border the wound, which rapidly undergo hyperplasia. The migrating basal cells proliferate, spreading in attempt to bridge the wound, and some of these cells differentiate; however, once the cells differentiate, they cease to proliferate and migrate. The proliferation phase can last up to 3 to 4 weeks or longer depending on the size of the wound. This phase is characterized by the generation of new endothelium (angiogenesis), epithelium (epithelialization), and connective tissue stroma (fibroplasia/desmoplasia) to restore normal structure and function to the injured tissue. The healing of skin after third-degree burns or severe ulcerations is an excellent example of this process. The return to normal structure and function depends on (1) the retention of normal stromal elements of the ECM to provide the structural framework for repair, and (2) normally functioning fibroblasts, myofibroblasts (contractile fibroblasts), endothelial cells, pericytes (nonendothelial components of blood vessels), and epithelial cells. Initial deposition of collagen and other key ECM molecules begins after fibroblasts have proliferated and fortified regions of the wound. Collagen fiber deposition alone is not sufficient for complete matrix repair without proliferative and functional fibroblasts.

The role of stem cells of epithelia and mesenchymal stroma in wound healing is increasingly understood. For epithelia, stem cells reside along the basal layer and are more clustered in specific regions. In the cornea of the eye, stem cells are located in the limbus. In skin, clusters are present in the bulge region of the hair follicle (roughly half-way down the follicular wall in the dermis). In lung, stem cells are present along the bronchiole-alveolar junction. In intestine, stem cells are present within the crypts. The stem cells are often in a quiescent (senescent) stage by the influence of bone morphogenic protein (BMP), which inhibits proliferation. Beta catenin (wnt) released from active stem cells in the dermal papilla of hair follicles, for example, induces proliferation of the quiescent cells that form new structures. Mesenchymal stromal cells subjacent to epithelia also undergo proliferation and communicate between epithelial cells and the subjacent inflammatory cells and stroma. The mesenchymal stromal cells function similarly to those of embryonic blastema cells.

The remodeling (maturation, contraction) phase begins approximately 3 to 4 weeks after injury, but only after the inflammation and proliferation phases have been successfully completed. This phase includes remodeling of granulation tissue by immature connective tissue and the conversion of immature connective tissue to mature connective tissue through extracellular collagen formation. Remodeling can last for 2 or more years. It essentially provides the time some tissues and organs, such as bone, need to return to the near-normal tensile strength required for normal axial and appendicular skeletal function.

A key component of wound repair is the ECM and stromal stem cells (fibroblasts, myofibroblasts). In mild or moderate injury, partially degraded collagen, proteoglycans, and elastin are completely degraded by MMPs and other enzymes removed by macrophages and then resynthesized by surviving fibroblasts. Simultaneously, fibroblasts and endothelial cells proliferate to fill tissue defects (granulation tissue) and epithelial cells, endothelial cells, and some parenchymal cells proliferate along basement membranes to restore the normal structure of the tissue. If basement membranes are degraded in the injury and the healing process disrupted, then complete healing is delayed because of a requirement for a new basement membrane to be deposited by endothelial cells that attach to and line the contiguous remaining basement membrane. Should healing be continually delayed (infection) or prevented (large tissue defect with loss of stroma and basement membrane), then dysregulated healing can occur in the form of extensive fibrosis (scars and hypertrophic scars) with haphazard arrangement and/or metaplasia of the overlying epithelial cells.

The four phases of wound healing described are applicable to all tissues and organ systems, but each system has its unique mesenchymal and parenchymal cell types that influence the process of healing. Bone healing with callus formation and skin healing with reepithelialization are good examples of healing and the specialization of cell types involved (see Chapters 16 and 17). Overall, the success of wound healing, especially in the skin, is often determined by whether the process occurs via first or second intention healing. Healing in other tissue is similar. In bone, for example, optimal healing occurs in bone fragments that are stabilized and in direct apposition.

FIRST AND SECOND INTENTION HEALING

First intention healing in skin occurs when the edges of a wound site are directly apposed and reattach and heal to each other rapidly (Fig. 3-35). Wounds lacking such close, intimate apposition are termed *second intention healing*. In the simplest type of wound, such as a cut or incision in the skin by a surgeon, there is initial hemorrhage from the damaged vasculature and retraction and constriction of blood vessels. In the wound area, there is deposition of fibrin, leakage of plasma proteins, clot formation, platelet aggregation, and neutrophil infiltration. The nature of repair depends on several factors, including the proximity of the cut edges to each other, the presence or absence of foreign bodies or infectious microbes, and the general health capacity of the animal to repair wounds. Under ideal conditions, such as in surgery, first intention healing is desired (see Fig. 3-35). First intention healing occurs in nonseptic wounds, whereas second intention healing occurs in septic wounds, with foreign bodies, or gaping wounds with nonopposed edges. If the wound healing process is disrupted or delayed, the process is shifted to second intention healing. First and second intention healing are also discussed in Chapter 17.

FIRST INTENTION HEALING

First intention healing occurs in 2 to 3 days in the skin, if the cut edges of a nonseptic wound are positioned in close proximity to each other by sutures or bandages. During this time, the hemorrhage, plasma proteins, and cell debris within the wound are phagocytosed and removed by macrophages, new blood vessels sprout and grow into the lesion, and the ECM is synthesized to fill the gap between the apposed tissue edges. With time (weeks), this stable interconnection in the dermis is replaced by collagen fibers that undergo continual maturation, thus providing the skin with near-normal tensile strength after wound healing. Concurrently, basal cells of the squamous epithelium will undergo hyperplasia and cover the defect in 3 to 5 days. This type of repair leaves little trace of the wound, except for perhaps mild fibrosis in the superficial dermis and loss of adnexa (e.g., hair follicles, sebaceous glands, and sweat glands) at the site of the wound. The tensile strength is nearly the same as that of adjacent tissue. First intention healing is the goal of the surgeon for repair of incision sites made during surgery.

SECOND INTENTION HEALING

Second intention healing occurs when the cut edges of the skin, for example, are not brought into appropriate apposition for healing (see Fig. 3-35). In such wounds, connective tissue is haphazardly synthesized and arranged and there is little or no organization in the healing process; however, fibrous connective tissue fills the defect in the superficial and deep dermis. This disorganization can also delay or prevent the migration of epithelial cells that attempt to cover the surface of the wound and disrupt the orderly deposition of ECM in the wound. In addition, new fibrous connective tissue lacks adnexa (hair follicles, sebaceous and sweat glands). In some cases, fibrous connective tissue can form into granulation tissue (see later section) in which histologically, proliferating fibroblasts are arranged perpendicular to new capillaries, and the long axes of the new capillaries are arranged perpendicular to the surface of the skin (Fig. 3-36). Tensile strength of granulation tissue is diminished and the lesions can tear or split. Thus with second intention healing, the site can remain ulcerated, lack hair, and in some cases, the fibrous connective tissue can undergo continuous proliferation and protrude from the skin surface as a hyperplastic scar.

IMPAIRED WOUND HEALING

In addition to spontaneously occurring impairments of wound healing, such as foreign bodies, infection, and neoplasms, certain other conditions can prevent or impair wound healing, even first intention healing. For example, altered deposition of collagen and ECM proteins can occur with osteogenesis imperfecta because of impaired production of type I collagen. Similarly, impaired synthesis, cross-linking, hydroxylation, or posttranslational processing of collagen can delay wound healing in individuals with Ehlers-Danlos syndrome. Hyperglycosylation of proteins, which can occur with prolonged diabetes mellitus, can alter the vasculature, lead to diabetic ulcers, and inhibit wound healing.

Chemotherapeutic drugs can also prevent cellular proliferation and may reduce healing. Several new chemotherapeutic drugs specifically target endothelial cell proliferation, which may greatly influence the process of neovascularization so vital to efficient wound repair. In humans, guinea pigs, and other species that require dietary vitamin C, deficiencies in intake can lead to scurvy, a disease in which there is decreased collagen hydroxyproline synthesis and poor wound healing. Extreme starvation, malnutrition, and cachexia from cancer or severe weight loss from chemotherapy can impair the synthesis and deposition of ECM proteins as a result of negative energy balance and a lack of amino acid substrates, normally synthesized in the liver. Additionally, such individuals and severe burn victims often lack adequate levels of serum proteins such as albumin, which results in lowered osmotic plasma pressure, impaired fluid resorption from the wound site, and enhanced edema fluid accumulation.

EXPRESSION OF GENES RESPONSIBLE FOR WOUND REPAIR

Wound repair requires activation of genes of the viable cells such as macrophages, fibroblasts, and endothelial cells adjacent to the sites of tissue injury. As indicated, macrophages internalize through phagocytosis cell debris to "clean-up" an area and degrade the ECM. In concert with fibroblasts, macrophages release growth factors that enhance the proliferation of (1) endothelial cells for neovascularization, (2) fibroblasts for deposition of a new ECM, (3) myofibroblasts for wound contraction, and (4) parenchymal cells for return to normal structure and function of the affected tissue.

Gene expression by cells in a wound is regulated to a large degree by oxygen levels (Fig. 3-37; Web Fig. 3-22). In the milieu of a wound, there is generally a reduced oxygen tension caused by vascular damage. Normal tissues have oxygen levels >90% oxygen saturation, and there is increased activity of non-heme iron-containing 2-oxglutarate (2-OG)-dependent oxygenases that sense oxygen levels and use dioxygen as a cosubstrate. These include prolyl hydroxylase domain-containing protein-1 (PHD-1), PHD-2, PHD-3, and factor-inhibiting HIF (FIH). These enzymes place a hydroxyl group on proline and asparagine amino acids in HIF-1α protein. Hydroxylated HIF-1α is degraded by the ubiquitin pathway when oxygen levels are high. In hypoxic tissue, however, as occurs in wounds, within neoplastic masses, and areas of inflammation, there is reduced activity of PHDs and FIH and thereby less hydroxylation of HIF-1α. Nonhydroxylated HIF-1α aggregates with HIF-1β and induces transcription of hypoxia-responsive elements (HREs) in the genome.

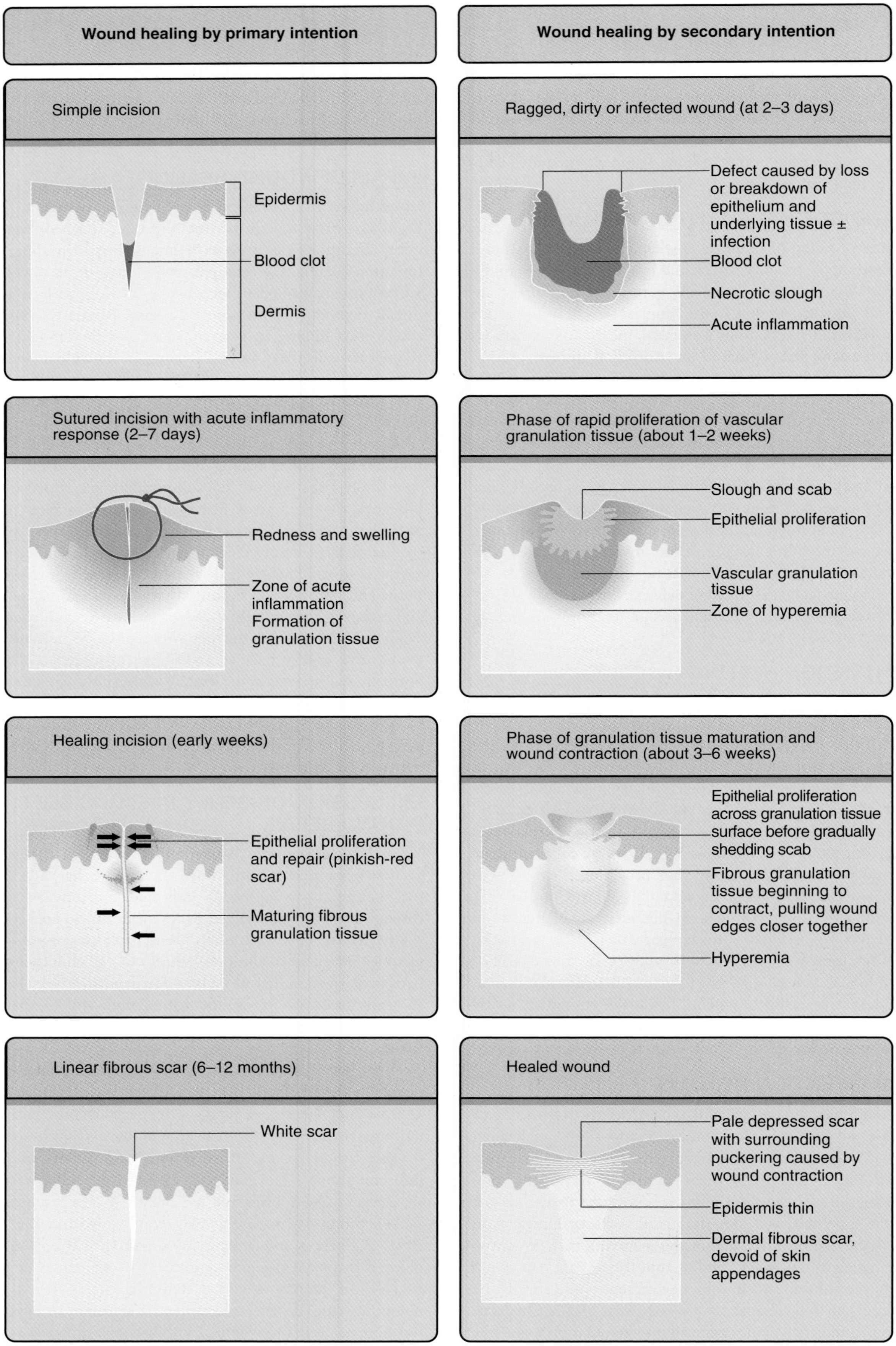

Fig. 3-35 Wound healing.

Steps in wound healing by primary intention *(left)* and secondary intention *(right)*. Note large amounts of granulation tissue and wound contraction in the healing by second intention. (From Young B, O'Dowd G, Stewart W: *Wheater's basic pathology: a text, atlas and review of histopathology*, ed 5, New York, 2010, Churchill Livingstone.)

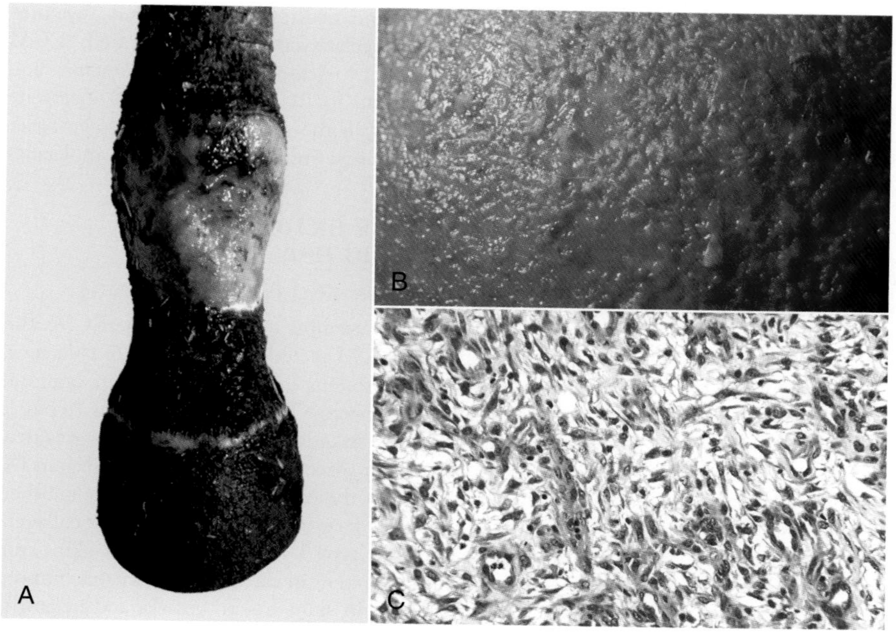

Fig. 3-36 Granulation tissue, nonhealing ulcer, skin, distal limb, horse.
A, In the bed of the ulcer, there is extensive fibrosis and granulation tissue. **B,** Gross photograph of the surface of the granulation tissue. Note the fine nodules or "granulations" on the surface that gave rise to the term *granulation tissue.* These are a mixture of newly formed blood vessels, extracellular matrix (ECM), and fibroblasts, with minimal or no collagen deposition. It provides the support for wound repair and remodeling via fibroplasia and reepithelialization. **C,** Photomicrograph of granulation tissue. Note how the new fibroblasts are arranged perpendicularly to the newly formed blood vessels in a rich bed of ECM *(clear spaces).* (Courtesy Dr. M.D. McGavin, College of Veterinary Medicine, University of Tennessee.)

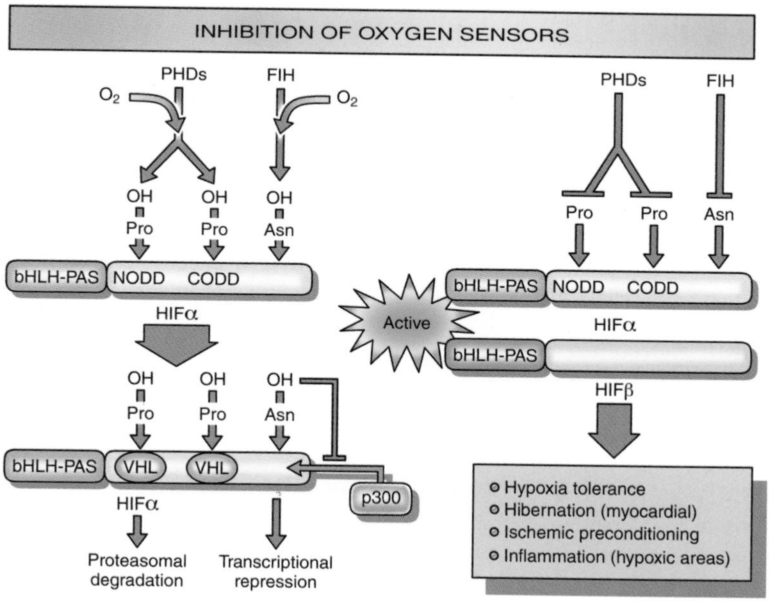

Fig. 3-37 Regulation of hypoxia-inducible factor (HIF) transcriptional activity by prolyl hydroxylase protein domain-containing proteins (PHDs) and factor-inhibiting HIF (FIH).
With sufficient oxygen *(left),* HIF-1α protein is hydroxylated by PHDs and FIH resulting in degradation. With insufficient oxygen *(right)* HIF-1α protein is not hydroxylated and forms an active complex with HIF-1β resulting in transcriptions of genes that contribute to wound healing an angiogenesis, including the transcription of vascular endothelial growth factor (VEGF). (Modified from Fraisl P, Aragones J, Carmeliet P: *Nat Rev Drug Discovery* 8(2):139-151, 2009.)

The HREs include genes for growth factors, including VEGF, iron-binding proteins, regulators of apoptosis, erythropoiesis, angiogenesis, pH regulation, and glucose and energy metabolism. Early growth response gene-1 (EGR-1) is another transcription factor activated in wounds that leads to expression of growth factors and cytokines. Therefore both HIF-1α and EGR-1 activity in hypoxic conditions lead to increased cellular transcription that upregulates genes for energy (glucose transporters, hexokinase 1 and 2, lactate dehydrogenase, phosphofructokinase), endothelial and fibroblast proliferation (TGF-β, VEGF), and iron sequestration (ceruloplasmin, transferring receptor). These genes promote cell survival in hypoxic conditions, enhance cell proliferation, especially of cells vital to repair (endothelial cells, fibroblasts), and delay or alter differentiation of other cells (epithelia or parenchymal cells) until endothelial and fibroblast proliferation is well established.

DEGRADATION OF CELLS AND TISSUE COMPONENTS IN WOUNDS

Wounds generally have a central core composed of (1) degenerate and/or necrotic cells, such as parenchymal cells, fibroblasts, and endothelial cells, as well as infiltrating leukocytes, such as neutrophils, platelets, lymphocytes, mast cells, and macrophages; (2) inflammatory products (cytokines, eicosanoids, chemokines, and their respective receptors); (3) serum proteins (albumin, acute phase proteins, complement); (4) clotting proteins (fibrin); and (5) ECM proteins and substances. Many of these cells and mediators need to be removed before optimal healing takes place. Phagocytic cells, such as neutrophils and macrophages, are very important in the clean-up process through phagocytosis of particulate matter and subsequent lysosomal degradation and the release of digestive enzymes into the tissue. In addition, macrophages have a major role in the uptake of apoptotic cells that form in response to TNF-α or other proapoptotic inflammatory stimuli. The ECM can be especially difficult to degrade. However, macrophages and fibroblasts are key to this process through the release of matrix metalloproteinases that degrade the ECM.

Degradation of the Extracellular Matrix In Wounds

The ECM is composed of (1) proteins and (2) the hydrated gel of proteoglycans in which they lie. It surrounds and interconnects cells in connective tissue such as fibroblasts, blood vessels, lymphatic vessels, resident mast cells, macrophages, dendritic cells, and nearby parenchymal cells and/or epithelia (Web Fig. 3-23). The ECM influences cellular development, polarity (organization), and function of epithelial cells (Web Fig. 3-24). Soluble proteoglycans and fragments of glycosaminoglycans can activate Toll-like receptors and proteoglycans and hyaluronan can facilitate leukocyte adhesion. Also, ECM binds and sequesters cytokines, chemokines, and growth factors that are released during ECM degradation.

With tissue injury, there is often destruction and degradation of the ECM. This process occurs through physical separation or tearing, dilution from plasma proteins, infiltration by inflammatory cells, and degradation by enzymes, largely the MMPs (Web Fig. 3-25). Macrophages, fibroblasts, mast cells, and most leukocytes produce MMPs (Table 3-11). Many MMPs were initially named after the type of ECM protein that they were found to degrade (e.g., collagenase), but because the MMPs are now known not to be uniquely specific for a particular ECM substrate, they have been reclassified in a numeric manner, MMP-1 through MMP-20.

For example, collagenase is MMP-1, gelatinase is MMP-2, stromelysin is MMP-3, and matrilysin is MMP-7. MMPs degrade collagen, gelatin, elastin, aggrecan, versican, proteoglycan, tenascin, laminin, fibronectin, and other ECM components. The MMP enzymatic domain contains three histidine residues that form a complex with zinc. A regulatory domain is responsible for latency and allows activation in the presence of zinc. MMP activity is also regulated by tissue inhibitors of MMP (TIMP). ADAM (a disintegrin and metalloproteinase) are zinc proteinases capable of degrading matrix molecules as can cathepsin G, tissue plasminogen-activator (tPA), and urokinase plasminogen activator (uPA) (Web Box 3-2). Fragments of proteins degraded by MMP, tPA, uPA, and other degradative processes are removed from wounds by lymphatic drainage and phagocytosis by macrophages and neutrophils. Proteoglycans are largely degraded by lysosomal enzymes of macrophages and neutrophils that include hyaluronidases, heparinases, and galactosidases. As indicated, ECM degradative enzymes also (1) release latent growth factors and other latent molecules bound to ECM molecules, (2) inactivate some molecules present within the region, (3) break down basement membranes, and (4) cleave intercellular adhesion molecules between epithelial cells.

TABLE 3-11 Matrix Metalloproteinase (MMP) Activity, Regulation, and Cellular Production

Function: Degrade basement membrane and extracellular matrix proteins
Co-factors necessary: Zinc (Zn^{2+})
Regulation: Cellular synthesis, lysosomal degradation and release, and tissue inhibitors of metalloproteinases

Type of MMP	Cell Type
MMP 1, 2, 3, 11, 14	Fibroblasts
MMP 9, 12	Macrophages
MMP 9	Neutrophils
MMP 2, 3, 9	Endothelial cells
MMP 9	Pericytes
MMP 1, 3, 7, 9, 13	Some cancer cells

RESYNTHESIS OF THE EXTRACELLULAR MATRIX WITH WOUND HEALING

Synthesis of Collagen and Matrix Proteins

As wounds repair, the body attempts to reestablish the ECM. The structural proteins of the ECM include several types of collagens, elastin, and adhesive type proteins including fibronectin, laminin, versican, tenascin, and vitronectin. The fibrillar collagens (types I, II, III, V, and XI) are triple-stranded helical structures aggregated into fibrils in the extracellular space and surrounded by collagens IX and XII, which interconnect the collagen fibrils with one another and the ECM. Most tissues have a predominance of one collagen type. For example, collagen type I is present in bone, skin, and tendon; collagen type II is present in cartilage and vitreous humor; collagen type III is present in skin, around vessels, and in newly formed wounds; collagens type V and VI are present in interstitial tissues; collagen type VI is present near epithelia; collagen type VIII is present near endothelial cells; and collagens type X and XI are present in cartilage.

Collagen type IV is largely present in basal lamina along with laminin, entactin, a heparin sulfate proteoglycan, and perlecan. Throughout the ECM are molecules of elastin, which stretch, recoil, and allow flexibility in the tissue. Collagen fibers, laminin, fibronectin, tenascin, and other ECM proteins bind to cells in the connective tissue via extracellular domain of integrin molecules of cells by means of a specific amino acid sequence, the RGDS sequence. For example, laminin binds $\alpha_2\beta_1$-integrins of endothelial cells, some collagens bind $\alpha_6\beta_1$-integrins of epithelial cells, and fibronectin and vitronectin bind $\alpha_5\beta_3$-integrins. The intracellular portion of integrin molecules interact with the cellular cytoskeleton (i.e., actin assembly) and thereby link the extracellular milieu with cellular activities such as cell growth, differentiation, proliferation, and senescence.

Collagen Production by Fibroblasts

Collagen deposition within a site of wound repair provides a scaffold for reestablishment of the ECM and stroma (Web Fig. 3-26). Fibroblasts are induced by TGF-β and other cytokines to synthesize collagen. Ribosomes in fibroblasts produce approximately 30 types of collagen α-chains that are composed of repetitive glycine-x-y segments. Although within the RER, praline and lysine residues in these chains are hydroxylated, and this hydroxylation process requires vitamin C. The chains are then glycosylated, arranged in a triple helix, and eventually released into the extracellular space as procollagen. The ends of procollagen are cleaved enzymatically resulting in the formation of fibrils termed *tropocollagen.* Cross-linkages between collagen fibrils occur at lysine and hydroxylysine residues through the activities of the enzyme lysyl oxidase, and this cross-linking process provides the tensile strength of collagen.

Synthesis of Proteoglycans

Proteoglycans are produced by fibroblasts. They retain water and are vital to the hydration of the ECM. Proteoglycans have a protein backbone surrounded by a network of glycosaminoglycan (GAG) chains (Web Fig. 3-27). The GAGs are negatively charged, often highly sulfated, polysaccharide chains covalently linked to the serine residues on a protein backbone. Most GAGs contain high concentrations of *N*-acetylglucosamine (Web Table 3-11). Hyaluronic acid lacks sulfation and is not connected to the protein backbone. GAGs are key to the water retention properties of proteoglycans and thus, hydration of the extracellular milieu. Proteoglycan hydration of the ECM allows tissues to be pliable and have elasticity.

Heparin sulfate proteoglycans, such as syndecan, decorin, and perlecan, encircle and surround cells and basal laminae. Syndecan is an integral transmembrane protein that can bind chemokines. With inflammation, syndecan can release the chemokine, which then induces leukocyte infiltration.

FIBROBLASTS AND THE MECHANISTIC BASIS OF FIBROSIS

Fibroblasts align along planes of tissue stress during development (Langer's lines or tension lines). In quadrupeds, these lines are generally dorsoventral over the thorax and abdomen (axial body plane) and parallel to the long axis of the limbs (appendicular body plane). Surgical incisions along Langer's lines extend between, rather than transect, bands of fibrous connective tissue and tend to pull the margins of surgical skin incisions together. Such incisions reduce the degree of postsurgical scar formation.

Fibroblasts of cats appear to be especially responsive to injury and inflammation. In fact, injury of fibroblasts has been associated with their neoplastic transformation in cats. For example, traumatic lens rupture can lead to intraocular inflammation and fibroblast proliferation, and in some cases, fibrosarcomas. In addition, fibroblast proliferation and fibrosarcomas are common in cats at vaccination sites.

Initially during the hemostasis and inflammation phases of wound repair, fibrin and serum proteins form a loose gel-like framework for the migration of fibroblasts and endothelial cells into the wound to form granulation tissue. Simultaneously, leukocytes and other cells, such as fibroblasts and endothelial cells, are stimulated by HIF-α and epidermal growth factor (EGF) to synthesize and release a variety of growth factors that result in fibroblast proliferation and migration. These factors include FGF-1 and FGF-2, PDGF, EGF, and TGF-β1, 2, and 3. FGF, PDGF, IL-13, and TGF-β induce fibroblasts to produce collagen, whereas FGF, VEGF, TGF-β, angiopoietin, and mast cell tryptase induce endothelial cells to proliferate and migrate and produce basement membrane for formation of new capillaries (Web Fig. 3-28).

With time, the newly formed, provisional connective tissue is remodeled into a more mature matrix. In the entire process, TGF-β has a central role in fibroblast activity and collagen deposition, because it is produced by platelets and macrophages and induces macrophage chemotaxis, fibroblast migration and proliferation, and synthesis of collagen and ECM proteins. TGF-β binds TGF-β receptor II (TGF-βRII), which dimerizes with TGF-βRI. The TGF receptor then phosphorylates R-SMAD and Co-SMAD to overcome inhibition of SMAD 7. This signaling process induces fibroblast activity, and regulation of the signaling may be useful in therapeutic strategies to control scarring and/or fibrosis (Web Fig. 3-29).

In addition to producing collagen, fibroblasts can migrate to a certain degree, and this process is mediated by adhesion molecules that bind to the ECM. This binding is a complicated event in which the adherence process is essential for migration of the cell and its anchoring to extracellular proteins. During wound repair, proliferating fibroblasts often align themselves parallel with lines of tension stress.

MORPHOLOGY OF GRANULATION TISSUE AND FIBROUS CONNECTIVE TISSUE

Granulation Tissue

Some lesions develop a distinctive type of arrangement of connective tissue fibers, fibroblasts, and blood vessels termed *granulation tissue.* Granulation tissue is the exposed connective tissue that forms within a healing wound. It is often red and hemorrhagic and bleeds easily when bumped or traumatized because of the fragility of the newly formed capillaries (see Fig. 3-36). It is especially common in horses. When viewed with a magnifying glass, the surface of granulation tissue has a granular appearance and thus the term granulation tissue arose. In granulation tissue, fibroblasts and connective tissue fibers grow parallel to the wound surface and are arranged perpendicularly to the proliferating capillaries. Often, the penetrating blood vessels are evenly spaced. Excessive granulation can lead to a type of hypertrophic scar called *proud flesh.* In cats, fasciotomy and fascial excision induce formation of early granulation tissue in cutaneous wounds and may be effective in enhancing closure of secondary wounds.

Hypertrophic Scars

Hypertrophic scars occur as a result of exuberant proliferation of fibroblasts and collagen in wounds that fail to heal properly. The best example of this condition occurs in skin wounds of the distal limbs of horses and is known as "proud flesh," as indicated proliferating connective tissue forms a large cauliflower-like mass that cannot be covered by epithelium (Fig. 3-38). Why this lesion most commonly occurs in horses is unclear; however, the epidermis of horses is often very "tight" with limited elasticity.

Keloid is a special type of excessive connective tissue deposit that occurs in humans. It has an incidence of 5% to 16% after skin trauma in high-risk populations, such as blacks, Hispanics, and Asians. Clinical management of hypertrophic scars, proud flesh, and keloids can be difficult but includes intralesional corticosteroids, compression, occlusive dressings, pulsed-dye laser therapy, cryosurgery, surgical excision, radiation, fluorouracil chemotherapy, topical silicone, interferons, and drugs, such as imiquimod, that induce IFN-γ.

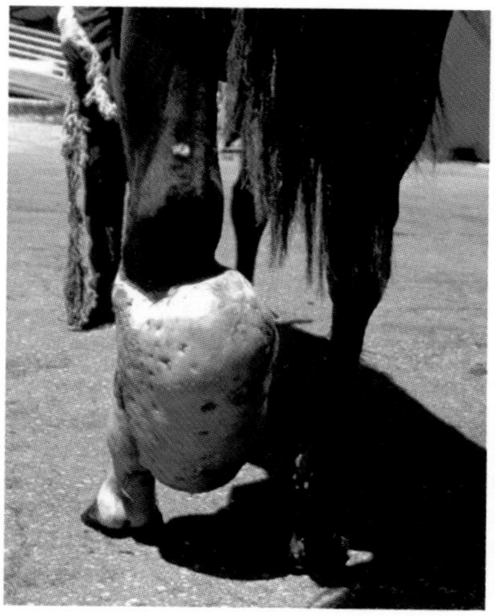

Fig. 3-38 Exuberant granulation tissue (proud flesh), chronic ulcer, skin, distal hindlimb, horse.

Note the large proliferating mass of fibrous tissue on the lower portion of the left hindlimb. It often lacks superficial epithelium. (Courtesy Dr. M.D. McGavin, College of Veterinary Medicine, University of Tennessee.)

Fibrous Connective Tissue

Fibrous connective tissue is the dense accumulation of fibroblasts and collagen formed within a wound site. Histologic characteristics depend on wound severity and duration. Fibrous connective tissue contains variable numbers of fibroblasts and collagen along with inflammatory cells (Fig. 3-39). In recently formed wounds, the collagen can be very immature and edematous with a variety of inflammatory cells, perhaps neutrophils. With time, the fibrous connective tissue progresses into mature, densely packed collagen with few inflammatory cells. Once formed and matured, fibrous connective tissue often persists for years, perhaps life.

WOUND CONTRACTION

The Scirrhous Reaction

With severe thermal/chemical burns or extensive abrasions of a large surface area of the skin, the healing process and the formation of connective tissue becomes extensive. In time, these areas of connective tissue contract and place tension on the surrounding normal skin, resulting in a scirrhous reaction that can cause immobility of the surrounding skin and perhaps limbs along with pain and deformation. Contraction of such wounds is mediated largely by myofibroblasts.

Similarly, within areas of necrosis and/or inflammation in the liver, lung, spleen, and kidney, excessive fibrosis in parenchymal areas can result in the formation of connective tissue tracts between the healing area and capsular and interstitial connective tissue. When this new connective tissue contracts during the healing process, it grossly results in local indentation or pitting on the organ surface, such as occurs with chronic renal cortical infarcts. If there are multiple such areas, the organ surface develops an undulating and/or nodular appearance such as occurs in a cirrhotic liver. Contraction of such wounds is again mediated largely by myofibroblasts.

Myofibroblasts

Myofibroblasts are specialized fibroblasts with contractile activity. They form within wounds in response to tissue plane stress and the secretion of TGF-β by platelets and macrophages as wounds develop, and they increase in number with time and severity. Their function is to contract the wound and thus bring together injured tissue separated by edema and inflammation. Physiologically, myofibroblasts also occur in tissues with contractility such as uterine submucosa, intestinal villi, testicular stroma, the ovary, periodontal ligament, bone stroma, capillaries, and pericytes.

Myofibroblasts have stress fibers, actin and myosin fibers, gap junctions, and a fibronexus. The fibronexus is a mechanotransduction region of the plasma membrane, which is rich in integrin molecules. The fibronexus interconnects intracellular actin fibers with extracellular proteins such as fibronectin. This connection provides an anchor point during myofibroblast contraction. In contrast, fibroblasts lack contractile myofilaments and a fibronexus. Actin polymerization and contractility in myofibroblasts is stimulated by Rho GTPases. The Rho signaling that induces contractility in myofibroblasts results in continual contraction of filaments in myofibroblasts. Continual contraction by myofibroblasts differs from the periodic contractility that occurs in smooth muscle cells. Such contractions condense wound sites and are frequently beneficial to repair. But excess, as in severe burns, induces excessive contraction and sometimes loss of mobility of nearby joints requiring patients to undergo physical therapy to maintain the range of motion for limbs extending from affected joints.

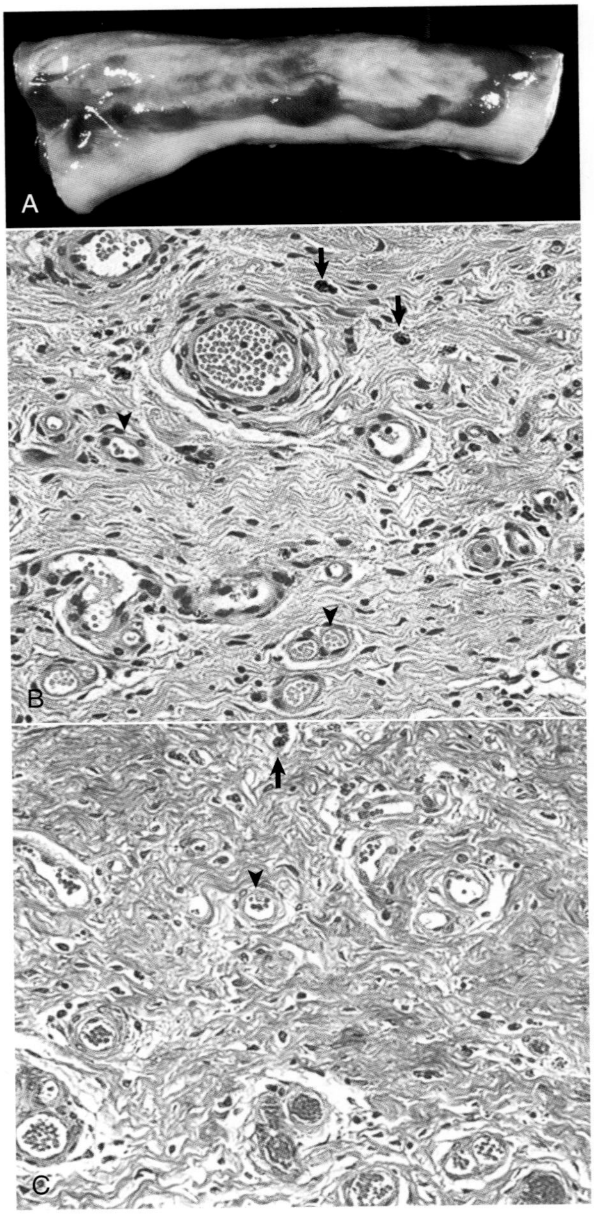

Fig. 3-39 Fibrous connective tissue.
A, Hemomelasma ilei, ileum, antimesenteric serosal surface, horse. This lesion is approximately 1 to 2 weeks old. *Strongylus edentatus*-induced injury to the serosal vasculature results in hemorrhage followed by wound healing. Note the raised areas of fibrosis *(raised gray-white areas),* hemosiderosis *(yellow-brown areas),* and hemorrhage *(red-brown areas).* **B,** Healing response in hemomelasma ilei. Note the abundant newly formed capillaries *(arrowheads)* and intervening fibrous connective tissue *(bands of red fibers).* This healing response is the next step following the granulation tissue phase demonstrated in Fig. 3-35. Hemosiderin *(arrows)* is present in the connective tissue and is indicative of hemorrhage having occurred in the injury at an earlier time (weeks). H&E stain. **C,** Fibrous connective tissue in the healing response. Collagen is readily demonstrated in fibrous connective tissue by a Trichrome stain *(blue-stained fibers).* Masson trichrome stain. (Courtesy Dr. J.F. Zachary, College of Veterinary Medicine, University of Illinois.)

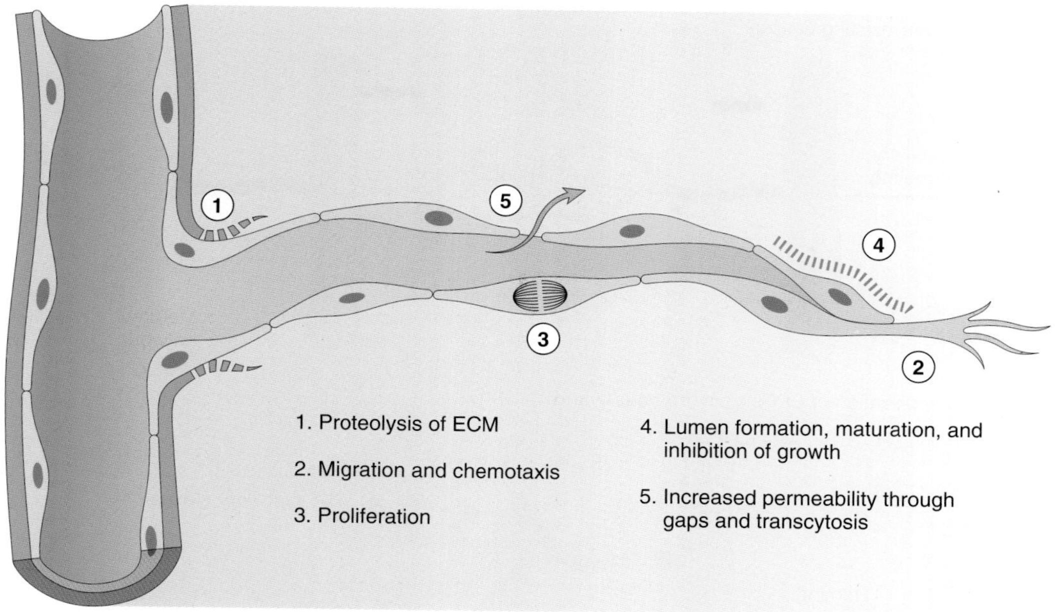

Fig. 3-40 Steps in the process of angiogenesis.
Extracellular matrix (ECM). (Modified from Motamed K, Sage EH: *Kidney Int* 51:1383, 1997.)

ANGIOGENESIS IN WOUND REPAIR

Angiogenesis is the formation of new blood vessels from preexisting vessels. It is a process essential for all living organisms with a cardiovascular system and involves a series of steps, as illustrated in Fig. 3-40, for the formation of new capillaries, including the following:

- Proteolysis of the ECM and basement membrane of parental vessels at the margins of the wound so a new capillary "bud" can form and initiate cellular migration
- Migration of immature endothelial cells into the wound
- Proliferation of endothelial cells to form solid "endothelial tubes"
- Maturation of endothelial tubes into new capillaries with the formation of lumina
- Formation of stalk cells (proliferative endothelial cells lining developing vessels) and tip cells at the end of vascular buds
- Establishment of endothelial cell adhesion to adjacent cells and basal lamina and expression of the receptors/ligands responsible for the leukocyte adhesion cascade along the luminal surface of the endothelial cells
- Recruitment of pericytes and smooth muscle cells to support the final differentiation stage of the newly formed vessel

This process occurs because as wounds heal, new vessels are necessary to supply the injured site with oxygen, remove carbon dioxide and other waste products, drain excess fluid, and provide a vascular pathway for cells and stem cells into the wound. This same beneficial process has also been adapted by primary and metastatic neoplastic cells to grow and spread throughout tissues of the body.

Initiation of Endothelial Cell Proliferation

Endothelial Cell Growth Factors

The formation of new blood vessels in wounds begins from the proliferation of endothelial cell buds from blood vessels in viable tissue adjacent to the wound or can be derived from bone marrow endothelial precursor cells (EPCs) (Fig. 3-41). These buds grow into the "healing" wound, form elongated vascular tubular structures within the wound, interconnect and revascularize the wound, and then eventually differentiate into mature vessels. Initially, endothelial cell buds form, and cells migrate into wounds under the autocrine influence of HIF-α and EGF (see section on Expression of Genes Responsible for Wound Repair), which enhance expression of genes that improve cell survival in hypoxic conditions.

Concurrently, growth factors such as PDGF, FGF, VEGF-A, angiogenins, and ephrins released from macrophages, endothelial cells, and fibroblasts bind receptors on endothelial cells and induce vascular formation (Fig. 3-42). VEGF A and its various isoforms stimulate the initial stages of endothelial cell proliferation through binding the VEGF-R2 receptor on endothelial cells. Proliferative effects of VEGF are regulated by Notch ligands and receptors. VEGF enhances expression of DII4, a ligand in vascular tip cells produced by tip cells that bind to Notch receptors expressed by stalk cells. DII4 binding of Notch receptor leads to expression of genes by the stalk cells that reduce VEGF-R expression and cellular proliferation. The secondary stages of endothelial cell proliferation involve angiopoietin 1 and its receptor, Tie2, both of which establish vascular stabilization through the recruitment of pericytes and smooth muscle cells and deposition of ECM proteins. Vascular stabilization is further advanced by PDGF and TGF-β. Recent work has shown that specific microRNA molecules, such as microRNA-92a (MiR-92a), control angiogenesis in mice. MiR-92a targets mRNAs with pro-angiogenic activity, binds these, and reduces their activity.

Endothelial Cell Migration Is Mediated by Integrins

Newly formed endothelial cells and fibroblasts migrate into wound sites and bind to fibrinogen and plasma proteins, as well as newly deposited ECM substances, such as heparin sulfate, chondroitin sulfate, type III collagen, laminin, vitronectin, and fibronectin. This adherence is mediated by adhesion molecules expressed by new endothelial cells and fibroblasts. These adhesion molecules include α_5- and β_3-integrins, which bind fibrin and fibronectin. It is interesting that for wound repair, enhancement of angiogenesis is beneficial and vital; however, in neoplasia, inhibition of angiogenesis and thus the growth of the tumor have potential therapeutic benefits.

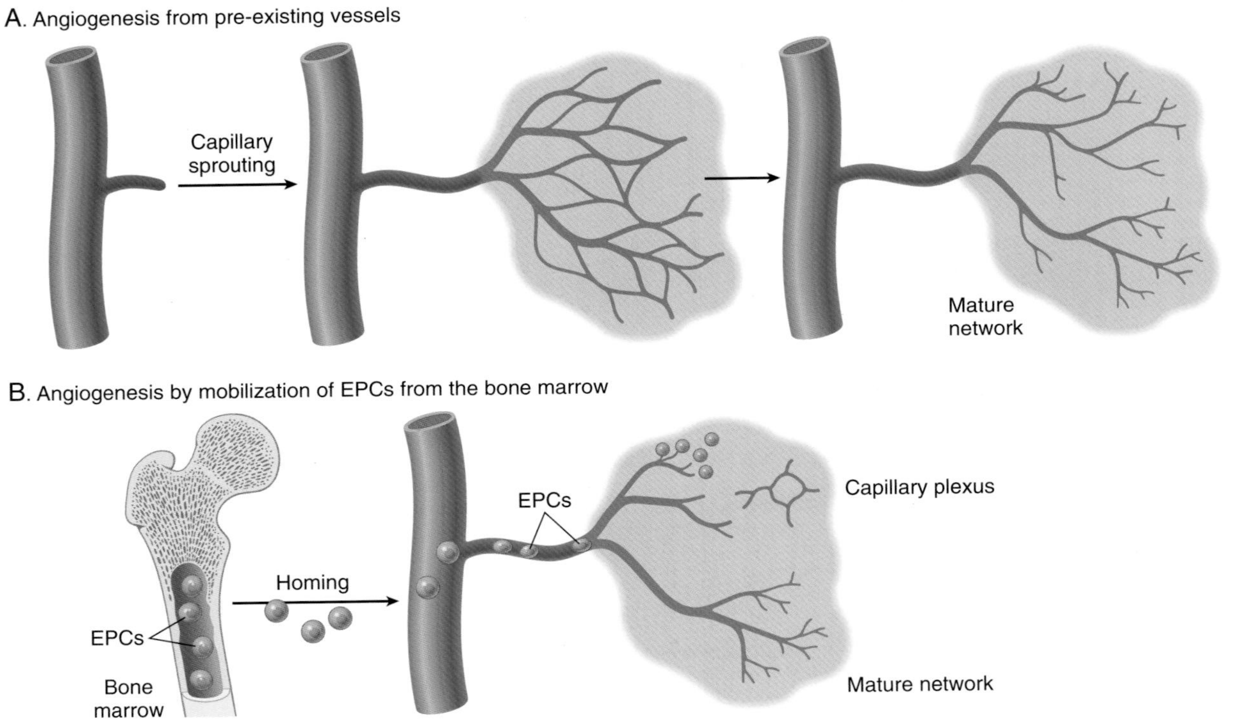

Fig. 3-41 Angiogenesis by mobilization of endothelial cell precursors (EPCs). **A,** Bone marrow. EPCs are mobilized from the bone marrow and may migrate to a site of injury. The homing mechanisms have not yet been defined. At these sites, EPCs differentiate and form a mature network by linking with existing vessels. **B,** Preexisting vessels (capillary growth). In angiogenesis from preexisting vessels, endothelial cells from these vessels become motile and proliferate to form capillary sprouts. Regardless of the initiating mechanism, vessel maturation (stabilization) involves the recruitment of pericytes and smooth muscle cells to from the periendothelial layer. (From Kumar V, Abbas A, Fausto N, et al: *Robbins & Cotran pathologic basis of disease*, ed 8, Philadelphia, 2009, Saunders.)

Vascular Remodeling

Once blood vessels are initially formed, they are loosely arranged and require remodeling to become mature. With remodeling, endothelial cells produce a mature basement membrane. In addition, smooth muscle cells and pericytes can form within the wall, and fibroblasts can form adventitial fibers, depending on whether the vessel is a capillary, artery, vein, or lymphatic vessel. Other endothelial cell growth factors and receptors involved with vascular remodeling include angiopoietin 2, which also binds Tie2 and ephrin B2 (EphB2) and its receptor, EphB4. Proliferation of lymphatic endothelial cells is mediated largely by VEGF-C and its receptor, VEGF-R3, as well as prox 1 gene expression.

Regulators/Inhibitors of Endothelial Cell Growth

Inhibitors of angiogenesis are produced by endothelial cells, macrophages, and fibroblasts. These inhibitors balance the proliferative healing responses of angiogenesis and prevent overexuberant proliferation of endothelial cells. These inhibitors include angiostatin, endostatin, thrombospondin, and specialized CXC chemokines (lacking ELR motif). In addition, certain isoforms of VEGF can bind VEGF receptors and reduce VEGF signaling and activity. Such inhibitors of angiogenesis are being studied intensely for their potential chemotherapeutic role against certain types of cancer and for exuberant vascularization that can occur in the retina, for example. Avastin (bevacizumab, Genetech, Inc., San Francisco) is an inhibitor of VEGF and can reduce vascularization in cancer and in the retina.

EPITHELIALIZATION IN WOUND REPAIR

Epithelialization (reepithelialization) is the process by which the skin and mucous membranes replace superficial epithelial cells damaged or lost in a wound. Epithelial cells at the edge of a wound proliferate almost immediately after injury to cover the denuded area. Under normal conditions, this process is rapid, and first intention healing occurs in 3 to 5 days to repair the wound. During wound repair, keratinocytes and mucosal epithelial cells must move laterally across the wound surface to fill the void. Before this lateral movement can occur, epithelial cells must disassemble their connections to the underlying basement membrane and their junctional complexes with neighboring cells. They must also express surface receptors that permit movement over the ECM of the wound surface.

Intact Basement Membranes Enhance Reepithelialization

The presence or rapid deposition of basement membrane into the wound greatly facilitates proliferation of viable epithelial cells at the margins of the wound. For example, with initial loss of enterocytes that cover the surface of intestinal villi or renal tubular cells that line proximal convoluted tubules, the immediate response is for the adjacent normal epithelial cells to extend over the denuded basement membrane and to cover the area, if it is larger, by becoming thin, elongated cells. At the same time, there is proliferation (mitosis) of viable adjacent epithelial cells, and these cells migrate along the basement membrane to cover the denuded surface and

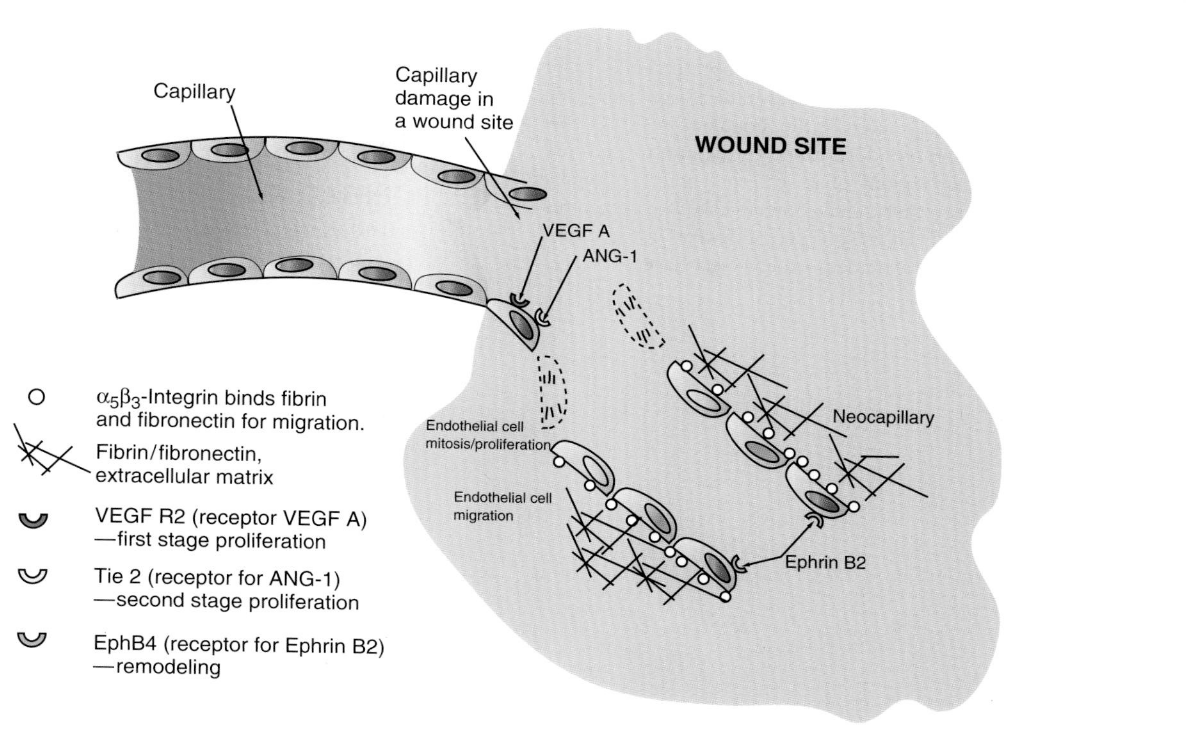

Fig. 3-42 Molecular mechanisms of angiogenesis.
Growth factors, such as vascular endothelial growth factor (VEGF-A) and angiopoietin (ANG-1), bind receptors on endothelial cells that induce proliferation and migration. The migration is mediated by $\alpha_5\beta_3$-integrins expressed by endothelial cells that bind molecules such as fibrin and fibronectin. Factors such as Ephrin B2 bind endothelial cell receptors Ephrin B4 and mediate vascular remodeling. (Redrawn from Dr. M.R. Ackermann, College of Veterinary Medicine, Iowa State University.)

replace lost cells. Without a basement membrane, proliferative cells lack a clear path of migration. The immature cells may loiter at the site of proliferation and fuse, thus forming syncytial cells, as can be seen with renal tubular injury and the failure of the tubular epithelium to migrate.

Similarly, regenerating skeletal muscle cells and transected axons will regenerate inside a tube surrounded by basal lamina and endoneurium. Components of the basement membrane, including laminin, type III collagen, and the associated proteoglycans, provide a substratum for epithelial and other cells to bind the basement membrane via integrins, proliferate, and migrate along the basement membrane surface.

Initiation of Cell Proliferation in Epithelia

Growth factors are vital for the proliferation of keratinocytes, mucosal epithelia, renal tubular cells, and other parenchymal epithelial cells. In skin and other surface epithelia, for example, keratinocyte growth factor (KGF) and EGF bind receptors on epithelial cells and induce signal transduction, which activates MAPK that induces cells in the nonproliferating G_o phase of the cell cycle to enter the cycle and proliferate (see Chapter 6). Hepatocyte growth factor (HGF) induces proliferation of hepatocytes, and nerve growth factor (NGF) enhances growth of nerve fibers. Cell proliferation is regulated by (1) the amount of growth factor produced; (2) the level of expression of the growth factor receptor; (3) inhibitory signals from other growth factors; (4) the microenvironment, including the availability of oxygen and nutrients; and (5) integrin attachment to an established basement membrane. Although TGF-β induces fibroblast proliferation and collagen deposition, TGF-β inhibits proliferation of epithelial cells in many parenchymal organs.

Differentiation of Epithelia

Once epithelial cells have filled in a gap in the epithelium of a tissue or an organ, cellular differentiation is required for return of the tissue or organ to normal function. FGF-10 is a key initiator of wound repair in skin and lung epithelia. FGF-10 binds FGF-RIII, which through BMP4 and sonic hedgehog (a signaling protein for developmental patterning) enhances expression of several transcription factors, including GATA-6, thyroid transcription factor-1 (TTF-1), hepatocyte nuclear factor-β (HNF-β), and hepatocyte factor homolog-4 (HFH-4). Each of these transcription factors enhances expression of genes, which regulate a specific function for a particular cell (Web Fig. 3-30). In the lung, for example, TTF-1 induces production of surfactant proteins A, B, and C, and HFH-4 stimulates cilia formation. Activity of these transcription factors is reduced in the presence of NF kappa B, an important mediator of inflammation. Therefore concurrent inflammation can impair differentiation of epithelial and parenchymal cells and thus inhibit or delay reepithelialization.

Metaplasia in Wound Repair

Some wounds do not heal properly and can turn into hypertrophic scars that impair epithelial and parenchymal cell growth. Such wounds may remain ulcerated or in parenchymal organs; the injured site may be replaced by fibroblasts and inflammatory cells rather than parenchymal cells. In either case, epithelial and parenchymal stem cells may continually attempt to cover or fill wound defects. With time, these cells may convert to another cell or tissue type. For example, regions of the lung constantly exposed to smoke can change from pseudostratified epithelium to stratified squamous epithelium, or regions of lower esophagus continually exposed to gastric acidity can undergo metaplasia into squamous cells. Osseous and chondroid metaplasia can occur in persistent wounds. In general, cells that undergo metaplasia have either (1) enhanced expression of an altered set of transcription factors and/or (2) decreased expression of transcription factors generally active for the affected tissue. The result is conversion of the cell's phenotype into a new phenotype. Often, if the initiating stimulus is removed, cells can revert to the original phenotype.

SUGGESTED READINGS

Suggested Readings are available at evolve.elsevier.com/Zachary/McGavin/.

CHAPTER 4

Mechanisms of Microbial Infections

James F. Zachary

The goal of this chapter is to provide a mechanistic overview of the key steps involved in understanding the pathogenesis of infectious diseases. Coverage is not intended to be encyclopedic nor will every fine distinction of individual microbial strains, genera, or families be discussed. Because the knowledge base for some veterinary diseases is limited, some sections of this chapter are based on (1) extrapolations from known experimental systems, (2) established mechanisms of injury covered in the basic pathology chapters of this book, and (3) assumptions anchored in the characteristics of macroscopic and microscopic lesions that arise with each disease. This chapter assumes that students have prior experiences with infectious diseases through coursework in microbiology, virology, mycology, and parasitology and with innate and adaptive defense mechanisms through coursework in immunology. Subject matter presented in this chapter changes rapidly, often daily, through new discoveries; nevertheless, every attempt has been made to assure that material presented is current. However, new discoveries that occur between the writing of this chapter and the publication of this book may not be included in this chapter. Although every effort has been made to minimize errors, this chapter is an attempt to meld information from many different disciplines, often with conflicting conclusions and/or differing terminologies and interpretations of how cells and tissues respond to injury. Errors in interpretation, although inadvertent, may occur.

This chapter will also discuss and illustrate selected "especially dangerous and contagious microorganisms" because diseases caused by these pathogens can have disastrous impact on livestock health and production and on the economies of affected countries. The location in this textbook of coverage of these diseases considered by the USDA/APHIS and the World Organization for Animal Health (OIE) as "Foreign Animal Diseases" or "OIE Reportable Diseases" is listed in Table 4-1.

SYNOPSIS

Infectious microorganisms like bacteria, viruses, fungi, protozoa, and prions cause many of the diseases common to the practice of veterinary medicine. For convenience, this chapter discusses individual diseases using an organ system approach under the headings: Bacterial Diseases, Viral Diseases, Fungal Diseases, Protozoal Diseases, and Prion Diseases. Students are advised to initially read (1) the opening portions of this chapter that discuss and illustrate background information about mechanisms of disease and (2) the opening portions of the sections covering bacterial diseases and viral diseases that discuss and illustrate background information about the chronologic sequences of events in disease processes. These materials provide the context for understanding individual animal diseases.

Infectious microorganisms follow chronologic sequences of events regulated by virulence determinates to infect target cells unique to specific organ systems and cause disease (Fig. 4-1). They most commonly enter the body through ingestion, inhalation, or cutaneous penetration and interact with mucosae or skin. If their target cell is not in mucosae or skin, they may spread to submucosal and subcutaneous lymphoid nodules such as in tonsils or Peyer's patches, then to regional lymph nodes, and then systemically in the circulatory and/or lymphatic systems to other organ systems. They often infect macrophages, lymphocytes, and/or dendritic cells and use these cells to spread via leukocyte trafficking to target cells in organ systems as they migrate through these systems as part of their normal immunologic surveillance activities. Cell and tissue specificity is based on ligand-receptor interactions in which proteins (ligands) expressed on the surface of infectious organisms bind to receptors on membranes of host target cells, mucus associated with these cells, vascularized extracellular matrix (ECM) tissues beneath these cells, or macrophages, lymphocytes, and dendritic cells supporting these cells. Once bound to receptors, a sequence of events facilitated by virulence determinates is initiated that colonizes the surface of these cells or invades the cells through phagocytosis or endocytosis. The organism then establishes control of normal metabolic systems of these cells and uses them to replicate in and spread to other organ systems. The outcome of this process is usually cell dysfunction and/or death and thus clinical disease.

PORTALS OF ENTRY

Except for contact with carrier animals, the chronologic sequence of events leading to disease caused by infectious organisms are not random events. Contact places susceptible animals in close proximity to infected animals, where infectious organisms can

TABLE 4-1 Location in this Textbook of the Coverage of Especially Dangerous and Contagious Microorganisms

Disorders of	Chapters
HORSES	
African horse sickness	4, 9, and 10
Anthrax	4, 7, 9, and 10
Glanders	4, 9, and 10
RUMINANTS (CATTLE, SHEEP, GOATS)	
Anthrax	4, 7, 9, and 10
Brucellosis	4, 18, and 19
Contagious bovine pleuropneumonia	4 and 9
Foot and mouth disease	4, 7, and 17
Rinderpest	4 and 7
Sheep and goat pox	4 and 17
PIGS	
African swine fever	4 and 10
Anthrax	4, 7, 9, and 10
Brucellosis	4, 18, and 19
Classical swine fever	4 and 10
Foot and mouth disease	4, 7, and 17

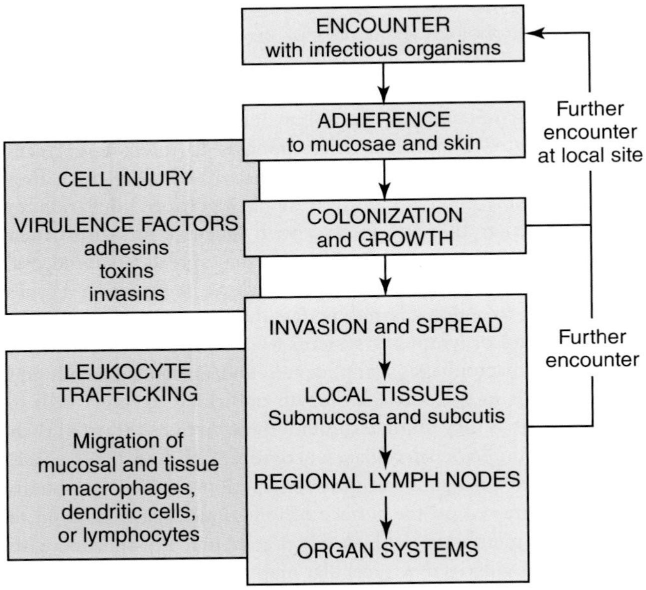

Fig. 4-1 Sequence of events in infection.
The chronologic sequence of events used by infectious microorganisms to colonize and invade mucosae and skin, spread to local tissues and regional and systemic organ systems, and cause disease. (Courtesy Dr. J. F. Zachary, College of Veterinary Medicine, University of Illinois.)

be spread through direct contact, grooming, licking, bite wounds, sneezing, and other normal physiologic body processes in fomites from body fluids, water droplets, snot, sputum, urine, and feces. Infection depends on creating an initial beachhead to establish, sustain, and spread the infection when organisms first encounter tissues of the body. Generally, the initial beachhead is established in one of two tissue types: (1) mucosae of the respiratory system (nasal cavity, nasal pharynx, conductive system [see Chapter 9]), alimentary (small intestine) system (see Chapter 7), lower urinary system (see Chapter 11), reproductive systems (see Chapters 18 and 19), or ear and eye (conjunctiva) (see Chapter 20) or (2) skin and subcutaneous tissues, including muscle and endothelial cells (Fig. 4-2). In these beachheads, organisms gain access and attach to, enter, and/or replicate in mucosal- and connective tissue-associated macrophages, lymphocytes, and dendritic cells. It is from these beachheads that they then spread locally (submucosae and subcutis), regionally (lymph nodes), and/or systemically (organ systems) to other target cells to sustain and amplify the infection and cause disease (Fig. 4-3).

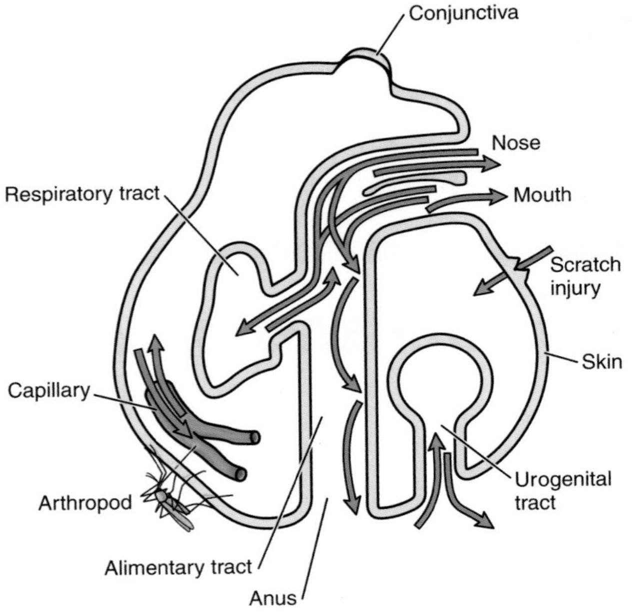

Fig. 4-2 Portals of entry.
Infectious microorganisms commonly enter the body through ingestion (alimentary portal), inhalation (respiratory portal), cutaneous penetration (skin portal), and ascending infection (lower urinary and reproductive portals) and interact with epithelial cells, macrophages, dendritic cells, and lymphocytes of the mucosae or skin. (Modified from Goering R, Dockrell H, Roitt I, et al: *Mims' medical microbiology*, ed 4, St. Louis, 2008, Mosby.)

A concept central to the pathogenesis of disease is the ability of an infectious organism to reach a site in the body suitable for growth and replication. Ingestion, inhalation, cutaneous penetration, and ascending infection are the most common portals of entry for infectious organisms to gain access to mucosae of the respiratory and alimentary systems; the epidermis, dermis, and subcutis of the integumentary system; and the lower urinary system and reproductive systems (see Fig. 4-2). The mucosae of the alimentary and respiratory systems are covered by a protective mucus gel composed predominantly of mucin glycoproteins synthesized and secreted by goblet cells (Fig. 4-4). The mucus layer forms a barrier system that attempts to do the following:

1. Block infectious organisms from reaching target cells.
2. Trap infectious organisms so they can be phagocytosed by mucosal macrophages and neutrophils.
3. Trap infectious organisms so they can be exposed to bacteriostatic and bacteriocidal molecules sequestered in the mucin matrix.
4. Facilitate phagocytosis of infectious organisms via mucosa-associated macrophages, mucosal dendritic cells, and microfold (M) cells.
5. Deliver microbial antigens to local lymphoid tissues like Peyer's patches or bronchial-associated lymphoid tissues

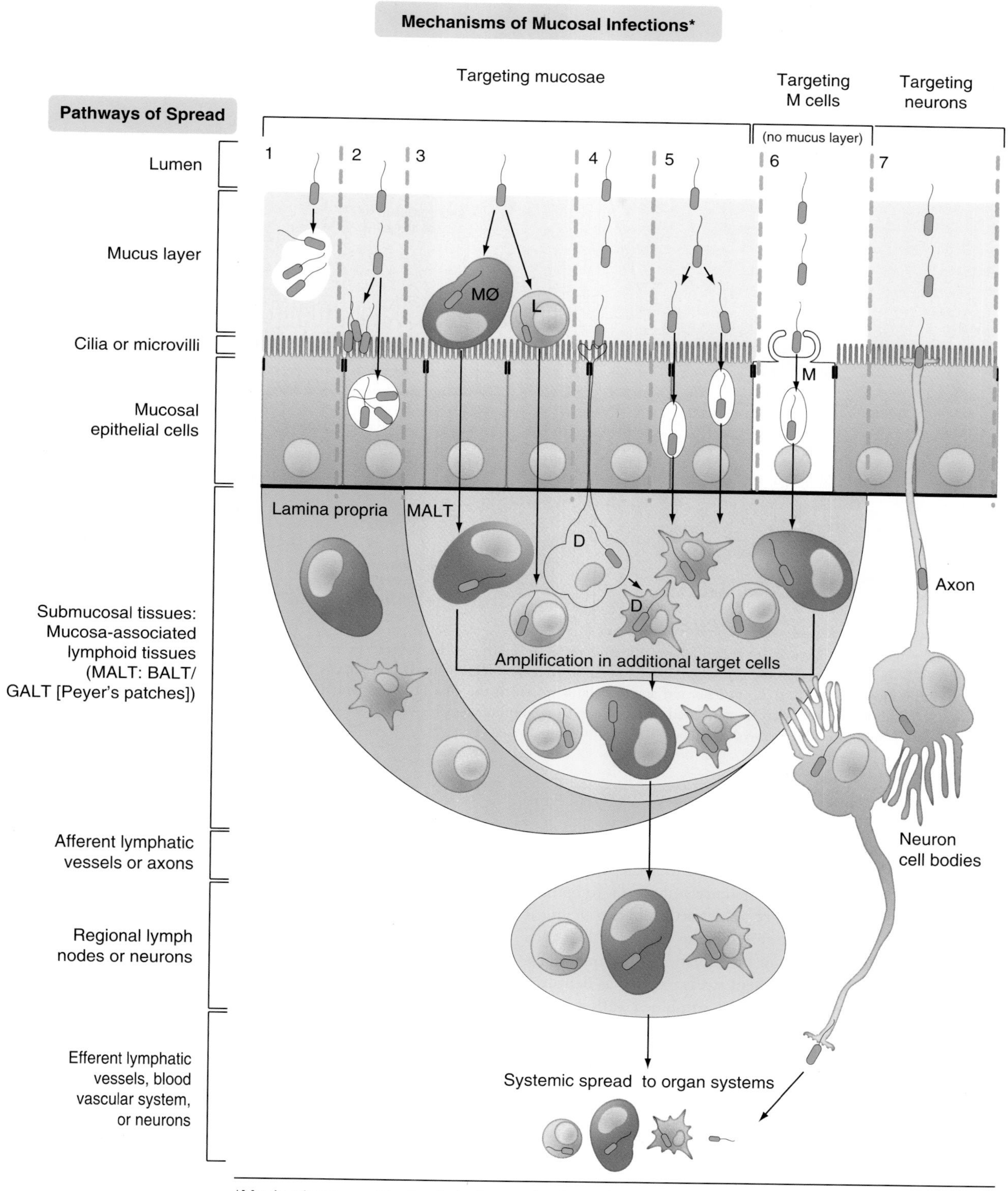

Fig. 4-3 Mechanisms of Microbial Infections and Pathways of Spread.
Pathway 1: Bacteria target the mucus layer.
Pathway 2: Bacteria target cilia or microvilli and/or mucosal epithelial cells.
Pathway 3: Bacteria target MALT via mucosal macrophages (MØ) and/or lymphocytes (L).
Pathway 4: Bacteria target MALT via dendritic cells (D).
Pathway 5: Bacteria target MALT via transcytosis or intercellular (junctional complexes) spread.
Pathway 6: Bacteria target MALT via M cells and transcytosis.
Pathway 7: Bacteria target nerve endings in mucosa and enter the brain via retrograde axonal transport. (Courtesy Dr. J. F. Zachary, College of Veterinary Medicine, University of Illinois.)

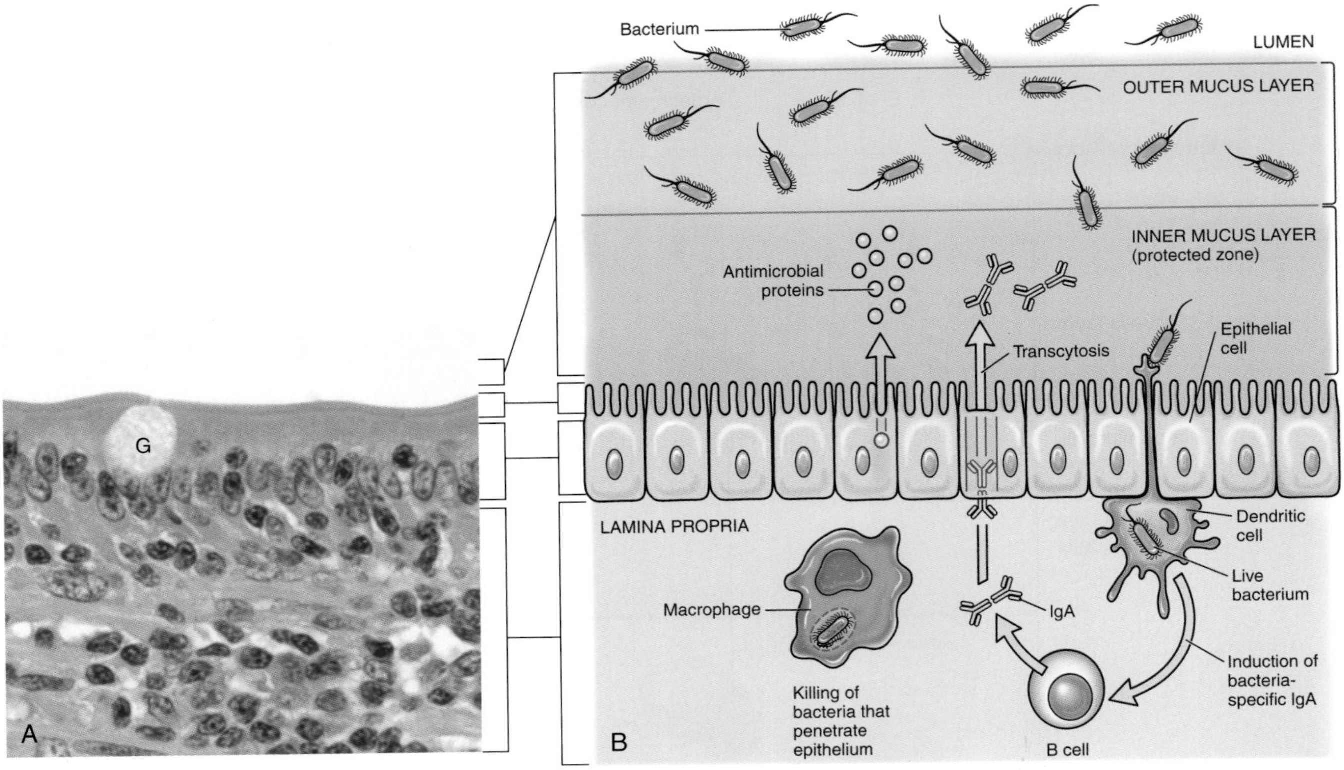

Fig. 4-4 Mucus layer of alimentary and respiratory mucosae.
A, Mucosa of the intestine (shown here) and of the conductive respiratory airways are covered by a mucus layer (not visible in H&E sections) secreted by goblet cells *(G)*. The mucus covers the microvilli or cilia of these systems. H&E stain. **B,** The mucus layer has an outer layer that traps microorganisms (infectious and noninfectious) and other particles and an inner layer in which the cilia beat and which contains antimicrobial substances that diffuse into the outer layer. Dendritic cells and mucosa-associated macrophages and lymphocytes play central roles in preventing infection of mucosa. (**A** courtesy Dr. J. F. Zachary, College of Veterinary Medicine, University of Illinois.)

(BALT) and then to regional lymph nodes via afferent lymphatic drainage.

Normal microflora such as bacteria are observed within the outer luminal zone of the mucus layer, indicating the importance of mucus gel in preventing direct adherence of bacteria to epithelial cells. Changes in the function of goblet cells and the chemical composition of mucus can occur through the release of bioactive factors from infectious organisms or by activation of immune cells. Additionally, predisposing management stressors, such as dehydration, shipping, humidity, and ventilation, combined with weather changes can also change the function of goblet cells and the chemical composition of mucus, making mucosae more susceptible to infection.

Infectious organisms use three mechanisms to penetrate the mucus layer and gain access to target cells. More information is known about the interactions of bacteria with the mucus layer, when compared to other infectious organisms, especially viruses. These mechanisms include penetrating motility, digestion of mucus via enzymes and its consumption as an energy source, and evasion of the mucus layer in areas around Peyer's patches and M cells, areas devoid of mucus. Mucus also provides pathogenic advantages to bacteria as follows: (1) mucin oligosaccharides represent a direct source of carbohydrates, peptides, and exogenous nutrients, including vitamins and minerals; (2) bacteria that colonize mucus avoid rapid expulsion out of the alimentary system by peristalsis; and (3) adhesion to specific molecules within the mucin facilitates colonization of the mucus layer by infectious organisms. Microbial mucolysis, the ability to enzymatically degrade mucus, appears to be a common trait among bacteria and provides access to readily available sources of carbon and energy and enables bacteria to reach the surface of epithelial cells. Mucins are classified as neutral and acidic types, with the latter being further categorized as sulfated (sulfomucins) or nonsulfated (sialomucins). These biochemical differences likely explain some of the segmental target cell specificity (i.e., localization in one area of the organ over another) of some diseases of the alimentary and respiratory systems. Localization and colonization of specific zones of mucus by certain organisms likely occurs through the expression of adherence molecules unique to specific types of mucins.

INGESTION

Organisms enter the alimentary system (see Chapter 7) by ingestion of infectious fomites. Through the processes of mastication, swallowing, and peristalsis, infectious organisms gain access to and are trapped in the mucus layer of the oral pharynx and intestines. Mucosae most commonly involved include tonsillar epithelium, villus epithelium, crypt epithelium, and epithelium containing M cells overlying Peyer's patches. Infectious organisms then must penetrate the mucus layer to reach targets such as mucosal epithelial cells, dendritic cells, and tissue macrophages. M cells are also targets but lack a mucus covering. Mucus in the alimentary system is produced by goblet cells distributed among mucosal epithelial cells in the villi and crypts where it covers and protects microvilli (see Fig. 4-4). The mucus layer is a (1) physical and (2) biologic barrier protecting the intestine against infectious organisms via (1) its thickness and viscosity, (2) binding to bacterial adhesins, (3)

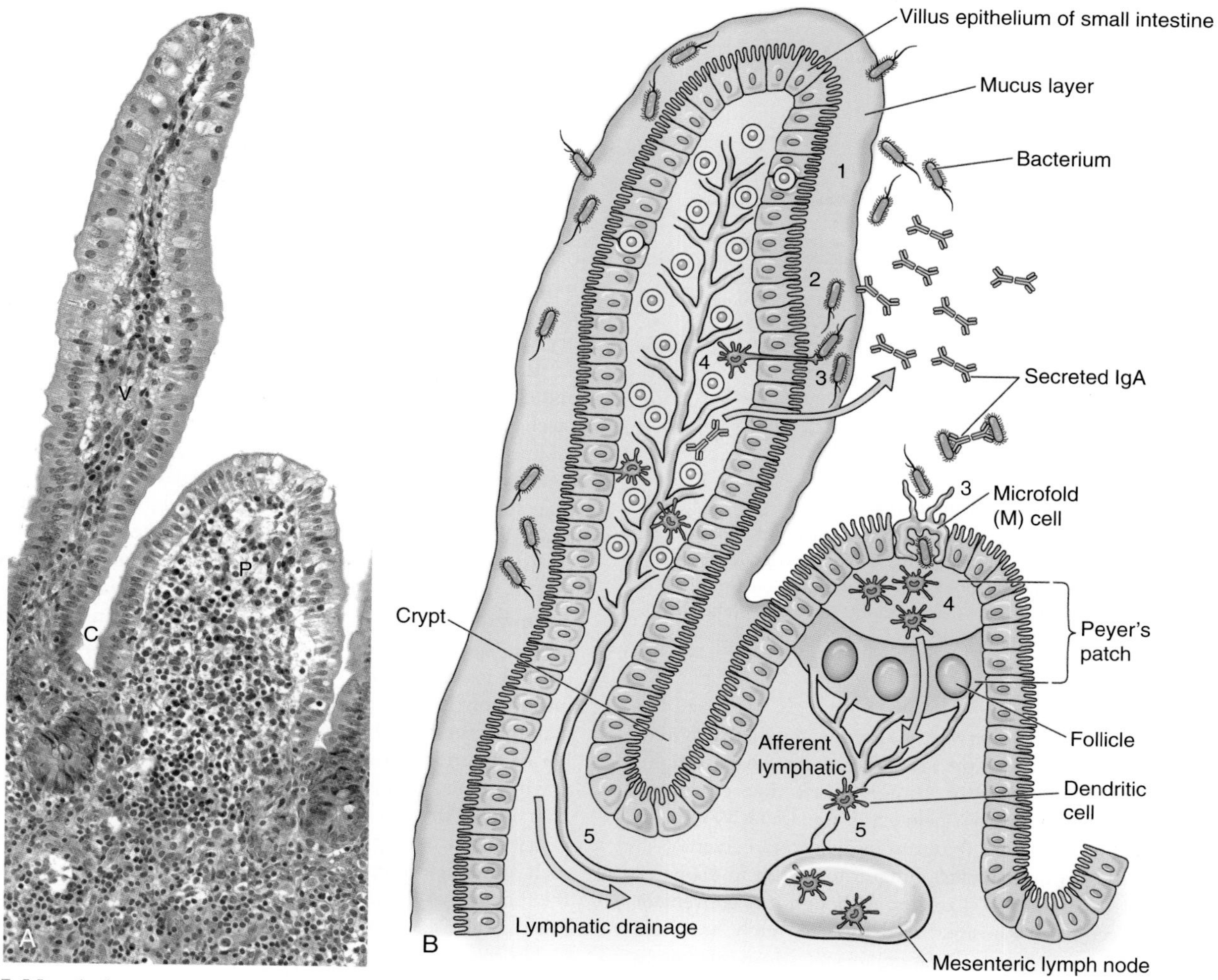

Fig. 4-5 **Microbial interactions with a barrier system: intestinal mucosa.**
A, Mucosa that cover intestinal villi *(V)* and Peyer's patches *(P)* and line crypts *(C)* form a barrier system that attempts to prevent the spread of infectious organisms into the underlying lamina propria. H&E stain. **B,** Schematic diagram of the responses of bacteria (or viruses) trapped in the mucus layer *(1)*. Bacterial proteins (virulence determinates) act to allow them to penetrate the mucus layer and come into contact with the mucosal epithelium *(2)*. IgA secreted by mature plasma cells in the lamina propria passes through mucosal epithelial cells into the lumen and can act as an "opsonizing" defense mechanism thus preventing infection. Bacteria then interact with mucosal epithelial cells, dendritic cells *(D)*, or M cells *(3)*. They then encounter lymphoid cells in the lamina propria or Peyer's patches *(4)* and spread in lymphocytes or as free virus in lymph from this location via efferent lymphatic vessels to regional lymph nodes *(5)*. Note the absence of a mucus layer over M cells and follicle-associated epithelium. Also see Fig. 4-7 for an example of barrier system: respiratory mucosae. (**A** courtesy Dr. J. F. Zachary, College of Veterinary Medicine, University of Illinois.)

serving as a reservoir for immunoglobulin A (IgA) and lysozyme, and (4) acting as a free radical scavenger. Additionally, the mucus layer is a habitat for beneficial enteric microflora.

Generally, there are more goblet cells in the large intestine than the small intestine, more in crypts than in villi, and more in the ileum than in the jejunum or duodenum. It appears that mucus covers all intestinal epithelial surfaces to varying degrees of thickness and viscosity and is composed of an inner gel layer and an outer soluble layer. The mucus layer is thickest in the colon (≈830 μm) and thinnest in the jejunum (≈123 μm). It is less prominent over absorptive enterocytes with microvilli when compared to crypt enterocytes. M cells are not covered by a mucus layer; therefore infectious organisms can readily interact with their cell membranes. Once entrapped in the mucus layer, infectious organisms must then penetrate it to gain access to target cells for infection. Additionally, infectious organisms also encounter mucosal fluids, such as gastric acid, mucins, secretions such as lysozyme, and humoral mediators such as immunoglobulins, and also compete with normal microflora for resources. Mucosae-associated lymphoid tissues (MALT), such as Peyer's patches (Fig. 4-5), are submucosal lymphoid nodules located in the distal jejunum and ileum that surround groups of intestinal crypts. Nodules are composed of lymphocytes, macrophages, and dendritic cells. They are covered by modified epithelial cells of intestinal crypts called M cells that transfer antigens in the lumen of the intestine across the mucosa to dendritic cells and immune cells like T lymphocytes in the nodule. M cells are the interface between materials in the lumen of intestinal crypts and the lymphoid nodules (see Fig. 4-5). Peyer's patches have afferent lymphatic vessels that drain to regional mesenteric lymph nodes.

INHALATION

In the respiratory system (see Chapter 9), infectious organisms are inhaled through the nostrils and are deposited on mucosae of

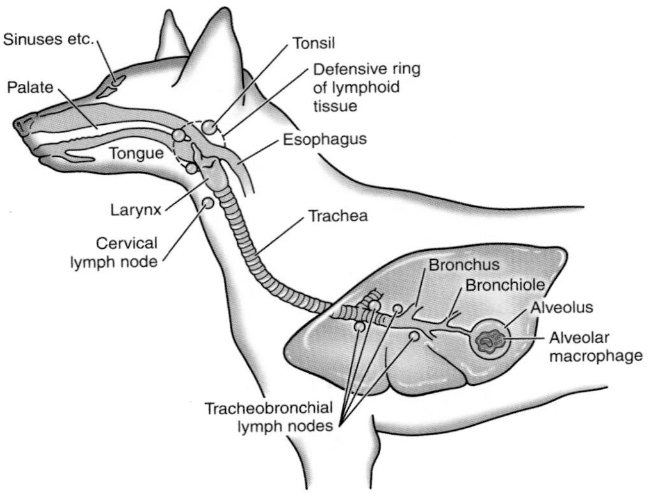

Fig. 4-6 Deposition of infectious microorganisms. Infectious microorganisms inhaled through the nostrils are deposited on mucosa of the nasal turbinates, nasal pharynx, and/or the conductive system of the respiratory tract. The site of deposition depends on the physical properties of the agent such as size, shape, weight, and electrostatic charge. (Modified from Goering R, Dockrell H, Roitt I, et al: *Mims' medical microbiology,* ed 4, St. Louis, 2008, Mosby.)

the nasal turbinates, nasal pharynx, and/or the conductive system based on physical properties of the agent such as size, shape, weight, and electrostatic charge (Fig. 4-6). Groups of infectious organisms ranked from smallest to largest include: viruses (5 to 300 nm [1×10^{-9} m] in diameter), prions (≈16 nm in diameter), bacteria (0.5 to 5 μm [1×10^{-6} m] in diameter), fungi 5 to 60 μm in diameter, and protozoa 1 to 300 μm in diameter. Although it is convenient to compare infectious organisms based on size, rarely are these organisms inhaled as free infectious organisms. Most commonly, they are enclosed in fomites (i.e., inanimate objects or substances capable of carrying infectious organisms) such as dust particles, soil, septum, or body fluids. Thus the physical properties of infectious fomites determine where they are deposited on mucosal surfaces of the respiratory system and cause disease. When inhaled, larger infectious fomites, such as bacteria and fungi, are deposited and trapped in the nasal turbinates, whereas in a gradient of descending size, smaller ones are able to reach the pharynx, larynx, trachea, and bronchi before they are deposited and trapped in the mucosae. The nasal cavity and turbinates trap 70% to 80% of particulate matter 3 to 5 μm or greater in diameter; 60% of particulate matter 2 μm or greater but cannot trap particles with sizes <1 μm in diameter. In a normal functioning respiratory system, only infectious fomites of 1 μm or less in diameter, such as viruses and some bacteria, can be inhaled into bronchioles, alveolar ducts, and alveoli, which are the oxygen-carbon dioxide (O_2-CO_2) exchange portion of the respiratory system.

When infectious fomites are inhaled, they first encounter the nasal turbinates. The movement of air through the turbinates causes centrifugal turbulence that forces them against the mucosae where they are trapped in its overlying mucus layer for removal. If the size of fomites allows them to pass through the turbinates and be carried to the pharynx, larynx, trachea, or bronchi, inertial turbulence forces fomites against airway mucosae where they are trapped in the mucus layer for removal. Inertial turbulence occurs when a laminar stream of airflow is disrupted by a septum within the conductive portion of the respiratory system when airways branch. When the flow is split by a septum, the flow rotates centrifugally on either side of the septum and forces fomites against the mucosae. Depending on the species, airways can branch 23 times en route from the trachea to the alveoli. The O_2-CO_2 exchange portion of the respiratory system (the bronchioles, alveolar ducts, and alveoli) are not ciliated and have no protective mucus layer because of their gas exchange function. The outcome of these turbulence mechanisms is to trap infectious fomites in the mucus layer overlying ciliated mucosal epithelial cells. When infectious fomites are trapped in the mucus layer, they are (1) acted on by other components of the innate immune system, such as phagocytes like alveolar macrophages and neutrophils, and microbicidal molecules, such as lysozyme and immunoglobulins, and (2) removed by the mucociliary apparatus (see Chapter 9).

The mucociliary apparatus is composed of the mucus layer and ciliated mucosal epithelial cells and is an important defensive mechanism in the respiratory system (Fig. 4-7). The mucus layer, produced by goblet cells and submucosal glands, is biphasic and consists of a luminal viscoelastic or gel layer used to trap infectious fomites and a serous inner layer in which the cilia of ciliated mucosal epithelial cells beat (see Fig. 4-7). The tips of the cilia just slightly enter the gel layer and their beating moves the gel and fomites. In the nasal cavity and sinuses, cilia move mucus and debris downward toward the pharynx for swallowing; in the conductive portion of the respiratory system, cilia move mucus and debris upward toward the pharynx for swallowing. The directionality of mucus flow is determined by the rhythmic unidirectional beating pattern of the cilia. The conductive portion of the respiratory system has an anterior and ventral flow pattern of distribution such that gravity influences the deposition of infectious fomites, if the mucus layer and/or the mucociliary apparatus are dysfunctional. Therefore injury to mucosal epithelial cells by specific infectious organisms, such as influenza and bovine rhinotracheitis viruses, can disrupt the function of the mucociliary apparatus, thereby exacerbating an existing disease or creating an opportunity for a secondary microbial infection of dependent lung usually prevented by this clearance mechanism. Swallowing of infectious organism-infected mucus may be a mechanism to clear certain bacteria; however, it provides other bacteria, such as *Rhodococcus equi,* the opportunity to gain access to the alimentary system and cause disease. The mucosae of the conductive portion of the respiratory system also contain dendritic cells and alveolar and tissue macrophages that commonly migrate through the mucosae and the mucus layer during their normal patterns of leukocyte trafficking (see Chapters 5 and 13). Because these cells can phagocytose and kill infectious organisms, they serve as a primary defense mechanism against infections. However, certain infectious organisms have virulence determinates that allow them to evade killing by phagocytes and use them like a "Trojan horse" to spread the agent and infect other cells and tissues. These cells are common targets for infectious organisms and along with mucosal epithelia serve as the initial beachhead infection before organisms spread locally often to the tonsil, regionally to lymph nodes, and systemically to other organ systems. bronchial-associated lymphoid tissues (BALTs) are submucosal lymphoid nodules located subjacent to ciliated mucosae, usually in areas in which inertial turbulence deposits foreign material on mucosae (see Fig. 4-5). Nodules are composed of lymphocytes, macrophages, and dendritic cells and function much like Peyer's patches. BALTs have afferent lymphatic vessels that drain to regional tracheobronchial lymph nodes.

CUTANEOUS PENETRATION

Infectious organisms enter the skin, dermis, and subcutaneous tissues (see Chapter 17) via penetration through abrasions,

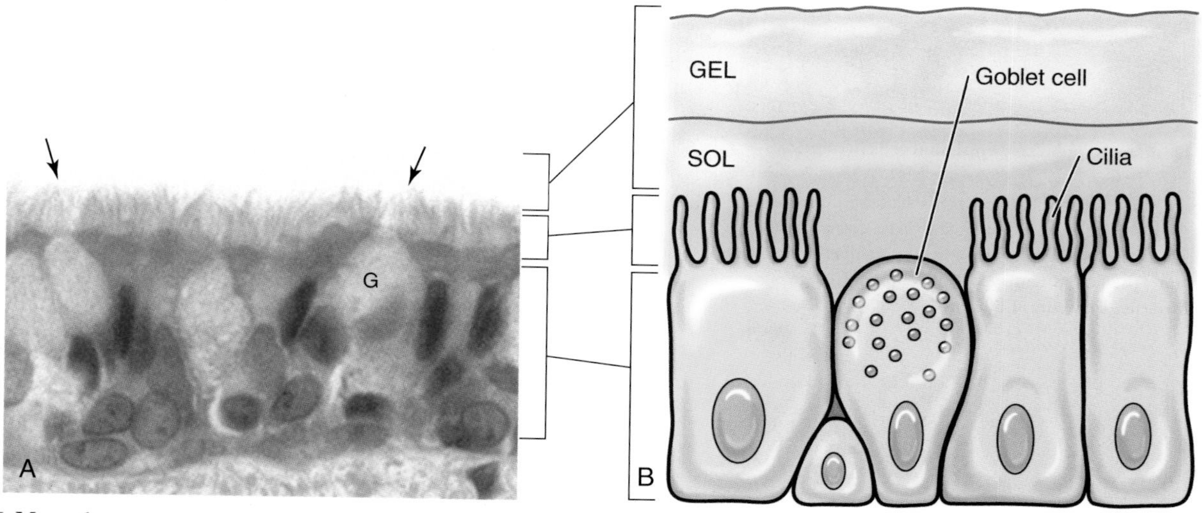

Fig. 4-7 Mucociliary apparatus.
A, Cilia *(arrows)* of the bronchiole mucosal epithelial cells and the mucus layer (not visible) form the mucociliary apparatus of the conductive component of the respiratory system. The mucus layer is not visible because it has been removed during histologic processing of tissue. H&E stain. **B,** Diagram of the mucociliary apparatus. The mucus layer is biphasic and consists of a luminal viscoelastic or gel layer used to trap bacteria and a serous inner layer in which the cilia of ciliated mucosal epithelial cells beat unidirectionally to move bacteria upward in the airways to be swallowed or expectorated. *G,* Goblet cell. (Courtesy Dr. J. F. Zachary, College of Veterinary Medicine, University of Illinois.)

scratches, and bite wounds or through bites of insect vectors such as mosquitoes that spread the agent into subcutaneous tissues such as muscle, blood vessels, and connective tissue (see Fig. 4-2). In these tissues, organisms encounter a limited range of host target cells such as epithelial cells in the skin, dendritic cells (Langerhans' cells), tissue macrophages, endothelial cells of the vascular system, and connective tissues and muscle of the dermis and subcutis. They may also be deposited directly in the blood vascular system via penetration of a capillary or venule by an insect proboscis. Additionally, organisms encounter body fluids, such as blood and plasma proteins, that serve as resources for survival, infection, and replication.

ASCENDING INFECTION

Infectious organisms can enter the lower urinary system and reproductive systems via ascending infection from coitus or the use of contaminated instruments, insemination straws, or semen. Traumatic injury of mucosae resulting in abrasions or penetrating wounds increases the likelihood of colonization by infectious microorganisms. The mechanisms of colonization and infection are similar to those discussed above.

DEFENSE MECHANISMS

HOST BARRIER SYSTEMS

Mucosal and cutaneous epithelia of the respiratory, alimentary, integumentary, lower urinary, and reproductive systems are the interface between the outside and inside of the body and are held together by occluding junctions such as tight junctions, desmosomes, and adherens junctions and to the basement membrane and ECM by anchoring junctions. Thus these cells form barrier systems that protect the body against entry by infectious organisms. In the respiratory and alimentary systems (and likely in other mucosae), the surface of an epithelial cell located above its junctional complexes and exposed to the lumen is called the *apical domain,* whereas the surface below junctional complexes on the sides and base make up the basolateral domain (Fig. 4-8). This relationship establishes a polarity to the cell, and it has been shown experimentally that such polarity is often reflected in the expression of different sets of cell membrane receptors that can potentially be used by infectious organisms to attach to and enter the cells. As examples, parvoviruses use receptors expressed only on the basolateral surfaces to infect small intestinal crypt cells via Peyer's patches, whereas influenza viruses use receptors expressed only on apical surfaces to infect respiratory epithelial cells via the airway. Infectious organisms enter cells through a process called *receptor-mediated endocytosis* most commonly at the apical surface and exit the cell from the basolateral surface via a mechanism called *exocytosis.*

INNATE AND ADAPTIVE IMMUNE RESPONSES

The innate and adaptive immune responses are covered in detail in Chapters 3 and 5.

MONOCYTE-MACROPHAGE SYSTEM

The monocyte-macrophage system is covered in detail in Chapter 5. In summary, cells of the monocyte-macrophage system form a network of phagocytic and immune cells like alveolar macrophages, mucosal macrophages, and tissue macrophages (Fig. 4-9) that migrate throughout the body in the circulatory and lymphatic systems looking for foreign matter and infectious organisms and return to local, regional, and systemic lymphoid tissues to share antigens with resident immune effector cells. These cells are important in phagocytizing and killing infectious organisms (Fig. 4-10) and commonly encounter infectious organisms, such as bacteria and viruses, in mucosae and the mucus layer. They migrate through the mucus layer, phagocytizing infectious organisms and material they recognize as foreign and carry it via cell migration through the mucosal epithelium to local lymphoid tissue using a mechanism called *leukocyte trafficking* (Fig. 4-11). Local lymphoid tissues, such as Peyer's patches and BALT, contain lymphocytes and macrophages that can be infected with organisms present in trafficking macrophages (see Fig. 4-5). From these local sites, infected lymphocytes and macrophages spread via lymphatic vessels to regional lymph nodes where additional cells are infected and then

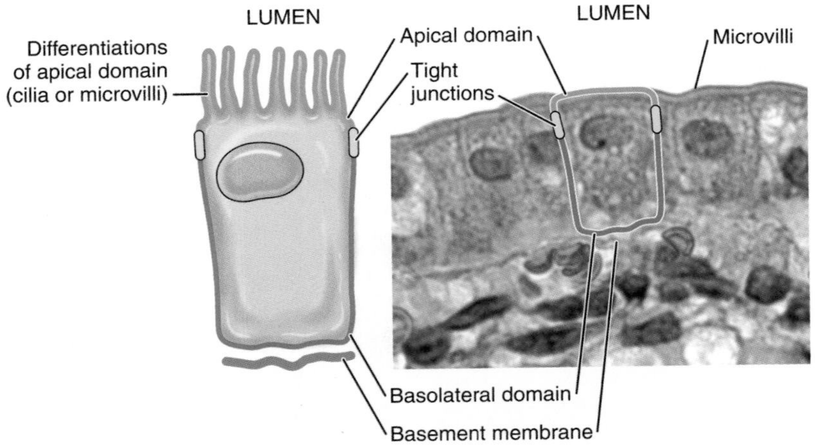

Fig. 4-8 Domains of polarized epithelial cells in mucosal barriers.
Infectious organisms use the apical or basolateral domains of mucosal epithelial cells to enter and exist from these cells. Apical or basolateral cell surface receptors may facilitate entry into the cell. (Courtesy Dr. J. F. Zachary, College of Veterinary Medicine, University of Illinois.)

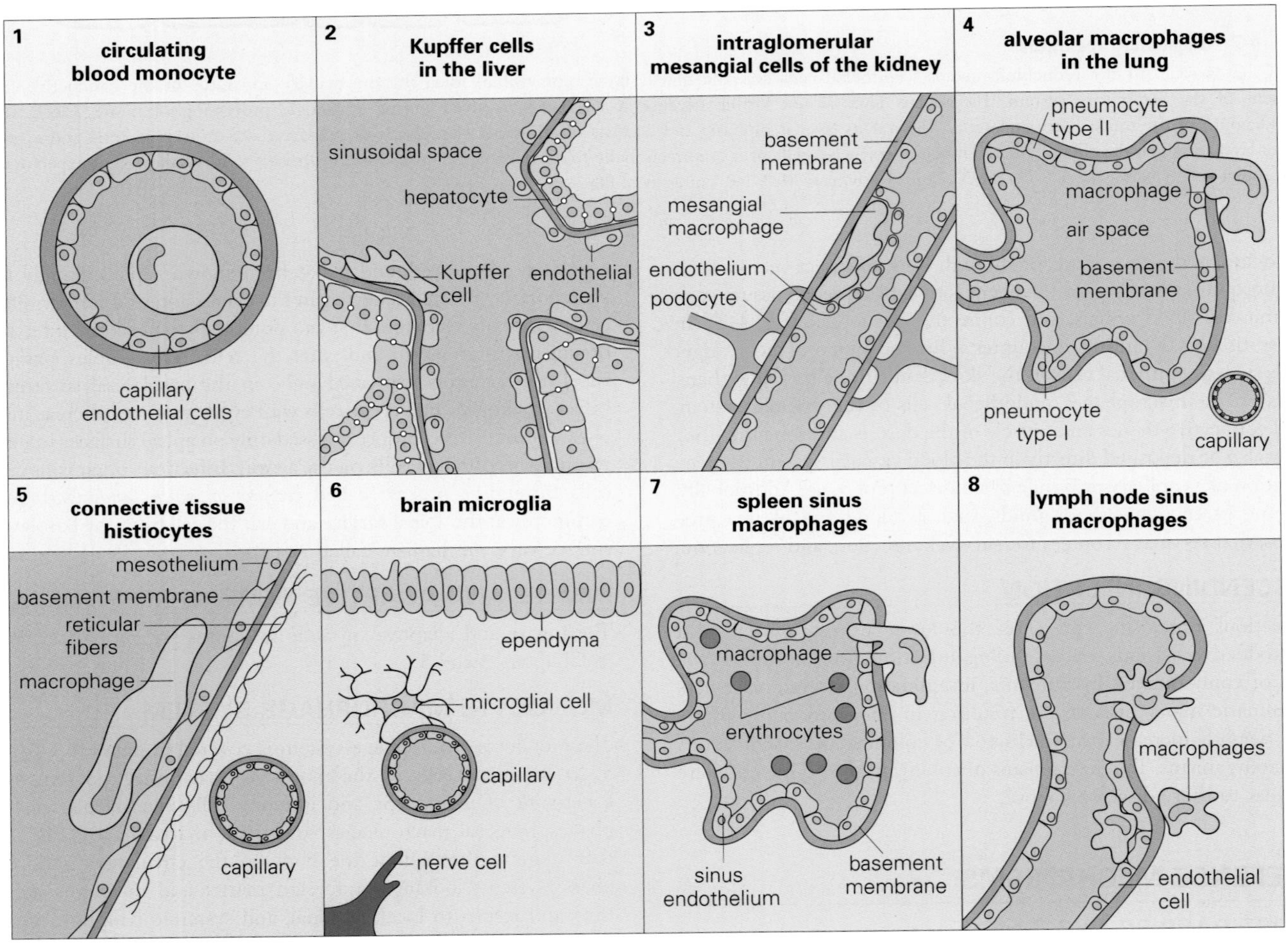

Fig. 4-9 Tissue locations of cells of the monocyte-macrophage system.
(From Goering R, Dockrell H, Roitt I, et al: *Mims' medical microbiology*, ed 4, St. Louis, 2008, Mosby.)

spread via lymphatic vessels to the thoracic duct and the circulatory system. From here, infected cells spread systemically to other organ systems in which specific target cells are infected, including lymphoid organs such as the spleen, lymph nodes, and bone marrow. Under normal conditions, tissue macrophages are derived from two sources: blood monocytes and tissue macrophage progenitor cells that are distributed throughout body tissues during organogenesis of the embryo. Precursor monocytes in bone marrow are capable of providing monocytes that migrate to and differentiate into macrophages in tissues. Tissue macrophages are also replenished locally and in large numbers by proliferation of tissue macrophage progenitor cells. These two populations of cells give rise to tissue macrophages that form the functional basis for innate and adaptive responses to microbes in tissues and organs (see Chapters 5 and 13). Tissues and organs that utilize cells of the monocyte-macrophage system include (1) lung (alveolar macrophages), (2) liver sinusoids (Kupffer cells), (3) lymph nodes (free and fixed macrophages), (4) spleen (free and fixed macrophages), (5) bone marrow (fixed

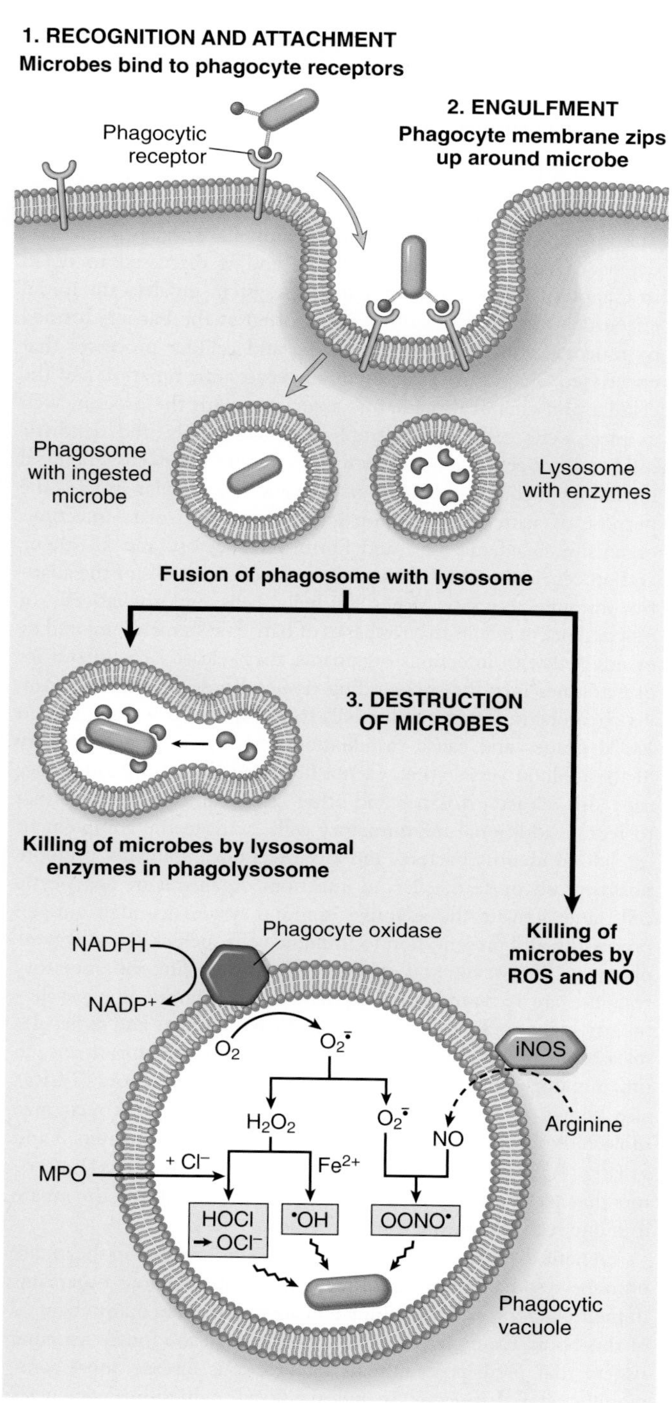

Fig. 4-10 **Phagocytosis and intracellular destruction of microbes.** Phagocytosis of a particle (e.g., infectious microorganism) involves binding to receptors on the leukocyte membrane, engulfment, and fusion of lysosomes with phagocytic vacuoles. This process is followed by destruction of ingested particles within the phagolysosomes by lysosomal enzymes and by reactive oxygen and nitrogen species. The microbicidal products generated from superoxide are hypochlorite (HOCl·) and hydroxyl radical (·OH), and from nitric oxide (NO) it is peroxynitrite (OONO·). During phagocytosis, granule contents may be released into extracellular tissues (not shown). *MPO,* Myeloperoxidase; *iNOS,* inducible NO synthase. (From Kumar V, Abbas A, Fausto N, et al: *Robbins & Cotran pathologic basis of disease,* ed 8, Philadelphia, 2009, Saunders.)

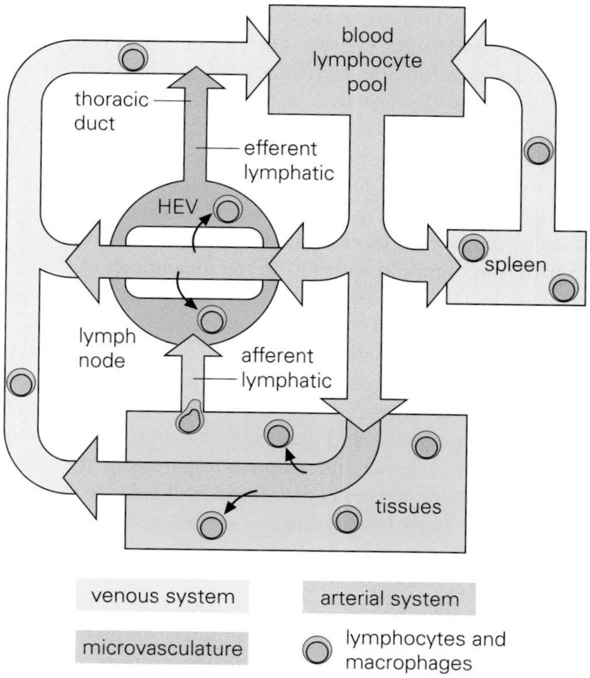

Fig. 4-11 **Leukocyte trafficking.** Infectious microorganisms often use macrophages, lymphocytes, and/or dendritic cells to spread themselves to other organ systems as these cells migrate through these systems as part of their normal immunologic surveillance activities. As an example, lymphocytes move through the circulation and enter lymph nodes via specialized endothelial cells of postcapillary venules (HEVs), leave through efferent lymphatic vessels and pass through other nodes, finally entering the thoracic duct, which empties into the circulation. Lymphocytes enter white pulp of the spleen, then pass into sinusoids of the red pulp and leave via the splenic vein. (From Goering R, Dockrell H, Roitt I, et al: *Mims' medical microbiology,* ed 4, St. Louis, 2008, Mosby.)

macrophages), (6) connective tissue (histiocytes), (7) serous fluids (pleural and peritoneal macrophages), and (8) skin (histiocytes, Langerhans' cells) (see Fig. 4-9).

DENDRITIC CELLS

Dendritic cells are covered in detail in Chapters 3 and 5. In summary, dendritic cells are migratory phagocytic antigen-processing and -presenting cells of mucosae (see Fig. 4-5) and skin (e.g., Langerhans' cells) that are commonly found intermixed with epithelial cells. Infected dendritic cells can migrate from mucosae and skin to local and regional lymphoid tissues via lymphatic vessels. Infectious organisms through their surface proteins are able to bind to receptors expressed on the apical domains of these cells and infect them, then exit via the basolateral domain via exocytosis, gain access to lymphoid nodules (tissues commonly associated with dendritic cells), and establish a local infection in lymphocytes and macrophages. Infected lymphocytes and macrophages spread the agent via leukocyte trafficking from local sites to regional lymph nodes and then systemically to other organ systems as discussed for the monocyte-macrophage system.

GENETIC RESISTANCE OF ANIMALS TO INFECTIOUS DISEASES

The resistance of animals to disease depends on the effective interplay of many structural and functional (physiologic) components of the body, including cutaneous and mucosal barrier systems and the immune system, respectively. Distinct networks of genes play central roles in structural and functional activities of the body. They control the development, maturation, and maintenance of epithelial cells, mucus, and supporting ECM tissues, such as collagen, that form the barrier systems. Additionally, they control similar structural activities for a variety of cell lineages of the innate and adaptive immune systems like T lymphocytes, macrophages, neutrophils, and dendritic cells and the expression of proteins that form pattern recognition receptors in the membranes of these cells (see Chapter 5). These receptors recognize pathogen-associated molecular patterns (PAMPs) expressed by infectious organisms and are discussed in greater detail in Chapters 3 and 5. Genes also play a central role in functional processes of cells, including adhesion, chemotaxis, phagocytosis, phagosome-lysosome fusion, intracellular killing of microbes, and antigen processing (see Chapters 3 and 5) involved in innate and adaptive responses of the immune system. Thus genetic resistance to infectious diseases is a polygenic trait regulated mainly by the immune system and its interactions with barrier systems and environmental factors such as weather conditions and nutritional status.

In animals, the genetics of disease resistance is most closely associated with the major histocompatibility complex (MHC), a tightly linked group of genes that encode proteins involved in immune responses. This genetic region in cattle has been given the abbreviated name *BoLA,* and similar regions have been identified in other animal species. Few specific genes or *genetic markers related to disease resistance have been identified in domestic animals;* however, genes involved in antigen processing appear to be important in resistance to infectious diseases.

DISORDERS OF BARRIER SYSTEMS

Barrier systems most commonly involved in infectious diseases of animals include mucosae and the skin and were discussed previously. Additionally, mucosae of the conjunctiva and urinary systems also serve as barriers to infectious organisms. These systems and their physical barriers develop embryologically under strict genetic control and when mature are functionally maintained, regulated, and repaired through processes dependent on transcription and translation of genes. Structural and/or functional alterations in these barriers can make animals more susceptible to infectious organisms.

An example of a genetic disorder that predisposes animals to infectious disease that occurs because of an alteration in the development of the basic structure of a barrier is epitheliogenesis imperfecta. It is an autosomal recessive hereditary disease of young horses, cattle, and pigs characterized by loss of epithelium affecting the skin and mucosae of the oral cavity and tongue likely caused by alterations in the subbasal plate and its hemidesmosomes and laminin-5 (see Chapter 17). Loss of the skin or mucosae exposes underlying vascularized ECM tissues to environmental contamination with feces and other matter allowing bacterial pathogens access to matrix tissues and capillary beds.

An example of a genetic disorder that predisposes animals to infectious disease that occurs because of an alteration in the function of a barrier is primary ciliary dyskinesia of the dog. It appears to be an autosomal recessive hereditary disease of young dogs, but an autosomal dominant mutation has not been excluded. This disorder is caused by ciliary dysfunction attributable to immotile or dyskinetic cilia caused by defects of proteins in the outer and/or inner dynein arms of cilia, which give them their motility. This outcome leads to dysfunction of the mucociliary apparatus and the retention of infectious organisms in the respiratory system leading to bacterial bronchitis and pneumonia. Other examples of genetic alterations of barrier systems that predispose animals to increased susceptibility to infectious disease are discussed in the organ system chapters of this book.

DISORDERS OF THE INNATE IMMUNE RESPONSE

The innate immune system provides animals with an immediate defense against infectious organisms and is discussed in detail in Chapters 3 and 5. In summary, this system involves the initial encounter with infectious organisms often at the barriers formed by mucosae and skin and the fluidic and cellular processes that ensue (see Chapter 3). It is essentially acute inflammation and the cellular and chemical mediators associated with the process, such as phagocytic cells like macrophages, neutrophils, and dendritic cells; effector cells, such as T lymphocytes and mast cells; chemical mediators of the complement system; and the vascular system. The purpose of acute inflammation is to dilute and isolate infectious organisms in edema fluid and fibrin, phagocytose and kill them, and process and present their antigens to effector cells of the adaptive immune response. When epithelial cells, endothelial cells, or mucosal or cutaneous macrophages of barrier systems are injured by or infected with infectious organisms, they release large quantities of cytokines into the surrounding tissues. These cytokines recruit, via chemotaxis, inflammatory cells from capillaries in vascularized ECM tissues and cause vasodilation and increased permeability of these blood vessels (i.e., edema fluid and fibrin). Inflammatory cells also release cytokines and other chemical mediators that act to recruit additional inflammatory cells, activate the complement cascade to identify bacteria and kill infectious organisms, promote phagocytosis of dead cells and infectious organisms by phagocytic cells, and activate the adaptive immune system through antigen processing and presentation to immune cells such as T and B lymphocytes. Phagocytic and effector cells of the acute inflammatory response are recruited from capillaries and migrate along a chemoattractant gradient formed by chemical mediators and molecules released from infectious organisms to the inflammatory focus. In inflammatory foci, these cells express Toll-like receptors (TLRs), also known as *pattern-recognition receptors* (PRRs) that recognize molecules on infectious agents called PAMPs (see Chapters 3 and 5) (Fig. 4-12). These cells also express interleukin-1 (IL-1) receptors that act in concert with PRRs to initiate and sustain the innate immune response through phagocytosis.

Genetic disorders can affect all of the steps involved in the innate immune response from initial recognition of infectious organisms to their phagocytosis and killing and are discussed in many chapters of this book. Examples of genetic disorders of the innate immune system that predispose animals to infectious disease, most commonly bacterial diseases, include leukocyte adhesion deficiencies and granulocytopathy syndromes. Leukocyte adhesion deficiency occurs in dogs and cattle and has an autosomal recessive mode of inheritance. It is characterized by alterations in the leukocyte adhesion cascade (see Chapter 3) involving deficiencies or dysfunction of integrins and selectins resulting in the inability of neutrophils to adhere to endothelial cells in the wall of blood vessels and migrate into sites of bacterial infection. Granulocytopathy syndrome occurs in dogs and cattle and has an autosomal recessive mode of inheritance. It is characterized by alterations in the ability of neutrophils to kill bacteria in phagosomes and is linked to reduced nicotinamide adenine dinucleotide phosphate (NADPH) concentrations that may arise from a metabolic anomaly in the hexose monophosphate shunt (see Fig. 4-10). This deficiency may lead to reduced concentrations of hydrogen peroxide in phagosome-lysosome

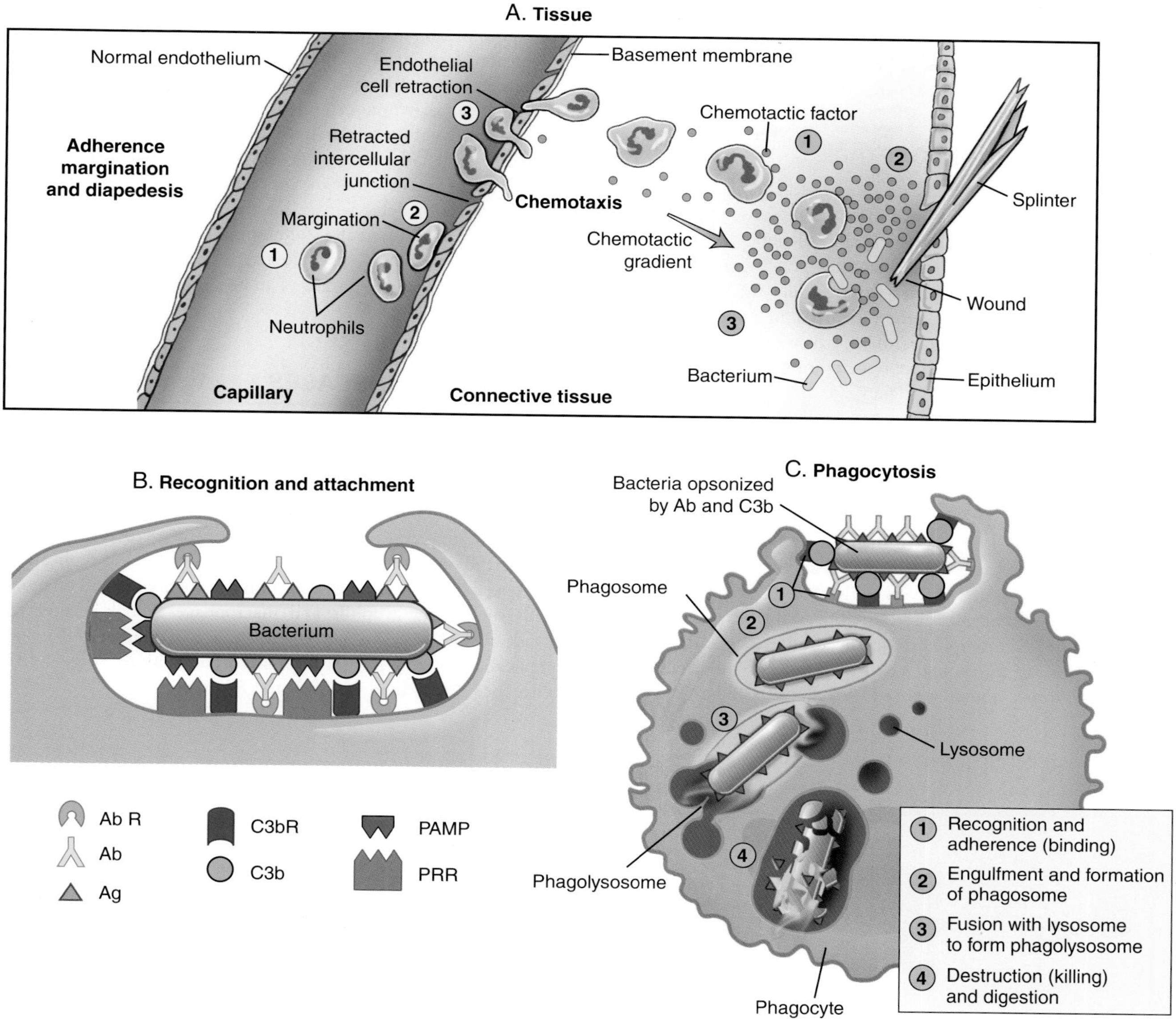

Fig. 4-12 Toll-like receptors in the process of phagocytosis.

The process that results in phagocytosis is characterized by three interrelated steps: adherence and diapedesis, tissue invasion by chemotaxis, and phagocytosis. **A,** Adherence, margination, diapedesis, and chemotaxis. The primary phagocyte in the blood is the neutrophil, which usually moves freely within the vessel *(1)*. At sites of inflammation, the neutrophil progressively develops increased adherence to the endothelium, leading to accumulation along the vessel wall (margination or pavementing) *(2)*. At sites of endothelial cell retraction the neutrophil exits the blood by means of diapedesis *(3)*. Chemotaxis: In the tissues, the neutrophil detects chemotactic factor gradients through surface receptors *(1)* and migrates towards higher concentrations of the factors *(2)*. The high concentration of chemotactic factors at the site of inflammation immobilizes the neutrophil *(3)*. **B,** Specific receptors for recognition and attachment. **C,** Phagocytosis. Opsonized microorganisms bind to the surface of a phagocyte through specific receptors *(1)*. The microorganism is engulfed (ingested) into a phagocytic vacuole, or phagosome *(2)*. Lysosomes fuse with the phagosome, resulting in the formation of a phagolysosome *(3)*. During this process the microorganism is exposed to products of the lysosomes, including a variety of enzymes and products of the hexose-monophosphate-shunt (e.g., H_2O_2, O_2^-). The microorganism is killed and digested *(4)*. *Ab,* Antibody; *AbR,* antibody receptor; *C3b,* complement component C3b; *C3bR,* complement C3b receptor; *PAMP,* pathogen-associated molecular pattern; *PRR,* pattern recognition receptor. (From McCance KL: *Pathophysiology: the biologic basis for disease in adults and children,* ed 6, St. Louis, 2010, Mosby.)

fusion and the bactericidal capability of the neutrophil. The process of phagocytosis is usually normal. Affected animals have shortened lifespan, long-term febrile disease, dermatitis, oral ulcers, lymphadenitis, and poor healing, attributable to irresolvable and repeated bacterial infections.

Genetic disorders of the innate immune system can also be caused by failure of leukocytes to correctly develop and mature in the bone marrow. Cyclic hematopoiesis occurs in dogs and has an autosomal recessive mode of inheritance. It is caused by an abnormality of stem cells in the bone marrow resulting in periodic declines, every 10 to 12 days, in neutrophil concentrations followed by hyperplasia and a return to normal. Abnormal concentrations of purine and pyrimidine metabolites in affected stems cells suggest that a metabolic derangement in purine or pyrimidine metabolism may be the cause of this genetic disorder. This outcome increases susceptibility to bacterial infection, often leading to periodic fever, joint pain, or other signs of ocular, respiratory, or skin infections. Other examples of genetic alterations of the innate immune response that predisposes animals to increased susceptibility to infectious disease are discussed in the organ system chapters of this book.

DISORDERS OF THE ADAPTIVE IMMUNE RESPONSE

Genetic disorders of the adaptive immune response are disorders in which affected animals are incapable of generating antigen-specific immune responses (see Chapter 5). Such genetic diseases are closely associated with genes that regulate the expression of the MHC, especially those genes involved in antigen processing and presentation. Examples of this type of disorder include agammaglobulinemia (a B lymphocyte immunodeficiency) and severe combined immunodeficiency (a B and T lymphocyte immunodeficiency). T lymphocyte, macrophage, and complement immunodeficiencies also occur but are not discussed here. Agammaglobulinemia has a X-linked recessive mode of inheritance and thus is a disorder of young colts. It is likely caused by dysfunction of cytoplasmic tyrosine kinase resulting in blockage in the differentiation of B lymphocyte lineages and a nearly complete absence of B lymphocytes and plasma cells. Clinically, this type of immunodeficiency results in colts with chronic bacterial diseases leading to pneumonia, enteritis, dermatitis, arthritis, and laminitis. Severe combined immunodeficiency occurs in dogs and Arabian horses and has an autosomal recessive mode of inheritance. In dogs, an X chromosome–linked mode of inheritance has also been indentified. Affected animals produce no antibodies after infection or immunization because of an absence of B lymphocytes and have no or nonfunctional T lymphocytes when present. This genetic disorder occurs when lymphocyte precursors fail to differentiate into mature T or B lymphocytes, which is likely because of the result of mutations within recombinase-activating genes or within genes encoding DNA-dependent protein kinase or when differentiated lymphocytes are incapable of completing signal transduction pathways because of defects in cell surface receptors for interleukins. Other examples of genetic alterations of the adaptive immune response that predisposes animals to increased susceptibility to infectious disease are discussed in the organ system chapters of this book.

BACTERIAL DISEASES

PATHOGENICITY

The pathogenicity (i.e., ability to cause disease) of a bacterium is regulated by its virulence determinates. Virulence determinates are molecules, often glycoproteins or glycolipids, derived from bacterial genes. Their expression establishes the processes used by bacteria to successfully colonize mucosae, infect cells, grow and replicate, and cause cell death. Virulence determinates are used to kill phagocytic cells such as neutrophils and macrophages, block phagocytosis, evade fusion with lysosomes and microbial killing, and enhance replication within phagocytes. Important actions (Fig. 4-13) of virulence determinates include the following:

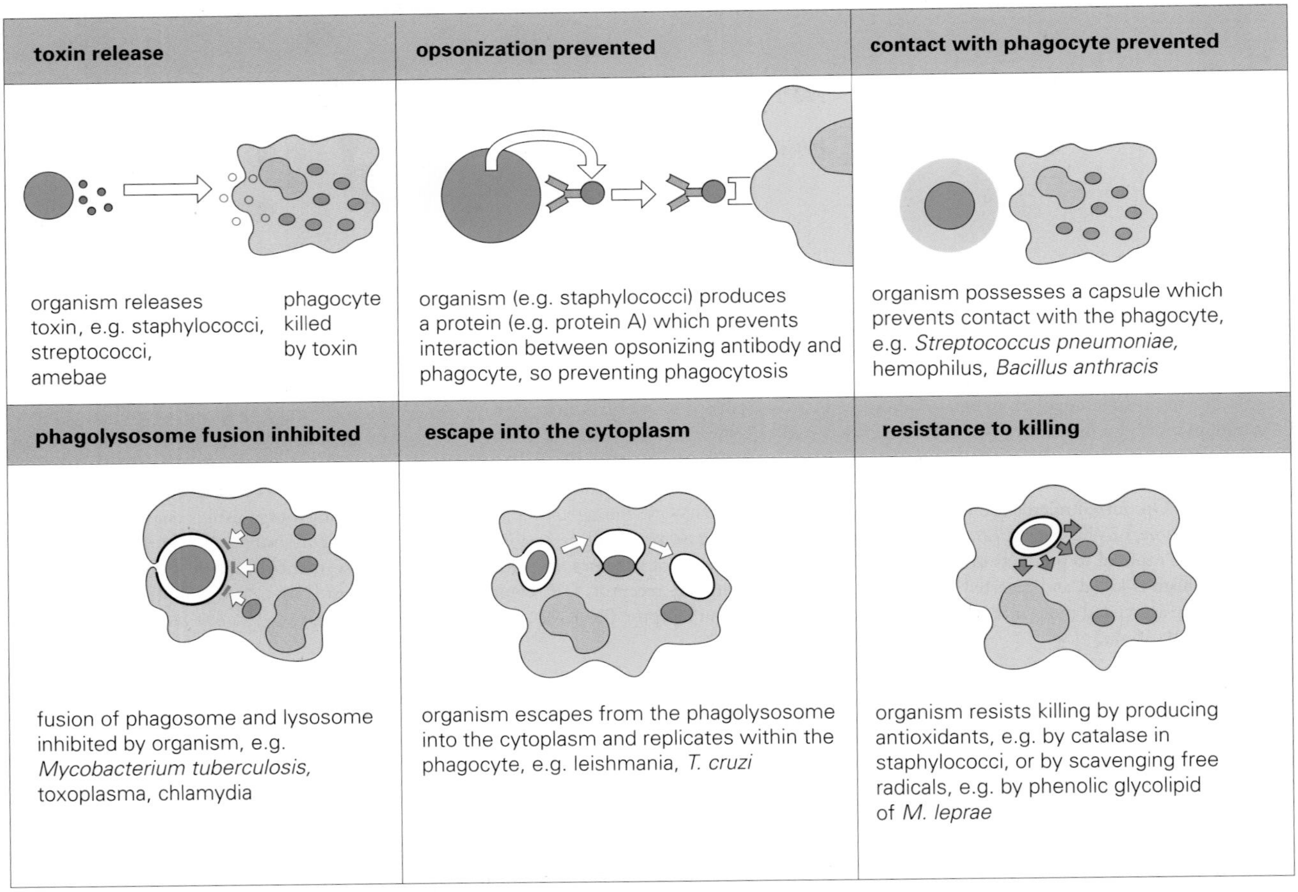

Fig. 4-13 Mechanisms adopted by infectious microorganisms to avoid phagocytosis.
(From Kumar V, Abbas A, Fausto N, et al: *Robbins & Cotran pathologic basis of disease,* ed 8, Philadelphia, 2009, Saunders.)

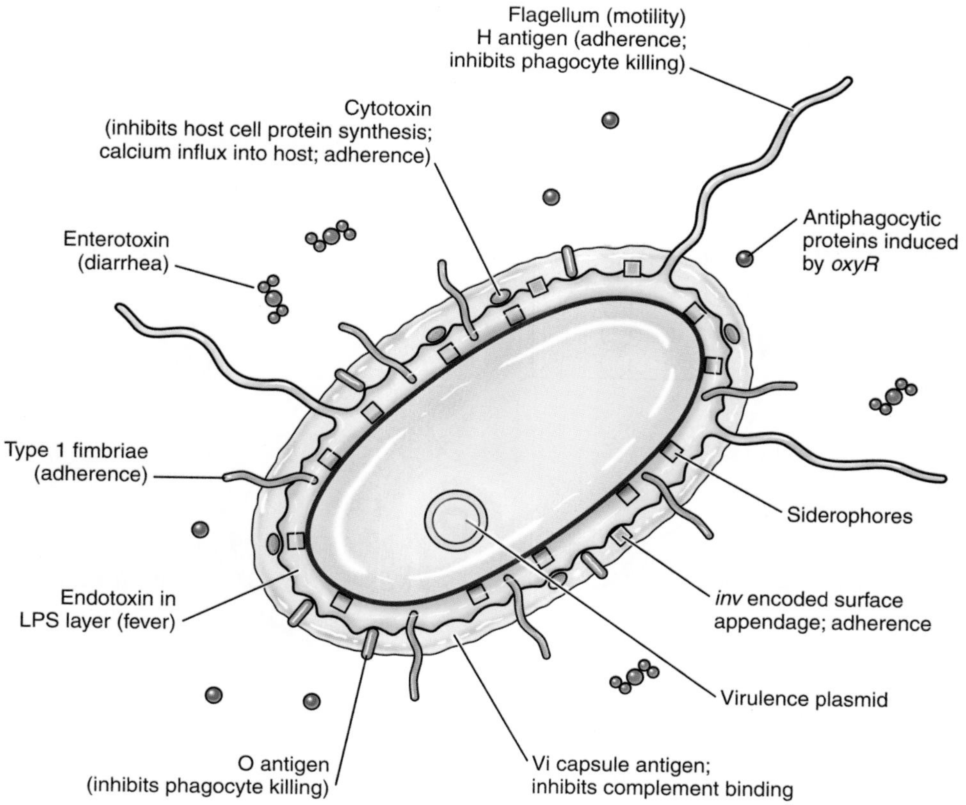

Fig. 4-14 Virulence determinates used by bacteria to cause disease.

1. Production of bacterial toxins that kill phagocytes.
2. Synthesis of bacterial proteins that prevent phagocytosis by blocking the interaction of opsonins with phagosomes.
3. Synthesis of a bacterial capsule that can block contact with the microbe and prevent phagocytosis.
4. Inhibition of fusion of the phagosome containing microbes with lysosomes.
5. Facilitate escape of the microbe into the cytoplasm before the microbe is killed in the phagolysosome.
6. Production of bacterial antioxidants (i.e., catalase) that block killing in phagolysosomes.

The interaction between an animal and a bacterial pathogen is back and forth, each acting to influence the activities and functions of the other. The outcome depends on the virulence of the pathogen and the resistance or susceptibility of the animal. Resistance or susceptibility to disease in healthy animals is derived from (1) innate defenses such as cellular and mucus barrier systems, acute inflammation (including neutrophil phagocytosis), the monocyte-macrophage system (phagocytosis), and normal bacterial flora and (2) adaptive defenses provided by the immune system such as passive immunity via colostrum and active immunity via T and B lymphocytes. In general, bacterial pathogenicity is determined by two characteristics: (1) its ability to infect cells and (2) its ability to produce toxins and damage cells and their ECM tissues such as collagen. To infect cells, infectious organisms use mechanisms such as adhesion, multiplication, colonization, tissue invasion, and circumvention of animal defense mechanisms. To damage cells via toxins, infectious organisms use mechanisms such as cytolysis and invasion of vascularized ECM tissues (locally or systemically) incited by bacteria-derived exotoxins (Gram-positive bacteria) and endotoxins (Gram-negative bacteria). Virulence determinates determine the sum of the characteristics that allow bacteria to cause disease and thus provide a pathogenicity profile or fingerprint for each bacterium.

VIRULENCE DETERMINATES

Bacterial virulence determinates are molecules that influence interactions between bacteria and cells, including events such as adherence to cell membranes; mucosal colonization; cell entry via endocytosis or phagocytosis; growth and replication; local, regional, and systemic spread; and cell disruption, inflammation, injury, or death by acting as toxins (Fig. 4-14). In general, they are coded for by more than one microbial gene. Furthermore, they inhibit immune responses and allow the organism to hide from defense mechanisms and proliferate in harsh environments. Bacterial virulence is determined in part by the type and number of factors the bacterium expresses to successfully complete its life cycle in an animal. Other things that can indirectly influence the success of these virulence determinates include physical and environmental issues, such as weather, access to food and water, and management (shipping) or housing stressors (ventilation, humidity, or overcrowding).

Initial Encounters

Before infecting cells, bacteria must often penetrate the mucus layer of mucosal barrier systems to gain access to mucosal epithelial cells, submucosal cells, and vascularized ECM tissues. Bacteria that are trapped in the mucus layer of mucosae may be phagocytosed by macrophages and dendritic cells that migrate in, on, and through the mucus layer and the mucosae. These cells may carry bacteria to mucosal epithelial cells and cells in submucosal lymph nodules, regional lymph nodes, and other organ systems. However, in many

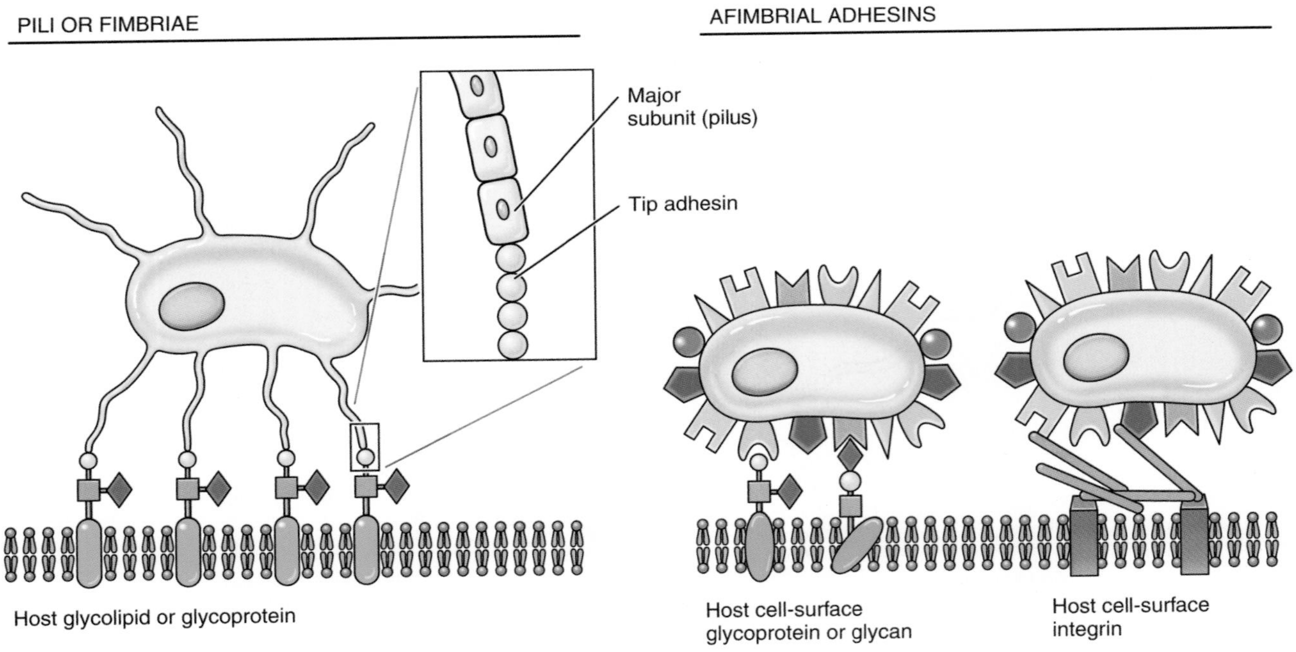

Fig. 4-15 **Fimbrial (pilus) and afimbrial adhesins.**
These structures are used by infectious microorganisms to attach and bind to protein receptors on membranes of target cells (especially mucosal epithelial cells) or to molecules of the mucus layer or vascularized extracellular matrix (connective) tissues.

diseases, it is unclear how bacteria ultimately invade or penetrate the mucus layer to gain access to mucosal epithelial cells (target cells). Several mechanisms are likely used, including (1) motility, (2) digestion and consumption of the mucus layer, and (3) random discovery of mucosae lacking a mucus layer. As examples in the alimentary system, some bacteria, such as the spirochetes, are motile and can penetrate the mucus layer and reach target cells. Other bacteria, such as *Clostridium septicum,* digest the mucus layer with bacterial enzymes and then consume oligosaccharides such as *N*-acetylglucosamine, galactose, and *N*-acetylgalactosamine in the mucus layer as a carbon source during intense periods of replication. Finally, some bacteria use M cells to gain access to target cells; these cells are not covered by mucus and their surface membranes and receptors are available to passing infectious organisms.

ADHESION, COLONIZATION, AND INVASION

Some virulence determinates mediate adhesion, colonization, and invasion; others act indirectly to minimize the animal's defense mechanisms by providing resistance to antibiotics, antiphagocytic properties, and weakened immune responses by acting as inhibitors. Adhesion, colonization, and invasion factors include bacterial membrane proteins, polysaccharide capsules, secretory proteins, cell wall and outer membrane components, and other miscellaneous molecules. Specific virulence determinates derived from membrane proteins assist the bacterium in adhering to, colonizing, and invading epithelia of barrier system portals of entry as in the alimentary, respiratory, integumentary, urinary, and reproductive systems. Because these epithelial cells are replaced continually (≈48 hour lifespan) and these systems have defensive mechanisms such as peristalsis, unidirectional mucociliary undulations, and urination, pathogenic bacteria must be able to adhere to, colonize (replicate), and/or invade into or between these epithelial cells to avoid being swept away. Attachment occurs when membrane proteins called *adhesins* (a broad term) bind to receptors on cell membranes. Attachment is a typical ligand-receptor interaction; a protein on the bacterium binds to a receptor on a host target cell. Some bacteria express adhesins, such as microbial surface cell recognition adhesion matrix molecules, that bind the bacterium to the surface of the cell. Other bacteria utilize extensions of their cell membranes called *fimbriae* or *pili* to bind to animal cells. Fimbriae and pili have adhesins, such as pilus-associated proteins, fimbrial antigens, or fimbrial adhesins, that bind to receptors on microvilli of the glycocalyx or in the mucus layer (Fig. 4-15). Fimbriae and pili may also act to inhibit phagocytosis. For example, uropathogenic and enterotoxic *Escherichia coli*, causes of urinary tract infections and diarrhea in animals, express fimbrial (type I, P, and S/F1C) and pilus (K99) adhesins, respectively. In the urinary tract, P-fimbriae is an important attachment adhesin and allows the bacterium to attach to the transitional epithelium and initiate the disease known as acute necrohemorrhagic urocystitis. Other virulence determinates, such as α-hemolysin and cytotoxic necrotizing factor type 1, cause necrosis and hemorrhage later. In the small intestine, K99 pilus adhesin allows *E. coli* to adhere to enterocytes and reduces their loss in number via peristalsis. When large numbers of *E. coli* are attached to the small intestine, they produce other virulence determinates, such as enterotoxin, that act directly on enterocytes, leading to diarrhea.

Ligand-receptor interactions are likely common to most bacterial diseases; however, in many veterinary diseases, specific bacterial ligands and their host cell receptors have not been identified. The attachment of sufficient numbers of bacteria at the appropriate portal of entry initiates an early stage of bacterial infection termed *colonization.* After colonization, another group of virulence determinates called *invasins,* or spreading factors, are produced by infectious organisms. These factors include hyaluronidase, collagenase, kinases, lecithinase, and phospholipase and act to break

TABLE 4-2 Biological Actions of Invasins or Spreading Factors

Virulence Determinate	Action
Hyaluronidase	Depolymerizes hyaluronic acid in the extracellular matrix
Collagenase	Breaks down collagen fibers especially in muscle tissue
Neuraminidase	Degrades neuraminic acid (sialic acid) that serves to keep epithelial cells attached to basement membrane in the mucosa
Kinases	Digest fibrin and prevent clotting of the blood needed to wall-off bacteria
Lecithinase	Punch holes through or break down cell membranes
Phospholipase	Punch holes through or break down cell membranes

down barrier systems formed by mucosae (mucus layer) and skin, cell junctional complexes, and ECM molecules like collagen (Table 4-2). This process allows bacteria to spread rapidly into and through intercellular spaces and protect itself in safe areas isolated from unfavorable host environments or host-derived defensive molecules. As examples, *Clostridium chauvoei,* the bacterium that causes blackleg in cattle, produces sufficient lecithinases and phospholipases to punch holes in cell membranes and cause death of myocytes and endothelial cells. *Listeria monocytogenes,* the cause of listeriosis in the nervous system of cattle, produces invasins that induce endocytosis of the bacterium for colonization by acting on host cell actin filaments. Other proteins of bacteria, such as surface components and polysaccharide capsules, are virulence determinates that allow bacteria to avoid phagocytosis and evade recognition by cells of the innate and/or adaptive immune systems. They disrupt or block one or more steps used by neutrophils, monocytes, or macrophages in the phagocytic process such as initial contact, engulfment, phagosome formation, phagosome-lysosome fusion, and killing and digestion. As examples, *Streptococcus pyogenes,* a cause of bovine mastitis, utilizes M-protein and a hyaluronic acid capsule to inhibit phagocytosis and the same hyaluronic acid capsule to evade recognition of the immune system.

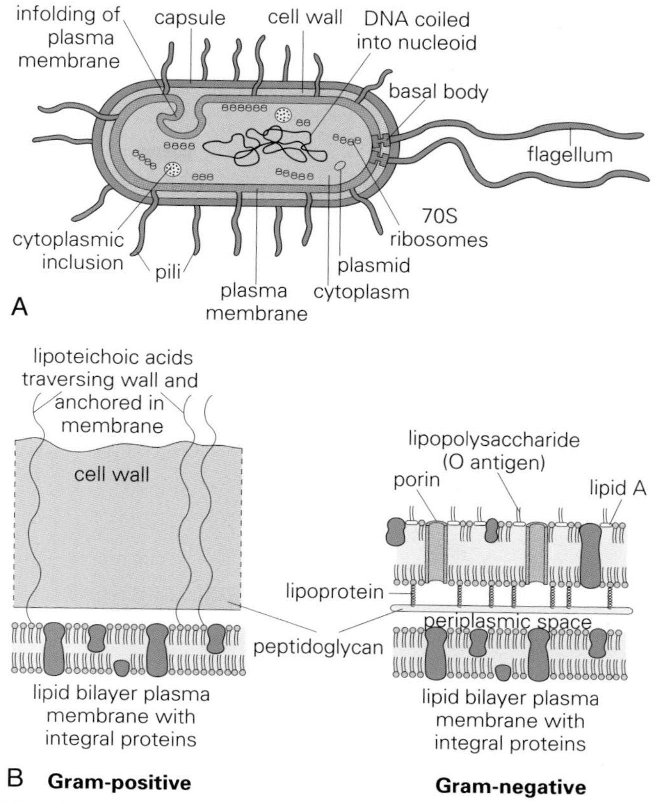

Fig. 4-16 Morphology and molecules of Gram-positive and Gram-negative bacteria.

Molecules like exotoxins, lipoteichoic acid, and endotoxins (lipopolysaccharide [LPS]) that form the structure of bacterial cell walls are often toxic. They act as virulence determinates that damage cells and their extracellular matrices such as collagen. **A,** Morphology of a typical bacterium. **B,** Gram-positive bacteria have a thick layer of peptidoglycan *(left).* Gram-negative bacteria have a thin peptidoglycan layer and an outer membrane of LPS *(right).* (**A** and **B** from Goering R, Dockrell H, Roitt I, et al: *Mims' medical microbiology,* ed 4, St. Louis, 2008, Mosby.)

Toxins

Certain virulence determinates are toxins like exotoxins, lipoteichoic acid, and endotoxins (lipopolysaccharide [LPS]) that damage cells, and their ECMs, such as collagen, are expressed by Gram-negative and Gram-positive bacteria (Fig. 4-16). Functionally, these molecules act to kill cells via cytolysis cells or through activation of the inflammatory cascade, often initiated via the complement pathway. In certain diseases, these toxins are named (and grouped) according to their biologic activity such as leukotoxins and neurotoxins.

Exotoxins and Lipoteichoic Acid

Exotoxins (usually from Gram-positive bacteria) are secreted from viable bacteria and are potent toxins (Fig. 4-17, *A*). Some act directly on cells to cause cytolysis; others act via the A-B toxin system and bind to cell membranes with a receptor (B subunit) and deliver a second toxic molecule (A subunit) into the cytoplasm. As examples, A-B toxin systems are used in botulism *(Clostridium botulinum),* tetanus *(Clostridium tetani),* and diseases caused by *Corynebacterium* spp. Another virulence determinate, lipoteichoic acid, is located in the cell wall of Gram-positive bacteria like *Staphylococcus aureus*. It behaves as a Gram-positive endotoxin because its actions mimic LPS. Lipoteichoic acid binds to endothelial cells, interacts with circulating antibodies, activates the complement cascade, and triggers the release of reactive oxygen and nitrogen species, acid hydrolases, highly cationic proteinases, bactericidal cationic peptides, growth factors, and cytotoxic cytokines from neutrophils and macrophages. Vacuolating toxin of *Helicobacter pylori*, *E. coli* hemolysin, and superantigens belonging to *Streptococcus pyogenes* and *Staphylococcus aureus* are surface-acting toxins. Surface-acting toxins bind to cell membranes and form pores through which cell death occurs. *Staphylococcus aureus* also has pore-forming cytotoxins called *α-toxin.*

Endotoxins

Endotoxins (usually from Gram-negative bacteria) are toxic to most animal cells (especially endothelial cells and macrophages), tissues, and organs and can be lethal if large quantities are released into the circulatory system, causing the activation of proinflammatory cytokines and nitric oxide (NO) from macrophages and endothelial cells. This result leads to the activation of the complement and coagulation cascades and endotoxic shock (Fig. 4-17, *B*). Pathogenic bacteria, such as *E. coli*, *Salmonella* spp., *Pseudomonas* spp., *Haemophilus* spp., and *Bordetella* spp., can release endotoxins into tissue when they die.

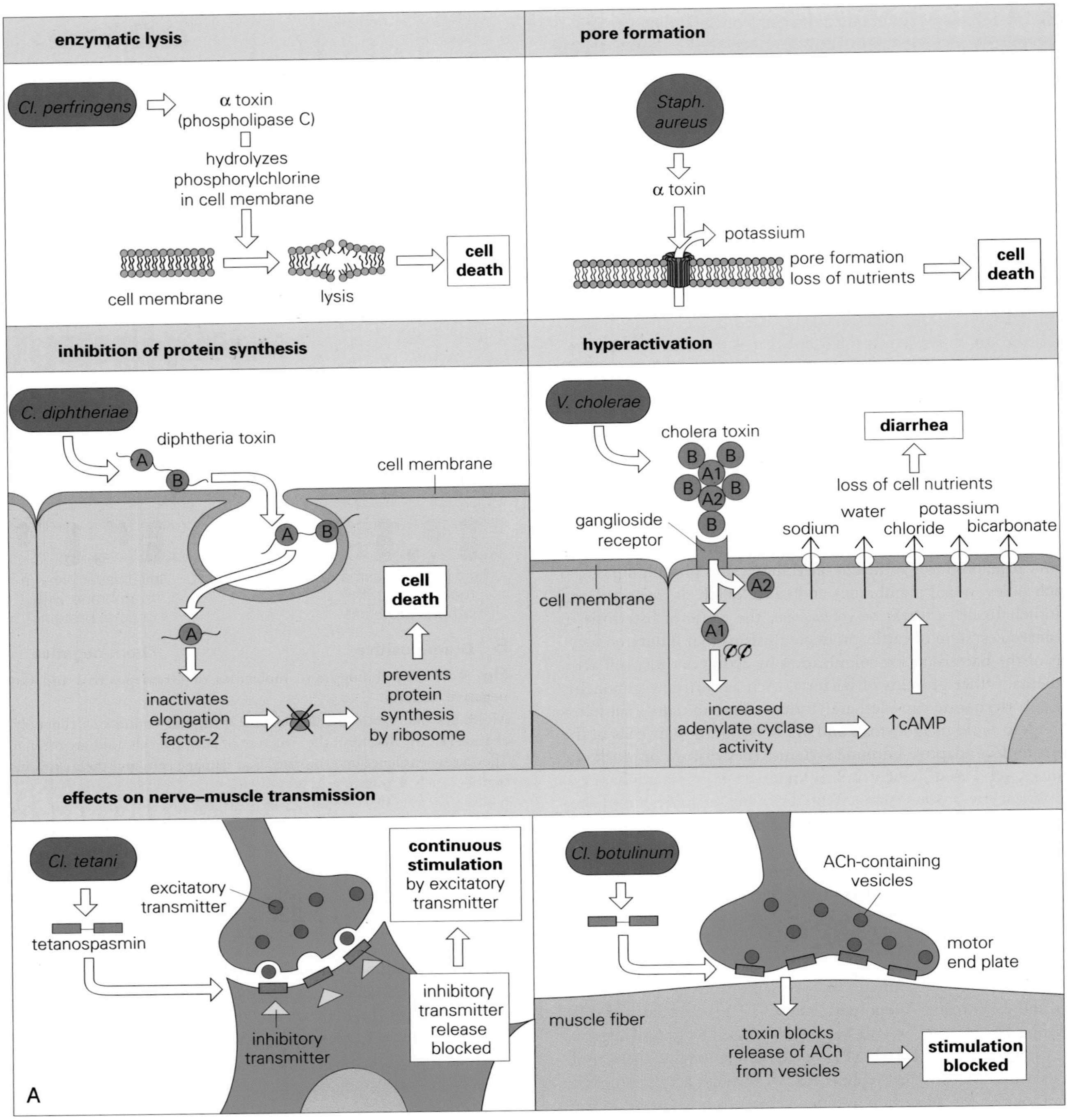

Fig. 4-17 **Actions of bacterial toxins (virulence determinates) on the structure and function of target cells.**
A, The mode of action of some exotoxins. Bacterial toxins act in a variety of ways. Often the toxin is a two-chain molecule, one chain being concerned with entry into cells while the other has inhibitory activity against some vital function. *ACh,* Acetylcholine; *cAMP,* cyclic adenosine monophosphate; *C, Corynebacterium*; *Cl, Clostridium*; *Staph, Staphylococcus*; *V, Vibrio.*

Other Virulence Determinates

Secretion Systems

Secretion systems, of which six types (type I to VI) have been described, are bacterial organelles that secrete or inject bacterial-derived toxins into the cytoplasm of host target cells. The type III secretion system is best known and occurs in some Gram-negative bacteria such as *Salmonella* spp. and *E. coli.* It injects, like a needle, specialized bacterial protein toxins like exotoxins into the cytoplasm of cells. These protein toxins often disrupt cell signal transduction and other cellular processes leading to cell death.

Siderophores

Some pathogenic bacteria require iron for colonization of mucosae. Iron is plentiful in cells but unavailable to bacteria because it is tightly bound in heme, ferritin, transferrin, or lactoferrin molecules. Siderophores are virulence determinates that mediate the release of iron from intracellular iron stores (see Fig. 4-14). An example

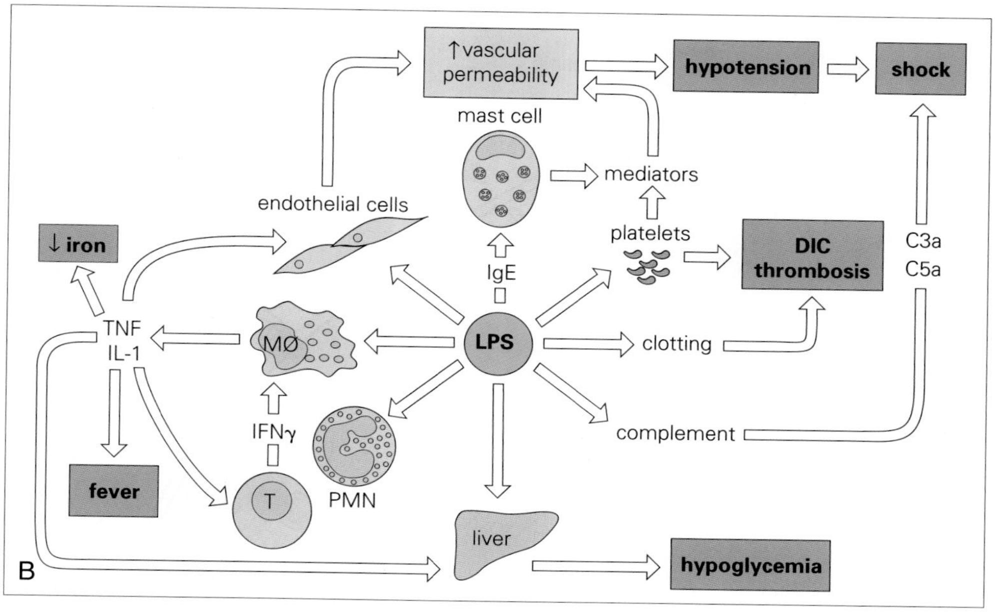

Fig. 4-17, cont'd
B, The activities of bacterial endotoxin. Lipopolysaccharide (LPS) activates almost every immune mechanism, as well as the clotting pathway, and as a result, LPS is one of the most powerful immune stimuli known. *DIC,* Disseminated intravascular coagulation; *IFN,* interferon; *IL,* interleukin; *M,* macrophage; *PMN,* polymorphonuclear leukocyte; *TNF,* tumor necrosis factor. (**A** and **B** from Goering R, Dockrell H, Roitt I, et al: *Mims' medical microbiology,* ed 4, St. Louis, 2008, Mosby.)

is enterochelin from *E. coli* and *Salmonella* spp.; this molecule scavenges bound iron from animal cells and makes it available for the bacteria.

Biofilms/Intracellular Bacterial Communities

Bacterial colonization and commensalism often occur through virulence determinates that form an exopolysaccharide matrix called a *biofilm* on mucosal surfaces lining, for example, the oral and nasal cavities and the mammary duct system. Bacteria embedded in biofilms are not susceptible to phagocytosis by macrophages and embedded bacteria can become resistant to antibiotics. For example, a surface protein, biofilm-associated protein (Bap), has been implicated in the formation of a *Staphylococcus aureus* biofilm in chronic bovine mastitis. Similarly, infections caused, for example, by certain strains of uropathogenic *E. coli* can result in the formation of intracellular bacterial communities affecting mucosal epithelial cells of the urinary bladder, which behave functionally much like a biofilm.

ROLE OF BACTERIAL GENES IN SUSCEPTIBILITY AND/OR RESISTANCE TO DISEASE

Virulence Determinates

Virulence determinates are encoded in and translated from genes in chromosomal DNA, bacteriophage DNA, or plasmids of bacteria. They can be readily transferred horizontally between bacteria (e.g., virulence determinates for antibiotic resistance) via pathogenicity islands and/or virulence plasmids. Pathogenicity islands are clusters of genes that code for virulence determinates found in bacterial chromosomes. Virulence plasmids are clusters of self-replicating extrachromosomal genes for virulence determinates located in plasmids within the cytoplasm of the bacteria. Most bacteria have only one chromosome but may contain hundreds of copies of a specific virulence plasmid. Plasmids replicate independently of cell division, and when a bacterium containing plasmids divides, the plasmids distribute randomly between the two resulting bacteria. Chromosomal or plasmid genes express virulence determinates such as bacterial adhesins, colonization factors, protein toxins like hemolysins, other types of toxins, and molecules that affect the innate and adaptive immune responses. Strains of bacteria lacking pathogenicity islands and/or virulence plasmids usually do not cause disease. The number and type of virulence determinates in a given bacterial strain are constantly changing, usually through genomic selection of those factors that favor the survival of the bacterium in the animal host. Each bacterial genera and strains within genera have their own unique virulence determinate profile; therefore the total number of determinates that have been identified in all bacteria genera combined are in the hundreds. As an example, strains of *Rhodococcus equi* that cause disease have chromosomal virulence determinates for capsular polysaccharide, cholesterol oxidase, phospholipase C, lecithinase, and cell wall mycolic acids and plasmid virulence determinates for virulence-associated protein (VAP).

Antibiotic Resistance

Antibiotic resistance, the ability of bacteria to withstand the static or lytic affects of antibiotics, evolves via natural selection of randomly mutated bacterial genes. These genes code for bacterial molecules (i.e., virulence determinates) that cause resistance through the following four key mechanisms (Fig. 4-18):

1. Enzymatic deactivation (antibiotic inactivation or modification) as occurs with β-lactamases and extended-spectrum β-lactamases (resistant to cephalosporins and monobactams) produced by bacteria such as *Klebsiella pneumoniae, Pseudomonas aeruginosa, E. coli,* and *Salmonella typhimurium.*
2. Alteration of antibiotic binding sites (penicillin-binding proteins [PBPs]) such as occurs in infections with methicillin-resistant *Staphylococcus aureus* (MRSA) and other penicillin/methicillin/oxacillin-resistant bacteria such as *Streptococcus pneumoniae*, vancomycin-resistant enterococci (VRE), and penicillin-resistant *Streptococcus pneumoniae* (PRSP).
3. Alteration of a metabolic pathway, such as occurs with some sulfonamide-resistant bacteria that utilize preformed folic

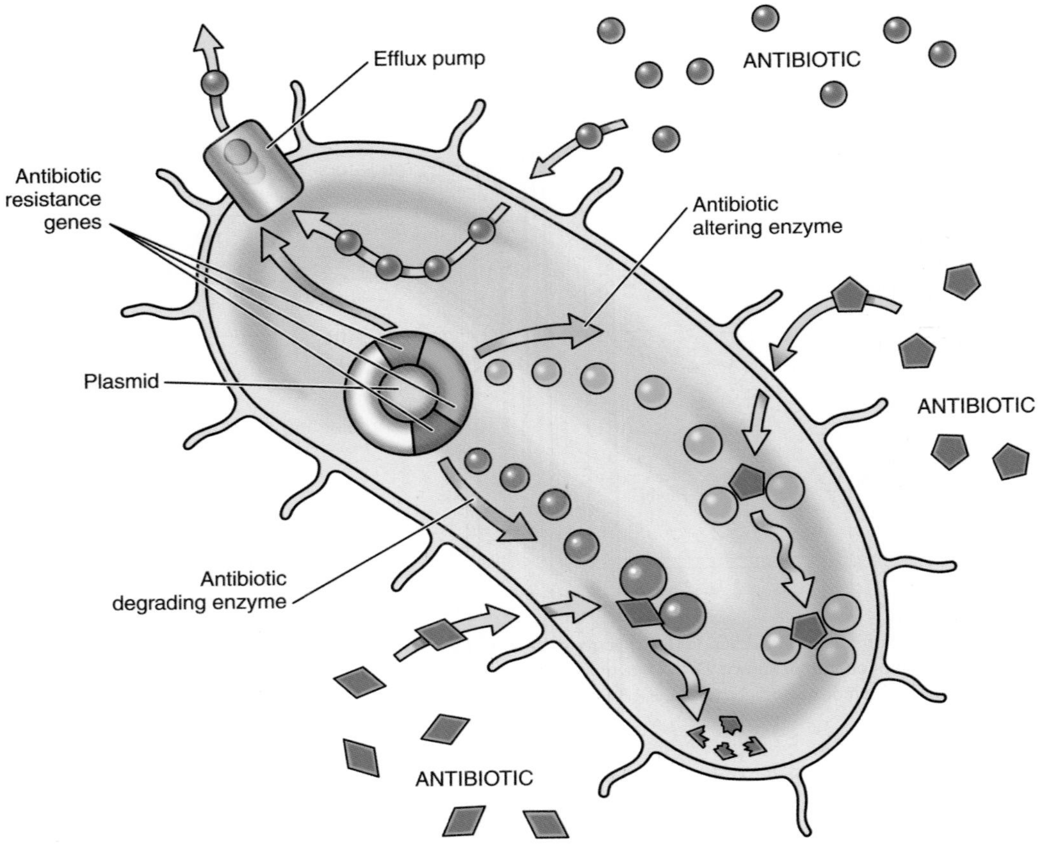

Fig. 4-18 Mechanisms used by bacteria to establish resistance to antibiotics.

acid in place of *para*-aminobenzoic acid (PABA), a precursor for the synthesis of folic acid in bacteria inhibited by sulfonamides.

4. Reduced antibiotic accumulation in bacteria through decreased membrane permeability to the antibiotic and/or enhanced efflux via membrane pumps.

Bacterial Transfer of Antibiotic Resistance

If a bacterium contains several antibiotic resistance genes, it is called a multiresistant pathogen. Although a human disease, MRSA infections are beginning to appear in animals. Such pathogens have multiple resistance genes that protect them from most if not all broad-spectrum antibiotics commonly used to treat the disease. These resistance genes are transferred between and among bacteria of related and different genera by vertical and horizontal gene transfer.

Bacterial Gene Transfer

Vertical Gene Transfer

The time required for bacteria to divide or a colony of bacteria to double in number is called the *generation time* and can be as short as 15 minutes. Although gene mutations for antibiotic resistance in bacteria are very rare events, because of fast generation times and the ability to reach extremely high absolute numbers of bacteria via binary fission in short periods of time, if unchecked it does not take long before antibiotic resistance develops. The spontaneous mutation rate for antibiotic resistance is approximately 1×10^8 to 1×10^9; this means that one out of every 100 million to 1 trillion bacteria in an infection develops resistance through a mutation. The use of antibiotics is a form of environmental pressure on bacteria; those having a favorable genetic mutation (i.e., virulence determinate for antibiotic resistance) survive therapy and continue to reproduce. Through vertical gene transfer, they then pass this virulence determinate for antibiotic resistance during DNA replication to their offspring, resulting in a fully resistant colony. As a result, the overuse of broad-spectrum antibiotics in humans and animals is a serious concern.

Horizontal Gene Transfer

Bacteria can also transfer antibiotic resistance genes between bacteria via horizontal gene transfer (Fig. 4-19) as follows:

1. Direct bacteria-bacteria contact (conjugation) via plasmids (the most common form).
2. Chromosomal DNA (transformation) in which pieces of DNA coded for antibiotic resistance and free in extracellular fluid as a result of death of its host bacterium are taken up by a viable bacteria.
3. Bacteria-specific viruses (bacteriophages) that transfer DNA (transduction) between two closely related bacteria.

BACTERIAL DISEASES BY BODY SYSTEMS

Although the same bacterial disease often affects several different organ systems, diseases in this section are placed into a specific organ system based on which organ system demonstrates the primary gross lesion or lesions that are most commonly used to initially recognize and identify the disease. Bacterial diseases are identified by a primary mechanism of injury in Table 4-3.

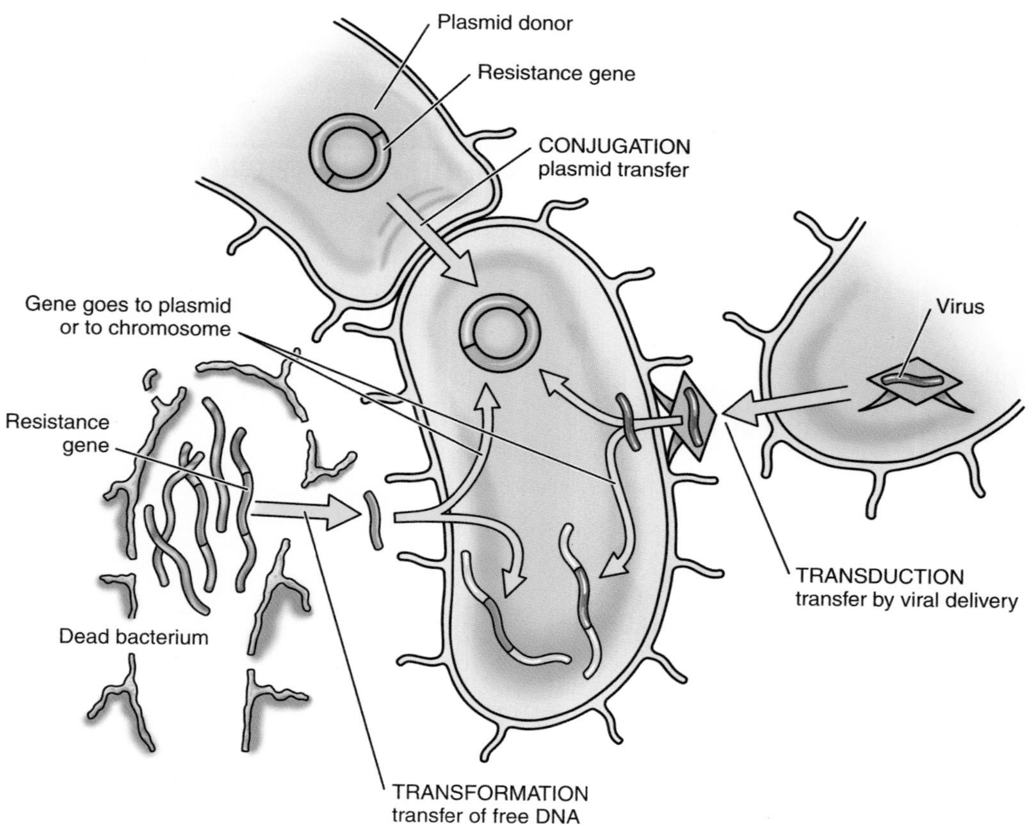

Fig. 4-19 Horizontal gene transfer.
Mechanisms used by bacteria to transfer resistance to an antibiotic to other bacteria.

Alimentary System and the Peritoneum, Omentum, Mesentery, and Peritoneal Cavity

Enteric Colibacillosis (Escherichia coli)

E. coli strains that cause disease in animals have been named enterotoxigenic, enteropathogenic, and enterohemorrhagic based on the mechanisms and virulence determinates that they use to cause diarrhea. The mechanisms of injury in enteric colibacillosis are (1) nonstructural alterations in the function of cell membrane ion and fluid transport systems (enterotoxigenic bacterial strains) and (2) acute coagulative necrosis of cells caused by bacterial toxins and by acute inflammation and its mediators and degradative enzymes (enteropathogenic and enterohemorrhagic bacterial strains). Enterotoxigenic and enteropathogenic strains do not invade enterocytes; enterohemorrhagic strains do invade enterocytes. Enterotoxigenic strains secrete toxins that functionally, but not structurally, affect enterocytes causing alterations in electrolyte and fluid secretion that result in a secretory diarrhea. Enteropathogenic strains structurally affect the microvillus border of enterocytes causing alterations in electrolyte and fluid secretion that result in an osmotic diarrhea (malabsorption) and a less significant secretory diarrhea. Enterohemorrhagic strains structurally affect the enterocytes of the colon causing cell death (necrosis), inflammation, and hemorrhage that leads to reduced absorption of colonic fluids and a malabsorption diarrhea. Endotoxins (LPS) likely directly or indirectly play a role in diseases caused by these three strains. There are no gross lesions in enterotoxigenic colibacillosis, whereas in enteropathogenic and enterohemorrhagic colibacillosis, the mucosae are rough and granular (enterocyte necrosis, villus atrophy) with areas of hemorrhage, acute inflammation, and fibrin exudation (see Fig. 7-157).

Animals encounter *E. coli* through ingestion of bacteria in fomites contaminated with fecal material. The bacterium is swallowed and gains access via peristalsis to the mucus layer and mucosae of the intestines. It is likely that flagella expressed by some strains of *E. coli* facilitate their penetration of the mucus layer to gain access to microvilli of enterocytes. Enterotoxigenic *E. coli* expresses K99 (F5) or F41 fimbrial adhesins that allow it to bind to receptor molecules in the mucus layer and to ganglioside and glycoprotein receptors on cell membranes of microvilli of enterocytes. When the mucosa is colonized, large numbers of bacteria are produced (Fig. 4-20), and they secrete heat labile (LT) and heat stable (ST) enterotoxins that diffuse in the mucus layer and microvilli, bind to specific receptors on the microvillus border of enterocytes, disrupt the function of cell membrane electrolyte and fluid transport systems, and cause secretory diarrhea. This process results in a functional lesion; no structural changes are observed grossly. LT and ST enterotoxins bind to glycolipid receptors on apical surfaces of enterocytes. After binding, these complexes are endocytosed and interact with a series of second messenger systems (epithelial cell signal transduction systems) that ultimately results in increased concentrations of intracellular cyclic adenosine monophosphate (cAMP, LT enterotoxin) and cyclic guanosine monophosphate (cGMP, ST enterotoxin). These molecules operate to open chloride channels (cystic fibrosis transmembrane regulator) in enterocyte cell membranes, thus acting irreversibly to move intracellular chloride ions extracellularly into the lumen of the intestine. Excessive chloride ion secretion also pulls water with it into the lumen of the intestine, thereby increasing the volume of fluid in the intestine. This volume ultimately exceeds the ability of the intestine to absorb the excessive fluid.

TABLE 4-3 Mechanisms of Injury in Diseases Caused by Bacteria

Inflammation	Toxins	Structural Injury	Disruption of Neurotransmitter Exocytosis	Alterations of the Cell Cycle	Dysfunction of Electrolyte/Fluid Pumps
ALIMENTARY SYSTEM AND THE PERITONEUM, OMENTUM, MESENTERY, AND PERITONEAL CAVITY					
• Enteric colibacillosis • Wooden tongue • Salmonellosis • Swine dysentery • Johne's disease • Rhodococcal enteritis • Bovine intestinal tuberculosis	• Alimentary anthrax • Salmonellosis • Swine dysentery • Enterotoxemia	• Enteric colibacillosis		• Proliferative enteritis	• Enteric colibacillosis
HEPATOBILIARY SYSTEM AND EXOCRINE PANCREAS					
• Hepatic leptospirosis	• Tyzzer's disease • Bacillary hemoglobinuria • Infectious necrotic hepatitis • Hepatic leptospirosis	• Hepatic leptospirosis			
RESPIRATORY SYSTEM, MEDIASTINUM, AND PLEURAE					
• Porcine polyserositis • *Streptococcus zooepidemicus* • Bovine enzootic pneumonia • Bovine pneumonic pasteurellosis/ Mannheimiosis • Porcine pleuropneumonia • Rhodococcal pneumonia • Contagious bovine pleuropneumonia • Bovine tuberculosis	• Porcine polyserositis • *Streptococcus zooepidemicus* • Atrophic rhinitis • Bovine pneumonic pasteurellosis/ Mannheimiosis • Porcine pleuropneumonia • Respiratory anthrax	• Porcine enzootic pneumonia			
CARDIOVASCULAR SYSTEM AND LYMPHATIC VESSELS					
• Embolic vasculopathy/ vasculitis • Vascular leptospirosis • Glanders (Farcy, Malleus, Droes)	• Edema disease • Embolic vasculopathy/ vasculitis • Septicemic anthrax • Vascular leptospirosis	• Vascular leptospirosis			
URINARY SYSTEM					
• "Necrohemorrhagic" urocystitis • Contagious bovine pyelonephritis • Renal leptospirosis	• Pulpy kidney (overeating) disease • "Necrohemorrhagic" urocystitis • Contagious bovine pyelonephritis • Renal leptospirosis	• Renal leptospirosis			
BONE MARROW, BLOOD CELLS, AND LYMPHATIC SYSTEM					
• Strangles • Caseous lymphadenitis • Brucellosis					
NERVOUS SYSTEM					
• Listeriosis • Thrombotic meningoencephalitis • Rhodococcal mesenteric lymphadenitis • Meningitis	• Edema disease • Focal symmetrical encephalomalacia		• Botulism • Tetanus		

TABLE 4-3 Mechanisms of Injury in Diseases Caused by Bacteria—cont'd

Inflammation	Toxins	Structural Injury	Disruption of Neurotransmitter Exocytosis	Alterations of the Cell Cycle	Dysfunction of Electrolyte/Fluid Pumps
SKELETAL MUSCLE					
	• Blackleg • Malignant edema • Big head, black disease				
BONE, JOINTS, TENDONS, AND LIGAMENTS					
• Lumpy jaw					
INTEGUMENTARY SYSTEM					
• Greasy pig disease • Canine pyoderma • Diamond skin disease	• Greasy pig disease • Canine pyoderma				
FEMALE REPRODUCTIVE SYSTEM AND MAMMARY GLAND					
• Brucellosis • Bovine mastitis	• Bovine mastitis				
MALE REPRODUCTIVE SYSTEM					
• Brucellosis					

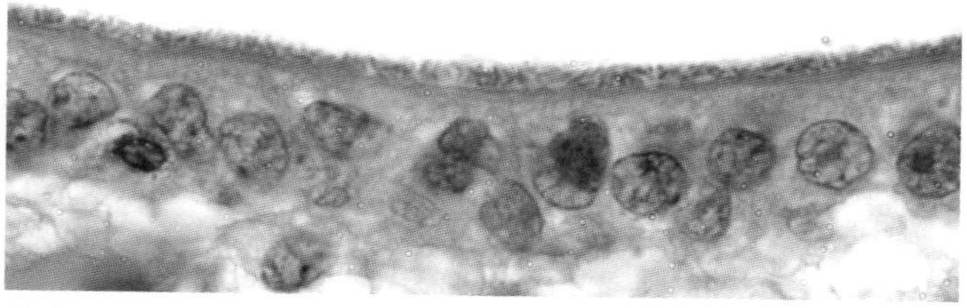

Fig. 4-20 Colonization of mucosa in enteric colibacillosis. *Escherichia coli* attach to microvilli, thus forming a uniform layer of blue-staining (hematoxylin) coccobacilli. Note the lack of epithelial cell injury. H&E stain. (Courtesy Dr. J. F. Zachary, College of Veterinary Medicine, University of Illinois.)

Enteropathogenic *E. coli* (EPEC) colonize the mucosae in a manner similar to that used by enterotoxigenic *E. coli*. EPEC do not produce LT or ST enterotoxins but do express adhesins such as fimbriae, EPEC adherence factor, and intimin (nonfimbrial outer membrane protein). Integrins may serve as host cell membrane receptors for intimin, and this interaction appears to produce a tight bond between the bacterium and the enterocyte. After colonization and growth, bacterial virulence determinates injure the brush border, leading to the loss of microvilli at the site of colonization. Such virulence determinates appear to involve processes that disrupt cytoskeletal functions of the microvilli through interference with actin filaments, actin polymerization, and other cytoskeletal components and by causing alterations in intracellular calcium concentrations. This type of change has been called *attaching and effacing injury* and has resulted in naming the bacterium attaching and effacing *E. coli*. Injury to and loss of microvilli leads to decreased digestive enzyme activity in the glycocalyx (osmotic diarrhea) and disruption of ion transport systems (secretory diarrhea). EPEC also secretes bacterial proteins and likely injects them into the cytoplasm of enterocytes through a type-III secretion system. These proteins, EspA, EspB, and EspD, activate a number of signal transduction pathways in the host cell, which appear to be involved in the pathogenesis of microvillus disruption. Additionally, acute inflammation occurs at the site of binding between the bacterium and the microvillus, likely contributing to the attaching and effacing lesion. Some attaching and effacing strains also secrete a virulence determinate called *verotoxin*, which kills enterocytes and cells of the lamina propria (vascularized ECM tissues), leading to mucosal erosions and ulcers, intestinal edema and hemorrhage, and increased denuded mucosal surfaces for the absorption of endotoxins.

Enterohemorrhagic *E. coli* appear to colonize the mucus layer and mucosae in a manner similar to that used by the other two strains of the bacterium; however, enterocytes of the colon are the primary target cells. This specificity could be mediated through ligand-receptor interactions, and bacterial fimbriae have been shown to act as adhesins and attach to enterocyte cell membranes. Chemical gradients, such as the concentration of iron in target cells, could also provide the basis for colonic specificity. Once attached to colonic enterocytes, the bacterium replicates in large numbers and secretes a verotoxin that elicits an intense acute inflammatory response. It is also able to invade enterocytes, and verotoxin kills the cells. Enterohemorrhagic *E. coli* do not produce LT or ST enterotoxins. Thus mucosal lesions (hemorrhagic colitis) characteristic of this strain of *E. coli* appear to result from a combination of inflammatory enzymes and mediators and toxins, all of which cause cell death and expose the underlying denuded lamina propria to a variety of harmful luminal molecules such as LPS that are readily available for absorption. Endotoxin, especially when in the blood, can lead to inflammation, capillary damage, vasculitis, thrombosis, intravascular coagulation, tissue degradation and infarction, endotoxic shock, and death. These mechanisms likely underlie the occurrence of acute adrenal cortical hemorrhage and necrosis (see Fig. 12-25) observed in endotoxemia with *E. coli* and other coliform infections. Septicemic colibacillosis, likely resulting from an enteropathogenic strain of *E. coli*, may begin as an alimentary manifestation and then progress to enterotoxemic colibacillosis or septicemic colibacillosis. In these forms, the bacterium and its enterotoxins most likely gain access to the circulatory system via invasion into and absorption through capillary beds in the lamina propria of injured mucosae. Enterotoxemic colibacillosis and its toxins cause edema disease of the nervous system (see section on Nervous System; also see Chapter 14) leading to fibrinoid arteriopathy/arteriolopathy of the brain and ischemia and malacia, whereas septicemic colibacillosis and its bacterium and toxins cause disease of the cardiovascular system (see Chapter 10) leading to death via toxic and endotoxic shock and cardiovascular collapse.

Wooden Tongue (Actinobacillus lignieresii)

The mechanism of injury in wooden tongue is incessant pyogranulomatous inflammation and fibrotic reparative responses. Gross lesions include a firm enlarged tongue that protrudes from the oral cavity. Cut surfaces have numerous randomly distributed yellow-white granulomas intermixed with broad bands of fibrous connective tissue (see Fig. 7-27). *Actinobacillus lignieresii* is a normal commensal bacterium of mucosae of the oral cavity of cattle and sheep. During chewing, the bacterium is carried through the mucosae into submucosal connective tissues via penetrating wounds such as those caused by sharp foreign bodies like sticks or wires. The bacterium colonizes submucosal connective tissue, and LPS of the bacterial cell wall, in part, likely plays a role in the pyogranulomatous inflammatory and concurrent fibrotic responses that occur. Little is known about how virulence determinates, ligand-receptor interactions, target cells, toxins, capsule antiphagocytic molecules, or other factors contribute to the pathogenicity of this bacterium. However, it appears likely that the bacterium is able to evade killing by neutrophils and macrophages, thus colonizing itself in abscesses in tissues of the tongue and oral cavity. Repeated cycles of phagocytosis, bacterial growth and replication, death of macrophages, release of large numbers of new bacteria, recruitment of additional naïve inflammatory cells, and reparative responses like fibrosis likely perpetuate and expand the scope of the disease process. Fibrosis and encapsulation occur concurrently and appear to represent a last ditch attempt to isolate and wall of the bacterium and exudate from the vascularized tissue in the tongue and oral cavity. *Actinobacillus lignieresii* can spread via lymphatic vessels to regional lymph nodes and cause a similar inflammatory response in these nodes.

Alimentary Anthrax (Bacillus anthracis)

The mechanism of injury in alimentary anthrax is acute coagulative necrosis of cells caused by bacterial toxins. Gross lesions include segments of the small intestine or the entire small intestine that are dark red to purple-black (hemorrhagic enteritis) and accompanied by mucosal, submucosal, and serosal edema and hemorrhage (see Fig. 7-135). Additionally, mesenteric lymph nodes can be enlarged, edematous, and hemorrhagic. These toxins are produced by bacteria that are lined up in a laminar fashion along the surfaces of the mucosae, and as toxins are produced, they diffuse into the mucosa and lamina propria, causing in addition to necrosis, thrombosis of mucosal and submucosal vessels. This latter lesion leads to ischemic necrosis of tissues supplied by these blood vessels. Inflammation usually does not occur.

Animals, most commonly cattle, encounter *Bacillus anthracis* through the ingestion of fomites contaminated with endospores and/or vegetative forms of the bacterium. The bacterium exists most commonly in soil and water as an endospore, a dormant, nonreproductive form that is resistant to UV radiation, dehydration, extremely cold and hot temperatures, and chemical disinfectants. These conditions are harmful to the vegetative form, the form of the bacterium that produces toxin and causes disease. Animals can ingest endospores that subsequently germinate into vegetative forms in the alimentary tract. However, animals can also ingest vegetative forms as the result of environmental conditions that allow the vegetative form to persist for a limited period of time. Heavy rain after a drought can cause the germination of endospores in areas contaminated with endospores and the multiplication of vegetative forms. Endospores present in undercooked or poorly processed meat wastes and by-products can germinate into vegetative forms, persist for a limited period of time, and then be ingested when fed to animals.

Endospores and/or vegetative forms are swallowed, evade destruction by gastric acidity, and gain access to the mucosae of the small intestine via peristalsis. The sequence of events from ingestion of endospores or vegetative forms to the occurrence of lesions is largely unknown. It has been suggested that endospores can gain access to the mucosae and lamina propria via ulcers, cuts, and puncture wounds of the alimentary system, geminate into vegetative forms, colonize the tissue, and secrete toxins causing disease. It is also likely that vegetative forms gain access to regional mesenteric lymph nodes via afferent lymphatic vessels as cell-free bacteria or within macrophages that migrate via leukocyte trafficking in lymphatic vessels to these nodes. Vegetative forms probably use mechanisms discussed next to cause disease in the injured mucosae. Alternatively, the need for mucosal injury as an initiating event in the disease is open to discussion. Hypothetically, three possible mechanisms could result in the production of vegetative forms, toxins, and lesions:

1. Endospores* could be trapped in the mucus layer of the mucosa, endospores germinate to vegetative forms, vegetative forms use mucus to grow and replicate, and vegetative forms produce toxins that diffuse into the mucosa and submucosa, resulting in lesions.
2. Endospores* could be trapped in the mucus layer of the mucosa, phagocytosed by macrophages or dendritic cells and carried to Peyer's patches where they germinate into vegetative forms, and vegetative forms produce toxins that diffuse into the mucosa and submucosa, resulting in lesions.
3. Endospores* are phagocytosed by M cells and carried to Peyer's patches where they germinate into vegetative forms, and vegetative forms produce toxins that diffuse into the mucosa and submucosa resulting in lesions.

Primary virulence determinates produced by *Bacillus anthracis* are in plasmid genes and include those that form the capsule and anthrax toxins. The capsule is important in establishing the infection, whereas anthrax toxins cause the lesions, disease, and death. The capsule consists of poly-D-glutamic acid that is nontoxic, protects the bacterium from destructive antibodies and bactericidal components of plasma, and inhibits phagocytosis, killing, and digestion of vegetative forms of the bacterium by macrophages and neutrophils. Anthrax toxins consist of three exotoxins that act together to cause cell death. One exotoxin, called *protective antigen*, facilitates the entry of itself into cells via endocytosis and then creates a pore in the cell membrane through which the remaining two toxins, *edema and lethal factors*, can enter the cell. Exotoxins must first bind to receptors on target cells. Protective antigen binds to two different cell surface receptors, tumor endothelial marker 8 (TEM8) and capillary morphogenesis protein 2 (CMG2). These receptors appear to explain the vascular orientation of the disease and the circulatory system collapse that results. In addition to vascular tissues, these receptors are also commonly expressed on cells in many other organ systems, likely accounting for the various

*If vegetative forms are ingested, three similar mechanisms are proposed to occur in animals, but the time course of disease would likely be shortened.

forms (inhalation, cutaneous, and gastrointestinal) of anthrax. Once inside cells, protective antigen combines with edema factor to form edema toxin, which disrupts cell membrane water and electrolyte transport systems, resulting in edema and also blocks phagocytosis of vegetative forms by neutrophils and macrophages. Additionally, protective antigen combines with lethal factor to form lethal toxin. This toxin stimulates the production of a variety of cytokines that act to cause cell death, especially affecting phagocytic cells such as macrophages and endothelial cells of capillaries. Because of injury to the mucosae and lamina propria, capillary beds in the ECM can absorb edema and lethal toxins, as well as a variety of intestinal endotoxins. Cytokines, anthrax toxins, and endotoxins have profound systemic effects on the cardiovascular system, all of which contribute to cardiogenic and circulatory shock and death. Chromosomal genes of the vegetative form of the bacterium also express a capsule virulence determinate, which makes it resistant to phagocytosis by mucosae-associated tissue macrophages. Additionally, the bacterium has several chromosomal virulence determinates for hemolysins, phospholipases, and iron acquisition proteins that can contribute to or cause cell death.

*Salmonellosis (*Salmonella *spp.)*

The mechanism of injury in salmonellosis is acute coagulative necrosis of cells caused by bacterial toxins and by acute inflammation and its mediators and degradative enzymes. Three forms of salmonellosis occur: peracute, acute, and chronic. Gross lesions in the peracute form include petechiation and a blue discoloration (cyanosis) of the skin, fibrinous polyserositis, and disseminated intravascular coagulopathy (see Fig. 7-128). These lesions are rooted in injury of the vascular system with vasculitis and thrombosis caused by bacterial toxins. In the acute form, lesions affect the mucosae of the small intestine, large intestine, and cecum (fibrinonecrotic ileotyphlocolitis) and are characterized by a rough and granular mucosal surface (necrosis) mixed with mucus, fibrin, and occasionally blood (see Fig. 7-128). The content is malodorous (septic tank odor). This pattern of injury is caused by bacterial toxins, acute inflammation, and their effects on enterocytes and blood vessels within the lamina propria. Bacteria can spread via the portal vein to the liver leading to the formation of foci of bacteria-induced necrosis and inflammation (paratyphoid nodules) (see Fig. 8-49). This spread likely occurs via leukocyte trafficking and infection of Kupffer cells, but bacteremia may also occur. Leukocyte trafficking also spreads the bacteria to mesenteric and systemic lymph nodes and the gall bladder (fibrinous cholecystitis). In the chronic form, injury is associated with discrete foci of necrosis and ulceration of the mucosae (button ulcers). These lesions are rooted in injury of the vascular system with vasculitis and thrombosis caused by bacterial toxins diffusing within the submucosa of the intestine.

Animals encounter *Salmonella* spp. through ingestion of bacteria in fomites contaminated with fecal material. The bacterium is swallowed and gains access via peristalsis to the mucus layer and mucosae of the intestines. *Salmonella* spp. appear to use two mechanisms to colonize the mucosae and gain access to the lamina propria and its capillary beds. The first mechanism uses M cells in intestinal crypts. Because a mucus layer is absent over M cells, the bacteria have direct contact with apically positioned cell membranes of M cells. The second mechanism uses apically positioned cell membranes of enterocytes to gain access to cells; however, these cells are covered with a mucus layer. Because *Salmonella* spp. are motile bacteria, they can penetrate through the mucus layer and gain access to these membranes. The bacterium must adhere to the apical surfaces of M cells and enterocytes to begin the process of colonizing the intestine, which is a process mediated through ligand-receptor interactions. Although unproved, it is likely that one or some of the fimbria possessed by *Salmonella* spp. are involved in the initial adherence between the bacterium and these cells. Which fimbriae are used to bind to host cells may vary depending on whether the target cell is an M cell or an enterocyte. Once bound to host cell membrane, a type III secretion system is used to inject bacterial proteins into the host cell that stimulate phagocytosis through the mobilization of actin filaments in the cytoplasm. It is thought, though unproved, that fimbria may determine susceptibility of the various strains of *Salmonella* spp. for animal species and for specific target cells within each species. Colonization of the mucosae only occurs if bacterial LPS is present in the bacterial cell, and it likely plays a role in adherence to target cells through its participation in bacterial cell wall stability and resistance to bile salts, cell surface hydrophobicity, and the correct insertion and folding of membrane proteins such as those that occur in fimbria. *Salmonella* spp. that enter the mucosa via M cells have direct access to macrophages and lymphoid cells in Peyer's patches, whereas those that enter via enterocytes are likely phagocytized by mucosal macrophages and carried via leukocyte trafficking in afferent lymphatic vessels to Peyer's patches. *Salmonella* spp. are able to inhibit phagosome-lysosome fusion, thereby blocking their killing within macrophages. If phagosome-lysosome fusion occurs, bacteria are able to block the effects of lysosomal enzymes, acidity, and free radicals. In fact, the bacterium resides and replicates in a phagosome and/or phagolysosome until released from the macrophage after the death of the macrophage caused by toxins produced by the bacterium. Once in Peyer's patches, macrophages infected with bacteria die and release bacteria that will infect additional macrophages through ligand-receptor interactions. *Salmonella* spp. can kill macrophages via apoptosis using a type I secretory system that leads to activation of caspase-1 in macrophages. These macrophages are often recruited as monocytes from the systemic circulation as a component of the acute inflammatory response. Once infected with the bacterium, macrophages migrate in efferent lymphatic vessels via leukocyte trafficking to regional mesenteric lymph nodes using mechanisms similar to those described in Peyer's patches and then systemically via the thoracic duct and circulatory system. Macrophages also likely gain access to the systemic circulatory system through capillaries and postcapillary venules in lymph nodes. It also appears that dendritic cells in the intestinal mucosa are infected by the bacterium and these cells likely spread the bacterium to Peyer's patches.

In all of these situations, acute inflammation occurs concurrently in response to bacterial toxins and antigens, resulting in vascular permeability changes and injury, and in the recruitment of neutrophils and their degradative enzymes, which can cause additional tissue injury. As part of this response, the interaction of M cells and enterocytes with bacteria appear to cause the release of chemokines and other chemoattractants for neutrophils into surrounding vascularized ECM. It appears that the form of disease (peracute, acute, or chronic) that occurs depends on which steps used in the chronology (as described previously) are emphasized through the expression of virulence determinates by different strains of *Salmonella* spp. The peracute form likely favors spread to regional lymph nodes and then systemically with the release of toxins leading to vascular injury, failure of the circulatory system, and death. The acute form likely favors mucosal adherence and colonization leading to mucosal necrosis mediated by bacterial toxins. Through this process and the acute inflammation that ensues, capillary beds in the lamina propria are permeable and likely bacteria, bacterial toxins, and bacteria-infected macrophages enter the venous circulatory system and spread via the portal vein to the liver. The chronic form likely favors invasion of the lamina propria and submucosa (motile bacteria) with direct effects on the vasculature that supplies the intestine with blood. However, it is possible that button ulcers observed in this form are a manifestation of septicemia with attachment of bacteria to vascular endothelium resulting in vasculitis, thrombosis, ischemia, and infarction. The lesions and clinical signs that occur in diseases caused by *Salmonella* spp. are in part attributable to (1) an enterotoxin (exotoxin) that produces a secretory diarrhea, (2) a cytotoxin that inhibits protein synthesis, and (3) endotoxins and LPSs that cause membrane injury and cell death. Acute inflammation and cell and tissue injury that ensue are also important causes of the lesions.

Enterotoxemia (Clostridium perfringens)

The mechanism of injury in enterotoxemia is acute coagulative necrosis of cells and tissues caused by bacterial toxins. Gross lesions include segments of the small intestine or the entire small intestine that are dark red to purple-black (hemorrhagic enteritis) and accompanied by mucosal, submucosal, and serosal edema and hemorrhage (see Figs. 7-131, 7-132, and 7-147). *Clostridium perfringens* attach in a laminar fashion to mucosal surfaces, and as toxins are released, they diffuse into the mucosa and lamina propria, causing in addition to necrosis, thrombosis of mucosal and submucosal vessels. Inflammation usually does not occur. *Clostridium perfringens* causes disease syndromes that are categorized based on bacterial type (type A-E), toxin type (α-, β-, ε-, and ι-toxins), species affected, and/or age of the animal affected.

Cattle, sheep, goats, pigs, and horses encounter *Clostridium perfringens* through ingestion of bacterial spores in the soil or from contact with fomites contaminated with the vegetative form of the bacterium from carrier animals. The vegetative form of *Clostridium perfringens* can be a normal inhabitant of the alimentary system of domestic animals. It appears that under the proper conditions in the intestine that are usually linked to changes in the diet or the ingestion of an energy source rich in carbohydrates, spores germinate into vegetative forms and proliferate or the ingested vegetative form proliferates. It has been shown experimentally that dietary trypsin can inactivate β-toxin, thus it is thought that diets deficient in trypsin may increase the likelihood of disease. Additionally, sudden dietary change can also alter the composition of normal intestinal microflora providing opportunities for the vegetative form of the bacterium to proliferate and produce toxins. Vegetative forms are nonmotile and gain access to mucosae via random motion from peristalsis. They colonize the mucus layer by using bacterial proteases to expose receptors in mucus and then use bacterial adhesins to bind to these receptors. Within the mucus layer, bacteria are protected from acids and enzymes in intestinal content. The bacterium also consumes mucus as an energy source for bacterial growth and replication, and this process is thought to activate bacterial genes that regulate the production of toxins. Once the mucus layer is colonized, bacteria then interact with microvilli of enterocytes by attachment and retraction of type IV pili (gliding motility) and eventually attach to the apical surfaces of enterocytes. Attachment is likely mediated by ligand-receptor interactions.

Experimental studies suggest that toxins may first injure endothelial cells in capillaries of the lamina propria before the attachment of bacteria to the apical surfaces of enterocytes and that attachment may require changes in the membranes of apical enterocytes that are induced directly by the effect of toxins at the apical surfaces of enterocytes and indirectly by ischemia. At this phase of the disease, injury is primarily limited to enterocytes. Once mucosae are colonized, bacteria replicate in immense numbers and the disease enters a second phase characterized by the production of abundant potent cytotoxins, which spread via diffusion as a wave into the mucosae, lamina propria, submucosa, and muscle layers. Some clinical forms of enterotoxemia remain in the first phase of the disease; others progress into the second phase. Discussion of these various clinical forms is outside of the scope of this chapter. Potent cytotoxins produced by the bacteria include α-, β-, ε-, and ι-toxins, which behave as enterocyte membrane toxins (α, β), such as phospholipases, lecithinases, and pore-forming toxins, as well as ECM toxins, such as collagenase, hyaluronidase, and sialidase. ε-Toxin has the unique ability to increase enterocyte and endothelial cell permeability by acting on the cytoskeleton and probably altering the function of junctional complexes, thus affecting the absorption of toxins by the vascular system resulting in systemic effects. Iota toxin disrupts the cytoskeleton, which leads to cell death. Because of the abundance of toxins produced in the second phase of enterotoxemia, toxins freely move in the intestinal lumen via peristalsis to interact with uncolonized normal enterocytes, thus the lesions are quickly spread to other areas within the intestine. Toxins cause death and sloughing of enterocytes of villi and crypts followed by further colonization by bacteria, additional proliferation and toxin production, and toxin-induced massive necrosis resulting in structural breakdown and hemorrhage of the entire intestinal wall. Because ε-toxin is a permease that alters cell permeability, the vascular beds in affected intestinal tissues readily absorb toxins from the lumen of the intestine into the circulatory system. Toxins are then carried to the brain, kidney, and other tissues in which the increase in vascular permeability leads to the release of blood plasma containing toxins into the interstitium and body cavities, resulting in edema and effusions. In the brain and kidney, these toxins cause focal symmetric encephalomalacia and pulpy kidney disease, respectively. However, it appears that the mechanisms leading to these two diseases occur in the first phase or early in the second phase of enterotoxemia before toxin-induced massive necrosis of the intestine occurs.

Proliferative Enteritis/Hemorrhagic Bowel Syndrome (Lawsonia intracellularis)

Although proliferative enteritis/hemorrhagic bowel syndrome is most commonly recognized as a disease of pigs, a syndrome resembling the proliferative form of this disease in pigs also occurs in horses and the pathogenesis is likely similar to that described in pigs. *Lawsonia intracellularis* appears to cause two distinct disease syndromes in a single disease continuum. The mechanism of injury of the first syndrome is characterized by biologic events that result in cell proliferation (i.e., proliferative enteritis), whereas the mechanism in the second syndrome is characterized by biologic events that result in cell death and hemorrhage (i.e., hemorrhagic bowel syndrome). It seems that the first syndrome can occur and resolve without transitioning into the second syndrome. The reverse scenario does not appear to occur. The proliferative form of this disease is also known as *porcine intestinal adenomatosis, proliferative ileitis, regional ileitis, garden hose disease,* and other similar names. The hemorrhagic form of this disease is also known as *necrotic enteritis* or *acute proliferative hemorrhagic enteropathy*. The mechanism of injury is initially cellular hypertrophy and hyperplasia (proliferation) that can be followed by cell death resulting from ischemia and necrosis. Gross lesions in proliferative enteritis include a circumferentially firm and thickened ileum with a mucosa that fills the lumen and bulges into the lumen on cut surface (see Fig. 7-153). Gross lesions in hemorrhagic bowel syndrome include segmental necrosis and hemorrhage with fibrinous diphtheritic membranes attached to the mucosa, luminal blood clots, and thinned intestinal walls (see Fig. 7-155).

Pigs encounter *Lawsonia intracellularis* through ingestion of the bacterium in manure-contaminated fomites from the environment. It is swallowed and gains access via peristalsis to the mucosae of the small intestine. It is unclear how the bacterium initially colonizes the mucus layer and mucosae and why it targets epithelial cells in the ileum. Ligand-receptor interactions are likely involved in this ileal specificity; however, specific bacterial adhesins or cell membrane receptors have not been identified. Alternatively, possibly in conjunction with ligand-receptor interactions, ileal specificity may be attributed to unidentified metabolic or growth factors required by the bacterium that are provided only by intestinal crypt cells (see later section for more detail). In addition, it is unclear how the bacterium is able to penetrate the mucus layer and gain direct access to the luminal membrane of epithelial cells. *Lawsonia intracellularis* is regarded as a nonmotile bacterium; however, there is scant experimental evidence suggesting that the bacterium develops a transient bacterial appendage that behaves as flagellum and could provide motility into and through the mucus layer. Colonization also appears to be enhanced by the presence of other anaerobic bacterial species in the mucus layer. The significance of these findings is unclear, but could be related to these species providing molecules required by *Lawsonia intracellularis* for colonization and replication. *Lawsonia intracellularis* infects cells of the crypts located in the proliferative zone (Fig. 4-21). Following colonization, the bacterium interacts with the brush border and then is taken into the cell via endocytosis and resides in a phagosome within the cytoplasm. The bacterium rapidly escapes from the phagosome before phagosome-lysosome fusion occurs and resides free in cell cytoplasm. A phospholipase bacterial virulence determinate, mediated through a type III secretion system, may be involved in the escape mechanism. Once free in the cytoplasm, bacteria remain in close proximity to the apical (luminal) cell membrane where they grow and replicate within the cytoplasm (see Fig. 7-156). In this location, bacteria appear to aggregate near mitochondria; thus it has been suggested that they may need preformed triphosphates for growth.

A unique feature of the pathogenesis of proliferative enteritis is the finding that proliferation of bacteria intracellularly (growth and replication) occurs concurrently with proliferation of crypt enterocytes (hypertrophy and hyperplasia) (see Fig. 7-154). One process does not occur without the other and vice versa. Under normal conditions, crypt cells within the proliferative zone are dividing cells that differentiate into nondividing cells of the differentiative zone as these cells migrate along basement membrane up the villus to its apex (see Fig. 4-21). It appears that once crypt cells of the proliferative zone are infected with bacteria, the bacterium is able to inhibit the normal maturation of crypt cells, probably through disruption of the cell cycle. Additionally, infection of crypt cells by bacteria dramatically increases the rate of crypt cell division. Therefore, when crypt cells are infected, they do not mature but remain in an undifferentiated proliferative state and divide continuously, thus resulting in massive thickening of the mucosal surface by proliferating crypt cells. Proliferating cells continue to migrate to the apices of villi where they die and are extruded into the lumen of the intestine. This outcome provides a source of bacteria to infect additional uninfected crypt enterocytes and spread through feces into the environment. Normal villus structure is lost and replaced by a branching glandular pattern, where cells lining the hyperplastic glands are crowded into a mucosal layer of up to 10 to 15 epithelial cells in thickness. Mitotic activity is prominent. Inflammation does not occur.

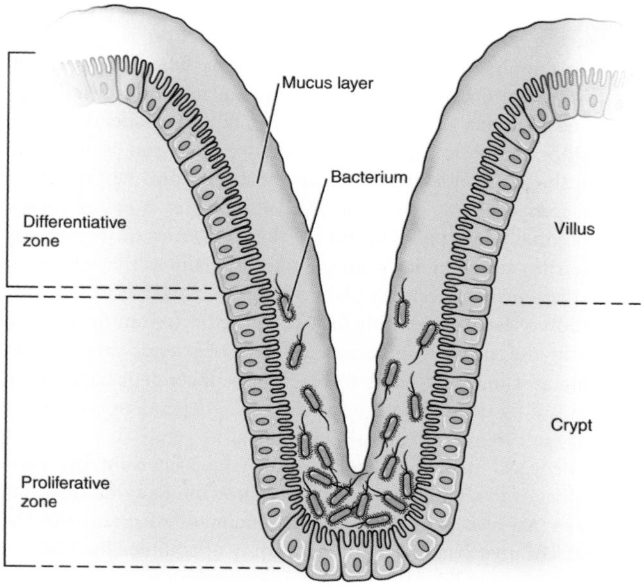

Fig. 4-21 Pathogenesis of proliferative enteritis in pigs. *Lawsonia intracellularis* infects cells of the crypts located in the proliferative zone.

The literature does not provide any discussion of the relationship between proliferative enteritis and hemorrhagic bowel syndrome and how the former transitions into the latter or if it does. Histologically, it has been shown that lesions occurring in necrotic enteritis (hemorrhagic bowel syndrome) include acute coagulative necrosis of the proliferating crypt epithelium. This lesion is consistent with ischemia or the direct effects of toxins (burnlike injury). Necrotic enteritis may simply be a manifestation of proliferating cells outgrowing an available blood supply, becoming ischemic, and then dying via acute coagulative necrosis. No cell in the body can survive if it is farther than 100 μm away from a source of oxygen, either from a capillary or highly oxygenated body fluid. Additionally, *Lawsonia intracellularis* is a Gram-negative bacterium, and endotoxin or other toxic molecules may directly cause injury and cell death consistent with acute coagulative necrosis. Acute inflammation with hemorrhage and fibrinogenesis commonly occur concurrently with acute coagulative necrosis.

Swine Dysentery (Brachyspira hyodysenteriae)

The mechanism of injury in swine dysentery is death of mucosal epithelial cells of the colon and cecum caused by bacterial hemolysins and proteases and from inflammation and its mediators and degradative enzymes. Gross lesions include a mucohemorrhagic necrofibrinous colitis and typhlitis with diphtheritic membranes covering intestinal mucosae formed by abundant mucus, hemorrhage, fibrin, plasma proteins, and cellular debris arising from necrotic mucosal epithelial cells and inflammatory cells (see Fig. 7-151).

Pigs encounter *Brachyspira hyodysenteriae* through ingestion of the bacterium in manure-contaminated fomites in the environment. The bacterium is swallowed and gains access via peristalsis to the intestine, especially the cecum and colon. Goblet cell mucus is important as a physical matrix and chemical substrate for colonization of the mucus layer by the bacterium, thus goblet cells play a central role in the pathogenesis of lesions affecting mucosal epithelial cells and their junctional complexes. *Brachyspira hyodysenteriae*, an anaerobic motile spirochete, is able to actively move through the mucus layer to gain access to mucosal epithelial and goblet cells. It is unclear why the bacterium infects the cecum and colon, but it appears that it prefers to initially replicate in mucigen droplets within goblet cells. Mucigen droplets fill the apical cytoplasm of goblet cells, and the nucleus is displaced to the basal region of the cell. Because the relative number of such cells is much greater in the cecum and colon when compared to other segments of the alimentary system, this quantitative difference may account for the location of the lesions. Additionally, mucins (e.g., the fucose and L-serine components) are strong chemoattractants for spirochetes, and because there are significant biochemical and pH differences in mucins, such as those that are synthesized and released from goblet cells, it is plausible that the chemical composition of the mucins may account for the locations of the lesions. Once the bacterium infects mucigen droplets within goblet cells, it appears to be able to activate the goblet cell to increase the production of mucus. Thus there is a large increase in the volume of mucus secreted by these cells so that mucosal surfaces are covered with a thick grayish gelatinous layer. It is unclear how the bacterium activates the goblet cell to produce and release large quantities of mucus. It is plausible that one or more bacterial virulence determinates influence the cellular processes of transcription, translation, assembly, and packaging of mucigen droplets thereby producing abundant quantities of mucus to enhance its opportunity to colonize the mucosa. Concurrently with infecting goblet cells, the bacterium begins the process of colonizing the thickened mucus layer covering the mucosal epithelium. It appears that mucus and their mucins are central to both the colonization and replication processes and result in the accumulation of large numbers of bacteria in close proximity to cell membranes and junctional complexes of mucosal epithelial cells.

Recently, it has been demonstrated experimentally that more virulent strains of the bacterium express increased numbers of genes for carbohydrate and amino acid metabolism and transport that potentially could be linked to energy and carbon sources that are available in the mucus layer. Additionally, highly fermentable feeds favor colonization of the mucus layer by bacteria. Fermentation may provide the bacterium with an energy source or other molecules required for colonization and replication. Colonization is also enhanced by the presence of other anaerobic bacterial species in the mucus layer. The significance of this finding is unclear, but again could be related to these species providing molecules required by *Brachyspira hyodysenteriae* for colonization and replication. Finally, because the bacterium is an anaerobe, it synthesizes high concentrations of nicotinamide adenine dinucleotide hydrogen (NADH) oxidase (a virulence determinate) that is used to protect itself from oxidative stress and toxic oxygen molecules in the oxygen-rich environment of the mucus layer.

The bacterium does not attach to luminal (apical) membranes of colonic and cecal epithelial cells; however, experimental studies have reported that the bacterium invades the epithelium and the lamina propria because they have been identified in these areas. The largest quantity of bacteria appears to exist in the mucus layer just overlying the epithelium. Therefore it is unclear as to whether this invasion is a direct and targeted process or merely an innocent bystander phenomenon, where the motility of the bacterium carries it into these locations to cause injury. Injury and death of colonic and cecal epithelial cells (enterocytes), as well as penetration through junctional complexes into the superficial lamina propria, are likely caused by one or more proteases and hemolysins and endotoxic effects of lipooligosaccharide (LOS) from the cell wall of the bacterium. Death and loss of the mucosal epithelium results in hemorrhage and the opportunity for infectious organisms, such as other anaerobic bacteria and the protozoan *Balantidium coli,* to invade the lamina propria. Additionally, denuded mucosa also provides a mechanism for the absorption of endotoxins, cytotoxins from inflammatory cells, and other toxic molecules that could cause endotoxic shock locally and systemically via the blood vascular system.

Johne's Disease (*Mycobacterium avium ssp. paratuberculosis*)

The mechanisms of injury in Johne's disease are (1) dysfunction and death of the epithelial cells and ECM proteins forming the junctional barrier systems of mucosae of the small intestinal, (2) dysfunction of the drainage of afferent lymphatic vessels in the lamina propria of villi of the small intestine, and (3) death of cells of the monocyte-macrophage system and of all cell populations in the lamina propria of intestinal villi from inflammation and its mediators and degradative enzymes. Gross lesions include granulomatous enteritis and mesenteric granulomatous lymphadenitis, lymphangitis, and lymphangiectasia (see Fig. 7-146). Granulomatous enteritis is characterized by a thickened intestinal wall, most commonly affecting the ileum and ileal-cecal junction with a yellow-white exudate exemplified by infiltrating granulomatous inflammatory cells. Mesenteric granulomatous lymphadenitis is characterized by enlarged mesenteric lymph nodes that on cut surfaces have discrete and coalescing areas of yellow-white caseous exudate, occasionally mineralized, infiltrating, and compressing contiguous parenchyma.

The young of cattle, sheep, and goats encounter *Mycobacterium avium* ssp. *paratuberculosis* through ingestion of the bacterium in manure-contaminated fomites in the environment. The bacterium is swallowed and gains access via peristalsis to the alimentary system. Bacteria appear to bind to receptors on luminal (apical) surfaces of M cells and are likely translocated in endocytotic vesicles or phagosomes to the basal membranes of the cell and are released into Peyer's patches where they can be phagocytosed by tissue macrophages. Unlike most other regions of the intestine, the luminal surface of M cells lacks a covering of mucus. Therefore bacteria have direct access to M cells. Lesions appear to have a segmental pattern of occurrence most commonly affecting the ileocecal intestine. Although attachment and phagocytosis of the bacterium by M cells likely involves ligand-receptor interactions, this mechanism does not explain why the lesions are most severe in ileocecal intestine.

Mycobacterium avium ssp. *paratuberculosis* requires iron for growth inside phagosomes of tissue macrophages. For an unknown reason, the concentration and availability of iron is greatest in tissue macrophages of the ileocecal intestine when compared to the concentration in other types of tissue macrophages. Therefore this gradient of iron appears to establish tissue specificity for lesions in Johne's disease. In macrophages, iron is stored as ferritin, but it is not accessible by the bacterium. Mycobacteria secrete iron-chelating proteins called exochelins, iron-reductases, and potentially siderophores and use these enzymes to acquire iron from ferritin stored in macrophages. Additionally, as the severity of inflammation increases, there is a concurrent increase in the concentration of ferritin available for use by the bacterium in cells and tissues in the areas of inflammation. Mycobacterial siderophores or reductases may also serve to block iron-dependent bactericidal reactions of tissue macrophages such as Fe^{3+}-dependent conversion of H_2O_2 into highly toxic hydroxyl radicals.

In ileocecal tissues, phagocytosis of the bacterium by tissue macrophages likely involves ligand-receptor interactions. Toll-like receptors may also be involved in attachment and phagocytosis. The cell walls of mycobacteria contain a variety of complex lipoglycans, glycoproteins, and lipoproteins such as lipoarabinomannan (LAM), 19-kDa lipoprotein, and the mycolyl-arabinogalactan-peptidoglycan complex that can serve as ligands. The cell membranes of tissue macrophages express receptors for these specific molecules and they are probably involved in the recognition, attachment, and adherence of the bacterium to the macrophage cell membrane. Additionally, complement receptors and other receptors, including mannose and CD14 receptors, expressed on tissue macrophages are the major receptors involved in phagocytosis of the bacterium, whereas integrin receptors, Toll-like receptors (TLRs), mannose receptors, CD14 receptors, scavenger receptors, and immunoglobulin Fc receptors are involved in early recognition and cell signaling in response to interaction with the bacterium. Generally, these signaling pathways initiate production of a variety of cytokines, chemokines, and antimicrobial metabolites that control mycobacterial infections; however, the bacterium through these signaling pathways is able to attenuate macrophage activation responses induced by interferon-γ (IFN-γ) and the secretion of IFN-γ. These interactions do not involve opsonin-mediated phagocytosis, thus the induction of a respiratory burst to kill the internalized bacteria does not occur and the bacterium persists in the phagosome. Receptors for opsonins expressed by tissue macrophages might also play a role in phagocytosis of the bacterium. Fibronectin may bind to the surface of macrophages and serve as a ligand to facilitate phagocytosis by macrophages. However, when employing opsonization as a means of entry into a phagosome, the bacterium must also use a mechanism to inhibit the respiratory burst to prevent its death.

The time from initial encounter with the bacterium to the expression of clinical disease is usually 12 months or longer. An explanation for this extended delay is unknown; it may simply be a slow-growing bacterium. However, bacterial growth likely involves the (1) interplay of bacterium-infected tissue macrophages and cells of the immune system mediated by proinflammatory and antiinflammatory cytokines, (2) migration of tissue macrophages locally from Peyer's patches into the lamina propria and submucosal tissues, (3) time it takes the bacterium to replicate in sufficient quantities to activate the adaptive immune response, and (4) progression of severity resulting from the death of bacterium-infected macrophages leading to the recruitment of additional macrophages.

After phagocytosis by tissue macrophages in Peyer's patches, the bacterium is confined within phagosomes and phagolysosomes. It appears to be able to disrupt phagosome-lysosome fusion and if fusion occurs, block the degradative actions of lysosomal enzymes and molecules via the structure and composition of its cell envelope and through the production of peroxidases. When a phagolysosome forms, the fused lysosome releases an acidic cytosol; proteases; and antibacterial substances, such as defensins and toxic oxygen and nitrogen intermediates, into the phagosome, all of which can injure and kill the bacterium. In general, mycobacterial species can (1) inhibit acidification of the phagosome, phagosome-lysosome fusion, and lysosomal enzyme activities; (2) block injury from toxic oxygen and nitrogen intermediates; and (3) suppress the ability of macrophages to be activated by cytokines such as INF-γ. Although highly probable, it is not known which or if any of these mechanisms are used by *Mycobacterium avium* ssp. *paratuberculosis*. Tissue macrophages, once infected with the bacterium, are activated and begin to secrete proinflammatory cytokines that act to recruit and activate additional macrophages. Additionally, because the lifespan of fully differentiated tissue macrophages is approximately 10 to 30 days, death of these cells related to aging and bacterial-induced injury releases bacterium into adjacent tissue where they are phagocytosed by newly recruited macrophages only to endlessly repeat this process. The severity and extent of the inflammatory response, concurrently with tissue injury, grows through the recruitment of additional monocytes and tissue macrophages from the circulatory system and regional lymph nodes. Bacteria-infected tissue macrophages can also spread via leukocyte trafficking in afferent lymphatic vessels within the intestinal mesentery to mesenteric lymph nodes (ileocecal lymph nodes) leading to a pyogranulomatous lymphadenitis and lymphangiectasia through the same progressive mechanism of inflammation.

Rhodococcal Enteritis (Rhodococcus equi)

See the section on the Respiratory System, Mediastinum, and Pleurae for discussion of the early pathogenesis of the alimentary form of rhodococcal enteritis. Gross lesions include (1) chronic active pyogranulomatous lymphadenitis (see Fig. 7-137) characterized by enlarged firm lymph nodes that on a cut surface have discrete and coalescing areas of yellow-white exudate infiltrating and compressing contiguous parenchyma and (2) ulcerative enteritis (see Fig. 7-136) characterized by discrete foci of ulceration and hemorrhage centered over Peyer's patches.

In the alimentary system, foals encounter *Rhodococcus equi* by swallowing mucus (sputum), exudate, and cellular debris contaminated with bacteria that move into the oral pharynx via the positive pressure of coughing and the upward rhythmic movement of cilia in the mucociliary apparatus. The bacterium then gains access to the alimentary system via intestinal peristalsis. Bacteria probably bind to receptors on luminal surfaces of M cells and are then transported in endocytotic vesicles to the basal membranes of the cell and released into the Peyer's patches where they can be phagocytosed by tissue macrophages or dendritic cells. Unlike most other regions of the intestine, the luminal surface of M cells lacks a covering of mucus. Therefore bacteria have direct access to M cells. It is likely that ligand-receptor mechanisms (as discussed in the section on the Respiratory System, Mediastinum, and Pleurae) are applicable to M cells and tissue macrophages in Peyer's patches. Once tissue macrophages are infected, the pathogenesis of the disease appears to progress much like that which occurs in the lung resulting in pyogranulomatous lymphadenitis. Ulcerative enteritis, characteristic of the alimentary form of the disease, occurs over affected Peyer's patches. Although unknown, it is probable that mediators and degradative enzymes from inflammation diffuse into contiguous tissues, causing direct injury to the mucosae or indirectly via vascular injury and occlusion leading to infarction and ulceration. Bacteria-infected tissue macrophages can also spread via leukocyte trafficking in afferent lymphatic vessels within the intestinal mesentery to mesenteric lymph nodes leading to a pyogranulomatous lymphadenitis and then systemically to lymph nodes and lymphoid tissues such as the spleen.

Bovine Intestinal Tuberculosis (Mycobacterium bovis)

Because the pathogenesis and lesions of bovine intestinal tuberculosis are identical to those observed in the pneumonic form, see the section on the Respiratory System, Mediastinum, and Pleurae. Also, the section on Johne's disease should be reviewed because it mimics intestinal tuberculosis. It appears that intestinal tuberculosis commonly begins as the pneumonic form and is spread to the intestine by (1) coughing up and swallowing sputum containing macrophages infected with bacteria and/or "free" bacteria and (2) hematogenous or lymphatic spread of infected macrophages via leukocyte trafficking to intestinal lymph nodes and Peyer's patches. Via the alimentary route, intestinal M cells and possibly dendritic cells are used to phagocytose bacteria and then release them via exocytosis from basolateral surfaces into Peyer's patches where they are phagocytosed by macrophages and granulomatous inflammation and granuloma formation follow. Intestinal tuberculosis is associated with mucosal ulceration overlying Peyer's patches. Ulceration appears to result from vasculitis, thrombosis, ischemia, and infarction secondary to inflammation in Peyer's patches, but could also be caused directly by inflammatory mediators released from granulomas diffusing to and acting on blood vessels or mucosae.

Tyzzer's Disease (Clostridium piliforme [Bacillus piliformis])

See Tyzzer's disease in the section on the Hepatobiliary System and Exocrine Pancreas.

Hepatobiliary System and Exocrine Pancreas

*Tyzzer's Disease (*Clostridium piliforme *[*Bacillus piliformis*])*

The mechanism of injury in Tyzzer's disease is necrosis of hepatocytes, intestinal mucosal epithelial cells, and adjacent vascular and stromal tissues. Gross lesions include hepatomegaly and numerous white-gray-yellow foci (<2-mm diameter) of hepatocyte necrosis distributed at random, usually throughout all lobes of the liver (see Fig. 8-48). In severe cases, the center of these foci may be depressed and red (hemorrhage).

The young of all animal species can contract Tyzzer's disease; however, foals appear to be the most susceptible and encounter *Clostridium piliforme*, an obligate intracellular bacterium, through ingestion of spores present in soil or vegetative forms in fecal fomites from infected animals. The disease is less common in dogs, cats, and calves. Although the bacterium uses the intestinal mucosa as an initial beachhead, it ultimately infects, replicates in, and injures the liver. The mechanism of spread from ingestion to the liver is unclear. In other diseases caused by *Clostridium* spp., such as blackleg, cells of the monocyte-macrophage system and M cells are probably used to spread spores and/or vegetative forms and hide (sequester) spores. After ingestion, it is likely that spores or vegetative forms are carried by normal peristaltic activities through the oral pharynx, esophagus, and stomach to their final destination, the small intestine. It is unknown if and how the bacterium interacts with and gains access to intestinal mucosal epithelial cells and/or mucosal macrophages. Vegetative forms of the bacterium are motile and may be able to penetrate the mucus layer and encounter mucosal epithelial cells of the small intestine. How they enter these cells is unknown, although direct penetration or receptor-mediated endocytosis through ligand-receptor interactions could be involved. Spores could be taken up through endostosis by intestinal mucosal epithelial cells, but how the spores penetrate the mucus layer and gain access to epithelial cells is unknown. They could be phagocytosed by mucosal macrophages in the mucus layer and carried to or through the mucosae by leukocyte trafficking. Additionally, spores could bind with receptors on the surface of M cells, which lack a mucus layer, enter though endocytosis, germinate into vegetative forms, infect and replicate in these cells, and then spread to adjacent mucosal epithelial cells.

In either case, spores or vegetative form are able to infect mucosal epithelial cells of the intestine through their apical surfaces and then replicate in the cells. It is not known what type of ligand-receptor interactions are involved in this process of entry into the cell. The bacterium appears to adhere to the apical cell membrane, be phagocytosed, and then escape the phagosome to reside and replicate in the cytoplasm of the cell.

It has not been shown how the bacterium spreads from mucosal epithelial cells or from M cells systemically to the liver. Because *Clostridium piliforme* is a motile bacterium, it has been suggested that it leaves epithelial cells of the intestine (possibly via their basal surfaces) and enters the circulatory system, likely by penetrating capillaries in the lamina propria that drain through the portal system to the liver. The bacterium could also potentially be transported to the liver by macrophages (leukocytic trafficking). If the bacterium is able to infect and replicate in M cells, the integration of M cells with Peyer's patches provides the opportunity for the bacterium to interact with macrophages or gain access to capillaries within submucosal ECM tissues. Macrophages could phagocytose the bacterium using ligand-receptor interactions and carry it via leukocyte trafficking in afferent lymphatic vessels to mesenteric lymph nodes and then systemically via the thoracic duct and venous system into the circulatory system and ultimately the liver via the hepatic artery. However, in a mouse model of Tyzzer's disease, depletion of macrophages did not change the course of infection. This outcome suggests that leukocyte trafficking may not be involved in the spread of the bacterium from the intestine to the liver.

The bacterium encounters endothelial cells lining hepatic sinusoids through spread in the circulatory system, likely via the portal vein. As a motile bacterium, it is free in the circulatory system and could (1) directly penetrate the endothelium and enter and infect hepatocytes, (2) infect and replicate in endothelial cells and then spread to adjacent hepatocytes, or (3) infect and replicate in Kupffer cells and then spread to adjacent hepatocytes. Hemorrhage occurs in Tyzzer's disease, and this lesion suggests that vascular injury occurs either from direct penetration of the blood vessels or by lysis of the endothelial cells after replication of the bacterium. Although direct penetration of endothelial cells and hepatocytes is a possible mechanism of entry into these cells, typical ligand-receptor interactions may also be involved. The bacterium enters hepatocytes probably via receptor-mediated endocytosis and then escapes the phagosome to reside and replicate in the cytoplasm. The replication of *Clostridium piliforme* in hepatocytes eventually results in hepatocellular necrosis. The mechanisms causing necrosis are unknown. Bacterial cytotoxic proteins and several cellular cytokines like interleukin and tumor necrosis factor (TNF) have been implicated as the cause of hepatocellular necrosis, but experimental results are inconclusive. It appears that the bacterium first causes hepatocyte necrosis, which then incites an acute inflammatory response with abundant neutrophils and occasional macrophages in affected tissues. In the same mouse model of Tyzzer's disease, the number of bacteria in hepatocytes and the severity of lesions were much worse in mice depleted of neutrophils and NK cells. This outcome suggests that the acute inflammation plays an important role as an innate defense mechanism in the disease.

Bacillary Hemoglobinuria (Clostridium haemolyticum)

The mechanism of injury in bacillary hemoglobinuria has a local and a systemic component. Local injury is cell death (necrosis) of hepatocytes (necrotizing hepatitis), whereas systemic injury is death of erythrocytes in the blood vascular system. Injury in both components is caused by phospholipase C and other toxins released from *Clostridium haemolyticum.* Gross lesions include vasculitis, infarction, coagulative necrosis, and hemorrhage in the liver (see Fig. 8-68) and hemoglobinuria in the urinary system.

Cattle and sheep probably encounter *Clostridium haemolyticum* through ingestion of spores present in the soil. Although the bacterium ultimately resides in and injures the liver, the mechanism of spread from ingestion to the liver is unknown. In other diseases caused by *Clostridium* spp., such as blackleg, cells of the monocyte-macrophage, M cells, and dendritic systems are likely used to spread and hide spores. It is plausible that after ingestion, spores are carried by normal peristaltic activities through the oral pharynx, esophagus, abomasum, and rumen to their final destination, the small intestine.

It is unknown how spores interact with and gain access to epithelial cells and mucosal macrophages. The mucus layer of the small intestine probably presents a significant barrier to spores; therefore spores could bind with receptors on the surface of M cells or dendritic cells and through transcytosis gain access to macrophages and lymphocytes located in Peyer's patches contiguous with these cells. Macrophages could also phagocytose spores using ligand-receptor interactions and carry the spores via leukocyte trafficking in afferent lymphatic vessels to mesenteric lymph nodes and then systemically via the thoracic duct and venous system into the circulatory system. Although unproved, spores are likely the form of the bacterium that spreads systemically to liver. Trafficking macrophages could enter the sinusoids of the liver and transfer spores to Kupffer cells embedded in the endothelium. Spores then hide in Kupffer cells until they are activated to germinate and produce vegetative bacteria. Tropism for Kupffer cells is probably mediated by ligand-receptor interactions.

The occurrence of bacillary hemoglobinuria follows injury to the liver caused by migration of liver flukes *(Fasciola hepatica, Fascioloides magna)*. Thus bacillary hemoglobinuria only occurs in geographic locations that have these flukes. The flukes migrate through the liver and injure intrahepatic veins, causing thrombosis, ischemia, and infarction of associated hepatocytes. Infarcted areas of liver are anaerobic and have a lowered oxidation-reduction (redox) potential required for germination of spores released from dead Kupffer cells. Spores germinate into vegetative bacteria and they produce large quantities of phospholipase C (also known as *lecithinase C,* an α-toxin) and hemolysins that destroy cell membranes and cause hepatocyte death. These toxins are also absorbed into the venous system within viable liver, resulting in entry into the systemic circulation leading to erythrocyte membrane injury, death of erythrocytes, release of hemoglobin, and hemoglobinuria.

Infectious Necrotic Hepatitis (Clostridium novyi)

The pathogenesis and lesions of infectious necrotic hepatitis are similar to those of bacillary hemoglobinuria; however, the disease lacks hemoglobinuria, which is likely attributable to the absence of toxins that injure erythrocyte membranes.

Hepatic Leptospirosis (Leptospira *spp.)*

The pathogenesis of hepatic leptospirosis begins as vascular leptospirosis caused by *Leptospira* spp., and this disease of the cardiovascular system and lymphatic vessels should be reviewed. The mechanisms used by *Leptospira* spp. to infect the liver are likely similar to those used in the kidney and are covered in the urinary system section of this chapter. Gross lesions include discrete and coalescing white-to-gray foci of hepatic necrosis scattered at random throughout hepatic parenchyma that are intermixed with hemorrhage.

Respiratory System, Mediastinum, and Pleurae

Porcine Polyserositis (Haemophilus suis/parasuis, Actinobacillus suis, Streptococcus suis, Escherichia coli)

Several bacteria cause porcine polyserositis, but it is most commonly associated with *Haemophilus suis/parasuis*, the bacterium that causes Glasser's disease. Gross lesions include vasculitis leading to variable quantities of a gray-white friable material (fibrin) on serosal surfaces (fibrinous polyserositis) of the lungs (fibrinous pleuritis), heart (fibrinous pericarditis), and abdominal cavity (fibrinous peritonitis) (see Fig. 7-157). The cavities formed by these anatomic structures may also contain a fibrinous exudate and edema fluid. Opposing serosal surfaces are often loosely attached to each other by fibrinous exudate, making normal physiologic processes like respiration more difficult. The serosa and cavities of meninges, joints, and testis can also be affected. Information about the mechanisms used by these bacteria to cause porcine polyserositis is limited. Thus portions of this section are speculative and based on (1) what is known mechanistically about other diseases of the respiratory system caused by the *Pasteurellaceae* family of bacteria and (2) a reasonable probability that inflammation, responses to injury, and lesions that have been described in porcine polyserositis are the result of underlying and known pathobiologic mechanisms.

Pigs likely encounter *Haemophilus suis/parasuis*, *Actinobacillus suis*, and *Streptococcus suis* through inhalation of these bacteria in contaminated fomites or fluid droplets. They appear to be commensal organisms of respiratory mucosae existing in biofilms in the nasopharynx and tonsil of healthy pigs. Environmental stressors, such as overcrowding, poor ventilation and humidity, or abrupt changes in ambient air temperature, alter the mucus layer and the commensal relationship, allowing bacteria to replicate in sufficient numbers to begin colonization of respiratory mucosae and to spread to other animals. Preceding or concurrent viral infections could also damage the mucociliary apparatus, allowing bacteria to colonize the mucus layer or mucosae. In the respiratory system, the bacteria are deposited on mucosae of the conductive component by centrifugal and inertial turbulence and trapped in the mucus layer. The bacterium is nonmotile, and it has not been clearly shown how it penetrates the mucus layer; gains access to cilia of mucosal epithelial cells; expresses virulence determinates such as adhesins, capsular molecules, fimbriae, and outer membrane proteins required for ligand-receptor interactions; and colonizes the mucosae. Once the mucus layer and/or mucosae are colonized and nonciliated and ciliated epithelial cells are injured by LPS, potentially by a neuraminidase, and by a suggested bacterial toxin, focal acute inflammation ensues and is followed to a limited extent by the death of these cells. In fact, receptors necessary for colonization of the mucus layer and/or mucosae or for the invasion of host cells may be exposed by the "potential" neuraminidase.

It has also been suggested that bacteria gain access to the lamina propria by altering the function of junctional complexes, allowing them to move between adjacent mucosal epithelial cells. The outcome of these processes is the loss of normal mucosal barriers, which provide the bacteria with direct access to the vascularized ECM of the lamina propria. It has not been determined how the bacteria actually cross this altered barrier, reach the capillary beds, penetrate the endothelium, and spread into the blood vascular system. Mechanisms, such as a cell-free bacteremia or leukocyte trafficking in alveolar or intravascular macrophages, lymphocytes, or dendritic cells, are hypothetic possibilities. A study of *Haemophilus suis* has shown that mucosal macrophages contain structures resembling phagolysosomes indicative of phagocytic activity. Lesions suggest these bacteria may have a tropism for vascular endothelial cells of serosae. It is unclear why this occurs, but it is probably linked to the expression of bacterial virulence determinates and ligand-receptor interactions with host endothelial cells. Additionally, it is thought that bacterial endotoxins may contribute to vascular injury and permeability changes leading to the leakage of fibrinogen and its polymerization to fibrin on serosal surfaces and in some cases to microthrombus formation and disseminated intravascular coagulation (DIC) in other organ systems.

Strep Zoo (Streptococcus equi *ssp.* zooepidemicus)

The mechanism of injury in "strep zoo" is injury and death of mucosal epithelial cells and vascular endothelial cells from bacterial toxins and from inflammation and its mediators and degradative enzymes. Gross lesions include vasculitis leading to (1) a lung with a firm texture attributable to the leakage of variable quantities of fibrin into alveoli and alveolar septa (fibrinous pneumonia) from injured blood vessels and (2) the appearance of variable quantities of a gray-white friable material (fibrin) often mixed with hemorrhage on serosal surfaces (fibrinous polyserositis) of the lungs (fibrinous pleuritis), heart (fibrinous pericarditis), and abdominal cavity (fibrinous peritonitis) (see Fig. 10-14). The cavities formed by these anatomic structures may contain a fibrinous exudate and edema fluid mixed with hemorrhage. Opposing serosal surfaces are often loosely attached to each other by fibrinous exudate making normal physiologic processes such as respiration more difficult. The serosa and cavities of meninges, joints, and testis can also be affected. Information about the mechanisms used by this bacterium is limited. Some of this section is speculative and based on (1) what is known about virulence determinates used by other members of the *Streptococceae* family, especially *Streptococcus equi* ssp. *equi*, to cause disease and (2) a reasonable probability that inflammation, responses to injury, and lesions that have been described in strep zoo are the result of underlying and known pathobiological mechanisms.

Streptococcus equi ssp. *zooepidemicus* is a zoonosis. Horses and dogs likely encounter *Streptococcus equi* ssp. *zooepidemicus* through inhalation of the bacterium in fomites or fluid droplets. The bacterium appears to be a commensal organism of mucous membranes of the nasal and oral pharynxes, probably existing in biofilms of healthy animals. Environmental stressors, such as overcrowding, poor ventilation and humidity, or abrupt changes in ambient air temperature, alter the mucus layer and the commensal relationship, allowing the bacteria to replicate in sufficient numbers to colonize the respiratory mucosae and spread the bacterium to other animals. Preceding or concurrent viral infections could also damage the mucociliary apparatus, allowing these bacteria to colonize the mucus layer or mucosae. In the respiratory system, the bacteria are deposited on mucosae of the conductive component by centrifugal and inertial turbulence and trapped in the mucus layer. Although *Streptococcus equi* ssp. *zooepidemicus* can express many of the virulence determinates expressed by *Streptococcus equi* ssp. *equi*, a causal link of these factors to disease is unclear. The bacterium is nonmotile, and it has not been clearly shown how it penetrates the mucus layer; gains access to mucosal epithelial cells or cilia; expresses virulence determinates such as adhesins, capsular molecules, fimbriae, and outer membrane proteins required for ligand-receptor interactions; and colonizes the mucosae. Once mucosae are colonized and epithelial cells are injured, acute inflammation ensues, leading to death of these cells and loss of the ciliated mucosal barrier. Injury to ciliated epithelial cells likely alters the function of the mucociliary apparatus, allowing the bacteria to gain access to terminal bronchioles and alveoli by dependent settling due to gravity. Herein, bacteria colonize mucosae of the terminal bronchioles and alveoli, spread into vascularized ECM tissues, interact with and injure blood vessels of the air-blood barrier, and leak fibrinogen into the alveoli (fibrinous pneumonia). This process accounts for a fibrinous pneumonia but may not satisfactorily account for the fibrinous polyserositis so characteristic of this disease.

By an undetermined mechanism, bacteria likely gain access to the lamina propria of the respiratory system and have direct access to the vascularized ECM. It has not been determined how bacteria actually cross this altered barrier, reach the capillary beds, penetrate the endothelium, and spread into the blood vascular system. Mechanisms, such as a cell-free bacteremia or leukocyte trafficking in alveolar or intravascular macrophages, lymphocytes, or dendritic cells, are hypothetical possibilities. The characteristic gross lesions of fibrinohemorrhagic polyserositis suggest these bacteria may have a tropism for vascular endothelial cells of serosae. It is unclear why this occurs, but it is probably linked to the expression of bacterial virulence determinates and ligand-receptor interactions with host endothelial cells. Additionally, it is possible that bacterial toxins may contribute to vascular injury and permeability changes leading to the leakage of fibrinogen and its polymerization to fibrin on serosal surfaces and in some cases to microthrombus formation and DIC in other organ systems.

Disease caused by *Streptococcus equi* ssp. *zooepidemicus* in dogs appears to follow the same chronologic sequence of events as in horses, but virulence determinates involved in the disease appear to cause more severe lesions to the vascular system and a greater degree of hemorrhage.

Strangles (Streptococcus equi *ssp.* equi)

See the section on Bone Marrow, Blood Cells, and the Lymphatic System for a discussion of strangles.

Porcine Enzootic Pneumonia (Mycoplasma hyopneumoniae)

The mechanism of injury in porcine enzootic pneumonia is injury of ciliated epithelial cells of the bronchi and bronchioles, causing dysfunction and death of these cells. This outcome results initially in dysfunction of cilia, loss of cilia, and then cell death followed by a secondary bacterial infection leading to additional cell death of all cell types in the lung from chronic inflammation and its mediators and degradative enzymes. The susceptibility to and severity of porcine enzootic pneumonia can be enhanced by environmental stressors (abrupt or long-term changes in ventilation, temperature, and/or humidity) and earlier or concurrent viral (porcine reproductive and respiratory virus, swine influenza virus) or bacterial (*Pasteurella multocida*) infections. Gross lesions characteristic of this disease are firm (consolidation) yellow-tan-gray anterior-ventral lung lobes (see Fig. 9-83). Pleural surfaces are usually not involved, indicating that vascular injury and permeability changes and their association with the expression of bacterial virulence determinates are not significant in the pathogenesis of the disease.

Pigs encounter *Mycoplasma hyopneumoniae* through inhalation of the bacterium in fomites or fluid droplets. The bacterium is deposited on mucosae of the conductive component by centrifugal and inertial turbulence and trapped in the mucus layer. The bacterium is nonmotile, and it has not been clearly shown how it penetrates the mucus layer, gains access to cilia of mucosal epithelial cells, and colonizes the mucosae. Colonization of the respiratory system appears to probably involve adherence and binding of the bacterium to cell membrane receptors, using fimbria and pili by ligand-receptor interactions, because it has been shown that the bacterium attaches to cilia and line up in parallel rows along the surface of the cells. A molecule called *cilium adhesin* expressed on the surface of the bacterium appears to be involved in the attachment and binding process, where it is thought to interact with glycosaminoglycan and heparin on cell membranes. Additionally, the bacterium probably expresses glycosaminoglycans, such as heparin, heparin sulfate, and chondroitin sulfate B, or coats itself with such molecules that bind to ECM molecules, such as fibronectin, vitronectin, laminin, and collagen, but little is actually known about this process. This interaction ultimately results in dysfunction of cilia (ciliostasis) and death of the epithelial cells and reduced function of the mucociliary apparatus. Virulence determinates used by the bacterium to cause dysfunction and death of these cells have not been determined. *Mycoplasma hyopneumoniae* does not produce toxins, but some mildly toxic molecules do occur. Because of dysfunction of the mucociliary apparatus, *Mycoplasma hyopneumoniae* and other bacteria are able to reach distal aspects of terminal bronchioles and alveoli by dependent settling caused by forces of gravity. The bacteria replicate in these sites and cause chronic anterior-ventral bronchopneumonia.

*Atrophic Rhinitis (*Bordetella bronchiseptica *and* Pasteurella multocida*)*

Although *Bordetella bronchiseptica* and *Pasteurella multocida* can each separately cause clinical forms of atrophic rhinitis in pigs, the classic form of the disease from a pathologist's perspective appears to be caused by these two bacteria interacting synergistically. Information about the mechanisms used by *Bordetella bronchiseptica* and *Pasteurella multocida* to cause atrophic rhinitis in pigs is limited. Thus portions of this section are speculative and based on (1) what is known mechanistically about other diseases of the respiratory system caused by *Pasteurella* spp. and (2) a reasonable probability that inflammation, responses to injury, and lesions that have been described in atrophic rhinitis are the result of underlying and known pathobiologic mechanisms. The mechanism of injury is (1) death of ciliated epithelial and stromal cells of turbinate mucosae and (2) concurrent activation and suppression of osteoclasts and osteoblasts, respectively resulting in osteolysis of bone of the turbinates leading to turbinate atrophy. Gross lesions include varying degrees of loss (atrophy) and remodeling of turbinate scrolls and the nasal septum, with ventral scrolls usually being most severely affected (see Fig. 9-21).

Pigs encounter *Bordetella bronchiseptica* and *Pasteurella multocida* through inhalation of the bacteria in fomites or fluid droplets. These bacteria are likely commensal organisms that reside in the nasopharynx of healthy pigs, but environmental stressors, such as overcrowding, poor ventilation and humidity, or abrupt changes in ambient air temperature, alter the commensal relationship, allowing the bacteria to replicate in sufficient numbers to colonize the mucosae and spread the bacterium to other animals. Colonization appears to be a two-stage process; a *Bordetella bronchiseptica* phase followed by a *Pasteurella multocida* phase. When inhaled, *Bordetella bronchiseptica* is deposited on and trapped in the mucus layer of mucosae. The bacterium is nonmotile and it has not been clearly shown how the bacterium penetrates the mucus layer, gains access to cilia of mucosal epithelial cells, and colonizes the mucosae. *Bordetella bronchiseptica* does produce a dermonecrotic toxin (virulence determinate) and possibly adenylate cyclase-hemolysin toxin that likely affect the mucus layer and ciliated epithelial cells, making them more susceptible to colonization. The types of adhesins (ligands) and receptors used in colonization have not been determined but may include adhesins such as filamentous hemagglutinin, pertactin, and fimbriae proteins. The bacterium has an outer membrane protein called *pertactin* that may act as an adhesin, allowing the bacterium to colonize turbinate mucosae that have been injured by dermonecrotic toxin. Receptors for pertactin on mucosal epithelial cells have not been identified, but once in contact with cell membranes, bacteria likely adhere and bind to cell membrane receptors using fimbria and pili. This process results in colonization of mucosae by *Bordetella bronchiseptica*.

Under normal conditions, *Pasteurella multocida* has limited and weak virulence determinates for attaching to and colonizing turbinate mucosae. Initial colonization by *Bordetella bronchiseptica* leads to disruption of the mucus layer and the mucosal barrier system and results in mucosae that are more suitable for colonization by *Pasteurella multocida* in the second phase of infection. Mucosal lesions begin as focal erosions and ulcerations accompanied by acute inflammation (neutrophils), which subsequently spread into underlying lamina propria, ECM tissues, and bone of the turbinates. These lesions result in altered clearance mechanisms of ciliated epithelial cells and exposure of its lamina propria, where *Pasteurella multocida* can adhere to and colonize vascularized ECM tissues. Once the mucosae and lamina propria are colonized, the primary virulence determinate expressed by the bacterium is *Pasteurella multocida* toxin (PMT), a dermonecrotic toxin. The toxin, a typical A-B toxin, causes turbinate atrophy and snout deformation through chronic inflammation leading to bone remodeling and fibrous osteodystrophy of periosteal fibroblast origin. Mechanistically, the toxin initially acts to stimulate osteoblasts, which in turn act to increase the numbers (hyperplasia) and activity of osteoclasts. As toxin concentrations increase, it acts by blocking the function of osteoblasts, and cell degeneration and death may ensue. Overall, *Pasteurella multocida* toxin causes turbinate atrophy by increasing osteoclast numbers and activities through osteolysis of existing turbinate bone, as well as by inhibiting osteoblastic activities and the formation of new bone, both resulting in turbinate atrophy.

*Bovine Enzootic Pneumonia (*Pasteurella multocida *ssp.* multocida *serogroup A)*

Mechanistically, the virulence determinates and mechanisms used by *Pasteurella multocida* ssp. *multocida* to cause bovine enzootic pneumonia are very similar functionally to those used by *Mannheimia haemolytica* to cause bovine pneumonic Mannheimiosis. However, in bovine enzootic pneumonia, bacterial pathogenicity is noticeably reduced and reflected by a slow onset and insidious inflammatory response and a nearly complete absence of cell necrosis, vasculitis, permeability changes, and fibrinogenesis. The mechanism of injury in bovine enzootic pneumonia is injury of all cell populations in the respiratory system attributable to inflammation and its mediators and degradative enzymes. The susceptibility to and severity of bovine enzootic pneumonia can be enhanced by environmental stressors and earlier or concurrent viral infection such as those caused by bovine respiratory syncytial virus, bovine viral diarrhea virus, infectious bovine rhinotracheitis virus, or parainfluenza III virus. Gross lesions include firm (consolidation) yellow-gray anterior-ventral lung lobes (see Fig. 9-56). Pleural surfaces are usually not involved, indicating that vascular injury and permeability changes and their association with the expression of bacterial virulence determinates are not significant in the pathogenesis of the disease.

Bovine Pneumonic Pasteurellosis/Mannheimiosis (Mannheimia [Pasteurella] haemolytica)

The mechanism of injury in bovine pneumonic pasteurellosis/Mannheimiosis is injury and death (coagulative necrosis) of all cell populations in the respiratory system. In addition to injury caused by bacterial toxins (leukotoxin), acute inflammation and its mediators and degradative enzymes significantly contribute to the pathogenesis of the disease. *Mannheimia haemolytica* can cause severe pneumonic disease independent of other contributory factors; however, the susceptibility to and severity of disease can be enhanced by environmental stressors and earlier or concurrent viral infection. Gross lesions include severe fibrinonecrotic (often hemorrhagic) pneumonia and vasculitis attributable to necrosis and apoptosis, especially affecting type I pneumocytes and capillary endothelial cells forming the air-blood barrier of alveolar septa and the vascular system (severe necrotizing vasculitis) (see Figs. 9-58, 9-71, and 9-72).

Cattle (and probably sheep and goats) encounter *Mannheimia haemolytica* through inhalation of the bacterium in fomites or fluid droplets. The bacterium is a commensal organism that resides in the nasopharynx and tonsils of healthy animals, but environmental stressors, such as weaning, adverse weather conditions, changes in diet, and shipping, can alter the commensal relationship, allowing the bacteria to replicate in sufficient numbers to colonize the respiratory mucosae and spread the bacterium to other animals. Colonization appears to be a two-stage process, first affecting the conductive component (terminal bronchioles and alveoli), then affecting the O_2-CO_2 (terminal bronchioles and alveoli) exchange component. When inhaled, bacteria are deposited on and trapped in the mucus layer of the mucosae of the conductive component by centrifugal and inertial turbulence. *Mannheimia haemolytica* is a nonmotile bacterium, and it has not been clearly shown how the bacterium penetrates the mucus layer to gain access to cilia of mucosal epithelial cells. Neuraminidase produced by *Mannheimia haemolytica* reduces the viscosity of the mucus, making it less dense and a more fluidic layer, thus allowing the bacterium better access to cell membranes via gravity and random Brownian movement. Additionally, neuraminidase cleaves sialic acid from the surface of cell membranes, thus decreasing the net negative surface charge and allowing closer contact of the bacterium with membranes. Once in contact with cell membranes, bacteria adhere and bind to receptors using fimbria and pili by ligand-receptor interactions. This process results in bacterial colonization of the mucosae. The types of adhesins (ligands) and receptors used in colonization have not been determined. Once colonization occurs, the bacteria replicate in large numbers in the conductive component of the respiratory system and produce enzymes, such as neuraminidase, and toxins, such as leukotoxin and LPS that injure and disrupt the function of the mucociliary apparatus.

Additionally, polysaccharides of the bacterial capsule (virulence determinate) inhibit phagocytosis of the bacterium by neutrophils and mucosal macrophages. Because of mucociliary dysfunction, bacteria spread via gravity to dependent portions of the lung, including terminal bronchioles and alveoli of the O_2-CO_2 exchange component. Once bacteria arrive in this location, the second stage of the process, which is more severe than the first stage, begins. The difference in severity is, in part, based on three factors: (1) extensive replication of bacteria in stage one that settle into the O_2-CO_2 exchange component and their subsequent amplification through replication, (2) the large surface area of lung tissue affected, and (3) the greater vulnerability of the air-blood barrier and septa in the O_2-CO_2 exchange component to injury. All of these factors contribute to the severity of the acute inflammatory responses and tissue injury.

The single most important virulence determinate in bovine pneumonic Mannheimiosis is leukotoxin. Leukotoxin, a member of the RTX group of toxins, is a cytotoxin that causes death and apoptosis of alveolar macrophages and neutrophils. RTX toxins attach to cells through passive adsorption and cell surface receptors, the latter being the transmembrane receptor CD18. At high concentrations, it causes necrosis by creating pores in cell membranes leading to cell swelling and death, whereas at lower concentrations, it causes apoptosis. Additionally, at lower concentrations, it activates neutrophils and induces the production of proinflammatory cytokines. When bacteria are phagocytosed by alveolar macrophages, leukotoxin is used to kill the macrophages and release the bacteria back into vascularized ECM tissue and alveolar spaces. Iron is also required for optimal growth of the bacterium and production of leukotoxin. LPS and leukotoxin also activate the complement system and the release of proinflammatory cytokines resulting in vascular injury and severe acute inflammation. Vascular injury leads to permeability changes with edema and the release of fibrinogen that polymerizes to fibrin in alveolar spaces, interalveolar septa, interlobular and interlobar septa, and on pulmonary serosal surfaces (fibrinonecrotic pneumonia). Vascular injury can also lead to pulmonary hemorrhage.

Acute inflammation is characterized by the recruitment of large numbers of neutrophils from the circulation into affected lung tissue followed by activation of these cells via a respiratory burst and the release of degradative enzymes. The bacterium has several mechanisms (see later) to minimize the effects of neutrophils, but innocent bystander lung tissue, such as terminal bronchioles and cells that form the air-blood barrier, are severely injured by the molecules and enzymes released from activated neutrophils. Capsular polysaccharides, outer membrane proteins, and LPS of the bacterium are also important in the pathogenesis of the disease, especially as related to acute inflammation and vascular injury. Polysaccharides are virulence determinates that facilitate adherence, colonization, and likely invasion of respiratory mucosae; inhibit phagocytosis by neutrophils; and disrupt complement-mediated death of bacteria. Outer membrane proteins are chemotactic for neutrophils, but when in contact with neutrophils, they disrupt phagocytosis and intracellular killing of bacteria. LPS binds with cell membrane CD14, β2-integrins, and TLRs on alveolar macrophages inducing the synthesis of proinflammatory cytokines, arachidonic acid metabolites, and NO that injure cells in inflammation. LPS may also injure endothelial cells directly and through molecules released from macrophages such as those listed in the previous sentence.

Pulmonary Histophilosis (Histophilus somni)

The pathogenesis of pulmonary histophilosis is likely very similar to the mechanisms as described previously for bovine pneumonic pasteurellosis/Mannheimiosis.

Porcine Pleuropneumonia (Actinobacillus pleuropneumoniae)

The mechanism of injury in porcine pleuropneumonia is injury and death (coagulative necrosis) of all cell populations in the respiratory system, especially those of the vascular system (severe necrotizing vasculitis), secondary to the effects of bacterial toxins and to acute inflammation and its mediators and degradative enzymes. Gross lesions, attributable to vascular injury affecting lung and regional lymph nodes, include (1) edema and alterations in vascular permeability; (2) hemorrhage; and (3) fibrinous and hemorrhagic pneumonic, pleural, and pericardial effusions and acute necrotizing inflammation and pneumonia (see Fig. 9-84).

Pigs encounter *Actinobacillus pleuropneumoniae* through inhalation of the bacterium in fomites or fluid droplets. In the respiratory system, the bacterium is deposited on mucosae of the conductive system and probably on the exchange system by centrifugal and inertial turbulence. The characteristic distribution pattern (dorsal-diaphragmatic) of gross lesions may reflect the fact that droplet size and inertial turbulence results in the initial deposit being near branch points of conductive airways. The bacterium must first colonize the mucosae by adhering and binding to the membranes of epithelial cells using ligand-receptor interactions mediated through fimbriae. Following colonization, *Actinobacillus pleuropneumoniae* requires iron to grow and replicate and is capable of utilizing porcine transferrin as a source of iron. However, it appears that iron is also obtained from blood and the death of red blood cells caused by bacterial hemolysins and proteases. After the death of red blood cells, LPS and outer membrane proteins of the bacterial cell wall can bind hemoglobin and assist in the transfer of the iron molecule required for growth and replication into the bacterium. In part, this requirement may explain the severe hemorrhage that occurs in this disease.

It has been shown that the bacterium binds poorly to cilia and the epithelium of the trachea and bronchi, whereas it binds strongly to cilia and membranes of terminal bronchioles and membranes of alveolar epithelial cells. This selective pattern of binding and inertial turbulence (see previous discussion) may account for the distribution of lesions observed in porcine pleuropneumonia. LPS and LOS are known to play important roles in the pathogenesis of Gram-negative infections; however, their role in porcine pleuropneumonia is unclear and may involve acting as ligands for adherence to host cell surfaces. Glycosphingolipids present in membranes of epithelial cells may serve as receptors for these ligands. It has not been determined if and how *Actinobacillus pleuropneumoniae* penetrates the mucus layer to gain access to cilia and cell membranes of epithelial cells. The suppression of mucus production and ciliary activity increase the severity of porcine pleuropneumonia by decreasing clearance of the bacteria through the mucociliary apparatus mechanism. Once *Actinobacillus pleuropneumoniae* is bound to cilia and cell membranes of terminal bronchioles and alveolar epithelial cells, the bacterium is positioned to be phagocytosed by alveolar, interstitial, and intravascular macrophages. Although all of these types of macrophages are phagocytic, intravascular macrophages also have strong cytolytic activities that may also account, in part, for the hemorrhage characteristic of pulmonary vascular lesions.

Neutrophils are not involved in the initial phagocytic response to the bacterium, but once the process has been started by macrophages and chemokines are released from activated macrophages, neutrophils are recruited from the vasculature into the inflammatory response to phagocytose the bacteria. After phagocytosis, it has been shown that neutrophils can immediately kill *Actinobacillus pleuropneumoniae,* whereas macrophages cannot. In fact, the bacterium can survive for more than 90 minutes in a phagosome of a macrophage, during which it grows, replicates, and synthesizes and releases Apx toxins, leading to the death of these macrophages and release of the bacterium. Additionally, during this time, infected macrophages can move into alveolar and lobular septa, alveolar lumina, and perivascular and peribronchiolar tissues. Thus, when an infected macrophage is killed, large numbers of bacteria are released into vascularized ECM, leading to more inflammation, recruitment of neutrophils and macrophages, and exacerbation of injury to surrounding tissues.

Actinobacillus pleuropneumoniae has several virulence determinates that allow it to survive in phagosomes and resist the effects of phagosome-lysosome fusion, including a capsule, cell-wall LPS, copper-zinc superoxide dismutase, stress proteins, and ammonia. The capsule, cell-wall molecules, and superoxide dismutase participate in removing oxygen free radicals. The bacterium produces ammonia within phagosomes through the release of a potent urease, which inhibits phagosome-lysosome fusion and disrupts acid hydrolase activity in lysosomes. Finally, at low concentrations probably early in the disease process, RTX toxins (ApxI-III) produced by the bacterium also impair chemotaxis and phagocytosis by macrophages and neutrophils by likely acting to disrupt actin-myosin–directed movements of the cell or its organelles. At higher concentrations, such as those that occur after the bacteria has gone through several replication and kill cycles in macrophages, ApxI and ApxIII are highly toxic and ApxII is moderately toxic for macrophages and neutrophils. Additionally, ApxI-III are highly toxic to surrounding tissues, such as blood and lymphatic vessels, and ECM tissues, resulting in loss of barrier systems, increased vascular permeability with fibrin leakage and polymerization, hemorrhage, and vasculitis. In fact, it should be remembered that all of these infected cells and innocent bystander cells and tissues are within several hundred micrometers of one another and the vascular system. In particular, vascular injury appears to result from the activation and killing of intravascular macrophages and endothelial cells by Apx toxins and LPS. Activation results in the release of oxygen free radicals (superoxide anion, hydrogen peroxide, and hydroxyl radical) as well as proteolytic enzymes and various cytokines, all of which can injure endothelial cells of capillaries and postcapillary venules. Injury leads to activation of the coagulation, fibrinolysis, and kinin systems with concurrent hemorrhage, edema, effusions, platelet activation, and the formation of thrombi, ischemia, and subsequent coagulative necrosis of lung.

Rhodococcus Pneumonia (Rhodococcus equi)

The mechanism of injury in rhodococcal pneumonia is death of cells of the monocyte-macrophage system and of all cell populations in the respiratory system secondary to inflammation and its mediators and degradative enzymes. Gross lesions include (1) cranioventral chronic active pyogranulomatous pneumonia characterized by consolidated firm yellow-white lung parenchyma attributable to infiltrating inflammatory cells, abscesses, and granulomas in the affected lung tissue (see Fig. 9-67) and (2) necrotizing pyogranulomatous lymphadenitis of tracheobronchial lymph nodes of the lung exemplified by enlarged firm lymph nodes that on a cut surface have discrete and coalescing areas of yellow-white exudate infiltrating and compressing contiguous parenchyma (see Fig. 7-137). The latter lesion occurs through leukocyte trafficking of bacteria-infected alveolar macrophages as described below.

Foals encounter *Rhodococcus equi* through inhalation of the bacterium in manure-contaminated fomites or water droplets from the environment. It is a common bacterium of the soil, grows optimally at 30° C in the manure of most animal species, and has a very rapid generation time. When inhaled, the bacterium is deposited on the mucosae of the conductive and exchange systems by centrifugal and inertial turbulence. Here, bacteria encounter cells of the monocyte-macrophage system, including alveolar macrophages and dendritic cells, which phagocytose bacteria in the mucus layer of the mucociliary apparatus. These cells carry bacteria via leukocyte trafficking to local lymphoid tissues, such as BALT, through peribronchiolar and alveolar septal connective tissue, and to regional lymph nodes via afferent lymphatic vessels. *Rhodococcus equi* replicates intracellularly in alveolar and other tissue macrophages. Alveolar macrophages phagocytize *Rhodococcus equi* through ligand-receptor interactions. The bacterium must initially adhere to macrophages and requires that the bacterium be opsonized with either antibody or complement fragments that occur through complement fixation and the activation of the alternative complement pathway. In nonimmune foals, complement is the primary opsonin. The bacterium also expresses uncharacterized surface molecules that bind to membrane receptors expressed on alveolar macrophages before phagocytosis can occur. Leukocyte complement receptor, Mac-1, other complement receptors, mannose receptors, and potentially TLRs are expressed on alveolar macrophages.

Opsonized bacteria and the products of complement fixation facilitate the process of adhesion and invasion through phagocytosis into alveolar macrophages. Phagocytosis is mediated by bacterial virulence determinates that appear to restrict tropism to specific types of phagocytic cells. After phagocytosis by alveolar macrophages, the bacterium is confined within phagosomes. Experimental results from studies on fusion of phagosomes with lysosomes to form phagolysosomes are contradictory. Some studies suggest that *Rhodococcus equi* can block the fusion of lysosomes with phagosomes, which allows for the survival, persistence, and replication of bacteria intracellularly. Other studies suggest that *Rhodococcus equi* is not able to block phagosome-lysosome fusion; however, the bacterium is able to produce molecules that suppress acidification of phagolysosomes, resulting in their survival and replication in alveolar macrophages. The mechanism used to block fusion is unknown but appears to involve bacterium-directed compartmentalization of the fusion process so that they are selectively isolated from lysosomal effector molecules, such as acid, reactive oxygen, NO compounds, and lysosomal hydrolases within phagosomes. Other proteins and molecules appear to contribute to persistence and replication in alveolar macrophages. For example, strains of *Rhodococcus equi* that cause disease have chromosomal virulence determinates for capsular polysaccharide, cholesterol oxidase, phospholipase C, lecithinase, and cell-wall mycolic acids and plasmid virulence determinates for virulence-associated protein (VAP). It is also likely that mycolic acids from the bacterial cell wall are involved in the pathogenesis of the pyogranulomatous pneumonia characteristic of the disease.

Because *Rhodococcus equi* is able to disrupt normal phagosome-lysosome killing in alveolar macrophages and the generation of an oxidative burst that could kill the bacterium, it is able to persist and replicate. Studies suggest that rapid replication of bacterium within phagosomes and molecules such as cholesterol oxidase produced by the bacterium contribute to premature death of alveolar macrophages, leading to the release of large numbers of infectious organisms into adjacent tissue. Additionally, because the lifespan of fully differentiated alveolar macrophages is approximately 10 to 30 days, death of these cells related to aging and bacteria-induced injury releases large numbers of bacteria into adjacent tissue where they are phagocytosed by macrophages only to endlessly repeat the process. The severity and extent of the inflammatory response, concurrently with tissue injury, grows through the recruitment of additional monocytes and tissue macrophages from the circulatory system and regional lymph nodes. Neutrophils are active in the acute inflammatory response against *Rhodococcus equi*. They are able to phagocytose the bacterium, fuse the phagosome with the lysosome to form a phagolysosome, initiate an oxidative burst, and kill the bacterium. However, this process is an ineffective mechanism in controlling the disease and results in extensive tissue destruction through the release of lysosomal enzymes and reactive oxygen species, thus contributing to the cyclic and progressive destruction of pulmonary parenchyma. This damage allows large numbers of bacteria to gain access to the alveoli and bronchioles and encounter mucus of the mucous membranes and the mucociliary apparatus. In general, the mucociliary apparatus is not directly affected by *Rhodococcus equi*, thus the bacterium is moved up the conductive system to the nasopharynx where it is swallowed and gains access via peristalsis to the alimentary system.

Respiratory Anthrax (Bacillus anthracis)

The mechanism of injury in respiratory anthrax is cell death caused by bacterial toxins that act directly on cell membranes leading to acute coagulative necrosis. Gross lesions include pulmonary and lymph node edema, hemorrhage, and necrosis.

Animals encounter *Bacillus anthracis* through inhalation of fomites contaminated with endospores from soil. Fomites containing endospores must be less than 5 μm in diameter to reach the O_2-CO_2 exchange portion of the respiratory system. Infected fomites are deposited on the mucosae, where they are then phagocytosed either by alveolar macrophages migrating through and on the surface of the mucosae or by dendritic cells. Infected macrophages and dendritic cells spread the bacterium to regional lymph nodes (bronchiolar and mediastinal) via afferent lymphatic vessels through leukocyte trafficking. During the migration process, endospores germinate into vegetative bacteria, so on arrival at the lymph nodes, bacteria are already producing anthrax toxins, which kill infected cells and release the bacteria into the ECM of the lymph nodes. In lymph nodes, bacteria continue to replicate and produce anthrax toxins killing additional lymphoid and endothelial cells, leading to edema and hemorrhage. The bacterium and its toxins enter lymphatic vessels and spread via the thoracic duct into the circulatory system as a septicemia, where endothelial cells and cells of other organ systems are injured, leading to edema, hemorrhage, and cell necrosis.

Contagious Bovine Pleuropneumonia (Mycoplasma mycoides *var.* mycoides *Small Colony)*

Little is known about the mechanisms used by *Mycoplasma mycoides* var. *mycoides* small colony (SC) to cause disease in the respiratory system of cattle, thus much of this section is speculative and based on a reasonable probability that lesions that occur are the result of underlying and known pathobiologic mechanisms. The mechanism of injury in contagious bovine pleuropneumonia is cell death likely caused by inflammation and its mediators and degradative enzymes and by vasculitis leading to thrombosis, ischemia, and infarction of lung tissue. Gross lesions include (1) fibrinous pleural effusion and fibrinous pleuritis with hemorrhage and (2) fibrinous pleuropneumonia with prominent interlobular septa filled with fibrinous effusion and fibrin thrombi (Fig. 4-22). Infarcts occur in affected lung tissues probably arising from vascular injury leading to permeability changes, vasculitis with activation of clotting cascades, thrombosis, and infarction. Infarcted lung often appears as sequestra likely arising from reparative mechanisms that isolate the dead infarcted tissue via fibrosis. It is unclear how infarcts occur in lung tissue when it has a dual blood supply, unless infarcts occur in areas that lack a dual supply or vasculitis and thrombosis concurrently affect vessels of each arterial source.

Cattle (and probably sheep and goats) encounter *Mycoplasma mycoides* var. *mycoides* SC through inhalation of fomites and fluid droplets. These droplets are deposited on mucosae of the conductive component of the respiratory system by centrifugal and inertial turbulence where they are trapped in the mucus layer and are subsequently phagocytosed by alveolar macrophages. Ligand-receptor interactions are probably involved in target cell specificity. Alveolar macrophages in all probability spread the bacterium to local lymphoid tissue such as BALT, in which the bacterium replicates and kills infected macrophages releasing bacterium into bronchiolar and alveolar interstitium, causing severe acute inflammation and the characteristic fibrinous lesions and vasculitis. How the bacterium evades killing by phagosome-lysosome fusion, produces toxic molecules that injure and kill cells, spreads to blood vessels, and causes vasculitis and thrombosis is unknown. Bacterial membrane lipoprotein LppQ, a common antigen of *Mycoplasma mycoides* ssp. *mycoides*, could be involved in some of these processes. Highly virulent strains of the bacterium are known to produce and release large quantities of H_2O_2 that are cytotoxic for all cells. H_2O_2 release appears to be correlated with adhesion of the bacterium to host cell membranes. It also appears that macrophages may spread the bacterium via leukocyte trafficking systemically to lymph nodes and synovium and joint space of joints such as the carpus where inflammation characteristic of the disease also occurs.

Bovine Tuberculosis (Mycobacterium bovis)

The mechanism of injury in bovine tuberculosis is death of cells of the monocyte-macrophage system and of all cell populations in the lung and associated regional lymph nodes secondary to

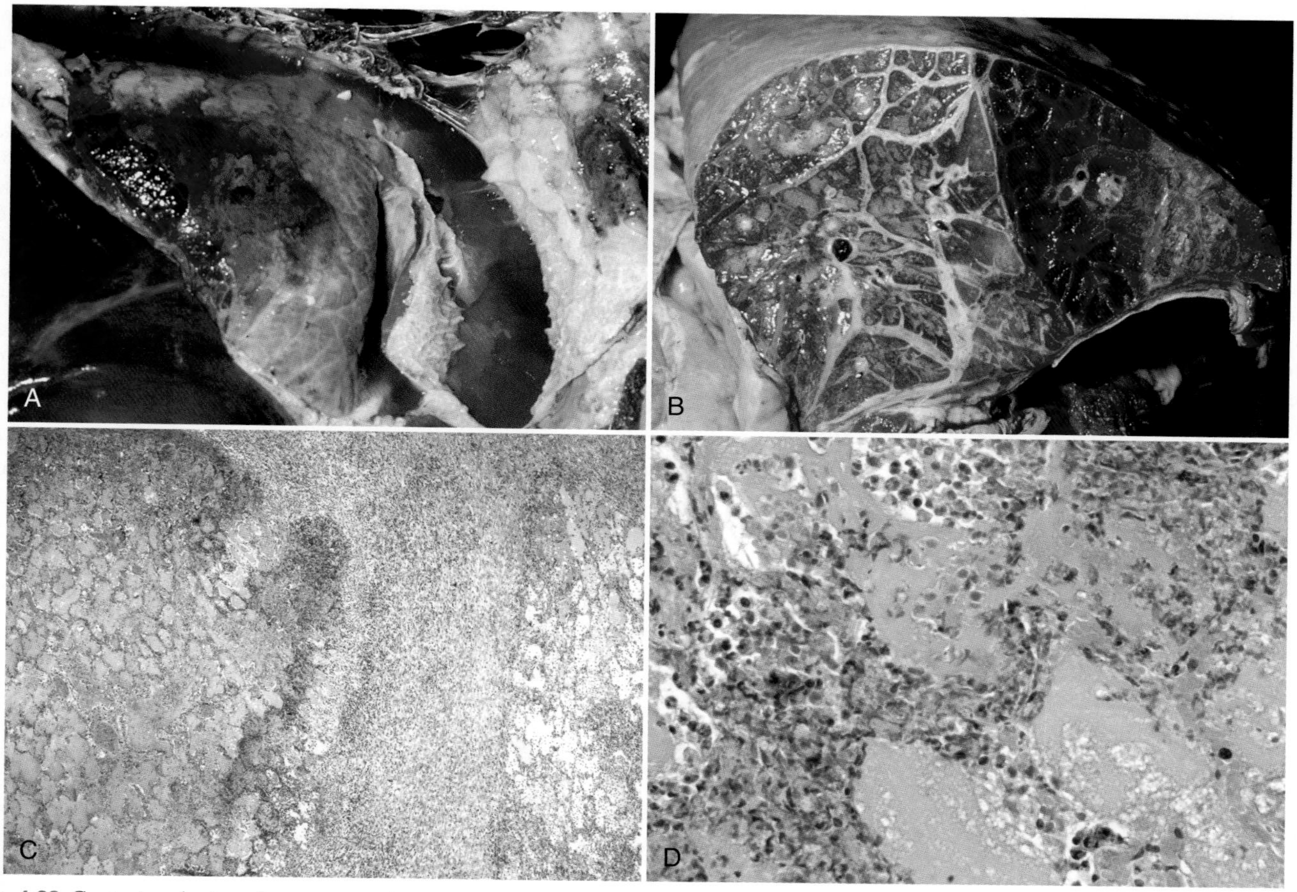

Fig. 4-22 Contagious bovine pleuropneumonia.
A, Thoracic cavity. The thoracic cavity is filled with a fibrinous pleural effusion and the visceral and parietal pleurae are covered by fibrin (fibrinous pleuritis). Also note the areas of hemorrhage affecting the pleurae and the subjacent lung. **B,** Transverse section of lung. Note the prominent interlobular septa filled with fibrinous effusion and fibrin thrombi and additionally the area of hemorrhage (right half of the section). Infarcts with pulmonary sequestra (not shown here) can occur in affected lung tissues likely arising from vascular injury leading to infarction. **C,** The interlobular septum *(center)* is filled with acute inflammatory cells mixed with a fibrinous effusion. Alveoli are filled with highly proteinaceous edema fluid, fibrinous effusion, and acute inflammatory cells. There is extensive necrosis of all tissues at the interface between alveoli and the interlobar septum *(dark blue staining band)*. H&E stain. **D,** Higher magnification of **C.** The dark blue color is attributable to necrosis of cells, including neutrophils leading to escape and coagulation of nucleic acids from degenerate nuclei in the inflammatory exudate. Alveoli are filled with edema fluid and acute inflammatory cells. H&E stain. (**A** and **B** courtesy Dr. D. Gregg, Plum Island Animal Disease Center and Noah's Arkive, College of Veterinary Medicine, The University of Georgia. **C** and **D** courtesy Dr. J. F. Zachary, College of Veterinary Medicine, University of Illinois.)

granulomatous inflammation and its mediators and degradative enzymes. Gross lesions include (1) enlarged lymph nodes that contain discrete and coalescing granulomas (tubercles) formed by dry and gritty (mineralized) yellow-white to green-white caseous exudate often encapsulated by fibrous connective tissue (see Fig. 1-19) and (2) lung parenchyma that contains similar granulomas distributed at random in some or all lung lobes (see Figs. 9-65 and 9-68).

Cattle (and probably sheep and goats) encounter *Mycobacterium bovis* through inhalation of fomites and fluid droplets contaminated with the bacterium. These droplets are deposited on mucosae of the conductive component of the respiratory system by centrifugal and inertial turbulence where they are trapped in the mucus layer and are subsequently phagocytosed by alveolar and tissue macrophages. Macrophages appear to use several routes to spread the bacterium across mucosal barriers and then to regional lymph nodes and the lung. Macrophages in the pharynx cross the mucosal barrier, migrate to the tonsil, and spread the bacterium to infect naïve macrophages in tonsillar tissues. Macrophages in other regions of mucosae encounter and phagocytose bacteria and spread them via lymphatic vessels to local lymphoid tissues and then via lymphatic vessels to regional lymph nodes such as the retropharyngeal and parotid nodes to infect naïve macrophages in these nodes.

Bacteria that are deposited in the mucus layer of mucosae of bronchi and bronchioles are phagocytosed by alveolar macrophages and spread via lymphatic vessels to local lymphoid tissues (BALT) and then via lymphatic vessels to regional lymph nodes, such as the tracheobronchial and mediastinal nodes, to infect naïve macrophages in these nodes. The primary goal of *Mycobacterium bovis* is to be phagocytosed by macrophages. In the mucus layer, macrophages encounter trapped bacteria via random movement. Once bacteria are in contact with macrophages, bacteria adhere and bind to pathogen PRRs on macrophage cell membranes. The process used by macrophages to phagocytose *Mycobacterium bovis* involves ligand-receptor interactions. In fact, the bacterium appears to utilize multiple membrane pathogen PRRs such as those for complement (CR1, 3, and 4), mannose, surfactant protein, and CD14 protein to enter macrophages. Some receptors are probably used in the early mucosal phases of infection when inflammation is minimal, whereas other receptors, such as those for complement, are used when vascular changes in lymph nodes and lung induced by acute inflammation result in permeability changes and the release of plasma proteins and complement into inflamed tissues.

Mycobacterium bovis is able to activate the alternative pathway of complement and use C3b and C3bi fragments to opsonize its surface and then bind to complement receptors CR1, 3, and/or 4 on cell membranes of macrophages. This binding results in phagocytosis of the bacterium in phagosomes. Mannose receptors, surfactant proteins and receptors, and lipoarabinomannan (LAM) and CD14 receptors are also involved in phagocytosis. It appears that the use of multiple ligands and pathogen PRRs ensures that the bacterium once inhaled or ingested can be phagocytosed by monocytes, macrophages, and/or even neutrophils that migrate to the site of local infection in response to chemokines secreted by infected macrophages. Subsequently, these cells can then be used to spread the infection to other regional or systemic sites, such as the liver, spleen, lymph nodes, and intestines, via leukocyte trafficking in the blood or lymphatic vascular systems.

Once present in a phagosome, *Mycobacterium bovis* is able to disrupt phagosome-lysosome fusion and prevent activation of macrophage antimicrobial mechanisms such as production of reactive oxygen or nitrogen intermediates and phagosome acidification. The bacterium is able to grow and replicate in the phagosome, but with cellular aging, infected macrophages die and release bacteria into the vascularized ECM tissues. This outcome results in repetitive cycles of inflammation and the recruitment of additional monocytes, macrophages, and neutrophils into the granuloma (tubercle). The formation of granulomas (tubercles) is covered in detail in Chapter 3, but components of the poorly digestible, waxy cell wall of the bacterium, such as sulpholipids and LAM, appear to contribute to the type of inflammatory response that ensues and the formation of granulomas.

Cardiovascular System and Lymphatic Vessels

Edema Disease (Escherichia coli)

The pathogenesis of edema disease begins as an alimentary enterotoxemia and ends as a fibrinoid arteriopathy/arteriolopathy of the vascular system, especially of the brain, leading to ischemia and malacia. The enterotoxemia phase is discussed in the section on the Alimentary System; the nervous system phase is discussed in the section on the Nervous System. The mechanism of injury is injury and death (coagulative necrosis) of endothelial and smooth muscle cells of arteries and arterioles caused by Shiga toxin 2e (also known as *verotoxin 2e*) produced by hemolytic strains of *E. coli.* After colonization of the intestinal mucosae, the toxin is absorbed from the alimentary system and circulates in the blood vascular system. Cells susceptible to the affects of this toxin include endothelial and smooth muscle cells of arteries and arterioles that express receptors for the toxin such as globotetraosylceramide, galactosylgloboside, and globotriaosylceramide. Toxin acts to disrupt protein synthesis leading to vascular permeability changes and cell death and thus edema of affected organs, most notably the eyelids, ventral neck (jowls), the gastric and colonic mesenteries, and the nervous system (see Figs. 7-126 and 7-127). Additionally, endothelial injury caused by this toxin may lead to hemorrhage, intravascular coagulation, microthrombosis, and infarction.

*Embolic Vasculopathy/Vasculitis (*Actinobacillus equuli, Escherichia coli, Staphylococcus *spp.,* Streptococcus *spp.,* Fusobacterium necrophorum*)*

This section covers a variety of diseases in which the key component of the underlying pathogenesis is embolization through the blood vascular system, leading to vasculitis and potentially thrombosis and ischemia. Such embolic diseases most commonly begin in the skin/subcutis or mucosae but end in a wide variety of highly vascularized organ systems. Examples of embolic diseases include white spotted kidney disease (*E. coli*), embolic nephritis (foal shigellosis [*Actinobacillus equuli*]), milk spots in the liver (*E. coli*), bacterial endocarditis (*E. coli*), and bacterial hepatitis (*Fusobacterium necrophorum*). Embolization also occurs in diseases caused by angioinvasive fungi, and they are covered in the section on fungal diseases. The mechanism of injury in embolic vasculopathy/vasculitis is cell death, probably acute coagulative necrosis, caused by bacterial toxins and inflammation and its mediators and degradative enzymes. Gross lesions include gray-white foci of necrosis and inflammation distributed at random (vascular embolization pattern) in tissue such as occur in renal actinobacillosis of foals (see Fig. 11-42).

Bacteria are able to enter and spread in the vascular system by two mechanisms: (1) direct entry into a blood vessel or (2) establishment of a local infection followed by invasion of the vascular system. The former category usually results from bacteria gaining direct access to blood vessels secondary to penetrating trauma, bite wounds, or lacerations, whereas the latter category usually is caused by similar traumatic injury that leads to local inflammation and often abscess formation. In the direct entry mechanism, access to the vascular system, embolization, and entrapment in capillary beds are likely physical interactions based on the anatomy of vascular distribution patterns, physiology of vascular flow and pressures, and pathobiology of endothelial cell surface molecules. As an example in the cerebral cortices, lesions caused by bacterial emboli tend to be observed at the interface between gray and white matter. Anatomically, at this location, capillaries penetrate through the gray matter from the overlying meninges and as they run into the white matter they make abrupt turns (90-degree), so capillaries can run parallel to fiber tracts in the white matter. This flow change causes vascular turbulence and endothelial cell surface perturbations, and under the proper conditions, activation of Virchow's triad can result in the formation of vascular endothelial surfaces that may be sticky or have attached fibrin that can entrap bacteria. Many of the bacterial virulence determinates discussed throughout this chapter, as well as ligand-receptor interactions, probably are involved to some extent in the origination and entrapment and growth of bacterial emboli in the direct entry mechanism.

In the establishment of a local infection mechanism, contamination of the umbilicus at birth and the skin/subcutis through management practices, such as tail docking, castration, and ear notching, are the common means of establishing local infections. Injury of mucosae, such as occurs in the abomasum from lactic acidosis in grain overload, also provides opportunities for bacteria to enter the portal blood vascular system and then embolize to and colonize the liver. Finally, bacteria that induce biofilms or cause irresolvable inflammatory processes, such as in a dermatitis, otitis, cellulitis, periodontal disease, arthritis, or abscesses, can serve as a site for intermittent bacteremia and embolization. Many of the bacterial virulence determinates discussed throughout this chapter, as well as ligand-receptor interactions, probably are involved to some extent in the origination and entrapment and growth of bacterial emboli in the local infection mechanism.

Septicemic Anthrax (Bacillus anthracis)

The sections in this chapter on alimentary and inhalation anthrax should be reviewed for background information pertinent to understanding septicemic anthrax (see Fig. 7-135). Once vegetative forms of the bacteria enter the circulatory system from the respiratory or alimentary systems, septicemia ensues and vascular collapse occurs, resulting from massive release of toxins into the blood plasma. Septicemic anthrax is characterized by animals found dead unexpectedly, often in a classic sawhorse stance and with hemorrhage (unclotted) from body orifices (Fig. 4-23). If inadvertently opened, the spleen will be enlarged and unclotted blood will exit from cut surfaces; lymph nodes will be enlarged, edematous, and hemorrhagic; and body tissues and serosal surfaces will be edematous and hemorrhagic (see Fig. 4-23). Necropsies should not be performed on animals that are suspected of dying from anthrax because the vegetative form proliferates in large numbers in blood; when they are released from lacerated blood vessels onto the ground, they form endospores, which contaminate the area long-term.

In the circulatory system, vegetative forms proliferate in large numbers and are arranged in long chains in the capillary beds of many organ systems, including the spleen (see Fig. 13-53). Large quantities of edema toxin and lethal toxin are released into the blood, causing dysfunction and cell death of endothelial cells and their barrier systems, thus the toxins increase the permeability of the capillary wall, leading to edema, vasodilation, and hemorrhage in infected organ systems. Anthrax toxins also disrupt the clotting cascade likely through massive activation of DIC and consumption of clotting factors, resulting in unclotted blood at body orifices and within tissues and organs.

*Vascular Leptospirosis (*Leptospira *spp.)*

The mechanism of injury in vascular leptospirosis is cell death caused by (1) physical properties (penetrating movements) of bacteria that disrupt functions of endothelial cells and (2) bacterial toxins that act directly on membranes of endothelial cells of small blood vessels, including capillaries of the systemic vasculature in all organ systems, leading to coagulative necrosis of affected cells. Gross lesions include acute vasculitis (endothelial cell necrosis) with systemic petechial and ecchymotic hemorrhages, edema, and DIC affecting all organ systems and serosal surfaces (see Fig. 2-18).

Animals encounter *Leptospira* spp. through direct contact of their oral or conjunctival mucous membranes or skin with leptospira-infected urine or with water from reservoirs or ponds into which infected urine drains. Ingestion may also serve as a portal of entry if water contaminated with leptospira is consumed and the bacteria encounter mucosae of the intestine. During mastication and swallowing, it is likely that the mucosae of the oral pharynx trap the bacteria in its mucus layer. After swallowing and through intestinal peristalsis, the bacteria are moved into contact with villi and crypts, where they are probably trapped in the mucus layer and encounter enterocytes. In the conjunctiva, it is also likely that the mucosae trap the bacteria in a mucus layer. For infection to occur, it has been suggested that the skin and mucosae must have small cuts or abrasions that allow the bacteria to penetrate into the vascularized submucosal or subcutaneous connective tissues and gain access to capillaries and/or postcapillary venules. However, the bacteria are motile and likely able to penetrate mucus layers and invade mucosae by moving directly through mucosal epithelial cells or between the cells through intracellular junctional complexes. In all three of these portals of entry, the goal is for the bacteria to reach well-vascularized ECM tissues. As a group, these spirochetes are highly motile and invasive and using its invasive motility (virulence determinate), it is able to penetrate the vascular wall and endothelial cells of capillaries and postcapillary venules to gain access to the circulatory system. *Leptospira* spp. may also invade lymphatic vessels and through this system and the thoracic duct eventually gain access to the circulatory system. *Leptospira* spp. are able to grow and replicate in the circulatory system and then spread systemically to all organ systems. To infect other organs such as the kidney and

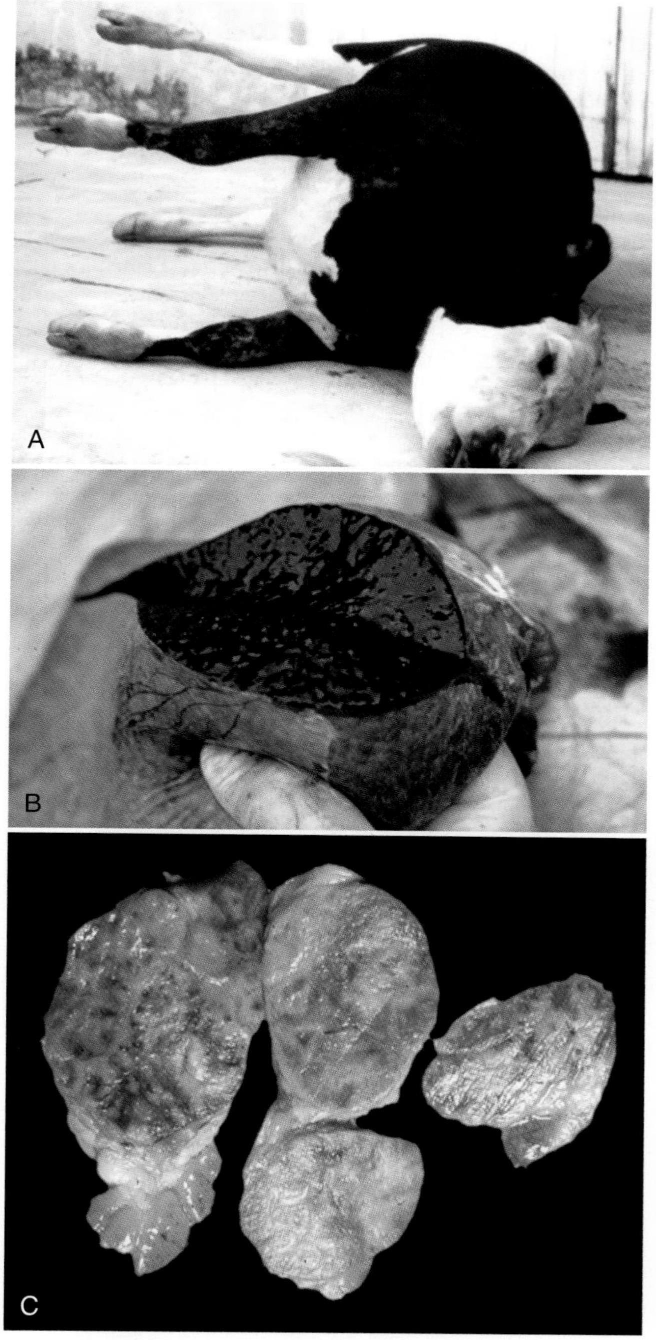

Fig. 4-23 Anthrax, ox.
A, Because of the high fever, cadavers of cattle dying of anthrax decompose rapidly with the usual result of excessive gas formation in the GI tract, abdominal distention and resultant "saw horse" position of the legs. **B,** The spleen is enlarged and bloody (splenomegaly, bloody spleen). A postmortem examination should not be performed on an animal suspected of dying from anthrax. Air-dried impression smears of blood from external orifices or from an ear vein can be stained and the bacterium identified (see Fig. 7-135). **C,** Lymph nodes are also enlarged and bloody as a result of anthrax toxins that destroy vascular endothelial cells (see Fig. 13-53). Anthrax toxin can also cause severe injury to the intestines (see Fig. 7-135) and lungs. (**A** courtesy Dr. D. Driemeier, Federal University of Rio Grande do Sul, Brazil. **B** and **C** courtesy Dr. J. King, College of Veterinary Medicine, Cornell University.)

liver, it appears that the bacteria must first attach to endothelial cell membranes via adhesins before invading these cells and their underlying vascularized tissues and then interact with renal tubular epithelial cells and hepatocytes.

Leptospira spp. initially spread through the vascular system to all tissues of the body and do not appear to specifically target the kidney or liver via a tropism (attraction to a specific cell type or tissue) mechanism. However, once epithelial cells are infected, the reason for dominance of lesions in these organs is unclear and may be related to some essential trophism (nourishment of tissues) provided by these cells to the bacteria for colonization and proliferation.

In the context of interacting with capillary endothelial cells and probably renal epithelium, surface-associated proteins (outer membrane leptospiral protein) appear to be involved in ligand-receptor interactions that facilitate adhesion to host cell receptors like cell-adhesion molecules and ECM proteins (Len protein family). Adhesion to cells also appears to cause an increased expression of adhesion receptors such as E-selectin on endothelial cells resulting in additional adhesion of bacteria, platelets, and neutrophils (acute inflammatory response). This response may be attributable to bacteria wall LPS, peptidoglycans, and outer membrane proteins, thus promoting inflammation in capillaries leading to vasculitis and hemorrhage. Bacterial LPS likely activates cells by binding to TLRs on host cell membranes. *Leptospira* spp. also produce pore-forming hemolysins, proteases, sphingomyelinases, and collagenases that may assist in this process, but their role in causing endothelial cell injury remains to be determined.

Glanders (Burkholderia mallei; *Farcy, Malleus, Droes*)

The mechanism of injury in glanders is cell death caused by pyogranulomatous inflammation and its mediators and degradative enzymes. It is a disease of lymphatic vessels (and surrounding integument) and of the respiratory system. Gross lesions include ulcers, pustules, and nodules that can affect any part of the body but most frequently involve the skin and lymphatic vessels of the legs and flanks (Fig. 4-24). Nodules typically occur along the course

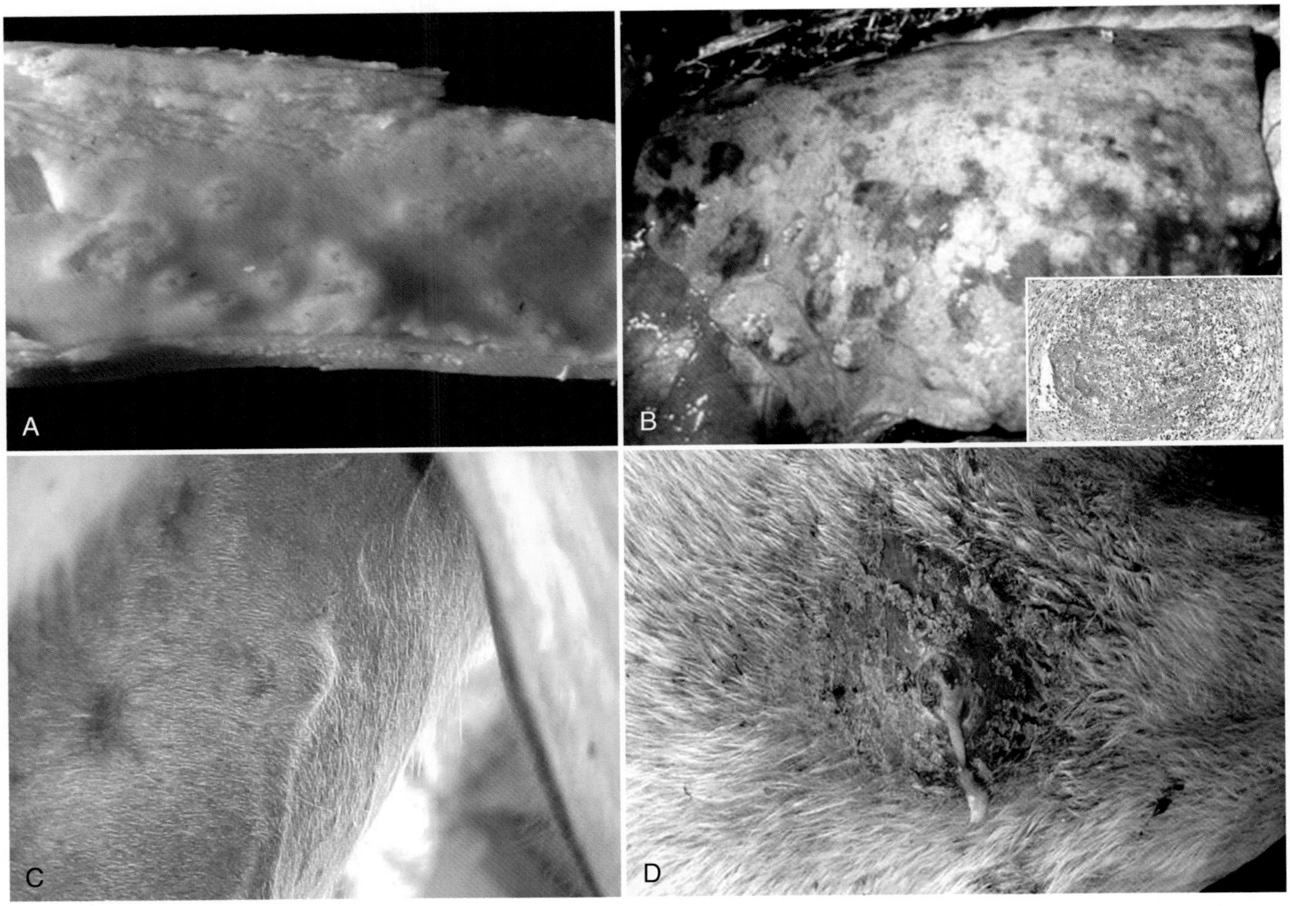

Fig. 4-24 Glanders disease.

A, Mucosa, nasal turbinates, multiple nasal ulcers, and granulomas. *Burkholderia mallei* colonizes the nasal turbinates resulting in pyogranulomatous inflammation, necrosis, and ulceration of the mucosa. **B,** When the bacterium colonizes the mucosae of the conductive system of the lung, it spreads into pulmonary parenchyma resulting in the formation of pyogranulomas *(inset)* throughout the lung. *Inset,* H&E stain. **C,** When the bacterium spreads to the skin, it colonizes subcutaneous lymphatic vessels resulting in the formation of pyogranulomatous nodules that typically occur along the course of lymphatic vessels (pyogranulomatous lymphangitis) resulting in a raised beaded appearance of the skin. **D,** These nodules frequently rupture because of trauma to the skin or from pressure necrosis due to the expanding volume of exudate within the nodules. This process results in crater-like ulcers of the skin that discharge a thick yellowish-white viscid and sticky purulent material containing abundant bacteria. (**A** courtesy Dr. D.D. Harrington, School of Veterinary Medicine, Purdue University; and Noah's Arkive, College of Veterinary Medicine, The University of Georgia. **B** courtesy United States Animal Health Association, St. Joseph, MO. **B inset** courtesy Dr. Tyler, College of Veterinary Medicine, University of Georgia and Noah's Arkive, College of Veterinary Medicine, University of Georgia. **C** courtesy Dr. D. Driemeier, Federal University of Rio Grande do Sul, Brazil. **D** courtesy Dr. R. Mota, Universidad Federal Rural de Pernambuco, Recife, Brazil and Dr. M. Brito, Universidad Federal Rural do Rio de Janeiro, Brazil.)

of lymphatic vessels resulting in a raised beaded appearance of the skin. These nodules often rupture because of trauma to the skin or from pressure necrosis caused by the expanding volume of exudate within the nodules. This process results in craterlike ulcers of the skin that discharge a thick yellowish-white viscid and sticky purulent material containing abundant bacteria (see Fig. 4-24), and the outcome has been called *farcy pipes.* In the respiratory system, pyogranulomas can occur in mucosae of the nasal cavity and in all lobes of the lungs (random pattern).

Horses, mules and donkeys encounter *Burkholderia mallei*, a facultative intracellular bacterium that resides in the soil, via fomites that (1) penetrate the skin by trauma or foreign objects or (2) are inhaled and/or ingested. In either case, these fomites are contaminated with bacteria-laden exudate derived from other infected animals with cutaneous lesions or nasal discharge. It appears that cutaneous glanders can occur through two mechanisms: (1) direct penetration of the skin or (2) through systemic spread to the skin via a systemic bacteremia or leukocytic trafficking from an initial infection of the respiratory or intestinal mucosae. For direct penetration, the skin apparently must have small cuts or abrasions that allow the bacterium to penetrate the subcutaneous connective tissues, gain access to lymphatic vessels, and cause infection and inflammation. Target cells for infection in the cutaneous lymphatic vessels and skin are unknown. Additionally, the role of ligand-receptor interactions in this process has not been determined. It appears that lesions characteristic of glanders probably result from inflammatory responses directed against a variety of molecules within the bacterium, resulting in pyogranulomatous inflammation.

For systemic spread to the skin, the bacterium appears to encounter mucosae of the nasal cavity and conductive component of the respiratory system. It is likely trapped in the mucus layer and then colonizes the mucosae. The development of a biofilm (virulence determinate) may be important in the colonization process. Once mucosae are colonized, the bacterium could then be phagocytosed by mucosal macrophages and/or dendritic cells and carried through mucosae to MALTs such as BALT. It is also possible, but unknown, that the bacterium has a mechanism to penetrate the mucus layer, enter the apical surfaces of mucosal epithelial cells via endocytosis or transcytosis, and exit the lateral-basal surfaces to gain access to mucosal-associated lymphoid tissues. In these lymphoid tissues, the target cells for infection and the role of ligand-receptor interactions have not been determined but appear to result in the nasal and pulmonary pyogranulomas characteristic of the disease. Cells of the monocyte-macrophage system and possibly mucosal dendritic cells probably play a role in the infection, replication, and spread of the bacterium. Once in MALTs, the bacterium could spread to regional lymph nodes in lymphatic vessels (1) as a cell-free bacteremia or (2) via leukocytic trafficking in macrophages, and after infection of and replication in lymphoid tissues, the bacterium could then spread systemically via lymphatic vessels and the thoracic duct to the circulatory system. Via the circulatory system, the bacterium ultimately arrives (cell free or in macrophages) at capillary beds of the skin, passes through the endothelial cells (leukocytic trafficking, endocytosis, or transcytosis), enters the subcutaneous tissues, encounters cutaneous lymphatic vessels, and elicits a pyogranulomatous inflammatory response in these tissues. Pyogranulomas have also been described in the spleen and liver.

Lesions in the respiratory system probably arise from an extension of the processes involved in colonizing mucosae as previously described, with secondary spread into adjacent interstitial tissues and alveoli. Additionally, it is possible that pyogranulomas in the lung could arise from spread of the bacterium through the circulatory system as a cell-free bacteremia or in macrophages as described. The existence of this mechanism of spread has not been determined.

Through ingestion and gastrointestinal peristalsis, *Burkholderia mallei* can also potentially reach the alimentary system. Herein, they could encounter the mucus layer of intestinal mucosae or M cells overlying Peyer's patches. How the bacterium could penetrate the mucus layer is unknown, but it could involve mucosae-associated macrophages as discussed previously in respiratory system mucosae. Bacteria could also infect M cells via endocytosis, undergo endocytosis or transcytosis, and exit the basal surfaces via exocytosis to gain access to macrophages within Peyer's patches. For either of these two pathways, macrophages within Peyer's patches could then be infected with bacteria and be used to spread bacteria systemically. The likely goal of these types of mucosal encounters is to provide the bacterium with the opportunity to infect the local lymphoid tissues and then gain access to local, regional, and systemic lymph nodules and the circulatory system directly or via macrophages.

How and if the bacterium evades killing by phagosome-lysosome fusion, replicates, and spreads to cutaneous lymphatic vessels via the circulatory system are unknown. Type III and IV secretion systems (virulence determinates) may be possible mechanisms for the invasion, escape from lysosomes or phagolysosomes, and survival in target cells. The bacterium is surrounded by a type I O-antigenic polysaccharide (capsular) antigen, a virulence determinate, that may also block phagocytosis or phagosome-lysosome fusion. LPS, which likely contains a lipid A component, may play a role in tissue injury. Additionally, an interaction of the bacterium with cell membranes is a prerequisite for infection to occur. A type IV pilin-like protein may be involved in the adherence of the bacterium to target cells.

Urinary System

Pulpy Kidney (Overeating) Disease (Clostridium perfringens)

The pathogenesis of pulpy kidney disease begins as an enterotoxemia caused by *Clostridium perfringens,* and this disease in the section on the alimentary system should be reviewed. Because ε-toxin is a permease that alters cell permeability, the vascular beds in affected intestinal tissues readily absorb toxins into the circulatory system. It appears that the sequence of events leading to pulpy kidney disease occur in the first phase or early in the second phase of alimentary enterotoxemia before toxin-induced massive necrosis of the intestine occurs. The mechanism of injury in pulpy kidney disease is cell death caused by ε-toxin that acts directly on renal endothelial and tubular epithelial cell membranes leading to vascular permeability changes and acute coagulative necrosis of tubular cells. Microthrombosis and ischemia from capillary endothelial injury are plausible but unproved mechanisms of tubular cell death. Gross lesions include soft pliable kidneys with hemorrhages; however, the lesions are often attributed to postmortem change. Experimental data suggest that vascular endothelial cells, such as those in the renal cortex supplying epithelial cells of renal tubules, express receptors (ligand-receptor interactions) for ε-toxin. Because ε-toxin is an angiotoxic permease, it increases the permeability of targeted endothelial cells, allowing plasma containing ε-toxin to leak into the ECM surrounding renal tubules. Renal tubular epithelial cells also express receptors for ε-toxin, and toxin binding may lead to membrane-mediated cytotoxicity and cell death.

Necrohemorrhagic Urocystitis (Escherichia coli, Corynebacterium renale, Pseudomonas *spp.*, Proteus vulgaris, or Klebsiella pneumoniae)

Necrohemorrhagic urocystitis is a term used to group bacteria whose virulence determinates can cause acute inflammation and hemorrhage of the mucosae of the urinary bladder, especially affecting transitional epithelial cells and the lamina propria and its capillary beds. Because more is known about virulence determinates for uropathogenic *E. coli,* it is discussed in greater detail; however, the other bacteria listed in this group likely use similar or related mechanisms to cause disease. The mechanism of injury is probably cell death (coagulative necrosis) caused by bacterial toxins that act directly on mucosal epithelial cells and capillaries in the lamina propria of the bladder and acute and chronic inflammation and their effector molecules and degradative enzymes. Gross lesions of the bladder include mucosal edema and mucosae that are rough and granular, red to dark red, and covered with white-gray flecks of fibrin mixed with cellular debris (see Fig. 11-64). Blood vessels in the wall and serosa of the bladder are prominent; this change is due to active hyperemia of the fluidic vascular phase of acute inflammation.

Animals encounter these bacteria through contact with them in fomites or fluid droplets of urinary or fecal origin. They commonly become commensal organisms that reside in the mucous membranes of the vagina and prepuce. Physical changes in pressure across the tubular components of the urinary and reproductive systems caused by parturition and breeding appear to force these commensal bacteria via reflux mechanisms into the urethra and urinary bladder. The length of the urethra, in part, appears to determine why females have cystitis more commonly than males. Environmental stressors, such as peak lactation, traumatic mucosal injury, and a high-protein diet that increases the pH of the urine, make mucosae more susceptible to colonization and alter the commensal relationship, allowing the bacteria to replicate in sufficient numbers to colonize the mucosae of the urinary and reproductive systems and spread bacteria to other animals. Once in the lumen of the urinary bladder, bacteria gain access to mucosal surfaces via random movement of the urine. The urinary mucosae lacks goblet cells, thus there is no mucus layer to penetrate. These bacteria encounter the apical surface of transitional epithelial cells, and using ligand-receptor interactions characteristic of other bacterial diseases, begin the process of adherence, binding, and colonization of the mucosae. Uropathogenic *E. coli* expresses adhesins, such as type 1 fimbriae, P fimbriae, and S fimbriae, that are involved in this process. These fimbriae (also known as *pili*) bind to hexagonal arrays of mannosyl-glycoprotein receptors known as *uroplakins.* They are expressed on the apical (and luminal) surfaces of specialized transitional epithelial cells called *umbrella cells.* The tips of the type 1 fimbriae express a ligand called *FimH adhesin* that binds to these uroplakin receptors.

Once bound, the bacteria begin a complicated process of entering and colonizing the cells and mucosae, respectively, through a series of conformational changes in the apical surface of the umbrella cells, leading to cytoskeletal rearrangements and cell entry by a zipper mechanism. Bacterial flagella may also have a role in this mechanism. This process results in colonization of the mucosae and the development of a biofilm-like arrangement affecting the mucosae (also known as *biomasses of bacteria* or *intracellular bacterial communities*). After formation of intracellular bacterial communities, bacteria kill infected umbrella cells via hemolysins that produce pores in membranes, thus releasing bacteria into the lumen of the bladder where they colonize new umbrella cells and repeat the infective process or are released into the environment during urination. The edema, hemorrhage, and necrosis characteristic of necrohemorrhagic urocystitis appear to be caused by acute inflammation and a variety of virulence determinates in highly pathogenic strains of uropathogenic *E. coli* and likely the other bacteria listed previously. Acute inflammation is probably induced via TLRs that recruit neutrophils from the vascular system into the lamina propria and mucosae and in response to cell necrosis, loss of the mucosal barrier, and interaction of the vascularized lamina propria with bacterial toxins. In umbrella cells infected by bacteria, bacterial toxins, such as LT and ST toxins, Shiga-like toxin, cytotoxins, and endotoxin, likely diffuse through the mucosae and cause membrane injury, leading to cell death (necrosis) and loss of the mucosal barrier system. These toxins may also stimulate apoptotic cell death, leading to release of bacteria into the urine. Once dead, these cells slough into the urine and endotoxins and other toxic molecules can be absorbed into the highly vascularized lamina propria, resulting in injury to the capillaries and acute vasculitis with active hyperemia.

Other virulence determinates that contribute to the pathogenesis of necrohemorrhagic urocystitis include bacterial surface molecules such as capsular K antigens and LPS that block phagocytosis and killing of the bacteria by neutrophils and macrophages. Uropathogenic *E. coli* usually produces siderophores that play a role in iron acquisition for the bacteria during and after colonization. The lytic actions of hemolysins also increase the availability of iron and other nutrients for bacterial growth in colonized mucosae. Hemolysins also can kill lymphocytes and block phagocytosis and chemotaxis by phagocytic cells. Some strains of uropathogenic *E. coli* have a virulence determinate for the production of urease, which hydrolyzes ammonia in urine into urea, resulting in an alkaline urine that causes additional injury to mucosae. Finally, these bacteria can readily exchange genetic information with less virulent bacterial strains by transduction and conjugation using drug resistance, toxin, and other virulence plasmids. These factors are a few of the reasons why it is often difficult to treat and resolve certain types of acute and chronic bladder infections.

Contagious Bovine Pyelonephritis (Corynebacterium renale *or* Escherichia coli)

Contagious bovine pyelonephritis is most commonly caused by *Corynebacterium renale*, but *E. coli* may also cause this disease. These bacteria are likely commensal organisms that reside in the mucous membranes of the vagina and prepuce. Mechanisms that contribute to the occurrence of cystitis that preceded pyelonephritis are discussed in the previous section. Information about the mechanisms used by *Corynebacterium renale* or *E. coli* to cause contagious bovine pyelonephritis in cattle is limited. Thus portions of this section are speculative and based on (1) what is known mechanistically about other diseases of the respiratory system caused by *Corynebacterium* spp. or *E. coli* and (2) a reasonable probability that inflammation, responses to injury, and lesions that have been described in contagious bovine pyelonephritis are the result of underlying and known pathobiologic mechanisms. The mechanism of injury in contagious bovine pyelonephritis is probably cell death (acute coagulative necrosis) caused by (1) bacterial toxins that act directly on transitional mucosal and tubular epithelial cells of the urinary system possibly by inducing tubular cell and collecting duct cell apoptosis and (2) acute and chronic inflammation and their effector molecules and degradative enzymes. Gross lesions include white-tan streaks often mixed with narrow red streaks (hemorrhage) that radiated from the pelvis, through the medulla, often extending to the cortical medullary junction or deeper into the cortex (see Fig.

11-53). In many ways, these lesions resemble inverted renal cortical infarcts with their bases against the pelvis and their apices extending into the medulla.

Cattle (and probably sheep and goats) encounter these bacteria through contact with them in fomites or fluid droplets of urinary or fecal origin. Environmental stressors such as parturition, peak lactation, traumatic mucosal injury, and a high-protein diet that increases the pH of the urine, making the mucosae more suitable to colonization, could alter the commensal relationship, allowing the bacteria to replicate in sufficient numbers to colonize the mucosae of the urinary and reproductive systems and spread the bacterium to other animals. It has been proposed that contagious bovine pyelonephritis occurs secondary to a chronic and often insidious cystitis that ascends in the lower urinary tract and reaches the renal pelvis via the ureters to then spread though the mucosal barrier formed by transitional epithelium of the renal pelvis into the interstitium of the renal medulla. The mechanism of ascension may be caused by the reflux of infected urine from the ureters and urinary bladder into the renal pelvis. In the pelvis, it may occur via spread of bacteria through the mucosal barrier formed by the transitional epithelium of the pelvis and into vascularized ECM connective tissues supporting the tubules. How each of the events occurs has not been specifically determined; however, ligand-receptor interactions characteristic of other bacterial diseases and their interaction with mucosae likely occur in contagious bovine pyelonephritis.

Although *Corynebacterium renale* is a nonmotile bacterium, more pathogenic strains of *E. coli* are motile and this virulence determinate may help in ascension of the bacterium up the ureter to the kidney. It has been shown that pili are required for *Corynebacterium renale* to adhere to transitional epithelium of the urinary system and to attach to and colonize mucosae of the reproductive system. Additionally, pili may serve to disrupt phagocytosis of the bacteria by neutrophils and macrophages. Binding is strongest to the mucosal epithelial cells of the vulva and vagina. The receptors used to bind to mucosae have not been determined; however, once bound, colonization of the mucosae begins. Once bacteria replicate to sufficient numbers, they then spread by ascending in the lower urinary tract to encounter and colonize the mucosae of the urethra and bladder and then by vesicoureteral reflux to ascend to the ureters and renal pelvis. The development of a chronic insidious urocystitis is often an intervening stage in the disease that serves to produce large numbers of bacteria. After colonization, it is not known how these bacteria cross mucosae to gain access to the medullary interstitium at the pelvis. Degradative enzymes and inflammatory mediators combined with bacterial virulence determinates, such as Renalin, which is an extracellular cytolytic protein produced by *Corynebacterium renale*, may facilitate spread across mucosal barriers and inflammation and cell death within the medulla. It has been suggested that lesions in the medulla (resembling inverted renal cortical infarcts) may actually begin as a vasculitis from inflammation resulting in thrombosis, ischemia, and necrosis. It has been shown that toxins from *E. coli* may stimulate apoptotic cell death in renal tubular cells in pyelonephritis.

Renal Leptospirosis (*Leptospira* spp.)

The pathogenesis of renal leptospirosis begins as vascular leptospirosis (see the section on the Cardiovascular System and Lymphatic Vessels) caused by *Leptospira* spp. The mechanism of injury in renal leptospirosis is cell death caused by (1) physical properties (penetrating movements) of bacteria that disrupt functions of endothelial cells, (2) bacterial toxins that act directly on membranes of tubular epithelial cells, and (3) acute and chronic inflammation and their effector molecules and degradative enzymes. Gross lesions include discrete and coalescing, often linear to radiating white to gray foci of tubular cortical necrosis and acute inflammation intermixed with hemorrhage (see Fig. 11-73). In chronic renal leptospirosis, lesions include discrete and coalescing, often linear to radiating white to gray foci of chronic inflammation and fibrosis (see Fig. 11-20). In the kidney, primary target cells for infection appear to be epithelial cells of the proximal convoluted tubules (cortex) (Fig. 4-25, *A*) and then later, epithelial cells of the loops of

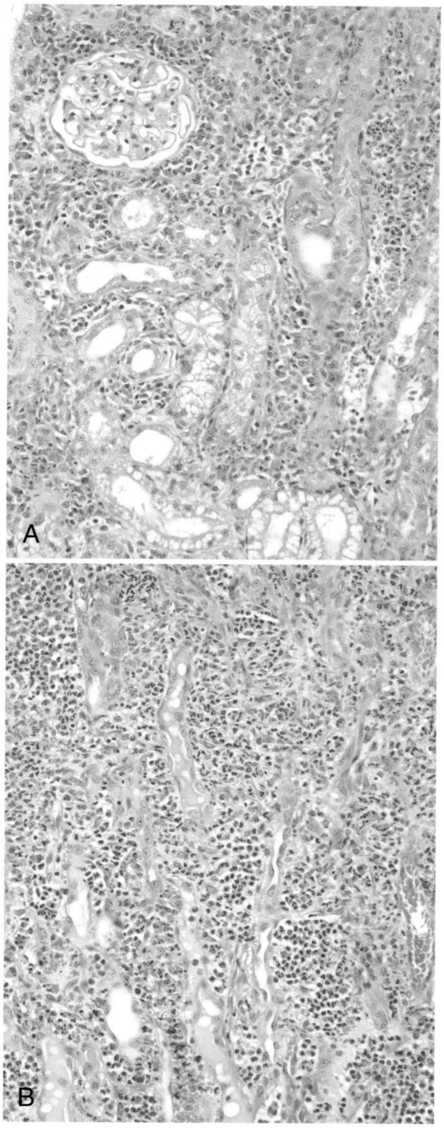

Fig. 4-25 Renal leptospirosis.
A, Kidney, outer cortex. Note the infiltration of mononuclear cells, chiefly macrophages, lymphocytes and plasma cells in the interstitium between the proximal convoluted tubules, the result of the leptospires infecting the proximal tubule cells after exiting the intertubular capillaries. **B,** Kidney (same as **A**), inner cortex. Numerous neutrophils distend the interstitium between the loops of Henle. This acute inflammatory response further down the nephron from the area in **A**, supports the concept that the cells of the loop of Henle are infected later than those in the proximal convoluted tubule. H&E stain. (**A** and **B** courtesy Dr. J. F. Zachary, College of Veterinary Medicine, University of Illinois.)

Henley (medulla) (Fig. 4-25, *B*). Once *Leptospira* spp. gain access to the circulatory system, they disseminate in glomerular capillaries and then intertubular capillaries of proximal convoluted tubules. Bacteria could access proximal tubular cells via their apical or basolateral surfaces by two routes, vascular by glomerular capillaries and migration into the lumen of the urinary space (apical) or vascular via intertubular capillaries and migration into the interstitium (basolateral). Because glomerular changes are usually unremarkable and bacteria and inflammation are observed in the interstitium, it appears that epithelial cells of the proximal convoluted tubules are infected via the basal-lateral surfaces of the cells via migration through intertubular capillaries.

The bacteria likely attach to endothelial cell membranes of intertubular capillaries via adhesins then penetrate the vessel wall by moving directly through the cells or through their junctional complexes to gain access to the interstitium. In reality, the distance in the interstitium between capillaries and proximal tubular epithelial cells is probably no more than 100 μm and it is likely that the flagella of these motile bacteria propel them to the epithelial cells. It is unclear why the bacteria target proximal tubular epithelial cells for infection. Although undetermined, such specificity could be attributed to ligand-receptor interactions or to a chemical gradient, such as an iron concentration, that could be required for bacterial growth and replication. The bacteria are present in the cytoplasm of these cells; endocytosis and phagosome-lysosome fusion are not involved in cell entry. It appears that the bacteria are able to directly enter these cells via their motility.

The cause of death of proximal tubular cells is probably multifactorial, involving vasculitis and ischemia, trauma from physical injury caused by bacterial motility, inflammatory mediators and degradative enzymes, and bacterial toxins. The inflammatory cells in this lesion progress from neutrophils (suppurative) to lymphocytes, macrophages, and plasma cells (chronic). Epithelial cells lining the loop of Henle could also be infected by an intertubular capillary-interstitial route. This mechanism has not been confirmed. Additionally and based on inflammatory cell responses, it is unclear why cells of the proximal tubules appear to be infected at an earlier point in the disease than those of the loop of Henle. When proximal tubular cells die, they release bacteria into the urinary lumen where they are carried in urine and spread into the environment via urination. During this luminal transit, the bacteria also encounter the apical surfaces of epithelial cells lining the loop of Henle. It is plausible that *Leptospira* spp. infect epithelial cells of the loop of Henle via their apical surfaces projecting into the urinary lumen, using mechanisms similar to those previously described. Infection appears to result in the same cascade of cell alterations and inflammatory responses as those described for proximal tubular cells. Biofilms (virulence determinate) formed by *Leptospira* spp. may also play a role in tubular injury. These outcomes in both proximal tubular and loop of Henle cells serve as the basis for characterizing this disease as tubulointerstitial nephritis.

Bone Marrow, Blood Cells, and Lymphatic System

*Strangles (*Streptococcus equi *ssp.* equi*)*

The mechanism of injury in strangles is death (coagulative necrosis) of cells of lymphatic vessels, lymph nodes, and the monocyte-macrophage system attributable to acute suppurative inflammation and its mediators and degradative enzymes. Gross lesions include the formation of acute abscesses within regional lymph nodes resulting in enlarged firm lymph nodes that on a cut surface have discrete and coalescing areas of yellow-white suppurative exudate infiltrating and compressing contiguous parenchyma (see Fig. 13-74). Affected retropharyngeal and mandibular lymph nodes may also have draining fistulous tracts between affected nodes and the surface of the skin, the guttural pouches, and the nasal cavities and sinuses, resulting in release of bacteria into the environment. This outcome occurs because degradative enzymes released from dead neutrophils in abscesses digest the capsule of the lymph node and the structures of all contiguous tissues until a fistulous tract is formed.

Foals encounter *Streptococcus equi* ssp. *equi* through inhalation or ingestion of fomites or body fluids contaminated with the bacterium. It is deposited on mucosae of the nasal (centrifugal turbulence) and oral pharynx and trapped in the mucus layer. The bacterium is nonmotile and it has not been clearly shown how it penetrates the mucus layer and gains access to mucosal epithelial cells. Mucosal epithelial cells of the tonsils and tonsillar crypts appear to be important target cells for adherence and binding, and this specificity may be determined by unique ligand-receptor interactions. Once in contact with cell membranes, several bacterial cell wall surface proteins, such as M-like proteins (SeM, SzPSe), may act as adhesins and attach to receptors expressed on the membranes of these cells. The characteristics of these receptors are unknown. It has not been determined if the bacterium needs to first colonize the mucosal surface before spreading into subjacent local lymphoid tissues. Additionally, it has not been determined how the bacterium crosses the mucosal barrier of the tonsil. Mucosal macrophages could phagocytose the bacteria in the mucus layer and carry it via leukocyte trafficking through the mucosal barrier into the local lymphoid tissues, or once bound to host cell receptors, it could be transported through the cell via transcytosis and released via exocytosis from the basal membranes of the cells into local lymphoid tissues of the tonsil. Dendritic cells could also be involved in the spread of bacteria across the mucosal barrier and into local and regional lymphoid tissues and lymph nodes. In local lymphoid tissues of the tonsil, the bacterium is able to replicate extracellularly and then spread to regional nodes such as the mandibular or retropharyngeal. Although unknown, the bacterium could spread by means of lymphatic vessels to these regional nodes in macrophages via leukocyte trafficking or through cell-free migration. The bacterium multiplies extracellularly in the lymph tissues and nodes, and the exudate contains large numbers of viable bacteria.

Mechanistically, several bacterial virulence determinates contribute to the character of this exudate (suppurative) and the large number of viable bacteria. Bacterial virulence determinates that act as chemoattractants for neutrophils and that disrupt phagocytosis and killing by neutrophils appear to explain the abundance of exudate and viable bacteria, respectively. Early in the sequence of events when bacteria encounter mucosal and tissue macrophages in local and regional lymphoid tissues and nodes, a bacterial cell wall protein, SeeH, interacts with these cells, resulting in the release of proinflammatory cytokines, increased vascular permeability, and edema. The occurrence of acute suppurative inflammation is facilitated by several virulence determinates. When peptidoglycan of the bacterial cell wall interacts with C3 of complement in the edema fluid via the alternative complement pathway, it produces complement-derived chemotactic factors that attract large numbers of neutrophils from capillary beds into local vascularized connective tissues. Furthermore, bacterial streptokinase interacts with plasminogen in the edema fluid to form active plasmin, which hydrolyzes fibrin. This process appears to increase the spread and dispersion of bacteria in tissue. Normally, fibrin confines bacteria by isolating them within its polymerized fibrillar meshwork so they can be phagocytosed and killed by neutrophils and macrophages, but when fibrin is hydrolyzed, large numbers of bacteria can accumulate in the exudate of an abscess and be readily available for release into the environment (see later). The outcome of these processes also contributes to the initiation of the cellular (leukocytic) phase of acute inflammation.

The surface of *Streptococcus equi* ssp. *equi* is coated with numerous protein virulence determinates, such as hyaluronic acid, SeM, and Se18.9 proteins that disrupt phagocytosis and killing. The bacterium also secretes leukocidal toxin and streptolysin S, a cell membrane pore-forming toxin, which kills leukocytes and disrupts phagocytosis. These processes lead to the accumulation of large numbers of viable bacteria in the exudate of lymphoid tissues and nodes and in abscess formation. Additionally, hyaluronic acid in the capsule appears to block interactions between bacteria and neutrophils by increasing the negative charge and hydrophobicity of the bacterial surface and by producing a localized oxygen-reduced environment that protects the activity of oxygen-labile proteases and toxins such as streptolysin S. It is likely but undetermined that bastard strangles occurs because of spread of the bacterium to systemic lymph nodes and organ systems by leukocyte trafficking or cell-free migration via efferent lymphatic vessels and/or capillaries or postcapillary venules in lymph nodes to gain access to the systemic circulatory system.

Caseous Lymphadenitis (Corynebacterium pseudotuberculosis)

The mechanism of injury in caseous lymphadenitis is cell death attributable to inflammation and its mediators and degradative enzymes affecting cells of the monocyte-macrophage system and cell populations in lymph nodes and other organ systems. Gross lesions include chronic active pyogranulomatous lymphadenitis (see Figs. 11-75 and 11-76) with enlarged firm lymph nodes that on a cut surface have discrete and coalescing areas of yellow-white caseous exudate infiltrating and compressing contiguous parenchyma and abundant connective tissue. In other organs, such as the lung, abscesses encapsulated by dense bands of fibrous connective tissue and containing yellow-white caseous exudate are common findings.

Sheep and goats encounter *Corynebacterium pseudotuberculosis* through penetrating wounds and potentially ingestion. The bacterium is a common contaminate of the environment usually from animals that have the cutaneous form of caseous lymphadenitis leading to fistulous tracts from draining cutaneous lymph nodes. Penetrating wounds most commonly involve the skin and mucous membranes of the oral cavity. Management practices, such as shearing, may cause skin abrasions, whereas objects like wire, sticks, and protruding barn or fence nails may puncture the skin. Similar types of injury may occur in the oral cavity by similar objects and mechanisms. Once the bacterium reaches the submucosa or subcutis, it is phagocytosed by neutrophils and macrophages and spread via leukocyte trafficking to regional lymph nodes via lymphatic vessels. The bacterium replicates in the lymph nodes and the inflammatory response results in multiple pyogranulomas (abscesses) that grow in size and with time, notably enlarge and affect the entire lymph node. Macrophages infected with bacteria leave the node via leukocyte trafficking and spread via lymphatic vessels and probably the thoracic duct to the systemic circulation system or spread by entering the capillary or venous circulation within the node to gain access to the systemic circulatory system. Via leukocyte trafficking, macrophages then spread the bacterium to other visceral lymph nodes, especially the mediastinal and bronchial, and to tissues in a wide variety of organ systems, especially the lung. Because the bacterium is able to replicate in large numbers in macrophages and neutrophils, the death of these cells attributable to mycolic acid or cell aging results in the release of bacteria into vascularized ECM tissues. This process activates integrins and adhesins in vascular endothelium and causes massive recruitment of additional neutrophils and macrophages into the tissues as part of a chronic active inflammatory response, thus repeating the inflammatory process of forming pyogranulomas (abscesses). The mechanisms used by *Corynebacterium pseudotuberculosis* to gain access to lymph nodes via ingestion (if it occurs) are unknown. Two potential pathways could be used and both focus on macrophages and leukocyte trafficking. First, bacteria could interact with the mucus layer and mucosae of the oral pharynx, be phagocytized by macrophages and carried to the tonsils, then to regional lymph nodes, and then systemically. Second, bacteria could be swallowed and via alimentary peristalsis encounter M cells of small intestinal crypts, spread via M cells to macrophages in contiguous Peyer's patches, then to regional lymph nodes, and then systemically. It is likely that the mechanisms and responses to injury described for the penetrating wounds portal of entry would also apply to these two scenarios.

Corynebacterium pseudotuberculosis has two known bacterial virulence determinates, phospholipase D and mycolic acid, that allow it to colonize tissues and produce pyogranulomas. Phospholipase D increases vascular permeability, which is thought to assist macrophages in migrating in and out of tissues infected with the bacterium, thus favoring the systemic spread of the bacterium. As a potent exotoxin, it also injures cell membranes leading to macrophage and neutrophil dysfunction, disruption, and death and interferes with neutrophil chemotaxis. *Corynebacterium pseudotuberculosis* does not have a protective capsule but has a waxy mycolic acid coat on the cell wall surface. Mycolic acid induces acute inflammation, has a role in the formation of granulomas, is toxic for macrophages, and prevents killing of the bacterium with phagosome-lysosome fusion likely by protecting against hydrolytic enzymes present within lysosomes.

*Brucellosis (*Brucella *spp.)*

The mechanism of injury in brucellosis is cell death caused by inflammation and its mediators and degradative enzymes. *Brucella* spp. do not have virulence determinates for exotoxins or endotoxins that cause direct injury to cells. Gross lesions include chronic active pyogranulomatous lymphadenitis with enlarged firm lymph nodes that on a cut surface have discrete and coalescing areas of yellow-white exudate infiltrating and compressing contiguous parenchyma.

Animals encounter *Brucella* spp. through inhalation or ingestion of bacteria in fomites contaminated with infected exudates from other body systems such as the female reproductive tract. The bacterium encounters mucosae and their mucus layers through centrifugal turbulence and entrapment in the mucus layer of the nasal pharynx and through mastication, gravity, and entrapment in the mucus layer of the oral pharynx. Bacteria are phagocytosed by macrophages or dendritic cells migrating through, on, or in the mucosae and spread to local lymphoid tissues via leukocyte trafficking by lymphatic vessels, to regional lymph nodes via lymphatic vessels, and then systemically to superficial and visceral lymph nodes and other organs such as spleen, liver, bone marrow, mammary glands, and reproductive organs. *Brucella* spp. can also cross the mucosal barrier via endocytosis, exit the basal surface of mucosal epithelial cells through exocytosis, and spread cell free in lymphatic vessels to local and regional lymph nodules and nodes where they are phagocytosed by macrophages and then spread systemically as discussed above. Through ingestion and peristalsis, *Brucella* spp. can also reach the alimentary system where they encounter M cells. Bacteria infect M cells via endocytosis, undergo transcytosis, and exit the basal surfaces via exocytosis to gain access to macrophages within Peyer's patches. Macrophages within Peyer's patches are then infected with the bacteria and used to spread bacteria systemically. The goals of these three types of mucosal encounters are to provide *Brucella* spp. with ample opportunity to infect macrophages and subsequently gain access to local, regional, and systemic lymph nodules and nodes.

In lymph nodes, bacteria-infected macrophages are killed by the bacterium or die through aging and the bacteria are released into vascularized ECM. These bacteria elicit an acute inflammatory response that is quickly replaced by a pyogranulomatous inflammation because of LPS in the bacterial cell wall. The material is not readily degradable, and macrophages (as monocytes) are recruited from the systemic circulation to phagocytose and degrade such material and kill the bacteria. *Brucella* spp. are able to evade the killing mechanisms when phagocytosed by neutrophils and macrophages. Additionally, they are able to grow and replicate in macrophages and dendritic cells. Once *Brucella* spp. encounter cell membranes of macrophages, they use ligand-receptor interactions to attach to and enter cells; however, the details remain unclear. Outer membrane protein of the bacterial cell wall and class A scavenger receptors on host target cells are likely involved but not necessarily with each other. TLRs are also likely involved in attachment and entry into macrophages. Entry occurs via endocytosis through a phagosome, but phagosome-lysosome fusion does not occur because bacteria are able to block fusion through rapid acidification of the phagosome. LPS (a PAMP]), a type IV secretion system, and a long list of other putative virulence determinates such as cyclic β-1,2-glucan and heat shock proteins may also be involved in blocking phagosome-lysosome fusion and promoting bacterial growth and replication. The virulence of *Brucella* spp. strains appears related to the LPS composition of its capsule, with the encapsulated smooth phenotypes generally being more virulent. Additionally, the presence of a smooth capsule enhances bacterial growth and replication in phagosomes.

When *Brucella* spp. spread via leukocyte trafficking systemically in macrophages, they are able to gain access to tissues in the male and female reproductive systems and the mammary gland (Fig. 4-26; see also Fig. 19-18). In summary, infected macrophages interact with and infect placental trophoblasts in placentomas and epithelial cells of other reproductive tissues. Once such cells are infected, the bacteria likely infect fetal macrophage-like cells that serve to spread the bacteria through the fetus and to other lymphoid tissues in reproductive organs (see Fig. 4-26, *C* and *D*). *Brucella* spp. also survive in macrophages of these tissues by inhibiting the phagosome-lysosome fusion. Bacterial growth and replication with concurrent death of bacteria-infected macrophages results in pyogranulomatous inflammation of these tissues and organ systems.

Rhodococcal Mesenteric Lymphadenitis (Rhodococcus equi)

The pathogenesis of rhodococcal mesenteric lymphadenitis begins as an infection of the respiratory system (see section on the Respiratory System, Mediastinum, and Pleurae), followed by infection of the alimentary system (see section on the Alimentary System and the Peritoneum, Omentum, Mesentery, and Peritoneal Cavity). The mechanism of injury in rhodococcal mesenteric lymphadenitis is death of cells of the monocyte-macrophage system and of all cell populations in the lymph node secondary to inflammation and its mediators and degradative enzymes. Gross lesions include chronic active pyogranulomatous lymphadenitis (see Fig. 7-137) with enlarged firm lymph nodes that on a cut surface have discrete and coalescing areas of yellow-white exudate infiltrating and compressing contiguous parenchyma. *Rhodococcus equi* enters the alimentary system through M cells and is released into Peyer's patches where it is phagocytosed by tissue macrophages. Bacteria-infected tissue macrophages spread via leukocyte trafficking in lymphatic vessels within the intestinal mesentery to mesenteric lymph nodes, leading to pyogranulomatous lymphadenitis, and then systemically via the thoracic duct and the blood vascular system to additional lymph nodes and lymphoid tissues such as the spleen. The pathogenesis of pyogranulomatous lymphadenitis appears to progress much like that which occurs in the lung.

Nervous System

Edema Disease (Escherichia coli)

The pathogenesis of edema disease begins as an enterotoxemia of the alimentary system (see section on the Alimentary System and the Peritoneum, Omentum, Mesentery, and Peritoneal Cavity). This disease is caused by a specific strain of hemolytic *E. coli* having virulence determinates for a bacterial toxin called *Shiga toxin 2e* (also known as *verotoxin 2e*). It was initially called *edema disease principle*. The mechanism of injury is death of endothelial and smooth muscle cells of arterioles (fibrinoid arteriopathy/arteriolopathy), thus the toxin biologically behaves as an angiotoxin. In the brain, vascular lesions are followed by secondary ischemia and necrosis of neural cells, particularly neurons in brainstem nuclei. Gross lesions include symmetric areas of yellow-gray malacia in the brainstem overlying affected nuclei (see Web Fig. 10-24). Pigs encounter *E. coli* through ingestion and colonization of the intestinal mucosae. The enterotoxemia phase is discussed in the section on the Alimentary System and the Peritoneum, Omentum, Mesentery, and Peritoneal Cavity. Shiga toxin 2e is absorbed in the alimentary system and circulates systemically in the blood vascular system. Endothelial and smooth muscle cells of arteritis and arterioles express receptors for this toxin. This toxin causes vascular permeability changes and edema followed by endothelial injury and death leading to hemorrhage, intravascular coagulation, microthrombosis, and infarction (grossly malacia). Shiga toxin 2e acts to disrupt protein synthesis in affected cells leading to cell death.

Focal Symmetric Encephalomalacia (Clostridium perfringens)

The pathogenesis of focal symmetric encephalomalacia begins as an enterotoxemia caused by *Clostridium perfringens*. Because ε-toxin is a permease that alters cell permeability, the vascular beds in affected intestinal tissues readily absorb toxins into the circulatory system. It appears that the sequence of events leading to focal symmetric encephalomalacia occurs in the first phase or early in the second phase of enterotoxemia before toxin-induced massive necrosis of the intestine occurs. The mechanism of injury is cell death caused by bacterial toxins that act directly on endothelial cell membranes causing permeability changes leading to acute coagulative necrosis of affected cells, including endothelial cells and neurons. Gross lesions include bilaterally symmetric malacia (acute coagulative necrosis of neuron cell bodies) and liquefactive necrosis of the basal ganglia, internal capsule, thalamus, and substantia nigra with edema and hemorrhage. Cerebral edema causes indistinct sulci and flattened gyri and in severe cases, coning of the cerebellar vermis through the foramen magnum. Because ε-toxin is a permease that alters cell permeability of the microvascular system, in the nervous system, it behaves as an angiotoxin. The vascular beds in affected intestinal tissues with enterotoxemia readily absorb toxins into the circulatory system. They are then carried to the brain via the blood vascular system where they act to increase the permeability

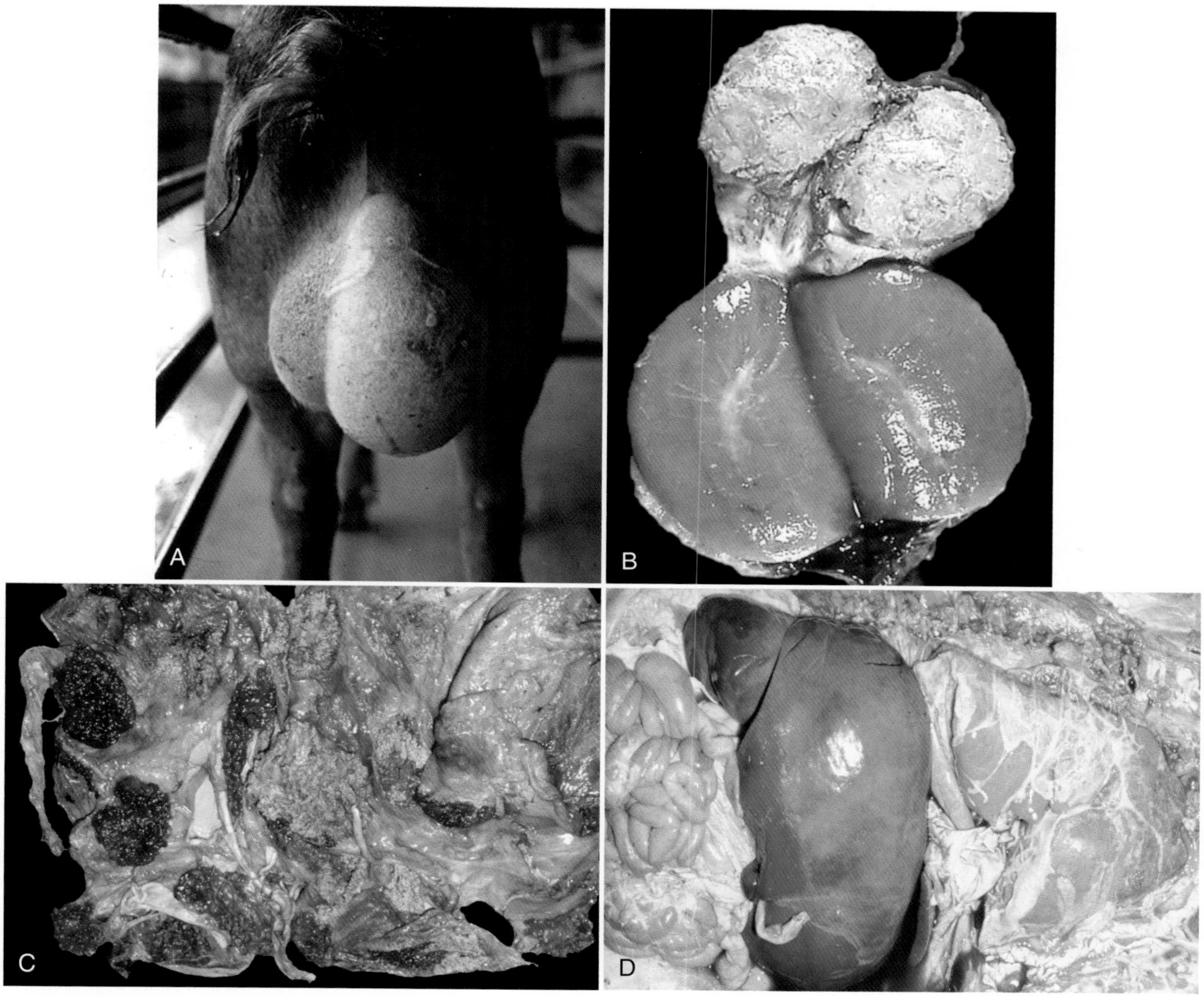

Fig. 4-26 Brucellosis.

Brucellosis is a disease in which the bacterium initially targets lymphocytes and macrophages in mucosae-associated lymphoid tissues, regional lymph nodes, systemic lymph nodes, and the spleen to replicate and grow in number. It uses macrophages to spread to and through these tissues and then systemically to infect cells and tissues in the placenta, sex organs of males and females, and fetuses. Therefore brucellosis is initially and long term characterized by a chronic active pyogranulomatous lymphadenitis with sequelae that affect the reproductive systems. **A,** Boar, swollen testis. The testis in enlarged due to chronic active pyogranulomatous inflammation. *Brucella* spp. spread in macrophages via leukocyte trafficking from lymphoid tissues systemically to the testis. **B,** The epididymis can be filled with pyogranulomatous exudate, which obstructs the flow of spermatozoa and causes infertility. Infected animals can also serve as carriers and spread the bacterium via sexual contact (also see Fig. 19-18). **C,** Fetal cotyledons. Note the roughened granular yellow-brown surface of cotyledons *(arrows)* infected with the bacterium. This lesion is caused by pyogranulomatous inflammation leading to severe necrosis of the affected cotyledons. Normal cotyledons are dark red and have a smooth shiny surface. **D,** Fetal brucellosis, hepatomegaly and fibrinous polyserositis. The bacterium is thought to be spread from infected cotyledons to fetal organs via leukocytic trafficking in fetal macrophage-like cells. The bacterium causes extensive injury of the vascular system and organs through inflammatory responses induced in the fetus. (**A** courtesy Dr. C. Wallace, College of Veterinary Medicine, The University of Georgia; and Noah's Arkive, College of Veterinary Medicine, The University of Georgia. **B** courtesy Dr. K. McEntee, Reproductive Pathology Collection, University of Illinois; and Dr. J. King, College of Veterinary Medicine, Cornell University. **C** and **D** courtesy Dr. K. McEntee, Reproductive Pathology Collection, University of Illinois.)

of capillary beds leading to the release of blood plasma containing toxins into the neuropil, resulting in severe generalized vasogenic cerebral edema. Circulating ε-toxin accumulates preferentially in the brain via ligand-receptor interactions. It is likely that receptors expressed on different populations of endothelial cells in the body and within the brain determine in part the specificity for certain neurons and nuclear groups within the nervous system. The cell membrane of cerebral endothelial cells is the probable site of toxin binding, and it appears that toxin-induced injury of endothelial cells leads to the expression of more receptors for circulating ε-toxin. Injury to the endothelium disrupts the integrity of the blood-brain barrier, leading to increased vascular permeability, vasogenic edema, and the diffusion of toxin into the neuropil where it encounters neuron cell bodies. Acute coagulative necrosis of neuron cell bodies has been attributed to toxin-induced microthrombosis of capillaries, resulting in neuronal ischemia and by direct cytotoxic action on neurons and other neural cells. The selective nature of neuronal death caused by ε-toxin may be explained by ligand-receptor interactions, selective metabolic vulnerability of specific populations of neurons, or the concentration of ε-toxin.

Botulism and Tetanus (Clostridium botulinum, Clostridium tetani)

The mechanism of injury in botulism is disruption of neurotransmitter vesicle exocytosis at myoneural (flaccid paralysis) junctions (i.e., synapses) by botulinum *(Clostridium botulinum)* neurotoxin. The mechanism of injury in tetanus is disruption of neurotransmitter vesicle exocytosis at neural-neural (spastic paralysis) junctions (i.e., synapses) by tetanus *(Clostridium tetani)* neurotoxin (tetanospasmin). These neurotoxins are produced in anaerobic microenvironments (a lowered oxidation-reduction [redox] potential) such as in necrotic tissue occurring in traumatic wounds (e.g., nail penetrating sole of the hoof, gastric ulcers in foals, muscle necrosis). Gross or microscopic lesions are not observed in the nervous system with these diseases.

Animals encounter these bacteria through contact with bacterial endospores present in soil and on environmental objects. Spores are carried into wounds and germinate to vegetative forms, and when this latter form dies, neurotoxins are released into dead tissue. Examples of such wounds include penetration of the skin or sole of the hoof or gastric ulcers. In addition, botulinum neurotoxin can also be released from lysed vegetative forms in the anaerobic environment of decaying vegetable matter (e.g., spoiled silage, hay, grain) and decomposing carcasses and absorbed into the circulatory system from the alimentary system with their ingestion. From a wound (or the alimentary system), neurotoxins access myoneural (botulinum neurotoxin) and neural-neural (tetanus neurotoxin) junctions by two routes, either hematogenously (botulinum neurotoxin) or via retrograde axonal transport (tetanus neurotoxin).

Botulinum neurotoxin enters the blood from (1) wounds as it diffuses via a concentration gradient to the periphery of the wound to areas with adequate circulation in which it is absorbed into the blood via capillaries and (2) absorption through intestinal villi and transfer to capillary beds within the lamina propria of the villi. Botulinum neurotoxin gains access to myoneural junctions via capillary beds that supply muscular tissues. On its release from capillaries, the neurotoxin diffuses in interstitial fluids until contacting the cell membrane of peripheral nerves (e.g., lower motor neuron), where it enters the cytoplasm of the neuron through the formation of endocytotic vesicles.

In contrast, tetanus neurotoxin (tetanospasmin) enters the nervous system and gains access to neural-neural junctions by initially entering the cytoplasm of distal processes of neurons through the formation of endocytotic vesicles in viable nerve endings located in tissue surrounding the site of the wound. The endocytotic vesicles are transported into the central nervous system (CNS) by retrograde axonal transport, and tetanus neurotoxin is released into the interstitial fluid of the neural-neural junctions by exocytosis. Free tetanus neurotoxin binds to the cell membrane of inhibitory interneurons of the spinal cord, is internalized via endocytosis, and acts to disrupt the release of inhibitory neurotransmitters via the same mechanism as used by botulinum toxin: disruption of the synaptic fusion complex. Presynaptic neurons (upper motor neurons) excite postsynaptic neurons (lower motor neurons) on a nearly continuous basis. Inhibitory interneurons acting on lower motor neurons serve to counterbalance and smooth the excitatory effects of acetylcholine released from presynaptic neurons (upper motor neurons) to excite the same lower motor neurons. Thus skeletal muscle groups (opposing flexor and extensor muscles) are given time to relax; as a result, skeletal muscle contractions initiated by lower motor neuron are well regulated and coordinated. Failure to have adequate inhibitory interneuron regulation of lower motor neurons leads to the spastic paralysis observed in tetanus.

Although botulinum and tetanus toxins gain access to targets in the nervous system by different mechanisms, from this point forward in the pathogenesis, both botulinum and tetanus neurotoxins share a common mechanism of injury, the disruption of neurotransmitter vesicle exocytosis by disrupting the synaptic fusion complex. The mechanisms are demonstrated in Figs. 4-27 and 4-28 for botulinum toxin and tetanus toxin, respectively. Thus diseases (clinical signs) that occur are the direct result of disruption of the function of myoneural (flaccid paralysis) and neural-neural (spastic paralysis) junctions. Botulinum and tetanus toxins have heavy and light chains and behave as typical A-B toxins (i.e., diphtheria, cholera, pertussis, and shigellae toxins) composed of two units: a binding B-domain (heavy chain) that mediates transport via endocytosis and exocytosis and an enzymatically active A-domain (light chain) that serves to cleave proteins within the target cell. The heavy chain binds to the neuronal membrane of myoneural junctions (botulinum toxin) and nerve endings (tetanus toxin), and the entire toxin molecule enters the neuron via receptor-mediated endocytosis. The A-domain is cleaved from the B-domain within the target cell endocytotic vesicle and then released into the cytoplasm where it is active. The A-domain (light chain), a zinc-containing endopeptidase, leaves the endocytotic vesicle and enters the cytoplasm of the neuron and acts to cleave proteins that form the synaptic fusion complex. This complex, formed by fusion of synaptic vesicle proteins with presynaptic plasma membrane proteins, serves to bring neurotransmitter vesicles into contact with the neuronal cell membrane at the myoneural (botulinum toxin) and neural-neural (tetanus toxin) junctions and facilitates membrane fusion and release of excitatory (acetylcholine) and inhibitory neurotransmitters (glycine and γ-aminobutyric acid [GABA]), respectively.

Different types of glycosylphosphatidylinositol-anchored protein(s) may be expressed on different types of neurons, which may explain why B-domain of tetanus toxin only binds to inhibitory interneurons and not other types motor neurons. Disruption of the synaptic fusion complex prevents the neurotransmitter vesicles from fusing with the membrane, which in turn prevents release of neurotransmitters into the synaptic cleft. Proteins that form the synaptic fusion complex (SNARE proteins) include neurotransmitter vesicle proteins (such as vesicle-associated membrane proteins [VAMPs]/synaptobrevin) and presynaptic plasma membrane proteins (syntaxin, synaptosomal-associated protein [SNAP-25]). Different types of *Clostridium botulinum* produce different types of toxins (toxin type A to G), and these types target and cleave specific types of SNARE proteins, synaptobrevin (cleaved by toxin types B, D, F, and G), syntaxin (cleaved by toxin type C), and synaptosomal-associated protein (cleaved by toxin types A, C, and E). Botulinum toxin seemingly does not cross the blood-brain barrier; therefore neural-neural junction functions in the CNS remain intact. Notwithstanding the profound neurologic signs of spastic paralysis and flaccid paralysis that occur with tetanus (*Clostridium tetani*) and botulism (*Clostridium botulinum*), respectively, macroscopic or microscopic lesions are not observed in the nervous system.

Listeriosis (Listeria monocytogenes)

The mechanism of injury in listeriosis is cell death that is uniquely localized to the brainstem caused by acute inflammation and its mediators and degradative enzymes. Gross lesions are often not observed, but when present consist of nodules and linear bands of gray-yellow exudate (perivascular microabscesses formed by neutrophils) mixed with active hyperemia and/or hemorrhage commonly arranged in a perivascular pattern (see Fig. 14-88).

Cattle, sheep, and goats encounter *Listeria monocytogenes* in soil, animal feed, water, and feces; however, the greatest risk of

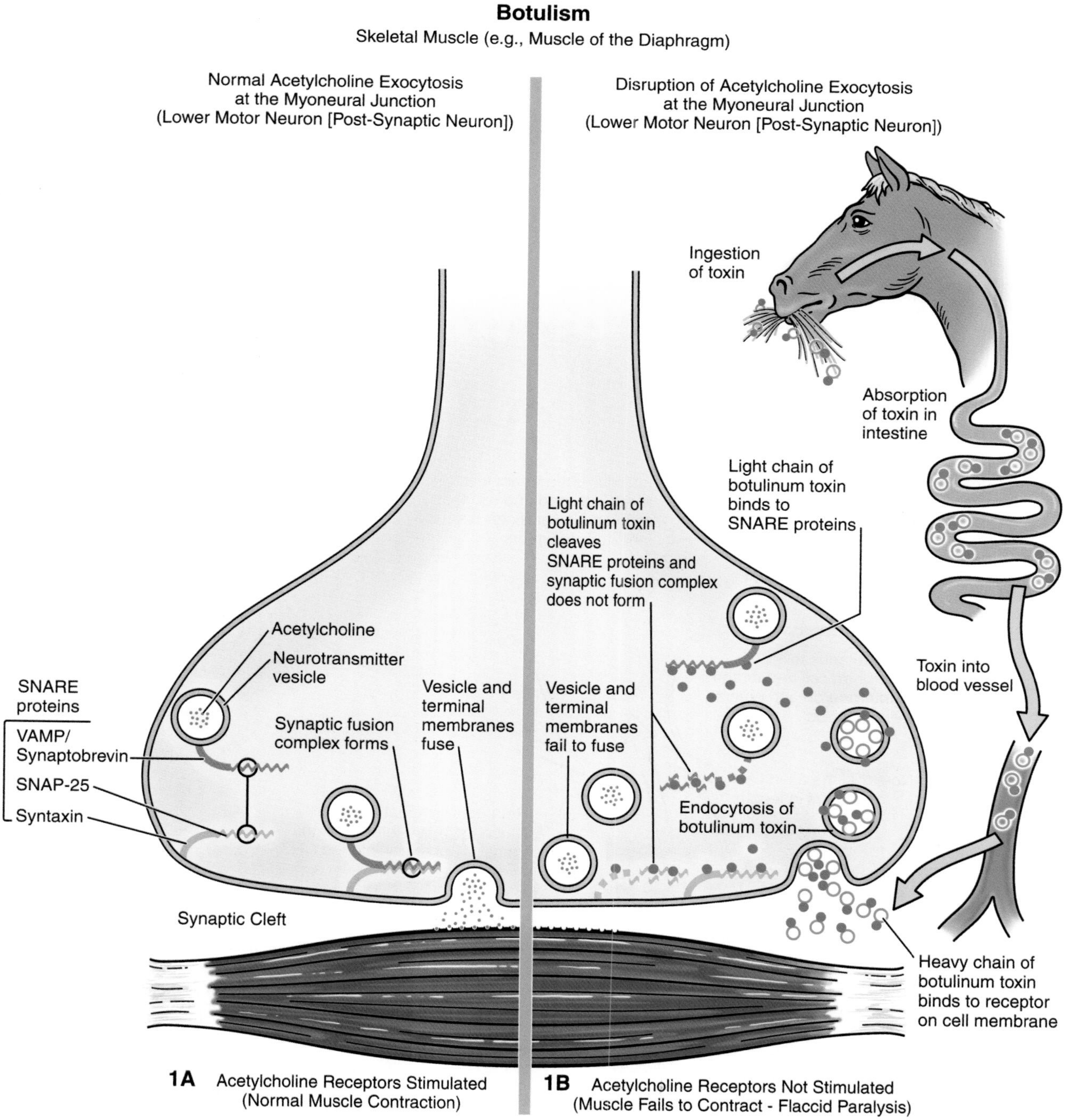

Fig. 4-27 Mechanism of myoneural junction dysfunction in botulism.
Note that botulinum toxin reaches the myoneural junction via the circulatory system. (Courtesy Dr. J. F. Zachary, College of Veterinary Medicine, University of Illinois.)

contracting the disease occurs when ruminants are fed improperly stored silage in which the pH is not acidic enough to prevent overgrowth of the bacterium. Consumption of *Listeria monocytogenes*–contaminated silage is not sufficient to cause CNS disease, unless it occurs with a penetrating injury of the oral cavity caused by a stick or other sharp object (nail) that carries the bacterium in the silage into the submucosal connective tissue of the oral cavity or tongue. At this point, the bacterium colonizes oral tissues, enters nerve endings in the oral cavity, and ascends into the CNS via retrograde axonal transport in cranial nerves. The oral cavity is primarily innervated by the trigeminal and other cranial nerves that terminate in the brainstem. Thus *Listeria monocytogenes* ultimately localizes to the brainstem (i.e., pons, medulla oblongata, and proximal cervical spinal cord). The mechanism of entry into nerve endings is unknown; however, it has been shown experimentally in cell culture systems that *Listeria. monocytogenes* gains entry into typically nonphagocytic cells through endocytosis and endocytic vesicles. Bacterial internalization, the entry process, is mediated by internalins (type A and B) that utilize host cell receptor E-cadherin, a transmembrane glycoprotein. Because *Listeria monocytogenes* resides intracellularly within cell bodies of neurons when it arrives in the brainstem, it initially does not disrupt the

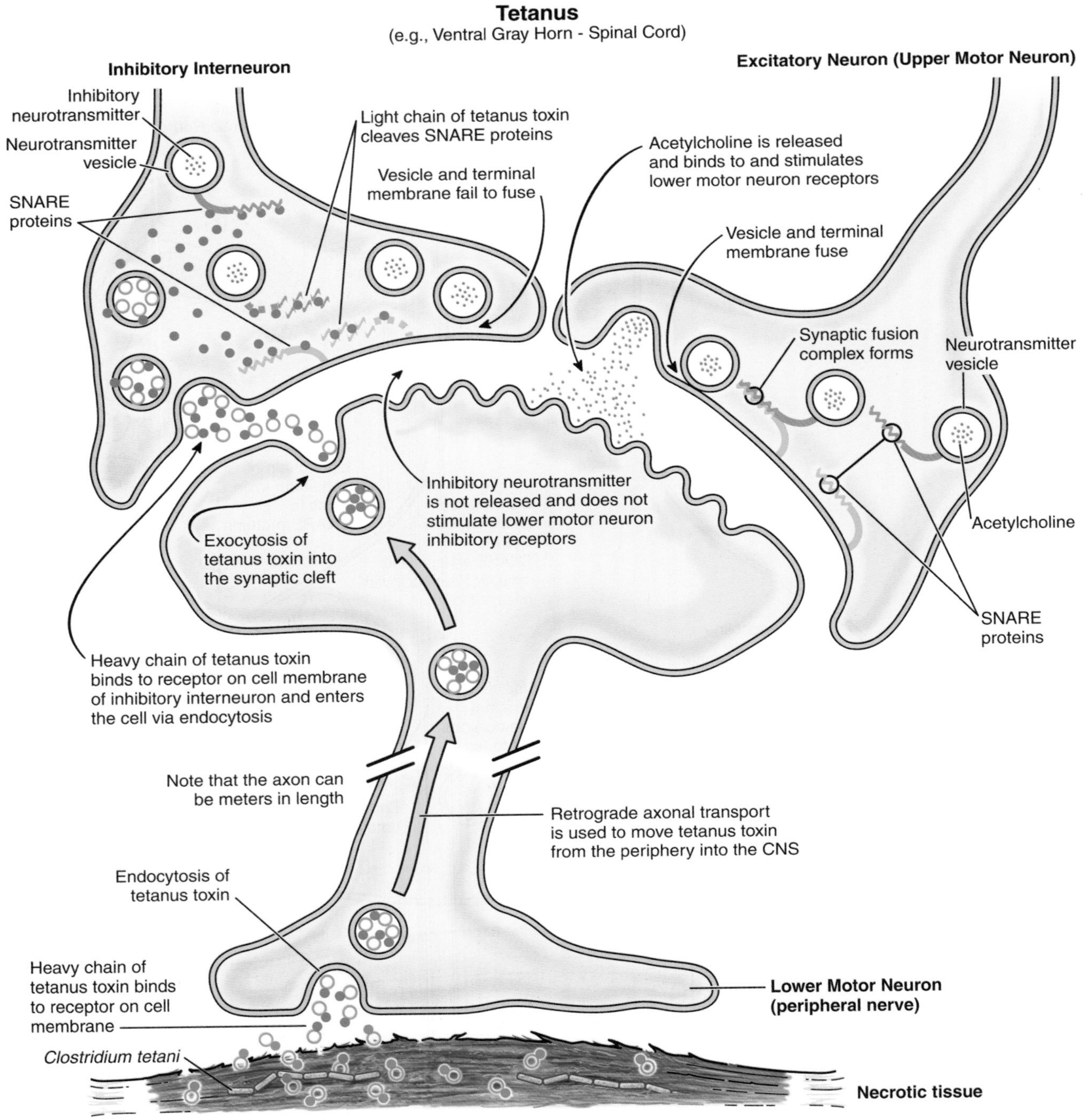

Fig. 4-28 Mechanism of neural-neural junction dysfunction in tetanus. Note that tetanus toxin reaches the neural-neural junction via retrograde axonal transport. The selectivity of tetanus toxin for inhibitory interneurons is likely mediated by the expression of different glycosylphosphatidylinositol-anchored protein(s) on different types of neurons. The B-domain of tetanus toxin appears to bind only to the type of glycosylphosphatidylinositol-anchored protein expressed on inhibitory interneurons. (Courtesy Dr. J. F. Zachary, College of Veterinary Medicine, University of Illinois.)

blood-brain barrier and thus does not activate defense mechanisms provided by the innate (inflammation) and adaptive immune responses. The cytoplasm of infected neuron cell bodies appears to be permissive and allows free proliferation of the bacterium. This permissive environment also appears to be promoted by a bacterial virulence determinate called *listeriolysin O* that inhibits immune responses and allows infected cells to hide from defense mechanisms.

Once free in the cytoplasm, the bacterium replicates to sufficient numbers and then begins the process of infecting other cells. In the cytoplasm, the bacterium has a doubling time of approximately 1 hour. When the number of bacterium in the cytoplasm reaches a level sufficient to facilitate infection of adjacent cells, bacteria move themselves, facilitated by a virulence determinate in the cytoplasm, to the inner side of the cell membrane via polymerization and depolymerization of host cell actin filaments. Once near

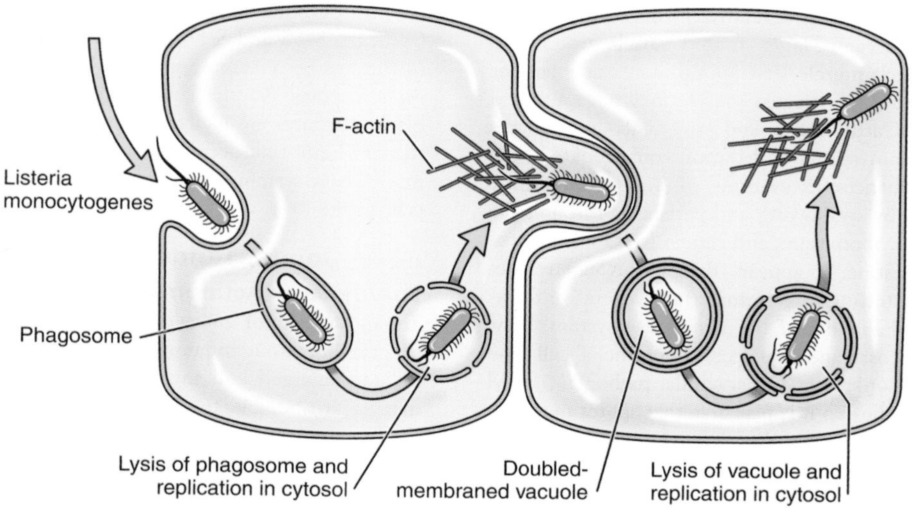

Fig. 4-29 **Mechanism of infection in listeriosis.**
Listeria monocytogenes propels itself via actin polymerization (*Listeria* actin-based motility) within a membrane pseudopod into cell membranes of adjacent neural cells forming invaginations of the membrane that ultimately result in double-membrane endocytotic phagocytic vesicles.

the cell membrane, aggregates of bacteria use a bacterial surface protein called *surface protein actA* to propel themselves via actin polymerization (listerial actin-based motility) and a pseudopod into cell membranes of adjacent cells, forming invaginations of the membrane that ultimately result in double-membrane endocytotic phagocytic vesicles (Fig. 4-29). This process is random, so it does not appear to target specific cells in the nervous system only neighboring cells. These double-membrane endocytotic phagocytic vesicles are lysed by listeriolysin O, phospholipase C, and lecithinase, and the bacteria are released into the cytoplasm of newly infected cells. Experimentally, *Listeria monocytogenes* has been shown to infect neutrophils, macrophages, fibroblasts, endothelial cells, and various types of nerve cells, including neurons and microglial cells. It appears that infection of and injury to endothelial cells of capillaries initiates the inflammatory process. Once initiated, the blood-brain barrier is disrupted and activation of the entire inflammatory cascade ensues. Neutrophils are the primary effector cells utilized by animal defense mechanisms to kill the bacterium. Experimentally, *Listeria monocytogenes* infected endothelial cells express exuberant endothelial adhesion molecules (P- and E-selectin, intercellular adhesion molecule-1 [ICAM-1], and vascular cell-adhesion molecule-1 [VCAM-1]) resulting in activation of the neutrophil adhesion cascade and neutrophil binding, both components of the acute inflammation. The bacterium can also spread from macrophages to endothelial cells.

Thrombotic Meningoencephalitis (Histophilus somni)

The pathogenesis of thrombotic meningoencephalitis (TME) begins as pulmonary histophilosis (see the section on Respiratory System, Mediastinum, and Pleurae). The mechanism of injury in the nervous system is infarction secondary to occlusive ischemia by bacterial-induced arteritis (vasculitis) and subsequent thrombosis caused by acute inflammation and its mediators and degradative enzymes. Gross lesions are red hemorrhagic infarcts of varied sizes distributed at random throughout nervous tissue, especially in the cerebral cortices (see Fig. 14-89).

Cattle encounter *Histophilus somni* (formerly *Haemophilus somnus*) via inhalation of fomites or water droplets contaminated with the bacterium. It likely exists in nasal or oral biofilms as a commensal bacterium of mucosae. Environmental stressors, such as overcrowding, combined with other factors, such as poor ventilation and humidity or abrupt changes in ambient air temperature, could alter the commensal relationship, allowing the bacteria to replicate in sufficient numbers to colonize mucosae and spread the bacterium to other animals. After colonization of the respiratory mucosae, the bacterium spreads to the lung (see the section on Pulmonary Histophilosis, Respiratory System, Mediastinum, and Pleurae) and then gains access to the vascular system in areas of inflammation, embolizes to the CNS (septicemia), and colonizes and infects small arterioles likely via ligand-receptor interactions. The first encounter with endothelial cells of arterioles occurs at anatomic sites in the brain in which there are abrupt changes in the laminar flow of blood resulting in turbulence, such as occurs at the interface between gray and white matter in the cerebral cortex. Turbulence favors perturbation of the endothelium and contact of the bacterium with platelets and the endothelium. Experimentally, *Histophilus somni* and its membrane LOS (a truncated form of LPS) have been shown to activate bovine platelets and increase the expression of adhesion molecules, such as ICAM-1 and E-selectin and tissue factor (factor III) on endothelial cells. Tissue factor is a protein necessary for activation of blood coagulation cascades. Thus, because strains of *Histophilus somni* have virulence determinates that enhance the adherence of the bacterium to endothelial cells, such areas are prone to endothelial injury, exposure of collagen, platelet aggregation and activation, activation of clotting cascades, arterial thrombosis and obstruction, and infarction (the lesion of TME).

*Meningitis (*Escherichia coli *and Other Bacterial Species)*

The pathogenesis of meningitis shares many of the mechanisms discussed for porcine polyserositis (see the section on the Respiratory System, Mediastinum, and Pleurae) and embolic vasculopathy/vasculitis (see the section on the Cardiovascular System and Lymphatic Vessels).

Muscle

Blackleg (Clostridium chauvoei)

The mechanism of injury in blackleg is necrosis (acute gangrenous myositis) of muscle, connective, and nervous tissues caused by α- and β-toxins released from vegetative forms of *Clostridium chauvoei*. Gross lesions occur in large striated muscle groups and include dark red to black muscle that appears dry and contains gas bubbles (see Fig. 15-38). Affected muscle may have a rancid (spoiled butter) smell. Cattle, sheep, and goats encounter spores through ingestion of plant matter and topsoil contaminated with spores often after disturbances (excavations) of the soil and pasture bed. Spores are carried by swallowing and peristalsis through the oral pharynx, esophagus, abomasum, and rumen to their final destination, the small intestine. It appears that spores can remain dormant in the small intestine or germinate into vegetative forms and become normal inhabitants of the alimentary system. How spores interact with mucosae and gain access to epithelial cells and mucosal macrophages is unknown. Other similar pathogens use M cells to enter Peyer's patches, so it is plausible that spores may gain access to and infect macrophages in Peyer's patches via this mechanism. Although suggested but unproved, spores are likely the form of the bacterium that spreads systemically to muscle. However, it is possible that vegetative forms of the bacterium spread to muscle and produce spores in dendritic cells and macrophages of muscle after their phagocytosis.

Spread to muscle could also occur via leukocyte trafficking followed by interaction with and infection of endothelial cells and then dendritic cells and macrophages of muscle. If it occurs, tropism for dendritic cells and macrophages of muscle is probably mediated by ligand-receptor interactions. Blackleg often follows some form of traumatic injury to muscle. It is thought that injury creates a microenvironment suitable with lowering of the oxidation-reduction (redox) potential (anaerobic environment) required for germination of spores. Such a hypothesis also assumes that the injury has damaged the dendritic cells and macrophages of muscle, allowing them access to this microenvironment. Spores germinate into vegetative forms of the bacterium and produce large quantities of a variety of α- and β-toxins such as oxygen-stable hemolysin, deoxyribonuclease (DNase), hyaluronidase, oxygen-labile hemolysin, and neuraminidase. These toxins diffuse out from the site of bacterial replication and coagulate muscle tissue and its vascular supply, resulting in acute gangrenous myositis.

Malignant Edema (Clostridium septicum)

The pathogenesis of malignant edema is similar to that of blackleg (see previous section) regarding bacterial replication, the production of toxins, tissue injury, and gross lesions affecting striated muscle and blood vessels. However, the mechanism of spread to muscle is different. Cattle, sheep, and goats encounter spores through wounds caused by penetrating objects, such as a wire, which carries spores into the wound. Wounds caused by castration, tail docking, unsanitary vaccination, and other management practices can also be infected with spores. The injury must be sufficient to create an anaerobic microenvironment in the wound with lowering of the oxidation-reduction (redox) potential suitable for germination of spores. Once spores germinate, vegetative forms release toxins that injure and coagulate muscles and vascular tissues resulting in necrosis and edema much like in blackleg.

Big Head and Black Disease (Clostridium novyi)

The pathogeneses of big head and black disease are very similar to malignant edema and blackleg, respectively. In big head of sheep, penetrating wounds of the skin of the head caused by horns during fighting establish the initial anaerobic microenvironment for spores to germinate. The resulting pathogenesis is similar to that which occurs in malignant edema. Black disease of cattle and sheep occurs because of fluke migration (*Fasciola hepatica*) through the liver (see Figs. 8-55 and 8-56) that causes hepatocellular necrosis and establishes an anaerobic microenvironment suitable for germination of spores. Kupffer cells likely contain dormant spores. As in blackleg, spores are likely ingested, enter through the mucosae of the small intestine, become phagocytosed by cells of the monocyte-macrophage system, and spread via leukocyte trafficking to Kupffer cells of the liver.

Bone, Joints, Tendons, and Ligaments

Lumpy Jaw (Actinomyces bovis)

The mechanism of injury in lumpy jaw is cell death attributable to pyogranulomatous inflammation and its mediators. Gross lesions include enlarged and misshapen bones of the mandible and/or maxilla attributable to abscesses, fibrosis, and fistulous tracts in the bone with secondary remodeling of the bone (i.e., pyogranulomatous alveolar osteomyelitis). The cut surface has numerous randomly distributed discrete and coalescing yellow-white granulomas surrounded by remodeled bone intermixed with bands of fibrous connective tissue (see Fig. 16-58). *Actinomyces bovis* is a commensal bacterium of mucosae of the oral cavity of cattle and sheep, likely existing in a biofilm. The bacterium can infect bone by several routes: (1) genetic or developmental defects of the tooth root and/or socket that provide access to bone, (2) injury to a tooth and its socket opening a pathway into the bone, and (3) penetrating wounds that give the bacterium access to the bone and its periosteum. During chewing, the bacterium is carried by direct extension through the mucosae into submucosal connective tissues via penetrating wounds such as those caused by sharp foreign bodies like sticks or wires. The object may penetrate the periosteum and the bone, giving the bacterium direct access to these tissues. The bacterium colonizes submucosal connective tissue, and LPS of the cell wall, in part, likely plays a role in the type of inflammatory response that occurs. Little is known about virulence determinates, ligand-receptor interactions, target cells, toxins, capsule antiphagocytic molecules, or other factors that may contribute to the pathogenicity of this bacterium. *Actinomyces bovis* can spread via lymphatic vessels to regional lymph nodes and cause a similar inflammatory response in these tissues.

Integumentary System

Greasy Pig Disease (Staphylococcus hyicus)

The mechanism of injury in greasy pig disease is cell death and exfoliation of cells of the skin secondary to inflammation and its mediators and degradative enzymes. Gross lesions include areas of patchy red skin (active hyperemia of acute inflammation) followed by thickening of the reddened skin and the formation of reddish brown macules, vesicles, and pustules first around the eyes, nose, lips, and ears and then the flanks and abdomen (see Fig. 17-47). Affected skin, mostly through inflammation, exudes large quantities of a greasy exudate consisting of serum and sebum mixed with inflammatory cells, degradative enzymes, and cell debris. This exudate is the basis for naming the disease.

Pigs encounter *Staphylococcus hyicus* through fomites and body fluids contaminated with the bacterium. This bacterium is likely a commensal organism that resides in the skin and hair follicles of healthy pigs. Environmental stressors, such as skin trauma caused by overcrowding combined with other factors such as poor ventilation and humidity or abrupt changes in ambient air temperature, could alter the commensal relationship, allowing bacteria to replicate in sufficient numbers to colonize the skin, spread the bacterium to other animals, and cause disease. Infected droplets are deposited on the surface of the skin, but the bacterium under most conditions is not able to infect and colonize intact skin. It appears that skin trauma is usually a prerequisite for colonization because abrasions on the feet and legs or lacerations on the body precede the onset of the disease.

The role of virulence determinates, ligand-receptor interactions, and cells of the monocyte-macrophage system, such as Langerhans' cells, are poorly understood in the pathogenesis of the disease. An exfoliative toxin that induces separation of epithelial cells of the stratum corneum and spinosum aids in the invasion of the bacterium into the skin. It serves to expose vascularized ECM tissues in traumatized skin. Fibronectin-binding proteins expressed on the surface of the bacteria appear to act as adhesins, allowing the bacteria to bind to the fibronectin present in collagen, fibrin, and heparin sulfate proteoglycans of traumatized skin. Fibronectin is a glycoprotein of vascularized ECM tissues and is produced by cells such as fibroblasts. Once the skin is colonized, the infection appears to spread to the hair follicles leading to suppurative inflammation and sebaceous gland hyperplasia and hypersecretion (i.e., greasy pig). It also appears that acute inflammation and its effector cells, such as neutrophils, play a central role in the onset and progression of the skin lesions. Capsule polysaccharides and protein A in the bacterial wall appear to block phagocytosis of the bacterium by neutrophils and increase the ability of bacteria to survive and replicate in vascularized ECM tissues of the skin.

Canine Pyoderma (Staphylococcus intermedius)

The pathogenesis of canine pyoderma appears to be similar to that of greasy pig disease (see previous section). Skin trauma arising from pruritus and scratching or from existing skin disease leads to the exposure of vascularized ECM tissues and its colonization by bacteria. Although incompletely characterized, it is likely that a variety of virulence determinates are involved in canine pyoderma, including surface proteins (colonization of host tissues); invasins such as leukocidin, kinases, hyaluronidase (promote bacterial spread in tissues); surface factors such as capsule polysaccharides and protein A (inhibit phagocytosis); and exotoxins and exfoliative toxins such as hemolysins, leukotoxin, and leukocidin (cause cell death).

Diamond Skin Disease (Erysipelothrix rhusiopathiae)

The mechanism of injury in diamond skin disease is cell death and infarction of skin secondary to cutaneous vasculitis. Gross lesions include active hyperemia and red-purple skin affecting the ears, ventral abdomen, and legs followed by thrombosis, ischemia, and infarction resulting in rhomboidal (diamond) red-purple areas of skin (cutaneous infarcts) (see Figs. 17-51 and 10-81).

Pigs encounter *Erysipelothrix rhusiopathiae* through ingestion of fomites and body fluids contaminated with the bacterium. This bacterium is likely a commensal organism that resides in a biofilm of the mucosae of the pharynx and tonsillar epithelia of healthy pigs. Environmental stressors, such as overcrowding combined with other factors such as poor ventilation and humidity or abrupt changes in ambient air temperature, can alter the commensal relationship, allowing the bacteria to replicate in sufficient numbers to colonize mucosae and spread the bacterium to other animals. Infected droplets are deposited on pharyngeal mucosae, where bacteria encounter the mucus layer and mucosal epithelial cells. It is unclear how this nonmotile bacterium is able to penetrate the mucus layer and gain direct access to the luminal membrane of epithelial cells. Additionally, it is unclear if and how the bacterium colonizes the mucus layer and mucosae. It appears that neuraminidase may be a virulence determinate for *Erysipelothrix rhusiopathiae* potentially involved in initial interactions with and invasion of the mucus layer of pharyngeal mucosae. It acts to remove sialic acid from glycoproteins, glycolipids, and oligosaccharides expressed on host cells, potentially exposing new receptors for the bacterium. It is also probably important later in the disease process in the attachment, colonization, and invasion of endothelial cells by the bacterium leading to vasculitis, thrombosis, infarction, and DIC.

Other virulence determinates involved in mucosal colonization and systemic spread of the bacterium include capsular polysaccharides (antiphagocytic properties), surface proteins (adhesins, antiphagocytic properties, biofilm formation), invasins such as hyaluronidase (invade ECM tissues), and enzymes such as superoxide dismutase and catalase (block the effects of the respiratory burst of phagocytosis and oxygen free radicals). Transcytosis could move bacteria through mucosal cells to the basal surface of mucosal epithelial cells to encounter local macrophages and lymphoid cells in the tonsils. Alternatively, mucosal macrophages could phagocytose bacteria in the mucus layer, migrate through the mucosal barrier, and spread them via leukocyte trafficking to the same cells.

Macrophages within the tonsil are likely used by the bacterium for replication and growth and then to spread them via leukocyte trafficking in lymphatic vessels to regional lymph nodes to infect additional macrophages. Ligand-receptor interactions are likely involved and bacterial surface proteins appear to serve as adhesins to macrophage and endothelial cell membrane receptors. Specific bacterial adhesins and host cell receptors for them on macrophages and endothelial cells have not been identified. Once bound to cell membrane, the bacterium is phagocytosed and retained in a phagosome within the cell cytoplasm. *Erysipelothrix rhusiopathiae* grows and replicates intracellularly in phagosomes and phagolysosomes. Capsular polysaccharides are able to inhibit phagocytosis of the bacterium by neutrophils and to a limited extent by macrophages. However, macrophages are used by the bacterium to isolate it from host innate and adaptive immune responses. Although it appears that phagosome-lysosome fusion occurs, capsular polysaccharides appear to block the oxidative burst and prevent killing of the bacterium by molecules present in the lysosome. Although undetermined, bacteria-infected macrophages in regional lymph nodes could spread the bacterium systemically via leukocyte trafficking using lymphatic vessels and the thoracic duct or postcapillary venules and the venous system to the systemic circulatory system and then to capillary beds within the skin. Cutaneous infarcts (also vascular-related lesions in other organs such as the kidney) suggest these bacteria may have tropisms for vascular endothelial cells. It is unclear why this occurs but is likely linked to the expression of bacterial virulence determinates and ligand-receptor interactions with host endothelial cells. In addition to cell death attributable to direct infection of endothelial cells by the bacterium, bacterial neuraminidase may also activate the alternative complement pathway and induce thrombocytopenia, producing complement-derived chemotactic factors that could contribute to injury of capillary beds in local vascularized connective tissues. These mechanisms may contribute, in part, to the development of vegetative valvular endocarditis and arthritis that occurs in the chronic septicemic form of this disease.

Female Reproductive System

*Brucellosis (*Brucella *spp.)*

The pathogenesis of Brucellosis begins as an infection of the regional and systemic lymph nodes (see the section on Bone Marrow, Blood Cells, and Lymphatic System) facilitated by entry through mucosae of the respiratory and alimentary systems. The mechanism of injury is cell death caused by pyogranulomatous inflammation and its mediators and degradative enzymes. Gross lesions include aborted fetuses; necrosis, inflammation, and fibrinoid exudation of uterine caruncles and fetal cotyledons (see Fig. 4-26); and a yellow-white uterine exudate. Bacteria spread in macrophages via leukocyte trafficking from regional lymph nodes to the caruncular side of placentomas when they likely leave the vascular system to migrate into and through these tissues. Although it is unclear what additional cells in the placentoma are infected during transplacental spread to the fetus, trophoblasts are infected with bacteria. Other cell types may be involved. Bacteria then could spread in fetal macrophage-like cells within the fetal circulatory system to the fetus via the umbilical cord or within the allantoic and amniotic membranes and infect the fetus via contact with fetal mucosae of the respiratory or alimentary systems, but if this occurs or what cells facilitate this spread are unclear.

Bovine Mastitis (Staphylococcus aureus, Streptococcus agalactiae, Streptococcus dysgalactiae, and Escherichia coli)

The mechanism of injury in bovine mastitis is death of all cell populations in the mammary gland from (1) bacterial toxins, (2) inflammation and its mediators and degradative enzymes, and (3) induced reparative responses such as fibrosis. Gross lesions in acute mastitis include firm, swollen, edematous, and occasionally hemorrhagic glands and ectatic ducts and sinuses containing yellow-white exudate (see Figs. 18-53 to 18-55, 18-57, and 18-58). In chronic mastitis, tissues are firm and consist of large zones of fibrous connective tissue that have replaced and displaced remaining normal glands (see Fig. 18-59). Inflammatory exudate is difficult to observe unless abscesses have formed. Ducts and sinuses may be ectatic.

Animals encounter these bacteria through physical contact in fomites or fluid droplets from mammary gland, uterine, or fecal origin on milking equipment and human hands. They commonly become commensal organisms that reside in biofilms of the mucous membranes of the teat canal and mammary duct and sinuses. Trauma to mucosae in the gland induced by pressure changes acting on the duct system caused by milking likely makes the mucosae more suitable for colonization and alters the commensal relationship, allowing the bacteria to replicate in sufficient numbers to spread the bacterium within the gland and to other animals mechanically during milking. Mastitis is an ascending infection, and milk in canals and sinuses is a suitable culture media for initial growth of bacteria. This environment is not suitable in the long-term for survival of the bacteria, thus they attempt to colonize mucosae to sustain the infection. Ligand-receptor interactions are likely involved in the adherence of these bacteria to receptors on mucosal epithelial cells; however, specific bacterial adhesins and host cell receptors have not been clearly identified. Once mucosae are colonized, bacteria employ mechanisms to sustain the infection. For example, *Staphylococcus aureus* produces toxins, such as superantigens, leukocidins, hemolysins, coagulase, and likely α-, β-, and δ-toxins (virulence determinates) that result in cell membrane injury and cell death and the activation of mucosal macrophages. The severity of this lesion and its progression to gangrenous mastitis in the peracute and acute forms are dependent on the type and quantity of toxins secreted by the bacterium as determined by its virulence determinates. Additionally, activated mucosal macrophages secrete proinflammatory cytokines resulting in the recruitment of neutrophils from the systemic circulation, through the mucosae, and ultimately into the milk, thus increasing the somatic cell count. With the focus of inflammation on the mucosae, epithelial cells and subjacent basement membrane are injured, killed, and sloughed, providing bacteria with access to vascularized ECM tissues of the gland. Using bacterial surface proteins, they are able to adhere to and colonize ECM tissues likely using receptors expressed on molecules such as fibronectin, vitronectin, laminin, and collagen in the matrix. This process allows bacteria to evade many of the harmful actions of the innate and adaptive immune responses. Additionally, capsular polysaccharides block phagocytosis by neutrophils and macrophages. As a result, acute inflammation progresses with time to chronic inflammation with fibrosis (see Chapter 3), which is a common manifestation of mastitis caused by *Staphylococcus aureus*.

Chronic mastitis is often linked with the formation of mucosal biofilms. In mastitis caused by *Streptococcus agalactiae* and *Streptococcus dysgalactiae*, the bacteria use most of the mechanisms employed by *Staphylococcus aureus* with one important exception. They lack virulence determinates that injure the mucosae and allow the bacterium to invade vascularized ECM tissues and colonize this area. Thus the bacterium is limited to colonizing the mucosae and causing inflammation at the mucosal barrier. The outcome of this process is loss of mucosal epithelial cells lining glands, collapse of the glands, and replacement of the glands with fibrous connective tissue. In mastitis caused by *E. coli* and other coliforms, the bacterium uses most of the mechanisms as discussed previously. However, in the initial phases of colonizing the mucosae, endotoxins (LPS) and other toxic molecules released from Gram-negative bacteria cause tissue injury and cell death, affecting the mucosae, submucosae, and capillary beds. The concurrent acute inflammatory response with neutrophils and their degradative enzymes exacerbate the severity of the injury. This outcome leads to tissue necrosis, edema, and hemorrhage. Endotoxin is also absorbed by the capillaries and can cause endotoxic shock of the circulatory system and death of affected animals (see Chapters 2 and 3).

Male Reproductive System

Brucellosis (Brucella *spp.)*

The pathogenesis of Brucellosis begins as an infection of regional and systemic lymph nodes (see the sections on Bone Marrow, Blood Cells, and Lymphatic Systems and Female Reproductive System) facilitated by entry through the mucosae of the respiratory and alimentary systems. The mechanism of injury is cell death caused by pyogranulomatous inflammation and its mediators and degradative enzymes. *Brucella* spp. spread in macrophages via leukocyte trafficking from regional lymph nodes to the testes, epididymides, and other male reproductive tissues. Gross lesions include enlarged and deformed testes and epididymides attributable to a yellow-white pyogranulomatous exudate against the bacteria in the tissues (see Fig. 4-26).

VIRAL DISEASES

Viruses are about a hundred times smaller than bacteria, and viruses, like bacteria, are genetically programmed to replicate endlessly, if all growth factors, metabolic needs, and microenvironments for replication are satisfactorily met. However, viruses are unable to produce energy and contain a limited number of enzymes; therefore they are completely dependent on animal cells for such resources and are obligate intracellular parasites. They have evolved to specifically utilize target cells in animals that are susceptible to and suitable for completion of their viral replication cycle. The term *target cell* assigns specificity to which cells are infected by viruses, and this process is based on the typical ligand (viral envelope or capsid proteins)-receptor (host cell membrane proteins) interactions common to all cells (Fig. 4-30). The phrase *virus replication*

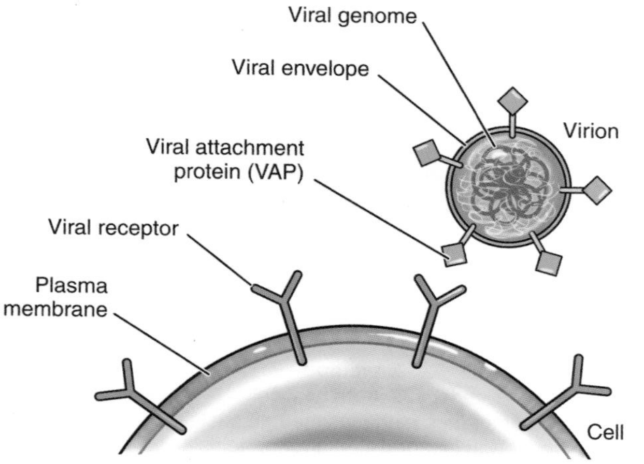

Fig. 4-30 Ligand-receptor interactions.
Ligand (viral envelope or capsid proteins)-receptor (host cell membrane proteins) interactions common to all cells are used by viruses to attach to and infect specific target cells.

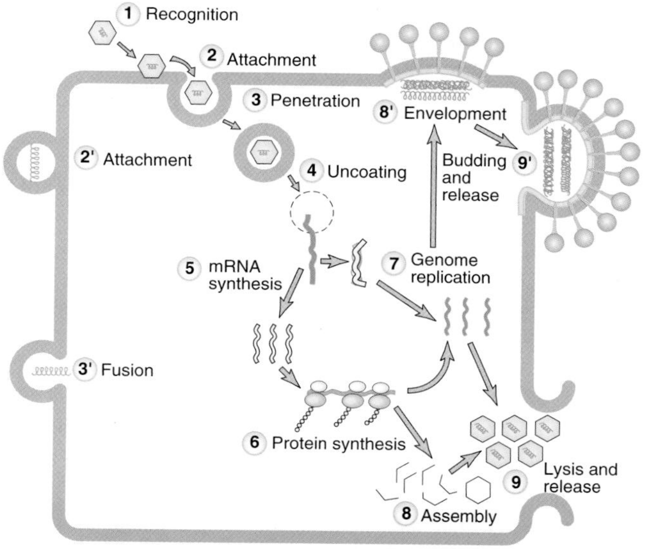

Step Inhibited	Antiviral Drugs
1 Recognition	Receptor antagonists, antiviral antibody
2 Attachment	Receptor antagonists, antiviral antibody
4 Uncoating	Amantadine, rimantadine
5 mRNA synthesis	Interferon, antisense oligomers
6 Protein synthesis	Interferon
7 Genome replication	Nucleoside analogues (e.g., acyclovir, ganciclovir, AZT); non-nucleoside analogs (e.g., phosphonoformate)
8 Assembly	Protease inhibitors (e.g., saquinavir)

Fig. 4-31 Virus replication cycle.
Stages in the infection, replication, and egress of a virus in a target cell. Several thousand virus particles may be formed within each infected cell. (From Rosenthal KS, Tan JS: *Rapid review microbiology and immunology,* ed 2, St. Louis, 2007, Mosby.)

cycle is used here to merge under a single key concept the chronologic sequence of the events that occurs when a virus encounters and enters cells, hijacks the functions of cellular organelles and metabolic processes, produces new virus, and ultimately injures or kills cells and causes disease.

TARGET CELLS, VIRAL PATHOGENICITY, AND VIRAL REPLICATION CYCLE

Target cells that allow replication of the virus are called *permissive cells,* whereas those that do not are called nonpermissive cells. Generally, virus-infected permissive cells are usually killed by the virus (cell death), whereas virus-infected nonpermissive cells are not killed. For example, the pathogenesis of the lentivirus disease, maedi-visna, is determined, in part, by nonpermissive cells (immature progenitor monoblasts and promonocytes in bone marrow) and permissive cells (mature monocytes and macrophages in the blood vascular system and tissues). Infection of nonpermissive progenitor cells in bone marrow is used to provide a reservoir of immunologically protected virus-infected cells that become permissive when they mature into monocytes and macrophages in the vascular system and when they migrate into specific tissues and organs. These permissive macrophages are ultimately killed by virus replication, and the cell is lysed to release new virus from the cell.

Viral pathogenicity is a phrase used to convey the severity of disease, clinical signs, and lesions caused by viruses. It is determined, in large part, by the expression of viral genes that are used to produce structural or functional proteins needed to sustain or enhance the virus replication cycle. Similar to bacteria, these viral genes and proteins biologically behave as viral virulence determinates; however, the occurrence of viral virulence determinates is nowhere near the complexity and diversity expressed by bacteria. As would be anticipated, viral virulence determinates focus on attachment, replication, and shedding of viruses and on the processes of modulating and/or evading host defense mechanisms. Thus the type, quantity, and arrangement of nucleic acid in viruses provide the basis for genomic diversity and the transfer of virulence determinates among viruses. The encounter between viruses with virulence determinates and host cells with innate and adaptive defense mechanisms determines the occurrence and severity of disease.

The severity of disease, and in large part the life or death of the host cell, is determined by how a virus (1) utilizes and truncates the processes of host cell organelles and transcriptional and translational processes in virus replication and (2) escapes from virus-infected host cells. The organ system specific clinical symptomatology of diseases caused by viruses is mechanistically linked to the following three key stages in the replication cycle of a virus (Fig. 4-31):

- Attachment and Entry Stage
  - Determines what organs are infected, thus determining the clinical signs of disease.
  - Viruses bind to receptors normally expressed on host cell membranes and these receptors are used to infect target cells.
- Replication Stage
  - Determines the utilization of cellular biologic processes, thus determining the characteristics of cellular dysfunction or death.
  - Viruses hijack cell organelles, genomes, and biologic processes to complete the viral replication cycle.
- Shedding (Release or Egress) Stage
  - Determines if the cell will live or die, thus determining the clinical signs of the disease.
  - Viruses that escape from cells by killing or lysing cells create more severe disease processes.

Once viruses encounter host cells, they attach to them via cell membrane receptors. Attachment is the process through which binding occurs between ligands (viral attachment proteins) on the surface of the virus and receptors on the host cell membrane.

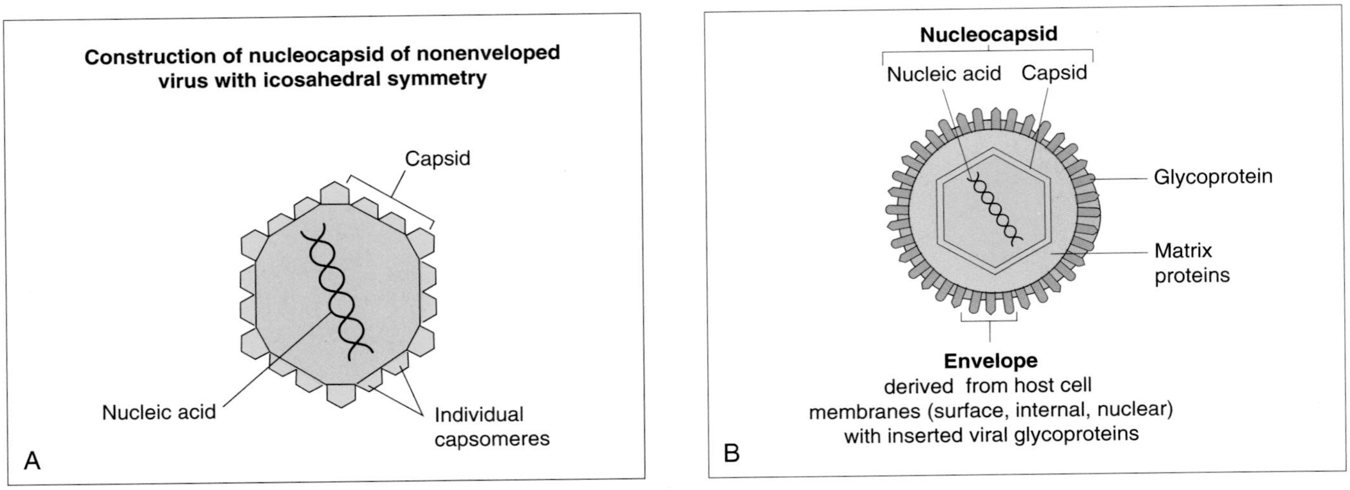

Fig. 4-32 Morphology of viruses.
A, Nonenveloped viruses. They attach to host cells using a protein coat (viral coat, capsid, capsomeres) and usually kill infected cells to release newly formed virus. **B,** Enveloped viruses. They attach to host cells using a viral envelope and usually do not kill infected cells to release newly formed virus. (From Goering R, Dockrell H, Roitt I, et al: *Mims' medical microbiology,* ed 4, St. Louis, 2008, Mosby.)

Receptors are often expressed in unique patterns on target cells, and these patterns appear to frequently determine the route used by viruses to infect target cells. For example, parvoviruses and herpesviruses use specific receptors with specific distribution patterns to attach to and enter target cells. Parvovirus (canine parvovirus enteritis) infects intestinal crypt epithelial cells through receptors expressed on the basolateral surface of the cells, thus using a circuitous route via leukocyte trafficking to Peyer's patches and M cells to gain access to this surface. Although this route is not likely the most direct route to intestinal epithelial cells, it may be advantageous for survival of the virus to avoid contact with gastric acids, bile, and other potentially toxic molecules in the alimentary lumen. Additionally, junctional complexes of intestinal epithelial cells would probably prevent the virus from reaching, and thus encountering, basolateral cell surfaces. Bovine herpesvirus 1 (infectious bovine rhinotracheitis) infects epithelial cells of the respiratory system through receptors expressed on the apical and lateral surface of the cells. These receptors are distributed above junctional complexes formed with adjacent epithelial cells; therefore virus in the lumen of the respiratory tract can encounter appropriate receptors on mucosae. Receptors on host target cells used by viruses include those for complement, growth factors, neurotransmitters, integrins, adhesion molecules, complement regulatory proteins, phospholipids, and carbohydrates. In general, specific viruses use one of these receptor types to infect a specific type of cell; however, some viruses use several receptors (coreceptors), which allows for invasion of a variety of cell types (i.e., pantropic viruses such as canine distemper virus). Experimental studies suggest that there are approximately 10^4 to 10^6 receptors for a virus expressed on a single target cell. Attachment is accomplished through the interaction of the host cell membrane receptors with the outermost layer of the virus.

Specific groups of viruses (nonenveloped viruses) attach to host cells using a protein coat (viral coat, capsid, or capsomeres) (Fig. 4-32, *A*); others attach via a viral envelope (enveloped viruses) (Fig. 4-32, *B*). Protein molecules, derived from viral genes and expressed in the protein capsid or envelope, are called *attachment proteins.* Attachment proteins are viral virulence determinates that provided a basis for genomic diversity among viruses. Once attachment occurs, viruses can enter target cells by one of two main mechanisms: receptor-mediated endocytosis or fusion. Once inside target cells, viruses initiate a variety of virus-specified processes to complete their replication cycles, such as replication of its genome, core proteins, and capsid and envelope proteins; assembly of new viruses; and release of new viruses from the cell (Fig. 4-33). When a DNA virus enters a cell and its components are released into the cytoplasm, the DNA genome is transferred into the nucleus where it utilizes host cell nuclear organelles to transcribe viral messenger RNA (mRNA) and later replicate new viral DNA. Viral mRNA leaves the nucleus and in the cytoplasm is translated into structural and nonstructural proteins of the virus by host cell organelles. After all viral proteins are translated in the host cell cytoplasm, new viral DNA is replicated (transcribed) and transferred into the cytoplasm where it is assembled with structural and nonstructural proteins to form new virus.

When a RNA virus enters a cell and its components are released into the cytoplasm, the RNA genome, depending on the virus, can (1) replicate new viral RNA from the cytoplasmic viral RNA via its own viral RNA-dependent RNA polymerase or (2) make viral DNA from viral RNA via RNA-dependent DNA polymerase (viral reverse transcriptase) and then use host cell nuclear and cytoplasmic organelles to transcribe and translate new proteins and viral RNA. Thus the genome of RNA viruses must express genes that code for enzymes such as RNA-dependent RNA polymerase and RNA-dependent DNA polymerase. Detailed coverage of these processes is outside of the scope of this chapter and can be reviewed in virology textbooks; however, these replicative processes often lead to injury and cell death. Generally, nonenveloped viruses (viral protein coats or capsids) are released from host target cells only when the cell death occurs.

Enveloped viruses (viral envelope glycoproteins) must acquire an envelope by budding through cellular membranes such as the plasma membrane, membranes of the Golgi complex or rough endoplasmic reticulum, or nuclear membrane. Viral envelope glycoproteins localize to zones in the membrane where the virus buds from the membrane. Most viruses that bud from the cell membrane do not cause cell lysis except for those that bud from the Golgi complex or rough endoplasmic reticulum (flavivirus, coronavirus, Arterivirus, and bunyavirus) or the nuclear membrane (herpesvirus).

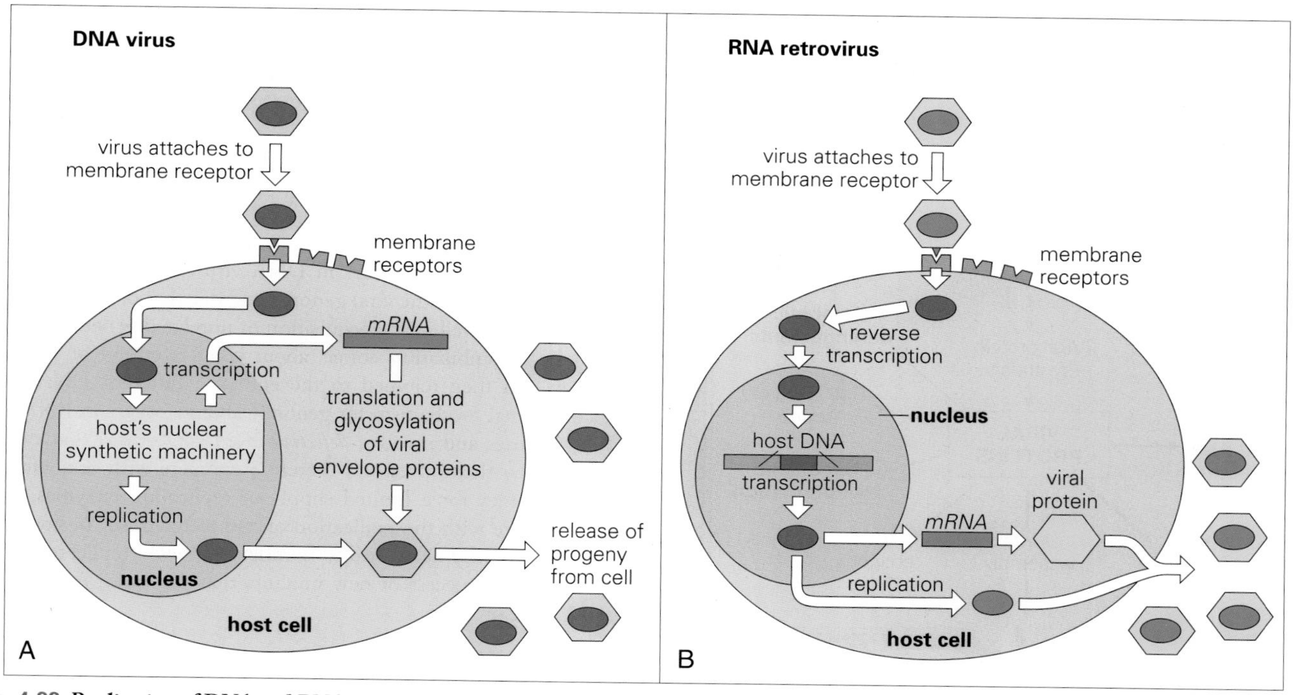

Fig. 4-33 Replication of DNA and RNA viruses.
(From Goering R, Dockrell H, Roitt I, et al: *Mims' medical microbiology*, ed 4, St. Louis, 2008, Mosby.)

Virus capsid proteins and envelope glycoproteins are used immunologically as a means to clinically prevent (e.g., vaccination) or control (e.g., pharmaceutical products) diseases caused by viruses by developing strategies to block one of more of the steps in the viral attachment or replication cycle. Antibiotics have no effect on viruses; however, fortunately, viral infections (viral antigens) usually activate host innate and adaptive defense mechanisms and cause an immune response (cell-mediated), which can completely eliminate a virus or prevent an infection by a virus (vaccination). However, these defensive responses can also injure and kill host cells leading to disease. The list of structural and biochemical effects that viruses have on the host cell is extensive. These effects are often called *cytopathic effects,* and as a general rule, many viral infections result in death of the host cell. Depending on the virus and its replication cycle, injury to and death of the host cell can occur at any point during the attachment, fusion, penetration, synthesis, assembly, or release phases. Generally, viruses cause injury and death most commonly by two mechanisms: (1) as a result of taking over cell transcriptional and translational processes and (2) when they exit from infected cells. Additionally, causes of cell death include alterations in cell membrane function, including ion transport and secondary messenger systems; alterations in metabolic processes, including activation cascades leading to altered cellular activities; alterations of host cell antigenic or immune properties, shape, and growth characteristics; inhibition of the synthesis of host cell macromolecules, including DNA, RNA, and protein; and direct (protein messenger molecules) and indirect (inflammatory mediators) activation of cell lysis and apoptosis cascades.

VIRULENCE DETERMINATES

Virulence determinates also have been identified for viruses. The purpose of these determinates is to improve a virus's ability to complete its replication cycle in the host cell, thus spreading and propagating the virus to naïve animals. Virulence determinates control the processes involved in (1) replication, including attachment to, replication in, and release of virus from host cells and (2) escaping, modulating, or suppressing the host innate and adaptive immune responses. For example, feline immunodeficiency virus hides within the immune system and replicates and spreads within macrophages and T lymphocytes. Other viruses have evolved mechanisms to evade cytotoxic T lymphocyte and natural killer (NK) cell killing of virus-infected cells, disrupt complement activation, synthesize cytokine homologs that interfere with normal immunologic functions, and synthesize molecules that inhibit interferon responses or block the induction of apoptosis in virus-infected cells. Other viral virulence determinates include viral proteins, as well as by-products of virus replication, such as caspases and caspase-like molecules, that accumulate in the cell and have toxin-like activities on host cells (Fig. 4-34). As an example of a viral toxin, rotavirus-infected enterocytes secrete a viral-directed toxin called *NSP4* into the intestinal lumen. Adjacent enterocytes not infected with virus absorb this toxin and it acts on a cytoplasmic messenger system to cause a secretory diarrhea. This diarrhea occurs before there is death of virus-infected enterocytes.

The number of virulence determinates for viruses when compared to bacteria is extremely small and is directly related to the number of genes in the respective microbes. The number of genes in viruses range between 10^1 to 10^2, whereas the range in bacteria is 10^3 to 10^4 genes. Correspondingly, the number of virulence determinates is low in viruses and much higher in bacteria. The introduction of a new viral virulence determinate to a viral family results from genomic variation through genetic drift, reassortment, recombination, or defective interfering viruses. Breaks in protection normally provided by commercial vaccines or the reemergence of a vaccinated/protected disease in certain regions of the country are often the result of genomic variation in the street virus and the introduction of a new viral strain such as has occurred with canine distemper and parvovirus infections.

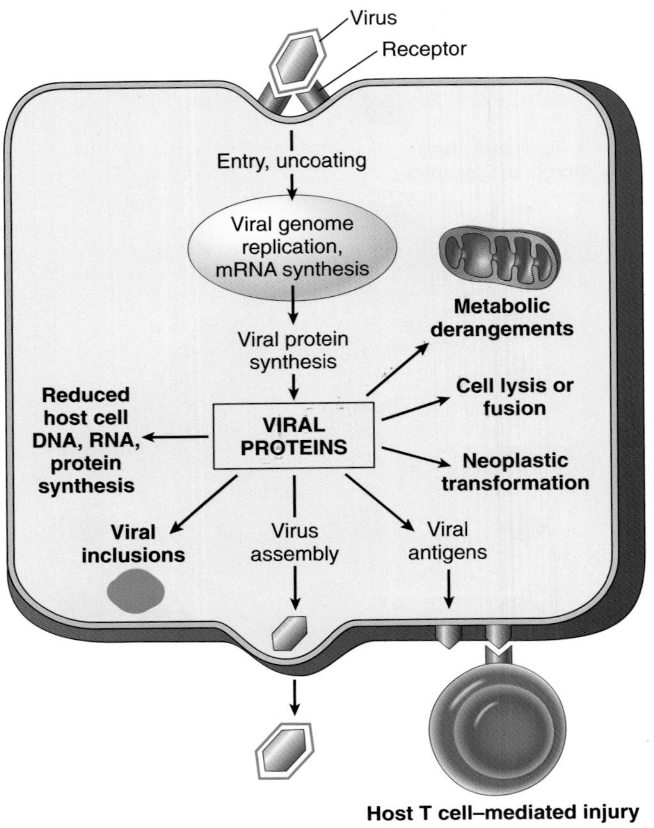

Fig. 4-34 Actions of viral proteins.
Proteins synthesized by viruses can affect normal cell function through mechanisms illustrated here. (From Kumar V, Abbas A, Fausto N, et al: *Robbins & Cotran pathologic basis of disease,* ed 8, Philadelphia, 2009, Saunders.)

MECHANISMS OF GENOMIC CHANGE

Viruses are often classified as DNA or RNA viruses based on the nucleic acid used to form their genes. In general, the competitive advantages for infecting host cells favor RNA viruses because they have an extremely high mutation rate, which increases their chances of expressing virulence determinates that improve their ability to complete their replication cycle. However, it is likely that this advantage is counterbalanced by their slower replication speed allowing host defense mechanisms to intervene in the replication process and kill the virus or virus-infected cell. *Genomic variation* is a broad term used to categorize a group of biologic processes that allow viruses to acquire new virulence determinates (genetic diversity) that favor their survival through infective and replicative mechanisms in host cells. The most common form of genomic variation, called *genetic drift,* is caused by a spontaneous point mutation of individual nucleic acid bases in viral DNA or RNA. These point mutations are usually silent and do not change the protein encoded by the affected gene; however, some mutations can result in a new protein (e.g., capsid or envelop proteins), thus providing an opportunity for the virus to improve its chances of infectivity, replication, and spread during its replication cycle. During virus replication, mutation of RNA viruses occurs at a much higher frequency than in DNA viruses and thus RNA viruses have the ability to more rapidly adapt to new situations and host environments via point mutations when compared to DNA viruses. *Antigenic shift* also leads to genomic variation and results in major changes in the genome of a virus. It occurs because of reassortment or recombination of viral genes. *Reassortment* occurs only in RNA viruses because they have discrete genomic segments, much like chromosomes, that behave independently of one another. These genomic segments can undergo reassortment during virus replication, resulting in new viruses with genomes different from the original infecting virus. Segmented genomes confer evolutionary advantages to RNA viruses. Reassortment is a powerful initiator of divergence, especially among viruses that can exchange genetic material between animals and humans like influenza viruses (Fig. 4-35). *Recombination* occurs in DNA viruses and results in rearrangements within the viral genome and deletion or duplication of viral genes, as well as the acquisition of unrelated genetic material. Genetic recombination comes about when a strand of DNA is broken and then rejoined to the end of a different DNA molecule. A final mechanism for genomic change occurs in RNA and DNA viruses and involves *defective interfering viruses* that cannot replicate by themselves and therefore compete with nondefective viral genomes for a limited supply of replication enzymes. They can interfere with the replication of complete viruses in host cells and significantly decrease the numbers of newly replicated virus, thus favoring success of new mutants that may arise in the virus replication process.

DEFENSE MECHANISMS

Defense mechanisms include many of the systems, biologic processes, and molecules described in Chapters 3 and 5. Host genes probably determine susceptibility to some viral infections via expression of or lack of expression of viral membrane receptors or through effects on the immune system. Stress (overcrowding), nutritional status, and environmental factors, such as temperature, humidity, and ventilation, also affect the susceptibility of animals to viral infections. Innate and adaptive mechanisms are actively involved in protection against viruses. However, it is important to remember that actions of the innate and adaptive immune systems, especially of T lymphocytes, against viral infections have both beneficial and harmful outcomes (Fig. 4-36). Beneficial outcomes include the return to normal structure and function of infected host cells and tissues and a host animal that is free of and fully protected (vaccinated) against the virus. Harmful outcomes include the failure to return to normal structure and function of infected host cells because the cells and tissues, their stem cells, supporting stroma, basement membrane, and vascularized ECM tissues have been degraded by enzymes from neutrophils of acute inflammation or macrophages of chronic inflammation and replaced by fibrous connective tissue. The innate immune system and TLRs, in response to viral antigens, induce inflammatory responses, cause secretion of cytokines and interferon, and activate the adaptive immune system. Cell-mediated immunity is the most important adaptive defense mechanism against viral infections. The monocyte-macrophage system, through phagocytosis, is active in containing the spread of viruses, whereas phagocytosis by neutrophils does not play an important role. Antibody deficiencies usually do not affect the outcome of viral infections, whereas antibodies are important in preventing reinfection (autoimmunization or vaccination). Although viruses are obligate intracellular parasites that have evolved sophisticated mechanisms to hijack host cell transcriptional and translational processes, this approach to replication results in alteration of host cell membranes that are recognized as foreign by lymphocytes of the adaptive immune system.

Virus replication and spread are abruptly stopped when virus-infected host cells are killed by cytotoxic NK cells and cytotoxic T lymphocytes. Interferons, a group of molecules that act on virus-infected cells to inhibit virus replication, function by inducing the

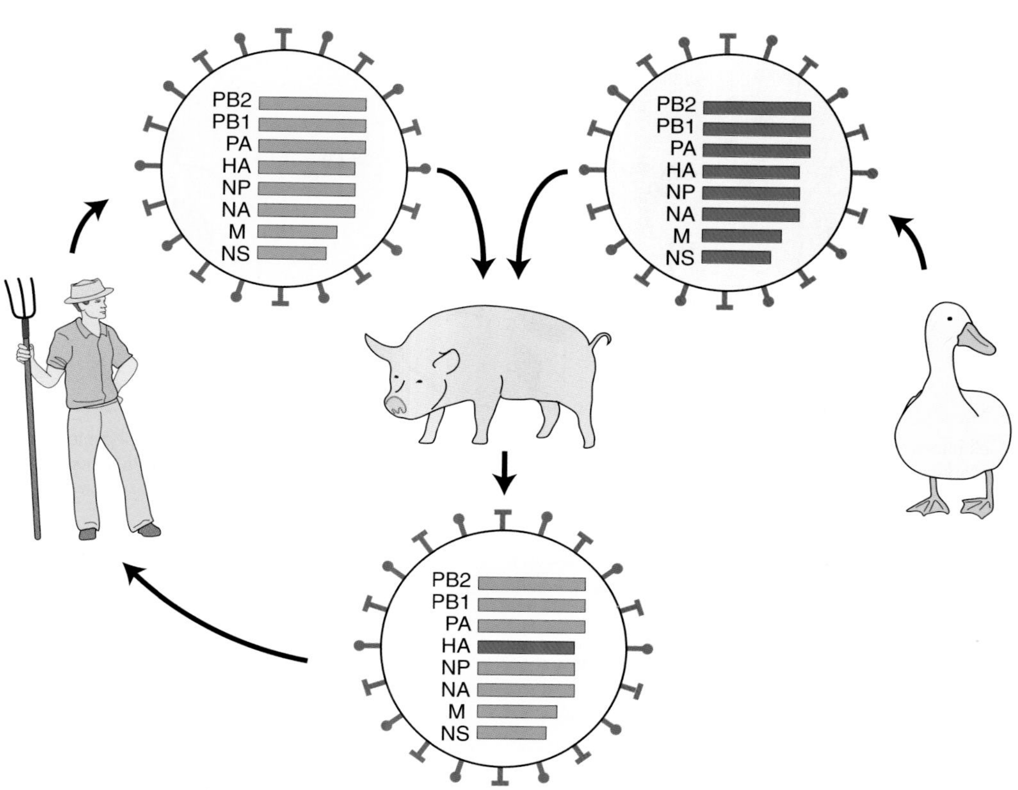

Fig. 4-35 Antigenic shifts in influenza virus.
One theory proposes that antigenic shifts occur when a human influenza virus *(blue)* and an avian influenza virus *(red)* coinfect a species that is permissive for both. The 8 ssRNA strands are co-expressed in the same infected cell, resulting in mixing of the strands so that a hybrid virus can be produced. The hybrid virus indicated here contains all the genetic information of the original virus that infected humans, but contains a new hemagglutinin (HA)-containing strand from the avian virus. This virus expresses a new HA antigen and will be less susceptible to residual immunity that normally provides partial protection against yearly influenza infections. (From McCance KL: *Pathophysiology: The biologic basis for disease in adults and children,* ed 6, St. Louis, 2010, Mosby.)

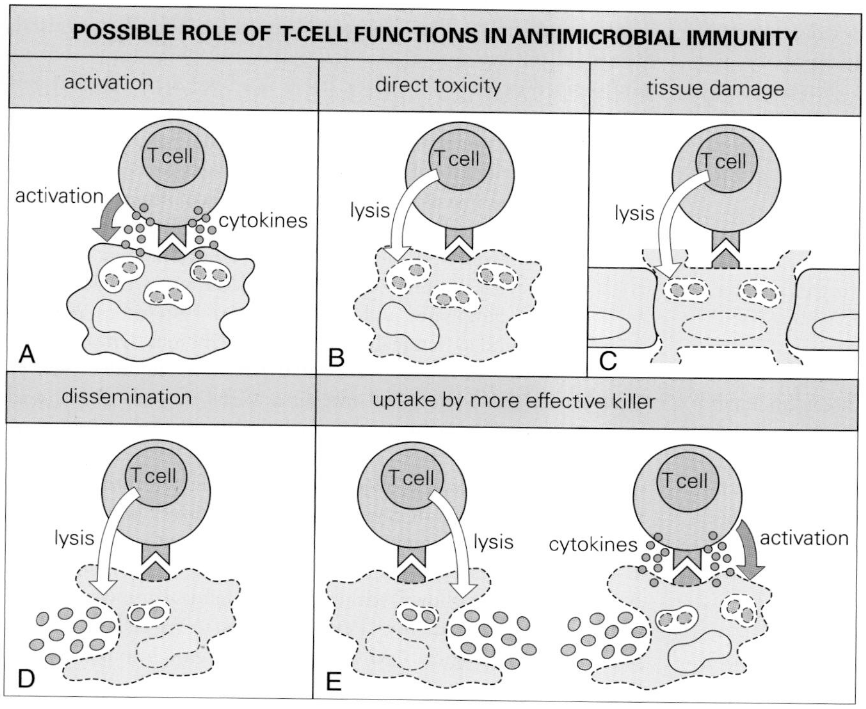

Fig. 4-36 Possible roles for T lymphocytes in immunity to intracellular microorganisms.
A, The T lymphocyte activates intracellular killing mechanisms by secretion of cytokines such as IFNγ, e.g., in a macrophage. **B,** The T lymphocyte directly kills cell and parasite. **C,** The T lymphocyte destroys vital tissue in the process of killing the parasite. **D,** By lysing cells the T lymphocyte allows still-living parasites to disseminate. **E,** Parasites released in this way may be phagocytosed by a more effective host cell. (From Goering R, Dockrell H, Roitt I, et al: *Mims' medical microbiology,* ed 4, St. Louis, 2008, Mosby.)

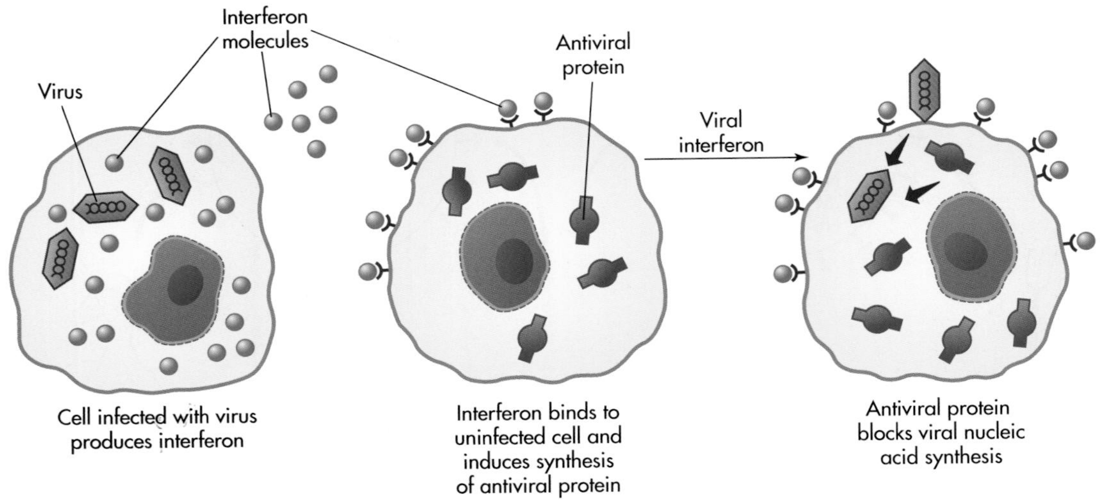

Fig. 4-37 Actions of interferon (IFN) in viral infection of target cells.
(From McCance KL: *Pathophysiology: The biologic basis for disease in adults and children,* ed 6, St. Louis, 2010, Mosby.)

synthesis of host cell proteins that inhibit translational activities of the virus (Fig. 4-37). The synthesis of interferon is induced by virus infection of host cells and by the action of proinflammatory molecules on host cells. Viral infection of host cells can also activate complement cascades independent of an antibody response. Complement components also act as opsonins (e.g., phagocytosis of viruses) and can cause death of viruses or virus-infected cells. Many of the viruses discussed in this chapter are able to infect cells of the lymphoid and monocyte-macrophage systems and dendritic cells. Under normal conditions, such cells are migratory immunosurveillance cells, behaving as sentinel cells for the adaptive immune system and monitoring for the presence of foreign antigens expressed by microbes or microbe-infected cells throughout the body. As part of their normal immunosurveillance functions, these cells migrate via lymphatic and blood vascular systems throughout all tissues and organs of the body, including the brain. It is through these normal migratory pathways that viruses within these infected cells are able to spread to other tissues and organs. This process is termed *cell-associated viremia* or *leukocyte trafficking.* Viruses can also spread to other cells as a cell-free viremia in the blood vascular or lymphatic systems.

VIRAL DISEASES BY BODY SYSTEMS

Although viral diseases often affect several different organ systems, diseases in this section are placed into a specific organ system based on which organ system demonstrates the primary gross lesion (or lesions) that is most commonly used to initially recognize and identify the viral disease. The heading for each viral disease includes information on whether the virus is enveloped or nonenveloped (type of injury) and the type of nucleic acid (virulence determinates, genomic diversity) it contains. This information is useful in understanding the mechanisms of injury in specific viral diseases. Viral diseases are identified by a primary mechanism of injury in Table 4-4.

Alimentary System and the Peritoneum, Omentum, Mesentery, and Peritoneal Cavity

Parvovirus Enteritis (Parvovirus, Nonenveloped DNA Virus)

Parvovirus enteritis is a general name used to group two closely related strains of parvovirus that cause canine parvovirus enteritis and feline panleukopenia (feline parvovirus enteritis). The mechanism of injury is death of crypt epithelial cells and lymphocytes, including those in the bone marrow. Specificity for these mitotically active cells occurs because parvoviruses require a host cell–derived duplex transcription template, which is only available when cells divide during the S-phase of the cell cycle. Parvoviruses are unable to turn on DNA synthesis in host cells, so they must wait for host cells to enter the S-phase of the cell cycle before infecting these cells. Gross lesions include segmental areas of the mucosae that are rough and granular (enterocyte necrosis, villus atrophy) with areas of hemorrhage, acute inflammation, and fibrin exudation (see Fig. 7-160).

Dogs and cats encounter parvoviruses in fomites from body fluids contaminated with virus-infected fecal matter through direct contact with virus-infected animals. The virus is inhaled or ingested; deposited on mucosae of the oral, nasal, and pharyngeal cavities; and trapped in the mucus layer. It has not been determined if and how virus penetrates the mucus layer to gain access to mucosal epithelial cells, mucosal macrophages, lymphocytes, and/or dendritic cells. Virus probably infects macrophages or dendritic cells migrating in the mucus layer and on the surface of mucosae. Virus replicates in these cells and is then spread via leukocyte trafficking to the lamina propria of the tonsils. Here, additional macrophages and lymphocytes are infected and spread the virus via leukocyte trafficking in lymphatic and blood vascular systems to regional lymph nodes and systemically to the spleen, thymus, lymph nodes, bone marrow, and mucosa-associated lymphoid nodules such as Peyer's patches of the small intestine. Virus may also be spread as a cell-free viremia in lymph via lymphatic vessels to regional lymph nodes.

In these diseases, the majority of virus-infected intestinal epithelial cells are found in crypts neighboring Peyer's patches in the small intestine. Experimental studies demonstrate that virus arrives at Peyer's patches before it reaches contiguous crypt enterocytes. Although not yet shown with canine or feline parvovirus, other similar viruses spread from Peyer's patches to M cells in Peyer's patches. Morphologically, M-cell processes extend into the mucosa and are contiguous with crypt enterocytes forming intestinal crypts. Additionally, virus entry into intestinal epithelial cells has a polarized pattern in which entry is restricted to the basolateral areas of crypt enterocytes, the areas nearest Peyer's patches and M cells.

TABLE 4-4 Mechanisms of Injury in Diseases Caused by Viruses

Cell Lysis	Cell Proliferation	Inflammation	Neoplastic Transformation	Cell Dysfunction
ALIMENTARY SYSTEM AND THE PERITONEUM, OMENTUM, MESENTERY, AND PERITONEAL CAVITY				
• Parvovirus enteritis • Bovine viral diarrhea and mucosal disease complex • Rinderpest • Blue tongue • Transmissible gastroenteritis • Rotavirus enteritis • Contagious ecthyma • Bovine papular stomatitis • Vesicular stomatitis • Swine vesicular disease • Vesicular exanthema of pigs • Foot and mouth disease	• Contagious ecthyma			
HEPATOBILIARY SYSTEM AND EXOCRINE PANCREAS				
• Infectious canine hepatitis • Wesselsbron disease • Rift valley fever				
RESPIRATORY SYSTEM, MEDIASTINUM, AND PLEURAE				
• Infectious bovine rhinotracheitis • Equine viral rhinopneumonitis • Feline viral rhinotracheitis • Feline calicivirus • Equine influenza • Bovine influenza • Swine influenza • Canine influenza • Canine infectious tracheobronchitis • Bovine respiratory syncytial virus • Inclusion body rhinitis		• Porcine reproductive and respiratory syndrome • Maedi • Caprine pneumonia		
CARDIOVASCULAR SYSTEM AND LYMPHATIC VESSELS				
• Parvovirus myocarditis • Canine herpesvirus infection • Equine viral arteritis • Bovine malignant catarrhal fever • Classical swine fever • African swine fever • African horse sickness		• Feline infectious peritonitis		
BONE MARROW, BLOOD CELLS, AND LYMPHATIC SYSTEM				
• Feline acquired immunodeficiency syndrome • Postweaning multisystemic wasting syndrome		• Equine infectious anemia	• Feline leukemia • Enzootic bovine lymphoma	
NERVOUS SYSTEM				
• Canine distemper • Equine encephalitis-encephalomyelitis • West Nile virus encephalitis-encephalomyelitis • Bovine herpesvirus meningoencephalitis • Equine herpesvirus myeloencephalopathy • Parvovirus-induced cerebellar hypoplasia • Pseudorabies		• Visna • Caprine encephalitis		• Rabies
BONE, JOINTS, TENDONS, AND LIGAMENTS				
		• Caprine arthritis		

Continued

TABLE 4-4 Mechanisms of Injury in Diseases Caused by Viruses—cont'd

Cell Lysis	Cell Proliferation	Inflammation	Neoplastic Transformation	Cell Dysfunction
INTEGUMENTARY SYSTEM				
• Pox • Contagious ecthyma • Bovine papular stomatitis • Vesicular stomatitis • Swine vesicular disease • Vesicular exanthema of pigs • Foot and mouth disease	• Viral papillomas			
FEMALE REPRODUCTIVE SYSTEM AND MAMMARY GLAND				
• Porcine reproductive and respiratory syndrome • Bovine herpesvirus abortion • Infectious pustular vulvovaginitis • Coital exanthema • Equine herpesvirus abortion • Porcine parvovirus abortion				
MALE REPRODUCTIVE SYSTEM				
• Infectious pustular balanoposthitis • Coital exanthema				
EAR AND EYE				
• Feline herpetic keratitis				

Collectively, these findings suggest that virus initially spreads to the intestine via the blood vascular system and not in ingesta via peristalsis. It is unclear whether a virus arrives as a cell-free viremia or within cells of the monocyte-macrophage and/or lymphoid systems; however, (1) virus infects such cells in the oral, nasal, pharyngeal mucosa, and tonsil and regional lymph nodes and (2) leukocyte trafficking is commonly used by other viruses to spread virus systemically to lymphoid and other organ systems, suggesting that parvovirus is spread to the intestine via leukocyte trafficking.

Infection is initiated through capsid-mediated attachment to one or more glycosylated receptors on target cell membranes and is followed by entry via receptor-mediated endocytosis. Parvoviruses appear to use coreceptors for the attachment and entry processes. Attachment receptors may assist in aggregating virus near the cell membrane, and entry receptors may assist the virus in penetrating the cell membrane. In the dog, this process requires capsid proteins to bind to transferrin receptors, whereas in the cat, the process requires capsid proteins to bind to neuraminic acid and transferrin receptors. These receptors appear to determine which cells and which species of animal are infected by parvovirus strains. Parvoviruses are released from infected crypt enterocytes when the cell is killed after the replication cycle is completed. Because of this outcome, parvovirus enteritis causes an osmotic malabsorption-maldigestion diarrhea. Diarrhea occurs because of the failure of replacement of absorptive enterocytes covering villi that are lost through normal turnover (≈48-hour lifespan). As a result, affected villi collapse, are atrophic, and all absorptive and digestive surfaces are lost; thus dietary carbohydrates are available for fermentation by intestinal bacteria. Under normal conditions, enterocytes covering villi are replaced by dividing crypt epithelial cells that move up and cover the villus. The loss of enterocytes covering villi also functionally opens a barrier system that normally prevents endotoxins from being absorbed by capillary beds in the lamina propria of the villi. Endotoxic shock and DIC can result and kill the affected animal. Panleukopenia also occurs because of virus-induced cytolysis of rapidly dividing stem cells in the bone marrow. The effects of parvovirus on organs of the lymphatic system are discussed in the section on Bone Marrow, Blood Cells, and Lymphatic System.

Bovine Viral Diarrhea and Mucosal Disease (BVD Virus, Pestivirus, Enveloped RNA Virus)

The range of diseases caused by BVD virus is diverse and complex. Some of these diseases will be discussed in this chapter and other chapters of this book. Bovine viral diarrhea and mucosal disease as discussed herein refers to the disease that affects mucosae of the alimentary system from the oral cavity to the small intestine. The mechanism of injury in bovine viral diarrhea and mucosal disease is dysfunction and death of mucosal epithelial cells of the oral cavity and esophagus (stratified squamous epithelium) and of the small intestines (enterocytes) preceded by dysfunction and death of submucosal lymphocytes in MALT, such as those in Peyer's patches. Gross lesions include erosion, ulceration, and hemorrhage of mucosae of oral/nasal cavities and pharynx, esophagus, and small intestine (see Figs. 7-3, 7-142, 7-143, and 7-144).

The typical pathogenesis of mucosal disease involves two forms of BVD virus, a noncytopathic form and a cytopathic form, acting synergistically to cause lesions. The *noncytopathic form* of the virus is likely introduced into the herd in new stock, commingling of cattle, semen, or other management practices that allow contact with carrier cattle. The *cytopathic form* of the virus commonly arises from a noncytopathic form that exists in the herd through mutations of its viral genome or it is introduced into the herd as discussed above. Under the proper conditions as discussed below, the noncytopathic form makes cattle immunotolerant to cytopathic forms of BVD virus. Mucosal disease occurs when immunotolerant cattle are exposed to a cytopathic form of the virus (1) most likely originating through mutations on the same farm or (2) introduced into the herd by means discussed above. When cattle with a normal adaptive immune response (i.e., not immunotolerant) are exposed to the cytopathic form of the virus, they are usually able to prevent or limit the severity of mucosal disease that occurs unless the viral strain has several highly pathogenic virulence determinates.

Immunotolerant calves occur when fetuses of naïve (normal immune responses, unvaccinated, no prior exposure) pregnant cows are infected with the noncytopathic form of the virus. Infected cows are asymptomatic, but functionally serve as a means for the virus to infect the fetus and establish "persistently infected (PI)" calves (noncytopathic form of the virus) in the herd. These calves, present in small numbers, usually die before a year of age, but serve as farm reservoirs for noncytopathic virus as they constantly shed virus in body secretions (saliva, tears) and feces into the environment.

For convenience, let's begin the mechanistic sequence of events that ultimately leads to mucosal disease with the exposure of pregnant cows to the noncytopathic form on the farm and *in utero* transplacental spread of this form from infected cows to their calves. Cows encounter the noncytopathic form in fomites from contaminated body fluids or wastes through direct contact with PI calves or carrier animals. The noncytopathic form is inhaled or ingested and deposited on mucosae of the oral, nasal, and pharyngeal cavities; especially favored are mucosae overlying the tonsil. It has not been determined if and how virus penetrates the mucus layer to gain access to mucosal epithelial cells or submucosal macrophages, lymphocytes, and/or dendritic cells, but this process could be facilitated via phagocytosis in the mucus layer by mucosa-associated macrophages, lymphocytes, and/or dendritic cells migrating through the mucosae. Noncytopathic virus probably infects and replicates in monocytes, macrophages, lymphocytes, and dendritic cells and is spread via leukocyte trafficking in lymphatic vessels from tonsil and submucosal lymphoid nodules to regional lymph nodes and then systemically to the caruncular side of placentomas. Trophoblasts in the placentoma can be infected by noncytopathic virus, likely allowing virus to complete a replication cycle, migrate into and through the cotyledons, and infect fetal macrophage-like cells that enter the fetal vascular system and spread to the fetus. Additionally, noncytopathic virus can infect and spread within the allantoic and amniotic membranes and then infect the fetus, but it is unclear which cells facilitate this spread.

Bovine fetuses, infected *in utero*, become immunotolerant (see Chapter 5) to the noncytopathic form of the virus. They also do not recognize antigens from cytopathic forms of the virus as foreign, and as a result they fail to develop an effective adaptive immune response. When exposed to cytopathic virus, mucosal disease ensues in these calves. Mechanistically, the sequence of events that ultimately leads to mucosal disease begins when these immunotolerant calves inhale or ingest cytopathic virus and it is deposited on mucosae of the oral, nasal, and pharyngeal cavities, and the tonsil. The mechanism of infection and spread of the virus from the mucus layer systemically to MALT of the alimentary system, especially Peyer's patches, is similar to that described above for the noncytopathic virus. Herein, the cytopathic virus infects follicular dendritic cells and B lymphocytes in MALT and spreads to, infects, and kills overlying stratified squamous epithelial cells and/or crypt enterocytes, resulting in mucosal erosions, ulcerations, and hemorrhage. In the small intestine because of the death of crypt enterocytes, there is a failure of replacement of sloughed villus enterocytes after normal enterocyte turnover at the villus tip. This outcome may in part explain the mucosal lesions and initiate the formation of ulcers. Hemorrhage occurring with the ulcers could be the result of exposure of capillary beds to endotoxins or other toxic molecules absorbed through an open intestinal barrier system (cell junctions). Diarrhea could also occur secondary to the absorption of large quantities of endotoxins into the lamina propria and deeper supporting stroma that contains the enteric nervous system, resulting in an acquired dysautonomia (see Chapter 14). It has been recently reported that certain molecules released from lymphocytes and/or monocytes infected with cytopathic virus can initiate apoptosis in bystander lymphocytes and monocytes not infected with virus. The role of apoptosis in ulceration of mucosae has not been determined. Additionally, a vasculopathy involving arterioles and small arteries in submucosal tissue of Peyer's patches has been reported and is characterized by segmental necrosis of vascular walls and lymphohistiocytic perivasculitis. Potentially, such lesions could cause endothelial injury and occlusive thrombi, resulting in infarction of the mucosal enterocytes overlying Peyer's patches. Lymphoid cells in Peyer's patches initially proliferate when infected, but infection is followed by massive death of lymphocytes as part of the viral replication cycle, likely caused by a virus-induced apoptotic mechanism.

Rinderpest (Cattle Plague, Morbillivirus, Enveloped RNA Virus)

Because of similarities in clinical presentations, lesions, causative virus, and mechanisms of infection and spread between Rinderpest and other viral diseases, the following materials should be reviewed: (1) morbilliviruses—local, regional, and systemic infection and spread and their target cells in the section on canine distemper; (2) bovine viral diarrhea-mucosal disease—clinical presentation and lesions; and (3) parvoviruses—mechanisms used to infect and spread between cells.

The mechanism of injury in Rinderpest is dysfunction and death of mucosal epithelial cells, dendritic cells (Langerhans' cells [oral cavity]), M cells, lymphocytes, and macrophages of the alimentary system from the oral cavity to the small intestine. Gross lesions include erosions, ulcerations, and hemorrhages of the oral cavity, including the gums, lips, hard and soft palate, cheeks, and base of the tongue, the esophagus, and the small intestine over Peyer's patches (Fig. 4-38). Lymph nodes, especially mesenteric nodes, are enlarged, hemorrhagic, and edematous.

Cattle (and likely sheep and goats) encounter the virus in fomites from body fluids and wastes, such as nasal-ocular fluids, salvia, urine, and feces, through direct contact with virus-infected cattle. Virus is inhaled, deposited on, and trapped in mucosae of the conductive and exchange components of the respiratory system through centrifugal and inertial turbulence. It has not been determined if and how virus penetrates the mucus layer to gain access to mucosal epithelial cells, mucosal macrophages, and/or dendritic cells. Virus probably infects and replicates in mucosal macrophages and dendritic cells as they migrate through the mucus layer and mucosae and then is spread by these cells locally through leukocyte trafficking to the submucosa where they infect and replicate in tissue macrophages, lymphocytes, and dendritic cells. These cells then spread virus via leukocyte trafficking through lymphatic vessels to regional lymph nodes. Herein, similar cells are infected and used to spread the virus systemically via lymphatic vessels, the thoracic duct, and the blood vascular system systemically to lymph nodes, and other organ systems, including the alimentary and respiratory systems. Systemically, primary cell targets for infection include those cells in Peyer's patches of the small intestine and in lymphoid nodules including Langerhans' cells of the Malphigian layer of stratified squamous epithelium of the oral cavity and esophagus.

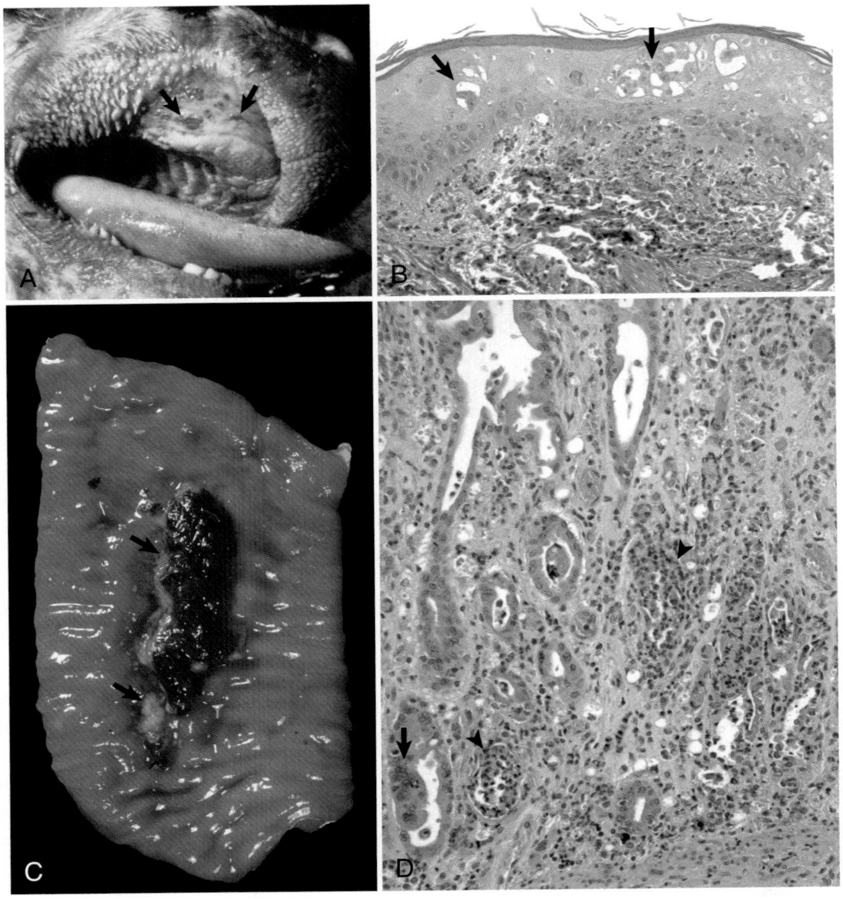

Fig. 4-38 Rinderpest.
A, Oral mucosa, dental pad. Note the erosions and ulcers *(arrows)* adjacent to the dental pad caused by Rinderpest virus. **B,** Oral mucosa. Focal aggregates of epithelial cells in the mucosa are swollen, necrotic, and some are detached *(arrows)*. When abraded by ingesta or other trauma, the mechanical force applied to the lesion in **A** can separate the epithelium overlying the lesion and it will grow and lead to ulcers or abrasions, depending on depth of the epithelial loss. Note the acute inflammatory response in the lamina propria. H&E stain. **C,** Ileum. The mucosa overlying Peyer's patches is ulcerated and covered with fibrin mixed with hemorrhage *(arrows)*. This lesion appears to result from spread of the virus from underlying lymphocytes in Peyer's patches to epithelial cells of the crypts. **D,** Epithelial cells of the crypts are hyperplastic and form syncytia *(arrow)*. In other areas, crypt enterocytes and cells in the adjacent lamina propria are necrotic *(arrowhead)* and accompanied by acute inflammation. This process leads to ulceration of the intestinal mucosa. H&E stain. (**A** and **C** courtesy Dr. C. Brown, College of Veterinary Medicine, The University of Georgia. **B** and **D** courtesy Dr. J.F. Zachary, College of Veterinary Medicine, University of Illinois.)

Erosive lesions in the oral-pharyngeal-lingual mucosae begin in the Malpighian layer (stratum basale [germinativum], stratum spinosum, and stratum granulosum). Langerhans' cells (dendritic cells) are located in the Malpighian layer and are sentinel cells that migrate in and out monitoring for foreign antigens. Although unproved, Langerhans' cells are likely infected with Rinderpest virus via encounters with virus-infected macrophages migrating through these mucosae. Infected oral Langerhans' cells also spread virus to contiguous squamous epithelial cells. Herein, the virus replication cycle results in lysis of infected squamous epithelial cells (oral-pharyngeal-lingual mucosal ulceration) and release of virus into the alimentary system. Erosive lesions in intestinal mucosae likely occur via a similar mechanism facilitated by the infection and migration of macrophages, monocytes, and dendritic cells systemically and into and through Peyer's patches and then to enterocytes. The entry of Rinderpest virus into mucosal enterocytes has a polarized pattern restricted to the their basolateral areas, the areas nearest Peyer's patches and M cells. The virus replication cycle results in lysis of infected enterocytes (small intestine mucosal ulceration) and release of virus into the alimentary system.

Similar to distemper virus, the Rinderpest virus has envelope and hemagglutinin/fusion surface glycoproteins for attachment and fusion, respectively, to host cell membrane glycoprotein receptor CD150 (signaling lymphocyte activation molecule [SLAM]). SLAM has been demonstrated in membranes of lymphocytes, monocytes, and macrophages and of epithelial cells of the respiratory, alimentary, and integumentary systems.

Feline Infectious Peritonitis (Feline Infectious Peritonitis Virus; Nonenveloped RNA Virus)

See the section on the Cardiovascular System and Lymphatic Vessels.

Bluetongue (Orbivirus, Nonenveloped RNA Virus)

The mechanism of injury in bluetongue is dysfunction and death of endothelial cells. Gross lesions include systemic hemorrhage, edema, and vasculitis. Such lesions are more severe in sheep when compared to cattle, apparently because there are species differences in the susceptibility of endothelial cells to infection and the severity of endothelial injury. Bluetongue is a noncontagious disease of sheep, cattle, and other ruminants (deer). The virus is encountered in fluids from hematophagous *Culicoides* (biting midges), which is the insect vector for the virus. After skin penetration, virus gains access to cutaneous blood and fluids, as well as cutaneous dendritic cells (Langerhans' cells), monocytes, and tissue macrophages. Although unproved, virus probably infects these cells, and virus-infected monocytes and macrophages migrate to local lymph nodules and/or aggregates, then to regional lymph nodes via lymphatic vessels. Here, virus infects lymphocytes and additional dendritic cells, monocytes, and macrophages. Macrophages then enter the blood vascular and lymphatic systems (blood vascular via the thoracic duct) and migrate in the vascular system to all organ systems. Herein, they adhere to, migrate through, and reside in the walls of blood vessels and thus are in direct contact with endothelial cells. Virus lyses and escapes from these macrophages and binds to receptors on endothelial cells.

Bluetongue virus has two attachment proteins, capsid structural proteins (VP2 and VP5). These proteins bind to glycosaminoglycans in host cell membranes and facilitate attachment and penetration of virus into macrophages and likely into endothelial cells. Systemically, the attachment of virus-infected macrophages to endothelial cells is likely facilitated by molecules of the leukocyte adhesion cascade (see Chapter 3). Virus in infected monocytes/macrophages that are adhered to endothelial cells escape (via cell lysis) from these monocytes/macrophages and adhere to, infect, and replicate in endothelial cells, leading to endothelial cell injury and death (necrosis-vasculitis). Depending on the severity of endothelial cell injury, vasculitis can be followed by hemorrhage and edema (increased vascular permeability) affecting the lung, vascular thrombosis leading to oral mucosal ulcerations, tissue infarction, and DIC, which kills the affected animal.

Transmissible Gastroenteritis (Coronavirus, Enveloped RNA Virus)

The mechanism of injury in transmissible gastroenteritis is dysfunction and death of epithelial cells (villus enterocytes) covering tips and sides of intestinal villi (Fig. 4-39, *A*). Gross lesions include congestion and thinning of the wall of the small intestine and shortening (atrophy) of villi (Fig. 4-39, *B*, see 7-148, 7-149, and 7-150). Piglets encounter virus in feces through direct contact with virus-infected pigs. Virus is ingested and by swallowing and peristasis it is carried through the oral pharynx, esophagus, and stomach to the small intestine where it is trapped in the mucus layer. The mucus layer has mucins and mucin-like glycoproteins that contain sialic acid. The viral envelope expresses S protein, which binds to sialic acid in the mucus layer, but it has not been determined how the virus penetrates the mucus layer to gain access to enterocytes. When in contact with cell membrane, S protein also binds to a glycoprotein receptor, aminopeptidase N, which is expressed on apical surfaces of villus enterocytes. This interaction facilitates the attachment and entry of virus into villus enterocytes where the virus replicates. Virus then lyses villus enterocytes and escapes into the lumen of the small intestine to be passed in the feces. Injured and killed villus enterocytes are sloughed, resulting in collapse (atrophy) of the villus. Basement membranes are not injured, and crypt enterocytes divide and migrate up the denuded villus to cover exposed basement membrane. Early in the reparative process, these migrating cells are flattened squamous-like cells stretched over the basement membrane. As the cells increase in density and maturity, they regain a more columnar morphology. Additionally, the loss of enterocytes allows endotoxins and other potentially harmful molecules in the digesta to gain access via diffusion to the capillary and lymphatic vessels in the lamina propria of villi and through absorption cause systemic cardiovascular and hemodynamic effects. A malabsorption osmotic diarrhea also occurs because of the loss of intestinal epithelial cells and the failure to digest carbohydrates (impaired hydrolysis) and other molecules in the digesta. This

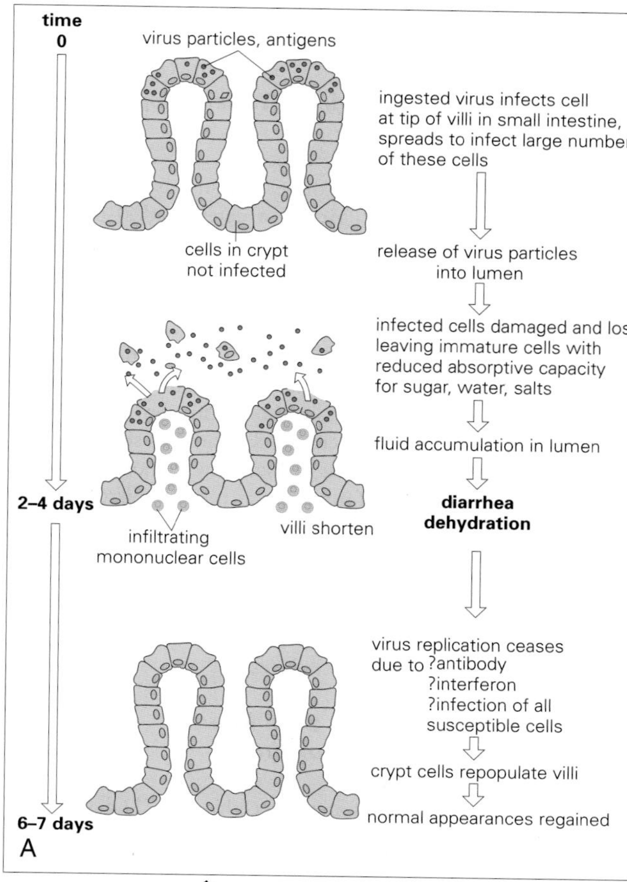

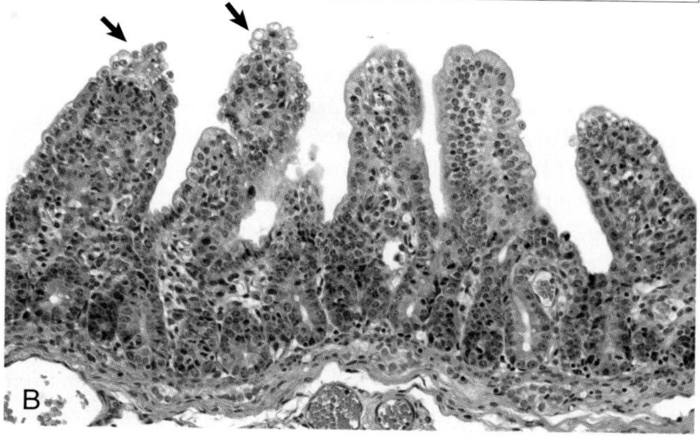

Fig. 4-39 Mechanism of viral infections that target villus absorptive enterocytes.

A, Transmissible gastroenteritis virus and rotavirus use similar mechanisms to infect villus enterocytes and cause disease. **B,** Small intestine, villus atrophy. Following the initial loss of tip enterocytes *(arrows)*, the villi contract, reducing the surface area to be reepithelialized. Note the crypt epithelium becomes hyperplastic with numerous mitoses and the villi are covered by a less specialized, usually low cuboidal epithelium. The villus lamina propria is infiltrated by acute inflammatory cells. H&E stain. (**A** from Goering R, Dockrell H, Roitt I, et al: *Mims' medical microbiology*, ed 4, St. Louis, 2008, Mosby. **B** courtesy Dr. J. F. Zachary, College of Veterinary Medicine, University of Illinois.)

outcome leads to bacterial fermentation of substrates like glucose and an osmotic diarrhea.

Rotavirus Enteritis (Rotavirus, Nonenveloped RNA Virus)

The mechanism of injury, pathogenesis, and clinical outcomes of rotavirus enteritis are similar to those of transmissible gastroenteritis, but the pathogenicity (virulence determinates) of rotavirus is much less severe (see Fig. 4-39). Viral capsid attachment proteins, VP4 and VP7, appear to be involved in the attachment and entry of virus into villus enterocytes through a multistage receptor-mediated process by binding to host cell membrane proteins such as sialic acids, integrins, heat shock proteins, and gangliosides located on apical surfaces. The replication of rotavirus in villus enterocytes results in the production of NSP4, an enterotoxin that (1) induces a secretory diarrhea, (2) stimulates the enteric nervous system and causes intestinal hypermotility, and (3) increases the concentration of intracellular calcium, disrupting the cytoskeletal system and tight junctions, and results in increased mucosal permeability. NSP4 appears to cause dysfunction of cell membrane systems modulating electrolyte and water movement such as calcium ion-dependent chloride secretion, sodium-glucose transport proteins, brush-border membrane disaccharidases, and calcium ion-dependent secretory reflexes.

Contagious Ecthyma (Orf, Sore Mouth, Pustular Dermatitis: Parapoxvirus; Enveloped DNA Virus)

The mechanism of injury in contagious ecthyma is (1) dysfunction and death of squamous epithelial cells of oral mucosae and/or skin by viral replication and cytolysis and (2) exuberant hyperplasia (proliferation) of squamous epithelial cells of oral mucosal and/or skin through modulation of regulatory activities in the cell-division cycle by virulence determinates expressed in the viral genome. Gross lesions include (1) macules, papules, vesicles, pustules, scabs, and scars and in cases having extensive injury resulting from vesicles and pustules (2) a reparative response with proliferation of mucosal squamous epithelial cells resulting in a thickened and granulation tissue–like appearance of affected mucosae (see Figs. 7-8 and 17-48). Lesions are most easily observed on wool-free or hair-free areas such as the muzzle (lips and mouth) and udder (teats) but also can occur in the skin of the perineum, groin, prepuce, scrotum, axilla, and vulva. This disease is zoonotic.

Sheep and goats encounter the virus in fomites of fluids from ruptured macules, vesicles, and pustules and from skin debris and scabs through direct contact with virus-infected animals. The virus can also be spread through mechanical contact with contaminated clothing, instruments, and clippers. Virus gains access to the Malpighian layer of the squamous mucosae through traumatic abrasions, lacerations, or burns and infects Langerhans' cells (dendritic cells) and capillary endothelial cells. Infection of additional Langerhans' cells occurs when these dendritic cells migrate through the subcutis of the Malpighian layer. Infection of endothelial cells may be facilitated by the migration of dendritic cells through the capillary wall. Virus appears to use F1L envelope protein as an attachment protein to bind to glycosaminoglycan heparin sulfate receptor proteins on the surface of host cells. Endothelial cells are injured and lysed (killed) by virus, and injury is accompanied by vascular dilatation, leakage (edema), and active hyperemia, likely contributing to formation of macules, vesicles, and papules. Reparative and regenerative responses contribute to proliferative lesions (hyperplasia) of squamous mucosae and skin. Hyperplasia is apparently caused by (1) synthesis of vascular endothelial growth factor molecules from virus-infected capillary endothelial cells, (2) proliferation of new capillaries as occurs in angiogenesis, and (3) the concurrent proliferation of mucosal epithelial cells much like in the formation of granulation tissue. Virus also infects cells of the stratum basale (germinativum) that are regenerating (actively dividing [mitotic]) as a reparative response to the initial injury of mucosae; however, the relationship between infection of these epithelial cells and the proliferative response that ensues is unclear.

Bovine Papular Stomatitis (Parapoxvirus, Enveloped DNA Virus)

The pathogenesis and mechanism of injury in bovine papular stomatitis are similar to those of contagious ecthyma. The disease occurs primarily in cattle and also in sheep and goats (see Figs. 7-6 and 7-7).

Vesicular Stomatitis (Vesiculovirus, Enveloped RNA Virus)

The mechanism of injury in vesicular stomatitis is cell dysfunction and death leading to intercellular edema (vesiculation) of mucosae and skin, followed by rupture of the vesicles and subsequently erosion and ulceration. Gross lesions include vesicles, erosions, and ulcerations on the mucous membranes and skin of the tongue, oral cavity, hoof coronary bands and interdigital skin, and teats. The pathogenesis has not been determined to an extent that results in an understanding of the chronologic sequence of events leading to disease. The virus, an arbovirus, is spread to cattle, horses, and pigs primarily by sandflies and blackflies and rarely by instruments or equipment. Animals encounter the virus through the bite wounds of these insects, where the biting process injures blood vessels and capillaries, resulting in virus being deposited directly into plasma of blood vessels and/or into interstitial fluids (also containing plasma leaked from vasopuncture) within vascularized submucosal and subcutaneous ECM (connective) tissues. It appears that vesicular lesions occur at or near the sites of insect bites, suggesting that the virus infects target cells locally and there is no systemic spread of virus to mucosae or skin through leukocyte trafficking or viremia. Squamous epithelial cells of mucosae and skin are the primary target cells for viral infection, but Langerhans' cells (dendritic cells) and cells of the monocyte-macrophage system, although likely target cells for infection with virus, have not been clearly identified as target cells. In addition, it is likely but unproved that local migration of dendritic cells and cells of the monocyte-macrophage system spread virus to additional local target cells as described below. Lesions suggest that epithelial cells of the stratum basale and/or spinosum must be targets for virus infection, replication, and escape (through cell lysis). Death of these cells results in the formation of intercellular spaces that fill with fluid and form vesicles. Trauma likely ruptures the vesicles and leads to erosion/ulceration of the overlying mucosa or skin; however, acute inflammation may also contribute to the process. Virus appears to use envelope glycoprotein G as an attachment protein to bind to host target cells; however, receptors on host cells have not been clearly identified.

Swine Vesicular Disease (Enterovirus, Nonenveloped RNA Virus)

The mechanism of injury in swine vesicular disease is cell dysfunction and death leading to intercellular edema (vesiculation), rupture of vesicles, and subsequent erosion and ulceration of mucosae and skin. Gross lesions include vesicles, erosions, and ulcers on the mucosae and skin of the snout, mouth, tongue, hoof coronary bands and interdigital skin, and teats (see Figs. 7-2 and 7-3). Pigs encounter virus through (1) contact with infected vesicular fluid, (2) contact with contaminated clothing or instruments, or (3) ingestion of contaminated pig offal, by-products, or meat products.

It appears that the virus can enter the body through inhalation, ingestion, or contact with abraded skin.

Through inhalation or ingestion, the virus encounters oronasal-pharyngeal mucosae, especially of the tonsil. It has not been determined if and how the virus penetrates the mucus layer to gain access to mucosal epithelial cells, mucosal macrophages, and/or dendritic cells. The role of mucosal epithelial cells in infection is unclear. The virus probably infects and replicates in mucosal macrophages, lymphocytes, and/or dendritic cells as they migrate through the mucus layer and mucosae and then is spread by these cells locally through leukocyte trafficking to the submucosa where they infect and replicate in submucosal tissue macrophages, lymphocytes, and dendritic cells of limpid nodules and aggregates. From here, the virus spreads via lymphatic vessels to regional lymph nodes and infects similar cells, spreads systemically in these cells to other organ systems, including mucosae and skin via lymphatic vessels, the thoracic duct, and the blood vascular system.

Through ingestion, the virus encounters mucosae of the small intestine especially overlying Peyer's patches. Although unproved, the virus likely infects M cells, which spread virus to tissue macrophages, dendritic cells, and other cells in Peyer's patches. Here, similar cells are infected and then migrate to spread virus via lymphatic vessels to regional lymph nodes and then systemically to other organ systems, including mucosae and skin.

Finally, it has been suggested that virus can infect Langerhans' (dendritic cells) or other cells of the Malpighian layer if the skin of the coronary band of the hooves is traumatized and epithelial cells of the stratum basale and/or spinosum are exposed to the environment. Virus can replicate in these squamous epithelial cells and also likely in Langerhans' cells. Thus they may serve as a site of local infection, followed by spread to regional lymph nodes via lymphatic vessels, and systemic spread to other organ systems, including mucosae and skin.

No matter the route used to establish, sustain, and amplify the systemic infection, it appears that virus can infect, injure, and lyse squamous epithelial (mucosae) and dendritic cells of the skin, resulting in vesicle formation. The mechanisms involved in vesicle formation have not been identified but could be similar to those used in poxvirus infections and swine vesicular disease. It is unclear whether spread is via a cell-free viremia or leukocyte trafficking; both mechanisms of virus spread have been demonstrated in enterovirus infections. Virus appears to use capsid proteins, VP1-4, as attachment proteins to bind to glycoprotein receptors, such as ICAM, expressed on the surface of host cells. When interacting with cell receptors, viral capsid proteins undergo conformational changes leading to fusion of virus to cell membrane and internalization of virus within the host target cell. The diversity of ICAM receptors expressed on a variety of host cell membranes probably determines target cell specificity. Additionally, coxsackievirus-adenovirus receptor and sulfated glycosaminoglycans, such as heparin sulfate, may also be used as receptors on host cells.

Vesicular Exanthema of Pigs (Calicivirus [Waikavirus], Nonenveloped RNA Virus)

The pathogenesis and mechanisms of injury in vesicular exanthema of pigs are likely similar to those of swine vesicular disease. Capsid proteins used by the virus to attach and bind to host target cells and receptors for virus on host cells have not been clearly identified. Vesicles are shown in Figs. 7-2 and 7-3.

Foot-and-Mouth Disease (Aphthovirus, Nonenveloped RNA Virus)

The pathogenesis and mechanisms of injury in foot-and-mouth disease in cattle and pigs (less common in sheep and goats) are likely similar to that of swine vesicular disease and vesicular exanthema of pigs. In summary, virus encounters target cells through inhalation or ingestion; establishes a local infection in the oronasal-pharyngeal mucosae especially of the tonsil and in submucosal lymphoid cells, macrophages, and dendritic cells; spreads via lymphatic vessels to regional lymph nodes to sustain and amplify the infection; and then spreads systemically to infect, replicate in, and lyse epithelial cells of the stratum spongiosum of mucosae and skin resulting in vesicles (Fig. 4-40). Capsid proteins used by the virus to attach and bind to host target cells appear to include VP1-4 attachment proteins, whereas α integrins (Vβ1, Vβ3, and Vβ6) expressed on host cells are used are receptors.

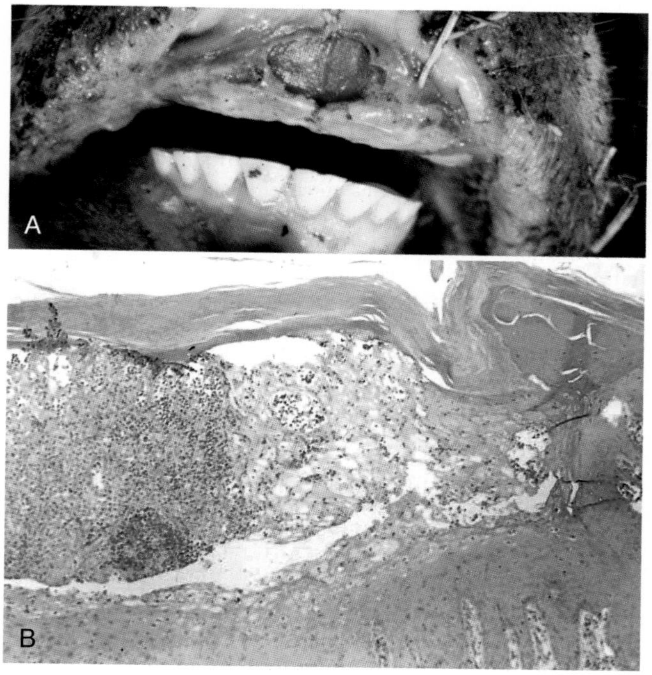

Fig. 4-40 Foot-and-mouth disease.
A, Ox. Note the ulcer on the mucosa of the upper dental pad. Such ulcers begin as fluid-filled vesicles that rupture usually from the trauma of mastication or prehension. Vesicles and ulcers that result from their rupture may occur on all mucosae of the body including the dental pad, tongue, gingiva, coronary bands, and teats as examples. **B,** The mucosa has a large focus of a previous vesicle, which is now partially filled with edema fluid, fibrin, cellular debris, and acute inflammatory cells forming a pustule. H&E stain. (**A** courtesy Dr. M. Adsit, College of Veterinary Medicine, The University of Georgia and Noah's Arkive, College of Veterinary Medicine, The University of Georgia. **B** courtesy Dr. C. Brown, College of Veterinary Medicine, The University of Georgia.)

Hepatobiliary System and Exocrine Pancreas

Infectious Canine Hepatitis (Canine Adenovirus Infection, Canine Adenovirus Type 1, Nonenveloped DNA Virus)

The mechanism of injury in infectious canine hepatitis is cell death (cytolysis) affecting epithelial cells of the liver and kidney and endothelial cells of all organ systems. Gross lesions include randomly distributed white-gray foci (≈1 mm in diameter) of miliary necrosis, as well as mucosal and serosal hyperemia and hemorrhage, and edema of multiple organ systems, including the liver, kidney, lymph nodes, thymus, gastric serosa, pancreas, and subcutaneous tissues (see Fig. 8-74). Edema of the gallbladder wall is prominent and is likely the result of injury of vascular endothelial cells leading to changes in permeability. Tonsillar enlargement, characteristic of the disease, probably results from proliferation of lymphocytes as part of the innate and/or adaptive immune responses against virus-infected cells through hyperplasia of uninfected lymphocytes in response to inflammatory mediators or through recruitment of lymphocytes from other lymphoid tissues and organs.

Dogs encounter the virus in fomites from body fluids such as saliva, urine, or feces. Virus enters the body through ingestion and likely inhalation and is trapped in the mucus layer of oral and pharyngeal mucosae, especially of the tonsils. It has not been determined if and how virus penetrates the mucus layer to gain access to mucosal epithelial cells, mucosal macrophages, and/or dendritic cells. Virus probably infects and replicates in mucosal macrophages and dendritic cells as they migrate through the mucus layer and mucosae. It is then spread by these cells locally through leukocyte trafficking to the submucosa and tonsil where they infect and replicate in additional tissue macrophages, lymphocytes, and dendritic cells and then spread via lymphatic vessels to regional lymph nodes and infect similar cells. A cell-free viremia has also been proposed as a mechanism of spread.

Although undetermined, virus may also be swallowed and through peristalsis encounter and infect M cells and spread and infect macrophages, dendritic cells, and lymphocytes in Peyer's patches and then be spread to regional mesenteric lymph nodes. A virus capsid protein called *fiber protein* has been identified and may serve as an attachment protein that binds to host cell receptors such as coxsackievirus-adenovirus or integrin receptors.

Using either the inhalation or ingestion route of infection and spread, virus spreads from regional lymph nodes, systemically to infect endothelial cells and their contiguous epithelial cells in many organ systems, including liver, kidneys, spleen, and lungs. Infection of, replication in, and release from these cells cause their lysis and subsequent necrosis. The attachment of virus or virus-infected macrophages to endothelial cells is likely facilitated by molecules of the leukocyte adhesion cascade (see Chapter 3). Virus infects and replicates in endothelial cells leading to endothelial cell injury and death (necrosis-vasculitis). Depending on the severity of endothelial cell injury, vasculitis can be followed by hemorrhage and edema (increased vascular permeability) and DIC. Infection of epithelial cells of the liver and kidney are likely facilitated by ligand-receptor interactions, although none have been identified, Infection and death of lymphocytes in lymphoid tissues and likely bone marrow may account for the leukopenia occurring early in the infection.

Wesselsbron Disease (Flavivirus, Enveloped RNA Virus)

The mechanism of injury in Wesselsbron disease is disruption and death of hepatocytes affecting young to very young sheep, cattle, and goats (ruminants). Gross lesions include an enlarged yellow to orange-brown liver (hepatomegaly) with randomly distributed white-gray foci (≈1 mm in diameter) of miliary necrosis of hepatocytes. Ruminants encounter this arbovirus through bite wounds from virus-infected mosquitoes; domestic herbivores likely serve as the animal reservoir. Seasonal variations in temperature and precipitation influence the population density of mosquitoes and thus the occurrence of disease. Virus can enter the circulatory system through direct penetration of a blood vessel during a bite wound, in which virus infects monocytes. It can also be deposited in vascularized ECM (connective) tissues, in which virus gains access to cutaneous blood and fluids, as well as Langerhans' cells (dendritic cells) and trafficking tissue macrophages.

Through either route, virus-infected monocytes, macrophages, and/or dendritic cells spread virus via lymphatic vessels to regional lymph nodes where similar cells are infected. These cells then spread virus systemically via lymphatic vessels and the thoracic duct or postcapillary venules to the blood vascular system and other lymphoid tissues, such as the spleen, and other organ systems, such as the liver and in this example use hepatocytes and Kupffer cells (part of the monocyte-macrophage system) as target cells. Hypertrophy and hyperplasia of Kupffer cells has been reported experimentally; however, their role in the pathogenesis of Wesselsbron disease has not been determined. The virus may also possibly spread via cell-free viremia. Although unidentified at this time, viral envelope glycoproteins probably serve as attachment proteins for receptors expressed on specific populations of host target cells, thus probably determining cellular tropism for the virus.

Rift Valley Fever (Phlebovirus, Enveloped RNA Virus)

The pathogenesis and mechanisms of injury in Rift Valley fever are similar to those of Wesselsbron disease.

Respiratory System, Mediastinum, and Pleurae

Infectious Bovine Rhinotracheitis (Bovine Herpesvirus, Alphaherpesvirus, Enveloped DNA Virus)

Bovine herpesvirus targets cells of the respiratory system, but can also infect cells of the nervous system. The mechanism of injury in infectious bovine rhinotracheitis is death of nonciliated and ciliated (mucociliary apparatus) epithelial cells of the oral, nasal, pharyngeal, and respiratory mucosae (Fig. 4-41). Gross lesions include active hyperemia, hemorrhage, edema, and necrosis leading to large areas of mucosal erosions and ulcers often covered with a fibrinous membrane (see Figs. 9-14 and 9-18).

Cattle encounter bovine herpesvirus in fomites of body fluids contaminated with virus through direct contact with virus-infected animals. Virus can be inhaled or ingested and deposited on and trapped in the mucus layers of oral, nasal, and pharyngeal mucosae. Virus can also be inhaled and deposited and trapped in the mucus layer of the mucosae of the conductive component of the respiratory system through centrifugal and inertial turbulence. Additionally, virus can be deposited on conjunctiva. It has not been determined if and how virus penetrates mucus layers of these mucosae to gain access to epithelial cells or if mucosal macrophages and/or dendritic cells are involved in carrying virus to the membranes of epithelial target cells. Viral envelope glycoproteins B, C, and D are used to attach to and enter a variety of host target cells via an array of glycosaminoglycan receptors, such as herpesvirus entry mediator A, nectin-1 and -2 (herpesvirus entry proteins C and B), and 3-*O*-sulfated heparin sulfate, most commonly expressed on mucosal epithelial cells and also on the sensory nerve endings that innervate the mucosa. These receptors have a polarized pattern of expression and are present only on apical and lateral surfaces of mucosal epithelial cells above junctional complexes; therefore inhalation of virus provides it with optimal opportunities for interactions with appropriate receptors. Virus enters nonciliated and ciliated mucosal epithelial cells, completes its replication cycle in these epithelial cells, and causes cell death through cytolysis as a means of releasing progeny virus into the environment.

Bovine herpesvirus can also gain access to sensory nerve endings in the respiratory mucosae. It infects, replicates, and spreads in the trigeminal and olfactory nerves via retrograde axonal transport and spreads via this mechanism to other neurons in the CNS. Neurons serve as reservoir cells in which virus establishes a latent infection. Additionally, because neurons express no MHC class II molecules and low concentrations of MHC class I molecules,

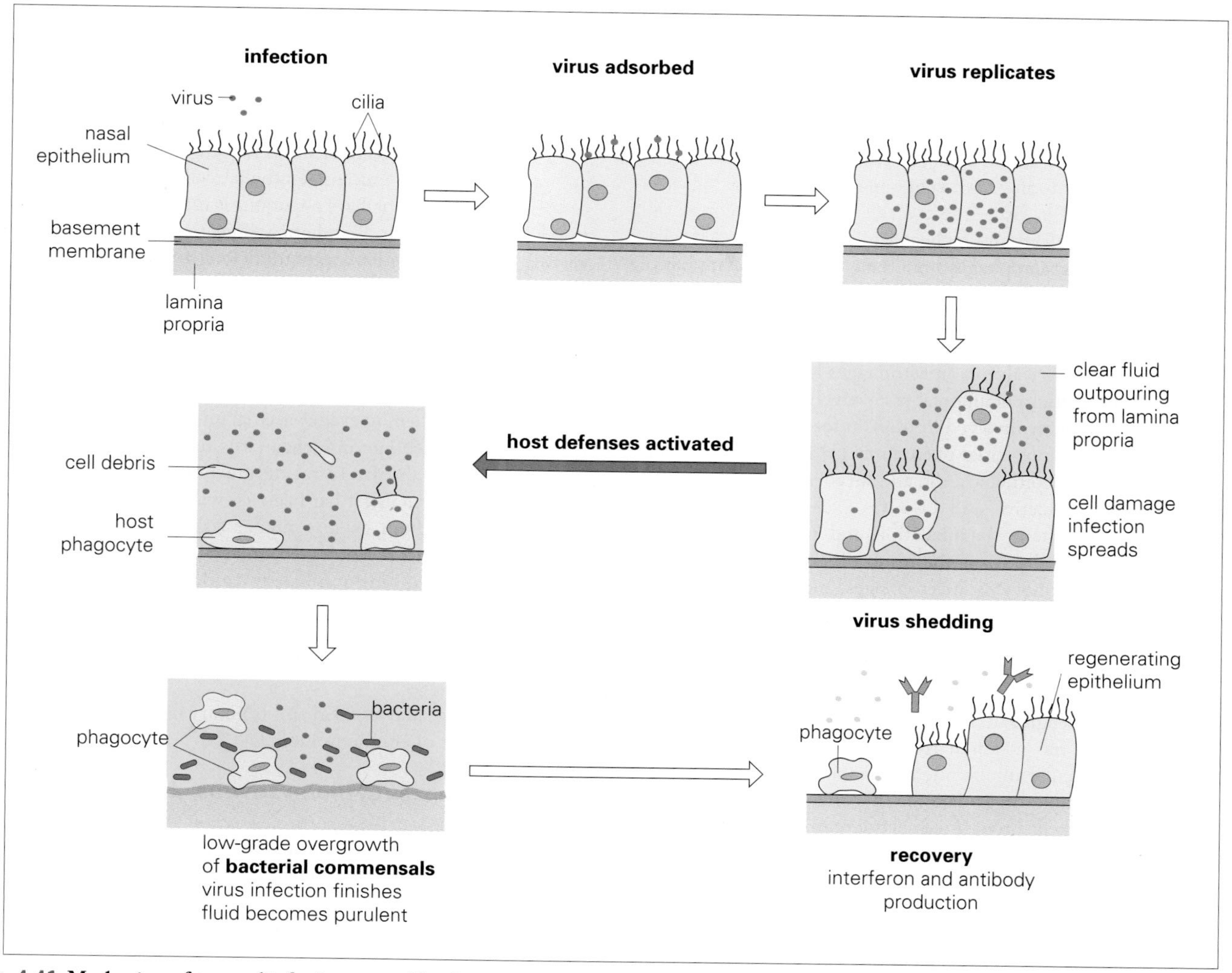

Fig. 4-41 Mechanism of mucosal infections caused by rhinotracheitis viruses.
For simplification, the epithelium is represented as one cell thick. (From Goering R, Dockrell H, Roitt I, et al: *Mims' medical microbiology,* ed 4, St. Louis, 2008, Mosby.)

they are less likely, even when infected with virus, to be recognized by and acted on by cytotoxic and helper T lymphocytes, macrophages trafficking through the nervous system, and by resident microglial cells. During latency, viral genomes are present in the nucleus of infected neurons, but no viral proteins (antigens) are synthesized. With activation, the virus reestablishes its replication cycle and through axonal transport mechanisms spreads back to nerve endings in mucous membranes to be released and potentially infect adjacent mucosal epithelial cells and transmit the disease. Bovine herpesvirus produces proteins that (1) disrupt the synthesis of interferon, (2) block the recognition of virus-infected cells by cytotoxic T lymphocytes, and (3) block the homing of T lymphocytes to virus-infected cells. Virus can also infect and induce high levels of apoptosis in T helper lymphocytes, thus suppressing the adaptive immune response to the virus. It is likely that a combination of these immunosuppressive mechanisms and disruption of the mucociliary apparatus through death of virus-infected ciliated mucosal epithelial cells make affected animals more susceptible to many secondary bacterial diseases of the respiratory system, such as Pasteurellosis or Mannheimiosis, that follow an outbreak of infectious bovine rhinotracheitis.

Equine Viral Rhinopneumonitis (Equine Herpesvirus, Alphaherpesvirus, Enveloped DNA Virus)

The pathogenesis and mechanisms of injury in equine viral rhinopneumonitis are similar to those of infectious bovine rhinotracheitis.

Feline Viral Rhinotracheitis (Feline Herpesvirus, Alphaherpesvirus, Enveloped DNA Virus)

Feline viral rhinotracheitis and feline calicivirus infections often occur concurrently and thus are termed the *feline upper respiratory disease complex.* The pathogenesis and mechanisms of injury in feline viral rhinotracheitis are similar to those of infectious bovine rhinotracheitis and equine viral rhinopneumonitis. Additionally, virus also infects mucosal macrophages and spreads to and infects similar cells in regional lymphoid nodes and then systemically via leukocyte trafficking or cell-free viremia to infect bone, eye, and lung, resulting in death of osteoblasts and osteocytes in the turbinates, necrosis of conjunctival and corneal epithelial cells, and necrosis of alveolar macrophages, respectively. Viral envelope glycoprotein G has been shown to attach and bind to chemokine receptors on host target cells.

Feline Calicivirus (Calicivirus, Nonenveloped RNA Virus)

The pathogenesis and mechanisms of injury in feline calicivirus infection are similar to those of feline viral rhinotracheitis, infectious bovine rhinotracheitis, and equine viral rhinopneumonitis. Although the mechanism of injury is probably necrosis and cell death, experimental studies have suggested that synthesis of caspases can be induced in virus-infected cells, resulting in apoptosis of these cells. Virus infects and replicates in mucosal epithelial cells and likely mucosal macrophages and then spreads in lymphatic vessels to regional lymph nodes via leukocyte trafficking (or cell-free viremia) to infect additional lymphocytes and macrophages. These cells then spread virus systemically to infect synovial macrophages and pulmonary alveolar macrophages leading to synovitis and probably interstitial pneumonia, respectively. Ligand-receptor interactions are probably involved in tropism for specific cell types. It is unclear whether interstitial pneumonia (1) results from direct infection of mucosal epithelial cells and alveolar macrophages of mucosae of the conductive and O_2-CO_2 exchange components of the respiratory system via inhalation and infection of apical membranes of these cells, (2) is the result of leukocyte trafficking of virus-infected lymphocytes, macrophages, and monocytes back to the lung after infecting and being amplified in regional and systemic lymph nodes and lymphoid organs, or (3) is attributable to a combination of both mechanisms.

Recently, a syndrome termed *virulent systemic feline calicivirus infection* has been recognized. In addition to epithelial cell tropism, this virulent strain has acquired tropism for endothelial cells. It causes systemic vascular injury, microthrombosis, DIC, and death attributable to multiple-organ failure. This change in viral pathogenicity likely occurred through reassortment of viral capsid genes leading to enhanced virulence determinates that modulate attachment and entry and likely replication in endothelial cells. Furthermore, an additional virulence determinate appears to contribute to an exuberant host cell cytokine response as a defense mechanism against virus-infected epithelial and endothelial cells. Thus vascular lesions may, in part, be immune-mediated.

Equine Influenza (Orthomyxovirus, Enveloped RNA Virus)

The mechanism of injury in equine influenza is death of epithelial cells of the oral, nasal, pharyngeal, and respiratory mucosae. Gross lesions include active hyperemia, hemorrhage, edema, and necrosis leading to mucosal erosions and ulcers often covered with a fibrinous membrane.

Horses encounter virus in fomites from body fluids contaminated with virus through direct contact with virus-infected animals. Virus is inhaled and deposited on and trapped in the mucus layer of mucosae of the nasal and pharyngeal cavities and of the conductive component of the respiratory system through centrifugal and inertial turbulence. Virus must penetrate the mucus layer to gain access to ciliated epithelial cells (mucociliary apparatus); however, mucus contains glycoprotein receptor molecules that bind to virus and prevent it from attaching to these cells. This defense mechanism allows virus to be removed via the mucociliary apparatus and phagocytosis and killing by mucosal macrophages. To counteract this defense mechanism, virus expresses a viral neuraminidase that destroys receptors that mimic viral glycoprotein receptors in the mucus. However, it has not been determined how virus penetrates the mucus layer to gain access to mucosal epithelial cells. When virus encounters these cells, hemagglutinin and neuraminidase glycoproteins in its viral envelope bind to host cell membrane receptors composed of sialyloligosaccharides. This ligand-receptor binding allows virus to attach to and enter ciliated epithelial cells. The overall structure of sialyloligosaccharide receptors, in part, determines the target specificity at the cellular and the species levels. Early in the encounter before cell death affects function, the mucociliary apparatus spreads virus to additional target cells. This mechanism of spread becomes less effective as virus kills ciliated and nonciliated mucosal epithelial cells and the physiologic continuity of the mucociliary apparatus is disrupted. It also appears that virus can spread in lymphatic vessels to regional lymph nodes via cell-free viremia or leukocyte trafficking and infect lymphocytes and macrophages. It is likely that death of lymphoid cells (immunosuppression) and ciliated epithelial cells and disruption of the mucociliary apparatus makes horses more susceptible to secondary bacterial diseases of the respiratory system. Antigenic drift, creating antigenically heterologous viruses, occurs commonly in influenza viruses, allowing them to evade vaccinal immunity. Recently, viruses closely related to equine influenza virus have caused outbreaks of severe respiratory disease in racing greyhounds and English foxhounds. Experimentally, it has been shown that canine and equine respiratory epithelium express similar sialyloligosaccharides. This finding suggests that receptors recognized by equine influenza virus are expressed on canine respiratory epithelial cells; nevertheless, subtle differences in receptor specificity may exist.

Bovine Influenza (Orthomyxovirus, Enveloped RNA Virus)

The pathogenesis and mechanisms of injury in bovine influenza are similar to those of equine influenza.

Swine Influenza (Orthomyxovirus, Enveloped RNA Virus)

The pathogenesis and mechanisms of injury in swine influenza are similar to those of equine influenza.

Canine Influenza (Orthomyxovirus, Enveloped RNA virus)

The pathogenesis and mechanisms of injury in canine influenza are similar to those of equine influenza.

Porcine Reproductive and Respiratory Syndrome (Mystery Swine Disease; PRRS Virus; Arterivirus; Enveloped RNA Virus)

The mechanism of injury in porcine reproductive and respiratory syndrome (PRRS) is death of all cell populations in the lung and associated regional lymph nodes secondary to acute inflammation (interstitial pneumonia) and its mediators and degradative enzymes. Gross lesions include lung lobules distributed at random throughout all lung lobes that are firm (consolidation) and red tan to beige with septal edema. Lymph nodes, especially those draining the lungs, are enlarged, firm, and edematous and have a beige-white cut surface that bulges. These lesions may, in part, be attributable to secondary infection with a bacterium like *Pasteurella multocida*.

PRRS occurs in two sequential stages: an acute stage followed by a persistent stage. In the acute stage, pigs encounter virus in fomites from body fluids through direct contact with virus-infected pigs. It is inhaled, deposited on, and trapped in the mucus layer of the mucosae of the conductive and O_2-CO_2 exchange components of the respiratory system through centrifugal and inertial turbulence. Pulmonary alveolar macrophages probably phagocytose the virus in the mucus layer and then spread it to BALT and to tissue macrophages of alveolar septa, pneumocytes of alveoli, and epithelial cells of bronchioles via leukocyte trafficking, where infection and replication occur and acute inflammation (acute interstitial pneumonia and alveolitis) ensue. In this context, virus appears to be able to escape being killed in these cells. Potential mechanisms are discussed below. Concurrently, virus-infected macrophages migrate via lymphatic vessels to regional lymph nodes (tracheobronchial) and infect macrophages and lymphocytes. It has also been suggested, but unproved, that porcine dendritic cells may be infected and spread the virus. Infection causes hypertrophy and hyperplasia of these cells, leading to enlarged lymph nodes; production of proinflammatory cytokines, resulting in cell death, acute inflammation, and edema; and the initiation of an adaptive immune response. Spread to other systemic organ systems (potentially the reproductive system) occurs at this stage, but it is unclear if spread is cell free or cell associated in macrophages (the latter being the most likely). In these organ systems, virus also likely infects cells of the monocyte-macrophage system.

In the persistent stage, virus via leukocyte trafficking establishes reservoirs in tissues, such as the tonsil, spleen, lymph nodes, and lung and in cells of the monocyte-macrophage system, such as alveolar macrophages. In part, infection of cells of the monocyte-macrophage system is likely determined by ligand-receptor interactions and may be related to the presence of sialoadhesin, a glycoprotein macrophage-specific receptor, expressed on cells of monocyte-macrophage lineage as well as scavenger receptor CD163 and heparan sulfate receptors. As an enveloped virus, PRRS virus escapes from cells without causing cell death, but infected alveolar macrophages release proinflammatory cytokines, leading to acute inflammation and the recruitment of additional inflammatory cells followed by cell death attributable to mediators and degradative enzymes of the inflammatory response. As a result, alveoli become filled with neutrophils, necrotic cell debris arising from killing of cells by the degradative activities of inflammatory cell enzymes, and edema fluid. Acute inflammation may also cause limited injury of the mucociliary apparatus leading to increased opportunities for pulmonary infections caused by other bacteria.

It appears that PRRS virus, possibly mediated via nucleocapsid proteins, has both suppressive and stimulatory activities on cells it infects in the immune system. On the one hand, it is able to alter functions of the innate and adaptive immune systems, specifically of cells of the monocyte-macrophage system, by suppressing the ability of these cells to (1) kill virus infected cells, (2) phagocytose, kill, and present antigens to effector cells, (3) stimulate other effector cells, and (4) secrete cytokines such as IFN-α, and TNF-α that are necessary to implement an effective immune response. On the other hand, during the acute phase of infection virus is able to stimulate cells to significantly increase the production of IL-10 from infected cells. This cytokine is immunosuppressive and interacts with a wide array of immune cells, including the cells of the monocyte-macrophage system and lymphocytes, resulting in inhibition of innate and adaptive immunity, particularly the cell-mediated immune responses.

Canine Infectious Tracheobronchitis (Canine Parainfluenza Virus, Enveloped RNA Virus)

Canine infectious tracheobronchitis is an example of a disease in which there is primary injury caused by canine parainfluenza virus leading to increased susceptibility secondarily to infection with *Bordetella bronchiseptica* (or other bacteria). Other viruses (canine adenovirus type 2, canine respiratory coronavirus, reovirus, canine herpesvirus, canine distemper virus) and bacteria (*Mycoplasma* spp., *Streptococcus zooepidemicus*) have been implicated in canine infectious tracheobronchitis, thus the phrase *canine infectious respiratory disease complex* has been used to categorize this multifactorial pathogenesis. The mechanism of injury is dysfunction and death of ciliated epithelial cells of the mucociliary apparatus primarily from virus-induced cytolysis and secondarily from acute inflammation (bronchitis/bronchiolitis) and its mediators and degradative enzymes. Gross lesions include active hyperemia and granularity (necrosis) of the respiratory mucosae and concurrent inflammation of mucosae and submucosae (see Fig. 9-88).

Dogs encounter parainfluenza virus in fomites of oronasal-pharyngeal fluids through direct contact with virus-infected dogs. It is inhaled, deposited on, and trapped in the mucus layer of the mucosae of the conductive component of the respiratory system through centrifugal and inertial turbulence, but it has not been determined if and how virus penetrates mucus layers of these mucosae to gain access to epithelial cells or if mucosal macrophages and/or dendritic cells are involved. Virus infects and replicates in all epithelial cells; however, ciliated mucosal cells are the primary target cells. It appears that virus attaches to and enters cells via viral attachment glycoproteins (HN and F glycoproteins) that bind to sialic acid receptors on host cell membranes. When the mucociliary apparatus is dysfunctional, its cells are more susceptible to secondary infection with bacteria, especially *Bordetella bronchiseptica*. It is inhaled, deposited on, and trapped in the mucus layer of the mucosae of the conductive component of the respiratory system through centrifugal and inertial turbulence. The bacterium colonizes ciliated epithelium via fimbrial and nonfimbrial adhesins such as filamentous hemagglutinin and pertactin. It has not been determined if and how it penetrates mucus layers to gain access to epithelial cells or if mucosal macrophages and/or dendritic cells are involved. Once ciliated cells are colonized, *Bordetella bronchiseptica* releases exotoxins, such as adenylate cyclase-hemolysin and dermonecrotic toxin and endotoxins, that further impair function of the mucociliary apparatus, allowing for additional colonization of the mucosae at new sites. This damage results in an acute inflammatory response that further injures the mucosa. Toxins may also disrupt phagocytosis and/or killing of bacteria by alveolar macrophages and neutrophils and suppress cellular and humoral immune responses. *Bordetella bronchiseptica* can also invade epithelial cells, evade immunologic defense mechanisms, and establish a persistent infection.

Ovine Progressive Pneumonia, (Maedi; Maedi-Visna Virus [Ovine Lentivirus]; Enveloped RNA Virus)

The mechanism of injury in ovine progressive pneumonia is dysfunction and death of cells of the respiratory system from infection with virus and from chronic-active granulomatous interstitial inflammation and its mediators and degradative enzymes. Ovine lentivirus persistently infects monocyte precursor cells, systemic monocytes, and alveolar and tissue macrophages. Gross lesions include dense, rubbery, and enlarged lung lobes that are uniformly affected and grayish-yellow to grayish-blue (see Figs. 9-61 and 9-79). Cut surfaces bulge and are rubbery and are not edematous or exudative, but excessive mucus may be present in airways.

Sheep most likely encounter virus in fomites from respiratory fluids through direct contact with virus-infected animals. In the fluid, virus may be free or in macrophages. However, any condition that facilitates mechanical transfer of infected blood to the circulatory system or mucosae of uninfected animals can also serve to spread virus. It is inhaled, deposited on, and trapped in the mucus layer of the mucosae of the conductive component of the respiratory system through centrifugal and inertial turbulence. Free virus is likely phagocytosed by alveolar macrophages in the mucus layer, whereas virus-infected macrophages likely release virus and/or die (or are killed) and release virus into mucus and mucosae; migrate to local lymphoid tissues (BALT) and release virus and/or die (or are killed) and release virus; or are killed by host immune cells in mucosae and release virus that is phagocytosed by host alveolar macrophages. Virus-infected alveolar macrophages migrate to local lymphoid tissues (BALT) and then via leukocyte trafficking in lymphatic vessels to regional lymph nodes where additional macrophages are infected. Macrophages then spread virus via leukocyte trafficking to immature monocyte precursor cells (monoblasts or promonocytes) in the bone marrow (and likely similar cells in spleen and lymph nodes) where small numbers of infected precursor cells serve as biological reservoirs for the distribution (via the circulatory and lymphatic systems) of virus-infected monocytes back into the blood. Virus likely uses envelope glycoproteins to attach, bind to, and fuse with alveolar macrophages and other target cells that express small ruminant lentivirus receptors A or B or some other membrane receptor. All cells infected with virus are permanently infected (persistent infection) because virus inserts its genome into chromosomal DNA of host cells.

The ability of virus to replicate in a cell is directly related to the maturity of the permanently infected cell. In bone marrow, virus integrates into precursor monocytes (monoblasts or promonocytes) and persistently infects a very small number of such cells. It is not able to replicate in these cells. These cells differentiate into monocytes, migrate to tissues and organ systems that utilize the services of the monocyte-macrophage system, and then differentiate into macrophages. Virus-infected monocytes in the peripheral blood do not produce virus. When infected monocytes mature and differentiate into macrophages in tissues, virus is able to replicate in these cells and express viral proteins and proinflammatory chemokine and cytokine molecules leading to inflammation. These macrophages can then infect and activate other susceptible and differentiated tissue macrophages, such as alveolar macrophages, and this interaction initiates and sustains the chronic active granulomatous inflammatory process. The lifespan of tissue macrophages ranges from 6 to 16 days. Thus the effective lifespan for virus-infected mature tissue macrophages capable of sustaining the infection is shortened because a portion of the lifespan must include time for integration of its genome, replication, and assembly of virus in tissue macrophages. As tissue macrophages infected with virus die off, a cyclic process evolves in which infected monocytes arrive from bone marrow to infect naïve tissue macrophages that replicate locally or arrive and differentiate from uninfected blood monocytes. This cyclic process, often characteristic of lentiviral-induced diseases, combined with genetic variation is used to sustain and enhance the severity of the interstitial pneumonia. Virus-infected monocytes travel throughout all tissues and organ systems of the body; however, chronic-active inflammation only occurs in specific tissues. It appears that selectivity and specificity of lung, brain, mammary gland, and synovia occur in tissues where macrophages are permissive to genome integration. Kupffer cells in the liver are not permissive and do not allow transcription of viral RNA, and the liver does not develop lesions. Based on this mechanism, Maedi-visna should occur in the same sheep at the same time; however, this outcome is not common. The mechanism for this outcome is unknown.

Interstitial pneumonia results from virus-infected alveolar macrophages expressing high concentrations of proinflammatory chemokine, IL-8, that recruits inflammatory cells (not infected with virus) into the lung. These uninfected and recruited lymphocytes, plasma cells, macrophages, and neutrophils produce additional proinflammatory cytokines capable of sustaining inflammation and propagating the interstitial pneumonia. Thus a small number of virus-infected alveolar macrophages, responding to molecules through specific cell-membrane receptors, utilize a cascade of membrane, cytoplasmic, and nuclear messenger systems to control and sustain a large inflammatory response. Additionally, several studies suggest that lesions in ovine progressive pneumonia are in part immune mediated and that cytotoxic T-lymphocytes may be important effector cells. Virus-infected macrophages present viral antigens to T lymphocytes, and activated T lymphocytes in turn release cytokines that lead to differentiation of monocytes to macrophages and recruitment of additional inflammatory cells. Host defense mechanisms are ineffective in ending virus infection because (1) the viral genome becomes part of the host cell genome; (2) viral infection of cells of the monocyte-macrophage system results in dysfunction of this system and an ineffective adaptive immune response (see Chapter 3); and (3) the parental virus can modify its progeny through repeated cycles of gene reassortment (genetic variation) so that these progeny are able to escape an effective adaptive immune response (cyclical [recurring] infection).

Caprine Pneumonia (Caprine Arthritis-Encephalitis Virus, Enveloped RNA Virus)

The pathogenesis and mechanism of injury in caprine pneumonia are similar to those of ovine progressive pneumonia (Maedi) and caprine encephalitis of goats.

Bovine Respiratory Syncytial Virus Pneumonia (Pneumovirus, Enveloped RNA Virus)

The mechanism of injury in bovine respiratory syncytial virus pneumonia is dysfunction and death of cells of the respiratory mucosa, including ciliated cells of the conductive system and alveolar type II pneumocytes from infection by virus and from acute inflammation and its mediators and degradative enzymes. Gross lesions include active hyperemia, interstitial edema and inflammation (proliferative and exudative bronchiolitis), and subpleural and interstitial emphysema. Syncytial cells with intracytoplasmic inclusion bodies are observed in the microscopic lesions (see Fig. 9-69).

Cattle encounter bovine respiratory syncytial virus in fomites from body fluids contaminated with virus through direct contact with virus-infected animals. It is inhaled, deposited on, and trapped in the mucus layer of the mucosae of the conductive component of the respiratory system through centrifugal and inertial turbulence, but it has not been determined if and how virus penetrates mucus layers of these mucosae to gain access to epithelial cells or if mucosal macrophages and/or dendritic cells are involved. Virus infects and replicates in all epithelial cells; however, ciliated cells are the primary target cells. When virus encounters ciliated cells, it attaches and binds to membrane glycosaminoglycan receptors via heparin-binding domains on envelope glycoprotein G (attachment protein) and enters via envelope glycoprotein F (fusion protein). It has also been shown that virus can infect and replicate in lung dendritic cells and alveolar macrophages and cause the synthesis of interferons and interleukins. Infection of all of the cell types as previously mentioned appears to induce the synthesis of a cascade of proinflammatory chemokines and cytokines that recruit neutrophils, lymphocytes, and macrophages and lead to tissue injury. Additionally, TLR3 and TLR4 may initiate this cascade. In tissue culture experiments, virus appears to cause little or no injury to ciliated epithelial cells, suggesting that lesions may result in part from host defense mechanisms such as those modulated by the innate and adaptive immune responses. Bovine respiratory syncytial virus is part of bovine respiratory disease complex (shipping fever). This complex is characterized chronologically by (1) environmental or management stressors that suppress protective mechanisms in the respiratory system such as the production of protective mucus, (2) a primary viral infection that injures structural protective mechanisms such as the mucociliary apparatus, and (3) a secondary bacterial infection that causes severe inflammation often with fibrin exudation.

Inclusion Body Rhinitis–Porcine Cytomegalovirus Infection (Herpesvirus-Cytomegalovirus; Enveloped DNA Virus)

The pathogenesis of porcine cytomegalovirus infection has not been studied in sufficient detail to provide an evidence-based discussion of the chronologic sequence of events characteristic of the disease. The mechanism of injury is probably dysfunction and death of epithelial cells of the nasal and respiratory mucosa via infection with virus, especially the epithelial cells that form the mucous glands of the nasal cavity and from acute inflammation and its mediators and degradative enzymes. Gross lesions can include active hyperemia, congestion, and excessive mucus covering mucosal surfaces of the nasal septum and turbinates.

Pigs encounter porcine cytomegalovirus in fomites from body fluids contaminated with virus through direct contact with virus-infected animals. It is inhaled, deposited on, and trapped in the mucus layer of the mucosae of the conductive component of the respiratory system through centrifugal and inertial turbulence, but it has not been determined if and how virus penetrates mucus layers of these mucosae to gain access to epithelial cells or if mucosal macrophages and/or dendritic cells are involved. The conjunctiva may also be a source of infectious virus that later infects the nasal turbinates and septum via the lacrimal duct. Envelope attachment and fusion glycoproteins and cell membrane receptor proteins are likely involved in host cell infection, virus replication, and spread of virus to other cells and tissues. It is unclear how virus spreads systemically from the nasal cavity to other organ systems; however, in other animal models and humans, leukocyte trafficking and cells of the monocyte-macrophage system are involved in the spread of similar viruses.

Cardiovascular System and Lymphatic Vessels

Feline Infectious Peritonitis (Feline Infectious Peritonitis Virus; Nonenveloped RNA Virus)

The mutation of feline enteric coronavirus to feline infectious peritonitis virus is central to the pathogenesis of this disease. The mechanism of injury is chronic-active pyogranulomatous inflammation (vasculitis and perivasculitis) and its mediators and degradative enzymes. Gross lesions include gray-white nodules of varied sizes that have a perivascular pattern of distribution and in some cases a linear pattern following blood vessels in serosa and mesenteries (see Figs. 7-161, 11-75, and 14-105). Body cavities may contain a thick yellow exudate containing fibrin and pyogranulomatous inflammatory cells (see Fig. 7-161).

Cats encounter feline enteric coronavirus by ingestion of virus-contaminated fomites through two routes: (1) contact with virus-contaminated feces in litter boxes and (2) contact with carrier cats, usually queens. Fomites from saliva or respiratory droplets probably serve as a source of the virus to infect naïve cats via ingestion; therefore grooming behavior increases the likelihood that virus will enter the oral cavity. Feline enteric coronavirus is swallowed and moved to the alimentary system via intestinal peristalsis where it gains access to mucosae. The replication of enteric coronavirus is primarily restricted to mature intestinal epithelial cells (terminally differentiated cells with a lifespan of 3 to 8 days); however, the virus can enter a carrier state and persist in unidentified cells of the intestinal mucosa. These cells are likely progenitor cells (i.e., crypt stem cells) with infinite lifespans, so cell death through normal enterocyte turnover does not affect the carrier state of the virus. Feline enteric coronavirus spreads from enterocytes and carrier cells into the lamina propria and then to macrophages in Peyer's patches. It has not been determined if and how virus penetrates the mucus layer to gain access to mucosal epithelial cells or if mucosal macrophages, dendritic cells, or M cells are involved. Leukocyte trafficking to the submucosa by these cells would explain how virus spreads to macrophages in Peyer's patches. Feline enteric coronavirus likely uses capsid proteins, such as S protein, and other glycoproteins to bind to feline aminopeptidase-*N*, a cell membrane receptor on monocytes and macrophages. In mucosal macrophages of Peyer's patches and in blood monocytes, feline enteric coronavirus mutates into feline infectious peritonitis virus. Thus the genome of each new feline infectious peritonitis virus variant is unique to an individual cat. When feline enteric coronavirus mutates to feline infectious peritonitis virus, feline infectious peritonitis virus acquires virulence determinates that allow it to infect and replicate in cells of the monocyte-macrophage system, resulting in rapid dissemination of the virus throughout the body.

Monocytes and macrophages infected with feline infectious peritonitis virus spread from Peyer's patches to regional lymph nodes via leukocyte trafficking in lymphatic vessels and infect additional macrophages. They then migrate in lymphatic vessels through the thoracic duct into the circulatory system and to all tissues of the body and infect additional populations of free and fixed tissue macrophages. Virus-infected macrophages appear to target small and medium-sized veins of serosal membranes and tissues, cause damage to endothelial cells, and are recognized as foreign by the cat's innate (inflammation) and adaptive (cell-mediated and humoral) defense mechanisms (see Chapters 3 and 5). This process likely involves activation of the leukocyte adhesion cascade and binding of macrophages and monocytes to endothelial cells facilitated by ligand-receptor interactions and the activation of acute inflammation via proinflammatory cytokines released from activated macrophages and monocytes. All of these processes result in injury of vascular and perivascular tissues (vasculitis). Cats with a strong cell-mediated response do not develop feline infectious peritonitis. Cats with a weak cell-mediated response have the dry (noneffusive) form; cats with no cell-mediated response have the wet form (effusive). An effective humoral response appears to increase the severity of disease. Tissue macrophages provide a source of viral antigens in and around venules, and if adequate antibody is present, antigen-antibody complexes form and a type III hypersensitivity response ensues. Where immune complexes are formed (i.e., basement membrane of endothelial cells) or whether they are free or cell associated is not clearly understood. These complexes activate complement resulting in chemotaxis and accumulation of neutrophils via the leukocyte adhesion cascade. Additionally, they also activate tissue macrophages, leading to the secretion of a variety of proinflammatory cytokines that act on endothelial cells to increase neutrophil and mononuclear cell chemotaxis into the area and open tight junctions of endothelial cells (increased permeability), thereby allowing leakage of plasma and fibrin into body cavities. These mechanisms result in the vasocentric pyogranulomas and pyogranulomatous inflammation, fibrinous effusions, and fibrinous polyserositis (feline coronaviral polyserositis) so characteristic of feline infectious peritonitis. A type IV hypersensitivity reaction may be involved in the pathogenesis of some pyogranulomas. It appears that the commonly used categories of wet and dry forms and type III and type IV hypersensitivities are based more on clinical characteristics and immunologic tests, respectively, than on any morphologic criteria. Experimental studies have shown that there are no distinct histopathologic lesions that distinguish wet from dry cases, type III from type IV hypersensitivities, or acute/subacute cases from chronic cases.

Parvovirus Myocarditis (Parvovirus, Nonenveloped DNA Virus)

See parvovirus enteritis in the section on the Alimentary System and the Peritoneum, Omentum, Mesentery, and Peritoneal Cavity for information on the pathogenesis of viral spread and replication before spreading to the heart. The mechanism of injury in parvovirus myocarditis is cell death (necrosis of rhabdomyocytes) attributable to infection with virus. Gross lesions include gray-white areas of varied sizes distributed in the myocardium (see Fig. 10-82). It is likely that virus spreads via leukocyte trafficking or cell-free viremia in lymphatic or blood vessels from Peyer's patches to regional lymph nodes and then systemically in the circulatory system to capillaries and rhabdomyocytes in the heart. Endothelial cells are dividing cells, and studies suggest that in the heart, virus initially infects and replicates in these cells and then spreads to infect contiguous cardiac rhabdomyocytes. Rhabdomyocytes are actively dividing cells in dogs under 15 days of age; therefore they can be infected with virus and are lysed with release of virus. This outcome results in necrosis of rhabdomyocytes and ectopic irritable foci, cardiac arrhythmias, and unexpected death. If dogs survive this stage, healing mechanisms cause cardiac fibrosis that can contribute clinically to dysfunction of the conduction system and contraction of the cardiac musculature later in life. Specificity for these mitotically active cells occurs because parvoviruses require a host cell–derived duplex transcription template, which is only available when cells divide during the S-phase of the cell cycle. Ligand-receptor interactions are also probably involved.

Canine Herpesvirus Infection (Canine Herpesvirus Type 1, Enveloped DNA Virus)

The mechanism of injury in canine herpesvirus infection is death of endothelial cells systemically and epithelial cells of multiple organ systems (pantropic). Gross lesions include mucosal and serosal hemorrhage and randomly distributed white-gray foci (≈1 mm in diameter) of miliary necrosis within organ systems, especially the kidneys (see Fig. 11-74). Miliary necrosis can also be observed in spleen, lymph nodes, lung, and liver.

Puppies ingest and inhale virus in fomites from body fluids of the birth canal or nasal-oral cavity of bitches through grooming. It is deposited on mucosae of the nasal and oral pharynx, especially those of the tonsil, and is thought to infect mucosal epithelial cells. It has not been determined if and how virus penetrates the mucus layer to gain access to mucosal epithelial cells. Although it appears that virus infects lymphocytes in the tonsil, it has not been determined if and how virus spreads from mucosal epithelial cells to lymphocytes or if leukocyte trafficking or dendritic cells are involved. It is also unclear if or how virus migrates to regional or systemic lymphoid nodes, thymus, or spleen before it spreads systemically to infect endothelial and epithelial cells of other organ systems; however, virus appears to be spread systemically in lymphocytes via leukocyte trafficking. It has not been satisfactorily determined (1) how virus-infected lymphocytes interact with endothelial and epithelial cells or if this interaction is facilitated by molecules of the leukocyte adhesion cascade (see Chapter 3); (2) how virus infects and replicates in endothelial cells, leading to injury and cell death; and (3) if injury results in vasculitis and vascular thrombosis, leading to tissue infarction and DIC. Canine herpesvirus expresses envelope glycoproteins B, C, and D; however, their role in attaching and binding to target cells has not been clearly defined. Heparin sulfate may serve as a target cell receptor for canine herpesvirus.

Equine Viral Arteritis (Arterivirus, Enveloped RNA virus)

The mechanism of injury in equine viral arteritis is death of endothelial cells, myocytes, and pericytes of small muscular arterioles and venules of multiple organ systems. Gross lesions include (1) congestion, edema, and hemorrhage in subcutaneous tissues of the limbs and abdomen; (2) hydroperitoneum, hydropericardium, and hydroabdomen; and (3) edema and hemorrhage in lymph nodes and intestines.

Horses inhale virus in fomites of body fluids, most commonly urine, through direct contact with virus-infected animals. It is deposited on mucosae of the conductive and O_2-CO_2 exchange systems through centrifugal and inertial turbulence and trapped in the mucus layer. Virus is likely phagocytosed by bronchiolar and alveolar macrophages as they migrate through the mucus layer and mucosae and spread locally through leukocyte trafficking to the submucosa (BALT) where they infect additional tissue macrophages. From here, macrophages spread virus to regional lymph nodes via lymphatic vessels where additional macrophages are infected. Ligand-receptor interactions are probably involved in tropism for specific cell types. Virus expresses envelope glycoproteins and a nucleocapsid protein; however, their role in binding to target cells has not been clearly defined. Additionally, membrane receptors for the virus have not been identified. Macrophages leave regional lymph nodes and enter the circulatory system via postcapillary venules or lymphatic vessels and the thoracic duct. During vascular migration, infected macrophages encounter endothelial cells, myocytes, and pericytes of small arterioles (and venules) and their interactions are facilitated by molecules of the leukocyte adhesion cascade (see Chapter 3). Monocytes containing viral antigens have been observed adhering to endothelial cells, and virus appears to spread from monocytes to endothelial cells, myocytes, and pericytes of these vessels.

Migrating monocytes also encounter and infect hepatocytes, adrenal cortical cells, seminiferous tubular cells, and thyroid follicular cells. Virus-induced vascular injury leads to cell death characterized by endothelial swelling, degeneration, and necrosis, acute and chronic (lymphomonocytic) inflammation, necrosis of myocytes, and thrombus formation, leading to edema and hemorrhage in many tissues and organs. Virus replication occurs in endothelial cells, and the expression of envelope glycoproteins in endothelial cells likely activates acute inflammation, fibrinogenesis, the complement cascade, and the recruitment of neutrophils into vascular intima and tunica media and in severe cases results in fibrinoid necrosis and vasculitis. The role of proinflammatory chemokines and cytokines in vascular injury has not been defined. A lymphomonocytic inflammatory cell population is also commonly found in the tunica media and adventitia suggesting that cytolytic T lymphocytes could induce cytolysis of virus-infected endothelial cells. Why death of endothelial cells and myocytes dominates over death of epithelial cells, such as those in renal tubules, is unknown. However, infection and death of renal tubular epithelial cells with release of virus into urine appears to be the mechanism by which virus is spread to naive horses.

Bovine Malignant Catarrhal Fever (Ovine Herpesvirus-2 and Alcelaphine Herpesvirus-1 [γ-Herpesviruses], Enveloped DNA virus)

The mechanism of injury in bovine malignant catarrhal fever is dysfunction and death of vascular endothelial cells and hyperplasia, dysfunction, and death of lymphocytes in lymphoid tissues. Gross lesions include (1) erosive, ulcerative, and hemorrhagic lesions of mucosae of gingiva, tongue, oral papillae, hard and soft palate, oral pharynx, esophagus, turbinates, trachea, rumen, reticulum, and omasum (see Fig. 7-4); (2) enlargement of lymphoid organs and tissues followed by atrophy; and (3) increased size of visceral organs and tissues resulting from perivascular accumulations of lymphocytes (lymphoproliferative vasculitis). Worldwide, sheep are the reservoir animal for sheep-associated ovine herpesvirus-2 (OvHV-2) that causes malignant catarrhal fever in cattle, bison, pigs, and deer. In Africa, blue wildebeest are the reservoir animal for wildebeest-associated Alcelaphine herpesvirus-1 (AlHV-1) that causes malignant catarrhal fever in cattle. These viruses persist in carrier animals without ill effects. The chronologic sequence of events leading to malignant catarrhal fever have not been clearly determined.

Animals probably encounter these viruses through inhalation and ingestion of fomites from oronasal-pharyngeal-ocular fluids (also seminal fluid) from reservoir animals that are actively shedding virus. In reservoir animals, OvHV-2 is shed predominantly through nasal secretions derived from turbinates and shedding episodes are stress-induced and occur more frequently in lambs than adult sheep. Virus is deposited on mucosae of the oral, nasal, and pharyngeal cavities; the conjunctiva; or the conductive component of the respiratory system through centrifugal and inertial turbulence. It is trapped in the mucus layer and apparently phagocytosed by mucosal macrophages and spread to submucosae and BALT via leukocyte trafficking. It has not been determined if dendritic cells are involved. In submucosae, virus infects lymphocytes (possibly B lymphocytes), macrophages, and monocytes and spreads in $CD8^+$ T lymphocytes via leukocyte trafficking to regional lymph nodes and then systemically to other organ systems and lymphoid tissues. Ligand-receptor interactions are probably involved in tropism for specific cell types, but viral envelope glycoproteins or cell receptors have not been identified.

Virus-infected $CD8^+$ T lymphocytes are distributed in intimal, medial, and adventitial tissues of blood vessels (vascular and perivascular pattern) in organ systems. This tropism may be determined by (1) ligand-receptor interactions or (2) permissiveness of specific vascular cells to viral infection and replication. As part of this tropism, virus-infected $CD8^+$ T lymphocytes produce proinflammatory cytokines and express viral glycoproteins in their cell membranes. Proinflammatory cytokines can act as cytotoxic molecules and may injure and kill bystander cells, such as those in the vasculature, and viral glycoproteins may recruit lymphocytes, macrophages, and monocytes and lesser numbers of neutrophils and plasma cells into perivascular and vascular tissues, leading to lymphoproliferative necrotizing vasculitis and vascular wall necrosis. Atrophy of lymphoid tissues after viral infection is not likely caused by virus-induced cell death. Because lymphocytes are short-lived effector cells, atrophy is likely the result of normal cell aging and turnover that follows massive proliferation. It is not known if virus can infect, injure, and kill endothelial cells directly. Additionally, virus-infected large granular lymphocytes and other recruited cytotoxic lymphocytes and macrophages may play roles in vascular injury because they have been shown to be cytotoxic for vascular endothelial cells. The cause of the erosive, ulcerative, and hemorrhagic lesions has not been determined; however, infarction of mucosal blood vessels secondary to thrombosis induced by necrotizing vasculitis could potentially lead to these outcomes. Apparently, there is a lack of spread between susceptible animals because they are dead-end hosts for these viruses. Virus spread appears to require cell-free virus in body fluids, and in susceptible animals, the virus replicates in a cell-associated manner (lymphocytes, macrophages, monocytes) and cell-free virus is not produced. Because virus-infected host cells do not produce infectious virus during the virus replication cycle, these species are unable to transmit virus to other animals (see carrier animals above).

Classical Swine Fever (Hog Cholera, Pestivirus, *Enveloped RNA Virus)*

The mechanism of injury in classical swine fever is death of endothelial cells of multiple organ systems and of hemopoietic cells. Gross lesions include a red-blue discoloration of the skin, hydropericardium, hydrothorax, and hydroperitoneum; hemorrhage and necrosis of the palatine tonsil; and petechial and ecchymotic hemorrhages in most organs of the body, especially the kidney (Fig. 4-42).

Pigs encounter virus through (1) ingestion and likely inhalation of fomites from body fluids, body waste, or offal or other virus-contaminated pork products and (2) mechanical transfer on virus-contaminated vehicles, clothes/boots, instruments, and needles. Virus is deposited on mucosae of the oral and nasal pharynx, especially of the tonsil, where it infects and replicates in epithelial cells of tonsillar crypts. Although unknown, virus likely buds from basal surfaces of tonsillar epithelial cells and infects subjacent mucosal macrophages in lymphoid nodules. It has not been determined how virus penetrates the mucus layer to gain access to mucosal epithelial cells or if mucosal macrophages or dendritic cells phagocytose virus in the mucus layer and spread it through leukocyte trafficking to the submucosa. E^{rns} and E2 envelope glycoproteins and other envelope glycoproteins appear to be involved in binding to and entering mucosal epithelial cells and macrophages via cell surface glycosaminoglycan receptors such as heparin sulfate. Infected macrophages migrate via leukocyte trafficking in lymphatic vessels to regional lymph nodes such as the submandibular and pharyngeal. Here, they infect and likely recruit additional macrophages and induce lymphoid hyperplasia through release of proinflammatory chemokines and cytokines. Lymph nodes become edematous and hemorrhagic because of injury (necrosis) to endothelial cells after infection with virus from tissue macrophages. Subsequently, macrophages leave regional lymph nodes and enter the circulatory system via postcapillary venules or lymphatic vessels and the thoracic duct to migrate systemically to other organ systems.

Infected macrophages likely interact with endothelial cells of these organs by adhering to and migrating through the endothelium, likely by activating the leukocyte adhesion cascade (see Chapter 3). Virus spreads from macrophages and infects and replicates in endothelial cells, resulting in direct injury and inducing an acute inflammatory response. Vascular lesions are probably lytic and characterized by endothelial swelling, degeneration, and necrosis; acute and chronic (lymphomonocytic) inflammation; necrosis of myocytes; and thrombus formation leading to edema and hemorrhage in many tissues and organs. This pattern of injury serves as the basis for hemorrhage observed in the kidney. Macrophages also spread virus to lymphoid tissues and bone marrow, where it infects and kills these cells, resulting in severely impaired adaptive immune responses with decreased neutralizing antibody production, decreased numbers of phagocytes, and decreased cell-mediated immune responses. The impairment or loss of these defense mechanisms makes pigs more susceptible to other infectious diseases.

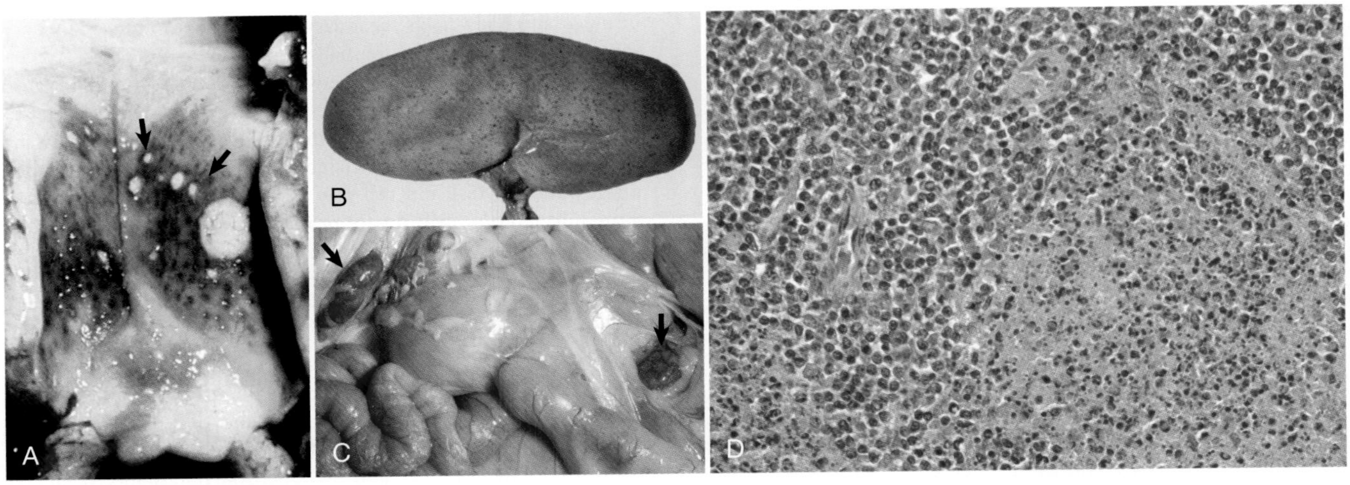

Fig. 4-42 Classical swine fever (hog cholera).
Lesions in classical swine fever are similar to those observed in African swine fever, but usually less severe. See Fig. 4-43 for lesions of African swine fever. **A,** The tonsil *(of the soft palate)*, a tissue of choice for isolation and identification of the virus, contains foci of hemorrhage and necrosis *(arrows)*, the result of necrosis of mucosal epithelial cells in tonsillar crypts and necrosis of the adjacent endothelial cells and lymphocytes in the lamina propria from infection with virus. **B,** Kidney. The cortical surface has numerous randomly distributed petechia caused by injury to and subsequent necrosis of endothelial cells following their infection with classical swine fever virus. **C,** Mesenteric lymph nodes *(arrows)* are enlarged and congested due to vascular injury caused by virus, resulting in blood in the subcapsular sinuses. **D,** Tonsillar crypt lymphoid nodules. Note the focal necrosis of lymphocytes *(right lower half of image)* in the nodules caused by infection with virus. H&E stain. (**A** courtesy Dr. R. Breeze, Plum Island Animal Disease Center and Noah's Arkive, College of Veterinary Medicine, The University of Georgia. **B** courtesy Dr. D. Gregg, Plum Island Animal Disease Center and Noah's Arkive, College of Veterinary Medicine, The University of Georgia. **C** courtesy Dr. M.D. McGavin, College of Veterinary Medicine, University of Tennessee. **D** courtesy Dr. J.F. Zachary, College of Veterinary Medicine, University of Illinois.)

*African Swine Fever (*Asfivirus*, Enveloped DNA Virus)*

The pathogenesis, mechanisms of injury, and clinical outcomes of African swine fever are very similar to those of classical swine fever, but the pathogenicity (virulence determinates) of and thus the disease and lesions caused by African swine fever virus are much more severe (Fig. 4-43). Additionally, African swine fever virus can gain access to the blood vascular system and directly infect macrophages through bites of ticks. Virus envelope glycoproteins p12, p54, and p30 appear to be involved in attaching and binding to and entering host target cells via cell receptors. Target cell receptors have not been clearly identified. DIC, leading to collapse of the circulatory system and shock, is likely the cause of death in virus-infected pigs.

*African Horse Sickness (*Orbivirus*, Nonenveloped RNA Virus)*

The pathogenesis and mechanism of injury in African horse sickness are similar to those of bluetongue disease. The mechanism of injury is endothelial cell barrier dysfunction and virus-induced dysfunction and death of endothelial cells. There are four clinical forms of African horse sickness; however, in each form the gross lesions are characteristic of vascular (endothelial cell) injury and include edema (pulmonary, systemic, subcutaneous, intramuscular, supraorbital fossae, eyelids, lips, cheeks, tongue, intermandibular space, and larynx), active hyperemia, petechial and ecchymotic hemorrhages (serosal [epicardial, endocardial], subcapsular [spleen], cortical [kidney], and mucosal [intestines]), hydrothorax, hydropericardium, and ascites, and rhabdomyocytic necrosis (Fig. 4-44). The expression of these forms may be related to differences in viral tropism for different types of vascular endothelial cells within organ systems of the body or the permissiveness of different types of endothelial cells in allowing the virus to replicate efficiently or in large numbers. African horse sickness virus also infects cells of the dendritic, lymphoid, and monocyte-macrophage systems. African horse sickness is a noncontagious disease of horses, donkeys, and mules.

Animals encounter virus in bite wounds from midges. After skin penetration, virus can enter the circulatory system or be deposited in vascularized ECM (connective) tissues. If a blood vessel is penetrated, virus can enter the circulatory system and infect macrophages and lymphocytes or be carried cell free to systemic lymphoid tissues. If deposited in connective tissue, virus gains access to cutaneous blood and fluids, as well as cutaneous dendritic cells (Langerhans' cells) and tissue macrophages. Although unproved, it is likely that virus infects these cells and virus-infected macrophages or dendritic cells spread the virus via leukocyte trafficking and lymphatic vessels to regional lymph nodes. Here, virus infects lymphocytes and additional dendritic cells and macrophages. African horse sickness virus has two attachment proteins, capsid structural proteins (VP2 and VP5). These proteins bind to glycosaminoglycans on host cell membranes and facilitate attachment and entry of virus.

From regional lymph nodes, virus spreads systemically in macrophages via leukocyte trafficking to the circulatory system, through postcapillary venules and/or lymphatic vessels and the thoracic duct, to infect, injure, and kill vascular endothelial cells in the lungs, heart, spleen, lymph nodes, liver, and kidney. Infected macrophages likely interact with endothelial cells of these organs by adhering to and migrating through the endothelium, likely by activating the leukocyte adhesion cascade (see Chapter 3). Virus spreads from macrophages and infects and replicates in endothelial cells, resulting in direct injury and inducing an acute inflammatory response. Vascular lesions are probably lytic and characterized by endothelial swelling, degeneration, and necrosis and depending on the severity of injury, vasculitis can be followed by hemorrhage and edema (increased vascular permeability) affecting the lung and vascular thrombosis leading to tissue infarction. Necrosis of

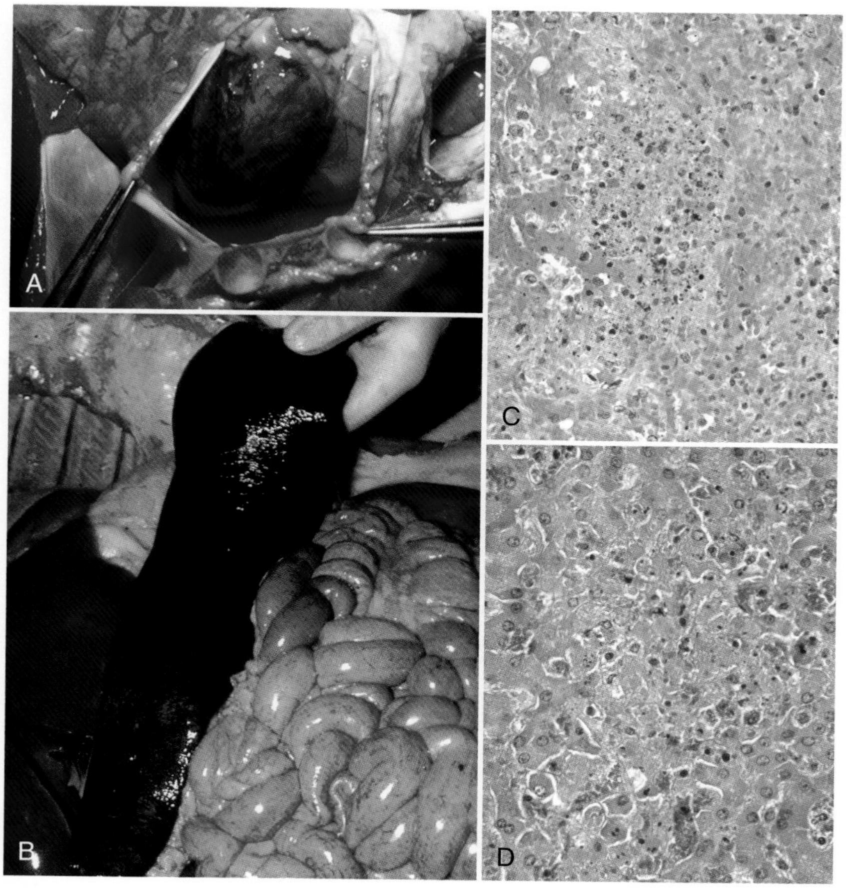

Fig. 4-43 African swine fever.
Lesions in African swine fever are similar to those observed in classical swine fever, but usually much more severe. See Fig. 4-42 for lesions of classical swine fever. **A,** Epicardium and pericardial cavity. The epicardium and subjacent myocardium have numerous randomly distributed ecchymoses caused by injury to and subsequent necrosis of endothelial cells from infection with African swine fever virus. Note the accumulation of a fibrinous effusion in the pericardial cavity. **B,** Splenomegaly, bloody spleen. The spleen is congested with blood and friable as a result of vascular damage caused by the virus. Lymph nodes (not shown here) are also congested and edematous (see classical swine fever). **C,** Endothelial cells and lymphoid cells of white pulp of the spleen are necrotic (e.g., pyknosis, karyolysis). H&E stain. **D,** Endothelial cells lining sinusoids of the liver are necrotic (e.g., pyknosis, karyolysis). Also note the necrosis of some hepatocytes. H&E stain. (**A** courtesy Dr. C. Brown, College of Veterinary Medicine, The University of Georgia. **B** courtesy Dr. D. Gregg, Plum Island Animal Disease Center and Noah's Arkive, College of Veterinary Medicine, The University of Georgia. **C** and **D** courtesy Dr. J.F. Zachary, College of Veterinary Medicine, University of Illinois.)

rhabdomyocytes in the heart has been attributed to the release of endogenous catecholamines, but experimental findings suggest that necrosis is caused by microthrombosis of myocardial capillaries likely resulting in myocyte ischemia. Rarely, DIC has been reported in African horse sickness. Additionally, NS3, a viral protein inserted in the host cell membrane, may be cytotoxic (acting as a viroporin that alters host cell membrane permeability) and involved in the release of virus from infected endothelial cells and membrane damage.

Bone Marrow, Blood Cells, and Lymphatic System

Canine Distemper (Morbillivirus; *Enveloped RNA Virus)*

See the section on the Nervous System.

Equine Infectious Anemia (Equine Infectious Anemia Virus; Enveloped RNA Virus)

The mechanism of injury in equine infectious anemia is inflammation (and proliferation [hypertrophy and hyperplasia]) of the monocyte-macrophage and lymphoid systems, particularly in the spleen and lymph nodes, resulting in chronic-active splenitis and lymphadenitis. Virus does not cause cell death. Gross lesions include an enlarged spleen (splenomegaly) and lymph nodes (lymphadenomegaly) with abundant white-gray lymphoid tissue arranged in follicles and solid sheets of cells that often bulge from cut surfaces.

Horses initially encounter virus through penetrating wounds of the blood vascular system, either from fly or mosquito bites or needles. In the blood, virus infects monocytes, but because they are not fully differentiated macrophages, virus cannot fully replicate. Thus monocytes spread virus via leukocyte trafficking in the circulatory system to all organ systems and migrate through blood vessel walls. After monocytes enter tissue, they differentiate into tissue macrophages and virus can replicate in these cells and serve to infect other macrophages and lymphocytes, especially in lymphoid tissues such as spleen and lymph nodes. Infected macrophages produce proinflammatory chemokines and cytokines that recruit additional monocytes and lymphocytes into organs, thus splenomegaly and lymphadenomegaly ensue. Virus does not cause cell death. It appears virus expresses an envelope glycoprotein (gp90 and likely other proteins) that attach and bind to equine lentivirus receptor-1 present in cell membranes of monocytes and macrophages.

The two clinical phases of equine infectious anemia are acute and chronic. In the acute phase, horses have recurring fever, anemia, thrombocytopenia, and petechia with interspersed periods of quiescence. Fever is likely attributable to release of proinflammatory cytokines and endogenous pyrogens from activated macrophages during the leukocyte trafficking stages of the disease. Anemia occurs from phagocytosis and complement-mediated lysis of erythrocytes that have had their membranes altered by virus, antibody, complement, and/or fibrinogen. Pulmonary intravascular macrophages, Kupffer cells, and fixed macrophages lining vascular sinusoids in the spleen and lymph nodes are reservoirs for virus and release it into the bloodstream. Cell-free virus adsorbs onto the surface of red blood cells (and likely platelets) in the circulatory system. Adsorbed viral proteins act as haptens that are recognized as foreign by cells of the monocyte-macrophage system and are phagocytosed. Additionally, the hapten is processed and presented to lymphocytes, leading to a humoral immune response and the generation

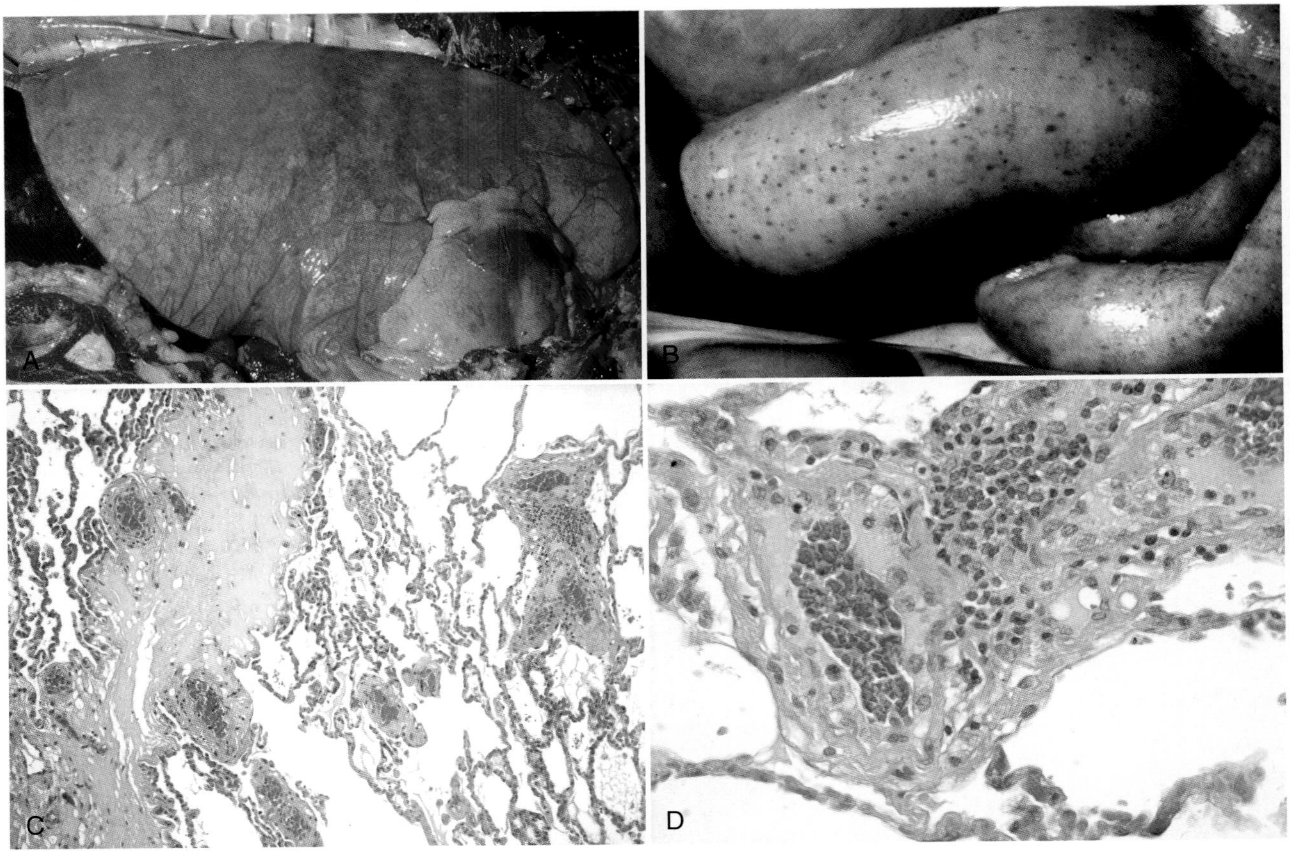

Fig. 4-44 African horse sickness.
A, Pulmonary edema. The interlobular septa are widely separated and distended with edema fluid. Edema fluid is also present in alveoli and alveolar septa. Also note the suffusive hemorrhage of the visceral pleura. These lesions are caused by infection of endothelial cells of the capillaries of the interlobular and alveolar septa by African horse sickness virus resulting in endothelial cell barrier malfunction and death of endothelial cells. **B,** Colonic serosa, petechial and ecchymotic hemorrhages. These lesions are also caused by infection of and damage to endothelial cells. **C,** Lung, interlobular edema. The interlobular septum and alveoli contain edema fluid. Capillaries and venules are surrounded by bronchiole-associated lymphoid tissue (BALT). H&E stain. **D,** Higher magnification of **C.** The endothelial cells of venules are swollen, have vacuolated and reticulated cytoplasm, and large reactive nuclei consistent with responses to injury caused by infection of these cells by African horse sickness virus, but is not pathognomonic. Note the bronchiole-associated lymphoid tissue (BALT). (**A** courtesy Dr. D. Gregg, Plum Island Animal Disease Center and Noah's Arkive, College of Veterinary Medicine, The University of Georgia. **B** courtesy Dr. R. Breeze, Plum Island Animal Disease Center and Noah's Arkive, College of Veterinary Medicine, The University of Georgia. **C** and **D** courtesy Dr. J. F. Zachary, College of Veterinary Medicine, University of Illinois.)

of plasma cells that secrete antibody against the hapten and other antigens on the red blood cell membrane (type II hypersensitivity response). If the hapten-antibody complex fixes complement, red blood cells are lysed intravascularly. If complement is not fixed, red blood cells are phagocytosed by cells of the monocyte-macrophage system and lysed extravascularly. Both of these mechanisms result in severe anemia. The cause of thrombocytopenia is less clear and is thought to occur because of activation of platelets and concurrent binding of fibrinogen to the surface of platelets during acute viremic phases of the disease. It is likely that activated platelets are quickly phagocytosed by the monocyte-macrophage system leading to thrombocytopenia. Petechial hemorrhages may be attributable to vascular injury caused by direct infection of endothelial cells by virus or more likely by a secondary response to injury induced by innate and adaptive defense mechanisms.

In chronic equine infectious anemia, recurrence of disease is caused by antigenic variation of surface glycoproteins of the virus. This genetic variation results in virus that expresses new surface glycoproteins, thus beginning anew the process of developing effective cell-mediated and humoral responses. Long-lasting control of equine infectious anemia appears to require that the adaptive immune response controls the disease before antigenic variation occurs. Large quantities of virus are replicated in cells of the monocyte-macrophage system, and virus is not eliminated from these cells during the acute phase of the disease. As adaptive immune responses develop, cytotoxic T lymphocytes are thought to control a limited extent viremia and virus replication in infected monocytes and macrophages. However, it appears that control of the disease (no or minimal anemia and thrombocytopenia) is linked to an effective antibody response against the virus that takes 6 to 8 months to develop.

Enzootic Bovine Lymphoma (Lymphosarcoma, Bovine Leukosis Virus-Associated Malignant Lymphoma, Deltaretrovirus: *Bovine Leukemia Virus, Enveloped RNA Virus)*

The mechanism of injury in enzootic bovine lymphoma is provirus-induced malignant transformation of B lymphocytes. Gross lesions include proliferation of neoplastic cells and their infiltration into perivascular spaces in organ systems resulting in (1) generalized enlargement of affected organs with increased pallor or (2) the formation of one or more solid white nodules distributed at random in the affected tissue (see Figs. 7-81, 10-54, 10-55, 13-56, *B*, 13-80, and 13-86). Additionally, cells can occupy and proliferate in confined spaces causing compressive atrophy of tissue in these spaces such as axons in the spinal cord, hemopoietic cells in the bone marrow, and the retina in the eye. Organ systems commonly having lesions include superficial and visceral lymph nodes and thymus, skin, abomasum, heart, spleen, kidneys, uterus (caruncles), spinal meninges, retrobulbar lymphatic tissue, bone, and bone marrow. Malignant transformation is a sequence of events in which normal cells acquire the biologic behaviors of neoplastic cells such as uncontrolled growth, tissue invasion, and metastasis. In cattle, it takes several years for this transformation to occur and be manifested in overt lymphoma. This long prodromal period is likely caused by the complexity and interplay of injurious and reparative processes induced by the provirus that eventually result in dysfunction or mutation of regulatory cell cycle genes. Bovine leukemia virus infects B lymphocytes and thus is not free as a virus in blood or body fluids but is a provirus, cell-associated, and integrated into the host cell's genome. When its replication cycle is completed, new virus is released from provirus-infected B lymphocytes. New virus serves to sustain and amplify the infection by infecting naïve B lymphocytes and cells of the monocyte-macrophage system.

Cattle and calves encounter provirus-infected B lymphocytes in blood, inflammatory exudates, and colostrum or milk. Provirus-infected B lymphocytes must gain access to the blood vascular and/or lymphatic systems and eventually to tissues and target cells suitable for infection. When it gains access to tissues, it is unclear whether B lymphocytes (1) behave as trafficking leukocytes and migrate into the vascular and/or lymphatic systems to spread new virus to other cells and tissues or (2) undergo cytolysis and release virus into tissues to infect local tissue macrophages, lymphocytes, or dendritic cells such as Langerhans' cells. The use of needles or surgical instruments contaminated with blood (provirus-infected B lymphocytes) can transfer these cells directly into the vascular system or place them in vascularized subcutaneous tissues or muscle in close proximity to capillary and lymphatic vascular beds. Such exposure may require traumatic injury to skin or mucous membranes. Insect bites can apparently result in the same outcome. In either case, provirus-infected B lymphocytes deposited in these locations encounter cells of the monocyte-macrophage and lymphoid systems and dendritic cells. It has been shown that virus can infect these cells, but whether these cells spread virus or provirus to regional lymph nodes and then systemically via leukocyte trafficking in these cells or in B lymphocytes is unknown.

Transplacental spread of bovine leukemia virus from cows to calves also occurs through the blood. Provirus-infected B lymphocytes can also be present in inflammatory exudates, such as those occurring with postpartum metritis or vaginitis, and must gain access to capillary and lymphatic beds in host animals as previously described. Finally, provirus-infected B lymphocytes can be present in colostrum or milk, and it has been suggested that enzootic bovine lymphoma can result from virus entering the body via the alimentary system and gaining access to the blood vascular system. However, the role, as examples, of alimentary peristalsis, gastric acidity, mucosal mucus barrier systems, mucosal epithelial barrier systems, mucosal immunity, and M cells has not been adequately addressed in experimental studies.

It appears that by whatever route used by provirus-infected B lymphocytes to enter the body, it must gain access to the blood vascular system to establish, sustain, and amplify an infection regionally and systemically. Although hypothetical, provirus-infected B lymphocytes could behave as typical trafficking leukocytes and thereby attach to and migrate through mucosae of the oral and nasal pharynx and gain access to local MALTs, lymphatic vessels, regional lymph nodes, and systemic lymphoid tissues. Virus uses bovine leukemia virus envelope glycoproteins (gp51, gp30) to attach to and enter naïve host B lymphocytes that express a novel membrane protein called *bovine leukemia virus–binding receptor*. Other studies have shown that B lymphocytes expressing surface immunoglobulin M and cell surface markers CD5 and CD11b are more susceptible to infection with virus; however, the role of these molecules as receptors is unclear.

The mechanism of B lymphocyte transformation has not been established. Transformation may be linked to a mechanism called *gene transactivation*. When the genome of bovine leukemia virus (provirus) is integrated into the genome of a B lymphocyte, the provirus asserts control over the transcriptional and translational organelles and processes of the host cell. Genes of the bovine leukemia provirus express a protein called bovine leukemia virus Tax protein (p34tax) that appears to stimulate the proliferation (increased mitoses) of B lymphocytes and increases viral replication in host cells. Tax protein also interacts with host cell genes and appears to transactivate genes that express proteins modulating host cell growth, such as cell division and differentiation, and are involved in regulatory steps of cell proliferation and longevity. Experimentally, Tax protein has been shown to be able to immortalize rat embryo fibroblasts in tissue culture and to cooperate with an oncogene to transform tissue culture cells that can then be grown as tumors in live animals. Collectively, these findings suggest that transformation of B lymphocytes, leading to bovine lymphoma, is linked to the likely long-term actions of p34tax on host cell regulatory genes, but the chronologic stages of transformation are uncertain. Studies suggest that transformation may also result from Tax protein forming complexes with proteins expressed by tumor-suppressor genes such as p53, whereas other studies suggest that point mutations in the p53 gene is one of the critical events leading to lymphoma. The proteins translated from tumor-suppressor genes have an inhibitory effect on the regulation of the cell cycle and function to inhibit cell division, inhibit division of cells with damaged DNA, initiate apoptosis of cells with damaged DNA, and amplify cell adhesion (metastasis suppressors). When the activities of the p53 gene and its protein gene products are perturbed or inhibited, transformation of affected cells could occur.

Feline Leukemia (Feline Leukemia Virus, Retrovirus, Enveloped RNA Virus)

The mechanism of injury in feline leukemia is virus-induced dysfunction and death and neoplastic transformation of lymphoid (hemopoietic) cells leading to (1) lymphoma (lymphosarcoma) and leukemia, (2) dysfunction of visceral organ systems, lymphoid tissues, or bone marrow, usually through compressive atrophy of parenchymal cells, in which the neoplastic cells proliferate, and (3) immunosuppression, resulting in increased susceptibility to other microbial diseases. Gross lesions include proliferation of neoplastic cells and their infiltration into perivascular spaces in organ systems resulting in (1) generalized enlargement of affected organs with increased pallor or (2) the formation of one or more solid white nodules distributed at random in the affected tissue (see Figs. 7-79, 13-79, and 13-85). Additionally, cells can occupy and proliferate in confined spaces, causing compressive atrophy of tissues such as axons in the spinal cord, hemopoietic cells in the bone marrow, and the retina in the eye.

Cats encounter virus in fomites from body fluids, such as salivary and nasal secretions, through direct contact with virus-infected cats. Virus is ingested or inhaled and is deposited on mucous members of the oral and nasal pharynx (preferentially the tonsils) and attaches to, infects, and replicates locally in mucosal epithelial cells and mucosa-associated lymphocytes and macrophages

(MALT). It has not been determined how virus penetrates the mucus layer to gain access to mucosal epithelial cells or if mucosal macrophages and/or dendritic cells are involved in infection or spread locally. Virus spreads via leukocyte trafficking in lymphocytes and macrophages through lymphatic vessels to regional pharyngeal lymph nodes where it infects and replicates in additional lymphocytes and macrophages. B lymphocytes appear to be the primary cells used to spread virus via leukocyte trafficking, whereas T lymphocytes appear to be the primary target cell for infection and T lymphocyte dysfunction is involved in the symptomatology of the disease. From regional lymph nodes, virus spreads systemically in B lymphocytes via leukocyte trafficking to the circulatory system, through postcapillary venules or lymphatic vessels and the thoracic duct to lymph nodes and lymphoid organs, such as the spleen and Peyer's patches, and then to bone marrow and mucosae of the salivary glands. Salivary gland secretions are an important mechanism to spread the virus. There are four subgroups of feline leukemia virus (FeLV) designated FeLV-A, FeLV-B, FeLV-C, and FeLV-T. FeLV-A is the subgroup transmitted between cats through saliva.

Once cats are infected with subgroup FeLV-A, the virus establishes a persistent infection (but not integrated in the genome) of bone marrow cells, which are most likely T lymphocytes or their precursor cells. Because viral replication occurs incessantly in these cells, there is greater opportunity for genomic variation to occur and new viral virulence determinates to be introduced. Subgroup FeLV-B appears to have arisen through recombination of endogenous genes of subgroup FeLV-A, whereas subgroup FeLV-C appears to have arisen through point mutations of endogenous genes of subgroup FeLV-A. Cats may be infected with only subgroup FeLV-A or a combination of subgroup FeLV-A with FeLV-B and/or FeLV-C. In general, subgroup FeLV-A causes immunosuppression and is found in approximately 100% of virus-infected cats; subgroup FeLV-B causes neoplastic transformation and is found in approximately 50% of virus-infected cats; and subgroup FeLV-C causes anemia and is found in approximately 1% to 2% of virus-infected cats. Recently, FeLV-T has been identified. It arises through genomic variation of FeLV-A, infects T lymphocytes, and causes an immunodeficiency syndrome.

Consideration of the encyclopedic listings of specific lesions and syndromes caused by feline leukemia virus is outside of the scope of this chapter; however, virus-induced lesions and syndromes include (1) lymphoma (lymphosarcoma) and all of its forms (alimentary, thymic, anterior mediastinal, multicentric, atypical) based on anatomic distribution, (2) leukemia, (3) myeloproliferative disorders, (4) nonregenerative anemia, (5) panleukopenia-like syndrome, and (6) glomerulonephritis. For successful replication, virus requires rapidly dividing cells such as lymphocytes. These syndromes arise from persistent infection of T lymphocytes in the bone marrow. Persistent infections result from modulation of virus and cellular gene expression and modification of the cat's immune response by the virus. Persistence lasts for long periods, often the life of the cat, and occurs when the virus is not eliminated by the adaptive immune response because of dysfunction of cytotoxic T lymphocytes.

Immunosuppression and lymphopenia coincide with systemic involvement of lymphoid tissues, specifically T lymphocytes. Persistently infected cats commonly die of secondary bacterial and viral opportunistic infections. Subgroups A, B, C, and T use envelope surface glycoproteins to attach to receptors and enter T lymphocytes, other lymphocytes, and mucosal epithelial cells. Receptors for viral glycoproteins on these cells include (1) feline thiamine transport protein (FeTHTR1) as a receptor for FeLV-A; (2) feline phosphate transporter proteins 1 and/or 2 (FePit1 or FePit2) as receptors for FeLV-B; and (3) FeLV-C cellular receptor (FeLVCR), a heme transporter protein, as a receptor for FeLV-C. FeLV-T uses two proteins to attach to, enter, and infect cells. FePit1 is used as a receptor, whereas FeLIX, a protein secreted primarily by T lymphocytes, is used to restrict tropism to T lymphocytes. Retroviruses also have envelope glycoproteins that form multiple membrane-spanning glycoprotein systems that attach to and bind with multiple membrane-spanning receptors on lymphocytes. To infect T lymphocytes, FeLV-T expresses in its viral envelope a multiple membrane-spanning glycoprotein that attaches to and binds with a host cell multiple membrane-spanning receptor molecule (FePit1). It also appears that expression of a specific host cell receptor, the total number of receptors expressed on the cell, and the use of soluble cofactors play roles in determining which host cells are infected by FeLVs. Additionally, persistent infection of bone marrow cells by FeLV-A provides many opportunities for mutations in the envelope gene that result in the expression of new viral subgroups through viral envelope glycoproteins that recognize new host cell membrane receptors. It is likely that the clinical scenarios caused by these virus subgroups are related to genomic variation through the expression of envelope surface glycoproteins that determine and restrict which host cells they can attach to, enter, and infect.

Immunosuppression, targeted primarily to the cell-mediated immune system, appears to result from (1) a reduction in the number of lymphocytes, especially cytotoxic and helper cell T lymphocytes, through virus-induced cell death; (2) suppression of lymphokines (interferon-δ and interleukin secreted by activated T lymphocytes that could eliminate virus and virus-infected cells; (3) production of FeLV protein p15 that suppresses lymphocyte function (controversial); (4) dysfunction of lymphokine-induced activation of macrophages; and (5) dysfunction of neutrophil phagocytosis. Estimates suggest that about 50% of cats with certain bacterial infections and hemobartonellosis *(Mycoplasma haemofelis)* and 75% of cats with toxoplasmosis *(Toxoplasma gondii)* are infected with and suppressed by FeLV. Additionally, virus-induced immunosuppression has also been associated with feline infectious peritonitis, chronic oral and gingival diseases, poor reparative responses in inflammation, recurrent abscesses and skin infections, respiratory diseases, acute enteritides, otitis, and virus-induced malignancies such as sarcomas.

Neoplastic transformation follows persistent infection of T lymphocytes usually in bone marrow. Virus produces reverse transcriptase that transcribes viral RNA into proviral DNA and facilitates the insertion of proviral DNA into chromosomal DNA of T lymphocytes or other bone marrow cells. When virus has integrated its genome into the host cell DNA, viral genome is passed to all new generations of cells when the infected and integrated host cell is mitotic. Reverse transcriptase is carried by the virus and is released into host cell cytoplasm along with its viral RNA genome after the attachment and entry phase of the virus during its replication cycle. Neoplastic transformation of T lymphocytes or other bone marrow cells occurs when DNA provirus integrates into chromosomal DNA at critical regions that (1) contain oncogenes such as the cellular gene c-myc or (2) are near genes influencing the expression of c-myc genes. Activation of these genes and the expression of their gene products result in a series of alterations to the cell regulatory environment that leads to irreversible changes in cell behavior characteristic of neoplastic transformation (see Chapter 6). Feline oncornavirus-associated cell membrane antigen (FOCMA) is expressed on the cell membranes of transformed cells and is not found on normal (nontransformed) cells, even if they are infected with virus.

Feline Acquired Immunodeficiency Syndrome (Feline Immunodeficiency Virus, Lentivirus, Enveloped RNA Virus)

The mechanism of injury in feline acquired immunodeficiency syndrome is provirus-induced dysfunction and death of CD4⁺ T lymphocytes leading to immunosuppression. Gross lesions include transient lymph node enlargement (lymphadenomegaly) followed by the occurrence of secondary opportunistic microbial infections. Feline immunodeficiency virus causes persistent and gradual depletion of CD4⁺ T lymphocytes (T helper (T_H) lymphocytes, effector T lymphocytes, T_H lymphocytes), resulting in an immunodeficiency syndrome characterized by chronic stomatitis and gingivitis, wasting syndrome (malnutrition), neurologic manifestations, and an increased incidence of lymphoma. The cause of CD4⁺ T lymphocyte depletion is unknown. It may have a multifactorial basis, including death of cells caused directly by viral infection, death (turnover) after massive and rapid replication of virus-infected and noninfected cells stimulated by viral antigen and/or inflammatory molecules, provirus-induced suppression of cell proliferation, death of provirus-infected CD4⁺ T lymphocyte by adaptive immune responses, or apoptosis of provirus-infected cells.

Cats encounter the virus in blood, most commonly as a provirus in infected CD4⁺ T lymphocytes, and much less commonly as free virus in fomites from saliva. During fights that result in bite wounds that bleed, blood contaminated with provirus-infected CD4⁺ T lymphocytes encounters (1) oral mucosae (macrophages and dendritic cells), especially of the tonsils through surface contamination and (2) macrophages and dendritic cells (Langerhans' cells) of the skin through penetrating wounds. It appears that virus is able to establish a local infection in mucosal dendritic cells, macrophages, and lymphocytes; however, it is not clear how virus penetrates the mucus layer to gain access to mucosal epithelial cells, mucosal macrophages, and/or dendritic cells and migrates through the mucosal epithelium to reach cells in the submucosa (MALT). Hypothetically, several mechanisms of spread could be involved (1) migration (leukocyte trafficking) of provirus-infected CD4⁺ T lymphocytes through the epithelium into the submucosa, (2) infection of mucosal epithelial cells via the typical envelope-host cell receptor mechanism by virus released from provirus-infected CD4⁺ T lymphocytes, (3) infection of mucosal epithelial cells via the typical envelope-host cell receptor mechanism by cell-free virus, or (4) transfer of cell-free virus via viral transcytosis, the process by which virus is transported across the interior of a cell in vesicles to be released from the basal surface on the abluminal side. Blood in a skin wound would have direct access to Langerhans' cells and tissue macrophages.

It appears that by whatever route used by virus to enter the body, it must gain access to local mucosal (MALT) or skin-associated lymphoid tissues (SALT) and CD4⁺ T lymphocytes, macrophages, and dendritic cells to establish an infection. Once these cells are infected, virus is then spread by leukocyte trafficking via lymphatic vessels to regional lymph nodes and then systemically via leukocyte trafficking to the spleen and other lymphoid tissues through postcapillary venules or lymphatic vessels and the thoracic duct. Some studies suggest that virus may also spread to the oral cavity and tonsillar mucosa via saliva either by provirus-infected CD4⁺ T lymphocytes or a cell-free viremia, especially if cats with chronic stomatitis and gingivitis are involved in grooming behavior or cat fights. Target cells for infection include CD4⁺ T lymphocytes, CD8⁺ T lymphocytes, B lymphocytes, cells of the monocyte-macrophage system, dendritic cells, megakaryocytes, and astrocytes. Virus envelope glycoproteins bind to host cell membrane receptors and serve to facilitate infection through virus attachment and entry into target cells. Little is known about the characteristics of envelope glycoproteins. Different stains of virus appear to express different envelope glycoproteins (and other proteins), thus these molecules likely contribute to viral pathogenicity. Target cells express feline CD134 receptor and CXCR4 cofactor in their membranes, both of which act as coreceptors and are needed for virus attachment, binding, and entry into host cells.

Postweaning Multisystemic Wasting Syndrome (Porcine Circovirus Type 2, Nonenveloped DNA Virus)

The mechanism of injury in postweaning multisystemic wasting syndrome is virus-induced dysfunction and death of lymphocytes leading to lymphocyte depletion and immunosuppression. Virus appears to require dividing cells, like lymphocytes, in the S-phase of the cell cycle for infection and replication. Gross lesions include systemic enlargement of lymph nodes, normal size lymph nodes, and small atrophic lymph nodes, which are a continuum of changes in the response of lymphocytes to viral infection, replication, and release. Initial infection is likely correlated with viral replication and intense hyperplasia (lymphadenomegaly). Hyperplasia is followed by release of virus from infected lymphocytes, a process that kills lymphocytes and results in atrophy. Microscopic lesions are unique in the fact that inflammation is granulomatous with macrophage-derived syncytial giant cells.

Pigs encounter virus in fomites from oronasal-pharyngeal body fluids, feces, and urine from infected animals. Virus is inhaled or ingested and deposited on mucosae. In the respiratory system, virus is deposited on and trapped in the mucus layer by centrifugal and inertial turbulence and encounters mucosae of the tonsils. It has not been determined if and how virus penetrates the mucus layer to gain access to mucosal epithelial cells, mucosal macrophages, and/or dendritic cells. In the alimentary system, it is swallowed, gains access to the small intestine through peristalsis, and encounters M cell overlying Peyer's patches. M cells lack a mucus layer, and virus has direct access to cell membranes.

It appears that virus establishes an infection in lymphoid tissues of the tonsil and Peyer's patches by infecting mucosal dendritic cells, macrophages, and lymphocytes. Except for M cells, it is not clear how virus spreads through the mucosal epithelium to reach cells in submucosae (MALT), but leukocyte trafficking is likely involved. Spread through the mucosal epithelium could also occur through ligand-receptor interactions followed by viral transcytosis to the basal surfaces with release on the abluminal side. Once macrophages, dendritic cells, and lymphocytes are infected locally, virus spreads by leukocyte trafficking in macrophages and dendritic cells via lymphatic vessels to regional lymph nodes and then systemically through postcapillary venules or lymphatic vessels and the thoracic duct to the circulatory system to lymphocytes in the spleen, lymph nodes, and other lymphoid tissues.

Virus uses a viral capsid protein to attach to glycosaminoglycan receptors, heparin sulfate and chondroitin sulfate B, on macrophages, dendritic cells, and lymphocytes to enter and infect these cells. Macrophages are nonpermissive to virus and appear to serve primarily as trafficking cells to spread virus to other locations, whereas lymphocytes are permissive to virus and allow viral replication. Lymphocytes are injured and killed during replication. Although virus-induced necrosis has been suggested as the mechanism for cell death, apoptosis may actually be the main cause through a viral protein that activates caspase pathways. Other studies suggest that lymphoid loss may result from reduced production of lymphoid cells in the bone marrow or reduced proliferation in secondary lymphoid tissues, resulting in depletion of all types of T and B lymphocytes, immunosuppression, and increased susceptibility to secondary opportunistic infections. Although there is no proof that it is the causal agent, porcine circovirus type 2 (PCV2) has also been linked to several other conditions, including PCV2 pneumonia, PCV2 enteritis, PCV2 reproductive failure, and PCV2 porcine dermatitis and nephropathy syndrome. Many of these conditions have concurrent infections caused by other microbes. These conditions have been grouped under the term PCV2–associated diseases and will not be covered in this chapter because of limited information.

Nervous System

Canine Distemper (Morbillivirus, *Enveloped RNA Virus)*

The mechanism of injury in canine distemper is dysfunction and death of epithelial, mesenchymal, neuroendocrine, and hematopoietic cells in many different tissues and organ systems. Gross lesions are not observed in the nervous system. In the bone marrow, blood cells, and lymphatic systems, they include lymphadenopathy followed by atrophy. Lymph nodes are initially enlarged, hemorrhagic, and edematous but are followed rapidly by cell death, resulting in loss of T and B lymphocytes in the spleen, lymph nodes, MALT, tonsil, and thymus. Alterations in bone marrow are minimal and nonspecific.

Dogs encounter virus in fomites from body fluids of the nasal and oral cavities, through direct contact with infected dogs. Virus is inhaled and deposited on mucosae of the conductive and O_2-CO_2 exchange systems through centrifugal and inertial turbulence. In the mucus layer of the oronasal pharynx, virus is phagocytosed by mucosal lymphocytes and macrophages and likely dendritic cells and spread via leukocyte trafficking to the tonsils. Here, lymphocytes and macrophages are infected and migrate in lymphatic vessels to regional lymph nodes, then systemically through postcapillary venules or lymphatic vessels and the thoracic duct to the circulatory system to lymphocytes in the spleen, thymus, lymph nodes, bone marrow, mucosa-associated lymphoid nodules and Peyer's patches, and to Kupffer cells of the liver. Infection of cells may also occur via a cell-free viremia and through platelets. After infection of systemic lymphoid tissue, infected cells or virus spreads to parenchymal organs, including the nervous, respiratory, alimentary, and urinary systems. It infects a wide variety of epithelial and mesenchymal cells (pantropic virus) and kills these cells as it replicates and escapes from them.

In the respiratory system, virus kills pneumocytes, bronchiolar epithelium, and alveolar macrophages, thereby disrupting the function of the air-blood barrier, the mucociliary apparatus, and innate and adaptive immune responses resulting in poor oxygenation of blood, disrupted removal of particulate debris and secondary bacteria, and phagocytosis and antigen presentation by macrophages, respectively. These mechanisms contribute to suppurative bronchopneumonia. In the alimentary system, virus kills enterocytes (and likely M cells), leading to diarrhea. Virus also gains access to ameloblasts during the development of adult teeth, infects and kills these cells, and results in a condition known as *enamel hypoplasia* (see Fig. 7-17). Virus uses two viral envelope proteins: an attachment protein called *viral H protein* and a fusion protein called *viral F protein* bind to cell membrane glycoprotein receptors. Viral fusion proteins are involved in the penetration of virus into uninfected lymphocytes, spread of virus from cell-to-cell, and formation of syncytial cells (e.g., CD9 transmembrane protein) characteristically seen in the lungs. It has been shown experimentally that when virus-infected lymphocytes encounter uninfected lymphocytes and other cell types, they are induced to express new and/or increased numbers of SLAM receptors. Molecules secreted by virus-infected lymphocytes likely mediate this process and thus may serve as a means to amplify virus infection in dogs. Glycoprotein receptor CD150 (SLAM) occurs in membranes of lymphocytes, monocytes, macrophages, transitional epithelial cells, endothelial cells, and unspecified cells in the stomach, small intestine, and lung.

Vaccination status, adaptive immune system viability, and viral pathogenicity determine whether polioencephalomyelitis, demyelinating leukoencephalomyelitis, or both occur in the CNS. Virus-infected lymphocytes and macrophages spread distemper virus via the blood vascular system to the CNS through leukocyte trafficking and cell-free viremia. Cells and virus likely interact via the leukocyte adhesion cascade (see Chapter 3) with endothelial cells by adhering to and migrating through the endothelium. Virus also infects and replicates in endothelial cells of capillaries and postcapillary venules, resulting in a perivascular lymphomonocytic inflammatory response characteristic of viral infections. Virus then infects and replicates in vascular pericytes, microglial cells, and perivascular astrocytic foot processes, as well as in choroid plexus epithelium. Virus escapes from choroid plexus epithelium and spreads in the cerebral spinal fluid (CSF) to infect ependymal cells and oligodendroglial cells in the subependymal white matter. The clinical signs caused by virus are likely related to injury of neurons and oligodendroglial cells. The virus can cause disease in both gray matter (neurons: polioencephalomyelitis) and white matter (oligodendroglial cells: demyelinating leukoencephalomyelitis). Neuronal infection likely arises after spread of virus to neurons from virus-infected pericytes and perivascular astrocytic foot processes. Virus-infected astrocytes may also serve as a reservoir for spreading virus within the CNS. Viral infection of neurons results in neuronal necrosis and subsequent neuronophagia via resident microglial cells and trafficking monocytes, macrophages, and lymphocytes. Spread of virus to oligodendroglial cells probably arises from infection of ependymal cells; however, infection through the blood vascular system, capillaries and postcapillary venules, and virus-infected pericytes and perivascular astrocytic foot processes has not been excluded as a potential infective mechanism.

Involvement of oligodendroglial cells results in demyelinating leukoencephalomyelitis, which has an acute phase and a chronic phase. Two mechanisms have been proposed for the acute phase of demyelinating leukoencephalomyelitis: (1) death of oligodendroglial cells from infection or (2) a type II hypersensitivity reaction against proteins such as myelin basic protein and myelin-associated glycoprotein. For a cell death mechanism, there is no evidence of virus-induced apoptosis or necrosis of oligodendroglial cells, and although virus can infect oligodendroglial cells, no viral proteins are present in these cells. Astrocytes and microglial cells can be infected and show activation such as hypertrophy and hyperplasia. It has been hypothesized that toxic molecules, such as proinflammatory cytokines produced by these glial cells, act to disrupt the function of oligodendroglial cells and kill the cells. For a hypersensitivity reaction mechanism, microscopic lesions of vacuolization (intramyelinic edema) of myelin lamellae surrounding axons in white matter accompanied by reactive astrocytes, macrophages (monocytes), resident microglial cells, and occasional multinucleated giant cells are consistent with this type of immune-mediated injury. As this injury progresses, the inflammatory response becomes more intense and is characterized by perivascular mononuclear infiltrations. Myelin is phagocytosed by macrophages (monocytes) and microglial cells and the lesion is repaired by proliferation of astrocytic processes, thus forming dense plaques (astrocytic scars). The chronic phase of demyelinating leukoencephalomyelitis appears to be a bystander mechanism involving inflammation and virus-induced immune responses, such as antibody dependent cell-mediated reactions (cytotoxic T lymphocytes) against viral proteins expressed in oligodendroglial cell membranes leading to macrophage-mediated separation, damage, and phagocytosis of myelin lamellae. Myelin damage is likely the result of proteolytic enzymes, oxygen free radicals, and cytokines from activated macrophages, monocytes, and resident microglia. Lipids from damaged lamellae stimulate an intense phagocytic response and likely initiate recruitment of additional monocytes and macrophages into the lesions. Disruption of the blood-brain barrier by proteolytic enzymes appears to play a role in the influx of inflammatory cells probably mediated by viral infection of astrocytes through their foot process involved in the structure and function of the blood-brain barrier.

Rabies (Lyssavirus, *Enveloped RNA Virus*)

The mechanism of injury in rabies is neuronal dysfunction likely caused by several proposed mechanisms such as viral takeover of RNA transcription and translation in neurons, disruption of neurotransmitter functions, dysfunction of ion channels, and/or induction of the synthesis of nitric oxide. Rabies virus infects neurons of all mammalian species. Gross lesions are not present in nervous tissue; however, inclusion bodies (Negri bodies) and a chronic lymphomonocytic perivascular inflammation characteristic of viral infections are observed (see Figs. 1-49,*C* and 14-45). In addition to neurons, the virus infects glial cells in the nervous system and epithelial cells such as those in the salivary glands.

Animals encounter virus in fomites from saliva through a skin-penetrating bite wound from a rabid animal. Virus gains access to interstitial (extracellular) body fluids and plasma (bite wound hemorrhage); diffuses at random in this fluid; and encounters, attaches to, and enters striated muscles cells via binding of rabies virus envelope G protein to neurotransmitter receptors, such as an acetylcholine receptors, in cell membranes. Envelope G protein is an important determinate of rabies neurovirulence and which neuron pathways are infected with virus in the nervous system. Virus replicates in muscle, buds from cell membranes, enters interstitial fluids of myoneural junctions, and randomly encounters and binds to acetylcholine receptors, neuronal cell-adhesion molecule receptors, neurotrophin receptors, or other types of gangliosides in cell membranes of unmyelinated axon terminals (nerve endings) of lower motor neurons or sensory neurons of peripheral nerves. Similar processes are also used to spread and replicate virus in cranial nerves after bite wounds to the face. Once bound, virus enters the cytoplasm of nerve endings through pinocytosis via clathrin-coated pits and the formation of vesicles. Virus in vesicles spreads centripetally from myoneural junctions to the cell body of the nerve via retrograde fast axonal transport, likely using the dynein light chain microtubule-based transport system. Virus replicates in the cell body of neurons and travels to dendrites via axonal transport where it buds from cell membrane of dendritic processes into synaptic clefts of neural-neural junctions. It randomly encounters receptors on sensory and motor nerve endings within the spinal cord and brain in gray horns of the spinal cord. Mechanistically, viral replication and spread in sensory and motor neurons within the spinal cord and brain are identical to that in peripheral spinal nerves. The exact mechanism that facilitates transsynaptic spread of rabies virus is unknown. It may be linked in part to viral assembly where M-protein encapsulates the virus and assists in moving the virus to cell membranes such as those in synapses that contain glycoproteins essential for formation of the viral envelope and viral budding. Envelope G protein is also required for attachment to cell membrane and transsynaptic spread of the virus to the next neuron in the neural pathway.

Virus uses axonal transport mechanisms to spread throughout the body via afferent and efferent neural pathways to infect the epithelial cells of the salivary glands (see Fig. 14-44). Rabies virus, through these neural pathways, can also infect other cells such as those in taste buds, nasal cavity, skin and hair follicles, adrenal gland, pancreas, kidney, heart muscle, and the retina and cornea. In fact, the "furious" and "dumb" forms of rabies in domestic animals are likely attributable to infection of specific neuronal populations and pathways such as those in the hippocampal formation or cerebellum, respectively. Virus spreads to salivary glands through axonal transport using parasympathetic nerves present in the facial (VII) and glossopharyngeal (IX) cranial nerves and sympathetic nerves in the thoracic segments of T1-T3 spinal cord segments. In addition to spreading virus to the salivary glands, viral infection of parasympathetic and sympathetic nerves also results in increased salivary gland secretions: (1) directly through stimulating β-adrenergic receptors on the salivary acinar and ductal cells, leading to an increase in cAMP concentrations and the corresponding increase of saliva secretion, and (2) indirectly through stimulating nerves innervating blood vessels that supply the salivary glands. Virus buds from the cell membrane of these nerve terminals, infects salivary acinar cells through the envelop G protein-specific cell surface receptor mechanism, and replicates in and is amplified to large quantities in salivary acinar cells. Virus then buds from apical (luminal) surfaces of acinar cell membranes, mixes with saliva, and can be transmitted in a bite wound. The apical specificity of viral budding is established during the assembly stage of viral replication. Viral genome and proteins form complexes in the acinar cell cytoplasm that congregate at areas of the cell membrane that contain matching glycoprotein receptors and then bud from this membrane into the acinar lumen.

Equine Polioencephalitis-Polioencephalomyelitis (Alphavirus, Enveloped RNA Virus)

The mechanism of injury in equine polioencephalitis-polioencephalomyelitis is disruption and death of neurons in the CNS. Gross lesions include active hyperemia, vasculitis, hemorrhage, and yellow-white-gray areas of necrosis in gray matter of the nervous system, especially the spinal cord (see Fig. 14-79). Because neurons are the primary target, lesions are most commonly observed in gray matter, areas in which neuron cell bodies are located, and these diseases are classified as polioencephalitides or polioencephalomyelitides. Equine polioencephalitis-polioencephalomyelitis is used to group three closely related strains of alphaviruses that cause Eastern equine encephalomyelitis, Western equine encephalomyelitis, and Venezuelan equine encephalomyelitis. St. Louis encephalomyelitis is the human counterpart to these horse diseases. Such diseases have also been called *arbovirus polioencephalitis-polioencephalomyelitis*. The term *arbovirus* is derived from the fact that these viruses are *ar*thropod-*bo*rne; the term was shortened and is used as a disease acronym.

Horses encounter viruses through skin penetrating bite wounds from virus-infected mosquitoes. Mosquitoes are infected by biting birds, the reservoir for the virus. Seasonal variations in temperature and precipitation greatly influence the population density of mosquitoes and thus the occurrence of disease. After skin penetration, virus can either directly enter the circulatory system and infect monocytes or be deposited in vascularized ECM (connective) tissue and infect dendritic cells (Langerhans' cells) and tissue macrophages (Fig. 4-45). In these cells, virus is spread via leukocyte trafficking to regional lymph nodes either by the circulatory system or lymphatic vessels where it infected lymphocytes. It may also spread to regional lymph nodes via cell-free viremia in lymphatic

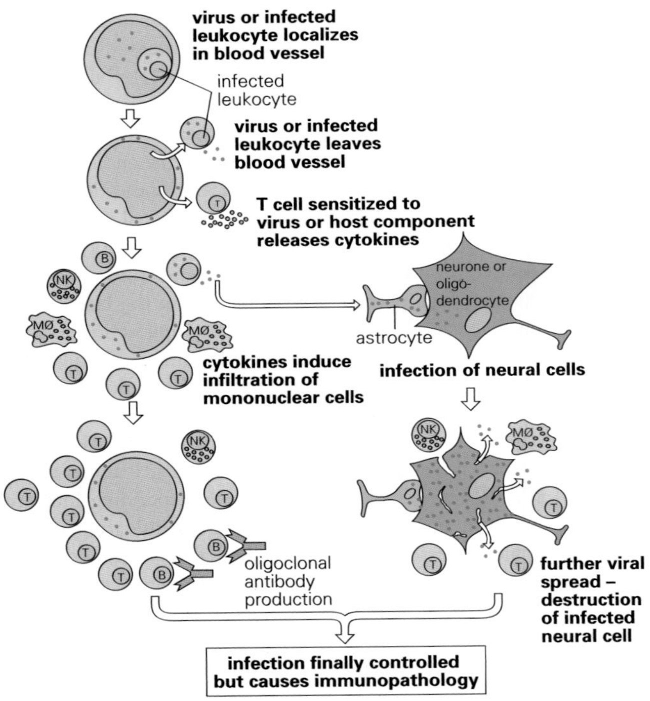

Fig. 4-45 Mechanism of arbovirus and West Nile virus infections. *M/O,* Macrophage; *NK,* natural killer cell. (From Goering R, Dockrell H, Roitt I, et al: *Mims' medical microbiology,* ed 4, St. Louis, 2008, Mosby.)

vessels. Viral envelope contains two membrane-anchored glycoproteins, E1 and E2. Attachment protein E2 is used to attach to target cell receptor, whereas viral envelope fusion protein E1 is used to enter cells via endocytosis. Receptors for E1 and E2 proteins occur on a variety of cell types and probably determine which organ systems, such as the nervous system, are targeted for infection by virus. Virus then spreads systemically via leukocyte trafficking in lymphocytes and macrophages through postcapillary venules or lymphatic vessels and the thoracic duct to the circulatory system to systemic lymph nodes, spleen, thymus, bone marrow, Peyer's patches, pancreas, and skeletal muscle. Infection results in necrosis of myeloid cells in bone marrow and lymphocytes in lymph nodes and spleen. Proinflammatory cytokines, such as IFN-γ, and antiinflammatory cytokines, such IL-10 produced by infected lymphocytes, may cause cell death. Cytokines released into the blood vascular system may also act on the blood-brain barrier, making it more susceptible to infection. In Eastern equine encephalomyelitis, osteoblasts appear to be the systemic population of target cells used to amplify virus so it can spread to the nervous system, whereas dendritic cells, lymphoid cells, and cells of the monocyte-macrophage system are not as susceptible to infection and thus systemic lymph nodes and spleen are infected to a limited degree with minimal injury. Although it is unclear how virus spreads to and enters the CNS, leukocyte trafficking by lymphocytes and macrophages (monocytes) appears to be the probable mechanism. Cell-free viremia may also occur.

West Nile Virus Polioencephalitis-Polioencephalomyelitis (Flavivirus, *Enveloped RNA Virus)*

The pathogenesis and mechanism of injury in West Nile virus polioencephalitis-polioencephalomyelitis are similar to those of equine polioencephalitis-polioencephalomyelitis (see Fig. 4-45).

Bovine Herpesvirus Meningoencephalitis (Bovine Herpesvirus 5: Alphaherpesvirus*, Enveloped DNA Virus)*

Bovine herpesvirus 5 infects cells, spreads, and behaves much like bovine herpesvirus 1, except it is more neurovirulent and induces a severe often fatal encephalitis. See infectious bovine rhinotracheitis in the section on the Respiratory System, Mediastinum, and Pleurae. The mechanism of injury is dysfunction and death of neurons and astrocytes caused by viral replication and likely the actions of cytotoxic T lymphocytes on virus-infected neural cells through proinflammatory chemokines and cytokines as part of lymphomonocytic inflammation (innate and adaptive immune responses). Gross lesions include randomly distributed cerebral edema, active hyperemia, hemorrhage, and malacia.

Cattle encounter virus in fomites from body fluids through direct contact with virus-infected animals. It is inhaled or ingested and deposited on mucosae of the oral, nasal, and pharyngeal cavities and of the conjunctiva or inhaled and deposited on mucosae of the conductive component of the respiratory system through centrifugal and inertial turbulence. Viral envelope glycoproteins B, C, D, and E are used to attach to receptors on sensory nerve endings that innervate these mucosae. They can also attach to receptors on a variety of other target cells. These receptors are glycosaminoglycan receptors such as herpesvirus entry mediator A, nectin-1 and -2 (herpesvirus entry proteins C and B), and 3-*O*-sulfated heparin sulfate. It has not been determined how virus penetrates the mucus layer to gain access to mucosal sensory nerve endings. Through these nerve endings, virus enters neurons, such as the trigeminal and olfactory nerves, and spreads via retrograde axonal transport to other neurons and glial cells within the nervous system. It appears that envelope glycoprotein E and 3-*O*-sulfated heparin sulfate receptors may amplify viral attachment, entry, and spread within the CNS. The mechanism of malacia remains unknown but apparently is not caused by obvious vascular injury. Neuronal lesions are consistent with necrosis, likely caused by virus-induced injury and cell death. However, overproduction of nitric oxide in virus-infected neurons and astrocytes could result in their dysfunction and death and that of contiguous non-infected cells.

Bovine herpesvirus 5 can enter latency in the nervous system, through mechanisms likely identical for bovine herpesvirus 1.

Equine Herpesvirus Myeloencephalopathy (Equine Herpesvirus 1: Alphaherpesvirus, Enveloped DNA Virus)

The mechanism of injury in equine herpesvirus myeloencephalopathy is dysfunction and death of endothelial cells in small arterioles of the brain and spinal cord; however, the means is uncertain but most likely caused by virus replication. Immune-complexes (type III hypersensitivity reaction) and the fixation of complement (immune complex-induced vasculitis) have also been suggested. Gross lesions include randomly distributed foci of edema, hemorrhage, and vasocentric malacia (yellow-white-gray areas) consistent with vascular occlusion, resulting in infarction (see Fig. 14-80).

Horses encounter virus in fomites from body fluids through direct contact with virus-infected animals. It is inhaled or ingested and deposited on mucosae of the oral, nasal, and pharyngeal cavities or inhaled and deposited on mucosae of the conductive component of the respiratory system through centrifugal and inertial turbulence. Virus infects and replicates in mucosal epithelial and endothelial cells, then in contiguous mucosal and submucosal lymphocytes and likely macrophages, monocytes, and dendritic cells (MALT), and then spreads via leukocyte trafficking in lymphatic vessels to regional lymph nodes. It has not been determined if and how virus penetrates the mucus layer to gain access to mucosal epithelial and endothelial cells or if or how mucosal macrophages and/or dendritic cells are involved, although very likely. Although specific ligands and receptors have not been identified, viral envelope glycoproteins likely attach to glycosaminoglycan receptors on host cell membranes and use this binding to enter the cells listed above. Infection appears to be sustained and amplified in lymphocytes and likely macrophages and monocytes of regional lymph nodes and then is spread systemically through blood and lymphatic vessels in these cells via leukocyte trafficking into the circulatory system. Infected cells probably use envelope adhesion molecules to bind to receptors on vascular endothelium and during migration through the vessel wall, interact with these cells, allowing virus to infect and replicate in endothelial cells, myocytes, and pericytes of small arterioles in the brain and spinal cord causing vasculitis and thrombosis. It is not known why these cells are targets for virus infection; however, typical ligand-receptor interactions or permissiveness of these cells are likely involved. Activation of endothelial and leukocyte adhesion molecules is an important step in spreading virus to endothelial cells and thus may contribute to endothelial cell tropism for viral infection.

Parvovirus-Induced Cerebellar Hypoplasia (Parvovirus, Nonenveloped DNA Virus)

See parvovirus enteritis in the section on the Alimentary System and the Peritoneum, Omentum, Mesentery, and Peritoneal Cavity for information about local and regional stages of viral spread and replication before spread to the CNS. In pregnant cats, parvovirus is able to cross the placenta and infect dividing cells in the developing cerebellum in kittens, resulting in cerebellar hypoplasia (see Fig. 14-35). Whether by leukocyte trafficking or cell-free viremia, parvoviruses are able to gain access to cells in the placenta. Virus infects and replicates in placental trophoblasts and spreads to, infects, and replicates in cytotrophoblasts and cells of the mesenchymal stroma of the fetal placenta. From these cells, virus gains access to the fetal vascular system and spreads to, infects, and replicates in hematopoietic cells and other dividing cells. It has also been suggested that placental macrophages and fetal endothelial cells are likely involved in the replication and spread of the virus in the fetus. Although the virus can infect a large number of different cells in the fetus, it is unclear why fetal infection is clinically dominated by injury to cells of the cerebellum and cerebellar hypoplasia. Ligand-receptor interactions could contribute to specificity; however, other unknown mechanisms are likely involved.

Parvoviruses only infect and replicate in dividing cells. Cells of the external granular layer of the cerebellum are dividing cells, whereas Purkinje cells are nondividing cells. However, cell death is observed in both of these cell types, when only one of them is a dividing cell population. Granule precursor cells of the cerebellar external granular layer are the major target cells for parvovirus replication during the perinatal period because they are able enter the S-phase of the mitotic cycle. Purkinje cells are also infected, but they are nondividing postmitotic cells. It appears that virus infects Purkinje cells via a host cell membrane transferrin receptor that is commonly used by parvovirus for entering other types of host cells. Virus is unable to replicate in postmitotic Purkinje cells, but transcription of viral proteins does occur. It has been suggested that a nonstructural parvovirus protein NS1 is produced at low concentrations during the G0 and G1 phases of the cell cycle. Because NS1 is known to be highly cytotoxic and able to induce cytoskeleton alterations, this effect could result in injury and cytolysis of Purkinje cells during *in utero* infection with virus. Although cerebellar hypoplasia is not commonly thought to occur from *in utero* infection of female dogs by canine parvovirus, a recent study has identified parvovirus DNA in brain tissue from puppies with the disease. However, the significance of this information remains unclear because parvovirus structural proteins were not identified in the same tissues. A similar syndrome, probably involving similar mechanisms, occurs in calves infected *in utero* with bovine viral diarrhea–mucosal disease virus (see Fig. 14-36).

Visna (Maedi-Visna Virus [Ovine Lentivirus], Enveloped RNA Virus)

The chronologic sequence of events that characterizes the pathogenesis of injury in visna is similar to those that occur in progressive ovine pneumonia (Maedi) of sheep. The mechanism of injury is chronic-active (granulomatous) inflammation of the CNS resulting in demyelinating encephalitis. Gross lesions include foci of yellow-white malacia distributed at random in the CNS. Ovine lentivirus persistently infects cells of the monocyte-macrophage system including microglial cells (local tissue macrophages in the CNS) and all of these cell types are central to the genesis of the inflammatory response in the CNS.

Caprine Encephalitis (Caprine Arthritis-Encephalitis Virus, Enveloped RNA Virus)

The pathogenesis and mechanism of injury in caprine encephalitis are similar to those that occur in progressive ovine pneumonia (Maedi) of sheep (see section on the Respiratory System, Mediastinum, and Pleurae); however, the initial route of exposure is different. The mechanism of injury is chronic-active (granulomatous) inflammation of the CNS resulting in demyelinating myelitis. Gross lesions include foci of yellow-white malacia distributed at random in the CNS, especially the spinal cord (see Fig. 14-90). Caprine arthritis-encephalitis virus persistently infects cells of the monocyte-macrophage system, thus microglial cells (local tissue macrophages) and trafficking monocytes serve as the cell type central to the genesis of the inflammatory response. Kid goats are primarily exposed to virus through the ingestion of virus-infected milk or colostrum. Although not proven, virus likely infects M cells overlying Peyer's patches. Once infected, virus is transferred to and released from basilar surfaces of M cells to gain access to macrophages and lymphocytes within Peyer's patches. It is here that macrophages are infected with virus and then serve to spread virus to monocyte precursor cells in the bone marrow and ultimately to the CNS.

Pseudorabies (Aujeszky Disease) (Alphaherpesviruses, Enveloped DNA Virus)

The mechanism of injury in pseudorabies is disruption and death of neurons likely caused by the actions of cytolytic immune cells interacting with virus-infected neurons. Because neurons are the primary target of viral infection, lesions are most commonly observed in gray matter and as a result, this disease is a polioencephalitis or polioencephalomyelitis. Gross lesions characteristic of injury are usually not observed but in severe cases could include active hyperemia and hemorrhage.

Pigs encounter virus in fomites from oronasal-pharyngeal body fluids most commonly through inhalation and potentially through contamination of skin-penetrating bite wounds. When inhaled, virus is deposited on mucosae of the oral, nasal, and pharyngeal cavities, especially of the tonsil or on mucosae of the conductive component of the respiratory system through centrifugal and inertial turbulence. In the tonsil, virus may infect and replicate in mucosal epithelial cells, mucosal and submucosal macrophages, and dendritic cells (MALT). In the lung, virus also infects and replicates in similar cells (BALT), including alveolar macrophages, which it kills, resulting in a secondary bronchopneumonia. Virus attachment and entry is likely mediated by binding of viral envelope glycoproteins to host cell membrane receptors. In the nasal and pharyngeal mucosae and submucosae, especially of the tonsil, virus encounters and infects sensory nerve endings of the olfactory, glossopharyngeal, and trigeminal cranial nerves and uses retrograde axonal transport to enter the brain. Virus can spread transsynaptically throughout the CNS by using mechanisms similar to those described in rabies and infect and replicate in many types of neurons. Viral envelope glycoproteins C, B, D, H, and L are used to attach to, fuse with, and enter membranes of nerve endings. These glycoproteins are also involved in transsynaptic spread to other neurons in the CNS and to other neural cells, such as astrocytes, microglial cells, ependymal cells, and trafficking monocytes/macrophages, as well as in the formation of syncytial cells and the modulation of innate and adaptive immune responses. Virus cannot replicate in these cells, thus they are incapable of infecting other cells in the CNS. This outcome may represent a local intrinsic and/or innate immune defense mechanism that isolates through phagocytosis the virus in astrocytes, monocytes-macrophages, and microglial cells and restricts spread of virus to other cells. Latent infections involve the trigeminal nerves and ganglia, but tonsillar lymph nodules may also be involved. Potentially, peripheral nerve endings in the skin, subcutis, and muscle may be exposed to infection via bite wounds and can be used by virus to gain access to and enter the CNS by mechanisms similar to those described in rabies.

Viral envelope glycoproteins in membranes of infected neurons are targets for neutralizing antibodies, cytotoxic T lymphocytes, and lymphokine-activated killer cells and are part of the chronic perivascular lymphomonocytic inflammatory response characteristic of viral infections. These cells may contribute in a large manner to neuronal injury and death in pseudorabies. Hypertrophy and hyperplasia of astrocytes, microglia, and monocytes-macrophages occur spatially and temporally with the severity of neuronal injury; however, the potential role of biologically active molecules, such as cytokines (e.g., TNF-α), from these cells is unclear.

Bone, Joints, Ligaments, and Tendons

Caprine Arthritis (Caprine Arthritis-Encephalitis Syndrome, Enveloped RNA Virus)

The mechanism of injury in caprine arthritis is chronic-active (granulomatous) inflammation of the synovium, resulting in proliferative synovitis. The chronologic sequence of events that characterizes the pathogenesis of injury in caprine arthritis is similar to those that occur in progressive ovine pneumonia (Maedi) of sheep (see section on the Respiratory System, Mediastinum, and Pleurae).

Integumentary System

Pox (Cowpox [Orthopoxvirus], Sheeppox and Goatpox [Capripoxvirus], Swinepox [Suipoxvirus], Enveloped DNA Virus)

The term pox is used to group diseases, such as bovine cowpox, sheeppox, goatpox, swinepox, and lumpy skin disease, that are caused by closely related strains of poxviruses. The mechanism of injury is dysfunction and death of dendritic and epithelial cells of the skin. Gross lesions include macules, papules, vesicles, pustules, scabs, and scars (see Figs. 17-31, 17-42, and 17-44). Lesions are most easily observed on wool-free or hair-free areas (Fig. 4-46). In general, sheeppox and goatpox are more virulent and cause

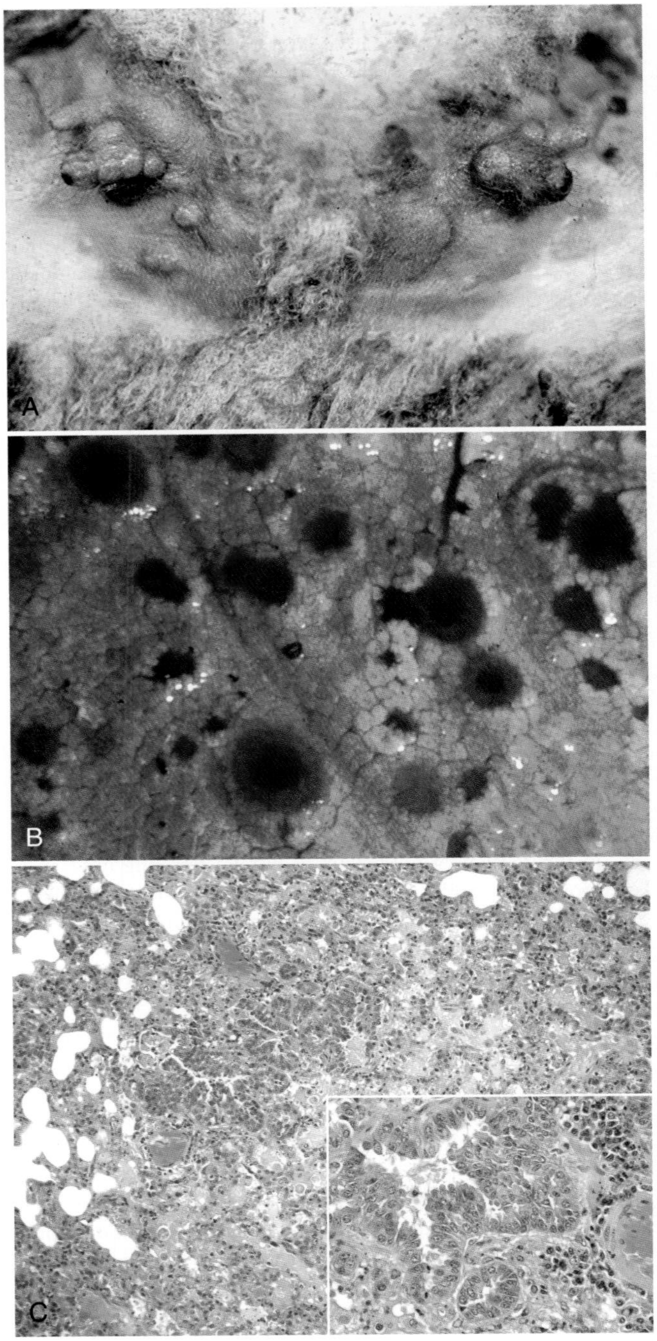

Fig. 4-46 **Sheeppox and goatpox.**
A, Skin, teats, inguinal area. Macules, papules, vesicles, crusts (scabs), and papillomas (epidermal hyperplasia) are present on the skin of the inguinal area and teats. Additional information about the development and progression of pox virus-induced lesions is schematically illustrated in Fig. 17-31 and macroscopically and microscopically in Figs. 17-42 (sheeppox) and 17-44 (swinepox). **B,** Lung, pox lesions. These circumferentially expanding dark red to plum-colored lesions of varied sizes are areas of proliferating bronchial and bronchiolar mucosal epithelial cells, necrotic epithelial cells, cell debris, and inflammation demonstrated in **C. C,** Lung, bronchiole. There is proliferation of mucosal epithelial cells of the lung's conductive system that are infected with poxvirus. Note the mononuclear inflammatory likely bronchiole-associated lymphoid tissue (BALT) in adjacent supporting stroma. *Inset,* Higher magnification of **C.** H&E stain. (**A** courtesy Dr. D. Gregg, Plum Island Animal Disease Center and Noah's Arkive, College of Veterinary Medicine, The University of Georgia. **B** courtesy Dr. R. Breeze, Plum Island Animal Disease Center and Noah's Arkive, College of Veterinary Medicine, The University of Georgia. **C** courtesy Dr. J. F. Zachary, College of Veterinary Medicine, University of Illinois.)

systemic disease, whereas bovine cowpox and swinepox usually do not cause systemic disease. In these latter species, spread of virus is the result of animal-to-animal contact or contact with clothing or tools/instruments contaminated with virus-infected skin, scabs, or other skin debris. It appears that skin must be injured (traumatic abrasions) so that capillary endothelial cells, trafficking leukocytes, or Langerhans' cells (dendritic cells) are exposed and can encounter virus.

As examples, bovine cowpox most commonly occurs on the teats of dairy cows, the areas most commonly injured by milking trauma in a diary herd. Insect bites result in penetrating skin wounds that can also carry virus into contact with susceptible target cells. However, in sheeppox and goatpox, animals encounter virus through the oronasal pharynx via inhalation or ingestion. It is deposited on mucosae, especially of the tonsil, and infects and replicates in epithelial cells, mucosal lymphocytes and macrophages, and dendritic cells (MALT). It has not been determined how virus penetrates the mucus layer to gain access to mucosal epithelial cells, macrophages, and/or dendritic cells, but it is likely virus is phagocytosed by leukocytes trafficking in the mucus layer when these cells encounter virus during migration. Submucosal macrophages are infected, and virus spreads in them via lymphatic vessels to regional lymph nodes, such as the submandibular and pharyngeal. Here, naïve lymphocytes and macrophages are recruited through the release of proinflammatory chemokines and cytokines and are infected with virus. Virus then spreads systemically via leukocyte trafficking in these lymphocytes and macrophages through postcapillary venules or lymphatic vessels and the thoracic duct to the circulatory system and then to systemic lymph nodes, spleen, and bone marrow and infects and replicates in similar cells. Virus then spreads from systemic lymphoid tissues via leukocyte trafficking to the skin (see below), lung, liver, and other organ systems.

In the skin, virus spreads from migrating macrophages and lymphocytes and infects and replicates in endothelial cells, resulting in direct injury and an acute inflammatory response. Endothelial cell injury accompanied by vascular dilation, active hyperemia, and acute inflammation in part likely account for macules and papules observed in early skin lesions. Langerhans' cells (dendritic cells) are in close contact with endothelial cells in the Malpighian layer of the skin. It appears that virus from capillary endothelial cells and trafficking leukocytes is able to infect Langerhans' cells and then spread virus to contiguous skin epithelial cells of the stratum basale and spinosum. All of these cells allow virus to replicate, thus when epithelial cells of the stratum basale and spinosum are killed, the space formerly occupied by these cells coalesces and is filled with cell debris and intercellular edema, forming vesicles. With injury, acute inflammation ensues, as does the pustular stage. Through adaptive immune responses, viral infection is resolved and pustular lesions heal as scabs over granulation tissue that become scars.

It is likely that both humoral and cell-mediated immunity are important in protecting against and resolving pox diseases; however, these responses can cause injury and death of virus-infected host cells. Similar lesions and lesion progression may affect oral mucous membranes. Pneumonia has been reported in systemic poxvirus-induced disease. Affected lungs have variable sized and randomly distributed pock lesions in the form of large, irregularly shaped lobular areas of consolidation (see Fig. 4-46). This pattern is consistent with hematogenous spread of the virus via leukocyte trafficking in virus-infected macrophages to pulmonary endothelial cells and then to bronchiolar and alveolar epithelial cells followed by cell death and acute inflammation. Although reservoir hosts for poxvirus are wild rodents, cats are now the most commonly recognized reservoir. Cats are infected with virus through their skin by an indirect mechanism when hunting virus-infected rodents; however, infection, as previously described, via a direct mechanism (inhalation) and systemic spread in monocytes and macrophages has been reported.

Poxviruses use attachment proteins to bind to glycosaminoglycan receptor proteins on the surface of the host target cells. Because of the volume of information related to attachment proteins and receptors in poxvirus diseases, discussion of these protein molecules is outside of the scope of this chapter.

Contagious Ecthyma (Orf Virus: Parapoxvirus, Enveloped DNA Virus)

See contagious ecthyma in the section on the Alimentary System and the Peritoneum, Omentum, Mesentery, and Peritoneal Cavity.

Bovine Papular Stomatitis (Parapoxvirus, Enveloped DNA Virus)

See bovine papular stomatitis in the section on the Alimentary System and the Peritoneum, Omentum, Mesentery, and Peritoneal Cavity.

Vesicular Stomatitis (Vesiculovirus, Enveloped RNA Virus)

See vesicular stomatitis in the section on the Alimentary System and the Peritoneum, Omentum, Mesentery, and Peritoneal Cavity.

Swine Vesicular Disease (Enterovirus, Nonenveloped RNA Virus)

See swine vesicular disease in the section covering the Alimentary System and the Peritoneum, Omentum, Mesentery, and Peritoneal Cavity.

Vesicular Exanthema of Pigs (Calicivirus [Waikavirus], Nonenveloped RNA Virus)

See vesicular exanthema of pigs in the section on the Alimentary System and the Peritoneum, Omentum, Mesentery, and Peritoneal Cavity.

Foot-and-Mouth Disease (Aphthovirus, Nonenveloped RNA Virus)

See foot-and-mouth disease in the section on the Alimentary System and the Peritoneum, Omentum, Mesentery, and Peritoneal Cavity.

Viral Papillomas (Warts, Sarcoids, Papillomaviruses, Nonenveloped DNA Virus)

The mechanism of injury in viral papillomas is dysfunction of host cell genes that regulate cell proliferation, differentiation, and adhesion, resulting in benign neoplastic transformation of virus-infected epithelial cells. Cells of stratum basale (germinativum) play a central role in the pathogenesis of neoplastic transformation. Gross lesions include the formation of exophytic and occasionally endophytic papillomatous fronds that arise from mucosae or skin (see Fig. 17-45). Papillomaviruses are species specific and in (1) cattle cause warts of the skin and papillomas of mucosae of the alimentary system, teats and udder, and penis; (2) horses, donkeys, and mules cause sarcoids of the skin; and (3) dogs cause papillomas of the mucosal epithelium of the oral cavity and reproductive system.

Animals encounter virus through direct contact with animals of the same species having warts, papillomas, or sarcoids. Viral infection is preceded by injury of the superficial layers of the stratified epithelium of mucosae or skin, resulting in exposure of target cells in the stratum basale. Epithelial cells of mucosae have short lifespans and with aging are shed from their surfaces into a lumen of the alimentary system or into the environment as a means of spreading the virus. Thus these cells are constantly being turned over and replenished by dividing stem cells located in their basal layers. Maturation of these cells begins with the least differentiated layer, the stratum basale, and progresses outwardly through the suprabasilar layers, the strata spinosum, granulosum, lucidum, and corneum. Stem cells of the stratum basale are continuously dividing to replace cells in the suprabasilar layers; cells of the suprabasilar layers do not divide. Virus likely uses capsid proteins, such as bovine L1 major capsid protein and L2 minor capsid protein, to attach and bind to and enter cells of the stratum basale. Viral receptors on cells of the stratum basale have not been clearly identified; however, heparin sulfate proteoglycans mediate the initial attachment of virions to cells in some experimental systems. Dividing cells of the stratum basale are target cells for viral infection and it replicates its genome to a limited extent within the nucleus of these cells. Stem cells of the stratum basale have a lifespan for the life of the animal and serve as reservoirs for virus-infected cells. They also are nonpermissive cells, and virus is not able to produce infective virions. As cells of the stratum basale mature through differentiation into cells of the strata spinosum, granulosum, lucidum, and corneum, these differentiated cells become permissive and allow virus to complete its replication cycle and produce infective virions. Virus is released from cells of the strata lucidum and corneum into the environment to spread the disease. A similar process likely occurs in infected mucosae of the alimentary system.

Neoplastic transformation of epithelial cells by papillomaviruses can result in the formation of benign tumors, such as papillomas, warts, and sarcoids, and malignant tumors, such as carcinomas. When virus infects stems cells of the stratum basale, the expression of viral genes is maintained at low numbers (approximately 20 to 100 extrachromosomal copies of viral DNA per cell) where it replicates in synchrony with the cell cycle as the cell divides. Normally, as epithelial cells leave the stratum basale and mature (differentiate), they turn off endogenous genes and the synthesis of proteins required for cell division. When virus-infected stem cells of the stratum basale divide, viral genomes are carried in cells that differentiate into cells of the suprabasilar layers. Viral proteins prevent these differentiated cells from stopping the cell cycle, thus cells of suprabasilar layers, especially the strata spinosum and granulosum, are now capable of division. Because cells of the suprabasilar layer are permissive and allow virus to complete its replication cycle and produce infective virions, large quantities of viral genes and regulatory proteins are present within these dividing host cells. As a general rule, neoplastic transformation of virus-infected epithelial cells appears to be linked to the quantitative and qualitative expression of viral genes and gene products, such as oncoproteins, and how these molecules interact with host cell genes and gene products regulating cell proliferation, differentiation, and adhesion. It looks as if strains of papillomavirus unable to integrate into host genes are most likely to cause benign transformation (papillomas, warts, and sarcoids) of virus-infected epithelial cells, whereas strains able to integrate into host genes are most likely to cause malignant transformation (carcinomas) of virus-infected epithelial cells. Benign transformation is most likely to occur in cells of the stratum basale. In these cells, virus does not integrate into host cell genes and viral genes and gene products like oncoproteins are expressed in low numbers. Thus the likelihood of virus activating growth-promoting genes (oncogenes) in host cell DNA, inactivating suppressor genes that would inhibit cell proliferation, and altering the functional expression of genes that regulate apoptosis is extremely limited. Malignant transformation is most likely to occur in suprabasilar cells where virus integrates into host cell genes and viral genes and gene products, such as oncoproteins, are expressed in high numbers. Thus the likelihood of virus activating growth-promoting genes (oncogenes) in host cell DNA, inactivating suppressor genes that would inhibit cell proliferation, and altering the functional expression of genes that regulate apoptosis is extremely high. A similar process likely occurs in infected mucosae of the alimentary system.

Female Reproductive System

Porcine Reproductive and Respiratory Syndrome (PRRS Virus, Enveloped RNA Virus)

The pathogenesis of the initiating phases of PRRS is discussed in the section on the Respiratory System, Mediastinum, and Pleurae. Although unknown, the mechanism and type of injury that occurs in the lung also probably affects a wide variety of cells in the placenta, fetal membranes, and fetus. Injury can be observed in fetal myocytes; however, it is unclear as to whether loss of myocytes is attributable to necrosis, apoptosis, or atrophy. Gross lesions include abortions (born weak) and fetal deaths (mummification, stillbirths). Virus probably spreads to the placenta in virus-infected macrophages within the circulatory system via leukocytic trafficking from an initial site of virus replication in another body system such as the lung or uterus. It is likely that virus-infected macrophages transfer virus to fetal macrophage-like cells in the placentome, which then spread virus to all organ systems in the fetus. Although all fetuses in a litter may not be infected, it has been shown that pig fetuses in all stages of gestation can be infected with and support replication of virus resulting in normal, born weak, stillborn, and mummified fetuses.

Bovine Herpesvirus Abortion (Bovine Herpesvirus 1: Alphaherpesvirus, Enveloped DNA Virus)

See infectious bovine rhinotracheitis in the section on the Respiratory System, Mediastinum, and Pleurae. Gross lesions include abortions (born weak) and fetal deaths (mummification, stillbirths). Virus-infected mucosal macrophages, lymphocytes, or dendritic cells migrate in lymphatic vessels via leukocyte trafficking and spread virus to regional lymph nodes such as the tracheobronchial. Here, it infects macrophages and lymphocytes, which spread it to the circulatory system and placenta via cell-free viremia or leukocyte trafficking through postcapillary venules or lymphatic vessels and the thoracic duct. It is not clear how virus spreads from the uterus, to the placenta, and then to the fetus, but some form of a fetal macrophage-like cell probably intervenes in the placentome. Cell types and injury involved are undetermined.

Equine Herpesvirus Abortion (Equine Herpesvirus 1 and 4: Alphaherpesvirus, Enveloped DNA Virus)

See equine viral rhinopneumonitis in the section on the Respiratory System, Mediastinum, and Pleurae. Gross lesions include abortions (born weak) and fetal deaths (mummification, stillbirths). Virus-infected mucosal macrophages, lymphocytes, or dendritic cells migrate in lymphatic vessels via leukocyte trafficking and spread virus to regional lymph nodes such as the tracheobronchial. Here, it infects macrophages and lymphocytes, which spread it to the circulatory system and placenta via cell-free viremia or leukocyte trafficking through postcapillary venules or lymphatic vessels and the thoracic duct. It is not clear how virus spreads from the uterus, to the placenta, and then to the fetus, but some form of a fetal macrophage-like cell probably intervenes in the placentome. Cell types and injury involved are undetermined.

Infectious Pustular Vulvovaginitis/Balanoposthitis (Bovine Herpesvirus 1: Alphaherpesvirus, Enveloped DNA Virus)

See infectious bovine rhinotracheitis in the section on the Respiratory System, Mediastinum, and Pleurae. Gross lesions include erosion and ulcerations with hemorrhage of reproductive mucosae (see Fig. 18-46). Virus-infected mucosal macrophages, lymphocytes, or dendritic cells migrate in lymphatic vessels via leukocyte trafficking and spread virus to regional lymph nodes such as the tracheobronchial. Here, it infects macrophages and lymphocytes, which spread it to the circulatory system and placenta via cell-free viremia or leukocyte trafficking through postcapillary venules or lymphatic vessels and the thoracic duct. Virus then spreads to epithelial cells of the mucous membranes of the penis, prepuce, vulva, or vagina via cell-free viremia or leukocyte trafficking. Because virus causes death of infected cells and thus erosions and ulcerations of mucosae, it may also be spread via direct contact (venereal disease) of virus-infected mucosae from the penis or prepuce with mucosae of the vulva or vagina, or vice-versa, during breeding.

Coital Exanthema (Equine Herpesvirus 3: Alphaherpesvirus, Enveloped DNA Virus)

The mechanism of injury in coital exanthema is dysfunction and death of mucosal epithelial cells of the male and female reproductive systems. Gross lesions include active hyperemia, hemorrhage, erosions, and ulceration of affected mucosae, leading to an acute inflammatory response (see Fig. 18-48). Horses encounter virus through direct contact (venereal disease) with infected horses during breeding. Mucosae do not need to be injured for virus to infect cells. Virus can also spread mechanically via hands, gloves, instruments, palpation sleeves, and sponges, if contaminated with virus. Although unidentified, equine herpesvirus 3 probably expresses attachment proteins in its envelope that attach and bind to specific receptors on cells of reproductive mucosae.

Equine Viral Arteritis (Arterivirus, Enveloped RNA Virus)

See equine viral arteritis in the section on the Cardiovascular System and Lymphatic Vessels. Gross lesions include abortions (born weak) and fetal deaths (mummification, stillbirths). Virus-infected macrophages spread virus to mucosal lymphocytes and macrophages of the endometrium and then to blood vessels of the endometrium leading to endothelial cell and myocyte necrosis and a necrotizing vasculitis. Trophoblasts can also be infected with virus. Abortion probably results from placenta-endometrial dysfunction (likely vascular necrosis and vasculitis), potentially resulting in detachment. The migration of virus in the placenta or the fetus and the cell types and injury involved are undetermined, but some form of a fetal macrophage-like cell is probably involved. Stallion semen is also a likely source of virus (accessory sex glands). It is deposited on mucosae and virus likely infects and replicates in mucosal macrophages and as they migrate through the mucosae and then is spread by these cells locally through leukocyte trafficking to submucosae where they infect and replicate in tissue macrophages and lymphocytes. These cells then migrate to blood vessels and injure endothelial cells of the endometrium as described previously.

Porcine Parvovirus Abortion (Parvovirus, Nonenveloped DNA Virus)

See canine parvovirus enteritis and parvovirus-induced cerebellar hypoplasia in the sections on the Alimentary System and the Peritoneum, Omentum, Mesentery, and Peritoneal Cavity and the Nervous System, respectively. The mechanism of injury is dysfunction and potentially death of placental and fetal cells. Gross lesions include reproductive failure, embryonic death, fetal resorption, stillbirths, and mummified fetuses (see Fig. 18-44).

Pigs encounter virus through direct contact with fomites from fluids or tissues of the reproductive system, placenta, or aborted fetuses. Virus can also be transferred mechanically via hands, gloves, and instruments, if they are contaminated with virus-infected body fluids. It is ingested or inhaled and deposited on mucosae of the oral, nasal, and pharyngeal cavities, especially of the tonsil. It has not been determined if and how virus penetrates the mucus layer to gain access to tonsillar mucosal epithelial cells. Virus likely infects and replicates in mucosal macrophages and dendritic cells as they migrate through the mucus layer and mucosae and then is spread by these cells locally through leukocyte trafficking to the submucosa where they infect and replicate in tissue macrophages, lymphocytes, and dendritic cells of the tonsil (MALT). A cell-free viremia may also occur. These cells spread virus in lymphatic vessels via leukocyte trafficking to regional lymph nodes where they infect and replicate in similar cells, and spread virus to the circulatory system and systemically to lymph nodes through postcapillary venules or lymphatic vessels and the thoracic duct. From the circulatory system, it is unclear how virus spreads from the uterus, to the placenta, and then to the fetus; however, studies suggest the spread of virus to the fetus occurs via leukocyte trafficking of placental fetal macrophage-like cells. Although unidentified, porcine parvovirus probably has capsid attachment proteins that bind to glycosylated cell membrane receptors (likely sialic acid-bearing cell surface receptors) of host target cells in the uterus, placenta, and fetus. Virus has been identified in placental and fetal endothelial cells and in most tissues of virus-infected fetuses. Parvoviruses only infect and replicate in dividing cells because they require a host cell derived duplex transcription template (see Chapter 6), which is available when cells divide during S-phase of the cell cycle. Parvoviruses are unable to turn on DNA synthesis in host cells, so they must wait for host cells to enter the S-phase of the cell cycle before they can infect cells. It is likely that the high mitotic rate of developing and growing fetal tissues is conducive to infection by virus. Virus-induced death of cells likely causes injury resulting in embryonic death, fetal resorption, stillbirths, and mummified fetuses.

Male Reproductive System

See the section on the Female Reproductive System.

Ear and Eye

Feline Herpetic Keratitis (Feline Herpesvirus 1: Alphaherpesvirus, Enveloped DNA Virus)

See feline viral rhinotracheitis, equine viral rhinopneumonitis, and infectious bovine rhinotracheitis in the section on the Respiratory System, Mediastinum, and Pleurae. The mechanism of injury is death of epithelial cells of the cornea. Gross lesions include corneal ulcerations; however, with severe injury involvement of the underlying corneal stromal can occur leading to edema, neovascularization, collagenization, and inflammation. These secondary lesions are attributable to inflammation and its mediators especially those derived from cytotoxic T lymphocytes. Cats encounter virus in fomites from body fluids, such as saliva and eye and nasal secretions, contaminated through direct contact with virus-infected cats. Virus is deposited on mucosae of conjunctiva where it infects and replicates in the epithelium. Viral envelope glycoproteins are used to attach to and enter these cells via glycosaminoglycan receptors on conjunctival epithelial cells. Virus replicates in mucosal epithelial cells and with cell death virus is released to spread in conjunctival fluids to corneal epithelial cells where the processes are repeated and the corneal epithelium becomes ulcerated and inflamed.

FUNGAL DISEASES (MYCOSES)

Fungi, infectious organisms common in the environment and as microflora of mucosae, exist as branched filamentous forms (molds) or yeasts. Most organisms discussed in this section have both forms in their life cycle and are known as *dimorphic fungi* (Fig. 4-47). They can also be classified as superficial mycoses (candidiasis, aspergillosis) and systemic or deep mycoses (histoplasmosis, coccidioidomycosis, blastomycosis, angioinvasive fungi, and cryptococcosis).

FUNGAL DISEASES BY BODY SYSTEMS

Alimentary System and the Peritoneum, Omentum, Mesentery, and Peritoneal Cavity

Candidiasis (Candida albicans)

The mechanism of injury in candidiasis is disruption and death of cells in mucosae caused by inflammation and the concurrent proliferation and invasion of filamentous pseudohyphae and hyphae. *Candida albicans* persists in two forms: yeast (commensal) and filamentous pseudohyphae and hyphae (pathogenic). Gross lesions include acute pseudomembranous glossitis with extensive white to yellow pseudomembrane consisting of desquamated epithelial cells, fibrin, and fungal hyphae over the dorsal surface of the tongue (see Figs. 7-28 and 7-29). Animals encounter yeast through ingestion where it persists as a commensal yeast that colonizes mucosae without causing injury or disease and becomes part of the normal microbial flora associated with mucosal surfaces. Yeast persists in the oropharyngeal cavity by adhering to and colonizing mucosae via ligand-receptor and/or hydrophobic interactions. Yeast ligands include cell wall components, such as mannose, C3d receptors, and mannoproteins, whereas mucosal receptors include fibrinogen, fibronectin, thrombin, collagen, laminin, and vitronectin-binding proteins. The balance between commensalism and disease is tenuous and perturbations of the mucosae and/or changes in the physiologic status of the animal may shift this balance in favor of disease (filamentous pseudohyphal and/or hyphal forms).

Through a process called morphologic (phenotypic) switching, the yeast phase switches to the invasive filamentous phase. Switching appears to occur through inducible chromosomal rearrangements in the genome of the yeast in response to changes in the mucosal environment. Switching is reversible. Under normal conditions, the temperature of mucosae in the oral cavity is near room temperature (25° C). This temperature favors the growth of yeast, whereas growth of the filamentous phase prefers 37° C. Yeast is able to switch this temperature dependence for growth so that the filamentous phase can grow at 25° C. Switching is attributable to virulence determinates selectively expressed under suitable predisposing conditions in the yeast combined with the breakdown of mucosae, excessive use of broad-spectrum antibiotics and corticosteroids, hyperglycemia, tissue damage secondary to chemotherapy or radiation, or immunosuppression. Additionally, innate (phagocytosis by neutrophils and macrophages) and adaptive (cell-mediated) immunity are important defense mechanisms in controlling candidiasis, and if one or more of these immune

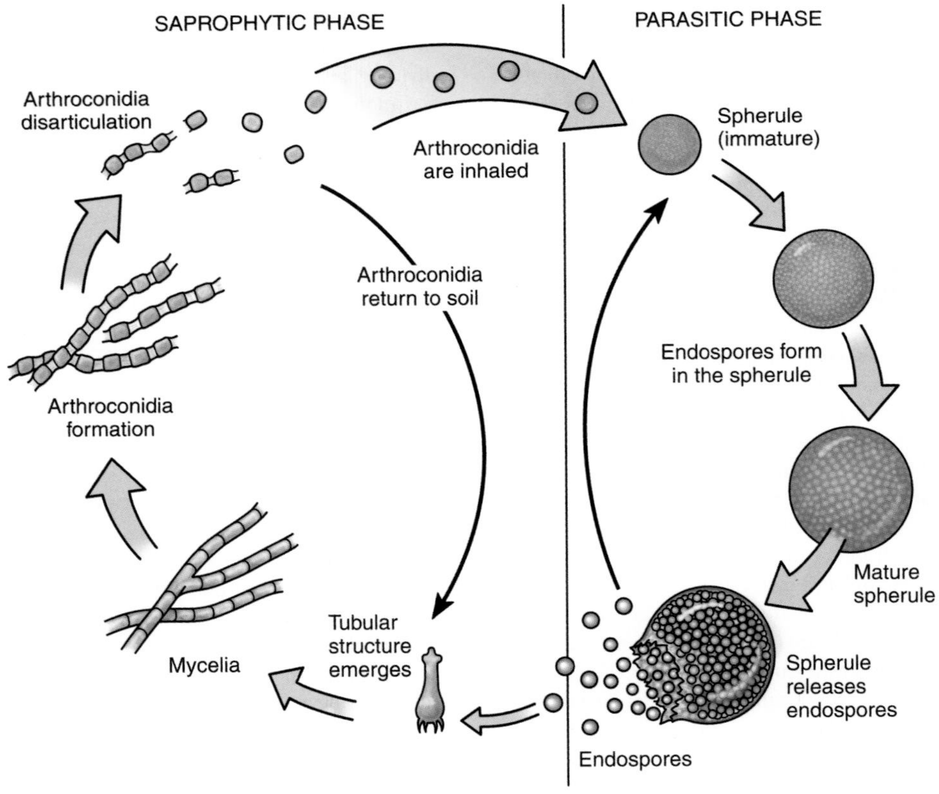

Fig. 4-47 Life cycle of *Coccidioides immitis* and other dimorphic fungi.

processes is disrupted, switching is favored. Pseudohyphae and hyphae of the filamentous phase express new adhesin ligands, secret hydrolytic aspartyl proteinases that injure the mucosa, and invade the mucosae and submucosae in which new groups of adherence receptors are encountered. It appears that a large group of virulence determinates are involved in the process of infection and invasion, but no single factor accounts for virulence and not all expressed virulence determinates may be necessary for a particular stage of infection.

Histoplasmosis (Histoplasma capsulatum)

The mechanism of injury in histoplasmosis is cell death via chronic granulomatous to pyogranulomatous inflammation and its effector molecules and degradative enzymes. *Histoplasma capsulatum* has a dimorphic life cycle; the mycelial (microconidia) phase occurs in extracellular environments (25° C), whereas the yeast phase occurs intracellularly within cells of the monocyte-macrophage system (37° C). Gross lesions include thickened walls of the small intestine and enlargement of the liver, lung, spleen, and mesenteric lymph nodes (see Figs. 7-163, 8-51, 13-84, and 14-48,*C*). Lesions are caused by the accumulation of inflammatory cells in perivascular spaces resulting in (1) generalized enlargement of affected organs with increased pallor or (2) the formation of one or more solid white-yellow nodules distributed at random in the affected tissue. Lesions are most prominent in the small intestine where inflammatory cells accumulate in the lamina propria of villi and the submucosa resulting in thickened walls and ulcerated mucosae. Systemic lymph nodes, bone marrow, and eyes may also become infected with fungus via leukocyte trafficking and acquire a granulomatous inflammatory response.

Dogs and cats encounter fungus through inhalation of microconidia (2- to 5-μm diameter spores), which can reach the lower respiratory tract. They are present in soil-derived aerosols from moist and humid environments. Microconidia are deposited on mucosae of the nasopharyngeal cavity and the conductive components of the respiratory system through centrifugal and inertial turbulence. Neutrophils and alveolar macrophages phagocytose microconidia trapped in the mucus layer of mucosae. Because microconidia can be killed by macrophages and neutrophils, there is a rapid transition to the yeast form because it provides protection against innate and adaptive immune responses. Recognition, attachment, and internalization of microconidia by phagocytes are likely mediated by ligand-receptor interactions, but specific molecules have not been identified. After phagocytosis and if not killed, microconidia germinate in phagosomes into the yeast form. Transitioning from mold to yeast is a requirement for fungal pathogenicity. Phagosomes attempt to kill the yeast by fusing with cellular lysosomes to form phagolysosomes. Lysosomes have an acidic pH and acid hydrolases that kill or restrict the growth of yeast. The yeast is able to prevent its death by synthesizing proteins that inhibit acidification of the phagolysosome and the activities of lysosomal proteases. The yeast form is protected against host defenses as long as it is hidden in phagosomes of viable macrophages; however, the lifespan of macrophages is short, 6 to 16 days. Yeast are spread in alveolar macrophages via leukocyte trafficking to local lymphoid tissues like BALT where additional macrophages are infected. From here, infected macrophages spread via afferent lymphatic vessels to regional lymph nodes and then systemically via the lymphatic and vascular systems to mesenteric lymph nodes and Peyer's patches. It is likely that macrophages spread from Peyer's patches into contiguous lamina propria and submucosa of the small intestine and via lymphatic vessels to mesenteric lymph nodes.

The ligand-receptor interactions that determine location specificity have not been identified. The innate immune system identifies fungi, in part, by recognition of pathogen-associated molecular patterns (see Chapters 3 and 5) formed by α- and β-glucan surface polysaccharides in yeast cell walls. Macrophages recognize these patterns through Toll-like receptors and other PRRs expressed on macrophages and use the information to develop an appropriate immune response. Fungi have developed mechanisms to evade and/or neutralize detection by PRRs on macrophages, neutrophils, and dendritic cells leading to modifications in surface polysaccharides through genomic variation. Because macrophages have short lifespans (6 to 16 days), yeast and yeast-derived surface polysaccharide antigens are released from dead macrophages into the lamina propria of the small intestine. These polysaccharides and the chemokines and cytokines secreted by infected macrophages lead to recruitment of additional macrophages and pyogranulomatous inflammatory cells into the lamina propria. This process is repetitive, thus the volume of inflammatory exudate grows with time resulting in a thickened intestinal wall, disruption of lymphatic vascular drainage, and disturbances of junctional complexes of villus epithelial cells, all resulting in the protein-losing enteropathy characteristic of histoplasmosis, clinically.

Respiratory System, Mediastinum, and Pleurae

Aspergillosis (Aspergillus fumigatus)

The pathogenesis of aspergillosis has many similarities to other fungal diseases discussed in this section. The mechanism of injury is disruption and death of mucosae in the nasal cavity and respiratory system caused by inflammation, its mediators and degradative enzymes, and concurrent proliferation and invasion of fungal hyphae. Gross lesions include acute pseudomembranous rhinitis and sinusitis with extensive gray-black pseudomembrane consisting of desquamated epithelial cells, fibrin, and fungal hyphae covering the mucosal surfaces of turbinates, sinuses, and airways or forming granulomas in the lungs (see Web Fig. 9-3,*A*). The underlying bone and cartilage may become necrotic as hyphae invade these tissues (see Web Fig. 9-3,*B*).

Animals, especially dogs, encounter fungus through inhalation of conidia (2 to 3 μm in diameter) that are deposited on mucosae of the nasopharynx and the conductive component of the respiratory system through centrifugal and inertial turbulence. Fungus is a saprophyte of dead or decaying matter. Conidia are present in aerosols derived from these materials and when inhaled are trapped in the mucus layer of mucosae. They interact with the mucociliary apparatus and defensive molecules (see Chapter 3) released from mucosal epithelial cells and are ultimately phagocytosed by neutrophils and alveolar and mucosal macrophages. Recognition, attachment, and internalization by phagocytes are likely mediated by ligand-receptor interactions such as sialic acid residues on conidia. When phagocytosed by healthy animals, conidia are killed by neutrophils and macrophages migrating in the mucus layer. If animals are unable to phagocytose and kill conidia, they germinate in the mucus layer and mucosae and begin the processes of colonizing mucosae of the nasal cavities and sinuses. Conidia secrete proteases, gliotoxin, fumagillin, verruculogen, and helvolic acid that slow the beat of cilia in the mucociliary apparatus, affect the viability of ciliated mucosal epithelial cells, and lead to detachment and loss of ciliated epithelial cells and exposure and damage of basement membrane (laminin). When conidia germinate into hyphae, a denuded and disrupted basement membrane may assist hyphae in their invasion of mucosae. Fibrinogen and fibronectin that cover exposed basement membrane as a reparative response can serve as receptors for sialic acid and other conidial and hyphal glycoproteins, thus contributing to fungal pathogenicity by enhancing adhesion to and colonization of injured mucosae and basement membrane. Through these mechanisms, fungus is able to invade and spread in affected tissue and extensively damage normal tissues.

In dogs, aspergillosis occurs in the nasal cavities, paranasal sinuses, or the respiratory system. In other animal species, aspergillosis begins as an infection of the respiratory system, often asymptomatic, and then spreads to other sites likely via leukocyte trafficking of fungus-infected macrophages. These sites include the lung, mammary gland, and placenta in cattle; guttural pouches in horses; and lungs in cats. The ability to disseminate and spread systemically to other organs is modulated in part by the ability of conidia and hyphae to block immune responses and evade killing by phagocytes. Alveolar macrophages phagocytose conidia and hyphae through a process mediated by the recognition of pathogen-associated molecular patterns by PRRs (TLRs) expressed on alveolar macrophages and other phagocytic cells as discussed in histoplasmosis. *Aspergillus fumigatus* uses β-glucans, melanin, and other molecules to block killing by reactive oxygen species, phagolysosomal acidification, and other mechanisms in macrophages and neutrophils. It can also disseminate via the circulatory system to other organ systems through a process called angioinvasion. Hyphae may invade endothelial cells lining capillaries, gain access to the circulatory system, break off into the bloodstream, circulate, and attach to and invade endothelium at other sites. Ligand-receptor interactions are probably involved in this process, determining which organ system and tissue types are targeted by the fungus.

Coccidioidomycosis (Coccidioides immitis)

The pathogenesis of coccidioidomycosis is similar to histoplasmosis. The mechanism of injury is cell death via chronic granulomatous to pyogranulomatous inflammation and its effector molecules and degradative enzymes. It has a dimorphic life cycle (see Fig. 4-47). Gross lesions include pyogranulomatous interstitial pneumonia with yellow-white granulomas of varied sizes distributed at random (embolic pattern) in the lungs and similar appearing expansile granulomas in lymph nodes. Bone marrow and eyes may be infected via leukocyte trafficking and have granulomatous inflammation. Fungus is present in the soil and with suitable growing conditions, produces arthroconidia (3 to 6 μm in diameter) that are carried into the air by disruption of the soil, such as during construction or farming.

Animals encounter arthroconidia through inhalation, and they are deposited on and trapped in the mucus layer of mucosae of airways through centrifugal and inertial turbulence. In the mucus layer, arthroconidia can be phagocytosed and killed by neutrophils and alveolar macrophages, but there is a rapid transition to spherules because it provides protection against phagocytosis. Change into spherules also causes acute inflammatory and mucosal injury. Neutrophils and eosinophils are present in the inflammatory exudate. Spherules grow to 20 to 60 μm in diameter (occasionally up to 100 μm) and form a small number of intraspherular endospores (1 to 5 μm in diameter) through a process called *endosporulation.* Spherules appear to escape phagocytosis because they are too large to be phagocytosed by neutrophils, macrophages, and dendritic cells. Spherules release endospores onto mucosae when mature or when they are damaged by inflammatory cells and mediators. These endospores then grow into second-generation spherules, which are now capable of producing an average of 200 to 300 endospores. Endospores are 1 to 5 μm in diameter and are capable of being phagocytosed by alveolar macrophages, mucosal macrophages, and dendritic cells. Because endosporulation and cell death become a repetitive process, chemokines and cytokines recruit additional macrophages and other granulomatous inflammatory cells into the lung. Macrophages infected with endospores likely spread via leukocyte trafficking in lymphatic vessels and the circulatory system locally to lymphoid tissues, regionally to lymph nodes, and systemically to other tissues such as the skin, bone, muscle, lymph nodes, adrenal glands, and CNS. A primary skin infection can also rarely occur by direct infection of damaged skin. Virulence determinates include the (1) production of a spherule outer wall glycoprotein that modulates the immune response and compromises cell-mediated immunity, (2) depletion of spherule outer wall glycoprotein on the surface of endospores which prevents their phagocytosis, and (3) production of host tissue arginase I and coccidioidal urease, which contribute to tissue damage at sites of infection.

Blastomycosis (Blastomyces dermatitidis)

The pathogenesis and mechanism of injury in blastomycosis are similar to those of histoplasmosis and coccidioidomycosis. Gross lesions include pyogranulomatous interstitial pneumonia with yellow-white granulomas of varied sizes distributed at random (embolic pattern) in the lungs (see Fig. 9-91) and similar appearing expansile granulomas in lymph nodes. In the disseminated form, lymph nodes, skin, subcutaneous tissues, eyes, brain, and bone may also become infected by spread via leukocyte trafficking of yeast-infected macrophages and acquire a pyogranulomatous inflammatory response. A primary skin infection can also rarely occur by direct infection of damaged skin. Fungus is present in the soil and with suitable growing conditions, produces conidia (2 to 10 μm in diameter) that are carried into the air by disruption of the soil. Animals inhale conidia, which are deposited on and trapped in the mucus layer of mucosae of airways through centrifugal and inertial turbulence. In the mucus layer, conidia are readily phagocytosed and killed by neutrophils and macrophages, whereas yeast cells are more resistant to phagocytosis and killing during the acute inflammatory response. On mucosal surfaces, conidia have surface adhesins to adhere to macrophages. After spreading to deeper tissues in macrophages, they shed their adhesin molecules or produce masking capsules to avoid phagocyte recognition. In the yeast phase, it has an immune-modulating virulence determinate in its cell wall and other virulence determinates that provide resistance to phagocytosis and killing. Yeast evades the adaptive immune system by changing surface polysaccharides and by hiding in phagosomes. Additionally, yeast has an adhesion-promoting protein termed *WI-1* that mediates adherence to CR3 and CD14 receptors on cell membranes of macrophages.

Cardiovascular System and Lymphatic Vessels

Angioinvasive Fungi

Angioinvasive fungi include a group of infectious organisms that have the ability to invade the vascular system, spread to organ systems, and cause disease. Fungi in this group include *Aspergillus* spp., *Candida* spp., *Fusarium* spp., *Absidia* spp., *Rhizopus* spp., and *Mucor* spp. The spores or conidia of these fungi are common microflora of the skin, body fluids, mucosal surfaces, and intestinal content. They are able to gain access to the vascular system via injury to the barrier system provided by skin or mucosae. Injury results in the loss of epithelial cells and the exposure of basement membrane and subjacent vascularized ECM connective tissue. Similar to what occurs with *Aspergillus fumigatus,* hyphae invade vascularized tissues and gain access to the circulatory system by growing in and invading through vessel walls, gain access to the circulatory system, break off into the bloodstream, circulate, and attach to and invade endothelium at other sites. Leukocyte trafficking could also be used to spread the fungus systemically. Ligand-receptor interactions are likely involved in this process, determining which organ system and tissue types are targeted by fungi. For example, granulomatous hepatitis attributed to fungal infection occurs in feedlot cattle. These animals are fed increasing quantities of grain that serves as a carbohydrate source for ruminal microflora that convert it, in part, to lactic acid. Excessive grain in the diet (grain overload) increases the quantity of lactic acid (lactic acidosis) in the rumen, and if such animals are deprived of water, lactic acid can accumulate and result in a drop of the pH of fluids covering ruminal mucosae. This outcome results in acid burns followed by loss of the epithelium and exposure of the basement membrane and subjacent vascularized connective tissue of the lamina propria. This denudation provides angioinvasive fungi the opportunity to infect locally (mycotic rumenitis and/or abomasitis) and spread regionally to other organ systems such as the liver (granulomatous fungal hepatitis) (see Figs. 8-46 and 14-51).

Nervous System

Cryptococcosis (Cryptococcus neoformans)

The pathogenesis of cryptococcosis has many similarities to those of histoplasmosis, coccidioidomycosis, and blastomycosis. The mechanism of injury is cell death likely caused by atrophy secondary to tissue distortion and compression from expanding cryptococcal cysts in brain parenchyma. There is little or no inflammation in this disease. *Cryptococcus neoformans* has a dimorphic life cycle. The mycelial (basidiospores) phase occurs in extracellular environments (25° C), whereas the yeast phase occurs intracellularly within cells of the monocyte-macrophage system (37° C). Gross lesions include the formation of expansile cystic spaces filled with a gelatinous matrix (the capsule) within the brain and spinal cord leading to compression and distortion of the tissue (see Figs. 14-49 and 14-50).

Animals encounter *Cryptococcus neoformans* (dimorphic fungus) through inhalation of basidiospores or poorly encapsulated yeast cells (1.8-3.0 μm in diameter), which can reach the lower respiratory tract and alveoli. They are present in soil-derived aerosols from moist and humid environments. Basidiospores are deposited on the surface of mucosae of the nasopharyngeal cavity and of the conductive component of the respiratory system through centrifugal and inertial turbulence. They are readily phagocytosed and killed by neutrophils and alveolar macrophages. For survival, basidiospores quickly germinate in mucosae or phagosomes to yeast. Yeast-derived glucosylceramide synthase is essential for survival in mucosae but is not needed after phagocytosis by alveolar macrophages. Yeast cells also produce phospholipases that injure alveolar epithelial cells and hinder the production and function of surfactant, thereby enhancing adhesion to pneumocytes and improving chances of being phagocytosed by alveolar macrophages. Recognition, attachment, and internalization by macrophages are likely mediated by ligand-receptor interactions, but specific molecules have not been identified. The polysaccharide capsule of yeast has antiphagocytic properties and may be immunosuppressive. The degree of encapsulation provides resistance to phagocytosis and killing by macrophages. In mucosae, unencapsulated or poorly encapsulated yeast cells are readily phagocytosed and killed, whereas encapsulated yeast is more resistant to phagocytosis and killing. The capsule's negative charge inhibits phagocytosis and killing by neutrophils and macrophages and causes complement depletion, antibody unresponsiveness, and dysregulation of cytokine secretion by monocytes and macrophages. The capsule can also inhibit recognition of yeast by macrophages and neutrophils and chemotaxis of leukocytes from the bloodstream into areas of inflammation. This latter response may account for the lack of inflammation in cysts. After phagocytosis and phagosome-lysosome fusion, yeast synthesizes additional polysaccharide capsule within the phagolysosome of the macrophage. Capsule dilutes lysosomal hydrolases and other toxic content and provides a physical separation between the yeast and the membrane of the phagosome in which microbicidal compounds are located. This process continues until macrophages are grossly distended with capsule (>30 μm in diameter) and is the underlying mechanism of the formation of expansile cysts filled with a gelatinous matrix observed grossly in the brain. The capsule is composed primarily of two polysaccharides, glucuronoxylomannan and galactoxylomannan, and a smaller quantity of mannoprotein. These molecules also suppress the immune response.

Yeast cells appear to spread to the CNS by direct extension into the meninges and neuropil, following compressive remodeling and osteolysis of the cribriform plate from a local infection of the nasal sinuses or by leukocyte trafficking via yeast-infected macrophages in the circulatory system with spread into the neuropil. The latter mechanism is hypothetical but is mostly probable based on what is known about the biology of the fungus. It is likely that yeast-infected macrophages interact through ligand-receptor interactions with endothelial cells of capillaries in the CNS. Capsule polysaccharides are also used to adhere and bind to brain endothelial cells and mediate endocytosis across the blood-brain barrier into the neuropil. Once in tissue, macrophages migrate through the neuropil. Because macrophages have short lifespans, yeast, yeast-derived antigens, and polysaccharide capsule are released from dead macrophages into the neuropil. This outcome and its associated chemokines and cytokines recruit additional macrophages into the nervous system. This process is repetitive, thus the volume of polysaccharide capsule increases and expansile cystic spaces filled with a gelatinous matrix are observed grossly in the brain. Additionally, melanin is an important cryptococcal virulence determinate, which facilitates yeast survival during infection of the CNS. It acts as an antioxidant and eliminates reactive oxygen species that could kill the yeast. In the nervous system, yeast may use neurotransmitters, such as dopamine, norepinephrine, and epinephrine, as substrates for melanin production.

PROTOZOAN DISEASES

PROTOZOAN DISEASES BY BODY SYSTEMS

Alimentary System and the Peritoneum, Omentum, Mesentery, and Peritoneal Cavity

Cryptosporidiosis (Cryptosporidium parvum)

The mechanism of injury in cryptosporidiosis is dysfunction and death of epithelial cells covering tips and sides of intestinal villi, resulting from dysfunction of microvilli of the brush border, from cytolysis after being released from infected cells, and from degradative effects of inflammation. Gross lesions are not observed; however, microscopic lesions include necrosis of epithelial cells, atrophy of villi, and mucosal inflammation (see Web Fig. 7-21).

Animals encounter *Cryptosporidium parvum* in water and food contaminated with oocysts through direct contact with feces from infected animals. Oocysts are ingested and carried through the oral pharynx, esophagus, stomach, and small intestine by normal peristaltic activities where they interact with gastric acids, pancreatic enzymes, and bile salts and undergo a process called *excystation.*

In the proximity of intestinal villi, sporozoites are released from oocysts and randomly encounter the apical brush-borders (microvilli with glycocalyx) of villus enterocytes covering tips and sides of intestinal villi. Sporozoites have a tropism for villus enterocytes of the jejunum and ileum that is apparently mediated by ligand-receptor interactions involved in attachment, invasion, and intracellular development of the protozoan. An apical complex and surface proteins expressed by sporozoites act as ligands, whereas *Cryptosporidium parvum* sporozoite ligand (CSL) and probably other cell membrane proteins expressed on the apical surfaces of villus enterocytes act as receptors. The apical ends of sporozoites adhere to the microvilli of brush borders of villus enterocytes via sporozoite-specific lectin adherence factor such as GP900. Sporozoites also expresses other surface glycoproteins that are virulence determinates in the pathogenicity of the organism. Once bound to cell membrane, sporozoites infect villus enterocytes by a mechanism dependent on parasite motility and secretion of enzymes from its apical organelles. Sporozoites are surrounded by the cell membranes of microvilli to form parasitophorous vacuoles. Such vacuoles are retained in the microvillus layer and do not enter, but directly communicate with, the cytoplasm of the cell through a feeding organelle. Once in parasitophorous vacuoles, sporozoites differentiate into trophozoites and then undergo asexual multiplication to form schizonts that contain six to eight merozoites. Schizonts rupture to release merozoites and infected villus enterocytes are lysed. Merozoites spread via alimentary peristalsis in the small intestine to infect additional villus enterocytes through ligand-receptor interactions. It is likely that such ligand-receptor interactions determine which populations of epithelial cells in what segment of the small intestine are infected. New schizonts are formed through (1) asexual multiplication to form schizonts and (2) sexual reproduction (gametogony) by differentiating into male microgamonts or female macrogamonts. Microgamonts release microgametes that fertilize macrogametes inside macrogamonts, resulting in the formation of oocysts with sporozoites that reinfect villus enterocytes or are passed in the feces to spread the infection. These processes cause additional cell death and villus atrophy and amplify the severity of the injury. It has been suggested that death of cells and villus atrophy are caused by (1) cell death from parasite invasion, multiplication, and extrusion and/or (2) cell dysfunction and damage from cytokines and inflammatory molecules from T lymphocyte and macrophage-mediated inflammation. This latter mechanism causes increased intercellular permeability and may alter secretory functions and impair absorption of villus enterocytes. Infection, injury, and loss of villus enterocytes result in diarrhea likely caused by a combination of mechanisms, including osmotic diarrhea (malabsorption), secretory diarrhea, and increased intercellular permeability from inflammation. Enterotoxins may be involved in the secretory diarrhea, but none have been identified.

Malabsorption likely occurs from dysfunction of digestive enzymes present in the brush border of villus enterocytes infected by sporozoites and the subsequent death of these cells, both leading to failure to digest carbohydrates (impaired hydrolysis) and other molecules in the ingesta. This outcome leads to bacterial fermentation of substrates and an osmotic diarrhea. Sporozoite-injured villus enterocytes are sloughed from the villi, resulting in collapse (atrophy) of the structure of the villus, whereas the basement membrane from under the sloughed villus enterocytes is unaffected and functionally normal. Because the basement membrane is not injured and remains structurally intact, villus enterocytes derived from regenerative crypt enterocytes can divide and replace sloughed cells. These regenerative cells migrate up the villus from the crypts to initially cover exposed basement membranes; thus they are recognized early in the reparative process as flattened squamous-like cells stretched over the basement membrane. As the cells increase in density and maturity, they regain a more normal columnar morphology. Additionally, the loss of enterocytes allows endotoxins and other potentially harmful molecules to gain access to the capillary and lymphatic vessels in the lamina propria of the villi and through absorption cause systemic cardiovascular and hemodynamic effects.

*Coccidiosis (*Eimeria *spp.,* Isospora *spp.)*

The pathogenesis of coccidiosis is similar in many ways to that of cryptosporidiosis. The mechanism of injury is adenomatous proliferation (hypertrophy and hyperplasia) of infected villus enterocytes covering tips and sides of small intestinal villi, followed by death resulting from release of organisms from infected cells. Gross lesions include mucosae that are focally raised with an adenomatous to cerebriform pattern and active hyperemia, hemorrhage, and necrosis often with fibrinous and/or fibrinohemorrhagic casts formed within the lumen of the intestine (see Figs. 7-168 through 7-172).

Animals (cattle, sheep, goats, and pigs) encounter the protozoan in grass, soil, and/or floors or surfaces contaminated with unsporulated oocysts from feces of infected animals. Coccidian oocysts are not infective (unsporulated) and therefore survive in pastures and other holding areas. Under the proper conditions (oxygen concentrations, humidity, and temperature), oocysts sporulate and become infective. Sporulated oocysts are ingested and carried through the oral pharynx, esophagus, stomach, and small intestine by normal peristaltic activities where they excyst. In proximity of intestinal villi, sporozoites are released from oocysts and randomly encounter mucosal villus enterocytes covering tips and sides of intestinal villi. Sporozoites have a tropism for villus enterocytes of specific segments of the small intestine; however, it is not known if tropism is mediated by ligand-receptor interactions involved in attachment, invasion, and intracellular development of the protozoan. Sporozoites go through one or more asexual generations and a (single) sexual generation in different segments of the small intestine (see section on Cryptosporidiosis). The replication and release of generations of these organisms in and from mucosal villus enterocytes, respectively, account for the lesions observed grossly.

Nervous System

Protozoal Encephalomyelitis (Sarcocystis neurona)

The mechanism of injury in protozoal encephalomyelitis is disruption and death of neurons and neural cells from replication of the organism and from inflammation and its mediators and degradative enzymes. Gross lesions include yellow-white areas of malacia mixed with hemorrhage in gray and white matter of the brain and spinal cord (see Figs. 14-81 and 14-82).

Horses and other animals encounter sporocysts in feed, water, grass, or soil, and/or on floors or surfaces contaminated with feces from infected opossums. They are ingested and swallowed and through peristalsis gain access to mucosae of the intestines. From this point, little is known about the mechanism of spread to the brain and spinal cord. It has been hypothesized that sporozoites released from sporocysts penetrate mucosae, lamina propria, and arterial walls to gain access to endothelial cells in intestinal villi. Schizonts containing merozoites may develop in endothelial cells, which eventually rupture and release merozoites into the blood. They infect adjacent endothelial cells, repeat the replicative process, and then spread in the circulatory system, systemically. It is not known how merozoites enter the CNS, but it has been hypothesized that infected leukocytes or endothelial cells are involved in spreading merozoites into the neuropil where schizonts are again formed. Although this hypothesis is plausible, it has many disjointed components and is not a well-integrated chronologic sequence of events. Based on known mechanisms used by *Toxoplasma gondii, Cryptosporidium parvum,* and other protozoans and the need to evade innate and adaptive immune responses, it seems more likely that sporozoites would attempt to gain access to intracellular locations in mucosal epithelial cells or mucosal macrophages as early as possible in the disease. Sporozoites in the mucosae could invade subjacent lamina propria, infect cells of the monocyte-macrophage system, and enter lymphatic vessels or could be phagocytized and carried via leukocyte trafficking through mucosae by macrophages to Peyer's patches and/or via lymphatic vessels to regional lymph nodes. From here, infected macrophages could migrate via lymphatic vessels and the thoracic duct and/or capillaries or postcapillary venules to gain access to the circulatory system. In blood vessels of the CNS, macrophages could interact with endothelial cells, allowing sporozoites or merozoites to infect endothelial cells and form schizonts containing merozoites. This process could injure endothelium, leading to inflammation, vasculitis and thrombosis, hemorrhage, and malacia.

Ligand-receptor interactions are probably involved in tropism for endothelial cells and macrophages and other cell types in the nervous system. If macrophages spread the protozoan (probably as merozoites) to the neuropil, the protozoan would likely infect and asexually replicate in neurons and other neural cells forming schizonts and merozoites, leading to cell death and acute inflammation. Other variations of this scenario could include replication in mucosal epithelial cells or M cells before infection of macrophages and infection and replication in endothelial cells in Peyer's patches or regional lymph nodes before migrating in macrophages to the nervous system. One additional mechanism, although unlikely because the protozoan has not been observed in peripheral nerves, must be considered. In intermediate hosts, the asexual stages of the protozoan through an unknown mechanism (likely macrophages and leukocyte trafficking) migrates to and encysts in striated muscle cells. Horses are aberrant or dead-end intermediate hosts, and it is possible, though unlikely, that macrophages carry an asexual stage of the protozoan to striated muscle, but here, through ligand-receptor interactions, it can only infect and enter nerve endings and spread via retrograde axonal transport to the CNS.

Reproductive System

Toxoplasmosis (Toxoplasma gondii)

The mechanism of injury in toxoplasmosis is dysfunction and death of epithelial cells of the placenta and the fetus resulting in abortion, neonatal mortality, and fetal malformation predominately in sheep and goats and less commonly in cattle. Toxoplasmosis in cats is usually inconsequential and will not be discussed here. Gross lesions include active hyperemia, rough and granular mucosae consistent with necrosis, and mineralization of caruncles of the uterus and cotyledons of fetal membranes (see Fig. 18-42). A component of this lesion includes acute inflammation. Intercaruncular and intercotyledonary tissues are unaffected.

Animals, other than cats, and humans are intermediate hosts and encounter oocysts in contaminated soil. Cats are the definitive host for *Toxoplasma gondii,* thus cat feces are the source of oocysts. Oocysts are resistant to degradation and may survive in the environment for years. Under the proper conditions (oxygen concentrations, humidity, and temperature), oocysts sporulate and become infective. Sporulated oocysts are ingested and carried by normal peristaltic activities through the oral pharynx, esophagus, and stomach to the small intestine where they excyst and release sporozoites into the intestinal lumen in close proximity to intestinal mucosal villus enterocytes. Infections are characterized by the ability of the organism to cross barrier systems such as the intestinal mucosae, blood-brain barrier, blood-retina barrier, and placenta. This process appears to involve parasite motility and interactions between parasite adhesins and target cell receptors that facilitate transfer of the organism through the mucosae. Mounting evidence also suggests that *Toxoplasma gondii* uses migrating leukocytes to disseminate throughout the host while avoiding adaptive immune defenses. Sporozoites infect and complete an asexual replication in parasitophorous vacuoles to form tachyzoites in mucosal villus enterocytes. Tachyzoites are released via cell death and infect and replicate in additional intestinal mucosal villus enterocytes and then invade subjacent lamina propria, infect cells of the monocyte-macrophage system, and enter lymphatic vessels. They spread locally to lymphoid tissues (likely Peyer's patches) and regionally to mesenteric lymph nodes via lymphatic vessels and then systemically via lymphatic vessels and the thoracic duct or capillaries or postcapillary venules to the circulatory system and then to caruncular epithelial cells and cotyledonary trophoblasts.

It is unclear if leukocyte trafficking or cell-free protozoemia is used to spread the organism to systemic target cells in the blood vascular system. *Toxoplasma gondii* requires an intracellular site for growth and replication. Tachyzoites and likely sporozoite tropism for target cells appears to be mediated by ligand-receptor interactions. Infection of intestinal villus enterocytes by sporozoites and tachyzoites is a well-studied process that involves six steps that begin with the recognition of target cells and end with the formation of a parasitophorous vacuole within the same cell. Parasitophorous vacuoles are a mechanism used to modulate host cell functions in support of parasite replication and infection. Tachyzoites (and likely sporozoites) express glycosylphosphatidylinositol-linked surface proteins (SAGs) that serve as ligands, whereas intestinal villus enterocyte membrane receptors appear to include laminin, lectin, and SAG1 receptor proteins. Proteins, such as SAG1, are abundant on tachyzoites and function in host cell attachment and immune modulation and may also cause direct injury to intestinal epithelium. Tachyzoites spread systemically from lymphoid tissues to other tissues such as the placenta via leukocyte trafficking or cell-free protozoemia in the blood vascular system. When they encounter cells of the uterine caruncle, they probably utilize ligand-receptor interactions and the six-step process described previously to infect cells of the caruncles and then spread to adjacent trophoblasts of the cotyledons. Tachyzoites replicate in these placental cells eventually causing their death (necrosis). Death leads to alterations in placental structure (necrosis and mineralization of caruncles and cotyledons), disturbances of vascular flow, and placental dysfunction that injures developing fetuses. Lesions caused by tachyzoites have also been described in the brain (inflammation and congenital malformations) and other tissues of the fetus. How and by what mechanism they spread from the placenta to the fetus is unknown (likely fetal macrophage-like cells); however, they appear to infect diverse populations of fetal cells resulting in injury and death. If infection occurs early in gestation, fetal death and resorption occur. Infection in mid-gestation causes fetal death, leading to mummification mixed with live but weak fetuses. Infection in late gestation does not usually injure the fetus because of a good adaptive immune response.

Neosporosis (Neospora caninum)

The pathogenesis and mechanisms of injury in neosporosis are similar to those of toxoplasmosis. The dog is the definitive host for

Neospora caninum; all other animals are intermediate hosts. Much like in toxoplasmosis, abortion is the primary disease caused by *Neospora caninum* in cattle, sheep, goat, and pigs.

PRION DISEASES

PRION DISEASES BY BODY SYSTEMS

Nervous System

Transmissible Spongiform Encephalopathies (Prion Diseases)

The mechanism of injury in transmissible spongiform encephalopathies is metabolic dysfunction of neurons and neural cells caused by the conversion of normal cellular prion protein (PrP^C) to an abnormal form (PrP^{Sc}) and the accumulation of PrP^{Sc} in neurons and neural cells (Fig. 4-48). Gross lesions are not observed except in chronic cases in which atrophy of the brain may occur. Microscopic lesions characteristic of injury include intracytoplasmic vacuoles in neurons (spongiform change), neuronal loss, gliosis, and an absence of leukocytic inflammation. These diseases in animals include scrapie (sheep), bovine spongiform encephalopathy (BSE), chronic wasting disease (CWD) in deer and elk, transmissible mink encephalopathy, feline spongiform encephalopathy, and ungulate spongiform encephalopathy. The source of prions that spread transmissible spongiform encephalopathies among animals and the natural routes of transmission of prions between animals have not been determined. Soil may serve as a prion reservoir.

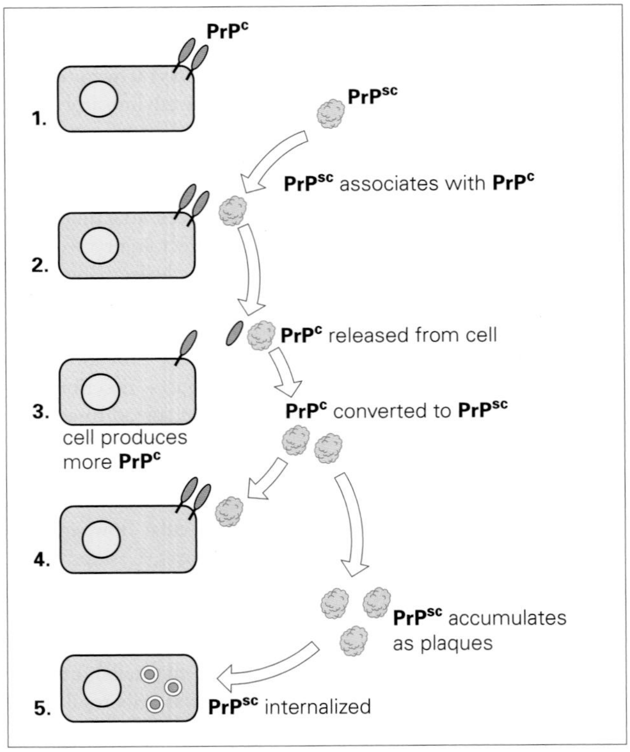

Fig. 4-48 How prions injure cells.
1, Normal cells express cellular prion protein (PrP^c) at the cell membrane as linear proteins. *2,* Abnormal form (PrP^{Sc}) exists as a free globular glycoprotein, which can interact with PrP^c. *3,* PrP^c is released from the cell membrane and is converted into PrP^{Sc}. *4,* Cells produce more PrP^c and the cycle is repeated. *5,* PrP^{Sc} accumulates as plaques and is internalized by cells. (From Goering R, Dockrell H, Roitt I, et al: *Mims' medical microbiology,* ed 4, St. Louis, 2008, Mosby.)

Animals probably encounter prions most commonly by ingestion. Alternatively, inhalation or direct contact (conjunctival mucous membranes) may also be important routes of spread in specific prion diseases such as scrapie and chronic wasting disease. Prions can be found in a tissue-free environment (urine, saliva, blood, and body waste) as a direct source of the microbe or in a tissue-associated environment (offal [i.e., entrails and internal organs of butchered animals], placentas, or decaying carcasses) as an indirect source of the microbe. This latter source appears to be the route that occurs primarily in cattle and mink. In the United Kingdom, cattle were infected with prions by ingesting offal derived from prion-infected sheep or cattle that had not been properly treated to kill the microbe. Mucosae of the oral pharynx especially the tonsil, small intestine, nasal pharynx, and conjunctiva are thought to be the probable locations of initial encounters with prions. It is unclear if and how prions are trapped in the mucus layer and, if so, how they gain access to mucosal epithelial cells, macrophages, and/or dendritic cells in the mucus layer. It appears that prions are able to attach to apical surfaces of mucosal epithelial cells, M cells, and possibly dendritic cells in tonsillar, alimentary, and respiratory mucosae, respectively. Transcytosis or dendritic cell migration (also potentially via macrophage migration) is probably used by prions to pass through mucosal epithelial cells and M cells to their basolateral surfaces and to gain access to and infect B and T lymphocytes, macrophages, and dendritic cells in Peyer's patches (GALT) or lymphoid nodules and aggregates like BALT. Prions are then probably spread systemically via leukocyte trafficking in lymphocytes, monocytes, and dendritic cells to other lymphoid organs such as the spleen and systemic lymph nodes. In lymphoid tissue, follicular dendritic cells and B lymphocytes are essential for prion replication and accumulation in large numbers before spread to the nervous system.

Prions are able to infect nerve endings of the vagus nerve, sympathetic nerves, and sensory nerves that innervate lymphoid tissues and organs and then use retrograde axonal transport to gain access to the CNS and spread in the nervous system via synaptically-linked neurons (Fig. 4-49). It is thought that prion-infected macrophages and dendritic cells deliver prions to these nerve endings; however, it is not known if endocytosis is involved in the entry of prions into nerve endings or in their spread between cell membranes in synapses. In macrophages and dendritic cells, prions are located in multivesicular endosomes and may be transferred between cells in exosomes. Such a mechanism may be involved in interneuronal spread within the nervous system. Attachment proteins of prions or membrane receptors on host target cells have not been identified. However, Toll-like PRRs may serve as receptors for prion entry into cells. Prions have tropisms for different animal species that are likely determined by the tertiary and quaternary structure of prions, resulting in their binding to or interaction with different molecules (receptors) and thus different host cells. Cellular tropism may also be restricted to those cells that express a cofactor compatible with the respective prion strain.

Most cells in the body have PrP^C; however, the highest concentrations are present in the nervous system, especially in synaptic membranes as a neuronal membrane glycoprotein. PrP^C is also expressed in cells of the immune system (see Fig. 4-48). The function of PrP^C is unknown, but its physiologic function may include immunoregulation, signal transduction, copper binding, synaptic transmission, induction of apoptosis, or protection against apoptotic stimuli. In neurons, PrP^{Sc} serves as a translation template that

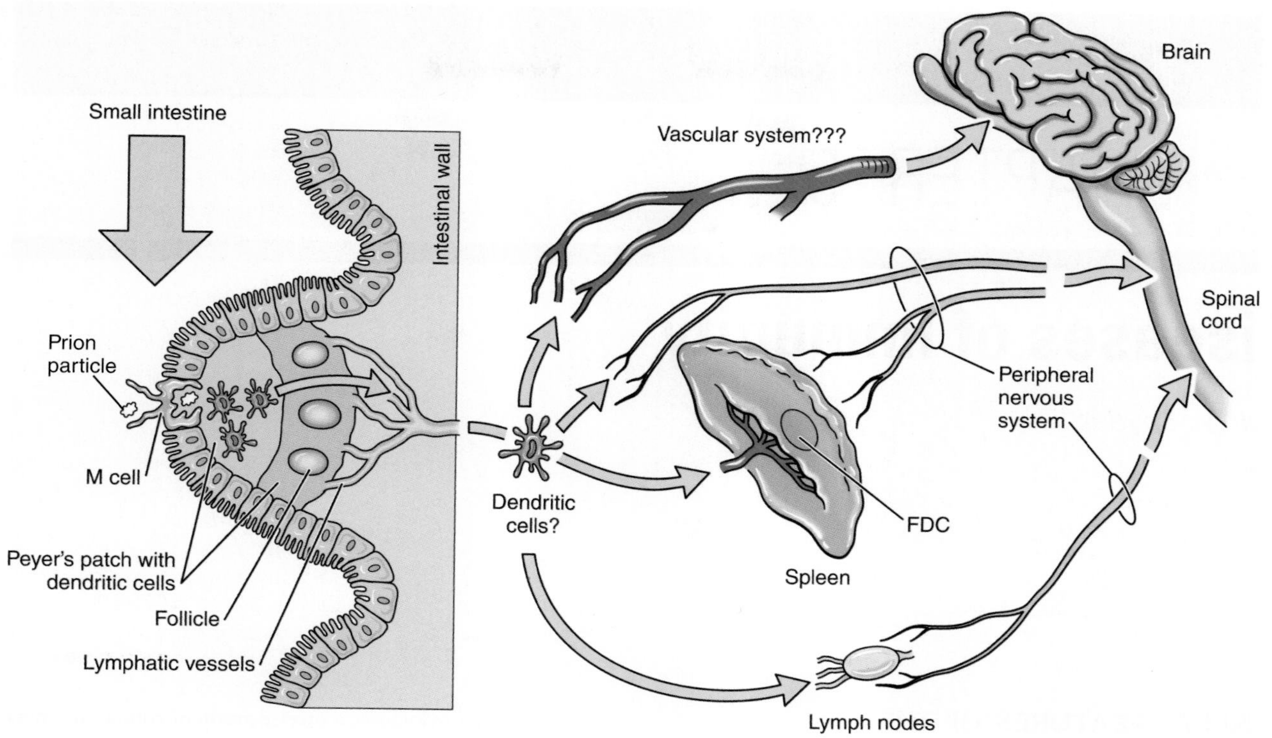

Fig. 4-49 Pathogenesis of transmissible spongiform encephalopathies. Prions appear to use M cells (also macrophages) to enter Peyer's patches and infect dendritic cells as well as macrophages and lymphocytes. Dendritic cells (and likely macrophages) then spread prions through leukocyte trafficking in lymphatic vessels to local, regional, and systemic lymphoid nodules, lymph nodes, and/or spleen where infection is sustained and amplified, especially in follicular dendritic cells (FDC) of the spleen and B lymphocytes. Prions released from dendritic cells are able to enter nerve endings in lymphoid tissues, and by retrograde and anterograde nerve transport they spread throughout the CNS. It has been hypothesized that prions may also spread to the CNS hematogenously, but the existence of this route is uncertain.

converts (conformational change) normal PrP^{C} to PrP^{Sc}, a misfolded and aggregated β-sheet–rich isoform of PrP^{C}. This folding pattern makes PrP^{Sc} resistant to the action of proteases and causes it to aggregate and accumulate as an insoluble amyloid in neurons in the form of large amyloid and fibrous plaques. It is not known how PrP^{Sc} causes neuronal degeneration; however, reduced antioxidant protection, increased oxidative stress, loss of function of normal PrP^{C}, or toxicity caused by PrP^{Sc} all related to the accumulation of amyloid plaque have been proposed. The activation (hypertrophy and hyperplasia) of microglial cells may also suggest that their biologic activities and effector molecules are involved in neuronal degeneration.

SUGGESTED READINGS

Suggested Readings are available at evolve.elsevier.com/Zachary/McGavin/.

CHAPTER 5

Diseases of Immunity

Paul W. Snyder

GENERAL FEATURES OF THE IMMUNE SYSTEM

The immune system is a defensive system whose primary functions are to protect against infectious organisms, such as bacteria, viruses, fungi, and parasites, and the development of cancer. The complexity by which these functions occur is evidenced not only by the cell types, recognition molecules, and soluble factors involved and interactions with other systems (e.g., endocrine, nervous) but also by the ability to recognize virtually any foreign antigen. Immunologic responses result in pathologic processes, primarily inflammatory responses, as a result of either normal immune responses to foreign antigens (e.g., microbial pathogens) or from aberrations of the immune system as in the case of hypersensitivity reactions and autoimmune diseases. Finally, the importance of a normal functional immune system cannot be more evident than in instances in which it is deficient as the result of a genetic defect or as the result of an acquired immunodeficiency disease.

Immunity is the result of nonspecific (innate) and specific (adaptive) responses that together provide effective protection. The immune system's recognition and response functional capabilities are key components of both innate and adaptive immune responses. The recognition capabilities are highly specific and allow immune responses to develop against a diverse group of foreign (nonself) antigens and prevent the development of immune responses to self-antigens. Innate and adaptive immune responses feature effector mechanisms for eliminating or neutralizing the antigen, whereas adaptive immunity has the additional feature of memory. The emphasis of this chapter is on diseases that are the result of inadequate or inappropriate immune responses. Before one can understand the pathogenic mechanisms of these diseases, one must first have an understanding of the basic elements of the immune system. The chapter begins with an overview of our current understanding of innate and adaptive immunity, cells of the immune system, cytokines, and major histocompatibility complex (MHC) molecules. This overview facilitates the discussion of disorders of the immune system that includes hypersensitivity reactions, autoimmunity, and immunodeficiency. This chapter concludes with a discussion of amyloidosis, a diverse group of conditions characterized by the deposition of a pathologic extracellular protein. One of the conditions is associated with the deposition of immunoglobulin components. Although the focus of this text is on the pathologic basis of veterinary diseases, with an emphasis on domestic species, in this chapter we use the vast knowledge base regarding human and rodent immunology (applicable to most mammalian species studied to date) as our basis and interject major known relevant species differences as appropriate.

INNATE IMMUNITY (NONSPECIFIC IMMUNITY)

As stated previously, the function of the immune system is to protect against infectious pathogens and the development of cancer. There are two categories of immune responses that are based in part on their specificity for the antigen: (1) innate immunity and (2) adaptive immunity (Fig. 5-1). Innate immune responses are considered the first-line defense mechanisms, are not specific to the antigen, and lack memory. These defense mechanisms are the result of anatomic (e.g., skin, mucosal epithelia, cilia) and physiologic (e.g., stomach pH, body temperature) properties, and phagocytic and inflammatory responses. Major components of innate immunity are intact epithelial barriers, phagocytic cells, natural killer (NK) cells, and a number of plasma proteins, the most important of which are the proteins of the complement system. Phagocytic cells are recruited to sites of infection during an inflammatory response where they have a number of functions, two of which are to ingest and destroy pathogenic organisms and neutralize toxins. Neutrophils, monocytes, and tissue macrophages are the major cells involved in phagocytosis. These cells recognize components of microbial pathogens through the expression of several membrane receptors, including receptors for mannose residues and *N*-formyl-methionine containing peptides and a family of pattern recognition receptors (PRRs) that, when activated by microbial components, signal the activation of transcription factors that facilitate the microbicidal mechanisms of the phagocytic cell and are

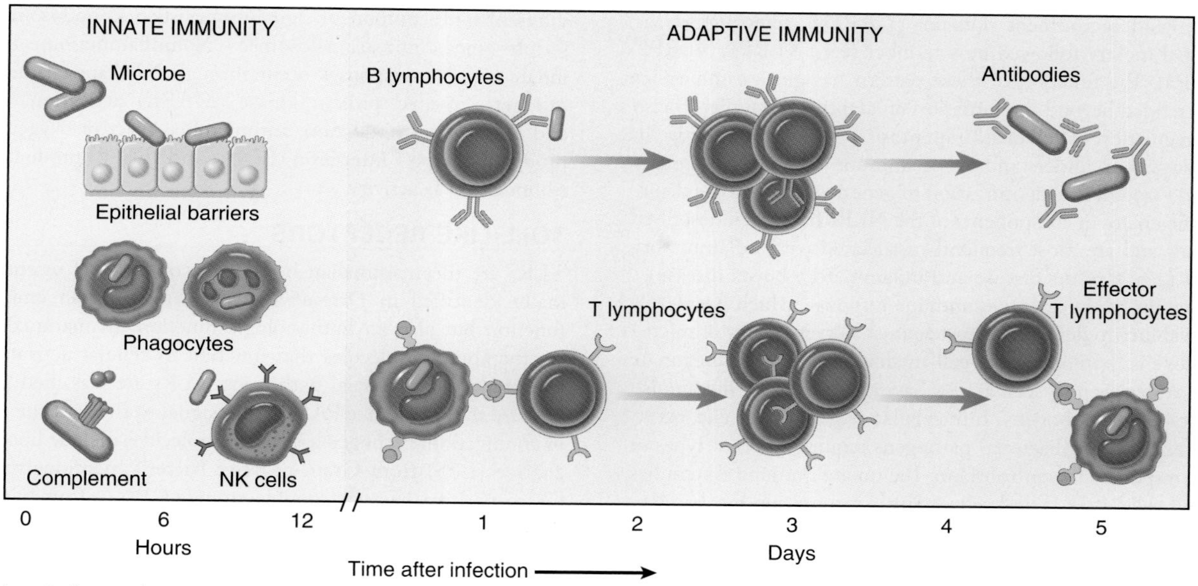

Innate Immunity

Physiologic barriers	→	pH, temperature, etc.
Anatomic barriers	→	intact epithelium (skin, mucous membranes)
↓		
Phagocytic barriers and	→	mononuclear phagocytic cells
Inflammatory barriers	→	delivery of cells and proteins
↓		

Adaptive Immunity

B lymphocytes	→	antibodies
T lymphocytes	→	cytotoxic cells and helper cells

Fig. 5-1 **Innate (nonspecific) and adaptive (specific) immunity are depicted in relation to the time course of an infection.** *NK,* Natural killer. (From Kumar V, Abbas AK, Fausto N: *Robbins & Cotran pathologic basis of disease,* ed 7, Philadelphia, 2005, Saunders.)

discussed later. NK cells are the cytotoxic cells of innate immunity and are also discussed later. The complement system, discussed in Chapter 3, is a complex cascade of proteins that has a number of biologic functions, including the formation of the membrane attack complex that efficiently lyses plasma membranes of microbial pathogens. The complement system can be activated by either the innate immune system (alternative and mannose/lectin pathways) or the adaptive immune system (classical pathway). Other important plasma proteins of the innate immune system include mannose-binding protein and C-reactive protein; two of the functions of these proteins are to facilitate phagocytosis through opsonization of pathogens and complement activation. Inflammatory responses comprise vascular, permeability, and cellular phases that act in response to damage to vascularized tissue. The features of the inflammatory response are also presented in Chapter 3.

RECOGNITION MOLECULES OF INNATE IMMUNITY

The recognition molecules of innate immunity provide an opportunity to recognize pathogens by cells other than lymphocytes. These germline-encoded molecules function to sense molecular structures shared by microbes and endogenous molecules associated with inflammation. The recognition molecules associated with microbes are generally referred to as *pathogen-associated molecular patterns* (PAMPs). The function of the innate immune system extends beyond microbial pathogen recognition to include endogenous molecules associated with cell damage and inflammation which are generally referred to as danger or damage associated molecular patterns (DAMPs). The activation of the innate immune system through these invariant PRRs not only precedes lymphocyte activation but also is required to initiate the adaptive immune responses. PRRs molecular patterns are associated with microbial pathogens and classified as secreted, transmembrane, and cytosolic forms. Collectins and pentraxin are examples of secreted PRRs that largely function to bind to microbial surfaces and activate the complement system. Collectins, having properties of collagen and lectins, include mannose binding lectins and pulmonary surfactants A and D. Pentraxin is comprised of five identical subunits to form a pentamer and include C-reactive protein, an activator of the classical pathway of complement. Toll-like receptors (TLRs) and C-type lectins are examples of the transmembrane PRRs, and they have limited cellular distribution, including macrophages, NK cells, and dendritic cells. TLRs are expressed on the plasma membrane or in endosomal/lysosomal organelles. The cytosolic PRRs are more widely distributed, including all nucleated cells, and include retinoic acid–inducible gene (RIG)-1–like receptors (RLRs) and nucleotide-binding domain (NOD) and leucine-rich repeat–containing receptors (NLRs). These recognition molecules provide the host with the ability to sense "danger" either through PAMPs in the case of microbial infections or through DAMPs in the presence of cellular damage or stress. This allows the innate immune system to detect and initiate immune responses in response to infectious and noninfectious causes. NLR molecules as immune sensors are not unique to mammals because they have been found in plants and urchins. The molecules are designated based on the structure of the molecule NLR with a suffix of P (pyrin domain) or C (caspase activation and recruitment domains [CARD]), referring to the N-terminal moiety followed by a number (e.g., NLRP1, NLRP2, or NLRP3). The function of these pattern recognition molecules is also extended beyond the initiation of adaptive immunity to also include regulation of cell death (apoptosis). As is often the case in immunology, our understanding of immune responses is greatly enhanced through the identification of genetic immunologic disorders. Deficiencies in components of the NLRs have been described in humans and are most frequently associated with inflammatory disorders (e.g., Crohn's disease and inflammatory bowel disease).

Analogous to the adaptive immune response, which has developed the ability to defend the host against a diverse array of microbial pathogens (humoral versus cell-mediated responses), the innate immune system is now seen as also having an ability to distinguish specific types of pathogens. Intracellular (e.g., viruses) and extracellular (extracellular bacteria) pathogens require different types of immune responses to control them. The innate immune system has developed cell-intrinsic and cell-extrinsic recognition mechanisms dependent on if it is mediated by an infected cell or an uninfected cell. Cell-extrinsic recognition mechanisms are a way in which an uninfected cell can participate in the immune response and are mediated through transmembrane receptors (e.g., TLRs) on specialized cells of the innate immune system such as macrophages and dendritic cells. Cell-intrinsic recognition mechanisms are essential for recognizing intracellular pathogens and involve type I interferon (IFN) gene transcription signaling by members of the RLRs. Three members of the RLR family are RIG-1, melanoma differentiation-associated gene-5 (MDA-5), and laboratory of genetics and physiology gene 2 (LPG-2). In viral sensing, the RLRs are highly discriminating with regards to the cytoplasmic localization and sensing of specific RNAs. They specifically detect RNA molecular patterns not normally present in the cytoplasm. Abnormal RNA patterns include chemical modifications, secondary or tertiary RNA conformations, specific RNA sequences, or double-stranded RNA. While much of what is currently known about RLRs is centered around the sensing of RNA viruses, there is preliminary evidence that similar intracellular mechanisms may exist for sensing DNA viruses and some intracellular bacteria.

Members of the NLR are central regulators of immunity and inflammation largely through activation of transcription factors like nuclear factor (NF) kappa B, interferon regulatory factor (IRF), or nuclear factor of activated T lymphocytes (NFAT). Some members of the NLR family form multiprotein complexes with the cysteine protease pro-caspase-1 and the adapter molecule ASC (apoptosis-associated speck-like protein containing a CARD) referred to as *inflammasomes* (also see Fig. 3-12). The inflammasome is a multiprotein complex that activates caspase-1. PAMPs and DAMPs are sensed through activation of the inflammasome complex, resulting in activation of caspase-1, which elicits effector functions through proteolytic cleavage of cytosolic proinflammatory cytokines (e.g., pro-interleukin [IL]-1β and pro-IL-18), which are then secreted in their active form. The inflammasome model is analogous to the model for the activation of the apoptotic caspases by CD95/Fas death–inducing signaling complex (DISC) and the Apaf-1 apoptosome. IL-1β functions in localized and systemic responses to infections and injury, to cause fever, activation of lymphocytes, and the extravasation of leukocytes at sites of injury or infection. IL-18 functions to induce IFN-γ by activated T lymphocytes and NK cells during a T_H1 response and to induce secondary inflammatory cytokines, chemokines, cell adhesion molecules, and nitric oxide (NO) synthesis. Other members of the NLR family are involved in inflammasome-independent (noninflammasome) innate immune responses and signal through different multicomponent signalosomes such as nodosomes, transcriptosomes, mito-signalosomes. Noninflammasome-mediated innate immune responses occur through NF kappa B activation, mitogen-activated protein kinase (MAPK) activation, cytokine and chemokine production, antimicrobial reactive oxygen species production, type I interferon (IFN-α and IFN-β) production, and ribonuclease L activity.

TOLL-LIKE RECEPTORS

TLRs are the mammalian homologue of the Toll receptor originally identified in *Drosophila.* It has not only an embryologic function but also an immunologic function. In mammals, TLRs are membrane molecules that function in cellular activation by a wide range of microbial pathogens. TLRs are classified as PRRs because they recognize PAMPs and signal to the host the presence of an infection. Pathogen associated molecules include lipopolysaccharide (LPS) from Gram-negative bacteria, peptidoglycan from Gram-positive bacteria, double-stranded RNA from viruses, or α-glucans from fungi (Table 5-1). In general, TLRs 1, 2, 4, and 6 recognize unique bacterial products that are found on the cell surface, and TLRs 3, 7, 8, and 9 are involved in viral detection and nucleic acid recognition within endosomes. The specificity of TLRs for microbial products depends on interactions between TLRs and non-TLR adapter molecules. All TLRs contain an extracellular domain characterized by a leucine-rich repeat motif flanked by a cysteine-rich motif (Fig. 5-2). They also contain a conserved intracellular signaling domain, Toll/IL-1 receptor (TIR), that is identical to the cytoplasmic domain of the IL-1 and IL-18 receptors. Fig. 5-2 illustrates how TLRs function in the recognition of LPS. In the blood or extracellular fluid, the binding of LPS to LPS-binding protein (LBP) facilitates the binding of LPS to CD14, a plasma protein and glycophosphatidylinositol-linked membrane protein present on most cells. The binding of LPS to CD14 results in the dissociation of LBP and the association of the LPS-CD14 complex with TLR4. An accessory protein, MD2, complexes with the LPS-CD14-TLR4 molecule and results in LPS-induced cell signaling.

TABLE 5-1 Toll-Like Receptors (TLRs) and TLR Ligands and Their Microbial Source

TLR	Ligand	Microbial Source
TLR2	Lipoproteins	Bacteria
	Peptidoglycan	Gram-positive bacteria
	Zymosan	Fungi
	LPS	*Leptospira*
	GPI anchor	Trypanosomes
	Lipoarabinomannan	*Mycobacterium* spp.
	Phosphatidylinositol dimannoside	*Mycobacterium* spp.
TLR3	Double-stranded RNA	Viruses
TLR4	LPS	Gram-negative bacteria
	HSP60	Chlamydia
TLR5	Flagellin	Various bacteria
TLR6	CpG DNA	Bacteria, protozoans
TLR7	Single-stranded RNA	Viruses
TLR8	Single-stranded RNA	Viruses
TLR9	CpG DNA	Bacteria, viruses

Modified from Kumar V, Abbas AK, Fausto N: *Robbins* & *Cotran pathologic basis of disease*, ed 7, Philadelphia, 2005, Saunders.

CpG, Cytosine and guanine linked oligonucleotide; *GPI,* glycosyl phosphatidyl inositol; *HSP60,* heat shock protein 60; *LPS,* lipopolysaccharide.

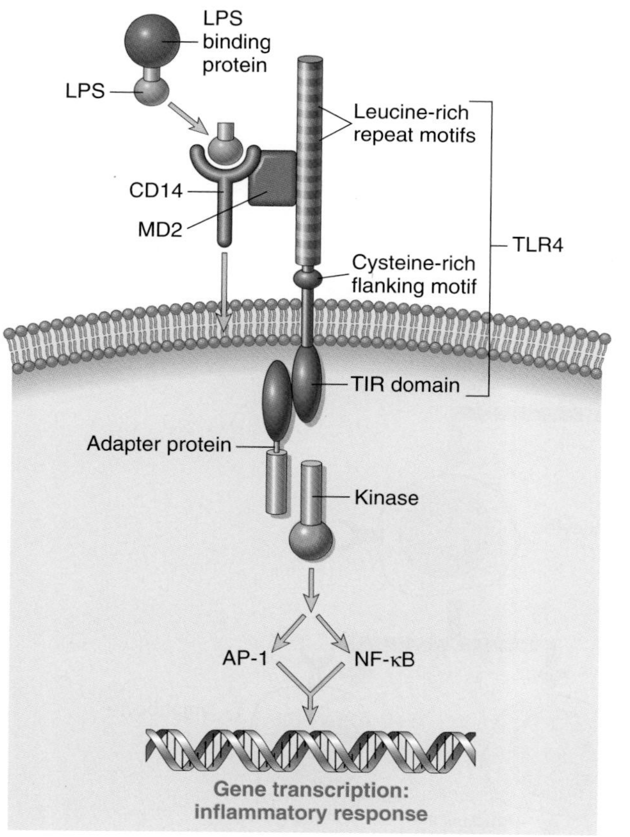

Fig. 5-2 **Signaling pathway for Toll-like receptor 4 (TLR4) in response to bacterial lipopolysaccharide (LPS).**
The binding of LPS to TLR4 results in activation of a signal transduction pathway, leading to gene transcription and the elicitation of an inflammatory response. *AP-1,* Activating protein 1; NF-κB, nuclear factor-kappa B; *TIR,* Toll/interleukin-1 receptor. (From Kumar V, Abbas AK, Fausto N: *Robbins & Cotran pathologic basis of disease,* ed 7, Philadelphia, 2005, Saunders.)

Briefly, TLR signaling through the binding of PAMP to a TLR leads to the activation of TIR, which forms a complex with the cytoplasmic adapter protein MyD88, an IL-1 receptor-associated kinase (IRAK), and tumor necrosis factor (TNF) receptor–associated factor 6 (TRAF6). Activated TRAF then activates the MAPK cascade leading to the activation of NF kappa B, a transcription factor. MyD88 is a universal signaling molecule for NF kappa B activation, and MyD88-deficient mice are incapable of activation by TLR, IL-1, and IL-18. Recent information suggests that there are also signaling mechanisms unique to individual TLRs.

TLRs and their pathogen-associated ligands are important recognition molecules for the innate immune system and trigger a number of antimicrobial and inflammatory responses. Up to 15 different TLR genes have been identified. The importance of these receptors in immunity is further supported by the observation of polymorphisms in the genes encoding them.

Although the individual TLRs exhibit ligand specificity, they differ in their cellular expression patterns and the signal pathways they activate, similar to that described for cytokines, which exhibit pleiotropy, redundancy, synergy, and antagonism. There are constitutively and inducibly expressed TLRs in different tissues. TLRs regulate cell recruitment to sites of infection through the upregulation of the expression of adhesion molecules, chemokines, and chemokine receptors during an inflammatory response. TLRs activate leukocytes (primarily neutrophils and NK cells of the innate immune system) and epithelial, endothelial, and hematopoietic cells. TLRs are also hypothesized to be essential for linking the innate immune response to the adaptive immune responses. Central to this hypothesis is the TLR-dependent dendritic cell-mediated control of T lymphocyte activation. Dendritic cells are important antigen-presenting cells for T lymphocyte activation. Dendritic cells uptake microbial antigens in the peripheral tissues and migrate to regional lymph nodes where they present peptide fragments, in the context of MHC molecules, to naïve T lymphocytes. In addition to the expression of the peptide-MHC signal, dendritic cells are also required to provide a second, co-stimulatory signal through the expression of B7, the ligand for the CD28 molecule on naïve T lymphocytes. The activation and maturation pathway related to the co-stimulatory signal occurs through TLR recognition of PAMPs.

There are species differences in the ligand specificity of TLRs and in the cellular responses elicited. Although sequences for canine, feline, and chicken TLR4 have been identified, no functional data have been published. With regard to domestic animals, a significant body of literature exists on TLRs of cattle.

Finally, TLRs have been implicated in "innate autoimmunity," with several reports of TLRs recognizing fibrinogen, heat-shock proteins, or DNA. There are also reports of TLR binding of DNA as a factor in directing antibody production by autoreactive B lymphocytes contributing to the pathogenesis of rheumatoid arthritis and systemic lupus erythematosus (SLE). Further studies are necessary to more fully understand these observations and the underlying immunopathogenesis.

ADAPTIVE IMMUNITY (SPECIFIC IMMUNITY)

Adaptive immunity in general consists of cell-mediated immunity, mediated by T lymphocytes against intracellular pathogens, and humoral immunity, mediated by B lymphocytes against extracellular pathogens and toxins (Fig. 5-3). The adaptive immune response is the second-line defense mechanism and is characterized by antigen specificity, diversity, memory, and self-/nonself-recognition. Antigen specificity and self-/nonself-recognition are the result of distinct membrane molecules. Mature B lymphocytes are activated by a specific antigen-binding molecule on its membrane. The antigen receptor is membrane-bound immunoglobulin. Mature T lymphocytes express a specific antigen-binding molecule, the T lymphocyte receptor (TCR), on their membrane. Unlike membrane-bound immunoglobulin on the B lymphocyte, which can recognize antigen alone, TCRs can recognize only antigens that are associated with cell membrane proteins called *MHC molecules.* Self-/nonself-recognition is the result of MHC molecules. There are two major classes of MHC molecules. Class I molecules are present on all nucleated cells, and class II molecules are present primarily on antigen-presenting cells. T lymphocytes and B lymphocytes are the major cells of adaptive immunity.

CELLS AND TISSUES OF THE IMMUNE SYSTEM

T Lymphocytes

T lymphocytes are small nongranular cells that constitute 50% to 70% of the peripheral blood mononuclear cells. They originate in the bone marrow and migrate to the thymus (thus the "T" designation), where they undergo differentiation, selection, and maturation processes before exiting to the periphery as effector lymphocytes. In secondary lymphoid tissues, they are located primarily in the

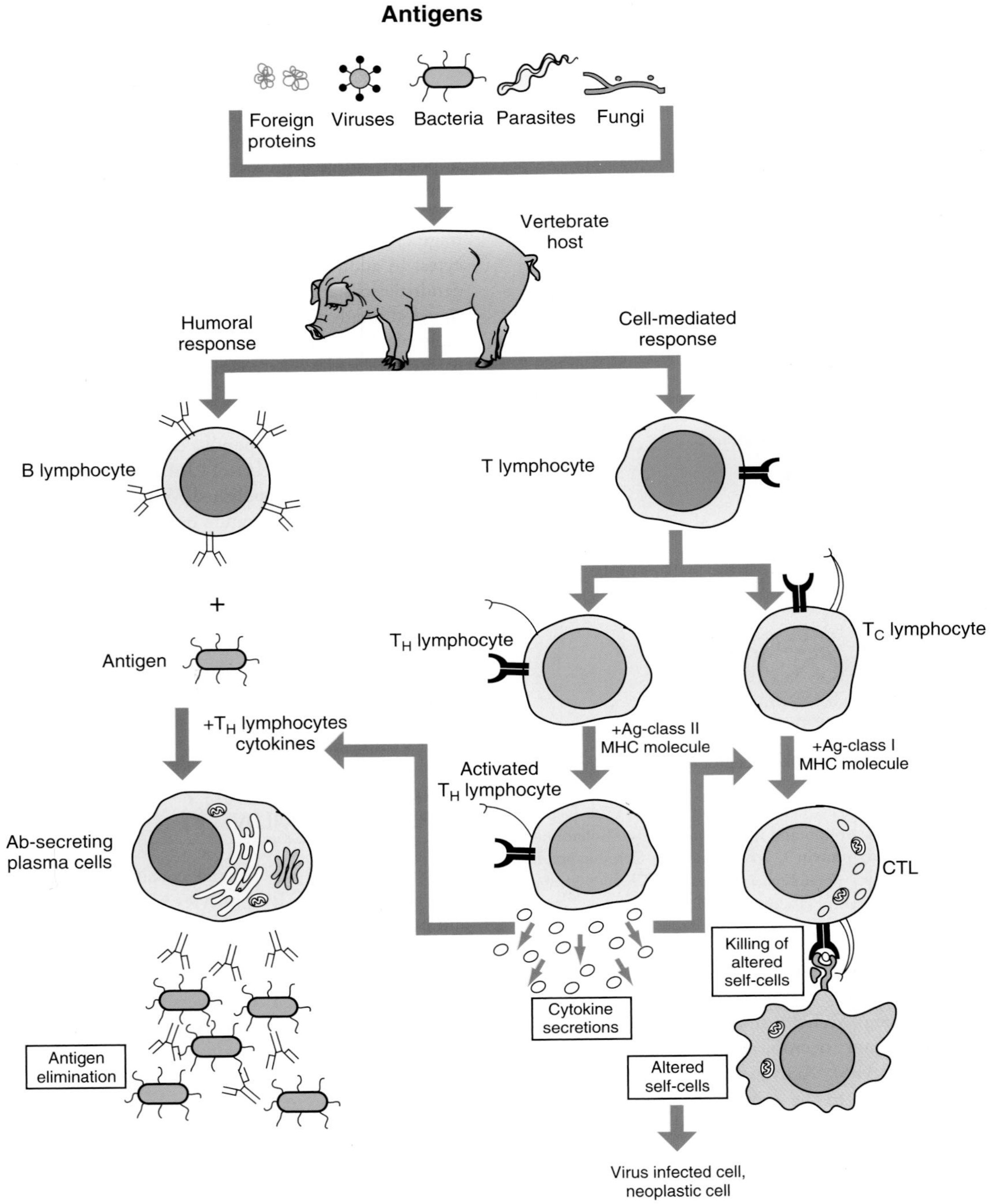

Fig. 5-3 Overview of humoral and cell-mediated arms of adaptive immunity.
CTL, Cytotoxic T lymphocyte. (Adapted from Goldsby RA, Kindt TJ, Osborne BA: *Kuby immunology,* ed 4, New York, 2000, WH Freeman.)

paracortical regions of lymph nodes and the periarteriolar sheaths (PALS) of the spleen. These specific anatomic sites elaborate chemoattractant cytokines (chemokines), for which the T lymphocytes express receptors. The definitive marker for T lymphocytes is the TCR, the polymorphic antigen-binding molecule. The antigen specificity of individual lymphocytes is attributed to their respective TCR, which is genetically determined. TCRs are classified as either αβ-TCR or γδ-TCR based on the composition of their disulfide-linked heterodimers. The individual polypeptide chains of the heterodimers contain variable (antigen-binding) and constant regions. In mammals, most peripheral blood T lymphocytes express αβ-TCR; however, in ruminants and swine, these lymphocytes make up only 10% to 50%, and 10% of peripheral blood T lymphocytes, respectively. Both TCRs are associated with CD3, and together they form the TCR-CD3 complex. There are significant activation and functional differences between αβ-TCR– and γδ-TCR–expressing lymphocytes. Unlike membrane-bound immunoglobulin on B lymphocytes that can recognize soluble antigen, the αβ-TCR can only recognize antigen after it has been processed into peptide fragments and associated with MHC molecules (the MHC is discussed later). In most instances, the antigen is associated with the MHC on the surface of an antigen-presenting cell, a virally infected cell, a neoplastic cell, or a cell of a foreign tissue graft. Individual αβ-TCRs are covalently linked to a cluster of five polypeptide chains, three comprising the CD3 molecule and two comprising the β-chain. The CD3 molecule and the β-chain are invariant, and although they do not bind antigen, they do function in the signal transduction after antigen binding by the TCR. Each T lymphocyte expresses a unique TCR with regard to structure and antigen specificity. The genes that encode α-, β-, γ-, and δ-chains of the TCR can undergo somatic rearrangements during their development in the thymus, resulting in tremendous diversity for antigen recognition. Not only are these rearrangements important for diversity, but also they can be used to molecularly phenotype proliferating populations of T lymphocytes as a diagnostic tool for the identification of clonal populations (neoplastic) and polyclonal populations (nonneoplastic) (see Chapter 6).

In most species, a minority of T lymphocytes express γδ-TCR. The γδ-TCR lymphocytes develop in the thymus and migrate to the epithelium of the skin and intestine, mammary gland, and reproductive organs. Although these cells can be found within regional lymph nodes and the lamina propria, in these organs they primarily reside as intraepithelial lymphocytes (IELS). As stated, in some species, notably ruminants, γδ-TCR lymphocytes are the predominant circulating population of T lymphocytes. In contrast to the αβ-TCR lymphocytes, γδ-TCR lymphocytes can recognize native antigen in the absence of MHC binding and they do not rely exclusively on the δ-chain as a signal transducer. Most γδ-TCR lymphocytes use the γ-chain for signal transduction after activation. The diversity of antigens recognized by γδ-TCR is limited in most species except ruminants and swine, indicating their importance in these species. Some have suggested that they may provide early cell-mediated immune responses in neonates. The precise function of γδ-TCR lymphocytes remains unknown. Another small subset of T lymphocytes, called *NK-T lymphocytes,* expresses molecules found on NK cells in addition to a limited diversity of TCRs. NK-T lymphocytes primarily recognize glycolipids that are associated with an MHC-like molecule, CD1. The function of NK-T lymphocytes remains unknown.

Although all T lymphocytes express the TCR-CD3 complex, they are further classified according to accessory CD4 and CD8 molecules. These nonpolymorphic accessory molecules include CD4, CD8, CD2, integrins, and CD28. CD4 and CD8 functionally subdivide T lymphocytes into CD8$^+$ cytotoxic T lymphocytes (CTL [T_C]) and CD4$^+$ helper T lymphocytes (T_H). During antigen presentation, CD4$^+$ lymphocytes only recognize antigen bound to MHC class II molecules (Fig. 5-4), whereas CD8$^+$ lymphocytes only recognize antigen bound to MHC class I molecules. This coreceptor requirement is commonly referred to as *MHC class I and MHC class II restriction,* the basis for positive selection in the thymus. Although there have been reports in some species of CD4 lymphocytes that are functionally cytotoxic and CD8 lymphocytes that are functionally "helper"-like, these appear to be anomalies and for the purposes of this text are excluded. In most species, peripheral blood T lymphocytes express either CD4 or CD8. Except for ruminants and swine, lymphocytes negative for both CD4 and CD8—"double negative" lymphocytes—are rare in the peripheral blood. So-called "double positive" lymphocytes, positive for both CD4 and CD8, are rare, except in swine, where they can approach 25% of the T lymphocytes in the peripheral circulation. T lymphocytes require two signals for activation. Signal 1 is provided by the TCR and the MHC-antigen complex and the CD4 or CD8 MHC complex. Signal 2 is provided by another accessory molecule expressed by T lymphocytes, the CD28 molecule. The ligands for CD28 are B7-1 (CD80) and B7-2 (CD81) expressed on activated

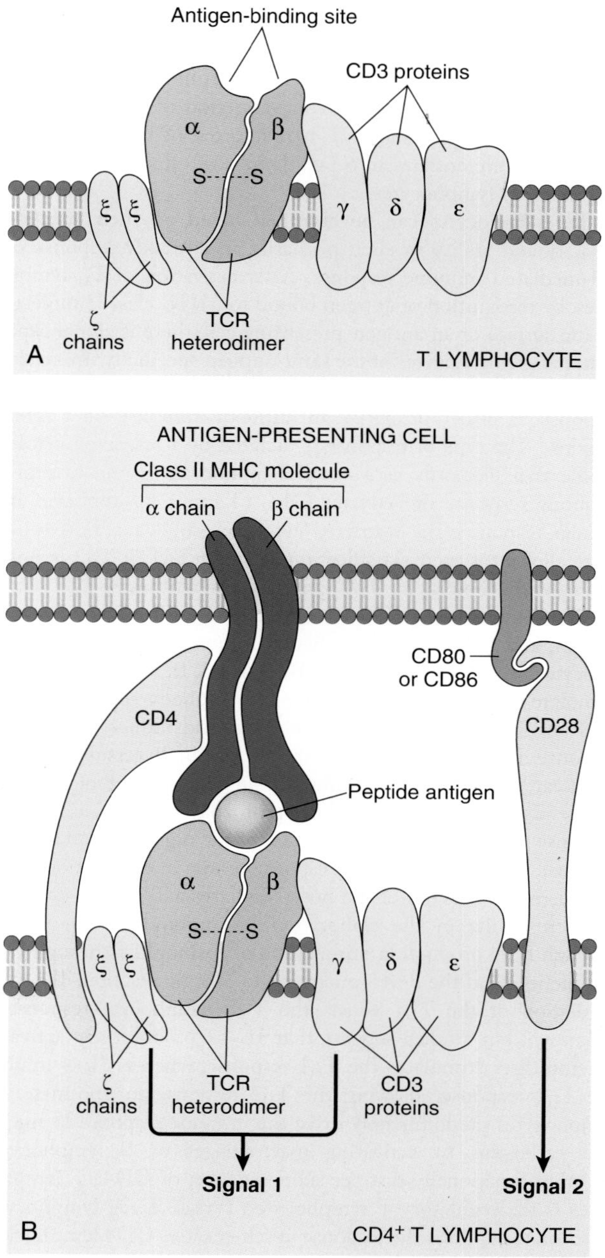

Fig. 5-4 The T lymphocyte receptor complex (T lymphocyte receptor [TCR]).

A, TCR-α and TCR-β chains complexed with CD3 γ-, δ-, and ε-chains and the invariant, ζ-chains. **B,** Illustrating how the TCR recognizes antigen in the context of major histocompatibility complex on the antigen-presenting cell (top) and how the ζ-chains and CD3 γ-, δ-, and ζ-chains deliver one of the two required signals for activation of the T lymphocyte. The second required signal is delivered by the co-stimulator molecules CD28 on the T lymphocyte and B_7 on the antigen-presenting cell. *MHC,* Major histocompatibility complex. (**A** from Kumar V, Abbas AK, Fausto N: *Robbins & Cotran pathologic basis of disease,* ed 7, Philadelphia, 2005, Saunders. **B** from Kumar V, Abbas AK, Fausto N, et al: *Robbins & Cotran pathologic basis of disease,* ed 8, Philadelphia, 2009, Saunders.)

dendritic cells, B lymphocytes, and macrophages (see Fig. 5-4). An inability to deliver the second signal results in an unresponsive T lymphocyte that either undergoes apoptosis or remains anergic. These molecules provide an important co-stimulatory signal for T lymphocyte activation, and are discussed in more detail later in the chapter regarding anergy and the development of tolerance with regard to autoimmunity. When T lymphocytes are activated by antigen and receive the appropriate co-stimulatory signals, they clonally expand as a result of their secretion of IL-2. This clonally expanded population of T lymphocytes, of the same antigen specificity, differentiates into populations of effector lymphocytes and memory lymphocytes.

T_H lymphocytes can be classified based on their functional capacity and ability to elicit primarily an antibody response or a cell-mediated immune response. After activation of T_H lymphocytes, by recognition of antigen bound to MHC class II molecules on the surface of an antigen-presenting cell, there is clonal expansion of T_H lymphocytes of the same antigen specificity. These clonally expanded lymphocytes are important in directing the immune response as either primarily an antibody response or a cellular response. The type of response is dictated by a restricted cytokine profile that primarily activates B lymphocytes in the case of an antibody response or activates CTL (T_c) and macrophages in a cellular response. The restricted cytokine profile for T_H lymphocytes allows for their classification as either T_H1 or T_H2 lymphocytes (Web Table 5-1). T_H1 lymphocytes synthesize and secrete IL-2 and interferon-γ (IFN-γ), stimulating CTL (T_c) and macrophages, and induce a cell-mediated immune response. T_H2 lymphocytes synthesize and secrete IL-4, IL-5, IL-6, and IL-13 that stimulate B lymphocytes to develop into antibody-secreting plasma cells and inhibit macrophage functions, and induce an antibody response. The type of immune response (antibody versus cell-mediated) can have a profound influence on the outcome of a disease. In the instance of an intracellular protozoal infection, a T_H2 type response results in rapid proliferation of the organism and death of the host, whereas a T_H1 type response results in elimination of the organism and survival of the host. Similarly, a T_H2 response to an allergen results in the elaboration of immunoglobulin (Ig) E, through IL-4 production, stimulation of eosinophils, through IL-5 production, and the development of an allergic reaction. The exact regulation of the T_H1 versus the T_H2 lymphocyte response is unknown, but studies suggest that IL-12 produced by activated macrophages stimulates the T_H1 response, whereas IL-4 inhibits the T_H1 response, allowing the T_H2 response to dominate. T_H lymphocytes predominately drive the immune response to microbial pathogens by activating macrophages or B lymphocytes. Another functionally distinct subpopulation of $CD4^+$ T lymphocytes is the regulatory T lymphocyte (T reg). T reg lymphocytes function to suppress the response of self-reactive CD4 lymphocytes that have escaped the negative selection process in the thymus. They are distinguished from other CD4 T lymphocytes by the expresson of CD25 on the cell surface. Like T_H1 and T_H2 lymphocytes, T reg lymphocyte differentiation is driven by cytokine environments; however, where T_H1 and T_H2 lymphocyte activation occurs through transcripional activators T-bet and GATA-3, respectively, T reg lymphocytes are activated through the transcriptional repressor FoxP3 (Fig. 5-5). This subpopulation of T reg lymphocytes are often referred to as Fox3P lymphocytes and produce the immunosuppressive and antiinflammatory cytokines IL-4, IL-10 and TGF-β. FoxP3 lymphocytes are an intense area of investigation for their role as suppressor lymphocytes of immunity and inflammation. T reg lymphocytes have been shown to have a role in the prevention of organ-specific autoimmune diseases and in modulation of immune responses to microbial pathogens to prevent overwhelming inflammatory reactions. Finally, a subpopulation of CD4 lymphocytes characterized by the ability to produce IL-17 is designated as T_H17 lymphocytes. T_H17 lymphocyte differentiation is driven by TGF-β, IL-6, IL-1, and IL-23. T_H17 lymphocytes, through production of chemokines IL-17 and IL-22, induce the recruitment of monocytes and neutrophils to sites of inflammation. Again, one must recognize that this is an oversimplification of a complex regulatory mechanism and that as additional knowledge is gained about T_H1, T_H2, T reg, and T_H17 lymphocyte responses, we will be able to understand pathogenic mechanisms of diseases, which will lead to the development of more specific therapeutic targets.

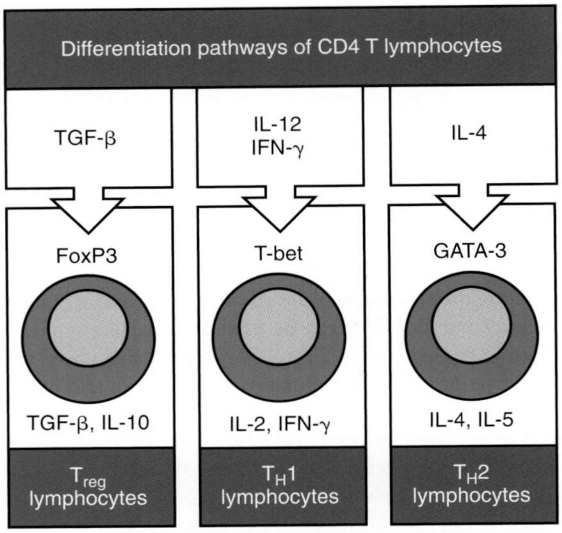

Fig. 5-5 Differentiation and expression of CD4 T lymphocytes. Cytokines in the extracellular tissue fluids direct the differentiation of CD4 T lymphocytes to specific secretory types, such that they secrete specific cytokines that have specific functions on other lymphocytes in the environment. (Adapted from Parham P: *The immune system*, ed 3, 2009, Garland Science.)

B Lymphocytes

B lymphocytes constitute 5% to 20% of the peripheral blood mononuclear cells. B lymphocyte development occurs in two phases, an antigen-independent phase in the primary lymphoid tissues, followed by an antigen-dependent phase in secondary lymphoid tissues. B lymphocytes can be found in primary lymphoid tissues, such as the bone marrow and ileal Peyer's patches (a primary lymphoid tissue in some species because it is the site of B lymphocyte development, rather than the bone marrow), and in secondary lymphoid tissues, such as the spleen, lymph nodes, tonsils, and Peyer's patches. Within secondary lymphoid tissues, B lymphocytes are aggregated in the form of distinct lymphoid follicles, which on activation expand to form prominent pale regions called *germinal centers* (Fig. 5-6). This anatomic localization, similar to T lymphocytes in the PALS and paracortex, is the result of elaboration of chemokines for which the B lymphocyte has receptors. The antigen receptor of the B lymphocyte is the membrane bound immunoglobulin. After the antigen-independent phase of development, B lymphocytes express IgM and IgD on their surface that signifies a mature B lymphocyte. In the antigen-dependent phase, antigen-activated mature B lymphocytes differentiate into IgM-secreting plasma cells or switch to another antibody isotype. Immunoglobulins can be generated against an almost unlimited number of antigenic determinants through the rearrangement of genes encoding the light chain and heavy chain components. As in the case of the TCR, an evaluation of the rearranged genes of a B lymphocyte can be used to molecularly phenotype B lymphocyte neoplasms (see Chapter 6).

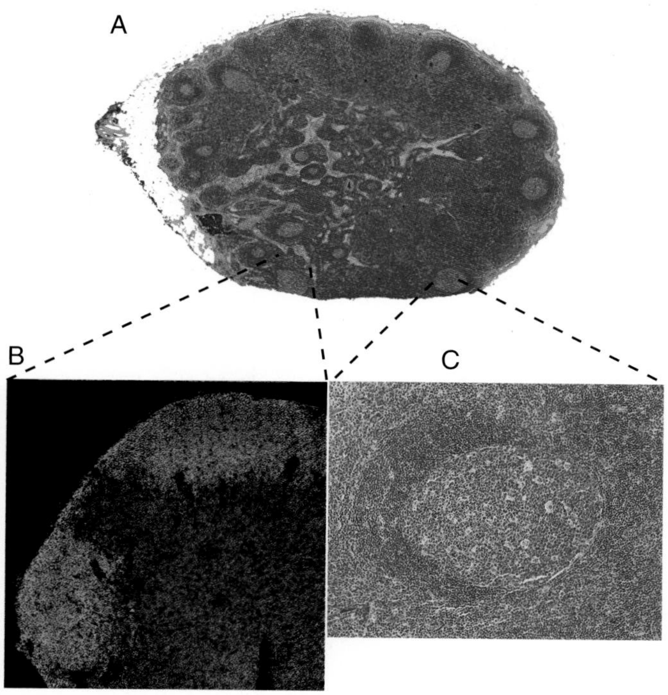

Fig. 5-6 Histology of a hyperplastic lymph node.
A, Outer cortex, containing numerous secondary lymphoid follicles with characteristic pale centers, and inner medulla are easily identifiable. **B,** Localization of B lymphocytes (labeled with a B lymphocyte marker conjugated with a green fluorochrome) and T lymphocytes (labeled with a T lymphocyte marker conjugated with a red fluorochrome). Immunofluorescence photomicrograph. **C,** Higher magnification of a secondary lymphoid follicle illustrating the central pale, germinal center, which contains primarily proliferating B lymphocytes, CD4$^+$ lymphocytes and dendritic cells, surrounded by densely packed small B lymphocytes. H&E stain. (**A, B,** and **C** from Kumar V, Abbas AK, Fausto N: *Robbins & Cotran pathologic basis of disease,* ed 7, Philadelphia, 2005, Saunders.)

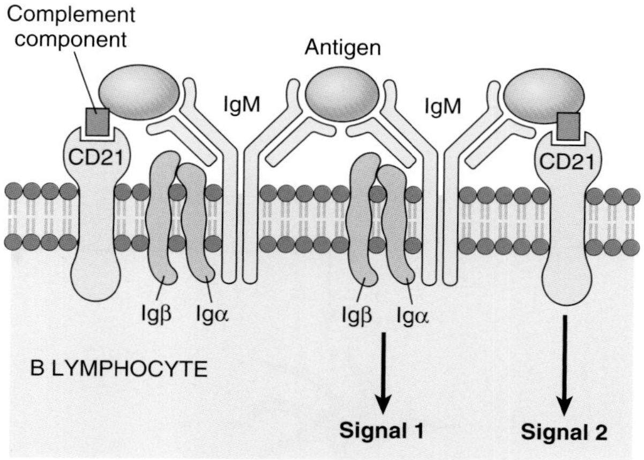

Fig. 5-7 The B lymphocyte antigen receptor complex.
Membrane *IgM* (or IgD, not shown) and the signaling molecules *Igα* and *Igβ. CD21,* also known as *complement receptor-2,* binds complement components and activates B lymphocytes. *Ig,* Immunoglobulin. (Courtesy Dr. Alex McPherson, University of California, Irvine.)

Like the T lymphocyte, the B lymphocyte also has accessory molecules that function to form the antigen receptor complex (Fig. 5-7). These nonpolymorphic molecules are nonpolymorphic heterodimers composed of Ig-α (CD79a) and Ig-β (CD79b) that do not bind antigen but do interact with the transmembrane portion of surface immunoglobulin involved in cell activation. B lymphocytes, unlike T lymphocytes, can recognize soluble antigens. Additional nonpolymorphic molecules that are important to B lymphocyte functions are CD21 and CD40. The CD21 molecule is the complement receptor-2 molecule whose ligands are C3b and C3d. B lymphocyte responses to protein antigens are dependent on cytokines produced by activated T lymphocytes (CD4$^+$). The CD40 molecule interacts with CD40 ligand on the surface of T_H lymphocytes and functions to allow B lymphocyte development into antibody-secreting plasma cells. A failure to express CD40 ligand has been associated with an inability to isotype switch, resulting in a hyper-IgM syndrome. B lymphocytes activated by antigen develop into antibody secreting plasma cells and memory lymphocytes of the same antigenic specificity.

Mononuclear Phagocytic System (Monocyte-Macrophage System)

The preferred term today for the functionally and phenotypically diverse population of mononuclear phagocytic cells is the *mononuclear phagocytic system* (MPS). It is also referred to as the monocyte-macrophage system. These cells have a broad range of functions contributing to immunity, inflammation, and tissue remodeling and repair. A brief history on the recognition of the defensive mechanism of phagocytosis not only facilitates our current understanding of how these cells play a crucial role in innate and adaptive immunity but also explains some of the terminology that often leads to confusion for students. Elie Metchnikoff (1845-1916), a comparative developmental zoologist, is credited with recognizing and establishing the process of phagocytosis, an important defensive mechanism for organisms. He recognized the association between the systemic clearance of microorganisms and the presence of the microorganisms in the spleen and liver. Subsequent studies evaluating the systemic clearance of dyes suggested that Kupffer cells and endothelial cells lining the sinusoids of the liver were responsible because both cell types internalized the dyes. Because the investigators considered macrophages (Kupffer cells) and endothelial cells to have a common biologic function, phagocytosis, they proposed that they be encompassed as a system, the reticuloendothelial system. We now understand that the mechanism of uptake by endothelial cells is not by phagocytosis and as a result the term *reticuloendothelial system* is no longer used. The term *mononuclear phagocytic system* was developed to differentiate lymphoid cells (mononuclear T and B lymphocytes), granulocytes (polymorphonuclear leukocytes), and endothelial cells from the lineage-committed precursors in the bone marrow, blood monocytes and tissue macrophages, and dendritic cells that currently comprise the MPS. It is very likely that as we learn more about the precursors and differentiated cells that constitute the MPS, there will be proposals for new, more specific classification schemes.

In general, a circulating MPS cell in the blood is designated as a monocyte, whereas the tissue-based cell is designated as a macrophage. The blood monocyte-to-tissue macrophage is well recognized, although the mechanisms that allow for differentiation of the circulating monocyte pool into the tissue-based pool are still largely unknown. The monocyte is a bone marrow–derived cell of the myeloid lineage that is the precursor cell to the terminally differentiated macrophage that has limited recirculation and replication capacity. The myeloid dendritic cell represents a specific type of mononuclear cell present in nonlymphoid tissues with unique migratory properties and is discussed separately. As

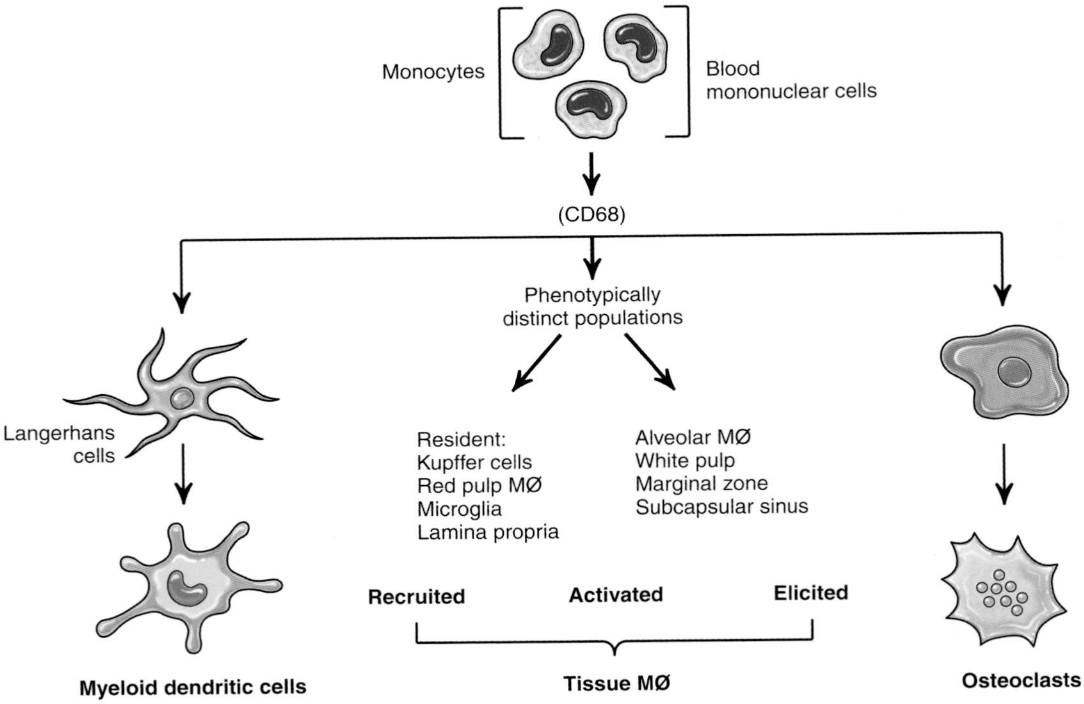

Fig. 5-8 Differentiation of mononuclear phagocytes based on antigen markers.
(Adapted from Paul WE: *Fundamental immunology*, ed 6, Philadelphia, 2008, Lippincott Williams & Wilkins.)

opposed to granulocytic myeloid cells, macrophages are long-lived (days to months) and can exist as quiescent "resident" cells widely distributed throughout the body. It is becoming increasingly clear that there is heterogeneity in the circulating monocyte pool that corresponds with the ultimate tissue localization of resident macrophages. The phenotypic characterization of the cells the MPS contains is often used in an attempt to identify specific populations of MPS (Fig. 5-8). Morphologically, monocytes are variably sized with an irregular shape, oval or kidney-shaped nucleus, prominent cytoplasmic vesicles, and a high cytoplasm to nucleus ratio. These features are not unique to monocytes, and as a result, they are difficult to distinguish from circulating dendritic cells, activated lymphocytes, and NK cells based on morphology or by light scatter (flow cytometry). This section covers basic concepts attributable to monocytes, tissue macrophages, and myeloid dendritic cells and refers to specific organ systems. See additional chapters in the section on pathology of organ systems for details on organ-specific cells of the MPS. Certain organ systems have specific names for their resident macrophages, whereas other organ systems only refer to them as macrophages (Table 5-2).

TABLE 5-2 Nomenclature and Location of Nonlymphoid Monocyte-Macrophage Cell Types

Organ/Tissue	Name	Location
Lung	Alveolar macrophages	Alveolar spaces
	Pulmonary intravascular macrophages	Capillaries of the lung
Connective tissues	Histiocytes	Interstitium
Kidney	Mesangial cells	Glomerular tuft
Brain	Microglial cells	Neuroparenchyma and perivascular areas
Bone	Osteoclasts	Bone marrow
Blood	Monocytes	Circulation
Liver	Kupffer cells	Hepatic sinusoids

Growth and differentiation of monocytes is regulated by specific growth factors, such as IL-3, colony-stimulating-factor-1 (CSF-1), granulocyte-macrophage CSF (GM-CSF), IL-4, and IL-13, and inhibitors such as type I interferons and transforming growth factor-β (TGF-β). CSF-1 is the most important because it controls the proliferation, differentiation, and survival of the monocyte. Monocytes represent approximately 4% to 10% of blood leukocytes and are identified in mammals, birds, amphibians, and fish. They are largely viewed as accessory cells that importantly link inflammation and innate immune responses to adaptive immunity. Hematopoietic stem cells (HSC) give rise to the common myeloid progenitor (CMP), the precursor cell to the granulocyte/macrophage progenitor (GMP) and macrophage/dendritic cell progenitor (MDP). The MDP is the common progenitor cell for monocytes, macrophages, and conventional dendritic cells. Monocytes express the CSF-1 receptor (CD115) and the chemokine receptor CX3CR1, are differentiated from polymorphonuclear cells (PMNs), NK cells, and lymphoid cells, and do not express CD3, CD19, or CD15. Monocyte heterogeneity based on surface marker expression and function has identified subsets that are an area of intense investigation and are best characterized in humans and rodents. Subpopulations of blood monocytes can be phenotyped based on the expression of surface markers CD14 and CD 16 (FcγR-III). Two additional subpopulations of blood monocytic cells are the myeloid blood dendritic cells, which are negative for CD14 and CD16. In the mouse, the main subset of $CD115^{+}$ monocytes are characterized as large cells expressing Ly6C, the chemokine receptor CCR2 and the adhesion molecule L-selectin (CD62L), and CX3CR1 (Fig. 5-9). These are referred to as inflammatory monocytes or inflammatory-monocyte-derived macrophages that are preferentially recruited to

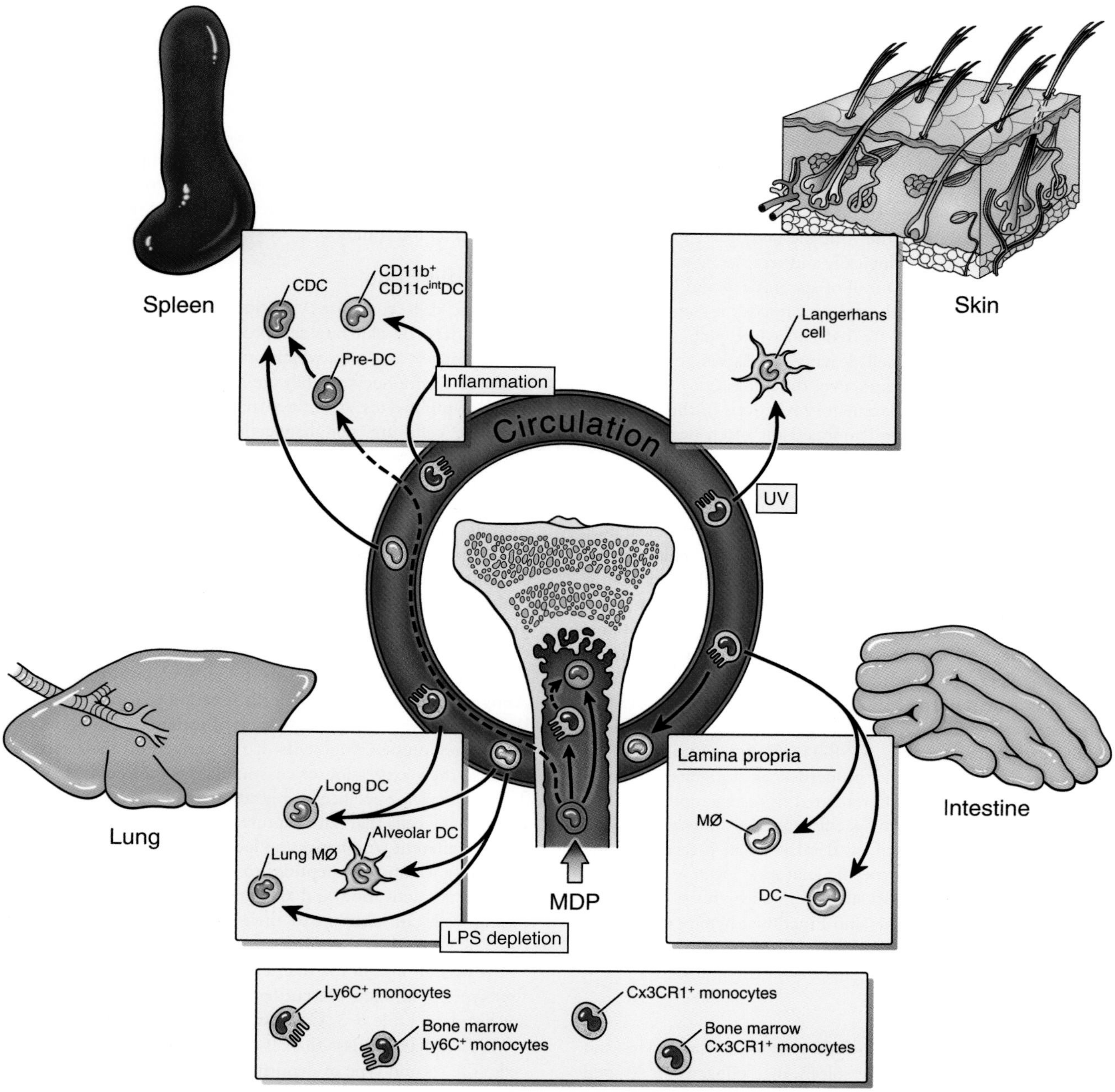

Fig. 5-9 Monocyte differentiation into dendritic cells and tissue macrophages. (Adapted from Serbina NV, Jia T, Hohl HM, et al: *Ann Rev Immunol* 26:421-452, 2008.)

inflamed tissues and lymph nodes where they produce high levels of TNF-α and IL-1. The emigration of Ly6C+ monocytes from the bone marrow to the periphery depends on the chemokine receptor CCR2 and its ligands CCL7 and CCL2. Ly6C negative monocytes have less of an influence on inflammatory reactions and appear to function more importantly as tissue resident cells and as cells involved in healing and regeneration associated with vascular injury. In those species characterized to date, there appear to be two major functional subpopulations of monocytes, one that is recruited and differentiated into macrophages at the site of inflammation and expresses higher levels of MHC class II and adhesion molecules and one that is responsible for repopulating resident tissue macrophages. Both populations can give rise to dendritic cells (see Fig. 5-8). Classification schemes are forever evolving, and there are definite species differences that may explain species differences in rates of infection and types of clinical disease associated with specific microbial agents. Similar phenotypic and functional heterogeneity exists with tissue-based macrophages.

The MPS of hematopoietic and lymphoid organs is diverse with functionally and phenotypically distinct parallel subpopulations in humans, rodents, and pigs. In primary lymphoid organs, mature macrophages are involved in the production, differentiation, and destruction of all lineages of hematopoietic cells in the bone marrow, and in positive and negative selection processes in the thymus. In secondary lymphoid organs, macrophages are uniquely positioned to enhance their phagocytic properties to endogenous and exogenous material and to influence other cell types through their products. The resident macrophages in the spleen differ in microscopic localization, phenotype, and function. The reason for this complexity is largely attributable the spleen's role as a hematopoietic organ and as a secondary lymphoid organ. Distinct subpopulations of macrophages are present in the red pulp, white pulp, and marginal zone with some recognized species differences (see Chapter 13). The red pulp macrophage functions in the phagocytosis of hematogenous pathogens and senescent erythrocytes. Erythrophagocytosis primarily occurs in the spleen and liver and allows for the removal of senescent erythrocytes and recycling of iron, often evident as cytoplasmic accumulations of pigments. The white pulp macrophages are also actively phagocytic, and a morphologically distinct cell, the "tingible body macrophage," can often be easily identified histologically and represents macrophages involved in the uptake and removal of apoptotic T and B lymphocytes. The marginal zone of the spleen provides a complex environment for the interface for the red and white pulp, specifically an important transit area for cells leaving circulation and entering the white pulp, and for B lymphocyte differentiation. The development of granulomatous inflammatory reactions in the spleen as a response to hematogenous microorganisms often begins in the marginal zone. The two subpopulations of macrophages present in the marginal zone are the metallophilic macrophage and the marginal zone macrophage. Marginal zone macrophages express high levels of PRRs and scavenger receptors that facilitate the clearance of pathogens from the circulation. The function of metallophilic macrophages is unknown. Tissue macrophages are derived from a combination of precursors in the blood (monocytes) and from local proliferation of precursors that varies for individual organ systems.

Much has been written about the relationship between monocytes, macrophages, and dendritic cells. The inclusion of dendritic cells as a component of the MPS is in part attributable to the fact that they are derived from a common myeloid precursor, influenced by similar growth factors (e.g., CSF-1), express common surface markers, and have no unique properties as antigen-presenting cells that allow them to be differentiated from macrophages. Like macrophages, dendritic cells in specific organ systems may have a specific name or designated only as dendritic cells preceded by the organ or in some instances a specific anatomic location within an organ. Dendritic cell subsets are also an intense area of investigation with regards to phenotypic and functional heterogeneity. The so-called conventional dendritic cells are present as immature cells in the interstitial tissues of all organs except the brain.

Macrophages

Mononuclear phagocytic cells include circulating monocytes and tissue-based macrophages. In the spleen, macrophages are located in the marginal zone, white pulp, and red pulp, where they function primarily as phagocytic cells. In the lymph node, macrophages are located in the subcapsular sinus, which is analogous to the marginal zone of the spleen, and the medulla. These physical locations, the subcapsular sinus of lymph nodes and marginal zone of the spleen, facilitate their exposure to potential antigens. Nonlymphoid tissue-based macrophages have different functions and are named according to the tissue in which they reside (see Table 5-2). One primary function of these cells is phagocytosis, as discussed in Chapter 3. Macrophages express Fc receptors (FcR) for antibody and can phagocytose antigens opsonized by antibody or complement components. Another primary function is their involvement in the immune response as antigen-presenting cells. In this instance, they phagocytose antigen and process it into peptide fragments, which are then presented to T lymphocytes, and the induction of cell-mediated immune responses. Although all nucleated cells express MHC class I molecules and could be considered antigen-presenting cells, only three cell types normally express MHC class II molecules and are regarded as the major antigen-presenting cells. They are the macrophage, dendritic cell, and B lymphocyte. Whereas B lymphocytes and dendritic cells constitutively express MHC class II molecules, macrophages express MHC class molecules on activation.

Macrophages also have an important role in the generation of a cell-mediated immune response and are essential to type IV hypersensitivity reactions. Activated T_H1 lymphocytes synthesize IFN-γ, a potent activator of macrophages. Under the influence of IFN-γ, macrophages have increased phagocytic activity and are more efficient at killing.

Dendritic Cells

Dendritic cells comprise a distinct population of cells that are characterized by elongate cell processes. Most dendritic cells are antigen-presenting cells, which process antigens and present fragments to T lymphocytes. They are more efficient than macrophages and B lymphocytes at antigen presentation. Antigen-presenting dendritic cells are nonphagocytic, bone marrow–derived cells. They are the most important antigen-presenting cell for initiating primary immune responses to protein antigens (Fig. 5-10). Antigen-presenting dendritic cells express a number of molecules, such as TLRs and mannose receptors, that make them efficient at capturing and responding to antigens. They also express high concentrations of MHC class II molecules and B7 co-stimulatory molecules. By expressing chemokine receptors similar to T lymphocytes, they have the ability to localize in T lymphocyte regions of lymphoid tissue. By colocalizing to these areas, they are uniquely positioned to present antigens to recirculating T lymphocytes. Antigen-presenting dendritic cells function to capture antigen and then migrate to T lymphocyte areas of secondary lymphoid organs, where they present fragments of the antigen on their surface and increase their expression of co-stimulatory molecules that activate T lymphocytes. Specifically, migrating dendritic cells, derived from Langerhans' cells that have captured antigen, enter the lymph node through efferent lymphatics and localize in lymphoid organs, where they present antigenic peptides to T lymphocytes that facilitate B lymphocyte activation and the production of antibody-secreting plasma cells. In addition to their function as antigen-presenting cells, they are also important in the process of negative selection in the thymus and in the maintenance of peripheral tolerance. The four types of antigen-presenting dendritic cells and their locations are listed in Table 5-3. Circulating dendritic cells, also known as *veiled cells,* make up less than 1% of peripheral blood mononuclear cells. The second type of dendritic cell, the follicular dendritic cell, is primarily located in lymphoid follicles. These cells are not derived from the bone marrow, do not express MHC class II molecules, and do not function as an antigen-presenting cell. Follicular dendritic cells have FcR and receptors for C3b. They store antigen-antibody and antigen-C3b complexes and are thought to be involved in the development and maintenance of memory B lymphocytes.

Natural Killer Cells

NK cells are nonspecific cytotoxic cells that are important in early responses to tumor cells and viral infections. NK cells are bone marrow–derived, large granular lymphocytes that make up 5% to 15% of the peripheral blood mononuclear cells. Their size, slightly larger than that of a small lymphocyte, and the presence of abundant granular cytoplasm distinguish them from T lymphocytes (Fig. 5-11). They are commonly referred to as large granular lymphocytes. The cytoplasm of NK cells and CTL (T_c) is characterized by cytotoxic granules that contain perforin and granzymes, two potent pathways mediating lysis of the target cell. NK cells and T lymphocytes express numerous similar surface molecules and kill

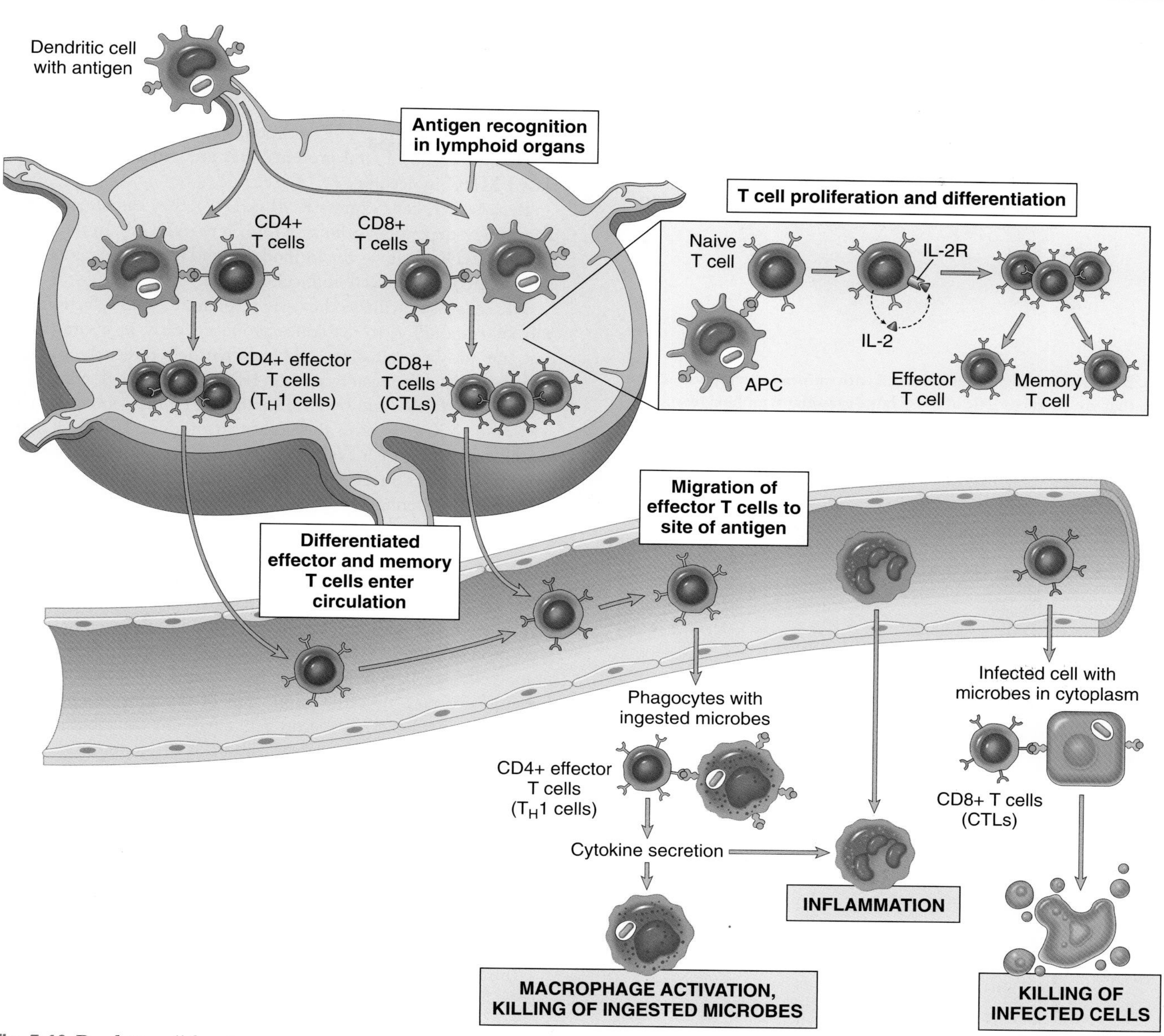

Fig. 5-10 Dendritic cell functions.
Specialized dendritic cells in the epidermis (Langerhans' dendritic cells) capture antigen via phagocytosis or endocytosis and migrate to regional lymph nodes, where they present peptide fragments of the antigen to naïve T lymphocytes. (From Kumar V, Abbas AK, Fausto N, et al: *Robbins & Cotran pathologic basis of disease*, ed 8, Philadelphia, 2009, Saunders.)

TABLE 5-3 Antigen-Presenting Dendritic Cells and Their Primary Location

Dendritic Cells	Location
Langerhans' cells	Skin, mucous membranes, iris, ciliary body
Interstitial dendritic cells	Most major organs
Interdigitating dendritic cells	T lymphocyte area of secondary lymphoid tissue and thymic medulla
Circulating dendritic cells	Peripheral blood

virus infected cells and tumor cells by similar mechanisms. Two membrane molecules, CD16 and CD56, are commonly used to identify NK cells. NK cells express FcγR (CD16) and the β-subunit of the IL-2 receptor (CD2). They do not express antigen-specific TCR or CD3 molecules. In contrast to cytotoxic lymphocytes, NK cells are not MHC restricted, are constitutively cytolytic, and do not develop memory cells. Because NK cells are activated early in an immune response and do not require a previous sensitization phase to develop memory cells after activation, they are the cytotoxic cell of innate immunity, the counterpart to the adaptive immune response's CTL (T_c).

Although NK cells do not express any antigen-specific molecules, they are very efficient at recognizing and killing altered or virally infected cells. NK cell activity is regulated through activating and inhibitory receptor molecules expressed on their cell surface (Fig. 5-12). These NK cell receptor molecules fall into two distinct categories: the immunoglobulin-like NK receptors and the C-type lectin-like NK receptors. Ligands for these receptors are cell surface molecules whose expression has been altered as a result of infection or damage. Ligands for activating receptors that stimulate NK cell activity commonly include viral and stress-induced proteins. Ligands for inhibitory receptors that block NK cell activity most

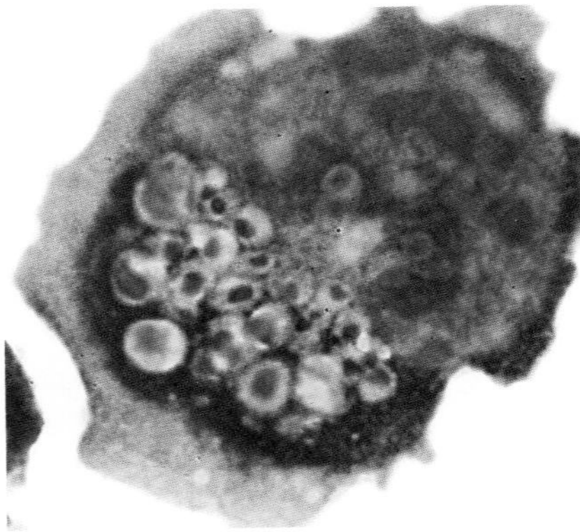

Fig. 5-11 Activated natural killer cell with numerous cytoplasmic granules that are characteristic of these large granular lymphocytes.
(Courtesy Dr. Noelle Williams, Department of Pathology, University of Texas Southwestern Medical School, Dallas.)

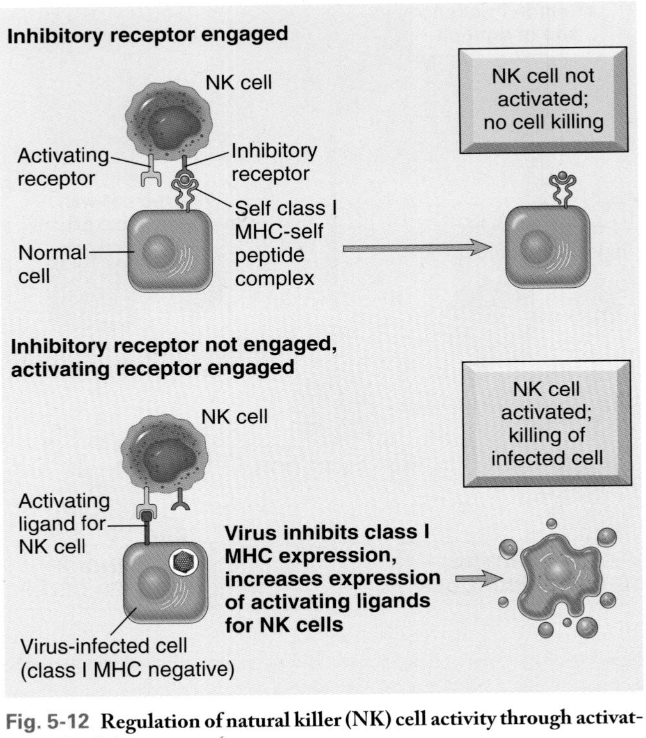

Fig. 5-12 Regulation of natural killer (NK) cell activity through activating and inhibitory receptors.
MHC, Major histocompatibility complex. (From Kumar V, Abbas AK, Fausto N, et al: *Robbins & Cotran pathologic basis of disease,* ed 8, Philadelphia, 2009, Saunders.)

commonly involve class I MHC molecules. A decreased expression of class I MHC molecules makes cells susceptible to NK cell–mediated lysis. A decrease in MHC class I expression often occurs in virus-infected cells and in neoplastic cells, making them susceptible to attack by NK cells. Normal cells are protected from NK cell killing because all nucleated cells express class I MHC molecules. This is an oversimplification of the "opposing-signals" model of NK cell regulation of how cytotoxic activity is limited to altered self-cells. Recent studies on the molecular mechanisms of NK cell regulation indicate that the absence of an inhibitory stimulus by itself is insufficient for triggering NK cell killing. NK cells also require triggering of activating receptors. Several activating receptors have been identified. One is the NKG2D receptor, a C-type lectin-like molecule that recognizes a number of stress-induced proteins. These stress-induced proteins are normally only constitutively expressed in the intestinal epithelium or as a result of cellular distress caused by infection or neoplastic transformation. There are a number of additional activating receptors, some of which recognized viral proteins, that are structurally similar to class I MHC molecules.

Because NK cells express FcγR (CD16), they can also function in antibody-dependent cellular cytotoxicity (ADCC). In the case of NK cells, ADCC allows for antibody-bound targets to be identified and targeted for NK cell–induced lysis.

NK cells also facilitate the early response to viral infections not only by responding to cytokines produced early in a viral infection, but also by producing cytokines that help direct the immune response. NK cells are activated by IFN-α and IFN-β, released by virus-infected cells, and by IL-12, released by macrophages. After activation, NK cells have the ability to produce IFN-γ, a major cytokine directing the development of T_H1-type immune response early in the infection. IL-2 and IL-15 stimulate NK cell proliferation, and IL-12 enhances NK cell killing.

CYTOKINES: MESSENGER MOLECULES OF THE IMMUNE SYSTEM

General Properties of Cytokines

Cytokines make up a vast group of low molecular weight soluble glycoprotein proteins that are produced by immune and nonimmune cells, are largely produced locally, and act locally to direct the immune response. The expression of cytokine receptors and their respective ligands is highly regulated and contributes to the complexity of the systemic organization of the immune response. Cytokines are involved in every aspect of leukocyte biology and the immune response and are essential to leukocyte development, recirculation, differentiation, and activation and in maintaining self-tolerance. Cytokines can influence the cytokine-producing cell itself (autocrine), other cells present locally (paracrine), or distant cells (endocrine) (see Fig. 12-1). Cytokines use common signal transducing pathways, converting an extracellular signal through a cell surface receptor to activate or inhibit the target cell.

The nomenclature of cytokines has evolved from a system that originally named them according to their cellular source (e.g., lymphokine from lymphocytes and monokines from monocytes) to one that named them according to not only the cellular source but also the target cell (e.g., interleukin, a cytokine produced by a leukocyte that influences another leukocyte) or to the primary function (e.g., chemokine, a cytokine that affects chemotaxis). As cytokines were characterized, it became apparent that they have pleiotropic, redundant, synergistic, and antagonistic features that do not allow for such a simplistic classification scheme. More recently, cytokines and their receptors have been classified based on their molecular structure and common signaling pathways. Many cytokines share a similar, α-helix structure that is also shared by their respective receptors and are classified as type I cytokines and receptors. As is discussed later, the classification of cytokines and cytokine receptors according to their structural similarities allowed for the identification of the cause of the profound cytokine defects associated with X-linked severe combined immunodeficiency disease in humans and dogs. Unfortunately, type I cytokines also have now been found to include other regulatory proteins such as growth hormone, prolactin, erythropoietin, thrombopoietin, and leptin. Type II cytokines include type I interferons (IFN-α and IFN-β), type II interferon (IFN-γ), and the IL-10 family of cytokines.

The breadth and depth of knowledge regarding the function, regulation, and control of cytokines is overwhelming; however, an overview of the major cytokines and their primary functions is important for understanding the pathogenic mechanism of many disease processes. Some of the major cytokines and their primary biologic activities are presented here and in Chapter 3 as they pertain to acute and chronic inflammatory responses.

Cytokines that broadly influence innate and adaptive immune responses include IL-1, interferons (type 1), IL-6, and TNF-α. These cytokines are produced and influence a wide array of cell types. Cytokines that are involved in hematopoiesis and lymphocyte development include IL-2, IL-3, IL-4, IL-5, IL-12, IL-15, TGF-β, and GM-CSF to mention a few. Chemokines are a large group of cytokines that influence leukocyte development, trafficking, and function. They are organized into subfamilies, with distinct functions, based on the position of cysteine residues. The C-X-C subfamily of chemokines is primarily produced by activated macrophages and tissue cells (e.g., endothelium), and the C-C subfamily is largely produced by activated T lymphocytes. Chemokines are responsible for the anatomic localization ("homing") of lymphocytes within lymphoid and nonlymphoid tissue. Chemokines and the other proinflammatory cytokines are more thoroughly covered in Chapter 3. The most important functional group of cytokines related to the pathogenesis of a number of diseases of immunity are those involved in the regulation of T_H lymphocytes. As discussed previously, T_H lymphocytes are classified based on their functional capacity and ability to elicit primarily an antibody response or a cell-mediated immune response rather than on their expression of specific cell markers (Fig. 5-13). T_H1 lymphocytes are activated by IL-12 and IL-18 and produce primarily IL-2, IFN-γ, and TNF-β to direct a cell-mediated immune response. T_H2 lymphocytes are activated by IL-4 and produce primarily IL-3, IL-4, IL-5, IL-6, IL-10, and IL-13 to direct a humoral immune response. As discussed later in the chapter, the type of response (T_H1 versus T_H2 type) may determine if a diseased state will occur. IL-15 regulates the growth and activity of NK cells. As indicated in Fig. 5-13, some cytokines, such as IL-10 and TGF-β, downregulate immune responses. In summary, cytokines produced by the T_H1 or T_H2 subset of lymphocytes not only promote the activation and functional capacities of the subset that produces them (autocrine effect) but also inhibit the development and activity of the other subset. This is known as cross-regulation and has important implications with regard to protective immune responses and adverse immune responses, as is discussed later.

Finally, a number of cytokine inhibitors were identified, and one of the more studied ones includes a factor called IL-1 receptor antagonist, which is produced by macrophages, hepatocytes, and keratinocytes. This factor inhibits the local and systemic effects of IL-1 by blocking the IL-1 receptor. Another group of inhibitors are the soluble cytokine receptors, which are the enzymatic product of cleavage of the extracellular domain of cytokine receptors that bind their respective cytokines, preventing interaction with the membrane-bound receptor form. The best characterized soluble cytokine receptor is the soluble IL-2 receptor. A number of pathogenic organisms have adapted this as an evasion strategy by producing cytokine-binding proteins or mimics to influence the development of the immune response. Although soluble receptors have been identified in a number of human diseases, their exact role remains to be determined.

STRUCTURE AND FUNCTION OF HISTOCOMPATIBILITY ANTIGENS

The MHC represents a complex of genes that encode specialized molecules involved in intercellular recognition and the distinguishing of self from nonself. These cell surface molecules have immunologic and nonimmunologic functions. The histocompatibility designation originated from the identification of these molecules in determining the compatibility of transplanted tissues. The MHC is an essential component in humoral and cell-mediated immunity. Most T lymphocytes only recognize fragments of antigen when they are bound to MHC molecules, and this requirement is the basis for MHC restriction. The repertoire of MHC molecules is genetically controlled and determines an individual's ability or inability to respond to specific antigens. MHC molecules are present throughout vertebrates and are maintained in gene clusters, each of which encodes different MHC products, which are linked. The primary function of cell surface MHC molecules is to bind peptide fragments of foreign proteins for presentation to antigen-specific T lymphocytes. There are three major classes of genes, and these encode for MHC molecules that are grouped according to their structure, tissue distribution, and function. Class I and class II genes encode cell surface molecules. Class III genes encode components of the complement system, enzymes 21-hydroxylase A and B, cytochrome p450, TNF-α and TNF-β, and heat shock protein 70.

MHC class I molecules are present on all nucleated cells (and platelets in some species). Their major function is the presentation of peptide fragments of antigens to CTL (T_c) ($CD8^+$). This requirement results in $CD8^+$ lymphocytes being MHC class I restricted. MHC class I molecules are further subdivided into highly polymorphic loci, referred to as Ia, and relatively nonpolymorphic loci, referred to as Ib, Ic, and Id. Each class I molecule is composed of a heterodimer consisting of a polymorphic α-chain that is linked to a nonpolymorphic β_2-microglobulin. The extracellular region of the α-chain consists of three domains (α_1, α_2, and α_3). The α_1 and α_2 domains form a groove where the peptide fragments bind the MHC molecule (Web Fig. 5-1). Although MHC class I molecules differ in their ability to bind peptide fragments, they are not as restrictive as antibodies and TCRs. The intracellular processing of antigen into peptide fragments, the association of those fragments with MHC class I molecules, and their transport to the cell surface is a complex process.

Antigen uptake by antigen-presenting cells is by phagocytosis or endocytosis. Antigen processing is the degradation of an antigen into peptide fragments, which are complexed with MHC molecules. Antigen presentation is the transport of the peptide-MHC complex to the membrane, where they are displayed. Antigens can arise intracellularly (endogenous) and extracellularly (exogenous), and the immune system most effectively eliminates these antigens through the elaboration of CTL (T_c) or secretion of antibody. The immune system uses two different processing pathways for antigen processing and antigen presentation. Intracellular antigens are processed in a cytosolic pathway and presented in association with MHC class I molecules (Fig. 5-14). Extracellular antigens are processed in an endocytic pathway and presented in association with MHC class II molecules. Endogenous antigens are degraded into small peptide fragments within the cytoplasm by the proteasome complex. Peptide fragments are transported to the endoplasmic reticulum (ER) by an adenosine triphosphate–binding peptide transporter (TAP). Within the ER, the newly synthesized MHC class I α-chain and associated β_2-microglobulin bind the antigenic peptide and form a complex that is transported from the ER to the Golgi and then to the plasma membrane for presentation to $CD8^+$ CTL (T_c). The antigen recognition molecule of the cytotoxic T lymphocyte (T_C) recognizes the MHC-peptide complex by means of its CD8 molecule, which functions as a co-receptor, binding to the nonpolymorphic α_3 domain of the MHC class I heavy chain. Because CTL (T_c) only recognize peptides when

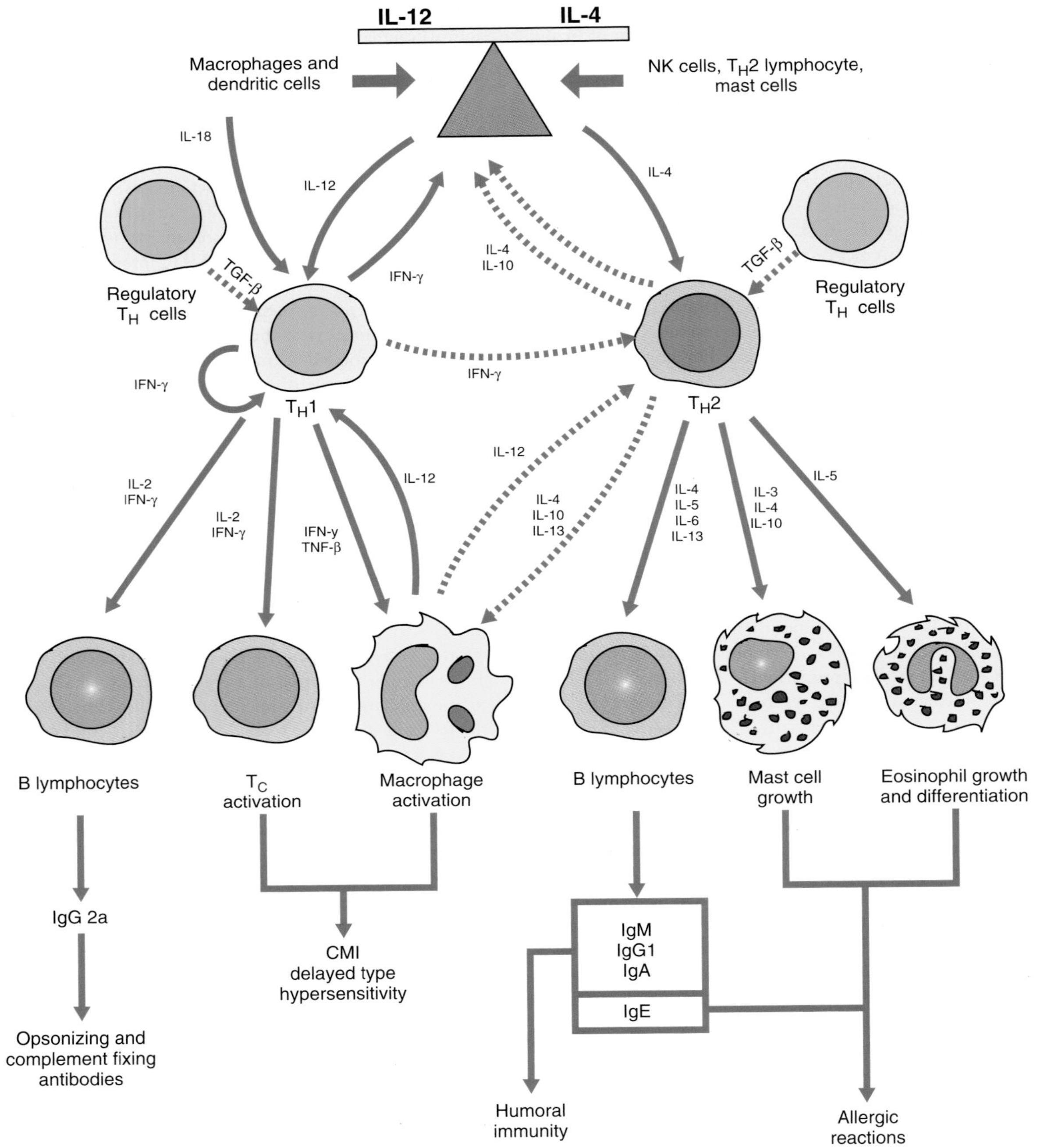

Fig. 5-13 Cross-regulation of immunity.
Cross-regulation of T_H1 and T_H2 lymphocytes in part determines if an immunity is primarily a cell-mediated response or a humoral response. T_H1 lymphocytes, activated primarily by IL-12 and IL-18, promote cell-mediated immunity *(CMI)* by activating macrophages and cytotoxic T lymphocytes. T_H2 lymphocytes, activated primarily by IL-4, promote humoral immunity by producing cytokines that activate B lymphocytes to develop into antibody-secreting plasma cells. T_H2 lymphocytes also produce cytokines that activate mast cells and eosinophils in the pathogenesis of allergic diseases. The cross-regulation of T_H1 and T_H2 lymphocytes provides an inverse relationship between cell-mediated and humoral immunity. *IFN-γ,* Interferon-γ; *Ig,* immunoglobulin; *IL,* interleukin; *NK,* natural killer; *TNF-β,* tumor necrosis factor-β. (Adapted from Goldsby RA, Kindt TJ, Osborne BA: *Kuby immunology,* ed 4, New York, 2000, WH Freeman.)

they are presented as a complex with MHC class I molecules, they are referred to as being MHC class I restricted. MHC restriction is the result of positive selection of lymphocytes during T lymphocyte development in the thymus. Portions of some antigens, those portions not processed for presentation, and in some cases, entire antigens are completely degraded by exopeptidases of the antigen-presenting cell into amino acids and do not initiate an immune response. Endogenous antigens are most frequently encountered during viral infections and thus CTL (T_c) are an important defense mechanism for eliminating virally infected cells.

Class II molecules have a variable tissue distribution depending on the species of domestic animal, but in general they are present on antigen-presenting cells (B lymphocytes, dendritic cells, and macrophages) and can be induced on T lymphocytes, keratinocytes, and endothelial cells by IFN-γ. There are significant species differences with regard to the constitutive expression of MHC molecules. The

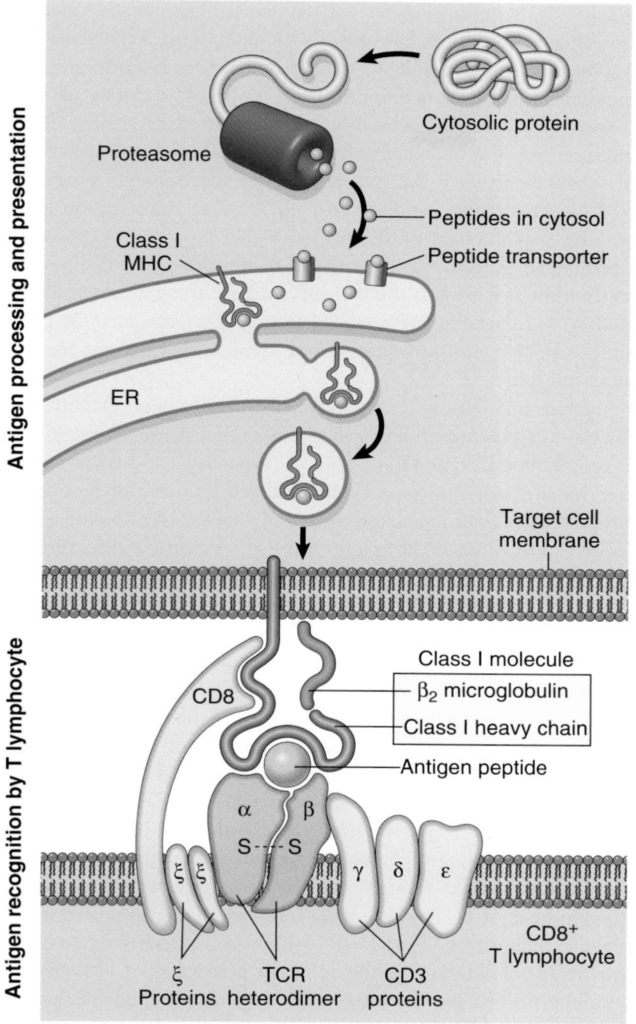

Fig. 5-14 Antigen processing and presentation by an antigen-presenting cell, and antigen recognition by T lymphocytes.
A class I major histocompatibility complex *(MHC)*–restricted $CD8^+$ lymphocyte is depicted. *ER,* Endoplasmic reticulum; *TCR,* T lymphocyte receptor. (From Kumar V, Abbas AK, Fausto N: *Robbins & Cotran pathologic basis of disease*, ed 7, Philadelphia, 2005, Saunders.)

major function of MHC class II molecules is the induction of T_H lymphocytes. Class II MHC molecules are heterodimers consisting of an α-chain and a β-chain. The antigen-binding site of the class II molecule, unlike that of the class I molecule, is formed by portions of both the α_1 and β_1 domain. Additionally, as with the class I MHC molecules, polymorphism of the class II MHC molecules is associated with determining an individual's response to antigens of infectious organisms (see next section). Peptides that bind to class II MHC molecules are in general derived from exogenous antigens, which have been internalized and processed within endosomes and lysosomes of antigen-presenting cells. Antigen-presenting cells can internalize antigen by phagocytosis or endocytosis (receptor mediated or pinocytosis). Macrophages are the only cell type capable of both because other antigen-presenting cells are poorly phagocytic. Extracellular antigens are processed into peptide fragments in an endocytic pathway and presented in association with MHC class II molecules on the cell membrane. During the synthesis of a class II molecule within the ER, it associates with another protein called the *invariant chain,* which prevents the molecule from binding endogenously derived peptides. The complex is then transported from the ER to the Golgi complex and into an endocytic compartment (vesicles) that contains the antigenic peptide fragments derived from exogenous antigens. Proteolytic cleavage of the invariant chain allows for the association of the peptide fragment with the class II MHC molecule. The peptide-class II MHC complex is then transported to the cell surface for presentation to $CD4^+$ T_H lymphocytes. The CD4 molecule acts as a coreceptor for induction of T_H lymphocyte activation. Because T_H lymphocytes only recognize peptides when they are presented as a complex with class II MHC molecules, they are referred to as *class II MHC restricted.* It is worth mentioning that of the two scientists, Peter Doherty and Rolf Zinkernagel, who received the Nobel Prize in Medicine in 1996 for discovering MHC restriction, Dr. Doherty is an Australian veterinarian.

MHC molecules are important in regulating T lymphocyte development in the thymus and in the peripheral lymphoid tissues determining specific responses to different forms of antigens. During the development and maturation process in the thymus, only T lymphocytes capable of recognizing self-MHC molecules are selected (positive selection) for export to the peripheral lymphoid tissues. These developmental processes influence an individual's T lymphocyte repertoire, which is the functional population that influences immunity. An individual's ability to mount an effective immune response is determined in part by his or her ability to recognize endogenous and exogenous antigens and their MHC haplotype. Thus, in one case, the association of an antigenic peptide fragment with a specific MHC molecule may result in a protective antibody response with elimination of an infectious agent, whereas in another case, the association of an antigenic peptide fragment with a specific MHC molecule may result in an inappropriate immune response to an innocuous antigen, producing an allergic reaction.

The organization (chromosomal location) and characterization (e.g., number of loci) of the MHC of each species of domestic animals appears to be fairly conserved and present in higher vertebrates and mammals. Most mammalian species studied have class I, II, and III genes, with differences between species being the arrangement and number of genetic loci comprising the MHC. In general, class I genes are more closely related within a species than between species, and the avian MHC is smaller and less complex, with many genes found in the mammalian MHC being absent. Although it is beyond the scope of this chapter to discuss the details regarding the differences between domestic species, the preceding overview is relevant to most domestic species.

Major Histocompatibility Complex and Disease Association

The MHC influences transplant acceptance or rejection, immune responsiveness, and the pathogenesis of a number of diseases. The MHC represents a complex of genes that encode specialized molecules involved in antigen presentation and thus regulate immune responses. The ability of the immune system to respond to an antigen is determined in part by the binding of peptide fragments to MHC molecules, which are then presented on the surface of antigen-presenting cells. There is a growing body of information associating certain MHC alleles with increased or decreased susceptibility to certain diseases (Web Table 5-2). Because the MHC genes of most domestic species are not well characterized, it is difficult to distinguish if the observed effects are due to the MHC itself or to other tightly linked genes. These conclusions are generally the result of an observation that some MHC alleles occur at a higher frequency among individuals affected with the disease, as compared with the general population. The association of an increased risk with certain MHC alleles is never the sole basis for determining if an individual will develop the disease, as often other hereditary and environmental factors also play an important role. The diseases most often associated with certain MHC alleles have a pathogenesis that incorporates a significant immunologic component. The types of diseases identified are diverse; however, they frequently include autoimmune, infectious, and allergic diseases. Additionally, MHC diversity may increase or decrease the susceptibility to infectious diseases. There is evidence that MHC polymorphisms may significantly impact disease resistance and is best illustrated in species in which there is a loss of MHC diversity attributed to a limited breeding pool of animals. In the case of the cheetah and Florida panther, the current breeding stocks of both species are derived from a limited genetic pool, thus resulting in reduced MHC diversity. In both species, there is an increased susceptibility to infectious agents that is not seen in other species of big cats.

Although there are a number of hypotheses to account for the role of MHC molecules in disease susceptibility, the actual mechanisms remain elusive. The most often hypothesized mechanism is attributed to the role of MHC alleles in determining responsiveness or nonresponsiveness to a particular pathogen. On the one hand, through antigen presentation and activation of cytotoxic or T lymphocytes, it determines whether a protective immune response is generated to a particular pathogen. On the other hand, certain MHC alleles may encode molecules that are used by infectious agents, as in the case of receptors for viruses or bacterial toxins, and facilitate their infectivity or pathogenicity.

DISORDERS OF THE IMMUNE SYSTEM

As has been discussed, immunity is a complex defensive system of recognition and effector mechanisms for protecting the host from infectious pathogens and cancer. During the normal immune response, there are mechanisms for eliminating the inciting foreign antigen, and associated with this is some degree of tissue damage that elicits an inflammatory response of appropriate duration and severity for the antigen. However, there are a number of instances in which the immune response elicits an inflammatory response that is not appropriate to the inciting antigen and these fall into three general categories. The largest category is the hypersensitivity reactions, which are associated with a large number of diseases covered throughout this text. The second category is the autoimmune diseases, in which the immune response is inappropriately directed at a self-antigen, resulting in damage to normal organs or tissue. The third category is the immunodeficiency diseases, in which a genetic or acquired defect results in an inability to mount an immune response and thus control infections, resulting in severe systemic inflammation. The chapter now focuses on general features of immunologic tissue injury, with discussion of some specific immunologic diseases that are attributable to disorders of the immune system. Finally, we conclude with a discussion of amyloidosis, a condition that is the result of a number of mechanisms, some of which have an immunologic basis.

MECHANISMS OF IMMUNOLOGIC TISSUE INJURY: HYPERSENSITIVITY REACTIONS

A hypersensitivity reaction is defined as the altered reactivity to a specific antigen that results in pathologic reactions upon the exposure of a sensitized host to that specific antigen. The designation of these immune responses as "hyper" is somewhat of a misnomer because the reactions elicited are better characterized as inappropriate or misdirected responses. An immune response can be either beneficial or harmful. By characterizing hypersensitivity responses as inappropriate or misdirected, we are not implying that these responses are any different from those that occur as a normal "beneficial" defense mechanism. To state it more clearly: If the immune response is beneficial it is immunity and if it is harmful, it is hypersensitivity. All hypersensitivity reactions are characterized by sensitization and effector phases. The sensitization phase requires that the host must have had either a previous exposure or a prolonged exposure to the antigen so that he or she can develop an immune response to the inciting antigen. The pathology associated with hypersensitivity reactions occurs in the effector phase and is most commonly manifested as an inflammatory reaction or as cell lysis.

Hypersensitivity reactions have historically been classified on the basis of the immunologic mechanism that mediates the disease as type I, type II, type III, or type IV. Types I, II, and III are mediated by antibody, and type IV is mediated by macrophages and T lymphocytes. Type I is also known as *immediate type hypersensitivity* and most often is the result of an IgE response that is directed against an environmental or exogenous antigen (also known as an *allergen*). The result is the release of vasoactive mediators from IgE-sensitized mast cells, and these mediators produce an acute inflammatory response. Type II is also known as cytotoxic hypersensitivity and most often occurs when IgG or IgM is directed against either an altered self-protein or a foreign antigen bound to a tissue or cell. The result can lead to either destruction of the tissue or cell by ADCC, complement-mediated lysis, or altered cellular function without evidence of tissue or cell damage. Type III is also known as *immune complex hypersensitivity* and is due to the formation of insoluble antibody-antigen complexes (also known as *immune complexes*). The result is activation of the complement system and the development of an inflammatory reaction at the sites of immune complex deposition. Type IV is also known as *delayed-type hypersensitivity* (DTH) and is the result of activation of sensitized T lymphocytes to a specific antigen. The resulting immune response is either mediated by direct cytotoxicity or by the release of cytokines that act primarily through macrophages. This original classification, as proposed by Gell and Coombs, was based largely on the primary initiating event involved in the individual reactions and not on the actual pathogenesis as it relates to what is seen clinically or pathologically. Although the original classification of hypersensitivity reactions is still valid, "newer" versions that are based on the pathogenesis better illustrate the complexity of these reactions and the specific pathology (lesions) associated with them. For the purposes of our discussion, we will use the original version of the Gell and Coombs classification presented in Table 5-4, understanding that many of the diseases associated with hypersensitivity reactions are actually complex and may involve more than one type. In humans, genetic mapping studies of most diseases characterized by a hypersensitivity reaction suggest that there are disease-associated susceptibility genes, further supporting the complex pathogenesis of these diseases. Finally, the pathogenesis of many diseases rarely involves a single hypersensitivity reaction, and in fact, some diseases may begin as an immediate hypersensitivity but progress to be predominantly DTH. For clarity, the hypersensitivity diseases are discussed in the context of their predominant mechanism except when it is appropriate to elaborate on the progression of a disease.

Type I Hypersensitivity (Immediate Hypersensitivity)

Type I hypersensitivity reactions are most commonly the result of an IgE-mediated immune response directed against environmental

TABLE 5-4 Mechanisms of Hypersensitivity Diseases

Type	Immunologic Component	Antigen	Prototype Disorder	Immune Mechanisms	Pathologic Lesions
Immediate (type I) hypersensitivity	IgE mediated	Allergens	Anaphylaxis; allergies (atopic forms)	Production of IgE antibody → Immediate release of vasoactive amines and other mediators from mast cells; recruitment of inflammatory cells (late-phase reaction)	Vascular dilation, edema, smooth muscle contraction, mucus production, inflammation
Antibody-mediated (type II) hypersensitivity	IgG and IgM mediated	Cell- or matrix-associated antigens Cell surface receptor	Autoimmune hemolytic anemia; neonatal isoerythrolysis; transfusion reactions; drug reactions; Pemphigus	Production of IgG, IgM → Binds to antigen on target cell or tissue → Phagocytosis or lysis of target cell by activated complement or Fc receptors; recruitment of leukocytes	Cell lysis; inflammation
Immune complex-mediated (type III) hypersensitivity	IgG and IgM mediated	Soluble antigen (e.g., bacterial and viral antigens)	Systemic lupus erythematosus; some forms of glomerulonephritis; serum sickness; Arthus reaction	Deposition of antigen-antibody complexes → Complement activation → Recruitment of leukocytes by complement products and Fc receptors → Release of enzymes and other toxic molecules	Necrotizing vasculitis (fibrinoid necrosis); inflammation
Cell-mediated (type IV) hypersensitivity	T lymphocyte mediated	Soluble antigen (e.g., bacterial and viral antigens) Contact antigens Cell-associated antigen	Contact dermatitis; transplant rejection; tuberculosis; chronic allergic diseases	Activated T lymphocytes → (i) Release of cytokines and macrophage activation (ii) T lymphocyte–mediated cytotoxicity	Perivascular cellular infiltrates; edema; cell destruction; granuloma formation

IgE, Immunoglobulin E; *IgG,* immunoglobulin G; *IgM,* Immunoglobulin M.

antigens (i.e., allergens) and parasite antigens. Harmful IgE-mediated responses to innocuous environmental antigens resulting in allergic reactions are termed *hypersensitivity,* whereas similar IgE-mediated protective responses to parasite antigens are considered immunity. This distinction emphasizes the fact that these are not unique immunologic reactions but rather misdirected or inappropriate "normal" immune responses. Type I hypersensitivity occurs in a previously sensitized host and is initially manifested as acute inflammatory process that occurs within minutes ("immediate hypersensitivity") of exposure to the specific antigen. In many instances, the reaction progresses from an early acute inflammatory response to a late-phase response and/or chronic inflammatory lesion that persists (Figs. 5-15 and 5-16). The basic pathogenesis involves a sensitization phase and an effector phase. The sensitization phase occurs during the initial exposure to an antigen when the host develops an antigen-specific IgE response, which results in sensitization of the host by the binding of the antigen-specific IgE to Fcε receptors on the surface of mast cells (Fig. 5-17). The host is now sensitized, and either through a second exposure or prolonged initial exposure to the IgE-specific antigen, there is cross-linking of two or more IgE molecules on the surface of the mast cell. This results in its activation and release of preformed and newly synthesized mediators, resulting in the effector phase. The effector phase can be limited to an acute inflammatory reaction (occurring within minutes), resulting primarily from the release of mast cell mediators, or can progress to a late-phase reaction (over a period of hours), or to a chronic reaction (persisting for days to years). The acute reaction is characterized by responses associated with release

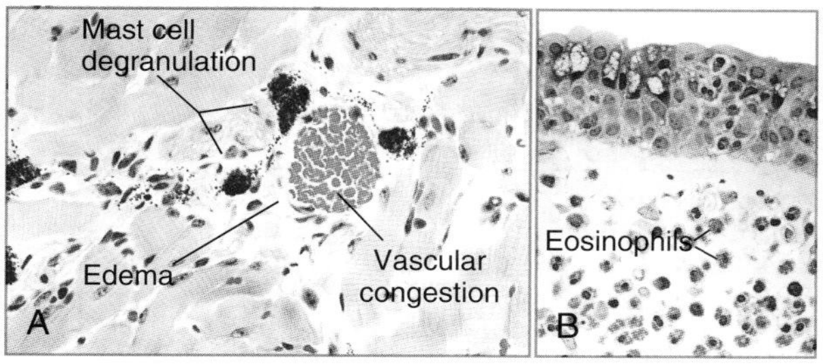

Fig. 5-15 Immediate hypersensitivity reaction.
A, Early reaction (minutes) is characterized by mast cell degranulation and release of preformed vasoactive substances that cause vasodilation and increased vascular permeability, resulting in edema of interstitial tissue. **B,** As the lesion progresses to the late phase (hours), the inflammatory infiltrate is primarily composed of eosinophils and fewer lymphocytes and neutrophils. (**A** and **B** courtesy Dr. Daniel Friend, Department of Pathology, Brigham and Women's Hospital, Boston.)

of preformed vasoactive amines from the mast cell and includes increased vascular permeability, smooth muscle contraction, and influx of inflammatory cells. The late-phase and chronic reactions, often associated with repeated or prolonged antigen exposures, are largely the result of a more intense inflammatory cell infiltration (primarily eosinophils, neutrophils, macrophages, and T lymphocytes) and tissue damage. Because the mast cell is central to the pathogenesis of a type I hypersensitivity reaction, their biologic features and primary functions are reviewed.

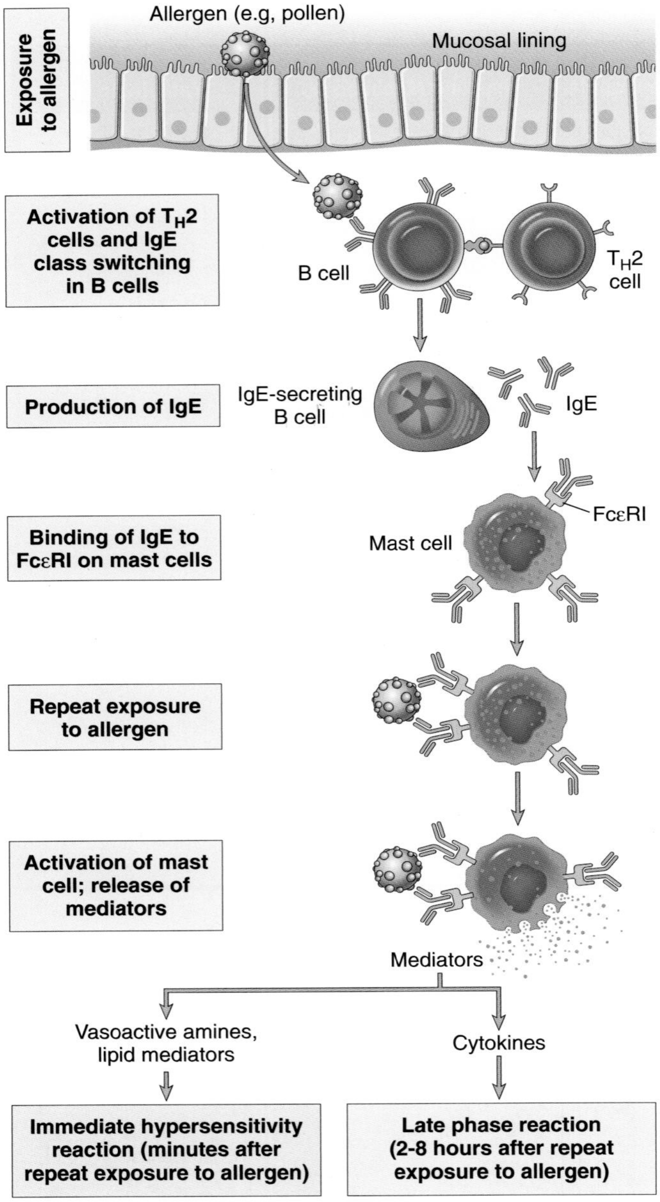

Fig. 5-16 Type I hypersensitivity reaction.
Pathogenesis of early and late responses of the type I hypersensitivity reaction. *IgE,* Immunoglobulin E. (From Kumar V, Abbas AK, Fausto N, et al: *Robbins & Cotran pathologic basis of disease,* ed 8, Philadelphia, 2009, Saunders.)

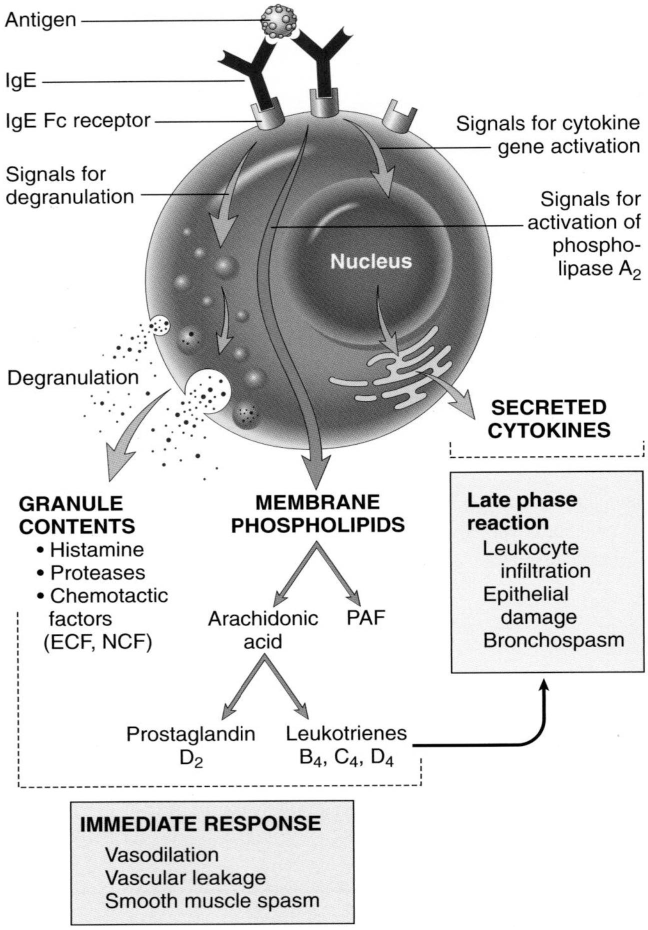

Fig. 5-17 Mast cell degranulation and activation.
Cross-linking of a sensitized (immunoglobulin E *[IgE]* bound to membrane Fcε receptors) mast cell by antigen results in mast cell activation and degranulation. Degranulation results in release of preformed mediators (histamine, proteases, and chemotactic substances). Activation results in synthesis of arachidonic acid from the plasma membrane and the production of prostaglandins and leukotrienes. *ECF,* Eosinophil chemotactic factor; *NCF,* neutrophil chemotactic factor; *PAF,* platelet-activating factor. (From Kumar V, Abbas AK, Fausto N, et al: *Robbins & Cotran pathologic basis of disease,* ed 8, Philadelphia, 2009, Saunders.)

Mast cells are a heterogeneous population of bone marrow–derived cells that reside in vascularized tissue. Mast cells are easily identified by their abundant metachromatic cytoplasmic granules. Metachromasia is defined as the staining of a tissue component so that the color (absorption spectrum) of the tissue-dye complex differs from the color of the original dye and of the other stained tissue. In other words, the metachromatic substance is a different color from those of the dye and the other stained tissue. For example, toluidine blue is a metachromatic dye, and it stains most tissues blue, but mast cell granules are purple. Other commonly used metachromatic dyes include methylene blue and thionine. Wright's and Giemsa stains are dye mixtures that include a metachromatic dye. Mast cells can be divided into mucosal and connective tissue subpopulations, not only based on their location but also on their phenotypic, morphologic, histochemical, and functional characteristics. This suggests that individual subpopulations of mast cells may have specific functions in normal and pathologic responses that are a result of their activation. The tyrosine kinase receptor, c-kit, expressed on mast cells, their precursors, and its ligand—stem cell factor (SCF)—is essential to mast cell development and function. Alterations in c-kit have been used to molecularly identify poorly differentiated mast cell tumors.

Mast cell activation can occur through a number of immunologic and nonimmunologic mechanisms. In addition to the activation of mast cells through cross-linking of membrane-bound IgE by antigen, other substances and stimuli can also activate mast cells. Mast cells can be activated by Fcε receptor–independent mechanisms, including cytokines (IL-8), complement products (the anaphylatoxins C3a and C5a), drugs (nonsteroidal antiinflammatory drugs, codeine, and morphine), and physical stimuli (heat, cold, and trauma). Non–IgE-mediated activation of mast cells is referred to as an *anaphylactoid reaction,* whereas the IgE-mediated activation is referred to as *type I hypersensitivity.* There are species and tissue differences in how type I reactions are manifested, and these are attributable to the types and proportions of mediators produced by the mast cell. Mast cells are a heterogeneous population of cells with regard to their structure and function. Although they are generally divided into mucosal-based and connective tissue–based populations, in either case they are primarily found adjacent to blood vessels and nerves where their mediators have their greatest influence. Mediators released by mast cells are broadly classified as preformed (primary) or newly synthesized (secondary), and as presented in Web Table 5-3 and Fig. 5-17, they influence local tissues and other cell types. Primary mediators are stored in cytoplasmic granules and include the vasoactive amines histamine, serotonin, and adenosine; chemotactic factors for eosinophils and neutrophils; enzymes, including neutral proteases and acid hydrolases; and proteoglycans, such as heparin and the chondroitin sulfates. Newly synthesized mediators consist largely of the lipid mediator products of cyclooxygenase and lipoxygenase metabolism of arachidonic acid (see Chapter 3), a number of cytokines and platelet-activating factor (PAF). The major products of arachidonic metabolism are the prostaglandins and leukotrienes, of which prostaglandin D_2 and leukotrienes C_4, D_4, and E_4 are most important. The major cytokines released from mast cells during a type I reaction include IL-4, IL-5, IL-6, and TNF-α. IL-4 and IL-5 contribute to B lymphocyte activation and IgE synthesis. IL-5 is chemotactic for eosinophils. IL-6 and TNF-α are involved in the pathogenesis of shock during a systemic type I (anaphylactic) reaction. The biochemical events involved in IgE-mediated activation and mediator release by mast cells are similar to those described for leukocyte activation in Chapter 3. The primary actions of preformed and newly synthesized mediators are attributable to cellular infiltration, vasoactive responses, and smooth muscle contraction. PAF, which was first identified as an initiator of platelet aggregation and degranulation, functions not only in the acute phase by increasing vasodilation and vascular permeability but is also important early in the late phase by recruiting and activating inflammatory cells. Finally, it is of note that recent studies have identified TLR pathways that mediate interactions between dendritic cells, T lymphocytes, and mast cells, thus modulating type I responses.

A type I reaction begins as an acute inflammatory reaction mediated largely by the vasoactive amines released by degranulation of mast cells. It is during this early stage that mast cells also release large quantities of chemotactic factors and cytokines. These mediators recruit and activate the inflammatory cells that will not only sustain the inflammatory response in the absence of antigen but also cause tissue damage. The immediate response is characterized by increased blood flow, increased vascular permeability (edema), and smooth muscle spasm. As the reaction progresses, additional leukocytes are recruited, and they release biologically active substances that cause cell damage. Of these leukocytes, eosinophils are particularly important.

Eosinophils are recruited to the sites of type I hypersensitivity reactions by chemokines, such as eotaxin, and their survival is influenced by IL-3, IL-5, and GM-CSF, which are largely derived from T_H2 lymphocytes. Eosinophils recruited during the early response play an active role in the late-phase response by releasing components of their granules, synthesizing lipid mediators, and producing cytokines. The basic proteins released by eosinophils are toxic to parasites and host tissue. In particular, eosinophil major basic protein is toxic not only to parasites but also to tumor cells and normal cells. These proteins contribute to the epithelial cell damage associated with chronic type I reactions. Lipid mediators synthesized by activated eosinophils include PAF, leukotrienes, and lipoxins. Cytokines produced and released by eosinophils include growth factors, chemokines, cytokines involved in inflammation and repair, and regulatory cytokines. Macrophages and lymphocytes also participate in the late-phase response to varying degrees.

Epithelial cells further contribute to the inflammation by becoming activated and producing factors that recruit and activate additional inflammatory cells. It is this complex series of cell activation, recruitment, and mediator release that amplifies the immune response and sustains the inflammatory reaction long after the antigen has gone.

The factors that determine whether a host will develop a type I hypersensitivity reaction are complex. The genetic makeup of the host and the dose and route of antigen exposure are most important. These factors influence whether the individual will have a T_H1 or T_H2 response. The development of an IgE-secreting B lymphocyte from an immature (naïve) B lymphocyte depends on activated $CD4^+$ lymphocytes of the T_H2 type. The cytokines that define a T_H2-lymphocyte response have important roles in regulating the cells involved in a type I hypersensitivity reaction. IL-3, IL-4, and IL-10 influence mast cell production; IL-4 is involved in isotype switching to IgE; and IL-3 and IL-5 influence eosinophil maturation and activation. IL-13 promotes the production of IgE. The major cytokine that defines a T_H1 response, IFN-γ, inhibits the T_H2 response. Thus an animal that develops predominantly a T_H2 response to a particular antigen would be more likely to develop a type I hypersensitivity reaction as compared with one that develops predominantly a T_H1 response. The $CD4^+$ T lymphocyte plays a central role in the pathogenesis of a type I hypersensitivity. In humans, additional genetic influences can be linked to the human leukocyte antigen (HLA)–linked immune response genes. These genes appear to control allergen-specific IgE responses. As mentioned previously, the association of specific class I MHC molecules with an increased susceptibility to atopy in the dog has been proposed. As with the mast cell and the eosinophil, a role for the $CD4^+$ T lymphocyte in the late-phase response has also been described. Studies suggest that the continued production of T_H2 cytokines contributes to the chronic inflammation associated with some chronic type I hypersensitivity reactions.

In summary, type I hypersensitivity is a complex disease process that occurs in sensitized hosts, which can result in three types of responses: (1) an acute inflammatory response, (2) a late-phase response, and (3) a chronic inflammatory response. In sensitized hosts, the cross-linking of IgE on the surface of mast cells results in the immediate release of mediators that influence local tissue and recruit additional inflammatory cells. The acute response is dependent on resident mast cells, whereas the late-phase and chronic responses are dependent on recruited cells, especially the eosinophil. Central to the pathogenesis of a type I hypersensitivity reaction are the T_H2 lymphocytes and the cytokines they produce, which influence IgE production and the recruitment and activation of leukocytes.

Systemic and localized type I hypersensitivity reactions occur in animals. The pathogenesis of many infectious and noninfectious diseases involves the production of IgE and the development of a type I hypersensitivity reaction. Type I hypersensitivity is an allergic reaction that occurs within minutes of exposure to an antigen to which the host has been previously sensitized. Allergy has become synonymous with type I hypersensitivity. By definition, type I hypersensitivity reactions are mediated by IgE. Systemic type I hypersensitivity reactions are called *anaphylaxis.* Atopy is the genetic predisposition to develop localized type I hypersensitivity reactions to innocuous antigens. Atopy is often limited to an organ or tissue such as in allergic dermatitis and rhinitis, food allergies, and asthma. Non–IgE-mediated allergic-like reactions are referred to as anaphylactoid reactions.

Systemic Type I Hypersensitivity (Anaphylaxis)

Anaphylaxis refers to an acute systemic hypersensitivity reaction to an antigen that is mediated by IgE and involves mast cell activation, resulting in a shocklike state often involving multiple organ systems. The clinical signs and pathology attributable to a systemic anaphylactic reaction vary by species and often correlate to the primary shock organ in its most severe manifestation—death. This variation reflects differences in the distribution of the mast cells, the mediator content of their granules that are unique to individual species, and the primary target tissue. The primary target tissues are blood vessels and smooth muscle. Blood vessel beds and smooth muscles vary in their histamine receptor content, and as such some are more susceptible than others to the influences of histamine. Because of the aforementioned, the early signs of anaphylaxis can be varied. Cutaneous signs include pruritus, hyperemia, and angioedema. Cardiovascular signs include hypotension and an accompanying sinus tachycardia (characteristic of a vasovagal response). Respiratory signs include bronchospasms, laryngeal edema, and dyspnea. As the anaphylactic reaction progresses, hypotension or hypoxia may lead to unconsciousness. Fatal anaphylaxis may occur as the result of asphyxiation secondary to edema of the upper airway, circulatory failure as a result of dilation of the splanchnic vascular bed, or hypoxemia as a result of severe bronchospasms. In humans, a body of evidence also implicates human heart mast cells (HHMCs) in myocardial anaphylaxis as a primary mechanism. Other than in cases with upper airway edema or pulmonary hyperinflation (emphysema), there are no pathognomonic lesions of anaphylaxis. The species most sensitive to the development of anaphylaxis is the guinea pig. The most common pathologic findings in most species are pulmonary edema and emphysema, except for dogs, for which the major shock organ is the liver, and severe hepatic congestion and visceral hemorrhage are the most common findings.

The types of antigens that can elicit a systemic anaphylactic reaction are diverse, but most commonly include drugs (especially penicillin-based antibiotics), vaccines, venom of stinging insects, and heterologous sera. Although the greatest risk for the development of an anaphylactic reaction occurs during parenteral administration, it must be noted that in some cases even a small quantity of antigen in a highly sensitized host can elicit a systemic response.

Localized Type I Hypersensitivity

In a localized type I hypersensitivity reaction, the clinical signs and pathologic findings are restricted to a specific tissue or organ. Localized reactions most commonly occur at epithelial surfaces such as the surfaces of the skin and mucosa of the respiratory and gastrointestinal tract. As discussed previously, species differences on the location of mast cells, the mediators contained within them, and the histamine receptor distribution on target tissue may explain the different spectra of diseases seen among individual species.

Allergic dermatitis is a cutaneous manifestation of a type I hypersensitivity reaction that results in inflammation of the skin. The route of exposure to the antigen may be by inhalation, ingestion, or percutaneous absorption. If the allergic dermatitis is thought to have a genetic predisposition, then the disease is referred to as atopic dermatitis. Dietary type I hypersensitivity reactions in the dog and cat more commonly present as a cutaneous disease rather than a gastrointestinal disease. Other common cutaneous manifestations of type I hypersensitivity are flea and other arthropod bites and urticaria and angioedema (hives). All of these diseases are characterized by an acute inflammatory reaction, often perivascular, caused by mediators released from sensitized mast cells. In some instances, as in atopic dermatitis, the lesion may progress to a late-phase response or chronic inflammation characterized by more intense inflammatory infiltrates (e.g., atopic dermatitis) or to a type IV hypersensitivity reaction (arthropod bites). Other secondary changes, such as acanthosis, hyperpigmentation, sebaceous gland metaplasia, and pyoderma, occur in long-standing cases or in animals that have significant trauma related to pruritus.

Allergic rhinitis is a respiratory manifestation of a type I hypersensitivity reaction that most commonly develops in ruminants. The most common antigens are grass and weed pollens and mold spores *(Micropolyspora faeni)*. This disease also frequently progresses from an acute inflammatory disease to a late-phase response and chronic inflammation. In cattle, long-standing allergic rhinitis may progress to a type IV hypersensitivity reaction with the formation of nasal granulomas. Mold spores *(Micropolyspora faeni)* are more frequently associated with a type III hypersensitivity reaction, resulting in an allergic pneumonitis (extrinsic allergic alveolitis).

Although an inherited predisposition has been implicated in some species, the exact mode of inheritance remains to be determined. In humans, a link to genes encoding IL-4 and certain MHC antigens, important components of allergic diseases, has been made.

Type II Hypersensitivity (Cytotoxic Hypersensitivity)

In the original Gell and Coombs classification, the type II hypersensitivity reaction was designated as antibody-mediated cytotoxic hypersensitivity. This type of hypersensitivity most often occurs as the result of the development of antibodies directed against antigens on the surface of a cell or in a tissue, with the result that the cell or tissue is destroyed. Antigens may be either endogenous (normal cellular or tissue protein) or exogenous (e.g., a drug or microbial protein adsorbed to the cell). In some instances, the antigen may be a cell surface receptor and the antibody may activate or block the activation of the cell rather than cause cytotoxicity. The pathogenesis of many immune-mediated and autoimmune diseases is centered on the development of antireceptor or antisurface antigen antibodies and a type II hypersensitivity reaction. The largest group of "cytotoxic" hypersensitivity reactions involves the hematologic diseases, with antibodies directed against antigens present on the surface of red blood cells and platelets. Type II hypersensitivity reactions are mediated by antibodies directed against antigens on the surface of tissue or cells so that the tissue or cell is destroyed or the function of the cell is altered. Type II hypersensitivity reactions most frequently involve IgM and IgG and occur within hours after exposure in a sensitized host.

There are three basic antibody-mediated mechanisms that result in type II hypersensitivity (Fig. 5-18). Complement-dependent reactions occur as a result of the complement activating capability of IgG and IgM. Complement activation can mediate cytotoxicity by either the formation of the membrane attack complex, resulting in cell lysis, or the fixation of C3b fragments (opsonization) to the surface facilitating phagocytosis (see Chapter 3). Antibody-dependent reactions can similarly opsonize cells, facilitating phagocytosis, or result in cell lysis by antibody-dependent cellular cytotoxicity. Opsonization of cells by antibody makes them susceptible to destruction by macrophages, neutrophils, NK cells, and eosinophils, all of which bear FcR. This is commonly referred to as *antibody-dependent cellular cytotoxicity* (ADCC). Finally, antibodies directed against surface receptors may result in altered cell or tissue function. The antireceptor antibodies can function

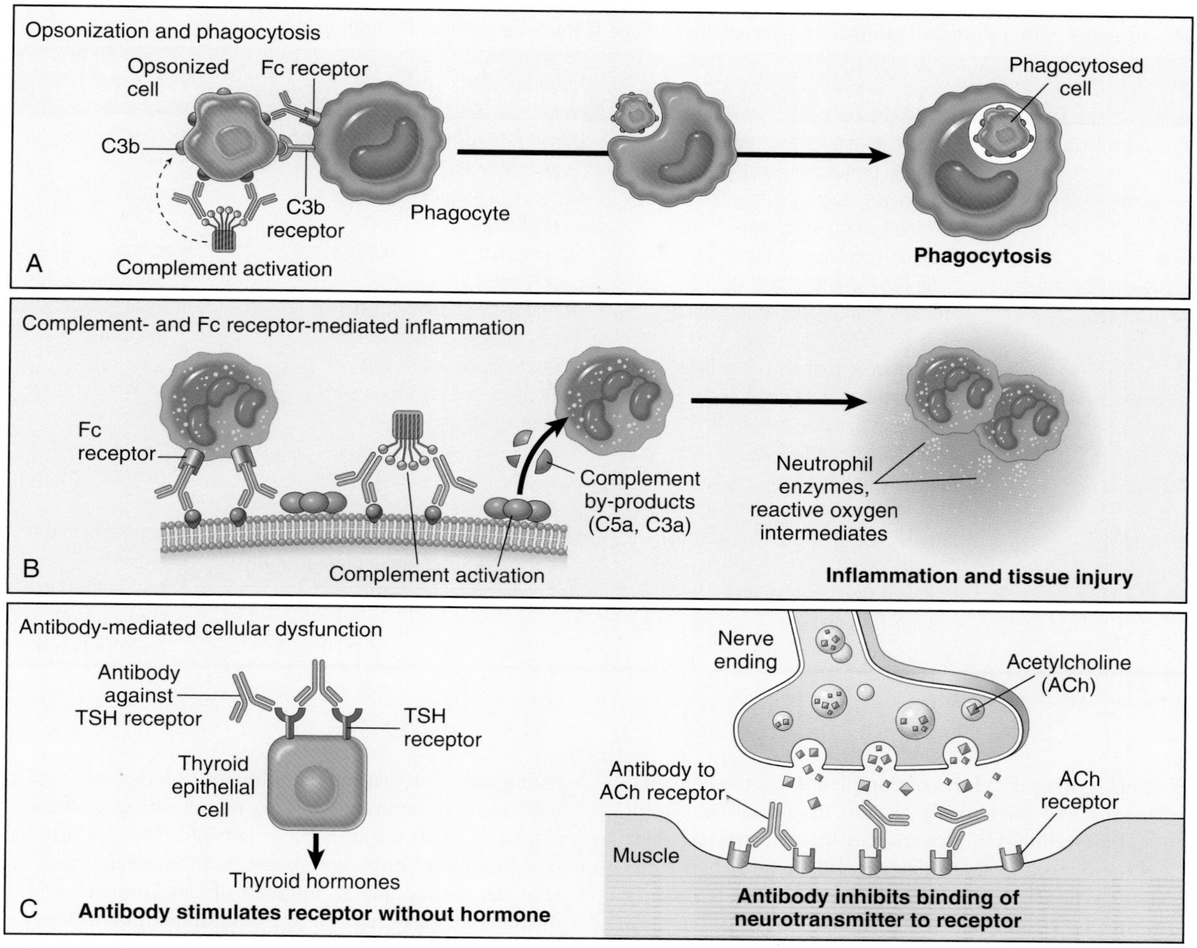

Fig. 5-18 Schematic depiction of the three major mechanisms of an antibody mediated injury. **A,** Opsonization by antibodies (or complement) enhances phagocytosis of antigen by monocyte-macrophage cells. **B,** Antibody can activate the complement system, via the classical pathway, resulting in the elaboration of inflammatory mediators, such as C5a and C3a. **C,** Antibodies against cell receptors can activate (depicted) or inhibit (not depicted) cell functions. *TSH,* Thyroid-stimulating hormone. (**A, B,** and **C** from Kumar V, Abbas AK, Fausto N, et al: *Robbins & Cotran pathologic basis of disease,* ed 8, Philadelphia, 2009, Saunders.)

as agonists, stimulating cell function, or as antagonists, blocking receptor function.

Diseases with a type II hypersensitivity pathogenesis are presented in Table 5-5. The physical and biochemical properties of red blood cells, platelets, and leukocytes make them susceptible to cytotoxic reactions. Two properties of red blood cells make them uniquely susceptible to being involved in type II reactions. First, their surface contains a complex array of blood group antigens that can become targets of antibody responses as is commonly the case in transfusion reactions or immune-mediated hemolytic disease of the newborn. Second, the biochemical properties of red blood cells make them prone to adsorb substances such as drugs or antigenic components of infectious agents or tumors. In these instances, the red blood cell may be either directly targeted because the substance alters a surface protein to an extent that it is now recognized as foreign, or indirectly targeted if there is an antibody response to the substance itself. Finally, in autoimmune forms of hemolytic anemia, agranulocytosis, and thrombocytopenia, there is a breakdown of tolerance and the subsequent development of antibodies to normal cells, and as a result they are destroyed.

The majority of cytotoxic type II diseases result in a decrease or loss of a population of cells (e.g., anemia, thrombocytopenia). Noncytotoxic type II diseases are initially characterized by activation or inhibition of cell or tissue function followed by inflammation, which may cause inflammatory damage to the targeted organ. In a type II reaction, the pathogenesis commonly begins with cell surface antigens eliciting an antibody response, whereby the antibodies bind to the cell and the cell is either lysed or complement components attract phagocytic cells that damage tissues by releasing proteolytic enzymes.

Type III Hypersensitivity (Immune Complex Hypersensitivity)

Type III hypersensitivity is designated as immune complex hypersensitivity. This reaction occurs through the formation of antigen-antibody complexes that activate complement and result in tissue damage (Fig. 5-19). The cell or tissue injury is similar to a type II hypersensitivity reaction, although the underlying pathogenesis is different. With a type III reaction, the cell or tissue is being destroyed not because the antibody is being directed against that cell or tissue, but rather because immune complexes either become "stuck" to that cell or are deposited in that tissue. Think of it as an "innocent bystander" reaction: The targeted tissue is not a direct target of the immune response. The pathogenesis begins with the formation of immune complexes that become lodged or are formed in or deposited in tissue and are capable of activating

TABLE 5-5 Diseases with a Primary Cytotoxic Hypersensitivity (Type II Hypersensitivity) Pathogenesis

Disease	Target Antigen	Mechanisms of Disease	Clinicopathologic Manifestations
Autoimmune hemolytic anemia	Erythrocyte membrane proteins (blood group antigens)	Opsonization and phagocytosis of erythrocytes	Hemolysis, anemia
Neonatal isoerythrolysis	Erythrocyte membrane proteins (blood group antigens)	Opsonization and phagocytosis of erythrocytes	Hemolysis, anemia
Autoimmune thrombocytopenic purpura	Platelet membrane proteins (gpIIb : IIIa integrin)	Opsonization and phagocytosis of platelets	Bleeding
Pemphigus diseases	Proteins in intercellular junctions of epidermal cells (e.g., the epidermal cadherin desmoglein 1)	Antibody-mediated activation of proteases, disruption of intercellular adhesions	Vesiculobullous (diseases of the skin)
Vasculitis caused by ANCA	Neutrophil granule proteins, presumably released from activated neutrophils	Neutrophil degranulation and inflammation	Vasculitis
Myasthenia gravis	Acetylcholine receptor	Antibody inhibits acetylcholine binding, downmodulates receptors	Muscle weakness, paralysis
Pernicious anemia	Intrinsic factor of gastric parietal cells	Neutralization of intrinsic factor, decreased absorption of vitamin B_{12}	Abnormal erythropoiesis, anemia
Bullous pemphigoid	Collagen type XVII within hemidesmosomes	Antibodies against basal cells	Subepidermal vesicles characterized by basement membrane clefts

ANCA, Antineutrophil cytoplasmic antibody.

the complement system. Products of complement activation such as anaphylatoxins and chemotactic factors result in neutrophil infiltration and activation. On activation, neutrophils release their enzymes and these result in tissue damage. Like type II hypersensitivity reactions, type III hypersensitivity reactions most frequently involve IgM and IgG and occur within hours after exposure in a sensitized host.

Antigen-antibody complexes form as a part of a normal immune response and usually facilitate the clearance of antigen by the phagocytic system without resulting in a type III hypersensitivity reaction. Although a number of factors determine whether a type III reaction will occur, the most important is the relationship of the antibody response to the quantity of antigen. When antibody is in great excess of antigen, the antigen-antibody complexes formed are large and insoluble, and easily removed by the phagocytic system. When antigen is in great excess of the quantity of antibody, the antigen-antibody complexes formed are too small to be capable of becoming lodged in tissues or of activating the complement system. However, when antigen is in slight excess of antibody, these small soluble complexes can become lodged in tissue and activate the complement system. When this type of small soluble antigen-antibody complex is formed in the circulation, their accumulation in tissue is essentially the result of anatomic and physiologic processes and has no immunologic basis. Finally, it has also been suggested that in some instances immune complex hypersensitivity may be the result of the normal phagocytic system being overwhelmed. Immune complex deposition can be localized to a tissue or generalized if the complexes are formed in circulation. Blood vessels, synovial membranes, glomeruli, and the choroid plexus are particularly vulnerable to deposition of immune complexes. The concentration and size of the complexes determine the sites of deposition.

Type III reactions can develop from antibody responses to endogenous or exogenous antigens and immune complexes can be deposited in a number of tissues (Table 5-6). Although a number of diseases of domestic species involve a type III hypersensitivity pathogenesis, a majority of diseases are the result of persistent infections, autoimmune disease, or inhalation of foreign antigen. Organisms that result in persistent infections are often characterized by a weak antibody response and the development of immune complex formation. A number of autoimmune and immune-mediated diseases result in the development of antibody responses to self-antigens or antigens complexed to self-proteins, and these are capable of generating complement-activating immune complexes. Immune complexes formed against commonly inhaled environmental antigens can lead to the development of an allergic alveolitis. Type III hypersensitivity reactions are mediated by the formation of antigen-antibody complexes, which results in complement activation leading to an influx of neutrophils and subsequent cell or tissue destruction. Antigen-antibody complexes may be formed in the circulation and lodge in tissue or may be formed in the tissue directly. The cell or tissue injury is largely determined by physiologic or anatomic properties rather than an immunologic basis. The pathogenesis of a number of diseases of domestic animals have a type III hypersensitivity basis.

Localized Type III Hypersensitivity

Localized type III hypersensitivity reactions are best exemplified by the Arthus reaction (see Fig. 5-19). The parenteral administration of an antigen to an animal that has a circulating antibody specific for that antigen results in a localized acute inflammatory response. The complexes are formed either within the tissue at the site of antigen deposition or localized within blood vessels, as the antigen and antibody diffuse into the vascular wall. Early, within hours, the reaction is characterized by margination and emigration of neutrophils to and from the blood vessels and progressively results in tissue and vascular damage. The quantity of antigen-antibody complexes formed in the wall of the vessel determines the extent of the tissue damage. Small quantities of complexes may result in only mild hyperemia and edema. Large quantities of complexes may result in tissue and vascular necrosis as a result of neutrophils releasing the contents of their granules. In some cases, the

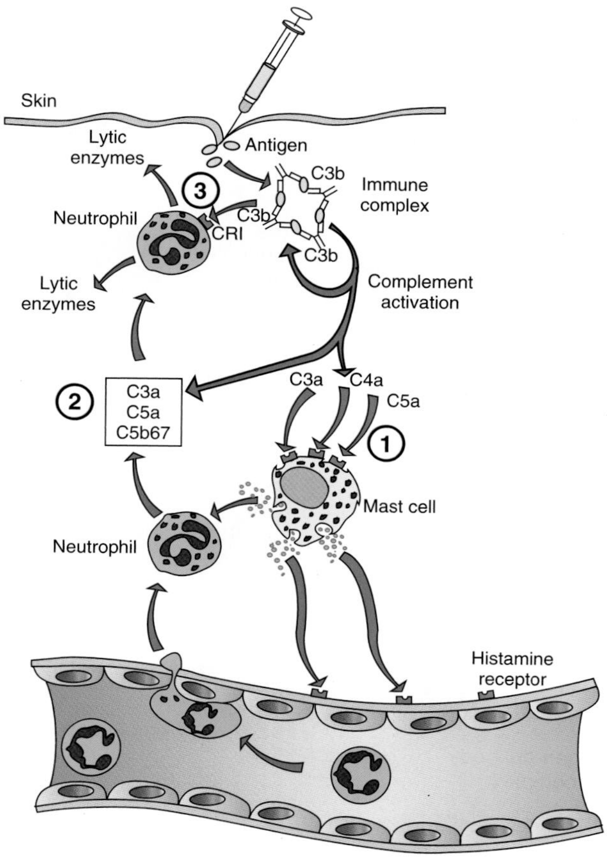

Fig. 5-19 A localized type III hypersensitivity reaction (Arthus reaction) in the dermis.

Antigen-antibody complexes, formed at the site of injection, activate the complement system to elaborate components that activate resident mast cells (1) and attract circulating neutrophils (2). Inflammation is the result of tissue damage caused by mediators and enzymes released from both cell types (3). *CRI,* Complement receptor 1. (Adapted from Goldsby RA, Kindt TJ, Osborne BA: *Kuby immunology,* ed 4, New York, 2000, WH Freeman.)

damage to the wall may be so severe as to cause thrombosis and localized ischemic injury. The Arthus reaction is still used today as an experimental model of a localized type III reaction. Recent studies, using the cutaneous Arthus reaction in complement-deficient mice, document the requirement of FcR activation for eliciting an inflammatory response and a revision of the hypothesis of the mechanism of immune complex-mediated inflammation. Complement components, such as C5a, are generated as a result of FcR activation. Conversely, the use of FcR-deficient mice and the Arthus reaction establish the requirement of this receptor because immune complexes and C3 alone are not sufficient to trigger an inflammatory response and tissue damage.

Many diseases have a progressive clinical course, and immune complex reactions often play a role, even though they may not be involved in the initial immunologic response. There are limited clinical examples of diseases characterized primarily by a localized immune complex reaction. One dramatic example is blue eye in the dog, which is an anterior uveitis that develops in a small percentage of dogs naturally infected with or vaccinated against canine adenovirus type I. Other organs commonly affected by localized immune complex disease include the lung and skin. In the lung, chronic exposure of the lower airways to inhaled antigens can lead to the development of antigen-specific antibodies that form complexes within alveolar walls. This form of allergic lung disease is commonly referred to as *allergic pneumonitis* (extrinsic allergic alveolitis). Common antigens include spore-forming organisms (e.g., some actinomycetes and fungi). Allergic diseases of the lower airways frequently lead to type II pneumocyte hyperplasia, emphysema, and fibrosis, which are all secondary to inflammation and tissue damage mediated by type III hypersensitivity. Chronic obstructive pulmonary disease (COPD) in horses may be caused in part by a localized type III reaction to spore-forming organisms or dust that results in bronchiolitis (see Chapter 9). In dogs, staphylococcal infections of the skin may develop a type I, III, or IV reaction. In the case of a type III reaction, a neutrophilic dermal vasculitis is often evident (see Chapter 17).

Generalized Type III Hypersensitivity

When antigen is present in the circulation at appropriate concentrations relative to circulating antibody concentrations (as discussed

TABLE 5-6 Diseases with a Primary Type III Hypersensitivity (Immune Complex Hypersensitivity) Pathogenesis

Disease	Antigen Involved	Clinicopathologic Manifestations
Systemic lupus erythematosus	DNA, nucleoproteins, others	Glomerulonephritis, arthritis, vasculitis
Blue eye	Canine adenovirus 1 antigen	Anterior uveitis
Equine infectious anemia	Viral antigens	Anemia, thrombocytopenia
Poststaphylococcal hypersensitivity	Staphylococcal cell wall antigens	Dermatitis
Cutaneous vasculitis	Bacterial antigens, viral antigens, drugs	Vasculitis
Poststreptococcal (*Streptococcus equi* ssp. *equi*) hypersensitivity	M protein	Purpura hemorrhagica, glomerulonephritis
Acute glomerulonephritis	Bacterial antigens; parasite antigens; viral antigens; tumor antigens	Nephritis
Reactive arthritis	Bacterial antigens	Acute arthritis
Arthus reaction	Various foreign proteins	Cutaneous vasculitis
Serum sickness	Various proteins (e.g., foreign serum)	Arthritis, vasculitis, nephritis
Hypersensitivity pneumonitis	Fungal spores, dust	Alveolitis, vasculitis
COPD	Fungal spores, dust	Bronchiolitis
Aleutian mink disease	Viral antigens	Glomerulonephritis, vasculitis
Rheumatoid arthritis	IgG	Erosive polyarthritis

COPD, Chronic obstructive pulmonary disease; *IgG,* immunoglobulin G.

previously), the result is the formation of immune complexes capable of generating a type III hypersensitivity reaction. Serum sickness is the prototypical disease with a type III hypersensitivity pathogenesis. Early examples of this disease were the result of the administration of heterologous serum, which led to the formation of circulating immune complexes that became lodged primarily in blood vessels, glomeruli, and joints. The blood vessel, glomerulus, or joint was not a target of the immune response but rather an "innocent bystander" because the resulting inflammation occurred as a result of the complement activating capacity of the immune complexes that lodged there.

The pathogenesis of a systemic immune complex disease is best illustrated in three phases as depicted in Fig. 5-20. The first phase, as discussed previously, occurs when the host develops an antibody response to an antigen so that the ratio of antigen to antibody is appropriate for the formation of small, soluble circulating complexes that are not adequately cleared by the monocyte-macrophage system. Because the formation of antigen-antibody complexes can be a normal component of an immune response, the presence of immune complexes in circulation by itself is not sufficient to diagnose an immune complex disease. In the second phase, the complexes adhere to cells or lodge in tissues that are uniquely susceptible to circulating immune complexes. The biochemical properties of the antigen-antibody complexes (e.g., overall quantity and size, charge) and the physiologic and anatomic characteristics of some cells and tissues account for their unique susceptibility to immune complex deposition. Other factors may also contribute to the formation or deposition of immune complexes in certain tissues. For example, in rheumatoid arthritis, it has been proposed that lymphocytes within the joint may produce an altered IgG molecule that stimulates the production of rheumatoid factor (anti-IgG). Complexes become lodged within blood vessel walls and extravascular tissues as a result of the increased vascular permeability caused by the anaphylatoxins and vasoactive amines released from neutrophils, activated through the binding of antigen-antibody complexes to complement and FcR on their surface. The result is phase three: the activation of the complement system and the development of an acute inflammatory reaction centered on the vasculature. Neutrophils and macrophages are activated similarly through FcR and produce a number of inflammatory cytokines that attract and activate additional inflammatory cells. The inflammatory cells and mediators have been thoroughly discussed in Chapter 3. Immune complexes that lodge in blood vessels, glomeruli, or joints result in vasculitis, glomerulonephritis, and arthritis, respectively. The damage to the vessels also results in damage to the intima and exposure of collagen, which initiates the formation of microthrombi by the activation of the coagulation cascade and platelets.

The two primary cell types involved in a type III hypersensitivity reaction are FcR–bearing neutrophils and macrophages (Fig. 5-21). Complement activation leads to the elaboration of factors (primarily C5a) that are chemotactic and attract neutrophils and macrophages to the site. These cells are activated and produce a number of proinflammatory cytokines. Early in the response, these cells release vasoactive amines that cause increased vascular permeability, allowing the immune complexes to lodge within the vessel wall. Many of these phagocytic cells are also stimulated to release their proteolytic enzymes and toxic free radicals, and these processes result in tissue and vascular damage. Platelets also contribute to the developing inflammatory reaction by releasing vasoactive amines and other proinflammatory constituents.

Diseases associated with type III hypersensitivity reactions are most commonly associated with a single exposure to a large quantity of antigen (e.g., administration of heterologous serum or from an immune response to systemic infections) or from continuous exposures to small quantities of antigen as in the case of autoimmune diseases (e.g., rheumatoid arthritis and systemic lupus erythematosus). In either of these instances, the development of type III hypersensitivity depends on antigen in excess of antibody.

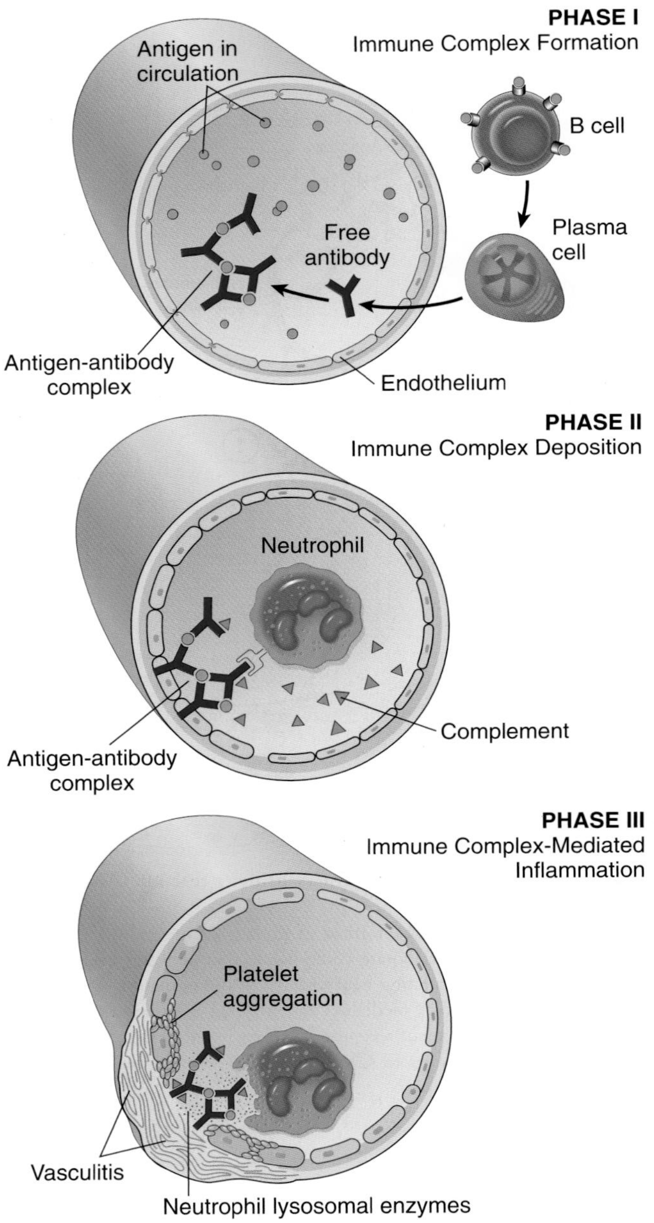

Fig. 5-20 Schematic depiction of the three phases of a systemic type III hypersensitivity reaction.
The first phase results in immune complex formation. In the second phase, the antigen-antibody complexes become lodged in the vessel wall and activate inflammatory cells. The end result, the third phase, is the elicitation of tissue damage and an inflammatory response. (From Kumar V, Abbas AK, Fausto N, et al: *Robbins & Cotran pathologic basis of disease*, ed 8, Philadelphia, 2009, Saunders.)

Type IV Hypersensitivity (Delayed-Type Hypersensitivity)

Type IV hypersensitivity is also known as *cell-mediated hypersensitivity* because it is the result of the interaction of T lymphocytes

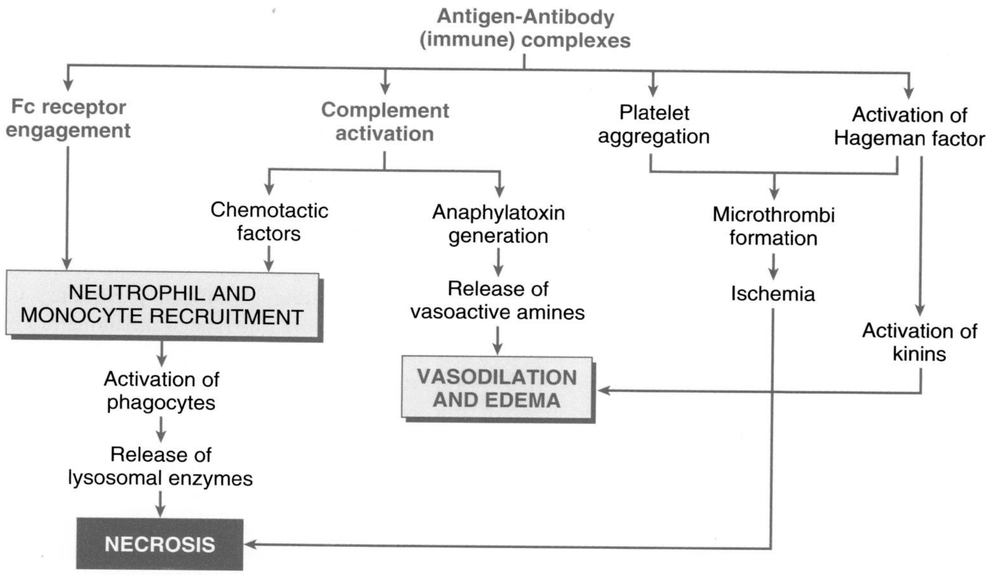

Fig. 5-21 Pathogenesis of type III hypersensitivity reactions and the morphologic consequences. Locally or systemically deposited immune complexes result in tissue damage and inflammation by activation of the complement system and through activation of neutrophils and macrophages through their Fc receptors. Activation of a component of the coagulation system also contributes to the tissue damage. (From Kumar V, Abbas AK, Fausto N: *Robbins & Cotran pathologic basis of disease,* ed 7, Philadelphia, 2005, Saunders.)

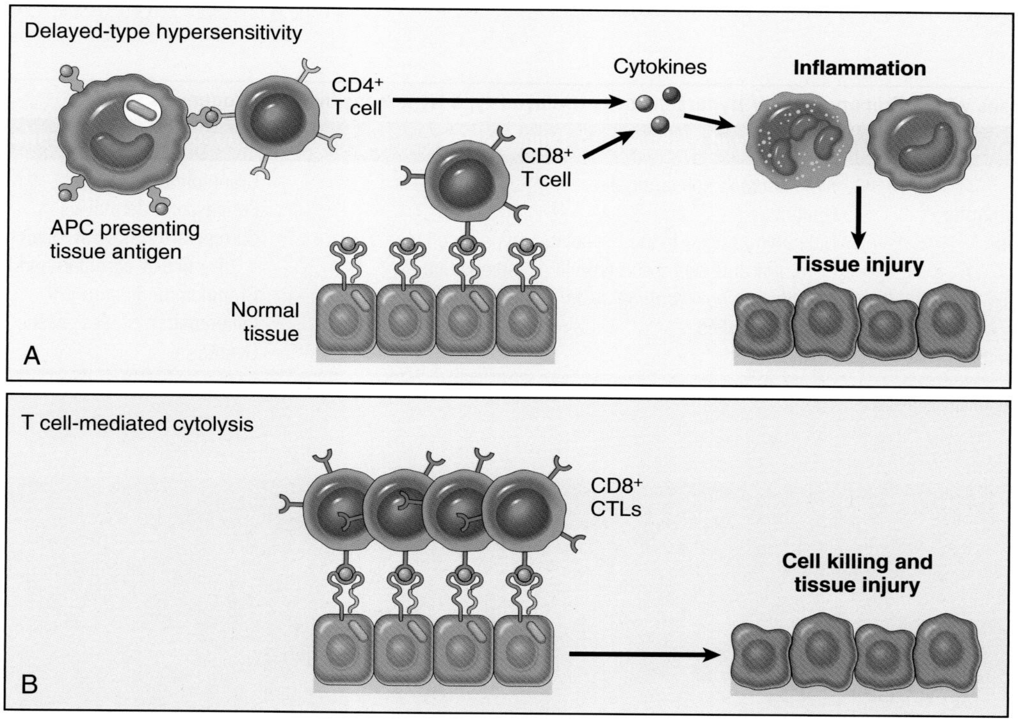

Fig. 5-22 The two primary mechanisms of T lymphocytes that cause type IV hypersensitivity reaction. **A,** $CD4^+$ T lymphocytes (and occasionally $CD8^+$ lymphocytes) are activated by antigen and produce cytokines that attract other cell types and promote an inflammatory response. **B,** $CD8^+$ T lymphocytes (cytotoxic T lymphocytes *[CTLs]*) are also activated by antigen and can cause inflammation by killing targeted cells and tissue. *APC,* Antigen-presenting cell. (**A** and **B** from Kumar V, Abbas AK, Fausto N, et al: *Robbins & Cotran pathologic basis of disease,* ed 8, Philadelphia, 2009, Saunders.)

and the specific antigen to which they have been sensitized. The resulting immune response is mediated either by direct cytotoxicity by $CD8^+$ T lymphocytes or by the release of soluble cytokines from $CD4^+$ lymphocytes, which act through mediator cells (primarily macrophages) to produce chronic inflammatory reactions (Fig. 5-22). Because these responses are dependent on sensitized T lymphocytes and require 24 to 48 hours to develop, they are also referred to as *delayed-type hypersensitivity* (DTH). Unlike type I, II, and III hypersensitivity reactions, type IV hypersensitivity is not dependent on an antibody. We first discuss the response mediated primarily by activated $CD4^+$ lymphocytes. The prototypical DTH reaction is the localized tuberculin response. After an intradermal exposure of tuberculin, a purified protein derivative (PPD) of the tubercle bacillus, a previously sensitized host will develop a localized type IV reaction at the site of inoculation at 24 to 72 hours. The intradermal antigens are taken up and processed by dendritic Langerhans' cells, which present antigenic peptides to antigen-specific CD4$^+$ lymphocytes that are activated to produce and secrete cytokines that attract and activate other inflammatory cells. Grossly the site appears as a swollen, firm nodule. Microscopically the nodule is composed of interstitial edema and a mononuclear infiltrate that is primarily centered around blood vessels. Early (<12 hours), the infiltrate is primarily neutrophilic, which is replaced largely by macrophages and lymphocytes (>12 hours). The DTH response is generally minimal and short lived because the concentration of PPD injected is small and rapidly degraded. A similar DTH reaction can be used to test for previous exposures to a number of intracellular organisms.

In addition to the tuberculin response, type IV hypersensitivity is the underlying pathogenesis for allergic contact hypersensitivity and granulomatous inflammatory responses. As mentioned with the other hypersensitivity reactions, the components of a type IV hypersensitivity reaction can be considered beneficial (protective immunity) when they occur as an appropriate response to intracellular organisms, or they can be considered harmful (hypersensitivity), for example, when they occur as an inappropriate response to exogenous chemicals or substances that are complexed with proteins, as in the case of allergic contact hypersensitivity.

In the tuberculin reaction, the quantity of antigen limits the extent of the inflammatory response, and resolution of the inflammation generally occurs in 5 to 7 days. This is in contrast to chronic infections with persistent intracellular organisms or poorly degradable intracellular antigens (Table 5-7) that develop into a specific type of chronic inflammatory response called *granulomatous inflammation*. DTH reactions frequently occur in response to intracellular organisms and cause extensive tissue damage. These diseases are characterized by granulomatous inflammation. In this type of response, the host is unable to destroy or eliminate the organism, resulting in antigen persistence. Compared with the tuberculin reaction, the type of inflammatory infiltrate is different. As discussed in Chapter 3, granulomatous inflammation designates that the inflammatory infiltrate has specific attributes, notably the presence of morphologically transformed macrophages into epithelial-like cells commonly called *epithelioid macrophages* (Figs. 5-23 and 5-24). Concurrently, there may be many multinucleated giant cells that represent fused macrophages. A number of fusion-related monocyte-macrophage surface proteins have been identified and include receptors for mannose and β_1 integrin, Src homology 2 domain-containing protein tyrosine phosphatase substrate 1 (SHPS-1), and the chemoattractant chemokine ligand 2. Lymphocytes can also represent a significant component of the inflammatory infiltrate. Generally, CD4$^+$ lymphocytes are interspersed with the macrophages, and CD8$^+$ lymphocytes are localized to the periphery. As these lesions progress, they may become

TABLE 5-7 Diseases with a Primary Type IV Hypersensitivity (Delayed-type Hypersensitivity) Pathogenesis

Disease	Specificity of Pathogenic T Lymphocytes	Clinicopathologic Manifestations
Tuberculosis	*Mycobacteria* spp. antigens	Granuloma formation
Allergic contact dermatitis	Haptens	Perivascular dermatitis
Rheumatoid arthritis	Unknown antigen in joint synovium (type II collagen?); role of antibodies and type III hypersensitivity?	Chronic arthritis with inflammation, destruction of articular cartilage and bone
Johne's disease	*Mycobacterium paratuberculosis* antigens	Granulomatous enteritis
Allograft rejection	MHC molecules	Inflammation of graft tissue
Equine recurrent uveitis	Unknown	Uveitis

MHC, Major histocompatibility complex.

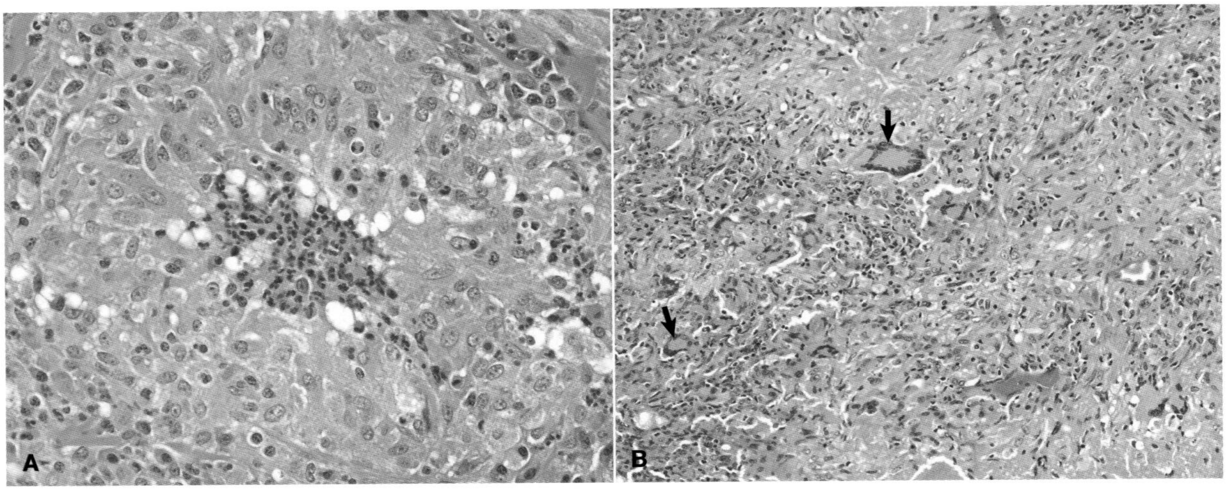

Fig. 5-23 Granulomatous inflammation associated with chronic infections.
A, Blastomycosis, skin, dog. Note the granuloma composed of sheets of epithelioid macrophages and the central focus of neutrophils. H&E stain. **B,** Mycobacteriosis, lung, gazelle. Numerous epithelioid macrophages and multinucleated Langhans'-type giant cells *(arrows)* constitute the granulomatous tissue that has replaced normal lung parenchyma. H&E stain. (**A** and **B** courtesy Dr. P.W. Snyder, School of Veterinary Medicine, Purdue University.)

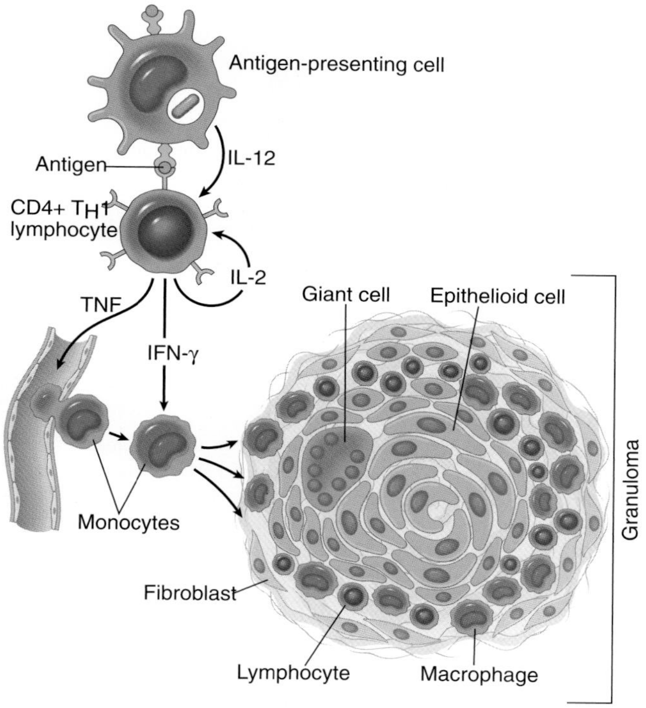

Fig. 5-24 Schematic depiction of granuloma formation in a type IV hypersensitivity reaction.

A T_H1 lymphocyte synthesizes cytokines in response to interleukin-12 production and antigen presentation by an antigen-presenting cell. The cytokines activate additional T_H1 lymphocytes (IL-2) and monocyte-macrophage cells *(IFN-γ),* and promote localized and systemic inflammatory responses (TNF-α). As the response develops, macrophages fuse to form multinucleated giant cells, and fibroblasts are stimulated to synthesize collagen, resulting in the formation of a granuloma. *IL,* Interleukin; *IFN-γ,* interferon; *TNF-α,* tumor necrosis factor-α. (From Kumar V, Abbas AK, Fausto N: *Robbins & Cotran pathologic basis of disease,* ed 7, Philadelphia, 2005, Saunders.)

organized into nodules commonly called *granulomas* (see Fig. 5-23, *A*). Depending on the inciting antigen, there may also be varying proportions of necrosis (often as a necrotic center), calcification of the necrotic tissue, and peripheral fibrous encapsulation. These features are largely the result of lytic enzymes released from activated macrophages. Nonimmunologic granulomas can occur in cases of foreign-body type granulomas, which typically have fewer lymphocytes. In either case, the body is trying to limit the spread or wall-off the inciting antigen.

The type IV hypersensitivity reaction is immunologically specific and like all the hypersensitivity reactions involves a sensitization phase and an effector phase. The sensitization phase occurs with the initial exposure to the antigen and results in the development of antigen-specific memory T lymphocytes. These $CD4^+$ lymphocytes recognize peptides presented in the context of class II molecules on the surface of antigen-presenting cells. In this context, the naïve $CD4^+$ T lymphocytes develop into functional T_H1 lymphocytes. These activated T_H1 lymphocytes are sometimes designated as T_{DTH} lymphocytes. Once the host is sensitized, a prolonged exposure or repeat exposure to the antigen results in the development of an effector phase. The effector phase can occur as a cytotoxic response mediated by $CD8^+$ lymphocytes or more commonly as a T_H1 response through the elaboration of cytokines by $CD4^+$ lymphocytes (see Fig. 5-24). T_H1 cytokines (most importantly, IL-2, IL-3, IFN-γ, and TNF-β) and chemokines (IL-8, macrophage chemotactic and activating factor, and macrophage-inhibition factor) enhance the function of cytokine-producing T lymphocytes (autocrine and paracrine fashion) and attract and activate macrophages. IL-2 induces the proliferation and long-term survival of T lymphocytes. IL-3 supports the growth and differentiation of T_H1 lymphocytes and NK cells. IFN-γ, the key mediator of type IV hypersensitivity, activates macrophages not only to enhance their phagocytic and killing mechanisms but also to enhance their ability to present antigen by inducing increased expression of class II MHC molecules. Activated macrophages and dendritic cells produce IL-12, which also facilitates the development of T_H1 lymphocytes. Activated macrophages also produce IL-1 and TNF-α, both of which act locally to increase the expression of adhesion molecules on endothelial cells, which further facilitates the extravasation of additional inflammatory cells. The production of cytokines and chemokines by the $CD4^+$ T_H1 lymphocytes influences macrophage function and mediates the production of cytokines that influence $CD4^+$ lymphocytes, resulting in a response that potentially goes from a beneficial protective response (immunity) to a harmful response that results in tissue damage (hypersensitivity).

The beneficial protective response of T lymphocyte–mediated hypersensitivity is not limited to intracellular organisms. It also can be a primary component of transplant rejection and immunity to cancer. There are other harmful T lymphocyte–mediated responses that result in disease. One example is allergic contact hypersensitivity. In allergic contact hypersensitivity, the antigen is often too small to elicit an immune response by itself. These antigens must be complexed with other, larger proteins to become antigenic and are specifically referred to as *haptens* or generally called *contact antigens* (Box 5-1). Allergic contact hypersensitivity also depends on processing and presentation of the antigen by dendritic Langerhans' cells to $CD4^+$ lymphocytes in regional lymph nodes. In the case of allergic contact dermatitis, the keratinocyte may also participate by producing a number of cytokines that activate Langerhans' cells, mast cells, and other inflammatory cells. In the sensitization phase, the protein-hapten complex is taken up and processed by Langerhans' cells that migrate to regional lymph nodes. In the paracortex region of the lymph node (T lymphocyte area), they present antigenic components to $CD4^+$ lymphocytes. The host develops a population of memory lymphocytes and is now sensitized to the antigen. In a sensitized host, continuous exposure to the antigen, or more commonly, repeat exposure to the antigen, results in an effector phase response seen as epidermal vesicle formation with dermal and epidermal infiltrates of mononuclear inflammatory cells. The result is tissue damage that is disproportionate to any beneficial effects of the immune response.

Finally, as mentioned earlier, another form of DTH can occur that is mediated by direct cytotoxicity by $CD8^+$ T lymphocytes. This response is most commonly associated with viral infections. $CD8^+$ T lymphocytes, bearing viral antigen-specific TCRs, kill antigen-expressing target cells. These cells are commonly referred to as CTL (T_c). The expression of viral proteins on the surface of an infected cell in association of class I MHC molecules serves as the recognition signal for the TCR-CD3 membrane complex. Following recognition of antigen by the CTL (T_c), there is upregulation of adhesion molecules on the CTL (T_c) and the target cell, resulting in a CTL (T_c)–target cell conjugate. This stimulates an activating signal pathway that results in death of the target cell by apoptosis. The two principal mechanisms of CTL (T_c)-mediated apoptosis are (1) the directional delivery of cytotoxic proteins and (2) the interaction of membrane-bound Fas ligand on the CTL (T_c), with the Fas receptor on the target cell. Both depend on the activation of caspases. Perforins and granzymes are preformed

BOX 5-1 Pathogens and Contact Antigens Commonly Associated with Type IV Hypersensitivity Reactions in Domestic Animals

SOURCES OF ANTIGEN

Infectious Agents

Bacteria
- *Mycobacterium tuberculosis*
- *Mycobacterium bovis*
- *Mycobacterium avium* ssp. *paratuberculosis*
- *Mycobacterium avium* ssp.
- *Listeria monocytogenes*
- *Yersinia* spp.

Viruses
- Lymphocytic choriomeningitis virus

Fungi
- *Blastomyces dermatitidis*
- *Histoplasma capsulatum*
- *Cryptococcus neoformans*

Protozoa
- *Toxoplasma gondii*
- *Leishmania* spp.

Contact Antigens (Haptens)

Components of insecticides in:
- Flea collars
- Sprays
- Dips

Chemical components of plastics, leather, metals, and dyes
Components of shampoos
Topically applied drugs
Pollens
House plants

Allograft Tissues and Cells

MHC molecules

Neoplastic Cells

Tumor-associated antigens
Tumor-specific antigens

MHC, Major histocompatibility complex.

cytotoxic proteins contained in the cytoplasmic granules of CTL (T_c). Perforin, released between the conjugated CTL (T_c) and the target cell, is polymerized in the presence of Ca^{2+} and forms pores in the plasma membrane of the target cell, not only causing lysis but also permitting the delivery of granzymes. Granzymes activate caspases, normally present in an inactive proenzyme form, that ultimately result in apoptotic death of the cell. The cross-linking of Fas by its ligand, membrane-bound Fas ligand, results in the activation of the extrinsic (death-receptor–initiated) pathway of apoptosis, which is covered in greater detail in Chapter 1.

CYTOKINE-RELATED DISEASES

A number of diseases are characterized by severe disruptions, either overproduction or underproduction, of cytokines or cytokine receptors. One of the most profound examples is the excessive elaboration of cytokines during bacterial septicemia and shock. The basic pathogenesis involves an infection with a Gram-negative, endotoxin-producing bacterium that stimulates macrophages to

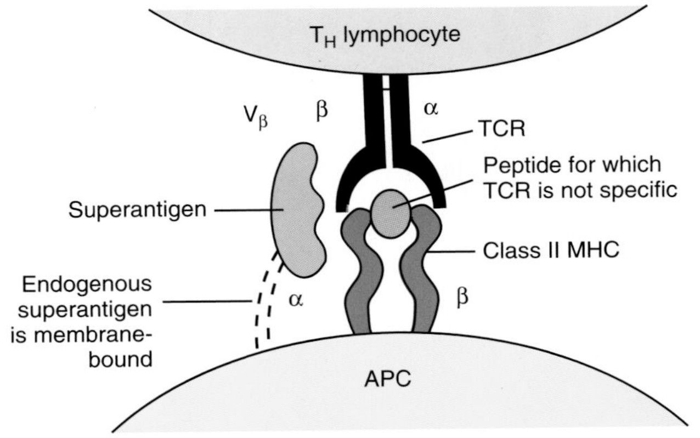

Fig. 5-25 Superantigens.
Schematic depiction of superantigens that bind to the V_β domain of the T lymphocyte receptor *(TCR)* and the α-chain of a class II major histocompatibility complex *(MHC)* molecule and activate large numbers of T lymphocytes irrespective of their antigen specificity. *APC,* Antigen-presenting cell. (Adapted from Goldsby RA, Kindt TJ, Osborne BA: *Kuby immunology,* ed 4, New York, 2000, WH Freeman.)

overproduce IL-1 and TNF-α. High concentrations of these two cytokines in circulation cause septic shock (see Chapters 2 and 3). A number of microbial pathogens also produce toxins or other antigenic molecules that are referred to as *superantigens.* Superantigens bind to class II MHC molecules and V_β domains of the TCR. This binding is outside the normal antigen binding site and activates all T lymphocytes expressing the same V_β domains, irrespective of their antigen specificity (Fig. 5-25). The result is the activation of numerous T lymphocytes (between 5% and 20% versus a normal response of $<0.01\%$) and the elaboration of cytokines. Superantigens are subclassified as exogenous or endogenous. Exogenous superantigens are produced by bacteria and include some enterotoxins, exfoliating toxin, and toxic shock syndrome toxin 1 (TSST-1). Endogenous superantigens are specific cell-membrane molecules produced during viral infections of cells. The best characterized is minor lymphocyte-stimulating (MLs) determinants associated with mouse mammary tumor virus infections. Similar to bacterial septic shock, increased serum concentrations of IL-1 and TNF-α cause systemic responses such as fever, disseminated intravascular coagulation (DIC), and shock.

TRANSPLANT REJECTION

Information on this topic, including Web Fig. 5-2, is available at evolve.elsevier.com/Zachary/McGavin/.

AUTOIMMUNE DISEASE

Autoimmunity is by definition a specific immune response to self-antigens. Autoimmunity reflects a loss of immunologic tolerance to self-tissue or cellular antigens and is characterized by abnormal or excessive activity of self-reactive immune effector cells. Autoimmunity can be organ specific, localized, or systemic. Autoimmunity can be mediated by both autoantibodies and by self-reactive T lymphocytes. The etiology of most autoimmune diseases remains elusive because they are often multifactorial and have a genetic and an environmental component. Criteria for diagnosing an autoimmune disease may include (1) direct proof, such as the fact that the disease can be transferred through cells or autoantibodies; (2) indirect proof, such as in identifying the antigen, then isolating the homologous antigen in an animal model, and reproducing the disease through administration of the antigen; (3) isolating self-reactive antibodies or T lymphocytes; and (4) circumstantial evidence, such as familial occurrence, lymphocyte infiltrate, MHC associations, and clinical improvement with immunosuppressive therapy. The complexity of autoimmune diseases is also supported by the fact that nonpathologic autoreactive T lymphocytes and antibodies can be found in normal individuals. Most autoimmune diseases have a tendency to be characterized by cyclic periods of alternating clinical disease and convalescence, an increased susceptibility of the female gender, and a predisposition to multiple autoimmune phenomena as in the case of the mixed connective tissue disorders.

How does a loss of self-tolerance occur? To understand the mechanisms related to a loss of self-tolerance, one must first understand the basic concepts of maintaining immunologic tolerance to self-antigens.

Immunologic Tolerance

When exposed to an antigen, the immune system can be responsive and develop an immune response or it can be nonresponsive and develop a state of tolerance. In either case, responsive or nonresponsive, the reaction is immunologically specific and has to be carefully regulated, as a response to a self-antigen or a nonresponse to a pathogen could be equally detrimental. Immunologic tolerance is an active physiologic process and is not simply the lack of an immune response. Immunologic tolerance is defined as a failure of the immune system to respond to a specific antigen after previous exposure to that antigen. It is an absence of a functional response rather than a lack of any response at all. The development of autoimmunity can be simply described as an escape from the mechanism by which self-tolerance is maintained.

Tolerance is maintained by a number of mechanisms including deletion, anergy, and suppression. Deletion, or self-tolerance, is the process of clonally eliminating self-reactive lymphocytes. For T lymphocytes, self-tolerance occurs as a developmental process of immature lymphocytes in the thymus, termed *central tolerance,* and as a component of mature effector cells on exposure to antigens in the peripheral tissues, known as *peripheral tolerance* (Fig. 5-26). Although immature B lymphocytes undergo selection processes in the bone marrow, independent of antigen, these are not referred to as central tolerance. Not all self-reactive B and T lymphocytes are deleted during their development. However, there are mechanisms of anergy and suppression that prevent the activation of self-reactive T or B lymphocytes outside the thymus and bone marrow.

Central Tolerance

Central tolerance occurs during T lymphocyte development in the thymus, where self-reactive T lymphocytes are clonally eliminated. Central tolerance has been most extensively studied in the thymus (see Fig. 5-26), where developing T lymphocytes undergo two selection processes that are essential for their development into mature effector cells and are based on the ability of developing lymphocytes to recognize self-peptides in association with MHC molecules. Positive selection is the clonal expansion of those cells capable of self-MHC restriction. Negative selection is the clonal deletion of those cells expressing TCRs capable of recognizing self-antigens in association with MHC molecules. Developing T and B lymphocytes expressing high avidity receptors for self-antigens are deleted from further development, resulting in a peripheral effector cell population lacking self-reactive cells. Self-reactive lymphocytes are eliminated by an apoptotic mechanism. For T lymphocytes, it is the interaction of an immature lymphocyte and an antigen-presenting cell that triggers the process of clonal deletion of self-reactive T lymphocytes. This process of clonal deletion involves an apoptotic pathway mediated by the Fas-Fas ligand. The exact molecular signals that trigger this apoptotic pathway remain elusive. The expression of peripheral antigens in the thymus is thought to be partially mediated by a protein called *autoimmune regulator* (AIRE), which is thought to be essential for the deletion of immature self-reactive T lymphocytes. Negative selection for developing B lymphocytes also occurs through a clonal deletion process involving an apoptotic pathway for those cells that have "excessive" stimulation of their antigen receptor molecules during development. Although the mechanisms regulating tolerance during lymphocyte development are very effective at identifying and eliminating self-reactive T and B lymphocytes, they are not perfect because self-reactive lymphocytes can be identified in normal individuals. Finally, the development of central tolerance requires exposure to the antigen during lymphocyte development, and many self-antigens are not present in the thymus or bone marrow. These self-antigens are commonly referred to as sequestered antigens because they are not seen by the developing lymphocytes. Some of the tissue antigens that fall into this class of antigens include myelin basic protein, lens proteins, and sperm protein, to mention a few. These antigens can be released as a result of infection or trauma and result in an immunologic response by self-reactive lymphocytes against myelin, lens, and sperm, respectively.

Because the development of self-reactive lymphocytes may escape the mechanisms of central tolerance, the immune system has developed peripheral tolerance mechanisms to prevent these cells from becoming activated and developing into effector cells capable of causing autoimmunity.

Peripheral Tolerance

In peripheral tolerance, self-reactive T lymphocytes that are not eliminated as a result of negative selection processes in the thymus have the potential to cause tissue injury when they exit the thymus and enter the peripheral tissues (see Fig. 5-26). Within the peripheral tissues, there are mechanisms to prevent the activation of these self-reactive lymphocytes, and these occur as a consequence of the normal immune response to antigen and involve the same signals required for activation of lymphocytes during an immune response. Regulation of cellular activation occurs primarily by three mechanisms, which are briefly discussed next.

Anergy

Anergy is the functional inactivation of lymphocytes that encounter antigen. As previously discussed, two signals are required for the activation of naïve T lymphocytes by antigen-presenting cells. The first is generated by interaction of peptide antigen in association with MHC molecules on the surface of antigen-presenting cells within the TCR-CD3 complex, and the second is generated by the presence of co-stimulatory molecules. Co-stimulatory molecules are essential for the activation of naïve T lymphocytes and involve the interaction between T lymphocyte molecules (CD28) and their ligands (B7-1 and B7-2) on antigen-presenting cells. The interaction of CD28 with B7 results in T lymphocyte activation and its survival. However, if an antigen-presenting cell does not provide the co-stimulatory signal, the T lymphocyte receives a negative signal, and the cell becomes anergic (see Fig. 5-26). Another mechanism for inducing anergy involves the delivery of a specific inhibitory signal by CTLA-4 molecules on T lymphocytes that also bind to B7 molecules. The interaction of CTLA-4 with B7 results in inhibition of activation by blocking IL-2 production.

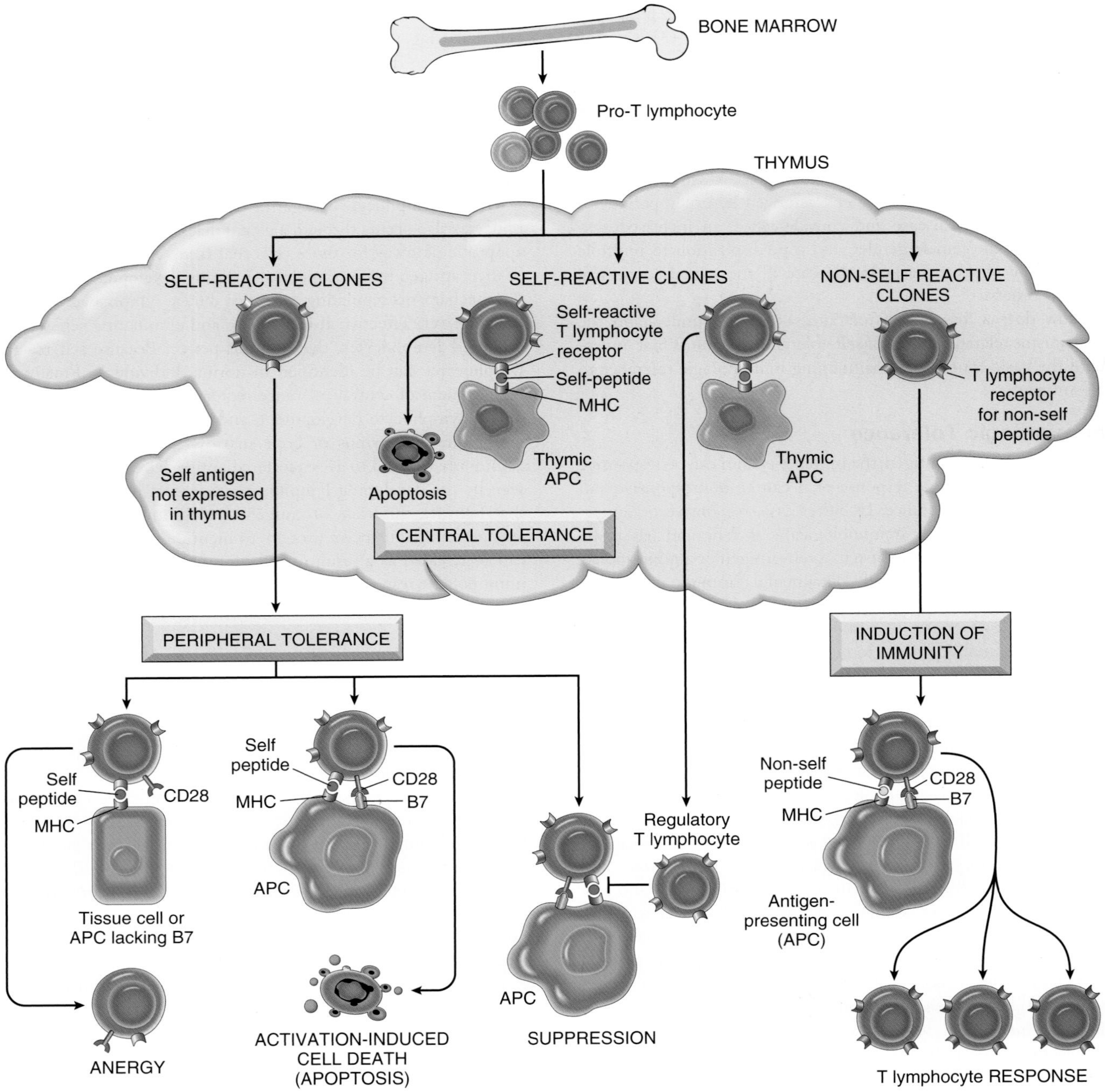

Fig. 5-26 Central and peripheral tolerance.
Schematic illustration of the mechanisms of central and peripheral tolerance of T lymphocytes. *APC,* Antigen-presenting cell; *FasL,* Fas ligand; *MHC,* major histocompatibility complex. (From Kumar V, Abbas AK, Fausto N, et al: *Robbins & Cotran pathologic basis of disease,* ed 8, Philadelphia, 2009, Saunders.)

The process of anergy is irreversible. The limited expression of co-stimulatory molecules by normal tissue facilitates the maintenance of peripheral tolerance to self-reactive lymphocytes. In general, CD28 is expressed on resting and activated T lymphocytes, whereas CTLA-4 is only expressed on activated T lymphocytes. What drives a T lymphocyte, expressing CD28 molecules, to recognize B7 molecules that lead to activation or to express CTLA-4 molecules that recognize the same B7 molecules that leads to anergy is unknown. Anergy of B lymphocytes occurs largely through the absence of specific T_H lymphocyte activation, although negative selection of mature self-reactive B lymphocytes is known to occur. An inability of B lymphocytes to receive appropriate signals from T_H lymphocytes, subsequent to antigen exposure, results in their deletion from lymphoid tissues.

Suppression by Regulatory T Lymphocytes

This mechanism of peripheral tolerance occurs through the activation of regulatory cells that prevent immune reactions to self-antigens. Suppression can occur as a result of cross-regulation of $CD4^+$ T_H1 lymphocytes by a specific population of $CD4^+$ T reg lymphocytes that were discussed previously. Specifically, $CD25^+$ and $CD4^+$ T reg lymphocytes producing IL-4, IL-10, and TGF-β downregulate T_H1 responses, effectively inhibiting lymphocyte activation and its effector function.

Clonal Deletion by Activation-Induced Cell Death

As discussed previously, one of the possible outcomes after lymphocyte activation as a result of antigen recognition during an immune response is lymphocyte proliferation. A second possible outcome after antigen exposure is cell death. For $CD4^+$ T lymphocytes, both outcomes—proliferation and death—are largely regulated by the expression of accessory co-stimulatory molecules. Activation-induced cell death (AICD) of T lymphocytes occurs by Fas-Fas ligand signaling following persistent stimulation by antigen-presenting cells expressing antigen. During the normal immune response, AICD functions to down-regulate immune responses and results in the return to immune homeostasis. Lymphocytes can be induced to express Fas (CD95), a member of the TNF-receptor family. The ligand for Fas, Fas ligand (FasL), is expressed primarily on activated T lymphocytes. The binding of Fas to FasL results in apoptosis of activated T lymphocytes. Antigens that are expressed to a high level in normal tissue would result in persistent stimulation of self-reactive T lymphocytes, thus resulting in deletion through Fas-FasL–mediated apoptosis. In the case of an autoreactive B lymphocyte exposed to soluble antigen in the periphery, the cell becomes anergic. If the anergic autoreactive B lymphocyte is recognized by a T lymphocyte specific for the autoantigen, the interaction of the Fas ligand on the T lymphocyte binding to the Fas molecule on the B lymphocyte results in activation-induced cell death of the B lymphocyte. Two strains of mice have been identified with a mutation in either the Fas molecule (lpr mice) or the FasL (gld mice). The lpr and gld strains have severe autoimmune disease develop with a phenotype similar to that of humans with SLE.

Antigen Sequestration

Antigens that are not expressed in the thymus or are "cryptic" in nature have the potential to induce a self-reactive immune response. Certain physiologic characteristics of some tissue (e.g., testis, eye, and brain) are considered to render them as "immunologically privileged sites" because of the difficulty in eliciting an immune response to antigens in these tissues. Antigens in these sites cannot be seen by the immune system because they are sequestered. The sequestering of antigens may occur through the blood-brain barrier, an absence of lymphatic drainage, or the limited ability to express MHC molecules. A mechanism for the eye is referred to as the anterior chamber–associated immune deviation (ACAID), thought in part to be the result of inhibitory cytokines, such as TGF-β, produced by the cells of the iris and ciliary body. However, if the antigens in these tissues are released as the result of trauma or infection, they have the potential to cause a severe immune response as a consequence of activating self-reactive lymphocytes. Posttraumatic uveitis and orchitis are thought to be the result of the release of sequestered antigens.

MECHANISMS OF AUTOIMMUNITY

Although central tolerance is important in lymphocyte development, it is the mechanisms of peripheral tolerance that have a greater influence on the development of autoimmunity. We have described the complexities of central and peripheral tolerance, and thus it is understandable that the mechanisms responsible for allowing autoreactive lymphocytes to become activated and develop into self-reactive T lymphocytes or autoantibody-producing plasma cells are equally diverse and complex (Fig. 5-27). Although autoantigens have been described for a number of autoimmune diseases, it is the identification of the initiating antigen that remains elusive. The cause of most autoimmune diseases remains unknown, as they often are multifactorial and have genetic and environmental components (Fig. 5-28).

Failure of Peripheral Tolerance

The mechanisms of self-tolerance, as previously discussed, serve as a basis for presenting how a failure to maintain those mechanisms can contribute to the pathogenesis of autoimmunity.

Genetic Factors in Autoimmunity

The majority of autoimmune diseases in humans have a strong genetic predisposition. The most well-studied genetic component centers around the MHC molecules. As previously discussed, MHC molecules are important in the development of lymphocytes and in the regulation of peripheral effector lymphocytes. Just as autoreactive lymphocytes have been identified in normal individuals without autoimmune disease, the presence of certain MHC molecules themselves is not sufficient to result in autoimmune disease. These observations would suggest that the expression of an autoimmune phenotype is not likely to be the result of a single-gene defect. Other genes that regulate proteins involved in other aspects of the immune response, or that are involved in the inflammatory or healing response, may also be involved. Additionally, experimental variations in the expression and activity of transcription factors can influence the expression of certain autoimmune diseases.

Several strains of mice with specific genetic mutations of factors involved in the maintenance of central and peripheral tolerance that results in autoimmune disease have been identified. Mice with defects of Fas or FasL have disruption of the activation-induced cell death signal in lymphocytes, resulting in autoimmune disease. Mice lacking the transcriptional factor AIRE, which is responsible for thymic expression of self-antigens, and mice defective in the expression of CTLA-4, the inhibitory receptor involved in T lymphocyte anergy, also develop autoimmunity. An important regulatory cytokine—IL-2, the major growth factor for lymphocytes—is also required for the development and function of regulatory T lymphocytes. Mice lacking either IL-2 or the IL-2 receptor develop autoimmune disease characterized by inflammatory bowel disease, anti-DNA antibodies, and autoimmune hemolytic anemia. The proposed mechanism of autoimmunity in these mice is thought to involve T lymphocytes and be a result of a failure of suppression by regulatory T lymphocytes and a failure of activation-induced cell death, two mechanisms of peripheral tolerance. These mouse models of autoimmune disease have facilitated the identification of pathogenic mechanisms of autoimmunity. Although all of these mechanisms have now been identified in human autoimmune diseases, it is likely only a matter of time before they are identified in other species.

Of the domestic species, there have been a number of autoimmune diseases in dogs documented to have a familial tendency, and the mechanism is in part attributed to certain MHC alleles. These recognized associations of specific autoimmune diseases and MHC molecules have been limited to a few specific breeds. It should also be noted that other diseases of immunity, for example, immunodeficiency and atopy, also have a higher incidence in some breeds.

Microbial Agents in Autoimmunity

The recognition that certain infections may result in the development of an autoimmune disease is the result of two observations. First, experimentally, one can induce autoimmunity in specific strains of mice by infection with certain strains of virus. Second, many spontaneous autoimmune diseases occur after viral infections, although attempts to isolate and identify viral agents in patients

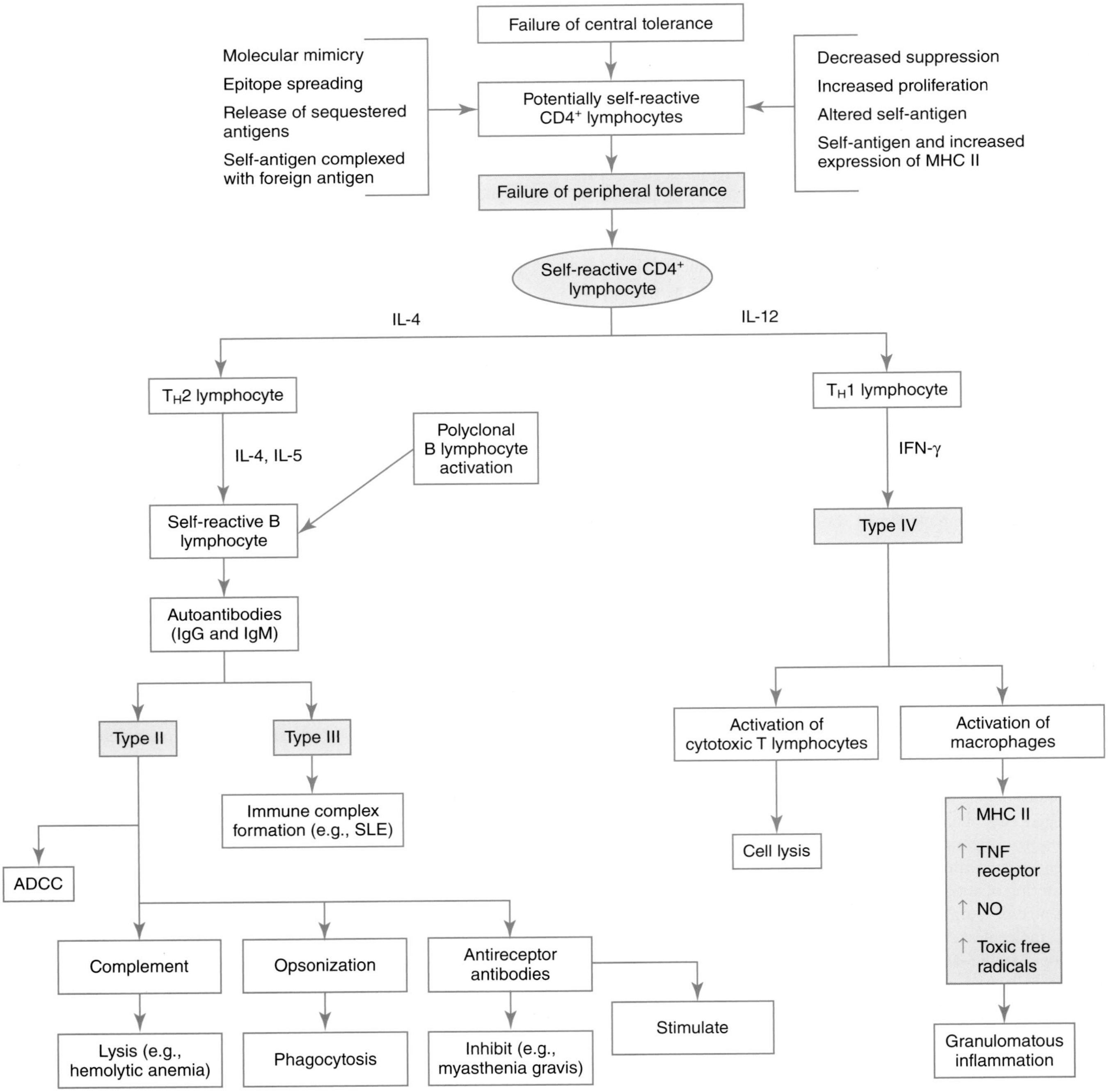

Fig. 5-27 Autoimmunity.
Pathogenetic mechanisms of autoimmunity mediated by activation of T lymphocytes ($CD4^+$). *ADCC,* Antibody-dependent cellular cytotoxicity; *IFN-γ,* interferon-γ; *Ig,* immunoglobulin; *IL,* interleukin; *MHC,* major histocompatibility complex; *NO,* nitric oxide; *SLE,* systemic lupus erythematosus; *TNF,* tumor necrosis factor.

with autoimmune diseases have been equivocal. Again, these observations would suggest that these diseases have a complex pathogenesis with a genetic and an environmental component.

The role of infections as environmental factors in the pathogenesis of autoimmune diseases may be explained by understanding how infectious agents may cause a breakdown of anergy to self-molecules (loss of self-tolerance). As discussed earlier, not all self-reacting B and T lymphocytes are eliminated during the differentiation and development process. These potentially self-reacting lymphocytes are regulated in the periphery by clonal anergy. Therefore a loss of this regulation could explain how autoimmune diseases develop. Plausible mechanisms of why infectious agents cause aberrations of peripheral clonal anergy are twofold (Fig. 5-29). One mechanism may be the result of nonspecific disruption of the regulatory cells, which results in the induction of co-stimulatory molecules on antigen-presenting cells that are expressing self-molecules. This mechanism is not specific to the antigens of the infectious agent and is likely the result of the overall inflammatory response to the pathogen. Additionally, during an inflammatory response, some cells are induced by the inflammatory

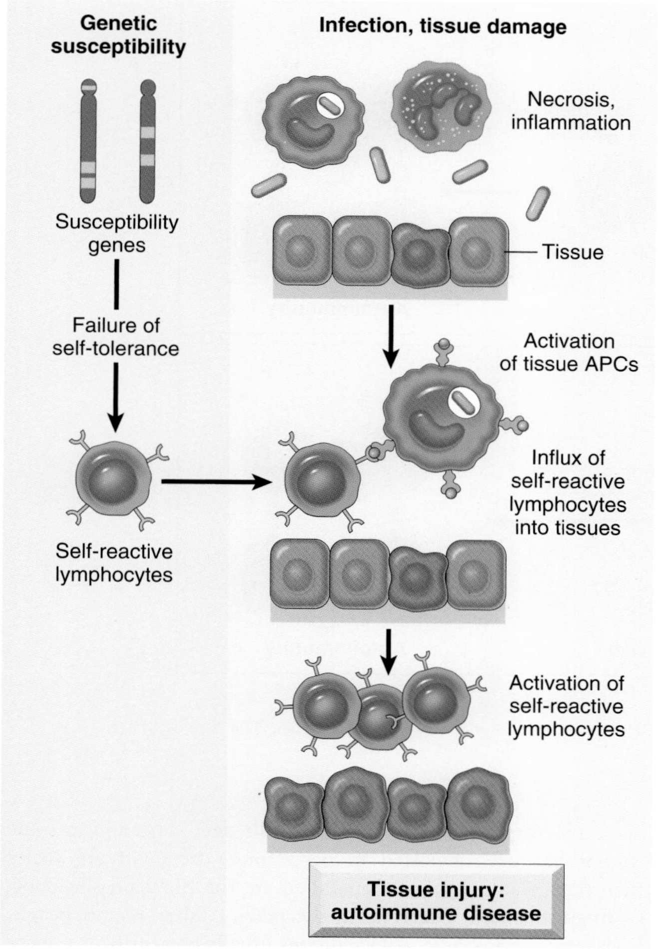

Fig. 5-28 Pathogenesis of autoimmunity.
APCs, Antigen-presenting cells. (From Kumar V, Abbas AK, Fausto N, et al: *Robbins & Cotran pathologic basis of disease,* ed 8, Philadelphia, 2009, Saunders.)

cytokine IFN-γ to increase their expression of MHC molecules. This can result in the expression of MHC molecules by cells that normally do not express them. Although the expression of MHC molecules in the absence of co-stimulatory molecules will not activate T lymphocytes, it does increase the potential to do so if co-stimulatory molecules are inappropriately expressed. The second mechanism is specific to the antigens of the infectious agent and is the result of cross-reactivity of T lymphocytes with an infectious agent's antigen and a self-antigen. Many infectious agents express antigens that have similar peptide sequences to those of normal peptides as a part of their immune evasion mechanism. Therefore the potential exists for any immune response to an infectious agent to cross-react with a normal peptide, resulting in an immune response directed against self-cells or self-tissues. This mechanism is called *molecular mimicry.* The result is the activation of T lymphocytes that recognize the infectious agent peptide–MHC complex. These T lymphocytes can potentially attack self-peptide–MHC complexes that are cross-reactive.

Once an autoimmune disease is initiated, the clinical course is generally progressive and characterized by cyclical periods of exacerbation and remission. As with any immune-mediated disease, antigen persistence is required to maintain the functional immune response. In autoimmune diseases, antigen persistence is thought in part to occur through epitope spreading. Epitope spreading is the process by which the immune response spreads from one epitope of an antigenic molecule to another, non–cross-reacting, epitope of the same antigenic molecule, or from one epitope of different peptides that are a part of a large complex. The epitopes involved are frequently ones that the immune response has not developed tolerance against because they are not normally presented by MHC molecules in sufficient concentrations. These so-called cryptic epitopes are normally not expressed at sufficient concentrations or are "hidden" during differentiation and development of lymphocytes. However, during an infection or inflammatory response, there may be tissue or cell damage that results in the release or expression of cryptic or hidden epitopes of self-antigens, and these become targets for the immune response. Because these epitopes were hidden, the immune system has not developed tolerance to them. Epitope spreading is thought to maintain the initiated immune response by means of the continued recruitment of autoreactive T lymphocytes specific for normal "cryptic" self-peptides.

With this basic understanding of self-tolerance and the possible molecular mechanisms involved in the pathogenesis of autoimmunity, we can present some of the more common autoimmune diseases of domestic species. Autoimmune diseases can be organ specific or systemic. With many of the organ-specific diseases, an immunologically mediated pathogenesis is suspected because of the finding of a lymphocytic inflammatory reaction within the affected tissue. Rarely, autoantibodies may be identified in the circulation. The organ-specific autoimmune diseases are discussed in the appropriate chapters covering individual organ systems. This chapter focuses on some of the systemic autoimmune diseases of domestic species, beginning with the multisystemic disease SLE.

SYSTEMIC LUPUS ERYTHEMATOSUS

SLE is one of the most well-studied systemic autoimmune diseases in humans and is characterized by the production of autoantibodies directed against a wide array of normal tissue and cellular components. The predominant autoantibody, commonly known as *antinuclear antibody* (ANA), is directed against nuclear antigens. The disease has been described in humans, nonhuman primates, mice, horses, dogs, cats, snakes, and iguanas. As with many autoimmune diseases, SLE has a highly variable and often progressive clinical course characterized by a variety of clinical and immunologic abnormalities. Unlike humans, in whom the disease predominantly affects women, there is no clear sex predilection in domestic species. There are certain breeds of dogs that have a higher incidence. The average age of diagnosis is approximately 5 years. Epidemiologic data on other species is limited.

Etiology and Pathogenesis

The cause of SLE remains undetermined, although the presence of autoantibodies directed against a number of tissues and cellular components suggests that the underlying immunologic abnormality is a failure to maintain self-tolerance. Antibodies against nuclear and cytoplasmic components, which are neither organ specific nor species specific, and those directed against cell surface antigens, particularly red blood cell antigens, are central to the pathogenesis of the disease. Detection of autoantibodies also facilitates the diagnosis and monitoring of human patients with SLE. The autoantibodies and self-antigens form immune complexes, which can be deposited in glomeruli (glomerulonephritis), blood vessels (vasculitis), skin (dermatitis), and joints (arthritis), resulting in the major clinical signs associated with the disease.

ANAs are found in a high percentage of patients with SLE. In humans, antinuclear antibodies are grouped into four categories: (1) antibodies against DNA, (2) antibodies against histones, (3)

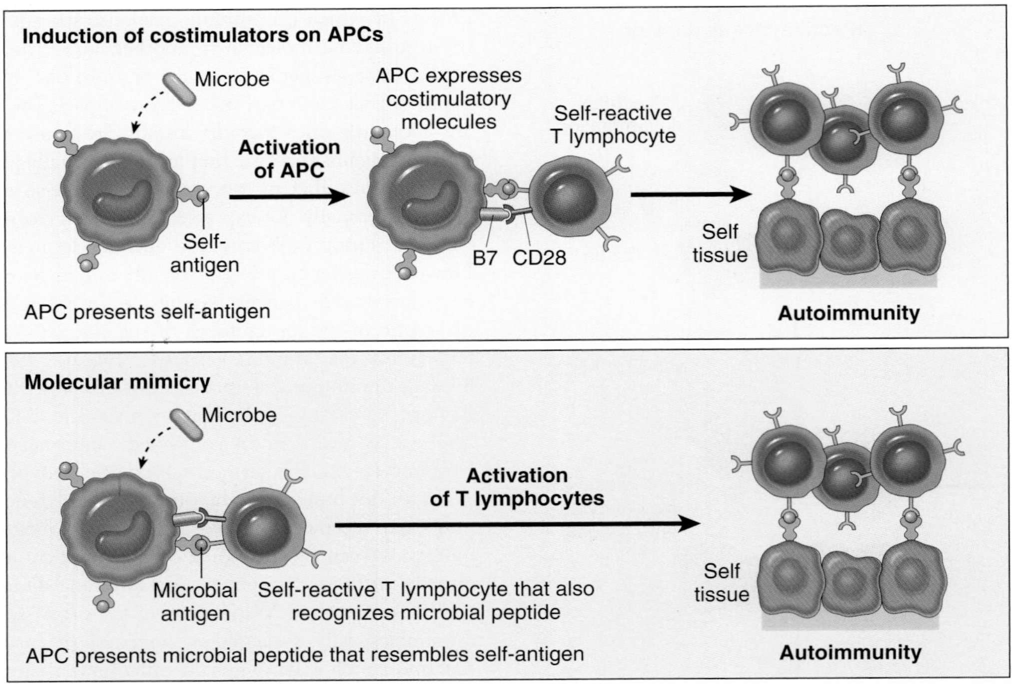

Fig. 5-29 Autoimmunity and the role of infections in its pathogenesis. *APC,* Antigen-presenting cell. (From Kumar V, Abbas AK, Fausto N, et al: *Robbins & Cotran pathologic basis of disease,* ed 7, Philadelphia, 2004, Saunders.)

antibodies to nonhistone proteins bound to RNA, and (4) antibodies against nucleolar antigens. The most common method of measuring antinuclear antibodies is indirect immunofluorescence. The pattern of immunofluorescence is used to help identify the type of autoantibody present. Other methods can be used to more specifically identify the target of ANA. In humans, the majority of ANAs are directed against nucleic acids in native double-stranded DNA, in contrast to the dog, in which the majority of ANAs are directed against nuclear proteins such as histones and extractable nuclear antigens (ENAs). ANAs are also found in normal patients and in patients with other diseases; however, their frequency is much lower. In the dog, the incidence of ANA in normal dogs and dogs with other canine diseases is 16% and 20%, respectively, compared with 97% to 100% in dogs with SLE. The indirect immunofluorescence test for ANA is sensitive but not specific because of the relatively high incidence in normal dogs and those with non-SLE diseases. Two anti-ENA antibodies appear to be specific for canine SLE. These are the anti-Sm and the anti-T1 antibodies.

Patients with SLE frequently have autoantibodies in an array of tissue and cells. Many patients have rheumatoid factors and thus have a positive Coombs' test for anti-IgG antibodies. Antibodies directed against cellular antigens on red blood cells, platelets, and lymphocytes are frequently noted. In these instances, they may lead to clinical signs of hemolytic anemia (anti-RBC antibodies), thrombocytopenia (antiplatelet antibodies), and immune system abnormalities (antilymphocyte antibodies). Other autoantibodies to components of muscle (myositis) and skin (dermatitis) are also frequently detected. While there can be an extensive number of autoantibodies identified in patients with SLE, the major clinical signs are attributed to the deposition of immune complexes in the joint, skin, and kidney and the elaboration of a type III hypersensitivity reaction. The tissues most frequently involved are in the joint, skin, and kidney.

Canine lupus primarily affects middle-aged dogs and in some studies has been reported to occur more frequently in males than females. Breeds overrepresented are the Shetland sheepdog, German shepherd, Old English sheepdog, Afghan hound, beagle, Irish setter, and poodle. Affected dogs usually present with a spectrum of clinical signs and the disease has a progressive clinical course. Common clinical findings include fever, nonerosive polyarthritis, glomerulonephritis, mucocutaneous lesions, lymph node and splenic enlargement, and hematologic abnormalities (e.g., anemia, thrombocytopenia, and leukopenia). ANAs are the most common immunologic finding. In some reports, up to 100% of affected animals have been positive for ANAs. Dogs can also have antierythrocyte antibodies (Coombs' positive), anti-IgG antibodies (rheumatoid factor positive), circulating immune complexes and deposits of these in the skin. Only the direct Coombs' test is valid in the dog. In the dog, as in other species, the immunologic abnormalities involve both humoral and cellular immunity. The abnormalities in humoral immunity are largely attributed to the already discussed presence of autoantibodies and are centered on the activation of self-reactive B lymphocytes. The abnormalities in cellular immunity include a lymphopenia that is characterized by a decrease in the percentage and absolute number of $CD8^+$ lymphocytes and a concurrent increase in the percentage and a decrease in the absolute number of $CD4^+$ lymphocytes. This translates into a high $CD4^+$:$CD8^+$ ratio (as high as 6 in dogs with SLE versus <2 in normal dogs).

Lesions of Systemic Lupus Erythematosus

A wide spectrum of morphologic lesions is associated with canine SLE. The most common finding, polyarthritis, is characterized as a nonerosive lesion that commonly affects the intervertebral, carpal, tarsal, and temporomandibular joints. The acute arthritis is characterized by exudation of neutrophils and fibrin into the synovial membrane and concurrent perivascular cuffing by mononuclear cells. The primary differential diagnosis for the arthritis is rheumatoid arthritis, which is an erosive lesion. The renal lesion, the result of immune complex deposition, involves the glomerulus, blood vessels, and the basement membranes of renal tubules (Web Fig. 5-3). The resulting glomerulonephritis is variable in appearance and ranges from slight mesangial alterations to diffuse proliferative lesions. The renal lesions have a common pathogenic mechanism that is a result of the deposition of immune complexes and the activation of complement (type III hypersensitivity). Glomerular lesions are often indicated by a persistent proteinuria (>0.5 g/dL).

Skin lesions are highly variable and nonspecific in canine SLE. The face, ears, and digital extremities are frequently involved and characterized by erythema, ulceration, and exfoliative dermatitis. The distribution of the lesions suggests that photosensitization may play a role. Histologically, the epidermis is characterized by basal cell vacuolation and necrosis, and the dermis is variably edematous with a superficial infiltration of mononuclear inflammatory cells at the dermal-epidermal junction (interface dermatitis). Additionally, there may be a panniculitis, composed primarily of lymphocytes and plasma cells, and vasculitis, with fibrinoid necrosis of the vessel wall. By indirect immunofluorescence, there are deposits of immunoglobulin and complement components at the dermal-epidermal junction. Other dermatologic variants of lupus are covered in Chapter 17. The definitive diagnosis of SLE is based on accepted criteria rather than pathognomonic findings. Using 11 established criteria for the dog, modified from the American Rheumatism Association criteria for humans, a definitive diagnosis requires the presence of four or more criteria. A "probable" diagnosis is based on the presence of three criteria or the presence of polyarthritis with the identification of ANAs. Other diagnostic schemes, using "major" and "minor" signs along with a positive ANA or SLE prep test, are also used to make definitive and probable diagnoses.

In the cat, SLE is less well recognized and manifests with fever, glomerulonephritis, dermatitis, and hemolytic anemia. The ANA test in cats is less reliable because many normal cats can have positive tests results. Horses with SLE similarly present with generalized skin disease and may also have glomerulonephritis, arthritis, and hemolytic anemia.

Genetic Factors

SLE in humans is characterized as a disease with a complex genetic component with MHC and multiple non-MHC genes involved. Extensive genetic studies in domestic animals are lacking, yet it is reasonable to suggest that the disease in other species is also characterized by involvement of multiple genes. The association of SLE with certain MHC alleles in human beings indicates that the MHC genes that regulate the production of specific antibodies are involved—specifically, MHC alleles that are linked to the production of anti–double-stranded DNA, anti-Sm, and antiphospholipid antibodies. Other than the observation of breed predilections for the dog and cat and the report of an association with the canine MHC allele DLA-A7, there are no definitive genetic studies similar to those reported in humans. Interestingly a low percentage of humans with SLE also have inherited deficiencies of complement components such as C2, C4, or C1q. Because complement components are important in the removal of circulating immune complexes by the monocyte-macrophage system, such a deficiency may contribute to the deposition of circulating complexes into tissue rather than to their removal. There is an increase in lupus-like autoimmunity in mice lacking certain complement components. Finally a well-described animal model of SLE is the NZB ∞ NZW mouse strain, in which a number of genetic loci have been identified as being associated with the development of the disease.

Environmental Factors

In addition to the genetic factors, SLE in humans has also been associated with a number of environmental factors. Specifically, drugs such as hydralazine, procainamide, and D-penicillamine can induce an SLE-like disease. In domestic animals, exposure to specific drugs and viral infections are suspected. Exposure to ultraviolet (UV) light is known to exacerbate the disease in the dog. These patients present with dermatologic manifestations localized to areas exposed to sunlight (e.g., face and dorsal regions) or areas lacking adequate hair coat (e.g., axillary region). A similar association has been noted in humans with SLE. The influence of UV radiation may be attributed to tissue damage and inflammation that result in activation of keratinocytes and the elaboration of IL-1, or the modification of DNA through the induction of apoptosis that renders the DNA immunogenic. The influence of sex hormones on the occurrence and manifestations of SLE in humans has not been documented in domestic species.

Immunologic Factors

As discussed previously, SLE is characterized by a number of immunologic abnormalities and is clinically noted to have manifestations attributable to specific immune components. It is therefore reasonable to suggest that the pathogenesis of SLE involves aberrations of humoral and/or cell-mediated immunity. Previously, as a result of the documentation of autoantibodies in patients with SLE, it was hypothesized that the pathogenesis centered on an intrinsic B lymphocyte defect. Additionally, polyclonal B lymphocyte activation is a common immunologic abnormality seen in patients with SLE and in animals that are models for the disease. Recent studies, however, indicate that the autoantibodies associated with the development of clinical SLE are not the result of polyclonal B lymphocyte activation but rather the result of antigen-specific T_H lymphocyte–dependent B lymphocyte responses. This observation is consistent with our overall understanding of autoimmunity, and the current hypothesis is that these diseases are more likely to be the result of an immunologic dysregulation centered on T_H lymphocytes. The currently proposed model for the pathogenesis of SLE is presented in Fig. 5-30. This model is an oversimplification of a complex disease with genetic and nongenetic factors that contribute to the development of a complex multisystemic disease with numerous clinical presentations, a progressive disease course, and an absence of specific cause.

Although the underlying cause of autoantibody production in SLE remains unknown, the elaboration of antibody-peptide complexes is central to the mechanism of tissue damage. The majority of lesions in SLE are the result of immune complex disease (type III hypersensitivity). Antibodies directed against cell surface antigens also lead to the destruction of leukocytes, red blood cells, and platelets through direct cell lysis and enhanced removal by opsonization and phagocytosis. ANAs bind to cell-free nuclei to produce characteristic hematoxylin bodies or lupus erythematosus (LE) bodies. These bodies are frequently found in the skin, kidney, lung, lymph node, spleen, and heart of patients with SLE. These ANAs can also lead to the formation of LE cells, which are typically present in the bone marrow and are a phagocytic cell (macrophage or neutrophil) that has engulfed an opsonized nucleus. This phenomenon is also used as an in vitro diagnostic test to demonstrate the presence of ANA (LE test or LE prep).

In summary, SLE represents the prototypical multiorgan autoimmune disease with a highly variable clinical presentation, a complex cause, and pathogenesis involving multiple genetic and environmental factors and a multitude of immunologic abnormalities. The

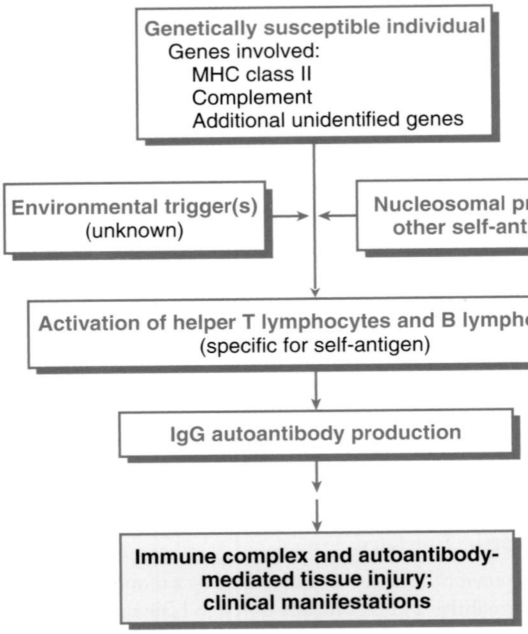

Fig. 5-30 Systemic lupus erythematosus.
Proposed model for the pathogenesis of systemic lupus erythematosus. *IgG,* Immunoglobulin G; *MHC,* major histocompatibility complex. (Modified from Kotzin BL: *Cell* 65:303-306, 1996.)

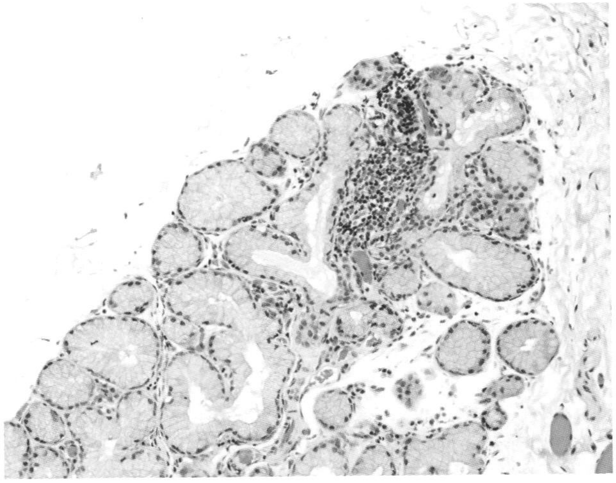

Fig. 5-31 Lymphoplasmacytic sialoadenitis, Sjögren syndrome, salivary gland, cat.
Note the focus of lymphocytes and macrophages around a group of salivary acini. H&E stain. (Courtesy Dr. P.W. Snyder, School of Veterinary Medicine, Purdue University.)

current pathogenesis suggests that these factors contribute to the activation of T and B lymphocytes, resulting in the production of autoantibodies directed against a number of self-constituents, namely molecules within the nucleus, in the cytoplasm, or on the cell surface.

RHEUMATOID ARTHRITIS

Rheumatoid arthritis is an autoimmune disease characterized by the presence of rheumatoid factors (anti-IgG antibodies) and is recognized in most species. The disease is discussed in Chapter 16.

SJÖGREN-LIKE SYNDROME

Sjögren-like syndrome is a systemic autoimmune disease characterized by keratoconjunctivitis sicca, xerostomia, and lymphoplasmacytic adenitis. In humans, Sjögren syndrome can manifest itself alone or in association with other autoimmune or immune-mediated diseases, such as rheumatoid arthritis, pemphigus, SLE, polymyositis, and immune-mediated thyroiditis. A Sjögren-like syndrome has been described in the dog and cat.

Etiology and Pathogenesis

The keratoconjunctivitis sicca (dry eyes) and xerostomia (dry mouth) result from the lymphocytic infiltration and fibrosis of lacrimal and salivary glands (lymphoplasmacytic sialoadenitis). In humans the infiltrate is primarily composed of activated $CD4^+$ lymphocytes and fewer B lymphocytes and plasma cells. Affected dogs are frequently hypergammaglobulinemic and less frequently have identifiable ANAs and rheumatoid factors. Many human patients have ANAs, rheumatoid factors, and nonorgan specific autoantibodies. Two autoantibodies specific to Sjögren syndrome in humans are directed against ribonucleoproteins, SS-A (Ro) and SS-B (La), which are considered serologic markers of the disease. Although autoantibodies can be identified, there is no direct evidence that they are the primary cause of tissue injury in any species evaluated to date. With the identification of autoantibodies and the presence of T lymphocytes within affected tissues, it is likely that the disease is the result of immunologic dysregulation centered on helper T lymphocytes. Sjögren syndrome in humans also is weakly correlated with certain MHC alleles, suggesting that as in SLE, the presence of certain MHC alleles may predispose the development of the disease.

As with many autoimmune diseases, viruses are suspected as potential causal agents. In most species in which viruses have been implicated, the evidence is largely circumstantial and Koch's postulates have rarely been satisfied. The mechanisms by which infectious agents can induce autoimmunity were discussed earlier.

Clinical Signs and Lesions

Dogs with Sjögren-like syndrome have an adult onset of conjunctivitis and keratitis. Other findings include gingivitis and stomatitis. A case reported in the cat was characterized by dry eyes and enlarged salivary glands. The keratoconjunctivitis frequently leads to blepharospasm and conjunctival hyperemia. The xerostomia leads to dysphagia. Involvement of tissues other than salivary and lacrimal glands, as is reported in about one-third of human cases, has not been documented in the dog and cat. Human patients have lymph node involvement that is characterized as a pleomorphic infiltrate with increased mitoses and are at a fortyfold increased risk for developing lymphoid malignancies. Microscopically the salivary and lacrimal glands are infiltrated predominately by lymphocytes (Fig. 5-31). In the cat, immunohistochemical analysis of lesions in these glands indicated that the predominant cell type was positive for CD79 (B lymphocyte marker) with fewer, scattered $CD3^+$ lymphocytes (T lymphocyte marker) and plasma cells. A mild interstitial fibrosis was also noted.

INFLAMMATORY MYOPATHIES

Inflammatory myopathies in domestic species comprise an uncommon, heterogeneous group of disorders that are characterized by skeletal muscle damage and inflammation. An immune-mediated pathogen is suspected. Four distinct disorders—masticatory muscle myositis, generalized inflammatory myositis, dermatomyositis, and extraocular myositis—are included in this category. They may occur alone or in association with other immune-mediated or autoimmune diseases. Of these diseases, only dermatomyositis is covered here; the remaining diseases are covered in Chapter 15.

Dermatomyositis

Dermatomyositis is an inflammatory disease of the skin, muscles, and vasculature affecting primarily young dogs. The cause and pathogenesis are unknown. The disease has a higher incidence in the collie and Shetland sheepdog breeds, and in these breeds, it is often referred to as *canine familial dermatomyositis,* an inheritable inflammatory disease of the skin and muscle. The disease has also been diagnosed in a number of other breeds. A sex predilection has not been reported. The clinical and pathologic findings suggest that an immune-mediated or an autoimmune mechanism is involved in the pathogenesis.

Lesions

The dermatologic manifestations of the disease are variable but generally begin at an early age (between 2 and 6 months) and are characterized by alopecia and erythematous dermatitis that involve the face, ears, and bony prominences of the distal extremities. Erosions and ulcers are common early in the disease and scarring and pigmentary changes are seen in chronic cases. Histopathologically, degeneration and necrosis of basal cells of the epidermis and follicular epithelium are characteristic. Frequently, vacuolation of the basal epithelium leads to subepidermal cleft formation. Infiltration of the superficial dermis is often composed of lymphocytes, plasma cells, and macrophages with fewer mast cells and neutrophils. Follicular atrophy and secondary ulceration and fibrosis can also be noted. The skeletal muscle manifestations of the disease are a myositis composed of a variable infiltrate of primarily mononuclear inflammatory cells and occasional neutrophils. There are varying degrees of myofiber degeneration characterized by myofiber fragmentation, vacuolation, and hyalinization. In chronic cases, there may be fibrosis and evidence of myofiber regeneration. The temporal and masseter muscles are commonly involved, although in severe cases there may be generalized muscle involvement. Involvement of the esophageal muscles can lead to the development of megaesophagus.

VASCULITIS

Vasculitis is inflammation of the walls of blood vessels. It is most often seen as a component of an underlying systemic disease process (e.g., infectious or neoplastic) or as an adverse reaction to drug or vaccine administration. In these instances, the pathogenesis involves a type III hypersensitivity reaction with the formation of immune complexes that are either formed in the vessel wall or formed in the circulation and lodge in the vessel wall. The inflammation of the blood vessel is not the result of an immunologic response to components of the blood vessel but rather an "innocent bystander" phenomenon with the formation or deposition of complexes in the wall and then activation of the complement system. The pathogenesis of a type III reaction was covered earlier in the chapter. An idiopathic febrile disease characterized by a systemic necrotizing vasculitis that occurs primarily in young (4 to 10 months of age) beagle dogs is suspected to be immune-mediated, based on clinical signs, immunologic abnormalities, and pathologic findings. The syndrome has been designated as juvenile polyarteritis or beagle pain syndrome, and there appears to be a familial predisposition in some colonies. A similar syndrome has been reported in other breeds. Males and females are equally affected.

Clinical Signs and Immunologic Abnormalities

The classic presentation is a febrile (104° F to 107° F) young dog with anorexia, hunched stance, cervical pain, and an unwillingness to move the head and neck. The disease has a cyclic course, with two to seven periods of signs that resolve. They have a moderate to notable leukocytosis, with neutrophilia, nonregenerative anemia, and hypoalbuminemia. Cerebral spinal fluid analysis indicates a neutrophilic pleocytosis with mild to moderate increases in microprotein. On serum protein electrophoresis, they have a high α_2-globulin fraction. ANA tests, LE preparations, and rheumatoid factor tests are generally negative. Immunologic abnormalities include an increase in serum IgA concentration, an increase in the percentage of peripheral B lymphocytes, and a decrease in the percentage of total peripheral T lymphocytes, a marked suppression of the blastogenic response to mitogenic stimulation, an inability to generate immunoglobulin-secreting plasma cells after polyclonal activation, and evidence of monocyte-macrophage activation. There are increased concentrations of IL-6 in the serum of acutely affected dogs, and these return to base-line concentrations during periods of remission or after corticosteroid therapy.

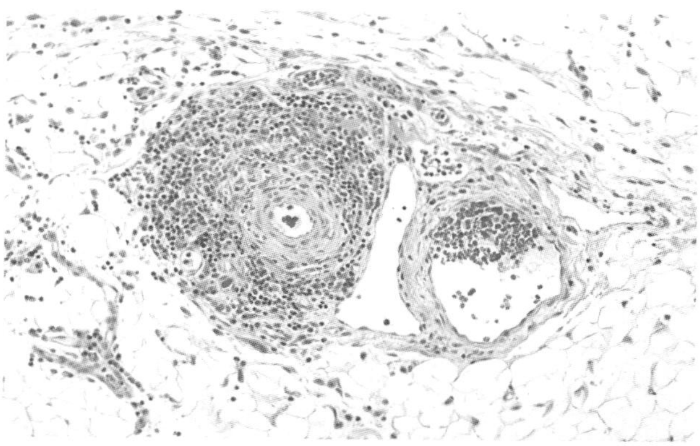

Fig. 5-32 Perivasculitis and vasculitis, polyarteritis, beagle dog. Note the accumulation of lymphocytes and macrophages around the arteriole. H&E stain. (Courtesy Dr. P.W. Snyder, School of Veterinary Medicine, Purdue University.)

Lesions

Severe necrotizing vasculitis and perivasculitis with thrombosis of small- to medium-sized blood vessels in the leptomeninges of the cervical spinal cord, cranial mediastinum, and heart are commonly seen (Fig. 5-32). In severe cases, a more widespread distribution of vascular lesions occurs and commonly involves the thyroid gland, small intestine, testes, diaphragm, esophagus, and urinary bladder. Most patients experience multiple episodes, but some may have only one to two episodes before becoming normal, and clinical signs appear to resolve in all but the most severely affected patients by 12 to 18 months of age. Some dogs that experience repeated acute episodes develop splenic, hepatic, and renal amyloidosis. The pathogenesis of amyloidosis is attributed to serum amyloidal A production and the development of reactive systemic amyloidosis secondary to the vascular inflammation.

IMMUNODEFICIENCY SYNDROMES

Immunodeficiency diseases occur when there is a failure of the immune system to protect the host from infectious organisms or the development of cancer. An immunodeficiency syndrome that is the result of a congenital or genetic defect in a component of the immune system is called a primary immunodeficiency. Although the defect may be present at birth, the disease may not be manifested until later in life. An immunodeficiency syndrome that is an acquired loss of immune function as a complication of infections, malnutrition, or aging or a side effect of immunosuppression, irradiation, or chemotherapy for cancer or autoimmune disease is called a *secondary immunodeficiency.* It is important to differentiate between a primary and secondary state of immunodeficiency with respect to treatment and prognosis. In some instances, it is useful to subclassify immunodeficiency diseases into those that affect adaptive (specific) or noninnate (nonspecific) immune responses. The study of immunodeficiency diseases has provided valuable insights and has enhanced our understanding of the complexities of the immune system. The ability to specifically identify the defective component provides great potential for the development of screening tests and of effective therapies. Naturally occurring and experimentally induced defects have made significant contributions to the field of immunology. There are a greater number of well-characterized immunodeficiency diseases in humans that likely have a domestic animal counterpart that have not yet been recognized. With the advent of new reagents and methodologies for characterizing cells and components of the immune system of domestic species, there should be a better chance in identifying immunodeficiency syndromes. Most primary immunodeficiency diseases are inherited, and the gene defect has been identified. There are additional forms of immunodeficiency that are the result of developmental defects that impair the function of an organ of the immune system. Finally, secondary immunodeficiency is a component of a large number of diseases of domestic species (ranging from malnutrition to viral infections that target lymphoid cells) and is beyond the scope of this chapter. This portion of the chapter covers some of the better characterized primary immunodeficiency diseases of domestic animals.

Primary Immunodeficiencies

Most primary immunodeficiency diseases are the result of a genetic defect (inherited or congenital) and affect specific (i.e., humoral and cell-mediated arms of the adaptive immune response) or nonspecific immunity (i.e., components of innate immune responses, such as complement, phagocytosis, NK cells, and so forth). Specific defects in adaptive immune responses can be divided into those affecting T lymphocytes or B lymphocytes or both (Fig. 5-33). As already discussed, interactions between B and T lymphocytes are necessary for the development of many immune responses. In some instances, the clinical distinction between a primary B lymphocyte defect and a T lymphocyte defect may not be obvious with respect to humoral immunity. For example, T lymphocyte defects almost always result in impaired antibody synthesis and as such are indistinguishable from B lymphocyte defects or combined B lymphocyte and T lymphocyte defects. In general, most primary deficiencies manifest themselves early in life and affected patients clinically have a failure to thrive and a susceptibility to recurrent infections. In many instances, the type of infection suggests to some extent the likely component of the immune system that is defective (Table 5-8). It is beyond the scope of this chapter to present all of the forms of human and rodent immunodeficiency, and thus only a few are referenced for clarity to facilitate understanding diseases that have been characterized in domestic species.

Primary Immunodeficiencies of Specific Immunity

Severe Combined Immunodeficiency Disease

Severe combined immunodeficiency disease (SCID) is a family of genetic defects that have in common deficiencies in both humoral and cell-mediated immunity. In its extreme form, SCID results from a defect in the common lymphoid stem cell that results in defective cell-mediated and humoral immune responses. More commonly, SCID defects affect either T lymphocytes or B and T lymphocytes and are best characterized in humans, mice, dogs, and horses. T lymphocyte defects often clinically have a combined immunodeficiency because there is a secondary impairment of humoral immunity that is the result of an inability of the T lymphocyte to provide the necessary signals for B lymphocyte activation. These defects result in an inability to generate a specific immune response and can have an autosomal recessive, X-linked, or sporadic inheritance pattern. The types of underlying defects are diverse and may involve enzyme systems or proteins necessary for lymphocyte development and differentiation, or signal transduction pathways involved in lymphocyte activation. Often the most common infectious manifestation of SCID is a viral or fungal infection. Immunity to viral and fungal infections is largely dependent on cell-mediated immunity. Immunity to most bacterial infections (especially extracellular bacteria) largely depends on humoral immunity, and neonates have adequate humoral immunity from the passive transfer of maternal antibodies that protect them.

SCID in horses is an autosomal recessive disorder described in the Arabian or Arabian-cross breed. The defect results in a severe lymphopenia (less than $1000/mm^3$) attributed to an inability to produce functional T and B lymphocytes. At birth, before they acquire maternal antibodies via colostrums, affected animals are deficient in serum IgM, and after catabolism of passively transferred antibodies, they have agammaglobinemia develop. Recurrent infections are typical and death is commonly the result of infection with equine adenovirus, *Pneumocystis carinii, Cryptosporidium parvum,* or a variety of common equine bacterial pathogens. Grossly the thymus is small and maybe undetectable. Microscopically, there is profound lymphoid hypoplasia of primary and secondary lymphoid tissue. Thymuses contain small lobules with no corticomedullary differentiation, few lymphocytes, Hassall's corpuscles, and occasional cysts. Spleens are characterized as having no lymphoid follicles, periarteriolar lymphoid sheaths, or plasma cells. Additionally, it has been noted that the lymphoid follicle sites in the spleen lack connective tissue stroma, and this characteristic can be used to differentiate hypoplasia from atrophy. Lymph nodes lack lymphoid follicles, plasma cells, and corticomedullary differentiation. The molecular basis for the defect has been identified as a spontaneous mutation in the gene encoding, the catalytic subunit of a DNA-dependent protein kinase (DNA-PKcs) that is located on chromosome 9. Affected foals have a complete absence of functional DNA-PKcs. DNA-PK is required for the recombination of immunoglobulin heavy chain and TCR genes during development, which when defective results in an inability to form functional V regions. Interestingly, as a result of the DNA-PKcs mutation, affected horses also are defective in their DNA repair mechanisms. The importance of DNA repair mechanisms in preventing the development of cancer (see Chapters 1 and 6) would suggest that affected foals and heterozygous carriers would be at an increased risk for cancer. Although affected foals rarely live beyond 5 months of age, heterozygous carriers do, and they have been observed to be at a greater risk for developing sarcoids, a locally aggressive fibroblastic cutaneous neoplasm.

SCID in dogs was first described in Basset hounds as an X-linked defect (XSCID) characterized by lymphopenia, with increased numbers of B lymphocytes and few to no T lymphocytes. The lymphopenia is not as profound as it is in foals with SCID. At approximately 6 to 8 weeks of age, as maternally-derived antibody concentrations decline, they develop recurrent infections of the skin, respiratory, or gastrointestinal system. Phenotypically, there is a decrease in the number of circulating $CD8^+$ lymphocytes resulting in a $CD4^+$:$CD8^+$ ratio of approximately 15:1 (compared with

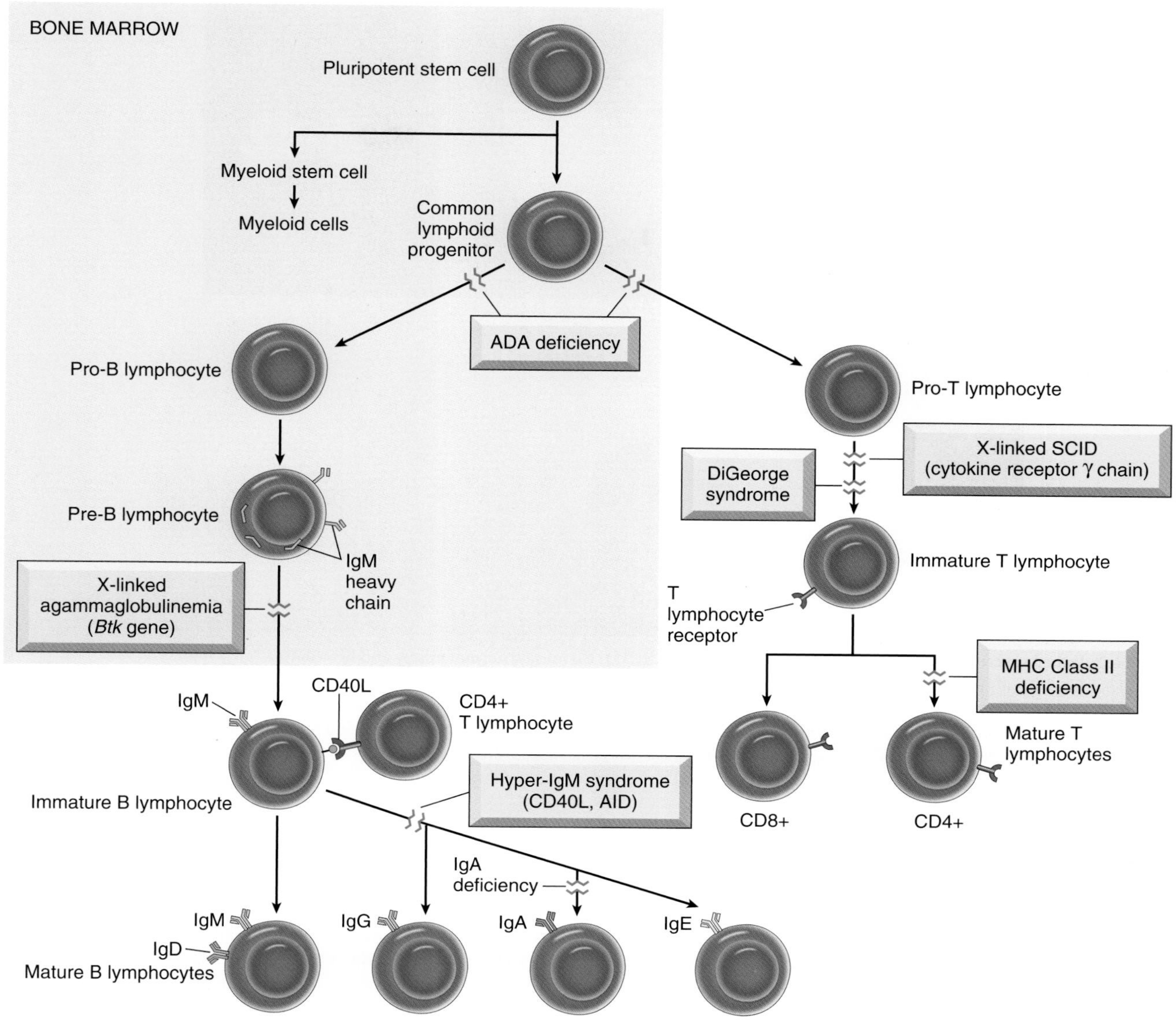

Fig. 5-33 **Primary immunodeficiency diseases.**
Schematic illustration of lymphocyte development and differentiation with known sites of disruption that cause primary immunodeficiency diseases. *ADA,* Adenosine deaminase; *Ig,* immunoglobulin; *MHC,* major histocompatibility complex; *SCID,* severe combined immunodeficiency disease. (From Kumar V, Abbas AK, Fausto N, et al: *Robbins & Cotran pathologic basis of disease,* ed 8, Philadelphia, 2009, Saunders.)

TABLE 5-8 Examples of Infections in Immunodeficiencies

Pathogen Type	T Lymphocyte Defect	B Lymphocyte Defect	Granulocyte Defect	Complement Defect
Bacteria	Bacterial sepsis	*Streptococcus* spp., *Staphylococcus* spp.	*Staphylococcus* spp., *Pseudomonas*	Pyogenic bacterial infections
Viruses	Cytomegalovirus, chronic infections with respiratory and intestinal viruses	Enteroviral encephalitis		
Fungi and parasites	*Candida, Pneumocystis carinii*	Intestinal giardiasis, aspergillosis	*Candida, Nocardia, Aspergillus*	
Special features	Aggressive disease with opportunistic pathogens, failure to clear infections, adverse reactions to attenuated vaccines	Chronic recurrent gastrointestinal infections, sepsis, meningitis	Neutrophilia	

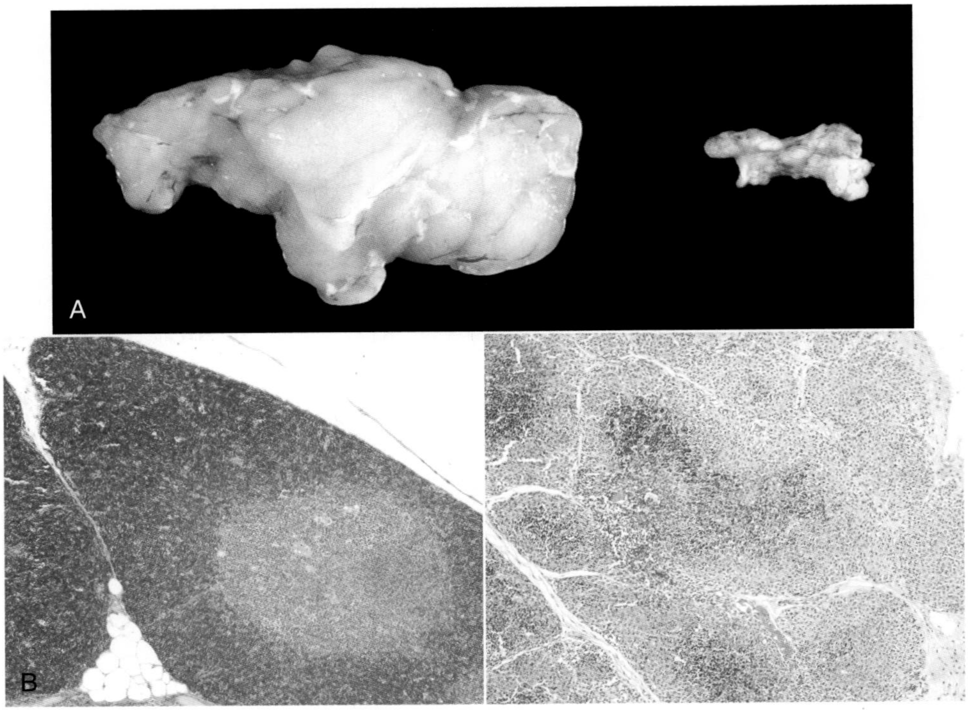

Fig. 5-34 X-linked severe combined immunodeficiency disease (XSCID) thymuses, normal puppy and littermate. **A,** The gland from the normal puppy *(left)* weighed 7.4 g, and the gland from the XSCID puppy *(right)* weighed 0.2 g. **B,** Thymus from a normal neonatal dog *(left)* and from a neonatal dog with XSCID *(right)*. The normal thymic lobule has a pale medullary region and a dark cortical region that is densely packed with small lymphocytes. The XSCID thymus has small lobules with no corticomedullary distinction and a paucity of small lymphocytes. H&E stain. (**A** and **B** courtesy Dr. P.W. Snyder, School of Veterinary Medicine, Purdue University.)

2:1 in normal dogs) and normal percentages of B lymphocytes. Dogs with XSCID are hypogammaglobulinemic with normal serum IgM concentrations and decreased concentrations of IgG and IgA. Affected dogs rarely live past 4 months of age, and death is frequently attributed to septicemia or systemic viral infections. At necropsy, lymph nodes, tonsils, Peyer's patches, and the thymus are extremely small and may be undetectable. Microscopically, there is severe lymphoid hypoplasia with similar characteristic features as described previously for lymphoid tissues of the foal with SCID. Thymuses of affected puppies are small (approximately 10% the weight of age-matched controls) and are characterized by a lack of corticomedullary demarcation and small lobules with few to no lymphocytes (Fig. 5-34). Thymuses have markedly increased percentages of CD8/CD4 lymphocytes (46% versus 16% in age-matched controls) compatible with a block in T lymphocyte differentiation. Canine XSCID is due to a mutation in the common gamma (γ_c) subunit of the IL-2, IL-4, IL-7, IL-9, and IL-15 receptors. These receptors, for five immunologically different cytokines, belong to the type I cytokine receptor family. A four-base pair deletion results in a stop codon that prevents full translation of the γ_c messenger RNA (mRNA). T lymphocytes are nonfunctional because of an inability to express a functional IL-2 receptor. B lymphocytes are only activated by T lymphocyte–independent antigens, and although they are capable of synthesizing IgM, they are incapable of class-switching to IgG. A similar molecular form of XSCID has also been described in the Cardigan Welsh Corgi breed. An insertional mutation, caused by the insertion of a cytosine in exon 4, also results in a stop codon preventing complete translation of γ_c mRNA. In human SCID, mutations of the γ_c are the most common molecular mechanism with numerous distinct point, insertion, and deletion mutations identified. An autosomal recessive form of SCID has been described in Jack Russell terriers that is the result of a mutation in DNA-PKcs similar to that described previously in the Arabian horse and the CB-17 mouse.

SCID in mice occurs in the CB-17 strain and is an autosomal recessive trait characterized by an absence of mature B and T lymphocytes. The molecular basis for the SCID phenotype is attributed to a defect resulting in decreased DNA-PK enzyme activity. Although mice are highly susceptible to opportunistic infections, they can be maintained in environments that minimize their exposure to pathogenic agents and kept alive for more than a year of age. An interesting, although poorly understood, immunologic finding in older (greater than 6 months of age) mice with SCID is the ability to produce small quantities of immunoglobulin and low numbers of mature T lymphocytes. This phenotype is referred to as *leaky SCID*. This leaky phenotype has not been described in other forms of SCID. As in other species with defective DNA repair mechanisms, there is an increased sensitivity to ionizing radiation damage.

Common Variable Immunodeficiency

Common variable immunodeficiency is a primary immunodeficiency disease characterized by an adult onset of hypogammaglobulinemia attributed to an intrinsic B lymphocyte defect, which results in an inability to produce much of the antibody. The disease has been described in a litter of miniature Dachshund dogs. The dogs were characterized as having an absence of B lymphocytes in lymphoid tissues and little to no serum immunoglobulins. At necropsy, the affected animals had lesions characterized as atrophy of lymphoid tissue and pneumonia. Lymph nodes were further characterized as lacking lymphoid follicles. The pneumonia was caused by *Pneumocystis carinii*, a common opportunistic pathogen in immunocompromised animals and humans. In humans, there have been a number of identified defects intrinsic to B lymphocytes that prevent their terminal differentiation and affect their ability to produce immunoglobulin, thus the designation as variable immunodeficiency. A similar disease has also been described in a 12-year-old Quarter Horse, which was characterized by hypogammaglobulinemia and an absence of B lymphocytes in circulation, bone marrow, and spleen.

Agammaglobulinemia

Agammaglobulinemia is a primary immunodeficiency characterized by an inability to produce immunoglobulins and an absence of mature B lymphocytes and plasma cells. The disease has been described in Thoroughbred, Quarter Horse, and Standardbred breeds of horses. To date, all cases have been males, suggesting that, as in the human disease, it is an X-linked trait. Microscopically, there was an absence of plasma cells, primary follicles, and germinal centers in lymph nodes. Affected horses commonly have extracellular bacterial infections of the joints and respiratory system. In humans, there is a mutation of the BTK gene located on the X chromosome that encodes a tyrosine kinase that results in an arrest of B lymphocyte development at the pre-B stage. The disease in humans is referred to as X-linked agammaglobulinemia (XLA).

Selective Immunoglobulin Deficiencies

Selective deficiencies are represented by a number of diseases characterized by a deficiency of an individual class of immunoglobulin. Forms of these diseases have been identified and described in horses and dogs. The most common forms are selective IgM deficiency and selective IgA deficiency, characterized by a serum level of IgM or IgA, respectively, that is at least two standard deviations below normal. Serum concentrations of other classes of immunoglobulin are normal, and B lymphocyte numbers are normal. These deficiencies may not result in clinical signs until there is degradation of passively transferred maternal antibody. In horses, there are distinct forms of selective IgM deficiency with most affected animals succumbing to septicemia or pneumonia by 10 months of age. A few affected foals live beyond 10 months and commonly die of recurrent respiratory infections before reaching adulthood. Some horses reach adulthood before they show clinical signs of selective IgM deficiency. Selective IgA deficiency has been described in a number of breeds of dogs, including the German shepherd, Shar-Pei, Irish setter, and beagle. Because of the importance of IgA in mucosal immunity, many affected animals have respiratory, gastrointestinal, and skin infections. Some affected dogs, like human patients with IgA deficiency, have a predisposition to developing atopic disease. In most instances there are normal numbers of IgA-producing plasma cells, suggesting an inability to synthesize or secrete IgA. Although the molecular basis for selective immunoglobulin deficiencies is unknown, they are thought to relate to the differentiation of naïve B lymphocytes into immunoglobulin-secreting plasma cells.

Thymic Hypoplasia

Thymic hypoplasia represents a number of immunodeficiency diseases characterized by a failure to develop a functional thymus, resulting in a T lymphocyte deficiency. Mice homozygous for the genetic trait nu (nu/nu) are hairless, and this athymic strain is commonly referred to as the nude mouse. Affected mice have a developmental arrest of the thymus, which occurs around day 12 of gestation and results in an absence of a functional thymus. Nude mice have defective cell-mediated immune responses and are unable to develop antibody responses. The immunologic abnormalities are attributed to a deficiency of T lymphocyte responses. Heterozygous (nu/+) animals are normal. The few circulating T lymphocytes in affected mice have TCRs of the γ/δ-type rather than the α/β-type. Under conventional housing conditions, mortality is high during the first 2 weeks of life; however, when maintained in germ-free environments, they can survive longer. This strain of mice is an important animal model, as they can tolerate allografts and xenografts. Similar, although less well-characterized, hairless and athymic conditions have been described in other species. A condition in humans characterized by thymic hypoplasia is referred to as *DiGeorge syndrome.* DiGeorge syndrome is a T lymphocyte deficiency resulting from an embryologic defect affecting the development of the third and fourth pharyngeal pouches. Affected humans have thymic (fourth pharyngeal pouch) and parathyroid (third pharyngeal pouch) defects. They have decreased circulating T lymphocytes, and T lymphocyte areas of lymphoid tissues (paracortical areas of lymph nodes and periarteriolar sheaths of the spleen) are depleted of lymphocytes. There is an absence of cell-mediated immune responses. DiGeorge syndrome is not familial but rather the result of the deletion of a specific gene that is a member of the T-box family of transcription factors. Specifically, how or why this transcription factor influences the development of the thymus and parathyroid is unknown.

Primary Immunodeficiencies of Nonspecific Immunity

Deficiencies of the Complement System

The complement system contains more than 30 soluble and cell-bound proteins that influence immune and inflammatory responses. The pathways of complement activation, regulation of the complement system, and biologic consequences of complement activation have been previously covered in Chapter 3. In humans, inherited deficiencies have been described for nearly all components and two of the inhibitors. Although a deficiency of C2 is the most common, humans with deficiencies in components of the classical pathway have little to no increased risk for infections, suggesting that the alternative and lectin pathways of activation are sufficient for controlling infections. Deficiencies of the classical pathway components are associated with an increased incidence of SLE-like autoimmune disease, which has been attributed to impaired clearance of immune complexes by the monocyte-macrophage system. Although deficiencies of components of the alternative pathway (properdin and factors D and H) are rare, when they do occur they are associated with recurrent pyogenic infections. A deficiency of C3, which is required for all three pathways of complement, is the most serious deficiency and results in serious recurrent infections. An autosomal recessive trait resulting in a genetically determined deficiency of C3 has been described in the Brittany spaniel dog. Homozygous dogs have serum concentrations of C3 and also opsonic and chemotactic activities that are severely decreased compared with normal dogs. Affected dogs are predisposed to recurrent infections and type 1 membranoproliferative glomerulonephritis. Bacterial infections with *Clostridium* spp., *Escherichia coli,* and *Klebsiella* spp. resulting in pneumonia, septicemia, and pyometra, respectively, are the most common clinical manifestations.

The molecular basis for the deficiency has been identified as a deletion mutation that results in a premature stop codon, preventing adequate translation and resulting in decreased concentrations of mRNA. Heterozygous dogs have serum concentrations of C3 that are approximately 50% of normal, but these dogs are clinically normal. C3 deficiency has also been described in guinea pigs and rabbits.

An autosomal recessive trait resulting in a deficiency of factor H, a component of the alternative pathway of complement, has been described in the Norwegian Yorkshire breed of pig. Factor H is a regulator of complement activation that blocks the formation of C3 convertase and is a cofactor for cleavage of C3b by factor I. Deficiencies of factor H result in unregulated elaboration of C3b on activation of the alternative pathway. The most common clinical manifestation is renal disease. Affected pigs develop a type II membranoproliferative glomerulonephritis characterized by glomerular changes consisting of thickened capillary walls, proliferation of mesangial cells, dense intramembranous deposits, and glomerular deposits of C3 components. The disease is commonly referred to as *porcine dense deposit disease.*

The molecular basis for the decreased serum concentrations of factor H has been reported to be the result of nucleotide sequence alterations in the factor H gene that cause a block in protein secretion. Hepatocytes of affected animals have increased intracellular concentrations of factor H. Hereditary factor H deficiency in humans can be characterized by a variety of clinical manifestations ranging from recurrent bacterial infections to glomerular disease to hemolytic uremic syndrome. Deficiencies of the terminal components (C5, C6, C7, C8, and C9), which are required for the formation of the membrane attack complex and the lysis of cell membranes, do occur and generally result in increased bacterial infections.

Deficiencies of C1 inhibitor and other complement regulatory proteins, although described in humans, have yet to be described in domestic animals. C1 inhibitor deficiency is an autosomal dominant trait that causes hereditary angioedema. C1 inhibitor is a protease inhibitor that targets C1r and C1s enzymes of the classical pathway of complement, Hageman factor (factor XII) of the coagulation pathway, and the kallikrein system. As indicated in Chapter 3, these three pathways are closely linked and result in the elaboration of vasoactive amines, notably bradykinin. Affected human patients develop episodes of edema involving the skin and mucosal membranes such as those of the larynx and gastrointestinal system. Deficiencies of membrane-bound regulator proteins, such as decay-accelerating factor and homologous restriction factor, result in paroxysmal nocturnal hemoglobinuria. In the absence of these regulatory factors, red blood cells can be more easily lysed by concentrations of complement that are much lower than normally required. The increased lysis of red blood cells causes chronic hemolytic anemia and hemoglobinuria.

Chédiak-Higashi Syndrome

Chédiak-Higashi syndrome is an inherited disease caused by defective lysosomes, melanosomes, platelet-dense granules, and cytolytic granules. The disease has been described in cats, cattle, killer whales, beige mice, rats, Aleutian mink, and humans. Common clinical manifestations of the disease may include hypopigmentation, a bleeding tendency, ocular abnormalities, and recurrent infections. Some species are more susceptible to recurrent infections than others. The hallmark of the disease is the presence of enlarged granules within melanocytes, neutrophils, eosinophils, and monocytes. The enlarged granules are melanosomes (melanocytes), lysosomes (many cell types), or cytoplasmic granules (e.g., fused primary and secondary granules of neutrophils). Neutrophils containing giant granules have impaired functions such as defective chemotaxis and intracellular killing. NK cells are also defective and may also contribute to the increased susceptibility to infections reported in some species. Mink with Chédiak-Higashi syndrome have an increased susceptibility to Aleutian mink disease virus. The hypopigmentation is the result of an inability of melanocytes, containing abnormally large melanosomes, to migrate and release their contents, resulting in a deficiency of pigment most commonly evident in the skin, hair, and eye. The bleeding tendency is a coagulopathy resulting from defective platelets. Platelet counts are generally normal. In most species studied, most recently cattle, there is insufficient platelet aggregation because of a decreased response to collagen. Research suggests that the GPIa/Iia ($\alpha_2\beta_1$-integrin) glycoprotein or rhodocytin pathway of platelet activation may be defective. Ocular abnormalities identified in cattle, cats, mink, mice, and humans are similar and are characterized by abnormal ocular pigmentation and an associated photophobia. Cats with Chédiak-Higashi syndrome frequently develop cataracts. The molecular basis for Chédiak-Higashi syndrome has been identified in some human forms and in beige mice and cattle to be a result of a mutation of the Lyst gene. The Lyst gene encodes a membrane-associated protein, which is thought to regulate intracellular protein trafficking. Exactly how the protein regulates intracellular trafficking remains unknown.

Leukocyte Adhesion Deficiency

Information on this topic is available at evolve.elsevier.com/Zachary/McGavin/.

AMYLOIDOSIS

Although there is no evidence to suggest that amyloidosis is always the result of a primary immunologic abnormality, the pathogenesis of amyloidosis may involve components of the immune system and as such is discussed here. Amyloidosis represents a broad spectrum of clinical and pathologic conditions that all have in common the deposition of amyloid material. Amyloid is a pathologic proteinaceous substance of different chemical entities with an identical conformational property of forming β-pleated sheets of nonbranching fibrils as identified by x-ray crystallography and infrared spectroscopy (Fig. 5-35). By light microscopy and standard hematoxylin and eosin (H&E) staining, amyloid appears as an amorphous, eosinophilic, hyaline, extracellular substance that with progressive accumulation results in pressure atrophy of adjacent cells and tissue (Fig. 5-36). Although amyloid can be derived from different chemical entities, all deposits have the same appearance and tinctorial characteristics. In humans, there are three major and several minor biochemical forms. Amyloidosis is a feature of

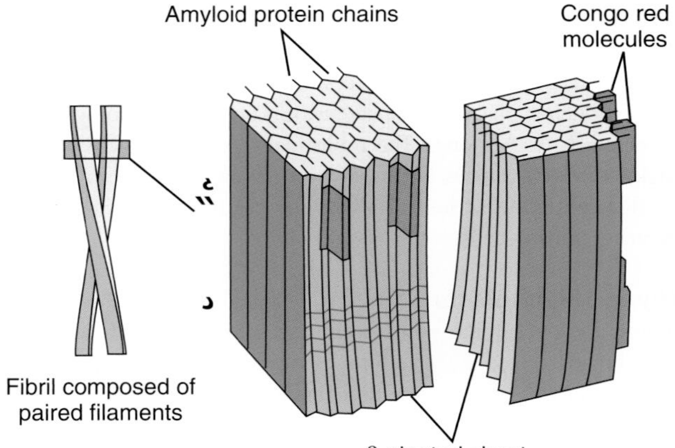

Fig. 5-35 Schematic depiction of amyloid fibrils, β-pleated sheets, and binding sites for Congo red dye.

(From Kumar V, Abbas AK, Fausto N, et al: *Robbins & Cotran pathologic basis of disease,* ed 8, Philadelphia, 2009, Saunders.)

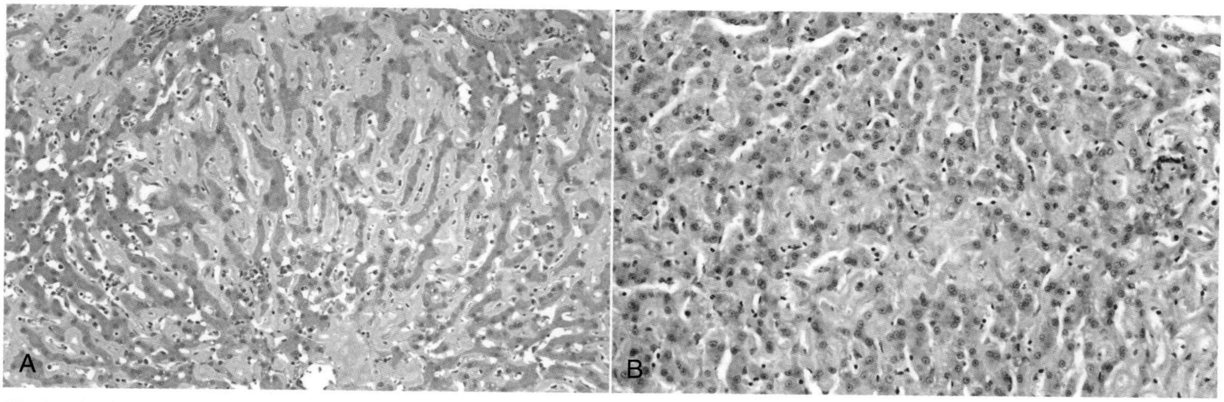

Fig. 5-36 **Amyloidosis, liver, dog.**
This dog had repeated episodes of vasculitis. The amyloid was attributed to systemic reactive amyloidosis (AA amyloid) caused by increased concentrations of serum amyloid A (SAA). **A,** Liver. The spaces of Disse are expanded by eosinophilic proteinaceous material (amyloid) that had caused atrophy of the hepatic cords. H&E stain. **B,** The deposits of amyloid are stained orange by the Congo red stain. (**A** and **B** courtesy Dr. P.W. Snyder, School of Veterinary Medicine, Purdue University.)

several different pathologic mechanisms and as such should not be considered a single disease but rather a group of diseases having in common the deposition of similar-appearing proteins. It is often necessary to differentiate amyloid from other similar-appearing extracellular deposits such as collagen and fibrin. Differentiating these proteins is readily accomplished using histochemical techniques. The most common technique for identifying amyloid is the Congo red stain, which does not have chemical specificity for amyloid but depends on the conformational property of being arranged in β-pleated sheets. Congo red stains amyloid an orange-to-red color, and when viewed by polarized light, reveals a characteristic green birefringent material (see Chapters 1, 8, and 11). A loss of Congo red staining by pretreating sections with potassium permanganate may suggest that the amyloidogenic protein is of amyloid-associated origin (see next section).

Chemical Nature of Amyloid

Amyloid contains approximately 95% fibrillar proteins and 5% P component and other glycoproteins. Of the 15 biochemically distinct forms of amyloid recognized in humans, 3 are most common: (1) amyloid light chain (AL), derived from immunoglobulin light chains of plasma cells; (2) amyloid associated (AA), derived from the acute phase protein serum amyloid A (SAA); and (3) Aβ amyloid, derived from amyloid precursor protein (APP). These forms of amyloid are also recognized in domestic species.

The AL form of amyloid can contain complete immunoglobulin light chains, the NH_2-terminus portion of immunoglobulin light chains, or both. Of the two immunoglobulin light chains, λ and κ, most AL forms consist of λ-light chains or their fragments. Immunoglobulin-secreting cells, B lymphocytes, and plasma cells are associated with deposition of AL amyloid.

The AA form of amyloid consists of a proteolytic fragment of a larger acute phase protein SAA, which is found in the plasma and synthesized in the liver and released during systemic inflammatory reactions.

The Aβ form of amyloid contains a proteolytic fragment of the APP and is associated with the cerebral amyloid angiopathy of Alzheimer's disease in humans and with some forms of neurodegeneration in the canine brain.

Of the large number of other biochemically distinct proteins that have been associated with the formation of amyloid in a number of human clinical diseases, only a few are relevant to domestic species. One of these is islet amyloidosis, affecting the feline pancreas. Islet amyloid is derived from islet amyloid polypeptide (IAPP), which is a hormone synthesized by the β cells of the pancreatic islets. All forms of amyloid contain other minor components, including serum amyloid P protein, proteoglycans, and glycosaminoglycans. Serum amyloid P may function to stabilize the fibrils and decrease their susceptibility to proteolysis.

Classification of Amyloidosis

In addition to the classification based on the primary biochemical constituent as discussed previously, it is also useful from a pathologist's perspective to categorize these conditions according to their clinical disease and pathogenesis (Table 5-9). Amyloid can be systemic (generalized), with deposits in many organ systems, or it can be localized, with deposits limited to a single organ. The systemic or generalized category can be further subclassified into primary amyloidosis (AL), when associated with immunocyte dyscrasia, or secondary amyloidosis (SAA), when associated with a chronic inflammatory or destructive tissue process. Hereditary or familial amyloidosis is in a separate heterogeneous category with several distinctive patterns of organ involvement that are primarily recognized in humans.

Primary Amyloidosis

Primary amyloidosis is the most common systemic form of amyloidosis in humans and is of the AL type. Many cases of AL amyloidosis are attributable to the presence of some type of immunocyte dyscrasias. The most common immunocyte dyscrasias associated with AL amyloidosis in domestic species is a neoplasm of plasma cells. Plasma cell–derived neoplasms include the extramedullary plasmacytoma and the myeloma or more common multiple myeloma that are most often limited to the bone marrow. Although neoplastic plasma cells often synthesize abnormal amounts of complete immunoglobulin or components of immunoglobulins (light or heavy chain only), only a small percentage of patients with these neoplasms develop amyloidosis. On serum protein electrophoresis, there may be a monoclonal gammopathy that is compatible with the presence of a single specific immunoglobulin. Additionally, in some cases, the serum may contain only the light chain component (referred to as *Bence-Jones protein*). Because an individual plasma cell can only synthesize either the λ- or κ-type of light chain and because plasma cell–derived neoplasms are of clonal origin, only

TABLE 5-9 Classification of Amyloidosis

Clinicopathologic Category	Associated Diseases	Major Fibril Protein	Chemically Related Precursor Protein
SYSTEMIC (GENERALIZED) AMYLOIDOSIS			
Immunocyte dyscrasias with amyloidosis (primary amyloidosis)	Multiple myeloma and other monoclonal B lymphocyte proliferations	AL	Immunoglobulin light chains, chiefly λ-type
Reactive systemic amyloidosis (secondary amyloidosis)	Chronic inflammatory conditions	AA	SAA
Familial amyloidosis	Some animals have systemic deposition of amyloid in addition to renal deposits	AA	
LOCALIZED AMYLOIDOSIS			
Amyloid of aging	Neurodegenerative disease, senile plaques, cerebral amyloid angiopathy	Aβ	APP
Endocrine tumors	—	A Cal	Calcitonin, polypeptide hormones or prohormones
Nonendocrine tumors	Amyloid-producing odontogenic tumor, ameloblastomas		
Islets of Langerhans	Diabetes mellitus	IAPP	Islet amyloid polypeptide
Pulmonary system	—	Apolipoprotein A-1	Apolipoprotein A-1 vasculature
Prion diseases	Various prion diseases of the CNS, spongiform encephalopathy	Misfolded prion protein (PrP^{sc})	Normal prion protein PrP
Familial amyloidosis of the dog	Renal disease	AA	Likely SAA
Familial amyloidosis of the cat	Renal disease	AA	Likely SAA
Gastrointestinal amyloidosis	Age-related finding		Unknown (not AA)

A Cal, Amyloid of hormone origin; *AA,* amyloid associated; *AL,* amyloid light chain; *APP,* amyloid precursor protein; *CNS,* central nervous system; *IAPP,* islet amyloid polypeptide; *SAA,* serum amyloid A.

one light chain type will be present. The λ-light chain is most often identified in AL-type amyloidosis. Because light chains are small proteins (approximately 50 kD), they are frequently detected in the urine of affected patients. The mere presence of Bence-Jones protein itself is not sufficient to produce AL amyloidosis because many cases of plasma cell neoplasms with identifiable Bence-Jones proteins occur in most domestic species without the development of amyloidosis. In contrast to amyloidosis in humans, in which the majority of patients with AL amyloid do not have any overt B lymphocyte or plasma cell neoplasm but do have monoclonal antibodies or light chains in their serum or urine, domestic species rarely have AL-type amyloid without evidence of an immunocyte dyscrasias. A more complete discussion of these neoplasms may be found in Chapter 13.

Reactive Systemic Amyloidosis

Reactive systemic amyloidosis is the most common form in animals. This form of amyloidosis has a systemic distribution and is also referred to as *secondary amyloidosis* because it is often secondary to a chronic inflammation of the destructive tissue process. Reactive systemic amyloidosis in domestic animals is a form of AA amyloid, which is most often either secondary to chronic inflammatory or neoplastic (nonimmunocyte dyscrasias) conditions or idiopathic, where no underlying disease is found. A prolonged increased serum concentration of SAA protein is necessary but by itself insufficient for the development of AA amyloid. This form of amyloidosis is recognized in most species. A form of the disease is also recognized in captive cheetahs and closely related Siberian tigers. In the cheetahs, in which renal deposits were primarily in the medullary interstitium, inflammatory conditions, most often gastritis, were found in all affected cats.

Familial Amyloidosis

Familial amyloidosis is a systemic form of AA amyloidosis that is hereditary in some breeds of cats and dogs. Familial AA amyloid has been described in the Abyssinian and Siamese breeds of cat and the Shar-Pei breed of dog. The organ systems affected are varied, but deposits most commonly occur in the kidney (primarily a glomerular deposition in the Abyssinian cat and medullary interstitium deposition in the Shar-Pei dog) and liver (Siamese cat). The amyloid fibrils consist of AA proteins, suggesting that this form may be related to chronic inflammatory conditions. Preliminary analysis of the different isoforms of SAA in the cat suggests that certain SAA genes may contribute to the development of this form of amyloid. Most domestic species have at least three isoforms of SAA.

Localized Amyloidosis

Occasionally, amyloid deposits are limited to a single organ or tissue. In many instances, the localized deposits are grossly visible as masses. Localized amyloidosis is present in calcifying epithelial odontogenic tumors (amyloid-producing odontogenic tumor) of the cat and dog. Of the prominent features of these rare neoplasms, one is the presence of amyloid, which often calcifies. Some forms of naturally occurring transmissible spongiform encephalopathies, such as chronic wasting disease (CWD), are characterized by amyloid plaques in the brain in addition to the intraneuronal vacuolation. The lesions of CWD and other prion diseases are discussed in Chapter 14.

Endocrine Amyloidosis

Deposition of amyloid in the pancreas of cats, nonhuman primates (macaques and baboons), and humans can lead to the development

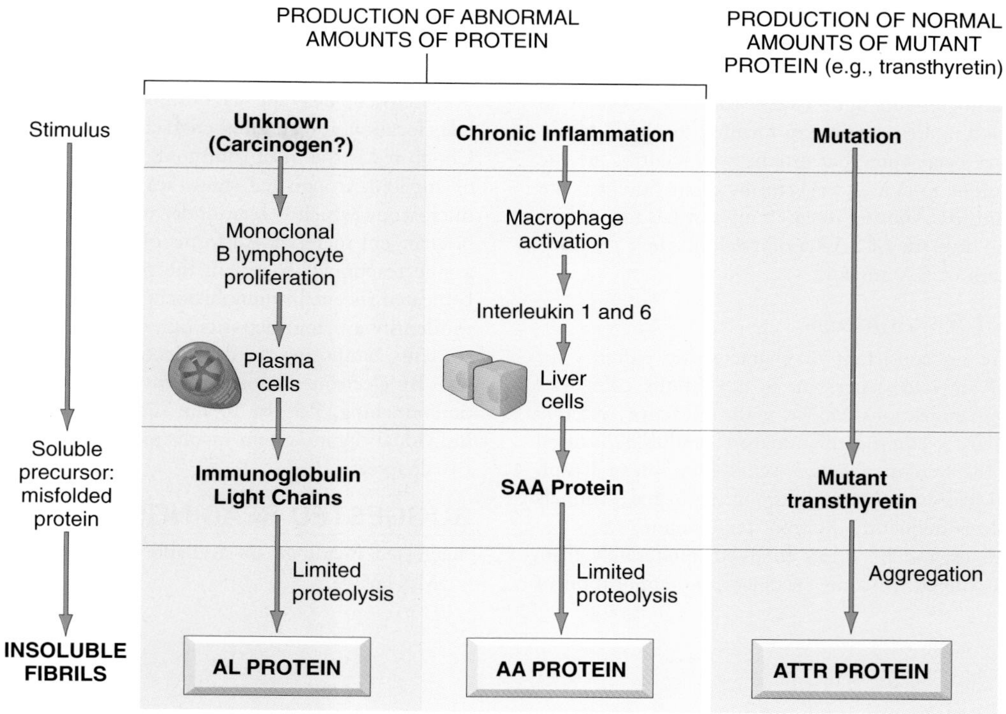

Fig. 5-37 Pathogenesis of the major forms of amyloidosis.
(From Kumar V, Abbas AK, Fausto N, et al: *Robbins & Cotran pathologic basis of disease,* ed 8, Philadelphia, 2009, Saunders.)

of type 2 diabetes mellitus. The amyloid is deposited in the pancreatic islets and is derived from islet amyloid polypeptide (IAPP), a normal protein secreted by the β cell of the pancreas. How a normal protein product becomes amyloidogenic in some instances remains unknown. It is not known if the deposition of amyloid and the development of clinical diabetes mellitus is the result of progressive loss of β cells from the amyloid or if the deposition of amyloid occurs as a result of prolonged stimulation of the β cells as a consequence of insulin resistance. The disease in cats is discussed in Chapter 12. Amyloid deposition can also occur in the cortex of the adrenal gland; however, it is not associated with any functional deficiencies.

Amyloid of Aging

Amyloid deposition can occur as an age-related change in a number of organ systems. Similar to senile systemic amyloidosis in humans, old dogs can develop neurodegenerative changes that may include cerebrovascular amyloidosis or the formation of senile plaques. These deposits can consist of a number of extracellular proteins but most commonly contain Aβ type amyloid. Other organ systems rarely containing amyloid deposits in the aged dog are heart, gastrointestinal tract, and lungs. The deposition of amyloid in the pulmonary vasculature of aged dogs was reported to be derived from apolipoprotein AI (Apo AI). These forms of amyloidosis are discussed in the appropriate chapters covering these respective organ systems.

Pathogenesis of Amyloidosis

Amyloid deposition is the result of abnormal folding of pathogenic proteins, deposited extracellularly as fibrils organized into β-pleated sheets. Although there are many diverse proteins associated with the formation of amyloid, they are all characterized by misfolded proteins leading to the formation of fibrils that are unstable and self-associated. Equally diverse are the number of conditions that can be associated with the formation of amyloid, and each of these conditions is characterized by excessive production of amyloidogenic proteins that are prone to misfolding. The two general categories of amyloidogenic proteins are (1) those that are normal proteins that have an inherent tendency to misfold and form fibrils when produced in excess quantities and (2) those that are abnormal protein products as a result of genetic mutations that are structurally unstable and form fibrils that self-associate. Misfolded proteins are normally degraded intracellularly within proteasomes or extracellularly by macrophages. In amyloidosis, these degradative processes are inadequate and may be responsible for the accumulation of misfolded proteins extracellularly. A simplified pathogenic scheme for the major forms of amyloidosis is presented in Fig. 5-37. As discussed previously, the overproduction of a precursor protein, although necessary, by itself is not sufficient to result in the formation of amyloid. In secondary reactive systemic amyloidosis, a component of a systemic inflammatory reaction results in the activation of macrophages that elaborate endogenous pyrogens IL-1 and IL-6, which stimulate hepatocytes to synthesize and secrete SAA.

During an inflammatory reaction, the quantity of SAA in the serum may increase several hundred times normal concentrations; however, not all systemic inflammatory reactions result in the formation of AA amyloid. Why is it that only some inflammatory reactions lead to amyloidosis? Two theories, one based on a defective degradation system for SAA and one based on abnormal SAA protein that is resistant to degradation, have been proposed. SAA is normally degraded to soluble protein products by enzymatic components of the monocyte-macrophage system. An enzymatic defect in this system may result in incomplete degradation and the production of insoluble AA molecules that form fibrils. Alternatively, a mutation of an SAA gene may result in the synthesis of an abnormal SAA protein that is resistant to degradation and prone to producing insoluble AA molecules that form fibrils. Finally, in the AL form of amyloidosis, plasma cells synthesize excessive quantities of immunoglobulin light chains that are resistant to complete degradation and susceptible to forming insoluble fibrils. Although there have been numerous attempts to identify specific sequence motifs unique to AA and AL forms of amyloid, to date none has been identified. Another research interest has focused on the existence of the diversity of SAA isoforms and their relationship to the formation of AA amyloid.

Morphology of Amyloidosis

Although there are no consistent or characteristic patterns for the distribution of amyloid deposition in any of the categories discussed, a few generalizations can be made. Reactive systemic amyloidosis, secondary to chronic inflammatory conditions, is often the most severe of the systemic forms. Liver, kidney, spleen, lymph nodes, and adrenal glands are most commonly affected. Animals with renal amyloidosis frequently die from renal failure.

Grossly affected organs are often enlarged, moderately firm, and abnormally discolored. In some instances, the application of an iodine solution (e.g., Lugol's iodine) to an affected tissue may stain the deposits brown, which develops into a blue-violet color when exposed to dilute sulfuric acid solution.

Microscopically the diagnosis of amyloid is based on its extracellular location and staining characteristics. As discussed previously, Congo red is the most commonly used stain for the identification of amyloid. Congo red stains amyloid orange to red under light microscopy, which is seen under polarized light as an apple-green birefringent material. All forms of amyloid stain with Congo red, as the reaction is based on the presence of fibril organized into β-pleated sheets. Immunohistochemistry can also be used not only to identify amyloid deposits but also to identify the specific constituents composing the deposits (e.g., anti–β-light chain antibodies). By electron microscopy, amyloid fibrils are characterized as nonbranching, 7.5- to 10-nm diameter tubules. Descriptions of individual organ system involvement are covered in their respective chapters.

SUGGESTED READINGS

Suggested Readings are available at evolve.elsevier.com/Zachary/McGavin/.

CHAPTER 6

Neoplasia and Tumor Biology*

Donna F. Kusewitt

Despite the relatively short lifespan of most animals, neoplasia is an important concern for veterinary practitioners, diagnosticians, and researchers. Tumor diagnosis and treatment for individual animals is becoming an increasingly prominent part of small animal practice. In food animals, infectious and environmental causes of cancer can have a major impact on herd or flock health. Furthermore, animal models provide important insights into the cause and treatment of human cancer.

DEFINITIONS

A neoplasm is a "new growth" composed of cells, originally derived from normal tissues, that have undergone heritable genetic changes allowing them to become relatively unresponsive to normal growth controls and to expand beyond their normal anatomic boundaries. Other common terms for neoplasms describe their clinical appearance or behavior: tumor ("swelling") and cancer ("crab"). Although the terms *neoplasm* and *tumor* may refer to benign or malignant growths, the term *cancer* always denotes a malignant growth. Oncology is the study of neoplasia; the term is derived from the Greek word *oncos* ("tumor").

Benign tumors do not invade surrounding tissue or spread to new anatomic locations within the body; thus these tumors are usually curable and rarely responsible for the death of the host. Malignant tumors, if left untreated, invade locally, may spread by metastasis ("change of place"), and ultimately kill the host. Interestingly, tumors of the nervous system very rarely metastasize; however, many of these tumors are notably invasive and kill their hosts, thus the tumors are malignant.

With the recognition that tumor development is a stepwise process, potentially preneoplastic changes have assumed new diagnostic and clinical significance. These changes include hyperplasia (increased cell number in a tissue), metaplasia (transformation of one differentiated cell type into another), and dysplasia (abnormal pattern of tissue growth) (Fig. 6-1). Hyperplasia, which is an increase in the number of cells in a tissue, should be distinguished from hypertrophy, which is an increase in individual cell size rather than number. Metaplasia is seen most commonly in epithelial tissue. In several species of animals, vitamin A deficiency is characterized by squamous metaplasia of respiratory and digestive epithelium. Dysplasia usually refers to disorderly arrangement of cells within epithelium. In general, preneoplastic changes are reversible. They arise in response to physiologic demands, injury, or irritation and resolve with the removal of the inciting factor. For example, epidermal hyperplasia is a normal part of wound repair, and skeletal muscle hypertrophy is an adaptive response to increased workload. Preneoplastic changes often indicate an increased risk for neoplasia in the affected tissue, and preneoplastic lesions may progress to neoplasia. The terms *dysplasia* and *metaplasia* can be applied to tumors to describe changes that persist during the transition from preneoplasia to neoplasia; however, the terms *hyperplasia* and *hypertrophy* are not appropriate in descriptions of true neoplasms.

NOMENCLATURE

Most tumors appear to consist of a single cell type, and the name of the neoplasm reflects the cell type (mesenchymal or epithelial) from which the tumor is presumed to arise.

MESENCHYMAL TUMORS

Mesenchymal tumors arise in cells of embryonic mesodermal origin. Benign tumors originating from mesenchymal cells are usually named by adding the suffix *-oma* to the name of the cell of origin. Thus a lipoma is a benign tumor derived from a lipocyte ("fat cell") (Fig. 6-2, *A*), and a fibroma is a benign tumor of fibroblast origin. A malignant tumor of mesenchymal origin is a sarcoma ("fleshy growth"). A prefix or modifier indicates the tissue of origin. For example, a liposarcoma is a malignant tumor of lipocyte origin (Fig. 6-2, *B*), and a fibrosarcoma is a tumor composed of malignant

*Dr. Laura J. Rush, Department of Veterinary Biosciences, The Ohio State University, made contributions to this chapter in the fourth edition.

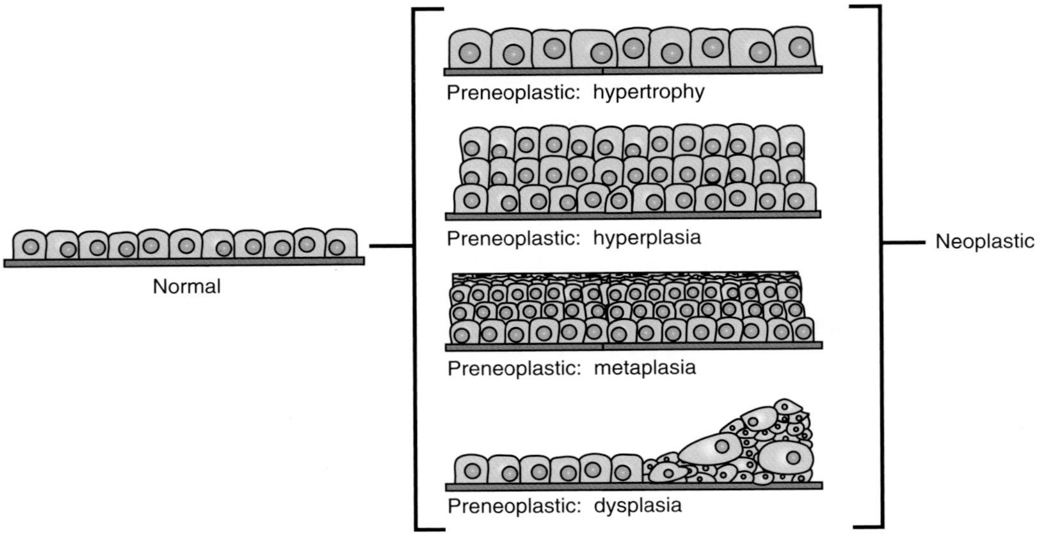

Fig. 6-1 Preneoplastic changes that may precede tumor emergence.
Preneoplastic changes in tissues include alterations in cell number, size, and organization. In this example, preneoplastic changes are illustrated in simple cuboidal epithelium, although such changes may also occur in other epithelial and mesenchymal cell types. (Redrawn with permission from Dr. D.F. Kusewitt, College of Veterinary Medicine, The Ohio State University.)

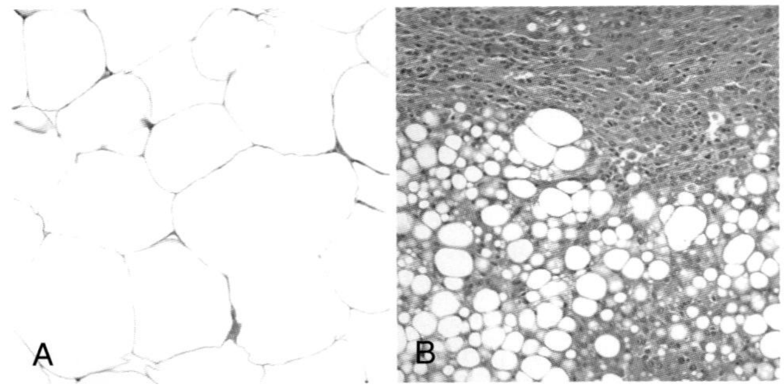

Fig. 6-2 Comparison of benign and malignant tumors of lipocyte origin, dog.
A, The benign lipoma is composed of mature fat cells indistinguishable from normal cells. H&E stain. **B,** The liposarcoma consists of poorly differentiated cells, many of which do not have the morphologic features characteristic of lipocytes. H&E stain. (Courtesy College of Veterinary Medicine, The Ohio State University.)

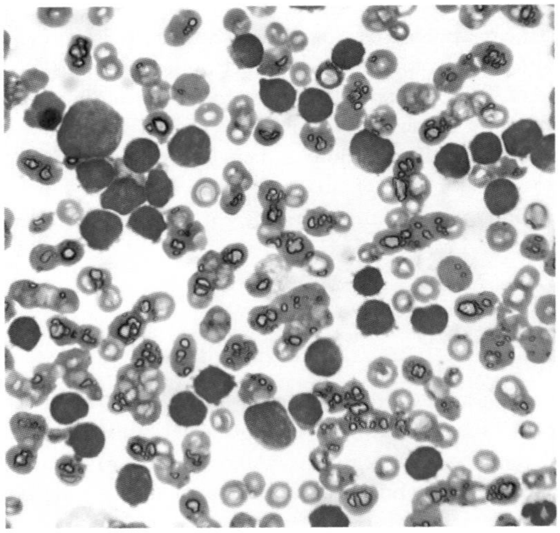

Fig. 6-3 Acute lymphoid leukemia, peripheral blood, dog.
The peripheral blood smear contains numerous neoplastic large lymphocytes. Flow cytometry identified these cells as B lymphocytes. The white blood cell count of this animal was 293,000 leukocytes/μL. Wright's stain. (Courtesy Dr. M.L. Wellman, College of Veterinary Medicine, The Ohio State University.)

fibroblasts. The cells of the hematopoietic system are mesenchymal. Tumors arising from circulating blood cells or their precursors are termed *leukemias* ("white blood"); neoplastic hematopoietic cells are usually found in large numbers in the bloodstream (Fig. 6-3), although they may also form solid tumor masses.

EPITHELIAL TUMORS

All of the three embryonic cell layers, endoderm, mesoderm, and ectoderm, can give rise to epithelial tissue and to tumors derived from this tissue. Terms for both benign and malignant epithelial tumors are frequently modified by prefixes or adjectives describing their appearance or the response they elicit in surrounding tissue. For instance, the adjective "squamous" is applied to an epithelial neoplasm that demonstrates squamous differentiation.

Benign tumors that arise from glandular epithelium are called *adenomas,* regardless of their microscopic appearance. However, the term is also applied to many tumors that are derived from nonglandular epithelial tissues but that have a tubular appearance such as renal adenomas. The term *papilloma* refers to a benign exophytic growth arising from an epithelial surface, whereas a polyp is a grossly visible, benign epithelial tumor projecting from a mucosal surface (Fig. 6-4).

All malignant tumors of epithelial origin are termed *carcinomas* ("cancers"). The general term carcinoma may be further modified to indicate the organ of origin, as in hepatocellular carcinoma. The prefix *adeno-* indicates a glandular pattern of tumor growth. Adenocarcinomas may be described as papillary, tubular, or cystic. Carcinomas and adenocarcinomas that stimulate the formation of abundant collagen in surrounding connective tissue (desmoplasia) may be termed scirrhous. The neoplastic epithelial cells of mucinous carcinomas and adenocarcinomas produce abundant mucin. Carcinoma in situ is a preinvasive form of carcinoma that remains

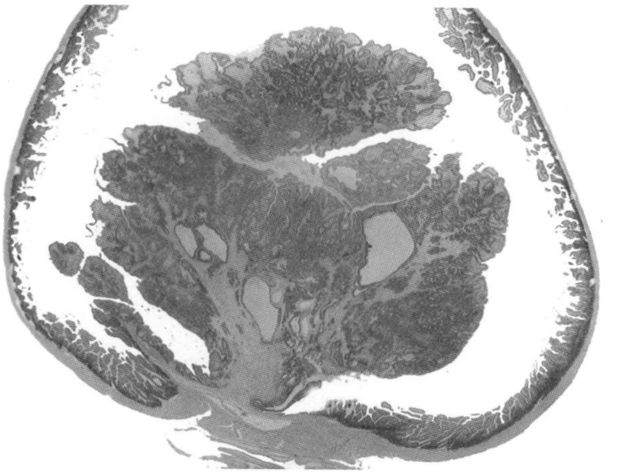

Fig. 6-4 Polyp, small intestine, mouse.
The neoplastic growth arises from the mucosa and extends into the lumen of the intestine. There is no invasion of the intestinal wall. H&E stain. (Courtesy College of Veterinary Medicine, The Ohio State University.)

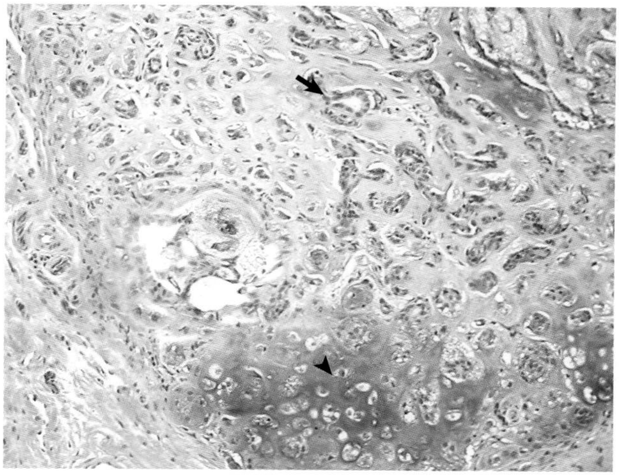

Fig. 6-5 Mixed mammary tumor, mammary gland, dog.
Mixed mammary tumors of dogs contain both epithelial structures *(arrow)* and mesenchymal elements, such as cartilage and bone *(arrowhead)*. H&E stain. (Courtesy College of Veterinary Medicine, The Ohio State University.)

within the epithelial structure from which it arises and does not penetrate the basement membrane to enter the stroma.

UNDIFFERENTIATED TUMORS

The appearance of some malignant tumors gives no clue to their cell of origin; thus they are termed *undifferentiated neoplasms.*

MIXED TUMORS

Mixed tumors contain multiple cell types derived from a single or multiple germ layers. Mixed tumors are believed to arise from a single pluripotent or totipotent cell capable of differentiating into a variety of more mature cell types. Teratomas and teratocarcinomas arise from totipotential germ cells; thus they contain tissue derived from all embryonic cell layers and consist of a bizarre mixture of adult and embryonic tissue types. The mixed mammary gland tumor of dogs is generally considered a mixed tumor. A mixed mammary tumor is composed of a variable admixture of neoplastic epithelial elements (luminal epithelium and myoepithelium) and mesenchymal elements (fibrous connective tissue, fat, cartilage, and bone) (Fig. 6-5).

TUMORLIKE LESIONS

Hamartomas are disorganized but mature mesenchymal or epithelial tissues found in their normal anatomic location. Many of the hamartomas identified in animals consist of abnormal proliferations of blood vessels. Hamartomas apparently represent the result of aberrant differentiation rather than true neoplasia, and their behavior is completely benign. Choristomas are composed of normal mature tissue located at an ectopic site. An example is the dermoid, a mass consisting of mature skin and its appendages, which may be found in a variety of unusual sites, including the cornea.

VETERINARY NOMENCLATURE

In Web Table 6-1, the names of common benign neoplasms in animals and their malignant counterparts are shown. The names given are those commonly employed in veterinary medicine. The terms used by veterinary pathologists to describe tumors in animals may differ from the terms used by medical pathologists to describe human tumors. This is partly because conventional usage plays an important role in tumor nomenclature; thus tumor nomenclature may be dictated by historic precedent rather than by logic. Moreover, attempts to standardize diagnostic terms for tumors in veterinary medicine have lagged far behind such efforts in the medical arena. A significant difference between veterinary and human nomenclature is that a benign tumor arising from melanocytes is termed a *benign melanoma* or *melanocytoma* by veterinary pathologists and a *nevus* by medical pathologists. Medical pathologists reserve the term *melanoma* for a malignant tumor of melanocyte origin, whereas veterinary pathologists term such tumors *malignant melanomas.*

TUMOR CHARACTERISTICS

BENIGN VERSUS MALIGNANT TUMORS

The most important distinction between benign and malignant tumors is that malignant tumors are able to invade locally and metastasize systemically, but benign tumors are not. The invasive capabilities of malignant tumors are associated with enhanced tumor cell motility, increased production of proteases, and altered tumor cell adhesion characteristics. Although benign tumors are ultimately distinguished from their malignant counterparts based on invasiveness, a variety of morphologic and behavioral features are generally considered to predict the potential for malignant behavior (Table 6-1). Although both benign and malignant tumors are composed of proliferating cells, malignant tumors have essentially unlimited replicative potential. The tumors are relatively independent of exogenous growth stimulatory molecules and are insensitive to growth inhibitory signals from their environment. Moreover, malignant cells are better able than benign cells to evade programmed cell death (apoptosis) and to escape the host's cytotoxic immune response. Compared with benign tumors, malignant tumors stimulate marked angiogenesis (the formation of new blood vessels), thus assuring adequate tumor nutrition.

Because some benign tumors evolve into malignant neoplasms and some malignant tumors develop increasingly aggressive behavior over time (a process termed *malignant progression*), tumors may

TABLE 6-1 Comparisons between Benign and Malignant Tumors

Characteristic	Benign	Malignant
Differentiation	Well-differentiated appearance	Usually some lack of differentiation
	Structure similar to tissue of origin	Structure often atypical
	Little or no anaplasia	Variable degree of anaplasia
Growth rate	Slow, progressive expansion	Slow-to-rapid growth; erratic growth rate
	Rare mitotic figures	Mitotic figures often numerous
	Normal-appearing mitotic figures	Mitotic figures sometimes abnormal
Local invasion	No invasion	Local invasion
	Cohesive and expansile growth	Infiltrative growth
	Capsule often present	Usually no capsule
Metastasis	No metastasis	Frequent metastasis (definitive criterion for malignancy)

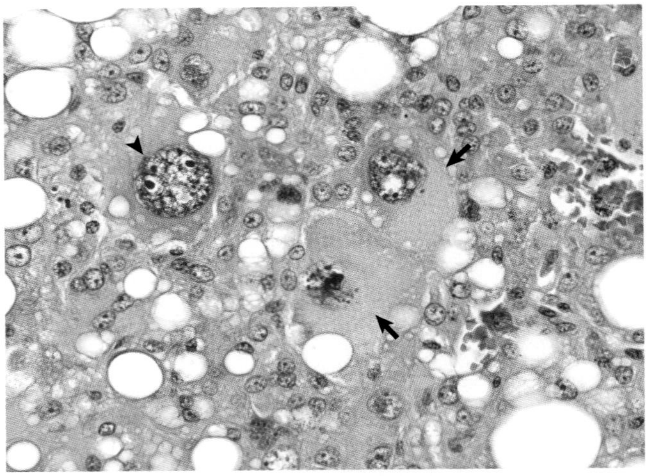

Fig. 6-6 **Anaplastic liposarcoma, subcutis, dog.** Anaplastic tumors of epithelial or mesenchymal cell origin often contain bizarre tumor giant cells such as the cells indicated by the arrows. Also, note the large nuclei with abundant coarsely aggregated chromatin and multiple nucleoli *(arrowhead)*. H&E stain. (Courtesy College of Veterinary Medicine, University of Illinois.)

be graded to reflect where they lie on the continuum from benign to highly malignant and/or staged to indicate the extent of tumor spread. Together, the grade and stage of the tumor indicate the risk the tumor poses to the host and help determine therapeutic strategy. It should be noted, however, that many benign tumors, such as equine sarcoids, have little or no malignant potential and rarely if ever evolve into malignant tumors.

DIFFERENTIATION

Hallmarks of Differentiation

Morphology

Each normal, fully differentiated, mature tissue type has a characteristic gross and microscopic appearance that varies little from individual to individual of a species. Neoplastic tissues lose these differentiated features of cellular morphology and organization to a variable extent. In general, malignant tumors appear less differentiated than benign tumors. Loss of morphologic hallmarks of tissue maturity is often accompanied by loss of functional capacity and development of aggressive behavior.

Neoplastic cells often show considerable morphologic variability compared with the normal tissue from which they are derived. Tumor cells, especially malignant tumor cells, may exhibit anaplasia (cellular atypia). Anaplastic cells are poorly differentiated cells that exhibit notable cellular and nuclear pleomorphism (variation in size and shape). In some tumors, bizarre tumor giant cells are seen (Fig. 6-6). Nuclei may exhibit extreme variability in number, size, shape, chromatin distribution, and nucleolar size and number (Fig. 6-7). Anaplastic nuclei are often hyperchromatic (darkly staining) because of increased DNA content; are disproportionately large relative to cell size, resulting in an increased nuclear:cytoplasmic ratio; and have prominent nucleoli. Mitotic figures in tumor cells may be numerous. Many of the nuclear changes seen in neoplastic cells reflect the frequent cell division, chromosomal abnormalities, and active metabolic state that characterize these cells.

Neoplastic cells often exhibit loss of characteristic cytoplasmic and nuclear features. For example, poorly differentiated mast cell tumors often lack the prominent cytoplasmic granules that are a hallmark of normal mast cells (Fig. 6-8). Special stains or

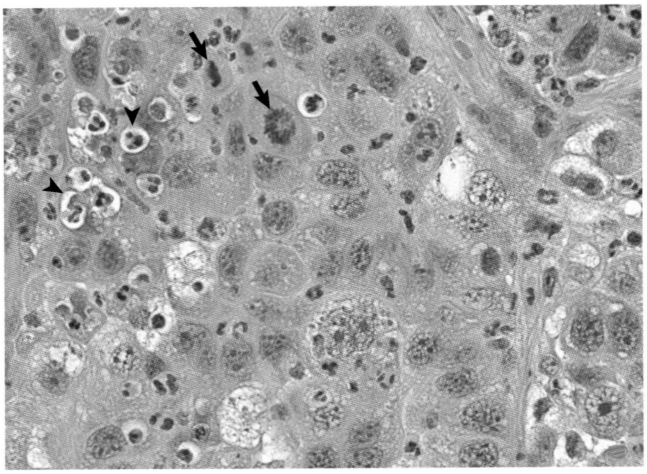

Fig. 6-7 **Anaplastic bronchioalveolar carcinoma, dog.** This tumor exhibits marked nuclear pleomorphism and has a fairly high mitotic index. Note the prominent mitotic figures *(arrows)* and phagocytosis of neutrophils by the tumor cells (emperipolesis) *(arrowheads)*. H&E stain. (Courtesy Dr. J. F. Zachary, College of Veterinary Medicine, University of Illinois.)

immunohistochemistry may be able to highlight some characteristic morphologic feature retained in at least a subpopulation of tumor cells. As an example, characteristic granules may be revealed in some cells of feline and canine mast cell tumors by staining with toluidine blue or Giemsa. Many tumor cells have noticeably basophilic cytoplasm as a result of the presence of large numbers of ribosomes required for rapid cell growth and frequent cell division.

In tumors, normal tissue organization is usually lost to some extent. Increasing loss of normal architecture in tumors correlates with increasing independence of tumor cells from their surrounding tissue. As an example, lymphomas arising in lymph nodes often consist of solid sheets of neoplastic cells that partially or completely efface normal lymph node architecture (Fig. 6-9). In tissue that normally undergoes continual renewal, such as the skin and oral mucosa, the normal maturation sequence may be altered. Thus in

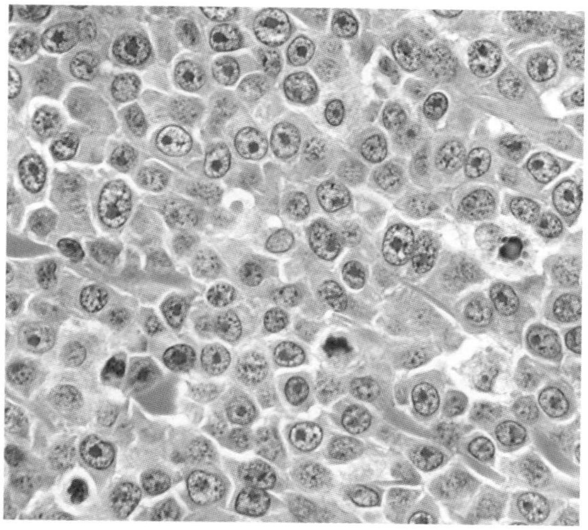

Fig. 6-8 Mast cell tumor, skin, cat.
With H&E staining, hallmark mast cell granules are not visible. To see these granules, the section must be stained with a metachromatic stain such as toluidine blue or Giemsa. Note the very large single nucleolus and marginated chromatin in the neoplastic cells. H&E stain. (Courtesy College of Veterinary Medicine, The Ohio State University.)

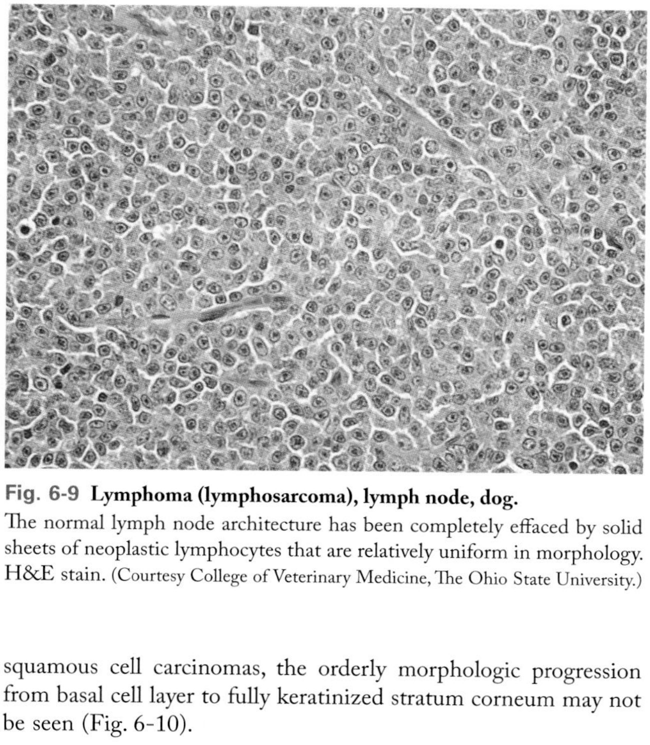

Fig. 6-9 Lymphoma (lymphosarcoma), lymph node, dog.
The normal lymph node architecture has been completely effaced by solid sheets of neoplastic lymphocytes that are relatively uniform in morphology. H&E stain. (Courtesy College of Veterinary Medicine, The Ohio State University.)

squamous cell carcinomas, the orderly morphologic progression from basal cell layer to fully keratinized stratum corneum may not be seen (Fig. 6-10).

Function

Loss of differentiated function frequently accompanies loss of differentiated morphology in tumors. Thus neoplastic cells arising from alveolar lining cells of the lung generally fail to perform normal respiratory functions and tumors of primitive germ cell origin do not form normal sperm or ova. Some aspects of normal function may be retained. Thyroid adenomas may continue to produce thyroid hormones, and plasma cell tumors may secrete immunoglobulins. However, in the majority of cases, these functions are no longer regulated appropriately because the neoplastic cells have lost responsiveness to and dependence on normal regulatory pathways.

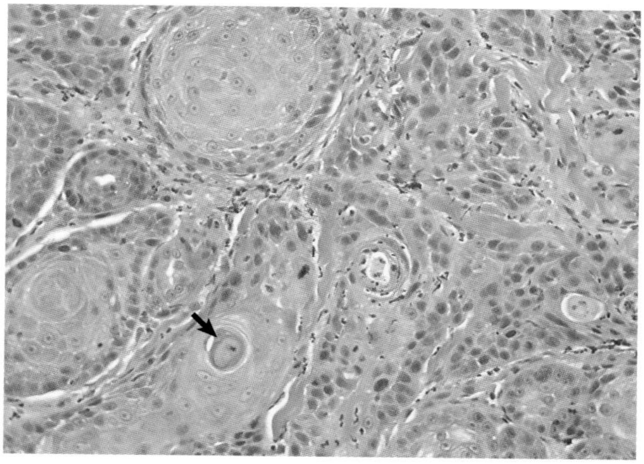

Fig. 6-10 Squamous cell carcinoma, tongue, cat.
The orderly pattern of epidermal maturation seen in normal oral mucosa is absent from this squamous cell carcinoma. An occasional "keratin pearl" *(arrow)* reveals the tissue of origin for this tumor. H&E stain. (Courtesy College of Veterinary Medicine, The Ohio State University.)

Thus thyroid adenomas may produce clinical hyperthyroidism, and plasma cell tumors may cause hypergammaglobulinemia.

Behavior

Benign tumors are generally expansile and may compress adjacent tissue, whereas malignant tumors have invasive and in many instances metastatic capabilities. In malignant tumors, alterations in adhesion, motility, and protease production allow tumor cells to leave the tumor mass and penetrate surrounding tissue. Moreover, for malignant cells to invade and ultimately metastasize, they must become completely independent of local growth regulatory controls and acquire an independent blood supply. Acquisition of these features allows tumors to spread well beyond their ordinary anatomic niches.

Stem Cells and Differentiation

Most tumors are composed of cells that lack fully differentiated morphologic, functional, and behavioral characteristics. Furthermore, many neoplastic cells share some features with the embryonic cells that gave rise to the mature tissue in which the tumor originated. This similarity between embryonic and neoplastic cells may be accounted for in two different ways. First, normal mature cells may undergo dedifferentiation as they evolve into tumor cells, leading to the reemergence of more primitive characteristics. Second, tumors may arise from the small population of stem cells found in all adult tissue; such stem cells are required for normal tissue renewal. The appearance and behavior of the tumor that develops from a neoplastic stem cell is determined by the stage of differentiation at which the malignant phenotype is manifested; the neoplastic stem cell is said to have undergone maturation arrest at that stage of its development. The diversity of cell types that can arise from a single progenitor stem cell is limited by the differentiation potential of that cell.

Totipotent stem cells, such as embryonic stem cells, can give rise to all tissues of the body, whereas multipotent or pluripotent stem cells can give rise to a smaller variety of tissue types. The plasticity of most adult stem cells is generally considered to be relatively restricted. Leukemias provide excellent examples of neoplasms arising from stem cells. A leukemia almost always arises from a single hematopoietic stem cell that has undergone heritable genetic change. The progeny of this stem cell all exhibit the same genetic change, although the cell type and degree of differentiation of the progeny may vary. Thus in myelogenous leukemia, a neoplastic multipotential stem cell may give rise to a combination of leukemic cells of the granulocytic, monocytic, and erythroid series (Fig. 6-11). The concept of a stem cell origin for cancer explains not only the embryonic characteristics of neoplastic cells but also the success of treatment strategies that use differentiating agents such as retinoids (vitamin A derivatives used to induce maturation of some human leukemia cells).

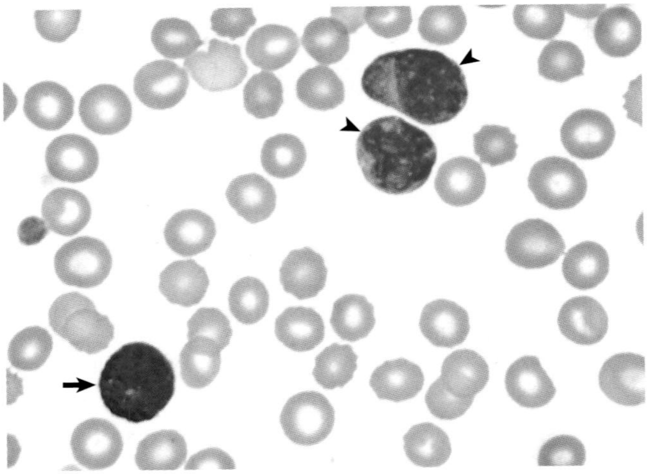

Fig. 6-11 Myelomonocytic leukemia, peripheral blood, dog. In this unusual case, leukemic cells of both monocytic *(arrowheads)* and granulocytic (basophil) *(arrow)* origin were present in peripheral blood. The animal had a marked leukocytosis (103,000 white blood cells/μL) and thrombocytopenia. Wright's stain. (Courtesy Dr. M.J. Burkhard, College of Veterinary Medicine, The Ohio State University.)

PROLIFERATION

The Cell Cycle

The cell cycle consists of G_1 (presynthetic), S (DNA synthesis), G_2 (premitotic), and M (mitotic) phases (Fig. 6-12). Quiescent cells are in a physiologic state called *G0*. In adult tissue, many cells reside in G_0 and are unable to enter the cell cycle at all or do so only when stimulated by extrinsic factors. Moreover, in response to DNA damage, even actively dividing normal cells undergo cell-cycle arrest, usually at one of several cell-cycle checkpoints. Cell-cycle arrest is initiated by the multifunctional tumor suppressor gene product p53 and gives the cell time to repair DNA damage.

Proliferative Activity in Nonneoplastic Tissue

Although composed primarily of quiescent cells in G_0, most mature tissue contains some combination of continuously dividing cells, terminally differentiated cells, stem cells, and quiescent cells that can enter the cell cycle. The tissues of the body may be divided into three groups on the basis of their proliferative activity.

Continuously Dividing Tissues (Labile Tissues)

In continuously dividing tissues (also called *labile tissues*), cells proliferate throughout life, replacing those that are lost. These tissues include surface epithelia, such as stratified squamous surfaces of

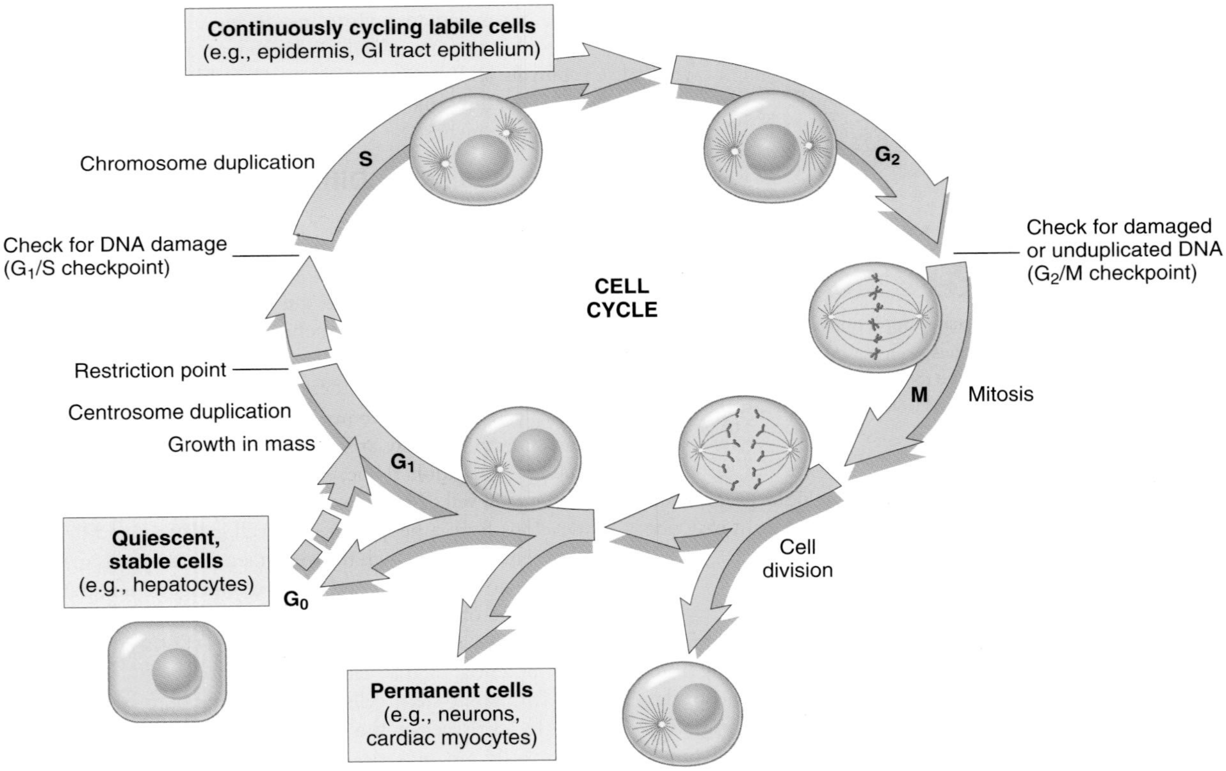

Fig. 6-12 Cell-cycle landmarks. The figure shows the cell-cycle phases (G_0, G_1, G_2, S, and M), the location of the G_1 restriction point, and the G_1/S and G_2/M cell-cycle checkpoints. Cells from labile tissues, such as the epidermis and the gastrointestinal *(GI)* tract, may cycle continuously; stable cells, such as hepatocytes, are quiescent but can enter the cell cycle; permanent cells, such as neurons and cardiac myocytes, have lost the capacity to proliferate. (Modified from Pollard TD, Earnshaw WC: *Cell biology*, Philadelphia, 2002, Saunders.)

the skin, oral cavity, vagina, and cervix; the lining mucosa of all the excretory ducts of the glands of the body (e.g., salivary glands, pancreas, and biliary tract); the columnar epithelium of the gastrointestinal tract and uterus; the transitional epithelium of the urinary tract; and cells of the bone marrow and hematopoietic tissue. In most of these tissues, mature cells are derived from stem cells, which have an unlimited capacity to proliferate and whose progeny may differentiate into a variety of mature cell types.

Quiescent Tissues (Stable Tissues)

Quiescent (or stable) tissues normally have a low level of replication; however, cells from these tissues can undergo rapid division in response to stimuli and are thus capable of reconstituting the tissue of origin. They are considered to be in the G_0 stage of the cell cycle but can be stimulated to enter G_1. This category includes the parenchymal cells of the liver, kidneys, and pancreas; mesenchymal cells, such as fibroblasts and smooth muscle; vascular endothelial cells; and resting lymphocytes and other leukocytes. The regenerative capacity of stable cells is best exemplified by the ability of the liver to regenerate after partial hepatectomy and after acute chemical injury. Fibroblasts, endothelial cells, smooth muscle cells, chondrocytes, and osteocytes are quiescent in adult mammals but proliferate in response to injury. Fibroblasts in particular may proliferate extensively.

Nondividing Tissues (Permanent Tissues)

Nondividing (permanent) tissues contain cells that have left the cell cycle and cannot undergo mitotic division in postnatal life. Neurons and skeletal and cardiac muscle cells belong to this group. If neurons in the central nervous system (CNS) are destroyed, the tissue is generally replaced by the proliferation of the CNS supportive elements, the glial cells. However, recent results demonstrate that limited neurogenesis from stem cells may occur in adult brains. Although mature skeletal muscle cells do not divide, skeletal muscle does have some regenerative capacity, through the differentiation of the satellite cells that are attached to the endomysial sheaths. If the ends of severed muscle fibers are closely juxtaposed, muscle regeneration in mammals can be excellent, but this is a condition that can rarely be attained under practical conditions. Cardiac muscle has very limited, if any, regenerative capacity, and extensive injury to the heart muscle, as may occur in myocardial infarction, is followed by scar formation.

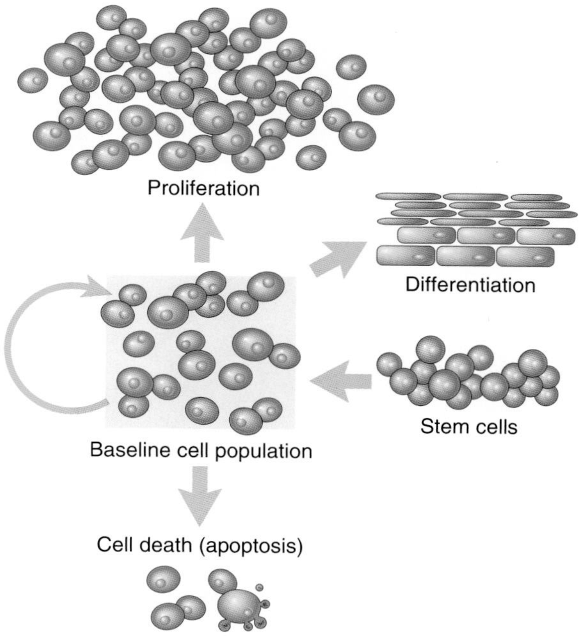

Fig. 6-13 Mechanisms regulating cell populations. Cell numbers can be altered by increased or decreased rates of stem cell input, by cell death due to apoptosis, or by changes in the rates of proliferation or differentiation. (Modified from McCarthy NJ, Smith CA, Williams GT: *Cancer Metastasis Rev* 11:157-178, 1992.)

Normal Tissue Growth

In adult tissues, the size of a cell population is determined by the relative rates of cell proliferation, differentiation, and death. Fig. 6-13 depicts these relationships and shows that increased cell numbers may result from either increased proliferation or decreased cell death.

Proliferation

Cell proliferation is largely controlled by signals (soluble or contact-dependent) from the microenvironment that either stimulate or inhibit cell proliferation. An excess of stimulators or a deficiency of inhibitors leads to net growth. Although accelerated growth can be accomplished by shortening the cell cycle, the most important mechanism of growth is the conversion of resting or quiescent cells into proliferating cells by making the cells enter the cell cycle. Both the recruitment of quiescent cells into the cycle and cell-cycle progression require stimulatory signals to overcome normal physiologic blocks to cell proliferation. Cell proliferation can be stimulated under both physiologic and pathologic conditions. The proliferation of mammary epithelium under hormonal stimulation during lactation is an example of physiologic proliferation. Pathologic conditions, such as tissue injury, cell death, and mechanical alterations, also stimulate cell proliferation. Excessive physiologic stimulation may create pathologic conditions, such as enlargement of the thyroid, as a consequence of increased serum levels of thyroid-stimulating hormone.

Differentiation

Differentiation also impacts the size of a cell population and its proliferative potential. For example, myocytes and neurons are terminally differentiated cells (i.e., they are at an end stage of differentiation and are not capable of replicating). In some adult tissues, such as liver and kidney, differentiated cells are normally quiescent but are able to proliferate when necessary. In proliferative tissue, such as bone marrow and the epithelia of the skin and gut, the mature cells are terminally differentiated, short-lived, and incapable of replication, but they may be replaced by new cells arising from stem cells. Thus in such tissues there is a homeostatic equilibrium between the proliferation of stem cells, their differentiation, and the death of fully differentiated cells.

Cell Death

A variety of cell death mechanisms, including senescence, apoptosis, and autophagy, eliminate irreversibly damaged or effete cells to maintain normal tissue homeostasis. In response to DNA damage, oxidative stress, and telomere shortening, proliferating cells may undergo a permanent arrest in the G_1 phase of the cell cycle termed *cellular senescence.* Senescence is mediated by activation of the p53 or retinoblastoma pathways of cell cycle arrest. Senescent cells often express senescence-associated β-galactosidase.

Apoptosis is a form of "programmed cell death" that serves both as a normal physiologic process and as a response to pathologic stimuli. In proliferative tissue, such as gut epithelium, terminally

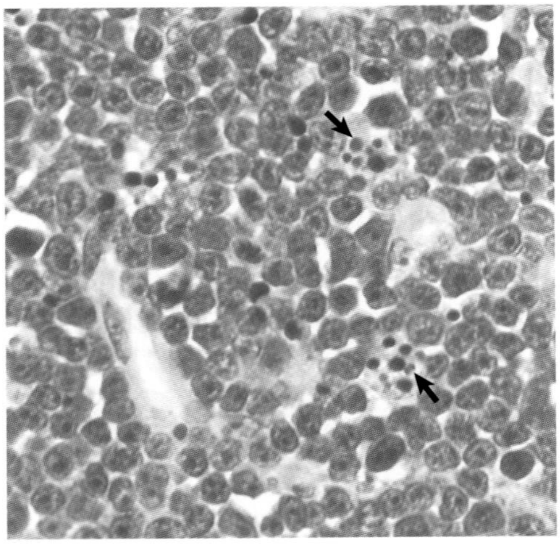

Fig. 6-14 Lymphoma, apoptosis, lymph node, horse.
The light microscopic appearance of apoptosis is characterized by condensation and fragmentation of nuclei *(arrows)*, cell shrinkage, engulfment of apoptotic bodies by surrounding cells, and lack of inflammation. H&E stain. (Courtesy Dr. R. Tan, College of Veterinary Medicine, University of Illinois.)

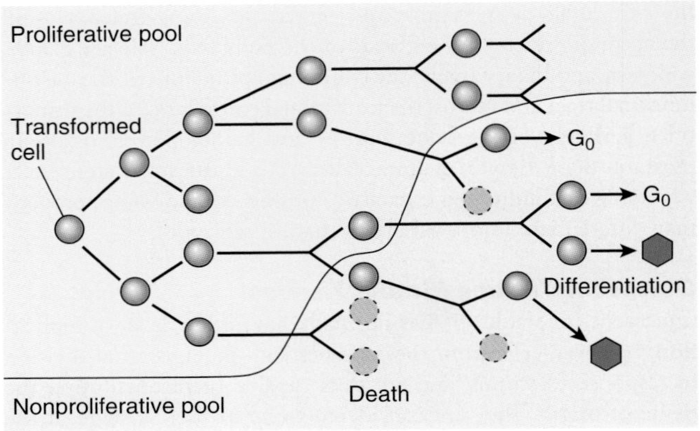

Fig. 6-15 Schematic representation of tumor growth.
As the cell population expands, a progressively higher percentage of tumor cells leave the replicative pool by reversion to G_0, differentiation, and death. (From Kumar V, Abbas A, Fausto N, et al: *Robbins & Cotran pathologic basis of disease*, ed 8, Philadelphia, 2009, Saunders.)

differentiated cells undergo apoptosis and are thus removed from the cell population. Apoptosis may occur in response to withdrawal of survival factors from the cell environment or by binding of death factors, such as Fas ligand and tumor necrosis factor-α (TNF-α) to cell surface receptors. Hypoxia and lack of essential nutrients may end in apoptosis. DNA damage may also induce apoptosis; in this case, apoptosis is triggered by p53. Apoptosis may be stimulated by the activity of cytotoxic immune cells, including T lymphocytes and natural killer (NK) cells. Signals for apoptosis activate a variety of signaling pathways, many of which ultimately result in the release of cytochrome C from mitochondria. The final effectors of apoptosis are the caspases, intracellular proteases that selectively destroy cellular organelles and degrade genomic DNA into nucleosome-sized fragments. The morphologic hallmarks of apoptosis include margination of chromatin, condensation and fragmentation of the nucleus, and condensation of the cell with preservation of organelles. Ultimately, the cell breaks into membrane-bound apoptotic bodies that are engulfed by surrounding cells without stimulating an inflammatory response (Fig. 6-14).

Autophagy refers to degradation of a cell's own organelles within autophagosomes. Autophagy can be a mechanism for cell survival in the face of nutrient deprivation, as it salvages important cellular components for reuse; however, extensive autophagy can also lead to a form of programmed cell death. The kinase mammalian target of rapamycin (mTOR) is the major cellular inhibitor of autophagy.

Tumor Growth

Essentially unlimited proliferative potential is a hallmark of neoplasia, especially of malignant neoplasms. Unlike normal cells, many tumor cells are immortal. This immortality is due to a combination of the alterations discussed later. In general, neoplastic cells escape normal limits on cell division, become independent of external growth stimulatory and inhibitory factors, and lose their susceptibility to apoptotic signals. This results in an imbalance between cell production and cell loss and a net increase in tumor size. However, it should be noted that the growth of a tumor is not completely exponential. A proportion of tumor cells is continually lost from the replicative pool because of irreversible cell-cycle arrest, differentiation, and death (Fig. 6-15).

Latency

As illustrated in Fig. 6-16, the latent period for a tumor is the time before a tumor becomes clinically detectable. The smallest clinically detectable mass is about 1 cm in diameter and contains about 10^9 cells. To form a tumor that size, a single transformed cell must undergo about 30 rounds of cell division, if all the progeny remain viable and capable of replication. Thus, by the time most tumors become clinically evident, they have probably been developing in the host for many years. However, once tumors reach a clinically detectable size, their growth may appear to be very rapid, because only 10 doubling cycles are required to convert a 1-g tumor into a 1-kg tumor. In fact, volume doubling times for tumors vary considerably, depending on the rate at which tumor cells divide, the fraction of tumor cells that are replicatively competent, and the rate at which tumor cells die. In general, benign neoplasms grow more slowly than malignant tumors, although there is considerable variation among tumors. Moreover, tumors may grow erratically, depending on their blood supply, the effect of extrinsic growth-regulating factors such as hormones, the efficacy of the host immune response, and the emergence of subpopulations of particularly aggressive tumor cells.

Proliferation

Many neoplastic cells no longer respond to extrinsic or intrinsic signals directing them into G_0 and no longer express functional p53. Thus the cells move continuously through the cell cycle. Moreover, because the tumor cells do not undergo cell-cycle arrest after DNA damage, they progressively accumulate potentially mutagenic DNA damage (Fig. 6-17). For homeostasis to be maintained, normal cells must engage in a continual dialogue with their environment. There is a constant exchange of information among cells via soluble mediators, including growth stimulatory factors, growth inhibitory factors, and hormones. These soluble mediators tightly control the growth of nonneoplastic cells. Neoplastic cells, on the other hand, often lose both their dependence on extrinsic growth stimulatory substances and their susceptibility to growth inhibitory signals from their environment. The mechanisms by which this occurs are discussed later. The end result is that tumor cells are no longer responsive to the needs of the organism as a whole and develop the capacity to drive their own replication.

The mitotic index is usually defined as the number of tumor cells in a microscopic field that contain condensed chromosomes

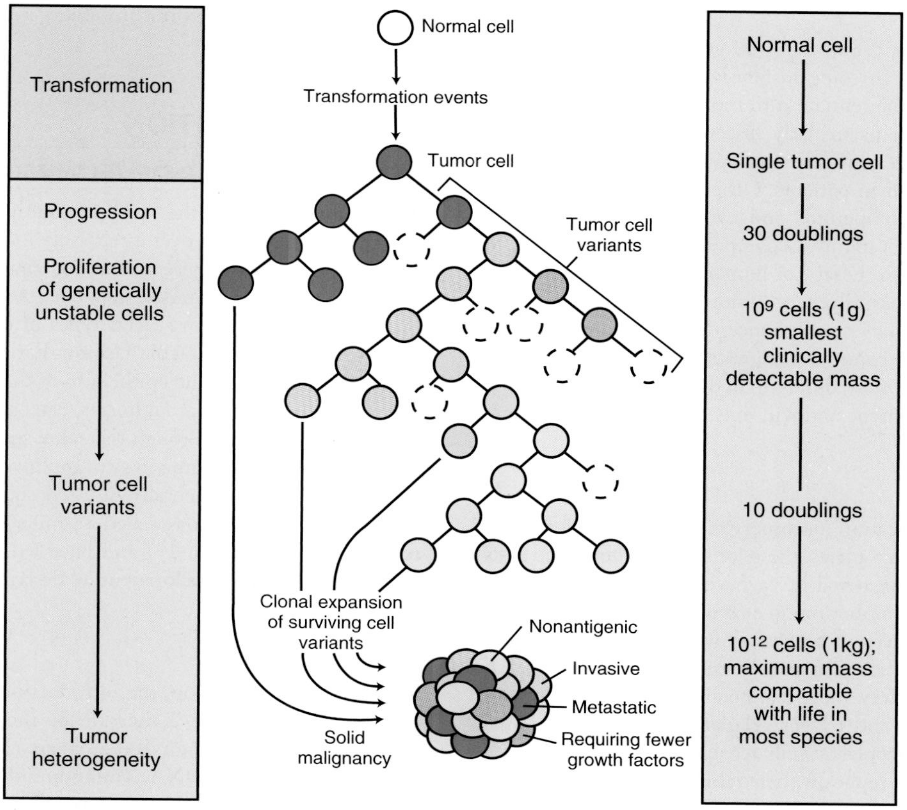

Fig. 6-16 Biology of solid tumor growth.
The center panel illustrates clonal evolution of a tumor and generation of tumor-cell heterogeneity. New subclones arise from descendents of the original transformed cell. With progressive growth, the tumor mass becomes enriched for those variants that are more adept at evading host defenses and are likely to be more aggressive. The left panel shows the corresponding stages of tumor progression, and the right panel depicts minimal estimates of tumor-cell doublings that precede the formation of a clinically detectable tumor mass. It is evident that by the time a solid tumor is detected, it has already completed a major portion of its life cycle, as measured by population doublings. The maximum tumor size compatible with life depends to some extent on the species affected. (Modified from Kumar V, Abbas A, Fausto N: *Robbins & Cotran pathologic basis of disease,* ed 7, Philadelphia, 2005, Saunders.)

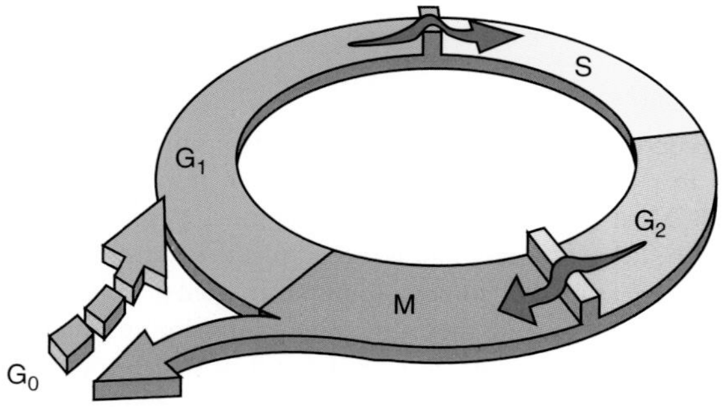

Fig. 6-17 Schematic representation of the cell cycle.
Many normal cells reside in G_0, a nonreplicative state. When they do enter the proliferative cycle, they can arrest at cell-cycle checkpoints at the G_1-S and G_2-M boundaries in response to a variety of stimuli, including DNA damage. In contrast, tumor cells spend little time in G_0 and often do not undergo cell-cycle arrest in response to DNA damage or lack of extrinsic growth stimuli. (Modified from Kumar V, Abbas A, Fausto N, et al: *Robbins & Cotran pathologic basis of disease,* ed 7, Philadelphia, 2005, Saunders.)

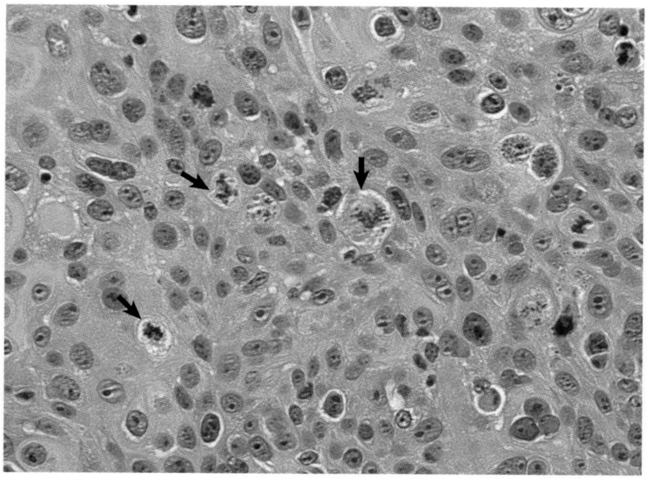

Fig. 6-18 Anaplastic neoplasm, dog.
The arrows indicate mitotic figures. This tumor has a high mitotic index. H&E stain. (Courtesy College of Veterinary Medicine, University of Illinois.)

and lack nuclear membranes (Fig. 6-18). Such cells are interpreted as being actively dividing, and the mitotic index of a tumor is considered to indicate its malignant potential. However, the mitotic index can be misleading. The fraction of tumor cells observed to be in mitosis depends not only on the number of cells undergoing mitosis but also on the length of time required to complete the process. In tumor cells, the time required for completion of the cell cycle is generally as long as or even longer than for normal cells. Mitotic figures may persist in cells unable to complete cell division and abnormal mitotic figures may be seen.

Differentiation

As discussed previously, tumor cells are generally less differentiated than normal cells. In some instances, however, some tumor cells can be forced to differentiate into more mature, near-normal cells. Leukemia cells are particularly susceptible to differentiation therapy, and retinoids are routinely employed to treat acute promyelocytic leukemia in human patients. Other differentiating agents, including vitamin D compounds and cytokines, have been less effective in this disease. Vitamin D compounds are showing some promise in differentiation therapy of human epithelial tumors, and compounds that epigenetically alter tumor cells by modifying the histones in chromatin may also enhance differentiation of tumor cells (discussed later). A common assumption underlying differentiation therapies is that more differentiated tumor cells will have a less stem cell-like phenotype and will thus have reduced proliferative potential.

Cell Death

Because the DNA replication machinery is unable to duplicate the extreme ends of DNA templates, the telomeres that form the ends of chromosomes are shortened at each cell division. Embryonic cells express telomerase, a riboprotein enzyme that allows telomeres to be replicated and even expanded; however, most adult cells do not express this protein and their telomeres shrink with each round of cell division. Very short telomeres are incompatible with continued cell division and trigger cellular senescence in normal cells. However, many neoplastic cells regain the ability to produce telomerase and thus to replicate their telomeres. Reexpression of telomerase appears to play an important role in the escape of tumor cells from senescence and their consequent immortality.

Although virtually all normal cells in the body can undergo apoptosis in response to appropriate physiologic signals, many cancer cells acquire resistance to apoptosis. This blocks a major route of tumor cell loss and enhances the overall growth rate of the tumor. Many tumor cells circumvent apoptosis by functional inactivation of the p53 gene, thus removing a key proapoptotic molecule. Additionally, tumor cells may constitutively activate survival signaling pathways, rendering the cells independent of exogenous survival factors. Finally, tumor cells may develop mechanisms for inactivating death factor signaling pathways, thus evading apoptosis in response to homeostatic signals from the cellular environment.

Autophagy plays a poorly understood and somewhat paradoxic role in tumor growth. In many tumors, authophagy is suppressed, thus presumably preventing autophagic tumor cell death. However, increased autophagy may also enhance tumor cell survival under the conditions of reduced nutrient availability that arise during therapy.

Genomic Instability

Evolving genomic instability is a hallmark of cancer. Many tumor cells fail to undergo cell-cycle arrest or apoptosis in response to DNA damage. They produce long and unstable telomeres subject to breakage, they lose the ability to carry out effective DNA repair, they demonstrate aberrant DNA methylation, and they exhibit increased rates of gene amplification, recombination, conversion, and transposition. These factors contribute to an increased rate of mutation and chromosomal aberration in neoplastic cells. Ultimately, this genomic instability results in aneuploidy, a chromosome complement that is not a simple multiple of the haploid chromosome content, or polyploidy, a chromosome complement more than twice the haploid chromosome number. The karyotypes of cancer cells may thus be notably abnormal and unstable. As a rule, increasing aneuploidy is correlated with increasingly malignant behavior. Genomic instability is discussed in more detail later in the chapter.

TUMOR EVOLUTION

STEPWISE TUMOR DEVELOPMENT

Neoplasms develop as the result of multiple genetic and epigenetic changes that occur over a relatively long time course. It is the cumulative effect of these alterations that creates a tumor. The stepwise evolution of tumors has been studied most thoroughly in carcinomas. There are several types of carcinoma that develop in an orderly and predictable fashion. For instance, squamous cell carcinoma arises from the epithelium of the eyelid in many species of animals, including cattle, horses, cats, and dogs. In all species, these tumors develop through the same sequence of steps: epidermal hyperplasia, carcinoma in situ, and invasive carcinoma. Extensive studies of experimentally induced squamous cell carcinomas in the skin of mice have revealed a similar morphologic pattern of tumor evolution (Fig. 6-19) and have led to a detailed model of stepwise carcinoma development as described in the next section (Fig. 6-20).

Initiation

The first step is initiation, the introduction of irreversible genetic change into basal cells of the skin by the action of a mutagenic initiating agent or initiator. Initiators are chemical or physical carcinogens that damage DNA. Mutation induction requires not only the introduction of a DNA lesion, but also mispairing of the DNA lesion during subsequent DNA replication to produce an altered complementary DNA strand. Thus at least a single round of DNA replication is necessary for fixation of the genetic change to occur. Initiated cells appear morphologically normal and may remain quiescent for many years. However, these cells harbor mutations that provide them with a growth advantage under special conditions. For example, the initiated cells may respond more vigorously to mitogenic signals or be more resistant to apoptosis-inducing stimuli than their neighbors.

Promotion

The second stage of tumor development is promotion. Promotion refers to the outgrowth of initiated cells in response to selective stimuli. Most of these selective stimuli, termed *promoting agents* or *promoters,* drive proliferation. For example, the skin irritant croton oil is an effective skin tumor promoter. In general, promoters are not mutagenic; instead, they alter gene expression in initiated and uninitiated cells to create an environment in which initiated cells have a growth advantage. Because promoters are nonmutagenic, their effects are usually reversible, and some papillomas can actually undergo regression. What emerges at the end of the promotion phase of tumor development is a papilloma, which is a benign tumor.

Progression

The final stage of tumor development, progression, includes the conversion of a benign tumor to an increasingly malignant tumor and ultimately to a metastatic tumor. Malignant conversion represents an irreversible change in the nature of the developing tumor. Progression is a complex and poorly understood process involving both genetic and epigenetic changes in tumor cells and their environment that select for increasingly malignant clones of tumor cells. Karyotypic instability in tumor cells and increasing tumor cell heterogeneity are hallmarks of progression.

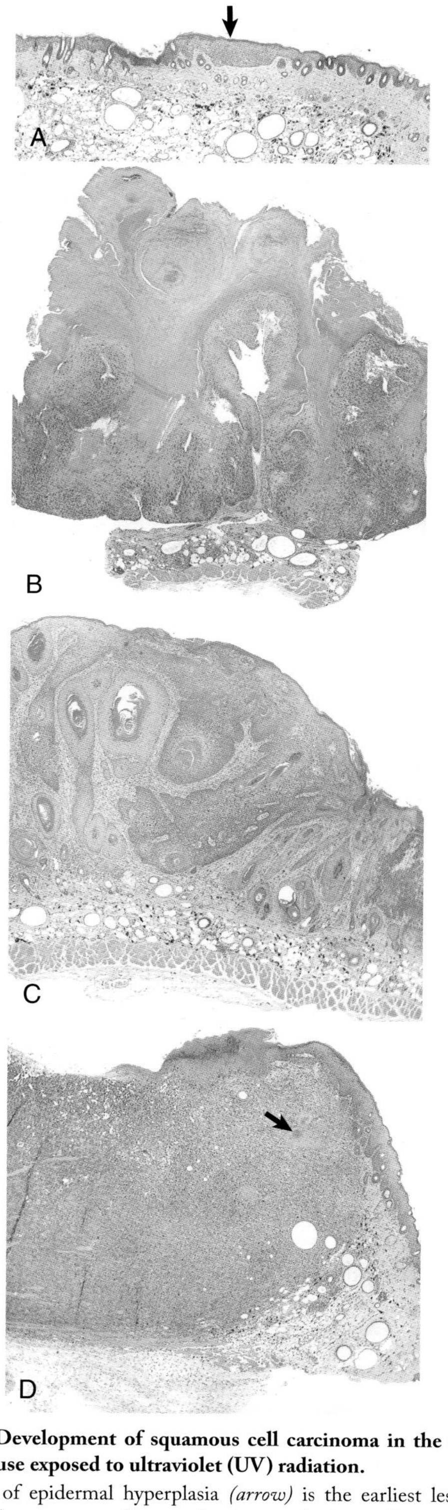

Fig. 6-19 Development of squamous cell carcinoma in the skin of a hairless mouse exposed to ultraviolet (UV) radiation.

A, A focus of epidermal hyperplasia *(arrow)* is the earliest lesion seen. **B,** This develops into a papilloma, a benign exophytic papillary growth that is highly keratinized and does not penetrate into the dermis. **C,** As the papilloma undergoes conversion into a malignant squamous cell carcinoma, it begins to invade the dermis and to lose the regular pattern of epithelial differentiation. **D,** A fully developed squamous cell carcinoma has lost most differentiated characteristics and extends deep into the dermis. Only a few keratin "pearls" *(arrow)* indicate the origin of this tumor from the epidermis of the skin. All figures were taken at the same magnification. H&E stain. (Courtesy Dr. T.M. Oberyszyn, The Ohio State University.)

TUMOR HETEROGENEITY AND CLONAL SELECTION

Most tumors are believed to be of clonal origin (i.e., they are ultimately derived from a single transformed cell). Tumor cell heterogeneity is generated during the course of tumor growth by the progressive accumulation of heritable changes in tumor cells (see Fig. 6-16). With each new genetic alteration, the progeny of the genetically altered tumor cell constitute a subclone of tumor cells. The generation of subclones is fostered by the marked genetic instability of tumor cells compared with normal cells. Successful subclones are those that have a high proliferative rate, are able to evade the host immune response, can stimulate the development of an independent blood supply, are independent of exogenous growth factors, and are able to escape from the primary tumor and spread to distant sites. These characteristics give successful subclones a selective advantage over other subclones of cells within the tumor. A tumor subclone with a selective advantage will eventually predominate.

MOLECULAR CHANGES UNDERLYING TUMOR PROGRESSION

In a few well-studied tumor types, such as chemically induced skin tumors in mice and colonic carcinomas in humans, the stepwise molecular changes that underlie morphologic changes in the tumors have been determined. Many of these genetic changes are associated with proliferation, DNA repair, angiogenesis, and invasiveness, as detailed later.

TUMOR SPREAD

FEATURES OF TUMOR SPREAD

Malignant tumors are often highly invasive. They do not respect anatomic boundaries, and they infiltrate adjacent normal tissue. Benign tumors, on the other hand, are generally expansile rather than infiltrative. The border between a benign tumor and adjacent tissue is usually distinct, and benign tumors of epithelial origin are often encapsulated (surrounded by a connective tissue capsule). Metastasis occurs when colonies of tumor cells take up residence at some distance from the parent tumor. Metastasis is the single most reliable hallmark of malignancy. Benign tumors do not metastasize. However, some malignant tumors, notably those of the CNS, are also nonmetastatic. Metastatic disease is believed to be responsible for 90% of human cancer deaths. Moreover, it is estimated that approximately 30% of solid cancers in humans have already metastasized by the time of initial diagnosis, greatly reducing the possibility of successful therapy. Cancer may metastasize by seeding the body cavities and surfaces (transcoelomic spread), by lymphatic spread, or by hematogenous spread.

PATHWAYS OF TUMOR METASTASIS

Transcoelomic

When cancers arise on the surface of an abdominal or thoracic structure, they encounter few anatomic barriers to spread. Thus mesotheliomas may be confined to the abdominal or pleural cavities, but the tumor cells within these cavities readily spread to cover all visceral and parietal surfaces (Fig. 6-21). In both humans and dogs, ovarian adenocarcinomas preferentially spread transcoelomically. Although such tumors are rare in dogs, they are commonly encountered in women. Even in the absence of invasion into the underlying organs, tumors such as mesotheliomas and ovarian adenocarcinomas are extremely difficult to treat and are generally fatal.

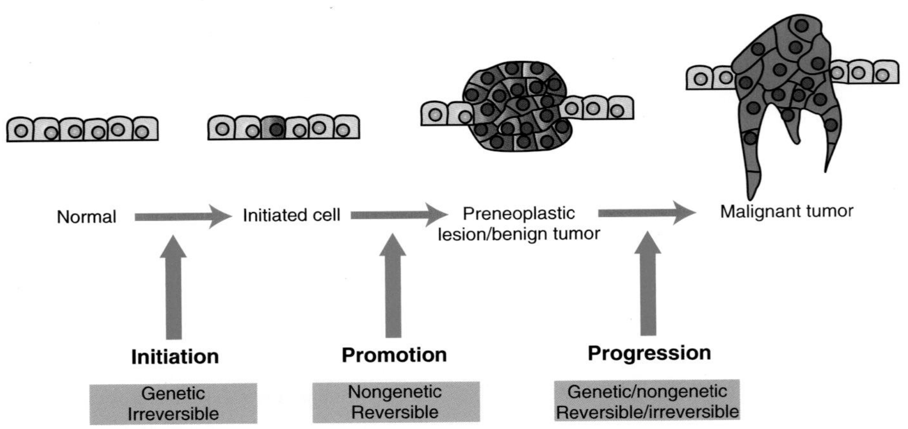

Fig. 6-20 Illustration of stepwise tumor development.
Initiated cells have irreversible genetic damage. In the presence of a promoter, these initiated cells expand to form a preneoplastic lesion or benign tumor. With further genetic and epigenetic alterations, a malignant tumor emerges from a subclone of cells within the benign precursor lesion. (Redrawn with permission from Dr. D.F. Kusewitt, College of Veterinary Medicine, The Ohio State University.)

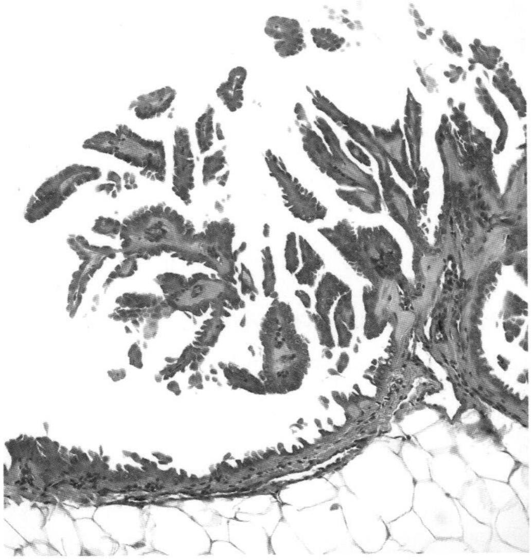

Fig. 6-21 Mesothelioma, peritoneum of the abdominal cavity, dog.
Mesotheliomas spread extensively within body cavities, but rarely metastasize by lymphatic or hematogenous routes. Note in the figure that neoplastic mesothelial cells cover the serosal surfaces and form papillary fronds, but they do not infiltrate underlying tissue. H&E stain. (Courtesy College of Veterinary Medicine, The Ohio State University.)

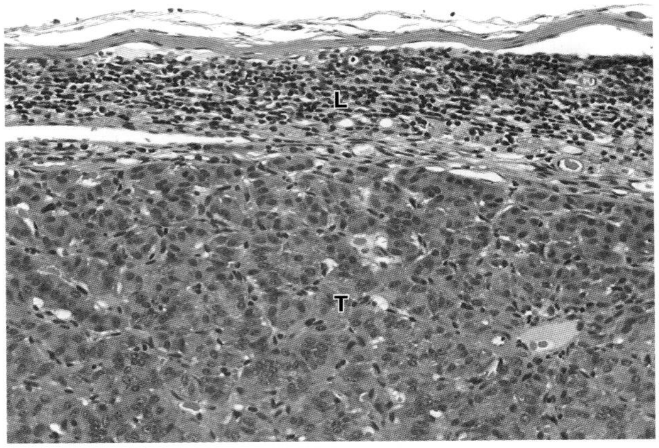

Fig. 6-22 Pancreatic carcinoma, metastatic, hepatic (portal) lymph node, dog.
Tumor cells *(T)* have almost completely replaced the normal architecture of the lymph node, except for a thin subcapsular rim of lymphocytes *(L)*. The tumor was confirmed by immunohistochemistry to be a functional pancreatic islet β-cell carcinoma. H&E stain. (Courtesy College of Veterinary Medicine, The Ohio State University.)

Lymphatic

In general, most carcinomas metastasize via the lymphatic system, although sarcomas may also employ this route of spread. The pattern of lymph node involvement is usually dictated by preexisting routes of regional lymphatic drainage. The lymph nodes closest to the tumor are usually colonized earliest and develop the largest metastatic tumor masses (Fig. 6-22). Thus adenocarcinomas of the intestine in all species usually metastasize first to the mesenteric lymph nodes and later to other lymph nodes within and outside the abdominal cavity. For many years, it was assumed that cancers spread in a stepwise manner from the primary site to regional lymph nodes, then to distant sites, such as the lung, and that regional lymph nodes actually represented a mechanical barrier to the spread of cancer. Thus removal of regional lymph nodes containing tumor tissue was believed to protect the patient from further spread of the tumor. However, regional lymph nodes may be bypassed as a result of natural, tumor-related, or treatment-induced anomalies in lymphatic drainage. More recent studies suggest that lymphatic spread does not occur in an orderly fashion and that metastasis to regional lymph nodes indicates that neoplastic disease has become widely systemic.

Hematogenous

Because lymphatic vessels connect with the vascular system, the distinction between lymphatic and hematogenous spread is somewhat artificial. However, sarcomas do tend to use the hematogenous route of spread more frequently than carcinomas. Tumors generally invade veins rather than arteries because arterial walls are much thicker and more difficult to penetrate. Tumors that enter veins ultimately enter the vena cava and lodge in the lungs (Fig. 6-23) or enter the portal system and lodge in the liver. Neoplasms metastatic

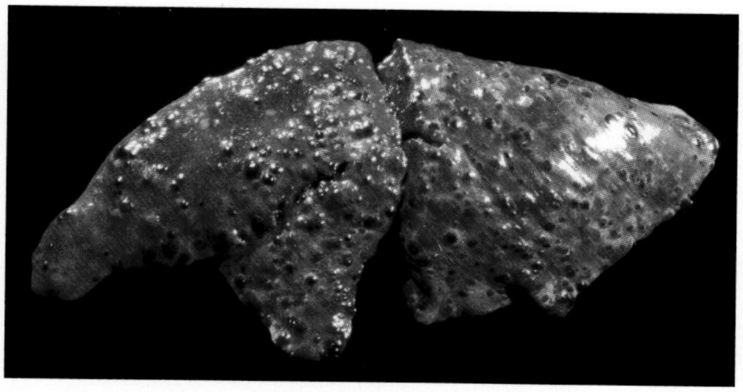

Fig. 6-23 Hemangiosarcoma, metastatic, lung, dog.
The multifocal (embolic) distribution of tumor nodules of relatively uniform size throughout the lung is characteristic of hematogenous metastasis. (Courtesy College of Veterinary Medicine, The Ohio State University.)

to the lungs may secondarily enter the arterial circulation. Some tumors have a notable predilection for veins. Pheochromocytomas of many species frequently enter the adrenal veins, where they may form large tumor masses extending into the vena cava.

MECHANISMS OF INVASION AND METASTASIS

Metastasis is a complex process requiring invasion of the extracellular matrix (ECM), entry into blood vascular or lymphatic vessels, extravasation of tumor cells, and colonization of the metastatic site (Fig. 6-24). These activities require many coordinated alterations in cell-cell and cell-matrix adhesion, motility, and invasiveness. Because of the complexity of the metastatic process and the heterogeneity of tumor cells, metastasis is inefficient. Of the many tumor cells that enter the circulation, only a few are able to produce metastases. Local invasion is a prerequisite for metastasis; thus the two processes share many features.

Adhesion

As a first event in invasion and metastasis, tumor cells must detach from the main tumor mass, penetrate the basement membrane, and enter the ECM. For cells to separate from each other, intercellular adhesion structures, including desmosomes and adherens junctions, must be dismantled. In many tumor cells of epithelial origin, this occurs because of the loss of cadherin or catenin function. These molecules are essential structural elements of intercellular junctions. At the same time that tumor cells detach from each other, they must also establish contacts with ECM components. Integrins and other specific receptors on the tumor cell membrane recognize and bind to a variety of ECM components such as fibronectin, laminin, collagen, and vitronectin. During invasion and metastasis, carcinoma cells often express increased numbers of these receptors. Moreover, instead of being localized to the basal surface of the tumor cell, the receptors are redistributed to cover the entire cell membrane. Tumor cells also appear to be able to modulate the types of ECM receptors that they express, allowing the cells to adapt to different microenvironments.

Invasion

Nonneoplastic epithelial cells generally rest on a specialized extracellular structure called the *basement membrane,* to which they are firmly attached by hemidesmosomes. In benign epithelial tumors, the basement membrane usually remains intact, whereas in malignant tumors the neoplastic epithelial cells penetrate the basement membrane to invade surrounding tissue. Tumor cells actively degrade basement membrane and ECM components by increasing

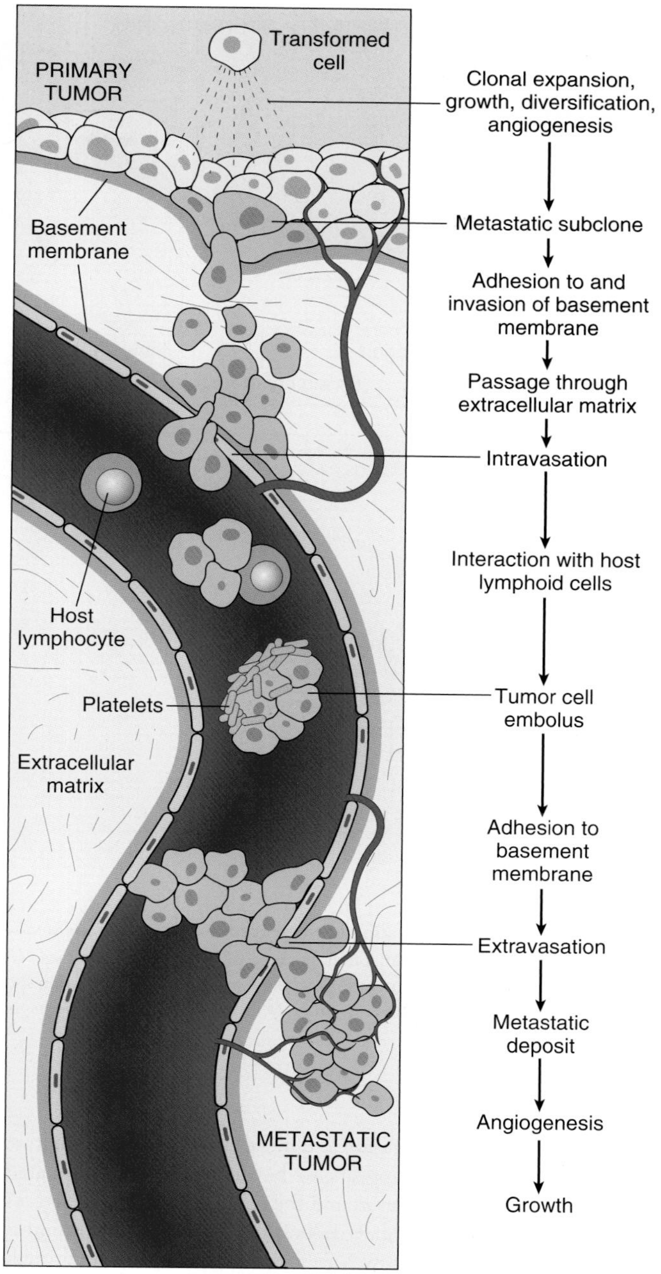

Fig. 6-24 The metastatic cascade.
This figure illustrates the sequential steps involved in the hematogenous spread of a tumor. Similar events occur during lymphatic spread. (From Kumar V, Abbas A, Fausto N, et al: *Robbins & Cotran pathologic basis of disease,* ed 8, Philadelphia, 2009, Saunders.)

the net protease activity in their vicinity (Fig. 6-25). Net protease activity is determined by a variety of interacting factors, including the rate of protease synthesis, the rate at which proteases are activated, and the rate at which protease inhibitors are produced. Proteases and antiproteases may be produced and activated by the tumor cells themselves, or tumor cells may induce nonneoplastic stromal cells to produce these enzymes. Proteases that appear to play an important role in tumor metastasis include matrix metalloproteinases, such as type IV collagenase, and urokinase, a serine protease.

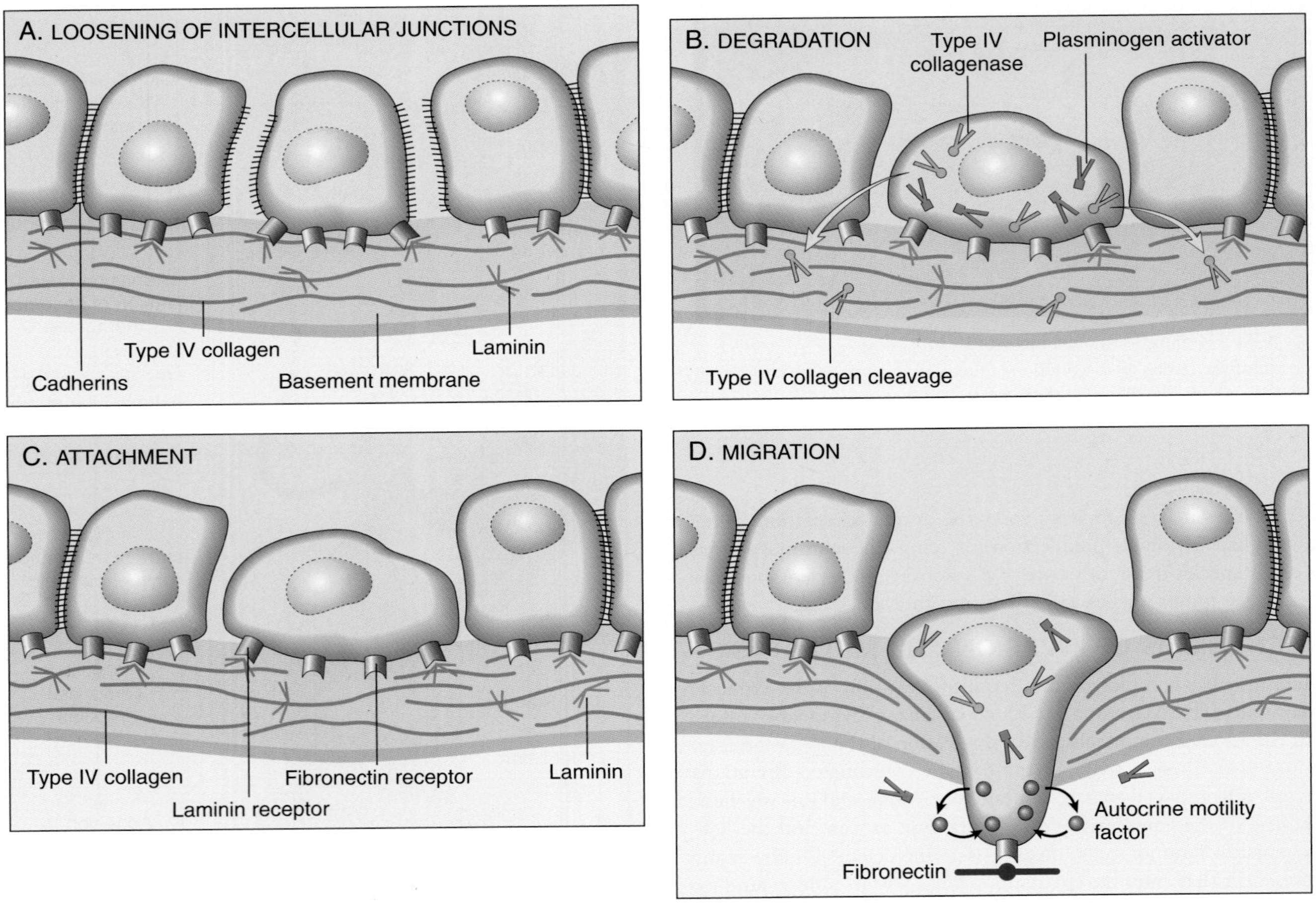

Fig. 6-25 Schematic illustration of the sequence of events in the invasion of epithelial basement membranes by tumor cells. Tumor cells detach from each other because of reduced adhesiveness **(A)**. Cells then attach to the basement membrane via laminin receptors **(B)** and secrete proteolytic enzymes, including type IV collagenase and plasminogen activator. Degradation of the basement membrane **(C)** and tumor cell migration **(D)** follow. (From Kumar V, Abbas A, Fausto N, et al: *Robbins & Cotran pathologic basis of disease,* ed 8, Philadelphia, 2009, Saunders.)

Migration

At many points during invasion and metastasis, tumor cells migrate actively. This migration appears to be mediated by coordinated alterations in the cytoskeleton and the cellular adhesion structures with which they are intimately associated. Tumor cell migration is stimulated by autocrine growth factors, such as hepatocyte growth factor, also called "scatter factor," and by cleavage products of ECM components, including fragments of collagen.

Tumor Emboli

The processes by which tumor cells invade blood and lymphatic vessels, extravasate from these vessels, and invade the ECM at a metastatic site are variations on those discussed earlier. Once inside a lymphatic or blood vessel, tumor cells tend to associate to form small emboli. In vessels, tumor cells may be recognized and attacked by host lymphocytes or may be surrounded by platelets. Interestingly, platelets may actually protect the tumor embolus and enhance tumor metastasis. The site at which tumor cells exit the blood vascular or lymphatic system is determined both by the pattern of lymphatic or vascular drainage of the primary tumor and by the ability of tumor cells to interact with adhesion molecules on endothelial cells. In addition, metastatic sites must provide a suitable microenvironment for tumor cell growth. Some tumors preferentially metastasize to specific sites. For example, prostate carcinomas in both humans and dogs frequently spread to bone (Fig. 6-26).

METASTASIS SUPPRESSION

A wide variety of genetic and epigenetic changes affect tumor cell adhesion, motility, and protease production. Thus metastatic potential is probably the cumulative effect of many different genetic alterations, and it seems unlikely that any individual genetic change single-handedly makes a tumor metastatic. On the other hand, a small number of genes have been identified that seem to function to suppress metastasis effectively. A good example of a candidate metastasis suppressor gene is the gene encoding E-cadherin, a component of adherens junctions, because loss of intercellular junctions appears to be essential for tumor metastasis.

TUMOR STROMA

COMPOSITION OF THE STROMA

A tumor consists of tumor cells proper, the tumor parenchyma, and nonneoplastic supporting structures, the stroma (Fig. 6-27, *A*). The stroma is composed largely of extracellular connective tissue and consists of proteins and glycoproteins, such as collagen, embedded in a complex matrix of proteoglycans. The stroma contains

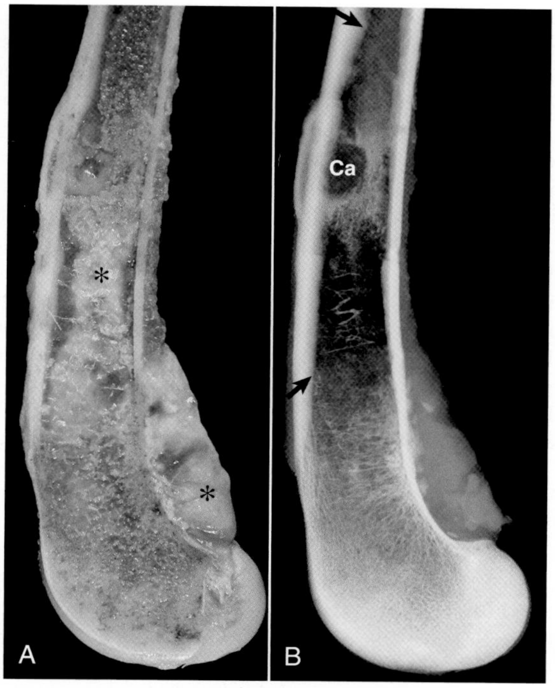

Fig. 6-26 Prostate carcinoma, metastasis, femur, dog.
A, The gross photograph of a sectioned femur reveals metastatic prostate carcinoma *(*)*. **B,** The radiograph illustrates an osteolytic bone metastasis *(Ca)*. In the regions between the arrows, extensive proliferation of new bone has occurred in response to the tumor. (Modified from Rosol TJ, Tannehill-Gregg SH, LeRoy BE, et al: Animal models of bone metastasis. In Keller ET, Chung LWK, editors: *Cancer treatment and research,* Boston, 2004, Kluwer Academic Publishers.)

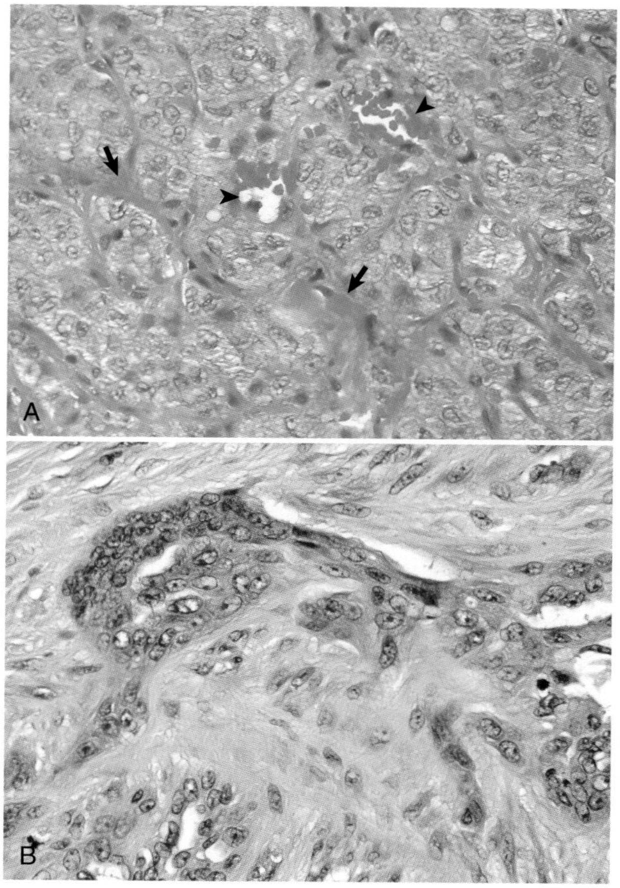

Fig. 6-27 Tumor stroma.
Tumor cells and the stroma in which they are embedded interact in a variety of ways that serve to modulate the growth rate, differentiation state, and behavior of both components. **A,** Pancreatic adenocarcinoma, pancreas, dog. The tumor parenchyma is divided into incomplete lobules by the tumor stroma *(arrows)* composed of collagen and extracellular matrix components in which blood vessels *(arrowheads),* fibroblasts, and inflammatory and immune cells are embedded. H&E stain. **B,** Scirrhous carcinoma, mammary gland, dog. Carcinomas and adenocarcinomas that stimulate the formation of abundant collagen in surrounding connective tissue *(desmoplasia)* may be termed scirrhous. Tumor-associated fibroblasts may secrete a fetal type of extracellular matrix (ECM) and co-evolve with adjacent tumor cells. Note how there is intimate interaction between the anaplastic malignant epithelial cells and the scirrhous connective tissue in which they are embedded, thus tumor stroma may both enhance and/or limit tumor development and spread. H&E stain. (**A** courtesy College of Veterinary Medicine, The Ohio State University. **B** courtesy of Dr. L. Borst, College of Veterinary Medicine, North Carolina State University.)

the blood vessels that supply nutrients to the tumor, fibroblasts, and a variety of inflammatory and immune cells. The amount of stroma associated with tumors can vary considerably. The extracellular material in the stroma of epithelial tumors is produced primarily by surrounding nonneoplastic mesenchymal cells (Fig. 6-27, *B*), whereas many mesenchymal tumors can produce the ECM in their stroma. For example, many osteosarcomas produce bone, a specialized form of connective tissue stroma. Stromal tissue may form a connective tissue capsule around epithelial tumors that limit neoplastic spread. In general, encapsulated epithelial tumors are considered to have a better prognosis than unencapsulated tumors (Fig. 6-28).

In the stroma of rare tumors, both mesenchymal and epithelial, there is an amorphous eosinophilic substance termed *amyloid.* Amyloid consists of one of a variety of abnormal proteins arranged in β-pleated fibrils. The proteins that form amyloid are usually secreted by the tumor cells themselves; for instance, λ-light chain protein secreted by neoplastic plasma cells forms the amyloid sometimes seen in the extramedullary plasmacytomas of various species.

TUMOR-STROMAL INTERACTIONS

Tumor cells interact with their stroma in a complex fashion, exchanging a wide variety of signaling molecules, including growth factors, cytokines, hormones, and inflammatory mediators (Fig. 6-29). These exchanges modulate the growth rate, differentiation state, and behavior of both stromal and tumor cells. Platelet-derived growth factor (PDGF) released by tumor cells stimulates tumor-associated fibroblasts to increase the production of collagen. In some cases, this process leads to an extensive fibrous reaction, termed a *scirrhous* or *desmoplastic response,* in the stroma. Transforming growth factor-α (TGF-α) of tumor origin can stimulate tumor-associated fibroblasts to differentiate into myofibroblasts, which are fibroblasts with contractile capabilities. Tumor-associated fibroblasts may acquire special characteristics that distinguish them from normal fibroblasts. Such fibroblasts may secrete a fetal type of ECM. In some tumors, tumor-associated fibroblasts acquire heritable genetic and epigenetic changes that allow them to co-evolve with adjacent tumor cells. Tumor cells may induce surrounding stromal cells to produce cytokines that promote tumor cell proliferation and motility. Furthermore, growth factors are sequestered in the ECM of the stroma, where they bind to proteoglycans. This interaction controls the bioavailability of these factors, which can

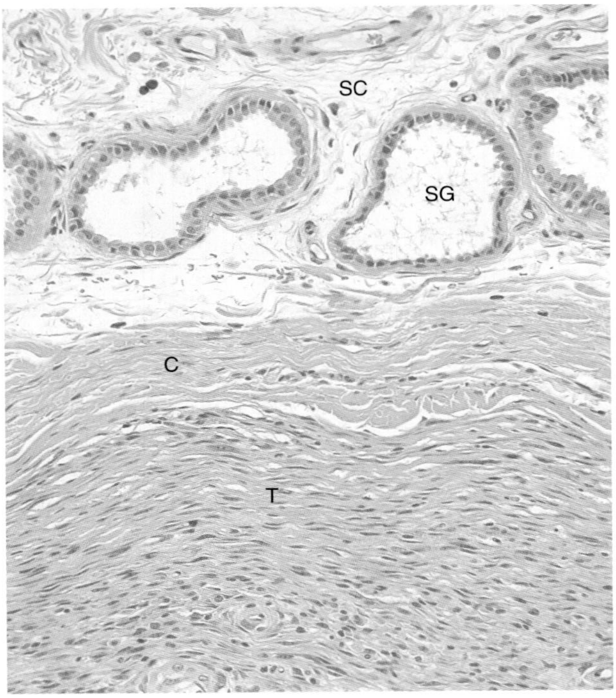

Fig. 6-28 Adnexal tumor, benign, skin, dog.
This tumor *(T)* lies within the subcutis *(SC)* and is surrounded by a thick connective tissue capsule *(C),* which is more frequently associated with benign than with malignant tumors. *SG,* Normal apocrine sweat glands of the subcutis. H&E stain. (Courtesy College of Veterinary Medicine, The Ohio State University.)

be released from the ECM by the activity of proteases secreted by tumor cells, stromal fibroblasts, or inflammatory cells.

ANGIOGENESIS

Continued growth of solid tumors absolutely depends on an adequate blood supply to provide oxygen and nutrients to tumor cells. Without the development of new blood vessels, a process termed *angiogenesis,* tumors are limited to a maximum diameter of 1 to 2 mm. At some point during tumor development, an angiogenic switch occurs that confers on tumor cells the ability to induce and sustain new tumor vasculature. Angiogenesis is a complex process involving recruitment of endothelial cells from preexisting blood vessels, endothelial cell proliferation, directed migration of endothelial cells through the ECM, and maturation and differentiation of the capillary sprout. Angiogenesis is controlled by the balance between a plethora of angiogenesis-stimulating and angiogenesis-inhibiting factors. Tumors induce angiogenesis by the production and release of angiogenic factors, such as vascular endothelial growth factor (VEGF), or by downregulating production of antiangiogenic factors, such as thrombospondin. In addition, angiogenic and antiangiogenic factors bound to ECM components can be released and activated by tumor protease activity. VEGF and acidic and basic fibroblast growth factors are among the most potent angiogenic factors produced by tumors. The tumor blood vessels that develop in response to angiogenic signals are usually more dilated, more tortuous, and more permeable than normal blood vessels (Fig. 6-30).

In addition to supplying nutrients, tumor vasculature plays other roles in tumor development. Vessel leakiness allows perivascular deposition of a fibrin network that promotes formation of collagenous tumor stroma. The endothelial cells of tumor blood vessels produce growth factors, such as PDGF and interleukin-1 (IL-1), that can stimulate the growth of tumor cells. Moreover, without access to the circulatory system, tumors cannot metastasize. Because solid tumor growth absolutely depends on an adequate blood supply, therapeutic strategies to inhibit angiogenesis are being developed.

Investigation of the development of lymphatic vasculature of tumors has demonstrated that tumor lymphangiogenesis shares many features with tumor angiogenesis. Tumor-associated lymphatic vessels sprout from preexisting lymphatic vessels in response to tumor-secreted factors such as VEGF. Tumor-associated lymphatics appear to be essential for metastasis of solid tumors to regional lymph nodes. In human tumors, there is a strong correlation between the levels of VEGF expression and lymphatic metastasis; and in genetically engineered mice that do not express VEGF, lymphatic metastasis does not occur.

INFLAMMATION

Many tumors are heavily infiltrated with neutrophils, eosinophils, mast cells, lymphocytes, histiocytes, or a combination of these cells. Inflammatory cells are attracted to tumors by chemokines and cytokines released by the tumor cells themselves or by mononuclear and polymorphonuclear cells infiltrating the tumor. Inflammatory cells serve as a source of prostaglandins, leukotrienes, and reactive oxygen species. In general, inflammation does not appear to protect against tumors. In fact, many chronic inflammatory conditions increase the risk of cancer in affected organs. As an example, the development of postvaccinal sarcomas in cats is clearly linked to the presence of inflammation at sites of inoculation. Moreover, in humans, epidemiologic studies suggest that nonsteroidal antiinflammatory drugs (NSAIDs) reduce the incidence of some cancers.

TUMOR IMMUNITY

TUMOR ANTIGENS

Tumor antigens are proteins, glycoproteins, glycolipids, or carbohydrates expressed on the tumor cell surface (Fig. 6-31). They include both tumor-specific antigens restricted to tumor cells and tumor-associated antigens present on both tumor cells and normal cells. Tumor antigens can be exploited both for diagnostic and therapeutic purposes. Tumor antigens released into the bloodstream allow noninvasive detection of tumors and monitoring tumor response to treatment. In combination with sophisticated imaging techniques, antibodies against tumor-restricted antigens can be used to localize tumors and detect metastases. Some tumor antigens can serve as the targets of effective immunosurveillance. However, many tumor antigens are not appropriate therapeutic targets. The antigens may not be restricted to tumor cells or may not elicit a strong cytotoxic response. Therapeutic strategies to enhance the immune response to tumor antigens are currently the subject of intense investigation.

Some tumor-specific antigens are newly expressed molecules, such as antigens derived from oncogenic viruses, or altered cellular products encoded by mutated genes. In these instances, productive viral infection or gene mutation is restricted to tumor cells and their progeny. Embryonic antigens or oncofetal antigens, normally not expressed in adult tissue but reexpressed in tumor tissue, may also behave as tumor antigens. For example, the developmental antigens, carcinoembryonic antigen and α-fetoprotein, are reexpressed in some tumors in a variety of species and may be released into the circulation. Serology for these antigens is widely used

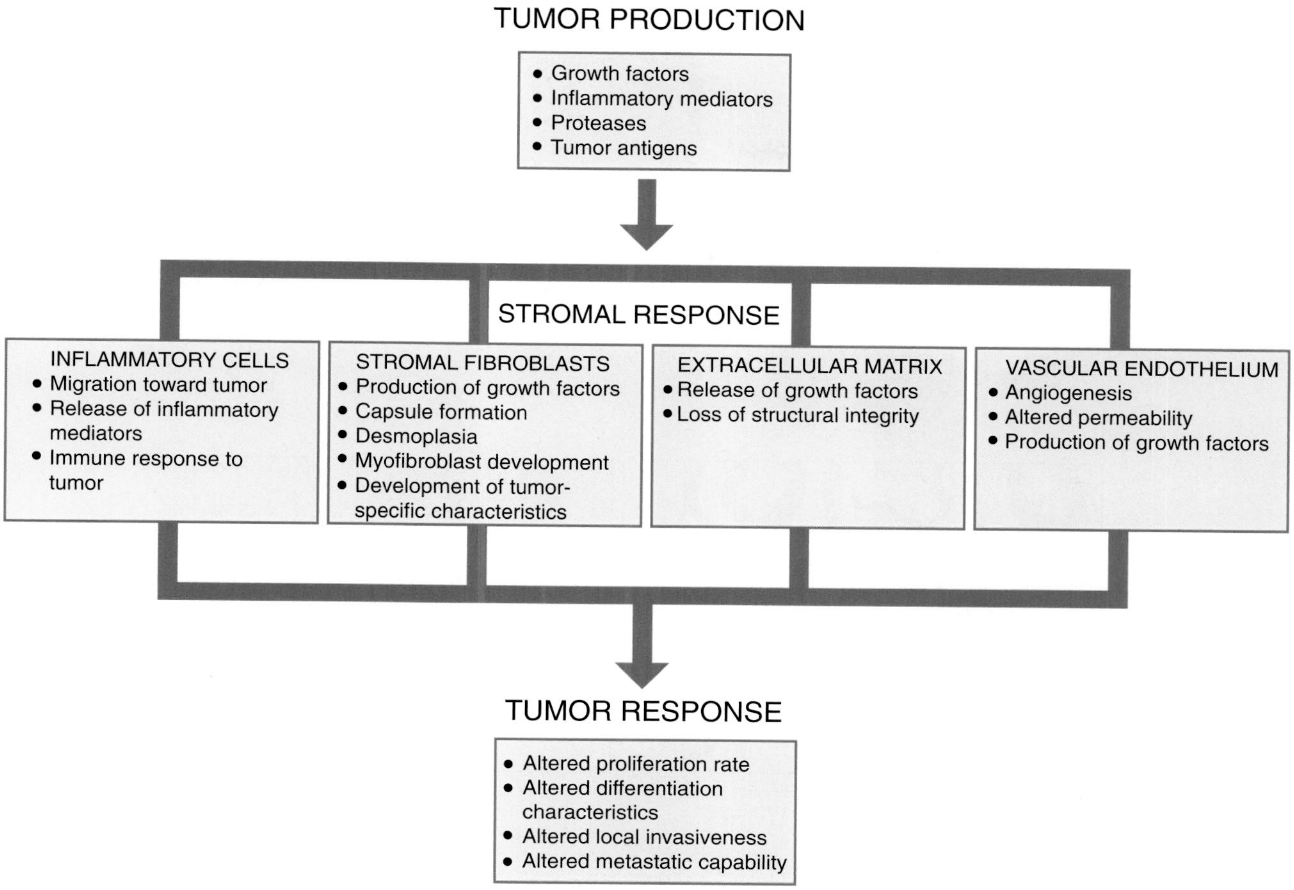

Fig. 6-29 Tumor-stromal interactions.
Tumor cells and the stroma in which they are embedded interact in a variety of ways that serve to modify the growth and behavior of both elements. Tumor stroma may both enhance and limit tumor development and spread. (Redrawn with permission from Dr. D.F. Kusewitt, College of Veterinary Medicine, The Ohio State University.)

to test for recurrence of liver and intestinal tumors in humans. Tumor-specific shared antigens are encoded by genes that have very limited expression in adult tissue but that are expressed by many types of tumor tissue. A striking example of useful tumor-specific shared antigens is the MAGE family of proteins, found in humans and other species. These antigens are not present on the surface of normal adult cells; however, they are expressed by a wide variety of tumor types and are promising candidates for antitumor immunotherapy. Tissue-specific antigens are shared by tumors and the normal tissues from which they arise. In some cases, these antigens are expressed only at specific stages of differentiation in the normal tissue and are thus termed differentiation antigens. When tissue-specific or differentiation antigens are expressed at considerably higher levels on tumor cells than normal cells, they may function much like tumor-specific antigens.

IMMUNOSURVEILLANCE

It is likely that the vertebrate immune system evolved primarily for the purpose of recognizing and destroying infectious organisms and the host cells they infect. However, the immune system also attacks tissue transplanted from genetically dissimilar animals of the same or different species. In special instances, the immune system can respond to self-antigens. It has been postulated that the immune system is capable of recognizing self-antigens on tumor cells as foreign and attacking antigen-bearing tumor cells as if they were microbially infected cells or foreign cells. This process is termed *immunosurveillance.* It is argued that effective immunosurveillance suppresses tumor development and that a failure of immunosurveillance allows tumors to emerge. The immunosurveillance hypothesis is supported by the dramatically increased tumor susceptibility of immunosuppressed transplant recipients. The inability of these individuals to mount effective antitumor responses apparently allows the emergence of many tumors usually eliminated by immunosurveillance. The presence of lymphocyte and macrophage infiltrates within and around tumors of many types in many species also suggests that tumors can elicit an immune response. Finally, there is abundant experimental evidence that mice can mount an effective immune response against chemically induced tumors. Much of our knowledge of tumor immunity comes from experimental studies employing mice.

ANTITUMOR EFFECTOR MECHANISMS

The body may mount a variety of immune responses against tumor antigens (Fig. 6-32). The type of immune response and its effectiveness against tumor cells is largely determined by the inherent immune responsiveness of the host and the characteristics of the tumor antigen under attack. The least specific immune response to tumor cells is carried out by the innate immune system. The innate immune response is believed to be the first line of defense against cancer cells. Antitumor effectors of the innate immune system, including NK cells and macrophages, do not require antigen-specific priming by dendritic cells. More specific immune responses

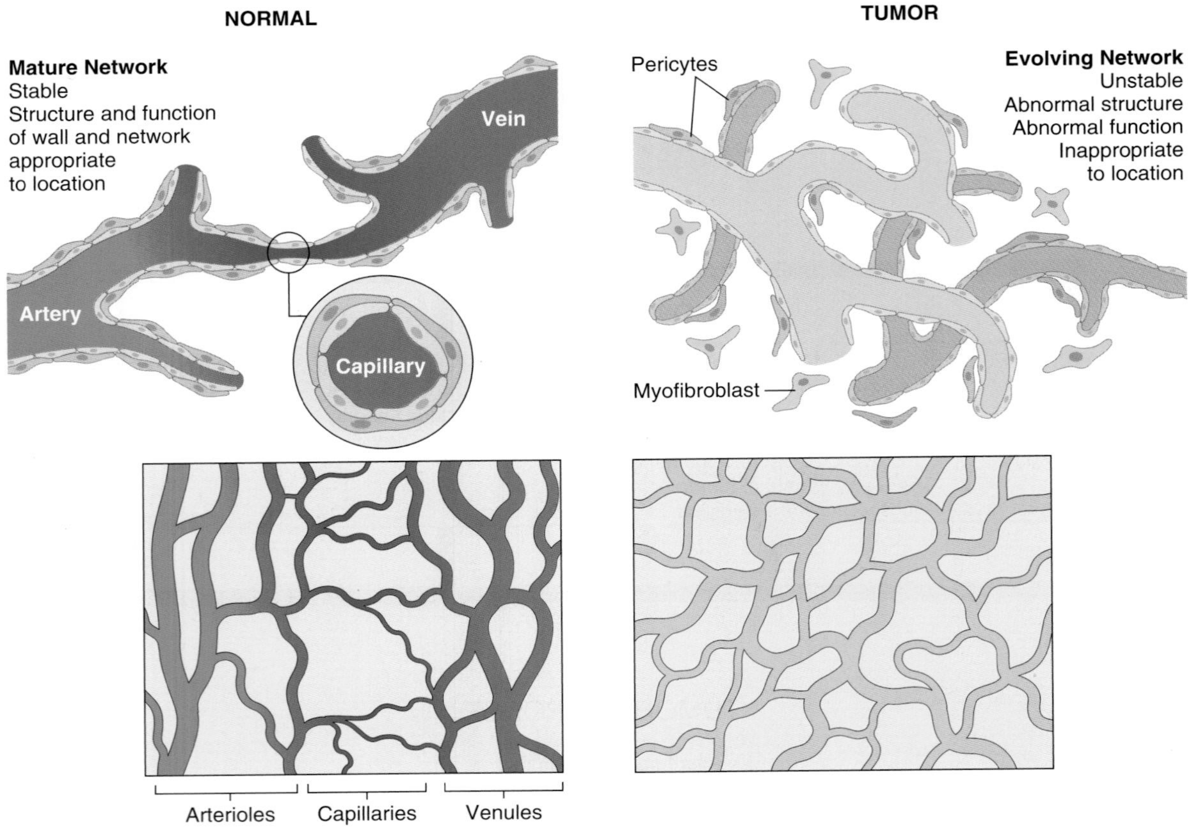

Fig. 6-30 Tumor angiogenesis.
Compared with normal vessels *(left panels),* tumor vessels are tortuous and irregularly shaped *(right panels).* The tumor vasculature is formed from circulating endothelial precursor cells and existing host vessels; myofibroblasts give rise to pericytes that surround vessels. In contrast to the stable vessel network of normal tissue, the networks formed by tumor vessels are unstable and leaky. Arterioles, capillaries, and venules are clearly distinguishable in normal vasculature; in the tumor, vessels are disorganized and specific vessel types cannot be identified. (Modified from Kumar V, Abbas A, Fausto N: *Robbins & Cotran pathologic basis of disease,* ed 7, Philadelphia, 2005, Saunders.)

are undertaken by the adaptive immune system, consisting of both cell-mediated and humoral components. The cell-mediated immune response is believed to mount the most effective antitumor defenses. Any adaptive antitumor immune response requires that tumor antigens be presented to immune cells in a recognizable context. Dendritic cells capture antigens that are secreted by viable tumor cells or released from dying tumor cells. The dendritic cells ingest these antigens, fragment them to a suitable size, link them to class I or class II major histocompatibility (MHC) antigens, and present them on the cell surface in association with appropriate co-stimulatory molecules. A dendritic cell can then interact with many different lymphocytes to prime their response to the specific tumor antigen presented by the dendritic cell. Antigen-activated $CD8^+$ and $CD4^+$ T lymphocytes develop into tumor-specific cytotoxic and T helper (T_H) lymphocytes, respectively, whereas B lymphocytes develop into immunoglobulin-secreting plasma cells. $CD8^+$ lymphocytes recognize tumor antigens in the context of MHC class I antigens, whereas $CD4^+$ cells recognize these antigens only in association with MHC class II molecules.

Natural Killer Cells

NK cells are lymphocytes that lack many of the usual markers of T or B lymphocytes. NK cells display a variety of receptors, both inhibitory and activating, that recognize MHC molecules and stress-induced ligands on tumor cells. NK cells can kill a wide variety of neoplastic and virally infected cells. Cells that express MHC class I molecules are preferentially spared by NK cells, whereas cells lacking MHC molecules are specifically targeted. After binding to a tumor cell, the NK cell releases lytic granules that activate apoptosis in the target cell. This mechanism of cell killing or cytolysis is shared with T lymphocytes and is discussed in more detail later.

Macrophages

Macrophages are migratory phagocytic cells capable of killing tumor cells by releasing reactive oxygen intermediates, lysosomal enzymes, nitric oxide, and tumor necrosis factor. Their antitumor activity is stimulated by interferon-γ (IFN-γ), which is produced by both T lymphocytes and NK cells. Macrophage-mediated tumor cell killing is independent of MHC antigens, tumor-specific antigens, and the type of transformed cell being targeted, but direct contact between the macrophage and tumor cell is required.

T Lymphocytes

Cytotoxic T lymphocytes (CTLs) are the primary effector cells of the adaptive antitumor immune response. Most CTLs are $CD8^+$ T lymphocytes that have been primed by dendritic cells to recognize and engage tumor antigens on the surface of tumor cells. When a CTL attaches to its target cell, a well-organized immunologic synapse is rapidly formed at the site of cell-to-cell contact and persists for more than an hour. Into this synapse, the CTL releases lytic granules containing perforin, a pore-forming

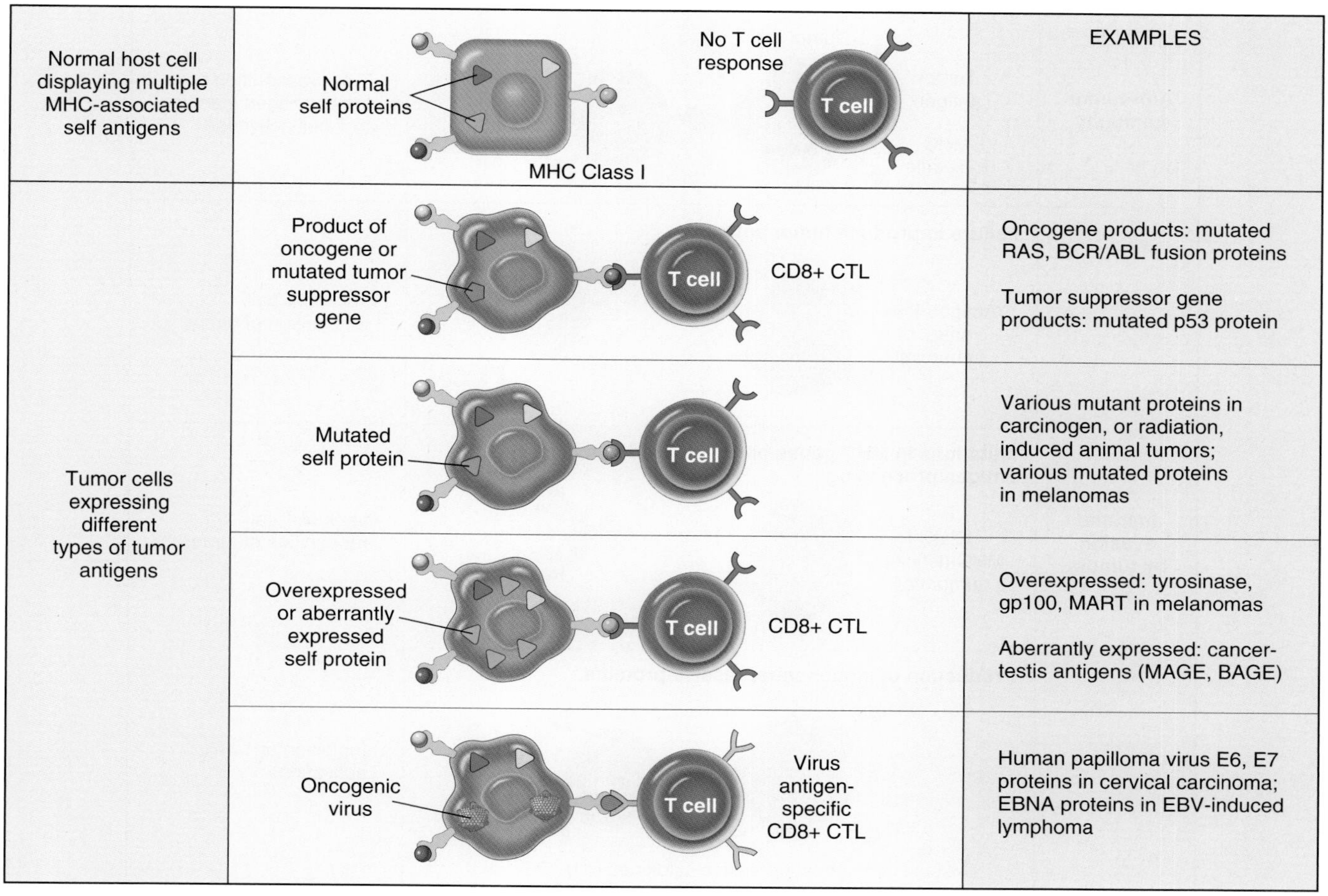

Fig. 6-31 Tumor antigens recognized by $CD8^+$ T lymphocytes.

Note that all tumor antigens are presented to $CD8^+$ T lymphocytes by major histocompatibility (MHC) class I molecules. *CTL,* Cytotoxic T lymphocyte. (From Kumar V, Abbas A, Fausto N, et al: *Robbins & Cotran pathologic basis of disease,* ed 8, Philadelphia, 2009, Saunders.)

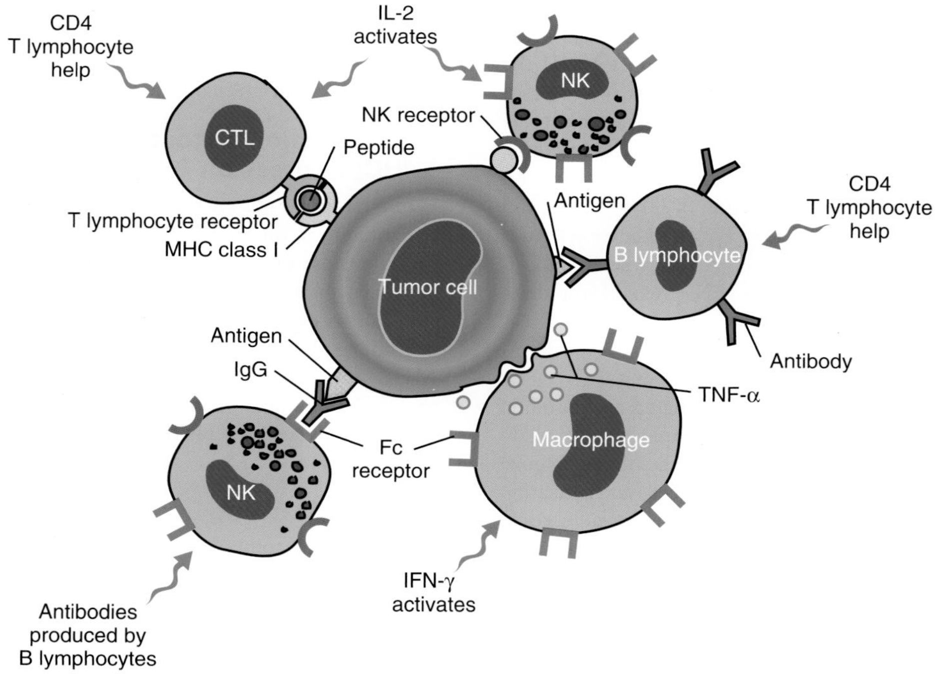

Fig. 6-32 Cells involved in immunosurveillance against tumors.

Antitumor responses involve cytotoxic $CD8^+$ and helper $CD4^+$ lymphocytes, natural killer (NK) cells, macrophages, B lymphocytes, and a variety of immunomodulatory cytokines. *CTL,* Cytotoxic T lymphocyte; *IFN-γ,* interferon-γ; *IgG,* immunoglobulin G; *IL-2,* interleukin-2; *MHC,* major histocompatibility complex; *TNF-α,* tumor necrosis factor-α. (Modified from Kumar V, Abbas A, Fausto N: *Robbins & Cotran pathologic basis of disease,* ed 7, Philadelphia, 2005, Saunders.)

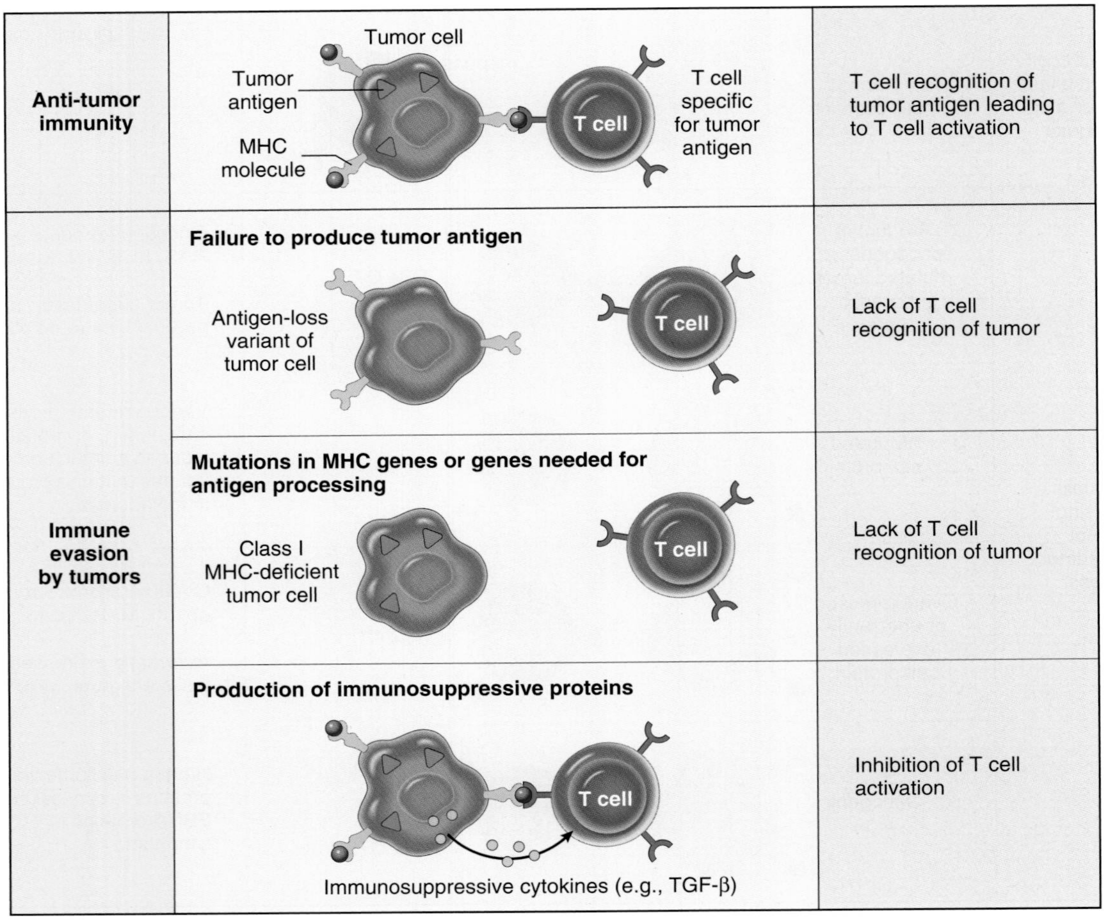

Fig. 6-33 Mechanisms by which tumors evade the immune system.
Tumor cells employ a variety of mechanisms to avoid attack by cytolytic T lymphocytes. *MHC,* Major histocompatibility complex; *TGF-β,* transforming growth factor-β. (From Kumar V, Abbas A, Fausto N, et al: *Robbins & Cotran pathologic basis of disease,* ed 8, Philadelphia, 2009, Saunders.)

protein, and granzymes, which are serine proteases. Perforin mediates the entry of granzymes into the target cell. Once inside the target cell, granzymes initiate both caspase-dependent and caspase-independent apoptosis. $CD4^+$ T lymphocytes do not appear to be essential for the generation or maintenance of a CTL response; instead, $CD4^+$ lymphocytes are generally considered to function as T_H lymphocytes that enhance the function of $CD8^+$ CTLs and antigen-producing B lymphocytes. $CD4^+$ T_H lymphocyte activities are largely mediated through secretion of cytokines, such as IL-2, which drives $CD8^+$ cell proliferation, and IFN-γ, which stimulates $CD8^+$ T lymphocyte differentiation.

B Lymphocytes

Many tumor antigens can incite both cell-mediated and humoral immune responses. Antibody-producing B lymphocytes mediate the humoral immune response to tumors. Antibodies that recognize tumor antigens kill tumor cells by binding to the cells and activating a local complement cascade. Activation of the complement cascade generates a membrane attack complex that induces loss of tumor cell membrane integrity and rapid cell death with the morphologic hallmarks of necrosis. In addition, antitumor antibodies may be bound by their constant regions to NK cells or macrophages, leaving the variable regions of the immunoglobulins available for specific recognition of tumor antigens. This allows the effector cells to recognize, attach to, and kill tumor cells by the mechanism of antibody-dependent cell-mediated cytotoxicity (ADCC).

EVASION OF THE IMMUNE RESPONSE

Many tumors are able successfully to evade immunosurveillance, using a variety of mechanisms (Fig. 6-33).

Altered Major Histocompatibility Complex (MHC) Expression

CTLs recognize tumor antigens only on tumor cells that display the antigens in the context of MHC class I molecules. Thus tumor cells that lose or downregulate expression of class I MHC antigens may have a distinct selective advantage. However, tumors that fail to express class I antigens are more susceptible to NK cell killing. Tumors may also downregulate expression of class II MHC antigens. Class II antigens are required for activation of the T_H lymphocytes that stimulate CTL differentiation, and loss of these antigens prevents the generation of an optimal antitumor CTL response.

Antigen Masking

Tumors may become invisible to the immune system by losing or masking tumor antigens. The outgrowth of clonal tumor variants that do not express tumor antigens is favored during tumor evolution. Tumor antigens on the cell surface may be hidden from the immune system if they are complexed with glycocalyx molecules, fibrin, or even antibodies. Some humoral responses to tumor antigens may therefore promote tumor survival by protecting tumor antigens from recognition by CTLs.

Tolerance

Although the immune system responds vigorously to non–self-antigens, it is tolerant to self-antigens. Thus tumor antigens shared with normal tissue usually are not able to evoke an immune response because the body has already been "tolerized" to the antigen. Tolerance can also result from presentation of non–self-antigens in a "tolerogenic" context (i.e., in the absence of co-stimulatory molecules required for effective T lymphocyte activation).

Immunosuppression

Tumor cells or their products may be immunosuppressive. Many tumors produce TGF-α, which inhibits the proliferation and function of lymphocytes and macrophages. Tumors may also produce Fas ligand. Fas ligand expressed by tumor cells binds to Fas receptors on nearby T lymphocytes and triggers their apoptosis. By this mechanism, T lymphocyte clones that recognize a tumor may be specifically deleted. Finally, tumor cells release tumor antigens into the circulation that form immune complexes with antibodies, and these immune complexes may be immunosuppressive.

TUMOR IMMUNOTHERAPY

The fact that the antitumor immune response attacks only the tumor cells and not normal tissue makes it an attractive candidate as a therapeutic modality. Moreover, effective immunotherapy would reduce or eliminate the need to use highly cytotoxic chemotherapeutic agents that indiscriminately target dividing cells. These drugs can cause significant morbidity and mortality in cancer patients. To date, immunotherapy results have been variable and disappointing; however, many new approaches are presently under investigation, some of which show promise.

In general, immunotherapeutic strategies are aimed at (1) providing the patient with mature effector cells or antibodies that recognize and destroy tumors (passive immunotherapy) or (2) stimulating the immune response of the host against the tumor (active immunotherapy).

Administration of monoclonal antibodies raised against tumor antigens or tumor-specific effector lymphocytes generated in vitro generates rapid but short-lived passive tumor immunity. Monoclonal antibodies raised in other species have a limited usefulness because the tumor host may develop an immune response to these antibodies that abrogates their effectiveness. However, coupling toxins to monoclonal antibodies may allow targeted delivery of therapeutic agents to tumor cells. Antitumor lymphocytes are generated by removing lymphocytes from the host or tumor and expanding them in vitro by incubation with IL-2; these autologous immune cells are then readministered to the patient. Many approaches to stimulate the active immunity of patients against their tumors have been attempted. These include vaccination with tumor cells or tumor antigens to generate antitumor CTLs, administration of cytokines to increase effector cell number and function, and nonspecific stimulation of the immune system by treatment with proinflammatory substances, such as bacterial products.

SYSTEMIC EFFECTS ON THE HOST

DIRECT EFFECTS VERSUS PARANEOPLASTIC SYNDROMES

Information on this topic, including Web Table 6-2, is available at evolve.elsevier.com/Zachary/McGavin/.

CACHEXIA

Information on this topic is available at evolve.elsevier.com/Zachary/McGavin/.

ENDOCRINOPATHIES

Information on this topic, including Web Fig. 6-1, is available at evolve.elsevier.com/Zachary/McGavin/.

SKELETAL SYNDROMES

Information on this topic, including Web Fig. 6-2, is available at evolve.elsevier.com/Zachary/McGavin/.

VASCULAR AND HEMATOLOGIC SYNDROMES

Information on this topic is available at evolve.elsevier.com/Zachary/McGavin/.

NEUROLOGIC SYNDROMES

Information on this topic is available at evolve.elsevier.com/Zachary/McGavin/.

CUTANEOUS SYNDROMES

Information on this topic is available at evolve.elsevier.com/Zachary/McGavin/.

MISCELLANEOUS SYNDROMES

Information on this topic is available at evolve.elsevier.com/Zachary/McGavin/.

GENETICS AND CANCER

Cancer is ultimately caused by heritable changes in the DNA of the tumor cells. These changes are manifested in enhanced expression of normal proteins, decreased or absent expression of normal proteins, and expression of abnormal proteins. For instance, tumor suppressor proteins, such as those encoded by p53, may fail to be expressed or may be expressed in an inactive form. Oncogene-encoded proteins may be overexpressed or expressed in constitutively active form. The altered protein repertoire of the tumor cell determines its phenotype. Such changes create cells with the features of neoplasia, including unlimited proliferative potential, growth factor independence, resistance to apoptosis, and invasive capabilities.

Genetic alterations in the coding region of a gene clearly may result in the production of an altered protein as a result of an altered coding sequence or premature protein termination. However, changes in other regions of the genome may also affect the sequence of the encoded protein and the level at which it is expressed. An alteration in splice site sequence can yield incorrectly spliced mRNA that is translated into an aberrant protein. Because the 5′ untranslated region of a gene generally contains its promoter and the 3′ untranslated region often contains messenger RNA (mRNA) stabilization motifs, sequence alterations in these regions of the genome may also have profound effects on gene expression level.

STEPWISE ACCUMULATION OF CHANGES

Cancer is associated with a progressive accumulation of genetic and epigenetic abnormalities. These defects lead to disruption of cell growth, cell death, apoptosis, differentiation, DNA repair, and other critical pathways. Some model systems demonstrate an orderly morphologic progression through premalignant to malignant to invasive and metastatic disease, and molecular genetic investigations of these various stages have made important contributions to our understanding of cancer biology. The molecular events that occur in the development of familial adenomatous polyposis, a form of human colorectal cancer, provide an excellent example of the genetic evolution that underlies progressive morphologic changes in cancer (Fig. 6-34). The initiating event is loss or mutation of the adenomatous polyposis coli (APC) tumor suppressor gene, leading to adenoma formation. This is followed by an activating mutation of a RAS oncogene and loss of genetic material harboring additional tumor suppressor genes. Ultimately, a malignant carcinoma emerges.

As illustrated in Fig. 6-35, DNA is susceptible to many types of chemical and physical alterations. Some of these changes are caused by injurious endogenous and exogenous agents. In addition, DNA alterations occur as part of normal processes of genome replication, repair, and rearrangement. Under some circumstances, these normal processes can lead to changes in DNA structure that contribute to the neoplastic phenotype. Furthermore, as tumors evolve, they often demonstrate reduced DNA repair capabilities and increased genomic instability. These developments accelerate the accumulation of genetic alterations in tumor cells.

Why do we study the molecular basis of cancer? Cancer is often treated using cytotoxic drugs and/or radiation therapy, neither of which discriminates between normal and tumor cells. Nonselective cell killing is responsible for many of the deleterious side effects of cancer treatment. More rational therapies would specifically target molecularly altered tumor cells, leaving nontumor cells lacking the molecular defect(s) relatively unharmed. Examples of molecularly targeted therapies used in humans include Gleevec, which is active against the BCR/ABL chromosomal translocation in chronic myeloid leukemia, and Iressa, which targets the epidermal growth factor receptor (EGF-R) in lung cancer. Specific molecular defects can also be exploited for early detection and/or early intervention at a stage when the tumor may be more responsive to treatment. Mutations in the BRCA1 gene are associated with a high risk for development of breast and/or ovarian cancer in women. Identification of the carrier status gives women the option of prophylactic mastectomy and/or oophorectomy. Mutations and other molecular defects can also be used to stratify patients for treatment and/or prognostic purposes.

GENETIC CHANGES IN CANCER

DNA Damage and Mutation

DNA damage, per se, does not constitute mutation. Mutation occurs during DNA replication, when the DNA strand containing unrepaired or misrepaired DNA damage is used as a template for the synthesis of a complementary DNA strand (see later discussion). At this time, unrepaired DNA lesions are misread by DNA polymerases, which insert incorrect bases in the newly synthesized DNA strand, and incorrectly repaired DNA lesions are reproduced in the daughter DNA strand. This process is known as *mutation fixation;* at least one and sometimes two rounds of replication are required for mutations to become fully fixed in the genome.

A chemical or physical change in an individual base may lead to the substitution of one base for another. The point mutation thus created can lead to altered protein sequence, if it is located

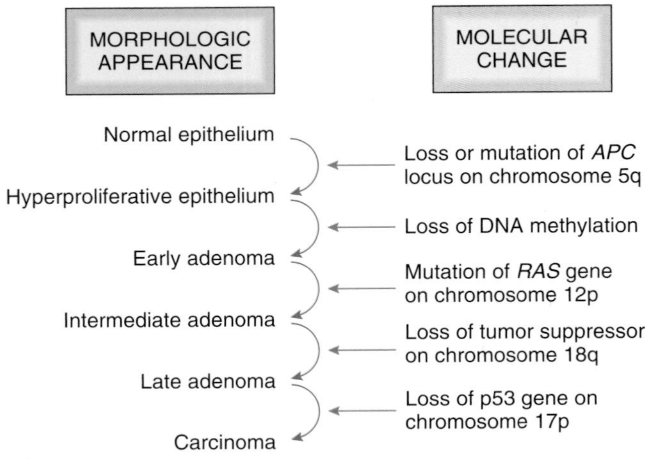

Fig. 6-34 Molecular model for the evolution of human colorectal cancers through the adenoma-carcinoma sequence.
Although adenomatous polyposis coli *(APC)* mutation is an early event and loss of p53 occurs late in the process of tumorigenesis, the timing for the other changes may show variations. Note also that individual tumors may not have all of the changes listed. (Adapted from Vogelstein B, Kinzler KW: Colorectal tumors. In Vogelstein B, Kinzler KW, editors: *The genetic basis of human cancer,* New York, 2002, McGraw-Hill.)

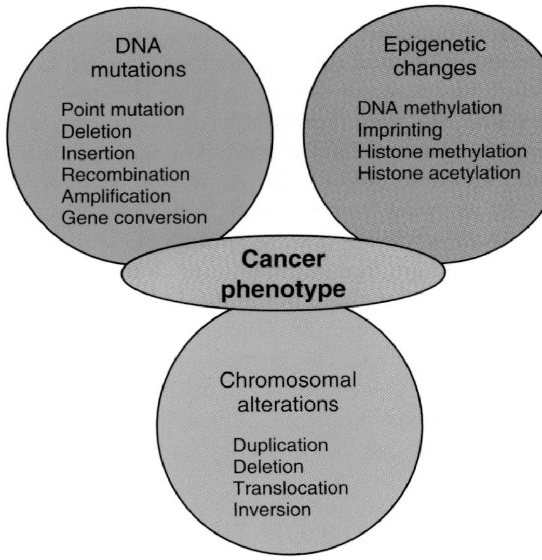

Fig. 6-35 Heritable alterations contributing to carcinogenesis.
Many genetic changes caused by extrinsic and intrinsic DNA-damaging agents, normal physiologic processes, and aging alter the amino acid sequences of encoded proteins and the levels at which these proteins are expressed. These changes in turn are responsible for the neoplastic phenotype. (Redrawn with permission from Dr. D.F. Kusewitt, College of Veterinary Medicine, The Ohio State University.)

in an exon or at a splice site, and to altered levels of expression, if it is located in the promoter or in the mRNA stabilization motif of a gene. Single- and double-strand breaks in DNA are caused by physical and chemical agents and viruses; they may also occur during normal physiologic processes such as recombination of immunoglobulin genes and T lymphocyte receptor genes. Although single-strand breaks are usually readily repaired, they can in some circumstances lead to gene conversion, the replacement of a gene or part of a gene by DNA derived from a closely related gene. Gene conversion is one mechanism by which organisms routinely generate diversity in large families of related genes, for example, MHC antigen genes. Double-strand breaks produce unprotected, recombinogenic DNA ends and often lead to major chromosomal anomalies, including deletions and translocations. Clearly, such large-scale chromosomal changes have the potential to alter the gene expression repertoire of a cell in a dramatic fashion. Insertions of DNA bases into the genome may be as small as a single base or larger than a viral genome. Insertion of individual bases by the enzyme terminal deoxynucleotide transferase is part of the system by which antibody diversity is normally generated. Retroviral genomes replicate only after insertion into the host genome, and these large insertions can interrupt the coding sequence of host genes, abrogating their expression. On the other hand, juxtaposition of viral promoter elements adjacent to cellular coding sequences can lead to dysregulated, often markedly increased, host gene expression. Unscheduled amplification of DNA segments is a poorly understood process by which multiple rounds of localized DNA replication produce hundreds or thousands of copies of DNA segments up to several megabases in length. Such amplified DNA segments may be visible in cytogenetic preparations as homogeneously staining regions in chromosomes or as episomal double minutes. Amplification of oncogenes or drug resistance genes may have significant effects on the life history of a tumor. Expansion or contraction of a small region of tandemly repeated DNA sequences can occur as the result of DNA polymerase slippage during replication. This process can introduce sequence alterations into protein encoding genes.

Chromosomal Instability

The karyotypes of many tumor cells are extremely abnormal because of changes in chromosome number and configuration. These alterations are the result of chromosomal instability. In tumors with notable chromosomal instability, each cell may have a different karyotype and exhibit a remarkable array of duplications, deletions, and reciprocal and nonreciprocal translocations. Such abnormalities can dramatically affect the levels of gene expression by altering the numbers of gene copies present and by juxtaposing regulatory and structural elements of unrelated genes. In some cases, specific chromosomal abnormalities are associated with specific disease entities. Probably the best studied example of such an association is the relationship between chronic myeloid leukemia in humans and a reciprocal translocation between chromosomes 9 and 22 that yields an abnormal chromosome called the *Philadelphia chromosome.* This translocation fuses portions of the BCR and ABL genes; the fusion gene thus produced encodes an abnormal protein that appears to be responsible for neoplastic transformation of myeloid cells.

Types of Genetic Alterations in Cancer Cells

Aneuploidy

The numeric aberrations in cancer can involve many different chromosomes or be limited to a single chromosome. Cytogenetic analysis can determine the copy number of each chromosome. *Monosomy* is the term used when only one copy of a chromosome exists. *Trisomy* is the term used when three copies of a chromosome exist. For example, one quarter of canine lymphomas show trisomy of chromosome 13. In mice, trisomy of chromosome 15 occurs in almost all T lymphocyte lymphomas and leukemias, suggesting that overexpression of a gene or genes on this chromosome plays an important role in tumor causation. Alterations in chromosome number (aneuploidy) are largely the result of mistakes in chromosome segregation caused by multipolar spindles, centrosome amplification, kinetochore malfunction, or abnormal cytokinesis.

Translocation

Translocations often occur when the cell response to DNA damage is dysregulated. When cells respond appropriately to DNA damage, multiple signaling cascades such as the p53 pathway are activated, leading to cell-cycle arrest, enhanced DNA repair, and apoptosis in the face of excessive DNA damage. However, if these pathways are no longer functional, chromosomal instability results. Dysfunctional telomeres also contribute to chromosomal instability (Fig. 6-36). The precise mechanisms by which an intact DNA damage response and normal telomerase activity maintain chromosomal integrity are unclear.

Mutation

In addition to abnormal numbers of chromosomes, mutations (heritable change in the DNA sequence) are also present in most tumors. Mutations can result in loss or inactivation of a protein. On the other hand, some mutations cause uncontrolled activation of a protein. One example is a point mutation of the RAS oncogene. This mutation causes constitutive and unregulated activation of the protein and gives the affected cell a growth advantage over surrounding normal cells. Another type of mutation is a dominant-negative mutation, in which the mutant gene product causes inactivation of the wild-type product, effectively eliminating

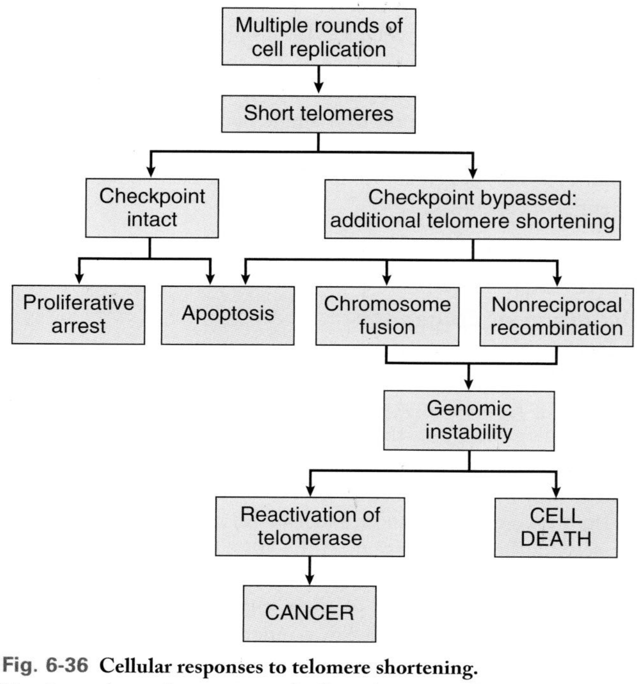

Fig. 6-36 Cellular responses to telomere shortening.
The figure shows the response of cells with intact cell-cycle checkpoints and those with checkpoint defects. (From Kumar V, Abbas A, Fausto N, et al: *Robbins & Cotran pathologic basis of disease,* ed 8, Philadelphia, 2009, Saunders.)

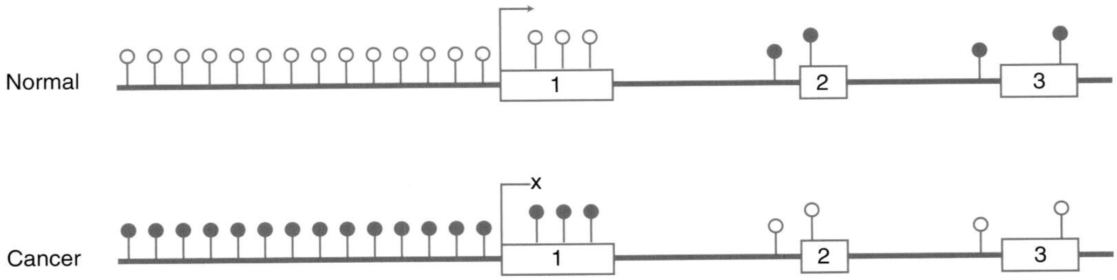

Fig. 6-37 CpG island methylation.
In most normal tissues, the dense clusters of CpG sites in the 5′ regions of genes (CpG islands) are unmethylated *(open lollipops),* whereas those in the body of the gene are methylated *(filled lollipops).* The reverse is often seen in cancer where 5′ CpG islands become hypermethylated, and there is concurrent hypomethylation of CpG sites in the body of the gene. Unmethylated 5′ CpG islands are associated with active transcription *(arrow),* whereas methylated 5′ CpG islands are associated with transcriptional repression *(x).* (Redrawn with permission from Dr. L.J. Rush, College of Veterinary Medicine, The Ohio State University.)

the cellular contribution of the normal gene. A missense mutation that changes a codon for one amino acid into a codon for a different amino acid has been identified in the Birt-Hogg-Dubé-(BHD) gene in German shepherd dogs with hereditary multifocal renal cystadenocarcinoma and nodular dermatofibrosis (see later discussion).

Deletion

Deletions involve loss of DNA from a chromosome and can be as small as one base pair or as large as an entire arm of a chromosome. Heterozygous deletions occur on only one chromosome, whereas homozygous deletions occur on both chromosomes. Small deletions of one or two base pair cause a shift in the reading frame during protein synthesis (frameshift mutation). One possible consequence is that the mutated sequence codes for a premature stop codon, resulting in a truncated protein. Large deletions often encompass chromosome regions that harbor tumor suppressor genes.

Amplification

Genomic amplifications result in the presence of more than one diploid copy of a DNA sequence. The amplified region can involve large segments of a chromosome and encompass millions of base pairs. Alternatively, the amplified region may be very small and contained within a portion of a single gene such as the internal tandem duplication (ITD) of the c-kit gene in canine mast cell tumors. Regions of genomic amplification are useful for identifying potential oncogenes.

Epigenetic Mechanisms of Altered Gene Expression

Definition of Epigenetic

Epigenetic alterations have recently come to light as being major players in tumor biology. The term *epigenetic* refers to a heritable change in gene expression in somatic cells resulting from something other than a change in the DNA sequence. The most frequently studied epigenetic changes are DNA cytosine methylation and histone modifications. These epigenetic modifications can enhance or suppress gene expression and can be transmitted to daughter cells during cell division. Although DNA methylation and histone modifications are carried out by normal cellular enzymes, the activity and specificity of these enzymes can be altered by exogenous agents acting through a variety of oncogenic pathways. And although epigenetic changes are stable for the most part, they can be modulated with various pharmacologic agents. This quality makes them attractive targets for therapeutic intervention designed to restore gene expression to its normal state.

Types of Epigenetic Changes in Cancer Cells

DNA Methylation

DNA methylation involves the addition of a methyl group to carbon 5 of cytosine, in cytosines located immediately 5′ to guanine (CpG dinucleotide). The methylation process is carried out by various methyltransferase enzymes. Methylation is essential for regulating gene expression in normal cells. Cancer cells, however, are characterized by an overall decrease in 5-methylcytosine in the bulk of the genome (global hypomethylation), with a paradoxic increase in gene-specific methylation of clusters of CpG sites located in the promoter and/or exon 1 of genes (CpG islands). In general, hypomethylation of genes, particularly of promoter regions, leads to gene activation, whereas hypermethylation results in gene silencing. Promoter methylation has been found in every type of human cancer studied (Fig. 6-37).

Imprinting

Another situation in which methylation plays a role is in imprinting. Genomic imprinting refers to the parent-of-origin, allele-specific expression of certain genes whereby only the maternal or paternal allele is expressed. This monoallelic expression is controlled in part by DNA methylation, but this regulation is sometimes lost in cancer. The loss of imprinting can allow a double dose of a growth-promoting gene product. For example, insulin-like growth factor-2 (IGF-2) is an imprinted gene that is expressed from only the paternal allele in most normal tissue. If a cancer cell undergoes relaxation of imprinting, the methylation-mediated silencing of one allele is lost, enabling biallelic expression and higher than normal levels of this growth-promoting gene product.

Histone Modification

In addition to DNA methylation, a second type of epigenetic regulation involves histone modification. DNA is wound around histones to form chromatin. Chromatin can exist in an open configuration in which DNA is accessible to transcription factors (euchromatin) or in a closed, compact configuration in which DNA is inaccessible to transcription factors (heterochromatin). Posttranslational modifications, such as acetylation, methylation, and phosphorylation, take place on the histone tails. In the aggregate, these modifications form the "histone code," which plays an important role in determining gene expression. For example, the addition of a negatively charged acetyl group (CH_3CO^-) to certain lysine residues in a histone tail results in a weaker bond between the DNA and the histone. This allows a relaxed chromatin configuration and increases transcription of the associated gene (Fig. 6-38).

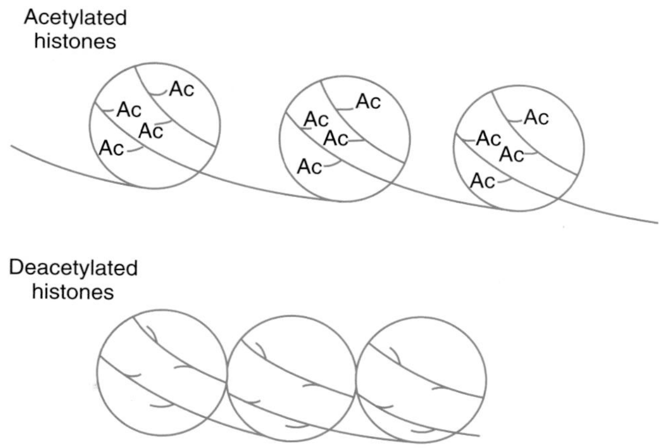

Fig. 6-38 Histone acetylation.
DNA is wound around histones. The presence of acetyl groups *(Ac)* on histone tails is associated with relaxed chromatin, which is permissive to gene transcription. Removal of acetyl groups by histone deacetylases results in a closed chromatin configuration that is less permissive to the transcription machinery. (Redrawn with permission from Dr. L.J. Rush, College of Veterinary Medicine, The Ohio State University.)

Posttranscriptional Regulation of Gene Expression by MicroRNAs

MicroRNAs (miRNAs) are small noncoding RNA molecules that posttranscriptionally regulate the expression of other genes. MiRNA genes are found throughout the genome, both within other genes and in intergenic regions. MiRNA genes are transcribed into large precursor RNAs that undergo extensive enzymatic processing within the nucleus and after export into the cytoplasm. Mature miRNAs are 18 to 25 nucleotides in length and bind to their target mRNAs as the result of sequence complementarity. Once bound, miRNAs either trigger degradation of their target mRNAs or prevent translation of these mRNAs into proteins.

Approximately 1000 miRNA genes are present in the human genome, and each miRNA can regulate translation of about 200 target mRNA species. Overall, miRNAs control translation of perhaps one-third of all protein-coding genes in the human genome. The pattern of miRNA expression is extensively dysregulated in cancers by a wide variety of genetic and epigenetic mechanisms. Altered patterns of miRNA expression in turn create extensive changes in cellular processes related to neoplasia, including proliferation, apoptosis, invasiveness, and genomic stability. Current research is focused on understanding how altered patterns of miRNA expression can be exploited for diagnostic and therapeutic purposes.

CANCER ETIOLOGY

The genetic alterations that contribute to cancer development include both heritable changes in germline sequences present in all cells within an organism and somatic changes that accumulate in individual cells and tissues of the body over time. Human families and genetically related animals that exhibit distinct Mendelian inheritance of specific types of cancer are said to have cancer syndromes. In these cases, a single germline mutation is generally responsible for tumor development. In contrast, sporadic tumors occur randomly in the population and are not associated with specific germline characteristics.

GERMLINE MUTATIONS AND CANCER SYNDROMES

Heritable genetic lesions undergo germline transmission from one generation to the next, and the affected individual is born with one defective copy of a gene in each cell. Heritable mutations may be linked to familial cancer syndromes. Characteristics of heritable familial cancers include an early age of onset compared with sporadic cases, the formation of bilateral tumors in paired organs, the occurrence of multiple primary tumors in nonpaired organs, and a family history of cancer. Although many of the familial cancer syndromes are the result of mutations in recessive tumor suppressor genes, the syndromes generally show a predominantly autosomal dominant pattern of inheritance. This apparent paradox is explained later in the discussion of hereditary retinoblastoma. Some cancer syndromes show a recessive mode of inheritance. In such syndromes, the affected individual must inherit the genetic defect from both parents. For instance, the mutant ter gene carried by strain 129/Sv-ter mice confers high susceptibility to testicular teratoma when present in the homozygous state but not when carried in the heterozygous condition. Interestingly, the role of germline mutations in oncogenes in hereditary cancer syndromes remains unclear.

The seminal work that identified the retinoblastoma (RB) tumor suppressor gene came about through the study of such inherited cancer syndromes (see later discussion). Other well-known inherited cancer syndromes in humans include germline mutations of p53 in Li-Fraumeni syndrome, mutations of NF1 and NF2 that lead to neurofibromatosis, mutations of BRCA1 and BRCA2 associated with breast and ovarian cancers, and mutations in MEN1 and RET, which are associated with multiple endocrine neoplasia. A well-documented veterinary cancer syndrome is the disease with the unwieldy name "hereditary multifocal renal cystadenocarcinoma and nodular dermatofibrosis" that occurs in the German shepherd dog. This disease is characterized by bilateral and multifocal renal tumors, uterine leiomyomas, and nodules in the skin (dermatofibrosis). The gene responsible has been mapped to a locus homologous to the human BHD locus; mutations in BHD cause a phenotypically similar human disease.

Although the inherited cancer syndromes account for less than 10% of all human cancers, they have led to the identification of a number of important tumor suppressor genes that also play a significant role in sporadic tumors. In dominant cancer syndromes, tumor risk is very markedly increased because of changes in a single gene; however, there are also a variety of tumor susceptibility genes that alter cancer incidence to a considerably lesser extent. A variety of cancer susceptibility patterns have been identified in the dog as shown in Table 6-2. The tumor susceptibility genes identified to date generally encode proteins involved in carcinogen metabolism or DNA repair. Their effects are substantially modified by interactions with each other and with the environment. For instance, the lack of pigmentation in white cats contributes to their susceptibility to squamous cell carcinoma of the ears; however, sun exposure makes a major contribution to tumor incidence in these animals.

ACQUIRED SOMATIC MUTATIONS

In contrast to germline mutations, acquired mutations occur in somatic cells and are restricted to individual cells and their progeny. These mutations are not passed through the germline but are required in the specific cells that give rise to the tumor. Somatic genetic alterations are caused both by intrinsic and extrinsic agents. These changes accumulate randomly over time, thus aging dramatically increases the risk of cancer. The graph shown

TABLE 6-2 Cancer Susceptibility in Dogs

Tumor Site	Tumor Type	Susceptible Breeds	Resistant Breeds
Hematopoietic system	Lymphoma	Boxer	Crossbreeds
	Malignant histiocytosis	Bernese mountain dog	
Brain	Various	Boston terrier, boxer, bulldog	
Skin	Mast cell tumor	Boxer, bulldog, retriever	
Vasculature	Hemangiosarcoma	German shepherd	
Mammary gland	Various	Boxer,* Brittany spaniel, dachshund, English setter, Labrador retriever, pointer, Springer spaniel	Boxer,* German shepherd, crossbreeds
Nose and sinuses	Various	Airedale, collie, Scottish terrier	
Oropharynx	Various	Boxer, cocker spaniel, golden retriever	Beagle, dachshund
Ovary	Carcinoma	Pointer	
Pancreas	Carcinoma, insulinoma	Airedale terrier, poodle	
Thyroid	Carcinoma	Beagle, boxer, retriever	Poodle
Skeleton	Osteosarcoma	Giant breeds, boxer, Danish dog, German shepherd, rottweiler	Crossbreeds
Testis		Boxer, collie, German shepherd	
Urinary bladder	Carcinoma	Beagle, collie, Scottish terrier	

Modified from McCullen JM, Page R, Misdorp W: An overview of cancer pathogenesis, diagnosis, and management. In Meuten DJ, editor: *Tumors in domestic animals,* Ames, 2002, Iowa State Press.
*Information obtained from two independent studies.

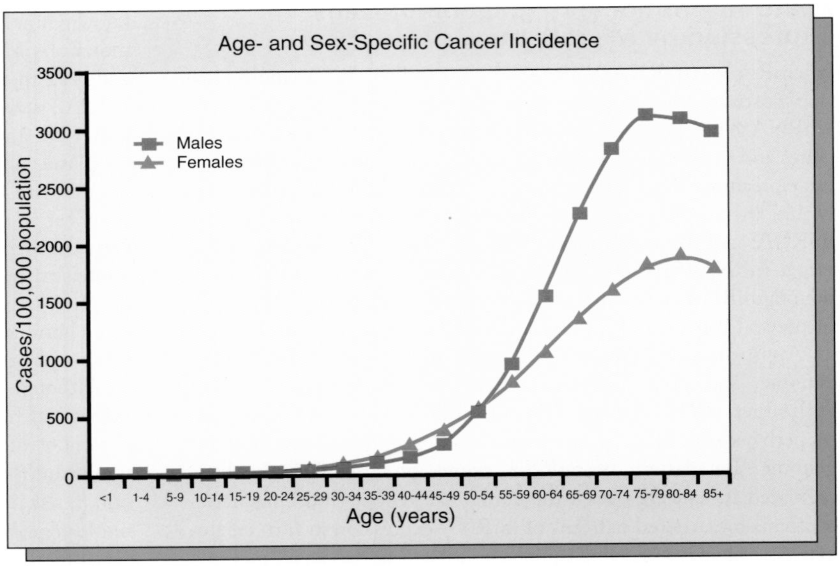

Fig. 6-39 Cancer incidence by age in the human population of the United States (US) for the year 2001. Cancer incidence is shown as the number of cases of invasive cancer per 100,000 persons. Data for all races and all cancer sites are combined. Basal and squamous cell carcinomas of sun-exposed skin and all in situ cancers except urinary bladder cancers are excluded. Data are from selected state and metropolitan area cancer registries and cover approximately 92% of the US population. (Compiled by Dr. D.F. Kusewitt from data released by the Centers for Disease Control and Prevention.)

in Fig. 6-39 illustrates the increased risk of cancer with age in the human population, for which solid epidemiologic data are available. Somatic mutations are responsible for the majority of cancers in humans and probably in animals.

Intrinsic Factors

As a by-product of ordinary metabolism, a variety of DNA damaging agents are produced, including reactive oxygen species. Moreover, DNA is susceptible to ordinary hydrolytic attack. These processes induce a variety of DNA lesions that can result in mutation. Additionally, in the course of many rounds of replication, DNA changes are introduced as a result of DNA polymerase errors. Illegitimate recombination, inappropriate nucleotide addition, and altered DNA methylation, activities carried out by normal cellular enzymes, can lead to the accumulation of DNA alterations. Chromosomal abnormalities also arise as a result of decreased telomere length, altered telomerase activity, and mistakes in chromosome segregation.

Extrinsic Factors

Extrinsic factors that interact with DNA to cause cancer include chemical, physical, and infectious agents. Mutagens are agents that create DNA damage that gives rise to mutations, whereas carcinogens are agents that cause cancer. Many mutagens are also carcinogens. However, there are carcinogens with unknown mechanisms of action; such carcinogens may or may not be mutagens.

Chemicals

Chemical carcinogens are widespread in the environment. All animals are exposed to low levels of carcinogens in air, water, food, and medications; accidental exposure to very high levels of carcinogens occasionally occurs. One notable chemical cause of cancer in animals is the bracken fern plant, the toxin of which causes urinary bladder cancer in cattle grazing pastures containing the plant. Unlike humans, however, animals do not voluntarily expose themselves to potent carcinogens such as tobacco smoke.

Radiation

Natural sources of radiation include the sunlight and cosmic rays that bombard the earth and naturally occurring radioisotopes, such as radon, in the soil. Medical procedures, including diagnostic radiographs and radiation therapy, can provide substantial radiation exposure. Radiant energy with wavelengths greater than 5×10^{-5} cm (visible light, infrared radiation, microwaves, radio waves, and electrical waves) is generally considered to be noncarcinogenic. However, shorter wavelength γ-rays, x-rays, and ultraviolet (UV) radiation can cause notable DNA damage and resultant mutation. In addition, high-energy particles, including α-particles (helium nuclei), β-particles (electrons), and neutrons, can be carcinogenic. Ionizing radiation includes those forms of radiation with enough energy to eject electrons from target molecules (γ-rays, x-rays, α-particles, β-particles, and neutrons). Because most animals have hair, UV radiation is generally not an important veterinary carcinogen. There are, however, two instances in which the UV radiation in sunlight poses a significant risk to animals: squamous cell carcinoma of the ears in white cats and ocular squamous cell carcinoma in Hereford cattle with nonpigmented eyelids.

Viruses as a cause of cancer were first identified and have been most thoroughly studied in animals. Virally induced tumors in animals often affect a relatively large number of animals in a flock or herd, frequently arise in relatively young animals, and generally show a pattern of occurrence consistent with an infectious cause. There are many types of oncogenic viruses that induce cancer by a large variety of mechanisms. Web Table 6-3 summarizes those viruses of significance to veterinary medicine. Oncogenic retroviruses are small RNA viruses that cause many neoplastic diseases of importance in animals, including avian leukosis, feline leukemia, and bovine leukosis. Oncogenic DNA viruses include papillomaviruses that cause skin cancer, hepadnaviruses associated with liver cancer, and herpesviruses that induce adenocarcinomas, lymphomas, and leukemias. Species of *Helicobacter* bacteria have been recently demonstrated to play a role in gastric carcinoma and gastric lymphoma in ferrets and mice and in hepatocellular carcinoma in mice.

MECHANISMS OF CARCINOGENESIS

Chemical

A very wide variety of chemicals can cause cancer. Direct-acting chemical carcinogens are effective in the form in which they enter the body, but most carcinogens are procarcinogens that require metabolic activation by cellular enzymes to form ultimate carcinogens. These are thus termed *indirect-acting carcinogens.* Despite their varied composition, the effective form of most carcinogens is an electrophilic compound that binds covalently to DNA to form DNA adducts. Fig. 6-40 illustrates the general mechanism of chemical carcinogenesis.

As discussed previously, experimental carcinogenesis studies have been critical in elucidating the stepwise development of cancer. Moreover, these studies have clearly defined the contribution of initiating versus promoting agents to cancer development (Fig. 6-41). In multistage tumorigenesis models, such as the

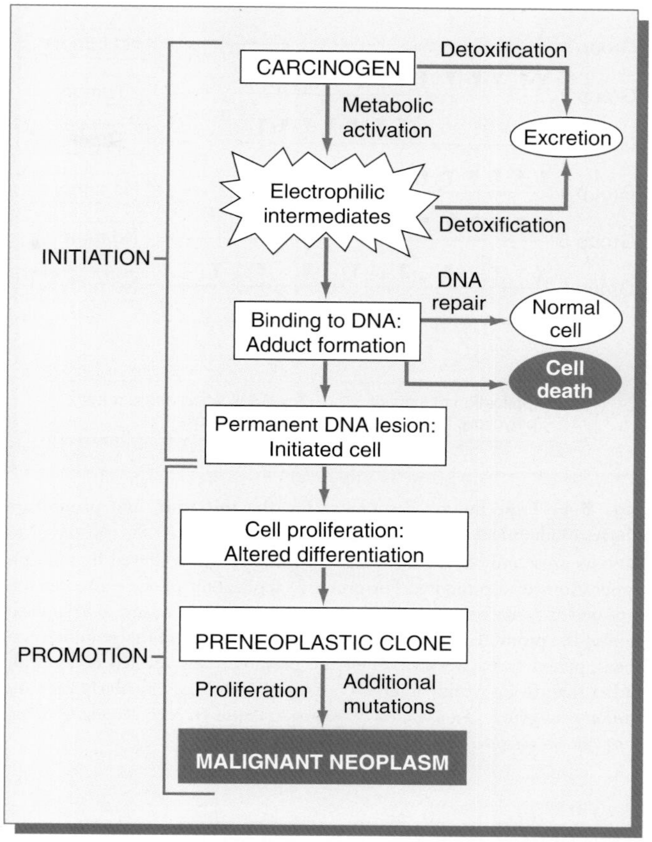

Fig. 6-40 General schema of events in chemical carcinogenesis. Note that promoters cause clonal expansion of the initiated cell, thus producing a preneoplastic clone. Further proliferation induced by the promoter leads to formation of a benign neoplasm. Accumulation of additional mutations during the phase of tumor progression results in emergence of a malignant tumor. (From Kumar V, Abbas A, Fausto N: *Robbins & Cotran pathologic basis of disease,* ed 8, Philadelphia, 2009, Saunders.)

skin carcinogenesis model in mice, the initiator must be administered before the promoting agent. The initiator is ineffective without subsequent application of a promoter. Moreover, multiple, closely spaced promoter treatments are required to drive tumor emergence.

Radiation

Unlike chemicals, all forms of radiation are complete carcinogens (i.e., they are able both to initiate and with continued exposure, to promote tumorigenesis). Direct DNA damage caused by ionizing radiation consists primarily of single- and double-strand breaks and base elimination. However, ionizing radiation also generates free radicals from many cellular molecules. The interactions of these highly reactive molecules result in many forms of DNA damage, including altered bases and DNA-protein cross-links. Absorption of UV radiation by DNA results in the formation of hallmark DNA adducts, pyrimidine dimers, which are potentially mutagenic. To a lesser extent, UV radiation generates reactive oxygen species, leading to indirect DNA damage like strand breaks and DNA-protein cross-links.

Viral

Oncogenic viruses employ a remarkable array of direct and indirect mechanisms to induce cancer.

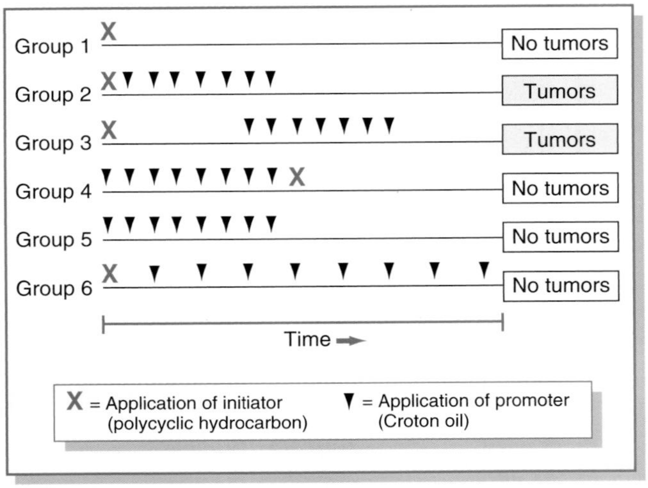

Fig. 6-41 Experiments demonstrating the initiation and promotion phases of chemical skin carcinogenesis in mice.
Tumors arose only if application of an initiator was followed by multiple applications of a promoter. For group 2, application of the promoter was repeated at twice-weekly intervals for several months. For group 3, application of the promoter was delayed for several months and the promoter was then applied twice weekly. When the promoter was applied at monthly rather than twice-weekly intervals (group 6), it did not effectively promote tumor emergence. (From Kumar V, Abbas A, Fausto N, et al: *Robbins & Cotran pathologic basis of disease,* ed 8, Philadelphia, 2009, Saunders.)

Dominant Oncogene

The genomes of many rapidly transforming viruses include a dominant oncogene that drives tumor development. Oncogenes may be of ancient or more recent host cell origin such as the fes, fgr, abl, fms, and kit genes transduced by oncogenic retroviruses of cats. Viruses may also contain oncogenes not of host cell origin. For example, papillomavirus genomes include the E6 and E7 genes that encode inhibitors of the p53 and pRb tumor suppressor proteins, respectively; some viruses contain genes that encode growth stimulatory molecules such as the small T antigen of SV40.

Insertional Mutagenesis

Viruses that do not possess their own oncogenes can instead activate expression of cellular oncogenes by a process of insertional mutagenesis. For example, most tumors caused by the avian leukosis virus exhibit a similar site of viral insertion, suggesting that virally induced alterations in genes at that site in the host genome are essential for tumorigenesis.

Hit and Run Mechanism

In the two mechanisms discussed previously, the viral genome or portions of the genome persist in the host cell. However, some viruses also cause tumors merely by transient residence in target cells. The precise mechanism by which this might occur has not been elucidated. Bovine papillomavirus uses such a hit and run mechanism of cell transformation.

Indirect Mechanisms

Viruses may also stimulate tumorigenesis by suppression of the host immune system or stimulation of target cell proliferation. The herpesvirus that causes Marek's disease is an example of a virus that suppresses the ability of the host to eliminate transformed cells, whereas hepatitis viruses exemplify viruses that stimulate cell proliferation.

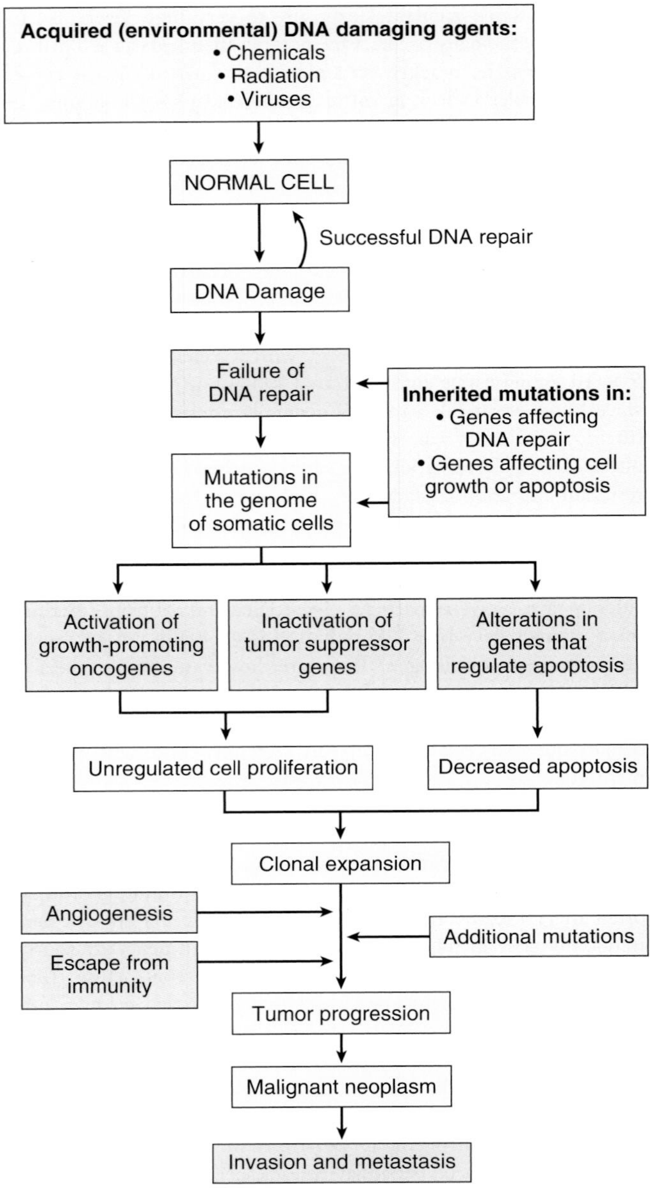

Fig. 6-42 Schematic diagram illustrating the molecular basis of cancer. (From Kumar V, Abbas A, Fausto N, et al: *Robbins & Cotran pathologic basis of disease,* ed 8, Philadelphia, 2009, Saunders.)

MOLECULAR DETERMINANTS OF CANCER

Fig. 6-42 illustrates the key steps in the molecular basis of cancer.

TUMOR SUPPRESSOR GENES

Cells receive signals that both stimulate and inhibit cell growth and must maintain the proper balance between these stimuli. The designation of tumor suppressor gene was originally given to genes that inhibited cell growth. Over time, the class of tumor suppressor genes has expanded to include many different types of cancer-related genes that, when inactivated through genetic and/or epigenetic means, allow uncontrolled proliferation or tumor growth. This includes genes that control cell cycle, apoptosis, DNA repair, and other fundamental pathways.

The pivotal concept of tumor suppressor genes was posited by Alfred Knudson in 1971, based on his observations of children with familial and sporadic retinoblastoma, an uncommon tumor arising in retinoblasts. According to Knudson's "two-hit" hypothesis, both alleles of a tumor suppressor gene must undergo mutation (i.e., a genetic "hit") for cancer to develop. In inherited cancer syndromes, the person is born with a mutation in one allele of all cells in the body (Web Fig. 6-3). The second hit is acquired as a somatic mutation of the remaining tumor suppressor allele in a single cell. In contrast, development of a sporadic tumor in those born with two normal tumor suppressor alleles requires that a cell sustain two hits, one on each allele of the tumor suppressor gene. Loss of both alleles in a single cell is a rare event; however, loss of only one allele occurs much more frequently. In cells with only a single copy of a tumor suppressor gene, loss of the second allele can occur by a variety of mechanisms, including point mutation in the allele, deletion of the allele or the chromosomal segment where it resides, deletion of the entire chromosome containing the allele, or mitotic recombination resulting in replacement of the normal allele by the mutant allele. When the normal allele has been completely lost, the cell and its progeny contain only a single abnormal allele. This condition is termed *loss of heterozygosity*.

Tumor suppressor genes are frequently located in areas of the genome that are deleted in cancer. The areas of chromosomal loss can be limited to small deletions of a few hundred base pairs or encompass a whole chromosome arm or even an entire chromosome. By examining a large number of tumors, the minimal region of loss can be defined as the common region deleted in all tumors of the type under investigation. Candidate tumor suppressor genes within the boundaries of this area can then be further interrogated for silencing of the remaining allele. In addition to loss of genetic material and inactivating mutations, it is now widely recognized that DNA methylation, as discussed earlier, is an alternative method of silencing tumor suppressor genes.

Although the classic definition of a tumor suppressor gene dictates that both alleles must be inactivated, recent evidence suggests that for certain genes inactivation of only one copy is sufficient for tumor growth (haploinsufficiency). Haploinsufficiency can contribute to tumor development by a number of mechanisms. One mechanism is a simple gene-dosage effect in which half the normal amount of a protein is insufficient to maintain the normal homeostatic balance in the cell. Alternatively, a mutation in one allele can give rise to a dominant-negative protein whereby the abnormal protein blocks the function of the normal protein produced by the remaining wild-type allele. A third mechanism occurs when a mutation in one allele of a tumor suppressor gene decreases the amount of normal protein in a cell, which may in turn influence other pathways that may have concurrent abnormalities.

Many tumor suppressor genes are key components of the cell cycle. One of the most widely studied tumor suppressor genes is p53, and it is inactivated most commonly by mutation in more than half of human cancers. It is a DNA-binding protein that regulates transcription of numerous genes and plays a critical role in cell-cycle arrest and induction of apoptosis after DNA damage. For these reasons, it has been entitled the "guardian of the genome." Levels of p53 are rapidly elevated in response to DNA damage. This leads to increased transcription of p53 target genes, such as p21 and GADD45, which function in cell-cycle arrest and DNA repair, respectively. The half-life of p53 is short (about 20 minutes) and it is rapidly degraded after completion of DNA repair. If the DNA repair is unsuccessful, p53 directs cell death by activating BCL2-associated X protein (BAX), a key component of the apoptotic cascade (Fig. 6-43). It is clear then that loss of functional p53 can have devastating consequences for maintaining integrity of the genome. Without p53, mutagenic DNA damage goes unrepaired, the cell proceeds through division, and the mutation becomes fixed in the genome.

Another widely studied tumor suppressor gene is the retinoblastoma gene. As described earlier, RB is a target for inactivation both in germline and somatic cells and like p53, plays an important role in cell-cycle control. In quiescent cells, RB is hypophosphorylated and active. When RB is hyperphosphorylated and inactive, the cell can proceed through the G_1/S transition. Control of proper RB function and phosphorylation status involves a host of other genes, including p16INK4a, cyclin D, and CDK4. Therefore a defect in any one of these gene products disrupts the RB pathway and leads to unregulated progression through the cell cycle.

ONCOGENES

Oncogenes are derived from proto-oncogenes, normal cellular genes that regulate cell growth and differentiation. Proto-oncogenes encode products involved in diverse pathways and include molecules such as growth factors and their receptors, cell-cycle regulators, DNA-binding proteins, transcription factors, protein kinases, and others. Oncogenes were first identified as RNA tumor virus proteins. Later it was discovered that normal cells have the equivalent gene products.

There are a number of ways in which oncogenes can be abnormally activated to promote tumor growth. The genomic region containing the gene can be amplified, resulting in dramatically increased copy number. For example, the N-MYC oncogene can be amplified up to 100 times in human neuroblastomas. Oncogenes can undergo mutations that cause constitutive activation of the gene. In these cases, the gene is always "turned on" and is unresponsive to inhibitory signals. This scenario is often the case for cell surface receptors such as the EGF-R in carcinomas. Many tyrosine kinase receptors have activating mutations that result in constitutive activation even in the absence of ligands. Tumor cells can also produce large amounts of stimulatory molecules along with their cognate receptors, forming a growth-promoting autocrine loop. All of these mechanisms serve to drive proliferation and render the cell unresponsive to normal inhibitory signals.

The prototype of signal transduction oncogenes is the RAS family of guanine triphosphate (GTP)-binding proteins (G proteins). There are several members of this family, including HRAS, KRAS, and NRAS. In normal cells, RAS transmits growth stimulatory signals from outside the cell to the nucleus, ultimately activating transcription of genes for cell-cycle progression. RAS alternates between an active and inactive state in its normal location on the cytoplasmic side of the cell membrane where it is closely associated with farnesyl transferase. Inactive RAS binds guanine diphosphate (GDP). Upon receiving a stimulatory signal from a growth factor, RAS exchanges GDP for GTP. RAS bound to GTP is the active form, which triggers the RAS–RAF–mitogen-activated protein kinase (MAPK) pathway and results in transcription of genes that promote cell division (Fig. 6-44). The activation of RAS is normally short lived, as RAS has an intrinsic GTPase that hydrolyzes GTP to GDP and converts RAS to its inactive state. In many cancers, RAS is constitutively activated either by mutations in RAS itself or by failure of the GTPase to inactivate RAS. RAS family members, the farnesyl transferase anchor to the plasma membrane, and other components of the signal transduction pathway are all attractive molecular targets for therapeutic intervention in cancer patients.

DEFECTS IN DNA REPAIR

Defects in DNA repair enzymes are one cause of mutations and genomic instability. If mutations inactivate tumor suppressor genes

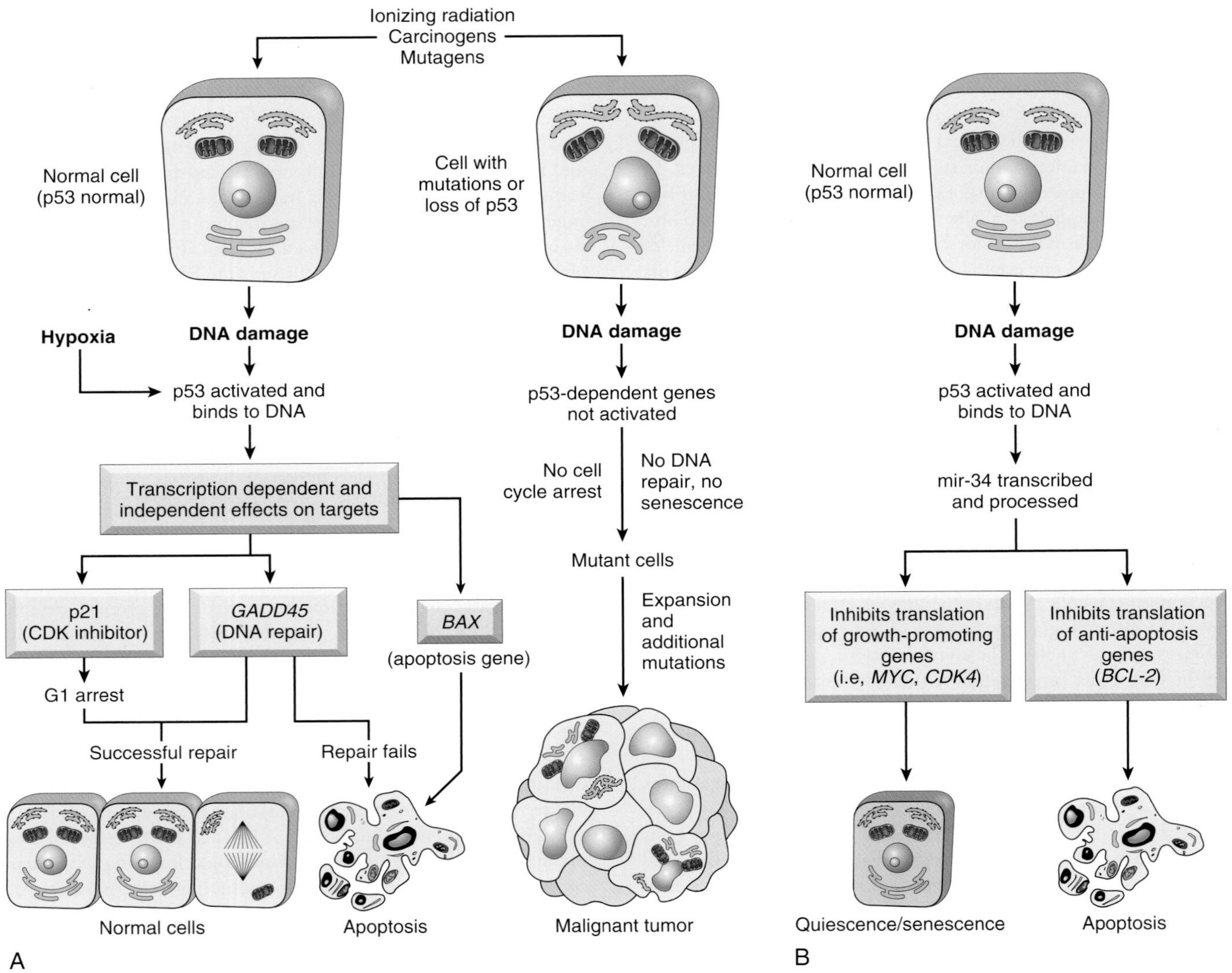

Fig. 6-43 The role of p53 in maintaining integrity of the genome.
DNA damage or hypoxia activate normal p53, leading to G_1 arrest and induction of DNA repair by upregulation of p21 and GADD45, respectively. Successful DNA repair allows cells to proceed through the cell cycle. If DNA repair fails, BCL2-associated X protein *(BAX)* promotes apoptosis. In cells with loss or mutation of p53, DNA damage does not induce cell-cycle arrest or DNA repair. The genetically damaged cells proliferate and may eventually give rise to malignant neoplasms. (From Kumar V, Abbas A, Fausto N, et al: *Robbins & Cotran pathologic basis of disease,* ed 8, Philadelphia, 2009, Saunders.)

and activate oncogenes, the cell has a selective growth advantage. Specific types of DNA repair mechanisms have evolved to repair specific DNA lesions. Mismatch repair enzymes, such as MLH1 and MSH2 proofread DNA, much like the "spell check" function on a computer, to locate and fix single nucleotide mismatches that occur on a regular basis. For example, if an adenine is mistakenly paired with a guanine during DNA replication, this error will be recognized and corrected.

It is well recognized that exposure to UV light leads to cross-linking of pyrimidine residues and formation of pyrimidine dimers. These lesions require a large cohort of DNA repair proteins to perform a nucleotide excision repair procedure. This process is similar to the "cut and paste" function of a computer in which the dimer is excised and the correct nucleotides are replaced and ligated in its stead. As discussed earlier, p53 levels rise in response to DNA damage from any number of agents and give the cell time to carry out the repair processes.

Additional DNA repair genes include ATM, BRCA1, and BRCA2 in humans. Failure of DNA repair of any type can lead to the mutation becoming fixed in the genome and passed on with subsequent rounds of cell division. When the DNA repair gene itself is defective, either through mutation, promoter methylation, or genomic loss, the result is a myriad of mutations throughout the genome with widespread genomic instability and increased cancer susceptibility.

ANIMALS AND CANCER

ANIMAL MODELS OF CANCER

Information on this topic is available at evolve.elsevier.com/Zachary/McGavin/.

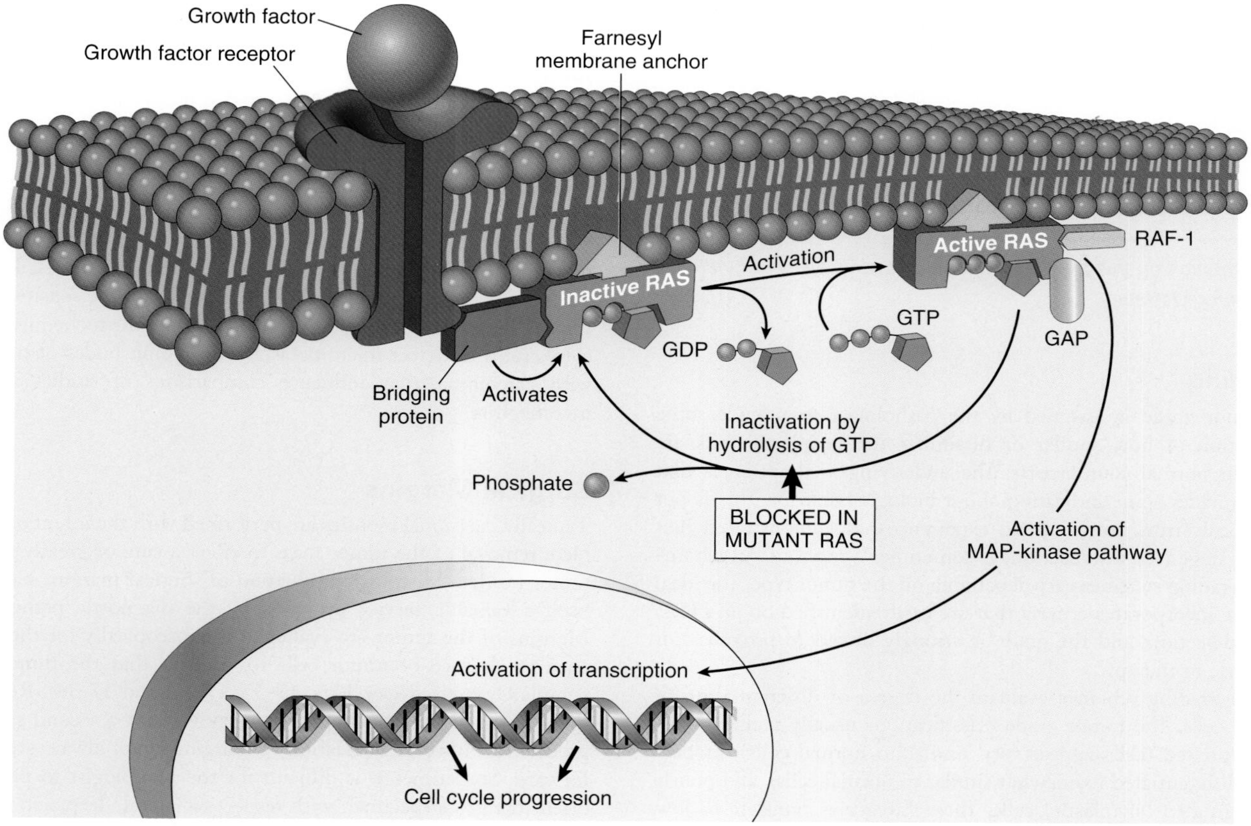

Fig. 6-44 Model for action of RAS genes.

When a normal cell is stimulated through a growth factor receptor, inactive (guanine diphosphate [GDP]-bound) RAS is activated to a guanine triphosphate (GTP)-bound state. Activated RAS recruits RAF and stimulates the mitogen-activated protein kinase (MAPK) pathway to transmit growth-promoting signals to the nucleus. In cancer, mutated RAS is permanently activated because of the inability to hydrolyze GTP, leading to continuous stimulation of cells in the absence of an external trigger. The anchoring of RAS to the cell membrane by the farnesyl moiety is essential for its action. *GAP,* GTPase-activating protein. (From Kumar V, Abbas A, Fausto N, et al: *Robbins & Cotran pathologic basis of disease,* ed 8, Philadelphia, 2009, Saunders.)

EXPERIMENTALLY-INDUCED TUMORS

Information on this topic is available at evolve.elsevier.com/Zachary/McGavin/.

NATURALLY OCCURRING TUMORS

Information on this topic is available at evolve.elsevier.com/Zachary/McGavin/.

Clinical Oncology

Histopathologic Diagnosis

A definitive diagnosis of cancer is frequently obtained by standard histopathology and/or cytology from incisional or excisional biopsies or aspirates. Biopsy specimens are analyzed by routine hematoxylin and eosin (H&E) staining for histopathologic evaluation and by Wright's stain or Diff-Quik for aspirates. Cells are scrutinized for features of malignancy, including abnormal morphology, evidence of invasion and/or metastasis, high mitotic index, presence of abnormal mitoses, high nuclear:cytoplasmic ratio, and absence of encapsulation. The degree of differentiation is evaluated. Malignant neoplasms are frequently poorly to moderately differentiated, and some may be so anaplastic that the cell of origin cannot be determined. Abnormal structures or cellular products may also provide clues to the presence of malignancy.

Special staining techniques may be used to aid in the diagnosis of some tumors. For example, immunohistochemistry can establish if a lymphoma originates from B or T lymphocytes (Web Fig. 6-4). This knowledge may be useful to the clinician in designing treatment or delivering a prognosis. The type of intermediate filaments present in an undifferentiated malignancy can indicate if the tumor is of epithelial (positive for cytokeratin staining) or mesenchymal (positive for vimentin staining) origin. Some neoplasms, such as mesotheliomas and synovial cell sarcomas, are often positive for both cytokeratin and vimentin. Squamous cell carcinomas that have undergone epithelial-to-mesenchymal transformation will have areas positive for one stain or the other, and the transition areas may be positive for both. An exhaustive list of antibodies is beyond the scope of this chapter, but immunohistochemical staining is becoming a widely used tool that assists the pathologist in providing a more complete diagnosis in cases in which routine H&E evaluation is limited.

Histochemical stains can also aid in diagnosis. Poorly differentiated canine mast cells may have granules that are not clearly visible by H&E staining. Staining with toluidine blue often highlights the granules and confirms the diagnosis in otherwise challenging cases.

Clonality Assays

Information on this topic, including Web Fig. 6-5, is available at evolve.elsevier.com/Zachary/McGavin/.

Other Molecular Diagnostic Techniques

Information on this topic is available at evolve.elsevier.com/Zachary/McGavin/.

Grading

A tumor grade is assigned by the pathologist to provide some indication of how similar or dissimilar the neoplastic cells are to their normal counterparts. The underlying assumption is that this provides some indication about biologic behavior. This is not universally true, however, and experience has demonstrated that tumor stage (see next section) is sometimes a more useful parameter. Grading schemes vary depending on the tumor type. The ideal scheme incorporates criteria that are easily identified on an H&E stained section, and the grade is strongly linked to prognosis or response to therapy.

All grading schemes evaluate the degree of differentiation of tumor cells. The tumor grade classifications usually include well-differentiated (cells appear very similar to normal cells), moderately differentiated (somewhat similar to normal cells), and poorly differentiated (anaplastic) cells. These categories translate to low, medium, and high grade, or grades I, II, and III, respectively. Other criteria that may be included in grading schemes include the mitotic rate (i.e., the number of mitotic figures in ten 40× fields), the degree of necrosis, location and invasiveness of the tumor, and overall cellularity. To be biologically relevant, the grading system for a particular tumor type should be based on objective criteria that can be assessed on routine sections with high concordance between different evaluators and provide the clinician with useful information. As such, criteria need to be periodically reevaluated in light of new discoveries and diagnostic capabilities.

Staging

Tumor stage gives an indication of the extent of tumor growth and spread. In general, staging guides the clinician in developing a therapeutic plan and offering an estimate of prognosis to the client. One of the most widely used schemes is the TNM system, which is based on the size of the primary tumor (T), degree of lymph node involvement (N), and extent of metastasis (M). Within each category, a number is assigned based on clinical, diagnostic, and histopathologic evaluation. A designation of T_0 is given to carcinoma in situ, whereas T_1 to T_4 indicate increasing size of the primary tumor. N_0 indicates the absence of detectable lymph node involvement, whereas N_1 to N_3 indicate progressive involvement. Similarly, M_0 signifies no detectable metastasis, whereas M_1 and M_2 indicate metastasis to one and two organs, respectively.

Overall, TNM staging provides a standard measurement by which the natural course of disease and impact of treatment modalities can be compared. Increased availability of more sophisticated diagnostic testing, such as computerized tomography (CT) and magnetic resonance imaging (MRI), as well as more sensitive histologic detection, such as the use of immunohistochemistry for cytokeratin to detect micrometastases in lymph nodes of patients with carcinoma, may influence comparisons of studies among investigators.

Surgical Margins

Typically, excisional biopsies are performed with the intent of complete removal of the tumor mass to effect a cure or greatly reduce tumor burden. Histologic evaluation of surgical margins has long been a valuable service provided by the diagnostic pathologist. Margins of the tumor are evaluated microscopically for the presence or absence of tumor cells to confirm that the tumor was completely excised (see Figs. 17-32, 17-33, and 17-34). Residual malignant cells at the surgical site may warrant a second surgical procedure. However, evaluation of margins is not always straightforward. Sometimes it is difficult for the pathologist to properly orient the gross specimen with respect to lateral, deep, and superficial margins. At other times it may be difficult to distinguish true surgical margins from those produced at trimming. It is important to realize that having clean surgical margins on a histologic slide does not guarantee that the patient is free of tumor. Neoplasms are three-dimensional lesions and only a portion of the mass is examined in any one section. In addition, multifocal or multicentric lesions may not be submitted to the pathologist. Lastly, lymphatic or hematogenous spread may not be evident on the section or sections examined.

Taken together, the tumor type, grade, stage, and completeness of excision are used by the clinician to develop the most appropriate treatment plan for the patient. As we learn more about the molecular pathogenesis of certain tumors, the need for specialized diagnostic tests will certainly increase. Targeted molecular therapies will be effective only if the target is present in the patient's tumor.

SUGGESTED READINGS

Suggested Readings are available at evolve.elsevier.com/Zachary/McGavin/.

SECTION 2

Pathology of Organ Systems

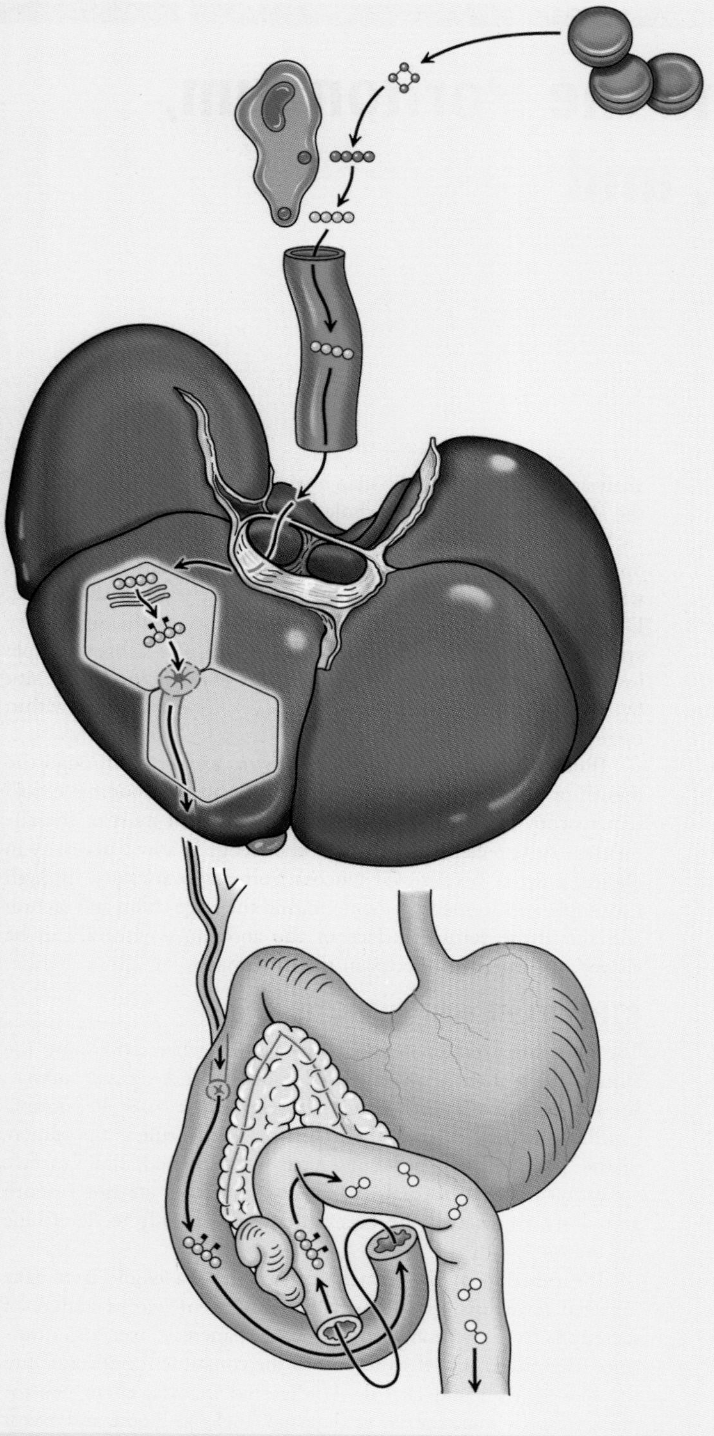

CHAPTER 7

Alimentary System and the Peritoneum, Omentum, Mesentery, and Peritoneal Cavity*

Howard B. Gelberg

INTRODUCTION

The alimentary system is a long and complex tube that varies in its construction and function among animal species. For example, herbivores need a fermentation chamber (either a rumen or an expanded cecum) for the digestion of cellulose, a feature not present in carnivores. Although a large variety of gastrointestinal (GI) disturbances are clinically important in all species of animals, the predominant form of disease varies from species to species. Pet carnivores, partly because of their long lifespan, effective vaccines, and a lifestyle and diet similar to that of humans, develop alimentary neoplasia far more often than herbivores. Meat, milk, and fiber-producing animals (ruminants and pigs) are host to a variety of infectious diseases that are largely resistant to vaccines. These pathogens may have evolved as a result of the herding instinct of these animals, giving the pathogens an opportunity to mutate within a large socially structured host population. Equids are most prone to displacements of alimentary viscera.

In general, the alimentary system, including the salivary glands, pancreas, and liver, functions by adding water, electrolytes, and enzymes to ingested matter and then mixing and grinding it to facilitate its breakdown to water-soluble nutrients for absorption across mucous membranes into the blood circulation and subsequent distribution through the body. Although the alimentary tract is open ended, most ingested substances and secretions produced by the GI system are absorbed.

A large part of the practice of veterinary medicine is devoted to the diagnosis and treatment of alimentary disorders. Many of the newer molecular and imaging methods have been designed specifically to increase the clinician's ability to make accurate diagnoses of the various conditions of the alimentary system. Additionally, every physical examination includes the opportunity for a fecal analysis that allows the clinician a window into the functioning of the alimentary system as a whole.

The polymerase chain reaction (PCR) is a tool that allows the opportunity to rapidly diagnose an infectious cause of enteritis without having to culture the organism in the traditional manner. Diagnosis of the cause of an infectious disease of the alimentary system can also be made from examination of a biopsy sample by histologic and immunohistochemical staining or by in situ hybridization that allows demonstration of the pathogen within target cells.

Through the use of fiberoptic endoscopes inserted through the mouth or anus or through a small incision in the abdominal wall (laparoscopy), a thorough clinical examination of most of the alimentary system can be made. This knowledge is now a necessity in clinical practice because GI mucosa from the oral cavity, through the esophagus, stomach, duodenum, and the large colon and rectum and the entire serosal surface of the abdominal viscera, can be viewed and sampled directly in the live animal.

STRUCTURE AND FUNCTION

The most important point to keep in mind when examining the alimentary system is that normal mucosal and serosal surfaces should be smooth and shiny (although there may be normal papilla, folds, and ridges). The exception to this rule is the rumen, whose papillae may normally have a roughened, dull, surface appearance. When serosal and mucosal surfaces are not smooth and shiny, animals should be examined thoroughly to determine the reason.

The function of the alimentary system as a whole is to take ingested feedstuffs, grind them and mix them with a variety of secretions from the oral cavity, stomach, pancreas, liver, and intestines (digestion), and then to absorb the constituent nutrients into the bloodstream and lacteals. Undigested ingesta, effete neutrophils, fresh (hematochezia) or digested (melena) blood, and excess secretions are passed from the body into the alimentary lumen and thus become a component of the feces. The quality and quantity of the feces and clinical signs, such as regurgitation and vomiting, are often early indicators of alimentary dysfunction.

*Dr. H. Van Kruningen of the Department of Pathobiology, University of Connecticut, made contributions to this chapter in the third edition.

BOX 7-1 Portals of Entry in the Alimentary System

- Ingestion
- Coughed up by the lungs and swallowed
- Systemic blood-borne infections
- Parasite migration

BOX 7-2 Defense Mechanisms in the Alimentary System

- Saliva
  Resident flora and fauna
  Gastric pH
  Secreted immunoglobulins
- Vomiting
- Extraintestinal secretions from the liver and pancreas
- Intestinal proteolytic enzymes
- Phagocytes and other effector cells within the submucosa
- High rate of epithelial turnover
- Increased peristalsis resulting in diarrhea
- Paneth cells
- Adaptive immune system

PORTALS OF ENTRY

There are limited numbers of ways that pathogenic agents gain entry into the alimentary system (Box 7-1). The most common, of course, is through ingestion. However, under certain circumstances, pathogens may be coughed up from the lungs into the pharynx and swallowed. Systemic blood-borne infections of viruses (viremia), bacteria (bacteremia), and systemic toxins (septicemia and toxemia) may make their way through the bloodstream and attach to specific receptors on the epithelial lining cells of the alimentary system. Parasites may migrate through various regions of the body to find a home within the mucosa or roam free in the lumen of the alimentary tract.

DEFENSE MECHANISMS

Considering the types of materials that are ingested by domestic animals, it is significant that they are not constantly ill. This resistance to disease occurs because the alimentary system is well suited to protect itself against most potentially pathogenic insults (Box 7-2). These protective mechanisms include oral secretions, such as saliva; "normal" resident flora and fauna; the gastric pH; opening of tight junctions between intestinal cells to allow macromolecules, such as immunoglobulins, into the lumen; vomiting; secretions from the liver and pancreas; intestinal proteolytic enzymes, macrophages, and other effector cells, such as neutrophils, within the submucosa, which are exuded into the alimentary lumen; the high rate of epithelial turnover; increased peristalsis resulting in diarrhea; Paneth cells; and the immune system. Paneth cells produce antimicrobial peptides and proteins, including lysozyme and secretory phospholipase A2. They also produce α-defensins (cryptdins).

ORAL CAVITY

The oral cavity is one of the places that can be examined directly by the clinician and pathologist and where they can use the same criteria for determining abnormality. The same can be said of the rectal mucosa.

BOX 7-3 Defense Mechanisms in the Oral Cavity

- Taste buds that reject potentially toxic materials based on taste and tongue feel
- Indigenous bacterial flora that occupy attachment sites of pathogens
- Saliva
- Flushing action so potential pathogens are cleared from the oropharynx
- Protective coating of the mucosa
- Contains antimicrobial lysozyme and immunoglobulins

Structure and Function

The physiologically normal oral mucosa is smooth, shiny, and pink. It is composed of variably keratinizing, stratified squamous epithelium (mucous membranes). In animals in which the oral mucosa is heavily pigmented (melanosis), assessment of circulatory function (capillary refill time) and color as an indicator of red blood cell concentration (packed cell volume) can be difficult. In these cases, examination of conjunctiva, rectal, and urogenital mucosa can be substituted. The oral cavity is where ingested materials are masticated; mixed with digestive enzymes, such as those in saliva; and passed on through the oropharynx to the esophagus.

Defense Mechanisms

Defense mechanisms of the oral cavity include the stratified epithelial surface that is resistant to trauma and some irritants; taste buds, which reject potentially toxic materials based on taste and tongue feel; an indigenous bacterial flora that occupy attachment sites that would otherwise be available to pathogens; and saliva (Box 7-3). Saliva provides a flushing action so potential pathogens are cleared from the oropharynx and swallowed. Saliva also forms a protective coating of the mucosa and contains antimicrobial lysozyme in the zymogen granules of serous cells and immunoglobulins, especially immunoglobulin A (IgA), in a manner analogous to cryptal enterocytes of the intestine, through the production of a secretory component. Migration through the alimentary tract, including the oral cavity, eliminates neutrophils at the end of their lifespan. In their absence, stomatitis results.

Developmental Anomalies

There are a wide variety of developmental abnormalities in the oral cavity. Some are incompatible with life unless surgically corrected. Only a few of these congenital lesions have a proven hereditary component. Most are idiopathic. Thorough physical examination of neonates must include examination of the oral cavity for these defects.

Palatoschisis, or cleft palate, and cheiloschisis, or cleft lip, are among the most common developmental abnormalities of the oral cavity. Cheiloschisis is sometimes referred to as *hare lip* because this is a normal feature of the rabbit. It is a failure of fusion of the upper lip along the midline or philtrum. Palatoschisis can be genetic or toxic in origin. It results from a failure of fusion of the lateral palatine processes. It can be caused by steroid administration during pregnancy in primates, including humans. Depending on the size of the defect, which may involve only the soft palate or both the soft and hard palates (Fig. 7-1), the lesion may be surgically correctable. It is a matter of some ethical concern whether to correct such defects without also sterilizing the patient because of the potential for cleft palate to have a genetic cause. Important sequelae to the host from cleft palate are starvation, as the result of the inability of

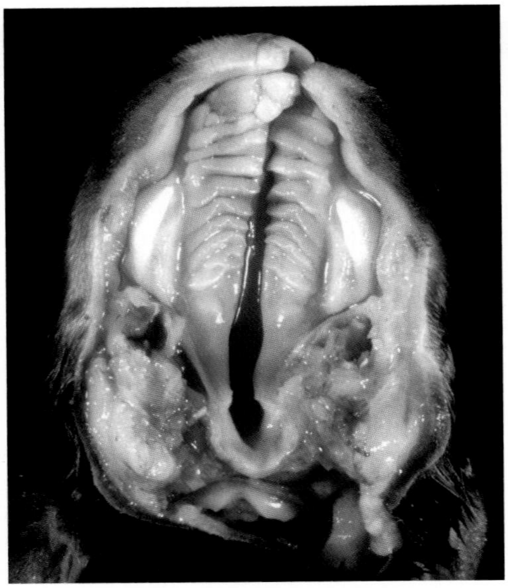

Fig. 7-1 Palatoschisis and cheiloschisis, hard and soft palate, puppy. The lateral palatine processes have failed to fuse during the first trimester of gestation (palatoschisis). In dogs, palatoschisis has been attributed to genetic abnormalities, excessive intake of vitamin A during gestation, and the administration of cortisone during gestation. The upper lip is also cleft (cheiloschisis). (Courtesy Dr. H. Gelberg, College of Veterinary Medicine, Oregon State University.)

the nursing animal to create a negative pressure in the mouth with a resultant failure to suckle, and aspiration pneumonia, since no effective separation is present between the oral and nasal cavities.

Stomatitis and Gingivitis

Stomatitis and gingivitis refer to inflammation of the mucous membranes of the oral cavity and gingiva, respectively. Because the oral cavity is constantly bombarded with ingested substances that are moved around by the tongue, the final result of a variety of insults to the lining of the oral cavity is a loss of mucosa—erosions, ulcerations, and necrosis. Thus, although inflammation is apparent, clues as to the initiating process may be absent. Lesions may be at different stages and are commonly classified as macules, papules, vesicles, erosions, abscesses, granulomas, and ulcers. These lesions can be caused by infectious agents, particularly viruses; chemical injury; trauma; intoxicants; or autoimmune or systemic disease. They often result in anorexia caused by painful mastication. Hypersalivation (ptyalism) is also apparent, whether from overproduction or a failure to swallow. In the cat, gingivitis is the first and most consistent sign of feline immunodeficiency virus (FIV) infection (immune system failure) associated with a reduction in CD4 lymphocytes, thymic atrophy, and lymph node atrophy.

Vesicular Stomatitides

Although vesicular stomatitis correctly refers to oral vesicles and blisters, the term is generally reserved for those lesions caused by epitheliotropic viruses. The vesicular stomatitides are listed in Table 7-1. Their genesis is from virus-induced epithelial cytolysis attended by fluid accumulation and subsequent rupture of the resultant vesicle. Blistering or vesiculation of the oral epithelium is present early in the course of these diseases. All of these diseases are virus-induced, and all have identical appearances at gross and histopathologic examination. None of these conditions is fatal. They produce great economic loss because of poor weight gain in

TABLE 7-1 Vesicular Stomatitides

Disease	Cause	Ruminant	Pigs	Horses
Foot-and-mouth disease	Picornavirus	+	+	–
Vesicular stomatitis	Rhabdovirus	++	+	+
Vesicular exanthema of swine	Calicivirus (vesivirus)	–	++	–
Swine vesicular disease	Enterovirus	–	++	–

+, Species in which disease occurs.
–, Species in which disease does not occur.

affected animals and sometimes abortions in gravid females. The exact cause of the abortions is unknown, but it is probably related to the stress induced by the painful oral, cutaneous, and pedal (hoof or foot) lesions. Secondary bacterial invaders, both Gram-negative and Gram-positive, of these lesions can result in endotoxemia. Several diseases, such as foot-and-mouth disease and vesicular exanthema, affect the coronary bands of the digits and interdigital clefts, resulting in lameness. Some of these diseases (foot-and-mouth disease, vesicular exanthema, and swine vesicular disease) are exotic to the United States (US) and thus are reportable to state or federal authorities, or both, if the clinician or pathologist suspects the disease. This requirement is due to the great expense involved in eradicating these diseases from the US and their potential use as agents of agroterrorism. Nontariff export/import barriers designed to prevent the introduction of highly contagious agents, such as foot-and-mouth disease, into animal populations of countries with which we trade are often put in place.

The gross lesions of the vesicular stomatitides are epithelial. Fluid-filled vesicles are present in the oral cavity, lips, rostral palate, and tongue (Fig. 7-2, *A*). Entry of virus in these cases is most likely oral into areas of temporary loss of mucosa as the result of normal mastication and trauma. The viruses are cytolytic, and the resultant release of virus from cells infects neighboring cells. The lesions enlarge centripetally, forming vesicles. Bullae result from coalescence resulting in erosions and ulcers. These ulcers are typically hyperemic (Fig. 7-2, *B*). Viremia, often transient, sometimes occurs.

Similar vesicular lesions occur in the nasal mucosa, particularly in pigs with vesicular exanthema and in the proximal epithelium of the alimentary system (esophagus and rumen) of cattle with foot-and-mouth disease. Some animals have conjunctivitis and vesicular dermatitis of the teats and vulva. Microscopically, the lesions of these four diseases (foot-and-mouth disease, vesicular stomatitis, vesicular exanthema, and swine vesicular disease) are similar. Virus-induced, intracellular edema progresses to swelling of the cells of the stratum spinosum, cell lysis and intercellular edema, and resultant vesicles. The epithelium overlying the virus-rich vesicular fluid is thin, and even slight friction can rupture vesicles and bullae, creating an ulcer. Healing of the ulcer progresses from the usual fibrin and/or neutrophil-rich acute stages (scab) to the more chronic stages of granulation.

Lesions and signs of the vesicular stomatitides include vesicles, bullae, and detachment of patches of epithelium with resultant raw ulcers, ptyalism, lameness, fever, and anorexia. Besides the lesions that develop from the initially infected cells, the virus spreads centripetally to adjacent susceptible epithelium, causing repeated episodes of this infectious, lytic cycle. The vesicular stomatitides are

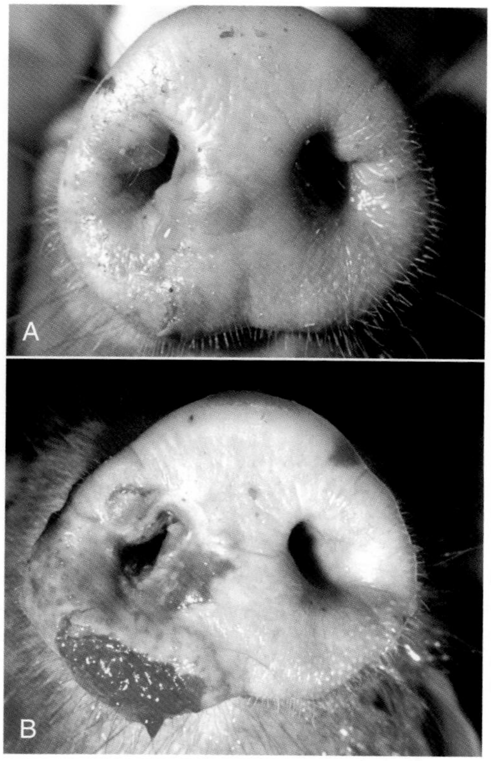

Fig. 7-2 Cutaneous vesicles, vesicular exanthema, snout, pig.
A, Vesicles, both intact (upper vesicle) and ruptured (lower vesicle), are present on the planum rostrale and are caused by the infection of injured mucosal epithelial cells with vesicular exanthema of swine virus, a calicivirus (vesivirus). **B,** Ruptured vesicles with cutaneous ulceration, vesicular exanthema (later stage of the disease). Note the ruptured vesicles which can cause pain resulting in inappetence. (**A** from Gelberg H, Lewis RM: *Vet Pathol* 19:424-443, 1982. **B** courtesy Dr. H. Gelberg, College of Veterinary Medicine, Oregon State University.)

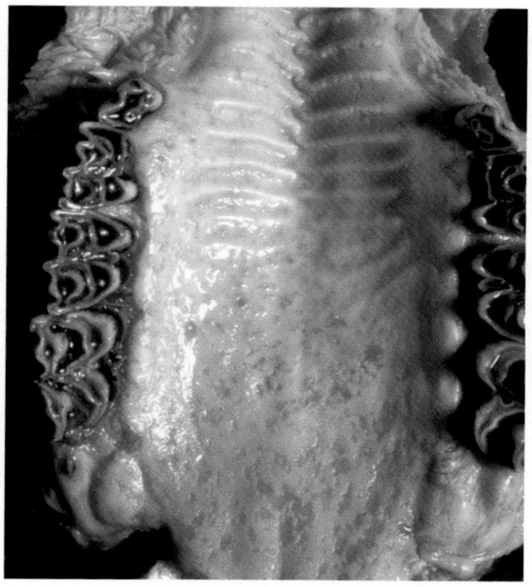

Fig. 7-3 Erosions and ulcers, bovine viral diarrhea virus infection, hard palate, cow.
Erosions and ulcers caused by this pestivirus are particularly evident on the mucosal epithelial surface of the caudal hard palate. These lesions are characteristic of the ulcerative stomatitides, which, unlike the vesicular disease viruses, do not form vesicles. (Courtesy Dr. M.D. McGavin, College of Veterinary Medicine, University of Tennessee.)

tentatively diagnosed based on the clinical signs and lesions resulting from oral and nasal ulceration, conjunctivitis, and ulceration of the genitalia and mammary glands. Lameness is secondary to hoof involvement that is focused at the coronary band. Definitive diagnosis is important and performed at federal laboratories equipped to rapidly respond to suspected outbreaks. Federal quarantine of infected herds is an important control mechanism, followed by eradication, slaughter, and carcass disposal.

Specific Vesicular Diseases

Foot-and-mouth disease is an extremely important disease and disease threat of arteriodactyls worldwide but has not appeared in US livestock since 1929, when it was eradicated after an outbreak in California. Virus spreads rapidly and principally by aerosol. The disease is characterized in its early stages by vesicles in the planum nasale, in the oral cavity, and tongue. The picornavirus of foot-and-mouth disease attaches to susceptible cells via integrins on the cell surface. Fluid from ruptured vesicles spreads to areas of abraded skin, for example, skin of a mammary gland. When coronary bands and hooves are affected, coronary band vesiculation may eventually lead to sloughing of the hoof. Although this disease is not fatal, the pain and accompanying inappetence lead to weight loss. If allowed to heal, the hoof will regrow into a ball-like structure. Young animals with foot-and-mouth disease frequently have a viral myocarditis without other signs. Vaccination is short-lived (6 months) and takes time to become effective in individual animals; thus immediate protection is not provided. Persistent infections occur in water buffalo and infected cattle that have been previously vaccinated.

Vesicular stomatitis is common in calves, pigs, and some wildlife species but does not occur in sheep or goats. It is the only vesicular disease to which horses are susceptible. In northern latitudes, it is generally a warm weather disease, suggesting that insects act as vectors. As the name implies, vesicles in the oral cavity characterize the disease. Clinically the disease is often recognized by inappetence in the affected animal, accompanied by ptyalism.

Vesicular exanthema is a specific disease of pigs that is indistinguishable clinically and pathologically from foot-and-mouth disease. This disease is uniquely American and was believed eradicated from pigs in 1956 through enactment of federal laws requiring the cooking of garbage fed to pigs. The evidence indicates that vesicular exanthema of swine serovars are variants of San Miguel sea lion virus. This latter marine calicivirus occurs in coastal sea lion and fur seal populations from California to Alaska (Web Fig. 7-1).

Swine vesicular disease is indistinguishable from the other vesicular diseases and is exotic to the US. Efforts are underway to develop DNA microarrays to facilitate rapid identification of specific vesicular diseases from a single sample.

Erosive and Ulcerative Stomatitides

Erosions are defined by a loss of part of the thickness of the surface epithelium, whereas ulcers are full-thickness epithelial losses exposing the basement membrane. Thus erosions may progress to ulcers, which in hollow organs may become perforating ulcers. Erosive and ulcerative stomatitis can have a variety of causes. Agents responsible include the viruses of bovine viral diarrhea (BVD) (Fig. 7-3), rinderpest, malignant catarrhal fever (Fig. 7-4), feline calicivirus, and bluetongue, and in equids, nonsteroidal antiinflammatory drugs (NSAIDs). Other causes include uremia (Fig. 7-5); ingested foreign bodies, such as foxtail awns; the feline eosinophilic granuloma complex; and vitamin C deficiency in primates and guinea pigs (Web Fig. 7-2). Often, the oral lesions must be evaluated in the

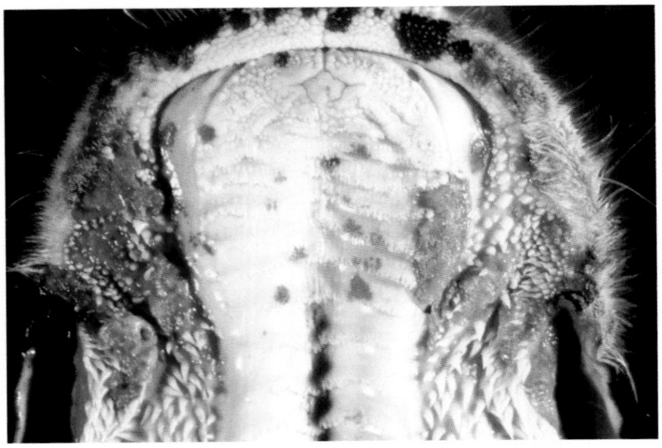

Fig. 7-4 Erosions and ulcers, malignant catarrhal fever, hard palate, dental pad and buccal papillae, cow.
The erosions and ulcers (red areas on mucosal surface) are due to malignant catarrhal fever virus, a herpes virus, but are characteristic of many ulcerative stomatitides. (Courtesy Dr. H. Gelberg, College of Veterinary Medicine, Oregon State University.)

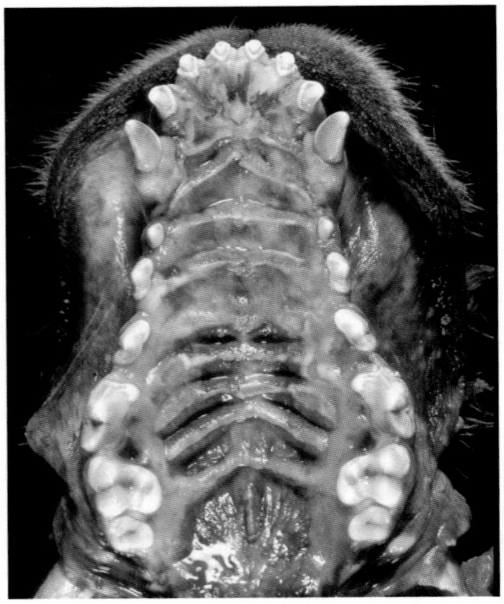

Fig. 7-5 Uremic ulcers, hard palate, dog.
Ulcers present on the transverse palatine ridges and periodontal gingiva are secondary to vascular damage associated with increased concentrations of plasma blood urea nitrogen and creatinine from kidney failure. Affected animals often have an ammoniacal or uremic odor to the breath. (Courtesy Dr. H. Gelberg, College of Veterinary Medicine, Oregon State University.)

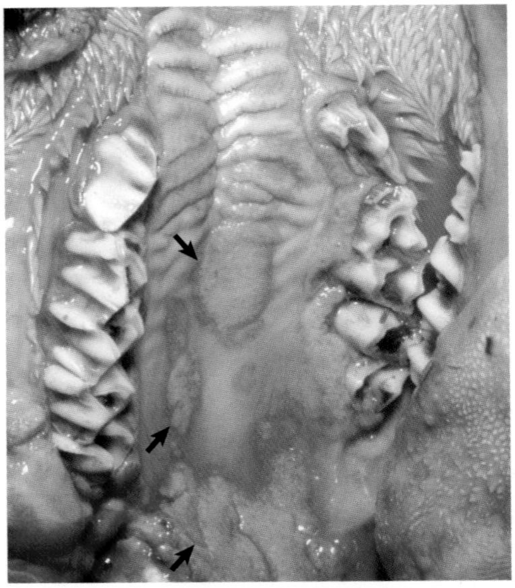

Fig. 7-6 Epithelial plaques, papular stomatitis, hard palate mucosa, calf.
Virus-induced (parapoxvirus) epithelial plaques and papules are present on the mucosal epithelium of the hard palate and adjacent gingiva *(arrows)*. (Courtesy Dr. M.D. McGavin, College of Veterinary Medicine, University of Tennessee.)

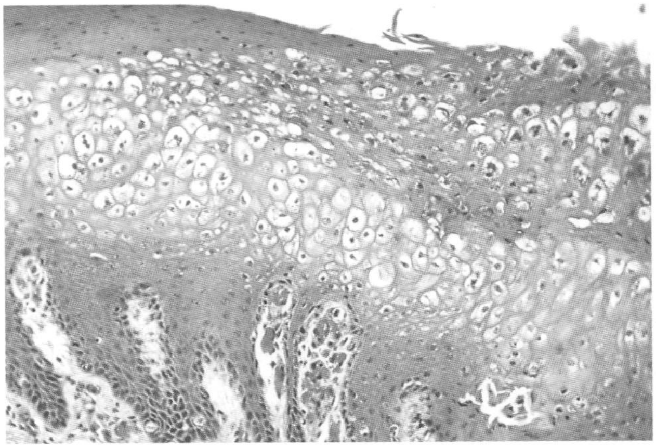

Fig. 7-7 Hydropic change, papular stomatitis, hard palate mucosa, cow.
There is massive cytoplasmic swelling of the epithelial cells of the stratum spinosum. At a later stage, these cells may contain intracytoplasmic eosinophilic parapoxvirus inclusions (not visible here). H&E stain. (Courtesy Dr. M.D. McGavin, College of Veterinary Medicine, University of Tennessee.)

context of the clinical signs, together with histopathologic findings and ancillary testing, to arrive at a definitive diagnosis. Additionally, the vesicular stomatitides can progress to ulceration secondary to abrasion to the point that they cannot be distinguished from the ulcerative stomatitides.

Parapox Stomatitides

The two major diseases in this category, bovine papular stomatitis and contagious ecthyma, are zoonotic. Bovine papular stomatitis is recognized by papules on the nares, muzzle, gingiva, buccal cavity, palate, and tongue (Fig. 7-6). Lesions also occur in the esophagus, rumen, and omasum. Microscopically, acantholysis is responsible for the macule and ballooning degeneration of these cells, which may contain intracytoplasmic eosinophilic parapoxvirus inclusions at a later stage (Fig. 7-7; also see Fig. 1-12). Erosion of the infected cells accompanied by a neutrophilic infiltrate heals readily from the unaffected basal epithelium. The disease is more common in immunosuppressed animals such as those persistently infected with BVD virus. In humans, the disease is called *milker's nodules* and is characterized by papules of the hands and arms.

Contagious ecthyma, sore mouth or infectious pustular dermatitis, is a condition of sheep and goats characterized by progression of the stages typical of pox viruses—macules, papules, vesicles, pustules, scabs, and scars in areas of skin abrasions, including the corners of the mouth (Fig. 7-8; also see Fig. 17-43), mouth, udder, teats, coronary bands, and anus. Occasionally, the mucosa of the esophagus and rumen also can be affected. The virus is quite hardy and can survive for 50 to 60 days in the summer and longer in

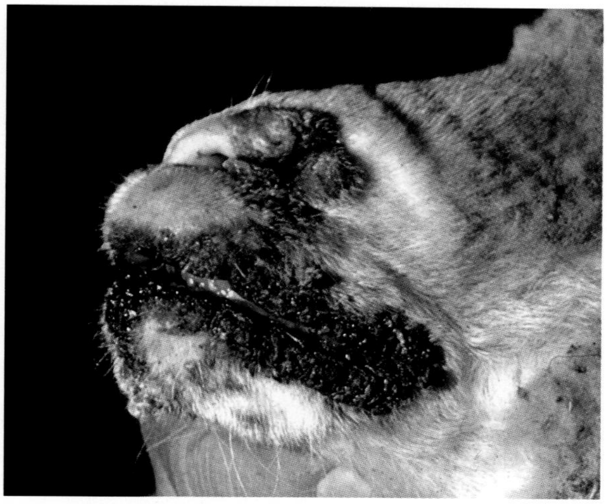

Fig. 7-8 Contagious ecthyma, oral mucous membranes, lamb. Note crusts around nose and lips. Multiple pustules and coalescing ruptured pustules covered by scabs are present on the skin. The parapoxvirus induces epithelial proliferation (acanthosis), followed by vesicle formation. These vesicles rupture and are quickly covered by scabs. Lesions develop at the sites of trauma, such as occur with a nursing lamb, where damage to the superficial oral epithelium allows entry of the virus into skin. (Courtesy Dr. M.D. McGavin, College of Veterinary Medicine, University of Tennessee.)

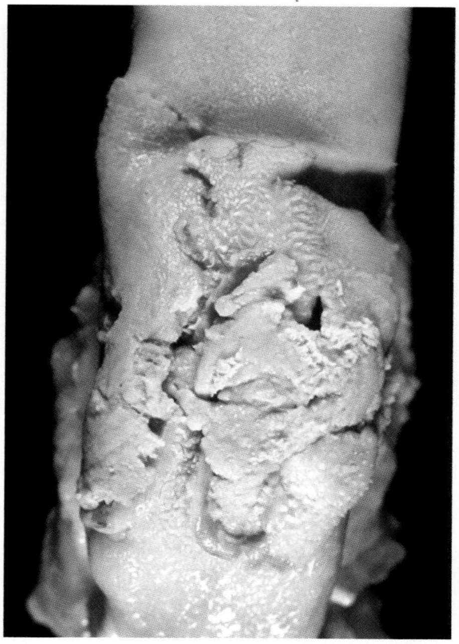

Fig. 7-9 Necrotizing stomatitis, calf diphtheria, tongue, calf. The dorsal surface of the tongue is ulcerated, and the ulcers are covered by a diphtheric membrane. Calf diphtheria is caused by infection with the bacterium *Fusobacterium necrophorum* secondary to abrasion and/or trauma to the mucosal epithelium of the oral cavity or larynx. (Courtesy Dr. M.D. McGavin, College of Veterinary Medicine, University of Tennessee.)

cold weather. At room temperature, scabs containing virus can be infective after 10 years. Eosinophilic cytoplasmic inclusion bodies are visible at microscopic examination of lesions early in the course of disease. The condition in humans is called *orf.*

Necrotizing Stomatitides

Necrotizing stomatitis occurs in cattle, sheep, and pigs. In cattle, it is sometimes referred to as *calf diphtheria* (Fig. 7-9). Necrotizing stomatitis is the end-stage of all other forms of stomatitis when they are complicated by infection with *Fusobacterium necrophorum,* a filamentous-to-rodlike-to-coccoid, Gram-negative anaerobe. Bacterial toxins are responsible for the extensive lesions. Necrotizing stomatitis is characterized by yellow-gray, round foci surrounded by a rim of hyperemic tissue in the oral cavity, larynx, pharynx, or tongue. Well-demarcated foci of coagulation necrosis typify the histologic appearance of necrotizing stomatitis. As might be expected in foci of inflammation, there is a circumferential rim of leukocytes and hyperemia. Clinical signs include swollen cheeks, inappetence, pyrexia, and halitosis. Infection may become systemic if severe, resulting in lesions throughout the alimentary system and associated lymphoid tissue.

Noma is a severe form of oral ischemic necrosis with lesional spirochetes and fusiform bacteria. Although rare, it is seen most often in primates, including humans, and dogs. It is characterized by severe necrotizing gingivitis that can extend into adjacent bone causing osteolysis and sometimes death.

Ulcerative gingivitis (trench mouth), caused by anaerobic spirochetes, affects humans, some nonhuman primates, and rarely, puppies. In addition to *Fusobacterium* spp., *Borrelia vincentii* may be causative. Debilitated animals and those with intercurrent infections are at increased risk for these secondary invaders, which may be part of normal oral flora. Similar clinically to necrotizing stomatitis, ulcerative gingivitis is characterized by acute inflammation and necrosis, oral ulceration and pain, halitosis, a fragile oral mucosa, and ptyalism. The morphologic diagnosis is an acute, necrotizing gingivitis. Unlike the case in necrotizing stomatitis, the causative agents are readily identified by tissue smears or by culture.

Eosinophilic Stomatitides

Oral granulomas or ulcers ("rodent ulcers") occur frequently in cats. Similar lesions occur sporadically in a variety of canine breeds. In cats, they are termed *oral eosinophilic granulomas.* Although the etiology of this condition is unknown, the histologic appearance of lesions suggests an immune-mediated mechanism, possibly a hypersensitivity reaction to an unknown antigen. Antibodies to intercellular material can often be demonstrated in affected cats. In the majority of cases of both dogs and cats, an increase in circulating eosinophils is present.

In cats, lip lesions are commonly visible near the philtrum and may extend through the adjacent haired skin. Oral lesions may occur anywhere in the mouth, including the gingiva, hard and soft palates, oral and nasal pharynx, tongue, and occasionally draining lymphoid tissues, excluding the tonsils, which do not have afferent lymphatic vessels (Fig. 7-10; also see Fig. 17-21, *C*). In dogs, eosinophilic granulomas typically are raised, fungating masses on the ventral and lateral lingual epithelium and palate. Collagenolysis (because collagen is acellular, it cannot undergo necrosis) is characteristically central in the lesion. The surrounding inflammatory tissue contains mixed inflammatory cells with increased numbers of eosinophils, mast cells, and multinucleated giant cells (see Web Fig. 3-14). Lesions grouped as the eosinophilic granuloma complex of cats include eosinophilic ulcer, linear (collagenolytic) granulomas, and eosinophilic plaques. The latter two lesions are strictly cutaneous and do not affect the oral cavity. No proven etiologic link has been established between these cutaneous conditions (linear granulomas and eosinophilic plaques) and oral eosinophilic granulomas. The cause of the canine lesions is unknown.

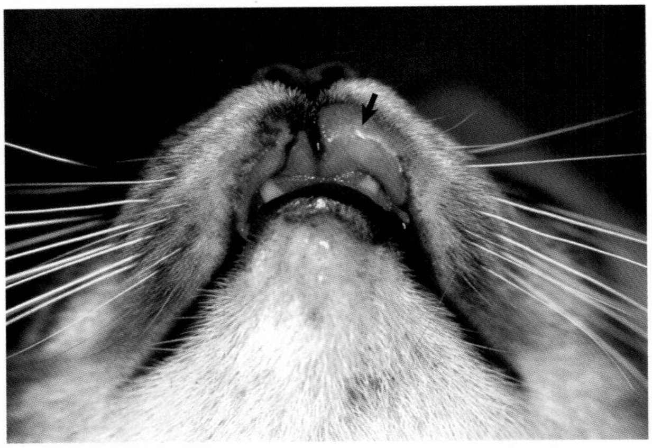

Fig. 7-10 Eosinophilic granuloma, skin, upper lip, cat.
Bilateral ulceration of the upper lip is present. The upper left lip is more extensively affected *(arrow)*. (Courtesy Dr. Ann M. Hargis, DermatoDiagnostics.)

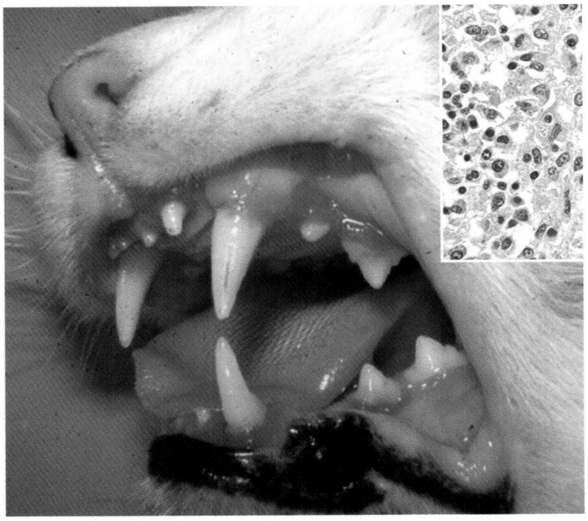

Fig. 7-11 Lymphoplasmacytic stomatitis, gingiva, cat.
This chronic condition of cats is characterized by red, inflamed gums, fetid breath, and inappetence. The oral mucosa can also be hyperplastic and ulcerated. *Inset,* There is a florid infiltrate of mixed inflammatory cells, including many lymphocytes and plasma cells in the submucosa beneath the epithelium. H&E stain. (Figure courtesy Dr. C. Patrick Ryan, Veterinary Public Health, Los Angeles Department of Health Services; and Noah's Arkive, College of Veterinary Medicine, University of Georgia. *Inset,* Courtesy Dr. J.F. Zachary, College of Veterinary Medicine, University of Illinois.)

Lymphoplasmacytic Stomatitis

Lymphoplasmacytic stomatitis is an idiopathic condition of the cat named on the basis of the histologic appearance of the lesions (Fig. 7-11). Associations have been hypothesized between this condition and the presence of bacteria or calicivirus associated with feline leukemia virus (FeLV) and/or FIV infection. It is a chronic condition characterized by red, inflamed gums, a fetid breath, and inappetence. The oral mucosa may be hyperplastic and ulcerated. An inefficient immune response may be responsible for the persistence of oral bacteria and the accumulation of lymphocytes and plasma cells.

Chronic Ulcerative Paradental Stomatitis

Chronic ulcerative paradental stomatitis, a condition of dogs also known as *ulcerative stomatitis* and *lymphocytic-plasmacytic stomatitis,*

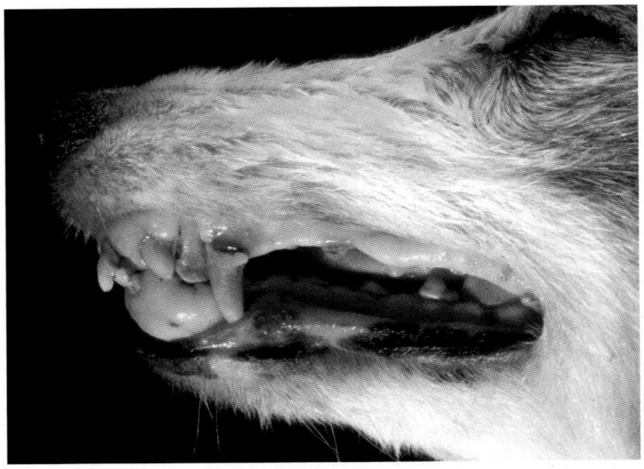

Fig. 7-12 Gingival hyperplasia, gingiva, dog.
Hyperplastic gingiva has enveloped the lower incisor teeth. Dental calculus (tartar, brown) is also present on both upper and lower incisor, canine and molar teeth. (Courtesy Dr. H. Gelberg, College of Veterinary Medicine, Oregon State University.)

is caused by apposition of "kissing ulcers" to dental plaque. The condition is painful with resultant inappetence and anorexia. Affected dogs drool and have halitosis. This condition occurs in older dogs of any breed, but Maltese dogs and cavalier King Charles spaniels are particularly susceptible. The lymphocytic-plasmacytic lesions noted on histologic examination are suggestive of an inflammatory rather than infectious etiology possibly caused by mediators released from the plaque. If untreated, bone resorption may occur.

Oral Mucosal Hyperplasia and Neoplasia

Hyperplastic Diseases

Gingival hyperplasia is a simple overgrowth of gum tissue, principally the fibrous submucosa. The hyperplasia can become so severe as to bury incisor teeth (Fig. 7-12). Gingival hyperplasia is most common in brachycephalic dog breeds and is present in 30% of boxer dogs older than 5 years.

Grossly, gingival hyperplasia can be indistinguishable from an epulis (Fig. 7-13). Epulis is a nonspecific term that designates a growth of the gingiva. The several kinds of epulides can only be distinguished by histopathologic examination. These include fibromatous epulis of periodontal ligament origin—a benign tumor of dental mesenchyme. This distinction is not just an academic exercise because, although all epulides are considered benign, one form, acanthomatous epulis or acanthomatous ameloblastoma, invades bone and can be quite destructive. This growth arises from the epithelial rests of Malassez or epithelial tooth germ. Fortunately, this type of epulis can be managed therapeutically. Whether the epulides represent fibrous and epithelial hyperplasia or benign neoplasms of tooth germ is controversial.

Neoplasia

In the dog, 70% of tumors of the alimentary system are in the oral cavity and oropharynx. These tumors run the gamut of biologic behavior from simple epithelial hyperplasia to malignant neoplasms with metastases to distant sites. Squamous cell carcinomas occur in the oral cavity, particularly in old cats, in which they account for 60% of oral neoplasms. They generally occur on the ventrolateral surface of the tongue and tonsils. Lingual squamous cell carcinomas occur more commonly in felids, and tonsillar squamous cell carcinomas are more common in canids. Although

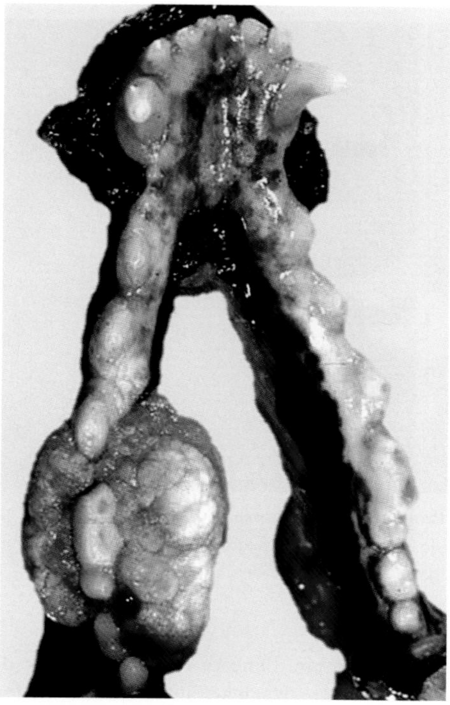

Fig. 7-13 Fibromatous epulis, left mandible, molar teeth, dog. This growth is an epulis (fibromatous type); however, epulides are often grossly indistinguishable from gingival hyperplasia. Epulis is a term used to designate a growth of the gingiva that is firm, periodontal, and usually solitary, in contrast to gingival hyperplasia. This distinction is not just an academic exercise because, although all epulides are considered benign, one form, acanthomatous ameloblastoma, is locally invasive. It invades bone and can be quite destructive. (Courtesy Dr. J. King, College of Veterinary Medicine, Cornell University.)

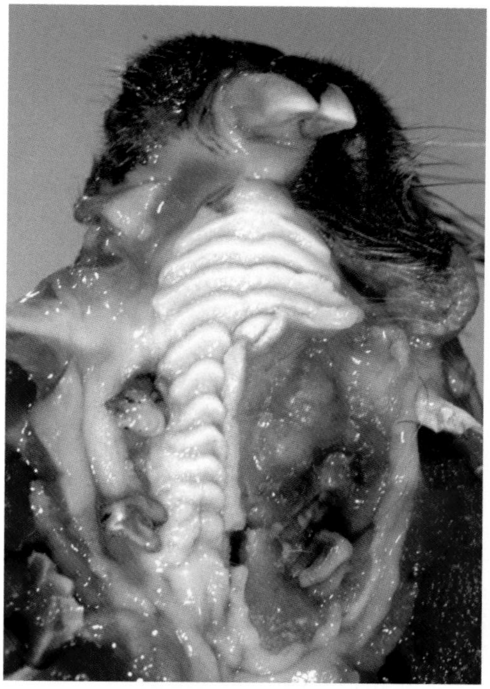

Fig. 7-14 Squamous cell carcinoma, palate, woodchuck. A mass of proliferating neoplastic squamous epithelial cells has displaced and replaced the mucosa and underlying tissue of the left hard palate and gingiva. (Courtesy Dr. H. Gelberg, College of Veterinary Medicine, Oregon State University.)

often appearing histologically aggressive, only a small percentage of lingual neoplasms metastasize, most commonly to draining lymph nodes, the mandibular and medial retropharyngeal. Unfortunately, most tonsillar carcinomas metastasize, initially to regional lymph nodes and then to distant sites.

Squamous cell carcinomas vary both in size and in gross appearance—from flat to proliferative (Fig. 7-14). These tumors are often quite aggressive locally, invading subjacent tissues. Some tumors contain more differentiated cells, keratin, often in whorls (keratin pearls) and visible desmosomes (intercellular bridges), whereas others are less well differentiated but with significant mitotic activity. In these latter cases, intracellular immunohistochemical markers for cytokeratin are useful in determining a definitive diagnosis. The amount of fibrous tissue within an individual tumor is variable. Some carcinomas induce a scirrhous response, whereas others have areas of necrosis caused by rapid tumor growth, "collision necrosis," of the tightly packed proliferating cells and loss of contiguity with the blood supply.

Ninety percent of melanomas of the oral cavities of dogs are malignant. A breed predilection exists for Scottish terriers, Airedales, cocker spaniels, golden retrievers, Bedlington terriers, Duroc pigs, and others. Most melanomas contain copious intracellular pigment and are visibly black. Some melanomas without pigment, termed *amelanotic melanomas,* present a greater diagnostic challenge to both the clinician and pathologist (Fig. 7-15). Immunohistochemical staining for tyrosinase-related proteins (TRP-1, TRP-2), Melan-A, and melanocytic antigen PNL2 are useful for immunohistochemically identifying amelanotic tumors. Melanomas are composed of melanocytes and are of neural crest origin. Cellular morphology within melanomas varies from spindloid to epithelioid. Thus some neoplasms are histologically difficult to differentiate from squamous cell carcinomas and others from fibrosarcomas.

Canine oral papillomatosis is a papovavirus-induced transmissible condition that usually occurs in animals younger than 1 year. The lesions usually regress spontaneously. Immunity is long lasting. The lesions are papilliform or cauliflower-like and can become quite numerous. They are generally white and friable and occur on the mouth, tongue, palate, larynx, and epiglottis. These oral tumors are usually multiple, white-to-gray, raised, and pedunculated with a keratinized surface and a stromal core. The epithelial cells comprising the lesion can be acanthotic, hyperplastic, and rest on a hyperplastic folded connective tissue stroma. The stratum spinosum is also hyperplastic and ballooned. Cytoplasmic inclusion bodies are sometimes present.

Oral extramedullary plasmacytomas may occur anywhere in the mucous membranes of the oral cavity, esophagus, or intestine. In the oral cavity, they are slow-growing neoplasms and in spite of often-recognized anisokaryosis, mitoses, and multinucleate cells, they rarely invade surrounding tissues and have not been reported to metastasize. Histologic examination is required for accurate diagnosis (see Fig. 13-33).

Fibrosarcomas arise from the collagen-producing cells (fibroblasts) of the oral cavity. Fibrosarcomas are most common in the cat, accounting for 20% of oral neoplasia in that species. They may occur anywhere in the oral cavity. In large breed dogs, histologically benign-appearing fibrosarcomas of the oral cavity invade bone and metastasize.

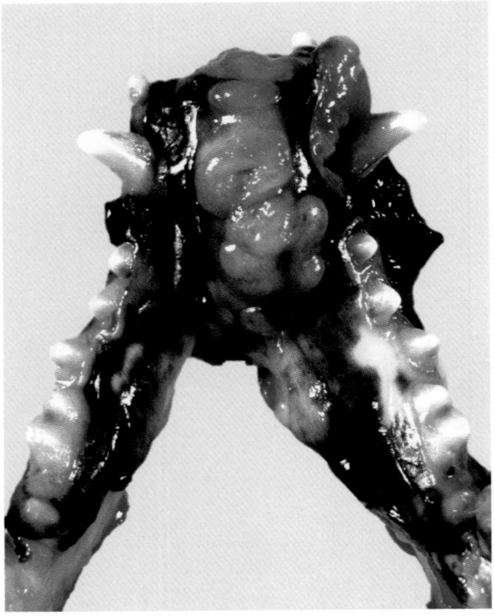

Fig. 7-15 Amelanotic melanoma, mandibular symphysis, dog.
A proliferative, ulcerated, nonpigmented mass is present on the oral mucosa at the mandibular symphysis and protrudes into the oral cavity, likely resulting in malocclusion. Incisor teeth have been lost. Note the absence of pigmentation (melanin) in this tumor. (Courtesy Dr. M.D. McGavin, College of Veterinary Medicine, University of Tennessee.)

TEETH*

Teeth provide mechanical advantage for prehension, tearing and/or mastication of food. Among domestic animals, there are differences in the growth pattern and numbers of teeth. Hypsodont teeth, such as in the horse, continue to grow throughout life, and appropriate leveling of the occlusive surfaces (floating) may be a necessary procedure to prevent malocclusion and sharp edges that can lacerate the adjacent buccal mucosa as the horse ages. Brachydont teeth, such as in carnivores, do not continue to grow after they are fully erupted. Most species of mammals have deciduous teeth that are replaced near maturity by permanent teeth. In many species, the approximate age of the animal may be determined by eruption date and examination of wear patterns and shape of the teeth.

Structure and Function

Molar teeth in general are designed for grinding feedstuffs, whereas incisors in ruminants (mandibular only) are for cropping forage. Canine teeth are designed for tearing flesh. Brachydont teeth consist of a crown, which is the portion above the gingiva (the neck that is slightly constricted), and just below the gingiva are the roots, which are embedded in the bony socket (alveolus) of the jaw. Enamel covers the crown, cementum covers the roots, and both cover the dentin. Besides carnivores, the incisor (lower) teeth of ruminants and porcine teeth, except the canines of the boar, are brachydontic.

Hypsodont teeth have an elongated body, but the neck and roots may form later in life. Cementum covers the tooth, and enamel is beneath the cementum. Beneath the enamel is the dentin. The cementum and enamel invaginate into the dentin, forming the infundibula. Enamel crests result from normal wear, with enamel being the hardest of the layers. The cheek teeth of ruminants and tusks of boars and the teeth of horses are hypsodont.

In simple-toothed animals, such as carnivores, the tooth root is not covered by enamel. Receding gum lines therefore expose the dentin, resulting in pain and invasion by bacteria. Domestic animal species seldom get caries, although buildup of plaque can result in gingival infections and tooth loss.

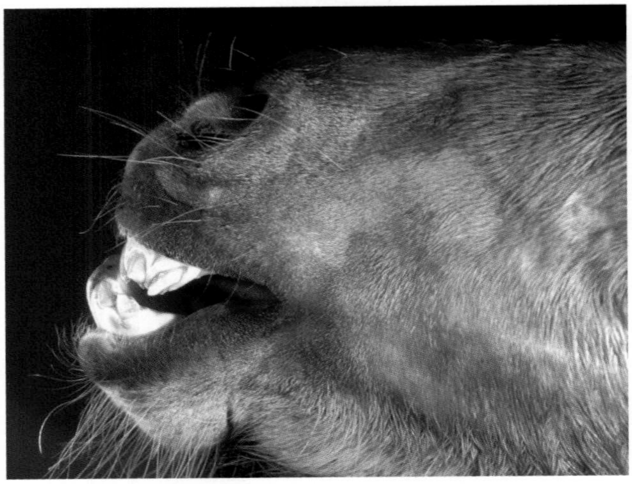

Fig. 7-16 Prognathia, head, horse.
The mandible is elongated compared with the maxilla. (Courtesy Dr. H. Gelberg, College of Veterinary Medicine, Oregon State University.)

Malocclusions

Abnormal development and positioning of the teeth may affect dental function. Malocclusion refers to a failure of the upper and lower incisors to oppose properly. This feature is "normal" for some dogs, particularly the brachycephalic breeds. In the extreme, malocclusions can lead to difficulty in the prehension and mastication of food. Malocclusions are named according to the position of the mandible. Protrusion of the lower jaw is termed *prognathia,* whereas a short lower jaw with resultant protrusion of the upper jaw is termed *brachygnathia* and sometimes *hypognathia* (Fig. 7-16). Sometimes these terms are incorrectly used, referring to brachygnathia as superior prognathia and prognathia as superior brachygnathia.

Malocclusions result from abnormal jaw conformation or rarely from abnormal tooth eruption patterns. In some animals, such as rodents and rabbits, the teeth continue to grow throughout the animal's lifetime. If these animals are not provided with sufficient roughage in their diets, the teeth (both incisors and cheek teeth) overgrow and either "lock" the jaw or because of a lack of occlusal grinding surfaces, prevent the animal from receiving proper nutrition (Web Fig. 7-3).

Anomalies of Tooth Development

In simple-toothed animals and rarely in other animals, agenesis of a tooth or teeth occurs and is generally of no clinical significance (see Fig. 17-35). Supernumerary tooth development is less common than tooth agenesis and is similarly of little clinical significance. Some animals, such as elasmobranches (sharks), continue to produce row on row of teeth as the outermost rows are lost.

*Dr. Richard Dubielzeg of the School of Veterinary Medicine, University of Wisconsin–Madison authored previous contributions to this section.

Dental dysgenesis may be primarily due to dysplasia of the enamel-forming organ or secondary to trauma, infection and hyperthermia, toxicosis, or other metabolic irregularities during odontogenesis.

Dentigerous cysts result from dental dysgenesis, and epithelial-lined, cystic structures in tissue, including the bone of the jaw result. Dentigerous cysts develop from abnormal proliferation of the cell rests of Malassez. They appear as variably sized, sometimes fluctuant swellings of the mandible or maxilla. In the maxilla, they sometimes invade the nasal sinuses. Although rare, dentigerous cysts are often painful, and while not usually neoplastic, they can destroy the jaw. Dentigerous cysts are epithelial-lined and may become impacted with keratin. Rudimentary, malformed teeth may be found within these cysts, and painful fistulas may develop, especially in horses. These draining tracts are seen most often rostral and ventral to the ear (ear tooth). Dentigerous cysts occur less frequently in otherwise normal, mature animals.

Segmental enamel hypoplasia occurs before eruption of the permanent teeth of dogs as a result of hyperthermia and viral infection, most often by canine distemper virus infection. Enamel is fully formed when the teeth erupt; therefore virus infection of ameloblasts must occur during enamel formation, which is before the dog is 6 months of age, if enamel hypoplasia is to occur. Canine distemper virus infection causes necrosis and disorganization of the enamel organ. After the virus is cleared, structure and function of the enamel organ return to normal. Thus segmental enamel hypoplasia results from the lack of enamel formation during the period of virus infection (Fig. 7-17). A similar condition in calves is caused by in utero BVD virus infection.

Chemicals, most notably tetracycline antibiotics ingested during the process of mineralization, can cause yellowish, permanent discoloration (see Fig. 1-58). Congenital porphyria, a defect in red blood cell production, may result in incorporation of porphyrins into dentin, resulting in pink discoloration of the teeth (pink tooth) (Web Fig. 7-4). Both tetracycline and porphyrins fluoresce under ultraviolet light, dramatically demonstrating these lesions.

Fluoride incorporation into the enamel and dentin occurs in fluoride toxicosis, particularly in cattle and sheep. A relationship exists in beef cattle between fluorosis and selenium supplementation, with selenium supplementation being protective in high fluoride areas such as those downwind from aluminum smelters or with high levels of fluoride in ground water. Excessive dietary concentrations of fluorine during odontogenesis (from 6 to 36 months of age) may result in incorporation of the fluoride in the enamel and dentin of the permanent teeth. The result is soft, chalky, discolored enamel, usually yellow, dark brown, or black (Web Fig. 7-5). Occlusal grinding of affected soft teeth against more normal enamel results in rapid dental wear to the extent that severely affected sheep may have almost completely worn down their incisors. One wonders therefore about the cumulative effect of fluoride supplementation in municipal drinking water, vitamins with added fluoride, fluoride-supplemented toothpaste, fluoride treatment of teeth, reconstituted and bottled soft drinks made with fluoridated water, and so forth. It is difficult to calculate the total fluoride load ingested by individuals or what the effects may be of that fluoride supplementation.

Lesions Caused by Attrition and Abnormal Wear

Loss of normal dental structure and function often results from rapid and irregular and/or abnormal wear of occlusal surfaces in many species of domestic animals. In those species with hypsodont teeth, attention to the dentition as the animal ages is often a major factor in overall body conditioning and health (Fig. 7-18). Aggressive treatment of occlusal surface irregularity by filing of high points in the dental arcade (floating) can notably prolong an animal's life. Rock chewing or other compulsive oral behaviors in dogs may result in accelerated dental wear. Similarly, cribbing in horses and herbivorous animals grazing on sandy soils can cause premature dental wear. In all species, exposure of dentin or the pulp canal may lead to dental infection with serious consequences.

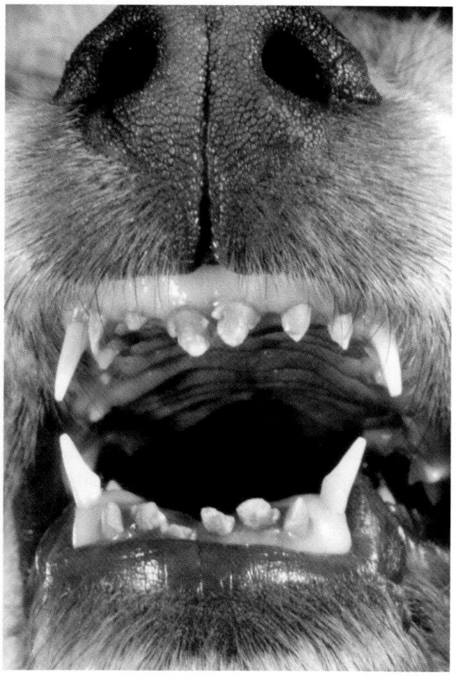

Fig. 7-17 Enamel hypoplasia, permanent incisor teeth, dog. There is a lack of enamel formation with resultant discrete deep pits and exposure of the dentin (light yellow to beige areas of the teeth), the result of infection with canine distemper virus and necrosis of the ameloblasts during enamel formation. Permanent adult teeth (shown in illustration) are infected with virus before their eruption and while they are still within their sockets (dental alveoli). (Courtesy Dr. H. Gelberg, College of Veterinary Medicine, Oregon State University.)

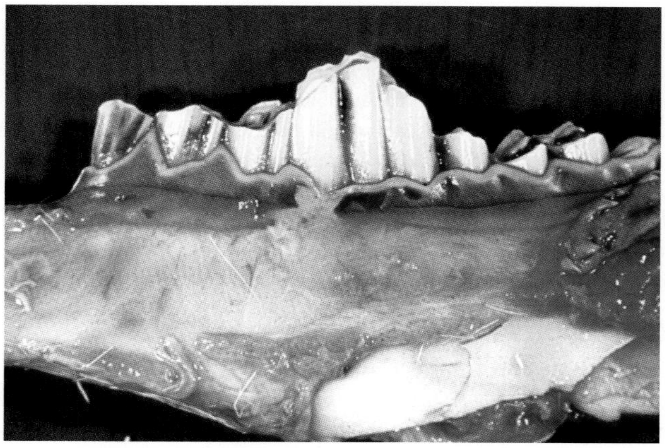

Fig. 7-18 Dental attrition, molar teeth, antelope. Age-associated dental wear results in improper mastication of feedstuffs and malnutrition. This condition occurs most commonly in horses and is referred to as "step-mouth" or "broken mouth." (Courtesy College of Veterinary Medicine, University of Tennessee.)

Miscellaneous Dental Lesions

Feline External Resorptive Neck Lesions

Cats suffering from feline external resorptive neck lesions often have pain upon chewing that may be reflected by inappetence and/or abnormal masticatory movements. External neck resorption of the cheek teeth of otherwise dentally normal cats is caused by odontoclastic resorption of cementum, particularly in the neck area or root of the tooth. Osteoclast ingrowths partially or completely line the resorption cavity. The resultant cavity may harbor bacterial plaque, resulting in intense inflammation and further osteoclastic resorption of dental tissue, including dentin and the root canal. The primary cause of this condition is not known.

Infundibular Impaction

Impaction of the infundibulum, also known as *infundibular necrosis* or *infundibular caries,* may cause serious dental disease in ruminants and more rarely in horses. Incomplete infundibular cementum formation before the tooth erupts likely predisposes to infundibular impaction. The pathogenic mechanism is comparable to dental caries in simple-toothed animals, which is uncommon in domestic animals. Feed material is ground into the infundibulum, where bacteria metabolize it to form acid, which causes demineralization. Bacterial enzymes digest the organic matrix of enamel and dentin. As a result of this destruction, the pulp cavity becomes exposed and infected, resulting in pulpitis and endodontitis. Dental abscesses and fistulous tracks may develop and rupture into the paranasal sinuses. The inflamed infundibular cavities often continue to become impacted with feed, creating a vicious cycle.

Periodontal Disease

More than 200 species of bacteria and fungi have been associated with dental plaque (a film of an organic matrix, food particles, and bacteria on the tooth surface). This plaque often becomes mineralized (tartar or dental calculus). The mineralized material contributes to atrophy and inflammation of the gingival mucosa and supporting stroma by acting as a nidus for additional plaque accumulation. Bacteria resident in films on the tooth surface produce acids and enzymes that may damage their enamel substrate (cavities) and also destroy the subjacent gingival tissue and periodontal ligament (periodontal disease).

The initial site for destructive inflammation is in the gingival crevice–forming pockets where bacteria lodge. With time, this inflammation spreads distally along the tooth, resulting in gingival-epithelial attachment only on the root of the tooth, deep in the alveolar socket. Progression of inflammation may destroy the connective tissue of the periodontal ligament, resulting in loosening of the tooth. The infection can spread causing alveolar osteomyelitis and pulpitis and can result in apical abscesses and bacteremia. There is significant oral pain, reluctance to masticate, and halitosis. Periodontal disease is common in carnivores and humans. Mildly abrasive diets and brushing of the teeth of pet carnivores, combined with regular dental examination, is preventive as it is in humans.

Dental Neoplasia

Proliferative, cystic, or neoplastic diseases of the dental arcade can originate from cell rests that form from the dental lamina or the enamel organ (the cell rests of Malassez). Dental neoplasms usually arise close to the teeth, either deeply in the jaw or from the oral epithelium. There is a relatively precise method of naming dental neoplasms based on the tissue or cell of origin and the extent of differentiation and odontogenesis present within the neoplastic tissue. The histologic appearance of these neoplasms is complex; pathologists with considerable experience in differentiating these uncommon neoplasms should be consulted when a precise diagnosis is indicated.

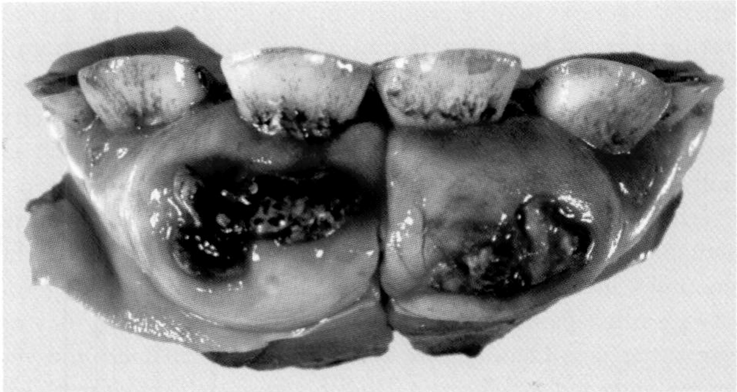

Fig. 7-19 Odontoma, incisor teeth, cow.
This is a hamartoma (a benign tumorlike nodule) of the enamel organ that in this case has expanded bilaterally on the rostral mandibles. There is extensive hemorrhagic ulceration over the tumor. Diagnosis can be confirmed by radiographic and histopathologic examination. (Courtesy Dr. M.D. McGavin, College of Veterinary Medicine, University of Tennessee.)

Odontomas are hamartomas originating in the enamel organ and are usually seen in puppies and foals (Fig. 7-19). They usually contain well-recognizable dentin and enamel, as well as ameloblasts, odontoblasts, and dental pulp.

Ameloblastoma is a term applied to epithelial neoplasms of enamel organ origin. Several subtypes, distinguished histologically, are ameloblastic fibroma, ameloblastic odontoma, calcifying epithelial odontogenic tumor, peripheral odontogenic fibroma, and other rare tooth neoplasms. Ameloblastoma appears randomly in the dental arcade, usually in adult dogs. They are often osteolytic and thus are locally invasive. Histologic examination by an expert is often necessary to distinguish ameloblastoma from acanthomatous epulis (acanthomatous ameloblastoma) and squamous cell carcinoma.

TONSILS

Structure and Function

The palatine tonsils are pharyngeal lymphoid structures covered by stratified squamous epithelium. Their function is uncertain, although it is likely they serve in lymphocyte production and antibody formation (see Chapter 13). In carnivores, they are found in crypts or recesses at the dorsolateral aspect of the caudal oropharynx. In pigs, they are flat and recognized by tiny pores in the surface epithelium of the caudal soft palate. Equids, ruminants, and pigs have lingual tonsils in addition to palatine tonsils.

Portals of Entry

Tonsils do not possess afferent lymphatic vessels and do not serve as lymph filters. Therefore only primary (or direct) or hematogenous infections occur (tonsillitis) (Fig. 7-20), as well as primary neoplasms of either the lymphoid (lymphoma) (Fig. 7-21) or epithelial (squamous cell carcinoma) (Fig. 7-22) components. In many viremias of mammals, such as pseudorabies of pigs, virus may be isolated from the tonsils.

SALIVARY GLANDS

Salivary glands are found in a variety of locations in the head and neck regions and vary in number and location from species to species. They arise from oral ectoderm. In all species, the major

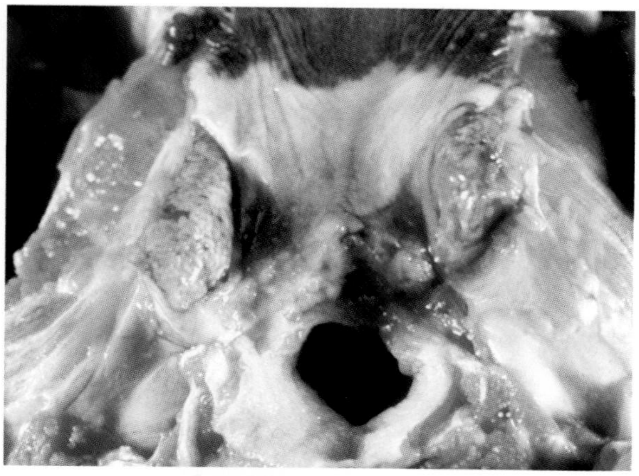

Fig. 7-20 Necrotizing tonsillitis, tonsils, dog.
The palatine tonsils are enlarged and discolored. The right tonsil is covered by a diphtheritic membrane, and the left tonsil is extensively ulcerated. Because there are no afferent lymphatics to the tonsils, infection is either primary (by direct spread) or hematogenous. (Courtesy Dr. M.D. McGavin, College of Veterinary Medicine, University of Tennessee.)

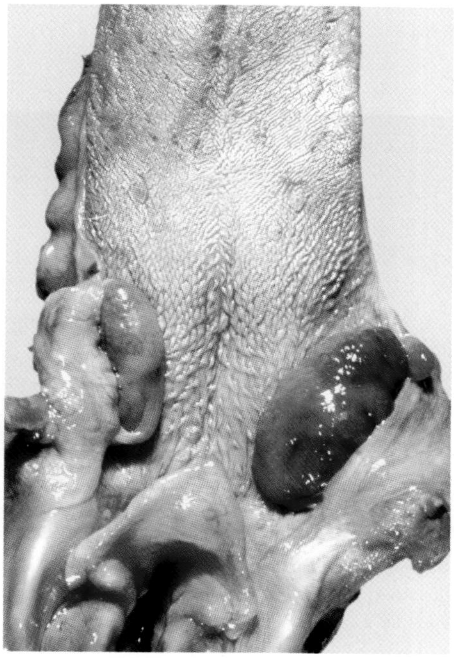

Fig. 7-21 Lymphoma (lymphosarcoma), tonsil, dog.
Proliferation of malignant lymphocytes has expanded the tonsils so that they now protrude beyond their crypts. (Courtesy Dr. M.D. McGavin, College of Veterinary Medicine, University of Tennessee.)

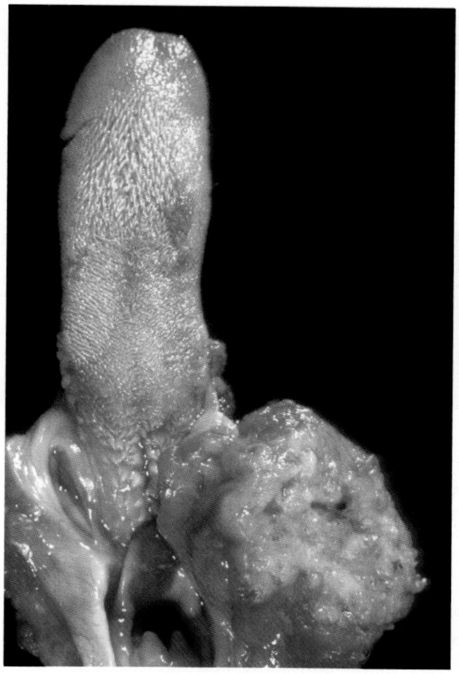

Fig. 7-22 Squamous cell carcinoma, tonsil, cat.
The right tonsil has been replaced by a large expansile neoplasm. The left tonsil is normal and remains in its crypt. (Courtesy Dr. R. Storts, College of Veterinary Medicine, Texas A&M University.)

salivary glands include the parotid, mandibular, and sublingual. Carnivores have a zygomatic gland as well. Minor salivary glands include buccal, labial, lingual, palatine, and others similarly named by location.

Structure and Function

Most salivary glands are discrete aggregates of compound tubuloalveolar tissue. Saliva is a mixture of serous and mucoid secretions. Saliva lubricates the mouth and esophagus and moistens ingesta. Saliva also dissolves water-soluble components of food so the taste buds can function. The mucus in saliva binds to masticated food and creates a bolus that is more easily swallowed. Salivary mucus also coats the epithelium of the mouth, preventing mechanical damage to the tissue. Saliva, through its flushing action, reduces bacterial populations. Saliva contains a lysozyme that lyses bacteria. Carbohydrate digestion begins in the oral cavity as a result of the presence of α-amylase, which changes starch into maltose. There are very small quantities of this enzyme in carnivores and cattle. Saliva also is an effective buffer, especially in ruminants, whose forestomachs have no glands. In carnivores, evaporation of saliva is a major mechanism of thermoregulation.

Portal of Entry

Salivary glands are generally affected by blood-borne pathogens, direct penetration by foreign objects, obstruction of the excretory ducts, or bite wounds. In humans, ascending infections from the salivary ducts occur, but there is no evidence that this occurs in domestic animals. The serous portions of the salivary glands are radiosensitive.

Response to Injury

Injury to the salivary gland is accompanied by incomplete regeneration, principally from ductular epithelium. There are often atrophy, fibrosis, and squamous metaplasia of secretory epithelium, sometimes resulting in blockage of ducts.

Inflammatory Diseases

Sialoadenitis, inflammation of a salivary gland, is relatively rare in veterinary medicine. Although diagnosis of systemic diseases is not made by examining the salivary gland, rabies and canine distemper are two very important diseases that cause inflammation of the salivary glands. Saliva is a particularly important medium of spread, by bite wounds, of the rhabdovirus that causes rabies. There are focal necrosis, mononuclear cell inflammation, and sometimes inclusions

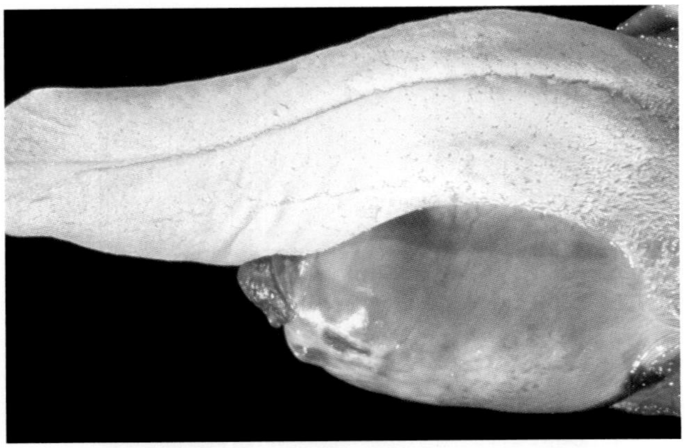

Fig. 7-23 **Ranula, mandibular salivary duct, dog.**
This is a cystic distention of the left mandibular salivary duct along the ventral-lateral aspect of the tongue. (Courtesy Dr. P. Stromberg, College of Veterinary Medicine, The Ohio State University.)

(Negri bodies) in the nuclei of ganglion cells. In the rat, a coronavirus termed *sialodacryoadenitis virus* is responsible for inflammation of the salivary gland and some adnexal ocular glands. *Salmonella typhisuis* has caused suppurative parotid sialoadenitis in pigs.

Gross lesions of sialoadenitis are subtle and include swelling and edema. Sialoadenitis can be accompanied by pain on palpation. Abscesses occasionally occur sometimes secondary to the migration of foreign bodies (grass awns) and are especially noticeable when they occur in the retrobulbar zygomatic gland where they may cause ocular protrusion (proptosis).

Miscellaneous Diseases or Conditions

Changes in the salivary glands are uncommon in domestic animal species. A ranula is a cystic saliva-filled distention of the duct of the sublingual or submaxillary salivary gland that occurs on the floor of the mouth alongside the tongue (Fig. 7-23). It is thus epithelial lined. The cause is generally unknown, although some cases are due to sialoliths. A salivary mucocele, in contrast, is a pseudocyst not lined by epithelium but filled with saliva. The cause of this lesion is also unknown, but it may occur secondary to traumatic rupture of the duct of a sublingual salivary gland with resultant leakage and encapsulation of saliva by reactive connective tissue.

Sialoliths are rare in domestic animal species. When they do occur, they are considered to be caused by inflammation of the salivary gland with sloughed cells or inflammatory exudate forming a nidus for mineral accretion (Fig. 7-24). Thus they are one cause of ranula formation.

Neoplasia

Salivary gland neoplasms, both benign and malignant, are uncommon but occur in all species (Fig. 7-25). They are composed of glandular or ductular elements or a combination of epithelial and mesenchymal components similar to those in mixed mammary neoplasms. A grossly appearing similar condition, salivary gland infarction, occurs infrequently in cats and rarely in dogs. The cause of the infarction is unknown. The gross appearance of firmness and swelling of an infarcted gland must be distinguished microscopically from neoplasia (Web Fig. 7-6). In salivary gland infarction, there are discrete foci of parenchymal necrosis with peripheral hemorrhage and inflammatory cells. Attempted incomplete regeneration of the gland from ductal epithelium can be mistaken for neoplasia unless one is familiar with the former condition.

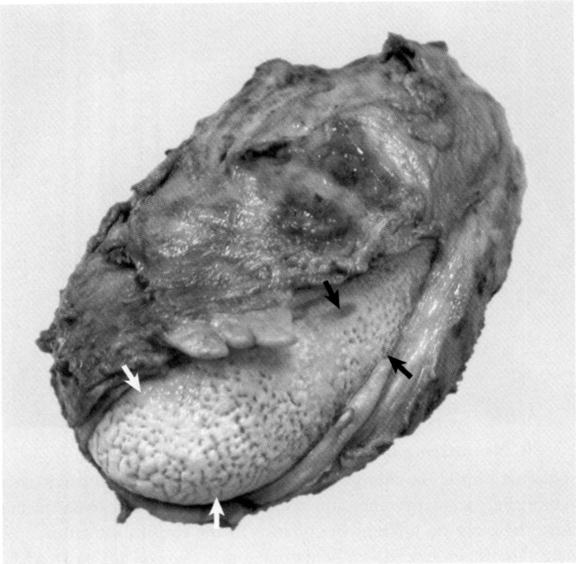

Fig. 7-24 **Sialolith, horse.**
Pressure necrosis from this large stonelike mass *(arrows)* has destroyed the gland in which it formed. (Courtesy Dr. B. Cooper, College of Veterinary Medicine, Oregon State University.)

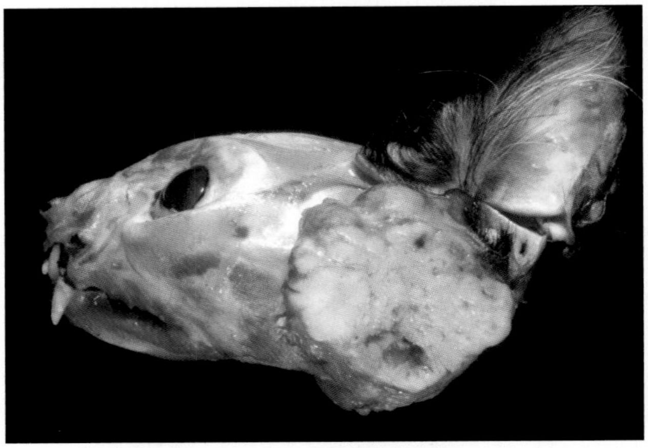

Fig. 7-25 **Salivary gland carcinoma, left parotid salivary gland, cat.**
A large proliferative carcinoma of the salivary gland has replaced the normal gland. (Courtesy Dr. H. Gelberg, College of Veterinary Medicine, Oregon State University.)

TONGUE

The tongue is a muscular organ covered by stratified epithelium and is functionally connected to the esophagus via the epiglottis.

Structure and Function

The tongue is necessary for prehension, mastication, and swallowing of feedstuffs and water. The epithelial covering of the tongue is stratified squamous with various degrees of keratinization dorsally, but ventrally the epithelium is not keratinized and the tongue attaches to the floor of the oral cavity by a frenulum. Keratinized papillae are most prominent in ruminants and cats. There are various types of papillae, some with secondary lamellae. Vallate papillae, for example, are on the dorsal surface of the tongue near its root and are flat structures completely surrounded by a cleft.

Some surface macroscopic papillae contain taste buds. The tongue is a highly vascular (functioning in heat loss in many animals, especially carnivores that have no sweat glands) and sensitive organ containing a variety of serous and mucus glands and sensory cells (taste buds). The muscular part of the tongue is striated in randomly arranged bundles. A cordlike structure enclosed in dense collagen extending lengthwise near the ventral central surface of the tongue of carnivores is called the *lyssa.* Porcine and equine tongues have a similar structure. The lyssa appears to be a structure without a function. Historically, the lyssa was removed as "prevention" for rabies. Lyssa bodies are synonymous with Negri bodies, and rabies used to be called lyssa. Adipose tissue becomes more abundant in the caudal part of the tongue in most species.

Developmental Anomalies

Congenital diseases of the tongue include epithelial defects such as fissures, epitheliogenesis imperfecta, macroglossia and microglossia, bifid tongue, and hair growing from the tongue (choristoma) (Web Fig. 7-7). Lethal glossopharyngeal defect, or bird tongue of dogs, is characterized by a pointed tongue that cannot wrap around a nipple and create the negative pressure required for nursing and without intervention, starvation results. Ventral ankyloglossia, fusion of the tongue to the floor of the oral cavity, has been reported in related Anatolian shepherd dogs. The cause of these congenital lesions is not known, but they sometimes occur in association with other defects. As in the case of other congenital defects, ingestion of unknown teratogenic substances by the dam during gestation is an etiologic possibility, as is mutation of T-box genes.

Systemic Disease: Primary Involvement of the Tongue

Disease agents that principally target the tongue are relatively rare. The exception to this rule is *Actinobacillus lignieresii,* a gram-negative bacillus that is a normal inhabitant of the oral cavity. It is an opportunistic invader of damaged lingual tissue, principally in bovids and occasionally in equids and small ruminants. The granulomas resulting from infection contain centrally located actinobacilli rimmed by radiating amorphic, eosinophilic, and clublike structures composed of immunoglobulin molecules from lesion plasmacytes (Fig. 7-26). Mixed mononuclear inflammatory cells, including multinucleated Langhans' giant cells, often surround these foci (Splendore-Hoeppli phenomenon), and infection may drain and cause similar inflammation in submaxillary and retropharyngeal lymph nodes. The amount of fibrous tissue present depends on the duration of the inflammation and the swelling. Inflammation and fibrosis cause increased firmness of the tongue and linguamegaly, or "wooden tongue" (Fig. 7-27). Horses are rarely affected by *Actinobacillus lignieresii* infections, but when they are, lesions are cutaneous or lymph node abscesses, mastitis, and occasional glossitis.

Systemic Disease: Secondary Involvement of the Tongue

Thrush is a *Candida albicans* (yeast) infection of intact mucous membranes of the tongue and esophagus (Fig. 7-28). It occurs principally in ungulates but has also been seen in carnivores. Thrush is not a primary disease but often indicates an underlying debility, particularly in young animals. It occurs as a result of antibiotic treatment that kills normal flora, increased serum glucose concentrations as a result of diabetes mellitus, a high-sugar diet, or intravenous glucose therapy. The availability of iron is a limiting factor for the indigenous bacteria, which compete with yeast for mucosal colonization. Immunodeficiency states also contribute to the development of thrush. All of these scenarios provide tissue conditions suitable for the proliferation of yeast forms. Rarely,

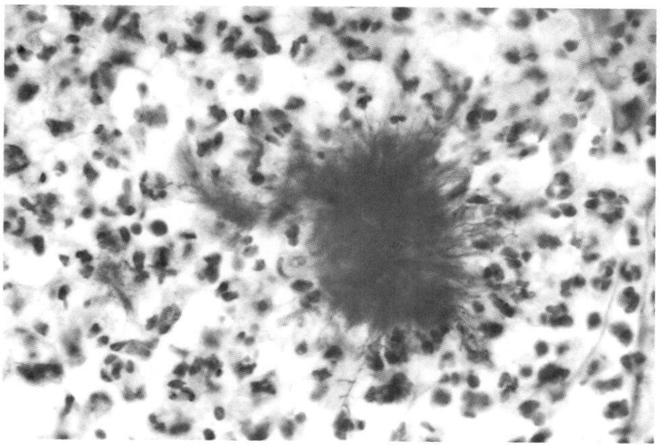

Fig. 7-26 Actinobacillosis (wooden tongue), tongue, cow.
Splendore-Hoeppli reaction (colony of bacteria with surrounding radiating "clubs" of immunoglobulin) is surrounded by suppurative inflammation. H&E stain. (Courtesy Dr. M.D. McGavin, College of Veterinary Medicine, University of Tennessee.)

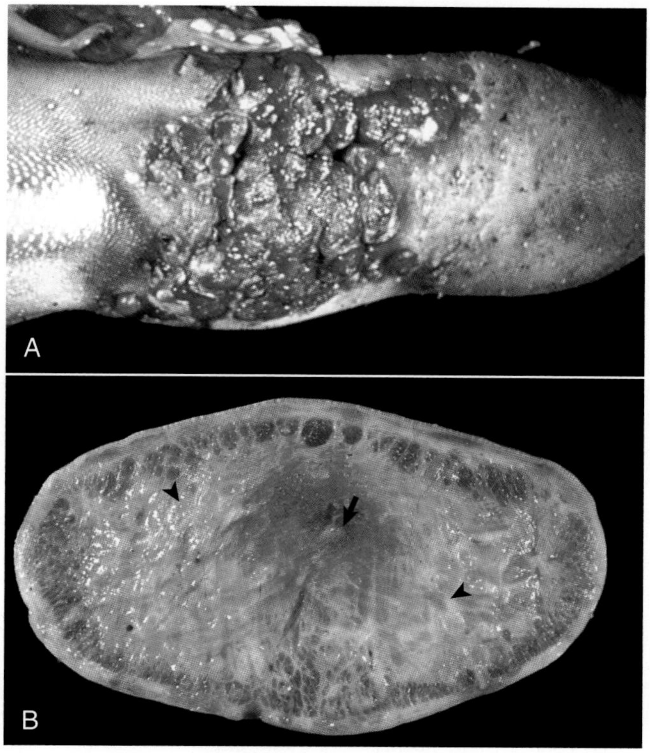

Fig. 7-27 Actinobacillosis, tongue, cow.
A, Dorsal surface. Proliferative and ulcerative chronic-active inflammatory lesions containing neutrophils mixed with mononuclear inflammatory cells (lymphocytes, macrophages, plasma cells) and fibrous tissue are present in the tongue. **B,** Chronic actinobacillosis (wooden tongue). Chronic inflammation results in loss of muscle of the tongue and its replacement by fibrous tissue during healing. Note the white interwoven bands of fibrous connective tissue *(arrowheads)* and the focus of granulomatous inflammation *(arrow).* (**A** courtesy Dr. M.D. McGavin, College of Veterinary Medicine, University of Tennessee. **B** courtesy Dr. R.J. Panciera, School of Veterinary Medicine, Oklahoma State University; and Noah's Arkive, College of Veterinary Medicine, The University of Georgia.)

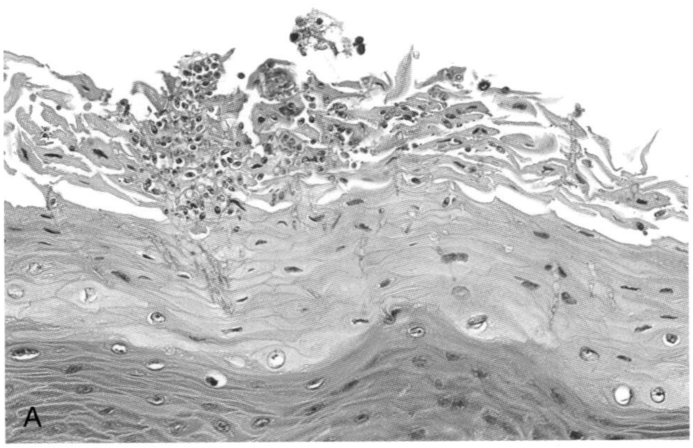

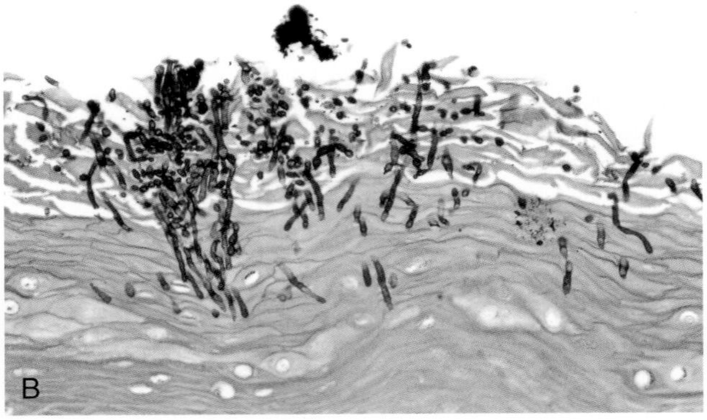

Fig. 7-28 Thrush (oral candidiasis), tongue, foal.
A, Hyphae of *Candida albicans* are growing in the superficial keratin of the tongue. H&E stain. **B,** Same specimen as **A.** Gomori's methenamine silver stain. (Courtesy Dr. J.F. Zachary, College of Veterinary Medicine, University of Illinois.)

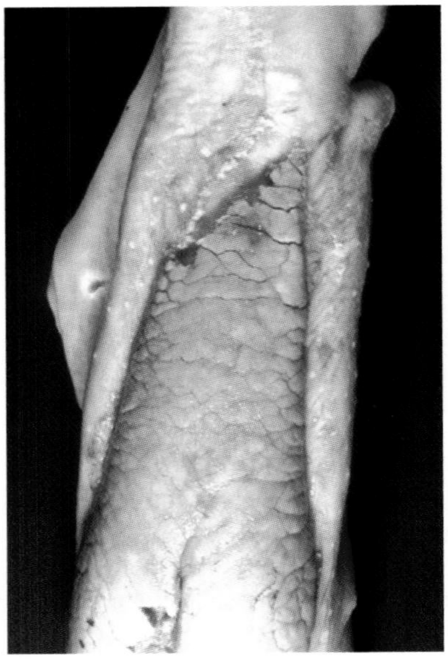

Fig. 7-29 Thrush, tongue, foal.
A pseudomembrane of hyphae of candida is present on the dorsal surface. It has been scraped off the rostral end of the tongue *(top)* to reveal normal mucosa beneath the fungal mat. (Courtesy Dr. H. Gelberg, College of Veterinary Medicine, Oregon State University.)

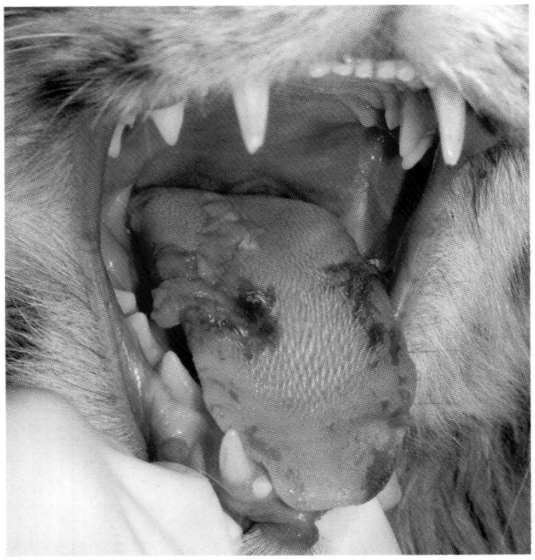

Fig. 7-30 Ulcerative glossitis, uremia (uremic glossitis), tongue, cat.
There is extensive ulceration of the mucosal epithelium of the tongue associated with increased concentrations of serum blood urea nitrogen and creatine from kidney failure. (Courtesy Drs. R.L. Fredrickson and R.A Doty, College of Veterinary Medicine, University of Illinois.)

systemic infection may result. Factors predisposing to systemic infections include multiple antibiotic usage, indwelling catheters, and endotracheal tubes. This infection presents as a gray-green pseudomembrane that is easily scraped off the intact underlying mucosal surface (Fig. 7-29).

Often, lingual lesions are manifestations of systemic diseases, such as BVD, foot-and-mouth disease, multisystemic amyloidosis, and uremia (Fig. 7-30; also see Fig. 11-27). These diseases are discussed in more detail in this and other chapters of this book.

Hyperplastic and Neoplastic Conditions

Epithelial hyperplasia of the lateral edges of the tongue is common in piglets before nursing, when the fringelike epithelium is rubbed off (Web Fig. 7-8).

Lingual (glossal) neoplasms are rare but when they occur are generally of epithelial origin. Squamous cell carcinomas are most common (Fig. 7-31; also see Fig. 6-10), but papillomas (Fig. 7-32), rhabdomyomas, rhabdomyosarcomas, fibrosarcomas, melanomas, and granular cell tumors have all been reported in domestic animals.

Parasites

Parasites of the tongue are uncommon, with the exception of those that reside in muscles such as *Sarcocystis* spp. in most species and *Trichinella spiralis* in pigs and occasionally in carnivorous wildlife such as polar bears. *Gongylonema* spp. can be present in the lingual mucosa of pigs and ruminants and are of no clinical significance.

ESOPHAGUS

Under normal circumstances, the esophageal lumen is a potential space. The wall collapses when the esophagus is not transporting ingesta.

Structure and Function

The esophagus extends from the aboral end of the oropharynx, passes through the mediastinum and the diaphragmatic hiatus, and ends at the stomach. The esophagus is lined by nonkeratinizing stratified squamous epithelium in carnivores and is keratinized in

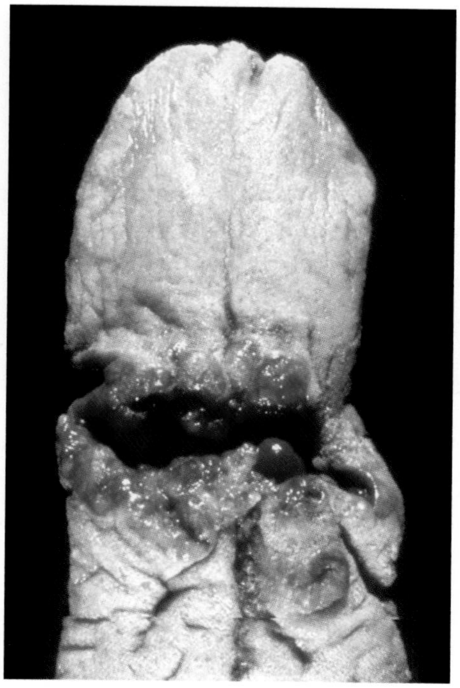

Fig. 7-31 Squamous cell carcinoma, tongue (dorsal surface), dog. Note the proliferative, ulcerated, and hemorrhagic neoplasm growing transversely across the surface of the tongue. (Courtesy Dr. H. Gelberg, College of Veterinary Medicine, Oregon State University.)

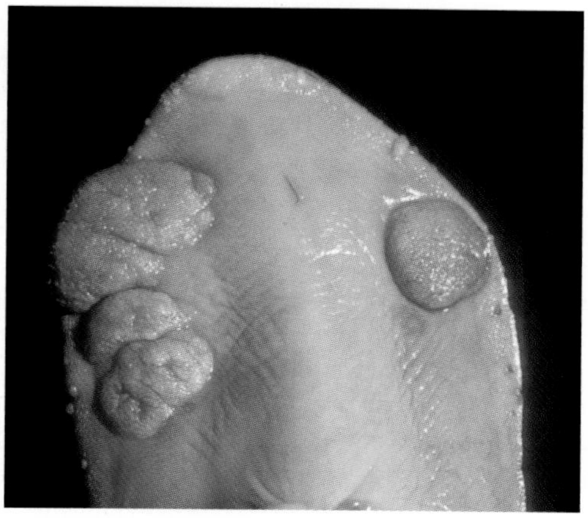

Fig. 7-32 Papillomas, tongue (ventral surface), cow. Papillomas, often caused by bovine papillomavirus, are present on the ventral surface of the tongue. The virus infects traumatized mucosal epithelial cells and induces epithelial cell proliferation. (Courtesy Dr. M.D. McGavin, College of Veterinary Medicine, University of Tennessee.)

pigs, horses, and ruminants. Keratinization is greatest in ruminants, less in horses, and least in pigs. Longitudinal and oblique mucosal folds are present to varying degrees. Transverse, herringbone-like folds are present in the cat.

The tunica muscularis is completely striated in ruminants and dogs. In the horse, the distal third of the esophagus contains smooth muscle. The pig is similar to the horse, except that the middle third of the esophagus contains a mixture of smooth and striated muscle. In cats, opossums, and primates, the distal two-thirds of the esophagus is composed of smooth muscle. The smooth muscle is arranged as an inner circular layer and an outer longitudinal layer.

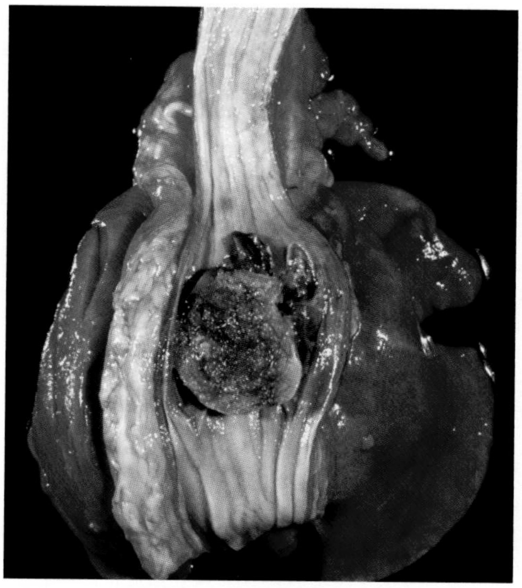

Fig. 7-33 Foreign body with necrosis, esophagus, dog. A ham bone lodged in this dog's esophagus dorsal to the base of the heart has caused esophageal dilation and pressure necrosis of the esophageal mucosa. (Courtesy Dr. C.S. Patton, College of Veterinary Medicine, University of Tennessee.)

Mixed mucinous glands are present in the tunica submucosa of pigs and dogs. In pigs, the glands are most abundant in the cranial half of the esophagus, and in dogs, they are present throughout. Glands are present in cats, horses, and ruminants only at the junction of the esophagus and pharynx.

It is important to remember that unlike the rest of the tubular digestive tract, the esophagus is unique in that it lacks a serosa in all but the abdominal portion. This means that there is no serosa to leak serum and fibrin to seal a puncture wound from a perforation of a foreign body or a surgical incision. Likewise, sutures are not likely to seal an incision. Combine this with the strong muscular peristaltic contractions that characterize this organ and it is easy to understand why esophageal surgery is not often performed and is even less often successful. For the same anatomic reasons, perforating foreign bodies of the esophagus do not seal themselves off.

Esophageal innervation is from the vagus nerves. Esophageal smooth muscle contains myenteric ganglia. Striated muscle is innervated by motor end-plates via efferent fibers of the hypoglossal nerve along with contributory neurofibers from cranial nerves 5, 9, and 10, which control voluntary lingual function.

Portals of Entry

Materials from the oral cavity pass via the esophagus to the stomach or rumen, including caustic chemicals. Penetration or obstruction by foreign objects is the most common portal of entry into the mediastinum (Fig. 7-33). Some parasites spend part or all of their life cycles in the esophagus. Iatrogenic puncture of the esophagus is a not uncommon sequela to passage of stomach tubes. Gastric reflux is an additional portal of entry into the esophagus.

Developmental Anomalies

Esophageal motility disorders are termed *achalasia*. In this condition, the sequential contractility of the esophagus is defective and the lower cricopharyngeal sphincter fails to function properly. Achalasia results in difficulty in swallowing and may be responsible for regurgitation and weight loss.

Cricopharyngeal achalasia is a congenital, possibly neurogenic, disorder of the upper esophageal (cricopharyngeal) sphincter. It occurs in young, small breed dogs, particularly terriers, cocker spaniels, and miniature poodles. Postweaning dysphagia and regurgitation after a meal of solid food is characteristic of this functional disorder. Liquids are generally swallowed without incidence. Gagging or choking behavior of the patient after swallowing is a good indicator in the appropriately aged dog of this condition.

Acquired canine achalasia is extremely uncommon. In this condition, there is often a visible abnormality of the musculature of deglutition (cricopharyngeus). There does not appear to be a characteristic change in the affected musculature. Esophageal myotomy of the appropriate cricopharyngeal sphincter muscle is palliative for these idiopathic conditions.

Megaesophagus

Megaesophagus or esophageal ectasia is dilation of the esophagus because of insufficient, absent, or uncoordinated peristalsis in the mid and cervical esophagus. It has been described in dogs, cats, cows, ferrets, horses, and new world camelids. Causes include innervation or denervation disorders and partial physical obstructions and stenosis, secondary to inflammatory diseases of esophageal musculature or persistence of the right aortic arch. Many cases are idiopathic.

Congenital megaesophagus is usually due to partial blockage of the lumen of the esophagus by a persistent right fourth aortic arch. Because of the persistence of the arch, a vascular ring forms around the esophagus and trachea, preventing full dilation of the esophagus. The ring is formed by the aorta, pulmonary artery, and ductus arteriosus. This form of megaesophagus is unique in that the esophageal obstruction, and thus dilation, occurs cranial to the heart because of the location of the obstructing vascular ring (Fig. 7-34; also see Fig. 10-64). Persistent right aortic arch is likely hereditary in German shepherds, Irish setters, and greyhounds. All other forms of megaesophagus result in dilation cranial to the stomach.

Congenital megaesophagus also occurs as an idiopathic denervation of the esophagus, most notably in great Danes, Irish setters, miniature schnauzers, Labrador retrievers, wire hair fox terriers, shar-peis, Newfoundlands, Siamese cats, and in some cases of vagal indigestion, in cattle. Some cases of myasthenia gravis (see later discussion) are congenital and may be of genetic origin.

Acquired megaesophagus (esophageal achalasia) is the result of failure of relaxation of the distal esophageal (cardiac) sphincter of the stomach. The obstruction and thus dilation occurs cranial to the stomach (Fig. 7-35). Although the gross appearance of acquired megaesophagus in animals is similar to that of humans, the cause of the condition in animals does not involve the cardiac sphincter. Causes are idiopathic or secondary to polymyositis (inflammation of the esophageal muscle), myasthenia gravis (a congenital or autoimmune disease directed against acetylcholine receptors of the neuromuscular junction), hypothyroidism (which can result in muscle atrophy and denervation disease), congenital myopathy, lead and thallium poisoning (via effect on innervation), peripheral neuropathies, vagal indigestion, esophagitis, and recurrent gastric dilation. Increased risk in dogs is seen in German shepherds, golden retrievers, and Irish setters.

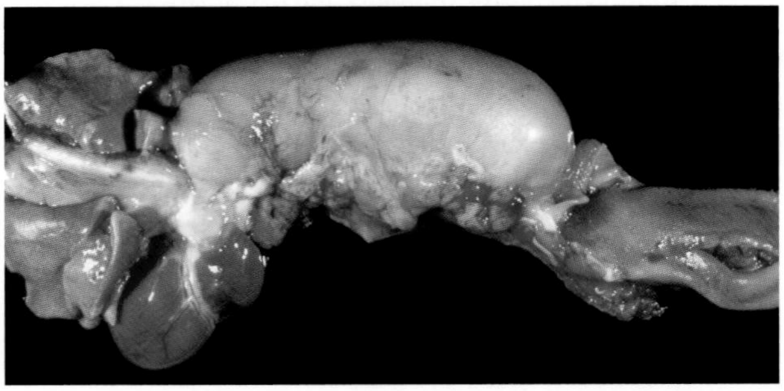

Fig. 7-34 Megaesophagus from a persistent right aortic arch, esophagus, dog.
Dilation of the esophagus cranial to the heart is the result of failure of the right fourth aortic arch to regress during embryonic life (vascular ring abnormality). (Courtesy Dr. C.S. Patton, College of Veterinary Medicine, University of Tennessee.)

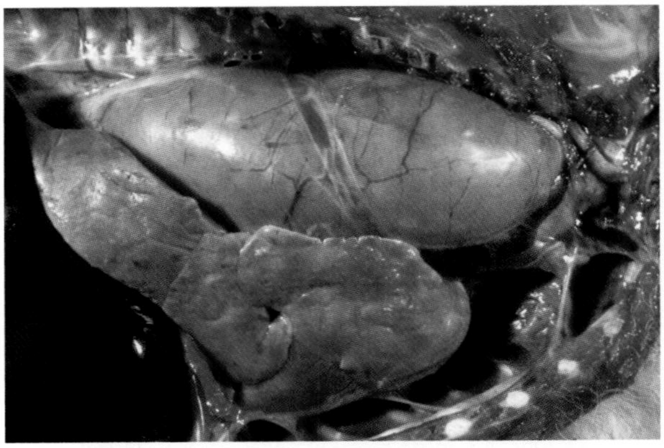

Fig. 7-35 Megaesophagus, thoracic esophagus, dog.
A notably dilated thoracic esophagus cranial to the diaphragm has displaced the right lung caudally and ventrally. This form of megaesophagus is often attributable to an abnormality (mass, foreign body, innervation disorder) affecting the cardiac sphincter. (Courtesy Dr. H. Gelberg, College of Veterinary Medicine, Oregon State University.)

Megaesophagus is recognized clinically by regurgitation after ingestion of solid food. Thus congenital megaesophagus is often recognized at weaning. Often, animals are thin and may have aspiration pneumonia. Radiographically, the esophagus is dilated anterior to the lesion and retains radiopaque dyes (Web Fig. 7-9). Dilation may vary from diffuse to locally extensive, depending on its cause. Putrid ingesta are sometimes found in the dilated, atonic portions of the esophagus. Although degenerate nerve fibers are occasionally found within vagus nerves, megaesophagus can occur without detectable histologic lesions.

Hiatal Hernia

Protrusion of the abdominal esophagus and cardia of the stomach through the diaphragm into the thoracic cavity is termed a *hiatal hernia.* This inversion is generally into the esophageal lumen and is self-reducing. Sometimes a gastroesophageal intussusception results.

Eosinophilic Esophagitis

Eosinophilic esophagitis is an emerging disease in humans; in a single dog, clinical signs include regurgitation, dysphagia, and cough, accompanying a diffusely affected, friable, hyperemic, ulcerated esophageal mucosa visible by endoscopy. Inflammation is dominated by granulocytes—half of which are eosinophils. Diagnosis is by elimination of other causes of inflammatory esophagitis. Seventy percent of humans and the single dog described had concurrent allergic skin disease.

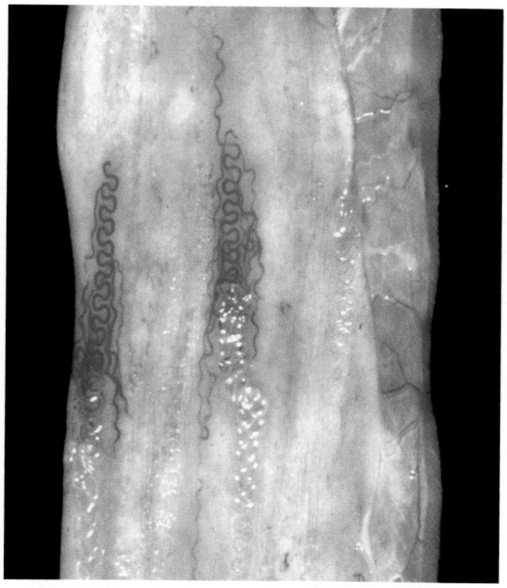

Fig. 7-36 Gongylonemiasis, esophagus, cow.
The serpentine intramucosal nematodes are characteristic of Gongylonema, a nematode of the superfamily Spiruroidea. (Courtesy Dr. M.D. McGavin, College of Veterinary Medicine, University of Tennessee.)

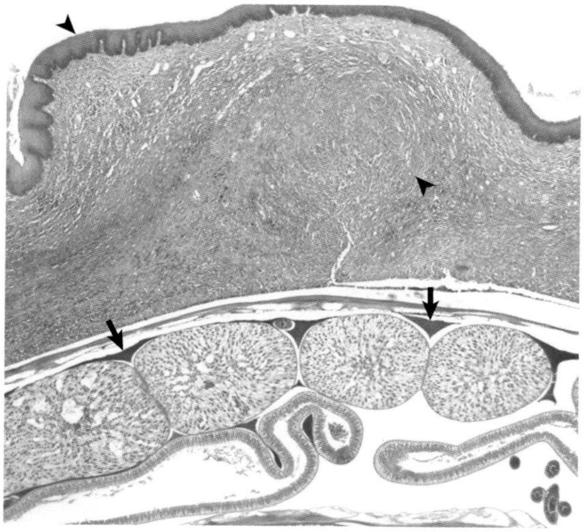

Fig. 7-37 Fibrosarcoma, esophagus, dog.
Spirocerca lupi (longitudinal section) *(arrows)* is present in the esophageal submucosa deep to the fibrosarcoma, which it has induced *(arrowheads)*. H&E stain. (Courtesy Dr. H. Gelberg, College of Veterinary Medicine, Oregon State University.)

Esophageal Parasites

With notable exceptions, parasitic diseases of the esophagus are generally of no clinical importance. The more common parasites of the esophagus are *Gongylonema* spp., which affect ruminants, pigs, horses, primates, and occasionally rodents. These nematodes reside in the esophageal mucosa and are characteristically thin, red, and serpentine. They can be 10 to 15 cm in length and are easily visible (Fig. 7-36). The intermediate hosts are cockroaches and dung beetles.

Gasterophilus spp. occur in equids. These fly larvae have interesting life cycles because their eggs are laid on the skin in varying locations. The warmth and moisture from licking activates them. The larvae burrow into the oral mucosa, molt, and then migrate down the esophagus. They occur both in the distal esophagus and stomach, where they attach to the mucosa via oral hooks. They eventually detach, leaving craters at the site of attachment, and pass in the feces.

Hypoderma lineatum is the larvae of the warble fly of ruminants. These parasites eventually migrate to the esophageal adventitia and then to the subcutaneous tissue of the back.

Spirocerca lupi of canids is probably the most pathogenic of the esophageal parasites. These nematodes reach the esophageal submucosa after migrating from the stomach. They penetrate through the gastric mucosa to reach the adventitia of arteries and then migrate in the adventitia to the abdominal aorta and aborally to the caudal aorta where they form a granuloma in the adventitia. From here they migrate to the adjacent esophageal submucosa. A passage forms between the esophageal lumen and the granuloma containing the parasite, allowing discharge of ova into the lumen of the alimentary system and eventually into the feces. Clinical sequelae of infestation include dysphagia, aortic aneurysms, hemothorax, and rarely esophageal fibrosarcomas or osteosarcomas (Fig. 7-37). Occasionally, chronic aortic granulomas will extend into the adjacent thoracic vertebral bodies of chronically affected canids to cause spondylosis deformans adjacent to the aortic granulomas. *Spirocerca lupi* infestations occur in warmer climates. The intermediate hosts are dung beetles, and the paratenic hosts are chickens, reptiles, and rodents.

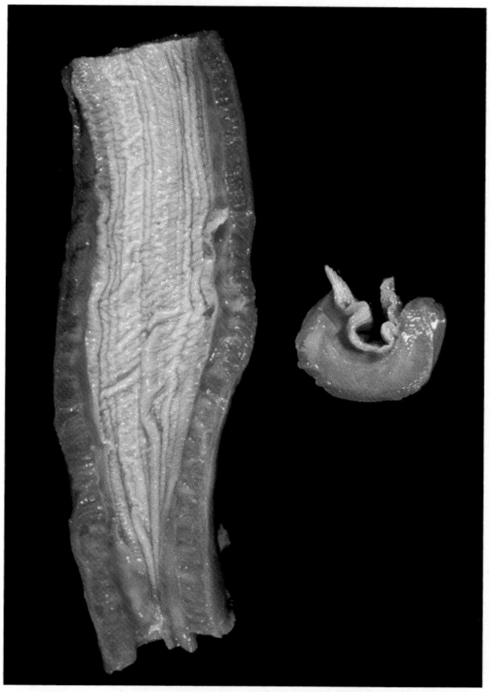

Fig. 7-38 Muscular hypertrophy, distal esophagus, horse.
Longitudinal *(left)* and transverse *(right)* sections of the esophagus demonstrate the marked increase in the thickness of the smooth muscle in the tunica muscularis of the distal esophagus. (Courtesy Dr. C.S. Patton, College of Veterinary Medicine, University of Tennessee.)

Miscellaneous Esophageal Lesions and Conditions

Idiopathic muscular hypertrophy of the distal esophagus is a lesion peculiar to horses and pigs that can be quite spectacular at necropsy (Fig. 7-38) but usually is of no clinical significance. The esophageal musculature can be several centimeters thick, and the lesion can extend along the distal quarter of the esophagus. Rarely this condition plays a role in esophageal impaction. Similarly, dilation of the esophageal glands present throughout the esophagus of aged dogs can be a spectacular gross lesion of no clinical consequence. It is therefore important to carefully evaluate these lesions either at necropsy or during fiberoptic viewing in the live animal to determine whether what appear to be erosions and ulcers are instead mucosal elevations caused by glands filled with mucus. Because the lesions are subepithelial, the overlying mucosa is smooth and shiny. Dilated esophageal glands vary in number and location but are generally only a few millimeters in diameter (Fig. 7-39). They are most numerous in the distal esophagus.

Esophageal erosions and ulcers are relatively common and have a variety of causes. One of the more common causes of esophageal erosions and ulcers is reflux of stomach acid. This reflux of gastric acids causes chemical burning of the distal or aboral esophagus and is commonly called *acid reflux esophagitis* (Fig. 7-40) or clinically, heartburn in humans. Other causes of esophageal ulcers include improper use of stomach tubes, which cause linear scraping on the crests of the longitudinal folds of the esophageal mucosa (Fig. 7-41), foreign bodies such as bones in dogs and infectious diseases, such as BVD (Fig. 7-42), which cause mucosal injury in other locations as well.

Leukoplakia of the esophagus and stomach is characterized by discrete, flat, white mucosal elevations (epithelial plaques) of no clinical significance and of unknown cause. They are sometimes mistaken for thrush lesions or neoplasia. Unlike thrush lesions, they do not scrape off easily, and their regularity, number, and location distinguish them from neoplasms. Histologically, the stratum basale and prickly cell layers are notably thickened, and the surface cells have pyknotic nuclei and some parakeratosis. In humans,

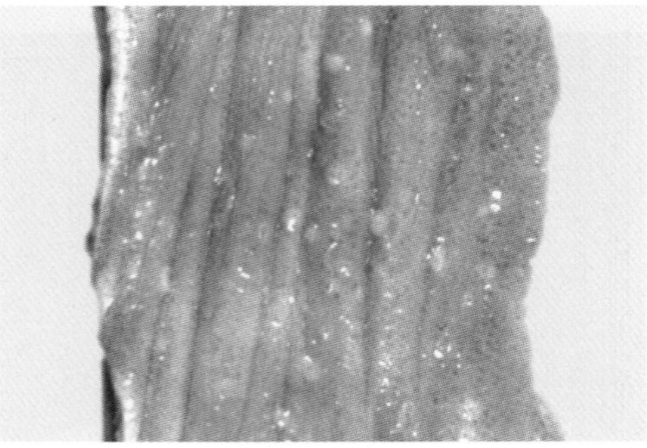

Fig. 7-39 Cystic esophageal glands, distal esophagus, dog.
Multiple white mucosal cysts are present in the esophageal glands of the mucosa and submucosa. These cysts are common and insignificant findings in aged dogs. (Courtesy Dr. H. Gelberg, College of Veterinary Medicine, Oregon State University.)

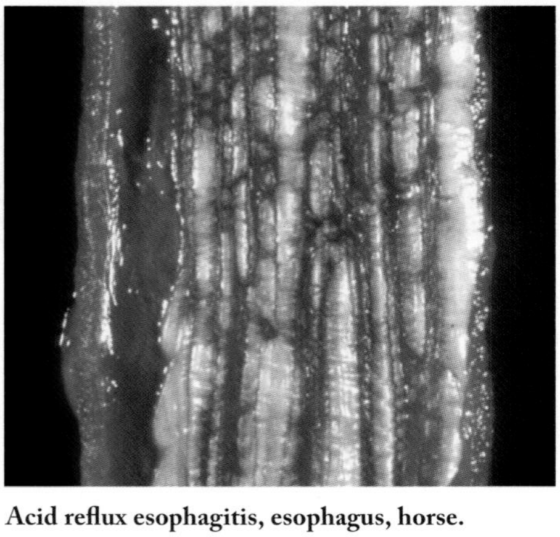

Fig. 7-40 Acid reflux esophagitis, esophagus, horse.
The dark red streaks on the surface of the esophagus are areas of epithelial loss secondary to gastric acid reflux. The white streaks and vertically linear areas on the surface of the esophagus are areas of unaffected and likely hyperplastic mucosal epithelium. As would be expected, erosions are most severe in the esophageal mucosa adjacent to the cardia and extend orad. This distribution is diagnostic of acid reflux esophagitis. (Courtesy Dr. H. Gelberg, College of Veterinary Medicine, Oregon State University.)

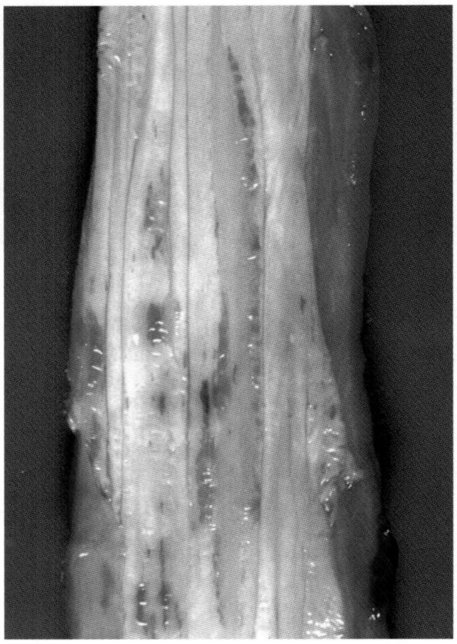

Fig. 7-41 Trauma-induced esophageal ulceration, esophagus, horse.
These red linear ulcers are the result of abrasion from improper stomach tubing, either from an overly large diameter tube, from a too-vigorous insertion, or from a tube with a roughened edge. (Courtesy Dr. H. Gelberg, College of Veterinary Medicine, Oregon State University.)

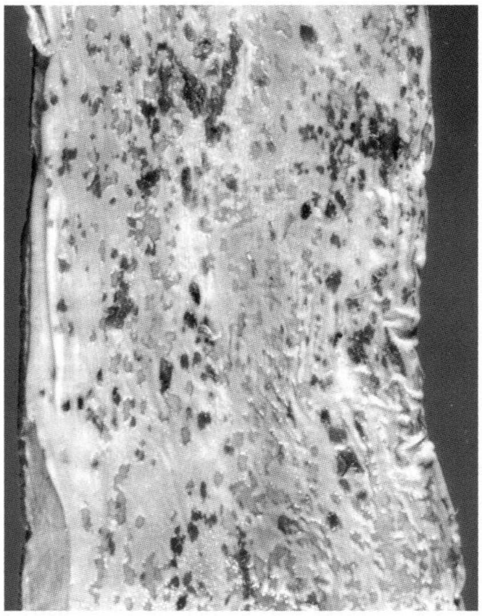

Fig. 7-42 Ulcerative esophagitis, bovine viral diarrhea (BVD), esophagus, cow.
Note the multiple variably sized (millimeter range) and variably shaped esophageal mucosal ulcers caused by the pestivirus of BVD. (Courtesy Dr. H. Gelberg, College of Veterinary Medicine, Oregon State University.)

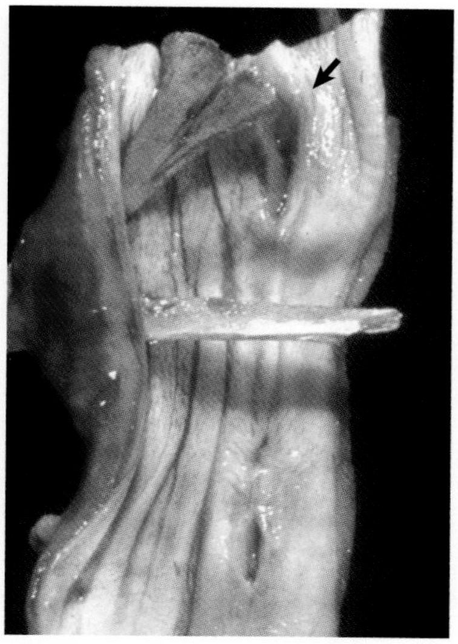

Fig. 7-43 Ulcers and perforation, foreign body, esophagus, dog. The esophagus has been perforated by an ingested chicken bone. Note that the end of the bone opposite the perforation site has caused a deep ulcer *(arrow)*. There are also several chronic ulcers caudal to the perforation, presumably from abrasion by other bones as they moved down the esophagus. (Courtesy Dr. C.S. Patton, College of Veterinary Medicine, University of Tennessee.)

about 5% of these lesions become cancerous. They are present in the oral cavity and esophagus of humans and are believed related to chronic irritation most often associated with smoking or chewing tobacco. Alcohol consumption and restorative dental amalgams may also predispose to leukoplakia.

Choke

Choke is a clinical term referring to esophageal obstruction subsequent to stenoses or blockage. Choke most often occurs in anatomic locations in which the esophagus cannot fully expand. These locations are dorsal to the larynx, cranial to the first rib at the thoracic inlet, the base of the heart, and the diaphragmatic hiatus. Choke occurs most frequently as a result of ingestion of large foreign bodies, such as potatoes, apples, bones (Fig. 7-43), or corn cobs (Fig. 7-44), or medicaments, such as large gelatin-filled capsules or tablets (dry boluses). If these bodies are lodged against the epithelium for longer than 2 days, the interaction often results in circumferential pressure necrosis of the esophageal mucosa (Fig. 7-45), which forms strictures during healing. These strictures then can cause reflex regurgitation after ingestion of food with possible starvation or aspiration pneumonia resulting.

In older horses, poor dentition causes feed to be incompletely masticated, resulting in impaction in the esophagus. Neoplastic or inflammatory lesions of the esophagus or periesophageal tissues also cause obstruction. Persistence of the right aortic arch has already been discussed as a cause of esophageal stenosis and megaesophagus.

Neoplasia

Neoplasms of the esophagus are rare. Bracken fern *(Pteridium aquilinum)* consumption sometimes in association with papilloma viruses has been associated with squamous cell carcinomas in bovids. The clinical signs are similar to those of other causes of esophageal blockage and include dysphagia, regurgitation, weight loss, and dilation of the esophagus proximal to the mass. Tumors of the esophagus are occasionally palpable but are most often intraluminal rather than mural. Epithelial tumors include papillomas (Fig. 7-46) and squamous cell carcinomas. The latter have wide metastatic potential. Smooth muscle tumors of the esophagus, whether benign or malignant, are also rare but may result in similar clinical signs (Fig. 7-47). Esophageal fibrosarcomas of dogs often develop in areas with *Spirocerca lupi* infestation. Esophageal lymphoma occurs sporadically in most species (Fig. 7-48).

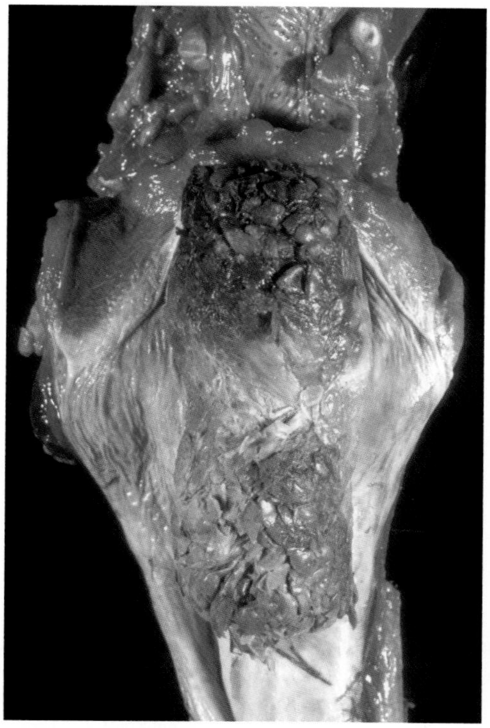

Fig. 7-44 Foreign body (choke), esophagus, cow. A corn cob has lodged in the esophagus subjacent to the larynx. (Courtesy Dr. H. Gelberg, College of Veterinary Medicine, Oregon State University.)

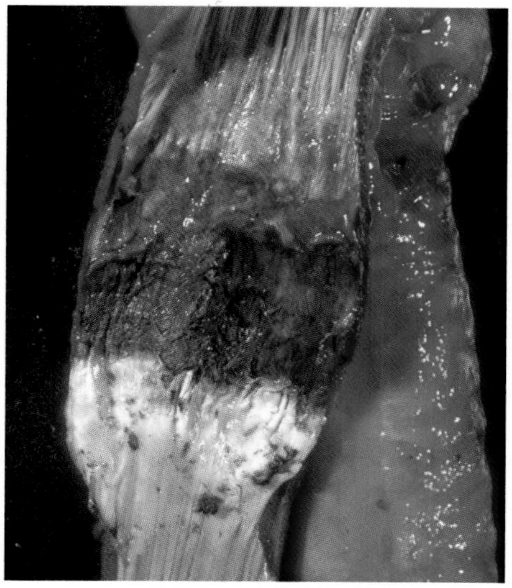

Fig. 7-45 Foreign body (choke), esophagus, horse. Pressure necrosis of the proximal esophageal mucosa, adjacent to the larynx has occurred secondary to lodgement of a foreign body (compacted chaff). As a general rule, pressure necrosis usually occurs if the foreign body remains in place against the mucosal epithelium for longer than 2 days. (Courtesy Dr. M.D. McGavin, College of Veterinary Medicine, University of Tennessee.)

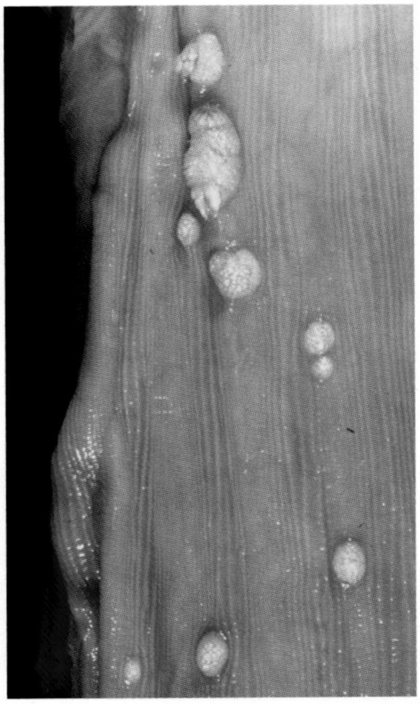

Fig. 7-46 Papillomatosis, bovine papilloma virus, esophagus, bull. Multiple papillomas, characteristic of this viral-induced disease, occur following trauma to the esophageal mucosa and infection of mucosal epithelial cells. Oral papillomas may be present concurrently. (Courtesy Dr. M.D. McGavin, College of Veterinary Medicine, University of Tennessee.)

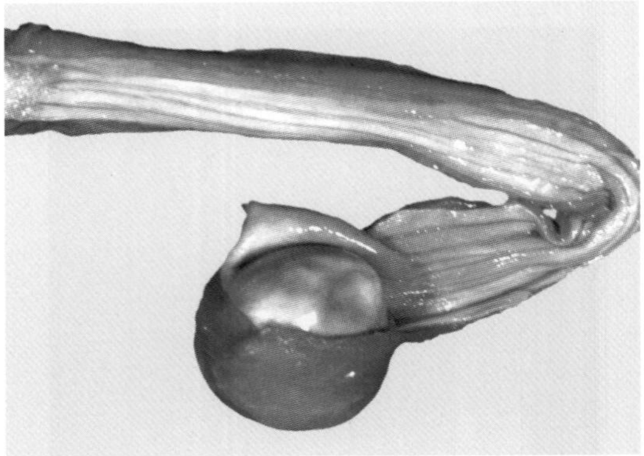

Fig. 7-47 Leiomyoma, esophagus, dog. A mass consisting of submucosal proliferation of smooth muscle cells bulges into the distal esophageal lumen causing obstruction. (Courtesy Dr. H. Gelberg, College of Veterinary Medicine, Oregon State University.)

RUMEN, RETICULUM, AND OMASUM

The three compartments of the ruminant forestomach are the reticulum, rumen, and omasum. Folds and compartments subdivide the forestomach. Normal forestomach motility, and thus innervation, is critical in maintaining digestive homeostasis. The forestomach is aglandular. The resident flora and fauna are responsible for digestion and fermentation of cellulose. In general, the rumen is a large fermentation vat where microorganisms break down ingesta by mechanical and chemical action into short-chain fatty acids, which are directly absorbed across the epithelial lining into the blood. These fatty acids supply more than half of the energy from nutrients absorbed by the alimentary tract. The reticulum and omasum act mechanically to further reduce the ingesta to fine particles.

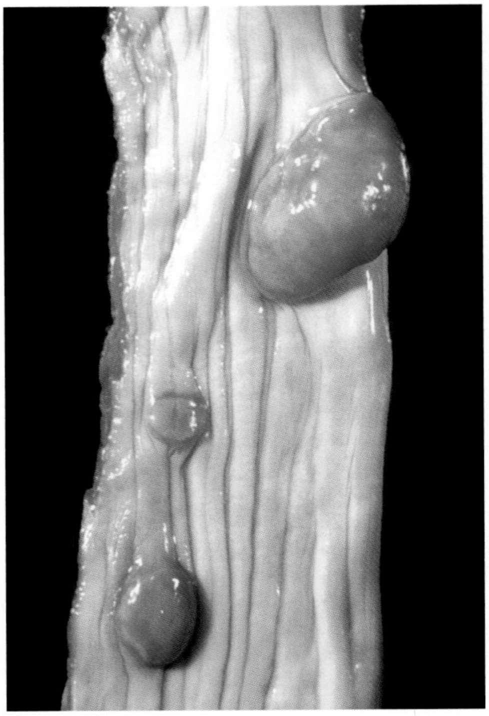

Fig. 7-48 Lymphoma (lymphosarcoma), esophagus, dog. Masses of submucosal proliferating malignant lymphocytes bulge into the esophageal lumen, causing partial obstruction. Note that the mucosal epithelium is intact (smooth and shiny). (Courtesy Dr. M.D. McGavin, College of Veterinary Medicine, University of Tennessee.)

Structure and Function

The rumen has small papillae that vary by diet up to 1.5 cm in length. Their length, shape, and degree of keratinization are affected by diet, and they are longer with high roughage diets and shorter with more concentrates in the ration. These changes are most obvious in the ventral compartment—the ventral ruminal sac. The reticulum has a honeycomb appearance, and the omasum consists of a series of about 100 longitudinal folds similar to the pages of a book. The nonglandular stratified squamous mucosa of the reticulum, rumen, and omasum can be acutely inflamed when their contents have an acid pH and the abnormal milieu permits bacterial and mycotic overgrowth.

The epithelial lining of the forestomach functions as a protective barrier for the forestomach and for the metabolism of ingesta and the absorption of volatile fatty acids. Because the reticulo-omasal orifice is more dorsal than the floor of the compartments, the reticulum can trap foreign bodies, especially dense metallic ones. These can irritate or penetrate the mucosa ("hardware disease"). Problems with motility and imbalances of rumen flora and fauna are the most frequent abnormalities of forestomach function. Often, the changes in flora and fauna are precipitated by a change in ingested substrate, promoting the growth of particular organisms. These changes alter ruminal pH and thus affect the integrity of the mucosal lining of the compartments of the forestomach or cause the production of excessive gas, resulting in ruminal distention.

Parts of compartment one (C1) and C2 and C3 of the camelid forestomach are lined by mucinous glandular epithelium. Concretions of ingesta are sometimes found within the saccules that contain the glands. The saccules are also the sites of water and other solutes. The nonglandular portions of C1 and C2 are lined by nonkeratinized stratified squamous epithelium without papillae.

The forestomach of new world camelids contracts at two to three times the rate of other ruminants (and in reverse order), and with each cycle, the saccules empty and refill. This results in high digestive efficiency across the saccules.

Bloat (Ruminal Tympany)

Ruminal tympany or bloat is by definition an overdistention of the rumen and reticulum by gases produced during fermentation. Mortality of affected animals is approximately 50%. A hereditary predisposition to bloat might exist in cattle because cases are on record of bloat in monozygotic twins. Bloat can be divided into primary tympany and secondary tympany.

Primary tympany is also known as *legume bloat, dietary bloat,* or *frothy bloat.* It generally occurs up to 3 days after animals begin a new diet. Certain legumes, such as alfalfa, ladino clover, and grain concentrates, promote the formation of stable foam. The nonvolatile acids of legume and ruminal fermentation lower the rumen pH to between 5 and 6, which is optimal for formation of bloat. Foam mixed with rumen contents physically blocks the cardia, preventing eructation and causing the rumen to distend with the gases of fermentation. Clinical signs include a distended left paralumbar fossa, a distended abdomen (see Fig. 1-27), increased respiratory and heart rates, and late in the disease, decreased ruminal movements. When death occurs, it is attributable to distention of the abdomen, which compresses the diaphragm, moving it cranially (orad), with resultant decreased pleural cavity size and respiratory embarrassment. There is also increased intraabdominal and intrathoracic pressure, resulting in decreased venous return to the heart and ultimately generalized congestion cranial to the thoracic inlet.

The lesions of primary tympany are often difficult to detect if there is an interval between death and postmortem examination because the foam can collapse. Conversely, fermentation can occur after death in a nonbloated animal, resulting in the production of abundant gas. The most reliable postmortem indicator of antemortem bloat is the sharp line of demarcation most evident in the mucosa between the pale, bloodless esophagus distal to the thoracic inlet and the congested proximal esophagus cranially (orad) to it. This line may sometimes form even after death before the blood clots. This division is known as a *bloat line* (Fig. 7-49).

Secondary tympany is caused by a physical or functional obstruction or stenosis of the esophagus resulting in failure to eructate. Examples of physical causes are esophageal papilloma, lymphoma, esophageal foreign bodies, and enlarged mesenteric or tracheobronchial lymph nodes, usually from lymphoma or tuberculosis. Vagus indigestion or other innervation disorders are examples of functional disorders.

It is questionable if new world camelids bloat.

Foreign Bodies

Foreign bodies can collect or lodge in the rumen. These include trichobezoars (hair balls) and phytobezoars (plant balls). Trichobezoars are sometimes a sequela to a habit of bucket-fed calves sucking on the skin of each other to satisfy their nursing instincts. Trichobezoars can form in utero because of hair circulating in the amniotic fluid and being swallowed by the fetus. Phytobezoars result from an excess of indigestible roughage.

Ingestion of nails and wire, common where straw and hay bales are bound by wire, can result in perforation of the wall of the reticulum with resultant reticulitis, peritonitis, or eventually possible pericarditis (hardware disease) (Fig. 7-50). Often, in areas in the US in which ruminants are at high risk of hardware disease because of farming practices, magnets are placed in rumens to prevent the ingested wires and nails from penetrating the reticular mucosa. Occasionally, ruminants ingest plates from storage batteries and suffer lead poisoning.

Inflammatory Diseases

Inflammation of the rumen, rumenitis, is generally considered synonymous with lactic acidosis. Lactic acidosis is synonymous with grain overload, rumen overload, carbohydrate engorgement, and chemical rumenitis. All ruminants are susceptible. The pathophysiology of lactic acidosis usually involves a sudden dietary change to an easily fermentable feed or a change in the feed volume consumed. The latter scenario is most likely to occur during weather changes, especially among feedlot cattle, when a sudden cooling rainstorm will stimulate food intake of cattle that had previously lost appetite because of high environmental temperatures and humidity.

Ruminal microflora is generally rich in cellulolytic gram-negative bacteria necessary for the digestion of hay. A sudden change to a highly fermentable, carbohydrate-rich feed promotes the growth of Gram-positive bacteria, *Streptococcus bovis,* and *Lactobacillus* spp. The lactic acid produced by the fermentation of ingested carbohydrates decreases the ruminal pH below 5 (normal = 5.5 to 7.5). This acidic pH eliminates normal ruminal flora and fauna and damages ruminal mucosa. Increased concentrations of

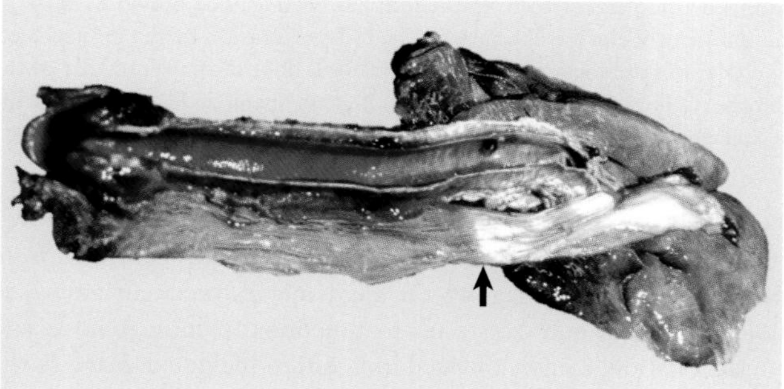

Fig. 7-49 Bloat line, esophagus and trachea at the thoracic inlet, cow. There is a sharp demarcation between the caudal (blanched) and the cranial (congested) mucosa of the esophagus *(arrow)*. This demarcation is caused by compromised venous return, the result of a grossly distended rumen displacing the diaphragm cranially and causing increased intrathoracic pressure, thus preventing the flow of venous blood into the thorax. In this illustration, a similar demarcation can be seen on the mucosa of the trachea. The subcutaneous tissues of the neck and head are also congested. (Courtesy Department of Veterinary Pathology, Cornell University.)

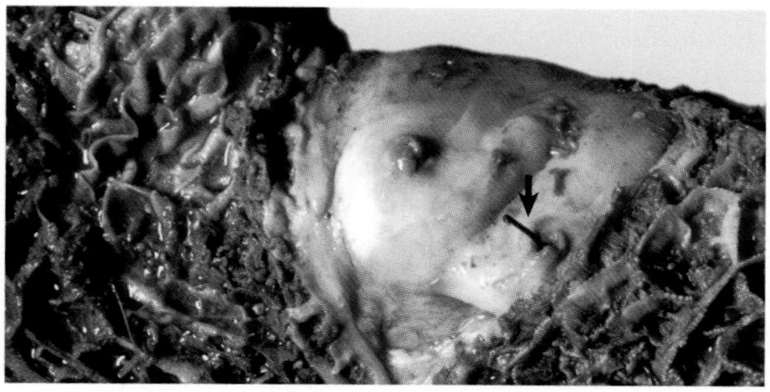

Fig. 7-50 Traumatic reticulitis, reticulum, cow. Several ingested wires have perforated the wall of the reticulum *(arrow)* and lodged in the tunica muscularis. Each wire is surrounded by a sinus tract draining to the surface of the reticulum. A chronic ulcer has formed around each area penetrated by the wires. (Courtesy Dr. M.D. McGavin, College of Veterinary Medicine, University of Tennessee.)

dissociated fatty acids lead to ruminal atony. When death occurs, it is due to dehydration secondary to the increased osmotic effect of ruminal solutes (organic acids), causing movement of fluids across the damaged ruminal mucosa into the rumen, acidosis (from absorption of lactate from the rumen), and circulatory collapse. Mortality among animals with lactic acidosis ranges from 25% to 90% and usually occurs within 24 hours.

At necropsy, the ruminal and intestinal contents are watery and acidic. Often, abundant grain is found in the rumen. The mucosa of the ruminal papillae is brown and friable and detaches easily, especially from the ventral ruminal sac. Caution must be exercised in interpreting this latter finding as a lesion because the ruminal mucosa often detaches easily in animals that have been dead for even a few hours at high environmental temperatures. Hydropic change and coagulative necrosis of the ruminal epithelium followed by an influx of neutrophils are common microscopic lesions. Animals surviving lactic acidosis develop stellate scars that are visible because of their color difference from the unaffected surrounding ruminal mucosa. Scars are pale; unaffected mucosa may be light to dark brown to black, depending on the original diet.

New world camelids appear to be more sensitive than ruminants to high carbohydrate diets. While their compartments do not have papillae, widespread ulceration of the squamous mucosa occurs in cases of lactic acidosis. New world camelids retain feed in their stomach longer than ruminants, possibly increasing fermentation and acid production. They rely on emptying of fluid to preserve milieu. High energy feeds may quickly impede motility promoting a drop in pH.

Bacterial rumenitis generally occurs secondary to lactic acidosis or mechanical injury to the ruminal mucosa. Bacteria that colonize the damaged ruminal wall can be transported into the portal circulation and to the liver, resulting in multiple abscesses. *Arcanobacterium (Actinomyces) pyogenes* is a common cause of bacterial abscesses in the liver. *Fusobacterium necrophorum,* also transported from the rumen to the liver, results in necrobacillosis, which has distinctive liver lesions.

Mycotic infections of the rumen also occur secondary to the damage to the ruminal mucosa caused by lactic acidosis and mechanical injury. Mycotic rumenitis also results from the administration of antibiotics, usually in calves but also in adult cattle, which reduce the numbers of normal flora and allow fungi to proliferate. In cases of mycotic rumenitis, lesions are generally circular and well delineated and are caused principally by infarction from thrombosis secondary to fungal vasculitis (Fig. 7-51). Offending fungi include *Aspergillus, Mucor, Rhizopus, Absidia,* and *Mortierella* spp. These fungi can spread to the placenta hematogenously and cause mycotic placentitis, which leads to abortions.

Ruminal candidiasis occurs as an incidental finding at necropsy. There is usually an underlying debilitating condition, glucose therapy, milk-replacer overload (sour rumen), or an antibiotic-induced kill-off of resident flora and fauna. Ruminal candidiasis is seldom diagnosed in a live animal.

Miscellaneous Diseases or Conditions

Ruminal papillae vary in length, becoming longer with high-roughage diets (Fig. 7-52). Such diets also can cause the papilla to become tongue- or leaf-shaped. Animals consuming diets with less than 10% roughage can develop ruminal parakeratosis. These rumens have hard, brown, often clumped, papillae. This lesion has little to no clinical consequence.

Ruminal papillomas are papilloma virus-induced in some cases, but in certain countries, bracken fern has been implicated as a cofactor in these forestomach neoplasms (Fig. 7-53).

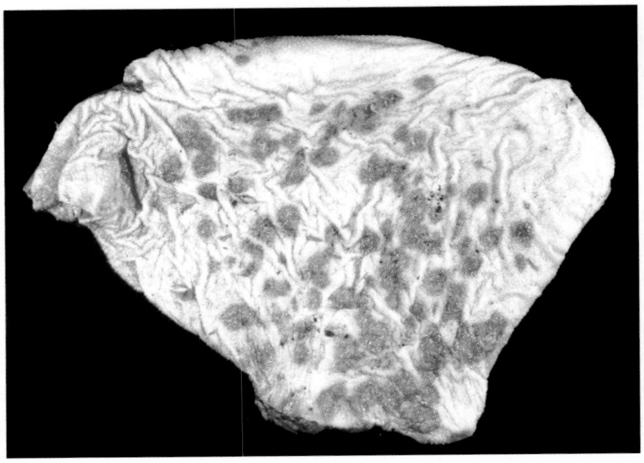

Fig. 7-51 Mycotic rumenitis, rumen, calf.
Note the numerous well-demarcated red foci of necrosis and hemorrhage (infarcts) in the ruminal mucosa that can be caused by angioinvasive fungi such as *Aspergillus, Mucor, Rhizopus, Absidia,* and *Mortierella* spp. This type of mycotic infection is usually preceded by a chemical (lactic acid) rumenitis (overeating). (Courtesy Dr. H. Gelberg, College of Veterinary Medicine, Oregon State University.)

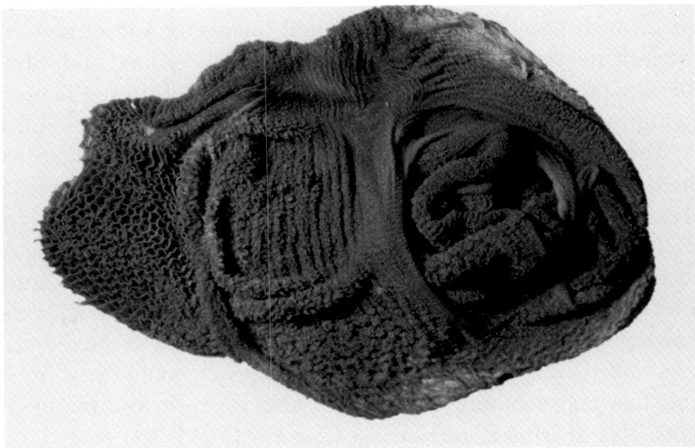

Fig. 7-52 Parakeratosis, reticulo-rumen, calf.
A diet that was almost devoid of roughage has resulted in atrophy and parakeratosis of ruminal papillae. Normal papillae are leaf shaped, but some of these papillae have become finger shaped, cauliflower shaped, or clumped. The parakeratotic epithelium has been stained brown to black by components of the feed because of the lack of abrasion by the ground feed. These lesions are most marked on the ventral floor of the ventral sac of the rumen. (Courtesy Dr. M.D. McGavin, College of Veterinary Medicine, University of Tennessee.)

Vagal indigestion results in a functional outflow problem from the forestomach. Damage to the vagus nerve can occur anywhere along its length and can result in functional pyloric stenosis and omasal dilation. Causes of vagal indigestion include damage to the vagus nerve due to traumatic reticuloperitonitis, liver abscesses with secondary peritonitis, volvulus of the abomasum, and bronchopneumonia. Mechanical obstruction of the forestomach or abomasal outflow can be due to abomasal lymphoma or papillomas or from blockage after ingestion of indigestible or foreign materials. Diet and dwarfism are sometimes associated with vagus indigestion. Many cases are idiopathic. Clinical signs include ruminoreticular distention. The presence of abomasal distention depends on the precise location of the damage to the vagus nerve. Vagal

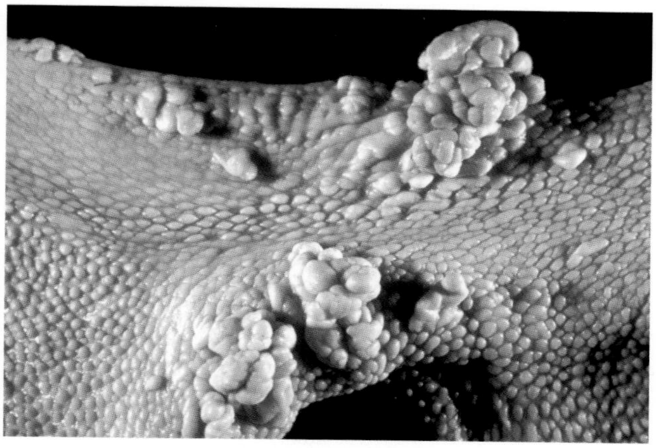

Fig. 7-53 Papillomas, rumen, cow.
Smooth-surfaced, squamous papillomas are present on the dorsal wall. (Courtesy Dr. H. Gelberg, College of Veterinary Medicine, Oregon State University.)

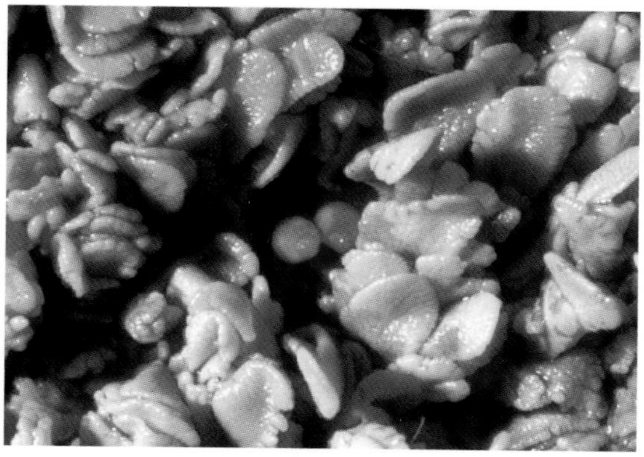

Fig. 7-54 Paramphistomiasis, rumen, cow.
The pink conical structures located in the center of the illustration are paramphistomes (ruminal flukes). They are considered to be innocuous, but massive numbers of immature flukes in the duodenum may cause a severe catarrhal duodenitis. Note the normal leaf-shaped ruminal papillae, indicative of a high-roughage diet. (Courtesy Dr. M.D. McGavin, College of Veterinary Medicine, University of Tennessee.)

indigestion is divided into the following four types, based on the anatomic location of the functional obstruction.

- Type I is usually caused by inflammatory lesions around the vagal nerve at any location and is a failure of eructation resulting in bloat.
- Type II is a functional or anatomic condition that results in failure of omasal transport into the abomasum. Usual causes are adhesions and abscesses on the medial wall of the reticulum associated with or secondary to traumatic reticuloperitonitis. Abomasal lymphoma and physical obstruction of the omasal canal (e.g., neoplasia or ingested placenta) may also be causative.
- Type III is caused by physical impaction of the abomasum by roughage and thus is dietary in origin. Abomasal displacements and volvulus are also potential causes.
- Type IV is pregnancy related, perhaps as a result of shifting of position of the abomasum secondary to the expanding uterus, causing compression of the abdominal branches of the vagus nerve.

Ruminal Parasitism

Paramphistomiasis is a fluke infestation of the ruminant forestomach in warmer latitudes around the world. These trematodes are in the genera *Paramphistomum, Calicophoron,* and *Cotylophoron.* They are similar in size and appearance to ruminal papillae (Fig. 7-54). Although the presence of adult organisms in the forestomach is usually of no clinical significance, heavy infestations of larvae in the proximal small intestine, before migration to the rumen and reticulum, can cause hypoproteinemia, anemia, and death. Larvae burrow deeply into and sometimes through the wall of the small intestine and can be found in the peritoneal cavity. The intermediate host is a snail. Cercariae encyst on aquatic vegetation and are eaten by the ruminant.

STOMACH AND ABOMASUM

Although some differences exist, the stomachs of the simple-stomached animals and the abomasum of ruminants (third compartment of new world camelids) are very similar in structure and function. A fundus and body make up the cranial portion lined by numerous spiral folds and produce acid and pepsin. The aboral portion, the pyloric part, is lined by epithelium with mucous-secreting glands and G cells that produce gastrin. Stomachs have an indigenous flora. Most of these organisms cannot be cultured by traditional methods. C3 of new world camelids is more tubular than the abomasum, with more peristalsis-like rather than mixing motility. The first two-thirds of C3 is fermentative with a pH around 6.5. At the caudal flexure, the mucosa thickens to 7 to 10 mm and the pH is around 2.0. The final portion surrounding the torus pyloricus has an alkaline pH.

Structure and Function

The gastric mucosa of simple-stomached animals contains numerous folds or rugae that are flattened when the stomach is distended. Foveolas or gastric pits communicate with the lumen of the stomach and transport gastric cell secretions. The glandular stomach functions in the enzymatic and hydrolytic digestion of ingested food substances. The epithelial covering is one cell thick, and the cell types include columnar mucus and bicarbonate-secreting surface epithelial cells, mucous neck cells arranged in tubuloalveolar glands, acid-secreting parietal cells, pepsinogen-secreting chief cells, and neuroendocrine (enterochromaffin, argentaffin) cells that secrete gastrin, enteroglucagon, and somatostatin (Fig. 7-55). The neuroendocrine cells do not communicate with the gastric lumen. The mucous neck cells are the precursor cells for all the other epithelial types in the stomach and are responsible for the replacement of surface epithelial cells as they are lost, either at the end of their normal lifespan or from some type of insult.

Multiple submucosal lymphoid patches are present in monogastric animals. In ruminants, a single lymphoid patch is present at the fold separating the omasum and abomasum.

In some species, such as the horse and rat, the cranial or orad part of the stomach (nonglandular part or pars nonglandularis) is lined by stratified squamous epithelium, whereas the distal portion (pars glandularis) is lined by glandular epithelium. In the horse, the dividing line between the two is called the *margo plicatus.* The pars nonglandularis in the pig is a small square to rectangular area of stratified squamous epithelium surrounding the esophageal opening.

Defense Mechanisms

The gastric mucosal barrier is significant in preventing autodigestion and bacterial overgrowth. There is, however, a resident

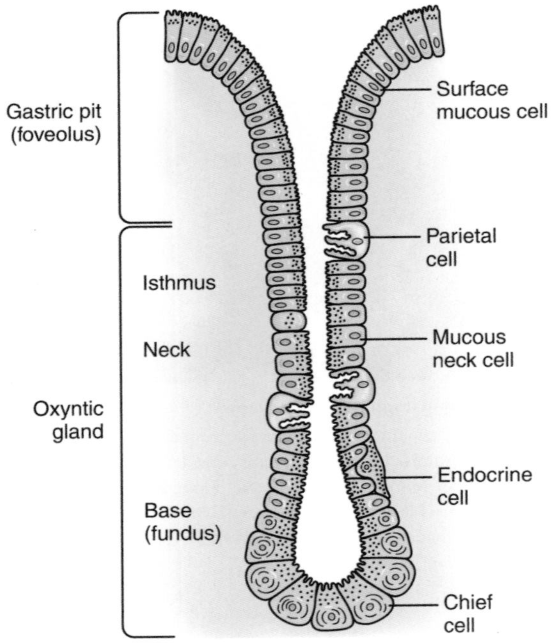

Fig. 7-55 Schematic illustration, microanatomy of the stomach.
(Adapted from Ito S, Winchester RJ: *J Cell Biol* 16:541, 1963.)

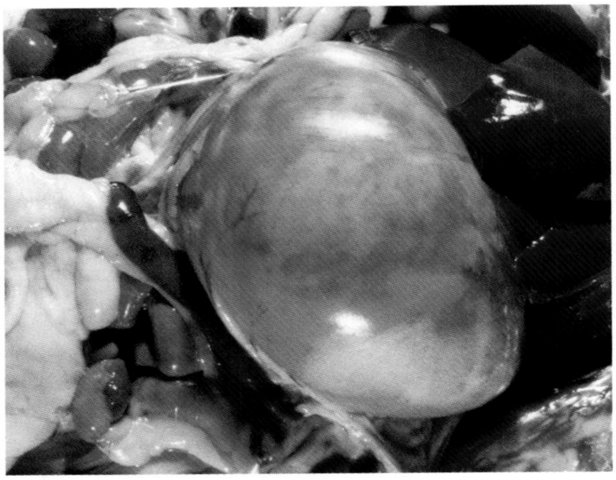

Fig. 7-56 Simple gastric dilation, stomach, rabbit.
The stomach is markedly dilated and filled with gas. Dilation occurs most commonly following aerophagia or overeating, and is relieved by eructation or vomiting. (Courtesy Dr. H. Gelberg, College of Veterinary Medicine, Oregon State University.)

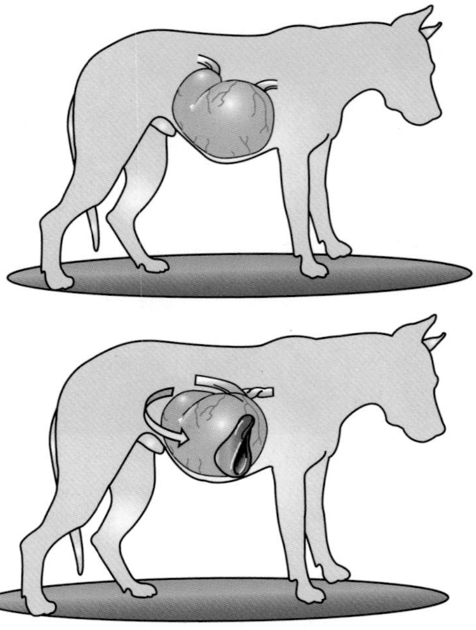

Fig. 7-57 Schematic illustration, gastric dilation and volvulus, stomach, dog.
The stomach is distended with food and gas *(top example)*. It rotates *(arrow)* on the mesenteric axis *(bottom example)* clockwise (180, 270, or 360 degrees on a ventrodorsal axis when the abdomen is viewed from the ventral surface), resulting in a gastric volvulus with an obstructed esophagus that prevents eructation and thus further contributes to gastric dilation. The spleen, attached to the stomach by the gastrosplenic ligament, rotates with the stomach and is thus folded back upon itself and located in the right cranial abdomen against the diaphragm *(bottom example)*. The splenic vein is compressed, resulting in a congested spleen, because the arterial blood supply remains patent longer than venous drainage. (Modified from Van Kruiningen HJ, Gregoire K, Meuten DJ: *J Am Anim Hosp Assoc* 10:294-324, 1974.)

flora that is difficult to grow on artificial media. Microorganismal overgrowth is prevented under normal physiologic conditions by abomasal or gastric motility, prostaglandin E_2 (PGE_2), a protective layer of mucus and bicarbonate, secretory IgA, transforming growth factor-α (TGF-α), epidermal growth factor, an extremely acid luminal pH, and an effective pyloric sphincter that prevents regurgitation into the stomach or abomasum of duodenal, hepatic, and pancreatic secretions. An intact epithelial layer and adequate blood flow also prevent acid-induced damage.

Gastric Dilation and Volvulus

Simple gastric dilation occurs in a variety of animals and in humans (Fig. 7-56). In dogs, particularly in the large, deep-chested breeds, the acute gastric dilation and volvulus syndrome occurs. This lesion is life-threatening and should not be confused with simple gastric dilation that is common in young puppies after overeating. Predisposing factors to acute gastric dilation include a source of distending gas, fluid, or feed; obstruction of the cardia that prevents eructation and emesis; and obstruction of the pylorus that prevents passage of gastric contents into the small intestine. The source of gas is not well understood. Theories include gas production by *Clostridium perfringens,* spores of which are present in the feed, carbon dioxide (CO_2) from physiologic mechanisms of digestion, or simple aerophagia.

The result of repeated episodes of gastric dilation is stretching and relaxation of the gastrohepatic ligament. Recurrent dilation, combined with overfeeding, postprandial exercise, and perhaps a hereditary predisposition, results in gastric rotation. Gastric rotation is recognized by splenic displacement and a twisted esophagus and results in vascular compression and decreased venous drainage and hypoxemia (Figs. 7-57 and 7-58). The stomach generally is rotated clockwise on the ventrodorsal axis when the abdomen is viewed from the ventral surface. Rotation is 180 to 360 degrees. The combination of gastric hypoxemia, acid-base imbalance, obstruction of the pylorus and cardia, and increased intragastric pressure leads to antiperistaltic waves followed by atony, cardiovascular ischemia, arrhythmias, and shock. Decreased portal venous return leads to pancreatic ischemia and release of myocardial depressant factor, cardiac collapse, and death.

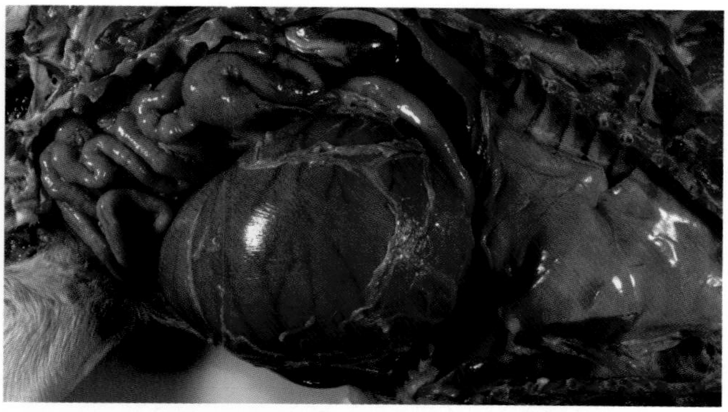

Fig. 7-58 Gastric dilation and volvulus, abdomen, dog.
The stomach is filled with gas and its serosa is congested. The duodenum and engorged spleen have been displaced to the right. (Courtesy Dr. M.D. McGavin, College of Veterinary Medicine, University of Tennessee.)

Epidemiologic evidence suggests that dry dog foods that list oils or fats among the first four ingredients increase the risk of the gastric dilation and volvulus syndrome. Gastric dilation and volvulus is sometimes associated with gastric eversion or intussusception into the distal esophagus. This latter condition can also occur independently of gastric dilation and volvulus.

Abomasal Displacement

Normally, the abomasum lies over the xiphoid process at the abdominal ventral midline. Abomasal displacement is usually to the left side, although right-sided displacements also occur (Fig. 7-59). Left-sided displacement of the abomasum is a generally nonfatal entity seen in high-producing dairy cattle during the 6 weeks after parturition. Strenuous activity can predispose nonpregnant cows to displacement. In the postcalving period, abomasal atony can occur as a result of heavy grain feeding (volatile fatty acids decrease motility) and hypocalcemia. Meanwhile, the gravid uterus may have displaced the rumen and abomasum cranially and to the left, rupturing the attachment of the greater omentum to the abomasum. The abomasum then occupies the cranial left quadrant of the abdomen and displaces the rumen medially. This change leads to partial obstruction of abomasal outflow. Metabolic alkalosis contributes to rumen atony and impaired movement of ingesta. The associated hypochloremia is a result of hydrogen chloride (HCl) secretion and is common along with hypokalemia. Abomasal ulcers and peritoneal adhesions can result in cases of chronic displacement.

Fifteen percent of abomasal displacements are right-sided. The abomasum can be overdistended, displaced dorsally, and rotated on its mesenteric axis, and 20% of these cases develop abomasal volvulus. Right-sided displacements occur in postparturient dairy cows and in calves.

Clinical features of displaced abomasums, whether right-sided or left-sided, include anorexia, cachexia, dehydration, lack of feces, ketonuria, and a characteristic high-pitched ping subsequent to percussion over the abomasum. Idiopathic abomasal volvulus occurs occasionally in ruminants and calves (Web Fig. 7-10).

Gastric Dilation and Rupture

Gastric dilation occurs in horses as a result of the ingestion of fermentable feeds or grain, a situation analogous to grain overload with lactic acidosis in cattle. Acute gastric dilation and rupture in equids occurs most frequently as a terminal event in intestinal obstruction and displacement. Because gastric dilation and rupture

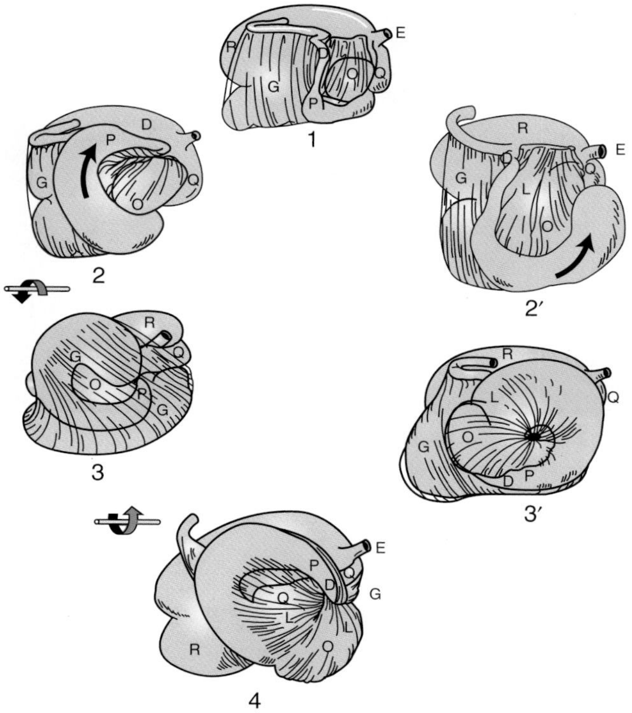

Fig. 7-59 Schematic diagrams illustrating two possible modes of rotation of the omasum, abomasum, and cranial part of the duodenum in volvulus.
1, Normal relations; *2,* simple dilation and displacement on the right; *3,* 180-degree volvulus around the longitudinal axis of the lesser omentum, counterclockwise as seen from the rear; *2′*, 90-degree rotation of the abomasum in a sagittal plane, counterclockwise as seen from the right; *3′*, 180-degree rotation of the abomasum and omasum around the transverse axis of the lesser omentum, drawing the duodenum cranially, medial to the omasum; *4,* 360-degree counterclockwise volvulus, final stage resulting from either mode of rotation. *D,* Duodenum; *E,* esophagus; *G,* greater omentum; *L,* lesser omentum; *O,* omasum; *P,* pylorus; *Q,* reticulum; *R,* rumen. (Modified from Habel RE, Smith DF: *J Am Vet Med Assoc* 179:447-455, 1981.)

can occur after death, the diagnostic challenge is to determine if the rupture occurred antemortem or postmortem. The only reliable indicator of the time of rupture, in relation to the death of the animal, is the presence of hemorrhage and evidence of inflammation, such as fibrin strands, along the margins of the rupture (usually the greater curvature) because such inflammatory responses occur only in live animals (Figs. 7-60 and 7-61).

In Northern Europe, acute gastric dilation occurs in horses on pasture as part of the syndrome called grass sickness or dysautonomia. The esophagus and stomach are often dilated and atonic. Although serologic evidence suggests an association of grass sickness with *Clostridium perfringens* type A enterotoxin, noninflammatory degeneration of associated autonomic ganglia have also been described. This condition can be experimentally produced in the horse with whole blood from affected animals, suggesting that a soluble toxin may be the cause.

Chronic gastric dilation is also associated with ingestion of poorly digestible substances. Habitual cribbing and aerophagia may also be contributory.

Dysautonomia also occurs in pet carnivores secondary to ganglionic death in cranial nerves, spinal nerves, and autonomic nerves. Associated ganglionic peptides are reduced in an amount consistent with the functional aberrations. Ganglioneuritis creates a similar

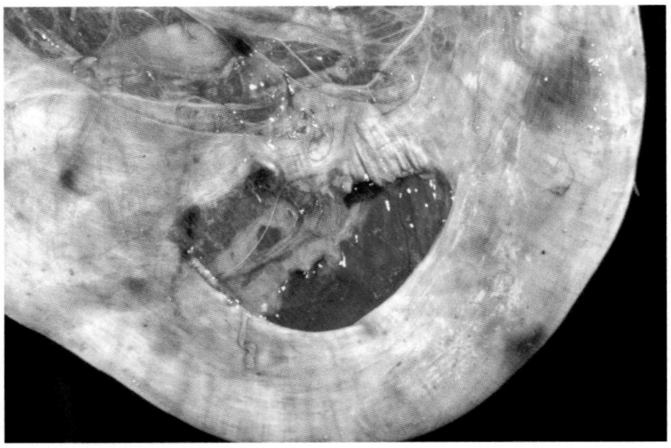

Fig. 7-60 Rupture, abomasum, calf.
Multifocal hemorrhages along the upper margin of the tear and subserosally adjacent to the greater curvature indicate that the rupture occurred antemortem. (Courtesy Dr. M.D. McGavin, College of Veterinary Medicine, University of Tennessee.)

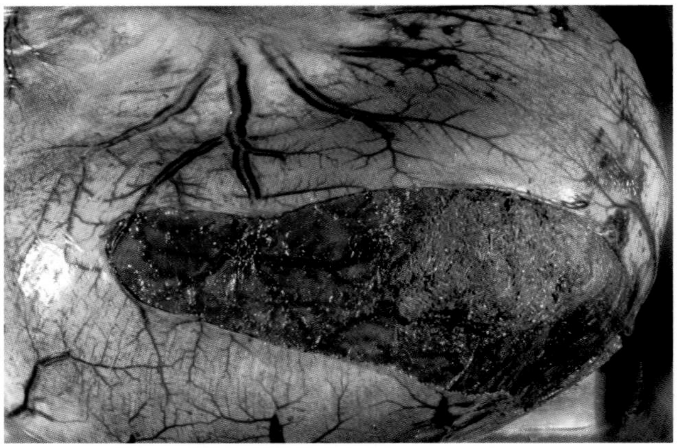

Fig. 7-61 Rupture, stomach, horse.
The hemorrhage visible on the right margin of the rupture indicates that the rupture occurred antemortem. Note also that the rent through the tunica muscularis is longer than that through the mucosa, which still covers the ingesta on the left and right sides. The mucosal and serosal surfaces are congested. (Courtesy Dr. H. Gelberg, College of Veterinary Medicine, Oregon State University.)

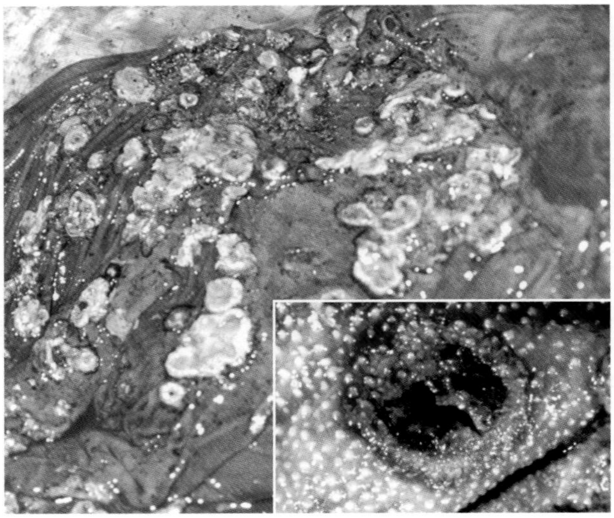

Fig. 7-62 Mycotic abomasitis and omasitis, calf.
The mucosal surface of the abomasum has discrete and coalescing ulcers covered by yellow-white diphtheritic membranes and a red outer margin of active hyperemia and inflammation. These lesions are indicative of infarcts and are likely secondary to vasculitis and thrombosis by angioinvasive fungi such as *Aspergillus, Mucor, Rhizopus, Absidia,* and *Mortierella* spp. The diphtheritic membranes are a mixture of necrotic cellular debris from the infarct, inflammatory cells, and hyphae from the inciting fungus. Inset: Mycotic omasitis. The lesion is similar to the one in the abomasum. The diphtheritic membrane has been lost due to omasal peristalsis, but the necrotic center (infarct) and red outer margin of active hyperemia and inflammation are prominent. (Figure courtesy College of Veterinary Medicine, University of Illinois. Inset courtesy Dr. H. Gelberg, College of Veterinary Medicine, Oregon State University.)

syndrome to dysautonomia in a variety of species and is infrequently diagnosed. GI signs of dysautonomia include xerostomia, decreased anal tone, vomiting, and regurgitation. See Chapter 14 for a description of the histologic lesions.

Chronic abomasal and/or ruminal dilation may occur in cows with overeating disease, dystocia, exhaustion, poor quality or frozen feedstuffs, abomasal ulcers with or without abomasal lymphoma, and vagal indigestion. A sequela of abomasitis may be a mycotic infection similar to that which occurs in the rumen (Fig. 7-62).

In monkeys, an increased frequency of acute gastric dilation often occurs during weekends, when there may be changes in feeding behavior secondary to unfamiliar keepers. Studies have implicated *Clostridium perfringens* overgrowth secondary to an increase in fermentable feed consumption in the pathogenesis of gastric dilation in primates.

Chronic gastric dilation in canids is usually secondary to gastric ulcer, mural gastric lymphomas, uremia affecting gastric structure and function, pyloric stenosis or obstruction, acute gastric dilation, intervertebral disc disease, or vagotomy. Chronic gastric dilation is characterized by reduced feed intake, diminished gastric motility, and increased gastric gas accumulation sometimes resulting in abdominal distention similar to that of bloat.

Abomasal Dilation and Tympany

Abomasal dilation and tympany is a syndrome of young cattle that occurs most commonly in dairy breeds with a history of one or more of the following: only a single milk feeding per day, cold milk or milk replacer, lack of free choice water, inconsistency of feeding time, dosing with high energy oral electrolyte solutions, and sometimes, failure of passive transfer of immunity. The pathophysiology is presumed to be abomasal fermentation of high energy ingesta by gas-producing bacteria. Hyperglycemia and a resultant glycosuria are present. Hemorrhage, edema, necrosis, and sometimes emphysema of the abomasum and other compartments of the forestomach are found at necropsy.

Impaction

Impaction of the monogastric stomach and abomasum has a variety of causes. Intrathoracic lesions, such as pneumonia, pleuritis, lymphadenopathy, and lymphoma of mediastinal lymph nodes, can infiltrate and damage the vagal nerves, resulting in a problem with abomasal/gastric motility and emptying. Roughage, hairballs, and other foreign materials also cause impaction. Gastric trichobezoars and phytobezoars of monogastric animals are similar to those that occur in the rumen (Web Fig. 7-11).

Abomasal emptying defect is principally a condition of Suffolk sheep 2 to 6 years of age. It is characterized by an impacted, dilated abomasum. Clinical signs include anorexia, weight loss, and increased ruminal chloride levels. The latter feature is believed to be secondary to abomasal reflux. Scattered chromatolysis and neuronal necrosis in the celiac and mesenteric ganglia are consistent changes from a neurotoxicosis. The process is likely mediated by excitotoxins, although viruses have not been ruled out. Clusters of affected animals in a single flock are suggestive of an environmental cause. Inflammation is minimal. Abomasal emptying defect may be a form of acquired dysautonomia.

Inflammatory Diseases

Inflammation of the simple stomach or abomasum is designated as gastritis and abomasitis, respectively, and must be differentiated from simple hyperemia and petechiae, which are often nonspecific agonal lesions. Gastritis is often associated clinically with vomiting, dehydration, and metabolic acidosis. Hemorrhage, edema, increased amounts of mucus, abscesses, granulomas, foreign body penetration, parasites, inflammatory cells of various types, erosions, ulcerations, and necrosis characterize the changes in the mucosal surface and subsequent inflammatory reaction.

Clostridium septicum is a cause of hemorrhagic abomasitis with submucosal emphysema of sheep and cattle, a disease known as *braxy*. Although this disease is most common in the United Kingdom and Europe, it occurs in North America as well. Generally, the disease follows ingestion of frozen feeds contaminated with the causative *Clostridium* spp. The lesions are produced by the exotoxin of the bacteria, and death therefore is due to an exotoxemia.

Sarcina-like organisms have been reported in association with abomasal bloat in several calves. Sarcinas are anaerobic, gram-positive, nonmotile cocci found in rafts or packets. They are suspected gastric pathogens in a variety of animal species. The lesions are similar to braxy.

In many septicemias of pigs, bacterial emboli lodge in the vessels of the gastric submucosa and cause thrombosis, resulting in hyperemia, hemorrhage, infarction, and ulceration. This occurs in salmonellosis, swine dysentery, Glasser's disease, and colibacillosis. Certain intoxicants such as vomitoxin produced by *Fusarium* spp. can cause similar lesions (Fig. 7-63).

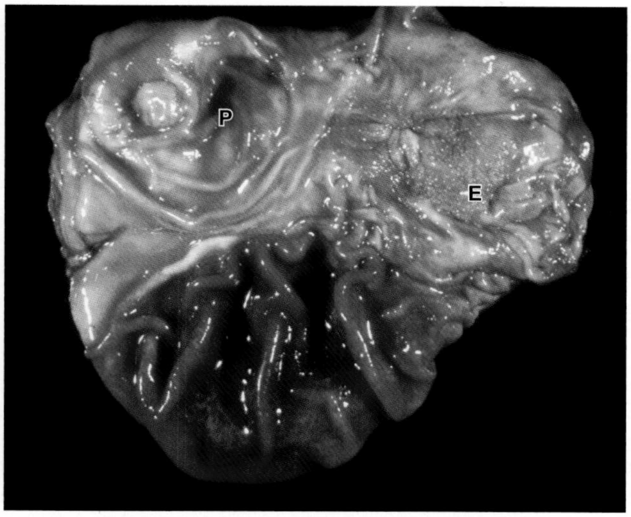

Fig. 7-63 Acute "hemorrhagic gastritis," stomach, pig. The fundus of the stomach is hemorrhagic. This type of gastric change is often seen in the pig in acute septicemia, for example, from salmonella, and the severe congestion is attributed to venous infarction from endotoxemia. *E*, Esophageal os; *P*, pylorus. (Courtesy Dr. H. Gelberg, College of Veterinary Medicine, Oregon State University.)

A deep mycosis that causes a granulomatous gastritis is due to *Histoplasma capsulatum* (see intestinal diseases of carnivores). Very rarely, *Mycobacterium tuberculosis* causes granulomatous gastritis in a variety of species. In granulomatous gastritis, epigastric discomfort after eating (postprandial), emesis, progressive cachexia, weakness, vomiting of blood (hematemesis), and pyloric obstruction caused by the space-occupying inflammatory reaction occur. In both histoplasmosis and tuberculosis, regional (gastric, splenic, and hepatic) lymph nodes may be affected. Nodular or diffusely thickened gastric and lymphoid lesions contain predominately macrophages. Mononuclear inflammatory cells, fibroblasts, granulocytes (including eosinophils), and multinucleate giant cells are also present. Often the causative organisms can be demonstrated within the granulomatous inflammation, but special stains, such as acid-fast for mycobacteria and periodic acid–Schiff (PAS) reaction, or Gomori's methenamine silver stain may be necessary to demonstrate fungi.

Eosinophilic gastritis is uncommon in all species of domestic animals but has been reported in pet carnivores and humans. In general, the etiologic basis for this condition is poorly understood. The three types of gastritis characterized by an influx of eosinophils are as follows:

- A characteristic focal eosinophilic infiltrate is sometimes associated with trapped, intramural nematode larvae, especially *Toxocara canis*. Larvae of *Toxocara canis* pass to nursing puppies through the milk, through fecal soiling of bedding, or from dirt or other fomites harboring eggs or larvae. After ingestion, the parasite's larval sheath, feces, and saliva are antigenic. In dogs and cats, tissue reaction to these larvae in the mucosal and submucosal intestine and gastric epithelial cell is hyperplasia, resulting in a polyp-like proliferation of the antral mucosa. Pyloric obstruction sometimes results.
- In other cases of eosinophilic gastritis, the infiltration of eosinophils is more diffuse and is believed to be a hypersensitivity reaction. The offending antigen is not known. In many of these cases, there is a peripheral eosinophilia, especially when associated with eosinophilic infiltration of the small intestine (eosinophilic gastroenteritis). This form of eosinophilic gastritis may become transmural, with necrosis and scarring.
- The third type, scirrhous eosinophilic gastritis of dogs and cats, for the most part has unknown causes. The fibrosis associated with scirrhous changes in the stomach and lymph nodes result in persistent emesis, weight loss, and malnutrition.

The gross lesions of eosinophilic gastritis are rather nonspecific and consist of diffuse or nodular mural thickenings. Microscopic lesions are characterized by infiltrates of eosinophils in the mucosa and the submucosa and are seen extensively through the muscularis of the stomach. Similar lesions are sometimes present in segments of the small intestine and colon. In the dog, there is sometimes necroproliferative eosinophilic perivasculitis and eosinophilic lymphadenopathy. In the scirrhous form, the eosinophilic infiltrate is followed by transmural fibroplasia and scarring.

Hypertrophic or Hyperplastic Enteritides

Hypertrophic gastritis, characterized by thickened rugae, is the result of hyperplasia of the gastric glands. This effect is believed to be a response to chronic retention of gastric fluid and reflux of intestinal bile. Similar mucosal glandular changes are seen in immune-mediated lymphoplasmacytic gastritis of dogs. Hypertrophic gastritis has also been described in primates, horses, pigs, and rodents. The nematode *Nochtia nocti* causes this lesion in the

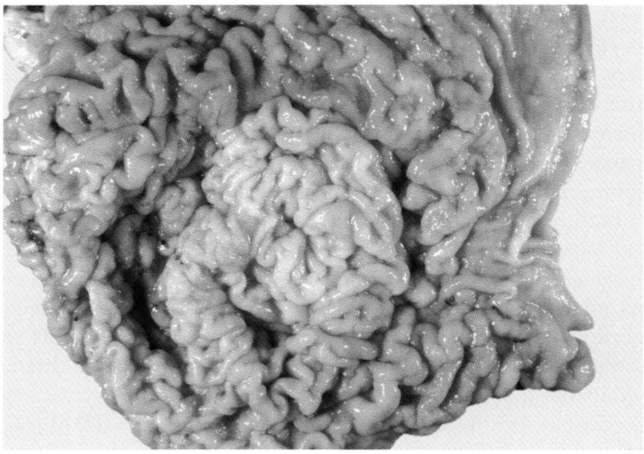

Fig. 7-64 Chronic giant hypertrophic gastropathy, stomach, dog. A cerebriform mass of redundant mucosa is present in the center of the gastric mucosa. Chronic inflammation in the mass results in increased mucosal permeability to serum proteins and a subsequent protein-losing gastropathy. (Courtesy College of Veterinary Medicine, Cornell University.)

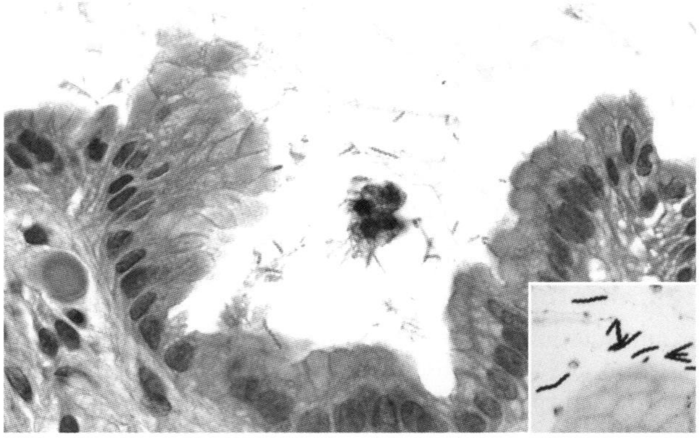

Fig. 7-65 *Helicobacter* spp. infection, stomach, cat. Numerous spiral bacteria are present in the superficial mucous layer. There is no inflammation in the adjacent mucosa; however, in some areas the epithelium is hyperplastic. H&E stain. Inset: The helical shape of the helicobacter organisms is demonstrated with a Steiner's silver stain. (Figure courtesy Dr. H. Gelberg, College of Veterinary Medicine, Oregon State University. Inset courtesy Dr. C.S. Patton, College of Veterinary Medicine, University of Tennessee.)

stomachs of monkeys. Equine hypertrophic gastritis is a focal lesion or more diffuse lesion associated with the nematodes, *Habronema* spp. and *Trichostrongylus axei*, respectively.

Chronic giant hypertrophic gastropathy of dogs affects the basenji, beagle, boxer, and bull terrier breeds, among others. The disease is similar to Ménétrier's disease in humans. Clinical signs include weight loss, diarrhea, vomiting, and hypoproteinemia. The chronic gastritis results in increased mucosal permeability to serum proteins with subsequent protein-losing gastropathy. Unlike normal gastric mucosal folds, in giant hypertrophic gastropathy, the mucosa does not flatten with distention of the organ (Fig. 7-64). Microscopically, the mucosa is hypertrophic and hyperplastic. The incorporation of folds of submucosa and muscularis mucosa is variable, as is the presence of inflammatory cells, principally lymphocytes and plasma cells. The cause of this condition is unknown.

An ulcer is a mucosal defect in which the entire epithelial thickness, down to or through the basement membrane, has been lost. Penetration through the remaining tissue layers to the peritoneal cavity is termed a perforating ulcer. Partial-thickness epithelial loss is termed an *erosion.* Chronic ulcers differ from acute ulcers by the presence of an indurated rim caused by fibrosis and attempts at epithelial regeneration. The identification of gastric ulcers is not challenging, either at necropsy or by endoscopy. They are sharply bordered cavities, often coated with exudate. Thrombosis of blood vessels is sometimes adjacent to ulcers in ruminants with mycotic vasculitis secondary to ruminal lactic acidosis. Thus it is an infarct.

The pathogenesis of most gastric and duodenal ulcers in humans has been demonstrated to be a result of infection with a helical bacterium, *Helicobacter pylori*. The same bacterium has been epidemiologically linked to gastric adenocarcinoma. *Helicobacter mustelae* acts similarly in ferrets. Although similar, gastric *Helicobacter*-like organisms (GHLOs) are readily demonstrated in dogs and cats, their relationship with ulcer formation or neoplasia is not established. It appears that the stomachs of as many animals without gastritis or ulcers are as heavily colonized by these bacteria as are those animals with ulcers (Fig. 7-65). More than 90% of cats are infected with two *Helicobacter* spp. *Helicobacter felis* can be cultured in vitro, but the noncultivatable *Helicobacter heilmannii* is the more frequent. Pathologic and clinical outcomes appear to depend on a number of bacterial virulence factors as well as on the host response to these agents. Investigations suggest there may be a link between the presence of *Helicobacter* and other diseases, including coronary and neurologic disease.

Theories abound as to the causes of most gastric ulcers in animals. None have been proved. There may be a heritable component to ulcer susceptibility. The conditions necessary for ulcer development boil down to an imbalance between acid secretion and mucosal protection. This imbalance occurs as a result of the following:

- Local disturbances or trauma to the mucosal epithelial barrier; this injury can be due to back flush of bile salts from the duodenum or ingestion of lipid solvents such as alcohol.
- Normal or high gastric acidity.
- Local disturbances in blood flow (stress-induced and sympathetic nervous system–mediated arteriovenous shunts) resulting in ischemia.
- Steroids and NSAIDs that depress prostaglandin formation (PGE_2, PGI_1) or concentration, thus decreasing phospholipid secretions, which are protective

All of these mechanisms allow pepsin and hydrochloric acid into the submucosa.

Severe gastric hyperacidity and gastric ulcers is sometimes associated with the presence of islet cell tumors producing gastrin. Some of these gastrin-producing tumors arise in the duodenum, but the majority originate in the pancreas. These neoplasms release histamine into the bloodstream, which binds to receptors on parietal cells of the stomach, increasing HCl secretion. The gastric ulceration produced associated with these tumors is known as *Zollinger-Ellison syndrome.*

In dogs, gastric ulceration causes vomiting, inappetence, abdominal pain, and anemia secondary to gastric bleeding (Fig. 7-66). Melena (digested blood in feces) may also be present if the ulceration persists, and significant amounts of blood are lost to the GI system. Gastric ulcers in dogs and cats are generally idiopathic but can occur in those animals with mast cell tumors that stimulate gastric HCl secretion through histamine release and its effect on the surrounding blood vessels or other neoplasia that infiltrate and weaken the gastric wall.

Ulcers are idiopathic in foals. Foals with gastric ulcers may have abdominal pain, bruxism (grinding of the teeth), ptyalism, and gastric reflux and may lie in dorsal recumbency. Gastric ulcers

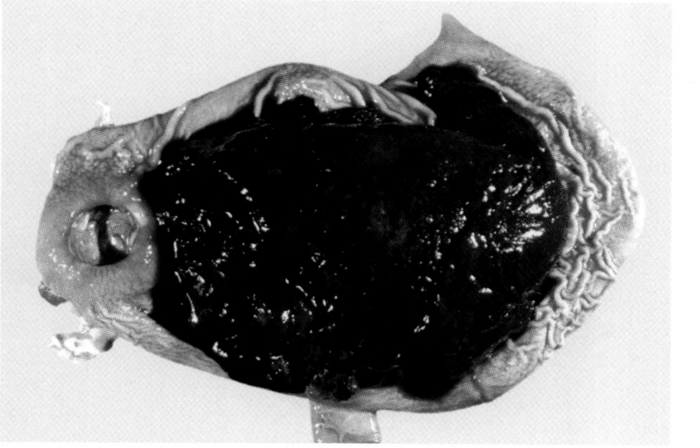

Fig. 7-66 Ulcer, stomach, dog.
The stomach contains a large volume of clotted and unclotted blood from a gastric ulcer (idiopathic) with rounded edges visible in the left side of the photograph. The hemorrhage was so severe that the dog died from exsanguination. (Courtesy Dr. H. Gelberg, College of Veterinary Medicine, Oregon State University.)

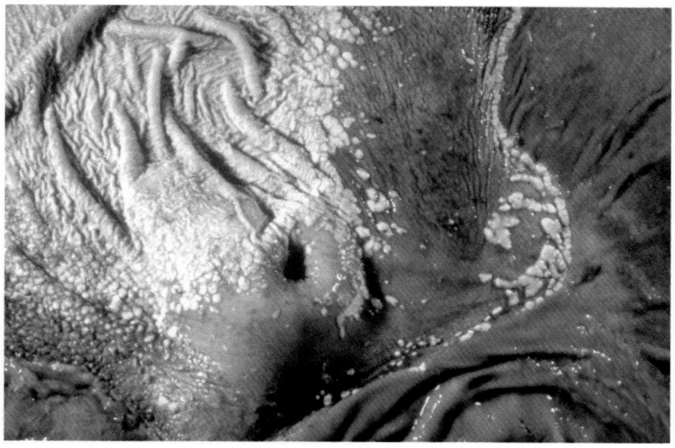

Fig. 7-67 Gastric ulcers, stomach, horse.
Administration of nonsteroidal antiinflammatory drugs (NSAIDs) has caused extensive ulceration of the stratified squamous epithelium of the nonglandular mucosa. The ulceration extends from the cardia *(center)* to the margo plicatus *(right)*. (Courtesy College of Veterinary Medicine, Cornell University.)

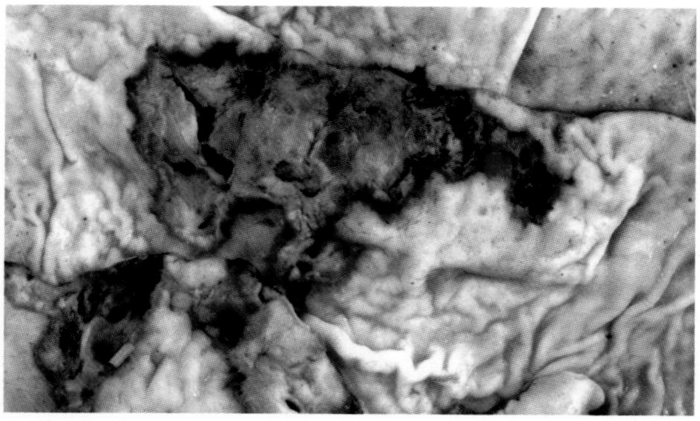

Fig. 7-68 Ulcers, abomasum, cow.
The ulcers consist of a central area of necrosis surrounded by an outer red margin characteristic of active hyperemia and inflammation. The discrete rounded outline of these ulcers suggests that they are infarcts, possibly from vasculitis and thrombosis caused by angioinvasive fungi. (Courtesy Dr. H. Gelberg, College of Veterinary Medicine, Oregon State University.)

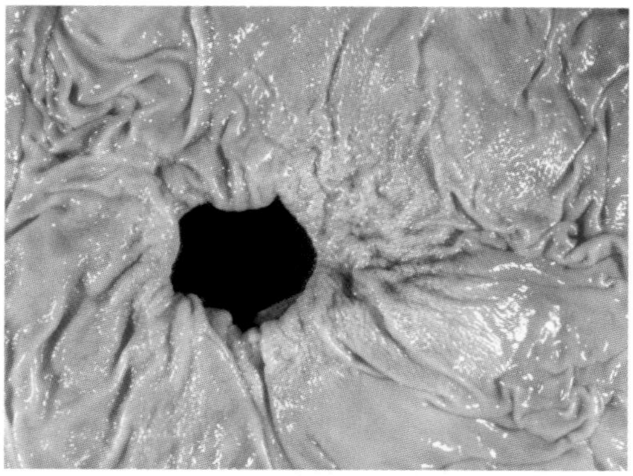

Fig. 7-69 Perforating ulcer, abomasum, cow.
The rounded borders of the ulcer indicate an attempt at repair and therefore chronicity. Death was due to peritonitis. (Courtesy Dr. H. Gelberg, College of Veterinary Medicine, Oregon State University.)

associated with administration of NSAIDs are common in horses and to a lesser extent in other species (Fig. 7-67). Equine gastric ulcer syndrome occurs in 40% to 90% of competitive and performance horses, with the most severe ulcers occurring in those animals that are worked the hardest. More than one-third of horses used less strenuously develop mild ulcers.

Cattle with abomasal ulcers have partial or complete anorexia, decreased milk production, palpable discomfort on pressure applied to the right xiphoid area, and melena. In any species, the vomiting of coffee grounds–like material (hematemesis) or passage of melena is highly suggestive of gastric ulcer disease. Abomasal ulcers of ruminants vary in significance from subclinical to fatal (Figs. 7-68 and 7-69). In calves, ulcers are associated with dietary changes or mechanical irritation of the abomasum by roughage. Dietary changes involve substitution of roughage for milk or milk replacer, together with the associated stress. In dairy cattle, ulcers are associated with heavy grain feeding (lactic acidosis) at the time of parturition, displacement of the abomasum, BVD, impaction, torsion, and gastric lymphoma. Because cattle have an effective omentum that seals abomasal ulcers, they may live for a long time unless a large perforation occurs, resulting in septic peritonitis.

In pigs, gastric ulcers are common and occur in penned pigs fed finely ground grain. These ulcers always are limited to the stratified squamous epithelium of the esophageal portion of the gastric mucosa that surrounds the cardia (Fig. 7-70). Death can result from exsanguination into the gastric lumen. Evidence suggests that a high-carbohydrate diet is not sufficient alone to produce erosions and ulcers but rather that the appropriate diet in combination with fermentative commensal bacteria, such as *Lactobacillus* and *Bacillus* spp., produces lesions. Lesions progress from parakeratosis to hyperkeratosis through keratolysis to erosive gastritis or perforation of the stomach

Miscellaneous Diseases and Conditions

Uremic gastritis occurs most frequently in carnivores as a result of chronic renal disease (Fig. 7-71; also see Fig. 1-54, Fig. 11-28, and Fig. 11-29). In ungulates, it is a rare event and is usually secondary to obstructive kidney disease (postrenal uremia). Uremic gastritis is characterized by mineralization of the glands, vessels, and lamina propria of the gastric mucosa and sometimes results in ulcer formation.

Amyloidosis occasionally is present in the stomach concomitant with systemic amyloid infiltrates. Generalized amyloid A (AA)

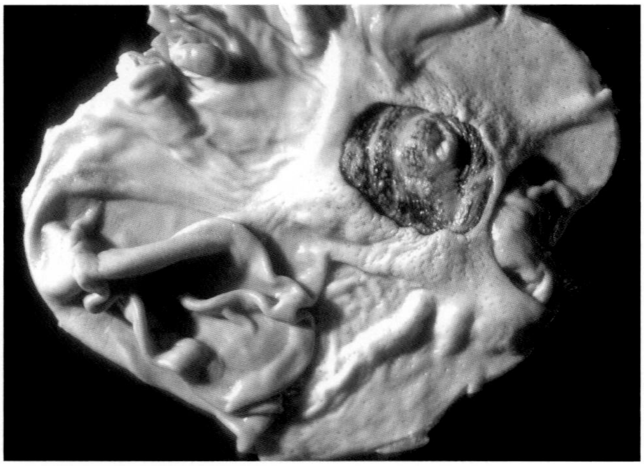

Fig. 7-70 Gastric ulcer (pars esophagea), stomach, pig.
This type of gastric ulcer occurs exclusively in pigs and most commonly in confined growing pigs. The lesion is limited to the stratified squamous epithelium surrounding the cardia (pars esophagea). Ulcers in this location characteristically have a multifactorial cause, including the ingestion of finely ground grain or pelleted feed (possibly deficient in vitamin E), fermentation of sugars in the feed, and stress of confinement rearing. These ulcers frequently bleed and can cause exsanguination. (Courtesy Dr. M.D. McGavin, College of Veterinary Medicine, University of Tennessee.)

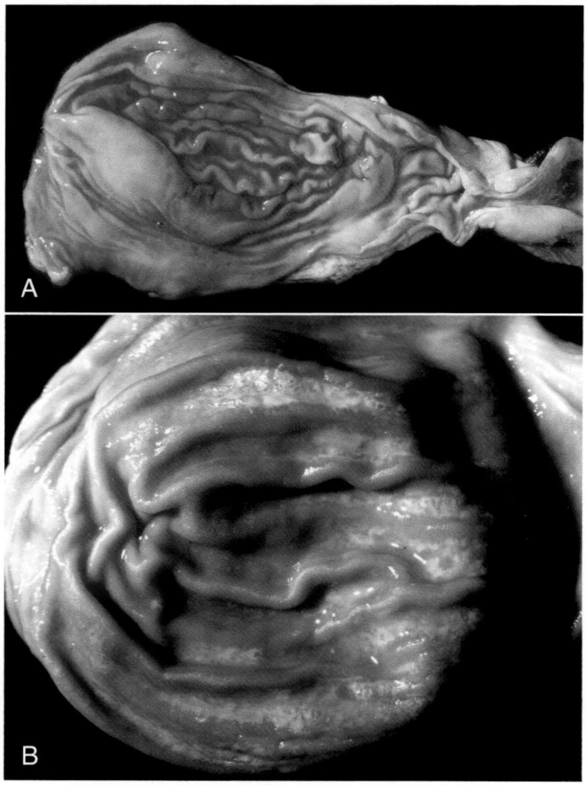

Fig. 7-71 Uremic gastropathy (also called uremic gastritis), stomach, cat.
A, The major lesion is congestion and edema of the gastric mucosa caused by injury to capillaries within the lamina propria associated with elevated concentrations of nitrogen-derived metabolic waste products in the systemic circulation from kidney failure. **B,** With chronicity, there is mineralization of the gastric mucosa, visible as fine white stippling and lines in the mucosa. (**A** courtesy Dr. C.S. Patton, College of Veterinary Medicine, University of Tennessee. **B** courtesy Dr. M.D. McGavin, College of Veterinary Medicine, University of Tennessee.)

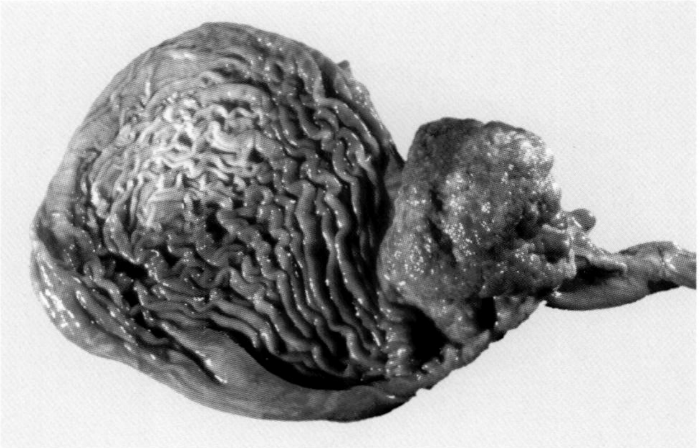

Fig. 7-72 Giant hypertrophic pyloric gastropathy, stomach, dog.
The mass of hyperplastic glandular tissue at the pylorus could be mistaken for a neoplasm. (Courtesy Dr. H. Gelberg, College of Veterinary Medicine, Oregon State University.)

amyloidosis with gastric deposits of amyloid has been reported in bats, Siamese and Abyssinian cats, goats, rhesus monkeys, sheep, and Siberian tigers.

Pyloric stenosis can be anatomic or physiologic because of an inability of the pyloric sphincter to function properly. This condition may be congenital or acquired. This lesion occurs most often in dogs (particularly brachycephalic breeds), Siamese cats, horses, and humans. Congenital pyloric stenoses may be hereditary, at least in humans. Pyloric stenosis is often first recognized in recently weaned animals by projectile vomiting, retention of gastric contents, gastromegaly, and the presence of strong gastric peristaltic waves (Web Fig. 7-12). Pyloric muscular hypertrophy, variable submucosal edema, vascular ectasia, and degeneration of myenteric ganglion cells (dysautonomia) may be identified histologically in some cases. Functional pyloric stenosis can be a feature of vagus indigestion of ruminants. In general, the many causes of pyloric stenosis are not well understood.

Giant hypertrophic pyloric gastropathy, not to be confused with giant hypertrophic gastropathy of basenjis and other dogs, is an idiopathic condition seen most often in older small breed dogs. To the uninitiated, the gross and microscopic features of this pyloric lesion strongly imitate those of carcinoma (Fig. 7-72). Microscopically, there is notable foveolar and glandular hyperplasia with variable hypertrophy of pyloric smooth muscle, small mucosal erosions, and ulcerations. There is usually a lymphoplasmacytic infiltrate of variable degree in the lamina propria.

Parasites

Horses

Many parasites cause disease of the stomach, especially in ungulates. Modern anthelmintics have made these diseases relatively easy to prevent and control both in individual animals and in herds.

Equine bots, *Gasterophilus intestinalis* and *Gasterophilus nasalis*, are commonly seen in animals on inadequate deworming regimens (Fig. 7-73). Both species migrate in the tissues of the oral cavity and often reside in infected spaces adjacent to teeth. *Gasterophilus intestinalis* colonizes the stratified portion of the stomach. The adult fly lays eggs on the hairs of the distal limbs of the horse. *Gasterophilus nasalis* lays its eggs around the nose of the horse. The larvae hatch after being moistened and warmed by licking. They are swallowed and live in the glandular stomach and duodenum. Both species attach to the mucosa via their anterior pincers. The larvae pass in the feces, pupate, and develop into flies.

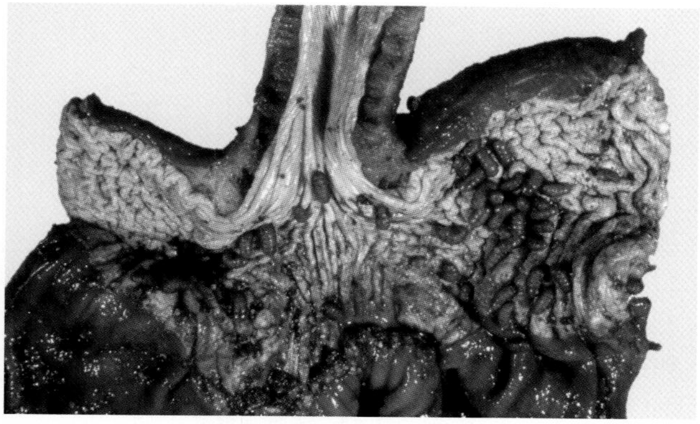

Fig. 7-73 Gasterophiliasis, stomach, horse.
Fly larvae (bots) of *Gasterophilus intestinalis* are attached to the epithelium of the nonglandular portion of the stomach. Note the muscular hypertrophy of the distal esophagus. Although not shown in this illustration, *Gasterophilus nasalis,* another similar equine gastric parasite, attaches to the epithelium of the glandular portion of the stomach. (Courtesy Dr. H. Gelberg, College of Veterinary Medicine, Oregon State University.)

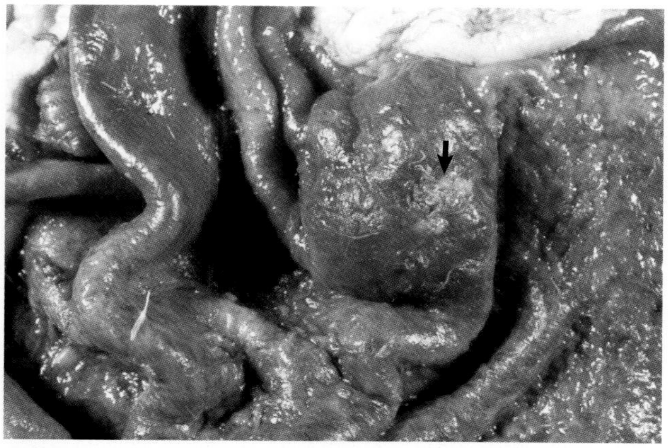

Fig. 7-74 Focal granulomatous gastritis, draschia brood pouch, stomach, horse.
A large parasitic brood pouch is present in the glandular mucosa adjacent to the margo plicatus *(right center of illustration).* Nematodes have been squeezed from the pouch and are visible on the surface *(arrow).* Histologically, the mucosa is expanded by focal granulomatous inflammation containing clusters of adult *Draschia megastoma.* (Courtesy Dr. H. Gelberg, College of Veterinary Medicine, Oregon State University.)

Draschia megastoma is found in "brood pouches" in the glandular mucosa adjacent to the margo plicatus (Fig. 7-74). Infection is sometimes referred to as *habronemiasis,* based on antiquated taxonomic nomenclature in which these nematodes were classified as *Habronema* spp. Eggs produced in the cysts are extruded through a pore in the brood pouch to the gastric lumen. The eggs pass out with the feces and are consumed by fly larvae that are the intermediate hosts. Both *Draschia* and *Gasterophilus* spp. can cause gastric ulcers. Considering their location and means of survival in the stomach, it is remarkable that they do not cause serious damage more often.

Ruminants (Cattle, Sheep, and Goats)

Haemonchus contortus, known as the *barber pole worm,* is relatively common in ruminant abomasums. The common name of this parasite is related to the macroscopically visible entwining of the blood-filled intestine and white uterus in the female worm (Fig. 7-75).

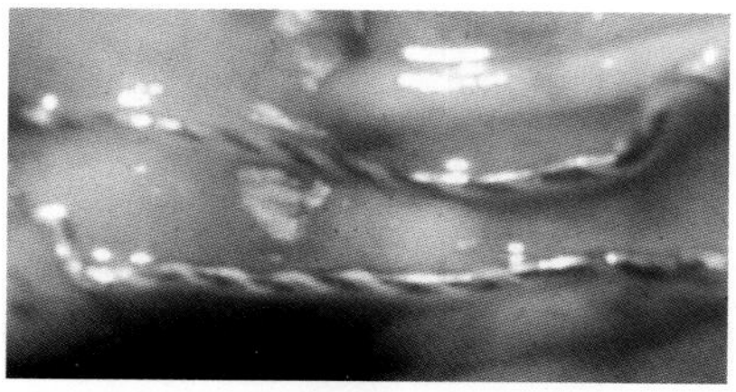

Fig. 7-75 *Haemonchus contortus*, abomasum, sheep.
The white spiral reproductive tract wrapped around the blood-filled intestine is responsible for the striped appearance, hence the common name "barber's pole worm." (Courtesy Dr. H. Gelberg, College of Veterinary Medicine, Oregon State University.)

Hyperinfested pastures containing numerous third-stage larvae are the source of infection. Lambs are particularly at risk. Larvae on grasses are ingested by the host and enter the abomasum, where they may lie dormant within the gastric glands. After development to adults, they exit to the abomasal surface and attach via a buccal tooth. Eggs pass in the feces, completing the life cycle. *Haemonchus* are blood feeders and can cause severe anemia, hypoproteinemia, and resultant edema. This edema is characteristically present in the intermandibular space, resulting in a physical resemblance to a bottle ("bottle jaw"). As with any process resulting in anemia and hypoproteinemia, there are pale mucous membranes, stunting, and diarrhea. Diagnosis is by fecal egg counts and at necropsy, by semiquantification of abomasal parasite load along with the attendant lesions of anemia and hypoproteinemia. At necropsy, the carcass is pale and has generalized edema and fluid in all body cavities secondary to hypoproteinemia. Abomasal contents are fluid and discolored from free blood. Foci of mucosal hemorrhage are present at sites of worm attachment.

In temperate climates, ostertagiosis is considered the most important parasitic disease in cattle *(Ostertagia ostertagia)* and small ruminants *(Ostertagia circumcincta)*. Affected animals are unthrifty. *Ostertagia* spp. have a direct life cycle similar to that of *Haemonchus* spp. The nematodes are smaller than those of *Haemonchus* and are uniformly brown. Third-, fourth-, and fifth-stage larvae reside in the abomasal gastric glands. *Ostertagia* spp. are often present along with *Trichostrongylus* spp. in other GI locations. Intercurrent GI parasitism with other trichostrongyles has an additive effect on the clinical signs. Unthriftiness, lack of proper mentation, diarrhea, hypoproteinemia, and ventral edema may result. The multinodular appearance of the abomasum of heavily infested animals resembles Morocco leather (Fig. 7-76). This cobblestone appearance is due to enlargement of the gastric glands because of mucous cell hyperplasia and hyperplasia of lymphoid nodules in the abomasal submucosa elevating the overlying mucosa. Abomasitis produced by *Ostertagia* spp. is characterized by an infiltration of mononuclear inflammatory cells and eosinophils in the lamina propria. There are also increased numbers of globule leukocytes, a decrease in the number of parietal and chief cells, and hyperplasia of abomasal mucous cells. Differential diagnoses include lymphoma.

Abomasal coccidiosis has been reported in a sheep. Mucosal lesions are nodular and hemorrhagic with hyperplasia of mucous neck cells, parietal cell atrophy, and lymphoplasmacytic fibrosis of the lamina propria associated with giant schizonts of uncertain taxonomy.

Pigs

Hyostrongylus rubidus of pigs is a gastric parasite that causes a thickening of the mucosa, with mucus accumulation and mucous cell hyperplasia and inflammation of the lamina propria by

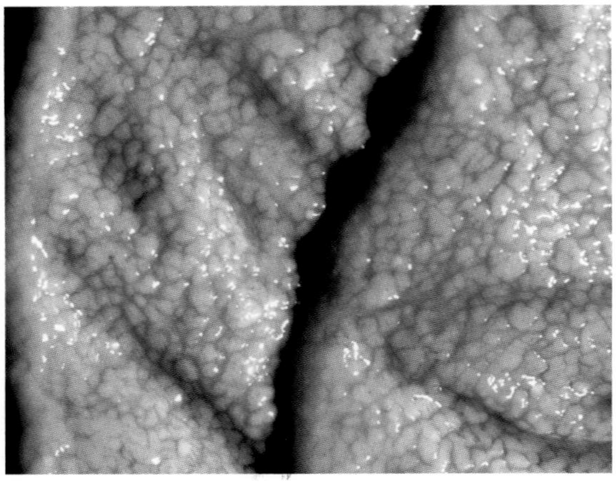

Fig. 7-76 Ostertagiosis, abomasum, cow.
The granular Moroccan leather appearance of the abomasal mucosa is characteristic of chronic ostertagiosis and is due to epithelial hyperplasia of the gastric glands, which may also contain ostertagia larvae. (Courtesy Dr. M.D. McGavin, College of Veterinary Medicine, University of Tennessee.)

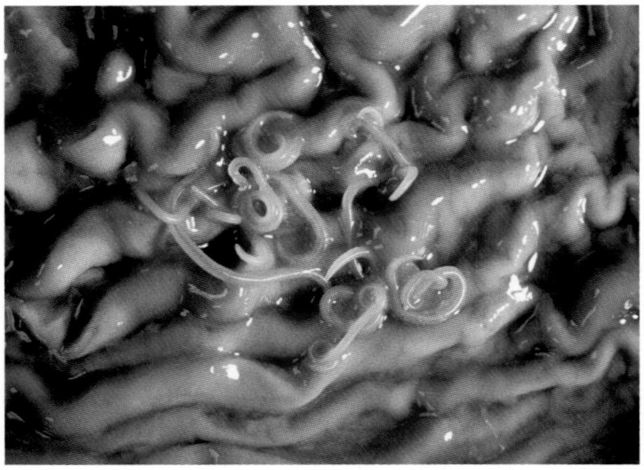

Fig. 7-77 Physalopteriasis, stomach, dog.
Stout coiled nematodes, *Physaloptera canis* are firmly attached to the gastric mucosa by dentate pseudolabia. (Courtesy Dr. M.D. McGavin, College of Veterinary Medicine, University of Tennessee.)

lymphocytes, plasma cells, and eosinophils. The parasite is threadlike and red. Clinically, hyostrongylosis is associated with the "thin sow syndrome." Grossly, the gastric mucosa is thickened, catarrhal, and somewhat cobblestone, similar to ostertagiosis of ruminants. Microscopically, there is mucous metaplasia of parasitized and adjacent gastric glands. Submucosal lymphoid follicles develop in chronic infections.

Carnivores (Dogs and Cats)

Several genera of nematodes, principally *Ollulanus, Gnathostoma, and Cylicospirura,* cause gastritis in dogs and cats, but these infections are rare.

Physaloptera spp. are often thought of as gastric parasites of carnivores because they are sometimes found in the stomach on endoscopic examination or at necropsy. They are occasionally responsible for vomiting. They appear similar to ascarids but generally attach by anterior hooks to the proximal duodenal mucosa at the gastric valve (Fig. 7-77). Intermediate hosts are coprophagous beetles.

Neoplasia

Gastric neoplasia, although uncommon, manifests in different ways in domestic animals. Leiomyoma and more rarely leiomyosarcoma arise from the tunica muscularis (Fig. 7-78). Lymphoma can be primary, metastatic, or multicentric in origin (Figs. 7-79 and 7-80; also see Fig. 13-85). In cattle, lymphoma is often caused by the bovine leukemia virus and has a predilection for the abomasum and the right atrium and uterus (Fig. 7-81). Squamous cell carcinoma of the stratified squamous (esophageal) portion of the stomach is relatively common in the horse (Fig. 7-82). Glandular neoplasms, adenomas, and adenocarcinomas occur in all species but are seen most often in dogs and cats. Dogs and rarely cats occasionally develop gastric mast cell tumors.

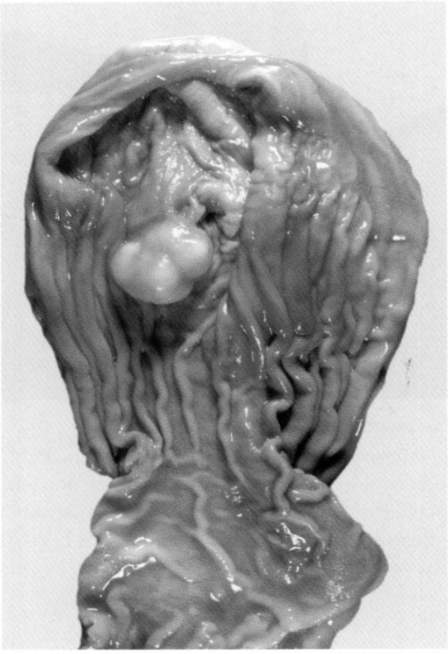

Fig. 7-78 Leiomyoma, stomach, dog.
This tumor arose from smooth muscle in the tunica muscularis and is covered by intact mucosa. (Courtesy Dr. H. Gelberg, College of Veterinary Medicine, Oregon State University.)

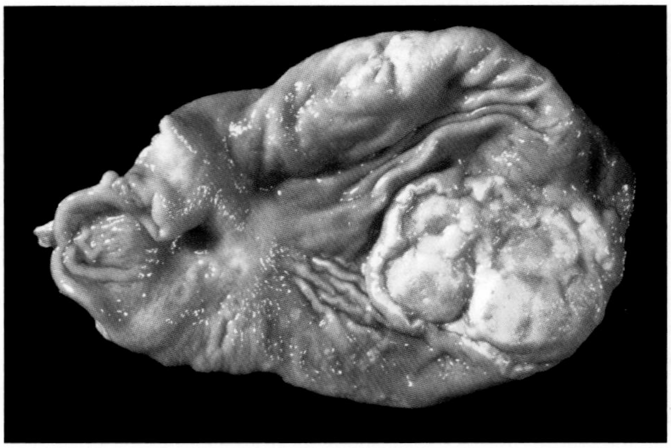

Fig. 7-79 Lymphoma, stomach, cat.
A large expansile mass is present in the submucosa of the stomach *(top edge)* and is covered by an intact mucosal epithelium. Note the other lymphomatous mass, which is ulcerated *(lower right).* This latter lesion is somewhat atypical of this disease, because ulceration is uncommon and occurs in late-stage disease when the mass is quite large and protrudes into the gastric lumen. In most cases of gastric lymphoma, the mucosal epithelium is intact and not ulcerated. (Courtesy Dr. C.S. Patton, College of Veterinary Medicine, University of Tennessee.)

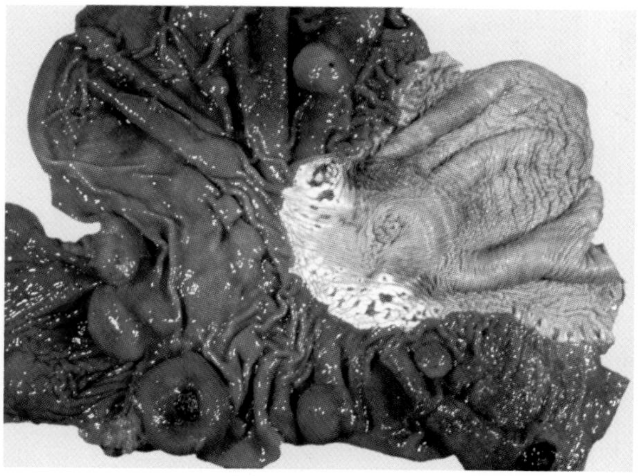

Fig. 7-80 **Lymphoma, stomach, horse.**
Large smooth-surfaced submucosal nodules, two of which have a central hemorrhagic ulcer, are present in the glandular portion of the stomach. Ulcers in the stratified squamous portion of the stomach are sites of *Gastrophilus intestinalis* attachment. (Courtesy Dr. H. Gelberg, College of Veterinary Medicine, Oregon State University.)

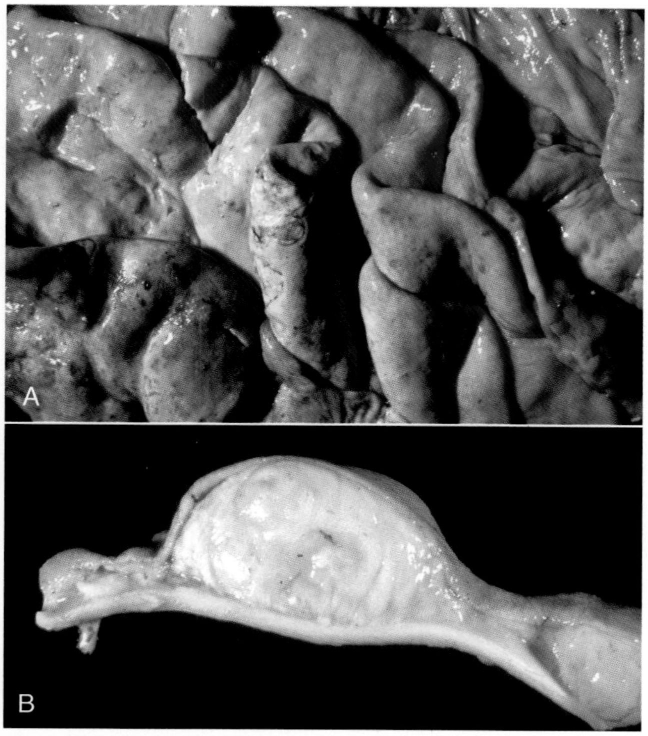

Fig. 7-81 **Lymphoma, abomasum, cow.**
A, Mucosal surface of abomasal folds. Note the folds are thickened and have a pale white-pink color resulting from the infiltration of neoplastic lymphocytes. Overlying mucosae are eroded and ulcerated. **B,** Transverse section. This cross-section demonstrates a white, space-occupying submucosal mass. The intact mucosa is located at the top of the specimen. (**A** courtesy Dr. M.D. McGavin, College of Veterinary Medicine, University of Tennessee. **B** courtesy Dr. H. Gelberg, College of Veterinary Medicine, Oregon State University.)

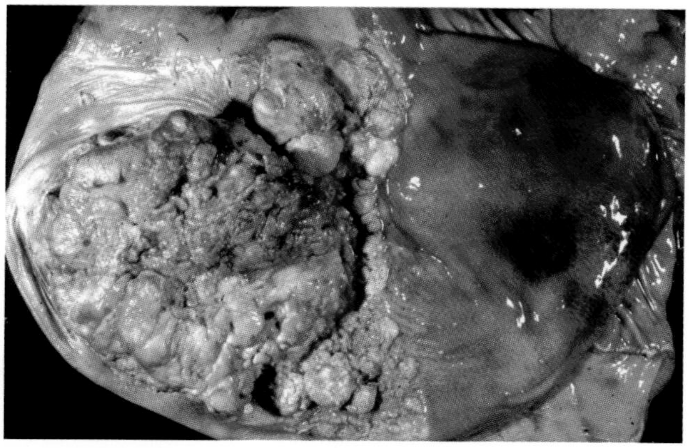

Fig. 7-82 **Squamous cell carcinoma, stomach, horse.**
A large proliferative, ulcerative mass has arisen from the epithelium of the nonglandular (squamous) mucosa of the stomach. (Courtesy Dr. A. Paulman, College of Veterinary Medicine, University of Illinois.)

INTESTINE

The intestines might be thought of as a tube within the body cavity that carries material (ingesta) through the body. The overall anatomic and histologic organization of this digestive tube is illustrated in Fig. 7-83. By the action of enzymes, resident flora, and added secretions from the liver and pancreas, ingesta are broken down, nutrients are absorbed into the body, and waste products are excreted. To perform these functions, the intestine needs a very large surface area, which is accomplished by the following three means:

1. Coiling the intestine in the abdomen.
2. Numerous intestinal folds that contain villi that notably increase the number of cells contacting the ingesta (Fig. 7-84).
3. Each enterocyte has a microvillous border, further increasing the surface area available for digestive and absorptive processes.

Herbivores have longer intestines than carnivores or omnivores and need a fermentation vat, either the rumen or cecum, to digest cellulose. Within the smooth muscle layers and villi are the neural network of the enteric nervous system.

Structure and Function

The intestinal mucosa is composed of three layers—a single-cell-thick layer of epithelial cells lining the intestinal lumen, mesenchymal cells of the lamina propria, and the muscularis mucosa. Damage to any of these structures can result in digestive dysfunction and resultant diarrhea.

These cells function as a selectively permeable barrier allowing nutrient, electrolyte, and water absorption, while excluding pathogens, toxins, and other antigens. An understanding of these cell types and their functional roles in digestion and absorption is important in understanding the mechanisms of intestinal disease. Similarly, an understanding of the biology of these cell types is important in predicting clinical outcomes and designing therapeutic strategies for treating intestinal disease.

Epithelial Cells

There are six major types of polarized epithelial cells lining the intestine. These epithelial cells are enterocytes, undifferentiated or crypt epithelial cells, goblet cells, Paneth cells, enterochromaffin (neuroendocrine, argentaffin) cells, and microfold (M) cells (Fig. 7-85).

Enterocytes are tall and columnar with luminal microvilli. They contain a surface glycocalyx that houses the digestive and absorptive enzymes. The mature cells do not proliferate, but they provide

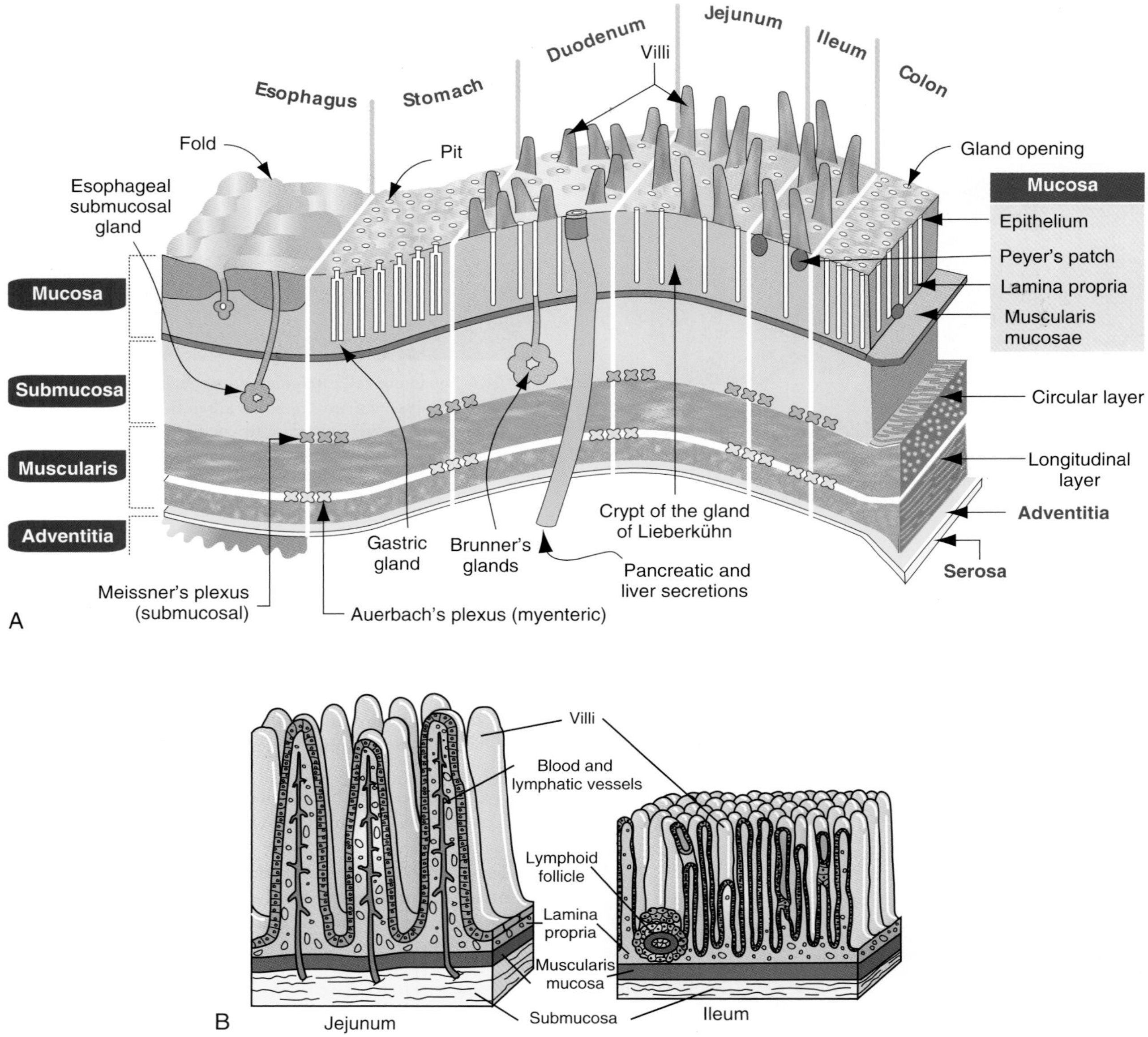

Fig. 7-83 Schematic diagram of the anatomic and histologic organization of the digestive tube. **A,** Entire digestive tube. **B,** Higher magnification of the jejunum and ileum. (**A** from Kierzenbaum AL: *Histology and cell biology: an introduction to pathology,* St Louis, 2002, Mosby.)

feedback inhibition of mitosis to the crypt cells by chalones. The cells are attached to each other by tight junctions composed of more than 40 proteins anchored to actin filaments, the most predominant of which are occludin, junctional adhesion molecules, and claudins. Many nutrients are absorbed through the lateral intercellular spaces between cells. Enterocytes move up the crypt and intestinal villus to the extrusion zone at the villus tip, where effete enterocytes are discarded into the fecal mass by an apoptotic mechanism called *anoikis.* The turnover rate for enterocytes is the most rapid of any fixed-cell population in the body. In neonatal pigs, for example, the turnover rate is 7 to 10 days. In 3-week-old pigs that have achieved a mature or climax flora, that rate accelerates to 2 to 3 days.

Undifferentiated crypt epithelial cells have little or no digestive capability. They are the progenitor cells that replace all of the other epithelial cell types. They have short, sparse microvilli. Crypt cells are the source of secretory component that acts as a receptor for IgA and IgM produced by plasmacytes in the intestinal lamina propria. The migration rate of crypt cells up the villus depends on several factors, one of which is an adaptation to gut microflora. In germ-free or gnotobiotic animals, the enterocyte replacement rate is similar to that of the neonate. Crypt cells are a source of chloride ion secretion into the intestinal lumen.

Goblet cells secrete mucus. They occur in both villous and crypt regions. Their numbers tend to increase aborally throughout the length of the intestine.

Paneth cells are located near the crypt base in some species, notably primates, horses, and rodents. It is not certain if Paneth cells are present in swine. Unlike all the other cells of the intestinal surface, these cells migrate toward the crypts rather than the villus tips. Paneth cells are considered to have both secretory and phagocytic functions. They produce cryptdin and lysins. These substances are toxic to bacteria and probably protect the proliferating crypt cells from infection. Paneth cells also act in a paracrine manner by opening anion channels in enterocytes causing chloride-secretion from crypt enterocytes. It has been suggested that Paneth cells play a role in elimination of heavy metals because they are selectively damaged by methylmercury. Collectively, Paneth cells comprise a cellular mass similar to that of the pancreas.

Enteroendocrine cells are also known as *enterochromaffin cells* and *argentaffin cells* because of their affinity for silver stains. They occur primarily in the crypts and produce serotonin, glucoinsulotropic peptide, catecholamines, gastrin, somatostatin, serotonin, cholecystokinin, secretin, bombesin, enteroglucagon, and likely others in response to chemical and mechanical stimuli. They secrete these products into the tissue rather than the gut lumen and thus are truly endocrine. Serotonin for example, activates both the intrinsic and extrinsic primary afferent neurons initiating peristalsis and secretory reflexes that are transmitted to the central nervous system (CNS). Occasionally, enteroendocrine cells form neoplasms called *carcinoids*.

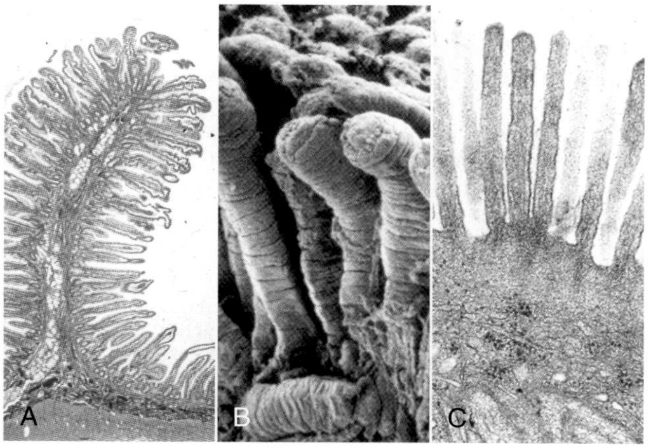

Fig. 7-84 Organization of the intestine.
The digestive and absorptive surfaces of the intestine are markedly increased by the presence of villi and microvilli on the enterocytes. **A,** Intestinal villus. Villus epithelial cells are present on a basement membrane (not seen) on a core of lamina propria. H&E stain. **B,** Small intestine, intestinal villi, scanning electron microscopy. Carbon sputter coat. **C,** Enterocyte microvilli. TEM. Uranyl acetate and lead citrate stain. (From Damjanov I, Linder J: *Anderson's pathology,* ed 10, St Louis, 1996, Mosby.)

M cells are so named because they have a microfolded or membranous surface. They form the dome epithelium that covers the gut-associated lymphoid tissue (GALT). They serve important functions in the uptake of protein and peptide antigens from the intestinal lumen and in the transport of these undigested antigens to the GALT where they are taken up by local dendritic cells and macrophages. Similarly, M cells also serve as a portal of entry for some pathogens, including bacteria, such as *Salmonella, Yersinia,* and *Rhodococcus* spp., and some viruses, such as BVD virus.

Mesenchymal Cells

Mesenchymal cells reside in the lamina propria. They arise from primitive mesenchyme rather than from ectoderm or endoderm. Their numbers increase with exposure to antigen, although there is a resident population of these cells in normal animals.

The intestinal lymphoid tissue is 25% of the body's lymphoid mass (Fig. 7-86) and consists of those in the lamina propria and the GALT. This volume is larger than that of the spleen. In spite of the fact that the average person ingests 700 tons of antigens in a lifetime, the gut is adept at not responding to these food antigens. Laminal propria lymphocytes also play a role in intestinal crypt cell differentiation. Data are beginning to accumulate identifying the different effector and regulatory T lymphocyte types in the lamina propria and the functional organization of the GALT (Fig. 7-87).

Neutrophils are transient within the lamina propria of the intestine. Neutrophils are short-lived in the blood and tissues; their normal route of removal from the body is to migrate through the wall of the alimentary tract to the lumen and be digested or excreted from the body via feces.

Eosinophils, when present in the intestinal lamina propria and submucosa, indicate a hypersensitivity reaction, often to food antigens or parasites.

Mast cells comprise 2% to 3% of the cells of the lamina propria and under normal conditions help regulate the intestinal epithelial barrier. They help control blood flow and coagulation, smooth muscle contraction, stimulation of the enteric nervous system, and

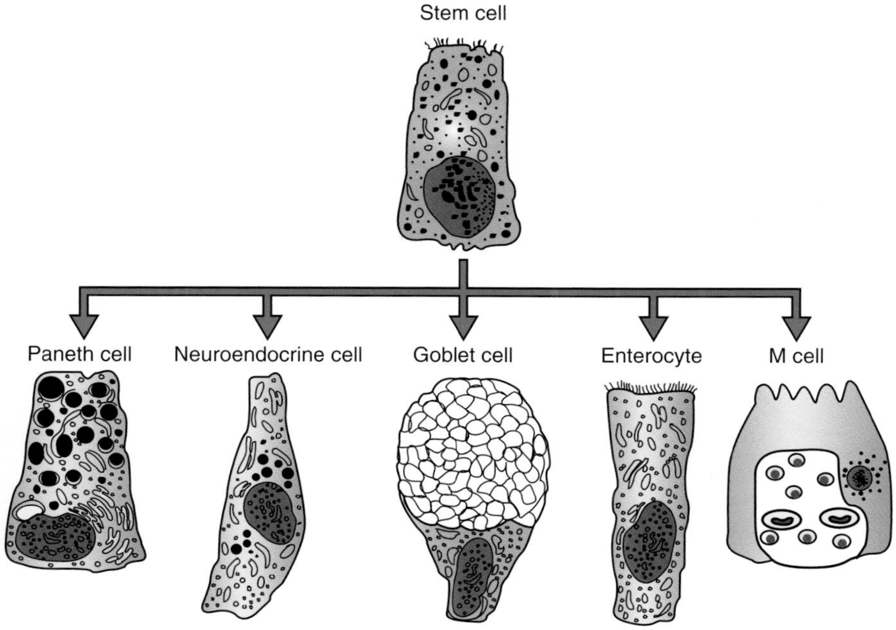

Fig. 7-85 Schematic illustration of the epithelial cell types of the small intestine.
Progenitor cells, located in the intestinal crypts, give rise to all other epithelial cell types lining the crypt and covering the villi. (From Damjanov I, Linder J: *Anderson's pathology,* ed 10, St Louis, 1996, Mosby.)

peristalsis. They also help regulate acid, electrolyte, and mucus production by enterocytes. They recognize parasites and microorganisms through antibody-dependent mechanisms and receptor recognition. Mast cells release proinflammatory mediators and attract inflammatory cells through cytokine release that acts in a paracrine manner.

Globule leukocytes are large granular lymphocytes that are interepithelial or within the lamina propria. They are found in all species and occasionally form neoplasms, most notably in the cat. The normal function of these cells is unknown.

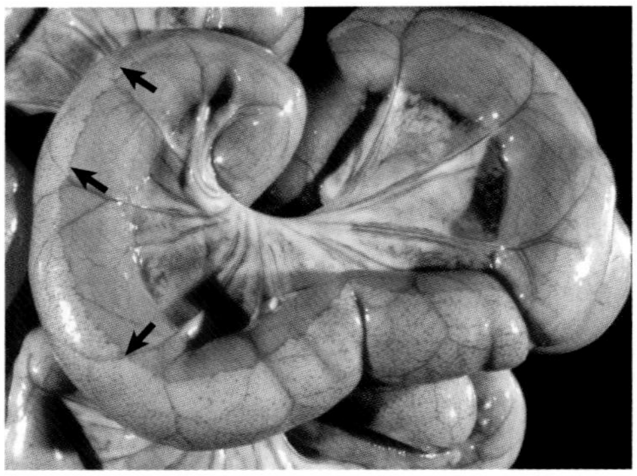

Fig. 7-86 Normal gut-associated lymphoid tissue (GALT), intestine, pig.
The lymphoid tissue on the antimesenteric surface of the intestine is outlined by arrows and makes up one quarter of the animal's total lymphoid mass. (Courtesy Dr. H. Gelberg, College of Veterinary Medicine, Oregon State University.)

Defense Mechanisms

Defense mechanisms of the intestinal tract are diverse. They include indigenous (nonpathogenic) bacterial flora, intestinal and extraintestinal secretions, gastric acidity, intestinal motility, epithelial cell turnover, bile salts, immunologic mechanisms, and although a secondary mechanism, the Kupffer cells of the liver.

Secretions of the oral cavity, saliva, and intestine, called mucins, inhibit the adherence of organisms to the mucosa of the alimentary system. In addition to physically trapping pathogens, intestinal mucus serves to cover glycolipid and glycoprotein receptors on the surface of enterocytes (unstirred layer), thus preventing pathogen attachment and damage by toxins. Mucins are viscous, thus aid in protecting the epithelium from the shear forces of particulates driven against them by peristaltic waves. Because they are extensively glycosylated, mucins can cross-link and trap bacteria, making them more amenable to clearance by passage through the alimentary system.

Normal gastric acidity kills many organisms before they have the chance to reach the small intestine. Very young animals are achlorhydric, thus they may be more susceptible to some organisms such as pathogenic *Escherichia coli.* Helical bacteria in the stomach are the single greatest cause of gastric ulcers in humans. Although similar organisms occur in the stomachs of domestic animals, particularly carnivores, their role in gastritis of animals is less certain. Normal gastric acidity apparently does not kill all potentially pathogenic bacteria (helical bacteria) in the stomach and proximal small intestine of domestic animals.

Indigenous (nonpathogenic) bacterial flora (microbiota) competitively bind to putative attachment sites on the enterocytes, thus

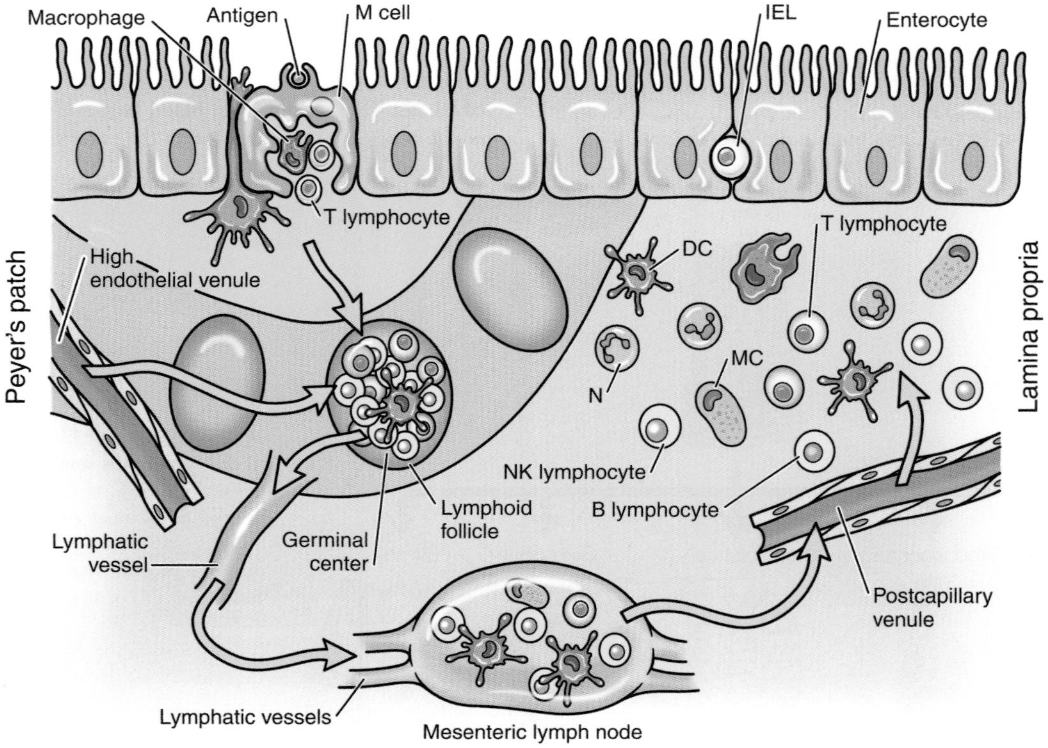

Fig. 7-87 Schematic illustration of GALT.
DC, Dendritic cell; *IEL,* intraepithelial lymphocyte; *M,* microfold cell; *MC,* mast cell; *N,* neutrophil. (Adapted from Cominelli F, Arseneau KO, Blumberg RS, et al: The mucosal immune system and gastrointestinal inflammation. In Yamata T, editor: *Textbook of gastroenterology,* ed 5, West Sussex, UK, 2009, Wiley-Blackwell.)

preempting pathogen attachment. These prokaryotic symbionts co-evolved with their hosts and are an integral part of homeostatic mechanisms. Killing of these bacteria through the use of antibiotics sometimes allows pathogens to colonize the intestine and produce disease. Thus gnotobiotic animals are more susceptible to infection. The microbiome enhances the host's genome in contributing to normal physiology and disease resistance and susceptibility. Bacteria in the intestine outnumber the total somatic and germ cells of the body by approximately a factor of ten. Probiotics are "friendly bacteria" that are sometimes used therapeutically or prophylactically in a variety of products and nutraceuticals. These "friendly bacteria" also compete for substrate with pathogens, alter the microenvironmental pH making the growth of competitive bacteria difficult, and produce short chain fatty acids and inhibitory growth substances (bacteriocins) that are toxic to other bacteria. Colicins are bacteriocins produced by *E. coli.* Bacterial growth is also inhibited by lactoferrin and peroxidase from the pancreas and lysozyme and defensins from Paneth cells. Transferrin in serum and lactoferrin produced by enterocytes and neutrophils at sites of infection serve to sequester iron that is necessary for bacterial growth.

Intestinal peristalsis is protective in that loss of motility may lead to bacterial overgrowth in the intestine and increased susceptibility of enterocytes to toxins that are not moved out of the gut. Diarrhea can be in part a defense mechanism that rids the body of bacteria and toxins. Conversely, some bacteria secrete toxins that impair intestinal motility thus allowing pathogens a greater opportunity to attach to enterocytes.

Epithelial cells of the intestine have the greatest turnover rate of any fixed cell population in the body. In effect, this means that pathogens with a life cycle that exceeds that of the enterocytes will likely not be successful because their host cell will slough before the pathogen can reproduce. In addition, experimental evidence indicates that enterocyte microvilli form unilaminar vesicles containing digestive enzymes such as catalase and alkaline phosphatase on their surface. These vesicles are shed into the intestinal lumen where they may interact with the pathogen(s), thus preventing contact of pathogens with enterocytes since these vesicles are passed in the feces.

Bile salts inhibit the growth of many organisms. Kupffer cells of the liver act as a secondary line of defense. Because all the blood from the intestine enters the portal vein and percolates through the hepatic sinusoids, the Kupffer cells are perfectly positioned to phagocytose bacteria and endotoxins with which they come in contact. In pigs, goats, and cattle (artiodactyls), these functions are performed by intravascular pulmonary macrophages.

Secretory IgA and IgM constitute very important mechanisms of humoral immunity and function largely to prevent attachment of pathogens to intestinal epithelium. Crypt epithelial cells produce the secretory component of IgA. IgA functions through adhesion to M cells that regulates transepithelial movement of antigens while masking certain other antigens (Fig. 7-88).

Although in its infancy, research indicates that genetic polymorphisms of the host, including human leukocyte antigen (HLA), likely play a role in disease susceptibility and resistance.

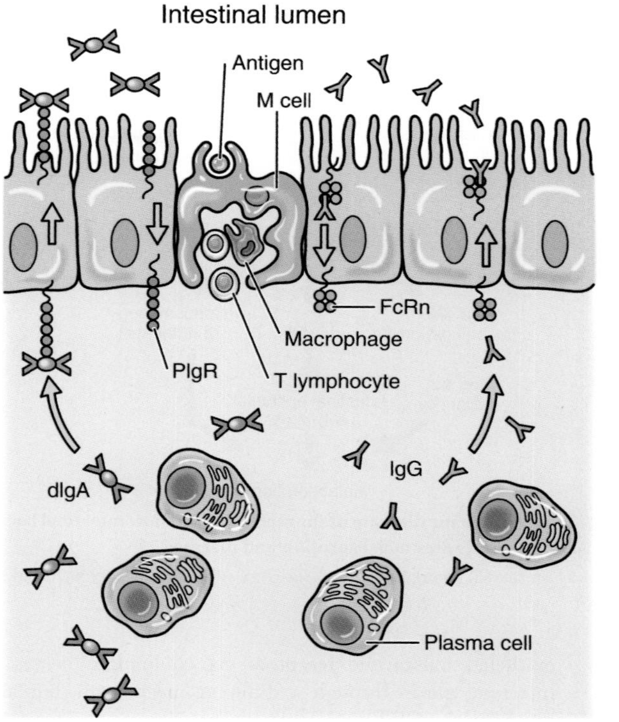

Fig. 7-88 Schematic diagram of immunoglobulin secretion in the intestine.

Dimeric IgA (dIgA), produced by plasma cells via interaction with polymeric IgR (PIgR) is transported across the intestinal epithelium in association with secretory component which is a portion of PIgR secreted into the intestinal lumen. IgG transport is mediated by MHC-I (FcRn). IgG transport is bidirectional, IgA is not. *M,* Microfold cell. (Adapted from Cominelli F, Arseneau KO, Blumberg RS, et al: The mucosal immune system and gastrointestinal inflammation. In Yamata T, editor: *Textbook of gastroenterology,* ed 5, West Sussex, UK, 2009, Wiley-Blackwell.)

Diarrhea

Response to Injury

Diarrhea is defined as secretion of abnormally fluid feces accompanied by an increased volume of feces and an increased frequency of defecation. Pathogens causing diarrhea fall into three major categories: those that induce intestinal secretion, such as enterotoxigenic *E. coli* (ETEC) (noninflammatory or secretory diarrhea); those that induce inflammation, such as *Lawsonia*; and those that are invasive, such as *Salmonella*. To simplify this further, there are two mechanistic "types" of diarrhea; noninflammatory and inflammatory. Noninflammatory diarrheas are produced by organisms that disrupt the absorptive or secretory mechanisms of the enterocytes without destroying the cells. Usually, but not always, noninflammatory diarrheas affect the more proximal portions of the bowel (ETEC, rotavirus, or *Cryptosporidium parvum*). Inflammatory diarrheas are produced by organisms that produce cytotoxins or are invasive and activate cytokines that initiate inflammatory cascades. The inflammatory diarrheas generally affect the ileum, cecum, or colon (*Salmonella, Brachyspira,* or *Lawsonia*). Combinations of mechanisms are present in specific diseases and are as follows:

- Malabsorption with or without bacterial fermentation leading to osmotic diarrhea. Generally, this is a problem of the small intestine, but secondary colonic malfunctions can occur because of malabsorption of bile salts and fatty acids that stimulate fluid secretion in the large intestine.
- Chloride (Cl^-) hypersecretion by the cystic fibrosis transmembrane regulator (CFTR) of a structurally intact mucosa. CFTR is regulated by kinases, which are dependent on cyclic adenosine monophosphate (cAMP), which acts as second messenger. Prostanoids, bacterial toxins, and protein kinases all increase cAMP, thus increasing Cl^- secretion. Calcium ion (Ca^{2+}) also plays a role in opening Cl^- channels through increases in acetylcholine interaction with

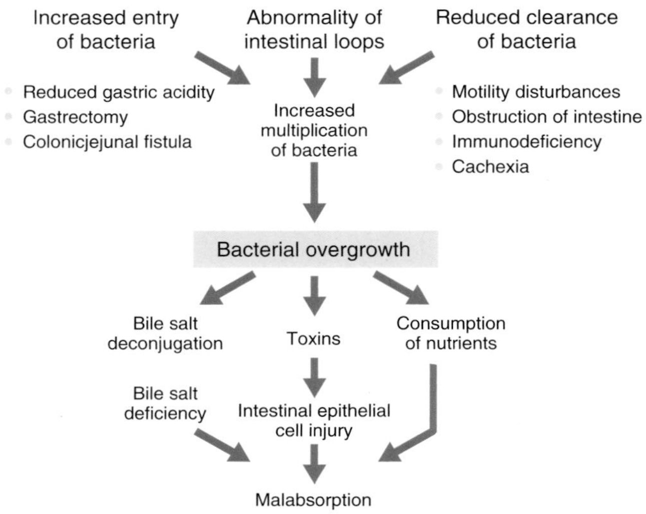

Fig. 7-89 Schematic diagram of the mechanism of how intestinal bacterial overgrowth causes malabsorption and diarrhea.

(From Damjanov I, Linder J: *Anderson's pathology,* ed 10, St Louis, 1996, Mosby.)

epithelial muscarinic receptors via cholinergic nerves in intestinal plexi. Through a different mechanism, but also involving the CFTR, bicarbonate secretion is also increased. This osmotic activity results in a net efflux of fluid and electrolytes independent of permeability changes, absorptive capacity, or exogenously generated osmotic gradients.

- Exudation caused by increased capillary or epithelial permeability (protein-losing enteropathy) by leaky tight junctions between enterocytes.
- Hypermotility generally is involved in diarrhea but usually not as a primary mechanism in domestic animals. Hypermotility is defined as an increased rate, intensity, or frequency of peristalsis. Theoretically, with decreased mucosal contact time, digestion and absorption of nutrients and water should be less efficient. It is suspected that decreased motility in some diseases allows for increased bacterial proliferation (Fig. 7-89). Conversely, some enterotoxins can stimulate intestinal motility. In some motility disorders of humans, such as achalasia, Hirschsprung's disease, inflammatory bowel disease (IBD) and others, there is an alteration in the network of interstitial cells of Cajal within the smooth muscle of the bowel wall. Whether this is a cause or effect of bowel motility disorders is not known.
- Toll-like receptors (TLRs) and their associated molecules produced by enterocytes and leukocytes are very important in the regulation of intestinal inflammation and in the host's response to intestinal pathogens.
- M cells regulate the presentation of antigens to GALT.
- Other factors (prostaglandins, leukotrienes, and platelet-activating factor) act on enteric nerves to induce neurotransmitter-mediated intestinal secretion by crypt cells.
- Cell damage is possibly a consequence of inflammation mediated by T lymphocytes or proteases and oxidants secreted by mast cells. T lymphocytes also may affect epithelial cell maturation, causing villous atrophy and crypt hyperplasia.
- Cell death can result from pathogen invasion into enterocytes, multiplication of the pathogen, and extrusion of the affected enterocytes. These changes lead to notable distortion of villous architecture with a lack of absorptive mature enterocytes accompanied by nutrient malabsorption and osmotic diarrhea.
- Mast cells of the lamina propria are in close association with enteric neurons and the enteric vasculature. They release histamine, prostaglandins, 5HT, and proteolytic enzymes that also play a role in diarrhea production.

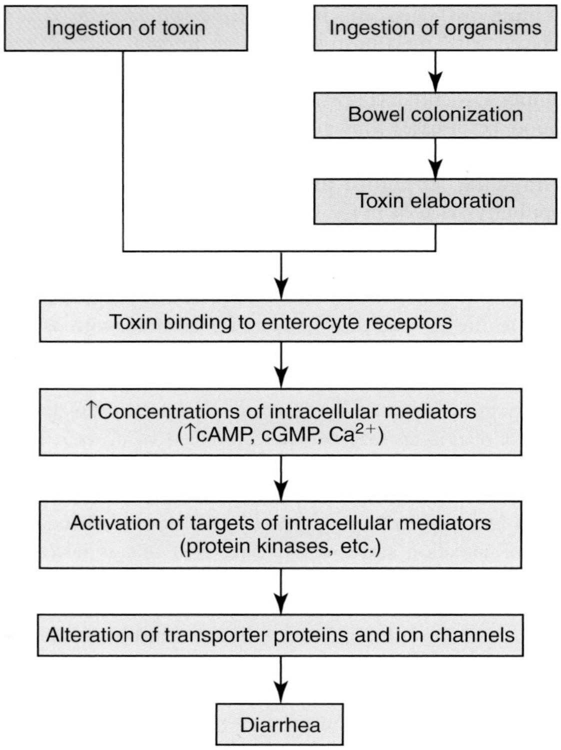

Fig. 7-90 Schematic diagram of the mechanism of action for enterotoxin-mediated bacterial diarrhea.

(Adapted from Cominelli F, Arseneau KO, Blumberg RS, et al: The mucosal immune system and gastrointestinal inflammation. In Yamata T, editor: *Textbook of gastroenterology,* ed 5, West Sussex, UK, 2009, Wiley-Blackwell.)

As might be expected, the pathogenesis of diarrhea is complicated, involving a complex interplay of cells and factors that are currently being elucidated by a variety of molecular techniques. For example, when a pathogen invades or attaches to an enterocyte, the pathogen can release an enterotoxin. This toxin causes the enterocyte to release cytokines, particularly interleukin-8 (IL-8). These cytokines activate resident macrophages and recruit new macrophages into the lamina propria from the blood. The activated leukocytes release soluble factors (histamine, serotonin, and adenosine) that increase intestinal secretion of chloride ions and water and inhibit absorption (Figs. 7-90 and 7-91). Recruitment of inflammatory cells to areas of injury results in release of a chemical soup of cytokines (Fig. 7-92).

Additionally, there are nonintestinal causes of diarrhea that must be considered in addition to diseases of the intestine. Among this group are hyperthyroidism, Addison's disease, pancreatic insufficiency, pancreatitis, chronic renal failure, and others. These diseases are discussed in their respective chapters of this book.

Consequences

Normal feces are 75% water. Diarrheal feces are greater than 85% water. The consequence of excess fluid loss in the feces through

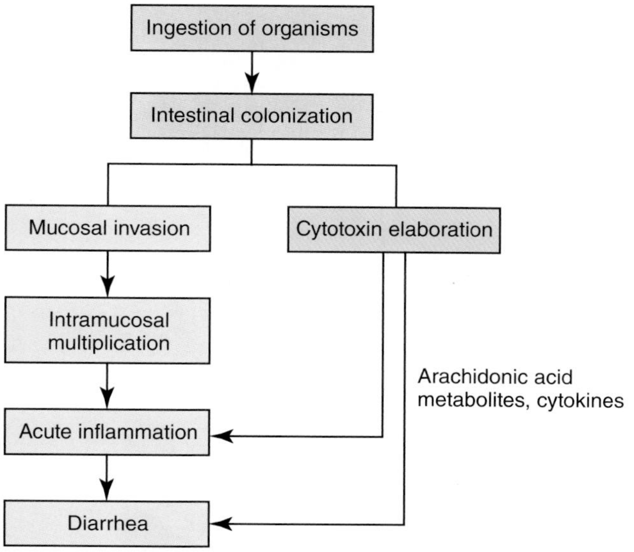

Fig 7-91 Schematic diagram of the mechanism of invasive and cytotoxin-mediated bacterial inflammation.
(Adapted from Cominelli F, Arseneau KO, Blumberg RS, et al: The mucosal immune system and gastrointestinal inflammation. In Yamata T, editor: *Textbook of gastroenterology,* ed 5, West Sussex, UK, 2009, Wiley-Blackwell.)

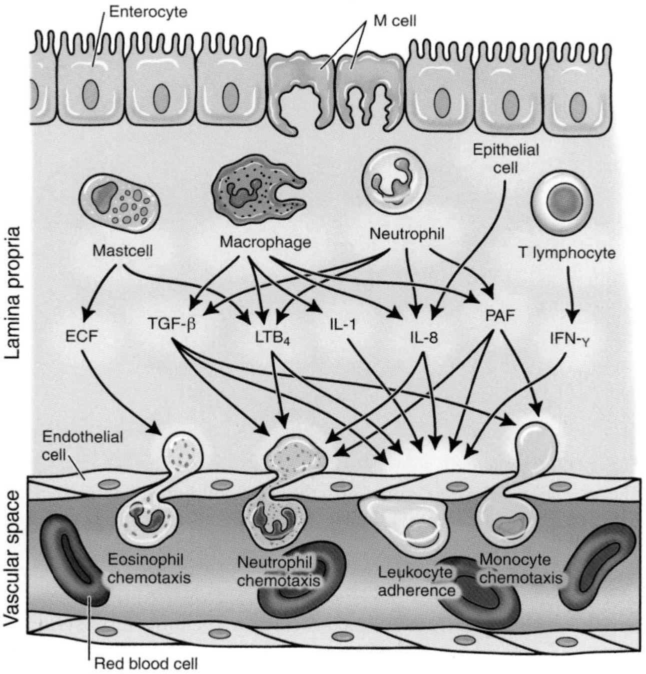

Fig 7-92 Schematic diagram of chemotactic factors during intestinal inflammation.
ECF, Eosinophil chemotactic factor; *IFN-γ,* interferon-γ; *IL,* interleukin; *LTB_4,* leukotriene B_4; *PAF,* platelet activating factor; *TGF-β,* transforming growth factor-β. (Adapted from Cominelli F, Arseneau KO, Blumberg RS, et al: The mucosal immune system and gastrointestinal inflammation. In Yamata T, editor: *Textbook of gastroenterology,* ed 5, West Sussex, UK, 2009, Wiley-Blackwell.)

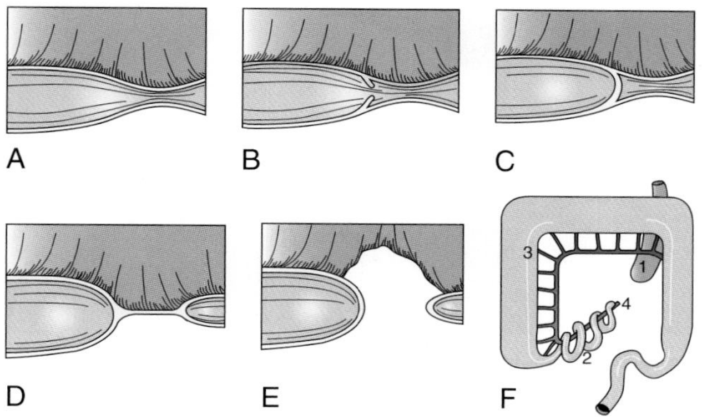

Fig. 7-93 Schematic illustration of the types of stenosis and atresia. **A,** Stenosis. **B,** Stenosis with partial membrane. **C,** Membrane atresia. **D,** Cord atresia. **E,** Blind end atresia. **F,** Christmas tree atresia (*1,* jejunum; *2,* ileum; *3,* colon; *4,* ileocolic artery). (From van der Gaag I, Tibboel D: *Vet Pathol* 17(5):565-574, 1980.)

diarrhea is dehydration. Dehydration results in hypovolemia. Hypovolemia results in hemoconcentration that results in inadequate tissue perfusion. Energy therefore is generated in tissue by anaerobic glycolysis. The resultant hypoglycemia leads to ketoacidosis. Acidosis is, by definition, a reduction in blood and tissue pH. Acidosis causes a reduction in pH-dependent enzyme system functions. Acidosis is compounded by fecal bicarbonate loss in diarrhea and the results of inadequate renal excretion of hydrogen ions and inadequate absorption of bicarbonate, which is a late effect of inadequate renal perfusion. The resultant electrolyte imbalance results in an increase in intracellular hydrogen ion concentration and a decrease in intracellular potassium ion concentration. The imbalances decrease neuromuscular control of myocardial contraction, leading to a further decrease in tissue perfusion. A vicious cycle results, culminating in hypovolemic shock.

Developmental Anomalies

Atresia

Occlusion of the intestinal lumen as the result of anomalous development of the intestinal wall is called *atresia* (Fig. 7-93). Atresia is generally named for the part of the bowel that is occluded such as atresia ani or atresia coli. The causes of atresia in domestic animals are not completely understood, but they can be a result of mechanical lesions to fetal blood vessels in a portion of the gut, such as caused by malpositioning, that compromises circulation and results in vascular accidents and ischemia. Release of meconium into the abdominal cavity of the fetus may result in sterile peritonitis and may be responsible for some cases of atresia such as in cystic fibrosis of humans. In still other cases, the embryonic cells that normally occlude the lumen fail to break down, resulting in atresia. The end result is segmental atresia in which a segment of the bowel is either entirely missing or completely occluded because of a lack of epithelial development and confluence between two contiguous portions (Figs. 7-94 and 7-95).

Meckel's Diverticulum

Meckel's diverticulum is a remnant of the omphalomesenteric duct. Generally, it disappears after the first trimester of gestation, but it can persist in all mammalian species. It is near the termination of the ileum, represents the stalk of the yolk sac, and because of its location and being blind-ended, can be confused with the cecum.

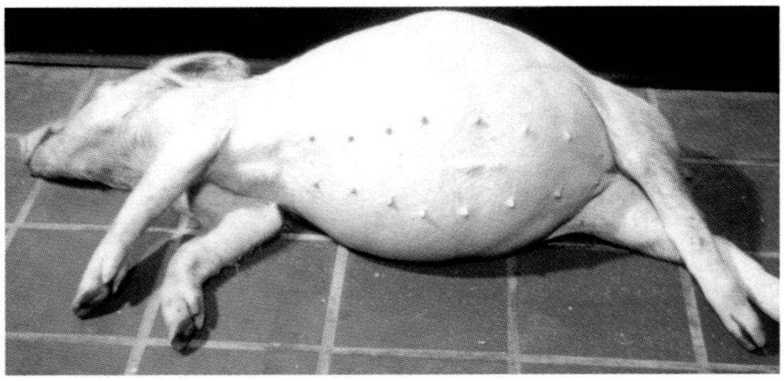

Fig. 7-94 Abdominal distention, atresia coli, feeder pig.
This pig has been unable to defecate since birth because of an atretic developmental malformation of the distal colon. Note the greatly distended abdomen. (Courtesy Dr. J. King, College of Veterinary Medicine, Cornell University.)

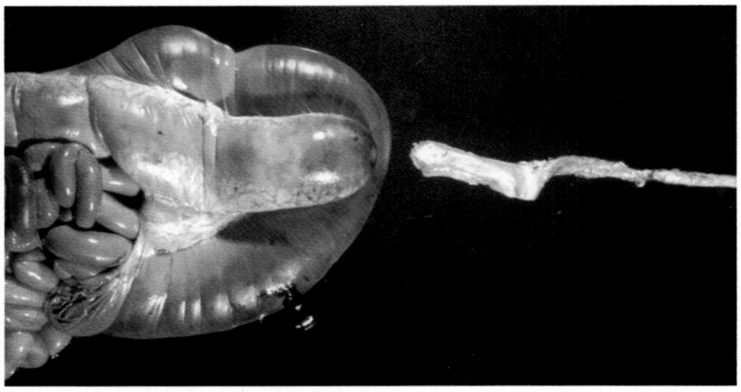

Fig. 7-95 Atresia coli, colon, cow.
There is a blind-ended atretic segment of the spiral colon. The smaller segment at the right of the photograph is distal, the terminal part of the colon. (Courtesy Dr. H. Gelberg, College of Veterinary Medicine, Oregon State University.)

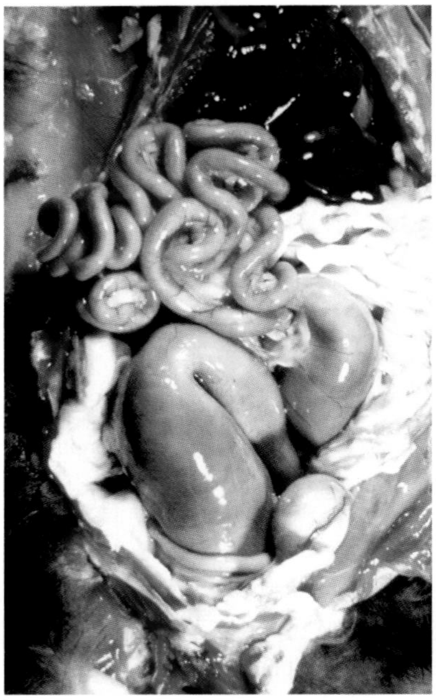

Fig. 7-96 Megacolon, colon, cat.
This disease may be congenital due to a lack of intestinal innervation or atresia of the distal colon or anus. It can also be acquired secondary to nerve injury. (Courtesy Dr. H. Gelberg, College of Veterinary Medicine, Oregon State University.)

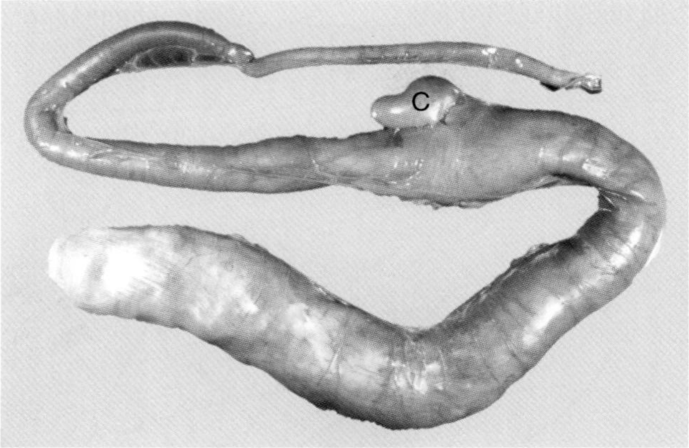

Fig. 7-97 Megacolon, colon, dog.
The large colon from the cecum *(C)* to the anus is dilated with feces. In dogs, this disease has pathogeneses similar to those described in cats (Fig. 7-96). (Courtesy Dr. H. Gelberg, College of Veterinary Medicine, Oregon State University.)

Megacolon

Megacolon, as its name implies, is a large, usually fecal-filled colon (Figs. 7-96 and 7-97) that can be congenital or acquired. The congenital form occurs in pigs, dogs, cats, overo foals, and humans from a developmental lack of myenteric plexuses (Hirschsprung's disease) secondary to the failure of migration of neuroblasts from the neural crest to the colorectal myenteric plexuses.

The equine overo pattern of spotting is defined by white patches of epidermis on the ventral or lateral abdomen and extends dorsally up to but not including, the dorsal midline. The epidermis is also nonpigmented on the lateral neck and flank. The overo pattern typically includes at least one pigmented leg. Affected foals are white and appear normal at birth. They do not pass meconium; subsequently, they develop colic and die usually by 72 hours after birth. These white foals are nonperistaltic because of absence of the myenteric (Auerbach's) plexus or submucosal (Meissner's) plexus, particularly in the colon and rectum. Thus these anomalies can be termed aganglionosis. A congenital aganglionic megacolon is contracted and nonperistaltic. Dilation or megacolon occurs proximal to the aganglionic section of the gut.

Acquired megacolon is secondary to damage to the colonic innervation. Such events are usually traumatic and most common in carnivores struck by automobiles. Atresia ani can also result in megacolon.

Intestinal Obstruction

Mechanical obstruction of the intestinal tract occurs in all species of domestic and wild animals. Although foreign bodies of all types have been removed from animals at surgery, the long-term systemic effects of some foreign bodies are also important. These include copper and zinc toxicosis from ingestion of coins in dogs, seals, ruminants, and horses and lead poisoning in cattle from ingestion of old batteries. Primates caged in outdated facilities with lead paint or lead bars can also succumb to lead poisoning. *Pythium insidiosum* infection has caused intestinal obstruction in a puppy because of inflammation associated with the infection.

Enteroliths and Impaction

Enteroliths are rare in species other than the horse. The Arabian breed has an increased incidence. Generally, affected animals are more than 4 years old. The stones are usually formed by ammonium magnesium phosphate (struvite) and collect around a small central nidus, often a metallic foreign body (Web Fig. 7-13). Enteroliths vary greatly in size from several centimeters in diameter to greater than 20 cm, and they can weigh several kilograms. They generally lodge at the pelvic flexure or transverse colon. Diets high in magnesium and phosphorus predispose to enterolith formation. In the past, millers' horses (grain and feed mills) had access to large amounts of inexpensive bran, and thus their horses were more prone to enteroliths. In California, the feeding of high-protein, magnesium-rich alfalfa hay may partially explain the higher incidence of enteroliths in California equids.

The presence of aggregated ingesta that cannot move along the intestinal tract (impaction) occurs in all species. It is especially common in horses after anthelmintic administration and is the result of the rapid die-off of large numbers of nematodes, particularly ascarids (Web Fig. 7-14). Cecal impaction occurs in old horses because of a high-roughage (indigestible) diet, debility, or poor dentition caused by a lack of mechanical leveling of the teeth (floating). Fibrous ingesta can also result in ileal impaction. Large amounts of ingested sand can accumulate anywhere in the equine colon, resulting in impaction (sand colic).

Strictures with Obstruction

Strictures are the result of narrowing of the lumen of a canal, which in the present case is the intestinal canal. They are generally the result of healing with scarring of penetrating and nonpenetrating wounds of all kinds or of a vascular injury causing infarction, followed by healing with fibrosis (Fig. 7-98). For example, rectal stricture is a sequela of salmonellosis in pigs and is the result in part of thrombosis of the cranial hemorrhoidal artery and lack of collateral circulation (Fig. 7-99) that could otherwise allow the intestinal segment to remain viable. They obstruct the intestine.

Intussusception

When one segment of intestine becomes telescoped into the immediately distal segment of intestine, the lesion is called an *intussusception* (Figs. 7-100 and 7-101). The intussusceptum is the trapped segment, and the intussuscipiens is the enveloping portion of the intestine. The cause is generally unknown but is thought to be associated with intestinal irritability and hypermotility. Irritability and hypermotility can occur secondary to enteritis, irritation caused by parasites of all sorts, and general debility. Foreign bodies, neoplasms, and some parasites, such as the nodular worm of sheep (*Oesophagostomum* spp.), by means of the subserosal nodules it produces, can provide a toehold for the intestine to telescope into itself. In the dog, intussusception of the intestine has been related to, or caused by, handling of the small intestine during surgery, hypertrophied lymphoid nodules, and granulomas secondary to inflammatory and parasitic diseases, linear foreign bodies (string) (Fig. 7-102, *A*), and ascarids.

In bovids and equids, tumors, abscesses, and granulomas may be causes of intussusceptions. In equids, verminous arteritis may uniquely cause intussusceptions. Ileoileal, ileocecal, cecocecal, and cecocolic intussusceptions are sometimes associated with *Anoplocephala perfoliata*. Rarely, duodenogastric and gastroesophageal intussusceptions occur.

Clinical features of intussusception are similar to those of intestinal obstruction. In small animals with thin abdominal walls, they can sometimes be palpated. Intussusceptions are enlarged, thickened segments of intestine that vary in length. Intussusceptions are grossly swollen, doughy-feeling segments of the intestine. They resemble the folds of an accordion (Fig. 7-102, *B*). Red to black discoloration depends on the degree of vascular compromise, ranging from congestion to hemorrhage and necrosis. The mesenteric attachment of the intussusceptum may be seen extending from the lesion. This occurs as the vascular mesentery gets pulled into the intussuscipiens compressing first the thinner walled veins and then the arteries. Fibrin exudation, ischemic necrosis, congestion, and edema may occur in both the intussusceptum and intussuscipiens. On rare occasions, antemortem intussusceptions spontaneously reduce by sloughing of the infarcted intussusceptum, which then passes in the feces. Often, the site of sloughing is replaced with fibrous tissue, and a circumferential scar or stricture forms.

Because peristalsis continues after death, intestinal invaginations can occur postmortem. Before attributing death to intestinal

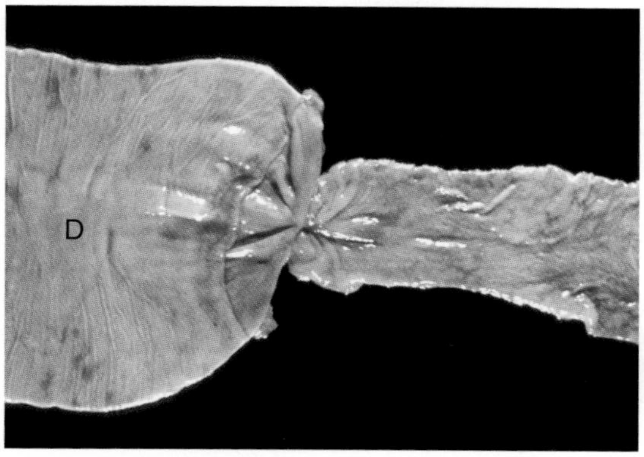

Fig. 7-98 Stricture, intestine, horse.
The dilated intestine *(D)* is proximal to the stricture. Such strictures can be caused by penetrating or nonpenetrating wounds of all kinds from the luminal surface or secondary to vascular injury. (Courtesy Dr. H. Gelberg, College of Veterinary Medicine, Oregon State University.)

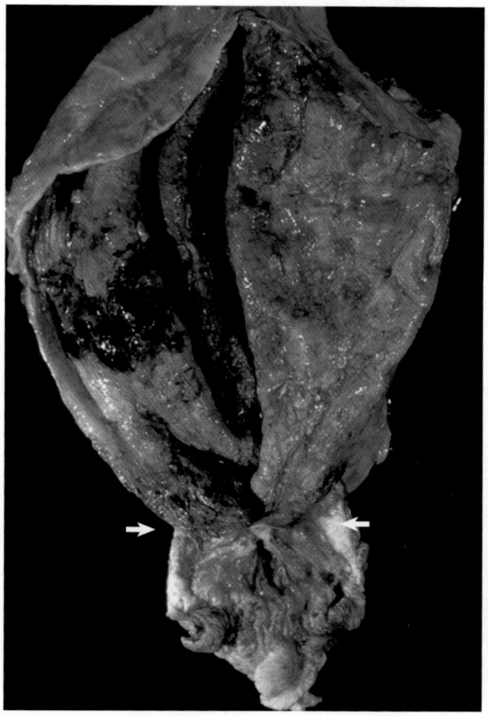

Fig. 7-99 Stricture, colon, pig.
This lesion *(between arrows)* in pigs has been attributed to thrombosis of the cranial hemorrhoidal artery from vasculitis and thrombosis caused by salmonella. (Courtesy Dr. C.S. Patton, College of Veterinary Medicine, University of Tennessee.)

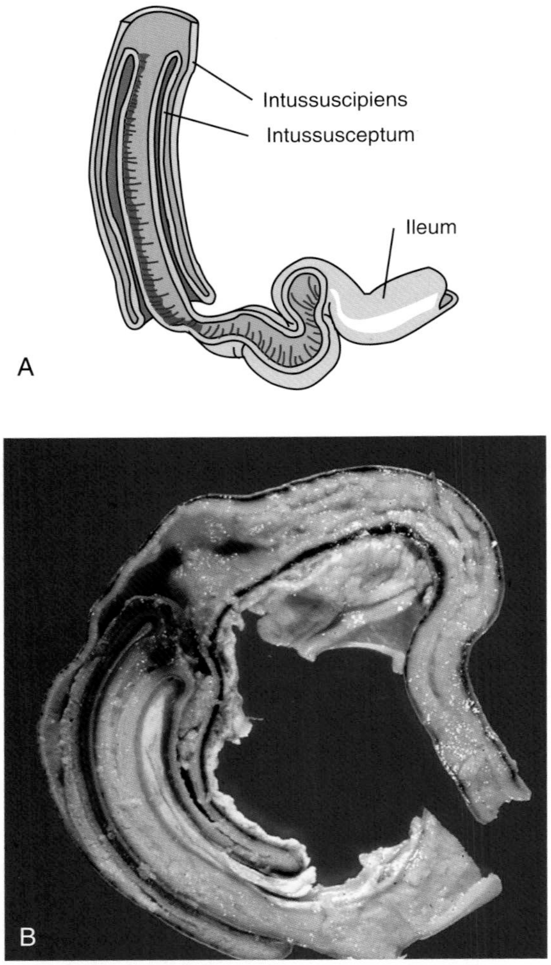

Fig. 7-100 Intussusception.
A, Schematic diagram showing the anatomic positioning of small intestinal segments in an intussusception. **B,** Longitudinal section of small intestinal intussusception demonstrating the position of the intussusceptum (trapped segment) and the intussuscipiens (the enveloping portion) of the small intestine. (**A** redrawn with permission from Dr. T. Boosinger; **B** courtesy Dr. T. Boosinger, College of Veterinary Medicine, Auburn University; and Noah's Arkive, College of Veterinary Medicine, The University of Georgia.)

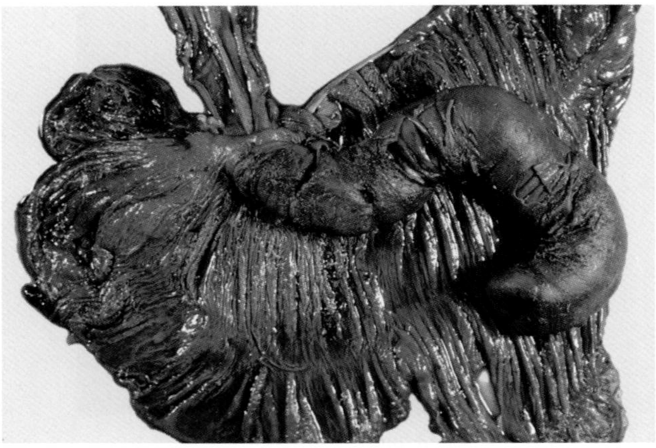

Fig. 7-101 Ileocecal intussusception, ileum, horse.
The necrotic intussuscipiens is present in the lumen of the opened cecum. (Courtesy Dr. M.D. McGavin, College of Veterinary Medicine, University of Tennessee.)

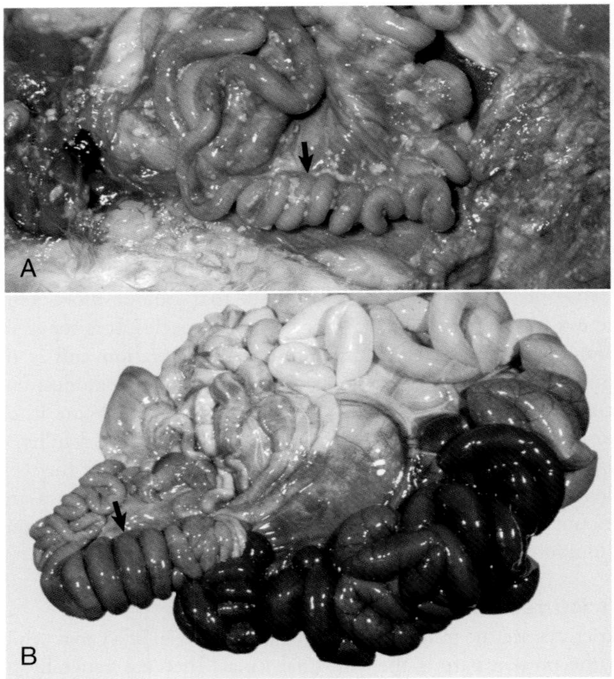

Fig. 7-102 Accordion-folded intestines.
A, Small intestine, cat. A linear foreign body (roast beef string) has caused the accordion-folded appearance of the small intestine *(arrow)*. Peristalsis of the intestine over the string, which is taut, in the intestinal lumen causes a sawing, abrasive effect and perforation of the intestine resulting in peritonitis, the white exudate seen on the serosal surfaces. **B,** Intussusception, intestine, pig. The accordion-folded intussusception *(arrow)* is contiguous with infarcted bowel, the result of vascular strangulation. (**A** courtesy College of Veterinary Medicine, University of Illinois. **B** courtesy Dr. H. Gelberg, College of Veterinary Medicine, Oregon State University.)

obstruction caused by intussusception, there is a need to determine if the intussusception took place before or after death. Because inflammation only occurs in the living organism, postmortem invaginations are easily reduced because there are no adhesions and they are not accompanied by hyperemia or fibrin on the peritoneal surfaces, which remain smooth and glistening.

Ileus

Paralytic ileus (adynamic ileus) is a nonmechanical hypomotility resulting in a functional obstruction of the bowel (pseudoobstruction). It can be due to paralysis of the bowel wall (generally the result of bowel manipulation at surgery), peritonitis from any cause, shock, severe pain, abnormal stimulation of splanchnic nerves, toxemia, electrolyte imbalances (especially hypokalemia), vitamin B–complex deficiency, uremia, tetanus, diabetes mellitus, or heavy-metal poisoning.

The gut is not paralyzed, but because of continuous nerve discharge, it becomes refractory, resulting in lack of tonic stimulation of the bowel musculature. In most cases of paralytic ileus, there are no gross lesions other than perhaps atonic dilation of the intestine. It occurs in most animal species.

Grass sickness of equids in Europe, southern South America, and rarely the US is associated with dysphagia, GI hypomotility, and subsequent colic. Degenerative lesions of this idiopathic condition are present in the autonomic ganglia, suggesting it is an acquired dysautonomia. An occasional outbreak in equids is associated with the temporospatial occurrence of similar lesions in

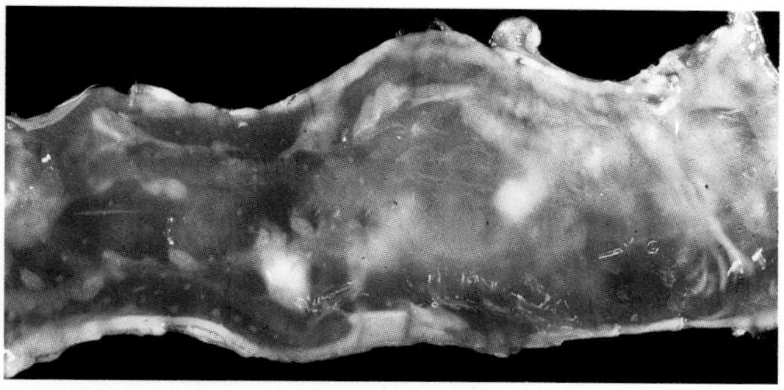

Fig. 7-103 Mucoid enteropathy, colon, rabbit.
Although *Escherichia coli* and *Clostridia perfringens* can often be isolated from the dilated, mucus-filled intestine, the cause of this condition is a dysautonomia of the intestinal plexi. (Courtesy College of Veterinary Medicine, Cornell University.)

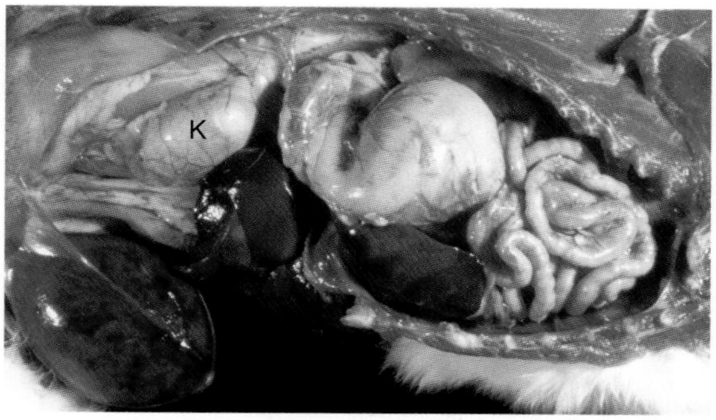

Fig. 7-104 Diaphragmatic hernia, abdomen, cat.
Traumatic rupture of the diaphragm has allowed intestines, stomach, and liver into the thoracic cavity, resulting in displacement and compression of the thoracic viscera and consequently compromise of cardiopulmonary function. *K,* Kidney. (Courtesy Dr. H. Gelberg, College of Veterinary Medicine, Oregon State University.)

rabbits. Ingestion of *Clostridium botulinum* type C with subsequent toxin production is suspected to be the cause of this condition.

Mucoid Enteropathy

Mucoid enteropathy is a subacute and fatal disease of young rabbits characterized by copious quantities of mucus in the feces concurrent with impaction of the cecum and sometimes the sacculated colon (Fig. 7-103). Although large numbers of coliform bacteria or *Clostridium perfringens* may be present in the affected intestine, dysautonomia (see Fig. 14-111) has been documented in rabbitries affected with this condition.

INTESTINAL DISPLACEMENTS

Intestinal displacements include herniations that lead to incarcerations (fixation) of the displaced bowel and finally strangulations (interference with blood flow) of the incarcerated segment of intestine and are categorized as internal or external.

Internal herniations are displacements of intestine through a normal or pathologic foramen in the abdominal cavity. The most common of these displacements occur in horses and include herniation through the epiploic foramen and through mesenteric tears. The dorsal border of the epiploic foramen is formed by the caudate lobe of the liver and the caudal vena cava. The ventral boundary is the right lobe of the pancreas, the gastropancreatic ligament, and the portal vein. The cranial boundary is the hepatoduodenal ligament, and the caudal boundary is the junction of the pancreas and mesoduodenum. The epiploic cavity is only a potential space. It is proposed that in older horses the caudate lobe of the liver atrophies, enlarging the foramen and allowing loops of intestine to slip through and become incarcerated and strangulated (Web Fig. 7-15).

External hernias are formed when a hernial sac, formed by a pouch of parietal peritoneum, penetrates outside the abdominal cavity. Types of external herniation include umbilical, ventral, diaphragmatic (Fig. 7-104), hiatal, inguinal, scrotal (Fig. 7-105), and perineal named for the location of the displaced viscera. Perineal hernias are seen in old male dogs with prostate gland enlargement and obstipation. Some of these herniations (diaphragmatic, perineal) are more correctly termed *eventrations* (protrusion of the intestine through the abdominal wall or diaphragm) because they are not accompanied by a peritoneal pouch. Postoperative wound dehiscence of a ventral abdominal incision also causes eventration.

It should be noted that umbilical hernias are generally caused by a defect in the abdominal wall and not by the chewing on the umbilical cord by the dam. Umbilical hernias may have a genetic

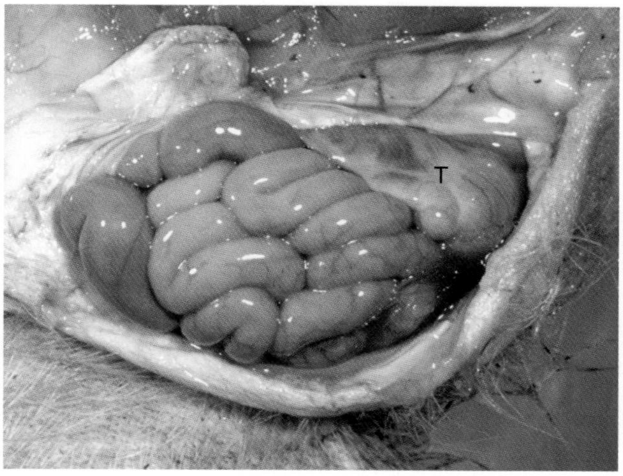

Fig. 7-105 Scrotal hernia, scrotum, pig.
Loops of intestine within the scrotum entered through the inguinal canal to lie in the scrotal cavity and have displaced the testis *(T)* caudally. (Courtesy Dr. H. Gelberg, College of Veterinary Medicine, Oregon State University.)

basis, so it may be a matter of some ethical concern whether to surgically repair these hernias in show and breeding animals. In calves, umbilical infections are also associated with an increased risk for hernia development.

Rectal prolapse may occur secondary to tenesmus or excessive postpartum straining (Fig. 7-106).

Volvulus and Torsion

A volvulus is a twisting of the intestine on its mesenteric axis. A torsion is a rotation of a tubular organ along its long axis. The latter is most common in the cecum of cattle and horses and occasionally of the abomasum of calves (see Web Fig. 7-10). Both volvulus and torsion result in compression of the mesenteric veins and arteries resulting in ischemia initially followed by obstruction—veins first and later as the pressure on the mesenteric vessels increases, the arteries. Infarction is a result of occlusion of the thin-walled mesenteric veins. Because the mesenteric arterial supply is anatomically more resistant to occlusion, blood is pumped into the twisted segment but cannot drain. Edema, congestion, hemorrhage, and eventual necrosis result (Figs. 7-107 and 7-108). It is probable that the mechanism of intestinal twisting is secondary to movement

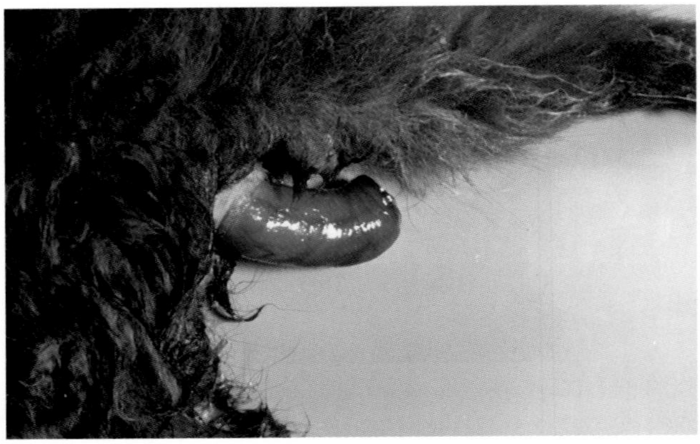

Fig. 7-106 Prolapsed rectum, anus, cat.
Tenesmus caused the rectum to prolapse. (Courtesy Dr. M.D. McGavin, College of Veterinary Medicine, University of Tennessee.)

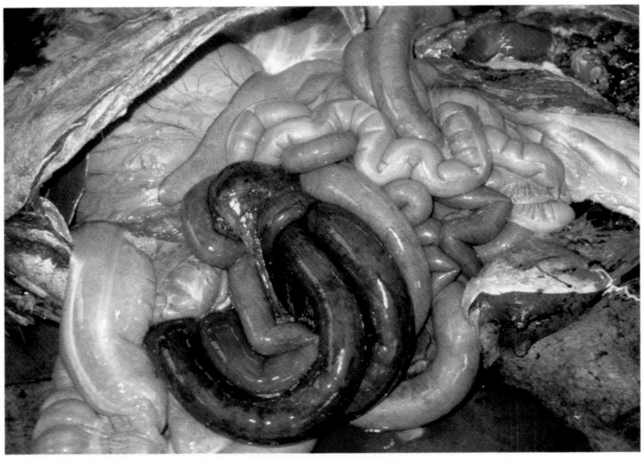

Fig. 7-107 Infarction, small intestine, horse.
Volvulus of the intestine has resulted in vascular compromise and infarction of several loops of bowel. (Courtesy Dr. M.D. McGavin, College of Veterinary Medicine, University of Tennessee.)

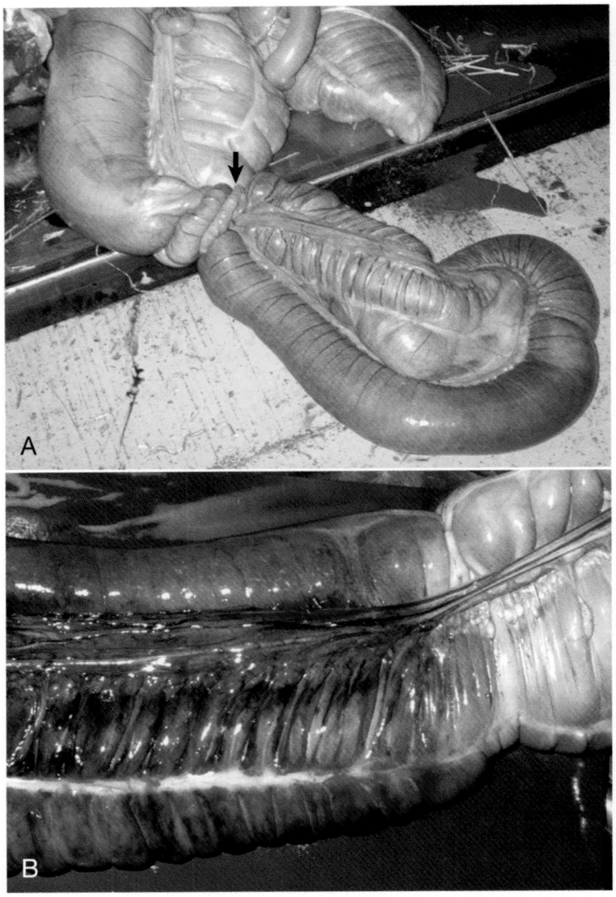

Fig. 7-108 Torsion, large colon, horse.
A, Rotation of the colon on its long axis has resulted in severe colic with strangulation *(arrow)*. Note the red to blue discoloration of the colon distal to the torsion caused by obstruction of venous blood flow. **B,** Note the sharp line of demarcation (point where the torsion occurred) between viable colon *(to the right)* and nonviable colon *(to the left)* caused by obstruction of venous blood flow. In this case, the torsion was not found at the time of necropsy; however, a torsion will commonly untwist itself (reduce itself) during transport of the dead animal to the postmortem room. (**A** courtesy Dr. H. Gelberg, College of Veterinary Medicine, Oregon State University. **B** courtesy Dr. M.D. McCracken, College of Veterinary Medicine, University of Tennessee.)

of the walls of the abdominal cavity (i.e., the intestine stays still and the horse rolls or otherwise moves around the static intestine).

At surgery or necropsy, the twisted segment of intestine is distended with gas and fluid and is discolored either dark red or black (see Fig. 2-42). There is usually a sharp line of demarcation between the affected and normal intestine. This line marks the site for surgical resection. A volvulus may result in a rotation of the intestine up to 720 degrees, either clockwise or counterclockwise on its mesenteric axis. Therefore surgical correction of a volvulus may be difficult and complex. It is very important to determine the viability of the bowel after reduction of a volvulus. The affected segment of intestine is often necrotic, congested, and hemorrhagic. Intestinal stasis and toxemia and/or bacteremia may result from bacterial overgrowth and anoxic bowel necrosis. Reperfusion injury may also occur. Toxemia and intestinal rupture may result in death.

Volvulus of the equine large intestine occurs most commonly in the left colon. In equids, the left ventral colon is an extension of the right ventral colon beginning at the sternal flexure. The left ventral colon doubles back on itself in the pelvic inlet to form the left dorsal colon. This pelvic flexure can be palpated rectally. The left dorsal colon becomes the right dorsal colon at the diaphragmatic flexure. The diaphragmatic flexure lies cranial to the sternal flexure and usually contacts the ventral body wall. The left dorsal colon is sacculated with one taenia; the left ventral colon is sacculated with four taeniae. When twisting occurs, it is usually clockwise around the mesocolon and is thus a volvulus. Torsion of the large colon of mares accounts for half of their intestinal displacements in the peripartum period.

A peculiar type of intestinal strangulation occurs in horses in which lipomas, which are pedunculated, wrap around the intestinal mesentery or the bowel, causing ischemia, colic, and death (Fig. 7-109). Pedunculated lipomas may rotate about their pedicle cutting off their own blood supply. When this occurs, they undergo mineralization and sometimes ossification. The stalk may become necrotic and break, leaving a free-floating lipoma within the abdominal cavity where it apparently does no harm. However, most mesenteric lipomas are of no clinical consequence. Rarely, intestinal strangulation by pedunculated lipomas has been reported in the dog.

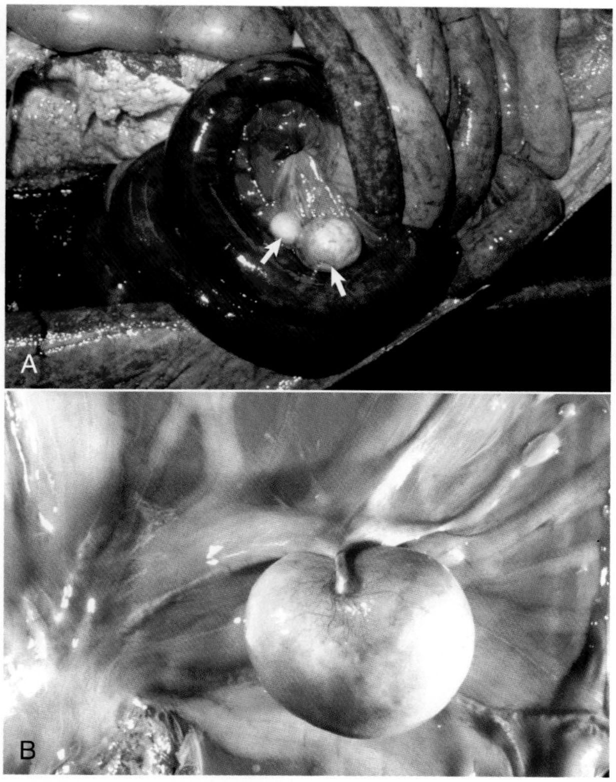

Fig. 7-109 Pedunculated lipomas.
A, Intestinal strangulation by pedunculated lipomas, small intestine, horse. Two lipomas *(arrows)* have wrapped around the mesentery and strangled the bowel resulting in infarction. **B,** Mesentery, horse. Closer view of a pedunculated lipoma. (**A** courtesy College of Veterinary Medicine, Cornell University. **B** courtesy College of Veterinary Medicine, University of Illinois.)

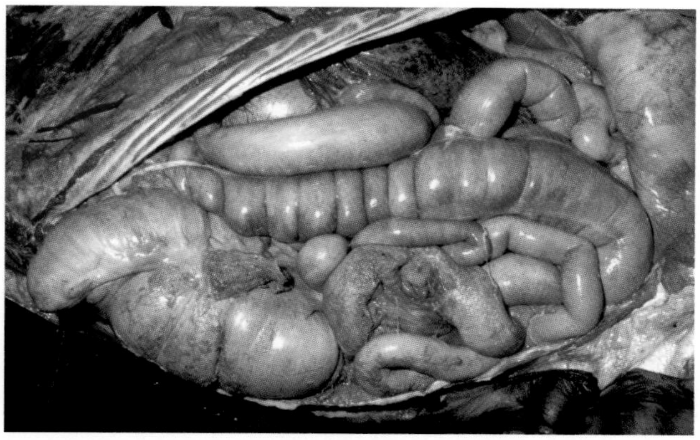

Fig. 7-110 Fibrinous peritonitis, abdomen, horse.
The presence of fibrin and ingesta adherent to serosal surfaces indicates antemortem perforation or rupture of the intestine. (Courtesy Dr. M.D. McGavin, College of Veterinary Medicine, University of Tennessee.)

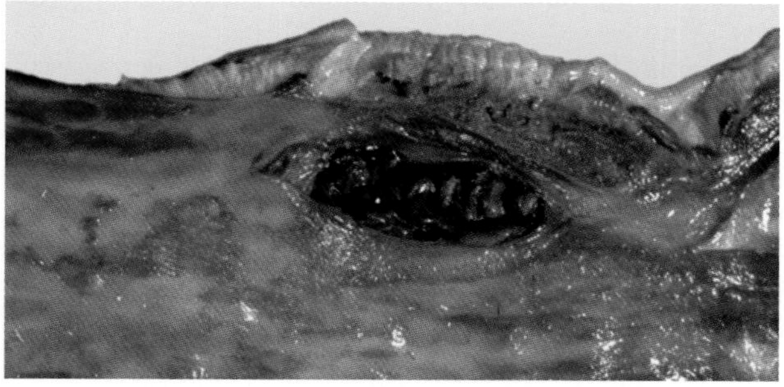

Fig. 7-111 Ulceration, rectum, horse.
Hemorrhage, ulcers, and tears in the rectum are often caused by inexperienced persons or overly vigorous rectal palpation. (Courtesy Dr. M.D. McGavin, College of Veterinary Medicine, University of Tennessee.)

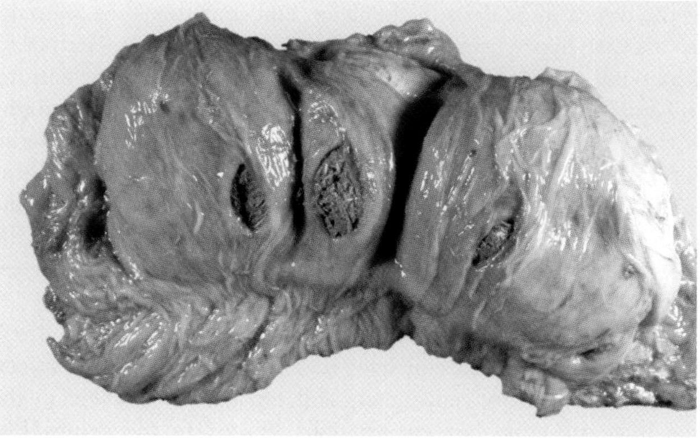

Fig. 7-112 Diverticula, cecum, horse.
Diverticula are mucosal outpouchings into the subjacent smooth muscle layers of the colon. They are filled with ingesta and lined by intact mucosa. (Courtesy Dr. H. Gelberg, College of Veterinary Medicine, Oregon State University.)

Renosplenic Entrapment

Renosplenic entrapment of the large colon in horses is due to left dorsal displacement of the left dorsal colon or left ventral colon between the spleen and left body wall. Entrapment occurs dorsally over the renosplenic ligament that runs between the left kidney and the spleen. The cause of the displacement is unknown but could occur secondary to rolling behavior in horses or gaseous distention of the large colon. If not corrected either by rolling the horse or by surgery, intestinal rupture and death may result.

Right Dorsal Displacement

In the equine condition, right dorsal displacement, the left dorsal and ventral colons are displaced to the right of the cecum and may result in torsion with signs of colic. It is a surgically correctable disease.

Miscellaneous Diseases and Conditions

Cecal or large intestinal rupture occurs most commonly in postparturient mares (Fig. 7-110) but can also result from impaction and as a complication of anesthesia. The sites of rupture vary, and the mechanisms are unknown. Iatrogenic rectal tearing may occur secondary to rectal palpation (Fig. 7-111). The presence of blood on a rectal sleeve after palpation is cause for concern because peritonitis may be the result of penetration of the peritoneal cavity, especially if the tear occurs ventrally.

Diverticula (singular, diverticulum) are epithelium-lined cavities that are derived from mucosal epithelium that extend through the muscularis mucosa, submucosa, and muscularis and often reach the serosa, where they sometimes rupture, causing peritonitis (Figs. 7-112 and 7-113; Web Fig. 7-16). This can occur in any part of the tubular gut, including the esophagus and cecum.

Muscular hypertrophy of the distal ileum is an idiopathic condition of horses and pigs. Although generally an incidental finding, hypertrophy of the tunica muscularis can lead to impaction and

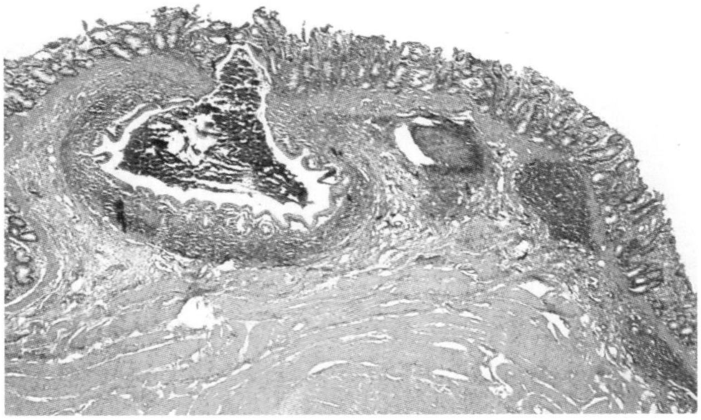

Fig. 7-113 Diverticulum, colon, cow.
A diverticulum lined by superficial mucosa has penetrated through the submucosa to lie next to the muscularis. H&E stain. (Courtesy Dr. M.D. McGavin, College of Veterinary Medicine, University of Tennessee.)

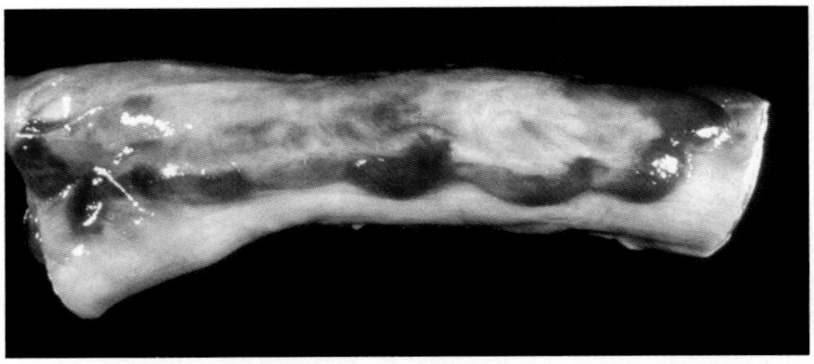

Fig. 7-114 Hemomelasma ilei, ileum, horse.
Hemorrhagic and siderotic fibrovascular plaques on the antimesenteric serosa are attributed to strongyle larval migration *(Strongylus edentatus)*, but this association has never been demonstrated. (Courtesy Dr. H. Gelberg, College of Veterinary Medicine, Oregon State University.)

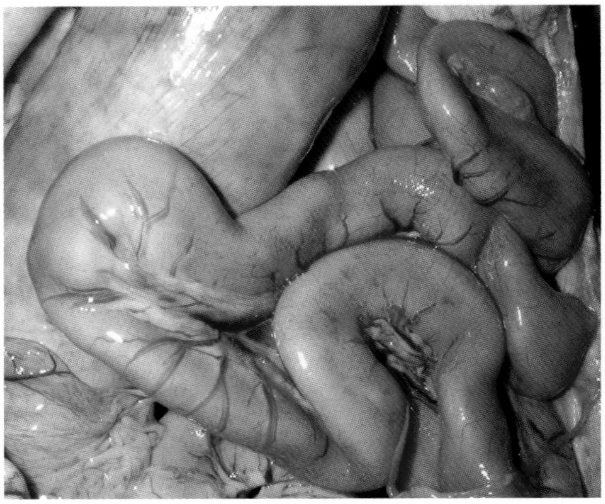

Fig. 7-115 Leiomyometaplasia, intestine, dog.
"Brown dog gut" is a rare condition caused by the accumulation of a brown pigment now known to be ceroid (formerly called *lipofuscin*) in the lysosomes of smooth muscle cells of the tunica muscularis. It is a dietary condition associated with vitamin E deficiency. (Courtesy Dr. L. Borst, College of Veterinary Medicine, University of Illinois.)

rupture of the ileum. The lesion in horses is sometimes segmental, affecting the ileum and variably the jejunum. Often, the lesion is a sequela of muscular hypertrophy caused by a damaged or stenotic ileocecal valve. Muscular hypertrophy of equids may also affect the duodenum and jejunum in association with diverticula in those gut segments. Horses with muscular hypertrophy of the distal ileum may have mild colic, occasional diarrhea, and weight loss. Often, muscular hypertrophy is asymptomatic. Muscular hypertrophy of the ileum in pigs generally occurs as an idiopathic, asymptomatic lesion. Muscular hypertrophy of the tunica muscularis associated with diverticulosis of the ileum has been recorded in young Yorkshire pigs and in Romney Marsh and Hampshire sheep. The lesion is suspected to be secondary to a functional obstruction of the ileocecal valve. Diverticulosis and/or intestinal rupture may result.

Cats can have a severe hypertrophy of the inner, circular layer of the tunica muscularis of the ileum and sometimes the jejunum. In cats with hypereosinophilic syndrome, a disease characterized by intramural eosinophil infiltrates, hypertrophy of the gastric antrum, and small intestinal musculature can occur. Muscular hypertrophy of the intestine and medial hyperplasia of the pulmonary arteries occur in cats given large oral doses of *Toxocara cati* larvae. These conditions are often accompanied by diarrhea and eosinophilic enteritis. Fibrosis of the lamina propria and hypertrophy of the inner layer of the tunica muscularis may result in a stiff, thickened intestine.

Another unique lesion in the horse is *Hemomelasma ilei*. These lesions are pink to black plaques that vary in length from several millimeters to many centimeters and can occur anywhere in the intestinal subserosa but are generally limited to the ileum (Fig. 7-114; also see Fig. 3-39). They are attributed to larval migrations of strongyles (usually *Strongylus edentatus*) and are located on the antimesenteric serosal surface. However, parasites have never been reported in the lesions and therefore the cause of hemomelasma ilei is unknown. They are generally of no clinical consequence but can on occasion lead to intestinal strictures and intermittent colic.

Intestinal ceroidosis or leiomyometaplasia is also called *brown dog gut*. The discolored intestinal smooth muscle may occur in association with chronic enteritis and pancreatitis. Experimentally, leiomyometaplasia can be produced in dogs by vitamin E deficiency, in association with excess dietary lipids. The canine and human intestinal pigmentation is the result of vitamin E deficiency. The dietary requirement for vitamin E is proportional to the concentration of polyunsaturated fatty acids in the diet. Intestinal ceroidosis probably does not cause clinical signs but may be an indicator of a metabolic or nutritional disorder. In this condition, the intestinal serosa varies from tan to dark brown (Fig. 7-115). The stomach and large bowel are variously affected, as is the small intestine. Accumulation of brown, granular, acid-fast–staining lipofuscin in the perinuclear lysosomes of the leiomyocytes is characteristic of this condition.

Amyloidosis occasionally is present in the intestinal and vascular walls of the lamina propria and muscularis in association with systemic amyloid AA infiltrations in a variety of animal species of all ages.

Tiger striping is a nonspecific congestion of colonic ridges secondary to diarrhea and/or tenesmus (Web Fig. 7-17). The red and pale longitudinal stripes are formed by the congested tips of the folds alternating with the uncongested mucosa between them.

Small Intestinal Intoxicants

Because most toxins enter the body through ingestion, those that are irritants can cause contact lesions in the oral cavity, esophagus, stomach, and intestine. The lesions that result are generally those of hemorrhage and inflammation. In many cases of intoxication, induction of vomiting is contraindicated because what burns going down will also burn coming up. For some intoxicants, multidrug resistance (MDR1) gene products of enterocytes are part of the detoxification process. In addition, P450 enzymes are present on villus enterocytes, although in much lesser amounts than in the liver. They are in highest concentration in the jejunum and decrease aborally. In humans, ingestion of grapefruit juice interferes with the function of these enzymes, sometimes resulting in enhanced oral drug availability.

The numbers and types of chemicals and intoxicants animals are exposed to make a listing of them a monumental undertaking. A few examples are phosphorus, arsenic, bracken fern (cattle), mercury, oak, copper, nitrate, thallium, and blister beetles. Blister beetles, a specific toxicity, are sometimes incorporated into crimped hay (Fig. 7-116). They contain a topical irritant called cantharidin. Lesions include sloughing of the epithelium of the stomach and enterocytes of the proximal small intestine (Fig. 7-117). In addition, cantharidin can cause hemorrhagic ulcers of the urinary bladder and myocardial necrosis.

Although not generally considered an intoxicant, corticosteroids cause colonic perforation in some treated dogs and can delay GI healing. They do this by decreasing cell turnover, decreasing mucus production, and stimulating gastrin secretion, leading to increased acid production. NSAIDs can cause *right dorsal colitis* in equids. This colitis is characterized by necrosis, resulting in erosions and ulcers. Epithelial loss may be severe, with only regenerating, rounded islands of normal mucosa remaining. The massive edema of the denuded intestine causes rupture of the submucosa in an elongated diamond-like pattern. The mechanism of injury is direct by topical application (oral administration) and through inhibition of prostaglandin synthesis. Neutrophils play a role by increasing synthesis of tumor necrosis factor-α, leukotriene B4, and upregulation of leukocyte adhesion molecules.

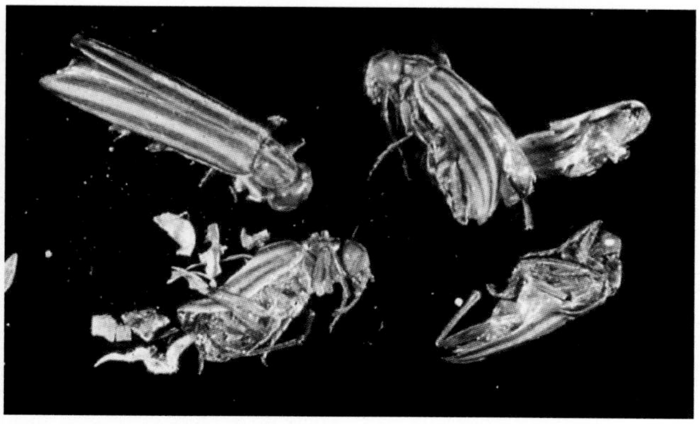

Fig. 7-116 Striped blister beetles.
Numerous species of blister beetles (*Epicauta* spp.), such as gray, black, and striped, can be found throughout the United States. They contain a vesicant (blister-causing substance) that causes inflammation and blistering of mucosal surfaces when they are ingested. Usually, these beetles are trapped and crushed in crimped hay. (Courtesy Dr. W. Crowell, College of Veterinary Medicine, University of Georgia; and Noah's Arkive, College of Veterinary Medicine, University of Georgia.)

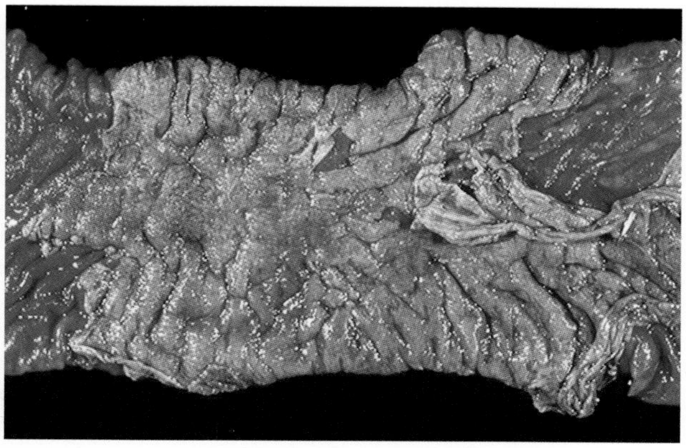

Fig. 7-117 Acute necrohemorrhagic enteritis, small intestine, horse.
The severe necrosis with sloughing of intestinal mucosa is the result of cantharidin, a toxin contained in ingested blister beetles. (Courtesy Dr. R. Panciera, School of Veterinary Medicine, Oklahoma State University; and Noah's Arkive, College of Veterinary Medicine, The University of Georgia.)

Vascular Diseases of the Intestine

Parasites

In horses, *Strongylus vulgaris* fourth-stage larvae are present in the wall of the cranial mesenteric artery, resulting in arteritis. So-called aneurysms (some with osseous metaplasia and bone marrow) and mural thromboses develop (Fig. 7-118; also see Fig. 10-71). In many cases, even complete occlusion of the anterior mesenteric artery (see Fig. 2-27) does not result in bowel infarction because collateral circulation will develop if the vascular occlusion develops slowly (Fig. 7-119). Therefore it is important to ascertain if the colonic arteries are thrombosed before assigning the cause of bowel death to *Strongylus vulgaris*. Severe colic and death often results from bowel infarction secondary to verminous arteritis and thrombosis.

Third-stage larvae are ingested and molt to fourth-stage larvae in the small intestine. They then invade small arterioles on their way to the anterior mesenteric artery. It takes 3 to 4 months in this location until fifth-stage larvae are produced and migrate through the blood vessels to the cecocolonic subserosa. They may be walled off similarly to *Oesophagostomum* spp. in ruminants and pigs. In the lumen of the large intestine, adults develop. The entire cycle takes up to 6 months or more. Thus the prepatent period in foals is considerable, and by the time ova appear in the feces, significant vascular damage may have occurred. Modern deworming regimens are quite effective and will hopefully succeed in making this disease of historic significance only.

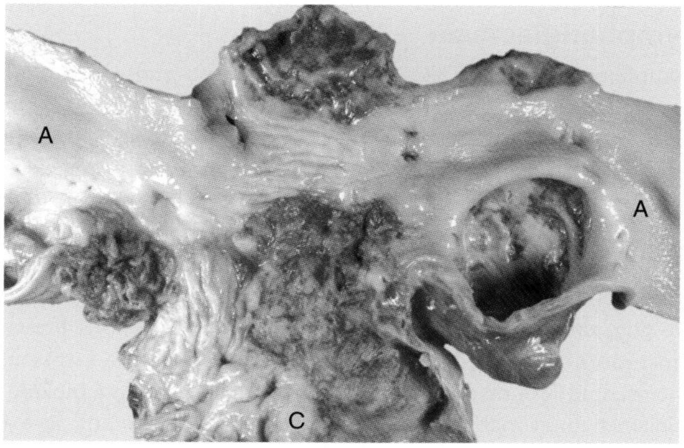

Fig. 7-118 Verminous arteritis, cranial mesenteric artery *(C)*, horse.
Chronic proliferative arteritis and mural thrombosis have resulted from the migration of *Strongylus vulgaris* fourth-stage larvae through and within the vessel wall at or near its origin from the aorta *(A)*. The arteritis can lead to mural thrombosis, formation of aneurysms *(lower right)*, arterial mineralization, and infarction of the bowel. (Courtesy Dr. H. Gelberg, College of Veterinary Medicine, Oregon State University.)

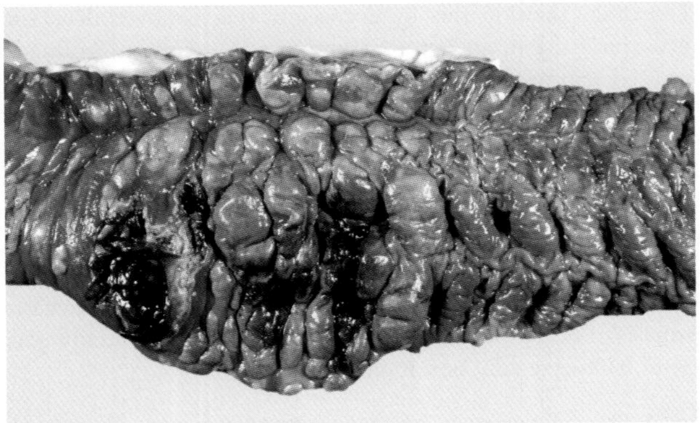

Fig. 7-119 Infarcts, small intestine, horse.
Thromboemboli from sites of verminous arteritis in the cranial mesenteric artery will often lodge in end arteries of segments of the small intestine, resulting in sudden vascular occlusion and bowel infarction. (Courtesy Dr. H. Gelberg, College of Veterinary Medicine, Oregon State University.)

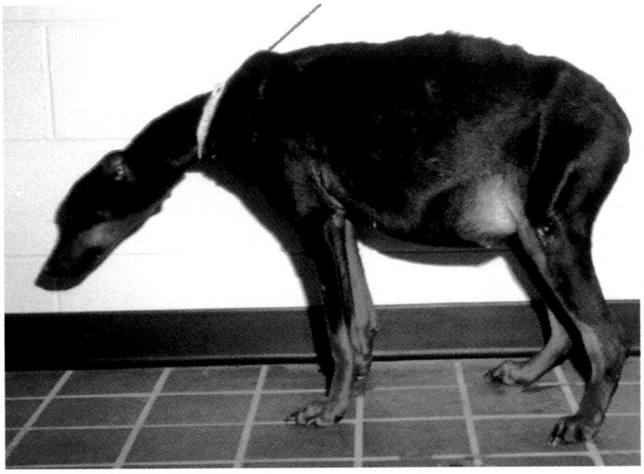

Fig. 7-120 Ascites, abdomen, emaciation, dog, Doberman pinscher.
Protein-losing enteropathy, secondary to idiopathic intestinal lymphangiectasia resulted in hypoproteinemia and then ascites. (Courtesy Dr. H. Gelberg, College of Veterinary Medicine, Oregon State University.)

Lymphangiectasia

Lymphangiectasia, or lacteal dilation, is the most commonly reported cause of protein-losing enteropathy in dogs. Clinical signs include diarrhea, steatorrhea, hypoproteinemia, and ascites (Fig. 7-120). Lymphangiectasia can be due to a congenital developmental disorder of the lymphatic vessels, or it can be acquired secondary to lymph vessel obstruction caused by granulomatous or neoplastic diseases. An inherited cause is suspected in some canine breeds. A special case is lipogranulomatous lymphangiectasia of the dog, the name of which is descriptive of the lesions present. Most cases of acquired lymphangiectasia are idiopathic. Gross and microscopic lesions are those of lymphangiectasia and include a thickened intestinal mucosa with dilated lymphatics and lacteals (Fig. 7-121). There are variable increases in lymphocyte and plasma cell numbers in affected tissue.

Targets for Microbial Colonization or Destruction of Intestinal Mucosae

Mucosal targets include absorptive enterocytes, undifferentiated crypt cells, microvilli and glycocalyx, apical junctional complexes, unknown or nonspecific structures, and the lamina propria as illustrated in Fig. 7-122 and discussed in detail later.

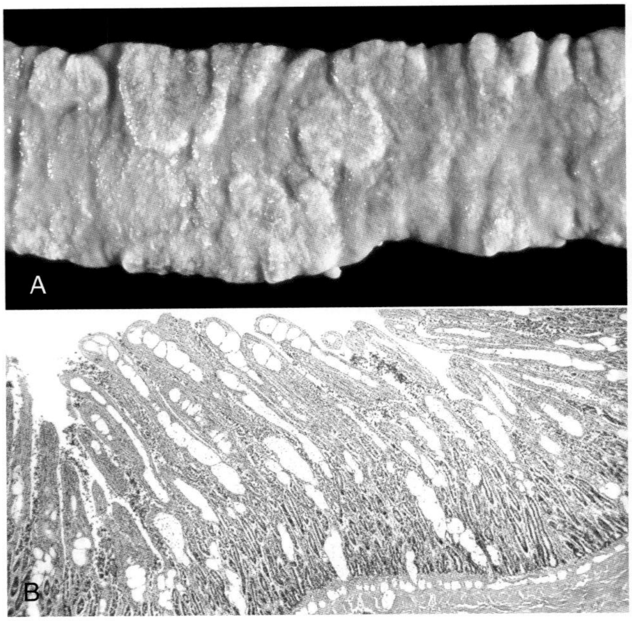

Fig. 7-121 Lymphangiectasia, jejunum, dog.
A, Intestinal villi are expanded by ectasia of the lymphatics *(raised white areas)*. Lymphangiectasia can be a congenital developmental disorder of the lymphatic vessels, or it can be acquired secondary to lymph vessel obstruction caused by granulomatous or neoplastic diseases. **B,** Lacteals are dilated, thus resulting in diminished lymph absorption by lacteals in the lamina propria and subsequent loss of protein (hypoproteinemia) and other nutrients into the intestinal lumen. H&E stain. (**A** courtesy College of Veterinary Medicine, University of Illinois. **B** courtesy Dr. H. Gelberg, College of Veterinary Medicine, Oregon State University.)

Diseases of the Intestinal Epithelium

A number of diseases are characterized by colonization or destruction of the epithelial components of the intestinal mucosa. Although the disease-producing effects of pathogens are complex and multifactorial, a simplified understanding of the principal cell under attack is helpful in predicting disease outcome and managing treatment.

Diseases of the Absorptive Enterocytes

A number of agents have a tropism for the absorptive cells lining the intestinal villi. These agents include viruses such as rotavirus, enteric coronavirus, and the coronavirus of transmissible gastroenteritis of pigs. Intracellular bacteria and parasites can likewise invade and multiply in absorptive epithelial cells. Examples include the agents of swine dysentery *(Brachyspira hyodysenteriae)*, coccidia, and cryptosporidium.

Some pathogens with a tropism for absorptive lining cells of the intestine cause destruction of these cells. This results in loss of enterocytes and at least temporary villous atrophy. The loss of the absorptive-digestive villous enterocytes causes maldigestion, and malabsorption results. Furthermore, because ingesta and normal alimentary secretions are unabsorbed, they are degraded further and fermented in the intestine by bacteria, increasing the osmolality of intestinal contents, with a subsequent increase in the fluid content of the bowel.

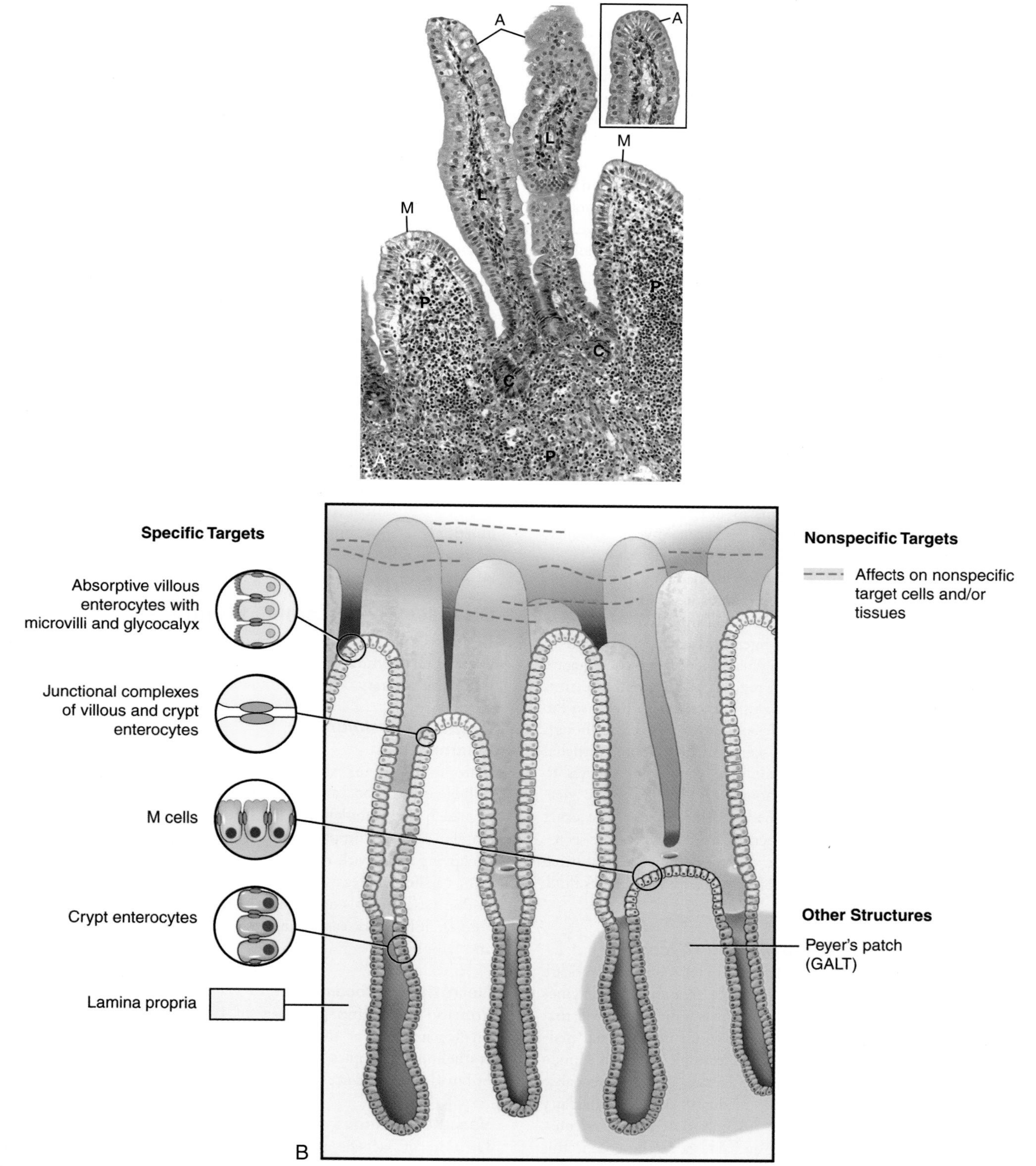

Fig. 7-122 Targets for microbial infection in the intestine.
A, Photomicrograph of small intestinal mucosae identifying targets for infection. Compare with schematic diagram illustrated in **B.** *A,* Absorptive enterocyte; *C,* undifferentiated crypt cells; *L,* lamina propria: *M,* M cells; *P,* Peyer's patch. *Inset,* Higher magnification of villus tip enterocytes with a microvillus border. **B,** Schematic diagram illustrating targets for infection. (**A** and **inset** courtesy Dr. J.F. Zachary, College of Veterinary Medicine, University of Illinois.)

Because the regenerative crypt cells are not attacked by pathogens with tropism for villous enterocytes, diseases with villous enterocyte damage are not necessarily fatal. The lost cells are replaced by the maturing cells migrating along the basement membrane from the crypt to the villus. The naked basement membrane contracts, causing villous atrophy. This contraction may be a function of the smooth muscle in the lamina propria. The functionally immature migrating crypt cells cover the villi. Often, these immature cells become squamoid in an effort to cover the maximum area of basement membrane. However, if naked basement membranes contact each other, they will adhere, resulting not only in villous blunting but also in villous fusion, preventing the reformation of normal villi.

Diseases of Undifferentiated Crypt Cells

Loss of the undifferentiated epithelial cells in the base of the crypts means loss of the cells capable of rapid mitosis, and thus regeneration of the epithelium is impaired. Therefore the clinical effect of crypt cell loss can be delayed for several days because the villi are initially still covered by enterocytes. This type of loss is more severe and often fatal, compared with villous enterocyte loss. Agents that target and destroy crypt cells are called *radiomimetic* because they mimic the effects of radiation on the rapidly dividing enterocytes. Examples of these agents include the parvoviruses of carnivores, BVD virus, rinderpest virus, and some mycotoxins such as vomitoxin.

Enterotoxic *Escherichia coli* infection of neonatal pigs, calves, lambs, and humans causes what is known as a secretory diarrhea. These bacteria are able to colonize the small intestinal enterocytes by way of their surface or pilus antigens, which anchor them to the enterocytes. Different pilus antigens adhere to glycoconjugate receptors on enterocytes in different regions of the small intestine. Thus these bacteria are not washed out by peristalsis. Because the enterocytes are not damaged, no lesions are observed, although microscopically the bacteria can be seen attached to the epithelial surface. The bacteria produce a toxin that causes enterocytes to secrete water and electrolytes. Although cAMP and cyclic guanosine monophosphate (cGMP) mediate this process, the exact mechanism by which this secretion occurs is unknown. Some secretions, especially those of Cl^-, occur via the crypt cells. Intestinal secretion exceeds the ability of the colon to absorb the surplus fluid. The net result is diarrhea.

Abnormalities of the Microvilli and Glycocalyx

Because the microvilli and glycocalyx on the villous enterocytes are largely responsible for the immense surface area and the enzymes responsible for nutrient digestion and absorption, it follows that damage to either of these structures can result in intestinal malfunction and resultant diarrhea. A prime example of this is human lactose intolerance. Such persons lack lactase in the glycocalyx. Because of this lack, they are unable to digest lactose from dairy products. The lack of lactase results in failure of uptake of milk sugar, and the lactose is fermented by bacteria in the colon. This results in an osmotic drain of fluid into the gut with resultant diarrhea. Thus the malabsorption in this case is limited to a single substrate. Histologically, the intestine is normal.

Some bacteria, such as attaching and effacing *Escherichia coli*, damage the microvilli by their attachment. This attachment disrupts enzyme systems housed in the microvilli and glycocalyx and causes diarrhea. The antibiotic neomycin can similarly cause fragmentation of microvilli and destruction of the glycocalyx with resultant diarrhea. Cessation of neomycin therapy results in a return to normal structure and function.

Diseases in which the Epithelial Targets are Unknown or Nonspecific

In a number of enteric diseases, the targeted epithelial cell is unknown or nonspecific. *Clostridium perfringens* type C is a pathogen of neonatal pigs, lambs, calves, and foals. Unlike the ETEC, which produces a toxin affecting enterocytes, *Clostridium perfringens* produces a nonspecific cytotoxin. This toxin causes necrosis of villous absorptive cells, which then extends to the lamina propria and blood vessels. The result is massive and acute necrohemorrhagic enteritis.

Separation of Apical Junctional Complexes

Apical junctional complexes, also called *tight junctions* or *zona occludens,* join enterocytes to each other. Transmembrane proteins, such as claudin, occludin, tricellulin, junction-associated molecules (JAMs), and the coxsackie virus and adenovirus receptor (CAR), form tight junctions. Normally, these junctions are a barrier to macromolecular transepithelial transport. In certain diseases, such as ostertagiosis, *Salmonella* Typhimurium in vitro, *Clostridium perfringens*, alimentary anthrax, and enterohemorrhagic *Escherichia coli,* these tight junctions are pathologically opened through effects of bacterial toxins and products on transmembrane proteins, allowing transport of macromolecules into the intestinal (abomasal) lumen. This opening of tight junctions is also important in allowing macromolecules, such as immunoglobulin, into the lumen where the pathogen can be attacked.

Diseases of the Lamina Propria

Lesions within the lamina propria can be infiltrative, necrotizing, or vascular, all of which can cause diarrhea even though the epithelium is not the primary cell type injured.

Response to Injury

Inflammation

Chronic injury of the lamina propria that results in dense cellular infiltration can cause diarrhea in a variety of ways, none of which are completely understood. These mechanisms include simple physical impairment of mucosal diffusion by space-occupying cells, with resultant disruption of the overlying epithelium causing increased permeability. Examples of these diseases in domestic animals are canine histiocytic ulcerative colitis (boxer colitis), Johne's disease (paratuberculosis) of cattle, amyloidosis, and lymphoma.

Necrotizing Processes

Primary necrotizing processes of the lamina propria generally involve necrosis of the GALT with extension to the overlying epithelium. Examples of diseases with these lesions include BVD of bovids and *Rhodococcus equi* infection of equids.

Vascular Changes and Lymphangiectasia

Dilation of lacteals is idiopathic or secondary to obstruction of flow. These lesions are seen most commonly as part of the syndrome resulting from space-occupying lesions of the lamina propria, such as occurs in Johne's disease and in lymphoma. In both cases, there is obstruction to outflow of lymph—a granulomatous lymphangitis and lymphadenitis in Johne's disease and tumor in the lamina propria and lymph node in lymphoma. Endotoxemia that results in vascular damage and disseminated intravascular coagulopathy can cause thromboemboli in small vessels and hemorrhage, necrosis, and ulceration of the intestine.

Diseases of Domestic Animals Caused by Specific Pathogens

A number of pathogens affect different animal species in similar ways. The mechanism of damage is similar among these animal species and pathogens. Therefore it is useful to discuss the diseases caused by these organisms across species. Specific diseases that do not have analogs in other species are described later in this chapter. Depending on the mechanism of injury and repair, the morphologic types of infectious enteritis include necrotizing, hemorrhagic, fibrosing, lymphoplasmacytic, eosinophilic granulomatous, proliferative, catarrhal, pseudomembranous, or combinations of these.

Viral Diseases

Group A Rotavirus Enteritis

Rotaviruses are ubiquitous pathogens present everywhere in the environment, including air and water. Each species of animal has its specific rotavirus, and although broad similarities exist in pathogenesis among viral infection of individual species, in general the viruses are not cross-infective among species. These viruses are important pathogens. Human group A rotavirus, for example, kills a million children a year in the developing countries of the world. In all species, these viruses cause disease in association with other enteropathogens of neonates.

In calves, the disease is most important during the first week of life and in piglets in the first 7 weeks of life. These ages correspond to the reduction of colostral and milk-associated antirotavirus antibody titers that occur after weaning. Specific diagnosis of these diseases is difficult for a variety of reasons. The virus is ubiquitous and therefore can be isolated or detected in many animals, most of whom do not have clinical disease. Additionally, because the viruses are cytolytic, some animals with viral diarrhea can be negative for viruses because the cells harboring the virus have been shed previously in the feces.

Rotaviruses are about 70 nm in diameter and are trilayered. Only the complete triple-layered virion is infectious. Rotaviruses have double-stranded RNA at their core, and protein spikes project from the surface. The complete particle looks like a wheel, thus the appellation *rotavirus*. The route of infection is oral, and the target cells are villus enterocytes. Piglets and calves with rotavirus disease are dehydrated, have yellow, watery diarrhea, and are weak and depressed. Production of clinical disease depends on the amount of villous epithelium that is lost. This varies by host species.

Pathogenesis

The epithelial cells over the upper two-thirds of the affected villi of the proximal small intestine are infected first in those species that suffer with severe diarrhea from rotavirus infection (Web Fig. 7-18). Sloughing of villous cells results in shortening and sometimes fusion of villi, if basement membranes are exposed (Fig. 7-123). Interestingly, besides causing a malabsorptive diarrhea, rotaviruses produce a secretory enterotoxin nonstructural protein (NSP4) that increases chloride secretion through a calcium-dependent mechanism. This toxin also activates the enteric nervous system and blocks the intestinal sodium/glucose cotransporter. All of these increase fluid and the rate of peristalsis in the intestinal lumen. Depending on the degree of enterocyte loss, recovery may be delayed or incomplete, depending on the amount of absorptive surface that is permanently lost. When death occurs, it is generally associated with intercurrent infections with those organisms that also target villous epithelial cells such as coronavirus, *Cryptosporidium, Escherichia coli*, coccidia, and others.

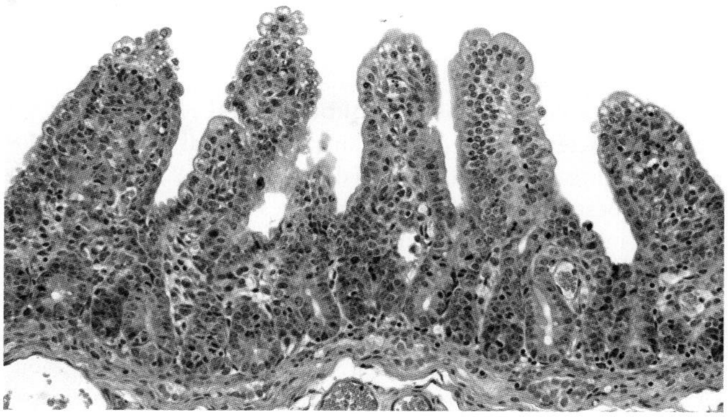

Fig. 7-123 Rotavirus enteritis, jejunum, piglet. There is notable blunting and fusion of intestinal villi secondary to virus-induced cytolysis of enterocytes covering the tips and sides of intestinal villi. H&E stain. (Courtesy Dr. J.F. Zachary, College of Veterinary Medicine, University of Illinois.)

Coronavirus Enteritis

Coronaviruses responsible for calfhood enteritis (at 100 to 120 nm) are larger than rotaviruses. Their genetic core is single-stranded RNA. Peplomers project from the surface, resulting in the appearance of a corona, such as created by the sun; hence the appellation *coronavirus*. The clinical course of the disease, histologic lesions, mechanism of diarrhea production, and age of affected calves are very similar to those of rotavirus enteritis, although somewhat prolonged. Virus infection is more virulent than in rotavirus enteritis, and death is more common. Colitis occurs in addition to small intestinal involvement, but the principal disease signs and pathogenicity are related to the small intestinal lesions. In the colon, similar to the small intestine, enterocytes when lost are initially replaced by less mature and often squamoid cells.

Pathogenesis

Unlike in rotavirus enteritis, crypt lumens contain cell debris and crypt cells may be focally hyperplastic, indicating attempts at enterocyte replacement and villous repair. The lamina propria and draining lymph nodes often contain increased numbers of inflammatory cells. A hemorrhagic form of the disease with extensive colitis has been reported.

Although generally a mild and self-limiting disease of neonates, feline enteric coronavirus has been associated with fatal enteritis in a series of cats. Lesions consist of degeneration and loss of enterocytes from jejunal villous tips. Cats 2 months to 7 years old are affected.

Adenovirus Enteritis

Adenoviral infection occurs in cattle, sheep, pigs, goats, Spanish ibex, cervids, horses, and inland bearded dragons. Each species-specific virus causes inapparent respiratory disease and under some circumstances, clinical enteric disease. Other organs may also be affected such as the liver and kidneys. Endothelial cells are often affected. In Arabian horses and Arabian crossbreeds, adenovirus enteritis occurs in association with combined immunodeficiency (CID). Adenovirus is transmitted by aerosols, feces, and fomites. When enteritis is produced, characteristic basophilic to amphophilic intranuclear inclusion bodies are present in villous enterocytes, usually in young animals that are immunosuppressed. Endothelial cells also are affected and have similar inclusions. Loss of enterocytes results in villous blunting and fusion. In general, adenovirus infection is subclinical, although severe enteric disease may occur in calves.

Bacterial Diseases

Escherichia coli Diseases (Colibacillosis)

Coliform bacteria arrive early among the normal flora that colonizes the intestinal tract of virtually all animals. Young animals are at highest risk for coliform diarrhea, especially pigs and calves. There is interplay of many intrinsic and extrinsic factors that act together to determine if disease will be produced by infection. Some of the factors are the genetic make-up of the host animals, the passive transfer of specific antibodies in the colostrums, the constant bathing of the intestine with milk-associated antibodies from nursing, environmental contamination, and the nutritional plane of the host. Environmental stressors predisposing to disease production include temperature extremes, crowding, and intercurrent infections with rotavirus, coronavirus, *Cryptosporidium,* coccidia, and others. The development of unique serotypes of *Escherichia coli* may cause problems in individual environments. In the past, autogenous vaccines, made to order for these environments, have been reasonably effective in controlling some disease outbreaks. Probiotics containing several *Escherichia coli* types and/or *Lactobacillus* spp. have shown promise as a preventive in calves. Lytic phages have also been promising in eliminating infection.

There are a variety of classification schemes for the *Escherichia coli* enteritides. They include enterotoxic (ETEC), septicemic (EIEC), edema disease (enterotoxemic), postweaning, enterohemorrhagic (EHEC), enteroinvasive, and enteropathogenic/attaching and effacing (EPEC/AAEC), among others (also see Chapter 4).

Escherichia coli attach to cells by a variety of pili or fimbriae (Fig. 7-124). ETEC may have fimbrial antigens F4 (K88), 5 (K99), 6 (987P), 18, or 41 and may also produce up to three enterotoxins and shigatoxins (STa, STb, LT). Fimbrial and nonfimbrial adhesins, such as adhesins involved in diffuse adherence (AIDA-1), may also be present. Many *Escherichia coli* produce verotoxins (verotoxic *E. coli* [VTEC]) important in disease pathogenesis. More than 200 serotypes of VTEC have been isolated from cattle alone. Diagnosis of toxin-producing *Escherichia coli* is by selective culture properties of the bacteria, immunomagnetic separation, and other monoclonal-based immunoassays for the Vero-Shiga toxins. A more recent development is the use of real-time PCR to detect pathogenic gene sequences. Many of the virulence factors of *Escherichia coli* can be exchanged among *E. coli* and other bacterial species by phages, as well as plasmids.

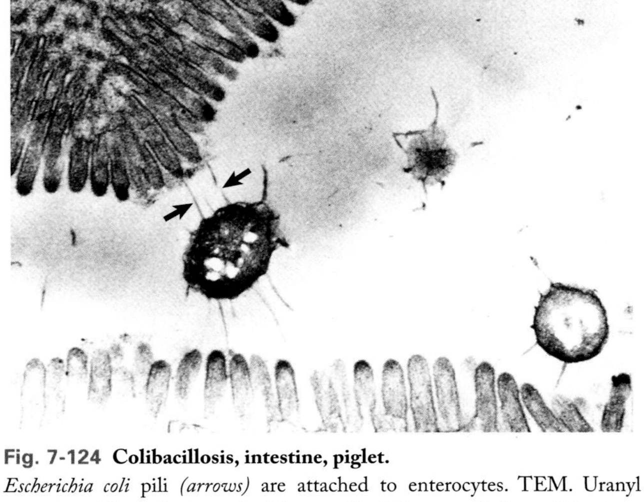

Fig. 7-124 Colibacillosis, intestine, piglet.
Escherichia coli pili *(arrows)* are attached to enterocytes. TEM. Uranyl acetate and lead citrate stain. (Courtesy Dr. R. Isaacson, College of Veterinary Medicine, University of Minnesota.)

Enterotoxic Colibacillosis (ETEC)

Enterotoxic, or enterotoxigenic, colibacillosis (F18ac) occurs most often in animals 2 days to 3 weeks of age. Calves and piglets are most often affected. Why enterotoxic colibacillosis is a disease of neonates is not well understood. Some speculation is that enteric bacterial colonization is a function of gastric acidity and that the low pH of the stomach of postneonatal animals kills the bacteria.

The diarrhea that occurs is largely a function of bacterial endotoxin-induced, cGMP- and cGAMP-dependent kinase-induced sodium and chloride secretion into the intestinal lumen. Water is drawn into the intestine to normalize the resultant sodium chloride (NaCl). Thus the diarrhea is termed *secretory.* Diarrhea is voluminous, yellow to white, and watery to pasty. At necropsy, the small intestine is dilated, flaccid, and filled with translucent, yellow fluid and sometimes gas. Chyle is present in the mesenteric lymphatic vessels similar to animals without enteric disease, indicating that unlike the malabsorptive diseases of the small intestine, absorption proceeds normally in cases of enterotoxic colibacillosis. Microscopically, the intestine is also normal. Diagnosis can be made by light microscopic examination in freshly dead animals by noting the presence of bacteria lining the luminal surface of the enterocytes (Fig. 7-125). Inflammation is absent. Affected animals are dehydrated, with a "tucked up" abdomen. Subsequent to dehydration, the eyes of affected animals may be recessed deeply into their sockets (sunken eyeballs). Animals that die from ETEC infection are often emaciated and have diarrheic feces pasted around their perineum.

Septicemic colibacillosis

Septicemic or enteroinvasive colibacillosis (EIEC) is a disease of newborn calves, lambs, and occasionally foals that have not received sufficient colostrum to develop immunity. Although the lesions produced are generally those of septicemia, similar to those caused by other organisms, infection can localize in the intestine, causing enteritis. Diagnosis is generally made by finding fibrin in any location in the body such as the eye, joints, abdomen, heart sac, meninges, and/or thorax. The bacteria gain entry to the body through the respiratory system, oral cavity, or umbilicus. Fibrinous arthritis, ophthalmitis, serositis, meningitis (polyserositis), and white-spotted kidneys (cortical abscesses) characterize the

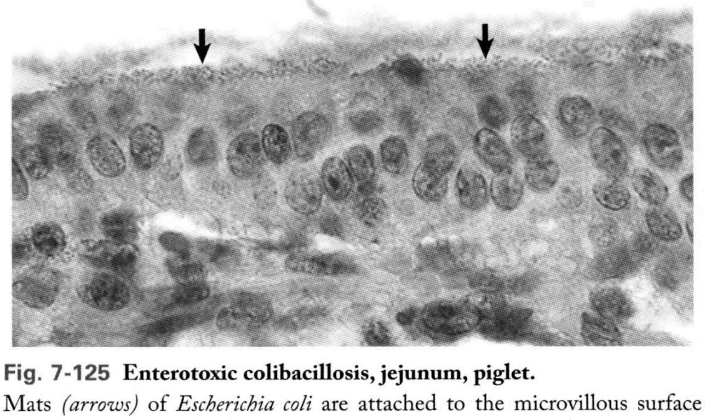

Fig. 7-125 Enterotoxic colibacillosis, jejunum, piglet.
Mats *(arrows)* of *Escherichia coli* are attached to the microvillous surface of the enterocytes. H&E stain. (Courtesy Dr. H. Gelberg, College of Veterinary Medicine, Oregon State University.)

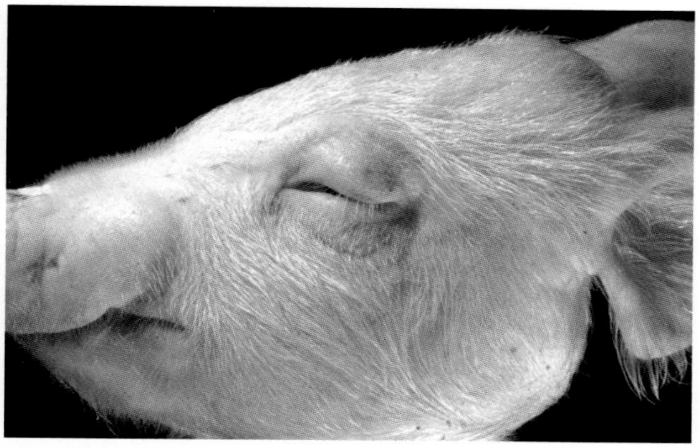

Fig. 7-126 Edema disease, head, pig.
The skin of the eyelids, snout, and submandibular area are edematous as a result of production of angiotoxin by *Escherichia coli,* which increases the permeability of capillaries. (Courtesy Dr. H. Gelberg, College of Veterinary Medicine, Oregon State University.)

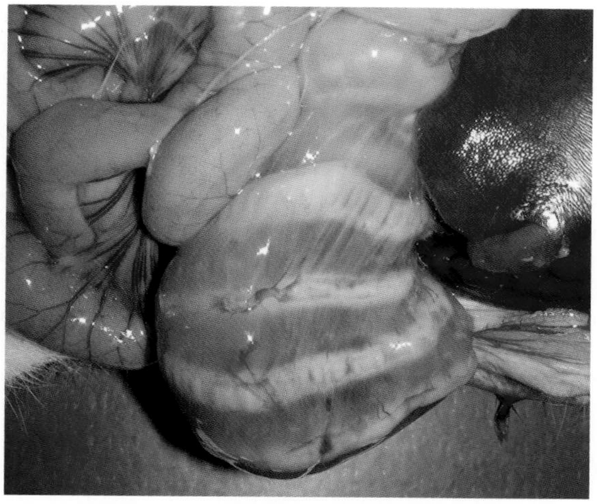

Fig. 7-127 Edema disease, spiral colon, pig.
Edema of the mesentery is a result of an angiotoxin produced by *Escherichia coli.* (Courtesy Dr. W. Hascheck-Hock and Dr. L. Borst, College of Veterinary Medicine, University of Illinois.)

septicemia (see Fig. 11-70). Mixed bacterial infections often occur with ETEC.

Edema disease

Edema disease, also known as *enterotoxemic colibacillosis,* is an *Escherichia coli* (F18ab) infection that is specific for pigs. Edema disease is caused by a bacterial enterotoxin (verotoxin) produced in the small intestine and spread hematogenously via induction of IL-8. This interleukin attracts neutrophils that carry the toxin throughout the body. It is generally a disease of pigs 6 to 14 weeks of age and is usually associated with dietary changes at weaning. It is often noted that the best pigs in a group are the ones affected. Edema disease is characterized by neurologic signs including incoordination, poor balance, weakness, tremors, and convulsions.

Hemolytic *Escherichia coli* proliferates in the small intestine subsequent to dietary changes and produces a heat-labile exotoxin called the *edema disease principle.* This systemic toxin (angiotoxin) causes generalized vascular endothelial injury of arterioles and arteries (see Fig. 10-42), resulting in fluid loss and edema. The edema can be found anywhere but is most characteristic in the gastric submucosa (see Fig. 10-80), eyelids (Fig. 7-126), forehead, gallbladder, and mesentery of the spiral colon (Fig. 7-127). In the brain, arterial damage causes focal malacia in the medulla, thalamus, and basal ganglia. These nervous tissue lesions are collectively known as focal symmetric encephalomalacia or swine cerebral angiopathy and are responsible for the variety of clinical signs. Death is due to an endotoxic shocklike syndrome. Some animals suffer from a Shwartzman-like bilateral renal cortical necrosis. Morbidity within a herd is approximately 35%, and all affected animals die.

Postweaning colibacillosis

Postweaning colibacillosis is another specific disease of pigs caused by a hemolytic *Escherichia coli.* The disease appears identical to enterotoxic colibacillosis of the neonate in that it produces a secretory diarrhea and therefore no lesions in the intestine, although gastric infarcts are common. It is a distinct strain of *Escherichia coli,* however, and is associated with feed and management changes at weaning.

Enterohemorrhagic colibacillosis

Enterohemorrhagic colibacillosis (EHEC) is described in humans, laboratory animals, and occasionally cattle and pigs. It has not been reported as a field problem in livestock. The pathogenesis of the disease is similar to that of other invasive bacteria such as *Salmonella* spp. In humans, the colon is affected. A Shiga toxin gene, a locus for enterocyte effacement, and a plasmid encoding for hemolysin are produced by *Escherichia coli,* which result in hemorrhagic colitis and sometimes the hemolytic-uremic syndrome. These strains are also called *VTEC,* which are strains based on the Vero (African green monkey kidney) cell line on which the bacteria are sometimes grown. Outbreaks of enteroinvasive colibacillosis in humans are often food-borne illnesses. These organisms are pathogenic because of their acid resistance and ability to survive transport through the stomach. Shiga toxin–producing enterohemorrhagic *Escherichia coli* O157:H7 rarely causes naturally occurring disease in domestic livestock but often contaminates ground beef. Surveys have indicated that the seroprevalence of *Escherichia coli* O157:H7 in dairy herds is 38.5%, with an individual cow prevalence of 6.5%, and is most often isolated from the skin surface. This finding is an important reason not to eat undercooked ground beef. Steaks are a different matter because bacterial contamination is only a surface phenomenon, and bacteria are killed by surface searing of meat.

Experimentally, calves may develop necrohemorrhagic or mucohemorrhagic diarrhea. Human disease can be serious, resulting in hemorrhagic colitis, thrombocytopenic purpura, and the hemolytic uremic syndrome. Deer, sheep, cattle, horses, dogs, and rabbits, including laboratory rabbits, may be carriers. Stable flies and fecal contamination of a variety of substances may create fomites.

Attaching and effacing Escherichia coli

Attaching and effacing *Escherichia coli* (AAEC), also called enteropathogenic *E. coli* (EPEC), has been infrequently reported in rabbits, calves, pigs, lambs, dogs, and humans. The actual incidence of this disease in domestic animals is unknown. Lesions are characterized by *Escherichia coli* attachment to the microvillous border of enterocytes and gallbladder epithelium via cups and pedestals (Web Fig. 7-19). Intimin, a bacterial outer membrane protein, facilitates bacterial attachment to the host cell's membrane, resulting in attachment and effacement. These bacteria also alter a variety of tight junction proteins and therefore cause leakage of enterocyte tight junctions. Gross lesions are not present except that the intestine is dilated and fluid-filled. Colonization of the epithelium by attaching and effacing *Escherichia coli* is relatively common; disease occurs most often in association with other enteropathogens of calves of this age, namely rotavirus, *Cryptosporidium parvum*, ETEC, coronavirus, BVD, and coccidia. In contrast to ETEC infection, in AAEC infection the brush border of the enterocytes is disrupted and can be seen on select enterocytes in hematoxylin and eosin (H&E) stained tissue sections. Microvillous disruption results in loss of the glycocalyx digestive enzymes, resulting in maldigestion, malabsorption, and diarrhea. AAEC also stimulates enterocyte apoptosis, Cl^- and mucus secretion, and toxin production. AAEC flagellin TLR-5 stimulates IL-8 release by enterocytes, which initiates an inflammatory response resulting in cell death and fluid secretion.

Extraintestinal pathogenic Escherichia coli

Extraintestinal pathogenic *Escherichia coli* (ExPEC) are gut inhabitants with virulence genes that differ from strains of *E. coli* that are enteropathogens or commensal organisms of the intestine. They contain fimbrial adhesins for attachment, cytotoxins and hemolysins responsible for tissue necrosis and hemorrhage, and siderophore receptors to sequester iron. ExPEC can be isolated from the feces of many healthy animals, particularly dogs and cats. When the animals are stressed, such as in group housing in shelters, aerosolized bacteria may be inhaled resulting in fulminating necrohemorrhagic pleuropneumonia. Septicemia can result in urogenital infections. In addition, meningitis has been reported in humans. There is concern about the zoonotic potential of these organisms.

Salmonellosis

Salmonella spp. are enteroinvasive bacteria. All known species of *Salmonella* are pathogenic, and salmonellosis is an important zoonosis and nosocomial infection. Salmonellosis is a significant cause of acute and chronic diarrhea and death in numerous animal species and in humans. *Salmonella* Typhimurium is the second most common food-borne pathogen in humans. In veterinary medicine, salmonellosis can occur epizootically, enzootically, or sporadically. The serovars most often isolated from diseased animals include *Salmonella* Typhimurium, *Salmonella* Enterica, *Salmonella* Dublin, *Salmonella* Choleraesuis, and *Salmonella* Typhosa.

The salmonellas are Gram-negative, aerobic to facultatively anaerobic, and motile. They survive and multiply within phagocytic cells, resulting in granulomatous inflammation. One way that they survive in the hostile environment of the phagosomes of professional phagocytes is by producing a nitrite transporter through their pathogenicity island (SPI-2) that neutralizes nitric oxide (NO) production by the phagocytosing cell. The form of salmonellosis that occurs—septicemic, acute enteric, or chronic enteric—depends on the challenge dosage of the bacterium, previous exposure to the bacterium, and stress factors such as overcrowding, transport, cold temperatures, feed changes, pregnancy, parturition, surgery, anesthesia, and antibiotic administration. Some recovered animals become carriers and shed the organism in their feces, particularly after stress. This may make diagnosis by culture difficult because carriers may not be ill. Conversely, antibiotic treatment of ill animals may create false-negative bacterial cultures. Although dogs and cats rarely get clinical salmonellosis, 10% are carriers and can infect their human companions. It has been documented that fatal salmonellosis may occur in cats in association with homemade, raw-meat diets.

The most common route of bacterial entry is fecal-oral. Effective handwashing is thus of paramount importance for food handlers ("typhoid Mary"). Besides being present in contaminated feed, water, and aerosols, flies and fomites can transmit salmonella. Transplacental infection may also occur. After ingestion, salmonella may colonize regional lymphoid tissue in the oral cavity and gut through dendritic cells by means of pathogenicity islands, which are clusters of plasmid genes coding for virulence factors such as fimbriae, motility, lipopolysaccharide (LPS), and other secreted proteins. Some species of *Salmonella* are enteroinvasive.

Salmonella Choleraesuis and Typhimurium in pigs have been shown to adhere to apical membranes of M cells, enterocytes, goblet cells, and sites of cellular extrusion. Salmonellas produce disease via enterotoxins, cytotoxins (verotoxins), and endotoxins, some of which block closure of Cl^- channels. In addition, inflammatory cells upregulate PGE_2, which results in hypersecretion of chloride. Secretory diarrhea results, as well as malabsorptive diarrhea from enterocyte death. Experimental infections of calves with *Salmonella* Typhimurium demonstrate upregulation of CXC chemokines (IL-8, growth-related oncogene-α [GRO-α], and granulocyte chemotactic protein-2 [GCP-2]), IL-1β, IL-1Rα, and IL-4 associated with a neutrophilic influx. Once in contact with macrophages of the lamina propria or Peyer's patches, the organisms are phagocytosed and transported to regional lymph nodes or by way of the portal circulation to the liver. The organisms colonize the small intestine, colon, mesenteric lymph nodes, and gallbladder, which may serve as reservoirs in carrier animals. Salmonellosis infects the young more frequently; the young are more severely affected than are adults; and the young are more likely to succumb to septicemia.

Peracute Salmonella *septicemia*

Peracute *Salmonella* septicemia is a disease of calves, foals, and pigs. Young animals are generally at greater risk than older animals, although the reasons for this difference are not understood. In foals, the feces of affected animals are typically green. The serovar of *Salmonella* most often involved in septicemic salmonellosis is *Salmonella* Choleraesuis. Gross lesions of animals dying of peracute *Salmonella* septicemia are minimal and are caused by fibrinoid necrosis of blood vessels (Fig. 7-128). Necrosis of blood vessels causes widespread petechiation and a blue discoloration (cyanosis) of the extremities and ventrum of white pigs. Fibrinous polyserositis may be present. Peracute *Salmonella* septicemia is usually fatal in animals 1 to 6 months of age. Death is usually attributable to disseminated intravascular coagulopathy secondary to the generalized Shwartzman reaction.

Acute enteric salmonellosis

Acute enteric salmonellosis is caused most frequently by *Salmonella* Typhimurium and occurs in cattle, pigs, and horses. Carnivores are rarely affected. Characteristic of the disease is diffuse catarrhal enteritis with diffuse fibrinonecrotic ileotyphlocolitis. Intestinal contents are malodorous and contain mucus, fibrin, and occasionally blood. The feces have a septic tank odor. *Salmonella* are enteroinvasive through specific surface bacterial fimbrial (pilus adhesin) antigens. Receptor-mediated endocytosis then occurs. Membrane bound vacuoles then translocate the bacteria to macrophages in the lamina propria. The intact *Salmonella* induce secretory diarrhea through interference with Cl^- channels. They also induce enterocyte apoptosis and recruit neutrophils. Endotoxins induce thrombosis. All these adherence and inflammatory changes are regulated by pathogenicity islands. Multiple foci of hepatocellular necrosis and hyperplasia of Kupffer cells (paratyphoid nodules), when present, are characteristic of acute enteric salmonellosis (see Fig. 8-49, *B*). Mesenteric lymphadenopathy is usually present.

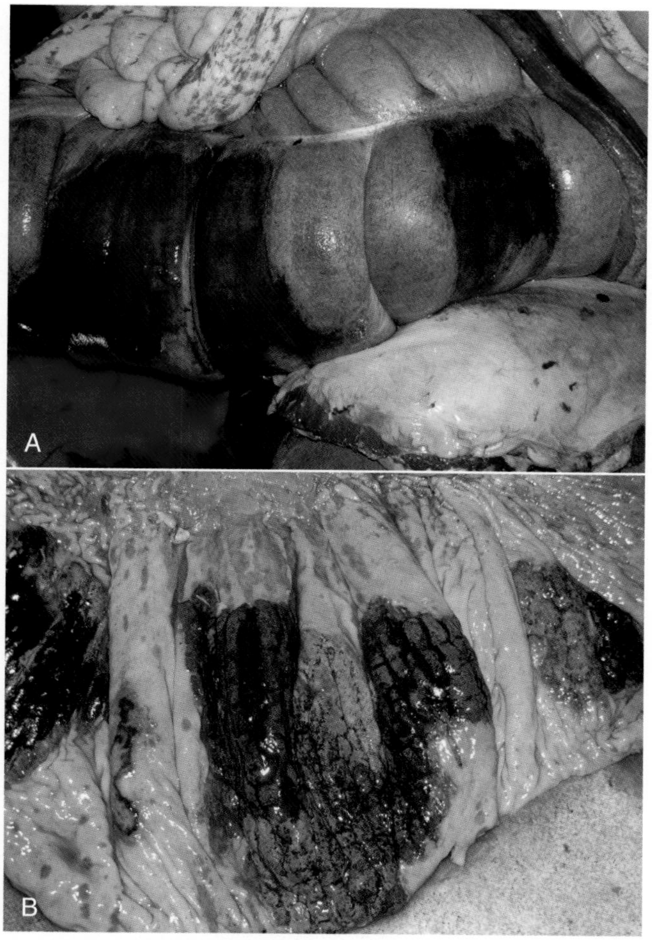

Fig. 7-128 Peracute to acute salmonellosis, colon, horse.
A, Serosal surfaces. Note the areas of hemorrhage and necrosis affecting multiple sacculations. This pattern is consistent with colonic infarcts secondary to ischemia caused by vascular thrombosis, which can occur with peracute and/or acute salmonellosis. **B,** Mucosal surfaces. Note the extensive mucosal edema and gray-white areas of mucosal necrosis. The green stained tissue is postmortem imbibition. Mucosal erosions and ulcerations are also present. (Courtesy Dr. A. Gillen, College of Veterinary Medicine, University of Illinois.)

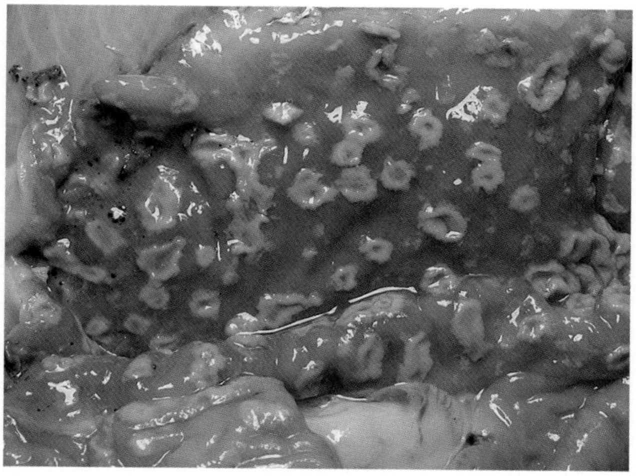

Fig. 7-129 Button ulcers, colon, pig.
Multiple foci of necrosis (infarcts) due to chronic enteric salmonellosis are termed *button ulcers* and are pathognomonic for this disease in North America and in other areas in which hog cholera has been eradicated. The morphology of this lesion is attributable to bacterial toxin-induced vasculitis and thrombosis of blood vessels in the lamina propria and submucosa resulting in focal intestinal infarcts. (Courtesy of Dr. D. Driemeier, Federal University of Rio Grande do Sul, Brazil.)

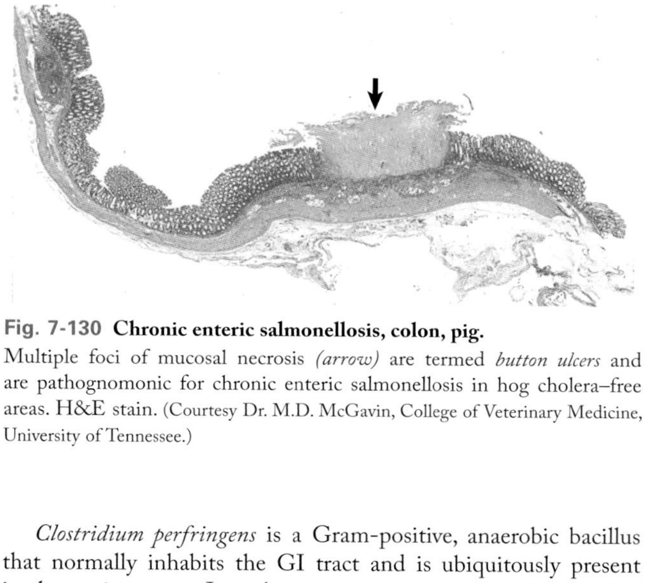

Fig. 7-130 Chronic enteric salmonellosis, colon, pig.
Multiple foci of mucosal necrosis *(arrow)* are termed *button ulcers* and are pathognomonic for chronic enteric salmonellosis in hog cholera–free areas. H&E stain. (Courtesy Dr. M.D. McGavin, College of Veterinary Medicine, University of Tennessee.)

Fibrinous cholecystitis at necropsy is pathognomonic for acute enteric salmonellosis in calves (see Fig. 8-78).

Chronic enteric salmonellosis

Chronic enteric salmonellosis occurs in pigs, cattle, and horses. Lesions are seen principally in pigs that have discrete foci of necrosis and ulceration, principally in the cecum and colon. These are termed *button ulcers* (Figs. 7-129 and 7-130). Because salmonellosis causes vascular thrombosis and pigs have poor or no collateral blood supply to the rectum (cranial hemorrhoidal artery), in affected animals, rectal strictures develop, with resultant abdominal distention secondary to fecal retention.

Clostridial Enteritis

Many diseases that affect animals and humans are caused by clostridial organisms. This discussion is limited to those clostridia that produce diarrheal disease. All clostridial enteritides produce enterotoxemias.

Clostridium perfringens is a Gram-positive, anaerobic bacillus that normally inhabits the GI tract and is ubiquitously present in the environment. It is the most important cause of clostridial enteritis in domestic animals. At least 17 exotoxins have been described, but only 4 are believed to be involved in the pathogenesis of disease. These spore-forming bacilli produce their toxins when circumstances provide them with an excess of nutrients that promotes bacterial growth in an anaerobic environment. The four major toxins—α (CPA), β (CPB), ε (ETX), and ι (ITX)—are used to classify the toxigenic types of *Clostridium perfringens* into five major groupings: A through E. The toxins are protein exotoxins, some of which are proenzymes while others have enzymatic activity. *Clostridium perfringens* type A produces the α-toxin responsible for necrotic enteritis of birds, enterotoxemia of calves and lambs, necrotizing enterocolitis of piglets, canine hemorrhagic enteritis, and possibly equine colitis. Type B produces α-, β-, and ε-toxins and the diseases lamb dysentery, hemorrhagic enteritis of neonatal calves and foals, and hemorrhagic enterotoxemia of sheep. Type C produces α- and β-toxins and necrotic enteritis of birds, hemorrhagic enterotoxemia of neonatal farm animal species, and struck of sheep. Type D produces α- and ε-toxins and pulpy kidney disease of lambs and enterocolitis of goats of all ages. Type E produces α- and ι-toxins and enteritis of lagomorphs and possibly enterotoxemia in calves and lambs.

Enterotoxigenic strains of *Clostridium perfringens*, particularly type A, are responsible for clostridial food poisoning. This generally occurs when cooked foods are improperly stored, and spores that survive the cooking environment germinate and produce enterotoxin.

Enterotoxemia

Enterotoxemia is produced by one of the five *Clostridium perfringens* types described previously. Type D occurs most often. Clostridial enterotoxemia most often affects the better-fleshed animals within a group. Outbreaks often follow an abrupt change in the amount or quality of feed such as occurs in an animal being "finished" for sale or slaughter. In foals, enterotoxemia has been associated with feeding materials rich in carbohydrates and proteins. This diet leads to a change in the intestinal microbial balance. *Clostridium perfringens* proliferates and produces abundant toxin. Clinical signs may be absent before death or may include diarrhea, sometimes with blood. Glycosuria occurs only in lambs with enterotoxemia and is a helpful feature in preliminary necropsy diagnosis. Enzyme-linked immunosorbent assay (ELISA) kits are available for toxin typing (CPA, CPB, ETX) and for the bacteria.

The small intestine, the target organ of clostridial enterotoxemia, typically has serosal and mucosal petechiae, ecchymoses, and paintbrush or diffuse hemorrhage similar in appearance to those of intestinal strangulation. The intestines are atonic and dilated. Emphysematous enteritis is variably present, as is coagulative necrosis of skeletal muscle. Congestive splenomegaly is present. On exposure to enterotoxin, villous tip enterocytes and mid-villous enterocytes degenerate and are sloughed into the intestinal lumen, leaving denuded basement membranes. The exposed basement membranes allow fluid leakage and attract leukocytes into the lamina propria. Death is usually rapid.

Clostridium perfringens *type A*

Clostridium perfringens type A is the most frequently occurring clostridium in mammals and birds. It is also the most common clostridium found in the environment. *Clostridium perfringens* type A produces enteric disease in a great variety of animals. These diarrheal diseases are generally mild with minimal damage to the intestinal mucosa. In addition to enteritis, infection produces gas gangrene and other anaerobic wound infections. In the western United States, it causes hemorrhagic abomasitis in young ruminants, often accompanied by severe diarrhea. In the Pacific Northwest, principally in Washington and Oregon, a condition called yellow lamb disease is associated with *Clostridium perfringens* type A. Death is rapid and accompanied by clinical and pathologic signs of hemolysis, hence the yellow discoloration of the carcass.

Clostridium perfringens *type B*

Clostridium perfringens type B is the cause of lamb dysentery. This is generally a disease of very young lambs, although older animals may be affected in prolonged disease outbreaks. Unexpected death is usual, but occasionally there is antecedent anorexia and abdominal pain with or without severe bloody diarrhea. Other young ruminants and foals may also be affected. This disease occurs sporadically in the US but is more common in Europe, South Africa, and the Middle East.

Clostridium perfringens *type C*

Enterotoxic hemorrhagic enteritis affects calves, lambs, and foals during the first few days of life and piglets during the first 8 hours of life. Adult horses may also be affected. Clinical signs vary from none to bloody diarrhea. When piglets are affected, the whole litter dies. Lesions at necropsy include hemorrhagic or necrotizing enteritis of the small intestines, sometimes with gas in the lumen and within the walls of the intestine (Figs. 7-131 and 7-132). Struck, which is also caused by *Clostridium perfringens* type C, affects adult sheep, goats, and feedlot cattle in winter and early spring and is characterized by hemorrhagic enteritis with ulceration, ascites, and peritonitis.

Clostridium perfringens *type D*

Clostridium perfringens type D affects fattening sheep, goats, and calves. The disease is diet-related and associated with grain overload or "overeating disease." The sudden change in diet promotes growth of organisms in the small intestine. The disease is often characterized by unexpected death, sometimes preceded by CNS signs or "blind staggers." Endothelial cell damage is produced by a bacterial toxin (angiotoxin). This lesion can result in bilateral symmetric encephalomalacia, which is similar in its regional distribution to edema disease of pigs (swine cerebral angiopathy)

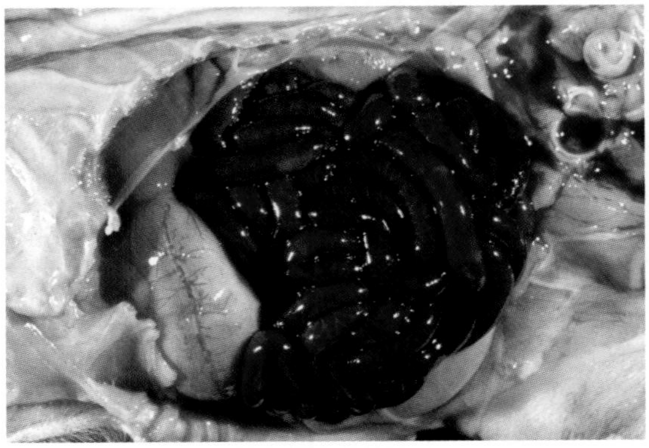

Fig. 7-131 Enterotoxemia, small intestine, pig.
The entire small intestinal mucosa is hemorrhagic. Necrosis can extend through the muscularis mucosa and is caused by toxins of the *Clostridium perfringens* type C group acting directly on the intestinal mucosa in the intestinal lumen. The entire litter of piglets was affected. (Courtesy Dr. H. Gelberg, College of Veterinary Medicine, Oregon State University.)

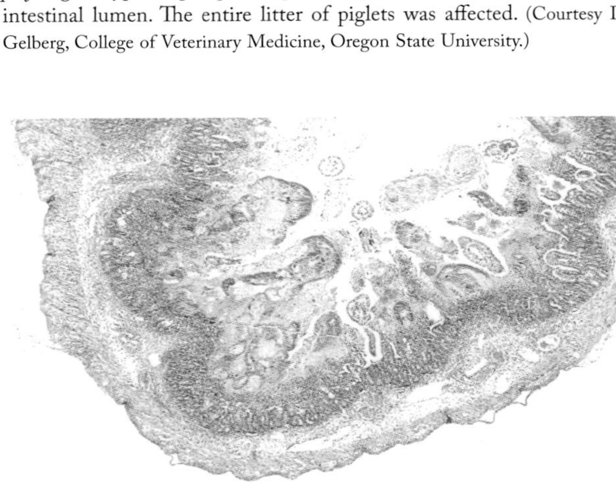

Fig. 7-132 Clostridial enteritis, small intestine, pig.
Nonspecific necrotizing enteritis results from the toxins produced by *Clostridium perfringens* type C. H&E stain. (Courtesy Dr. H. Gelberg, College of Veterinary Medicine, Oregon State University.)

(see Fig. 14-96). Lesions of *Clostridium perfringens* type D infection are multisystem hemorrhages, particularly of serosal surfaces. Fibrinonecrotic enterocolitis can also occur in association with the β-2 toxin, at least in goats. Pericardial effusion is present along with mild gastroenteritis. The angiotoxin produces "pulpy kidney disease" of sheep (see Fig. 11-49).

Clostridium perfringens *type E*

Case reports of necrohemorrhagic diarrhea associated with *Clostridium perfringens* type E infection are poorly documented. It is safest to state that *Clostridium perfringens* type E may rarely cause enterotoxemia of lambs, calves, and rabbits.

Peracute hemorrhagic gastroenteritis of dogs

The cause of peracute hemorrhagic gastroenteritis of dogs, also known as canine hemorrhagic gastroenteritis, is undiscovered but is considered likely a result of infection with *Clostridium perfringens* of unknown type. The disease most often occurs in dogs of toy and miniature breeds younger than 2 years. Blood is observed at the anus before death. As the name of the disease denotes, there is hemorrhagic necrosis of the GI mucosa anywhere from the stomach caudally. Numerous clostridial organisms are present in the intestinal debris but are not attached to intact mucosa. Unlike parvoviral enteritis in which crypts are preferentially destroyed, the crypts are spared in peracute hemorrhagic gastroenteritis.

Lincomycin or antibiotic enteritis

Lincomycin or antibiotic enteritis is associated with antibiotic administration and is seen most commonly in rabbits and horses; both are cecal fermenters. It has been suggested but not proved that antibiotic administration causes death of normal enteric flora, which allows overgrowth of *Clostridium perfringens* type A. Clinical signs and gross and microscopic lesions are similar to those observed in animals with *Clostridium* spp. enteritis, but bacterial organisms are often lacking.

Clostridium piliforme

Clostridium piliforme infects multiple mammalian species and is commonly called *Tyzzer's disease.* The target organs of *Clostridium piliforme* vary among affected animals. Although pathogen entry is usually via the intestine, the principal target is the liver, but lesions also occur in the intestine and heart. Intestinal involvement is variable and most common in rodents and rabbits. The enteric manifestations of Tyzzer's disease are generally in the distal small intestine, particularly the ileum. Colitis occurs in some cats. Mucosal necrosis and edema extend into the muscularis. Definitive diagnosis is made by finding the causative bacillus (best done with silver stains such as Dieterle's or Steiner's) in the characteristic hepatic (see Fig. 8-48) or intestinal lesions (Fig. 7-133).

Clostridium difficile

Clostridium difficile spores are common in the environment and in the intestinal tract of many mammals. They cause pseudomembranous colitis in primates, including humans, hemorrhagic necrotizing enterocolitis in foals, necrotizing typhlocolitis in horses (colitis X) and possibly cats, and enteritis in a variety of laboratory animals. *Clostridium difficile* also affects suckling pigs in outbreaks characterized by mesocolonic edema and typhlocolitis. Dogs, especially those hospitalized, may also shed the organism. The disease-producing ability of *Clostridium difficile* in the dog is not understood, but its zoonotic potential may be important. The induction of disease by *Clostridium difficile* is likely dose-related, but the reasons for bacterial overgrowth, apart from those caused by oral antibiotic administration, are not known. The lesions are similar to those produced by *Clostridium perfringens* infection.

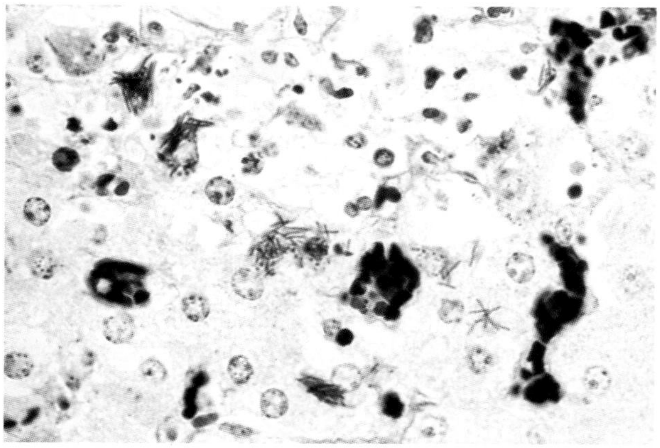

Fig. 7-133 Tyzzer's disease, intestine, foal.
Criss-crossed bacilli resembling Chinese characters or pickup sticks are diagnostic of infection with *Clostridium piliforme.* Warthin-Starry stain. (Courtesy Dr. H. Gelberg, College of Veterinary Medicine, Oregon State University.)

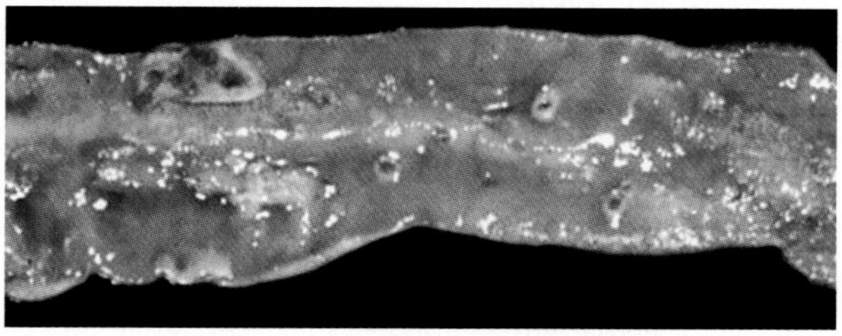

Fig. 7-134 Multifocal necroulcerative colitis, quail.
Sharply demarcated ulcers are present in the colon. Quail disease is caused by *Clostridium colinum.* (Courtesy College of Veterinary Medicine, Cornell University.)

Clostridium spiroforme

Clostridium spiroforme causes enterotoxemia in lagomorphs and rodents. The bacterium is semicircular *in vivo* and has a coiled appearance *in vitro* when bacteria are joined end to end. In the rabbit, weaning and/or antibiotic treatment with a concomitant change in cecal flora precede diarrhea and death. Lesions include a dilated cecum with liquid contents. As is the case with other clostridia, the cause is confirmed by mouse lethality studies or Vero cell cytotoxicity studies; the appropriate toxin may be isolated from intestinal contents soon after death of the animal.

Clostridium colinum

Clostridium colinum, also known as quail disease or quail enteritis, is an ulcerative colitis restricted to gallinaceous birds. The disease occurs in birds secondary to stress that is often a result of intercurrent infections. Classically, there is hemorrhagic enteritis of the small intestine often accompanied by necroulcerative enterotyphlitis. Necrohemorrhagic hepatosplenitis is often present. Death is rapid and losses are high, especially in quail (Fig. 7-134).

Lawsoniasis

Lawsonia intracellularis is the cause of a proliferative segmental enteropathy in a variety of species, including humans. *Lawsonia* are curved, Gram-negative, motile, and obligate intracellular bacteria that cannot be grown on artificial media. Lesions of proliferative enteropathy have been reported in pigs, dogs, horses, sheep, rabbits, guinea pigs, hamsters, rats, ferrets, foxes, cervids, monkeys, ostriches, and emus. In the dog, the majority of cases occur in puppies younger than 3 months. The mechanism of enterocyte proliferation may relate to *Lawsonia*-induced altered transcription of host "alarm response" genes that affect regulation of the cell cycle and cell differentiation. Lesions consist of surface erosions and proliferation of cryptal enterocytes with the presence of bacteria in the apical cytoplasm of affected cells. Diagnosis depends on characteristic histopathologic findings of crypt cell proliferation and by the presence of comma-shaped bacteria in the intestinal crypt epithelial cytoplasm. Clinically, diarrhea is of 5 to 15 days' duration. The diarrhea is mucoid or watery, with or without blood, and is accompanied by partial anorexia, vomiting, and a slight fever.

Campylobacter

Campylobacter infections from asymptomatic poultry (*Campylobacter jejuni*) and swine (*Campylobacter coli*) are an important issue in food safety and thus an important emerging zoonotic disease. Although *Campylobacter jejuni* is present in a high percentage of dogs without clinical signs, it has been associated with mild enterocolitis in kennels.

Yersiniosis

Yersinia are Gram-negative coccobacilli of the species *enterocolitica* and *pseudotuberculosis* that may cause mild-to-severe diarrhea, septicemia, or lymphadenitis, primarily in ruminants. Swine, cervids, and wild ungulates are also susceptible to infection and disease. Carrier states exist and cool climates support bacterial growth and environmental contamination. The bacteria invade the intestine through M cells overlying GALT via bacterial invasins and cell-associated β-1 integrins and then spread systemically. Microabscesses and granulomas, including giant cells, occur randomly in the intestinal lamina propria and crypts and there is widespread lymphoid necrosis. The bacteria are extracellular and intracellular, and there is massive recruitment of host neutrophils. Histologic diagnosis with bacterial isolation is definitive.

Intestinal Mycobacteriosis

Intestinal tuberculosis, caused by *Mycobacterium tuberculosis* and *Mycobacterium bovis*, is an uncommon disease in cattle, nursing calves, nonhuman primates, and humans. Although historically associated with drinking unpasteurized milk, more recently, intestinal tuberculosis is an important acquired immunodeficiency syndrome (AIDS)-associated disease in humans. The bacteria are ingested and then taken up by the M cells of the GALT, particularly in the distal ileum. Like Johne's disease of cattle, intestinal tuberculosis is a chronic wasting disease characterized by a roughened, rugae-like appearance to the intestine.

In small animals, it is sometimes clinically possible to palpate the thickened intestine. A thickened colon is sometimes palpable rectally in large animals. Granulomatous lymphadenopathy is often present, sometimes with mineralization and necrosis. The intestinal lamina propria and submucosa, as in Johne's disease, are enlarged and the architecture distorted by epithelioid macrophages and giant cells. Fewer acid-fast organisms are seen as compared with Johne's disease. In most cases of *Mycobacterium avium-intracellulare*–induced intestinal tuberculosis, lepromatous (noncaseating) granulomatous inflammation occurs similar to that of Johne's disease of small ruminants.

Pigs often contract intestinal tuberculosis as a result of the husbandry practice of feeding them avian litter as an inexpensive protein source. As might be expected, early lesions develop in the retropharyngeal lymph nodes.

Alimentary Anthrax

Anthrax occurs worldwide, principally in ruminants but any mammal, including humans, can be affected. In the US, it is a reportable disease and a potential agent of bioterrorism and agroterrorism. Most birds, along with amphibians, reptiles, and fish, are resistant to disease. Herbivores contact the disease by ingesting spore-contaminated vegetation, through a cutaneous wound or by inhaling spores, whereas carnivores are usually infected by ingesting contaminated carcasses. Biting flies can also transmit the causative bacterium, *Bacillus anthracis,* or its spores. In peracute disease, generally in ruminants, bacteremia and septicemia results and the blood may fail to clot because of toxin production from the bacteria. The spleen is often very large and bloody (blackberry jam spleen) and unclotted blood may ooze from any orifice. Blood or exudate smears often demonstrate the organisms as short chains of bacterial cells, thus avoiding the necessity of a necropsy. The spores are very resistant to environmental extremes and are infective. They have been known to survive the tanning process of hides. Pulmonary anthrax in humans is also called *woolsorter's disease.* The type of infection that occurs is directly related to the route of infection: cutaneous, respiratory, or GI.

Alimentary anthrax is most common in horses, pigs, dogs, and cats and may be oropharyngeal or intestinal. The oropharyngeal type is characterized by oral or esophageal ulcers with infection of associated lymph nodes. The clinical signs are swelling, dyspnea and dysphagia. The intestinal form is most severe in the terminal ileum or cecum and is characterized by abdominal pain, hematemesis, and fever. Mechanistically, alimentary infection requires that vegetative bacteria cross the intestinal epithelium. In vitro, anthrolysin O produced by *Bacillus anthracis,* disrupts the intestinal tight junction protein occludin. Cattle may develop ulcerative hemorrhagic abomasitis or small intestinal enteritis, as well as similar lesions in the large intestine (Fig. 7-135). The spleen and lymph nodes and mesentery are edematous and hemorrhagic. Swine are relatively resistant to anthrax; they generally develop pharyngeal and neck swelling, but necrohemorrhagic enteritis may occur. Live attenuated livestock vaccines are safe and generally provide about 9 months of immunity.

Algae

Chlorellosis and protothecosis

Unicellular and sometimes achlorophyllic algae have been reported to opportunistically cause cutaneous or widely disseminated granulomatous disease in a variety of species including humans, dogs, cats, dromedaries, gazelle, a beaver, cattle, and sheep. These algae are found in a variety of environmental locales, including both fresh and marine water. Primary infection is believed to be in the alimentary tract with chronic bloody diarrhea or through cutaneous wounds. Lesions are often tinted green if the algae contain chlorophyll. In the intestine, the transmural lesions are those of granulomatous enteritis and lymphadenitis. Intracellular algae measuring 5 to 11 μm, including those in giant cells, are visualized by Gomori methenamine silver (GMS) or PAS staining of the thick capsule. *Chlorella*, unlike *Prototheca,* which is considered to be its achlorophyllous mutant, contains starch bodies and chloroplasts that are birefringent in H&E sections, PAS positive, and diastase negative. Internal septation of the organisms is present with 2 to 20 sporangiospores.

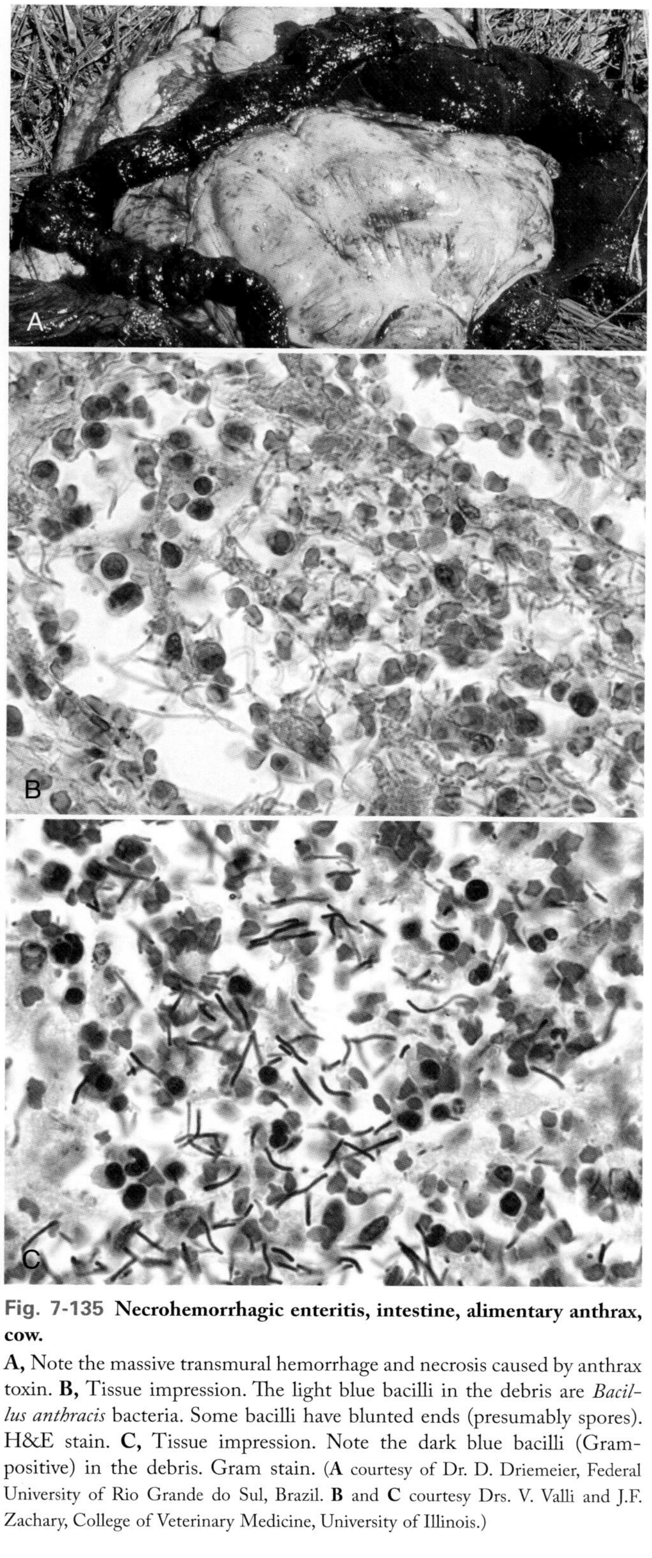

Fig. 7-135 Necrohemorrhagic enteritis, intestine, alimentary anthrax, cow.
A, Note the massive transmural hemorrhage and necrosis caused by anthrax toxin. **B,** Tissue impression. The light blue bacilli in the debris are *Bacillus anthracis* bacteria. Some bacilli have blunted ends (presumably spores). H&E stain. **C,** Tissue impression. Note the dark blue bacilli (Gram-positive) in the debris. Gram stain. (**A** courtesy of Dr. D. Driemeier, Federal University of Rio Grande do Sul, Brazil. **B** and **C** courtesy Drs. V. Valli and J.F. Zachary, College of Veterinary Medicine, University of Illinois.)

Disorders of Domestic Animals

Intestinal Disorders of Horses

Bacterial Diseases

Rhodococcus equi *Enteritis*

Rhodococcus equi is a soil saprophyte and a normal inhabitant of the equine intestine. The disease caused by this large, potentially zoonotic, Gram-positive, and facultatively anaerobic rod is often characterized by pulmonary pyogranulomas in foals under 6 months (see Fig. 9-67) and in immunocompromised adult horses and humans, or those with intercurrent disease (AIDS patients). The bacterium is not resistant to neutrophil-mediated destruction but can resist the intracellular environment of macrophages. All pathogenic *Rhodococcus equi* isolated from horses but not humans have a large plasmid and the encoded surface-expressed lipoprotein VapA, which is associated with virulence. The frequent intercurrence of helminths and *Rhodococcus equi* infection suggests that migrating larvae aid in distributing the bacterium through the body of the foal. Stringent control of helminth infections may therefore help to reduce or eliminate *Rhodococcus equi* infections.

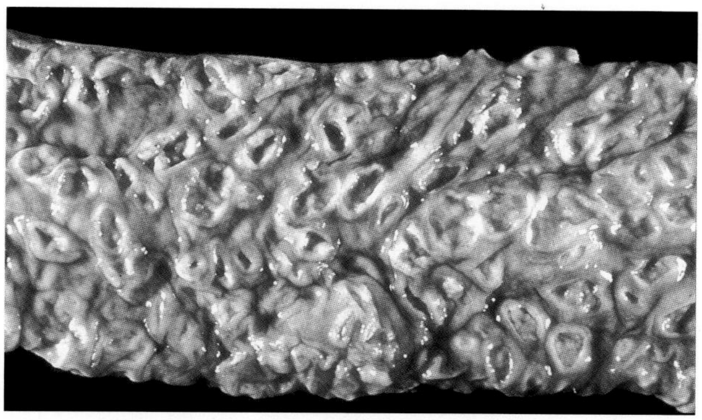

Fig. 7-136 Multifocal ulcerative colitis, colon, horse.
Rhodococcus equi infection causes multiple mucosal ulcers centered over gut-associated lymphoid tissue. (Courtesy Dr. H. Gelberg, College of Veterinary Medicine, Oregon State University.)

Equine abortion, pneumonia, and placentitis have been associated with infection, as have sporadic infections, sometimes fatal, of a wide variety of mammalian species. *Rhodococcus equi* can be isolated from a large number of otherwise healthy mammals of different species.

When coughed up and swallowed in large numbers, the bacteria enter the intestinal M cells overlying the GALT, resulting in pyogranulomatous lymphadenitis of GALT and lymph nodes and pyogranulomatous ulcerative enterotyphlocolitis.

Intestinal infection commences in Peyer's patches, which are ultimately replaced by granulomatous inflammation, abscess formation, and necrotic tissue, and the patches are ulcerated. Infection then spreads to mesenteric lymph nodes with a similar result. Macrophages, often laden with intact bacteria, fill the intestinal lamina propria and submucosa, resulting in a markedly thickened, corrugated intestine. The grossly observable abscesses and foci of necrosis and ulceration often correspond to the distribution of GALT (Fig. 7-136). Mesenteric, cecal, and colonic lymph nodes are enlarged, firm, and gray (Fig. 7-137). They, along with the spleen, may contain granulomas and abscesses (see Fig. 13-65). The large number of macrophages and multinucleated giant cells within the lamina propria and lymphoid tissue is characteristic of this infection. Bacteria may be seen within these cells with Giemsa and tissue Gram stains. The florid inflammatory infiltrate expands the intestinal villi and may distort the crypts of the entire intestinal tract.

Contamination of skin wounds by *Rhodococcus equi* may result in cutaneous ulcerative lymphangitis in horses. Swine cervical lymphadenopathy may also be a result of infection.

Rickettsial Diseases

Equine monocytic ehrlichiosis

Equine monocytic ehrlichiosis, also known as *Potomac horse fever,* was first reported in 1983. It appears that the disease was

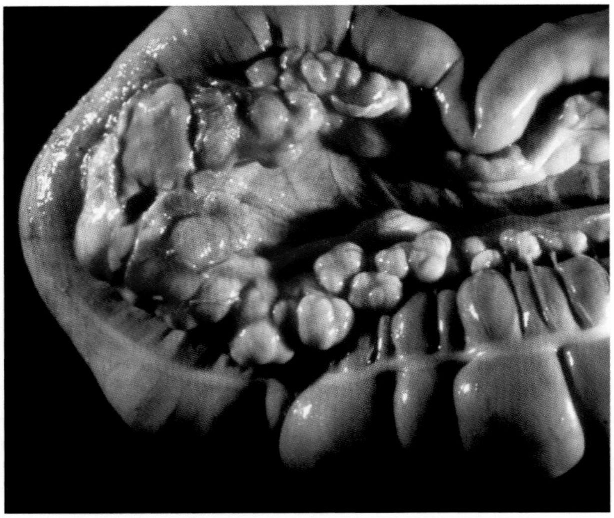

Fig. 7-137 Mesenteric lymphadenitis, colon, horse.
Infection of colic lymph nodes with *Rhodococcus equi* causes pyogranulomatous lymphadenomegaly. (Courtesy Dr. H. Gelberg, College of Veterinary Medicine, Oregon State University.)

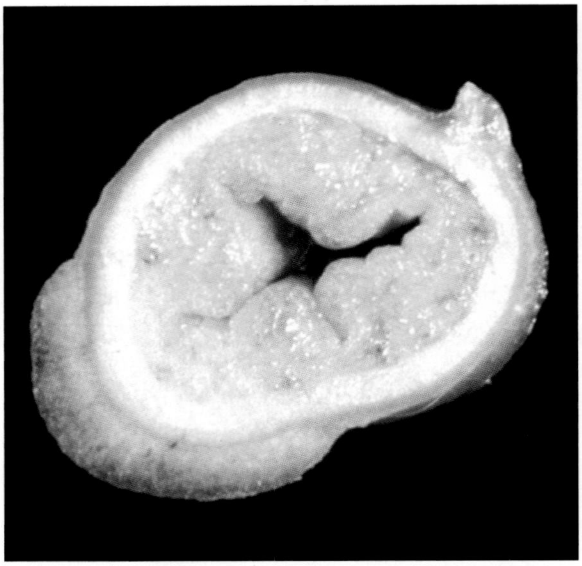

Fig. 7-138 Equine granulomatous enteritis, small intestine (formalin fixed), horse.
The lamina propria is greatly thickened by granulomatous inflammatory cells. (Courtesy Dr. H. Gelberg, College of Veterinary Medicine, Oregon State University.)

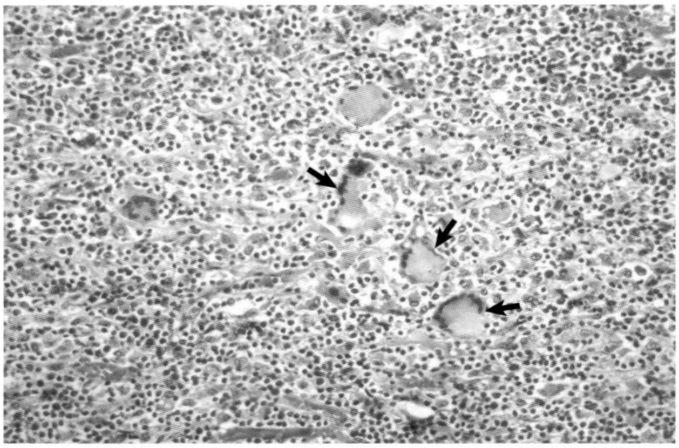

Fig. 7-139 Equine granulomatous enteritis, small intestine, horse.
Mononuclear inflammatory cells (macrophages, lymphocytes, plasma cells) and multinucleate giant cells *(arrows)* are present in the lamina propria and submucosa. H&E stain. (Courtesy Dr. H. Gelberg, College of Veterinary Medicine, Oregon State University.)

present for at least the previous 5 years. First described in the Potomac River valley of Maryland, Virginia, and Pennsylvania, it is now found throughout the US and elsewhere. The common denominator is a proximity of horses to slow-moving bodies of water.

The causative agent, *Neorickettsia risticii*—an intracytoplasmic rickettsial pathogen of epithelial cells, macrophages, and monocytes—is found in trematodes in freshwater snails. A reduction in pollution levels of the Potomac River basin is believed to have resulted in an increase in the number of freshwater snails. Mayflies and caddis flies have been implicated in transmission. Horses are believed to become infected by eating the dead flies that may accumulate in water buckets and feed troughs, particularly those under artificial light. *Rickettsia* are often transmitted by arthropods, and this disease is seasonal in northern latitudes (May through September). Without treatment, one-third of cases with diarrhea die as a result of dehydration.

Experimental evidence indicates that *Neorickettsia risticii* may be abortigenic. The gross lesions of Potomac horse fever are subtle, consisting of congestion, petechiae, and edema, primarily in the cecum and colon. There is a variable superficial necrotizing enterocolitis. Sometimes the small intestine is affected. Intestinal contents are tan, watery, and malodorous.

Because the experimental reproduction of clinical disease in germ-free animals has not been done, the microscopic appearance of lesions is not certain. Intercurrent bacteria may be responsible for some of the reported lesions. Interestingly, horses with Potomac horse fever have a mild necrotizing typhlocolitis similar in distribution to colitis X and enteric salmonellosis. The nature of the gross lesions is somewhat controversial because experimental infections produce variable results. Like hog cholera, Potomac horse fever is sometimes associated with concurrent *Salmonella* infection, perhaps accounting for the *Salmonella*-like lesions. Monocytes and macrophages in all layers of the intestine can be demonstrated with stains, such as Giemsa, to contain *Neorickettsia* organisms.

Clinical signs associated with Potomac horse fever include fever, watery diarrhea, depression, dehydration, variable colic, laminitis, and subcutaneous edema of the thorax, abdomen, and hind legs. Equine monocytic ehrlichiosis is apparently the same disease known as churrido equino (equine scours), which has been present for more than a century in Uruguay and Brazil.

Idiopathic Disorders

Equine granulomatous enteritis

Equine granulomatous enteritis is characterized by wasting and hypoalbuminemia and has been reported most often in thoroughbred and standardbred horses younger than 5 years. The pathogenesis of the disease is unknown. In a few cases, *Mycobacterium avium* was isolated from lesions. The disease is characterized by diffuse or segmental transmural noncaseating granulomatous inflammation of the small and occasionally large intestines. Giant cells are present in about half the cases. The result is a notably thickened bowel (Figs. 7-138 and 7-139).

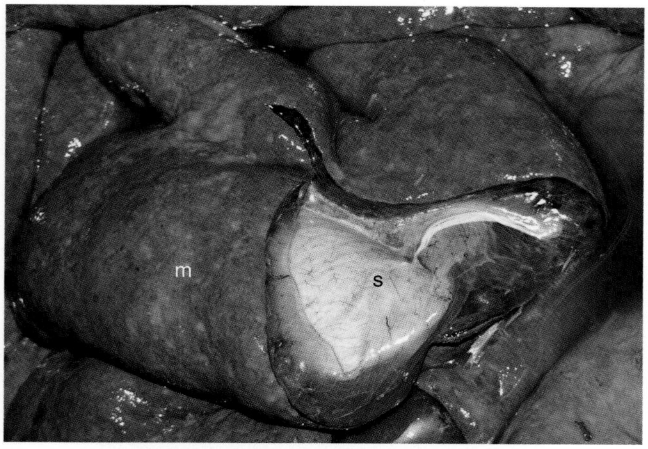

Fig. 7-140 Clostridial enteritis, colon, horse.
Commonly called *colitis X,* this disease is characterized by mucosal edema, congestion, and hemorrhage. The lesions are attributed to endotoxemia caused by several species of clostridia, most likely *Clostridium difficile.* Note the punctate mucosal erosions and ulcerations. *s,* Serosa; *m,* mucosa. (Courtesy Drs. V. Hsiao and A. Gillen, College of Veterinary Medicine, University of Illinois.)

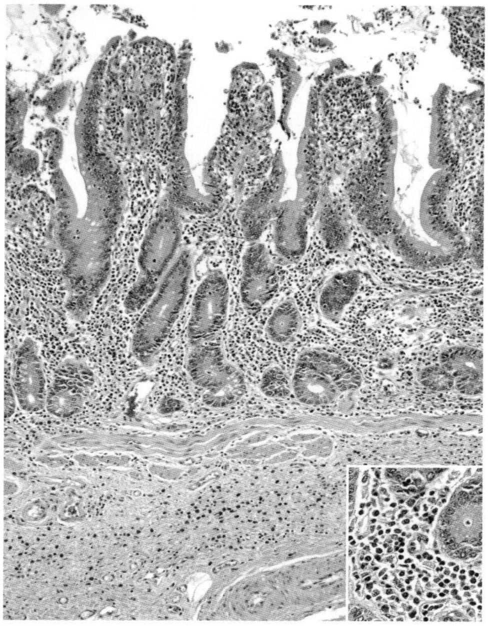

Fig. 7-141 Eosinophilic enteritis, small intestine, horse.
Eosinophils are numerous within the deep lamina propria, mucosal/submucosal interface, and superficial submucosa. Except in rare cases where an etiologic agent is diagnosed and treated successfully, affected horses die. H&E stain. (Courtesy Dr. H. Gelberg, College of Veterinary Medicine, Oregon State University.)

Clostridial enteritis (colitis X)

The severe diarrhea seen in cases of colitis X contains no blood and is rapidly fatal. The cause is unknown. However, the disease is associated with certain environmental and clinical variables. These include exhaustion; shock or other stressors; enterotoxemia, perhaps associated with overgrowth of *Clostridium perfringens* type A (antibiotic enteritis); *Clostridium cadaveris; Clostridium difficile*; anaphylaxis; or high protein-low cellulose diets. Lesions are limited to the mucosa of the cecum and colon and consist of edema, congestion, and hemorrhage (Fig. 7-140). The location and nature of these lesions overlap with those of acute enteric salmonellosis and equine monocytic ehrlichiosis. Therefore elimination of *Salmonella* spp. and *Neorickettsia risticii* as causes is necessary before a diagnosis of colitis X can be made. Thus colitis X is a diagnosis made by exclusion of other causes. At necropsy, in addition to the intestinal lesions, evidence of endotoxic shock, such as disseminated intravascular coagulopathy, thrombosis, and hemorrhage of the adrenal cortices (Waterhouse-Friderichsen syndrome) can be present, as in salmonellosis and other septicemic diseases.

Hemorrhagic fibrinonecrotic duodenitis-proximal jejunitis

In hemorrhagic fibrinonecrotic duodenitis-proximal jejunitis, also known as *anterior enteritis* and *gastroduodenojejunitis,* the morphologic description of the lesions is the same as the name of this idiopathic disease. The disease is characterized microscopically by submucosal edema and a neutrophilic infiltrate of the submucosa and lamina propria. *Salmonella* and clostridial infections are suspected as the cause. This disease occurs in horses older than 9 years, and the definitive diagnosis is made at necropsy by the characteristic hemorrhagic necrotizing lesions in the small intestine. The duodenum is always involved; jejunal involvement is variable.

Chronic eosinophilic gastroenteritis and multisystemic eosinophilic epitheliotropic disease

Soft stools accompanied by weight loss characterize chronic eosinophilic gastroenteritis and multisystemic eosinophilic epitheliotropic disease, which are uncommon conditions. The inflammatory reaction consists of eosinophils among other inflammatory cells in both nodular and diffuse accumulations within all portions and layers of the GI system, salivary glands, and mesenteric lymph nodes (Fig. 7-141). A circulating eosinophilia may be present. The histology of the condition, especially the presence of eosinophils, suggests a hypersensitivity reaction that in at least one instance was associated with *Pythium* spp. infection. With the exception of the rare cases with a specific etiologic agent, affected horses die. The disease is associated with an upregulated T_H2 response and increased IL-5 production.

Clinical signs relating to the GI system may include watery diarrhea and hypoproteinemia secondary to protein-losing enteropathy. In humans and occasionally in horses, the lymphoplasmacytic infiltrates in this condition are precursors to lymphoma.

Idiopathic focal eosinophilic enteritis

Idiopathic focal eosinophilic enteritis is characterized by infiltration of eosinophils along with macrophages and fibroblasts in the mucosa and transmurally to the serosa (see Fig. 7-141). The cause of the condition is unknown and is associated with obstructive colic. Resection of the affected portion of the intestine is curative in most cases.

Anaphylactoid purpura

Leukocytoclastic vasculitis associated with numerous discrete foci of necrosis and hemorrhage throughout the intestine and in the mucosa of the larynx and skeletal muscles is termed *anaphylactoid purpura* in the horse and *Henoch-Schönlein disease* in humans (see Fig. 15-33). Anecdotal evidence suggests that an Arthus-like hypersensitivity reaction to a streptococcal respiratory infection is the mechanism of lesion production.

Intestinal Diseases of Ruminants (Cattle, Sheep, and Goats)

Viral Diseases

Bovine viral diarrhea

Bovine viral diarrhea (BVD), also known as *mucosal disease,* affects cattle of all ages but is most common in animals 8 months to 2 years of age. In this respect, clinical cases are typically younger than in animals susceptible to Johne's disease. Animals, including new world camelids, infected in utero or early in life with noncytopathic BVD pestivirus develop a persistent infection. They shed virus throughout their lives. Later in life, if exposed to cytopathic pestivirus, they may develop disease. Multifocal, sharply demarcated erosions and ulcers in the tongue, gingiva, palate (see Fig. 7-3), esophagus (Fig. 7-142), rumen, abomasum, and coronary bands of the hooves characterize BVD. In the intestine, the characteristic lesion is sharply demarcated foci of necrosis in the epithelium over the GALT (Figs. 7-143 and 7-144). Lesions in the stratified squamous epithelium begin in the stratum spinosum. Necrosis of the epithelium is soon followed by the formation of erosions and ulcerations. Villous and crypt enterocytes become necrotic. There is lympholysis in the GALT. Follicular medullary regions of intestinal lymphoid tissue may be filled with cell debris and dead enterocytes. There is commonly a fibrinonecrotic pseudomembrane over the damaged GALT.

Clinical signs may include anorexia, depression, profuse watery diarrhea with staining of the perineum and tail, agalactia, pyrexia, rumen atony, ptyalism, lacrimation, and a mucopurulent nasal discharge. Calves infected in utero may have cerebellar hypoplasia, cataracts, microphthalmia, or renal dysplasia, and other congenital defects develop. Abortions, stillbirths, and mummified fetuses can also result from in utero infection in new world camelids, cervids, sheep, and goats, as well as cattle. Aborted calves often have enlarged hemal lymph nodes. Morbidity in a herd varies from 2% to 50%. All affected animals die.

A more common outcome from BVD infection occurs in immunocompetent animals that are seronegative at the time of exposure to either the cytopathic or noncytopathic virus. Variable signs develop, but they are mostly mild or subclinical. Most cattle in the US have serologic evidence of exposure to nonvaccine BVD. Exotic ruminants may also become infected. Under certain circumstances pigs may become subclinically infected. This is of interest because the viruses of BVD and hog cholera are antigenically closely related. This may cause confusing serologic results when testing hogs for cholera. New world camelids may also succumb to BVD infection, although infections are often subclinical. The diagnosis of persistent infection is by immunohistochemistry of skin biopsies because calves shed large amounts of virus through the skin. Feedlot cattle that are persistently infected are believed to be more susceptible to mannheimiosis, chronic pneumonia and polyarthritis syndrome, salmonellosis, infectious bovine rhinotracheitis, bovine respiratory syncytial virus, and mycoses. Other diagnostic means are virus isolation, reverse transcription PCR (RT-PCR), and antigen-capture ELISA.

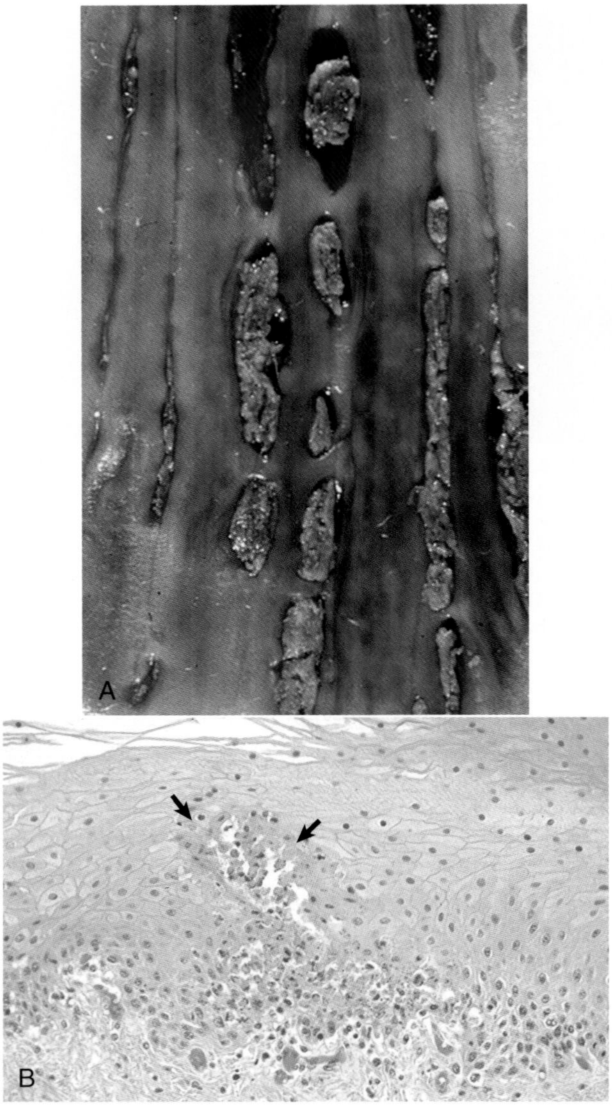

Fig. 7-142 Acute multifocal ulcers, esophagus, cow.
A, Grossly, there are multiple sharply demarcated ulcers *(vertically linear red streaks)* and similar areas covered by diphtheritic membranes *(vertically linear yellow-brown streaks).* The cause is the pestivirus of bovine viral diarrhea (BVD). **B,** Microscopically, there is a focus of necrosis *(arrows)* of cells of the stratum basale and stratum spinosum caused by the pestivirus of BVD. H&E stain. (**A** courtesy Department of Veterinary Biosciences, College of Veterinary Medicine, The Ohio State University; and Noah's Arkive, College of Veterinary Medicine, The University of Georgia. **B** courtesy Dr. J.S. Haynes, College of Veterinary Medicine, Iowa State University; and Noah's Arkive, College of Veterinary Medicine, The University of Georgia.)

Rinderpest

Lesions similar to those of BVD occur in cattle with rinderpest. The morbillivirus associated with rinderpest infects cattle, sheep, goats, pigs, water buffalo, giraffes, wildebeest, and other wild ruminants. Disease spread is via aerosolization and contact with other body secretions. Initial virus replication is in tonsils and pharyngeal and mandibular lymph nodes resulting in viremia. Acute necrosis is typically severe in all lymph nodes and the epithelial lining of the alimentary, respiratory, and reproductive systems, including erosions and ulcers of the oral cavity and nasal planum. These lesions are particularly severe in regions of GALT, similar to BVD. Pale eosinophilic, cytoplasmic, and perinuclear inclusion bodies surrounded by a halo are sometimes seen in epithelia and lymphoid tissue macrophages. Intranuclear inclusions are visible less often. The signature lesion is characteristic multinucleate enterocytes in epithelial tissues, including the intestinal lesions that do not occur in BVD. Postinfection immunity is likely lifelong. Rinderpest does not occur in the US or Europe but is a significant disease in Africa and Asia and is believed to be on the verge of eradication through

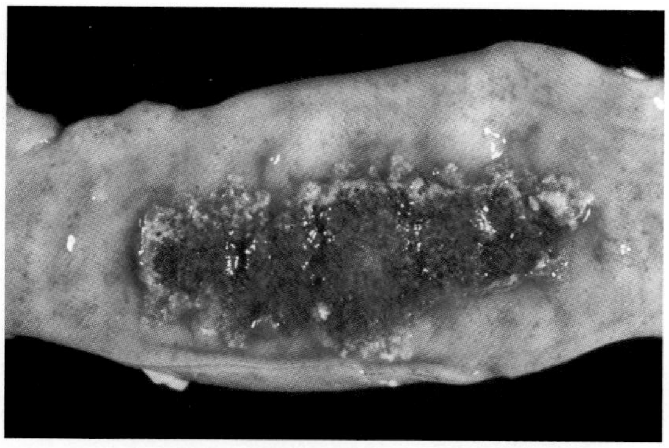

Fig. 7-143 Bovine viral diarrhea (BVD), ileum, mucosa, cow. Peyer's patches and the overlying epithelium are necrotic and covered with suppurative exudate. (Courtesy Dr. H. Gelberg, College of Veterinary Medicine, Oregon State University.)

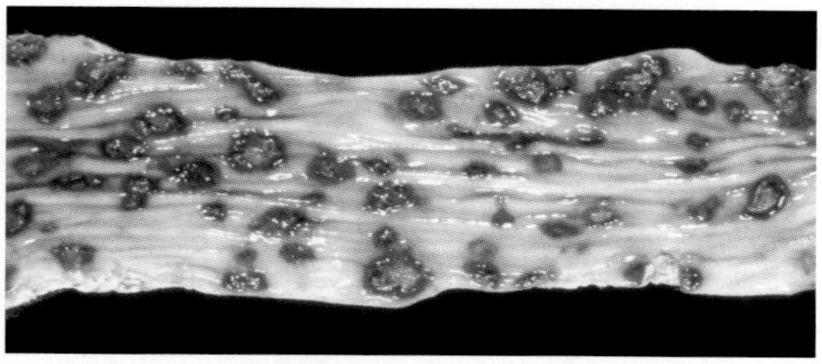

Fig. 7-144 Multifocal ulcerative colitis, bison, colon. Multiple mucosal ulcers were caused by bovine viral diarrhea (BVD) virus. (Courtesy Dr. H. Gelberg, College of Veterinary Medicine, Oregon State University.)

effective vaccination. In immunologically naïve populations of animals, morbidity and mortality may be high.

Peste des petits ruminants

Peste des petits ruminants is a distinct morbillivirus disease of sheep and goats that causes ulcerative and pseudomembranous lesions of the oral cavity, similar to rinderpest, along with necrotizing tonsillitis, fibrinohemorrhagic enteritis, and bronchointerstitial pneumonia. Syncytial cells and nuclear and cytoplasmic inclusion bodies of epithelial and lymphoid tissues similar to those found in rinderpest are also present. Peste des petits ruminants is enzootic in the Middle East, the Indian subcontinent, and North Africa.

Border disease

The pestivirus causing border disease in sheep and goats is antigenically related to the noncytopathic biotype of BVD virus. Border disease is usually a congenital infection associated with reproductive failure or birth of abnormal lambs and kids. When subsequently infected with a cytopathic virus, they develop lesions similar to BVD of cattle. Border disease has been reported in the British Isles, Australia, New Zealand, and the US.

Malignant catarrhal fever

Malignant catarrhal fever, which is caused by closely related rhadinoviruses (γ-herpesviruses), occurs in a variety of species of ruminants, including cervids and bison. Persistent infection is common in host species, and disease occurs as a result of cross-species transmission. The African form of the disease, caused by alcelaphine herpesvirus-1 (AHV-1) is common in wildebeests and other ruminants. In the US and worldwide, ovine herpesvirus-2 (OHV-2), caprine herpesvirus-2 (CpHV-2), and white-tailed deer herpesvirus (MCF-WTD) are most often reported in ruminants. The respiratory form of the disease, associated with keratoconjunctivitis, is most commonly seen in cattle in the US.

Lesions include widespread lymphadenomegaly, lymphoplasmacytic necrotizing arteritis and phlebitis of the subcutis, and especially in the rete mirabile surrounding the base of the pituitary gland. Hoof walls may be shed. Coagulation necrosis is found in lymph nodes, and lymphoplasmacytic infiltrates are present in the retina, myocardium, brain, spinal cord, and meninges. The alimentary form of the disease is characterized as multifocal ulcerative stomatitis (see Fig. 7-4), glossitis, esophagitis, abomasitis, and enterotyphlocolitis associated with vasculitis. Hemorrhagic cystitis may also be present.

Winter dysentery

Winter dysentery is a somewhat enigmatic, acute, generally nonfatal disease of adult cattle. Although its cause is unknown, a coronavirus has been implicated as causative and can sometimes be demonstrated immunohistochemically in colonic basal enterocytes of affected animals. As the disease progresses in a herd, virtually all members become ill. As the name implies, it is a seasonal disease and additionally occurs only in northern latitudes. Catarrhal ileitis and jejunitis characterize this highly contagious disease.

Mild lesions are noted in the rare animal that dies of winter dysentery. The intestinal mucosa is intact, but there is variable congestion and petechiae of the abomasum and small intestine. The intestine may be atonic. The colon may have congestion and hemorrhage of the colonic mucosal folds, a nonspecific lesion associated with tenesmus (tiger striping).

Acute onset of profuse diarrhea, decreased milk production in dairy cattle, variable depression, and anorexia are characteristic. Malodorous green to black (melena) diarrhea lasts for up to 4 days and may contain fresh blood and mucus. Immunity in dairy herds is protective for years. Older animals are more severely affected than are younger ones. Calves appear to be refractory to disease development. Diagnosis is generally made by epizootic information, clinical signs, its seasonal occurrence, and lack of significant mortality.

Bovine torovirus diarrhea

The shedding of bovine torovirus (BoTV), or bredavirus, has been associated with diarrhea of neonatal veal calves. BoTV is a single-stranded, enveloped RNA virus, which currently cannot be grown in cell culture. BoTV is associated with the presence of other enteropathogens of neonates, including rotavirus, coronavirus, *Cryptosporidium, Salmonella,* and *Giardia.* Although it is not uncommon to have intercurrent infections producing diarrhea in calves, especially in the presence of immunosuppression, malnutrition, and other stressors, BoTV may cause disease independently. Necrosis and sloughing of enterocytes on the middle and lower villi, extending into the crypts, are noted on histologic examination. Diagnosis is confirmed by antigen-capture ELISA or RT-PCR in feces in the absence of evidence of other enteric pathogens. Death, when it occurs, is due to dehydration.

Bacterial Diseases

Paratuberculosis

Paratuberculosis, or Johne's disease, has been described in numerous ruminant species. Ruminants are infected from feces-contaminated soil. In cattle, the disease is characterized by intractable diarrhea, emaciation, and hypoproteinemia in animals older than 19 months. In the average infected herd, 32% to 42% of

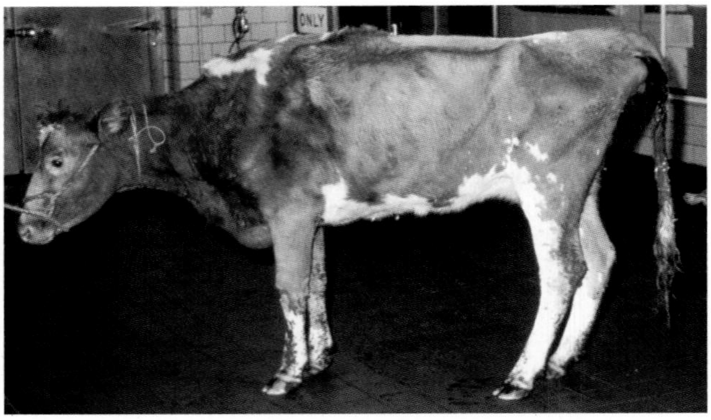

Fig. 7-145 Granulomatous enteritis, Johne's disease (*Mycobacterium avium* ssp. *paratuberculosis*), cow.
There is chronic wasting and diarrhea in this 18-month-old heifer. The age at which this cow showed clinical signs is not typical of the disease. Signs usually occur 2 or more years after initial infection. (Courtesy College of Veterinary Medicine, Cornell University.)

animals are infected. In small ruminants (sheep and goats), the clinical disease is similar to that observed in cattle except that diarrhea does not occur. The pygmy goat is an exception to the course of disease in small ruminants in that some pygmy goats develop explosive diarrhea and die unexpectedly. In other ruminants, the disease has a protracted course and is considered a wasting disease because of the loss of body mass (Fig. 7-145). Newer methods of bacterial classification suggest that the causative bacterium *Mycobacterium paratuberculosis* should be reclassified as *Mycobacterium avium* ssp. *paratuberculosis*.

The causative organisms are very resistant to environmental stressors, particularly in regions with acid soils. After ingestion, the bacilli are transported through M cells and taken up by macrophages. Lesions in the lamina propria of the intestines, particularly in the ileum, include the accumulation of macrophages. There is little correlation between the severity of the gross lesions and the severity of clinical disease. An age-related immune resistance to infection and disease develops in animals older than 2 months. Fetuses can be infected, but disease is delayed until the animals are much older. Isolation of newborns from fecal contamination is a useful measure to reduce the incidence of infection in a particular herd.

Diagnosis is made by observing clinical signs together with the signalment. The gross lesion in Johne's disease is a chronic, segmental thickening of the ileum, cecum, and proximal colon (Fig. 7-146). The ileocecal valve region is usually affected. Affected segments have a variably thickened, rough, rugose mucosa, often with multiple foci of ulceration. There is mesenteric lymphadenopathy.

Noncaseating granulomas contain numerous foamy macrophages with large numbers of acid-fast organisms (see Fig. 7-146; also see Figs. 3-25 and 13-78). In contrast, sheep, goats, and deer may have tuberculoid (caseating) granulomas in the intestines, lymphatics, and lymph nodes. These granulomas are sometimes mineralized and contain whorled accumulations of epithelioid macrophages with variable numbers of Langhans'-type giant cells. It is more difficult to find acid-fast mycobacteria in these mature granulomas.

Mycobacterium avium ssp. *paratuberculosis* can be isolated from feces of affected animals, from diseased intestines and regional lymph nodes, and sometimes from a variety of other tissues and fluids, including the liver, uterus, fetus, milk, urine, and semen.

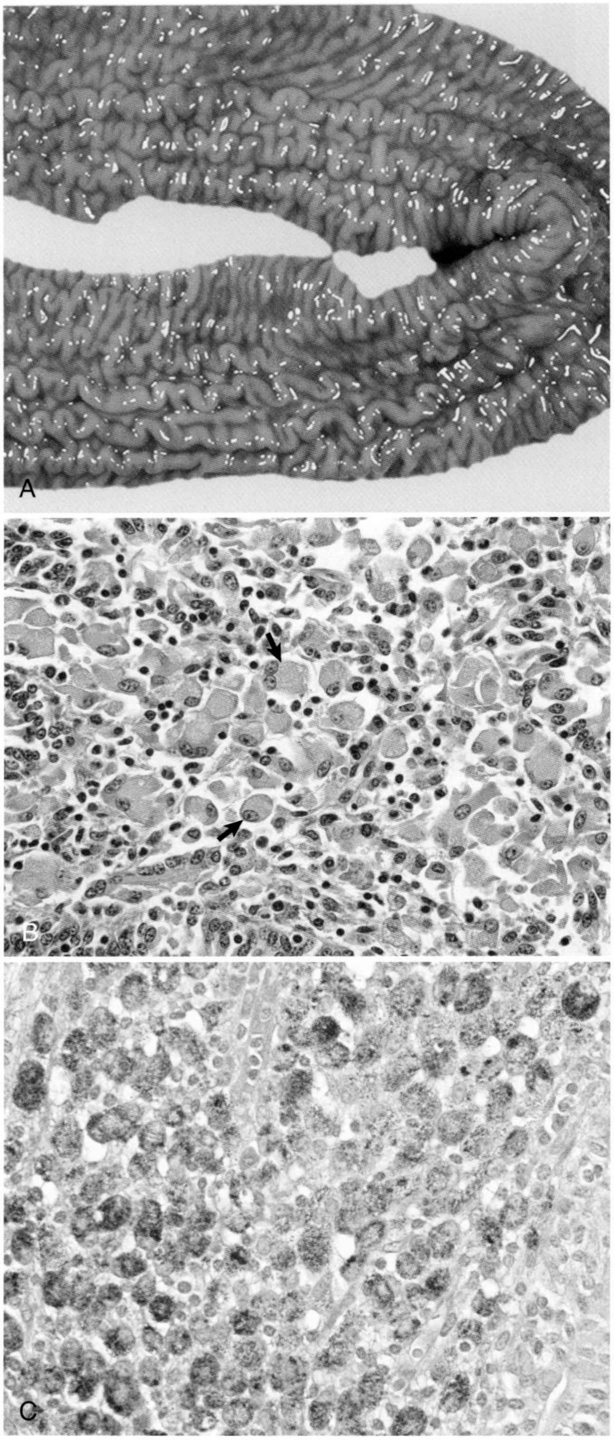

Fig. 7-146 Granulomatous enteritis, Johne's disease (*Mycobacterium avium* ssp. *paratuberculosis*).
A, Ileum, sheep. There is notable thickening of the mucosa, which is smooth and shiny (intact) and not ulcerated. **B,** Small intestine, cow. The lamina propria of the intestine is markedly expanded by granulomatous inflammatory cells (*arrows* = macrophages), which compress the crypts and eventually result in their loss (atrophy). H&E stain. **C,** Small intestine, cow. Mycobacterium-containing macrophages distend the lamina propria. Ziehl-Neelsen stain. (**A** courtesy Dr. M.D. McCracken, College of Veterinary Medicine, University of Tennessee; and Noah's Arkive, College of Veterinary Medicine, The University of Georgia. **B** and **C** courtesy Dr. J.F. Zachary, College of Veterinary Medicine, University of Illinois.)

Acid-fast bacteria in rectal mucosal scrapings are found in 60% of the cases. Hepatic microgranulomas occur in about 25% of affected animals. Aortic and endocardial mineralization (arteriosclerosis), when it occurs in association with the clinical signs and lesions of paratuberculosis, is specific for Johne's disease in cattle (see Figs. 10-32 and 10-39). The pathogenesis of this vascular lesion is not well understood but is associated with the severe cachexia associated with the disease. The epizootiology of Johne's disease leads many to believe it is one of the most important diseases facing the dairy industry. Speculation has existed for many years that Johne's disease is zoonotic and somehow causative of Crohn's disease in humans.

Hemorrhagic bowel syndrome of dairy cattle

Hemorrhagic bowel syndrome, also known as fatal jejunal hemorrhage syndrome and intraluminal-intramural hemorrhage of the small intestine, is characterized by intraluminal hemorrhage resulting in blood clots that lead to intestinal obstruction. It is characterized by dark, clotted blood in the feces; variable and multifocal distention of the small intestine; small intestinal ileus; and necrohemorrhagic jejunitis or enteritis (Fig. 7-147). The cause is unknown, but *Clostridium perfringens* type A is suspected. The mortality rate is high.

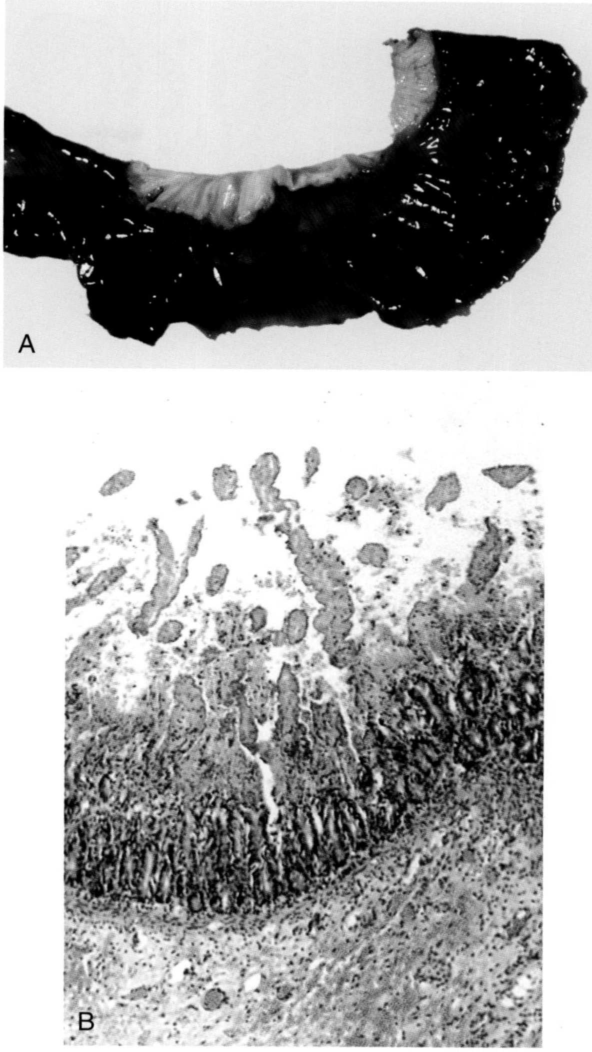

Fig. 7-147 Necrohemorrhagic enteritis, hemorrhagic bowel syndrome, small intestine, cow.
A, The massive small intestinal hemorrhage and necrosis is characteristic of clostridial infections of the intestine. **B,** Note the horizontal linear "band" of acute coagulative necrosis affecting the superficial half of the mucosa *(light pink zone)* of the intestine caused by clostridial toxins. H&E stain. (**A** courtesy Dr. M.D. McGavin, College of Veterinary Medicine, University of Tennessee. **B** courtesy Dr. C.W. Qualls, College of Veterinary Medicine, Oklahoma State University and Noah's Arkive, College of Veterinary Medicine, The University of Georgia.)

Miscellaneous diseases

Chlamydiosis

Bovine chlamydia (*Chlamydophila pecorum*) has been recovered from spontaneous enteritis of young calves. After experimental inoculation, newborn calves develop fever and diarrhea within 24 hours and become moribund within 4 to 5 days. Grossly the ileum is most severely affected, but the jejunum and large intestine also have lesions. In diseased segments, the mucosa is congested and marked with petechiae. The intestinal wall and mesentery are edematous. The lumen contains watery, yellow fluid mixed with a yellow, tenacious, fibrin-rich material attached to the surface. Colonic ridges are hyperemic and have small erosions. Bleeding from petechiae and ecchymoses of the colonic or rectal ridges occurs infrequently. Regional lymph nodes are enlarged. Microscopically, villous epithelial cells, enterochromaffin cells, goblet cells, macrophages, fibroblasts of the lamina propria, and endothelial cells of lacteals are parasitized by the chlamydia. The chlamydia are endocytosed and multiply in epithelial cell apices. They subsequently are liberated into the lamina propria. Villi are enlarged by dilated lacteals and infiltrates of mononuclear cells and neutrophils. Crypts of both small and large intestines are dilated and have sloughed epithelial cells and inflammatory exudate (colitis cystica superficialis). The centers of lymphoid follicles of Peyer's patches are necrotic. The mucosa and submucosa of the intestines are thickened by a diffuse granulomatous reaction. The abomasum also has lesions, and in some calves, foci of inflammation extend transmurally, thereby causing focal peritonitis. Affected calves have diarrhea, fever, anorexia, and depression.

Intestinal Disorders of Pigs

Enteric diseases of pigs are a major cause of economic loss. Rapid and accurate on-farm diagnosis is critical in controlling disease outbreaks. If one takes into account the epizootiology of the outbreak, the age of the affected animals and the location and nature of lesions, one can generally be fairly accurate in rendering an on-farm diagnosis, pending laboratory confirmation. This listing of specific infectious causes of enteritis in pigs is exclusive of those agents already discussed. When formulating a differential diagnosis, all causes of enteritis must be considered, including intestinal displacements, colibacillosis, rotavirus, *Salmonella,* clostridia, parasites, toxins, and so on.

Viral Diseases

Transmissible gastroenteritis

Transmissible gastroenteritis (TGE) is an important disease in pigs younger than 10 days. Older animals apparently can compensate for the small intestinal damage through fluid and short-chain fatty acid absorption in the large intestine. The coronavirus that causes this disease cross-reacts with but is distinct from the coronavirus that causes feline infectious peritonitis. The virus is inactivated by sunlight, therefore TGE disease occurs mostly in winter. Target cells for the virus are villous enterocytes, therefore lesions consist of notable atrophy of villi of the small intestine (Fig. 7-148). In piglets, epithelial replacement time is much longer than in more

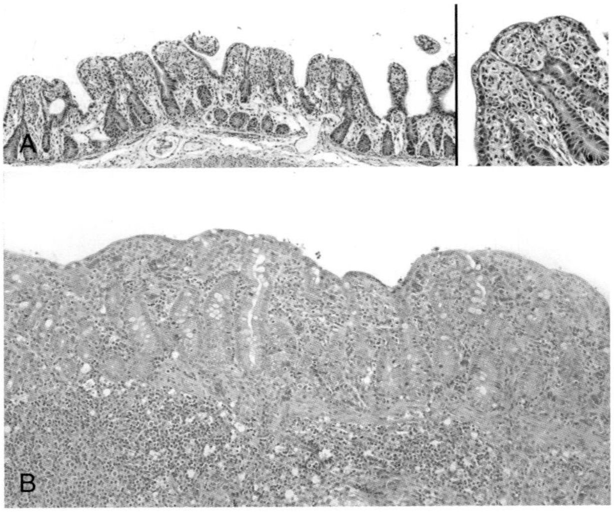

Fig. 7-148 Transmissible gastroenteritis, small intestine, piglet.
A, Early stage of the disease. Transmissible gastroenteritis virus targets epithelial cells of the tips and upper sides of intestinal villi causing necrosis of the enterocytes and atrophy of the villi. These cells are sloughed and replaced by flattened epithelial cells migrating up the basement membrane from progenitor cells in the crypts. *Inset,* Note the flattened epithelial cells covering the tips and sides of the atrophic villi and the fusion of the adjacent villi. Inflammation is minimal. H&E stain. **B,** Later stage of the disease. There is severe blunting (marked villus atrophy) of intestinal villi with fusion of their basement membranes. Chronic inflammation is prominent in the lamina propria and submucosa. H&E stain. (**A** courtesy Dr. B.G. Harmon, College of Veterinary Medicine, The University of Georgia and Noah's Arkive, College of Veterinary Medicine, The University of Georgia. **B** courtesy Dr. H. Gelberg, College of Veterinary Medicine, Oregon State University.)

mature animals, accounting for the high mortality. Diagnosis is by positive immunostaining of intestinal sections in piglets acutely ill with the disease.

Similar to rotavirus or non-TGE coronavirus infections, the virus is lytic and sloughed enterocytes carry virus into the feces. The difference in pathogenicity between rotavirus and non-TGE coronavirus infections and TGE is the number of villous enterocytes destroyed by a virus. In TGE, most of the villous enterocytes are destroyed and therefore the clinical disease is more severe.

The diarrhea contains odoriferous undigested milk. The loss of the majority of villous enterocytes results in continued significant intestinal malabsorption. Because of fusion of adjacent villi, the enterocyte mass may never fully be restored. Affected surviving animals remain chronic "poor doers."

Piglets dead from TGE are dehydrated and their perineum is stained with liquid, yellow, fecal material. The small intestine is dilated and thin walled because of the loss of enterocytes, and contains yellow fluid and gas (Fig. 7-149). Mesenteric lymph vessels are devoid of chyle as a result of malabsorption. The diagnosis is partially based on the presence of villous atrophy. The decrease in villous height: crypt depth ratio is marked and may be appreciated subgrossly (Fig. 7-150). Colibacillosis, coccidiosis, cryptosporidiosis, rotavirus infection, and non-TGE coronavirus infection are among the differential diagnoses.

Piglets suffer from acute diarrhea, weight loss, vomiting, and dehydration. Morbidity and mortality, especially in neonates, approach 100% in susceptible herds. Death occurs within 48 hours to 5 days after the commencement of clinical signs. In feeder pigs, transmissible gastroenteritis virus infection causes transient clinical signs with eventual recovery. Sows are susceptible to the virus, and

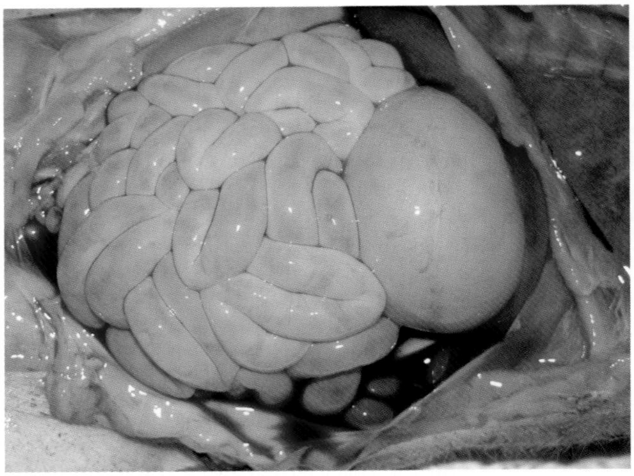

Fig. 7-149 Transmissible gastroenteritis, small intestine, piglet.
The small intestine is dilated by gas, is thin walled, and contains undigested milk. (Courtesy Dr. V. Hsiao, College of Veterinary Medicine, University of Illinois.)

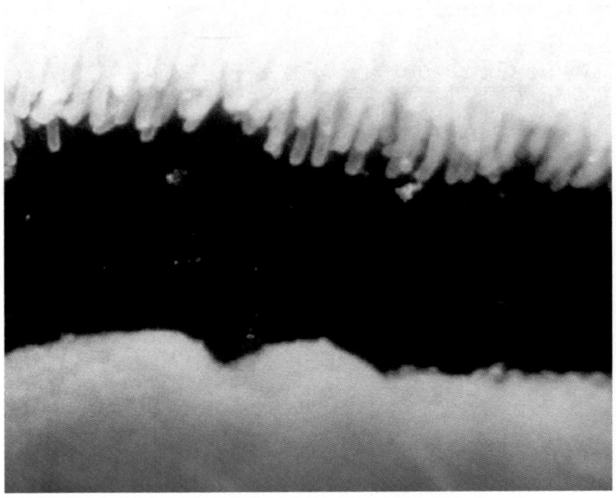

Fig. 7-150 Wet mount, intestinal villi, transmissible gastroenteritis, small intestine, piglet.
There is notable villous atrophy *(bottom)* compared with normal intestine *(top)*. (Courtesy Dr. H. Gelberg, College of Veterinary Medicine, Oregon State University.)

morbidity among the sows is 100%, but the clinical signs are mild and transient (fever, vomiting, inappetence, and agalactia), and none die. Immunity is solid.

Bacterial Diseases

Swine dysentery

Unlike most of the other diseases of the porcine gut, swine dysentery is generally confined to the large intestine. The causative bacterium, *Brachyspira hyodysenteriae*, previously known as *Treponema* and *Serpulina*, is a Gram-negative, flagellated, and anaerobic spirochete that acts synergistically with anaerobic colonic flora, such as *Fusobacterium necrophorum* or *Bacteroides vulgatus,* to produce disease. This synergism is believed to be partially responsible for the age restriction (8 to 14 weeks old) of the disease because neonatal animals have not yet developed the appropriate anaerobic gut flora. *Brachyspira hyodysenteriae* produces a cytotoxic hemolysin, which is a virulence determinant.

The gross lesions of the disease closely approximate those of acute enteric salmonellosis except that bloody feces are more usual in dysentery. Weanling pigs 8 to 14 weeks old are usually affected, and the disease spreads rapidly through a herd. Morbidity approaches 90%, and mortality is around 30%. Lesions of mucohemorrhagic enteritis are present in the spiral colon, colon, cecum, and rectum. The intestine often has a fibrinonecrotic pseudomembrane that correlates with the severe diarrheic feces that contains blood, mucus, and fibrin (Fig. 7-151). The diarrhea and electrolyte loss that occur are caused by colonic absorptive failure.

Brachyspira hyodysenteriae is identified by impression smear (Fig. 7-152), dark-field microscopy, immunolabeling techniques, and PCR. It is assumed that a carrier state exists because the disease is enzootic in affected herds.

Lawsonia *enteritis*

Lawsonia enteritis manifests in a variety of ways as indicated by the number of names applied to it: proliferative enteropathy, proliferative ileitis, intestinal adenomatosis, distal ileal hypertrophy, terminal ileitis, and proliferative hemorrhagic enteropathy. The genus of the causative agent has undergone several recent changes in nomenclature. For many years, this disease was believed to be caused by *Campylobacter* spp. (*Campylobacter sputorum mucosalis, Campylobacter jejuni, Campylobacter hyointestinalis*). Newer methods of bacterial classification caused the name to be changed to *Ileobacter* and now *Lawsonia*. Pigs older than 4 weeks of age are susceptible; thus this condition is a postweaning disease. Disease is believed to be caused by an unknown interaction of *Lawsonia* with normal gut flora. The nature of the lesions is a function of the extent of intestinal mucosal necrosis. The disease begins as a bacteria-induced stimulation of small intestinal crypt epithelial cells, particularly in the ileum (Figs. 7-153 and 7-154), where lesions are generally most severe. With time, the lesions progress to necrosis of the proliferating crypt cells with hemorrhage (Fig. 7-155). Thus the morphologic appearance of the lesions varies from case to case. The mechanism of lesion production is not well understood. Infection results in immunosuppression with a reduction

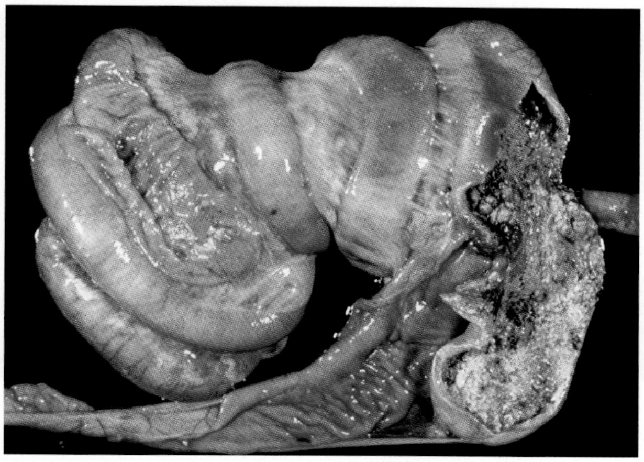

Fig. 7-151 Necrohemorrhagic enterocolitis, swine dysentery, spiral colon, pig.
There is marked necrosis and hemorrhage of the intestinal mucosa caused by the bacterium *Brachyspira hyodysenteriae.* (Courtesy Department of Veterinary Biosciences, College of Veterinary Medicine, The Ohio State University and Noah's Arkive, College of Veterinary Medicine, The University of Georgia.)

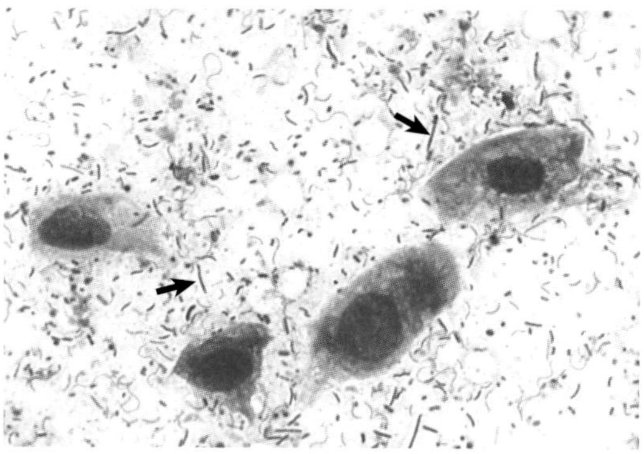

Fig. 7-152 Swine dysentery, colon, pig.
This impression smear contains a few enterocytes and numerous bacteria. Note the spiral bacteria *(arrows)* consistent with *Brachyspira* spp. Diff-Quik stain. (Courtesy Dr. H. Gelberg, College of Veterinary Medicine, Oregon State University.)

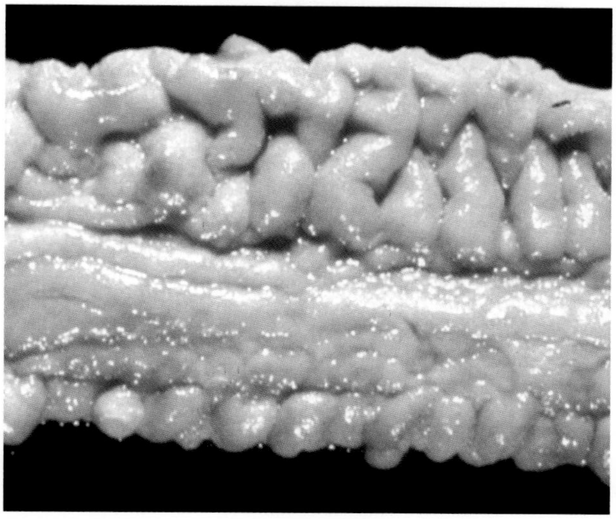

Fig. 7-153 Proliferative enteritis, ileum, pig.
Note the marked mucosal expansion, the result of *Lawsonia*-induced epithelial hyperplasia. (Courtesy Dr. H. Gelberg, College of Veterinary Medicine, Oregon State University.)

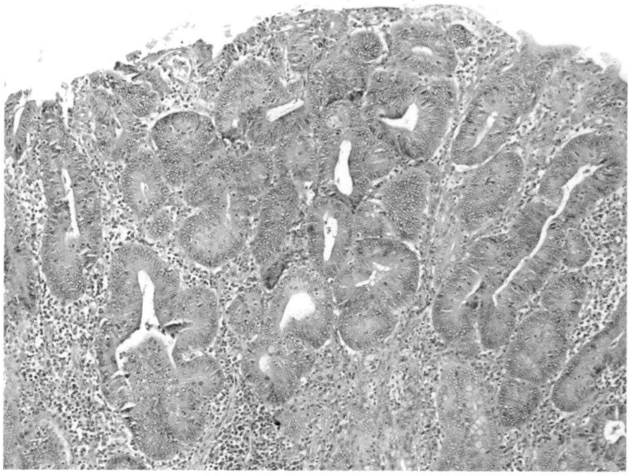

Fig. 7-154 *Lawsonia* enteritis, ileum, pig.
There is notable hyperplasia of enterocytes, resulting in distortion of normal architecture and "collision necrosis" of tightly packed proliferating enterocytes. H&E stain. (Courtesy Dr. J.F. Zachary, College of Veterinary Medicine, University of Illinois.)

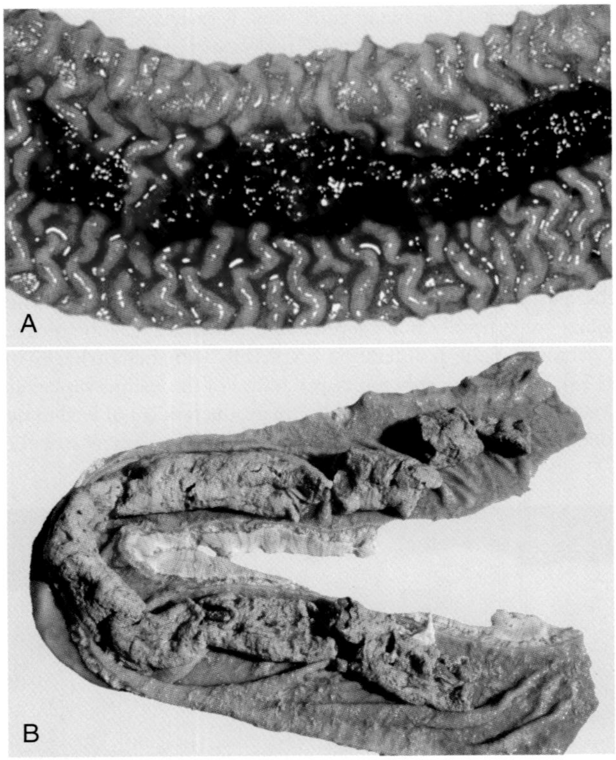

Fig. 7-155 ***Lawsonia* enteritis, ileum, pig.**
A, Hemorrhagic bowel form. Note the prominent folds of hyperplastic mucosa and the concurrent hemorrhage forming a luminal cast. **B,** Necroproliferative form. Note the prominent necrosis of the ileal mucosa and its diphtheritic membrane (cast) formed by cellular debris and inflammatory exudate. (**A** courtesy Dr. D.D. Harrington, School of Veterinary Medicine, Purdue University and Noah's Arkive, College of Veterinary Medicine, The University of Georgia. **B** courtesy of Dr. D. Driemeier, Federal University of Rio Grande do Sul, Brazil.)

in $CD8^+$ T and B lymphocytes. In the proliferative form of the disease, the causative bacteria may be seen in apical cytoplasm of enterocytes. The mechanism of enterocyte proliferation may relate to *Lawsonia*-induced altered transcription of host "alarm response" genes that affect regulation of the cell cycle and cell differentiation. The enterocyte hyperplasia that results may cause release of cytokines that attract macrophages. With severe disease, bacteria are present in macrophages in the lamina propria. This may cause release of tumor necrosis factor-α (TNF-α) resulting in vascular permeability and hemorrhage.

At clinical and necropsy examination, variable amounts of blood and intestinal casts are present in the feces. Microscopically, the comma-shaped bacteria are made visible with special stains, such as Steiner's, within the mitotically active cells of the small intestinal crypts (Fig. 7-156). The massive mitoses of crypt cells and resultant cryptal crowding and necrosis prevent maturation to absorbent villous enterocytes. There is resultant villous shortening. Mitosis can be so intense that the histologic features suggest neoplasia and a diagnosis of "intestinal adenomatosis."

Morbidity within a herd is 10% to 15%; mortality is around 50%. In fatal cases, affected pigs usually die within a day of the appearance of clinical signs. Pigs that recover are generally "poor-doers." A similar organism with associated intestinal proliferation is found in horses, hamsters, ostriches, cervids, and macaques.

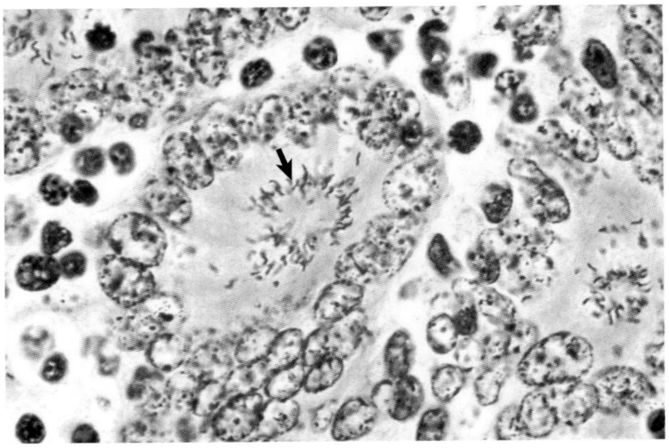

Fig. 7-156 **Proliferative enteritis, ileum, pig.**
Curved *Lawsonia* spp. bacteria *(arrow)* are present in the apical cytoplasm of enterocytes. There is proliferation of crypt enterocytes. Warthin-Starry stain. (Courtesy Dr. H. Gelberg, College of Veterinary Medicine, Oregon State University.)

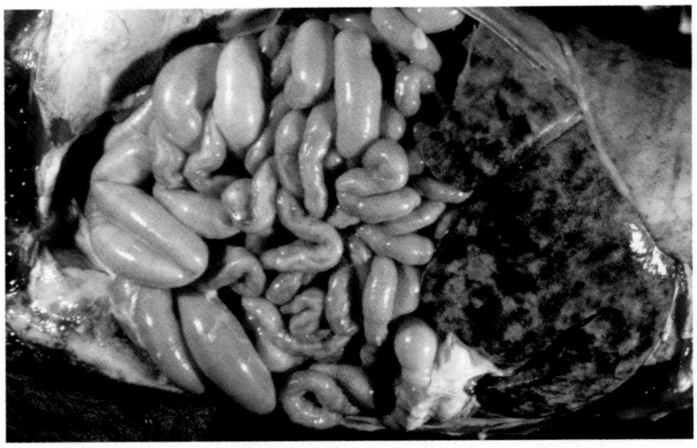

Fig. 7-157 **Fibrinous polyserositis, abdomen, pig.**
Strands and clumps of fibrin are scattered throughout serosal surfaces. A milk-spotted liver is also present. (Courtesy Dr. H. Gelberg, College of Veterinary Medicine, Oregon State University.)

Glasser's disease

Glasser's disease is characterized by fibrinous polyserositis (pleuritis, pericarditis, peritonitis, arthritis, and leptomeningitis). Although not generally a diarrheal disease, it causes inflammation of the intestinal serosa (serositis). Lesions range from arthritis to peritonitis to leptomeningitis, depending on the serous surface infected. Glasser's disease generally occurs in 5- to 12-week-old pigs. Mortality of affected animals within a herd is high, but morbidity is low. Although classic Glasser's disease is caused either by *Haemophilus suis* or *Haemophilus parasuis,* porcine polyserositis can be caused by *Mycoplasma hyorhinis*, *Streptococcus suis type II* (zoonotic), septicemic salmonellosis, and septicemic *Escherichia coli* (Fig. 7-157).

Miscellaneous Disorders

Chlamydia infection

Chlamydia has been found in enterocytes of normal pigs and pigs with diarrhea. In gnotobiotic pigs, *Chlamydia trachomatis* and *Chlamydia suis* infection result in villous atrophy and villous-tip necrosis. These lesions are most severe in the distal jejunum and ileum. Colonic infection has also been reported.

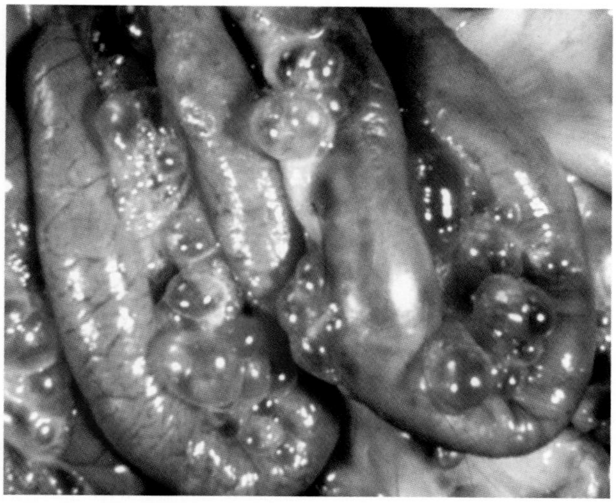

Fig. 7-158 Intestinal emphysema, intestines, pig. Gas bubbles dilate serosal and mesenteric lymphatics. (Courtesy Dr. H. Gelberg, College of Veterinary Medicine, Oregon State University.)

Intestinal emphysema

Intestinal emphysema (pneumatosis cystoides intestinalis) of pigs and rabbits translates to gas-dilated lymphatics of the intestinal serosa and mesentery. The cause of this condition is unknown, and it is not associated with clinical disease (Fig. 7-158).

Intestinal Disorders of Carnivores (Dogs and Cats)

Viral Diseases

Parvovirus enteritis

Parvovirus enteritis of dogs and cats is a severe, usually fatal disease. Because the target cells are those that are rapidly dividing, in the intestine the crypt cells are principally affected. This tropism is called *radiomimetic.* Identical crypt lesions in felids are sometimes associated with FeLV infection. Initial virus replication occurs in lymphoid tissue. Although there is much overlap in the disease syndrome in dogs and cats, the dissimilarities warrant independent discussion of each species. To complicate matters further, there is a high mutation rate among canine and feline parvoviruses and genetic recombination between the two viruses has been documented.

In the cat, mink, and raccoon, panleukopenia, cat distemper, feline enteritis, and mink enteritis are synonyms for this important disease. Early lesions in the course of the disease are lymphoid depletion and thymic involution. Later, lesions include flaccid, segmentally reddened intestine with serositis. Lesions are generally limited to the small intestine, but colitis occurs in some cats. Villous atrophy occurs secondary to crypt cell destruction (Fig. 7-159). Basophilic intranuclear inclusion bodies are present in enterocytes and lymphocytes early in infection. In germ-free cats with a low enterocyte turnover, the disease caused by feline parvovirus is much less severe. Intrauterine infection causes congenital cerebellar hypoplasia of kittens. The virus, as described previously, is cytolytic and infects dividing cells and thus alters the differentiation of layers in the cerebellum during organogenesis. The clinical disease is characterized by dehydration, depression, and diarrhea and vomiting. Because the bone marrow is a rapidly dividing tissue, panleukopenia dominates the clinical pathologic findings.

Canine parvovirus enteritis first appeared in Europe and the US in 1978. The disease was initially recognized because of the gross and microscopic lesions that were identical to those of feline parvovirus

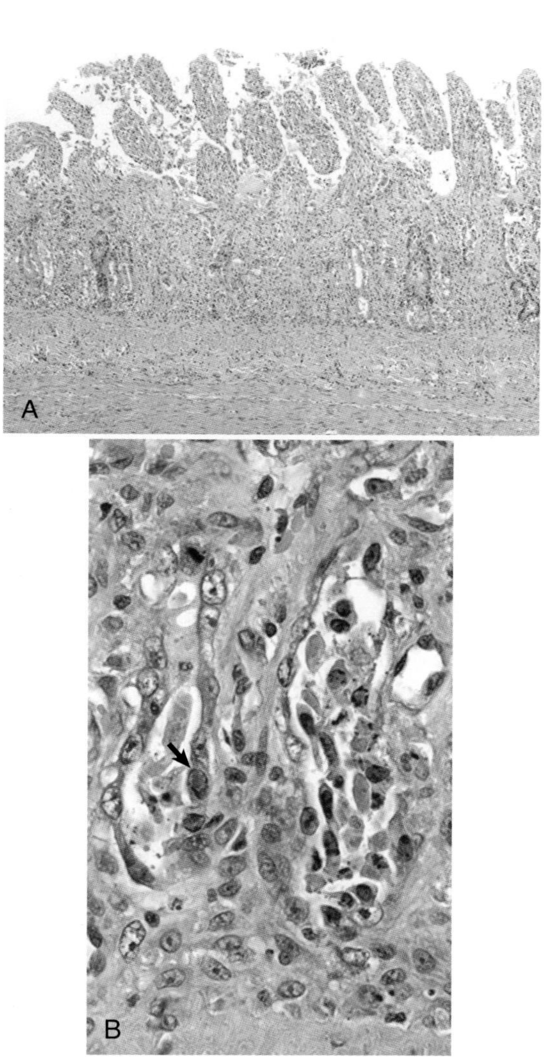

Fig. 7-159 Panleukopenia virus enteritis, small intestine, cat. **A,** Villi are denuded of epithelium and are atrophic. Note that because of the loss of epithelial cells in the crypts, they have collapsed, obliterating their lumens. Some crypts are dilated. H&E stain. **B,** Higher magnification of crypts. Note the sloughed necrotic epithelial cells in the crypt lumens and the lining of the crypts by squamoid epithelial cells and hyperplastic cells (some with intranuclear inclusion bodies) *(arrow),* all indicative of attempts at epithelial repair and regeneration. Chronic inflammatory cells are present in the lamina propria. H&E stain. (**A** and **B** courtesy Dr. J.F. Zachary, College of Veterinary Medicine, University of Illinois.)

enteritis. Panleukopenia vaccines were effective in preventing this disease in dogs and were used extensively until canine-specific parvovirus vaccines were developed. Rottweilers and Doberman pinschers, which are genetically related, are at increased risk for parvovirus disease even if properly vaccinated.

Canine parvovirus disease initially was described as occurring in three distinct syndromes. Puppies younger than 2 weeks of age had generalized disease with focal areas of virus-induced necrosis in those tissues with rapidly dividing cells. Thus multiple organs and tissues, such as the liver, kidney, heart, vessel, bone marrow, intestine, and lung, were affected. Puppies 3 to 8 weeks of age would sometimes have myocarditis develop for the same reason. Often, initial infection would go undetected, and these animals would die

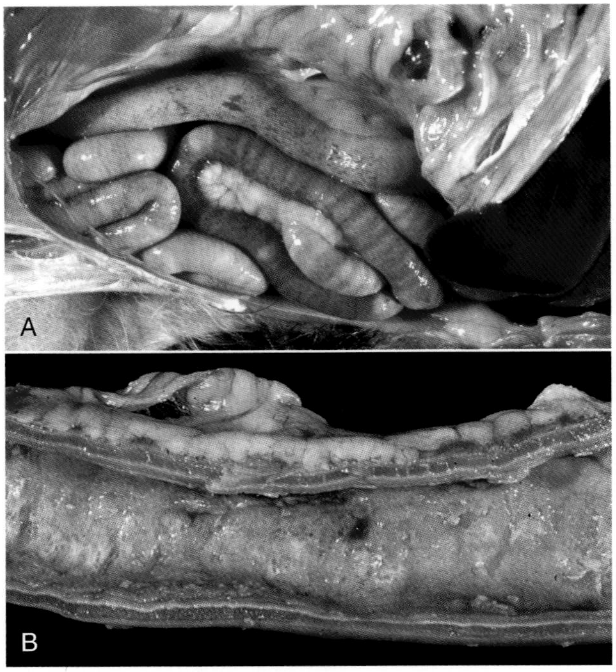

Fig. 7-160 Parvovirus enteritis, small intestine, dog.
A, Segments of the small intestine are diffusely reddened (active hyperemia of the mucosa), and the serosal surface is roughened, faintly granular, and petechiated. **B,** The mucosa of the small intestine is necrotic. Note the roughened, granular, focally petechiated, and focally sloughing mucosa. (**A** courtesy College of Veterinary Medicine, University of Illinois. **B** courtesy Department of Veterinary Biosciences, College of Veterinary Medicine, The Ohio State University and Noah's Arkive, College of Veterinary Medicine, The University of Georgia.)

unexpectedly up to 5 months later because of myocardial scarring and conduction failure (see Fig. 10-82). In puppies 8 weeks or older, the disease is identical to that in the cat. Cerebellar hypoplasia has not been induced in puppies.

At necropsy, the dilated, fluid-filled, flaccid, and hemorrhagic small intestine with serositis similar to that of panleukopenia is quite characteristic (Fig. 7-160, *A*). The contents of the small intestine are brown to red-brown and fluid with a fibrinous exudate, with or without hemorrhage (Fig. 7-160, *B*). Mesenteric lymphadenomegaly with variable hemorrhage is present. The bone marrow is depleted. Dogs but not cats may have coagulative lymphadenitis associated with severe lymphoid infection.

The intestinal lesion is necrosis of crypt epithelial cells. Surviving epithelial cells are not targets of the virus, but their morphology changes to squamoid to cover the surface of the denuded crypts and later to temporarily cover the denuded villous basement membrane, as replacement cells are not being produced, even though senile epithelial extrusion continues to occur from the villous tips. Severe lesions consist of partially denuded villi over debris-filled crypts, some of which lack an epithelial lining. Because the villous basement membrane is exposed during the continuing extrusion process, villous fusion occurs, resulting in lack of a scaffold for enterocyte replacement once the crypts recover and in permanent villous distortion and atrophy. Hyperplastic crypt epithelium may therefore be present. Inclusion bodies are not present in lymphoid tissue. In bone marrow, erythropoiesis is normal, but granulopoiesis is reduced. Necrotizing colitis may occur but is much less important than the small intestinal lesions. Dogs with hemorrhagic parvovirus enteritis have bloody diarrhea and die from shock within 24 hours.

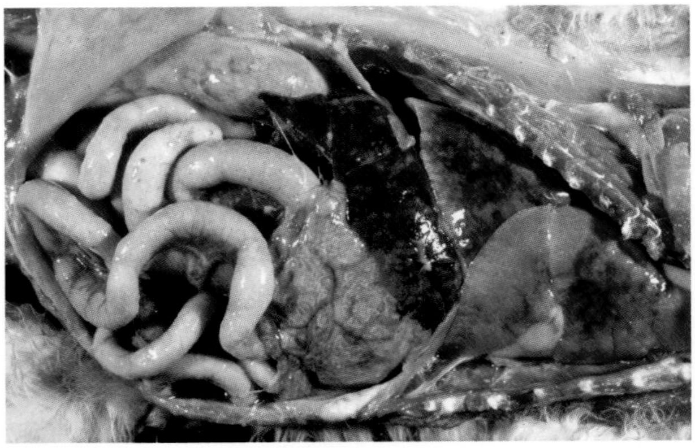

Fig. 7-161 Fibrinous polyserositis, abdomen, cat.
Fibrin strands between viscera and mats of fibrin on organ surfaces are characteristic of the "wet form" of feline infectious peritonitis. The mesentery *(below and left of the liver)* has numerous white linear serpentine tracts, which are inflamed (type III hypersensitivity, immune complex) capillaries and venules. Note the small nodules (pyogranulomas) on the intestinal serosa and on the surface of the kidney. (Courtesy Dr. H. Gelberg, College of Veterinary Medicine, Oregon State University.)

Secondary bacterial infections with endotoxemia are believed to be associated with this syndrome.

Minute virus of canids

Canine parvovirus type 1 produces myocarditis and respiratory disease in young pups. The virus is widely distributed in the canine population, but disease is only diagnosed sporadically. The virus is spread via the oronasal route. Fetal death and embryo absorption occur between 25 and 35 days of gestation. Microscopically, intestinal lesions consist of enterocyte hyperplasia with eosinophilic or amphophilic intranuclear inclusion bodies in the enterocytes of the villous tips of the duodenum and jejunum. Crypt necrosis characteristic of canine parvovirus type 2 infection is not present.

Feline infectious peritonitis

Feline infectious peritonitis (FIP) is a uniformly fatal disease of cats. A nearly identical coronaviral disease has been described in ferrets. Although it affects cats of all ages, the disease is principally found in the young and old. Twelve percent of feline deaths are associated with FIP. The cause of the disease is a coronavirus related to the coronavirus of transmissible gastroenteritis of pigs. The coronavirus of FIP in cats is believed to be a mutated enteric coronavirus. After entry into the body, the first round of viral replication takes place in the lymphoid system. Macrophages are infected and carry the virus systemically. Endothelial cells are activated secondary to upregulation of major histocompatibility complex II. Observations suggest that activated monocytes are critical for development of vasculitis. Lesions are multifocal and most organs, including the CNS, may be affected (see Figs. 14-105 and 14-106). The lesions in the vasculature of the eye are sometimes useful in making a tentative diagnosis of FIP in the live cat, but other diseases, such as toxoplasmosis and systemic fungi, may cause similar lesions (see Figs. 20-69 and 20-139). The "wet form" of the disease is characterized by fibrinous polyserositis (Fig. 7-161); the "dry form" is without the effusive process. Why one form develops rather than the other is not completely understood but may relate to the major type of immune effector cell. The disease often clusters in households, and virus spreads among cats by saliva on shared bowls and utensils or by mutation of an endogenous coronavirus.

Because of the presence of a nonneutralizing antibody, immune complexes develop and Arthus reactions localize in the vasculature. Complement is fixed, and inflammatory cell chemoattractants are produced. Vasculitis results in protein effusion. Thus lesions are vasocentric. The prodromal course of FIP is shortened, and the development and extent of lesions are accelerated in seropositive cats. FIP is usually characterized by progressive wasting because of protein loss. It is unusual for a virus to result in pyogranulomatous lesions, but in FIP the vasocentric deposition of immune complexes results in pyogranulomas. These lesions are single to multiple, white, and raised. On the surface of the kidney, they often are linear, clearly following the renal surface vasculature (see Fig. 11-75). In its "wet form," FIP is characterized by variable of amounts of thick, stringy, high-protein effusion in body cavities. When placed between gloved fingers, this transudate may be drawn out in strings as the fingers are separated. The transudate is sterile, eliminating most other causes of fibrinous peritonitis. The granulomas are translucent and less than 2 mm in diameter. The "dry form" of the disease is identical to the wet but contains only pyogranulomas and not the exudates.

Bacterial Diseases

Histiocytic ulcerative colitis

Because of its occurrence in boxer dogs and the genetically related French bulldog, histiocytic ulcerative colitis has been called *boxer colitis. Granulomatous colitis* is another term for this disease, although true granulomas are not present. It generally occurs in dogs younger than 2 years. Dogs can have soft feces, but often no diarrhea or weight loss is observed. In some cases, mucus and blood appear in the stool. The lesions, which are visible by proctoscopy, are raised ulcerative nodules (Fig. 7-162). Microscopically the colon is ulcerated and has marked infiltration by macrophages containing PAS-positive material.

Large macrophages with abundant foamy eosinophilic cytoplasm are present in the colonic lamina propria and submucosa early in the disease process. There may be lesser numbers of smaller, mononuclear inflammatory cells, principally lymphocytes and plasmacytes. The PAS-positive material in macrophages has been visualized by tissue Gram stains, electron microscopy, and immunohistochemistry. They likely contain bacteria and the phagolysosomal remnants of digested cells. Evidence suggests that the bacteria are probably *Escherichia coli.* The massive numbers of engorged macrophages within the lamina propria results in a space-occupying lesion that affects the overlying enterocytes. Enterocyte necrosis results in colonic erosion and ulceration. There is lymphadenopathy, both regional and generalized, characterized by an influx of foamy macrophages in the lymphatic sinuses.

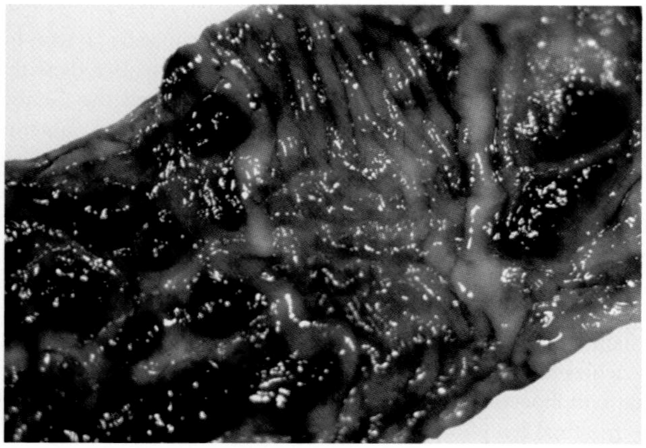

Fig. 7-162 Histiocytic ulcerative colitis, colon, boxer dog. There are numerous round and coalescing ulcers in the colon in this case of "boxer colitis." Research suggests *Escherichia coli* as the causative agent of boxer colitis. (Courtesy Dr. H. Gelberg, College of Veterinary Medicine, Oregon State University.)

Citrobacter freundii *enteritis*

Bacteremia and septicemia associated with *Citrobacter freundii* have been reported to cause mucohemorrhagic diarrhea in dogs with hemorrhagic lesions in the small intestine and colon. It is believed to be a condition of puppies and immunocompromised dogs. Being bacteremic and/or septicemic, many organs and tissues are affected besides the gut. The condition is more common in humans as a nosocomial infection with a high mortality rate. In humans, the route of infection is through the urinary tract, gallbladder, GI tract, or cutaneous wounds. *Citrobacter* infections should be considered potentially zoonotic.

Fungal Diseases

Canine histoplasmosis

Canine histoplasmosis occurs most often in the Ohio and Mississippi river valleys. This zoonotic systemic fungus can infect the intestine, but pneumonia is more common. Thus the route of infection is inhalation or ingestion. The reservoir is believed to be soil and bird feces. The yeast invades tissue, causes necrosis, and replicates in macrophages. Granulomatous lesions may be present in pulmonary, intestinal, lymphoid, hepatic, and other tissue. At necropsy or biopsy, the intestine has a thickened and corrugated mucosa with ulceration. There is hepatomegaly and mesenteric lymphadenopathy and lymphadenomegaly. Scattered pulmonary granulomas may be present.

In the affected ileum and colon, the lamina propria is widened by macrophages that contain *Histoplasma capsulatum* (Fig. 7-163). With time, infection may extend transmurally through the intestine and to the lymphoid system. There is hyperplasia of regional lymph nodes, and lymphoid sinuses contain numerous macrophages (see Figs. 13-55, 13-83, and 13-84). Multifocal granulomas with intracellular fungi are in the liver, presumably arriving via the portal vein (see Fig. 8-51).

Signs of intestinal histoplasmosis in the dog include intractable chronic diarrhea with anorexia and its attendant weight loss, lethargy, poor pelage, and anemia. Respiratory signs and peripheral lymphadenitis may be present.

Rickettsial Diseases

Salmon poisoning

Salmon poisoning is an acute and fatal hemorrhagic granulomatous enterocolitis of the dog and fox that results from consuming salmon carrying the fluke *Nanophyetus salmincola.* When this trematode harbors *Neorickettsia helminthoeca*, a 0.3-μm coccoid rickettsia, disease may result. Lesions may extend from the pylorus to the anus. The enteric lesions consist of hemorrhage at sites of GALT necrosis, especially near the ileocecal valves. In the small intestine, trematodes may be embedded in the mucosa. Diagnosis is confirmed by visualizing macrophages in many tissues, including the lymph nodes, lamina propria and brain, containing Giemsa- or Gram-stained elementary bodies (Web Fig. 7-20).

Six to eight days after eating parasitized fish, affected canids become febrile and depressed. There is an oculonasal discharge, severe diarrhea, emesis, anorexia, and splenolymphadenopathy characterized by enlarged tonsils, spleen, and lymph nodes. The mesenteric lymph nodes are often more severely affected

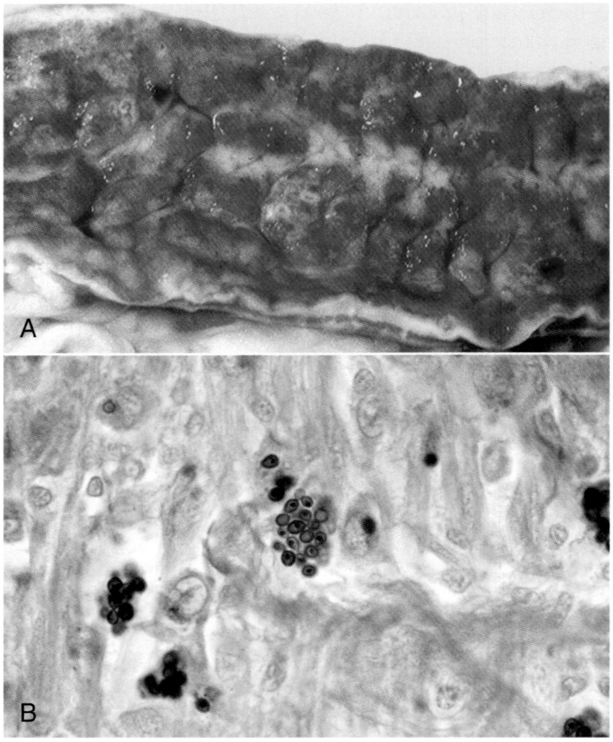

Fig. 7-163 Histoplasmosis, granulomatous enteritis, intestine, dog. **A,** The mucosa is congested and greatly thickened from granulomatous inflammation that has expanded the lamina propria. **B,** Clusters of 3- to 5-μm *Histoplasma capsulatum* organisms with a central nucleoid are in macrophages. Grocott-Gomori's methenamine silver stain. (**A** courtesy Dr. R. Panciera, School of Veterinary Medicine, Oklahoma State University; and Noah's Arkive, College of Veterinary Medicine, The University of Georgia. **B** courtesy Dr. H. Gelberg, College of Veterinary Medicine, Oregon State University.)

than peripheral nodes. Unless treated, affected animals die within 10 days.

Parasitic Diseases

Canine multifocal eosinophilic gastroenteritis

Canine multifocal eosinophilic gastroenteritis is an uncommon disease of dogs generally younger than 4 years. It is caused by migrating larvae of *Toxocara canis*. Therefore this disease occurs in association with poor parasite management.

Larvae of *Toxocara canis* are ingested, invade the mucosa of the stomach and small intestine, and then become trapped and localized in their self-induced inflammation. Dormant larvae migrate into the uterus and fetuses during late pregnancy. Postpartum, larvae are secreted in the milk of the bitch or ingested from environmental feces. Ingested larvae penetrate the gastric and small intestinal mucosa, enter lymph vessels or the portal vein, and travel to the liver and lungs. They then develop into third-stage larvae and are coughed up and swallowed. In the GI tract, they mature to adult ascarids. In the majority of puppies, ascarid larvae complete their life cycle in several weeks. Alternatively, the larvae are enveloped in granulomas that kill the parasite secondary to immune reactivity. These granulomas may occur anywhere along the parasite's migration tracts, including most abdominal organs, eyes, brain, and the lungs. Eosinophils are a prominent component of the inflammatory reaction and are attracted to the site of parasite entrapment by the waste products of the larvae. There may be subsequent mineralization of larvae, or they may remain viable for up to 4 years. This condition is especially common in aberrant host species and is called *visceral larval migrans*. It is an environmental danger where children play in sand or dirt contaminated by feces of infected animals. The ova are relatively resistant to environmental extremes.

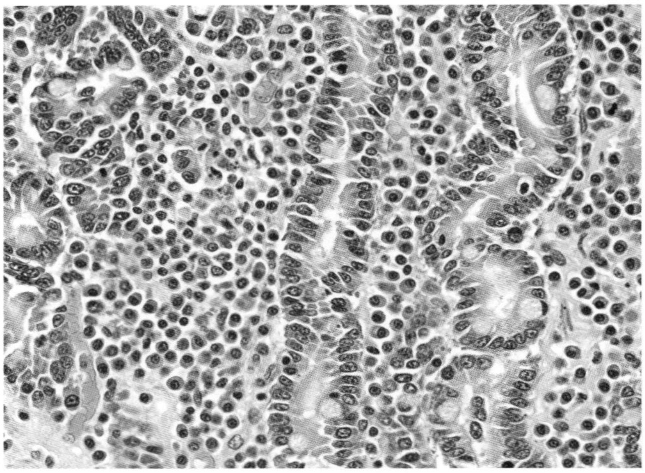

Fig. 7-164 Lymphoplasmacytic enteropathy, intestine, dog. The lamina propria is widened with lymphocytes and plasma cells. H&E stain. (Courtesy Dr. H. Gelberg, College of Veterinary Medicine, Oregon State University.)

Lesions are microscopic to macroscopic and may be quite numerous. As in other inflammatory diseases, there may be regional lymphadenopathy with or without nodules that vary from principally granulomatous to eosinophilic or a mix of the two. Larvae, when present, are surrounded by an eosinophilic, amorphous, fringed material that stains PAS-positive (the Splendore-Hoeppli phenomenon).

In general, canine multifocal eosinophilic gastroenteritis is asymptomatic. However, chronic diarrhea, moderate weight loss, intermittent or persistent eosinophilia, and elevated serum γ-globulin concentrations may characterize this disorder. Serum albumin concentration, absorption tests, and small bowel contrast radiographs usually are normal.

Immunologic Disorders

Inflammatory bowel disease

In dogs and cats, this disease is microscopically a lymphoplasmacytic enteritis. Diagnosis is made by biopsy. Breeds with a predilection for this disease include the basenji and the German shepherd. The cause is unknown, but the presence of numerous lymphocytes and plasma cells suggests an immunologic problem. Malabsorption and chronic protein-losing enteropathy can result from the marked infiltrate of lymphocytes and plasmacytes in the lamina propria. In dogs, there are increased numbers of both B and T lymphocytes in the lamina propria of the small intestine (Fig. 7-164). In cats but not dogs, dietary antigens cause some cases of inflammatory bowel disease; therefore control of the disease can be achieved by regulation of the diet. Anecdotal evidence suggests that lymphocytic plasmacytic enteritis in the cat can be a prelude to intestinal lymphoma.

Diffuse eosinophilic gastroenteritis

Although diffuse eosinophilic gastroenteritis has a predilection for the German shepherd breed, it occurs in other breeds of dogs and in cats. It is characterized by recurrent episodes of diarrhea

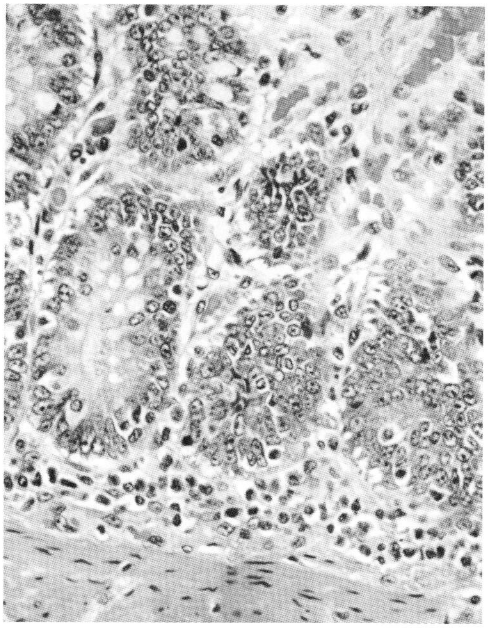

Fig. 7-165 Diffuse eosinophilic enteritis, small intestine, dog. Numerous eosinophils are present in the deep lamina propria and the mucosal-submucosal interface. The cause of this hypersensitivity reaction is not known. H&E stain. (Courtesy Dr. H. Gelberg, College of Veterinary Medicine, Oregon State University.)

associated with tissue and circulating eosinophilia. The increased concentration of eosinophils in the circulation and within lesions suggests a hypersensitivity reaction to some ingested substance or to parasites. The cause has not been identified. There are no gross lesions. Eosinophils, along with lymphocytes and plasma cells, heavily infiltrate all layers of the mucosa of the stomach and intestine (Fig. 7-165).

Wheat-sensitive enteropathy of Irish setters

Wheat-sensitive enteropathy, a hereditable condition similar to gluten-sensitive enteropathy of humans, is the first described dietary-induced enteropathy of dogs. It is characterized initially by increased numbers of intraepithelial lymphocytes and goblet cells and later by partial villous atrophy, particularly of the jejunum. Dietary therapy is palliative.

Idiopathic Disorders

Feline ulcerative colitis

Feline ulcerative colitis is grossly and histologically analogous to its canine counterpart, histiocytic ulcerative colitis (Fig. 7-166). The cause is unknown.

Canine senile gastrointestinal amyloidosis

Amyloid located in and around vessels of the submucosal and muscular layers of the alimentary tract and within the mesentery has been reported in dogs. The mechanism and chemical nature of the amyloid deposition has not been determined. Dysfunction of the alimentary tract has not been reported to occur with canine senile gastrointestinal amyloidosis.

Parasitic Enteritides

Parasites of the intestinal tract are legion in the various domestic animal species. Refer to a parasitology textbook for specific information regarding the life cycles and identification of the various species. Diagnosis of enteric parasitism is generally performed via fecal flotation or intestinal scrapings.

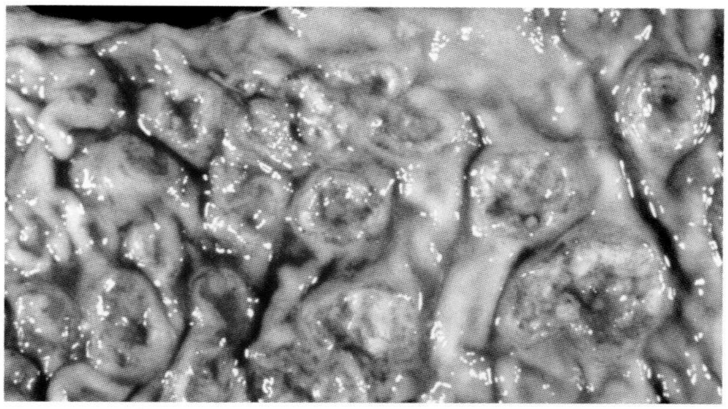

Fig. 7-166 Feline ulcerative colitis, colon, cat. There are numerous round ulcers in the mucosa of this idiopathic disease. (Courtesy Dr. H. Gelberg, College of Veterinary Medicine, Oregon State University.)

Amebiasis

Entamoeba spp. are obligate intracellular parasites with a direct life cycle. The portal of entry is oral. Trophozoites are produced that dwell in the intestinal lumen. They may also invade through the intestinal wall and go to many other organs, such as the liver, brain, and lung, especially in humans, in whom microabscesses may form. Cysts are excreted with formed feces and continue their life cycle when ingested by another host. Trophozoites are more likely seen in diarrheic feces. Because cysts are the infective form, diarrheic feces of dogs are not usually considered to be especially dangerous to humans or other animals. The trophozoites vary from 12 to 30 μm in diameter, and the cysts vary from 10 to 20 μm with four nuclei. Contact of ameba and host cells is likely mediated by adhesins. Soluble factors produced by the parasite mediate pathogenicity.

Entamoeba histolytica is zoonotic in humans, other primates, dogs, cats, and other animals. Disease is serious in humans. Lesions include colonic congestion, petechia, and ulceration (ulcerative colitis). This colitis may be acute or chronic, bloody or mucoid. In tissue, the amebas may be as large as 50 μm and often form typical flask-shaped ulcers spanning the mucosa and submucosa of the colon. After penetrating the surface mucus and adhering to the colonic enterocytes, *Entamoeba histolytica* releases amebophores (channel-forming peptides) that lyse the enterocytes without killing the ameba.

Balantidiasis (Balantidium coli)

Balantidium coli is a normal inhabitant of the cecum and colon of primates, including humans, and swine. It is large (50-60 μm × 25-45 μm) and ciliated. Dogs with whipworm infestation may become infested after contact with infected pigs. In general, *Balantidium* is an opportunistic pathogen associated with enteric disease (Fig. 7-167).

Trichomoniasis

Tritrichomonas foetus is a sexually transmitted pathogen of cattle. Cats, especially those less than a year of age housed in groups, have a tendency toward large bowel diarrhea when infected with this flagellate. Diagnosis is often made by visualization of motile flagellates on fecal wet mounts. Histologic diagnosis is most accurate when at least six biopsy sections of colon containing surface mucus are examined. PCR on paraffin-embedded tissue has also been successful, even in the absence of histologic evidence of the parasite. Infection occurs in the ileum, cecum, and colon. Lesions

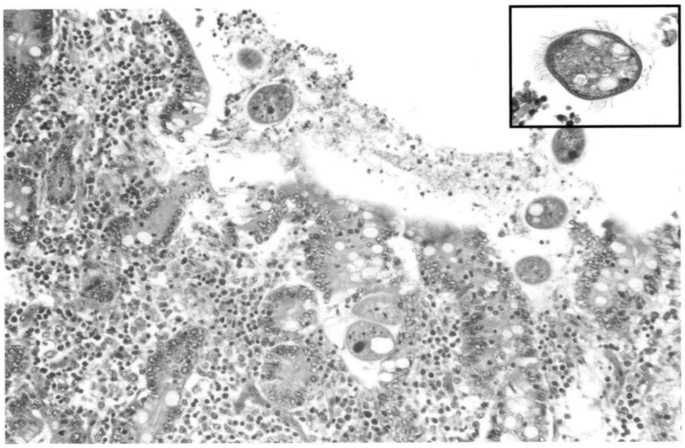

Fig. 7-167 *Balantidium coli*, colon, pig.
Balantidium coli is an opportunistic flagellated protozoan that is normally present in the pig intestine. This pig had concurrent proliferative *(Lawsonia)* enteritis. H&E stain. *Inset,* Higher magnification of *Balantidium coli.* H&E stain. (Courtesy of Dr. C. Löhr, College of Veterinary Medicine, Oregon State University. Insert, Courtesy Dr. J.F. Zachary, College of Veterinary Medicine, University of Illinois.)

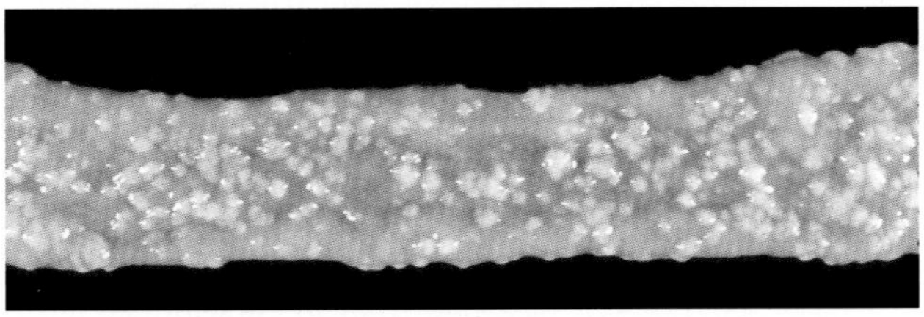

Fig. 7-168 Multifocal proliferative enteritis, small intestine, goat.
Proliferative nodules (also see Fig. 7-172) in the small intestinal mucosa are characteristic of ovine and caprine coccidiosis. Sporozoites and merozoites infect enterocytes and replicate, stimulating hyperplasia of enterocytes. (Courtesy Dr. H. Gelberg, College of Veterinary Medicine, Oregon State University.)

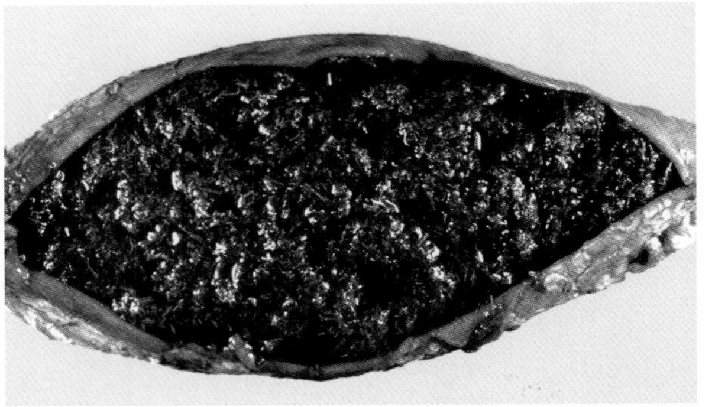

Fig. 7-169 Necrohemorrhagic enteritis, small intestine, calf.
Coccidiosis in cattle, dogs, and cats is characterized by intestinal hemorrhage. Hemorrhagic diarrheic feces may be visible on the perineum and hind legs. In severe cases, there may be anemia, which will be evident as pale external mucous membranes. (Courtesy College of Veterinary Medicine, Cornell University.)

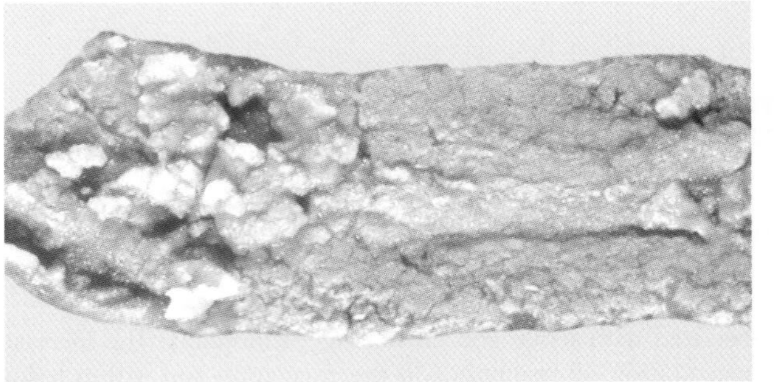

Fig. 7-170 Fibrinonecrotic enteritis, small intestine, pig.
Pseudomembranes are characteristic of porcine coccidiosis. (Courtesy Dr. H. Gelberg, College of Veterinary Medicine, Oregon State University.)

include mild-to-moderate colitis, with microabscesses and occasional extension of infection into the lamina propria. There may be colonic enterocyte attenuation and/or increased mitotic activity in the crypts. The 5 μm by 7 μm teardrop-shaped parasites can often been seen in surface mucus, within colonic glands, and occasionally within macrophages and lymphatics. Thus the parasite is enteroinvasive under certain circumstances. Flagella are not visible on H&E staining. There is no effective treatment. The diarrheal disease in cats generally resolves within 2 years of onset.

Coccidiosis

Coccidia are exquisitely host- and tissue-specific protozoa. They are obligate intracellular pathogens. Lesions vary from proliferative in sheep and goats (Fig. 7-168) to hemorrhagic in dogs, cats, and cattle (Fig. 7-169). In pigs, a fibrinonecrotic pseudomembrane, without blood, in 5- to 7-day-old animals is characteristic of enteric coccidiosis (Fig. 7-170). *Eimeria macusaniensis* is a relatively common cause of sickness and death in new world camelids of all ages. Gross lesions, even in heavily infested animals, are minimal to absent. In many cases, fecal examinations are negative.

Most species of *Eimeria* and *Isospora* infect villous or crypt epithelial cells, more rarely lacteals, the lamina propria, and regional lymph nodes. The coccidia undergo one or more asexual reproductive cycles within enterocytes. The resulting sporozoites produce schizonts containing merozoites, which infect additional enterocytes.

Merozoites produce gamonts that differentiate into microgametes and macrogametes (Fig. 7-171). Microgametes fertilize macrogametes, producing zygotes that develop into oocysts. When a small number of coccidia parasitize the intestine of otherwise healthy young growing animals, little disease results. However, when animals are in crowded conditions associated with poor sanitation, fecal-oral transmission of large numbers of organisms can occur. It is in these circumstances, compounded by malnutrition and intercurrent infections or parasitism, that clinical disease results. Enterocyte rupture occurs in all stages of the parasite's life cycle. Clinical disease depends on parasitic load and varies by animal species. Because of diminished epithelial turnover in young animals, they are most susceptible to disease.

Gross lesions of coccidiosis are variable by host species, parasite species, and intestinal location. Bleeding is variably present both within species and among species. Coccidiosis in sheep and goats is characterized by enterocyte proliferation that is visible grossly as mucosal nodules (Fig. 7-172). The large schizonts of some species are sometimes grossly visible as well. *Eimeria leuckarti* of equids is asymptomatic. In dogs and cats a slightly different organism, *Cystoisospora,* is responsible for disease. Intestinal toxoplasmosis of felids is an important zoonotic concern, especially for pregnant women.

"Poor doing" associated with diarrhea is characteristic of clinical coccidiosis. Depending on the host species and the region of

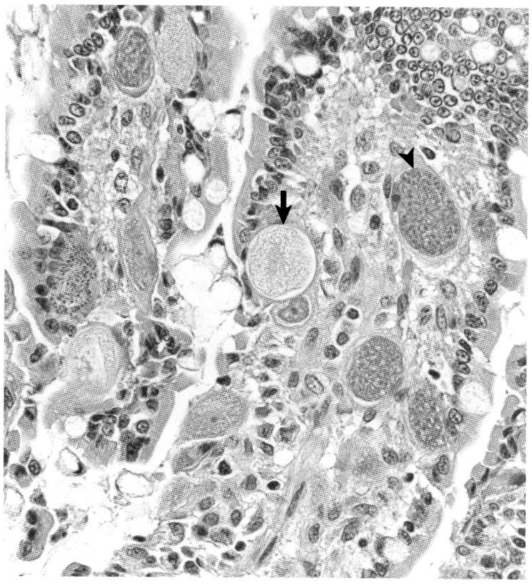

Fig. 7-171 Sexual stages of intestinal coccidiosis. small intestine, cow. Note that the mucosal epithelial cells are distended with microgametes *(arrow)* and macrogametes *(arrowhead)*. H&E stain. (Courtesy Dr. J.F. Zachary, College of Veterinary Medicine, University of Illinois.)

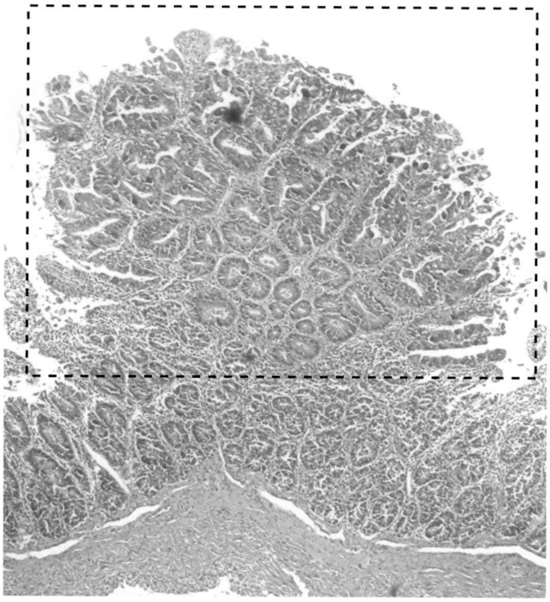

Fig. 7-172 Proliferative enteritis, small intestine, goat. Coccidia-induced enterocyte hyperplasia results in nodule formation *(area identified by dashed-lines)* as seen in Fig. 7-168. Note the hyperplastic enterocytes lining crypts within the nodule. H&E stain. (Courtesy Dr. H. Gelberg, College of Veterinary Medicine, Oregon State University.)

intestine that is affected, infected fresh blood may be present in the feces. The presence of tenesmus is variable. Oocysts are usually demonstrable in the feces.

Cryptosporidiosis

Cryptosporidium parvum is a ubiquitous protozoan pathogen of mammals. Often waterborne, it is a significant cause of municipal water contamination. Although it causes a self-limiting infection in immunocompetent animals, the very young or immunocompromised individuals, such as AIDS patients, suffer from intractable diarrhea. When treating calves, veterinarians and veterinary students are at particular risk for infection. Cryptosporidia attach to surface epithelial cells of the stomach, small intestine, or colon. The protozoa displace the microvilli and are enclosed by surface cell membranes. Thus the parasite lives in a unique environment described as intracellular but extracytoplasmic (Web Fig. 7-21). Microgametes, macrogametes, schizonts, trophozoites, meronts, merozoites, and oocysts can be demonstrated in the intestine adjacent to, or attached to, epithelial cells. Oocysts are 4 to 5 μm in diameter and are shed in the feces. Studies have indicated that there are species-specific tropisms or biotypes of cryptosporidia. Previously, fecal contamination of water supplies by ruminants was believed to be the cause of most human outbreaks. Molecular typing of the organism has shown in many disease outbreaks that contamination with human feces and human-specific cryptosporidia causes most human epidemics.

Oocysts can be identified in feces by Sheather's sucrose flotation and a modified acid-fast stain. Cryptosporidiosis causes subacute or chronic, sometimes bloody, watery diarrhea. The mechanism of diarrhea involves more than just cell loss. Prostaglandins, perhaps secreted by macrophages, increase anion (Cl^-) secretion through cAMP and inhibit sodium absorption and thus water absorption. In addition, *Cryptosporidium parvum* interferes with interferon-γ (IFN-γ) gene expression of host cells thus contributing to immune evasion by the parasite. There is associated dehydration and electrolyte loss. Although the disease can be fatal, particularly in the presence of other pathogens, it is often self-limiting in immunocompetent individuals. In these cases, the illness resolves spontaneously in about a week.

Affected portions of the GI tract are diffusely reddened and have fluid contents. The organisms appear as tiny blue (hematoxylinophilic) dots attached to the epithelial cells of affected segments. In addition to the dot forms, ring- and banana-shaped organisms are readily seen in Giemsa-stained sections. The lesions of enteritis or colitis consist of decreased mucosal (villous) height, irregular mucosal thickness, crypt necrosis, hyperemia, and an increase in lymphocytes and plasma cells in the lamina propria. Villous atrophy and fusion of the villi of the small intestine are the end result. Because of the intracellular, extracytoplasmic location of the parasite, chemotherapeutic intervention is ineffective. There are few chemicals that can decontaminate the environment. Clorox, for example, is used experimentally to purify the parasites.

Giardiasis

Giardiasis has been reported in many species, including humans, dogs, cats, horses, cattle, rabbits, guinea pigs, hamsters, rats, mice, chinchillas, and parakeets. In clinical veterinary practice, giardiasis is frequently recognized in puppies and kittens and causes concern among owners because of its zoonotic potential. Prevalence of the parasite in humans in the developed world is estimated at 2% to 5%. Giardiasis is caused by a pear-shaped protozoan with posterior flagella, a ventral sucker, and four nuclei, two of which resemble eyes (Fig. 7-173). *Giardia lamblia* parasitizes the small intestine, particularly the duodenum. *Giardia* attach to the microvillous border of epithelial cells, producing membrane damage. Although generally asymptomatic, diarrhea may result in very young animals or in animals otherwise immunologically deficient.

Giardia spp. have been shown to induce apoptosis of enterocytes thus increasing membrane permeability. In large numbers, the parasites decrease the absorption of simple sugars and disaccharides secondary to microvillous destruction. Ingesta are then fermented by bacterial flora, creating gas and osmotically drawing water into the intestinal lumen. An enterotoxin stimulates intestinal Cl^- secretion. Clinical cases of giardiasis have brown, fluid diarrhea, and

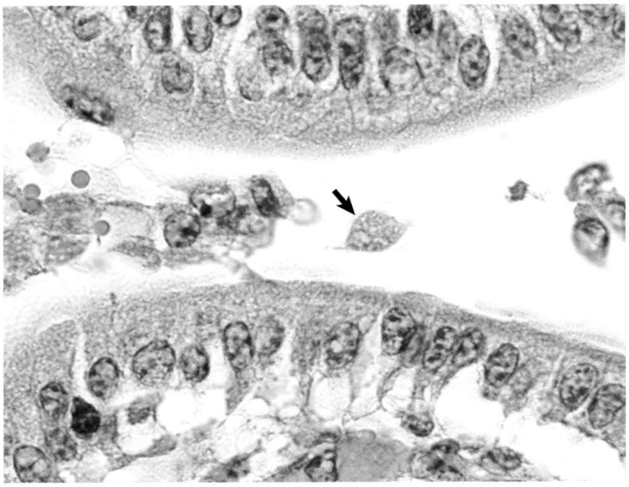

Fig. 7-173 Giardiasis, small intestine, dog.
A single pear-shaped flagellated protozoa is readily visible in the intestinal lumen *(arrow)*. H&E stain. (Courtesy Dr. J.F. Zachary, College of Veterinary Medicine, University of Illinois.)

abdominal discomfort without fever, weight loss, melena, and/or steatorrhea. The diagnosis is made by demonstrating *Giardia* in preparations of fresh feces or in histologic sections by identifying the organisms either with H&E or Giemsa stains.

Ascariasis

Ascarids are easily recognized as proximal-intestinal, luminal nematodes that are smooth and white. They are round on cross-section, thus giving them the appellation of roundworms together with the other nematodes. They vary greatly in length; the larger the host species, the larger the ascarids. They are 3 to 4 cm long in small animals and attain lengths of 40 to 50 cm in pigs and horses. Ascarids of domestic animals belong to the genera *Ascaris* (pigs), *Parascaris* (horses), and *Toxocara* (dogs, cats, and humans). The young of these species acquire larval ascarids by intrauterine transmission during the last 7 to 10 days of gestation, through the milk of the dam, and later in life through parasite ova contamination of the environment. After ingestion, infective larvae penetrate the intestine and migrate to the liver via the portal circulation. From there the larvae migrate via the caudal vena cava to the lungs. After leaving the circulation and entering the alveoli, the larvae undergo development, and are coughed into the pharynx and swallowed. Development to adults occurs in the intestine. Ova passed in the feces complete the life cycle.

Alternatively, *Toxascaris leonina* of canids and felids is ingested via an intermediate host. Hepatopulmonary migration does not occur. Lesions produced by ascarid larval migration include canine multifocal eosinophilic gastroenteritis and visceral larval migrans. Animals affected with heavy ascarid burdens lose weight, grow poorly as a result of competition for nutrients between luminal parasites and the host, and often have a pear-shaped abdomen when held vertically. Adult worms may be vomited or passed in the diarrheic feces. A hacking cough termed *thumping* is a sign of pulmonary larva migrans, especially in pigs. Anthelmintic administration can cause a rapid die off of adult ascarids, resulting in intestinal occlusion (see Web Fig. 7-14). Ascarids continue to migrate after the death of the host and may be found in aberrant locations such as the bile duct, stomach, oral cavity, pancreatic duct, and abdomen (Fig. 7-174).

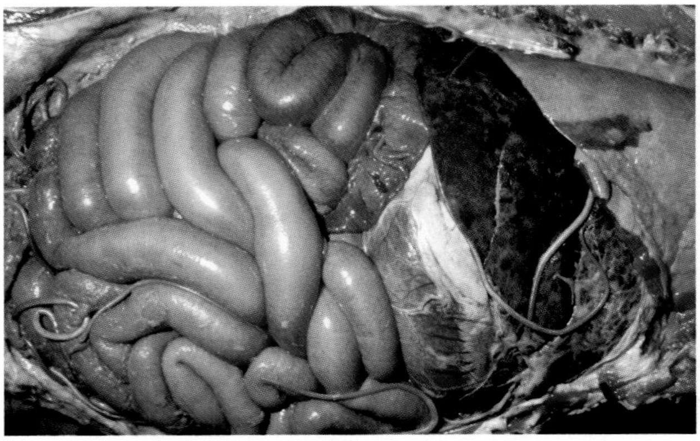

Fig. 7-174 Fibrinous peritonitis, abdomen, pig.
The presence of fibrin along with ascarids in this pig's abdomen indicates that the intestinal rupture occurred antemortem. (Courtesy Dr. M.D. McGavin, College of Veterinary Medicine, University of Tennessee.)

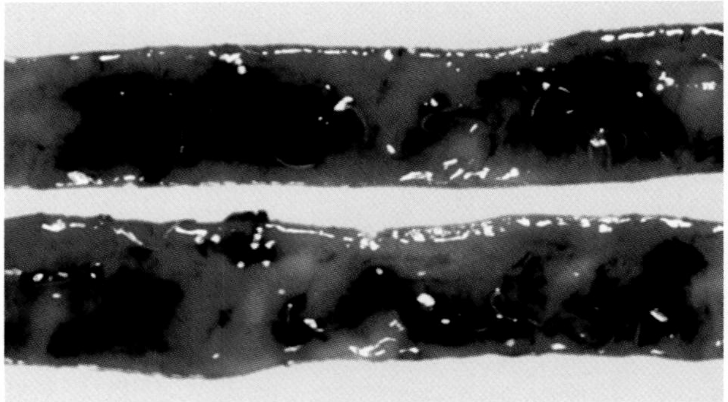

Fig. 7-175 Hookworms, hemorrhagic enteritis, small intestine, dog.
Where hookworms have detached, hemorrhage is present. (Courtesy Dr. H. Gelberg, College of Veterinary Medicine, Oregon State University.)

Hookworm Disease

Parasitism by hookworms varies from asymptomatic to fatal based on the challenge dose of parasites, the host's age, nutritional status, and likely its immunologic state. When death occurs, it is by exsanguination because hookworms are blood eaters (Fig. 7-175). Challenge dosage is often exacerbated by poor nutritional and sanitary conditions, mild climatic conditions, and moisture. Hookworms are generally small nematodes, 1 to 1.5 cm long. Their habitat is usually the proximal small intestine. Genera include *Ancylostoma* and *Uncinaria* in dogs, Bunostomum in ruminants, *Globocephalus* in pigs, and *Ancylostoma* and *Necator* in humans. *Ancylostoma caninum* in dogs has zoonotic potential. Environmental contamination occurs from the large number of eggs produced in the intestine. The first- through third-stage larvae feed on environmental bacteria. Third-stage larvae are infective and enter the host either by ingestion or direct dermal penetration. From either point of entry, they migrate through the pulmonary system, through somatic tissue to the uterus, or through mucosal tissue. Larvae may also be present in colostrum. The final destination is the intestine, where eggs are produced, completing the life cycle.

Because prenatal infections with hookworms do not become patent for 11 days, fecal examinations may be negative. Otherwise, fecal examination, especially in young animals with anemia, is diagnostic of this disease. Adult hookworms bury into the villous, ingesting tissue, mucus, and blood (Fig. 7-176). When the worm

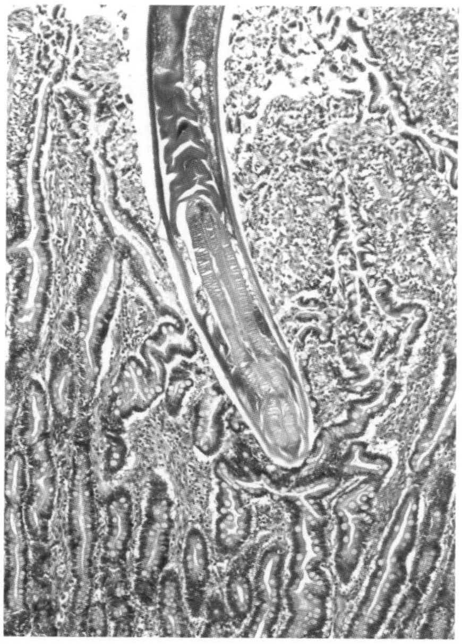

Fig. 7-176 Hookworm enteritis, intestine, dog.
A hookworm has burrowed deep into and attached to the mucosa. H&E stain. (Courtesy College of Veterinary Medicine, Cornell University.)

moves to another attachment site, blood may continue to flow from the wound for 30 minutes.

Trichuriasis

Trichurids, or whipworms, are long and slender at their anterior ends and may be numerous within the cecum and colon. Trichurids have a direct life cycle. The name *Trichuris* translates to "whip-tail," which is a misnomer because the parasite actually has a "whip-head" that invades and attaches to the mucosa of the cecum, colon, and rectum. Although the parasite ingests blood, anemia is rarely a clinical symptom. Bloody diarrhea may be present. Different species are parasites of carnivores, ruminants, pigs, and humans. The disease in each species is similar. The horse does not have a whipworm.

Trichuris eggs are elongate, or football-shaped, with an operculum at either end, and are very resistant to environmental conditions. Most infections are asymptomatic and the complete life cycle may take up to 3 months. Therefore repeated dewormings are necessary to eliminate infection, even in the absence of fecal ova. Symptoms may be vague, with only paroxysmal diarrhea. Gross enteric lesions vary from mild to erosive and ulcerative.

Strongyloidosis

Strongyloides spp. are unique in having free-living and parasitic forms. Rhabditiform larvae may develop parthenogenetically. Free-living parasites are both male and female and undergo sexual reproduction. Enteritis can be severe; larvae or larvated eggs are in the feces of infected animals.

Strongyloides stercoralis of dogs is zoonotic. *Strongyloides* spp. also infect horses, pigs, and cats. Geographic differences in parasite populations account for differences in virulence within host species. Hyperinfection and autoinfection may occur, adding to the parasite burden. Larvae may enter the host by skin penetration, or less often by ingestion. *Strongyloides* spp. infection may be acquired in utero and through colostrum and milk. Larvae migrate to the bloodstream and lungs. When they gain access to alveoli, they subsequently migrate to airways, where they are carried, via the mucociliary elevator, to the pharyngeal cavity and are swallowed. Small intestinal parasitism is characterized by larvae residing within superficial mucosa (Web Fig. 7-22). Epithelial destruction by the parasites may result in villous atrophy and crypt hyperplasia. The nonspecific clinical signs include diarrhea, hypoproteinemia, weight loss, and dehydration. Rhabditiform dermatitis may also occur.

Trichostrongylosis

Trichostrongyles are small nematodes that parasitize the small intestine of ruminants. Mild climates promote clinical disease. These parasites have a direct life cycle. Third-stage larvae are rendered infective in the acid environment of the abomasum. The larvae burrow in between crypt enterocytes, but do not generally penetrate the basement membrane. Paradoxically, crypt hyperplasia is followed by villous atrophy. As with most other parasitisms, crowding, poor sanitation, and inadequate nutrition potentiate disease. Protein leakage into the intestinal lumen together with absorptive enterocyte loss leads to diarrhea, cachexia, and its metabolic consequences, which can be severe and widespread through many organ systems.

Cyathostomiasis

In ponies and horses under 5 years of age in temperate climates, sudden emergence of massive numbers of fourth- and fifth-stage cyathostome larvae from the cecum and colon results in necroulcerative hemorrhagic typhlocolitis. Ova are generally not detected in feces but larvae are often visible.

Nematodirosis

Nematodirus nematodes are parasites of the cranial small intestine of ruminants. The life cycle is direct. Unlike the case with other strongyles, Nematodirus larvae within ova are resistant to cold temperatures. In fact, the ova must overwinter to be infective. This is evolutionally interesting because it allows for a new crop of susceptible hosts, particularly lambs and calves each year. Fourth- and fifth-stage larvae reside in deeper layers of the mucosa than do the trichostrongyles. Villous atrophy of the cranial small intestine is the predominant histologic lesion. *Nematodirus* spp. do not generally cause disease except in association with other parasites. Signs include green diarrhea, weight loss, and hypoproteinemia secondary to weight loss and inappetence.

Cooperiosis

A small intestinal parasite of ruminants, *Cooperia* nematodes—unlike other trichostrongyles—do not burrow into the intestine. Rather, they reside between villi, causing pressure necrosis. Their life cycle and clinical signs are similar to that of the other strongyles already described.

Oesophagostomum

The nodular worms of ruminants *(Oesophagostomum columbianum, Oesophagostomum radiatum)* and pigs *(Oesophagostomum dentatum)* cause subserosal mineralized nodules that are characteristic of the disease. These nodules generally are of no clinical significance, but they make the intestines unsuitable for use as sausage casings. Occasionally, they are associated with, and can be the cause of, intussusceptions.

Third-stage larvae of *Oesophagostomum columbianum* of sheep are ingested, penetrate deeply into the small intestinal wall, excyst, and molt to fourth-stage larvae, which mature in the colon. They may encyst in the colonic wall and become mineralized subserosal nodules or may mature to adults. Disease is more severe in

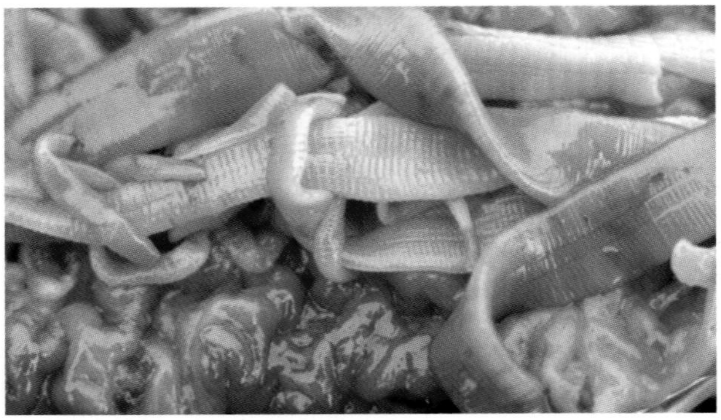

Fig. 7-177 **Cestodiasis, small intestine, fur seal.** Segmented tapeworms are present in this otherwise normal intestine. (Courtesy Dr. H. Gelberg, College of Veterinary Medicine, Oregon State University.)

nutritionally debilitated animals. Most infestations are asymptomatic. *Oesophagostomum radiatum* of cattle may produce inappetence, hypoproteinemia from damaged enterocyte tight junctions, and anemia and hemorrhage from consumptive coagulopathy induced by the parasites. Nodules may also form, as in sheep. Oesophagostomiasis in pigs is usually asymptomatic, although ill thrift and malaise secondary to typhlocolitis may occur.

Pinworms

Oxyuris equi is the most common pinworm of domestic animals. The parasites occupy the lumen of the distal intestine of horses and occasionally cause rectal pruritus by laying their eggs on the perineal region. *Enterobius vermicularis* is the pinworm of primates and great apes. It is not zoonotic and is generally of little clinical consequence.

Cestodes

Tapeworms, although frequently found in the alimentary system, are generally of little clinical significance. They require two and sometimes three hosts, often including arthropods and other invertebrates, to complete their life cycles. Tapeworms attach to the gut wall by means of their anterior scolex, which may have hooks in addition to four suckers (Fig. 7-177). Although they can cause some damage at the site of attachment, generally they compete with the host for nutrients. Lacking an alimentary system, they absorb nutrients through their surface. Tapeworms are flat, segmented, and hermaphroditic, reproducing by addition of segments or proglottids. Examples of tapeworms are *Anoplocephala* spp. in horses, *Moniezia* spp. in ruminants, and *Diphyllobothrium* and *Dipylidium* spp. in dogs and cats. *Mesocestoides* spp. can infect dogs and cats. In some cases, this parasite can perforate through the intestine and proliferate in the peritoneal cavity (Fig. 7-178).

Taenia and *Echinococcus* spp. are the most destructive of the cestodes. Although carnivores are the definitive hosts, the larval forms reside in the viscera and body cavities of the intermediate hosts, usually ruminants, pigs, horses, or rodents (see Fig. 8-54). Humans can also become infected, and sometimes it takes 20 or 30 years for clinical disease to appear. The damage in the intermediate hosts may be quite severe.

Trematodes

Trematodes are uncommon parasites of the alimentary tract. *Nanophyetus salmincola* uses a snail and a fish as intermediate hosts. It carries the rickettsia responsible for salmon poisoning in the Northwestern US. Lesions of the intestine are hemorrhagic enteritis.

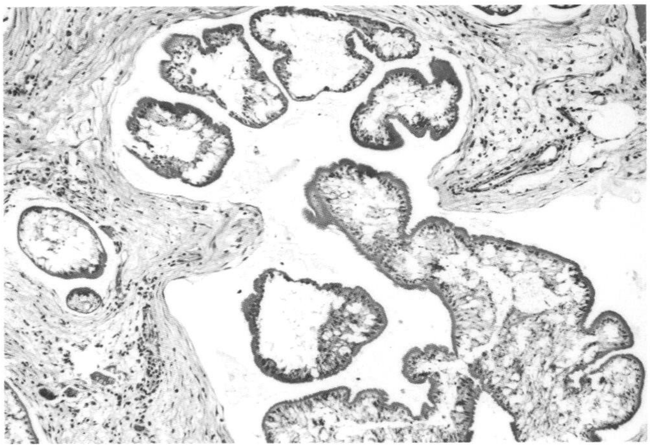

Fig. 7-178 **Mesocestoides infection, peritoneum, dog.** Encysted larval cestodes have elicited a granulomatous inflammatory reaction in the peritoneum of this dog. H&E stain. (Courtesy Dr. C. Löhr, College of Veterinary Medicine, Oregon State University.)

Alaria spp. can attach to the small intestine of dogs and cats, but are generally innocuous. The mesocercariae can cause tissue damage during their migrations through body organs of the host. Paratenic hosts are frogs, snakes, and mice.

Schistosomiasis of ruminants, pigs, horses, and dogs can cause granulomatous intestinal lesions with protein loss secondary to the parasite's presence in mesenteric veins after migration through the liver. Parasites are acquired by direct penetration of the skin by cercariae.

Acanthocephalans

The thorny-headed worm of pigs, *Macracanthorhynchus hirudinaceus,* is a small intestinal parasite with a soil-based arthropod intermediate host such as dung beetles. They are thus more common, as are many other parasites in a variety of mammalian species, in "free range" animals. They are occasionally misidentified as tapeworms, which they superficially resemble. However, they are not truly segmented parasites. They occasionally penetrate the bowel wall at the site of parasite attachment, causing peritonitis.

Prosthenorchis spp. are acanthocephalids of primates. Cockroaches are the intermediate hosts.

Intestinal Neoplasia

Neoplasms of various types occur in the GI system of domestic animals. Those of the oral cavity and stomach have already been discussed. Intestinal neoplasms are diagnosed most frequently in dogs and cats, in large part because of their longer lifespans. Additionally, pets live in close harmony with their human companions, and thus it is possible that some of the same environmental factors that cause human cancer may also cause similar problems in animals.

In dogs, benign neoplasms of the intestinal tract are most commonly adenomas or polyps (see Fig. 6-4), and their malignant counterparts adenocarcinomas. Dogs and cats infrequently develop intestinal mast cell tumors and plasmacytomas. Smooth muscle neoplasms termed leiomyomas and leiomyosarcomas arise from existing intestinal muscular layers. An important caveat in diagnosing these spindle cell tumors is that some of them when examined immunohistochemically are composed of undifferentiated cells with an uncertain histogenesis. These neoplasms have

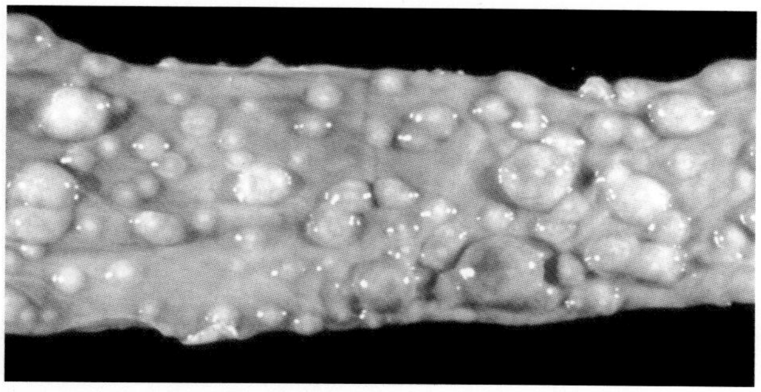

Fig. 7-179 **Lymphoma (lymphosarcoma), colon, cat.**
Numerous submucosal nodules contain neoplastic lymphocytes. Note that the mucosal epithelium is intact (smooth and shiny) and not ulcerated. (Courtesy Dr. H. Gelberg, College of Veterinary Medicine, Oregon State University.)

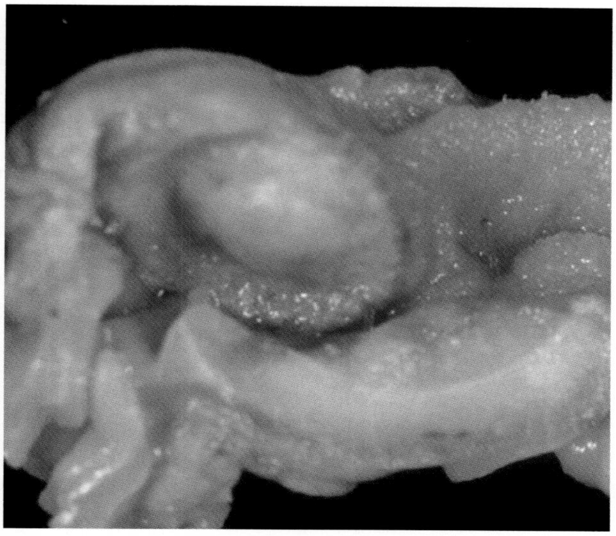

Fig. 7-180 **Mast cell tumor, small intestine, cat.**
The submucosal nodule contains neoplastic mast cells. (Courtesy Dr. H. Gelberg, College of Veterinary Medicine, Oregon State University.)

been reported in dogs, horses, rats and primates. They are termed *GI stromal tumors* (GIST). Supposition exists that these neoplasms arise from the interstitial cells of Cajal which normally become the pacemaker cells of the gut. Most are KIT (CD117) positive (proto-oncogene c-kit).

Lymphoma can be solitary, metastatic, or multicentric. In cats, the most common neoplasms include alimentary lymphoma (Fig. 7-179); mastocytomas (Fig. 7-180), which are associated with ulceration; adenomas; adenocarcinomas; and carcinoids. In canids, 5% to 7% of lymphomas are GI. Those of the GI tract are epitheliotropic and primarily T lymphocyte in origin. In humans, most GI lymphomas are B lymphocyte in origin. In sheep, adenocarcinomas of the intestine are fairly common and are virus-induced. In cows, alimentary lymphoma is most common. Horses rarely have intestinal neoplasms develop.

PERITONEUM, OMENTUM, MESENTERY, AND PERITONEAL CAVITY

Structure and Function

The peritoneum is a membrane composed of a connective tissue stroma and a mesothelial cell component separated by a basement membrane. Mesothelial cells are permeable and function as a dialysis membrane. Their rapid regeneration after injury may be misinterpreted as neoplasia. It is speculated that mesothelial regeneration occurs from stem cells in the subserosal tissues rather than proliferation of adjacent uninjured mesothelial cells. Thus repair of a damaged peritoneum occurs across the whole of the damaged surface rather than from the edges such as occurs on epithelial-lined mucous membranes and skin. The peritoneum lines the abdominal cavity (parietal peritoneum) and reflects around and covers the visceral organs and scrotal cavity (visceral peritoneum). The omentum, mesenteries, and ligaments are doubled sheets of peritoneum that connect the visceral peritoneum to the parietal peritoneum. Nerves and vessels course through these structures into the various visceral structures. The visceral and parietal peritoneum receive afferent innervation from different sources. The visceral innervation is autonomic responding with dull pain sensation to pressure and traction. In contrast, the parietal peritoneum receives afferent nerves from somatic and visceral sources resulting in sharp pain when stimulation occurs. The peritoneal structures are an important site of fat storage and a site of serous atrophy when the animal is in negative energy balance. The kidneys are only covered by peritoneum on one surface and are thus termed *retroperitoneal.* Like other serous surfaces, peritoneal structures are smooth and shiny when not diseased.

Omenta (greater and lesser) connect the stomach to other organs or to the body wall. Ligaments course from the body wall to an organ or from organ to organ. A mesentery in its broad definition runs from the abdominal wall to the intestine or female reproductive system. The peritoneum and its associated structures produce a small amount of fluid, which is useful in lubrication of mesothelial surfaces. This fluid does not contain fibrinogen and therefore does not clot on exposure to air, except in swine.

The omenta are capable of localizing infection and serve as an important source of revascularization of surgically altered tissues. Unfortunately, it also serves as a blood supply to metastatic tumors (i.e., carcinomatosis). Horses in general have a small omentum and thus are less able to wall off peritoneal infections than are ruminants. Omentectomy does not appear to have an adverse effect on general health.

Portals of Entry

Most infections of the peritoneal cavity are traumatic in origin from a rupture in the alimentary, urinary, or reproductive systems. Extension from organ infection or neoplasia is another common source of introduction of foreign agents into the peritoneum. Traumatic injury to a body wall, such as by a projectile, can introduce foreign material or air (pneumoperitoneum). Traumatic injury to a vessel or to an organ or rupture from a tumor or ingestion or administration of anticoagulants may cause hemoperitoneum. The liver is particularly prone to rupture when infiltrated by fat or amyloid.

Responses to Injury

Ascites

Ascites or hydroperitoneum is defined as excess fluid in the peritoneal cavity. The quality of the fluid varies by cause from thick and syrupy in FIP to thin and watery in cases of hypoproteinemia (see Fig. 3-3). Ascites is nonspecific and can result from any cause of hypoproteinemia such as heart (see Fig. 10-7 and Web Fig. 10-11), liver or kidney failure, protein-losing enteropathies such as Johne's disease, lymphangiectasia (see Figs. 7-120 and 7-121), lymphatic blockage, ruptured lymph ducts, bladder rupture (uroperitoneum), and hypertension. Evaluation of fluid obtained by abdominocentesis is very helpful in the live animal in sorting out the various etiologies.

Fat Necrosis

There are four main categories of fat necrosis. They are nutritional, pancreatic, traumatic and idiopathic, as follows:

- Nutritional fat necrosis, also called *steatitis* or *yellow fat disease,* results in peroxidation of lipids, including those in cell membranes. It is most common in felids but occurs in a variety of species. The free radicals produced evoke an inflammatory response. The inciting cause is generally a diet very high in lipids and low in vitamin E or other tocopherols. Although steatitis of felids has historically been a sequela of fish-based diets, anecdotal evidence suggests that it may also be caused by some unconventional diets being used today.
- Pancreatic or enzymatic fat necrosis is initiated by pancreatic enzyme release (lipase) associated with pancreatic necrosis (pancreatitis). Lipase converts triglycerides into fatty acids and glycerol. The fatty acids combine with calcium, magnesium and sodium ions forming soaps resulting in chalky white deposits (see Figs. 1-22 and 8-83). This is a painful condition, and free lipid droplets are sometimes seen in fluids recovered from abdominocentesis.
- Traumatic fat necrosis results from direct, usually blunt, trauma to adipose tissue and is a relatively uncommon occurrence. Rupture of adipocytes releases triglycerides which are hydrolyzed by tissue and/or serum lipases.
- Idiopathic fat necrosis can be focal or massive and occurs in all species of mammal but is seen primarily in large animal species, especially in sheep, horses (Fig. 7-181), and obese dairy cattle. With massive necrosis in cattle, the hard lumps of dense necrotic fat can envelop intestinal loops resulting in stricture and functional blockage of ingesta. The etiology of this condition is unknown but may relate in some way to nutritional imbalances.

Damaged and necrotic adipose tissue frequently has a white, chalky or gritty appearance and texture caused by saponification and mineralization. Inflammatory cell presence and density vary based on the various causes of tissue damage and the area of fat sampled.

Inflammation: Peritonitis

Inflammation of the peritoneum or peritonitis is caused by a variety of agents varying from viral (FIP) (see Fig. 7-161), to bacterial (see Fig. 7-157) to parasitic (ascarid migrations) (see Fig. 7-174) to mechanical (hardware disease) to sterile (bile peritonitis) to organ rupture (see Fig. 7-110). Peritonitis has also been called *serositis,* and when multiple serous membranes like those of the meninges, pleura, pericardium, peritoneum, and scrotum are affected, it is called a *polyserositis.* Glasser's disease of pigs is an example of a polyserositis (see Fig. 7-157). Different species vary in their stoicism and survival in the face of peritonitis, with equids showing the most pain and intolerance while cattle and cats may live a long time with severe disease. The nature of the exudate includes those covered in Chapter 2 that result in suppurative peritonitis (Fig. 7-182) or fibrinous peritonitis (Fig. 7-183) as examples. Cytologic examination and bacterial culture are instrumental in determining an etiology in the live animal. As in other diseases, the peritoneum responds to injury via acute inflammation (Fig. 7-184) and if needed, chronic inflammation (Fig. 7-185) and/or granulomatous inflammation (Fig. 7-186), if the source of the injury remains unresolved.

Pneumoperitoneum

Spontaneous pneumoperitoneum is secondary to perforation of the GI or reproductive tracts. Causes include neoplasia, NSAIDs, and steroids. Traumatic pneumoperitoneum is caused by penetrating projectiles (e.g., bullets, knives, arrows), vehicular trauma, penetrating bite wounds, iatrogenic (surgery, peritoneal dialysis, positive pressure ventilation, urinary catheterization with penetration, penetrating gastrotomy, or PEG tubes), and idiopathic causes. Unless removed mechanically, it takes approximately 30 days for the air to be absorbed.

Parasitic Diseases

Aberrant migration of nematodes and trematodes in most species of mammals can cause focal fibrosis when they travel through the abdominal cavity (see Fig. 8-26). Setaria are nematodes that are sometimes found in the peritoneal cavity of ungulates and rarely cause significant damage in this location. Mild focal peritonitis is

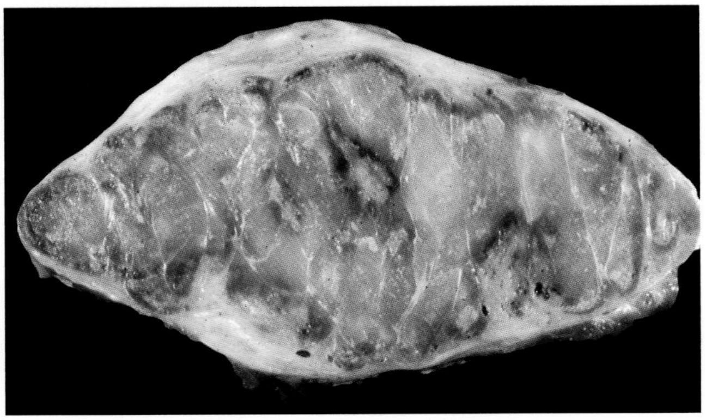

Fig. 7-181 Idiopathic fat necrosis, ventral parietal peritoneum, horse. This cross-section of necrotic fat is mottled by a mixture of areas of saponification and normal adipocytes. The cause of this sporadic condition is unknown. (Courtesy College of Veterinary Medicine, Cornell University.)

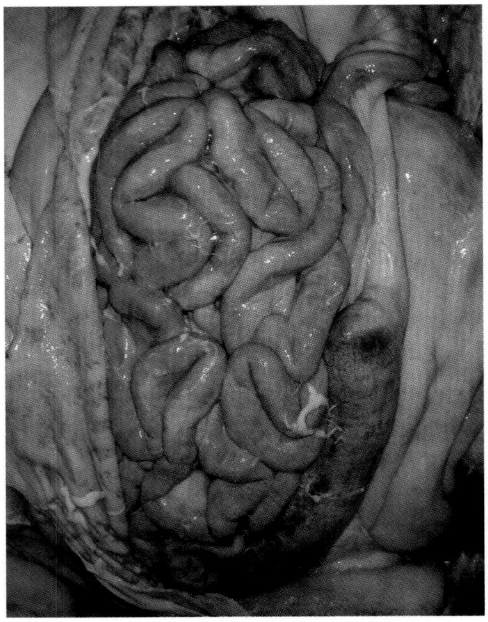

Fig. 7-182 Acute suppurative peritonitis, bacterial infection, pig. The surface of the peritoneum is rough and granular and covered with gray/white-yellow flecks of pus and fibrin. Red areas are indicative of active hyperemia and hemorrhage. (Courtesy College of Veterinary Medicine, University of Illinois.)

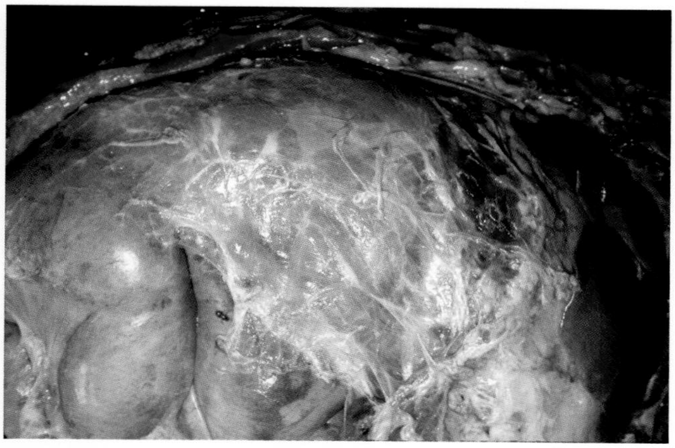

Fig. 7-183 Fibrinous peritonitis, acute inflammation, bacterial infection, cow.
This lesion was the result of extensive damage to capillaries in the peritoneum leading to leakage of fibrinogen and polymerization to fibrin on peritoneal surfaces. (Courtesy Dr. M.D. McGavin, College of Veterinary Medicine, University of Tennessee.)

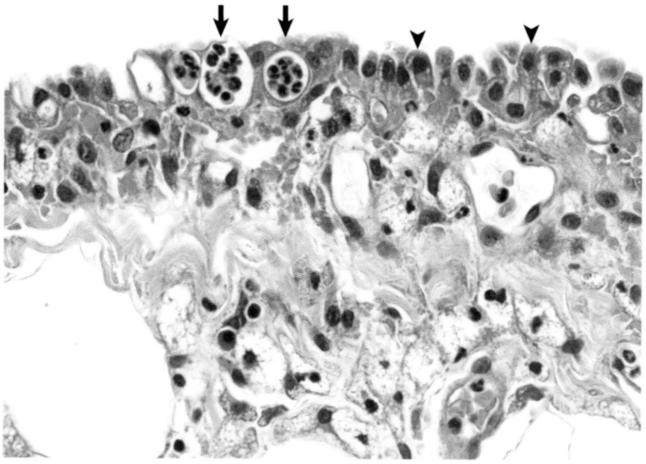

Fig. 7-184 Acute peritonitis, peritoneum, dog.
The mesothelial cells are swollen, vacuolated, and misshapen *(arrowheads)*, indicating their response to injury. Capillaries under the mesothelial cells are dilated (active hyperemia and leukocyte adhesion cascade). Neutrophils are migrating through endothelial cell junctions and in the interstitium to reach the inflammatory stimulus in the abdominal cavity. Note the microabscesses in junctional spaces *(arrows)*. H&E stain. (Courtesy Dr. J.F. Zachary, College of Veterinary Medicine, University of Illinois.)

sometimes the result of their travels. A variety of cestodes may be found in the abdominal cavity of many species of mammal. Some, such as *Echinococcus granulosus* (hydatid cysts) are zoonotic and may take 20 to 30 years to cause clinical signs in persons. *Mesocestoides* and *Porocephalus* (pentastomiasis) are found in carnivores in which their presence may induce a pyogranulomatous reaction (see Fig. 7-178).

Neoplasia

Primary neoplasms of the peritoneum are uncommon with the exception of lipomas, which may become pedunculated and result in intestinal strangulation (see Fig. 7-109). Mesotheliomas occur sporadically in animals and more commonly in humans (Fig. 7-187). In humans, mesotheliomas are associated with asbestosis

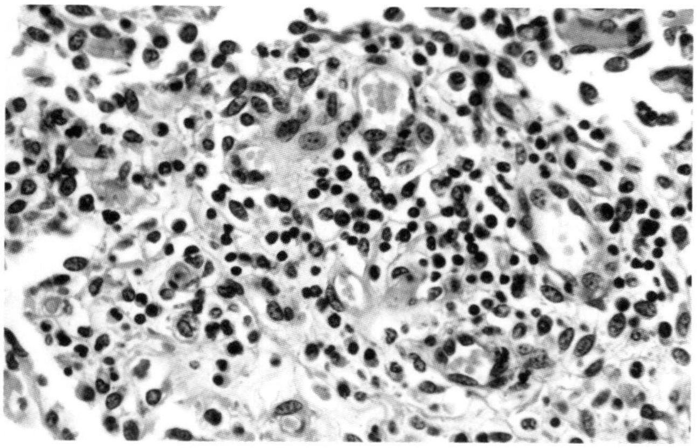

Fig. 7-185 Chronic peritonitis, peritoneum, cow.
Because the inflammatory stimulus in the abdominal cavity has persisted, the inflammatory response has shifted to a chronic exudate in an attempt to resolve the damage. Note the abundance of immature collagen fibers in the areolar tissue of the peritoneum. H&E stain. (Courtesy Dr. M.D. McGavin, College of Veterinary Medicine, University of Tennessee.)

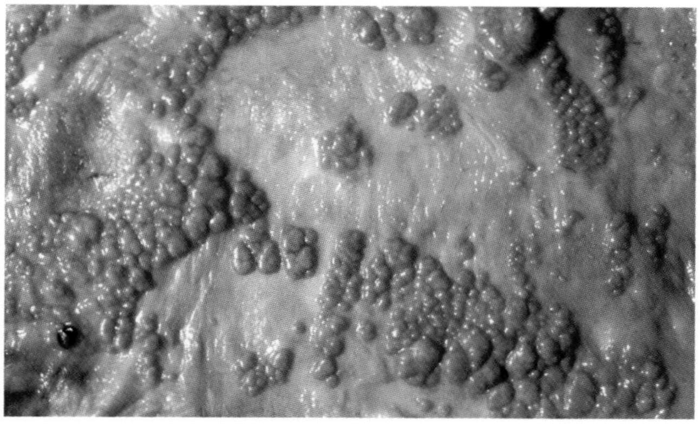

Fig. 7-186 Granulomatous peritonitis, peritoneum, tuberculosis, cow.
In long-standing cases of tuberculosis, granulomas can form on the peritoneum. (Courtesy Dr. M.D. McGavin, College of Veterinary Medicine, University of Tennessee.)

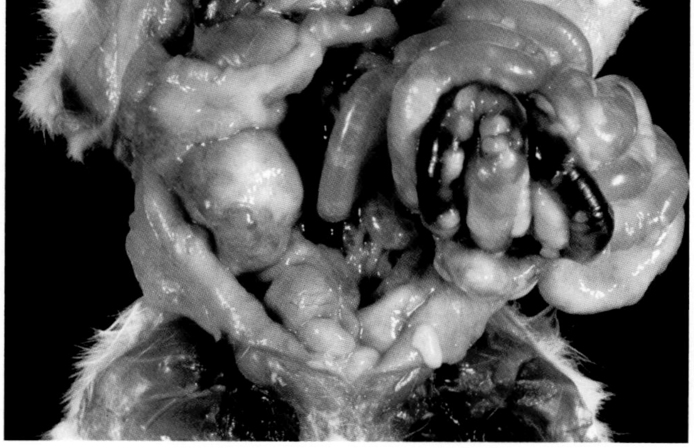

Fig. 7-187 Mesothelioma, abdominal cavity, rat.
Raised nodules of neoplastic mesothelial cells are present on serosal surfaces of the abdominal organs. (Courtesy College of Veterinary Medicine, University of Illinois.)

and other fibers with similar physicochemical properties and are considered an occupational hazard for some industries. Great efforts have been made to reduce occupational exposure to asbestos. Mesotheliomas have been reported in calves as a congenital disease. Tumors of mesothelial origin are all considered malignant because they may spread transcoelomically. They seldom metastasize to draining lymph nodes or distal sites. They are quite pleomorphic and vary from papillary and adenocarcinoma-appearing to spindloid and fibrosarcoma-like. It is extremely difficult to distinguish neoplastic mesothelium from hyperplastic, reactive mesothelium (see Fig. 6-21).

Pacinian Corpuscles

Pacinian corpuscles are baroreceptors that are commonly present in the pancreatic interstitium (see Fig. 8-82) and in the mesentery of felids. They are often visible macroscopically and may whorl in a fingerprint pattern (Web Fig. 7-23), or appear as solid masses resembling parasites (see Fig. 8-82).

SUGGESTED READINGS

Suggested Readings are available at evolve.elsevier.com/Zachary/McGavin/.

CHAPTER 8

Hepatobiliary System and Exocrine Pancreas

John M. Cullen and Danielle L. Brown

LIVER AND INTRAHEPATIC BILIARY SYSTEM

STRUCTURE AND FUNCTION

Development

Early in embryogenesis, the origins of the liver are evident. The hepatic diverticulum, also termed the *liver bud,* arises from embryonic endoderm as a hollow out-pouching of the primitive duodenum. Primitive hepatic epithelial cells of the hepatic diverticulum extend into the adjacent mesenchymal stroma and surround the vessels that form the vitelline venous plexus, a complex of vessels that drain the yolk sac. This relationship between the epithelial cells of the liver and the small-caliber vitelline vessels is the earliest developmental form of the hepatic sinusoids. The caudal part of the hepatic diverticulum develops into the gallbladder and the cystic duct. Hepatic connective tissue is derived from the septum transversum, a sheet of cells that incompletely separates the pericardial and peritoneal cavity, and an ingrowth of mesenchymal cells from the coelomic cavity.

The biliary epithelium also arises from the hepatic diverticulum. Intrahepatic ducts develop from a structure, termed the *ductal plate,* which is composed initially of a single row of hepatoblasts that surround the portal vein branches and ensheathe the mesenchyme of the primitive portal tract. A second discontinuous outer layer of primitive hepatoblasts forms subsequently, and the two-cell-thick regions remodel into tubules and become the intrahepatic biliary ductular system. Development of the ducts begins at the porta hepatis and extends to the margins of the liver until the later stages of gestation. The residual portion of the hollow outpouching of the hepatic diverticulum persists to become the extrahepatic bile ducts.

It is known that the hepatocytes and the biliary epithelial cells share a common embryonic origin, but the factors that lead to the final characteristic morphology of the primitive hepatoblasts are not well understood. Epithelial-mesenchymal interactions are believed to play a role. Primitive hepatic epithelial cells in contact with vascular endothelium are destined to become hepatocytes, and those in contact with the developing mesenchyme of the portal tracts develop into bile ducts.

Macroscopic and Microscopic Structure

The liver is the largest internal organ in the body. In adult carnivores, the liver constitutes 3% to 4% of the body weight. In adult omnivores, it is about 2% of body weight and about 1% of the body weight in herbivores. In the neonate of all species, the liver is a larger percentage of body weight than in the adult. In monogastric animals, the liver abuts the diaphragm and occupies the central area of the cranial abdomen. In ruminants the liver is displaced to the right side of the cranial abdominal cavity. A series of ligaments maintains the liver in its position. The coronary ligament attaches the liver to the diaphragm near the esophagus. The falciform ligament attaches the midline of the liver to the ventral midline of the abdomen. The round ligament, a remnant of the umbilical vein, is embedded within the falciform ligament. The liver is supplied with blood from two sources. The portal vein drains the digestive tract and provides 60% to 70% of the total afferent hepatic blood flow. The hepatic artery provides the remainder of hepatic blood flow. Blood leaves the liver via the hepatic vein, which is very short, and enters the caudal vena cava. The liver has a smooth capsular surface, and the parenchyma consists of friable red-brown tissue that is divided into lobes. Gross subdivision of the liver into lobes differs among the domestic species. At the periphery, the lobes taper to a sharp edge.

The classic functional subunit of the liver is the hepatic lobule, a hexagonal structure, 1 to 2 mm wide. At the center, the lobule has a central vein (also termed the terminal hepatic venule), which is a tributary of the hepatic vein, and at the angles of the hexagon, it has portal tracts (Fig. 8-1). The portal tracts contain bile ducts, branches of the portal vein, the hepatic artery, nerves, and lymph vessels, all supported by a collagenous stroma (Fig. 8-2). The limiting plate, a discontinuous border of hepatocytes, forms the outer boundary of the portal tract. Blood flows into the sinusoids from the terminal distributing branches of the hepatic artery and portal veins that leave the portal tracts and form an outer perimeter of the lobule (see Figs. 8-1 and 8-2). Portal blood and hepatic arterial

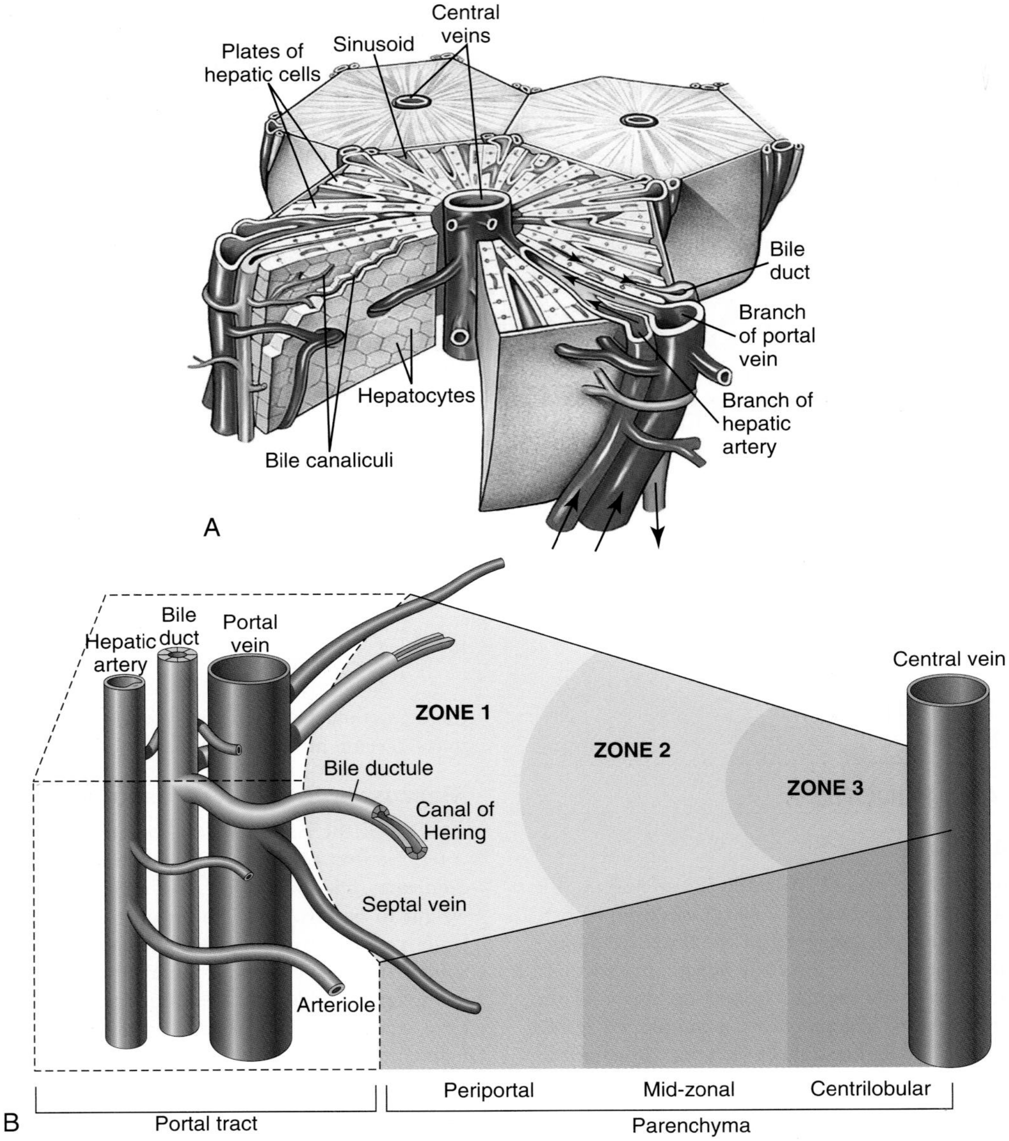

Fig. 8-1 Schematic views of the microscopic and functional organization of the liver.
A, Microscopic organization of the liver. A central vein is located in the center of the lobule with plates of hepatocytes arranged radially. Branches of the portal vein and hepatic artery are located on the periphery of the lobule, and blood from both perfuses the sinusoids. Peripherally located bile ducts drain the bile canaliculi that run between hepatocytes. **B,** Functional organization of the liver. Both the lobule and the acinus are represented. The lobule is a hexagonal unit with portal areas at the margin and a terminal hepatic vein (central vein) at the center. The lobule is divided into the periportal, midzonal, and centrilobular areas. The acinus is a diamond-shaped structure with the distributing branches of the vessels from the portal areas as the center of the structure. Zone 1 of the acinus is closest to the afferent blood supply, and zone 3 is at the tip of the diamond-shaped structure, close to the terminal hepatic vein. Zone 2 is between Zones 1 and 3. (**A** from McCance KL, Huether SE: *Pathophysiology: the biologic basis for diseases in adults and children,* ed 6, St Louis, 2010, Mosby. **B** from Kumar V, Abbas AK, Fausto N: *Robbins & Cotran pathologic basis of disease,* ed 7, Philadelphia, 2005, Saunders.)

blood mix in the sinusoids. Blood drains from the sinusoids into the central veins and to progressively larger sublobular veins and then into the hepatic veins.

Alternatively, when the liver is viewed as a bile-secreting gland, the acinus is the anatomic subunit of the hepatic parenchyma. Terminal afferent branches (penetrating vessels) of the portal vein and hepatic artery project into the parenchyma, like branches from the trunk of a tree, forming the long axis of the diamond-shaped acinus. Thus terminal afferent branches of the portal vein and hepatic artery are at the center of the acinus and the terminal hepatic venule is located at the periphery. Each terminal hepatic venule (central vein) receives blood from several acini. There are three zones within the acinus. Zone 1 is closest to the afferent blood coming from the hepatic artery and the portal vein. Zone 2 is peripheral to zone 1, and zone 3 borders the terminal hepatic venule (see Fig. 8-1). In this anatomic unit, bile flow begins in the canaliculi of the hepatocytes in zone 3 and flows through zones 2 and 1 then into the interlobular bile ducts in the portal areas.

The ultrastructural appearance of hepatocytes reflects the cell's active metabolism, bile secretion, and close contact with the plasma (Web Fig. 8-1). The surface of the hepatocyte that faces the lumen of the sinusoids contains an abundance of microvilli, which increase the hepatocytic surface area and facilitate uptake of plasma-borne substances, such as bilirubin and amino acids, and the secretion of

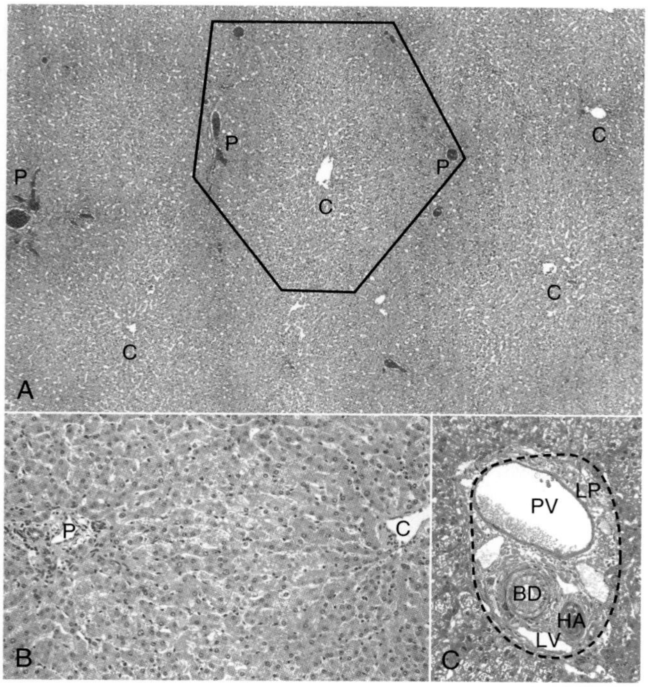

Fig. 8-2 Liver, hepatic lobules, normal dog.
A, Low magnification. A central vein *(C)* is located in the center of the lobule. Branches of the portal vein, hepatic artery, bile duct, and lymphatic vessels are located on the periphery of the lobule in portal tracts *(P)* (also Fig. 8-2, *C*). H&E stain. **B,** Higher magnification. Plates of hepatocytes arranged radially between portal tracts *(P)* to a central vein *(C)*. H&E stain. **C,** Higher magnification, portal tract. The normal portal tract contains the hepatic artery *(HA),* bile duct *(BD),* portal vein *(PV),* and several lymphatic vessels *(LV).* These structures are surrounded by a collagenous extracellular matrix that forms an abrupt border with a circumferential row of hepatocytes, termed the *limiting plate* (LP—*dotted line*). Note that the profile of the portal vein is typically larger than those of the hepatic artery and bile duct. H&E stain. (**A** and **C** courtesy Dr. J.M. Cullen, College of Veterinary Medicine, North Carolina State University. **B** courtesy Dr. J.F. Zachary, College of Veterinary Medicine, University of Illinois.)

products of hepatic metabolism, such as lipoproteins and clotting factors. Basolateral aspects of hepatocytes are characterized by the presence of canaliculi, modified portions of the cell membrane in two adjacent hepatocytes, which form a lumen for bile secretion. The cytoplasm contains glycogen and a variety of organelles, including numerous mitochondria, lysosomes, and abundant smooth and rough endoplasmic reticulum.

Within the liver, hepatocytes are arranged in one-cell-thick branching plates, which extend radially from the terminal hepatic venule. Hepatic plates are separated by vascular sinusoids. Blood from the terminal afferent branches of the hepatic artery and portal vein mixes in the hepatic sinusoids and flows to the terminal hepatic venule. Hepatic sinusoids differ from capillaries in that they are lined by discontinuous endothelial cells that lack a typical basement membrane (Fig. 8-3), whereas capillaries have a continuous endothelial lining and are ensheathed in the basement membrane. The sinusoids are critical for appropriate hepatic function. The architecture of the sinusoids enables efficient uptake of plasma constituents by hepatocytes and facilitates hepatocellular secretion. A fine scaffold of electron lucent basement membrane that contains collagen types III, IV, and XVIII, and other extracellular matrix (ECM) components supports the sinusoidal endothelial cells (Web

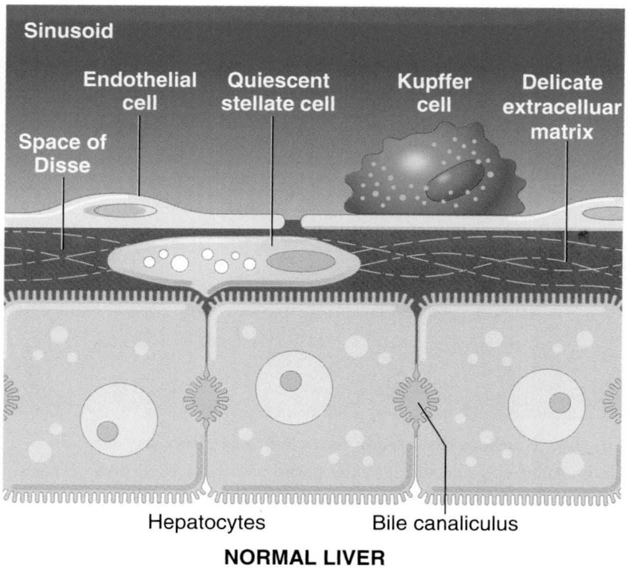

Fig. 8-3 Schematic diagram of the hepatic sinusoid.
The vascular lumen is lined by discontinuous capillaries. Kupffer cells rest on the endothelial cells and project into the sinusoid. Between the endothelial cells and the hepatocytes is a gap called the space of Disse. Microvilli extending from the luminal aspect of the hepatocytes are found in this space. Hepatic stellate cells are situated within the space of Disse and extend between hepatocytes. (Schematic based on concepts in Friedman SL: *J Biol Chem* 275:2247-2250, 2000; and Crawford JM: *Curr Op Gastroenterol* 13:175-185, 1997.)

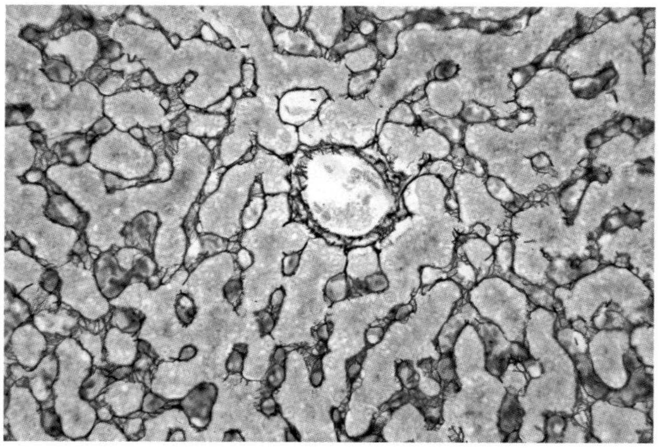

Fig. 8-4 Reticulin fibers (reticulin stain), hepatic extracellular matrix, liver, normal dog.
This stain reveals "reticulin" *(black),* composed of extracellular matrix found within the space of Disse that forms the scaffolding of the hepatic parenchyma. Note the radial arrangements of the hepatic plates and the single hepatocyte thickness of the plates. A central vein is evident in the center of the image. Gordon and Sweet's reticulin stain with a nuclear fast red counterstain. (Courtesy Dr. M.D. McGavin, College of Veterinary Medicine, University of Tennessee.)

Fig. 8-2; see Fig. 8-3). These elements collectively make up the "reticulin" of the liver (Fig. 8-4).

Although blood cells are normally excluded from the space of Disse because they are too large to pass through endothelial gaps, the modified endothelial cells and basement membrane permit plasma to pass freely into a gap between the endothelial cells and the hepatocytes (see Fig. 8-3). This critical anatomic feature of the liver is termed the space of Disse. Within this space, plasma

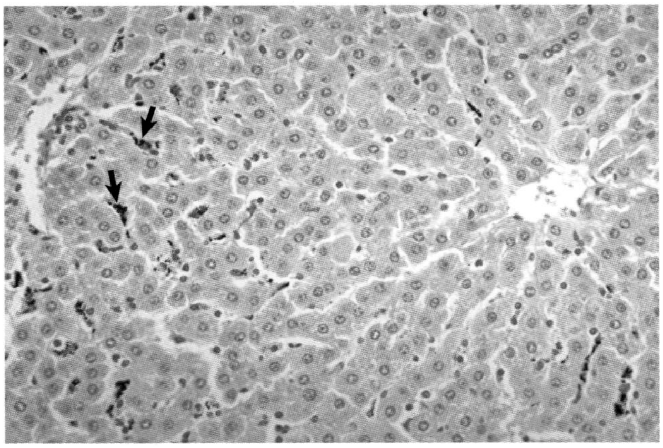

Fig. 8-5 Kupffer cells, carbon particle uptake, liver, normal calf. Carbon particles injected into the portal vein have been phagocytosed by Kupffer cells *(arrows),* making them more easily detectable along the sinusoids of the liver. Nuclear fast red stain. (Courtesy Dr. M.D. McGavin, College of Veterinary Medicine, University of Tennessee.)

constituents come into contact with the luminal surface of the hepatocytes. This surface of the hepatocytes is characterized by the presence of numerous microvilli, which increase the surface area of the hepatocytes and facilitate uptake of a variety of plasma-borne substances, as well secretion of synthesized products. Any damage to this area has significant impact on hepatic function.

The lumen of the sinusoids contains hepatic macrophages, termed *Kupffer cells* (Fig. 8-5). These cells are members of the monocyte-macrophage system, and they clear infectious agents and senescent cells, such as erythrocytes, particulate material, endotoxin, and other substances, from the sinusoidal blood. They are mobile and able to migrate along the sinusoids and into areas of tissue injury and regional lymph nodes. Kupffer cells are involved in cytokine-driven interactions with hepatocytes, endothelial cells, and the stellate cells discussed later. They can express class II histocompatibility antigens and function as antigen-presenting cells, although they are not as efficient as the macrophages in other tissue. Phagocytosis and clearance of immune complexes are the primary roles of Kupffer cells. Kupffer cells are derived from in situ replication and recruitment of blood-borne monocytes.

Hepatic stellate cells (also termed *lipocytes* or *Ito cells*) are found within the space of Disse and between hepatocytes at the edge of the space of Disse (Web Fig. 8-3). Normally, hepatic stellate cells are primarily responsible for storing vitamin A in their characteristic cytoplasmic vacuoles. During hepatic injury, hepatic stellate cells alter their morphology and their function. These activated hepatic stellate cells lose their vitamin A content and synthesize collagen and other ECM components that lead to hepatic fibrosis.

Bile flows within the lobule in the opposite direction to blood flow, which facilitates the concentration of bile. The biliary system commences as canaliculi within the centrilobular (periacinar) areas of the hepatic lobule. The walls of canaliculi are formed entirely by the cell membranes of adjacent hepatocytes. Just outside the limiting plate, canaliculi drain into the canals of Hering that are lined partially by hepatocytes and partially by biliary epithelium. These drain into cholangioles with low cuboidal biliary epithelium. The cholangioles converge into interlobular bile ducts that are lined with cuboidal epithelium and located in the portal areas. Bile then flows into the right and left hepatic ducts that unite to form the hepatic duct. The confluence of the common hepatic duct and the cystic duct from the gallbladder form the common bile duct by which bile is carried to the duodenum. The gallbladder is responsible for storage and concentration of bile in most species. It is absent in the horse, elephant, and rat.

Bipotential progenitor cells that have the ability to differentiate into hepatocytes or biliary epithelium are believed to reside in the area of the cholangiole, although their precise location and nature is not resolved. These cells may proliferate in circumstances in which mature hepatocytes or bile duct epithelium cannot replicate such as severe injury or nutritional deficits. When these cells proliferate, they form islands or crude tubules of small basophilic cells found initially at the margin of the limiting plate. This proliferation is termed the *ductular reaction* and is a hallmark of severe injury.

Both sympathetic and parasympathetic nerves running along the portal vein and the hepatic artery innervate the liver. The nerve fibers enter the liver at the hilus and ramify to the level of the portal tracts and then extend along the sinusoids. Nerve supply is believed to affect sinusoidal blood flow, the balance of hepatic blood flow from the portal vein and the hepatic artery, and metabolic functions of the liver.

Normal Function

The liver performs many critical functions, including the following:

- Bilirubin metabolism
- Bile acid metabolism
- Carbohydrate metabolism
- Lipid metabolism
- Xenobiotic metabolism
- Protein synthesis
- Immune function

Bilirubin Metabolism

Excretion of bile is the main exocrine function of the liver. Bile is composed of water, cholesterol, bile acids, bilirubin, inorganic ions, and other constituents. Bile formation is continuous, but the rate of secretion can vary significantly. There are three major purposes for bile synthesis. The first purpose is excretory; many of the body's waste products, such as surplus cholesterol, bilirubin, and metabolized xenobiotics, are eliminated in bile. The second purpose is the facilitation of digestion; bile acids secreted into the intestine aid in the digestion of lipids within the intestine. The third is to provide buffers to neutralize the acid pH of the ingesta.

Bilirubin, a major component of bile, is produced from the metabolic degradation of hemoglobin, and to a lesser extent, other heme proteins including myoglobin and the hepatic hemoproteins, such as cytochromes (Fig. 8-6). The majority of bilirubin is derived from normal extrahepatic breakdown of senescent erythrocytes in cells of the monocyte-macrophage phagocytic cell series. Senescent erythrocytes normally are phagocytosed by macrophages of the spleen, bone marrow, and liver. Within the phagocyte, the globin portion is degraded and the constituents are returned to the amino acid pool. The heme iron is transferred to iron-binding proteins, such as transferrin, for recycling. The remaining portion of heme is first oxidized by heme oxygenase to biliverdin. In the next metabolic step, biliverdin reductase converts biliverdin to bilirubin. Subsequently, the bilirubin, which is poorly soluble in an aqueous medium, is then released into the blood in its unconjugated form and bound to albumin to increase its solubility in plasma.

The process of bilirubin elimination can be divided into three phases: uptake, conjugation, and secretion. Uptake refers to the process by which hepatocytes remove the bilirubin bound to albumin from the circulation. Unconjugated bilirubin is separated

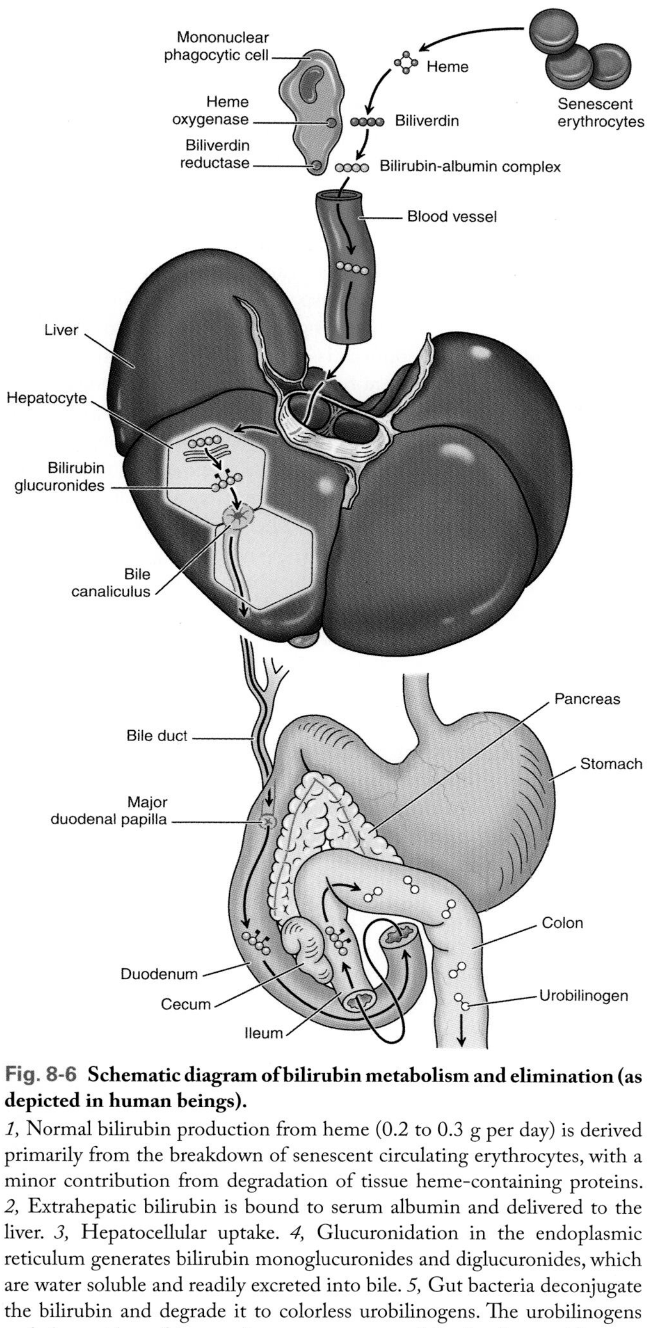

Fig. 8-6 Schematic diagram of bilirubin metabolism and elimination (as depicted in human beings).
1, Normal bilirubin production from heme (0.2 to 0.3 g per day) is derived primarily from the breakdown of senescent circulating erythrocytes, with a minor contribution from degradation of tissue heme-containing proteins. *2,* Extrahepatic bilirubin is bound to serum albumin and delivered to the liver. *3,* Hepatocellular uptake. *4,* Glucuronidation in the endoplasmic reticulum generates bilirubin monoglucuronides and diglucuronides, which are water soluble and readily excreted into bile. *5,* Gut bacteria deconjugate the bilirubin and degrade it to colorless urobilinogens. The urobilinogens and the residue of intact pigments are excreted in the feces, with some reabsorption and excretion into urine. Residual urobilinogen is metabolized by bacteria into the brown pigment stercobilin, imparting the typical color to feces.

from albumin at the sinusoidal surface and bilirubin is taken up by hepatocytes by a carrier-mediated process. In the second phase of bilirubin metabolism, bilirubin is conjugated, principally with glucuronic acid, by bilirubin UDP-glucuronyltransferase in the endoplasmic reticulum. After conjugation, bilirubin becomes water soluble and less toxic. It is then excreted, in the third phase of bilirubin metabolism, into the bile by active transport through specialized portions of hepatocyte membranes that form the margins of the bile canaliculi. The excretion phase is the rate-limiting step in most species.

Within the gastrointestinal tract, conjugated bilirubin is converted to urobilinogen by bacteria and a fraction of this is reabsorbed into the portal blood, a process called *enterohepatic circulation,* and returned to the liver. The majority of urobilinogen that is absorbed from the gastrointestinal tract is resecreted into bile. Urobilinogen has a small molecular weight and is freely filtered through the glomerulus, and small amounts are normally found in the urine. Urobilinogen that is not absorbed from the intestine becomes oxidized to stercobilin, which is responsible for the color of the feces.

Bile Acid Metabolism

The three principal functions of bile acids, important constituents of bile, are maintenance of cholesterol homeostasis, stimulation of bile flow and digestion, and absorption of fats and fat-soluble vitamins. Bile acids are synthesized in the liver from cholesterol and are conjugated to glycine or taurine to facilitate their interaction with other components of bile and to prevent precipitation into calculi when they are secreted into the bile. The major bile acids are cholic acid and chenodeoxycholic acid, but there are various types and proportions of bile acids found in different species. Bile acids are actively secreted into the bile canaliculi from the hepatocyte cytoplasm by specific intramembranous molecular pumps against a concentration gradient, which creates an osmotic gradient, stimulating the inflow of water and solutes into the bile canaliculi. Conjugated bile acids are therefore the principal physiologic stimulus for bile production through a process termed *bile acid–dependent flow.* Bile acids are effective detergents that assist in the digestion of lipids within the intestine and increasing the solubility of lipids secreted into the bile. The quantities of bile acids required far exceed the liver's capacity to produce them. For this reason, bile acids are avidly reabsorbed from the ileum, extracted from the portal blood, and resecreted into bile via a process known as enterohepatic circulation. This is a very efficient system. As much as 95% of secreted bile acids are recycled, and the proportion of reabsorbed bile acids in the liver greatly exceeds that of recently synthesized bile acids; bile acids may be recycled 15 times a day. Interruption of this process results in fat malabsorption and a deficiency of fat-soluble vitamins.

Carbohydrate Metabolism

The liver has an important role in the regulation of plasma glucose concentrations. After eating, the liver removes carbohydrates (i.e., glucose, fructose) from the plasma and stores them as glycogen or fatty acids. In periods of need, energy balance is maintained by glycolysis of stored glycogen or by gluconeogenesis. Production of energy by oxidative phosphorylation and β-oxidation of fatty acids in hepatic mitochondria is used to sustain the activities of the hepatocyte.

Lipid Metabolism

The liver plays a central role in lipid metabolism. It is involved in the production and degradation of plasma lipids such as cholesterol, triglycerides, phospholipids, and lipoproteins. Cholesterol is synthesized, secreted, and degraded by hepatocytes. Hepatocytes can synthesize fatty acids when energy levels are high, and they can oxidize fatty acids as an energy source when necessary.

Xenobiotic Metabolism

Foreign substances (xenobiotics), such as many therapeutic drugs, insecticides, and endogenous substances—such as steroids that are lipophilic—require conversion to water-soluble forms for elimination from the body. The cytochrome p450 enzymes of the smooth endoplasmic reticulum of the hepatocytes serve as the major site of metabolism of these substances in preparation for excretion in bile or urine. This process is discussed in detail in the section on toxic liver injury.

Protein Synthesis

Synthesis of the majority of plasma proteins, mainly within the rough endoplasmic reticulum, is a principal function of the liver. Proteins produced in the liver include plasma proteins, such as albumin; a variety of transport proteins; lipoproteins; clotting factors II, V, and VII to XIII; fibrinolysis proteins; some acute phase proteins; and components of the complement system. The liver is responsible for synthesis of approximately 15% of body proteins.

The liver is also the principal site of ammonia metabolism. Highly toxic ammonia is generated through catabolism of amino acids. Metabolic conversion of ammonia into urea, a far less toxic compound, occurs through the urea cycle, which occurs almost exclusively in the liver. Urea then enters the systemic circulation (blood urea nitrogen) and is excreted in the urine.

Immune Function

The liver has a significant immune function. It is involved in systemic, local, and mucosal immunity. Hepatocytes participate in the response to systemic inflammation through the synthesis and release of acute phase proteins. Approximately 10% of the cells in the liver belong to the adaptive immune system (T and B lymphocytes) or the innate immune system (Kupffer cells, natural killer lymphocytes, and natural killer T lymphocytes). Compared with other organs, the liver is particularly enriched with cells of the innate immune system, likely a result of the fact it is the site where foreign antigens from the gastrointestinal tract first encounter the innate immune system defenses. The liver contains the largest pool of mononuclear phagocytes and natural killer cells in the body in most species. The Kupffer cells lining the sinusoids provide the first line of defense against infectious agents, endotoxin, and foreign material absorbed from the intestines before they gain access to the systemic circulation. Most blood-borne foreign material is cleared by Kupffer cells in all domestic species, except members of the Order Artiodactyla (pigs, goats, and cattle), in which this function is performed by intravascular macrophages in the pulmonary alveolar capillaries. The liver is also involved in transport of secretory immunoglobulin A (IgA), the primary immunoglobulin of the mucosal surfaces, from plasma cells and recirculation into the biliary tree and intestine.

RESPONSE OF THE LIVER TO INJURY

Necrosis and Apoptosis

The epithelial cells of the liver, hepatocytes, and biliary epithelium are the principal targets of most liver diseases. Sublethal injury to hepatocytes is characterized by cell swelling (hydropic degeneration), steatosis, or atrophy. Cells that have sustained a sublethal injury often remove damaged organelles by forming autophagosomes. Material that cannot be digested further is retained as lipofuscin, which is why after sublethal injury, this pigment can often be found in affected cells and associated phagocytes.

By convention, cell death has been divided into two distinct processes. These are necrosis, which is characterized by cytoplasmic swelling, destruction of organelles, and disruption of the plasma membrane, and apoptosis, or programmed cell death, which is characterized by one of several active processes involving caspases that lead to cell shrinkage and an intact cell membrane. Necrosis is triggered by lethal injury. Necrotic cells typically exhibit karyorrhexis and fragmentation of the cell body. Coagulative necrosis results from sudden denaturation of hepatocytes and produces swollen hepatocytes with a preserved eosinophilic cytoplasmic outline and karyorrhexis or karyolysis. Lytic necrosis is characterized by a loss of hepatocytes and an influx of erythrocytes into the vacant space or condensation of the reticular connective tissue (collagen and other ECM) scaffolding of the liver that once supported the hepatocytes.

Classic apoptosis is triggered by an interaction between tumor necrosis factor-α (TNF-α) or Fas ligand and specific receptors on the cell membrane leading to caspase activation, although other pathways, including those involving mitochondrial cytochrome-c, have been identified. Apoptosis is recognized by the formation of acidophilic bodies, which are brightly eosinophilic, homogeneous, round structures that can be found between hepatocytes, within the lumen of sinusoids, or within macrophages or hepatocytes. A detailed review of cell death is beyond the scope of this section but is covered in Chapter 1. However, recent evidence reveals that there may some overlap between necrosis and apoptosis, depending on the cell type and the type and dose of injurious agent. Thus both hepatic necrosis and apoptosis can be produced by the same agent and can occur in the same liver.

Patterns of Hepatocellular Degeneration and Necrosis

Although the liver is subjected to a wide variety of different insults, the cellular degeneration and/or necrosis that results invariably occurs in one of following three morphologic patterns:

- Random hepatocellular degeneration and/or necrosis
- Zonal hepatocellular degeneration and/or necrosis
- Massive hepatocellular degeneration and/or necrosis

Random Hepatocellular Degeneration

Random hepatocellular degeneration and/or necrosis is characterized by the presence either of single cell necrosis throughout the liver or multifocal areas of necrotic hepatocytes. These areas are scattered randomly throughout the liver; there is no predictable location within a lobule. This pattern is typical of many infectious agents, including viruses, bacteria, and certain protozoa. Lesions may be obvious grossly as discrete, pale, or less often, dark red foci that are sharply delineated from the adjacent parenchyma (Fig. 8-7, *A*). The size of such foci is variable, ranging from tiny (<1 mm) to several millimeters. Hepatocytes in affected areas are either degenerated or necrotic because of the injurious effects of the infectious agents and the stage of the process (Fig. 8-7, *B*).

Zonal Hepatocellular Degeneration and/or Necrosis

Zonal hepatocellular degeneration and/or necrosis or as it is more simply termed, *zonal change,* affects hepatocytes within defined areas of the hepatic lobule. The zones are centrilobular (periacinar), midzonal (between centrilobular and periportal areas), or periportal (centroacinar) areas. Extensive zonal change within the liver, regardless of location within the lobule, typically produces a liver that is pale and modestly enlarged with rounded margins, has increased friability, and characteristically has an enhanced lobular pattern on the capsular and cut surface of the organ (Fig. 8-8). Degenerated hepatocytes swell and when the majority of hepatocytes in a zone are affected, that portion of the lobule appears pale. In contrast, once the hepatocytes in a particular zone of the lobule have become necrotic, this results in dilation and congestion of sinusoids so that the affected zone appears red. Although zonal change typically produces an enhanced lobular pattern, microscopic examination is usually required to determine

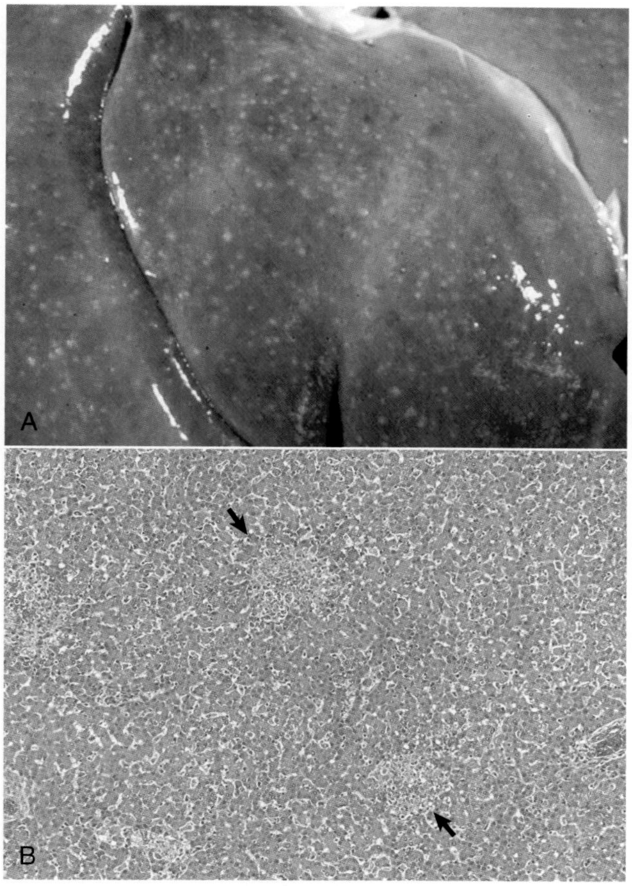

Fig. 8-7 Random hepatocellular injury, liver.
A, Equine herpes virus infection, foal. Random foci of viral-induced lytic necrosis. **B,** Salmonellosis, focal necrosis and inflammation, pig. The random pattern of hepatocellular necrosis and inflammation *(arrows)* caused by septicemic *Salmonella* spp. can also be seen within the hepatic lobules. H&E stain. (**A** courtesy Drs. J. King and L. Roth, College of Veterinary Medicine, Cornell University. **B** courtesy Dr. J.M. Cullen, College of Veterinary Medicine, North Carolina State University.)

the type of zonal change. Specific forms of zonal change are described next.

Centrilobular degeneration and necrosis

Centrilobular degeneration and necrosis of hepatocytes is particularly common (Fig. 8-9), as this portion of the lobule receives the least oxygenated blood and is therefore susceptible to hypoxia, and it has the greatest enzymatic activity (mixed-function oxidases) capable of activating compounds into toxic forms. Centrilobular necrosis can result from a precipitous and severe anemia or right side heart failure. Similarly, passive congestion of the liver results in hypoxia as a result of stasis of blood and produces atrophy of centrilobular hepatocytes.

Paracentral (periacinar) cellular degeneration

Paracentral (periacinar) cellular degeneration involves only a wedge around the central vein because only the periphery of one acinus is affected, typically reflecting the action of a direct-acting toxin that requires bioactivation (Fig. 8-10) or severe, acute anemia. As several acini border on a single central vein (terminal hepatic venule), changes induced by hypoxia may not be present equally in all acini, and thus hepatocytes at the periphery of one acinus can have more severe change than those in adjacent acini.

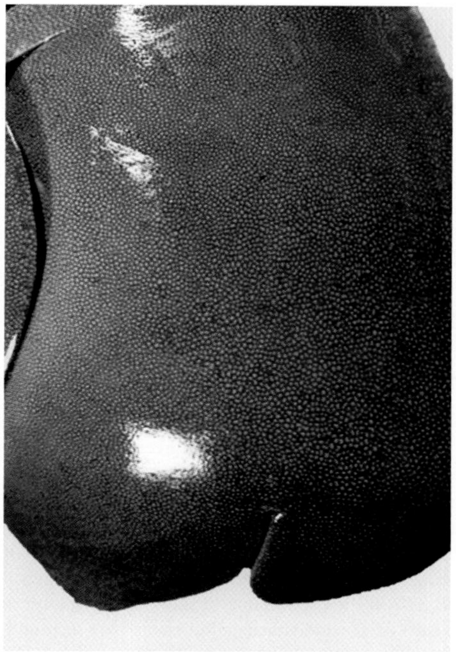

Fig. 8-8 Zonal hepatocellular injury, liver, horse.
Accentuation of the normal lobular pattern is evident on the capsular surface of the liver. This is not a specific change, as it may be associated with zonal hepatocellular degeneration and/or necrosis (regardless of lobular location), passive congestion, or diffuse cellular infiltration of the portal and periportal areas (often reflecting hepatic involvement of hematopoietic neoplasms, such as lymphoma and myeloproliferative disorders). (Courtesy Dr. J. King, College of Veterinary Medicine, Cornell University.)

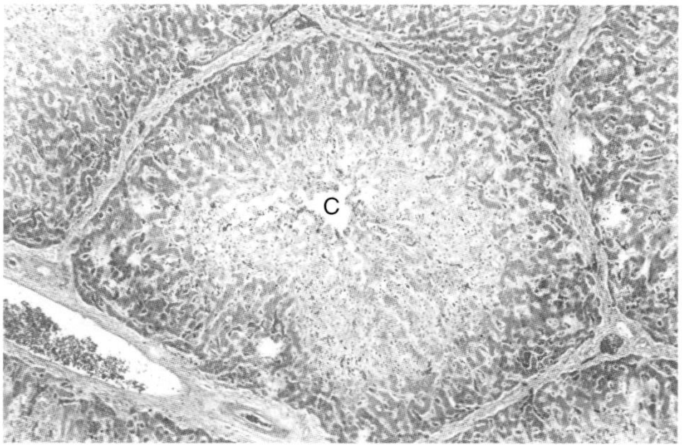

Fig. 8-9 Centrilobular necrosis, zonal hepatocellular injury, liver, pig.
Centrilobular necrosis (periacinar or zone 3) is characterized by a circumferential zone of hepatocellular necrosis surrounding the terminal hepatic venule (central vein *[C]*). H&E stain. (Courtesy Dr. M.D. McGavin, College of Veterinary Medicine, University of Tennessee.)

Midzonal degeneration and necrosis

Midzonal degeneration and necrosis are unusual lesions in domestic animals but have been reported in pigs and horses with aflatoxicosis and cats exposed to hexachlorophene (Fig. 8-11).

Periportal degeneration and necrosis

Periportal degeneration and necrosis are also uncommon but may occur following exposure to toxins, such as phosphorus, that do not require metabolism by mixed function oxidases (most

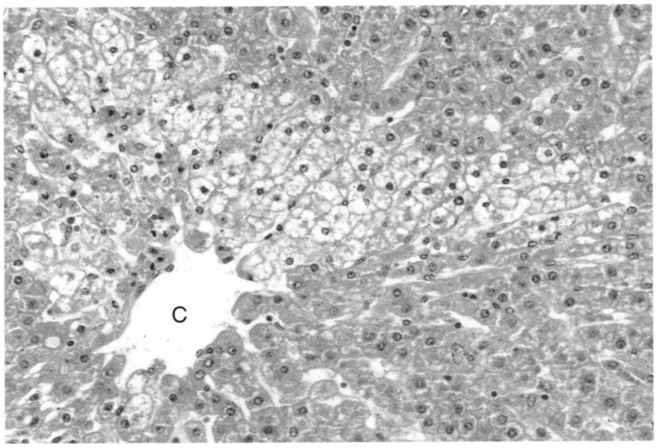

Fig. 8-10 Paracentral degeneration and necrosis, zonal hepatocellular injury, liver, cow.
Rather than a pattern of complete circumferential necrosis, a wedge-shaped area of hepatocytes is damaged. In this case, the paracentral lesion consists of necrotic hepatocytes to the left and other hepatocytes with hydropic degeneration. This wedge is the apex of the diamond-shaped liver acinus (zone 3) and reflects the partitioning of the lobule based on the inflow of blood from each of the individual portal tracts that surround the lobule. This change can be seen as an early manifestation of hepatic hypoxia in animals with anemia or right-sided heart failure and precedes centrilobular necrosis. *C,* Central vein. H&E stain. (Courtesy Dr. M.D. McGavin, College of Veterinary Medicine, University of Tennessee.)

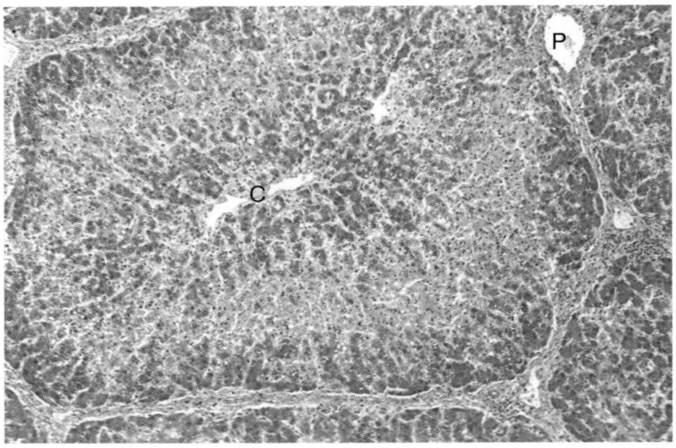

Fig. 8-11 Midzonal necrosis, zonal hepatocellular injury, liver, horse.
Midzonal necrosis is the least common pattern of hepatic injury. Hepatocytes in the middle portion of the lobule (zone 2) are affected and hepatocytes in the other regions are spared. *C,* Central vein; *P,* portal vein. H&E stain. (Courtesy Dr. M.D. McGavin, College of Veterinary Medicine, University of Tennessee.)

active in the centrilobular hepatocytes) to cause injury (Fig. 8-12). Some of these compounds may be metabolized to injurious intermediates by cytoplasmic enzymes found in periportal hepatocytes. Alternatively, some of these toxins may not require metabolism and produce hepatocyte injury in the first hepatocytes that they encounter as they flow from the portal areas.

Bridging necrosis

Bridging necrosis is the result of confluence of areas of necrosis. Bridging may link centrilobular areas (central bridging) or centrilobular areas to periportal areas (Fig. 8-13).

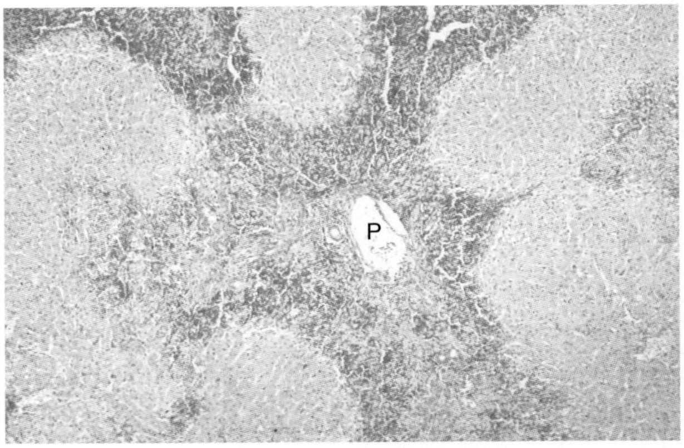

Fig. 8-12 Periportal necrosis, zonal hepatocellular injury, liver, horse.
Periportal (or zone 1) necrosis is an uncommon pattern of hepatocellular injury. Hepatocytes surrounding the portal tracts *(P)* are affected. H&E stain. (Courtesy Dr. M.D. McGavin, College of Veterinary Medicine, University of Tennessee.)

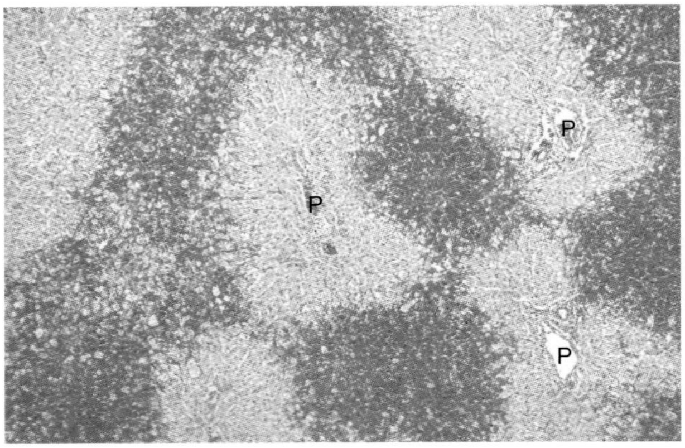

Fig. 8-13 Bridging necrosis, zonal hepatocellular injury, liver.
Bridging necrosis refers to a pattern characterized by connection of areas of necrosis between different lobules. Three patterns of bridging necrosis are recognized: central to central, as seen here; portal to portal; and central to portal. *P,* Portal area. H&E stain. (Courtesy Dr. M.D. McGavin, College of Veterinary Medicine, University of Tennessee.)

Massive Necrosis

Massive necrosis is not necessarily, as the name might be taken to imply, necrosis of the entire liver, but rather the term describes necrosis of an entire hepatic lobule or contiguous lobules (Fig. 8-14, *A*). All hepatocytes within affected lobules are necrotic. The gross appearance of the liver varies with the maturity of the lesion. If, in acute cases, the majority of the parenchyma is affected, the liver may initially be modestly increased in size with a smooth external surface and dark parenchyma because of extensive congestion. At first, necrotic hepatocytes lyse and the residual stroma becomes condensed. Regeneration does not occur because virtually all hepatocytes in the lobule are affected. Microscopically, affected areas consist of blood-filled spaces within a connective tissue stroma devoid of hepatocytes (Fig. 8-14, *B*). Later in the course of the process, stellate cells or other ECM–producing cells from the portal and centrilobular areas that may survive or migrate to the site of injury contribute new collagen (collagen I, in particular). The final result is collapse of the lobule and replacement of the lost hepatic parenchyma with a scar consisting of condensed stroma, including variable amounts and types of collagen. Grossly the

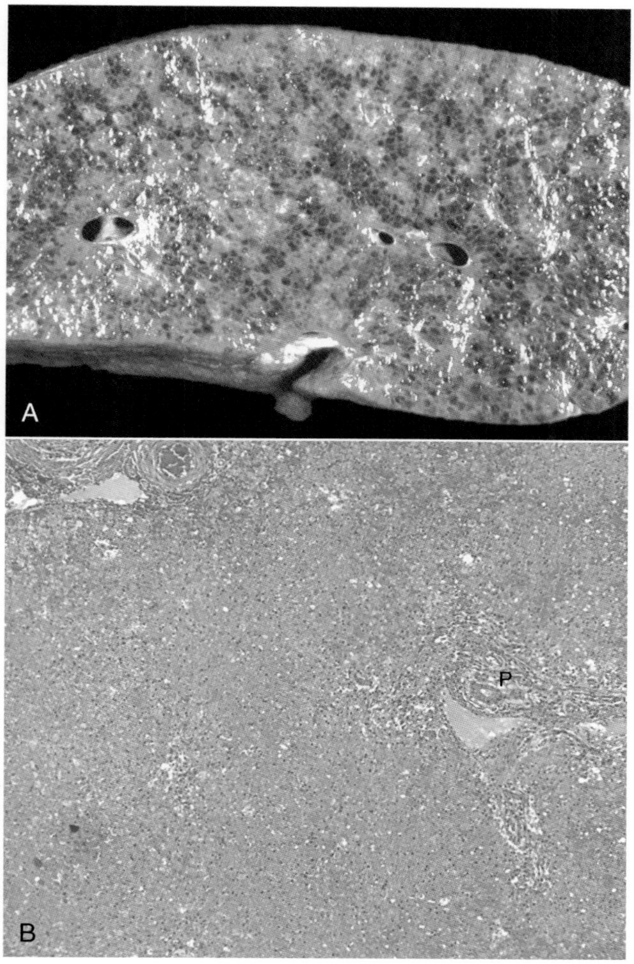

Fig. 8-14 Massive necrosis, liver.
A, Pig, cut surface. Massive necrosis refers to a pattern of necrosis that involves an entire hepatic lobule, as seen here. **B,** Dog. The entire population of hepatocytes within the lobule has undergone necrosis. *P,* Portal area. H&E stain. (**A** courtesy Dr. D. Cho, College of Veterinary Medicine, Louisiana State University; and Noah's Arkive, College of Veterinary Medicine, The University of Georgia. **B** courtesy Dr. J.M. Cullen, College of Veterinary Medicine, North Carolina State University.)

liver may be smaller than normal with a wrinkled capsule. Partial involvement of the liver is characterized by depressed areas of parenchymal necrosis and vascular congestion scattered throughout the organ.

Disturbances of Bile Flow and Icterus

Hepatic injury is frequently manifested as an increased concentration of conjugated or unconjugated bilirubin in blood called *hyperbilirubinemia.* High concentrations of bilirubin (>approximately 2 mg/dL) can produce jaundice (icterus), a yellow discoloration of tissue that is especially evident in tissue rich in elastin such as the aorta and sclera (Fig. 8-15). This concentration is within the reference range for horses, so horses may not be hyperbilirubinemic at this level. However, in other species, hyperbilirubinemia can occur once the concentration exceeds 0.5 mg/dL (dog) and therefore the patient is hyperbilirubinemic, but icterus will not be detected until it exceeds 2 mg/dL. Maximal accumulation of bilirubin in tissues takes about 2 days and explains why some animals with acute hepatic failure may have only slight icterus.

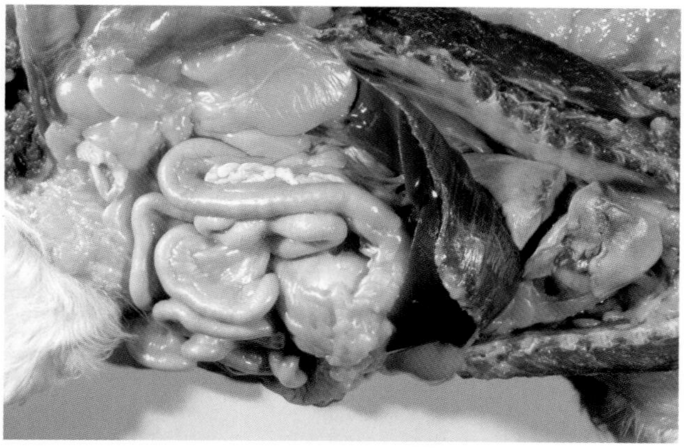

Fig. 8-15 Icterus, dog.
Icterus and jaundice are terms that refer to the yellow discoloration of tissue, by bilirubin, in this case evident in the fat and serosa. (Courtesy Dr. M.D. McGavin, College of Veterinary Medicine, University of Tennessee.)

The causes of hyperbilirubinemia include the following:

1. Overproduction of bilirubin as a consequence of hemolysis, particularly severe intravascular hemolysis, which overwhelms the liver's capacity to remove bilirubin from the plasma and to secrete conjugated bilirubin into bile. The destruction of damaged red blood cells by extravascular hemolysis can also increase the burden of bilirubin presented to the liver. Hypoxia secondary to anemia may also play a role. Decreased uptake, conjugation, or secretion of bilirubin by hepatocytes arising as a consequence of severe, diffuse hepatic disease, whether acute or chronic.
2. Reduced outflow of bile (cholestasis). Cholestasis is defined as a defect in bile secretory mechanisms that leads to an accumulation in the blood of substances normally excreted into the bile. Cholestasis occurs as a consequence of either obstruction of the biliary ducts (extrahepatic cholestasis) or impairment of bile flow within canaliculi (intrahepatic cholestasis).

Obviously, hepatic dysfunction is not the only cause of hyperbilirubinemia and icterus. In fact, icterus in ruminants is usually a consequence of severe intravascular hemolysis and less often a sequel to hepatic damage. Horses often manifest icterus with acute hepatic dysfunction, but icterus may or may not occur in horses with chronic hepatic disease. Interestingly, "physiologic icterus" is also common in the horse, and horses deprived of feed for several days can become icteric because uptake of bilirubin from the plasma by hepatocytes is decreased. Icterus in carnivores occurs as a consequence of either hemolysis or hepatic dysfunction. Inherited metabolic abnormalities can also lead to abnormal concentrations of serum bilirubin. In Southdown sheep with certain mutations, bile is ineffectively taken up from the circulation and a persistent unconjugated hyperbilirubinemia develops, although icterus is rarely apparent because there is sufficient excretion despite the mutation. Corriedale sheep may have a mutation that leads to deficient conjugated bilirubin excretion. Affected sheep have persistently elevated plasma bilirubin concentration, but jaundice is not apparent. Other compounds that are normally excreted through conjugation also accumulate in the liver of affected sheep. The livers are dark and discolored because of accumulated polymerized catecholamine metabolites that accumulate in lysosomes. These residues resemble lipofuscin histologically.

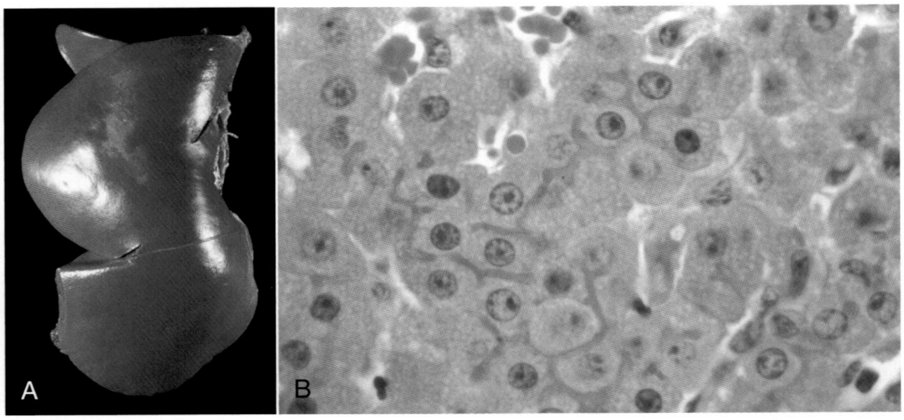

Fig. 8-16 Hepatic bilirubin retention, icterus, liver.
A, Cat. The liver is markedly yellowed by retained bilirubin. **B,** Canalicular bilirubin, acute hemolytic anemia, calf. Acute hemolysis caused by babesiosis has led to a dramatic increase in bilirubin production and distention of canaliculi, clearly demonstrating the location of canaliculi between hepatocytes. H&E stain. (**A** courtesy College of Veterinary Medicine, University of Illinois. **B** courtesy Dr. M.D. McGavin, College of Veterinary Medicine, University of Tennessee.)

Cholestasis can be divided into two types: intrahepatic and extrahepatic. Intrahepatic cholestasis can result from (1) a wide spectrum of liver injury affecting the ability of hepatocytes to metabolize and excrete bile; (2) hemolysis, which produces an abundance of bilirubin for excretion and diminishes the supply of oxygen for hepatocyte metabolism; or (3) inherited abnormalities of bile synthesis that inhibit the excretion of bile. Extrahepatic cholestasis is produced by obstruction of the extrahepatic bile ducts. This can occur by intraluminal obstruction (calculi or possibly parasites) or extraluminal means, including neoplasia or adjacent inflammation, often involving the pancreas. Cholestasis, if sufficiently severe, can produce a greenish brown discoloration to the liver (Fig. 8-16, *A*).

Histologically, acute intrahepatic cholestasis is characterized by formation of bile plugs within canaliculi (Fig. 8-16, *B*). As intrahepatic cholestasis becomes more chronic, bile that has been released from hepatocytes is taken up by Kupffer cells and can be detected within their cytoplasm.

Acute extrahepatic obstruction is characterized by edema of the portal areas, a mild neutrophilic inflammatory cell infiltrate, and a proliferative reaction by the biliary epithelium of the bile ducts. In chronic extrahepatic biliary obstruction, portal areas are enlarged by deposition of fibrosis, and there is a prominent laminar, circumferential fibrosis of bile ducts (Fig. 8-17). Biliary hyperplasia characterized by proliferation of small-caliber bile ducts is often prominent. Pigmented macrophages, containing bile, and mixed inflammatory infiltrates are also present. In severe cases, bridging fibrosis connecting portal tracts may develop.

Complete biliary obstruction leads to maldigestion of fats and a characteristic clay-colored stool termed *acholic feces* because of the lack of normal dark pigment, stercobilin, the bilirubin-derived pigment produced by bacterial metabolism (Fig. 8-18).

Regeneration

A characteristic feature of the liver is the ability to rapidly and efficiently regenerate lost hepatic mass. Experimentally, as much as two-thirds of the liver can be excised from a healthy animal without signs of hepatic dysfunction, and the liver is rapidly regenerated. In addition to replication of hepatocytes, there is a wave of replication in bile duct epithelium, endothelium, and sinusoidal lining cells that is coordinated with hepatocyte replication.

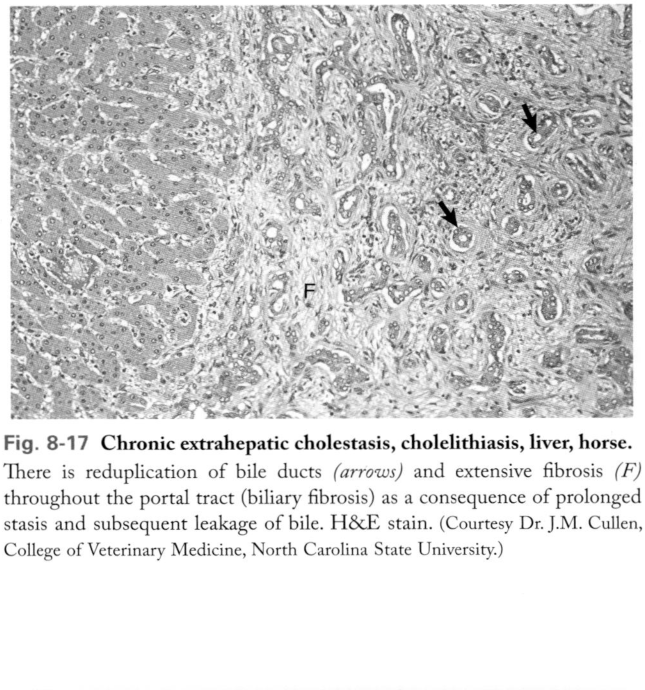

Fig. 8-17 Chronic extrahepatic cholestasis, cholelithiasis, liver, horse.
There is reduplication of bile ducts *(arrows)* and extensive fibrosis *(F)* throughout the portal tract (biliary fibrosis) as a consequence of prolonged stasis and subsequent leakage of bile. H&E stain. (Courtesy Dr. J.M. Cullen, College of Veterinary Medicine, North Carolina State University.)

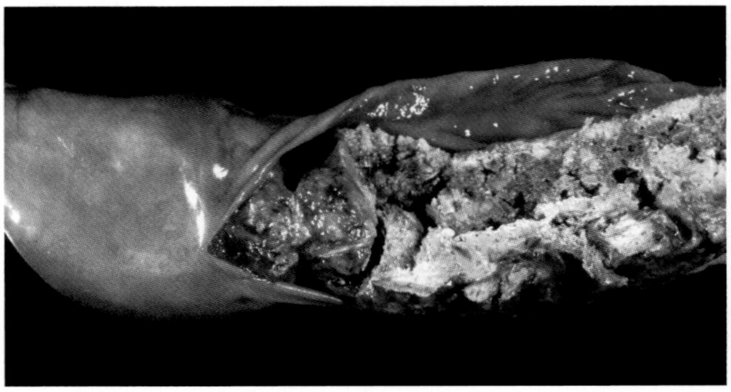

Fig. 8-18 Intrahepatic biliary obstruction, intestine, dog.
In cases of complete biliary obstruction, bile is unable to reach the intestine and as a result stool(s) lacks the characteristic dark color produced by bile pigments. (Courtesy College of Veterinary Medicine, North Carolina State University.)

Regeneration usually takes place by replication of mature hepatocytes. In most circumstances, this leads to an increase in the size of existing lobules; however, recent data suggest that some new lobule formation can also occur through subdivision of existing lobules. After removal of liver lobes only, the remaining liver lobes persist, and no new lobe formation occurs.

Individual cell necrosis leads to local proliferation by regeneration of adjacent hepatocytes. Scattered foci of necrotic hepatocytes are quickly replaced through cell division of adjacent hepatocytes. Necrosis in the centrilobular area of the lobule leads to a wave of hepatocyte proliferation in the hepatocytes in the remaining areas of the lobule, particularly the periportal hepatocytes. In some circumstances, such as necrosis of nearly all hepatocytes or exposure to certain chemical toxins that inhibit replication of mature hepatocytes, replacement of hepatocytes lost by necrosis occurs through proliferation of hepatocyte stem cells or oval cells. This process is most often observed in experimental manipulations of laboratory rodents but probably occurs in naturally occurring cases of hepatotoxicity also. These cells reside in the connective tissue of the portal tracts and have the ability to differentiate into hepatocyte or bile duct epithelium. Histologically, they are identified as small basophilic cells with an oval shape. They are not apparent in most circumstances of hepatic regeneration but can be abundant in experimental studies of hepatic regeneration.

The body carefully orchestrates hepatic regeneration to replace lost hepatocyte mass along with bile ducts and vessels without producing excess liver. A variety of growth factors, including transforming growth factor-α (TGF-α) and hepatocyte growth factor, stimulate hepatocyte replication. Once normal hepatic mass has been established, macrophages release TGF-β, which, in concert with other less well characterized factors, stops hepatic parenchymal cell proliferation.

A single episode of extensive hepatic necrosis is usually followed by parenchymal regeneration without scarring, as long as the normal ECM (reticulin) scaffolding of the affected portion remains intact and has not collapsed. However, repetitive injury or massive necrosis can disrupt the normal lobular architecture, and there may be parenchymal collapse after removal of the dead hepatocytes and/or stromal collapse with repair by collagen synthesis (postnecrotic scarring) (Fig. 8-19). Even when necrosis of hepatocytes is continuous, the liver attempts to regenerate its functional mass. However, prolonged regenerative effort with damage to the normal ECM scaffolding of the liver often results in nodular proliferations of parenchyma, which architecturally distort the liver. Although regenerative nodules may reconstitute a proportionately large amount of hepatic mass, adequate function is rarely attained. Blood flow into the regenerative nodules and bile flow out of the nodules is abnormal, and as a result, hepatic function cannot be reestablished. As the nodules develop, the portal tract vessels and the central veins develop communications within the fibrous septa between nodules, which leads to vascular shunts between the portal vein and the central vein that bypass hepatocytes within the nodules.

Fibrosis

Fibrosis is one of the more common manifestations of chronic liver injury. The pattern of fibrosis is frequently a useful indicator of the type of insult that produces the lesion. The significance of fibrosis depends on its effect on hepatic function and its reversibility. Despite the considerable regenerative capacity of the liver, hepatic fibrosis, when sufficiently severe, can be lethal.

In the normal liver, fibrillar collagens I and III are confined primarily to the connective tissue of the portal tracts and immediately around the terminal hepatic venule (central vein). Collagen IV is the most abundant collagen type in the reticulin framework of the sinusoids, but it is present in only small amounts. A delicate scaffolding of collagen and other ECM components, which are produced by stellate cells, endothelial cells, and hepatocytes, make up the normal framework of the sinusoid. This stroma in the space of Disse supports the endothelial cells and maintains their relationship to the hepatocytes.

Hepatic fibrosis is an overall increase in the ECM within the liver. In a fibrotic liver, there is an increase in the amount of ECM and a change in the types of collagen and their site of deposition. A severely fibrotic liver can contain up to six times as much collagen and proteoglycan as a normal liver. Hepatic fibrosis is characterized by an increase of fibrillar collagens, type I and type III, and nonfibrillar collagen XVIII within the space of Disse, the portal areas, and the area surrounding the central veins. In addition to an increase in collagens, there is also a commensurate increase in the ECM components, proteoglycans, fibronectin, and hyaluronic acid.

The stellate cells (Ito cells and lipocytes) have a central role in hepatic fibrosis, although it should be noted that there are myofibroblastic cells with similar capabilities found within the connective tissue of the portal areas and connective tissue surrounding the central vein. In the normal liver, stellate cells occupy the space of Disse (a subendothelial position in the sinusoid) nestled between hepatocytes. They are characterized by the presence of large lipid-containing vacuoles in their cytoplasm (see Web Fig. 8-3). The vacuoles are a primary storage site for retinyl esters, including vitamin A. Stellate cells are positioned in the space of Disse around the circumference of the endothelium of the sinusoids and have been likened to pericytes in other organs, such as the mesangial cells of the renal glomerulus. Hepatic stellate cells have been shown to have a role in the control of the diameter of the sinusoids and consequently the flow of blood through the sinusoids.

When the liver is injured, these cells go through a progressive phenotypic change from the typical lipid-storing cell to a cell with a myofibroblastic appearance (Fig. 8-20). When they are activated, they express smooth muscle actin and desmin, a marker usually found in muscle cells. Once these cells have switched to the myofibroblast phenotype, they begin synthesis of collagen types I, III, and IV. They also produce other ECM components, including laminin and chondroitin sulfate proteoglycans. Hepatocytes synthesize few or no matrix proteins, and the large sum of matrix proteins is derived from the hepatic stellate cells. The type of hepatic injury does not seem to be important in the genesis of hepatic fibrosis. Chemical injury, biliary obstruction, and iron overload produce similar patterns of activation of hepatic stellate cells.

The site in which collagen is deposited in the liver has a significant impact on liver function. Perisinusoidal fibrosis can have a severe effect on hepatic function. In addition to collagen and ECM deposits, there is a loss of gaps in the endothelial cells and a loss of microvilli on the luminal surface of the hepatocytes. These changes have been termed *capillarization of the sinusoids* because the alterations in the sinusoids result in a vascular structure that more closely resembles a capillary than a sinusoid. The functional effect of this microanatomic change is profound. The ability of the liver to carry out its synthetic, catabolic, and excretory roles is severely compromised by the reduced exposure of hepatocytes to plasma.

Within the hepatic lobule, the site of fibrosis can be indicative of the type of insult. Most often, chronic toxic injury produces centrilobular (periacinar) fibrosis. This region is affected because the centrilobular hepatocytes are the site of metabolism for most drugs. Long-standing right-sided heart failure can cause fibrosis in

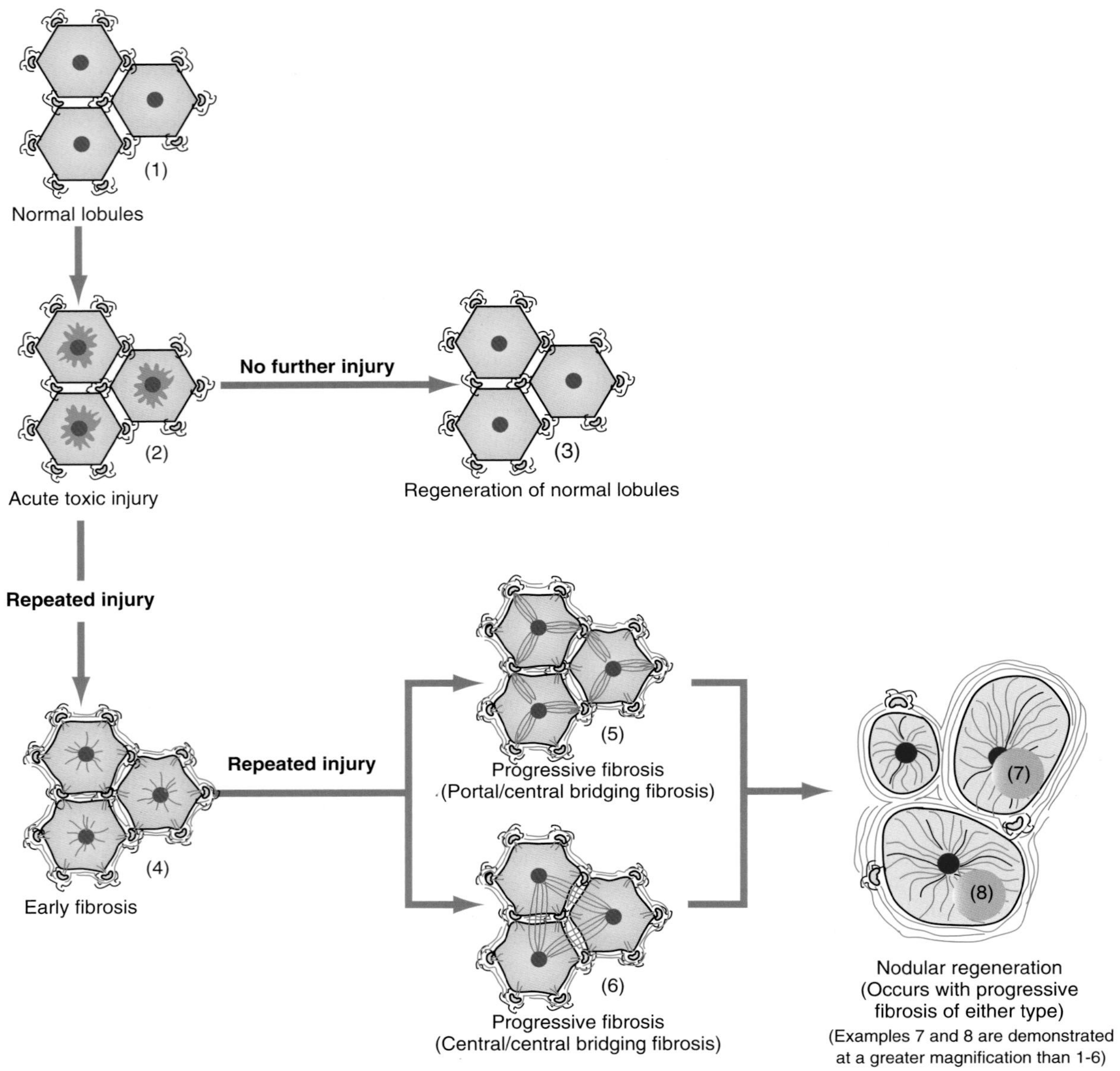

Fig. 8-19 Schematic diagram of the effects of hepatic injury on the development of fibrosis.
Acute hepatic centrilobular injury *(2)* that occurs only once usually resolves, and normal liver architecture returns *(1, 3)*. Repeated bouts of injury or severe injury can initiate hepatic fibrosis *(4)*. In the earliest stages, fibrosis may be reversible, but as fibrosis progresses it reaches a point at which repair is not likely. Fibrosis often starts as fine branches of collagen deposition between portal areas or central areas or dissecting into the hepatic parenchyma *(5, 6)*. Over time, greater amounts of collagen and other extracellular matrix are deposited and the lobular architecture becomes progressively distorted. In the end-stage liver, nodular regeneration *(7, 8)* and extensive, circumferential fibrosis are typical. The regenerative nodules shown here *(7, 8)* are at an early stage of regeneration. As shown in Fig. 8-21, they will regenerate to form nodules that will commonly exceed the size of normal hepatic lobules. These nodules will often compress *(7)* the central vein(s) of hepatic lobules within and adjacent to those from which they arose.

this site as well. Periportal (centroacinar) fibrosis can result from chronic inflammatory conditions or a small group of toxins that affect the periportal hepatocytes because they do not require metabolism by the cytochrome p450 enzymes to produce an injurious metabolite. Fibrosis may be limited to individual lobules, but in more severe injuries, the areas of fibrosis can be more extensive. Bridging fibrosis, which is analogous to bridging necrosis, implies fibrosis that extends from one portal tract to another or from portal tracts to central veins. Bridging fibrosis is more likely to impair hepatic function than focal forms of hepatic fibrosis; however, all forms of hepatic fibrosis, if sufficiently severe, lead to impaired hepatic function. However, because of the enormous reserve capacity of the liver, fibrosis is usually quite extensive before there are clinical signs of hepatic dysfunction.

A single event of widespread hepatocellular necrosis is sometimes followed, not by the usual regenerative response, but by fibrosis and condensation of the preexisting connective tissue stroma that results in formation of bands of dense connective tissue. This process is referred to as *postnecrotic scarring*.

Other patterns of hepatic fibrosis can occur, including biliary fibrosis (centered on bile ducts in the portal triads), focal or multifocal hepatic fibrosis (randomly scattered throughout the hepatic parenchyma)—which is produced, for example, by migrating nematode larvae—and diffuse hepatic fibrosis (affects all regions of the

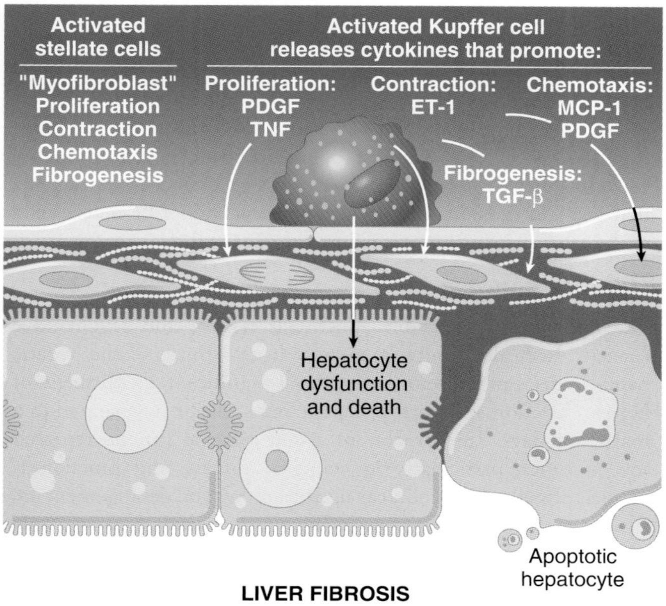

Fig. 8-20 Schematic diagram of a fibrotic hepatic sinusoid.
Sinusoidal fibrosis dramatically reduces contact between the plasma and the hepatocytes. The sinusoidal endothelial cells have lost their fenestrations. The space of Disse contains abundant collagen type I fibers that have been synthesized by activated hepatic stellate cells. The hepatic stellate cells have eliminated the lipid vacuoles and assumed a myofibroblastic morphology with cell extensions that often surround the endothelial cells (not shown here). Hepatocyte microvilli have been lost along the sinusoid, as shown on the apoptotic hepatocyte, and this loss begins with the onset of hepatocyte dysfunction and degeneration. *ET-1,* Endothelin-1; *MCP-1,* macrophage chemotactic protein-1; *PDGF,* platelet-derived growth factor; *TGF-α,* transforming growth factor-α; *TNF,* tumor necrosis factor. (Schematic based on concepts presented in Friedman SL: *J Biol Chem* 275:2247-2250, 2000; and Crawford JM: *Curr Op Gastroenterol* 13:175-185, 1997.)

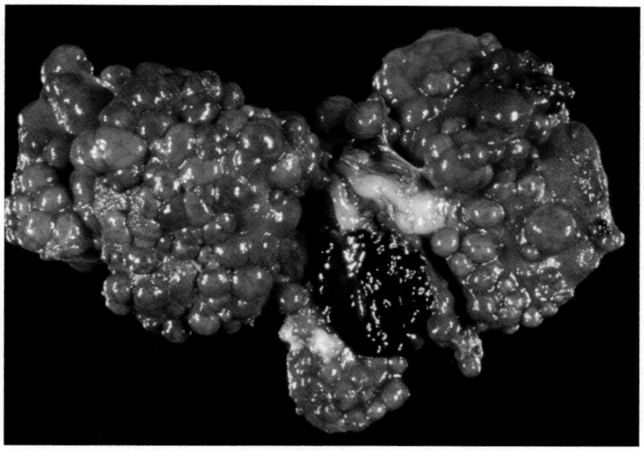

Fig. 8-21 End-stage liver (cirrhosis), dog.
End-stage liver from a dog that had received phenobarbital for many years. The liver is small, firm, and irregular with nodules of regenerative parenchyma separated by tracts of fibrous connective tissue. (Courtesy Dr. J.M. Cullen, College of Veterinary Medicine, North Carolina State University.)

BOX 8-1 Causes of End-Stage Liver

- Chronic toxicity (therapeutic agents or naturally occurring toxins)
- Chronic cholangitis and/or obstruction
- Chronic congestion (right side heart failure)
- Inherited disorders of metal metabolism (copper or iron)
- Chronic hepatitis
- Idiopathic

lobule and is present throughout the liver). Diffuse fibrosis with regenerative nodule formation is by definition cirrhosis. Different hepatic insults may produce different patterns of fibrosis, but when fibrosis is severe (end-stage liver disease), it frequently is impossible to determine either the cause or the initial pattern of fibrosis.

Biliary Hyperplasia

Biliary hyperplasia, which is proliferation of new biliary ducts within the portal areas and periportal regions, can be a relatively nonspecific response to a variety of insults to the liver. The mechanism responsible for this proliferation is unknown. In severe hepatic injury, proliferation of bipotential progenitor cells with the ability to differentiate into hepatocytes or biliary epithelium can form small caliber ducts and tubules in a response termed the *ductular reaction.* These cells can mature and replace adult biliary epithelium or hepatocytes. Biliary hyperplasia or ductular reaction can occur swiftly, particularly in young animals. Biliary hyperplasia is typically regarded as a lesion seen in long-standing hepatic injury. Biliary hyperplasia occurs particularly after diseases that obstruct normal bile drainage.

End-Stage Liver or Cirrhosis

The best accepted definition for cirrhosis was pronounced by the World Health Organization (WHO) in 1977 and is as follows: "a diffuse process characterized by fibrosis and the conversion of the normal liver architecture into structurally abnormal lobules (Fig. 8-21)." As it is the final, irreversible result of any one of several different hepatic diseases, the term *end-stage liver* is appropriate, particularly because the term *cirrhosis* is neither descriptive nor precise in meaning and originally meant "tawny yellow." Another authority states that the hallmark is the total absence of any normal lobular architecture. The architecture of the liver is altered by loss of hepatic parenchyma, condensation of reticulin framework, and formation of tracts of fibrous connective tissue. Regeneration of hepatic tissue between fibrous bands leads to the formation of variably sized regenerative nodules (Fig. 8-22). The entire liver is thus distorted and consists of nodules of regenerating parenchyma separated by fibrous bands, which appear as depressions on the surface (see Fig. 8-21).

Profound vascular abnormalities with serious consequences for the health of affected patients occur in this condition, including multiple abnormal vascular anastomoses between the portal vein and the systemic vasculature, as a consequence of the increased portal pressure. Also, venous shunts between the central veins and the portal veins and arteriovenous shunts between the hepatic arteries and the central veins can occur within the regenerative nodules.

The potential causes of an end-stage (cirrhotic) liver are numerous (Box 8-1). Chronic toxic insult results from the continued ingestion of any hepatotoxin (e.g., herbivores ingesting toxic plants, such as those that contain pyrrolizidine alkaloids, and the long-term administration of anticonvulsant drugs, such as primidone for dogs). Chronic extrahepatic biliary obstruction and cholestasis leads to extensive fibrosis, which primarily affects the portal triads, but the fibrosis can eventually extend into the adjacent hepatic parenchyma. Chronic inflammation of the liver (hepatitis) or

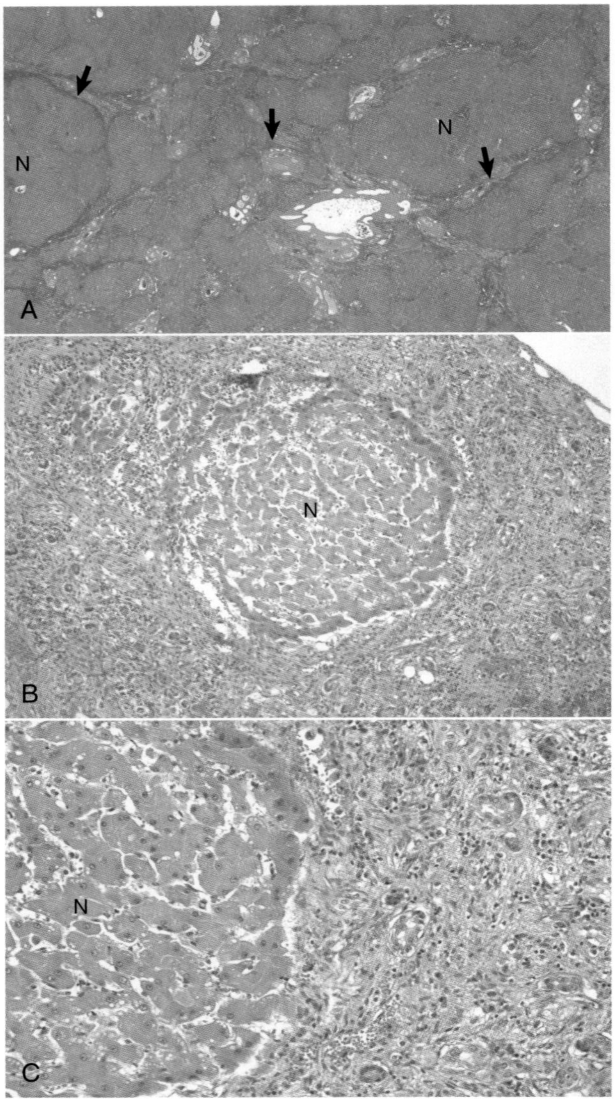

Fig. 8-22 End-stage, liver, dog.
A, Histologic appearance of end-stage liver disease. Nodules of regenerative parenchyma *(N)* are separated by septa of collapsed reticulin and fibrous connective tissue *(arrows),* which also contains numerous blood vessels and bile ducts. H&E stain. **B,** A single regenerative hepatic nodule *(N)* is surrounded by haphazardly arranged bands of fibrous connective tissue that contains numerous blood vessels and hypertrophied and hyperplastic bile ducts. H&E stain. **C,** Higher magnification of Fig. 8-22, *B.* Note the regenerative nodule *(N),* bands of fibrous connective tissue, hyperplastic bile ducts, and mononuclear inflammatory cells. H&E stain. (**A** courtesy Dr. J.M. Cullen, College of Veterinary Medicine, North Carolina State University. **B** and **C** courtesy College of Veterinary Medicine, University of Illinois.)

biliary tract (cholangitis) may lead to an end-stage liver. Although infection of the liver typically is focal or multifocal, diffuse hepatitis and subsequent fibrosis occurs in disease entities such as canine chronic hepatitis. Chronic passive hepatic congestion eventually leads to fibrosis near central veins, which is sometimes termed *cardiac sclerosis* and which can progress to cardiac cirrhosis. The actual amount of fibrosis is usually small. Abnormal storage or metabolism of metals, particularly copper, as occurs in Bedlington terriers and several other breeds, may produce chronic inflammation and an end-stage liver. Lobular dissecting hepatitis, a specific form of end-stage liver or cirrhosis, is usually seen in young dogs and is described further under specific diseases of dogs. A variety of more poorly defined disease entities can lead to progressive hepatocellular injury and hepatic fibrosis resulting in end-stage hepatic disease.

The end-stage liver obviously cannot perform its normal functions, so the clinical manifestations of hepatic failure invariably occur in affected animals. However, the cause of the hepatic damage that leads to the end-stage liver frequently cannot be determined at the time signs of hepatic failure are observed.

Hepatic Failure

The liver has considerable functional reserve and regenerative capacity. In healthy animals, more than two-thirds of the hepatic parenchyma can be removed without significant impairment of hepatic function and normal hepatic mass can be regenerated in a matter of days. This process of tissue removal can be repeated several times, particularly in younger animals, and function is retained. In all species, clinical signs from hepatic derangement are similar, regardless of their cause. These are manifest, however, only when the liver's considerable reserve and regenerative capacity are depleted or when biliary outflow is obstructed. Only lesions that affect the majority of the hepatic parenchyma are likely to produce the signs of hepatic failure because focal lesions rarely destroy sufficient parenchyma to deplete the liver's reserve. The term *hepatic failure* implies loss of adequate hepatic function as a consequence of either acute or chronic hepatic damage; however, all hepatic functions are not usually lost at the same time. The potential consequences of hepatic dysfunction and failure include (1) hepatic encephalopathy; (2) disturbances of bile flow with a resultant hyperbilirubinemia (discussed previously); (3) a variety of metabolic disturbances; (4) vascular and hemodynamic alterations, such as shunting of portal blood into the systemic circulation bypassing the hepatocytes; (5) cutaneous manifestations, such as epidermal necrosis in dogs and photosensitization in herbivores; and (6) immunologic manifestations.

Hepatic Encephalopathy

Information on this topic is available at evolve.elsevier.com/Zachary/McGavin/.

Metabolic Disturbances of Hepatic Failure

Hepatic failure can be manifested by a variety of metabolic disturbances. The type and duration of the hepatic disorder may influence the nature of the metabolic perturbation.

Bleeding Tendencies

Information on this topic is available at evolve.elsevier.com/Zachary/McGavin/.

Hypoalbuminemia

Information on this topic is available at evolve.elsevier.com/Zachary/McGavin/.

Vascular and Hemodynamic Alterations of Hepatic Failure

Chronic hepatic injury typically is accompanied by extensive diffuse fibrosis of the liver, which increases resistance to blood flow through the liver. This in turn elevates pressure within the portal vein (portal hypertension). With time, collateral vascular channels open to allow blood in the portal vein to bypass the abnormal liver (acquired portosystemic vascular anastomoses, which connect the portal vein and its tributaries to the systemic venous circulation). Shunting of portal vein blood directly to the central vein can also occur within the fibrous septa formed in the liver. In addition, the increased pressure within the hepatic vasculature causes transudation of fluid (modified transudate) into the peritoneal cavity to produce ascites in several species, except in most cases horses. Transudation of fluid into the peritoneal cavity can be enhanced by hypoalbuminemia because there is a decreased colloid osmotic pressure in plasma. Hypoalbuminemia and reduced plasma colloid osmotic pressure can arise as a consequence of accelerated albumin loss into the lumen of the intestines as a result of portal hypertension or because of reduced hepatic synthesis of albumin and other plasma proteins by the diseased liver. Ascites associated with hepatic fibrosis in chronic liver disease (end-stage liver) or other causes of portal hypertension, such as right-sided heart failure, occurs most commonly in the dog and cat, occasionally in sheep, and rarely in horses and cattle.

Cutaneous Manifestations of Hepatic Failure

Hepatocutaneous Syndrome (Necrolytic Migratory Erythema, Superficial Necrolytic Dermatitis)

Information on this topic, including Web Fig. 8-4, is available at evolve.elsevier.com/Zachary/McGavin/.

Photosensitization

Information on this topic, including Web Fig. 8-5, is available at evolve.elsevier.com/Zachary/McGavin/.

Primary photosensitization

Information on this topic is available at evolve.elsevier.com/Zachary/McGavin/.

Secondary photosensitization

Information on this topic is available at evolve.elsevier.com/Zachary/McGavin/.

Congenital porphyria

Information on this topic is available at evolve.elsevier.com/Zachary/McGavin/.

Immunologic Manifestations of Hepatic Failure

Chronic liver failure leads to an impairment of normal hepatic immune function. As a consequence, the affected patient frequently develops endotoxemia and an increased risk of systemic infection. For the most part, this impairment is manifest as a reduction of blood filtration by Kupffer cells, which is primarily a result of shunting of portal blood rather than reduced phagocytic activity of the Kupffer cells.

PORTALS OF ENTRY

The liver and biliary systems are exposed to infectious or otherwise injurious substances via three main routes: hematogenous, biliary, and direct penetration (Table 8-1). The liver receives the entire flow of the portal vein and as a consequence is bathed in potentially injurious microbes, which inhabit and penetrate the digestive system, and toxic substances that have been ingested or produced by the intestinal flora. The distribution of blood from the portal vein to the different lobes of the liver is most likely not uniform. So-called portal streaming refers to the differential flow of portal blood from one segment of the digestive tract to particular lobes of the liver. This explains why some lobes of the liver are more severely affected by toxins that are absorbed by the small intestine rather than the large intestine. Examples of this include the preponderance of injury to the left liver lobe of sheep that ingest the mycotoxin sporidesmin. Systemic infections or intoxications can also affect the liver through the blood from the hepatic artery. Neonates and fetal animals are also at risk from infections ascending the umbilical vein. Infectious agents, such as enteric

TABLE 8-1 Portals of Entry

	Liver	Biliary System	Exocrine Pancreas
DIRECT EXTENSION			
Penetrating trauma through the abdominal wall or rib cage	Yes	Yes	Yes
Penetrating trauma through the lumen of the gastrointestinal tract	Yes	Yes	Yes
HEMATOGENOUS			
Localization within the sinusoids via the portal vein, hepatic artery, or umbilical vein in neonates	Yes	No	No
Localization within Kupffer cells	Yes	No	No
Localization within capillary beds of the wall of the gallbladder or arteriolar rete of the biliary tree	No	Yes	No
Localization within capillary beds of the pancreatic parenchyma	No	No	Yes
RETROGRADE BILIARY TRANSPORT			
Ascending bacterial or parasitic infections gain access to the organ	Yes	Yes	No
RETROGRADE PANCREATIC DUCTULAR TRANSPORT			
Ascending bacterial or parasitic infections gain access to the organ	No	No	Yes

TABLE 8-2 Defense Mechanisms against Injury and Infectious Agents

	Liver	Biliary System	Exocrine Pancreas
STRUCTURAL AND FUNCTIONAL BARRIER			
Skin	Yes	Yes	Yes
Rib cage	Yes	Yes	Yes
Omentum (barrier that limits access of injurious material to the organ)	Yes	Yes	Yes
IMMUNOLOGIC RESPONSES			
Kupffer cells	Yes	No	No
Resident and migrating cells (recruited monocytes), which are part of the monocyte-macrophage system	Yes	No	No
Innate and adaptive immunologic responses (including secretory immunoglobulin A), which form the body's overall immune system	Yes	Yes	Yes
BIOCHEMICAL DEFENSES			
Enzyme inhibitors that reduce the risk of premature enzyme activation and tissue injury	No	No	Yes

bacteria and parasites, can also gain access to the liver through the biliary tree that is in direct connection with the duodenum and enteric bacteria. Finally, direct penetration of the body cavity or from the digestive tract (i.e., traumatic reticuloperitonitis or foreign bodies in the reticulum) can deliver infectious or traumatic insults.

DEFENSE MECHANISMS

The liver is well defended from blood-borne injury by the Kupffer cells, the fixed macrophages that are distributed intermittently throughout the lumen of the sinusoids on the surface of endothelial cells (Table 8-2). They actively ingest and degrade bacteria and other organisms; senescent cells, such as erythrocytes; and particulate matter in the sinusoidal blood. They are very efficient and able to clear virtually all particulate matter in a single pass through the liver. Kupffer cells are particularly important in the removal of endotoxin from the portal blood.

The biliary tree, like the upper gastrointestinal tract, is defended from infection by secreted IgA as part of mucosal immunity (see Table 8-2). The majority of biliary IgA is synthesized by gastrointestinal plasma cells. The majority of released IgA is taken into lymph and from there it enters the bloodstream. Hepatocytes in many species can transport IgA from blood across their cell membranes via a secretory component–mediated endocytosis. Subsequently, IgA molecules reach the bile by secretion into canaliculi. Concentrations of bile IgA are maintained by enterohepatic circulation. Within the biliary tree, IgA provides defense from infectious agents and clearance of harmful antigens as antibody-antigen complexes. In addition, the biliary tree is protected by the sphincter at the terminal end of the common bile duct, which provides a physical barrier to the ascent of enteric bacteria and the continuous flow of bile that assists in flushing bacteria out of the ducts.

The liver is protected from direct penetration by its anatomic location within the protection of the rib cage. The wall of the digestive tract also provides a certain degree of protection from penetration by ingested foreign bodies.

The high metabolic rate of hepatocytes renders them highly susceptible to metabolic disturbances that lead to cellular degeneration and necrosis (Box 8-2). This section will consider the patterns of hepatic degeneration, responses of the liver to injury, and inflammation of the liver.

BOX 8-2 Mechanisms of Liver Injury

- Metabolic bioactivation of chemicals via cytochrome P450 to reactive species
- Stimulation of autoimmunity
- Stimulation of apoptosis
- Disruption of calcium homeostasis leading to cell surface blebbing and lysis
- Canalicular injury
- Mitochondrial injury

Data from Lee W: *N Engl J Med* 349:474-485, 2003.

GALLBLADDER AND EXTRAHEPATIC BILE DUCTS

STRUCTURE AND FUNCTION

The structure of the gallbladder and major ducts of the biliary system is similar in all species (the gallbladder is absent in the horse, the rat, and the elephant). It consists of a muscular wall (tunica muscularis) and a mucosa lined by simple columnar epithelium. The epithelium and muscularis are separated only by the lamina propria because the gallbladder lacks a muscularis mucosa. Right and left hepatic ducts carry bile from different lobes of the liver; these ducts and the cystic duct from the gallbladder unite to form the common bile duct. Location of the opening of the common bile duct into the intestine differs somewhat among the domestic species; it is as little as 2 cm from the pylorus in the pig to as much as 70 cm from the pylorus in the cow. The gallbladder stores and concentrates bile. Considerable concentration (twentyfold to thirtyfold) of bile by active transport of sodium and anions across the gallbladder epithelial cells occurs in dogs and cats, whereas little concentration occurs in pigs and ruminants. The horse lacks a gallbladder and continuously releases bile into the duodenum.

Animals that have not eaten in 24 to 48 hours or that are starving or cachectic can have notably enlarged gallbladders (Fig. 8-23). The reason is that these animals lack the paracrine stimulus (i.e., cholecystokinin), and a number of other neural and hormonal stimuli, to contract the gallbladder and relax the sphincter at the

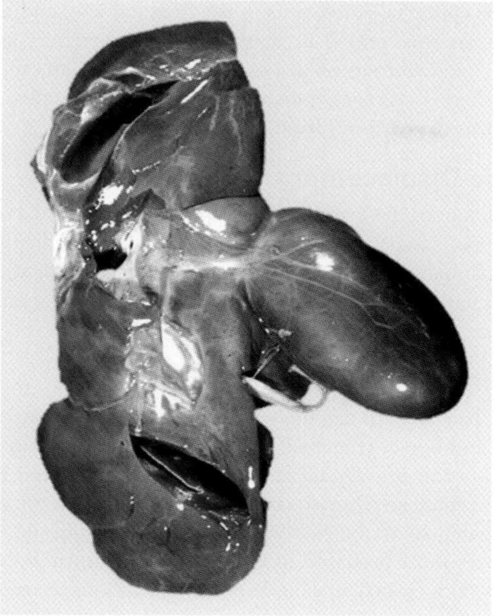

Fig. 8-23 Distended gallbladder, calf.
Note the distended gallbladder, which is common in all species after a prolonged period of fasting, because there is no stimulus for emptying the gallbladder. Thus they are frequently seen at necropsy of sick animals. (Courtesy Dr. J. King, College of Veterinary Medicine, Cornell University.)

termination of the common bile duct, which regulates flow of bile into the duodenum.

EXOCRINE PANCREAS

STRUCTURE AND FUNCTION

Development

The embryonic origin of the pancreas begins as a dorsal and a ventral bud of the duodenum. These buds fuse during embryogenesis to give rise to the entire pancreas. The major pancreatic duct arises from fusion of the ventral duct and the distal portion of the dorsal duct.

Macroscopic and Microscopic Structure

The pancreas is a lobulated, pink to gray, tubuloalveolar gland, a large portion of which is located in the mesentery immediately adjacent to the duodenum. The blood vessels, nerves, and lymph vessels that serve the pancreas are located within the delicate connective tissue septa that separate the lobules of pancreatic tissue. The pancreas contains both endocrine and exocrine elements, the endocrine portion being the islets of Langerhans. The exocrine portion constitutes the majority of the pancreas, up to 80% to 85% of the organ, and consists of acini composed of columnar to triangular secretory cells. The acinar cells have basally oriented nuclei and cytoplasm with a deeply basophilic basal margin and eosinophilic, granular zymogen granules occupying the apical portion. When the cells are appropriately signaled, the zymogen granules, containing the digestive enzymes of the pancreas, are released into the lumen of the acinus. The ductal system, in which secretions of the exocrine pancreas are conveyed to the intestinal tract, commences as fine radicals within acini and progresses to intralobular and interlobular ducts. These small ducts eventually drain into the main pancreatic duct or ducts. The arrangement of the major pancreatic ducts and how they empty into the duodenum varies among the domestic species. It is particularly variable in the dog, in which at least five different anatomic arrangements are recognized. In the cat, the major pancreatic duct enters the duodenum in close proximity to the common bile duct, and this may predispose the cat to pancreatic injury.

Normal Function

The exocrine pancreas produces secretions that contribute to digestion. The secretions contain a variety of enzymes that break down dietary lipids (lipase and phospholipase), proteins (trypsin and chymotrypsin), and carbohydrates (amylase). The secretions also contain electrolytes, which maintain the pH of the intestinal contents within a range that is optimal for enzymatic activity. Pancreatic enzymes act on the products of gastric digestion after they enter the duodenum. These enzymes often are released into secretions as inactive precursors (proenzymes), which helps prevent degradation of the pancreas by its own digestive enzymes. These are activated within the intestine. In addition, inhibitors of pancreatic enzymes are present in the pancreatic tissue. Secretion is controlled by neural stimulation regulated by the vagus nerve and by humoral factors. Secretin is one of the more important hormones involved in pancreatic secretion, and it stimulates water and bicarbonate secretion by duct cells. It is produced by neuroendocrine cells within the duodenal epithelium. The efflux of acid from the stomach and the presence of fatty acids in the duodenum stimulate its release. Cholecystokinin, another important hormone, stimulates the release of digestive enzymes from the acinar cells. It is produced by neuroendocrine cells of the duodenum in response to the presence of fatty acids, peptides, and amino acids.

RESPONSES TO INJURY

The pancreas possesses modest regenerative capacity after necrosis of pancreatic exocrine epithelial cells, although more robust regeneration after partial pancreatectomy has been shown. Acinar cells can undergo replication in cases of limited injury, and precursor cells arise from cells within or adjacent to ductal epithelium in more severe injury. After acute pancreatic injury, there is usually little evidence of regeneration of the exocrine pancreas if there has been sufficient tissue destruction, and fibrosis is the principal response. Proliferated ductules and atrophic exocrine pancreatic lobules are also found after significant pancreatic injury.

PORTALS OF ENTRY

Portals of entry into the exocrine pancreas are listed in Table 8-1.

DEFENSE MECHANISMS

Defense mechanisms for the exocrine pancreas are listed in Table 8-2. The pancreas is protected by the continuous flow of secretions into the duodenum, which prevents reflux of duodenal contents. The normal secretion of the pancreas contains trypsin, chymotrypsin, elastase, aminopeptidases, lipase, phospholipases, amylase, and nucleases. Trypsin is a critical enzyme because it has a role in the activation of several of the other pancreatic enzymes. Several mechanisms exist to protect the healthy pancreas from the effects of digestive enzymes it produces. Before secretion, enzymes are isolated from the acinar cell cytoplasm in membrane-bound zymogen granules. Most enzymes, except amylase and lipase, are secreted as proenzymes to prevent pancreatic injury. In particular, trypsin activation is tightly controlled because of its central role in activation of other enzymes. Consequently, the proenzyme trypsinogen is not normally activated until it enters the lumen of the duodenum through duodenal enteropeptidase. In addition, the chance of inappropriate trypsin activation in acinar cells or ducts of the pancreas is reduced by secretion of protective trypsin inhibitors. In circumstances in which trypsin or other enzymes are inappropriately activated, there are several other defenses in place. Acinar cells have an innate resistance to several of the digestive enzymes. Intrapancreatic release of active enzymes triggers the release of other enzymes that degrade the offending digestive enzymes, and lysosomal enzymes can degrade the zymogen granules when the pancreatic secretion is disturbed, reducing the burden of potentially injurious enzymes.

DISORDERS OF THE LIVER AND BILIARY SYSTEM OF DOMESTIC ANIMALS

DEVELOPMENTAL ANOMALIES AND INCIDENTAL FINDINGS

Developmental anomalies of the liver occur in domestic animals, although most are of little consequence.

Congenital Biliary Cysts

Congenital biliary cysts are found within the livers of dogs, cats, and pigs, but presumably all domestic species can be affected. The cysts are usually an incidental finding and can be found in animals of any age. Grossly, the cysts can be single or multiple and are filled with clear fluid (Fig. 8-24). Histologically, cysts have a thin wall lined by a single layer of biliary epithelium. Congenital cysts must be distinguished from parasitic cysts, particularly cysticerci, because they also have a thin wall and are fluid-filled. The presence of the larval cestode within parasitic cysts assists in distinguishing the two structures.

Multiple cysts that affect extensive areas of the liver occur in cats and occasionally dogs and are thought to represent developmental anomalies of the intrahepatic bile ducts. There are several types of these anomalies, which are collectively termed *ductal plate malformations.* Congenital polycystic disease, characterized by numerous epithelial-lined cysts in the liver, kidneys, and occasionally the pancreas, occurs in dogs, with Cairn terriers and West Highland white terriers predisposed; cats, with Persian cats believed to have a higher risk for the disorder; and goats and lambs. Affected animals can die of either liver or renal failure.

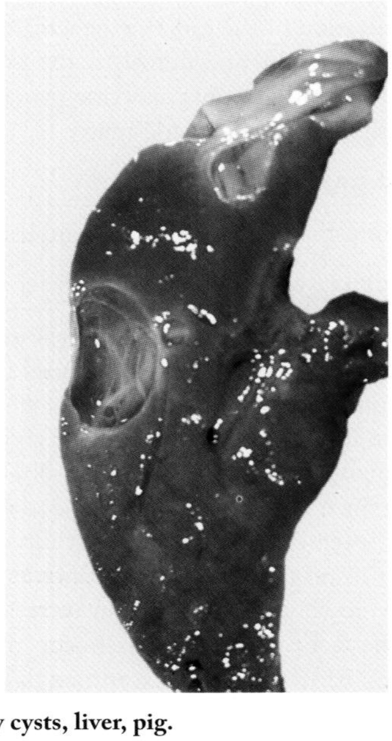

Fig. 8-24 Biliary cysts, liver, pig.
Multiple biliary cysts within the liver of a pig. Unilocular cysts replace a portion of the parenchyma in the affected portion of the liver. (Courtesy Dr. J. King, College of Veterinary Medicine, Cornell University.)

Hepatic Displacement

Displacement of the liver into the thoracic cavity, called a *diaphragmatic hernia,* can occur when there is a defect in the diaphragm. A congenital malformation that leaves an opening in the diaphragm or a traumatic event that ruptures the diaphragm can cause this condition.

Tension Lipidosis (Steatosis)

Discrete, pale areas of parenchyma at the liver margins are common in cattle and horses (Fig. 8-25). These foci typically occur adjacent to the insertion of a ligament (serosal) attachment, and it is proposed that these attachments impede blood supply to the subjacent hepatic parenchyma by exerting tension on the capsule. Affected hepatocytes most probably accumulate fat within their cytoplasm (steatosis) as a consequence of hypoxia. The lesions are of no functional significance.

Capsular Fibrosis

Discrete fibrous tags or plaques are frequently present on the diaphragmatic surface of the liver and on the adjacent diaphragm of the horse (Fig. 8-26). Larval nematode migration tracts were originally believed to be the cause of this lesion, but this pathogenesis seems less likely in view of the widespread use of anti-parasitic treatments and the continued evidence of the lesion. Resolution of nonseptic peritonitis, possibly as a result of contact between the diaphragm and the adjacent liver capsule, has now been proposed as the cause of these regions of capsular fibrosis.

Postmortem Change

Autolysis of the liver occurs rapidly and can be advanced before it is obvious in most other tissue. At or just before death, bacteria are released from the gastrointestinal tract into the portal circulation and reach the liver where they proliferate rapidly after death. This process is especially rapid in large animals during hot weather—particularly cattle, in which fermentation in the adjacent rumen produces heat—and in pigs, which are often well insulated by fat.

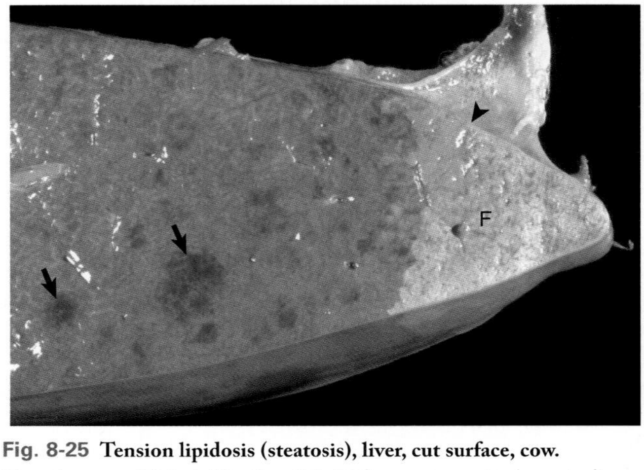

Fig. 8-25 Tension lipidosis (steatosis), liver, cut surface, cow.
Note the area of fatty infiltration *(F),* the ligamentous attachment adjacent to the affected portion *(arrowhead),* and the areas of telangiectasis *(arrows).* (Courtesy College of Veterinary Medicine, North Carolina State University.)

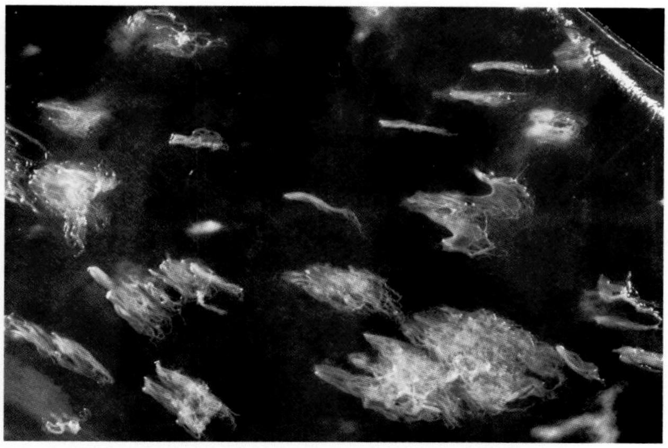

Fig. 8-26 Capsular fibrosis, liver, horse.
Numerous fibrous tags are present on the diaphragmatic surface of the liver. The cause of these tags is not clear. (Courtesy College of Veterinary Medicine, North Carolina State University.)

Pale areas appear on the capsular surface as bacterial degradation begins. In time, the organ becomes green-blue as bacteria degrade blood pigments to iron sulfide. The liver in contact with the gallbladder is quickly discolored by bile pigment, which passes through the wall of the gallbladder. The consistency of the organ becomes puttylike and gas bubbles may form beneath the capsule and in the parenchyma from bacterial fermentation. Postmortem changes are covered in detail in Chapter 1.

MORPHOLOGIC CLASSIFICATION OF HEPATOBILIARY DISEASE

The nature and distribution of inflammatory lesions in the liver are usually dictated by the route of entry, the host inflammatory response, the nature of the infectious agent (e.g., virus, bacterium, or fungus), and any predilection they have for involvement with a particular cell type in the liver. The hematogenous route of infection tends to cause a random multifocal distribution of lesions. Infections, usually bacterial, that ascend the biliary tract are typically centered in the bile ducts. Severe infections may affect the entire portal tract and extend into the adjacent parenchyma. Penetrating wounds cause discrete areas of inflammation with or without necrosis that are evident on the capsule and extend into the hepatic parenchyma. Liver injury should be characterized by the pattern of involvement (multifocal random, zonal, or massive), type of inflammatory cells involved (neutrophils, lymphocytes, plasma cells, eosinophils, or macrophages), evidence of necrosis or fibrosis, severity of these processes, evidence of regeneration, and the presence of an etiologic agent or agents. The type of inflammatory response and the duration of the injury can help identify the infectious agents.

Acute Hepatitis

Inflammation of the liver parenchyma is termed *hepatitis.* Acute hepatitis is characterized by inflammation, hepatocellular necrosis, and apoptosis. The proportion and type of inflammatory cells involved varies considerably, depending on the cause of inflammation, the host response, and the stage or age of the lesion. Characterization of the type of inflammation usually requires microscopic evaluation. In many forms of acute hepatitis, particularly bacterial and protozoal infections, neutrophils accumulate in response to the usual chemotactic stimuli. Random foci of neutrophilic hepatitis, as a consequence of embolic localization of bacteria, are relatively common in all species. In neonates—especially calves, lambs, and foals—bacteria, such as *Escherichia coli,* usually seed the liver via the umbilical veins or less often the portal venous or hepatic arterial systems. Acute hepatitis produced by viral infections, such as herpesvirus infection in many species, is more frequently characterized by a random distribution of necrosis and apoptosis with minimal inflammation or infiltrations of lymphocytes.

Chronic Hepatitis

Chronic hepatitis results when there is continued inflammation as a result of persistence of an antigenic stimulus. In the absence of such a stimulus, inflammation rapidly resolves. Chronic hepatitis is characterized by fibrosis; accumulation of mononuclear inflammatory cells, including lymphocytes, macrophages, and plasma cells, and frequently, regeneration. Neutrophils often are present in chronic unresolved hepatic inflammation such as that which characterizes some forms of canine chronic hepatitis. The proportion and distribution of each of these elements varies with the inciting cause and host response. Local variation within the liver can also occur.

Different terms are used to distinguish separate types of chronic hepatitis. Granulomatous hepatitis may be obvious grossly if it produces discrete granulomas of sufficient size. These may be focal or diffuse. Chronic suppurative hepatitis is usually manifested as discrete or multiple abscesses. Focal lesions, such as abscesses or granulomas, often are sufficiently localized so that they do not alter hepatic function. In contrast, diffuse and severe chronic hepatitis, as seen in dogs, usually leads to loss of hepatic parenchyma and architectural distortion of the liver as a consequence of fibrosis and nodular parenchymal regeneration. This process can proceed to end-stage hepatic disease with hepatic failure and its associated constellation of clinical signs. The form of chronic hepatitis that has been referred to as chronic active hepatitis is discussed in a separate section next.

Nonspecific Reactive Hepatitis

Nonspecific reactive hepatitis is a diffuse process distributed throughout the liver in response to some systemic illness, most often the gastrointestinal tract, or is the residuum of prior liver inflammation. Typically, there is a mild inflammatory infiltrate in the portal tract and possibly the parenchyma without evidence of necrosis. In acute cases, there is a minimal-to-mild infiltrate of neutrophils within the connective tissue of the portal tracts that may vary in intensity. Mononuclear cells, primarily lymphocytes and plasma cells, predominate in more chronic manifestations. Pigmented macrophages containing hemosiderin, lipofuscin, or both may be scattered throughout the parenchyma. Mononuclear inflammatory cells may also be evident within the hepatic parenchyma and at the periphery of central veins. Kupffer cells are usually reactive (i.e., they appear somewhat swollen because of abundant cytoplasm and display prominent nuclei as well).

Cholangitis

Inflammation of the biliary ducts (either intrahepatic or extrahepatic) is termed *cholangitis.* There are several patterns of cholangitis. The inflammatory cell population and the degree of fibrosis will vary with the type and duration of injury. Specific forms of cholangitis are discussed below.

Neutrophilic Cholangitis

Neutrophilic (suppurative) cholangitis is the most common type of cholangitis. It is characterized by the presence of neutrophils within

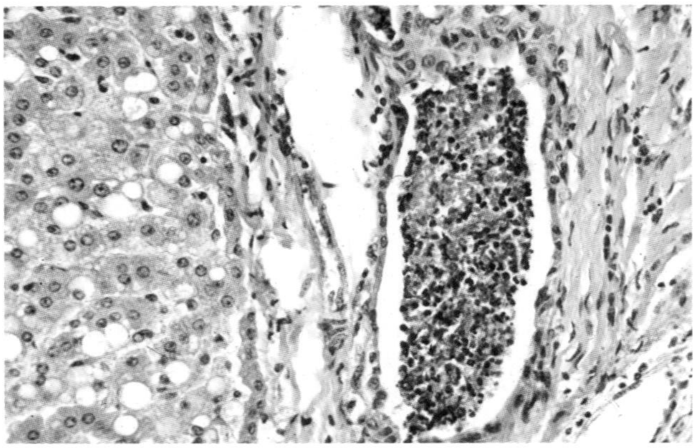

Fig. 8-27 Neutrophilic cholangitis (intrahepatic), liver, cat. This condition is characterized by the presence of degenerate neutrophils within the lumen or the walls of bile ducts in the portal areas. Ascending bacterial infection from the intestine via the common bile duct is the most common cause. H&E stain. (Courtesy Dr. M.D. McGavin, College of Veterinary Medicine, University of Tennessee.)

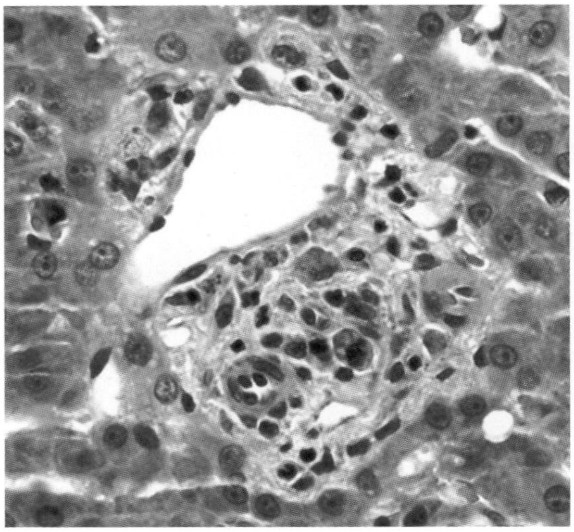

Fig. 8-28 Destructive cholangitis, liver, dog. This condition is an uncommon disorder characterized by the destruction of bile duct epithelium, followed by regeneration in some instances. Necrotic or absent biliary epithelium, pigmented macrophages, and small numbers of mononuclear inflammatory cells in portal tracts are the typical histologic findings. H&E stain. (Courtesy Dr. J.M. Cullen, College of Veterinary Medicine, North Carolina State University.)

the lumen or the epithelium of the bile ducts (Fig. 8-27). Acute and chronic forms of this process can occur. Fibrosis and the addition of mononuclear inflammatory cells are characteristic of the chronic form. Rupture of affected bile ducts can lead to hepatic abscess formation. Most neutrophilic cholangitis is believed to be caused by ascending bacterial infections from the intestine. Bacterial culture from bile most often reveals infection with *Escherichia coli, Enterococcus, Bacteroides, Streptococcus,* or *Clostridium.*

Lymphocytic Cholangitis

Lymphocytic cholangitis occurs most often in cats and is described in detail in the section on Disorders of Cats.

Destructive Cholangitis

Destructive cholangitis is an uncommon syndrome characterized by necrosis of the epithelium of bile ducts (Fig. 8-28). Inflammation is often present around the areas of biliary destruction, but within the portal area. Certain chemicals, such as trimethoprim sulfa, have been implicated in this syndrome in dogs.

Cholangiohepatitis

Inflammation that affects the biliary ducts and hepatic parenchyma is termed *cholangiohepatitis.* In most cases of intrahepatic disease, the primary focus of inflammation can be identified as affecting either the hepatocytes or the biliary tree, but on occasion, both components of the liver are affected, usually as an extension of biliary disease, such as neutrophilic cholangitis, to involve the periportal hepatocytes; in that circumstance the term *cholangiohepatitis* should be used.

CIRCULATORY DISORDERS

Disturbances of Outflow

Passive Congestion (Acute and Chronic)

Passive congestion of the liver can occur in any species and is almost always the consequence of cardiac dysfunction. Right-sided heart failure produces elevated pressure within the caudal vena cava that later involves the hepatic vein and its tributaries. Chronic passive congestion is particularly common in aged dogs and occurs secondary to endocardiosis (mucoid degeneration) of the right atrioventricular valve. Acute passive congestion, on the other hand, can

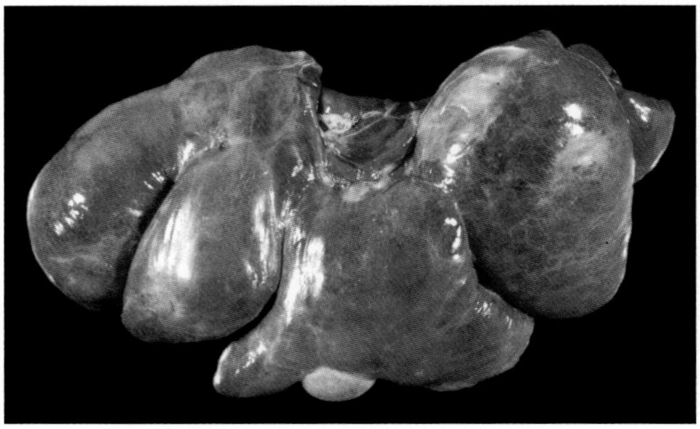

Fig. 8-29 Chronic passive congestion, liver, dog. Chronic passive hepatic congestion in the liver of a dog with a heart base tumor that impeded venous return to the heart. The liver is enlarged with rounded margins. (Courtesy College of Veterinary Medicine, North Carolina State University.)

occur as a consequence of acute right-sided heart failure, which has a wide variety of causes.

The appearance of the liver differs with the duration and severity of the congestion. Passive congestion initially causes distention of central veins and centrilobular sinusoids. Persistent centrilobular hypoxia leads to atrophy or loss of hepatocytes and eventually to centrilobular fibrosis. Fibrosis of the central vein (phlebosclerosis) may also occur.

Acute congestion of the liver produces slight enlargement of the organ, and blood flows freely from any cut surface. The intrinsic lobular pattern of the liver may be slightly more pronounced, particularly on the cut surface, because centrilobular areas are congested (dark red) in contrast to the more normal color of the remainder of the lobule.

Diffuse enlargement and rounded edges of liver lobes are the main features of chronic passive congestion (Fig. 8-29). Chronic

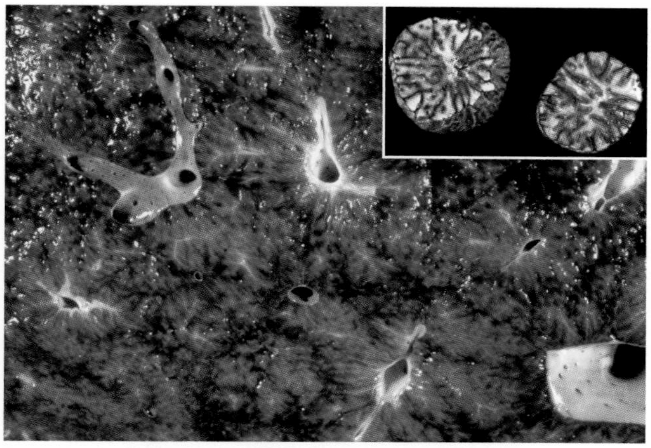

Fig. 8-30 **Chronic passive congestion (nutmeg liver), liver, cut surface, cow.**
The congestion in the centrilobular areas and the peripheral lipid accumulation give the liver a characteristic appearance that has been likened to that of the cut surface of a nutmeg, hence the term nutmeg liver. *Inset,* Cut surface of a nutmeg for comparison. (Figure courtesy Dr. D.A. Mosier, College of Veterinary Medicine, Kansas State University. Inset courtesy Dr. M.O. Howard, College of Veterinary Medicine, Iowa State University; and Noah's Arkive, College of Veterinary Medicine, The University of Georgia.)

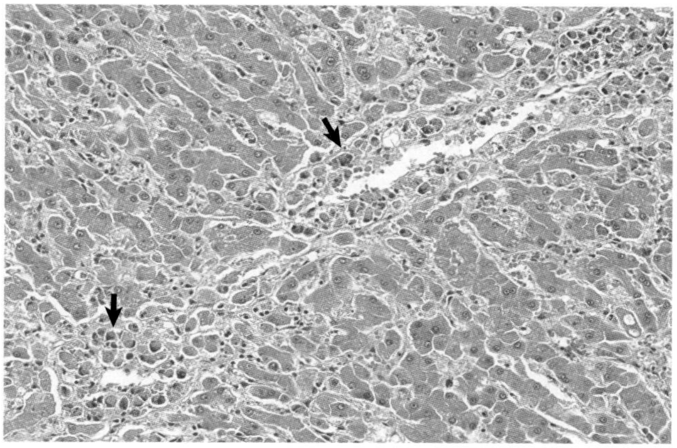

Fig. 8-31 **Chronic passive congestion, liver, dog.**
The liver is firm because of hepatic fibrosis that is most severe in centrilobular areas *(arrows).* The central vein is surrounded by a mild amount of connective tissue from which fine fibrous septa extend out into the lobule. Note the macrophages containing hemosiderin, the result of erythrocyte breakdown in this area as a result of chronic congestion. H&E stain. (Courtesy Dr. J.M. Cullen, College of Veterinary Medicine, North Carolina State University.)

passive congestion leads to persistent hypoxia in centrilobular areas and because of oxygen and nutrient deprivation, the centrilobular hepatocytes atrophy, degenerate, or eventually may undergo necrosis. As a result, sinusoids in these areas are dilated and congested and grossly appear red, whereas periportal hepatocytes frequently undergo steatosis (fatty degeneration) because of hypoxia, thereby causing this area of the lobule to appear yellow. The result is accentuation of the lobular pattern of the liver, referred to as an *enhanced lobular* or *reticular pattern.* It is especially evident on the cut surface of the liver, and the enhanced lobular pattern that occurs with severe chronic passive congestion has been likened to the appearance of the cut surface of a nutmeg and is termed *nutmeg liver* (Fig. 8-30). This pattern is not unique to passive congestion, however, and is encountered with other processes such as zonal hepatic necrosis. In addition to an enhanced lobular pattern, chronic passive congestion is characterized by focal fibrous thickening of the capsule and in severe cases, widespread hepatic fibrosis that bridges between central veins (Fig. 8-31).

Hepatic Veno-Occlusive Disease

Intimal thickening and occlusion of the central vein by fibrous connective tissue characterize the distinctive lesions of this syndrome. The consequence is passive hepatic congestion and resultant hepatic injury, which may progress to hepatic failure and its associated constellation of signs. The lesion is not etiologically specific but can follow pyrrolizidine alkaloid or aflatoxin-induced hepatic injury. An extremely high incidence is recognized in captive exotic cats, such as cheetahs, possibly because of the ingestion of large amounts of vitamin A, although the mechanism for this lesion is not known.

Disturbances of Blood Flow into the Liver

Anemia

The centrilobular (periacinar) regions of the lobule receive blood last; thus it is the least oxygenated, and the effects of hypoxia are usually manifested first in this area. Acute severe anemia, regardless of cause, can cause centrilobular or paracentral degeneration and even necrosis of hepatocytes. This typically occurs in severe anemias of precipitous onset. Chronic anemia can cause atrophy of centrilobular hepatocytes, which results in dilation and congestion of sinusoids (Fig. 8-32). Livers from animals with severe anemia, whether acute or chronic, typically have an enhanced lobular pattern that is evident on both the capsular and cut surfaces of the organ.

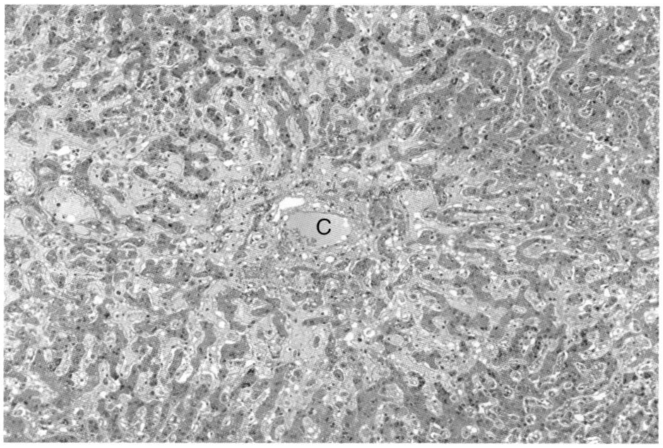

Fig. 8-32 **Centrilobular hepatocyte atrophy, liver, dog.**
In chronic anemia, centrilobular hepatocytes, which are the last hepatocytes in the lobule to receive oxygenated blood, become atrophic, and as a consequence, their sinusoids are more dilated. *C,* Central vein. H&E stain. (Courtesy Dr. J.M. Cullen, College of Veterinary Medicine, North Carolina State University.)

Congenital Portosystemic Shunts

A congenital portosystemic shunt is an abnormal vascular channel that allows blood within the portal venous system to bypass the liver and to drain into the systemic circulation. A congenital shunt can be either intrahepatic or extrahepatic in location but is usually limited to a single relatively large-caliber vessel (Fig. 8-33, *A*). A variety of different shunts have been described. Typically, intrahepatic portosystemic shunts involve failure of closure of the ductus

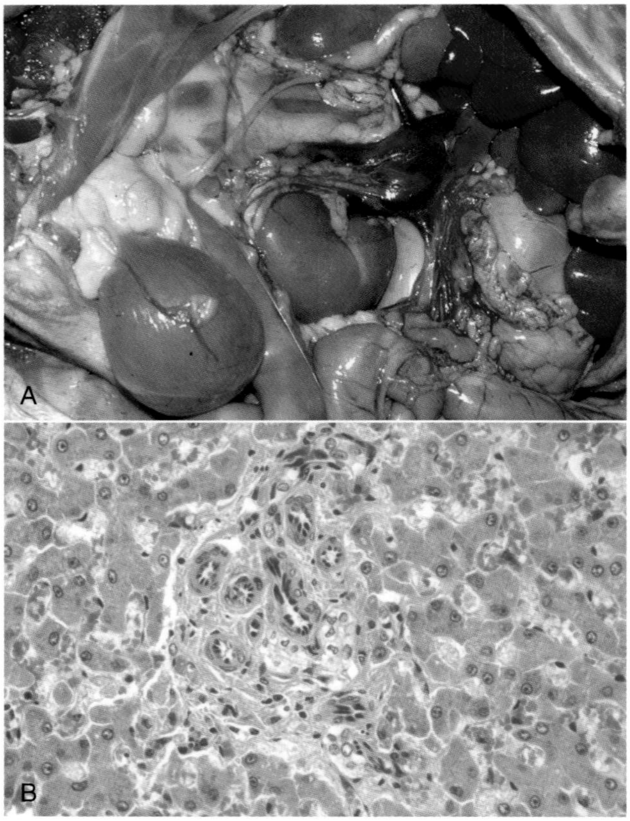

Fig. 8-33 Portosystemic shunts, liver, dog.
A, A single anomalous vessel that connects the portal circulation with the systemic circulation is the characteristic lesion of congenital portosystemic shunt. Note the small size but normal color of the liver (up under the rib cage). **B,** Congenital portosystemic shunt. Portal areas are abnormal because they lack a portal vein and contain numerous small-caliber arterioles. H&E stain. (**A** courtesy Dr. J. Sagartz, College of Veterinary Medicine, The Ohio State University; and Noah's Arkive, College of Veterinary Medicine, The University of Georgia. **B** courtesy Dr. J.M. Cullen, College of Veterinary Medicine, North Carolina State University.)

venosus at birth. The ductus venosus is a normal fetal vessel that conducts blood from the portal vein to the caudal vena cava. Intrahepatic shunts, such as the patent ductus venosus, are most often located in the left side of the liver and occur most commonly in large breed dogs. Extrahepatic congenital shunts, such as portal vein to caudal vena cava anastomoses and portal vein to azygous vein anastomoses, occur more often in small breeds of dogs and cats. Shunts have been described in several species but occur most commonly in the dog and cat. Affected animals are typically stunted and frequently develop signs of hepatic encephalopathy. The liver is small and may have a characteristic histologic appearance of lobular atrophy, reduplication of arterioles, and small or absent portal veins within the portal tracts (Fig. 8-33, *B*). Studies have shown that the histologic appearance of the liver in animals with congenital portosystemic shunts is not a good prognostic indicator. The portal vein pressure is normal in congenital shunts and ascites does not occur. Abnormal vascular anastomoses are often difficult to identify without benefit of antemortem imaging studies. Affected dogs frequently have abnormal plasma ammonia concentrations and as a consequence, pass ammonium biurate crystals in their urine (Fig. 8-34). It should be noted that the liver has a stereotypic response to inadequate portal vein perfusion. Thus the

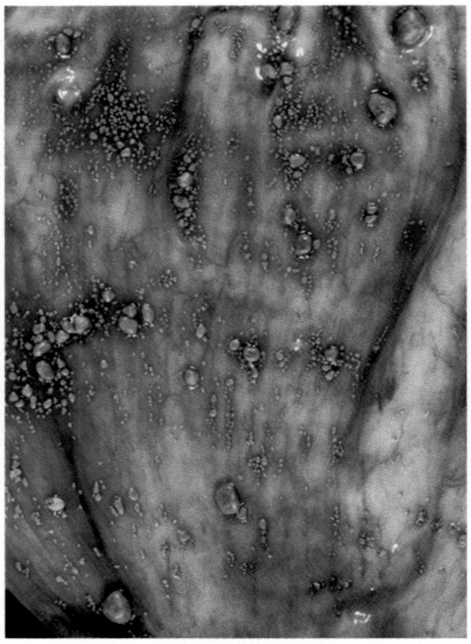

Fig. 8-34 Ammonium biurate crystals, urinary bladder, dog.
The bladder contains ammonium biurate crystals. These crystals can result from abnormal ammonia metabolism in dogs with portosystemic vascular anastomoses. (Courtesy College of Veterinary Medicine, North Carolina State University.)

histologic appearance of congenital portosystemic shunts and other vascular anomalies of the liver (discussed later) have considerable overlap. Clinical data, such as the presence or absence of shunt vessels and the determination of portal vein pressure, may be necessary to achieve a final diagnosis.

Portal Hypertension

Increased pressure within the portal vein can arise from disturbances of venous blood flow in any of the following three sites:

- Prehepatic
- Intrahepatic
- Posthepatic

Prehepatic portal hypertension is relatively uncommon and occurs when blood flow through the portal vein is impaired before it enters the liver. Portal vein thrombosis can be induced by damage to the portal vein, by local inflammatory disorders, including pancreatitis, or by hypercoagulable states. Tumor emboli can also obstruct the portal vein. External compression by tumors or abscesses can restrict or obstruct portal vein flow as well. Portal vein hypoplasia (discussed later) affecting the extrahepatic segment of the portal vein is another cause.

Intrahepatic portal hypertension arises from increased resistance to blood flow to or within the sinusoids. Chronic liver disease that typically results in bridging collagenous septa, loss of normal lobular architecture, and regenerative nodule formation is the most common intrahepatic cause of portal hypertension. Sinusoidal fibrosis from diseases, such as lobular dissecting hepatitis, is another cause. Disorders, such as veno-occlusive disease, amyloidosis, and schistosomiasis, and other granulomatous disease processes can also produce intrahepatic portal hypertension. Arteriovenous fistulae (discussed later) within the hepatic parenchyma can also lead to intrahepatic portal hypertension.

Posthepatic causes of portal hypertension are uncommon and include any abnormalities that lead to increased resistance to venous outflow in the hepatic vein or adjacent vena cava. Partial or complete thrombosis of the hepatic veins (Budd-Chiari syndrome) or of the adjacent caudal vena cava are the most likely, although

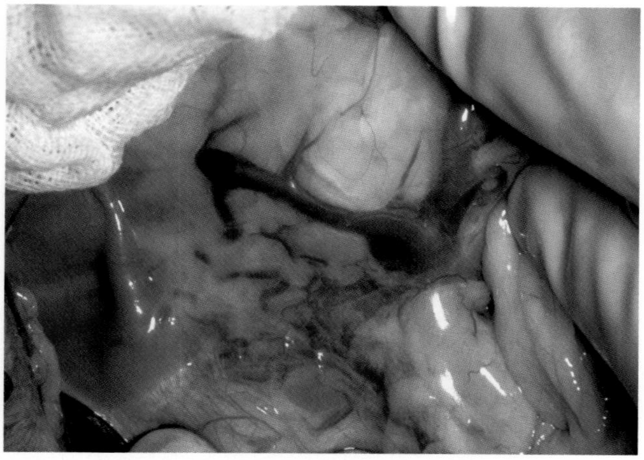

Fig. 8-35 Acquired portosystemic anastomoses, abdomen, dog. Acquired portosystemic anastomoses secondary to portal hypertension (in this case as a consequence of chronic hepatitis in a dog). The numerous prominent veins that are present over the surface of the kidney allow blood within the portal venous system to bypass the liver and directly enter the systemic circulation. (Courtesy Dr. L. Hardy, College of Veterinary Medicine, North Carolina State University.)

uncommon, causes of posthepatic portal hypertension. Congestive heart failure can also lead to portal hypertension.

Regardless of cause, persistent portal hypertension can lead to acquired portosystemic shunts with the exception of passive congestion, which rarely, if ever, results in the development of shunt vessels. These shunts are usually numerous and composed of distended thin-walled veins, which may connect the mesenteric veins and the caudal vena cava (Fig. 8-35). Ascites is common in conditions that develop acquired shunts because of the associated portal hypertension.

Vascular Anomalies that May Produce Portal Hypertension

Intrahepatic arteriovenous shunts (anastomoses)

Arteriovenous shunts, either acquired or congenital, occur in the dog and cat and are direct communications between the hepatic artery and branches of the portal vein. They may occur anywhere within the liver. Affected portions of the liver contain convoluted thick-walled arteries and distended portal vein branches. Shunting of blood may lead to portal hypertension or reversal of the direction of portal blood flow, subsequent development of acquired portocaval shunts, and ascites. Clinical signs vary in intensity, most likely in relationship to the caliber of vessels that are affected, and are probably the result of the degree of portosystemic shunting of blood.

Portal vein hypoplasia (microvascular dysplasia, noncirrhotic portal hypertension)

Portal vein hypoplasia is a congenital vascular anomaly that occurs in dogs and occasionally in cats. It is characterized by abnormally small extrahepatic or intrahepatic portal veins, which result in diminished hepatic perfusion by the portal vein blood flow and the potential for portal hypertension. Typically, affected animals have small livers and the typical histologic pattern of portal vein hypoperfusion: small or absent portal veins, proliferated hepatic arterioles (so-called reduplication), and hepatocyte atrophy. This disorder resembles portosystemic shunts histologically, but affected animals often have portal hypertension and resultant ascites. Portal

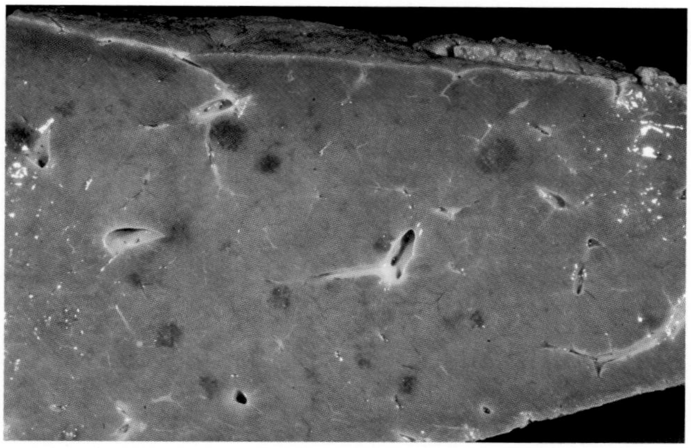

Fig. 8-36 Telangiectasia, liver, cut surface, cow. Telangiectasia is a condition in which hepatic sinusoids become dilated and filled with blood. These lesions can be seen as dark red areas on the cut and capsular surface of the liver. (Courtesy Dr. M.D. McGavin, College of Veterinary Medicine, University of Tennessee.)

fibrosis and biliary hyperplasia occur in about half of the cases. Because of the histologic similarities between portal vein hypoplasia and congenital portosystemic shunts, clinical data, such as imaging studies to determine the presence of a shunt vessel, are often required to make a final diagnosis from biopsy material.

Incidental Vascular Disorders

Telangiectasis

Telangiectasis is the notable dilation of sinusoids in areas where hepatocytes have been lost. Grossly, these areas appear as variably sized dark red-blue foci within the liver that vary from pinpoint to several centimeters in size (Fig. 8-36). Telangiectasis is particularly common in cattle and apparently is of no clinical significance. It also occurs in old cats, in which it can be mistaken for vascular tumors such as hemangioma or hemangiosarcoma. Histologically, there is ectasia of the sinusoidal space and a loss of hepatocytes. There is no evidence of inflammation or fibrosis associated with this lesion.

Infarction

Infarction of the liver occurs infrequently because of the organ's dual blood supply from the hepatic artery and portal vein. Infarcts are usually sharply delineated and may be either dark red when acute or pale as they age. They tend to occur at the margins of the liver, the terminal end of parenchymal perfusion, and can affect small wedges of only a few centimeters in length or larger portions of a lobe. The cut surface of infarcted liver tends to be dry and granular. Histologically, infarcted liver is characterized by a zone of coagulative necrosis bordered by a basophilic band of inflammatory cells and an outer band of hyperemia (Fig. 8-37). Torsion of individual lobes of the liver, which occurs infrequently, can result in vascular occlusion and infarction of the affected lobe.

METABOLIC DISTURBANCES AND HEPATIC ACCUMULATIONS

Hepatocellular Steatosis (Lipidosis)

Lipids are normally transported to the liver from adipose tissue and the gastrointestinal tract in the form of either free fatty acids or chylomicrons, respectively. Within hepatocytes, free fatty acids are esterified to triglycerides, converted to cholesterol or phospholipids. Some oxidation of fatty acids to ketone bodies for energy production occurs within hepatocytes. Triglycerides can be complexed

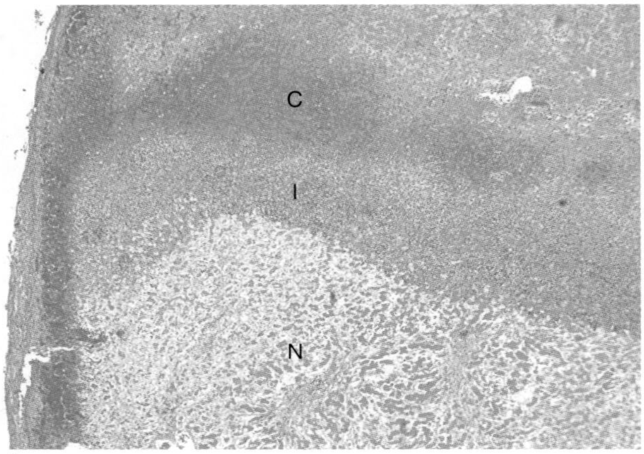

Fig. 8-37 Hepatic infarction, liver, dog.
Hepatic infarction is uncommon and usually occurs at the margins of the liver where the terminal divisions of the blood supply are found. Infarction of the liver is characterized by a zone of coagulative necrosis *(N)* rimmed with inflammatory cells *(I)* and an outer zone of congestion *(C)* in the viable liver. H&E stain. (Courtesy Dr. J.M. Cullen, College of Veterinary Medicine, North Carolina State University.)

with apoproteins to form low-density lipoproteins, and these are released into the plasma as a readily available energy source for use by a variety of tissues. With the exception of ruminants, the liver also actively produces lipids from amino acids and glucose.

The presence of excessive lipid within the liver is termed *lipidosis* or steatosis (also known as fatty liver or fatty change) and occurs when the rate of triglyceride accumulation within hepatocytes exceeds either their rate of metabolic degradation or their release as lipoproteins. Hepatocellular steatosis is obviously not a specific disease entity but can occur as a sequel to a variety of perturbations of normal lipid metabolism. The potential mechanisms responsible for excessive accumulation of fat within the liver include the following:

1. Excessive entry of fatty acids into the liver, which occurs as a consequence of excessive dietary intake of fat or increased mobilization of triglycerides from adipose tissue because of increased demand (e.g., lactation, starvation, and endocrine abnormalities).
2. Excessive dietary intake of carbohydrates results in the synthesis of increased amounts of fatty acids with formation of excessive triglycerides within hepatocytes.
3. Abnormal hepatocyte function leads to accumulation of triglycerides within hepatocytes as a result of decreased energy for oxidation of fatty acids as in hypoxia or mitochondrial damage impairing oxidation of fatty acids.
4. Increased esterification of fatty acids to triglycerides in response to increased concentrations of glucose and insulin, which stimulate the rate of triglyceride synthesis from glucose or from prolonged increases in dietary chylomicrons.
5. Decreased apoprotein synthesis and subsequent decreased production and export of lipoprotein from hepatocytes.
6. Impaired secretion of lipoprotein from the liver because of secretory defects produced by hepatotoxins or drugs.

It must be stressed that these are potential mechanisms (some being more significant than others, depending on the condition of the animal) and that more than one defect might occur in any given hepatic disorder. Regardless of cause, the gross appearance of the hepatocellular steatosis is highly characteristic. With progressive accumulation of lipid, the liver enlarges and becomes yellow (Fig. 8-38, *A*). In mild cases, lipids may only accumulate in specific portions of each lobule, such as centrilobular regions, thereby imparting an enhanced lobular pattern to the liver. In extreme cases, the entire liver is affected, and the organ may become considerably enlarged and have an extremely greasy texture. Histologically, hepatocellular lipid appears as a clear round vacuole. The vacuoles are clear because lipid is removed in routine processing of tissue for histologic review. Macrovesicular steatosis is most common and is characterized by large vacuoles that displace the nucleus of the hepatocyte (Fig. 8-38, *B*). Microvesicular steatosis has multiple small, round, and clear vacuoles that do not displace the nucleus and can be associated with significant hepatocellular dysfunction. Frozen sections and special stains, such as Oil Red O, are employed to identify lipid.

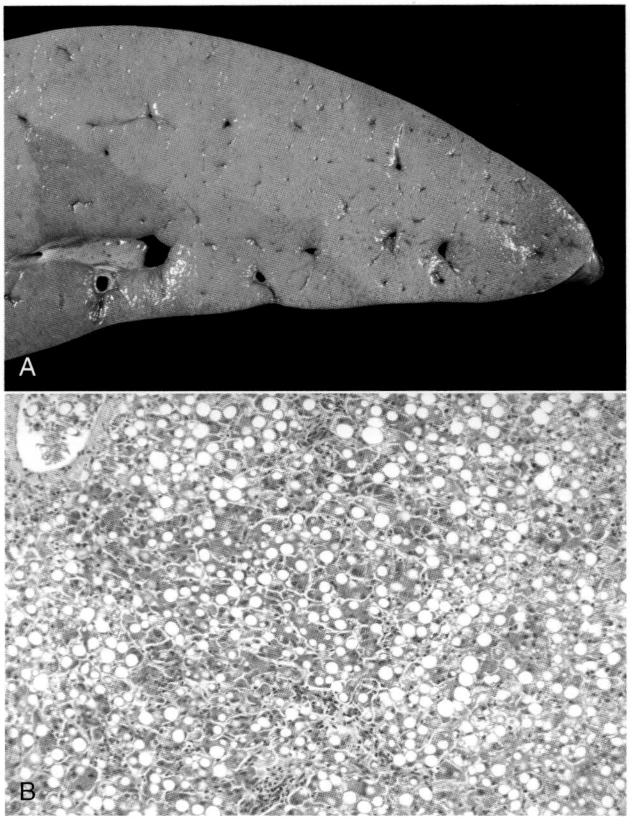

Fig. 8-38 Fatty liver syndrome (hepatic steatosis).
A, Cut surface, cow. The liver is swollen and yellow because of notable infiltration of lipid into hepatocytes. **B,** Steatosis or fatty degeneration, cat. Diffuse cytoplasmic accumulation of lipid is evident within the hepatocytes throughout the liver. H&E stain. (**A** courtesy Dr. M.D. McGavin, College of Veterinary Medicine, University of Tennessee. **B** courtesy Dr. J.M. Cullen, College of Veterinary Medicine, North Carolina State University.)

Specific causes and syndromes of hepatocellular steatosis in domestic animals include the following:

1. Dietary causes of hepatocellular steatosis include simple dietary excess in monogastric animals, such as a high-fat and/or high-cholesterol diet. Dietary deficiencies of cobalt and vitamin B_{12} have been implicated as causes of fatty liver in sheep and goats.
2. Toxic and anoxic causes of hepatocellular steatosis are common. Sublethal (reversible) injury to hepatocytes frequently results in accumulation of lipid within the affected cell.

3. Ketosis is a metabolic disease that results from impaired metabolism of carbohydrate and volatile fatty acids. In times of energy demand, free fatty acids are released from body fat stores, and the free fatty acids are esterified into fatty acyl CoA in the liver. Ketone bodies (acetoacetic acid and β-hydroxybutyric acid) are derived from fatty acyl CoA by oxidation in the mitochondria. In pregnant and lactating animals, there is a continuous demand for glucose and amino acids, and ketosis results when fat metabolism, which occurs in response to the increased energy demands, becomes excessive. Ketosis is characterized by increased concentrations of ketone bodies in blood (hyperketonemia), hypoglycemia, and low concentrations of hepatic glycogen. Ketosis is common in ruminants and usually occurs during peak lactation, whereas ketosis of sheep usually occurs in late gestation, particularly in ewes carrying twins; this latter disease is known as pregnancy toxemia.
4. Bovine fatty liver syndrome, also known as *fatty liver disease,* is mechanistically similar to ketosis and is especially common in ruminants with high energy demands. In dairy cattle, the disease is usually encountered in obese animals in late gestation, within a few days after parturition or peak lactation and is often precipitated by an event that causes anorexia such as retained placenta, metritis, mastitis, abomasal displacement, or parturient paresis. Typically, affected beef cattle are obese and the disease occurs within a few days before parturition. Accumulation of lipid within the liver is the result of both increased mobilization of lipids from adipose tissue, which results in increased influx of fatty acids to the liver, and in severe cases, defective hepatocytic function, which results in decreased export of lipoprotein from the liver.
5. Feline fatty liver syndrome is a distinct syndrome of idiopathic hepatocellular steatosis recognized in cats. Typically, affected cats are obese and anorectic and have no other diseases that could cause hepatocellular steatosis. Cats with this type of hepatocellular steatosis frequently develop hepatic failure, icterus, and subsequently hepatic encephalopathy.
6. Hepatocellular steatosis occurs in ponies, miniatures horses, and donkeys. Shetland ponies are predisposed. The condition usually occurs in overweight pregnant or lactating mares, characteristically after an event that causes stress or anorexia. In addition to notable hepatocellular steatosis, affected ponies are usually hyperlipemic and may also manifest signs of renal failure and hepatic rupture. In severe cases, hepatic encephalopathy and/or terminal DIC can occur.
7. Endocrine disorders, such as diabetes mellitus and hypothyroidism, can produce hepatocellular steatosis in a variety of species. In these cases, hepatocellular steatosis is obviously but one manifestation of abnormal metabolism. The accumulation of lipids in the liver in the diabetic animal is the result of increased fat mobilization and decreased use of lipids by injured hepatocytes.

Glycogen Accumulation

Glucose is normally stored within hepatocytes as glycogen and is often present in large amounts after feeding. Excessive hepatic accumulation of glycogen occurs with metabolic perturbations involving glucose regulation, including diabetes mellitus and the glycogen storage diseases. In these instances, hepatic involvement is just one manifestation of a systemic disease process. Excessive hepatic accumulation of glycogen is also observed in dogs secondary to excess glucocorticoids, and is explained further in the section on liver diseases in dogs.

Grossly, glycogen accumulation in the liver can lead to variable degrees of pallor and swelling. Microscopically, hepatocytes are swollen with lacy vacuolated cytoplasm. Unlike lipid vacuoles, glycogen vacuoles are poorly defined and hepatocyte nuclei are not displaced to the periphery of the cell.

LYSOSOMAL STORAGE DISEASES

Vacuolation of hepatocytes and Kupffer cells can be observed in several types of lysosomal storage diseases. This lesion is most often seen in addition to vacuolation of neurons, other macrophages and/or other cells. Affected animals are usually young and have an abnormal pattern of growth and development.

AMYLOIDOSIS

Hepatic amyloidosis occurs in most species of domestic animals. Amyloidosis is not a single disease entity but a term used for various diseases that lead to the deposition of proteins that are composed of β-pleated sheets of nonbranching fibrils. Affected livers are enlarged, friable, and pale (Fig. 8-39, *A*). Histologically, hepatic amyloid appears as bright eosinophilic amorphous deposits that are usually found in the space of Disse along the sinusoids but can be found in the portal tracts and within blood vessel walls (Fig. 8-39, *B*). Amyloid physical properties are responsible for its birefringence and characteristic apple green appearance in Congo red–stained sections viewed under polarized light. As many as 15 distinct amyloid proteins have been identified, but the hepatic amyloid is usually derived from one of three types. In primary amyloidosis, the amyloid fibril is designated AL (amyloid light

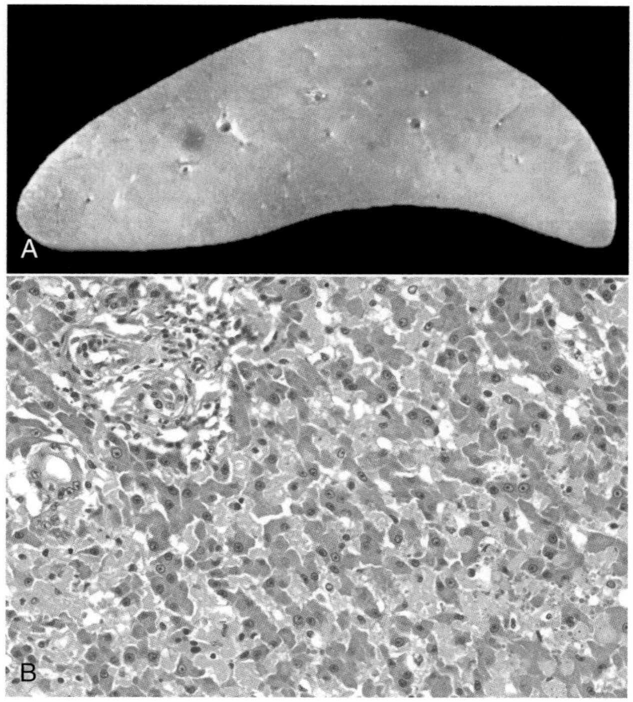

Fig. 8-39 Hepatic amyloidosis, liver.
A, Cut surface, duck. Hepatic amyloidosis has imparted a firm, waxy appearance and a pale brownish hue to the affected liver. **B,** Dog. The perisinusoidal spaces of Disse adjacent to the sinusoids are lined with a glassy eosinophilic (hyaline) material—amyloid. H&E stain. (**A** courtesy Drs. J. King and L. Roth, College of Veterinary Medicine, Cornell University. **B** courtesy Dr. J.M. Cullen, College of Veterinary Medicine, North Carolina State University.)

chain) and is composed of immunoglobulin light chains derived from the amino terminal variable region of κ- and λ-light chains synthesized by plasma cell neoplasms. Secondary or reactive amyloidosis occurs as a consequence of prolonged inflammation such as chronic infection or tissue destruction. In secondary amyloidosis, by far the most common type to occur in veterinary medicine, the fibrils are composed of amyloid A (AA). The precursor protein is serum amyloid–associated (SAA) protein, an apolipoprotein that is an acute phase protein synthesized by the liver. Inherited or familiar amyloidosis is uncommon in animals but occurs in Shar-Pei dogs and Abyssinian, Siamese, and other Oriental breeds of cats.

Regardless of its cause, amyloid can accumulate in more than one pattern. It may accumulate in vessel walls in the portal area, within the connective tissue of the portal area, and in the space of Disse, where it impairs the normal access of plasma to hepatocytes. Amyloid deposits can produce varying degrees of hepatomegaly, and extensive accumulations cause the liver to appear pale. In severe cases, affected animals may have clinical signs of either hepatic dysfunction or failure because the liver is more fragile; liver rupture and exsanguination may occur, especially in the horse. Frequently, amyloid is also deposited within the kidneys, particularly the glomeruli. Renal failure often occurs before signs of hepatic dysfunction are manifested.

Copper Accumulation

Copper poisoning is included as a metabolic disorder because hepatic injury in copper poisoning of domestic animals frequently is the result of progressive accumulation of copper within the liver. This occurs in domestic animals, especially sheep, in which storage of copper is poorly regulated. Also, disorders of copper metabolism have been described in various dog breeds and rarely cats.

Copper is an essential trace element of all cells, but even a modest excess of copper can be life threatening because copper must be properly sequestered to prevent toxicosis. Normally, serum copper is bound to ceruloplasmin and the majority of hepatic copper is bound to metallothionein and stored in lysosomes. Excess copper, like excess iron, can lead to the production of reactive oxygen species that initiate destructive lipid peroxidation reactions that affect the mitochondria and other cellular membranes. In domestic animals, copper toxicosis usually occurs as a consequence of one of the following:

1. Simple dietary excess in ruminants, particularly sheep, and pigs occurring, for example, because of excessive dietary supplementation as an overcorrection for copper deficiency or from contamination of the pasture with copper from sprays or fertilizer. It also occurs in sheep that have access to copper-containing mineral blocks formulated for cattle.
2. Grazing animals on pastures with normal concentrations of copper but with inadequate concentrations of molybdenum, which antagonizes copper uptake.
3. Pasturing herbivores on fields with plants that contain hepatotoxic phytotoxins, usually pyrrolizidine alkaloids. *Heliotropium, Crotalaria,* and *Senecio* species are common examples of such plants (Web Table 8-1). Pyrrolizidine alkaloids prevent hepatocellular DNA synthesis and mitosis. This failure to replace necrotic hepatocytes leads to an ever-increasing copper load in surviving hepatocytes because these hepatocytes take up the copper released by the dying cells.
4. Metabolic disorders of copper metabolism, as occur in dogs. The disorder is best characterized in Bedlington terriers that have an autosomal recessive inheritance of a mutation in the COMMD1 gene that leads to impaired biliary excretion of copper, which results in progressive accumulation within the liver.

The consequences of excessive accumulation of copper within the liver of domestic animals are species-dependent. See specific species disease sections for more information.

Pigment Accumulation

Pigments are colored substances, some of which are normal cellular constituents, whereas others accumulate only in abnormal circumstances. They are covered in detail in Chapter 1.

Bile Pigments

Bile pigments may accumulate in excessive amounts as a consequence of either extrahepatic or intrahepatic cholestasis and typically produce icterus and green discoloration of the liver.

Hemosiderin

Hemosiderin is an iron-containing, golden-brown, granular pigment derived from ferritin, the initial iron-storage protein. As iron accumulates within the cell, aggregates of ferritin molecules form hemosiderin (Web Fig. 8-6). Most hemosiderin in Kupffer cells and other macrophages located in tissues throughout the body is derived from the breakdown of erythrocytes, whereas most hepatocellular hemosiderin is derived from iron present in transferrin and to a lesser extent hemoglobin. Hemosiderin forms in the liver when there is local or systemic excess of iron, such as when erythrocytic breakdown is excessive (e.g., hemolytic anemia), and within areas of hepatic necrosis. An excessive systemic load of iron that is characterized by abundant hemosiderin in a variety of tissues without impairment of organ function is called hemosiderosis. In contrast, hemochromatosis is an abnormally increased storage of iron within the body that can cause hepatic dysfunction. Notable accumulation of iron can produce a dark brown or even a black liver.

Lipofuscin

Lipofuscin is an insoluble pigment that is yellow-brown to dark brown and is derived from incomplete oxidation of lipids such as those in cell membranes (Web Fig. 8-7). Lipofuscin is progressively oxidized with time; thus it actually is a group of lipid pigments, all of which consist of polymers of lipid, phospholipids, protein (and minimal carbohydrate in early forms). Amounts of lipofuscin present in the liver tend to increase with age.

Melanin

Melanin is an endogenous pigment that is dark brown or black. Benign disorders of melanin pigmentation are usually designated as melanosis. Congenital melanosis of the liver occurs in pigs and ruminants and produces variably sized areas of discoloration of the liver. Acquired "melanosis" of sheep has been described in Australia and is associated with the ingestion of certain plants, but the pigment has not been proved to be melanin and may be derived from a component of the ingested plants.

Parasite Hematin

Liver flukes specifically produce very dark excreta that contain a mixture of iron and porphyrin. These excreta produce the characteristic discoloration that occurs in fascioliasis *(Fasciola hepatica)* and is especially pronounced in the migratory tracts produced by *Fascioloides magna* in bovine livers (see Fig. 8-56).

INFECTIOUS DISEASES OF THE LIVER

Viral Diseases

Herpesvirus Infections

Herpesvirus infections of the liver typically occur in neonates or fetuses. A variety of abortigenic herpesviruses are described, each animal species being affected by a specific virus. Examples of these viruses include the abortigenic equine herpesvirus *(equine herpesvirus 1),* infectious bovine rhinotracheitis virus *(bovine herpesvirus 1),* caprine herpesvirus, canine herpesvirus *(canine herpesvirus 1),* feline viral rhinotracheitis virus *(feline herpesvirus 1),* and pseudorabies virus (suid herpesvirus 1).

Infection can occur via several routes, including transplacental exposure, passage through the birth canal, contact with infected littermates, and contact with oronasal secretions from the dam. In neonates, initial infection often occurs in the oronasal epithelium where virus replication first takes place. After local replication, the virus enters the bloodstream via infected mononuclear phagocytic cells. Viremia leads to dissemination of the virus to a variety of organs, and viral infection is cytolytic.

The abortigenic herpesviruses characteristically induce multifocal, randomly distributed, small (<1 mm) areas of necrosis in several fetal organs, including the liver (Fig. 8-40, *A*). Similar lesions occasionally are present in neonates infected with herpesviruses.

Histologically, herpesvirus can produce multifocal hepatic necrosis with scant inflammation in fetuses and neonates (Fig. 8-40, *B*). The liver is often affected, but foci of necrosis are more consistently present in the kidneys, lungs, and spleen. The virus most often affects neonates in the first 2 weeks of life and is most severe before they develop competent thermoregulation. Animals that are able to maintain a normal body temperature are less likely to be affected.

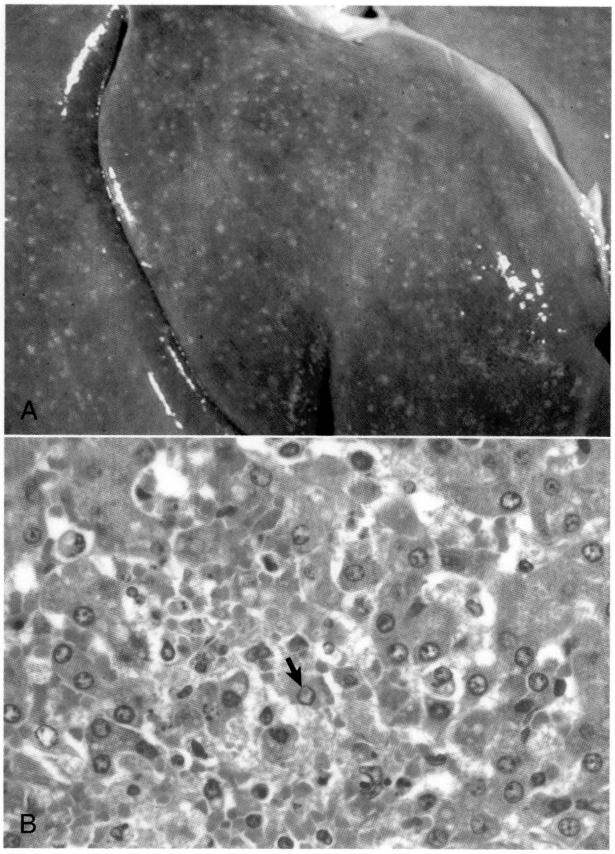

Fig. 8-40 Equine herpesvirus hepatitis, hepatic necrosis, liver, foal. **A,** Note the randomly distributed gray-to-white foci of random hepatocellular necrosis caused by equine herpesvirus. **B,** Infection of hepatocytes with equine herpesvirus produces characteristic acidophilic intranuclear inclusions surrounded by a clear zone that separates them from the marginated chromatin *(arrow).* Note the individual cell necrosis. H&E stain. (**A** courtesy Drs. J. King and L. Roth, College of Veterinary Medicine, Cornell University. **B** courtesy Dr. J.M. Cullen, College of Veterinary Medicine, North Carolina State University.)

Other Viral Infections

Infectious canine hepatitis, Rift Valley fever, and Wesselsbron disease are discussed under species-specific disease sections later in the chapter.

Certain viral diseases may involve the liver, but the hepatic involvement either does not occur invariably or it may be but one manifestation of a systemic process. Such diseases include feline infectious peritonitis (FIP) that is characterized by foci of pyogranulomatous vasculitis or perivascular accumulations of lymphocytes and plasma cells within multiple organs, sometimes including the liver. Subacute and chronic forms of equine infectious anemia are characterized by cellular accumulations, particularly lymphocytes, in sinusoids and the space of Disse. Systemic adenoviral infection of lambs, calves, and goat kids may produce multifocal areas of hepatocellular necrosis, cholangitis, and necrosis of biliary epithelium. *Porcine circovirus* type 2 injures hepatocytes and Kupffer cells and can cause mild-to-severe necrosis.

Bacterial Diseases

Liver Abscesses and Granulomas

Bacteria can reach the liver via a number of different routes and form abscesses (Figs. 8-41 to 8-43). Routes include the following:

- The portal vein
- The umbilical veins from umbilical infections in newborn animals
- The hepatic artery, as part of a generalized bacteremia
- Ascending infection of the biliary system
- Parasitic migration
- Direct extension of an inflammatory process from tissues immediately adjacent to the liver, such as the reticulum

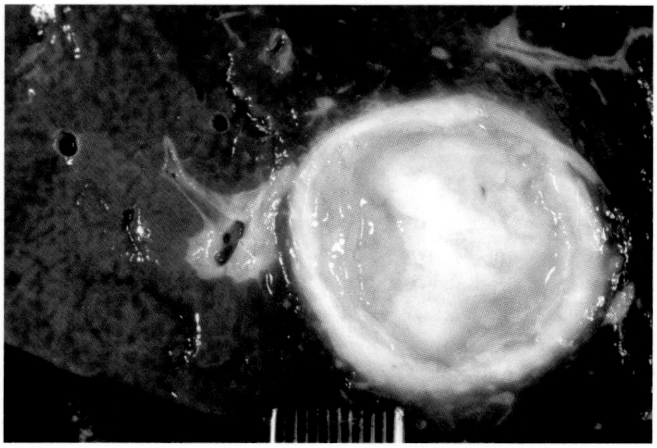

Fig. 8-41 Chronic hepatic abscesses, *Corynebacterium pseudotuberculosis*, liver, sheep. Note the thick fibrous capsule and the characteristic pale caseous exudate produced by *Corynebacterium pseudotuberculosis* in sheep. (Courtesy College of Veterinary Medicine, North Carolina State University.)

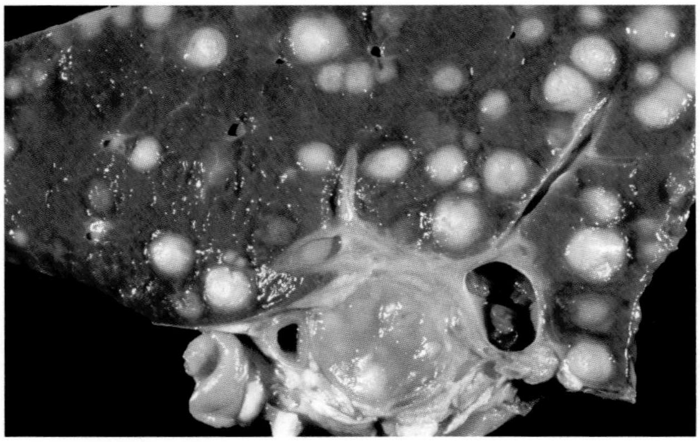

Fig. 8-42 Hepatic abscesses, *Rhodococcus equi*, liver, goat. Disseminated hepatic abscesses in a goat caused by *Rhodococcus equi.* This lesion is more commonly found in foals. (Courtesy Dr. P. Stromberg, College of Veterinary Medicine, The Ohio State University.)

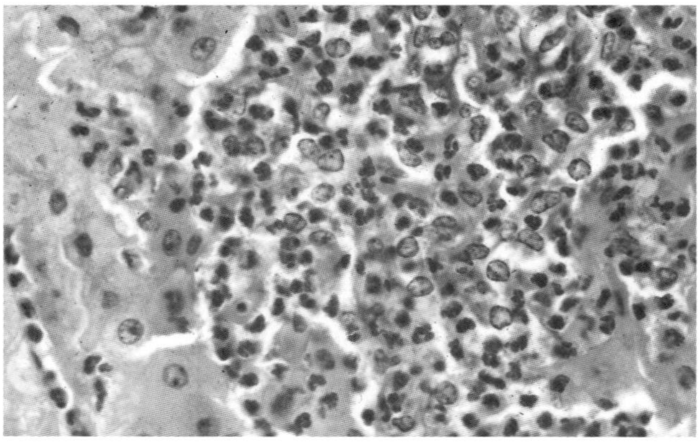

Fig. 8-43 Hepatic abscess, liver, cow. An abscess in the liver is similar to those in other tissues and consists of an infiltrate of neutrophils, degenerating neutrophils, and necrotic tissue debris. H&E stain. (Courtesy Dr. M.D. McGavin, College of Veterinary Medicine, University of Tennessee.)

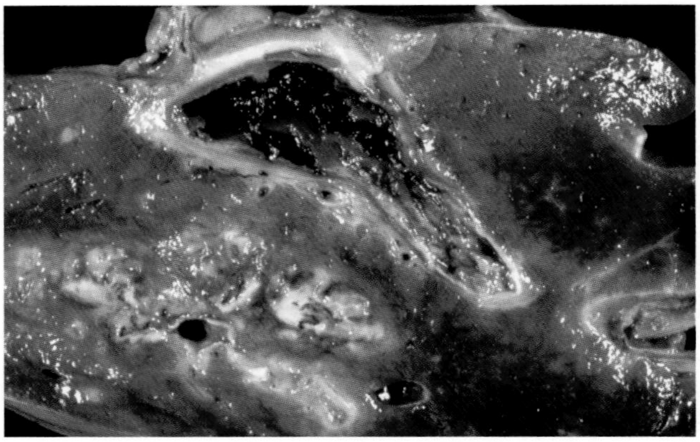

Fig. 8-44 Hepatic abscess, *Fusobacterium necrophorum*, liver, cow. Foci of necrosis and abscess formation. Abscesses, such as this one, can erode the wall of a hepatic vein or the caudal vena cava, rupture, and release their contents into the bloodstream. (Courtesy Dr. P. Stromberg, College of Veterinary Medicine, The Ohio State University.)

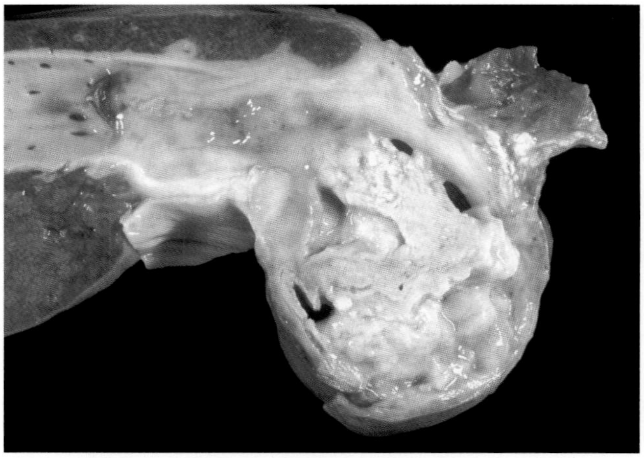

Fig. 8-45 Hepatic abscess, caudal vena cava, cow. A hepatic abscess has eroded the wall of the vena cava, ruptured, and released its contents into the caudal vena cava. (Courtesy College of Veterinary Medicine, North Carolina State University.)

Both Gram-positive and Gram-negative organisms can cause hepatic abscesses. In adult small animals, hepatic abscesses are often caused by any of a variety of enteric species, as well as *Francisella* spp., *Nocardia asteroides,* and *Actinomyces* spp. Bacterial infections of the liver and subsequent formation of hepatic abscesses or foci of necrosis are especially common in neonatal foals and ruminants, in addition to feedlot cattle. In feedlot cattle, hepatic abscesses usually occur as a sequel to toxic rumenitis because damage to the ruminal mucosa allows ruminal microflora, particularly *Fusobacterium necrophorum,* to enter the portal circulation. After initially localizing within the liver, bacteria proliferate and produce focal areas of hepatocellular necrosis and hepatitis that can in time develop into hepatic abscesses (Fig. 8-44). Liver abscesses of cattle frequently are incidental lesions, but they can cause weight loss and decreased milk production. Less commonly, a hepatic abscess encroaches on the lumen of either a hepatic vein or the caudal vena cava. This can cause phlebitis that results in mural thrombosis, and because of the obstruction of the outflow to the venous drainage of the liver, passive congestion of the liver and portal hypertension can occur (Fig. 8-45). Detachment of portions of these mural thrombi can produce septic thromboemboli that lodge in the lungs. Rupture of hepatic abscesses directly into the hepatic vein or into the caudal vena cava occurs sporadically in cattle and may result in fatal septic embolization of the lungs. Sometimes death can be sudden from the blockage of large areas of pulmonary capillaries by the exudate. Hepatic abscesses derived from bacteria arriving via the portal vein may not be evenly distributed throughout the liver, possibly because of selective distribution of portal blood into different liver lobes, termed *portal streaming.* Occasionally, fungi, such as *Mucor* sp., that proliferate in areas of ruminal ulceration invade the portal circulation and are carried to the liver and there cause extensive areas of necrosis and inflammation (Fig. 8-46).

Tuberculosis *(Mycobacterium bovis)* has been eradicated from almost all of the United States (US), but its occurrence in other countries varies with the effectiveness of control efforts. The primary site of the disease is pulmonary with subsequent dissemination to other organs, including the liver. Other domestic animal species can be infected with *Mycobacterium bovis,* and it is also a zoonotic microbe. *Mycobacterium avium-intracellulare* complex can occur in domestic animals, especially dogs, in the southern areas of the US. Granulomas are randomly distributed (i.e., hematogenous spread) in the liver. They have a central core of cell debris, caseation,

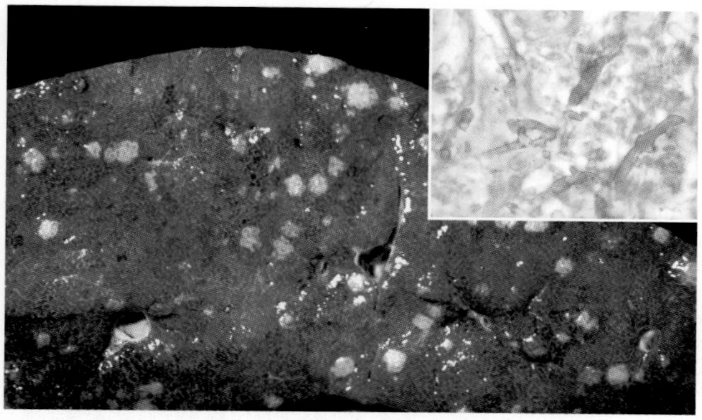

Fig. 8-46 Multiple necrotic foci, disseminated fungal infection (*Mucor* spp.), liver, cow.

Mucor spp. enter the portal blood after ulcerative rumenitis and cause focal necrosis and inflammation in the liver. *Inset,* The hyphae of the causative organism *(pink)* are usually evident within the granuloma. Periodic acid–Schiff (PAS) reaction. (Figure courtesy College of Veterinary Medicine, University of Illinois. Inset courtesy Dr. M.D. McGavin, College of Veterinary Medicine, University of Tennessee.)

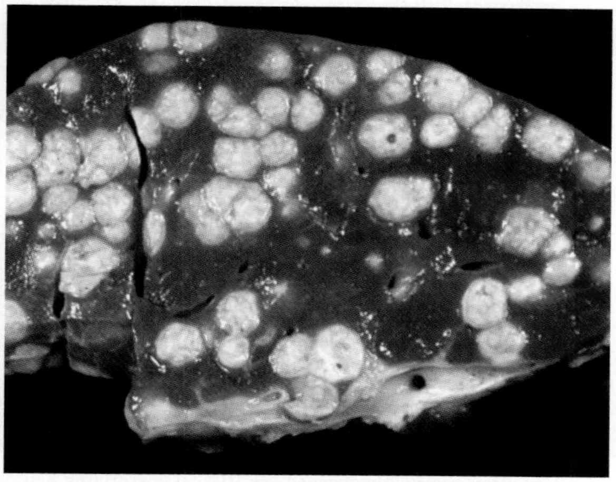

Fig. 8-47 Multiple caseous granulomas, tuberculosis, *Mycobacterium bovis,* liver, cow.

Hepatic tuberculosis is characterized by random multifocal pale white-to-yellow caseous granulomas on the capsular and cut surfaces. (Courtesy Dr. M. Domingo, Autonomous University of Barcelona; and Noah's Arkive, College of Veterinary Medicine, The University of Georgia.)

and granulomatous inflammation surrounded by a fibrous capsule (Fig. 8-47).

Tyzzer's Disease

This disease is caused by *Clostridium piliforme* (formerly *Bacillus piliformis*), a Gram-negative obligate intracellular parasite. It is well recognized in laboratory animals but occurs only sporadically in domestic animals. Infection is most common in foals but has been described in calves, cats, and dogs and many other species. Typically, only very young or immunocompromised animals are affected. The bacteria are found in the intestinal tract of rodents. Infection is most likely through the oral route. The mechanisms of attachment and entry into host cells are unknown. After colonization of the gastrointestinal tract, organisms penetrate into the portal venous drainage and enter the liver. The disease is characterized by enlarged, edematous, and hemorrhagic abdominal lymph nodes, hepatic enlargement, and the presence of randomly distributed, pale foci of hepatocellular necrosis surrounded by a variably intense inflammatory infiltrate of neutrophils and mononuclear cells (Fig. 8-48, *A*). Diagnosis requires the demonstration of the characteristic, elongated large bacilli within viable hepatocytes at the margins of necrotic foci (Fig. 8-48, *B*). Silver stains, such as Warthin-Starry or Gomori's silver stain, are frequently used for this purpose (Fig. 8-48, *C*).

Leptospirosis

Leptospirosis is caused by infection with the Gram-negative, thin, spiral, and motile bacterium of the genus *Leptospira.* There are two species, of which *Leptospira interrogans* is capable of causing disease in animals. The taxonomy of these organisms is complicated because there are more than 23 antigenically distinct pathogenic serogroups and 200 serovars. Each serovar can differ with respect to the species affected, organs affected, and severity of disease. Leptospires enter the body through the mucous membranes or through the skin if its barrier functions have been disrupted. Contaminated water, bedding, and soil are common sources of infection because the organism is shed in urine. Fetuses can develop transplacental infection and are often aborted. Infection can involve red blood cells, kidney, liver, and a number of other tissues, depending on the infecting serovar. The liver is often involved in acute, severe leptospirosis of all domestic species because a number of serovars cause intravascular hemolytic anemia leading to ischemic injury to centrilobular areas. Furthermore, organisms can be seen in large numbers in the liver after silver staining methods, although the direct effects of leptospira toxins on hepatocytes are less well established.

Gross lesions include icterus when animals are infected with serovars that produce hemolysis. Hepatic hemorrhage and ascites can occur, depending on the course of infection and the serovar involved. In some cases, acute infection can cause focal necrosis in addition to or instead of centrilobular necrosis. A common but nonspecific change in the liver of infected dogs is dissociation of hepatocytes. Affected cells become rounded and have eosinophilic granular cytoplasm and dark, shrunken hyperbasophilic nuclei. Bile casts in canaliculi are often apparent. Kupffer cells may contain abundant hemosiderin. Infection of dogs with *Leptospira grippotyphosa* has been reported to produce chronic (chronic-active) hepatitis, but it is unlikely that leptospira are involved in the pathogenesis of the majority of spontaneous cases of chronic hepatitis.

Other Bacterial Infections

These diseases are grouped together because they all arise from a bacteremia that occurs during a systemic infection. A comprehensive list of systemic infections that may produce hepatocellular necrosis and hepatitis is beyond the scope of this chapter, but examples include *Yersinia pseudotuberculosis, Salmonella* spp. (lesions present within the liver are discrete accumulations of mixed mononuclear inflammatory cells, which often are referred to as *paratyphoid nodules*) and *Brucella* spp. infection in many species (Fig. 8-49, *A* and *B*). *Haemophilus agni* and *Pasteurella haemolytica* can present as infections in sheep. Other infections include *Arcanobacter pyogenes (Actinomyces pyogenes)* of the bovine fetus and neonate, *Campylobacter fetus* ssp. fetus in fetal and neonatal lambs (Fig. 8-50), *Actinobacillus equuli* infection of neonatal foals, and *Nocardia asteroides* infection of dogs. *Yersinia tularensis (Francisella tularensis),* the cause of tularemia, can occur in cats and dogs. Bacterial infections such as these may produce lesions within the liver that range from small foci of hepatic necrosis to multiple, large abscesses. Determination of the specific causative agent often depends on bacterial isolation and characterization.

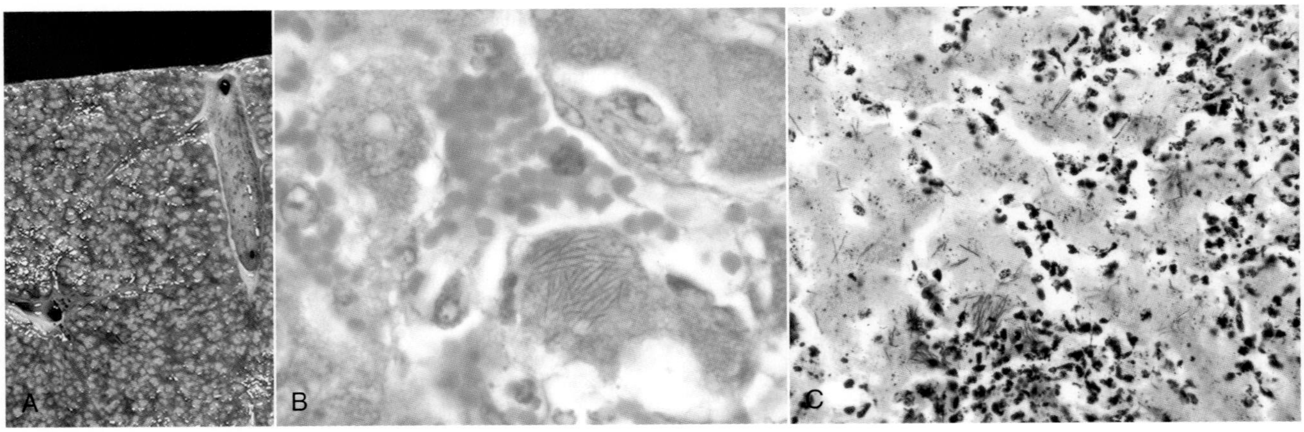

Fig. 8-48 Tyzzer's disease *(Clostridium piliforme).*
A, Liver, horse. Disseminated gray-white 1- to 2-mm foci of necrosis surrounded by suppurative inflammation. **B,** Foal. *Clostridium piliforme* can be identified by the haphazard distribution of filamentous bacteria in the cytoplasm of hepatocytes. Giemsa stain. **C,** Foal. *Clostridium piliforme* can be readily seen with special stains such as Giemsa and Warthin-Starry. Warthin-Starry stain. (**A** courtesy Dr. R.C. Giles, University of Kentucky; and Noah's Arkive, College of Veterinary Medicine, The University of Georgia. **B** and **C** courtesy Dr. M.D. McGavin, College of Veterinary Medicine, University of Tennessee.)

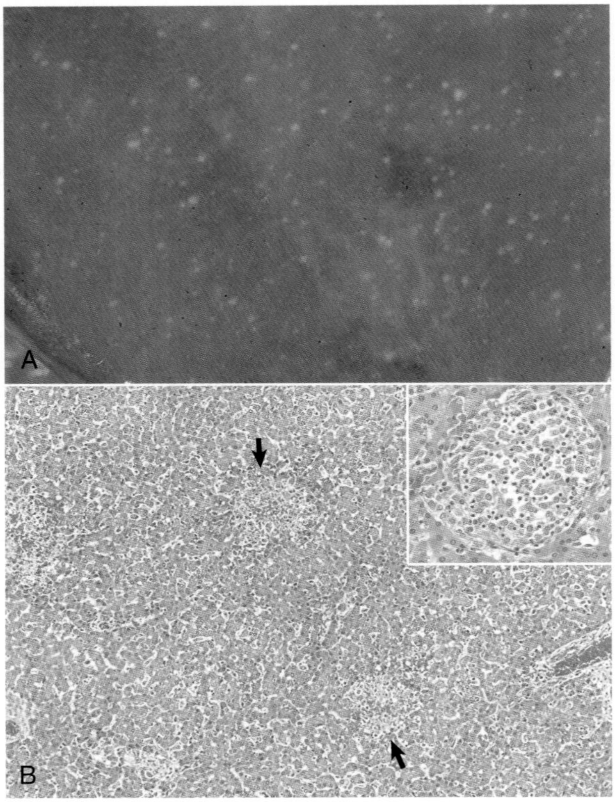

Fig. 8-49 Hepatic salmonellosis, liver.
A, Diaphragmatic surface, cow. Random 1- to 2-mm foci of focal necrosis in a cow with Salmonella septicemia. Multiple pale subcapsular foci of necrosis are evident. **B,** Pig, Later in the disease process, the necrotic foci are infiltrated by macrophages and form discrete granulomas termed paratyphoid nodules *(arrows).* H&E stain. *Inset,* Higher magnification of a paratyphoid nodule. H&E stain. (**A** courtesy Dr. M.D. McGavin, College of Veterinary Medicine, University of Tennessee. **B** courtesy Dr. M.D. McGavin, College of Veterinary Medicine, University of Tennessee. Inset courtesy Dr. J. Simon, College of Veterinary Medicine, University of Illinois.)

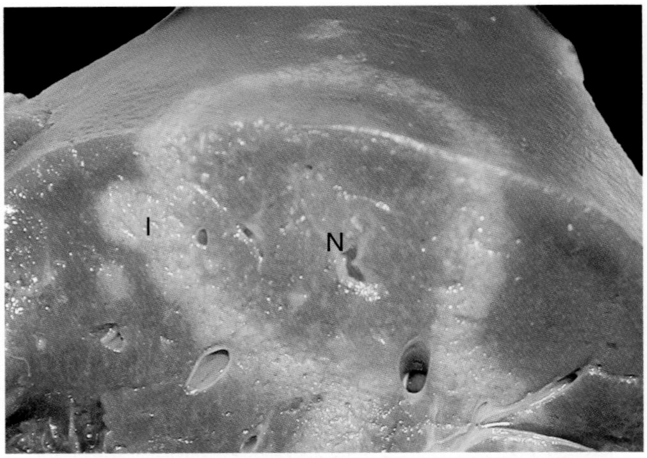

Fig. 8-50 Hepatic campylobacteriosis, multifocal necrotizing hepatitis, liver, capsular and cut surfaces, lamb fetus.
The lesion consists of a necrotic center (coagulation necrosis) *(N),* which in older lesions is distinctly tan and depressed. This center is surrounded by a white to gray rim of inflammatory cells *(I).* The cut surface *(lower)* illustrates the same changes and the extent of the necrosis into the hepatic parenchyma. (Courtesy Drs. C. Lichtensteiger and R. Doty, College of Veterinary Medicine, University of Illinois.)

Bacillary hemoglobinuria and infectious necrotic hepatitis, both due to species of *Clostridia,* are described in detail in the section on Disorders of Ruminants.

Protozoal Diseases

The liver can be involved in systemic infections with *Toxoplasma gondii, Neospora* sp., and other less common protozoa (Web Fig. 8-8). Liver lesions are usually characterized by multifocal necrosis and inflammation. Inflammatory cells include neutrophils, macrophages, and smaller numbers of other inflammatory cells. Free tachyzoites or cysts containing bradyzoites can be found within necrotic areas or adjacent to them. Although there are subtle physical differences between the organisms, immunologic testing, such as immunohistochemical staining, is a more reliable means to separate the two organisms.

Dimorphic Fungal Diseases

Systemic involvement with dimorphic fungi often includes the liver. There are several genera of fungi that may involve the liver including, *Blastomyces, Coccidioides, Aspergillus,* and *Histoplasma.* Histoplasmosis is a fungal disease that is endemic in the US and Canada and can occur occasionally in other areas. It is caused by *Histoplasma capsulatum,* a soil-dwelling organism. Dogs are affected most often. The route of infection is primarily through inhalation, although ingestion is also a possible route. In some circumstances pulmonary infections become disseminated and affect a variety of visceral organs, including the liver. Lesions in the liver consist of a multifocal distribution of granulomas with intralesional yeast forms of the organism. Numerous yeast forms can be found in the cytoplasm of macrophages and can be readily stained with the periodic acid–Schiff (PAS) reaction (Fig. 8-51, *A* and *B*).

Parasitic Diseases

Nematodes

Migration of larvae through the liver is a common component of a nematode's life cycle in domestic animals. As larvae travel through the liver, they produce local tracts of hepatocellular necrosis that are accompanied by inflammation. These tracts are eventually replaced with connective tissue that matures into fibrous scars and which are especially prominent on the capsular surface (Fig. 8-52). These capsular scars appear as pale areas, and the term *milk-spotted liver* has been used to describe livers in pigs scarred by migrating larvae of *Ascaris suum.* Larvae occasionally become entrapped within the liver or its capsule and are walled off within abscesses or granulomas. Examples of chronic hepatitis or hepatic scarring as a consequence of larval migration include migration of ascarids in several species of domestic animals, such as *Stephanurus dentatus* in pigs, and *Strongylus* sp. in the horse. Infection of the liver with adult nematodes is considerably less common than larval migration. *Calodium hepatica* occasionally may be found in the hepatic parenchyma of dogs and cats where the ova provoke granulomatous inflammation.

Dogs with heartworm infection *(Dirofilaria immitis)* occasionally develop vena caval syndrome, also known as the *postcaval syndrome,* which is characterized by DIC, intravascular hemolysis, and acute hepatic failure. The syndrome typically occurs in dogs with large numbers of adult worms in the vena cava and their more usual location within the right side of the heart and pulmonary artery (Fig. 8-53). The liver is engorged with blood as a consequence of severe passive congestion from the partial blockage of the caudal vena cava. It is proposed that mechanical factors

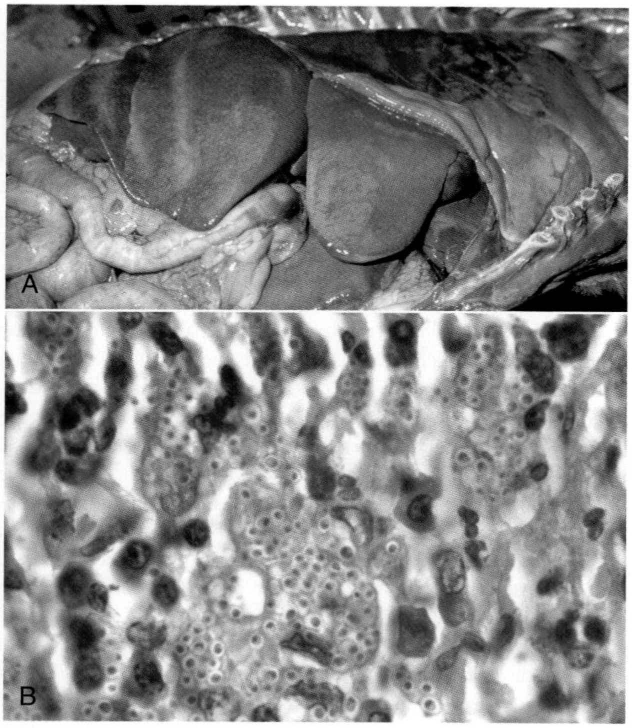

Fig. 8-51 Hepatic histoplasmosis, liver, dog.

A, In disseminated cases, *Histoplasma capsulatum* can involve the liver. Affected livers tend to be enlarged and pale mahogany from the diffuse hypertrophy and proliferation of Kupffer cells and macrophages. **B,** Note the yeast form of *Histoplasma* in the cytoplasm of Kupffer cells and macrophages. H&E stain. (**A** courtesy College of Veterinary Medicine, University of Illinois. **B** courtesy Dr. J. Simon, College of Veterinary Medicine, University of Illinois.)

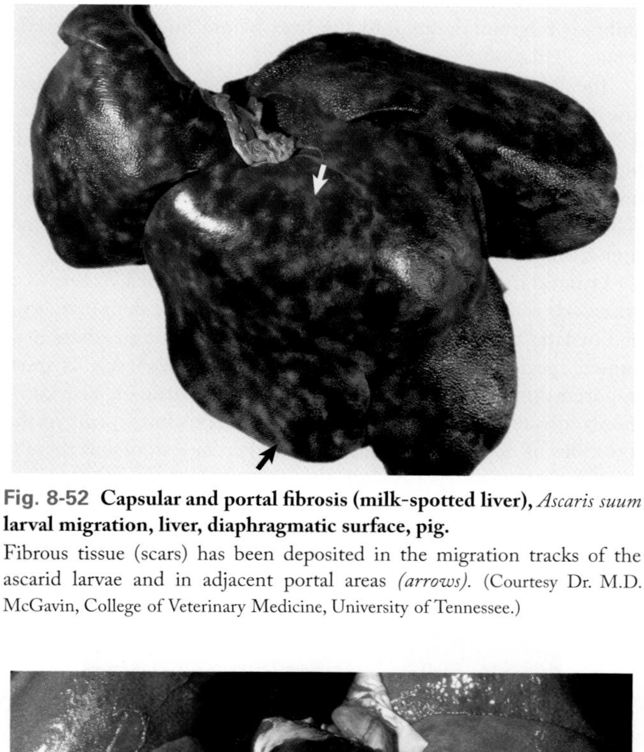

Fig. 8-52 Capsular and portal fibrosis (milk-spotted liver), *Ascaris suum* **larval migration, liver, diaphragmatic surface, pig.**

Fibrous tissue (scars) has been deposited in the migration tracks of the ascarid larvae and in adjacent portal areas *(arrows).* (Courtesy Dr. M.D. McGavin, College of Veterinary Medicine, University of Tennessee.)

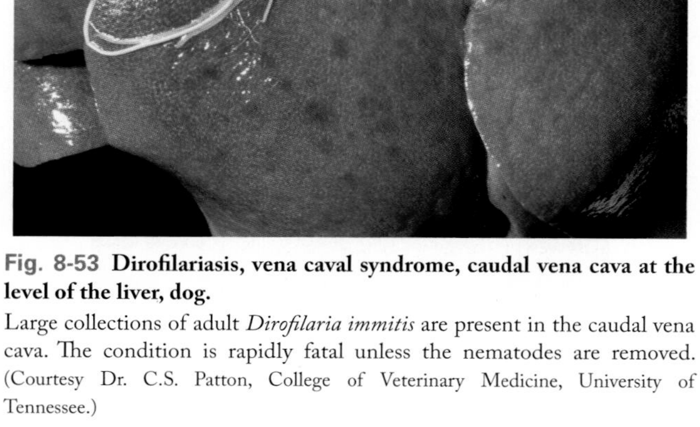

Fig. 8-53 Dirofilariasis, vena caval syndrome, caudal vena cava at the level of the liver, dog.

Large collections of adult *Dirofilaria immitis* are present in the caudal vena cava. The condition is rapidly fatal unless the nematodes are removed. (Courtesy Dr. C.S. Patton, College of Veterinary Medicine, University of Tennessee.)

produced by the presence of large numbers of worms in the right atrium or caudal vena cava are the cause of intravascular hemolysis, which characterizes vena caval syndrome, although other theories suggest that there may be a hypersensitivity reaction to antigens released by the worms.

Cestodes

A number of cestodes occur within the hepatobiliary system of domestic animals. Those cestode parasites of greatest clinical significance develop encysted forms within the liver of the intermediate hosts. The most important are larval cestodes of the genus *Taenia;* adults inhabit the gastrointestinal tract of carnivores and usually are innocuous to their definitive host. The ova ingested by an intermediate host develop into embryos, which penetrate the wall of the gut and then are distributed via the blood to virtually any site in the body. Parasitic cysts develop within the tissue of the intermediate host, and the life cycle of the parasite is completed when the cysts are ingested by the definitive host. Although the liver is but one organ in the intermediate host that may be affected, hepatic involvement is common because portal blood, in which embryos migrate, drains into the liver before flowing to the systemic circulation.

The adult cestode *Taenia hydatigena* shows up in the small intestine of dogs, whereas its intermediate stage, *Cysticercus tenuicollis,* appears in the peritoneal cavity of a variety of species, including horses, ruminants, and pigs (Fig. 8-54). Immature cysticerci migrate in the liver and can induce extensive damage if infection is heavy; lesions present are comparable to those induced by migration of immature *Fasciola hepatica.*

Hydatid liver disease is common in some countries. *Echinococcus granulosus* is a cestode that parasitizes canids as the definitive host, and hydatid cysts can develop in many different intermediate host animal species, including humans. The dog-sheep cycle is most important in many geographic areas. Pastured cattle are also commonly affected in other geographic locations. Adult worms in the intestines of dogs pass proglottids into the dog's stool and thereby contaminate pastures. Ova are then ingested by sheep, cattle, or other species. Embryos may develop into hydatid cysts in virtually any organ in the intermediate host, but the liver and lungs are commonly affected. These cysts are usually less than 10 cm in diameter but can attain quite a spectacular size, particularly in humans. Hydatid cysts, even when present in large numbers, rarely cause overt clinical signs of disease in domestic animals.

Cestode adults occurring within the hepatobiliary system include *Stilesia hepatica, Stilesia globipunctata,* and *Thysanosoma actinoides,* all of which can inhabit the bile duct of ruminants. Infections with these parasites may result in chronic inflammation of the biliary tract, but they usually do not produce clinical signs of hepatic dysfunction.

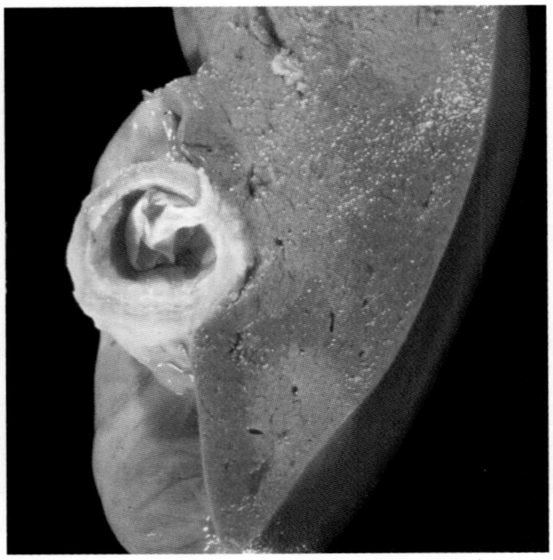

Fig. 8-54 Cysticercosis, liver, cut surface, sheep.
The thick fibrous capsule usually indicates the death of the larva. (Courtesy Dr. K. Read, College of Veterinary Medicine, Texas A&M University; and Noah's Arkive, College of Veterinary Medicine, The University of Georgia.)

Trematodes

The majority of parasitic hepatic injury caused by trematodes is produced by members of three major families. These include the families Fasciolidae, Dicrocoelidae, and Opisthorchidae.

The principal liver fluke disease of sheep and cattle and occasionally other species is caused by *Fasciola hepatica.* Hepatic fascioliasis occurs throughout the world in areas where climatic conditions, typically in low swampy areas, are suitable for the survival of aquatic snails, which serve as intermediate hosts for the parasites. Adult *Fasciola hepatica* are leaf-shaped parasites that inhabit the biliary system; their eggs pass via the bile to the intestinal tract and eventually are passed in the feces. Larvae (miracidium) then must develop in the snail intermediate host (genus *Lymnaea).* Cercariae that leave the snail encyst on herbage where they develop into infectious metacercariae. Metacercariae are ingested by the ruminant host and penetrate the wall of the duodenum to enter the peritoneal cavity and subsequently enter the liver. They migrate within the liver before taking up residence within the bile ducts. Migration of immature flukes through the liver produces hemorrhagic tracts of necrotic liver parenchyma. These tracts are grossly visible and in acute infection are dark red, but with time become paler than the surrounding parenchyma. Repair is often by fibrosis. A variety of untoward sequelae can follow these migrations, including acute peritonitis; hepatic abscesses; death of the host as a consequence of acute, widespread hepatic necrosis produced by a massive infiltration of immature flukes; and the proliferation of spores of *Clostridium haemolyticum* or *Clostridium novyi* in necrotic tissue, which causes the subsequent development of bacillary hemoglobinuria or infectious necrotic hepatitis, respectively.

Mature flukes reside in the larger extrahepatic and intrahepatic bile ducts and cause cholangitis. Chronic cholangitis and bile duct obstruction lead to ectasia and stenosis of the ducts and periductular fibrosis that thickens the walls so that the ducts become increasingly prominent. Mineralization may occur producing the classic "pipestem" appearance of diseased bile ducts. The contents of the bile ducts are often dark brown and viscous caused by a combination of abnormal bile, cellular debris, and the iron-porphyrin pigment excreted by the flukes. Obstruction of the ducts leads to cholestasis. Animals with chronic liver fluke disease are often in poor body condition.

Fasciola gigantica and *Fascioloides magna* are important causes of liver fluke disease of ruminants in some parts of the world. *Fasciola gigantica* is most common in areas of Africa and surrounding countries, and *Fascioloides magna* is found in North America. The adults of *Fasciola gigantica* and *Fasciola hepatica* reside in the bile ducts (Fig. 8-55). In contrast, adult *Fascioloides magna,* whose normal hosts are elk and white-tailed deer, reside in the hepatic parenchyma in aberrant hosts, such as cattle and sheep. In cattle, the immature *Fascioloides magna* flukes cause extensive tissue damage as they migrate through the liver (Fig. 8-56), but the adults are enclosed by fibrous connective tissue in cysts containing a black

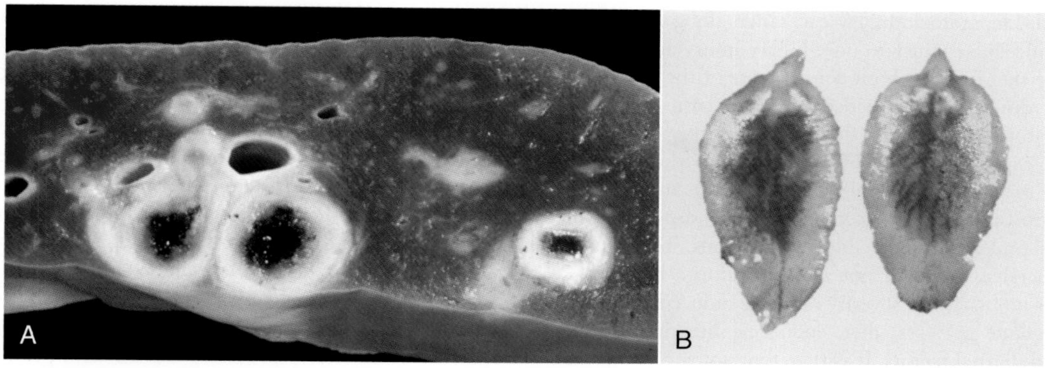

Fig. 8-55 ***Fasciola hepatica*** **infection.**
A, Chronic intrahepatic cholangitis *(Fasciola hepatica),* liver, cow. When *Fasciola hepatica* metacercariae are ingested, they migrate to the liver and then take up residence within the bile ducts. Mature flukes reside in the larger extrahepatic and intrahepatic bile ducts and cause chronic cholangitis and bile duct obstruction that lead to ectasia and stenosis of the ducts and periductular fibrosis that thickens the walls so that the ducts become increasingly prominent, as shown here. **B,** Adult *Fasciola hepatica* are leaf-shaped flukes that inhabit the biliary system; their eggs pass via the bile into the intestinal tract and eventually are passed in the feces. (**A** courtesy Dr. K. Read, College of Veterinary Medicine, Texas A&M University; and Noah's Arkive, College of Veterinary Medicine, The University of Georgia. **B** courtesy Dr. T. Boosinger, College of Veterinary Medicine, Auburn University; and Noah's Arkive, College of Veterinary Medicine, The University of Georgia.)

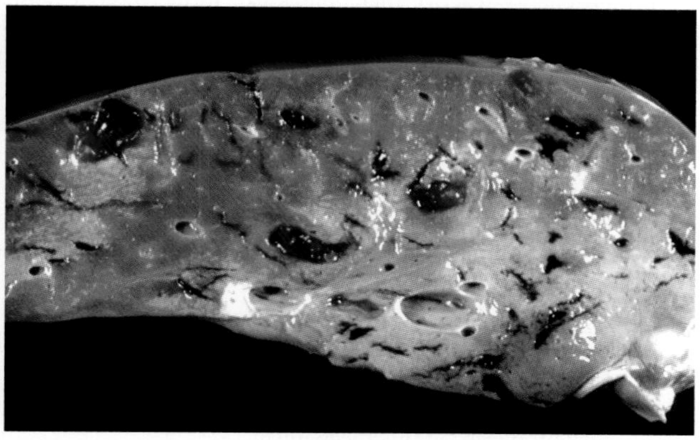

Fig. 8-56 **Fluke migration tracts, fascioloidiasis, liver, cow.**
Migration of *Fascioloides magna* through the bovine liver produces extensive parenchymal damage. A black excretory pigment deposited by the fluke discolors the migration tracks black. (Courtesy Dr. J. Wright, College of Veterinary Medicine, North Carolina State University; and Noah's Arkive, College of Veterinary Medicine, The University of Georgia.)

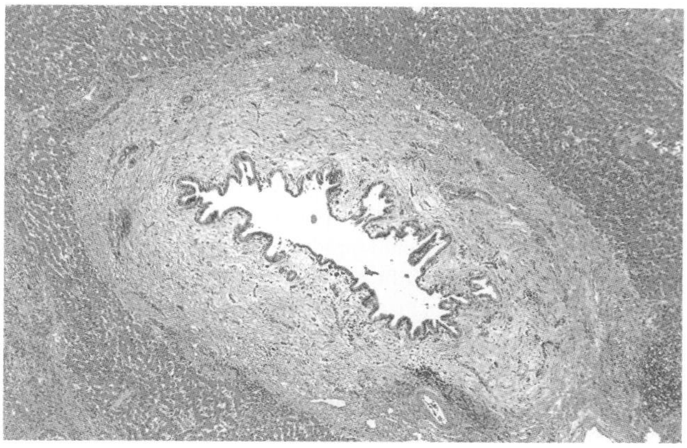

Fig. 8-57 **Chronic intrahepatic cholangitis, liver, cat.**
Fluke infections of the biliary tree of cats produce a characteristically pronounced periductular fibrosis, dilated bile duct, and papillary projections of biliary epithelium, although flukes may be difficult to find. H&E stain. (Courtesy Dr. J.M. Cullen, College of Veterinary Medicine, North Carolina State University.)

fluid. In sheep and goats, the flukes continuously migrate through the liver, causing extensive damage and eventual death.

Other trematodes that may inhabit the bile ducts include *Dicrocoelium dendriticum* in horses, ruminants, pigs, dogs, and cats; *Eurytrema pancreaticum* and *Eurytrema coelomaticum* in ruminants; *Opisthorchis tenuicollis* in pigs, dogs, and cats and *Opisthorchis felineus* in dogs and cats; *Pseudamphistomum truncatum, Metorchis conjunctus, Metorchis albidus, Parametorchis complexus, Concinnum procyonis,* and *Platynosomum fastosum* in dogs and cats. All are capable of inducing changes similar to but usually considerably milder than those caused by *Fasciola hepatica.* In addition, they occasionally cause obstruction of the biliary ducts.

Cats, and less often dogs, can develop pronounced chronic cholangitis from infections with flukes, most often Opisthorchiidae. Microscopically, larger intrahepatic bile ducts are dramatically thickened by concentric fibrosis and the duct lumen is usually dilated, often with papillary projections of biliary epithelium into the lumen (Fig. 8-57). A mild-to-moderate inflammatory infiltrate of neutrophils and macrophages is often found in and around the ducts, and the portal tracts are infiltrated by neutrophils, lymphocytes, and plasma cells. Eosinophils are generally uncommon. It is often difficult to detect adult flukes or ova in affected animals.

Dogs can be infected with the schistosome *Heterobilharzia americana,* which is normally a parasite in raccoons. Ova shed into water by infected raccoons release miracidia, which penetrate host snails. Dogs become infected when their skin is penetrated by cercariae, which are released from the intermediate snail hosts. Granulomatous lesions of the liver, pancreas, intestines, and mesentery result when ova released by adult schistosomes lodge in affected tissue and incite an inflammatory reaction.

TOXIN-INDUCED LIVER DISEASE

The liver is subjected to toxic injury more often than any other organ. This is not surprising because the portal vein blood that drains from the absorptive surface of the intestinal tract flows directly to the liver. Thus the liver is exposed to virtually all ingested substances, including plant, fungal, and bacterial products, and metals, minerals, drugs and other chemicals that are absorbed into the portal blood. Hepatotoxic injury can range along a spectrum from pure hepatocellular injury to pure biliary injury and a mixed pattern of injury that involves both components of the liver.

Hepatotoxic drugs can be divided into two basic categories. Predictable hepatotoxins are those that affect the large majority of animals that are exposed, and the effect is evident within a similar dose range. The majority of recognized hepatotoxins in veterinary medicine fall into this category; acetaminophen and pyrrolizidine alkaloids are examples of predictable hepatotoxins. Toxic injury, even with predictable toxins, is not always uniform, however. A variety of factors influence the severity of injury induced by a toxin; these factors include age, sex, diet, endocrine function, genetic constitution, and diurnal factors. It is therefore not surprising that responses of individual animals exposed to the same toxin can vary considerably. Idiosyncratic drug reactions are characterized as responses seen in only a small minority of exposed individuals. There are a number of possible mechanisms for idiosyncratic drug reactions, including atypical metabolism as a result of inheritance of rare genes encoding enzymes involved in drug metabolism or deletions of genes encoding certain enzymes or immunologic responses to drugs or modified hepatocyte proteins. Interactions with other drugs or effects of diet and health status can also play a role in idiosyncratic toxicity. Diazepam toxicity in cats is an example of an idiosyncratic toxicity.

The response of the liver to acute hepatotoxic injury depends on the mechanism and site of toxic insult. By far, the most common pattern of acute liver toxicity is centrilobular necrosis. The mechanisms for this pattern of injury involve metabolism by the cytochrome p450 system and are discussed later. Certain chemicals that are uncommonly encountered produce periportal necrosis. These chemicals are able to produce a toxic effect without requiring metabolism by the cytochrome p450 system and include white phosphorus (once used as a rodenticide) and allyl alcohol.

It should be kept in mind that a single episode of nonlethal hepatotoxic injury in an otherwise healthy animal is difficult to detect histologically within a few days after the episode. Within 48 to 72 hours, macrophages clear cell debris, and hepatocytes begin to undergo mitosis to replace the lost cells. Within a week or less, the liver regains a normal histologic appearance, unless there is massive necrosis, which can lead to collapse of the hepatic connective tissue scaffolding and subsequent fibrosis surrounding the central vein. Chronic toxic liver injury, manifest either as repeated bouts of toxin exposure or more consistent daily exposure (e.g., through dietary contamination) can lead to activation of hepatic stellate cells within the space of Disse or related myofibroblasts in the portal areas and the connective tissue of the central vein area, which may then initiate synthesis of ECM leading to hepatic fibrosis. In addition, chronic liver injury can lead to disruption of the normal framework that supports the hepatic architecture and leads to hepatic fibrosis. Sufficient injury also can produce nodules of regenerative hepatocytes that are surrounded by bands of fibrosis that connect central vein areas to each other, connect portal tracts to each other, or bridge portal tracts to centrilobular areas. This pattern is recognized as cirrhosis.

Hepatocytes are not the only cell type in the liver that can be affected by toxic drugs. The biliary epithelium is susceptible to injury from trimethoprim-sulfa and the mycotoxin, sporidesmin, Kupffer cells to endotoxin, sinusoidal endothelial cells to arsenicals and some pyrrolizidine alkaloids, and the hepatic stellate cells to vitamin A excess. Bile duct necrosis or proliferation can disrupt bile flow. Activated Kupffer cells can release cytokines that affect the type and degree of inflammation within the liver. Hepatic stellate cells play a central role in hepatic fibrosis, as is discussed later. Damage to endothelial cells can affect blood flow through the liver.

Hepatotoxic liver injury can be classified into the following six categories based on the cellular target involved:

1. The most frequent mechanism of hepatocellular injury involves production of injurious metabolites by the cytochrome p450 system. This family of enzymes is located in the smooth endoplasmic reticulum of hepatocytes primarily, although they are also found in many other cells of the body. A major role of cytochrome p450 enzymes is to metabolize lipid-soluble chemicals into water-soluble compounds for excretion from the body in bile or urine. In the first step of this three-step process, termed *biotransformation,* chemicals are bioactivated to a high-energy reactive intermediate molecule, termed *phase I,* in preparation for the second step, phase II, which involves formation of covalent bonds with polar molecules, such as glucuronic acid. This conjugation forms a water-soluble metabolite that can be excreted. Phase III involves the transport of these molecules across the cell membrane into the lumen of the canaliculus by molecular pumps. In some circumstances, such as an overdose, the high-energy reactive metabolites can form covalent bonds with other cellular constituents, such as proteins, and nucleic acids termed adducts. In acute toxicity, adducts with essential cellular enzymes may lead to cell injury or death. Toxic hepatocellular injury of this category occurs most often in the centrilobular area of the liver because this is the region of the liver with the highest concentration of cytochrome p450 enzymes. For example, acetaminophen is metabolized by cytochrome p450 enzymes to *N*-acetyl-*p*-benzo-quinone imine (NAPQI), a free radical that is responsible for the toxicity of the parent compound. Lesions induced by acetaminophen are most severe in the centrilobular (periacinar) areas, where the active form of the chemical is present in greatest concentration. Many plant toxicities are examples of injury produced by this mechanism.
2. Adduct formation between drugs and cellular enzymes, other proteins, or nucleic acids can alter the cellular constituents sufficiently that they become neoantigens, as may be the case with halothane toxicity. These neoantigens, like other foreign antigens, can be processed in the cytoplasm, transported to the cell surface, presented as antigens, and recognized by the immune system. Consequently, the immune system may develop an inflammatory response toward hepatocytes or biliary epithelium that contain the adducts. Both cellular and humoral immunity can be involved. Injury can occur through direct cellular cytotoxicity and antibody-dependent cellular cytotoxicity. Although this mechanism is not well characterized in clinical veterinary medicine, it is likely to occur on occasion.
3. Certain toxins, including retained or excess hydrophobic bile acids, can trigger apoptosis (individual cell necrosis), by direct stimulation of proapoptotic pathways in the hepatocytes. Alternatively, apoptosis can be stimulated by immune-mediated events, such as those discussed previously, which lead to the release of TNF-α or activate Fas pathways.
4. Injury that damages cell membranes and disables enzymes responsible for calcium homeostasis, as seen in carbon tetrachloride toxicity, can lead to an influx of calcium. One consequence of the increased intracellular calcium is activation of proteases that damage actin filaments. Blebbing and lysis of the cell membranes can result.

5. Chemicals that bind to and disrupt the molecular pumps that secrete bile constituents into the canaliculi, such as estrogen and erythromycin, can produce cholestasis. More extensive hepatocellular injury that affects canalicular pumps and hepatocytes may produce cholestasis by disrupting the actin filaments situated around the bile canaliculi and preventing the normal pulsatile contractions that move bile through the canalicular system to the bile ducts.
6. Hepatocyte injury or death can follow mitochondrial damage, as seen with some toxic antiviral nucleosides or intravenous tetracycline administration. Chemical or reactive oxygen species–induced injury to mitochondrial membranes, enzymes, or DNA can inhibit or disrupt mitochondrial function. Disruption of the electron transport chain can release reactive oxygen species, such as superoxide, which can produce widespread cellular damage. Damaged mitochondria do not produce sufficient adenosine triphosphate (ATP) to power the essential functions of the hepatocytes. Also, β-oxidation of lipids is reduced once the mitochondria are damaged, which leads to intrahepatic lipid accumulation (microvesicular steatosis) and diminished energy production. Damaged mitochondria may release cytochrome-c, triggering apoptosis, or if disruption of mitochondrial function is sufficient, hepatocyte necrosis ensues.

Hepatotoxic Agents

Hepatotoxic Bacteria Blue-Green Algae

Blue-green algae are classified in the phylum Monera, division Cyanophyta; are considered to be more closely related to bacteria; and are no longer considered members of the plant family. Several genera of blue-green algae, including *Anabaena, Aphanizomenon,* and *Microcystis,* can cause lethal poisoning of livestock and less commonly small animals such as dogs and cats. Algal blooms usually occur in late summer or early fall because of the warm temperatures, long hours of sunlight, and abundance of essential nutrients. Dead and dying algae, which contain preformed toxins, such as microcystin LR, a cyclic heptapeptide, accumulate on the surface of bodies of water and are ingested by livestock. Secondary bacterial growth in dying algae may contribute to toxin formation. Signs develop rapidly and include diarrhea, prostration, and death. Gross lesions include hemorrhagic gastroenteritis and a red, swollen, hemorrhagic liver. Histologically, centrilobular, or even massive, hepatic necrosis and hemorrhage is evident. Animals that survive the acute manifestations may develop clinical signs of chronic liver disease. Other preformed toxins that affect different organ systems, including the nervous system, have also been identified in blue-green algae.

Hepatotoxic Plants

Toxic plants of great variety cause hepatic injury in domestic animals. A comprehensive discussion of each is beyond the scope of this chapter.

Pyrrolizidine Alkaloid-Containing Plants

Pyrrolizidine alkaloids are found in many plant families, including Compositae, Leguminosae, and Boraginaceae, that occur throughout much of the world. The most important genera are *Senecio, Cynoglossum, Amsinckia, Crotalaria, Echium, Trichodesma,* and *Heliotropium.* Approximately 100 different alkaloids are recognized; toxic effects depend on which alkaloids are present within ingested plants. Ingested alkaloids are converted to pyrrolic esters by hepatic cytochrome p450 enzymes. These esters are alkylating agents, which react with cytosolic and nuclear proteins and nucleic acids. Pigs are particularly susceptible to pyrrolizidine alkaloid intoxication, sheep considerably less so, and cattle and horses are intermediate in susceptibility. Most cases of intoxication arise from chronic intoxication, and the gross lesion is typically hepatic fibrosis (Fig. 8-58, *A*). The characteristic histologic lesions of pyrrolizidine alkaloid intoxication are the megalocytes, which are hepatocytes with enlarged nuclei and increased cytoplasmic volume. Megalocytes may be many times the size of normal hepatocytes (Fig. 8-58, *B*). Megalocytes are the result of the antimitotic effects of pyrrolizidine alkaloids, which prevent cell division but not DNA synthesis because the hepatocytes attempt to divide to replace those that have undergone necrosis. This change, although indicative of pyrrolizidine alkaloid intoxication, is not pathognomonic because it occurs with other toxins such as aflatoxins and nitrosamines. Typically, chronic pyrrolizidine intoxication is accompanied by hepatic fibrosis, biliary proliferation, and in some circumstances, nodular regeneration of parenchyma. Nodular regeneration does not always occur because hepatocyte proliferation can be inhibited by pyrrolizidines; however, exposure is not likely to be constant, and there may be periods during which hepatocyte replication can occur, such as the

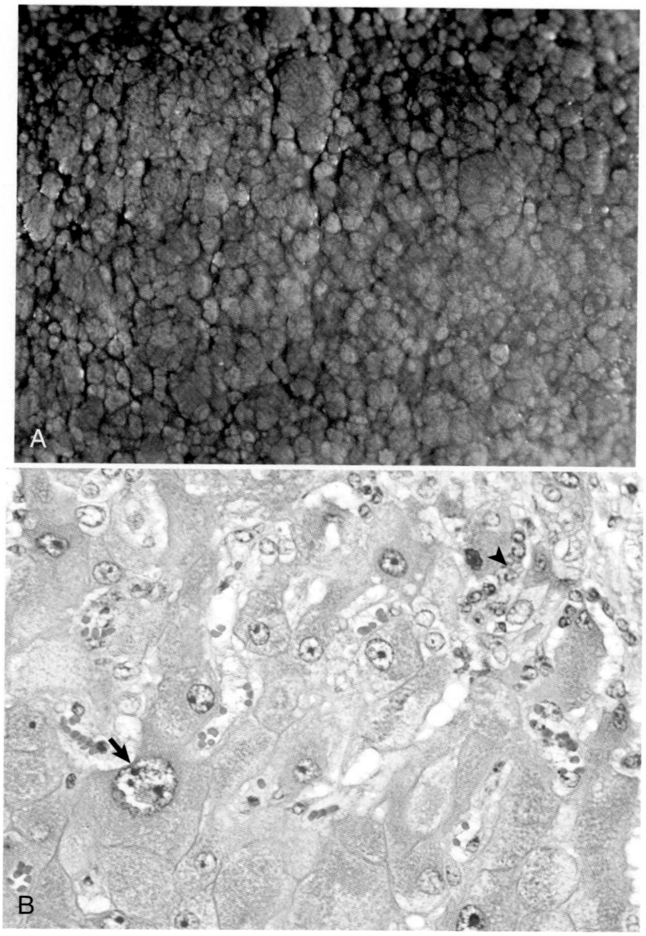

Fig. 8-58 Chronic pyrrolizidine hepatotoxicity, cow.
A, Chronic pyrrolizidine intoxication produces a fibrotic and sometimes distorted liver with an irregular capsular surface. **B,** Greatly enlarged hepatocytes (megalocytes) *(arrow)* and hyperplasia of biliary epithelium *(arrowhead)* in the persisting parenchyma are typical of pyrrolizidine toxicity. H&E stain. (**A** courtesy Dr. P. Carbonell, School of Veterinary Science, Melbourne. **B** courtesy Dr. M.D. McGavin, College of Veterinary Medicine, University of Tennessee.)

end of the dry season when more desirable plant species reappear. Species differences may also have an effect on the hepatic response to pyrrolizidines because cattle have regenerative nodules more often than horses. Chronic hepatic damage can lead to hepatic failure and its associated constellation of signs (described in detail earlier).

Cycads

Cycads are primitive palmlike plants that inhabit tropical and subtropical regions. They contain cycasin and macrozamin, nontoxic glycosides, which after ingestion are deconjugated by intestinal bacteria to release a toxic metabolite, methylazoxymethanol. After absorption into the portal vein, hepatic metabolism of this compound yields alkylating agents, leading to acute or chronic liver injury. Acute injury is manifested as acute centrilobular necrosis. Chronic hepatic lesions in cattle include hepatocellular megalocytosis caused by the mitoinhibitory effects of alkylating agents and nuclear hyperchromasia and varying degrees of hepatic fibrosis. Chronic cycad poisoning in cattle causes a nervous disease with progressive proprioceptive deficits in the hind legs because of "dying back" of axons in the dorsal funiculus and the spinocerebellar and corticospinal tracts. Acute intoxication is more common in sheep than in other species and produces acute gastrointestinal dysfunction and centrilobular hepatic necrosis. Dogs can also be intoxicated by cycads.

Cholestatic or Crystal-Associated Plant Intoxications

The ornamental shrub *Lantana camara* produces toxic pentacyclic triterpenes, lantadene A and B, that primarily produce a syndrome of chronic cholestasis in grazing animals. Bile accumulation is evident within the canaliculi, hepatocytes, and Kupffer cells.

Primarily in South Africa, *Tribulus terrestris* (puncture vine) ingestion by sheep can produce a fatal disorder (geeldikkop) characterized by icterus, biliary injury, and secondary photosensitization. Histologically, there is abundant crystalline material within and obstructing the bile ducts. Crystals may also be found in Kupffer cells. In various parts of the world, a similar pattern of crystal deposition can be seen in sheep and goats that graze a number of grass species, including *Panicum* sp., that contain steroidal saponins.

Secondary photosensitization and icterus can occur in all of these conditions as the result of impaired bile secretion.

Mycotoxins

Mycotoxins are secondary metabolites of fungi, that is, their production is not necessary for the survival of the fungus. The amount of toxin synthesized by a given strain of fungus reflects the genetic constitution of the particular strain, presence of appropriate substrate, temperature, humidity, and available nutrients. There are several hepatotoxic mycotoxins of veterinary significance.

Aflatoxin

The fungus *Aspergillus flavus* is the most important source of aflatoxins. Aflatoxin B_1 is the most common form and is also the most potent toxin and carcinogen. Aflatoxins are usually elaborated during storage of fungus-contaminated feed, particularly in humid conditions, and may be present in many crops, including corn, peanuts, and cottonseed. These can be incorporated into commercial food leading to significant outbreaks of acute toxicity in dogs. Aflatoxins are converted to toxic intermediates by hepatic cytochrome p450 enzymes. Carcinogenic, toxic, and teratogenic effects of aflatoxins reflect binding of the toxic intermediates to cellular DNA, RNA, or proteins. Pigs, dogs, horses, cattle, and ducks, especially younger animals, are sensitive to the toxic effects of aflatoxins, whereas sheep are more resistant. Acute aflatoxin intoxication is rare in horses and cattle because an inordinately large amount of contaminated feed would have to be ingested to achieve a sufficient dose. Acute aflatoxicosis in dogs is characterized by hemorrhagic central to massive necrosis. Steatosis and biliary proliferation also may occur. Chronic intoxication is more common than acute intoxication and results in ill-thrift, increased susceptibility to infection, and occasionally signs of hepatic failure. Affected livers are firm and pale and microscopically are characterized by steatosis and necrosis of hepatocytes, biliary hyperplasia, centrilobular to bridging fibrosis, and cellular atypia of hepatocytes, characterized by variable cell size and variable nuclear size (Fig. 8-59, *A* and *B*).

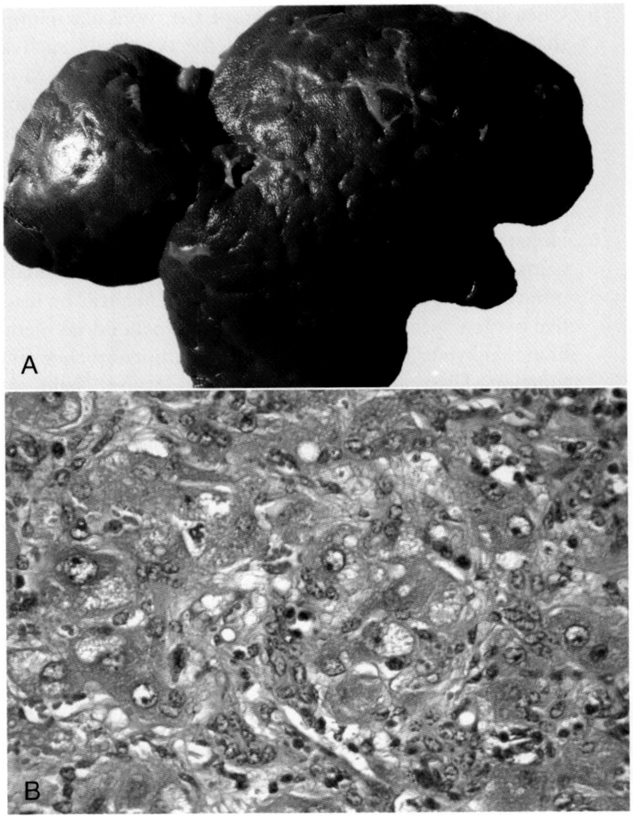

Fig. 8-59 Chronic hepatic aflatoxicosis.
A, Postnecrotic scarring, pig. Chronic aflatoxicosis produces a shrunken and fibrotic liver from collapse of areas of massive necrosis and condensation of the fibrous stroma. **B,** Histologic appearance. Chronic aflatoxicosis is characterized by variable amounts of steatosis (fatty change), biliary hyperplasia, and cellular atypia in hepatocytes. H&E stain. (**A** courtesy Dr. M.D. McGavin, College of Veterinary Medicine, University of Tennessee. **B** courtesy Dr. J. Simon, College of Veterinary Medicine, University of Illinois.)

Phomopsins

Phomopsins are toxic metabolites of the fungus *Phomopsis leptostromiformis*. The fungus grows on lupines (*Lupinus* sp.), and cattle, sheep, and occasionally horses that graze contaminated lupine stubble develop hepatic injury. Hepatic dysfunction is usually chronic, and the liver is atrophic and fibrotic. The microscopic appearance of affected livers is characterized by diffuse scattered hepatocyte necrosis with a background of mitotic figures, often appearing to be arrested in metaphase. Later in the course of the disease, diffuse fibrosis and biliary hyperplasia predominate. Signs of hepatic failure, including photosensitization, may occur in affected animals. This mycotoxicosis should not be confused with the condition known as *lupinosis,* which is caused by naturally occurring alkaloids in lupines that are capable of inducing skeletal deformities but not obvious hepatic injury.

Sporidesmin

The mycotoxin sporidesmin is produced by *Pithomyces chartarum,* a fungus that grows particularly well in dead rye grass *(Lolium perenne),* a common pasture plant in New Zealand and Australia. The majority of the toxin is concentrated into the fungal spores, and when a sufficient amount of the spores is ingested by sheep and to a lesser extent, cattle, the toxin is secreted into the biliary tree in an unconjugated form that produces necrosis of the epithelium of large intrahepatic and extrahepatic biliary ducts with minimal inflammation. Cholestasis with a concurrent failure to excrete phylloerythrin frequently leads to photosensitization with skin lesions predominantly on the head, thus the common name facial eczema. Acute cases are characterized by a bile-stained liver with prominent small-caliber bile ducts. These are dilated by bile in the lumens and surrounded by periductal edema. In chronic cases of facial eczema, the bile ducts become thickened by fibrosis secondary to biliary epithelial necrosis and subsequent inflammation (chronic cholangitis). Perhaps because of streaming of blood in the portal vein, the left lobe of the liver (although this lobe occupies the ventral portion of the ruminant liver), which may have an increased proportion of blood draining from the small intestine, is usually most severely affected and in severe cases undergoes atrophy and fibrosis.

Mushrooms

Poisonous mushrooms, such as *Amanita* sp. and others, can cause acute fatal liver necrosis. Intoxication by *Amanita phalloides,* known as the Death Cap, is caused by a group of toxins termed toxic cyclopeptides. This species is particularly toxic; a single gram of this mushroom is sufficient to kill a human, and even smaller amounts are likely to prove fatal to dogs. Amatoxin, an octapeptide, is in particular responsible for hepatocellular injury. The mechanism of injury is attributed to inhibition of RNA polymerase II function disrupting DNA and RNA transcription. Gross lesions usually consist of hepatic hemorrhage and a shrunken liver because of the loss of hepatocytes. Hepatocellular steatosis, hemorrhage, and centrilobular to massive necrosis are the typical lesions. Death from liver failure may occur 3 to 4 days after the onset of clinical signs. Phalloidin, a toxic heptapeptide found in *Amanita* sp., causes disruption of intracellular actin filaments, leading to cell injury or death. It is a less significant toxin in natural exposure because of the limited absorption from the digestive tract. Other mushroom species contain different toxic agents.

Hepatotoxic Chemicals

Xylitol

The artificial sweetener xylitol is used in various food items and snacks prepared for diabetics or dieters. Although innocuous to humans, xylitol can be acutely toxic to dogs. After ingesting as little as 0.5 gm/kg, affected dogs can develop hyperinsulinemia, hypoglycemia, icterus, and acute, severe centrilobular to massive hepatic necrosis.

Phosphorus

Phosphorus occurs in two forms: red phosphorus and white phosphorus. Red phosphorus is unimportant as a toxin, but white phosphorus was previously used as a rodenticide. The mechanism of phosphorus toxicity is unclear, although it apparently is directly toxic. Poisoning is first indicated by signs of gastroenteritis and subsequently by microscopic lesions of steatosis of hepatocytes and periportal necrosis. The pattern of periportal necrosis is unusual because most toxic liver injury occurs in the centrilobular region of the liver. This is explained by the fact that white phosphorus does not require metabolic transformation to a reactive intermediate by cytochrome p450 enzymes, which are most concentrated in the centrilobular region of the liver lobule.

Carbon Tetrachloride

Carbon tetrachloride is the classic example of a hepatotoxin that must be bioactivated by the mixed-function oxidase system to produce a toxic intermediate form. Although once used widely, it is only occasionally used as an anthelmintic. Carbon tetrachloride produces centrilobular hepatic necrosis and steatosis of surviving hepatocytes (see Chapter 1).

Metals

Several metals can cause toxic hepatic injury. Excessive iron supplementation in dogs and cats may result in excessive storage of iron and subsequently hepatic disease caused by iron overload, termed *hemochromatosis.* Two specific syndromes of iron poisoning are iron-dextran intoxication of piglets and ferrous fumarate intoxication of newborn foals. Severe cases of these two toxicities are characterized by massive hepatic necrosis. Intoxication of foals with ferrous fumarate occurred after its use as a component of a specific dietary supplement, and was characterized by massive necrosis and also a remarkable amount of hyperplasia of bile ducts and cholangioles, possibly with oval cell proliferation, despite the short clinical course of the disease. Iron-dextran is frequently administered intramuscularly to suckling pigs to prevent anemia, but administration of iron-dextran has occasionally resulted in significant mortality, and affected pigs die soon after injection.

Copper toxicity is discussed in separate sections on Disorders of Ruminants and Canine Chronic Hepatitis.

Hepatotoxic Therapeutic Drugs

There are a variety of drugs that have a proven therapeutic application but can cause significant acute or chronic hepatic injury in some animals. A partial list of hepatotoxic therapeutic drugs in dogs and cats is presented in Web Table 8-2. Clearly, these drugs would not be used if the proportion of injured animals was high, but it is important to keep in mind that many drugs have the potential to cause hepatic injury in some patients. The mechanisms by which these drugs cause injury vary by species and by individual. Some therapeutic drugs are predictable toxins, and all members of a particular species are susceptible to liver injury if a sufficient dose is given. But because the therapeutic effect occurs at a lower dose than the toxic dose, liver injury occurs only when overdoses are ingested. Hepatic metabolism (bioactivation) of these compounds is likely to be involved because the site of liver injury is typically centrilobular. Cats are more susceptible than dogs to intoxication by many chemicals because they are relatively deficient in hepatic glucuronyltransferase activity. This phase II enzyme forms conjugates between bioactivated (phase I) xenobiotics and glutathione. When phase II metabolism is overwhelmed, injurious bioactivated products cause liver injury. Cats are more sensitive to acetaminophen intoxication than dogs because of this relative enzyme deficiency. Other therapeutic drugs are idiosyncratic toxins, and they affect only a small minority of patients. The mechanism of injury is not known but may be a consequence of inherited differences in hepatic enzyme content and activity, atypical immune reactions to drug metabolites, or novel antigens created when drug metabolites bind to cellular proteins. For example, the antiinflammatory drug carprofen can occasionally cause acute hepatic necrosis in a variety of dogs, but certain breeds of dogs, such as Labrador retrievers, may be affected more often than others. The tranquilizer diazepam can cause acute fatal hepatic injury in some cats, but the majority of treated cats are unaffected, and dogs do not seem to be adversely affected.

Chronic liver toxicity has been described in dogs receiving any of the anticonvulsants, primidone, phenytoin, and phenobarbital for prolonged periods. The mechanism of hepatotoxicity is unknown. Only a small proportion of dogs receiving these drugs are affected, and these dogs frequently have signs of hepatic failure. The liver is small and has widespread hepatic fibrosis and nodular regeneration (end-stage liver).

HEPATIC INJURY AS A CONSEQUENCE OF SYSTEMIC DISEASE

A variety of extrahepatic disorders, usually affecting the gastrointestinal tract, can result in hepatocellular injury and hepatic dysfunction. Acute hemorrhagic pancreatitis of dogs, for example, sometimes is accompanied by icterus and increased activities of hepatic enzymes in serum. Release of various toxins and inflammatory mediators from the injured pancreas into the portal vein showers the liver with a variety of injurious substances. Similarly, movement of hepatotoxic substances, such as endotoxins, into the portal vein can occur as a consequence of diseases that disrupt the mucosal barrier of the intestine. Some cases of chronic inflammation of the colon can result in chronic hepatic inflammation as well. Accumulation of inflammatory cells within the portal triads may accompany blood-borne infection or abdominal sepsis (nonspecific reactive hepatitis).

The liver is particularly susceptible to the effects of hypoxia; thus any disease that causes anemia can produce centrilobular or paracentral degeneration and necrosis. Also, the hepatocytes in hemolytic anemias must remove and conjugate the increased amounts of circulating bilirubin and hemoglobin, and Kupffer cells must remove either erythrocytes during extravascular hemolysis or erythrocytic fragments during intravascular hemolysis.

PROLIFERATIVE LESIONS OF THE LIVER

Hepatocellular Nodular Hyperplasia

Hepatocellular nodular hyperplasia is common only in the dog. The incidence increases with age, starting around 6 years of age, without predilection for either sex or breed. Nodular hyperplasia is not the result or the cause of significant hepatic dysfunction, but nodular hyperplasia should be distinguished from regenerative nodules and hepatic neoplasms, with which they are often confused. Multiple hyperplastic nodules are frequently present. Nodules that can be seen on the capsular surface are typically raised and hemispherical, yellow to tan (although they can be dark red when congested), 0.5 to 3 cm in diameter, and are more friable than normal liver. On incision, the hyperplastic nodules are well demarcated from normal parenchyma and usually compress adjacent parenchyma (Fig. 8-60, *A* and *B*). Hyperplastic nodules contain all the elements of normal liver, but the lobular pattern is distorted. The lobules in areas of nodular hyperplasia contain an increased proportion of hepatocytes and decreased numbers of portal tracts and central veins compared with a normal liver. Hepatocytes are variably sized and frequently

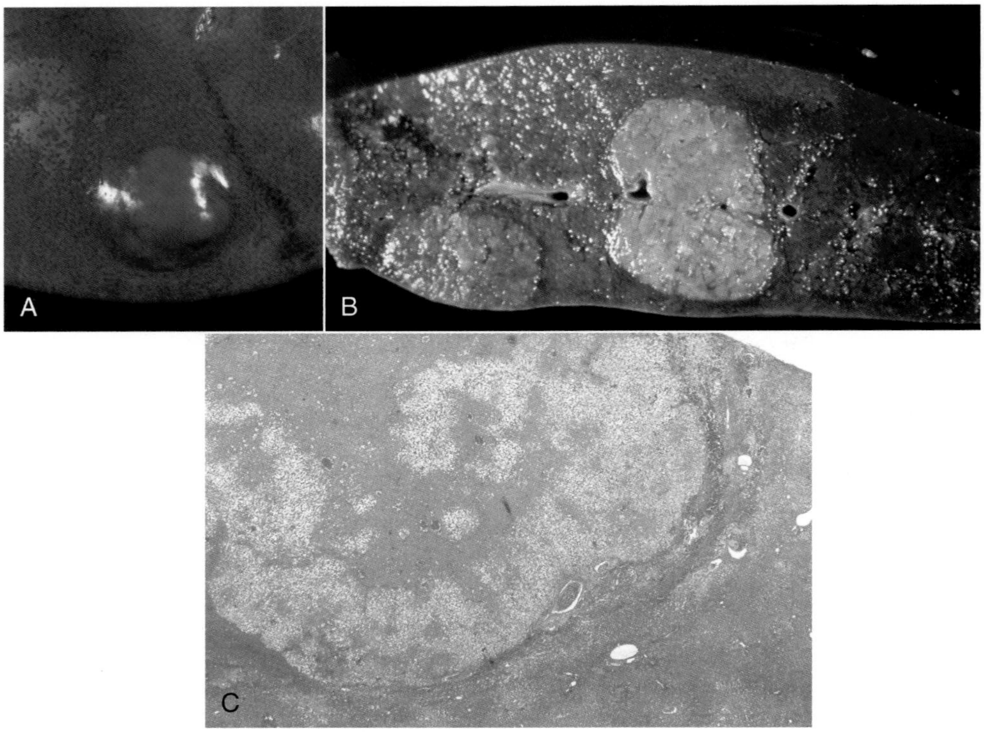

Fig. 8-60 Hepatic nodular hyperplasia, liver, dog.

A, A nodule protrudes above the surface of the adjacent, normal parenchyma. **B,** Nodular hyperplasia, cut surface of liver. Two hyperplastic nodules are shown. **C,** A hyperplastic nodule compresses adjacent hepatocytes, and the hepatocytes of the nodule can be prominently vacuolated as in this case. H&E stain. (**A** courtesy Dr. M.D. McGavin, College of Veterinary Medicine, University of Tennessee. **B** courtesy Dr. R. Fairley, Lincoln University. **C** courtesy Dr. J.M. Cullen, College of Veterinary Medicine, North Carolina State University.)

contain cytoplasmic lipid or glycogen-containing vacuoles (Fig. 8-60, *C*).

Regenerative Nodules

Regenerative nodules are another type of nodular hepatocellular lesion. Regenerative nodules are unlikely to be related to nodular hyperplasia because regenerative nodules arise from the proliferation of hepatocytes in response to loss of hepatocytes, and the incidence is not related to age. Often the insult is unknown, but the response of some dogs to anticonvulsant drugs, such as phenobarbital or phenytoin, is a well-recognized cause. Regenerative nodules are readily distinguished from nodular hyperplasia because the process occurs in the presence of significant fibrosis and disruption of normal hepatic parenchymal architecture. Because these lesions result from the outgrowth of surviving hepatocytes, there is usually only a single portal tract apparent in sections of the regenerative nodules.

Cholangiocellular (Bile Duct) Hyperplasia

Hyperplasia of biliary ductules commonly occurs as a nonspecific response to a variety of hepatic injuries and has been described in the Response of the Liver to Injury section. Reactive proliferation of the bile ductules of the liver must be distinguished from neoplastic proliferations.

Hepatic Neoplasia

Primary neoplasms of the hepatobiliary system can arise from epithelial elements, including hepatocytes, biliary epithelium of bile ducts or the gallbladder, and mesenchymal elements such as connective tissue and blood vessels. The liver is a common site of metastasis for many malignant tumors; in fact, the majority of neoplasms within the liver are metastases from other organs.

Hepatocellular Adenoma

Hepatocellular adenomas are benign neoplasms of hepatocytes. Hepatocellular adenomas have been described most commonly in young ruminants, although hepatic adenomas are likely underdiagnosed in older dogs where they may be diagnosed as well-differentiated hepatocellular carcinomas. The neoplasms usually are single, unencapsulated, variably sized, and red or brown masses that compress adjacent parenchyma. They are typically spherical but may be pedunculated (Fig. 8-61). They are composed of well-differentiated hepatocytes, which form uniform plates that may be two to three cells thick. Hepatic plates in adenomas tend to abut normal adjacent hepatocytes at right angles. Portal tracts and central veins are scarce within the neoplasm, if they can be found at all. Diagnostic criteria to distinguish hepatocellular adenomas from hepatocellular nodular hyperplasia can be somewhat subjective because both arise in livers with no background abnormality, unlike regenerative nodules that arise in damaged livers. Histologically, adenomas are characterized by only one or very few portal tracts, whereas hyperplastic nodules retain normal lobular architecture elements, although the portal tracts are more separated than normal. In other cases, it may be difficult to distinguish hepatocellular adenomas from well-differentiated hepatocellular carcinomas.

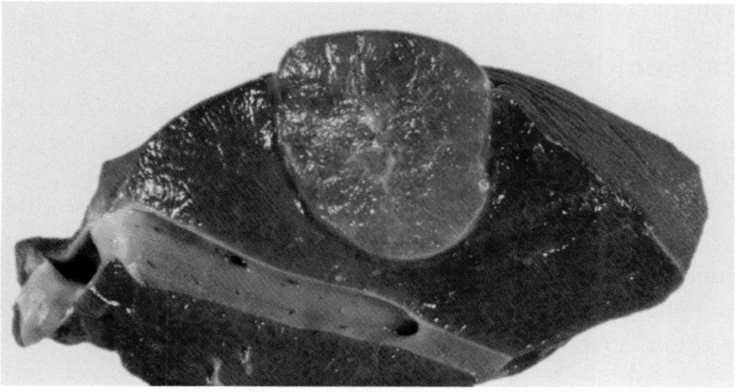

Fig. 8-61 Hepatocellular adenomas, liver, dog.
Hepatocellular adenomas form discrete masses of hepatocytes that compress adjacent normal parenchyma. (Courtesy Dr. J.M. Cullen, College of Veterinary Medicine, North Carolina State University.)

Hepatocellular Carcinoma

Hepatocellular carcinomas are malignant neoplasms of hepatocytes. They are uncommon in all domestic species but may occur more frequently in ruminants, particularly sheep. These neoplasms are often solitary, frequently involve an entire lobe, and are well demarcated. They typically consist of friable, gray-white or yellow-brown tissue, which is subdivided into lobules by multiple fibrous bands (Fig. 8-62, *A*). Malignant hepatocytes characteristically form irregular plates (trabeculae) three or more cells thick, and vascular spaces are present between the trabeculae (Fig. 8-62, *B*). Crude acini forming a pseudoglandular pattern of neoplastic cells are sometimes present. Within an individual tumor, trabecular,

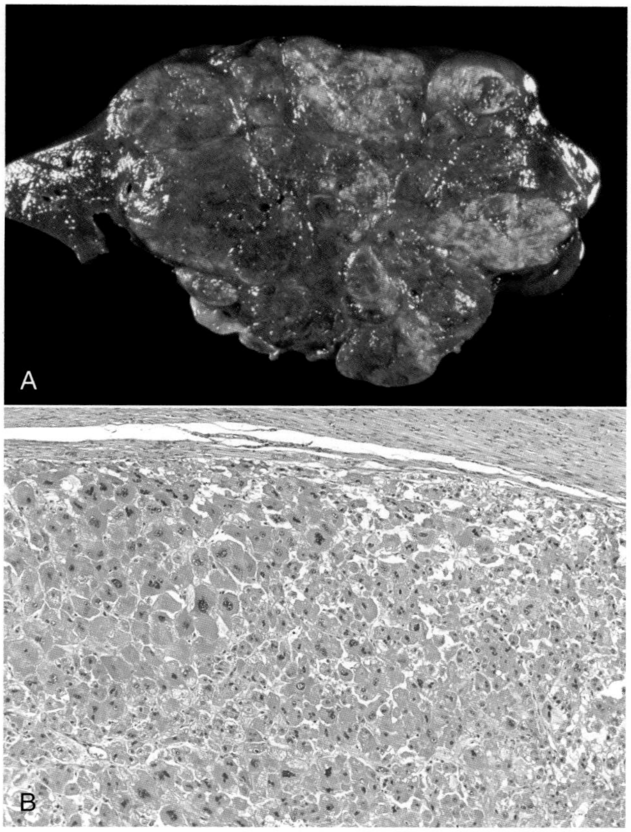

Fig. 8-62 Hepatocellular carcinoma, liver, dog.
A, A multilobular carcinoma has replaced much of the normal liver. **B,** Hepatocellular carcinomas contain pleomorphic hepatocytes that can form trabeculae, a glandular-like pattern or solid sheets of cells, as in this case. H&E stain. (**A** courtesy College of Veterinary Medicine, North Carolina State University. **B** courtesy Dr. J.M. Cullen, College of Veterinary Medicine, North Carolina State University.)

pseudoglandular, and solid patterns may be found. Cells present in the neoplasm range from well-differentiated hepatocytes to atypical or bizarre forms. In the absence of metastasis, which is obviously indicative of malignancy, distinction of well-differentiated carcinoma from adenoma can be difficult, although invasion by malignant hepatocytes at the margin of the adjacent compressed normal hepatocytes and hepatocellular atypia are useful indicators of malignancy. Metastasis to a variety of sites may occur, particularly to lymph nodes within the cranial abdomen, lungs, and seeding into the tissue of the peritoneal cavity. Some hepatocellular carcinomas extensively spread within the liver (intrahepatic metastasis).

Biliary Neoplasia

Cholangiocellular (Bile Duct) Adenoma

Adenomas of the biliary ducts are uncommon in most species but may be the most common primary hepatic neoplasm in cats. They are usually discrete, firm, and gray or white masses consisting of well-differentiated biliary epithelium. Cholangiomas are glandlike structures formed by tubules lined with cuboidal epithelium and moderate amounts of stroma. The tubules may have narrow lumens or may be distended by fluid-forming cystic structures of variable sizes. Cystic variants, termed *biliary cystadenomas,* typically have a nonencapsulated, multilocular cystic structure. Hepatocytes are usually compressed at the margins or may on occasion be entrapped by expanding cysts. The stroma of the cyst wall consists of fibrovascular tissue with moderate amounts of collagen. Cysts are lined with benign biliary epithelium (simple cuboidal to flattened). The lining epithelium tends to be more flattened in the biliary cystadenomas, presumably because of compression. Biliary epithelial cells may form papillary projections extending into the cystic spaces.

In cats, large cystic cavities that are lined with flattened biliary epithelium are regarded as adenomas or cystadenomas by some investigators, but it may be more appropriate to consider them to be congenital malformations. Congenital biliary cysts are multiloculated and can involve extensive areas of the liver. Typically, they have flattened epithelium and varying amounts of fibrous tissue, and islands of hepatocytes are often scattered between the cysts.

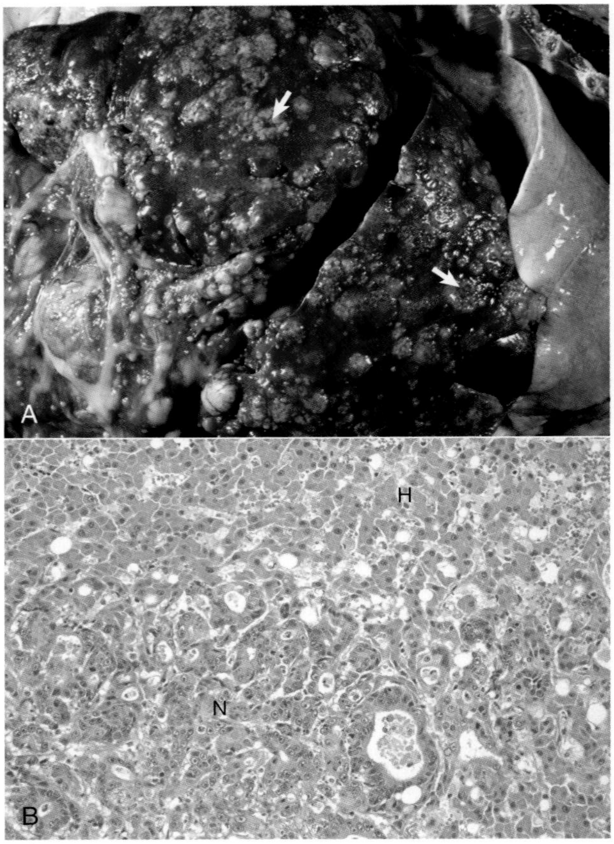

Fig. 8-63 Cholangiocellular carcinoma, liver.
A, Dog. Multiple nodules of tumor, some of which are umbilicated *(arrows)*. B, Cat. Cords and acini of neoplastic bile duct epithelial cells *(N)* invade the adjacent normal hepatic parenchyma *(H)*. H&E stain. (**A** courtesy Dr. M.D. McGavin, College of Veterinary Medicine, University of Tennessee. **B** courtesy Dr. J. Simon, College of Veterinary Medicine, University of Illinois.)

Cholangiocellular (Bile Duct) Carcinoma

Cholangiocellular carcinomas are malignant neoplasms of biliary epithelium, which usually arise from the intrahepatic ducts, but extrahepatic bile ducts can be affected. These neoplasms occur in all species. A large single mass or multiple nodules may be present within the liver; these typically are firm, raised, often with a central depression (umbilicated), pale gray to tan, and unencapsulated (Fig. 8-63, *A*). The tumors are composed of cells that retain a resemblance to biliary epithelium. Characteristically, well-differentiated carcinomas are organized into a tubular or acinar arrangement. In less differentiated neoplasms, some acinar arrangements can be detected among solid masses of neoplastic cells. Poorly differentiated carcinomas are composed of packets, islands, or cords, and areas of squamous differentiation can occur. The epithelial components of the neoplasms are usually separated by fibrous connective tissue (Fig. 8-63, *B*). The amount of connective tissue varies among tumors, but an abundant deposition of collagen, termed a *scirrhous response,* is relatively common and is responsible for the firm texture of these neoplasms. The margins of cholangiocarcinomas are characterized by multiple sites of local invasion by tumor cells of surrounding hepatic parenchyma. Multiple sites of hepatic necrosis are also common in the adjacent parenchyma.

Metastasis to extrahepatic sites is common, particularly to the adjacent lymph nodes of the cranial abdomen, lungs, or by seeding into the abdominal cavity. Metastasis into the peritoneal cavity can produce variably sized nodules within the mesentery and on the serosal surface of the abdominal viscera.

A unique cutaneous paraneoplastic syndrome can be observed in cats with pancreatic adenocarcinoma or cholangiocarcinoma. This manifests grossly as symmetric alopecia of the ventral trunk and limbs with a glistening appearance. Histologically, affected areas have marked follicular and adnexal atrophy and loss of the stratum corneum of the epidermis.

Carcinoids

Carcinoids are uncommon tumors that are believed to arise from neuroendocrine cells that lie within the biliary epithelium. They can form within the intrahepatic or extrahepatic biliary system. Often, they form a single mass, but multiple nodules can occur, probably secondary to intrahepatic metastasis. Cells tend to be small, elongated, or spindle-shaped and form ribbons or rosettes (Fig. 8-64). Immunohistochemical detection of neuroendocrine markers, such as chromogranin A, can be used to confirm the diagnosis.

Miscellaneous Primary Mesenchymal Neoplasms of the Liver

Primary neoplasms can arise from any of the cellular constituents of the liver, including mesenchymal neoplasms derived from the

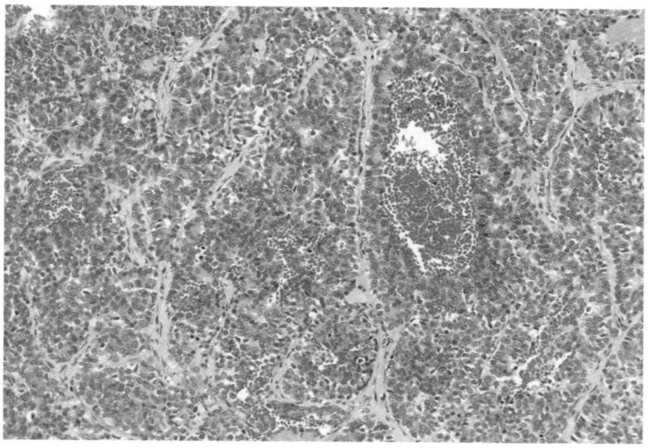

Fig. 8-64 Neuroendocrine tumors, carcinoid, liver, dog.
Carcinoids are malignant neoplasms of neuroendocrine cells, including those of the liver or bile ducts. Histologically, the tumor is composed of small elongated or spindle-shaped basophilic cells that form ribbons or rosettes and contain numerous vascular spaces. H&E stain. See Chapter 12 and Figs. 12-53, 12-54, and 12-55) for more information on carcinoids. (Courtesy Dr. J.M. Cullen, College of Veterinary Medicine, North Carolina State University.)

liver's connective tissue (fibrosarcoma, leiomyosarcoma, and osteosarcoma) and endothelium (hemangioma and hemangiosarcoma). Primary hepatic hemangiosarcoma is well recognized in dogs, although it is a relatively uncommon site of origin for this neoplasm as compared with the skin and spleen and heart. Primary mesenchymal neoplasms of the liver must be distinguished from metastases; the presence of disseminated masses throughout the liver is more typical of metastatic sarcomas than of primary hepatic sarcomas.

Metastatic Neoplasms

The liver and the lung are the two most common sites for metastatic spread of malignant neoplasms. Metastatic neoplasms must be distinguished from primary hyperplasia or neoplasia of the hepatobiliary tissue. It is important therefore when evaluating a neoplasm within the liver to determine if a neoplasm is present at some extrahepatic site that might be the primary neoplasm. The animal's medical history should also be reviewed to determine if masses have been removed previously. Malignant lymphoma is the most common metastatic neoplasm found in the liver of most, if not all, species.

Some metastatic neoplasms have a typical appearance within the liver; for example, melanomas frequently are black because of the presence of melanin, and hemangiosarcomas are usually dark red to brown because of blood. Hematopoietic neoplasms, such as lymphoma and the myeloproliferative disorders, can diffusely expand the liver and can be diffusely infiltrative (Fig. 8-65, *A*), producing hepatomegaly and an enhanced lobular pattern on the cut surface, or may have a nodular appearance (Fig. 8-65, *B*). This characteristic appearance of diffuse involvement is attributable to centrilobular hepatocellular degeneration because of anemia in both lymphoma and myeloproliferative disorders and because of the specific location of accumulations of neoplastic cells; locations include portal and periportal for lymphomas (Fig. 8-65, *C*) and sinusoidal for myeloproliferative disorders. Metastatic carcinomas often have an umbilicated appearance, similar to that seen with cholangiocellular carcinomas, but umbilication is rarely a feature of sarcomas.

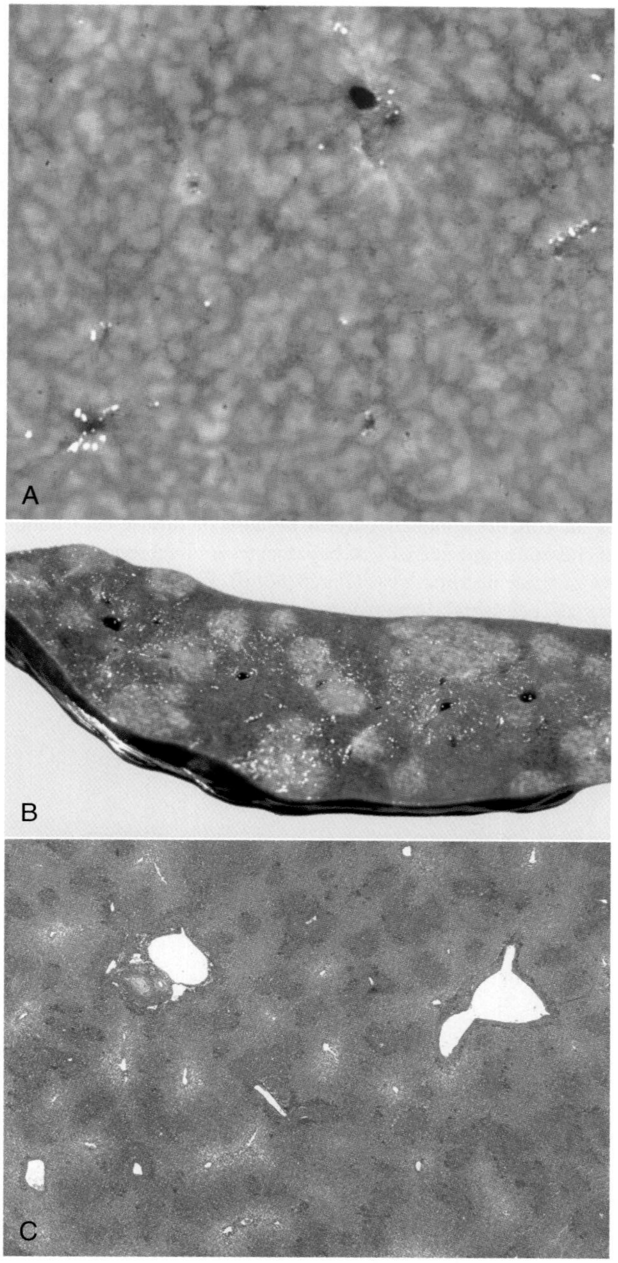

Fig. 8-65 Hepatic lymphoma, liver.
A, Cut surface, high magnification, dog. The entire liver is enlarged (not shown here), and there are multiple pale foci caused by infiltrating neoplastic lymphocytes. The regular distribution of neoplastic foci apparent on the cut surface is due to the preferential infiltration of the portal tracts by neoplastic cells. **B,** Cow. As shown here, hepatic lymphoma can have a nodular rather than a diffuse pattern, as seen in Fig. 8-65, *A*. **C,** Dog. Neoplastic lymphocytes *(blue areas)* are typically distributed within and around the portal tracts and central veins. H&E stain. See Chapter 6 and Fig. 6-9 for more information on lymphomas. (**A** and **C** courtesy Dr. J.M. Cullen, College of Veterinary Medicine, North Carolina State University. **B** courtesy College of Veterinary Medicine, University of Illinois.)

DISORDERS OF HORSES

EQUINE SERUM HEPATITIS

Equine serum hepatitis was first described by Theiler in South Africa at the beginning of the twentieth century but is now recognized in many countries. It occurs frequently but not invariably in horses that have received an injection of a biologic that contains equine serum; for example, equine antisera such as tetanus antitoxin or pregnant mare serum gonadotropin. It appears that an infectious agent is responsible, although none has been identified. The incubation period is prolonged, but the clinical course of the disease is very rapid and is invariably fatal. Affected horses typically have hepatic failure, which manifests as hepatic encephalopathy and icterus. Intravascular hemolysis occurs in the terminal stages of the disease. The livers of affected animals may be normal size or even enlarged but are typically small, flabby, and discolored greenish brown to dark brown (Fig. 8-66, *A*). The liver of affected animals has an enhanced lobular pattern because of diffuse centrilobular degeneration and necrosis of hepatocytes and subsequent congestion of these necrotic areas (Fig. 8-66, *B*). Frequently, only narrow rims of periportal hepatocytes survive and these cells may be prominently vacuolated with lipid. The centrilobular areas usually contain only remnants of necrotic hepatocytes, apoptotic bodies, pigmented Kupffer cells, and dilated sinusoids. Sometimes the portal areas contain proliferating tubules or columns of small basophilic cells, which are probably a regenerative response of bipotential hepatic precursor cells, termed a *ductual reaction.*

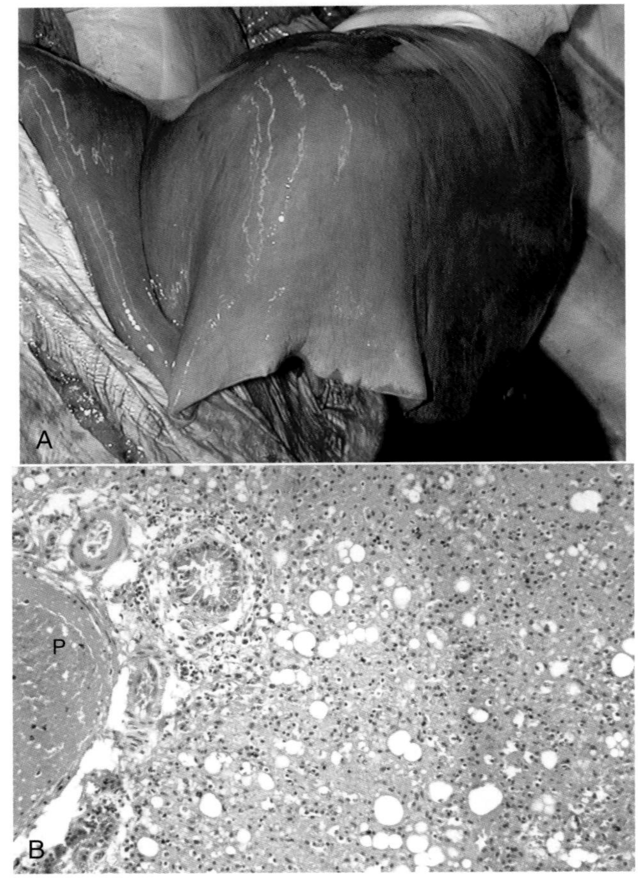

Fig. 8-66 Equine serum hepatitis, liver, horse.
A, Livers from horses affected with equine serum hepatitis can be small, flabby, and pale or discolored by bile pigment. **B,** In horses with equine serum hepatitis, most hepatocytes are necrotic, although there may be a few remaining hepatocytes with lipid-containing vacuoles in the periportal regions *(P)*. Inflammation consists of mononuclear cells predominantly. H&E stain. (**A** courtesy Dr. K. Bailey, College of Veterinary Medicine, University of Illinois. **B** courtesy Dr. J.M. Cullen, College of Veterinary Medicine, North Carolina State University.)

DISORDERS OF RUMINANTS (CATTLE, SHEEP, AND GOATS)

COPPER TOXICOSIS

In ruminants, particularly sheep, copper can accumulate within the liver over a period of time due to dietary excess or insufficient molybdenum to antagonize bioavailability of copper. When such sheep ingest hepatotoxins, such as pyrrolizidine-containing plants or mycotoxins, the resultant hepatocellular injury can, when sufficiently serious, trigger a sudden release of copper, which is followed by acute, severe intravascular hemolysis and additional hepatocellular necrosis, mostly because of acute anemia. Necrosis of the liver is extensive and affects centrilobular and midzonal regions most consistently because of hypoxia, but massive necrosis can occur in severe cases. Affected animals are icteric with swollen pale to orange livers, and hemoglobinuria is prominent. Despite the acute and fulminant nature of the terminal event, this process is referred to as *chronic copper poisoning* to distinguish it from disease caused by simple copper intoxication that causes gastroenteritis.

RIFT VALLEY FEVER

Rift Valley fever is an acute, arthropod (mosquito)-transmitted zoonotic viral disease that principally affects ruminants, causing extensive mortality among calves and lambs, and abortion in ewes and cows, although adults can also be affected. The causative virus is a member of the family Bunyaviridae in the genus *Phlebovirus.* The disease is enzootic in southern and eastern Africa, but significant outbreaks can spread throughout much of Africa and extend into the Middle East. It is especially prevalent after periods of unusually high rainfall. Disease manifestations are typically more severe in the epidemic outbreaks than in enzootic cases. In severe cases, affected animals are febrile, may abort, and have respiratory and gastrointestinal signs, including prominent diarrhea. Mortality is highest in sheep, with lambs most severely affected, but even in cattle up to a third of calves may die.

Hepatic involvement is consistently present in fulminant cases, typically in neonates, and is characterized by hepatomegaly with a yellow-orange discoloration. Areas of congestion may be present. In older animals, pale, 1 to 2 mm randomly scattered foci of hepatocellular necrosis impart a mottled appearance and sometimes an enhanced lobular pattern. Microscopic lesions are characterized by the presence of both randomly distributed foci of hepatocellular necrosis and apoptosis. Secondarily, more widespread zonal necrosis, which ranges from centrilobular to include the midzonal region can develop (Fig. 8-67). These lesions, particularly random hepatic necrosis, are more severe and widespread in young animals and aborted fetuses. Fibrin deposition within sinusoids is common, but cholestasis is not a consistent feature. Eosinophilic intranuclear inclusion bodies may be present in degenerate hepatocytes in areas of necrosis.

Diffuse petechiae and ecchymoses are also characteristic of the disease, as are edema and hemorrhages of the intestinal tract and the wall of the gallbladder. DIC probably contributes to the hemorrhagic diathesis and perhaps to the development of zonal hepatic necrosis.

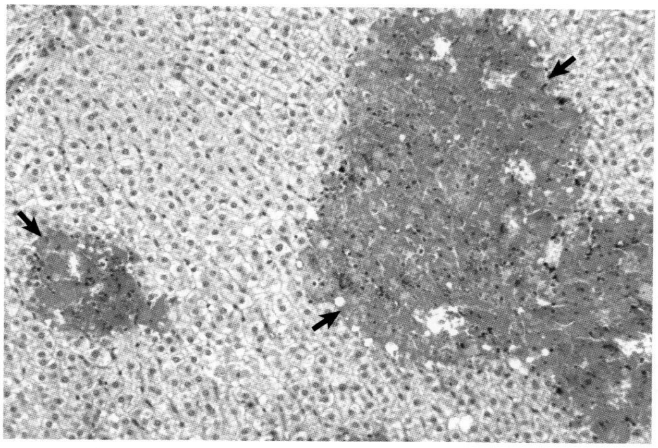

Fig. 8-67 Focal hepatic necrosis, Rift Valley fever, liver, sheep. This disease produces randomly distributed focal areas of necrosis *(arrows)* in the liver of lambs and fetuses, often with a central area of older necrosis surrounded by a rim of hepatocytes, which have been killed at a later stage in the infection. H&E stain. (Courtesy Armed Forces Institute of Pathology.)

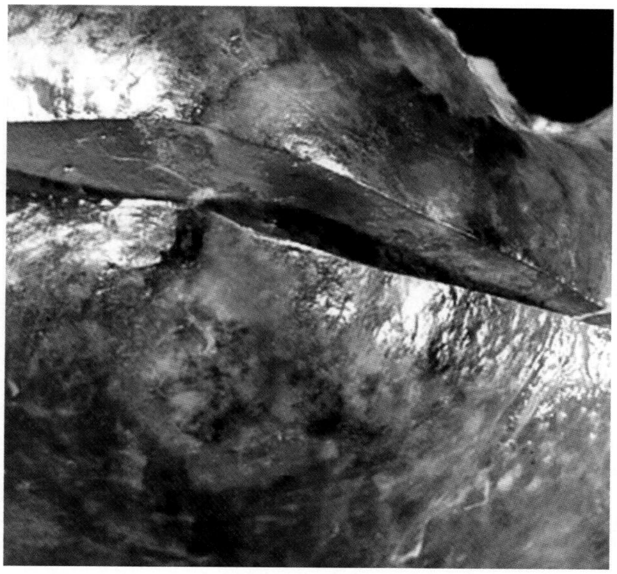

Fig. 8-68 Focal hepatic necrosis, *Clostridium haemolyticum* (bacillary hemoglobinuria), liver, cut surface, cow. These large areas of necrosis are sharply delineated from the adjacent parenchyma, usually pale, and surrounded by an intensely hyperemic zone of acute inflammation. (Courtesy Dr. J. King, College of Veterinary Medicine, Cornell University.)

WESSELSBRON DISEASE

Wesselsbron disease of sheep is caused by Wesselsbron virus, a flavivirus, and like Rift Valley fever, is a zoonotic arthropod (mosquito)-transmitted viral disease that occurs in Africa. The virus can cause disease in newborn lambs and abortion in ewes, but adults rarely have apparent clinical signs. Affected lambs have multifocal areas of generalized petechiae, intestinal hemorrhage, and an enlarged pale-to-orange liver. Icterus may develop. Canalicular cholestasis is often apparent and is occasionally prominent. Scattered individual hepatocyte and sinusoidal lining cell necrosis accompanied with pigmented macrophages and mononuclear inflammatory cells within the parenchyma are typical. Eosinophilic inclusions can be found in hepatocytes. In Wesselsbron disease, foci of hepatic necrosis are typically less extensive than in Rift Valley fever, although cholestasis is usually more prominent.

BACILLARY HEMOGLOBINURIA

Bacillary hemoglobinuria is an acute and highly fatal disease of cattle and sheep that occurs in various areas of the world and can be endemic in those regions in which liver fluke, particularly *Fasciola hepatica,* infection also occurs. Spores of *Clostridium haemolyticum,* the causative agent of bacillary hemoglobinuria, are ingested and come to reside within Kupffer cells, but they proliferate only in areas of low oxygen tension. Migration of immature liver flukes, or less commonly other parasites, or an event, such as liver biopsy, produces a nidus of necrotic hepatic parenchyma in which bacterial spores can germinate. Bacteria proliferate and release exotoxins, including the beta toxin, phospholipase C, that induces the hepatocellular necrosis, intravascular hemolysis, anemia, and hemoglobinuria that characterize the disease. Grossly, these foci (or often a large single lesion), which have been misnamed infarcts, are sharply delineated from the adjacent parenchyma, and usually are pale and surrounded by an intensely hyperemic zone (Fig. 8-68). The causative organisms, Gram-positive spore-containing rods, may be visible in histologic sections. Migration tracts of the immature flukes that typically precipitate the disease may be present. Serous cavities (pleura, peritoneum, and pericardium) can be flecked with fibrin.

INFECTIOUS NECROTIC HEPATITIS

Infectious necrotic hepatitis, also known as black disease, is most common in sheep and cattle but also occurs in pigs and horses. This disease is somewhat analogous to bacillary hemoglobinuria in that dormant spores of *Clostridium,* in this circumstance, *Clostridium novyi* (type B), germinate in areas of lowered oxygen tension and release exotoxins that produce discrete foci of coagulation necrosis and hemorrhage within the liver, hemolysis, and eventually death of the host. In endemic areas, germination of spores is usually initiated by hepatic necrosis caused by the migration of immature liver flukes; however, a variety of other initiating factors that produce low oxygen tension within the liver parenchyma have been described. Parasitic migration tracts are usually present within the affected liver. Other lesions that may be present include diffuse venous congestion and accumulation of fluid within the pericardial sac and pleural and peritoneal cavities. Affected animals typically have one or more areas of hepatocellular necrosis, which usually manifests as discrete, pale areas of variable size. A zone of intense hyperemia often surrounds these foci. Histologically, well-demarcated areas of necrosis with peripheral neutrophils and subjacent, abundant Gram-positive rods within the necrotic areas are found. The carcass of affected animals typically putrefies rapidly because of high fever before death.

WHITE LIVER DISEASE

White liver disease derives its name from the pale, fatty livers in sheep that develop from a nutritional deficiency caused by insufficient cobalt intake. Animals grazing on soil that is depleted in cobalt either by natural deficiency or previous use of the area for plants, such as potatoes, that deplete soil of cobalt are affected. Cobalt is a necessary cofactor in the synthesis of vitamin B_{12} and other enzymes. Deficiency of vitamin B_{12} can lead to anemia, and the liver lesions may be attributed to the effects of anemia.

DISORDERS OF PIGS

HEPATOSIS DIETETICA

Hepatosis dietetica (nutritional hepatic necrosis) is a syndrome of acute hepatic necrosis that occurs in young, rapidly growing pigs. This is but one manifestation of a variety of disorders that are likely to be at least in part caused by deficiency of vitamin E and/or selenium. The pathogenesis of hepatosis dietetica is incompletely defined. Although it is apparent that affected animals respond to the provision of vitamin E or selenium, it has been difficult, on an experimental basis, to produce the syndrome consistently by feeding diets deficient in vitamin E and selenium. Because vitamin E and selenium-containing enzymes are antagonists of free radical formation and are therefore important for the maintenance of stability and integrity of cellular membranes, it is believed that oxidative injury leads to hepatocyte necrosis.

Regions of massive necrosis in the affected liver are initially distended, deep red, and friable. Hepatosis dietetica is characterized by hemorrhagic centrilobular to massive hepatic necrosis (Fig. 8-69, *A* and *B*). The appearance of the liver reflects the extent of hepatic necrosis, the severity of the hemorrhage, and the duration of the deficiency. Later, in animals that survive the acute disease, parenchymal collapse and dense tracts of connective tissue (postnecrotic scarring) are usually evident.

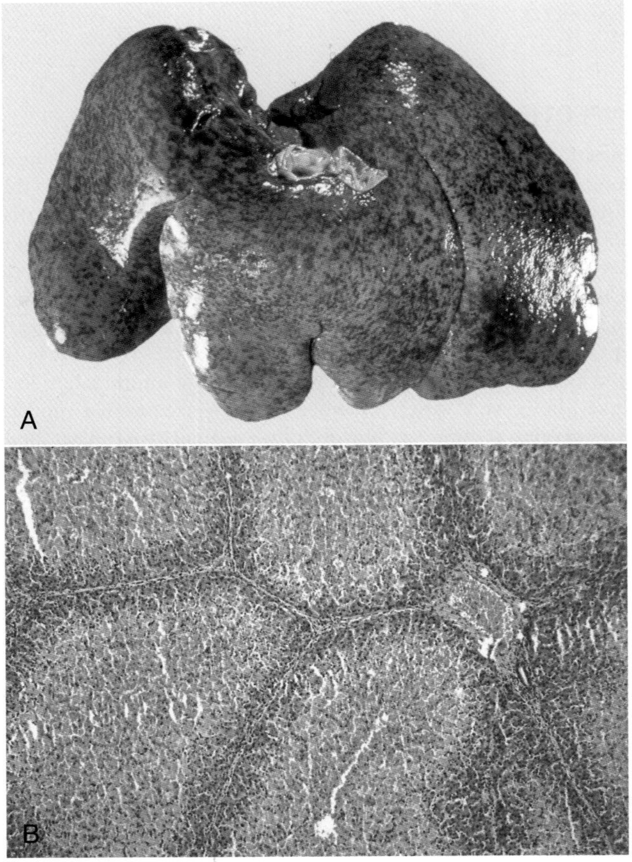

Fig. 8-69 **Massive necrosis, hepatosis dietetica, liver, pig.** **A,** Areas of hemorrhagic centrilobular necrosis and massive necrosis appear as dark regions of different size scattered throughout the liver. **B,** Acute centrilobular necrosis is the principal lesion of this disorder. (**A** courtesy Dr. R. Michel, College of Veterinary Medicine, University of Tennessee. **B** courtesy College of Veterinary Medicine, North Carolina State University; Dr. A.R. Doster, University of Nebraska; and Noah's Arkive, College of Veterinary Medicine, The University of Georgia.)

CRESOLS

Cresols once were incorporated in clay pigeons and asphalt shingles. If pigs ingest cresols, centrilobular to massive hepatic hemorrhage and necrosis result, a pattern that can also be seen in pigs with hepatosis dietetica or in those that ingest cottonseed meal.

DISORDERS OF DOGS

CANINE CHRONIC HEPATITIS (CHRONIC-ACTIVE HEPATITIS)

Chronic hepatitis in dogs is poorly understood. The terminology of this entity, in keeping with the inflammatory process, has been a persistent topic of dispute. *Chronic-active hepatitis* is a descriptive term that has been used to identify a particular pattern of inflammation in the human liver. Originally, the purpose of this classification was to identify hepatic lesions, regardless of cause, that were predictive of a progressive course of inflammation and fibrosis. This term was adopted by veterinary pathologists and used to indicate hepatic disorders of the dog that have microscopic changes similar to those seen in human livers. Based on usage, the term *chronic-active hepatitis* has incorrectly evolved from a morphologic description into a disease entity. The appropriateness and usefulness of this designation is conjectural in humans and dogs. Recent publications in the medical literature have argued that this terminology should be abandoned because it is no longer regarded as useful in predicting the course of liver disease, and it ignores the cause of the liver inflammation. Accordingly, the term *chronic hepatitis* is preferred to describe this entity in dogs.

Chronic hepatitis, with modifiers indicating the type and degree of inflammation and fibrosis, is used to fully characterize the activity and stage of the lesion. If the cause of the inflammation is known, it should be included in the diagnosis. The cause of most of the spontaneous cases of canine chronic hepatitis is uncertain. Some cases have been hypothesized to be caused by leptospira infection or experimental canine adenovirus I infection. Immune-mediated, toxin, or drug-related mechanisms and breed-associated metabolic abnormalities have also been described.

Excessive copper retention is the best characterized and the likely, most common recognizable cause of chronic hepatitis in dogs. Progressive chronic hepatitis has been described in cases of excessive copper retention leading to toxicosis in variety of breeds. Bedlington terriers are the only breed with a recognized mutation (COMMD1), although several breeds appear to have a familiar involvement with copper retention, including Skye terriers, West Highland white terriers, Labrador retrievers, and Dalmatians. Dobermans and American and English cocker spaniels are also recognized for their potential to accumulate excess copper. The cause of the abnormal concentrations of hepatic copper is not well understood. Although copper is excreted in bile, extrahepatic cholestasis does not seem to significantly increase hepatic copper levels. Copper can be detected within hepatocytes and in macrophage or Kupffer cell aggregates using special stains such as rhodanine. Copper accumulates first in the centrilobular hepatocytes in dogs with excessive copper storage.

The liver in cases of chronic hepatitis is usually small, often with an accentuated lobular pattern; severely affected livers are characterized by architectural distortion, which ranges from a coarsely nodular texture to an end-stage liver (Fig. 8-70, *A*). Chronic hepatitis, depending on the duration of inflammation and injury, is

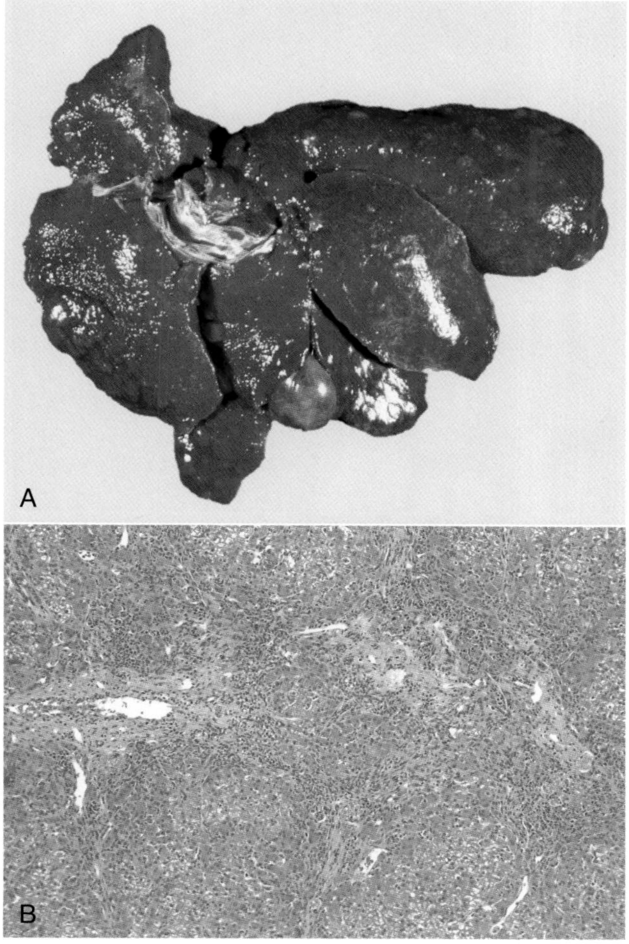

Fig. 8-70 Chronic hepatitis.
A, Liver, diaphragmatic surface, dog. The liver is characterized by scattered regenerative nodules of different sizes and extensive fibrosis that gives the liver an irregular surface. **B,** End-stage liver with chronic hepatitis (also see Fig. 8-22). The liver lobular architecture is replaced by irregular nodules of regenerative parenchyma separated by tracts of connective tissue with an inflammatory infiltrate and pigment accumulation. H&E stain. (**A** courtesy College of Veterinary Medicine, University of Illinois. **B** courtesy Dr. J.M. Cullen, College of Veterinary Medicine, North Carolina State University.)

characterized by portal and periportal mononuclear cell inflammation, intrahepatic cholestasis, and fibrosis of portal areas that may extend into adjacent periportal areas of the lobule, leading to the prominent lobular pattern (Fig. 8-70, *B*).

LOBULAR DISSECTING HEPATITIS

Lobular dissecting hepatitis is a form of cirrhosis usually seen in young dogs. The condition is frequently fatal and has no known cause. Affected livers tend to be smooth and small, rather than the multinodular livers seen in typical cirrhosis. Histologically, the livers are characterized by fine septa with increased fibrosis that dissect the hepatic plates, distort the lobular architecture, and isolate small aggregates or individual hepatocytes (Fig. 8-71). Inflammation in the tissue is usually mild to moderate, and the inflamed area contains mononuclear cell infiltrates.

COPPER TOXICOSIS

Copper accumulates continuously in the livers of Bedlington terriers shown to have a mutation (deletion of exon 2) or other mutations in the COMMD1 gene, which encodes a chaperone protein involved in copper excretion by hepatocytes. Copper accumulates in the centrilobular regions of the liver and leads to ongoing necrosis of hepatocytes, chronic inflammation, replacement fibrosis, and eventually to an end-stage liver and signs of hepatic failure (Fig. 8-72). Excessive concentrations of hepatic copper may be present in other breeds of dog including the Dalmatian, West Highland white terrier, Skye terrier, Doberman Pinscher, Anatolian shepherd dog, and Labrador retriever, although the significance or role of copper in the hepatic disease of these breeds of dog is uncertain. These diseases are discussed above in the section on Canine Chronic Hepatitis.

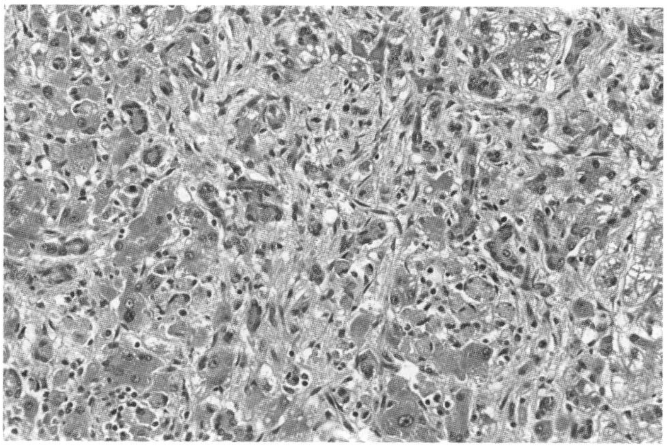

Fig. 8-71 Lobular dissecting hepatitis, liver, dog.
Lobular dissecting hepatitis is a form of end-stage liver characterized microscopically by fine septa of extracellular matrix (chiefly collagen) that divide hepatocyte plates into small clusters of individual hepatocytes. Because of the disruption of blood flow through the liver and the failure of hepatocytes to come in contact with blood, there is profound hepatic dysfunction. H&E stain. (Courtesy Dr. J.M. Cullen, College of Veterinary Medicine, North Carolina State University.)

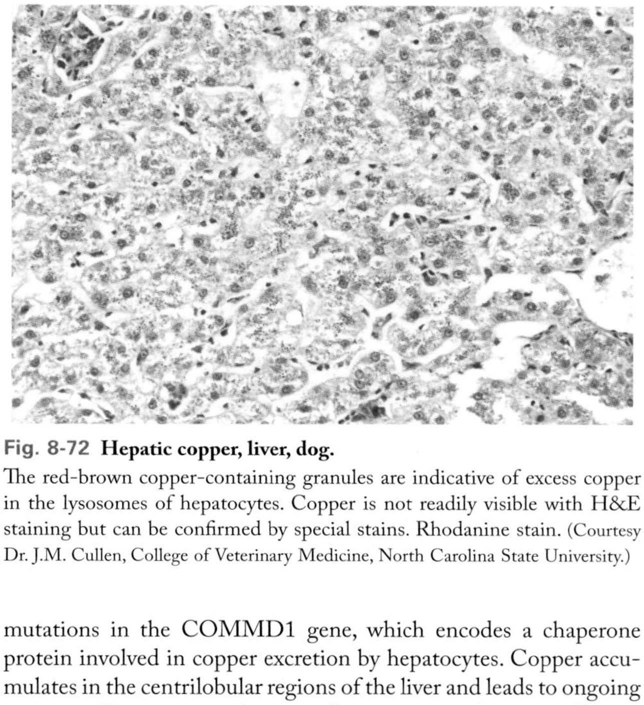

Fig. 8-72 Hepatic copper, liver, dog.
The red-brown copper-containing granules are indicative of excess copper in the lysosomes of hepatocytes. Copper is not readily visible with H&E staining but can be confirmed by special stains. Rhodanine stain. (Courtesy Dr. J.M. Cullen, College of Veterinary Medicine, North Carolina State University.)

GLUCOCORTICOID-INDUCED HEPATOCELLULAR DEGENERATION (STEROID HEPATOPATHY)

Glucocorticoid-induced hepatocellular degeneration is a specific disorder characterized by excessive hepatic accumulation

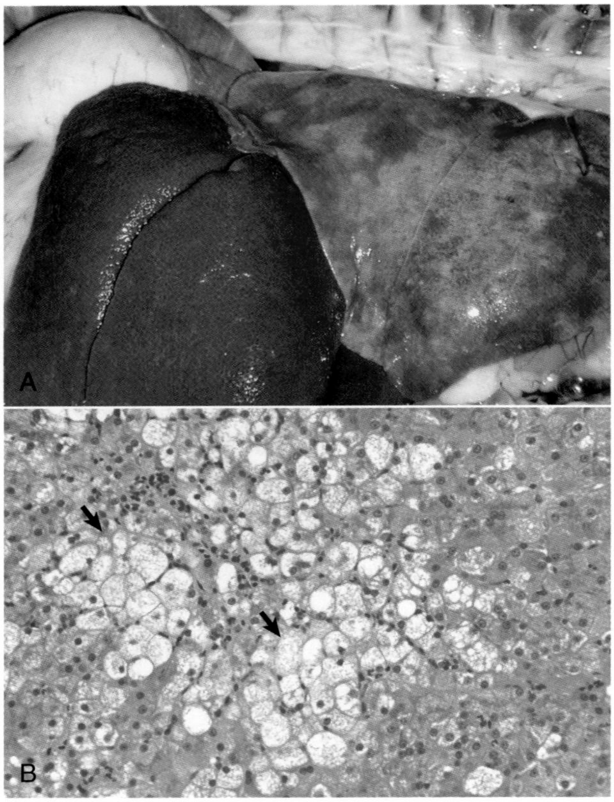

Fig. 8-73 Glucocorticoid-induced hepatopathy, liver, dog. **A,** In dogs with glucocorticoid excess (Cushing's disease) from endogenous or exogenous sources, an extensive accumulation of glycogen in hepatocytes results in an enlarged, pale-brown to beige liver. **B,** Note the swollen hepatocytes *(arrows)* with extensive cytoplasmic vacuolation from glycogen accumulation. H&E stain. (**A** courtesy Dr. K. Bailey, College of Veterinary Medicine, University of Illinois. **B** courtesy Dr. J.M. Cullen, College of Veterinary Medicine, North Carolina State University.)

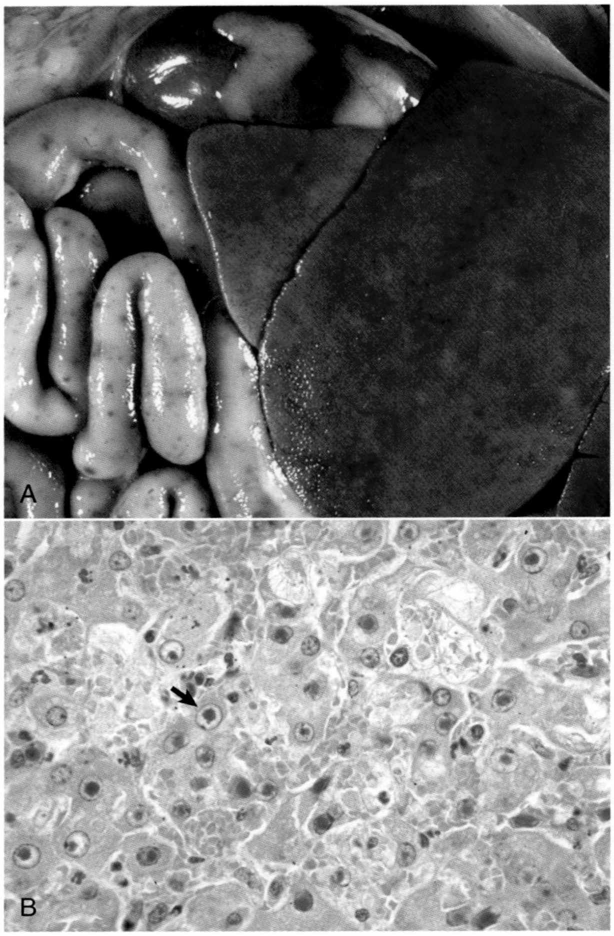

Fig. 8-74 Infectious canine hepatitis, hepatic necrosis, liver, dog. **A,** The liver from a dog infected with infectious canine hepatitis (ICH) can be slightly enlarged and friable with a blotchy yellow discoloration. Sometimes, fibrin is evident on the capsular surface. Note the petechiae on the serosal surface of the intestines caused by vascular damage from canine adenovirus type I infection. **B,** Infection of hepatocytes and endothelial cells with canine adenovirus type I produces characteristic deeply eosinophilic to amphophilic intranuclear inclusions surrounded by a clear zone that separates them from the marginated chromatin *(arrow).* H&E stain. (**A** courtesy Dr. W. Crowell, College of Veterinary Medicine, The University of Georgia; and Noah's Arkive, College of Veterinary Medicine, The University of Georgia. **B** courtesy Dr. M.D. McGavin, College of Veterinary Medicine, University of Tennessee.)

of glycogen (Fig. 8-73, *A*). Excessive amounts of endogenous or exogenous glucocorticoids cause extensive swelling of hepatocytes from the accumulation of glycogen. Glucocorticoids induce glycogen synthetase and so enhance hepatic storage of glycogen. Glycogen accumulation leads to pronounced swelling of hepatocytes (up to 10 times normal volume), particularly those in the midzonal areas (Fig. 8-73, *B*). In severe cases of glucocorticoid-induced hepatocellular degeneration (often referred to as *steroid-induced hepatopathy*), the liver is enlarged and pale but otherwise unremarkable. The disorder occurs in dogs and frequently is iatrogenic but can also be a consequence of hyperadrenocorticism. The diagnosis can be confirmed on the basis of the characteristic microscopic appearance of the liver and identification of the source of the excess glucocorticoids.

INFECTIOUS CANINE HEPATITIS

Infectious canine hepatitis is, as the name implies, a viral infection of the liver of dogs and other canids, including foxes and coyotes. The disease is caused by *canine adenovirus 1*. The majority of infections are asymptomatic, and infections that result in disease may not be fatal. Young dogs, in the first 2 years of life, are more likely to die of the infection than older dogs. The virus has a predilection for hepatocytes, vascular endothelium, and mesothelium; fulminant disease is characterized by hepatic necrosis and widespread serosal hemorrhage that can affect a variety of organs.

Exposure of susceptible dogs is most often via the oral route by contact with urine from infected dogs. Viremia lasts for 4 to 8 days, but virus is shed in the urine of infected dogs for prolonged periods. Virus multiplication initially occurs in the tonsils and produces tonsillitis, which can be severe, with spread to local lymph nodes and then to the systemic circulation. Viremia is associated with leukopenia and fever. Spread of virus to the liver, endothelial cells, and mesothelial cells follows. Infection of Kupffer cells may precede hepatocytic injury. Adenoviruses are cytolytic and cause necrosis of infected cells.

Lesions of infectious canine hepatitis include widespread petechiae and ecchymoses, accumulation of clear fluid in the peritoneal and other serous cavities, the presence of fibrin strands on the surface of the liver, and enlargement and reddening of the tonsils and lymph nodes (Fig. 8-74, *A*). The liver is moderately enlarged and friable and may contain small foci of hepatocellular necrosis centered on centrilobular areas. An enhanced lobular pattern is sometimes evident because of the centrilobular hepatic necrosis. Characteristically, the wall of the gallbladder is thickened by edema. Foci of hemorrhage in the lung, brain, kidneys, and the metaphysis of the long bones may also be evident.

The severity of microscopic lesions present in individual dogs may reflect the duration of the disease. Susceptible puppies rapidly succumb to infection and have only scattered foci of hepatocellular necrosis, whereas fulminant disease in more mature dogs often produces both randomly scattered foci of hepatocellular necrosis and widespread centrilobular necrosis. The predilection for centrilobular necrosis may be related to the virus's penchant for infection and necrosis of endothelial cells that may lead to vascular stasis and local hypoxia rather than to any increased propensity for the virus to damage centrilobular hepatocytes, although this issue is not resolved. Large deeply eosinophilic to amphophilic intranuclear inclusions are found in hepatocytes, vascular endothelium, and Kupffer cells (Fig. 8-74, *B*). Inflammation tends to be mild and neutrophils are the most abundant cell type. Virus-induced endothelial damage may lead to DIC and hemorrhagic diathesis, which contribute to the hemorrhage observed in affected dogs. Some dogs recovering from infectious canine hepatitis develop an immune-complex uveitis (type III hypersensitivity), which produces degeneration and necrosis of the corneal endothelium and resultant corneal edema clinically known as "blue eye."

DISORDERS OF CATS

LYMPHOCYTIC CHOLANGITIS

Lymphocytic cholangitis, a relatively common disorder of cats, is slowly progressive and chronic. Affected cats are usually older than 4 years of age and may have icterus as a consequence of intrahepatic cholestasis. Small lymphocytes infiltrate the portal tracts and usually center on bile ducts directly. The intensity of the infiltration can make it difficult to identify the original bile duct within an affected portal tract. Often, by the time a biopsy is obtained, the liver is characterized by extensive aggregations of inflammatory cells, typically lymphocytes and plasma cells in portal tracts, and surrounding numerous small bile ducts (Fig. 8-75). Inflammation usually is accompanied by bile duct proliferation, hepatic or biliary fibrosis, and intrahepatic cholestasis. The cause or causes of this syndrome are unknown. The disease might have an immunologic basis. The main differential diagnosis is lymphoma. Chronic lymphocytic cholangitis should be distinguished from suppurative cholangitis, which is caused most often by ascending bacterial infection of the biliary tree.

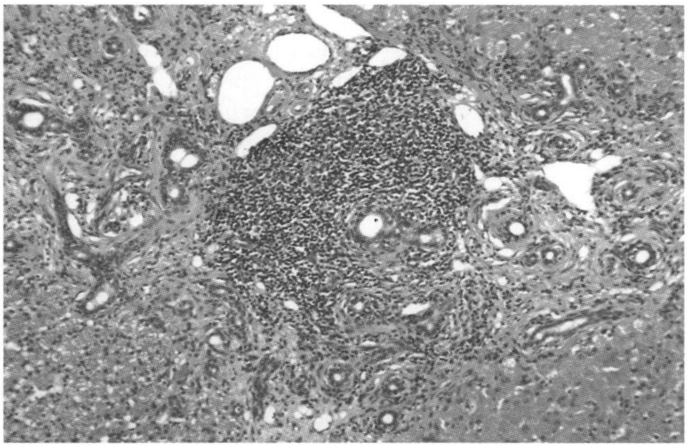

Fig. 8-75 Feline lymphocytic cholangitis, liver, cat.
Large numbers of lymphocytes surrounding bile ducts and biliary hyperplasia in portal areas are the hallmarks of this disease. The inflammation most often affects the periphery of the bile ducts and could be termed a *pericholangitis,* but the syndrome is referred to as cholangitis. H&E stain. (Courtesy Dr. J.M. Cullen, College of Veterinary Medicine, North Carolina State University.)

DISORDERS OF THE GALLBLADDER AND EXTRAHEPATIC BILE DUCTS

DEVELOPMENTAL ABNORMALITIES

Developmental anomalies of the gallbladder may be most common in the cat; bilobed and occasionally trilobed gallbladders can occur (Fig. 8-76). These anomalies usually are of no clinical significance but rarely can be associated with cholecystitis or cholelithiasis.

CHOLELITHIASIS

Choleliths, or *gallstones* as they are commonly called, occur infrequently in all the domestic species, but they are especially well described in ruminants. Choleliths are concretions of normally soluble components of bile (Fig. 8-77). They form when these components become supersaturated and precipitate. Choleliths in

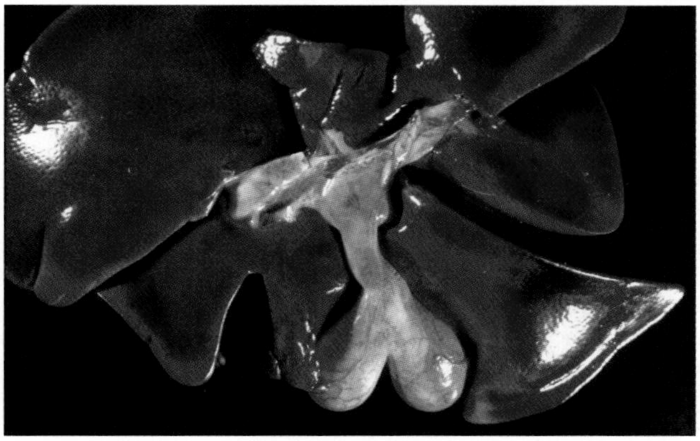

Fig. 8-76 Bilobed gallbladder, liver, cat.
Bilobed gallbladders are developmental anomalies that have little or no clinical significance and are found most often in cats. (Courtesy College of Veterinary Medicine, University of Illinois.)

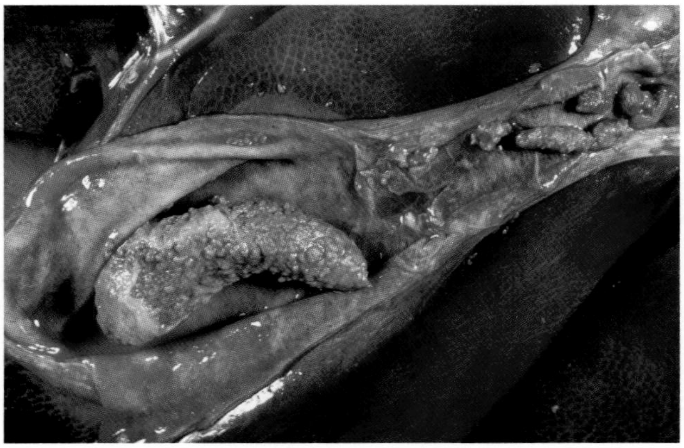

Fig. 8-77 Choleliths, gallbladder, pig.
Choleliths are concretions formed from the constituents of bile. (Courtesy Dr. M.D. McGavin, College of Veterinary Medicine, University of Tennessee.)

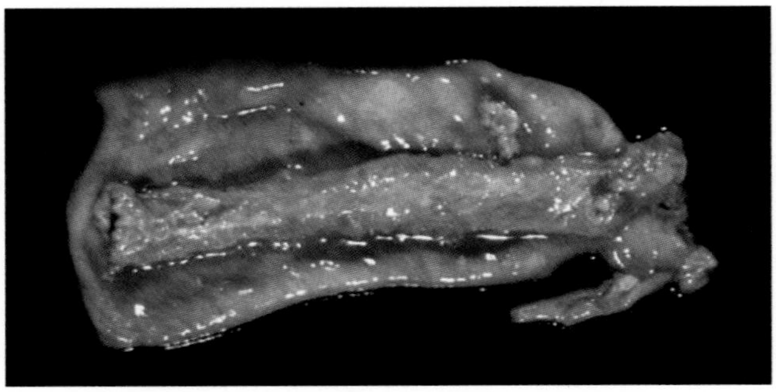

Fig. 8-78 Fibrinous cholecystitis, gallbladder, cow.
Fibrinous cholecystitis caused by *Salmonella enteritidis* serotype *Dublin* has produced a fibrinous cast, which is evident in the lumen of the gallbladder. (Courtesy Dr. D.A. Mosier, College of Veterinary Medicine, Kansas State University.)

the gallbladder usually do not become clinically significant unless they migrate and obstruct the extrahepatic bile ducts.

CHOLECYSTITIS

Cholecystitis is inflammation of the gallbladder and can be acute or chronic. Acute inflammation of the gallbladder may be produced by viral infections, such as Rift Valley fever in ruminants and infectious canine hepatitis, and produces characteristic edema and hemorrhage in the gallbladder. Fibrinous cholecystitis may occur in calves with acute salmonellosis, particularly that caused by *Salmonella enteritidis* serotype *Dublin* (Fig. 8-78). Other bacteria, either derived from the blood or ascended from the intestine, can cause acute or chronic cholecystitis. Chronic cholecystitis typically accompanies prolonged bacterial infection of the biliary tree, or ongoing irritation from choleliths or parasites of the gallbladder. Rupture of the gallbladder is rare but can occur as a result of acute or chronic infection. The resultant release of bile, with or without accompanying bacteria, can cause life-threatening peritonitis because of the irritating effect of bile on the serosal surfaces of the abdomen.

THROMBOSIS AND INFARCTION OF THE GALLBLADDER

Occasionally, infarction without significant inflammation of the gallbladder can be seen in dogs. Thrombi can be found in the arteries of the muscular wall of the affected gallbladders. Rupture of the gallbladder can occur secondarily to the infarction of the wall. The cause is not known.

GALLBLADDER MUCOCELE

Gallbladder mucocele refers to a syndrome in dogs characterized by a distended gallbladder filled with mucus that is often associated with signs of biliary obstruction and that can occasionally lead to gallbladder rupture. Small breed dogs appear to be most often affected. The mucosa of the gallbladder is usually hyperplastic. Occasionally, the common bile duct is similarly affected and cholestasis can develop. The pathogenesis of gallbladder mucocele is uncertain, although dogs with hyperadrenocorticism are reported to have a higher incidence of the disorder, as are Shetland sheepdogs, than other dogs.

HYPERPLASTIC AND NEOPLASTIC LESIONS

Cystic Mucinous Hyperplasia of the Gallbladder

Cystic mucinous hyperplasia of the gallbladder mucosa has only been reported in dogs and sheep. There are no apparent abnormalities evident from the exterior of the gallbladder, and the features of cystic hyperplasia can only be appreciated by opening the gallbladder and draining residual bile that may obscure the mucosa. When the bile is rinsed away, affected mucosa is gray-white and has a diffusely thickened, spongelike consistency. Sessile or polypoid masses or large cysts are occasionally found, and they are evident as papillary projections into the lumen of the gallbladder (Fig. 8-79). Numerous 1- to 3-mm cysts within the hyperplastic mucosa impart the characteristic appearance. Histologically, the hallmark of cystic hyperplasia of the gallbladder is the abundance of variably sized cystic spaces that distort and thicken the entire mucosa of the gallbladder. Most of the cysts contain a copious amount of mucus. The majority of the lining epithelial cells are typical of the normal gallbladder epithelium (i.e., tall columnar with abundant apical cytoplasmic mucus). The entire mucosa may be affected. These lesions are usually of no significance to the host. In all likelihood, cystic hyperplasia of the gallbladder frequently goes undetected visually. The cause is not known.

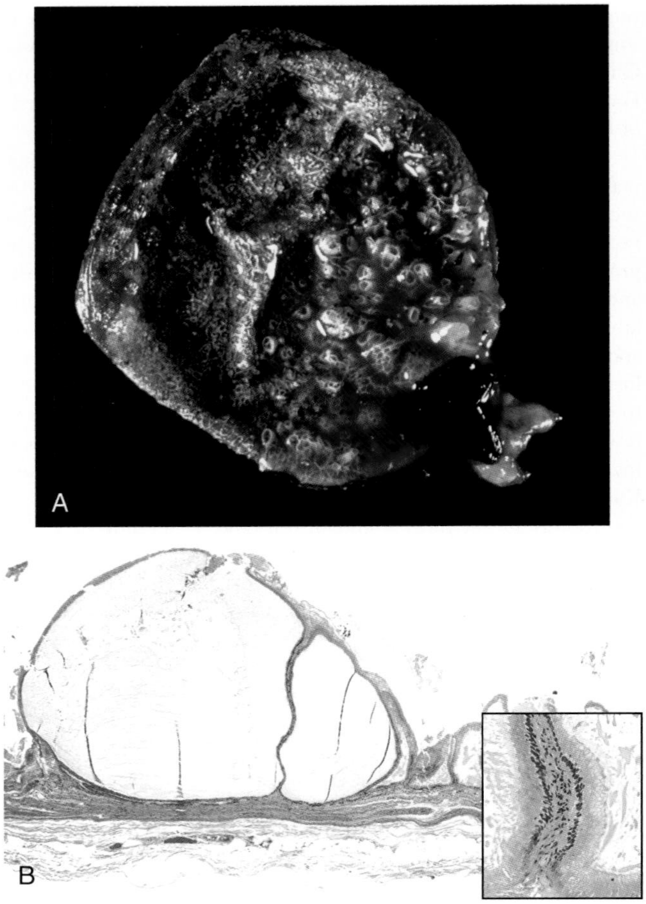

Fig. 8-79 Cystic mucinous hyperplasia, gallbladder, dog.
A, The gallbladder mucosa is thickened and contains multiple mucous cysts. **B,** The mucosa contains a mucous cyst. H&E stain. *Inset,* The mucosa is hyperplastic with prominent goblet cells that produce the mucus that fills the cysts. H&E stain. (**A** courtesy Dr. W. Crowell, College of Veterinary Medicine, The University of Georgia; and Noah's Arkive, College of Veterinary Medicine, The University of Georgia. **B** and inset courtesy Dr. M.D. McGavin, College of Veterinary Medicine, University of Tennessee.)

Adenoma

Adenomas of the gallbladder are rare neoplasms but are most common in young cattle and have also been described in dogs,

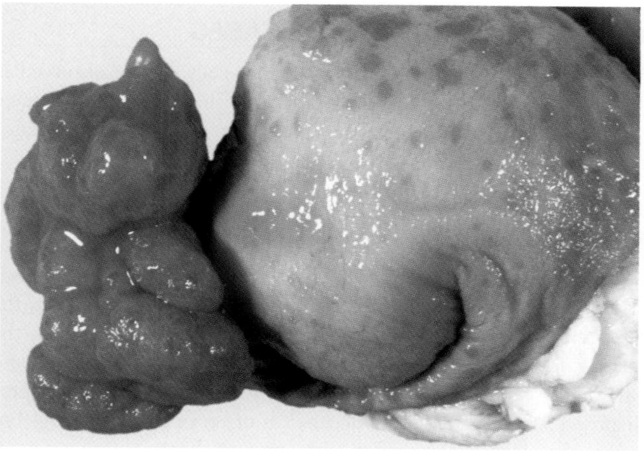

Fig. 8-80 Adenoma, gallbladder, dog.
Papillary projections of proliferating mucosa *(left third of the image)* bulge into the lumen of the gallbladder. (Courtesy Dr. M.D. McGavin, College of Veterinary Medicine, University of Tennessee.)

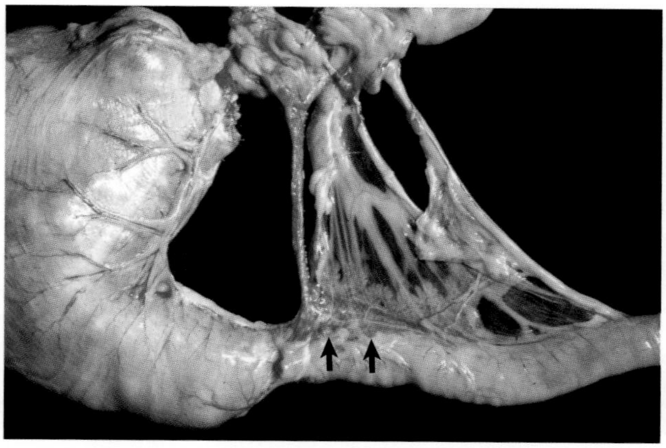

Fig. 8-81 Pancreatic atrophy/hypoplasia, pancreas, dog.
Virtually no pancreatic tissue is present in this case. Pancreatic remnants are indicated by arrows. (Courtesy Dr. M.D. McGavin, College of Veterinary Medicine, University of Tennessee.)

cats, and sheep. They are multinodular or papillary masses that protrude from the mucosal surface and consist of a loose connective tissue stalk that is lined with well-differentiated biliary epithelium (Fig. 8-80).

Carcinoma

Malignant neoplasms of the gallbladder epithelium are rare in domestic animals but have been described in dogs, cats, and cattle. They typically are composed of mucin-secreting epithelial cells and often have a papillary arrangement. Carcinoma of the gallbladder may invade the liver by direct extension and may metastasize to the hepatic lymph nodes and to more distant sites.

DISORDERS OF THE EXOCRINE PANCREAS

DEVELOPMENTAL ANOMALIES

Exocrine Pancreatic Atrophy (Juvenile Pancreatic Atrophy)

A distinct syndrome characterized by a dramatically diminished exocrine pancreas has been recognized in several breeds of dog. It is particularly common in the German shepherd dog and rough-coated collies, in which it appears to be inherited as an autosomal recessive trait. In German shepherd dogs, decreased expression of the gene gp25L is observed within the affected pancreas. This lesion is most likely one of atrophy rather than hypoplasia, given recent evidence that suggests that an autoimmune pancreatitis precedes the loss of normal pancreatic parenchyma. The pancreas in affected dogs is small (Fig. 8-81), but islands of normal exocrine pancreatic tissue usually remain. Histologically, there is marked depletion of exocrine pancreatic acinar cells with relative uninvolvement of endocrine islet cells. Young animals are affected, usually between 6 to 12 months of age. Affected dogs have signs typical of maldigestion secondary to exocrine pancreatic insufficiency and rapidly lose weight despite a voracious appetite.

There may be several conditions in which the pancreas is found to be smaller than expected, and the pathogenesis of the lesions may vary, depending on the species. A syndrome termed *hypoplasia of the exocrine pancreas* occurs sporadically in calves and is characterized by signs of exocrine pancreatic insufficiency. The distinction between atrophy and hypoplasia can be difficult to determine because both processes lead to an abnormally small organ with diminished function. Cells of the hypoplastic exocrine pancreas do not usually contain lipofuscin, which can be seen in atrophic cells.

A recent entity of juvenile pancreatic atrophy has been reported in Greyhounds, in which atrophy of both the exocrine and endocrine pancreas is observed.

Anomalies of the Duct System

The arrangement of the major pancreatic duct or ducts varies between and within species, so a variety of normal arrangements occur. Sheep, for example, have only one pancreatic duct that drains into the common bile duct, whereas cattle and horses typically have two ducts, and several distinct arrangements of the pancreatic ducts have been described in dogs. The pancreatic duct of cats enters the duodenum immediately adjacent to or confluent with the common bile duct. Specific anomalies include congenital stenosis of the pancreatic ducts and cystic dilation of the ducts. Congenital cysts within the pancreas occasionally occur in lambs. Congenital ductal cysts within the pancreas can also be observed in animals with polycystic kidney and/or liver disease.

INCIDENTAL FINDINGS

Ectopic Pancreatic Tissue

Nodules of ectopic pancreatic tissue sometimes are present in the duodenum or other sections of the small bowel, stomach, spleen, gallbladder, and mesentery of the dog and cat. This type of anomaly, normal tissue in an abnormal location, is termed a *choristoma.*

Pacinian Corpuscles

Pacinian corpuscles are normally present within the interlobular connective tissue of the pancreas and mesentery of the cat, and appear as discrete 1- to 3-mm nodules (Fig. 8-82 and Web Fig. 7-23). The corpuscles should not be mistaken for abnormal structures.

Autolysis

Autolysis of the pancreas is very rapid after death, particularly if the pancreas is traumatized. Postmortem release and activation of pancreatic proteolytic enzymes within the pancreas can hasten tissue breakdown. Thus autolysis may be advanced in the pancreas

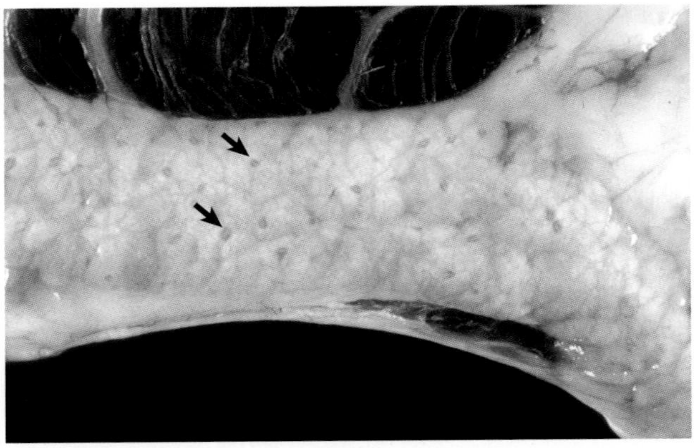

Fig. 8-82 Pacinian corpuscles, pancreas, cat.
The feline pancreas contains numerous pacinian corpuscles *(arrows)*, which may be visible grossly as about 1-mm clear foci. (Courtesy College of Veterinary Medicine, North Carolina State University.)

before it is evident in other organs. As autolysis progresses, the color of the gland may change from its normal pink to dark red or green. The metabolic activity of intestinal bacteria, which can easily gain access to the pancreas, can contribute to the discoloration of the pancreas through hemolysis and tissue decomposition.

Pancreatic Calculi

The formation of concretions or "stones" within the pancreatic duct system is termed pancreolithiasis, and occurs uncommonly in cattle. It is usually an incidental finding at slaughter, and apparently is slightly more common in cattle older than 4 years of age than in younger animals.

Stromal Fat Cell Infiltration

Fat cell infiltration of the interstitial connective tissue of the pancreas occurs occasionally, especially in obese cats. The pancreas itself is usually unaffected, so exocrine pancreatic function is normal, but the dispersion of the parenchyma creates the impression that the pancreas has been replaced by adipose tissue.

PANCREATIC DEGENERATION AND ATROPHY

Degeneration of the acinar cells of the exocrine pancreas is a nonspecific process that can occur as a consequence of a variety of local and systemic diseases. For example, starvation results in loss of zymogen granules within the cytoplasm of acinar cells of the exocrine pancreas because the rate of synthesis of the granules is diminished, and available protein is used to maintain serum protein concentrations when dietary protein is limited. Obstruction of the pancreatic ducts, whatever the cause, can also cause degeneration and atrophy of the exocrine pancreas. Obstruction of the pancreatic duct(s) can be caused by neoplasms or chronic inflammation and associated fibrosis that compress the duct, or by foreign bodies, such as parasites or pancreoliths, that occlude the ductal lumen. Exocrine pancreatic atrophy also may occur secondary to widespread interstitial fibrosis of the pancreas, as occurs, for example, in dogs with chronic pancreatitis.

PANCREATIC PSEUDOCYSTS

Pancreatic pseudocysts are fluid-filled nonepithelialized fibrous sacs containing cellular debris and pancreatic enzymes that form within the pancreas or adjacent to the organ following pancreatic inflammation. They are described in dogs and cats. They should be distinguished from abscesses, cystic neoplasms, and congenital cysts seen with polycystic disease.

LYSOSOMAL STORAGE DISEASES

Vacuolation of exocrine pancreatic acinar cells can be observed in several types of lysosomal storage diseases. This lesion is most often seen in addition to vacuolation of neurons, macrophages, hepatocytes, and/or other cells.

ACUTE PANCREATITIS/ACUTE PANCREATIC NECROSIS

Acute pancreatitis is a condition characterized primarily by necrosis and varying degrees of inflammation of the pancreas. In fact, the predominance of necrosis over inflammation supports using the term *acute pancreatic necrosis* over acute pancreatitis for dogs and cats in most instances. Obese, sedentary bitches are especially predisposed. Acute pancreatitis occurs less often in cats than dogs but more often in cats than most other species. Acute pancreatitis has been described in a variety of species, although the cause usually is different in each species. In dogs, an increased incidence of acute pancreatitis has been observed in cocker spaniels.

Pathogenesis

The three major proposed mechanisms of pancreatitis are as follows:

- Obstruction of the duct(s)
- Direct injury to acinar cells
- Disturbances of enzyme trafficking within the cytoplasm of acinar cells

Obstruction of ductal flow by calculi or parasites can lead to interstitial edema that compresses small-caliber vessels and compromises local blood flow, leading to ischemic damage to acinar cells. Direct damage to acinar cells can be caused by a few specific agents in animals, including compounds found in *Cassia occidentalis* and T-2 toxin, a trichothecene mycotoxin that affects pigs, and zinc toxicosis of dogs, veal calves, and sheep. Certain therapeutic drugs, such as sulfonamides and potassium bromide–phenobarbital combinations, can damage the pancreas in dogs, and other species are probably similarly affected. Ischemia to the pancreas from a variety of causes may also produce direct injury to the acinar cells. A third mechanism involves aberrant transport of proenzymes within the acinar cells, leading to inappropriate activation of the enzymes within the cells. The association between corticosteroid administration in dogs and an increased risk of acute pancreatitis could possibly be explained by this mechanism. However, many cases of acute pancreatitis commonly occur after dogs have consumed a meal high in fat or some other dietary indiscretion, and the specific mechanism triggering the disease remains unclear. Pancreatitis is occasionally initiated by trauma, usually in dogs and cats as a consequence of some accidental crushing or impact trauma to the abdomen or surgical trauma. Acute pancreatitis in dogs occurs as a consequence of release of activated pancreatic enzymes into the pancreatic parenchyma and adjacent tissue producing autodigestion. Trypsin is believed to be a key player in pancreatitis. Once activated, trypsin in turn can activate proelastase and prophospholipase into elastase and phospholipase A. These enzymes digest pancreatic tissue and adjacent fat and damage blood vessels. Trypsin also activates prekallikrein, leading to involvement of the kinin system, complement, and clotting cascades in affected tissue. These in turn amplify the process, promote thrombosis and hemorrhage, and attract inflammatory cells.

Acute Pancreatitis

The gross lesions of acute pancreatitis are referable to proteolytic degradation of pancreatic parenchyma, vascular damage and hemorrhage, and necrosis of peripancreatic fat by lipolytic enzymes of

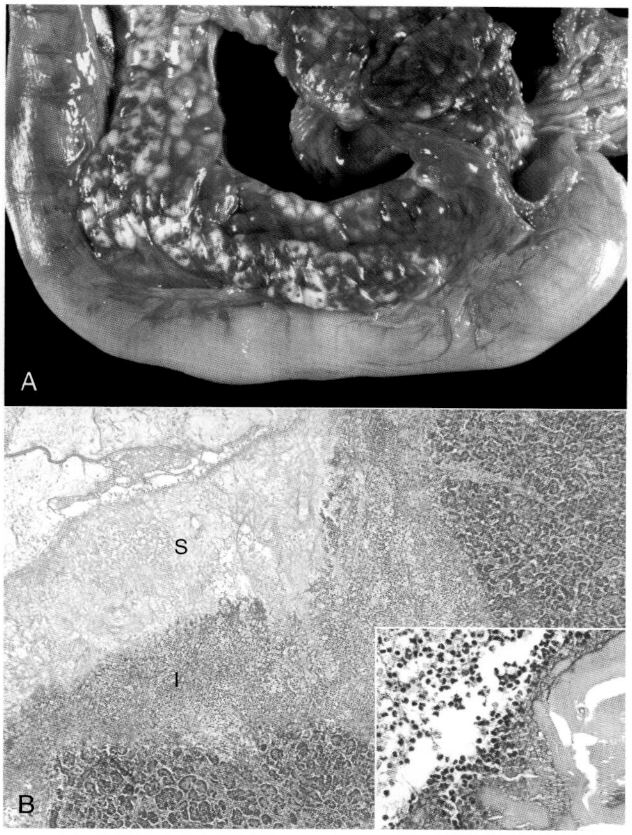

Fig. 8-83 Acute pancreatic necrosis, acute pancreatitis, pancreas, dog. **A,** Note the expansion of the pancreas by areas of hemorrhage and edema. **B,** Acute pancreatitis (histologic appearance of the pancreas depicted in **A**). Note the accumulation of fibrinous exudate and edema within the interlobular septa *(S)* and inflammatory cell infiltrate *(I)*. H&E stain. *Inset,* Higher magnification of acute pancreatitis. Note the abundant neutrophils and the area of "saponification" of fat *(lower right)*. H&E stain. (**A** courtesy Dr. R. Fairley. **B** courtesy Dr. J.M. Cullen, College of Veterinary Medicine, North Carolina State University. Inset courtesy Dr. M.D. McGavin, College of Veterinary Medicine, University of Tennessee.)

the pancreas. Mild cases of pancreatitis are characterized by edema of the interstitial tissue of the pancreas. Acute hemorrhagic pancreatitis is more severe, and characteristically, the pancreas is edematous and contains areas that are gray-white, the result of coagulation necrosis, and other areas that are dark red or blue-black, which are hemorrhagic (Fig. 8-83, *A*). Areas of fat necrosis are manifest as chalky-white foci as a result of saponification of necrotic adipose tissue in the mesentery adjacent to the pancreas. Portions of normal pancreatic parenchyma may be interspersed between affected portions. The peritoneal cavity frequently contains blood-stained fluid, which may contain droplets of fat in the early stage. Peritonitis is manifest by fibrinous adhesions between the affected portions of the pancreas and adjacent tissues.

The microscopic appearance of acute hemorrhagic pancreatitis reflects the gross lesions just described. Characteristic lesions include focally extensive areas of hemorrhage, influx of leukocytes, and coagulation necrosis of the pancreatic parenchyma; accumulation of fibrinous exudate in the interlobular septa; and necrosis and inflammation of fat in the mesentery adjacent to the affected portions of pancreas (Fig. 8-83, *B*).

Species differences in acute pancreatitis are recognized. For example, in cats, there appear to be two distinct syndromes of acute pancreatitis, one characterized by an acute pancreatic necrosis and a distinct suppurative pancreatitis that is most likely the consequence of ascending bacterial infection.

Acute pancreatitis is usually characterized by vomiting, diarrhea, anorexia, and abdominal tenderness. Acute, severe pancreatitis also produces systemic effects secondary to the release of inflammatory mediators and activated enzymes from the damaged pancreas; these effects include widespread vascular injury and subsequent hemorrhage, shock, and DIC. The liver also is affected in many cases of pancreatitis, as indicated by increased concentrations of serum hepatic enzymes (such as alanine aminotransferase), and sometimes, focal hepatic necrosis.

Acute pancreatitis sufficient to cause clinical disease apparently is considerably less common in species other than the dog and cat. Acute pancreatic necrosis and pancreatitis have been described in the horse, but the pathogenesis of pancreatitis in this species differs from that in the dog and cat. Necrosis and inflammation are the result of migration of strongyle larvae through the pancreas, which results in the release of pancreatic enzymes and enzymatic digestion of the pancreas and surrounding tissue.

Chronic Pancreatitis

Chronic pancreatitis is typically accompanied by fibrosis and parenchymal atrophy. It can occur in all species as a consequence of obstruction of the pancreatic ducts and presumably all of the other mechanisms associated with acute pancreatitis. In the dog, pancreatic fibrosis and chronic pancreatitis are the result of progressive destruction of the pancreas by repeated mild episodes of acute pancreatic necrosis and pancreatitis. An increased incidence of chronic pancreatitis has been reported in cocker spaniels, cavalier King Charles spaniels, collies, and boxer dogs. The pancreas has modest regenerative capacity and responds to injury with replacement fibrosis and atrophy of persisting parenchyma. Thus ongoing destruction of pancreatic tissue causes progressive loss of glandular tissue without replacement (Fig. 8-84). Grossly, the pancreas in affected animals is a distorted, shrunken, nodular mass with fibrous adhesions to adjacent tissue. If a significant portion of the pancreas is affected, dogs may develop signs of exocrine pancreatic insufficiency, with or without signs of endocrine pancreatic insufficiency (diabetes mellitus). However, destruction of pancreatic tissue frequently is not of sufficient magnitude to cause exocrine pancreatic insufficiency, and pancreatic fibrosis is sometimes found as incidental lesions at necropsy of dogs with apparently normal digestive function. In cats, chronic pancreatitis most always manifests as extensive fibrosis, with little inflammation. Fibrosis of the exocrine pancreas also occurs after the necrosis of exocrine pancreatic cells from zinc toxicosis in sheep. Ectasia of the pancreatic ducts with cyst formation also is relatively common in cats with interstitial pancreatic fibrosis.

Chronic pancreatitis and replacement fibrosis occurs sporadically in the horse, usually as a consequence of either parasitic migration or from ascending bacterial infection of the pancreatic ducts. In addition, pancreatitis may occur in horses with chronic eosinophilic gastroenteritis. However, chronic pancreatitis usually is not clinically apparent in the horse, as signs of exocrine pancreatic insufficiency rarely, if ever, occur in this species. Chronic inflammation of the pancreas, characterized by lymphoplasmacytic infiltrates, is most common and important in the dog, but does occur in the cat, horse, and cattle, in which it is rarely of clinical significance.

PARASITIC INFECTIONS

A variety of parasites may inhabit the pancreatic ducts of domestic animals. Parasitic infections of the pancreatic ducts are important

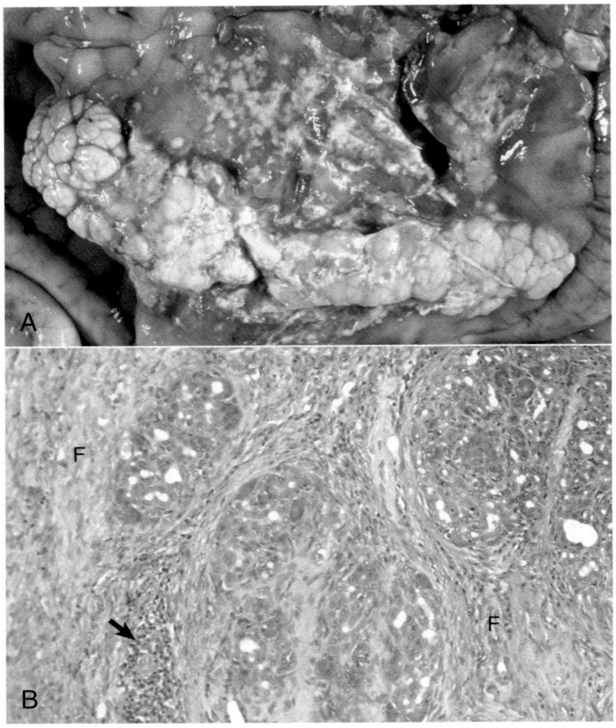

Fig. 8-84 Chronic pancreatitis, pancreas, dog.
A, Lobules are more prominent as the result of fibrosis, and the pancreas is paler than normal. The white, raised, granular areas in the pancreas and mesentery are foci of fat necrosis that result from enzymatic digestion of lipids that then become mineralized. **B,** Remaining exocrine pancreatic cells are separated into small lobules by abundant fibrous connective tissue *(F)*, which contains chronic inflammatory cells *(arrow)*. H&E stain. (**A** courtesy College of Veterinary Medicine, North Carolina State University. **B** courtesy Dr. J.M. Cullen, College of Veterinary Medicine, North Carolina State University.)

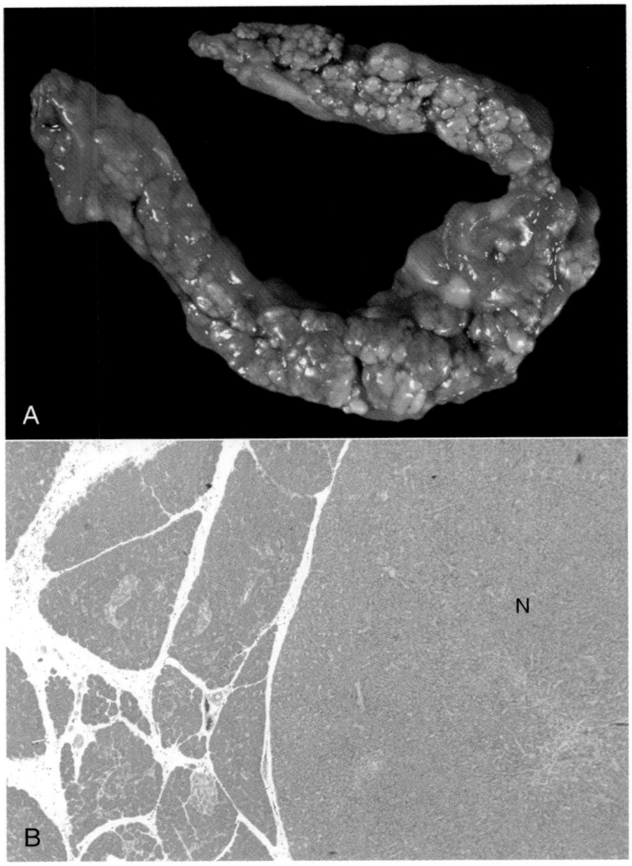

Fig. 8-85 Pancreatic nodular exocrine hyperplasia, pancreas, dog.
A, Hyperplastic nodules are pale beige to white and project above the surface. B, Microscopically hyperplastic nodules *(N)* are composed of numerous small acini, most of which, in this case, lack typical zymogen granules. H&E stain. (**A** courtesy Dr. M.D. McGavin, College of Veterinary Medicine, University of Tennessee. **B** courtesy Dr. J.M. Cullen, College of Veterinary Medicine, North Carolina State University.)

if they occlude the ducts, either by direct physical obstruction or by inducing inflammation within and around ducts. Examples include flukes of the families Opisthorchiidae *(Opisthorchis tenuicollis, Opisthorchis viverrini, Clonorchis sinensis, Metorchis albidus, Metorchis conjunctus)* and Dicrocoeliidae *(Eurytrema pancreaticum, Concinnum procyonis, Dicrocoelium dendriticum)*, which may inhabit the pancreatic ducts of a variety of animal species and occasionally cause fibrosis and/or pancreatitis. Nematodes, particularly ascarids, and cestodes are common gastrointestinal parasites of the domestic species; occasionally, they may lodge within the pancreatic ducts.

HYPERPLASIA AND NEOPLASIA

Pancreatic Nodular Hyperplasia

Nodular hyperplasia of the exocrine pancreas occurs in dogs, cats, and cattle. It is especially common in older dogs and cats. The lesion is of no clinical significance, but it must be distinguished from neoplasms of the endocrine and exocrine pancreas.

These hyperplastic nodules typically are multiple, raised, smooth, and a uniform gray or white on cut surface (Fig. 8-85, *A*). The nodules may be firmer than the adjacent normal pancreas. Microscopically, these nodules consist of unencapsulated aggregates of acinar cells that may lack zymogen granules or contain an abundance of them (Fig. 8-85, *B*). Some nodules contain a mixture of the two types of acinar cells. The distinction between hyperplasia and adenoma of the exocrine pancreas is poorly defined in domestic animals.

Pancreatic Adenoma

Adenomas of the exocrine pancreas are extremely rare but have been described in the cat. Those of acinar cell origin share all the features of hyperplastic nodules but are single and larger than normal pancreatic lobules, whereas hyperplastic nodules are not larger than normal lobules; this distinction clearly is somewhat arbitrary.

Pancreatic Carcinoma

Carcinoma of the ductular epithelium or acinar cells of the exocrine pancreas is uncommon in all species. It is most often reported in the dog and cat. The neoplasms may consist of single or multiple nodules of variable size within the pancreas, each of which consists of gray or yellow tissue. Lesions may consist of a single nodule or affect the organ diffusely. Tumors are typically grayish-white to pale yellow with a firm-to-hard consistency (Fig. 8-86, *A*). Tumors are often gritty when cut. Areas of hemorrhage, mineralization, or necrosis may be present within the neoplasm. The neoplasm is usually firmer than the adjacent pancreas because of proliferation of fibrous connective tissue. Adhesion of the affected pancreas to adjacent tissue may occur. This neoplasm often invades adjacent tissue and seeds the peritoneal cavity. Peritoneal implants form nodules over the mesentery, omentum, and serosa of the abdominal viscera. Metastasis to the regional lymph nodes

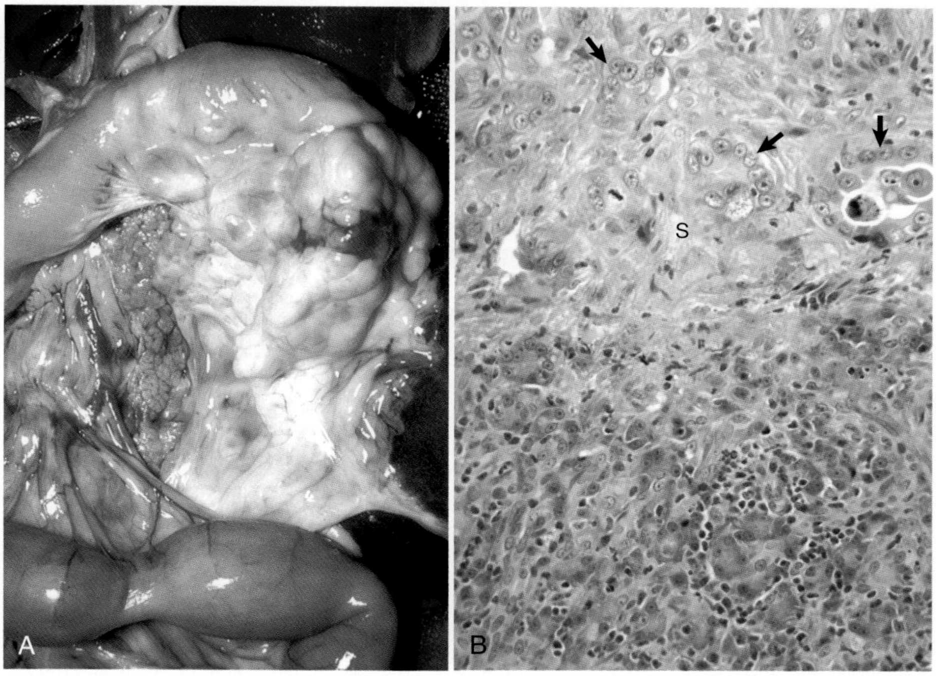

Fig. 8-86 **Pancreatic carcinoma.**

A, Stomach and pancreas *(center),* ventral-dorsal view, dog. Pancreatic carcinoma has invaded the mesentery, wall of the stomach, and gastrosplenic ligament. Note the lobulated appearance of the mass, which is formed by neoplastic exocrine pancreatic epithelial cells and scirrhous connective tissue. Proximal duodenum *(bottom),* liver *(top),* and spleen *(right [left anatomically]).* **B,** Pancreas, cat. Pancreatic carcinoma tends to form crude acini or tubules *(arrows)* that aggressively invade adjacent normal tissue. Prominent fibrosis, termed *scirrhous response (S),* is commonly caused by this type of tumor. H&E stain. (**A** courtesy College of Veterinary Medicine, University of Illinois. **B** courtesy Dr. M.D. McGavin, College of Veterinary Medicine, University of Tennessee.)

(pancreatoduodenal, which is inconstantly present and the right hepatic lymph node) is also common, and some carcinomas metastasize widely.

Microscopic features of carcinomas of the exocrine pancreas range from well-differentiated adenocarcinomas with tubular patterns to undifferentiated carcinomas with solid patterns. The amount of fibrous stroma varies considerably and usually is greatest in poorly differentiated neoplasms (Fig. 8-86, *B*). Zymogen granules similar to those present in normal acinar cells of the pancreas are often absent within the cytoplasm of the neoplastic cells. Mitotic figures are common.

A unique cutaneous paraneoplastic syndrome can be observed in cats with pancreatic adenocarcinoma or cholangiocarcinoma. This manifests grossly as symmetric alopecia of the ventral trunk and limbs with a glistening appearance. Histologically, affected areas have marked follicular and adnexal atrophy and loss of the stratum corneum of the epidermis.

SUGGESTED READINGS

Suggested Readings are available at evolve.elsevier.com/Zachary/McGavin/.

CHAPTER 9

Respiratory System, Mediastinum, and Pleurae

Alfonso López

Diseases of the respiratory system (respiratory apparatus) are some of the leading causes of morbidity and mortality in animals and a major source of economic losses. Thus veterinarians are routinely called to diagnose, treat, and implement health management practices to reduce the impact of these diseases. In companion animals, diseases of the respiratory tract are also common and, although of little economic significance, are important to the health of the animals and thus to clinicians and owners.

STRUCTURE AND FUNCTION

To facilitate the understanding of the structure and function, it is convenient to arbitrarily divide the respiratory system into conducting, transitional, and gas exchange systems (Fig. 9-1). The conducting system includes nostrils, nasal cavity, paranasal sinuses, nasopharynx, larynx, trachea, and extrapulmonary and intrapulmonary bronchi, all of which are largely lined by pseudostratified, ciliated columnar cells plus a variable proportion of secretory goblet (mucous) and serous cells (Figs. 9-2 and 9-3 and Web Fig. 9-1). The transitional system of the respiratory tract is composed of bronchioles, which serve as a transition zone between the conducting system (ciliated) and the gas exchange (alveolar) system (see Fig. 9-1). The disappearance of cilia in the transitional system is not abrupt; the ciliated cells in the proximal bronchiolar region become scarce and progressively attenuated, until the point where distal bronchioles no longer have ciliated cells. Normal bronchioles also lack goblet cells, but instead have other types of secretory cells, notably Clara and neuroendocrine cells. Clara cells, also referred to as secretory bronchiolar cells, contain numerous biosynthetic organelles that play an active role in detoxification of xenobiotics (foreign substances), similar to the role of hepatocytes (Fig. 9-4). Clara cells are also critical stem cells in the repair and remodeling of not only the bronchioles, but of most of the respiratory tract. In addition, Clara cells contribute to the innate immunity of the lung by secreting protective proteins (collectins) and pulmonary surfactant (Fig. 9-4, *B*). In carnivores and monkeys, and to a much lesser extent in horses and humans, the terminal portions of bronchioles are not only lined by cuboidal epithelium but also by segments of alveolar capillaries. These unique bronchioloalveolar structures are known as respiratory bronchioles (Fig. 9-5; also see Fig. 9-1). The gas exchange system of the respiratory tract in all mammals is formed by alveolar ducts and millions of alveoli (Fig. 9-6; also see Fig. 9-1). The surface of the alveoli is lined by two distinct types of epithelial cells known as type I pneumonocytes (membranous) and type II pneumonocytes (granular) (Fig. 9-7).

All three—the conducting, transitional, and exchange systems of the respiratory system—are vulnerable to injury because of constant exposure to a myriad of microbes, particles and fibers, and toxic gases and vapors present in the air. Vulnerability of the respiratory system to aerogenous (airborne) injury is primarily because of (1) the extensive area of the alveoli, which are the interface between the blood in alveolar capillaries and inspired air; (2) the large volume of air passing continuously into the lungs; and (3) the high concentration of noxious elements that can be present in the air (Table 9-1). For humans, it has been estimated that the surface of the pulmonary alveoli is approximately 200 m^2, roughly the area of a tennis court. It has also been estimated that the volume of air reaching the human lung every day is around 9000 L. The surface of the equine lung is estimated to be around 2000 m^2.

Lungs are also susceptible to blood-borne (hematogenous) microbes, toxins, and emboli. This fact is not surprising because the entire cardiac output of the right ventricle goes into the lungs, and approximately 9% of the total blood volume is within the pulmonary vasculature. The pulmonary capillary bed is the largest in the body, with a surface area of 70 m^2 in the adult human; this area is equivalent to a length of 2400 km of capillaries, with 1 mL of blood occupying up to 16 km of capillary bed.

NORMAL FLORA OF THE RESPIRATORY SYSTEM

The respiratory system has its own normal flora (microbiota), as does any other body system in contact with the external environment. If a sterile swab is passed deep into the nasal cavity of any healthy animal and cultured for microbes, yeasts, and fungi, many species of bacteria are recovered, such as *Mannheimia (Pasteurella) haemolytica* in cattle; *Pasteurella multocida* in cats, cattle, and pigs; and *Bordetella bronchiseptica* in dogs and pigs. The organisms that constitute the normal flora of the respiratory tract are restricted to

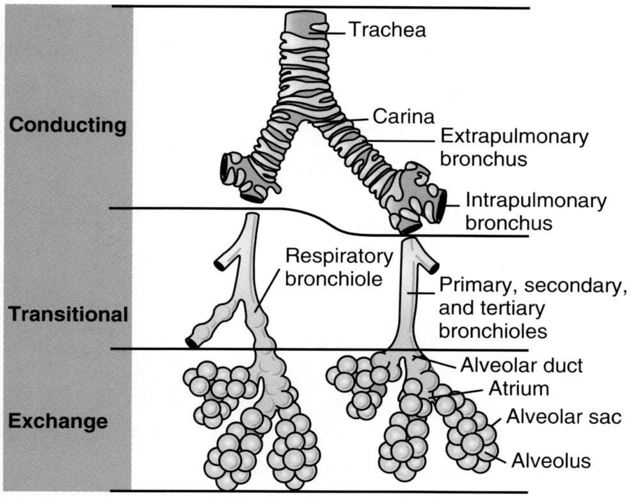

Fig. 9-1 Schematic diagram of airways from the trachea to the alveoli.
Conducting, transitional, and exchange components of the respiratory system. The transitional zone (bronchioles) is not as equally well developed in all species. (From Banks WJ: *Applied veterinary histology,* ed 3, St Louis, 1993, Mosby.)

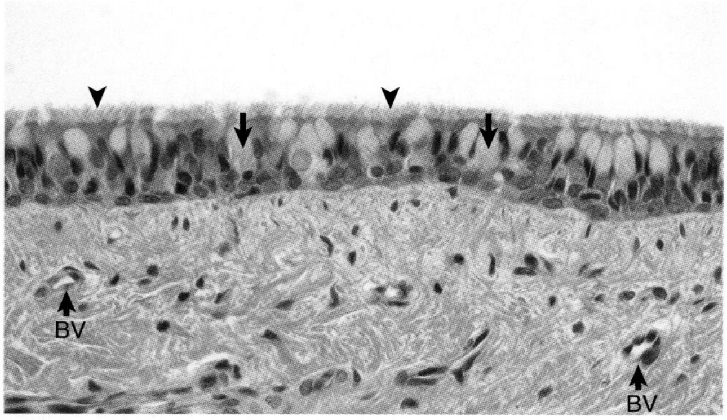

Fig. 9-2 Normal mucosa, trachea dog.
Mucosa consists of ciliated and nonciliated secretory cells. Goblet cells have a pale staining cytoplasm *(arrows).* The proportion of ciliated to nonciliated cells varies depending on the level of airways. Ciliated cells *(arrowheads)* are more abundant in proximal airways, whereas secretory cells are proportionally more numerous in distal portions of the conducting and transitional systems. The submucosa of the conducting system (nasal to bronchi) has abundant blood vessels *(BV).* (Courtesy Dr. J.F. Zachary, College of Veterinary Medicine, University of Illinois.)

the most proximal (rostral) region of the conducting system (nasal cavity, pharynx, and larynx). The thoracic portions of the trachea, bronchi, and lungs are considered to be essentially sterile. The types of bacteria present in the nasal flora vary considerably among animal species and in different geographic regions of the world. Some bacteria present in the nasal flora are pathogens that can cause important respiratory infections. For instance, *Mannheimia (Pasteurella) haemolytica* is part of the bovine nasal flora, yet this bacterium causes a devastating disease in cattle—pneumonic Mannheimiosis (shipping fever). Experimental studies have established that microorganisms from the nasal flora are continuously carried into the lungs via tracheal air. In spite of this constant bacterial bombardment from the nasal flora and from contaminated air, normal lungs remain sterile because of their remarkably effective defense mechanisms.

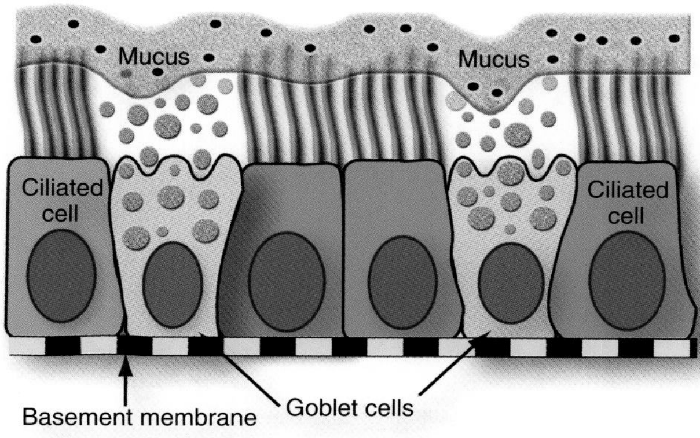

Fig. 9-3 Schematic representation of the mucociliary apparatus of the conducting system.
Both ciliated and goblet cells rest on the basement membrane. Mucus produced and released by goblet cells forms a carpet on which inhaled particles *(dots)* are trapped and subsequently expelled into the pharynx by the mucociliary apparatus. (Courtesy Dr. A. López, Atlantic Veterinary College.)

PORTALS OF ENTRY INTO THE RESPIRATORY SYSTEM

Microbes, toxins, and pneumotoxicants can gain access into the respiratory system by the following routes (also see Tables 9-1 and 9-2):

1. Aerogenous—Pathogens, such as bacteria, mycoplasmas, and viruses, along with toxic gases and foreign particles, including food, can gain access to the respiratory system via inspired air. This is the most common route in the transmission of most respiratory infections in domestic animals.
2. Hematogenous—Some viruses, bacteria, parasites, and toxins can enter the respiratory system via the circulating blood. This portal of entry is commonly seen in septicemias, bacteremias, and protozoa and viruses that target endothelial cells. Also, circulating leukocytes may release infectious organisms such as retroviruses and *Listeria monocytogenes* while traveling through the lungs.
3. Direct extension—In some instances, pathogenic organisms can also reach the pleura and lungs through penetrating injuries, such as gunshot wounds, migrating awns, or bites, or by direct extension from a ruptured esophagus or perforated diaphragm.

DEFENSE MECHANISMS OF THE RESPIRATORY SYSTEM

It is axiomatic that a particle, microbe, or toxic gas must first gain entry to a vulnerable region of the respiratory system before it can induce an adaptive immune response or have a pathologic effect. The characteristics of size, shape, dispersal, and deposition of particles present in inspired air are studied in aerobiology. It is important to recognize the difference between deposition, clearance, and retention of inhaled particles. Deposition is the process by which particles of various sizes and shapes are trapped within specific regions of the respiratory tract. Clearance is the process by which deposited particles are destroyed, neutralized, or removed from the mucosal surfaces. The difference between what is deposited and what is cleared from the respiratory tract is referred to as *retention.* The main mechanisms involved in clearance are sneezing, coughing,

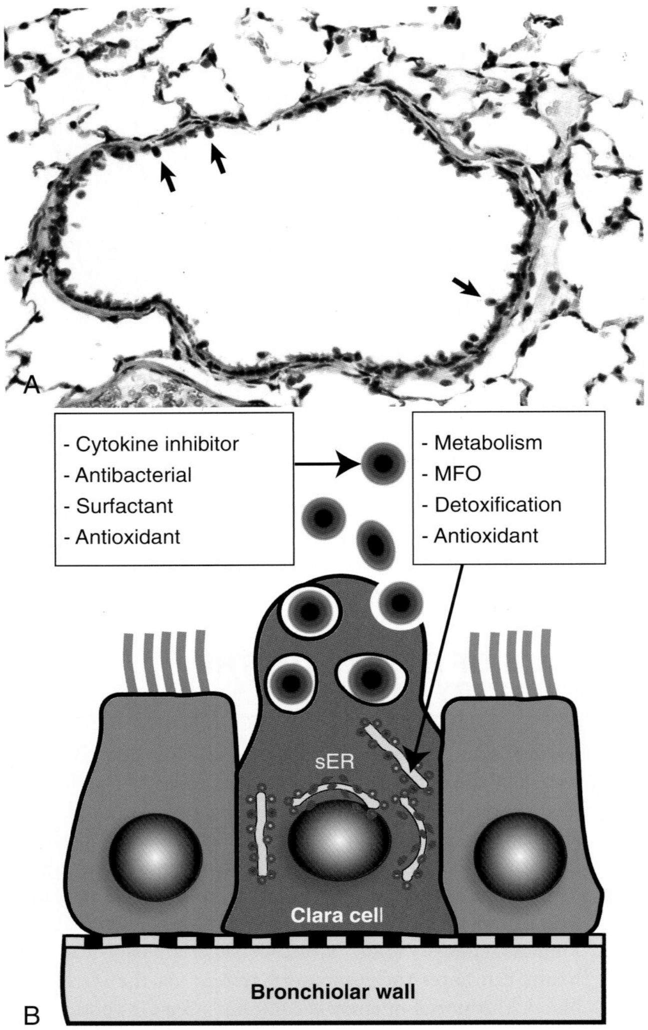

Fig. 9-4 Normal bronchiole, rat.
A, Bronchiole showing a thin wall composed of a basement membrane, smooth muscle, and connective tissue. On the luminal surface of the bronchiole note dome-shaped Clara cells *(arrows)* protruding into the lumen. H&E stain. **B,** Schematic representation of a Clara cell showing abundant smooth endoplasmic reticulum (SER) and cytoplasmic granules, which are extruded into the bronchiolar lumen. *MFO,* Mixed function oxidases. (Courtesy Dr. A. López, Atlantic Veterinary College.)

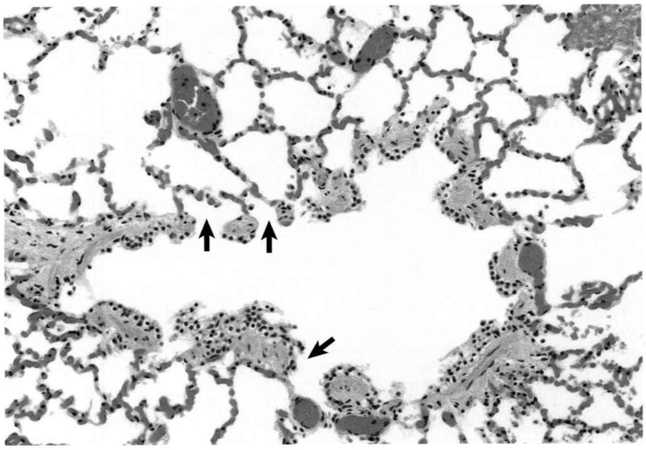

Fig. 9-5 Normal respiratory bronchiole, dog.
The wall of the bronchiole is covered by ciliated epithelium, which is supported by smooth muscle and connective tissue. Terminally, the wall becomes interrupted, forming lateral communications between the bronchiolar lumen and alveoli *(arrows)*. (Courtesy Dr. A. López, Atlantic Veterinary College.)

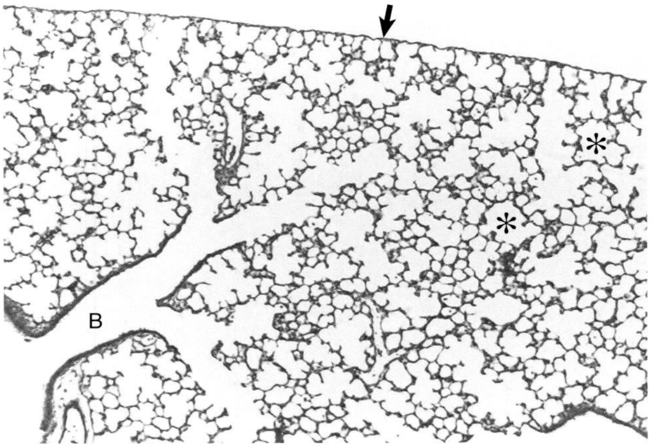

Fig. 9-6 Lung, rat.
Lungs were fixed by intratracheal perfusion of fixative to retain normal distention of airways. Note the dichotomous branching of the bronchioles and the thin visceral pleura *(arrow)* covering the surface of the lungs *(B)* that terminate as alveoli *(asterisks)*. H&E stain. (Courtesy Dr. J. Martinez-Burnes, Atlantic Veterinary College.)

mucociliary transport, and phagocytosis (Table 9-3). Abnormal retention of particles resulting from increased deposition, decreased clearance, or a combination of both is the underlying pathogenetic mechanism in many pulmonary diseases (Fig. 9-8).

The anatomic configuration of the nasal cavity and bronchi plays a unique role in preventing or reducing the penetration of noxious material into the lungs, especially into the alveoli, which is the most vulnerable portion of the respiratory system. The narrow nasal meatuses and the coiled arrangement of the nasal conchae generate enormous turbulences of airflow and as a result, physical forces are created that forcefully impact particles larger than 10 μm onto the surface of the nasal mucosa (Fig. 9-9). Although particles smaller than 10 μm could escape trapping in the nasal cavity, these medium-sized particles meet a second barrier at the tracheal and bronchial bifurcations. Here, abrupt changes in the direction of air (inertia), which occurs at the branching of major airways, cause particles in the 2- to 10-μm size range to collide with the surface of bronchial mucosa (see Fig. 9-1). Because the velocity of inspired air at the level of the small bronchi and bronchioles has become rather slow, inertial and centrifugal forces no longer play a significant role in the trapping of inhaled particles. Here, in the transitional (bronchiolar) and exchange (alveolar) regions, particles 2 μm or smaller may come into contact with the mucosa by means of sedimentation because of gravitation or by diffusion as a result of Brownian movement. Infective aerosols containing bacteria and viruses are within the size ranges (0.01 to 2 μm) that typically gain access to the bronchioloalveolar region.

In addition to size, other factors, such as shape, length, electrical charge, and humidity, play an important role in mucosal deposition, retention, and pathogenicity of inhaled particles. For example, particles longer than 200 μm may also reach the lower respiratory tract, provided their mean aerodynamic diameter is less than 1 μm. Asbestos is a good example of a large but slender fiber that can bypass the filtrating mechanisms by traveling parallel to the airstream. Once in the terminal bronchioles and alveoli, asbestos fibers cause asbestosis, a serious pulmonary disease in humans.

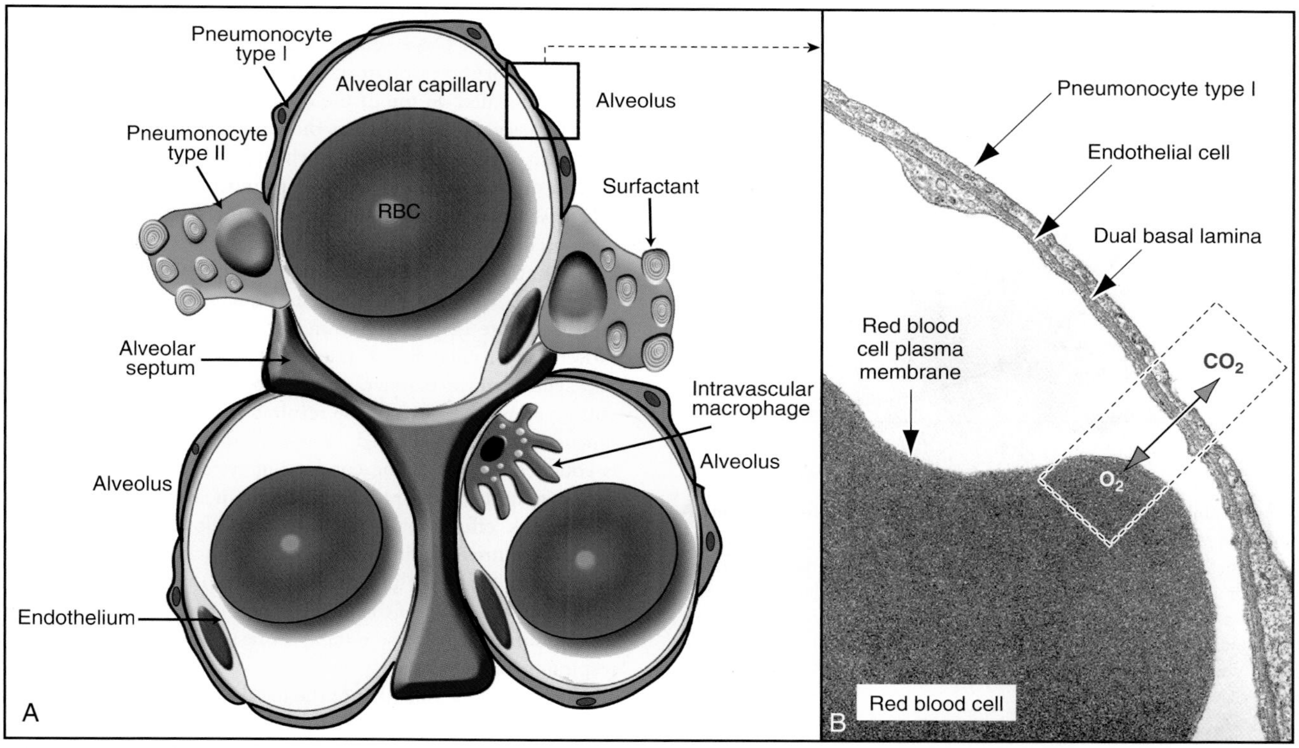

Fig. 9-7 **The blood-air barrier.**

A, In this schematic diagram, note the thin membrane (blood-air barrier) separating the blood compartment from the alveoli. Type I alveolar cells (membranous pneumonocytes) are remarkably thin and cover most of the alveolar wall. Note the endothelial cells lining the alveolar capillary. Alveolar interstitium supports the alveolar epithelium on one side and the endothelium on the other side of the blood-air barrier. Type II (granular) pneumonocytes appear as large cuboidal cells with lamellar bodies (surfactant) in the cytoplasm. A pulmonary intravascular macrophage, a component of the monocyte-macrophage system, is depicted on the wall of an alveolar capillary. A red blood cell (RBC) is present inside the lumen of the alveolar capillary. **B,** Alveolar wall. The blood-air barrier consists of cytoplasmic extensions of (1) type I alveolar cells (membranous pneumonocytes); (2) a dual basal lamina synthesized by type I alveolar cells; (3) cytoplasmic extensions of endothelial cells. TEM. Uranyl acetate and lead citrate stain. (**A** courtesy Dr. A. López, Atlantic Veterinary College. **B** from Kierszenbaum AL: *Histology and cell biology*, St Louis, 2002, Mosby.)

TABLE 9-1 Common Pathogens, Allergens, and Toxic Substances Present in Inhaled Air

Category	Agents
Microbes	Viruses, Chlamydophila, bacteria, fungi, protozoa
Plant dust	Grain, flour, cotton, wood
Animal products	Dander, feathers, mites, insect chitin
Toxic gases	Ammonia (NH_3), hydrogen sulfide (H_2S), nitrogen dioxide (NO_2), sulfur dioxide (SO_2), chlorine
Chemicals	Organic and inorganic solvents, herbicides, asbestos, nickel, lead

TABLE 9-2 Portals of Entry into the Respiratory System

Route	Agents
Aerogenous (inhalation)	Virus, bacteria, Chlamydophila, fungi, toxic gases, and pneumotoxicants
Hematogenous (blood)	Virus, bacteria, fungi, parasites, toxins, and pneumotoxicants
Direct extension	Penetrating wounds, migrating awns, bites, and ruptured esophagus or perforated diaphragm (hardware)

TABLE 9-3 Main Defense Mechanisms of the Respiratory System

Regions of the Respiratory System	Defense Mechanisms
Conducting system (nose, trachea, and bronchi)	Mucociliary clearance, antibodies, lysozyme, mucus
Transitional system (bronchioles)	Clara cells, antioxidants, lysozyme, antibodies
Exchange system (alveoli)	Alveolar macrophages (inhaled pathogens), intravascular macrophages (circulating pathogens), opsonizing antibodies, surfactant, antioxidants

In summary, the anatomic features of the nasal cavity and airways provide an effective barrier, preventing the penetration of most large particles into the lungs.

Once larger particles are trapped in the mucosa of conducting airways and small particles are deposited on the surface of the nasal, tracheal, or bronchioalveolar mucosa, it is crucial that these exogenous materials be removed to prevent or minimize injury to the respiratory system. For these purposes, the respiratory system is equipped with several defense mechanisms, all of which are provided by specialized cells operating in a remarkably well-coordinated manner.

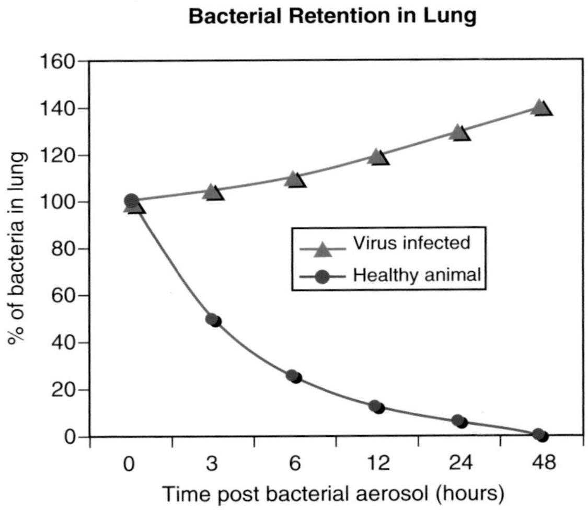

Fig. 9-8 Pulmonary clearance and retention of bacteria following inhalation of an experimental aerosol of bacteria.

When large numbers of bacteria are inhaled, the normal defense mechanisms promptly eliminate these microorganisms from the lungs *(blue line)*. However, when the defense mechanisms are impaired by a viral infection, lung edema, stress, and so forth, the inhaled bacteria are not eliminated but colonize and multiply in the lung *(red line)*. (Courtesy Dr. A. López, Atlantic Veterinary College.)

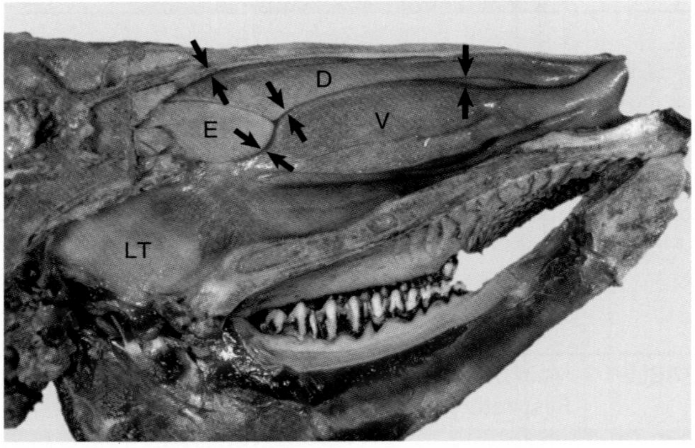

Fig. 9-9 Dorsal (D), ventral (V), and ethmoidal (E) conchae, midsagittal section of head, cow.

These meatuses *(*spaces between arrows) are narrow and the air turbulence produced in them by the coiled arrangement of the conchae causes suspended particles to impact on the mucus covering the surface of the nasal mucosa. These particles are then moved caudally by the mucociliary apparatus to the pharynx and finally swallowed. Note the abundant lymphoid tissue *(LT)* in the nasopharynx. (Courtesy Dr. R.G. Thomson, Ontario Veterinary College.)

DEFENSE MECHANISMS OF THE CONDUCTING SYSTEM (NOSE, TRACHEA, AND BRONCHI)

Mucociliary clearance is the physical unidirectional movement and removal of deposited particles and gases dissolved in the mucus from the respiratory tract. Mucociliary clearance, also referred to as the *waste disposal system,* is provided by the mucociliary blanket (mucociliary escalator) and is the main defense mechanism of the conducting system (nasal cavity, trachea, and bronchi) (see Figs. 9-2 and 9-3). Mucus acts primarily as a barrier and a vehicle and is a complex mixture of water, glycoproteins, immunoglobulins, lipids, and electrolytes produced by goblet (mucous) cells, serous cells, submucosal glands, and fluid from transepithelial ion and water transport. Once serous fluid and mucus are secreted onto the surface of the respiratory mucosa, a thin, double-layer film of mucus is formed on top of the cells. The outer layer of this film is in a viscous gel phase, whereas the inner layer, which is in a fluid or sol phase, is directly in contact with cilia (see Fig. 9-3). A healthy human produces around 100 mL of mucus per day. Each ciliated cell in the conducting system has around 100 to 200 motile and chemosensory cilia (6 μm long), beating metachronously (forming a wave) at a ciliary beat frequency of approximately 1000 strokes per minute, and in a horse, for example, mucus moves longitudinally at a rate of up to 20 mm per minute. Rapid and powerful movement of cilia creates a series of waves that, in a continuous and synchronized manner, propel the mucus, exfoliated cells, and entrapped particles out of the respiratory tract to the pharynx. The mucus is finally swallowed, or when present in large amounts, it is coughed up out of the conducting system. If mucus flow were to move at the same rate in all levels of a conducting system, a "bottleneck" effect would be created in major airways as the minor but more numerous airways enter the bronchi. For this reason, the mucociliary transport in proximal (rostral) airways is physiologically faster than that of the distal (caudal) ones. Ciliary activity and mucus transport increase notably in response to stimuli such as in respiratory infections.

The mucociliary blanket of the nasal cavity, trachea, and bronchi also plays an important role in preventing injury from toxic gases. If a soluble gas contacts the mucociliary blanket, it mixes with the mucus, thus reducing the concentration of gas reaching deep into the alveoli. In other words, mucus acts as a "scavenger system," whereby gases are solubilized and subsequently cleared from the respiratory tract via mucociliary transport. If ciliary transport is reduced (loss of cilia) or mucus production is excessive, coughing becomes an important mechanism for clearing the airways.

In addition to the mechanical barrier and physical transport provided by the mucociliary escalator, other cells closely associated with ciliated epithelium contribute to the defense mechanism of the conducting system. Among the most notable ones are the microfold (M) cells, which are modified epithelial cells covering the bronchial-associated lymphoid tissue (BALT), both of which are strategically situated at the corner of the bifurcation of bronchi and bronchioles, where inhaled particles often collide with the mucosa because of inertial forces. From here, inhaled particles and soluble antigens are phagocytosed and transported by macrophages, dendritic cells, and other professional antigen-presenting cells (APCs) into the BALT, thus providing a unique opportunity for B and T lymphocytes to enter into close contact with inhaled pathogenic substances. Pulmonary lymphocytes are not quiescent in the BALT but are in continual traffic to other organs and contribute to both cellular (cytotoxic, helper, suppressor T lymphocytes) and humoral immune responses. Immunoglobulin A (IgA), produced by mucosal plasma cells, and to a lesser extent, immunoglobulin G (IgG) and M (IgM) play important roles in the local immunity of the conducting system, especially with regard to preventing attachment of pathogens to the cilia. Chronic airway diseases, especially those caused by infection, such as those caused by mycoplasmas or retroviruses, are often accompanied by severe hyperplasia of the BALT.

The mucociliary clearance terminates at the pharynx, where mucus, propelled caudally from the nasal cavity and cranially from the tracheobronchial tree, is eventually swallowed and thus eliminated from the conducting system of the respiratory tract. Some respiratory pathogens, such as *Rhodococcus equi,* can infect the intestines after having been removed and swallowed from the respiratory tract into the alimentary system.

DEFENSE MECHANISMS OF THE EXCHANGE SYSTEM (ALVEOLI)

Alveoli lack ciliated and mucus-producing cells; thus the defense mechanism against inhaled particles in the alveolar region cannot be provided by mucociliary clearance. Instead, the main defense mechanism of alveoli (exchange system) is phagocytosis provided by the pulmonary alveolar macrophages (Fig. 9-10). These highly phagocytic cells, which are not to be confused with intravascular pulmonary macrophages, are derived largely from blood monocytes and to a much lesser extent, from a slowly dividing population of interstitial macrophages. After a temporary adaptive stage within alveolar interstitium, blood monocytes reduce their glycolytic metabolism and increase their oxidative metabolism to function in an aerobic rather than an anaerobic environment. Pulmonary alveolar macrophages contribute to the pulmonary innate and adaptive immune response rapidly attaching and phagocytosing bacteria and any other particle reaching the alveolar lumens. The number of free macrophages in the alveolar space is closely related to the number of inhaled particles reaching the lungs. This ability to increase, within hours, the number of available phagocytic cells is vital in protecting the distal lungs against foreign material, particularly when the inhaled particle load is high. Unlike that of tissue macrophages, the lifespan of alveolar macrophages in the alveoli is notably short, only a few days, and thus they are continuously being replaced by newly migrated blood monocytes.

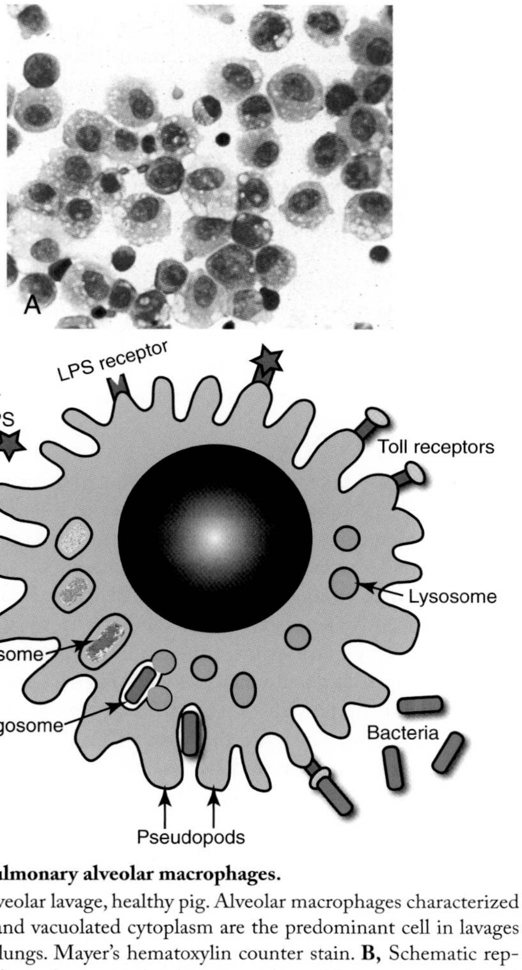

Fig. 9-10 Pulmonary alveolar macrophages.
A, Bronchoalveolar lavage, healthy pig. Alveolar macrophages characterized by abundant and vacuolated cytoplasm are the predominant cell in lavages from healthy lungs. Mayer's hematoxylin counter stain. **B,** Schematic representation of a pulmonary alveolar macrophage. Note receptors in cell membrane, attachment of bacteria to cell receptor, bacteria being engulfed by cytoplasmic projections (pseudopods), formation of cytoplasmic phagosomes, and fusion of lysosomes with phagosome (phagolysosomes) which finally kill the ingested bacteria. (**A** courtesy Dr. L.A. Rijana-Ludbit, Tübingen; **B** courtesy of Dr. A. López, Atlantic Veterinary College.)

Alveolar phagocytosis plays a prominent role in the innate defense mechanism against inhaled bacteria without the need of an inflammatory reaction. Bacteria reaching the alveoli are rapidly phagocytosed, and bactericidal enzymes present in lysosomes are discharged into the phagosome containing the bacteria (see Fig. 9-10). Except for some facultative pathogens that are resistant to intracellular killing (e.g., *Mycobacterium tuberculosis, Listeria monocytogenes, Brucella abortus,* and some *Salmonella* spp.), most bacteria reaching the lungs are rapidly destroyed by activated alveolar macrophages. Similarly, inhaled particles, such as dust, pollen, spores, carbon, or erythrocytes from intraalveolar hemorrhage, are all phagocytosed and eventually removed from alveoli by pulmonary alveolar macrophages. Most alveolar macrophages leave the alveoli by migrating toward the bronchiolar (transitional) region until the mucociliary blanket is reached. Once there, pulmonary macrophages are removed in the same way as any other particle: along the mucociliary flow to the pharynx and swallowed. In the cat, as many as 1 million macrophages per hour move out from the alveoli into the conducting system and pharynx.

Destruction and removal of inhaled microbes and particles by alveolar macrophages is a well-orchestrated mechanism that engages many cells, receptors (i.e., Toll-like receptors [TLRs]) and pulmonary secretions in the lung. The cell-to-cell interactions are complex and involve pulmonary alveolar macrophages, pneumonocytes, endothelial cells, lymphocytes, plasma cells, natural killer (NK) cells, and dendritic cells. Antibodies are also important in the protection (acquired immune response) of the respiratory tract against inhaled pathogens. IgA is the most abundant antibody in the nasal and tracheal secretions and prevents the attachment and absorption of antigens (immune exclusion). IgG and to a lesser extent IgE and IgM promote the uptake and destruction of inhaled pathogens by phagocytic cells (immune elimination). IgG is the most abundant antibody in the alveolar surface and acts primarily as an opsonizing antibody for alveolar macrophages and neutrophils. In addition to antibodies, there are several secretory products locally released into the alveoli that constitute the alveolar lining material and contribute to the pulmonary defense mechanisms. The most important of these antimicrobial products are transferrin, anionic peptides, and pulmonary surfactant (Table 9-4).

To facilitate phagocytosis and discriminate between "self" and "foreign" antigens, pulmonary alveolar macrophages are furnished with a wide variety of specific receptors on their cell surfaces. Among the most important ones are Fc receptors for antibodies; complement receptors (C3b, C3a, C5a); tumor necrosis factor (TNF) receptor; and CD40 receptors, which facilitate phagocytosis and destruction of opsonized particles. TLRs recognize microbial components, and FAS receptors are involved in apoptosis and in the phagocytosis of apoptotic cells in the lung. "Scavenger receptors," which are responsible for the recognition and uptake of foreign particulates, such as dust and fibers, are also present on pulmonary alveolar macrophages.

DEFENSE MECHANISMS AGAINST BLOOD-BORNE PATHOGENS (INTRAVASCULAR SPACE)

Lungs are also susceptible to hematogenously borne microbes, toxins, or emboli. The hepatic (Kupffer cells) and splenic macrophages are

TABLE 9-4 Defense Mechanisms Provided by Some Cells and Secretory Products Present in the Respiratory System

Cell/Secretory Product	Action
Alveolar macrophage	Phagocytosis, main line of defense against inhaled particles and microbial pathogens in the alveoli
Intravascular macrophage	Phagocytosis, removal of particles, endotoxin, and microbial pathogens in the circulation
Ciliated cells	Expel mucus and inhaled particles and microbial pathogens by ciliary action
Clara cells	Detoxification of xenobiotics (mixed function oxidases) and protective secretions against oxidative stress and inflammation; production of surfactant
Mucus	Physical barrier; traps inhaled particles and microbial pathogens and neutralizes soluble gases
Surfactant	Protects alveolar walls and enhances phagocytosis
Lysozyme	Antimicrobial enzyme
Transferrin and lactoferrin	Inhibition and suppression of bacterial growth
α_1-Antitrypsin	Protects against the noxious effects of proteolytic enzymes released by phagocytic cells; also inhibits inflammation
Interferon	Antiviral agent and modulator of the immune and inflammatory responses
Interleukins	Chemotaxis, upregulation of adhesion molecules
Antibodies	Prevent microbe attachment to cell membranes, opsonization
Complement	Chemotaxis; enhances phagocytosis
Antioxidants*	Prevent injury caused by superoxide anion, hydrogen peroxide, and free radicals (ROS) generated during phagocytosis, inflammation, or by inhalation of oxidant gases (ozone, nitrogen dioxide [NO_2], sulfur dioxide [SO_2])

*Superoxide dismutase, catalase, glutathione peroxidase, oxidant free radical scavengers (tocopherol, ascorbic acid).

the primary phagocytic cells responsible for removing circulating bacteria and other particles from the blood of dogs, some rodents, and humans. In contrast, the cell responsible for the removal of circulating particles, bacteria, and endotoxin from the blood of ruminants, cats, pigs, and horses is mainly the pulmonary intravascular macrophage, a distinct population of phagocytes normally residing within the pulmonary capillaries (see Fig. 9-7). In pigs, 16% of the pulmonary capillary surface is lined by pulmonary intravascular macrophages. In ruminants, 95% of intravenously injected tracer particles or bacteria are rapidly phagocytosed by these intravascular macrophages. Recent studies showed that an abnormally reduced number of Kupffer cells in diseased liver results in a compensatory increase in pulmonary intravascular macrophages, even in animal species in which these phagocytic cells are normally absent from the lung. In some abnormal conditions, such as sepsis, excessive release of cytokines by pulmonary intravascular macrophages may result in acute lung injury.

DEFENSE MECHANISMS AGAINST OXIDANT-INDUCED LUNG INJURY

Existing in an oxygen-rich environment and being the site of numerous metabolic reactions, the lungs also require an efficient defense mechanism against oxidant-induced cellular damage (oxidative stress). This form of damage is caused by inhaled oxidant gases (e.g., nitrogen dioxide, ozone, sulfur dioxide, or tobacco smoke), by xenobiotic toxic metabolites produced locally, by reaching the lungs via the bloodstream (e.g., 3-methylindole and paraquat), or by free radicals (reactive oxygen species) released by phagocytic cells during inflammation. Free radicals and reactive oxygen species (ROS) not only induce extensive pulmonary injury but also impair the defense and repair mechanisms in the lung. Oxygen and free radical scavengers, such as catalase, superoxide dismutase, ubiquinone, and vitamins E and C, are largely responsible for protecting pulmonary cells against peroxidation. These scavengers are present in alveolar and bronchiolar epithelial cells and in the extracellular spaces of the pulmonary interstitium.

In summary, the defense mechanisms are so effective in trapping, destroying, and removing bacteria that, under normal conditions, animals can be exposed to aerosols containing massive numbers of bacteria without any ill effects. If defense mechanisms are impaired, inhaled bacteria colonize and multiply in bronchi, bronchioles, and alveoli, and produce infection, which can result in fatal pneumonia. Similarly, when blood-borne pathogens, inhaled toxicants, or free radicals overwhelm the protective defense mechanisms, cells of the respiratory system are likely to be injured, often causing serious respiratory diseases.

IMPAIRMENT OF DEFENSE MECHANISMS IN THE RESPIRATORY SYSTEM

For many years, factors such as stress, viral infections, and pulmonary edema have been implicated in predisposing humans and animals to secondary bacterial pneumonia. There are many pathways by which the defense mechanisms can be impaired; only those relevant to veterinary species are discussed.

VIRAL INFECTIONS

Viral agents are notorious in predisposing humans and animals to secondary bacterial pneumonias by what is known as viral-bacterial synergism. A good example of this synergistic effect of combined virus-bacterial infections is documented from epidemics of humans with influenza virus in which the mortality rate has been significantly increased from secondary bacterial pneumonia. The most common viruses incriminated in predisposing animals to secondary bacterial pneumonia include influenza virus in pigs and horses; bovine herpesvirus 1 (BoHV-1), parainfluenza-3 (PI-3), and bovine respiratory syncytial virus (BRSV) in cattle; canine distemper virus in dogs; and herpesvirus and calicivirus in cats. The mechanism of the synergistic effect of viral-bacterial infections was previously believed to be the destruction of the mucociliary blanket and a concurrent reduction of mucociliary clearance, but in experimental studies, viral infections did not significantly reduce the physical removal of particles or bacteria out of the lungs. Now, it is known that 5 to 7 days after a viral infection, the mucociliary clearance and phagocytic function of pulmonary alveolar macrophages are notably impaired (see Fig. 9-8). Other mechanisms by which viruses impair defense mechanisms are multiple and remain poorly understood (Box 9-1). Immunization against viral infections in many cases prevents or reduces the synergistic effect of viruses and thus the incidence of secondary bacterial pneumonia

BOX 9-1 Postulated Mechanisms by Which Viruses May Impair the Defense Mechanisms of the Respiratory Tract

- Reduced mucociliary clearance
- Injured epithelium enhances attachment for bacteria
- Enhanced bacterial attachment predisposes to colonization
- Decreased mucociliary clearance prolongs resident time of bacteria favoring colonization
- Injured epithelium prevents mucociliary clearance and physical removal of bacteria
- Lack of secretory products facilitates further cell injury
- Break down the antimicrobial barrier in mucus and cells (β-defensins and anionic peptides)
- Ciliostasis caused by inflammation or by some pathogenic organism (mycoplasmas)
- Dysfunction of pulmonary alveolar macrophages and lymphocytes
- Consolidation of lung causes hypoxia resulting in decreased phagocytosis
- Infected macrophages fail to release chemotactic factors for other cells
- Infected macrophages fail to attach and ingest bacteria
- Lysosomes become disoriented and fail to fuse with phagosome-containing bacteria
- Intracellular killing or degradation is decreased because of biochemical dysfunction
- Altered cytokines and secretory products impair bacterial phagocytosis
- Viral-induced apoptosis of alveolar macrophages
- Altered CD4 and CD8 lymphocytes
- Toll-like receptors (TLRs) in virus-infected macrophages increase proinflammatory response to bacteria

TOXIC GASES

Certain gases also impair respiratory defense mechanisms, rendering animals more susceptible to secondary bacterial infections. For instance, hydrogen sulfide and ammonia, frequently encountered on farms, especially in buildings with poor ventilation, can impair pulmonary defense mechanisms and increase susceptibility to bacterial pneumonia. The effects of environmental pollutants on the defense mechanisms of humans and animals living in crowded and polluted cities remain to be determined.

IMMUNODEFICIENCY

Immunodeficiency disorders, whether acquired or congenital, are often associated with increased susceptibility to viral, bacterial, and protozoal pneumonias. For example, humans with acquired immunodeficiency syndrome (AIDS) are notably susceptible to pneumonia caused by proliferation of *Pneumocystis carinii.* This ubiquitous organism, which under normal circumstances is not considered pathogenic, is also found in the pneumonic lungs of immunosuppressed pigs, foals, dogs, and rodents. Pigs infected with the porcine reproductive and respiratory syndrome (PRRS) virus frequently develop *Pneumocystis carinii* infection. Arabian foals born with combined immunodeficiency disease easily succumb to infectious diseases, particularly adenoviral pneumonia. Combined infections with two respiratory viruses, such as canine distemper and canine adenovirus (CAV-2), are sporadically reported in immunosuppressed puppies. Also, large doses of chemotherapeutic agents, such as steroids and alkylating agents, cause immunosuppression in dogs, cats, and other animals, increasing susceptibility to secondary viral and bacterial infections.

OTHER CONDITIONS THAT PREDISPOSE TO SECONDARY BACTERIAL PNEUMONIA

Uremia, endotoxemia, dehydration, starvation, hypoxia, acidosis, pulmonary edema, anesthesia, ciliary dyskinesia, and stress are only some of the many conditions that have been implicated in impairing respiratory defense mechanisms and consequently predisposing animals to develop secondary bacterial pneumonia. The mechanisms by which each of these factors suppresses pulmonary defenses are diverse and sometimes not well understood. For example, hypoxia and pulmonary edema decrease phagocytic function of pulmonary alveolar macrophages and alter the production of surfactant by type II pneumonocytes. Dehydration is thought to increase the viscosity of mucus, reducing or stopping mucociliary movement. Anesthesia induces ciliostasis, with concurrent loss of mucociliary function. Ciliary dyskinesia, an inherited defect in cilia, causes abnormal mucus transport; starvation, hypothermia, and tress can reduce humoral and cellular immune responses.

EXAMINATION OF THE RESPIRATORY TRACT

POSTMORTEM

Information on this topic, including Web Fig. 9-2, is available at evolve.elsevier.com/Zachary/McGavin/.

HISTOPATHOLOGY AND BIOPSIES

Information on this topic is available at evolve.elsevier.com/Zachary/McGavin/.

BRONCHOALVEOLAR LAVAGE AND TRACHEAL ASPIRATES

Information on this topic is available at evolve.elsevier.com/Zachary/McGavin/.

DISEASES OF THE RESPIRATORY SYSTEM

NASAL CAVITY AND SINUS MUCOSA

Pattern of Injury and Host Response

The conducting portion of the respiratory system is lined by pseudostratified columnar ciliated epithelium (most of the nasal cavity, paranasal sinuses, part of the larynx, and all of the trachea and bronchi), olfactory epithelium (part of the nasal cavity, particularly ethmoidal conchae), and squamous epithelium (nasal vestibulum and parts of the larynx). The pattern of injury, inflammation, and host response (wound healing) is characteristic for each of these three types of epithelium and independent of its anatomic location.

Pseudostratified ciliated epithelium, which lines most of the nasal cavity and nasopharynx, part of the larynx, and all of the trachea and bronchi, is exquisitely sensitive to injury. When these cells are irreversibly injured, whether caused by a viral infection, trauma, or inhalation of toxic gases, ciliated cells swell, typically lose their attachment to underlying basement membrane, and rapidly exfoliate (Fig. 9-11). A transient and mild exudate of fluid, plasma proteins, and neutrophils covers the ulcer. In the absence of complications or secondary bacterial infections, a specific type of

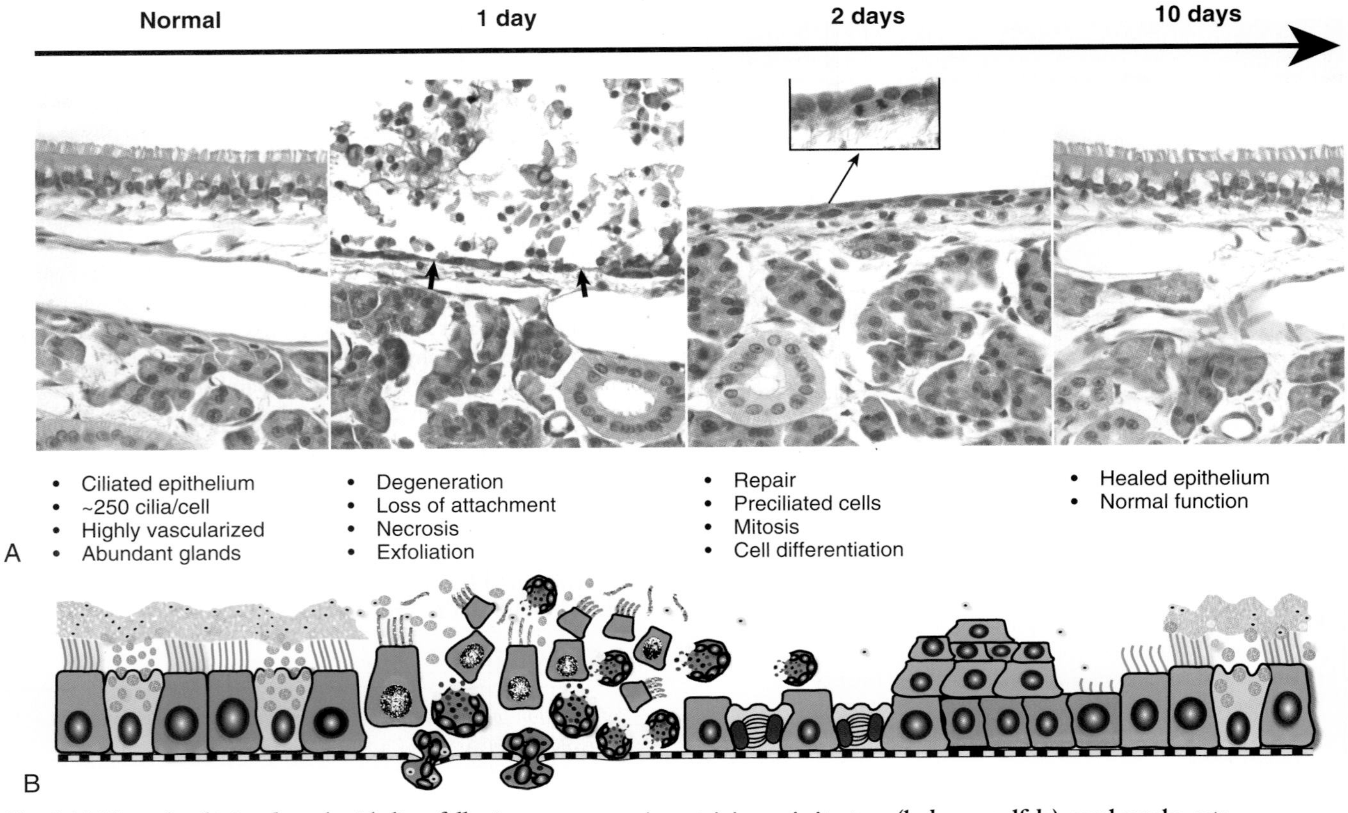

Fig. 9-11 Normal and injured nasal epithelium following exposure to air containing an irritant gas (hydrogen sulfide), nasal concha, rats. **A,** Normal ciliated epithelium composed of tall columnar cells with numerous cilia. Day 1. Note detachment and exfoliation of ciliated cells, leaving a denuded basement membrane *(arrows)*. This same type of lesion is seen in viral or mechanical injury to the mucosa of the conducting system. Two days after exposure, the basement membrane is lined by rapidly dividing preciliated cells, some of which exhibit mitotic activity *(inset)*. Ten days after injury, the nasal epithelium is completely repaired. H&E stain. **B,** Schematic representation of the events of injury and repair in the respiratory mucosa of the conducting system. Blue cell = ciliated mucosal epithelial cell; pink cell = goblet cell; red cell = neutrophil. (**A** from López A, Prior M, Yong S et al: *Am J Vet Res* 49:1107-1111, 1988; **B** courtesy of Dr. A. López, Atlantic Veterinary College.)

progenitor cell known as *nonciliated secretory cells,* which is normally present in the mucosa, migrates to cover the denuded basement membrane and undergoes mitosis, eventually differentiating into new ciliated epithelial cells (see Fig. 9-11). Cellular migration, proliferation, and attachment are regulated by locally released growth factors and extracellular matrix (ECM) proteins such as collagen, integrins, and fibronectin. The capacity of ciliated epithelium to repair itself is remarkably effective. For example, epithelial healing in an uncomplicated ulcer of the tracheal mucosa can be completed in only 10 days. This sequence of cell degeneration, exfoliation, ulceration, mitosis, and repair is typically present in many viral infections in which viruses replicate in nasal, tracheal, and bronchial epithelium, causing extensive mucosal ulceration. Examples of transient infections of this type include human colds (rhinoviruses), infectious bovine rhinotracheitis (bovine herpesvirus 1), feline rhinotracheitis (feline herpesvirus 1), and canine infectious tracheobronchitis (CAV-2 and canine parainfluenza-2).

If damage to the mucociliary blanket becomes chronic, goblet cell hyperplasia takes place, leading to excessive mucus production (hypersecretion) and reduced mucociliary clearance, and when there is loss of basement membrane, repair is by fibrosis and granulation tissue (scarring). In the most severe cases, prolonged injury causes squamous metaplasia, which together with scarring, causes airway obstruction and an impediment to mucociliary clearance. In laboratory rodents, hyperplastic and metaplastic changes, such as those seen in nasal polyps and squamous metaplasia, are considered a prelude to neoplasia.

The second type of epithelium lining the conducting system is the sensory olfactory epithelium, present in parts of the nasal mucosa, notably in the ethmoidal conchae. The patterns of degeneration, exfoliation, and inflammation in the olfactory epithelium are similar to those of the ciliated epithelium, except that olfactory epithelium has only limited capacity for regeneration. When olfactory epithelium has been irreversibly injured, olfactory cells swell, separate from adjacent sustentacular cells, and finally exfoliate into the nasal cavity. Once the underlying basement membrane of the olfactory epithelium is exposed, cytokines are released by leukocytes and endothelial cells, and inflammatory cells move into the affected area. When damage is extensive, ulcerated areas of olfactory mucosa are replaced by ciliated and goblet cells or squamous epithelium, or by fibrous tissue, all of which eventually cause reduction (hyposmia) or loss of olfactory function (anosmia). Repair of the olfactory epithelium is slower and less efficient than repair of the respiratory epithelium. Neurons in the olfactory mucosa have the unique ability to regenerate, a fact that is being explored as a potential source of new neurons in the treatment of spinal cord injury.

Squamous epithelium, located in the vestibular region of the nose (mucocutaneous junctions), is the third type of epithelium present in the nasal passages. Compared with ciliated and olfactory epithelia, nasal squamous epithelium is quite resistant to all forms of injury.

Anomalies of the Nasal Cavity

Information on this topic is available at evolve.elsevier.com/Zachary/McGavin/.

Metabolic Disturbances of the Nasal Cavity

Metabolic disturbances affecting the nasal cavity and sinuses are also rare in domestic animals. Amyloidosis, the deposition of amyloid protein (fibrils with a β-pleated configuration) in various tissues, has been sporadically reported in the nasal cavity of horses and humans. Microscopic lesions are similar to those seen in other organs and consist of a deposition of hyaline amyloid material in nasal mucosa that is confirmed by a histochemical stain, such as Congo red. Unlike amyloidoses in other organs of domestic animals where amyloid is generally of the reactive type (amyloid AA), equine nasal amyloidosis appears to be of the immunocytic type (amyloid AL). Affected horses with large amyloid masses have difficulty breathing because of nasal obstruction, and may exhibit epistaxis and reduced athletic performance; on clinical examination, large, firm nodules resembling neoplasms (amyloidoma) can be observed in the alar folds, rostral nasal septum, and floor of nasal cavity.

Circulatory Disturbances of the Nasal Cavity

Congestion and Hyperemia

The nasal mucosa is well vascularized and is capable of rather dramatic variation in blood flow, whether passively as a result of interference with venous return (congestion) or actively because of vasodilation (hyperemia). Congestion of the mucosal vessels is a nonspecific lesion commonly found at necropsy and presumably associated with the circulatory failure preceding death (e.g., heart failure, bloat in ruminants in which the increased intraabdominal pressure causes increased intrathoracic pressure impeding the venous return from the head and neck). Hyperemia of the nasal mucosa is seen in early stages of inflammation, whether caused by irritations (e.g., ammonia, regurgitated feed), viral infections, secondary bacterial infections, allergy, or trauma.

Hemorrhage

Epistaxis is the clinical term used to denote blood flow from the nose (nosebleed) regardless of whether the blood originates from the nasal mucosa or from deep in the lungs such as in horses with "exercise-induced pulmonary hemorrhage." Unlike blood in the digestive tract, where the approximate anatomic location of the bleeding can be estimated by the color the blood imparts to fecal material, blood in the respiratory tract is always red. This fact is due to the rapid transport of blood out of the respiratory tract by the mucociliary blanket and during breathing. Hemorrhages into the nasal cavity can be the result of local trauma, originate from erosions of submucosal vessels by inflammation (e.g., guttural pouch mycosis), or be caused by neoplasms. Hemoptysis refers to the presence of blood in sputum or saliva (coughing or spitting blood) and is most commonly the result of pneumonia, lung abscesses, ulcerative bronchitis, pulmonary thromboembolisms, and pulmonary neoplasia.

Ethmoidal (progressive) hematomas are important in older horses and are characterized clinically by chronic, progressive, often unilateral nasal bleeding. Grossly or endoscopically, an ethmoidal hematoma appears as a single, soft, tumorlike, pedunculated, expansive, dark red mass arising from the mucosa of the ethmoidal conchae (Fig. 9-12). Microscopic examination reveals a capsule lined by epithelium and hemorrhagic stromal tissue infiltrated with abundant macrophages, some of which are siderophages.

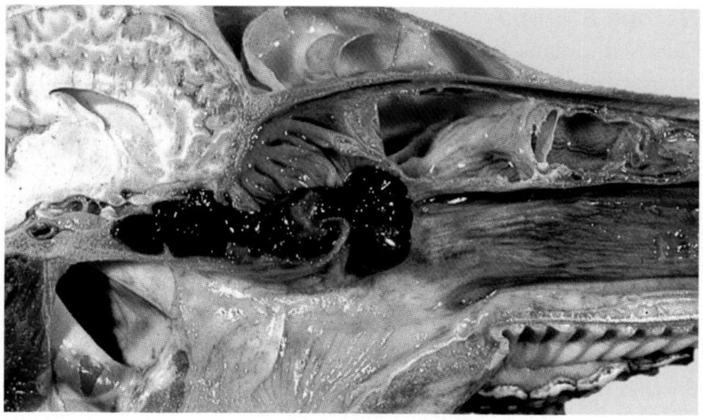

Fig. 9-12 Ethmoidal hematoma, midsagittal section of head, horse. A large amount of dark-red hemorrhage overlying the ethmoid conchae conceals an underlying hematoma in these conchae. (Courtesy Dr. J.M. King, College of Veterinary Medicine, Cornell University.)

Inflammation of the Nasal Cavity

Inflammation of the nasal mucosa is called *rhinitis,* and inflammation of the sinuses is called *sinusitis.* These conditions usually occur together, although mild sinusitis can be undetected. Clinically, rhinosinusitis is characterized by nasal discharge.

The occurrence of infectious rhinitis presupposes an upset in the balance of the normal microbial flora of the nasal cavity. Innocuous bacteria present normally and protect the host through a process called *competitive exclusion,* whereby potential pathogens are kept at a harmless level. Disruption of this protective mechanism can be caused by respiratory viruses, pathogenic bacteria, fungi, irritant gases, environmental changes, immunosuppression, local trauma, stress, or prolonged antibacterial therapy.

Inflammatory processes in the nasal cavity are not life threatening and usually resolve completely. However, some adverse sequelae in cases of infectious rhinitis include bronchoaspiration of exudate leading to bronchopneumonia. Chronic rhinitis often leads to destruction of the nasal conchae (turbinates), deviation of the septum, and eventually, craniofacial deformation. Also, nasal inflammation may extend into the sinuses causing sinusitis; into facial bones causing osteomyelitis; through the cribriform plate causing meningitis; into the Eustachian tubes causing otitis media; and even into the inner ear causing otitis interna and vestibular syndrome (abnormal head tilt and abnormal gait), which in severe cases may lead to emaciation.

Based on the nature of exudate, rhinitis can be classified as serous, fibrinous, catarrhal, purulent, or granulomatous. These types of inflammatory reactions can progress from one to another in the course of the disease (i.e., serous to catarrhal to purulent), or in some instances exudates can be mixed, such as those seen in mucopurulent, fibrinohemorrhagic, or pyogranulomatous rhinitis. Microscopic examination of impression smears or nasal biopsy, and bacterial or fungal cultures are generally required in establishing the cause of inflammation. Common sequels to rhinitis are hemorrhage, ulcers, and in some cases polyps (hyperplasia) arising from inflamed nasal mucosa. Rhinitis also can be classified according to the age of the lesions as acute, subacute, or chronic; to the severity of the insult as mild, moderate, or severe; and to the etiologic agent as viral, allergic, bacterial, mycotic, parasitic, traumatic, or toxic.

Serous Rhinitis

Serous rhinitis is the mildest form of inflammation and is characterized by hyperemia and increased production of a clear fluid locally manufactured by serous glands present in the nasal submucosa. Serous rhinitis is of clinical interest only. It is caused by mild irritants or cold air, and it occurs during the early stages of viral infections, such as the common cold in humans, upper respiratory tract infections in animals, or in mild allergic reactions.

Catarrhal Rhinitis

Catarrhal rhinitis is a slightly more severe process and has, in addition to serous secretions, a substantial increase in mucus production by increased activity of goblet cells and mucous glands. A mucous exudate is a thick, translucent, or slightly turbid viscous fluid, sometimes containing a few exfoliated cells, leukocytes, and cellular debris. In chronic cases, catarrhal rhinitis is characterized microscopically by notable hyperplasia of goblet cells. As the inflammation becomes more severe, the mucus is infiltrated with neutrophils giving the exudate a cloudy mucopurulent appearance. This exudate is referred to as *mucopurulent.*

Purulent (Suppurative) Rhinitis

Purulent (suppurative) rhinitis is characterized by a neutrophilic exudate, which occurs when the nasal mucosa suffers a more severe injury that generally is accompanied by mucosal necrosis and secondary bacterial infection. Cytokines, leukotrienes, complement activation, and bacterial products cause exudation of leukocytes, especially neutrophils, which mix with nasal secretions, including mucus. Grossly, the exudate in suppurative rhinitis is thick and opaque, but it can vary from white to green to brown, depending on the types of bacteria and type of leukocytes (neutrophils or eosinophils) present in the exudate (Fig. 9-13 and Web Fig. 9-3). In severe cases, the nasal passages are completely blocked by the exudate. Microscopically, neutrophils can be seen in the submucosa and mucosa and form plaques of exudate on the mucosal surface. Neutrophils are commonly found marginated in vessels, in the lamina propria, and in between epithelial cells in their migration to the surface of the mucosa.

Fibrinous Rhinitis

Fibrinous rhinitis is a reaction that occurs when nasal injury causes a severe increase in vascular permeability, resulting in abundant exudation of plasma fibrinogen, which coagulates into fibrin. Grossly, fibrin appears like a yellow, tan, or gray rubbery mat on nasal mucosa. Fibrin accumulates on the surface and forms a distinct film of exudate sometimes referred to as *pseudomembrane* (Fig. 9-14). If this fibrinous exudate can be removed, leaving an intact underlying mucosa, it is termed a *croupous* or *pseudodiphtheritic rhinitis.* Conversely, if the pseudomembrane is difficult to remove and leaves an ulcerated mucosa, it is referred to as *diphtheritic* or *fibrinonecrotic rhinitis.* The term *diphtheritic* was derived from human diphtheria, which causes a severe and destructive inflammatory process of the nasal, tonsillar, pharyngeal, and laryngeal mucosa. Microscopically, the lesions include a perivascular edema with fibrin, a few neutrophils infiltrating the mucosa, and superficial plaques of exudate consisting of fibrin strands mixed with leukocytes and cellular debris covering a necrotic and ulcerated epithelium. Fungal infections, such as aspergillosis, can cause a severe fibrinonecrotizing rhinitis.

Granulomatous Rhinitis

Granulomatous rhinitis is a reaction in the nasal mucosa and submucosa that is characterized by infiltration of numerous activated macrophages mixed with a few lymphocytes and plasma cells. In some cases, inflammation leads to the formation of polypoid nodules that in severe cases are large enough to cause obstruction of the nasal passages (Fig. 9-15). Granulomatous rhinitis is generally associated with chronic allergic inflammation or infection with specific organisms, such as those of the systemic mycoses (see the section on Lungs), tuberculosis, or rhinosporidiosis, and with foreign bodies. In some cases, the cause of granulomatous rhinitis cannot be determined.

Sinusitis

Sinusitis occurs sporadically in domestic animals and is frequently combined with rhinitis (rhinosinusitis), or it occurs as a sequela to penetrating or septic wounds of the nasal, frontal, maxillary, or palatine bones; improper dehorning in young cattle, which exposes the frontal sinus; or maxillary tooth infection in horses and dogs (maxillary sinus). Based on the type of exudate, sinusitis is classified as serous, catarrhal, fibrinous (rare), purulent, or granulomatous. Paranasal sinuses have poor drainage; therefore exudate tends to accumulate, causing mucocele (accumulation of mucus) or empyema (accumulation of pus) (Fig. 9-16). Chronic sinusitis may extend into the adjacent bone (osteomyelitis) or through the ethmoidal conchae into the meninges and brain (meningitis and encephalitis).

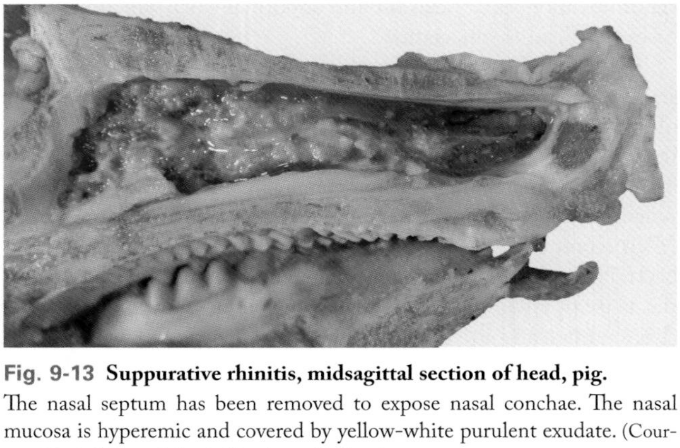

Fig. 9-13 Suppurative rhinitis, midsagittal section of head, pig. The nasal septum has been removed to expose nasal conchae. The nasal mucosa is hyperemic and covered by yellow-white purulent exudate. (Courtesy Dr. A. López, Atlantic Veterinary College.)

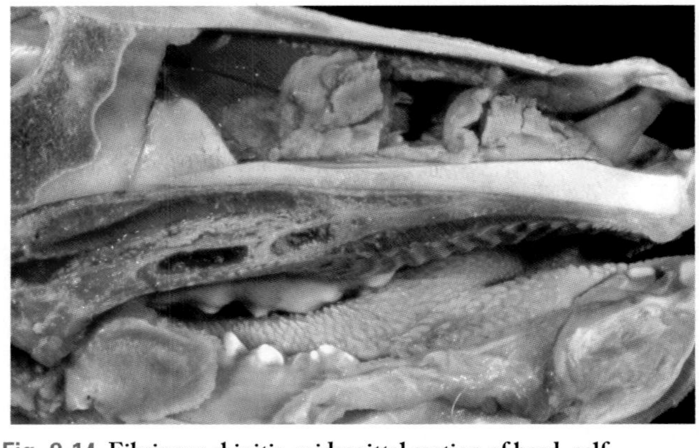

Fig. 9-14 Fibrinous rhinitis, midsagittal section of head, calf. Infectious bovine rhinotracheitis (IBR; bovine herpesvirus 1). The nasal septum has been removed to expose nasal conchae. The nasal mucosa is covered by diphtheritic yellow membranes consisting of fibrinonecrotic exudate. Removal of these fibrinous membranes reveals focal ulcers in the underlying mucosa. (Courtesy Dr. Scott McBurney, Atlantic Veterinary College.)

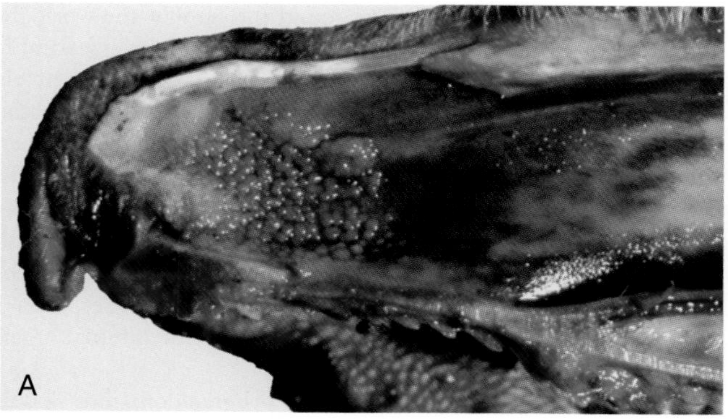

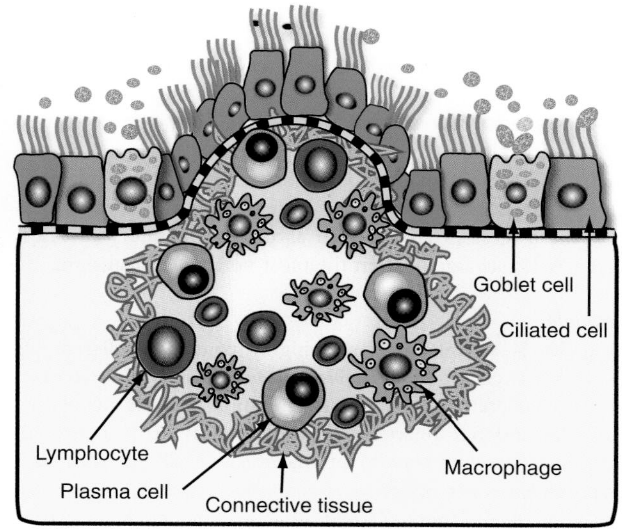

Fig. 9-15 Granulomatous rhinitis, midsagittal section of head, cow.
A, Note multiple and often confluent granulomas arising from the nasal mucosa. **B,** Schematic representation of a nasal granuloma showing the outer wall of the granuloma composed of connective tissue enclosing the center, which has been infiltrated with lymphocytes, plasma cells, and macrophages. (**A** courtesy Ontario Veterinary College. **B** courtesy of Dr. A. López, Atlantic Veterinary College.)

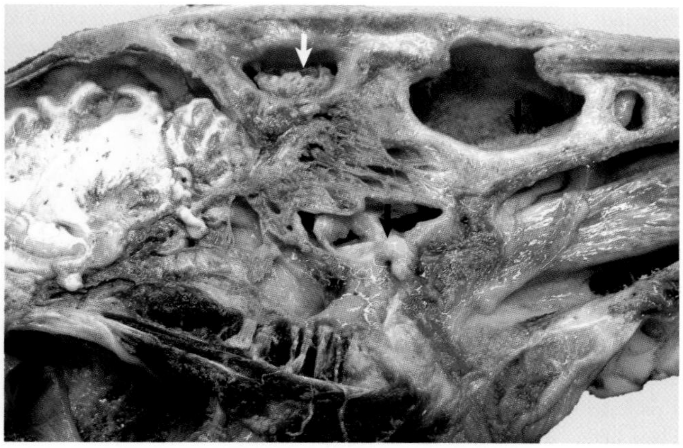

Fig. 9-16 Fibrinosuppurative sinusitis, midsagittal section of head, donkey.
Note that the paranasal sinuses are filled with fibropurulent exudate *(arrow)*. (Courtesy Facultad de Medicina Veterinaria y Zootecnia, Universidad Nacional Autónoma de México.)

Specific Diseases of the Nasal Cavity and Sinuses

Equine Nasal Diseases

Equine Viral Infections

Viruses, such as equine viral rhinopneumonitis virus, influenza virus, adenovirus, and rhinovirus, cause mild and generally transient respiratory infections in horses. The route of infection for these respiratory viruses is typically aerogenous. All these infections are indistinguishable clinically; signs consist mainly of malaise, fever, coughing, and nasal discharge varying from serous to purulent. Viral respiratory infections are common medical problems in adult horses.

Equine viral rhinopneumonitis

Equine viral rhinopneumonitis (EVR) is caused by two ubiquitous equine herpesviruses (EHV-1 and EHV-4) and may be manifested as a mild respiratory disease in weanling foals and young racehorses, as a neurologic disease (myeloencephalopathy), or as abortion in mares. The portal of entry for the respiratory form is typically aerogenous, and the disease is generally transient; thus the primary viral-induced lesions in the nasal mucosa and lungs are rarely seen at necropsy unless complicated by secondary bacterial rhinitis, pharyngitis, or bronchopneumonia. Studies with polymerase chain reaction (PCR) techniques have demonstrated that, like other herpesvirus, EHV-1 and EHV-4 persist latently in the trigeminal ganglia for long periods of time. Reactivation because of stress or immunosuppression and subsequent shedding of the virus are the typical source of infection for susceptible animals on the farm.

Equine influenza

Equine influenza is a common, highly contagious, and self-limiting upper respiratory infection of horses caused by aerogenous exposure to type A strains of influenza virus (H7N7 [A/equi-1] and H3N8 [A/equi-2]). Equine influenza has high morbidity (outbreaks) but low mortality, and it is clinically characterized by fever, conjunctivitis, and serous nasal discharge. It occurs mainly in 2- to 3-year-old horses at the racetrack. As with human influenza, equine influenza is usually a mild disease, but occasionally it can cause severe bronchointerstitial pneumonia with pulmonary edema. In some horses, impaired defense mechanisms caused by the viral infection are complicated by a secondary bacterial bronchopneumonia caused by opportunistic organisms (*Streptococcus zooepidemicus, Staphylococcus aureus,* or *Bacteroides* sp.) found in the normal flora of the upper respiratory tract. Uncomplicated cases of equine influenza are rarely seen in the postmortem room.

Other equine respiratory viruses

Equine rhinovirus, adenovirus, and parainfluenza virus produce mild and transient upper respiratory infections (nasopharynx and trachea) in horses, unless complicated by secondary pathogens. In addition to reduced athletic performance, infected horses may have a temporary suppression of cell-mediated immunity leading to opportunistic infections such as *Pneumocystis carinii* pneumonia.

Fatal adenoviral infections with severe pneumonia or enteritis occur commonly in immunocompromised horses, particularly in Arabian foals with inherited combined immunodeficiency disease.

Equine Bacterial Infections: Strangles, Glanders, and Melioidosis

Strangles, glanders, and melioidosis of horses are all systemic bacterial diseases that cause purulent rhinitis and suppuration in various organs. These diseases are grouped as upper respiratory diseases because nasal discharge is often the most notable clinical sign.

Strangles

Strangles is an infectious and highly contagious disease of Equidae that is caused by *Streptococcus equi* ssp. *equi* (*Streptococcus equi*). It is characterized by suppurative rhinitis and lymphadenitis (mandibular and retropharyngeal lymph nodes) with occasional hematogenous dissemination to internal organs. Unlike *Streptococcus equi* ssp. *zooepidemicus (Streptococcus zooepidemicus)* and *Streptococcus dysgalactiae* ssp. *equisimilis (Streptococcus equisimilis)*, *Streptococcus equi* is not part of the normal nasal flora. Infection occurs when susceptible horses come into contact with feed, exudate, or air droplets containing the bacterium. After penetrating through the nasopharyngeal mucosa, *Streptococcus equi* drains to the regional lymph nodes—mandibular and retropharyngeal lymph nodes—via lymphatic vessels. The gross lesions in horses with strangles (mucopurulent rhinitis) correlate with clinical findings and consist of copious amounts of mucopurulent exudate in the nasal passages with notable hyperemia of nasal mucosa. Affected lymph nodes are enlarged and may contain abscesses filled with thick purulent exudate (purulent lymphadenitis). The term *bastard strangles* is used in cases in which hematogenous dissemination of *Streptococcus equi* results in metastatic abscesses in such organs as the lungs, liver, spleen, kidneys, or brain or in the joints. This form of strangles is often fatal.

Common sequelae to strangles include bronchopneumonia caused by aspiration of nasopharyngeal exudate; laryngeal hemiplegia ("roaring"), resulting from compression of the recurrent laryngeal nerves by enlarged retropharyngeal lymph nodes; facial paralysis and Horner syndrome caused by compression of sympathetic nerves that run dorsal to the medial retropharyngeal lymph node; and purpura hemorrhagica as a result of vasculitis caused by deposition of *Streptococcus equi* antigen-antibody complexes in arterioles, venules, and capillaries of the skin and mucosal membranes. In severe cases, nasal infection extends directly into the paranasal sinuses or to the guttural pouches via the Eustachian tubes, causing inflammation and accumulation of pus (guttural pouch empyema). Rupture of abscesses in the mandibular and retropharyngeal lymph nodes leads to suppurative inflammation of adjacent subcutaneous tissue (cellulitis), and in severe cases the exudate escapes through cutaneous fistulas.

Strangles can affect horses of all ages, but it is most commonly seen in foals and young horses. It is clinically characterized by cough, nasal discharge, conjunctivitis, and painful swelling of regional lymph nodes. Some horses become carriers and a source of infection to other horses.

Glanders

Glanders is an infectious Office International des Epizooties (OIE)-notifiable disease of Equidae caused by *Burkholderia mallei (Pseudomonas mallei)* that can be transmitted to carnivores by consumption of infected horse meat. Humans are also susceptible, and the untreated infection is often fatal. This bacterium has been listed as a potential agent for biologic warfare and bioterrorism. In the past, *Burkholderia mallei* was found throughout the world, but today, glanders has been eradicated from most countries, except for some areas in North Africa, Asia, and Eastern Europe. There also have been some sporadic outbreaks reported in Brazil. The pathogenesis of glanders is not fully understood. Results from experimental infections suggest that infection occurs via the ingestion of contaminated feed and water and, very rarely, via inhalation of infectious droplets. The portals of entry are presumed to be the oropharynx or intestine, in which bacteria penetrate the mucosa and spread via lymph vessels to regional lymph nodes, then to the bloodstream, and thus hematogenously to the internal organs, particularly the lungs.

Lesions in the nasal cavity start as pyogranulomatous nodules in the submucosa; these lesions subsequently ulcerate, releasing copious amounts of *Burkholderia mallei*–containing exudate into the nasal cavity (see Fig. 4-24). Finally, ulcerative lesions in conchal mucosa heal and are replaced by typical stellate (star-shaped), fibrous scars. In some cases, the lungs also contain numerous gray, hard, small (2 to 10 mm), miliary nodules (resembling millet seeds), randomly distributed in one or more pulmonary lobes because of the hematogenous route. Microscopically, these nodules are typical chronic granulomas composed of a necrotic center, with or without calcification, surrounded by a layer of macrophages enclosed by a thick band of connective tissue infiltrated with macrophages, some giant cells, lymphocytes, and plasma cells. Cutaneous lesions, often referred to as equine farcy, are the result of severe suppurative lymphangitis characterized by nodular thickening of extended segments of lymph vessels in the subcutaneous tissue of the legs and ventral abdomen (see Fig. 4-24). Eventually, affected lymph vessels rupture and release large amounts of purulent exudate through sinuses to the surface of the skin.

Melioidosis (pseudoglanders)

Melioidosis (pseudoglanders) is an important, life-threatening disease of humans, horses, cattle, sheep, goats, pigs, dogs, cats, and rodents caused by *Burkholderia pseudomallei (Pseudomonas pseudomallei)*. This disease in horses is clinically and pathologically similar to glanders, hence the name *pseudoglanders*. In humans, this infection can cause severe sepsis and septic shock and has also been considered to have potential for biologic welfare. Melioidosis is currently present in Southeast Asia and to a much lesser extent in Northern Australia and some European countries where the causative organism is frequently found in rodents, feces, soil, and water. Ingestion of contaminated feed and water appears to be the main route of infection; direct transmission between infected animals and insect bites has also been postulated as a possible mechanism of infection. After gaining entrance to the animal, *Burkholderia pseudomallei* is disseminated by the bloodstream and causes suppuration and abscesses in most internal organs, such as nasal mucosa, joints, brain and spinal cord, lungs, liver, kidneys, spleen, and lymph nodes. The exudate is creamy or caseous and yellow to green. The pulmonary lesions in melioidosis are those of an embolic bacterial infection with the formation of pulmonary abscesses, which can become confluent. Focal adhesive pleuritis develops where abscesses rupture through the pleura and heal.

Other Causes of Equine Rhinitis

Information on this topic, including Web Fig. 9-4, is available at evolve.elsevier.com/Zachary/McGavin/.

Bovine Nasal Diseases

Infectious Bovine Rhinotracheitis

Infectious bovine rhinotracheitis (IBR), or "rednose," occurs worldwide and is a disease of great importance to the cattle industry because of the synergism of the IBR virus with *Mannheimia haemolytica* in producing pneumonia. The causative agent, bovine herpesvirus 1 (BoHV-1), has probably existed as a mild venereal disease in cattle in Europe since at least the mid-1800s, but the respiratory form was not reported until intensive management feedlot systems were first introduced in North America around the 1950s. Typically, the disease is manifested as a transient, acute, febrile illness, which only in very severe cases results in inspiratory dyspnea caused by obstruction of the airways by exudate. Other forms of BoHV-1 infection include ulcerative rumenitis; enteritis; multifocal hepatitis in neonatal calves; nonsuppurative meningoencephalitis; infertility; and in experimental infections, mastitis, mammillitis, and ovarian necrosis. Except for the encephalitic form, the type of disease caused by BoHV-1 depends more on the site of entry than the viral strain. Like other herpesviruses, BoHV-1 also can remain latent in nerve ganglia, with recrudescence after stress or immunosuppression. This virus also causes bovine abortion, systemic infections of calves, and genital infections such as infectious pustular vulvovaginitis (IPV) and infectious balanoposthitis (IBP).

The respiratory form of IBR is characterized by severe hyperemia and focal necrosis of nasal, pharyngeal, laryngeal, tracheal, and sometimes bronchial mucosa (Figs. 9-17 and 9-18 and Web Fig. 9-5). As in other respiratory viral infections, IBR lesions are microscopically characterized by necrosis and exfoliation of ciliated cells followed by repair. Secondary bacterial infections of these areas of necrosis result in the formation of a thick layer of fibrinonecrotic material (diphtheritic) in the nasal, tracheal, and bronchial mucosa (see Figs. 9-17 and 9-18). Intranuclear inclusion bodies, commonly seen in herpesvirus infections, are rarely seen in field cases because inclusion bodies occur only during the early stages of the disease.

The most important sequela to IBR is pneumonia, which is caused either by direct aspiration of exudate from airways or as a result of an impairment in pulmonary defense mechanisms, thus predisposing the animal to secondary bacterial infection, most frequently *Mannheimia haemolytica* (see pneumonic Mannheimiosis discussion). Postmortem diagnosis of IBR is confirmed by isolation of the virus or its identification by immunohistochemistry or PCR in affected tissues.

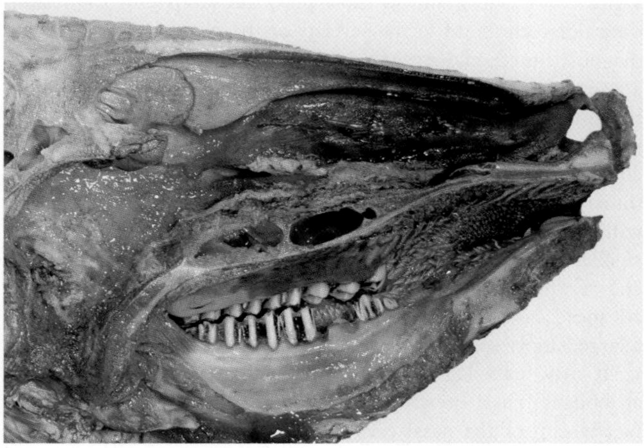

Fig. 9-17 Fibrinous rhinitis and pharyngitis, midsagittal section of head, steer.

The nasal and pharyngeal mucosae are covered by diphtheritic yellow membranes consisting of fibrinonecrotic exudate. The dorsal concha is markedly hyperemic. (Courtesy Dr. A. López Atlantic Veterinary College.)

Other Bovine Rhinitis

Information on this topic is available at evolve.elsevier.com/Zachary/McGavin/.

Ovine and Caprine Nasal Disease

Oestrus ovis (Diptera: Oestridae; nasal bot) is a brownish fly about the size of a honeybee that deposits its first-stage larvae in the nostrils of sheep in most parts of the world. Microscopic larvae mature into large bots (maggots), which spend most of their larval stages in nasal passages and sinuses, causing irritation, inflammation, and obstruction of airways. Matured larvae drop to the ground and pupate into flies. This type of parasitism in which living tissues are invaded by larvae of flies is known as *myiasis* (Fig. 9-19). Although *Oestrus ovis* is a nasal myiasis primarily of sheep, it sporadically affects goats, dogs, and sometimes humans (shepherds). The presence of the larvae in nasal passages and sinuses causes chronic irritation and erosive mucopurulent rhinitis and sinusitis; bots of *Oestrus ovis* can be found easily if the head is cut to expose the nasal passages and paranasal sinuses. Rarely, larvae of *Oestrus ovis* penetrate the cranial vault through the ethmoidal plate, causing direct or secondary bacterial meningitis.

Infectious rhinitis is only sporadically reported in goats, and most of these cases are caused by *Pasteurella multocida* or *Mannheimia haemolytica*. The lesions range from a mild serous to catarrhal or mucopurulent inflammation.

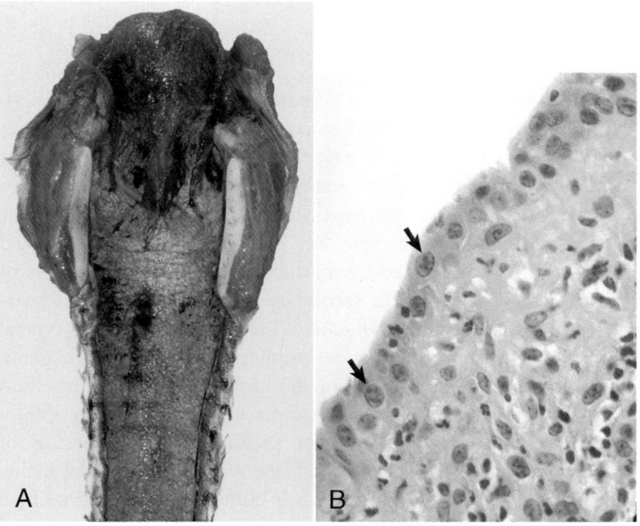

Fig. 9-18 Subacute fibrinonecrotic laryngitis and tracheitis, infectious bovine rhinotracheitis (IBR; bovine herpesvirus 1), longitudinal (dorsal) section of larynx and trachea, calf.

A, Thick plaques of fibrinonecrotic exudate cover the laryngeal and tracheal mucosae. **B,** Note the intranuclear inclusions *(arrows),* characteristic of herpesvirus infection, in a tracheal mucosal epithelial cell. Chronic inflammation is also present in the subjacent connective tissue. (**A** courtesy Dr. A. López, Atlantic Veterinary College. **B** courtesy College of Veterinary Medicine, University of Illinois.)

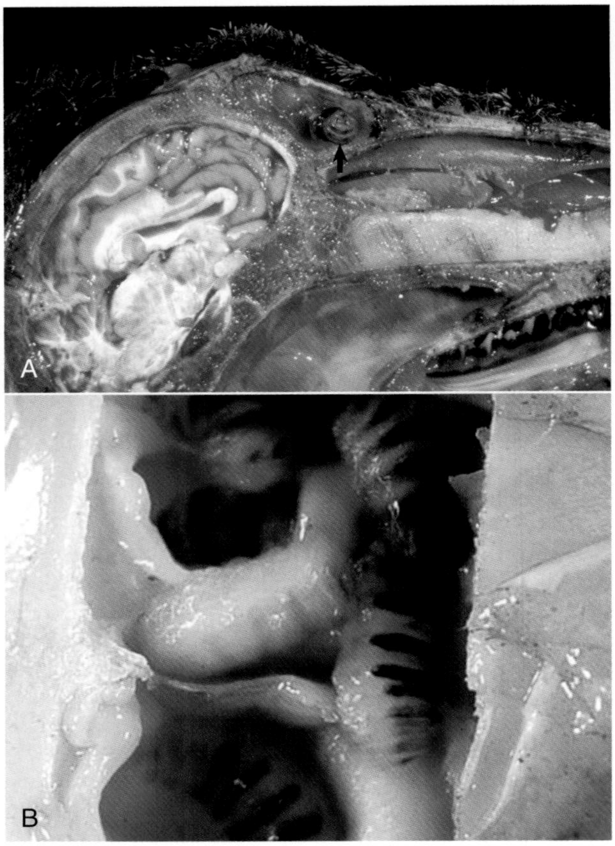

Fig. 9-19 *Oestrus ovis*, sheep.
A, Frontal sinus. Note the parasitic (fly) larvae in the frontal sinus *(arrow)*. **B,** Nasal cavity. Higher magnification view of larvae of *Oestrus ovis* in a nasal cavity. (**A** courtesy Dr. M.D. McGavin, College of Veterinary Medicine, University of Tennessee. **B** courtesy Dr. M. Sierra and Dr. J. King, College of Veterinary Medicine, Cornell University.)

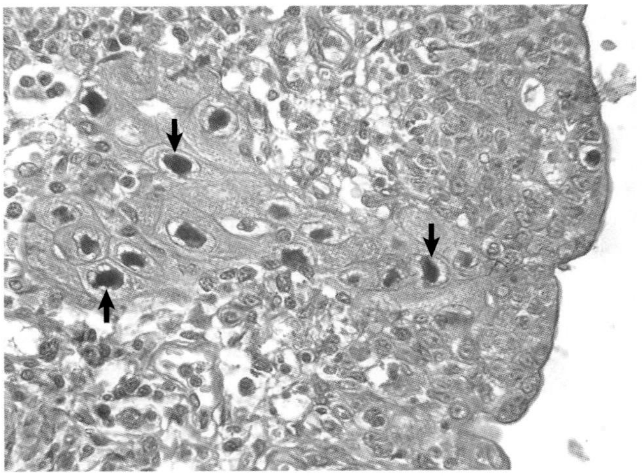

Fig. 9-20 Inclusion body rhinitis caused by Cytomegalovirus infection, nasal conchae, 3-week-old pig.
Epithelial cells of mucosal glands contain large basophilic intranuclear inclusion bodies *(arrows)*. H&E stain. (Courtesy Dr. A. López, Atlantic Veterinary College.)

Porcine Nasal Diseases

Inclusion Body Rhinitis

Inclusion body rhinitis is a disease of young pigs with high morbidity and low mortality caused by a porcine cytomegalovirus (herpesvirus) and characterized by a mild rhinitis. This virus commonly infects the nasal epithelium of piglets younger than 5 weeks and causes a transient viremia. Because this disease is seldom fatal, lesions are seen only incidentally or in euthanized animals. In uncomplicated cases, the gross lesion is hyperemia of the nasal mucosa, but with secondary bacterial infections, mucopurulent exudate can be abundant. Microscopic lesions are typical and consist of a necrotizing, nonsuppurative rhinitis with giant, basophilic, intranuclear inclusion bodies in the nasal epithelium and glands (Fig. 9-20). Immunosuppressed piglets can develop a systemic cytomegalovirus infection characterized by necrosis of the liver, lungs, adrenal glands, and brain with intralesional inclusion bodies. Inclusion body rhinitis is clinically characterized by a mild and transient rhinitis, causing sneezing, nasal discharge, and excessive lacrimation.

Atrophic Rhinitis

A common worldwide disease of pigs, atrophic rhinitis (progressive atrophic rhinitis) is characterized by inflammation and atrophy of nasal conchae (turbinates). In severe cases, atrophy of the conchae may cause a striking facial deformity in growing pigs because of deviation of the nasal septum and nasal bones. The etiopathogenesis of atrophic rhinitis is complex and has been a matter of controversy for many years. Pathogens historically associated with atrophic rhinitis include *Bordetella bronchiseptica, Pasteurella multocida, Haemophilus parasuis,* and viral infections such as porcine cytomegalovirus (inclusion body rhinitis). In addition, predisposing factors have included genetic makeup, environment, and nutritional deficiencies. The cause of atrophic rhinitis is currently believed to be a combined infection by specific strains of *Bordetella bronchiseptica* and toxigenic strains of *Pasteurella multocida* (types D and A). The only lesion associated with infection with *Bordetella bronchiseptica* alone is a mild-to-moderate turbinate atrophy (nonprogressive atrophic rhinitis), but this bacterium actively promotes the colonization of the nasal cavity by *Pasteurella multocida.* The toxigenic strains of *Pasteurella multocida* produce potent cytotoxins that inhibit osteoblastic activity and promote osteoclastic reabsorption in nasal bones, particularly in the ventral nasal conchae, where abnormal bone remodeling results in progressive atrophy of conchae.

The degree of conchal atrophy in pigs with atrophic rhinitis varies considerably, and in most pigs, the severity of the lesions does not correspond to the severity of the clinical signs. The best diagnostic method of evaluating this disease at necropsy is to make a transverse section of the snout between the first and second premolar teeth. In normal pigs, conchae are symmetric and fill most of the cavity, leaving only narrow air spaces (meatuses) between coiled conchae. The normal nasal septum is straight and divides the cavity into two mirror-imaged cavities. In contrast, the septum in pigs with atrophic rhinitis is generally deviated and the conchae appear smaller and asymmetric (Fig. 9-21). Conchal atrophy causes dorsal and ventral meatuses to appear rather enlarged, and in the most advanced cases, the entire nasal conchae may be missing, leaving a large, empty space.

It may seem logical to assume that after loss of conchae in an obligate nasal breather, such as the pig, the filtration defense mechanism of the nasal cavity would be impaired, thus enhancing the chances of aerogenous infections in the lung. However, the relationship between atrophic rhinitis, pneumonia, and growth rates in pigs is still controversial.

Osteoclastic hyperplasia and osteopenia of the conchae are the key microscopic lesions in atrophic rhinitis. Depending on the stage

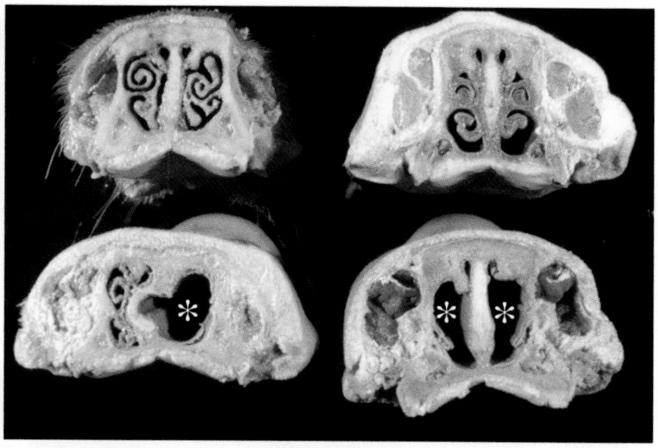

Fig. 9-21 **Atrophic rhinitis, transverse sections of nasal passages and sinuses, caudal surfaces, level of the first or second premolar teeth, pigs.** *Top left,* Normal nasal cavity showing complete conchae (turbinates) that fill most of the nasal cavity and form narrow air passages (meatuses). *Top right,* Mild, symmetric atrophy of nasal conchae. *Bottom left,* Severe, unilateral atrophy of the right ventral nasal concha *(asterisk)* with deviation of the nasal septum to the left and widening of the ventral meatus. *Bottom right,* Severe, bilateral atrophy with complete loss of nasal conchae and extensive widening of the meatuses *(asterisks).* (Courtesy Dr. A. López, Atlantic Veterinary College.)

of the disease, mucopurulent exudate may be found on the surface of the conchae. Hyperplastic or metaplastic changes can occur in the nasal epithelium and glands, and infiltrates of lymphoplasmacytic cells can be present in the lamina propria. In summary, atrophic rhinitis is an important disease in pigs worldwide; morphologic diagnosis is simple, but additional understanding of the pathogenesis will be necessary before effective preventive measures can be established.

Atrophic rhinitis is clinically characterized by sneezing, coughing, and nasal discharge as a result of inflammation and atrophy of nasal conchae (turbinates). Obstruction of the nasolacrimal duct is common and results in accumulation of dust and dried lacrimal secretions on the skin inferior to the medial canthus of the eye.

Canine Nasal Diseases

Dogs have no specific viral infections affecting exclusively the nasal cavity or sinuses. Acute rhinitis occurs as part of general respiratory disease caused by several distinct viruses, such as canine distemper virus, CAV-1 and -2, canine parainfluenza virus, reovirus, and canine herpesvirus. The viral lesions in the respiratory tract are generally transient, but the effect of the virus on other tissues and cells can be fatal, as in distemper encephalitis in dogs. As in other species, secondary bacterial rhinitis, sinusitis, and pneumonia are possible sequelae of respiratory viral infections; *Bordetella bronchiseptica, Escherichia coli,* and *Pasteurella multocida* are the most common isolates in dogs with bacterial rhinitis. A nonspecific (idiopathic) chronic lymphoplasmatic rhinitis is occasionally seen in dogs. Immotile cilia syndrome (ciliary dyskinesia), a congenital disease, reduces mucociliary clearance and is an important factor in recurrent canine rhinosinusitis, bronchitis, bronchiectasis, and pneumonia.

Other Causes of Canine Rhinitis

Information on this topic, including Web Figs. 9-6 and 9-7, available at evolve.elsevier.com/Zachary/McGavin/.

Feline Nasal Diseases

Feline Viral Rhinotracheitis

Feline viral rhinotracheitis (FVR) is a common, worldwide respiratory disease of cats caused by a feline herpesvirus (FHV-1). The disease causes an impairment of pulmonary defense mechanisms, predisposing cats to secondary bacterial pneumonia or to a co-infection with feline calicivirus. The virus also can remain latent in ganglia. The vast majority of cats that recover from FVR become carriers and shed FHV-1, either spontaneously or after stress. Susceptible animals, particularly kittens with low maternal immunity, become infected after exposure to a diseased or a carrier cat. Replication of FHV-1 in the nasal, conjunctival, pharyngeal, and to a lesser extent, tracheal epithelium causes degeneration and exfoliation of cells.

Lesions caused by FHV-1 are fully reversible, but secondary infections with bacteria, such as *Pasteurella multocida, Bordetella bronchiseptica, Streptococcus* spp., *and Mycoplasma felis,* can cause a chronic, severe suppurative rhinitis, and conjunctivitis. Intranuclear inclusion bodies are rarely seen in cats with FVR because inclusions are only present during the early stages of infection and have already disappeared by the time the cat is presented for diagnosis.

Respiratory sequelae to FVR can include chronic bacterial rhinitis and sinusitis with persistent purulent discharges; lysis of nasal bones, which can lead to conchal atrophy; permanent damage to the olfactory epithelium; and secondary bacterial pneumonia. In addition to rhinitis and interstitial pneumonia, FVR also causes ulcerative keratitis, hepatic necrosis, emaciation, abortion, and stillbirths. Clinical signs of FVR infection are characterized by lethargy, oculonasal discharges, severe rhinitis, and conjunctivitis.

Feline Calicivirus

Feline calicivirus rhinitis (FCR) is caused by different strains of feline calicivirus (FCV). It is an important infection of the respiratory tract of cats, and depending on the virulence of the strain, lesions vary from a mild oculonasal discharge to severe rhinitis, mucopurulent conjunctivitis, and ulcerative gingivitis and stomatitis. The lesions, in addition to rhinitis and conjunctivitis, include acute, diffuse interstitial pneumonia with necrotizing bronchiolitis (see the section on Pneumonias of Cats) and prominent ulcers of the tongue and hard palate. Primary viral lesions are generally transient, but secondary bacterial infections *(Bordetella bronchiseptica, Pasteurella multocida,* or *Escherichia coli)* are a common complication. Some kittens develop lameness after infection or vaccination with calicivirus because of an acute and self-limiting arthritis ("limping kitten syndrome"). Carrier state and virus shedding from oronasal secretions and feces are natural sequelae after recovery from the acute phase of the disease. Clinical and pathologic features of FCV disease are strikingly similar, but not identical to those of FVR; these two viral infections account for 80% of all cases of feline respiratory diseases. A febrile systemic hemorrhagic syndrome with high mortality (up to 50%) has been recently reported in cats infected with virulent strains of FCV.

Feline Chlamydiosis

Feline chlamydiosis is a persistent respiratory infection of cats caused by *Chlamydophila felis.* Infection results in a conjunctivitis (similar to the conjunctivitis seen in human trachoma caused by *Chlamydia trachomatis*) and serous or mucopurulent rhinitis. In the past, *Chlamydophila felis* was incriminated as the agent responsible for "feline pneumonitis," but its role in causing bronchointerstitial pneumonia in cats has been seriously challenged in recent years (see the section on Pneumonias of Cats).

Other Causes of Feline Rhinitis and Sinusitis

Information on this topic is available at evolve.elsevier.com/Zachary/McGavin/.

Neoplasia of the Nasal Cavity and Paranasal Sinuses

Neoplasms of the nasal cavity and paranasal sinuses may arise from any of the tissues forming these structures, including bone (osteoma or osteosarcoma), cartilage (chondroma or chondrosarcoma), connective tissue (fibroma or fibrosarcoma, myxoma or myxosarcoma), and blood vessels (hemangioma or hemangiosarcoma), and from all the different types of cells of glands and lining epithelium (adenoma, carcinoma, or adenocarcinoma). Nasal tumors originating from stromal tissues, such as bone, cartilage, and connective tissue, are morphologically indistinguishable from those seen in other sites. In general, nasal neoplasms are rare in domestic animals, except for endemic ethmoidal neoplasms (retroviral) in sheep and cattle, which can occur in several animals in a flock or herd (see the next section).

In companion animals, nasal neoplasms are most common in dogs, particularly in breeds such as the collie, Airedale terrier, basset hound, and German shepherd. The cat and the horse are less frequently affected. The main sites in order of frequency are the nasal passages and sinuses for dogs, the tip of the nose and nasal passages for cats, and the maxillary sinus and nasal passages for horses.

The majority of neoplasms in the nasal cavity are malignant. Benign nasal neoplasms (papilloma and adenoma) are rare and generally are either solitary or multiple, well-delineated nodules. In contrast, nasal carcinomas and nasal sarcomas are generally larger but vary in size and are often pale and multilobulated masses composed of fleshy to friable tissue (Fig. 9-22). Malignant neoplasms are locally invasive and tend to infiltrate sinuses, meninges, frontal brain, olfactory nerves, and vessels resulting in epistaxis. Carcinomas vary from anaplastic (poorly differentiated) to well differentiated, in which cell and tissue morphology retains some glandular (adenocarcinoma) or squamous cell patterns. Because nasal tumors in dogs and cats are usually large and invasive at the time of diagnosis, prognosis is usually poor and survival times are short. Sarcomas originating in the nasal cavity and paranasal sinuses are less common than carcinomas. Mesenchymal tumors can arise from bone (osteoma or osteosarcoma), cartilage (chondroma or chondrosarcoma), blood vessels (hemangioma or hemangiosarcoma), and connective tissue (fibroma or fibrosarcoma). Overall, benign epithelial and mesenchymal tumors are less common than their malignant counterparts. Secondary tumors in the nasal cavity are rare, with lymphoma being the most common metastatic tumor in the nasal cavity of domestic animals.

Nasal neoplasms become secondarily infected by bacteria, and clinical signs often overlap with those of infectious rhinitis and include catarrhal or mucopurulent nasal discharge, periodic hemorrhage, increased lacrimation as a result of obstruction of nasolacrimal ducts, and sneezing. In some instances, it is not possible to clinically or grossly differentiate neoplasms from hyperplastic nodules or granulomatous rhinitis. Some neoplasms may infiltrate adjacent bone structures and produce notable facial deformities, loss of teeth, exophthalmus, and nervous signs. Large neoplasms also project into the meatuses, narrow the lumen, and interfere with airflow, causing stertorous breathing (Fig. 9-23). Biopsies, as well as brush and imprint cytology, have proved effective in the antemortem diagnosis of nasal neoplasms, particularly in those of epithelial lineage.

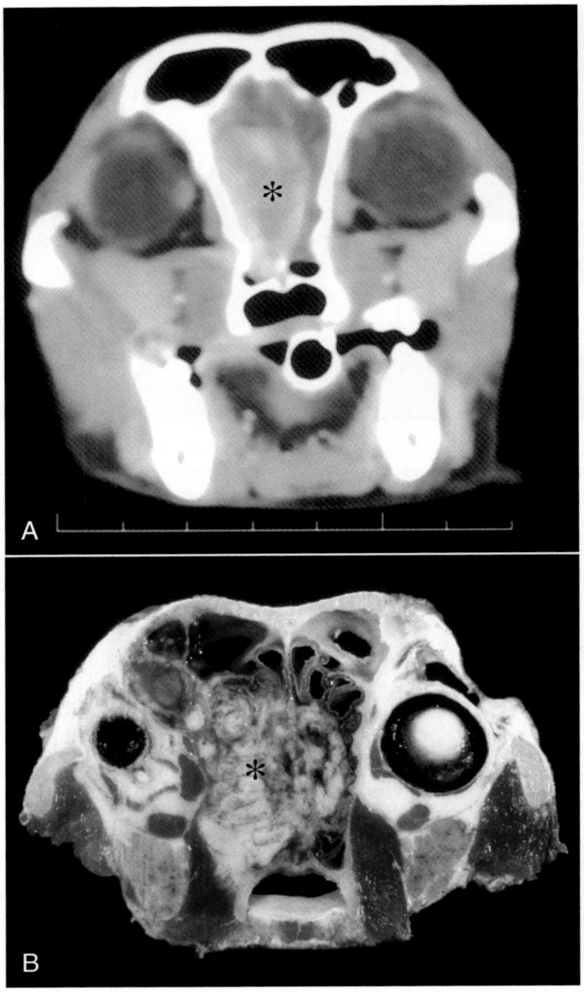

Fig. 9-22 Nasal carcinoma, transverse section of nasal passages and sinuses, 10-year-old dog.
A, Computerized tomography shows a large neoplastic mass *(asterisk)* infiltrating the nasal cavity and displacing the nasal septum laterally. Scale bar units in centimeters. **B,** Transverse section of head showing tumor diffusely infiltrating the nasal conchae and obliterating the meatuses *(asterisk).* (Courtesy Atlantic Veterinary College.)

Endemic Ethmoidal Tumors

A unique group of nasal carcinomas (enzootic nasal tumors, enzootic intranasal tumors, and enzootic nasal carcinoma) of sheep, goats, and cattle arise from the surface epithelium and glands of the ethmoidal conchae. These types of carcinomas are caused by an oncogenic retrovirus, and the neoplasm has been successfully transmitted to susceptible animals by inoculation of virus or infected tissues. Endemic ethmoidal tumors are typically invasive but do not metastasize (Fig. 9-24). In some regions of the world, ethmoid tumors have been reported in horses and pigs, particularly in those farms where the endemic nasal tumors of ruminants are known to occur.

Nasal Polyps and Nasal Cysts Resembling Neoplasms

Nonneoplastic exophytic masses that resemble neoplasms are commonly found in horses, cats, and to a lesser extent other species. In horses, polyps tend to form in the ethmoidal region, whereas in cats, polyps are most frequently found in the nasopharynx and Eustachian tubes. The pathogenesis of these benign growths is

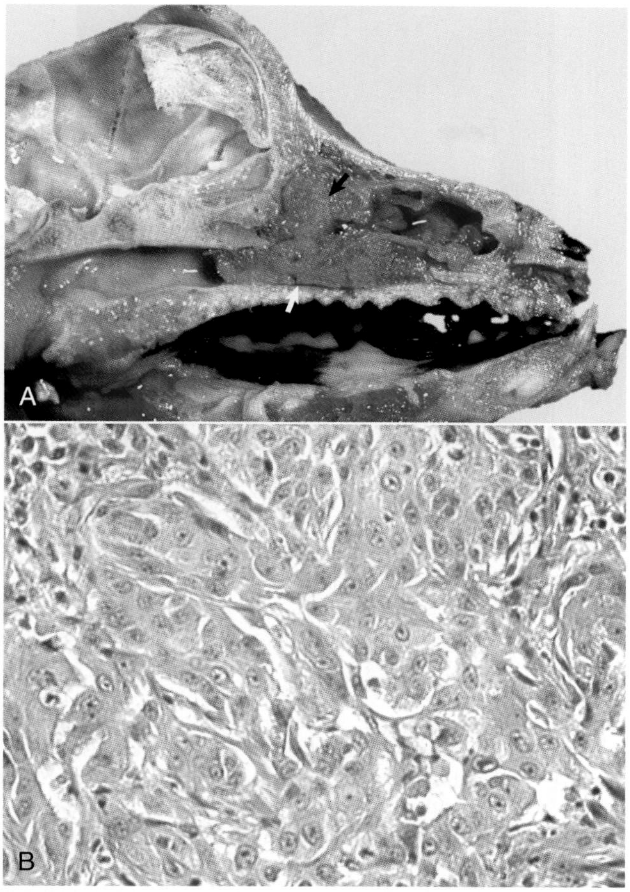

Fig. 9-23 Nasal adenocarcinoma, midsagittal section, head, adult dog.
A, A large neoplastic mass *(arrows)* has arisen from the ethmoidal concha and has infiltrated along the nasal passages. **B,** Multiple clusters of neoplastic epithelial cells with abundant eosinophilic cytoplasm and prominent nucleoli. H&E stain. (**A** courtesy Dr. J. M. King, College of Veterinary Medicine, Cornell University. **B** courtesy Dr. A. López, Atlantic Veterinary College.)

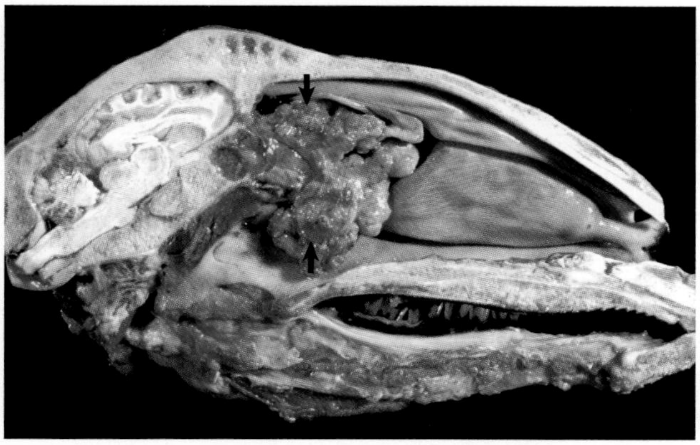

Fig. 9-24 Nasal adenocarcinoma *(arrows)*, midsagittal section of the head, sheep.
The tumor has occluded the right nasal passage and choanae. The location (ethmoturbinates) and type of tumor (carcinoma) are typical of retrovirus-induced "enzootic nasal carcinoma." (Courtesy Dr. L.E. Craig, College of Veterinary Medicine, University of Tennessee.)

uncertain, although in many cases they follow chronic rhinitis or sinusitis. Grossly, polyps appear as firm, pedunculated nodules of various sizes protruding from the nasal mucosa into the nasal passages; the surface may be smooth, ulcerated, secondarily infected, and hemorrhagic. Microscopically, polyps are characterized by a core of well-vascularized stromal tissue that contains inflammatory cells and are covered by pseudostratified or squamous epithelium.

Nasal and paranasal sinus cysts are common in horses and are medically important because they clinically mimic neoplasms or infections. Although not considered a neoplastic growth, cysts are expansive and cause deformation or destruction of the surrounding bone. These cysts are typically composed of an epithelial cell capsule filled with yellow or hemorrhagic fluid and do not recur after surgical removal. Ethmoidal hematomas also resemble nasal tumors in horses.

PHARYNX, GUTTURAL POUCHES, LARYNX, AND TRACHEA

Patterns of Injury and Host Response

The laryngeal mucosa is formed by pseudostratified columnar ciliated epithelium with goblet cells (mucociliary blanket) and squamous epithelium, whereas the trachea is exclusively lined by columnar ciliated epithelium. The pattern of injury and host response in the larynx and trachea is similar to those in the nasal mucosa (see the section on Defense Mechanisms of the Conducting System). The pharyngeal mucosa, composed of squamous epithelium, has similar patterns of necrosis and inflammation as the oral mucosa (see Chapter 7).

Anomalies

Congenital anomalies of this region are rare in all species. Depending on their location and severity, they may be inconsistent with postnatal life, pose little or no problem, interfere with quality of life, or manifest themselves in later life. If clinical signs of respiratory distress, such as stridor, coughing, dyspnea, or gagging, do occur, they are usually exacerbated by excitement, heat, stress, or exercise.

Brachycephalic Airway Syndrome

Information on this topic is available at evolve.elsevier.com/Zachary/McGavin/.

Hypoplastic Epiglottis, Epiglottic Entrapment, and Dorsal Displacement of the Soft Palate

Information on this topic is available at evolve.elsevier.com/Zachary/McGavin/.

Subepiglottic and Pharyngeal Cysts

Information on this topic is available at evolve.elsevier.com/Zachary/McGavin/.

Tracheal Agenesis and Tracheal Hypoplasia

Tracheal hypoplasia occurs most often in English bulldogs and Boston terriers; the tracheal lumen is decreased in diameter throughout its length.

Tracheal Collapse and Tracheal Stenosis

Tracheal collapse with reduction in tracheal patency occurs in toy, miniature, and brachycephalic breeds of dogs, in which the

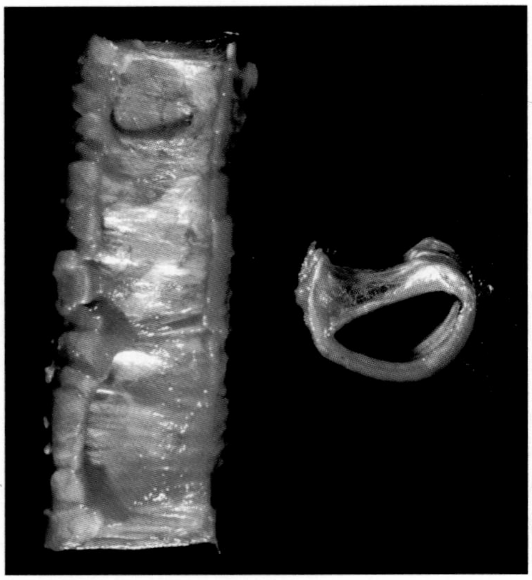

Fig. 9-25 Tracheal collapse, trachea, pony.
Left specimen, The dorsal surface of the trachea is flattened dorsoventrally, the dorsal ends of the C-shaped tracheal rings are widely separated, and the dorsal ligament between the two ends is lengthened and thinned. *Right specimen* (transverse section), The ends of the tracheal rings are widely separated, and the dorsal wall of the trachea is formed by the lengthened and thinned dorsal ligament. (Courtesy Dr. C.S. Patton, College of Veterinary Medicine, University of Tennessee.)

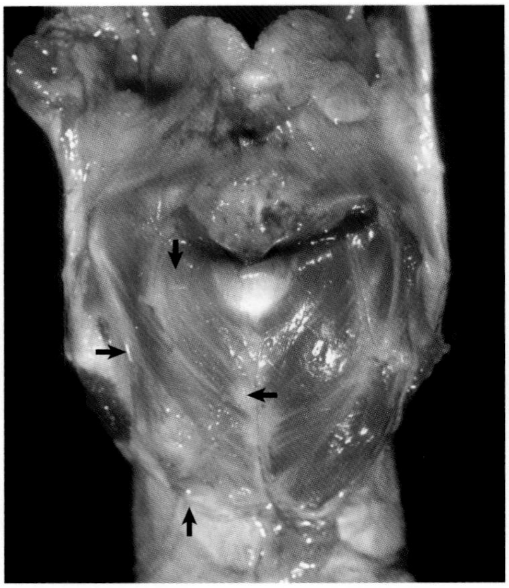

Fig. 9-26 Laryngeal hemiplegia, larynx, dorsal surface, 2-year-old horse. The left cricoarytenoideus dorsalis muscle is pale and atrophic *(arrows),* whereas the right cricoarytenoideus dorsalis muscle is normal. (Courtesy Dr. A. López, Atlantic Veterinary College.)

condition is also called *tracheobronchial collapse* or *central airway collapse.* The defect also occurs in horses, cattle, and goats. By radiographic, endoscopic, or gross examination, there is dorsoventral flattening of the trachea with concomitant widening of the dorsal tracheal membrane, which may then prolapse ventrally into the lumen (Fig. 9-25). Most commonly, the defect extends the entire length of the trachea and only rarely affects the cervical portion alone. Affected segments with a reduced lumen contain froth and even are covered by a diphtheritic membrane. In horses, the so-called scabbard trachea is characterized by lateral flattening, so that the tracheal lumen is reduced to a narrow vertical slit.

Segmental tracheal collapse causing stenosis has been associated with congenital and acquired abnormalities. In severe cases, abnormal cartilaginous glycoproteins and loss of elasticity of tracheal rings causes the trachea to collapse. In some other cases, it is an acquired tracheal lesion that follows trauma, compression caused by extraluminal masses, peritracheal inflammation, and flawed tracheotomy or transtracheal aspirate techniques.

Other tracheal anomalies include tracheoesophageal fistula, which is most commonly found in humans and sporadically in dogs and cattle. Congenital fistulas can occur at any site of the cervical or thoracic segments of the trachea. Acquired tracheoesophageal fistula can be a complication of improper intubation, tracheotomy, or esophageal foreign body.

Degenerative Diseases

Laryngeal Hemiplegia

Laryngeal hemiplegia (paralysis), sometimes called *roaring* in horses, is a common but obscure disease characterized by atrophy of the dorsal and lateral cricoarytenoid muscles (abductor and adductor of the arytenoid cartilage), particularly on the left side. Muscular atrophy is most commonly caused by a primary denervation (recurrent laryngeal neuropathy) of unknown cause (idiopathic axonopathy) and to a much lesser extent, secondary nerve damage (see the section on Denervation Atrophy in Chapters 14 and 15). Idiopathic laryngeal hemiplegia is an incurable axonal disease (axonopathy) of the cranial laryngeal nerve that affects mostly larger horses. Secondary laryngeal hemiplegia is rare and occurs after nerve damage caused by other pathologic processes such as compression or inflammation of the left recurrent laryngeal nerve. The medial retropharyngeal lymph nodes are located immediately ventral to the floor of the guttural pouches. As a result of this close anatomic relationship, swelling or inflammation of the guttural pouches and retropharyngeal lymph nodes often results in secondary damage to the laryngeal nerve. Common causes of secondary nerve damage (Wallerian degeneration) include guttural pouch mycosis, retropharyngeal abscesses, inflammation because of iatrogenic injection into the nerves, neck injury, and metastatic neoplasms involving the retropharyngeal lymph nodes (e.g., lymphosarcoma).

Grossly, the affected laryngeal muscle in a horse with laryngeal hemiplegia is pale and smaller than normal (muscle atrophy) (Fig. 9-26). Microscopically, muscle fibers have lesions of denervation atrophy (see Chapters 14 and 15). Atrophy of laryngeal muscles also occurs in dogs as an inherited condition (Siberian husky and Bouvier des Flandres), as a degenerative neuropathy in older dogs, secondary to laryngeal trauma in all species (e.g., choke chain damage), or to hepatic encephalopathy in horses.

The abnormal inspiratory sounds (roaring) during exercise in horses with laryngeal hemiplegia are caused by paralysis of the left dorsal and lateral cricoarytenoid muscles, which cause incomplete dilation of the larynx, obstructing of airflow, and vibration of vocal cords.

Circulatory Disturbances

Laryngeal and Tracheal Hemorrhages

Hemorrhages in these sites occur as mucosal petechiae and are most commonly seen in coagulopathies; inflammation; septicemia and sepsis, particularly in pigs with classical swine fever (hog cholera); African swine fever or salmonellosis; and horses with equine infectious anemia. Severe dyspnea and asphyxia before death can cause congestion, ecchymosis, and petechiae in the laryngeal and tracheal mucosa; this lesion must be differentiated from postmortem imbibition of hemoglobin in autolyzed carcasses (see Chapter 1).

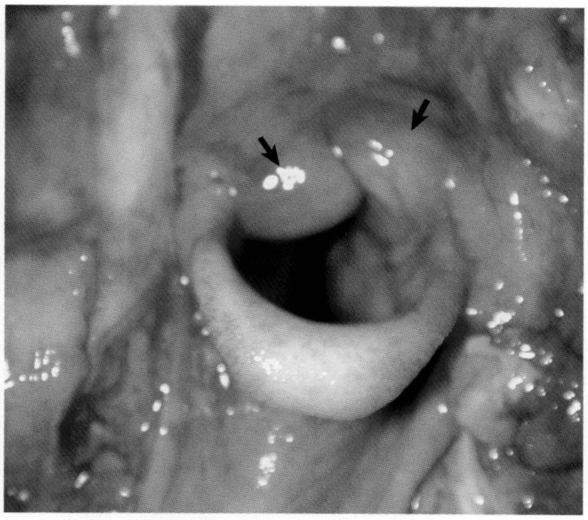

Fig. 9-27 Laryngeal edema, larynx, mature cow.
Note the edematous thickening of the laryngeal mucosa of the vocal cords *(arrows)*, which can cause respiratory distress due to the narrowing of the laryngeal lumen (rima glottidis). (Courtesy Dr. J. Andrews, College of Veterinary Medicine, University of Illinois.)

Laryngeal Edema

Laryngeal edema is a common feature of acute inflammation, but it is particularly important because swelling of the epiglottis and vocal cords can obstruct the laryngeal orifice, resulting in asphyxiation. Laryngeal edema occurs in pigs with edema disease; in horses with purpura hemorrhagica; in cattle with acute interstitial pneumonia; in cats with systemic anaphylaxis; and in all species as a result of trauma, improper endotracheal tubing, inhalation of irritant gases (e.g., smoke), local inflammation, and allergic reactions. Grossly the mucosa of the epiglottis and vocal cords is thickened and swollen, often protrudes dorsally onto the epiglottic orifice, and has a gelatinous appearance (Fig. 9-27).

Tracheal Edema and Hemorrhage

Tracheal edema and hemorrhage syndrome of feeder cattle, also known as the *honker syndrome* or *tracheal stenosis of feedlot cattle,* is a poorly documented acute disease of unknown cause, most often seen during the summer months. Severe edema and a few hemorrhages are present in the mucosa and submucosa of the dorsal surface of the trachea, extending caudally from the midcervical area as far as the tracheal bifurcation. On a cut section, the tracheal mucosa is diffusely thickened and gelatinous. Clinical signs include inspiratory dyspnea that can progress to oral breathing, recumbency, and death by asphyxiation in less than 24 hours.

Inflammation

Pharyngitis, Laryngitis, and Tracheitis

Inflammation of the pharynx, larynx, and trachea are important because of their potential to obstruct airflow and to lead to aspiration pneumonia. The pharynx is commonly affected by infectious diseases of the upper respiratory and upper digestive tracts, and the trachea can be involved by extension from both the lungs and larynx.

Intraluminal foreign bodies in the pharynx, such as medicament boluses, apples, or potatoes, can move down and obstruct the larynx and trachea. Also, pharyngeal obstruction can be caused by masses in surrounding tissue such as neoplasms of the thyroid gland, thymus, and parathyroid glands.

Pharyngeal Perforation

A number of nonspecific insults can cause lesions and clinical signs. Trauma may take the form of penetrating wounds in any species: perforation of the caudodorsal wall of the pharynx from the improper use of drenching or balling guns in sheep, cattle, and pigs; choking injury because of the use of collars in dogs and cats; and the shearing forces of bite wounds. The results of the trauma may be minimal (local edema and inflammation) or as serious as complete luminal obstruction by exudate. Foreign bodies may be lodged anywhere in the pharyngeal region; the location and size determine the occurrence of dysphagia, regurgitation, dyspnea, or asphyxiation. Pigs have a unique structure known as the *pharyngeal diverticulum* (4 cm long in adult pigs), which is located in the pharyngeal wall rostral and dorsal to the esophageal entrance. It is important because barley awns may lodge in the diverticulum, causing an inflammatory swelling that affects swallowing. The diverticular wall may be perforated by awns or drenching syringes, which results in an exudate that can extend down the tissue planes between muscles of the neck and even into the mediastinum. The pharynx of the dog may also be damaged by trauma from chicken bones, sticks, and needles, resulting in the formation of a pharyngeal abscess.

Equine Pharyngeal Lymphoid Hyperplasia

Equine pharyngeal lymphoid hyperplasia, or pharyngitis with lymphoid follicular hyperplasia, is a common cause of partial upper airway obstruction in horses, particularly in 2- and 3-year-old racehorses. Lymphoid hyperplasia is also seen in healthy horses as part of a response to mild chronic pharyngitis, which in many instances tends to regress with age in older animals. The cause is undetermined, but chronic bacterial infection combined with environmental factors may cause excessive antigenic stimulation and lymphoid hyperplasia. The gross lesions, visible endoscopically or at necropsy, consist of variably sized (1 to 5 mm) white foci located on the dorsolateral walls of the pharynx and extend into the openings of the guttural pouches and onto the soft palate. In severe cases, lesions may appear as pharyngeal polyps. Microscopically, the lesions consist of large aggregates of lymphocytes and plasma cells in the pharyngeal mucosa. Clinical signs consist of stertorous inspiration, expiration, or both.

Inflammation of Guttural Pouches

The guttural pouches of horses are large diverticula (300 to 500 mL) of the ventral portion of the auditory (eustachian) tubes. These diverticula are therefore exposed to the same pathogens as the pharynx and have drainage problems similar to the pathogens of sinuses. Although it is probable that various pathogens, including viruses, can infect them, the most common pathogens are fungi, which cause guttural pouch mycosis and guttural pouch empyema in the horse. Because of the close anatomic proximity of guttural pouches to the internal carotid arteries, cranial nerves (VII, IX, X, XI, and XII), and atlantooccipital joint, disease of these diverticula may involve these structures and cause a variety of clinical signs in horses.

Guttural pouch mycosis occurs primarily in stabled horses and is caused by *Aspergillus fumigatus* and other *Aspergillus* sp. Infection is usually unilateral and presumably starts with the inhalation of spores from moldy hay. Grossly, the mucosal surfaces of the dorsal and lateral walls of the guttural pouch mucosa are first covered by focal, rounded, raised plaques of diphtheritic (fibrinonecrotic) exudate, which with time can become confluent and grow into a large fibrinonecrotic mass (Fig. 9-28). Microscopically, the lesions are severe necrotic inflammation of the mucosa and submucosa

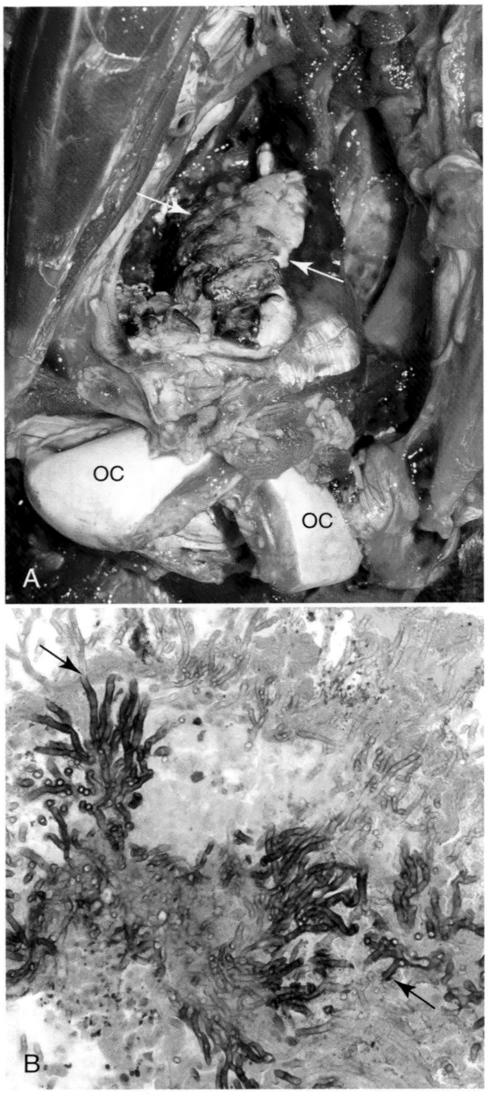

Fig. 9-28 Guttural pouch mycosis, ventral view of the head, horse.
A, Note the large mass filling the right guttural pouch *(arrows)*. It is firmly attached to the wall and composed of fibrinonecrotic exudate and surrounded by clotted blood. *OC,* Occipital condyles. **B,** Fungal hyphae *(arrows)* are admixed with necrotic exudate. H&E stain. (Courtesy of Dr. A. López, Atlantic Veterinary College)

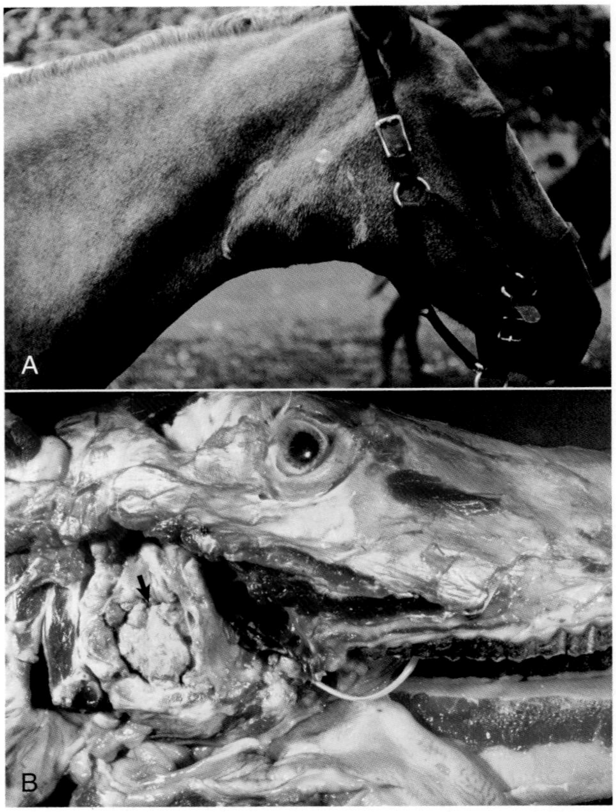

Fig. 9-29 Guttural pouch empyema, guttural pouch, horse.
A, Note the swollen right neck *(outlined in yellow)* in this horse with guttural pouch empyema. **B,** The guttural pouch is filled with masses of inspissated purulent exudate *(arrow)*. (**A** courtesy College of Veterinary Medicine, University of Illinois. **B** courtesy Dr. M.D. McGavin, College of Veterinary Medicine, University of Tennessee.)

with widespread vasculitis and intralesional fungal hyphae. Necrosis of the wall of the guttural pouches can extend into the wall of the adjacent internal carotid artery causing hemorrhage into the lumen of the guttural pouch and recurrent epistaxis. Invasion of the internal carotid artery causes arteritis, which can also lead to formation of an aneurysm and fatal bleeding into the guttural pouches. In other cases, the fungi may be angioinvasive, leading to the release of mycotic emboli into the internal carotid artery, generally resulting in multiple cerebral infarcts. Dysphagia, another clinical sign seen in guttural pouch mycosis, is associated with damage to the pharyngeal branches of the vagus and glossopharyngeal nerves, which lie on the ventral aspect of the pouches. Horner's syndrome results from damage to the cranial cervical ganglion and sympathetic fibers located in the caudodorsal aspect of the pouches. Finally, equine laryngeal paralysis (hemiplegia) can result from damage to the laryngeal nerves as previously described in the section on Laryngeal Hemiplegia.

Empyema of guttural pouches is a sequela to suppurative inflammation of the nasal cavities, most commonly from *Streptococcus equi* infection (strangles). In severe cases, the entire guttural pouch can be filled with purulent exudate (Fig. 9-29). The sequelae are similar to those of guttural pouch mycosis except that there is no erosion of the internal carotid artery. It is clinically characterized by nasal discharge, enlarged retropharyngeal lymph nodes, painful swelling of the parotid region, dysphagia, and respiratory distress.

Guttural pouch tympany develops sporadically in young horses when excessive air accumulates in the pouch from the one-way valve effect caused by inflammation or malformation of the Eustachian tube. It is generally unilateral and characterized by nonpainful swelling of the parotid region.

Necrotic Laryngitis

Necrotic laryngitis (calf diphtheria, laryngeal necrobacillosis) is a common disease of feedlot cattle and cattle affected with other diseases, with nutritional deficiencies, or housed under unsanitary conditions. It also occurs sporadically in sheep and pigs. Necrotic laryngitis, caused by *Fusobacterium necrophorum*, is part of the syndrome termed *laryngeal necrobacillosis,* which can include lesions of the tongue, cheeks, palate, and pharynx. An opportunistic pathogen, *Fusobacterium necrophorum* produces several exotoxins and endotoxins after gaining entry either through lesions of viral infections,

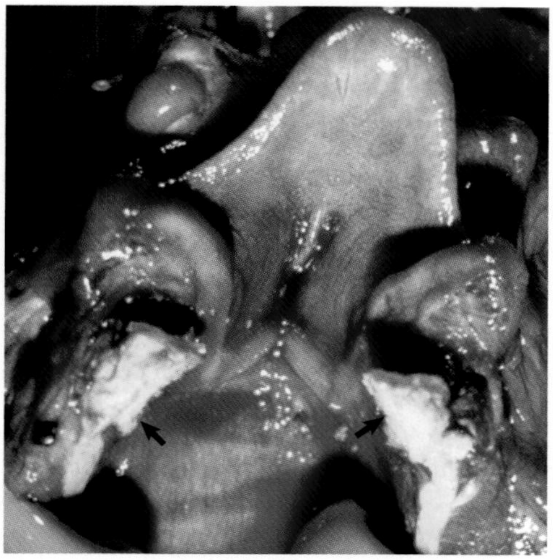

Fig. 9-30 Necrotic laryngitis, calf diphtheria *(Fusobacterium necrophorum)*, larynx, calf.
Plaques of fibrinopurulent exudate are present on the mucosa of the arytenoid cartilages *(arrows)*. Pieces of the exudate can be aspirated into the lungs and cause bronchopneumonia. (Courtesy Ontario Veterinary College.)

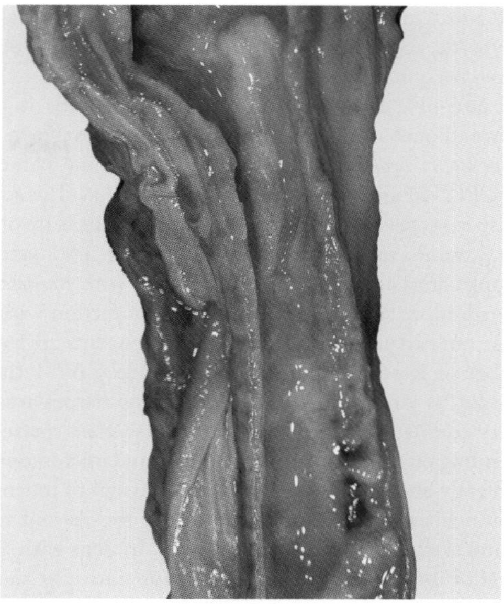

Fig. 9-31 Fibrinopurulent tracheitis, cat.
Note uniform plaque of fibrinopurulent exudate covering the entire tracheal mucosa. This cat also had suppurative bronchopneumonia and *Pasteurella multocida* was isolated from trachea and lung. (Courtesy Dr. L. Miller and Dr. A. López, Atlantic Veterinary College.)

such as IBR and vesicular stomatitis in cattle, or after traumatic injury produced by feed or careless use of specula or balling guns.

The gross lesions, regardless of location in the mouth or larynx (most common in the mucosa overlying the laryngeal cartilages), consist of well-demarcated, dry, yellow-gray, thick-crusted, and fibrinonecrotic exudate (Fig. 9-30) that in the early stages is bounded by a zone of active hyperemia. Deep ulceration develops, and if the lesion does not result in death, healing is by granulation tissue formation. Microscopically, the necrotic foci are first surrounded by hyperemic borders, then by a band of leukocytes, and finally the ulcers heal by granulation tissue and collagen (fibrosis). The lesions can extend deep into the submucosal tissue. Numerous bacteria are evident at the advancing edge.

There are numerous and important sequelae to calf diphtheria; the most serious is death from severe toxemia or overwhelming fusobacteremia. Sometimes, the exudate may be copious enough to cause laryngeal obstruction and asphyxiation or be aspirated and cause bronchopneumonia. The clinical signs of necrotic laryngitis are fever, anorexia, depression, halitosis, moist painful cough, dysphagia, and inspiratory dyspnea and ventilatory failure because of fatigue of the respiratory muscles (diaphragm and intercostal).

Laryngeal Contact Ulcers

Ulcerative lesions in the larynx are commonly found in feedlot cattle. Grossly, the laryngeal mucosa reveals circular ulcers (up to 1 cm in diameter), which may be unilateral or bilateral and sometimes deep enough to expose the underlying arytenoid cartilages. The cause has not been established, but causal agents, such as viral, bacterial, and traumatic, have been proposed, along with increased frequency and rate of closure of the larynx (excessive swallowing and vocalization) when cattle are exposed to market and feedlot stresses such as dust, pathogens, and interruption of feeding. Contact ulcers predispose a calf to diphtheria *(Fusobacterium necrophorum)* and laryngeal papillomas. Ulceration of the mucosa and necrosis of the laryngeal cartilages have also been described in calves, sheep, and horses under the term *laryngeal chondritis*. Laryngeal abscesses involving the mucosa and underlying cartilage occur as a herd or flock problem in calves and sheep, presumably caused by a secondary infection with *Arcanobacterium pyogenes (Actinomyces pyogenes; Corynebacterium pyogenes)*.

Tracheitis

The types of injury and host inflammatory responses in the trachea are essentially the same as those described for the nasal mucosa. Although tracheal mucosa is prone to aerogenous injury and necrosis, it has a remarkable capacity for repair. The most common causes of tracheitis are viral infections, such as those causing IBR (see Fig. 9-18), EVR, canine distemper, and feline rhinotracheitis. Viral lesions are generally mild and transient but often become complicated with secondary bacterial infections. At the early stages, the mucosa is notably hyperemic and can show white foci of necrosis. In the most severe cases, the affected mucosa detaches from the underlying basement membrane, causing extensive tracheal ulceration.

Chemical tracheitis is also commonly seen after aspiration (Fig. 9-31). Also, inhalation of fumes during barn fires can cause extensive injury and necrosis of the tracheal mucosa. In forensic cases, the presence of carbon pigment in the mucosal surface of trachea, bronchi, and bronchioles indicates that the burned animal was alive during the fire.

According to the exudate, tracheitis in all animal species is classified as fibrinous, catarrhal, purulent, or granulomatous. Chronic polypoid tracheitis occurs in dogs and cats, probably secondary to chronic infection.

Canine Infectious Tracheobronchitis

Canine infectious tracheobronchitis (kennel cough) is a highly contagious infection that is clinically characterized by an acute onset of coughing notably exacerbated by exercise. The term is nonspecific, much like the "common cold" in humans or bovine respiratory disease (BRD) in cattle. The infection occurs commonly as a result of mixing dogs from different origins such as occurs at commercial kennels, animal shelters, and veterinary clinics. Between bouts of coughing, most animals appear normal, although some have rhinitis, pharyngitis, tonsillitis, or conjunctivitis; some with secondary pneumonia become quite ill.

The cause of canine infectious tracheobronchitis is complex, and many pathogens and environmental factors have been incriminated. *Bordetella bronchiseptica,* CAV-2, and canine parainfluenza virus-2 (CPIV-2) are most commonly implicated. The severity of the disease is increased when more than one agent is involved or if there are extreme environmental conditions (e.g., poor ventilation). For example, dogs asymptomatically infected with *Bordetella bronchiseptica* are more severely affected by superinfection with CAV-2 than those not carrying the bacterium. Other agents are sometimes isolated but of lesser significance and include CAV-1 (infectious canine hepatitis virus), reovirus type 1, canine herpesvirus, canine respiratory coronavirus (CRCoV), and *Mycoplasma* species.

Depending on the agents involved, gross and microscopic lesions are completely absent or they vary from catarrhal to mucopurulent tracheobronchitis, with enlargement of the tonsils and retropharyngeal and tracheobronchial lymph nodes. In dogs with *Bordetella bronchiseptica* infection, the lesions are suppurative or mucopurulent rhinitis and tracheobronchitis, and suppurative bronchiolitis. In contrast, when lesions are purely viral, microscopic changes are focal necrosis of the tracheobronchial epithelium. Sequelae can include spread either proximally or distally in the respiratory tract, the latter sometimes inducing chronic bronchitis and bronchopneumonia.

Parasitic Diseases of the Larynx and Trachea

Parasitic infections of the larynx and trachea can cause obstruction with dramatic consequences, but burdens sufficient to cause such effects are not commonly seen in veterinary practice.

Besnoitiosis (Besnoitia Bennetti; Besnoitia Besnoiti)

Information on this topic is available at evolve.elsevier.com/Zachary/McGavin/.

Mammomonogamus (Syngamus) Laryngeus

Information on this topic is available at evolve.elsevier.com/Zachary/McGavin/.

Oslerus (Filaroides) Osleri

Information on this topic, including Web Fig. 9-8, is available at evolve.elsevier.com/Zachary/McGavin/.

Neoplasms of Guttural Pouches, Larynx, and Trachea

Information on this topic is available at evolve.elsevier.com/Zachary/McGavin/.

LUNGS

Species Differences

Each lung is subdivided into various numbers of pulmonary lobes. In the past, these were defined by anatomic fissures. However, in current anatomy, lobes are defined by the ramification of the bronchial tree. Following this criterion, the left lung of all domestic species is composed of cranial and caudal lobes, whereas the right lung, depending on species, is composed of cranial, middle (absent in horse), caudal, and accessory lobes. Each pulmonary lobe is further subdivided by connective tissue into pulmonary lobules, which in some species (cattle and pigs) are rather prominent and in others are much less conspicuous. From a practical point of view, identification of the lungs among different species could be achieved by carefully observing the degree of lobation (external fissures) and the degree of lobulation (connective tissue between lobules). Cattle and pigs have well-lobated and well-lobulated lungs; sheep and goats have well-lobated but poorly lobulated lungs; horses have both poorly lobated and poorly lobulated lungs and resemble human lungs; finally, dogs and cats have well-lobated but not well-lobulated lungs. The degree of lobulation determines the degree of air movement between the lobules. In pigs and cattle, movement of air between lobules is practically absent because of the thick connective tissue of the interlobular septa separating individual lobules. This movement of air between lobules and between adjacent alveoli (pores of Kohn) constitutes what is referred to as collateral ventilation. This collateral ventilation is poor in cattle and pigs and good in dogs. The functional implications of collateral ventilation are discussed in the section on Pulmonary Emphysema.

The lungs have an interconnecting network of stromal tissue supporting the blood and lymphatic vessels, nerves, bronchioles, and alveoli. For purposes of simplicity, the pulmonary interstitium can be anatomically divided into three contiguous compartments: (1) bronchovascular interstitium, where main bronchi and pulmonary vessels are situated; (2) interlobular interstitium separating pulmonary lobules and supporting small blood and lymph vessels; and (3) alveolar interstitium supporting the alveolar walls that contain pulmonary capillaries and alveolar epithelial cells (no lymphatic vessels here) (see discussion on the blood-air barrier in the section on Alveoli). Pulmonary changes, such as edema and emphysema, may affect one or more of these interstitial compartments.

Congenital Anomalies

Congenital anomalies of the lungs are rare in all species but are most commonly reported in cattle and sheep. Compatibility with life largely depends on the type of structures involved and the proportion of functional tissue present at birth. Accessory lungs are one of the most common anomalies and consist of distinctively lobulated masses of incompletely differentiated pulmonary tissue present in the thorax, abdominal cavity, or subcutaneous tissue virtually anywhere in the trunk. Large accessory lungs can cause dystocia. Ciliary dyskinesia (immotile cilia syndrome, Kartagener's syndrome) is characterized by defective ciliary movement, which results in reduced mucociliary clearance because of a defect in the microtubules of all ciliated cells and most importantly, in the ciliated respiratory epithelium and spermatozoa. Primary ciliary dyskinesia often associated with situs inversus has been reported in dogs, which as a result usually have chronic recurrent rhinosinusitis, pneumonia, and infertility. Pulmonary agenesis, pulmonary hypoplasia, abnormal lobulation, congenital emphysema, lung hamartoma, and congenital bronchiectasis are occasionally seen in domestic animals. Congenital melanosis is a common incidental finding in pigs and ruminants and is usually seen at slaughter (Fig. 9-32). It is characterized by black spots, often a few centimeters in diameter, in various organs, mainly the lungs, meninges, intima of the aorta, and caruncles of the uterus. Melanosis has no clinical significance, and the texture of pigmented lungs remains unchanged.

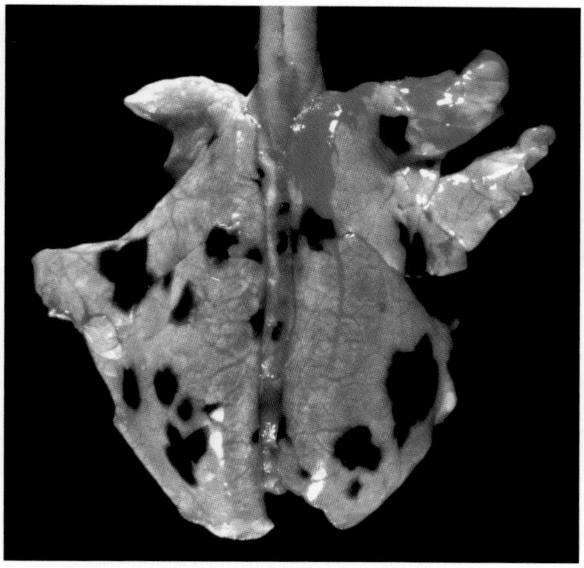

Fig. 9-32 Pulmonary melanosis, lungs, pig.
Note the areas of black (melanin pigment) discoloration of the pleural surface. This pigmentation extends into the lungs and is an incidental finding that has no clinical or pathologic significance. It is most common in "black-face" breeds of animals, especially sheep. (Courtesy College of Veterinary Medicine, University of Illinois.)

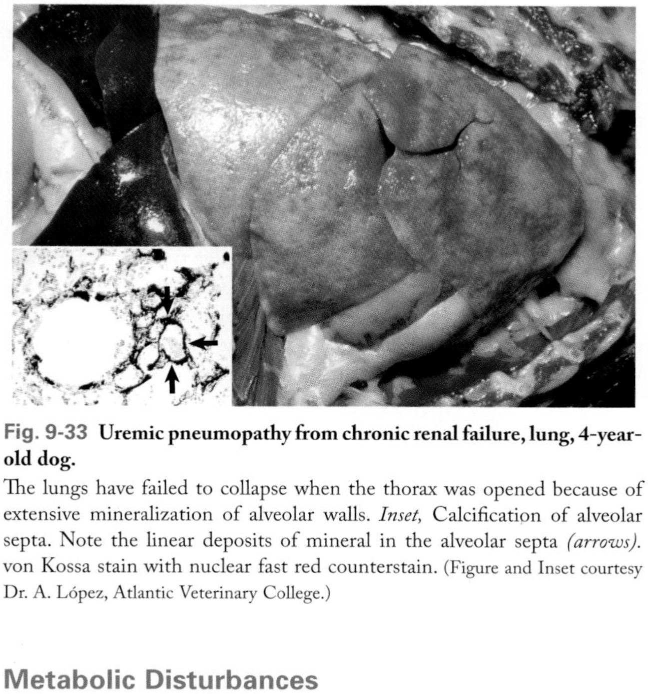

Fig. 9-33 Uremic pneumopathy from chronic renal failure, lung, 4-year-old dog.
The lungs have failed to collapse when the thorax was opened because of extensive mineralization of alveolar walls. *Inset,* Calcification of alveolar septa. Note the linear deposits of mineral in the alveolar septa *(arrows).* von Kossa stain with nuclear fast red counterstain. (Figure and Inset courtesy Dr. A. López, Atlantic Veterinary College.)

Metabolic Disturbances

Pulmonary Calcification ("Calcinosis")

Calcification of the lungs occurs in some hypercalcemic states, generally secondary to hypervitaminosis D or from ingestion of toxic (hypercalcemic) plants, such as *Solanum malacoxylon* (Manchester wasting disease) that contain vitamin D analogs. It is also a common sequela to uremia and hyperadrenocorticism in dogs and to pulmonary necrosis (dystrophic calcification) in most species. Calcified lungs may fail to collapse when the thoracic cavity is opened and have a characteristic "gritty" texture (Fig. 9-33). Microscopically, lesions vary from calcification of the alveolar basement membranes (see Fig. 9-33) to heterotopic ossification of the lungs.

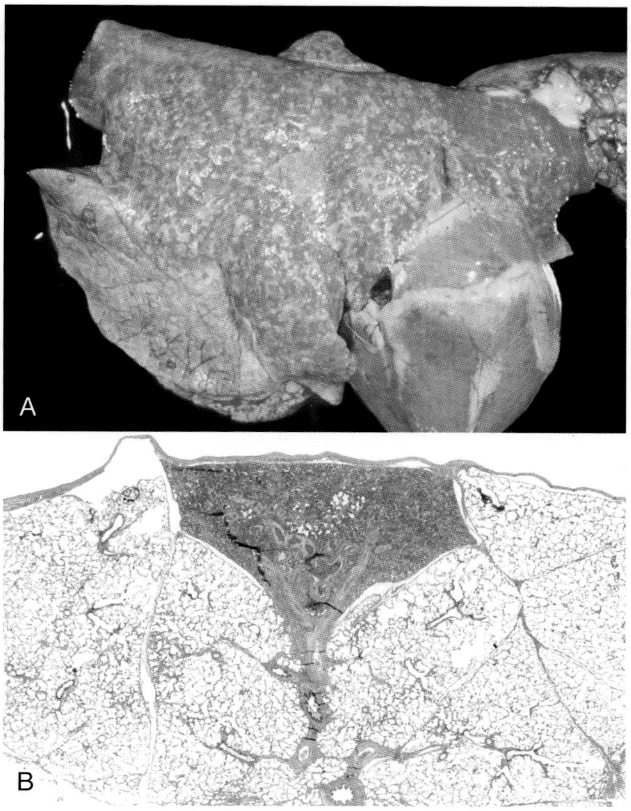

Fig. 9-34 Pulmonary atelectasis.
A, Multifocal neonatal atelectasis of the lung from 1-day-old calf. Note the prominent mosaic pattern of normally inflated *(light)* and atelectatic, uninflated *(dark)* lobules. Neonatal atelectasis is caused by aspiration of amniotic fluid, meconium, and squamous epithelial cells, causing obstruction of small bronchi and bronchioles at the time of birth. All pulmonary lobes are involved. Although focal lobular atelectasis is commonly seen in neonates, this lesion suggests that the fetus was acidotic and aspirated amniotic fluid. **B,** Atelectasis of a superficial pulmonary lobule in a cow. Note the absence of air in alveoli of this lobule that has resulted in its collapse and thus its darker beige color as shown in **A.** H&E stain. (**A** from López A, Bildfell R: *Vet Pathol* 29:104-111, 1992. **B** courtesy Dr. M.D. McGavin, College of Veterinary Medicine, University of Tennessee.)

In most cases, pulmonary calcification in itself has little clinical significance, although its cause (e.g., uremia or vitamin D toxicosis) may be very important.

Abnormalities of Inflation

To achieve gaseous exchange, a balanced ratio of the volumes of air to capillary blood must be present in the lungs (ventilation/perfusion ratio), and the air and capillary blood must be in close proximity across the alveolar wall. A ventilation-perfusion mismatch occurs if pulmonary tissue is either collapsed (atelectasis) or overinflated (hyperinflation and emphysema).

Atelectasis (Congenital and Acquired)

The term *atelectasis* means incomplete distention of alveoli and is used to describe lungs that have failed to expand with air at the time of birth (congenital atelectasis) or lungs that have collapsed after inflation has taken place (acquired atelectasis or alveolar collapse) (Figs. 9-34 and 9-35).

During fetal life, lungs are not fully distended, contain no air, and are partially filled with a locally produced fluid known as fetal

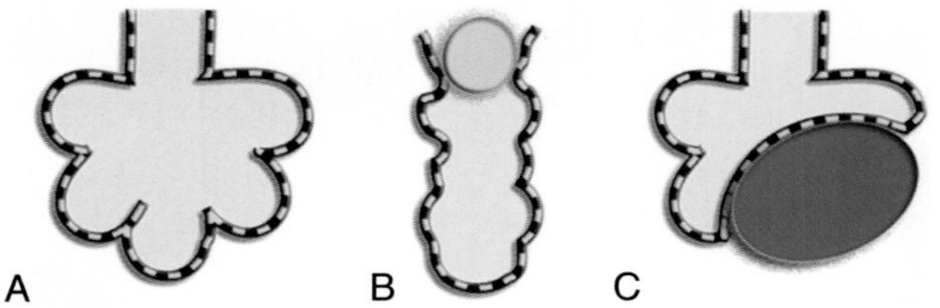

Fig. 9-35 Schematic representation of the types of atelectasis. **A,** Normal alveolar distention. **B,** Obstructive atelectasis; obstruction of airways (i.e., exudate or parasite) affecting airflow and causing alveolar collapse. **C,** Compressive atelectasis; mass (i.e., abscess or tumor) compressing the lung parenchyma and causing alveolar collapse. (Redrawn from Dr. A. López, Atlantic Veterinary College.)

lung fluid. Not surprisingly, lungs of aborted and stillborn fetuses sink when placed in water, whereas those from animals that have breathed float. At the time of birth, fetal lung fluid is rapidly reabsorbed and replaced by inspired air, leading to the normal distention of alveoli. Congenital atelectasis occurs in newborns who fail to inflate their lungs after taking their first few breaths of air; it is caused by obstruction of airways, often as a result of aspiration of amniotic fluid and meconium (described in the section on Meconium Aspiration Syndrome) (see Fig. 9-34). Congenital atelectasis also develops when alveoli cannot remain distended after initial aeration because of an alteration in quality and quantity of pulmonary surfactant produced by type II pneumonocytes and Clara cells. This form infant of congenital atelectasis is referred to in human neonatology as infant respiratory distress syndrome (IRDS) or as hyaline membrane disease because of the clinical and microscopic features of the disease. It commonly occurs in babies who are premature or born to diabetic or alcoholic mothers and is occasionally found in animals, particularly in foals and piglets. The pathetic, gasping attempts of affected foals and pigs to breathe have prompted the use of the name "barkers"; foals that survive may have brain damage from cerebral hypoxia (see Chapter 14) and are referred to as "wanderers," owing to their aimless behavior and lack of a normal sense of fear.

Acquired atelectasis is much more common and occurs in two main forms: compressive and obstructive (see Fig. 9-35). Compressive atelectasis has two main causes: space-occupying masses in the pleural cavity, such as abscesses and tumors, or transferred pressures, such as that caused by bloat, hydrothorax, hemothorax, chylothorax, and empyema (Fig. 9-36). Another form of compressive atelectasis occurs when the negative pressure in the thoracic cavity is lost because of pneumothorax. This form generally has massive atelectasis and thus is also referred to as lung collapse.

Obstructive (absorption) atelectasis occurs when there is a reduction in the diameter of the airways caused by mucosal edema and inflammation, or when the lumen of the airway is blocked by mucus plugs, exudate, aspirated foreign material, or lungworms (see Fig. 9-35). When the obstruction is complete, trapped air in the lung eventually becomes reabsorbed. Unlike the compression type, obstructive atelectasis often has a lobular pattern as a result of blockage of the airway supplying that lobule. This lobular appearance of atelectasis is more common in species with poor collateral ventilation, such as cattle and sheep. The extent and location of obstructive atelectasis depends largely on the size of the affected airway (large versus small) and on the degree of obstruction (partial versus complete).

Atelectasis also occurs when large animals are kept recumbent for prolonged periods, such as during anesthesia (hypostatic

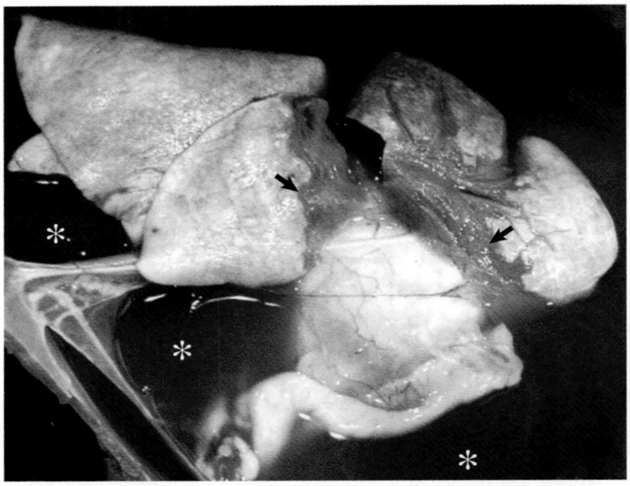

Fig. 9-36 Compressive atelectasis and hydrothorax, lungs, dog. Atelectatic lung appears as dark depressed pulmonary tissues *(arrows)*. Also note a large volume of transudate in the ventral pleural cavity *(*)*. (Courtesy Atlantic Veterinary College.)

atelectasis). The factors contributing to hypostatic atelectasis are a combination of blood-air imbalance, shallow breathing, airway obstruction because of mucus and fluid that has not been drained from bronchioles and alveoli, and from inadequate local production of surfactant. Atelectasis can also be a sequel to paralysis of respiratory muscles and prolonged use of mechanical ventilation or general anesthesia in intensive care.

In general, the lungs with atelectasis appear depressed below the surface of the normally inflated lung. The color is generally dark blue and the texture is flabby or firm; they are firm if there is concurrent edema or other processes, such as can occur in ARDS or "shock" lungs (see the section on Pulmonary Edema). Distribution and extent vary with the process, being patchy (multifocal) in congenital atelectasis, lobular in the obstructive type, and of various degrees in between in the compressive type. Microscopically, the alveoli are collapsed or slitlike and the alveolar walls appear parallel and close together, giving prominence to the interstitial tissue even without any superimposed inflammation.

Pulmonary Emphysema

Pulmonary emphysema, often simply referred to as *emphysema,* is an extremely important primary disease in humans, whereas in animals, it is always a secondary condition resulting from a variety of pulmonary lesions. In human medicine, emphysema is strictly defined as an abnormal permanent enlargement of airspaces distal to the terminal bronchiole, accompanied by destruction of alveolar walls (alveolar emphysema). This definition separates it from simple air space enlargement or hyperinflation, in which there is no destruction of alveolar walls and which can occur congenitally (Down syndrome) or be acquired with age (aging lung, sometimes misnamed "senile emphysema"). The pathogenesis of emphysema in humans is still controversial, but current thinking overwhelmingly suggests that destruction of alveolar walls is largely the result of an imbalance between proteases released by phagocytes and antiproteases produced in the lung as a defense mechanism (the protease-antiprotease theory). The destructive process is markedly accelerated by any factor, such as cigarette smoking, pollution, or defects in the synthesis of antiproteases in humans, that increases the recruitment of macrophages and leukocytes in the lungs. This theory originated when it was found that humans with homozygous α_1-antitrypsin deficiency were remarkably susceptible to emphysema and that proteases (elastase) inoculated intratracheally into the lungs of laboratory animals produced lesions similar to those found in the disease. More than 90% of the problem relates to cigarette smoking, and airway obstruction is no longer considered to play a major role in the pathogenesis of emphysema in humans.

Primary emphysema does not occur in animals, and thus no animal disease should be called simply emphysema. In animals, this lesion is always secondary to obstruction of outflow of air or is agonal at slaughter. Secondary pulmonary emphysema occurs frequently in animals with bronchopneumonia, in which exudate plugging bronchi and bronchioles causes an airflow imbalance where the volume of air entering exceeds the volume leaving the lung. This airflow imbalance is often promoted by the so-called one-way valve effect caused by the exudate, which allows air into the lung during inspiration but prevents movement of air out of the lung during expiration.

Depending on the localization in the lung, emphysema can be classified as alveolar or interstitial. Alveolar emphysema characterized by distention and rupture of the alveolar walls, forming variably sized air bubbles in pulmonary parenchyma, occurs in all species. Interstitial emphysema occurs mainly in cattle, presumably because of their wide interlobular septa, and lack of collateral ventilation in these species does not permit air to move freely into adjacent pulmonary lobules. As a result, accumulated air penetrates the alveolar and bronchiolar walls and forces its way into the interlobular connective tissue, causing notable distention of the interlobular septa. It is also suspected that forced respiratory movements predispose to interstitial emphysema when air at high pressure breaks into the loose connective tissue of the interlobular septa (Fig. 9-37). Sometimes these bubbles of trapped air in alveolar or interstitial emphysema become confluent, forming large (several centimeters in diameter) pockets of air that are referred to as *bullae* (singular: bulla); the lesion is then called *bullous emphysema*. This lesion is not a specific type of emphysema and does not indicate a different disease process, but rather is a larger accumulation of air at one focus. In the most severe cases, air moves from the interlobular septa into the connective tissue surrounding the main stem bronchi and major vessels (bronchovascular bundles) and from here it leaks into the mediastinum, causing pneumomediastinum first, and eventually exits via the thoracic inlet into the cervical and thoracic subcutaneous tissue causing subcutaneous emphysema.

It should be noted that mild and even moderate alveolar emphysema is difficult to judge at necropsy and by light microscopy unless special techniques are used to prevent collapse of the lung when the thorax is opened. These techniques include plugging of the trachea or intratracheal perfusion of fixative (10% neutral-buffered formalin) before the thorax is opened to prevent collapse of the lungs. Important diseases that cause secondary pulmonary emphysema in animals include small airway obstruction (such as heaves) in horses and pulmonary edema and emphysema (fog fever) in cattle (see Fig. 9-37) and exudates in bronchopneumonia.

Circulatory Disturbances of the Lungs

Lungs are extremely well-vascularized organs with a dual circulation provided by pulmonary and bronchial arteries. Disturbances in pulmonary circulation have a notable effect on gaseous exchange, which may result in life-threatening hypoxemia and acidosis. In addition, circulatory disturbances in the lungs can have an impact on other organs, such as the heart and liver. For example, impeded blood flow in the lungs because of chronic pulmonary disease results in cor pulmonale, which is caused by unremitting pulmonary hypertension followed by cardiac dilation, right heart failure,

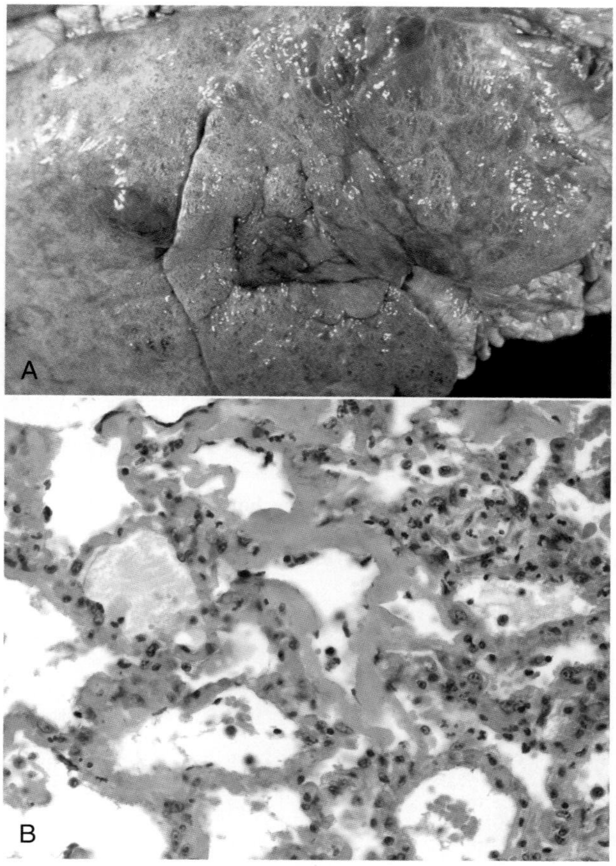

Fig. 9-37 Bovine pulmonary edema and emphysema (fog fever), lung, cow.
A, Emphysema, edema, and interstitial pneumonia involving all pulmonary lobes. Note the variably sized air bubbles in the interlobular septa and pulmonary parenchyma. The texture of these lungs would be notably crepitus as a result of the accumulation of air in pulmonary parenchyma. **B,** Note the thick eosinophilic hyaline membranes lining the alveoli. The alveoli are dilated and also contain some edema fluid, occasional pulmonary macrophages, and necrotic alveolar cells. H&E stain. (**A** courtesy Western College of Veterinary Medicine. **B** courtesy Dr. A. López, Atlantic Veterinary College.)

chronic passive congestion of the liver (nutmeg liver), and generalized edema (anasarca).

Hyperemia and Congestion

Hyperemia is an active process that is part of acute inflammation, whereas congestion is the passive process resulting from decreased outflow of venous blood, as occurs in acute congestive heart failure (Fig. 9-38). In the early acute stages of pneumonia, the lungs appear notably red, and microscopically, blood vessels and capillaries are engorged with blood from hyperemia. Pulmonary congestion is most frequently caused by heart failure, which results in stagnation of blood in pulmonary vessels, leading to edema and egression of erythrocytes into the alveolar spaces. As with any other foreign particle, erythrocytes in alveolar spaces are rapidly phagocytosed (erythrophagocytosis) by pulmonary alveolar macrophages. When extravasation of erythrocytes is severe, large numbers of macrophages with brown cytoplasm may accumulate in the bronchoalveolar spaces. The brown cytoplasm is the result of accumulation of considerable amounts of hemosiderin; these macrophages filled with iron pigment (siderophages) are generally referred to as *heart failure cells* (Fig. 9-39). The lungs of animals with chronic heart

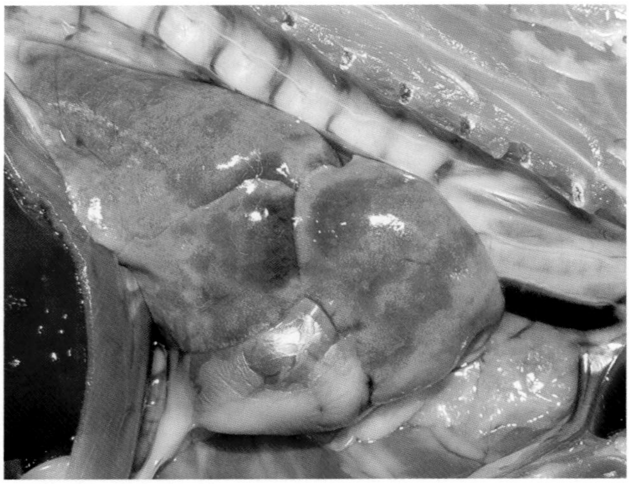

Fig. 9-38 Acute pulmonary congestion, lungs, dog.
The lung parenchyma is red because of congestion of pulmonary vasculature and alveolar capillaries. (Courtesy Dr. A. López, Atlantic Veterinary College.)

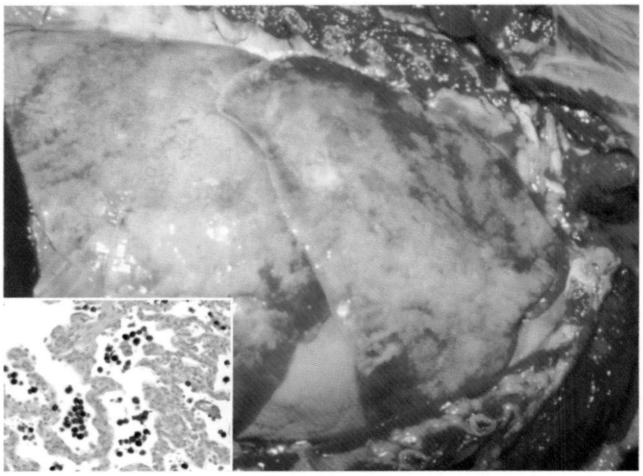

Fig. 9-39 Chronic pulmonary congestion and edema because of chronic heart failure (dilative cardiomyopathy), lungs, 5-year-old dog.
The lungs have failed to collapse (fibrosis) and have a mottled and brownish appearance (hemosiderosis). *Inset,* Microscopic view of alveoli. Large numbers of macrophages containing hemosiderin (heart failure cells) are present in alveoli. During heart failure, red blood cells gain access to alveoli where they are rapidly phagocytosed by pulmonary macrophages and the iron of the hemoglobin molecule is converted to hemosiderin. Hemosiderin gives a positive reaction for iron with the Prussian blue reaction. Prussian blue (iron) reaction with nuclear fast red counterstain. (Courtesy Dr. A. López, Atlantic Veterinary College.)

failure usually have a patchy red appearance with foci of brown discoloration because of accumulated hemosiderin. In severe and persistent cases of heart failure, the lungs fail to collapse because of edema and pulmonary fibrosis. Terminal pulmonary congestion (acute) is frequently seen in animals euthanized with barbiturates and should not be mistaken for an antemortem lesion.

Hypostatic congestion is another form of pulmonary congestion that results from the effects of gravity and poor circulation on a highly vascularized tissue, such as the lung. This type of gravitational congestion is characterized by the increase of blood in the lower side of the lung, particularly the lower lung, of animals in lateral recumbency, particularly horses and cattle. The affected

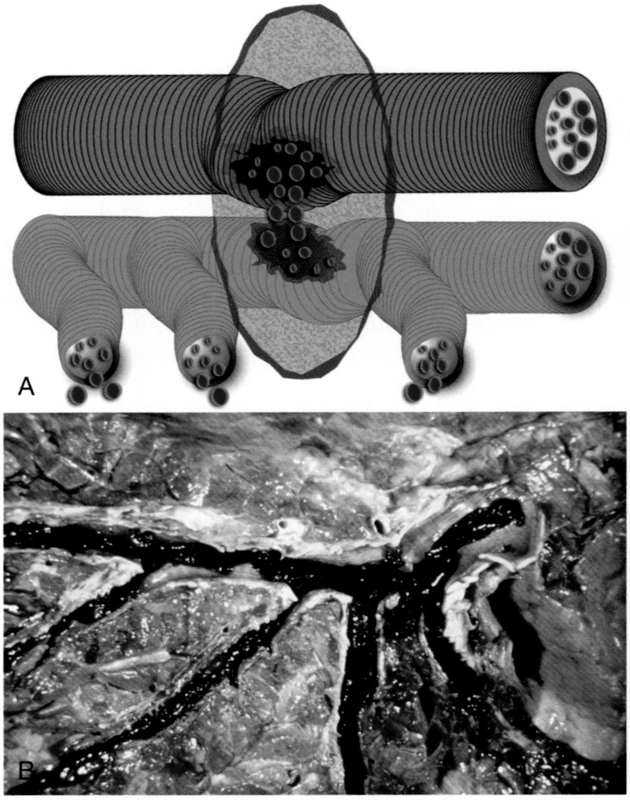

Fig. 9-40 Fatal pulmonary hemorrhage.
A, Schematic of an abscess *(green)* eroding the wall of a major pulmonary artery *(*red) and causing bleeding into the airways *(blue).* **B,** Cut surface of lung, cow. Major bronchi and the trachea are filled with clotted blood. This cow died unexpectedly, with severe respiratory distress and blood coming from the nose and mouth. A large abscess in the lung had eroded through the wall of a major pulmonary vessel. (**A** courtesy Dr. A. López, Atlantic Veterinary College. **B** courtesy Dr. R. Curtis, Atlantic Veterinary College.)

portions of the lung appear dark red and can have a firmer texture. In animals and particularly humans that have been prostrated for extended periods of time, hypostatic congestion may be followed by hypostatic edema, and hypostatic pneumonia as edema interferes locally with the bacterial defense mechanisms.

Pulmonary Hemorrhage

Pulmonary hemorrhages can occur as a result of trauma, coagulopathies, pulmonary thromboembolism from jugular thrombosis or from embolisms of exudate from a hepatic abscess that has eroded the wall and ruptured into the caudal vena cava (cattle), disseminated intravascular coagulation (DIC), vasculitis, or sepsis. A gross finding, often confused with intravital pulmonary hemorrhage is the result of severing both the trachea and carotid arteries simultaneously at slaughter. Blood is aspirated into the transected trachea and thence into the lungs and there forms a random pattern of scattered irregular red foci (1 to 10 mm), in one to more lobes. These red foci are readily visible on both the pleural and cut surfaces of the lung and free blood is visible in the lumens of bronchi and bronchioles.

Rupture of a major pulmonary vessel with resulting massive hemorrhage occurs occasionally in cattle when a growing abscess in a lung invades and disrupts the wall of a major pulmonary artery or vein (Fig. 9-40). In most cases, animals die rapidly, often with spectacular hemoptysis, and on postmortem examination, bronchi are filled with blood (see Fig. 9-40).

Exercise-induced pulmonary hemorrhage (EIPH) is a specific form of pulmonary hemorrhage in racehorses after exercise and clinically is characterized by epistaxis. Because only a small percentage of horses with bronchoscopic evidence of hemorrhage have clinical epistaxis, it is likely that EIPH goes undetected in many cases. The pathogenesis is still controversial, but current literature suggests laryngeal paralysis, bronchiolitis, extremely high pulmonary vascular and alveolar pressures during exercise, alveolar hypoxia, and preexisting pulmonary injury as possible causes. EIPH is seldom fatal; postmortem lesions in the lungs of horses that have been affected with several episodes of hemorrhage are characterized by large areas of dark brown discoloration, largely in the caudal lung lobes. Microscopically, lesions are alveolar hemorrhages, abundant alveolar macrophages containing hemosiderin (siderophages), and mild fibrosis of the alveolar walls.

Pulmonary Edema

In normal lungs, fluid from the vascular space slowly but continuously passes into the interstitial tissue where it is rapidly drained by the pulmonary and pleural lymphatic vessels. Recent investigations demonstrated that alveolar fluid clearance across the alveolar epithelium is also a major mechanism of fluid removal from the lung. Edema develops when the rate of fluid transudation from pulmonary vessels into interstitium or alveoli exceeds that of lymphatic and alveolar removal (Fig. 9-41). Pulmonary edema can be physiologically classified as cardiogenic (hydrostatic; hemodynamic) and noncardiogenic (permeability) types.

Hydrostatic (cardiogenic) pulmonary edema develops when there is an elevated rate of fluid transudation because of increased hydrostatic pressure in the vascular compartment or decreased osmotic pressure in the blood. Once the lymph drainage has been overwhelmed, fluid accumulates in the perivascular spaces, causing distention of the bronchovascular bundles and alveolar interstitium, and eventually leaks into the alveolar spaces. Causes of hemodynamic pulmonary edema include congestive heart failure (increased hydrostatic pressure); iatrogenic fluid overload; disorders in which blood osmotic pressure is reduced, such as in the hypoalbuminemia seen in some hepatic diseases; nephritic syndrome; and protein-losing enteropathy. Hemodynamic pulmonary edema also occurs when lymph drainage is impaired, generally secondary to neoplastic invasion of lymph vessels.

Permeability edema (inflammatory) occurs when there is excessive opening of endothelial gaps or damage to the cells that constitute the blood-air barrier (endothelial cells or type I pneumonocytes). This type of edema is an integral and early part of the inflammatory response, primarily because of the effect of inflammatory mediators, such as leukotrienes, platelet-activating factor (PAF), cytokines, and vasoactive amines released by neutrophils, macrophages, mast cells, lymphocytes, endothelial cells, and type II pneumonocytes. These inflammatory mediators increase the permeability of the blood-air barrier. In other cases, permeability edema results from direct damage to the endothelium or type I pneumonocytes, allowing plasma fluids to move freely from the vascular space into the alveolar lumen (Fig. 9-42). Because type I pneumonocytes are highly vulnerable to some pneumotropic viruses (influenza, BRSV), toxicants (nitrogen dioxide [NO_2], sulfur dioxide [SO_2], hydrogen sulfide [H_2S], 3-methylindole), and particularly to free radicals, it is not surprising that permeability edema commonly accompanies many viral or toxic pulmonary diseases. A permeability edema also occurs when endothelial cells in the lung are injured by bacterial toxins, sepsis, ARDS, DIC, anaphylactic shock, milk allergy, paraquat toxicity, and adverse drug reactions.

The concentration of protein in edematous fluid is greater in permeability edema (exudate) than in hemodynamic edema (transudate); this difference has been used clinically in human medicine to differentiate one type of pulmonary edema from another. Microscopically, because of the higher concentration of protein, edema fluid in lungs with inflammation or damage to the blood-air barrier tends to stain more intensely eosinophilic than that of the hydrostatic edema from heart failure.

Grossly the edematous lungs—independent of the cause—are wet and heavy; the color varies, depending on the degree of congestion or hemorrhage; and fluid may be present in the pleural cavity. If edema is severe, bronchi and trachea contain considerable amounts of foamy fluid, which originates from the mixing of edema fluid and air (Fig. 9-43). On cut surfaces, the lung parenchyma

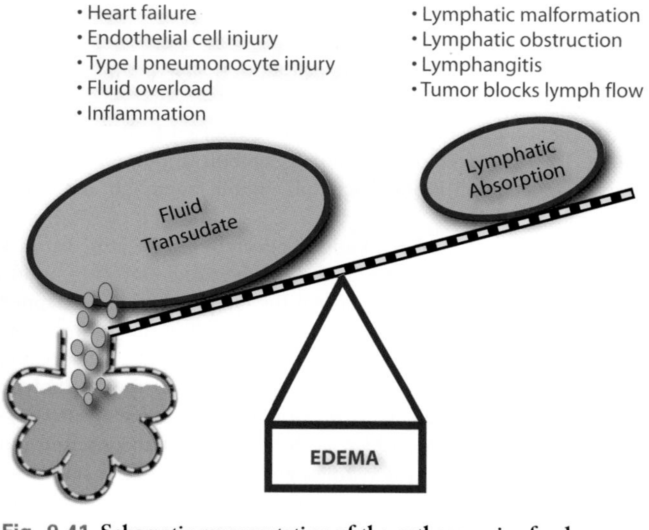

Fig. 9-41 Schematic representation of the pathogenesis of pulmonary edema.
(Courtesy Dr. A. López, Atlantic Veterinary College)

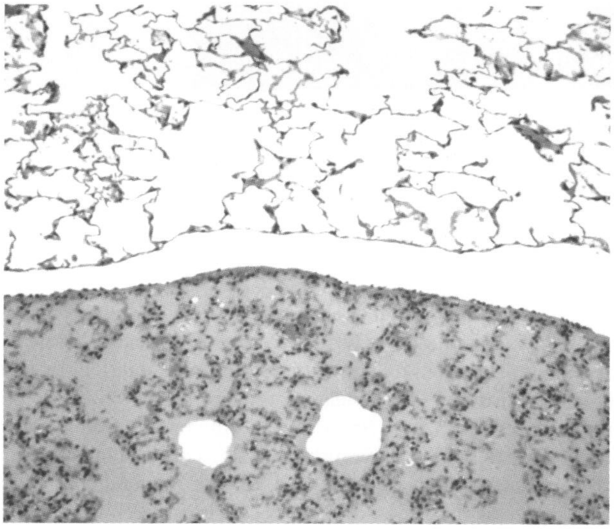

Fig. 9-42 Pulmonary edema, lung, rat.
Normal lung with alveoli filled with air *(top)* and lung with severe pulmonary edema characterized by transudation of protein-rich fluid (deeply eosinophilic) filling the alveoli and congested alveolar septa *(bottom)*. H&E stain. (Courtesy Dr. A. López, Atlantic Veterinary College.)

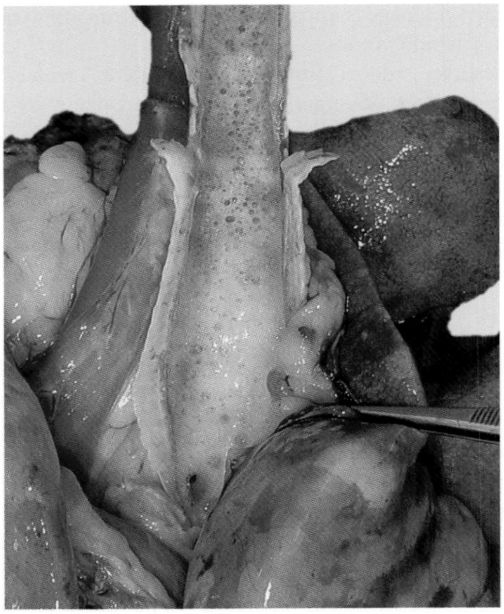

Fig. 9-43 Pulmonary edema, lungs and trachea, sheep. Note large amounts of foamy fluid in the trachea and uncollapsed lungs with wet appearance. (Courtesy Dr. C. Legge and Dr. A. López, Atlantic Veterinary College.)

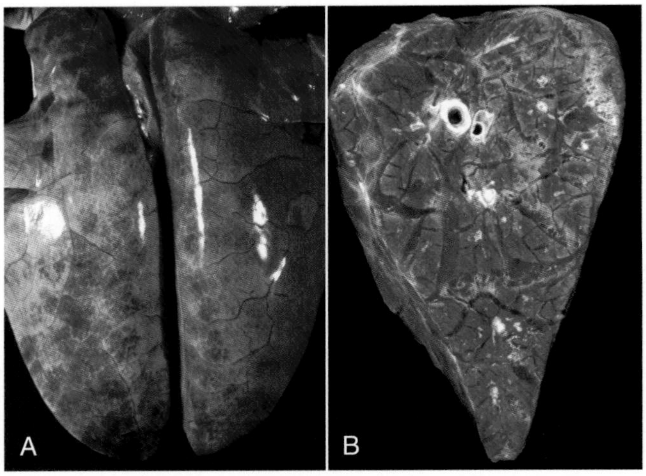

Fig. 9-44 Pulmonary edema, lungs, pig. **A,** The lungs are distended by edema fluid, which has resulted in rounded edges and edematous distention of the interlobular septa. **B,** The cut surface is wet and the interlobular septa are markedly distended with edema fluid. Lung lobules are also congested. (**A** and **B** courtesy College of Veterinary Medicine, University of Illinois.)

oozes fluid like a wet sponge. In cattle and pigs that have distinct lobules, the lobular pattern becomes rather accentuated because of edematous distentions of lymphatic vessels in the interlobular septa and the edematous interlobular septum itself (Fig. 9-44). Severe pulmonary edema may be impossible to differentiate from peracute pneumonia; this fact is not surprising because pulmonary edema occurs in the very early stages of inflammation. Careful observation of the lungs at the time of necropsy is critical because diagnosis of pulmonary edema cannot be reliably performed microscopically. This is due in part to the loss of the edema fluid from the lungs during fixation with 10% neutral-buffered formalin and in part to the fact that the fluid itself stains very poorly or not at all with eosin because of its low protein content (hemodynamic edema). A protein-rich (permeability) edema is easier to visualize microscopically because it is deeply eosinophilic in hematoxylin and eosin (H&E)-stained sections (see Fig. 9-42), particularly if a fixative, such as Zenker's solution, which precipitates protein, is used.

Acute Respiratory Distress Syndrome

Acute (adult) respiratory distress syndrome (ARDS; shock lung) is an important condition in humans and animals characterized by pulmonary hypertension, intravascular aggregation of neutrophils in the lungs, diffuse alveolar damage, permeability edema, and formation of hyaline membranes, which are a mixture of plasma proteins, fibrin, surfactant, and cellular debris from necrotic pneumonocytes. The pathogenesis is complex and multifactorial but in general terms can be defined as diffuse alveolar damage that results from lesions in distant organs, from generalized systemic diseases, or from direct injury to the lung. Sepsis, major trauma, aspiration of gastric contents, extensive burns, and pancreatitis are some of the disease entities known to trigger ARDS. All these conditions provoke "hyperreactive macrophages" to directly or indirectly generate overwhelming amounts of cytokines (mainly TNF-α, interleukin [IL]-1, IL-6, and IL-8). Some of these cytokines prime neutrophils previously recruited in the lung capillaries and alveoli to release enzymes and free radicals, thus causing diffuse endothelial and alveolar damage that culminates in a fulminating pulmonary edema (Fig. 9-45). ARDS occurs in domestic animals and explains why pulmonary edema is one of the most common lesions found in many animals dying of sepsis, toxemia, aspiration of gastric contents, and pancreatitis, for example. A familial form of ARDS has been reported in Dalmatians. The pulmonary lesions in this syndrome are further discussed in the sections on Interstitial Pneumonia and Aspiration Pneumonia in Dogs.

Neurogenic pulmonary edema is another distinctive but poorly understood form of life-threatening lung edema in humans that follows increased intracranial pressure (i.e., head injury, brain edema, brain tumors, or cerebral hemorrhage). This type of pulmonary edema can be experimentally reproduced in laboratory animals by injecting fibrin into the fourth ventricle. It involves both hemodynamic and permeability pathways presumably from massive sympathetic stimulation and overwhelming release of catecholamines. Neurogenic pulmonary edema has sporadically been reported in animals with brain injury or severe seizures or after severe stress and excitement.

Pulmonary Embolisms

With its vast capillary bed and position in the circulation, the lung acts as a safety net to catch emboli before they reach the brain and other tissues. However, this positioning is often to its own detriment. The most common pulmonary emboli in domestic animals are thromboemboli, septic (bacterial) emboli, fat emboli, and tumor cell emboli.

Pulmonary thromboembolism generally originates from a thrombus present elsewhere in the venous circulation (Fig. 9-46). Fragments released inevitably reach the lungs and become trapped in the pulmonary vasculature (Fig. 9-47). Small sterile thromboemboli are generally of little clinical or pathologic significance because they can be rapidly degraded and disposed of by the fibrinolytic system. Parasites, such as *Dirofilaria immitis* and *Angiostrongylus vasorum;* endocrinopathies, such as hyperadrenocorticism and hypothyroidism; glomerulopathies; and hypercoagulable states can be responsible for pulmonary arterial thrombosis and pulmonary thromboembolism in dogs. Pieces of thrombi breaking free from a jugular, femoral, or uterine vein can cause pulmonary thromboembolism. Pulmonary thromboembolisms occur in heavy horses

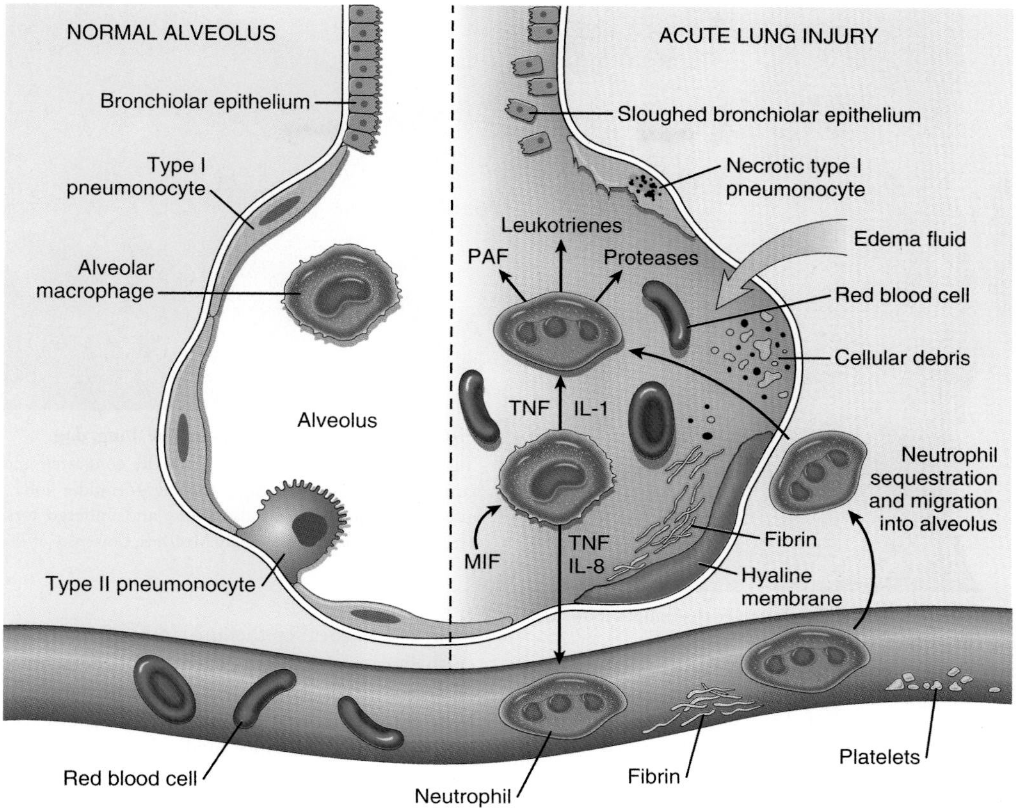

Fig. 9-45 Schematic representation of the cellular events leading to acute respiratory distress syndrome.
The normal alveolus *(left side)* compared to the injured alveolus in the early phase of acute lung injury and acute respiratory distress syndrome. Proinflammatory cytokines, such as interleukin-8 (IL-8) and interleukin-1 (IL-1) , and tumor necrosis factor (TNF) (released by macrophages), cause neutrophils to adhere to pulmonary capillaries and extravasate into the alveolar space, where they go activate. Activated neutrophils release a variety of factors such as leukotrienes, oxidants, proteases, and platelet-activating factor (PAF), which contribute to local tissue damage, accumulation of edema fluid in the airspaces, surfactant activation, and hyaline membrane formation. Macrophage migration inhibition factor (MIF) released into the local milieu sustain the ongoing pro-inflammatory response. Subsequently, the release of macrophage-derived fibrogenic cytokines such as transforming growth factor-β (TGF-β) and platelet-derived growth factor (PDGF) stimulate fibroblastic growth and collagen deposition associated with the healing phase of injury. (From Kumar V, Abbas A, Fausto N, et al: *Robbins & Cotran pathologic basis of disease,* ed 8, Philadelphia, 2009, Saunders.)

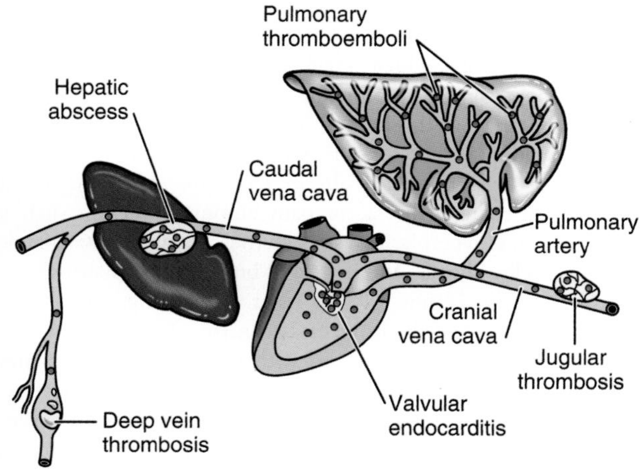

Fig. 9-46 Sources of pulmonary emboli.
Schematic diagram of pulmonary emboli *(red dots)* arising from: (1) rupture of a hepatic abscess into the caudal vena cava; (2) vegetative valvular endocarditis (tricuspid valve); (3) jugular thrombosis; and (4) deep vein thrombosis. Pulmonary infarcts are rare and often of little clinical significance because of the lung's dual arterial circulation (i.e., pulmonary and bronchial arteries). (Redrawn with permission from Dr. A. López, Atlantic Veterinary College.)

after prolonged anesthesia (deep vein thrombosis), recumbent cows ("downer cow syndrome"), or in any animal undergoing long-term intravenous catheterization in which thrombi build up in the catheter and then break off (see Fig. 9-47).

Septic emboli, pieces of thrombi contaminated with bacteria or fungi and broken free from infected mural or valvular thrombi in the heart and vessels, eventually become entrapped in the pulmonary circulation. These emboli originate most commonly from bacterial endocarditis (right side) and jugular thrombophlebitis in all species, hepatic abscesses that have eroded and discharge their contents into the caudal vena cava in cattle, and septic arthritis and omphalitis in farm animals (see Figs. 9-46 and 9-47). When present in large numbers, septic emboli may cause unexpected death because of massive pulmonary edema; survivors generally develop pulmonary arteritis and thrombosis and embolic (suppurative) pneumonia, which may lead to pulmonary abscesses.

Fat emboli can form after bone fractures or surgical interventions of bone. These are not as significant a problem in domestic animals as they are in humans. Brain emboli (i.e., pieces of brain tissue) in the pulmonary vasculature reported in severe cases of head injury in humans have recently been recognized in the bovine lung after strong pneumatic stunning at slaughter (captive bolt). Although obviously not important as an antemortem pulmonary

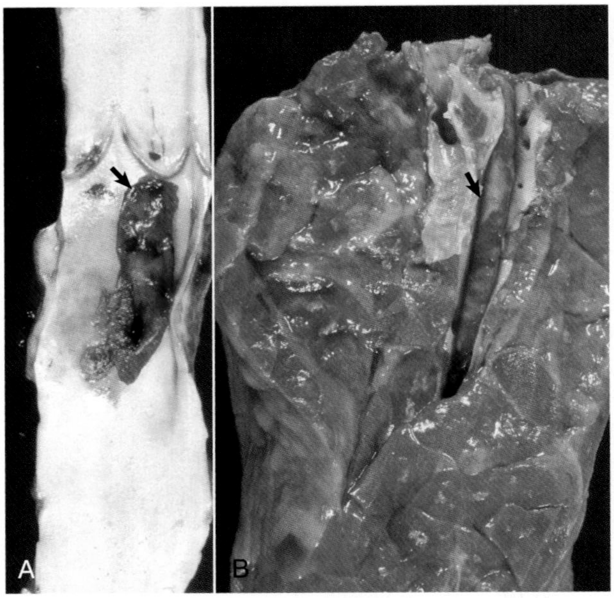

Fig. 9-47 Jugular thrombophlebitis and pulmonary thromboembolism, jugular vein and lung cut surface, cow.
A, The jugular vein has a large thrombus *(arrow)* attached to the wall at the site of prolonged catheterization. **B,** The pulmonary artery contains a large thrombus *(arrow),* presumably a thromboembolus that has broken off the jugular mural thrombus. Note that the pulmonary thromboembolus is not attached to the wall of the pulmonary artery. (Courtesy Dr. A. López, Atlantic Veterinary College.)

lesion, brain emboli are intriguing as a potential risk for public health control of bovine spongiform encephalopathy (BSE). Hepatic emboli formed by circulating pieces of fragmented liver occasionally become trapped in the pulmonary vasculature after severe abdominal trauma and hepatic rupture. Tumor emboli (e.g., osteosarcoma and hemangiosarcoma in dogs and uterine carcinoma in cattle) can be numerous and striking and the ultimate cause of death in malignant neoplasia. In experimental studies, cytokines released during pulmonary inflammation are chemotactic for tumor cells and promote pulmonary metastasis.

Pulmonary (Lung) Infarcts

Because of a dual arterial supply to the lung, pulmonary infarction is rare and generally asymptomatic. However, pulmonary infarcts can be readily caused when pulmonary thrombosis and embolism are superimposed on an already compromised pulmonary circulation such as occurs in congestive heart failure. It also occurs in dogs with torsion of a lung lobe (Fig. 9-48). The gross features of infarcts vary considerably, depending on the stage, and they can be red to black, swollen, firm, and cone or wedge shaped, particularly at the lung margins. In the early acute stage, microscopic lesions are severely hemorrhagic, and this is followed by necrosis. In 1 to 2 days, a border of inflammatory cells develops, and a few days later, a large number of siderophages are present in the necrotic lung. If sterile, pulmonary infarcts heal as fibrotic scars; if septic, an abscess may form surrounded by a thick fibrous capsule.

Patterns of Injury and Host Response in the Lungs

Bronchi

The patterns of necrosis, inflammation, and repair in intrapulmonary bronchi are similar to those previously described for the nasal and tracheal epithelium. In brief, injury to ciliated bronchial epithelium may result in degeneration, detachment, and exfoliation of necrotic cells. Under normal circumstances, cellular exfoliation is promptly followed by inflammation, mitosis, cell proliferation, cell differentiation, and finally by repair (Fig. 9-49). Depending on the type of exudate, bronchitis can be fibrinous, catarrhal, purulent, fibrinonecrotic (diphtheritic), and sometimes granulomatous. When epithelial injury becomes chronic, production of mucus is increased via goblet cell hyperplasia (chronic catarrhal inflammation). This form of chronic bronchitis is well illustrated in habitual smokers who continually need to cough out excessive mucus secretions (sputum). Unfortunately, in some cases, excessive mucus cannot be effectively cleared from airways, which leads to chronic obstructive bronchitis and emphysema (see Fig. 9-49). Chronic bronchial irritation causes squamous metaplasia of highly functional but vulnerable ciliated epithelium to nonfunctional, but more resistant, squamous epithelium. Squamous metaplasia has a calamitous effect on pulmonary clearance because it causes a structural loss and functional breakdown of portions of the mucociliary escalator. Hyperplasia of bronchial glands occurs frequently in chronic bronchitis, which translates to an increase of the Reid Index (bronchial-gland to bronchial-wall ratio). This index is less than 40% in the healthy human lung and in the lungs of most domestic species, except for cats, which generally have an index higher than 40%. The term *airway remodeling* encompasses all the structural changes that accompany chronic bronchitis such as hypertrophy and hyperplasia of smooth muscle, submucosal glands, and goblet cells; fibrosis; and increased bronchial vascularity.

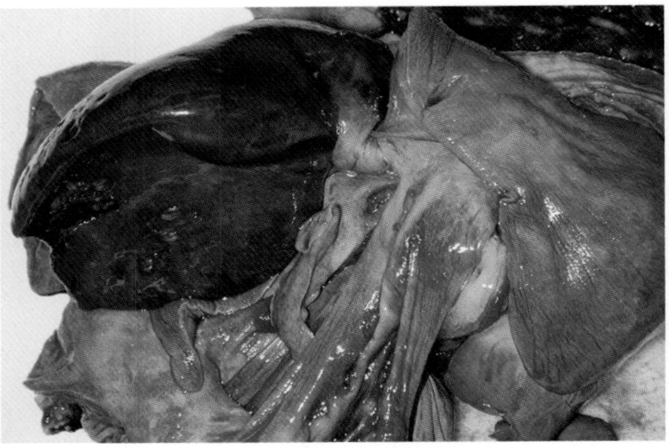

Fig. 9-48 Lobe torsion, middle lobe, lung, dog.
The right middle lung lobe is markedly congested and hemorrhagic from complete torsion. Although the right middle lobe is most frequently affected, other lobes can also rotate and undergo torsion. (Courtesy Dr. R. Fredrickson, College of Veterinary Medicine, University of Illinois.)

Bronchiectasis is one of the most devastating sequelae to chronic remodeling of the bronchi. It consists of a pathologic and permanent dilation of a bronchus with rupture of the bronchial wall as a result of obstruction or chronic inflammation. Destruction of walls occurs in part when proteolytic enzymes and oxygen radicals released from phagocytic cells during chronic inflammation degrade and weaken the smooth muscle and cartilage that help to maintain normal bronchial diameter (Fig. 9-50). Bronchiectasis may be saccular when destruction affects only a small localized portion of the bronchial wall or cylindric when destruction involves a large segment of a bronchus. Grossly, bronchiectasis is manifested by prominent lumps in the lungs (bosselated appearance or having rounded eminences) resulting from distention of bronchi

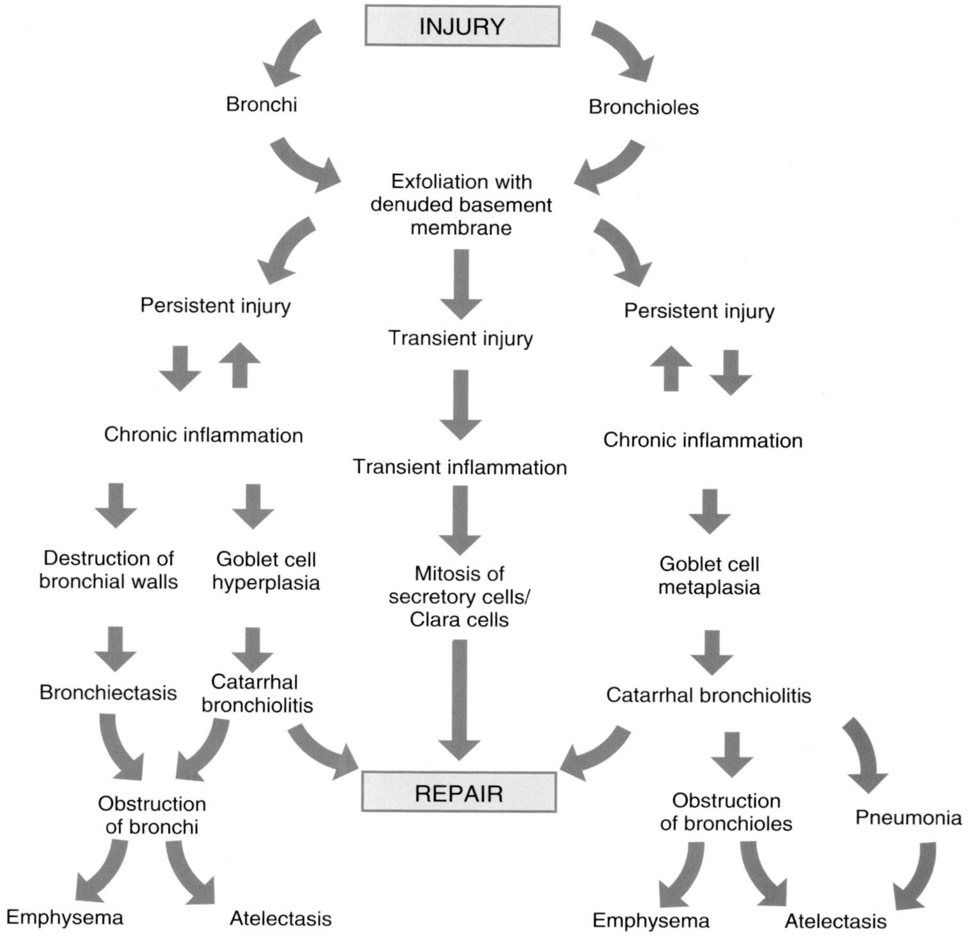

Fig. 9-49 Schematic diagram of the patterns of host response and possible sequelae to bronchial and bronchiolar injury. (Courtesy Dr. A. López, Atlantic Veterinary College.)

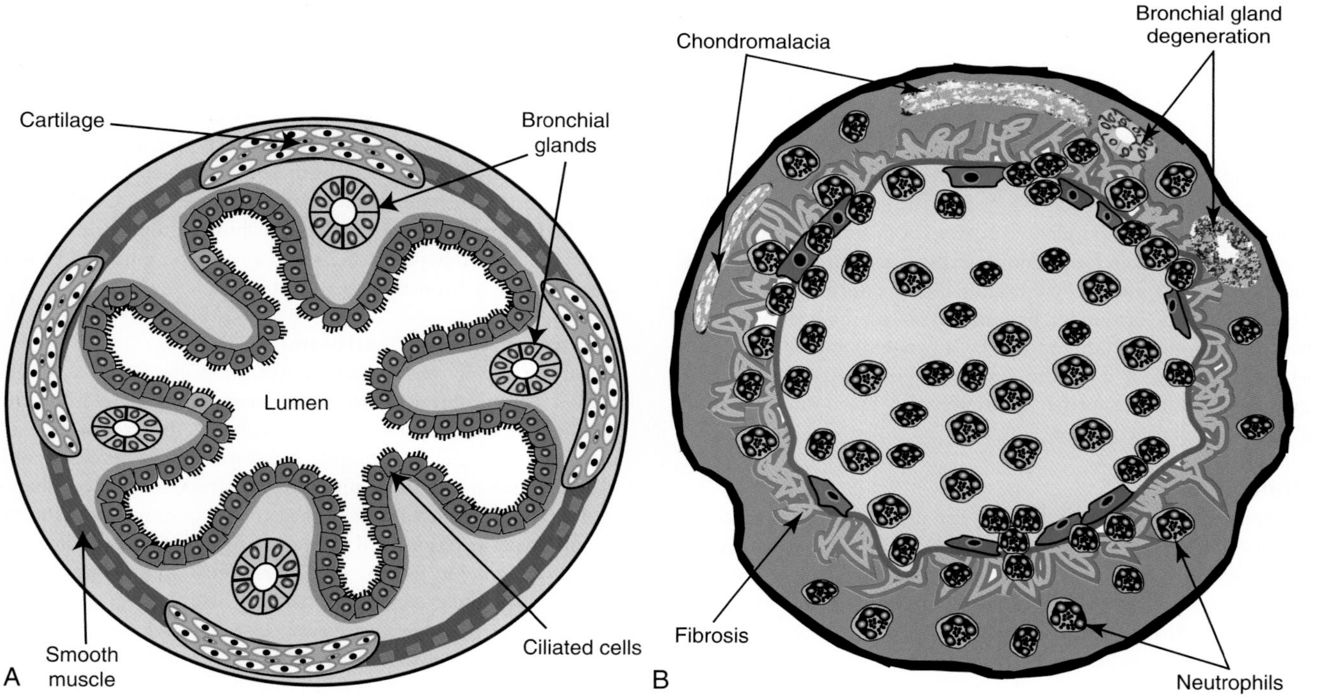

Fig. 9-50 Schematic representation of bronchiectasis.

A, Normal bronchus showing mucosa, submucosa, bronchial glands, and cartilage. **B,** Bronchiectasis. The affected bronchus is dilated and has lost its normal projections of the mucosa into the lumen. Note the inflammation, loss of mucosa, destruction of bronchial wall, and fibrosis with atrophy of cartilage and bronchial glands. (Courtesy Dr. A. López, Atlantic Veterinary College.)

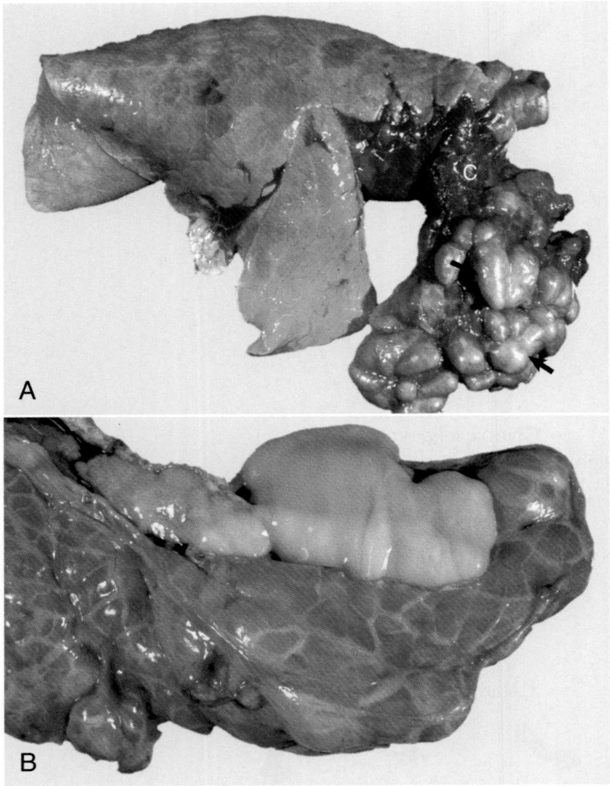

Fig. 9-51 Severe bronchiectasis with chronic bronchopneumonia, right lung, calf.
A, Note the segmentally distended (bosselated) bronchi *(arrows)* supplying the ventral portion of the cranial lung lobe. The lumens of affected bronchi are filled with purulent exudate. The surrounding lung parenchyma supplied by these bronchi is atelectatic *(C)*. Bronchiectatic bronchi resemble pulmonary abscesses, but unlike abscesses, which contain a pyogenic exudate, the "exudate" in bronchiectasis is composed of remnants of the bronchial wall mixed with mucus. **B,** These distended bronchi are filled with purulent exudate. (**A** courtesy Ontario Veterinary College. **B** courtesy Dr. M.D. McGavin, College of Veterinary Medicine, University of Tennessee.)

with exudate, which results in a concurrent obstructive atelectasis of surrounding parenchyma (Fig. 9-51). The cut surfaces of dilated bronchi are filled with purulent exudates; for this reason, bronchiectasis is often mistaken for pulmonary abscesses. Careful inspection, usually requiring microscopic examination, confirms that exudate is contained and surrounded by remnants of a bronchial wall lined by squamous epithelium and not by a pyogenic membrane (connective tissue) as it is in the case of a pulmonary abscess. The squamous metaplasia further interferes with the normal function of the mucociliary escalator.

Bronchioles

The epithelial lining of the bronchiolar region (transitional zone) is exquisitely susceptible to injury, particularly to that caused by some respiratory viruses (PI-3, adenovirus, BRSV, or canine distemper), oxidant gases (NO_2, SO_2, or ozone [O_3]), and toxic substances (3-methylindole, paraquat). The precise explanation as to why bronchiolar epithelium is so prone to injury is still not clear, but it is presumably due in part to (1) its high vulnerability to oxidants and free radicals; (2) the presence of Clara cells rich in mixed-function oxidases, which locally generate toxic metabolites; and (3) the tendency for pulmonary alveolar macrophages and leukocytes to accumulate in this region of the lungs. Depending on the types of injury and inflammatory response, bronchiolitis is classified as necrotizing, suppurative, catarrhal (mucous metaplasia), or granulomatous.

Repair in Acute and Mild Bronchiolar Injury

Once injury to the cells becomes irreversible, bronchiolar ciliated cells degenerate and exfoliate into the bronchiolar lumen, leaving a denuded basement membrane. Repair in the bronchiolar region is similar to but less effective than that in the tracheal or nasal mucosa. Under normal circumstances, recruited phagocytic cells remove exudate and cell debris from the lumina of affected bronchioles, thus preparing the basement membrane to be repopulated with new, undifferentiated cells originating from a rapidly dividing pool of Clara cells. After several days, these proliferating cells fully differentiate into normal bronchiolar ciliated cells (see Fig. 9-49).

Repair in Acute and Severe Bronchiolar Injury

In severe acute injury, such as that caused by aspiration pneumonia, exudate cannot be removed from the basement membrane of bronchioles. The exudate becomes infiltrated by fibroblasts, which form small masses of fibrovascular tissue that develop into well-organized, microscopic polyps inside the bronchiolar lumen. Their external surface eventually becomes covered by ciliated cells. This lesion is referred to as *bronchiolitis obliterans,* and the polyps may become so large as to cause airflow impairment (Fig. 9-52).

Repair in Chronic Bronchiolar Injury

In mild but persistent bronchiolar injury, goblet cells normally absent from bronchioles proliferate from basal cells, resulting in goblet cell metaplasia and causing a profound alteration in the physicochemical properties of bronchiolar secretions (Fig. 9-53). The normally serous bronchiolar fluid released by Clara cells becomes a tenacious material when mucus produced by goblet cells is added. As a result of increased viscoelasticity of the mucus, bronchiolar secretions cannot be removed effectively by ciliary action, leading to plugging and obstruction of distal airways. Under such conditions, often grouped as chronic obstructive pulmonary disease, coughing is required to clear mucus from obstructed bronchioles. Pulmonary emphysema and atelectasis are further sequelae to bronchiolar metaplasia and mucous hypersecretion blocking or partially blocking the lumens of these bronchioles. These two inflation abnormalities are characteristically present in COPD, which is called "heaves" in horses. Peribronchiolar proliferation of lymphocytes (BALT hyperplasia) is also a common microscopic lesion seen in chronic bronchiolitis.

Recurrent Airway Obstruction in Horses

Recurrent airway obstruction (RAO) of horses, such as COPD, heaves, chronic bronchiolitis-emphysema complex, chronic small airway disease, alveolar emphysema, and "broken wind," is a common clinically asthma-like syndrome of horses and ponies, characterized by recurrent respiratory distress, chronic cough, poor athletic performance, airway neutrophilia, bronchoconstriction, mucus hypersecretion, and airway obstruction. The pathogenesis is still obscure, but genetic predisposition, T_H2 (allergic) immune response, and the exceptional sensitivity of airways to environmental allergens (hyperreactive airway disease) have been postulated as the basic underlying mechanisms. What makes small airways hyperreactive to allergens is still a matter of controversy. Epidemiologic and experimental studies suggest that it could be the result of preceding bronchiolar damage caused by viral infections; ingestion of pneumotoxicants (3-methylindole); or prolonged exposure to

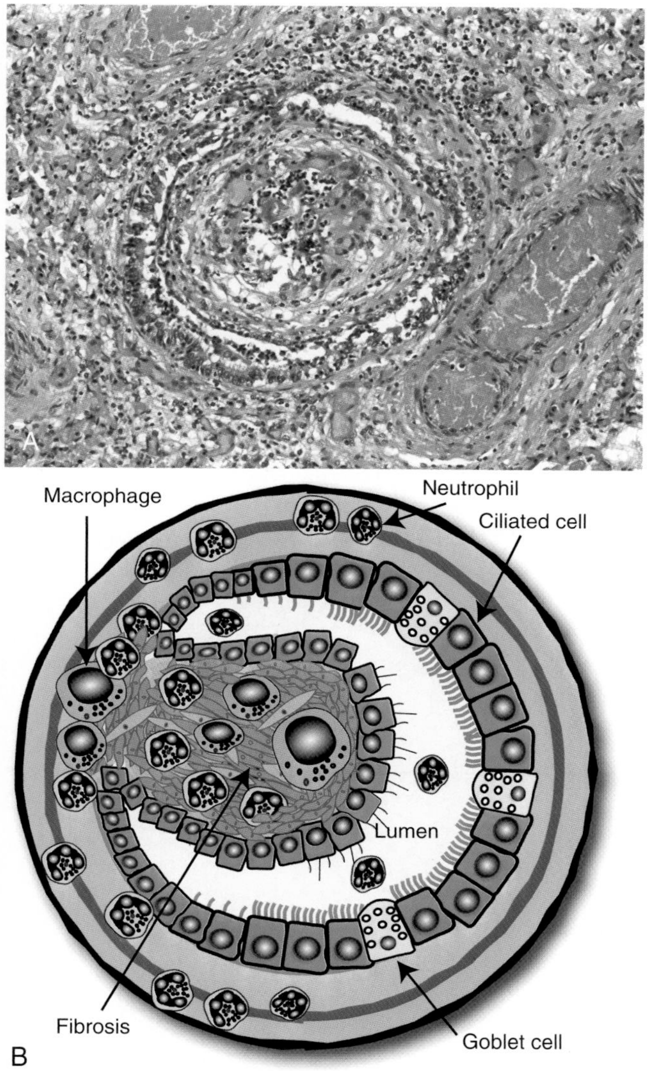

Fig. 9-52 Bronchiolitis obliterans.
A, Chronic inflammation in the bronchiolar wall resulting in the formation of a nodular mass of granulation tissue firmly attached to the airway wall and protruding into the bronchiolar lumen. H&E stain. **B,** Diagram illustrating organized exudate formed by connective tissue, macrophages, lymphocytes, and neutrophils, which is attached to the bronchiolar wall and covered by respiratory ciliated cells. (**A** courtesy Dr. A. López, Atlantic Veterinary College and Dr. Dominique Fournier, Ministère de l'Agriculture, des Pêcheries et de l'Alimentation, Quebec. **B** courtesy Dr. A. López, Atlantic Veterinary College.)

organic dust, endotoxin, and environmental allergens (molds). It has been postulated that sustained inhalation of dust particles, whether antigenic or not, up-regulates the production of cytokines (TNF-α, IL-8, and monokine-inducible protein [MIP-2]) and neuropeptides (neurokinin A [NKA], neurokinin B [NKB], and substance P), attracting neutrophils into the bronchioloalveolar region and promoting leukocyte-induced bronchiolar injury. Summer pasture-associated obstructive pulmonary disease (SPAOPD) is a seasonal airway disease also reported in horses with similar clinical and pathologic findings. More recently, the term *inflammatory airway disease* has been introduced in equine medicine to describe RAO-like syndrome in young horses 2 to 4 years old.

The lungs of horses with heaves are grossly unremarkable, except for extreme cases in which alveolar emphysema may be present. Microscopically, the lesions include goblet cell metaplasia in bronchioles; plugging of bronchioles with mucus mixed with a few eosinophils (see Fig. 9-53); peribronchiolar infiltration with lymphocytes, plasma cells, and variable numbers of eosinophils; and hypertrophy of smooth muscle in bronchi and bronchioles. In severe cases, accumulation of mucus leads to the complete obstruction of bronchioles and alveoli, and resultant alveolar emphysema characterized by enlarged "alveoli" from the destruction of alveolar walls.

Airway Hyperresponsiveness

Airway hyperresponsiveness, or hyperreactive airway disease, is another sequela of bronchiolar injury. It develops in humans and animals (experimentally) after a transient and often innocuous viral infection of the lower respiratory tract or from exposure to certain allergens. Experimental work has shown that airway hyperreactivity in postviral bronchiolitis is associated with increased expression of TLRs and unusual susceptibility to inhaled endotoxin. Hyperreactive animals typically have an increased number of mast cells, eosinophils, and T lymphocytes in the airway mucosa. Clinically, airway hyperresponsiveness is characterized by an exaggerated bronchoconstriction after exposure to mild stimuli, such as cold air, or after animals are exposed to aerosols of histamine or methacholine.

Feline Asthma Syndrome

Feline asthma syndrome, also known as *feline allergic bronchitis,* is a clinical syndrome in cats of any age characterized by recurrent episodes of bronchoconstriction, cough, or dyspnea. The pathogenesis is not well understood but is presumed to originate, as in human asthma, as a type I hypersensitivity (IgE–mast cell reaction) to inhaled allergens. Dust, cigarette smoke, plant and household materials, and parasitic proteins have been incriminated as possible allergens. This self-limited allergic disease responds well to steroid therapy; thus it is rarely implicated as a primary cause of death except when suppressed defense mechanisms allow a secondary bacterial pneumonia. Bronchial biopsies from affected cats at the early stages reveal mild-to-moderate inflammation characterized by mucosal edema and infiltration of leukocytes, particularly eosinophils. Increased numbers of circulating eosinophil leukocytes (blood eosinophilia) are present in some but not all cats with feline asthma. In the most advanced cases, chronic bronchoconstriction and excess mucus production may result in smooth muscle hyperplasia and obstruction of the bronchi and bronchioles and infiltration of the airway mucosa by eosinophils. A syndrome known as *canine asthma* has been reported in dogs but is not as well characterized as the feline counterpart.

Alveoli

Because of their extremely delicate structure, alveoli are quite vulnerable to injury once the local defense mechanisms have been overwhelmed. The alveolar wall is a thin membrane formed by a core of interstitium supporting an extensive network of alveolar capillaries. Fibroblasts (septal cells), myofibroblasts, collagen, elastic fibers, and few interstitial macrophages and mast cells constitute the alveolar interstitium. The wall of the alveolar capillaries facing the airspace is remarkably thin and has three layers composed of vascular endothelium, basal lamina, and alveolar epithelium. These three layers of the alveolar capillaries constitute what is customarily referred to as the *blood-air barrier* (see Fig. 9-7). The epithelial side of the alveolus is primarily lined by rather thin type I pneumonocytes, which are arranged as a very delicate continuous membrane extending along the alveolar surface (see Fig. 9-7). Type

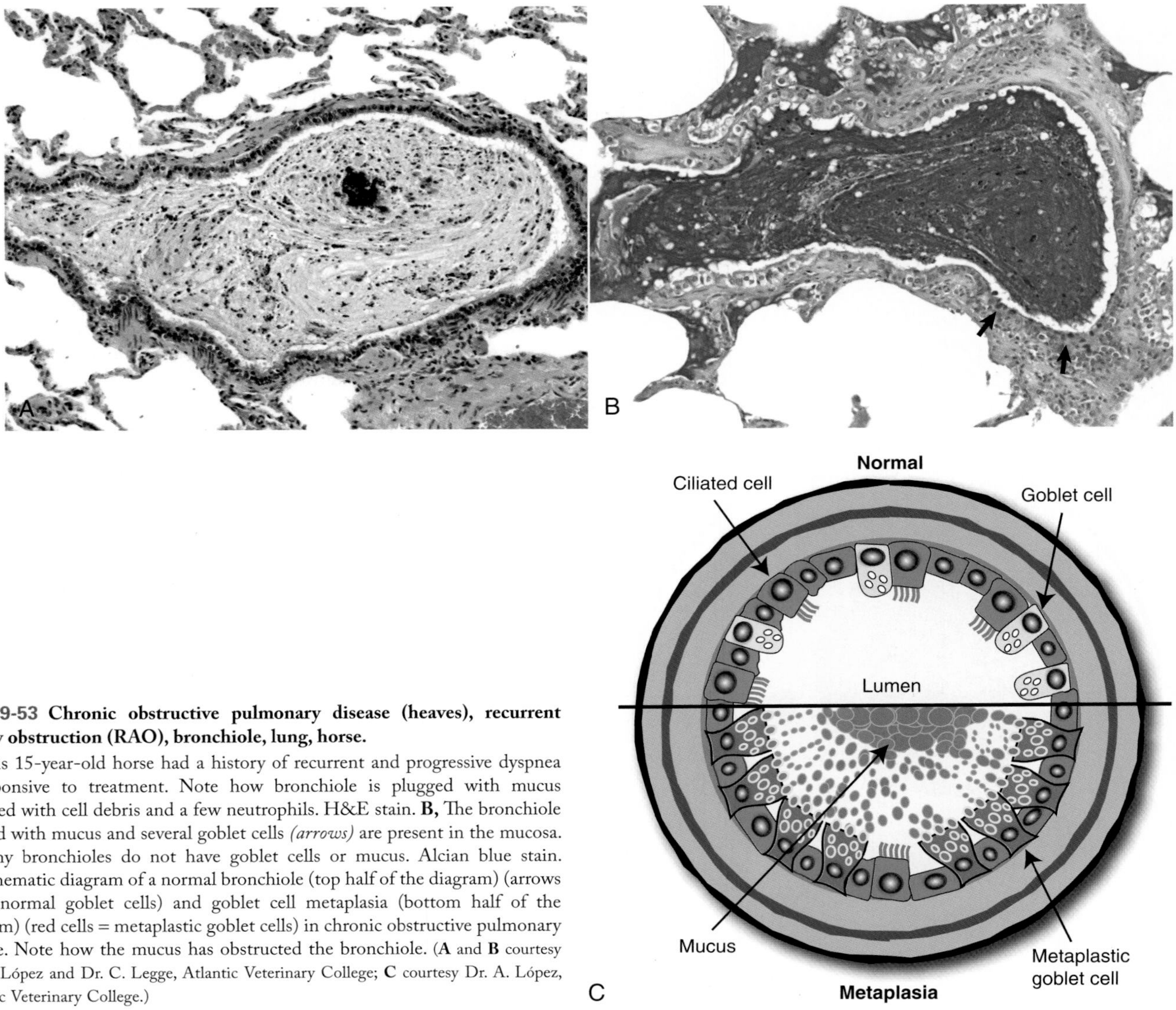

Fig. 9-53 Chronic obstructive pulmonary disease (heaves), recurrent airway obstruction (RAO), bronchiole, lung, horse.
A, This 15-year-old horse had a history of recurrent and progressive dyspnea unresponsive to treatment. Note how bronchiole is plugged with mucus admixed with cell debris and a few neutrophils. H&E stain. **B,** The bronchiole is filled with mucus and several goblet cells *(arrows)* are present in the mucosa. Healthy bronchioles do not have goblet cells or mucus. Alcian blue stain. **C,** Schematic diagram of a normal bronchiole (top half of the diagram) (arrows show normal goblet cells) and goblet cell metaplasia (bottom half of the diagram) (red cells = metaplastic goblet cells) in chronic obstructive pulmonary disease. Note how the mucus has obstructed the bronchiole. (**A** and **B** courtesy Dr. A. López and Dr. C. Legge, Atlantic Veterinary College; **C** courtesy Dr. A. López, Atlantic Veterinary College.)

I pneumonocytes are particularly susceptible to noxious agents that reach the alveolar region either aerogenously or hematogenously. Injury to type I pneumonocytes rapidly causes swelling and vacuolation of these cells. When cellular damage has become irreversible, type I cells detach, resulting in denudation of the basement membrane, increased alveolar permeability, and alveolar edema. Alveolar repair is possible as long as the basement membrane remains intact and lesions are not complicated by further injury or infection. Within 3 days, cuboidal type II (granular) pneumonocytes, which are the precursor cells and more resistant to injury, undergo mitosis and provide a large pool of new undifferentiated cells (Fig. 9-54). These new cells repave the denuded alveolar basement membrane and finally differentiate in type I pneumonocytes. When alveolar injury is diffuse, proliferation of type II pneumonocytes becomes so spectacular that the microscopic appearance of the alveolus resembles that of a gland or fetal lung; the lesion has been termed *epithelialization* or f*etalization.* Although it is part of the normal alveolar repair, hyperplasia of type II pneumonocytes can interfere in gas exchange and cause hypoxemia. In uncomplicated cases, type II pneumonocytes eventually differentiate into type I pneumonocytes, thus completing the last stage of alveolar repair. In some forms of chronic interstitial lung injury the surface of the alveolar basement membrane could become populated with migrating bronchiolar cells, a process known as alveolar *bronchiolization* or *lambertosis.* In severe cases, lambertosis, a metaplastic change, can be mistaken microscopically with alveolar adenomas.

Type I pneumonocytes are one of the three structural components of the blood-air barrier, so when these epithelial cells are damaged, there is an increase in alveolar capillary permeability and transient leakage of plasma fluid, proteins, and fibrin into the alveolar lumen. Under normal circumstances, these fluids are rapidly cleared from the alveolus by alveolar and lymphatic absorption, and necrotic pneumonocytes (type I) and fibrin strands are phagocytosed and removed by pulmonary alveolar macrophages. When there is persistent and severe injury, fibroblasts and myofibroblasts may proliferate in the alveolar walls (alveolar interstitium), causing alveolar fibrosis, whereas in other forms of severe injury, fibroblasts and myofibroblasts actively migrate from the interstitium into the alveolar spaces, causing intraalveolar fibrosis. These two types of alveolar fibrosis are most commonly seen in toxic and allergic pulmonary diseases, and this alveolar fibrosis has a devastating effect on lung function.

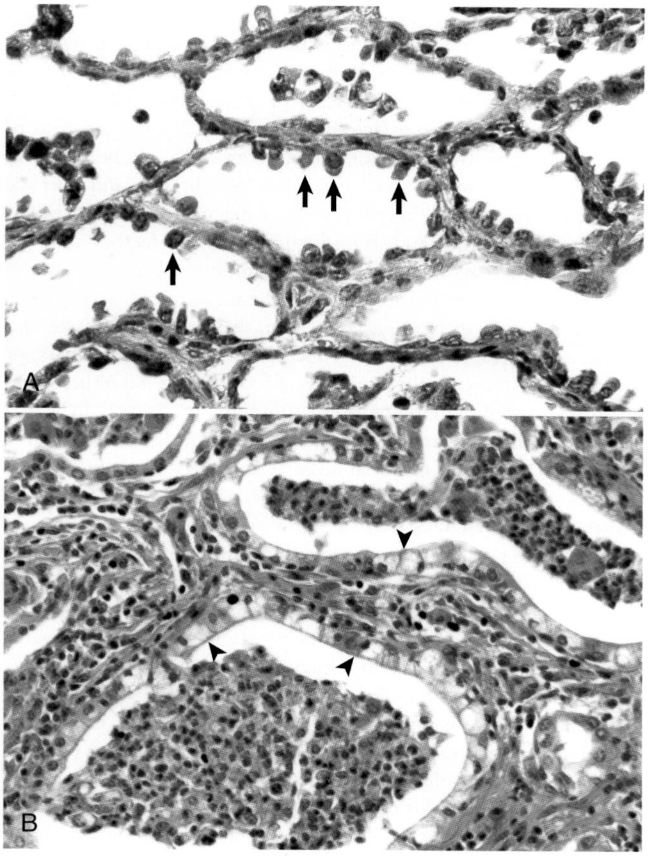

Fig. 9-54 Hyperplasia of type II pneumonocytes. **A,** Acute alveolar injury, crude oil aspiration, cow. Note proliferation of cuboidal epithelial cells (type II pneumonocytes) *(arrows)* along the luminal surface of the alveolar wall. During alveolar repair, type II pneumocytes are the precursor cell for necrotic and lost type I pneumonocytes. **B,** Chronic alveolar injury, interstitial pneumonia, horse. Note entire alveolar membrane lined with cuboidal type II pneumonocytes *(arrowheads)*. The alveolar interstitium is expanded with inflammatory cells and the alveolar lumens contain cell debris mixed with leukocytes. (**A** courtesy Dr. A. López, Atlantic Veterinary College. **B** courtesy Drs. G. Hines, Provincial Veterinary Laboratory, New Brunswick and A. López, Atlantic Veterinary College.)

Endothelial cells are also major players in the normal and abnormal physiology of the alveolus. These cells trap and share circulating antigens with intravascular and interstitial macrophages. The junction between alveolar endothelial cells is not as tight as that of the type I pneumonocytes, allowing some movement of fluid and small size molecular weight proteins into the alveolar interstitium. Endothelial cells maintain an intimate cell contact with erythrocytes and leukocytes passing through the lung, since the lumen of alveolar capillaries is slightly smaller (5.0 μm) than the diameter of red and white blood cells. Erythrocytes are easily deformable, so their transit time through the alveolar capillaries is shorter than leukocytes, which are less deformable cells. This longer transit time of leukocytes and their close cellular contact with alveolar endothelial cells has major impact in lung inflammation and ARDS.

On a minute-to-minute basis, the pulmonary defense mechanisms deal effectively with noxious stimuli and mild tissue injury without the need for an inflammatory response. However, if normal defense mechanisms are ineffective or insufficient (overwhelmed), the inflammatory process is rapidly turned on as a second line of defense.

General Aspects of Lung Inflammation

In the past three decades, an information explosion has increased the overall understanding of pulmonary inflammation, with so many proinflammatory and antiinflammatory mediators described to date that it would be impossible to review them all here (see Chapters 3 and 5).

Pulmonary inflammation is a highly regulated process that involves a complex interaction between cells imported from the blood (platelets, neutrophils, eosinophils, mast cells, and lymphocytes) and pulmonary cells (type I and II pneumonocytes; endothelial and Clara cells; alveolar and intravascular macrophages; and stromal interstitial cells, such as mast cells, interstitial macrophages, fibroblasts, and myofibroblasts). Blood-borne leukocytes, platelets, and plasma proteins are brought into the areas of inflammation by an elaborate network of chemical signals emitted by pulmonary cells and resident leukocytes. Long-distance communication between pulmonary cells and blood cells is largely done by soluble cytokines; once in the lung, imported leukocytes communicate with pulmonary and vascular cells through adhesion and other inflammatory molecules. The best known inflammatory mediators are the complement system (C3a, C3b, and C5a), coagulation factors (factors V, VII), arachidonic acid metabolites (leukotrienes and prostaglandins), cytokines (interleukins, monokines, and chemokines), adhesion molecules (ICAM, VCAM), neuropeptides (substance P, tachykinins, and neurokinins), enzymes and enzyme inhibitors (elastase, antitrypsin), oxygen metabolites (O_2•, OH•, H_2O_2), antioxidants (glutathione), and nitric oxide (Web Table 9-1). Acting in concert, these and many other molecules send positive or negative signals to initiate, maintain, and hopefully resolve the inflammatory process without causing injury to the lung.

Pulmonary macrophages (alveolar, intravascular, and interstitial), which have an immense biologic armamentarium, are the single most important effector cell and source of cytokines for all stages of pulmonary inflammation. These all-purpose phagocytic cells modulate the recruitment and trafficking of blood-borne leukocytes in the lung through the secretion of chemokines (see Web Table 9-1).

Before reviewing how inflammatory cells are recruited in the lungs, three significant features in pulmonary injury must be remembered: (1) leukocytes can exit the vascular system through the alveolar capillaries, unlike in other tissues, where postcapillary venules are the sites of leukocytic diapedesis (extravasation); (2) the intact lung contains within alveolar capillaries a large pool of resident leukocytes (marginal pool); and (3) additional neutrophils are sequestered within alveolar capillaries within minutes of local or systemic inflammatory response. These three pulmonary idiosyncrasies, along with the enormous length of the capillary network in the lung, explain why recruitment and migration of leukocytes into alveolar spaces develops so rapidly. Experimental studies with aerosols of endotoxin or Gram-negative bacteria have shown that within minutes of exposure, there is a significant increase in capillary leukocytes, and by 4 hours the alveolar lumen is filled with neutrophils. Not surprisingly, the BAL fluid collected from patients with acute pneumonia contains large amounts of inflammatory mediators such as TNF-α, IL-1, and IL-8. Also, the capillary endothelium of patients with acute pneumonia has increased "expression" of adhesion molecules, which facilitate the migration of leukocytes from capillaries into the alveolar interstitium and from there into the alveolar lumen. In allergic pulmonary diseases, eotaxin and IL-5 are primarily responsible for recruitment and trafficking of eosinophils in the lung (see Web Table 9-1).

Movement of plasma proteins into the pulmonary interstitium and alveolar lumen is a common but poorly understood phenomenon in pulmonary inflammation. Leakage of fibrinogen and plasma proteins into the alveolar space occurs when there is structural damage to the blood-air barrier. This leakage is also promoted by some types of cytokines that enhance procoagulant activity, whereas others reduce fibrinolytic activity. Excessive exudation of fibrin into the alveoli is particularly common in ruminants and pigs. The fibrinolytic system plays a major role in the resolution of pulmonary inflammatory diseases. In some cases, excessive plasma proteins leaked into alveoli mix with necrotic type I pneumonocytes and pulmonary surfactant, forming microscopic eosinophilic bands (membranes) along the lining of alveolar septa. These membranes, known as *hyaline membranes,* are found in specific types of pulmonary diseases, particularly in ARDS, and in cattle with acute interstitial pneumonias such as bovine pulmonary edema and emphysema and extrinsic allergic alveolitis (see Figs. 9-37 and 9-45).

In the last few years, nitric oxide has been identified as a major regulatory molecule of inflammation in a variety of tissues, including the lung. Produced locally by macrophages, pulmonary endothelium, and pneumonocytes, nitric oxide regulates the vascular and bronchial tone, modulates the production of cytokines, controls the recruitment and trafficking of neutrophils in the lung, and switches on/off genes involved in inflammation and immunity. Experimental work has also shown that pulmonary surfactant upregulates the production of nitric oxide in the lung, supporting the current view that pneumonocytes are also pivotal in amplifying and downregulating the inflammatory and immune responses in the lung (see Web Table 9-1).

As the inflammatory process becomes chronic, the types of cells making up cellular infiltrates in the lung change from mainly neutrophils to largely mononuclear cells. This shift in cellular composition is accompanied by an increase in specific cytokines, such as IL-4, interferon-γ (IFN-γ), and interferon-inducible protein (IP-10), which are chemotactic for lymphocytes and macrophages. Under appropriate conditions, these cytokines activate T lymphocytes, regulate granulomatous inflammation, and induce the formation of multinucleated giant cells such as in mycobacterial infections.

Inflammatory mediators locally released from inflamed lungs also have a biologic effect in other tissue. For example, pulmonary hypertension and right-sided heart failure (cor pulmonale) often follows chronic alveolar inflammation, not only as a result of increased pulmonary blood pressure but also from the effect of inflammatory mediators on the contractibility of smooth muscle of the pulmonary and systemic vasculature. Cytokines, particularly TNF-α, which are released during inflammation are associated, both as cause and effect, with the systemic inflammatory response syndrome (SIRS), sepsis, severe sepsis with multiple organ dysfunction, and septic shock (cardiopulmonary collapse).

As it occurs in any other sentinel system where many biologic promoters and inhibitors are involved (coagulation, the complement and immune systems), the inflammatory cascade could go into an "out-of-control" state, causing severe damage to the lungs. Acute lung injury (ALI), extrinsic allergic alveolitis, ARDS, pulmonary fibrosis, and asthma are archetypical diseases that ensue from an uncontrolled production and release of cytokines.

As long as acute alveolar injury is transient and there is no interference with the normal host response, the entire process of injury, degeneration, necrosis, inflammation, and repair can occur in less than 1 week. On the other hand, when acute alveolar injury becomes persistent or when the capacity of the host for repair is impaired, lesions can progress to an irreversible stage in which restoration of alveolar structure is no longer possible. In diseases, such as extrinsic allergic alveolitis, the constant release of proteolytic enzymes and free radicals by phagocytic cells perpetuates alveolar damage in a vicious circle. In other cases, such as in paraquat toxicity, the magnitude of alveolar injury can be so severe that type II pneumonocytes, basement membranes, and alveolar interstitium are so disrupted that the capacity for alveolar repair is lost. Fibronectins and transforming growth factors (TGFs) released from macrophages and other mononuclear cells at the site of chronic inflammation regulate the recruitment, attachment, and proliferation of fibroblasts. In turn, these cells synthesize and release considerable amounts of ECM (collagen, elastic fibers, or proteoglycans), eventually leading to fibrosis and total obliteration of normal alveolar architecture. In summary, in diseases in which there is chronic and irreversible alveolar damage, lesions invariably progress to a stage of terminal alveolar and interstitial fibrosis.

Alveolar Filling Disorders

Alveolar filling disorders are a heterogeneous group of lung diseases characterized by accumulation of various chemical compounds in the alveolar lumens. The most common are alveolar proteinosis in which the alveoli are filled with finely granular eosinophilic material; alveolar microlithiasis in which the alveoli contain numerous concentric calcified "microliths" or "calcospherites." A similar but distinct concretion is known as *corpora amylacea,* which is an accumulation of cholesterol (cholesterol pneumonitis) or lipids (endogenous lipid pneumonia; see the section on Other Pneumonias of Cats). There is often little host response, and in many cases, it is only an incidental finding. Some of the alveolar filling disorders originate from inherited metabolic defects in which alveolar cells (epithelial or macrophages) cannot properly metabolize or remove lipids or proteins while others result from an excessive synthesis of these substances in the lung.

Classification of Pneumonias

Few subjects in veterinary pathology have caused so much debate as the classification of pneumonias. Historically, pneumonias in animals have been classified or named based on the following:

1. Presumed cause, with names such as viral pneumonia, Pasteurella pneumonia, distemper pneumonia, verminous pneumonia, chemical pneumonia, and hypersensitivity pneumonitis
2. Type of exudation, with names such as suppurative pneumonia, fibrinous pneumonia, and pyogranulomatous pneumonia
3. Morphologic features, with names such as gangrenous pneumonia, proliferative pneumonia, and embolic pneumonia
4. Distribution of lesions, with names such as focal pneumonia, cranioventral pneumonia, diffuse pneumonia, and lobar pneumonia
5. Epidemiologic attributes, with names such as enzootic pneumonia, contagious bovine pleuropneumonia, and "shipping fever"
6. Geographic regions, with names such as Montana progressive pneumonia
7. Miscellaneous attributes, with names such as atypical pneumonia, cuffing pneumonia, progressive pneumonia, aspiration pneumonia, pneumonitis, farmer's lung, and extrinsic allergic alveolitis

Until a universal and systematic nomenclature for animal pneumonias are established, veterinarians should be acquainted with this heterogeneous list of names and should be well aware that one disease may be known by different names. In pigs, for instance,

TABLE 9-5 Morphologic Types of Pneumonias in Domestic Animals

Type of Pneumonia	Port of Entry (e.g., Pathogens)	Distribution of Lesions	Texture of Lung	Grossly Visible Exudate	Disease Example	Common Pulmonary Sequelae
Bronchopneumonia: Suppurative (lobular)	Aerogenous (bacteria and mycoplasmas)	Cranioventral consolidation	Firm	Purulent exudate in bronchi	Enzootic pneumonia	Cranioventral abscesses, adhesions, bronchiectasis
Bronchopneumonia: Fibrinous (lobar)	Aerogenous (bacteria and mycoplasmas)	Cranioventral consolidation*	Hard	Fibrin in lung and pleura	Pneumonic Mannheimiosis	BALT hyperplasia, "sequestra," pleural adhesions, abscesses
Interstitial pneumonia	Aerogenous or hematogenous (virus, toxin, allergen, sepsis)	Diffuse	Elastic with rib imprints	Not visible, trapped in alveolar septa	Influenza, extrinsic allergic alveolitis, PRRS, ARDS	Edema, emphysema, type II alveolar hyperplasia, alveolar fibrosis
Granulomatous pneumonia	Aerogenous or hematogenous (mycobacteria, systemic mycoses)	Multifocal	Nodular	Pyogranulomatous, caseous necrosis, calcified nodules	Tuberculosis, blastomycosis, cryptococcosis	Dissemination of infection to lymph nodes and distant organs
Embolic pneumonia	Hematogenous (septic emboli)	Multifocal	Nodular	Purulent foci surrounded by hyperemia	Vegetative endocarditis, ruptured liver abscess	Abscesses randomly distributed in all pulmonary lobes

ARDS, Adult respiratory distress syndrome; *BALT,* bronchial-associated lymphoid tissue; *PRRS,* porcine reproductive and respiratory syndrome.
*Porcine pleuropneumonia is an exception because it often involves the caudal lobes.

enzootic pneumonia, virus pneumonia, and *Mycoplasma* pneumonia all refer to the same disease caused by *Mycoplasma hyopneumoniae* (Table 9-5).

The word *pneumonitis* has been used by some as a synonym for pneumonia; however, others have restricted this term to chronic proliferative inflammation generally involving the alveolar interstitium and with little or no evidence of exudate. In this chapter, the word *pneumonia* is used for any inflammatory lesion in the lungs, regardless of whether it is exudative or proliferative, alveolar, or interstitial.

On the basis of texture, distribution, appearance, and exudation, pneumonias can be grossly diagnosed into four morphologically distinct types: bronchopneumonia, interstitial pneumonia, embolic pneumonia, and granulomatous pneumonia. By using this classification, it is possible to predict with some degree of certainty the likely cause (virus, bacteria, fungi, or parasites), routes of entry (aerogenous versus hematogenous), and possible sequelae. These four morphologic types allow the clinician or pathologists to predict the most likely etiology and therefore facilitate the decision as to what samples need to be taken and which tests should be requested to the diagnostic laboratory (i.e., histopathology, bacteriology, virology, or toxicology). However, overlapping of these four types of pneumonias is possible, and sometimes two morphologic types may be present in the same lung.

The criteria used to classify pneumonias grossly into bronchopneumonia, interstitial pneumonia, embolic pneumonia, and granulomatous pneumonia are based on morphologic changes, including distribution, texture, color, and general appearance of the affected lungs (see Table 9-5). Distribution of the inflammatory lesions in the lungs can be (1) cranioventral, as in most bronchopneumonias; (2) multifocal, as in embolic pneumonias; (3) diffuse, as in interstitial pneumonias; or (4) locally extensive, as in granulomatous pneumonias (Fig. 9-55). Texture of pneumonic lungs can be firmer or harder (bronchopneumonias), more elastic (rubbery) than normal lungs (interstitial pneumonias), or have a nodular feeling (granulomatous pneumonias). Describing in words the palpable difference between the texture of a normal lung compared with the firm or hard texture of a consolidated lung can be a difficult undertaking. An analogy illustrating this difference based on touching the parts of the face with the tip of your finger has been advocated by some pathologists. The texture of a normal lung is comparable to the texture of the center of the cheek. Firm consolidation is comparable to the texture of the tip of the nose, and hard consolidation is comparable to the texture of the forehead. The term *consolidation* is frequently used to describe a firm or hard lung filled with exudate.

Changes in the appearance of pneumonic lungs include abnormal color, presence of nodules or exudate, fibrinous or fibrous adhesions, and presence of rib imprints on serosal surfaces (see Fig. 9-55). On cut surfaces, pneumonic lungs may have exudate, hemorrhage, edema, necrosis, abscesses, bronchiectasis, granulomas or pyogranulomas, and fibrosis, depending on the stage.

Palpation and careful observation of the lungs are essential in the diagnosis of pneumonia. (For details, see the section on Examination of the Respiratory Tract.)

Bronchopneumonia

Bronchopneumonia refers to a particular type of pneumonia in which injury and the inflammatory process take place primarily in the bronchial, bronchiolar, and alveolar lumens. Bronchopneumonia is undoubtedly the most common type of pneumonia seen in domestic animals and is with few exceptions characterized by

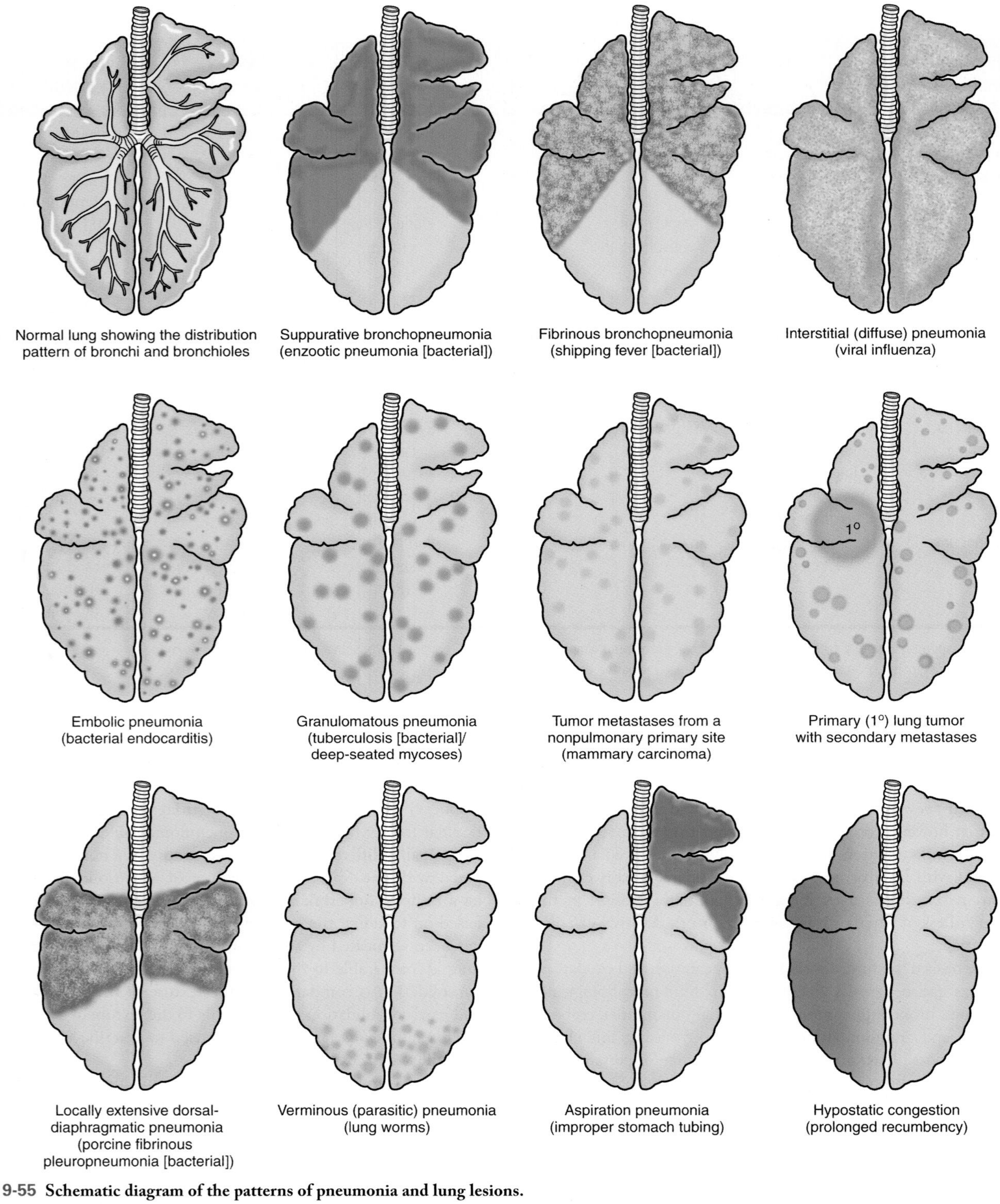

Fig. 9-55 Schematic diagram of the patterns of pneumonia and lung lesions.
A dorsal view of the bovine lung illustrates these patterns. They can readily be extrapolated to the lungs of other domestic animal species. (Courtesy Drs. A. López, Atlantic Veterinary College and J.F. Zachary, College of Veterinary Medicine, University of Illinois.)

craniovental consolidation of the lungs (Fig. 9-56). The reason why bronchopneumonias in animals are almost always restricted to the cranioventral portions of the lungs is not well understood. Possible factors contributing to this topographic selectivity within the lungs include (1) gravitational sedimentation of the exudate; (2) greater deposition of infectious organisms; (3) inadequate defense mechanisms; (4) reduced vascular perfusion; (5) shortness and abrupt branching of airways; and (6) regional differences in ventilation.

The term *cranioventral* in veterinary anatomy is the equivalent of "anterosuperior" in human anatomy. The latter is defined as "in front (ventral) and above (cranial)." Thus applied to the lung of animals, "cranioventral" means the ventral portion of the cranial lobe. However, by common usage in veterinary pathology, the term

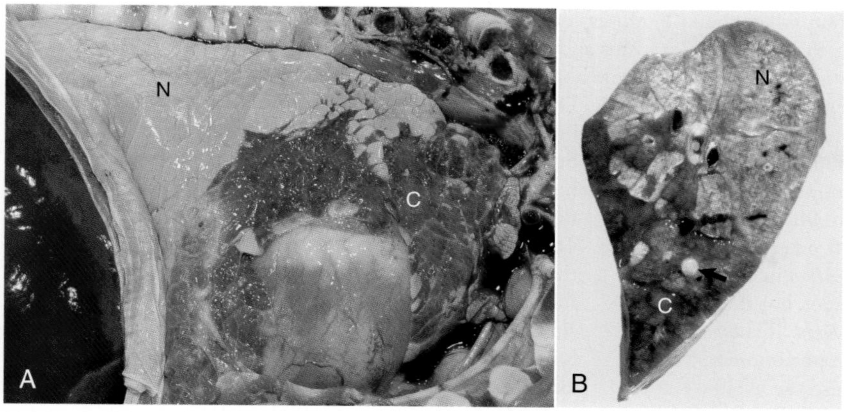

Fig. 9-56 Suppurative bronchopneumonia, enzootic pneumonia, lung, calf.
A, Cranioventral consolidation *(C)* of the lung involves approximately 40% of pulmonary parenchyma. Most of the caudal lung is normal *(N)*. **B,** Cut surface. Consolidated lung is dark red to mahogany *(C)*, and a major bronchus contains purulent exudate *(arrow)*. *N,* Normal. (**A** courtesy Dr. A. López, Atlantic Veterinary College. **B** courtesy Ontario Veterinary College.)

cranioventral used to describe the location of lesions in pneumonias has come to mean "cranial and ventral." Thus it includes pneumonias affecting not only the ventral portion of the cranial lobe (true cranioventral) but also those cases in which the pneumonia has involved the ventral portions of adjacent lung lobes—initially the middle and then caudal on the right and the caudal lobe on the left side.

Bronchopneumonias are generally caused by bacteria and mycoplasmas, by bronchoaspiration of feed or gastric contents, or by improper tubing. As a rule, the pathogens causing bronchopneumonias arrive in the lungs via inspired air (aerogenous), either from infected aerosols or from the nasal flora. Before establishing infection, pathogens must overwhelm or evade the pulmonary defense mechanism. The initial injury in bronchopneumonias is centered on the mucosa of bronchioles; from there, the inflammatory process can spread downward to distal portions of the alveoli and upward to the bronchi. Typically, for bronchopneumonias, the inflammatory exudates collect in the bronchial, bronchiolar, and alveolar lumina leaving the alveolar interstitium unchanged, except for hyperemia. Through the pores of Kohn, the lesions and exudate can spread centripetally to adjacent alveoli until most or all of the alveoli in an individual lobule are involved. If the inflammatory process cannot control the inciting cause of injury, the lesions spread rapidly from lobule to lobule through alveolar pores and destroyed alveolar walls, until an entire lobe or large portion of a lung is involved. The lesion tends to spread centrifugally, with the older lesions in the center, and exudate can be coughed up and then aspirated into other lobules, where the inflammatory process starts again.

At the early stages of bronchopneumonia, the pulmonary vessels are engorged with blood (active hyperemia) and the bronchi, bronchioles, and alveoli contain some fluid (permeability edema). In cases in which pulmonary injury is mild to moderate, cytokines locally released in the lung cause rapid recruitment of neutrophils and alveolar macrophages into bronchioles and alveoli (Fig. 9-57). When pulmonary injury is much more severe, proinflammatory cytokines induce more pronounced vascular changes by further opening endothelial gaps, thus increasing vascular permeability resulting in fibrinous exudates and sometimes hemorrhage in the alveoli. Alterations in permeability can be further exacerbated by structural damage to pulmonary capillaries and vessels directly caused by microbial toxins. The final result of these functional and structural changes is that blood vessels become notably permeable and allow substantial leakage of plasma fluid and proteins (fibrinogen) into the alveoli. Filling of alveoli, bronchioles, and small bronchi with inflammatory exudate progressively obliterates airspaces, and as a consequence of this process, portions of severely

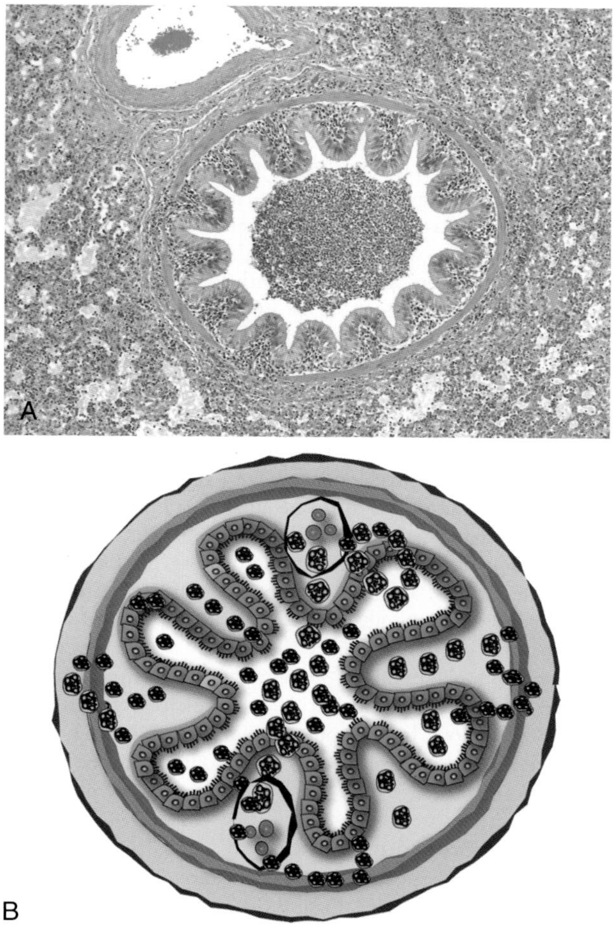

Fig. 9-57 Suppurative bronchopneumonia, lung, pig.
A, Note the bronchiole plugged with purulent exudate. The alveoli are filled with leukocytes and some edematous fluid. H&E stain. **B,** Schematic diagram of acute bronchiolitis. Note the neutrophils exiting the submucosal capillaries (leukocyte adhesion cascade; see Chapter 3) and moving into the walls of the bronchioles (blue cells = ciliated mucosal epithelium) and then into the bronchiolar lumen. (Courtesy Dr. A. López, Atlantic Veterinary College.)

affected (consolidated) lungs sink to the bottom of the container when placed in fixative. The replacement of air by exudate also changes the texture of the lungs, and depending on the severity of bronchopneumonia, the texture varies from firmer to harder than normal.

The term *consolidation* is used at gross examination when the texture of pneumonic lung becomes firmer or harder than normal as a result of loss of airspaces because of exudation and atelectasis. (For details, see the discussion of lung texture in the section on Classification of Pneumonias). Inflammatory consolidation of lungs has been referred to in the past as *hepatization* because the affected lung had the appearance and texture of liver. The process was referred to as *red hepatization* in acute cases in which there was notable active hyperemia with little exudation of neutrophils; conversely, the process was referred to as *gray hepatization* in those chronic cases in which hyperemia was no longer present, but there was abundant exudation of neutrophils and macrophages. This terminology, although used for and applicable to human pneumonias, is rarely used in veterinary medicine primarily because the evolution of pneumonic processes in animals does not necessarily follow the red-to-gray hepatization pattern.

Bronchopneumonias can be arbitrarily subdivided into *suppurative bronchopneumonia* if the exudate is predominantly composed of neutrophils, and *fibrinous bronchopneumonia* if fibrin is the predominant component of the exudate (see Table 9-5). It is important to note that some pathologists use the term *fibrinous pneumonia* or *lobar pneumonia* as a synonym for fibrinous bronchopneumonia and *bronchopneumonia* or *lobular pneumonia* as a synonym for suppurative bronchopneumonia. Human pneumonias for many years have been classified based on their etiology and morphology, which explains why pneumococcal pneumonia *(Streptococcus pneumoniae)* has been synonymous with lobar pneumonia. In the old literature, four distinct stages of pneumococcal pneumonia were described as (1) congestion, (2) red hepatization (liver texture), (3) grey hepatization, and (4) resolution. Because of the use of effective antibiotics and prevention, pneumococcal pneumonia and its four classic stages are rarely seen, thus this terminology has been largely abandoned. Currently, the term *bronchopneumonia* is widely used for both suppurative and fibrinous consolidation of the lungs because both forms of inflammation have essentially the same pathogenesis in which the pathogens reach the lung by the aerogenous route, injury occurs initially in the bronchial and bronchiolar regions, and the inflammatory process extends centrifugally deep into the alveoli. It must be emphasized that it is the severity of pulmonary injury that largely determines whether bronchopneumonia becomes suppurative or fibrinous. In some instances, however, it is difficult to discriminate between suppurative and fibrinous bronchopneumonia because both types can coexist (fibrinosuppurative bronchopneumonia), and one type can progress to the other.

Suppurative Bronchopneumonia

Suppurative bronchopneumonia is characterized by cranioventral consolidation of lungs (see Figs. 9-56 and 9-57), with typically purulent or mucopurulent exudate present in the airways. This exudate can be best demonstrated by expressing intrapulmonary bronchi, thus forcing exudate out of the bronchi (see Fig. 9-56). The inflammatory process in suppurative bronchopneumonia is generally confined to individual lobules, and as a result of this distribution, the lobular pattern of the lung becomes notably emphasized. This pattern is particularly obvious in cattle and pigs because these species have prominent lobulation of the lungs. The gross appearance often resembles an irregular checkerboard because of an admixture of normal and abnormal (consolidated) lobules (see Fig. 9-56). Because of this typical lobular distribution, suppurative bronchopneumonias are also referred to as lobular pneumonias.

Different inflammatory phases occur in suppurative bronchopneumonia where the color and appearance of consolidated lungs varies considerably, depending on the virulence of offending organisms and chronicity of the lesion. The typical phases of suppurative bronchopneumonia could be summarized as follows:

1. During the first 12 hours when bacteria are rapidly multiplying, the lungs become hyperemic and edematous.
2. Soon after, neutrophils start filling the airways and by 48 hours the parenchyma starts to consolidate and becomes firm in texture.
3. Three to 5 days later, hyperemic changes are less obvious, but the bronchial, bronchiolar, and alveolar spaces continue to fill with neutrophils and macrophages, and the affected lung sinks when placed in formalin. At this stage, the affected lung has a gray-pink color, and on cut surface, purulent exudate can be expressed from bronchi.
4. In favorable conditions where the infection is under control of the host defense mechanisms, the inflammatory processes begin to regress, a phase known as *resolution.* Complete resolution in favorable conditions could take 1 to 2 weeks.
5. In animals in which the lung infection cannot be rapidly contained, inflammatory lesions can progress into a chronic phase. Around 7 to 10 days after infection, the lungs become pale gray and take a "fish flesh" appearance. This appearance is the result of purulent and catarrhal inflammation, obstructive atelectasis, mononuclear cell infiltration, peribronchial and peribronchiolar lymphoid hyperplasia, and early alveolar fibrosis.

Complete resolution is unusual in chronic bronchopneumonia, and lung scars, such as pleural and pulmonary fibrosis; bronchiectasis as a consequence of chronic destructive bronchitis (see bronchiectasis); atelectasis; pleural adhesions; and lung abscesses may remain unresolved for a long time. "Enzootic pneumonias" of ruminants and pigs are typical examples of chronic suppurative bronchopneumonias.

Microscopically, acute suppurative bronchopneumonias are characterized by hyperemia, abundant neutrophils, macrophages, and cellular debris within the lumen of bronchi, bronchioles, and alveoli (see Fig. 9-57). Recruitment of leukocytes is promoted by cytokines, complement, and other chemotactic factors that are released in response to alveolar injury or by the chemotactic effect of bacterial toxins, particularly endotoxin. In most severe cases, purulent or mucopurulent exudates completely obliterate the entire lumen of bronchi, bronchioles, and alveoli.

If suppurative bronchopneumonia is merely the response to a transient pulmonary injury or a mild infection, lesions resolve uneventfully. Within 7 to 10 days, cellular exudate can be removed from the lungs via the mucociliary escalator, and complete resolution may take place within 4 weeks. In other cases, if injury or infection is persistent, suppurative bronchopneumonia can become chronic with goblet cell hyperplasia, an important component of the inflammatory process. Depending on the proportion of pus and mucus, the exudate in chronic suppurative bronchopneumonia varies from mucopurulent to mucoid. A mucoid exudate is found in the more chronic stages when the consolidated lung has a "fish flesh" appearance.

Hyperplasia of BALT is another change commonly seen in chronic suppurative bronchopneumonias; it appears grossly as conspicuous white nodules (cuffs) around bronchial walls (cuffing pneumonia). This hyperplastic change merely indicates a normal reaction of lymphoid tissue to infection. Further sequelae of chronic suppurative bronchopneumonia include bronchiectasis (see Fig. 9-51), pulmonary abscesses, pleural adhesions (from pleuritis), and atelectasis and emphysema from completely or partially obstructed bronchi or bronchioles (e.g., bronchiectasis).

Clinically, suppurative bronchopneumonias can be acute and fulminating but are often chronic, depending on the etiologic agent, stressors affecting the host, and immune status. The most common pathogens causing suppurative bronchopneumonia in domestic animals include *Pasteurella multocida, Bordetella bronchiseptica, Arcanobacterium (Actinomyces) pyogenes, Streptococcus* spp., *Escherichia coli*, and several species of mycoplasmas. Most of these organisms are secondary pathogens requiring a preceding impairment of the pulmonary defense mechanisms to allow them to colonize the lungs and establish an infection. Suppurative bronchopneumonia can also result from aspiration of bland material (e.g., milk). Pulmonary gangrene may ensue when the bronchopneumonic lung is invaded by saprophytic bacteria (aspiration pneumonia).

Fibrinous Bronchopneumonia

Fibrinous bronchopneumonia is similar to suppurative bronchopneumonia except that the predominant exudate is fibrinous rather than neutrophilic. With only a few exceptions, fibrinous bronchopneumonias also have a cranioventral distribution (Fig. 9-58; see Fig. 9-55). However, exudation is not restricted to the boundaries of individual pulmonary lobules, as is the case in suppurative bronchopneumonias. Instead the inflammatory process in fibrinous pneumonias involves numerous contiguous lobules and the exudate moves quickly through pulmonary tissue until the entire pulmonary lobe is rapidly affected. Because of the involvement of the entire lobe and pleural surface fibrinous bronchopneumonias are also referred to as lobar pneumonias or pleuropneumonias. In general terms, fibrinous bronchopneumonias are the result of more severe pulmonary injury and thus cause death earlier in the sequence of the inflammatory process than suppurative bronchopneumonias. Even in cases in which fibrinous bronchopneumonia involves 30% or less of the total area, clinical signs and death can occur as a result of severe toxemia and sepsis.

The gross appearance of fibrinous bronchopneumonia depends on the age and severity of the lesion and on whether the pleural surface or the cut surface of the lung is viewed. Externally, early stages of fibrinous bronchopneumonias are characterized by severe congestion and hemorrhage, giving the affected lungs a characteristically intense red discoloration. A few hours later, fibrin starts to accumulate on the pleural surface, giving the pleura a ground glass appearance and eventually forming plaques of fibrinous exudate over a red, dark lung (see Fig. 9-58). At this stage, a yellow fluid starts to accumulate in the thoracic cavity. The color of fibrin deposited over the pleural surface is also variable. It can be yellow when the exudate is formed primarily by fibrin, tan when fibrin is mixed with blood, and gray when a large number of leukocytes are part of the fibrinous plaque. Because of the tendency of fibrin to deposit on the pleural surface, some pathologists use the term *pleuropneumonia* as a synonym for fibrinous bronchopneumonia.

On the cut surface, early stages of fibrinous bronchopneumonia appear as simple red consolidation (see Fig. 9-58). In more advanced cases (24 hours), fibrinous bronchopneumonia is generally accompanied by notable dilation and thrombosis of lymph vessels and edema of interlobular septa. This distention of the interlobular septa gives affected lungs a typical marbled appearance. Distinct focal areas of coagulative necrosis in the pulmonary parenchyma are also common in fibrinous bronchopneumonia such as in shipping fever pneumonia and contagious bovine pleuropneumonia. In animals that survive the early stage of fibrinous bronchopneumonia, pulmonary necrosis often develops into pulmonary "sequestra," which are isolated pieces of necrotic lung encapsulated by connective tissue. Pulmonary sequestra result from extensive necrosis of lung tissue either from severe ischemia (infarct) caused by thrombosis of a major pulmonary vessel such as in contagious bovine pleuropneumonia, or from the effect of necrotizing toxins released by pathogenic bacteria such as *Mannheimia haemolytica.*

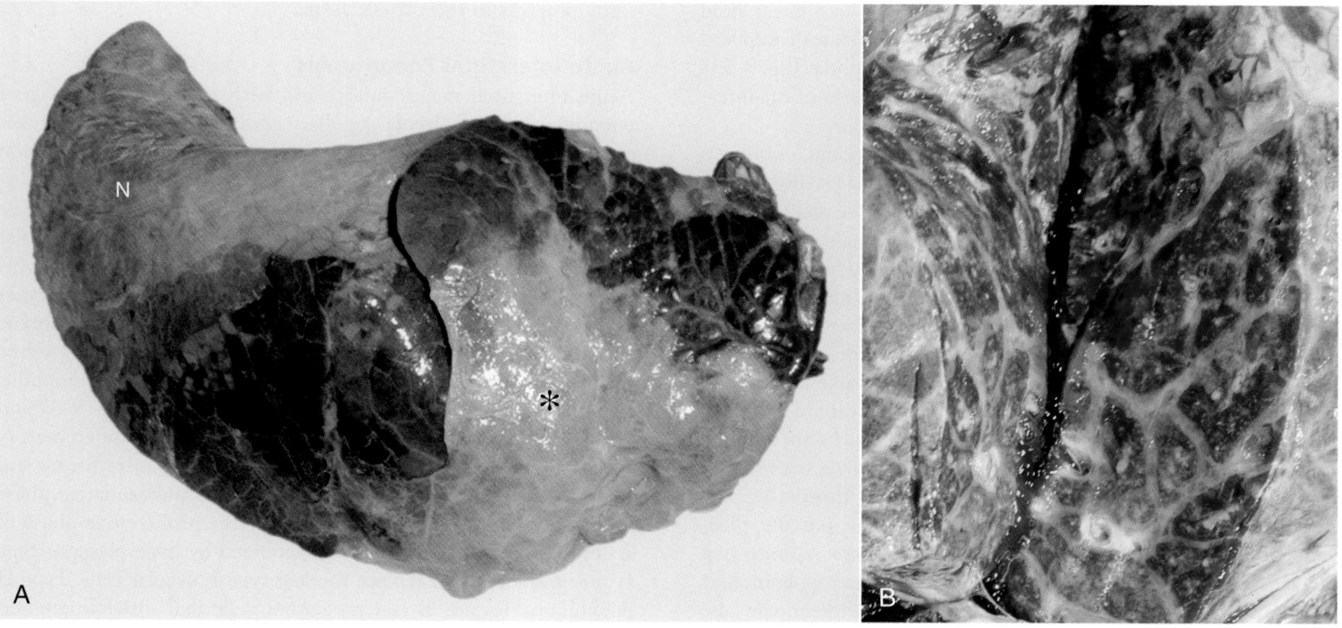

Fig. 9-58 Fibrinous bronchopneumonia (pleuropneumonia), right lung, steer.
A, The pneumonia has a cranioventral distribution that extends into the middle and caudal lobes and affects approximately 80% of the lung parenchyma. The lung is firm, swollen, and covered with yellow fibrin *(*)*. The dorsal portion of the caudal lung is normal *(N)*. **B,** Cut surface. Affected parenchyma appears dark and hyperemic as compared with more normal lung *(top quarter of figure)*. Interlobular septa are prominent (yellow bands) due to the accumulation of fibrin and edema fluid. This type of lesion is typical of *Mannheimia haemolytica* infection in cattle (shipping fever). (**A** courtesy Ontario Veterinary College. **B** courtesy Dr. A. López, Atlantic Veterinary College.)

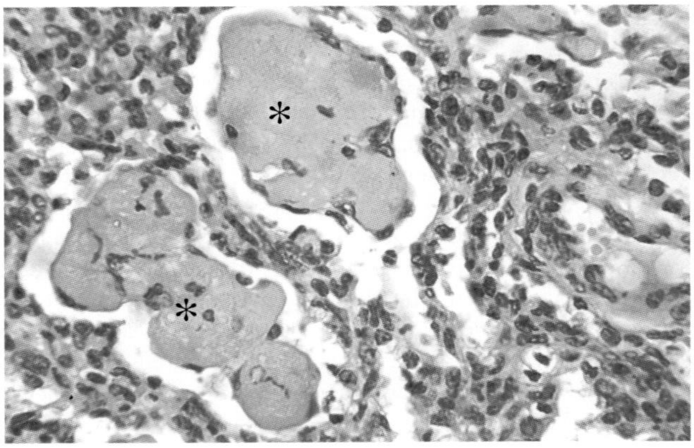

Fig. 9-59 Fibrinous bronchopneumonia, chronic, lung, calf. Note large aggregates of condensed fibrin *(asterisks)* surrounded and infiltrated by phagocytic cells. H&E stain. (Courtesy Dr. A. López, Atlantic Veterinary College.)

Sequestra in veterinary pathology should not be confused with "bronchopulmonary sequestration," a term used in human pathology to describe a congenital malformation in which whole lobes or parts of the lung develop without normal connections to the airway or vascular systems.

Microscopically, in the initial stage of fibrinous bronchopneumonia, there is massive exudation of plasma proteins into the bronchioles and alveoli, and as a result most of the airspaces become obliterated by fluid and fibrin. Leakage of fibrin and fluid into alveolar lumina is because of extensive disruption of the integrity and increased permeability of the blood-air barrier. Fibrinous exudates can move from alveolus to alveolus through the pores of Kohn. Because fibrin is chemotactic for neutrophils, these types of leukocytes are always present a few hours after the onset of fibrinous inflammation. As inflammation progresses (3 to 5 days), fluid exudate is gradually replaced by fibrinocellular exudates composed of fibrin, neutrophils, macrophages, and necrotic debris (Fig. 9-59). In chronic cases (after 7 days), there is notable fibrosis of the interlobular septa and pleura.

In contrast to suppurative bronchopneumonia, fibrinous bronchopneumonia rarely resolves completely, thus leaving noticeable scars in the form of pulmonary fibrosis and pleural adhesions. The most common sequelae found in animals surviving an acute episode of fibrinous bronchopneumonia include bronchiolitis obliterans, in which organized exudate becomes attached to the bronchiolar lumen; gangrene, when saprophytic bacteria colonize necrotic lung; pulmonary sequestra; pulmonary fibrosis; abscesses; and chronic pleuritis with pleural adhesions. In some cases, pleuritis can be so extensive that fibrous adhesions extend onto the pericardial sac. Pathogens causing fibrinous bronchopneumonias in domestic animals include *Mannheimia (Pasteurella) haemolytica* (pneumonic Mannheimiosis), *Histophilus somni* (formerly *Haemophilus somnus*), *Actinobacillus pleuropneumoniae* (porcine pleuropneumonia), *Mycoplasma bovis,* and *Mycoplasma mycoides* ssp. *mycoides* small colony type (contagious bovine pleuropneumonia). Fibrinous bronchopneumonia and pulmonary gangrene can also be the result of bronchoaspiration of irritant materials such as gastric contents.

Fulminating hemorrhagic bronchopneumonia can be caused by highly pathogenic bacteria such as *Bacillus anthracis.* Although the lesions in anthrax are primarily related to a severe septicemia and sepsis, anthrax should always be suspected in animals with sudden death and exhibiting severe acute fibrinohemorrhagic pneumonia, splenomegaly, and multisystemic hemorrhages. Animals are considered good sentinels for anthrax in cases of bioterrorism.

Interstitial Pneumonia

Interstitial pneumonia refers to that type of pneumonia in which injury and the inflammatory process take place primarily in any of the three layers of the alveolar walls (endothelium, basement membrane, and alveolar epithelium) and the contiguous bronchiolar interstitium. This type of pneumonia is the most difficult to diagnose at necropsy and requires microscopic confirmation as it is easily mistaken in the lung showing congestion, edema, hyperinflation, or emphysema.

The pathogenesis of interstitial pneumonia is complex and can result from aerogenous injury to the alveolar epithelium (type I and II pneumonocytes) or from hematogenous injury to the alveolar capillary endothelium or alveolar basement membrane. Aerogenous inhalation of toxic gases (i.e., ozone, NO_2) or toxic fumes (smoke inhalation) and infection with pneumotropic viruses (influenza, IBR, EVR, or canine distemper) can damage the alveolar epithelium. Inhaled antigens, such as fungal spores, combine with circulating antibodies and form deposits of antigen-antibody complexes (type III hypersensitivity) in the alveolar wall, which initiate a cascade of inflammatory responses and injury (allergic alveolitis). Hematogenous injury to the vascular endothelium occurs in septicemias (sepsis), DIC, larva migrans *(Ascaris suum),* toxins absorbed in the alimentary tract (endotoxin) or toxic metabolites locally generated in the lungs (3 methylindole, paraquat), release of free radicals in alveolar capillaries (ARDS), and viremias and infections with endotheliotropic viruses (CAV and classic swine fever [hog cholera]).

Interstitial pneumonias in domestic animals, like those in humans, are subdivided, based on some morphologic features, into acute and chronic. It should be kept in mind, however, that not all acute interstitial pneumonias are fatal and that they do not necessarily progress to the chronic form.

Acute Interstitial Pneumonias

Acute interstitial pneumonias begin with injury to either type I pneumonocytes or alveolar capillary endothelium, which provokes a disruption of the blood-air barrier and a subsequent exudation of plasma proteins into the alveolar space. This leakage of proteinaceous fluid into the alveolar lumen constitutes the exudative phase of acute interstitial pneumonia. In some cases of diffuse alveolar damage, exuded plasma proteins mix with lipids and other components of pulmonary surfactant and form elongated membranes that become partially attached to the alveolar basement membrane and bronchiolar walls. These membranes are referred to as hyaline membranes because of their hyaline appearance (eosinophilic, homogeneous, and amorphous) microscopically (see Figs. 9-37 and 9-45). In addition to intraalveolar exudation of fluid, inflammatory edema and neutrophils accumulate in the alveolar interstitium and cause thickening of the alveolar walls. This acute exudative phase is generally followed a few days later by the proliferative phase of acute interstitial pneumonias characterized by hyperplasia of type II pneumonocytes to replace the lost type I alveolar cells. Type II pneumonocytes are in fact progenitor cells that differentiate and replace necrotic type I pneumonocytes (see the section on General Aspects of Lung Inflammation). As a consequence, the alveolar walls become increasingly thickened. This process is in part the reason why lungs become rubbery on palpation, what prevents their normal collapse after the thorax is opened, and why the cut surface of the lung has a "meaty" appearance.

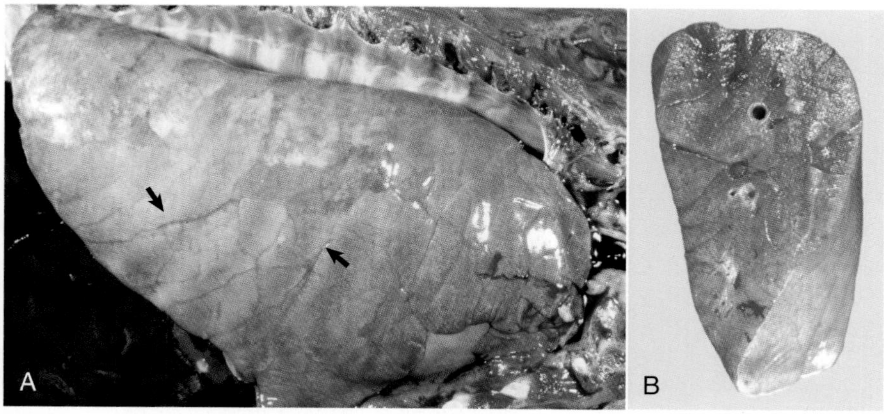

Fig. 9-60 Interstitial pneumonia, lung, feeder pig.
A, The lung is heavy, pale, and rubbery in texture. It also has prominent costal (rib) imprints *(arrows),* a result of hypercellularity of the interstitium and the failure of the lungs to collapse when the thorax was opened. **B,** Transverse section. The pulmonary parenchyma has a "meaty" appearance and some edema, but no exudate is present in airways or on the pleural surface. This type of lung change in pigs is highly suggestive of a viral pneumonia. (Courtesy Dr. A. López, Atlantic Veterinary College.)

Acute interstitial pneumonias are often mild and transient, especially those caused by some respiratory viruses, such as those responsible for equine and porcine influenza. These mild forms of pneumonia are rarely seen in the postmortem room because they are not fatal and do not leave significant sequelae (see the section on Defense Mechanisms of the Exchange System). In severe cases of acute interstitial pneumonias, animals may die of respiratory failure, usually as a result of diffuse alveolar damage, a profuse exudative phase (leakage of proteinaceous fluid) leading to a fatal pulmonary edema. Examples of this type of fatal acute interstitial pneumonia are bovine pulmonary edema and emphysema, and ARDS in all species.

Gross lesions

In contrast to bronchopneumonias, in which distribution of lesions is generally cranioventral, in acute or chronic interstitial pneumonias, lesions are more diffusely distributed and generally involve all pulmonary lobes, or in some cases, they appear to be more pronounced in the dorsocaudal aspects of the lungs. Three important gross features of interstitial pneumonia are (1) the failure of lungs to collapse when the thoracic cavity is opened, (2) the occasional presence of rib impressions on the lung's pleural surface indicating poor deflation, and (3) the lack of visible exudates in airways unless complicated with secondary bacterial pneumonia (Fig. 9-60; also see Fig. 9-55). The color of affected lungs varies from diffusely red in acute cases to diffusely pale gray to a mottled red, pale appearance in chronic ones. Pale lungs are caused by severe obliteration of alveolar capillaries (reduced blood-tissue ratio), especially evident when there is fibrosis of the alveolar walls. The texture of lungs with uncomplicated interstitial pneumonia is typically elastic or rubbery, but definitive diagnosis based on texture alone is difficult and requires histopathologic examination. On a cut surface, the lungs may appear and feel more "meaty" (having the texture of raw meat) and have no evidence of exudate in the bronchi or pleura (see Fig. 9-60). In acute interstitial pneumonias, particularly in cattle, there is frequently pulmonary edema (exudative phase) and interstitial emphysema secondary to partial obstruction of bronchioles by edema fluid and strenuous air gasping before death. Because edema tends to gravitate into the cranioventral portions of the lungs, and emphysema is often more obvious in the dorsocaudal aspects, acute interstitial pneumonias in cattle occasionally have a gross cranioventral-like pattern that may resemble bronchopneumonia, although the texture is different. Lungs are notably heavy because of the edema and the infiltrative and proliferative changes.

Chronic Interstitial Pneumonia

When the source of alveolar injury persists, the proliferative and infiltrative lesions of acute interstitial pneumonia can progress into a morphologic stage referred to as *chronic interstitial pneumonia* whose hallmark is fibrosis of the alveolar walls (with or without intraalveolar fibrosis) and infiltrative and proliferative changes. Infiltrative changes are characterized by the presence of lymphocytes, macrophages, fibroblasts, and myofibroblasts in the alveolar interstitium (Fig. 9-61). Proliferative changes are generally characterized by hyperplasia and persistence of type II pneumonocytes (see Fig. 9-54), and in rare cases, by squamous metaplasia of the alveolar epithelium. It should be emphasized again that, although the lesions in interstitial pneumonia are centered in the alveolar walls and its interstitium, a mixture of desquamated epithelial cells, macrophages, and mononuclear cells are usually present in the lumen of bronchioles and alveoli. Other, concurrent changes that can occur are microscopic granulomas and hyperplasia of smooth muscle in bronchioles and pulmonary arterioles. Ovine progressive pneumonia, hypersensitivity pneumonitis in cattle and dogs, and silicosis in horses are good veterinary examples of chronic interstitial pneumonia. Pneumoconioses (silicosis, asbestosis), paraquat toxicity, pneumotoxic antineoplastic drugs (bleomycin), and extrinsic allergic alveolitis (farmer's lung) are well-known examples of diseases that lead to chronic interstitial pneumonias in humans. Massive pulmonary migration of ascaris larvae in pigs also causes interstitial pneumonia (Fig. 9-62).

There is an insidious and poorly understood group of chronic interstitial diseases, both in humans and animals, that eventually progresses to terminal interstitial fibrosis. These were originally thought to be the result of repeated cycles of alveolar injury, inflammation, and fibroblastic/myoblastic response to an unknown agent. However, aggressive antiinflammatory therapy generally fails to prevent or reduce the severity of fibrosis. Now, it is proposed that a genetic mutation alters the cell-cell communication between epithelial and mesenchymal cell in the lung. This aberrant cellular communication leads to an overexpression of inflammatory and repair molecules (i.e., IL-4, IL-13, TGF-β1, and caveolin) leading to increased apoptosis and interstitial deposition of extracellular matrix (ECM). The chronic interstitial (restrictive) diseases in human medicine include "idiopathic pulmonary fibrosis," "nonspecific interstitial pneumonia," "unusual interstitial pneumonia," and "cryptogenic organizing pneumonia," also referred to as *bronchiolitis obliterans organizing pneumonia* (BOOP). Equine multinodular pulmonary fibrosis and feline idiopathic pulmonary fibrosis are examples of this type of progressive interstitial disease in veterinary

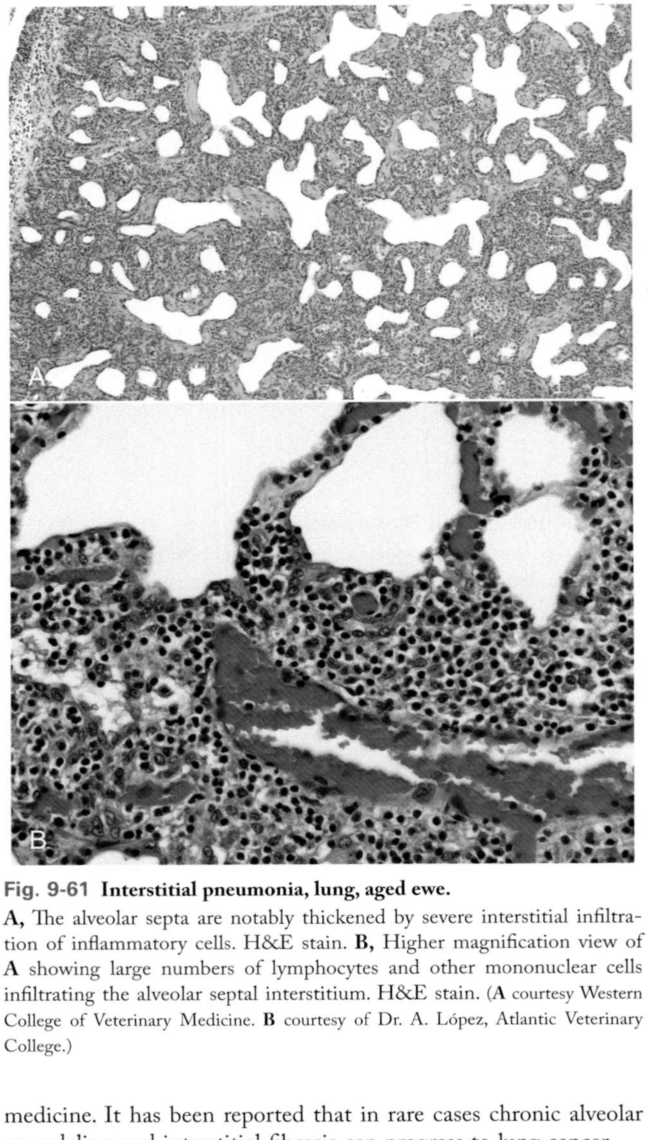

Fig. 9-61 Interstitial pneumonia, lung, aged ewe.
A, The alveolar septa are notably thickened by severe interstitial infiltration of inflammatory cells. H&E stain. **B,** Higher magnification view of **A** showing large numbers of lymphocytes and other mononuclear cells infiltrating the alveolar septal interstitium. H&E stain. (**A** courtesy Western College of Veterinary Medicine. **B** courtesy of Dr. A. López, Atlantic Veterinary College.)

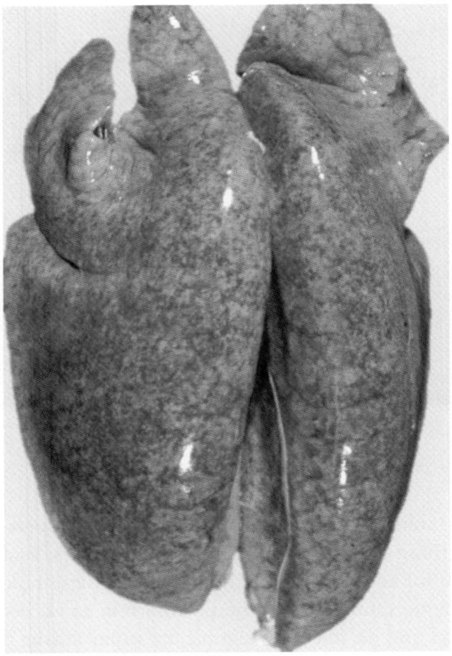

Fig. 9-62 Interstitial pneumonia, edema, and hemorrhages, lungs, pig. This pig had migrating *Ascaris suum* larvae. The lungs are heavy and wet and failed to collapse when the thorax was opened, as a result of pulmonary edema. The mottled appearance of lungs is due to the presence of numerous petechiae scattered in the pulmonary parenchyma. Petechiae are likely alveolar hemorrhages caused by migrating larvae. Larvae leave the bloodstream to enter the alveoli by penetrating and rupturing alveolar capillaries and thus damage the air-blood barrier of alveolar septa. (Courtesy Dr. J.M. King, College of Veterinary Medicine, Cornell University.)

medicine. It has been reported that in rare cases chronic alveolar remodeling and interstitial fibrosis can progress to lung cancer.

The term *bronchointerstitial pneumonia* has been introduced into veterinary pathology to describe cases in which pulmonary lesions share some histologic features of both bronchopneumonia and interstitial pneumonia. This combined type of pneumonia is in fact frequently seen in many viral infections in which viruses replicate and cause necrosis in bronchial, bronchiolar, and alveolar cells. Damage to the bronchial and bronchiolar epithelium causes an influx of neutrophils similar to that in bronchopneumonias, and damage to alveolar walls causes proliferation of type II pneumonocytes, similar to that which takes place in the proliferative phase of acute interstitial pneumonias. It is important to emphasize that bronchointerstitial pneumonia is a microscopic not a gross diagnosis. Examples include uncomplicated cases of respiratory syncytial virus infections in cattle and lambs, canine distemper, and influenza in pigs and horses.

Embolic Pneumonia

Embolic pneumonia refers to a particular type of pneumonia in which lung injury is hematogenous, and the inflammatory response is typically centered in pulmonary arterioles and alveolar capillaries. Lungs act as a biologic filter for circulating particulate matter. Sterile thromboemboli, unless extremely large, are rapidly dissolved and removed from the pulmonary vasculature by fibrinolysis, causing little if any ill effects. Experimental studies have confirmed that most types of bacteria when injected intravenously (bacteremia) are phagocytosed by pulmonary intravascular macrophages, or bypass the lungs and are finally trapped by macrophages in the liver, spleen, joints, or other organs. To cause pulmonary infection, circulating bacteria must first attach to the pulmonary endothelium with specific binding proteins or simply attach to intravascular fibrin and then evade phagocytosis by intravascular macrophages or leukocytes. Septic thrombi facilitate entrapment of bacteria in the pulmonary vessels and provide a favorable environment to escape phagocytosis. Once trapped in the pulmonary vasculature, usually in small arterioles or alveolar capillaries, offending bacteria disrupt endothelium and basement membranes, spread from the vessels to the interstitium and then to the surrounding lung, forming finally a new nidus of infection.

Embolic pneumonia is characterized by multifocal lesions randomly distributed in all pulmonary lobes (see Fig. 9-55). Early lesions in embolic pneumonia are characterized grossly by the presence of very small (1 to 10 mm), white foci surrounded by a discrete, red, hemorrhagic halo (Fig. 9-63 and Web Fig. 9-9). Unless emboli arrive in massive numbers, causing fatal pulmonary edema, embolic pneumonia is seldom fatal; therefore these acute lesions are rarely seen at postmortem examination. In most instances, acute lesions if unresolved rapidly progress to pulmonary abscesses. These are randomly distributed in all pulmonary lobes and are not restricted to the cranioventral aspects of the lungs, as is the case of abscesses developing from suppurative bronchopneumonia. The early microscopic lesions in embolic pneumonias are always

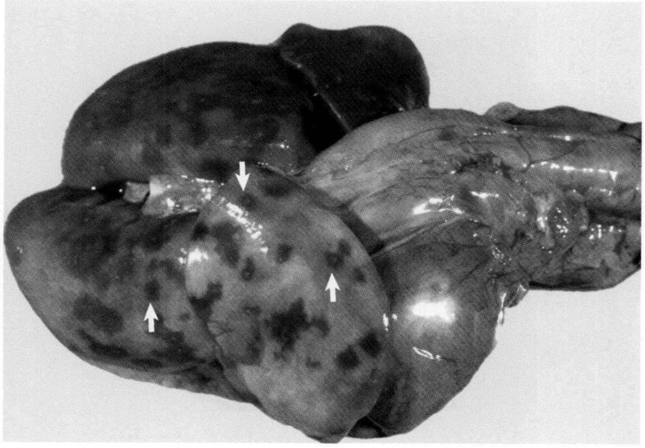

Fig. 9-63 Embolic pneumonia, lungs, 6-week-old puppy.
Large hemorrhagic foci are scattered relatively uniformly throughout all pulmonary lobes *(arrows)*. These hemorrhagic foci are the sites of lodgment of *Pseudomonas aeruginosa* emboli (septic) that originated from necrotizing enteritis. Note the multifocal distribution of the inflammatory foci, which is typical of embolic pneumonia. Septic emboli were also present in the liver. (Courtesy Atlantic Veterinary College.)

focal (Fig. 9-64); thus they differ from those of endotoxemia or septicemia, in which endothelial damage and interstitial reactions (interstitial pneumonia) are diffusely distributed in the lungs.

When embolic pneumonia or its sequelae (abscesses) is diagnosed at necropsy, an attempt should be made to locate the source of septic emboli. The most common are hepatic abscesses which can have ruptured into the caudal vena cava in cattle, omphalophlebitis in farm animals, chronic bacterial skin or hoof infections, and a contaminated catheter in all species (see Fig. 9-46). Valvular or mural endocarditis in the right heart is a common source of septic emboli and embolic pneumonia in all species. Most frequently, bacterial isolates from septic pulmonary emboli in domestic animals are *Arcanobacterium (Actinomyces) pyogenes* (cattle), *Fusobacterium necrophorum* (cattle, pigs, and humans), *Erysipelothrix rhusiopathiae* (pigs, cattle, dogs, and humans), *Streptococcus suis* type II (pigs), *Staphylococcus aureus* (dogs, humans), and *Streptococcus equi* (horses).

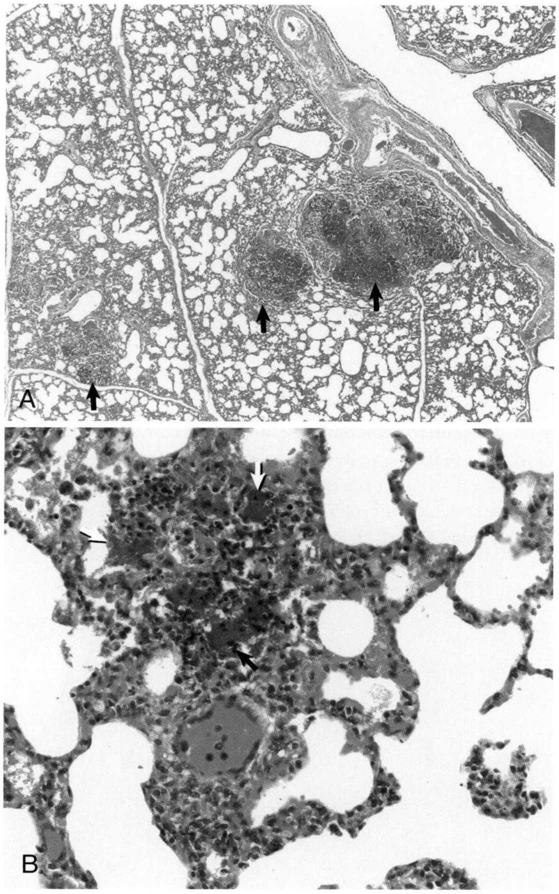

Fig. 9-64 Embolic pneumonia, lung, cow.
A, Foci of necrosis and infiltration of neutrophils *(arrows)* resulting from septic emboli. Note the multifocal distribution of the lesion, which is typical of embolic pneumonia. Vegetative endocarditis involving the tricuspid valve was the source of septic emboli in this cow. H&E stain. **B,** Embolic focus in the lung. Note bacterial colonies *(arrows)* mixed with neutrophils and cellular debris. H&E stain. (Courtesy Dr. A. López, Atlantic Veterinary College.)

Granulomatous Pneumonia

Granulomatous pneumonia refers to a particular type of pneumonia in which aerogenous or hematogenous injury is caused by organisms or particles that cannot be normally eliminated by phagocytosis and that evoke a local inflammatory reaction with numerous alveolar and interstitial macrophages, lymphocytes, a few neutrophils, and sometimes giant cells. The term *granulomatous* is used here to describe an anatomic pattern of pneumonia typically characterized by the presence of granulomas.

The pathogenesis of granulomatous pneumonia shares some similarities with that of interstitial and embolic pneumonias. Not surprisingly, some pathologists group granulomatous pneumonias within one of these types of pneumonias (e.g., granulomatous interstitial pneumonia). What makes granulomatous pneumonia a distinctive type is not so much the portal of entry or site of initial injury in the lungs, but the unique type of inflammatory response that results in the formation of granulomas, which can be easily recognized at gross and microscopic examination. The portal of agent entry into lungs can be aerogenous or hematogenous. As a rule, agents causing granulomatous pneumonia are resistant to intracellular killing by phagocytic cells and to the acute inflammatory response and persist in affected tissue for a long time.

The most common causes of granulomatous pneumonia in animals include systemic fungal diseases, such as cryptococcosis *(Cryptococcus neoformans)*, coccidioidomycosis *(Coccidioides immitis)*, histoplasmosis *(Histoplasma capsulatum)*, and blastomycosis *(Blastomyces dermatitidis)*. In most of these fungal diseases, the port of entry is aerogenous and from the lungs the fungi disseminate systemically to other organs, particularly the lymph nodes, liver, and spleen. Granulomatous pneumonia is also caused by some bacterial diseases, such as tuberculosis *(Mycobacterium bovis)* in all species, and inhaled foreign material (starch). Sporadically, aberrant parasites such as *Fasciola hepatica* in cattle and aspiration of foreign bodies can also cause granulomatous pneumonia. Feline infectious peritonitis is one of a few viral infections of domestic animals that result in granulomatous pneumonia. Lesions are caused by the deposition of antigen-antibody complexes in the vasculature of many organs, including the lungs, and subsequent vasculitis.

Granulomatous pneumonia is characterized by the presence of variable numbers of caseous or noncaseous granulomas randomly distributed in the lungs (Fig. 9-65; also see Fig. 9-55). On palpation, lungs have a typical nodular character given by well-circumscribed, variably sized nodules that generally have a firm texture, especially if calcification has occurred (see Fig. 9-65). During postmortem

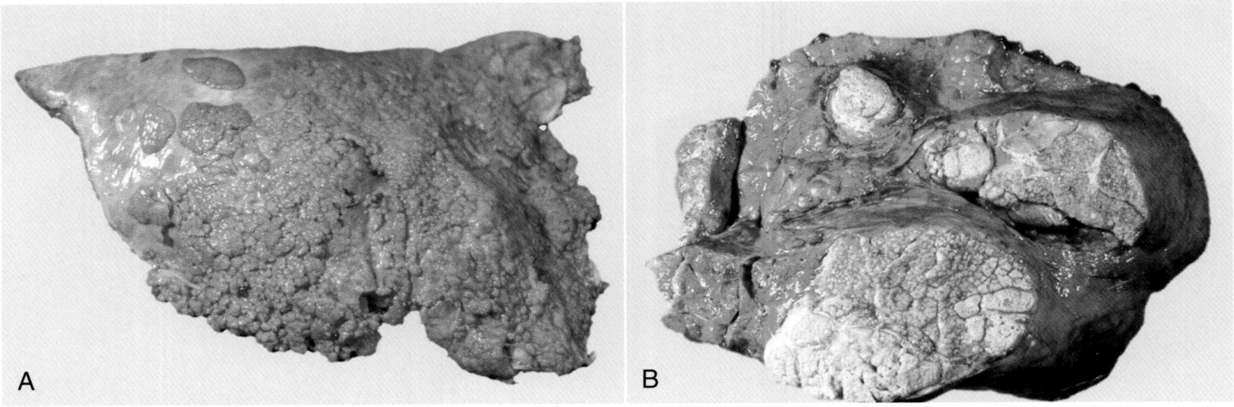

Fig. 9-65 Pulmonary tuberculosis, lung, aged cow.
A, Multifocal, coalescing granulomatous pneumonia involves most of the lung, except for the dorsal portion of the caudal lung lobe. **B,** Transverse section. Large multifocal to confluent caseating granulomas are present in the pulmonary parenchyma. Note the caseous ("cheesy," pale yellow-white) appearance of the granulomas, which is typical of bovine tuberculosis. (**A** courtesy Facultad de Medicina Veterinaria y Zootecnia, UNAM, México. **B** courtesy Dr. J.M. King, College of Veterinary Medicine, Cornell University.)

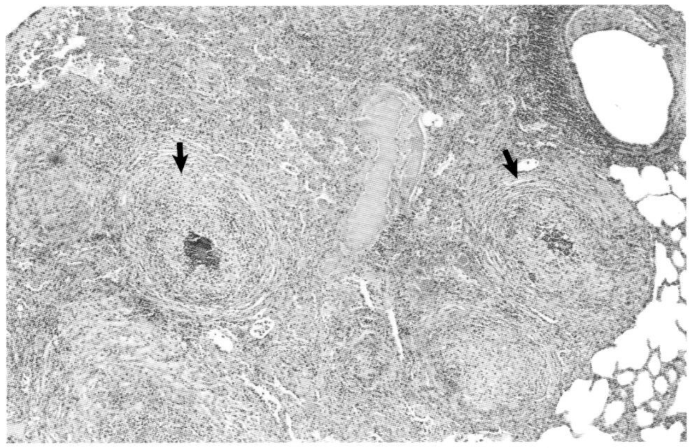

Fig. 9-66 Granulomatous pneumonia, lung, cow.
There are several noncaseous granulomas *(arrows),* each with a small necrotic center filled with neutrophils, surrounded by histiocytes and mononuclear cells, and with an outer rim of connective tissue. H&E stain. (Courtesy Western College of Veterinary Medicine.)

examination, granulomas in the lungs occasionally can be mistaken for neoplasms. Microscopically, pulmonary granulomas are composed of a center of necrotic tissue, surrounded by a rim of macrophages (epithelioid cells) and giant cells and an outer delineated layer of connective tissue commonly infiltrated by lymphocytes and plasma cells (Fig. 9-66). Unlike other types of pneumonias, the causative agent in granulomatous pneumonia can, in many cases, be identified microscopically in sections stained by PAS reaction or by Grocott-Gomori's methenamine silver (G-GMS) stains for fungi or the acid-fast stain for mycobacteria.

Species-Specific Pneumonias

Pneumonias of Horses

Viral infections of the respiratory tract, particularly equine viral rhinopneumonitis and equine influenza, are important diseases of horses around the world. The effects of these and other respiratory viruses on the horse can be manifested in three distinct ways. First, as pure viral infections, their severity may range from mild to severe, making them a frequent interfering factor in training and athletic performance. Second, superimposed infections by opportunistic bacteria, such as *Streptococcus* spp., *Escherichia coli, Klebsiella pneumoniae, Rhodococcus equi,* and various anaerobes, can cause fibrinous or suppurative bronchopneumonias. Third, it is possible but yet unproved that viral infections may also predispose horses to airway hyperresponsiveness and COPD.

Equine Influenza

Equine influenza is an important and highly contagious flulike respiratory disease of horses characterized by high morbidity and low mortality and explosive outbreaks in susceptible populations of horses. It is an OIE-notifiable disease. Two antigenically unrelated subtypes of equine influenza viruses have been identified (H7N7 [A/equi-1] and H3N8 [A/equi-2]). The course of the disease is generally mild and transient, and its importance is primarily because of its economic impact on horse racing. The types of injury and host response in the conducting system are described in the section on Equine Nasal Diseases. Uncomplicated lesions in the lungs are mild and self-limiting bronchointerstitial pneumonia. In fatal cases, the lungs are hyperinflated with dark red coalescing ares of dark red discoloration. Microscopically, there is a bronchointerstitial pneumonia characterized by necrotizing bronchiolitis that is followed by hyperplastic bronchiolitis, hyperplasia of type II pneumonocytes, hyaline membranes in alveoli, and sporadic multinucleated giant cell. The microscopic changes are ARDS in severe and fatal cases. The influenza virus antigen can be readily demonstrated in ciliated cells and alveolar macrophages. Clinical signs are characterized by fever, cough, abnormal lung sounds (crackles and wheezes), anorexia, and depression. Secondary bacterial infections (*Streptococcus equi, Streptococcus zooepidemicus, Streptococcus aureus,* and *Escherichia coli*) commonly complicate equine influenza.

Equine Viral Rhinopneumonitis

Equine viral rhinopneumonitis (EVR), or equine herpesvirus infection, is a respiratory disease of young horses that is particularly important in weanlings between 4 and 8 months of age and to a much lesser extent in young foals and adult horses. The causative agent is a ubiquitous equine herpesvirus (EHV-1 and EHV-4) that in addition to respiratory disease can cause abortion in pregnant mares and neurologic disease (equine herpes myeloencephalopathy) (see the section on Equine Nasal Diseases).

The respiratory form of EVR is a mild and a transient bronchointerstitial pneumonia seen only by pathologists when complications with secondary bacterial infections cause a fatal bronchopneumonia (*Streptococcus equi, Streptococcus zooepidemicus,* or *Staphylococcus aureus*). Uncomplicated lesions in EVR are seen only in aborted fetuses or in foals that die within the first few days of life. They consist of focal areas of necrosis (0.5 to 2 mm) in various organs, including liver, adrenal glands, and lungs. In some cases, intranuclear inclusion bodies are microscopically observed in these organs. Recent outbreaks of interstitial pneumonia in donkeys have been attributed to a novel strain of asinine (equine) herpesvirus (AHV-3). Clinically, horses and donkeys affected with the respiratory form of EVR exhibit fever, anorexia, conjunctivitis, cough, and nasal discharge.

Equine Viral Arteritis

Equine viral arteritis (EVA), a pansystemic disease of foals and horses caused by an arterivirus, occurs sporadically throughout the world, sometimes as an outbreak. This virus infects and causes severe injury to macrophages and endothelial cells. Gross lesions are hemorrhagic and edematous in many sites, including lungs, intestine, scrotum, and periorbital tissues and voluminous hydrothorax and hydroperitoneum,. The basic lesion is fibrinoid necrosis and inflammation of the vessel walls (vasculitis), particularly the small muscular arteries (lymphocytic arteritis), which is responsible for the edema and hemorrhage that explain most of the clinical features. Pulmonary lesions are those of interstitial pneumonia with hyperplasia of type II pneumonocytes and vasculitis with abundant edema in the bronchoalveolar spaces and distended pulmonary lymphatic vessels. Viral antigen can be detected by immunoperoxidase techniques in the walls and endothelial cells of affected pulmonary vessels and in alveolar macrophages.

Clinical signs are respiratory distress, fever, abortion, diarrhea, colic, and edema of the limbs and ventral abdomen. Respiratory signs are frequent and consist of serous or mucopurulent rhinitis and conjunctivitis with palpebral edema. Like most viral respiratory infections, EVA can predispose horses to opportunistic secondary bacterial pneumonias.

African Horse Sickness

African horse sickness is a vector-borne, "List A" OIE-notifiable disease of horses, mules, donkeys, and zebras that is caused by an orbivirus (family Reoviridae) and characterized by respiratory distress or cardiovascular failure. It has a high mortality rate—up to 95% in the native population of horses in Africa, the Middle East, India, Pakistan, and most recently Spain and Portugal. Although the virus is transmitted primarily by insects *(Culicoides)* to horses, other animals, such as dogs, can be infected by eating infected equine flesh. The pathogenesis of African horse sickness remains unclear, but this equine orbivirus has an obvious tropism for pulmonary and cardiac endothelial cells and to a lesser extent mononuclear cells. Based on clinical signs (not pathogenesis), African horse sickness is arbitrarily divided into four different forms: pulmonary, cardiac, mixed, and mild.

The pulmonary form is characterized by severe respiratory distress and rapid death because of massive pulmonary edema, presumably from viral injury to the pulmonary endothelial cells. Grossly, large amounts of froth are present in the airways, lungs fail to collapse, subpleural lymph vessels are distended, and the ventral parts of the lungs are notably edematous (see Fig. 4-44). In the cardiac form, recurrent fever is detected, and heart failure results in subcutaneous and interfascial edema, most notably in the neck and supraorbital region. The mixed form is a combination of the respiratory and cardiac forms. Finally, the mild form, rarely seen in postmortem rooms, is characterized by fever and clinical signs resembling those of equine influenza; it is in most cases transient and followed by a complete recovery. This mild form is most frequently seen in donkeys, mules, and zebras and in horses with some degree of immunity. Detection of viral antigen for diagnostic purposes could be done by immunohistochemistry in paraffin-embedded tissues.

Equine Henipavirus (Hendra Virus)

Fatal cases of a novel respiratory disease in horses and humans suddenly appeared around 1994 in Hendra, a suburb of Brisbane, Australia. This outbreak was attributed to a newly recognized zoonotic virus that was tentatively named equine *Morbillivirus* (Hendra virus) and is currently classified as a member of the Henipavirus (Hendra virus and Nipah virus), new members of the subfamily *Paramyxoviridae.* Fruit bats (flying foxes) act as natural reservoirs and are involved in the transmission by poorly understood mechanisms. The lungs of affected horses are severely edematous with gelatinous distention of pleura and subpleural lymph vessels. Microscopically, the lungs have diffuse alveolar edema associated with vasculitis, thrombosis, and presence of multinucleated syncytial cells in the endothelium of small pulmonary blood vessels and alveolar capillaries. The lymphatic vessels are notably distended with fluid. The characteristic inclusion bodies seen in other *Paramyxovirus* infections are not seen in horses; however, the virus can be easily detected by immunohistochemistry in pulmonary endothelial cells and alveolar epithelial cells. Clinical signs are nonspecific and include fever, anorexia, respiratory distress, and nasal discharge.

Rhodococcus Equi

Rhodococcus equi, formerly known as *Corynebacterium equi,* is an important cause of morbidity and mortality in foals around the world. It is a facultative intracellular Gram-positive bacterium that causes two major forms of disease: the first involves the intestine, causing ulcerative enterocolitis, and the second severe and often fatal bronchopneumonia. Although half of foals with pneumonia have ulcerative enterocolitis, it is rare to find animals with intestinal lesions alone. Occasionally, infection is disseminated to lymph nodes, joints, bones, genital tract, and other organs. Because *Rhodococcus equi* is present in soil and feces of herbivores (particularly foals), it is not unusual for the disease to become enzootic on farms where the organism has been shed earlier by infected foals. Serologic evidence of infection in horses is widespread, yet clinical disease is sporadic and largely restricted to young foals or to adult horses with severe immunosuppression. Virulence factors encoded by plasmids (virulence-associated protein A [VapA gene]) appear to be responsible for the survival of *Rhodococcus equi* in macrophages, thus determining the evolution of the disease. This bacterium also has been sporadically incriminated with infections in cattle, goats, pigs, dogs, and cats, and quite often in immunocompromised humans, for example, those infected with the AIDS virus, after organ transplantation, or undergoing chemotherapy.

It is still debatable whether natural infection starts as a bronchopneumonia (aerogenous route) from which *Rhodococcus equi* reaches the intestine via swallowed sputum or whether infection starts as an enteritis (oral route) with a subsequent bacteremia into the lungs. The results of experimental studies suggest that natural infection likely starts from inhalation of infected dust or aerosols. Once in the lung, *Rhodococcus equi* is rapidly phagocytosed by alveolar macrophages, but because of defective phagosome-lysosome fusion

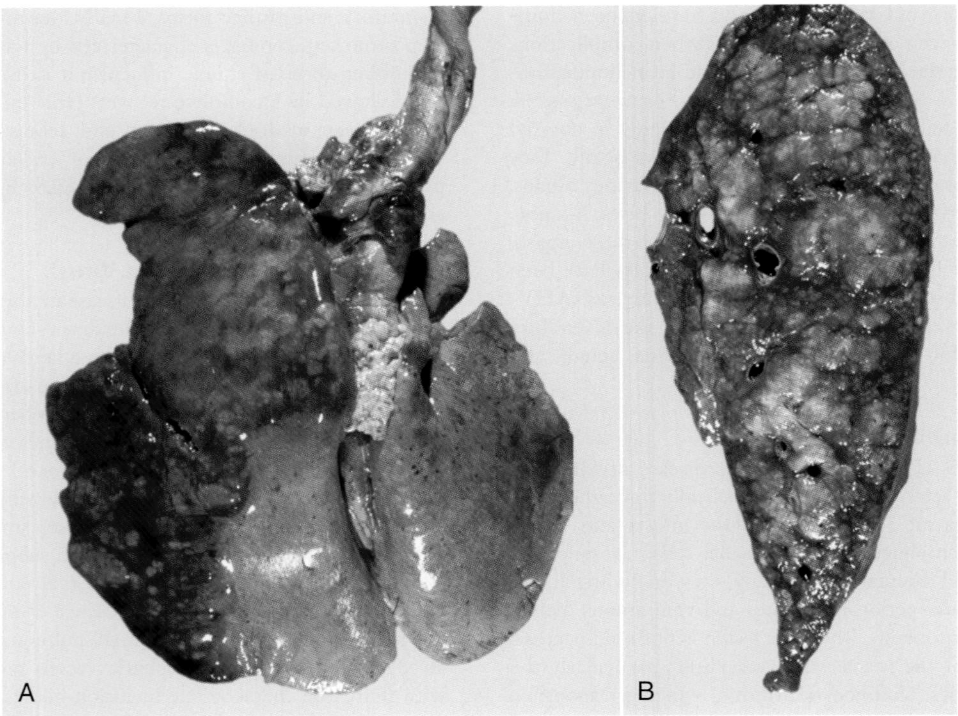

Fig. 9-67 Granulomatous pneumonia *(Rhodococcus equi)*, lungs, foal.
A, Cranioventral consolidation of the lungs with subpleural granulomas. Note that the pneumonic lesions in this foal are unilateral. This was an experimental case in which a foal was intratracheally inoculated with a suspension of *Rhodococcus equi.* **B,** Cut surface. Note the large, confluent, caseated granulomas. (Courtesy Drs. J. Yager and J. Prescott, Ontario Veterinary College.)

and premature lysosomal degranulation, bacteria survive and multiply intracellularly, eventually leading to the destruction of the macrophage. Interestingly, *Rhodococcus equi* appears to be easily killed by neutrophils but not macrophages. Released cytokines and lysosomal enzymes and bacterial toxins are responsible for extensive caseous necrosis of the lungs and the recruitment of large numbers of neutrophils, macrophages, and giant cells containing intracellular Gram-positive organisms in their cytoplasm.

Depending on the stage of infection and the immune status and age of affected horses, pulmonary lesions induced by *Rhodococcus equi* can vary from suppurative bronchopneumonia to granulomatous pneumonia. In young foals, the infection starts as a suppurative cranioventral bronchopneumonia, which progresses within a few days into small variable-size pulmonary abscesses. These abscesses rapidly transform into pyogranulomatous nodules some of which become confluent and form large masses of caseous exudate (Fig. 9-67). Microscopically the early lesion starts with neutrophilic infiltration, followed by an intense influx of alveolar macrophages into the bronchoalveolar spaces. This type of histiocytic inflammation tends to persist for a long period of time because *Rhodococcus equi* is a facultative intracellular organism that survives the bactericidal effects of equine alveolar macrophages. In the most chronic cases, the pulmonary lesions culminate with the formation of large necrotic masses with extensive fibrosis of the surrounding pulmonary parenchyma. PCR analysis of tracheal aspirates has successfully been used as an alternative to bacteriologic culture in the diagnosis of *Rhodococcus equi* infection in live foals.

Clinically, *Rhodococcus equi* infection can be acute, with rapid death caused by severe bronchopneumonia, or chronic, with depression, cough, weight loss, and respiratory distress. In either form, there may be diarrhea, arthritis, or subcutaneous abscess formation.

Other Pneumonias of Horses

Chlamydophila (Chlamydia) psittaci, an obligatory intracellular zoonotic pathogen, can cause systemic infection in many mammalian and avian species; in horses, it also causes keratoconjunctivitis, rhinitis, pneumonia, abortion, polyarthritis, enteritis, hepatitis, and encephalitis. Serologic studies suggest that infection without apparent disease is common in horses. Horses experimentally infected with *Chlamydophila psittaci* develop mild and transient bronchointerstitial pneumonia. There are unconfirmed reports suggesting a possible association between this organism and recurrent airway obstruction in horses. Detection of chlamydial organisms in affected tissue is not easy and requires special laboratory techniques such as PCR, immunohistochemistry, and fluorescent antibody tests.

Horses are susceptible to mycobacteriosis (*Mycobacterium avium complex, Mycobacterium tuberculosis*, and *Mycobacterium bovis*). The intestinal tract and associated lymph nodes are usually affected, suggesting an oral route of infection with subsequent hematogenous dissemination to the lungs (Fig. 9-68). The tubercles (granulomas) differ from those in ruminants and pigs, being smooth, gray, solid nodules without grossly visible caseous necrosis or calcification; they typically appear more like sarcomas. Microscopically, the tubercles are composed of macrophages, epithelioid cells, and multinucleated giant cells. Fibrosis increases with time, accounting in part for the sarcomatous appearance.

Adenovirus infections occur commonly in Arabian foals with combined immunodeficiency (CID), a hereditary lack of B and T lymphocytes. In cases of adenoviral infection, large basophilic or amphophilic inclusions are present in the nuclei of tracheal, bronchial, bronchiolar, alveolar, renal, and intestinal epithelial cells. As it occurs in other species, infection with a unique fungal pathogen

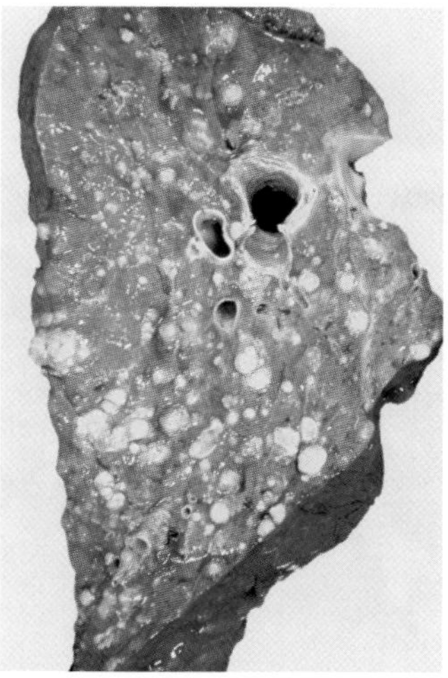

Fig. 9-68 Multifocal granulomatous pneumonia, tuberculosis *(Mycobacterium avium-intracellulare)*, lung, cut surface, aged horse. Note the large numbers of noncaseating granulomas scattered throughout the pulmonary parenchyma. In horses, granulomas caused by Mycobacteria often resemble sarcomatous nodules. (Courtesy Western College of Veterinary Medicine.)

known as *Pneumocystis carinii* typically occurs in immunosuppressed or immunoincompetent individuals such as Arabian foals with CID. Diagnosis of *Pneumocystis carinii* requires microscopic examination of lungs and special stains (see the section on Pneumonias of Pigs).

Interstitial and bronchointerstitial pneumonias of undetermined cause that can progress to severe pulmonary fibrosis have been reported in foals and young horses. The gross and microscopic lesions are reminiscent of those of bovine pulmonary edema and emphysema or ARDS. The lungs are notably congested and edematous and microscopically are characterized by necrosis of the bronchiolar epithelium, alveolar edema, hyperplasia of type II pneumonocytes, and hyaline membranes. The cause of this form of equine interstitial pneumonia is not known, but toxic and particularly viral causes have been proposed.

Equine multinodular pulmonary fibrosis characterized by progressive focal to coalescing fibrotic lesions in the lung has been described in adult horses. The pathogenesis is still under investigation, but equine herpes-5 virus has been proposed as the putative etiology.

Aspiration pneumonia is often a devastating sequela to improper gastric tubing of horses, particularly exogenous lipid pneumonia from mineral oil delivered into the trachea in treatment of colic. Gross and microscopic lesions are described in detail in the section on Aspiration Pneumonias of Cattle.

Parasitic pneumonias of horses

Parascaris equorum is a large nematode (roundworm) of the small intestine of horses; the larval stages migrate through the lungs as ascarid larvae do in pigs. It is still unclear whether migration of *Parascaris equorum* larvae can cause significant pulmonary lesions under natural conditions. Experimentally, migration of larvae results in coughing, anorexia, weight loss, and small necrotic foci and petechial hemorrhages in the liver, hepatic and tracheobronchial lymph nodes, and lungs. Microscopically, eosinophils are prominent in the interstitium and airway mucosa during the parasitic migration and in focal granulomas caused by dead larvae in the lung.

Dictyocaulus arnfieldi is not a very pathogenic nematode, but it should be considered if there are signs of coughing in horses that are pastured together with donkeys. Donkeys are considered the natural hosts and can tolerate large numbers of parasites without ill effects. *Dictyocaulus arnfieldi* does not usually become patent in horses, so examination of fecal samples is not useful; BAL is only occasionally diagnostic because eosinophils (but not parasites) are typically found in the lavage fluid. Mature parasites (up to 8 cm in length) cause obstructive bronchitis, edema, and atelectasis, particularly along the dorsocaudal lung. The microscopic lesion is an eosinophilic bronchitis similar to the less acute infestations seen in cattle and sheep with their *Dictyocaulus* species.

Pneumonias of Cattle

Bovine Respiratory Disease Complex and Acute Undifferentiated Respiratory Disease

Bovine respiratory disease (BRD) complex and acute undifferentiated respiratory disease are general terms often used by clinicians to describe acute and severe bovine respiratory illness of clinically undetermined cause. These terms do not imply any particular type of pneumonia and therefore should not be used in pathology reports. Clinically, the BRD complex includes enzootic pneumonia of calves (multifactorial etiology); pneumonic Mannheimiosis *(Mannheimia haemolytica);* respiratory histophilosis *(Histophilus somni),* previously known as respiratory hemophilosis *(Haemophilus somnus); Mycoplasma bovis;* respiratory viral infections, such as IBR/BoHV-1, PI-3 virus, and BRSV; and noninfectious interstitial pneumonias, such as bovine pulmonary edema and emphysema, reinfection syndrome, and many others.

Bovine Enzootic Pneumonia

Enzootic pneumonia, sometimes simply referred to as *calf pneumonia,* is a multifactorial disease caused by a variety of etiologic agents that produces an assortment of lung lesions in young, intensively housed calves. Morbidity is often high (up to 90%), but fatalities are uncommon (>5%) unless management is poor or unless new, virulent pathogens are introduced by additions to the herd. Enzootic pneumonia is also called *viral pneumonia* because it often begins with an acute respiratory infection with PI-3 virus, BRSV, or possibly with one or more of several other viruses (adenovirus, BoHV-1, reovirus, bovine respiratory coronavirus, and rhinovirus). Mycoplasmas, notably *Mycoplasma dispar, Mycoplasma bovis, Ureaplasma,* and possibly *Chlamydophila,* may also be primary agents. Following infection with any of these agents, opportunistic bacteria, such as *Pasteurella multocida, Arcanobacterium (Actinomyces) pyogenes, Histophilus somni, Mannheimia haemolytica,* and *Escherichia coli,* cause a secondary suppurative bronchopneumonia, the most serious stage of enzootic pneumonia. The pathogenesis of the primary invasion and how it predisposes the host to invasion by the opportunists are poorly understood, but it is likely that there is impairment of pulmonary defense mechanisms. Environmental factors, including air quality (poor ventilation), high relative humidity, and animal crowding, have been strongly incriminated. The immune status of the calf also plays an important role in the development and severity of enzootic pneumonia. Calves with bovine leukocyte adhesion deficiency (BLAD), which prevents the migration of neutrophils from the capillaries, are highly susceptible to bronchopneumonia.

Lesions are variable and depend largely on the agents involved and on the duration of the inflammatory process. In the acute phases, lesions caused by viruses are those of bronchointerstitial pneumonia, which are generally mild and transient, and therefore are seen only sporadically at necropsy. Microscopically, the lesions are necrotizing bronchiolitis, necrosis of type I pneumonocytes with hyperplasia of type II pneumonocytes, and mild interstitial and alveolar edema.

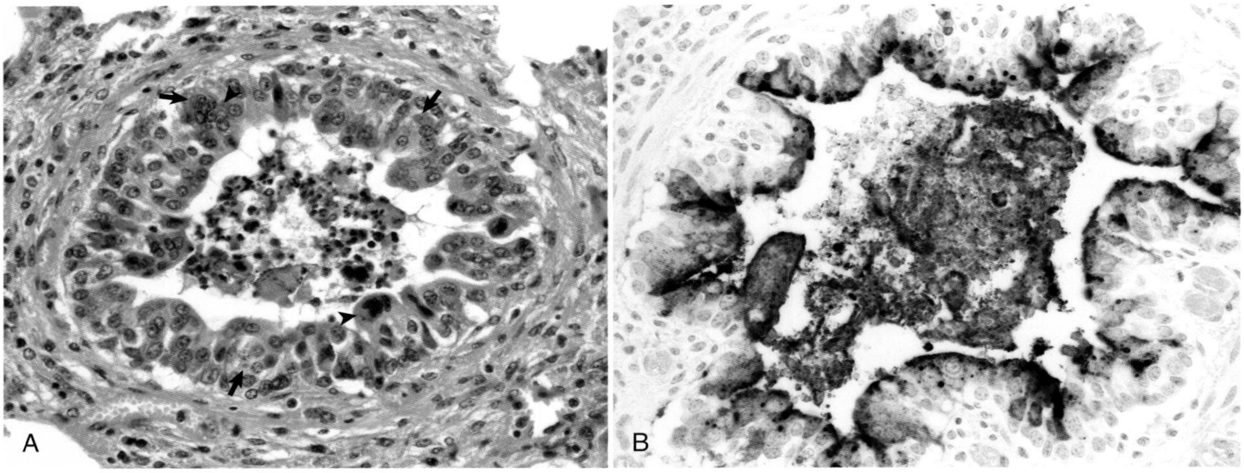

Fig. 9-69 Necrotizing bronchiolitis, bovine respiratory syncytial virus, lung, 5-week-old calf.
This is the reparative stage of necrotizing bronchiolitis and is characterized by epithelial hyperplasia and exfoliation of necrotic cells into the bronchiolar lumen. **A,** Epithelial cells are swollen, some are multinucleated *(arrowheads)* and the cytoplasm of some cells contains eosinophilic inclusion bodies surrounded by a clear halo *(arrows)*. Many of these hyperplastic bronchiolar cells eventually undergo apoptosis during the last stage of bronchiolar repair. H&E stain. **B,** Necrotizing viral bronchiolitis. Note positive staining for bovine respiratory syncytial virus antigen in bronchiolar cells and in exfoliated necrotic material in the bronchiolar lumen. Immunohistochemical stain. (**A** and **B** courtesy Dr. A. López, Atlantic Veterinary College.)

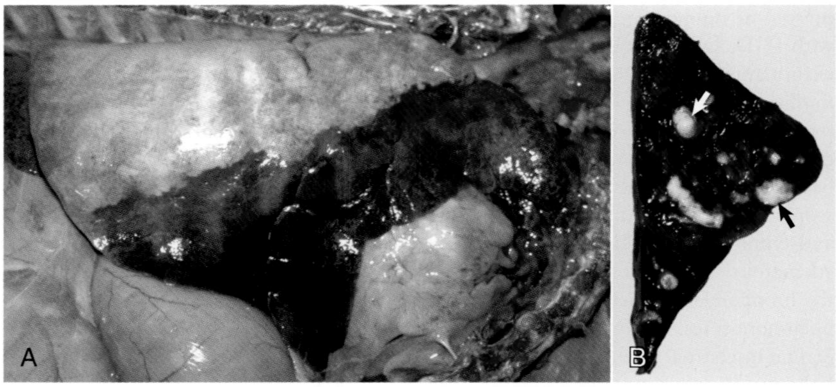

Fig. 9-70 Suppurative bronchopneumonia, right lung, calf.
A, Approximately 40% of the lung parenchyma is consolidated and includes most of the cranial lung lobe and the ventral portions of the middle and caudal lung lobes, a distribution often designated as cranioventral. Note the dark color of the consolidated lung and the normal appearance of the dorsal portion of the caudal lung lobe. **B,** Transverse section of the cranial lung lobe showing bronchi filled with purulent exudate *(arrows)*. (Courtesy Ontario Veterinary College.)

In the case of PI-3 and BRSV infection, intracytoplasmic inclusion bodies and the formation of large multinucleated syncytia, resulting from the fusion of infected bronchiolar epithelial cells, can also be observed in the lungs (Fig. 9-69). Airway hyperreactivity has been described in calves after BRSV infection; however, the significance of this syndrome in relation to enzootic pneumonia of calves is still under investigation.

The mycoplasmas also can cause bronchiolitis, bronchiolar and alveolar necrosis, and an interstitial reaction, but in contrast to viral-induced pneumonias, mycoplasmal lesions tend to progress to a chronic stage characterized by striking peribronchiolar lymphoid hyperplasia (cuffing pneumonia). When complicated by secondary bacterial infections (e.g., *Pasteurella multocida, Arcanobacterium pyogenes*), viral or mycoplasmal lesions change from a pure bronchointerstitial to a suppurative bronchopneumonia (Fig. 9-70). In late stages of bronchopneumonia, the lungs contain a creamy-mucoid exudate in the airways and later often have pulmonary abscesses and bronchiectasis (see Fig. 9-51).

It should be noted that the same viruses and mycoplasmas involved in the enzootic pneumonia complex can also predispose cattle to other diseases, such as pneumonic Mannheimiosis (*Mannheimia haemolytica*). Clinically, enzootic pneumonia is usually mild, but fatal cases are occasionally seen even in farms with optimal health management.

Pneumonic Mannheimiosis (Shipping Fever)

Shipping fever (transit fever) is a vague clinical term used to denote acute respiratory diseases that occur in cattle several days or weeks after shipment. The disease is characterized by a severe fibrinous bronchopneumonia, reflecting the fact that death generally occurs early or at an acute stage. Because *Mannheimia haemolytica* (formerly *Pasteurella haemolytica*) is typically isolated from affected lungs, the names pneumonic Mannheimiosis and pneumonic pasteurellosis have been used synonymously. It is known that pneumonic Mannheimiosis can occur in animals that have not been shipped and that organisms other than *Mannheimia haemolytica* can cause similar lesions. Therefore the term *shipping fever* should be relinquished in favor of more specific names such as pneumonic Mannheimiosis or respiratory histophilosis (hemophilosis).

Pneumonic Mannheimiosis (shipping fever) is the most important respiratory disease of cattle in North America, particularly in feedlot animals that have been through the stressful marketing and assembly processes. *Mannheimia haemolytica* biotype A, serotype 1 is the etiologic agent responsible for the severe pulmonary lesions.

A few investigators still consider that *Pasteurella multocida* and other serotypes of *Mannheimia haemolytica* are also causes of this disease.

Even after many years of intense investigation, from the gross lesions to the molecular aspects of the disease, the pathogenesis of pneumonic Mannheimiosis remains incompletely understood. Experiments have established that *Mannheimia haemolytica* A1 alone is usually incapable of causing disease because it is rapidly cleared by pulmonary defense mechanisms. These findings may explain why *Mannheimia haemolytica*, in spite of being present in the nasal cavity of healthy animals, only sporadically causes disease. For *Mannheimia haemolytica* to be established as a pulmonary infection, it is first required that stressors impair the defense mechanisms and allow the bacteria to colonize the lung (see section on Impairment of Defense Mechanisms). These stressors include weaning, transport, fatigue, crowding, mixing of cattle from various sources, inclement weather, temporary starvation, and viral infections. Horizontal transmission of viruses and *Mannheimia haemolytica* occurs during crowding and transportation of cattle.

Viruses that most commonly predispose cattle to pneumonic Mannheimiosis include BoHV-1, PI-3, and BRSV. Once established in the lungs, *Mannheimia haemolytica* causes lesions by means of different virulence factors, which include endotoxin, lipopolysaccharide, adhesins, and outer membrane proteins, but the most important is probably the production of a leukotoxin (exotoxin), which binds and kills bovine macrophages and neutrophils. The fact that this toxin exclusively affects ruminant leukocytes probably explains why *Mannheimia haemolytica* is a respiratory pathogen in cattle and sheep but not in other species. During *Mannheimia haemolytica* infection, alveolar macrophages, neutrophils, and mast cells release maximum amounts of proinflammatory cytokines, particularly TNF-α, IL-1, IL-8, adhesion molecules, histamine, and leukotrienes. By locally releasing enzymes and free radicals, leukocytes further contribute to the injury and necrosis of bronchiolar and alveolar cells.

The gross lesions of acute and subacute pneumonic Mannheimiosis are the prototypic fibrinous bronchopneumonia, with prominent fibrinous pleuritis (Fig. 9-71 and Web Fig. 9-10) and pleural effusion. Lesions are always cranioventral and usually ventral to a horizontal line through the tracheal bifurcation. The interlobular septa are distended by yellow, gelatinous edema and fibrin. The "marbling" of lobules is the result of intermixing areas of coagulation necrosis, interlobular interstitial edema, and congestion (Fig. 9-72).

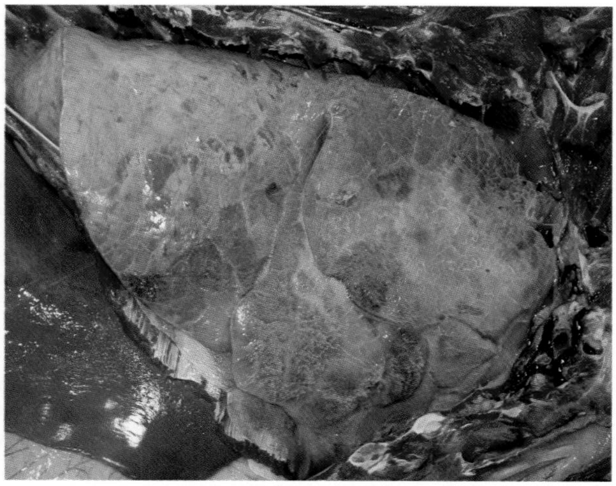

Fig. 9-71 Fibrinous bronchopneumonia (pleuropneumonia), pneumonic Mannheimiosis *(Mannheimia haemolytica)*, right lung, steer. Note the cranioventral pneumonia involving approximately 85% of the lung parenchyma. The lung is firm and swollen, and the pleura are covered with a thick layer of fibrin. (Courtesy Dr. A. López, Atlantic Veterinary College.)

Microscopically, lung lesions are evident 4 hours after experimental infection in which neutrophils fill the bronchial, bronchiolar, and alveolar spaces. Within 24 to 48 hours, the cytotoxic effect of *Mannheimia haemolytica* is manifested by necrosis of individual alveolar cells and fibrin begins to exude into the alveoli from increased permeability of alveolar capillaries. These changes are exacerbated by endothelial swelling, altered platelet function, increased procoagulant activity, and diminished profibrinolytic activity in the lungs. By 72 hours, alveolar macrophages start to appear in the bronchoalveolar space. At this time, large and irregular areas of coagulative necrosis are typically bordered by a rim of elongated cells often referred to as *swirling macrophages* or *oat-shaped cells,* now known to be degenerating neutrophils mixed with a few alveolar macrophages (see Fig. 9-72). In the early stages of the necrosis, there is no evidence of vascular thrombosis, suggesting that necrosis is primarily caused by the cytotoxin of *Mannheimia haemolytica* and is not the result of an ischemic change. The interlobular septae becomes distended with protein-rich edematous fluid and the lymphatic vessels contain fibrin thrombi. The trachea and bronchi can have considerable amounts of blood and exudate, which are transported by the mucociliary escalator or coughed up from deep within the lungs, but the walls of the trachea and major bronchi may or may not be involved. Because of the necrotizing process, sequelae to pneumonic Mannheimiosis can be serious and can include abscesses, encapsulated sequestra (isolated piece of necrotic lung), chronic pleuritis, fibrous pleural adhesions, and bronchiectasis.

Clinically, pneumonic Mannheimiosis is characterized by a severe toxemia that can kill animals even when considerable parts of the lungs remain functional and structurally normal. Cattle usually become depressed, febrile (104° to 106° F [40° to 41° C]), and anorexic and have a productive cough, encrusted nose, mucopurulent nasal exudate, shallow respiration, or an expiratory grunt.

Hemorrhagic Septicemia

Pneumonic Mannheimiosis should not be confused with hemorrhagic septicemia (septicemic pasteurellosis) of cattle and water buffalo *(Bubalus bubalis)* caused by inhalation or ingestion of serotypes 6:B and 6:E of *Pasteurella multocida.* This OIE-notifiable disease does not occur in North America and currently is reported only from some countries in Asia and Africa. In contrast to pneumonic Mannheimiosis, in which lesions are always confined to the lower respiratory tract, the bacteria of hemorrhagic septicemia always disseminates hematogenously to other organs. At necropsy, typically, generalized petechiae are present on the serosal surfaces of the intestine, heart, and lungs and in skeletal muscles. Superficial and visceral lymph nodes are swollen and hemorrhagic. Variable lesions include edematous and hemorrhagic lungs with or without consolidation, hemorrhagic enteritis, blood-tinged fluid in the thorax and abdomen, and subcutaneous edema of the head, neck, and ventral abdomen. Bacteria can be cultured from blood, and animals have high fever and die rapidly (100% case fatality).

Respiratory Histophilosis (Hemophilosis)

Respiratory histophilosis is part of the *Histophilus somni (Haemophilus somnus)* disease complex, which has at least eight different clinicopathologic forms, each one involving different organs. This complex includes septicemia, encephalitis (known as *thrombotic meningoencephalitis* [TME]), pneumonia (respiratory histophilosis

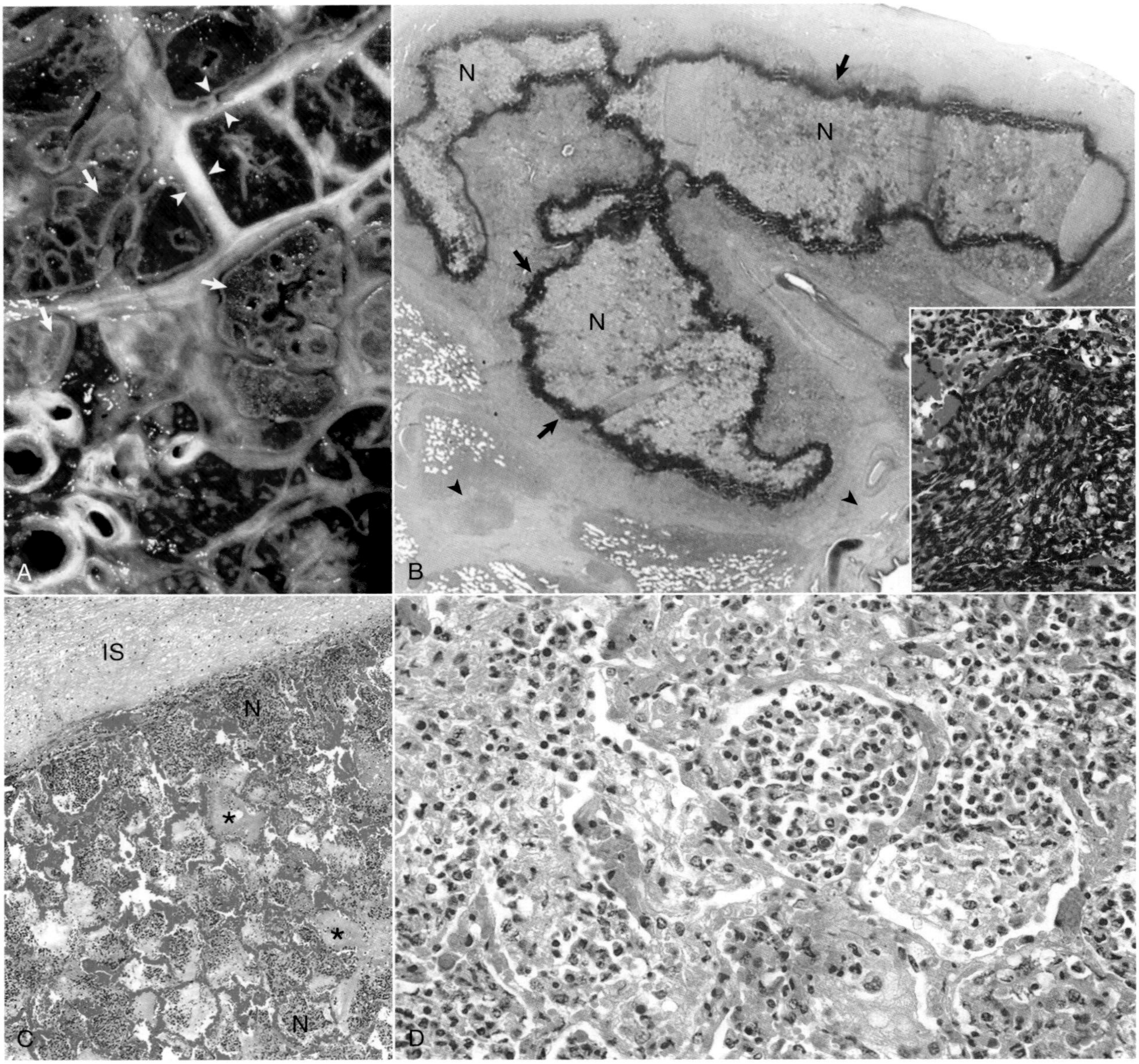

Fig. 9-72 Pneumonic Mannheimiosis *(Mannheimia haemolytica)*, lung, steer.

A, Cut surface. Interlobular septa *(arrowheads)* are notably distended by edema and fibrin. In the lung parenchyma are irregular areas of coagulative necrosis *(arrows)* surrounded by a rim of inflammatory cells. **B,** Note a large irregular area of necrosis *(N)* of the pulmonary parenchyma. Typically these necrotic areas are surrounded by an outer dense layer of inflammatory cells *(arrows)*. The interlobular septa are distended *(arrowheads)*. Inset *(bottom right corner)* shows the typical elongated and basophilic appearance of degenerated neutrophils known as oat-shaped cells. H&E stain. **C,** Note alveoli filled with fibrin *(asterisks)* and with neutrophils *(N)*. The interlobular septa *(IS)* is distended with proteinaceous fluid. H&E stain. **D,** *Mannheimia haemolytica* produces leukotoxin (cytotoxic for ruminant leukocytes) and lipopolysaccharide. Note the accumulation of cells, chiefly neutrophils, in the alveoli. Also note the active hyperemia of acute inflammation of the alveolar capillaries. H&E stain. (**A, B,** and **C** courtesy Dr. A. López, Atlantic Veterinary College. **D** courtesy Dr. J.F. Zachary, College of Veterinary Medicine, University of Illinois.)

[hemophilosis]), pleuritis, myocarditis, arthritis, ophthalmitis, conjunctivitis, otitis, and abortion. The portals of entry for the different forms of histophilosis have not been properly established.

The respiratory form of bovine histophilosis is the result of the bacterium's capacity to induce both suppurative and fibrinous bronchopneumonia. The latter is in some cases indistinguishable from that of pneumonic Mannheimiosis. The pathogenesis of respiratory histophilosis is still poorly understood, and the disease cannot be reproduced consistently by administration of *Histophilus somni* alone. Like *Mannheimia haemolytica,* it requires predisposing factors such as stress or a preceding viral infection. *Histophilus somni* is often isolated from the lungs of calves with enzootic pneumonia. The capacity of *Histophilus somni* to cause septicemia and localized infections in the lungs, brain, eyes, ear, heart, mammary gland, male and female genital organs, or placenta is perhaps attributable to specific virulence factors, such as immunoglobulin-binding proteins (IgBPs) and lipooligosaccharide (LOS). Also, *Histophilus somni* has the ability to undergo structural and antigenic variation, evade phagocytosis by promoting leukocytic apoptosis, inhibit intracellular killing, reduce transferrin concentrations, and induce endothelial apoptosis in the lungs of affected calves. Mixed pulmonary infections of *Histophilus somni, Mannheimia haemolytica,*

Pasteurella multocida, Arcanobacterium pyogenes, and mycoplasmas are fairly common in calves.

Mycoplasma Bovis Pneumonia

Mycoplasma bovis is the most common *Mycoplasma* sp. isolated from pneumonic lungs of cattle in Europe and North America. Pulmonary infection is exacerbated by stress or any other adverse factor (e.g., viral infection) that depresses the pulmonary defense mechanisms. Lung lesions are typically those of a chronic necrotizing bronchopneumonia with numerous well-delineated caseated nodules (Fig. 9-73 and Web Fig. 9-11). Microscopically, lesions are quite characteristic and consist of distinct areas of pulmonary necrosis centered around bronchi or bronchioles. The lesion is formed by a core of fine eosinophilic granular debris surrounded by a rim of neutrophils, macrophages, and fibroblasts (see Fig. 9-73). The diagnosis is confirmed by isolation or immunohistochemical labeling of tissue sections for *Mycoplasma* antigens. *Mycoplasma bovis* has also been incriminated in arthritis, otitis, mastitis, abortion, and keratoconjunctivitis.

Contagious Bovine Pleuropneumonia

Contagious bovine pleuropneumonia is a "List A" OIE-notifiable disease of historic interest in veterinary medicine because it was the object of early national control programs for infectious disease. It was eradicated from North America in 1892 and from Australia in the 1970s, but it is still enzootic in large areas of Africa, Asia, and Eastern Europe. The etiologic agent, *Mycoplasma mycoides* ssp. *mycoides* small colony type, was the first *Mycoplasma* isolated and is one of the most pathogenic of those that infect domestic animals. Natural infection occurs in cattle and Asian buffalo. Portal of entry is aerogenous, and infections occur when a susceptible animal inhales infected droplets. The pathogenic mechanisms are still inadequately understood but are suspected to involve toxin and galactan production, unregulated production of TNF-α, ciliary dysfunction, immunosuppression, and immune-mediated vasculitis. Vasculitis and thrombosis of pulmonary arteries, arterioles, veins, and lymphatics lead to lobular infarction.

The name of the disease is a good indication of the gross lesions. It is a severe, fibrinous bronchopneumonia (pleuropneumonia) similar to that of pneumonic Mannheimiosis (see Figs. 9-71 and 9-72) but having a more pronounced "marbling" of the lobules because of extensive interlobular edema and lymphatic thrombosis. Typically, 60% to 79% of lesions are in the caudal lobes (not cranioventrally), and pulmonary sequestra (necrotic lung encapsulated by connective tissue) are more frequent and larger than pneumonic Mannheimiosis. Unilateral lesions are common in this disease. Microscopically, the appearance again is like that of pneumonic Mannheimiosis, except that vasculitis and thrombosis of pulmonary arteries, arterioles, and capillaries are much more obvious and are clearly the major cause of the infarction and thrombosis of lymphatic vessels in interlobular septa. *Mycoplasma mycoides* ssp. *mycoides* small colony type remains viable in the sequestra for many years, and under stress (e.g., starvation), the fibrous capsule may break down, the mycoplasma is released into the airways, and it becomes a source of infection for other animals. Clinical signs are those of severe sepsis, including fever, depression, anorexia followed by severe respiratory signs such as opened-mouth dyspnea and coughing, and crepitation and pleural friction on thoracic auscultation. Vaccination is highly effective in preventing the disease.

Bovine Tuberculosis

Tuberculosis is an ancient, communicable, worldwide, chronic disease of humans and domestic animals. It continues to be a

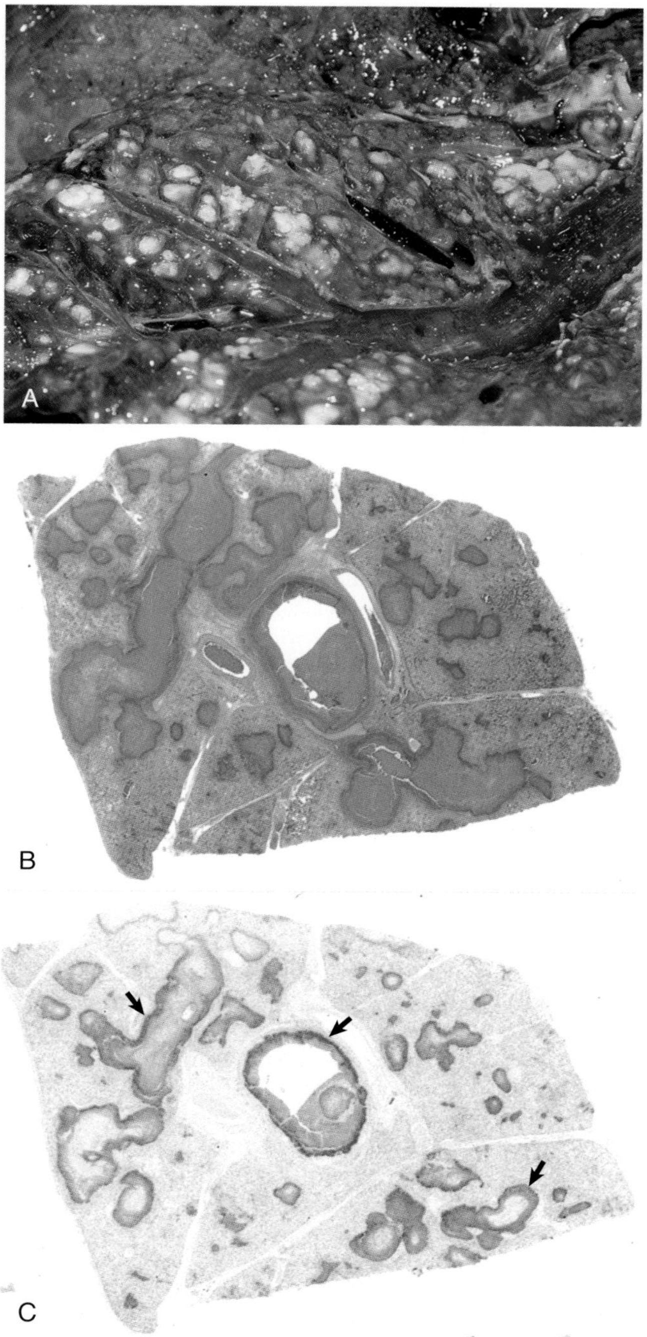

Fig. 9-73 Chronic bronchopneumonia *(Mycoplasma bovis)*, steer. **A,** The lung has numerous caseated granulomas scattered throughout the cranioventral lobes. **B,** Section of lung showing large rounded areas of necrosis filled with hypereosinophilic granular debris. **C,** Necrotizing bronchopneumonia, immunohistochemistry. Note positive staining for *Mycoplasma bovis* antigen in the margin of the necrotic lung (arrows). Immunoperoxidase stain. (**A** courtesy Dr. A. López, Atlantic Veterinary College; **B** and **C** courtesy Dr. A. López and Dr. C. Legge, Atlantic Veterinary College.)

major problem in humans in underdeveloped countries, and it is on the rise in some industrialized nations, largely because of the immunosuppressive effects of AIDS, immigration, and movement of infected animals across borders. The World Health Organization (WHO) estimated that 30 million people, mostly in developing countries, died of tuberculosis between 1990 and 1999. *Mycobacterium tuberculosis* is transmitted between humans, but where unpasteurized cow's milk is consumed, *Mycobacterium bovis* from the milk of cattle with mammary tuberculosis is also an important cause of human tuberculosis.

Bovine tuberculosis is primarily caused by *Mycobacterium bovis,* but infection with *Mycobacterium tuberculosis,* the pathogen of human tuberculosis, can occur sporadically. Tuberculosis can be acquired by several routes, but infection of the lungs by inhalation of *Mycobacterium bovis* is the most common in adult cattle, whereas ingestion of infected milk is more predominant in young animals. Organisms belonging to the *Mycobacterium avium-intracellulare complex* can also infect cattle, but for infection caused by these organisms, the term *mycobacteriosis* (not tuberculosis) is currently preferred.

Respiratory infection usually starts when inhaled bacilli reach the alveoli and are phagocytosed by pulmonary alveolar macrophages. If these cells are successful in destroying the bacteria, infection is averted. However, *Mycobacterium bovis,* being a facultative pathogen of the monocytic-macrophagic system, may multiply intracellularly, kill the macrophage, and initiate infection. From this first nidus of infection, bacilli spread aerogenously via airways within the lungs and eventually via the lymph vessels to tracheobronchial and mediastinal lymph nodes.

The initial focus of infection at the portal of entry (lungs) plus the involvement of regional lymph nodes is termed the *primary (Ghon) complex* of tuberculosis. If the infection is not contained within this primary complex, bacilli disseminate via the lymph vessels to distant organs and other lymph nodes by the migration of infected macrophages. Hematogenous dissemination occurs sporadically when a granuloma containing mycobacteria erodes the wall of a blood vessel, causes vasculitis, and allows the granuloma to discharge mycobacteria into the alveolar circulation. If dissemination is sudden and massive, mycobacteria are widely disseminated and numerous small foci of infection develop in many tissues and organs and the process is referred to as miliary tuberculosis (like millet seeds). The host becomes hypersensitive to the mycobacterium, which enhances the cell-mediated immune defenses in early or mild infections but can result in host-tissue destruction in the form of caseous necrosis. The evolution and dissemination of the pulmonary infection are closely regulated by cytokines and TNF-α production by alveolar macrophages.

Unlike abscesses that tend to grow rather fast, granulomas evolve slowly at the site of infection. The lesion starts with few macrophages and neutrophils ingesting the offending organism, but because mycobacterium organisms are resistant to phagocytosis, infected macrophages eventually die, releasing viable bacteria, lipids, and cell debris. Cell debris accumulates in the center of the lesion, whereas viable bacteria and bacterial lipids attract additional macrophages and a few lymphocytes at the periphery of the lesion. Some of these newly recruited macrophages are activated by local lymphocytes and become large phagocytic cells with abundant cytoplasm resembling epithelial cells, thus the term *epithelioid cells.* Multinucleated macrophages also appear at the edges of the lesion, and finally the entire focus of inflammatory process becomes surrounded by fibroblasts and connective tissue. It may take weeks or months for a granuloma to be grossly visible.

Bovine tuberculosis, the prototype for granulomatous pneumonia, is characterized by the presence of a few or many caseated granulomas (see Fig. 9-65). The early gross changes are small foci (tubercles) most frequently seen in the dorsocaudal, subpleural areas. With progression, the lesions enlarge and become confluent with the formation of large areas of caseous necrosis. Calcification of the granulomas is a typical finding in bovine tuberculosis. Single nodules or clusters occur on the pleura and peritoneum, and this presentation has been termed *pearl disease.* Microscopically the tubercle is composed of mononuclear cells of various types. In young tubercles, which are noncaseous, epithelioid and Langhans' giant cells are at the center, surrounded by lymphocytes, plasma cells, and macrophages. Later, caseous necrosis develops at the center, secondary to the effects of cell-mediated hypersensitivity and enclosed by fibrosis at the periphery. Acid-fast organisms may be numerous but more often are difficult to find in histologic section or smears.

Clinically, the signs relate to the dysfunction of a particular organ system or to general debilitation, reduced milk production, and emaciation. In the pulmonary form, which is more than 90% of bovine cases, a chronic, moist cough can progress to dyspnea. Enlarged tracheobronchial lymph nodes can contribute to the dyspnea by impinging on airways, and the enlargement of caudal mediastinal nodes can compress the caudal thoracic esophagus and cause bloating.

Interstitial Pneumonias of Cattle

Atypical interstitial pneumonia (AIP) is a vague clinical term well entrenched in veterinary literature, but one that has led to enormous confusion among veterinarians. It was first used to describe acute or chronic forms of bovine pneumonia that did not fit in any of the "classic" forms because of the lack of exudate and lack of productive cough. Microscopically, the criteria for diagnosis of AIP in cattle were based on the absence of obvious exudate and the presence of edema, interstitial emphysema (see the section on Pulmonary Emphysema), hyaline membranes, hyperplasia of type II pneumonocytes, and alveolar fibrosis with interstitial cellular infiltrates. At that time, any pulmonary disease or pulmonary syndrome that had a few of the above lesions was traditionally diagnosed as AIP, and grouping all these different syndromes together was inconsequential because their etiopathogenesis were then unknown.

Field and laboratory investigations have demonstrated that most of the bovine syndromes previously grouped under AIP have rather different causes and pathogeneses (Fig. 9-74). Further, what was "atypical" in the past has become so routine that it is fairly common nowadays to find "typical cases" of AIP. For all these reasons, investigators, largely from Britain, proposed that all these syndromes previously clustered into AIP should be named according to their specific cause or pathogenesis. The most common bovine syndromes characterized by edema, emphysema, hyaline membranes, and hyperplasia of type II pneumonocytes include (1) bovine pulmonary edema and emphysema (fog fever), (2) "extrinsic allergic alveolitis" (hypersensitivity pneumonitis), (3) "reinfection syndromes" (hypersensitivity to *Dictyocaulus* sp. or BRSV), (4) milk allergy, (5) ingestion of moldy potatoes, (6) Paraquat toxicity, and others.

Acute bovine pulmonary edema and emphysema (fog fever)

Acute bovine pulmonary edema and emphysema (ABPEE), known in Britain as fog fever (no association with atmospheric conditions), occurs in cattle usually grazing "fog" pastures (i.e., aftermath or foggage, regrowth after a hay or silage has been cut). Epidemiologically, ABPEE usually occurs in adult beef cattle in the fall when there is a change in pasture, from a short,

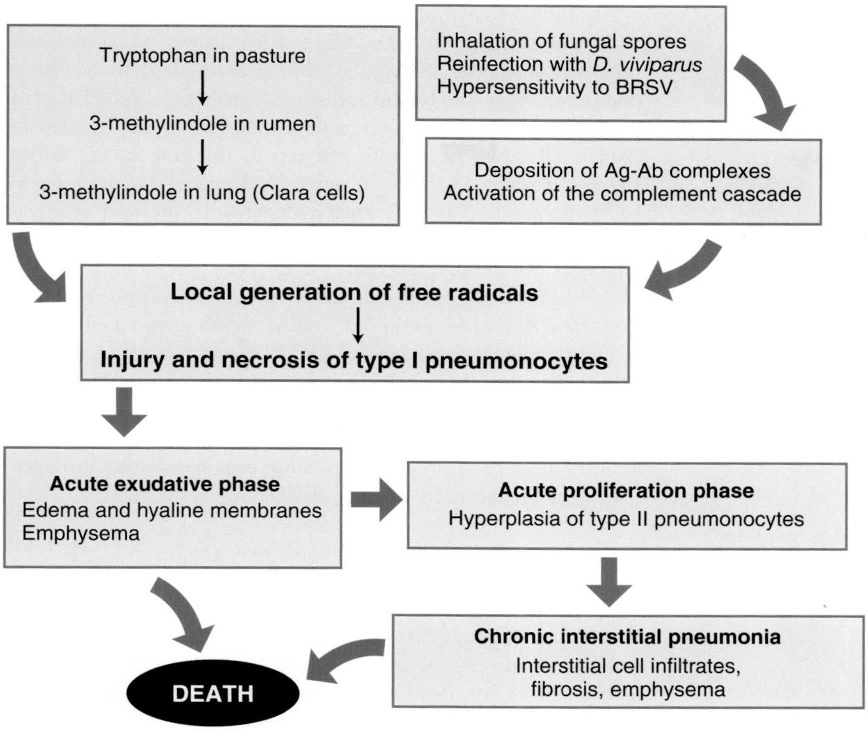

Fig. 9-74 Schematic diagram of the pathogenesis of toxic and allergic pneumonias ("atypical interstitial pneumonia") in cattle.
BRSV, Bovine respiratory syncytial virus. (Redrawn with permission from Dr. A. López, Atlantic Veterinary College.)

dry grass to a lush, green grass. It is generally accepted that L-tryptophan present in the pasture is metabolized in the rumen to 3-methylindole, which in turn is absorbed into the bloodstream and carried to the lungs. Mixed function oxidases present in the nonciliated bronchiolar epithelial (Clara) cells metabolize 3-methylindole into a highly pneumotoxic compound that causes extensive and selective necrosis of bronchiolar cells and type I pneumonocytes (see Figs. 9-74 and 9-75) and increases alveolar permeability, leading to edema, thickening of the alveolar interstitium, and alveolar and interstitial emphysema. 3-Methylindole also interferes with the lipid metabolism of type II pneumonocytes.

The gross lesions are those of a diffuse interstitial pneumonia with severe alveolar and interstitial edema and interlobular emphysema (see Fig. 9-37). The lungs are expanded, pale, and rubbery in texture, and the lesions are most notable in the caudal lobes. Microscopically, the lesions are alveolar and interstitial edema and emphysema, formation of characteristic hyaline membranes within alveoli (see Fig. 9-37), and in those animals that survive for several days, hyperplasia of type II epithelial cells and alveolar interstitial fibrosis.

Clinically, severe respiratory distress develops within 10 days of the abrupt pasture change, and cattle develop expiratory dyspnea, oral breathing, and evidence of emphysema within the lungs and even subcutaneously along the back. Experimentally, reducing ruminal conversion of L-tryptophan to 3-methylindole prevents the development of ABPEE.

A number of other agents cause virtually the same clinical and pathologic syndrome as is seen in ABPEE. The pathogenesis is assumed to be similar, although presumably other toxic factors are specific for each syndrome. One of these pneumotoxic factors is 4-ipomeanol, which is found in moldy sweet potatoes contaminated with the fungus *Fusarium solani.* Mixed-function oxidases in the lungs activate 4-ipomeanol into a potent pneumotoxicant capable of producing irreversible oxidative injury to type I pneumonocytes and bronchiolar epithelial cells, presumably through lipoperoxidation of cell membranes. Similarly, purple mint (*Perilla frutescens*), stinkwood (*Zieria arborescens*), and rapeseed and kale (*Brassica* species) also cause pulmonary edema, emphysema, and interstitial pneumonia.

Extrinsic allergic alveolitis

Extrinsic allergic alveolitis (hypersensitivity pneumonitis), one of the most common allergic diseases in cattle, is seen mainly in housed, adult dairy cows in the winter. This disease shares many similarities with its human counterpart known as *farmer's lung,* which results from a type III hypersensitivity reaction to inhaled organic antigens, most commonly fungal spores, mainly of the thermophilic actinomycete, *Saccharopolyspora rectivirgula (Micropolyspora faeni),* commonly found in moldy hay. This is followed by an antibody response to inhaled fungal spores and local deposition of antigen-antibody complexes (Arthus reaction) in the lungs (see Fig. 9-74). Because it affects only a few animals of the herd or the sporadic person working in a farm, it is presumed that intrinsic host factors, such as dysregulation of dendritic cells, T lymphocytes, IgG, interleukins, IFN-γ, and surfactant, are involved in the pathogenesis of the disease. Clinically, it can be acute or chronic; the latter has a cyclical pattern of exacerbation during winter months. Weight loss, coughing, and poor exercise tolerance are clinical features.

Grossly, the postmortem lesions vary from subtle, gray, subpleural foci (granulomatous inflammation) to severe lesions, in which the lungs are firm and heavy and have a "meaty appearance" because of type II alveolar epithelial hyperplasia, lymphocytic infiltration, and interstitial fibrosis. Characteristically, discrete noncaseous granulomas formed in response to the deposition of antigen-antibody complexes are scattered throughout the lungs. Chronic cases of extrinsic allergic alveolitis can eventually progress to diffuse fibrosing alveolitis. Full recovery can occur if the disease is recognized and treated early.

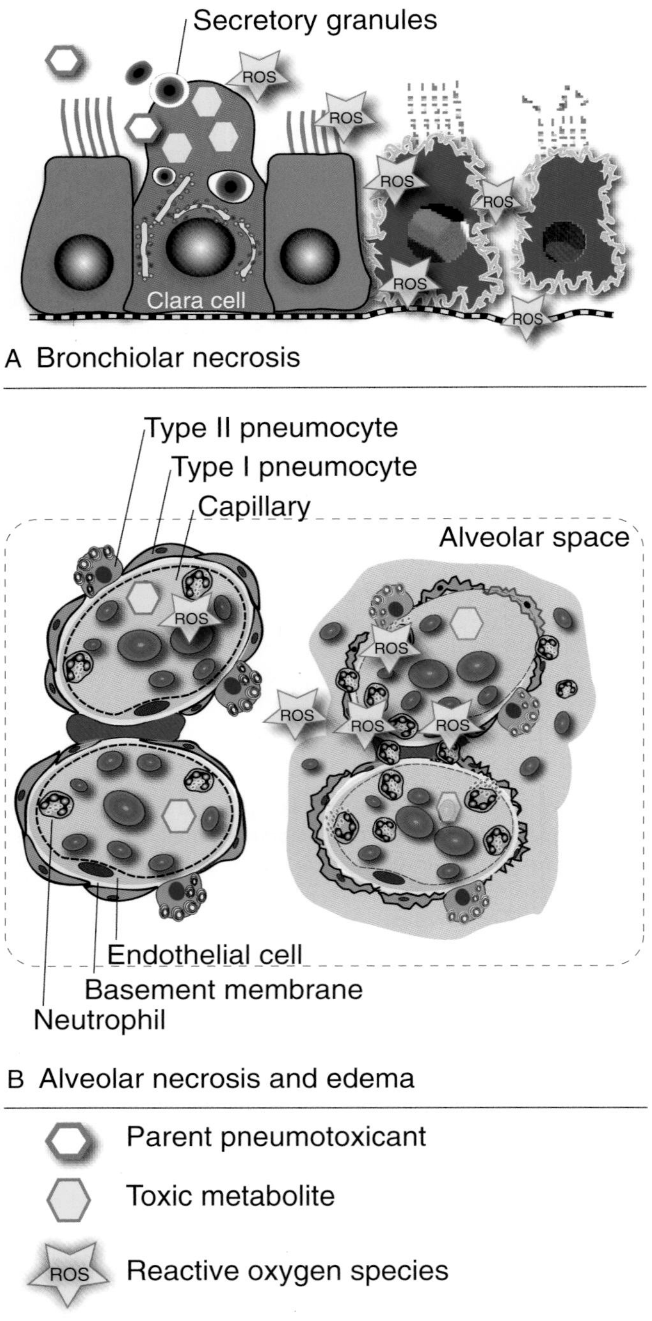

Fig. 9-75 Schematic representation of bronchiolar and alveolar injury caused by pneumotoxicants.

A, Inhaled pneumotoxicants, such as paraquat or 3-methyl-indole, are metabolized into highly reactive compounds (ROS) by bronchiolar Clara cells. ROS reach adjacent bronchiolar cells *(blue)* by diffusion and cause injury and necrosis (*right two cells*). Secretory granules contain several proteins such as surfactant-like protein, antiinflammatory protein (CC10) and bronchiolar lining proteins. **B,** ROS produced by Clara cells are also absorbed into capillaries within the lamina propria and are transferred by the circulatory system to pulmonary capillaries where they also disrupt the air-blood barrier, causing degeneration and necrosis of type I pneumocytes. This process leads to leakage of plasma fluid (alveolar edema *[pink color]*) and extravasation of erythrocytes (alveolar hemorrhage) and neutrophils (active hyperemia). Ingested pneumotoxicants can also be metabolized by the liver, leading to release of ROS into the circulatory system that then disrupts the air-blood barrier. (Courtesy Dr. A. López, Atlantic Veterinary College.)

Reinfection syndrome

Hypersensitivity to reinfection with larvae of *Dictyocaulus viviparus* is another allergic syndrome manifested in the lungs that causes signs and lesions indistinguishable from ABPEE, with the exception of eosinophils and possibly larvae in the alveolar exudate. The hypersensitivity reaction in the lung causes diffuse alveolar damage and edema, necrosis of type I pneumonocytes and hyperplasia of type II pneumonocytes. In the later stages of the disease there is formation of small granulomas with interstitial infiltrates of mononuclear cells.

It has been suggested that emphysema with diffuse proliferative alveolitis and formation of hyaline membranes can also occur sporadically in the late stages of BRSV infection in cattle. Presumably, this disease shares many similarities with "atypical" infections occasionally seen in children with respiratory syncytial virus (RSV human strain), in which a hypersensitivity to the virus or virus-induced augmentation of the immune response results in hypersensitivity pneumonitis (see Fig. 9-74).

Other Forms of Bovine Interstitial Pneumonia

Inhalation of manure ("pit") gases, such as NO_2, H_2S, and ammonia (NH_3), from silos or sewage can be a serious hazard to animals and humans. At toxic concentrations, these gases cause necrosis of bronchiolar cells and type I pneumonocytes, a fulminating pulmonary edema that causes asphyxiation, and rapid death (see Fig. 9-42). Like other oxidant gases, inhalation of NO_2 (silo gas) also causes bronchiolitis, edema, and interstitial pneumonia and in survivors, bronchiolitis obliterans ("silo filler's disease").

Smoke inhalation resulting from barn or house fires is sporadically seen by veterinarians and pathologists. In addition to skin burns, animals involved in fire accidents suffer extensive thermal injury produced by the heat on the nasal and laryngeal mucosa, and severe chemical irritation caused by inhalation of combustion gases and particles in the lung. Animals that survive or are rescued from fires frequently develop nasal, laryngeal, and tracheal edema, and pulmonary hemorrhage and alveolar edema, which are caused by chemical injury to the blood-air barrier or by ARDS caused by the excessive production of free radicals during the pulmonary inflammatory response. Microscopic examination of the lungs often reveals carbon particles (soot) on mucosal surfaces of the conducting system.

Parasitic Pneumonias of Cattle

Verminous pneumonia (Dictyocaulus viviparus)

Pulmonary lesions in parasitic pneumonias (the word is used here in its restricted sense to mean helminth infestations of the lungs) vary from interstitial pneumonia caused by migrating larvae to chronic bronchitis from intrabronchial adult parasites, to granulomatous pneumonia, which is caused by dead larvae, aberrant parasites, or eggs of parasites. In many cases, an "eosinophilic syndrome" in the lungs is characterized by infiltrates of eosinophils in the pulmonary interstitium and bronchoalveolar spaces and by blood eosinophilia. Atelectasis and emphysema secondary to the obstruction of airways by parasites and mucous secretions are also common findings in parasitic pneumonias. The severity of these lesions relates to the numbers and size of the parasites and the nature of the host reaction, which sometimes includes hypersensitivity reactions (see re-infection syndrome). A common general term for all of these diseases is *verminous pneumonia,* and the adult nematodes are often visible grossly in the airways (Fig. 9-76).

Dictyocaulus viviparus is an important pulmonary nematode (lungworm) responsible for a disease in cattle referred to as *verminous pneumonia* or *verminous bronchitis.* Adult parasites live in

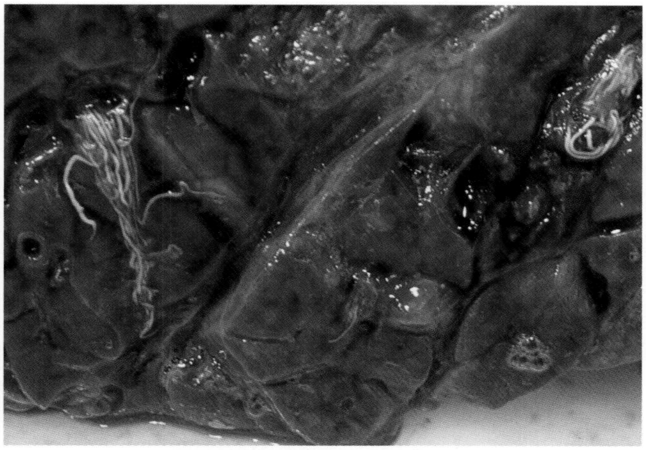

Fig. 9-76 Verminous pneumonia *(Dictyocaulus viviparus),* bronchus, calf.
The bronchi contains numerous slender lungworms and large amounts of clear foamy fluid, indicative of pulmonary edema. (Courtesy Dr. A. López and Dr. L. Miller, Atlantic Veterinary College.)

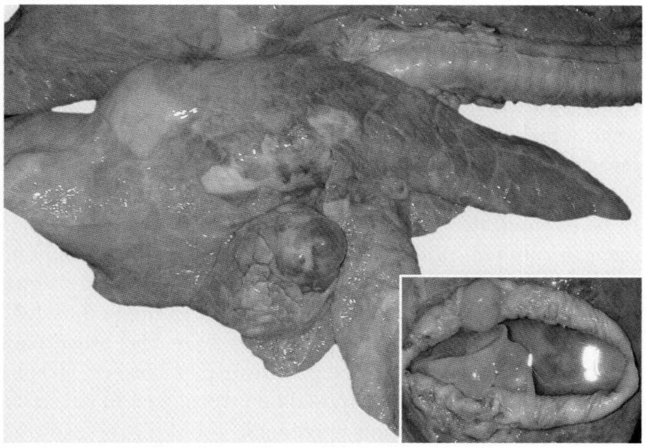

Fig. 9-77 Hydatidosis (echinococcosis), lung, sheep.
A large hydatid cyst is present in the pulmonary parenchyma. *Inset,* Hydatid cyst, cut-open section. The cyst contains fluid and larvae and is often enclosed by a fibrous capsule. (Courtesy Dr. Manuel Quezada, Universidad de Concepción, Chile.)

the bronchi of cattle, mainly in the caudal lobes and cause severe bronchial irritation, bronchitis, and pulmonary edema, which in turn is responsible for lobular atelectasis and interstitial emphysema. Atelectasis is confined to the lobules of the lungs ventilated by the obstructed bronchi (dorsocaudal). Interstitial emphysema (interlobular) is caused by forced expiratory movements against a partially obstructed single bronchus. In addition to the inflammation of bronchial mucosa, bronchoaspiration of larvae and eggs also causes an influx of leukocytes into the bronchoalveolar space (alveolitis). Verminous pneumonia is most commonly seen in calves during their first summer grazing pastures that are repeatedly used from year to year, particularly in regions of Europe that have a moist, cool climate. The parasite can overwinter in pastures, even in climates as cold as Canada's, and older animals may be carriers for a considerable length of time.

At necropsy, lesions appear as dark or gray, depressed, wedge-shaped areas of atelectasis involving few or many lobules usually along the dorsocaudal aspect of the lungs. On a cut surface, edematous foam and mucus mixed with white, slender (up to 80-mm long) nematodes are visible in the bronchi (see Fig. 9-76). In the most severe cases, massive numbers of nematodes fill the bronchial tree. Microscopically the bronchial lumens are filled with parasites admixed with mucus because of goblet cell hyperplasia, and there is also squamous metaplasia of the bronchial and bronchiolar epithelium because of chronic irritation. There is also alveolar edema; hyperplasia of BALT caused by persistent immunologic stimuli; hypertrophy and hyperplasia of bronchiolar smooth muscle because of increased contraction and decreased muscle relaxation; and a few eosinophilic granulomas around the eggs and dead larvae. These granulomas, grossly, are gray, noncaseated nodules (2 to 4 mm in diameter) and may be confused with those seen at the early stages of tuberculosis.

The clinical signs (coughing) vary with the severity of infection, and severe cases can be confused clinically with interstitial pneumonias. Expiratory dyspnea and death can occur with heavy parasitic infestations when there is massive obstruction of airways.

A different form of bovine pneumonia, an acute allergic reaction known as *re-infection syndrome,* occurs when previously sensitized adult cattle are exposed to large numbers of larvae *(Dictyocaulus viviparus).* Lesions in this syndrome are those of a hypersensitivity pneumonia as previously described.

Other lung parasites

Ascaris suum is the common intestinal roundworm of pigs; larvae cannot complete their life cycle in calves, but the larvae can migrate through the lungs and cause severe pneumonia and the death of calves within 2 weeks of infection, usually acquired from the soil in which infested pigs were previously kept. Pigs, the natural host, also can be killed if exposed to an overwhelming larval migration. Clinical signs as a result of migration of larvae through the lungs include cough and expiratory dyspnea to the point of oral breathing. The gross lesions are a diffuse interstitial pneumonia with hemorrhagic foci, atelectasis, and interlobular edema and emphysema, similar to what is seen in the lungs of pigs (see Fig. 9-62). Microscopically, there are focal intraalveolar hemorrhages caused by larvae migrating through the alveolar walls. Some larvae admixed with edematous fluid and cellular exudate (including eosinophils) may be visible in bronchioles and alveoli. The alveolar walls are thickened because of edema and a few inflammatory cells.

Hydatid cysts, the intermediate stage of *Echinococcus granulosus,* can be found in the lungs and liver and other viscera of sheep and to a lesser extent in cattle, pigs, goats, horses, and humans. The adult stage is a tapeworm that parasitizes the intestine of Canidae. Hydatidosis is still an important zoonosis in some countries, and perpetuation of the parasite life cycle results from animals being fed uncooked offal from infected sheep and consumption of uninspected meat. Hydatid cysts are generally 5 to 15 cm in diameter, and numerous cysts can be found in the viscera of affected animals (Fig. 9-77). Each parasitic cyst is filled with clear fluid; numerous daughter cysts attach to the wall, each containing several "brood capsules" with protoscolices inside. Hydatid cysts have little clinical significance in animals but are economically important because of carcass condemnation.

Aspiration Pneumonias of Cattle

The inhalation of regurgitated ruminal contents or iatrogenic deposition of medicines or milk into the trachea can cause severe and often fatal aspiration pneumonia. Bland substances, such as mineral oil, may incite only a mild suppurative or histiocytic bronchopneumonia, whereas some "home remedies" or ruminal contents are highly irritating and cause a fibrinous, necrotizing bronchopneumonia. The right cranial lung lobe tends to be more severely affected because the right cranial bronchus is the most cranial branch and enters the ventrolateral aspect of the trachea. However, the distribution may vary when animals aspirate while in lateral recumbency. In some severe cases, pulmonary necrosis can be complicated by infection with saprophytic organisms present in ruminal contents, causing fatal gangrenous pneumonia. Aspiration pneumonia should always be considered in animals whose swallowing has been compromised, for example those with cleft palate or hypocalcemia (milk fever). On the other hand, neurological diseases such as encephalitis (e.g., rabies) or encephalopathy (e.g., lead poisoning) should be investigated in animals in which the cause of aspiration pneumonia could not be explained otherwise. Depending on the nature of the aspirated material, histopathologic evaluation generally reveals foreign particles such as vegetable cells, milk droplets, and large numbers of bacteria in bronchi, bronchioles, and alveoli. Vegetable cells and milk typically induce an early neutrophilic response followed by a histocytic reaction with "foreign body" multinucleated giant cells. Special stains are used for the microscopic confirmation of aspirated particles in the lung (e.g., PAS for vegetable cells and O-red oil for oil or milk droplets).

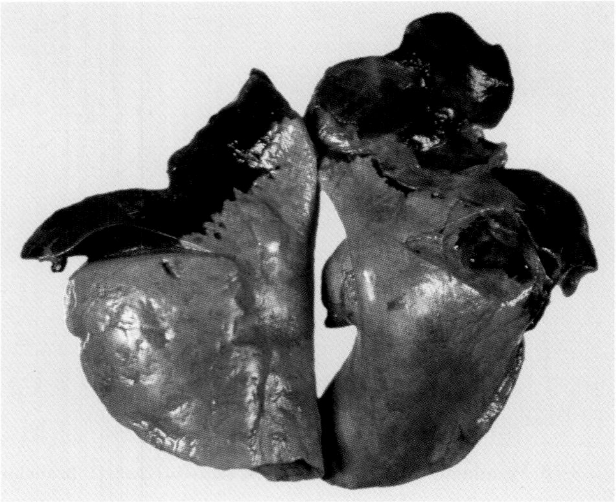

Fig. 9-78 Acute fibrinous bronchopneumonia (pleuropneumonia), pneumonic Mannheimiosis *(Mannheimia haemolytica)*, lungs, lamb. The cranioventral aspects of the lung are red, swollen, and very firm (consolidated) with some fibrin on the pleural surface. Note that the consolidated lung resembles liver, a change that was previously referred to as "hepatization." (Courtesy Ontario Veterinary College.)

Pneumonias of Sheep and Goats

In the past, *Pasteurella haemolytica* was incriminated in four major ovine diseases known as (1) *acute ovine pneumonic pasteurellosis* (shipping fever), (2) *enzootic pneumonia* (nonprogressive chronic pneumonia), (3) *fulminating septicemia,* and (4) *mastitis.* Under the new nomenclature, *Mannheimia haemolytica* is responsible for ovine pneumonia resembling shipping fever in cattle (ovine pneumonic Mannheimiosis), septicemia in young lambs (under 3 months of age), and ovine enzootic pneumonia and sporadic severe gangrenous mastitis in ewes. *Bibersteinia (Pasteurella) trehalosi* (formerly *Pasteurella haemolytica* biotype T) is the agent incriminated in septicemia in lambs 5 to 12 months old.

Ovine Pneumonic Mannheimiosis

Ovine pneumonic Mannheimiosis is one of the most common and economically significant diseases in most areas where sheep are raised. It is caused by *Mannheimia haemolytica* and has pathogenesis and lesions similar to those of pneumonic Mannheimiosis of cattle. Colonization and infection of lungs are facilitated by stressors, such as changes in weather, handling, deworming, or dipping, and viral infections, such as PI-3 virus, RSV, adenovirus, and probably chlamydia and *Bordetella parapertussis.* Lesions are characterized by a severe fibrinous bronchopneumonia (cranioventral) with pleuritis (Fig. 9-78). Subacute to chronic cases progress to purulent bronchopneumonia, and sequelae include abscesses and fibrous pleural adhesions.

Chronic Enzootic Pneumonia

In sheep, this entity is a multifactorial disease complex that, in contrast to ovine pneumonic Mannheimiosis, causes only a mild-to-moderate pneumonia, and it is rarely fatal. It generally affects animals younger than 1 year of age. Significant costs associated with chronic enzootic pneumonia include reduction of weight gain, labor costs, veterinary fees, and slaughterhouse waste. The modifier "chronic" is used here to avoid any confusion with pneumonic Mannheimiosis ("acute enzootic pneumonia"). It is also sometimes called atypical pneumonia, chronic nonprogressive pneumonia, proliferative pneumonia, or other names.

Chronic enzootic pneumonia is a clinical epidemiologic term and does not imply a single causal agent but is the result of a combination of infectious, environmental, and managerial factors. The list of infectious agents involved in ovine enzootic pneumonia includes *Mannheimia haemolytica, Pasteurella multocida,* PI-3, adenovirus, reovirus, RSV, chlamydia, and mycoplasmas *(Mycoplasma ovipneumoniae).*

In the early stages of the disease, a cranioventral bronchointerstitial pneumonia is characterized by moderate thickening of alveolar walls because of hyperplasia of type II pneumonocytes. In some cases, when lungs are infected with secondary pathogens, such as *Pasteurella multocida,* pneumonia may progress to fibrinous or suppurative bronchopneumonia. One might expect some specific evidence pointing to the infectious agents (e.g., large intranuclear inclusion bodies in epithelial cells with adenoviral infection), but this is often not the case, either because examination is seldom done at the acute stage when the lesions are still present or because secondary bacterial infections mask the primary lesions. In the late stages, chronic enzootic pneumonia is characterized by hyperplastic bronchitis, atelectasis, alveolar and peribronchiolar fibrosis, and marked peribronchial lymphoid hyperplasia (cuffing pneumonia).

Septicemic Pasteurellosis

Septicemic pasteurellosis, a common ovine disease, is caused by *Bibersteinia trehalosi* (formerly *Pasteurella trehalosi or Mannheimia haemolytica* biotype T) in lambs 5 months or older, or by *Mannheimia haemolytica* (biotype A) in lambs younger than 2 months of age. Both organisms are carried in the tonsils and oropharynx of clinically healthy sheep, and under abnormal circumstances, bacteria can invade adjacent tissues, enter the bloodstream, and cause septicemia, particularly under stress from dietary or environmental changes. Affected animals usually die within few hours of infection, and these animals only rarely have clinical signs such as dullness, recumbency, and dyspnea. Gross lesions include a distinctive necrotizing pharyngitis and tonsillitis, ulcerative esophagitis, severe congestion and edema of the lungs, focal hepatic necrosis, and petechiae in the mucosa of the tongue, esophagus, and intestine and particularly in the lungs and pleura. Microscopically, the hallmark lesion is a disseminated intravascular thrombosis often with bacterial colonies in the capillaries of affected tissues. The alveolar capillaries contain bacteria and microrhombi, and the alveolar lumens have fibrin and red blood cells. *Mannheimia haemolytica* and *Bibersteinia trehalosi* are readily isolated from many organs.

Contagious Caprine Pleuropneumonia

Contagious caprine pleuropneumonia in goats is the counterpart of contagious bovine pleuropneumonia in cattle; sheep do not have a corresponding disease. The etiopathogenesis and geographic distribution of contagious caprine pleuropneumonia are yet to be determined. Three mycoplasmas, namely *Mycoplasma mycoides* ssp. *mycoides* large colony type, *Mycoplasma mycoides* ssp. *capri*, and *Mycoplasma capricolum* ssp. *capripneumoniae*, can produce respiratory tract infections; however, only the last is considered to cause typical contagious caprine pleuropneumonia.

Caprine pleuropneumonia (OIE-notifiable disease) is important in Africa, the Middle East, and parts of Asia but is also seen elsewhere. *Mycoplasma mycoides* ssp. *mycoides* large colony type and *Mycoplasma mycoides* ssp. *capri* are present in North America and have been isolated from respiratory diseases of goats.

The gross lesions caused by *Mycoplasma capricolum* ssp. *capripneumoniae* are similar to those of the bovine disease and consist of a severe, often unilateral fibrinous bronchopneumonia and pleuritis; however, distention of the interlobular septa (which are normally not as well developed in sheep as in cattle) and formation of pulmonary sequestra are less obvious than in the bovine disease. Fibrinous polyarthritis, septicemia, meningitis, mastitis, peritonitis, and abortion are other possible manifestations of disease caused by *Mycoplasma mycoides* ssp. *mycoides* large colony type and *Mycoplasma mycoides* ssp. *capri*. The pathogenicity of other mycoplasmas, such as *Mycoplasma ovipneumoniae, Mycoplasma arginini,* and *Mycoplasma capricolum* ssp. *capricolum,* in sheep and goats is still being defined, and specific description of the lesions would be premature. These organisms probably cause disease only in circumstances similar to those for enzootic pneumonia, where host, infectious, and environmental factors create a complex interaction in the pathogenesis of the disease. Most recently, it has been suggested that IgG antibodies directed against ovine mycoplasmal antigens cross-react with ciliary proteins, causing inflammation and ciliary dysfunction, a condition in lambs referred to as *coughing syndrome.* Clinically, contagious caprine pleuropneumonia is similar to contagious bovine pleuropneumonia, with high morbidity and mortality, fever, cough, dyspnea, and increasing distress and weakness.

Maedi (Maedi-Visna)

Maedi is an important, lifelong, and persistent viral disease of sheep and occurs in most countries, except Australia and New Zealand. Maedi means "shortness of breath" in the Icelandic language, and it is known as *Graaff-Reinet disease* in South Africa, *Zwoegerziekte* in The Netherlands, *La bouhite* in France, and *ovine (Montana or Marsh's) progressive pneumonia* (OPP) in the US. More recently, the disease has also been referred to as *ovine lentivirus-induced lymphoid interstitial pneumonia* or simply, *lymphoid interstitial pneumonia* (LIP).

Maedi is caused by a nononcogenic small ruminant lentivirus (ovine lentivirus) of the family Retroviridae antigenically related to the lentivirus causing caprine arthritis-encephalitis. Seroepidemiologic studies indicate that infection is widespread in the sheep population, yet the clinical disease seems to be rare.

The pathogenesis is incompletely understood, but it is known that transmission occurs largely through ingestion of infected

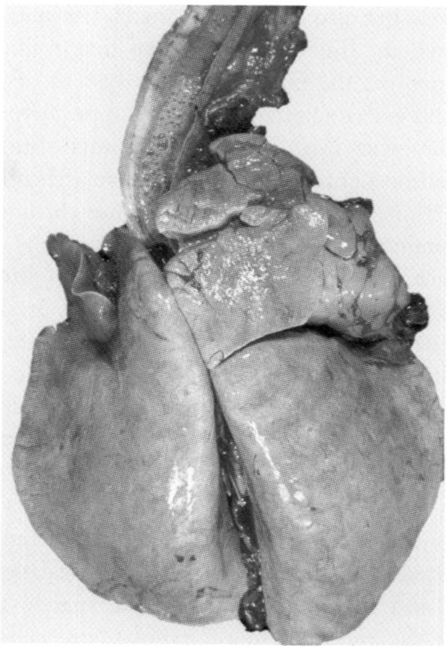

Fig. 9-79 Interstitial pneumonia (unknown etiology), lung, sheep. The lungs are heavy, rubbery, and show costal (rib) imprints on the visceral pleural surface. The diffuse distribution is typical of interstitial pneumonia. The trachea contains some edema fluid. (Courtesy Western College of Veterinary Medicine.)

colostrum and to a lesser extent by close contact between infected and susceptible sheep. Once in the body, the ovine lentivirus remains for long periods of time within monocytes and macrophages, including alveolar and pulmonary intravascular macrophages; clinical signs do not develop until after a long incubation period of 2 years or more.

Pulmonary lesions at the time of death are a severe interstitial pneumonia, and the lungs fail to collapse when the thorax is opened. Notable rib imprints, indicators of uncollapsed lungs, are often present on the pleural surface (Fig. 9-79). The lungs are pale and mottled and typically heavy (2 to 3 times normal weight), and the tracheobronchial lymph nodes are enlarged. Microscopically, the interstitial pneumonia is characterized by BALT hyperplasia and thickening of alveolar walls and peribronchial interstitial tissue by heavy infiltration of lymphocytes, largely T lymphocytes (see Fig. 9-61). Recruitment of mononuclear cells into the pulmonary interstitium is presumably the result of sustainable production of cytokines by retrovirus-infected pulmonary macrophages and lymphocytes. Hyperplasia of type II pneumonocytes is not a prominent feature of maedi likely because in this disease there is no injury to type I pneumonocytes, but there is some alveolar fibrosis and smooth muscle hypertrophy in bronchioles. Secondary bacterial infections often cause concomitant bronchopneumonia. Enlargement of regional lymph nodes (tracheobronchial) is because of severe lymphoid hyperplasia, primarily of B lymphocytes. The virus also can infect many other tissues, causing nonsuppurative encephalitis (visna), lymphocytic arthritis, lymphofollicular mastitis, and vasculitis.

Maedi is clinically characterized by dyspnea and an insidious, slowly progressive emaciation despite good appetite. Death is inevitable once clinical signs are present, but may take many months.

Caprine Arthritis-Encephalitis

Caprine arthritis-encephalitis (CAE) is a retroviral disease of goats (small ruminant lentivirus) that has a pathogenesis remarkably similar to that of maedi-visna in sheep. It was first described in the

US in the 1970s, but also occurs in Canada, Europe, Australia, and probably elsewhere. This disease has two major clinicopathologic forms: One involves the central nervous system of goat kids and young goats and is characterized by a nonsuppurative leukoencephalomyelitis; the other form involves the joints of adult goats and is characterized by a chronic, nonsuppurative arthritis-synovitis. In addition, infection with CAE virus can cause chronic lymphocytic interstitial pneumonia.

The lentivirus of CAE is closely related to the maedi-visna virus, and, in fact, cross infection with CAE virus in sheep has been achieved experimentally. Similar to maedi, CAE infection presumably occurs during the first weeks of life when the doe transmits the virus to her offspring through infected colostrum or milk. Horizontal transmission between infected and susceptible goats has also been described. After coming into contact with mucosal cells at the portal of entry, the virus is phagocytized by macrophages which migrate to the regional lymph nodes. Infected macrophages are disseminated hematogenously to the central nervous system, joints, lungs, and mammary glands. Like maedi, there is some evidence that the recruitment of lymphocytic cells results from dysregulation of cytokine production by infected macrophages and lymphocytes in affected tissues. It can take several months before serum antibodies can be detected in infected goats.

Grossly, the interstitial pneumonia is diffuse and tends to be most severe in the caudal lobes. The lungs are gray-pink and firm in texture with numerous, 1- to 2-mm, gray-white foci on the cut surface (Fig. 9-80). The tracheobronchial lymph nodes are consistently enlarged. Microscopically, the alveolar walls are thickened by lymphocytes and conspicuous hyperplasia of type II pneumonocytes. One important difference between the pneumonias of CAE and maedi is that in CAE the alveoli is filled with proteinaceous eosinophilic material, which in electron micrographs has structural features of pulmonary surfactant. The pulmonary form of CAE can be mistaken for parasitic pneumonia (*Muellerius capillaris*) because these two diseases have lymphocytic interstitial pneumonia and can coexist in the same goat.

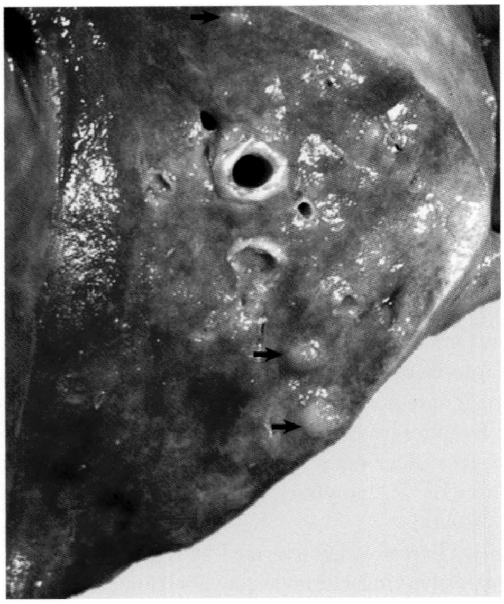

Fig. 9-80 Interstitial pneumonia with alveolar proteinosis, lung, cut surface, sheep.
Note the gray nodules (*arrows*) and meaty appearance of the lung. These lesions are seen in sheep with the caprine arthritis-encephalitis-pneumonia disease complex. (Courtesy Dr. J.M. King, College of Veterinary Medicine, Cornell University.)

Clinically, goats are active and afebrile but progressively lose weight in spite of normal appetites. The encephalitic or arthritic signs tend to obscure the respiratory signs, which are only evident on exertion. Secondary bacterial bronchopneumonia is common in affected animals.

Tuberculosis

Tuberculosis is uncommon in sheep and goats, but infection with *Mycobacterium bovis* or with the *Mycobacterium avium* complex does occur when the disease is prevalent in other species in the locality. The pulmonary form, similar to that seen in cattle, is characterized by a granulomatous pneumonia with multiple, large, caseous, calcified, and well-encapsulated granulomas scattered throughout the lungs. Intralesional acid-fast organisms within macrophages are not as abundant as in bovine tuberculosis.

Parasitic Pneumonias of Sheep and Goats

Dictyocaulus filaria is a serious, worldwide, parasitic disease of the lungs, most commonly of lambs and goat kids, but occurring in adults as well. The life cycle and lesions are similar to those of *Dictyocaulus viviparus* of cattle. As seen in cattle with *Dictyocaulus viviparus*, areas of atelectasis secondary to bronchiolar obstruction are present, particularly along the dorsal caudal aspects of the caudal lung lobes. Microscopically, affected lungs are characterized by a catarrhal, eosinophilic bronchitis, with peribronchial lymphoid hyperplasia and smooth muscle hyperplasia of bronchi and bronchioles. Bronchioles and alveoli can contain edematous fluid, eosinophils, and parasitic larvae and eggs. Microscopic granulomas caused by aspirated eggs can be observed in the distal lung. The clinical signs (cough, moderate dyspnea, and loss of condition) and lesions relate mainly to obstruction of the small bronchi by adult worms and filaria. Anemia of undetermined pathogenesis and secondary bacterial pneumonia are common in small ruminants with this parasitic disease.

Muellerius capillaris, also called the *nodular lungworm,* occurs in sheep and goats in most areas of the world and is the most common lung parasite of sheep in Europe and Northern Africa. It requires slugs or snails as intermediate hosts. The lesions in sheep are typically multifocal, subpleural nodules that tend to be most numerous in the dorsal areas of the caudal lung lobes (Fig. 9-81). These nodules are soft and hemorrhagic in the early stages but later become gray-green and hard or even calcified. Microscopically, a focal, eosinophilic, and granulomatous reaction occurs in the subpleural alveoli where the adults, eggs, and coiled larvae reside (see Fig. 9-81). Clinical signs are usually not apparent.

Goats differ from sheep by having diffuse interstitial rather than focal lesions, and the reaction to the parasites seen microscopically varies from almost no lesions to a severe interstitial pneumonia with heavy infiltrates of mononuclear cells in alveolar walls resembling CAE or mycoplasmal infections. Secondary effects of *Muellerius capillaris* infection in sheep and goats include decreased weight gain and possibly secondary bacterial infections.

Protostrongylus rufescens is a worldwide parasite of sheep, goats, and wild ruminants. It requires an intermediate snail as a host. Infection is usually subclinical, but *Protostrongylus rufescens* can be pathogenic for lambs and goat kids and can cause anorexia, diarrhea, weight loss, and mucopurulent nasal discharge. The adult parasite lives in bronchioles as *Dictyocaulus* spp., but it causes pulmonary nodules similar to those of *Muellerius capillaris.*

Pneumonias of Pigs

Porcine pneumonias are unequivocally a major component of the problems facing the contemporary swine industry. The incidence,

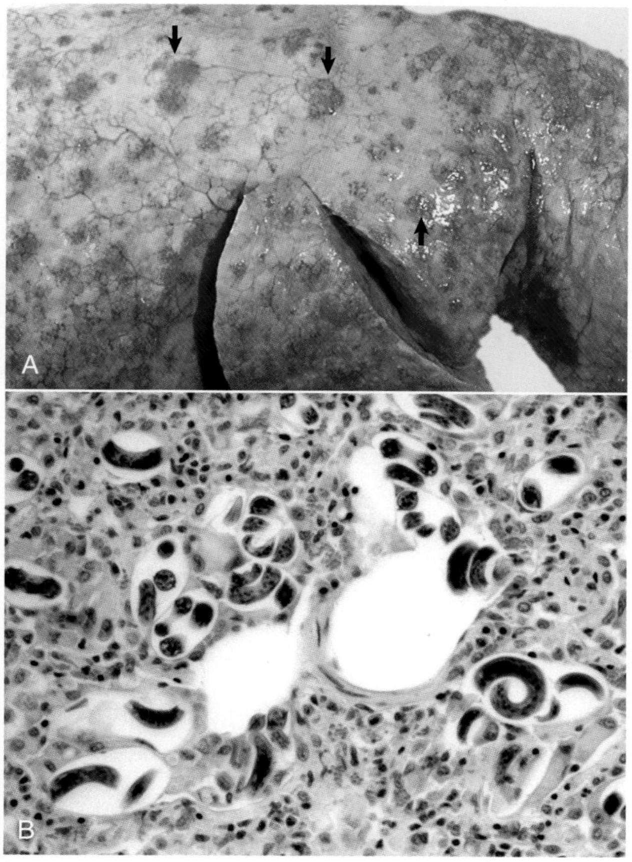

Fig. 9-81 Multifocal granulomatous pneumonia, lungworms (*Muellerius* spp.), lungs, sheep.
A, Multiple gray nodules (granulomas) *(arrows)* are scattered throughout the pulmonary parenchyma. On palpation, the lungs have a nodular texture. **B,** Coiled larvae of *Muellerius* spp. in the lung. Note also mononuclear cells extending into the surrounding pulmonary interstitium. H&E stain. (**A** courtesy Dr. J. Edwards, Texas A&M University, Olafson Short Course, Cornell Veterinary Medicine. **B** courtesy Dr. A. López, Atlantic Veterinary College.)

prevalence, and mortality rates of pneumonias in pigs depend on a series of complex, multifactorial interactions. Among the most commonly recognized elements linked to porcine pneumonias are the following:

- Host (age, genetic makeup, immune status)
- Infectious agents (viruses, bacteria, mycoplasmas)
- Environmental determinants (humidity, temperature, ammonia concentrations)
- Management practices (crowding, mixing of animals, air quality, nutrition, stress)

Because of the nature of these multifactorial interactions, it will become obvious in the following paragraphs that more often than not a specific type of pneumonia frequently progresses to or coexists with another one. The term *porcine respiratory disease complex* (PRDC) has been introduced in clinical practice to describe pigs with signs of respiratory infection involving one or more viruses, bacteria, and mycoplasmas.

Swine Influenza (Swine Flu)

It is generally accepted that swine influenza resulted from adaptation of the type A influenza virus, the cause of the human influenza pandemic during World War I. Swine influenza is enzootic worldwide and is known to infect humans who are in close contact with sick pigs. In 2009, an outbreak of swine-human influenza (H1N1), presumably transmitted from pigs to humans, emerged in Mexico and rapidly spread to many countries around the world. This new "pandemic" was attributed to a triple-reassortant of influenza A virus containing gene segments of swine, Eurasian avian, and human strains. Human infection with this novel strain affected mainly children and young adults, as well as individuals of any age with an underlying debilitating condition.

Transmission between influenza-infected and susceptible pigs occurs mainly by aerosols or oral route. The infection of epithelial cells spreads rapidly throughout the nasal, tracheal, and bronchial mucosa, with the more severe outbreaks reflecting more involvement of intrapulmonary airways and secondary infection with *Pasteurella multocida, Arcanobacterium pyogenes,* or *Haemophilus* spp. Although uncommon, humans infected with swine influenza (H1N1) can pass the virus back to pigs, therefore it is important that veterinarians or workers with influenza-like illness should stay away from pig farms. Natural transmission of H1N1 and H5N1 from humans to ferrets (*Mustela putorius furo*) and from humans to cats and dogs has been recently reported.

Pulmonary lesions caused by influenza virus alone are rarely seen in the postmortem room because this disease has very low mortality rate unless complicated with secondary bacterial infections. Grossly a copious catarrhal to mucopurulent inflammation extends from the nasal passages to the bronchioles, the volume of mucus being sufficient to plug small airways and cause a lobular or multilobular atelectasis in the cranioventral regions of the lungs. The appearance can be quite similar grossly, although not microscopically, to that of *Mycoplasma pneumoniae.* Fatal cases have severe alveolar and interstitial pulmonary edema. Microscopically, the lesions in uncomplicated cases are typical of a virus-induced, necrotizing bronchitis-bronchiolitis, which in severe cases extends into the alveoli as bronchointerstitial pneumonia. It is characterized by thickening and infiltration of the alveolar wall with mononuclear cells and aggregates of macrophages, neutrophils, mucus, and some necrotic cells within the alveolar lumen. If these changes are extensive enough, the lumen of bronchioles can be occluded by exudate, causing lobular atelectasis. Viral antigen can be demonstrated in infected epithelial cells by immunoperoxidase techniques. In the later stages of alveolar inflammation, neutrophils are progressively replaced by intraalveolar macrophages, unless the pneumonia is complicated by secondary bacterial infections. Recent serologic surveys indicate that infection is also prevalent in wild pigs.

Clinically, a sudden onset of painful and often paroxysmal coughing is followed by respiratory distress, nasal discharge, high fever, stiffness, and weakness or even prostration in most or the entire herd, including animals of all age groups. The outbreak subsides virtually without mortality within a week; the clinical appearance is much more alarming than the pathologic changes, unless the pigs have secondary infection with bacteria. Infection can be confirmed using PCR in secretions collected with nasal swabs. The most important effect of most outbreaks of influenza is severe weight loss, but pregnant sows also abort or give birth to weak piglets.

Porcine Reproductive and Respiratory Syndrome

A disease originally named *mystery disease of swine* was first recognized in the US in 1987. In 1990, it was also seen in Europe, and since then, PRRS has been reported in many Latin American and Asian countries. In 1991, Dutch investigators isolated a virus as the etiologic agent, which is currently classified under the *Arterivirus* group.

As its name implies, PRRS is characterized by late-term abortions and stillbirths and respiratory problems in young pigs. The respiratory form is generally seen in nursing or young pigs. The pathogenesis has not been completely elucidated, but it is presumed that there is a mucosal portal of entry with virus replication in local macrophages, followed by transient viremia and finally dissemination of infected macrophages to the lungs and other organs, such as the thymus, liver (Kupffer cells), spleen, all lymph nodes, and intestine. The PRRS virus induces apoptosis in many cells including the pulmonary intravascular macrophages, The virus also deregulates the adaptive immune response and interferes with the normal defense mechanisms predisposing pigs to septicemia and bacterial pneumonia. The most common opportunistic organisms are *Streptococcus suis, Haemophilus parasuis, Bordetella bronchiseptica, Pasteurella multocida,* and *Pneumocystis carinii.* Dual viral infections with PRRS virus and porcine circovirus-2 (PCV-2) are quite commonly found in pigs.

On postmortem examination, pulmonary lesions vary from very mild changes characterized by failure of the lung to collapse when the thorax is opened and the presence of rib imprints (see Fig. 9-61) to severe changes manifested by consolidation of the lung in cases that have been complicated with bacterial pneumonia. Tracheobronchial and mediastinal lymph nodes are typically enlarged. Microscopically, pulmonary changes are those of interstitial pneumonia characterized by thickening of alveolar walls by infiltrating macrophages and lymphocytes and mild hyperplasia of type II pneumonocytes. Necrotic cells are scattered in the alveolar lumens. Unlike some other viral infections, bronchiolar epithelium does not appear to be affected. Diagnosis of PRRS in tissue collected at necropsy can be confirmed by immunohistochemistry and PCR techniques. Infected pigs may become carriers and transmit the infection through body fluids and semen. Clinically, PRRS is characterized by anorexia, dyspnea, cough, and occasional death. Some piglets develop severe cyanosis of the abdomen and ears, which explains why this syndrome when first described in Europe was named *blue ear disease.*

Postweaning Multisystemic Wasting Syndrome

Another emerging porcine syndrome, characterized clinically by progressive emaciation in weaned pigs, was originally described in the 1990s in Canada, the US, and Europe. Since then, it has disseminated to many countries, causing economic devastation in pig farms worldwide. Because of the clinical signs and lesions in many organs, this syndrome was named *postweaning multisystemic wasting syndrome* (PMWS); a PCV-2 has been incriminated as the etiologic agent.

At necropsy, affected pigs are in poor body condition, and the most remarkable changes, not considering other possible secondary infections, are enlargement of the superficial and visceral lymph nodes and a mild interstitial pneumonia characterized by failure of the lungs to collapse when the thorax is opened. Jaundice is occasionally observed. Microscopically, the lymph nodes show necrosis of lymphoid follicles, depletion of lymphocytes, and notable proliferation of follicular macrophages, some of which fuse and form syncytial cells (granulomatous lymphadenitis). In many cases, large basophilic botryoid inclusion bodies resembling grapes are present in the cytoplasm of macrophages, particularly in Peyer's patches, spleen, and lymph nodes. Similar inclusions are occasionally seen in bronchial and renal epithelial cells. The lungs show thickening of the alveolar walls because of hyperplasia of type II pneumonocytes and interstitial infiltrates of mononuclear cells, some of which may contain intracytoplasmic inclusion bodies. Circovirus antigen can be confirmed in affected tissue by immunohistochemical or PCR techniques.

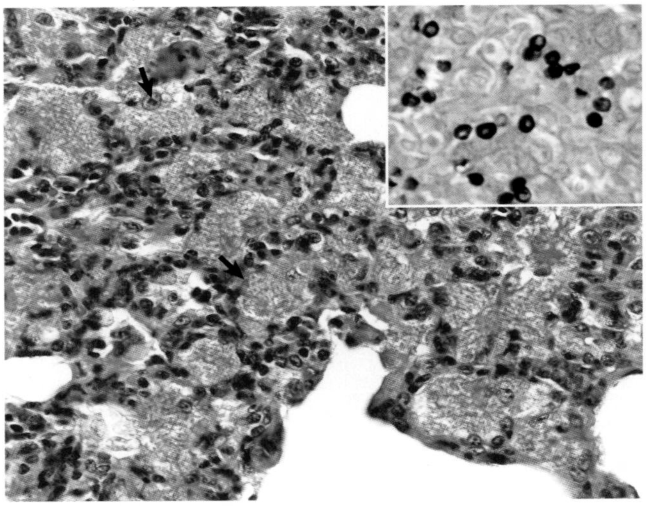

Fig. 9-82 Pneumocystosis *(Pneumocystis carinii),* lung, pig. Alveoli are filled with a foamy eosinophilic proteinaceous material in which numerous punctiform organisms *(arrows)* are present. H&E stain. *Inset,* Silver-stained oval bodies typical of *Pneumocystis carinii.* Pneumocystosis is generally a microscopic diagnosis because this condition does not cause remarkable gross lesions. Gomori's methenamine silver stain. (Courtesy Dr. A. López, Atlantic Veterinary College.)

Secondary infections with *Pneumocystis carinii* are commonly seen in pigs with PRRS and PMWS. Characteristically, alveoli are filled with a distinctive foamy exudate, which contains the organism not visible in H&E-stained sections but easily demonstrated with Gomori's methenamine silver stain (Fig. 9-82). In humans, *Pneumocystis carinii* pneumonia (pneumocystosis) is one of the most common and often fatal complications in AIDS patients. As in AIDS patients, in foals and pigs, abnormal populations of $CD4^+$ and $CD8^+$ T lymphocytes have been incriminated as the underlying mechanism leading to pneumocystosis.

Porcine Enzootic Pneumonia (Mycoplasmal Pneumonia of Pigs)

Porcine enzootic pneumonia, a highly contagious disease of pigs caused by *Mycoplasma hyopneumoniae,* is grossly characterized by suppurative or catarrhal bronchopneumonia (Fig. 9-83 and Web Fig. 9-12). When its worldwide prevalence and deleterious effect on feed conversion are taken into account, this disease is probably the most economically significant respiratory disease of pigs. Although an infectious disease, it is very much influenced by immune status and management factors, such as crowding (airspace and floor space), ventilation (air exchange rate), concentrations of noxious gases in the air (ammonia, hydrogen sulfide), relative humidity, temperature fluctuations, and mixing of stock from various sources. It has been demonstrated with PCR technique that *Mycoplasma hyopneumoniae* is present in the air of infected farms.

The cause of porcine enzootic pneumonia remained unclear for many years, and so the disease was mistakenly known as "virus pneumonia of pigs" based on the assumption that if the agent was hard to find, it must be a virus. The causative agent, *Mycoplasma hyopneumoniae,* is a fastidious organism and very difficult to grow; thus the final diagnosis is frequently based on interpretation of lesions alone, or supported by ancillary tests to detect this mycoplasma in affected lungs by immunohistochemical, immunofluorescence,

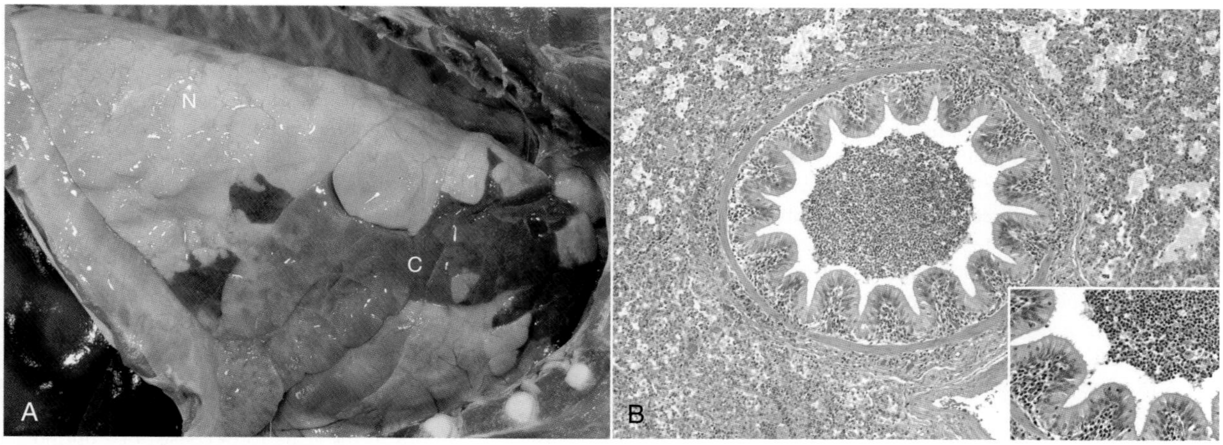

Fig. 9-83 Chronic-active (suppurative) bronchopneumonia (enzootic pneumonia), lung, pig.
A, Cranioventral consolidation of 40% to 50% of pulmonary parenchyma. Consolidated lung *(C)* is firm, and the outlines of the lobules are accentuated by edema of the interlobular septa. *N,* Normal lung. **B,** The bronchiole and alveoli contain numerous neutrophils and macrophages. Some of the neutrophils are migrating from the capillaries of the lamina propria of the bronchiole into its lumen. Alveoli are edematous and contain similar inflammatory cells. Alveolar septa are also widened by inflammation. H&E stain. *Inset,* Higher magnification of wall of bronchiole in **B.** H&E stain. (Courtesy Dr. A. López, Atlantic Veterinary College.)

enzyme-linked immunosorbent assay (ELISA), or PCR techniques. The bronchopneumonic lesions of porcine enzootic pneumonia are in most cases mild to moderate, and thus mortality is low unless complicated with secondary pathogens, such as *Pasteurella multocida, Arcanobacterium pyogenes, Bordetella bronchiseptica, Haemophilus* spp., *Mycoplasma hyorhinis,* and other mycoplasmas and ureaplasmas. Although the pathogenesis of porcine enzootic pneumonia is not completely elucidated, it is known that *Mycoplasma hyopneumoniae* first adheres to the cilia of the bronchi by means of a unique adhesive protein, produces ciliostasis, and finally colonizes the respiratory system by firmly attaching to the ciliated epithelial cells of the trachea and the bronchi of the cranioventral regions of the lungs. Once attached to the respiratory epithelium, it provokes an influx of neutrophils into the tracheobronchial mucosa, causes extensive loss of cilia (deciliation), stimulates an intense hyperplasia of lymphocytes in the BALT, and attracts mononuclear cells into the peribronchial, bronchiolar, and alveolar interstitium. Additional virulence factors include the ability of *Mycoplasma hyopneumoniae* to cause immunosuppression, reduce the phagocytic activity of neutrophils in the lung, and change the chemical composition of mucus. All of these functional alterations can predispose the lung to secondary bacterial infections.

The lesions caused by *Mycoplasma hyopneumoniae* start as a bronchointerstitial pneumonia microscopically characterized by mononuclear infiltrates in the alveolar walls and a few macrophages and neutrophils in bronchiolar and alveolar lumens. This inflammatory reaction progresses to a suppurative or mucopurulent bronchopneumonia once secondary pathogens, such as *Pasteurella multocida, Bordetella bronchiseptica,* or *Arcanobacterium pyogenes,* are involved (commonly seen at necropsy). In most pigs, gross lesions affect only portions of the cranial lobes, but in more severely affected pigs, lesions involve 50% or more of the cranioventral portions of the lungs (see Fig. 9-83). The affected lungs are dark red in the early stages but have a homogeneous pale-gray ("fish flesh") appearance in the more chronic stages of the disease. On the cut surface, exudate can easily be expressed from airways, and depending on the stage of the lesions and secondary infections, the exudate varies from purulent to mucopurulent to mucoid. Microscopic lesions are characterized by an influx of macrophages and neutrophils into the bronchi, bronchioles, and alveoli, and with time there is also notable BALT hyperplasia. In some cases, accumulation of exudate can be severe enough to cause occlusion of bronchioles and atelectasis of their lobules (see Fig. 9-83). The suppurative bronchopneumonia may be accompanied by a mild fibrinous pleuritis, which is often more severe if other organisms, such as *Mycoplasma hyorhinis, Pasteurella multocida,* or *Actinobacillus pleuropneumoniae,* are also involved. Abscesses and fibrous pleural adhesions are sequelae of chronic complicated infections.

Clinically, enzootic pneumonia occurs as a herd problem in two disease forms. A newly acquired infection of a previously clean herd causes disease in all age groups, resulting in acute respiratory distress and low mortality. In a chronically infected herd, the mature animals are immune and clinical signs are usually apparent only in growing pigs at times of particular stress such as at weaning. In such herds, coughing and reduced rate of weight gain are the most notable signs.

Porcine Pasteurellosis

Porcine pasteurellosis is an infectious disease complex with unclear pathogenesis that includes primary infections by *Pasteurella multocida* alone, or more frequently, after the defense mechanisms are impaired and a secondary bacterium colonizes the lung (porcine pneumonic pasteurellosis). In some rare cases, *Pasteurella multocida* causes acutely fatal septicemias in pigs. It is important to remember that *Pasteurella multocida* serotypes A and D are both part of the normal nasal flora and are also causative agents of bronchopneumonia, pleuritis, and atrophic rhinitis in pigs.

Pasteurella multocida is one of the most common secondary pathogens isolated from the lungs of pigs with porcine influenza, PRRS, PCV-2 infection, pseudorabies, classic swine fever (hog cholera), enzootic pneumonia, and porcine pleuropneumonia. Secondary infections with *Pasteurella multocida* notably change the early and mild bronchointerstitial reaction of enzootic and viral pneumonias into a severe suppurative bronchopneumonia with multiple abscesses and sometimes pleuritis. The other important role of *Pasteurella multocida* in porcine pneumonias is as a cause of a fulminating, cranioventral, fibrinous bronchopneumonia (pleuropneumonia) after influenza virus infection or stress from inadequate ventilation resulting in high levels of ammonia in the air. The nature of the lesion and the predisposing factors of poor management or coexisting viral infections suggest that fulminating porcine pasteurellosis has a pathogenesis similar to that of pneumonic Mannheimiosis of cattle. Pharyngitis with subcutaneous cervical edema, fibrinohemorrhagic polyarthritis, and focal lymphocytic interstitial nephritis are also present in porcine pneumonic pasteurellosis. Whether this disease is a separate form of pasteurellosis (septicemic) or a change to bronchopneumonia needs to be elucidated. Sequelae of porcine pneumonic pasteurellosis include fibrous pleuritis and pericarditis, pulmonary abscesses, so-called sequestra, and usually death. In contrast to ruminants, *Mannheimia haemolytica* is not a respiratory pathogen for pigs, but in some instances, it can cause abortion in sows.

Porcine Pleuropneumonia

Porcine pleuropneumonia is a highly contagious, worldwide disease of pigs caused by *Actinobacillus pleuropneumoniae (Haemophilus pleuropneumoniae),* which is characterized by a severe, often fatal, fibrinous bronchopneumonia with extensive pleuritis (pleuropneumonia). Survivors generally develop notable residual lesions and become carriers of the organisms. Porcine pleuropneumonia is an increasingly important cause of acute and chronic pneumonias, particularly in intensively raised pigs (2 to 5 months old). Transmission of *Actinobacillus pleuropneumoniae* occurs by the respiratory route, and the disease can be reproduced experimentally by intranasal inoculation of the bacterium. Considered as a primary pathogen, *Actinobacillus pleuropneumoniae* can sporadically produce septicemia in young pigs and otitis media and otitis interna with vestibular syndrome in weaned pigs. Twelve serotypes of the organism, most of which can cause the disease, have been identified. The pathogenesis is not yet well understood, but specific virulence factors, such as RTX and Apx toxins, capsular factors, fimbriae and adhesins, lipopolysaccharide, hemolysins, cytotoxins, and permeability factors, have been identified. These factors allow *Actinobacillus pleuropneumoniae* to attach to cells; produce pores in cell membranes; damage capillaries and alveolar walls, resulting in vascular leakage and thrombosis; impair phagocytic function; and elicit failure of clearance mechanisms.

The gross lesions in the acute form consist of a fibrinous bronchopneumonia characterized by severe consolidation and a fibrinous exudate on the pleural surface. Although all lobes can be affected, a common site is the dorsal area of the caudal lobes. In fact, a large area of fibrinous pleuropneumonia involving the caudal lobe of a pig's lung is considered almost diagnostic for this disease (Fig. 9-84). On the cut surface, consolidated lungs have notably dilated interlobular septa and irregular but well-circumscribed areas of necrosis caused by potent cytotoxins produced by *Actinobacillus*

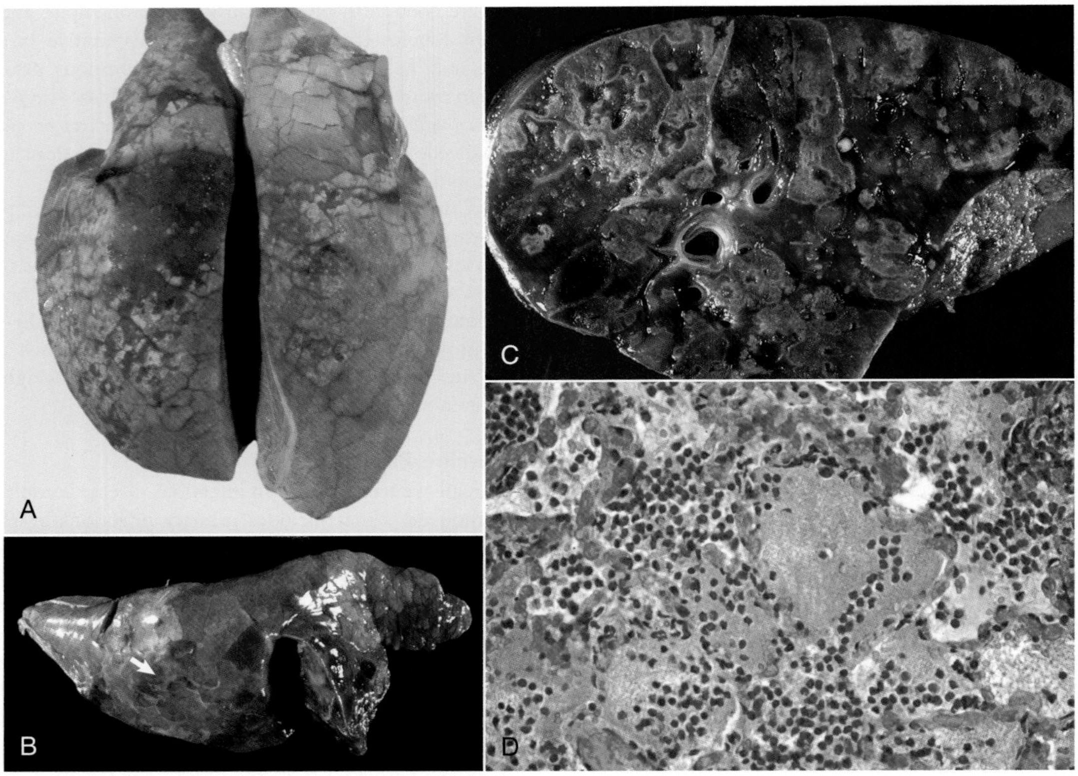

Fig. 9-84 Porcine pleuropneumonia *(Actinobacillus pleuropneumoniae)*, lung, pig.
A, In peracute porcine pleuropneumonia, the pneumonic lesions are locally extensive in the dorsal aspects of the caudal lung lobes. There is lobular congestion, consolidation, and interlobular edema. **B,** As the disease progresses and becomes acute to subacute, the lesions expand in size and severity. Note the large area of hemorrhagic necrotizing fibrinous bronchopneumonia. Fibrin is abundant *(arrow)* on the pleural surface and in interlobular septa. **C,** The cut surface has numerous discrete and coalescing zones of lobular inflammation and necrosis *(upper left),* which are pale pink to white and often surrounded by a white margin (inflammation). There is extensive congestion (active hyperemia) and hemorrhage throughout the section. **D,** Alveoli are filled with fibrin, edema fluid, and neutrophils. Capillaries in alveolar septa are congested (active hyperemia), and in many cases, there is necrosis of alveolar septa (not visible at this magnification). (**A** courtesy Dr. A. López, Atlantic Veterinary College. **B** courtesy Dr. J. Render, College of Veterinary Medicine and Animal Health Diagnostic Laboratory, Michigan State University; and Noah's Arkive, College of Veterinary Medicine, The University of Georgia. **C** and **D** courtesy Dr. A.R. Doster, University of Nebraska; and Noah's Arkive, College of Veterinary Medicine, The University of Georgia.)

pleuropneumoniae. Except for the distribution, pulmonary lesions of porcine pleuropneumonia are identical to those of pneumonic Mannheimiosis of cattle. The microscopic lesions are also very similar and include areas of coagulative necrosis surrounded by a thick cluster of "streaming (oat-shaped) leukocytes" and a notable distention of the interlobular septa because of severe edema and lymphatic thrombosis. Bronchioles and alveoli are filled with edematous fluid, fibrin, neutrophils, and few macrophages (see Fig. 9-84). Pigs with the chronic form have multiple pulmonary abscesses and large (2 to 10 cm) pieces of necrotic lung encapsulated by connective tissue (sequestra), changes frequently seen in slaughterhouses.

Clinically, porcine pleuropneumonia can vary from an acute form with unexpected death and blood-stained froth at the nostrils and mouth to a subacute form characterized by coughing and dyspnea accompanied by clinical signs of sepsis such as high fever, hypoxemia, anorexia, and lethargy. A chronic form is characterized by decreased growth rate and persistent cough. Animals that survive often carry the organism in the tonsils, shed the organism, and infect susceptible pigs.

Haemophilus Pneumonia

In addition to Glasser's disease characterized by polyserositis (pericarditis, pleuritis, peritonitis, polyarthritis, and meningitis), some serotypes of *Haemophilus parasuis* (originally *Haemophilus parasuis suis*) can also cause suppurative bronchopneumonia that in some severe cases can be fatal. The causal organism, *Haemophilus parasuis,* is usually carried in the nasopharynx of normal pigs and requires abnormal circumstances such as those following stress (weaning, cold weather) or viral infections (swine influenza or PCV-2). Specific pathogen-free (SPF) pigs seem to be particularly susceptible to Glasser's disease (arthritis and serositis) but not to pulmonary infection (bronchopneumonia).

Streptococcal Pneumonia

Streptococcus suis is a common cause of porcine disease worldwide and a serious zoonosis capable of causing death by septic shock or meningitis and residual deafness in butchers, veterinarians, and pig farmers. Typically, *Streptococcus suis* gains entrance to the susceptible young pig through the oropharyngeal mucosa and is carried in the tonsils, nasal mucosa, and mandibular lymph nodes of healthy animals, particularly in survivors of an outbreak. Infected sows can abort or vertically transmit the infections to their offspring. Some serotypes of *Streptococcus suis* cause neonatal septicemia, and this can result in suppurative meningitis, otitis, arthritis, polyserositis, myocarditis, valvular endocarditis, and embolic pneumonia (Fig. 9-85). Other serotypes of *Streptococcus suis* can reach the lung by the aerogenous route and cause a suppurative bronchopneumonia, in combination with *Pasteurella multocida, Escherichia coli,* or *Mycoplasma hyopneumoniae,* or in combination with *Actinobacillus pleuropneumoniae,* which causes a fibrinous bronchopneumonia.

Tuberculosis

Tuberculosis is an important disease in domestic and wild pigs that has a much greater prevalence in pigs than in cattle or other domestic mammals in many countries, including those in North America. Porcine tuberculosis is attributed to infection with *Mycobacterium bovis* and porcine mycobacteriosis to *Mycobacterium avium-intracellulare* complex. A common scenario in small mixed-farming operations is the diagnosis of avian tuberculosis at the time that pigs are slaughtered, and the source is ingestion of tuberculous chickens or contaminated litter. As would be expected, granulomas are found in the mesenteric, mandibular, and retropharyngeal

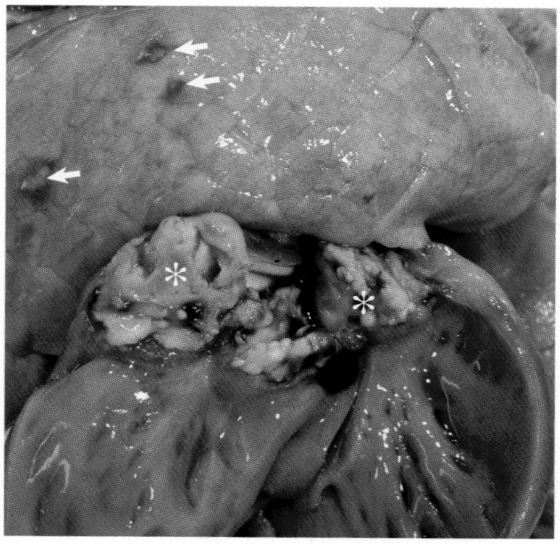

Fig. 9-85 Vegetative endocarditis, heart and multiple embolic lesions, lung, pig.
Note large vegetative (cauliflower-like) mass attached to the tricuspid valve *(asterisks).* The lung *(top half of figure)* shows multifocal well-circumscribed nodules *(arrows)*, the result of emboli being released from the tricuspid valve. (Courtesy Dr. A. López, Atlantic Veterinary College.)

lymph nodes, to a lesser extent in the intestine, liver, and spleen, and only in rare cases in the lung. The route of infection in pulmonary tuberculosis and mycobacteriosis of pigs is most often hematogenous after oral exposure and intestinal infection. Lung lesions are those of a granulomatous pneumonia. The microscopic lesions are basically those of tubercles, but the degree of encapsulation, caseation, and calcification varies with the type of mycobacterium, age of the lesion, and host immune response.

Other Infectious Pneumonias of Pigs

Porcine respiratory coronavirus (PRCV) is sporadically incriminated in pneumonia in pigs. This viral pneumonia is generally mild, and most pigs fully recover if the pneumonia is not complicated with other infections. Lesions in the lung are those of interstitial pneumonia with necrotizing bronchiolitis. Interestingly, infections with porcine and other respiratory coronaviruses have been used to investigate the pathogenesis of severe acute respiratory syndrome (SARS), an emerging and highly contagious condition recently reported in humans and attributed to a novel human coronavirus (SARS-CoV). The relationship between SARS-CoV and animal coronavirus is still under investigation.

Septicemias in pigs often cause petechial hemorrhages in the lung and pulmonary edema, and these lesions may be present in African swine fever, classic swine fever (hog cholera), pseudorabies, and other diseases. *Salmonellae, Escherichia coli,* and *Listeria monocytogenes* can cause severe interstitial pneumonia in very young animals. *Salmonella choleraesuis* causes a necrotizing fibrinous pneumonia similar to porcine pleuropneumonia, and *Salmonella typhisuis* causes a chronic suppurative bronchopneumonia.

Foreign body granulomatous pneumonia occurs frequently in pigs after inhalation of vegetable material (starch pneumonia), presumably from dusty (nonpelleted) feed. Lesions are clinically silent but are often mistaken for other pneumonic processes during inspection at slaughterhouses. Microscopically, pulmonary changes are typical of foreign body granulomatous inflammation in which variably sized feed particles are surrounded by macrophages and neutrophils, and often have been phagocytosed by multinucleated giant cells. Feed (vegetable) particles appear as thick-walled polygonal cells that stain positive with PAS because of their rich carbohydrate (starch) content.

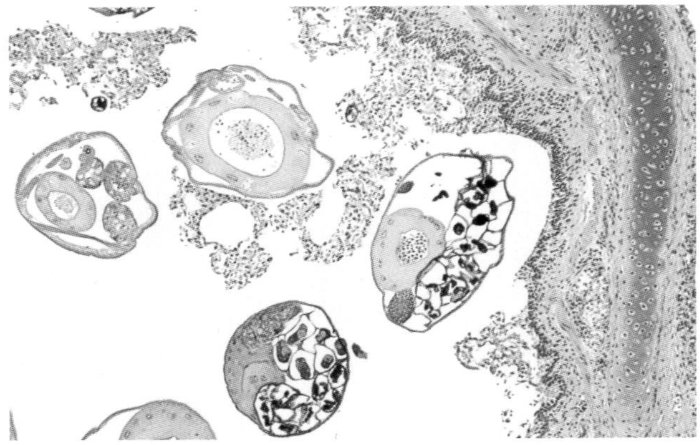

Fig. 9-86 Acute verminous bronchitis *(Metastrongylus apri)*, bronchus, cross section, pig.
Several sections of nematodes *(Metastrongylus apri)* admixed with mucus, neutrophils, and eosinophils (not visible at this magnification) are present in the lumen of the bronchus. H&E stain. (Courtesy Armed Forces Institute of Pathology and Dr. G. Conboy, Atlantic Veterinary College.)

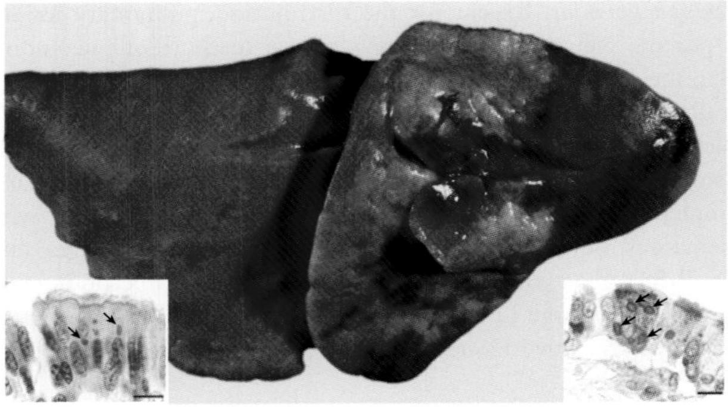

Fig. 9-87 Interstitial pneumonia, canine distemper, lungs, dog.
The lungs are heavy, edematous, and rubbery, with costal (rib) imprints on the pleural surface. *Inset, left*: Bronchial epithelium contains intracytoplasmic eosinophilic inclusion bodies *(arrows)*. H&E stain. *Inset, right*: Immunoperoxidase stain revealing canine Morbillivirus antigen *(arrows)* in the cytoplasm and apical borders of bronchial epithelial cells. Immunoperoxidase stain. Bars = 20 μm. (From Berrocal A, López A: *J Vet Diagn Invest* 15:292-294, 2003.)

Parasitic Pneumonias of Pigs

Metastrongylus apri (elongatus), Metastrongylus salmi, and *Metastrongylus pudendotectus* (lungworms) of domestic and feral pigs occur throughout most of the world and require earthworms as intermediate hosts for transmission. Lungworms may transmit the virus of swine influenza. The importance of pig lungworms is mainly because infection results in growth retardation of the host. Clinical signs include coughing because of parasitic bronchitis.

The gross lesions, when noticeable, consist of small gray nodules, particularly along the ventral borders of the caudal lobes. The adult worms are grossly visible in bronchi, and microscopically, the parasites cause a catarrhal bronchitis with infiltration of eosinophils and lobular atelectasis (Fig. 9-86).

The larvae of *Ascaris suum* can cause edema, focal subpleural hemorrhages, and interstitial inflammation (see Fig. 9-62). Along their larval migration tracts, hemorrhages also occur in the liver, and after fibrosis, they become the large, white "milk spots" seen so frequently as incidental findings at necropsy. It has recently been reported that *Ascaris suum* may cause immunosuppression in severely affected pigs.

Pneumonias of Dogs

In general, inflammatory diseases of the lungs are less of a problem in dogs than in food-producing species and can be subdivided in two major groups, infectious and noninfectious pneumonias. Of the infectious type, two diseases account for most cases: infectious tracheobronchitis (kennel cough), which was discussed previously, and canine distemper. Uremia and paraquat toxicity are perhaps the two most notable noninfectious causes.

Canine Distemper

Canine distemper is an important and ubiquitous infectious disease of dogs, other Canidae, wild Felidae, Mustelidae, and marine mammals around the world. It is caused by a Morbillivirus that is antigenically related to the human measles, rinderpest, "peste de petit ruminants," and phocine distemper viruses. Distemper virus is transmitted to susceptible puppies through infected body fluids. The virus invades through the upper respiratory tract and conjunctiva, proliferates in regional lymph nodes, becomes viremic, and in dogs with an inadequate antibody response, infects nearly all body tissues (pantropic), particularly the epithelial cells. Distemper virus hampers the immune response and appears to downregulate cytokine production and persist for a long time in some tissues. This virus can target the lungs either directly as a viral pneumonia or by its immunosuppressive effects rendering the lungs susceptible to secondary bacterial and protozoal infections, or as a co-infection with other viruses such as CAV.

Gross lesions in the acute stages include serous to catarrhal to mucopurulent nasopharyngitis and conjunctivitis. The lungs are edematous and have a diffuse interstitial pneumonia (Fig. 9-87) microscopically characterized by necrotizing bronchiolitis, necrosis and exfoliation of pneumonocytes, mild alveolar edema, and several hours later, thickening of the alveolar walls because of interstitial mononuclear cell infiltrates and hyperplasia of type II pneumonocytes. Secondary infections with *Bordetella bronchiseptica* and mycoplasmas are common and induce life-threatening suppurative bronchopneumonia. The thymus may be small relative to the age of the animal because of viral-induced lympholysis.

Microscopically, eosinophilic inclusions are present in the epithelial cells of many tissues, in the nuclei or cytoplasm, or in both (see Fig. 9-87). They appear early in the bronchiolar epithelium but are most prominent in the epithelium of the lung, stomach, renal pelvis, and urinary bladder, making these tissues good choices for diagnostic examination. Viral inclusions are rarely seen in the later stages of this disease. The suppurative secondary bronchopneumonias often hinder the detection of viral lesions in the lung, particularly because bronchiolar cells containing inclusion bodies exfoliate and mix with the neutrophils recruited by the bacterial infection. Distemper virus antigens can be readily demonstrated in infected cells by the immunoperoxidase technique (see Fig. 9-87), which can also be used in skin biopsies for the antemortem diagnosis of canine distemper.

Distemper virus also has a tendency to affect developing tooth buds and ameloblasts, causing enamel hypoplasia in dogs that recover from infection. Of all distemper lesions, demyelinating encephalomyelitis, which develops late, is the most devastating (see Chapter 14). Sequelae to distemper include the nervous and pneumonic complications mentioned previously and various systemic infections, such as toxoplasmosis and sarcocystosis, because of depressed immunity. Persistent viral infection occurs in some dogs that survive the disease, and they may become carriers and the source of infection for other susceptible animals.

Clinical signs consist of biphasic fever, diarrhea, vomiting, weight loss, mucopurulent oculonasal discharge, coughing, respiratory distress, and possible loss of vision. Weeks later, hyperkeratosis of foot pads ("hard pad") and the nose are observed, along with nervous signs, including ataxia, paralysis, convulsions, or residual myoclonus (muscle twitches, tremors, and "tics").

Canine Adenovirus Type 2 Infection

CAV-2 is a common but transient contagious disease of the respiratory tract of dogs, causing mild fever, oculonasal discharge, coughing, and poor weight gain. The portal of entry is generally by inhalation of infected aerosols followed by viral replication in pneumonocytes. Pulmonary lesions are initially those of a bronchointerstitial pneumonia, with necrosis and exfoliation of bronchiolar and alveolar epithelium and edema, and a few days later, proliferation of type II pneumonocytes, mild infiltration of neutrophils and lymphocytes in alveolar interstitium, and hyperplastic bronchitis and bronchiolitis. Large basophilic intranuclear viral inclusions are typically seen in bronchiolar and alveolar cells (Fig. 9-88). The disease is sometimes associated or may be confused with the infectious tracheobronchitis complex (kennel cough). The infection with CAV is clinically mild unless complicated with a secondary bacterial infection or co-infections with other viruses such as distemper virus. Experimental work suggests CAV-2 reinfection may lead to hyperreactive airways, a nonspecific condition in which the bronchial mucosa becomes highly "responsive" to irritation such as that caused by cold air, gases, or cigarette smoke. However, it is not clear if this outcome is true in natural infections.

Canine Herpesvirus 1

Canine herpesvirus 1 (CHV-1) can cause fatal generalized disease in newborn puppies, and it is probably part of the variety of factors that result in the "fading puppy syndrome." Hypothermia has been suggested as a pivotal component in the pathogenesis of fatal infections in puppies. Many dogs are seropositive, suggesting that transient or subclinical infections are more common than realized; the virus remains latent in the trigeminal and other ganglia and can be reactivated after stress, resulting in asymptomatic transmission of CHV-1 virus to offspring via the placenta, resulting in abortion or stillbirths. In puppies, CHV-1 causes ulcerative tracheitis, interstitial pneumonia, and focal necrosis and inflammation in kidneys, liver, and brain. CHV-1 has also been identified as a cause of ulcerative keratoconjunctivitis in older dogs.

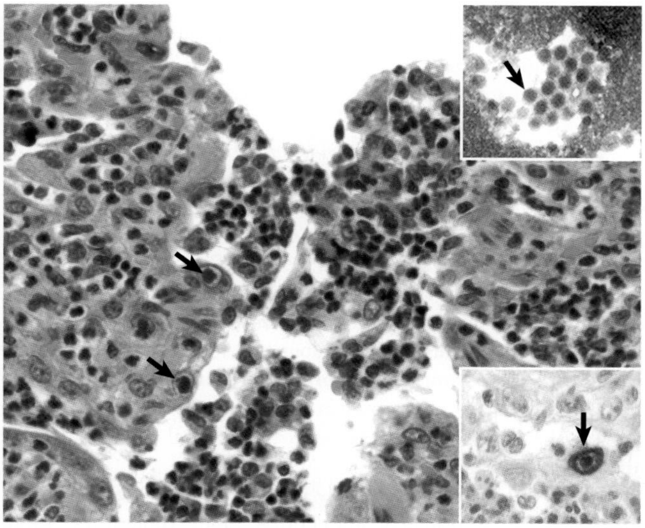

Fig. 9-88 Necrotizing bronchiolitis, canine adenovirus-2 (CAV-2), puppy.
Note necrosis and exfoliation of bronchiolar epithelial cells and the neutrophil infiltrates in the mucosa and bronchiolar lumen. Large basophilic inclusion bodies are present in nuclei of some bronchiolar cells (*arrows*). H&E stain. *Inset right bottom corner,* Immunopositive staining for CAV-2 antigen *(arrow)*. Immunoperoxidase stain. *Inset top right corner,* Paracrystalline arrays of electron dense particles typical of adenovirus *(arrow)* in a transmission electron photomicrograph. Uranyl acetate and lead citrate stain. (From Rodríguez LE, Ramírez-Romero R, Valdez-Nava Y, et al: *Can Vet J* 48:632-634, 2007.)

Canine Influenza (Canine Flu)

Canine influenza is an emerging contagious respiratory infection of dogs that has been recently described in the US. It has a high morbidity (close to 100%), but the mortality, as with most other influenza infections, is relatively low (less than 8%). This disease first diagnosed in greyhounds is caused by a novel influenza-A virus that appears to be a mutation from a previously recognized strain of equine influenza virus, the H3N8 strain. Dog-to-dog transmission does occur and therefore this infection must be distinguished from kennel cough. Pulmonary lesions are generally mild and transient, but infected dogs are susceptible to secondary bacterial bronchopneumonia. The most relevant lesions in dogs dying unexpectedly from canine influenza are pleural and pulmonary hemorrhages. Microscopically, there is necrotizing tracheitis, bronchitis, and bronchiolitis with exudation of neutrophils and macrophages. Vasculitis and thrombosis are occasionally observed in the lungs. Influenza antigen can be demonstrated by immunohistochemistry in airway epithelium and alveolar macrophages. Clinically, dogs with canine influenza are lethargic, inappetent, and hyperthermic and frequently cough and show nasal discharge. These signs resemble those seen in dogs with kennel cough or secondary bacterial pneumonia. In addition, there are confirmed cases of canine influenza caused by the porcine H1N1 presumably transmitted from infected pet owners.

Bacterial Pneumonias of Dogs

Dogs generally have bacterial pneumonias when the pulmonary defense mechanisms have been impaired. *Pasteurella multocida, Streptococcus* spp., *Escherichia coli, Klebsiella pneumoniae,* and *Bordetella bronchiseptica* can be involved in pneumonia secondary to distemper or after aspiration of gastric contents (Fig. 9-89 and Web Fig. 9-13). *Streptococcus zooepidemicus* also causes acute and fatal hemorrhagic pleuropneumonia with hemorrhagic pleural effusion in dogs. Death is generally a consequence of severe sepsis and septic shock or from β-hemolytic *Streptococci* bacteremia causing bacteremia and embolisms affecting the lungs, liver, brain, and lymph nodes. The primary source of the infection cannot be determined in most cases. Dental disease in dogs may be a source of systemic and pulmonary infection, which is not a new concept, as it has been recognized in human medicine for many years. The role of mycoplasmas in canine pneumonia is still uncertain because these organisms are frequently isolated from normal nasopharyngeal flora.

Tuberculosis is uncommon in dogs because these animals appear to be quite resistant to infection; most cases occur in immunocompromised dogs or in dogs living with infected humans. Dogs are susceptible to the *Mycobacterium tuberculosis, Mycobacterium bovis,* and *Mycobacterium avium-intracellulare* complex strains, and therefore canine infection presupposes contact with human or animal tuberculosis. The clinicopathologic manifestation is pulmonary after inhalation or alimentary after oral exposure, but in most cases infection is disseminated to lymph nodes and visceral

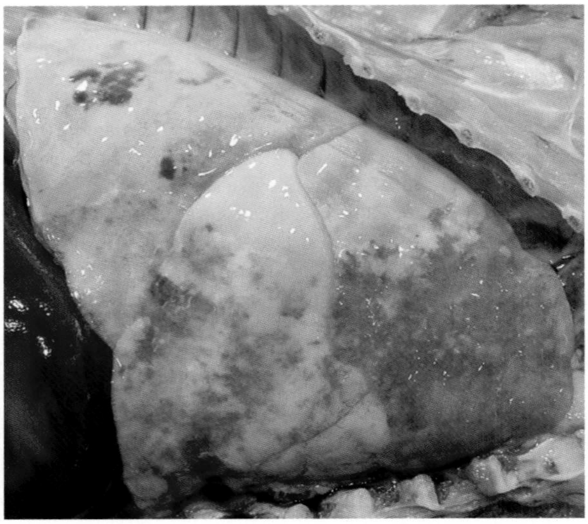

Fig. 9-89 Aspiration pneumonia, bronchopneumonia, right lung, dog. Subacute to chronic bronchopneumonia. The cranioventral portions of the lung are firm and contain purulent exudate *(yellow areas)*. Aspiration pneumonia starts as an acute necrotizing bronchitis and bronchiolitis caused by aspiration of irritant materials such as gastric acid or a caustic material administered by mouth. The aspirate also contains potentially pathogenic bacteria, and because the mucociliary apparatus is damaged and these bacteria are not removed, they settle into the ventral portions of the lung (from gravity) and provoke a fibrinosuppurative bronchopneumonia. (Courtesy Dr. A. López, Atlantic Veterinary College.)

organs. The gross lesions are multifocal, firm nodules with necrotic centers, most often seen in the lungs, lymph nodes, kidneys, and liver. Diffuse granulomatous pleuritis and pericarditis with copious serofibrinous or sanguineous effusion are common. Microscopically, granulomas are formed by closely packed macrophages, but with very little connective tissue.

Mycotic Pneumonias of Dogs

Mycotic pneumonias are serious diseases seen commonly in animals in some areas. There are two main types: those caused by opportunistic fungi and those caused by a group of fungi associated with systemic "deep" mycoses. All these fungi affect humans and most domestic animals but are probably not transmitted between species.

Opportunistic fungi, such as *Aspergillus fumigatus,* are important in birds, but in domestic animals, they mainly affect immunosuppressed animals or those animals on prolonged antibiotic therapy. The pulmonary lesion is a multifocal, nodular, pyogranulomatous, or granulomatous pneumonia. Microscopically, there is necrosis and infiltrates of neutrophils, macrophages and lymphocytes, and proliferation of fibroblasts eventually leads to encapsulation of the granuloma. Fungal hyphae are generally visible in the core of the lesion and in the walls of blood vessels.

Systemic (deep) mycoses are caused by *Blastomyces dermatitidis, Histoplasma capsulatum, Coccidioides immitis,* and *Cryptococcus neoformans* (Fig. 9-90). Blastomycosis mainly affects dogs and is discussed here, whereas cryptococcosis is discussed in the section on Pneumonias of Cats. In contrast to other fungi, such as *Aspergillus* spp., organisms of the systemic mycosis group are all primary pathogens of humans and animals and thus do not necessarily require a preceding immunosuppression to cause disease. These fungi have virulence factors that favor hematogenous dissemination and evasion of immune and phagocytic responses. Systemic dissemination is often exacerbated by the administration of immunosuppressant drugs such as corticosteroids. These fungi are usually detected by cytological evaluation of affected tissues.

Blastomycosis occurs in many countries of the North American continent, Africa, the Middle East, and occasionally in Europe. In the US, it is most prevalent in the Atlantic, St. Lawrence, and Ohio-Mississippi River Valley states, as compared with the Mountain-Pacific region. *Blastomyces dermatitidis* is a dimorphic fungus (mycelia-yeast) seen mainly in young dogs and occasionally in cats. This fungus is present in the soil, and inhalation of spores is considered the principal route of infection; thus it most frequently affects outdoor and hunting dogs. From the lung, infection is disseminated hematogenously to other organs, mainly bone, skin, brain, and probably eyes.

Pulmonary lesions are characterized by multifocal to coalescing granulomatous pneumonia, generally with firm nodules (pyogranulomas) scattered throughout the lungs (see Fig. 9-66). Microscopically, nodules are granulomas with numerous macrophages (epithelioid cells), some neutrophils, multinucleated giant cells, and thick-walled yeasts (see Fig. 9-91; also see Fig. 9-90, *A*). Yeasts are 5 to 25 μm in diameter and are much better visualized when they are stained with PAS reaction or Gomori's methenamine silver stain. Nodules can also be present in other tissues, chiefly lymph nodes, skin, spleen, liver, kidneys, bones, testes, prostate, and eyes. This fungus can be easily identified in properly prepared and stained transtracheal washes or lymph node aspirates.

Clinical signs can reflect involvement of virtually any body tissue; pulmonary effects include cough, decreased exercise tolerance, and terminal respiratory distress.

Coccidioidomycosis (San Joaquin Valley fever), caused by the dimorphic fungus *Coccidioides immitis,* occurs mainly in animals living in arid regions of the southwestern US, Mexico, and Central and South America. It is a primary respiratory tract (aerogenous) infection commonly seen at slaughterhouses in clinically normal feedlot cattle. In dogs, coccidioidomycosis also has an aerogenous portal of entry and then disseminates systemically to other organs. Clinical signs relate to the location of lesions, so there can be respiratory distress, lameness, generalized lymphadenopathy, or cutaneous lesions, among others.

The lesions caused by *Coccidioides immitis* consist of focal granulomas or pyogranulomas that can have suppurative or caseated centers. The fungal organisms are readily seen in histologic or cytologic preparation as large (10 to 80 μm in diameter), double-walled, and highly refractile spherules (see Fig. 9-90, *D*).

Histoplasmosis is a systemic infection that results from inhalation of another dimorphic fungus, *Histoplasma capsulatum*. Histoplasmosis occurs sporadically in dogs and humans and to a lesser extent, in cats and horses. Bats often eliminate *Histoplasma capsulatum* in the feces, and droppings from bats and birds, particularly pigeons, heavily promote the growth and survival of this fungus in the soil of enzootic areas.

Pulmonary lesions are grossly characterized by variably sized, firm, poorly-encapsulated granulomas, and, sometimes, more diffuse involvement of the lungs. Microscopically, granulomatous tissue typically has many macrophages filled with small (1 to 3 μm), punctiform, intracytoplasmic, dark oval bodies (yeasts), and best demonstrated with PAS reaction (Fig. 9-90, *C*) or Gomori's methenamine silver stain. Similar nodules can be present in other tissues, chiefly lymph nodes, spleen, intestines, and liver.

Parasitic Pneumonias of Dogs

Toxoplasmosis is a worldwide disease caused by the obligate intracellular, protozoal parasite *Toxoplasma gondii*. Cats and other

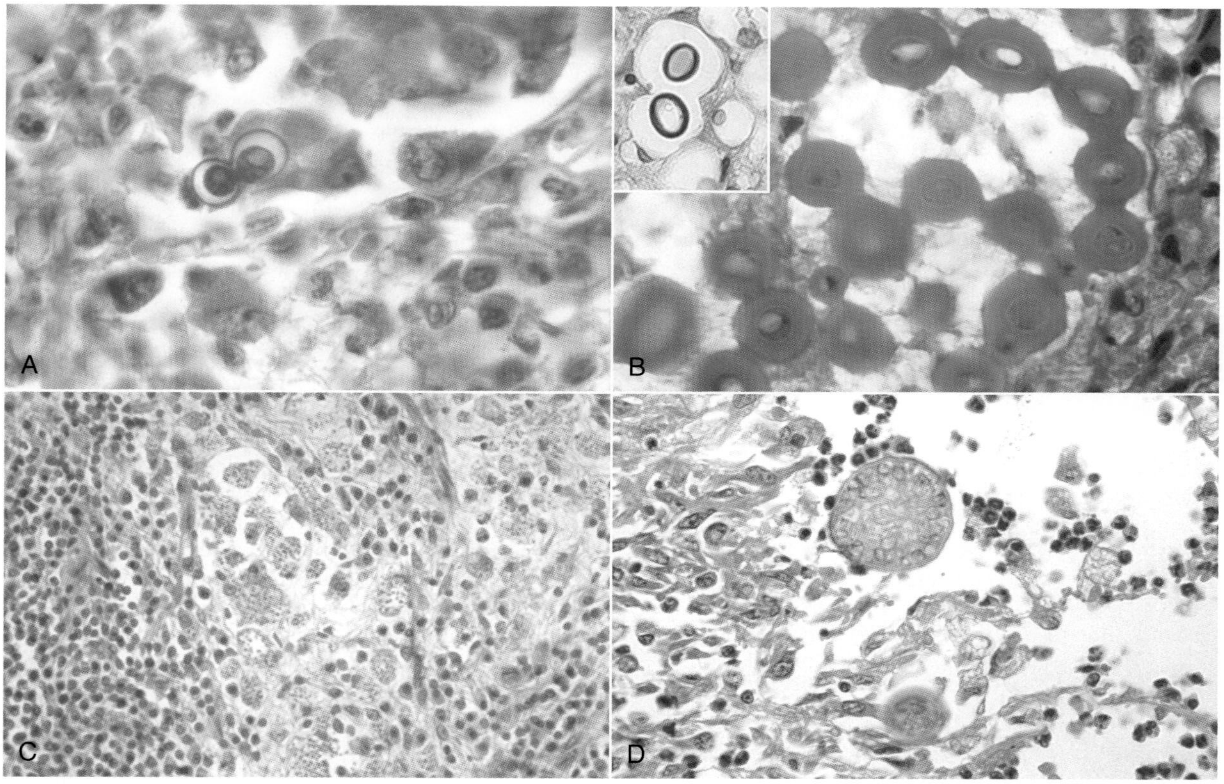

Fig. 9-90 Systemic (deep) mycoses.
A, *Blastomyces dermatitidis,* 8 to 25 μm in diameter, broad-based budding spherical yeastlike organisms, intracellular or extracellular location. H&E stain. **B,** *Cryptococcus neoformans,* spherical, 2 to 10 μm in diameter, usually surrounded by a thick mucus capsule, which can increase the overall diameter up to 30 μm, intracellular or extracellular location. The mucus capsule does not stain with H&E *(inset)* but is stained by mucicarmine. With routine mountants, the capsule shrinks and distorts, but this effect has been prevented here by using an aqueous mounting medium. Mayer's mucicarmine stain, aqueous mounting medium. *Inset,* In H&E–stained sections, the capsule is not visible but appears as a halo around the cell body. **C,** *Histoplasma capsulatum,* located intracellularly, is spherical to slightly elongated, 5 to 6 μm in diameter. H&E stain. **D,** *Coccidioides immitis,* spherules, 20 to 30 μm in diameter, containing endospores (<5 μm in diameter), intracellular or extracellular location. H&E stain. **(A, B, C,** and Inset courtesy Dr. M.D. McGavin, College of Veterinary Medicine, University of Tennessee. **D** courtesy College of Veterinary Medicine, University of Illinois.)

Felidae are the definitive host where the mature parasite divides sexually in the intestinal mucosa. Humans, dogs, cats, and many wild mammals can become intermediate hosts after accidental ingestion of fertile oocysts shed in cat feces, or fetuses can be infected transplacentally from an infected dam. In most instances, the parasite infects many cells of different tissues and induces an antibody response (seropositive animals) but does not cause clinical disease. Toxoplasmosis is often triggered by immunosuppression, such as that caused by canine distemper virus. Toxoplasmosis is characterized by focal necrosis around the protozoan.

Pulmonary lesions are severe, multifocal necrotizing interstitial pneumonia with notable proliferation of type II pneumonocytes and infiltrates of macrophages and neutrophils. Other lesions in disseminated toxoplasmosis include focal necrotizing hepatitis, myocarditis, splenitis, myositis, encephalitis, and ophthalmitis. The parasites appear microscopically as small (3 to 6 μm) basophilic cysts that can be found free in affected tissues or within the cytoplasm of many epithelial cells and macrophages. Similar findings can be seen sporadically in dogs infected with *Sarcocystis canis,* and immunohistochemistry would be required to differentiate those protozoal organisms from *Toxoplasma gondii.*

Pneumocystis carinii has also been reported as a sporadic cause of chronic interstitial pneumonia in dogs with a compromised immune system (see Pneumonias of Horses; also see Fig. 9-82).

Filaroides hirthi, a lungworm of the alveoli and bronchioles of dogs, has long been known as a cause of mild subclinical infection in large colonies of beagle dogs in the US. However, it can on occasion cause severe and even fatal disease in individual pets, presumably as a result of immunosuppression. Clinical signs may include coughing and terminal respiratory distress. Grossly, the lesions are multifocal subpleural nodules, often with a green hue because of eosinophils, scattered throughout the lungs. Microscopically, these nodules are eosinophilic granulomas arising from the alveolar interstitium associated with larvae or dead worms, as little reaction develops to the live adults.

Crenosoma vulpis is a lungworm seen commonly in foxes and sporadically in dogs with access to the intermediate hosts—slugs and snails. The adult lungworms live in small bronchi and bronchioles in the caudal lobes, causing eosinophilic and catarrhal bronchitis manifested grossly as gray areas of inflammation and atelectasis. In some animals, *Crenosoma vulpis* causes bronchiolar goblet cell metaplasia and mucous obstruction, resulting in lobular atelectasis due to the valve effect of the mucous plug.

Eucoleus aerophilus (Capillaria aerophila) is a nematode parasite typically found in the trachea and bronchi of wild and domestic carnivores. In some cases, this parasite may also involve the nasal passages and sinuses. Although generally asymptomatic, some dogs cough because of the local irritation caused by the parasites on the tracheal or bronchial mucosa.

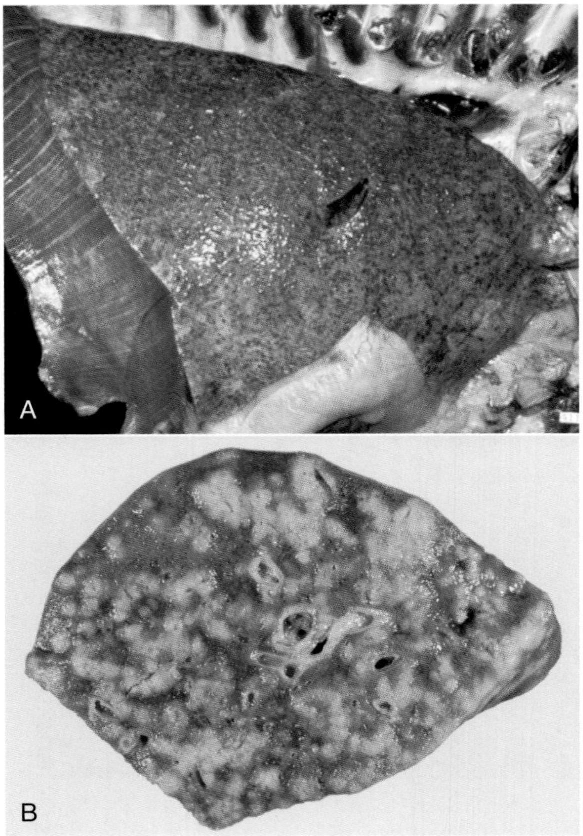

Fig. 9-91 Granulomatous pneumonia, blastomycosis *(Blastomyces dermatitidis)*, right lung, dog.

A, The lung contains large numbers of small granulomas distributed throughout all pulmonary lobes. **B,** The cut surface of the lung shows multiple discrete and coalescing gray-white granulomas distributed randomly throughout the lung. (Courtesy College of Veterinary Medicine, University of Illinois.)

Paragonimus kellicotti in North America and *Paragonimus westermani* in Asia are generally asymptomatic fluke infections in fish-eating species; cats and dogs acquire it in North America by eating crayfish. Gross lesions include pleural hemorrhages when the metacercariae migrate into the lungs. Later, multifocal eosinophilic pleuritis, and subpleural cysts up to 7 mm long containing pairs of adult flukes, are found along with eosinophilic granulomas around clusters of eggs. Like many other parasitic pneumonias, lesions and scars are more frequent in the caudal lobes. Pneumothorax can occur if a cyst that communicates with an airway ruptures to the pleural surface.

Angiostrongylus vasorum and *Dirofilaria immitis* are parasites of the pulmonary arteries and right ventricle and, depending on the stage, can produce different forms of pulmonary lesions. Adult parasites can cause chronic arteritis that leads to pulmonary hypertension, pulmonary arterial thrombosis, interstitial (eosinophilic) granulomatous pneumonia, pulmonary interstitial fibrosis, congestive right-sided cardiac failure, and eventually caudal vena caval syndrome. Other lesions include pleural petechial hemorrhages, and in later stages, diffuse pulmonary hemosiderosis, parasitic granulomas around eggs and larvae, and multifocal pulmonary infarcts. Larvae also cause alveolar injury, thickening of the alveolar walls with eosinophils and lymphocytes (interstitial pneumonia), and multifocal or coalescing granulomas with giant cells.

Aspiration Pneumonia in Dogs

Aspiration pneumonia is an important form of pneumonia in dogs when vomit or regurgitated materials are aspirated into the lungs, or when drugs or radiographic contrast media are accidentally introduced into the airways. As in other animal species, aspiration pneumonia may be unilateral or may more often affect the right cranial lobe (see Fig. 9-89). The severity of lesions depends very much on the chemical and microbiologic composition of the aspirated material. In general, aspiration in monogastric animals, particularly in dogs and cats, is more severe because of the low pH of the gastric contents (chemical pneumonitis). In severe cases, dogs and cats die rapidly from septic shock and ARDS (see Fig. 9-45), which is microscopically characterized by diffuse alveolar damage, protein-rich pulmonary edema, neutrophilic alveolitis, and formation of typical hyaline membranes along the alveolar walls (Fig. 9-92). In animals that survive the acute stages of aspiration,

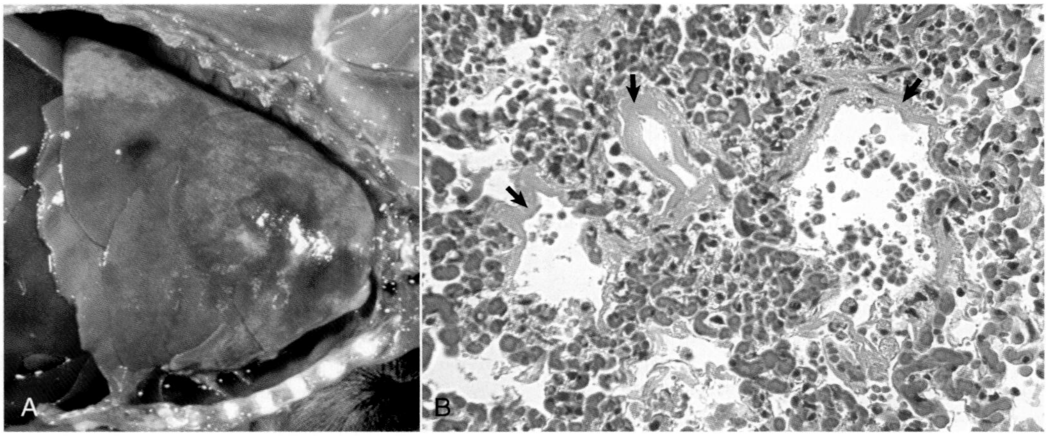

Fig. 9-92 Acute hemorrhagic bronchopneumonia, acute respiratory distress syndrome (ARDS), lungs, 4-week-old puppy.

A, Note that the lungs did not collapse when the thorax was opened (loss of negative pressure) and as a result fill almost the entire thoracic cavity. The cranioventral aspects of the lung are consolidated with hemorrhage. **B,** Alveolar capillary congestion, thick hyaline membranes along the alveolar septa *(arrows)*, and intraalveolar hemorrhage. These microscopic changes are typical of the diffuse alveolar damage seen in lungs with ARDS. H&E stain. (Courtesy Dr. A. López, Atlantic Veterinary College.)

pulmonary lesions progress to bronchopneumonia. Aspiration pneumonia is a common sequela to cleft palate, and in dogs with megaesophagus secondary to either myasthenia gravis or persistent right aortic arch. It is also an important complication of anesthesia or neurologic diseases affecting laryngeal function.

Toxic Pneumonias in Dogs

Paraquat, a broad-spectrum herbicide widely used in gardening and agriculture, can cause severe and often fatal toxic interstitial pneumonia (pneumonitis) in dogs, cats, humans, and other species. After ingestion or inhalation, this herbicide selectively accumulates in the lung and paraquat metabolites are produced by Clara cells. These metabolites promote local release of free radicals in the lung, which cause extensive injury to Clara cells and to the blood-air barrier, presumably through lipid peroxidation of type I and II pneumonocytes and alveolar endothelial cells (see Fig. 9-75). Paraquat toxicity has been used experimentally as a model of oxidant-induced alveolar injury and pulmonary fibrosis. Soon after poisoning, the lungs are heavy, edematous, and hemorrhagic because of extensive necrosis of epithelial and endothelial cells in the alveolar walls. The lungs of animals that survive acute paraquat toxicosis are pale, fail to collapse when the thorax is opened, and have interstitial emphysema, bullous emphysema, and may have pneumomediastinum. Microscopic findings in the acute and subacute phases include necrosis of type I pneumonocytes, interstitial and alveolar edema, intraalveolar hemorrhages, and proliferation of type II pneumonocytes. In the chronic stages (4 to 8 weeks later), the lesions are typically characterized by severe interstitial and intraalveolar fibrosis.

Uremic pneumonopathy (pneumonitis) is one of the many extrarenal lesions seen in dogs with chronic uremia. Lesions are characterized by a combination of pulmonary edema and calcification of vascular smooth muscle and alveolar basement membrane. In severe cases, alveolar calcification prevents lung collapse when the thorax is opened. In the more advanced cases, the lungs appear diffusely distended, pale red or brown in color, and show a rough pleural surface with rib imprints (see Fig. 9-33). On palpation, the pulmonary parenchyma has a typical "gritty" texture because of mineralization of the alveolar and vascular walls, which is best visualized microscopically by using special stains such as von Kossa (see Fig. 9-33). Because this is not primarily an inflammatory lesion, the term *pneumonitis* should not be used.

Pneumonias of Cats

Although upper respiratory tract infections are common and important in cats, pneumonias are uncommon except when there is immunosuppression or aspiration of gastric contents. Viral infections such as feline rhinotracheitis and calicivirus may cause lesions in the lungs, but unless there is secondary invasion by bacteria, they do not usually cause a fatal pneumonia (see Specific Diseases of the Nasal Cavity and Sinuses).

Feline Pneumonitis

The term *feline pneumonitis* is a misnomer because the major lesions caused by *Chlamydophila (psittaci) felis* are a severe conjunctivitis and rhinitis (see Specific Diseases of the Nasal Cavity and Sinuses). The elucidation of the importance of feline viral rhinotracheitis and feline calicivirus has removed *Chlamydophila felis* from its previously overstated importance as a lung pathogen.

Bacterial Pneumonias of Cats

Bacteria from the nasal flora such as *Pasteurella multocida* and Pasteurella-like organisms are occasionally associated with secondary bronchopneumonia in cats (Fig. 9-93). *Pasteurella multocida* also causes otitis media and meningitis, but its role as a respiratory pathogen is mainly associated with pyothorax. Interestingly, there are reports of *Pasteurella multocida* pneumonia in older or immunosuppressed humans acquired through contact with domestic cats. Mycoplasmas are often isolated from the lungs of cats with pulmonary lesions but are not definitively established as primary pathogens in feline pneumonias.

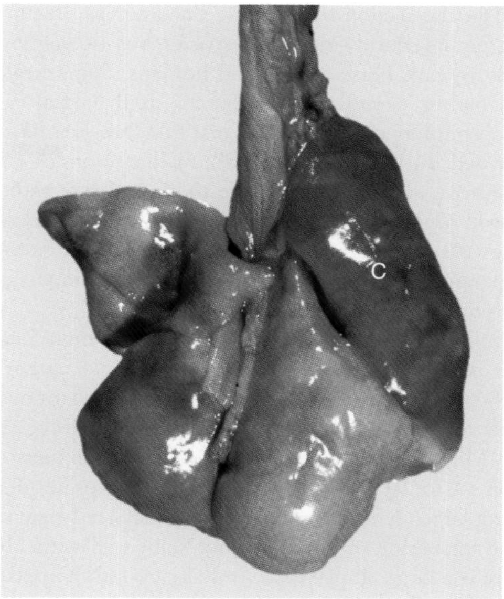

Fig. 9-93 Fibrinopurulent bronchopneumonia, lungs, 5-month-old kitten with history of conjunctivitis, rhinitis, and bacterial pneumonia. Cranioventral consolidation *(C)* of the right lung involves approximately 40% of its parenchyma. The consolidated lung is firm, and on the cut surface, some exudate is present in major bronchi. (Courtesy Dr. S. McBurney, Atlantic Veterinary College.)

Cats are susceptible to three types of mycobacterial infections: classic tuberculosis, feline leprosy, and atypical mycobacteriosis. Classic tuberculosis in cats is rare and generally caused by *Mycobacterium bovis*, but also to a lesser extent by *Mycobacterium tuberculosis* and *Mycobacterium avium*. The usual route of infection for feline tuberculosis is oral, through unpasteurized milk or infected meat, so the granulomatous lesions are mainly in the intestine and mesenteric lymph nodes where they may disseminate through infected phagocytes to other organs. The solid and noncaseated appearance of tuberculous nodules is grossly similar to that of neoplasms, so they must be differentiated from pulmonary neoplasms (e.g., lymphosarcoma). Classic tuberculosis with dermal lesions in cats should be differentiated from feline leprosy (localized skin granulomas) caused by *Mycobacterium lepraemurium* and other nonculturable species of acid-fast bacilli. Atypical mycobacteriosis is caused by contamination of a skin wound with saprophytic and nonsaprophytic mycobacteria such as those of the *Mycobacterium avium-intracellulare* complex. Advances in PCR techniques have notably reduced the time required for etiologic diagnosis of mycobacteriosis in veterinary diagnostic laboratories.

Mycotic Pneumonias of Cats

Cryptococcosis (pulmonary *Cryptococcus neoformans*) is the most frequent systemic mycosis in cats, and lesions are akin to those discussed in the section on Mycotic Pneumonias, Pneumonias of Dogs. It occurs worldwide in all species but is diagnosed most frequently in cats, horses, dogs, and humans. Some healthy dogs and cats harbor *Cryptococcus neoformans* in the nasal cavity and become asymptomatic carriers. Cats that are immunologically compromised, such as by FeLV, FIV, malnutrition, or corticosteroid treatment, are most susceptible to clinical infection. Lesions can occur in nearly any tissue, resulting in a wide variety of clinical signs. However, granulomatous rhinitis, sinusitis, otitis media and interna, pneumonia, ulcerative dermatitis, and meningoencephalitis are most common.

The pulmonary lesion in cryptococcosis is a multifocal granulomatous pneumonia and, like those occurring in other internal organs, they are small, gelatinous, white foci. The gelatinous appearance is because of the broad mucous capsule around the yeast (Fig. 9-90, *B*). Microscopically, lesions contain great numbers of fungal organisms (4 to 10 μm in diameter without capsule) and only a few macrophages, lymphocytes, and multinucleated giant cells. This thick polysaccharide capsule does not stain well with H&E, and thus there is a large empty space or halo around the yeast.

Other Pneumonias of Cats

Endogenous lipid (lipoid) pneumonia

Endogenous lipid pneumonia is an obscure, subclinical pulmonary disease of cats and occasionally of dogs, which is unrelated to aspiration of foreign material. Although the pathogenesis is not understood, it is presumed that lipids from pulmonary surfactant and from degenerated cells accumulate within alveolar macrophages, some of which exit the lung via the mucociliary escalator. The gross lesions are multifocal, white, firm nodules scattered throughout the lungs. Microscopically, the alveoli are filled with foamy, lipid-laden macrophages accompanied by interstitial infiltration of lymphocytes and plasma cells, fibrosis, and alveolar epithelialization.

Lipid (lipoid) pneumonia occurs frequently in the vicinity of cancerous lung lesions in humans, cats, and dogs. The reason for this association remains unknown and frequently unrecognized by pathologists. Recent investigations suggest that lipids are the breakdown products of neoplastic cells.

Exogenous lipid pneumonia

Another form of lipid pneumonia occurs accidentally in cats given mineral oil by their owners in attempts to remove hairballs (aspiration pneumonia).

Aspiration pneumonias

Aspiration pneumonias are common in cats as a result of vomiting, regurgitation, dysphagia, or anesthetic complication or after accidental administration of food, oral medicaments, or contrast media into the trachea (iatrogenic). Pulmonary lesions are similar to those described for dogs, and the type of lung lesion depends on the chemical and bacterial composition of the aspirated material (see the section on Aspiration Pneumonia in Dogs).

Feline idiopathic pulmonary fibrosis

Feline idiopathic pulmonary fibrosis is a rare disease of cats of uncertain etiology characterized by fibrotic nodules in the lung and subpleurally resulting in the pleural surface resembling nodular cirrhosis of the liver (Fig. 9-94). Microscopically, affected alveolar and peribronchiolar interstitium is thickened by excessive fibrosis and abundant deposition of ECM. The alveolar walls are diffusely lined by cuboidal hyperplastic type II pneumonocytes and the alveolar lumen often contains exfoliated cells and necrotic debris.

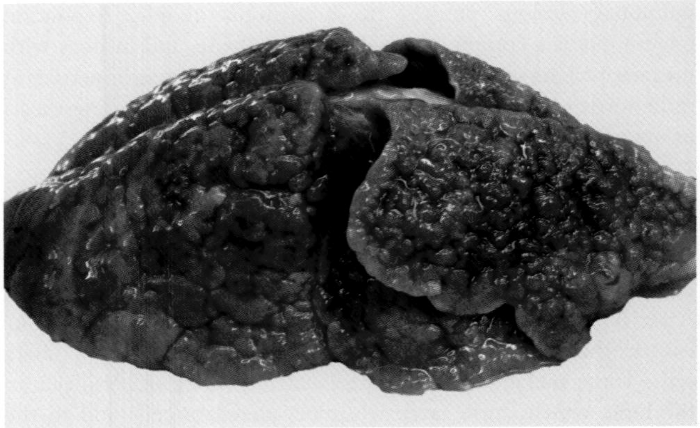

Fig. 9-94 Idiopathic nodular pulmonary fibrosis, lung, cat. The lung contains large numbers of nodules distributed throughout all pulmonary lobes. These nodules are formed by focal areas of fibrosis with retraction of the pulmonary parenchyma admixed with focal areas of pulmonary hyperinflation. This cat had a history of chronic respiratory problems. (Courtesy Facultad de Medicina Veterinaria y Zootecnia, Universidad Nacional Autónoma de México.)

This feline condition has morphologic features similar to "equine multinodular pulmonary fibrosis" and "cryptogenic pulmonary fibrosis" in humans.

Parasitic Pneumonias of Cats

Aelurostrongylus abstrusus, known as *feline lungworm,* is a parasite that occurs in cats wherever the necessary slug and snail intermediate hosts are found. It can cause chronic respiratory disease with coughing and weight loss and, sometimes, severe dyspnea and death, particularly if there are secondary bacterial infections. The gross lesions are multifocal, amber, and subpleural granulomatous nodules up to 1 cm in diameter throughout the lungs. On incision, these nodules may contain viscous exudate. Microscopically, the parasites and their eggs and coiled larvae are in the bronchioles and alveoli where they cause catarrhal bronchiolitis, hyperplasia of submucosal glands, and later, granulomatous alveolitis, alveolar fibrosis, and fibromuscular hyperplasia. During routine examination of feline lungs, it is quite common to find fibromuscular hyperplasia in bronchioles and arterioles in otherwise healthy cats. It was alleged in the past that this fibromuscular hyperplasia was a long-term sequela of subclinical infection with *Aelurostrongylus abstrusus.* However, this view has been challenged, thus the pathogenesis and significance of pulmonary fibromuscular hyperplasia in healthy cats remains uncertain.

Toxoplasma gondii, Paragonimus kellicotti, and *Dirofilaria immitis* can also affect cats (see the section on Parasitic Pneumonias of Dogs).

Fetal and Perinatal Pneumonias

Fetal Pneumonias

Pneumonia is one of the most frequent lesions found in fetuses submitted for postmortem examination, particularly in foals and food-producing animals. Because of autolysis, lack of inflation, and the lungs being at various stages of development, fetal lesions are often missed or misdiagnosed. In the nonaerated fetal lung, the bronchoalveolar spaces are filled with a viscous, locally produced fluid known as *lung fluid* or *lung liquid.* It has been estimated that an ovine fetus produces about 2.5 mL of "lung fluid" per kilogram of body weight per hour. In the fetus, this fluid normally moves along the tracheobronchial tree, reaching the oropharynx, where a fraction is swallowed into the gastrointestinal tract, and a small portion is released into the amniotic fluid. At the time of birth, the lung fluid is rapidly reabsorbed from the lungs by alveolar absorption and lymphatic drainage.

Aspiration of amniotic fluid contaminated with meconium and bacteria from placentitis is the most common route by which microbial pathogens reach the fetal lungs. This form of pneumonia is secondary to fetal hypoxia and acidosis ("fetal distress"), which cause the fetus to relax the anal sphincter, release meconium into the amniotic fluid, and in the terminal stages inspire deeply with open glottis, resulting in the aspiration of contaminated fluid (see Web Fig. 9-14). Gross lesions are only occasionally recognized, but microscopic changes are similar to those of a bronchopneumonia. Microscopically, bronchoalveolar spaces contain variable numbers of neutrophils, macrophages, and pieces of meconium that appear as bright yellow material because of its bile content. In contrast to postnatal bronchopneumonia, lesions in fetuses are not restricted to the cranioventral aspects of the lungs but typically involve all pulmonary lobes.

In cattle, *Brucella abortus* and *Arcanobacterium (Actinomyces) pyogenes* are two of the most common bacteria isolated from the lungs of aborted fetuses. These bacteria are usually present in large numbers in the amniotic fluid of cows with bacterial placentitis. Inflammation of the placenta interferes with oxygen exchange between fetal and maternal tissue, and the resultant fetal hypoxia induces the fetus to "breathe" with an open glottis and aspirate the amniotic fluid. *Aspergillus* spp. (mycotic abortion) and *Ureaplasma diversum* cause sporadic cases of placentitis, which results in fetal pneumonia and abortion.

In addition to the respiratory route (aspiration), pathogens, such as bacteria and viruses, can also reach the lungs via fetal blood and cause interstitial pneumonia. Listeriosis *(Listeria monocytogenes)*, salmonellosis (*Salmonella* spp.), and chlamydiosis *(Chlamydophila psittaci)* are the best known examples of blood-borne diseases that cause fetal pneumonia in farm animals. Gross lesions in the lungs are generally undetected, but microscopic lesions include focal necrotizing interstitial pneumonia and focal necrosis in the liver, spleen, or brain. Fetal bronchointerstitial pneumonia occurs also in some viral abortions, such as those caused by IBR virus and PI-3 virus in cattle and EVR in horses. Fetal pneumonias in dogs and cats are infrequently described, perhaps because aborted puppies and kittens are rarely submitted for postmortem examination. With advancements in molecular biology techniques, the etiologic diagnosis of abortions and their association with pulmonary fetal lesions is rapidly improving.

Neonatal Pneumonias and Septicemias

These entities are rather common in newborn animals lacking passive immunity from hypogammaglobulinemia because of the lack of either ingestion or absorption of maternal colostrum (failure of passive transfer). In addition to septicemias causing interstitial pneumonia, farm animals with hypogammaglobulinemia can develop bronchopneumonia by inhalation of bacterial pathogens. These include *Histophilus somni* and *Pasteurella multocida* in calves, *Streptococcus* spp. in foals, and *Escherichia coli, Listeria monocytogenes, and Streptococcus suis* in pigs.

Meconium Aspiration Syndrome

Information on this topic is available at evolve.elsevier.com/Zachary/McGavin/.

Neoplasms of the Lungs

General Considerations

Lung cancer in animals is rare, unlike in humans in which the incidence is alarming and continues to be the number one cause of cancer deaths in Canada, the US, and Europe. Interestingly, prostatic and breast cancers, so much feared by men and women, are a distant second. To say that cigarette smoking is responsible for this epidemic of lung cancer is unnecessary. Although dogs have been proposed as valuable "sentinels" for environmental hazards, such as exposure to passive smoking, asbestos, dyes, and insecticides, it is not known if the prevalence of canine lung tumors has increased in geographical areas with high contamination. Alterations in genes (oncogenes) and chromosomes and changes in biologically active molecules have been linked to lung cancer in recent years. As with many other forms of cancer, epidemiologic studies indicate that the incidence of pulmonary neoplasms increases with age, but there are still insufficient data to confirm that particular canine or feline breeds have a higher predisposition to spontaneous lung neoplasms.

A standard nomenclature of pulmonary neoplasms in domestic animals is lacking, and as a consequence, multiplicity of names and synonyms occur in the veterinary literature. Some classifications are based on the primary site, whereas others emphasize more the histomorphologic type. The most common types of benign and malignant pulmonary neoplasms in domestic mammals are listed in Box 9-2.

BOX 9-2 Classification of Pulmonary Neoplasms

PRIMARY EPITHELIAL ORIGIN

Benign

Papillary adenoma
Bronchiolar-alveolar adenoma

Malignant

Adenocarcinoma (acinar or papillar)
Squamous cell carcinoma
Adenosquamous carcinoma
Bronchiolar-alveolar carcinoma
Small cell and large cell carcinomas
Anaplastic (undifferentiated) carcinoma
Carcinoid tumor (neuroendocrine)
Ovine (retroviral) pulmonary carcinoma

PRIMARY MESENCHYMAL ORIGIN

Benign

Hemangioma

Malignant

Osteosarcoma, chondrosarcoma
Hemangiosarcoma
Malignant histiocytosis
Lymphomatoid granulomatosis
Granular cell tumor
Mesothelioma

SECONDARY (METASTATIC) LUNG TUMORS

Any malignant tumor metastatic from another body location (e.g., osteosarcoma in dogs, uterine carcinoma in cows, malignant melanoma in horses)

Clinically, the signs of pulmonary neoplasia vary with the degree of invasiveness, the amount of parenchyma involved, and locations of metastases. Signs may be vague such as cough, lethargy, anorexia, weight loss, and perhaps dyspnea. In addition, paraneoplastic syndromes, such as hypercalcemia, endocrinopathies, and pulmonary hypertrophic osteoarthropathy, have been associated with pulmonary neoplasms.

Primary Neoplasms of the Lungs

Primary neoplasms of the lungs arise from cells normally present in the pulmonary tissue and can be epithelial or mesenchymal, although the latter are rare. Primary benign neoplasms of the lungs, such as pulmonary adenomas, are highly unusual in domestic animals. Most primary neoplasms are malignant and appear as solitary masses of variable size that, with time, can metastasize to other areas of the lungs and to distant organs. It is sometimes difficult on gross and microscopic examination to differentiate primary lung cancer from pulmonary metastasis resulting from malignant neoplasms elsewhere in the body.

It is often difficult to determine the precise topographic origin of a neoplasm within the lungs—for example, whether it originates in the conducting system (bronchogenic carcinoma), transitional system (bronchiolar carcinoma), exchange system (alveolar carcinoma), or bronchial glands (bronchial gland carcinoma). According to the literature, pulmonary carcinomas in animals arise generally from Clara cells or type II pneumonocytes of the bronchioloalveolar region, in contrast to those in humans, which are mostly bronchogenic. Tumors located at the hilus generally arise from major bronchi and tend to be a solitary large mass with occasional small metastasis to the periphery of the lung. In contrast, tumors arising from the bronchioloalveolar region are often multicentric with numerous peripheral metastases in the lung parenchyma. Because of histologic architecture and irrespective of their site of origin, many malignant epithelial neoplasms are frequently classified by the all-encompassing term of pulmonary adenocarcinomas.

Dogs and cats are the species most frequently affected with primary pulmonary neoplasms, largely carcinomas, generally in older animals. The mean age for primary lung tumors is 11 years for dogs and 12 years for cats. Pulmonary carcinomas in other domestic animals are less common, possibly because fewer farm animals are allowed to reach their natural life span. These neoplasms can be invasive or expansive, vary in color (white, tan, or gray) and texture (soft or firm), and often have areas of necrosis and hemorrhage, which result in a "craterous" or "umbilicate" appearance. This umbilicate appearance is frequently seen in rapidly growing carcinomas in which the center of the tumoral mass undergoes necrosis as a result of ischemia. Some lung neoplasms resemble pulmonary consolidation or large granulomas. Cats with moderately differentiated neoplasms had significantly longer survival time (median, 698 days) than cats with poorly differentiated neoplasms (median, 75 days). Dogs with primary lung neoplasms, grades I, II, and III, had survival times of 790, 251, and 5 days, respectively.

Ovine Pulmonary Adenocarcinoma (Ovine Pulmonary Carcinoma)

Ovine pulmonary adenocarcinoma, also known as *pulmonary adenomatosis* and *jaagsiekte* (from the South African Afrikaans word for "driving sickness"), is a transmissible, retrovirus-induced neoplasia of ovine lungs. It occurs in sheep around the world, with the notable exception of Australia and New Zealand; its incidence is high in Scotland, South Africa, and Peru and unknown but probably low in North America. This pulmonary carcinoma behaves very much like a chronic pneumonia, and the "Jaagsiekte sheep retrovirus" shares many epidemiologic similarities with the ovine lentivirus responsible for Maedi and the retrovirus responsible for enzootic nasal carcinoma in ruminants. Pulmonary adenomatosis has been transmitted to goats experimentally but is not known to be a spontaneous disease in that species.

This disease affects mainly mature sheep but can occasionally affect young stock. Intensive husbandry probably facilitates horizontal transmission by the copious nasal discharge and explains why the disease occurs in Iceland as devastating epizootics with 5% to 80% mortality. Differential diagnosis between maedi and pulmonary adenomatosis can prove difficult because both diseases often coexist in the same flock or in the same animal. Death is inevitable after several months of the initial onset of respiratory signs, and a specific humoral immune response to the Jaagsiekte sheep retrovirus is undetectable in affected sheep.

During the early stages of ovine pulmonary carcinoma, the lungs are enlarged, heavy, and wet and have several firm, gray, variably-sized nodules that tend to be located in the cranioventral lobes (Fig. 9-95, *A*). In the later stages, the nodules become confluent, and large segments of both lungs are diffusely, but not symmetrically, infiltrated by neoplastic cells. On cross-section, edematous fluid and a copious mucoid secretion are present in the trachea and bronchi (Fig. 9-95, *B*). Microscopically, the nodules consist of cuboidal or columnar epithelial cells lining airways and alveoli and forming papillary or acinar (glandlike) structures (Fig. 9-95, *A inset*). Because the cells have been identified ultrastructurally as originating from both type II alveolar epithelial cells and Clara cells, the neoplasm is considered a "bronchioloalveolar" carcinoma. Sequelae often include secondary bronchopneumonia, abscesses, and fibrous pleural adhesions. Metastases occur to tracheobronchial and mediastinal lymph nodes and to a lesser extent to other tissues such as pleura, muscle, liver, and kidneys.

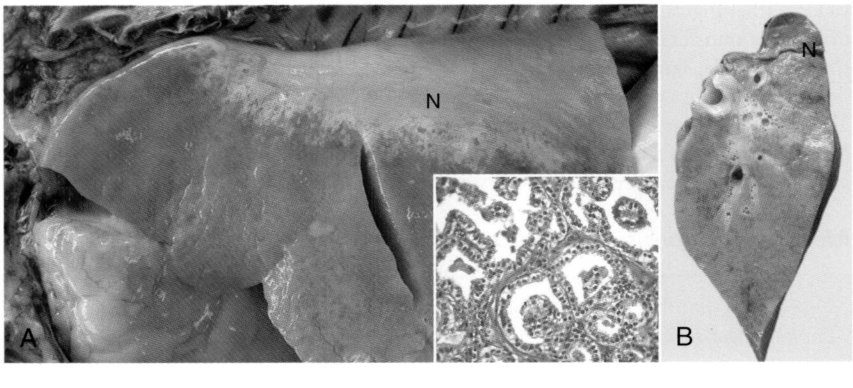

Fig. 9-95 Ovine pulmonary carcinoma (pulmonary adenomatosis, jaagsiekte), lung, 3-year-old sheep. **A,** Neoplastic cell infiltration involving the cranial and ventral portions of the lung and mainly sparing the dorsal portions of the caudal lung lobe *(N)*. The affected lung is enlarged and firm. *Inset,* Papillary proliferation of cuboidal epithelial cells (presumed type II pneumonocytes). H&E stain. **B,** Transverse section of the cranial lobe. Note the solid appearance of the ventral portion *(bottom)* of the lung and the frothy fluid (edema) that originates in the alveolar walls. *N,* Normal lung. (Courtesy Dr. M. Heras, Facultad de Veterinaria, Universidad de Zaragoza, Spain.)

Clinically, pulmonary adenomatosis is characterized by a gradual loss of condition, sometimes coughing, and respiratory distress, especially after exercise (such as herding or "driving"). Appetite and temperature are normal, unless there are secondary bacterial infections. An important differentiating feature from maedi (interstitial pneumonia) can be observed if the animals with pulmonary adenomatosis are raised by their hind limbs; copious, thin, mucoid fluid, produced by neoplastic cells in the lungs, pours from the nostrils of some animals.

Carcinoid (Neuroendocrine) Tumor of the Lungs

Carcinoid tumor of the lungs is a neoplasm presumably arising from neuroendocrine cells that is sporadically seen in dogs as multiple, large, firm pulmonary masses close to the mainstem bronchi. It has also been reported in the nasal cavity of horses. Tumor cells are generally polygonal with finely granular, pale, or slightly eosinophilic cytoplasm. Nuclei are small, and mitotic figures are absent or rare.

Granular Cell Tumor

Granular cell tumor is a rare and locally invasive tumor that has been reported mainly in humans and older horses. The cell origin of this tumor was thought to be the myoblast, but it is currently presumed to be Schwann cells, which are normally present in the bronchovascular bundles of the lung. Microscopically, neoplastic cells are large, polyhedron-shaped with abundant cytoplasm containing numerous acidophilic granules, which are positive for S-100 protein. Although this tumor can caused bronchial obstruction and respiratory signs, in most cases, it is an incidental finding in older horses submitted for postmortem examination.

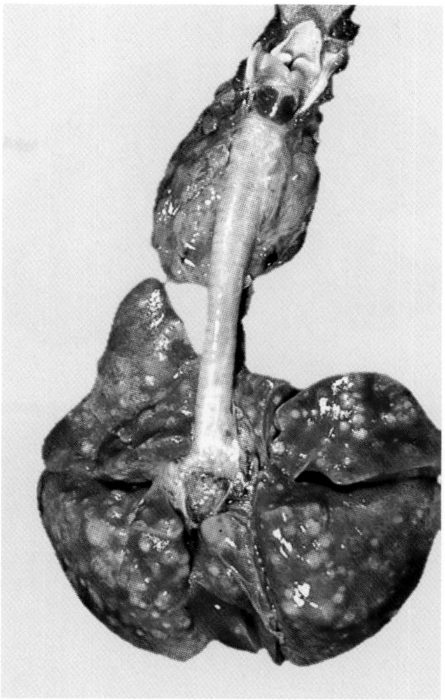

Fig. 9-96 Metastatic thyroid carcinoma, lungs, adult dog. The lungs contain multiple randomly distributed metastatic nodules, which originated from the enlarged and neoplastic left thyroid gland. (Courtesy Dr. J.M. King, College of Veterinary Medicine, Cornell University.)

Lymphomatoid Granulomatosis

Lymphomatoid granulomatosis is a rare but interesting disease of humans, dogs, and cats characterized by nodules or large solid masses in one or more lung lobes. These frequently metastasize to lymph nodes, kidneys, and liver. Microscopically, tumors are formed by large pleomorphic mononuclear (lymphomatoid) cells with a high mitotic rate and frequent formation of binucleated or multinucleated cells. Tumor cells have a distinct tendency to grow around blood vessels and destroy the vascular walls. Lymphomatoid granulomatosis has some resemblance to lymphomas, and phenotypic marking confirms that neoplastic cells are a mixed population of plasma cells, B and T lymphocytes, and histiocytes.

Secondary Neoplasms of the Lungs

Secondary neoplasms of the lungs are all malignant by definition because they are the result of metastasis to the lungs from malignant neoplasms elsewhere. Because the pulmonary capillaries are the first filter met by tumor emboli released into the vena cava or pulmonary arteries, secondary neoplasms in the lung are relatively common in comparison to primary ones. Also, secondary tumors can be epithelial or mesenchymal in origin. Common metastatic tumors of epithelial origin are mammary, thyroid (Fig. 9-96), and uterine carcinomas. Tumors of mesenchymal origin are osteosarcoma (Fig. 9-97, *A*); hemangiosarcoma (see Fig. 9-97, *B* and Web Fig. 9-15); malignant melanoma in dogs; malignant lymphoma in cows, pigs, dogs, and cats (Fig. 9-98); and the recently reported vaccination-site fibrosarcoma in cats. Usually, secondary pulmonary neoplasms are multiple, scattered throughout all pulmonary lobes (hematogenous dissemination), of variable size, and according to the growth pattern, can be nodular, diffuse, or radiating.

The appearance of metastatic neoplasms differs according to the type of neoplasm. For example, dark red cystic nodules containing blood indicate hemangiosarcoma; dark black solid nodules indicate melanoma; and hard solid nodules (white, yellow, or tan color) with bone spicules indicate osteosarcoma. The gross appearances of metastatic carcinomas are generally similar to the primary neoplasm and sometimes have umbilicated centers. Proper diagnoses of pulmonary neoplasms in live animals require history, clinical signs, radiographs, cytologic analysis of BAL fluid, and when necessary, a lung biopsy. Identification of a specific lineage of neoplastic cells in biopsy or postmortem specimens is often difficult and requires electron microscopy or immunohistochemical techniques. Electron microscopy allows identification of distinctive cellular components such as osmophilic lamellar phospholipid nephritic bodies in alveolar type II epithelial cells or melanosomes in melanomas. Immunohistochemical staining of intermediate filaments is also helpful in identifying tumor cells, for example, a metastatic neurofibrosarcoma can be distinguished from an anaplastic hemangiosarcoma by the presence of S-100 protein and factor VIII–related markers.

THORACIC CAVITY AND PLEURA

The thoracic wall, diaphragm, and mediastinum are lined by the parietal pleura, which reflects onto the lungs at the hilum and continues as the visceral pleura, covering the entire surface of the lungs, except at the hilus where the bronchi and blood vessels enter. The space between the parietal and visceral pleura (pleural space) is only minimal and under normal conditions contains only traces of clear fluid, which is a lubricant, and a few exfoliated cells. Samples of this fluid are obtained by thoracocentesis, a simple procedure in which a needle is passed into the pleural cavity. Volumetric, biochemical, and cytologic changes in this fluid are routinely used in veterinary diagnostics.

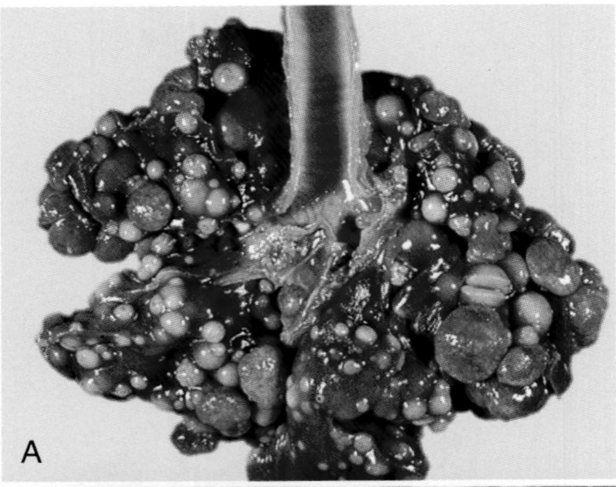

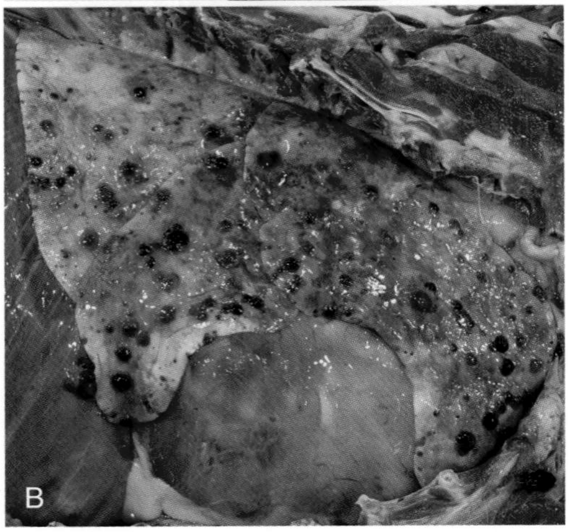

Fig. 9-97 Lung, dog.
A, Metastatic sarcoma (primary site unknown). Large numbers of metastatic nodules are randomly distributed throughout all lung lobes. **B,** Metastatic hemangiosarcoma. Note the red to dark red masses throughout the lung parenchyma. If these masses were black, metastatic melanoma would be the likely diagnosis. (**A** courtesy Dr. J.M. King, College of Veterinary Medicine, Cornell University. **B** courtesy Dr. A. Bourque and Dr. A. López, Atlantic Veterinary College.)

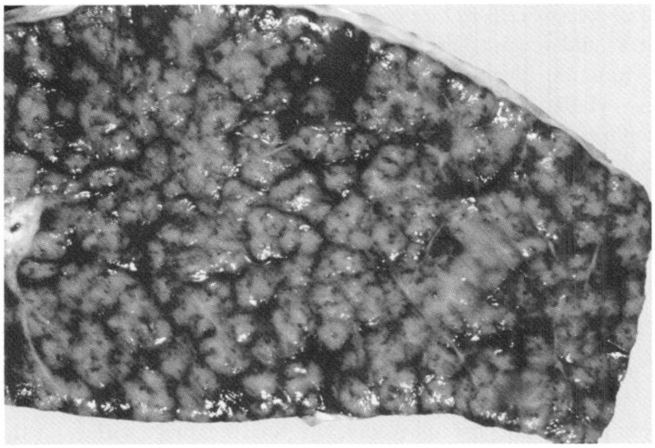

Fig. 9-98 Metastatic lymphoma (lymphosarcoma), lungs, cut surface, cow.
Note the numerous discrete and confluent metastatic nodules with the smooth texture and gray color characteristic of lymphoma. (Courtesy College of Veterinary Medicine, University of Illinois.)

Anomalies

Congenital defects are rare and generally of little clinical significance. Cysts within the mediastinum of dogs can be large enough to compromise pulmonary function or mimic neoplasia in thoracic radiographs. These cysts may arise from the thymus (thymic branchial cysts), perinephric tissue (perinephric pseudocyst), bronchi, or from remnants of the branchial pouches and are generally lined by epithelium and surrounded by a capsule of stromal tissue. Anomalies of the thoracic duct cause some cases of chylothorax.

Degenerative Disturbances

Pleural Calcification

Pleural calcification is commonly found in dogs with chronic uremia. Lesions appear as linear white streaks in parietal pleura, mainly over the intercostal muscles of the cranial part of the thoracic cavity. The lesions are not functionally significant but indicate a severe underlying renal problem. Vitamin D toxicity (hypervitaminosis D) and ingestion of hypercalcemic substances, such as vitamin D analogs, can also cause calcification of the pleura and other organs.

Pneumothorax

Pneumothorax is the presence of air in the thoracic cavity where there should normally be negative pressure to facilitate inspiration. Humans have a complete and strong mediastinum so that pneumothorax is generally unilateral and thus not a serious problem. In dogs, the barrier varies, but in general is not complete, so often some communication exists between left and right sides.

There are two main forms of pneumothorax. In spontaneous pneumothorax, air leaking into the pleural cavity from the lungs occurs without any known underlying disease or trauma. In secondary pneumothorax, movement of air into the pleural cavity results from an underlying pulmonary or thoracic wall disease. Most common causes of secondary pneumothorax in veterinary medicine are penetrating wounds to the thoracic wall, ruptured esophagus, iatrogenic trauma to thorax and lung during a transthoracic lung biopsy or thoracoscopy, tracheal rupture from improper intubation, and rupture of emphysematous bullae or parasitic pulmonary cysts (*Paragonimus* spp.) that communicate with the thoracic cavity. Pneumothorax and pneumomediastinum caused by high air pressure (barotrauma) are also well documented in cats after equipment failure during anesthesia. Clinical signs of pneumothorax include respiratory distress, and the lesion is simply a collapsed, atelectatic lung. The air is readily reabsorbed from the cavity if the site of entry is sealed.

Circulatory and Lymphatic Disturbances

Pleural Effusion

Pleural effusion is a general term used to describe accumulation of any fluid (transudate, modified transudate, exudate, blood, lymph, or chyle) in the thoracic cavity. Cytologic and biochemical evaluations of pleural effusions are sometimes helpful in suggesting a possible pathogenesis. Based on protein concentration and total numbers of nucleated cells, pleural effusions are cytologically divided into transudates, modified transudates, and exudates.

Hydrothorax

When the fluid is serous, clear, and odorless and fails to coagulate when exposed to air, the condition is referred to as *hydrothorax (transudate).* Causes of hydrothorax are the same as those involved in edema formation in other organs: increased hydrostatic

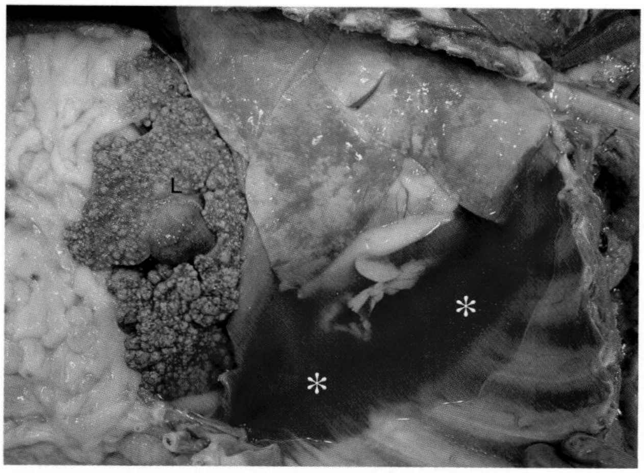

Fig. 9-99 Hydrothorax, pleural cavity, 8-year-old dog.
The pleural cavity contains a large amount of deep yellow transudate *(asterisks)* (ventrally). Scattered foci of atelectasis are visible on the surface of the lung. Fluid in the pleural cavity usually compresses the ventral portions of the lung, resulting in a compressive atelectasis. Also note the nodular surface of the cirrhotic liver *(L)*. (Courtesy Dr. S. McBurney, Atlantic Veterinary College.)

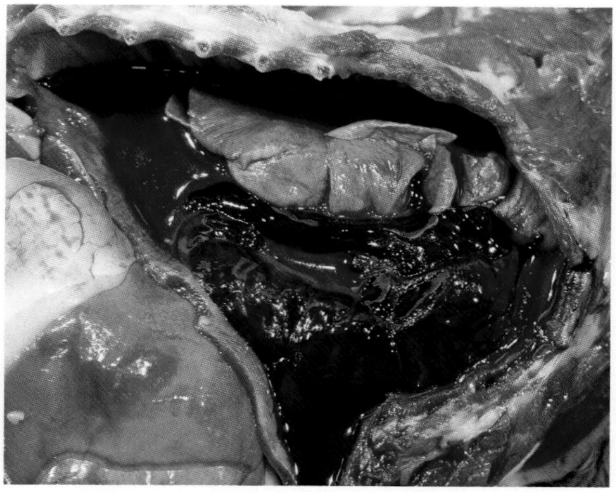

Fig. 9-100 Hemothorax, right pleural cavity, dog.
The right pleural cavity is filled with a large clot of blood from a ruptured thoracic aortic aneurysm, which caused unexpected death. Canine aortic aneurysms are associated with migration of *Spirocerca lupi* larvae along the aortic wall before their final migration into the wall of the adjacent esophagus. In other cases like this dog, the cause remains unknown (idiopathic aortic aneurysm). (Courtesy Dr. L. Gabor and Dr. A. López, Atlantic Veterinary College.)

pressure (heart failure), decreased oncotic pressure (hypoproteinemia, as in liver disease), alterations in vascular permeability (α-naphthylthiourea [ANTU] toxicity), or obstruction of lymph drainage (neoplasia). In cases where the leakage is corrected, if the fluid is a transudate, it is rapidly reabsorbed. If the fluid persists, it irritates the pleura and causes mesothelial hyperplasia and fibrosis, which thickens the pleura.

In severe cases, the amount of fluid present in the thoracic cavity can be considerable. For instance, a medium-size dog can have 2 L of fluid, and a cow may accumulate 25 L or more. Excessive fluid in the thorax causes compressive atelectasis, resulting in respiratory distress (see Fig. 9-36). Hydrothorax is most commonly seen in cattle with right-sided heart failure or cor pulmonale (hydrostatic); dogs with congestive heart failure (hydrostatic) (see Web Fig. 9-16), chronic hepatic disease (hepatic hydrothorax) (Fig. 9-99) or nephrotic syndrome (hypoproteinemia); pigs with mulberry heart disease (increased vascular permeability); and horses with African horse sickness (increased vascular permeability).

Hemothorax

Blood in the thoracic cavity is called *hemothorax,* but the term has been used for exudate with a sanguineous component. Causes include rupture of a major blood vessel as a result of severe thoracic trauma (e.g., hit by car); erosion of a vascular wall by malignant cells or inflammation (e.g., aortitis caused by *Spirocerca lupi*); ruptured aortic aneurysms; clotting defects, including coagulopathies; warfarin toxicity; disseminated intravascular coagulation (consumption coagulopathy); and thrombocytopenia caused by bone marrow suppression. Hemothorax is generally acute and fatal. On gross examination, the thoracic cavity can be filled with blood, and the lungs are partially or completely atelectatic (Fig. 9-100).

Chylothorax

The accumulation of chyle (lymph rich in triglycerides) in the thoracic cavity (Fig. 9-101) is a result of the rupture of major lymph vessels, usually the thoracic duct or the right lymphatic duct. The clinical and pathologic effects of chylothorax are similar to those of the other pleural effusions. Causes include thoracic neoplasia (the most common cause in humans, but a distant second to idiopathic cases in dogs), trauma, congenital lymph vessel anomalies, fungal infections in the lymphatics, dirofilariasis, and iatrogenic rupture of the thoracic duct during surgery. The source of the leakage of chyle is rarely found at necropsy. When the leakage of chyle occurs

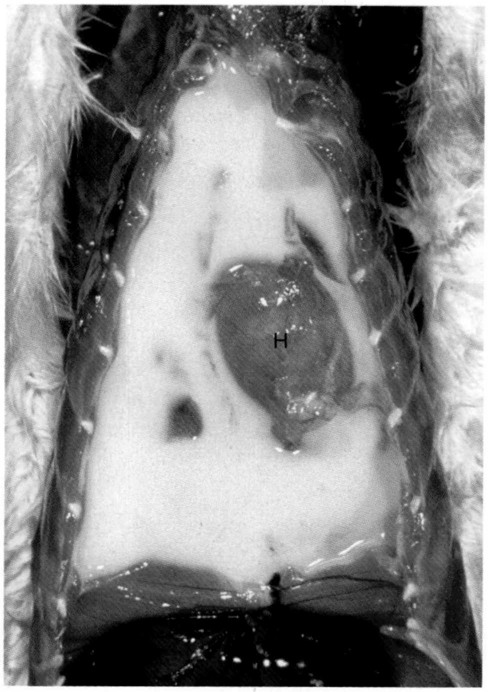

Fig. 9-101 Chylothorax (cause unknown), thoracic (pleural) cavity, mink.
Lymph (chyle) fills both the left and right pleural cavities. The heart *(H)* and pericardium are essentially normal because the chyle does not adhere to the outer surface of the pericardial sac, as typically happens with suppurative and fibrinous exudates in the thoracic cavity. (Courtesy Western College of Veterinary Medicine.)

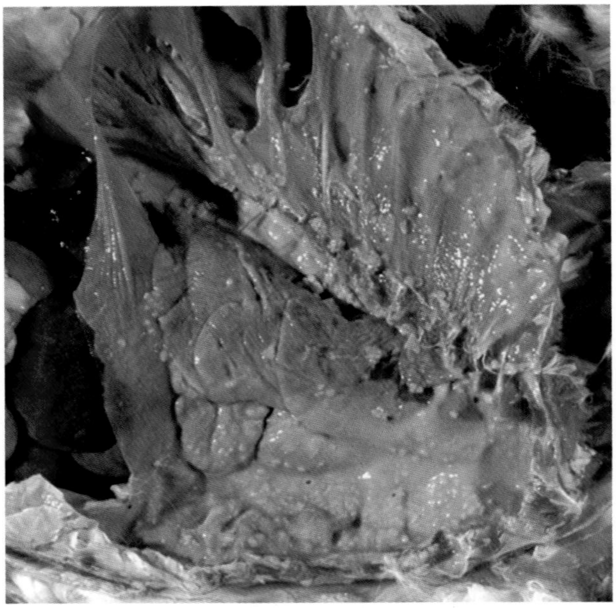

Fig. 9-102 Pyothorax *(Pasteurella multocida)*, right pleural cavity, cat. Pus in the thoracic cavity is called pyothorax or empyema. Purulent exudate also covers the visceral and parietal pleurae. This lesion is also referred to as *suppurative pleuritis.* (Courtesy Dr. A. López, Atlantic Veterinary College.)

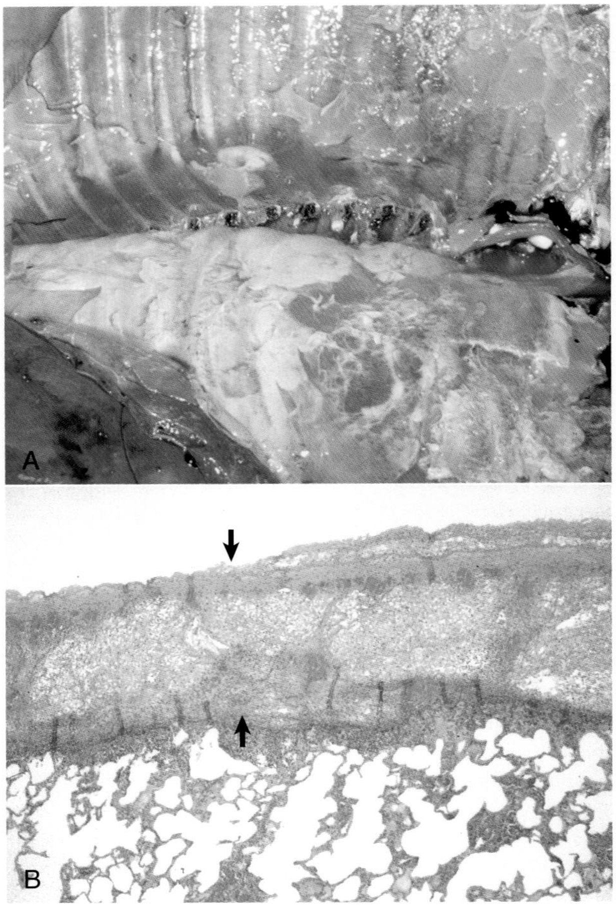

Fig. 9-103 Fibrinous pleuritis, right pleural cavity, horse. **A,** Large masses of yellow fibrin cover the visceral and parietal pleurae. The lungs are normal. **B,** The visceral pleura is covered by a thick layer of fibrin (between arrows). Subjacent alveoli are essentially normal. H&E stain. (**A** courtesy Dr. A. López, Atlantic Veterinary College. **B** courtesy College of Veterinary Medicine, University of Illinois.)

in the abdominal cavity, the condition is referred to as *chyloabdomen.* Cytologic and biochemical examination of fluid collected by thoracocentesis typically reveals large numbers of lymphocytes, few neutrophils in chronic cases, and a high triglyceride content.

Inflammation of the Pleura

Pleural tissue is readily susceptible to injury caused by direct implantation of an organism through a penetrating thoracic or diaphragmatic wound, by hematogenous dissemination of infectious organisms in septicemias, or by direct extension from an adjacent inflammatory process, such as in fibrinous bronchopneumonia or from a perforated esophagus. Chronic injury typically results in serosal fibrosis and tight adhesions between visceral and parietal pleurae. When extensive, these adhesions can obliterate the pleural space.

Pleuritis or Pleurisy

Inflammation of the visceral or parietal pleurae is called *pleuritis,* and according to the type of exudate, it can be fibrinous, suppurative, granulomatous, hemorrhagic, or a combination of exudates. When suppurative pleuritis results in accumulation of purulent exudate in the cavity, the lesion is called *pyothorax* or *thoracic empyema* (Fig. 9-102). Clinically, pleuritis causes considerable pain, and in addition, empyema can result in severe toxemia. Pleural fibrous adhesions (between parietal and visceral pleura) and fibrosis are the most common sequelae of chronic pleuritis and can significantly interfere with inflation of the lungs.

Pleuritis can occur as an extension of pneumonia, particularly in fibrinous bronchopneumonias (pleuropneumonia), or it can occur alone, without obvious pulmonary involvement (Fig. 9-103). Bovine and ovine pneumonic Mannheimiosis and porcine and bovine pleuropneumonia are good examples of pleuritis associated with fibrinous bronchopneumonias. Polyserositis in pigs and pleural empyema, particularly in cats and horses, are examples of pleural inflammation in which involvement of the lungs may not accompany the pleuritis. Pleural inflammation is most frequently caused by bacteria, which cause polyserositis reaching the pleura hematogenously. These bacteria include *Haemophilus parasuis* (Glasser's disease), *Streptococcus suis* type II, and some strains of *Pasteurella multocida* in pigs; *Streptococcus equi* ssp. *equi* and *Streptococcus zooepidemicus* ssp. *zooepidemicus* in horses; *Escherichia coli* in calves; and *Mycoplasma* spp. and *Haemophilus* spp. in sheep and goats. Contamination of pleural surfaces can be the result of extension of a septic process (e.g., puncture wounds of the thoracic wall and in cattle traumatic reticulopericarditis) and ruptured pulmonary abscesses (e.g., *Arcanobacterium [Actinomyces] pyogenes*).

In dogs and cats, bacteria (such as *Nocardia, Actinomyces,* and *Bacteroides*) can cause pyogranulomatous pleuritis, characterized by accumulation of blood-stained pus ("tomato soup") in the thoracic cavity. This exudate usually contains yellowish flecks called *sulfur granules* (Fig. 9-104), although these are less common in nocardial empyema in cats. Many species of bacteria, such as *Escherichia coli, Arcanobacterium pyogenes, Pasteurella multocida,* and *Fusobacterium necrophorum,* can be present in pyothorax of dogs and cats. These bacteria occur alone or in mixed infections. The pathogenesis of pleural empyema in cats is still debatable, but bite wounds or

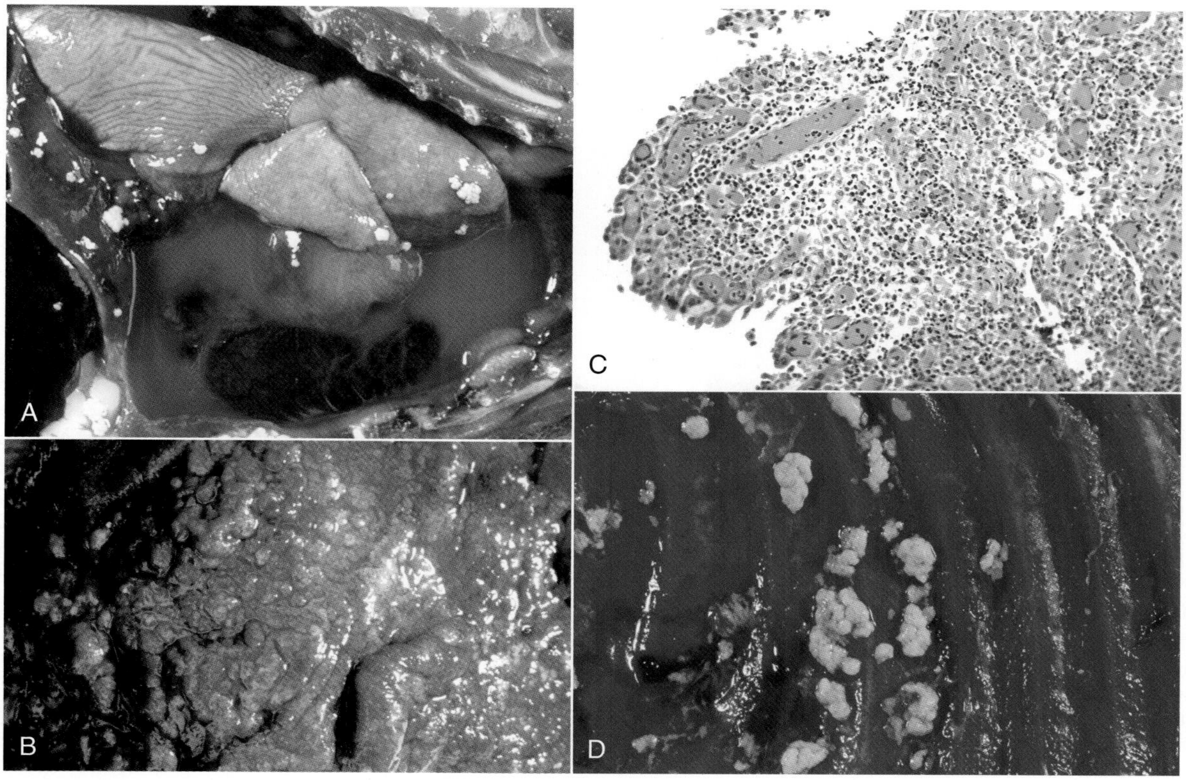

Fig. 9-104 Nocardiosis.
A, Chronic pleuritis *(Nocardia asteroides),* pleural cavity, cat. The pleural cavity holds abundant red-brown exudate ("tomato soup"). Once considered to be pathognomonic of *Nocardia* infection, it is no longer regarded as being diagnostic of nocardiosis. The fluid contains granulomatous inflammatory cells and sulfur granules. **B,** Chronic pleuritis *(Nocardia asteroides),* visceral pleura, dog. The thickened pleura has a granular appearance because of granulomatous inflammation and the proliferation of fibrovascular tissue of the pleura. **C,** Chronic pleuritis *(Nocardia asteroides),* thoracic cage, dog. The pleura has been thrown up into villous-like projections composed of abundant fibrovascular tissue and granulomatous inflammation. Leakage from the neocapillaries of the fibrovascular tissue is responsible for the hemorrhagic appearance of the pleural exudate. H&E stain. **D,** Chronic pleuritis *(Nocardia asteroides),* parietal pleura, cat. Large pieces of exudate, which contain sulfur granules, are present on the thickened pleura. (**A, B,** and **C** courtesy Dr. M.D. McGavin, College of Veterinary Medicine, University of Tennessee. **D** courtesy College of Veterinary Medicine, University of Illinois.)

penetration of foreign material (migrating grass awns) are likely. Pyogranulomatous pleuritis with empyema occurs occasionally in dogs, presumably associated with inhaled small plant material and penetrating (migrating) grass awns. Because of their physical shape (barbed) and assisted by the respiratory movement, aspirated grass awns can penetrate airways, move through the pulmonary parenchyma, and eventually perforate the visceral pleura causing pyogranulomatous pleuritis.

Cats with the noneffusive ("dry") form of feline infectious peritonitis frequently have focal pyogranulomatous pleuritis, in contrast to those with the effusive ("wet") form, in which thoracic involvement is primarily that of a pleural effusion. Cytologic evaluation of the effusion typically shows a high cellularity with many degenerated leukocytes, lymphocytes, macrophages, and mesothelial cells, and a pink granular background as a result of the high protein content.

Pleuritis is also an important problem in horses. *Nocardia asteroides* and *Nocardia brasiliensis* can cause fibrinopurulent pneumonia and pyothorax with characteristic sulfur granules. Although *Mycoplasma felis* can be isolated from the respiratory tract of normal horses, it is also isolated from horses with pleuritis and pleural effusion, particularly during the early stages of infection. The portal of entry of this infection is presumably aerogenous, first to the lung and subsequently to the pleura.

Neoplasms

The pleural surface of the lung is often involved in neoplasms that have metastasized from other organs to the pulmonary parenchyma and ruptured the visceral pleura to seed the pleural cavity. Mesothelioma is the only primary neoplasm of the pleura.

Mesothelioma

Mesothelioma is a rare neoplasm of the thoracic, pericardial, and peritoneal mesothelium of humans that is seen most commonly in calves, in which it can be congenital. In humans, it has long been associated with inhalation of certain types of asbestos fibers (asbestos mining, ship building) alone or with cigarette smoking as a probable cocarcinogen; no convincing association between the incidence of mesothelioma and exposure to asbestos has been made in domestic animals. In animals, there may be pleural effusion with resulting respiratory distress, cough, and weight loss.

Mesothelioma initially causes a thoracic effusion, but cytologic diagnosis can be difficult because of the morphologic resemblance of malignant and reactive mesothelial cells. During inflammation, mesothelial cells become reactive and not only increase in number but also become pleomorphic and form multinucleated cells that may be cytologically mistaken for those of a carcinoma.

Grossly, mesothelioma appears as multiple, discrete nodules or arborescent, spreading growths on the pleural surface (Fig. 9-105).

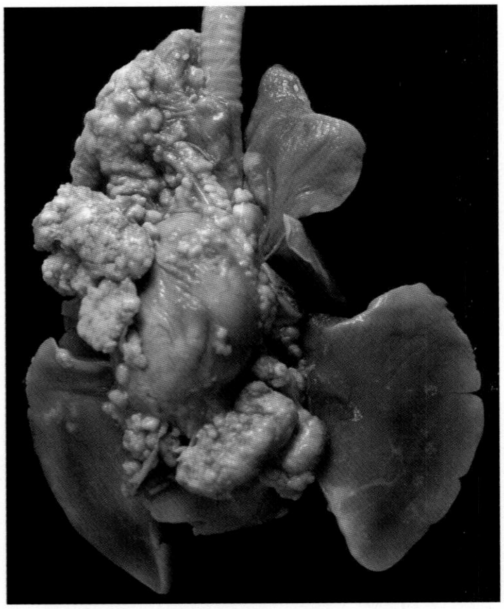

Fig. 9-105 Mesothelioma *(M)*, lungs and heart, cat.
The tumor *(upper left)* has proliferated and extended over the ventral parietal pleurae and pericardium. The pericardial sac was subsequently opened (not shown here), and the epicardium appeared normal, indicating that the tumor, although on the pericardium, had not invaded the pericardial sac to involve the epicardium. (Courtesy Facultad de Medicina Veterinaria y Zootecnia, Universidad Nacional Autónoma de México.)

Microscopically, either the mesothelial covering cells or the supporting tissue can be the predominant malignant component, so the neoplasm can microscopically resemble a carcinoma or a fibrosarcoma. Although considered malignant, mesotheliomas rarely metastasize to distant organs.

Secondary tumors may also spread into the visceral and parietal pleura. Thymomas are rare neoplasms that grow in the cranial mediastinum of adult or aged dogs, cats, pigs, cattle, and sheep. Thymomas are composed of thymic epithelium and lymphocytes (see Chapter 13).

ACKNOWLEDGMENTS

I thank Dr. William Yates (Canadian Food Inspection Agency) for having provided the basis of this chapter; all pathologists at the Atlantic Veterinary College for providing case material; Dr. Julio Martinez-Burnes, University of Tamaulipas, Mexico, for his suggestions; and Dr. Shannon Martinson, Atlantic Veterinary College, for reviewing the text. Finally, I acknowledge Dr. Reginald G. Thomson (deceased), former Dean of the Atlantic Veterinary College, and Dr. M. Grant Maxie, University of Guelph, for years of advice and inspiration, and Rosalie and Adriana for their support.

SUGGESTED READINGS

Information on this topic is available at evolve.elsevier.com/Zachary/McGavin/.

CHAPTER 10

Cardiovascular System and Lymphatic Vessels

*Lisa M. Miller, John F. Van Vleet, and Arnon Gal**

STRUCTURE

DEVELOPMENT OF THE HEART AND GREAT VESSELS

The heart is a conical, muscular organ that in mammals has evolved into a four-chambered pump with four valves. During early fetal development, it is converted from an elongated muscular tube into a C-shaped structure by a process termed *looping* (Fig. 10-1). Subsequently, septation occurs to produce the right and left atrial and ventricular chambers and separation of the common truncus arteriosus into the aorta and pulmonary artery, respectively. The heart is interposed as a pump into the vascular system, with the right side supplying the pulmonary circulation and the left side the systemic circulation (Web Fig. 10-1; also see Chapter 2). The vascular system is subdivided into arterial, capillary, venous, and lymphatic segments. The arteries are classified into three types: elastic arteries, muscular arteries, and arterioles. The venous vessels are termed *venules* and *veins.* The lymphatic vasculature includes lymphatic capillaries and lymphatic vessels. Interposed between the arterial and venous segments are the capillary beds. A vascular segment termed the *microcirculation* (systemic capillary beds) includes arterioles, capillaries, and venules and is the major area of exchange between the circulating blood and the peripheral tissue (see Web Fig. 10-1; also see Chapter 2).

MACROSCOPIC STRUCTURE

The heart lies within a fibroelastic sac called the *pericardium,* and the wall of the heart is composed of three layers: the epicardium, the myocardium, and the endocardium (Fig. 10-2). Structurally, the heart contains in order of blood flow four major blood vessels (vena cava, pulmonary artery, pulmonary vein, and aorta), four chambers (right atrium/auricle, right ventricle, left atrium/auricle, and left ventricle), and four valves (tricuspid, pulmonic semilunar, mitral, and aortic semilunar) (Fig. 10-3).

Pericardium and Epicardium

The pericardium, which normally contains a small amount of clear, serous fluid (see Fig. 10-2), is composed of an outer fibrous component and an inner serous layer, which form the sac surrounding the heart. The outer component is continuous with the mediastinal pleura. The base of the fibrous pericardium surrounds and blends with the adventitia of the greater arteries and veins exiting and entering the heart. The serous pericardium forms a closed sac surrounding the heart.

The epicardium (also known as *visceral pericardium*), the outermost layer of the heart, is continuous at the cardiac base with the parietal pericardium. The parietal pericardium is fused with the fibrous pericardium. The entire inner surface of the pericardial cavity is covered by mesothelium. The subepicardial layer is attached to the myocardium and consists of a thin layer of fibrous connective tissue, variable but generally abundant amounts (in well-nourished animals) of adipose tissue, and numerous blood vessels, lymphatic vessels, and nerves.

Myocardium

The myocardium is the muscular layer of the heart. It consists of cardiac muscle cells (cardiac myocytes [also known as *cardiac rhabdomyocytes*]) arranged in overlapping spiral patterns. These sheets of cells are anchored to the fibrous skeleton of the heart, which surrounds the atrioventricular valves and the origins of the aorta and pulmonary artery. The myocardial thickness is related to the pressure present in each chamber; thus the atria are thin walled and the ventricles are thicker. In adult animals, the thickness of the left ventricular free wall is approximately threefold that of the right ventricle, measured in a transverse section across the middle of the ventricles, because the pressure is greater in the systemic circulation than in the pulmonary circuit.

The arterial supply to the heart is the left and right coronary arteries, which arise from the aorta at the sinus of Valsalva behind the left and right cusps of the aortic valves. The arteries course over the heart in the subepicardium and give off perforating intramyocardial arteries that supply a rich capillary bed throughout the myocardium. Extensive anastomoses occur between the capillaries

*Dr. Gal contributed the sections on the cardiac conduction system.

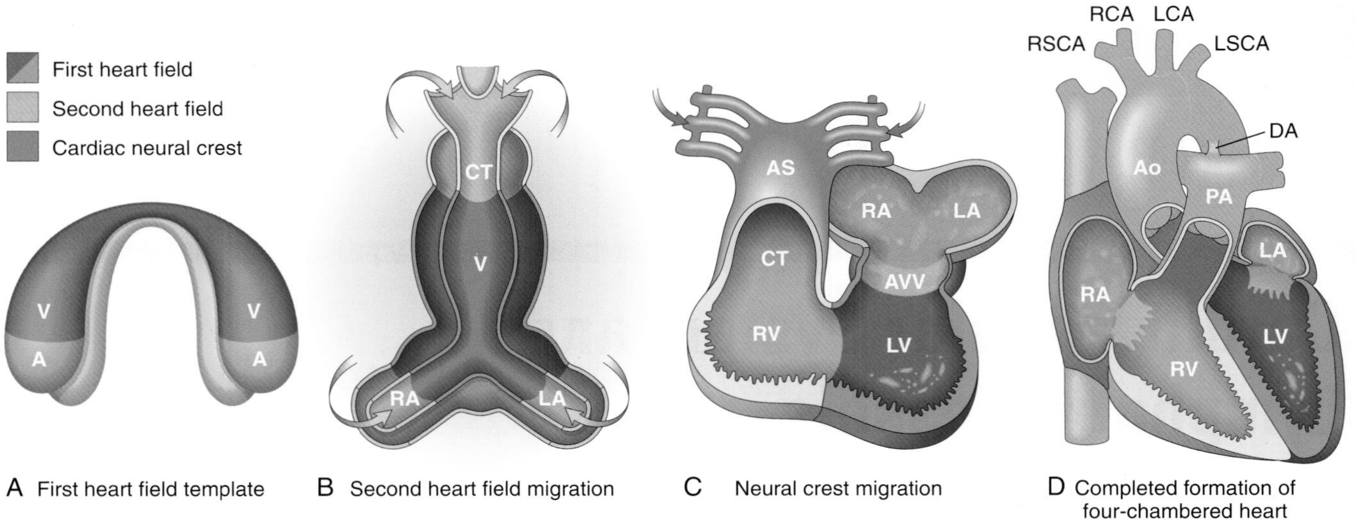

Fig. 10-1 Heart development, emphasizing the three sources of cells.
A, Day 15. First heart field *(FHF)* cells *(shown in red)* form a crescent shape in the anterior embryo with second heart field *(SHF)* cells *(shown in yellow)* near the FHF. **B,** Day 21. SHF cells lie dorsal to the straight heart tube and begin to migrate *(arrows)* into the anterior and posterior ends of the tube to form the right ventricle *(RV),* conotruncus *(CT),* and part of the atria *(A).* **C,** Day 28. Following rightward looping of the heart tube, cardiac neural crest cells *(shown in blue)* also migrate *(arrow)* into the outflow tract from the neural folds to septate the outflow tract and pattern the bilaterally symmetric aortic arch arteries (III, IV, and VI). **D,** Day 50. Septation of the ventricles, atria, and atrioventricular valves *(AVV)* results in the appropriately configured four-chambered heart. *Ao,* Aorta; *AS,* aortic sac; *DA,* ductus arteriosus; *LA,* left atrium; *LCA,* left carotid artery; *LSCA,* left subclavian artery; *LV,* left ventricle; *PA,* pulmonary artery; *RA,* right atrium; *RCA,* right carotid artery; *RSCA,* right subclavian artery; *V,* ventricle. (Modified from Srivastava D: Making or breaking the heart: from lineage determination to morphogenesis, *Cell* 126:1037, 2006. In Kumar V, Abbas A, Fausto N et al: *Robbins & Cotran pathologic basis of disease,* ed. 8, Philadelphia, 2009, Saunders.)

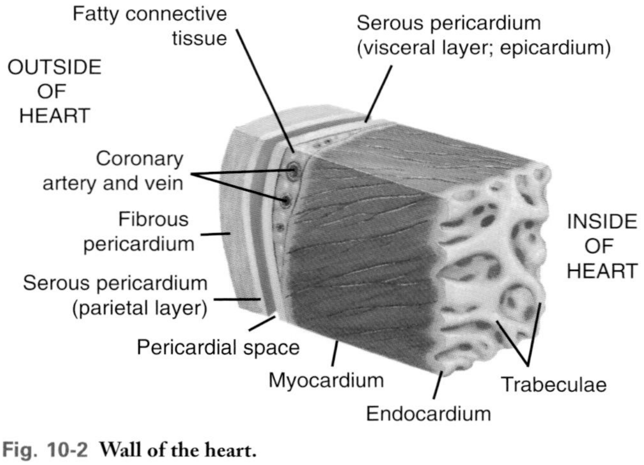

Fig. 10-2 Wall of the heart.
This section of the heart wall shows the fibrous pericardium, the parietal and visceral layers of the serous pericardium (with the pericardial space between them), the myocardium, and the endocardium. Note the fatty connective tissue between the visceral layer of the serous pericardium (epicardium) and the myocardium. Note also that the endocardium covers beamlike projections of myocardial muscle tissue called *trabeculae.* (From Huether SE, McCance KL: *Understanding pathophysiology,* ed 4, St Louis, 2007, Mosby.)

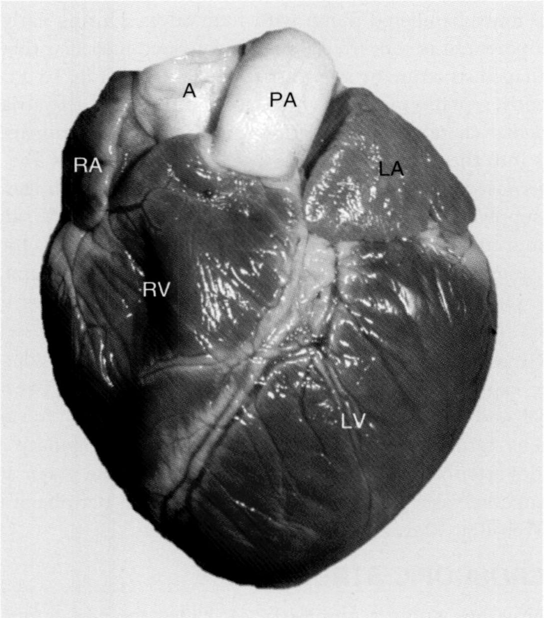

Fig. 10-3 Normal heart, pig.
A, Aorta; *LA,* left atrium; *LV,* left ventricle; *PA,* pulmonary artery; *RA,* right atrium; *RV,* right ventricle. (Courtesy School of Veterinary Medicine, Purdue University.)

that tend to run parallel to the elongated cardiac muscle cells. The ratio of the area of capillaries to that of muscle cells is approximately 1:1, a fact evident when the myocardium is viewed histologically in cross-section.

Cardiac Conduction System

The heart is a muscular four chamber pump that simultaneously supplies blood to the pulmonary and systemic circulatory beds (see Web Fig. 10-1 and Fig. 2-1). Mechanical pumping is composed of sequential contraction (systole) and relaxation (diastole) that must be preceded by an electrophysiologic process that triggers a coordinated chronologic sequence of electrical events that result in muscle contractions. This electrophysiologic process is made possible by a network of special conducting fibers that are collectively referred to as the *cardiac conduction system.*

The cardiac conduction system is infrequently examined in animals because it is a labor-intensive process. Exceptions are cases with documented electrocardiographic alterations of undetermined origin. Components include (1) the sinoatrial node (SAN) at the junction of the cranial vena cava and the right atrium, (2) the atrioventricular node (AVN) located above the septal leaflet of the tricuspid valve and the atrioventricular (AV) bundle traversing the lower atrial septum onto the dorsal portion of the muscular interventricular septum, and (3) the right and left bundle branches that descend on each side of the muscular interventricular septum and eventually ramify in the ventricular myocardium as the Purkinje fiber network.

The major pacemaker of the cardiac conduction system is the SAN. This disk-shaped structure lies between the wall of the cranial vena cava and the external wall of the right auricular appendage. Four internodal pathways connect the SAN with the AVN. The AVN is present in the wall of the right atrium dorsal to the septal cusp of the tricuspid valve. For the atria to be electrically insulated from the ventricles, so that an unwarranted ectopic conduction wave will not activate the ventricles (or vice versa) and disrupt the synchronous events of the cardiac cycle, a fibrous cardiac skeleton composed of a layer of dense collagen (central fibrous body [CFB]), as well as occasional plates of chondroid and osseous metaplasia, separates the atrial from the ventricular myocardium. This skeleton forms two fibrous rings around the AV orifices and the aortic and pulmonic orifices. Conduction fibers arising from the AVN, known as the *bundle of His* or *AV bundle,* pierce through the CFB into the ventricles and continue along the subendocardium of the interventricular septum. The AV bundle then splits into the right and left bundle branches that further split and ramify into many other smaller branches that blend into the ventricular myocardium. Purkinje fibers constitute the AV bundle and downstream conduction pathways.

Endocardium and Heart Valves

The endocardium is the innermost layer of the heart and lines the chambers and extends over projecting structures such as the valves, chordae tendineae, and papillary muscles. The endocardium of the atria is thicker than that of the ventricles and thus normally appears white to gray on gross examination. The surface of the endocardium is endothelium that lies on a thin layer of vascularized connective tissue; the subendocardial layer contains blood vessels, nerves, and connective tissue. Purkinje fibers are distributed in the subendocardium throughout both ventricles. The heart valves (tricuspid valve [right AV valve], mitral valve [left AV valve], aortic valve, and pulmonary valve) are attached to fibrous rings and have thin avascular cusps. The valves open and close to regulate blood flow through the heart. During embryogenesis, endocardial cushions (mesenchymal tissue covered by endothelium) are precursors of the valve cusps. By remodeling, growth, and elongation, the cushions become thin mature cusps composed of connective tissue with an endothelial covering.

Blood and Lymphatic Vascular Systems

Blood Vessels

The aorta originates from the left ventricle and provides oxygenated blood to the entire body via arteries. In a treelike manner, arteries branch and become smaller arterioles as they approach capillary beds (see Web Fig. 10-1; also see Chapter 2). These beds and postcapillary venules provide the site for exchange of oxygen, carbon dioxide, nutrients, and waste. Small venules return the exchanged fluid and blood to larger veins and eventually the postcava and precava drain into the right atrium. The poorly oxygenated blood enters the pulmonary artery from the right ventricle. Oxygen exchange occurs in the capillaries of the lung, and oxygenated blood is returned to the heart via the pulmonary veins into the left atrium.

Lymphatic Vessels

Lymphatic vessels are thin walled, endothelial-lined channels that originate near the capillary beds and serve as a drainage system for returning interstitial tissue fluid and inflammatory cells to the blood. Afferent lymphatic vessels drain lymph into regional lymph nodes, which then filter and provide immunologic surveillance of the lymph, its cells, and the foreign matter it contains. The filtered lymph continues into larger efferent lymphatic vessels, which eventually drain into the caval blood via the thoracic duct. Both lymphatic vessels and veins have valves to prevent backflow of fluid. A more complete description can be found in Chapter 2.

MICROSCOPIC STRUCTURE

Pericardium and Epicardium

The pericardial sac is composed of parietal and visceral pericardium, both of which are covered by mesothelium. Beneath the visceral mesothelium is a thin layer of fibrous connective tissue, adipocytes, and vascular structures. This organization forms the subepicardium and interdigitates with the myocardium. The parietal pericardium is composed of an inner layer of mesothelium that interdigitates with the dense connective tissue forming the outer pericardial sac.

Myocardium

The myocardium consists of cardiac muscle cells surrounded by interstitial components that include blood and lymphatic vessels, nerves, and connective tissue cells, such as fibroblasts, histiocytes, mast cells, pericytes, primitive mesenchymal stem cells, and extracellular matrix elements of connective tissue, including collagen fibrils, elastic fibers, and acid mucopolysaccharides. Cardiac muscle cells can be divided into two populations: the contracting myocytes and the specialized fibers of the conduction system. The contracting myocyte is a cross-striated branching fiber of an irregular cylindric shape that measures 60 to 100 μm in length and 10 to 20 μm in diameter, with centrally located, elongated nuclei. Myocytes in young animals are smaller and have small amounts of sarcoplasm. Atrial myocytes are smaller than ventricular myocytes. Adjacent myocytes are joined end-to-end by specialized junctions known as *intercalated disks* and less frequently by side-to-side connections termed *lateral junctions.* Multinucleated fibers with nuclei arranged in central rows are frequently seen in hearts of growing pigs (Fig. 10-4). The myocytes of old animals commonly have large polyploid nuclei. The cytoplasm (sarcoplasm) of myocytes is largely occupied by the contractile proteins that are highly organized into sarcomeres, the repeating contractile units of the myofibril (see Figs. 15-3 and 15-8). Myofibrils are formed by end-to-end attachment of many sarcomeres. The cross-striated or banded appearance of myocytes is the result of sarcomere organization into A bands composed of myosin in the form of "thick" filaments (12 to 16 nm in diameter), I bands composed of actin in the form of "thin" filaments (5 to 8 nm in diameter), and dense Z bands at the end of each sarcomere. Thick and thin filaments interdigitate and provide the basis for the sliding mechanism of muscle contraction. Myocytes are enclosed by the sarcolemma, which consists of the plasma membrane and the covering basal lamina (external lamina). Other important components of cardiac muscle cells are generally only apparent in electron micrographs and include abundant mitochondria, a highly organized network of intracellular tubules termed the *sarcoplasmic reticulum,* cylindric invaginations of the plasma membrane called *T tubules,* ribosomes, cytoskeletal filaments, glycogen particles, lipid droplets, Golgi complexes, atrial granules (contain atrial natriuretic factor), lysosomes, and residual bodies (Web Fig. 10-2).

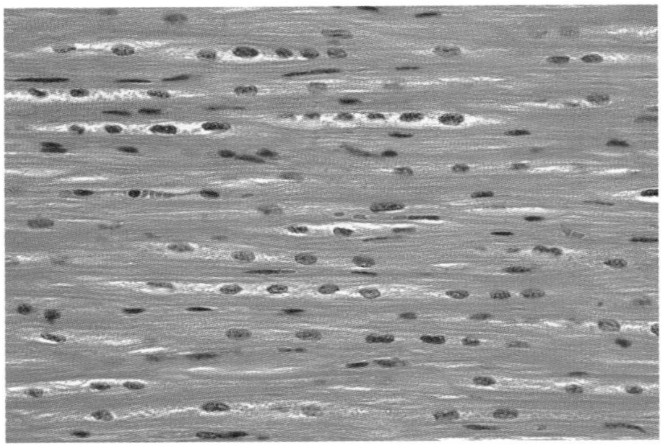

Fig. 10-4 Normal cardiac muscle.
Left ventricular myocardium, longitudinal section, normal young pig. The multiple nuclei in a myocyte are readily seen and evaluated in a longitudinal section. H&E stain. (Courtesy School of Veterinary Medicine, Purdue University.)

Cardiac Conduction System

The morphologic features of the cardiac muscle cells that form specialized conduction tissues, including the SAN, AVN, AV bundle (bundle of His), and bundle branches, vary greatly at different sites and among animal species but generally are thin, branching nodal muscle cells with scarce myofibrils separated by highly vascularized connective tissue (Fig. 10-5; Web Fig. 10-3). Autonomic nerve fibers are contained within the SAN. The Purkinje fibers (cardiac conduction fibers) are distinguished by their large diameters (in horse, ox) and abundant pale eosinophilic sarcoplasm rich in glycogen and poor in myofibrils.

Sinoatrial Node

The SAN is positioned adjacent to the epicardial adipose tissue and is often centered around a branch of the right coronary artery (Fig. 10-5, *A*). Several large autonomic nervous system ganglions can occasionally be seen clustering in the epicardium adjacent to the node. The SAN lacks discrete structure, and its ill-defined borders merge with the adjacent atrial wall. It structurally consists of a collection of haphazardly oriented myofibers that appear as a pseudosyncytium and are embedded within abundant loose collagenous and elastic connective tissue, with rare cores of epicardially oriented dense collagen fibers (Fig. 10-5, *A1*). The nodal myofibers have discrete cell borders, a moderate amount of wavy sarcoplasm with

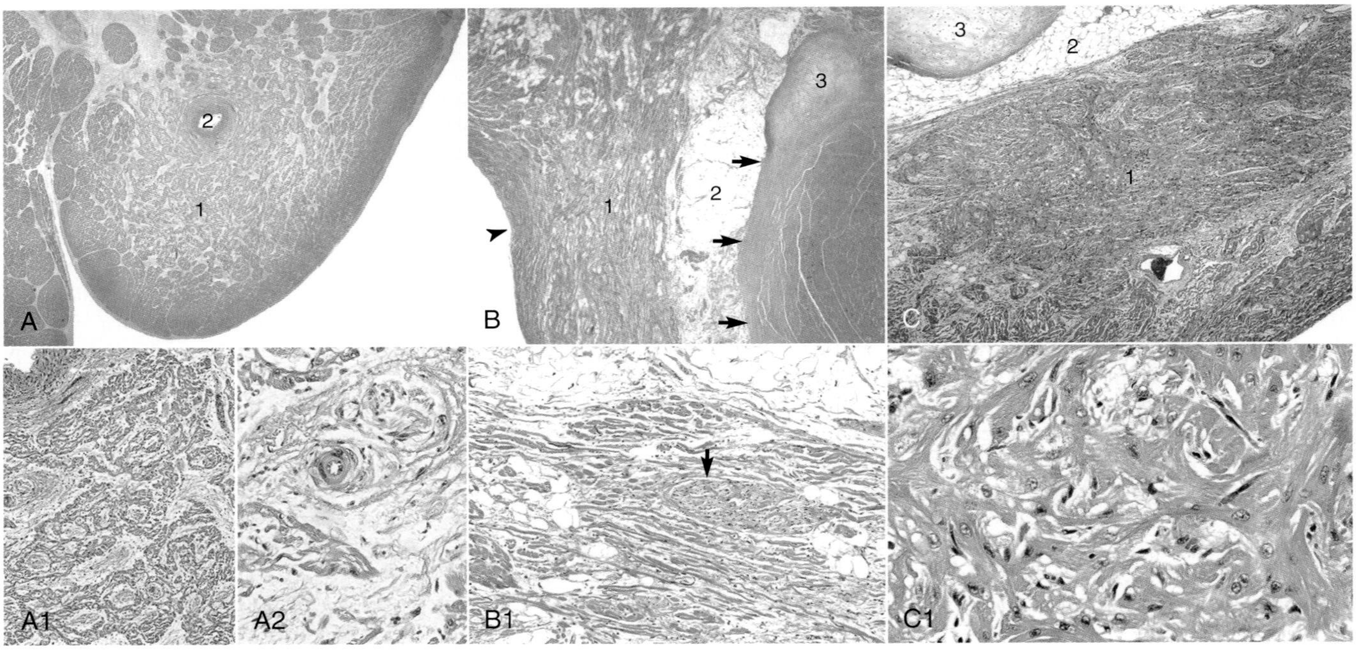

Fig. 10-5 Cardiac conduction system.
A, Sinoatrial *(SA)* node, foal. The center of the SA node *(1)* contains a nodal artery *(2).* H&E stain. **A1,** Higher magnification. Haphazardly oriented myofibers are embedded within abundant loose collagenous and elastic connective tissue. H&E stain. **A2,** Higher magnification. Nodal myofibers have discrete cell borders, a moderate amount of wavy sarcoplasm and an elongated nucleus. H&E stain. **B,** Atrioventricular *(AV)* node, goat. The AV node *(1)* is composed of interconnecting nodal myofibers that are supported by loose collagenous and elastic fibrous stroma. The node is embedded in adipose tissue *(2).* Note that in this illustration the AV node (1) is a poorly demarcated region (see *B1* for greater detail) that is elongated *(flattened)* from top to bottom and that it and its surrounding adipose tissue are positioned adjacent to the cardiac fibrous skeleton *(arrows)* that has undergone focal chondroid metaplasia *(3).* The position and overall shape of the AV node in a histologic section is dependent upon the plane of section. Endocardium *(arrowhead).* H&E stain. **B1,** AV node, goat. In this higher magnification of *B,* AV nodal myofibers have a characteristic pale eosinophilic and thin sarcoplasm, with abundance of distinct striations and a short oval to elongated nucleus with dispersed chromatin. An autonomic myelinated nerve is present in the AV node *(arrow).* H&E stain. **C,** AV bundle, goat. The AV bundle *(1)* travels diagonally through the center of the figure from the lower left to the upper right margins. It is formed by an interweaving pseudosyncytium of cardiac myofibers supported by a loose to dense intervening collagenous stroma (see *C1* for greater detail) and may be surrounded by adipose tissue *(2).* Cardiac cartilaginous skeleton *(3).* H&E stain. **C1,** Higher magnification. The AV bundle myofibers of the pseudosyncytium have moderate to large, pale eosinophilic sarcoplasm with prominent striations and large nuclei with fine stippled chromatin. H&E stain. (Courtesy Drs. A. Gal and J.F. Zachary, College of Veterinary Medicine, University of Illinois.)

sparse myofibrils, and an elongated nucleus that contains clumps of coarse chromatin (Fig. 10-5, *A2*).

Atrioventricular Node, Atrioventricular Bundle, and Bundle Branches

The AVN lies within the right atrial subendocardium and consists of a discrete, compact to loose mass of interconnecting myofibers that are often embedded within adipose tissue. A small nodal artery, parasympathetic ganglia, and large myelinated autonomic nerves are often present adjacent to the AVN. The nodal myofibers that have characteristic pale eosinophilic and thin sarcoplasm generally run parallel to each other but occasionally have an interweaving pattern with intervening loose collagen fibers. These myofibers contain a moderate amount of sarcoplasm with abundance of distinct striations and a short oval to elongated nucleus with dispersed chromatin.

The AV bundle (Fig. 10-5, *B*) emerges from the cranial pole of the AVN (Fig. 10-5, *B1*) and pierces through the CFB, approximately at the level of the annuli of the aortic and mitral valves (Fig. 10-5, *B2*), to become the left and right bundle branches. The size of an AV bundle myofiber progressively enlarges and its cytomorphology transitions from a pale eosinophilic, small and thin (AVN-like morphology) myofiber to a pale eosinophilic, foamy to waxy, large, and somewhat rectangular myofiber that lacks cross striations (a Purkinje-like cellular morphology) (Fig. 10-5, *C*).

Autonomic Nervous System

The nerve supply to the heart is autonomic and includes sympathetic, parasympathetic, and nonadrenergic noncholinergic innervation. Histologically, large nerves can be seen in the epicardium and adjacent to the coronary blood vessels, whereas special staining techniques are required for demonstration of neural tissue elsewhere. Electron microscopy and immunohistochemistry allow differentiation between sympathetic and parasympathetic nerves that are otherwise indistinguishable with H&E stain. Preganglionic parasympathetic fibers pass to the heart through the cardiac branch of the vagal nerve and synapse with parasympathetic ganglionic neurons. Postganglionic neurons are distributed to the SAN and AVN, as well as to atrial and, to a much lesser extent, ventricular myocardium (however, the ventricular conduction system is well supplied by cholinergic innervation). Postganglionic sympathetic fibers arising from the cervicothoracic and middle cervical ganglia intensely innervate the SAN and AVN and to lesser extent the AV bundle. The atrial endocardium, myocardium, and epicardium are evenly innervated, whereas the ventricles are considerably less innervated with epicardium more densely populated by neural tissue than the endocardium.

Endocardium and Heart Valves

The endocardium, lining the atrium and ventricles, consists of a continuous endothelium, subendothelium, and subendocardium. The subendothelial layer contains dense irregular fibroblasts intermixed with collagen and elastic fibers and occasional smooth muscle cells. Elastic fibers are abundant within the subendocardium of the atria. The subendocardial layer contains vascular structures, elastic and collagen bands, and fibroblasts and is continuous with the myocardium. Purkinje fibers are located in the subendocardium. The heart valves are poorly vascularized, endocardial folds covered by endothelium. The subendothelial layer is composed of fibroblasts with abundant elastic and collagen fibers. The AV valves (AVVs) consist of a layer of stratum spongiosum and stratum fibrosum. The stratum spongiosum consists of loosely arranged fibroblasts with moderate amounts of collagen and elastin fibers and vascular structures. The stratum fibrosis contains fibroblasts and collagen, which are continuous with the annulus fibrosis and chordae tendineae.

Blood and Lymphatic Vascular Systems

The overall design of the blood and lymphatic vessels is similar, except that luminal diameter, wall thickness, and the presence of other anatomic features, such as valves, vary between the different segments. The luminal surface of all vessels is lined by longitudinally aligned endothelial cells covering a basal lamina. Vessel walls are divided into three layers or tunics: intima, media, and adventitia. However, some of the layers can be absent or all of the layers can be thinned in some segments of the vascular system, depending on the intravascular pressures. The large elastic arteries, such as the aorta, have (1) an intima composed of endothelium and subendothelial connective tissue, (2) a very thick tunica media composed of fenestrated elastic laminae with interposed smooth muscle cells and ground substance and bordered internally by the internal elastic lamina and externally by the external elastic lamina, and (3) an outer tunica adventitia layer composed of collagen and elastic fibers and connective tissue cells with penetrating blood vessels, termed the *vasa vasorum,* supplying nutrients to the adventitia and the outer half of the media. In muscular arteries and arterioles, the tunica media is composed largely of smooth muscle cells arranged in a circumferential pattern. Arterioles are the smallest arterial channels and are generally less than 100 μm in diameter and with one to three layers of smooth muscle cells in the tunica media.

Capillaries are 5 to 10 μm in diameter, and their endothelium is one of three types: (1) continuous, (2) fenestrated (as in the endocrine glands), or (3) porous (as in renal glomeruli). The endothelium rests on an external lamina surrounded by pericytes. Pericytes are located abluminally to capillaries and postcapillary venules and because of their location, contractility, and cytoskeletal proteins may play a role in regulating capillary and venular blood flow. Lesions of the endothelium might not be evident by light microscopy, and electron microscopy is required for characterization.

Veins have thin walls in relation to their luminal size when compared with those of arteries, in which blood pressure is greater. The adventitia is the thickest layer. Valves are present to prevent retrograde blood flow (i.e., away from the heart).

Lymphatic capillaries lack a basal lamina. Large lymphatic vessels are similar in structure to veins and generally have large lumina, thin walls, and intimal valves but contain lymph.

The morphology of large arteries, veins, microvasculature, and lymphatic vessels is described in Chapter 2 and is not discussed further in this chapter.

NECROPSY ASSESSMENT OF HEART AND VASCULAR STRUCTURES

Information on this topic including Web Appendix 10-1 and Web Figs. 10-4 and 10-5 is available at evolve.elsevier.com/Zachary/McGavin/.

EXAMINATION OF THE CARDIOVASCULAR SYSTEM AND LYMPHATIC VESSELS AT NECROPSY AND TISSUE SAMPLING FOR HISTOPATHOLOGIC EVALUATION

Information on this topic including Web Appendix 10-2 and Web Fig. 10-6 is available at evolve.elsevier.com/Zachary/McGavin/.

FUNCTION

The primary function of the cardiovascular and lymphatic systems is to maintain an adequate and steady supply of nutrients to and facilitate the removal of waste products from all organs and tissues of the body. Cardiac myocytes provide the force of contraction; the conduction system and the nervous system control the flow and volume.

PERICARDIUM AND EPICARDIUM

The pericardium contains a small amount of serous fluid, which allows frictionless cardiac movement of the mesothelial surfaces of the pericardium and epicardium on each other. The pericardial sac can adapt to changes in the heart size provided adequate time. The pericardium functions to provide a protective environment for cardiac function. Rapid, abnormal filling with blood (hemopericardium), fluid (hydropericardium), or exudate (pyopericardium) can result in compression of the heart (cardiac tamponade), particularly the large veins, right atrium, and right ventricle. Animals can survive without a pericardial sac.

MYOCARDIUM

The results of normal cardiac function include the maintenance of adequate blood flow, called cardiac output, to peripheral tissues that provide delivery of oxygen and nutrients, the removal of carbon dioxide and other metabolic waste products, the distribution of hormones and other cellular regulators, and the maintenance of adequate thermoregulation and glomerular filtration pressure (urine output). The normal heart has a threefold to fivefold functional reserve capacity, but this capacity can eventually be lost in cardiac disease and the result is impaired function.

Cardiac Pathophysiology: Myocardial Dysfunction

Cardiovascular dysfunction is the result of one or more of six basic pathophysiologic mechanisms (Box 10-1). Compensatory mechanisms operate in both normal and diseased hearts in an attempt to meet both the short- and long-term demands for adequate cardiac output. These mechanisms include cardiac dilation, myocardial hypertrophy, increase in heart rate, increase in peripheral resistance, increase in blood volume, and redistribution of blood flow. These compensatory mechanisms can maintain cardiac output that is adequate for some time, even in animals with severe cardiac disease sufficient to compromise cardiac function from loss of myocardial contractility, sustained pressure overload, or sustained volume overload. Cardiac dilation can occur as a terminal lesion in many cardiac diseases (Fig. 10-6, *A*). As a compensatory response to achieve increased cardiac output, dilation allows stretching of cardiac muscle cells to increase contractile force according to the Frank-Starling phenomenon and increased stroke volume is the result. However, stretching beyond certain limits decreases contractile strength. Myocardial hypertrophy is an important long-term compensatory response of the heart to maintain adequate cardiac output in the face of increased pressure or volume overload (see the discussion on the myocardium in the section on Responses to Injury) (Fig. 10-6, *B*).

BOX 10-1 Basic Pathophysiologic Mechanisms of Cardiovascular Dysfunction

- Pump failure: Weak contractility and emptying of chambers, impaired filling of chambers
- Obstruction to forward blood flow: Valvular stenosis, vascular narrowing, systemic or pulmonary hypertension
- Regurgitant blood flow: Volume overload of chamber behind failing affected valve
- Shunted blood flows from congenital defects: Septal defects in heart, shunts between blood vessels
- Rupture of the heart or a major vessel: Cardiac tamponade, massive internal hemorrhage
- Cardiac conduction disorders (arrhythmias): Failure of synchronized cardiac contraction

Modified from Schoen FJ, Mitchell RN: The heart. In Kumar V, Abbas AK, Fausto N et al, editors: *Robbins & Cotran pathologic basis of disease,* ed 8, Philadelphia, 2009, Saunders, p. 532.

Syndromes of Cardiac Failure or Decompensation

Information on this topic including Web Table 10-1 is available at evolve.elsevier.com/Zachary/McGavin/.

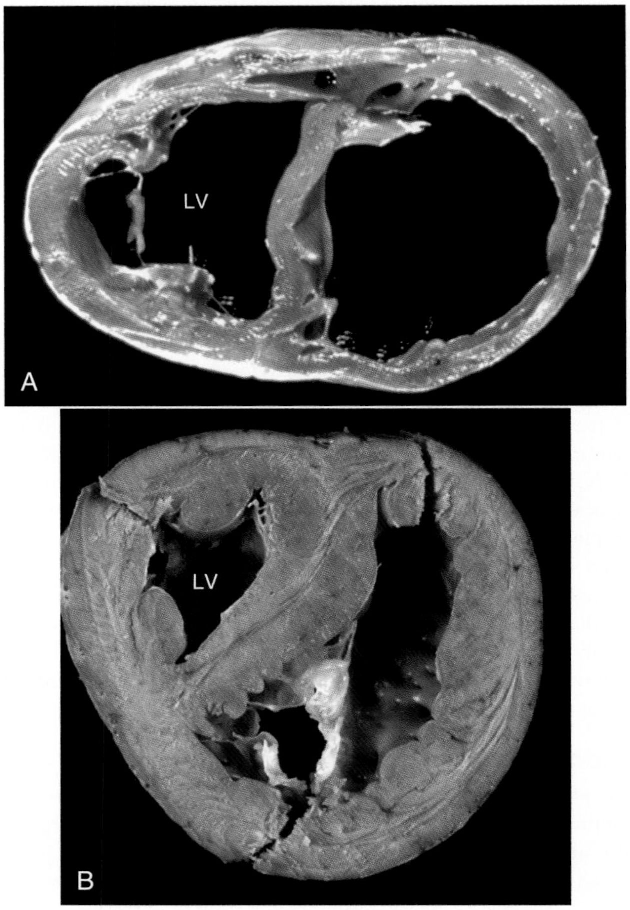

Fig. 10-6 Cardiac dilation and hypertrophy, heart, transected ventricles, dog.
A, Cardiac dilation. Note the thin walls of both dilated ventricles. *LV,* Left ventricle. **B,** Cardiac hypertrophy *(fixed tissue).* Note that the right ventricular and left ventricular *(LV)* walls are approximately the same thickness, indicating that there is right ventricular hypertrophy. (**A** courtesy Dr. Y. Niyo, College of Veterinary Medicine, Iowa State University; and Noah's Arkive, College of Veterinary Medicine, The University of Georgia. **B** courtesy College of Veterinary Medicine, University of Florida; and Noah's Arkive, College of Veterinary Medicine, The University of Georgia.)

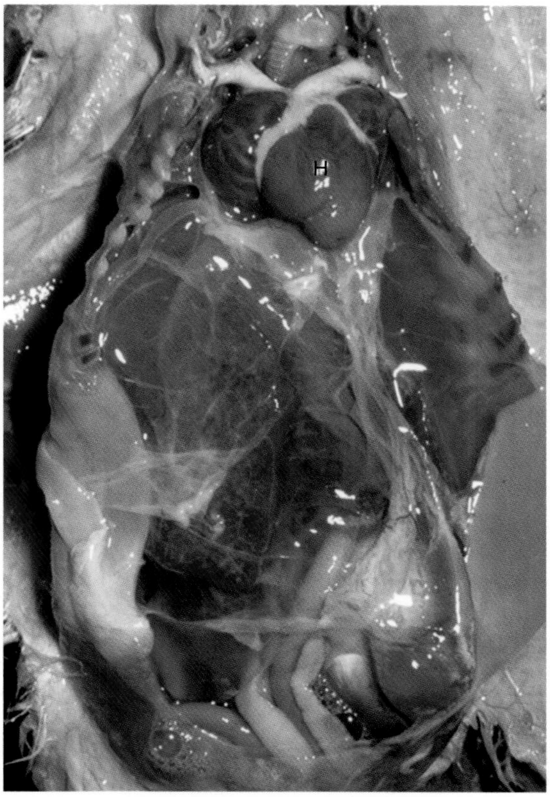

Fig. 10-7 Ascites, congestive heart failure, furazolidone cardiotoxicity, heart and liver, duckling.
Note prominent accumulations of serous fluid in the abdomen and fibrin deposits over the surface of the liver. The heart *(H)* is dilated. (Courtesy School of Veterinary Medicine, Purdue University.)

Cardiac Syncope

Cardiac syncope, an acute expression of cardiac disease, is characterized clinically by collapse, loss of consciousness, and extreme changes in heart rate and blood pressure, and with or without demonstrable lesions. Syncope can be caused by massive myocardial necrosis, ventricular fibrillation, heart block, arrhythmias, and reflex cardiac inhibition (e.g., that associated with high intestinal blockage).

Types of Heart Failure

A wide variety of experimental animal models of heart failure exist (see Web Table 10-1). The models have been used to develop an understanding of human cardiac diseases.

Congestive Heart Failure

Congestive heart failure usually develops slowly from gradual loss of cardiac pumping efficiency coupled with either pressure or volume overload or myocardial damage (Figs. 10-7 and 10-8; also see Figs. 8-29, 8-30, and 9-39). Pathophysiologically, congestive heart failure is initiated by development of cardiac disease (e.g., myocardial, valvular, congenital) or increased workload associated with pulmonary, renal, or vascular disease leading to loss of cardiac reserve and development of decreased blood flow to peripheral tissue (forward failure) and accumulation of blood behind the failing chamber (backward failure). Reduced renal blood flow creates hypoxia in the kidneys and increases renin release from the juxtaglomerular apparatus, resulting in stimulation of aldosterone release from the zona glomerulosa of the adrenal cortex. Sodium

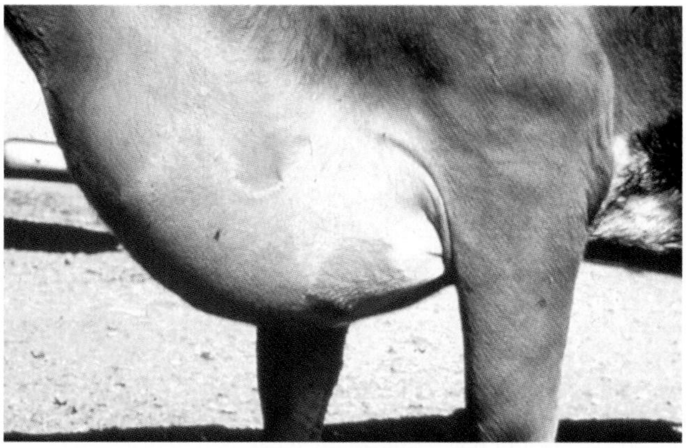

Fig. 10-8 Subcutaneous edema, high altitude disease with congestive heart failure ("brisket disease"), presternal, sternal, and caudal sternocephalic regions (brisket), cow.
The extensive subcutaneous edema is the result of chronic congestive heart failure. (Courtesy School of Veterinary Medicine, Purdue University.)

and water retention are the results of the action of aldosterone on the renal tubules; increased plasma volume follows, as does accumulation of edema fluid (mainly in body cavities). Hypoxia also stimulates increased erythropoiesis in bone marrow and extramedullary organs, such as the spleen, causing polycythemia and thus increased viscosity of the blood. The hypervolemia from aldosterone-induced water retention increases the workload on the already failing heart. Thus a vicious cycle of cardiac decompensation is initiated that eventually leads to death from cardiac failure unless therapeutic intervention occurs. Cardiac dilation, hypertrophy, and increased heart rate can provide some compensation for the increased workload.

Acute and Chronic Left-Sided Heart Failure

Acute left-sided heart failure is manifested by pulmonary congestion and edema, whereas chronic left-sided heart failure is manifested by chronic passive pulmonary congestion, chronic pulmonary edema, hemosiderosis ("heart failure cells"; see Fig. 9-39), and fibrosis. The most common causes are (1) myocardial contractility loss associated with myocarditis, myocardial necrosis, or cardiomyopathy; (2) dysfunction of the mitral or aortic valves; and (3) several congenital heart diseases.

Acute and Chronic Right-Sided Heart Failure

Acute right-sided heart failure results in acute passive congestion (see Fig. 2-35) leading to hepatomegaly and splenomegaly (see Figs. 2-35 and 13-50, *A*), whereas chronic right-sided heart failure (see Fig. 2-36) results in hepatic congestion (nutmeg liver) (see Fig. 8-30) and more severe sodium and water retention than in left-sided heart failure. Edema is evident predominantly as ventral subcutaneous edema in horses and ruminants (see Fig. 10-8), ascites in dogs, and hydrothorax in cats. Causes of right-sided failure include (1) pulmonary hypertension, (2) cardiomyopathy, and (3) disease of the tricuspid and pulmonary valves. (See Chapters 8 and 9 for further details on hepatic and pulmonary lesions, respectively, associated with congestive heart failure.)

Clinical Diagnostic Procedures

Information on this topic including Web Appendix 10-3 is available at evolve.elsevier.com/Zachary/McGavin/.

CARDIAC CONDUCTION SYSTEM

Cells of the cardiac conduction system are modified cardiac myofibers that are able to spontaneously depolarize, which is also called *autoexcitation,* and function to (1) coordinate the sequence of events required for efficient ventricular filling during diastole and ejection during systole and (2) maintain the pressure in the pulmonary and systemic circuits (see Web Fig. 10-1).

Depolarization of the membrane of these pacemaker cells is due to a transiently increased rapid permeability to sodium ions and a slightly longer lasting increase in permeability to calcium ions that results in their influx into the myofiber sarcoplasm, thus changing the membrane potential (see Chapter 14). As this transient permeability is lost, membranal potassium channels open, and rapid outward potassium flux results in myofiber membranal hyperpolarization (along with sodium and calcium efflux), ultimately bringing the membrane potential back to a "normal" steady state (resting potential). During this period of time (refractory period), the myocyte cannot depolarize again because of a special conformation of membrane sodium channels that is transiently lost with depolarization and regained only with hyperpolarization. Intrinsically, the resting membrane potential of pacemaker cells is more positive than that of contracting cardiomyocytes and slightly more negative than the membrane threshold potential. This difference is due to leakiness of the pacemaker cell membrane to sodium and calcium ions and a steady low-grade influx of these ions.

Once one pacemaker cell depolarizes, a wave of depolarization propagates through the surrounding myocytes because these cells are connected to each other by special membranal pores (gap junctions), which allow for ionic exchange between adjacent cells. The number of gap junctions between cells of the conduction system is therefore a property that affects conduction velocity. Because the heart cycle must be strictly coordinated so that both atria and both ventricles contract and relax at the same time, and atrial contraction occurs simultaneous to the late ventricular relaxation, the depolarization wave has to be conducted fast at certain points along the conduction pathway and slower at others. Therefore, at different anatomic regions along the conduction pathway, the degree of cell-to-cell interaction dictates a slightly different cellular morphology.

When an electric signal (a propagating depolarization front) is generated in the SAN and spreads throughout the atria from cell to cell and eventually reaches the AVN, it is also conveyed through the specialized internodal conducting fibers. The conduction in these fibers is approximately three times faster than that of the atrial myofibers. By conveying the signal through these fibers, both atria can contract simultaneously and in a coordinated manner that allows the process of pushing of blood into the ventricles. Correlating with their special fast conducting function, these cells have a Purkinje-like morphology. The conduction velocity is then slowed down when propagating through the AVN. The time it takes to conduct the signal through the AVN and penetrating AV bundles is approximately four times longer than the time it takes for it to be conducted from the SAN to the AVN. This delay in conduction serves to empty the atria from blood before the ventricles start to contract. It also contributes to the unidirectional blood flow between the atria and the ventricles, above and beyond the similar role played by the AVVs.

Finally, the signal is delivered through the AV bundle, bundle branches, and Purkinje fibers in a velocity approximately 150 times faster than that of the AVN. The bundle branches run along the subendocardium of the interventricular septum and free ventricular walls and give rise to Purkinje fibers that supply the myocardium in a subendocardial-to-epicardial direction. This organization allows for a rapid and synchronous contraction of both ventricles at an order that ultimately enables blood to be "squeezed" from apex-to-base, toward both outflow tracts.

Cardiac myofibers have a unique property of intrinsic coupling of the electrical stimulation with mechanical contraction, which is fundamental for cardiac function. Diastole starts immediately at the end of ventricular contraction, as the cardiac muscle (myocardium) starts to relax. For a brief moment, relaxation leads to a rapid fall in ventricular pressure, without change in ventricular volume as the AVVs are still sealed off (isovolumetric relaxation). Because of the fall in ventricular pressure, the blood that has pooled in the atria during systole, along with incoming blood that constantly flows from systemic and pulmonary veins through the atria, pushes the AVV open and rapidly and passively fills the ventricles (rapid-filling phase). Next, because of the resultant pressure rise in the ventricles, the flow of blood that continues to enter the ventricles through the atria abruptly ends (diastasis phase). The last phase of diastole is active contraction of the atria, which pushes blood into the (now somewhat less compliant) ventricles and further raises their pressure ("atrial kick").

In systole, the myocardium contracts, leading to a rapid increase in intraventricular pressure. Since the aortic and pulmonary valves are shut during diastole, the sudden rise in pressure leads to closure of the AVVs. In this brief period, which is termed *isovolumetric contraction,* the change in ventricular pressure has not led to a change in ventricular volume, since the blood had not yet been ejected into the aorta and pulmonary arteries. When the pressure in the ventricles exceeds the pressure in the great arteries, the aortic and pulmonary valves (semilunar valves) open and the ejection of the blood through the right and left side outflow tracts ensues (ejection phase). Simultaneously with the ejection phase, the atria relax, atrial pressure falls, and blood enters the atria and pools within it passively.

An additional level of complexity is brought about by the innervation of the autonomous nervous system (ANS). In general, the ANS influences heart rate (chronotropy), alters the rate of conduction (dromotropy), and controls myocardial contractility (inotropy) and the rate of mechanical relaxation (lusitropy). Parasympathetic postganglionic nerve terminals secrete acetylcholine that affects muscarinic (M2) receptors, whereas sympathetic postganglionic nerve terminals secrete norepinephrine that predominantly acts on the β_1-adrenergic receptors. The latter, when stimulated by catecholamines, lead to a chain of intracellular events that increases calcium influx, increases the magnitude of potassium and chloride repolarization, and shortens the refractory period. Therefore adrenergic agonists are said to be positive chronotropes, inotropes, dromotropes, and lusitropes, whereas parasympathetic agonists have the opposite effects. Heart rate is primarily regulated by opposing effects of adrenergic and cholinergic nerve terminals on the SAN and at the same time by modulation of conduction velocity of the AVN and AV bundle. Physiologically, the force of contraction represents the sum of interactions between myocardial contractility, which is positively modulated by adrenergic nerve terminals that act on β_1 receptors on ventricular myocardial myofibers (positive inotropic effect), and by the volume of blood that is present in the ventricles just before contraction (preload), as well as by the resistance in front of which contraction actually takes place (afterload).

ENDOCARDIUM AND HEART VALVES

The endocardium lines the myocardium and contains Purkinje nerve fibers, which transmit a rhythmic action potential throughout the myocardium leading to contraction. The endocardium is lined by endothelial cells, which modulate many aspects of normal hemostasis. In normal states, the endothelial cells are antithrombotic preventing circulating cells from attaching and thus allowing normal flow of blood through the heart and blood vessels. The endocardium is continuous with the endothelium of blood and lymphatic vessels. Normal flow of blood through the heart depends on functional valves (see Chapter 2). Properly functioning valves serve as one-way valves, allowing blood to flow either from one chamber to another (AVVs) or exiting from the heart to either the pulmonary circulation (pulmonic valve) or the systemic circulation (aortic valve).

BLOOD AND LYMPHATIC VASCULAR SYSTEMS

Blood and lymphatic vessels have several important functions. Blood vessels regulate the differential distribution of blood flow to tissues. Blood vessels actively synthesize and secrete vasoactive substances that regulate vascular tone and antithrombotic substances, which maintain the fluidity of the blood. Blood and lymphatic vessels play an important role in transporting and controlling inflammation and thrombosis. Blood and lymphatic vessels also constitute an important pathway for disease dissemination through transport of bacteria and tumor cells to distant sites.

PORTALS OF ENTRY

Routes used to enter the cardiovascular system and lymphatic vessels are numerous and listed in Box 10-2. Toxic chemicals and pathogenic organisms can enter via ingestion, inhalation, cutaneous contact, trauma, or iatrogenic injection and gain access to the cardiovascular system. Microorganisms and toxins penetrate and enter deeper tissues, dermis, lamina propria, subcutis, or submucosa, triggering an acute inflammatory reaction. All three of the major components of acute inflammation may be responsible for entry of the toxin or organism into the vascular or lymphatic system. The increase in the vascular caliber increasing blood flow increases the number of capillary beds exposed to the agent. Changes in the microvasculature that allow the exit of plasma proteins and leukocytes also increase the entry of an agent. Finally, the increase in leukocytes can result in vascular injury and phagocytosis of material. Organisms that are not diluted, but are denatured by molecules from lysosomes of neutrophils, or restricted in movement by being trapped in fibrin at the site of inflammation can gain entry into the lymphatic vessels, thin-walled capillaries, or venules. Entry into lymphatic vessels allows invading microorganisms to be carried in lymph to draining regional and systemic lymph nodes and eventually via the thoracic duct to the circulatory system. Microorganisms that gain access to veins spread with the circulation and can localize in the lungs. In occurrences in which severe pulmonary inflammation leads to the formation of AV fistulas, microorganisms can gain access to pulmonary veins, be pumped through the left heart, and enter the systemic arterial circulation. The circulatory system can distribute organisms and materials to other organs and tissues (see Web Fig. 10-1, also see Chapter 2).

EPICARDIUM AND PERICARDIUM

Bacteria and viral agents can enter the pericardial sac via endothelial damage to capillaries on visceral (epicardium) and parietal (pericardium) surface. Bacteria can enter by direct penetration. In cattle, foreign bodies exiting the reticulum and penetrating the diaphragm carry bacterial pathogens into the pericardial cavity. Direct entry from bacterial or viral infections in the pleura or mediastinum can also occur.

BOX 10-2 Portals of Entry for the Cardiovascular System

PERICARDIUM
- Hematogenous dissemination
- Foreign body penetration from reticulum (cattle)
- Direct extension from pleura or mediastinum

ENDOCARDIUM
- Hematogenous dissemination
- Parasitic migration
- Intravenous and intracardiac catheters (long-term placement)
- Uremia-induced vascular damage and secondary endocardial ulceration (dog, left atrium)

MYOCARDIUM
- Hematogenous dissemination
- Embolic dissemination of infective material fragments from vegetative endocarditis lesions into coronary arterial tree
- Direct extension from endocardium or pericardium

ARTERIES
- Hematogenous dissemination
- Local extension of suppurative and necrotizing inflammatory processes
- Immune-mediated arterial injury
- Parasitic migration

VEINS
- Hematogenous dissemination
- Local extension of severe inflammatory processes
- Intravenous injections and indwelling catheters
- Parasitic migration
- Immune-mediated venous injury

LYMPHATIC VESSELS
- Hematogenous dissemination
- Local extension of severe inflammatory processes
- Parasitic migration

MYOCARDIUM

Pathogens gain entry to the myocardium through the vascular system from the coronary arteries, which provide blood flow to the myocardium. Coronary arteries originate in the sinus of Valsalva at the origin of the aorta and travel in the coronary grooves to the apex of the heart supplying blood to both ventricles. Branches of the coronary arteries bifurcate and send smaller arteries on the outer surface of the heart within the visceral pericardium. These smaller arteries then penetrate the myocardium, becoming arterioles and finally a rich network of capillaries in which there is nearly one vessel adjacent to each cardiac muscle cell. This rich network of capillaries provides an opportunity for bacteria or virus to gain entrance into the myocardium once they have entered the circulatory system. As a result many bacterial and viral infections may result in myocarditis. Bacteria within fibrin and inflammatory debris loosely attached to affected valves (bacterial valvular endocarditis) may detach and lodge in coronary arteries. This septic emboli damages endothelial cells and initiates acute inflammation resulting in myocarditis. Toxins or toxic byproducts can directly damage endothelial cells or diffuse through the endothelium to affect myocardial fibers. In addition, the myocardium is susceptible to direct extension of pathogens located within the endocardium or pericardium.

ENDOCARDIUM AND HEART VALVES

The endocardium and the cardiac valves are in direct contact with any pathogen that enters the circulatory system, including parasites, bacterial and viral pathogens, and toxins. The endocardium, particularly the left atrial endocardium, is particularly susceptible to toxins resulting from renal failure in the dog.

BLOOD AND LYMPHATIC VASCULAR SYSTEMS

The circulatory systems are intrinsically susceptible to microbial organisms and toxins because of the primary role of providing oxygen and nutrients to and removing waste from tissues. Hematogenous, lymphogenous dissemination of microbial pathogens and toxins directly exposes the corresponding vasculature to these hazards. Parasitic migration and local extension of an inflammatory process can directly result in entry into the circulatory or lymphatic system and directly damage these tissues.

DEFENSE MECHANISMS

Defense mechanisms used by the cardiovascular system and lymphatic vessels are listed in Box 10-3. These structures are fortunate in that most of the components of the innate and humoral immunity are present within the lumen. A review of inflammation (see Chapter 3) and circulatory disturbances (see Chapter 2) is invaluable in understanding the defense mechanisms of the cardiovascular and lymphatic systems. The constant flow of blood and lymph through intact circulatory and lymphatic systems, respectively, provides the surface endothelium of the chambers and vessels with constant exposure to nutrients, plasma proteins such as immunoglobulins, preformed chemical mediators, and circulating leukocytes.

RESPONSES TO INJURY

Common responses of the cardiovascular system and lymphatic vessels to injury are listed in Box 10-4. The key characteristics of these responses are summarized next. The specific diseases that result from these responses are discussed in greater detail in the sections covering diseases that occur in all domestic animal species or are unique to one species.

BOX 10-3 Defense Mechanisms

CONSTANT BLOOD FLOW
Endocardium, blood and lymphatic vascular components
Endothelium-facilitated barrier systems (see Chapters 2 and 14)

INNATE RESPONSES
Inflammation
Complement
Chemical mediators of inflammation

PHAGOCYTOSIS
Monocyte-macrophage system
Intravascular macrophages
Adaptive immune system

HUMORAL RESPONSES

CELL-MEDIATED RESPONSES

PERICARDIUM AND EPICARDIUM

Disturbances of Circulation

Hemorrhage

Hemorrhage involving the pericardium and epicardium (Fig. 10-9; Web Fig. 10-7) results from stretching, tearing, lacerating, or crushing blood vessels in these structures and may be caused by penetrating wounds (foreign objects, bullets, or knives), lacerations from fractured bone, shear forces that stretch and ultimately tear vessels in tissues (blunt force trauma), and tears and rupture of tissue resulting from loss of structural integrity attributable to invasive and destructive properties of neoplasms such as hemangiosarcomas (see Chapter 2).

BOX 10-4 Responses to Injury

DISTURBANCES OF CIRCULATION
Hemorrhage
Effusions
Thrombosis and embolism

DISTURBANCES OF GROWTH
Atrophy (dilation)
Hypertrophy
Agenesis (aplasia), hypoplasia, dysplasia (dysgenesis)
Developmental errors, congenital anomalies
Neoplasia (neoplastic transformation)

CELL DEGENERATION AND DEATH
Cell and metabolic dysfunction
Oncotic necrosis
Apoptosis

INFLAMMATION

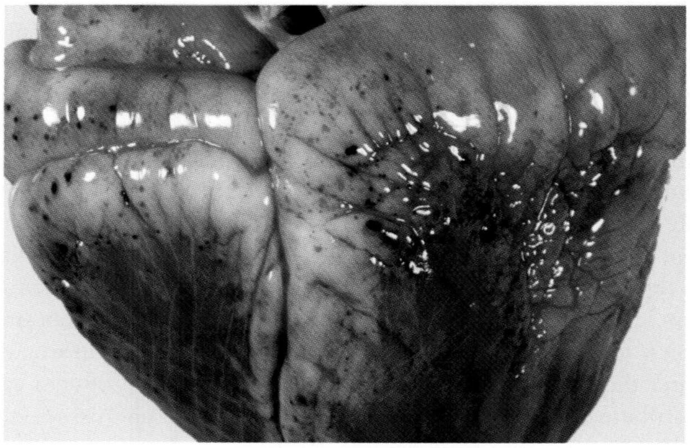

Fig. 10-9 **Epicardial hemorrhage, petechiae and ecchymoses, endotoxemia, heart, cow.**

Note the epicardial and subepicardial hemorrhages in the fat of the coronary groove (a common site). Petechiae and ecchymoses are often attributable to severe septicemia, endotoxemia, anoxia, or electrocution. In this case, the hemorrhage resulted from injury to the endothelium from endotoxin (component of the cell wall of Gram-negative bacteria). The smaller, pinpoint hemorrhages (1 to 2 mm) are petechiae. The larger hemorrhages (3 to 5 mm) are ecchymoses. (Courtesy Dr. M.D. McGavin, College of Veterinary Medicine, University of Tennessee.)

Effusions

See the discussions on the mechanisms of edema formation and Fig. 2-6 in Chapter 2 and on the formation of transudates and exudates and Figure 3-3 in Chapter 3.

Hemopericardium

Hemopericardium is an accumulation of whole blood in the pericardial sac (Figs. 10-10 and 10-11; also see the section on Disorders of Domestic Animals). Death often occurs unexpectedly from cardiac tamponade, a condition in which the compression of the heart caused by the accumulation of blood in the pericardial sac leads to reduced cardiac output and poor perfusion of vascular beds in all organ systems. As examples, hemopericardium may be caused by blunt force trauma (impact with an automobile) or from rupture of the wall of the right atrium after invasion by a hemangiosarcoma.

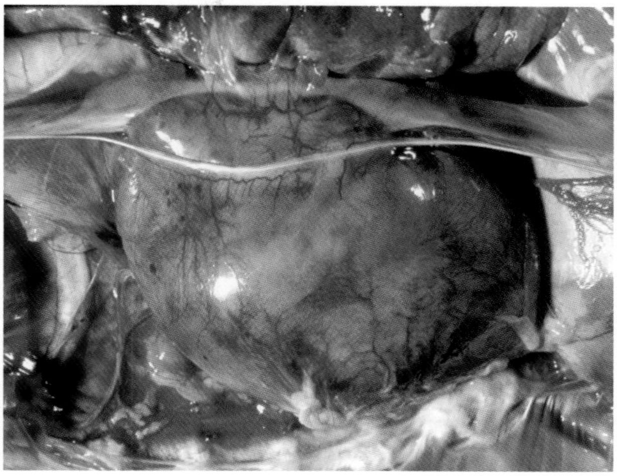

Fig. 10-10 Hemopericardium (cardiac tamponade), right atrium, hemangiosarcoma, heart, dog.
The pericardium is distended and dark blue because it contains whole blood secondary to rupture of an atrial hemangiosarcoma. Hemopericardium can cause death if it is sudden and is of sufficient volume to compress the heart and thus reduce cardiac output, a condition known as cardiac tamponade. On clinical examination, heart sounds are muffled. (Courtesy College of Veterinary Medicine, University of Illinois.)

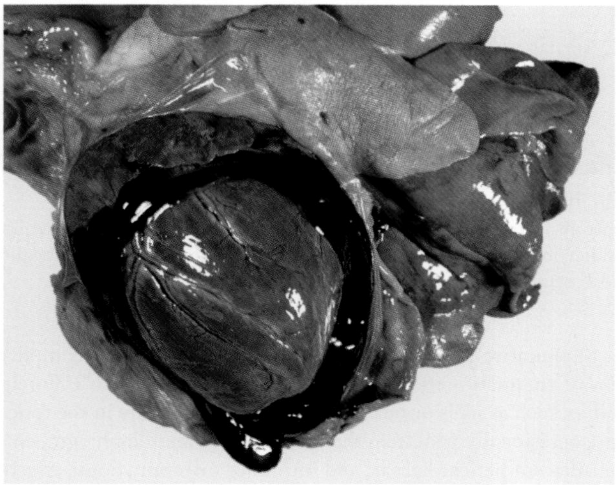

Fig. 10-11 Hemopericardium, heart, dog.
The pericardial sac is filled with clotted blood. Hemorrhage into a body cavity results in pooling of coagulated or uncoagulated blood within that cavity. (Courtesy Dr. D.A. Mosier, College of Veterinary Medicine, Kansas State University.)

Hydropericardium

Hydropericardium is the accumulation of clear, light yellow, watery, serous fluid (i.e., transudate) in the pericardial sac (Fig. 10-12; Web Fig. 10-8; also see the section on Disorders of Domestic Animals). As examples, hydropericardium can occur in animals with (1) hypoproteinemia (decreased colloid osmotic pressure) caused by liver disease or protein-losing nephropathy/enteropathy, (2) heart failure (increased hydrostatic pressure) where there is poor venous return to the heart, and (3) vascular injury, where damage to the barrier function of the vascular wall can result in leakage of small quantities of plasma proteins. In this latter example, a few fibrin strands can be present and the fluid could clot after exposure to air. The pericardial surfaces are smooth and glistening in acute cases, but in chronic cases, the epicardium becomes opaque because of mild fibrous thickening and can appear roughened and granular when there is villous proliferation of fibrous tissue, especially over the atria. The mechanisms involved in these fluid shifts are discussed in Chapters 2 and 3.

Disturbances of Growth

Serous Atrophy

Serous atrophy of fat is readily identified by the gray gelatinous appearance of epicardial fat deposits (Fig. 10-13). Healthy animals normally have abundant white or yellow epicardial fat deposits, especially along the AV junction. Microscopically, lipocytes are atrophic and edema is present in the interstitial tissue. Serous atrophy of epicardial fat occurs rapidly during anorexia, starvation, or cachexia because fat is catabolized to maintain energy balance.

Pericardial Dilatation

The pericardium responds to excess fluid in the pericardial space by dilation. However, this outcome requires adequate time to allow adjustments in size. In hemopericardium, blood rapidly fills the pericardial cavity and death often occurs unexpectedly from cardiac tamponade, a condition with compression of the heart caused by blood accumulation leading to reduced cardiac output. Hydropericardium is the accumulation of clear, light yellow, watery, serous

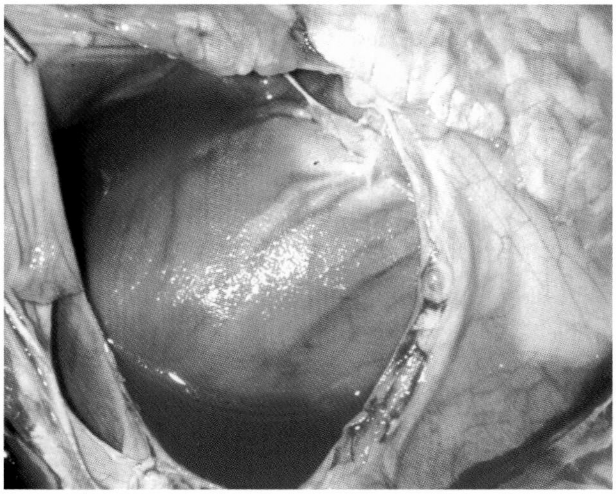

Fig. 10-12 Hydropericardium, pericardial sac, pig.
The thin-walled dilated pericardial sac contains serous fluid that has accumulated secondary to alterations in hydrostatic pressure between the pericardial cavity, circulatory system, and lymphatic system. (Courtesy College of Veterinary Medicine, University of Illinois.)

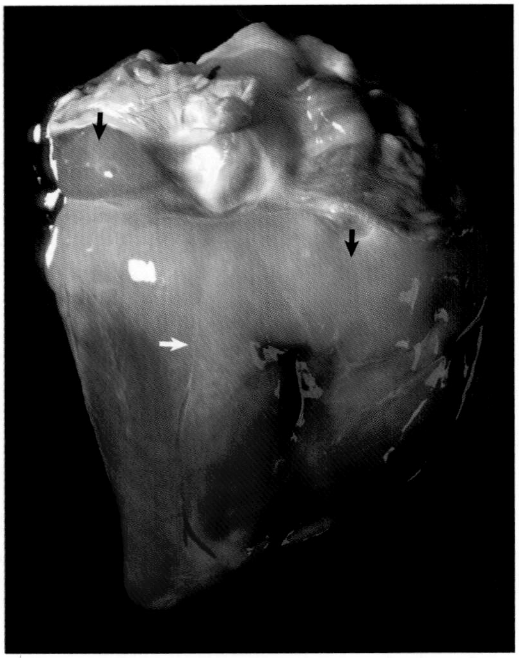

Fig. 10-13 Serous atrophy of fat, heart, epicardium, cow. The epicardial fat deposits are gray and gelatinous *(arrows),* indicating that fat has been catabolized, for example as in the early stages of starvation. (Courtesy Dr. M.D. McGavin, College of Veterinary Medicine, University of Tennessee.)

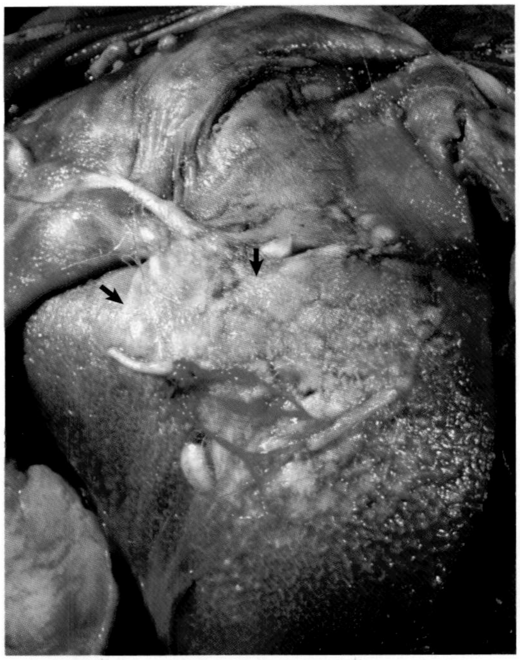

Fig. 10-14 Fibrinous pericarditis, heart, epicardium, horse. The epicardium is covered dorsally by a thick, yellow layer of fibrin *(arrows)* and ventrally by granulation tissue *(finely granular surface),* thus indicating the chronicity of the inflammatory process. The apposing parietal pericardium (not shown) was also covered with fibrin. This lesion commonly occurs in horses with *Streptococcus equi* ssp. *zooepidemicus* septicemia causing vasculitis. (Courtesy Dr. M.D. McGavin, College of Veterinary Medicine, University of Tennessee.)

fluid (i.e., transudate) in the pericardial sac (see Fig. 10-12; see Web Fig. 10-8). In cases associated with vascular injury, a few fibrin strands are present, and the fluid could clot after exposure to air.

Cell Degeneration and Death

Epicardial Calcification

Epicardial calcification is a feature in hereditary calcinosis in mice and cardiomyopathy in hamsters (Web Fig. 10-9). Myocardial mineralization (discussed later) may be visible on the epicardial surface in vitamin E–selenium deficiency in sheep and cattle, vitamin D toxicity in several species, calcinogenic plant toxicosis in cattle ("Manchester wasting disease"), and spontaneous myocardial calcification in aged rats and guinea pigs.

Gout

Visceral gout has not been reported in domestic animals but does occur in birds and reptiles (Web Fig. 10-10; see Chapter 1).

Inflammation

Pericarditis

Inflammation of the pericardium is frequently seen with bacterial septicemias and typically results in fibrinous pericarditis. Grossly, both the visceral and parietal pericardial surfaces are covered by variable amounts of yellow fibrin deposits, which can result in adherence between the parietal and visceral layers. When the pericardial sac is opened the attachments are torn away (so-called bread-and-butter heart) (Fig. 10-14). Microscopically, an eosinophilic layer of fibrin with admixed neutrophils lies over a congested epicardium (Fig. 10-15).

The outcome of fibrinous pericarditis varies. Early death is frequent because many of these lesions result from infection by highly virulent bacteria and concurrent septicemia. When survival is prolonged, adhesions form between the pericardial surfaces after fibrous organization of the exudate.

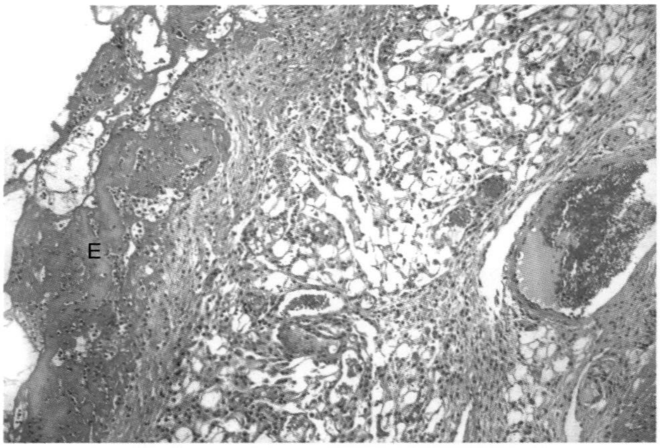

Fig. 10-15 Fibrinous pericarditis, heart, epicardium, pig. Note eosinophilic fibrin deposits *(E) (left)* on the epicardial surface. This lesion commonly occurs with septicemias by bacteria that cause vasculitis. H&E stain. (Courtesy School of Veterinary Medicine, Purdue University.)

Suppurative pericarditis is seen mainly in cattle as a complication of traumatic reticuloperitonitis ("hardware disease"). Foreign bodies, such as nails or pieces of wire that accumulate in the reticulum, occasionally penetrate the reticular wall and diaphragm, enter the adjacent pericardial sac, and introduce infection. Some affected cattle survive for weeks to months until death ensues from congestive heart failure or septicemia. Grossly, the pericardial surfaces are notably thickened by white, often rough, shaggy-appearing masses of fibrous connective tissue that enclose an accumulation of white to gray, thick, foul-smelling, purulent exudate (Fig. 10-16).

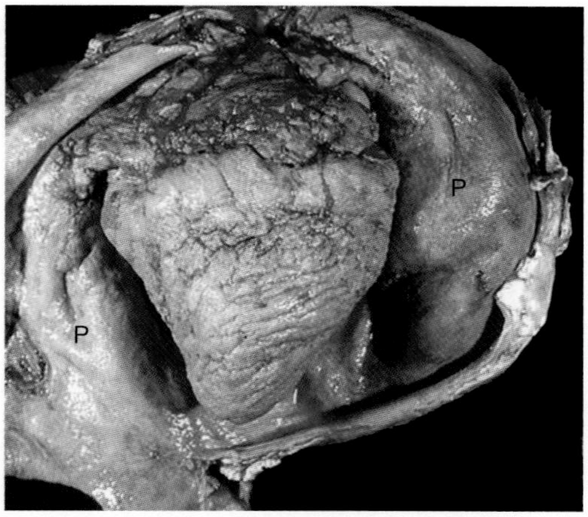

Fig. 10-16 Chronic suppurative (active) pericarditis, traumatic reticuloperitonitis ("hardware disease"), heart, pericardial sac (opened), cow. The exposed epicardial and parietal surfaces are notably thickened by fibrous connective tissue and covered by a fibrinopurulent exudate. On clinical examination, heart sounds are muffled. *P,* Reflected parietal pericardium. (Courtesy Dr. J. King, College of Veterinary Medicine, Cornell University.)

Constrictive pericarditis is a chronic inflammatory lesion of the pericardium accompanied by extensive fibrous proliferation and eventual formation of fibrous adhesions between the surfaces of the visceral and parietal pericardium. The condition is seen in some cases of suppurative pericarditis in cattle and pigs with chronic fibrinous pericarditis. Severe lesions obliterate the pericardial sac and constrict the heart with fibrous tissue and can interfere with cardiac filling and thus cardiac output. Compensatory myocardial hypertrophy can result in diminished ventricular chamber volumes and contribute to the eventual development of heart failure.

MYOCARDIUM

The involvement of specific areas of the heart with major myocardial diseases is illustrated in Fig. 10-17.

Disturbances of Circulation

Hemorrhage: Trauma (Physical Injury)

See the discussion on hemorrhage in the section on Pericardium and Epicardium, Disturbances of Circulation, and the discussion on hemorrhage in Chapter 2.

Disturbances of Growth

See the discussion on hypertrophy in Chapter 1.

Hypertrophy

Hypertrophy of the myocardium represents an increase in muscle mass, which is the result of an increase in the size of cardiac muscle cells (Fig. 10-18; see Fig. 10-6, *B*). Hypertrophy is generally secondary and is the result of a compensatory response to increased workload; it is usually reversible on removal of the cause. However, primary hypertrophy also occurs, as in cats and dogs with idiopathic hypertrophic cardiomyopathy (see later discussion), and is not reversible. Two anatomic forms of hypertrophy are recognized. Eccentric hypertrophy results in a heart with enlarged ventricular chambers and walls of normal to somewhat decreased thickness; it is produced by lesions that increase blood volume load such as valvular insufficiencies and septal defects. In concentric hypertrophy the heart is characterized by small ventricular chambers and thick walls; it results from lesions that increase pressure load such as valvular stenosis, systemic hypertension, and pulmonary disease. Some cats with hyperthyroidism have a cardiac hypertrophy that is mediated by enhanced production of myocardial contractile proteins under the influence of increased concentration of circulating thyroid hormones (Fig. 10-19). The hypertrophy is reversible on return to euthyroidism.

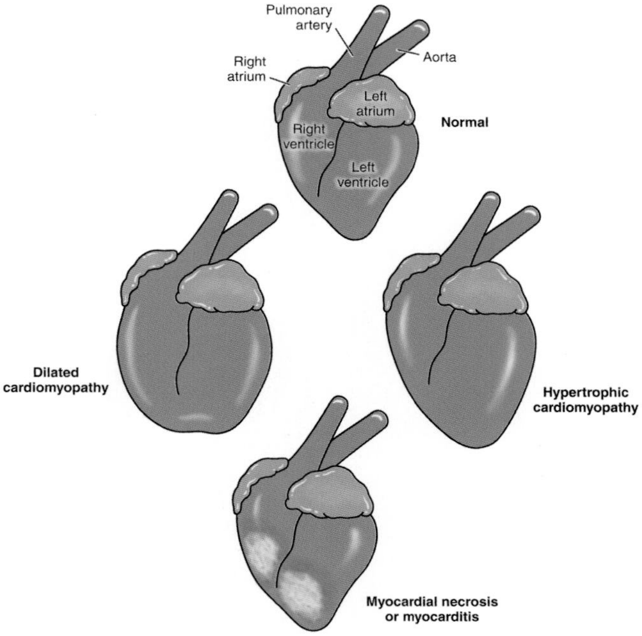

Fig. 10-17 Schematic diagram of the major myocardial diseases. (Redrawn with permission from School of Veterinary Medicine, Purdue University.)

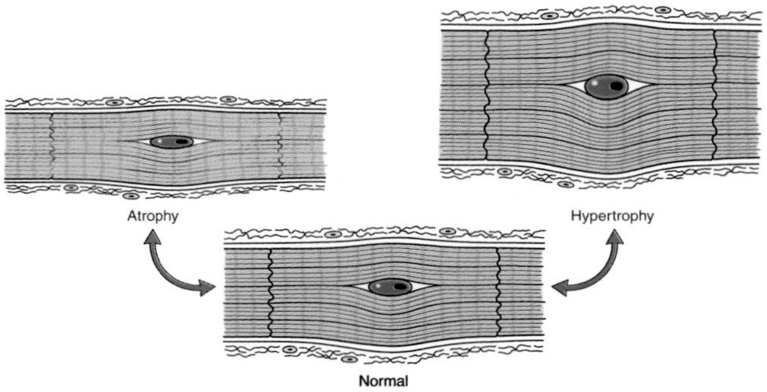

Fig. 10-18 Schematic diagram of cardiac muscle cells. Growth disturbances of atrophy and hypertrophy. (Redrawn with permission from School of Veterinary Medicine, Purdue University.)

Stages of Myocardial Hypertrophy

Three stages of myocardial hypertrophy are recognizable: (1) initiation, (2) stable hyperfunction, and (3) deterioration of function associated with degeneration of hypertrophied myocytes. Microscopically, in myocardial hypertrophy, the myocytes are enlarged and have large nuclei (Fig. 10-20).

Right Ventricular Hypertrophy

Right ventricular hypertrophy is structurally or functionally caused by pulmonary stenosis or pulmonary hypertension, respectively. The former diseases include congenital pulmonic stenosis in dogs (see Fig. 10-59); the latter include dirofilariasis in dogs and cats (Fig.

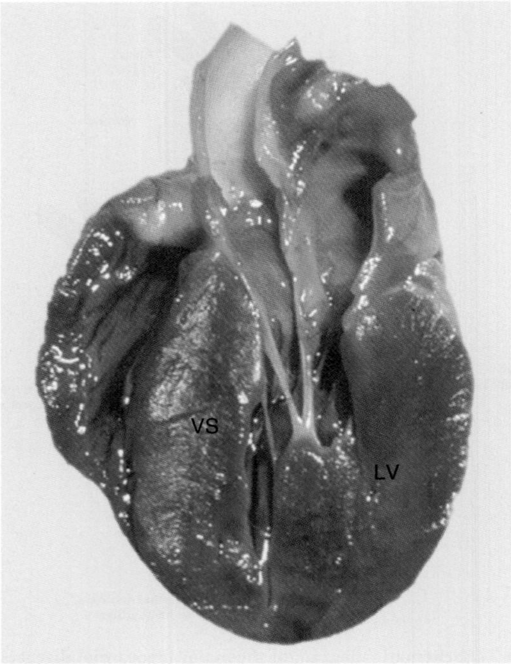

Fig. 10-19 Left ventricular hypertrophy, hyperthyroidism, heart, bisected, cat.
Note prominent thickening of the left ventricular *(LV)* free wall. The ventricular septum *(VS)* is also thickened. (Courtesy School of Veterinary Medicine, Purdue University.)

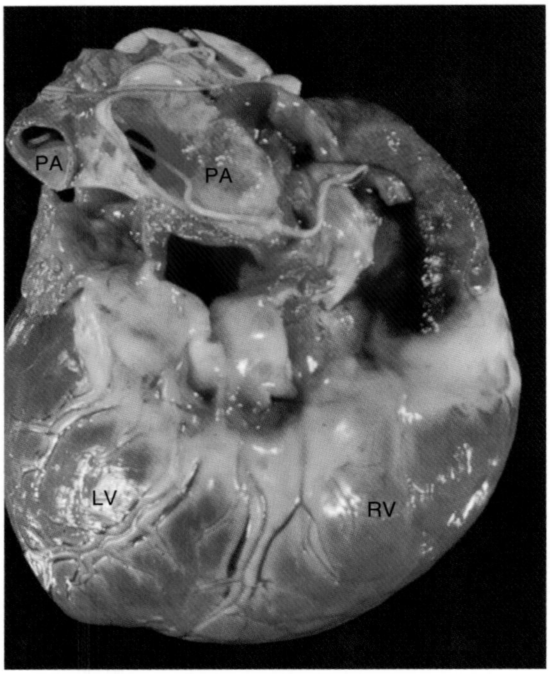

Fig. 10-21 Dirofilariasis, heart, dog.
Note the hypertrophy of the right ventricle *(RV)* and adult *Dirofilaria immitis* in the pulmonary artery and its branches *(PA)*. *LV,* Left ventricle. (Courtesy Dr. K. Read, College of Veterinary Medicine, Texas A&M University; and Noah's Arkive, College of Veterinary Medicine, The University of Georgia.)

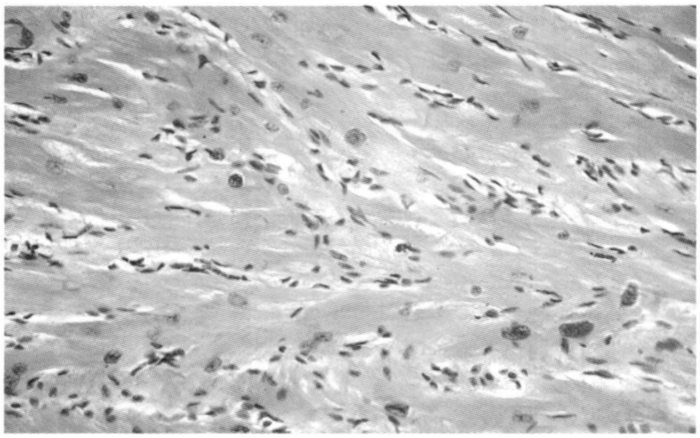

Fig. 10-20 Hypertrophic cardiomyopathy, myocyte hypertrophy, heart, myocardium, cat.
Cardiac myocytes are hypertrophied, and there is an increase in interstitial fibroblasts. H&E stain. (Courtesy School of Veterinary Medicine, Purdue University.)

10-21), "brisket disease" ("high-altitude disease") in cattle (see Fig. 10-8), and chronic alveolar emphysema ("heaves") in horses (see Fig. 9-53). Dirofilariasis (heartworm disease) may occur in 35% to 45% of dogs and 2% of cats in areas of high infection rates such as within 150 miles of the Atlantic and Gulf coasts from Texas to New Jersey and along the Mississippi River and its major tributaries. The extent of cardiac alterations is related to the numbers of adult parasites present. Initially, the parasites accumulate in the pulmonary arteries (see Figs. 10-21 and 10-90), and as the numbers increase, they are present in the right ventricle, then in the right atrium, and finally may occupy the vena cavae. Pulmonary hypertension results from vascular blockage and pulmonary vascular lesions produced by the parasites and right ventricular hypertrophy follows. Right-sided heart failure may eventually develop. Dogs with massive adult parasite loads may suffer acute collapse from caval syndrome, characterized by shock, intravascular hemolysis, and hepatic and renal failure. In "brisket disease," cattle maintained under the hypoxic conditions that exist at altitudes above 7000 feet above sea level develop pulmonary hypertension and subsequent right-sided heart failure with subcutaneous edema, chronic passive congestion of the liver (nutmeg liver), and right ventricular hypertrophy. Exposure to certain poisonous plants (*Oxytropis* spp. and *Astragalus* spp.) increases the severity of the disease.

Left Ventricular Hypertrophy

Left ventricular hypertrophy occurs in dogs with congenital subaortic stenosis, in cats with hyperthyroidism, and in dogs and cats with systemic hypertension. Systemic hypertension tends to be associated with hyperthyroidism and chronic renal failure in cats, and with chronic renal failure, hyperadrenocorticism, and pheochromocytomas in dogs. Affected animals may have ocular lesions secondary to damage to retinal vessels.

Biventricular Hypertrophy

Biventricular hypertrophy can occur with hypertrophic cardiomyopathy and various congenital cardiac anomalies. Eccentric hypertrophy develops in the late stages of diseases that initially cause concentric hypertrophy as cardiac dilation is superimposed.

The appearance of cardiac hypertrophy and dilation is summarized in Fig. 10-22.

Physiologic Atrophy

Physiologic atrophy of heart muscle may occur in confined animals and also occurs as a result of decompensation of cardiac myocytes

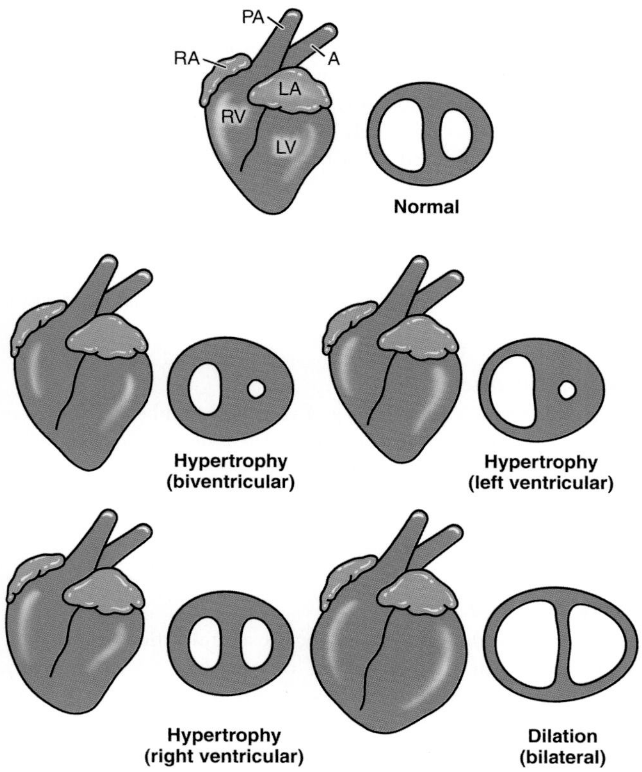

Fig. 10-22 Schematic diagram of the types of myocardial hypertrophy and dilation.

Left lateral view and midventricular cross section *(not drawn to same scale)*. *A*, Aorta; *LA*, left atrium; *LV*, left ventricle; *PA*, pulmonary artery; *RA*, right atrium; *RV*, right ventricle. (Redrawn with permission from School of Veterinary Medicine, Purdue University.)

in chronic congestive heart failure (see Fig. 10-6, *A*). Initially, these myocytes respond through hypertrophy with increased contractile force according to the Frank-Starling phenomenon. However, stretching beyond certain limits decreases contractile strength and eventually leads to loss of contractile proteins within these cells or loss of these cells resulting in atrophy of the affected myocardium (see Fig. 10-18).

Neoplastic Transformation

Rhabdomyomas and rhabdomyosarcomas are primary tumors that originate from the myocardium in domestic animals (see Chapter 6). Fibrosarcomas also occur rarely. Numerous types of secondary tumors, such as lymphosarcomas, metastasize to the myocardium and are discussed in this chapter and other chapters of this book. Hemangiosarcomas are tumors of blood vessels of the myocardium of the right atrium and are discussed later.

Cell Degeneration and Death

Histopathologic study of sections of the myocardium is substantially limited in respect to specific diagnoses and only rarely can an etiologic diagnosis be made from the morphologic alterations. This inadequacy exists because the spectrum of pathologic reactions is limited, and many agents that damage the heart produce similar lesions. Myocardial necrosis can be confused with myocardial inflammation with secondary necrosis because both lesions have substantial leukocytic infiltration. Some animals that die peracutely from cardiac failure lack detectable microscopic alterations and are presumed to have suffered from an arrhythmic episode resulting in syncope. Hearts with long-standing myocardial damage have foci of fibrosis, regardless of the cause of the loss of myocytes. Correlation between the severity of clinical cardiac disease and the severity of myocardial injury can be poor: a small lesion at a critical site, such as a portion of the conduction system, can be fatal, whereas a widespread myocardial lesion, such as myocarditis, can be asymptomatic (Fig. 10-23; see Chapter 1).

Cardiac myofibers can respond to toxins in a variety of ways—apoptosis, myofibrillar lysis, and coagulation necrosis are but a few mechanisms that may result from toxic exposure. A long list of toxins (included in Box 10-5) are responsible for causing myocardial injury; some of the most frequently observed current examples are ionophore toxicity in horses and ruminants, vitamin E–selenium deficiency in the young of many species, "heart-brain syndrome" of dogs (see Fig. 10-83), anthracycline toxicity in dogs,

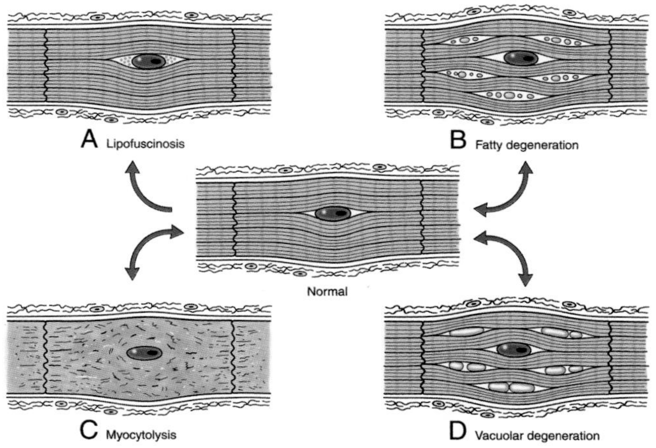

Fig. 10-23 Schematic diagram of various sublethal cardiac muscle cell injuries.

A, Lipofuscinosis. **B**, Fatty degeneration. **C**, Myocytolysis. **D**, Vacuolar degeneration. (Redrawn with permission from School of Veterinary Medicine, Purdue University.)

BOX 10-5 Causes of Myocardial Necrosis in Animals

NUTRITIONAL DEFICIENCIES

Vitamin E–selenium, potassium, copper, thiamine, magnesium

TOXICITIES

Cobalt, catecholamines, vasodilator antihypertensives, methylxanthines (theobromine, theophylline, caffeine), ionophores (monensin, lasalocid, salinomycin, maduramicin, narasin), vitamin D and calcinogenic plants *(Cestrum diurnum, Trisetum flavescens, Solanum malacoxylon, Solanum torvum)*, other poisonous plants *(Acacia georginae, Gastrolobium* spp., *Oxylobium* spp., *Dichapetalum cymosum, Persea americana, Cassia occidentalis, Cassia obtusifolia, Karwinskia humboldtiana, Ateleia glazioviana, Eupatorium rugosum, Adonis aestivalis, Pachystigma pygmaeum, Fadogia homblei, Pavetta harborii)*, blister beetles *(Epicauta)*, high-erucic-acid rapeseed oil, brominated vegetable oils, gossypol, T-2 mycotoxin, uremia

PHYSICAL INJURIES AND SHOCK

Central nervous system lesions and trauma ("heart-brain syndrome"), gastric dilation and volvulus, stress, overexertion, electrical defibrillation, hemorrhagic shock

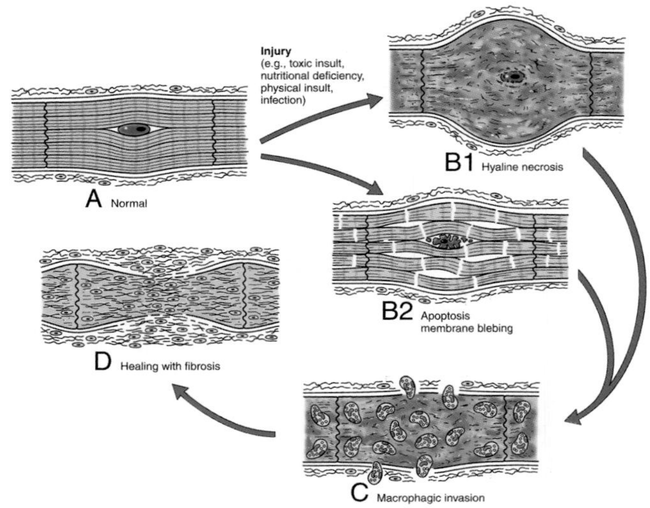

Fig. 10-24 Schematic diagram of the sequential events in myocardial necrosis.

A, Various injuries lead to **(B1)** hyaline necrosis or **(B2)** apoptosis membrane blebbing. **C,** Healing with phagocytosis of cellular debris by macrophages, and **(D)** subsequent healing with fibrosis, rather than by regeneration. (Redrawn with permission from School of Veterinary Medicine, Purdue University.)

and gossypol toxicosis in pigs. In various localized areas throughout the world, numerous deaths in ruminants have resulted from consumption of poisonous plants such as *Acacia georginae* and *Dichapetalum cymosum*.

Cardiotoxicity has emerged as a significant clinical entity in veterinary medicine in recent years with the growing use of antineoplastic drugs in small animal practice and the widespread use of growth promotants in ruminants (see Fig. 10-69). The mechanisms of cardiotoxicities include (1) exaggerated pharmacologic action of drugs acting on cardiovascular tissues, (2) exposure to substances that depress myocardial function, (3) direct injury of cardiac muscle cells by chemicals, and (4) hypersensitivity reactions.

Oncotic Necrosis

Necrosis of cardiac muscle cells is generally followed by leukocytic invasion and phagocytosis of sarcoplasmic debris (Fig. 10-24; see Figs. 15-15 and 15-16). The end result is persistence of collapsed sarcolemmal "tubes" of basal lamina surrounded by condensed interstitial stroma and vessels. Lesions with severe disruption of the myocardium have residual changes of fibroblastic proliferation and collagen deposition to form scar tissue. Regeneration of cardiac muscle cells generally does not occur, except in less evolved animals, such as amphibians and fish, and in certain inbred mouse strains. The continual contraction of intact cardiac muscle cells impairs the mechanisms for regeneration. Also, in hearts of neonatal animals and more often in avian hearts, a limited amount of myocyte regeneration has been reported. Recent studies indicate that stem cells exist in adult animal and human hearts, and with myocardial injury, these cells may differentiate into cardiac muscle cells. However, the extent of myocyte regeneration is probably minimal. Hyperplasia of myocytes is a normal component of cardiac growth in the first several months of life. Then proliferation ceases. Normal growth then is the result of hypertrophy of myocytes until cell sizes normal for the species are reached.

Apoptosis

Apoptosis (programmed cell death of cardiac myocytes) is increasingly recognized for its role in the development of various myocardial lesions and cardiac diseases (see Chapter 1). These conditions include cardiac development, ischemic injury, several types of experimentally induced heart failure (ischemia-reperfusion, hypoxia, pressure-overload hypertrophy), and cardiotoxicity. In some cell systems, apoptosis can be triggered by the presence of excessive amounts of oxygen free radicals. Cells dying by apoptosis shrink and form apoptotic bodies. In contrast to cell death by necrosis, apoptosis is not accompanied by an inflammatory reaction and fibrosis.

Fatty Infiltration

Fatty infiltration is the presence of increased numbers of lipocytes interposed between myocardial fibers. The lesion is associated with obesity and age and appears as abundant epicardial and myocardial deposits of adipose tissue. Grossly, the myocardium has irregular layers of adipose tissue infiltrating normal myocardium. The atria and right ventricle are most often affected.

Fatty Degeneration

Fatty degeneration (fatty change) is the accumulation of abundant lipid droplets in the sarcoplasm of myocytes. Microscopically, affected myocytes have numerous variably sized spherical droplets that appear as empty vacuoles in paraffin sections but stain positively for lipids with lipid-soluble stains in frozen sections. This lesion occurs with systemic disorders, such as severe anemia, toxemia, and copper deficiency, but is seen much less often in the heart than in the liver and kidneys (also see Chapter 1).

Hydropic Degeneration

Hydropic degeneration, a distinctive microscopic alteration in cardiac muscle cells, is associated with chronic administration of anthracyclines, a group of antineoplastic drugs. Chronic passive congestion with ascites and cardiac dilation may result (Web Figs. 10-11 and 10-12; see Figs. 10-6, *A* and 10-7). Affected fibers have extensive vacuolization of sarcoplasm that is initiated by distention of elements of sarcoplasmic reticulum and eventually ends in lysis of contractile material (Web Figs. 10-13 and 10-14).

Hydropic degeneration of cardiac muscle cells may also result from drug-induced injury to mitochondria. Antiretroviral drugs, such as nucleoside reverse transcriptase inhibitors (zidovudine or AZT), are linked to this distinctive lesion. Scattered cardiac muscle cells appear swollen with pale sarcoplasm by light microscopy. Electron microscopy reveals extensive mitochondrial swelling and disruption of cristae with subsequent formation of myelin figures from the membrane debris of damaged mitochondria.

Myofibrillar Degeneration

Myofibrillar degeneration (myocytolysis) represents a distinctive sublethal injury of cardiac muscle cells. Affected fibers have pale eosinophilic sarcoplasm and lack cross-striations. Ultrastructurally, myofibrils have a variable extent of dissolution (myofibrillar lysis). This lesion has been described in furazolidone cardiotoxicity in birds (Fig. 10-25; Web Fig. 10-15) and potassium deficiency in rats.

Lipofuscinosis

Lipofuscinosis (brown atrophy) of the myocardium occurs in aged animals and in animals with severe cachexia, but it also has been described as a hereditary lesion in healthy Ayrshire cattle. Severely affected hearts appear brown and microscopically have clusters of

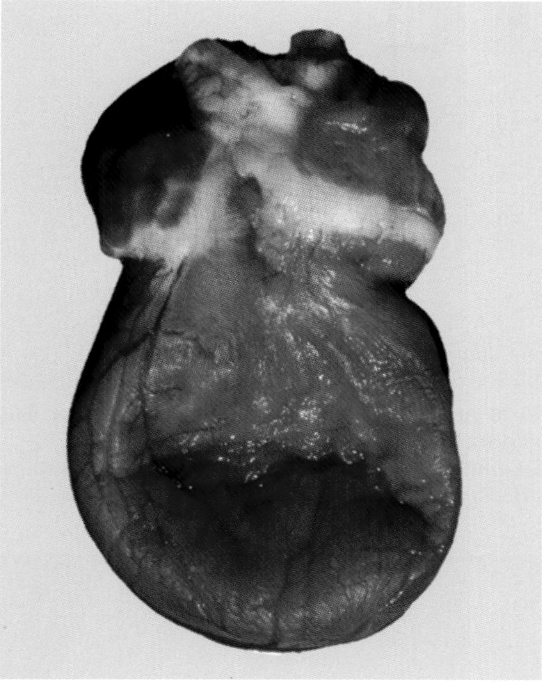

Fig. 10-25 Ventricular dilation, furazolidone cardiotoxicity, heart, duckling.
Note that the dilated ventricles have collapsed once the blood was removed. (Courtesy School of Veterinary Medicine, Purdue University.)

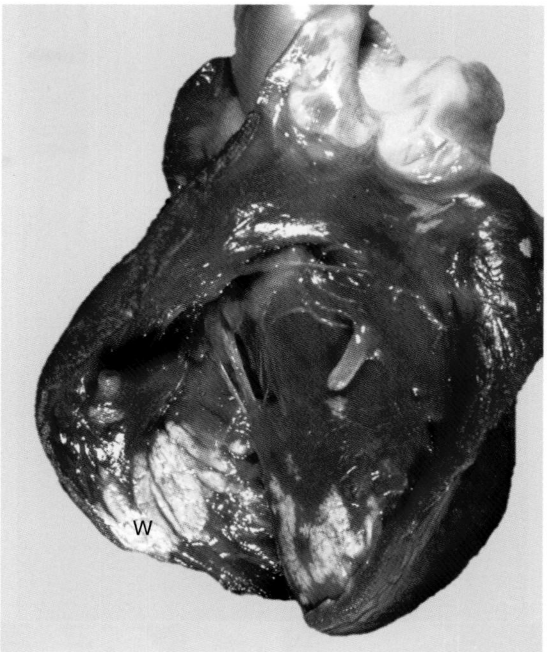

Fig. 10-26 Calcification, vitamin E–selenium deficiency, myocardial necrosis, heart, right ventricle, lamb.
The multiple white *(W)* subendocardial lesions are areas of calcified necrotic cardiac myocytes. (Courtesy Dr. M.D. McGavin, College of Veterinary Medicine, University of Tennessee.)

yellow-brown granules at the nuclear poles of myocytes. These granules represent intralysosomal accumulation of membranous and amorphous debris (residual bodies).

Mineralization

Myocardial mineralization (calcium) is a prominent feature in several diseases, such as hereditary calcinosis in mice, cardiomyopathy in hamsters, vitamin E–selenium deficiency in sheep and cattle (Fig. 10-26; see Web Fig. 10-9), vitamin D toxicity in several species, calcinogenic plant toxicosis in cattle ("Manchester wasting disease"), and spontaneous myocardial calcification in aged rats and guinea pigs.

Myocardial Necrosis

Myocardial necrosis can result from a number of causes, including nutritional deficiencies, chemical and plant toxins, ischemia, metabolic disorders, heritable diseases, and physical injuries (see Box 10-5). Grossly, affected areas appear pale initially, and some progress to prominent yellow to white (see Fig. 10-69), dry areas made gritty by dystrophic mineralization. The lesions are focal, multifocal, or diffuse. The most frequent sites of focal lesions are the left ventricular papillary muscles and the subendocardial myocardium, especially when such lesions are related to transient reduction of vascular perfusion. These lesions can be overlooked at necropsy unless multiple incisions are made in the ventricular myocardium. In diseases with diffuse cardiac necrosis, such as white muscle disease of calves and lambs due to vitamin E–selenium deficiency, the discrete white lesions can be readily observed beneath the epicardial and endocardial surfaces (Fig. 10-27).

Microscopically, the appearance depends on the age of the lesions. Fibers in areas of recent necrosis often appear swollen and hypereosinophilic (hyaline necrosis). Striations are indistinct, and nuclei are pyknotic. Necrotic fibers often have scattered basophilic granules (Fig. 10-28) that represent calcified mitochondria and can be confirmed by electron microscopy (Web Fig. 10-16). In a second pattern of necrosis, affected myocytes have a "shredded" appearance because of hypercontraction and the formation of multiple transversely oriented bars of disrupted contractile material (often termed *contraction band necrosis*) (Web Fig. 10-17). A third pattern is seen in necrotic myocytes in large areas of ischemic necrosis (infarcts). These myocytes have features of coagulation necrosis and have relaxed rather than hypercontracted contractile elements.

Within 24 to 48 hours after injury, necrotic areas are infiltrated by inflammatory cells, mainly macrophages and a few neutrophils; these phagocytose and lyse the necrotic cellular debris (Web Fig. 10-18). In early stages of healing of necrosis, it is often difficult to distinguish the lesions from those found in some types of myocarditis (see later discussion). Later, when necrosis has progressed somewhat, lesions consist of persistent stromal tissue (interstitial fibroblasts, collagen, and capillaries) and empty "tubes" of basal laminae formally occupied by necrotic myocytes (see Chapter 15). The healing phase is characterized by proliferation of connective tissue cells (fibroblasts) (Fig. 10-29) and by deposition of connective tissue products (collagen and elastic tissue and acid mucopolysaccharides). Grossly, these areas with healing of myocardial necrosis appear as white, firm, contracted scars.

The outcome of myocardial necrosis varies, depending on the extent of the damage:

- Many animals die unexpectedly of acute cardiac failure if the myocardial damage is extensive.
- Early deaths from necrosis-related arrhythmias also occur when cardiac conduction is disrupted.
- Some cases eventually develop cardiac decompensation and die with cardiac dilation, scarring, and lesions of chronic congestive failure.

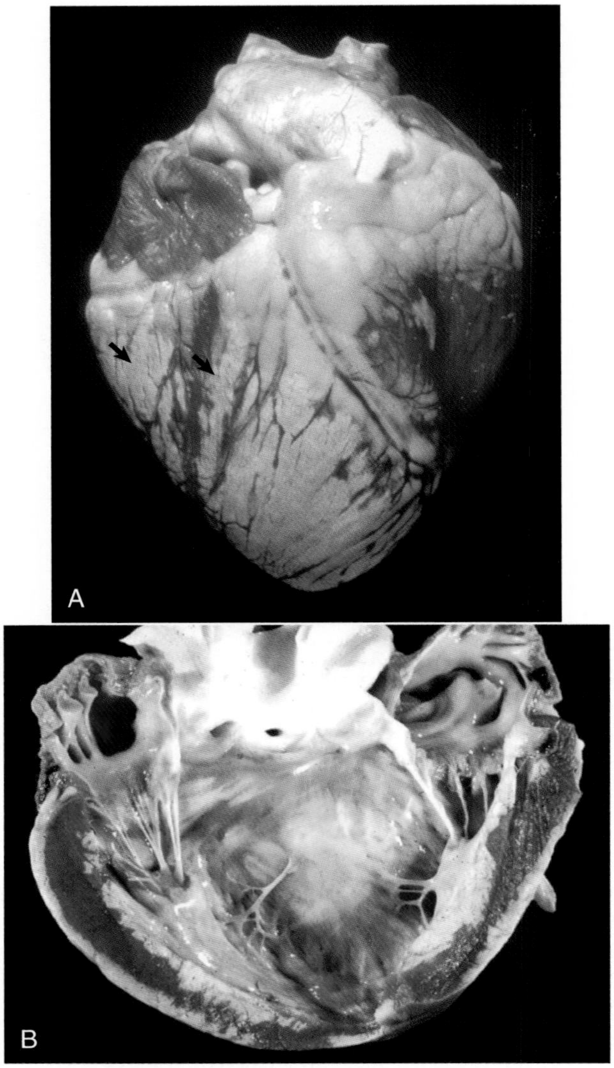

Fig. 10-27 Myocardial necrosis, vitamin E–selenium deficiency, heart, left ventricular myocardium, calf.
A, Note the prominent white chalky areas of necrosis with mineralization *(arrows)* of the myocardium. **B,** Similar necrosis is subepicardially and subendocardially in the sectioned free walls of the left ventricle and subendocardially in the myocardium of the ventricular septum *(center)*. (**A** courtesy School of Veterinary Medicine, Purdue University. **B** courtesy Dr. P.N. Nation, Animal Pathology Services; and Noah's Arkive, College of Veterinary Medicine, The University of Georgia.)

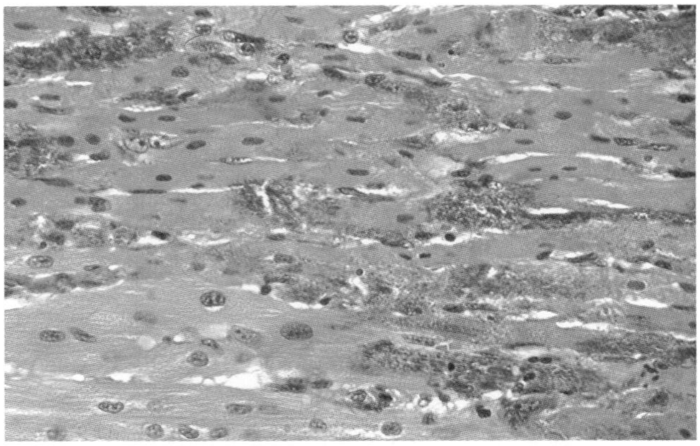

Fig. 10-28 Acute myocardial necrosis with mineralization, minoxidil cardiotoxicity, heart, ventricular myocardium, pig.
The darker red myocytes are necrotic, and some are mineralized *(purplish areas)*. H&E stain. (Courtesy School of Veterinary Medicine, Purdue University.)

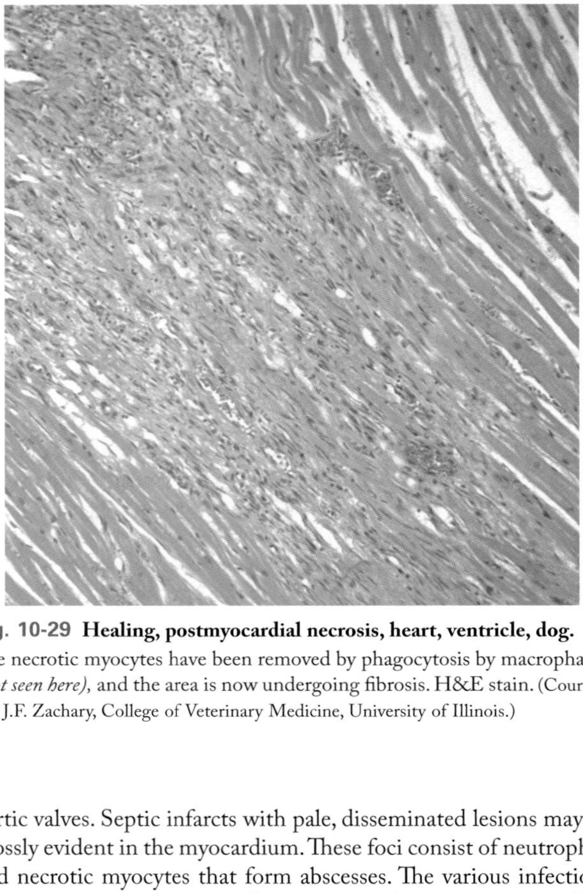

Fig. 10-29 Healing, postmyocardial necrosis, heart, ventricle, dog.
The necrotic myocytes have been removed by phagocytosis by macrophages *(not seen here)*, and the area is now undergoing fibrosis. H&E stain. (Courtesy Dr. J.F. Zachary, College of Veterinary Medicine, University of Illinois.)

Hearts with minimal damage have only microscopically detectable myocardial fibrosis when death eventually occurs from other diseases.

Inflammation

Myocarditis

Myocarditis generally is the result of infections spread hematogenously to the myocardium and occurs in various systemic diseases. Infrequently, the heart is the primary location in affected animals and responsible for death. Types of inflammation provoked by infectious agents that produce myocarditis include suppurative, necrotizing, hemorrhagic, lymphocytic, and eosinophilic. Suppurative myocarditis results from localization of pyogenic bacteria in the myocardium (Fig. 10-30) that are trapped in thromboemboli originating from vegetative valvular endocarditis on the mitral and aortic valves. Septic infarcts with pale, disseminated lesions may be grossly evident in the myocardium. These foci consist of neutrophils and necrotic myocytes that form abscesses. The various infectious diseases that cause myocarditis in animals are summarized in Box 10-6.

The pathogenesis and expected outcome of cases of myocarditis remain an important area of research because of the severity of this lesion in cardiac failure in humans. The sequelae to myocarditis include (1) complete resolution of lesions, (2) scattered residual myocardial scars, or (3) progressive myocardial damage with acute or, in some cases, chronic cardiac failure as secondary dilated (congestive) cardiomyopathy. In experimental studies of myocarditis induced in mice by coxsackie B virus, the severity of myocarditis was influenced by the virulence of the virus and mouse strain and was enhanced by host factors such as young age, male sex,

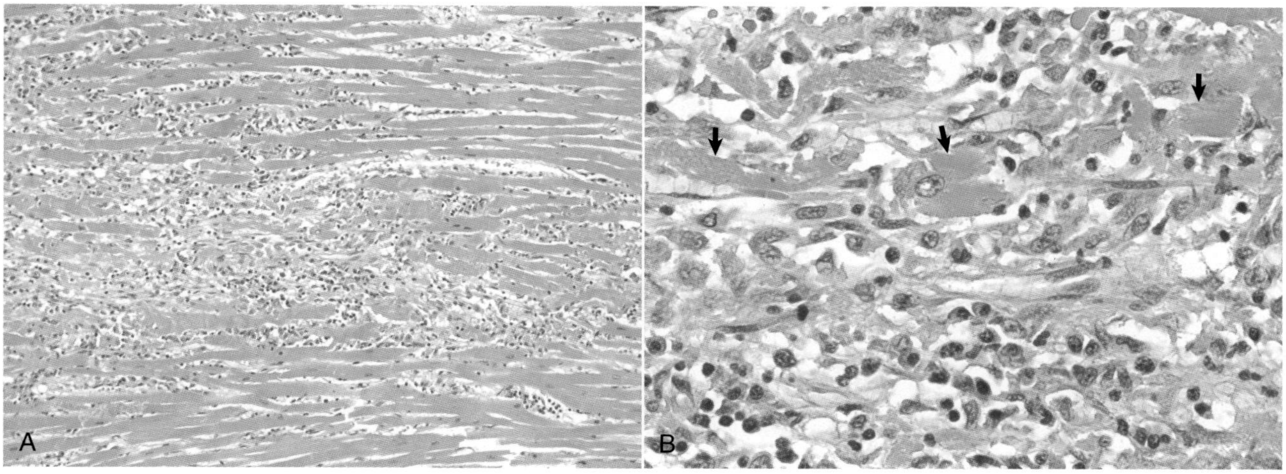

Fig. 10-30 **Acute myocarditis, horse.**
A, The parallel arrays of myofibers are disrupted by acute inflammatory cells, edema fluid, and fibrin. **B,** Higher magnification of **A**. Note the myocardial fiber degeneration and necrosis with loss of cross striations *(arrows)*; fragmentation of cardiac rhabdomyocytes (cardiomyocytes); and hypereosinophilia, coagulation, and clumping of the sarcoplasm. Neutrophils are the predominant inflammatory cell in the exudate. H&E stain. (Courtesy Dr. J.F. Zachary, College of Veterinary Medicine, University of Illinois.)

BOX 10-6 Diseases that Cause Myocarditis in Animals

VIRAL
Canine parvovirus, encephalomyocarditis, foot-and-mouth disease, pseudorabies, canine distemper, cytomegalovirus, Newcastle disease, avian encephalomyelitis, Eastern and Western equine encephalomyelitis, West Nile Virus

BACTERIAL
Blackleg *(Clostridium chauvoei)*, listeriosis *(Listeria monocytogenes)*, Tyzzer's disease *(Bacillus piliformis)*, necrobacillosis *(Fusobacterium necrophorum)*, tuberculosis (*Mycobacterium* spp.), caseous lymphadenitis *(Corynebacterium pseudotuberculosis)*, Lyme disease *(Borrelia burgdorferi)*, disseminated infections by *Actinobacillus equuli, Staphylococcus* sp., *Corynebacterium kutscheri, Arcanobacter pyogenes, Histophilus somni, Pseudomonas aeruginosa, Streptococcus equi*, and *Streptococcus pneumoniae*

PROTOZOAN
Toxoplasmosis *(Toxoplasma gondii)*, sarcocystosis (*Sarcocystis* sp.), neosporosis *(Neospora caninum)*, encephalitozoonosis *(Encephalitozoon cuniculi)*, trypanosomiasis (Chagas' disease *[Trypanosoma cruzi]*), East Coast fever *(Theileria parva)*

PARASITIC
Cysticercosis *(Cysticercus cellulosae)*, trichinosis *(Trichinella spiralis)*

IDIOPATHIC
Eosinophilic myocarditis

pregnancy, poor nutrition, whole-body ionizing radiation, cold environmental temperatures, alcohol ingestion, exercise, and cortisone administration. Much of the myocardial damage in coxsackie B virus infection is induced by immunologic reactions (with T lymphocyte involvement) rather than by direct viral injury.

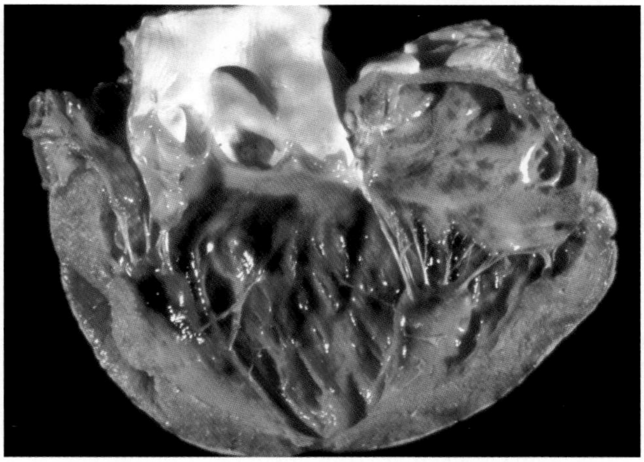

Fig. 10-31 **Endocardial suffusive hemorrhage, heart, left ventricle, calf.** A red to dark-red sheet of suffusive hemorrhage is present in the endocardium of the left ventricle. Suffusive hemorrhage is often attributed to severe septicemia, endotoxemia, anoxia, or electrocution. (Courtesy College of Veterinary Medicine, University of Illinois.)

CARDIAC CONDUCTION SYSTEM

In domestic animals, the responses to injury of the cardiac conduction system are poorly understood but likely involve forms of cell degeneration and death, as well as inflammation as discussed in other sections.

ENDOCARDIUM AND HEART VALVES

Disturbances of Circulation

Hemorrhage

Endocardial hemorrhages are commonly seen and may be the result of trauma or septicemias, especially those with endotoxins, or can occur agonally at death (Fig. 10-31). See the previous sections on the Pericardium and Epicardium and the Myocardium and also Chapter 2.

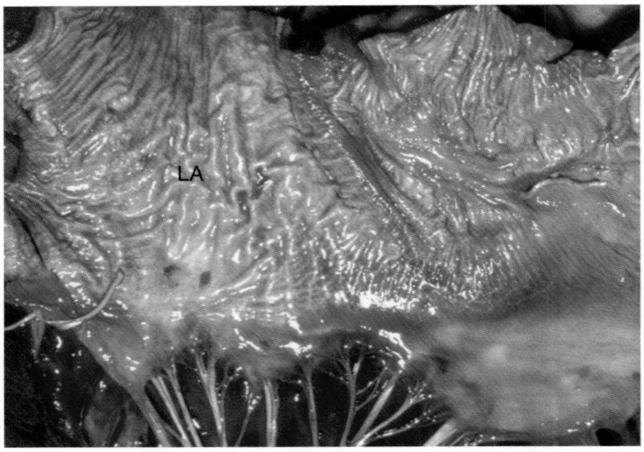

Fig. 10-32 Endocardial mineralization, Johne's disease, heart, left atrial endocardium, cow.
The left atrial *(LA)* endocardium is white, thick, and wrinkled from mineralization. (Courtesy School of Veterinary Medicine, Purdue University.)

Disturbances of Growth

Valvular Anomalies and Dysplasia

See the discussion on valvular anomalies and dysplasia in the section on Endocardium and Heart Valves, Disturbances of Growth, Disorders of Domestic Animals.

Cellular Degeneration and Death

See Chapter 1.

Myxomatous Valvular Degeneration (Endocardiosis)

See the discussion on myxomatous valvular degeneration (endocardiosis) (see Fig. 10-84) in the section on Disorders of Dogs.

Mineralization

Mineralization of the endocardium is seen with Vitamin D toxicity, calcinogenic plant toxicosis in cattle, and calcium phosphorus imbalance, as well as in Johne's disease (Fig. 10-32; see Chapter 7). The endocardium and large elastic arteries are prone to mineralization because of their abundant elastic fibers.

Inflammation

See Chapter 3.

Vegetative Valvular and Mural Endocarditis

Endocarditis is usually the result of bacterial infections, except for lesions produced by migrating *Strongylus vulgaris* larvae in horses and rarely in mycotic infections. The lesions are often very large by the time of death and are present on the valves (valvular endocarditis), although some lesions originate from the underlying myocardium or extend from the affected valve to the adjacent wall (mural endocarditis). Grossly, the affected valves have large, adhering, friable, yellow-to-gray masses of fibrin termed *vegetations,* which can occlude the valvular orifice (see Figs. 10-73, *A,* and 10-76). In chronic lesions, the fibrin deposits are organized by fibrous connective tissue to produce irregular nodular masses termed *verrucae* (wartlike lesions). Microscopically, the lesion consists of accumulated layers of fibrin and numerous embedded bacterial colonies underlain by a zone of infiltrated leukocytes and granulation tissue (see Fig. 10-73, *B*). Relative frequency of valvular involvement with endocarditis in animals is mitral > aortic > tricuspid > pulmonary.

The pathogenesis of endocarditis is complicated and incompletely understood, but the components of Virchow's triad in thrombogenesis—endothelial injury, turbulence, and hypercoagulability—are involved. Affected animals often have preexisting extracardiac infections, such as gingivitis, mastitis, hepatic abscesses or dermatitis, that have resulted in one or more bouts of bacteremia. Turbulent intracardiac blood flow associated with congenital anomalies or the presence of intracardiac and vasculature devices, such as catheters, may contribute to initiation of the lesion. Focal trauma–induced endothelial disruption on the surface of the normally avascular valves allows bacteria to adhere, proliferate, and initiate an inflammatory reaction that results in subsequent deposition of masses of fibrin. Death is the result of cardiac failure from valvular dysfunction or the effects of bacteremia. In some animals, septic emboli lodge in organs such as the heart and kidneys, leading to infarction and localized inflammation or abscess formation. Also see the discussion of vegetative valvular and mural endocarditis in the section on Endocardium, Disorders of Domestic Animals.

Atrial Thrombosis

Atrial thrombi may occur with valvular or myocardial disease and are the result of hemostatic abnormalities resulting from stasis or turbulence.

BLOOD AND LYMPHATIC VASCULAR SYSTEMS

Blood Vessels

The response of blood vessels to injury involves a complex interaction among the cellular and noncellular elements of the vessel wall and the cellular and noncellular elements of the blood. The key cells of vessels in these reactions are endothelial cells and smooth muscle cells. Endothelial cells are metabolically active and provide a thromboresistant monolayer at the interface of blood and the vessel wall unless damaged. Endothelial cells play an important role in fluid distribution, inflammation, angiogenesis, and hemostasis (see Chapter 2). Responses of blood vessels to a variety of toxins are listed in Web Box 10-1.

Key functions of endothelial cells include prostacyclin production, macromolecular transport, and recruitment of inflammatory cells. Injury of endothelial cells is followed by separation from the underlying basement membrane and increased permeability to movement of plasma proteins into the subendothelium. Necrosis of endothelium exposes subendothelial collagen and elicits thrombus formation. Endothelial cells at the margin of denuded areas proliferate and re-endothelialize the damaged area. The arterial intima has regional differences in the uptake of macromolecules, as well as other unique structural and functional features that result in lesion-prone areas of the vasculature. Bilirubin staining of the intima results in yellow discoloration in jaundiced animals (Fig. 10-33).

The other major cellular component of vessels involved in reaction to injury is the smooth muscle cell. These cells have important functions, including production of extracellular components, such as collagen, elastin, and proteoglycans; maintenance of vascular tone; monocyte recruitment; lipoprotein metabolism; production of bioactive lipids, such as prostaglandins; and formation of oxygen-free radicals. These functions are regulated by a wide variety of biochemical mediators such as various growth factors, cytokines, and inflammatory mediators.

Disturbances of Circulation

Hemorrhage

Hemorrhage resulting from vascular injury is a frequent lesion of the epicardium, endocardium, and myocardium. Hemorrhages vary

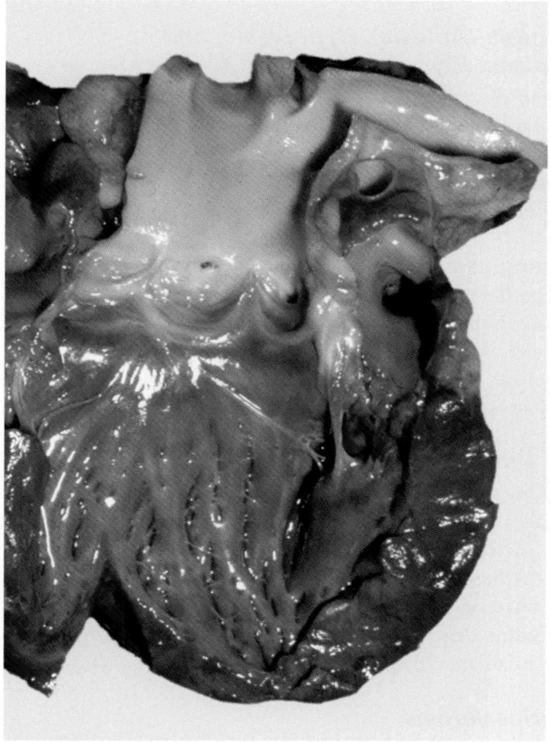

Fig. 10-33 Jaundice, heart, aorta, dog.
Note yellow discoloration of the aortic intima. (Courtesy School of Veterinary Medicine, Purdue University.)

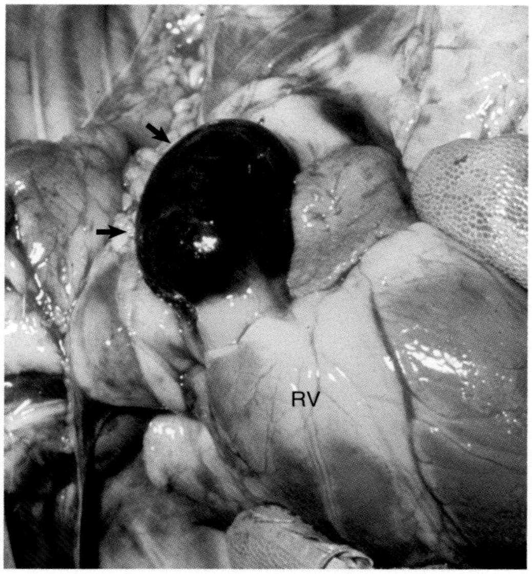

Fig. 10-34 Dissecting aneurysm, copper deficiency, heart, pulmonary artery, right ventricle *(RV)*, pig.
The dark, blood-filled, bulging segment of the wall of the pulmonary artery *(arrows)* has resulted from disruption of elastic fibers. (Courtesy School of Veterinary Medicine, Purdue University.)

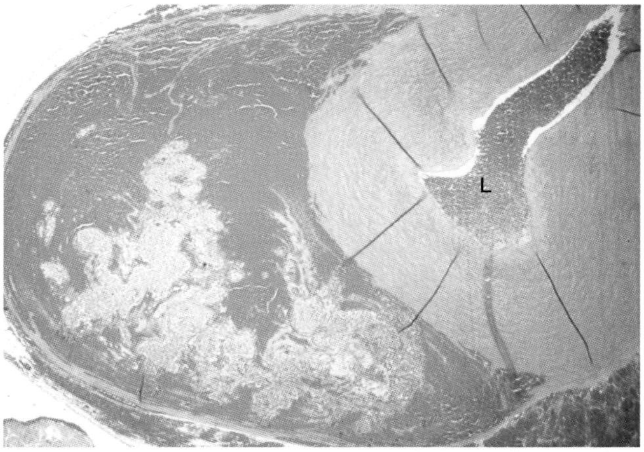

Fig. 10-35 Dissecting aneurysm, aorta, turkey.
Blood has dissected through the tunica media (in a nearby section of the aorta) and in this section has come to lie in the outer layers of the tunica media and adventitia. *L,* Vessel lumen. H&E stain. (Courtesy School of Veterinary Medicine, Purdue University.)

in size from petechiae (1- to 2-mm diameter), to ecchymoses (2- to 10-mm diameter), to suffusive (diffuse). Animals dying from septicemia, endotoxemia, anoxia, or electrocution often have prominent epicardial (see Fig. 10-9) and endocardial (see Fig. 10-31) hemorrhages. Horses dying of any cause usually have agonal hemorrhages on the epicardial and endocardial surfaces. A distinctive example of a specific disease with cardiac hemorrhage is mulberry heart disease, associated with vitamin E–selenium deficiency in growing pigs. In these pigs, hydropericardium accompanies severe myocardial hemorrhage that results in a red, mottled (mulberry-like) appearance of the heart. Also see the previous discussions on disturbances of circulation in the sections on the Pericardium and Epicardium and the Myocardium in the Responses to Injury section.

Effusions

See the previous discussion on disturbances of circulation in the section on the Pericardium and Epicardium.

Hemopericardium

See the previous discussion on hemopericardium under Effusions in the section on Disturbances of Circulation, Pericardium and Epicardium, Responses to Injury and the later discussion on the hemopericardium under Effusions in the section on Disturbances of Circulation, Pericardium and Epicardium, Disorders of Domestic Animals.

Hemothorax and Hemoabdomen

Hemothorax and hemoabdomen arise from spontaneous or traumatic rupture of large arteries or veins or from rupture of aneurysms located in the thoracic or abdominal cavity, respectively. An aneurysm is a localized dilation or outpouching of a thinned and weakened portion of a vessel. Usually, arteries are affected, especially large elastic arteries, but the lesion can also occur in veins. Known causes include copper deficiency in pigs (Fig. 10-34) because copper is necessary for normal development of elastic tissue and damage from infection with *Spirocerca lupi* in dogs or *Strongylus vulgaris* in horses. Most cases are idiopathic. Dissecting aneurysms are infrequent but have been seen in birds, most notably turkeys (Fig. 10-35). They result from disruption of the intima, which allows entry of blood into the media, and this dissects along the wall. Aneurysms can rupture. Usually the consequences are rapidly fatal, as rather large arteries typically are involved. See the later discussion on hemopericardium under Effusions in the section on Disturbances of Circulation, Pericardium and Epicardium, Disorders of Domestic Animals.

Disturbances of Growth

See Chapter 1.

Hypertrophy

Arterial hypertrophy is a response to sustained increases in pressure or volume loads. Affected vessels are generally muscular arteries, and the increase in wall thickness is predominantly caused by hypertrophy (and to some degree, hyperplasia) of smooth muscle cells of the tunica media. Muscular pulmonary arteries of cats are frequently affected, and the lesion has been associated with infection by several parasites, including *Aelurostrongylus abstrusus* (the lungworm of cats), *Toxocara* sp., and *Dirofilaria immitis* (Fig. 10-36). However, the lesions often occur in the absence of parasitic infections (Fig. 10-37). Often, no clinical disease is associated with the lesion in cats, but asthmatic signs have been seen in cats with these parasitic infections. Similar hypertrophy of muscular pulmonary arteries occurs in cattle with hypoxia-induced pulmonary arterial vasoconstriction and subsequent pulmonary hypertension associated with right-sided heart failure from exposure to high altitudes (so-called high-altitude disease or "brisket disease") (see the previous section on Stages of Myocardial Hypertrophy). Also, animals with cardiovascular anomalies that shunt blood left to right result in pulmonary hypertension and have hypertrophy of the muscular pulmonary arteries and can result in plexogenic pulmonary arteriopathy. Uterine arteries in pregnant animals also are hypertrophic.

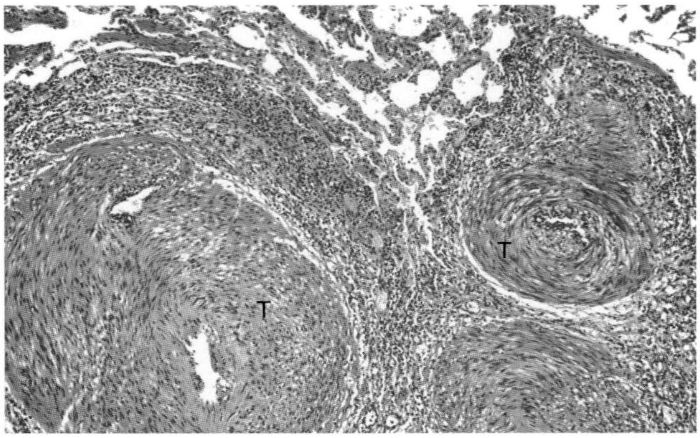

Fig. 10-36 Medial hypertrophy, periarteritis, dirofilariasis, lung, small pulmonary arteries, cat.
Note the massively thickened tunica media *(T)* of the small branches of the pulmonary arteries and their periarterial cuff of chronic inflammatory cells and some eosinophils. H&E stain. (Courtesy School of Veterinary Medicine, Purdue University.)

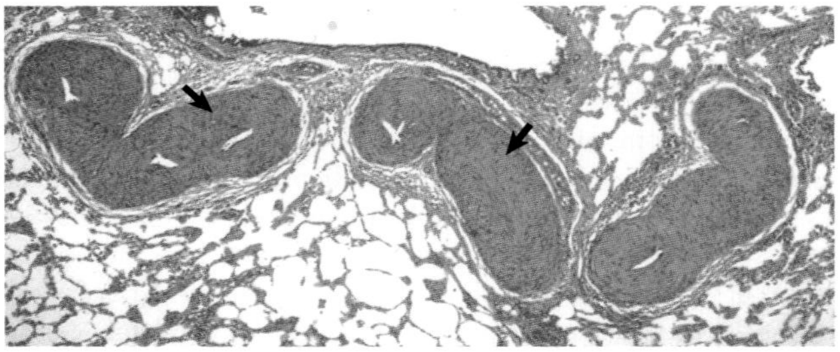

Fig. 10-37 Medial hypertrophy, lung, small pulmonary arteries, cat.
Proliferation of smooth muscle cells *(arrows)* has resulted in marked thickening of the tunica media. Note luminal narrowing. H&E stain. (Courtesy School of Veterinary Medicine, Purdue University.)

Agenesis (Aplasia), Hypoplasia, and Dysplasia (Dysgenesis)

See the discussion on Developmental Errors in the section on Endocardium and Heart Valves, Disorders of Domestic Animals.

Neoplastic Transformation

See Chapter 6; also see the section on Disorders of Dogs.

Hemangiosarcoma

Cardiac hemangiosarcoma is an important neoplasm of dogs and can arise either in the heart (primary) or by metastasis (secondary) from sites such as the spleen. This neoplasm is usually seen in the wall of the right atrium and only occasionally involves the right ventricle (see the section on Disorders of Dogs).

Cell Degeneration and Death

See Chapter 1. Generalized vascular degenerative diseases in animals are classified into the following three principal groups:

- Arteriosclerosis
- Atherosclerosis
- Arterial medial calcification

Hyaline degeneration, fibrinoid necrosis, and amyloidosis also occur in all animal species.

Arteriosclerosis

Arteriosclerosis is characterized by intimal fibrosis of large elastic arteries, atherosclerosis is characterized by intimal and medial lipid deposits in elastic and muscular arteries, and arterial medial calcification has characteristic mineralization of the walls of elastic and muscular arteries.

Arteriosclerosis is an age-related disease that occurs frequently in many animal species but rarely causes clinical signs. The disease develops as chronic degenerative and proliferative responses in the arterial wall and results in loss of elasticity ("hardening of the arteries") and less often luminal narrowing. The abdominal aorta is most frequently affected, but other elastic arteries and peripheral large muscular vessels may be involved. Lesions are often localized around the orifices of arterial branches. Etiologic factors in the development of arteriosclerosis are not well defined, but the significant role of hemodynamic influences is suggested by the frequent involvement at arterial branching sites, in which blood flow is turbulent. Grossly, the lesions are seen as slightly raised, firm, white plaques. Microscopically, initially the intima is thickened by accumulation of mucopolysaccharides and later by the proliferation of smooth muscle cells in the tunica media and fibrous tissue infiltration into the intima. Splitting and fragmentation of the internal elastic lamina are common.

Atherosclerosis

Atherosclerosis, the vascular disease of greatest importance in humans, occurs only infrequently in animals and rarely leads to clinical disease such as infarction of the heart or brain. The principal alteration is accumulation of deposits (atheroma) of lipid, fibrous tissue, and calcium in vessel walls, which eventually results in luminal narrowing. Many studies have established that the pig, rabbit, and chicken are susceptible to the experimental disease produced by the feeding of a high-cholesterol diet; the dog, cat, cow, goat, and rat are resistant. Lesions of the naturally occurring disease have been detected in aged pigs and birds (especially parrots) and in dogs with hypothyroidism and diabetes mellitus that develop an accompanying hypercholesterolemia. Arteries of the heart, mesentery, and kidneys are prominently thickened, firm,

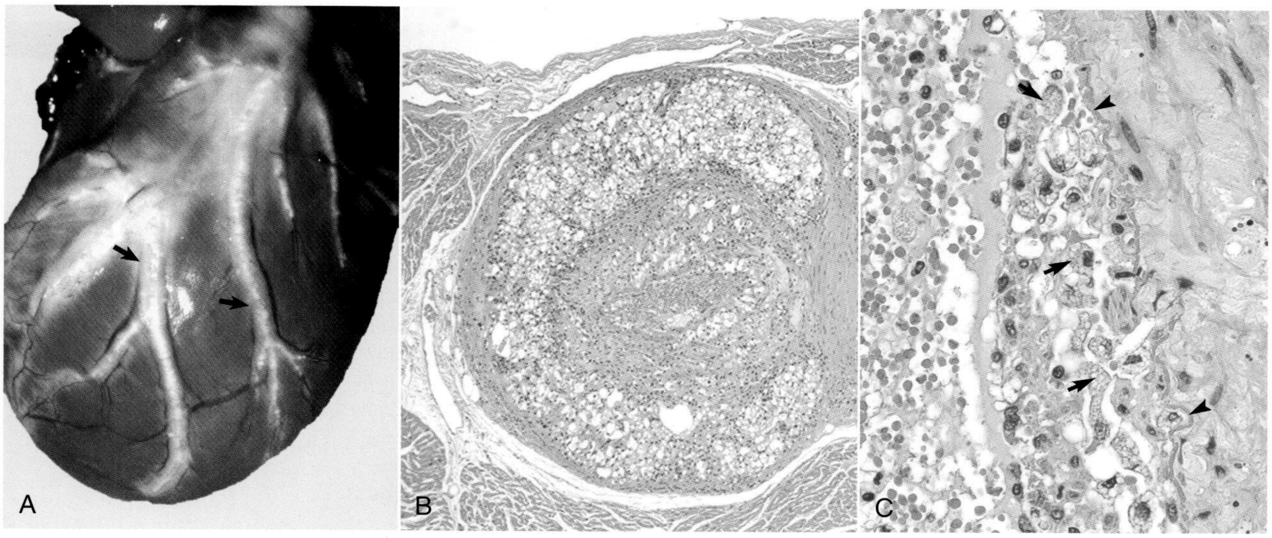

Fig. 10-38 Coronary atherosclerosis, hypothyroidism, heart, left ventricle, dog.
A, The affected coronary arteries are prominent and cordlike *(arrows)* with thickened walls. The diffuse and focal yellow areas in the walls of the arteries are the sites of atheromatous deposits. **B,** Note the extensive accumulation of lipid-laden (clear vacuoles) macrophages termed "foam cells" throughout the thickened tunica intima and media of this branch of the coronary artery. H&E stain. **C,** Higher magnification of **B.** The tunica intima contains abundant lipid-laden macrophages *(arrows).* Note the disruption of the endothelium and the plasma proteins and fibrin on their surfaces. This condition is highly unstable and is prone to activation of Virchow's triad and the coagulation cascade with the formation of mural thrombi and infarction of myocardium supplied by this artery. The arrowheads identify the internal elastic lamina of the tunica intima. H&E stain. (**A** courtesy School of Veterinary Medicine, Purdue University. **B** and **C** courtesy College of Veterinary Medicine, University of Illinois.)

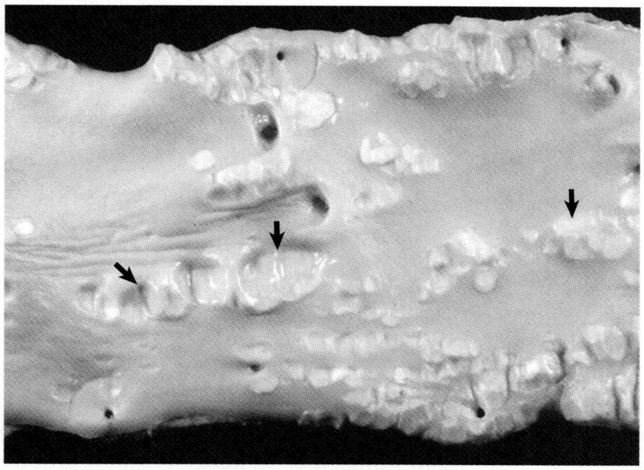

Fig. 10-39 Johne's disease, arteriosclerosis, aorta, cow.
Multiple prominent, white, mineralized foci are in the tunica intima and media *(arrows).* (Courtesy College of Veterinary Medicine, University of Illinois.)

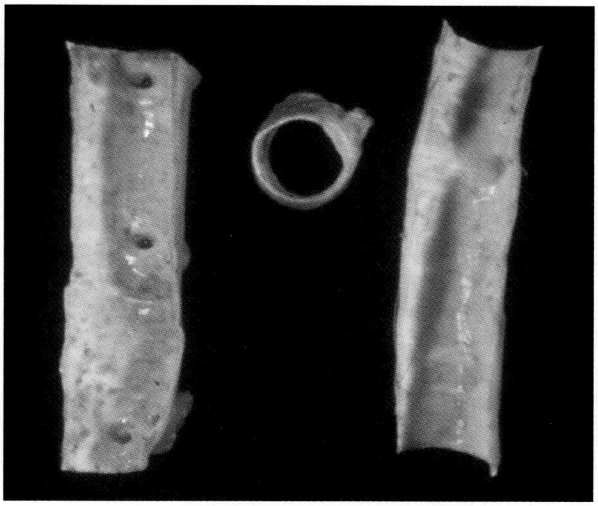

Fig. 10-40 Calcification, vitamin D toxicosis, aorta, rabbit.
The aorta is firm and inelastic because of the calcium deposits in the tunica intima and media. (Courtesy School of Veterinary Medicine, Purdue University.)

and yellow-white (Fig. 10-38, *A*). Microscopically, lipid globules accumulate in the cytoplasm of smooth muscle cells and macrophages, often termed *foam cells,* in the media and intima (Fig. 10-38, *B* and *C*; also see Fig. 3-10). Necrosis and fibrosis develop in some arterial lesions.

Arterial Medial Calcification

Arterial medial calcification is a frequent lesion in animals that often have concurrent endocardial mineralization and involves both elastic and muscular arteries. The causes of arterial medial calcification include calcinogenic plant toxicosis, vitamin D toxicosis, renal insufficiency, and severe debilitation, as seen in cattle with Johne's disease (Fig. 10-39). Medial calcification occurs spontaneously in horses, rabbits, aged guinea pigs, and in rats with chronic renal disease. Affected arteries, such as the aorta, have a unique gross appearance; they appear as solid, dense, pipelike structures with raised, white, solid intimal plaques (Fig. 10-40). Microscopically, in elastic arteries, prominent basophilic granular mineral deposits are present on elastic fibers of the media, but in muscular arteries, they can form a complete ring of mineralization in the tunica media (Fig. 10-41). Siderocalcinosis (so-called iron rings), the result of deposition of both iron and calcium salts, occurs in the cerebral arteries of aged horses. Lesions in the surrounding brain tissue are generally absent. Siderocalcinosis lesions are considered incidental.

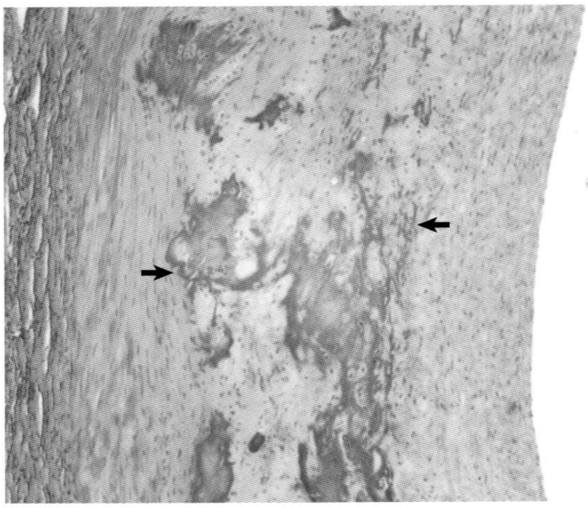

Fig. 10-41 Medial calcification, aorta, cow.
Note the layer of mineralization *(between arrows)* in the middle of the tunica media. H&E stain. (Courtesy Dr. M.D. McGavin, College of Veterinary Medicine, University of Tennessee.)

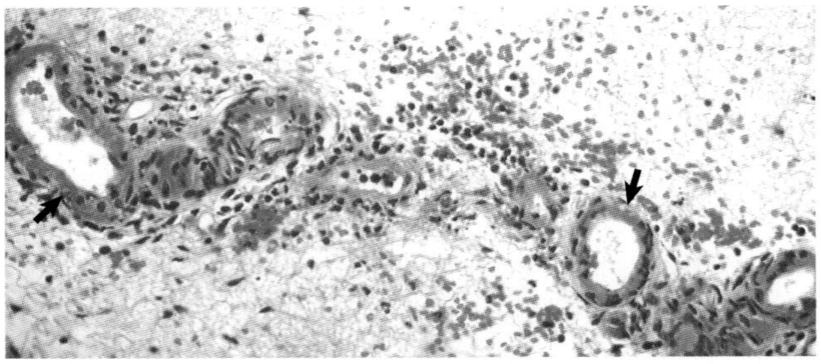

Fig. 10-42 Fibrinoid necrosis of small arteries, edema disease, stomach, submucosa, pig.
Note the circumferential eosinophilic *(arrows)* material in the walls of the arterioles and the extensive edema and mild hemorrhage in surrounding submucosa. H&E stain. (Courtesy School of Veterinary Medicine, Purdue University.)

Hyaline Degeneration, Fibrinoid Necrosis, and Amyloidosis

Hyaline degeneration, fibrinoid necrosis, and amyloidosis are vascular lesions of small muscular arteries and arterioles and occur in all animal species. These lesions are generally not detected grossly, but in some diseases with fibrinoid necrosis of vessels, hemorrhages and edema are seen in affected organs at necropsy. The microscopic feature shared by these lesions is the formation of a homogeneous eosinophilic zone in the vessel wall (Fig. 10-42; also see Fig. 10-79). Special stains allow differentiation into three types: (1) amyloid confirmed by Congo red and methyl violet; (2) fibrinoid deposits, positive by the periodic acid–Schiff technique; and (3) negative staining of hyaline deposits by these stains. Amyloidosis and hyaline degeneration are often observed in small muscular arteries of the myocardium, lungs, and spleen of old dogs. Lesions in the intramyocardial arteries can cause small foci of myocardial infarction.

Fibrinoid necrosis of arteries is associated with endothelial damage and is characterized by entry and accumulation of serum proteins followed by fibrin polymerization in the vessel wall. These materials form an intensely eosinophilic collar that obliterates cellular detail. This lesion is frequent in many acute degenerative and inflammatory diseases of small arteries and arterioles. Fibrinoid necrosis is seen frequently in dogs with uremia and in dogs with hypertension, although hypertension is an uncommon finding in animals.

BOX 10-7 Diseases that Cause Arteritis in Animals

VIRAL
Equine viral arteritis, African horse sickness, equine infectious anemia, equine morbillivirus, malignant catarrhal fever, bovine virus diarrhea, bovine ephemeral fever, bluetongue, hog cholera, African swine fever, feline infectious peritonitis

BACTERIAL
Bartonella henselae, leptospirosis, Salmonellosis, erysipelas *(Erysipelothrix rhusiopathiae)*, *Haemophilus* spp. infections *(Haemophilus suis, Haemophilus somnus, Haemophilus parasuis)*, heartwater *(Ehrlichia ruminantium)*, Rocky Mountain spotted fever *(Rickettsia rickettsii)*, Lyme disease *(Borrelia burgdorferi)*

MYCOTIC
Phycomycosis, aspergillosis

PARASITIC
Equine strongylosis *(Strongylus vulgaris)*, dirofilariasis *(Dirofilaria immitis)*, French heartworm *(Angiostrongylus vasorum)*, spirocercosis *(Spirocerca lupi)*, onchocerciasis, elaeophoriasis (*Elaeophora* sp.), filariasis in primates, aelurostrongylosis

IMMUNE-MEDIATED
Canine systemic lupus erythematosus, rheumatoid arthritis, Aleutian mink disease, polyarteritis nodosa, lymphocytic choriomeningitis, drug-induced hypersensitivity

Inflammation

See Chapter 3.

Arteritis and Vasculitis

Arteritis occurs as a feature of many infectious and immune-mediated diseases (Box 10-7). Often, all types of vessels are affected rather than only arteries, and then *vasculitis* or *angiitis* (a term that includes blood and lymphatic vessels) is the term applied to the lesions. The vascular system serves as the major mechanisms for transport of organisms, e.g. *Bacillus anthracis.* In inflamed vessels, leukocytes are present within and surrounding the walls, and damage to the vessel wall is evident as fibrin deposits or necrotic endothelial and smooth muscle cells. As a result of endothelial damage, thrombosis, which can result in ischemic injury or infarction in the circulatory field, may be present. Arteritis and vasculitis can develop from endothelial injury caused by either infectious agents or immune-mediated mechanisms or may be caused by local extension of suppurative and necrotizing inflammatory processes in adjacent tissues. Arteritis is a prominent feature of several parasitic diseases.

Systemic infections with phlebitis as a lesion include salmonellosis in several species and feline infectious peritonitis. In pigs with various septicemias, such as salmonellosis and colibacillosis, the gastric fundic mucosa is often severely congested and hemorrhagic because of venous endothelial damage and thrombosis. In severe local infections, such as in metritis or hepatic abscesses, inflammation extends into the walls of adjacent veins and produces phlebitis, with or without thrombosis. Intravenous injections of irritant solutions, injecting solutions into the vascular wall, or intimal trauma produced by indwelling venous catheters result in vascular damage and create an opportunity for localization and proliferation of infectious agents and development of phlebitis and thrombosis (Fig. 10-43). Animals with phlebitis complicated by thrombosis have the additional risk of septic embolism, which can cause endocarditis and pulmonary abscesses or pulmonary infarcts.

Many reportable foreign animal diseases are viral diseases, which are endotheliotropic and result in vasculitis; examples include classic swine fever (hog cholera), African horse sickness, and African swine fever (see the sections on disorders of specific animal species).

Thrombosis and Embolism

Coronary and Other Arteries

Thrombosis or embolism of the coronary arteries can result in myocardial infarction (Fig. 10-44) and cardiac failure. These lesions are much less common in animals than in humans. Affected animals generally have one of several types of coronary arterial disease, including atherosclerosis, arteriosclerosis, or periarteritis. In atherosclerosis associated with hypothyroidism or diabetes mellitus (discussed previously), severe lesions are present in the extramural (epicardial) coronary arteries of dogs, but this only rarely leads to thrombosis and myocardial infarction. In contrast, severe arteriosclerosis of intramural cardiac arteries in aged dogs can cause small multifocal myocardial infarcts (see Fig. 10-44). Affected dogs often also have myxomatous valvular degeneration (valvular endocardiosis), which is also an age-related disease. Thrombosis of or embolism to other large arteries, such as the interlobular artery of the kidney, can lead to infarction of the tissue supplied by the artery (Web Fig. 10-19; also see Chapter 2).

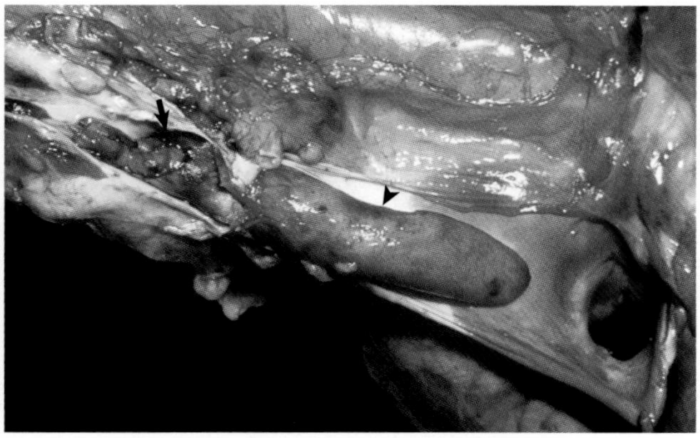

Fig. 10-43 **Thrombus (mural), jugular vein (opened), dog.** Note the nodular mural thrombus *(left [arrow])* in the jugular vein. This thrombus likely occurred at a site of venipuncture and a subsequent phlebitis. The smooth-surfaced red-tan thrombus *(right [arrowhead])* extending toward the heart is a trailing thrombus, a continuation of the mural thrombus. (Courtesy School of Veterinary Medicine, Purdue University.)

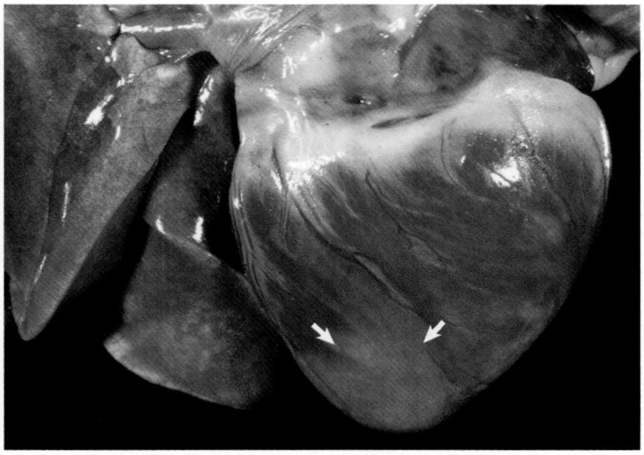

Fig. 10-44 **Myocardial infarction, heart, left and right ventricles, dog.** Pale, necrotic, circumscribed areas *(arrows)* are present in the ventricular walls and are most prominent at the apex. (Courtesy Dr. M.D. McGavin, College of Veterinary Medicine, University of Tennessee.)

LYMPHATIC VESSELS

Disturbances of Circulation

Effusions

Rupture of the Thoracic Duct

Rupture of the thoracic duct, either as a result of trauma or from spontaneous disruption, causes chylothorax in dogs and cats (see Fig. 9-101). However, many cases of chylothorax occur without injury to the thoracic duct and have been attributed to lesions that interfere with central venous return or produce obstruction of the thoracic duct (right-sided heart failure, neoplasms, granulomas, cranial vena cava thrombosis, or dirofilariasis) or that are idiopathic.

Disturbances of Growth

Agenesis (Aplasia), Hypoplasia, Dysplasia (Dysgenesis)

See the discussion on Developmental Errors: Congenital Anomalies in the section on Disturbances of Growth, Lymphatic Vessels, Disorders of Domestic Animals.

Neoplastic Transformation

Tumors arising from lymphatic vessels are benign (lymphangioma) and malignant (lymphangiosarcoma). See Chapter 6 and also the section on Disorders of Dogs.

Inflammation

The endothelial cells lining the lymphatic vessels are subject to the same reactions to injury and inflammation as the vascular system. Inflammation of the lymphatic vessels is called *lymphangitis* and may be seen with specific diseases such as septicemias caused by bacteria like *Salmonella* spp. (Box 10-8). Lymphangitis may be acute, subacute, granulomatous, or chronic resulting in lymphedema. See Chapter 3 and also see the discussion on Glanders

BOX 10-8 Diseases that Cause Lymphangitis in Animals

BACTERIAL

Porcine anthrax *(Bacillus anthracis)*, Johne's disease *(Mycobacterium paratuberculosis)*, tuberculosis (*Mycobacterium* spp.), actinobacillosis *(Actinobacillus lignieresii)*, glanders (farcy) *(Pseudomonas mallei)*, cutaneous streptothricosis *(Dermatophilus congolensis)*, bovine farcy, ulcerative lymphangitis of horses, sporadic lymphangitis of horses, ulcerative lymphangitis *(Corynebacterium pseudotuberculosis, Pseudomonas aeruginosa)*

MYCOTIC

Epizootic lymphangitis of horses *(Histoplasma farciminosum)*, sporotrichosis *(Sporothrix schenckii)*

PARASITIC

Brugia spp. infection of dogs and cats

disease and other cutaneous lymphangitides in the section on Disorders of Horses.

DISORDERS OF DOMESTIC ANIMALS

The most common cardiac diseases in horses, ruminants, pigs, dogs, and cats are summarized in Boxes 10-9 and 10-10. The appearance of the heart with major neoplastic diseases is illustrated in Fig. 10-45. Cardiovascular diseases with known or suspected heritability are listed in Web Box 10-2.

PERICARDIUM AND EPICARDIUM

See the discussion on the pericardium and epicardium in the section on Responses to Injury.

Disturbances of Circulation

Effusions

Hydropericardium

Hydropericardium occurs in those diseases that have generalized edema (see Fig. 10-12). Thus ascites and hydrothorax often occur concurrently with hydropericardium. Congestive heart failure is an important mechanism of hydropericardium and is usually the result of primary myocardial, valvular, congenital, or neoplastic diseases. Common specific diseases include dilated cardiomyopathy of dogs and cats and "ascites syndrome" of poultry. Hydropericardium can also accompany pulmonary hypertension (e.g., "brisket disease" or "high-altitude disease" of cattle), renal failure, and hypoproteinemia from various chronic debilitating diseases. Hydropericardium can also occur in various systemic diseases with vascular injury, such as septicemia in pigs, "heartwater" *(Cowdria ruminantium* infection) in small ruminants, African horse sickness, and bovine ephemeral fever.

Hemopericardium

Bleeding into the pericardial sac can result from spontaneous atrial rupture in dogs, atrial rupture in dogs with hemangiosarcoma, rupture of the intrapericardial aorta or pulmonary artery in horses, or as a complication of intracardiac injections (see Figs. 10-10 and 10-11).

BOX 10-9 Most Common Cardiac Diseases of Horses and Production Animals

HORSES

Fibrinous pericarditis
Toxic cardiomyopathy (ionophores, white snakeroot)
Endocardial fibrosis and calcification
Endocarditis

RUMINANTS (CATTLE, SHEEP, AND GOATS)

White muscle disease (vitamin E–selenium deficiency)
Cardiotoxicity (ionophores, gossypol, *Cassia occidentalis, Karwinskia humboldtiana*)
Brisket disease (high altitude disease)
Pericarditis
Endocarditis
Malignant lymphoma

PIGS

Mulberry heart disease (vitamin E–selenium deficiency)
Pericarditis
Endocarditis

BOX 10-10 Most Common Cardiac Diseases in Dogs and Cats

DOGS

1. Myxomatous valvular degeneration (valvular endocardiosis)
2. Congenital heart disease
3. Dilated cardiomyopathy
4. Hemorrhagic pericardial effusion
5. Cardiac neoplasia
6. Dirofilariasis

CATS

1. Hypertrophic cardiomyopathy
2. Dilated cardiomyopathy
3. Hyperthyroidism-associated hypertrophy
4. Congenital heart disease

Disturbances of Growth

Developmental Errors: Congenital Anomalies

Peritoneopericardial Diaphragmatic Hernias

Peritoneopericardial diaphragmatic hernias occur in cats and dogs with incomplete development of the diaphragm. Abdominal viscera can be located in the pericardial sac.

Pericardial Agenesis

The absence of a pericardial sac has been reported rarely in animals.

Atrophy

See the previous discussion on serous atrophy of fat in the section on the Pericardium and Epicardium, in the Responses to Injury section.

Inflammation

Pericarditis

See the discussion on pericarditis in the section on the Pericardium and Epicardium, Responses to Injury.

Fibrinous Pericarditis

Hematogenous spread of specific organisms may result in fibrinous pericarditis. Mannheimiosis, blackleg, coliform septicemias,

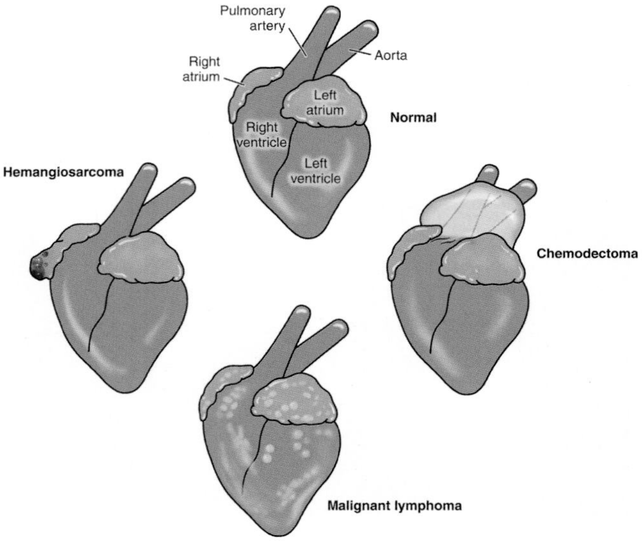

Fig. 10-45 Schematic diagram of the locations of the major cardiac neoplasms.
(Redrawn with permission from School of Veterinary Medicine, Purdue University.)

contagious bovine pleuropneumonia, sporadic bovine encephalomyelitis, and in utero *Brucella* spp. and *Arcanobacter pyogenesis* fetal septicemias may all produce fibrinous pericarditis. In sheep, Mannheimiosis and streptococcal infections most commonly result in fibrinous pericarditis. Sterile swabs of the pericardial exudates are recommended to identify the causative organism.

MYOCARDIUM

See the discussion on the myocardium in the section on Responses to Injury.

Disturbances of Growth

Developmental Errors: Congenital Anomalies

The complex events involved in the embryologic development of the heart and great vessels allow substantial opportunities for congenital anomalies to develop (see Fig. 10-1). The functional significance of these anomalies varies widely. Animals with the most extreme defects are unable to survive in utero, and those with the mildest lesions could have no clinical signs of disease during life. However, animals with defects of intermediate severity are most likely to be presented to a veterinarian because of gradually developing signs of cardiac failure, including poor exercise tolerance, cyanosis, and stunted body growth. Ectopia cordis is a congenital development of the heart at an abnormal site outside of the thoracic cavity. In cattle, cases in healthy adult animals have been described in which the heart was located subcutaneously in the caudoventral neck area. The most frequently observed cardiovascular anomalies in domestic animals are listed in Box 10-11.

BOX 10-11 Most Common Cardiovascular Anomalies in Domestic Animal Species

HORSES
Ventricular septal defect
Patent ductus arteriosus
Persistent truncus arteriosus

RUMINANTS (CATTLE, SHEEP, AND GOATS)
Valvular hematomas
Patent foramen ovale
Ventricular septal defect
Transposition of aorta and pulmonary artery

PIGS
Subaortic stenosis
Endocardial cushion defects

DOGS
Patent ductus arteriosus
Pulmonic stenosis
Subaortic stenosis
Persistent right aortic arch
Ventricular septal defect

CATS
Endocardial cushion defects
Mitral malformation
Ventricular septal defect
Endocardial fibroelastosis
Patent ductus arteriosus

The causes of congenital cardiovascular anomalies are varied. Most animal species have a low background frequency of spontaneous cardiac malformations. In many species, especially in dogs, these defects are heritable and can be attributed to either single or multiple gene effects. Under experimental conditions, cardiovascular congenital defects can be elicited by exposure of pregnant dams to various chemicals and drugs, physical agents, toxins, or nutritional deficiencies. Chemical compounds implicated include thalidomide, ethanol, salicylates, griseofulvin, and cortisone. Prenatal exposure to x-irradiation or fetal hypoxia can induce defects. Maternal nutritional deficiencies of vitamin A, pantothenic acid, riboflavin, or zinc and excess intake of vitamin A, retinoic acid, or copper can result in cardiovascular anomalies in newborn animals. Infectious diseases have been incriminated, but not confirmed, in cardiovascular defects; they include bluetongue infections in sheep, bovine virus diarrhea in cattle, and parvoviral infections in dogs and cats.

Sites of the major cardiovascular anomalies in the dog are shown in Fig. 10-46.

Failure of Closure of Fetal Cardiovascular Shunts

Interventricular Septal Defect

A ventricular septal defect indicates failure of complete development of the interventricular septum and allows the shunting of blood between the ventricles (Fig. 10-47). The defect occurs in many species and more commonly in the upper, membranous portion of the interventricular septum rather than in the lower, muscular septum. Among breeds of dogs, the greatest frequency has been observed in the English bulldog, English springer spaniel, and West Highland white terrier.

Atrial Septal Defect

An atrial septal defect could represent the failure of closure of the foramen ovale, which is an interatrial septal shunt that allows blood to bypass the lungs of the fetus, or it can be the result of true septal defects at another site because of faulty development of the interatrial septum (Fig. 10-48). Although this defect occurs in all domestic animal species, dog breeds with greatest frequency of this defect are the Boxer, Doberman pinscher, and Samoyed.

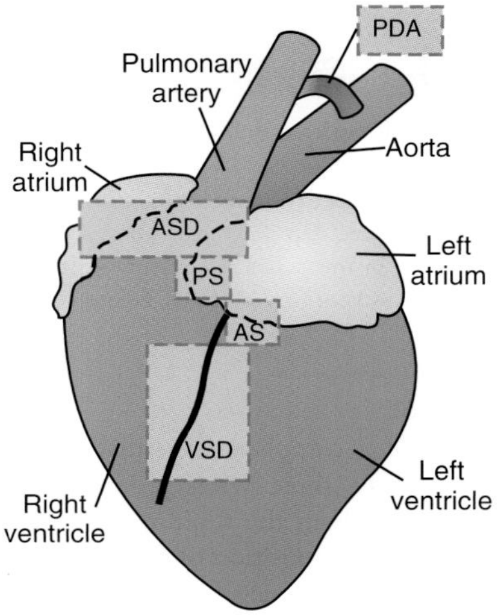

Fig. 10-46 Schematic diagram of the sites of the major cardiovascular anomalies of the dog.
AS, Aortic stenosis; *ASD,* atrial septal defect; *PDA,* patent ductus arteriosus; *PS,* pulmonic stenosis; *VSD,* ventricular septal defect. (Redrawn with permission from School of Veterinary Medicine, Purdue University.)

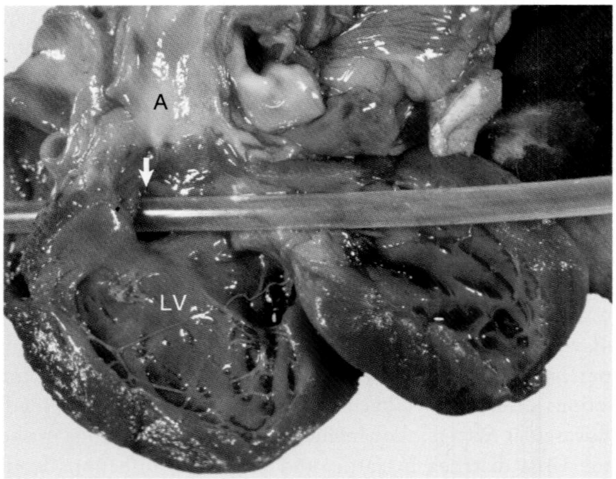

Fig. 10-47 Ventricular septal defect (high defect), heart, opened left side, calf.
Note the large opening in the basal portion of the ventricular septum *(arrow)* immediately below the aortic valve through which the tube has been passed. *A,* Aorta; *LV,* left ventricle. (Courtesy Dr. M. D. McGavin, College of Veterinary Medicine, University of Tennessee.)

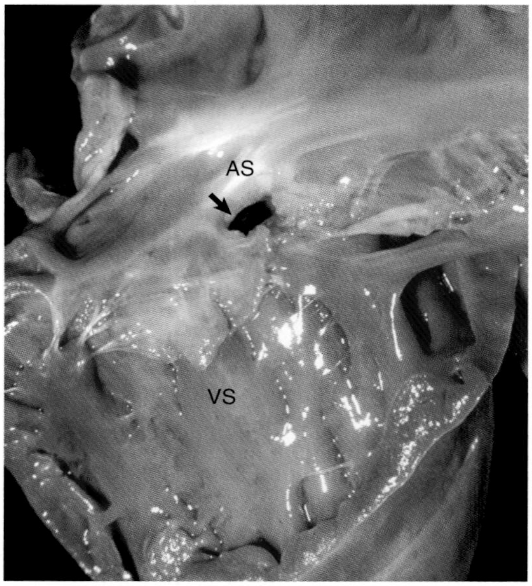

Fig. 10-48 Endocardial cushion defect and tricuspid dysplasia, heart, opened right side, pig.
The endocardial cushion defect (prominent opening *[arrow]*) can be mistaken as an atrial septal defect but not the location and presence of abnormal valves incorporated in the defect. *AS,* Atrial septum; *VS,* Ventricular septum. (Courtesy School of Veterinary Medicine, Purdue University.)

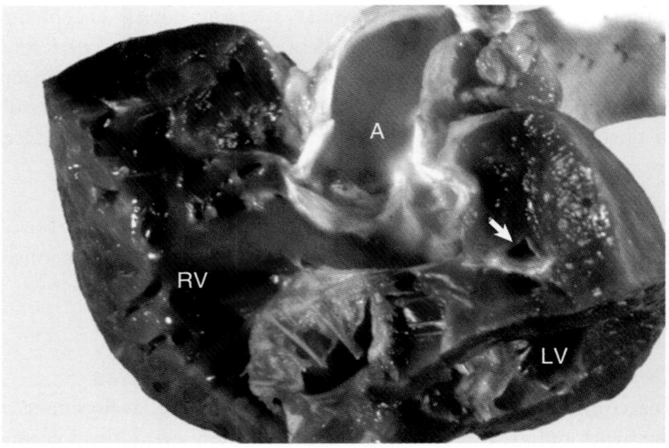

Fig. 10-49 Tetralogy of Fallot, heart, dissected, dog.
Above the large membranous ventricular septal defect is an overlying, straddling aorta *(A).* There is also severe pulmonic stenosis *(arrow)* with massive right ventricular hypertrophy. *LV,* Left ventricle; *RV,* right ventricle. (Courtesy School of Veterinary Medicine, Purdue University.)

BOX 10-12 Cardiomyopathies in Animals

PRIMARY CARDIOMYOPATHIES (IDIOPATHIC)

Hypertrophic: Cat, dog, rat, pig
Dilated (congestive): Cat, dog, hamster, turkey, pig, cow, sea otters, sea lions, cynomolgus monkeys
Restrictive: Cat
Arrhythmogenic right ventricular cardiomyopathy: Dog, cat

SECONDARY CARDIOMYOPATHIES (SPECIFIC HEART MUSCLE DISEASES)

Heritable (known or suspected): Hereditary cardiomyopathy of hamsters, mice, rats, turkeys, and cattle; Duchenne's type, x-linked muscular dystrophy of golden retriever dogs with dystrophin deficiency; glycogenoses
Nutritional deficiencies: See list in Box 10-5; other examples include taurine deficiency in cats and foxes
Toxic: See list in Box 10-5; other examples include anthracycline toxicity, furazolidone toxicity, NaCl toxicity
Physical injuries and shock: See list in Box 10-5
Endocrine disorders: Hyperthyroidism, acromegaly (hypersomatotropism), hypothyroidism, glucocorticoid excess, functional pheochromocytoma, diabetes mellitus
Infections: See lists in Boxes 10-6, 10-7, and 10-8
Neoplastic infiltration: Malignant lymphoma
Systemic hypertension in cats and dogs: Spontaneous or associated with chronic renal disease, hyperthyroidism, diabetes mellitus, acromegaly, primary aldosteronism

Tetralogy of Fallot

Tetralogy of Fallot is a complicated cardiac anomaly with four lesions (Fig. 10-49). The three primary defects are a ventricular septal defect located high in the septum, pulmonic stenosis (see later discussion), and dextroposition of the aorta (see later discussion). The fourth defect, which develops secondarily, is hypertrophy of the right ventricular myocardium. This complex anomaly is inherited in Keeshond dogs and is frequent in English bulldogs. Cyanosis is often an associated clinical sign. The anomaly is one of the most common cardiac abnormalities seen in hearts of humans (so-called blue babies). In genetic and pathologic studies of Keeshond dogs, the basic defect has been determined to be hypoplasia and malpositioning of the conotruncal septum. Wide variability in the severity of the lesions has been observed. The inheritance pattern in Keeshonds is a simple autosomal locus with partial penetration in heterozygotes and complete penetrance in homozygotes.

Hypertrophy and Atrophy

Cardiomyopathies

Primary and secondary cardiomyopathies (Box 10-12) represent important, sometimes inherited, generalized myocardial diseases of either idiopathic or known causation that can result in either hypertrophy or atrophy of the affected myocardium. Primary or idiopathic cardiomyopathies are progressive cardiac diseases. These diseases affect cats, dogs, and cattle and resemble some diseases of humans. These diseases are divided into three morphologic types: hypertrophic, dilated, and restrictive cardiomyopathies. Secondary cardiomyopathies (also termed *specific heart muscle diseases*) are generalized myocardial diseases of known cause.

Hypertrophic cardiomyopathy (hypertrophy)

Hypertrophic cardiomyopathy occurs frequently in cats, especially in young adult to middle-aged males (1 to 3 years old), and is seen infrequently in dogs, usually affecting males of large breeds. Cats usually have congestive heart failure, and approximately 10% to 20% have posterior paresis from concurrent thromboembolism of the caudal abdominal aorta ("saddle thrombosis") secondary to left atrial thrombosis. Hypertrophic cardiomyopathy is inherited as an autosomal dominant trait with complete penetrance in Maine coon cats. The occurrence of clusters of cases in Persians, American shorthairs, and ragdoll cat breeds strongly suggests heritability of the disease in some cases. Some cats and dogs die unexpectedly as the only clinical expression of the disease. This clinical presentation also is often seen in humans with the disease. In both cats and dogs, the hearts are enlarged and have prominent hypertrophy of the left ventricle and interventricular septum (Fig. 10-50). The left ventricular cavity is small and the left atrium is dilated. In a few cases, the interventricular septum is disproportionately hypertrophied in relation to the remainder of the myocardium. Microscopically, the lesions of the myocardium are prominent disarrays or disorganizations of myocytes, with interweaving rather than parallel arrangement of fibers (Fig. 10-51; Web Fig. 10-20). Myocyte hypertrophy, various degenerative alterations in myocytes, and interstitial fibrosis also are present.

Dilated or congestive cardiomyopathy

Dilated or congestive cardiomyopathy is an important cause of congestive heart failure in cats and dogs. Many affected cats and some dogs have low tissue concentrations of taurine, and supplementation of cats with taurine has reversed the clinical signs of cardiac failure. Routine taurine supplementation of feline commercial diets has resulted in a dramatic reduction in cases of dilated cardiomyopathy. Taurine-deficient foxes also develop cardiac failure. Cattle with dilated cardiomyopathy in Switzerland and Japan have an autosomal recessive mode of inheritance.

Affected cats often are middle-aged males, and affected dogs often are males of large breeds such as Doberman pinschers, Portuguese water dogs, dalmatians, Scottish deerhounds, Irish wolfhounds, Saint Bernards, Afghan hounds, Newfoundland dogs, Old English sheepdogs, Great Danes, and boxers, although smaller breeds, such as English cocker spaniels, may be affected. The disease often has a familial pattern in the affected breeds and appears to be inherited as an autosomal recessive or X-linked recessive trait. Some cats also develop aortic thromboembolism. At necropsy, lesions of congestive heart failure are present and the hearts are rounded because of biventricular dilation (Figs. 10-52 and 10-53). The dilated cardiac chambers often have a diffusely white, thickened endocardium. Microscopic and ultrastructural alterations are nonspecific, can be either mild or absent, and may include interstitial fibrosis and fatty infiltration and changes of myocyte degeneration, including the occurrence of so-called attenuated wavy fibers.

Restrictive cardiomyopathy

Restrictive cardiomyopathy occurs infrequently. It occurs in cats as one of two types of endocardial lesions that result in impaired ventricular filling. In one type, the left ventricular endocardium has diffuse notable fibrosis. Available evidence suggests that the fibrotic lesion is preceded by endomyocarditis. The second type results from excessive moderator bands that traverse the left ventricular cavity. Other examples of restrictive cardiomyopathy in animals include endocardial fibrosis in certain strains of aged rats and congenital endocardial fibroelastosis in Burmese cats (Fig. 10-54).

Molecular mechanisms of hereditary cardiomyopathies

Our understanding of the molecular mechanisms of the hereditary cardiomyopathies is developing rapidly. In humans with familial hypertrophic cardiomyopathy inherited in an autosomal

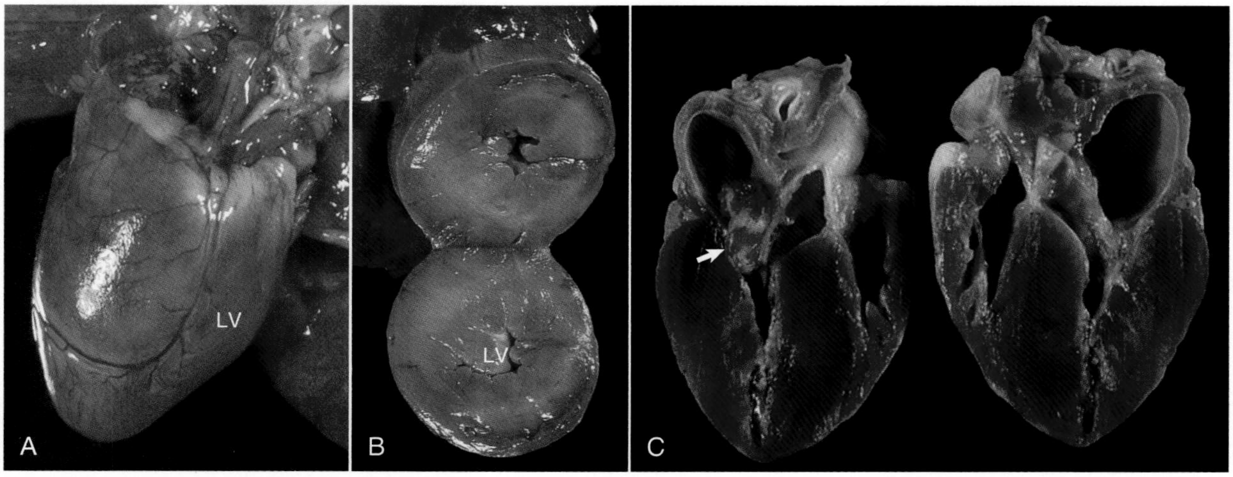

Fig. 10-50 Hypertrophic cardiomyopathy, heart, cat.

A, Note the thickened left ventricular wall *(LV)*. **B,** The thickened left ventricular free wall and septum have markedly reduced the lumen of the left ventricle *(LV)*. **C,** There is severe diffuse concentric hypertrophy of the left ventricular free wall, interventricular septum, and papillary muscles. Left atrial dilation is present. There is a fibrotic plaque *(arrow)* of the midinterventricular septum where the hypertrophied papillary muscle contacts the septum. (**A** and **B** courtesy Dr. W. Crowell, College of Veterinary Medicine, The University of Georgia; and Noah's Arkive, College of Veterinary Medicine, The University of Georgia. **C** courtesy Ettinger SJ, Feldman EC (eds): *Textbook of veterinary internal medicine. Diseases of the dog and cat,* vol 2, ed 7, Philadelphia, 2010, Saunders.)

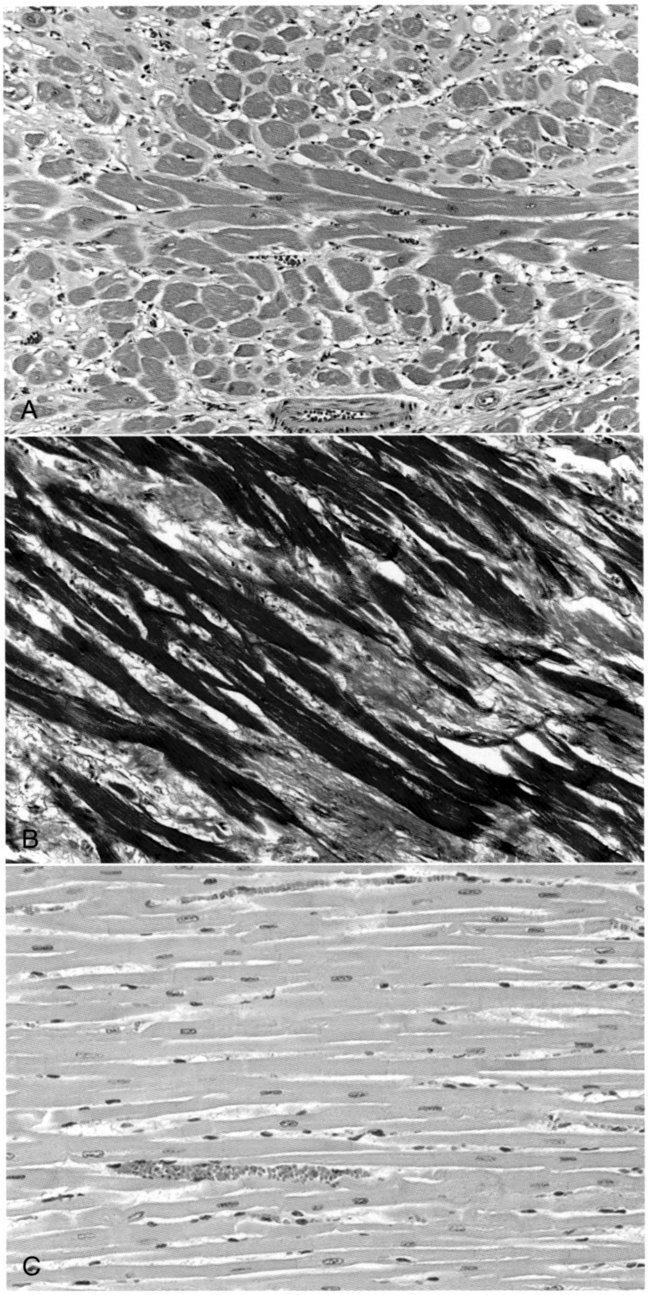

Fig. 10-51 Hypertrophic cardiomyopathy, heart, ventricular myocardium, cat.

A, Cardiac myocytes are hypertrophied and in disarray. H&E stain. **B,** Masson's trichrome stain demonstrates abundant amounts of interstitial collagen *(blue)* produced by fibroblasts. **C,** Normal cardiac myocytes arranged in parallel bundles. H&E stain. (**A** and **B** courtesy Atlantic Veterinary College, University of Prince Edward Island. **C** courtesy Dr. L. Borst, College of Veterinary Medicine.)

dominant manner, a variety of single-gene mutations have been documented. The mutations affect genes that encode sarcomere proteins of cardiac myocytes. Altered cardiac proteins include cardiac α- and β-myosin heavy chain, cardiac troponin T and I, and Ca-tropomyosin, actin, titin, ventricular myosin essential light chain, ventricular myosin regulatory light chain, and cardiac myosin-binding protein C. It remains unclear how these mutant proteins result in functional and structural alterations of cardiac

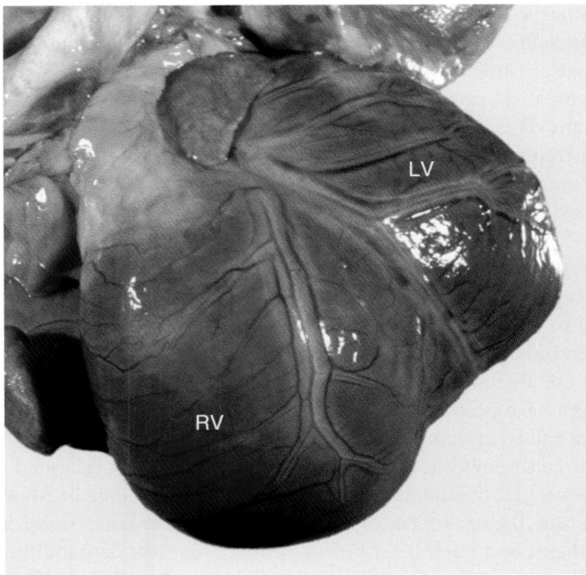

Fig. 10-52 Dilated (congestive) cardiomyopathy, heart, left ventricle *(LV)* and right ventricle *(RV)*, dog.

Biventricular dilation has resulted in the heart having a double apex. (Courtesy Dr. T. Boosinger, College of Veterinary Medicine, Auburn University; and Noah's Arkive, College of Veterinary Medicine, The University of Georgia.)

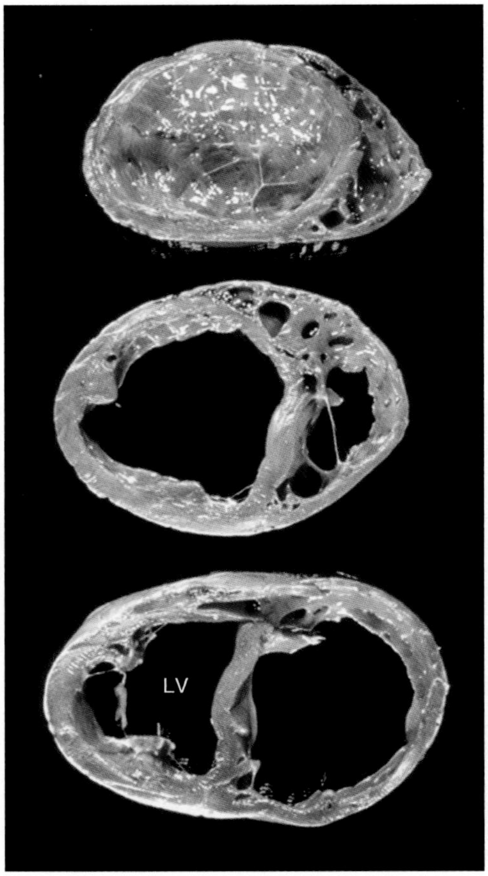

Fig. 10-53 Dilated (congestive) cardiomyopathy, heart, ventricles, cross-section, dog.

The left ventricle *(LV)* and right ventricle have thin walls, dilated chambers, and white fibrotic endocardium. (Courtesy Dr. Y. Niyo, College of Veterinary Medicine, Iowa State University; and Noah's Arkive, College of Veterinary Medicine, The University of Georgia.)

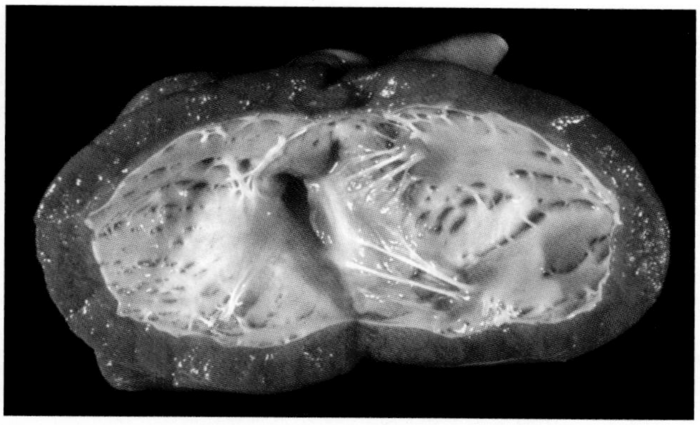

Fig. 10-54 Subendocardial fibroelastosis, heart, left ventricle, dog. The endocardium is opaque because increased amounts of collagen and elastic fibers were deposited in the subendocardium secondary to turbulence of blood flow within the ventricles. This dog had a persistent ductus arteriosus. This lesion may have a hereditary basis in Burmese cats and is often a sequela to turbulence within ventricles in cardiac disease. (Courtesy College of Veterinary Medicine, University of Illinois.)

muscle cells. However, recent studies suggest that shortening of telomeres (structures that cap the ends of chromosomes) triggers apoptosis of cardiac muscle cells and may explain the end-stage finding of myocardial fibrosis in heart failure of various causes, including cardiomyopathy. Some similar gene mutations and altered proteins were recently discovered in the various heritable cardiomyopathies of animals (e.g. cardiac myosin-binding protein C in Maine Coon cats and Ragdoll cats with hypertrophic cardiomyopathy). Also, a portion of cases of dilated cardiomyopathy in humans appears to be inherited. In these patients, alterations in several myocytic proteins, including dystrophin, actin, desmin, troponin T, β-myosin heavy chain, lamin, and taffazin, and alterations in the cardiac calcium regulating protein phospholamban have been documented.

Neoplastic Transformation

Various primary and secondary neoplasms develop either in or near the heart. Primary neoplasms include rhabdomyoma, rhabdomyosarcoma, schwannoma, and hemangiosarcoma. Rhabdomyomas and rhabdomyosarcomas are rare in animals and form white to gray nodules in the myocardium that often project into the cardiac chambers. Congenital rhabdomyomatosis in pigs and guinea pigs is a nonneoplastic hamartoma (i.e., malformation often resembling a neoplasm that is composed of an overgrowth of mature cells and tissues that normally occur in the affected organ). Single or multiple, pale, poorly circumscribed areas are scattered in the myocardium and are composed of large glycogen-laden myocytes.

Malignant lymphoma (lymphosarcoma) is the most common secondary neoplasm occurring in the heart and often causes lesions in the hearts of cattle, which can be severe enough to cause death from cardiac failure. Cardiac lesions may be present in dogs and cats with malignant lymphoma. The neoplastic cell infiltration can be diffuse or nodular and involve the myocardium, endocardium, and pericardium. Lymphomatous tissue appears as white masses that may resemble deposits of fat (Fig. 10-55). Microscopically, extensive infiltrations of neoplastic lymphocytes are present between myocytes (Fig. 10-56). Other neoplasms, such as malignant melanomas, occasionally have metastatic lesions in the heart.

Heart-based tumors are primary neoplasms of extracardiac tissues in dogs and rarely cats. They arise at the base of the heart and can produce vascular obstruction and cardiac failure. The most

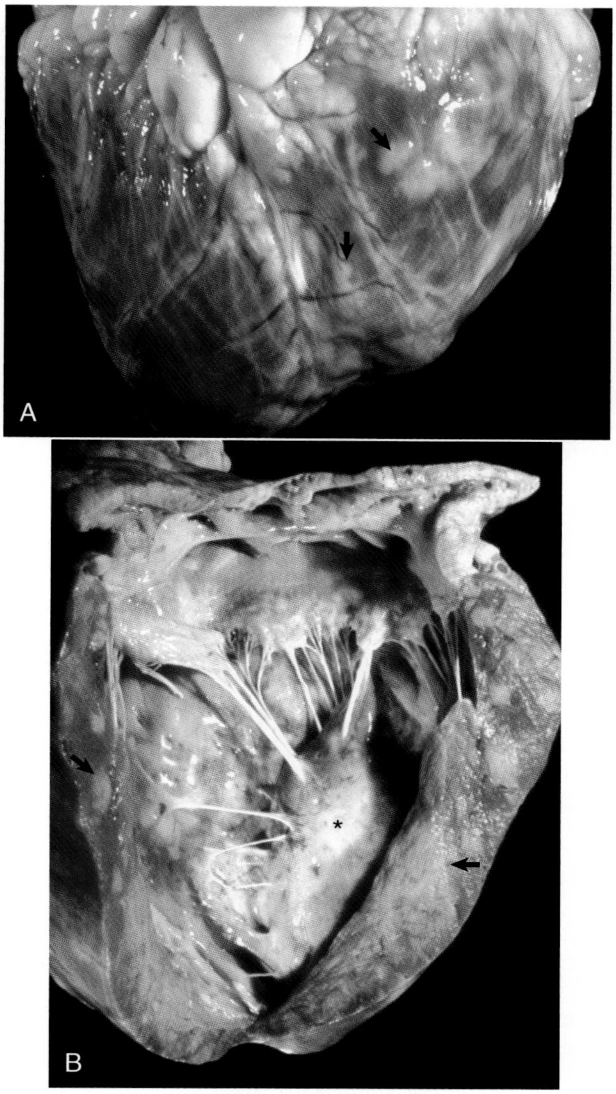

Fig. 10-55 Lymphosarcoma, heart, myocardium, cow. **A,** Sites of infiltrating neoplastic lymphocytes in the ventricular myocardium are evident as numerous white areas and nodules *(arrows)*. **B,** Similar white areas of tumor are visible in the section of the left ventricular wall *(arrows)* and subendocardially *(asterisk)* in the ventricular septum. (Courtesy College of Veterinary Medicine, University of Illinois.)

common neoplasm arising at this location is the aortic body tumor or paraganglioma (chemodectoma), but occasionally, ectopic thyroid or parathyroid tissue gives origin to neoplasms in this area. The aortic body is a chemoreceptor organ. In some cases, aortic body tumors become large, white, firm masses that surround and compress the great vessels and atria (Fig. 10-57). Brachycephalic dog breeds are most frequently affected. Microscopically, the neoplastic cells are polyhedral with vacuolated cytoplasm and are supported by a fine connective tissue stroma (see Fig. 12-55).

Cell Degeneration and Death

Toxicoses

The mechanisms of cardiotoxicities include (1) exaggerated pharmacologic action of drugs acting on cardiovascular tissues, (2) exposure to substances that depress myocardial function, (3) direct injury of cardiac muscle cells by chemicals, and (4) hypersensitivity reactions.

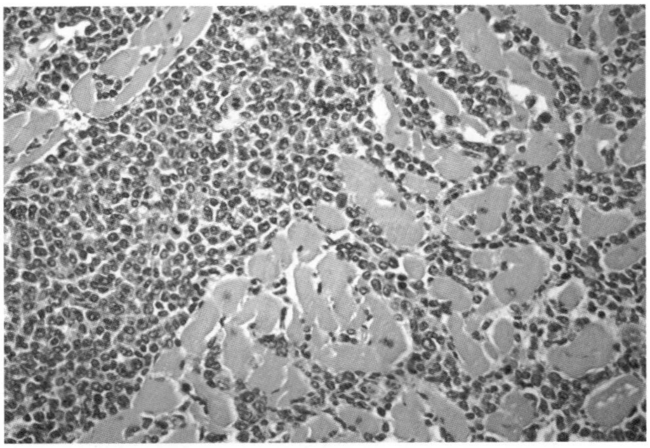

Fig. 10-56 Lymphosarcoma, heart, section of myocardium, cow. Neoplastic lymphocytes have extensively infiltrated between the cardiomyocytes. Extensive infiltration can result in myocyte atrophy and loss. H&E stain. (Courtesy School of Veterinary Medicine, Purdue University.)

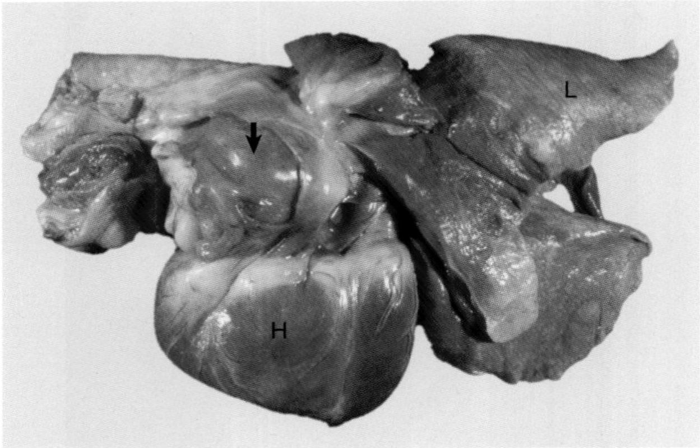

Fig. 10-57 Chemodectoma (heart base tumor), aortic body, dog. Note the large mass *(arrow)* at the base of the heart *(H)*. *L*, Lungs. (Courtesy College of Veterinary Medicine, University of Illinois.)

Plant Toxins

White snakeroot–induced myocardial degeneration

See the discussion on white snakeroot–induced myocardial degeneration in the section on Disorders of Horses.

Chemical Toxins

Ionophore-induced myocardial degeneration

See the discussion on ionophore-induced myocardial degeneration in the section on Disorders of Horses.

Gossypol-induced myocardial degeneration

See the discussion on gossypol-induced myocardial degeneration in the section on Disorders of Ruminants.

Chemotherapeutic agent-induced myocardial degeneration

Cardiotoxicity has emerged as a significant clinical entity in veterinary medicine in recent years with the growing use of antineoplastic drugs in small animal practice and the widespread use of growth promotants in ruminants (see Fig. 10-69).

Myocardial Necrosis and Mineralization

Myocardial necrosis and mineralization can result from a number of causes, including nutritional deficiencies, chemical and plant toxins, ischemia, metabolic disorders, heritable diseases, and physical injuries (see Box 10-5). From this large list of causes of myocardial injury, some of the most frequently observed current examples are ionophore toxicity in horses and ruminants, vitamin E–selenium deficiency in the young of all species, "heart-brain syndrome" of dogs (see Fig. 10-83), anthracycline toxicity in dogs, and gossypol toxicosis in pigs. In various localized areas throughout the world, numerous deaths in ruminants have resulted from consumption of poisonous plants such as *Acacia georginae* and *Dichapetalum cymosum*.

Mulberry Heart Disease

See the discussion of mulberry heart disease in the section on Disorders of Pigs.

Brain-Heart Syndrome

See the discussion on brain-heart syndrome in Chapter 14.

Inflammation

Myocarditis

See the discussion on inflammation in the section on Myocardium, Responses to Injury.

Bacterial Septicemias

See the discussion on bacterial septicemias in Chapter 4.

CARDIAC CONDUCTION SYSTEM

See the discussion on the cardiac conduction system in the section on Responses to Injury.

Disturbances of Growth

Neoplastic Transformation

Schwannomas

Schwannomas involve cardiac nerves in cattle and appear as single or multiple white nodules detected as incidental findings at slaughter (see Fig. 14-115).

Cell Degeneration and Death

Conduction system diseases have been described mainly in dogs and horses, probably because clinical cardiac evaluations are done most frequently in these species. Secondary conduction system disorders result from myocardial disease (inflammation, neoplasia, or degeneration) near the conduction system. Specific presumably inherited diseases in dogs include (1) syncope in pug dogs with lesions of the bundle of His; (2) intermittent sinus arrest in deaf dalmatian dogs, presumably associated with lesions in the sinus node; (3) sinoatrial syncope (sick sinus dysfunction) in female miniature schnauzers, West Highland white terriers, cocker spaniels, and dachshunds; (4) inherited ventricular arrhythmia and sudden unexpected death in German shepherds, and (5) widespread conduction pathology in Alaskan sled dogs that died suddenly and unexpectedly in a race. Other arrhythmias in dogs and horses are atrial fibrillation and heart block. Dogs with atrial fibrillation often have concurrent congestive heart failure and have atrial dilation with AV valve insufficiency, but most horses live a normal or near-normal lifespan, may respond to cardioversion, and at necropsy have atrial myocardial fibrosis. Heart block of the first degree (delay of impulse through AV node), second degree (intermittent failure to conduct through the AV node with dropped beats), and third degree (complete) has been associated with myocardial lesions, such as areas of scarring, in horses and dogs. Second-degree heart block is considered to be a normal phenomenon in horses.

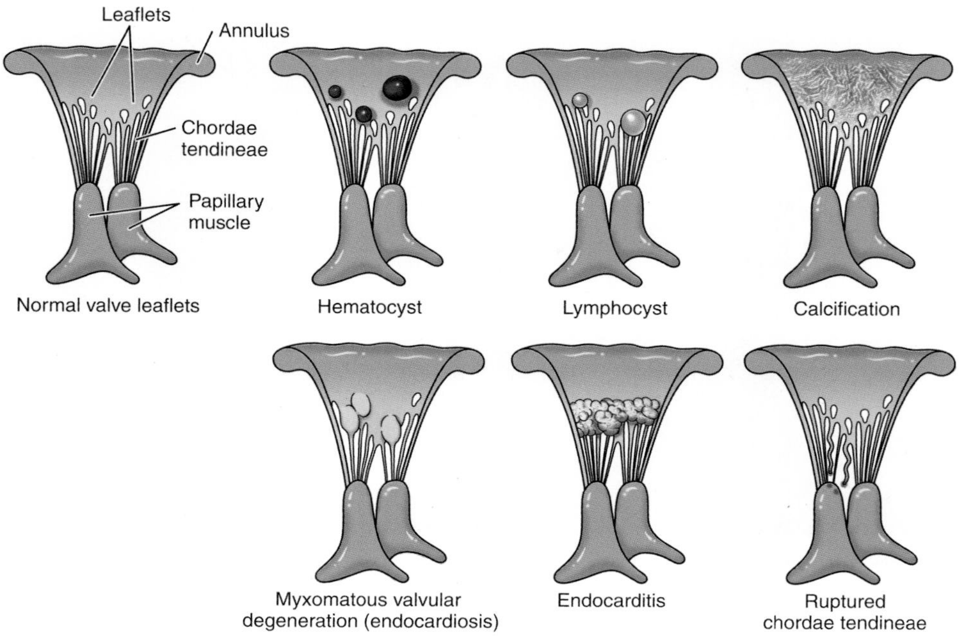

Fig. 10-58 Schematic diagram of the major types of cardiac atrioventricular valvular disease. (Redrawn with permission from School of Veterinary Medicine, Purdue University.)

Persistent atrial standstill (silent atria, AV myopathy) is a progressive cardiac disease of English springer spaniels and cats characterized by notable atrial dilation and fibrosis.

Atrial fibrillation occurs in cattle in association with right atrial dilation and fibrosis and alterations in the SA mode. Also, sudden (unexpected) cardiac death is described in racehorses with right atrial myocardial fibrosis, fibrosis of the upper ventricular septum, and arteriosclerosis of intramyocardial arteries.

ENDOCARDIUM AND HEART VALVES

See the discussion of the endocardium and heart valves in the section on Responses to Injury. The major types of AV valvular diseases are shown in Fig. 10-58.

Disturbances of Growth

Developmental Errors: Congenital Anomalies

Failure of Normal Valvular Development

Pulmonic stenosis

Pulmonic stenosis has been recognized as a frequently occurring anomaly in dogs and is inherited in the beagle (Fig. 10-59). Other breeds in which this lesion is frequent are basset hound, boxer, Chihuahua, Chow chow, cocker spaniel, English bulldog, Labrador retriever, mastiff, Newfoundland, Samoyed, schnauzer, and terrier. Several types of valvular lesions have been described and include formation of a circumferential band of fibrous or muscular tissue beneath the valve (subvalvular stenosis) or malformation of the valve (valvular stenosis), with a small central orifice in a dome of thickened valvular tissue. Notable concentric hypertrophy (see the discussion on hypertrophy in the section on Disturbances of Growth, Myocardium, Responses to Injury) of the right ventricle develops from the resulting pressure overload.

Aortic and subaortic stenoses

True stenoses of the aortic valve are uncommon. Subaortic stenosis is a cardiac anomaly frequently observed in pigs and dogs. It apparently is inherited in Newfoundland, boxer, and German shepherd dogs (Fig. 10-60). The lesion is also observed in the German shorthair pointer, golden retriever, Great Dane, Rottweiler, Samoyed, and bull terrier breeds. In clinical cases, the stenosis is produced by the presence of a thick zone of endocardial fibrous tissue that encircles the left ventricular outflow tract below the valve. In mild cases, often subclinical, the lesion is limited to white nodules on the ventricular septum immediately below the valve. Microscopically, the altered endocardial tissue can contain proliferated mesenchymal cells, mucinous ground substance, and foci of metaplastic cartilage. Other cardiac lesions develop as a result of the altered left ventricular outflow; these include left ventricular concentric hypertrophy, disseminated foci of myocardial necrosis, fibrosis in the inner left ventricular wall, and thickening of the walls of intramyocardial arteries.

Valvular dysplasias: endocardial cushion defects

Other valvular developmental anomalies include endocardial cushion defects (persistent AV canal) in pigs, sheep, and cats; mitral dysplasia in cats and dogs; and tricuspid dysplasia in cats and dogs (see Fig. 10-48). Tricuspid dysplasia is inherited as an autosomal dominant trait with reduced penetrance in Labrador retrievers. The tricuspid valve is abnormal with shortened and thickened chordae tendineae resulting in an incompetent valve and right-sided heart failure.

Other Endocardial Anomalies

Endocardial fibroelastosis

Endocardial fibroelastosis in animals was historically recognized as a primary cardiac defect in Burmese and Siamese cats. Affected animals had prominent, white, thickened endocardium, especially of the left ventricle, because of the proliferation of fibroelastic tissue (see Fig. 10-54). Endocardial fibroelastosis is a reaction of the endocardium to hypoxia and often associated with heart disease, which results in dilated cardiac chambers. It is unclear whether this is a true congenital anomaly or a response to left atrial dilation.

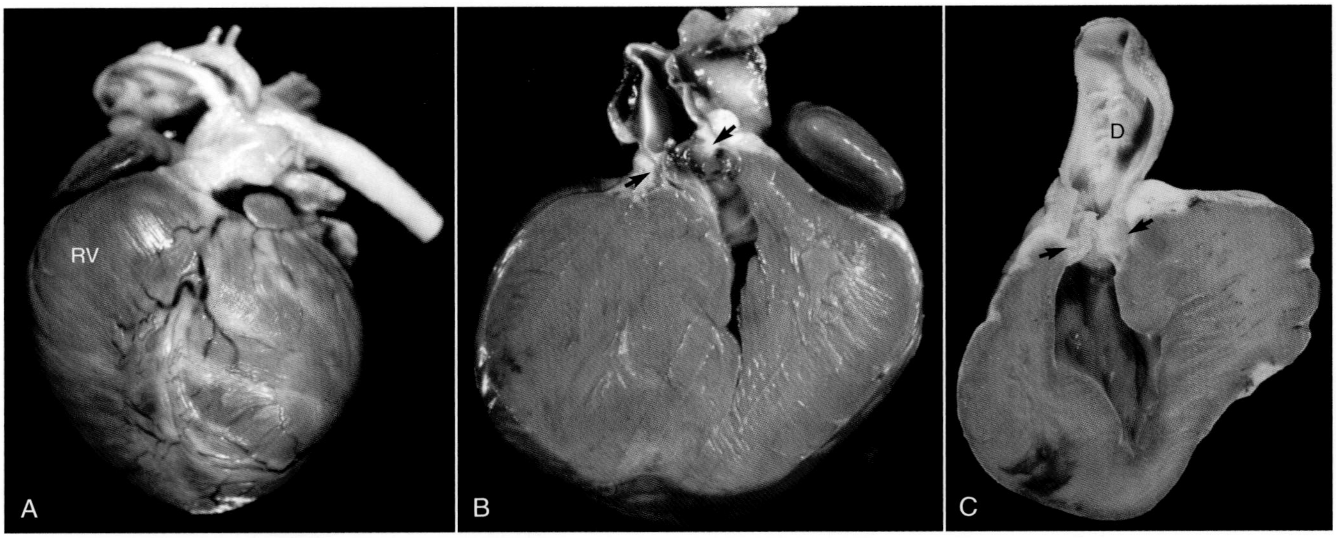

Fig. 10-59 Pulmonic stenosis, heart, pulmonary artery, dogs.
A, Closed heart, and **B,** sectioned heart. Note the prominent concentric right ventricular *(RV)* hypertrophy resulting from pressure overload. The orifice of the pulmonic valve *(arrows)* is markedly narrowed. **C,** sectioned heart, there is poststenotic dilation *(D)* of the pulmonary artery with irregular intimal thickenings (jet lesions). (Courtesy Atlantic Veterinary College, University of Prince Edward Island.)

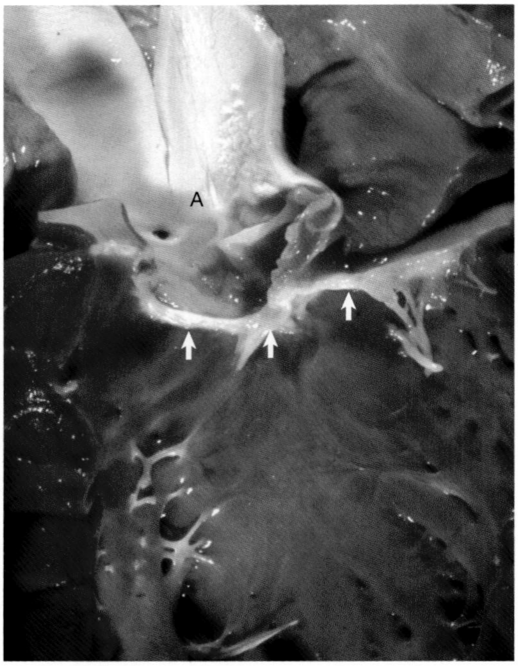

Fig. 10-60 Subaortic stenosis, heart, opened left side, dog.
A thick, white, broad band of fibrous connective tissue *(arrows)* encircles the left ventricular outflow tract below the aortic valve. The force of the blood ejected through the stenotic lesion is responsible for the "jet lesions" in the overlying aorta (A) (right half: roughened surface; left half: dilation [note the *gray* area]). (Courtesy College of Veterinary Medicine, University of Illinois.)

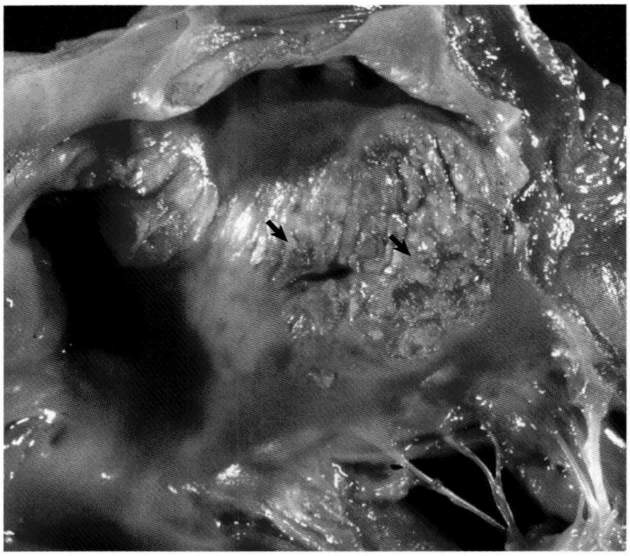

Fig. 10-61 Ulcerative endocarditis (uremia), heart, endocardium of left atrium, dog.
Note the white-red, thick, wrinkled area *(arrows)* of endocarditis, mineralization, and fibrous tissue *(scar)* formation caused by uremia in this dog with chronic renal failure. (Courtesy Dr. K. Read, College of Veterinary Medicine, Texas A&M University; and Noah's Arkive, College of Veterinary Medicine, The University of Georgia.)

Valvular hematomas

See the discussion on valvular hematomas in the section on Disorders of Ruminants.

Valvular lymphocysts

See the discussion on valvular lymphocysts in the section on Disorders of Ruminants.

Cell Degeneration and Death

Uremic Endocarditis

Uremic endocarditis is most commonly a disorder in dogs that follows acute or repeated episodes of uremia. These episodes cause ulcerative endocarditis (injury of the endothelium) of the left atrium that is resolved via healing characterized by fibrosis, with or without mineralization and chronically dilated atria (Fig. 10-61).

Myxomatous Valvular Degeneration (Valvular Endocardiosis)

Degenerative changes in the valves are frequently seen in older dogs and the process that leads to this lesion is termed *myxomatous valvular degeneration* (valvular endocardiosis). Also see the section on Disorders of Dogs; also see Fig. 10-84).

Endocardial Mineralization

Endocardial mineralization occurs from intake of excessive amounts of vitamin D and from intoxication by calcinogenic plants *(Cestrum diurnum, Trisetum flavescens, Solanum malacoxylon, Solanum torvum)* that contain vitamin D analogs. These plant-induced syndromes of cattle have been called by different names in various areas of the world, such as "Manchester wasting disease" in Jamaica, "enzootic calcinosis" in Europe, "Naalehu disease" in Hawaii, "enteque seco" in Argentina, and "espichamento" in Brazil. Multiple, large, white, rough, firm plaques of mineralized fibroelastic tissue are present in the endocardium and intima of large elastic arteries. Fibrosis, with or without mineralization, occurs in chronically dilated hearts, in hearts of debilitated cattle with Johne's disease (see Figs. 10-32 and 10-39), in dogs with healed lesions of left atrial ulcerative endocarditis associated with a prior uremic episode (see Fig. 10-61), and in the so-called jet lesions produced by the trauma of refluxed blood in valvular insufficiencies.

Inflammation

Valvular Endocarditis

See the discussion on vegetative valvular and mural endocarditis in the section on Inflammation, Endocardium, Responses to Injury, as well as the discussion on valvular endocarditis in Chapter 3.

BLOOD AND LYMPHATIC VASCULAR SYSTEMS

See the discussion on blood and lymphatic vascular systems in the section on Responses to Injury. The major arterial diseases are shown in Fig. 10-62.

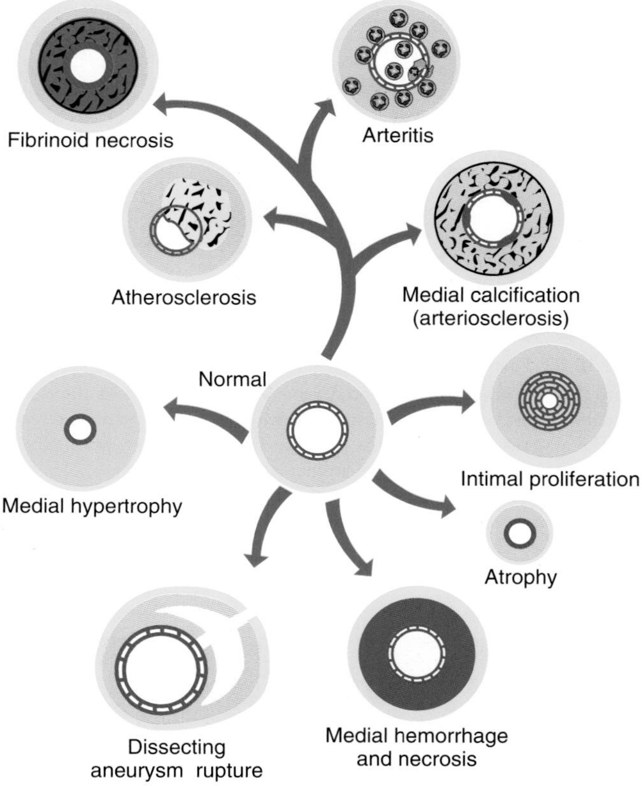

Fig. 10-62 Schematic diagram of the major arterial diseases. (Redrawn with permission from School of Veterinary Medicine, Purdue University.)

Blood Vessels

Disturbances of Circulation

Effusions

See the discussion on effusions in the section on Disturbances of Circulation, Pericardium and Epicardium, Responses to Injury and Disorders of Domestic Animals.

Aortic rupture and rupture of large arteries

Aortic rupture and rupture of large arteries can be the sequela of severe trauma or occur spontaneously (see Figs. 10-34 and 10-35). Sudden rupture of the ascending aorta or pulmonary artery near the pulmonic valve in horses is associated with notable exertion and severe trauma to the ventral thorax from falling. Death ensues rapidly from cardiac tamponade, as the tear is in that portion of the aorta or pulmonary artery within the pericardial sac. In horses, the internal carotid artery can rupture into the adjacent guttural pouch, with subsequent epistaxis. This is a consequence of deep mycotic infection of the guttural pouch. Rupture of the middle uterine artery may occur during parturition in mares and with uterine torsion or prolapse in cows. Aortic rupture, with or without dissection, is an important cause of death in male turkeys. The most common vascular diseases with rupture are listed in Box 10-13.

BOX 10-13 Most Common Vascular Diseases with Rupture

Aortic rupture: Horse, turkey
Carotid artery rupture: Horse
Thoracic duct rupture: Dog and cat

Gastric Dilation and Volvulus

See the discussion on gastric dilation and volvulus in Chapter 7.

Disturbances of Growth

Developmental Errors: Congenital Anomalies

Failure of closure of fetal cardiovascular shunts

Patent ductus arteriosus. See the discussion of patent ductus arteriosus in the section on Diseases of Dogs.

Portacaval shunts. Portacaval shunts occur in animals, particularly in the dog. The normal flow from the portal vein is diverted, either partially or completely, to the systemic circulation, thus bypassing the liver (Fig. 10-63). Normal hepatic detoxification of portal flow is incomplete and may result in neurologic signs and elevated circulating bile acids. The resulting nervous system syndrome is termed *hepatic encephalopathy*. Specifically, the shunts represent retained fetal vascular structures, as in persistent ductus venosus, or arise from prominent dilation of various portosystemic shunts that normally are quite small vessels. See Chapter 8 on diseases of the liver for further details.

Malpositioning of great vessels

Persistent right aortic arch. Persistent right aortic arch occurs in dogs; German shepherd, Irish setter, and Great Dane dogs are predisposed (Fig. 10-64). This defect arises because the right fourth aortic arch, rather than the normal left fourth aortic arch, develops and ascends on the right side of the midline so that

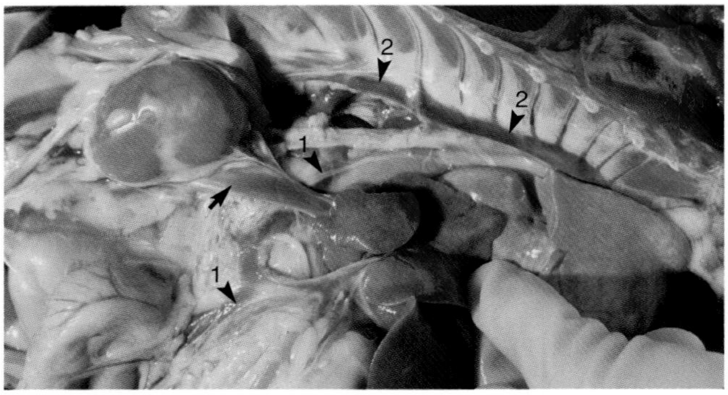

Fig. 10-63 Portacaval shunt, dog.
Note that the branch of the portal vein *(arrowhead 1)* passes under the caudal vena cava *(arrow)* and anastomoses with the azygous vein *(arrowhead 2)*. The azygous vein returns the blood to the caudal vena cava near the heart and thus this blood and its ammoniacal and protein metabolites are shunted away from processing to blood urea nitrogen (BUN) in the liver. The liver is normal color but extremely small, which is typical of these types of shunts (see Chapter 8). (Courtesy Dr. M.D. McGavin, College of Veterinary Medicine, University of Tennessee.)

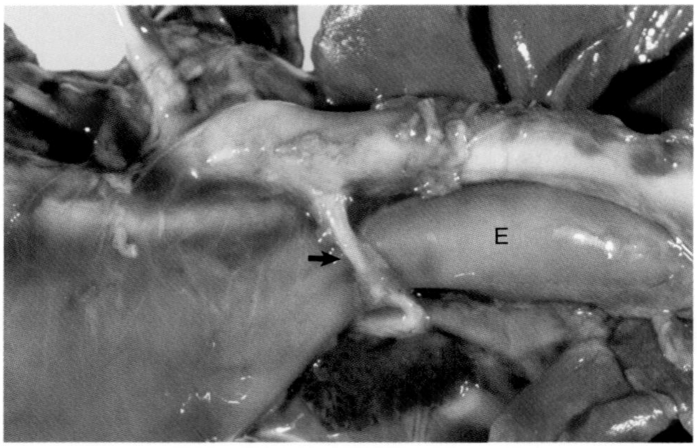

Fig. 10-64 Persistent right aortic arch, ligamentum arteriosum, megaesophagus, calf.
During embryogenesis the aorta was formed from the right aortic arch instead of the left one, thus the aorta is now on the right. For the ligamentum arteriosum *(arrow)* to connect the aorta with the pulmonary artery, it has to pass dorsally over the esophagus and trachea. The ligamentum, together with the aorta and pulmonary artery, form a vascular ring that constricts the esophagus *(E)*, which is dilated cranial to the constriction. (Courtesy Dr. S. Snyder, College of Veterinary Medicine, Colorado State University; and Noah's Arkive, College of Veterinary Medicine, The University of Georgia.)

the ligamentum arteriosum forms a vascular ring over the esophagus and trachea. This arrangement eventually results in esophageal obstruction and proximal dilation (megaesophagus), which often results in aspiration pneumonia as the animal matures and consumes solid feed.

Transposition of the aorta and pulmonary artery. Transposition of the aorta and pulmonary artery are severe anomalies, of which there are several types. In complete transposition, the aorta serves as the outflow from the right ventricle and the pulmonary artery is the left ventricle primary outflow. Other congenital anomalies, including ventricular septal defect, often accompany this anomaly.

Vascular Melanosis
See the discussion on vascular melanosis in Chapters 1 and 2.

Neoplastic Transformation
See the discussion on neoplastic transformation in the section on Disorders of Dogs.

Cell Degeneration and Death
Toxicants that affect vessels are listed in Web Box 10-1.

Vitamin E–Selenium Deficiency
See the discussion on vitamin E–selenium deficiency in the section on Disorders of Pigs.

Inflammation
Omphalophlebitis ("Navel Ill")
Omphalophlebitis ("navel ill") is inflammation of the umbilical vein that often occurs in neonatal farm animals because of bacterial contamination of the umbilicus immediately after parturition. Bacteria from this site can cause septicemia, suppurative polyarthritis, hepatic abscesses (the umbilical vein drains into the liver), and umbilical abscesses.

Jugular Thrombophlebitis
Jugular thrombophlebitis may be associated with indwelling jugular catheters and is reported to be increased with several concurrent disease conditions such as hypoproteinemia, salmonellosis, endotoxemia, and large intestinal disease (see Fig. 10-43).

Lymphatic Vessels
Disturbances of Circulation
Effusions
Rupture of the thoracic duct
Rupture of the thoracic duct, either as a result of trauma or from spontaneous disruption, causes chylothorax in dogs and cats (see Fig. 9-101). However, many cases of chylothorax occur without injury to the thoracic duct and have been attributed to lesions that interfere with central venous return or produce obstruction of the thoracic duct (right-sided heart failure, neoplasms, granulomas, cranial vena cava thrombosis, or dirofilariasis) or that are idiopathic.

Disturbances of Growth
Developmental Errors: Congenital Anomalies
Lymphangiectasia
Lymphangiectasia is dilation of lymphatic vessels. The cause may be a congenital anomaly (Fig. 10-65) or caused by obstruction of lymph drainage by invading masses of malignant neoplasms or inflammation (Fig. 10-66).

Hereditary lymphedema
Hereditary lymphedema has been described in dogs, Ayrshire and Angus calves, and pigs. Affected animals have prominent subcutaneous edema that, in calves, often causes severe swelling of the tips of the ears. Interference with lymph drainage results from defective development of the lymphatic vessels that are aplastic or hypoplastic.

Neoplastic Transformation
Lymphangioma is a rare benign neoplasm composed of lymphatic channels. Lymphangiosarcoma, the malignant counterpart, occurs more often than the benign neoplasm. Vascular spaces formed by neoplastic lymphatic endothelial cells contain lymph rather than blood. Lymphatic vessels are frequently invaded by primary

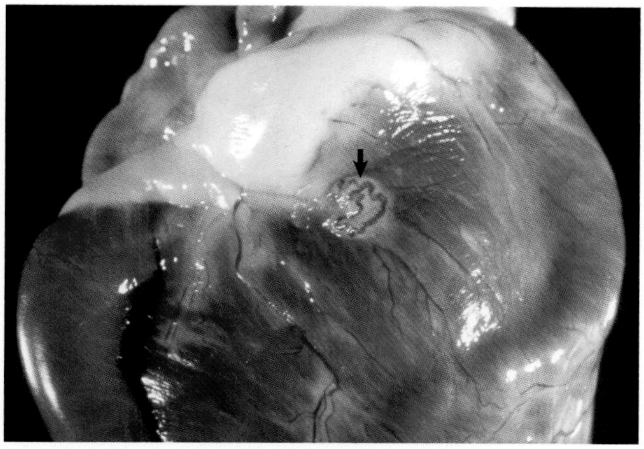

Fig. 10-65 Congenital lymphangiectasia, epicardium, young horse. Note the tortuous appearance of the epicardial lymphatic vessel *(arrow)*. In congenital lymphangiectasia, lymphatic vessels fail to make connections with other vessels or are obstructed because of anomalous development. (Courtesy College of Veterinary Medicine, University of Illinois.)

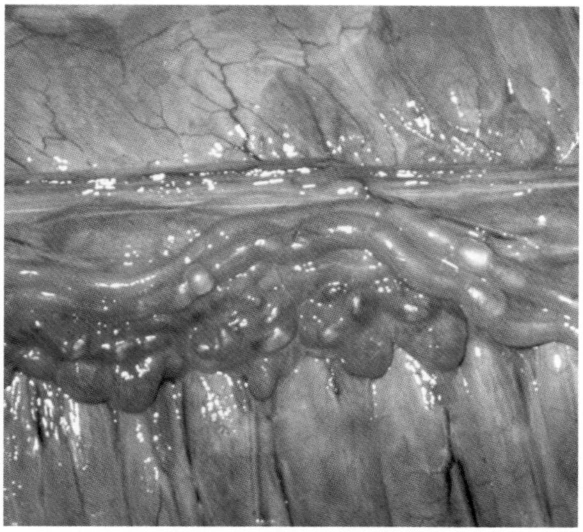

Fig. 10-66 Acquired lymphangiectasia, lymphoma (lymphosarcoma), mesoccolon, horse. Note the distended lymphatics on the serosal surface of the large colon, the result of impeded lymph flow through the colic lymph nodes, caused by compression of their cortical and medullary sinuses by proliferating neoplastic lymphocytes. (Courtesy College of Veterinary Medicine, University of Illinois.)

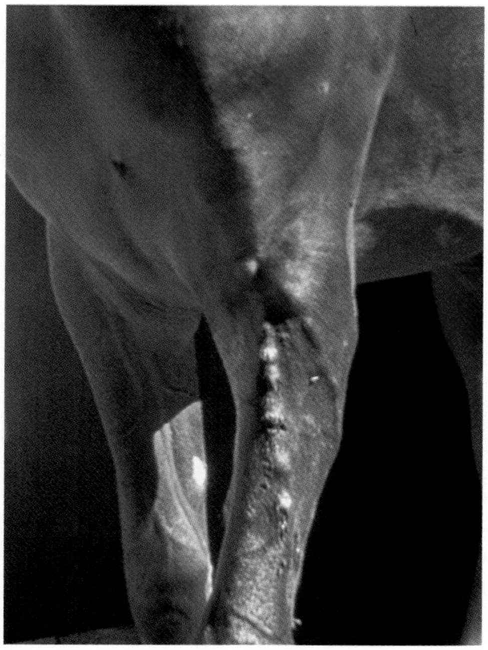

Fig. 10-67 Lymphangitis, forelimb, lymphatic vessels, horse. Note the multiple swellings (cordlike) of the afferent lymphatics in the skin. These lymphatics lie in the subcutis and empty into the caudal superficial cervical (prescapular) lymph node. (Courtesy School of Veterinary Medicine, Purdue University.)

carcinomas and are a common route of metastasis (see the section on Disorders of Dogs).

Inflammation

The most common diseases with thrombosis and embolism are listed in Box 10-14.

BOX 10-14 Most Common Diseases with Thrombosis and/or Embolism in Animals

Pulmonary thromboembolism: Dogs and cats
Aortic thromboembolism in cats and dogs with cardiomyopathy: "Saddle" thrombi
Aortoiliac thrombosis in horses: Verminous or idiopathic
Verminous arteritis in horses; *Strongylus vulgaris*
Septic embolism from lesions of vegetative endocarditis
Fibrocartilaginous emboli: Dogs
Conditions accompanied by DIC (e.g., hog cholera, ICH, FIP, Gram-negative endotoxemia)
Thrombosis of caudal vena cava: Cattle

DIC, Disseminated intravascular coagulation; *ICH,* infectious canine hepatitis; *FIP,* feline infectious peritonitis.

Lymphangitis

Lymphangitis is a feature of many diseases (see Box 10-8). The affected vessels are often located in the distal limbs and are thick, cordlike structures (Fig. 10-67). Lymphedema can be present. Nodular suppurative lesions of lymphangitis often ulcerate and discharge pus onto the surface of the skin. In Johne's disease, the mesenteric lymphatic vessels are often prominent because of granulomatous lymphangitis, an extension of the enteric infection producing a granulomatous enteritis and lymphangitis (Fig. 10-68).

DISORDERS OF HORSES

PERICARDIUM AND EPICARDIUM

Fibrinous Pericarditis

Hematogenous spread of specific organisms may result in fibrinous pericarditis in the horse. These include streptococcal and mycoplasma infections. Sterile swabs of the pericardial exudates are recommended to identify the causative organism.

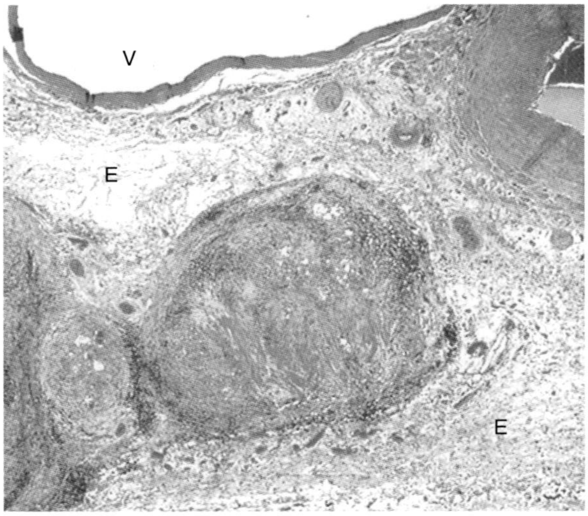

Fig. 10-68 Granulomatous lymphangitis, Johne's disease, mesenteric lymphatic vessel, sheep.
The lymphatic is occluded by a fibrinous thrombus secondary to the destruction of the endothelium by inflammatory cells including macrophages. Early proliferating fibrous tissue and extensive edema *(E)* surround the lymphatic vessel. The adjacent artery *(upper right)* and vein *(V)* are unaffected. H&E stain. (Courtesy School of Veterinary Medicine, Purdue University.)

MYOCARDIUM

Ionophore-Induced Myocardial Degeneration

Ionophores, such as monensin, lasalocid, salinomycin, and narasin, are toxic to horses at extremely low concentrations. They are used as feed additives to increase feed efficiency and weight gain of beef and dairy cattle and control coccidiosis in poultry. Horses gain access to ionophores when they consume (1) ruminant feed containing ionophores, (2) horse feed accidentally mixed with ionophores, and (3) horse feed accidentally contaminated in a mill producing poultry, cattle, and horse feeds. Ionophores cause acute cardiac rhabdomyocyte degeneration and necrosis; this type of injury is discussed in detail in the section on Responses to Injury. Ionophores form complexes with monovalent cations, such as Na^+ and Ca^+, and cross cell membranes and enter the cell via ion transport systems in exchange for H^+ and K^+ ions. Increases in the concentrations of intracellular Ca^+ and possible Na^+ are thought to cause cell membrane injury and dysfunction resulting in mitochondrial swelling and decreased adenosine triphosphate (ATP) production. Additionally, they cause lipid peroxidation of cell membranes leading to loss of cell membrane integrity, fluid and ion shifts, and oncotic necrosis. Macroscopic and microscopic lesions are similar to those that occur with white snakeroot–induced myocardial degeneration described next (Fig. 10-69).

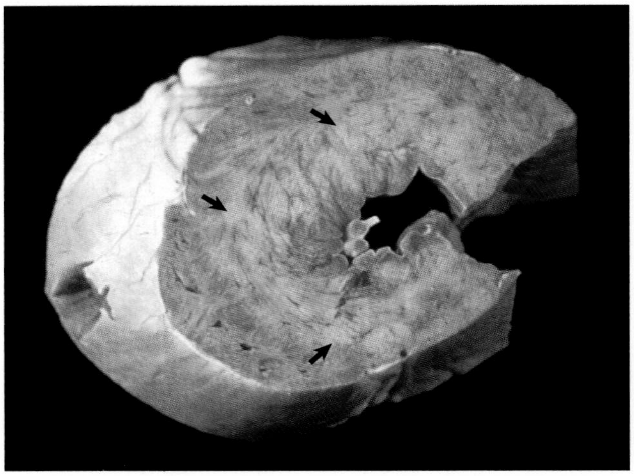

Fig. 10-69 Myocardial necrosis, acute monensin toxicosis, heart, cross-section, left ventricular myocardium, calf.
Note the pale, mottled, necrotic areas *(arrows)* distributed throughout the ventricular myocardium. (Courtesy School of Veterinary Medicine, Purdue University.)

White Snakeroot–Induced Myocardial Degeneration

After ingestion, white snakeroot *(Eupatorium rugosum)* causes myocardial degeneration and necrosis (acute injury) followed by fibrosis (reparative response). Tremetol is the toxic compound in white snakeroot; it becomes toxic after microsomal activation of a precursor compound by cytochrome P-450 enzymes in the liver. The mechanism used by tremetol to cause injury is unclear, but dysfunction of mitochondrial oxidative phosphorylation by inhibiting the tricarboxylic acid cycle has been suggested. Acute cardiac rhabdomyocyte degeneration and necrosis are discussed in detail in the section on Responses to Injury and also in Chapter 15. Reparative responses are discussed in Chapter 3. Macroscopic lesions include pale white to tan areas and linear streaks throughout the myocardium; microscopic lesions include multifocal myocardial degeneration and necrosis with vacuolation of myocardial cytoplasm; loss of cross striations; fragmentation of rhabdomyocytes; hypereosinophilia, coagulation, and clumping of the sarcoplasm; and nuclear pyknosis and karyolysis. The pericardium may contain a modified transudate with fibrin.

Gossypol-Induced Myocardial Degeneration

Gossypol-induced myocardial degeneration can follow the ingestion of cottonseed or cottonseed products that contain excess free gossypol. Gossypol is a potentially toxic pigment in the cotton plant; however, it is toxic only when in a free form (not bound to protein). Gossypol causes myocardial degeneration and necrosis and cardiac conduction failure (see later). The macroscopic and microscopic characteristics of the lesions are in many ways similar to those caused by ionophore-induced and white snakeroot–induced myocardial degeneration in horses. Additionally, acute rhabdomyocytic degeneration and necrosis are discussed in detail in the section on Responses to Injury and also in Chapter 15. Horses are more sensitive to gossypol-induced myocardial degeneration and necrosis than ruminants and pigs. In summary, macroscopic lesions include pale white to tan areas throughout a "flabby" myocardium; microscopic lesions include multifocal myocardial degeneration and necrosis.

BLOOD AND LYMPHATIC VASCULAR SYSTEMS

Blood Vessels

Equine Viral Arteritis

Equine viral arteritis is a systemic viral infection with a tropism for vascular endothelial cells. In this disease, affected small muscular arteries have lesions of fibrinoid necrosis, extensive edema, and leukocytic infiltration (Fig. 10-70). Grossly the vascular injury is reflected by hemorrhage and severe edema of the intestinal wall and mesentery accompanied by notable accumulation of

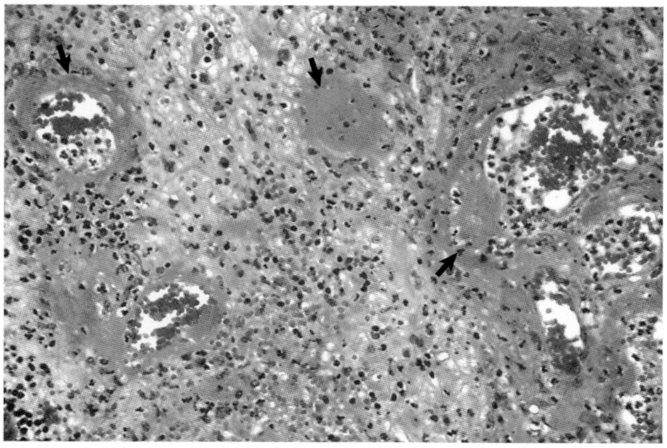

Fig. 10-70 Acute arteritis, equine viral arteritis, small intestine, submucosa, horse.
Small arteries have fibrinoid degeneration (circumferential eosinophilic material *[arrows]*) with leukocytic infiltration of the tunica media. The surrounding loose connective tissue is edematous and infiltrated by numerous leukocytes. H&E stain. (Courtesy School of Veterinary Medicine, Purdue University.)

serous fluids in body cavities and pulmonary edema (see Chapter 14).

African Horse Sickness: Subacute Cardiac Form

African horse sickness is an insect-borne (*Culicoides* spp.) viral disease of *Equidae* that is endemic in Africa, the Middle East, India, and Spain. The occurrence is seasonal because the insect vectors thrive in hot wet conditions. The febrile disease may produce high mortality (up to 95%) and appears in several clinical forms, including the subacute cardiac form described here, as well as an acute respiratory form with massive pulmonary edema. The pathogenesis is initiated by the introduction of the virus by bites of the insect vector. The virus proliferates in local lymph node, and viremia ensues. The virus has a tropism for endothelial cells, monocytes, and macrophages and increased vascular permeability, edema, hemorrhage, and microthrombosis are produced. The gross lesions are extensive subcutaneous and intermuscular edematous swelling of the head and neck. Massive hydropericardium is present with accompanying epicardial and endocardial ecchymotic hemorrhages. Histopathologically, endothelial degeneration and necrosis occur with the edema. In the myocardium, hemorrhage, edema, and focal myocardial necrosis with inflammatory cell infiltrates are present (see Chapter 4 and Fig. 4-44).

Cranial Mesenteric Arteritis and Thrombosis

Cranial mesenteric arteritis and thrombosis results from fourth stage larval migration from *Strongylus vulgaris* (Fig. 10-71). Infection of horses by *Strongylus vulgaris* is now less common because of widespread use of highly efficacious antiparasitic drugs. During its larval development, the parasite migrates through the intestinal arteries, and the most severe lesions are generally found in the cranial mesenteric artery near its origin. The affected vessel is enlarged, and its wall is firm and fibrotic. The intimal surface often has an adhering thrombus admixed with larvae. Microscopically, the affected vessel has extensive infiltration of inflammatory cells and proliferation of fibroblasts throughout the wall. As a consequence, thromboembolism of the intestinal arteries frequently occurs and can produce colic, but the abundant collateral circulation to the equine intestinal tract makes intestinal infarction an unusual event.

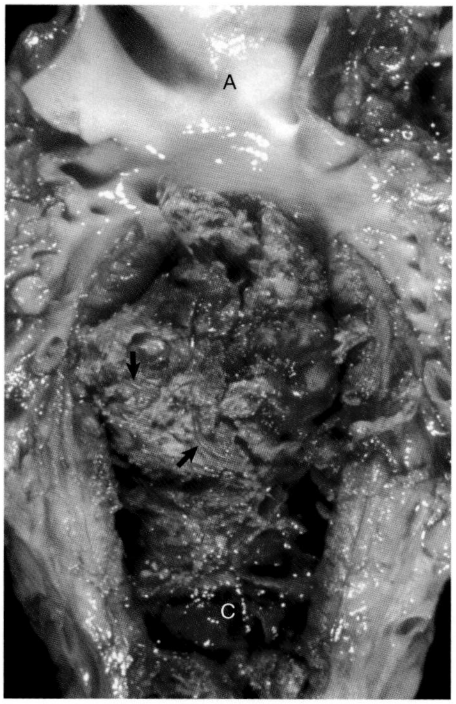

Fig. 10-71 Verminous arteritis and mural thrombosis, strongylosis, abdominal aorta *(A)* and cranial mesenteric artery, horse.
A pale friable thrombotic mass, in which several *Strongylus vulgaris* larvae *(arrows)* are embedded, is attached to the wall of the cranial mesenteric artery *(C)*. (Courtesy College of Veterinary Medicine, University of Illinois.)

Aortoiliac Thrombosis

Aortoiliac thrombosis is thought to be caused by migration of fourth stage larval migration from *Strongylus vulgaris.* See the previous section on cranial mesenteric arteritis and thrombosis.

Jugular Thrombophlebitis

See the discussion on jugular thrombophlebitis in the section on Inflammation, Blood and Lymphatic Vessels, Disorders of Domestic Animals.

Arterial Intimal Calcification

Arterial intimal calcification (intimal bodies) are distinctively small, mineralized masses within the subendothelium in small muscular arteries and arterioles of horses (Web Fig. 10-21). They have no deleterious effect.

Lymphatic Vessels

Glanders Disease (Farcy): Cutaneous Form

Glanders disease (Farcy) is a contagious disease of horses caused by infection with *Burkholderia (Pseudomonas) mallei.* Once worldwide in distribution, it is now seen in Eastern Europe, Asia, and northern Africa. The disease occurs in several clinical forms, and the cutaneous form with involvement of lymphatic vessels is described here. The pathogenesis is initiated by ingestion of contaminated food and water. The organisms enter through the pharynx and are disseminated to the skin hematogenously. The gross lesions of the skin appear as multiple ulcerated nodules that follow infected lymphatic vessels. Most frequent in the limbs, the ulcerated lesions discharge suppurative exudate onto the skin surface. Swollen tortuous cutaneous lymphatic vessels are visible between the ulcerative lesions. Microscopically, the skin nodules represent pyogranulomatous inflammation extending from cutaneous lymphatic vessels with suppurative lymphangitis (see Fig. 4-24).

Miscellaneous Cutaneous Lymphangitides (See Box 10-8)

The cutaneous lesions affecting lymphatic vessels in the diseases are as follows:

1. Ulcerative (likely caused by *Corynebacterium pseudotuberculosis* and other cutaneous bacteria)
2. Sporadic (cause unknown)
3. Epizootic lymphangitis *(Histoplasma farciminosum)*
4. Melioidosis *(Burkholderia pseudomallei)*

These lesions mimic those of Glanders disease, and differentiation occurs by impression smears and microbiologic cultures and analyses. The skin of the legs, head, neck, and/or flanks has raised firm nodules (≈1 to 2 cm in diameter), draining nodules, and draining fistulous tracts, often arranged in linear bands (beaded appearance) that follow the flow of lymphatic vessels. These lesions contain or drain pus, which is often thick and white-yellow in color. Microscopically, lesions are characterized by suppurative to pyogranulomatous inflammation. Infectious microorganisms are often present in the exudate (see Fig. 4-24).

DISORDERS OF RUMINANTS (CATTLE, SHEEP, AND GOATS)

PERICARDIUM AND EPICARDIUM

Suppurative Pericarditis (Traumatic Reticulopericarditis)

Suppurative pericarditis is seen mainly in cattle as a complication of traumatic reticuloperitonitis ("hardware disease"). Foreign bodies, such as nails or pieces of wire that accumulate in the reticulum, occasionally penetrate the reticular wall and diaphragm, enter the adjacent pericardial sac, and introduce infection. Some affected cattle survive for weeks to months until death ensues from congestive heart failure and septicemia. Grossly the pericardial surfaces are notably thickened by white, often rough, shaggy-appearing masses of fibrous connective tissue that enclose an accumulation of white to gray, thick, foul-smelling, purulent exudate (see Fig. 10-16). See the discussion on pericarditis in the section on Epicardium and Pericardium, Disorders of Domestic Animals and also Chapters 7 and 9.

Fibrinous Pericarditis

Hematogenous spread of specific organisms may result in fibrinous pericarditis. Mannheimiosis, blackleg, coliform septicemias, contagious bovine pleuropneumonia, sporadic bovine encephalomyelitis, and in utero *Brucella* spp. and *Arcanobacter pyogenesis* fetal septicemias may all produce fibrinous pericarditis. In sheep, Mannheimiosis and streptococcal infections most commonly result in fibrinous pericarditis. Sterile swabs of the pericardial exudates are recommended to identify the causative organism. See the discussion on pericarditis in the section on Epicardium and Pericardium, Disorders of Domestic Animals and also Chapters 7, 9, 14, 18, and 19.

MYOCARDIUM

Gossypol-Induced Myocardial Degeneration

See the discussion on gossypol-induced myocardial degeneration in Disorders of Horses.

Dilated Cardiomyopathy

Dilated cardiomyopathy in red Holstein-Friesian and Simmental-Red Holsteins occurs frequently in Switzerland. Affected cattle develop right-sided heart failure with cardiac dilation. Histopathologic findings are loss of cardiac muscle cells and replacement fibrosis. Occasional cases in Holsteins were also reported in Japan, Canada, Australia, Denmark, Sweden, and the Netherlands. Congenital cardiomyopathy occurs in Poll Hereford cattle in association with wooly haircoat syndrome. Inherited as an autosomal recessive trait, affected calves usually die from congestive heart failure by 12 weeks of age (also see the discussion on cardiomyopathies in the section on Myocardium, Disorders of Domestic Animals).

Blackleg Myocarditis

Hemorrhagic myocarditis occurs together with the hemorrhagic inflammation typically found in skeletal muscle of cattle with blackleg *(Clostridium chauvoei)* (Fig. 10-72). See the discussion on

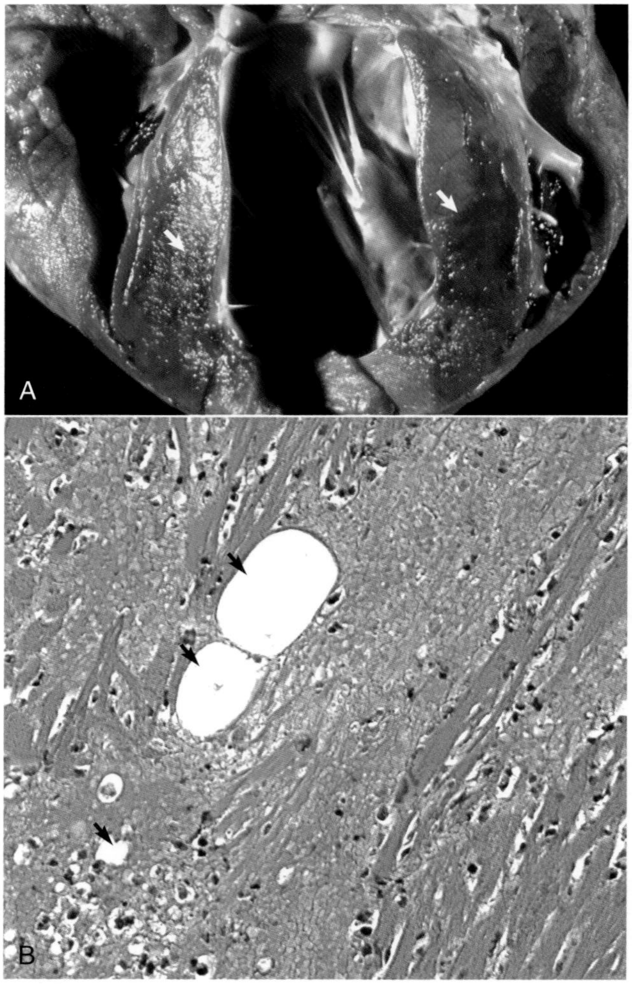

Fig. 10-72 **Necrohemorrhagic myocarditis, "blackleg," heart, steer.** **A,** Note the area of hemorrhagic myocarditis *(arrows)* in the wall of the ventricular myocardium. This disease is caused by *Clostridium chauvoei*, and lesions are most common in skeletal muscle. **B,** Necrohemorrhagic myocarditis, heart, cow. Note the myocardial necrosis, serocellular interstitial debris, and the clear spaces *(arrows)* representative of gas bubbles. (**A** courtesy Dr. J. Simon, College of Veterinary Medicine, University of Illinois. **B** courtesy Atlantic Veterinary College, University of Prince Edward Island.)

myocarditis in the section on Myocardium, Disorders of Domestic Animals and also Chapter 15.

East Coast Fever *(Theileria parva)*

East Coast fever is a tick-transmitted protozoal disease of cattle in Africa caused by *Theileria parva,* which causes myocardial necrosis and inflammation (Web Fig. 10-22).

Eosinophilic Myocarditis

Eosinophilic myocarditis and the accumulation of eosinophils in the inflammatory response are the result of some parasitic infections such as sarcocystosis (see Chapter 15).

Excess Vitamin D and Calcinogenic Plants

See the discussion on mineralization in the section on Cell Degeneration, Myocardium, Responses to Injury and also Chapters 1 and 15.

Lymphoma (Lymphosarcoma)

See the discussion on neoplastic transformation in the section on Disturbances of Growth, Myocardium, Disorders of Domestic Animals.

ENDOCARDIUM AND HEART VALVES

Vegetative Valvular Endocarditis

Endocarditis is usually the result of bacterial infections in which the affected valves have large, adhering, friable, yellow-to-gray masses of fibrin termed *vegetations,* which can largely occlude the valvular orifice (Fig. 10-73, *A*). Microscopically, the lesion consists of accumulated layers of fibrin and numerous embedded bacterial colonies underlain by a zone of infiltrated leukocytes and granulation tissue (Fig. 10-73, *B*). See the discussion on vegetative valvular and mural endocarditis in the section on Inflammation, Endocardium, Responses to Injury and also Chapter 3.

Endocardial Mineralization

See the discussion on mineralization in the section on Cell Degeneration, Endocardium, Responses to Injury and also Chapters 1 and 15.

Valvular Hematomas

Valvular hematomas (hematocysts) frequently are observed on the AV valves of postnatal ruminants (Fig. 10-74, *A*). These lesions, which generally regress spontaneously by the time the animals are several months of age, do not produce any functional abnormalities. Lesions are bulging, blood-filled cysts, several millimeters in diameter, on the AV valves.

Valvular Lymphocysts

Valvular lymphocysts may also occur and appear as yellow serum-filled cysts on the AV valve cusps (Fig. 10-74, *B*).

BLOOD AND LYMPHATIC VASCULAR SYSTEMS

Blood Vessels

Thrombotic Meningoencephalitis

Histophilus somni (formerly *Haemophilus somnus*) causes a systemic vasculitis in cattle resulting in meningoencephalitis. Mural thrombi from local vascular injury rather than thromboemboli from distal sites of vascular injury, such as the lungs, are the major type of thrombus in this disease. Gross lesions in the central nervous system (CNS) are characteristic of infarcts (see Fig. 14-89, *A*). Microscopic lesions are initially vasculitis and vascular necrosis, which are followed by thrombosis and infarction (see Fig. 14-89, *B*). Septic vasculitis, the initial event, is followed by edema and an influx of neutrophils and macrophages in and around vessel walls and adjacent parenchyma. Colonies of small Gram-negative bacilli are frequent in thrombi, in and around affected vessels, and in areas of necrosis. *Histophilus somni* can also cause a necrotizing myocarditis.

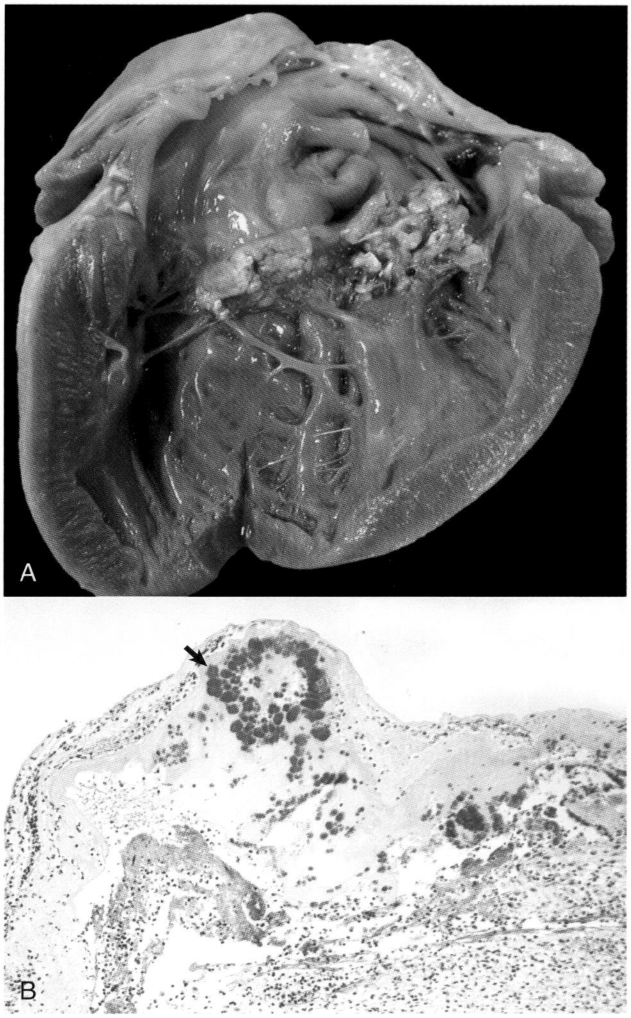

Fig. 10-73 Vegetative valvular endocarditis.
A, Mitral valve, heart, calf. Multiple, large, raised, friable, yellow-red thrombotic masses are attached to cusps of the mitral valve. The roughened and granular surface of the valve leaflets is attributable to fibrin, platelets, and trapped bacteria and erythrocytes. **B,** Bacterial infection, heart, tricuspid valve, cow. Note abundant masses of fibrin and bacterial colonies *(arrow).* H&E stain. (**A** courtesy Atlantic Veterinary College, University of Prince Edward Island. **B** courtesy Dr. M.D. McGavin, College of Veterinary Medicine, University of Tennessee.)

Thrombosis of the Caudal Vena Cava

Thrombosis of the caudal vena cava occurs in association with rupture of hepatic abscesses into either the hepatic vein or the caudal vena cava. The hepatic abscess inflammation extends into the adjacent large hepatic veins and results in formation of a septic thrombus in the caudal vena cava. Rupture and release of the contents of the abscess into the lumen can cause multiple septic emboli in the pulmonary capillaries and unexpected death of the affected animal, often preceded by severe hemoptysis.

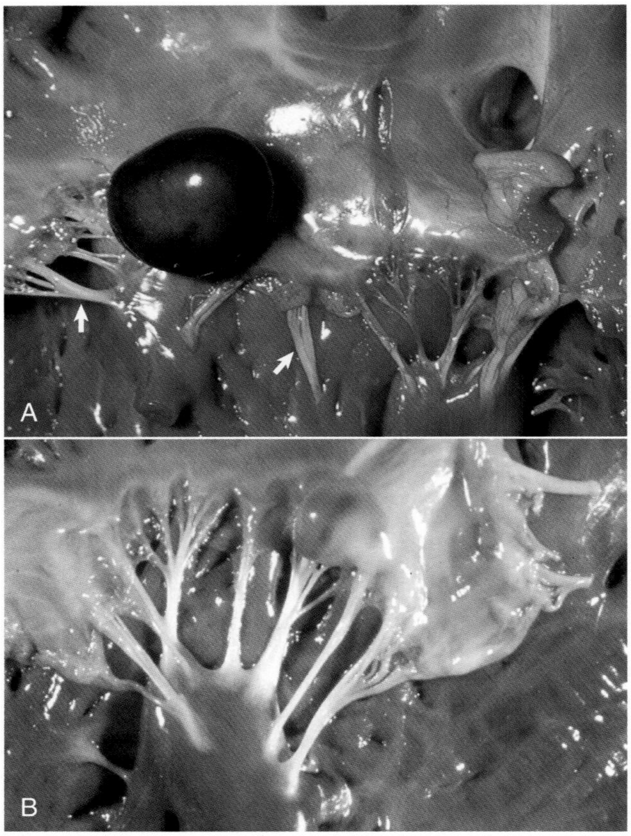

Fig. 10-74 Hematocysts and lymphocysts, calf.
A, Valvular hematocyst, heart, opened left side, mitral valve, postnatal calf. A dark, blood-filled cyst protrudes from a cusp of the mitral valve. *Arrows* indicate chordae tendineae. Hematocysts usually occur in ruminants, do not cause any functional abnormality, and usually regress within a few months of birth. **B,** Valvular lymphocyst, heart. A lymph-filled cyst is on a cusp of the atrioventricular valve. Like hematocysts, lymphocysts usually occur in ruminants, do not cause any functional abnormality, and usually regress within a few months of birth. (**A** courtesy Dr. M.D. McGavin, College of Veterinary Medicine, University of Tennessee. **B** courtesy College of Veterinary Medicine, University of Illinois.)

Foreign Parasitic Diseases

Foreign parasitic diseases important in tropical regions of the world are characterized by presence of parasites in the lumens of veins. These diseases in cattle include schistosomiasis (blood fluke infection—*Schistosoma* spp.) in which adult parasites are present in the mesenteric and portal veins, and the resulting phlebitis is characterized by intimal proliferation and thrombosis.

Omphalophlebitis ("Navel Ill")

See the discussion on omphalophlebitis ("navel ill") in the section on Inflammation, Blood and Lymphatic Vessels, Disorders of Domestic Animals, and also Chapters 8 and 16.

Johne's Disease

Lesions of Johne's disease affecting blood and lymphatic vessels and characterized by intimal mineralization and granulomatous lymphangitis, respectively, are discussed in greater detail in Chapters 4, 7, and 13.

Anthrax

Anthrax in herbivores often occurs as an acute febrile highly fatal septicemic disease. Although global in distribution, the disease is enzootic in certain areas. The etiology is *Bacillus anthracis,* a large rod-shaped spore-forming bacterium. The pathogenesis of the disease in affected herbivores is exposure by ingestion of contaminated food (especially bone meal) and water. The organisms produce a variety of lethal toxins that provoke local edema and tissue necrosis and increased vascular permeability associated with lymphangitis and lymphadenitis. Herbivores that die from septicemic anthrax have dark thick unclotted blood oozing from body orifices. These cases should NOT be subjected to necropsy to avoid massive contamination of the environment by the spores of the organism. Instead, a blood smear should be collected and examined for the presence of the diagnostic bacilli. If a case is necropsied by mistake, the diagnostic findings are massive splenomegaly (so-called blackberry jam spleen), disseminated serosal hemorrhages, and swollen edematous lymph nodes. Microscopic findings (histopathologic evaluation is NOT recommended) include massive numbers of typical large rod-shaped organisms in the blood, congestion, hemorrhage, lymphangitis, and lymphadenitis (see Chapter 4, Fig. 4-23, and Chapter 7, Fig. 7-135).

Neospora caninum

See the discussion on *Neospora caninum* in Chapter 4.

Malignant Catarrhal Fever

See the discussion on malignant catarrhal fever in Chapter 4.

Bovine Virus Diarrhea

See the discussion on bovine virus diarrhea in Chapters 4 and 7.

Bluetongue

See the discussion on bluetongue in Chapters 4 and 7.

DISORDERS OF PIGS

PERICARDIUM AND EPICARDIUM

Fibrinous Pericarditis

Fibrinous pericarditis may accompany Glasser's disease *(Haemophilus parasuis)* (Fig. 10-75), streptococcal infections, enzootic mycoplasma pneumonia, and salmonellosis. Sterile swabs of the pericardial exudates are recommended to identify the causative organism. See the discussion of pericarditis in the section on Pericardium and Epicardium, Disorders of Domestic Animals and also Chapters 3, 7, and 9.

Porcine Polyserositis (Glasser's Disease, *Streptococcus suis II*)

See Fig. 10-75; also see the discussion in Chapters 4 and 7.

ENDOCARDIUM AND HEART VALVES

Endocarditis

Endocarditis is commonly found in pigs and results from a bacterial septicemia. The most commonly isolated organisms are *Streptococcus* spp. and *Erysipelothrix rhusiopathiae.* Confirmation of the definitive organism requires bacterial isolation. Affected valves have large, adhering, friable, yellow-to-gray masses of fibrin termed *vegetations,* which can largely occlude the valvular orifice (Fig. 10-76). Microscopically, the lesion consists of accumulated layers of fibrin and numerous embedded bacterial colonies underlain by a zone

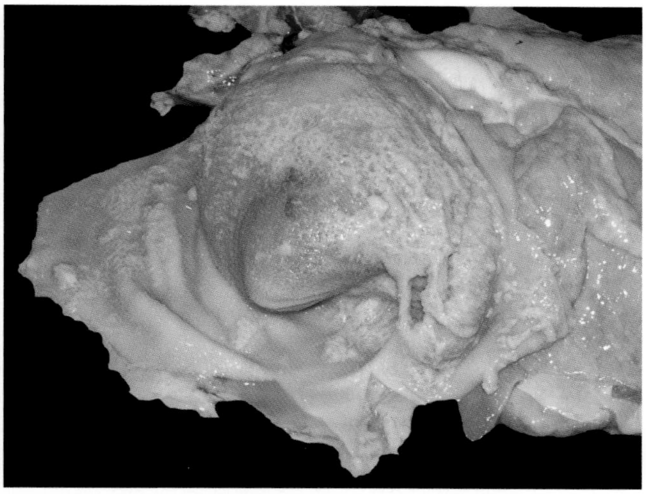

Fig. 10-75 Fibrinous porcine polyserositis, Glasser's disease, pericardium and epicardium (pericardial cavity), pig.
A fibrinous pericarditis is typical of Glasser's disease (*Haemophilus parasuis*). Streptococcal infections, enzootic mycoplasma pneumonia, and salmonellosis can also cause this lesion. (Courtesy Dr. D. Driemeier, Federal University of Rio Grande do Sul, Brazil.)

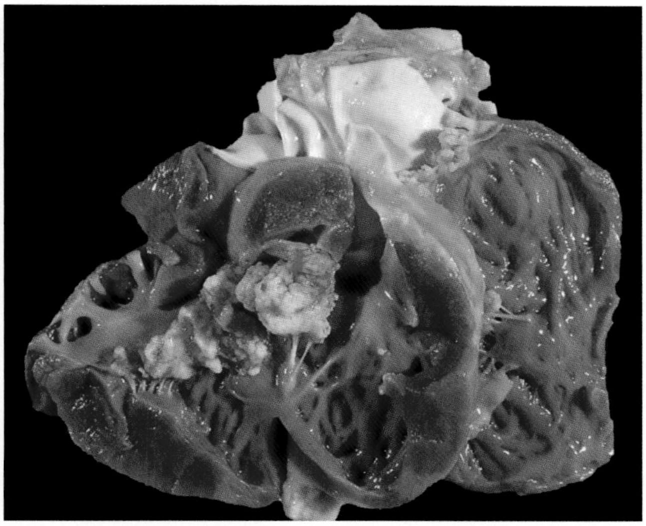

Fig. 10-76 Valvular endocarditis, *Streptococcus suis*, heart mitral and pulmonic valves, pig.
Note the friable, yellow material adhering to and replacing some of the normal left atrioventricular valve. The left ventricular chamber is dilated due to failure of normal function of the valve (eccentric hypertrophy). (Courtesy Atlantic Veterinary College, University of Prince Edward Island.)

of infiltrated leukocytes and granulation tissue (see Fig. 10-73, *B*). See the discussion on valvular and mural endocarditis in the section on Inflammation, Endocardium, Responses to Injury and also Chapter 3.

MYOCARDIUM

Mulberry Heart Disease

See the discussion on mulberry heart disease in the next section on Dietary Microangiopathy.

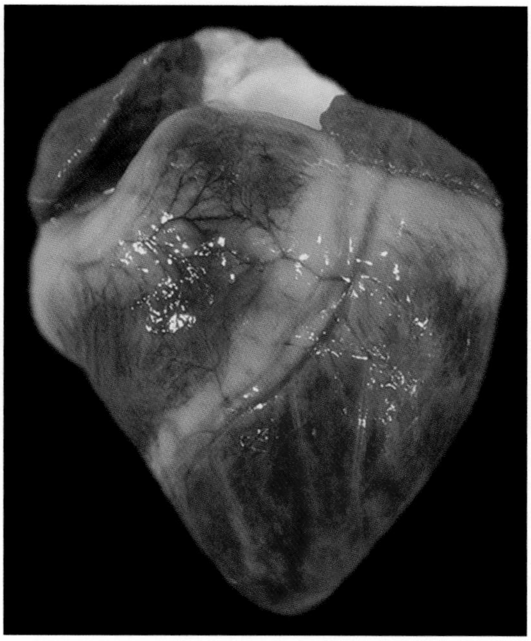

Fig. 10-77 Mulberry heart disease, suffusive hemorrhage, epicardium, right ventricle, heart, pig.
Red areas of suffusive hemorrhage ("mulberry-like") are present on the epicardial surfaces of the ventricles. (Courtesy Dr. L. Miller, Atlantic Veterinary College.)

BLOOD AND LYMPHATIC VASCULAR SYSTEMS

Blood Vessels

Dietary Microangiopathy: Mulberry Heart Disease

Dietary microangiopathy of pigs or "mulberry heart disease" is produced by a deficiency of vitamin E and/or selenium and the resultant effect on the microvasculature, which is characterized by fibrinoid necrosis, and thromboses of small vessels resulting in microhemorrhages. The hemorrhage results in major discoloration of the epicardial surface of the heart, particularly the right atrium said to resemble a mulberry (Figs. 10-77 and 10-78). In addition to the epicardial hemorrhages, hydropericardium often ensues. Massive hemorrhagic hepatic necrosis (hepatosis dietetica) is also produced with vitamin E and/or selenium deficiency (see Fig. 8-69). With either form of the disease, fibrinoid necrosis of small muscular arteries and arterioles is widespread and is accompanied by endothelial damage and fibrin thrombi in capillaries, especially capillaries of the myocardium (Fig. 10-79; Web Fig. 10-23). This complex of vascular lesions has been termed *dietary microangiopathy.*

Cerebrospinal Angiopathy (Edema Disease)

Cerebrospinal angiopathy in pigs is characteristically sporadic in pigs with signs of nervous system disease. Fibrinoid necrosis is consistently present in arteries of the CNS. Similar lesions occur in the arteries of the gastric submucosa of pigs with edema disease, a form of colibacillosis, and many researchers believe that cerebrospinal angiopathy represents a subacute form of edema disease (Fig. 10-80; Web Fig. 10-24; also see Fig. 10-42; Chapters 4, 7, and 11; and Figs. 7-126 and 7-127).

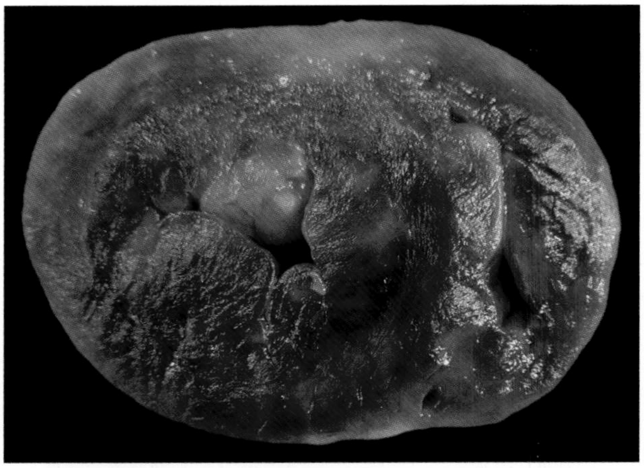

Fig. 10-78 Mulberry heart disease, hemorrhage and necrosis, left and right ventricular myocardium, transverse section, pig.
Red and pale mottled areas are caused by hemorrhage and necrosis, respectively. (Courtesy Dr. L. Miller, Atlantic Veterinary College.)

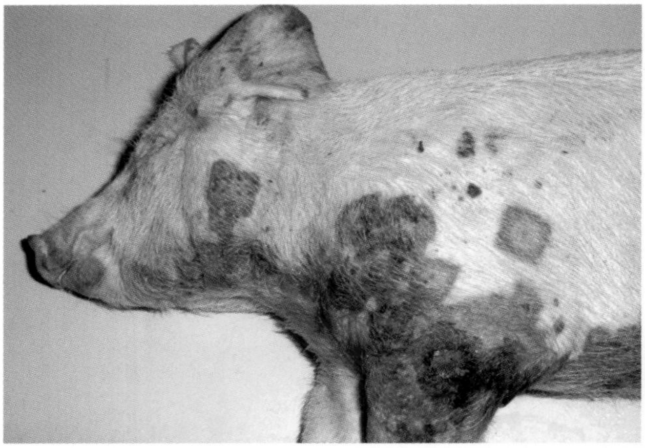

Fig. 10-81 Cutaneous infarcts, diamond skin disease, ***Erysipelothrix rhusiopathiae*** **septicemia, skin, pig.**
Emboli of Erysipelothrix rhusiopathiae have lodged in cutaneous vessels and caused a localized vasculitis, which has resulted in thrombosis followed by ischemia and cutaneous infarction. (Courtesy Dr. M.D. McGavin, College of Veterinary Medicine, University of Tennessee.)

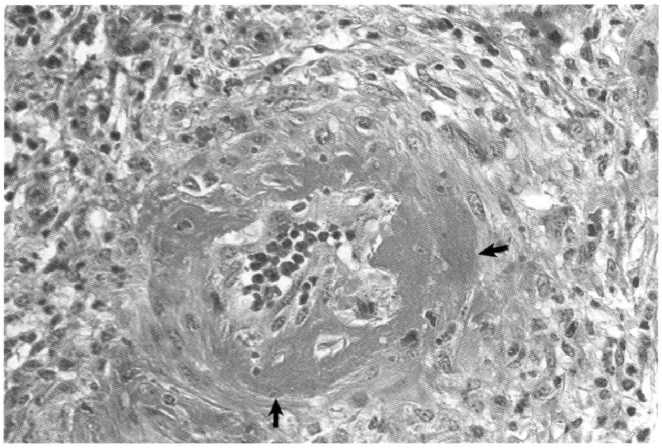

Fig. 10-79 Vitamin E–Selenium deficiency ("mulberry heart disease"), fibrinoid necrosis, myocardial arteriole, heart, pig.
Note the circumferential eosinophilic deposits *(arrows)* in the wall of the arteriole. H&E stain. (Courtesy Dr. J. Simon, College of Veterinary Medicine, University of Illinois.)

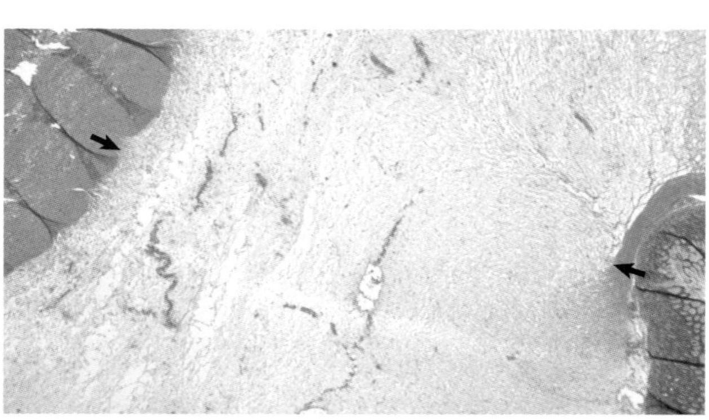

Fig. 10-80 Submucosal edema, edema disease, stomach, submucosa, pig.
The submucosa *(between arrows)* is distended with edema fluid. H&E stain. (Courtesy School of Veterinary Medicine, Purdue University.)

Fibrinoid Necrosis of Blood Vessels

Fibrinoid necrosis of arteries and veins (see Fig. 10-42) is particularly frequent in pigs and is an important diagnostic feature in cases of vitamin E–selenium deficiency (heart), edema disease (gastric submucosa), cerebrospinal angiopathy, porcine circovirus II vasculopathy, and organic mercury toxicosis (meninges). See the previous section on Dietary Microangiopathy: Mulberry Heart Disease.

Erysipelosis (Erysipelelothrix rhusiopathiae)

Cutaneous lesions in erysipelosis are caused by *Erysipelothrix rhusiopathiae* and are the result of bacterial embolization to the skin during sepsis. Lesions consist of square to rhomboidal, firm, raised, pink to dark purple areas (Fig. 10-81, see Fig. 17-51) caused by vasculitis, thrombosis, and ischemia (infarction). The rhomboidal shape likely represents an area of skin supplied by a thrombosed vessel (see Chapter 17).

Porcine Polyserositis (Streptococcus suis II)

Streptococcus suis II is one of several bacteria that can cause the disease porcine polyserositis. Gross lesions include vasculitis leading to variable quantities of a gray-white friable material (fibrin) on serosal surfaces (fibrinous polyserositis) of the lungs (fibrinous pleuritis), heart (fibrinous pericarditis [see Fig. 10-75]), and abdominal cavity (fibrinous peritonitis). The bacterium gains access to and spreads systemically through the blood vascular system. Lesions suggest this bacterium may have a tropism for vascular endothelial cells of serosae and bacterial endotoxins may contribute to vascular injury and permeability changes leading to the leakage of fibrinogen and its polymerization to fibrin on serosal surfaces and in some cases to microthrombus formation and disseminated intravascular coagulation (DIC) in other organ systems (see Chapters 4, 7, and 9).

African Swine Fever (Wart Hog Disease, African Pig Disease)

African swine fever (ASF) is a highly contagious febrile hemorrhagic disease of pigs associated with a DNA virus. The clinical and pathologic features are very similar to those of classic swine fever (hog cholera). The disease is enzootic in Africa, and outbreaks have occurred in Europe, South America, and the Caribbean region. The pathogenesis of the disease is via entry in the upper respiratory tract. The virus proliferates in the tonsils and lymph nodes of the head and neck with subsequent viremia and dissemination to the entire body. Transmission to domestic swine is via ingestion of infected tissues of warthogs and bush pigs, which develop an inapparent infection, or by the bite of infected soft ticks *(Ornithodoros moubata).* The distinctive hemorrhagic lesions are attributed to disruption of the clotting mechanism and thrombocytopenia. The gross lesions are characterized by widespread congestion, edema, and hemorrhage. Hemorrhagic visceral lymph nodes and splenomegaly are present along with petechial hemorrhages of the renal cortices, epicardium, and other serosal surfaces. Pulmonary edema and hydrothorax also occur. Microscopically, viral-induced vascular alterations include congestion, hemorrhage, and edema with fibrin microthrombi (Web Fig. 10-25). The virus produces widespread necrosis of lymphocytes and macrophages (see Fig. 4-42).

Hog Cholera/Classic Swine Fever (Swine Fever, Swine Plague, Schweinpest)

Hog cholera (also termed *classic swine fever*) is a highly contagious febrile hemorrhagic disease of swine produced by an RNA virus. The disease is enzootic in South America, Central America, Caribbean countries, Asia, and Europe. The pathogenesis of the disease is initiated by inhalation of the virus from direct contact with infected pigs or by ingestion of uncooked infected pork. The virus traverses the oral mucosa, replicates in the tonsils, and initiates viremia. The virus selectively damages endothelial cells, cells of the immune system (lymphoreticular cells and macrophages) and epithelial cells. The characteristic hemorrhagic lesions are associated with increased vascular permeability, thrombocytopenia, and DIC (see Web Fig. 10-25). The gross lesions are characterized by widespread petechial hemorrhages, especially of the renal cortices, urinary bladder, larynx, gastric mucosa, and epicardium with accompanying hemorrhage in lymph nodes and skin. A distinctive finding is hemorrhagic infarction of the spleen and "button ulcers" of the colonic mucosa. Microscopically, endothelial damage is evident as hydropic degeneration and cellular proliferation. Affected vessels may have fibrinoid necrosis with fibrin deposition in the media and intima. Circulatory alterations include congestion, hemorrhage, thrombosis, and infarction. The brain has a diffuse nonsuppurative encephalitis (see Fig. 4-43).

Porcine Anthrax

See the discussion on anthrax in the section on Blood and Lymphatic Vascular Systems, Disorders of Ruminants, and also Chapter 4.

DISORDERS OF DOGS

PERICARDIUM AND EPICARDIUM

Hemorrhagic Pericardial Effusion

Hemorrhagic pericardial effusion of unknown cause is frequently seen in dogs. Large or giant breeds, such as the Great Dane, Saint Bernard, Great Pyrenees, German shepherd, and golden retriever, are most often affected. The preferred treatment for the condition is pericardiectomy. See the discussion on effusions in the section on Disturbances of Circulation, Pericardium and Epicardium, Disorders of Domestic Animals, and also Chapters 3, 7, and 9.

MYOCARDIUM

Developmental Errors: Congenital Anomalies

See the discussion of developmental errors in the section on Disturbances of Growth, Myocardium, Disorders of Domestic Animals.

Cardiomyopathies

Dilated (Congestive) Cardiomyopathy

Dilated or congestive cardiomyopathy is an important cause of congestive heart failure in dogs. Some affected dogs have low tissue concentrations of taurine, but supplementation has not proved beneficial. Affected dogs often are males of large breeds, such as Doberman pinschers, Portuguese water dogs, dalmatians, Scottish deerhounds, Irish wolfhounds, Saint Bernards, Afghan hounds, Newfoundland dogs, Old English sheepdogs, Great Danes, and Boxers, although smaller breeds, such as English cocker spaniels, may be affected. The disease often has a familial pattern in the affected breeds and appears to be inherited as an autosomal recessive or X-linked recessive trait. At necropsy, lesions of congestive heart failure are present and the hearts are rounded because of biventricular dilation (see Figs. 10-52 and 10-53). The dilated cardiac chambers often have a diffusely white, thickened endocardium. Microscopic and ultrastructural alterations are nonspecific, can be either mild or absent, and may include interstitial fibrosis and fatty infiltration and changes of myocyte degeneration, including the occurrence of so-called attenuated wavy fibers. See the discussion on cardiomyopathies in the section on Disturbances of Growth, Myocardium, Disorders of Domestic Animals.

Arrhythmogenic Right Ventricular Cardiomyopathy

Arrhythmogenic right ventricular cardiomyopathy (ARVC) is an important cardiac disease of Boxer dogs, and rare cases are seen in cats. Other names for the disease include Boxer cardiomyopathy and familial ventricular arrhythmias of Boxers. Inherited as an autosomal dominant trait in Boxers, most dogs present with arrhythmias and enlargement of the right ventricular chamber. The distinctive histopathologic findings are similar to those of the disease in humans and include thinning of the right ventricular free wall with fibrofatty replacement of cardiac muscle cells.

Canine Parvovirus

Lymphocytic myocarditis is usually a lesion of viral infections and is well illustrated by the lesions of parvoviral myocarditis of puppies. Dogs with parvoviral myocarditis die unexpectedly and have generalized lesions of acute congestive heart failure but lack lesions in the intestine, the primary site of viral damage in approximately 95% of clinical cases. The heart is pale and flabby and has disseminated interstitial lymphocytic infiltrations and scattered myocytes with large, basophilic, intranuclear viral inclusion bodies in dogs that survive fibrosis (Fig. 10-82).

Neurogenic Cardiomyopathy (Heart-Brain Syndrome)

Neurogenic cardiomyopathy (heart-brain syndrome) is a syndrome in dogs characterized by unexpected death 5 to 10 days after diffuse CNS injury (usually hit by car). Affected dogs die of cardiac arrhythmias caused by myocardial degeneration and necrosis. Grossly, the myocardium has numerous discrete and coalescing pale white streaks and/or poorly defined areas of myocardial necrosis—most often involving the papillary muscles of the left ventricle (Fig. 10-83). Neurogenic cardiomyopathy is thought to be caused by overstimulation of the heart by autonomic neurotransmitters and

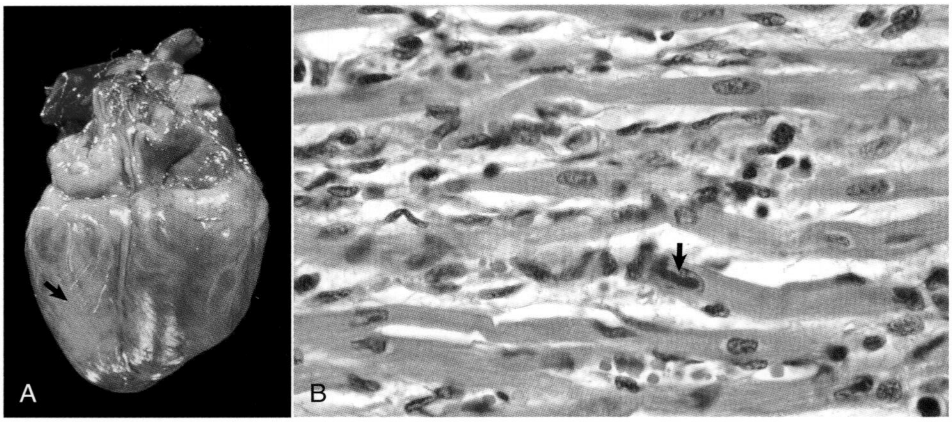

Fig. 10-82 Parvovirus myocarditis, heart, dog.
A, Note the multifocal pale areas *(arrow)* in the ventricular myocardium. **B,** Parvovirus infection, section of myocardium. An intranuclear basophilic inclusion body is in a myocyte *(arrow)*. H&E stain. (**A** courtesy Dr. B. Weeks, College of Veterinary Medicine, Texas A&M University; and Noah's Arkive, College of Veterinary Medicine, The University of Georgia. **B** courtesy School of Veterinary Medicine, Purdue University.)

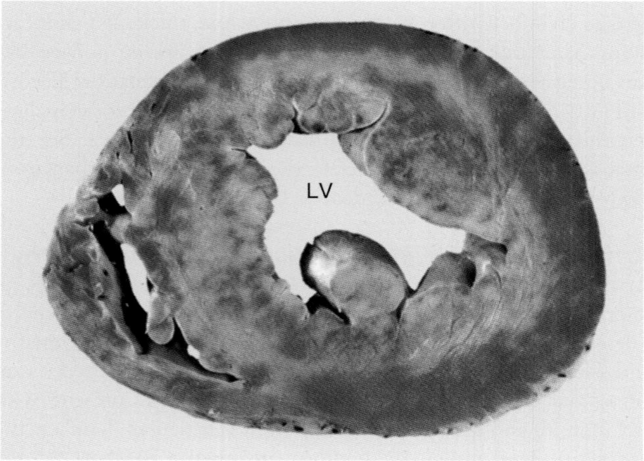

Fig. 10-83 Myocardial necrosis, "heart-brain syndrome," heart, transverse section of ventricles, dog.
Necrotic areas are pale beige to white and are concentrated in the inner half of the wall of the left ventricle *(LV)* and in the ventricular septum. (Courtesy School of Veterinary Medicine, Purdue University.)

systemic catecholamines released at the time of trauma. It is unknown why there is a 5- to 10-day delay in the development of myocardial necrosis. See Chapter 14 for a discussion of heart-brain syndrome.

ENDOCARDIUM AND HEART VALVES

Endocarditis

Endocarditis is occasionally observed in dogs (see Fig. 10-73). Bacterial septicemias result in location and inflammation of cardiac valves. Bacteria most commonly isolated include *Streptococcus* spp., *Bartonella* spp., and *Escherichia coli*. Infections with *Bartonellosis* may only have inflammatory changes involving the aortic valve leaflets. *Erysipelothrix rhusiopathiae* is occasionally isolated. Confirmation of the definitive organism requires bacterial isolation. See the discussion on vegetative valvular and mural endocarditis in the section on Inflammation, Endocardium and Heart Valves, Responses to Injury, and also Chapter 3.

Myxomatous Valvular Degeneration (Valvular Endocardiosis)

Myxomatous valvular degeneration (valvular endocardiosis) is an important age-related cardiac disease of middle-aged to old dogs, especially small, toy, and medium-sized breeds, associated with degeneration of valvular collagen. Other names for this disease include *valvular fibrosis, degenerative mitral valve disease,* and *myxomatous* or *mucoid valvular degeneration.* This disease, the most common cause of congestive heart failure in old dogs, appears to have a polygenic inheritance. Males of affected breeds develop the disease at an earlier age than females. The cavalier King Charles spaniel breed has a unique susceptibility, with more than 50% prevalence by 4 years of age and 100% prevalence by 10 years of age. Other breeds with high incidence include the cocker spaniel, beagle, dachshund, poodle, papillon, Pomeranian, schnauzer, Chihuahua, Doberman pinscher, fox terrier, Boston terrier, bull terrier, Pekingese, deerhound, and wolfhound. Lesions occur most frequently (about two-thirds of cases) on the mitral valve only, less commonly (about one-third of cases) on the mitral and tricuspid valves, and infrequently on the aortic and pulmonary valves. The lesions become progressively worse with age. Affected valves are shortened and thickened (nodular), either focal or diffusely, and appear smooth and shiny (Fig. 10-84) rather than rough and granular, as is usual in cases of valvular endocarditis. These lesions result in valvular insufficiency with subsequent atrial dilation and development of atrial "jet lesions." The jet lesion is a raised, rough, firm streak of endocardial fibrosis resulting from long-term trauma by a jet of blood leaking through the damaged valve in the closed position. Other more severe complications of myxomatous valvular degeneration (valvular endocardiosis) include occasional rupture of the chordae tendineae and occasional splitting or rupture of the left atrial wall. Microscopically, the thickened valves have notably increased myofibroblastic proliferation and deposition of acid mucopolysaccharides (Fig. 10-85). Frequent accompanying myocardial alterations include arteriosclerosis of intramyocardial arteries and multifocal myocardial necrosis and fibrosis.

Valvular Anomalies and Dysplasia

See the discussion on valvular anomalies and dysplasia in the section on Disturbances of Growth, Disorders of Domestic Animals.

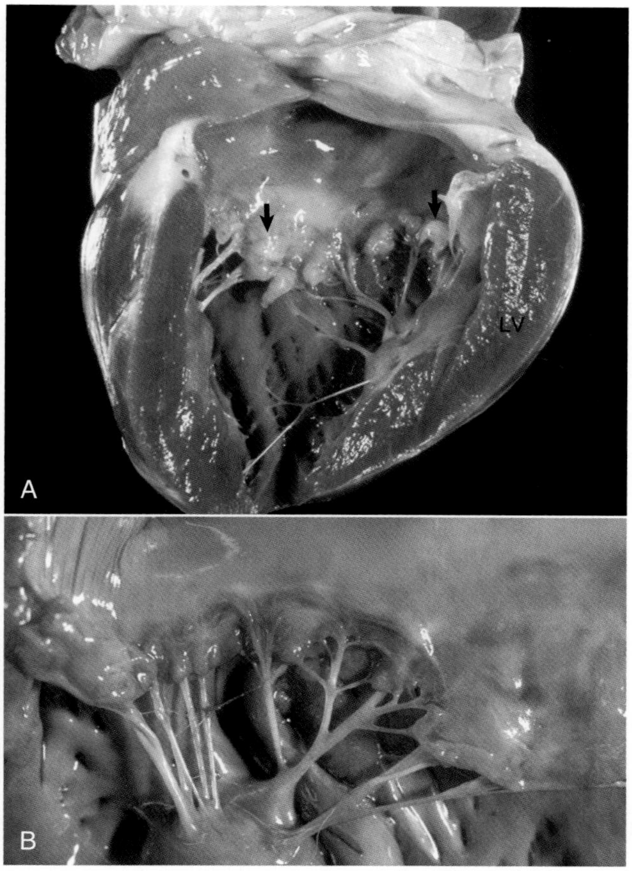

Fig. 10-84 Myxomatous valvular degeneration (valvular endocardiosis), left atrioventricular valve, heart, dog.
A, The cusps of the mitral valve are thickened by white, smooth nodules *(arrows). LV,* Left ventricular free wall. **B,** Note the characteristic smooth and shiny (endocardial) surface of the valve and nodules. This differentiates myxomatous valvular degeneration (endocardiosis) from the rough and granular surface of chronic bacterial endocarditis. The pink staining of the valve is caused by postmortem imbibition of hemoglobin. (**A** courtesy Dr. J. Wright, College of Veterinary Medicine, North Carolina State University; and Noah's Arkive, College of Veterinary Medicine, The University of Georgia. **B** courtesy Dr. M.D. McGavin, College of Veterinary Medicine, University of Tennessee.)

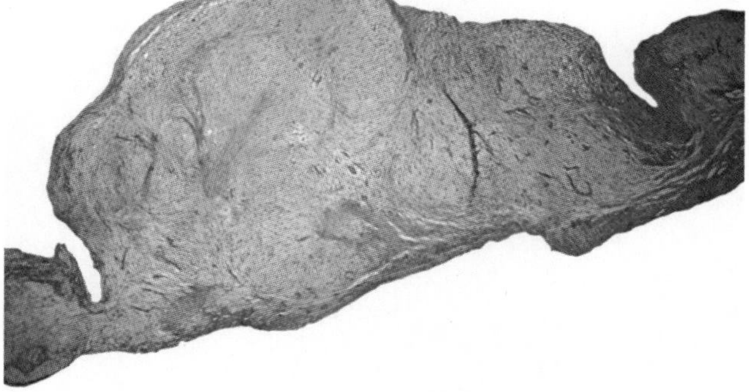

Fig. 10-85 Myxomatous valvular degeneration (valvular endocardiosis), cusp of right atrioventricular valve, heart, dog.
The valve is thickened and nodular from an increase in myxomatous tissue supported by a fibrous stroma. H&E stain. (Courtesy School of Veterinary Medicine, Purdue University.)

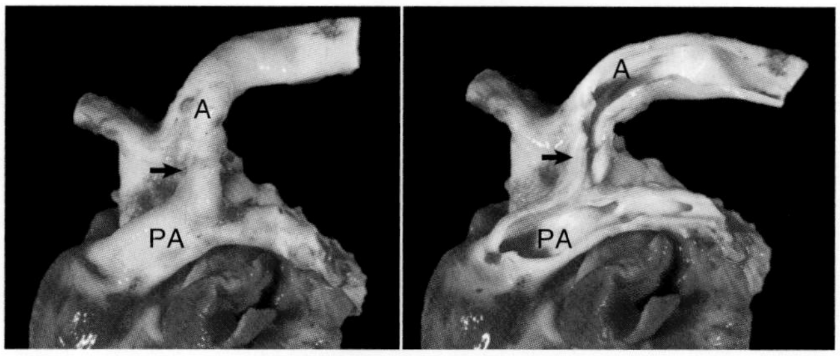

Fig. 10-86 Patent ductus arteriosus, heart, neonatal animal.
Note the prominent ductus arteriosus *(arrow)* between the pulmonary artery *(PA)* and the aorta *(A)* in the undissected *(left)* and dissected vessels *(right).* (Courtesy Dr. D.D. Harrington, School of Veterinary Medicine, Purdue University; and Noah's Arkive, College of Veterinary Medicine, The University of Georgia.)

BLOOD AND LYMPHATIC VASCULAR SYSTEMS

Blood Vessels

Developmental Errors: Congenital Anomalies

Patent Ductus Arteriosus

Patent ductus arteriosus is a frequent anomaly in poodle, collie, Pomeranian, Chihuahua, cocker spaniel, English springer spaniel, German shepherd, Keeshond, Maltese, Yorkshire terrier, bichon frise, and Shetland sheepdog breeds (Fig. 10-86). In poodles, it is an inherited polygenic trait. Female dogs have a greater incidence. This vascular channel between the pulmonary artery and aorta allows blood to bypass the lungs during fetal life and normally is converted to the solid ligamentum arteriosum postnatally. It remains patent in dogs with this anomaly. Generally, blood is shunted from the left to the right ventricle, resulting in overperfusion of the pulmonary vascular, subsequent pulmonary hypertension, and increased preload to the left ventricle.

Medial Necrosis and Hemorrhage

Medial necrosis and hemorrhage is a distinctive lesion produced in muscular arteries and arterioles of dogs and rats by a wide variety of vasoactive drugs. These vascular lesions, detected during evaluations of new compounds, produce grossly apparent hemorrhage, especially in the epicardium. Microscopically, acute damage is evident as necrosis of smooth muscle cells in the tunica media with surrounding erythrocytes. Healing lesions have fibrosis of the vessel wall and perivascularly.

Fibrocartilaginous Embolism

Fibrocartilaginous embolism of the spinal cord vasculature and resultant infarction of the spinal cord supplied or drained by the obstructed blood vessel lead to posterior paresis or paralysis. Affected dogs are typically middle-aged large or giant breeds, but occurrence in young Irish wolfhounds has been reported. The mechanism of formation of the arterial or venous emboli is still unclear, but movement within the spinal vasculature of fibrocartilaginous fragments from degenerated intervertebral disks is generally considered to underlie the presence of these unusual emboli (Fig. 10-87; Web Fig. 10-26).

Pulmonary Artery Thromboembolism

Pulmonary artery thromboembolism is often life threatening and occurs in dogs and cats (Fig. 10-88). A wide variety of predisposing conditions that may result in altered blood flow, hypercoagulability, or endothelial damage includes sepsis, immune-mediated

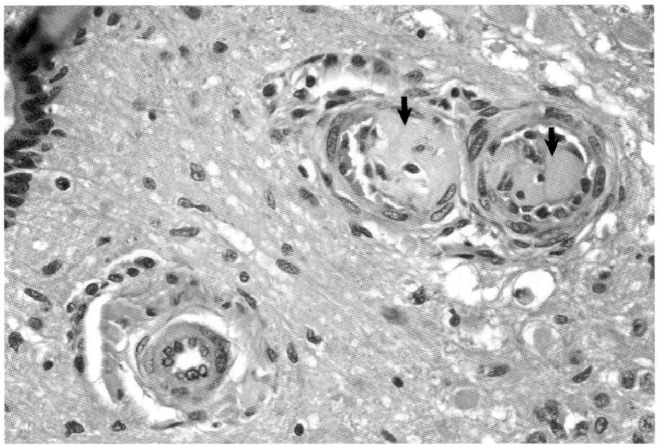

Fig. 10-87 Fibrocartilaginous emboli, spinal cord, pig.
The basophilic masses *(arrows)* occluding small arteries *(cross-sections)* in the spinal cord gray matter adjacent to the central canal *(top left margin)* are fibrocartilaginous emboli. H&E stain. (Courtesy School of Veterinary Medicine, Purdue University.)

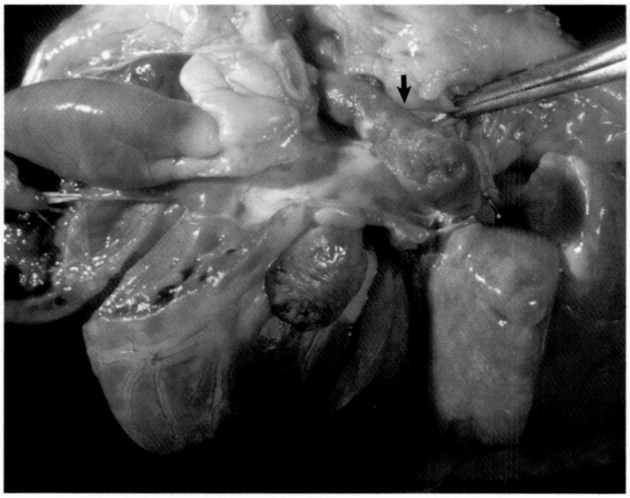

Fig. 10-88 Arterial mural thrombus, pulmonary artery, dog.
Arterial thrombi are composed primarily of platelets and fibrin because the rapid flow of blood tends to exclude erythrocytes from the thrombus, and thus arterial thrombi are usually pale beige to gray *(arrow)*. (Courtesy Dr. D.A. Mosier, College of Veterinary Medicine, Kansas State University.)

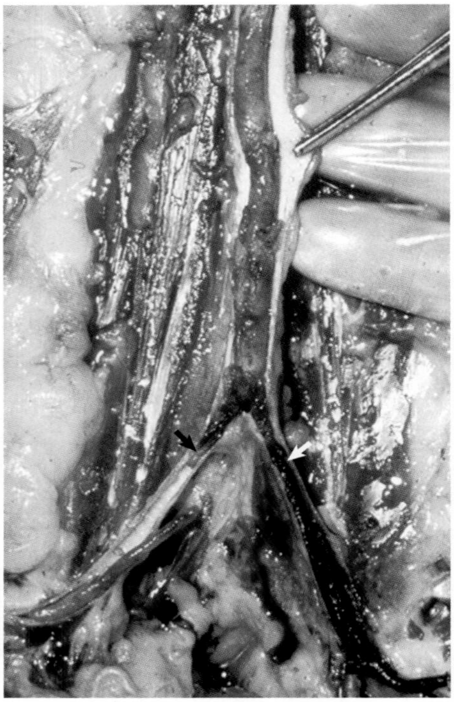

Fig. 10-89 Aortic thrombosis, aorta and external iliac arteries, dog.
The tan thrombus occluding the caudal abdominal aorta is a cranial extension of the red saddle thromboembolus at the aortic bifurcation and in the external iliac arteries *(arrows)*. (Courtesy School of Veterinary Medicine, Purdue University.)

hemolytic anemia, protein-losing nephropathy or enteropathy, disseminated intravascular coagulation, cardiac disease, neoplastic disease, hyperadrenocorticism, dirofilariasis, amyloidosis, and use of intravenous catheters.

Aortoiliac Thromboembolism and Thrombosis

Aortoiliac thromboembolism and thrombosis occurs in dogs (Fig. 10-89), cats (see Disorders of Cats), and horses (see Disorders of Horses). They arise from injury to vascular endothelium, propagate via the coagulation cascade (see Chapter 2), and ultimately occlude the caudal abdominal aorta and the external iliac arteries at the aortic bifurcation.

Thrombosis of the Femoral Artery

Thrombosis of the femoral artery, with resulting partial to complete occlusion, has been reported in cavalier King Charles spaniels. The condition may share a common etiopathogenesis with myxomatous valvular degeneration (valvular endocardiosis), which is frequent in this breed, through a genetically mediated connective tissue disorder. Affected dogs generally do not develop hindlimb ischemia, in contrast to human patients with this condition, because of extensive collateral circulation.

Heartworm Dirofilariasis (Dirofilaria immitis)

In canine dirofilariasis (heartworm infection), maturation of adult parasites occurs in the pulmonary arteries and may extend into the right atrium and ventricle. The pulmonary arteries containing parasites initially have an infiltration of the intima (termed *endarteritis*) by eosinophils, with subsequent development of an irregular fibromuscular proliferation of the intima visible grossly as a rough granular or shaggy appearance of the luminal surface (Fig. 10-90; Web Figs. 10-27 and 10-28). Live or dead parasites can be present within these vascular lesions and be accompanied by thromboembolism and pulmonary infarction. The presence of a massive number of adult worms may result in filling the right heart extending into venae cavae resulting in venal caval syndrome. This syndrome results in sudden collapse, liver failure, hemolytic anemia, shock, and death if the adult worms are not removed surgically.

Polyarteritis: "Beagle Pain Syndrome"

Polyarteritis is a disease that occurs sporadically in many animal species and is an important disease of aged rats (Web Fig. 10-29). Many recent reports have described the occurrence of polyarteritis in a disease termed *idiopathic necrotizing polyarteritis* (idiopathic canine polyarteritis, juvenile polyarteritis syndrome) involving multiple arteries including the coronary and meningeal arteries in dogs, most often pet and laboratory beagle dogs ("beagle pain

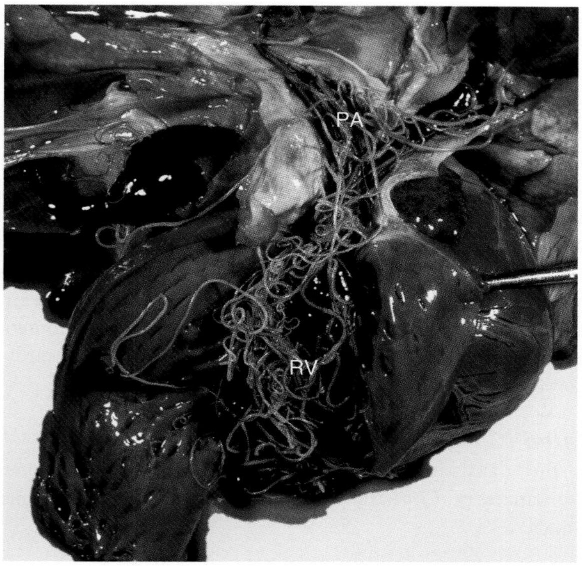

Fig. 10-90 Dirofilariasis, heart, opened right ventricle, and pulmonary artery, dog.
Numerous adult *Dirofilaria immitis* are present in the right ventricle *(RV)*, right atrium, and pulmonary artery *(PA)*. (Courtesy Dr. M.D. McGavin, College of Veterinary Medicine, University of Tennessee.)

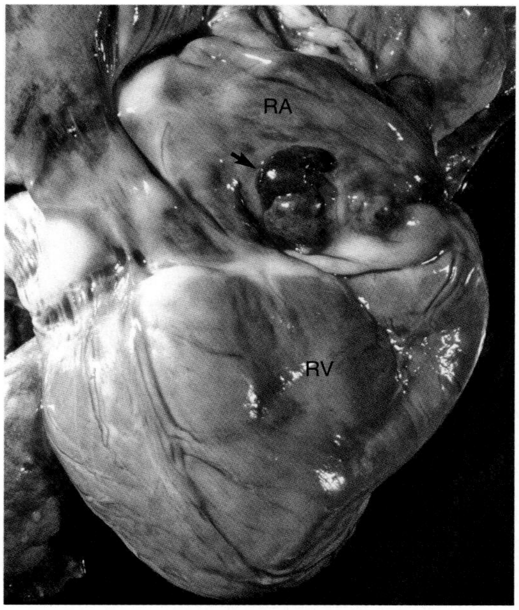

Fig. 10-91 Hemangiosarcoma, heart, right atrium, dog.
A dark-red hemangiosarcoma protrudes from the wall of the right atrium *(RA)*, a predilection site in the dog for this tumor *(arrow)*. *RV*, Right ventricle. (Courtesy Dr. M.D. McGavin, College of Veterinary Medicine, University of Tennessee.)

syndrome"). Clinically, affected dogs typically show recurrent episodes of fever, body weight loss, and occasionally cervical pain manifested by a still gait and stiff neck with a hunched body posture. However, some affected dogs do not display clinical signs of disease. The lesions are usually attributed to an immune-mediated vascular injury. Medium-sized muscular arteries in a wide variety of organs, including the heart and meninges, are selectively involved and grossly appear thick and tortuous, have associated focal hemorrhage, and develop aneurysms and thrombosis. Microscopically the early lesions include fibrinoid necrosis and leukocytic invasion of the intima and media (Web Fig. 10-30). In chronic lesions, inflammatory cells and fibrosis involve all layers of the vascular wall.

Hemangiosarcoma and Hemangioma

Cardiac hemangiosarcoma is an important neoplasm of dogs and can arise either in the heart (primary) or by metastasis (secondary) from sites such as the spleen. This neoplasm is usually seen in the wall of the right atrium and only occasionally involves the right ventricle. Grossly, protruding red to red-black blood-containing masses are located on the epicardial surface (Fig. 10-91) and may also protrude into the atrial lumen. Rupture can produce fatal hemopericardium and cardiac tamponade. Microscopically, the neoplasms are composed of scattered, elongated, plump neoplastic endothelial cells, which may or may not form vascular spaces containing blood (Fig. 10-92). Pulmonary metastases are frequent. Immunohistochemistry staining for Factor VIII-related antigen confirms the tumor cells are endothelial in origin. Hemangiomas are benign neoplasms often found in the skin of dogs (Fig. 10-93). These red, blood-filled masses are well circumscribed.

Heart-Base Tumors

See the discussion on neoplastic transformation in the section on Disturbance of Growth, Myocardium, Disorders of Domestic Animals and also Fig. 10-57.

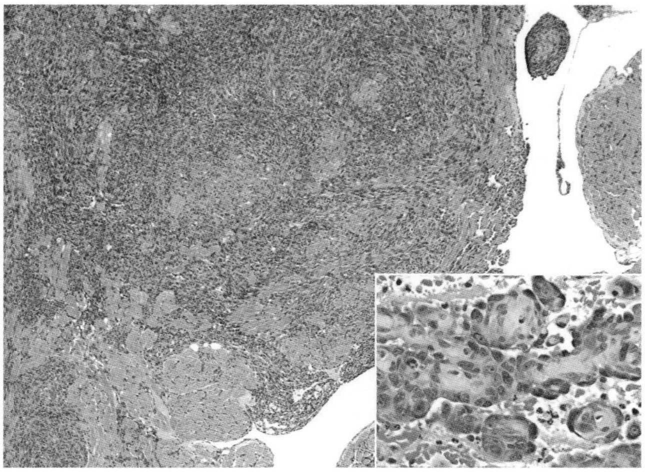

Fig. 10-92 Hemangiosarcoma, heart, right atrium, dog.
Malignant endothelial cells have invaded the myocardium of the right atrium, thus giving it the bluish granular appearance (cell nuclei) at low magnification. The high magnification *(inset)* shows these endothelial cells with large, round-to-oval nuclei forming poorly delineated and haphazardly arranged vascular channels. These cells can also "pile up" and be arranged in clusters or solid sheets. Mitotic figures can be prominent and numerous (not shown here). A golden-brown pigment (hemosiderin) can form secondary to erythrophagocytosis of damaged or effete erythrocytes (not shown here). H&E stain. (Courtesy Dr. J.F. Zachary, College of Veterinary Medicine, University of Illinois.)

Lymphatic Vessels

Intestinal Lymphangiectasia

Intestinal lymphangiectasia is an important disease of dogs in which there is a protein-losing enteropathy. Lacteals in the intestinal villi are prominently dilated, and lymphatic vessels throughout the wall of the bowel and the mesentery are distended (see Fig.

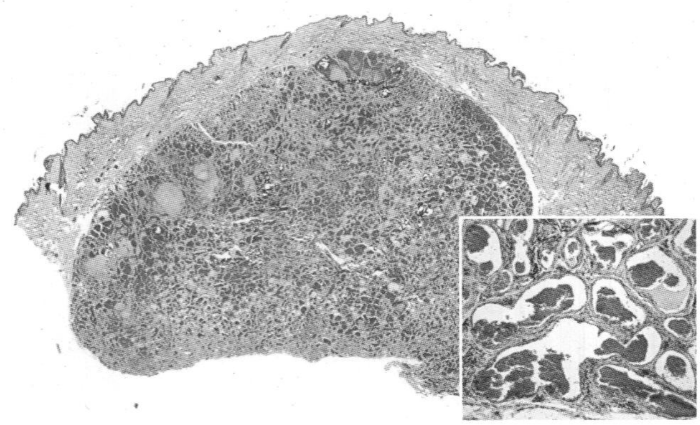

Fig. 10-93 Cutaneous hemangioma, skin, dog.
The subcutis contains a well-demarcated mass formed by vascular channels lined by a single layer of well-differentiated endothelial cells. *Inset,* Higher magnification of the well-differentiated endothelial cells lining the vascular channels. H&E stain. (Courtesy Dr. M.D. McGavin, College of Veterinary Medicine, University of Tennessee.)

7-121). The role of obstruction of lymphatic vessels in the pathogenesis of this disease is still unclear. Many diseases with severe acute inflammatory alterations accompanied by vascular damage, as with the pneumonia of bovine pasteurellosis, have prominently dilated lymphatic vessels.

Lymphangioma and Lymphangiosarcoma

Lymphangioma represents a rare benign neoplasm composed of lymphatic channels. Lymphangiosarcoma, the malignant counterpart, occurs more often than the benign neoplasm. Endothelial-lined vascular spaces contain lymph rather than the blood. Lymphatic vessels are frequently invaded by primary carcinomas and are a common route of metastasis.

DISORDERS OF CATS

MYOCARDIUM

Developmental Errors: Congenital Anomalies

See the discussion on developmental errors in the section on Disturbances of Growth, Myocardium, Disorders of Domestic Animals.

Cardiomyopathies

Hypertrophic Cardiomyopathy

Hypertrophic cardiomyopathy occurs frequently in cats (65% of cases), especially in young adult to middle-aged males (1 to 3 years old). Cats usually have congestive heart failure, and approximately 10% to 20% have posterior paresis from concurrent thromboembolism of the caudal abdominal aorta ("saddle thrombosis") secondary to left atrial thrombosis. Hypertrophic cardiomyopathy is inherited in an autosomal dominant manner in Maine coon cats. The occurrence of clusters of cases in Ragdoll, Norwegian Forest, and sphinx cat breeds suggests heritability of the disease as an autosomal dominant trait. Some cats die unexpectedly, which is the only clinical expression of the disease. This clinical presentation is often seen in humans with the disease. Affected hearts are enlarged and have prominent hypertrophy of the left ventricle and interventricular septum (see Fig. 10-50). The left ventricular cavity is small, and the left atrium is dilated. In a few cases, the interventricular septum is disproportionately hypertrophied in relation to the remainder of the myocardium. Microscopically the lesions of the myocardium are prominent disarray or disorganizations of myocytes, with interweaving rather than parallel arrangement of fibers (see Fig. 10-51). Myocyte hypertrophy, various degenerative alterations in myocytes, and interstitial fibrosis are present. Caudal aortic thromboembolism is seen in 10% of cats with primary hypertrophic cardiomyopathy (see Fig. 10-89). Current research in cats with the inherited disease and in human patients has documented mutated genes that encode for sarcomere proteins. To date, eleven altered genes are described in the human disease and one in cats (cardiac myosin-binding protein C). See the discussion on cardiomyopathies in the section on Disturbances of Growth, Myocardium, Disorders of Domestic Animals.

Dilated (Congestive) Cardiomyopathy

See the discussion on cardiomyopathies in the section on Disturbances of Growth, Myocardium, Disorders of Domestic Animals.

Endocardium and Heart Valves

Endomyocarditis

Endomyocarditis is a disease of cats of undetermined cause. The affected areas are thickened and often in the area of the outflow of the left ventricle. Lesions consist of a mixed population of inflammatory cells, which extends into the adjacent myocardium. Chronic lesions have marked, often visible fibrous connective tissue with fewer inflammatory cells within the endocardium.

Valvular Anomalies and Dysplasia

See the discussion on valvular anomalies and dysplasia in the section on Disturbances of Growth, Disorders of Domestic Animals.

Blood and Lymphatic Vascular Systems

Blood Vessels

Pulmonary Artery Thromboembolism

See the discussion on pulmonary artery thromboembolism in the section Blood Vessels, Blood and Lymphatic Vascular Systems, Disorders of Dogs.

Feline Infectious Peritonitis

Feline infectious peritonitis is a severe viral infection, which produces phlebitis in various organs. This lesion appears to result from deposition of immune complexes, which subsequently induce an inflammatory reaction in affected vessels (see Chapters 4, 7, and 11).

Medial Hypertrophy of Pulmonary Arteries

Medial (tunica media) hypertrophy of pulmonary arteries is a disorder of cats of unknown cause (see Fig. 10-37); however, a response to antigens during nematode infections may be involved.

Foreign Parasitic Diseases

Foreign parasitic diseases important in tropical regions of the world are characterized by presence of parasites in the lumens of veins. These diseases include infection of cats in South America by *Gurltia paralysans*. Affected cats have spinal cord damage from thrombophlebitis in the lumbar veins, associated with the presence of adult parasites in affected vessels.

SUGGESTED READINGS

Suggested Readings are available at evolve.elsevier.com/Zachary/McGavin/.

CHAPTER 11

The Urinary System*

Shelley J. Newman

STRUCTURE OF THE KIDNEY

Mammalian kidneys are paired organs present in the retroperitoneum, ventrolateral and adjacent to the lumbar vertebral bodies and their corresponding transverse processes. These complex organs, which function in excretion, metabolism, secretion, and regulation, are susceptible to disease insults that affect the four major anatomic structures of the kidney: the glomeruli, tubules, interstitium, and vasculature. Because of the limited ways that renal tissue can respond to injury and the limited patterns of injury, in severe and prolonged disease the endpoint will be similar—chronic renal disease and failure. Interdependence between components of the nephron also are responsible for producing a narrow range of repeatable injury patterns, which students can come to recognize on gross or histologic assessment.

Macroscopically, kidneys are organized functionally and anatomically into lobules. Each lobule represents collections of nephrons separated by the medullary rays (Fig. 11-1). Renal lobules should not be confused with renal lobes. Each lobe is represented by a renal pyramid (see Fig. 11-1). Among domestic animals, carnivores and horses have unilobar (or unipyramidal) kidneys. Porcine and bovine kidneys are multilobar (or multipyramidal), but only bovine kidneys have external lobation (Fig. 11-2). A diffuse fibrous capsule that in normal kidneys can be easily removed from the renal surface covers the kidneys. The renal parenchyma is divided into a cortex and medulla (Fig. 11-3). The corticomedullary ratio is usually approximately 1:2 or 1:3 in domestic animals. The ratio varies among species; for example, those adapted to the desert have a far larger medulla and thus a corticomedullary ratio that can approach 1:5. Normally the cortex is radially striated and dark red-brown except in mature cats, in which the cortex is often yellow because of the large lipid content of tubular epithelial cells. The renal medulla is pale gray and has either a single renal papilla, as in cats; a fused, crestlike papilla (renal medullary crest), as in dogs, sheep, and horses; or multiple renal papillae, as in pigs and cattle. The medulla generally can be subdivided into an outer zone, that portion of the medulla close to the cortex, and an inner zone, that portion closer to the pelvis. Papillae are surrounded by minor calyces that coalesce to form major calyces, which empty into the renal pelvis, where urine collects before entry into the ureters.

Microscopically, for ease of discussion, the kidney (and nephron) can be divided into four structural units: renal corpuscle (glomerulus and Bowman's capsule), tubules, interstitium, and vasculature. The functional unit of the kidney is the nephron, which includes the renal corpuscle and renal tubules (the tubular system includes the proximal convoluted tubules, the loop of Henle, and the distal convoluted tubule). The uriniferous tubule is composed of the nephron and the collecting ducts, which are embryologically distinct from the renal tubules (Fig. 11-4). The uriniferous tubule is embedded structurally in the renal interstitium formed by a meshwork composed of stromal cells such as fibroblasts. The interstitium also contains the renal vasculature, which supplies blood first to the glomerulus and then to the renal tubules.

GLOMERULUS (GLOMERULAR TUFTS)

Macroscopically, glomeruli are difficult to detect in the normal kidney but can be accentuated by lesions that allow them to be identified on cut section as randomly distributed granular foci or as red dots throughout the cortex. Microscopically, the glomerulus is a complex, convoluted tuft of fenestrated endothelial-lined capillaries held together by a supporting structure of cells in a glycoprotein matrix, the mesangium (Fig. 11-5). The entire glomerulus is supported by mesangial matrix that is secreted by the mesangial cells, a type of modified pericyte (Fig. 11-6). Mesangial cells are pluripotential mesenchymal cells, which are contractile and phagocytic and capable of synthesizing collagen and mesangial matrix, as well as secreting inflammatory mediators.

Glomerular Filtration Barrier

The glomerular filtration barrier is composed of (1) pedicles of podocytes (visceral epithelium of Bowman's capsule), (2) basal

*Dr. Anthony W. Confer and Dr. Roger J. Panciera of the Center for Veterinary Health Sciences, Oklahoma State University made contributions to this chapter in the fourth edition.

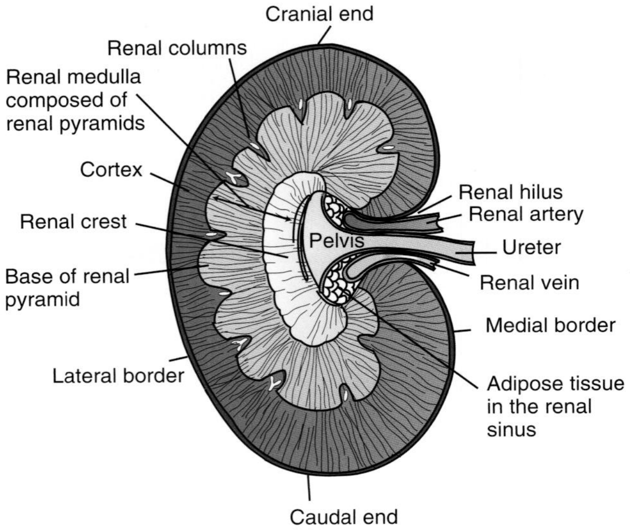

Fig. 11-1 Schematic diagram, kidney, dorsal section, dog.
(Based on Schaller O, Constantinescu GM, eds: *Illustrated veterinary anatomical nomenclature,* Stuttgart, Germany, 2007, Enke Verlag.)

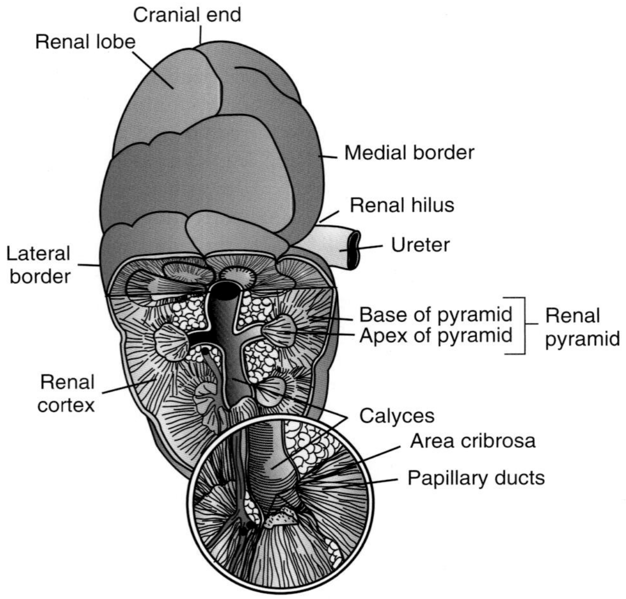

Fig. 11-2 Schematic diagram, kidney, dorsal surface and partial dorsal section, cow.
(Based on Schaller O, Constantinescu GM, eds: *Illustrated veterinary anatomical nomenclature,* Stuttgart, Germany, 2007, Enke Verlag.)

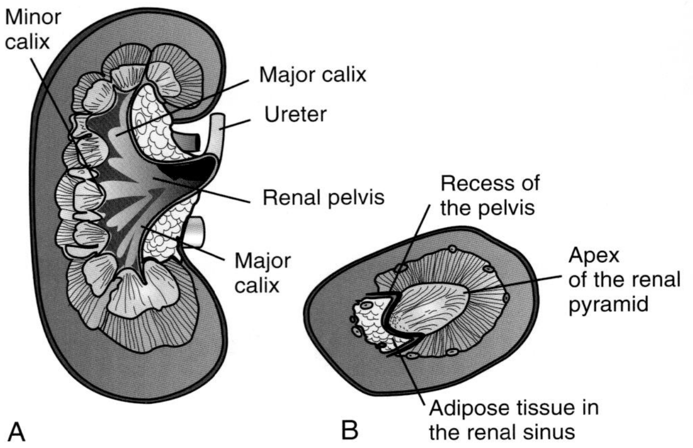

Fig. 11-3 Schematic diagram, kidney.
A, Dorsal section through hilus, pig. **B,** Transverse section through hilus, dog. (Based on Schaller O, Constantinescu GM, eds: *Illustrated veterinary anatomical nomenclature,* Stuttgart, Germany, 2007, Enke Verlag.)

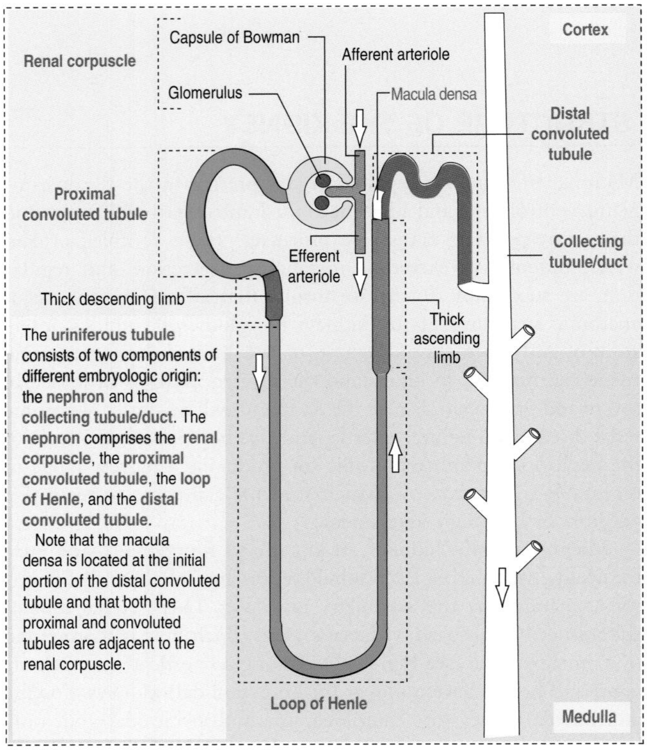

Fig. 11-4 Schematic diagram of the uriniferous tubule.
(From Kierszenbaum AL: *Histology and cell biology: an introduction to pathology,* ed 2, St Louis, 2007, Mosby.)

lamina (produced by both endothelial and epithelial cells), and (3) the fenestrated endothelium of glomerular capillaries (Fig. 11-7).

Visceral Epithelium (Podocytes)

Visceral epithelial cells (podocytes), aligned on the external surface of the basement membrane, are responsible for synthesis of basement membrane components and have special cytoplasmic processes (foot processes) that are embedded in the lamina rara externa. Negatively charged glycoproteins overlying the endothelial cells and the podocytes contribute to the charge differential of the glomerular basement membrane (GBM). Foot processes from adjacent visceral epithelium interdigitate to form filtration slits between them. Filtration slit diaphragms are composed of nephrin, a cell adhesion molecule of the immunoglobulin superfamily, which controls slit size by its connection to podocyte actin (see Fig. 11-7). The glomerular filtration barrier selectively filters molecules based on size (70,000 Da), electrical charge (the more cationic, the more permeable), and capillary pressure. In summary, both size-dependent and charge-dependent filtration is possible because of the porous structure of capillary walls, which is a function of endothelial fenestrations, a basement membrane formed of

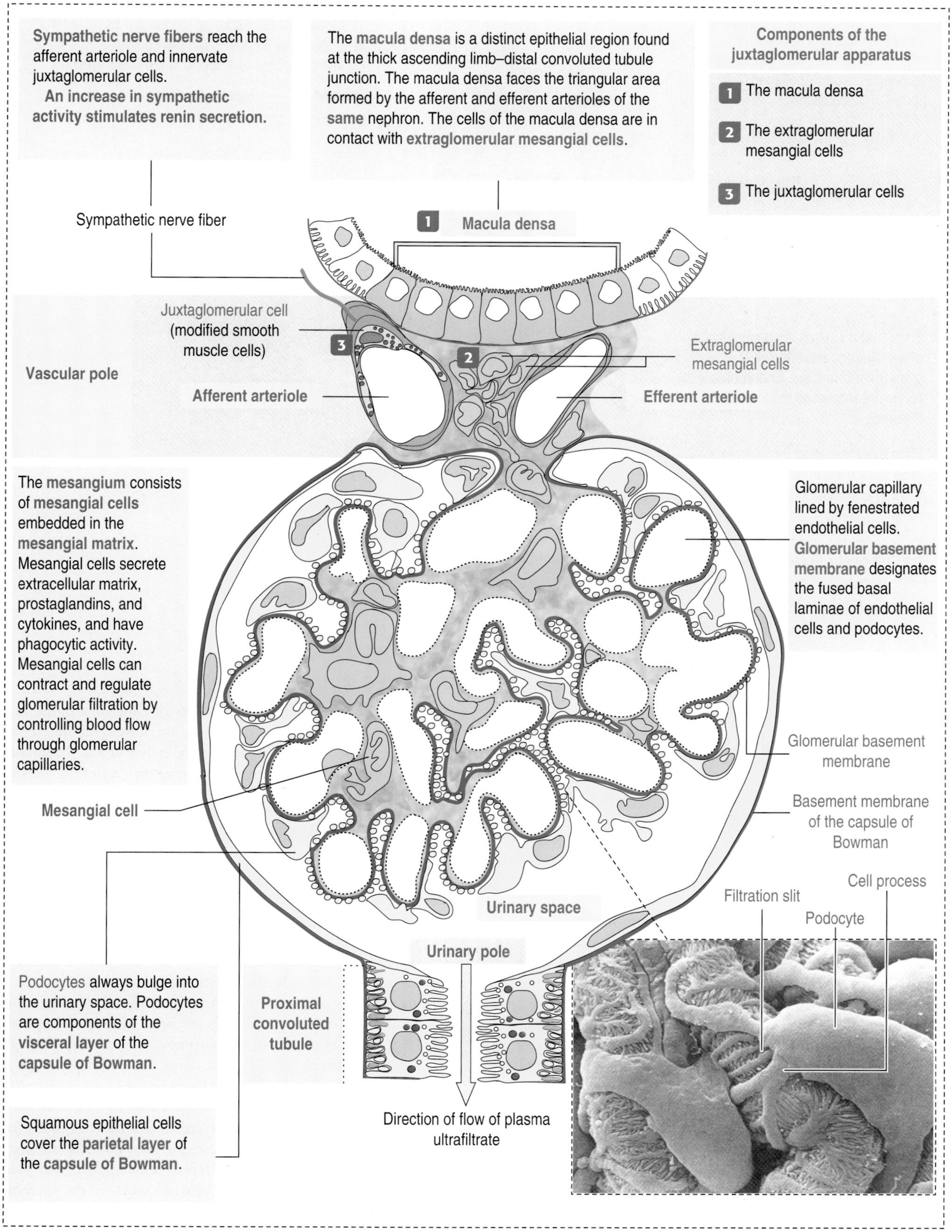

Fig. 11-5 Schematic diagram of the renal corpuscle.

(From Kierszenbaum AL: *Histology and cell biology: an introduction to pathology,* ed 2, St Louis, 2007, Mosby. Scanning electron micrograph from Kessel RG, Kardon RH: *Tissues and organs,* New York, 1979, WH Freeman.)

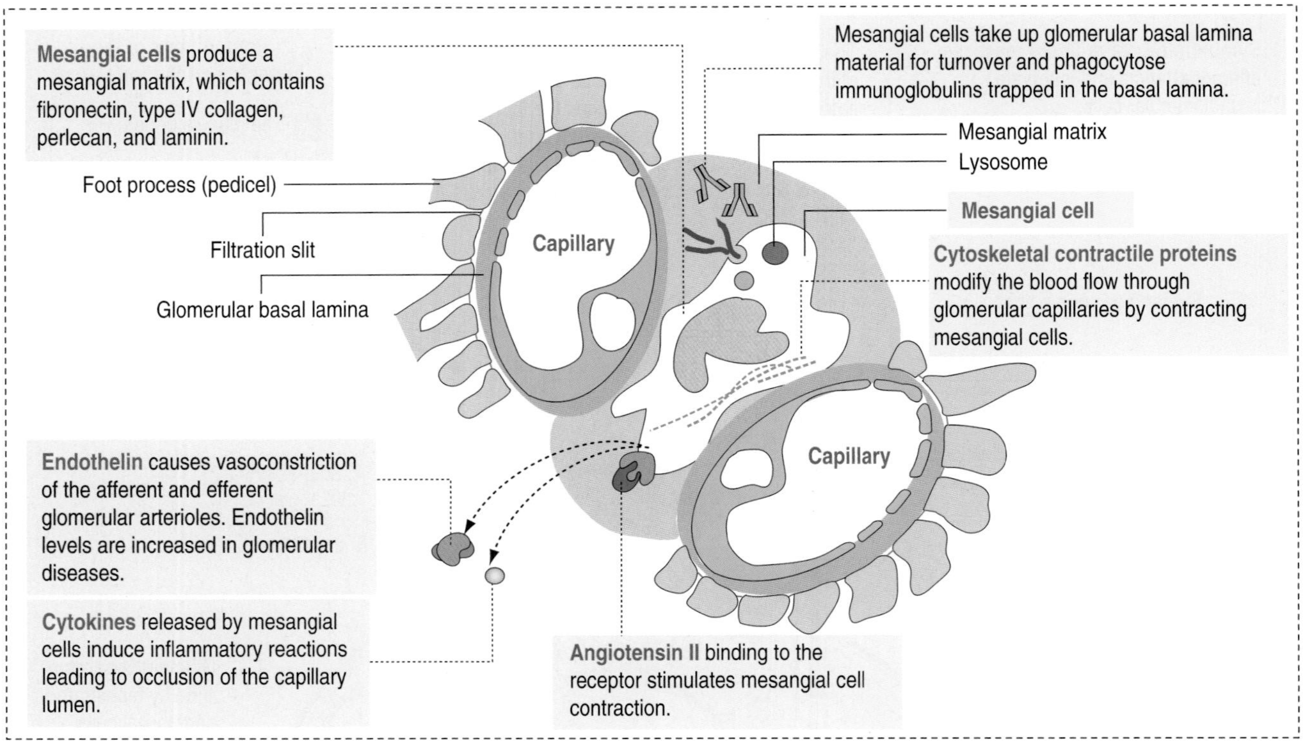

Fig. 11-6 Schematic diagram of the functions and organization of the mesangium.
(From Kierszenbaum AL: *Histology and cell biology: an introduction to pathology,* ed 2, St Louis, 2007, Mosby.)

type IV collagen, basement membrane anionic glycoproteins, and filtration slits of the visceral epithelium.

Glomerular Basement Membrane (Basal Lamina)

The glomerular basement membrane has a thick, dense central layer, the lamina densa, which is covered by thinner, more electron-lucent inner and outer layers, the lamina rara interna and lamina rara externa, respectively. The basement membrane has a network of type IV collagen, which forms a tetrameric porous infrastructure. Numerous glycoproteins, such as acidic proteoglycans and laminin, together with the collagen fibers form the complete structure of the membrane.

Glomerular Capillaries

The glomerular capillaries exist between the afferent and efferent arterioles and form the glomerular tuft. Glomerular capillaries interdigitate with the visceral lining of Bowman's space. The capillary endothelium is fenestrated and covered by a complete basal lamina.

BOWMAN'S CAPSULE

Bowman's capsule is a cup-shaped sac at the beginning of the nephron that encloses the glomerulus (see Fig. 11-4).

Parietal Epithelium

The capillary tuft (glomerulus) is covered by visceral epithelial cells (podocytes) and is contained within the membranous "cap" (Bowman's capsule) that is lined by parietal epithelial cells resembling squamous epithelium (see Fig. 11-5).

TUBULES

The renal tubular system (in the order of flow of urine) consists of a proximal tubule, loop of Henle, and distal tubule (see Fig. 11-4). The tubules connect to the renal pelvis at the distal end of the collecting ducts, and the whole structure, including the renal corpuscle, renal tubules, and collecting ducts is referred to as the *uriniferous tubule* (see Fig. 11-4). Macroscopically, the proximal and distal convoluted tubules are linked by the loop of Henle, which is divided into a descending and an ascending limb. The wall of the descending limb and initial portion of the ascending limb is thin (permeable), whereas the cortical portion of the ascending limb is thick (impermeable). Microscopically, the proximal tubule is lined by columnar epithelial cells that have a microvillous (brush) border. This arrangement greatly increases their absorptive surface, and their numerous intracellular mitochondria supply energy for the various secretory and absorptive functions. Distal tubules, collecting tubules, and the loop of Henle are lined by cuboidal epithelial cells that contribute to the concentration of urine by absorptive and secretory activities.

INTERSTITIUM

Macroscopically, the interstitium consists of a relatively scant connective tissue stroma, primarily present as a reticular meshwork found around and between uriniferous tubules. Microscopically, fibroblasts and connective tissue provide most of the interstitial tissue support. Glycosaminoglycans secreted as part of the extracellular matrix (ECM) increase with age and ischemic damage. Cells in the interstitium, particularly in the medulla, are responsible for local production of prostaglandins. Blood vessels, nerves, and lymphatic vessels are present in the renal interstitium.

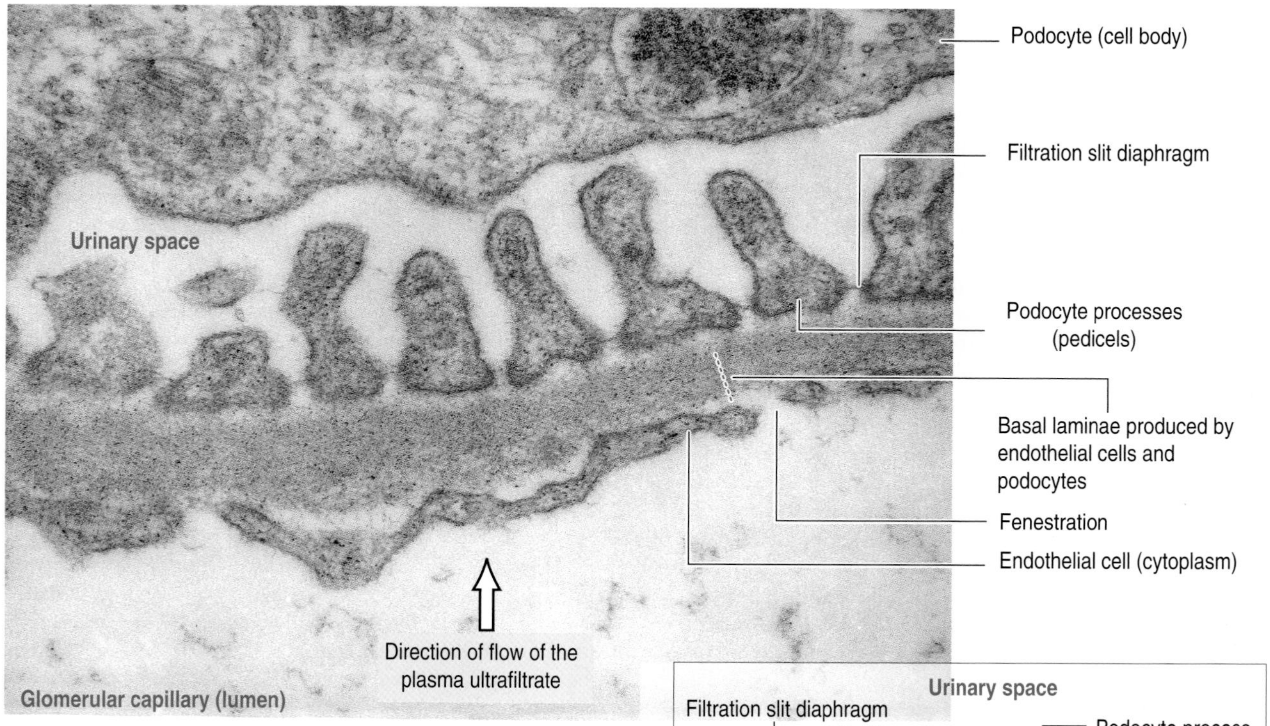

Components of the filtration barrier

1 The **endothelium** of the glomerular capillaries is **fenestrated** and permeable to water, sodium, urea, glucose, and small proteins. Endothelial cells are coated by **negatively charged glycoproteins** (heparan sulfate), which slow down the filtration of large anionic proteins.

2 The **basal lamina**, a product of endothelial cells and podocytes, contains type IV collagen, laminin, fibronectin, and proteoglycans rich in the glycosaminoglycan heparan sulfate—which also slows down the filtration of anionic proteins.

3 The pedicels are interdigitating cell processes of podocytes covering the basal lamina and coated by a negatively charged glycoprotein coat. The space between adjacent pedicels is called the **filtration slit**. A **filtration slit diaphragm** links adjacent pedicels.

The diaphragm consists of **nephrin**, a cell adhesion molecule of the immunoglobulin superfamily, anchored to actin filaments within the pedicel by the proteins CD2AP, zonula occludens (ZO)-1, and podocin.

A mutation of the gene encoding nephrin causes **congenital nephrotic syndrome**, characterized by massive proteinuria (leakage of albumin in urine) and edema.

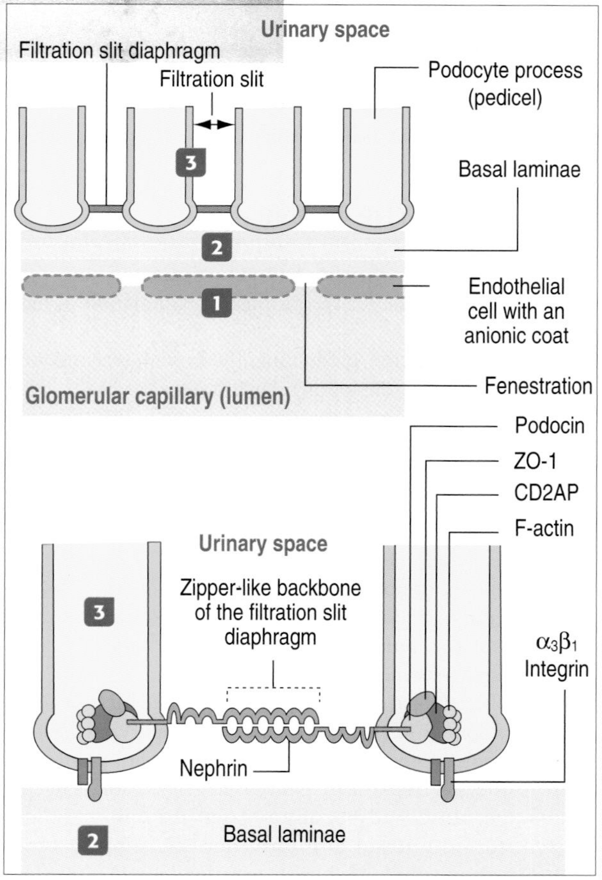

Fig. 11-7 Schematic diagram of the filtration barrier.

(From Kierszenbaum AL: *Histology and cell biology: an introduction to pathology,* ed 2, St Louis, 2007, Mosby.)

VASCULATURE

Macroscopically, knowledge of the normal renal blood supply is important in understanding the pathogenesis and distribution of various renal lesions, especially renal infarcts. The kidneys receive blood primarily through the renal artery. An interlobar artery extends along the boundary of each renal lobe (renal column) and then branches at right angles to form an arcuate artery that runs along the corticomedullary junction (Fig. 11-8). Interlobular arteries branch from the arcuate artery and extend into the cortex. They have no anastomoses, making them susceptible to focal ischemic necrosis (infarct) as in any organ with end arteries.

Microscopically, interlobular arteries have small branches that become afferent glomerular arterioles, which enter the renal corpuscle and subsequently exit at the vascular pole as efferent glomerular arterioles (see Fig. 11-8). Efferent arterioles supply the blood for the extensive network of capillaries that surround the cortical and medullary tubular system of the kidneys, known as the *peritubular capillary network*. The latter surrounds cortical segments of the tubules and then drains into the interlobular vein, arcuate vein, interlobar vein, and ultimately the renal vein. Additionally, the vasa recta are formed from the deeper portions of the peritubular network and descend into the medulla and around the lower portions of the loop of Henle before ascending to the cortex and emptying into venous vessels that connect to the interlobular and arcuate veins. The vasa recta parallel the descending and ascending limbs of the loop of Henle and the collecting ducts (see Fig. 11-4). Hence the blood supply to the tubules depends on passage through the glomerular vessels.

FUNCTION OF THE KIDNEY

The kidney has the following five basic functions:

- Formation of urine for the purpose of elimination of metabolic wastes.
- Acid-base regulation, predominantly through reclamation of bicarbonate from the glomerular filtrate.
- Conservation of water through reabsorption by the proximal convoluted tubules, the countercurrent mechanism of the loop of Henle, antidiuretic hormone (ADH) activity in the distal tubules, and the urea gradient in the medulla. The tubular system is capable of absorbing up to 99% of the water in the glomerular filtrate.
- Maintenance of normal extracellular potassium ion concentration through passive reabsorption in the proximal tubules and tubular secretion in the distal tubules under the influence of aldosterone.
- Control of endocrine function through three hormonal axes: renin-angiotensin (see Fig. 11-8), most importantly, but also erythropoietin and vitamin D. Erythropoietin, produced in the kidneys in response to reduced oxygen tension, is released into the blood and stimulates bone marrow to produce erythrocytes. Vitamin D is converted in the kidneys to its most active form (1,25-dihydroxycholecalciferol [calcitriol]), which facilitates calcium absorption by the intestine.

FUNCTION OF THE GLOMERULAR BASEMENT MEMBRANE

The GBM is structurally adept at separating substances based on size and charge. Additionally, the glomerulus is equipped with its own specialized mesangial cells, a component of the monocyte-macrophage system (see Figs. 11-6 and 11-7). Both size-dependent and charge-dependent filtration is possible because of the porous structure of capillary walls, which is a function of endothelial fenestrations, a basement membrane formed of type IV collagen, basement membrane anionic glycoproteins, and filtration slits of visceral epithelium. In addition to the principal glomerular function of plasma filtration, glomerular functions also include regulation of blood pressure by means of secreting vasopressor agents and/or hormones, regulation of peritubular blood flow, regulation of tubular metabolism, and removal of macromolecules from circulation by the glomerular mesangium. Integral to these functions is the juxtaglomerular apparatus, which functions in tubuloglomerular feedback by autoregulating renal blood flow and glomerular filtration rate. The juxtaglomerular apparatus is composed of four components: (1) an afferent arteriole whose smooth muscle is modified to form myoepithelial cells, which are the juxtaglomerular cells that secrete renin; (2) an efferent arteriole; (3) the macula densa; and (4) the extraglomerular mesangium. Renin, produced by cells of the juxtaglomerular apparatus, stimulates the production of angiotensin I from circulating angiotensinogen. The angiotensin-converting enzyme in the macula densa converts angiotensin I to angiotensin II, which then functions to constrict afferent renal arterioles; maintain renal blood pressure; stimulate aldosterone secretion from the adrenal gland, thus increasing sodium (Na^+) reabsorption; and stimulate ADH release (Fig. 11-9). ADH principally increases the permeability of collecting tubules to water and increases the permeability of the medullary region to urea.

FUNCTION OF THE PROXIMAL TUBULES

A key function of the proximal tubules is to reabsorb Na^+, chloride (Cl^-), potassium (K^+), albumin, glucose, water, and bicarbonate. This is facilitated by luminal brush border, basolateral infoldings, magnesium-dependent Na^+ and K^+ pumps, and transport proteins. The proximal tubule is continuous with the loop of Henle that is in close physiologic and anatomic association with the peritubular capillary network (within the cortex) and the vasa recta (within the medulla). The loop of Henle, via a countercurrent mechanism and Na^+/K^+-adenosine phosphatase (ATPase) pumps, absorbs Na^+ and Cl^- ions, producing a hypotonic filtrate that flows into the next portion of the nephron—the distal convoluted tubule. Here, water is reabsorbed from the tubule into the interstitium because of a solute concentration gradient and by the effects of ADH. The filtrate is further concentrated in the collecting ducts by water and sodium reabsorption by a Na^+/K^+-ATPase pump and additional water reabsorption into the medullary interstitium by a urea gradient. Intercalated cells of the collecting tubule regulate acid-base balance and reabsorb potassium. Thus the final excretory product, urine, is formed (Fig. 11-10).

Renal Failure (Loss of Function)

Renal failure occurs when one or more of the functions previously listed are altered. When renal functional capacity is abruptly impaired (loss of 75%), such that the kidneys fail to carry out their normal metabolic and endocrine functions, acute renal failure can ensue. It is important to remember that the glomerulus, tubules, collecting ducts, and capillary blood supply in each nephron are closely interrelated, both anatomically and functionally. The fluid that filters through the glomerulus into Bowman's space is called *glomerular filtrate,* and it arises after passage through the glomerular filtration barrier. This ultrafiltrate of plasma (primary urine), which contains water, salts, ions, glucose, and albumin, passes into the capsular space (Bowman's space) and then empties into the proximal convoluted tubule at the urinary pole to traverse through and be acted on by the tubular system. Alterations in tubular structure

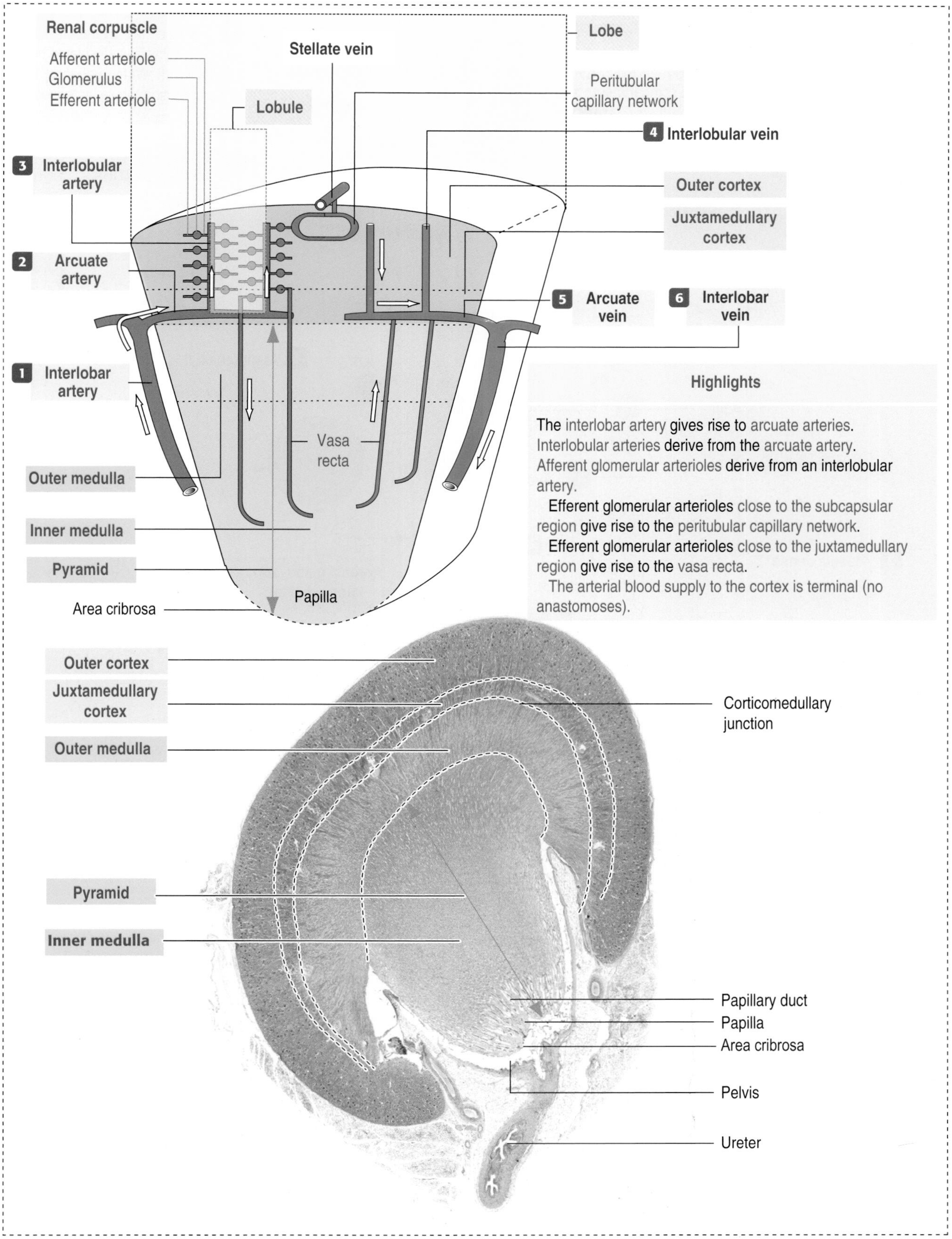

Fig. 11-8 Schematic diagram of the vasculature of the kidney.
(From Kierszenbaum AL: *Histology and cell biology: an introduction to pathology,* ed 2, St Louis, 2007, Mosby.)

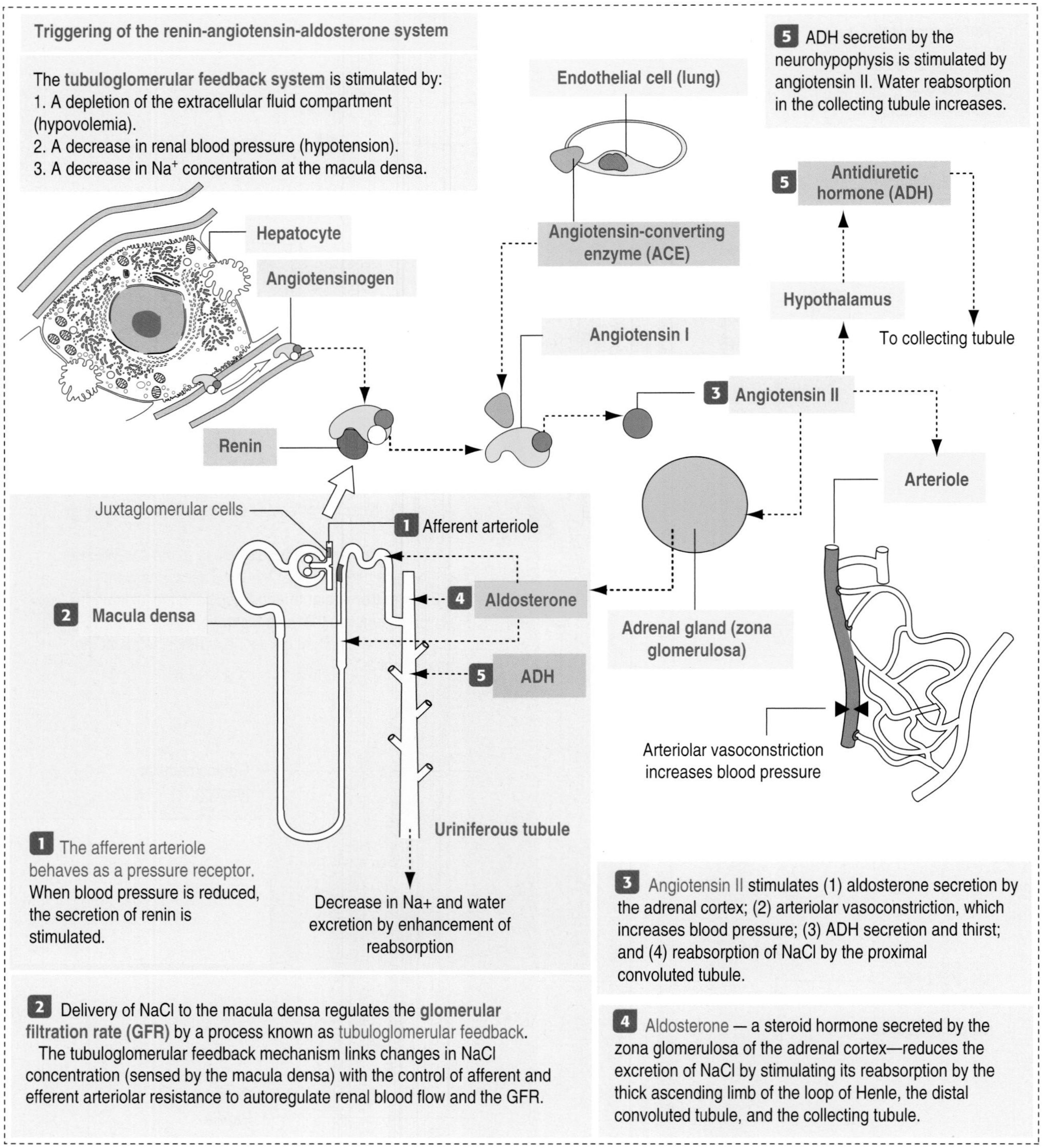

Fig. 11-9 Schematic diagram of the renin-angiotensin-aldosterone system.
(From Kierszenbaum AL: *Histology and cell biology: an introduction to pathology,* ed 2, St Louis, 2007, Mosby.)

or function influence glomerular structure and function and vice versa. For example, necrosis or atrophy of renal tubules results in loss of function of the affected nephrons and secondary atrophy of the glomerulus. In addition, because most of the capillary blood supply to tubules is through postglomerular capillaries, a reduction in glomerular blood flow consequently reduces the blood supply to the tubules.

Acute Renal Failure

Acute renal failure can be caused by (1) tubular necrosis from infectious agents, such as bacteria (*Leptospira* spp., *Escherichia coli*, *Streptococcus* spp., *Staphylococcus* spp., and *Proteus* spp.) or viruses (infectious canine hepatitis virus, canine distemper virus, and canine herpesvirus); (2) obstructive nephropathy from urolithiasis, transitional cell neoplasms of the lower urinary system, or

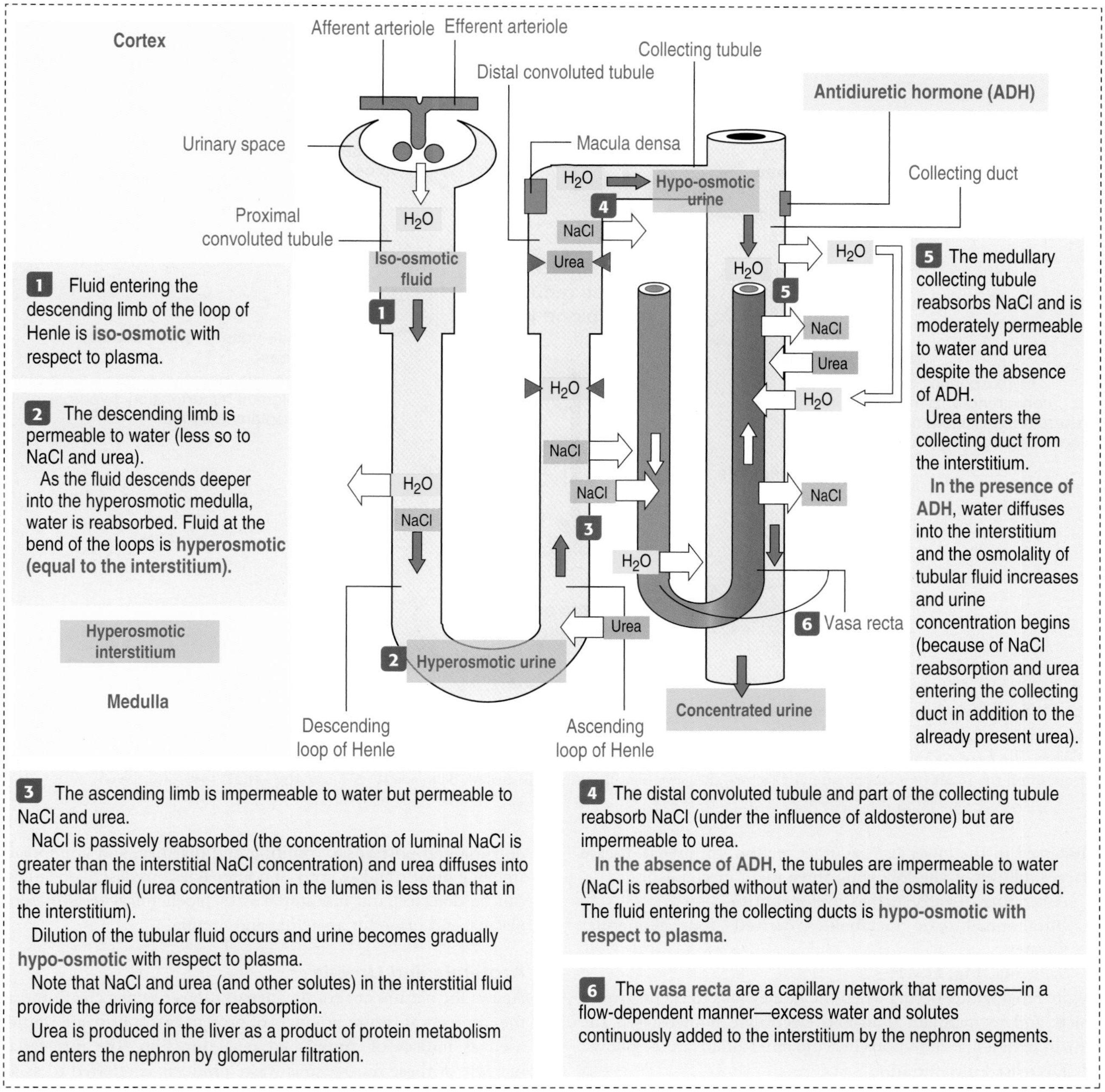

Fig. 11-10 Schematic diagram of the counter-current multiplier and exchanger.
(From Kierszenbaum AL: *Histology and cell biology: an introduction to pathology,* ed 2, St Louis, 2007, Mosby.)

trauma; (3) renal ischemia with tubular necrosis from occlusive vasculitis/vasculopathy caused by bacteria, bacterial toxins, or tumor emboli; (4) tubular necrosis from nephrotoxic drugs, such as aminoglycoside-based antimicrobial drugs or antineoplastic drugs; and/or (5) tubular necrosis from chemicals, such as ethylene glycol and heavy metals.

Functionally, acute renal failure can be caused by prerenal (compromised renal perfusion), intrarenal (compromised kidney function), or postrenal (obstruction of the urinary tract) factors. Prerenal factors include reduced renal blood flow, whether secondary to circulatory collapse (shock, severe hypovolemia) or local obstruction of vascular supply (thrombus or lodgement of embolus). Acute tubular necrosis, a form of intrarenal acute renal failure, induces clinical oliguria (decrease in urine production) or anuria (absence of urine production) by one or several mechanisms. These mechanisms include the following:

- Leakage of tubular ultrafiltrate from damaged tubules across disrupted basement membranes into the renal interstitium.
- Intratubular obstruction resulting from sloughed necrotic epithelium.

The latter mechanism is less well accepted, but both mechanisms result in decreased glomerular filtration rate.

Prerenal and intrarenal factors are most responsible for episodes of acute renal failure, with prerenal azotemia and ischemic tubular damage actually being a continuum. Postrenal obstructive diseases

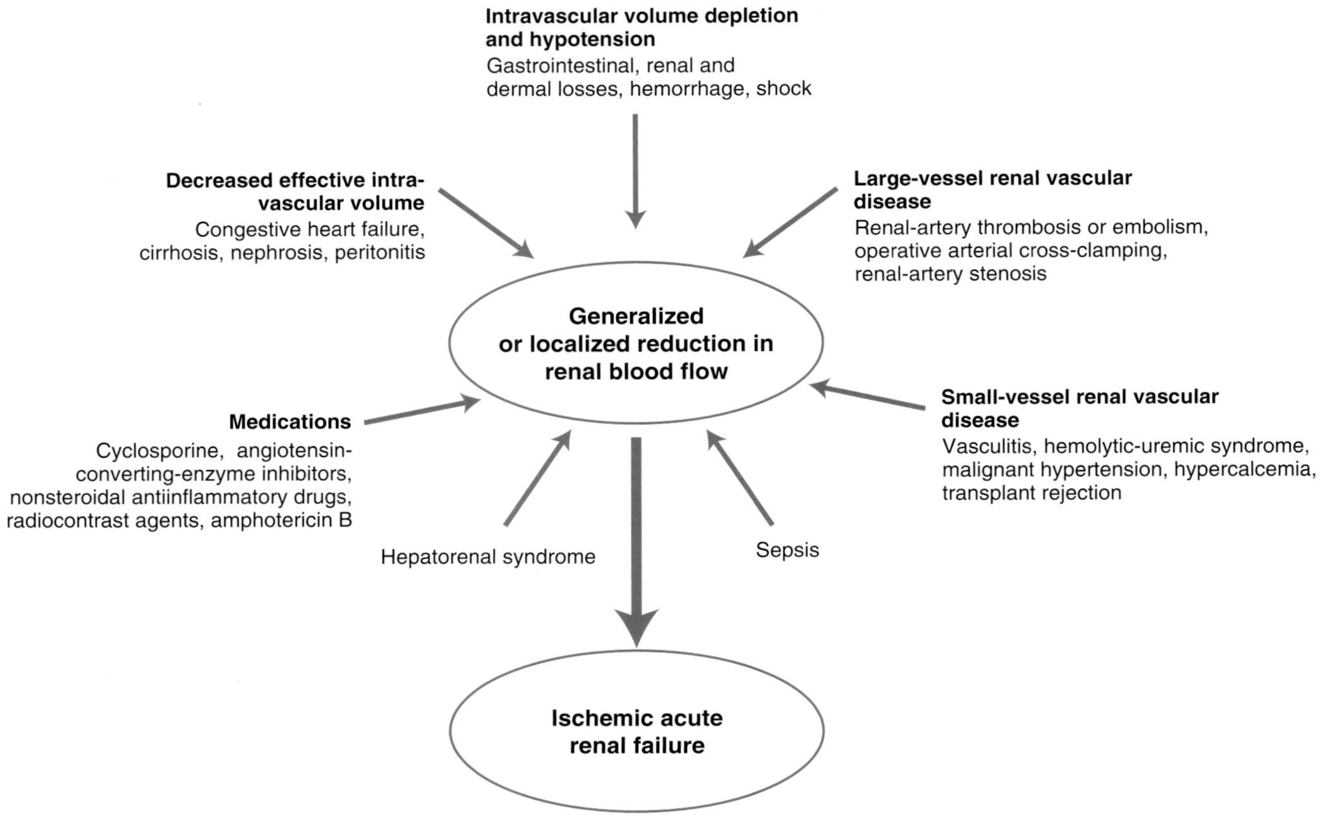

Fig. 11-11 Schematic diagram of ischemic renal failure.
A wide spectrum of clinical conditions can result in a generalized or localized reduction in renal blood flow, thus increasing the likelihood of ischemic acute renal failure. The most common condition leading to ischemic acute renal failure is severe and sustained prerenal azotemia. Kidney ischemia and acute renal failure are often the result of a combination of factors. (Redrawn from Thadhani R, Pascual M, Bonventre JV: *N Engl J Med* 334(22):1448-1460, 1996.)

are discussed in the lower urinary tract section. Intrarenal disease can target tubules by the following three main mechanisms:

- Ascending disease, such as pyelonephritis
- Intraluminal toxic metabolites derived from glomerular filtrate
- Ischemia (Fig. 11-11)

Acute renal failure occurs when the kidney fails to excrete waste products and to maintain fluid and electrolyte homeostasis. The four main pathologic alterations in acute renal failure are as follows:

- Decreased ultrafiltration
- Intratubular obstruction
- Fluid back leak
- Intrarenal vasoconstriction

These alterations can occur after many insults, including the following:

- Decreased renal perfusion
- Decreased glomerular filtration
- Ischemic tubular damage
- Toxic tubular damage
- Obstructive renal tubular damage
- Tubulointerstitial inflammation, edema, or fibrosis

Animals that die of acute renal failure often do so because of the cardiotoxicity of elevated serum potassium, metabolic acidosis, and/or pulmonary edema. Hyperkalemia results from decreased filtration, decreased tubular secretion, and decreased tubular sodium transport. Cell lysis and the extracellular shift of fluid in acidic environments also contribute to the increased serum potassium concentrations. These alterations are reflected clinically by signs, such as polyuria and polydipsia, vomiting and diarrhea, and ammoniacal-smelling breath, and an array of nonrenal lesions described later and can be detected and monitored with biochemical tests of serum, plasma, and urine for azotemia and uremia.

Azotemia and Uremia

Assays for plasma or serum concentrations of urea, creatinine, and the nitrogenous waste products of protein catabolism, are routinely used as indices of diminished renal function. The intravascular increase of these nitrogenous waste products is referred to as azotemia. Renal failure can result in the following:

- Intravascular accumulation of other metabolic wastes such as guanidines, phenolic acids, and large molecular weight alcohols (example: myoinositol)
- Reduced blood pH (metabolic acidosis)
- Alterations in plasma ion concentrations, particularly potassium, calcium, and phosphate
- Hypertension

The result of renal failure is a toxicosis called *uremia.* Uremia can therefore be defined as a syndrome associated with multisystemic lesions and clinical signs because of renal failure. These multisystemic lesions are discussed in greater detail in the section on Disorders of Domestic Animals.

Chronic Renal Failure

Similar to acute renal failure, chronic renal failure occurs over a longer time duration and results in several additional hematologic and biochemical alterations. In the diseased kidney, production of erythropoietin, a stimulant of erythropoietic maturation, is reduced and contributes to nonregenerative anemia, as does uremia-associated increased erythrocytic fragility. Most animals in renal failure have hyperphosphatemia and low to normal calcium levels, although variations exist, depending on species and stage of the disease. Alterations in calcium-phosphorus metabolism in the uremic animal are a hallmark of chronic renal failure and result from a complex set of events as outlined in the following:

- When the glomerular filtration rate is chronically reduced to less than 25% of normal, phosphorus is no longer adequately secreted by the kidneys and hyperphosphatemia results.
- Because of the mass law interactions between serum calcium and phosphorus, ionized calcium concentration in serum is reduced as a result of precipitation of calcium and phosphorus.
- Reduced ionized serum calcium stimulates parathyroid hormone (PTH) secretion, causing calcium release from the readily mobilizable calcium stores in the bone and from osteoclastic bone resorption.

These changes in calcium-phosphorus metabolism are made more severe by the reduced ability of the diseased kidneys to hydroxylate 25-hydroxycholecalciferol to the more active 1,25-dihydroxycholecalciferol (calcitriol), resulting in decreased intestinal absorption of calcium. Calcitriol production is further inhibited by hyperphosphatemia. In addition, calcitriol normally suppresses PTH secretion; therefore reduced calcitriol production further increases PTH secretion. With time, these events lead to parathyroid chief cell hyperplasia (renal secondary hyperparathyroidism), fibrous osteodystrophy (renal osteodystrophy), and soft tissue calcification.

Renal secondary hyperparathyroidism is further thought to perpetuate and enhance renal disease by stimulating nephrocalcinosis (see Fig. 11-31; also see Chapter 12), the process by which renal tubular epithelium is damaged by an increase in intracellular calcium. Calcium is precipitated in mitochondria and in tubular basement membranes. Soft tissue calcification associated with uremia occurs in numerous sites and represents both dystrophic and metastatic calcification. These lesions are discussed in greater detail in the section on Disorders of Domestic Animals.

PORTALS OF ENTRY

KIDNEY AS A WHOLE

The urinary system and especially the kidney can be exposed to injurious stimuli and agents via a number of routes (Box 11-1), including the following:

- Hematogenous
- Ascending from ureter
- Glomerular filtrate
- Direct penetration

RENAL CORPUSCLE

Hematogenous

As in all visceral organs, the sustaining blood supply can provide a portal of hematogenous entry for infectious organisms, which in the kidney can lead to glomerular localization or embolic nephritis.

TUBULES

Glomerular Filtrate

Substances secreted into the glomerular filtrate can produce localized trauma to tubular lining cells such as crystalline salt oversaturation (e.g., oxalate crystals). Filtered preformed toxins or metabolized substances processed by the tubular lining epithelium exert their effect principally on the proximal tubular epithelium.

BOX 11-1 Portals of Entry to the Kidney

ASCENDING FROM URETER

- Extension from lower urinary tract secondary to gastrointestinal content contamination (diarrhea) (females primarily)
- Extension from lower urinary tract secondary to genital tract contamination (pyometra) (females exclusively)
- Extension from lower urinary tract secondary to dermal contamination (perivulvar dermatitis)
    - Targets tubules and interstitium primarily

HEMATOGENOUS

- Localization within corticomedullary vessels
    - Septic—embolic nephritis
    - Nonseptic necrosis with infarction
- Localization within large renal vasculature
    - Massive infarction
- Localization within glomerular tufts
- Localization within interstitial vessels
    - Targets glomeruli, tubules, interstitium, and vasculature

DIRECT PENETRATION

- Activation of products in proximal tubules—necrosis
- Presence of heavy metal—mercury, cadmium
- Crystalline oversaturation
- Direct toxic action—cisplatin
    - Targets tubules

Ascending Injury

Ascension from the exterior via the urethra and urinary bladder is relatively unique in that few body systems have an opening to the exterior, and these are rarely blind-ended as in the urinary system. Thus ascending infection from the exterior can localize and be perpetuated in the kidneys. Common etiologic agents in this process, such as bacteria, may originate from the exterior skin surface and the adjacent orifices of the intestinal tract or the genital tract.

Hematogenous (Interstitial Capillaries and Vasa Recta)

The luminal and abluminal surfaces of epithelial cells lining renal tubules can be exposed to systemic blood-borne (hematogenous) toxins that are secreted via peritubular capillaries into the interstitial and/or luminal fluid, respectively.

INTERSTITIUM

Hematogenous

The interstitium can be entered most successfully by the associated interstitial blood supply, allowing for interstitial localization of blood-borne pathogens, similar to those seen with glomerular blood-borne infections.

Ascending Injury

See previous section on Tubules.

Lymphoid Nodules

Although often present as aggregates or less commonly as nodules, lymphoid infiltrates within the interstitium are not normal but the result of previous insults typically from infectious etiologies, such as *Leptospirosis,* or as a result of ascension secondary to long-standing pyelonephritis.

VASCULATURE

As in all visceral organs, the sustaining blood supply can provide a portal of hematogenous entry for infectious organisms, which in the case of the kidney principally leads to arterial localization at one of several gradated sites as follows:

- Localization within large renal vasculature. Massive infarction of the kidney is the result of large-bore renal vessel disease.
- Localization within corticomedullary vessels. In the case of associated bacterial spread, septic embolic nephritis can occur. In those examples in which the embolus is nonseptic, the result is infarctive necrosis.
- Localization within glomerular tufts. In this example, the lesions are localized to the vasculature of the small vessels within the glomerular tuft.
- Localization within interstitial vessels. In this example, the lesions are localized to necrosis of interstitial tissues and tubules.

DEFENSE MECHANISMS

Defense mechanisms unique to the renal system have evolved to counteract the routes of typical exposure to injurious agents and include those localized to the renal corpuscle, tubules, interstitium, and vasculature (Box 11-2).

RENAL CORPUSCLE

Glomerular Basement Membrane

The most important of these barrier systems is the glomerular filtration membrane (see Fig. 11-7). The glomerular membrane is structurally adept at separating substances based on size and charge. Both size-dependent and charge-dependent filtration is possible because of the porous structure of capillary walls, which is a function of endothelial fenestrations, a basement membrane formed of type IV collagen, basement membrane anionic glycoproteins, and filtration slits of visceral epithelium. This inherent function of the glomerulus can also protect other regions of the nephron from damage by circulating inflammatory cells and their cytokines, as well as infectious agents that are present in the systemic circulation (i.e., bacteria in bacteremia).

Glomerular Mesangium

Additionally, the glomerulus is equipped with its own specialized mesangial cells, a component of the monocyte-macrophage system (see Fig. 11-6), which can remove macromolecules from circulation.

BOX 11-2 Renal Defense Mechanisms Against Injury and Infectious Agents

- Barrier system—glomerular basement membrane (GBM)
- Monocyte-macrophage system—glomerular mesangium
- Immune system
  - Innate responses
  - Humoral responses
  - Cellular responses

TUBULES

The most effective barrier system associated with the tubules is the tubular basement membrane. Intact basement membranes prevent intraluminal organisms, such as ascending bacteria, from gaining easy access to the interstitium. They also provide the scaffolding for reepithelialization of the tubule, which follows tubular necrosis in association with many toxic principles but not in instances of renal ischemia.

INTERSTITIUM

Innate humoral and cellular responses by the immune system contribute to protection of the kidney. Humoral antibodies may protect mucosal surfaces such as those of the renal pelvis and less commonly the tubular epithelial cell lining, especially against insults such as ascending bacterial infections. Cell infiltrates are typically localized to the interstitial tissues. Lymphocytes and plasma cells within the interstitium provide either cell-mediated surveillance against invasive pathogens (i.e., *Leptospira*) and in the case of plasma cells, can produce local antibodies.

VASCULATURE

Intact endothelial lining of the renal vasculature functions as a localized defense mechanism (barrier system) to prevent access by intravascular pathogens, many of which produce toxic by-products that can damage endothelium and allow for localized vasculitis and colonization. The result is often embolic septic nephritis. Intact endothelium also prevents activation of the clotting cascade and thus reduction in the likelihood of thrombus formation.

RESPONSES TO INJURY

The response of the urinary system to injury is the response of each of its components—kidney, ureter, bladder, and urethra—to injury. Additionally, components within the kidney, such as the renal corpuscle, tubules, interstitium, and vasculature, have their own unique responses to injury. Responses to injury are described sequentially in this section and are summarized in Box 11-3.

RESPONSES OF THE KIDNEY TO INJURY

The functional unit of the kidney is the nephron, and damage to any component of the nephron (renal corpuscle and tubules) results in diminished function and progressive damage to the kidney. Renal disease can be best summarized by dividing it into general tissue responses that affect the primary anatomic components: glomeruli, tubules, interstitium, and vasculature. In the early stages of disease, specific anatomic components may be targeted by specific insults: glomeruli in immune-mediated disease and tubules in toxin-induced necrosis. But in the more chronic stages of disease, the kidney undergoes changes related to nephron loss that are not specific to the original cause but are considered common end-stage responses to many injurious stimuli.

Renal Corpuscle

Primary glomerular damage often occurs as a result of deposition of immune complexes, entrapment of thromboemboli and bacterial emboli, or direct viral or bacterial infection of glomerular components. Such insults are reflected morphologically by necrosis, thickening of membranes, or infiltration of leukocytes, and functionally by reduced vascular perfusion. Continued or severe injury can result in chronic changes characterized at first by atrophy and fibrosis of the glomerular tuft (sclerosis) and secondarily by atrophy

BOX 11-3 Renal Responses to Injury

GLOMERULI
Acute inflammation
Endothelial proliferation
Hypertrophy
Inclusion bodies
Necrosis
Mesangial cell proliferation
Amyloid deposition
Glomerular cell proliferation
Glomerular basement membrane proliferation
Increased vascular permeability
Atrophy of the glomerular tuft
Fibrosis of the glomerular tuft

TUBULES
Cell degeneration
Cell necrosis
Basement membrane rupture
Basement membrane thickening
Cell regeneration
Renal fibrosis

INTERSTITIUM
Hyperemia
Edema
Inflammation
Fibrosis

VASCULATURE
Hyperemia and congestion
Hemorrhage and thrombosis
Embolic nephritis
Infarction

of renal tubules, as the nephron dies. Similar chronic glomerular changes can result from reduced blood flow or chronic loss of tubular function.

Damage to the glomerular filtration barrier can result from several causes and produce a variety of clinical signs. The major clinical finding of glomerular disease is the leakage of various low molecular weight (small molecule size) proteins, such as albumin, into the glomerular filtrate. As a result, large quantities of albumin overload the protein reabsorption capabilities of the proximal convoluted tubular epithelium to such an extent that protein-rich glomerular filtrate accumulates in the variably dilated tubular lumina and protein subsequently appears in the urine. Renal diseases that result in proteinuria are called *protein-losing nephropathies.* Protein-losing nephropathy is one of several causes of severe hypoproteinemia in animals. Prolonged, severe renal protein loss results in hypoproteinemia, reduced plasma colloid osmotic (oncotic) pressure, and loss of antithrombin III. The nephrotic syndrome is further characterized by generalized edema, ascites, pleural effusion, and hypercholesterolemia.

The functions of the glomerulus listed in the following are affected by processes that injure it in disease:

- Plasma ultrafiltration
- Blood pressure regulation
- Peritubular blood flow regulation
- Tubular metabolism regulation
- Circulating macromolecule removal

The pathophysiologic mechanisms of glomerular injury from infectious or chemical insults have been summarized by the following three theories:

- Intact nephron hypothesis
- Hyperfiltration hypothesis
- The theory of complex deposition

The intact nephron hypothesis proposes that damage to any portion of the nephron affects the entire nephron function. This is seen when glomerular damage interferes with peritubular blood flow and results in decreased tubular resorption or secretion. Not all nephron damage is irreversible, for example, renal tubular epithelium can regenerate but whole nephrons are not capable of regeneration. Thus the outcomes for the nephrons vary from hypertrophy to repair.

Unlike the intact nephron hypothesis, the hyperfiltration hypothesis helps explain the progressive nature of glomerular disease. Glomerular hyperfiltration is a result of increased hydrostatic pressure that damages delicate glomerular capillaries and in cases of prolonged hypertension produces a sustained repeating deleterious effect on the glomerulus, ultimately resulting in glomerulosclerosis. Increased dietary protein can produce a transient increase in glomerular hyperfiltration and if persistent can result in glomerulosclerosis. There may be a species effect, as dogs that undergo experimental hyperfiltration are much less prone to development of progressive glomerular disease than are rats.

The theory of complex deposition is derived from the fact that glomeruli are the primary site for removal of macromolecules (principally immune complex) from the circulation. Complexes may be deposited in subepithelial, subendothelial, or mesangial locations. These immune complexes are capable of triggering a sequence of inflammatory responses including the following:

- Recruitment and localization of inflammatory cells at the site.
- Release of inflammatory mediators and enzymes.
- Destruction of glomerular structures such as the basement membrane.
- Further compromise of nephron function.
- Continuing damage by altered transglomerular hyperfiltration and perfusion shifts between nephron populations, so the less affected become overworked and succumb to the same fate.

Kidney lesions differ slightly, depending on the duration of the glomerular disease. Acute disease may be identified by pallor of the parenchyma and accentuation of the glomerular tufts as fine red dots. Accompanying petechial hemorrhages may be noted. In the more chronic stage, the kidney can be shrunken and show a fine granularity to the cortical cut section. The capsule may be adherent.

RESPONSES OF TUBULES TO INJURY

Renal tubular epithelial cells can respond to injury by undergoing degeneration, necrosis, apoptosis, and/or atrophy. The basement membrane can respond by rupturing or thickening. Tubular disease occurs as a result of tubular epithelial damage from the following:

- Blood-borne infections (innocent bystander effect)
- Ascending infections (intratubular pathogens)
- Direct damage from toxins (intratubular effects)
- Ischemia, infarction

When nephrons are lost because of injury, remaining tubules can undergo compensatory hypertrophy in an attempt to maintain overall renal function, but there is no regeneration of nephrons. In many instances of tubular epithelial cell necrosis, particularly as a response to toxins, tubular epithelium has an incredible capacity to regenerate and contribute to restoration of function, providing the tubular basement membrane scaffolding remains intact. Severe damage to or loss of tubular basement membranes, as occurs after ischemic damage, results in necrosis and loss of tubular segments, failure of functional repair, and permanent loss of function of the entire nephron, despite the potential for tubular epithelial hyperplasia.

Atrophy

Tubular atrophy can occur secondary to the following:

- External compression of tubule by a space-occupying mass, neoplasm, or abscess
- Interstitial fibrosis as the end result of ischemia
- Intratubular obstruction and backpressure
- Diminished glomerular perfusion and filtration
- Reduced oxygen tension such as with hypoxia

If the insult to the renal tubules is not lethal and is removed, some forms of acute tubular degeneration are reversible. The success of reparative regeneration is affected by several variables, including severity of degeneration.

Apoptosis

Single cell loss (apoptosis) from the tubular epithelial lining is handled efficiently by adjacent viable tubular epithelial cells, which by mitotic division fill the epithelial gap. The cells that are lost slough into the lumen to form cellular casts within the lumens of renal tubules.

Acute Tubular Degeneration

More severe generalized loss of tubular epithelial lining cells is repaired by proliferation of the remaining viable epithelial cells over an intact tubular basement membrane to form a low cuboidal rather than a mature columnar epithelial lining. This appears as an ectatic proximal tubule. Restitution of renal function eventually results, despite the presence of replacement low cuboidal epithelium, which is not identical to the tubular lining cell (with microvilli) present before the injury. The exact mechanism of this return to function is not entirely known. The main determinant of this regenerative ability is the viability of tubular basement membranes, which are retained more consistently after toxic rather than ischemic insults.

Tubular Regeneration

Because the regenerative process is reliant on many factors for its success, things often go awry. Examples of adverse outcomes include the following:

- Focal loss of basement membrane scaffolding allows for a bulge defect to occur where the regenerative population of proliferating tubular epithelial cells coalesce to form well-differentiated syncytial cells (giant cells) at certain levels of the tubule.
- Regenerative epithelial cells fail to regain all cytoplasmic structural aspects of the original columnar epithelial cells (e.g., microvilli and luminal enzymes) because of a failure to fully differentiate, and thus function may be affected.
- If there is excessive tubular epithelial loss, the potential for regeneration is lost and repair proceeds by replacement fibrosis and scarring.
- Reperfusion is necessary for cell viability following ischemia, but reperfusion injury occurs when activated endothelial cells produce proinflammatory mediators, such as reactive oxygen species, proteolytic enzymes, and cytokines, which result in further renal injury. Recent evidence indicates that epidermal growth factor secreted by distal convoluted tubules mediates the tubular repair process. The sequence of events in tubular regeneration after necrosis has been well documented in experimental model systems using mercuric chloride in mice, rats, and rabbits. In that system, morphologic evidence of regeneration of proximal convoluted tubules is seen within 3 days after a toxic dose. At this time, basement membranes are partially covered with low cuboidal to flattened and elongated epithelial cells that are more basophilic than normal because of the increased concentrations of cytoplasmic ribosomes and rough endoplasmic reticulum producing protein for repair. Nuclei are hyperchromatic and mitotic figures are present. Regenerating tubules do not function normally because they lack both a brush border and normal tubular membrane function, and this is evident clinically as polyuria. Normal-appearing tubular epithelium subsequently reappears between 7 and 14 days after toxin exposure. Normal renal structure without residual evidence of tubular damage is restored between 21 and 56 days after exposure to the nephrotoxin. Similar time frames for tubular regeneration have been described through sequential renal biopsies from human patients naturally exposed to inorganic mercury and in experimental systems using other nephrotoxins.

Acute Tubular Necrosis

Acute tubular necrosis is the single most important cause of acute renal failure. Acute tubular degeneration and necrosis, often referred to as *nephrosis, lower nephron nephrosis, tubular nephrosis, tubular dysfunction,* or *acute cortical necrosis,* is principally the result of nephrotoxic injury to the renal tubular epithelial cells or ischemia (Box 11-4). This was borne out by a recent study of cats with renal failure in which 18 of 32 cases were the result of nephrotoxin exposure and four of 32 cases were the result of ischemia.

Acute tubular necrosis induces clinical oliguria (decrease in urine production) or anuria (absence of urine production) by one or several mechanisms. These mechanisms include the following:

- Leakage of tubular ultrafiltrate from damaged tubules across disrupted basement membranes into the renal interstitium
- Intratubular obstruction resulting from sloughed necrotic epithelium

The latter mechanism is less well accepted, but both mechanisms result in decreased glomerular filtration rate.

Nephrotoxic Injury

Nephrotoxic injury can be caused by a large group of substances that are called *nephrotoxins.* They preferentially damage kidneys because (1) 20% to 25% of cardiac output goes to the kidney, (2) the substance is filtered into the urine by the glomerulus, and (3) the toxin or its metabolites within the renal tubular lumens are concentrated. Nephrotoxins can do the following:

- Directly damage renal epithelial cells, particularly those of the proximal convoluted tubules, after their intracellular conversion via enzyme pathways to reactive metabolites.
- Produce reactive metabolites in the tubular filtrate, which can cause renal tubular epithelial necrosis after reabsorption.
- Cause renal tubular epithelial necrosis after diffusion through the intertubular capillary walls and basement membranes into the tubule epithelial cell.
- Indirectly stimulate vasoconstriction of the intertubular capillaries, thus causing ischemia, which further compromises renal function.
- Result in nephrotoxin-associated ischemia.

BOX 11-4 Causes of Ischemic Acute Renal Failure in Small Animals

INTRAVASCULAR VOLUME DEPLETION
Dehydration
Vomiting
Diarrhea
Sequestration or shock
Thermal burns
Blood loss
Trauma
Surgery
Hypoalbuminemia
Hypoadrenocorticism
Hyponatremia (nondilutional)

DECREASED CARDIAC OUTPUT
Congestive heart failure
Low output
Restrictive pericardial disease
Tamponade
Arrhythmia
Positive-pressure ventilation
Prolonged resuscitation after cardiac arrest

INCREASED BLOOD VISCOSITY
Multiple myeloma
Polycythemia (absolute or relative)

ALTERED RENAL AND SYSTEMIC VASCULAR RESISTANCES
Renal vasoconstriction
Circulating catecholamines
Renal sympathetic nervous stimulation
Vasopressin
Angiotensin II
Hypercalcemia
Amphotericin B
Hypothermia
Myoglobinuria
Hemoglobinuria
Systemic vasodilation
Arteriolar or mixed vasodilator therapy
Anaphylaxis
Gaseous anesthesia
Sepsis
Heatstroke

INTERFERENCE WITH RENAL AUTOREGULATION DURING HYPOTENSION
Nonsteroidal antiinflammatory drugs

WARM OR COLD ISCHEMIA

Modified from Chew D, DiBartola S: Diagnosis and pathophysiology of renal disease. In Ettinger SJ, ed: *Textbook of veterinary internal medicine,* ed 7, vol 2, Philadelphia, 2010, Saunders.

One of the first events in renal tubular cell damage is altered ion transport at the luminal surface (uptake). This process results in decreased sodium absorption and increased sodium ions in the lumens of the distal tubules, which stimulate the renin-angiotensin mechanism, causing vasoconstriction and reduced blood flow that result in ischemia and tubular cell damage. Nephrotoxins usually do not damage the tubular basement membranes, and thus regeneration (repair) of tubules can occur in an orderly and expeditious manner. The intact basement membrane acts as a scaffold over which regenerating epithelial cells may slide. Exposure to a variety of nephrotoxins, either from the vasculature (including certain chemicals [glycolaldehyde, glycolic acid, and glyoxylic acid]) or from the tubular lumen (including certain antibiotics [aminoglycosides], pigments [hemoglobin], metals [lead], or chemicals [ethylene glycol–induced calcium oxalate crystals]), or their metabolites cause cells to undergo degeneration followed by necrosis and desquamation into the tubular lumen.

Cell death results from decreased adenosine triphosphate (ATP) production, which is central to many of the secondary metabolic derangements, including calcium ion influx, purine depletion, metabolic acidosis, and generation of oxygen radicals. Increased intracellular calcium is associated with degenerative changes in renal tubular cells, smooth muscle cells, and mesangial cells. Oxygen radicals activate phospholipase, which subsequently increases membrane permeability. Because mitochondrial respiration is disrupted, further cell membrane damage occurs.

Notably reduced renal perfusion from any cause can result in tubular necrosis. Severe hypotension associated with shock results in preglomerular vasoconstriction and reduced glomerular filtration. The resulting renal ischemia can produce sublethal tubular cell injury and dysfunction or cause cell death by necrosis or apoptosis. Following less severe insults and within different portions of the renal tubule, apoptosis may occur in lieu of necrosis. The apoptotic pathway can be triggered by the following:

- Binding of ligands to the tumor necrosis factor (TNF) superfamily
- Deficiency of cellular growth factors
- Imbalance between proapoptotic and antiapoptotic oncogenes
- Alteration of other mediators of apoptotic signaling pathways such as reactive oxygen metabolites, caspases, and ceramide

Proximal tubular epithelium has a microvillous border, which amplifies absorptive surface area and cellular junctional complexes that structurally polarize the cell so that membrane phospholipids and specialized proteins remain in the appropriate domains. The integrity of these cellular structures is critical to absorption and secretion. Early structural changes after ischemic insult include formation of apical blebs, loss of brush border, loss of cellular polarity, disruption of tight junctions, and sloughing of cells, which result in intratubular cast formation (Fig. 11-12).

Damage to the cellular cytoskeleton modifies cell polarity, cell-to-cell interactions, and cell-matrix interactions. Initially, ischemic damage modifies cell polarity by disruption of the terminal web and disassembly of the microvillar actin cores. This is followed by conversion of G actin to F actin and its redistribution from the apical cell component to form diffuse aggregates throughout the cytoplasm (Figs. 11-13 and 11-14). Cells are attached to each other by junctional complexes, tight junctions, and adherens junctions and to the ECM by integrins. Several mechanisms

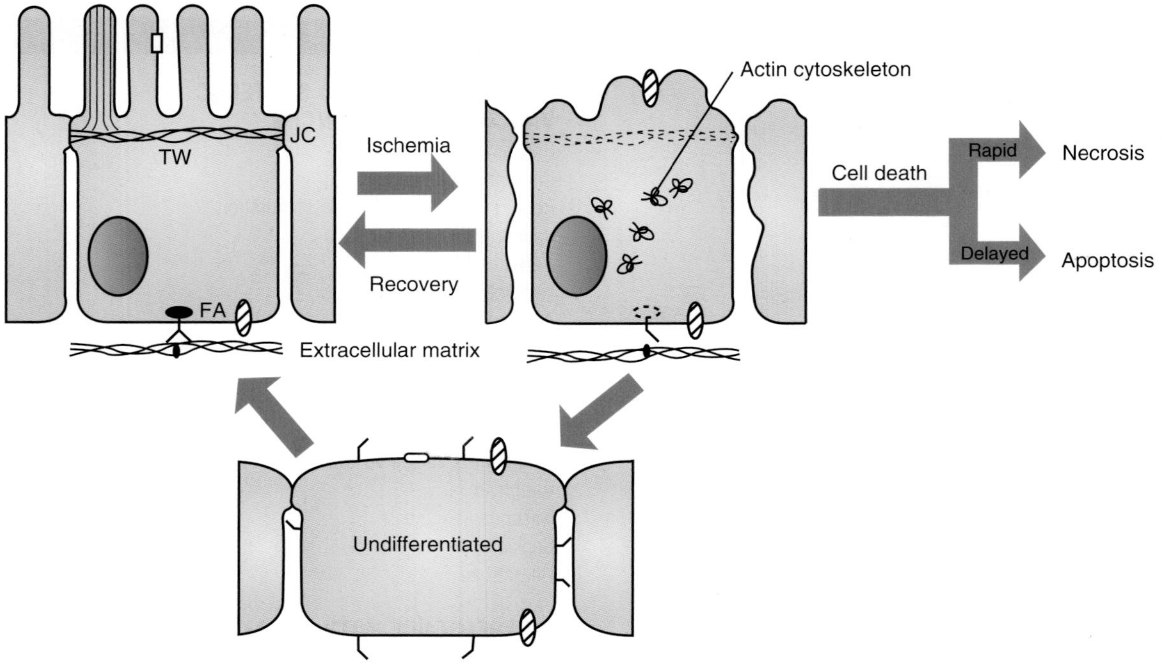

Fig. 11-12 Schematic diagram of the effect of ischemia on cell structure and function.
A polarized renal proximal tubule cell with a well-developed actin cortical cytoskeleton is shown on the left. Also shown is attachment to the extracellular matrix (ECM) via integrins. Following ischemic injury there is extensive disruption, redistribution, and aggregation of the actin cytoskeleton resulting in loss of microvilli structure, blebbing of microvilli into the lumen, detachment of cells from the ECM, and opening of junctional complexes *(JC).* Injured proximal tubule cells can undergo primary repair and recover directly into a polarized epithelial cell. Cells can also go through an undifferentiated phase followed by redifferentiation, or cells can die either rapidly via necrosis or in a much slower programmed fashion known as apoptosis. The primary route of cellular repair involves direct recovery. The percentage of cells reverting to an undifferentiated state or dying depends on the severity of the injury and the location within the kidney. *FA,* Focal adhesions; *TW,* terminal web. (Redrawn from Molitoris BA, Marrs J: *Am J Med* 106:583-592, 1999.)

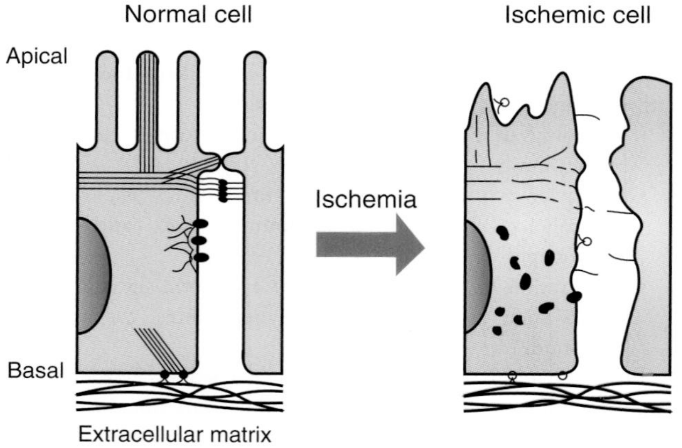

Fig. 11-13 Schematic diagram of the effect of ischemia on the actin cytoskeleton and the cytoskeletal-surface membrane interactions in proximal tubule cells.
During ischemia, alterations in the actin cytoskeleton involve disruption of the actin cytoskeleton with redistribution and aggregation of actin throughout the cytoplasm. Consequently, notable alterations occur in cytoskeletal-surface membrane interactions. Loss of cell-cell adhesion, cell-matrix adhesion, and polarity of surface membrane proteins during ischemia play a role in the diminished glomerular filtration rate that is the hallmark of ischemic acute renal failure. See Fig. 11-14 for more detail about the actin cytoskeleton and the cytoskeletal-surface membrane. (Redrawn from Sutton TA, Molitoris BA: *Sem Nephr* 18(5):490-497, 1998.)

contribute to tight junction disruption, which is manifested as alteration in cellular permeability and cell polarity. The contributing mechanisms include redistribution of membrane lipids and proteins, such as Na^+/K^+-ATPase, to the apical membrane after alteration of the actin cytoskeleton and redistribution of integrins to the apical cell surface so that cell desquamation occurs. The former results in deranged sodium handling by the proximal tubular cell.

Animals with severe tubular necrosis have accompanying functional derangements of vascular, tubular, and/or glomerular origin. Vascular derangements include the following:

- Afferent arteriolar constriction
- Efferent arteriolar dilation
- Loss of autoregulation of renal blood flow

Prolonged ischemia can produce a paradoxic response of the autoregulatory system, where increased glomerular capillary resistance from tubular fluid stasis results in activation of afferent arteriolar vasoconstriction. Decreased production of or response to vasodilative factors, such as prostaglandin and atrial natriuretic peptide, also contribute. Afferent arteriole vasoconstriction, back leak of fluid, and tubular obstruction account for decreased glomerular filtration rate (GFR) (Fig. 11-15).

Tubuloglomerular feedback is the mechanism by which GFR is matched to the solute load and the solute handling characteristics of the tubules. Because of altered sodium handling, increased levels reach the macula densa, and activation of the renin-angiotensin system occurs. This is followed by intrarenal vasoconstriction, particularly affecting outer cortical nephrons, and results in decreased glomerular blood flow, decreased filtration, and reduced formation of urine.

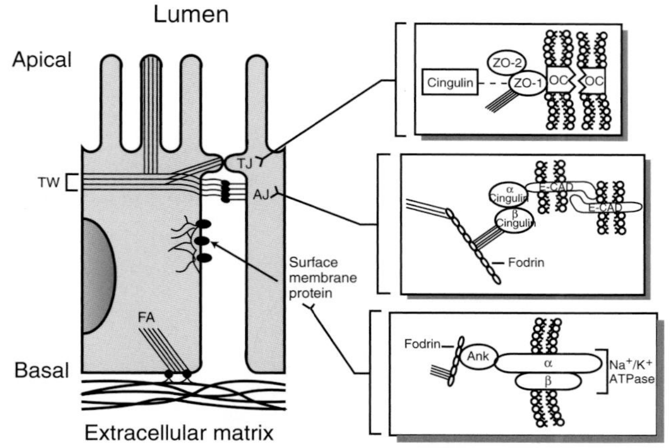

Fig. 11-14 Schematic diagram of the actin cytoskeleton and the cytoskeletal-surface membrane interactions in proximal tubule cells. Microvillar F-actin filaments extend into the apical actin network termed the terminal web *(TW)* and are bound together by villin and attached to the surface membrane by myosin and ezrin to form the structural core of the apical microvilli. The actin cytoskeleton associates with junctional complexes involved in cell-cell interactions, including the tight junction and the adherens junction. More detailed schematics of the tight junction *(TJ)* and the adherens junction *(AJ)* appear to the right and demonstrate the interaction of F-actin filaments with TJ and AJ protein complexes. *OC* represents occludin in the schematic of the TJ, and *E-CAD* represents E-cadherin in the schematic of the AJ. The cortical actin network associates with surface membrane proteins, such as the sodium-potassium adenosinetriphosphatase, which is demonstrated by the detailed schematic to the lower right. *Ank* represents ankyrin in this schematic. Finally the actin cytoskeleton associates with structures involved in cell-matrix interactions, including focal adhesions *(FA)*. F-actin filaments (stress fibers) possibly bundled together by myosin II associate with a protein complex at sites where integrins bind to the extracellular matrix (ECM). (Redrawn from Sutton TA, Molitoris BA: *Sem Nephr* 18(5):490-497, 1998.)

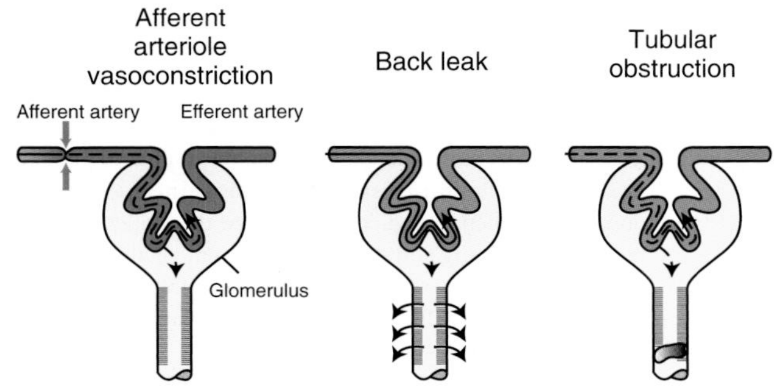

Fig. 11-15 Schematic diagram of the mechanisms of decreased glomerular filtration rate (GFR) during ischemic acute renal failure. Proposed mechanisms for the decrease in GFR that occurs during ischemic acute renal failure include afferent arteriole vasoconstriction, back leak of glomerular filtrate, and tubular obstruction. All three of these mechanisms relate to ischemia-induced alterations in proximal tubule cells. Deranged proximal tubule handling of sodium leads to a high delivery of sodium to the macula densa, which in turn causes afferent arteriole vasoconstriction via tubuloglomerular feedback. Afferent arteriole vasoconstriction reduces glomerular capillary pressure and therefore GFR. Altered cell-cell adhesion results in an open tight junction that leads to increased paracellular permeability and subsequent back leak of glomerular filtrate from the tubular lumen into the extracellular space and ultimately into the bloodstream. Disrupted cell-matrix adhesion and abnormal cell-cell adhesion leads to cellular cast formation, which obstructs the tubular lumen and causes increased tubular pressure resulting in diminished or no GFR. (Redrawn from Sutton TA, Molitoris BA: *Sem Nephr* 18(5):490-497, 1998.)

Gross Lesions of Acute Tubular Necrosis

On gross necropsy, the recognition of acute tubular necrosis is often difficult. Nevertheless, initially the cortex is swollen, pale mahogany to beige, and with a slightly translucent smooth, thinned, capsular surface. The cut surface of the renal cortex bulges and is excessively moist; striations are muted or accentuated by radially oriented opaque, white streaks, presumably related to the stage of the necrosis, with coagulation necrosis being responsible for the white streaks. The medulla is either pale or diffusely congested.

Microscopic Lesions of Acute Tubular Necrosis

The microscopic appearance of kidneys with acute tubular necrosis varies, depending on the following:

- The extent of the tubular necrosis
- The duration of exposure to the damaging agent
- The length of time between the injury and death, in other words the stage of necrosis or dissolution of necrotic epithelium

Initially, tubular necrosis is randomly distributed in nephrons, but the proximal convoluted tubules are most severely affected because of their high metabolic demands and first line of exposure (Fig. 11-16). Prolonged ischemia can produce necrosis of epithelium of the proximal and distal convoluted tubules, the loops of Henle, and the collecting ducts throughout the cortex and to a lesser extent, the medulla. Glomeruli are resistant to ischemia and often remain morphologically normal, even when ischemia is prolonged. Initially, proximal tubular epithelium is swollen, and the cytoplasm is vacuolated or granular and intensely eosinophilic, all features indicative of necrosis (Fig. 11-17). In such cells, the nuclear changes are pyknosis, karyorrhexis, or karyolysis. Necrotic tubular epithelium is subsequently sloughed into tubular lumens resulting in dilated, notably hypocellular tubules that contain necrotic cellular debris and hyalinized or granular casts.

A characteristic histologic lesion of ischemic tubular necrosis is possible disruption of the tubular basement membranes, referred to as tubulorrhexis (Fig. 11-18). Tubular repair in these kidneys is imperfect because regenerating epithelial cells do not have their normal scaffolding. Tubules that remain in an affected site are less functional in resorption, can be dilated and lined by flattened epithelium, or are notably atrophic, appearing shrunken with a collapsed lumen lined by flattened epithelium and fail to heal completely by regeneration, resulting in tubular atrophy.

Nephrosis

Nephrosis is a form of acute tubular injury that is not caused by inflammation. Most commonly, it is caused by tubular ischemia or nephrotoxins as described in the sections on acute tubular necrosis and is often exacerbated by hemoglobin (hemoglobinuric nephrosis) or myoglobin pigments (myoglobinuric nephrosis).

Miscellaneous Responses to Injury of Renal Tubules

Lipofuscinosis

Fine golden granules of brown iron free pigment with the staining characteristics of lipofuscin ("wear and tear pigment") can accumulate in renal epithelial cells of old cattle and in striated muscle, resulting in lipofuscinosis. Grossly, the renal cortex can have streaks of brown discoloration, but renal function is not affected. Microscopically, the accumulations are noted most prominently within the proximal convoluted epithelial cells. The direct cause is not known, but it is suspected that accumulations result from previous cell membrane breakdown and subsequent storage of end-product in the tubular epithelial cells.

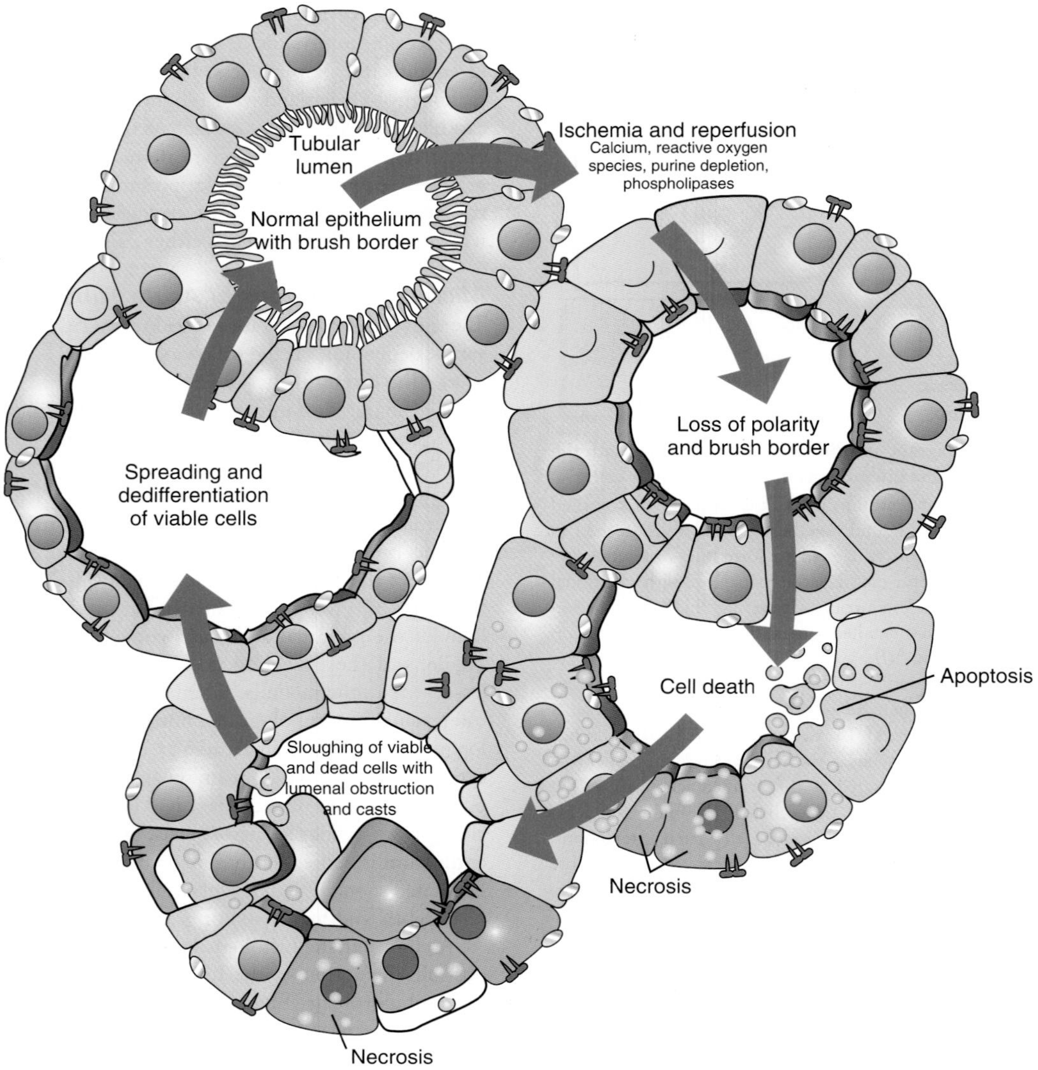

Fig. 11-16 Schematic diagram of the effects of ischemia and reperfusion.
After ischemia and reperfusion, morphologic changes occur in the proximal tubules, including loss of the brush border, loss of polarity, and redistribution of integrins and sodium-potassium adenosinetriphosphatase to the apical surface. Calcium, reactive oxygen species, purine depletion, and phospholipases probably have a role in these changes in morphology and polarity and in the subsequent cell death that occurs as a result of necrosis and apoptosis. There is a sloughing of viable and nonviable cells into the tubular lumen, resulting in the formation of casts and luminal obstruction and contributing to the reduction in the glomerular filtration rate. The severely damaged kidney can completely restore its structure and function. Spreading and dedifferentiation of viable cells occur during recovery from ischemic acute renal failure, which duplicates aspects of normal renal development. A variety of growth factors probably contribute to the restoration of a normal tubular epithelium. (Redrawn from Thadhani R, Pascual M, Bonventre JV: *N Engl J Med* 334(22):1448-1460, 1996. Color from Molitoris BA, Finn WF, eds: *Acute renal failure: a companion to Brenner and Rector's the kidney,* Philadelphia, 2001, Saunders.)

Hydropic Degeneration

Hydropic degeneration is defined as cloudy swelling and because it is a degenerative change can sometimes be reversed. While rare in the kidney, a severe hydropic degeneration of the proximal convoluted tubules and the ascending loop of Henle, has been observed after intravenous administration of hypertonic solutions such as dextrose.

Glycogenic Degeneration

Abundant cytoplasmic vacuolation of tubular epithelium of the outer medulla and inner cortex is seen in dogs and cats with diabetes mellitus. Glycogen can be demonstrated as the accumulating compound within the cells of the ascending limb. Treatment with insulin relieves the deposition. The change is not thought to affect renal function.

Fat

Proximal tubular epithelial cell cytoplasm is often expanded by accumulations of lipid especially in cats. This is a normal storage location and is recognized as large clearings within the renal tubular epithelial cells, most prominently the proximal tubules. There is not thought to be any significant alteration to renal function.

Hemosiderin and Ferritin

Pigment can be present in the renal tubules. The origin of hemosiderin pigment is most likely from degradation of hemoglobin resorbed from the glomerular filtrate by proximal tubular epithelium. However, a history or concurrent lesions of a prior hemolytic crisis are often lacking. In dogs, microscopic granules of hemosiderin are frequent incidental findings in the cytoplasm of proximal

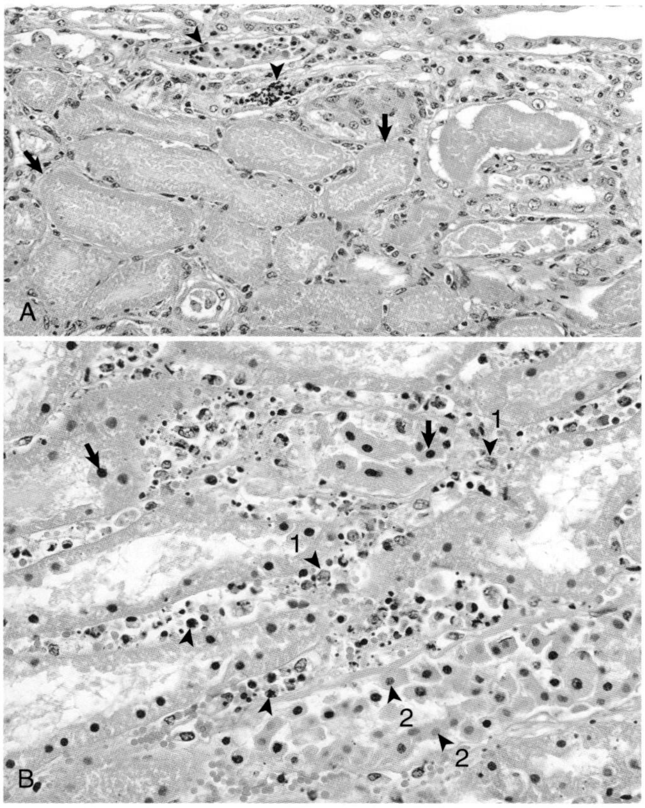

Fig. 11-17 Acute tubular necrosis, kidney, proximal tubules, cat.
A, This lesion is characterized primarily by coagulation necrosis of tubular epithelial cells *(arrows)* and nuclear pyknosis and intratubular nuclear and proteinaceous debris *(arrowheads)*. H&E stain. **B,** This lesion is characterized primarily by nuclear pyknosis *(arrows)*, karyorrhexis *(arrowheads)*, and karyolysis *(arrowheads 1)* with intratubular nuclear and proteinaceous debris and coagulation necrosis with detachment of the epithelium from the tubular basement membrane *(arrowheads 2)*. H&E stain. (Courtesy Dr. J. F. Zachary, College of Veterinary Medicine, University of Illinois.)

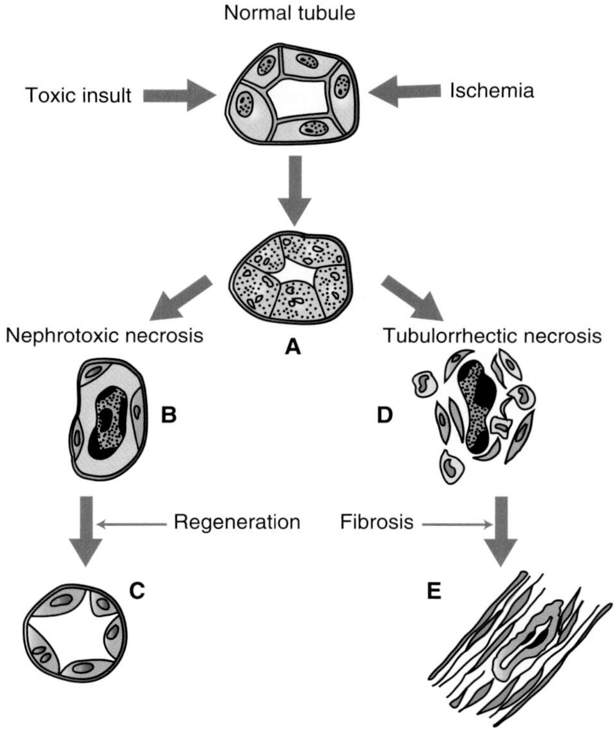

Fig. 11-18 Schematic diagram of acute tubular necrosis, kidney, proximal tubules.
Acute tubular necrosis results from a nephrotoxin or ischemia. **A,** Both insults cause acute necrosis characterized by cellular swelling, pyknosis, karyorrhexis, and karyolysis. **B,** Subsequent to nephrotoxic necrosis, there is sloughing of necrotic epithelium into the tubular lumina. The basement membranes remain intact and act as a scaffold for **(C)** tubular epithelial regeneration to occur. **D,** Ischemia may result in tubulorrhexis. Necrotic epithelial cells slough into the tubular lumen, the basement membrane is disrupted, macrophages infiltrate, and fibroblasts proliferate. **E,** Fibrosis with tubular atrophy results.

convoluted tubular epithelial cells in kidneys that are otherwise normal.

Cloisonné kidneys, which occur in goats, are the result of proximal tubular basement membrane thickening as a result of deposits of ferritin and hemosiderin. Grossly, these kidneys have diffuse, intense, black or brown discoloration of the cortex (Fig. 11-19). The medulla is spared. Although this lesion is striking, renal function is normal.

Other causes of incidental tubular changes include the following:

- Vacuolation of renal tubular epithelium in the lysosomal storage diseases, such as feline sphingomyelinosis and ovine GM1 gangliosidosis
- Intranuclear eosinophilic crystalline pseudoinclusions (so-called crystalloids), which occur in renal tubular epithelium of old dogs. These can be round or rectangular and often greatly distort the nuclei.

RESPONSES OF THE INTERSTITIUM TO INJURY

Hyperemia

In instances of acute interstitial nephritis, especially those caused by septicemia, there can be an accompanying hyperemia of renal vasculature within the interstitium.

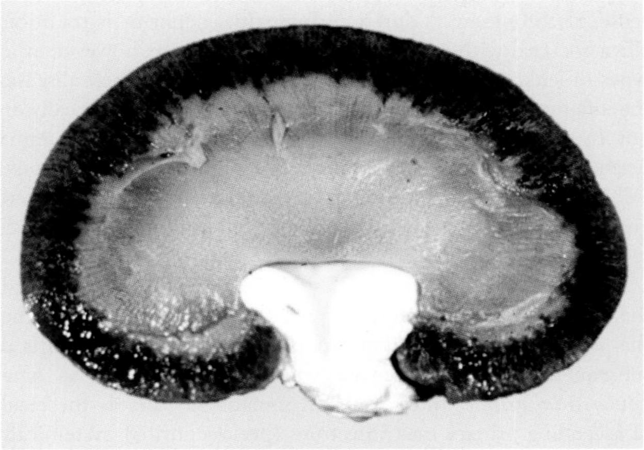

Fig. 11-19 Cloisonné kidney, dorsal section, goat.
The cortex is diffusely black; the medulla is unaffected. (Courtesy Dr. J. King, College of Veterinary Medicine, Cornell University.)

Edema

Similarly, in instances of acute inflammation targeting the interstitium, vascular leakage of high protein fluid (edema) can be the end result. Additionally, tubular damage, especially with basement membrane breach, allows for more extensive interstitial edema accumulation.

Inflammatory Infiltrates

Interstitial inflammation is a consistent component of injury to the interstitium, whether acute or chronic, focal or generalized, or suppurative or nonsuppurative. Suppurative interstitial inflammation is typically seen in instances of hematogenous bacteremia. A variety of renal insults result in release of a wide array of cytokines and growth factors that stimulate interstitial inflammation, particularly monocyte infiltration. Fibroblasts often become activated and fibrosis ensues.

Fibrosis

Once interstitial fibroblasts become activated, fibrosis can ensue. Often, at this stage, the underlying or inciting pathogen is not present and thus its role is not determined. Recurrent bouts of fibrosis continue and set up a vicious cycle of loss and scarring, so that the result is a common endpoint, known as *end-stage kidney.*

Lymphofollicular Inflammation

Lymphofollicular inflammation is the most common response to *Leptospira* infection of the kidney. Severe multinodular lymphocytic inflammatory reaction is confined to the cortex. The reaction subsides slowly and inflammatory cells decrease in numbers and the degree of fibrosis increases. Similarly, with chronic recurrent bouts of pyelonephritis, lymphocyte-rich inflammatory infiltrates are noted within the interstitium.

Interstitial Nephritis

When interstitial inflammation, mounted against the veins, arteries, lymphatic vessels, or connective tissues of kidneys appears to be a primary lesion, it has traditionally been called *interstitial nephritis* and may have an infectious or noninfectious cause and is acute, subacute, or chronic in its duration. Interstitial nephritis is traditionally associated with a lymphoplasmacytic infiltrate; however, other types of leukocytes can also be present. In many of these diseases, the inflammatory cell infiltrates are visible only microscopically, are not associated with renal failure, and are generally inconsequential (examples are canine ehrlichiosis and equine infectious anemia). When the renal interstitium is the site of moderate-to-severe, grossly visible, interstitial inflammatory cell infiltrates and fibrosis, renal failure can occur.

The renal interstitium is the fibrovascular stroma that surrounds the nephron and is significantly involved in renal diseases, whether this is of primary interstitial origin as in interstitial nephritis or subsequent to tubular damage, when it is referred to as *tubulointerstitial disease.* Interstitial inflammation occurs as the result of ascending urinary tract infections (pyelonephritis), systemically derived infections of tubules and interstitium, toxins, or secondary to injury of tubules or glomeruli. Common acute lesions of the interstitium in response to toxins and tubular necrosis include edema, hemorrhage, and inflammation characterized by infiltration of neutrophils. As lesions become subacute to chronic, neutrophils become less prominent, and in several diseases, infiltrates of macrophages, lymphocytes, and plasma cells predominate. With chronic injury to or after atrophy of nephrons, fibrosis of the interstitium can be severe, resulting in notable reduction in nephron function and accentuation of renal disease.

BOX 11-5 Causes of Interstitial Nephritis

HORSES
Equine viral arteritis

CATTLE
Escherichia coli septicemia, "white spotted kidney"
Leptospira interrogans serovar *canicola*
Malignant catarrhal fever

SHEEP
Sheeppox

PIGS
Leptospira interrogans serovar *pomona*
Porcine reproductive and respiratory syndrome

DOGS
Leptospira interrogans serovars *canicola, icterohaemorrhagiae,* and others
Infectious canine hepatitis virus, recovery phase
Theileria parva

Tubulointerstitial Nephritis

More recently, the term *tubulointerstitial* nephritis has been used to characterize a group of inflammatory diseases that involve the interstitium and tubules. Acute tubulointerstitial disease includes a group of processes, namely, inflammation secondary to acute tubular necrosis, whereas chronic tubulointerstitial processes include the progression with time or instances in which the interstitium is the primary target.

Tubulointerstitial nephritis can result from bacterial or viral septicemias, in which these infectious agents first infect the kidney tubules and damage them, which then incites an inflammatory response in the interstitium (Box 11-5). Acute tubulointerstitial nephritis is characterized by the presence of inflammatory cells (principally neutrophils) within the interstitium and may result from toxicoses or from acute infection with agents such as *Leptospira* (see Fig. 11-73), adenoviruses, lentiviruses, or herpesviruses. Chronic tubulointerstitial nephritis (Fig. 11-20, *A*) is a less well-characterized entity in dogs, but atrophy of tubular segments is a significant feature of this syndrome along with sparse mononuclear cell infiltration, cortical and medullary fibrosis (Fig. 11-20, *B* and *C*), variable degrees of tubular and glomerular atrophy and/or sclerosis, and compromised nephron function.

The pathogenesis of leptospirosis is discussed as an example of acute bacterial tubulointerstitial nephritis, the most well-understood causes of which include the following serovars of *Leptospira interrogans* (Fig. 11-20, *D*):

- Serovars *canicola* and *icterohaemorrhagiae* are the most common causes of canine leptospirosis (see the section on Disorders of Dogs).
- Serovar *pomona* is the most common cause of the lesion in pigs and less consistently in cattle (see the section on Disorders of Ruminants).
- Other serovars, such as *grippotyphosa* and *bratislava,* have also been associated with renal leptospirosis in several animal species.

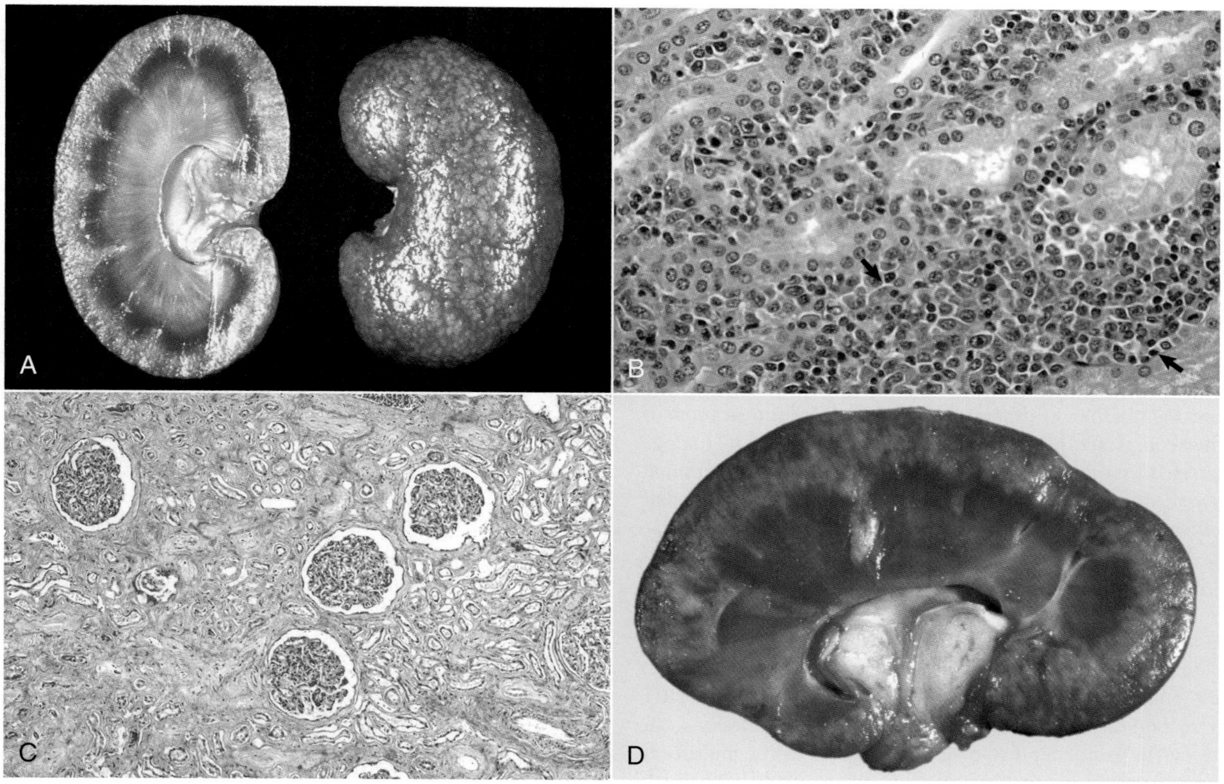

Fig. 11-20 Chronic tubulointerstitial nephritis.
A, Kidney, dorsal surface and dorsal section, dog. Note the nodularity of the capsular surface (right) from cortical interstitial fibrosis and the reduced width of the cortex (atrophy) *(left)*. **B,** Kidney, dorsal section, dog. There is an intense lymphoplasmacytic interstitial infiltrate *(arrows)*. H&E stain. **C,** Exotic zoo animal. This lesion is characterized by cortical and medullary fibrosis, variable degrees of tubular atrophy, and mononuclear cell interstitial infiltrate. Masson trichrome stain. **D,** Leptospirosis, dog. The pale streaks and foci in the cortex are chiefly interstitial lymphoplasmacytic infiltrates. (**A** and **C** courtesy Dr. A. Confer, College of Veterinary Medicine, Oklahoma State University. **B** courtesy Dr. Abdy, College of Veterinary Medicine, The University of Georgia; and Noah's Arkive, College of Veterinary Medicine, The University of Georgia. **D** courtesy Dr. M.D. McGavin, College of Veterinary Medicine, University of Tennessee.)

Mechanism of Injury of Tubulointerstitial Nephritis

Three theories on the cause of chronic tubulointerstitial nephritis are (1) focal acute interstitial nephritis evolves into the chronic form, (2) it is produced as a secondary manifestation of chronic glomerulonephritis (GN) or chronic pyelonephritis, or (3) it is produced after immune-mediated damage to the renal tubules and interstitium. There are few acute tubulointerstitial diseases to account for the large number of cases of chronic tubulointerstitial nephritis seen in dogs, and thus the first theory cannot account for a high percentage of the cases. As diagnostic techniques improve, some cases of chronic tubulointerstitial nephritis may be reclassified more specifically as either chronic pyelonephritis or secondary to chronic GN.

The mechanism of injury is known in a few instances, most specifically with Leptospira infections. After exposure to the organism, leptospiremia occurs and then organisms do the following:

- Localize in the renal interstitial capillaries
- Migrate through vascular endothelium
- Persist in the interstitial spaces
- Migrate via the lateral intercellular junctions of tubular epithelial cells to reach renal tubular lumina
- Associate with epithelial microvilli
- Persist within phagosomes of the epithelial cells of the proximal and distal convoluted tubules
- Induce tubular epithelial cells to undergo degeneration and necrosis as a result of either direct toxic effects of the leptospires or the accompanying interstitial inflammatory reaction

Although neutrophils can be present in tubular lumina, the predominant chronic lesion is an infiltrate of monocytes, macrophages, lymphocytes, and plasma cells in the interstitium (chiefly cortical) (see Fig. 11-20, *D*). In affected dogs, interstitial plasma cells secrete *Leptospira*-specific antibodies. However, the role of those antibodies in pathogenesis or resolution of the lesion is not known.

Another well-documented mechanism for the production of tubulointerstitial nephritis is the immune response that develops secondary to canine adenoviral infection. The sequence of events includes the following:

- Localization of virus in the glomeruli (viral glomerulitis) during the viremic phase of the disease
- Production of a transient immune-complex GN
- Recovery from the acute phase of the disease
- Onset of the systemic immune response
- Disappearance of virus from the glomeruli only to reappear in tubular epithelial cells in various portions of the nephron in basophilic intranuclear viral inclusions
- Persistence of virus in tubular epithelium for weeks to months
- Production of tubular epithelial necrosis as a result of viral-induced cytolysis
- Production of chronic lymphocytic, plasmacytic, and less commonly histiocytic interstitial nephritis

Infection with equine arteritis virus or porcine reproductive and respiratory syndrome (PRRS) virus often results in multifocal lymphohistiocytic chronic tubulointerstitial nephritis with interstitial edema. Lesions can involve any area of the cortex but are especially intense in the medulla and at the corticomedullary junction. A severe vasculitis, characterized by fibrinoid necrosis and lymphohistiocytic infiltrates that involve the adventitial and medial layers of cortical and medullary arteries and veins, is present. Virus can be found in endothelium and in macrophages.

Deposition of immune complexes in or interactions between antibasement membrane antibodies and tubular basement membranes can initiate immune-mediated tubulointerstitial disease in humans and laboratory animals. Depositions of immunoglobulin (Ig) and complement have rarely been identified in renal tubular basement membranes in domestic animals, but administration of preformed complexes (bovine serum albumin and antibody) to dogs demonstrated that these complexes interacted with proximal renal tubules not glomeruli. Damaged tubules respond with epithelial cell proliferation, basement membrane thickening, and peritubular fibrosis. At present, the role of immune-mediated mechanisms in tubulointerstitial nephritis in domestic animals is unclear.

Gross Lesions of Tubulointerstitial Nephritis

Gross lesions can be classified as acute, subacute, or chronic; chronic tubulointerstitial nephritis is discussed in more detail later (see the section on Renal Fibrosis). The distribution of lesions can be diffuse as in canine leptospirosis (see Fig. 11-73) or multifocal as in "white spotted kidneys" of calves as the result of *Escherichia coli* septicemia (see Fig. 11-70), infectious canine hepatitis (see Fig. 11-43), canine herpesvirus infection (see Fig. 11-74), malignant catarrhal fever, or porcine and bovine leptospirosis (see Fig. 11-73). In diffuse tubulointerstitial nephritis, kidneys can be swollen and pale tan with a random gray mottling of the capsular surface. The cut surface bulges; gray infiltrates of varying sizes and intensities obscure the normal radially striated cortical architecture. These renal lesions usually are manifested as coalescing gray foci that are particularly intense in the inner cortex. Focal lesions of tubulointerstitial nephritis are less extensive and composed of more discrete gray areas in the cortex and outer medulla.

Microscopic Lesions of Tubulointerstitial Nephritis

Microscopically, aggregates of lymphocytes, plasma cells, monocytes, and fewer neutrophils are randomly scattered or intensely localized throughout the edematous interstitium. Tubular epithelial cells within severely inflamed areas can be degenerate, necrotic, or both, and profound tubular loss is usually accompanied by eventual replacement fibrosis.

Renal Fibrosis (Scarring)

The alternative to regeneration is irreparable damage that results in functional tubular loss when cuboidal epithelium is replaced by nonabsorptive cuboidal or squamous cells or actual physical loss of tubules so that the nephron is lost. This can occur after either an ischemic insult or exposure to a limited number of nephrotoxins. The ultimate result is replacement fibrosis/scarring. This is seen most commonly if the following occur:

- The toxin is not removed.
- The basement membrane does not remain intact.
- Adequate tubular epithelium does not survive the toxic dose to allow for complete repair.

Fibrosis with a finely granular pattern can occur subsequent to widespread necrosis of renal tubular epithelium (acute tubular necrosis). An example is oak poisoning of cattle (see Fig. 11-69), in which severe tubular necrosis extends to the level of the renal tubular basement membrane, resulting in leakage of tubular contents. The loss of the continuity of the basement membrane prevents orderly tubular epithelial cell regeneration, which can be followed by interstitial fibrosis. Recent experimental studies have demonstrated that after severe nephrotoxin-induced tubular epithelial cell injury, the remaining cells undergo accelerated apoptosis resulting in tubular atrophy, interstitial fibroblast proliferation, and eventual fibrosis.

Renal fibrosis is the replacement of renal parenchyma, including tubules, glomeruli, and interstitium with mature fibrous connective tissue. It can occur as a primary event, but more frequently is a manifestation of the healing phase of a preexisting tubular or glomerular lesion. It is the common endpoint of all reparative stages and results when conditions are not conducive for healing of the tubular epithelium by regeneration. Regeneration of nephrons as a whole is not possible. Renal fibrosis follows many renal lesions, including primary inflammation of glomeruli (GN), tubules, or interstitial tissue (tubulointerstitial nephritis) (Fig. 11-21) and necrosis of renal tubules. Its severity usually parallels the intensity of the primary renal disease. The mechanisms by which fibrosis is induced are related to destruction and loss of nephron components by inflammatory or less commonly noninflammatory processes. T lymphocytes and interleukin-6 (IL-6) play important roles in renal fibrosis. Renal fibrosis is seen commonly following any number of renal insults and includes the following:

- Infarction
- GN/amyloidosis
- Tubulointerstitial disease/chronic pelvic diseases

Renal fibrosis may manifest in a multitude of grossly recognizable forms as described previously. Generally, fibrotic kidneys are recognized grossly by the pale, tan-to-white, shrunken, pitted, and firm consistency, along with excessive adhesions of the capsule to the underlying cortex. Fibrosis can be diffuse and finely stippled with pinpoint dimpling and granularity on the capsular surface, or it can be coarser as seen by deep and irregularly shaped depressions of the capsular surface in either a diffuse, multifocal, or patchy distribution. In addition to these changes of the capsular surface, the cut surface of the cortex is thinned beneath the capsular surface depressions, and these fibrotic areas are pale tan when compared with more normal parenchyma.

Microscopically, renal fibrosis is characterized by an increase in interstitial connective tissue and absence of renal tubules (Fig. 11-22, *A*). Remaining tubules are usually atrophic and have a reduced luminal diameter or can appear ectatic because they are lined by flattened epithelium, producing an enlarged luminal diameter. A thickened hyalinized basement membrane and a lining of flattened epithelium (squamous or low cuboidal) are also characteristic. Multiple acquired cysts can be present throughout the cortex and medulla and can be a result of either dilated Bowman's capsules and associated atrophic glomerular tufts or nephrons whose tubules have segments compressed by connective tissue (Fig. 11-22, *B*). Even in fibrotic lesions that are not the result of an infectious disease or inflammation, foci of lymphocytes and plasma cells can be seen randomly scattered throughout the interstitium (Fig. 11-22, *C*). In areas of severe interstitial fibrosis, glomerulosclerosis (as an end-stage of isolated glomeruli) is common. Calcification of vessels, tubular basement membranes, Bowman's capsules, and degenerate tubular epithelium are common in fibrotic kidneys because of alterations in calcium-phosphorus metabolism associated with chronic renal failure.

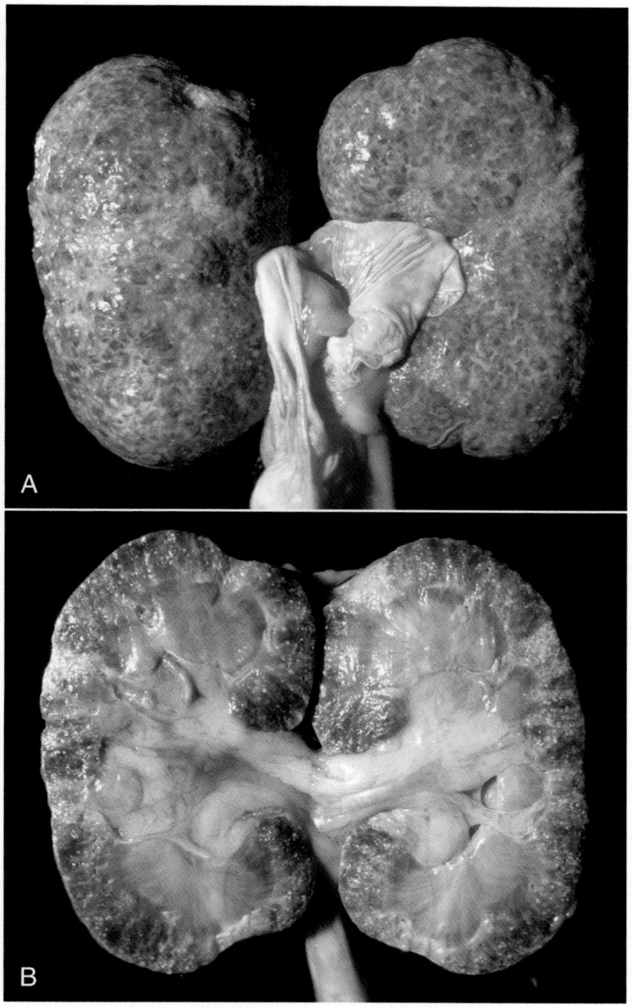

Fig. 11-21 Chronic interstitial nephritis, kidney, dog.
A, Diffuse interstitial fibrosis is responsible for the fine pitting of the capsular cortical surface, which is stippled red, the result of bands of fibrous tissue *(gray)* surrounding islands of renal cortex. **B,** Dorsal section. The cortex is pitted and granular because of multiple linear and focal scars, and it is also thinner than normal (atrophic). (Courtesy Dr. M.D. McGavin, College of Veterinary Medicine, University of Tennessee.)

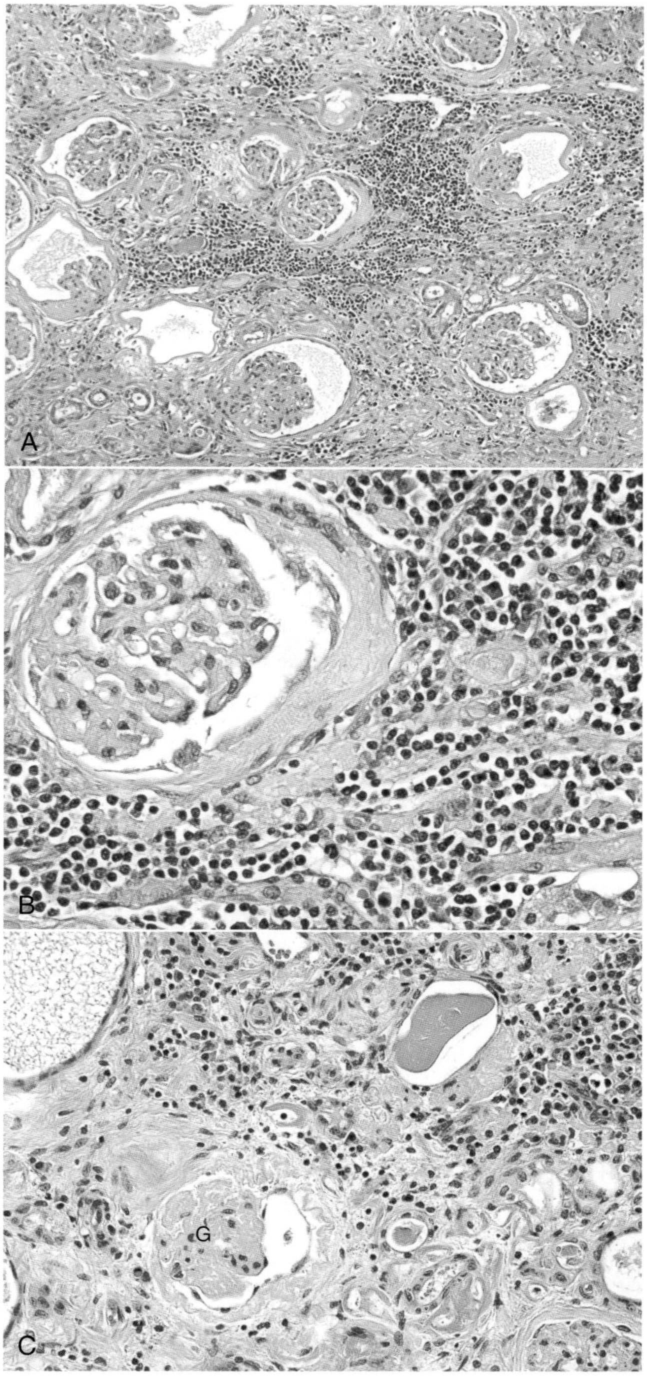

Fig. 11-22 Chronic interstitial nephritis, kidney, dog.
A, Dorsal section, cortex. This lesion is characterized by interstitial fibrosis, tubular atrophy, and interstitial inflammatory cell (lymphocytes and plasma cell) infiltration. The renal corpuscles have contracted glomeruli with increased volume of mesangial matrix and thickened Bowman's capsules. H&E stain. **B,** Higher magnification of **A.** H&E stain. **C,** Cortex. Higher magnification showing interstitial fibrosis, lymphocytic inflammatory infiltrates, sclerotic glomerular tufts *(G)*, and ectatic tubules and Bowman's spaces. H&E stain. (**A** and **B** courtesy Dr. J.F. Zachary, College of Veterinary Medicine, University of Illinois. **C** courtesy Dr. M.D. McGavin, College of Veterinary Medicine, University of Tennessee.)

Renal fibrosis and chronic renal disease are the most frequently recognized renal pathologic processes in mature or aging domestic animals, particularly dogs and cats. When renal fibrosis and loss of nephrons are severe, these lesions can be manifested clinically as chronic renal failure and uremia. One of the most common expressions of this chronic disease is the inability of an animal to concentrate urine, resulting in frequent urination (polyuria) of dilute urine (isosthenuria). Polyuria is accompanied by dehydration and excessive water drinking (polydipsia). Hypoplastic anemia occurs as a result of the kidneys' failure to synthesize and secrete erythropoietin. Fibrous osteodystrophy can develop because of abnormal calcium-phosphorus metabolism and renal secondary hyperparathyroidism.

End-Stage Kidneys

Without careful attention to the pattern of resultant fibrosis, such kidneys can be indiscriminately termed as *end-stage kidneys;*

however, fibrosis generally follows a pattern characteristic of the antecedent injury and is described here for tubulointerstitial disease.

A coarser pattern of diffuse renal fibrosis occurs in chronic interstitial nephritis and certain progressive juvenile nephropathies of dogs. Both cortex and medulla can be fibrotic, cortical striations are severely distorted or effaced, and the formation of multiple cortical cysts is common. End-stage kidneys are those referred to as a result of fibrosis, mineralization, sclerotic glomeruli, and foci of hyperplastic and hypertrophic tubules. Progressive interstitial fibrosis is thought to be the final common pathway to chronic renal failure.

RESPONSES OF THE VASCULATURE TO INJURY

Hyperemia and Congestion

Hyperemia refers to an increase in arterial blood flow, and congestion is an increase in venous blood pooling within the vasculature of the kidney. Renal hyperemia is an active process usually secondary to acute renal inflammation.

Renal congestion can be the following:

- Physiologic
- Passive
- Secondary to hypovolemic shock
- Secondary to cardiac insufficiency
- Hypostatic

Hyperemic kidneys are darker red than normal, can be perceptibly swollen, and ooze blood from the cut surface. Congested kidneys are dark purple and ooze blood from the cut surface as the result of the accumulation of unoxygenated blood in the renal venous system. At necropsy, unilateral renal hypostatic congestion is present in animals that die in lateral recumbency, after which the force of gravity pulls the unclotted blood downward. Microscopically, the arterial and venous vessels are distended with blood, and if there has been sufficient time for the blood to clot, serum and blood cells may be present.

Hemorrhage and Thrombosis

Hemorrhage occurs when red blood cells extend beyond the vessel walls. Large intrarenal hemorrhages can result from direct trauma, renal needle biopsy, and systemic bleeding disorders, such as factor VIII deficiency. Subcapsular and renal cortical hemorrhages occur in association with septicemic diseases, vasculitis, vascular necrosis, thromboembolism, and disseminated intravascular coagulation (DIC). Perirenal hemorrhage has been noted with ovine herpesvirus arteritis (malignant catarrhal fever [MCF]) and of course, abdominal trauma.

Petechial hemorrhages are commonly seen on the surface and throughout the cortex of kidneys from pigs that die of viremia or septicemia caused by diseases such as hog cholera (swine fever), African swine fever, erysipelas (see Fig. 11-71), streptococcal infections, salmonellosis, and other embolic bacterial diseases (e.g., *Actinobacillus* spp.). Renal cortical ecchymotic hemorrhages associated with multifocal tubular and vascular necrosis are salient and diagnostically important lesions of viremia in neonatal puppies infected with herpesvirus. Portions of thrombus that break free from affected heart valves in valvular endocarditis can lodge in the glomeruli or interstitial capillaries in any species.

When DIC causes widespread thrombosis in the glomerular capillaries (Fig. 11-23), the afferent arterioles and most importantly the interlobular arteries, widespread cortical infarction results and is designated renal cortical necrosis. This lesion is not to be confused with ischemic acute tubular necrosis discussed in this chapter (see the section on Acute Tubular Necrosis). Partial or complete renal cortical necrosis is usually a bilateral lesion that occurs in all animal species, especially as a result of Gram-negative septicemias or endotoxemias, and is related to the following:

- Endotoxin-induced endothelial damage
- Activation of the extrinsic clotting mechanism
- Widespread capillary thrombosis

The lesion can be induced experimentally in animals by two endotoxin injections 24 hours apart and is a manifestation of the generalized Shwartzman reaction. The resulting microthrombosis of vessels throughout the renal cortex results in widespread ischemia and small and large infarcts of coagulation necrosis and hemorrhage. The renal cortex can be diffusely pale with a zone of hyperemia separating the necrotic cortex from the viable medulla, or more often the cortex is a mosaic of large, irregular hemorrhagic areas, resembling hemorrhagic infarcts interspersed with large yellow-gray areas resembling pale infarcts. The necrotic tissue can involve the full width of the cortex or only the outer portion. Thrombi are demonstrable mainly in the interlobular arteries.

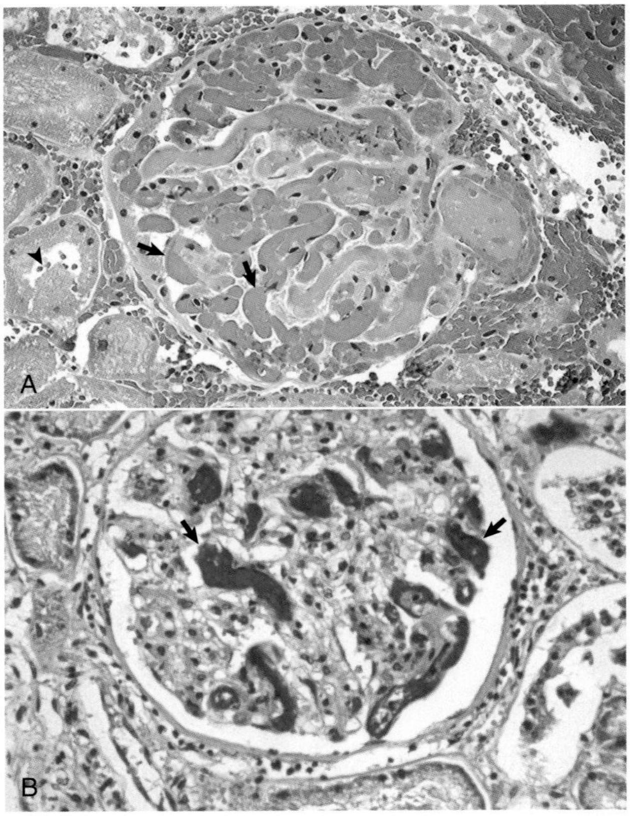

Fig. 11-23 Glomerular capillary thrombosis, kidney, glomerulus, dog. **A,** Microthrombi. Capillary lumens are occluded by microthrombi *(arrows)* caused by disseminated intravascular coagulation. Adjacent cortical tubular epithelial cells are undergoing coagulation necrosis with nuclei undergoing pyknosis and karyolysis *(arrowhead),* the result of ischemia from reduced blood flow to the peritubular capillaries, which are downstream from the glomerulus. H&E stain. **B,** Fibrinous microthrombi. A glomerulus similar to the one shown in Fig. 11-23,*A,* stained to demonstrate fibrinous thrombi *(arrows).* Fibrin is red. Lendrum-Fraser stain for fibrin. (**A** courtesy Dr. W. Crowell, College of Veterinary Medicine, The University of Georgia; and Noah's Arkive, College of Veterinary Medicine, The University of Georgia. **B** courtesy College of Veterinary Medicine, University of Illinois.)

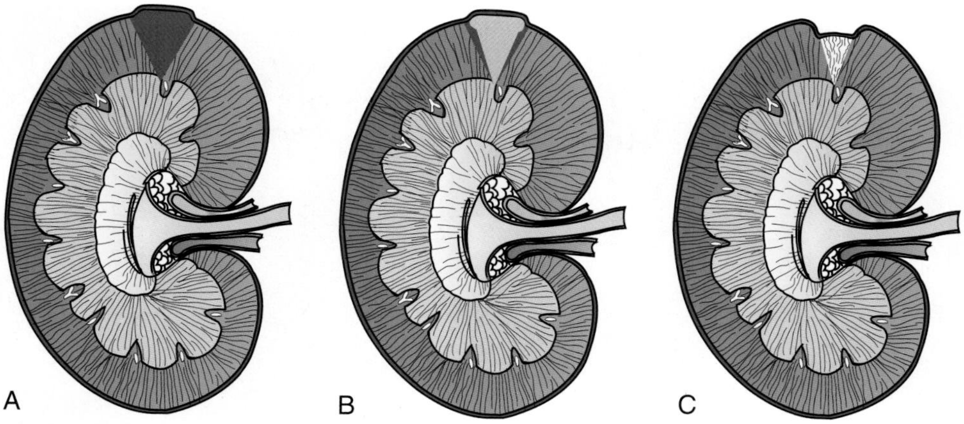

Fig. 11-24 Schematic diagram of renal infarction.
The normal progression of renal infarcts is outlined. **A** and **B,** Acute renal infarcts. Initially, renal infarcts are swollen and hemorrhagic **(A).** In 2 to 3 days, infarcts become pale **(B),** surrounded by a zone of hyperemia and hemorrhage. **C,** Chronic infarcts are pale, shrunken, and fibrotic, resulting in distortion and depression of the renal contour.

Infarction

Renal infarcts are areas of coagulative necrosis that result from the local ischemia of vascular occlusion and usually are due to thromboembolism.

Renal emboli are derived from the following:

- Thromboemboli
- Mural thrombi on heart valves in valvular endocarditis
- Endarteritis in parasitic diseases such as canine dirofilariasis and equine strongylosis
- Arteriosclerosis in cattle (rare)
- Neoplastic cell emboli
- Bacterial emboli

Because of the high circulating blood volume (20% to 25% of cardiac output) through the kidney, renal infarcts from thromboemboli derived from lesions of mitral or aortic valvular vegetative endocarditis or mural endocarditis are common in many species, especially in cattle with *Arcanobacterium* colonization, in pigs with *Erysipelas* or in cats with left atrial thrombosis associated with cardiomyopathy. Rarely, emboli may occlude the renal artery, causing infarction of the entire kidney. Sometimes, emboli occlude the interlobar/arcuate arteries, causing infarction of triangular (in cross-section of the kidney) segments of the cortex and medulla. Most commonly, emboli obstruct many smaller vessels (e.g., interlobular arteries), causing multiple smaller infarcts involving only the renal cortex. In general, renal infarction can occur because of thrombosis resulting from endothelial damage of glomerular capillaries associated with a vascular disease (as in Alabama rot in greyhounds; see Fig. 11-44). Renal infarcts in horses can result from emboli lodging in the renal vasculature after mural thrombosis of the aorta, from aortic wall damage, caused by migrating larvae of *Strongylus vulgaris.* Thrombosis of pulmonary, coronary, splenic, or renal arteries and the resultant infarction are common in dogs with glomerular amyloidosis, which results in loss of plasma anticoagulants, such as antithrombin III, through damaged glomeruli. Endotoxin-mediated arterial or capillary thromboemboli are a common cause of infarction in association with Gram-negative sepsis or endotoxic shock. Septic emboli, particularly those from bacterial valvular endocarditis, caused by *Arcanobacterium pyogenes* in cattle, *Erysipelothrix rhusiopathiae* in pigs, and *Staphylococcus aureus* in small animals, can cause renal infarcts and can progress to microabscesses or granulomas, depending on the microorganism involved.

Grossly, renal infarcts appear red or pale white depending on several factors, including the interval after vascular occlusion (i.e., age of infarct) (Figs. 11-24 and 11-25). Occlusion of small interlobular arteries results in infarcts that are initially slightly swollen and red because of hemorrhage (Fig. 11-25, *A*) and later become pale yellow-gray within 2 to 3 days because of lysis of erythrocytes and loss of hemoglobin (Fig. 11-25, *B*). Initially, large infarcts develop when an embolus lodges in the interlobular artery closer to its origin from the arcuate artery. These larger infarcts have a central area of pallor (coagulative necrosis) and are usually surrounded by a peripheral red zone of congestion and hemorrhage along with a pale margin because of a surrounding zone of leukocytes (Fig. 11-25, *C*). Because of the loss of parenchyma, during healing infarcts are depressed below the cortical surface and later become pale and shrunken as a result of fibrosis (Fig. 11-25, *D*).

The scarring that follows infarction is related to several variables, including the size of the ischemic area caused by vascular compromise. Healing is by fibrosis and results in large, deeply depressed wedge-shaped (on cross-section of the kidney) scars that involve primarily the cortex but can extend into the medulla. Obstruction of smaller arterioles results in smaller areas of more superficial coagulative necrosis that heal as small-diameter pits in the renal surface, which correspond to pale white, linear scars on the cut surface.

Infarcts are often wedge-shaped in a cross-section of kidney, with the base against the cortical surface and the apex pointing toward the medulla, conforming to a zone of cortical parenchyma supplied by the site of the obstruction. Usually, infarcts are the result of blockage of an interlobular artery and exactly how large that infarct depends on where the artery is blocked. Blockage of the interlobular artery at its point of origin causes the largest infarcts, blockage toward its end in the outer cortex causes the smallest. Infarcts can involve the cortex only or the cortex and medulla depending on the size of the occluded vessel and the site of obstruction. For example, thrombosis of an arcuate artery, which supplies both cortex and medulla, would result in an infarct involving the cortex and extending partway into the medulla (see Fig. 11-8). Thrombosis of a cortical interlobular artery, which supplies mainly the cortex, would result in an infarct of the cortex only (see Fig. 11-8). Although less common, hypoxic renal necrosis as the result of venous occlusion and/or infarction is seen occasionally, and they retain their hemorrhagic appearance longer than infarcts

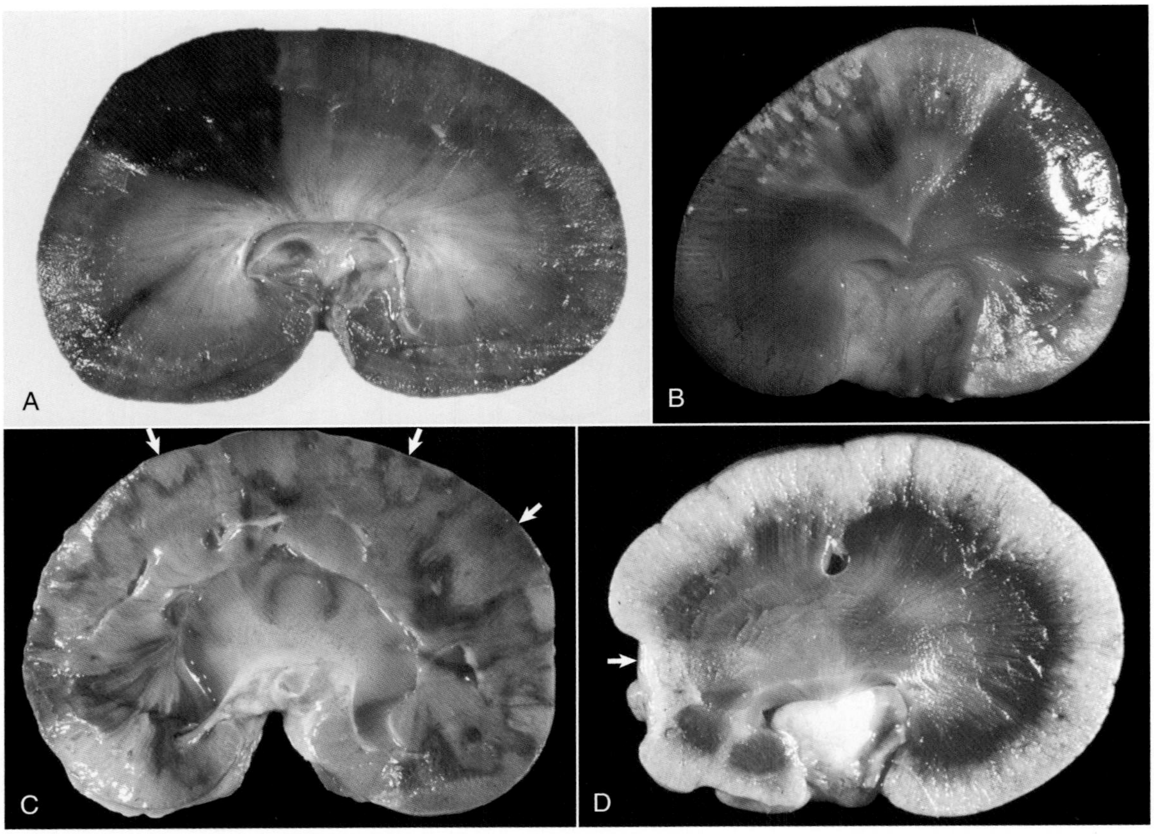

Fig. 11-25 Gross appearance of renal cortical infarcts with age, kidney, dorsal sections.
A, Acute (early) hemorrhagic infarct, dog. Focal wedge-shaped area of cortical necrosis. Note how the infarct bulges above the capsular surface due to cell swelling and hemorrhage. **B,** Acute pale infarcts, rabbit. There are two pale white to tan wedge-shaped infarcts *(top, lower right)*. Note how the infarct *(top)* bulges above the capsular surface, indicating cell swelling. **C,** Subacute infarcts, dog. Multiple renal cortical infarcts are pale and surrounded by a red rim of active hyperemia *(arrows)*. The cortical surface of many, but not all, of the infarcts is even with that of the adjacent unaffected cortex, indicating that cell swelling has subsided. **D,** Chronic infarct, cat. A focal pale truncated wedge-shaped scar of fibrous connective tissue has replaced the pole *(arrow)* of the renal cortex. Note that the surface of the infarct is below that of the adjacent normal kidney because of the loss of tissue, fibrosis, and contraction of the fibrous scar. (**A** courtesy Dr. W. Crowell, College of Veterinary Medicine, The University of Georgia; and Noah's Arkive, College of Veterinary Medicine, The University of Georgia. **B** courtesy Dr. M.D. McGavin, College of Veterinary Medicine, University of Tennessee. **C** courtesy Dr. K. Read, College of Veterinary Medicine, Texas A&M University; and Noah's Arkive, College of Veterinary Medicine, The University of Georgia. **D** courtesy Dr. J. Sagartz, College of Veterinary Medicine, The Ohio State University; and Noah's Arkive, College of Veterinary Medicine, The University of Georgia.)

resulting from arterial occlusion because of the continued arterial blood flow into the area.

Microscopically, in an acute infarct, nephrons (including tubules, glomeruli, and interstitium) in the central zone of the infarct become necrotic (Fig. 11-26). At the periphery of the infarct, only the proximal tubules, because of their high metabolic rate, are necrotic; the glomeruli tend to be spared. After a couple of days, the margin of the necrotic zone contains an inflammatory infiltrate consisting largely of neutrophils and fewer macrophages and lymphocytes. Capillaries adjacent to the necrotic area are notably engorged with blood (hyperemia). Healing of the infarcted area occurs by lysis and phagocytosis of the necrotic tissue and replacement by fibrous connective tissue, which matures to a discrete scar. Scars range from linear to broad depending on the size of the acute infarct. Septic infarcts are initially hemorrhagic, but because of the presence of pyogenic bacteria, the necrotic tissue undergoes liquefactive necrosis and the infarcts can eventually develop into abscesses and ultimately into substantial scars. Septic infarcts often fail to respect a solely cortical or medullary pattern of distribution caused by the extensive local inflammation that they generate.

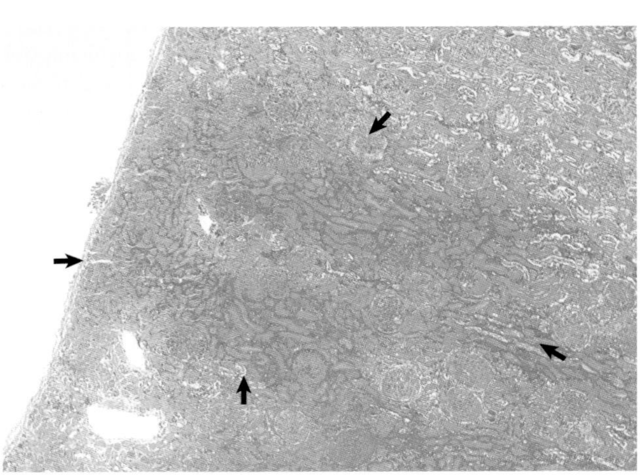

Fig. 11-26 Acute infarct, kidney, cortex, dog.
Note the acute infarct with a central zone of coagulation necrosis surrounded by a zone of hyperemia and hemorrhage *(arrows)*. H&E stain. (Courtesy Dr. S.J. Newman, College of Veterinary Medicine, University of Tennessee.)

Papillary (Medullary Crest) Necrosis

See the section on Disorders of Domestic Animals for a discussion of papillary necrosis.

Embolic Nephritis

Acute suppurative glomerulitis, or bacterial (embolic) nephritis, is discussed in the section on Disorders of Domestic Animals.

STRUCTURE OF THE LOWER URINARY TRACT

The lower urinary tract is the conduit for the transport of urinary waste from the kidney to the exterior through paired ureters, the urinary bladder, and the urethra.

URETERS

Macroscopically, the ureters enter the bladder wall obliquely and are covered by a mucosal flap, the vesicoureteral valve, which is an important structure because it normally prevents reflux of urine from the bladder into the ureter and renal pelvis. The normal mucosa of the ureter should be smooth and glistening. Microscopically, the ureters are lined by transitional epithelium. Histologically, the ureteral mucosa is folded longitudinally; there are poorly defined internal and external longitudinal muscle layers, a prominent middle circular muscle layer and externally, either adventitia or peritoneal serosa.

URINARY BLADDER

Macroscopically at death, the urinary bladder can contract to such a degree that the normal bladder wall appears thick on necropsy. The normal mucosa of the urinary bladder should be smooth and glistening. Urine should be clear except in horses, where it is cloudy because of the normal presence of mucus and crystalline material produced by the branched tubuloalveolar mucous glands in the submucosa of the renal pelvis and proximal ureter. Microscopically, as in other mucous membranes, the lamina propria has small lymphoid follicles, which, after inflammation or antigenic stimulation, can be large enough to be seen grossly as discrete, circular, white foci (1 to 2 mm) in the mucosa. Histologically, the bladder is an expanded ureter, lined by pseudostratified transitional epithelium ranging from 3 to 14 cells thick, depending on the species and degree of distention. Histologically, the urinary bladder wall is composed of poorly defined internal and external longitudinal muscle layers, a prominent middle circular muscle layer, and externally either adventitia or peritoneal serosa.

URETHRA

Macroscopically, during continence, the bladder is relatively flaccid and the urethra acts as a valve. Microscopically, the urethra is lined by transitional epithelium cranially and stratified squamous epithelium immediately cranial to or at the urethral orifice.

FUNCTION OF THE LOWER URINARY TRACT

URETERS

The function of the ureters is to propel urine from the kidney to the urinary bladder by peristalsis.

BOX 11-6 Portals of Entry into Lower Urinary System

ASCENDING

Extension from exterior secondary to contamination from the gastrointestinal tract
Extension from exterior secondary to contamination from the genital tract
Extension from exterior secondary to contamination from the dermis

DESCENDING

Extension from disease processes that occur within the kidney and renal pelvis

DIRECT PENETRATION FROM THE LUMEN

Accumulation of toxic levels in urine due to stasis and collection
Urinary tract calculi formation

DIRECT PENETRATION FROM THE ABDOMEN

URINARY BLADDER AND URETHRA

The urinary bladder stores urine and, in concert with the urethra, expels it. During micturition, contraction of the detrusor muscle (the urinary bladder musculature) pumps urine through the relaxed urethra.

PORTALS OF ENTRY

Common portals of entry for the lower urinary tract are shown in Box 11-6.

ASCENDING INFECTION

Extension from the exterior secondary to contamination from the gastrointestinal tract, the genital tract, or severe bacterial dermatitis can result in damage secondary to ascension of bacteria. This represents a distinctly unique mechanism because the lower urinary tract represents a tubular system that is blind-ended and has only one exit to the exterior (i.e., through the urethra), unlike the intestinal system, which is a continuous tubular system. This predisposes to bacterial ascension and colonization by adherent bacteria, especially in females. In males, end-stage obstruction is due partially to the narrow diameter and length of the urethra. Etiologic agents, such as bacteria, may originate from the exterior skin surface or the closely located openings of the intestinal tract and the female genitourinary tract. Bacteria with adhesion capabilities may overcome peristalsis and periodic urine flushing. Regular complete emptying will minimize risks of pathologic changes, in contrast to stasis, retention of urine, and infrequent urinations, which predispose to ascending disease.

DESCENDING INFECTION

Extension from disease processes that occur within the kidney and renal pelvis, such as pyelonephritis, may account for extension of inflammation into the lower urinary tract. The presence of renal pelvic calculi may also be seen concurrently.

DIRECT PENETRATION FROM THE LUMEN

When toxic principles are excreted in the urine, they may accumulate to toxic levels because urine is stored in the urinary bladder for extended periods of time. These agents may produce lesions to the lower urinary tract as a result. Additionally, the presence of a

BOX 11-7 Defense Mechanisms against Injury and Infectious Agents

- Urine flow—flushing
- Peristalsis
- pH control
- Urothelial cell protective mucus coat
- Immune system
  - Innate responses
  - Humoral responses
  - Cellular responses

urolith anywhere within the lower urinary tract can result in trauma to the mucosa, with accompanying edema, hemorrhage, ulceration, and in the most severe cases, rupture caused by pressure necrosis.

DIRECT PENETRATION FROM THE ABDOMEN (CYSTOCENTESIS)

Although rare as a portal of entry, it is possible for surface skin bacteria to be transmitted to the urinary bladder lumen through direct penetration of the abdomen after diagnostic procedures such as cystocentesis.

DEFENSE MECHANISMS

Defense mechanisms unique to the lower urinary system have evolved to counteract the typical forms of injury (Box 11-7). The most notable of these defense mechanisms of the lower urinary tract, which includes the ureters, urinary bladder, and urethra are as follows:

- The flushing action of urine minimizes risks of ascension of bacteria
- Peristalsis acts to eliminate bacteria with adhesion capabilities
- Inhospitable environment for bacterial growth controlled by urine pH
- Protective urothelial mucus coating
- Innate immune response
- Humoral immune response
- Cellular immune response

RESPONSES TO INJURY

URETER, URINARY BLADDER, AND URETHRA

The predominant responses to injury include dilation and pressure necrosis caused by obstruction to the lower urinary tract system, inflammation after exposure to infectious etiologies, and/or neoplastic transformation. Additionally, concentration of excreted urinary substances, such as drug metabolites, pesticides, and other toxins, can damage the surface of the lower urinary system and predispose it to infection, secondary hyperplasia, or neoplastic responses.

DISORDERS OF DOMESTIC ANIMALS

NONRENAL LESIONS OF UREMIA

Nonrenal lesions of uremia identified clinically or at necropsy are useful indicators of renal failure (Table 11-1). The severity of nonrenal lesions of uremia depends on the length of time that the animal has survived in the uremic state. Therefore, in acute renal failure, nonrenal lesions are few, whereas many lesions can be present in chronic renal failure. Typically, nonrenal lesions can be attributed to either one of the following mechanisms:

- Endothelial degeneration and necrosis, resulting in vasculitis with secondary thrombosis and infarction in a variety of tissues (i.e., intestinal tract).
- Caustic injury to epithelium of the oral cavity and stomach, which results in ulcer formation, is secondary to the production of large concentrations of ammonia after splitting of salivary or gastric urea by bacteria.

Systemic nonrenal lesions of uremia include one or more of the following:

- Ulcerative and necrotic glossitis/stomatitis characterized by a brown, foul-smelling, mucoid material adherent to the eroded and ulcerated lingual and oral mucosa; ulcers are most commonly bilateral (symmetric) and present on the underside of the tongue (Fig. 11-27).

TABLE 11-1 Nonrenal Lesions of Uremia

Lesion	Mechanism
Pulmonary edema	Increased vascular permeability
Fibrinous pericarditis	Increased vascular permeability
Ulcerative and hemorrhagic gastritis	Ammonia secretion and vascular necrosis
Ulcerative and necrotic stomatitis	Ammonia secretion in saliva and vascular necrosis
Atrial and aortic thrombosis	Endothelial and subendothelial damage
Hypoplastic anemia	Increased erythrocyte fragility and lack of erythropoietin production in the kidney
Soft-tissue mineralization	Altered calcium-phosphorus metabolism (stomach, lungs, pleura, kidneys)
Fibrous osteodystrophy	Altered calcium-phosphorus metabolism
Parathyroid hyperplasia	Altered calcium-phosphorus metabolism

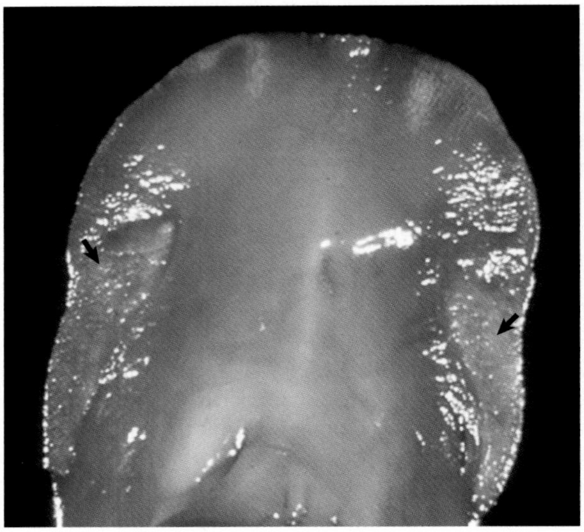

Fig. 11-27 Ulcerative glossitis, uremia, tongue, ventral surface, cat. Bilaterally symmetrical ulcers *(arrows)* are present on the rostrolateral borders of the ventral surface of the tongue. (Courtesy Dr. M.D. McGavin, College of Veterinary Medicine, University of Tennessee.)

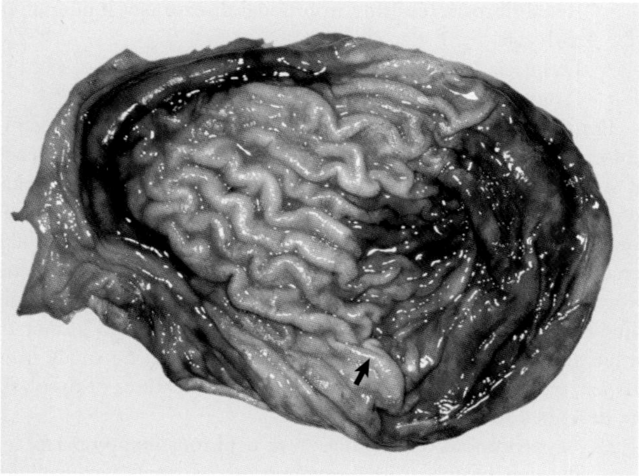

Fig. 11-28 Uremic gastritis, stomach, dog.
Because of uremia, the stomach wall is hemorrhagic *(right)* and the stomach contents may contain blood and mucus (not shown here). Note the edematous mucosal thickening *(arrow)*. (Courtesy Dr. A. Confer, College of Veterinary Medicine, Oklahoma State University.)

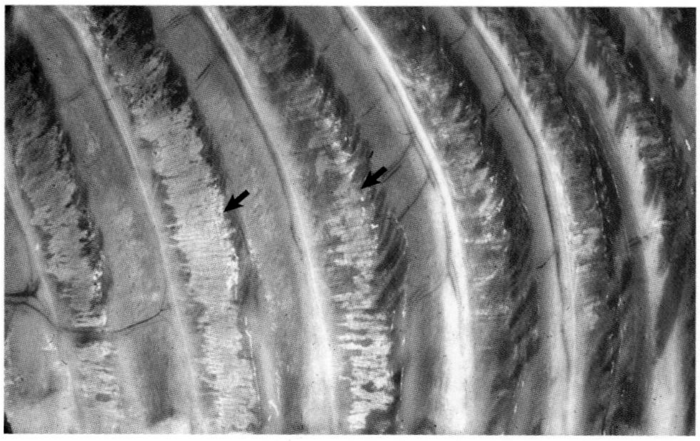

Fig. 11-30 Thoracic cavity, parietal pleura, cat.
Horizontally oriented streaks *(arrows)* of mineral (intercostal mineralization) are present in the subpleural intercostal connective tissue as a result of chronic uremia. (Courtesy Dr. J. King, College of Veterinary Medicine, Cornell University.)

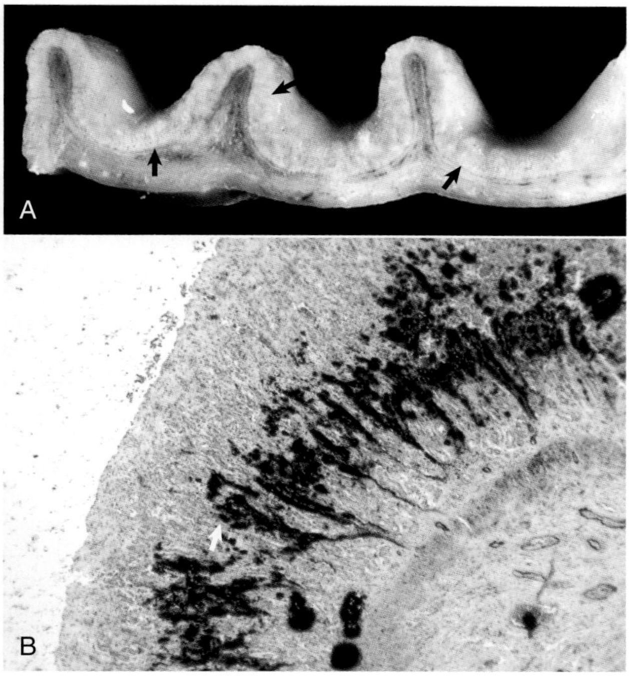

Fig. 11-29 Uremic gastritis, stomach, dog.
A, There is accentuation of the gastric rugae and calcification in the deep mucosa *(arrows)*. **B,** The mucosa has laminar mineralization *(black color)* of gastric glands *(arrow)*, von Kossa stain. (**A** courtesy Dr. J. King, College of Veterinary Medicine, Cornell University. **B** courtesy Dr. M.D. McGavin, College of Veterinary Medicine, University of Tennessee.)

- Ulcerative and hemorrhagic gastritis in dogs and cats (Fig. 11-28), often with secondary midzonal mineralization (Fig. 11-29). The gastric wall can be gritty when cut because of calcification of the inner and middle layers of the mucosa and the submucosal arterioles. This lesion is less commonly seen in horses and cattle, in which intestinal lesions predominate.
- Ulcerative and hemorrhagic colitis in horses and cattle, in which large areas of colonic mucosa are often edematous and dark red because of hemorrhage. The gastrointestinal contents can be bloody and smell of ammonia. Microscopically, coagulative necrosis, hemorrhage, and a neutrophilic infiltrate occur in the intestinal mucosa. Degeneration, necrosis, and mineralization of the arteriolar intima and media are often present in the gastric mucosa and submucosa (Fig. 11-29, *B*).
- Intercostal mineralization/uremic mineralization is characterized, particularly in dogs, by calcification of the subpleural connective tissue of the cranial intercostal spaces (Fig. 11-30). These lesions are white-gray granular pleural thickenings with a horizontal "ladderlike" arrangement. The intercostal muscles are only superficially calcified. Patchy or diffuse pulmonary calcification of the lungs results in their failure to collapse, areas of paleness, and mild-to-moderate firmness and crunchiness and can occur occasionally in conjunction with the lesions of uremic pneumonitis and localized emphysema.
- Fibrinous pericarditis is characterized by fine granular deposits of calcium on the epicardium (visceral pericardium).
- Diffuse pulmonary edema is characterized by alveoli that contain fibrin-rich fluid and often a mild infiltrate of macrophages and neutrophils. This lesion is also called *uremic pneumonitis.* The underlying lesion is a vasculitis affecting the alveolar capillaries, which results in increased vascular permeability and high protein effusion.
- Arteritis is characterized macroscopically by finely granular roughened plaques within the left atrial endocardium and less frequently in the proximal aorta and pulmonary trunk. Arteritis in conjunction with loss of the anticoagulant antithrombin III by glomerular leakage is conducive to the formation of large mural thrombi at these sites.
- Nephrocalcinosis (calcification), although usually not visible at necropsy and not a true nonrenal lesion of uremia, occurs in the kidneys (Fig. 11-31). The kidneys can be gritty when cut because of calcification of tubular basement membranes, Bowman's capsules, and necrotic tubular epithelium, especially in the medulla and inner cortex.

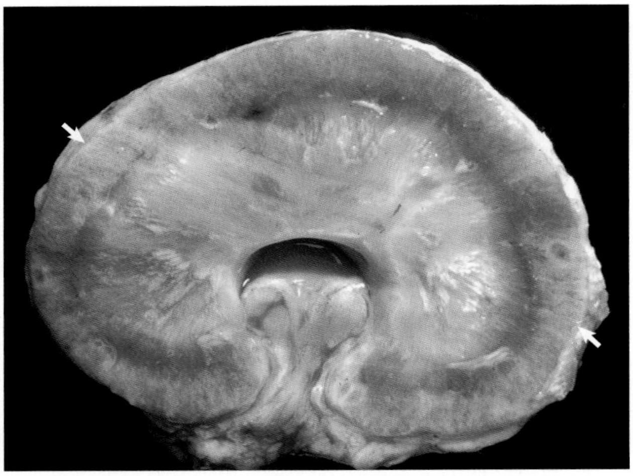

Fig. 11-31 Nephrocalcinosis, kidney, dorsal section, dog. Note the white streaks *(arrows)* in the cortex and medulla attributable to mineralization of the interstitium, basement membranes, and tubules. This lesion results from diseases that increase plasma calcium concentrations (e.g., hyperparathyroidism). Renal tubular epithelium is damaged by an increase in intracellular calcium, which is initially precipitated in mitochondria and tubular basement membranes. (Courtesy Dr. M.D. McGavin, College of Veterinary Medicine, University of Tennessee.)

DISEASES OF THE KIDNEY

Developmental Abnormalities

Renal Aplasia, Hypoplasia, and Dysplasia

Renal aplasia (agenesis) is the failure of development of one or both kidneys so that there is no recognizable renal tissue present. In these cases, the ureter may be present or absent. If present, the cranial extremity of the ureter begins as a blind pouch. A familial tendency for renal aplasia has been observed in Doberman pinscher and beagle dogs. Because life can be sustained when more than one-fourth of renal function is maintained, unilateral aplasia is compatible with life, provided that the other kidney is normal. Unilateral aplasia can go unnoticed during life and be recognized at necropsy. Bilateral aplasia is obviously incompatible with life and occurs sporadically.

Renal hypoplasia designates incomplete development of the kidneys in a variety of species so that fewer than normal nephrons are present at birth. Renal hypoplasia has been documented as an inherited disease of purebred or crossbred Large White pigs in New Zealand and described in foals of various breeds, as well as in dogs (Fig. 11-32, *A*) and cats (Fig. 11-32, *B*). Hypoplasia can be unilateral (Fig. 11-32, *B*) or bilateral; it is rare and difficult to diagnose subtle cases at necropsy or microscopically. In cattle and pigs, the number of renal papillae in the hypoplastic kidney can be compared with those in a normal kidney. Hypoplastic kidneys from pigs and foals have a notable reduction in the number of glomeruli. In foals, for example, 5 to 12 glomeruli are present per low-power field in affected kidneys compared with 30 to 35 glomeruli per low-power field in normal adult kidneys. Unless significant renal mass is compromised by this condition, hypoplasia is clinically silent.

Occasionally, some bovine kidneys are found to have reduced numbers of external lobes, but these kidneys are not hypoplastic and are microscopically and functionally normal; the reduction in external lobes merely represents fusion of the lobes. The shrunken, pitted kidneys in young animals, particularly dogs, are often diagnosed as hypoplastic. However, in most of these cases, these small kidneys are due to the following:

- Renal fibrosis, resulting from renal disease developing at an early age
- Dysplasia
- Progressive juvenile nephropathy

Renal dysplasia is an abnormality of altered structural organization resulting from abnormal differentiation and the presence of structures not normally present in nephrogenesis. Cystic renal dysplasia has been described in sheep and is inherited as an autosomal dominant trait. Renal dysplasia occurs infrequently and like renal hypoplasia, must be differentiated from renal fibrosis and progressive juvenile nephropathy. Dysplastic changes can be unilateral or bilateral and can involve much of an affected kidney or occur only as focal lesions. Dysplastic kidneys can be small, misshapen, or both. Microscopically, five primary features of dysplasia are described as follows:

- Asynchronous differentiation of nephrons inappropriate for the age of the animal—aggregates of small hypercellular glomeruli in the cortex
- Persistence of primitive mesenchyme so that the interstitial connective tissue has a myxomatous appearance
- Persistence of metanephric ducts
- Atypical (adenomatoid) tubular epithelium
- The presence of cartilaginous and/or osseous tissue

Interstitial fibrosis, renal cysts, and a few enlarged hypercellular glomeruli (compensatory hypertrophy) are changes seen secondarily to the primary dysplastic changes. The number of nephrons, lobules, and calyces are normal. Bilateral renal dysplasia characterized by persistent mesenchyme and atypical tubular development has been described in foals.

Progressive juvenile nephropathy (familial renal disease) of Lhasa Apso, Shih Tzu, golden retriever dogs, and perhaps other canine breeds could be examples of renal dysplasia (Fig. 11-32, *C* to *E*). Asynchronous differentiation is often seen and to a lesser extent several other features of dysplasia. However, until these hereditary lesions of dogs are better characterized, it is probably best to retain the diagnostic term of progressive juvenile nephropathy (see the section on Disorders of Dogs).

Ectopic and Fused Kidneys

Ectopic kidneys are misplaced from their normal sublumbar location because of abnormal migration during fetal development. Ectopic kidneys occur most frequently in pigs and dogs and usually involve only one kidney. Ectopic locations often include the pelvic cavity or inguinal position. Although ectopic kidneys are usually structurally and functionally normal, malposition of the ureters predisposes them to obstruction, which results in secondary hydronephrosis. Fused (horseshoe) kidneys result from the fusion of the left and right cranial or left and right caudal poles of the kidneys during nephrogenesis. This fusion results in the appearance of one large kidney with two ureters. The histologic structure and function of the fused kidneys are usually normal.

Renal Cysts

Renal cysts are spherical, thin-walled, variably sized distentions principally of the cortical or medullary renal tubules and are filled with clear, watery fluid. Congenital renal cysts can occur as a primary entity or in cases of renal dysplasia. The pathogenesis of primary renal cysts is not entirely understood. Cysts are likely derived from normal or noncystic segments of the nephron, most commonly the renal tubules, the collecting ducts, and Bowman's (uriniferous) space. Although genetic mechanisms can be involved in the pathogenesis of renal cysts, experiments with toxic chemicals indicate that genetic predisposition is not a requirement. The

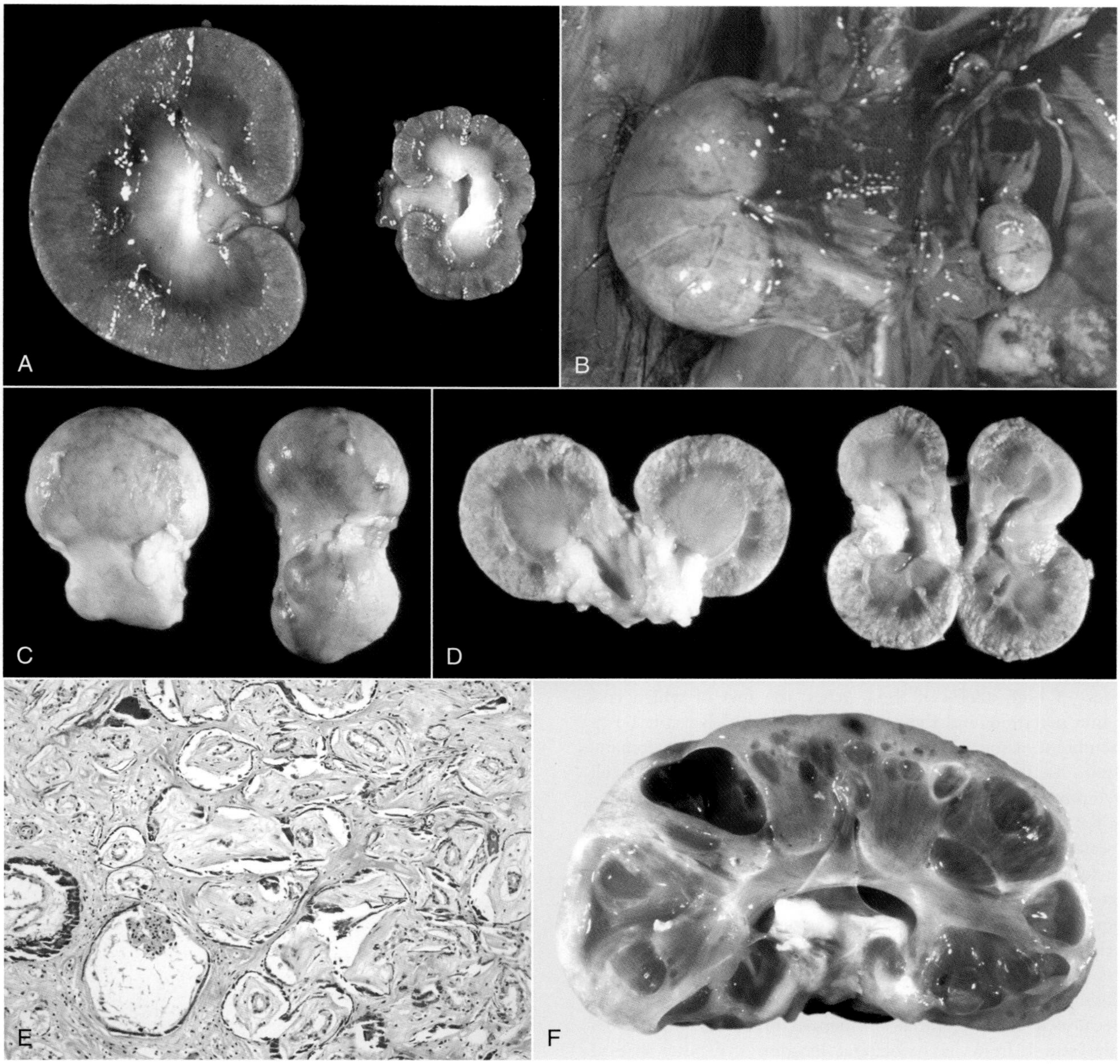

Fig. 11-32 Types of congenital developmental anomalies, kidney.
A and **B,** Unilateral hypoplastic kidneys, young dogs. **A,** Dorsal sections. **B,** The grossly affected right kidney is nearly identical in structure to the left kidney but smaller (hypoplasia). **C,** Juvenile progressive nephropathy, young dog. Bilateral abnormally shaped firm kidneys. **D,** Juvenile progressive nephropathy, dorsal sections, dog. Section of the kidneys from **C. E,** Juvenile progressive nephropathy, chronic, dog. Note the interstitial fibrosis, tubular atrophy, dilated urinary space, and mineralization. H&E stain. **F,** Polycystic disease, dorsal section, cat. Numerous variably sized tubular cysts are present in the cortex and medulla. The cysts contain clear colorless fluid. This condition is hereditary, and Persian cats are predisposed. (**A** courtesy Dr. B. Weeks, College of Veterinary Medicine, Texas A&M University; and Noah's Arkive, College of Veterinary Medicine, The University of Georgia. **B** courtesy Dr. M. Miller, College of Veterinary Medicine, University of Missouri; and Noah's Arkive, College of Veterinary Medicine, The University of Georgia. **C** and **D** courtesy College of Veterinary Medicine, University of Illinois. **E** courtesy Dr. S.J. Newman, College of Veterinary Medicine, University of Tennessee. **F** courtesy Dr. A. Confer, College of Veterinary Medicine, Oklahoma State University.)

following four mechanisms of renal cystic dilation are considered plausible:

- Obstruction of nephrons can cause increased luminal pressure and secondary dilation (called *cystic dilation* when it is well-developed).
- Modifications in ECM and cell-matrix interactions result in weakened tubular basement membranes allowing saccular dilation of tubules.
- Focal tubular epithelial hyperplasia with production of new basement membranes, increased tubular secretion, and increased intratubular pressure causes development of enlarged, dilated tubules.
- Dedifferentiation of tubular epithelial cells results in loss of polarity of cells with abnormal cell arrangements in tubules, reduced tubular fluid absorption, increased intratubular pressure, and dilation of tubules.

These mechanisms are not mutually exclusive, and several mechanisms often work in concert to create renal cysts.

Cysts range in size from barely visible to several centimeters in diameter. Cysts are usually spherical, delineated by a thin fibrous connective tissue wall lined by flattened epithelium, and are filled with clear, watery fluid. The sources of fluid are glomerular filtrate, transepithelial secretions, or both. When viewed from the renal surface, the cyst wall is pale gray, smooth, and translucent. Cysts can arise anywhere along the nephron and be located in either cortex or medulla. Kidneys can have single or multiple cysts. Some cysts cause no alteration in renal function and therefore are considered incidental findings. Such incidental renal cysts are common in pigs and calves and must be differentiated from hydronephrosis. Acquired renal cysts can occur as a result of renal interstitial fibrosis or other renal diseases that cause intratubular obstruction. These cysts are usually small (1 to 2 mm in diameter) and occur primarily in the cortex.

Polycystic Kidneys

Polycystic kidneys have many cysts that involve numerous nephrons. Congenital polycystic kidneys occur sporadically in many species but can be inherited as an autosomal dominant lesion in pigs and lambs and inherited along with cystic biliary disease in Cairn and West Highland white terriers. The lesion, termed *polycystic kidney disease* (PKD), is inherited as an autosomal dominant trait in families of Persian cats and bull terriers. Although less well characterized in animals than in humans, this autosomal dominant, high penetrance, heritable condition is thought to be related to mutations in one or more genes (PKD-1 and/or PKD-2) and altered function of the related proteins, principally polycystin-1 and polycystin-2. Manifestation of tubular cysts occurs after mutation of both alleles of these genes, the first of which is a germ-line mutation, and the second is somatic. Polycystin-1 is a cell membrane–associated protein with a large extracellular domain. Polycystin-1, the product of PKD-1, is involved in normal cell proliferation and apoptosis pathways. Although the exact mechanisms for cyst formation are not known, polycystin-1 mutations allow cells either to enter a differentiation pathway that results in tubule formation or to become susceptible to apoptosis. PKD-1 regulates tubular morphology throughout life, but the pathologic consequences are defined by developmental status of the organ with those incurred before the end of terminal renal maturation process, resulting in more severe lesions. Additionally, polycystin-1 is known to be important in both cell adhesion and cell signaling because it is an essential component of desmosomes. Loss of polycystin-1 from its basolateral location may alter critical pathways controlling normal tubulogenesis, thus contributing to cyst formation. Similarly, polycystin-2 functions principally as a localized plasma membrane calcium channel. Additionally, reduced levels of renal cyclic adenosine monophosphate (cAMP) are known to inhibit growth of renal cysts in animal models of PKD so there is an energy-dependent process involved in cyst formation. Further study of these mutated proteins will allow us to narrow the mechanistic pathway of the inherited form and potentially extrapolate to the acquired and sporadic congenital cystic lesions documented. A polycystic renal disease with cysts arising from glomeruli has been described in collie puppies. The gross appearance of the cut surface of a polycystic kidney has been described as "Swiss cheese" (Fig. 11-32, *F).* As cysts enlarge, they compress the adjacent parenchyma. When extensive regions of renal parenchyma are polycystic, renal function can be impaired.

Diseases of the Glomerulus

Immune-Mediated Glomerulonephritis

GN most often results from immune-mediated mechanisms, most notably after the deposition of soluble immune complexes within the glomeruli and less commonly after the formation of antibodies directed against antigens within the GBM. Antibodies to the basement membrane (anti-GBM disease) bind and damage the glomerulus through fixation of complement and resulting leukocyte infiltration. This mechanism of GN has been well documented in humans and nonhuman primates but only rarely in other domestic animals. To confirm the diagnosis of anti-GBM disease, Ig and complement (C3) must be demonstrated within glomeruli. Antibodies must be eluted from the kidneys and found to bind to normal GBMs of the appropriate species.

Immune-complex GN occurs in association with persistent infections or other diseases that characteristically have a prolonged antigenemia that enhances the formation of soluble immune complexes. In domestic animals, immune-complex GN occurs most commonly in dogs and cats. Immune-complex GN is associated with specific viral infections, such as feline leukemia virus (FeLV) or feline infectious peritonitis (FIP) virus; chronic bacterial infections, such as pyometra or pyoderma; chronic parasitism, such as dirofilariasis; autoimmune diseases, such as canine systemic lupus erythematosus; and neoplasia (Box 11-8). In addition to the role

BOX 11-8 Diseases with Immune-Complex Glomerulonephritis

HORSES
Equine infectious anemia
Streptococcus sp.

CATTLE
Bovine viral diarrhea
Trypanosomiasis

SHEEP
Hereditary hypocomplementemia in Finnish Landrace lambs

PIGS
Hog cholera
African swine fever

DOGS
Infectious canine hepatitis
Chronic hepatitis
Chronic bacterial diseases
Endometritis (pyometra)
Pyoderma
Prostatitis
Dirofilariasis
Borreliosis (Lyme disease)
Systemic lupus erythematosus
Polyarteritis
Autoimmune hemolytic anemia
Immune-mediated polyarthritis
Neoplasia—mastocytoma
Hereditary C3 deficiency

CATS
Feline leukemia virus (FeLV) infection
Feline infectious peritonitis (FIP)
Feline immunodeficiency virus (FIV)
Progressive polyarteritis
Neoplasia
Progressive membranous glomerulonephritis (GN)

of persistent infections, a familial tendency for development of immune-complex GN has been described in a group of related Bernese mountain dogs.

Immune-complex GN is initiated by the formation of soluble immune complexes (antigen-antibody complexes) in the presence of antigen-antibody equivalency or slight antigen excess, which then do the following:

- Selectively deposit in the glomerular capillaries.
- Stimulate complement fixation with formation of C3a, C5a, and C567, which are chemotactic for neutrophils.
- Damage the basement membrane through neutrophil release of proteinases, arachidonic acid metabolites (such as thromboxane), and oxidants, particularly oxygen-derived free radicals and hydrogen peroxide.
- Continue to damage the glomeruli by the release of biologically active molecules from monocyte infiltrations in the later stages of inflammation (Fig. 11-33, *A*).

Although circulating immune complexes may contribute to this process, antibody binding to endogenous glomerular antigens or entrapped nonspecific antigens is more common. Direct action of C5b to C9 on the glomerular components results in activation of both glomerular epithelial cells and mesangial cells to produce damaging mediators, such as oxidants and proteases.

Many specific factors determine the extent of deposition of soluble immune complexes in the glomerular capillary walls. These include persistence of appropriate quantities of immune complexes in the circulation, glomerular permeability, the size and molecular charge of the soluble complexes, and the strength of the bond between the antigen and antibody (avidity). Small or intermediate complexes are the most damaging because large complexes are removed from circulation through phagocytosis by cells of the monocyte-macrophage system in the liver and spleen. An increase in local glomerular vascular permeability is necessary for immune complexes to leave the microcirculation and deposit in the glomerulus. This process is usually facilitated via vasoactive amine release from mast cells, basophils, or platelets (see Fig. 11-33, *A*). Mast cells or basophils release vasoactive amines as a result of the interaction of the immune complexes with antigen-specific IgE on the surface of these cells, by stimulation of the mast cells or basophils by cationic proteins released from neutrophils, or by the anaphylatoxin activity of C3a and C5a. Platelet-activating factor (PAF) is released from immune complex–stimulated mast cells, basophils, or macrophages and causes platelets to release vasoactive amines.

Localization of the complexes within the various levels of the basement membrane or in subepithelial locations depends on their molecular charge and avidity. Once small, soluble immune

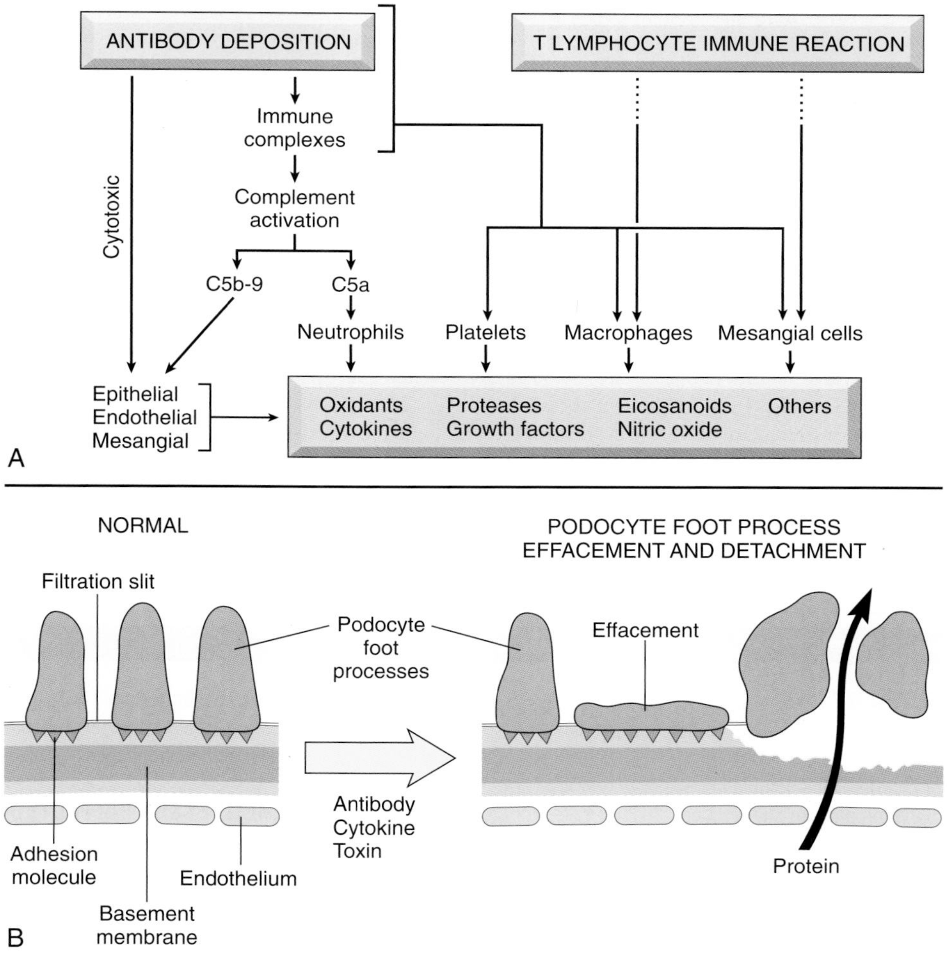

Fig. 11-33 Schematic diagram of the mediators of immune glomerular injury and epithelial cell injury.
A, Mediators of immune glomerular injury. **B,** Epithelial cell injury. The postulated sequence is a consequence of antibodies to epithelial cell antigens, with subsequent toxins, cytokines, or other factors causing injury and detachment of epithelial cells, resulting in protein leakage through the defective glomerular basement membrane and filtration slits. (From Kumar V, Abbas AK, Fausto N, et al: *Robbins & Cotran pathologic basis of disease,* ed 8, Philadelphia, 2009, Saunders.)

complexes are deposited within the capillary wall, they can become greatly enlarged as a result of interactions of immune complexes with free antibodies, free antigens, complement components, or other immune complexes.

After immune-complex deposition, glomerular injury can also occur from the aggregation of platelets and activation of Hageman factor, which results in the formation of fibrin thrombi that produce glomerular ischemia. Furthermore, glomerular epithelial cell and ECM damage can result directly from the terminal membrane attack complex of the activated complement cascade (C5 to C9). This can result in epithelial detachment (causing proteinuria) and GBM thickening subsequent to upregulation of epithelial cell receptors for transforming growth factor (Fig. 11-33, *B*). Cell-mediated cytotoxic responses (from sensitized T lymphocytes) to glomerular antigens or complexes may exacerbate renal lesions. Complexes themselves may modulate the immune response through interaction with receptors on various cells.

Finally, if exposure of the glomerulus to immune complexes is short lived, as in a transient infection, such as infectious canine hepatitis, glomerular immune complexes will be phagocytosed by macrophages or mesangial cells and removed, and the glomerular lesions and clinical signs may resolve. Conversely, continual exposure of glomeruli to soluble immune complexes, such as in persistent viral infections (e.g., FeLV infection) and chronic heartworm disease, can produce progressive glomerular injury, with severe lesions and clinical manifestation of glomerular disease (Box 11-9).

Ultrastructurally, immune complexes either in the GBM or in a subepithelial location appear as electron-dense bodies. Complexes that are poorly soluble, fairly large, or of high avidity often enter the mesangium, where they can be phagocytosed by macrophages and appear ultrastructurally as dense granular deposits within the mesangial stroma or within macrophages. Other ultrastructural changes commonly seen are loss or effacement of visceral epithelial cell foot processes, cytoplasmic vacuolation, retraction and detachment of visceral epithelium, and infiltrates of neutrophils and monocytes within the mesangium.

A diagnosis of immune-mediated GN can be made by immunofluorescent or immunohistochemical demonstration of immunoglobulin and complement components, usually C3, in glomerular tufts. In dogs, IgG or IgM are the most common immunoglobulin isotypes demonstrated in GN; however, combinations of IgG, IgM, and IgA also occur in the glomeruli of some dogs. In one study, IgA was the only immunoglobulin found in three dogs with immune-complex GN. Both Ig and C3 are usually demonstrated in a granular ("lumpy-bumpy") pattern using immunofluorescent or immunohistochemical techniques (Fig. 11-34); however, in anti-GBM disease, as reported in humans and horses, the antibody deposits have a linear distribution conforming to the basement membranes. It is important to remember that fluorescing deposits indicate the presence of immunoglobulin or complement but do not specifically indicate the presence of disease. Additionally, immunofluorescence may be negative when all reactive binding sites are occupied, thus complicating diagnosis of this condition.

The diagnosis of preformed immune-complex GN can be confirmed only by demonstrating that the antibodies from the immune complexes, eluted from glomeruli, are not capable of binding to normal glomerular elements and hence represent deposition of preformed circulating complexes. Once this has been done, the ideal situation would be to identify the causative antigen present in the immune complexes. This process is accomplished by eluting antibodies from diseased glomeruli and attempting to identify their specificity for suspected antigens. For example, antibodies eluted from the glomeruli of dogs with GN associated with severe heartworm disease bind to several *Dirofilaria immitis* antigens, including the body wall of adult worms, parasitic uterine fluid, and microfilaria. In most cases of immune-complex GN, the specific causative antigen usually escapes determination. Demonstration of electron-dense deposits in mesangial, subepithelial, or subendothelial locations by electron microscopy is also supportive of the diagnosis of immune-mediated GN.

Gross lesions of acute immune-complex GN are usually subtle. The kidneys are often slightly swollen, have a smooth capsular surface, are of normal color or pale, and have glomeruli that are visible as pinpoint red dots on the cut surface of the cortex (Fig. 11-35). The normal glomeruli of horses are usually visible, so this feature of pinpoint red dots for glomeruli cannot be used for diagnosis in that species. If lesions do not resolve but become subacute to chronic, the renal cortex becomes somewhat shrunken and the capsular surface has a generalized fine granularity. On cut surface, the cortex can be thinned and its surface granular, and glomeruli can appear as pinpoint pale gray dots. With time, more severe scarring can develop throughout the cortex (see the section on Renal Fibrosis).

Microscopically, immune-complex GN has several histopathologic forms. Although various classifications of GN have been published, the following simple classification is well understood among veterinary pathologists. Lesions in glomeruli may be described as proliferative, membranous, or membranoproliferative (Fig. 11-36). Glomerular lesions can be distributed diffusely, when most of the

BOX 11-9 Progression of Glomerular Immune-Complex Deposition

DEPOSITION AFFECTED BY

Appropriate quantities of immune complexes in the circulation
Glomerular permeability
The size and molecular charge of the soluble complexes
Strength of the bond between antigen and antibody

GLOMERULAR PERMEABILITY AFFECTED BY

Release of vasoactive amines from mast cells, basophils, or platelets

- Immune complexes interact with antigen-specific immunoglobulin E on surface of mast cells or basophils
- Cationic proteins from neutrophils stimulate release of vasoactive amines from mast cells and basophils
- C3a and C5a cause release of vasoactive amines
- Platelets release vasoactive amines following release of platelet-activating factor from immune-complex stimulated mast cells, basophils, and macrophages

GLOMERULAR PROGRESSION AFFECTED BY

Aggregation of platelets, activation of Hageman factor, fibrin thrombi formation, and glomerular ischemia
Terminal membrane active complex of activated complement cascade damages glomerular epithelial cells and extracellular matrix (ECM) resulting in epithelial cell detachment and basement membrane thickening
Cell-mediated cytotoxic responses from T lymphocytes sensitized to glomerular antigens or complexes may exacerbate renal lesions

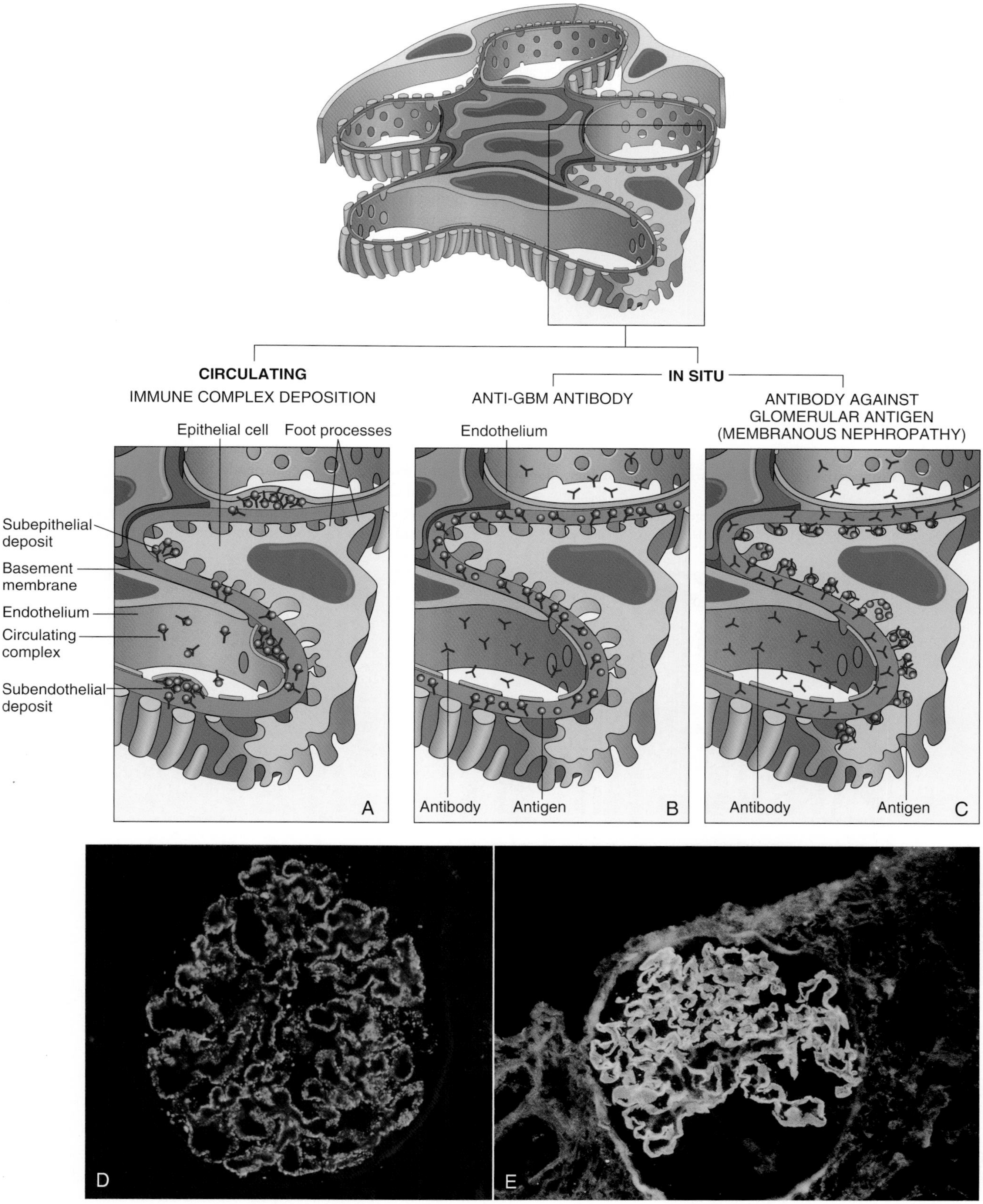

Fig. 11-34 Schematic diagrams of the antibody-mediated glomerular injury.
Antibody-mediated glomerular injury can result either from the deposition of circulating immune complexes **(A)** or from formation of complexes in situ (**B** and **C**). Antiglomerular basement membrane (anti-GBM) disease **(B)** or antitubular deposits **(C)** are characterized by linear immunofluorescence patterns, whereas lesions caused by immune complexes reveal granular patterns. **D** and **E**, Two patterns of deposition of immune complexes as seen by immunofluorescence microscopy: granular, characteristic of circulating and in situ immune complex nephritis **(D)**; and linear, characteristic of classic anti-GBM disease **(E).** (From Kumar V, Abbas AK, Fausto N, et al: *Robbins & Cotran pathologic basis of disease,* ed 8, Philadelphia, 2009, Saunders.)

glomeruli are involved; focally, when only a certain proportion of glomeruli are involved; globally, when an entire glomerular tuft is involved; and segmentally, when only a portion of the glomerular tuft is affected. Most of the lesions in immune-complex GN are diffuse, but within an individual affected glomerulus, the lesions can be either global or segmental.

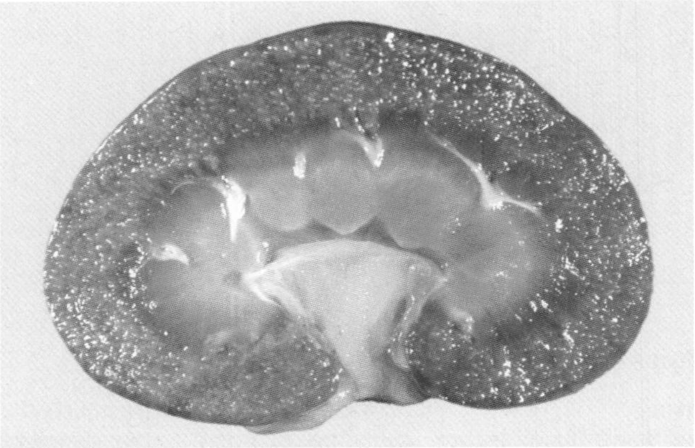

Fig. 11-35 Proliferative glomerulonephritis (GN), kidney, dorsal section, dog.

The small, white, round foci in the cortex are enlarged glomeruli. (Courtesy Dr. S.J. Newman, College of Veterinary Medicine, University of Tennessee.)

In the more chronic form, a variety of glomerular tuft changes will be noted, depending on whether the damage is related to mesangial proliferation, membranous proliferation, or both. There is typically enlargement of the tuft by the presence of abundant mesangial matrix, a reduction in cellularity, enhancement of the capillary outlines within the tuft, proliferation of the parietal epithelial cells, expansion of Bowman's space by high protein ultrafiltrate, and variable thickening of Bowman's capsule. Glomerulosclerosis is the stage where there is a reduction in the number of functional glomeruli with replacement by large amounts of fibrous connective tissue and subsequent obliteration of Bowman's space due to capsular fibrosis.

Additionally, in protein-losing diseases, the proximal tubular cells often have microscopic eosinophilic intracytoplasmic bodies referred to as *hyaline droplets,* which represent accumulations of intracytoplasmic protein absorbed from the filtrate.

Microscopic details of each type of glomerular disease are outlined in the next sections.

Proliferative Glomerulonephritis

Proliferative GN is a form of immune-complex glomerular disease characterized by increased cellularity of the glomerular tufts caused by proliferation of glomerular endothelial, epithelial, and mesangial cells and an influx of neutrophils and other leukocytes and involves both the capillary loops and the mesangium (see Fig. 11-36, *A*). This form is the most common variant in horses but only rarely

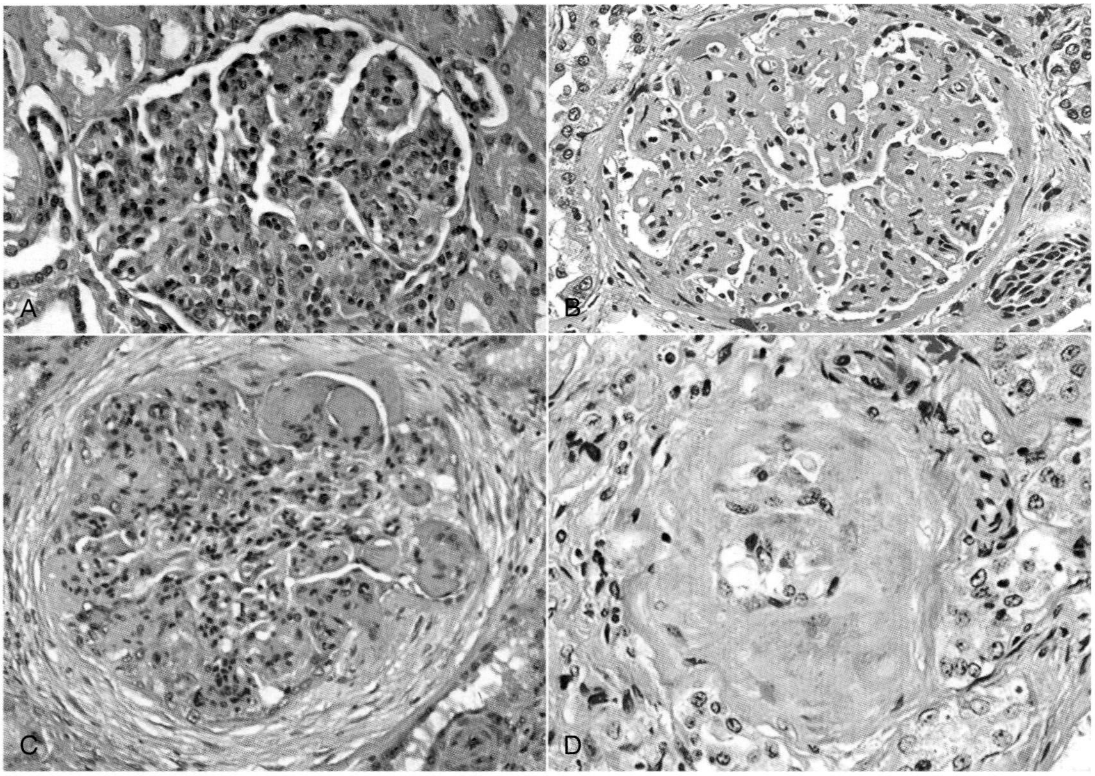

Fig. 11-36 Types of glomerulonephritis (GN).

A, Proliferative GN, pig. The lesion is characterized principally by hypercellularity of the glomerulus due to increased numbers of mesangial cells. H&E stain. **B,** Membranous GN, dog. The lesion is characterized by generalized hyaline thickening of glomerular capillary basement membranes. It can occur in dogs with dirofilariasis. H&E stain. **C,** Membranoproliferative GN, horse. Membranoproliferative GN has histologic features of both proliferative GN and membranous GN. Abundant periglomerular fibrosis surrounds this hypercellular glomerulus (mesangial cells). Mesangial matrix is prominent in the top-right area of the glomerulus. H&E stain. **D,** Glomerulosclerosis, dog. Note the hypocellularity, shrinkage, and hyalinization due to an increase in fibrous connective tissue and mesangial matrix and almost complete loss of glomerular capillaries. In glomerulosclerosis (the end-stage of chronic GN), glomeruli are essentially nonfunctional. H&E stain. (**A** and **C** courtesy Dr. W. Crowell, College of Veterinary Medicine, The University of Georgia; and Noah's Arkive, College of Veterinary Medicine, The University of Georgia. **B** and **D** courtesy Dr. S.J. Newman, College of Veterinary Medicine, University of Tennessee.)

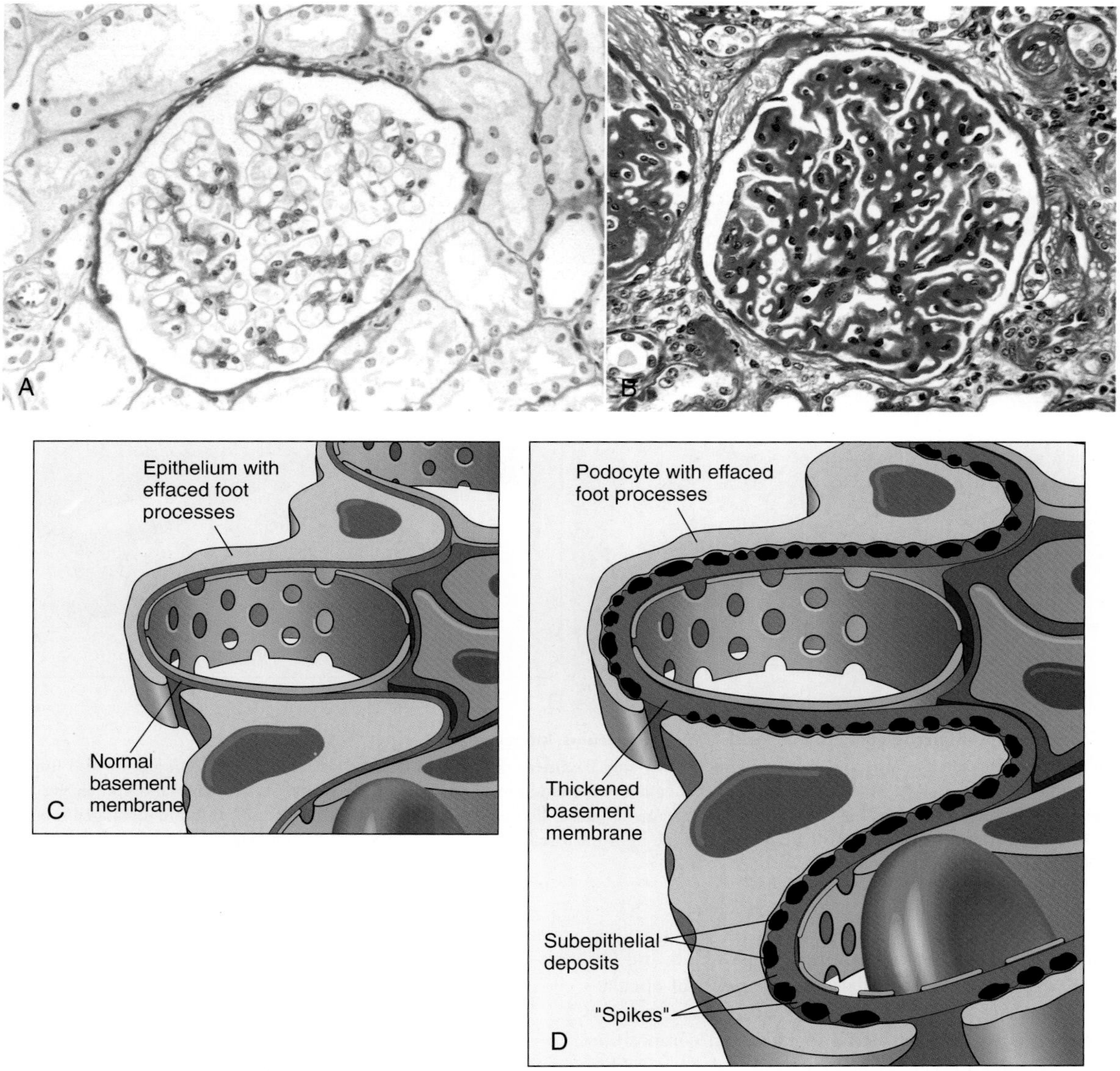

Fig. 11-37 Lupoid nephrosis (A and C) and membranous glomerulonephritis (GN) (B and D).
A, Lupoid nephrosis. The glomerulus appears normal, with a thin basement membrane. PAS reaction. **B,** Membranous GN. The glomerular basement membrane is diffusely thickened. PAS reaction. **C,** Schematic diagram of lupoid nephrosis. Diffuse loss of foot processes of visceral epithelial cells. **D,** Schematic diagram of membranous GN. Membranous GN is characterized by subepithelial deposits, which by transmission electron microscopy are electron dense, and by loss of foot processes. (From Cotran RS, Rennke H, Kumar V: *The kidney and its collecting system,* ed 7, Philadelphia, 2002, Saunders.)

does it result in chronic renal failure. Equine infectious anemia and streptococcal antigen are the only antigens in horses proved to be associated with proliferative GN.

Membranous Glomerulonephritis

Membranous GN is characterized by diffuse glomerular capillary basement membrane thickening because of the presence of subepithelial immunoglobulin deposits, as the predominant change (Fig. 11-37; also see Fig. 11-36, *B*). These deposits are separated by protrusions of GBM matrix that eventually encompass these deposits. After removal of the deposited material, cavities are left in the GBM and later these fill with GBM-like material, which results in sclerotic change within the glomerular tuft. This is characterized by increased deposition of positive material (periodic acid–Schiff [PAS]) and a lesser amount of fibrosis. This variation is the most common form of immune-complex GN in cats.

Membranoproliferative Glomerulonephritis

Membranoproliferative GN (mesangioproliferative, mesangiocapillary) is characterized by hypercellularity following proliferation of glomerular cells and thickening of the capillary basement membrane and mesangium (Fig. 11-38; also see Fig. 11-36, *C*). This variant appears to be the most common morphologic form of immune-complex GN in the dog. Light microscopy fails to detect differences evident by immunofluorescent and electron microscopy. The latter allows subcategorization of membranoproliferative GN into type I and type II (see Fig. 11-38). Type I is characterized by the presence of subendothelial deposits and a granular pattern

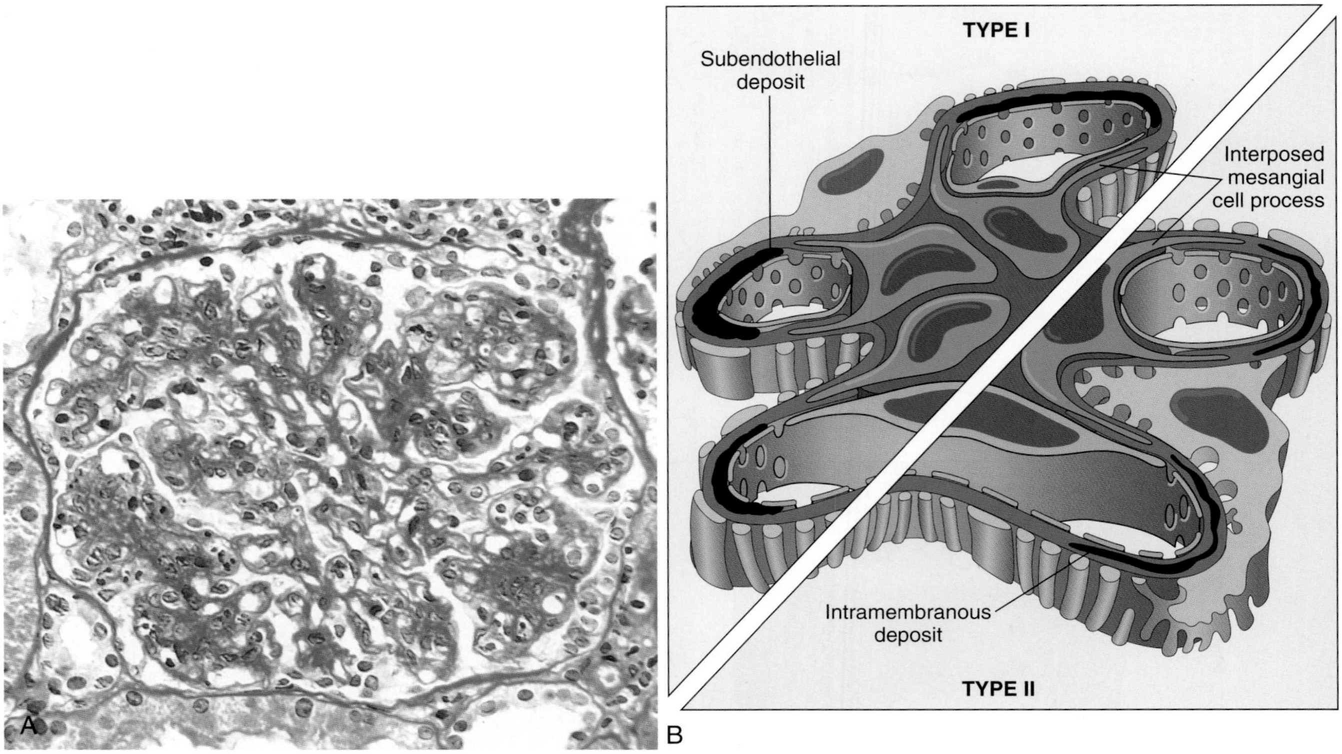

Fig. 11-38 Membranoproliferative glomerulonephritis (GN), glomerulus, kidney.
A, Note the increased mesangial matrix and thickened and focally split basement membranes (stained dark red). The glomeruli are also infiltrated by leukocytes (not visible here). Periodic acid Schiff reaction. **B,** Schematic representation of patterns in the two types of membranoproliferative GN. In type I there are subendothelial deposits; type II is characterized by intramembranous dense deposits (dense deposit disease). In both, mesangial interposition gives the appearance of split basement membranes when viewed in the light microscope. (From Cotran RS, Rennke H, Kumar V: *The kidney and its collecting system,* ed 7, Philadelphia, 2002, Saunders.)

after deposition of C3 and lesser quantities of IgG, C1q, and C4. Type I disease appears to be secondary to deposition of circulating immune complexes. Type II is also referred to as *dense deposit disease* because electron-dense material of unknown composition and smaller quantities of C3 form an irregular deposit within the subendothelial space and the lamina densa. Type II disease appears to be a form of autoimmune disease, but its pathogenesis is not clear.

Several other changes in the glomerulus and Bowman's capsule usually accompany the lesions discussed previously. These changes include adhesions between the epithelial cells of the glomerular tuft and Bowman's capsule (synechiae; singular = synechia), hypertrophy and hyperplasia of the parietal epithelium lining Bowman's capsule, deposition of fibrinogen and fibrinous thrombi in glomerular capillaries, secondary to or as a result of the glomerular damage, and dilated renal tubules filled with homogeneous proteinaceous fluid. An increase in mesangial matrix is often also present. If the damage is mild and the cause is removed, glomeruli can heal without obvious or with minimal residual lesions. However, if the lesion is severe and prolonged, subacute to chronic glomerular changes develop. Bowman's capsule can become thickened, hyalinized, and reduplicated. In severe cases, proliferation of parietal epithelium, an influx of monocytes, and deposition of fibrin can occur within Bowman's capsule, resulting in the formation of a semicircular, hypercellular, intraglomerular lesion known as a *glomerular crescent.* The glomerular crescent can also undergo fibrosis, and if Bowman's capsule ruptures, glomerular fibrosis can become continuous with interstitial fibrosis. Interstitial and periglomerular fibrosis, foci of interstitial lymphocytes, and plasma cells and glomerulosclerosis may be present in chronic GN.

Glomerulosclerosis

In chronic GN, severely affected glomeruli shrink and become hyalinized because of an increase in both fibrous connective tissue and mesangial matrix and a loss of glomerular capillaries (Fig. 11-36, *D*) and additionally there is periglomerular fibrosis. These glomeruli are hypocellular and essentially nonfunctional. This process is referred to as *glomerulosclerosis.* There is a specific nomenclature for describing the numbers of glomeruli involved and the location of the lesion in the glomerulus. Glomerulosclerosis can be diffuse, involving all glomeruli, or multifocal. In addition, glomerulosclerosis can involve a whole glomerular tuft (global) or only portions of the tuft (segmental), thus appearing as a nodular or segmental hyalinized thickening in affected glomeruli. Because tubules receive their blood supply from the vasa recta, derived from the glomerular efferent arteriole, glomerulosclerosis reduces the blood flow through the vasa recta, thus decreasing oxygen tension in the tubules. The resulting hypoxia is responsible for tubular epithelial cell death via apoptosis and results because of failure to regenerate to columnar cells. The tubules are lined instead by cuboidal or squamous cells, which lack a brush border and the functions of the normal columnar cells. In addition, chronic proteinuria often accompanies glomerulosclerosis and has been reported to promote tubular epithelial cell loss through apoptosis.

Numerous factors are associated with and accelerate glomerulosclerosis. These factors include the following:

- Unrestricted protein in the diet
- Increased glomerular capillary pressure in the remaining functional glomeruli
- Cytokines from local GN-induced inflammation
- Platelet-derived growth factors (PDGFs)

These factors have the following effects:

- Alter cellular components of the functional glomerular tufts
- Cause hypertension and transglomerular hyperfiltration with resultant damage to endothelium
- Activate mesangial cells to proliferate
- Increase mesangial matrix production
- Accelerate visceral epithelial cell loss, which allows synechiae (i.e., adhesions between visceral and parietal epithelial cell layers in the glomerulus) to form

Glomerulosclerosis is not only the end-stage of GN but also can develop in any chronic disease in which severe damage to nephrons or loss of nephron function occurs. Mild multifocal glomerulosclerosis of unknown cause is often an incidental finding in aged animals. Glomerulosclerosis has been reported occasionally in animals with hypertension and diabetes mellitus. In these cases, global or nodular eosinophilic glycoprotein material (hyaline material) is deposited in the glomerular mesangium.

Glomerular Amyloidosis

Amyloid, an insoluble fibrillar protein with a β-pleated sheet conformation, is produced after incomplete proteolysis of several soluble amyloidogenic proteins. Amyloid deposits in patients with plasma cell myelomas or other B lymphocyte dyscrasias (called *AL amyloidosis*) are composed of fragments of the light (λ) chains of immunoglobulins. In domestic animals, spontaneously occurring amyloidosis is usually an example of what is called *reactive amyloidosis* (AA amyloidosis). This form of the disease is often associated with chronic inflammatory diseases; the amyloid deposits are composed of fragments of a serum acute-phase reactant protein called *serum amyloid–associated* (SAA) *protein.* Amyloid fibrils from either source are deposited in tissue along with a glycoprotein called *amyloid P component.*

Glomeruli are the most common renal sites for deposition of amyloid in most domestic animal species, although the medullary interstitium is a common site in cats, particularly in Abyssinian breeds. Renal amyloidosis commonly occurs in association with other diseases, particularly chronic inflammatory or neoplastic diseases. However, idiopathic renal amyloidosis (i.e., amyloidosis in which an associated disease process is not recognized) is also described in dogs and cats. The underlying pathogenic mechanisms of idiopathic renal amyloidosis are not known. In a recent study, 23% of dogs that presented with proteinuria had renal amyloidosis. A hereditary predisposition for the development of reactive amyloidosis (AA) has been found in Abyssinian cats and Chinese Shar-Pei dogs. A familial tendency is suspected in Siamese cats, English foxhounds, and beagle dogs. In cattle, renal amyloidosis is nearly always due to chronic systemic infectious disease. Glomerular amyloidosis is responsible for many cases of protein-losing nephropathy in animals that have notable proteinuria and uremia. It can, like immune-complex GN, result in the nephrotic syndrome. Long-standing glomerular amyloidosis results in diminished renal blood flow through the glomeruli and the vasa recta. Such reduced renal vascular perfusion can lead to renal tubular atrophy, degeneration, and diffuse fibrosis and in severe cases, renal papillary necrosis. Medullary amyloidosis is usually asymptomatic unless it results in papillary necrosis.

Kidneys affected with glomerular amyloidosis are often enlarged, pale, and increased in consistency, and have a smooth to finely granular capsular surface (Fig. 11-39). Amyloid-laden glomeruli may be visible grossly as fine translucent dots on the capsular surface. Similarly, the cut surface of the cortex can have a finely granular appearance with scattered glistening foci, less than 0.5 mm diameter in the cortex (see Fig. 11-39). Treatment of kidneys with an iodine solution, such as Lugol's iodine, in many cases results in red-brown staining of glomeruli, which become purple when treated with dilute sulfuric acid (Fig. 11-40).

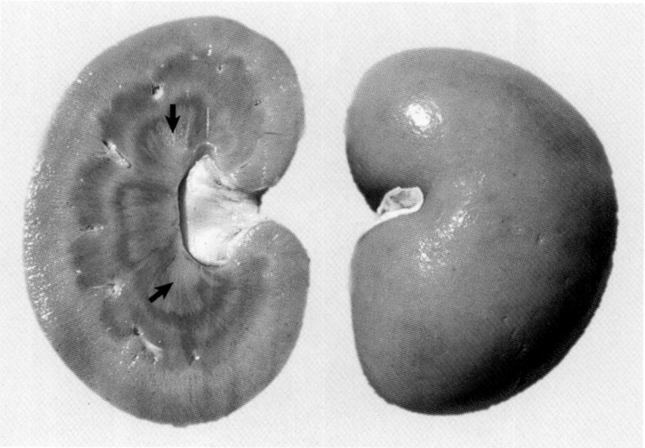

Fig. 11-39 Amyloidosis, kidney, dog.
Grossly, kidneys affected by amyloid deposition are diffusely tan, waxy (firm), and of normal size or slightly enlarged. Affected glomeruli are not grossly visible in this specimen, unlike in advanced cases of glomerular amyloidosis or chronic GN. In advanced cases of amyloidosis, glomeruli may be visible as pinpoint, glistening, round, cortical foci. In cats and Shar-Pei dogs, amyloid is deposited in the medullary interstitium, not in the glomeruli. There are also multiple foci of medullary crest necrosis (yellowish-green *[arrows]*). (Courtesy Dr. G.K. Saunders, The Virginia-Maryland Regional College of Veterinary Medicine; and Noah's Arkive, College of Veterinary Medicine, The University of Georgia.)

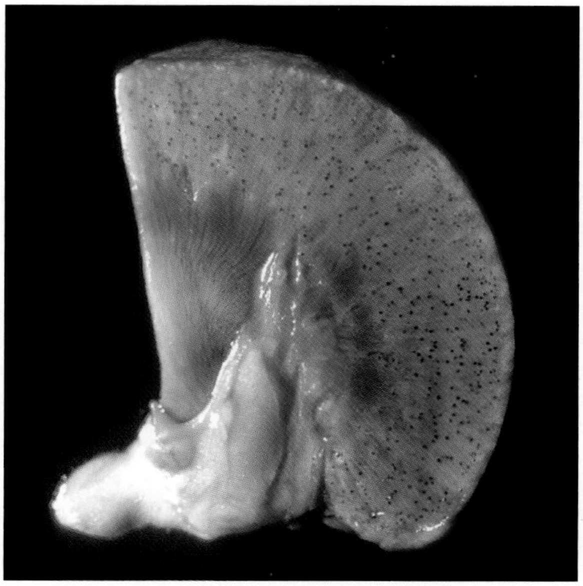

Fig. 11-40 Amyloidosis, kidney, transverse section, dog.
On the cut surface of fresh kidney treated with Lugol's iodine followed by dilute sulfuric acid, glomeruli containing amyloid are visible as multiple dark blue dots in the cortex. Lugol's iodine treatment. (Courtesy Dr. M.D. McGavin, College of Veterinary Medicine, University of Tennessee.)

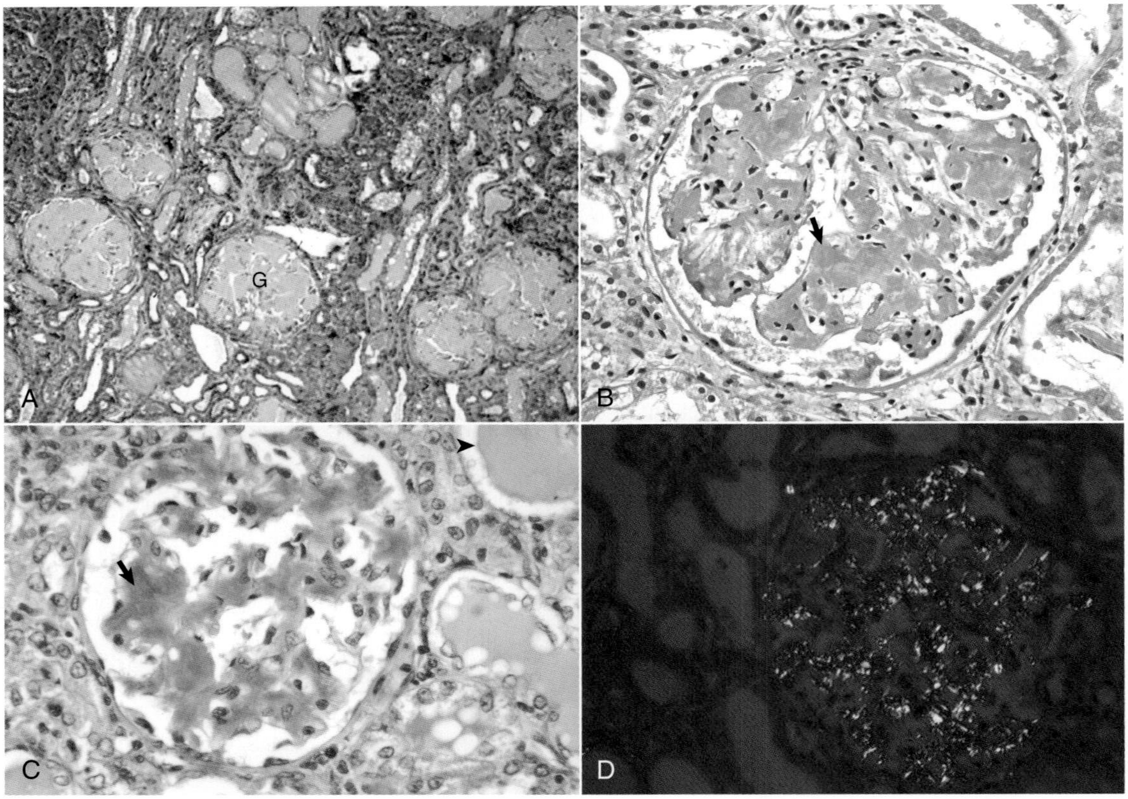

Fig. 11-41 Amyloidosis, glomerulus, kidney, dog.
A, All glomerular tufts *(G)* are diffusely and notably expanded by amyloid (pale eosinophilic homogeneous deposits), with the result that they are relatively acellular. H&E stain. **B,** Amyloid, the pale eosinophilic homogeneous hyalinized deposits, expands the mesangium of the glomerulus *(arrow)*. H&E stain. **C,** Amyloid stains orange with Congo red staining *(arrow)*, a technique used to confirm it. Note the proteinaceous casts in tubular lumina *(arrowhead)*, a consequence of glomerular damage allowing leakage of proteins into the filtrate (protein-losing nephropathy). Congo red stain. **D,** Congo red–stained amyloid deposits. These deposits have a light-green (often called apple green) birefringence when viewed under polarized light. Polarized light microscopy. (**A** courtesy Dr. B.C. Ward, College of Veterinary Medicine, Mississippi State University; and Noah's Arkive, College of Veterinary Medicine, The University of Georgia. **B** courtesy Dr. S.J. Newman, College of Veterinary Medicine, University of Tennessee. **C** courtesy Dr. M.D. McGavin, College of Veterinary Medicine, University of Tennessee. **D** courtesy Dr. W. Crowell, College of Veterinary Medicine, The University of Georgia; and Noah's Arkive, College of Veterinary Medicine, The University of Georgia.)

This technique provides a rapid presumptive diagnosis of renal amyloidosis. Medullary amyloidosis is usually not grossly recognizable.

Microscopically, glomerular amyloid is deposited in both the mesangium and subendothelial locations. Amyloid is relatively acellular and can accumulate segmentally within glomerular tufts; thus a portion of the normal glomerular architecture is replaced by eosinophilic, homogeneous to slightly fibrillar material (Fig. 11-41, *A*). When amyloidosis involves the entire glomerular tuft, the glomerulus is enlarged, capillary lumina become obliterated, and the tuft can appear as a large hypocellular eosinophilic hyaline sphere (Fig. 11-41, *B*). Amyloid can be present in renal tubular basement membranes, and these membranes appear hyalinized and thickened. Additionally, in cases of glomerular amyloid deposition, secondary changes may be present in renal tubules, which are usually markedly dilated, have variably atrophic epithelium and contain proteinaceous and cellular casts. Amyloid is confirmed microscopically by staining with Congo red stain (Fig. 11-41, *C*). When viewed with polarized light, amyloid has a green birefringence (Fig. 11-41, *D*). Loss of Congo red staining after treatment of a section of affected kidney with potassium permanganate suggests amyloid is AA (i.e., of acute-phase reactant protein origin).

Acute Suppurative Glomerulitis: Bacterial (Embolic) Nephritis

Embolic nephritis, which can also be referred to as *acute suppurative glomerulitis,* is the result of a bacteremia in which bacteria lodge in random glomerular capillaries and to a lesser extent in interstitial capillaries and cause the formation of multiple foci of inflammation (microabscesses) throughout the renal cortex. While the glomeruli appear targeted, this is really a manifestation of renal vascular disease. A specific example of embolic GN is *Actinobacillosis* of foals caused by *Actinobacillus equuli,* although many emboli may also affect vasculature within the interstitium (Fig. 11-42). These foals usually die within a few days of birth and have small abscesses in many visceral organs, especially the renal cortex. Embolic nephritis also occurs commonly in the bacteremia of pigs infected with *Erysipelothrix rhusiopathiae* or sheep and goats infected with *Corynebacterium pseudotuberculosis. Arcanobacterium pyogenes* was the most common isolate (26/31) from cases of embolic nephritis in necropsy cattle. *Staphylococcus aureus*, *Mannheimia haemolytica,* and *Streptococcus bovis* were also represented.

Grossly, multifocal random, raised, tan pinpoint foci are seen subcapsularly and on the cut surface throughout the renal cortex. Microscopically, glomerular capillaries contain numerous bacterial colonies intermixed with necrotic debris and extensive infiltrates

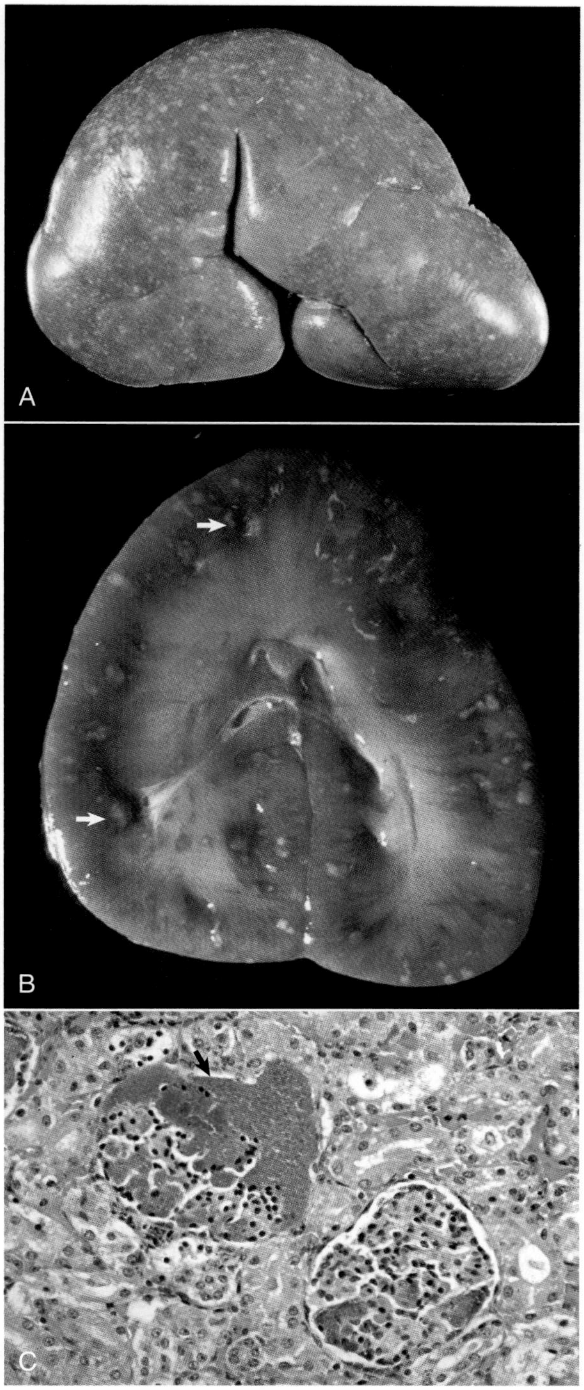

Fig. 11-42 Embolic nephritis (suppurative glomerulitis), kidney, horse. **A,** Multiple, small pale white necrotic foci and abscesses are present subcapsularly. **B,** Dorsal section. Variably sized abscesses are scattered throughout the cortex *(arrows).* **C,** Causative bacteria *(arrow)* enter the kidney via the vasculature (bacteremia) and lodge in the capillaries of glomeruli, where they replicate and induce necrosis and inflammation. H&E stain. (**A** courtesy Dr. A. Confer, College of Veterinary Medicine, Oklahoma State University. **B** courtesy Dr. M.D. McGavin, College of Veterinary Medicine, University of Tennessee. **C** courtesy Dr. W. Crowell, College of Veterinary Medicine, The University of Georgia; and Noah's Arkive, College of Veterinary Medicine, The University of Georgia.)

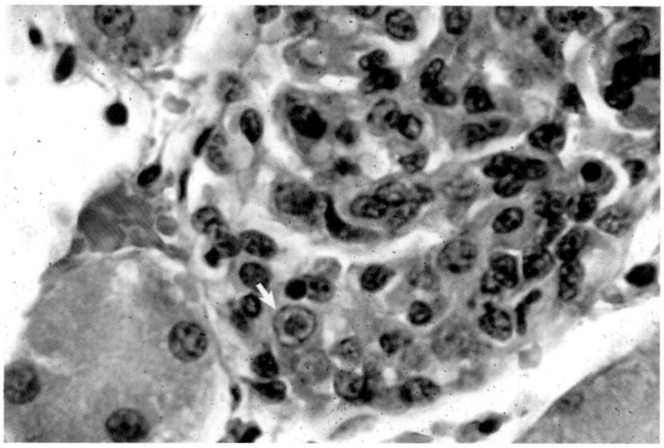

Fig. 11-43 Infectious canine hepatitis, kidney, cortex, dog. Renal glomerular endothelial cells contain intranuclear inclusion bodies *(arrow).* H&E stain. (Courtesy Dr. W. Crowell, College of Veterinary Medicine, The University of Georgia; and Noah's Arkive, College of Veterinary Medicine, The University of Georgia.)

of neutrophils that often obliterate the glomerulus. Glomerular or interstitial hemorrhage can occur as well. As with many other inflammatory diseases, if the affected animal survives, the neutrophilic infiltrates either persist as focal residual abscesses or are progressively replaced by increasing numbers of lymphocytes, plasma cells, and macrophages; reactive fibroblasts; and ultimately coalescing scars.

Viral Glomerulitis

Glomerulitis, caused by a direct viral insult to the glomerulus, occurs in acute systemic viral diseases, such as acute infectious canine hepatitis (Fig. 11-43), equine arteritis virus infection, hog cholera, avian Newcastle disease, and neonatal porcine cytomegalovirus infection. The lesions are mild, usually transient, and result from viral replication in capillary endothelium. Acute viral GN produces the following gross lesions:

- Kidneys are often slightly swollen.
- Renal capsular surface is smooth.
- Kidneys are normal color or pale.
- Glomeruli are visible as pinpoint red dots on the cut surface of the cortex.

Viral-induced intranuclear inclusions are present in glomerular capillary endothelium from viremias of infectious canine hepatitis and cytomegalovirus infections. The inclusions of each disease are similar and are usually large, basophilic to magenta, and either fill the nucleus or are separated from the nuclear membrane by a clear halo. In the other diseases (equine arteritis, hog cholera, maedi-visna, porcine circovirus, and avian Newcastle), viral antigens can be demonstrated in endothelium, epithelium, or mesangial cells by immunofluorescence, immunohistochemistry or polymerase chain reaction (PCR). In cases of viral glomerulitis, lesions include endothelial hypertrophy, hemorrhages, necrosis of endothelium, and a thickened and edematous mesangium. Clinically, animals are systemically ill from the viral infection, but the glomerular signs are specifically those of a transient proteinuria.

Chemical Glomerulonephritis

Although much less common than the immune-mediated forms of GN, chemically induced glomerular disease occurs in a variety of different ways. Chemicals typically induce glomerular injury by any of the following:

- Direct injury to glomerular epithelial cells
- Direct injury to endothelial cells of the glomerulus
- Altered renal blood flow
- Induction of immunologic reactions and inflammatory responses, which may occur with any of the following:
  - Incorporation of drugs into immune complexes
  - The formation and targeted deposition of antigen-antibody complexes
  - The formation of antinuclear antibodies
  - The formation of anti-GBM antibodies within the glomerular tuft

Puromycin aminonucleoside, adriamycin, and histamine-receptor antagonists all induce proteinuria through targeted damage to glomerular epithelial cells. The immunosuppressive drug, cyclosporine A, alters renal perfusion and ultimately the glomerular filtration rate by damaging glomerular endothelial cells. Examples of foreign substances capable of producing immune complexes include injectable hyperimmune serum, gold, and D-penicillamine. Procainamide and hydralazine result in production of antinuclear antibodies, and occupational exposure to hydrocarbon solvents can create anti-GBM antibodies. Often, drug-induced lesions lead to irreversible nephron loss and compensatory cellular and functional hypertrophy of other nephrons. The continuing physical loss of nephrons sets up a cycle for an increase in glomerular hypertension and hyperfiltration, which results in glomerulosclerosis, progressive nephron loss, and interstitial fibrosis.

Miscellaneous Glomerular Lesions

Glomerular Lipidosis

Glomerular lipidosis, characterized by small aggregates of lipid-laden foamy macrophages in glomerular tufts, is an occasional incidental finding in dogs. A similar but more extensive glomerular lipidosis has been described in cats with inherited hyperlipoproteinemia, which is a generalized disease characterized by hyperchylomicronemia, atherosclerosis, and xanthogranulomas in numerous parenchymatous organs, including the kidneys (see the section on Granulomatous Nephritis). Microscopically, glomeruli contain foamy macrophages, characteristic of glomerular lipidosis, as well as increased mesangium and thickened Bowman's capsule.

Glomerular Vasculopathy

An idiopathic renal glomerular vasculopathy and cutaneous vasculopathy occurs in greyhounds. The cause of this disease is unknown, but renal lesions are similar to those seen in DIC, thrombotic thrombocytopenic purpura, and hemolytic-uremic syndrome in humans. At necropsy, kidneys from affected dogs are swollen and congested and show cortical petechiae (Fig. 11-44, *A*). Microscopically, numerous glomeruli have segmental or global fibrinous thrombi, hemorrhage, and necrosis (Fig. 11-44, *B*). At the glomerular vascular pole, the walls of afferent arterioles have fibrin deposits and foci of necrosis. Affected greyhounds have multifocal erythematous and ulcerated skin lesions and distal limb edema. Variable systemic signs of uremia often accompany the cutaneous lesions.

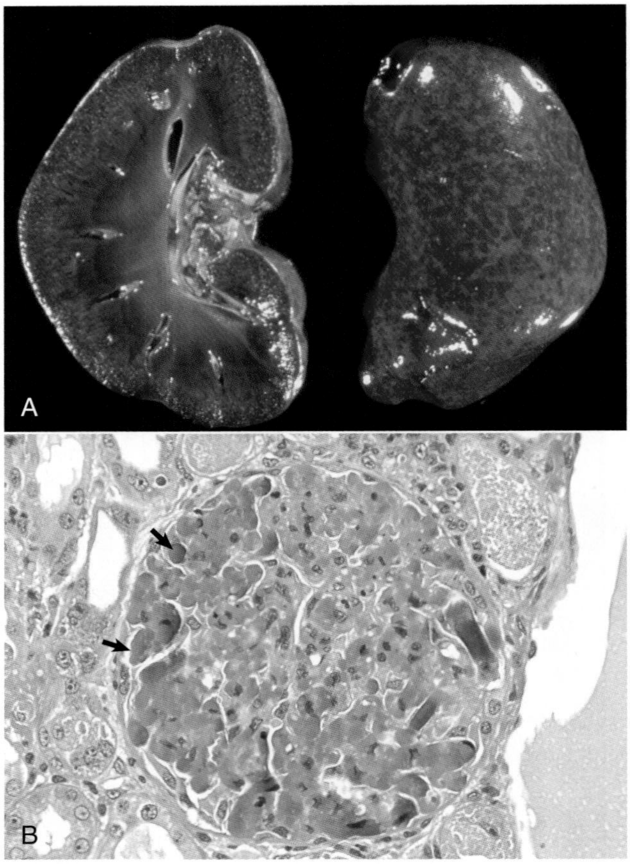

Fig. 11-44 Vasculopathy, renal (and cutaneous) vasculopathy syndrome, glomerulus, kidney, dog, greyhound.
A, The fine white dots in the cortex (both on the capsular and cut surfaces) are glomeruli with extensive glomerular capillary thrombosis. **B,** Necrotic glomerular endothelial cells and extensive glomerular capillary thrombosis *(arrows)* are typical of idiopathic glomerular (and cutaneous) vasculopathy syndrome in greyhound dogs. H&E stain. (**A** courtesy Dr. B. Weeks, College of Veterinary Medicine, Texas A&M University; and Noah's Arkive, College of Veterinary Medicine, The University of Georgia. **B** courtesy Dr. B.W. Fenwick, Virginia Tech.)

Diseases of the Tubules

Inherited Abnormalities in Renal Tubular Function

Inherited abnormalities in tubular metabolism, in transport, or in reabsorption of glucose, amino acids, ions, and proteins have been described in dogs. Primary renal glucosuria, an inherited disorder in Norwegian elkhounds and sporadically occurring in other dog breeds, occurs when the capacity of tubular epithelial cells to reabsorb glucose is significantly reduced. Gross and histologic lesions are not seen because this is a functional disorder. Glucosuria most commonly results from diabetes mellitus, acromegaly, or catecholamine release and predisposes dogs to the following:

- Bacterial infections of the lower urinary tract
- Urinary bladder emphysema, secondary to splitting of glucose molecules by bacteria (principally *Escherichia coli, Clostridium perfringens,* and rarely with *Candida* yeasts), with subsequent release of carbon dioxide (CO_2) into the bladder lumen and absorption of gas into the bladder lymphatocele (Fig. 11-45).

A hereditary generalized defect in tubular reabsorption similar to the Fanconi syndrome in humans has been described in Basenji dogs. The underlying tubular defect appears to be abnormal membrane structure of the proximal tubular epithelial cell brush borders because of altered lipid content in the cell membrane. Gross lesions are not identifiable in the early stages. Histopathologic changes in the kidneys are initially minimal, consisting of irregularly sized tubular epithelial cells in the convoluted tubules and loops of Henle. With time, dogs with Fanconi syndrome develop progressive renal insufficiency and associated renal fibrosis. Aminoaciduria, glucosuria, proteinuria, increased phosphaturia, metabolic acidosis,

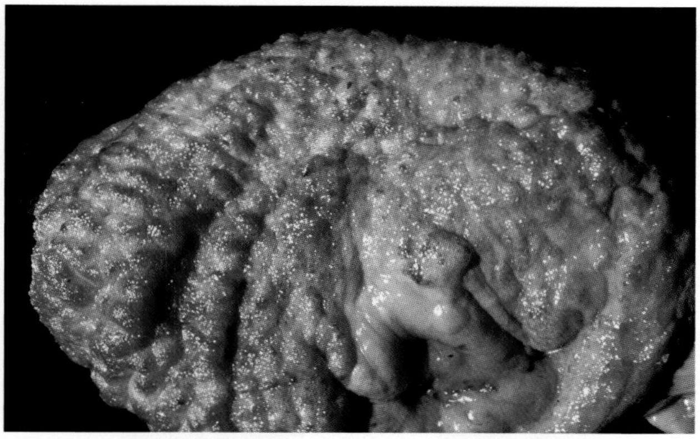

Fig. 11-45 Emphysema, urinary bladder mucosa, cow. The multiple "nodules" are mucosal gas bubbles that have expanded the mucosa and are secondary to bacterial infections of the lower urinary tract (principally by *Escherichia coli, Clostridium perfringens,* and rarely *Candida* yeasts). Microorganisms split glucose molecules to release CO_2 into the bladder lumen, from where the gas can be absorbed into bladder lymphatics. This animal was injected with calcium borogluconate as a calcium source to treat milk fever. Following intravenous injection, calcium ions readily dissociate from the parent molecule, and the resulting gluconate provides a sugar source for resident urinary bacteria. (Courtesy Dr. M.D. McGavin, College of Veterinary Medicine, University of Tennessee.)

and multiple endocrine abnormalities characterize this disease clinically. Transient acquired forms have been noted in association with copper storage hepatopathy.

The excretion of large quantities of cystine in the urine (cystinuria) is a sex-linked inherited tubular dysfunction seen occasionally in purebred and mongrel male dogs. It is important because it predisposes affected dogs to calculus formation and obstruction of the lower urinary tract (see the section on Urolithiasis).

Acute Tubular Necrosis

Acute tubular necrosis, as described in the section on tubular response to injury, can be seen following exposure to any of the following nephrotoxins (Box 11-10):

- Pigments
  - Hemoglobin
  - Myoglobin
  - Bile/bilirubin
- Heavy metals
  - Lead
  - Mercury
- Pharmaceutical agents (e.g., chemotherapeutic and antimicrobial agents)
  - Cisplatin
  - Aminoglycosides (see the section on Disorders of Dogs)
  - Oxytetracycline
  - Amphotericin B
  - Sulfonamides
  - Monensin
- Nonsteroidal antiinflammatory drugs
- Fungal toxins
  - Ochratoxins
- Plant toxins
  - Pigweed
  - Oxalate-containing plants
  - Oak tannins
- Antifreeze
  - Ethylene glycol

BOX 11-10 Common Nephrotoxins of Domestic Animals

HEAVY METALS
Mercury
Lead
Arsenic
Cadmium
Thallium

ANTIBACTERIAL AND ANTIFUNGAL AGENTS
Aminoglycosides:
- Gentamicin
- Neomycin
- Kanamycin
- Streptomycin
- Tobramycin

Tetracyclines
Amphotericin B

GROWTH-PROMOTING AGENTS
Monensin

NONSTEROIDAL ANTIINFLAMMATORY DRUGS
Aspirin
Phenylbutazone
Carprofen
Flunixin meglumine
Ibuprofen
Naproxen

MYCOTOXINS
Ochratoxin A
Citrinin

PLANTS
Pigweed *(Amaranthus retroflexus)*
Oaks (*Quercus* sp.)
Isotropis sp.
Yellow wood tree *(Terminalia oblongata)*

OXALATES
Ethylene glycol (antifreeze)
Halogeton *(Halogeton glomeratus)*
Greasewood *(Sarcobatus vermiculatus)*
Rhubarb *(Rheum rhaponticum)*
Sorrel, dock (*Rumex* sp.)

VITAMIN D
Vitamin D supplements
Calciferol-containing rodenticides
Cestrum diurnum
Solanum sp.
Trisetum sp.

ANTINEOPLASTIC COMPOUNDS
Cisplatin

- Vitamins and Minerals
  - Vitamin D
  - Hypercalcemia
- Bacterial toxins
  - Shiga toxin
- Pet food contaminants (see the section on Disorders of Dogs)
  - Melamine
  - Cyanuric acid

These nephrotoxins are covered in greater detail in the next section.

Nephrotoxic Pigments

Hemoglobinuric nephrosis

A set of events leading to ischemic tubular necrosis frequently occurs in hypoperfused kidneys complicated by hemoglobinuria. Hemoglobinemia results in hemoglobinuria when the renal threshold for resorption is exceeded. Hemoglobinuria may occur in the following:

- Chronic copper toxicity in sheep
- Leptospirosis or babesiosis in cattle
- Red maple toxicity in horses
- Babesiosis or autoimmune hemolytic anemia in dogs

In these diseases, serum concentrations of hemoglobin are increased. Hemoglobin passes into the glomerular filtrate, producing greatly increased intraluminal concentrations that cause hemoglobinuric nephrosis. Hemoglobin attaches to a carrier haptoglobin for transportation, but the latter is too big to pass through the glomerulus. Hemoglobin is not excreted in the urine until supplies of the carrier molecule are depleted and hemoglobin becomes free in the plasma. Hemoglobin is not nephrotoxic itself, and intravenous infusions of hemoglobin into healthy animals produce no recognizable lesions. However, large concentrations of hemoglobin in the glomerular filtrate can increase the tubular necrosis that occurs as a result of renal ischemia, for example, in chronic copper toxicity in sheep, renal ischemia is secondary to hypovolemic shock or severe anemia. Hemoglobinuria can have an additive deleterious affect on tubular epithelium already undergoing ischemic necrosis.

At necropsy, the renal cortices in severe hemoglobinuria are diffusely stained red-brown to blue-black and have intratubular hemoglobin casts (Fig. 11-46, *A*). These hemoglobin casts appear as a red-black stippling of the capsular surface and continue into the cortex as radially oriented, dark red streaks. The medulla is diffusely dark red or has patchy red streaks. Classically, kidneys from sheep with chronic copper toxicity are diffusely, uniformly, and strikingly blue-black and described as "gunmetal blue." Microscopically, proximal tubular epithelial degeneration and necrosis are severe and tubular lumens are filled by abundant orange-red granular refractile material, the characteristic appearance of a heme compound (Fig. 11-46, *B*).

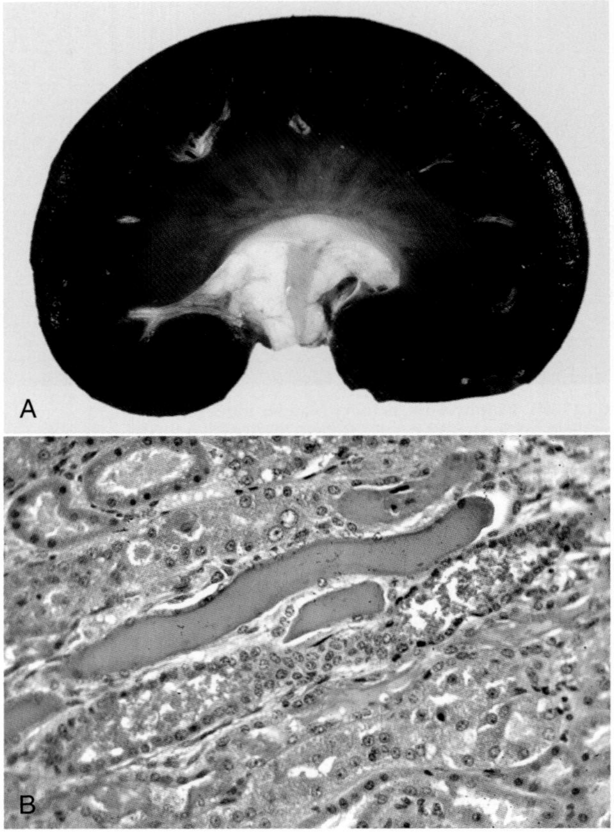

Fig. 11-46 Hemoglobinuric nephrosis, kidney. **A,** Dog. Severe diffuse hemoglobin staining of the cortex and medulla is secondary to hemoglobinemia from an acute intravascular hemolytic crisis. Note the yellow staining (jaundice) of the pelvic fat and the intima of cross sections of the arcuate artery at the corticomedullary junction. **B,** Sheep. Several distal tubules contain hyaline and coarsely granular hemoglobin casts that occurred following intravascular hemolysis (hemoglobinemia) from chronic copper toxicosis. H&E stain. (**A** courtesy Dr. A. Confer, College of Veterinary Medicine, Oklahoma State University. **B** courtesy Dr. A.R. Doster, University of Nebraska; and Noah's Arkive, College of Veterinary Medicine, The University of Georgia.)

Myoglobinuric nephrosis

Myoglobinuria results from acute and extensive muscle necrosis and occurs in the following:

- Azoturia ("Monday morning disease") of horses (see the section on Disorders of Horses)
- Capture myopathy of exotic or wild animals
- Severe direct trauma to muscle (e.g., traffic accident)

A set of events leading to ischemic tubular necrosis frequently occurs in hypoperfused kidneys complicated by myoglobinuria. In these diseases, serum concentrations of myoglobin are increased, as these products pass into the glomerular filtrate, producing greatly increased intraluminal concentrations that cause myoglobinuric nephrosis. Myoglobin does not use a carrier protein for transportation, and because it is a small molecule, it more freely passes through the glomerulus and is excreted in the urine. Myoglobin is not nephrotoxic in itself, and intravenous infusions into healthy animals produce no recognizable lesions. However, large concentrations of myoglobin in the glomerular filtrate can increase the tubular necrosis that occurs as a result of renal ischemia; for example, in rhabdomyolysis in horses, renal ischemia is secondary to hypovolemic shock or severe anemia. Myoglobinuria can have an additive deleterious effect on tubular epithelium already undergoing ischemic necrosis.

At necropsy, the renal cortices in myoglobinuria are diffusely stained red-brown to blue-black and have intratubular myoglobin casts (Fig. 11-47).

Cholemic Nephrosis

Increased serum concentrations of bilirubin, as in young lambs, calves, and foals with immature hepatic conjugating mechanisms, can be associated with proximal tubular cellular swelling, degeneration, and yellow-brown-green pigmentation of the proximal tubular epithelial cells. The term *cholemic nephrosis* has been applied to this lesion; however, its significance is doubtful. Acute tubular

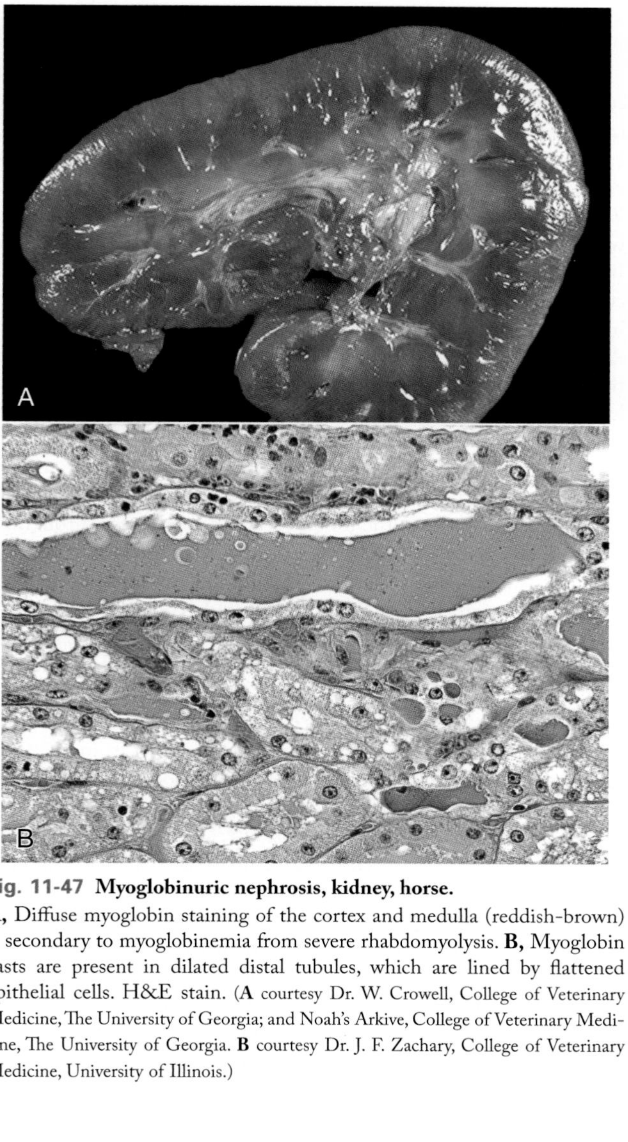

Fig. 11-47 Myoglobinuric nephrosis, kidney, horse.
A, Diffuse myoglobin staining of the cortex and medulla (reddish-brown) is secondary to myoglobinemia from severe rhabdomyolysis. **B,** Myoglobin casts are present in dilated distal tubules, which are lined by flattened epithelial cells. H&E stain. (**A** courtesy Dr. W. Crowell, College of Veterinary Medicine, The University of Georgia; and Noah's Arkive, College of Veterinary Medicine, The University of Georgia. **B** courtesy Dr. J. F. Zachary, College of Veterinary Medicine, University of Illinois.)

necrosis, when seen in association with severe bilirubinemia, the so-called hepatorenal syndrome, probably is not caused by bile acid or bilirubin retention per se but by ischemia from prerenal causes such as constriction of renal vessels related to shock or catecholamine release.

Heavy Metals

Nephrotoxic tubular necrosis is caused by several classes of naturally occurring or synthetic compounds. Inorganic arsenic and certain heavy metals, including inorganic mercury, lead, cadmium, and thallium, are nephrotoxins. Common sources of heavy metals for oral exposure include herbicides (arsenic), old paints (lead), batteries (lead), automobile components (lead), impure petroleum distillates, and other environmental contaminants. Acute tubular necrosis from mercury is caused by the following:

- Damage to membranes of proximal convoluted tubular epithelial cells.
- Mitochondrial damage produced by these toxins; damage is often related to the interaction of these metals with protein sulfhydryl groups.

In mercury toxicosis, mercuric ions enter the proximal tubular cells both from the luminal side because the ions are present in the glomerular filtrate and from the peritubular side, where the mercuric ions diffuse from the capillary blood, traverse the interstitium and tubular basement membrane, and enter the tubular epithelium. Mercuric ions become concentrated in the rough endoplasmic reticulum and cause early tubular changes that include loss of brush border and dispersion of ribosomes. These changes are followed by mitochondrial swelling and cellular death. Recently, cadmium has been reported to cause cell death in proximal convoluted tubules by apoptosis.

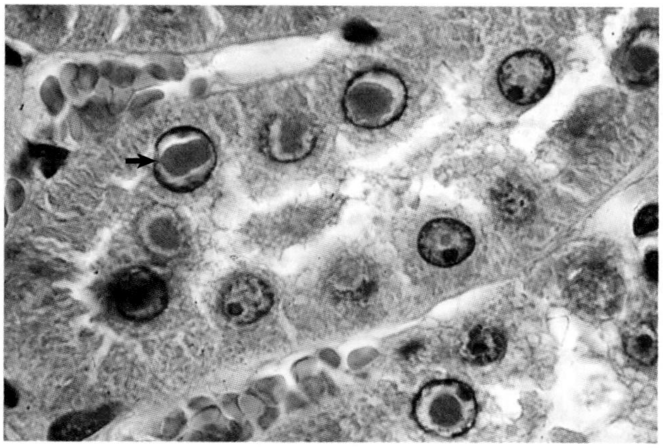

Fig. 11-48 Nephrosis, lead toxicosis, kidney, cortex, rat.
Acid-fast intranuclear inclusion bodies *(arrow)* present in the proximal convoluted tubular epithelium are diagnostic of lead poisoning. Acid-fast stain with H&E counterstain. (Courtesy Dr. J. King, College of Veterinary Medicine, Cornell University.)

The specific metal involved in toxic tubular injury cannot be identified by the renal lesions alone. The exception is lead toxicity, in which the endothelial and epithelial cells of affected glomeruli and proximal tubules, respectively, sometimes have acid-fast intranuclear inclusions composed of a lead-protein complex (Fig. 11-48).

Pharmaceutical Agents

These agents are nephrotoxic and cause acute tubular necrosis when administered at excessive doses or too frequently. Cisplatin, a platinum-containing cancer chemotherapeutic agent, causes tubular necrosis by the following:

- Direct tubular epithelial damage.
- Reducing renal blood flow via vasoconstriction mediated by the renin-angiotensin mechanism.

Oxytetracycline is occasionally nephrotoxic in cattle and dogs. The mechanism of tubular damage has not been determined, but it is known that large concentrations of tetracycline antibiotics are necessary and are thought to inhibit protein synthesis in tubular epithelial cells.

Amphotericin B, an antifungal polyene antibiotic, is nephrotoxic by either vasoconstriction and/or the direct disruption of cellular membranes; this membrane damage interferes with normal cholesterol-lipid interactions and causes potassium ion loss, intracellular hydrogen ion accumulation, acute cellular swelling, and necrosis of proximal and distal tubules. These renal changes are not confined to cases of an overdose of the drug but can occur in animals given the recommended therapeutic dosage.

Sulfonamide-induced tubular necrosis, a common entity in years past, occurs infrequently today because the presently used sulfonamides have greater solubility than those used in the past. Sulfonamides produce tubular epithelial cell necrosis most readily in dehydrated animals. Crystals form in tubules and cause necrosis of the renal tubular epithelium by direct toxicity and by mechanical damage. Fine granular yellow crystalline deposits can be seen grossly in the medullary tubules of affected animals, but the crystalline deposits are dissolved during fixation in aqueous fixatives such as 10% buffered neutral formalin.

Monensin is an ionophore antibiotic used as a feed additive to control coccidiosis and stimulate weight gains in poultry and cattle. Horses are particularly susceptible to toxicosis with monensin. Although necrosis of striated muscle is the major lesion, renal tubular degeneration or necrosis occurs concurrently.

Nonsteroidal Antiinflammatory Drugs

Ingestion of nonsteroidal antiinflammatory drugs (NSAIDs), such as phenylbutazone, aspirin, carprofen, flunixin meglumine, ibuprofen, and naproxen, have been associated with acute renal failure in small animals, especially dogs. The mechanism of acute renal failure is related to NSAIDs decreasing the synthesis of renal prostaglandins. Because prostaglandins are responsible for maintaining normal renal blood flow, NSAID administration results in afferent arteriolar constriction that decreases renal perfusion, resulting in acute tubular degeneration and medullary papillary necrosis and acute renal failure. The overall incidence of NSAID-induced renal failure in small animals is low and is seen most commonly in animals that ingest excessive amounts of the drug or have a concomitant disorder such as dehydration, congestive heart failure, or chronic renal disease.

Fungal Toxins

Naturally occurring nephrotoxins can originate from plants (ochratoxins and citrinins, castor beans) or from fungal organisms (mycotoxins produced by *Aspergillus* sp. and *Penicillium* sp). Ochratoxin A is nephrotoxic for monogastric animals, particularly pigs, in which the lesions are tubular degeneration and necrosis. In addition, long-term ingestion results in diffuse renal fibrosis presumably as the result of continual damage to the tubule epithelial cells and thus allowing no time for regeneration.

Plant Toxins

Several species of pigweed, particularly *Amaranthus retroflexus*, can be responsible for acute tubular necrosis and perirenal edema in pigs and cattle. The toxic principle has not been identified. Oxalate-induced tubular necrosis also occurs in sheep and cattle after ingestion of toxic quantities of oxalates that accumulate in plants of various genera such as *Halogeton, Sarcobatus, Rheum,* and *Rumex.* After absorption from the intestine, calcium oxalates precipitate in either vessel lumens or walls or within renal tubules, where they cause obstruction and epithelial cell necrosis. Illness in oxalate poisoning occurs not only because of renal disease but also because of neuromuscular dysfunction, the result of the hypocalcemia produced by chelation of serum calcium by oxalates. Recently, an oxalate-induced nephrosis was described in Tibetan spaniels with an inherited hyperoxaluria. A chronic oxalate nephrosis in Ragdoll cats of unknown inheritance and etiology is also reported.

Tannins

See the section on Disorders of Cattle for a discussion of tannins as a nephrotoxin.

Chemicals

Antifreeze

See the section on Disorders of Dogs for a discussion of antifreeze as a nephrotoxin.

Vitamins and Minerals

Vitamin D

Vitamin D given as multiple excessive doses (vitamin D intoxication [vitamin D nephropathy]) or by accidental ingestion of calciferol-containing rodenticides can cause nephrosis in dogs and cats. In livestock, chronic ingestion of plants, such as *Cestrum diurnum* in the southern United States (US) or *Solanum* sp. or *Trisetum* sp. in other countries, each of which contains a chemical with vitamin D–like biologic activity, can also cause nephrosis. Ingestion of excessive amounts of vitamin D can induce hypercalcemia. Hypercalcemia results in decreased cAMP formation, which impairs sodium resorption and interferes with ADH receptors. Additionally, if the hypercalcemia persists, progressive mineralization of tubular and GBMs occurs (see Fig. 11-31). Development of lesions depends on the length of time between exposure to rodenticides and death or the duration of continued exposure to vitamin D. In acute cases, the kidneys have a smooth capsular surface. Microscopically, tubular epithelium is necrotic and atrophic with a few calcified deposits in the tubules scattered randomly throughout the cortex. In more chronic cases, the surface of the kidney is finely granular as a result of fibrosis. White, chalky deposits can be seen within the cortex. Interstitial fibrosis, tubular dilation, glomerular atrophy, and extensive calcification of tubular basement membranes are seen microscopically.

Interstitial calcification (hypercalcemic nephropathy)

Hypercalcemia from a variety of causes results in inactivation of adenyl cyclase, decreased AMP so that sodium transport is impaired in the ascending limb of the loop of Henle, distal tubule, and collecting ducts. Hypercalcemia interferes with ADH receptors in the collecting ducts, resulting in renal diabetes insipidus. Mineralization of the basement membrane and epithelium initially in the outer zone of the medulla and then involving the interstitium, vessels, and glomeruli is seen when hypercalcemia persists. The leading cause of hypercalcemia in dogs and cats is hypercalcemia of malignancy, a paraneoplastic syndrome. PTH-related peptide (PTHrp), a peptide that resembles PTH, results in bone resorption. It is produced most commonly by lymphosarcomas or carcinomas of the apocrine glands of the anal sac. Additionally, excess vitamin D either from rodenticides or excess dietary sources (toxic plants) can result in a similar syndrome. Less common causes of hypercalcemia include primary hyperparathyroidism and secondary renal hyperparathyroidism.

Bacterial Toxins

Bacterial toxins, such as the epsilon exotoxin, produced after marked enteric proliferation by *Clostridium perfringens* type D in small ruminants, can result in grossly recognizable bilateral renal lesions termed *pulpy kidney* (Fig. 11-49, *A*). The pulpy texture of the kidney is due to acute tubular epithelial degeneration and/or necrosis and interstitial edema and hemorrhage (Fig. 11-49, *B*). Epsilon toxin binds to receptors on distal renal tubular epithelium causing this degeneration. Autolysis can produce similar changes, and this finding should be interpreted with caution, especially with a long necropsy interval.

Pet Food Contaminants

See the section on Disorders of Dogs for a discussion of pet food contaminants.

Diseases of the Renal Pelvis

Hydronephrosis

Hydronephrosis refers to dilation of the renal pelvis because of obstruction of urine outflow and is principally caused by a slow or

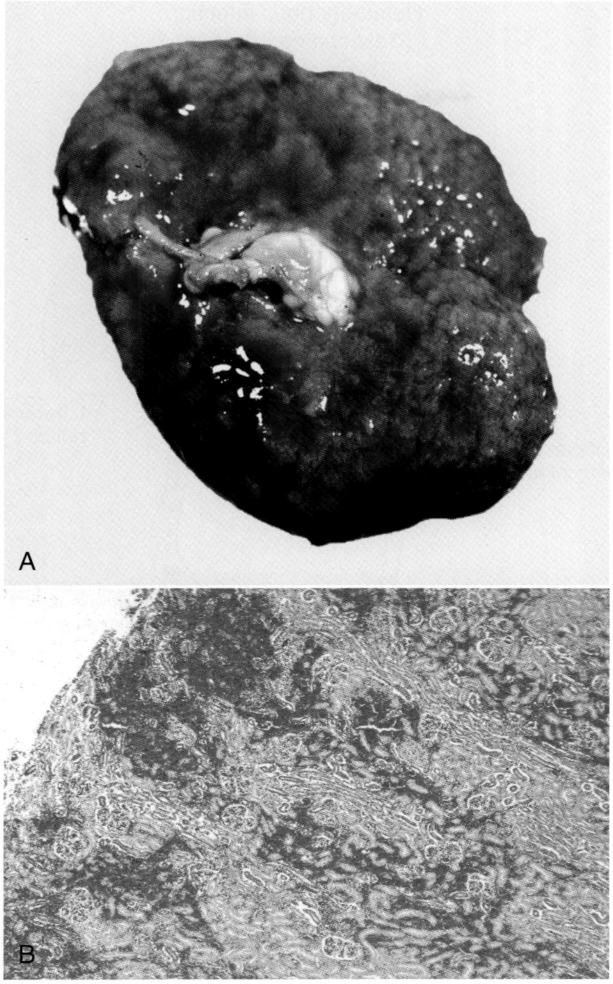

Fig. 11-49 Pulpy kidney disease, *Clostridium perfringens* type D toxin, kidney, lamb.
A, The Epsilon exotoxin from an enteric overgrowth of *Clostridium perfringens* type D causes soft, swollen, and pale kidneys, often with hemorrhage, and are termed *pulpy kidneys.* **B,** The soft pulpy nature of the kidney is the result of acute tubular epithelial cell degeneration and/or necrosis, interstitial edema, and hemorrhage. H&E stain. (**A** courtesy Dr. J. King, College of Veterinary Medicine, Cornell University. **B** courtesy Dr. M.D. McGavin, College of Veterinary Medicine, University of Tennessee.)

intermittent increase in pelvic pressure. Abrupt increases in pressure, such as those associated with inadvertent surgical ligation of a ureter, more commonly result in a decline in filtration rate in the affected kidney and a lesser propensity to develop hydronephrosis.

Obstruction leading to hydronephrosis can occasionally be caused by congenital malformation of the ureter, vesicoureteral junction, or urethra or from congenitally malpositioned kidneys with secondary kinking of the ureter. The more common causes of hydronephrosis are as follows:

- Ureteral or urethral blockage due to urinary tract calculi (see the section on Lower Urinary Tract)
- Chronic inflammation
- Ureteral or urethral neoplasia
- Neurogenic functional disorders

Hydronephrosis occurs in all domestic animals. Depending on the location of the obstruction, hydronephrosis can be unilateral (ureteral) or bilateral (both ureters, bladder trigone, or urethra). Unilateral hydronephrosis is caused by obstruction of the ureters anywhere throughout its length or at its entrance into the urinary bladder. Bilateral hydronephrosis can be caused by urethral obstruction, bilateral ureteral obstruction, or extensive urinary bladder lesions centered on the trigone. When hydronephrosis is unilateral, pelvic enlargement of the kidney can become extensive, even cystic, before the lesion is recognized clinically. If the obstructive process causes partial or intermittent blockage, bilateral hydronephrosis can become notable because of continual urine production and pooling of urine in the expanding pelvis. When obstruction is complete and bilateral, death as a result of uremia occurs before pelvic enlargement becomes extensive.

When the increase in intrapelvic pressure is substantial and sustained, the following occur:

- Intratubular pressure is increased and results in microscopic renal tubular dilation.
- Glomeruli remain functional, and even with complete obstruction, glomerular filtration does not stop completely and soon overwhelms tubular reabsorption pathways.
- Much of the glomerular filtrate diffuses into the interstitium, where it is initially removed via lymphatic vessels and veins.
- As intrapelvic pressure increases, the interstitial vessels collapse and renal blood flow is reduced, resulting in hypoxia, tubular atrophy, and if the pressure increase is continued, interstitial fibrosis.
- The glomeruli have a relatively normal morphologic appearance for a prolonged period, but they eventually become atrophic and sclerotic.

Early changes of hydronephrosis include dilation of the pelvis and calyces and blunting of the renal crest and papillae (Fig. 11-50). When pelvic dilation is progressive, the kidney silhouette is enlarged and rounder than normal, and the cortex and medulla are progressively thinned (Fig. 11-51). Interstitial vascular obstruction from compression produces an expanding front of medullary and later cortical ischemia and necrosis. The continued pelvic dilation causes loss of tubules by degeneration and atrophy, followed by condensation of interstitial connective tissue and fibrosis of the renal parenchyma. In its most advanced form, the hydronephrotic kidney is a thin-walled (2- to 3-mm), fluid-filled sac. This sac is lined by flattened transitional epithelium, which is spared during lesion development. Occasionally, a severely hydronephrotic kidney becomes contaminated by bacteria and the thin-walled sac becomes filled with pus instead of urine. This lesion, referred to as *pyonephrosis,* is likely the result of blood-borne bacteria lodging in a hydronephrotic kidney.

Pyelonephritis

Bacterial infection of the pelvis with extension into the renal tubules and a concomitant interstitial inflammation is referred to as *pyelonephritis.* Because of differences in pathogenesis, lesion distribution, and microscopic appearance, pyelonephritis is considered a form of tubulointerstitial nephritis.

Although pyelitis refers to inflammation of the renal pelvis, pyelonephritis is inflammation of both the renal pelvis and renal parenchyma and is an excellent example of suppurative tubulointerstitial disease. The condition usually originates as an extension of a bacterial infection affecting the lower urinary tract that ascends the ureters to the kidneys and establishes an infection in the pelvis and inner medulla (Fig. 11-52). Rarely, pyelonephritis can result from descending bacterial infections, wherein bacterial infection of the kidneys occurs via the hematogenous route (i.e., embolic nephritis). In human pathology, the term *pyelonephritis* is used to include both ascending and descending infections. Ascending infection, however, is by far the most common cause of pyelonephritis in animals.

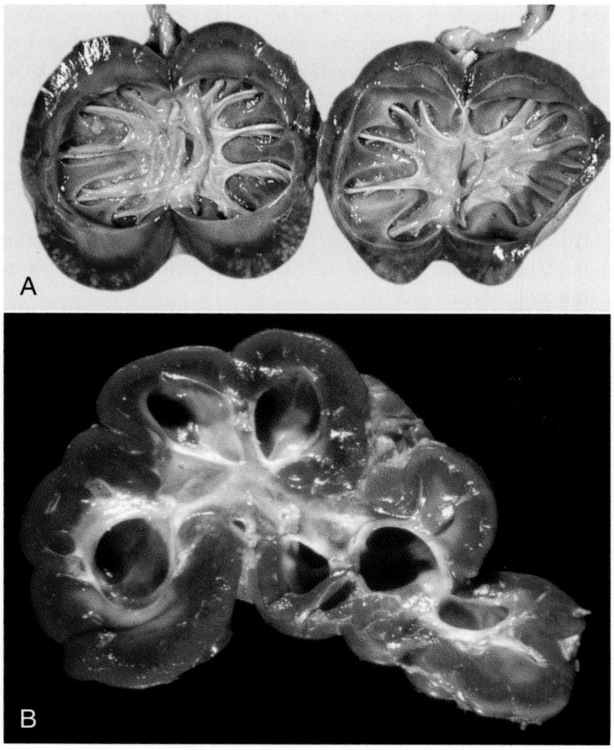

Fig. 11-50 Hydronephrosis, kidney, dorsal section.
A, Sheep. The pelvis of each kidney is markedly dilated. **B,** Cow. Bovine kidneys are lobulated, and each lobule has its own renal papilla surrounded by a calyx, an extension of the pelvis. Thus in early hydronephrosis, each of these calyces is distended, and these distended calyces should not be confused with the cysts of a cystic or polycystic kidney. (**A** courtesy Dr. J. King, College of Veterinary Medicine, Cornell University. **B** courtesy College of Veterinary Medicine, University of Illinois.)

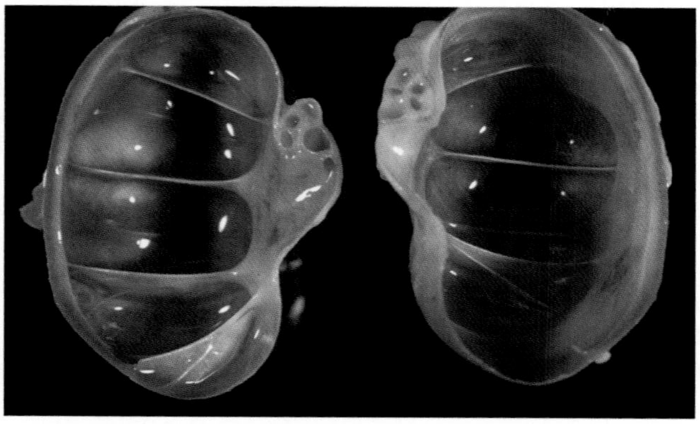

Fig. 11-51 Chronic hydronephrosis, kidney, dorsal section, cat.
Advanced hydronephrosis is characterized by loss of medullary tissue and atrophy or even loss of the entire cortex in response to elevated pelvic fluid pressure. Note that this case was so severe that only the renal capsule, which contains clear yellow fluid, remains. (Courtesy Dr. M.D. McGavin, College of Veterinary Medicine, University of Tennessee.)

The pathogenesis of ascending pyelonephritis depends on the abnormal reflux of bacteria-contaminated urine from the lower tract to the renal pelvis and collecting ducts (vesicoureteral reflux). Normally, little vesicoureteral reflux occurs during micturition. Vesicoureteral reflux occurs more readily when pressure is increased within the urinary bladder, as with urethral obstruction. Most

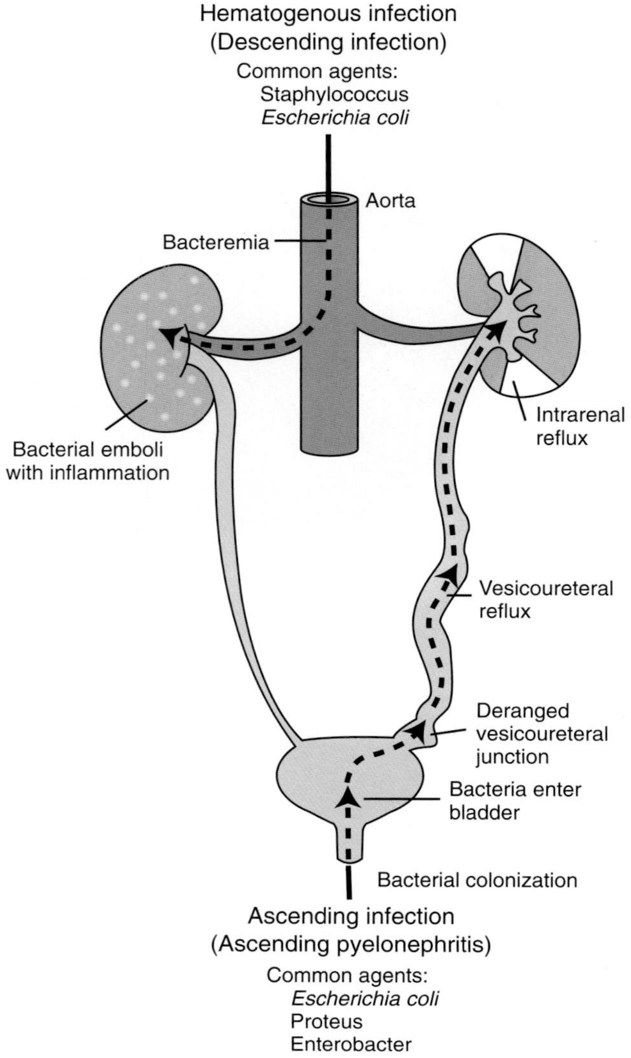

Fig. 11-52 Schematic diagram of the pathways of renal infection.
Hematogenous infection results from bacteremia. More common is ascending infection, which results from a combination of urinary bladder infection, vesicoureteral reflux, and intrarenal reflux. (From Kumar V, Abbas AK, Fausto N: *Robbins & Cotran pathologic basis of disease,* ed 8, Philadelphia, 2010, Saunders.)

recently, this mechanism has been postulated for end-stage pyelonephritis with mild dysplasia seen in young Boxer dogs in Norway. Bacterial infection of the lower urinary tract can enhance vesicoureteral reflux by several other mechanisms as follows:

- When the bladder wall is inflamed (cystitis), the normal competency of the vesicoureteral valve can be compromised, allowing greater opportunity for urine to reflux.
- Endotoxin, liberated from Gram-negative bacteria infecting the ureter and bladder, can inhibit normal ureteral peristalsis, increasing reflux.

The urinary tract has a number of protective features in place to help prevent bacterial colonization and these include the following:

- Mucoproteins in the surface urothelial mucosal lining that prohibit bacterial adherence
- Desquamation of superficial urothelial cells to minimize surface colonization
- Goblet cell metaplasia
- Phagocytosis by superficial mucosal urothelial cells

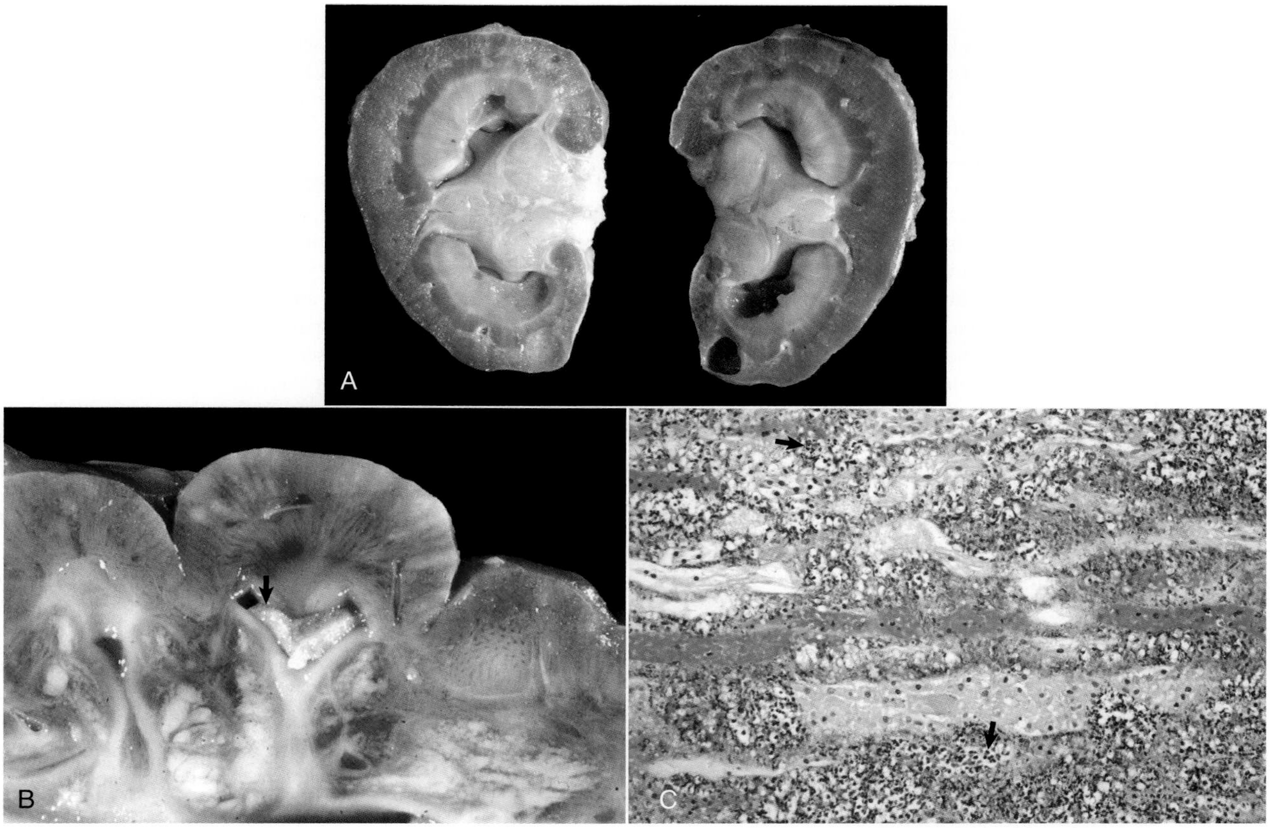

Fig. 11-53 **Pyelonephritis, kidney.**
A, Dorsal section, dog. Extensive pelvic inflammation has destroyed areas *(gray-white)* of the inner medulla and extends focally into the outer medulla. **B,** Dorsal section, cow. Renal calyces in the cow contain suppurative exudate *(arrow)*. **C,** Dog. There is both intratubular and interstitial inflammation with tubular necrosis, characterized by infiltrates of principally neutrophils *(arrows)*. H&E stain. (**A** courtesy Dr. M.D. McGavin, College of Veterinary Medicine, University of Tennessee. **B** courtesy Dr. K. Read, College of Veterinary Medicine, Texas A&M University; and Noah's Arkive, College of Veterinary Medicine, The University of Georgia. **C** courtesy Dr. J. F. Zachary, College of Veterinary Medicine, University of Illinois.)

Bacteria that colonize the pelvis can readily infect the inner medulla. The medulla is highly susceptible to bacterial infection because of the following:

- Its poor blood supply
- Its great interstitial osmolality and/or osmolarity that inhibits neutrophil function
- Its large ammonia concentration that inhibits complement activation

Thus bacteria can infect and ascend collecting ducts, cause tubular epithelial necrosis and hemorrhage, and incite a notable inflammatory response. Bacterial infection can progressively ascend within tubules and the interstitium until the inflammatory lesions extend from pelvis to capsule. Chronic pyelonephritis may result from infection superimposed on conditions that result in recurrent obstructive disease or reflux (reflux nephropathy). Recurrent infections lead to recurrent bouts of inflammation that result in scarring.

Because most occurrences of pyelonephritis are ascending infections and because females are more susceptible to lower urinary tract infections, pyelonephritis occurs more frequently in females. *Escherichia coli*, especially uropathogenic strains that produce virulence factors such as α-hemolysin, adhesions, and P fimbria, is one of the most common causes of lower urinary tract disease and pyelonephritis. *Proteus* sp., *Klebsiella* sp., *Staphylococcus* sp., *Streptococcus* sp., and *Pseudomonas aeruginosa* are also common causes of lower urinary tract infection and pyelonephritis in all species. *Corynebacterium renale*, *Arcanobacterium pyogenes,* and *Eubacterium (Corynebacterium) suis* are specifically pathogenic for the lower urinary tract of cattle and pigs, respectively, and are common causes of pyelonephritis. Recent or multiple catheterizations may be a predisposing factor.

A gross diagnosis of pyelonephritis is accomplished by recognizing the existence of pelvic inflammation with extension into the renal parenchyma (Fig. 11-53, *A*). Pyelonephritis can be unilateral, but it is often bilateral and most severe at the renal poles. The pelvic and ureteral mucous membranes can be acutely inflamed, thickened, reddened, roughened, or granular and coated with a thin exudate. The pelvis and ureters can be markedly dilated and have purulent exudate in the lumina (Fig. 11-53, *B*). The medullary crest (papilla) is often ulcerated and necrotic. Renal involvement is notable by irregular, radially oriented, red or gray streaks involving the medulla extending toward and often reaching the renal surface. Occasionally, inflammation extends through the surface of the kidneys to produce extensive subcapsular inflammation and localized peritonitis.

Microscopically, the most severe acute lesions of pyelonephritis are usually in the inner medulla. The transitional epithelium is usually focally or diffusely necrotic and sloughed. Necrotic debris, fibrin, neutrophils, and bacterial colonies can be adherent to the denuded surface. Medullary tubules are notably dilated, and their lumina contain neutrophils and bacterial colonies. Focally the tubular epithelium is necrotic. An intense neutrophilic infiltrate, present in the renal interstitium, can be accompanied by notable interstitial hemorrhages and edema (Fig. 11-53, *C*). If obstruction of vasa recta has occurred, coagulative necrosis of the inner medulla (papillary necrosis) can be severe. Similar tubular and interstitial lesions, although less severe, extend radially into the cortical tubules and interstitium. When the lesions become subacute, the severity of the neutrophilic infiltrates diminishes, and lymphocytes, plasma cells, and monocytes infiltrate the interstitium. Chronic lesions have severe fibrosis. If active bacterial infection persists or is untreated, an intense infiltrate of all inflammatory cell types interspersed with tubular necrosis and fibrosis can be seen. All stages of disease progression can occur in a single kidney.

The renal lesions of chronic pyelonephritis, in which an active bacterial infection exists, include most of the elements of acute inflammation described previously and extensive necrosis of the medulla, patchy fibrosis in the outer medulla and cortex, and variable amounts of pelvic inflammatory exudates. Chronic pyelonephritis often produces a grossly visible deformity of the renal parenchyma because of extensive interstitial inflammation and scarring (Fig. 11-54). Fibrosis secondary to the tubulointerstitial inflammation of pyelonephritis follows the pattern of the acute

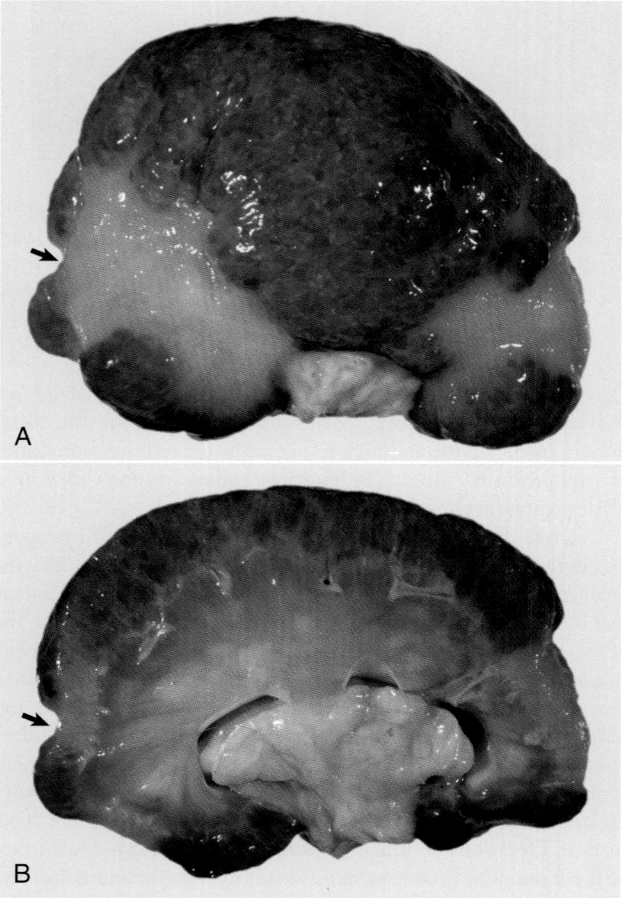

Fig. 11-54 Chronic pyelonephritis, kidney, dog.
A, Note the two large polar scars visible as large indentations on the capsular surface *(arrow)*. The fine gray spots are regions of chronic inflammatory infiltrates and fibrosis. **B,** Dorsal section. The cortical scars are localized to the renal poles *(arrow)*, but there is a finely stippled pattern of nodularity and fibrosis in the remaining kidney. This polar pattern of scarring suggests previous bouts of pyelonephritis. (Courtesy Dr. A. Confer, College of Veterinary Medicine, Oklahoma State University.)

disease (targeting the renal poles), and results in irregularly distributed, patchy scarring that is seen as deeply depressed regions on the renal capsular surface and linear areas extending through both the cortex and medulla to the pelvis. Such lesions often resemble chronic polar infarcts.

Papillary (Medullary Crest) Necrosis

Necrosis of the renal papillae, or their counterpart, the medullary crest, is a response of the inner medulla to ischemia. Papillary necrosis can be a primary or secondary lesion. Papillary necrosis occurs as a primary disease in animals treated with NSAIDs and is analogous to analgesic nephropathy in humans. The primary disease occurs quite frequently in horses treated for prolonged periods with phenylbutazone or flunixin meglumine. It is important in dogs and cats because of accidental ingestion of or treatment with ibuprofen, aspirin, or acetaminophen at excessive dosages. Drugs associated with papillary necrosis are sometimes referred to as *papillotoxins.* The medullary interstitial cells are the primary targets of papillotoxins. These cells have a key role in synthesis of prostaglandins, antihypertensive factors, and the glycosaminoglycan matrix of the medullary interstitium. Interstitial cell damage decreases prostaglandin synthesis, which reduces normal blood flow and causes ischemia, increases tubular transport, and modifies the interstitial matrix; the net effect is degenerative changes in tubular epithelial cells in the inner medulla. In addition to its inhibition of prostaglandin biosynthesis, acetaminophen also causes direct oxidative damage to medullary tubular epithelium after covalent binding to the cells, further enhancing necrosis of the renal papillae.

Secondary papillary necrosis results from the following:

Reduced blood flow in vasa recta:

- Glomerular lesions restricting blood flow—amyloid, hyalinization
- Compression of vasa recta—within the medulla
  - Interstitial fibrosis—chiefly in the outer medulla, secondary to ischemia (see later discussion)
  - Interstitial renal medullary amyloidosis (cats)
  - Pyelitis—ascending tubular and interstitial inflammation, edema, and fibrosis

Compression of renal papilla by:

- Increased intrapelvic pressure secondary to:
  - Pelvic calculi
  - Lower urinary tract obstruction
  - Vesicoureteral reflux

The outer medulla and the cells of the thick ascending loop of Henle in particular are the least well perfused of any zones of the kidneys. This is because the medulla has little direct perfusion; instead, most of the medullary blood supply comes from the cortex after passing through the glomeruli and entering the vasa recta. Because of this limited blood flow, in addition to the high metabolic medullary cellular demand, any lesion or disease process that further reduces medullary blood flow can cause ischemic necrosis (infarction) of the papillae. Additionally, the high metabolic demand for cell transport and the maintenance of an ion gradient to enhance urinary concentration makes this area particularly vulnerable. This is most evident after ischemic tubular damage where swollen endothelial and tubular epithelial cells, in conjunction with neutrophil adhesion in small vessels, upset the balance of oxygenation and energy demand by the outer medullary tubular cells. Medullary blood flow is ultimately balanced through levels of vasodilators, such as prostaglandin, nitric oxide, and adenosine, and vasoconstrictors, such as endothelin and angiotensin II.

Typically, acute lesions are irregular, discolored areas of necrotic inner medulla sharply delineated from the surviving medullary

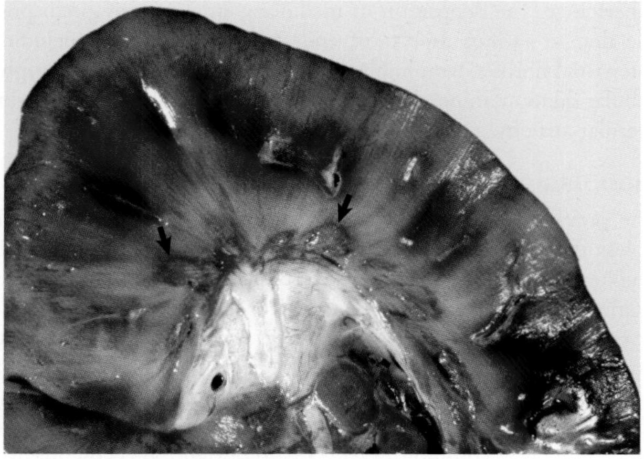

Fig. 11-55 Papillary (medullary crest) necrosis, chronic nonsteroidal antiinflammatory drug treatment, kidney, dorsal section, horse. Acute coagulation necrosis of the medullary crest and inner medulla *(green areas [arrows])*. There is also hemorrhage of the outer medulla. The term *papillary necrosis* is retained for all animals, although only the pig and cow have distinct renal papillae. In other animals, these have fused to form the medullary crest. (Courtesy Dr. A. Confer, College of Veterinary Medicine, Oklahoma State University.)

tissue (Fig. 11-55). The affected tissue, which initially undergoes coagulation necrosis, is yellow-gray, green, or pink. With time, the necrotic tissue sloughs, resulting in a detached, friable, and discolored tissue fragment in the pelvis. The remaining inner medulla is usually attenuated and on cross-section is narrowed. Overlying cortex can be somewhat shrunken because of atrophy of some of the nephrons caused by blockage of their tubules in the affected medulla. Small pieces of sloughed necrotic medullary tissue pass inconsequentially into the ureter. However, large pieces can obstruct the ureter, causing hydronephrosis, or form a nidus for precipitation of minerals, resulting in the formation of pelvic or ureteral calculi. Papillary necrosis is usually an incidental finding at necropsy and rarely leads to progressive renal damage and failure.

Diseases of the Interstitium

Granulomatous Nephritis

Granulomatous nephritis is an interstitial disease that often accompanies chronic systemic diseases that are characterized by multiple granulomas in various organs. In domestic animals, granulomatous nephritis has been associated with a variety of infectious agents, including viruses (feline coronavirus [see the section on Disorders of Cats], porcine circovirus), bacteria (mycobacteria), fungi (*Aspergillus* sp.), and parasites (*Toxocara* sp. and *Angiostrongylus vasorum* larvae/eggs). Common to each, however, is the formation of grossly visible granulomas randomly scattered throughout the kidneys, especially in the cortex.

Granulomatous nephritis is also caused by a variety of granuloma-inducing infectious agents, including fungi such as *Aspergillus* sp., *Phycomycetes*, or *Histoplasma capsulatum*; algae, such as *Prototheca* sp.; Rickettsia such as *Ehrlichia canis*; protozoa such as *Encephalitozoon cuniculi*; and bacteria such as *Mycobacterium bovis*. Small, gray-white, granulomatous foci (2 to 5 mm) or larger nodules (up to 10 cm in diameter) can be scattered randomly throughout the kidneys of animals with granulomatous nephritis. These foci are white to tan, dry, and granular and can have calcified, caseous centers. Microscopically, lesions are characterized by central foci of necrosis surrounded by epithelioid macrophages, variable minerals, and giant cells that contain acid-fast bacteria.

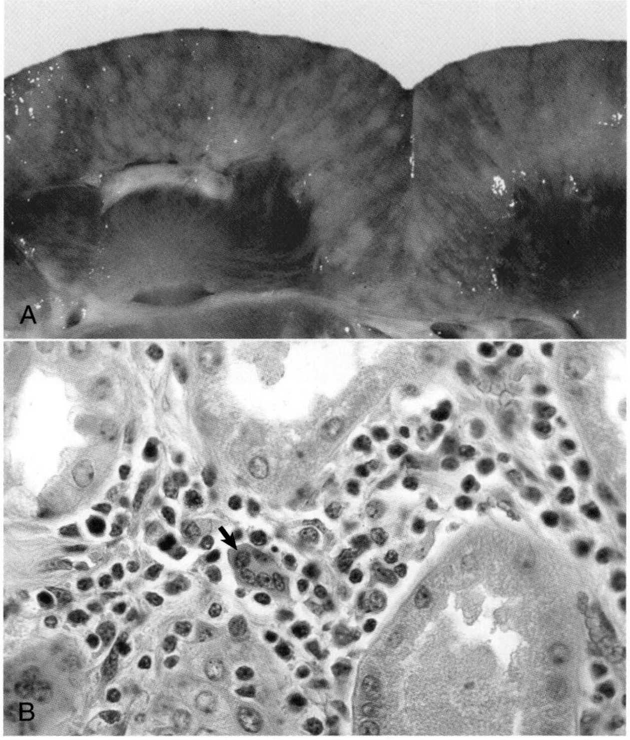

Fig. 11-56 Granulomatous nephritis, hairy vetch toxicosis, kidney, cow. **A,** Cortical striations are obliterated by coalescing granulomatous foci associated with hairy vetch toxicosis. **B,** Cortex. Lesions associated with hairy vetch toxicosis are characterized by a mixed cell interstitial inflammatory infiltrate (macrophages, lymphocytes, and occasional multinucleated giant cell *[arrow]*) with renal tubular atrophy. It is specifically known as an unusual type of poisoning because of its ability to induce granulomatous inflammation in addition to the necrosis. The kidney is not the primary organ affected. H&E stain. (**A** courtesy Dr. J. King, College of Veterinary Medicine, Cornell University; and Dr. J. Edwards, College of Veterinary Medicine, Texas A&M University. **B** courtesy Dr. R. Panciera, College of Veterinary Medicine, Oklahoma State University.)

In cattle, granulomatous nephritis is part of the multisystemic granulomatous disease caused by hairy vetch *(Vicia villosa)* toxicosis (see the section on Disorders of Ruminants). Lesions are characterized by multifocal to coalescing cortical granulomas (Fig. 11-56, *A*). Microscopically, infiltrates of monocytes, lymphocytes, plasma cells, eosinophils, and multinucleated giant cells are seen primarily within the interstitium of the renal cortex (Fig. 11-56, *B*).

Migratory *Toxocara canis* larvae can induce small, gray-to-white granulomas (2 to 3 mm) randomly scattered throughout the subcapsular renal cortex of dogs (Fig. 11-57, *A*). Such lesions probably are due to cell-mediated foreign body immune response to the migrating larvae and are composed of aggregates of macrophages, lymphocytes, and eosinophils surrounded by fibroblasts within concentrically arranged fibrous connective tissue (Fig. 11-57, *B*). In recently acquired lesions, nematode larvae can often be seen in the center of these lesions (see Fig. 11-57, *B*). Following death, the larvae become fragmented and the debris is either phagocytosed and eliminated or less commonly retained with a resultant granulomatous response. Lesions heal by fibrosis, leaving a few finely pitted (contracted) foci on the capsular surface.

Xanthogranulomas

Cats with inherited hyperlipoproteinemia have xanthogranulomas in various organs, including the kidneys. We have observed

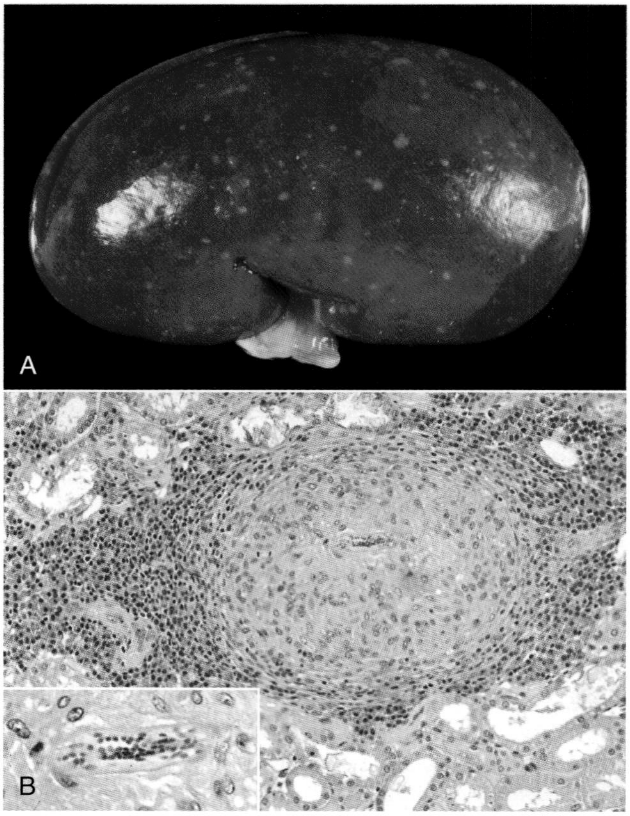

Fig. 11-57 Granulomatous nephritis, kidney, cortex, dog. **A,** Multiple subcapsular, cortical, tan, raised granulomas caused by migrating ascarid larvae. **B,** A mature granuloma composed of a central ascarid larva surrounded by epithelioid macrophages and concentrically arranged fibrous connective tissue and inflammatory cells. H&E stain. *Inset,* Ascarid larva. (Courtesy Dr. W. Crowell, College of Veterinary Medicine, The University of Georgia; and Noah's Arkive, College of Veterinary Medicine, The University of Georgia.)

similar renal xanthogranulomas in dogs with hypothyroidism and severe atherosclerosis. These lesions are characterized by foamy, lipid-laden macrophages, lymphocytes, plasma cells, and fibrosis interspersed with cleftlike spaces typical of cholesterol deposits (cholesterol clefts).

Renal Interstitial Amyloidosis

Although glomeruli are the most common renal sites for deposition of amyloid in most domestic animal species, the medullary interstitium is a common site in cats, particularly in Abyssinian breeds. Renal amyloidosis commonly occurs in association with other diseases, particularly chronic inflammatory or neoplastic diseases. However, idiopathic renal amyloidosis (i.e., amyloidosis in which an associated disease process is not recognized) is also described in dogs and cats. The underlying pathogenic mechanisms of idiopathic renal amyloidosis are not known. A hereditary predisposition for the development of reactive amyloidosis (AA) has been found in Abyssinian cats and a familial tendency is suspected in Siamese cats. Medullary amyloidosis is usually asymptomatic unless it results in papillary necrosis. Similarly, Shar Pei dogs represent one of the most commonly affected canine breeds to have systemic AA amyloidosis that accumulates preferentially in the renal interstitium, and it is thought to be autosomal recessive in its familial inheritance. The deposition of medullary amyloid may predispose the dog to various aspects of end-stage renal disease, including interstitial fibrosis, lymphoplasmacytic infiltration, tubular atrophy, tubular dilation, mineralization, deposition of oxalate crystals, glomerular atrophy, and glomerulosclerosis.

Neoplasia

The prevalence of primary renal neoplasms in domestic animals is less than 1% of the total neoplasms reported. They are usually unilateral and can be epithelial, mesenchymal, or embryonal in origin. A recent study of canine cases revealed carcinomas (49/82), sarcomas (28/82), and nephroblastomas (5/82) with a 4% bilateral involvement. Median survival for carcinomas was 16 months, for sarcomas was 9 months, and for nephroblastoma 6 months, helping confirm that primary renal tumors are highly malignant and metastatic disease is common (77%). Inappropriate polycythemia is a paraneoplastic condition seen in association with excess erythropoietin production by renal adenocarcinomas.

Epithelial Tumors

Renal adenomas are rare, benign, epithelial neoplasms comprised of proliferations of renal cortical epithelial cells, most often reported in dogs, cats, and horses. They are incidental findings at necropsy and usually appear as a small (1 to 3 cm), white-to-yellow, solitary, well-circumscribed, nonencapsulated mass in the cortex. Microscopically, adenomas are composed of solid sheets, tubules, or papillary proliferations of cuboidal epithelial cells that are uniform in size and have granular eosinophilic cytoplasm and small, round-to-oval nuclei. Mitotic figures, necrosis, and fibrosis are rare. These incidental tumors are clinically asymptomatic.

Oncocytomas are rare benign epithelial tumors that can occur in a variety of tissues. Grossly, renal oncocytomas are tan, homogeneous, well-encapsulated masses composed of oncocytes. Histologically, they are composed of large eosinophilic granular round cells with condensed round nuclei. Ultrastructurally, they are characterized by numerous prominent cytoplasmic mitochondria. Their origin in the kidney is speculated to be from the intercalated cells of the collecting ducts. These tumors are clinically asymptomatic.

Renal carcinomas are the most common primary renal neoplasms and occur most frequently in older dogs. The specific causes of renal adenocarcinomas in humans are well determined compared with those in animal species, but several mechanisms have been proved in natural animal disease or experimental models. These include the following:

- Viruses—herpesvirus oncogenes are known to play a major role in formation of virally induced adenocarcinoma (Lucke's tumor) in the kidney of frogs, and avian erythroblastosis virus [strain ES4] induces renal adenocarcinomas in chickens.
- Chemical carcinogens—these have been postulated to be causative and typically exert their neoplastic influence by direct DNA damage or inhibition of DNA synthesis or repair.
- Autosomal dominant gene mutations in Eker rats—these predispose these rats to bilateral renal cell carcinoma and a variety of other secondary cancers, resembling the human von Hippel-Lindau disease.

These neoplasms are usually large (up to 20 cm in diameter), spherical to oval, and firm. They often are pale yellow and contain dark areas of hemorrhage and necrosis and foci of cystic degeneration. The masses usually occupy and obliterate one pole of the kidney and grow by expansion, compressing the adjacent normal

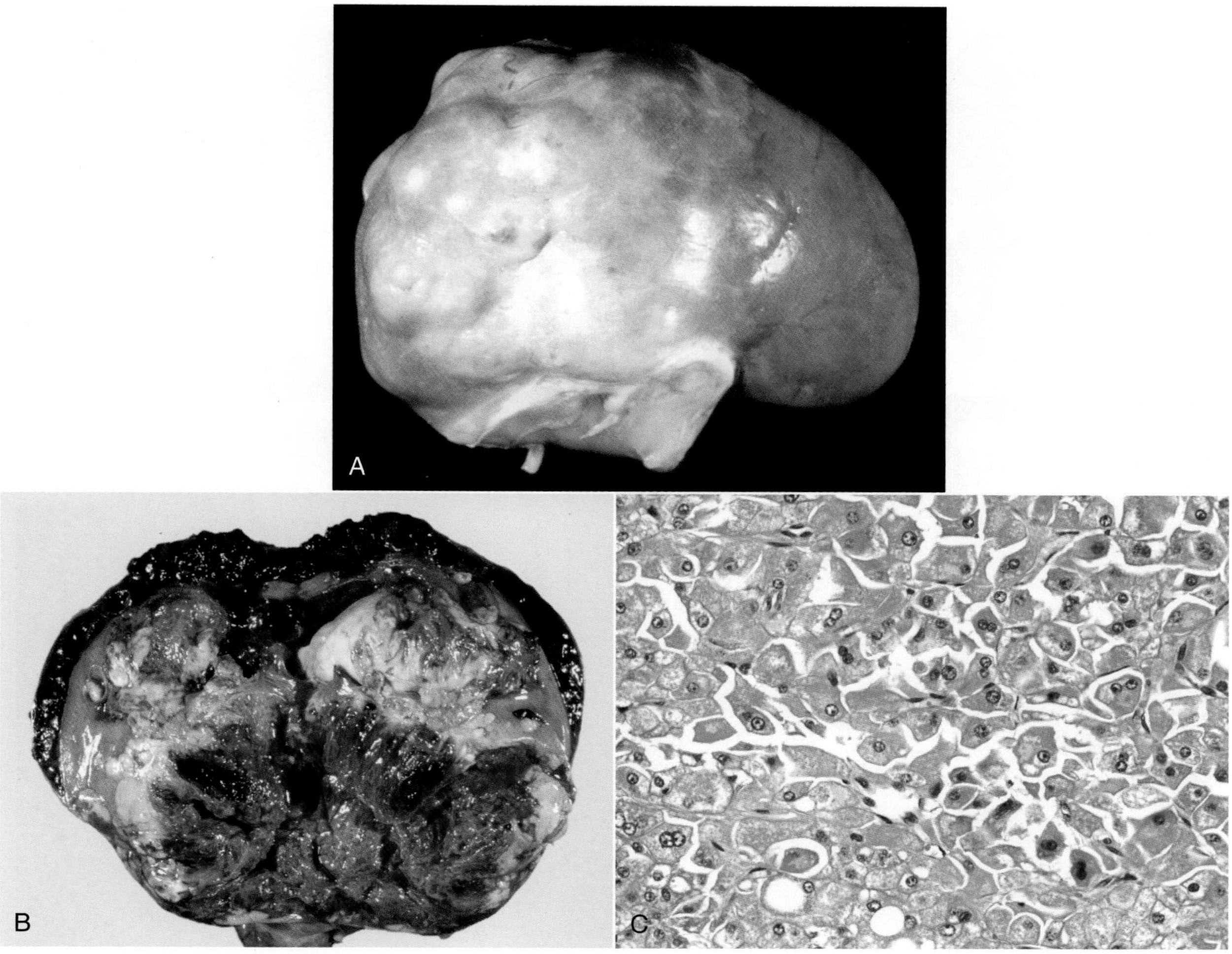

Fig. 11-58 Renal carcinoma, kidney, dog.
A, The neoplasm is pale white with reddish areas, lobulated, and has infiltrated and replaced one pole of the kidney. **B,** Dorsal section. The normal architecture of the cranial half of the kidney has been obliterated by the tumor, which has hemorrhaged caudally into the adjacent kidney and subcapsularly. **C,** The tumor consists of anaplastic renal epithelial cells, typical of the solid, more poorly differentiated variant of renal carcinoma. H&E stain. (**A** and **B** courtesy College of Veterinary Medicine, University of Illinois. **C** courtesy Dr. S.J. Newman, College of Veterinary Medicine, University of Tennessee.)

renal tissue (Fig. 11-58, *A* and *B*). Histologic types include papillary, tubular, and solid (Fig. 11-58, *C*), with solid variants being the most poorly differentiated. Metastasis to the lungs, lymph nodes, liver, and adrenal occur frequently. Renal carcinoma has been associated with paraneoplastic conditions, principally polycythemia. This is because of concurrent overexpression of erythropoietin, which increases bone marrow production of red blood cells.

A variant of the typical renal carcinoma has been seen in German shepherd dogs in conjunction with nodular dermatofibrosis. The lesions are hereditary and consist of multifocal, bilateral, renal cystadenomas or cystadenocarcinomas. Grossly, these resemble the adenocarcinomas described previously, but cysts are much more prominent. The neoplastic cells form solid sheets, tubules, or papillary growth patterns, and the cells in the carcinomas are more atypical and anaplastic. Cells vary in shape from cuboidal and columnar to polyhedral, vary in size, and have clear or granular eosinophilic cytoplasm. Nuclei range from small, round, granular, and uniform to large, oval, vesicular, and pleomorphic. Mitotic figures are numerous. These neoplasms have a moderate fibrovascular stroma.

Transitional cell papillomas and transitional cell carcinomas arise in the renal pelvis and lower urinary tract and when large, can obstruct urinary outflow. Such carcinomas can invade into the kidney and typically carry a poor prognosis. The morphologic features of transitional cell neoplasms are discussed later with the urinary bladder neoplasms (see the section on the Lower Urinary System).

Mesenchymal Tumors

Occasionally, fibromas, fibrosarcomas, or hemangiosarcomas originate in the kidneys. Primary renal sarcomas are rare. Microscopically, in hemangiosarcomas (HAS), neoplastic spindle cells are arranged in solid interlacing bundles and whorls or as variable channels lined by neoplastic endothelium. Cellular pleomorphism and mitotic rate are relatively low. Dogs with renal HAS have protracted disease progression with improved 1-year survival rates and longer median survival times compared to dogs with splenic carcinoma or retroperitoneal HAS.

Metastatic Tumors

Carcinomas and sarcomas (metastatic tumors) arising in other organs can metastasize to the kidneys and are characteristically composed of randomly scattered multiple nodules, usually involving both kidneys (Fig. 11-59). Renal lymphosarcoma occurs with

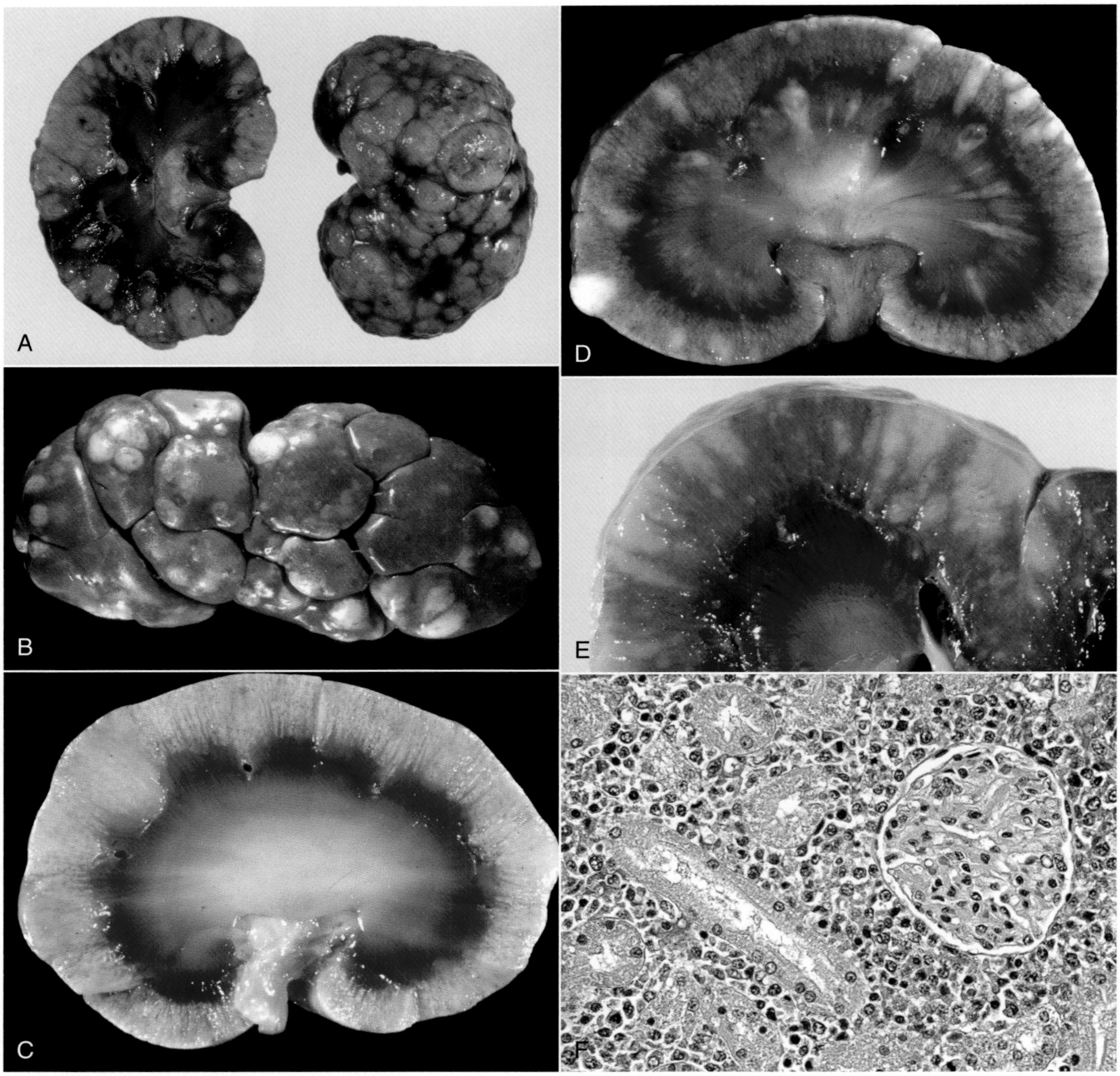

Fig. 11-59 Primary and metastatic renal tumors, kidney.
A, Metastatic mast cell tumor, dorsal section, dog. Multiple pale tan, raised nodules are randomly scattered throughout the renal cortex. **B,** Lymphoma (lymphosarcoma), cow. Multifocal raised pale white nodules are typical of nodular renal lymphosarcoma. **C,** Lymphoma (lymphosarcoma), dorsal section, cat. Note the pale white areas in the cortex, which bulge from the surface. This lesion can be confused with the granulomatous vasculitis of renal feline infectious peritonitis, thus warranting histologic evaluation. **D,** Systemic cryptococcosis *(Cryptococcus neoformans),* cat. This is not a neoplasm, but the multiple pale, occasionally raised nodules can be confused with the nodular form of lymphoma **(C),** thus requiring histologic examination. **E,** Lymphoma (lymphosarcoma), dorsal section, bovine. Multiple coalescing pale white nodules are present throughout the cortex. **F,** Lymphoma (lymphosarcoma), cow. Neoplastic lymphocytes infiltrate and distend the renal interstitium. H&E stain. (**A** courtesy Dr. A. Confer, College of Veterinary Medicine, Oklahoma State University. **B** courtesy College of Veterinary Medicine, University of Illinois. **C** courtesy Dr. K. Read, College of Veterinary Medicine, Texas A&M University; and Noah's Arkive, College of Veterinary Medicine, The University of Georgia. **D** courtesy Dr. S.J. Newman, College of Veterinary Medicine, University of Tennessee. **E** courtesy Dr. J. King, College of Veterinary Medicine, Cornell University; and Dr. J. Edwards, College of Veterinary Medicine, Texas A&M University. **F** courtesy Dr. J.F. Zachary, College of Veterinary Medicine, University of Illinois.)

some frequency in cattle and cats, particularly as part of generalized or multicentric lymphosarcoma, which is secondary to retrovirus infection. These neoplastic foci appear as single or multiple homogeneous gray-white nodules (Fig. 11-59, *B* and *E*) or as diffuse lymphomatous infiltrates that cause uniform enlargement and pale discoloration of the kidney (Fig. 11-59, *C*). In cats, renal lymphosarcoma must be differentiated histologically from the necrotizing, fibrinous, and granulomatous renal vasculitis of feline infectious peritonitis and less commonly systemic cryptococcosis (Fig. 11-59, *E*). Microscopically, neoplastic lymphocytes form obliterative sheets of cells within the renal parenchyma, unrelated to the vasculature (Fig. 11-59, *F*). Neoplastic lymphocytes have distinct cellular borders, moderate amounts of basophilic cytoplasm, and large round vesicular nuclei with variable prominence to the nucleoli. Lymphosarcoma of the kidney can be treated with some success with chemotherapeutics.

Tumors of Embryonal Origin

Nephroblastomas (embryonal nephroma or Wilms tumor) are common renal neoplasms of pigs and chickens, and are usually recognized as incidental findings at slaughter. They occur in cattle and dogs as well, but less frequently. These neoplasms arise from metanephric blastema and thus occur in young animals. It is speculated that neoplasms result from malignant transformation during normal nephrogenesis or from neoplastic transformation of nests of embryonic tissue that persists in the postnatal kidneys. At necropsy, nephroblastomas can be solitary or multiple masses that often reach a great size and in which recognizable renal tissue can be difficult to detect. They usually are soft to rubbery and gray with foci of hemorrhage. On a cut surface, they are often lobulated. Because nephroblastomas arise from primitive pluripotential tissue, histologic features vary but are morphologically similar to the developmental stages of embryonic kidneys. Characteristically, three components, including primitive, loose myxomatous mesenchymal tissue interspersed with primitive tubules lined by elongated, deeply staining cells and structures that resemble primitive glomeruli, are present. Nests of cells resembling the metanephric blastema can be present. Nephroblastomas also have mesenchymal components such as cartilage, bone, skeletal muscle, and adipose tissue. Clinically, these are usually incidental findings, except in dogs, in which they rarely present as spinal dysfunction, the result of spread to the vertebral canal with secondary spinal cord compression.

LOWER URINARY SYSTEM

Developmental Anomalies

Aplasia and Hypoplasia

Ureteral aplasia (agenesis) is the lack of formation of a recognizable ureter, and hypoplasia is the presence of a notably small-diameter ureter. Agenesis of the ureters is the result of failure of the ureteral bud to form and may be unilateral or bilateral. Both conditions are rare. If these defects occur alone, then there is disruption of urinary flow from the kidney to the urinary bladder, resulting in obstructive diseases such as hydronephrosis. If these defects occur with concurrent renal aplasia, then they are clinically silent when unilateral and life-threatening when bilateral.

Ectopic Ureters

Ectopic ureters are ureters that may empty into the urethra, vagina, neck of the bladder, ductus deferens, prostate, or other secondary sex glands. The two possible causes are as follows:

- The ureteral bud arises too far craniad to be incorporated into the urogenital sinus.
- The differential growth of the sinus is abnormal, and the ureter fails to migrate to its usual location.

Ectopic ureters are more subject to obstruction or infection, and thus they predispose animals to pyelitis and pyelonephritis. Otherwise, histologically these are normal. This condition is found most frequently in dogs and certain breeds, especially the Siberian husky, are at greater risk. Affected animals present clinically with urinary incontinence and consequent urine dribbling.

Patent Urachus

The most common malformation of the urinary bladder is patent urachus (pervious urachus). This lesion develops when the fetal urachus fails to close and therefore forms a direct channel between the bladder's apex and the umbilicus. Failure of the urachal remnant and the umbilical arteries and vein to involute is frequently observed in cases of "neonatal" omphalitis, in which abscess formation may result in a patent urachus. Patent urachus has also occurred because of congenital urethral obstruction. Increased bladder pressure, because of the obstruction, forces urine out into the urachus. Rupture of the urachus causes uroperitoneum. The condition must be differentiated from perinatal rupture of the bladder. Foals are affected most often and animals with this defect dribble urine from the umbilicus. Diverticula of the bladder may be primary or acquired and secondary to partial obstruction of the outflow of urine or the result of pressure changes exerted during normal contractions. Occasionally, during urachal closure, the mucosa closes but closure of the bladder musculature is incomplete. When this occurs, a bladder diverticulum (outpouching) at the apex of the bladder can develop. Urine stasis can occur in the diverticulum, predisposing the animal to cystitis or urinary calculi.

Hydroureter and Hydrourethra

Hydroureter and hydrourethra refer to dilation of the ureter and urethra, respectively, and are caused by obstruction of urine outflow by blockage of the ureter(s) or urethra by calculi, chronic inflammation, or luminal or intramural neoplasia. Hydroureter can be unilateral or bilateral. Depending on the location of the obstruction, hydronephrosis, hydroureter, and hydrourethra can occur concurrently (see the previous section on Hydronephrosis). Histologic findings demonstrate little change except for a greater cross-sectional diameter of the ureter or urethra and compression of their lining epithelium. The clinical signs of these conditions are related to obstruction.

Urolithiasis (Obstructive Disease)

Urolithiasis is a syndrome that occurs when familial, congenital, and pathophysiologic factors occur together and increase the risk of precipitation of excretory metabolites in urine to form stones. Urinary calculi (uroliths) are concretions formed anywhere in the urinary collecting system, and although some clearly originate in the lower urinary tract or as microscopic calculi in the renal collecting tubules, the point of development of most is not known. Uroliths are commonly found in the ureter, followed by any portion of the lower urinary tract and least commonly in the renal pelvis (accounting for 1% to 4% of canine uroliths). The diseases caused by uroliths are among the most important urinary tract problems of domesticated animals, especially cattle, sheep, dogs, and cats, and are of lesser importance in horses and pigs.

Mechanistically, factors that are important either in predisposing to calculus formation or in precipitating disease include the following:

- Calculus precursor material in urine in quantities sufficient to be precipitated.
- Substances metabolized in an unusual way, as is uric acid in Dalmatian dogs.
- Substances processed abnormally by the kidney (hereditary defects), as with cystine or xanthine.
- Substances are encountered in the diet in abnormally high levels such as the following:
  - Silicic acid in native pastures
  - Phosphate in milo or sorghum products (struvites)
  - Estrogen in subterranean clover (clover stones [benzocoumarin] or carbonates)
  - Magnesium in commercial dry cat food
  - Oxalate in oxalate-accumulating plants (oxalates)
- Abnormally low levels of a substance are encountered in the diet such as the following:
  - Vitamin A (equivocal evidence that vitamin A deficiency may produce metaplastic change in the urinary tract epithelium

that creates a nidus of calculus formation following desquamation of epithelium)

Regardless of the type of calculus, certain factors are more or less important in calculus formation; these are as follows:

- Urinary pH, in terms of its optimum for solute precipitation (oxalates at acid pH and struvites and carbonates at alkaline pH)
- Reduced water intake, in relation to the degree of urine concentration and mineral supersaturation
- Bacterial infection of the lower urinary tract (struvite calculi in dogs)
- Obstruction
- Structural abnormalities of the lower urinary system
- Foreign bodies (suture, grass awn, catheter, or needle), or a conglomerate of bacterial colonies, exfoliated epithelium, or leukocytes, which can serve as a nidus for precipitation of mineral constituents
- Drugs excreted in the urine, which may act as a nidus for calculus formation (e.g., sulfonamides and tetracyclines)

Supersaturation of urine with respect to the components of stone-forming salts is the essential precursor to initiation of urolith formation (nucleation). Supersaturation may be in the unstable range, in which precipitation occurs spontaneously (homogeneous nucleation), or the metastable range, in which precipitation occurs by epitaxy (one type of crystal grows on the surface of another type; heterogeneous nucleation).

Although it was formerly thought that urinary proteins, such as uromucoid, which make up 5% to 20% or more of some calculi, were preeminent initiators of crystal formation in the metastable range, it is now believed that in many cases either co-precipitation of proteins and minerals occurs or that proteins are adsorbed onto formed crystals. It is possible that crystals of one salt, for which urine is supersaturated in the unstable range, cause induction of crystals of another salt for which supersaturation is apparently stable.

Crystals are much more common in urine than are calculi. Even though equine urine is normally supersaturated with calcium carbonate, and crystalluria is normal, horses experience a low prevalence of calculi. The factors, which promote or prevent crystal growth and crystal aggregation, are poorly understood. Experimentally, high concentrations of urinary inorganic pyrophosphate and magnesium are important inhibitors of calcium phosphate and calcium oxalate crystallization. Pyrophosphate also inhibits aggregation of calcium phosphate crystals. Certain urinary macromolecules, probably glycosaminoglycans, are also strong inhibitors of crystal aggregation in experimental systems. Deficiency of inhibitors of crystallization may be important in calcium oxalate and calcium phosphate calculogenesis (crystallization-inhibition theory of urolith initiation).

Macroscopically, calculi are grossly visible aggregations of precipitated urinary solutes, principally mineral admixed with urinary proteins and proteinaceous debris. Calculi typically are hard spheres or ovoids, with a central nidus, surrounded by concentric laminae ("stone"), an outer shell, and surface crystals. Many calculi contain significant quantities of "contaminants" such as calcium oxalates in "silica" calculi; few are relatively pure. Large renal pelvic calculi classically have a "staghorn" appearance because they take the shape of the renal calyces in animal species that have true calyces (Fig. 11-60). These calculi predispose affected animals to pyelitis and pyelonephritis. Urinary bladder calculi can be single or multiple, variable in size (2 to 10 cm), and sometimes are composed of a fine, sandlike material, which causes cloudy urine (Fig. 11-61). Calculi can have smooth or rough surfaces and may be solid, soft, or friable. Calculi vary in color, depending on their composition; however,

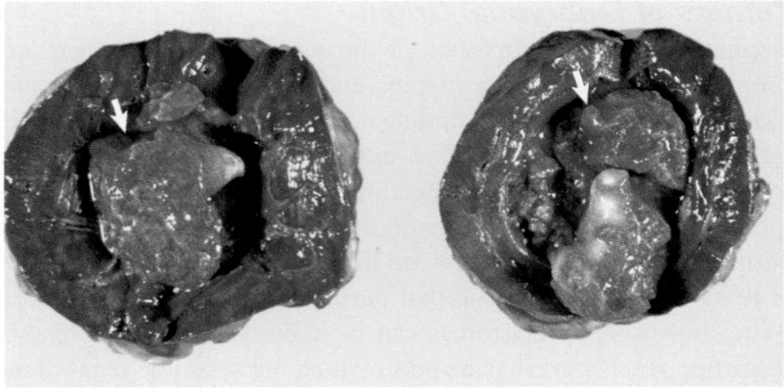

Fig. 11-60 Urolithiasis, kidney, dorsal section, dog.
A calculus fills and distends the renal pelvis *(arrows)* and has caused pressure atrophy of the medulla. (Courtesy Dr. M.D. McGavin, College of Veterinary Medicine, University of Tennessee.)

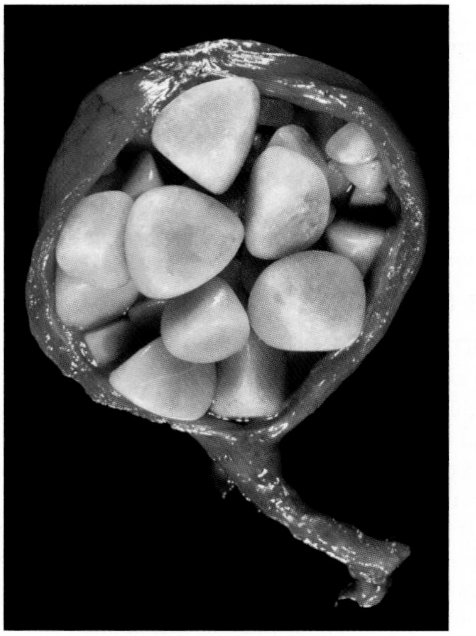

Fig. 11-61 Urolithiasis, urinary bladder, dog.
Multiple smooth calculi are present in the urinary bladder. The bladder wall is diffusely thickened. (Courtesy Dr. A. Confer, College of Veterinary Medicine, Oklahoma State University.)

color is variable among calculi, even of the same composition. The calculi can be white to gray (e.g., struvite and oxalate), yellow (e.g., urate, cystine, benzocoumarin, and xanthine), or brown (e.g., silica, urate, and xanthine), depending on their composition.

Small calculi may be voided in the urine, but typically calculi cause urinary obstruction. This is more common in males because of their long and narrow-diameter urethra. The most common sites of lodgement of urethral calculi vary with the animal species. In male cattle, calculi lodge in the urethra at the ischial arch and at the proximal end of the sigmoid flexure; in rams and wethers, the urethral process (vermiform appendage) is the most common site (Fig. 11-62, *A*); and in dogs, calculi lodge proximal to the base of the os penis (Fig. 11-62, *B*). At the site in which calculi lodge, there is local pressure necrosis, ulceration of the mucosa, and acute hemorrhagic urethritis. Because the urethral sites are prone to rupture, hydronephrosis after urethral obstruction is less common than with unilateral long-standing ureteral impaction. In cats, fine struvite crystals (sand) in a rubberlike protein matrix can fill the entire urethra, and such calculi are typical for the disease

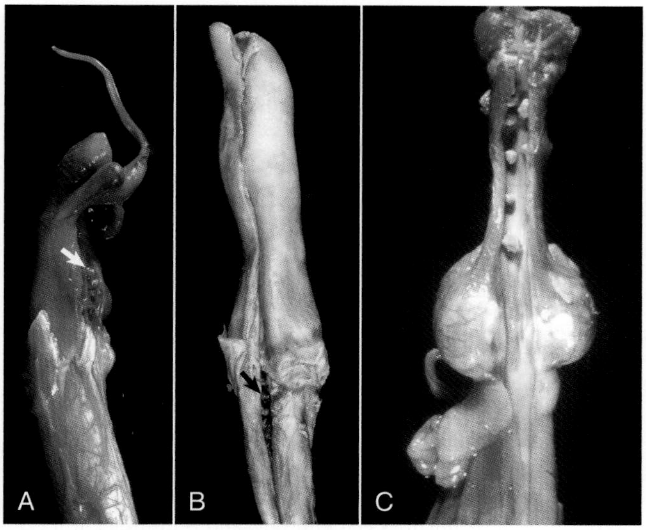

Fig. 11-62 Urolithiasis, penile urethra.
A, Sheep. Multiple calculi are present in the penile urethra *(arrow)* and the urethral process (vermiform appendage). **B,** Ventral aspect, dog. Calculi have lodged in the urethra proximal to the caudal end of the os penis *(arrow)*. **C,** Cat. Calculi are present throughout the penile urethra, several just caudal to the external urethral orifice at tip of the penis. (**A** and **B** courtesy Dr. M.D. McGavin, College of Veterinary Medicine, University of Tennessee. **C** courtesy College of Veterinary Medicine, University of Illinois.)

called *feline urologic syndrome* (Fig. 11-62, *C*). When obstruction or dysuria occurs in females, calculi are usually large and located in the renal pelvis or urinary bladder.

At necropsy, animals that have died of urinary obstruction have greatly distended (Fig. 11-63, *A*), turgid, or ruptured bladders and dilated ureters and renal pelves. The bladder wall is thin and often has mucosal to transmural ecchymoses or diffuse hemorrhage (Fig. 11-63, *B*). When urine is released from the bladder, either because of rupture or incision at surgery or necropsy, the wall of the bladder is flaccid, the mucosa is often ulcerated, and the urine contains blood clots. Mucosal ulceration, localized lamina propria hemorrhage, and mucosal necrosis are usually present in the ureter, bladder, or urethra adjacent to an obstructive calculus. If the bladder ruptures antemortem, blood clots and fibrin are at the site of rupture, and in some cases there is an acute, localized chemical (urine-induced) peritonitis.

Microscopically, inflammation and hemorrhage are present in the lower urinary tract. Lesions are most severe in cases in which obstruction has been complete. The mucosa is usually ulcerated, and areas of hyperplastic transitional epithelium are interspersed with goblet cells. The lamina propria is usually infiltrated with inflammatory cells. Neutrophils are present at foci of ulceration, and lymphocytes and plasma cells infiltrate perivascularly or uniformly throughout the lamina propria. Hemorrhage is transmural but is most evident in the mucosa and can cause separation of the smooth muscle bundles. Degeneration and necrosis of smooth muscle occurs in severe cases.

Clinically, urolithiasis can cause urinary obstruction or traumatic injury to the urinary bladder mucosa. Lesions of the urinary bladder are manifested clinically as difficult or painful urination (stranguria; dysuria), with or without hematuria. Small calculi may be voided in the urine, but typically calculi cause urinary obstruction. In males, dysuria can result from large calculi, but urinary tract obstruction with uremia most commonly occurs because of obstruction of the urethra with small calculi.

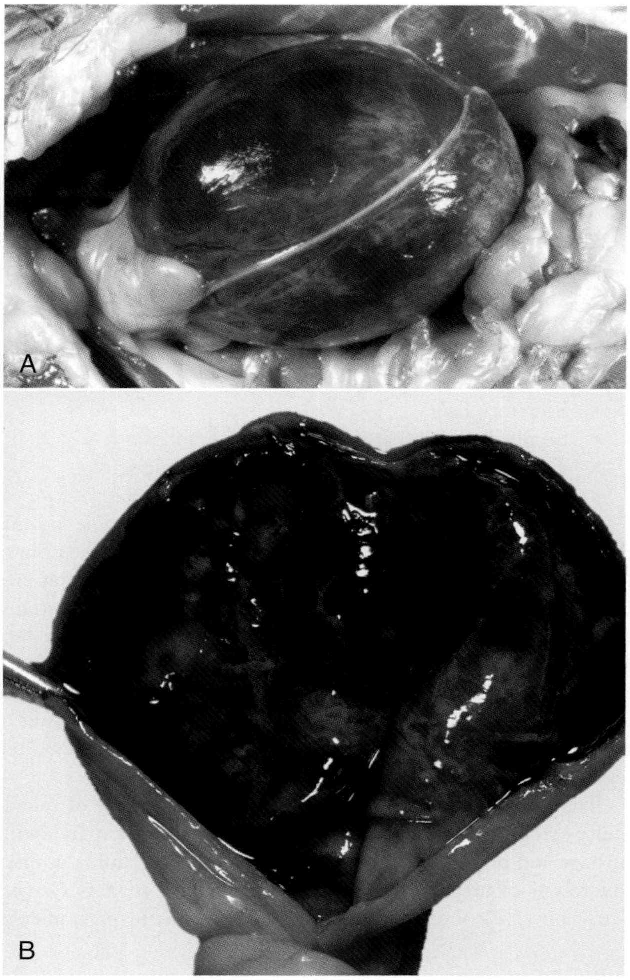

Fig. 11-63 Hemorrhagic urocystitis (feline urologic syndrome) urinary bladder, cat.
A, Obstructive urolithiasis. The bladder is overdistended and turgid as the result of urethral obstruction. Note the serosal and intramuscular ecchymotic and suffusive hemorrhages at the neck and apex of the bladder. **B,** Urolithiasis, acute hemorrhagic cystitis. The severe diffuse transmural hemorrhage throughout the urinary bladder wall is secondary to blockage of the urethra by calculi and distention of the urinary bladder. (Courtesy Dr. M.D. McGavin, College of Veterinary Medicine, University of Tennessee.)

Inflammatory Diseases

Acute Cystitis

Inflammation of the urinary bladder (cystitis) is common in domestic animals. Because inflammation of the ureter (ureteritis) or urethra (urethritis) in the absence of cystitis is rare, this discussion concentrates on cystitis. The causes of acute cystitis are varied; however, for all animal species, bacterial infection is the most common cause. Cystitis may be acute or chronic. Normally, the bladder is resistant to infection, and contaminating bacteria are quickly eliminated by the normal flow of normal urine. Predisposition to urinary tract infection (UTI) occurs when there is stagnation of urine because of obstruction, incomplete voiding at micturition, or urothelial trauma. Other risk factors for UTI include catheterization, vaginoscopy, vaginitis, urinary incontinence, or prolonged administration of medications such as antibiotics that induce bacterial resistance. Bacterial cystitis is more common in females because their relatively short urethra provides a shorter barrier to ascending infections than the longer, narrow diameter of the male urethra. The bacterial species most commonly associated with cystitis are uropathogenic *Escherichia coli* (α-hemolysin–producing strains) in all animal species; *Corynebacterium renale* in cattle; *Actinobaculum suis (Eubacterium suis)* in pigs; *Enterococcus faecalis* in cats; and *Klebsiella* sp. in horses. In addition, *Proteus* sp., *Streptococcus* sp., and *Staphylococcus* sp. have been isolated from cases of cystitis in several animal species.

Except for the distal urethra, the lower urinary tract is normally free of bacteria. Sterility of the urinary bladder is maintained through normal repeated voiding of urine and because of the antibacterial properties of urine. These antibacterial properties are attributed to the following:

- The acidic urine of carnivores
- Secretory IgA
- Secreted mucin that inhibits bacterial adhesion
- The large concentration of urea and organic acids
- High urine osmolality

Cystitis occurs when bacteria are able to overcome normal defense mechanisms and adhere to or invade (colonize) the urinary bladder mucosa. Several factors can enhance colonization and predispose animals to cystitis. Colonization is more likely for strains of bacteria that express molecules on their surfaces that enhance adhesion (e.g., the P and type 1 fimbriae of certain strains of *Escherichia coli* and *Actinobaculum suis* and the pH-dependent adherence by pili of *Corynebacterium renale*). Retention of urine as a result of obstruction or neurogenic causes, such as spinal cord diseases, often leads to cystitis.

Trauma to the urinary bladder mucosa as the result of calculi, faulty catheterization, or other causes can cause erosion and hemorrhage and predispose to bacterial invasion of the lamina propria. Hydrolysis of urea by urease-producing bacteria, such as *Corynebacterium renale* in cattle and *Actinobaculum suis* in pigs, releases excessive ammonia that can damage the mucosa and result in urine alkalinity. Bacterial growth can be enhanced when glucosuria is present, such as in diabetes mellitus. Compromise of the host immune system as found with infection by the feline immunodeficiency virus (FIV) can increase susceptibility to bacterial cystitis. Other bacterial virulence factors, such as the *Escherichia coli* hemolysin, enhance pathogenicity and help bacteria overcome antibacterial factors of the urinary bladder and urine.

Once bacteria gain access to the lamina propria, they cause vascular damage and inflammation. Acute cystitis is often grossly described as hemorrhagic, fibrinopurulent, necrotizing, or ulcerative, and these changes are often sequential over time. Vascular damage predisposes to hemorrhage, leakage of fibrin, and if severe, ischemic necrosis of the bladder. This is often accompanied by mucosal ulceration. Neutrophils are present as a component of vascular damage and in any lesion with accompanying bacterial colonization. However, in each case, components of several of these processes are present. The urinary bladder wall often is thickened by edema, an inflammatory cell infiltrate, and is diffusely or focally hemorrhagic. Hemorrhage is most common when obstruction is concurrently present or after direct trauma from catheterization. Urine in such cases is described as cloudy, flocculent, foul smelling, and red-tinged. The mucosa can have foci of erosion or ulceration, patches or sheets of adherent exudate and necrotic debris, or adherent blood clots (Fig. 11-64, *A*). *Corynebacterium urealyticum* in dogs and cats and *Corynebacterium matruchotii* in a horse were implicated in a condition known as *encrusted cystitis,* in which plaques and accumulation of sediment predominate. Rarely, surgical debridement in addition to appropriate antimicrobial therapy is required.

Microscopically, acute cystitis is characterized by epithelial denudation with bacterial colonies present on the surface. The lamina propria is intensely edematous and has a diffuse neutrophilic

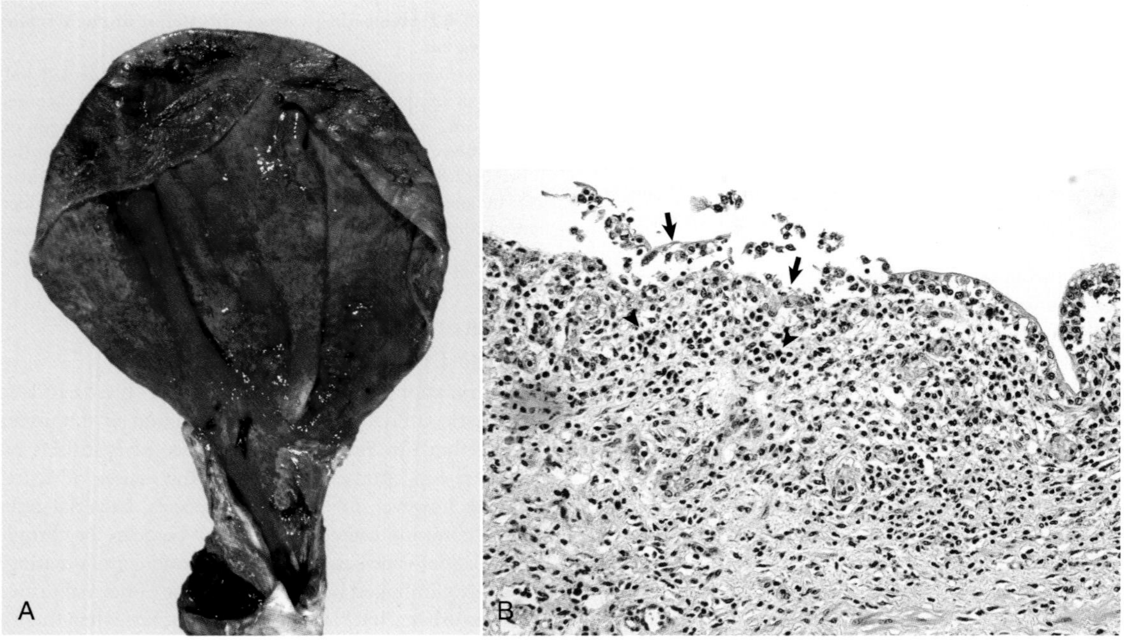

Fig. 11-64 Acute cystitis, urinary bladder.

A, Mucosal and serosal surfaces, calf. Patchy areas of ulcerated mucosa are interspersed with areas of hemorrhagic mucosa. Note the subserosal hemorrhages *(top).* **B,** Mucosal and serosal surfaces, dog. The mucosa has been partially denuded of transitional epithelium *(arrows).* There are mucosal and submucosal infiltrates of neutrophils *(arrowheads),* which extend into the adjacent tunica muscularis. Note the congested vessels with active hyperemia in the lamina propria. H&E stain. (**A** courtesy Dr. A. Confer, College of Veterinary Medicine, Oklahoma State University. **B** courtesy Dr. J.F. Zachary, College of Veterinary Medicine, University of Illinois.)

infiltrate. Superficial hyperemia and hemorrhage are usually present (Fig. 11-64, *B*). A mild perivascular leukocytic infiltrate can occur in the tunica muscularis.

Clinically, dysuria, stranguria, and hematuria characterize acute onset of bacterial cystitis. An inflammatory sediment is detected on urinalysis, and bacteria can be grown in pure culture from urine samples.

Viral causes of acute cystitis are relatively rare in veterinary medicine. In cats, a cell-associated herpesvirus has been found in some cases of mild cystitis. Hemorrhagic cystitis sometimes occurs in malignant catarrhal fever in cattle and deer and occasionally is the dominant gross feature in the disease.

Acute cystitis can result from several chemical causes. Active metabolites of cyclophosphamide, a drug used to treat neoplastic and immune-mediated diseases of dogs and cats, can cause a sterile hemorrhagic cystitis. Cantharidin toxicosis in horses results from ingestion of blister beetles (*Epicauta* spp.) in alfalfa hay, and hemorrhagic and necrotic cystitis develops from cantharidin excreted through the urinary tract. Chronic ingestion of bracken fern *(Pteridium aquilinum)* by cattle can result in the syndrome of enzootic hematuria, which can be manifested as acute urinary bladder hemorrhage, chronic cystitis, or urinary bladder neoplasia.

Chronic Cystitis

Chronic cystitis presents as several forms based on the pattern and type of inflammatory response noted. These forms include diffuse, follicular, and polypoid variants. Diffuse variants reveal an irregularly reddened and usually thickened mucosa. There is some epithelial desquamation, and the submucosa is heavily infiltrated with mononuclear inflammatory cells; there are few neutrophils. In addition, there is often connective tissue thickening of the submucosa and hypertrophy of the muscularis layer.

Follicular variants reveal disseminated, nodular, submucosal lymphoid proliferations (2 to 4 mm in diameter) so that the mucosa has a cobblestone appearance (follicular cystitis) (Fig. 11-65). This response is particularly common when cystitis is associated with chronic urolithiasis. These white-gray lymphoid foci are often surrounded by a zone of hyperemia. Often, the lesions are a diffusely thickened, hyperplastic mucosa with goblet cell hyperplasia and a chronic lymphoplasmacytic infiltrate and fibrosis in the lamina propria. Hypertrophy of the tunica muscularis can be observed.

Polypoid masses (chronic polypoid cystitis), seen predominantly in female dogs, likely develop from inflammatory and hyperplastic responses secondary to chronic irritation, which most often arises from persistent bacterial urinary tract infection or uroliths. These hyperplastic transitional epithelial responses are called cystitis cystica, cystitis glandularis, and Brunn's epithelial nests. Inflammation, epithelial proliferation, and development of a nonneoplastic mass occur most typically in the cranioventral bladder wall. The mucosa has single or multiple nodular mucosal masses (Fig. 11-66) composed of fibrous connective tissue and infiltrated with neutrophils and mononuclear leukocytes. The masses are broad-based or pedunculated, ulcerated, or covered by hyperplastic epithelium with goblet cell metaplasia. Chronic polypoid cystitis is characterized by clinical hematuria.

Toxic Cystitis

Bracken Fern–Induced Hemorrhagic Urocystitis

Information on this topic is available at evolve.elsevier.com/Zachary/McGavin/.

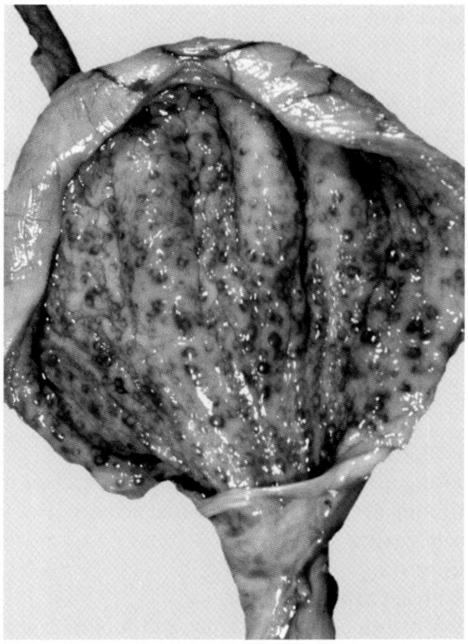

Fig. 11-65 Chronic follicular cystitis, urinary bladder, mucosal surface, dog.
Multiple small raised red nodules are present on the mucosal surface. These nodules are hyperplastic lymphoid cells surrounded by hyperemia and hemorrhage. (Courtesy Dr. A. Confer, College of Veterinary Medicine, Oklahoma State University.)

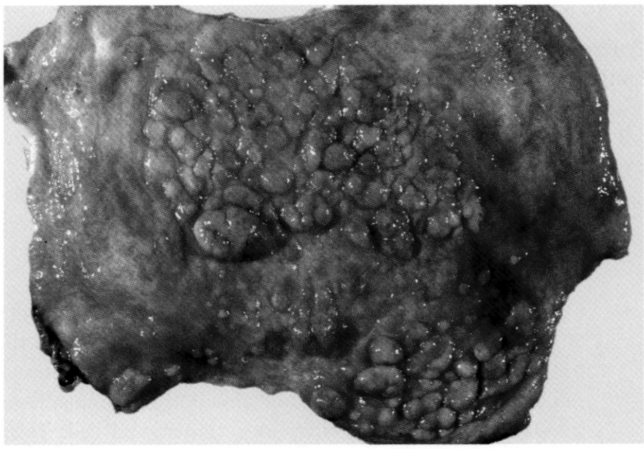

Fig. 11-66 Chronic polypoid cystitis, urinary bladder, mucosal surface, dog.
This type of cystitis is characterized by multiple masses composed of proliferative nodules of connective tissue (polyps) mixed with neutrophils and lymphocytes. (Courtesy Dr. A. Confer, College of Veterinary Medicine, Oklahoma State University.)

Bracken fern–induced neoplasia is discussed later in more detail in the section on Disorders of Ruminants.

Mycotic Cystitis

Mycotic cystitis is occasionally seen in domestic animals when opportunistic fungi, such as *Candida albicans* or *Aspergillus* sp., colonize the urinary bladder mucosa. Such fungal infections usually occur secondary to chronic bacterial cystitis, especially when animals are immunosuppressed or subjected to prolonged antibiotic therapy. Occasionally, *Blastomyces dermatitidis* can produce lower urinary tract lesions in dogs. The urinary bladder is usually ulcerated with proliferation of underlying lamina propria; a generalized thickening of the urinary bladder wall is the result of extensive inflammation consisting of neutrophils, lymphocytes, plasma cells, macrophages and edema, and fibrosis.

Neoplasia

Neoplasms of the lower urinary tract occur predominantly in the urinary bladder. Neoplasms are much more common in the bladder than the urethra and are rare in the ureter. They are observed most frequently in dogs, occasionally in cats, and rarely in other species. Urinary bladder neoplasms comprise less than 1% of total canine neoplasms. Most occur in old dogs, without a sex predisposition.

Risk factors associated with bladder cancer in dogs include the following:

- Topical insecticides
- Exposure to marshes sprayed with chemicals for mosquitoes
- Environments with high industrial activity
- Female gender
- Obesity
- Breed (e.g., Scottish terrier)

Retention of urine in the bladder and longer exposure of the epithelium to carcinogens results in a higher incidence of tumors in the urinary bladder. Many chemicals, including intermediate components of aniline dyes, aromatic hydrocarbons, and tryptophan metabolites, have been found experimentally or epidemiologically to induce urinary bladder neoplasms. Chemically induced and spontaneous tumors progress through a series of histologic stages from hyperplasia, squamous metaplasia, papilloma, adenoma, dysplasia, carcinoma in situ, to carcinoma.

Epithelial Tumors

Epithelial neoplasms are by far the most common of the urinary system and are classified as transitional cell papillomas, transitional cell carcinomas, squamous cell carcinomas, adenocarcinomas, and undifferentiated carcinomas, as follows:

- Papillomas have a papilliferous or pedunculated appearance. Microscopically, they have a papillary growth pattern consisting of multiple papilliferous fibrous cores covered by well-differentiated transitional epithelium.
- Carcinomas are focal, raised nodules or diffuse thickenings of the urinary bladder wall that are most common in the trigone region of the bladder (Fig. 11-67, *A*). Transitional cell carcinomas are composed of pleomorphic to anaplastic transitional epithelium. Neoplastic transitional cells cover the mucosal surface as irregular layers, readily invade the lamina propria in the form of solid nests and acini, and are found within lymphatic vessels of the submucosal and muscle layers (Fig. 11-67, *B*). Terriers may be at a slightly elevated risk for development, and there has been an association made between occurrence of these tumors and exposure to lawn pesticides. This neoplasm in cats is rare but aggressive when present. Males are more commonly affected. Unlike dogs, the trigone area is not the predilection site for development.
- Squamous cell carcinomas, adenocarcinomas, and unclassified carcinomas most likely arise from transitional epithelium. In the bitch, carcinomas are multicentric in origin, develop not only in the urinary bladder but also in the urothelium of the ureters, urethra, and renal pelvis, and often extend to the vagina and vestibule.

Metastasis of urinary bladder carcinomas is most often first seen in regional lymph nodes adjacent to the aortic bifurcation, including the deep inguinal, medial iliac, and sacral lymph nodes. Other potential sites of metastasis include lungs and kidneys, with metastasis to other parenchymatous organs occurring later.

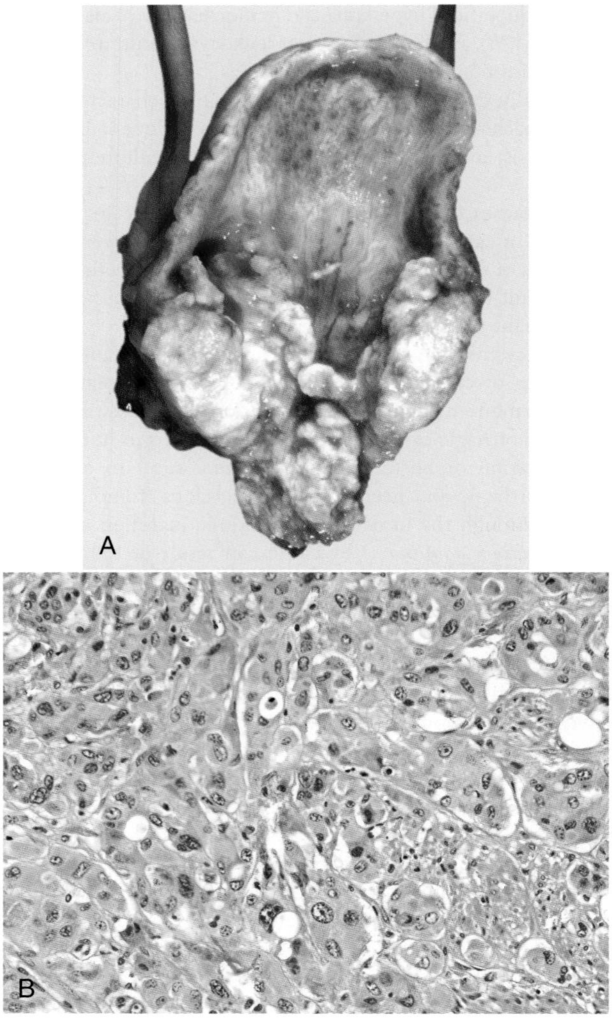

Fig. 11-67 Transitional cell carcinoma, urinary bladder, dog. **A,** Transitional cell carcinomas are typically adjacent to the trigone (as here), where they can become large enough to obstruct the opening of a ureter or ureters and result in secondary hydroureter and/or hydronephrosis. **B,** Lamina propria. The tumor is formed by anaplastic cells grouped in small islands and clusters. Nuclei are vesicular with prominent nucleoli, and some nuclei show remarkable anisokaryosis. H&E stain. (**A** courtesy Dr. A. Confer, College of Veterinary Medicine, Oklahoma State University. **B** courtesy Dr. S.J. Newman, College of Veterinary Medicine, University of Tennessee.)

Mesenchymal Tumors

Mesenchymal tumors, including fibromas, fibrosarcomas, leiomyomas, leiomyosarcomas, rhabdomyosarcomas, lymphosarcomas, hemangiomas, and hemangiosarcomas, occur in the lower tract. Primary fibrosarcomas, leiomyosarcomas, hemangiomas, and hemangiosarcomas are rare. Mesenchymal tumors are classified as follows:

- Leiomyomas are the most common neoplasms and are solitary or multiple, circumscribed, firm, and pale white-to-tan masses in the urinary bladder wall. Leiomyomas have the macroscopic consistency and microscopic appearance of normal smooth muscle. Malignant counterparts

(leiomyosarcoma) are much more rarely identified. These are locally infiltrative but only rarely show metastatic spread.
- Fibromas arise from lamina propria connective tissue and project into the bladder lumen as solitary nodules.
- Lymphosarcoma occasionally infiltrates the wall, not only of the bladder but also of the ureters and renal pelves in cattle, pigs, dogs, and/or cats. Common complications include hydronephrosis and hydroureter.
- Rhabdomyosarcomas are rare but occur in the bladder and urethra of young large breed dogs (younger than 18 months old), suggesting an embryonal origin. The cell of origin is speculated to be embryonic myoblasts from the urogenital ridge. These masses are described as botryoid (grapelike) masses (4 to 18 cm in diameter) that protrude into the bladder lumen. Local invasion and occasional metastasis to lymph nodes characterize the typical behavior. Microscopically, the neoplasms are composed of sheets of fusiform cells interspersed with pleomorphic cells. Microscopic demonstration of cross-striations typical of skeletal muscle or immunohistochemical demonstration of the intermediate filament, desmin, are useful to confirm the diagnosis of rhabdomyosarcoma. Clinical presentation includes hematuria, urinary obstruction, hydroureter, hydronephrosis, and hypertrophic osteopathy.

DISORDERS OF HORSES

EMBOLIC NEPHRITIS *(ACTINOBACILLUS EQUULI)*

Actinobacillus equuli is a normal inhabitant of the mucous membranes of the alimentary tract. Fecal contamination or extension from oral mucous membranes is the method of inoculation. Umbilical contamination in foals is the most common route of infection. Microabscesses occur in a variety of organs, including the kidney, as multifocal random, raised, tan pinpoint foci on the cut surface throughout the renal cortex (see Fig. 11-42, *A* and *B*). Microscopically, glomerular capillaries contain numerous bacterial colonies intermixed with necrotic debris and extensive infiltrates of neutrophils that often obliterate the glomerulus (see Fig. 11-42, *C*). As with many other inflammatory diseases, if the affected animal survives, the neutrophilic infiltrates will either persist as focal residual abscesses or be progressively replaced by increasing numbers of lymphocytes, plasma cells, macrophages, reactive fibroblasts, and ultimately coalescing scars.

MYOGLOBINURIC NEPHROSIS (RHABDOMYOLYSIS)

A set of events leading to ischemic tubular necrosis frequently occurs in hypoperfused kidneys complicated by myoglobinuria. In these diseases, serum concentrations of myoglobin are increased, as these products pass into the glomerular filtrate, producing greatly increased intraluminal concentrations that cause myoglobinuric nephrosis. Myoglobin does not use a carrier protein for transportation and because it is a small molecule, it freely passes through the glomerulus and is excreted in the urine. Myoglobin is not nephrotoxic in itself, and intravenous infusions into healthy animals produce no recognizable lesions. However, large concentrations of myoglobin in the glomerular filtrate can increase the tubular necrosis that occurs as a result of renal ischemia; for example, in rhabdomyolysis in horses, renal ischemia is secondary to hypovolemic shock or severe accompanying anemia. Myoglobinuria can have an additive deleterious effect on tubular epithelium already undergoing ischemic necrosis. At necropsy, the renal cortices in myoglobinuria are diffusely stained red-brown to blue-black and have intratubular myoglobin casts (see Fig. 11-47).

The pathophysiology of this condition is not known. Predisposing and triggering factors are required in this multifactorial disorder and yet the combination may be different in different individuals. Possible predisposing factors include carbohydrate overload, local hypoxia, thiamine deficiency, vitamin E and selenium deficiency, metabolic pathway abnormalities, alterations in reproductive hormones, thyroid hormones and cortisol, viruses, and electrolyte imbalances. Triggering factors include temperament, management, nutrition, concurrent disease, weather, time of year, hormonal imbalances. Clinical signs tend to occur intermittently during or after exercise. Syndrome has been divided into three forms: (1) a mild acute form, (2) an intermediate form, and (3) a severe form. Dark urine occurs when myoglobin level exceeds 40 mg/100 mL. Renal damage may occur as the result of circulatory damage and precipitation of myoglobin in the renal tubules. Mechanism of pigment-induced renal injury is still not understood, but increased hydroxyl radical formation associated with reduction of ferrous iron compounds and tubular obstruction by casts of myoglobin proteins are likely contributing factors.

PAPILLARY NECROSIS

Hypovolemia during NSAID administration can predispose to papillary necrosis. It is often seen on necropsy examination in horses with a clinical history of administration but rarely does it produce clinical signs.

Necrosis of the renal papillae, or their counterpart, the medullary crest, is a response of the inner medulla to ischemia. Papillary necrosis can be a primary or secondary lesion. Papillary necrosis occurs as a primary disease in animals treated with NSAIDs and is analogous to analgesic nephropathy in humans. The primary disease occurs quite frequently in horses treated for prolonged periods with phenylbutazone or flunixin meglumine. Drugs associated with papillary necrosis are sometimes referred to as *papillotoxins*. The medullary interstitial cells are the primary targets of papillotoxins. These cells have a key role in synthesis of prostaglandins, antihypertensive factors, and the glycosaminoglycan matrix of the medullary interstitium. Interstitial cell damage and inhibition of cyclooxygenase decreases prostaglandin synthesis, which reduces normal blood flow and causes ischemia/hypoxia, increases tubular transport, and modifies the interstitial matrix; the net effect is degenerative changes in tubular epithelial cells in the inner medulla.

The outer medulla and the cells of the thick ascending loop of Henle in particular are the least well-perfused of any zones of the kidneys. This is because the medulla has little direct perfusion; instead, most of the medullary blood supply comes from the cortex. After passing through the glomeruli, blood enters the vasa recta. Because of this limited blood flow, in addition to the high metabolic medullary cellular demand, any lesion or disease process that further reduces medullary blood flow can cause ischemic necrosis (infarction) of the papillae. Additionally, the high metabolic demand for cell transport and the maintenance of an ion gradient to enhance urinary concentration makes this area particularly vulnerable. This is most evident after ischemic tubular damage in which swollen endothelial and tubular epithelial cells, in conjunction with neutrophil adhesion in small vessels, upset the balance of oxygenation and energy demand by the outer medullary tubular cells. Medullary blood flow is ultimately balanced through levels of vasodilators, such as prostaglandin, nitric oxide, and adenosine, and vasoconstrictors, such as endothelin and angiotensin II.

Typically, acute lesions are irregular, discolored areas of necrotic inner medulla sharply delineated from the surviving medullary tissue (see Fig. 11-55). The affected tissue, which is undergoing coagulation necrosis, is yellow-gray, green, or pink. With time, the necrotic tissue sloughs, resulting in a detached, friable, and discolored tissue fragment in the pelvis. The remaining inner medulla is usually attenuated and on cross-section is narrowed. Overlying cortex can be somewhat shrunken because of atrophy of some of the nephrons caused by blockage of their tubules in the affected medulla. Small pieces of sloughed necrotic medullary tissue pass inconsequentially into the ureter. However, large pieces can obstruct the ureter, causing hydronephrosis, or form a nidus for precipitation of minerals, resulting in the formation of pelvic or ureteral calculi. Papillary necrosis is usually an incidental finding at necropsy and rarely leads to progressive renal damage and failure.

PATENT URACHUS

The most common malformation of the urinary bladder is patent urachus (pervious urachus). This lesion develops when the fetal urachus fails to close, therefore forming a direct channel between the bladder's apex and the umbilicus. Failure of the urachal remnant and the umbilical arteries and vein to involute is frequently observed in cases of "neonatal" omphalitis, in which abscess formation may result in a failure to close and hence a patent urachus. Patent urachus has also occurred because of congenital urethral obstruction. Increased bladder pressure because of the obstruction forces urine out into the urachus and ultimately, the rupture of the urachus causes uroperitoneum. The condition must be differentiated from perinatal rupture of the bladder. Foals are affected most often, and animals with this defect dribble urine from the umbilicus.

Occasionally, during urachal closure, the mucosa closes, but closure of the bladder musculature is incomplete. When this occurs, a bladder diverticulum (outpouching) of the apex of the bladder can develop. Urine stasis can occur in the diverticulum, predisposing the animal to cystitis or urinary calculi.

KLOSSIELLA EQUI INFECTION

Klossiella equi is a sporozoan parasite of the horse, which has various stages of development in the kidney after oral infection. No gross lesions are noted. Various stages of schizogony can be found microscopically in proximal convoluted tubular epithelium and to a lesser extent in glomerular endothelium (Fig. 11-68). Stages of sporogony are present in the epithelial cells of the loop of Henle, but different coccidial stages occur multifocally in affected tubules. Occasionally, however, *Klossiella equi* has been associated with multifocal lesions of mild tubular necrosis and in the case of tubular rupture, with interstitial infiltrates of lymphocytes and plasma cells. Renal function is typically normal.

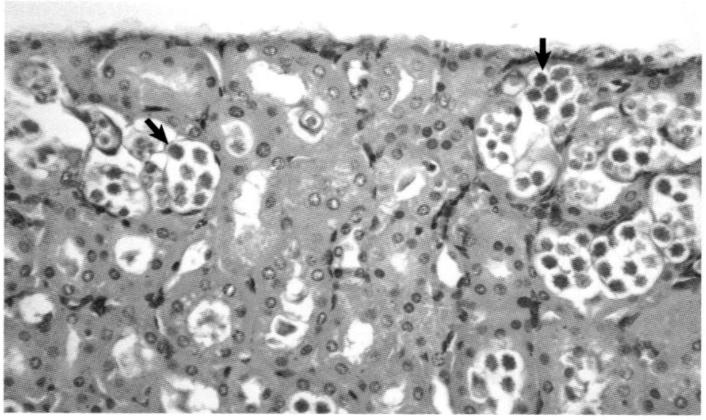

Fig. 11-68 *Klossiella equi* infection, kidney, horse.
Tubular epithelium containing various developmental stages of *Klossiella equi (arrows)*. H&E stain. (Courtesy Dr. J. Simon, College of Veterinary Medicine, University of Illinois.)

DISORDERS OF RUMINANTS (CATTLE, SHEEP, AND GOATS)

OAK TOXICITY: ACUTE TUBULAR NECROSIS (*QUERCUS* SPP.)

Ruminants develop tubular necrosis after ingestion of leaves, buds, or acorns from oak trees and shrubs (*Quercus* spp.). The toxic substances are metabolites of tannins and include tannic acid, gallic acid, and pyrogallol; however, the mechanism of tubular damage is unknown. Acutely affected cattle often have swollen, pale kidneys that occasionally have cortical petechial hemorrhages (Fig. 11-69). Perirenal edema is a common lesion and the body cavities contain excessive amounts of a clear fluid. Endothelial cells are a target for the binding of the toxic metabolites, subsequently resulting in vascular leakage. The kidneys are swollen and pale, and there are hemorrhages on capsular and cortical surfaces. Microscopically, acute proximal tubular necrosis with casts and intratubular hemorrhage are characteristic and chronic cases develop chronic interstitial nephritis with the usual changes of fibrosis, atrophy, thinned cortex, and a finely pitted surface.

PULPY KIDNEY DISEASE

Pulpy kidney disease is a unique condition caused by *Clostridium perfringens* type D whose epsilon toxin binds to renal tubular epithelial cells and causes selective degeneration of distal tubules. The critical predisposing factor is access to excessive starch in the small intestine, which allows for excessive bacterial proliferation there. Hyperglycemia and glucosuria can occasionally be detected. Although postmortem interval is critical for assessment of "pulpiness," the classic necropsy lesions are medullary congestion, hemorrhage, and tubular degeneration (see Fig. 11-49, *A*). Histologic lesions include mild degeneration and necrosis of epithelium of the proximal convoluted tubules with edema, congestion, and interstitial hemorrhage in the renal cortex and congestion of the medulla (see Fig. 11-49, *B*).

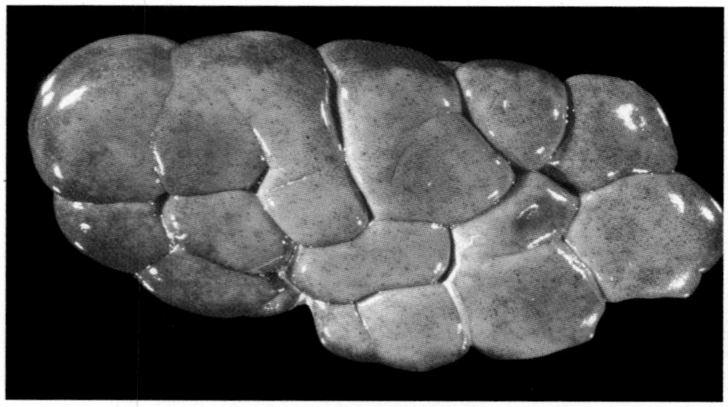

Fig. 11-69 Acute tubular necrosis, oak toxicity, kidney, cow.
Ingestion of leaves, buds, or acorns from oak trees produces cortical petechiation, acute tubular necrosis, and perirenal edema. The toxic principle is a metabolite of oak tannins and causes acute tubular necrosis, which heals by scarring. (Courtesy Dr. K. Read, College of Veterinary Medicine, Texas A&M University; and Noah's Arkive, College of Veterinary Medicine, The University of Georgia.)

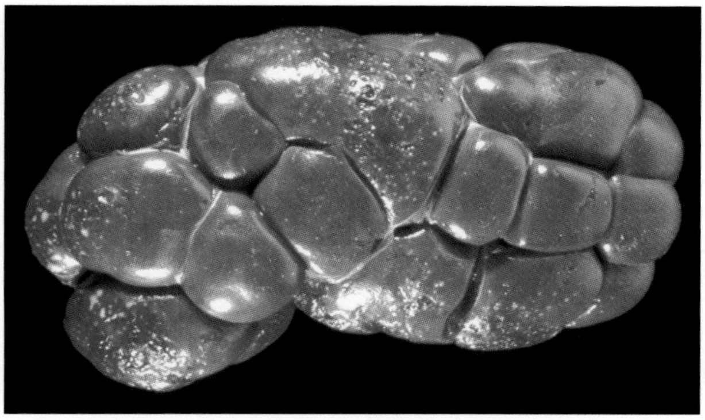

Fig. 11-70 Multifocal interstitial nephritis (white-spotted kidney), kidney, calf.
Multiple pale-yellow to white 2- to 5-mm foci of inflammatory cells (usually neutrophils) are scattered randomly throughout and over the surface of the kidney (as shown here). (Courtesy College of Veterinary Medicine, University of Illinois.)

EMBOLIC NEPHRITIS (WHITE SPOTTED KIDNEY)

Embolic nephritis, or white spotted kidney, is the best-known example of nonsuppurative interstitial nephritis. It occurs as a result of abscess formation and occurs when bacteria (*Escherichia coli, Salmonella* spp., or *Brucella* spp.) seed the kidneys. Bacteria lodge in glomerular tufts and peritubular capillaries and produce multiple small white nodules of varying sizes throughout the cortex (Fig. 11-70). Histologically, the lesions are consistent with microabscesses, which are soon replaced by lymphocytes, plasma cells, and macrophages. If healing occurs, it is by scar formation and atrophy. Capsular adhesions may be present.

INTERSTITIAL NEPHRITIS (LEPTOSPIROSIS)

The pathogenesis of leptospirosis is discussed as an example of acute bacterial tubulointerstitial nephritis, the most well-understood causes of which include serovars of *Leptospira interrogans*. Although neutrophils can be present in tubular lumina, the predominant chronic lesion is in the interstitium, which becomes infiltrated with monocytes, macrophages, lymphocytes, and plasma cells. Serovars *hardjo, pomona,* and *grippotyphosa* are the most commonly implicated in renal infection in cattle. Small ruminants are relatively resistant to infection. Infection with the adapted serovar *hardjo* rarely causes overt dysfunction. Nonadapted serovars create renal lesions from direct damage to the vascular endothelium, hypoxia caused by anemia, tubular epithelial damage from intratubular hemoglobin accumulation, and interstitial nephritis. The range of lesions is from few to mild interstitial nephritis to diffuse severe lymphocytic interstitial nephritis with fibrosis (see Fig. 11-73).

Chronic interstitial nephritis has mononuclear cell infiltrates, interstitial fibrosis, and generalized tubular atrophy. In the case of exposure to gamma herpesvirus of malignant catarrhal fever, lesions of a chronic interstitial nephritis are characterized by chronic ongoing inflammatory infiltrates composed of lymphocytes and fewer plasma cells within the interstitium accompanied by variable amounts of fibrosis. Occasionally, with this condition, vasculitis can be detected in vessels around which much of the interstitial inflammation occurs and can help differentiate the two agents.

GRANULOMATOUS NEPHRITIS: HAIRY VETCH TOXICOSIS (*VICIA* SPP.)

Hairy vetch is a legume used throughout regions with extensive farming and can be fed as pasture, hay, or silage. Hairy vetch toxicosis is a unique manifestation of a toxic plant ingestion that can result in lesions of eosinophilic and granulomatous inflammation within the kidney, skin, and other viscera. The toxic mechanism is not clearly determined for the visceral disease. It has been postulated that the visceral inflammation is similar to a type IV hypersensitivity reaction and may be caused by antigen formation in the form of a hapten or a complete antigen that sensitizes lymphocytes. Although gross lesions at necropsy can involve multiple organs, the kidney contains multifocal to radiating cortical infiltrates (see Fig. 11-56, *A*). These are often oriented around the vasculature. Histologically, the infiltrates are mixed and include monocytes, lymphocytes, plasma cells, multinucleated giant cells, and eosinophils (see Fig. 11-56, *B*). The clinical syndrome develops several weeks after ingestion of the plant and the dermal manifestation of pruritus is consistently seen concurrently. Mortality can result 10 to 20 days after illness begins, and older cattle and those of Holstein or Angus breeds are the most susceptible. Diagnosis is often made by exclusion.

PYELONEPHRITIS

After colonization of the lower urinary tract with bacteria of bowel or skin origin, local defense mechanisms can be overcome and allow for colonization of the pelvis and subsequent infection of the kidney. Thus pyelonephritis is often bilateral. *Corynebacterium renale* is a recognized obligate urinary mucosal organism and a potential pathogen in bovine cases because this organism has pili to accommodate adhesion and resist shedding from the lower urinary tract.

Acute pyelonephritis is uncommon in cattle and often seen as an incidental finding at necropsy (see Fig. 11-53). Chronic pyelonephritis of the bovine is described as a slowly progressive suppurative tubulointerstitial nephritis with either excessive targeting to the medulla and pus accumulation in the calyces, such that a thin rim of cortex may be all that remains, or more commonly as radially distributed interstitial infiltrates with or without fibrosis (see Fig. 11-54). As fibrosis progresses, there is contraction of scars that extend from the cortical surface throughout the medulla to the level of the pelvis.

RENAL LYMPHOSARCOMA

Renal lymphosarcoma is common in cattle since the neoplasm is one of the most common bovine tumors. The cause is bovine leukosis virus (BLV), a retrovirus, known to be spread by blood contact between animals. Gross lesions may be seen as diffuse renomegaly or more commonly as multiple poorly defined tan, soft, raised cortical nodules (see Fig. 11-59, *E* and *F*). Peripelvic and periureteral infiltrates are common in cattle and can produce concurrent hydronephrosis. Focal or diffuse infiltrates of neoplastic lymphocytes efface interstitium and/or tubules.

UROLITHIASIS

In cases of urolithiasis in cattle, the sigmoid flexure is most commonly affected. The obstruction can be caused by a large discrete mineral aggregate or by accumulation of fine sandlike material. Hemorrhage and necrosis of the urethral mucosa is typical at the site of urolith lodgement. In more severe cases, with subsequent rupture, there can be subcutaneous accumulation of urine in the inguinal area, prepuce and ventral abdomen. Uroliths would be found most commonly in males and castrated males. Silica uroliths (calculi) are a problem for sheep and cattle grazing native rangeland grasses of western North America. Unpolymerized silicic acid is dissolved in rumenal fluid and excreted in high concentrations in urine under the proper conditions.

Silica calculi (75% silica dioxide) are very common in pastured ruminants. Certain grasses contain as much as 4% to 5% silica;

most of the silica is insoluble, except that which is in the cell sap (unpolymerized silicic acid). After absorption, silica is returned to the gut in digestive secretions; less than 1% of dietary silica is excreted in urine and up to 60% is resorbed from the filtrate. However, when urine production is very low, the concentration of silicic acid excretion in urine may reach five times the saturation level. Precipitation from solution requires other substances in the urine. Silica calculi are hard, white to dark-brown, radiopaque, often laminated, large-diameter stones and are a major cause of urinary tract obstruction. Calculus formation is reduced to subclinical levels by adding sodium chloride to the ration, acidifying the diet, or reducing the dietary calcium to phosphorus ratio. Struvites develop in ruminants on cereal-grain rations, particularly those that are pelleted and high in phosphorus.

See the section on Disorders of Domestic Animals for illustrations.

ENZOOTIC HEMATURIA

Information on this topic is available at evolve.elsevier.com/Zachary/McGavin/.

BRACKEN FERN–INDUCED NEOPLASIA

Information on this topic is available at evolve.elsevier.com/Zachary/McGavin/.

AMYLOIDOSIS

Amyloidosis is a sporadic protein-losing nephropathy of cattle. Chronic diarrhea, poor productivity and weight loss are common. Amyloid is classified as AA type, which is associated with chronic inflammation, and such conditions are often seen concurrently. AA fibrils are created through abnormal catabolism of serum amyloid A (SAA). On gross necropsy examination, kidneys are yellow tan and appear waxy on cut section. Histologic deposition of amyloid occurs in the glomerulus, interstitium, and tubular lumens.

DISORDERS OF PIGS

GLOMERULONEPHRITIS OF PIGS

Although an uncommon entity in pigs, GN is seen as a sequel to chronic infections with hog cholera, African swine fever, systemic cytomegalovirus, and group A streptococcal abscesses. Additionally, inherited forms of membranoproliferative GN in Yorkshire pigs are due to an autosomal recessive deficiency of the complement inhibitory protein factor H. GN can be observed in systemic vasculitis in cases of porcine dermatitis and nephropathy syndrome. Kidney lesions in the acute form of this syndrome are exudative and occasionally necrotizing and have an accompanying vasculitis. It is thought that this response is an immune-mediated (type III) hypersensitivity response. PRRS and circovirus are both implicated as viremia may coexist with the presence of antibodies, a situation that facilitates the formation of immune complexes. A similar porcine dermatitis and nephropathy syndrome characterized by GN with intralesional fibrin and interstitial nephritis is associated with high antibody titers to PCV2, which are thought to trigger the glomerular and dermal lesions in these cases. In acute GN, grossly, there is enlargement, pallor, edema, and cortical petechiation. Eventually, this produces granular cortical infiltrates and the kidney may appear shrunken and contracted due to cortical fibrosis.

TOXIC NEPHRITIS

Ingestion of several species of pigweed may cause acute renal failure in pigs. Gross lesions include marked perirenal edema and blood-tinged serous effusions elsewhere in the body. Histologically, swelling and necrosis of the lining epithelial cells, the presence of casts, dilated tubules and mild interstitial edema are characteristic.

LEPTOSPIROSIS

Host-adapted *Leptospira* serovars *pomona, tarassovi,* and *australis* cause significant disease in pigs. Preferential localization of the organism occurs in the renal proximal tubules and passage to the interstitium results in multifocal interstitial nephritis, similar to that seen in cattle and dogs. Grossly, poorly circumscribed white foci of various shapes and sizes that correspond to infiltrates of lymphocytes, plasma cells, and macrophages in the interstitial tissues are present. Additionally, in chronic cases, concurrent interstitial fibrosis occurs.

CIRCOVIRUS (VIRAL INTERSTITIAL NEPHRITIS)

Porcine circovirus infection results in postweaning multisystemic wasting syndrome (PMWS) and can produce a variety of lesions. Grossly, there are white foci seen within the renal parenchyma. These correspond to inflammatory renal lesions, including lymphoplasmacytic tubulointerstitial nephritis and/or granulomatous interstitial nephritis. Additionally, multifocal interstitial nephritis can be seen with cytomegalovirus, adenovirus, and PRRS.

UROLITHIASIS

Urinary calculi (uroliths) are concretions formed anywhere in the urinary collecting system, and although some clearly originate in the lower urinary tract or as microscopic calculi in the renal collecting tubules, the point of development of most is not known. Urinary bladder calculi can be single or multiple, variable in size (2 to 10 cm), and sometimes are composed of a fine, sandlike material, which causes cloudy urine. Pigs most commonly have calcium carbonate, calcium phosphate, struvite, and uric acid or urate uroliths. As with other species, obstructive disease and/or rupture can occur at sites of lodgement, which is more commonly seen in males.

See the section on Disorders of Domestic Animals for illustrations.

KIDNEY WORM

In North America, the kidney worm *(Stephanurus dentatus)* is found most often in adult pigs in southern regions of the US. The parasite is also a problem in other countries with warm climates. *Stephanurus dentatus* is a strongyloid worm that migrates to the kidney after cycling through the liver. Adult worms normally encyst in perirenal fat; however, some parasites may reside in the kidney. Peripelvic cysts often communicate with the renal pelvis and ureter, and fibrosis and chronic granulation tissue can enclose the parasite. Occasionally, shed nematode eggs are present in the urine sediment.

ERYSIPELOTHRIX

Erysipelothrix rhusiopathiae is the most common bacterial cause of embolic nephritis in pigs. The organism may spread to the kidney after cutaneous involvement or much more commonly as a result of bacteremia related to the development of septic valvular endocarditis. Grossly, the disease presents as either glomerular hemorrhages seen as multifocal regions of pinpoint hemorrhage throughout the

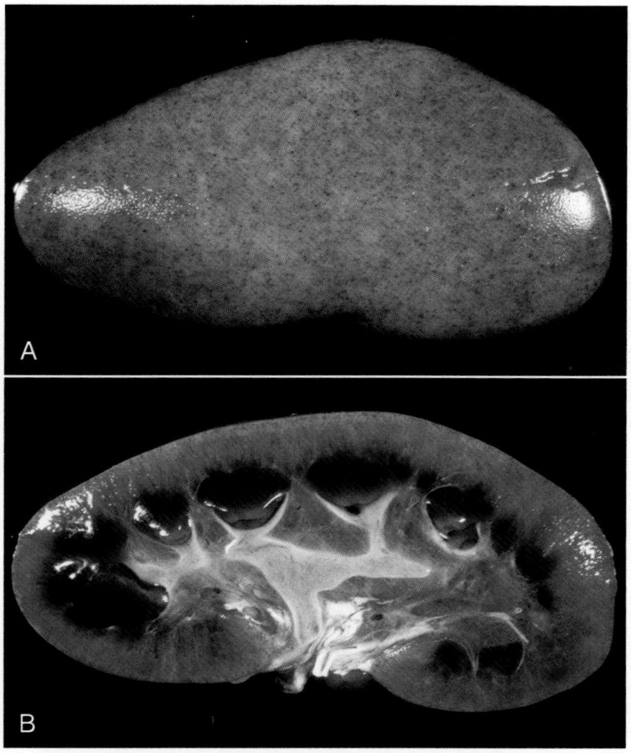

Fig. 11-71 Bacterial-induced septicemic renal cortical hemorrhages, erysipelas, kidney, pig.
A, Petechial hemorrhages caused by septic emboli of *Erysipelothrix rhusiopathiae* are randomly scattered over the capsular surface of the kidney. **B,** Dorsal section. Similar petechiae are present on the cut surface of the renal cortex. (Courtesy Dr. M.D. McGavin, College of Veterinary Medicine, University of Tennessee.)

renal cortex or as multiple foci of tan-to-white inflammatory infiltrates within the renal interstitium (Fig. 11-71). Histologically, the change described in the former situation is characteristic of septic embolic GN with fibrin and neutrophil aggregates noted within glomerular capillary tufts or as small abscesses within the interstitium.

DISORDERS OF DOGS

GREYHOUND VASCULOPATHY

An idiopathic renal glomerular and cutaneous vasculopathy, formerly known as *Alabama rot,* occurs in greyhounds and is a potentially fatal disease of unknown etiology. As the name suggests, it typically affects the skin and kidneys of racing- and training-age Greyhounds. Typically, there are characteristic, well-demarcated cutaneous ulcers of the extremities, with concurrent thrombocytopenia and acute renal insufficiency. The cause of the disease is unknown, but renal lesions are similar to those seen in acute DIC, thrombotic thrombocytopenic purpura, and hemolytic uremic syndrome in humans. At necropsy, kidneys from affected dogs are swollen and congested and show cortical petechiae (see Fig. 11-44, *A*). Microscopically, numerous glomeruli have segmental or global fibrinous thrombi, hemorrhage, and necrosis (see Fig. 11-44, *B*). At the glomerular vascular pole, the walls of afferent arterioles have fibrin deposits and foci of necrosis. Additionally, there are multifocal erythematous and/or ulcerated skin lesions, commonly accompanied by distal limb edema as the result of a similar cutaneous vasculitis. Electron microscopy findings indicate that glomerular endothelial damage is an important early event in the pathogenesis of this condition.

ETHYLENE GLYCOL INTOXICATION

Ethylene glycol (antifreeze) ingestion is one of the most common causes of intoxication and acute tubular necrosis in dogs, cats, and occasionally pigs. Ethylene glycol, the major constituent of antifreeze, is readily absorbed from the gastrointestinal tract, and a small percentage is oxidized by hepatic alcohol dehydrogenase to the toxic metabolites glycolaldehyde, glycolic acid, glyoxalate, and oxalate. Ethylene glycol and its toxic metabolic products are filtered by the glomeruli, and acute tubular necrosis is caused by the direct interaction of these toxic metabolites, especially glycolic acid, on the tubular epithelium (Fig. 11-72, *A* and *B*). Of particular significance is that large numbers of pale yellow foci of calcium oxalate crystals precipitate in renal tubular lumens, tubular epithelial cells, and the interstitium (Fig. 11-72, *C*). These crystals cause intrarenal obstruction and degeneration and necrosis of tubular epithelium, postulated to be the direct effect of mechanical damage. With polarized light, the microscopic image is one of large numbers of birefringent, round-to-pyramidal crystals arranged in rosettes or sheaves within renal tubules that are virtually pathognomonic for ethylene glycol ingestion in dogs and cats (Fig. 11-72, *D*).

ACUTE TUBULAR NECROSIS (AMINOGLYCOSIDES)

Aminoglycoside antimicrobials, such as gentamicin, neomycin, kanamycin, tobramycin, amikacin, and streptomycin, are nephrotoxic. Relative renal toxicity varies among the different aminoglycoside drugs and correlates with the concentration of the compound in the renal cortex. Neomycin, which is highly nephrotoxic, concentrates to the greatest extent in the renal cortex, whereas streptomycin, the least nephrotoxic, does not concentrate appreciably in the renal cortex. Although gentamicin is intermediate in its nephrotoxicity between neomycin and streptomycin, tubular damage from gentamicin occurs with some frequency because it is a commonly used drug in veterinary medicine.

The susceptibility of animal species to the nephrotoxic effects of these drugs is variable and is related to differences in susceptibility of renal tubules and differences in the rate of excretion or inactivation of the drug among animal species. Aminoglycosides become concentrated in lysosomes, and their toxic effects occur after release of large concentrations of the drugs from these organelles. Toxic levels of aminoglycosides produce the following changes:

- Become concentrated in lysosomes.
- Subsequently escape from lysosomes to accumulate in the cytoplasm.
- Alter tubular cell membrane transport by the inhibition of Na^+/K^+-ATPase, causing an intracellular influx of hydrogen, sodium ions, and water.
- Inhibit phospholipase activity so that phospholipids accumulate intracellularly.
- Alter mitochondrial function.
- Inhibit protein synthesis.

These biochemical changes are responsible for the lesions of acute swelling of proximal tubular epithelial cells, mitochondrial swelling, rupture of lysosomes, dilation of endoplasmic reticulum, shedding of the tubular brush border, and cellular death.

LEPTOSPIROSIS

Dogs are susceptible to several serovars of *Leptospira,* although *L. icterohaemorrhagiae* and *L. canicola* are determined to be the

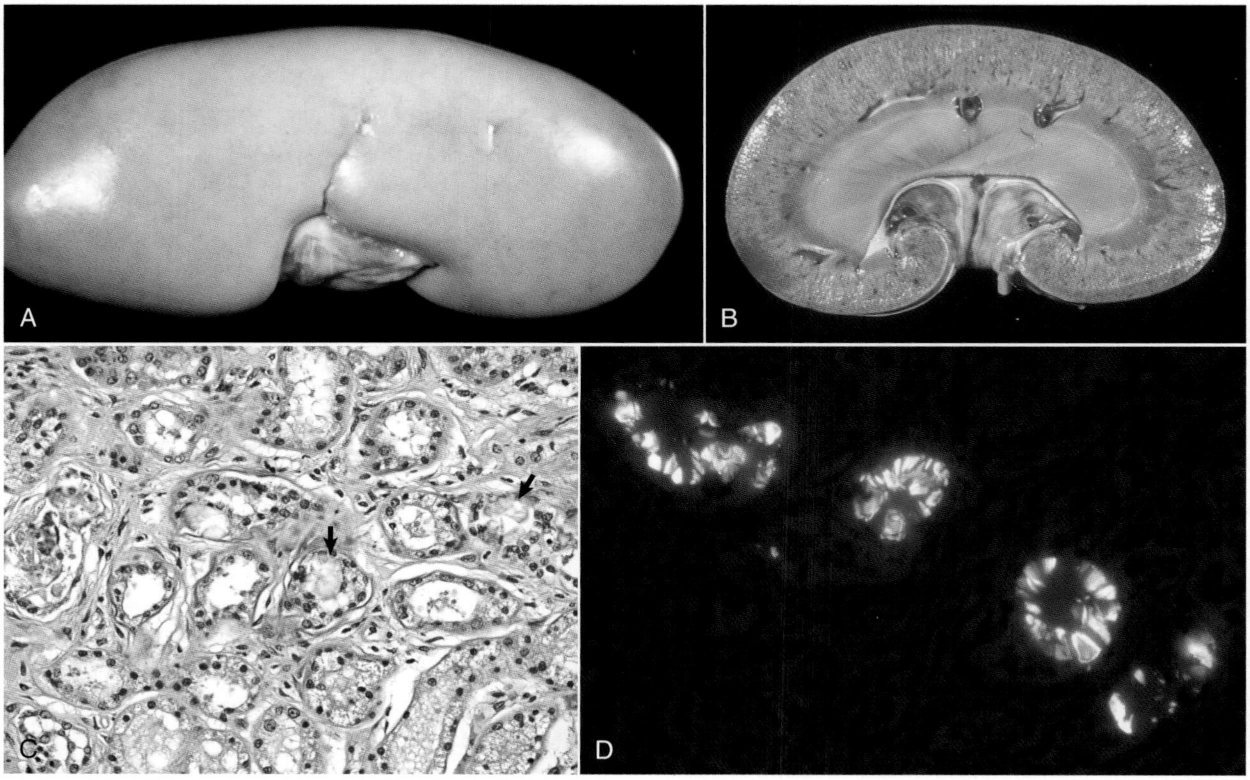

Fig. 11-72 Oxalate nephrosis, kidney.
A, Pig. Oxalate nephrosis following ingestion of oxalate-containing plants. The kidney is diffusely pale beige and swollen. **B,** Dorsal section, dog. The cortex is beige and finely mottled due to the deposition of multiple small foci of oxalate crystals in the renal tubules. **C,** Dog. Tubular dilation, necrosis, and early regeneration (increased numbers of epithelial cells lining several tubules). Numerous tubules contain oxalate crystals *(arrows),* which have dilated the tubules and compressed their epithelium. H&E stain. **D,** Cat. Birefringent radiating sheaves of calcium oxalate crystals in renal tubules. Polarized light. H&E stain. (**A** and **B** courtesy Dr. M.D. McGavin, College of Veterinary Medicine, University of Tennessee. **C** courtesy Dr. S.J. Newman, College of Veterinary Medicine, University of Tennessee. **D** courtesy Dr. J.F. Zachary, College of Veterinary Medicine, University of Illinois.)

most common canine isolates. Leptospires enter the body through breaches in the mucous membranes, multiply and spread to the kidney where they persist in the renal tubular cells. Affected dogs may exhibit fever, anorexia, vomiting, dehydration, icterus, muscle pain, and evidence of coagulopathy. In the more chronic infections, fever, anterior uveitis, anorexia, and weight loss are noted. Grossly, inflammatory infiltrates that extend from the cortical medullary junction to the capsular surface are present (Fig. 11-73, *A*). In the more acute stages, in which tubular damage is prominent, there will be neutrophilic infiltrates, but this rapidly changes to lymphocytes and plasma cells. In more chronic cases, variable amounts of fibrosis and subcapsular scarring occur (Fig. 11-73, *B*). Leptospires may often be identified within the cytoplasm and the lumen of affected tubules when special silver stains are used (Fig. 11-73, *C*).

INFECTIOUS CANINE HEPATITIS

Glomerulitis, caused by a direct viral insult to the glomerulus, occurs in acute systemic viral diseases such as acute infectious canine hepatitis. The lesions are mild, usually transient, and result from viral replication in capillary endothelium. Acute viral GN produces the following gross lesions:

- Kidneys are often slightly swollen.
- Renal capsular surface is smooth.
- Kidneys are normal color or pale.
- Glomeruli are visible as pinpoint red dots on the cut surface of the cortex.

Viral-induced intranuclear inclusions are present in glomerular capillary endothelium in cases of infectious canine hepatitis. The inclusions are usually large, basophilic to magenta, and either fill the nucleus or are separated from the nuclear membrane by a clear halo. In cases of viral glomerulitis, lesions include endothelial hypertrophy, hemorrhages, necrosis of endothelium, and a thickened and edematous mesangium. Clinically, animals are systemically ill from the viral infection, but the glomerular signs are specifically those of a transient proteinuria.

CANINE HERPESVIRUS

In young puppies less than 4 to 6 weeks of age, intrauterine or neonatal infections can occur with insults being directed to the kidney. Typically, there is acute tubular necrosis with hemorrhage and the presence of intraepithelial intranuclear eosinophilic to amphophilic inclusions (Fig. 11-74). Once the puppies are older, typically more than 12 to 16 weeks, herpesvirus infections fail to induce renal lesions.

PYELONEPHRITIS

Dogs with acute pyelonephritis can exhibit fever, depression, arched back from lumbar or renal pain, polydipsia, and polyuria. The most common causes of bacterial pyelonephritis in order of frequency include infection with *Escherichia coli, Staphylococcus aureus, Proteus mirabilis, Streptococcus* sp., *Klebsiella pneumoniae, Pseudomonas aeruginosa,* and *Enterobacter* sp. For the most part, these organisms take

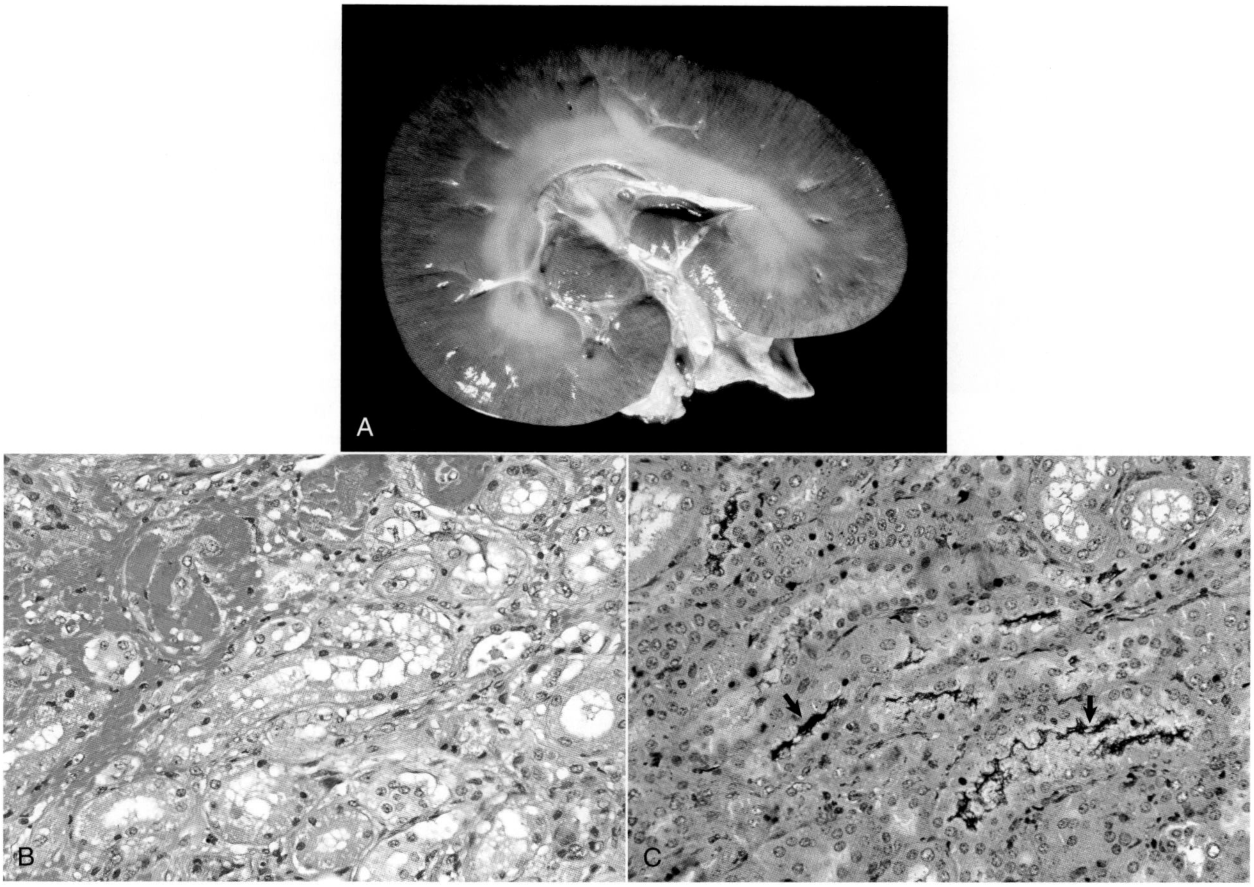

Fig. 11-73 Acute leptospirosis, kidney.
A, Interstitial nephritis, acute leptospira infection, dorsal section, dog. Radiating pale streaks are caused by cortical tubular necrosis, and acute interstitial inflammatory infiltrates. The hilar fat and medulla are yellow from jaundice. **B,** Acute tubular necrosis, early regeneration, dog. Note the segments of tubular epithelium devoid of nuclei (coagulation necrosis) *(top left)* and the hemorrhage. At this early stage, there is an almost complete lack of inflammatory cells in the interstitium, but later in the subacute stage of leptospirosis there are interstitial infiltrates of lymphocytes and plasma cells, which tend to be near the corticomedullary junction. H&E stain. **C,** Leptospira, cow. Numerous leptospira *(arrows)* are present in the lumens of tubules. Leptospira colonization of tubule epithelial cells is typical of this bacterium. Warthin Starry silver stain. (**A** and **C** courtesy Dr. M.D. McGavin, College of Veterinary Medicine, University of Tennessee. **B** courtesy Dr. S.J. Newman, College of Veterinary Medicine, University of Tennessee.)

advantage of altered lower urinary tract defense mechanisms and ascend from the lower urinary tract to colonize the renal pelvis. Grossly, there can be accumulation of suppurative exudate in the pelvis with variable extension of tan cellular infiltrates from the medulla to variable portions of the overlying cortex (see Fig. 11-53, *A* and *B*). Histologically, there is tubular necrosis and loss with extension of bacterial colonies and variable amounts of neutrophils within tubules and the interstitium (see Fig. 11-53, *C*). In the more chronic forms, neutrophil numbers are reduced and lymphocytes and plasma cells predominate.

PROGRESSIVE JUVENILE NEPHROPATHY

The development of severe bilateral renal fibrosis has been described in young dogs of several breeds and referred to as *progressive juvenile nephropathy* or *familial (hereditary) renal disease.* In many dog breeds, a familial tendency is demonstrated (Box 11-11), but the mode of inheritance has been determined with certainty in only a few dog breeds. In Samoyeds, the lesion is gender-linked; in bull terriers, it is autosomal dominant; and in the Shih Tzu, the disease appears to have a simple autosomal recessive inheritance.

BOX 11-11 Breeds of Dogs with Progressive Juvenile Nephropathy

- American cocker spaniels
- English cocker spaniels
- Norwegian elkhounds
- Samoyeds
- Doberman pinschers
- Lhasa Apsos
- Shih Tzus
- Soft-coated Wheaten terriers
- Bull terriers
- Standard poodles
- Alaskan malamutes
- Miniature schnauzers
- German shepherds
- Keeshounds
- Chow chows
- Weimaraners
- Golden retrievers

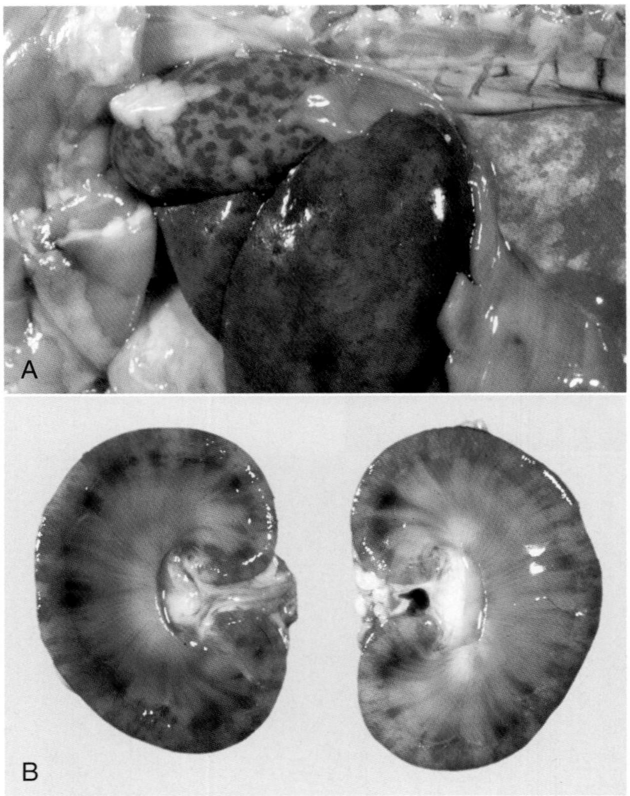

Fig. 11-74 Canine herpesvirus nephritis (canine herpesvirus type I), kidney, neonatal puppy.

A, Abdominal viscera. Multifocal renal cortical hemorrhages are grossly characteristic of this disease. **B,** Dorsal sections. Multifocal cortical hemorrhages are due to viral-induced vasculitis with necrosis and secondary hemorrhage. (Courtesy Dr. M.D. McGavin, College of Veterinary Medicine, University of Tennessee.)

Progressive juvenile nephropathy is a syndrome in which the morphologic manifestations can be the result of any of several chronic pathologic processes. The main manifestations include the following:

- Membranoproliferative GN
- Tubular disease of unknown cause with tubular atrophy and interstitial fibrosis
- Renal dysplasia

Gross renal lesions of progressive juvenile nephropathy are variable among affected breeds and among affected dogs within a breed. Generally, kidneys are notably shrunken, pale tan to white, and firm (see Fig. 11-32, *C* and *D*). The renal surface can be diffusely pitted and have a fine granular pattern, particularly in those dogs in which glomerular disease is the primary event. In cases of juvenile nephropathy that are tubular or dysplastic, the renal surface can have patchy, deeply depressed areas of cortical scarring. On the cut surface, the cortex is thin and has linear radial scars. The medulla is usually diffusely fibrotic. Small (1 to 2 mm), variably sized cysts are seen often in the cortex and the medulla.

In the Doberman pinscher, the primary lesion is a glomerulopathy that appears microscopically as a membranoproliferative GN. Later in the clinical course of the disease, the lesions include extensive periglomerular fibrosis, tubular atrophy, and cystic dilation of Bowman's (urinary) space and tubules. In affected Samoyeds and English cocker spaniels, multilamellar splitting of the GBM is caused by inherited abnormalities in basement membrane collagen. These lesions progress to severe glomerulosclerosis.

In Norwegian elkhounds, a tubular disorder of unknown cause has been described and is characterized by progressive tubular atrophy, periglomerular and interstitial fibrosis, and glomerulosclerosis without any indication of a primary glomerular disease.

Progressive juvenile nephropathy has been described in Lhasa Apsos, Shih Tzus, Wheaten terriers, Standard poodles, and Golden retrievers as a condition resembling renal dysplasia, defined as an abnormality of renal development as a result of anomalous differentiation. Small, shrunken, fetal-like glomeruli composed of small cells with dense nuclei, minimal mesangial tissue, and nonpatent capillaries can be seen interspersed with normal, sclerotic, or hypertrophied glomeruli. Other lesions include marked interstitial fibrosis and tubular dilation. Most of the kidneys have minimal lymphoplasmacellular interstitial cell infiltrates.

Juvenile nephropathy in boxer dogs is characterized by pericapsular and interstitial fibrosis, inflammatory cell infiltration, dilated tubules, sclerotic glomeruli, and dystrophic calcification.

Although variations exist in gross and microscopic lesions (see Fig. 11-32, *E*), as well as in the pathogenesis of progressive nephropathy among the different breeds, a typical case is a dog 4 months to 2 years of age that has polyuria, polydipsia, and uremia. The clinical presentation, gross lesions, and microscopic changes are identical to those of chronic renal disease and renal fibrosis in mature or aging dogs.

RENAL CARCINOMA

Renal carcinomas are the most common primary renal neoplasms and occur most frequently in older dogs. The specific causes of renal adenocarcinomas in humans are well determined compared with those in animal species, and little is specifically known about the pathogenesis of this entity in dogs. These renal neoplasms are usually large (up to 20 cm in diameter), spherical to oval, and firm. They often are pale yellow and contain dark areas of hemorrhage and necrosis and foci of cystic degeneration. The masses usually occupy and obliterate one pole of the kidney and grow by expansion, compressing the adjacent normal renal tissue (see Fig. 11-58). Histologic types include papillary, tubular, and solid (see Fig. 11-58, *C*), with solid variants being the most poorly differentiated. Metastasis to the lungs, lymph nodes, liver, and adrenals occurs frequently. Renal carcinoma has been associated with paraneoplastic conditions, principally polycythemia. This is because of concurrent overexpression of erythropoietin, which increases bone marrow production of red blood cells.

A variant of the typical renal carcinoma has been seen in German shepherd dogs in conjunction with nodular dermatofibrosis. The lesions are hereditary and consist of multifocal, bilateral, renal cystadenomas or cystadenocarcinomas. Grossly, these resemble the adenocarcinomas described previously, but cysts are much more prominent. The neoplastic cells form solid sheets, tubules, or papillary growth patterns, and the cells in the carcinomas are more atypical and anaplastic. Cells vary in shape from cuboidal and columnar to polyhedral, vary in size, and have clear or granular eosinophilic cytoplasm. Nuclei range from small, round, granular, and uniform to large, oval, vesicular, and pleomorphic. Mitotic figures are numerous. These neoplasms have a moderate fibrovascular stroma.

UROLITHIASIS

See the section on Disorders of Domestic Animals for illustrations.

Struvite Calculi

Information on this topic is available at evolve.elsevier.com/Zachary/McGavin/.

Uric Acid and Urate Calculi

Information on this topic is available at evolve.elsevier.com/Zachary/McGavin/.

Xanthine Calculi

Information on this topic is available at evolve.elsevier.com/Zachary/McGavin/.

Cystine Calculi

Information on this topic is available at evolve.elsevier.com/Zachary/McGavin/.

CHRONIC UROCYSTITIS

Several manifestations of chronic urocystitis exist in the canine and include those with prominent follicular lymphoid proliferation in the submucosa (follicular cystitis) and those with prominent polypoid epithelial change (polypoid). Follicular cystitis (see Fig. 11-65) has a grossly recognized cobblestone appearance as a result of the presence of disseminated, nodular, submucosal lymphoid proliferations (2 to 4 mm in diameter).This form of response is particularly common when cystitis is associated with chronic urolithiasis. These white-gray lymphoid foci are often surrounded by a zone of hyperemia. Additionally, the lesions can be associated with a diffusely thickened, hyperplastic mucosa with goblet cell hyperplasia, chronic lymphoplasmacytic infiltrate, and fibrosis in the lamina propria. Hypertrophy of the tunica muscularis can be observed.

Polypoid masses (chronic polypoid cystitis), seen predominantly in female dogs, typically develop from inflammatory and hyperplastic responses secondary to chronic irritation, which most often arise from persistent bacterial urinary tract infection or uroliths. These hyperplastic transitional epithelial responses are called cystitis cystica, cystitis glandularis, and/or Brunn's epithelial nests. Inflammation, epithelial proliferation, and development of a nonneoplastic mass occur most typically in the cranioventral bladder wall. The mucosa has single or multiple, nodular mucosal masses (see Figs. 11-65 and 11-66) composed of fibrous connective tissue and infiltrated with neutrophils and mononuclear leukocytes. The masses are broad-based or pedunculated, ulcerated, or covered by hyperplastic epithelium with goblet cell metaplasia. Chronic polypoid cystitis is characterized by clinical hematuria.

TRANSITIONAL CELL CARCINOMA

Carcinomas are focal, raised nodules or diffuse thickenings of the urinary bladder wall, most common in the trigone region of the bladder (Fig. 11-67, *A*). Transitional cell carcinomas are composed of pleomorphic to anaplastic transitional epithelium. Neoplastic transitional cells cover the mucosal surface as irregular layers, readily invade the lamina propria in the form of solid nests and acini, and are found within lymphatic vessels of the submucosa and muscle layers (Fig. 11-67, *B*). Terriers may be at a slightly elevated risk for development, and there has been an association made between occurrence of these tumors and exposure to lawn pesticides.

TOXIC TUBULOINTERSTITIAL NEPHRITIS

Melamine and Cyanuric Acid

Recently, pet food contaminated with melamine and cyanuric acid to artificially elevate the dietary protein content produced large-scale outbreaks of renal failure–related mortality in dogs and cats in the US and Korea. Sick animals had inappetence, vomiting, polyuria, polydipsia, and lethargy. Azotemia was recorded in many affected animals. The unique aspects of this food toxicity outbreak included necrosis that was localized to the distal rather than the proximal tubules. Unique intratubular rough and irregular brown birefringent crystals were noted in the more distal tubular portions of the nephron and these may have been mistaken for oxalates in some early cases. In contrast, these crystals failed to stain with von Kossa calcium stains or alizarin Red S. A combination of both melamine and cyanuric acid was required to produce the ultimate renal failure in these cases.

GRAPE INGESTION

Similarly, ingestion of grapes or raisins as part of the diet or inadvertently by dogs can lead to a syndrome of acute renal failure and uremia accompanied by vomiting, lethargy, anorexia, and diarrhea. The mechanism for induction of acute proximal renal tubular necrosis is unclear but tannins, similar to those in oak poisoning, are implicated as a toxic principle in these cases. The gross changes are those of an enlarged pale tan bulging kidney, and the histologic changes are not characteristic but are represented by acute proximal tubular necrosis.

PARASITES

The giant kidney worm *(Dioctophyma renale)* is seen infrequently in dogs from temperate and cold countries worldwide. It is endemic in Canada and in northern regions of the US. Because of a prolonged and complex life cycle, this nematode is seen only in dogs 2 years old or older. The adult nematode is red and cylindric; the females measure 20 to 100 cm long and 4 to 12 mm in diameter and the males measure 14 to 45 cm long and 4 to 6 mm in diameter. This nematode resides in the renal pelvis where it causes severe hemorrhagic or purulent pyelitis, subsequent ureteral obstruction, and destruction of the renal parenchyma, resulting in a hydronephrotic kidney that appears as a cyst containing the nematode and purulent exudate.

Capillaria plica and *Capillaria feliscati* have been identified infrequently in dogs and cats worldwide. Typically, these nematodes are attached to the renal pelvis, ureter, or bladder of animals of various ages. Microscopically, inflammatory cells infiltrate and focal hemorrhages are associated with sites of attachment in the underlying submucosa. Clinical effects usually are not present, but hematuria and dysuria are produced occasionally.

DISORDERS OF CATS

GRANULOMATOUS NEPHRITIS

Cats with FIP, particularly the noneffusive (dry) form, often have multifocal pyogranulomatous nephritis, secondary to the severe primary vasculitis. The pathogenesis of this lesion is thought to be related to a cell-mediated hypersensitivity (type IV) reaction to FIP virus (feline coronavirus). The immune response causes a granulomatous necrotizing vasculitis and development of interstitial pyogranulomas. The renal lesions are characterized grossly by multiple,

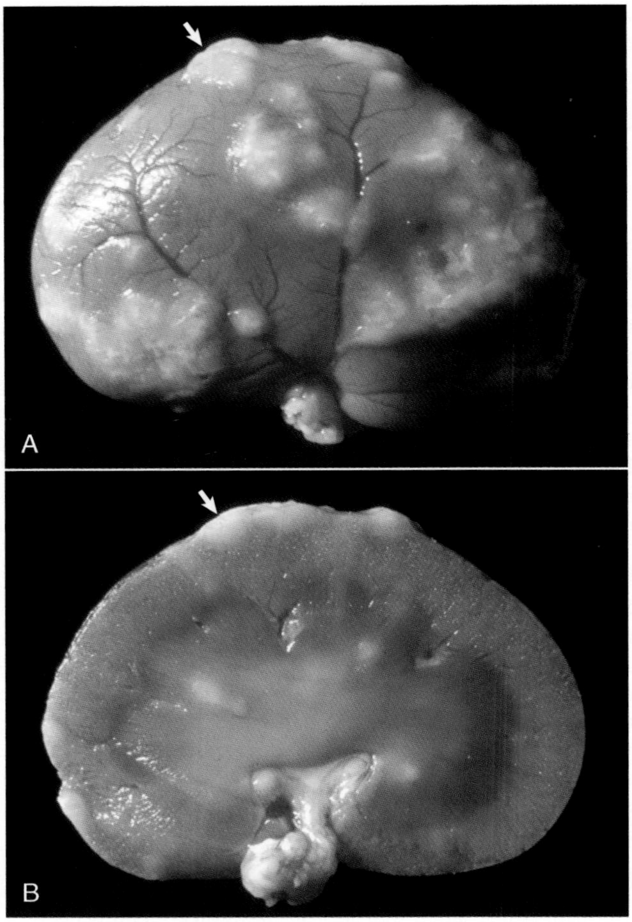

Fig. 11-75 Granulomatous nephritis, feline infectious peritonitis, kidney, cat.

A, Lesions are typical of the noneffusive (dry) form of feline infectious peritonitis. There are multifocal, coalescing white to gray granulomas *(arrow)*, which can be confused with the nodular form of lymphosarcoma, thus warranting histologic examination. **B,** Dorsal section. Multifocal, coalescing white to gray granulomas extend into the cortical parenchyma *(arrow)*. The pathogenesis of this lesion is determined by the effectiveness and/or ineffectiveness of both humoral and cellular immune responses. Depending on the immune response, the pathogenesis can involve a primary immune complex vasculitis (type III hypersensitivity [effusive form]) and/or delayed hypersensitivity response (type IV hypersensitivity [noneffusive form]); thus the lesions are oriented around blood vessels (primarily capillaries and venules) and are granulomatous. (Courtesy Dr. M.D. McGavin, College of Veterinary Medicine, University of Tennessee.)

large, irregular, and pale gray subcapsular cortical foci (Fig. 11-75, *A*) that are firm and granular on cut surface (Fig. 11-75, *B*). These lesions are somewhat circumscribed and bulge from the capsular surface. They may be misinterpreted as neoplastic infiltrates, such as those associated with renal lymphosarcoma, which tend not to have such a vascular orientation to the infiltrates. Microscopically, extensive accumulations of macrophages interspersed with lymphocytes, plasma cells, and neutrophils (pyogranulomas) surround foci of necrotizing fibrinoid vasculitis.

RENAL LYMPHOSARCOMA

Lymphosarcoma is one of the most common neoplasms in cats and can affect the kidney as part of a systemic syndrome or involve the kidney alone. The gross appearance is that of diffuse renomegaly or multinodular enlargement (see Fig. 11-59). The multiple masses are variably sized and present on capsular and cut surface as white to tan and homogeneous. Unlike with FIP-induced renal granulomas, the orientation of these neoplastic infiltrates does not typically center around vessels. Histologically, sheets of neoplastic lymphocytes are diffuse or nodular infiltrates that often obliterate normal renal architecture. Immunophenotyping for T or B lymphocyte origin can be performed.

UROLITHIASIS

Struvite Calculi

Information on this topic is available at evolve.elsevier.com/Zachary/McGavin/.

HEMORRHAGIC UROCYSTITIS (FELINE UROLOGIC SYNDROME)

Interstitial cystitis is a condition diagnosed in cats which some imply is similar to the condition of a similar name in humans. However, FLUTD has little in common with human interstitial cystitis other than an undetermined etiology, a variety of clinical manifestations, and lack of effective treatment. Unlike in humans, FUS as a component of FLUTD is more common in males, and urethral obstruction by calculi and obstructive uropathy are seen consistently. Recent literature strongly cautions against overdiagnosing interstitial cystitis in cases of cats with dysuria and hematuria. Clearly, a syndrome of idiopathic dysuria with and without bacteria, calculi, and mucosal ulceration is diagnosed by histopathology, but until more is known it should not be likened to human interstitial cystitis, whether the ulcerative or nonulcerative variant. Feline interstitial cystitis is diagnosed when all three of the following criteria are met: chronic irritation while voiding, sterile cytologically negative urine, and submucosal hemorrhages. It also is consistent with idiopathic cystitis, a noninfectious inflammatory lower urinary tract disease of cats. Little is recorded about histologic lesions, but they are nonspecific and include submucosal edema, dilation of blood vessels with neutrophil margination, and submucosal hemorrhage. Surprisingly, ulceration is not specifically listed, although in the human form, there is an ulcerative and nonulcerative variant of interstitial cystitis. Several other alterations that may reflect pathogenesis are usually noted in affected cats. These include an increase in submucosal mast cells, a decrease in glycosaminoglycans, specifically GP-51, an increase in urinary bladder permeability, and neurogenic inflammation. It is possible that mast-cell degranulation contributes to inflammation. Decreased GP-51 may allow urine to penetrate and induce submucosal inflammation. Disruption of the tight junctions between urothelial cells results in increased permeability. Neurogenic inflammation may occur after local release of neurotransmitters that results in vasodilation and leakage. Thus there may be abnormalities in local, sensory, central, and efferent nervous systems so that this syndrome has complex interactions between the bladder and the nervous system.

TOXIC TUBULOINTERSTITIAL NEPHRITIS

Melamine and Cyanuric Acid

Cats were similarly affected by the methamine/cyanuric acid contamination of pet foods as dogs (see previous section on Disorders of Dogs).

Lily Toxicity

Cats are prone to a species-specific toxicity associated with ingestion of leaves or flowers of lily plants. This is often seasonal when Easter Lily *(Lilium longiflorum)* plants are purchased and brought into the cat's environment. Day lily (*Hemerocallis* spp.), tiger lily (*Lilium* sp.), Japanese show lily *(Lilium hybridum),* and rubrum lily (*L. rubrum*) can all cause renal toxicosis in cats. Vomiting and lethargy within 1 to 5 days of ingestion is common. The toxic ingredient is not known, but renal damage in the form of acute tubular necrosis from exposure seems particularly severe in these cases.

SUGGESTED READINGS

Suggested Readings are available at evolve.elsevier.com/Zachary/McGavin/.

CHAPTER 12

Endocrine System*

Krista M.D. La Perle

STRUCTURE AND FUNCTION

Endocrine glands are collections of specialized cells that synthesize, store, and directly release their secretions, such as polypeptides, steroids, and amino acid derivatives—including catecholamines and thyroid hormones—into the bloodstream, resulting in physiologic effects on target cells distant from the glands. They are sensing and signaling devices located in the extracellular fluid compartment that are capable of responding to changes in the internal and external environments to coordinate a multiplicity of activities that maintain homeostasis.

Signaling molecules are grouped into three general categories according to the source of the signal and the location of the target on which the signal has an effect (Fig. 12-1). In autocrine signaling, cells respond to signals that they themselves secrete. Molecules produced by one cell that act on a neighboring cell are characteristic of paracrine signaling. The final pattern of signaling, which is the focus of this chapter, is endocrine signaling, whereby hormones produced by cells of endocrine organs are released into the circulation and act on distant target cells.

Endocrine cells that produce polypeptide hormones have a well-developed, rough endoplasmic reticulum that assembles the hormone, and a prominent perinuclear Golgi apparatus that packages the hormone into granules for intracellular storage and transport. Secretory granules are unique to polypeptide hormone- and catecholamine-secreting endocrine cells and provide a mechanism for intracellular storage of substantial amounts of preformed active hormone. When the cell receives a signal to secrete a hormone, secretory granules are moved to the periphery of the endocrine cell, most likely by the contraction of microfilaments. After release of the peptides into the bloodstream, they bind to receptors on the surface of target cells, activating a series of intracellular events often mediated by second messengers such as cyclic adenosine monophosphate (cAMP), protein kinases, or calcium.

Steroid hormone–secreting cells are characterized by large cytoplasmic lipid bodies that contain cholesterol and other precursor molecules. The lipid bodies are in close proximity to an extensive smooth endoplasmic reticulum and large mitochondria. The latter have hydroxylase and dehydrogenase enzyme systems that attach various side chains to the basic steroid nucleus. Steroid-producing cells lack secretory granules and do not store significant amounts of preformed hormone. They depend on continued biosynthesis to maintain the normal secretory rate of a particular hormone. Steroid hormones enter target cells by diffusion across the plasma membrane and then bind to nuclear or cytosolic receptors.

In general, endocrine organs are composed of islands of secretory epithelial cells delineated by a fine fibrovascular stroma rich in capillaries. With the exception of thyroid follicular epithelial cells, endocrine cells are arranged in cords or packets. Endocrine cells that secrete polypeptide hormones and catecholamines typically contain abundant, lacy to finely granular, pale eosinophilic cytoplasm, which is immunoreactive for chromogranins and synaptophysin that are present in secretory granules and microvesicles, respectively. Steroid hormone–secreting endocrine cells also contain abundant cytoplasm that appears foamy because of the presence of numerous lipid vacuoles.

PITUITARY GLAND (HYPOPHYSIS)

The adenohypophysis consists of three portions: the pars distalis, pars tuberalis, and pars intermedia (Fig. 12-2). In many animal species, the adenohypophysis completely surrounds the pars nervosa of the neurohypophyseal system. The pars distalis is the largest and is composed of several different endocrine cell populations surrounded by abundant capillaries to facilitate secretion of their trophic hormones (Web Fig. 12-1).

The pars tuberalis is an extension of the adenohypophysis and consists of dorsal projections of parenchymal cells along the infundibular stalk. It primarily functions as a scaffold for the capillary network of the hypophyseal portal system as it courses from the median eminence to the pars distalis. The pars intermedia is located between the pars distalis and pars nervosa; it lines the residual lumen of Rathke's pouch and has two populations of cells in certain

*In memory of Dr. Charles C. Capen, Department of Veterinary Biosciences, The Ohio State University, who made contributions to this chapter in the fourth edition.

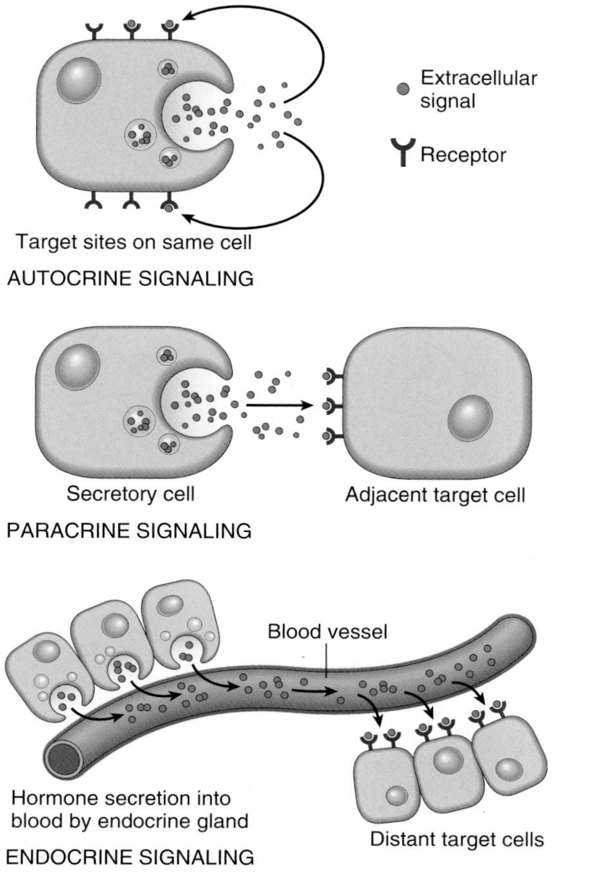

Fig. 12-1 Schematic diagram of the patterns of intercellular signaling (see text).

(Modified from Lodish H, Baltimore D, Berk A, et al, editors: *Molecular cell biology*, ed 3, New York, 1995, WH Freeman.)

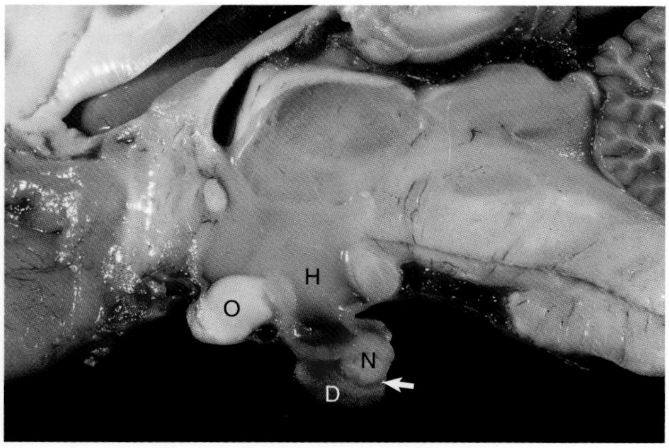

Fig. 12-2 Pituitary gland and brainstem, normal dog.

Longitudinal section of the pituitary region illustrating the close relationship to the optic chiasm *(O)*, hypothalamus *(H)*, and overlying brain. The pars distalis *(D)* forms a major part of the adenohypophysis and completely surrounds the pars nervosa *(N)*. The residual lumen of Rathke's pouch *(arrow)* separates the pars distalis and pars nervosa and is lined by the pars intermedia. (Courtesy Dr. C. Capen, College of Veterinary Medicine, The Ohio State University.)

species. In the dog, one of these cell types (B cell) synthesizes and secretes adrenocorticotropic hormone (ACTH).

A specific population of endocrine cells is present in the pars distalis (and also in the pars intermedia of dogs for ACTH secretion) that synthesizes, processes, and secretes each of the pituitary trophic hormones (Fig. 12-3). Secretory cells in the adenohypophysis are classified as acidophils, basophils, and chromophobes based on the reactions of their secretory granules with pH-dependent histochemical stains (Fig. 12-4). Based on contemporary specific immunohistochemical staining, acidophils can be further subclassified functionally into somatotrophs that secrete growth hormone (GH; somatotrophin) and lactotrophs that secrete prolactin. Basophils include gonadotrophs that secrete luteinizing hormone (LH) and follicle-stimulating hormone (FSH), thyrotrophs that secrete thyrotrophic hormone (thyroid-stimulating hormone [TSH]), and ACTH-secreting corticotrophs. Chromophobes are pituitary cells that by light microscopy lack stainable cytoplasmic secretory granules. They include the pituitary cells involved with the synthesis of ACTH and melanocyte-stimulating hormone (MSH) in some species, nonsecretory follicular (stellate) cells, degranulated chromophils (acidophils and basophils) in the actively synthesizing phase of the secretory cycle, and undifferentiated stem cells of the adenohypophysis.

Each type of endocrine cell in the adenohypophysis is under the control of a specific releasing hormone or factor from the hypothalamus (see Fig. 12-3). These releasing hormones are small peptides synthesized and secreted by neurons of the hypothalamus. They are transported by axonal processes to the median eminence, where they are released into capillaries and conveyed by the hypophyseal portal system to specific endocrine cells in the adenohypophysis. Each hormone stimulates the rapid release of secretory granules containing a specific preformed trophic hormone.

The neurohypophysis is subdivided into three anatomic parts. The pars nervosa (posterior lobe) represents the distal component of the neurohypophyseal system. The infundibular stalk joins the pars nervosa to the overlying hypothalamus and is composed of axonal processes from neurosecretory neurons. It also has numerous capillaries, supported by modified glial cells or pituicytes, which are termination sites for the nonmyelinated axonal processes of neurosecretory neurons in the hypothalamus. The neurohypophyseal hormones, oxytocin and antidiuretic hormone (ADH) or vasopressin, are synthesized in the cell body of hypothalamic neurons, packaged into secretory granules, transported by long axonal processes of the hypothalamohypophyseal tract to axons in the pars nervosa, and released into the capillary bed of the hypothalamohypophyseal portal system.

Neurosecretory neurons in the hypothalamus secrete hormone in response to neural input from higher centers, resulting in hormonal secretion. ADH and oxytocin are nonapeptides synthesized by neurons situated either in the supraoptic or paraventricular nuclei of the hypothalamus. ADH and its corresponding neurophysin appear to be synthesized as part of a common larger biosynthetic precursor molecule, termed *propressophysin*. The hormones are packaged with a corresponding binding protein (i.e., neurophysin) into membrane-limited neurosecretory granules and transported to the pars nervosa for release into the circulation.

ADRENAL GLAND

Adrenal Cortex

The adrenal glands of mammals consist of two distinct parts that differ not only in morphology and function but also in embryologic origin. Because of their close structural relationships, the outer cortex and inner medulla of the adrenal glands usually have been

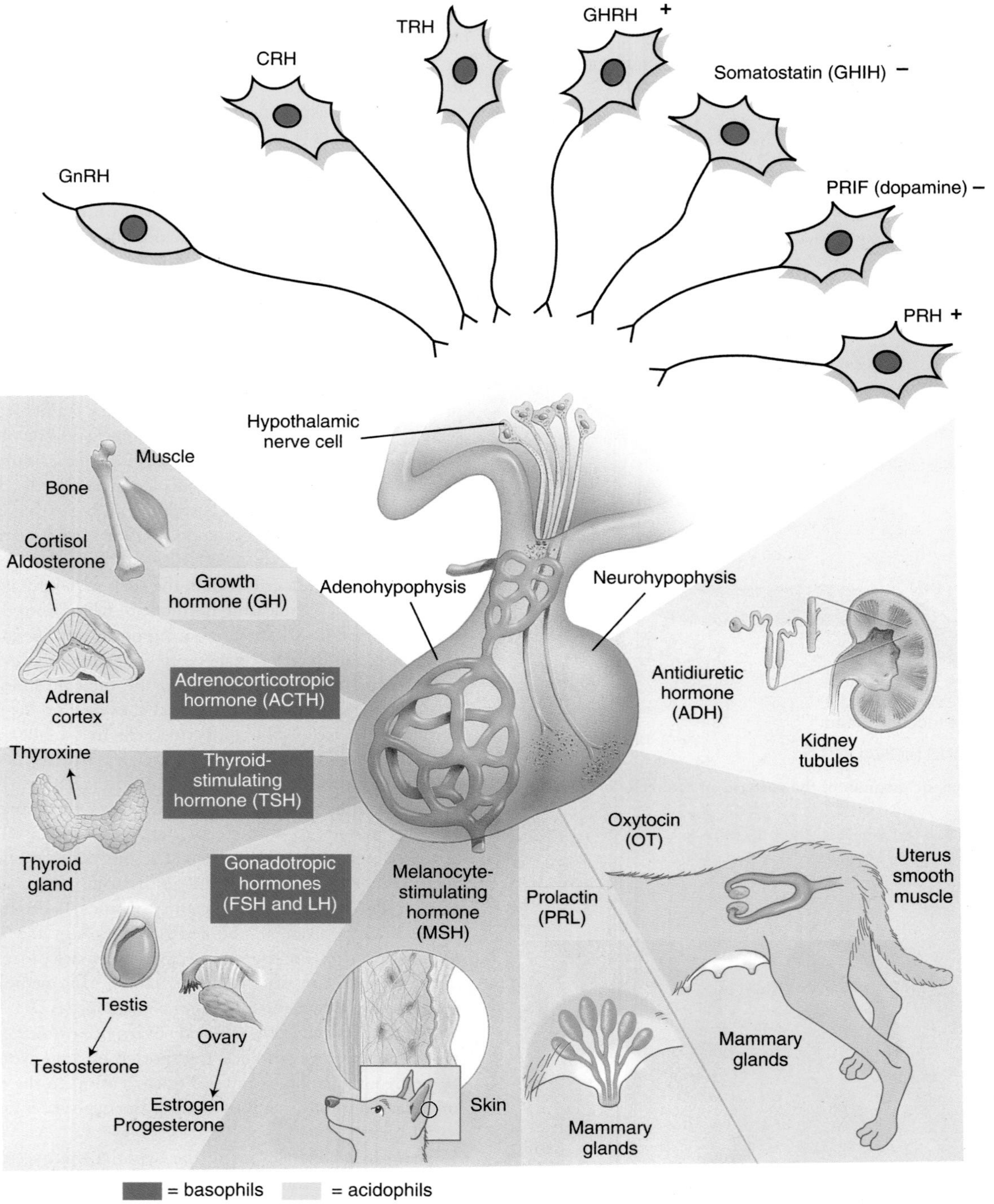

Fig. 12-3 Hypothalamic-pituitary-target gland axis.

Releasing hormones produced by the hypothalamus act on anterior or posterior portions of the pituitary gland to release trophic hormones. Trophic hormones act on specific endocrine glands, stimulating them to produce hormones that exert ultimate actions on downstream tissues. *CRH,* Corticotropin-releasing hormone; *FSH,* follicle-stimulating hormone; *GHIH,* growth hormone–inhibiting hormone; *GHRH,* growth hormone–releasing hormone; *GnRH,* gonadotropin-releasing hormone; *LH,* luteinizing hormone; *PRH,* prolactin-releasing hormone; *PRIF,* prolactin release–inhibiting factor; *TRH,* thyrotropin-releasing hormone. (Modified from Huether SE, McCance KL: *Understanding pathophysiology,* ed 2, St Louis, 2000, Mosby; and Squire L, Bloom F, McConnell S: *Fundamental neuroscience,* ed 2, San Diego, 2003, Academic Press.)

considered parts of one organ (Fig. 12-5). The adrenal cortex develops from cells of the coelomic epithelium that are of mesodermal origin. The chromaffin tissue and sympathetic ganglion cells of the adrenal medulla are derived from ectoderm of the neural crest.

The adrenal cortex of normal dogs is firm, yellow, and nearly uniformly thick. The soft, brown medulla is surrounded by the cortex. In normal dogs, the cortical-to-medullary ratio is approximately 2:1. The adrenal glands are richly vascularized, and a sinusoidal network, which demarcates the cell columns of the adrenal cortex, empties into the venous tree at the periphery of the medulla.

The adrenal cortex microscopically and functionally is subdivided into three layers or zones, although the demarcation between

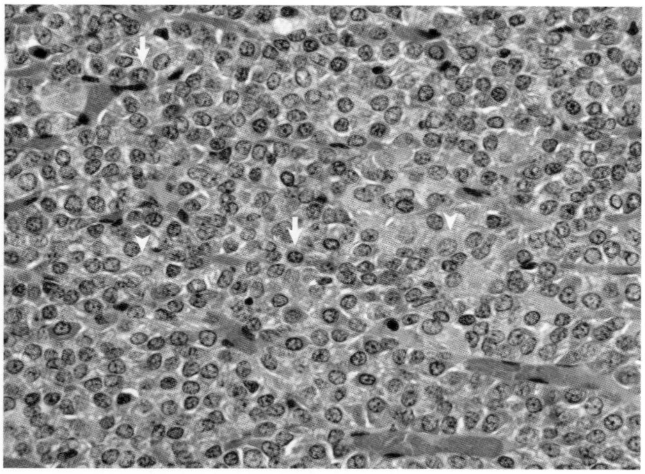

Fig. 12-4 Pars distalis, normal dog.
The pars distalis is composed of acidophils *(arrows)*, basophils (none shown here) and chromophobes *(arrowheads)*. H&E stain. (Courtesy Dr. J.F. Zachary, College of Veterinary Medicine, University of Illinois.)

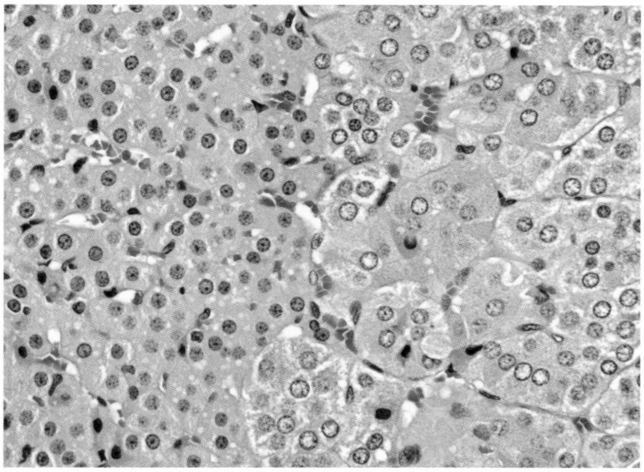

Fig. 12-5 Adrenal gland, normal dog.
Interface between the finely vacuolated (lipid droplets) cells of the adrenocortical zona reticularis *(left)* and chromaffin cells of the adrenal medulla *(right)*. H&E stain. (Courtesy Dr. J.F. Zachary, College of Veterinary Medicine, University of Illinois.)

zones often is not distinct. The zona glomerulosa or multiformis (outer zone) adjacent to the capsule is composed of columns of cells that have a sigmoid or arclike arrangement. It represents about 15% of the cortical volume and is responsible for the secretion of mineralocorticoid hormones. The secretory cells of the zona fasciculata (middle zone) are arranged in long anastomosing cords separated by numerous small capillaries. This zone constitutes about 80% of the cortical volume, is composed of cells that contain abundant cytoplasmic lipid, and is responsible for the secretion of the glucocorticoid hormones. The zona reticularis (inner zone) accounts for the remaining 5% of the cortical volume. The secretory cells, arranged in small groups surrounded by capillaries, are responsible for the secretion of sex steroids.

Mineralocorticoids are adrenal steroids that principally affect ion transport by epithelial cells and cause excretion of potassium and conservation of sodium. The most potent and important naturally occurring mineralocorticoid is aldosterone. Enzymatically controlled electrolyte pumps in epithelial cells of the renal tubule

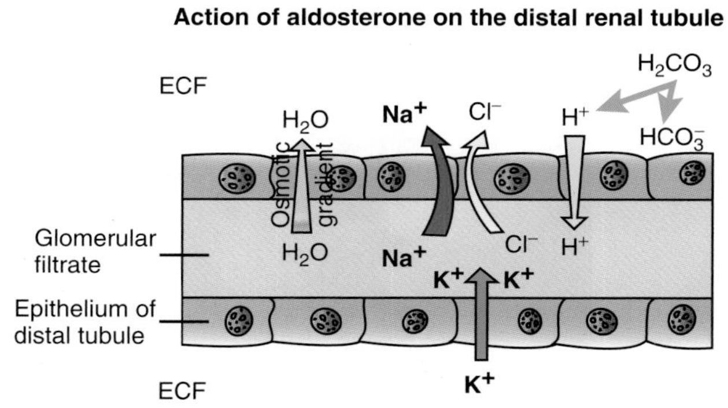

Fig. 12-6 Aldosterone secreted by the zona glomerulosa of the adrenal cortex acts on the distal portions of the nephron to increase tubular excretion of potassium and increase resorption of sodium (and secondarily of chloride).
The resulting osmotic gradient facilitates movement of water from the glomerular filtrate into the extracellular fluid *(ECF)*. (Redrawn with permission from Dr. C. Capen, College of Veterinary Medicine, The Ohio State University.)

and sweat glands respond to mineralocorticoids by conserving sodium and chloride and by excreting potassium. In the distal convoluted tubule of the mammalian nephron, a cation-exchange mechanism is responsible for the resorption of sodium from the glomerular filtrate and secretion of potassium into the lumen (Fig. 12-6). These reactions are accelerated by mineralocorticoids but still proceed, although at a much slower rate in their absence. Lack of mineralocorticoid secretion, such as in the Addison's-like disease of dogs, can result in lethal retention of potassium and loss of sodium.

Cortisol and lesser amounts of corticosterone are the most important naturally occurring glucocorticoid hormones secreted by the adrenal glands in many animal species. In general, the actions of glucocorticoids on carbohydrate, protein, and lipid metabolism result in sparing of glucose, a tendency to hyperglycemia, and increased glucose production. In addition, glucocorticoids decrease lipogenesis and increase lipolysis in adipose tissue, which results in release of glycerol and free fatty acids.

Glucocorticoids also function to suppress both inflammatory and immunologic responses, thereby reducing the necrosis and fibroplasia that can occur with these responses. However, under the influence of increased concentrations of glucocorticoids, an animal has reduced resistance to bacteria, viruses, and fungi. Glucocorticoids can impair the immunologic response at any stage from the initial interaction and processing of antigens by cells of the monocyte-macrophage system through the induction and proliferation of immunocompetent lymphocytes and subsequent antibody production. Inhibition of a number of functions of lymphoid cells by glucocorticoids forms part of the basis for immunosuppression.

Glucocorticoids exert a profound negative effect on wound healing. Dogs with hypercortisolism can have wound dehiscence (Fig. 12-7). The basic mechanism is inhibition of fibroblast proliferation and collagen synthesis, leading to a decrease in scar tissue formation.

Sex hormones (e.g., progesterone, estrogens, and androgens) are synthesized in small amounts by secretory cells of the zona reticularis of the adrenal cortex. Excessive adrenal sex steroids secreted by a neoplasm arising in the zona reticularis can occur infrequently, resulting in clinical manifestations of virilism, precocious sexual development, or feminization (effects depend on which steroid is secreted in excess, the sex of the patient, and the age at onset).

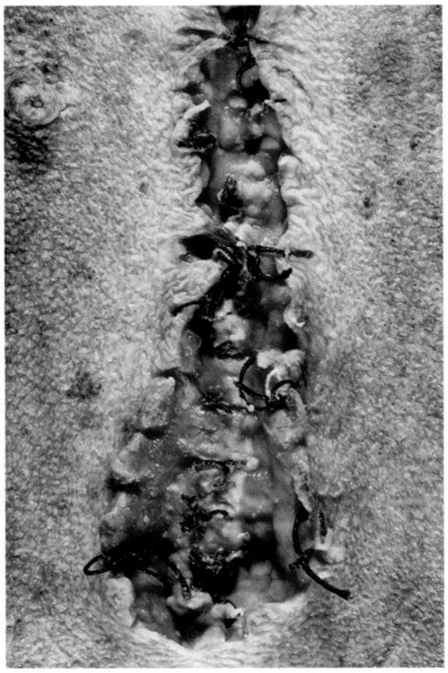

Fig. 12-7 Dehiscence of surgical wound, skin, ventral abdomen, dog. Wounds heal slowly in dogs with cortisol excess because of an inhibition of fibroblastic proliferation. (Courtesy Dr. C. Capen, College of Veterinary Medicine, The Ohio State University.)

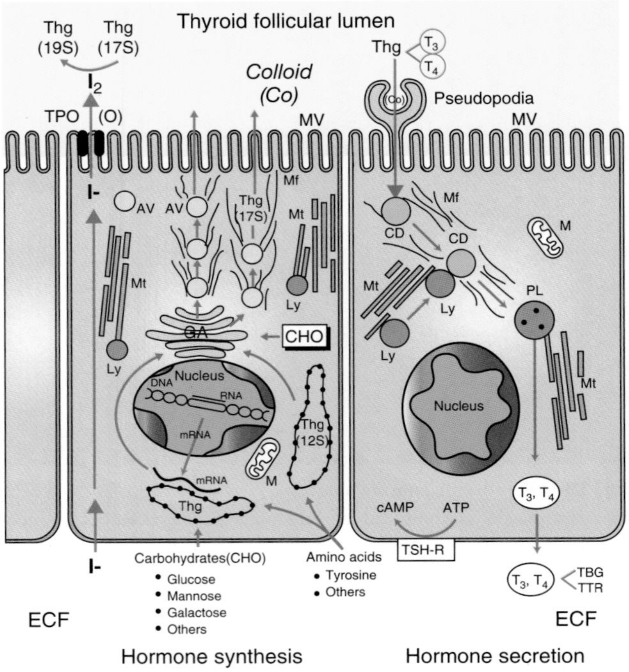

Fig. 12-8 Thyroid follicular cells illustrating two-way traffic of materials from capillaries into the follicular lumen. Raw materials, such as iodide, are concentrated by follicular cells and rapidly transported into the lumen *(left side of drawing).* Amino acids (tyrosine and others) and sugars are assembled by follicular cells into thyroglobulin *(Thg),* packaged into apical vesicles *(AV)* and released into the lumen. The iodination of tyrosyl residues with the thyroglobulin molecule to form thyroid hormones occurs within the follicular lumen. Elongation of microvilli *(MV)* and endocytosis of colloid *(Co)* by follicular cells occur in response to thyroid-stimulating hormone *(TSH)* stimulation *(right side of drawing).* The intracellular colloid droplets *(CD)* fuse with lysosomal bodies *(Ly),* active thyroid hormone is enzymatically cleaved from thyroglobulin, and free T4 and T3 are released into the circulation. *ATP,* Adenosine triphosphate; *cAMP,* cyclic adenosine monophosphate; *CHO,* carbohydrates; *ECF,* extracellular fluid; *GA,* Golgi apparatus; *M,* mitochondrion; *Mf,* microfilaments; *Mt,* microtubules; *PL,* phagolysosome; *TBG,* thyroid-binding globulin; *TPO,* thyroid peroxidase; *TSH-R,* thyroid-stimulating hormone receptor; *TTR,* transthyretin. (From Capen CC: Pathophysiology of the thyroid gland. In Dunlop RH, Malbert C-H, editors: *Veterinary pathophysiology,* Ames, IA, 2004, Blackwell Publishing.)

Adrenal Medulla

The adrenal medulla is derived from neuroectoderm of the neural crest and produces catecholamine hormones. The main biosynthetic pathway for catecholamines in mammals starts with tyrosine that is converted first to 1-dihydroxyphenylalanine (dopa) by tyrosine hydroxylase. Dopa is then decarboxylated by 3,4-amino acid decarboxylase to 3,4-dihydroxyphenylethylamine (dopamine), which subsequently undergoes β-hydroxylation by dopamine β-oxidase to form norepinephrine. In mammals the medulla is completely surrounded by the adrenal cortex, and venous blood from the cortex bathes the medullary cells. This blood has the greatest concentration of corticosteroids of any fluid in the body. This close anatomic association between the adrenal cortex and medulla in mammals is not fortuitous because the *N*-methylating enzyme, phenylethanolamine-*N*-methyl transferase, which converts norepinephrine to epinephrine, is corticosteroid hormone dependent.

THYROID GLAND

Thyroid Follicular Cells

The thyroid gland in most animal species has two lobes, one on each lateral surface of the trachea. In pigs, the main lobe of the thyroid gland is on the midline in the ventral cervical region with dorsolateral projections from each side. In dogs, the right lobe of the thyroid gland is situated slightly cranial to the left lobe and almost touches the caudal aspect of the larynx.

The thyroid gland is the largest of the endocrine organs that function exclusively as endocrine glands. The basic histologic structure of the thyroid gland is unique among endocrine glands and consists of follicles of varying size (20 to 250 μm), which contain colloid produced by the follicular cells. The follicular cells are cuboidal to columnar and are orientated so that their secretory pole is directed toward the lumen of the follicle. An extensive network of interfollicular and intrafollicular capillaries provides the follicular cells with an abundant blood supply. Follicular cells have extensive profiles of rough endoplasmic reticulum for synthesis and a large Golgi apparatus for packaging of substantial amounts of protein, which are then transported into the follicular lumen. The luminal side of follicular cells in contact with the colloid has numerous microvilli (Web Fig. 12-2).

The synthesis of thyroid hormones is unique among those of the endocrine glands because the final assembly of hormone occurs extracellularly within the follicular lumen. Follicular cells trap essential raw materials, such as iodide from the blood, by a sodium-iodide symporter in the basolateral plasma membrane and then transport them rapidly against a concentration gradient to the lumen, where the iodide is oxidized by thyroid peroxidase in the microvilli to iodine (I_2) (Fig. 12-8). The assembly of thyroid hormones within the follicular lumen is made possible by a unique protein, thyroglobulin. Thyroglobulin is a high molecular weight (600,000 to 750,000 Da) glycoprotein synthesized in successive subunits on the ribosomes of the endoplasmic reticulum in follicular cells. The constituent amino acids (tyrosine and others) and carbohydrates (e.g., mannose, fructose, galactose) are derived from the circulation. Recently synthesized thyroglobulin (17S) leaves the Golgi apparatus and is packaged into apical vesicles that are extruded into the follicular lumen (see Fig. 12-8). The amino acid tyrosine, an essential component of thyroid hormones, is incorporated within the molecular structure of thyroglobulin. Iodine is bound to tyrosyl residues in thyroglobulin at the apical surface of follicular cells to form monoiodotyrosine (MIT) and diiodotyrosine (DIT) (see Fig. 12-8). The resulting MIT and DIT combine to form the two biologically active iodothyronines, T_4 and T_3, secreted by the thyroid gland.

The secretion of thyroid hormones into the bloodstream from colloid is initiated by elongation of microvilli and formation of pseudopodia on the luminal surface of follicular cells. In response to TSH, these extend into the follicular lumen and indiscriminately phagocytose the adjacent colloid. Colloid droplets within follicular cells fuse with numerous lysosomes. T_3 and T_4 are released from the thyroglobulin molecule, diffuse across the follicular cell basement membrane, and enter into adjacent capillaries. Negative feedback control of thyroid hormone secretion is accomplished by the coordinated response of the adenohypophysis and certain hypothalamic nuclei to concentrations of T_4 and T_3 in the blood.

TSH is delivered to thyroid follicular cells where it binds to the basilar aspect of the cell, activates adenyl cyclase, and increases the rate of all biochemical reactions concerned with the biosynthesis and secretion of thyroidal hormones. If the secretion of TSH is sustained (hours or days), thyroid follicular cells become more columnar and follicular lumina become smaller as a result of increased uptake of colloid by endocytosis (Fig. 12-9). Numerous periodic acid–Schiff (PAS)-positive colloid droplets are present in the luminal aspect of the hypertrophied follicular cells. The converse occurs in the thyroid gland in response to increases in circulating T_4 and T_3, which cause a corresponding decrease in TSH. Thyroid follicles become enlarged and distended with colloid as a result of decreased TSH-mediated endocytosis of colloid. Follicular cells lining the involuted follicles become low cuboidal, with only a few endocytic vacuoles at the interface between the colloid and follicular cells (Fig. 12-10).

T_4 and T_3, once released into the circulation, act on many different target cells in the body. The overall functions of T_4 and T_3 are similar, although much of the biologic activity appears to be the result of monodeiodination of T_4 to 3,5,3′-triiodothyronine (T_3) before they interact with high-affinity nuclear receptors in target cells. In certain conditions, such as protein starvation during the neonatal period, hepatic and renal disease, and fever, T_4 is preferentially monodeiodinated to 3,3′,5′-triiodothyronine (reverse T_3). Because reverse T_3 produced by target cells is biologically inactive, monodeiodination to form reverse T_3 provides a mechanism by which the overall metabolic effects of thyroid hormones are attenuated. The subcellular mechanism of action of thyroid hormones resembles that of steroids, in that free hormone enters target cells and binds initially to cytosol-binding proteins and subsequently to high-affinity nuclear receptors. Binding of thyroid hormone to receptors on the inner mitochondrial membrane is responsible for the early activation of energy metabolism and increased oxidative phosphorylation.

Thyroid C (Parafollicular) Cells

Calcitonin is secreted by a second endocrine cell population, C or parafollicular cells, in the mammalian thyroid gland. These cells are situated either in the follicular wall, within the basement membrane between follicular cells, or in small groups adjacent to interfollicular capillaries between follicles (Web Fig. 12-3). C cells do not border the follicular colloid directly, and their secretory pole is oriented toward the interfollicular capillaries. The distinctive feature of C cells is the presence of numerous small, membrane-limited, cytoplasmic secretory granules, which are immunoreactive for calcitonin.

Calcitonin is a polypeptide hormone secreted according to the calcium ion concentration in plasma and extracellular fluids. The rate of calcitonin secretion is upregulated in response to increased blood calcium concentrations.

C cells store substantial amounts of calcitonin in their cytoplasm, and the hormone is discharged rapidly into interfollicular capillaries in response to hypercalcemia (Fig. 12-11). C cells respond to long-term hypercalcemia by hyperplasia. When the blood calcium concentration is reduced, the stimulus for calcitonin secretion is diminished, and numerous secretory granules accumulate in the cytoplasm of C cells (see Fig. 12-11). Calcitonin exerts its function by interacting with target cells located primarily in bone and kidneys. The actions of parathyroid hormone (PTH) and

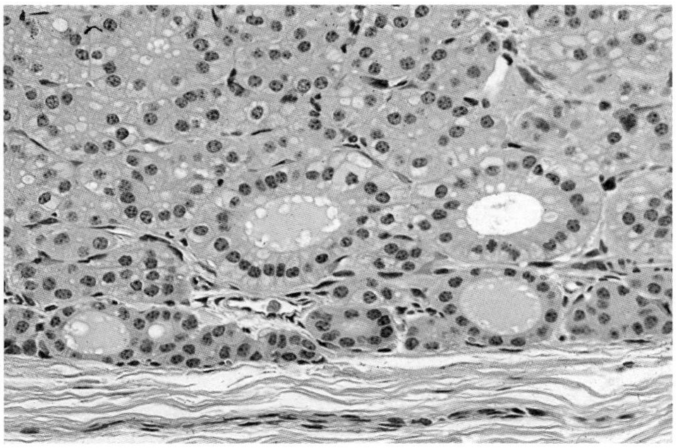

Fig. 12-9 Hyperplasia, thyroid gland, horse.
Follicular epithelial cells following prolonged thyroid-stimulating hormone stimulation are columnar. Note the many collapsed follicles. The lumens of remaining follicles contain pale pink colloid and have numerous endocytic vacuoles at the epithelial cell-follicular lumen interface. H&E stain. (Courtesy Dr. B. Harmon, College of Veterinary Medicine, The University of Georgia; and Noah's Arkive, College of Veterinary Medicine, The University of Georgia.)

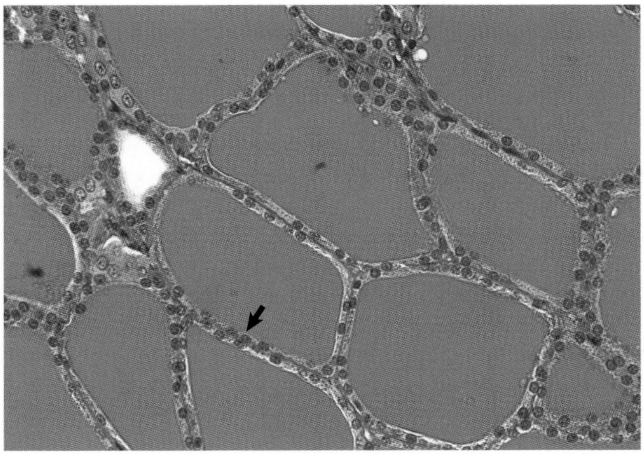

Fig. 12-10 Atrophy, thyroid gland, dog.
Thyroid follicular epithelial cells *(arrow)* after long-term administration of exogenous thyroxine are cuboidal and follicular lumens are distended with dense colloid. Periodic acid–Schiff reaction. (Courtesy Dr. C. Capen, College of Veterinary Medicine, The Ohio State University.)

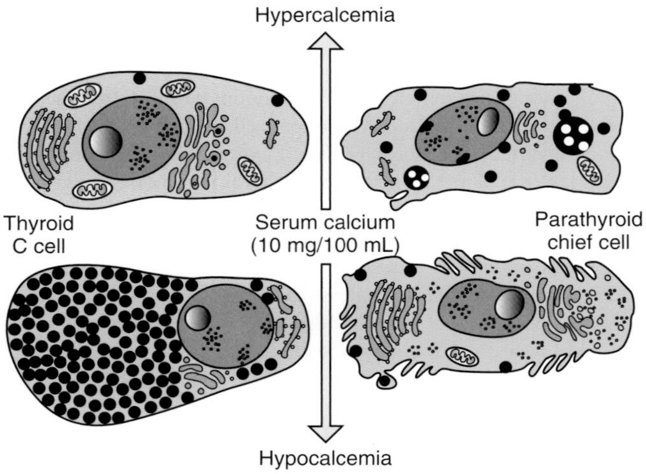

Fig. 12-11 Response of thyroid C cells and parathyroid chief cells to hypercalcemia and hypocalcemia.
C cells accumulate secretory granules in response to hypocalcemia, whereas chief cells are nearly degranulated but have an increased development of synthetic and secretory organelles. In response to hypercalcemia, C cells are degranulated and parathyroid chief cells are predominantly in the inactive stage of the secretory cycle. (Redrawn with permission from Dr. C. Capen, College of Veterinary Medicine, The Ohio State University.)

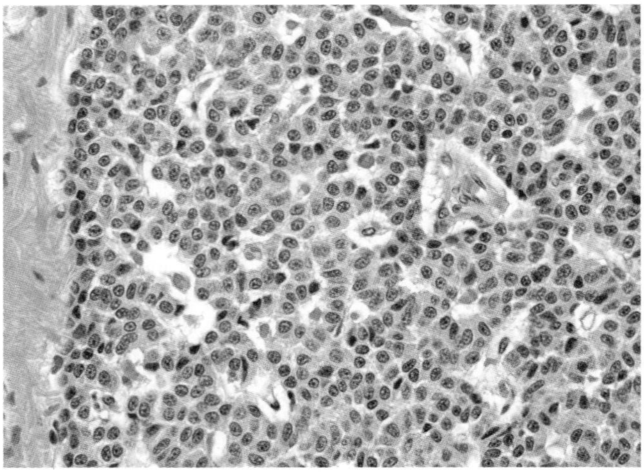

Fig. 12-12 Parathyroid gland, normal dog.
Numerous chief cells are separated and supported by a fine fibrovascular stroma. H&E stain. (Courtesy Dr. J.F. Zachary, College of Veterinary Medicine, University of Illinois.)

calcitonin are antagonistic on bone resorption, but synergistic in decreasing the renal tubular reabsorption of phosphorus.

PARATHYROID GLANDS

Parathyroid glands in most animal species consist of two pairs of glands situated in the cranial cervical region. The dog and cat have both external and internal parathyroid glands located near the thyroid gland. Other animal species, such as the pig, have only a single pair of parathyroid glands cranial to the thyroid gland, embedded either in the thymus in young animals or in adipose connective tissue in adult animals. In cattle and sheep, the larger external parathyroid gland is located a considerable distance cranial to the thyroid gland in the loose connective tissue along the common carotid artery. The smaller internal parathyroid glands are situated on the dorsal and medial surface of the thyroid gland. In horses, the larger ("lower") parathyroid gland is located a considerable distance from the thyroid gland in the caudal cervical region, near the bifurcation of the bicarotid trunk at the level of the first rib, whereas the smaller ("upper") parathyroid gland is situated near the thyroid gland.

The parathyroid glands of animals are composed predominantly of chief cells in different stages of secretory activity (Fig. 12-12). Oxyphil cells, often forming nodules, are also present in parathyroid glands of senile horses and cattle. They are larger than chief cells, and their abundant cytoplasm is filled with numerous large, often bizarre-shaped mitochondria and few secretory granules. Although their presence has been associated with hyperparathyroidism in certain species, the extent of their functional capacity remains controversial.

Biologically active PTH secreted by chief cells is a straight-chain polypeptide consisting of 84 amino acid residues, with a molecular weight of approximately 9500 Da. Secretory cells in the parathyroid glands of most animals store relatively small amounts of preformed hormone but are capable of responding to minor fluctuations in calcium ion concentration rapidly, by altering the rate of hormonal secretion, and more slowly, by altering the rate of hormonal synthesis (Fig. 12-13). In contrast to most endocrine organs that are under complex control, the parathyroid glands have a unique feedback control system based primarily on the concentration of calcium and, to a lesser extent, of magnesium ions in blood. Calcium ion concentration controls not only the rate of biosynthesis and secretion of PTH but also other metabolic and intracellular degradative processes within chief cells. Increased calcium ion concentration in extracellular fluids rapidly inhibits the uptake of amino acids by chief cells, and consequently synthesis of proPTH, its conversion to PTH, and secretion of stored PTH (see Fig. 12-13).

PTH is the principal hormone involved in the minute-to-minute, fine regulation of blood calcium concentration (total and ionic calcium) in mammals. It does this by directly influencing the function of target cells located primarily in bone and the kidneys, and indirectly acting in the intestine to maintain plasma calcium concentration sufficient to ensure the optimal functioning of a wide variety of body cells. The overall action of PTH on bone is to mobilize calcium into extracellular fluids (Fig. 12-14). Bone responds to PTH by increasing the activity of osteoclasts and osteocytes existing in bone.

PTH has a rapid (within 5 to 10 minutes) and direct effect on renal tubular function, leading to decreased reabsorption of phosphorus and consequently the development of phosphaturia. The site of action where PTH blocks tubular reabsorption of phosphorus has been determined to be the proximal tubule. The ability of PTH to enhance the renal absorption of calcium also is of considerable importance in the maintenance of calcium homeostasis. This effect of PTH on tubular reabsorption of calcium appears to be a result of a direct action on the distal convoluted tubule. Calcitonin and PTH, acting in concert, provide a dual negative feedback control mechanism to maintain the concentration of calcium in extracellular fluids within narrow limits.

The third major hormone involved in the regulation of calcium metabolism and skeletal remodeling is cholecalciferol or vitamin D_3 (see Fig. 12-14). Cholecalciferol is ingested in small amounts in the diet and can be synthesized in the epidermis from precursor molecules (e.g., 7-dehydrocholesterol) through a provitamin D_3 intermediate form in response to ultraviolet light. The active metabolites of vitamin D increase the absorption of calcium and phosphorus from the intestine and thereby maintain adequate concentrations

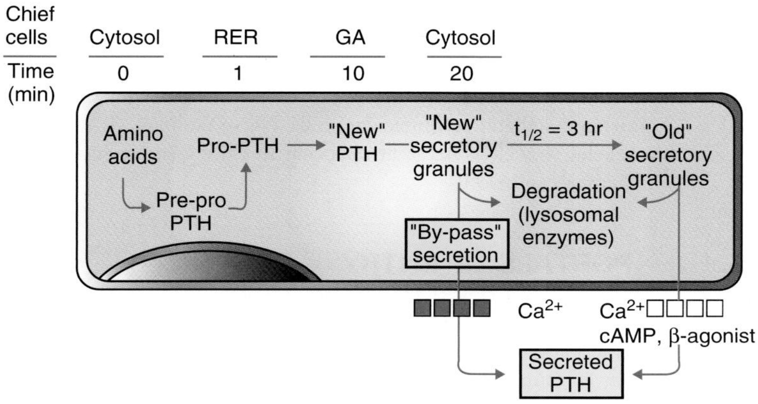

Fig. 12-13 Bypass secretion of parathyroid hormone *(PTH)* in response to increased demand signaled by decreased blood calcium ion concentration.

Recently synthesized and processed active PTH can be released directly without entering the storage pool of mature ("old") secretory granules in the cytoplasm of chief cells. PTH from the storage pool can be mobilized by cyclic adenosine monophosphate *(cAMP)* and β-agonists, such as epinephrine, norepinephrine, and isoproterenol, and by lowered blood calcium ion, whereas secretion from the pool of recently synthesized PTH can be stimulated only by a decreased calcium ion concentration. *RER,* Rough endoplasmic reticulum; *GA,* Golgi apparatus. (Redrawn with permission from Dr. C. Capen, College of Veterinary Medicine, The Ohio State University.)

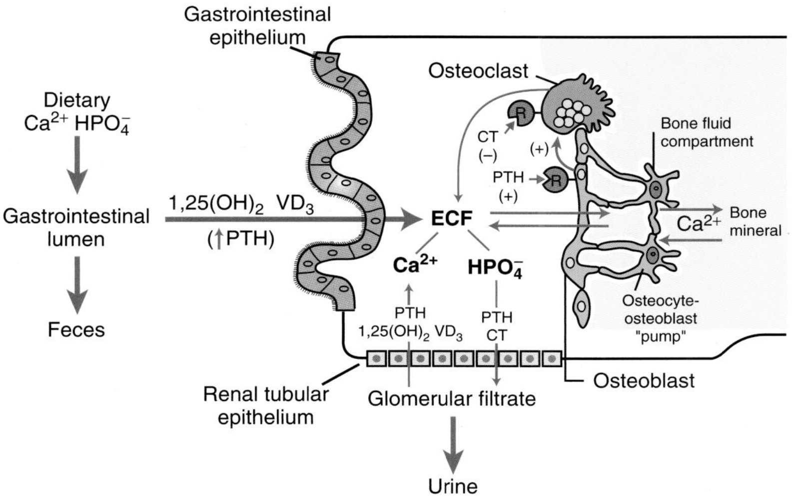

Fig. 12-14 Interrelation of parathyroid hormone *(PTH),* calcitonin *(CT),* and 1,25-dihydroxycholecalciferol *(1,25-[OH]$_2$ VD$_3$)* in hormonal regulation of calcium and phosphorus in extracellular fluids *(ECF).*

(Redrawn with permission from Dr. C. Capen, College of Veterinary Medicine, The Ohio State University.)

of these electrolytes in the extracellular fluids as required for the appropriate mineralization of bone matrix. From a functional point of view, vitamin D brings about the retention of sufficient mineral ions to ensure mineralization of bone matrix, whereas PTH maintains the proper ratio of calcium to phosphorus in extracellular fluids. The major target tissue for 1,25-$(OH)_2D_3$ is the mucosa of the small intestine, where it increases the active transcellular transport of calcium (cranial small intestine) and phosphorus (caudal small intestine).

PANCREATIC ISLETS

The endocrine function of the pancreas is performed by small groups of cells, the islets of Langerhans (Fig. 12-15), which are completely surrounded by acinar or exocrine cells that produce digestive enzymes. During embryonic development of the pancreas, a close relationship exists between the endocrine and exocrine portions. Evidence suggests that islet, acinar, and ductal cells arise from a common multipotential precursor cell. In early embryonic development, the endocrine cells are integrated within the exocrine matrix of the pancreatic bud. They subsequently accumulate in nonvascularized clusters and later become separated from the exocrine tissue and then independently vascularized.

The pancreatic islets of normal animals contain multiple types of cells. The predominant secretory cells are the β cells, which function in the biosynthesis of insulin but co-secrete islet amyloid polypeptide. The glucagon-secreting α cells are less numerous than β cells. δ Cells and F, or PP, cells in the islets secrete somatostatin and pancreatic polypeptide, respectively. The different cell types of the endocrine pancreatic cells can be differentiated by cytochemical and immunohistochemical techniques, and by electron microscopy (Web Fig. 12-4). The α, β, and δ cells have well-developed rough endoplasmic reticulum and Golgi complexes that participate in

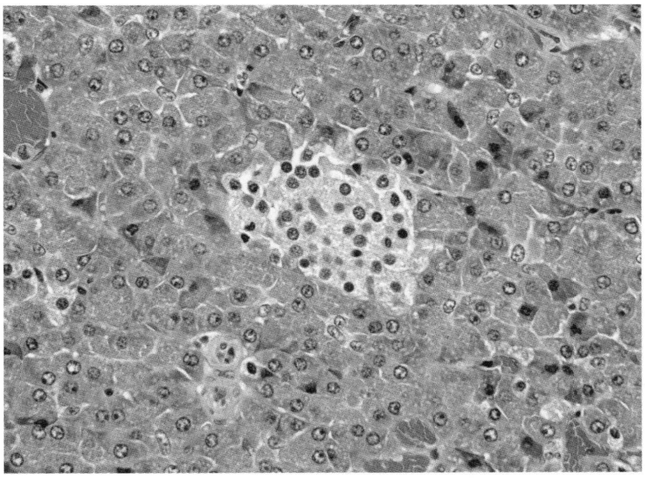

Fig. 12-15 Pancreatic islet, normal dog.

The islet is surrounded by the exocrine pancreas. H&E stain. (Courtesy Dr. J.F. Zachary, College of Veterinary Medicine, University of Illinois.)

the biosynthesis of polypeptide hormones, as well as numerous secretory granules in the cytoplasm. Each type of endocrine cell in the pancreatic islets has secretory granules with distinct ultrastructural characteristics, which can be used to identify the cell types; however, immunohistochemical identification of the specific islet hormone is a more accurate method of identifying different cell types in the pancreatic islets.

The major physiologic stimulus for the release of insulin from β cells is glucose. An appropriate concentration of calcium ion in extracellular fluids is required for induction of insulin release from β cells. Insulin is a powerful hormone with broad biologic influences that either directly or indirectly affects the structure and function of every organ in the body. Tissues especially responsive to insulin include skeletal and cardiac muscle, adipose tissue, fibroblasts, hepatocytes, leukocytes, mammary glands, cartilage, bone, skin, aorta, pituitary gland, and peripheral nerves. The principal function of insulin is to stimulate anabolic reactions involving carbohydrates, lipids, proteins, and nucleic acids. It catalyzes the formation of macromolecules used in cell structure, energy stores, and regulation of many cell functions. Hepatocytes, adipose cells, and muscle are three principal target sites for insulin. In general, insulin increases the transfer of glucose and certain other monosaccharides, some amino acids and fatty acids, and potassium and magnesium ions across the plasma membrane of target cells. In addition, it enhances glucose oxidation and glycogenesis and stimulates lipogenesis and the formation of adenosine triphosphate (ATP), DNA, and RNA. Insulin also decreases the rate of lipolysis, proteolysis, ketogenesis, and gluconeogenesis.

Glucagon is a hormone that stimulates energy release from target cells and is secreted in response to a reduction in blood glucose concentration. It mobilizes stores of energy-yielding nutrients by increasing glycogenolysis, gluconeogenesis, and lipolysis, thereby increasing the blood concentration of glucose. At physiologic concentrations, glucagon increases both hepatic glycogenolysis and gluconeogenesis. Insulin and glucagon act in concert to maintain the concentration of glucose in extracellular fluids within relatively narrow limits. A glucose sensor in the pancreatic islets controls the relative proportion of these two biologic antagonists. Glucagon controls glucose influx into the extracellular space from the hepatocytes, and insulin controls glucose efflux from the extracellular space into such insulin-sensitive cells as adipocytes, myocytes, and hepatocytes.

PINEAL GLAND

The pineal gland is a neuroendocrine organ that influences circadian rhythm and is intimately associated with the brain. It is composed of loose neuroglial stroma containing nests of pinealocytes and scattered calcified bodies known as *brain sand* or *corpora arenacea.* Pinealocytes secrete the hormone-like compound melatonin during periods of darkness. In addition to its role in circadian rhythms, melatonin is thought to influence seasonal reproductive activity in mammals through inhibition of gonadotropin-releasing hormone (GnRH).

CHEMORECEPTOR ORGANS

Chemoreceptor tissue is present at several sites in the body, including the carotid body, aortic bodies, nodose ganglion of the vagus nerve, ciliary ganglion in the orbit, pancreas, bodies on the internal jugular vein below the middle ear, and glomus jugular along the recurrent branch of the glossopharyngeal nerve. The chemoreceptor organs are sensitive indicators of changes in the blood carbon dioxide content, pH, and oxygen tension, thereby aiding in the regulation of respiration and circulation. Carotid and aortic bodies can initiate an increase in the depth, minute volume, and rate of respiration via parasympathetic nerves, and an increase in heart rate and elevation of arterial blood pressure via the sympathetic nervous system. The bodies are composed of parenchymal (chemoreceptor) and stellate (sustentacular) cells. Nerve endings with synaptic vesicles, as well as nerve fibers, occur in close association with the chemoreceptor cells.

PORTALS OF ENTRY

The portals of entry for the inflammatory agents affecting endocrine glands include hematogenous spread and direct extension. Autoimmune and infectious inflammatory diseases affect various endocrine glands. The pathogenesis of autoimmune diseases typically involves autoreactive T lymphocytes and autoantibodies, both of which gain access to the endocrine gland via the blood. Bacterial, viral, and fungal diseases preferentially restricted to individual endocrine glands rarely occur; however, endocrine glands are equally vulnerable to involvement in systemic diseases. Endocrine glands, such as the pituitary and pineal glands and the thyroid and parathyroid glands, can also become secondarily involved through direct extension from the meninges and larynx, respectively.

The endocrine system is unique in the fact that many of the disease processes affecting it involve disturbances of growth such as hyperplasia and neoplasia. The histopathologic differentiation among nodular hyperplasia, adenoma, and carcinoma is often more difficult in endocrine glands than in most other organs of the body. However, criteria used to differentiate these proliferative lesions should be established and applied in a uniform manner in the evaluation of proliferative lesions in endocrine glands. For many endocrine glands, there appears to be a continuous spectrum of proliferative lesions derived from a specific population of secretory cells between focal or nodular hyperplasia and adenomas.

Excessive focal growth of endocrine cells is the consequence of aberrant secretion of growth- and/or function-stimulating hormone(s) and has been referred to as *nonneoplastic endocrine hyperplasia.* Nodules arising in hyperplastic endocrine glands can be polyclonal and of clonal origin. Hyperfunction and cellular hypertrophy caused by nonneoplastic endocrine hyperplasia are considered to be largely reversible on cessation of the inciting stimulus; however, chronic and severe hyperplasia of endocrine tissues is not always fully reversible.

Endocrine glands appear predisposed to the development of an increased incidence of neoplasms after prolonged stimulation of a population of secretory cells. Long-continued stimulation can lead to the development of clones of cells within the hyperplastic endocrine glands that grow more rapidly and are consequently more susceptible to genetic alterations, resulting in neoplastic transformation on exposure to the appropriate combination of promoting agents.

RESPONSES TO INJURY

PATHOGENIC MECHANISMS OF ENDOCRINE DISEASES

Although injury of cells in endocrine glands is often attributable to processes, such as necrosis, inflammation, and autoimmunity, discussed in Chapters 1, 3, and 5, respectively, many diseases of endocrine glands are characterized by dramatic functional disturbances and characteristic clinicopathologic alterations affecting one or more body systems. The affected animal can have changes primarily involving the skin (alopecia caused by hypothyroidism), nervous system (seizures caused by hyperinsulinism), urinary system (polyuria caused by diabetes mellitus, diabetes insipidus, and hyperadrenocorticism), or skeletal system (fractures induced by hyperparathyroidism). There are several mechanisms that can disrupt normal endocrine function, with the majority of processes resulting in insufficient or excessive hormone production.

Primary Hypofunction of an Endocrine Gland

Hormone secretion is subnormal because of extensive destruction of secretory cells by a disease process, the failure of an endocrine gland to develop properly, or the result of a specific biochemical defect in the synthetic pathway of a hormone. In animals, immune-mediated injury characterized by notable infiltration of lymphocytes and plasma cells and deposition of electron-dense immune complexes along basement membranes causes hypofunction via progressive destruction of secretory parenchyma in one or more endocrine glands.

Failure of development also results in primary hypofunction of an endocrine gland. The classic example of this mechanism in animals is the failure of oropharyngeal ectoderm to differentiate completely into trophic hormone–secreting cells of the adenohypophysis in dogs, resulting in pituitary dwarfism (see the section on Disorders of Dogs).

Secondary Hypofunction of an Endocrine Gland

In secondary hypofunction of an endocrine gland, a destructive lesion in one organ, such as the pituitary gland, interferes with the secretion of a trophic hormone. This results in hypofunction of the target endocrine gland. Large, endocrinologically inactive pituitary neoplasms in adult dogs, cats, and other animals can interfere with the secretion of multiple pituitary trophic hormones and result in clinically detectable hypofunction of the adrenal cortex (Fig. 12-16), follicular cells of the thyroid gland, and gonads.

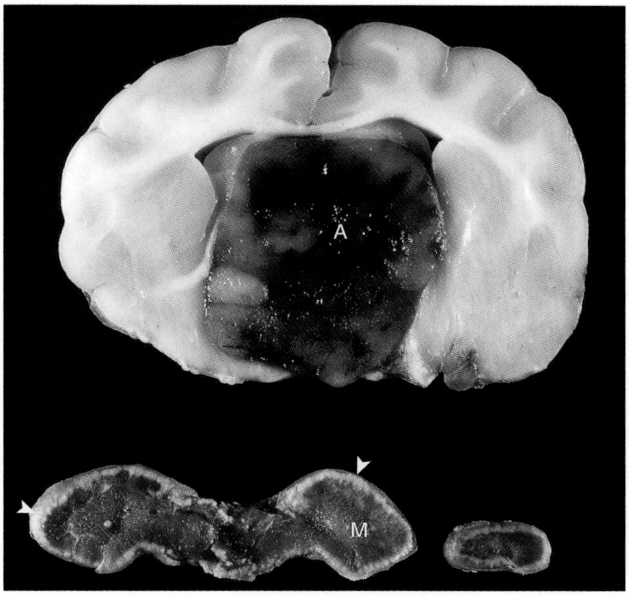

Fig. 12-16 **Secondary hypofunction of adrenal glands, brain, pituitary gland and left *(longitudinal section)* and right *(cross section)* adrenal glands, dog.**
A large nonfunctional chromophobe adenoma *(A)* has invaded and completely destroyed the adenohypophysis and hypothalamus, and infiltrated into the thalamus. Destruction of the adenohypophysis has resulted in a lack of secretion of thyrotropin, adrenocorticotropin, and other pituitary trophic hormones, resulting in severe bilateral (symmetrical) trophic atrophy of the adrenal cortex *(arrowheads),* especially the adrenocorticotropic hormone–dependent zona fasciculata and zona reticularis, and consequently, in a relatively more prominent medulla *(M).* (Courtesy Dr. C. Capen, College of Veterinary Medicine, The Ohio State University.)

Primary Hyperfunction of an Endocrine Gland

Primary hyperfunction of an endocrine gland is one of the most important pathologic mechanisms of endocrine disease in animals. The cells of a lesion, often a neoplasm derived from endocrine cells, autonomously synthesize and secrete a hormone at a rate in excess of the body's ability to use and degrade it, thereby resulting in a syndrome caused by hormone excess. Examples are summarized in Table 12-1.

TABLE 12-1 Primary Hyperfunction of an Endocrine Gland

Neoplasia	Hormone	Lesion/Sign
Acidophil adenoma (pituitary gland)	Growth hormone	Acromegaly
Adrenal cortical adenoma/carcinoma	Estrogen	Feminization
Pheochromocytoma (adrenal medulla)	Norepinephrine	Hypertension
Thyroid follicular cell adenoma	T_4, T_3	↑Basal metabolic rate
C-cell adenoma/carcinoma (thyroid gland)	Calcitonin	Osteosclerosis
Parathyroid gland chief cell adenoma	Parathyroid hormone	Fibrous osteodystrophy
Pancreatic β-cell adenoma/carcinoma	Insulin	Hypoglycemia

Secondary Hyperfunction of an Endocrine Gland

In this mechanism of endocrine disease, a lesion in one organ (e.g., adenohypophysis) secretes an excess of a trophic hormone that leads to long-term stimulation and hypersecretion of a hormone by a target organ. The classic example in animals is the ACTH-secreting neoplasm derived from pituitary corticotrophs in dogs and cats (Fig. 12-17). The functional disturbances and lesions are caused by increased blood cortisol concentrations resulting from the ACTH-stimulated hypertrophy and hyperplasia of the cells of the zonae fasciculata and reticularis of the adrenal cortex. In some aging dogs with notable adrenal cortical enlargement and functional disturbances of cortisol excess, no gross or histopathologic evidence of a neoplasm is present in the pituitary gland. These animals can have a change in negative feedback control as the result of an age-related increase in monoamine oxidase-β in the hypothalamus and increased metabolism of dopamine. The outcome is reduced inhibition of ACTH production by the pars intermedia of the pituitary gland leading to severe corticotroph hyperplasia, increased ACTH concentration in the blood, and long-term stimulation of the adrenal cortex, resulting in the syndrome of cortisol excess.

Hypersecretion of Hormones or Hormonelike Factors by Nonendocrine Neoplasms

Certain neoplasms of nonendocrine tissue in animals secrete either new humoral substances or hormones that share chemical and/or biologic characteristics with the "native" hormones secreted by an endocrine gland. Most of the recently discovered humoral

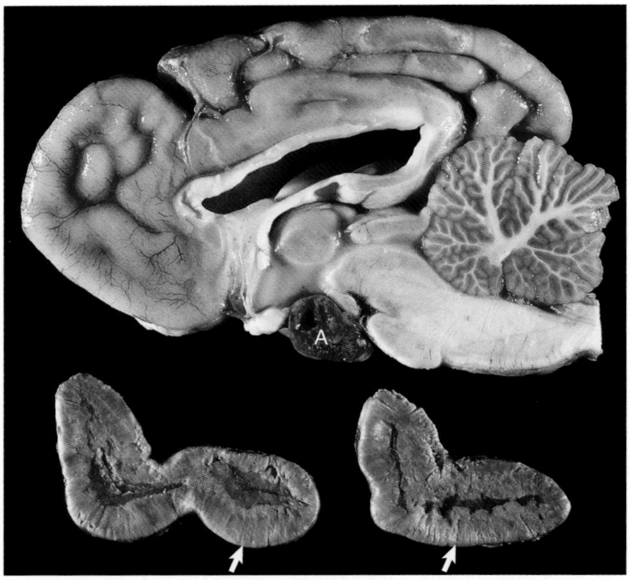

Fig. 12-17 **Secondary hyperfunction of adrenal glands, brain, pituitary gland and left and right adrenal glands, dog.**
Corticotroph (adrenocorticotropic hormone [ACTH]-secreting) chromophobe adenoma *(A)* in the pituitary gland and bilateral (symmetrical) enlargement of the adrenal glands. The chronic secretion of ACTH has resulted in bilateral (symmetrical) hypertrophy and hyperplasia of secretory cells of the zona fasciculata and zona reticularis in the adrenal cortex *(arrows)* and excessive secretion of cortisol. (Courtesy Dr. C. Capen, College of Veterinary Medicine, The Ohio State University.)

substances secreted by nonendocrine neoplasms are peptides rather than steroids, iodothyronines, or catecholamines. The nonpeptide hormones require more complex biosynthetic pathways and are infrequently produced by cancer cells. Pseudohyperparathyroidism or humoral hypercalcemia of malignancy is a clinical syndrome primarily produced by the autonomous hypersecretion of PTH–related peptide (PTHrP) by cancer cells. PTHrP interacts with the parathyroid hormone receptor in target cells (e.g., bone and kidneys) and results in persistent, often life-threatening hypercalcemia. A well-characterized example of this disease mechanism in animals is the adenocarcinoma of the apocrine glands of the anal sac in dogs (see the section on Disorders of Dogs). These neoplasms produce PTHrP, which mimics the action of PTH and results in an accelerated mobilization of calcium from bone by osteoclasts leading to the development of persistent hypercalcemia. Serum PTH concentrations are lower in dogs with apocrine carcinomas than in controls, and PTH concentrations are undetectable in neoplastic tissue.

Endocrine Dysfunction Caused by Failure of Target Cell Response

Failure of target cells to respond to a hormone can be caused by a lack of adenyl cyclase in the cell membrane or to an alteration in hormone receptors on the cell surface. Hormone is secreted in normal or increased amounts by the cells of the endocrine gland. For example, insulin resistance in obese animals can result from a decrease or downregulation of receptors on the surface of target cells. Receptor downregulation develops in response to a chronic increase in insulin stimulated by the hyperglycemia resulting from excessive food intake. Secretory cells in the corresponding endocrine gland (i.e., pancreatic islets) undergo compensatory hypertrophy and hyperplasia in an attempt to secrete additional hormone.

Endocrine Hyperactivity Caused by Diseases of Other Organs

The best-characterized example of endocrine hyperactivity caused by disease of other organs is the hyperparathyroidism that develops as a result of chronic renal failure or nutritional imbalance. In the renal form, hyperphosphatemia occurs because of a decreased glomerular filtration rate, resulting in a reciprocal decline in serum calcium and parathyroid stimulation. Subsequently the progressive destruction of cells of the proximal convoluted tubules interferes with the metabolic activation of vitamin D by 1α-hydroxylase in the kidneys, leading to decreased intestinal calcium absorption and continued parathyroid stimulation. This rate-limiting step in the metabolism of vitamin D is controlled by multiple factors, including levels of PTH, serum phosphorus, and several other hormones. The intestinal absorption of calcium is impaired and results in the development of progressive hypocalcemia; the hypocalcemia leads to long-term parathyroid gland stimulation and subsequently to the development of generalized demineralization of the skeleton. Nutritional hyperparathyroidism develops in animals fed abnormal diets that are either too low in calcium, too high in phosphorus, or deficient in cholecalciferol.

Endocrine Dysfunction Resulting from Abnormal Hormone Degradation

A decreased rate of hormonal degradation resulting in persistently elevated blood concentrations that simulate a syndrome of hypersecretion is the most common mechanism reported in domestic animal species. The classic example of this mechanism is the syndrome of hyperestrogenism-induced feminization secondary to decreased hepatic degradation of estrogens in patients with cirrhosis. Hypercalcemia, caused in part by a decrease in the ability of proximal convoluted tubular epithelial cells in the diseased kidneys to degrade PTH (along with a decrease in urinary excretion of calcium), is occasionally reported in dogs with chronic renal disease.

Iatrogenic Syndromes of Hormone Excess

The administration of an exogenous hormone can influence the activity of target cells either directly or indirectly and result in important functional disturbances. It is well recognized that the chronic administration of potent preparations of adrenal cortical steroids at inappropriately large daily doses (for the symptomatic treatment of various diseases) can produce most of the functional disturbances that are secondary to an endogenous hypersecretion of cortisol. Increased concentrations of exogenous cortisol result in notable atrophy of the adrenal cortex, particularly the ACTH-dependent zonae fasciculata and reticularis (Fig. 12-18). Similarly the administration of excessively large doses of insulin can result in hypoglycemia, and an excess of T_4 or T_3 can result in hyperthyroidism, especially in certain species, such as cats, which have limited capacities to conjugate T_4 with glucuronic acid and thus enhance its biliary excretion.

The administration of progestogens to dogs indirectly results in a syndrome of growth hormone excess. For example, the injection of medroxyprogesterone acetate for the prevention of estrus in dogs stimulates the expression of the growth hormone gene in the mammary glands and results in elevated circulating growth hormone concentrations, producing many of the clinical manifestations of acromegaly. The excessive skinfolds (Fig. 12-19), expansion of interdigital spaces, and abdominal enlargement in dogs with iatrogenic acromegaly are related to the protein anabolic effects of growth hormone. Elongation of bones in response to exogenous

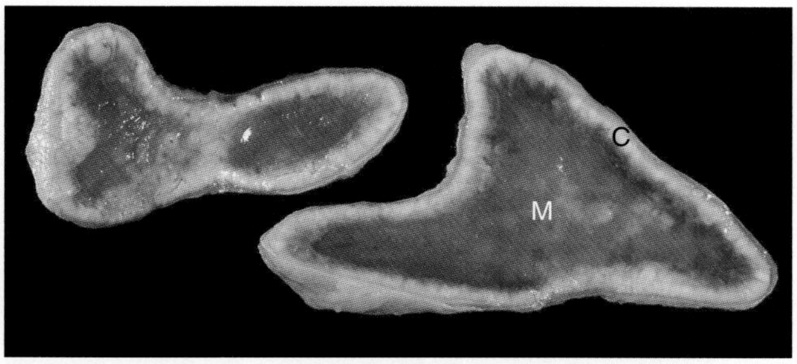

Fig. 12-18 Iatrogenic hyperadrenocorticism, left and right adrenal glands, dog.
Hyperadrenocorticism, caused by long-term administration of exogenous corticosteroids, has resulted in notable trophic atrophy of the adrenocorticotropic hormone–dependent zona fasciculata and zona reticularis of the adrenal cortex *(C)*. The adrenal medulla *(M)* comprises a relatively greater percentage of the atrophic adrenal gland than of a normal adrenal gland. (Courtesy Dr. C. Capen, College of Veterinary Medicine, The Ohio State University.)

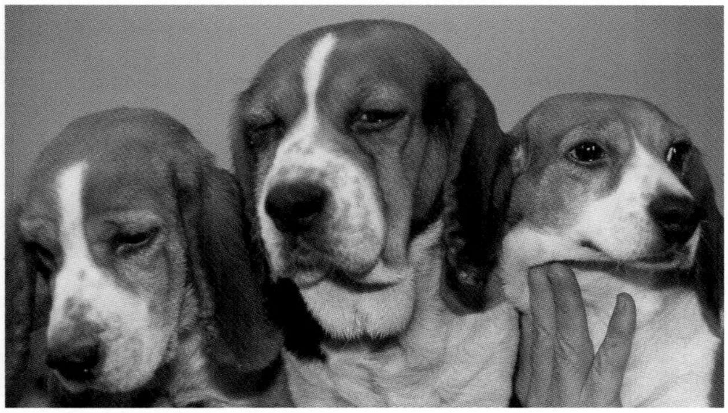

Fig. 12-19 Iatrogenic acromegaly, beagle *(center)* compared with unaffected littermates *(left and right)*.
Note the coarseness of the facial features and the markedly thick folds of the skin of the face. These characteristic changes are the result of the protein anabolic effects of somatotropin (produced by hyperplastic mammary ductular epithelial cells), which have been stimulated by the administration of exogenous medroxyprogesterone acetate. (Courtesy Dr. P. Concannon, College of Veterinary Medicine, Cornell University.)

progestogens requires functional growth plates and osteogenic surfaces.

DEFENSE MECHANISMS

The primary defense mechanism employed by the endocrine system is the hierarchy of hormonal regulation known as the *hypothalamic-pituitary-target gland axis* (see Fig. 12-3). The hypothalamus produces a number of releasing and inhibitory hormones in response to sensory input from the central nervous system (CNS). These releasing and inhibitory hormones act on anterior or posterior portions of the pituitary gland to stimulate or prevent the release of trophic hormones. Trophic hormones act on specific endocrine glands, stimulating them to produce hormones that exert ultimate actions on downstream tissues. Under normal circumstances, the action of a hormone is self-limiting because of the existence of negative feedback loops for each hormone series in which secretion of a particular hormone ultimately leads to inhibition of its subsequent secretion. Negative feedback from target endocrine glands can be directed at the hypothalamus, the pituitary gland, or both.

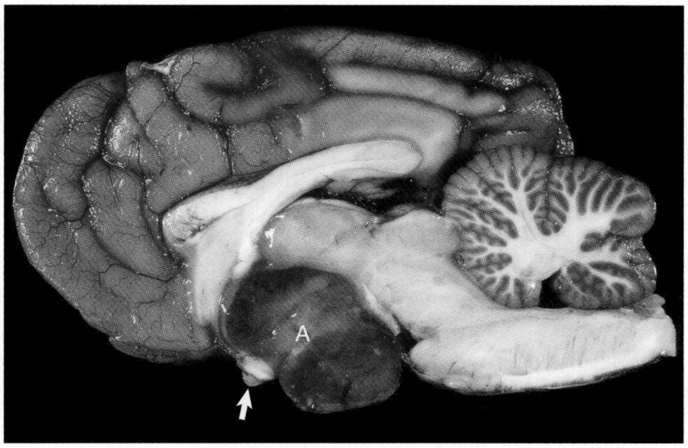

Fig. 12-20 Adenoma, pituitary gland, dog.
A large pituitary adenoma *(A)* has extended dorsally and compresses the overlying brain. The optic chiasm *(arrow)* is also severely compressed. The adenohypophysis, neurohypophysis, and hypothalamus have been destroyed by the neoplasm. (Courtesy Dr. C. Capen, College of Veterinary Medicine, The Ohio State University.)

DISORDERS OF DOMESTIC ANIMALS

Disorders known or thought to have a genetic basis and/or be inherited are listed in Web Table 12-1.

DISORDERS OF THE ADENOHYPOPHYSIS

Hypopituitarism and Neoplasms of the Adenohypophysis

Aplasia and Prolonged Gestation

See the section on Disorders of Ruminants for a discussion of aplasia and prolonged gestation.

Pituitary Cysts and Pituitary Dwarfism

See the section on Disorders of Dogs for a discussion of pituitary cysts and pituitary dwarfism.

Endocrinologically Inactive Chromophobe Adenomas

Nonfunctional pituitary neoplasms occur in dogs and cats but are uncommon in other species. Although chromophobe adenomas seem endocrinologically inactive, they can cause significant functional disturbances and clinical signs by compressing and causing atrophy of adjacent portions of the pituitary gland, as well as dorsal extension into the overlying brain (Fig. 12-20). The clinical disturbances result either from the lack of secreted pituitary trophic hormones and subsequent diminished target organ function (e.g., adrenal cortex; see Fig. 12-16) or from dysfunction of the CNS. Affected animals often have decreased spontaneous activity, incoordination, and disturbances of balance; are weak; and sometimes collapse after exercise. Chronically affected animals are blind and have dilated and fixed pupils because of compression and disruption of the optic nerves by dorsal extension of the pituitary neoplasms (see Fig. 12-20). Endocrinologically inactive pituitary adenomas often become large before they cause clinical signs or kill the animal (see Figs. 12-16 and 12-20).

Clinical signs reported with nonfunctional pituitary adenomas and hypopituitarism are not specific and could be confused with other disorders of the CNS, such as brain neoplasms and encephalitis, or with chronic renal disease. There is no effect on body stature secondary to compression of the pars distalis and interference with growth hormone secretion because these neoplasms usually arise in adult animals that have already completed their growth. However, atrophy of the skin and loss of muscle mass could be related in part to a lack of the protein anabolic effects of growth hormone. Impaired secretion of pituitary trophic hormones often leads to a reduced basal metabolic rate because of decreased TSH secretion and hypoglycemia secondary to trophic atrophy of the adrenal cortex (see Fig. 12-16).

Pituitary Gland Carcinomas

Pituitary gland carcinomas are uncommon neoplasms compared with adenomas but have been seen in older dogs and cattle. They usually are endocrinologically inactive but can cause significant functional disturbances by destroying the pars distalis and neurohypophyseal system, leading to panhypopituitarism and diabetes insipidus. Carcinomas are large and invade extensively into the overlying brain, along the ventral aspect of the cranial cavity, and into the basisphenoid bone where they cause osteolysis. Metastases occur infrequently to cervical lymph nodes or distant sites such as the spleen or liver. Carcinomas are highly cellular and often have large areas of hemorrhage and necrosis. Giant cells, nuclear pleomorphism, and mitotic figures are encountered more frequently than in adenomas.

Craniopharyngiomas (Intracranial Germ Cell Tumors)

Craniopharyngiomas are benign neoplasms derived from epithelial remnants of the oropharyngeal ectoderm of the craniopharyngeal duct (Rathke's pouch). They often occur in animals younger than those with other types of pituitary neoplasms and are present in either suprasellar or infrasellar locations. Craniopharyngioma is associated with dwarfism in young dogs because it causes subnormal secretion of somatotrophin and other trophic hormones at an early age, before closure of the growth plates.

The reclassification of some pleomorphic neoplasms in the suprasellar region of younger dogs from craniopharyngiomas to germ cell tumors has recently been proposed. The diagnosis of germ cell tumors was based on three criteria: (1) midline suprasellar location, (2) presence within the tumor of several distinct cell types (one population resembles a seminoma or dysgerminoma and others suggest teratomatous differentiation into secretory glandular and squamous elements), and (3) α-fetoprotein immunoreactivity.

Craniopharyngiomas and suprasellar germ cell tumors often are large and grow along the ventral aspect of the brain, where they can surround several cranial nerves. In addition, they extend dorsally into the hypothalamus and thalamus (Fig. 12-21). The resulting clinical signs often occur because of a combination of the following:

- A lack of secretion of pituitary trophic hormones resulting in trophic atrophy and subnormal function of the adrenal cortex and thyroid gland, atrophy of the gonads, and failure to attain somatic maturation because of a lack of secretion of growth hormone
- Disturbances in water metabolism (polyuria, polydipsia, low urine specific gravity, and osmolality) resulting from an interference in the synthesis and release of ADH by the large neoplasm
- Deficits in cranial nerve function
- CNS dysfunction caused by extension into the overlying brain

Microscopically, craniopharyngiomas have alternating solid and cystic areas. The solid areas are composed of nests of cuboidal, columnar, or squamous epithelial cells with focal areas of mineralization. The cystic spaces are lined by either columnar or squamous cells and contain keratin debris and colloid.

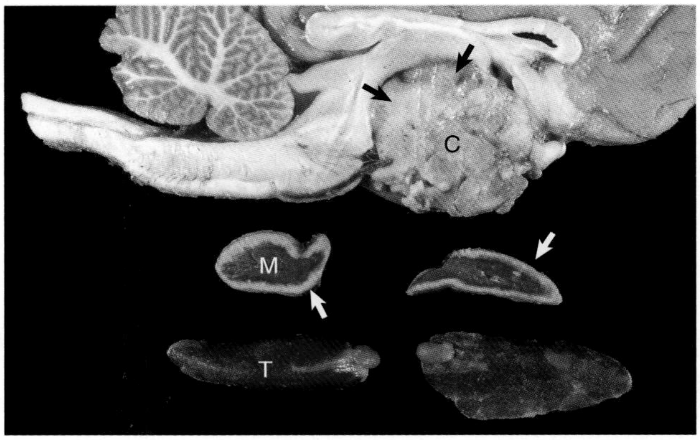

Fig. 12-21 Craniopharyngioma *(C)*, pituitary area, left and right adrenal glands, left and right thyroid glands, dog.
The neoplasm has extended dorsally through the hypothalamus and compressed the thalamus *(black arrows)*. The neoplasm has also destroyed the adenohypophysis and neurohypophysis, resulting in severe bilateral (symmetrical) trophic atrophy of the adrenal cortices *(white arrows)*. The adrenal glands consist predominantly of medulla *(M)* surrounded by a thin rim of cortex (capsule plus zona glomerulosa). Although the thyroid follicular cells are atrophic, the overall gland *(T)* size is within normal limits because of colloid involution of the follicles. (Courtesy Dr. C. Capen, College of Veterinary Medicine, The Ohio State University.)

Hyperpituitarism and Neoplasms of the Adenohypophysis

Pars Intermedia Adenomas

Adenomas derived from cells of the pars intermedia are the most common type of pituitary gland neoplasm in horses and the second most common type in dogs, but they are rare in other species. Adenomas develop in older horses, more frequently in females. Nonbrachycephalic breeds of dogs have adenomas of the pars intermedia more often than brachycephalic breeds.

Adenomas of the pars intermedia in dogs are either functionally inactive and result in varying degrees of hypopituitarism and diabetes insipidus, or endocrinologically active and secrete excessive levels of ACTH, leading to bilateral adrenal cortical hyperplasia and a syndrome of cortisol excess. Endocrinologically active (ACTH-secreting) adenomas of the pars intermedia in dogs have prominent groups of corticotrophs that have abundant eosinophilic cytoplasm and more widely scattered follicles.

Two cell populations have been identified in the pars intermedia of normal dogs by immunohistochemistry. The predominant cell type (A cell) is strongly immunoreactive for α-MSH, as in the pars intermedia of other species, whereas the second cell type (B cell) in the canine pars intermedia is strongly immunoreactive for ACTH. This second cell population accounts for the high bioactive ACTH concentration found in the pars intermedia of dogs and most likely gives rise to corticotroph adenomas of the pars intermedia in dogs with the syndrome of cortisol excess.

The clinical syndrome reported with neoplasms of the pars intermedia in horses is characterized by polyuria, polydipsia, polyphagia, muscle weakness, somnolence, intermittent hyperpyrexia, and generalized hyperhidrosis. The affected horses often develop hirsutism because of a failure to seasonally shed hair. The hair over most of the trunk and extremities is long (up to 10 to 12 cm), abnormally thick and wavy, and often matted (Fig. 12-22). Horses with larger neoplasms sometimes have insulin-resistant hyperglycemia and glycosuria, probably resulting from the downregulation of insulin receptors on target cells induced by chronic excessive intake of feed and hyperinsulinemia. The disturbances in

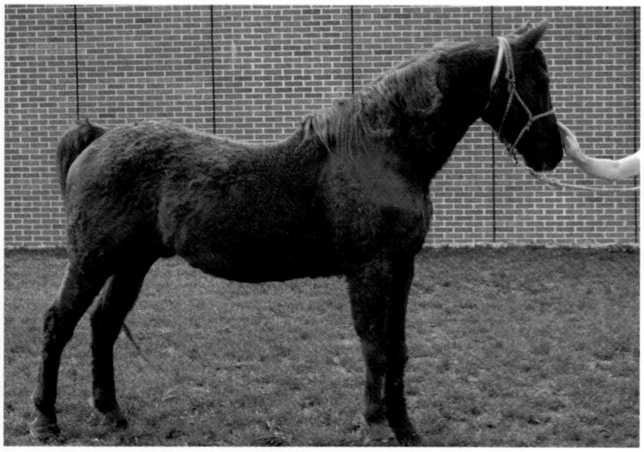

Fig. 12-22 Hirsutism, skin, horse.
The hirsutism is the result of a failure to shed hair because of hypothalamic compression by an adenoma of the pars intermedia. (Courtesy Dr. C. Capen, College of Veterinary Medicine, The Ohio State University.)

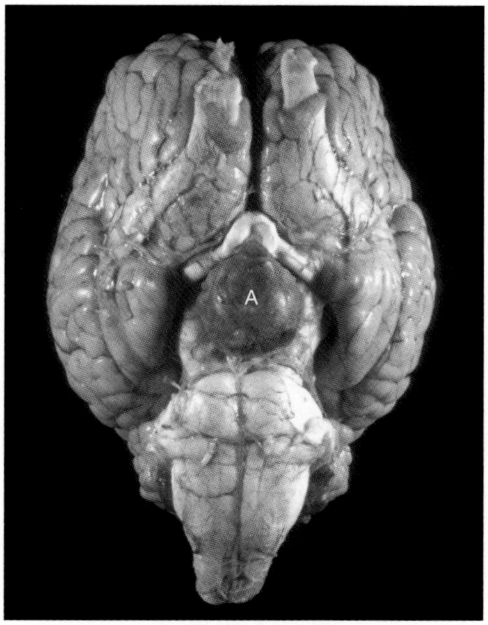

Fig. 12-23 Adenoma, brain, pituitary gland, horse. The pituitary gland is notably enlarged because of an adenoma *(A)* of the pars intermedia. (Courtesy College of Veterinary Medicine, University of Illinois.)

carbohydrate metabolism, ravenous appetite, hypertrichosis, and hyperhidrosis reflect deranged hypothalamic function caused by compression of the overlying hypothalamus by the large pituitary neoplasms. The hypothalamus is the primary center for homeostatic regulation of body temperature, appetite, and cyclic shedding of hair.

In addition to their space-occupying effects, some adenomas of the pars intermedia are endocrinologically active. Plasma cortisol and immunoreactive adrenocorticotropin (iACTH, molecular weight 4500 Da) concentrations can be modestly elevated in horses with pars intermedia adenomas. The cortisol concentrations often lack normal diurnal rhythm and are not suppressed by either large or small doses of dexamethasone. The modest increases of plasma iACTH appear to be caused by the different processing of proopiomelanocortin (POMC) in neoplasms derived from cells of the pars intermedia. This could explain the normal or slightly increased blood cortisol concentrations and normal or mildly hyperplastic adrenal cortices observed in some horses with adenomas of the pars intermedia. The concentrations of ACTH in the neoplasm have been reported to be six times that of the normal pars intermedia and only approach the concentrations found in the pars distalis of normal horses. The plasma and neoplasm concentrations of pars intermedia–derived peptides (corticotrophin-like intermediate lobe peptide [CLIP], α-MSH, β-MSH, and β-endorphin [β-END]) are disproportionately increased (40 times or more) compared with those of ACTH, apparently as the result of selective posttranslational processing of POMC in a manner similar to that of the normal pars intermedia.

Adenomas of the pars intermedia have immunohistochemical staining similar to that of the nonneoplastic equine pars intermedia. The findings include a strong, diffuse cytoplasmic reaction for POMC, a moderately strong reaction for α-MSH and β-END, a weak reaction for ACTH, and negative immunostaining for prolactin, glial fibrillary acidic protein, and neuron-specific enolase. Two antisera directed against different parts of the *N*-terminal fragment of human (h) POMC differ in their immunoreactivity. Immunostaining of neoplastic cells was stronger with anti-$h^{1\text{-}48}$ *N*-POMC antisera than with anti-$h^{1\text{-}76}$ *N*-POMC antisera. These immunohistochemical findings support the biochemical studies that suggest horses with pituitary adenomas derived from the cells of the pars intermedia develop a unique clinical syndrome that is the result of hypothalamic and neurohypophyseal derangement and an autonomous production of excess amounts of POMC-derived peptides. Although many of the functional disturbances in horses with pituitary adenomas (e.g., diabetes insipidus, polyphagia, hyperpyrexia, hyperhidrosis, and hirsutism) appear to be the result of hypothalamic or neurohypophyseal dysfunction, other behavioral signs (e.g., docility and diminished responsiveness to painful stimuli) could be related to increased plasma and cerebrospinal fluid concentrations of β-END. The clinical syndrome in horses with pituitary neoplasms is distinctly different from that of Cushing's disease in dogs and cats.

In dogs, adenomas of the pars intermedia result in only a moderate enlargement of the pituitary gland. The pars distalis is readily identifiable and sharply demarcated from the anterior margin of the neoplasm, usually by an incomplete layer of condensed stroma. The neoplasm can extend across the residual hypophyseal lumen and result in compression atrophy, but it usually does not invade the pars distalis. The posterior lobe is incorporated within the neoplasm, but the infundibular stalk is intact. Histologically, canine pars intermedia adenomas are composed of numerous large colloid-filled follicles lined by partially ciliated simple columnar epithelium scattered among nests of variably sized chromophobic cells.

In horses, adenomas of the pars intermedia often are large neoplasms that extend out of the fossa hypophysialis and severely compress the overlying hypothalamus (Fig. 12-23). The adenomas are yellow to white and multinodular and enclose the pars nervosa. When the neoplasm is incised, the pars distalis usually can be identified as a compressed subcapsular rim of tissue on the anterior margin. A sharp line of demarcation remains between the neoplasm and the compressed pars distalis. The neoplastic cells are arranged in cords and nests along the capillaries and connective tissue septae and are large, cylindrical, spindle-shaped, or polyhedral with oval hyperchromatic nuclei (Fig. 12-24). The pattern is often reminiscent of that of the prominent pars intermedia of normal horses. Ribbons of more cuboidal to columnar neoplastic cells occasionally form follicular structures that have dense eosinophilic colloid.

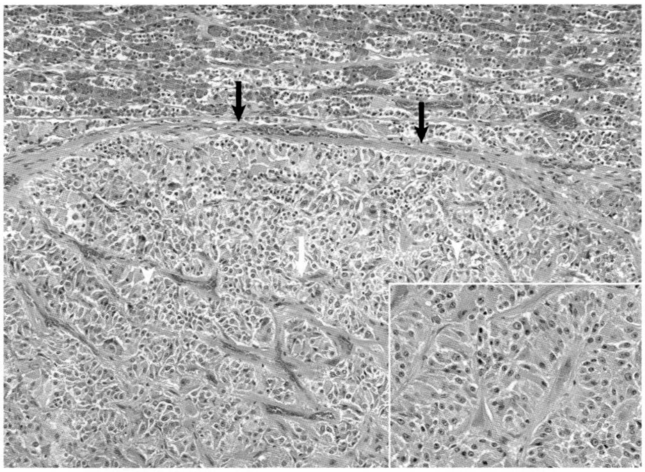

Fig. 12-24 Adenoma, pituitary gland, pars intermedia, horse. The adenoma is composed of cords and ribbons of well-differentiated, tall cuboidal to columnar cells with ample amounts of granular basophilic cytoplasm. Note the normal pituitary gland *(top quarter of figure)* that is demarcated from the adenoma by a band of connective tissue *(arrows)*. The expanding volume of the adenoma has compressed the normal gland. *Inset,* Higher magnification of the cells of the adenoma. H&E stain. (Courtesy Dr. J.F. Zachary, College of Veterinary Medicine, University of Illinois.)

Adrenocorticotropic Hormone-Secreting (Corticotroph) Adenomas

Functional (endocrinologically active) neoplasms arise in the pituitary gland of dogs, particularly boxers, Boston terriers, and dachshunds, and increasingly in cats. They are derived from corticotroph (ACTH-secreting) cells in the pars distalis but can also arise from the pars intermedia. These neoplasms cause a clinical syndrome of cortisol excess (Cushing's disease), resulting in gluconeogenic, lipolytic, protein catabolic, and antiinflammatory activities.

The pituitary gland is consistently enlarged (see Fig. 12-17); however, neither the occurrence nor the severity of functional disturbances appears to be directly related to the size of the neoplasm. Because the diaphragma sellae is incomplete in these species, the line of least resistance is dorsal expansion of the gradually enlarging pituitary mass. This results in invagination into the infundibular cavity, dilation of the infundibular recess and the third ventricle with eventual compression or replacement of the hypothalamus, and possible extension of the neoplasm into the thalamus (see Fig. 12-16).

Bilateral enlargement of the adrenal glands occurs with functional corticotroph adenomas (see Fig. 12-17). This enlargement is due to cortical hyperplasia, primarily of the zonae fasciculata and reticularis. Nodules of yellow-orange cortical tissue are often found outside the capsule and extending down into and compressing the adrenal medulla.

Pituitary corticotroph adenomas are composed of well-differentiated, large or small, chromophobic cells supported by fine connective tissue septa. The cytoplasm of the neoplastic cells usually is devoid of secretory granules but demonstrates immunoreactivity for ACTH +/− MSH, and hormone-containing secretory granules can be demonstrated by electron microscopy.

DISORDERS OF THE NEUROHYPOPHYSIS

Diabetes Insipidus

Diabetes insipidus results when inadequate ADH is produced (hypophyseal form) or when target cells in the kidneys lack the biochemical pathways necessary to respond to the secretion of normal or increased circulating concentrations of ADH (nephrogenic form). The hypophyseal form of diabetes insipidus results from compression and destruction of the pars nervosa, infundibular stalk, or supraoptic nucleus in the hypothalamus. The disruption of ADH synthesis or secretion in hypophyseal diabetes insipidus can be a result of a large pituitary neoplasm, a dorsally expanding cyst, inflammatory granuloma, or traumatic injury to the skull with hemorrhage and glial proliferation in the neurohypophyseal tissue. Compression or disruption of the posterior lobe, infundibular stalk, and hypothalamus by neoplastic cells interrupts the transport of ADH in nonmyelinated axons from the site of production, primarily in the supraoptic nucleus of the hypothalamus, to the site of release in the capillary plexus of the pars nervosa.

Animals with diabetes insipidus excrete large volumes of hypotonic urine, which in turn necessitates the ingestion of large amounts of water to prevent dehydration and hyperosmolality of body fluids. Urine osmolality is decreased below normal plasma osmolality (approximately 300 mmol/L) in both hypophyseal and nephrogenic forms of diabetes insipidus. In response to water deprivation, urine osmolality still remains below that of the plasma in both forms of diabetes insipidus in contrast to increased osmolality observed in normal animals. Urine osmolality is increased above that of plasma in response to exogenous ADH in the hypophyseal form, but this increase does not occur in nephrogenic diabetes insipidus, a useful feature in differential diagnosis.

DISORDERS OF THE ADRENAL CORTEX

Hypoadrenocorticism (Addison's Disease)

Adrenal cortical insufficiency was the first recognized endocrine disease and is a common endocrinopathy in dogs; however, it can occur in all animal species. Heritable hypoadrenocorticism has been reported in standard poodles, Portuguese water dogs, bearded collies, and Nova Scotia duck tolling retrievers. Clinical signs are a result of deficient production of any or all classes of corticosteroids (mineralocorticoids, glucocorticoids, and adrenal sex steroids). The synthesis and secretion of mineralocorticoids are reduced, resulting in marked alterations of serum potassium, sodium, and chloride concentrations (see Fig. 12-6). Less potassium is excreted by the kidneys (hypokaluria), resulting in severe hyperkalemia. Less sodium and chloride are reabsorbed from renal tubules, leading to varying degrees of hypernaturia and hyperchloriduria and a corresponding decline in blood concentrations of these ions. The severe hyperkalemia frequently produces notable cardiovascular disturbances. The pronounced bradycardia that develops in some dogs (heart rate of 50 or fewer beats per minute) does not change with exercise but does predispose to weakness and circulatory collapse after minimal exertion.

A decreased production of glucocorticoids results in several characteristic functional disturbances of hypoadrenocorticism. A failure of gluconeogenesis and increased sensitivity to insulin contributes to the development of moderate hypoglycemia. Hyperpigmentation of the skin occurs in some dogs with long-standing adrenocortical insufficiency. This lesion results from a lack of negative feedback to the pituitary gland and the increased release of ACTH (and possibly MSH). The plasma cortisol concentrations in dogs with hypoadrenocorticism are low and range from 0.1 to 1.5 μg/dL. Because of the severe atrophy of the adrenal cortex, little or no increase in blood cortisol concentration results after the administration of ACTH.

Adrenalitis

Bacterial and parasitic agents frequently localize in the adrenal glands and produce varying degrees of inflammation and necrosis.

Focal inflammatory processes usually are suppurative, arising in the course of bacterial septicemias. The adrenal capsule provides an effective barrier against direct invasion by inflammatory reactions in adjacent tissue. Granulomatous adrenalitis caused by *Histoplasma capsulatum, Coccidioides immitis,* or *Cryptococcus neoformans* occasionally occurs in dogs and cats. Multiple granulomas with central areas of necrosis and calcification can destroy nearly the entire adrenal cortex. *Toxoplasma gondii* produces necrosis with an infiltration of histiocytes in the adrenal cortex of many species of animals. Experimental evidence suggests that large local concentrations of antiinflammatory steroids in the adrenal cortex (e.g., cortisol and corticosterone) suppress local cell-mediated immunity and permit the progressive growth of certain fungi (e.g., *Histoplasma capsulatum, Coccidioides immitis*), protozoa (e.g., *Babesia darlingi, Babesia jellisoni,* or *Toxoplasma gondii*), and bacteria (e.g., *Mycobacterium tuberculosis*).

Adrenocortical Hemorrhage (Waterhouse-Friderichsen Syndrome)

Massive, diffuse, often bilateral adrenal cortical hemorrhage, a condition known as *Waterhouse-Friderichsen syndrome,* is an uncommon but fatal consequence of overwhelming sepsis (Fig. 12-25). Although frequently seen in conjunction with endotoxic shock, Waterhouse-Friderichsen syndrome can also result from Gram-positive organisms and noninfectious causes such as anticoagulant therapy and trauma.

Idiopathic Adrenocortical Atrophy

See the section on Disorders of Dogs for a discussion of idiopathic adrenocortical atrophy.

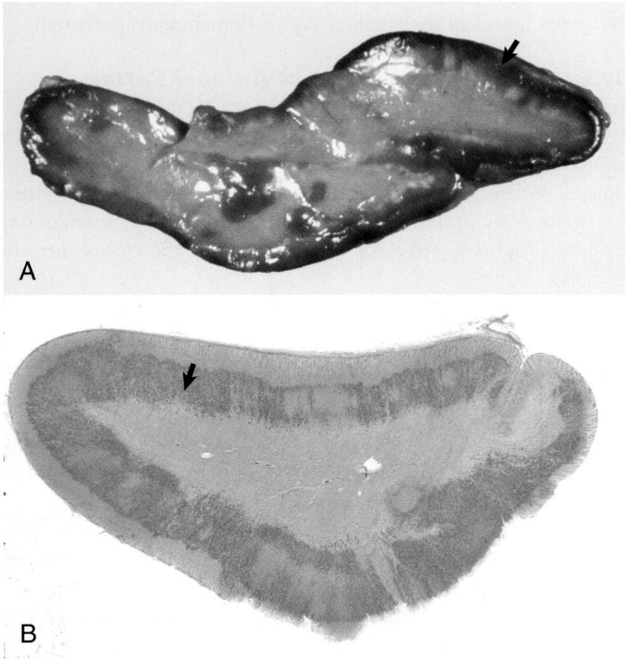

Fig. 12-25 Adrenocortical hemorrhage (Waterhouse-Friderichsen syndrome), adrenal gland, horse.

A, Diffuse hemorrhage *(arrow)* affecting the adrenal cortex is frequently seen in endotoxic shock. **B,** Subgross photomicrograph of diffuse hemorrhage *(arrow)* affecting the adrenal cortex. H&E stain. (Courtesy College of Veterinary Medicine, University of Illinois.)

Hyperadrenocorticism (Cushing's Syndrome or Disease)

Cortisol excess, or Cushing's syndrome, is one of the most common endocrinopathies in adult and aged dogs, increasingly in cats and rarely in other domestic animals. The clinical manifestations and lesions characteristic of the syndrome of hyperadrenocorticism result primarily from chronic overproduction of cortisol by hyperactive cells of the adrenal cortex. Affected animals develop a spectrum of functional disturbances and lesions resulting from the combined glyconeogenetic, lipolytic, protein catabolic, and antiinflammatory effects of the glucocorticoid hormones on many organs. The disease is insidious and slowly progressive. The increase in circulating cortisol concentrations in dogs with hyperadrenocorticism can result from one of several different pathogenic mechanisms. The most common cause of Cushing's syndrome is Cushing's disease in which a functional corticotroph (ACTH-secreting) adenoma of the pituitary gland causes bilateral adrenal cortical hypertrophy and hyperplasia (Fig. 12-26). The cortex of each adrenal gland is widened considerably as a result of diffuse and nodular hyperplasia, primarily in the zona fasciculata. Functional adrenal gland neoplasms are an infrequent (10% to 15% of cases) cause of Cushing's syndrome in the dog. Many of the clinical signs and lesions of naturally occurring hyperadrenocorticism can be induced by the long-term, daily administration of large doses of corticosteroids. To accurately separate the different pathogenetic mechanisms responsible for cortisol excess, plasma cortisol concentrations must be evaluated with the animal in the basal state and then after dexamethasone (large or small dose) suppression and ACTH stimulation.

Appetite and food intake often are increased as a direct result of either the hypercortisolism or damage caused by compression of the hypothalamic appetite centers by a large, dorsally expanding pituitary gland neoplasm. The muscles of the extremities and abdomen are weakened and atrophied, resulting in gradual abdominal enlargement (Fig. 12-27), lordosis, muscle trembling, and a straight-legged, skeletal-braced posture assumed to support the body's weight. Hepatomegaly caused by increased deposits of lipid and glycogen (steroid hepatopathy; see Fig. 8-73) can contribute to the development of the distended, often pendulous, abdomen. The muscular asthenia and wasting are the result of increased catabolism of structural proteins combined with diminished protein synthesis in skeletal myocytes from the influence of long-term cortisol excess. Cutaneous lesions occur frequently with hyperadrenocorticism. The initial changes in the skin often are observed over points of wear (e.g., neck, flanks, or behind the ears) and bony prominences. These initial cutaneous changes spread in a bilaterally symmetric pattern to involve a significant percentage of the body surface (see Fig. 12-27). Cutaneous lesions caused by excessive cortisol include atrophy of the epidermis and pilosebaceous units, combined with loss of collagen and elastin in the dermis and subcutis. Cutaneous calcification or calcinosis cutis is a characteristic lesion and occurs in up to 30% of dogs with hypercortisolism. Numerous calcium crystals are deposited along collagen and elastin fibers in the dermis and can penetrate through the atrophic and thinned epidermis, primarily in dogs and often with normal blood calcium and phosphorus concentrations. This manifestation of hypercortisolism is most likely related to the glyconeogenetic and protein catabolic action of cortisol, which results in the rearrangement of the molecular structure of such proteins as collagen and elastin, and the formation of an organic matrix that attracts and binds calcium. Severe calcification also occurs in other tissues such as lungs, active skeletal muscle, and the stomach.

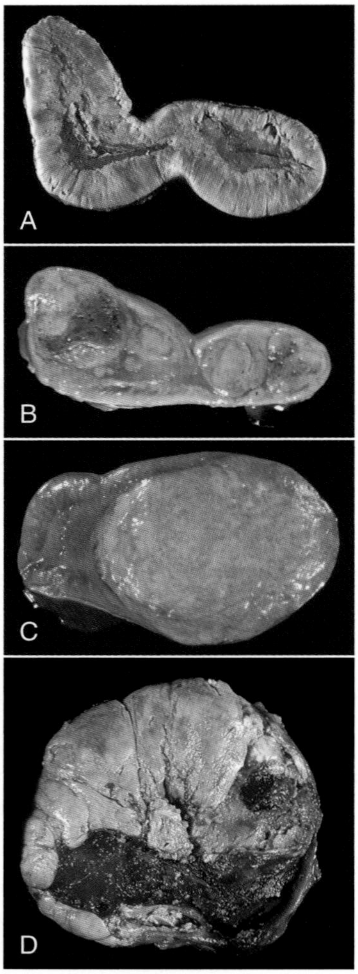

Fig. 12-26 Adrenal cortices, disturbances of growth, adrenal glands, dogs.
A, Laminar hyperplasia: diffuse thickening of the zona fasciculata and zona reticularis secondary to the effects of a "functional" corticotroph adenoma in the pituitary gland. **B,** Nodular hyperplasia: multiple discrete hyperplastic nodules extending from the cortex into the medulla. **C,** Adenoma: note the well-demarcated, large, yellow-tan adenoma compressing the adjacent medulla. **D,** Adenocarcinoma: large carcinoma with hemorrhage and necrosis. (**A** courtesy Dr. C. Capen, College of Veterinary Medicine, The Ohio State University. **B** courtesy Dr. W. Crowell, College of Veterinary Medicine, The University of Georgia and Noah's Arkive, College of Veterinary Medicine, The University of Georgia. **C** courtesy Dr. B. Weeks, College of Veterinary Medicine, Texas A&M University and Noah's Arkive, College of Veterinary Medicine, The University of Georgia. **D** courtesy Dr. C. Capen, College of Veterinary Medicine, The Ohio State University.)

Hyperaldosteronism (Conn's Syndrome)

Hyperaldosteronism is an increasingly recognized entity in cats and rarely in dogs because of unilateral or bilateral aldosterone-secreting adrenocortical neoplasms or adrenal hyperplasia. Unilateral adrenal adenomas are more common in cats. An adrenocortical carcinoma concomitantly secreting aldosterone, corticosterone, and cortisol has been reported. Older cats present with systemic hypertension and polymyopathy associated with hypernatremia and hypokalemia, respectively.

Congenital Adrenal Hyperplasia (Adrenogenital Syndrome)

Congenital adrenal hyperplasia is a condition of hypoadrenocorticism and hyperadrenocorticism. Affected individuals are deficient

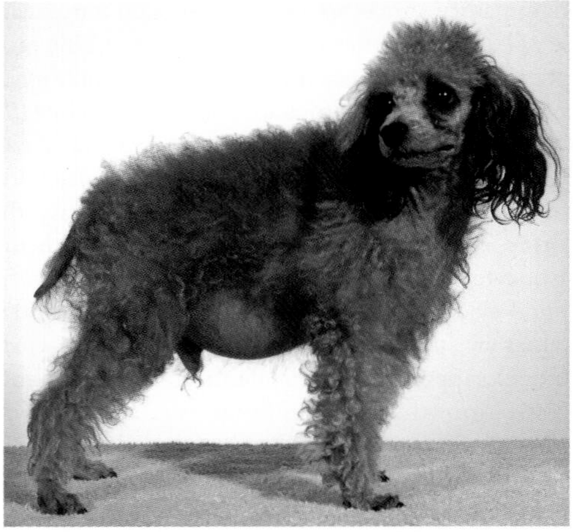

Fig. 12-27 Cushing's-like disease, hypercortisolism, dog, poodle. Hypercortisolism after exogenous corticosteroid administration for the treatment of idiopathic adrenal cortical hyperplasia. Muscle asthenia is the cause of the pendulous abdomen. Note the alopecia of the skin of the abdomen, ventral cervical region, and tail. (Courtesy Dr. C. Capen, College of Veterinary Medicine, The Ohio State University.)

in an enzyme, such as 21-hydroxylase, which is involved in both mineralocorticoid and glucocorticoid synthesis. As a consequence of reduced cortisol levels, there is a compensatory increase in ACTH secretion resulting in adrenal cortical hyperplasia. Subsequent steroid synthesis is diverted to the androgenic pathway, which is independent of 21-hydroxylase. Excessive androgen production leads to virilization and sexual ambiguity in newborns and premature closure of epiphyses. Pomeranians are predisposed to a congenital adrenal hyperplasia–like syndrome and associated dermatosis; however, no mutations in the 21-hydroxylase enzyme have been found in the small group of Pomeranians evaluated.

Hyperplasia and Neoplasia of Adrenal Cortex

Accessory Adrenal Tissue

Accessory or ectopic adrenal cortical tissue is common in the adrenal glands of adult to aged animals and can be found in the capsule, cortex, and medulla. Many of these nodules arise either as evaginations of the cortex into the capsule and surrounding periadrenal adipose tissue or invaginations of the cortex into the medulla.

Hyperplasia

Nodular hyperplasia is common in the adrenal glands as well-defined spherical nodules in the cortex or attached to the capsule (see Fig. 12-26). Hyperplastic nodules are usually multiple, bilateral and yellow, and involve any of the three zones of the cortex. Histologically, the nodules near the capsule resemble the zona glomerulosa and sometimes the zona fasciculata. The lipid content in these hyperplastic nodules is retained in circumstances that reduce the amount of lipid in the normal adrenal cortex. Hyperplastic cortical nodules are most common in older horses, dogs, and cats. Nodular hyperplasia of the zona reticularis has been seen in animals with functional disturbances suggestive of androgen excess (e.g., greater muscle mass, well-developed crest, clitoral hypertrophy, and mammary gland involution).

Diffuse cortical hyperplasia results in a uniform, usually bilateral, enlargement of the adrenal cortices (see Fig. 12-26). Notable hypertrophy and hyperplasia of cells of the zonae fasciculata and reticularis occur in response to an autonomous hypersecretion of

ACTH by a corticotroph adenoma of the pituitary gland (see Fig. 12-17). The cytoplasm of the hyperplastic cells of the zona fasciculata is vacuolated because of the lipid content. Cells of the outer zona glomerulosa can be compressed by the expansion of the inner two zones. Nodular hyperplasia can be present in a diffusely hyperplastic cortex.

Cortical Adenomas and Carcinomas

Adenomas of the adrenal cortex occur most frequently in older dogs and only sporadically in horses, cattle, and sheep. Castrated male goats have a greater incidence of cortical adenomas than intact males. Although these neoplasms are usually incidental findings at necropsy, they are occasionally endocrinologically active. Cortical adenomas are well demarcated and usually are a single, unilateral nodule (see Fig. 12-26). Larger cortical adenomas are yellow to red, distort the contour of the gland, compress the adjacent cortical parenchyma, and are partially or completely encapsulated. Cortical adenomas often develop in an adrenal gland with multiple nodules of hyperplasia and can be difficult to differentiate grossly from hyperplastic nodules. However, these hyperplastic nodules consist of multiple small foci, usually in both adrenal glands, without encapsulation, and often with extracapsular nodules of hyperplastic cortical tissue. Cortical adenomas are composed of well-differentiated cells that resemble secretory cells of the normal zona fasciculata or zona reticularis. The cytoplasm of neoplastic cells is abundant and lightly eosinophilic and filled with lipid droplets. Adenomas are partially or completely surrounded by a fibrous connective tissue capsule of varying thickness and a rim of compressed cortical parenchyma.

Adrenal cortical carcinomas occur less frequently than adenomas and have been reported most often in cattle and older dogs, but they also occur infrequently in other species. Carcinomas develop in adult to older dogs with no apparent breed or sex prevalence. Adrenal carcinomas are larger than adenomas, more likely to be bilateral, and frequently obliterate the affected gland(s). In dogs, they are composed of variegated, yellow-red, friable tissue (see Fig. 12-26) and can invade extensively into surrounding structures, such as the wall of the caudal vena cava, resulting in thrombus formation. Carcinomas attain considerable size in cattle (up to 10 cm or more in diameter) and have multiple areas of calcification or ossification.

Carcinomas are composed of more highly pleomorphic secretory cells than adenomas and are subdivided by a fine fibrovascular stroma. The growth pattern of neoplastic cells varies between neoplasms and within the same carcinoma and can be trabecular, lobular, or focal. Neoplastic cells usually are large and polyhedral, and they have prominent nucleoli and densely eosinophilic or vacuolated cytoplasm.

Carcinomas and adenomas of the adrenal cortex in dogs occasionally are functional and secrete excessive amounts of cortisol. The clinical syndrome produced by excessive secretion by adrenal cortical carcinomas can be complicated by signs produced by compression of adjacent organs when the neoplasm is large; by invasion into the aorta or caudal vena cava, which can lead to intraabdominal hemorrhage; and by metastases to distant sites (e.g., liver, kidneys, mesenteric lymph nodes, and lungs). Functional cortical adenomas and carcinomas are responsible for severe atrophy of the contralateral adrenal cortex because of negative feedback inhibition of pituitary ACTH secretion by the increased blood cortisol concentrations (Fig. 12-28). The atrophic cortex consists primarily of the adrenal capsule and zona glomerulosa. Atrophy is also present in the remnants of the adrenal cortex compressed by functional adenomas. Because of the lack of cortical tissue, the adrenal medulla appears more prominent (see Fig. 12-28).

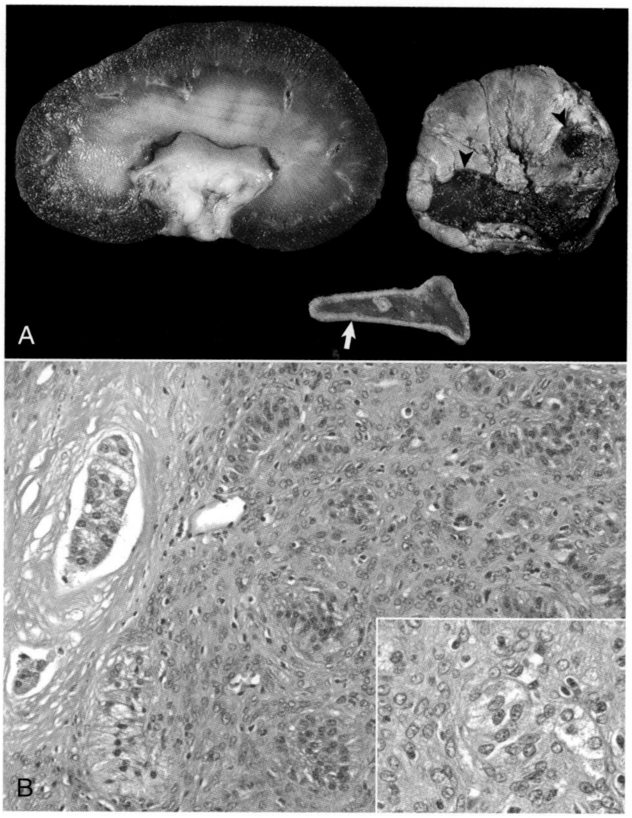

Fig. 12-28 **Adrenocortical carcinoma and contralateral cortical atrophy, adrenal glands, dog.**
A, The adrenal gland *(right)* has a large adrenocortical carcinoma that is almost half the size of an adult kidney *(left)*. Multifocal to coalescing areas of hemorrhage and necrosis are apparent *(arrowheads)* in this tumor. The cortex of the contralateral adrenal gland *(lower)* is notably thinned *(arrow)* because of severe trophic atrophy of the zona fasciculata and zona reticularis. Also see Fig. 12-31. **B,** Note the invasive adrenocortical carcinoma *(right)* and the vascular invasion characteristic of this tumor in the left margin of the figure. *Inset:* Cells are haphazardly arranged and there is marked variation of cellular and nuclear size, typical of the cells that form anaplastic neoplasms. H&E stain. (**A** courtesy Dr. C. Capen, College of Veterinary Medicine, The Ohio State University. **B** courtesy Dr. J.F. Zachary, College of Veterinary Medicine, University of Illinois.)

Functional Proliferative Lesions in Ferrets

Information on this topic is available at evolve.elsevier.com/Zachary/McGavin/.

DISORDERS OF THE ADRENAL MEDULLA

Proliferative Lesions

Adrenal Medullary Hyperplasia

Diffuse or nodular adrenal medullary hyperplasia appears to precede the development of pheochromocytoma in bulls with C-cell neoplasms of the thyroid gland. The proliferated chromaffin cells are nonencapsulated but compress the surrounding adrenal cortex (Fig. 12-29). Hyperplastic cells are round to oval and have pale basophilic cytoplasm. Some bulls with prominent diffuse medullary hyperplasia also often have a few small proliferative nodules. Medullary hyperplasia is diagnosed on the basis of the following criteria: an increased adrenal weight, a decrease in cortical to medullary

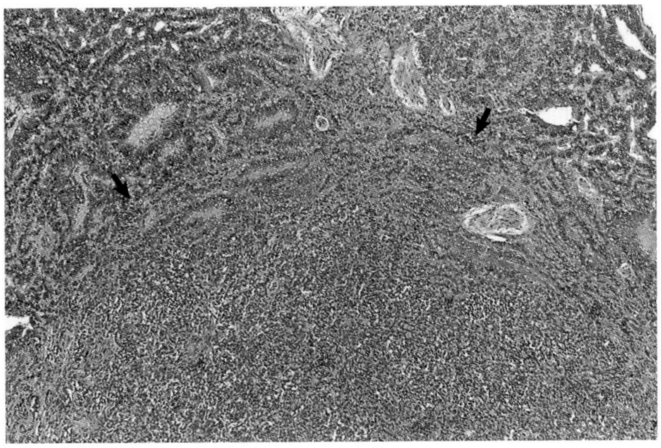

Fig. 12-29 Hyperplasia, adrenal medulla, bull.
Bilateral diffuse hyperplasia of adrenal medulla in a bull with a concomitant C-cell carcinoma of the thyroid gland. The expanded adrenal medulla *(bottom)* has compressed the adjacent adrenal cortex *(arrows)*. H&E stain. (Courtesy Dr. C. Capen, College of Veterinary Medicine, The Ohio State University.)

ratio because of an increase in the size and number of medullary cells, and numerous mitotic figures in the adrenal medulla.

Neoplasms

Neuroblastomas and Ganglioneuromas

Neuroblastomas usually occur in young animals, arise from primitive neuroectodermal cells, and form large intraabdominal masses. The tumors are composed of small neoplastic cells that have hyperchromatic nuclei and scant amounts of cytoplasm and resemble lymphocytes. Neoplastic cells tend to aggregate around blood vessels, forming pseudorosettes. Neurofibrils or unmyelinated nerve fibers can be demonstrated in neuroblastomas.

Ganglioneuromas are benign neoplasms composed of multipolar ganglion cells and neurofibrils and have a prominent fibrous connective tissue stroma. The surrounding adrenal cortex is often severely compressed. Occasionally, neoplastic cells in adrenal medullary neoplasms differentiate into two cell lines, resulting in pheochromocytoma and ganglioneuroma in the same adrenal gland.

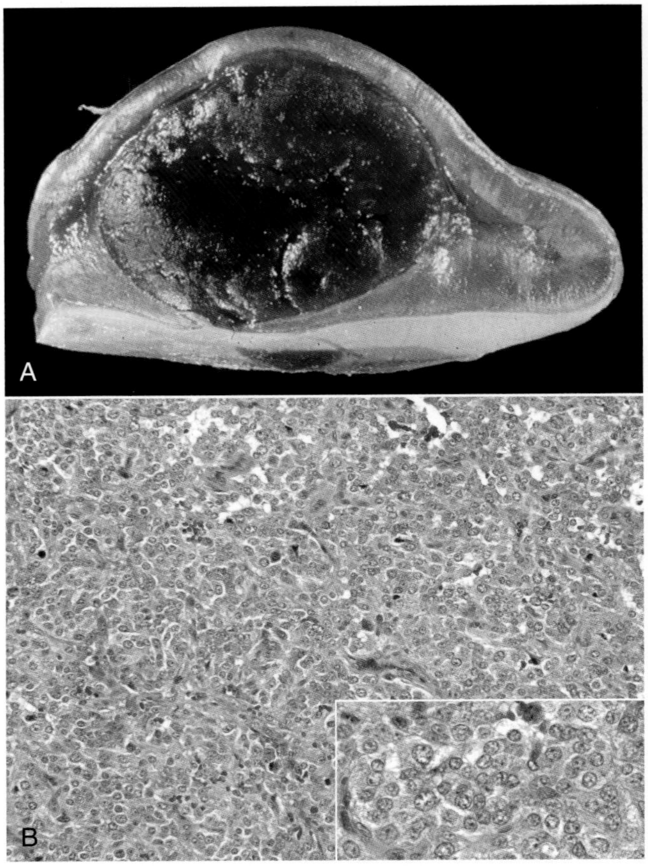

Fig. 12-30 Pheochromocytoma, adrenal gland, horse.
A, Pheochromocytoma compressing the adjacent unaffected adrenal cortex. Note the yellow color of the adrenal cortex attributable to the accumulation of intracellular lipids used to synthesize cortisol. Also see Fig. 12-31. **B,** Neoplastic chromaffin cells are haphazardly arranged in poorly demarcated lobules of varied sizes. There is moderate variation in cellular and nuclear size and shape. *Inset:* Higher magnification of the chromaffin cells. H&E stain. (**A** courtesy Dr. B. Weeks, College of Veterinary Medicine, Texas A&M University and Noah's Arkive, College of Veterinary Medicine, The University of Georgia. **B** courtesy Dr. J.F. Zachary, College of Veterinary Medicine, University of Illinois.)

Pheochromocytomas

Pheochromocytomas are the most common neoplasms in the adrenal medullas of animals, occurring most often in cattle and dogs and infrequently in other species. Calcitonin-secreting C-cell neoplasms of the thyroid gland occasionally develop concurrently with pheochromocytomas in bulls. Extraadrenal pheochromocytomas, referred to as *paragangliomas,* also occur infrequently in the abdomen.

Pheochromocytomas often are large (10 cm or more in diameter) and replace most of the affected adrenal gland. Smaller neoplasms are completely surrounded by a thin, compressed rim of adrenal cortex (Fig. 12-30). Large pheochromocytomas are multilobular and variegated light brown to yellow-red as a result of areas of hemorrhage and necrosis. Malignant pheochromocytomas invade through the capsule of an adrenal gland into adjacent structures, such as the caudal vena cava (Fig. 12-31), and metastasize to distant sites, including the liver, regional lumbar aortic and renal lymph nodes, or lungs. Histologically, neoplastic cells vary from small, round to polyhedral cells to large, pleomorphic cells with multiple hyperchromatic nuclei. The cytoplasm is lightly eosinophilic, finely granular, and often indistinct.

Functional pheochromocytomas composed of epinephrine- and/or norepinephrine-secreting cells have been reported infrequently in animals. Tachycardia, edema, and cardiac hypertrophy observed in several dogs and horses with pheochromocytomas were attributed to excessive catecholamine secretion. Arteriolar sclerosis and widespread medial hyperplasia of arterioles have been reported in dogs with pheochromocytomas and clinical signs suggestive of paroxysmal hypertension. Hypertension was detected in 43% of dogs with pheochromocytomas; all hypertensive dogs had concurrent diseases that could have contributed to the increase in blood pressure. Infrequently, hyperadrenocorticism occurs concurrently in dogs with pheochromocytoma and could contribute to the development of hypertension, particularly during digital manipulation of the affected adrenal gland during surgery.

Norepinephrine is the predominant catecholamine extracted from pheochromocytomas in dogs. This is similar to the finding in normal pups, in which norepinephrine is the predominant catecholamine; in adult dogs, epinephrine predominates in adrenal medullary tissues. The catecholamine content of pheochromocytomas in bulls with concurrent C-cell neoplasms of the thyroid gland

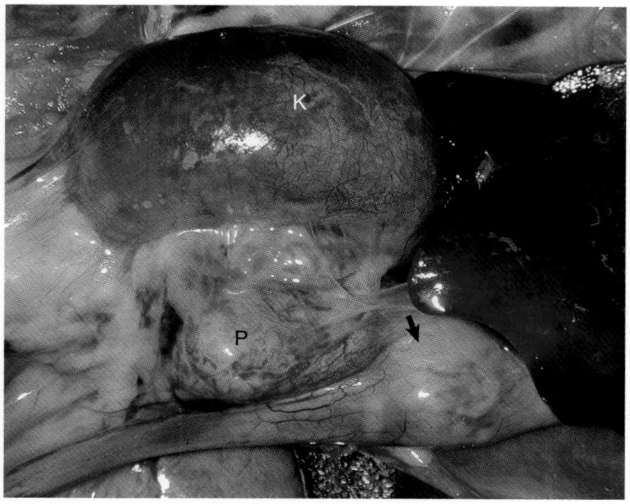

Fig. 12-31 Pheochromocytoma, kidney, adrenal gland, caudal vena cava, dog.
A large pheochromocytoma *(P)* has obliterated the adrenal gland medial to the kidney *(K)* and has extensively invaded into the lumen of the caudal vena cava *(arrow)*. (Courtesy Dr. A. Paulman, College of Veterinary Medicine, University of Illinois.)

is greater than in the normal adrenal medulla. Urinary excretion of free unconjugated catecholamines and metabolites of catecholamines, such as vanillylmandelic acid, are increased in bulls with pheochromocytomas.

DISORDERS OF THE THYROID GLAND

Developmental Disturbances

Accessory Thyroid Tissue

The thyroid gland originates embryologically as a thickened plate of epithelium in the ventral aspect of the pharynx. The complex embryogenesis of the thyroid frequently leads to the formation of accessory thyroid tissue. This accessory thyroid tissue is most typically located in the mediastinum but can be located anywhere from the base of the tongue to the diaphragm. About 50% of adult dogs have nodules of accessory thyroid tissue embedded in the adipose around the base of the heart and the origin of the aorta. The follicular structure and function are the same as those of the main thyroid lobes. Attempts to induce hypothyroidism in the dog by surgical thyroidectomy are usually unsuccessful because the accessory thyroid tissue readily responds to the prompt increase in endogenous TSH secretion and can undergo sufficient hyperplasia to sustain adequate hormone production. This accessory thyroid tissue can also undergo neoplastic transformation.

Thyroglossal Duct Cysts

Thyroglossal duct cysts develop most frequently in dogs and pigs and are present occasionally in other animals. They form as a result of persistence of portions of the midline embryologic primordia of the thyroid gland, which migrate caudally from the ventral aspect of the primitive pharynx to form the thyroid lobes postnatally. These cysts are present in the ventral aspect of the cervical region in dogs and are fluctuant masses that can rupture and form a tract to the exterior. Their lining epithelium consists of multiple layers of follicular cells in which colloid-containing follicles are found occasionally. These cells sometimes undergo neoplastic transformation and give rise to papillary carcinomas.

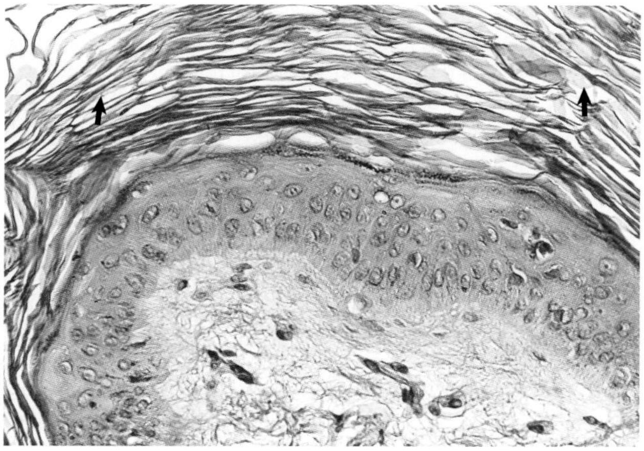

Fig. 12-32 Hypothyroidism, skin, dog.
Hyperkeratosis *(arrows)* has resulted in thickening of the epidermis of the skin. H&E stain. (Courtesy Dr. C. Capen, College of Veterinary Medicine, The Ohio State University.)

Hypothyroidism

Hypothyroidism is a well-recognized and clinically important disease in dogs but is encountered only occasionally in other animals. Although the disease occurs in many adult purebred and mixed breed dogs, certain breeds, such as the golden retriever, Doberman pinscher, dachshund, Shetland sheep dog, Irish setter, miniature schnauzer, cocker spaniel, and Airedale, are more commonly affected. Hypothyroidism in dogs is usually the result of primary lesions in the thyroid gland, particularly idiopathic follicular collapse and lymphocytic thyroiditis. Less common causes of hypothyroidism include bilateral nonfunctional follicular cell neoplasms and severe iodine-deficient goiter. Hypothyroidism caused by long-standing pituitary gland or hypothalamic lesions, which prevent the release of either TSH or thyrotropin-releasing hormone, is encountered infrequently in the dog. In these cases, the thyroid gland is moderately reduced in size and composed of colloid-distended follicles, lined by flattened follicular cells.

Many functional disturbances reported with hypothyroidism occur because of a reduction in basal metabolic rate. A gain in body weight without an associated change in appetite occurs in some hypothyroid dogs. Thinning of the hair coat is often accompanied by bilaterally symmetric alopecia. Areas affected initially by hair loss are those receiving frictional wear such as the tail and cervical area.

Hyperkeratosis is a consistent finding in hypothyroidism and results clinically in an increased scaliness of the skin. When severe, it occurs as circular scaly patches resembling seborrhea. Microscopically, hyperkeratosis (Fig. 12-32) involves the external root sheath, resulting in follicular keratosis. Hyperpigmentation, especially in such localized areas of alopecia as the dorsal aspect of the nose and distal portion of the tail, occurs in many dogs with hypothyroidism. Myxedema may also develop because of the accumulation of glycosaminoglycans and hyaluronic acid in the dermis and subcutis. These substances bind considerable amounts of water, which results in notable thickening of the skin. Microscopically, mucins appear as granular or fibrillar material in hematoxylin and eosin (H&E)-stained sections.

Reproductive abnormalities include lack of libido, reduced sperm count, abnormal or absent estrus cycles, and reduced conception rates. In chronic hypothyroidism, spermatogenic epithelium in the testes is often notably atrophic.

Hypothyroidism in dogs is accompanied by decreased circulating thyroidal hormone concentrations and decreased ^{131}I uptake by the thyroid gland. In dogs with hypothyroidism, the concentration of T_4 is usually below 0.8 μg/dL (normal 1.5 to 3.4 μg/dL) and that of T_3 is below 50 ng/dL (normal 48 to 150 ng/dL). In the euthyroid dog, T_4 concentrations will at least double 8 hours after intravenous or intramuscular injection of TSH. In dogs with hypothyroidism, the T_4 concentrations do not change significantly after injection of TSH.

Serum cholesterol concentrations are often greatly increased (300 to 900 mg/dL) in many hypothyroid dogs (normal 40 to 80 mg/dL). The marked hypercholesterolemia in long-standing and severe hypothyroidism results in a variety of secondary lesions, including atherosclerosis, hepatomegaly, and glomerular and corneal lipidosis. Atherosclerosis of coronary (Web Fig. 12-5; also see Fig. 10-38) and cerebral vessels develops in dogs that have severe hypothyroidism and long-standing hyperlipidemia.

Congenital Dyshormonogenetic Goiter

Congenital dyshormonogenetic goiter in sheep (Corriedale, Dorset Horn, Merino, and Romney breeds), Afrikaner cattle, Saanen dwarf goats, dogs (rat and toy fox terriers), and cats (Abyssinian and Japanese) is inherited as an autosomal recessive trait. Indications that affected young are clinically hypothyroid include subnormal growth rate, abnormal wool or guard hair development, subcutaneous myxedematous swellings, lethargy, and abnormal mentation.

Thyroid lobes are symmetrically enlarged at birth because of an intense diffuse hyperplasia of follicular cells (Fig. 12-33). Thyroid follicles are often collapsed because of lack of colloid resulting from the notable endocytic activity. Follicles are lined by tall columnar follicular cells, which have dilated profiles of rough endoplasmic reticulum, large mitochondria, and dense lysosomal granules associated with the Golgi apparatus, but have few thyroglobulin-containing apical vesicles near the luminal plasma membrane. Numerous long microvilli extend into the follicular lumen.

Although thyroid scintigraphy can be normal, circulating T_3 and T_4 concentrations after TSH stimulation are consistently low. The lack of a defect in iodide uptake or organification, plus an absence of normal 19S thyroglobulin in goitrous thyroids and only minute amounts of thyroglobulin-related antigens (0.01% of normal) suggest impaired thyroglobulin biosynthesis in sheep, cattle, and goats. Organification defects caused by mutations in thyroid peroxidase have been documented in dogs and cats.

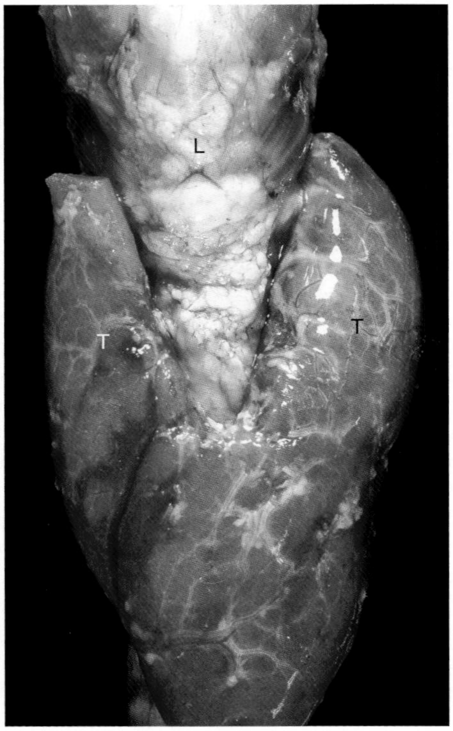

Fig. 12-33 Congenital dyshormonogenetic goiter, thyroid gland, lamb. The symmetrically enlarged thyroid *(T)* lobes are fused at the midline ventral to the larynx *(L)* and trachea. (Courtesy Dr. C. Capen, College of Veterinary Medicine, The Ohio State University.)

Idiopathic Follicular Atrophy

In follicular atrophy, or "collapse," the loss of follicular epithelium and disruption of follicles is progressive and the gland is replaced by adipose connective tissue with only a minimal inflammatory response. The gland usually is smaller and lighter in color than normal (Fig. 12-34). The early lesion in dogs with mild clinical signs of hypothyroidism appears to be confined to one part of the thyroid gland. The affected part is composed of small follicles that contain little colloid and are lined by tall columnar follicular cells. A more advanced form of follicular atrophy is present in dogs with clinical hypothyroidism and low blood concentrations of thyroidal hormones. These thyroid glands are notably reduced in size and are composed predominantly of adipose connective tissue with only a few clusters of small follicles containing vacuolated colloid.

Lymphocytic (Immune-Mediated) Thyroiditis

Lymphocytic thyroiditis in dogs and a large European population of horses closely resembles Hashimoto's disease of humans with evidence suggesting a polygenic mode of inheritance, particularly in affected breeds such as laboratory beagles, giant schnauzers, Doberman pinschers, and Labrador retrievers. The immunologic basis of the development of chronic lymphocytic thyroiditis is through production of autoantibodies, usually directed against thyroglobulin or a microsomal antigen such as thyroperoxidase and infrequently against the TSH receptor, a nuclear antigen, or a second colloid antigen from thyroid follicular cells.

Microscopic lesions consist of multifocal to diffuse infiltrates of lymphocytes which occasionally form nodules, plasma cells, and macrophages. Thyroid follicles are small and lined by columnar

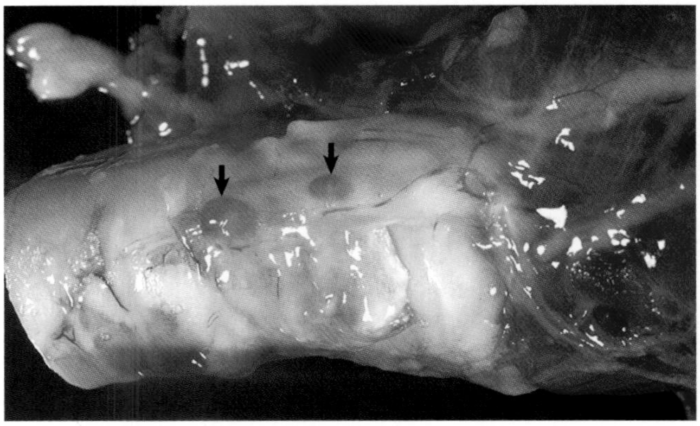

Fig. 12-34 Atrophic thyroid gland, dog. The thyroid gland on the lateral surface of the trachea is very small and pale tan. As a result, the two parathyroid glands are very prominent *(arrows)*. (Courtesy Dr. W. Crowell, College of Veterinary Medicine, The University of Georgia and Noah's Arkive, College of Veterinary Medicine, The University of Georgia.)

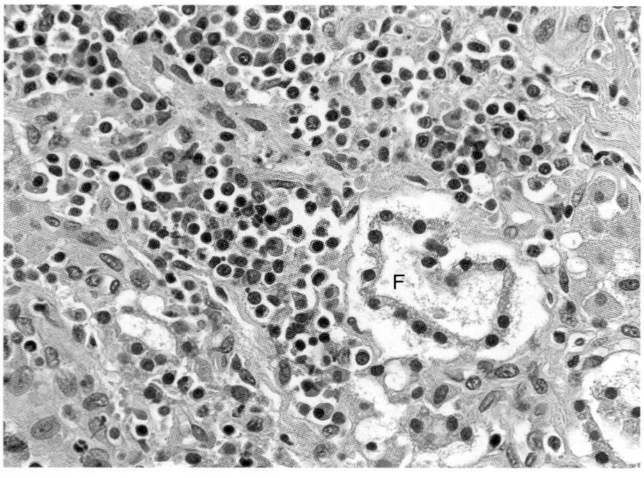

Fig. 12-35 Lymphoplasmacytic thyroiditis, severe hypothyroidism, dog. Numerous lymphocytes, plasma cells, and a few macrophages have infiltrated the thyroid gland. Only occasional follicles *(F)* remain. (Courtesy Dr. J.F. Zachary, College of Veterinary Medicine, University of Illinois.)

epithelial cells; lymphocytes, macrophages, and degenerate follicular cells are often present in the colloid, which is vacuolated (Fig. 12-35; also see Web Fig. 12-6). Thyroid C cells are present as small nests or nodules between follicles and often are more prominent than those in normal dogs. Some remaining follicular cells appear to be transformed into large oxyphilic cells with densely eosinophilic granular cytoplasm.

Hyperthyroidism

Hyperthyroidism, or thyrotoxicosis resulting from elevated circulating levels of T_4 and T_3, commonly occurs in middle-aged to older cats and rarely in dogs. The condition in cats is associated with a spectrum of functional proliferative lesions, whereas in dogs it results from thyroid neoplasms.

Clinical signs result from an increased rate of basal metabolism. Consequently, animals are polyuric and polydipsic and frequently lose weight despite a voracious appetite. Weakness and fatigue, nervousness or hyperexcitability, and hyperthermia and heat intolerance are also present. In addition, cardiac manifestations of hyperthyroidism, such as tachycardia and dysrhythmias, are well documented in animals; however, secondary hypertrophic cardiomyopathy characterized by concentric hypertrophy is primarily restricted to cats.

In general, the likelihood of animals developing clinical hyperthyroidism secondary to thyroid neoplasms depends on (1) the capability of neoplastic cells to synthesize T_4 and T_3 (e.g., well-differentiated thyroid neoplasms that form follicles and produce colloid are more likely to synthesize thyroid hormones than poorly differentiated solid neoplasms) and (2) the extent of the increase in circulating concentrations of T_4 and T_3, which depends on a balance between the rate of secretion of thyroid hormones by the neoplasm, and the rate of degradation of thyroid hormones. Dogs have a much more efficient enterohepatic excretory mechanism for thyroid hormones, which are difficult to overload, than cats; therefore clinical hyperthyroidism in dogs with functional thyroid follicular cell neoplasms is infrequent. Cats are very sensitive to phenol and phenol derivatives and have a poor ability to conjugate phenolic compounds, such as T_4, with glucuronic acid and excrete the T_4 glucuronide into the bile. The capacity of conjugation of T_3 with sulfate is limited and easily overloaded in cats.

Functional Proliferative Lesions in Cats

A spectrum of proliferative lesions that secrete excess thyroidal hormones (e.g., adenomas and multinodular hyperplasia) is common in the thyroid glands of adult and aged cats. Since the late 1970s, there has been a dramatic increase in the incidence of neoplasms and other focal proliferative lesions in the thyroid glands of cats and these have resulted in hyperthyroidism. Hyperthyroidism is one of the two most common endocrine diseases in adult to aged cats (diabetes mellitus is the other). Before 1980, clinical hyperthyroidism was infrequently diagnosed in cats. The reason for the apparently increased incidence is uncertain but appears to be related in part to (1) a larger population of geriatric cats receiving veterinary medical care, (2) improved assays for thyroid hormones, (3) detailed characterization of the clinical syndrome, and (4) increased awareness by veterinary clinicians of its common occurrence in adult to aged cats. In addition, there does appear to be a real increase in the incidence of feline hyperthyroidism over the past 30 years. Potential risk factors that have been reported include a predominantly indoor environment, regular treatment with flea powders, exposures to herbicides and fertilizers, a diet primarily of canned food, and non-Siamese breeds (10 times greater occurrence). It has been suggested that wide variations (excessive to inadequate) in dietary iodine intake over prolonged periods could play a role in the pathogenesis of hyperthyroidism in cats.

The disease in cats is mechanistically different from that of Graves' disease in human patients in that hyperthyroid cats do not have increased concentrations of circulating thyroid-stimulating immunoglobulins, which are comparable to long-acting thyroid stimulator (LATS) in humans (LATS is an autoantibody that binds to the TSH receptor and activates follicular cells). Purified immunoglobulin G (IgG) prepared from hyperthyroid cats significantly increases ^{3}H-thymidine incorporation into DNA and stimulates thyroid follicular cell proliferation fifteenfold but does not stimulate intracellular cAMP production. The ^{3}H-thymidine incorporation can be completely inhibited by a specific TSH receptor blocking antibody. These data suggest that increased titers of thyroid growth-stimulating immunoglobulins are present in cats with hyperthyroidism and most likely act by the TSH receptor. In cats, the disease most closely resembles toxic nodular goiter in human patients with mutations in genes encoding for either the TSH receptor or the $G_{s\alpha}$ protein. Mutations in $G_{s\alpha}$ that correspond to the mutations in humans have been reported in a small group of hyperthyroid cats. $G_{s\alpha}$ is a G protein that mediates cAMP-dependent TSH signaling. Follicular cell proliferation, differentiation, and secretion of thyroid hormone result from constitutive activation of TSH signaling. In a separate study, all cases of feline follicular hyperplasia and adenomas evaluated by immunohistochemistry demonstrated overexpression of the c-ras oncogene. As was the case for activating $G_{s\alpha}$ mutations, overexpression of c-ras results in constitutive mitogenesis of thyroid follicular epithelial cells. Hyperplastic and neoplastic thyroid tissue from cats is transplantable into athymic (nude) mice and continues to overproduce T_4 and T_3 in a subcutaneous location.

Follicular cell adenomas, which often develop in a thyroid gland with multinodular hyperplasia, are more common than thyroid carcinomas. Follicles in the rim of thyroid tissue around a functional adenoma are notably enlarged and distended with colloid (colloid involution). The follicular cells are low cuboidal and atrophic with little evidence of endocytic activity in response to the increased concentrations of circulating thyroid hormones. In cats with solitary adenomas, the opposite thyroid lobe should be examined carefully for evidence of nodular hyperplasia or microadenomas. These small foci of multinodular follicular cell hyperplasia can be the

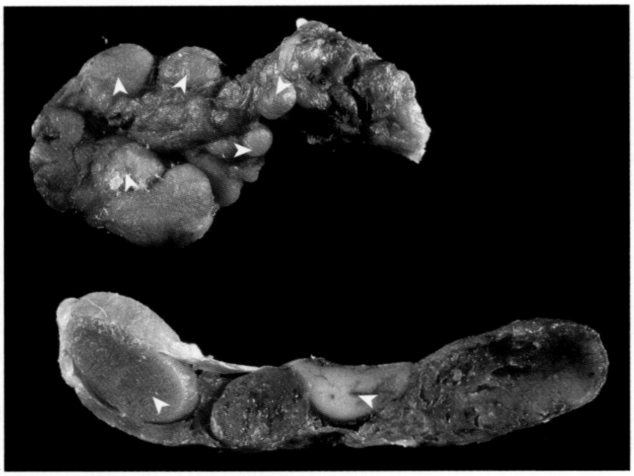

Fig. 12-36 **Hyperplasia, hyperthyroidism, left and right thyroid glands, cat.**
Multinodular follicular cell hyperplasia *(arrowheads)* involves both thyroid lobes. (Courtesy Dr. C. Capen, College of Veterinary Medicine, The Ohio State University.)

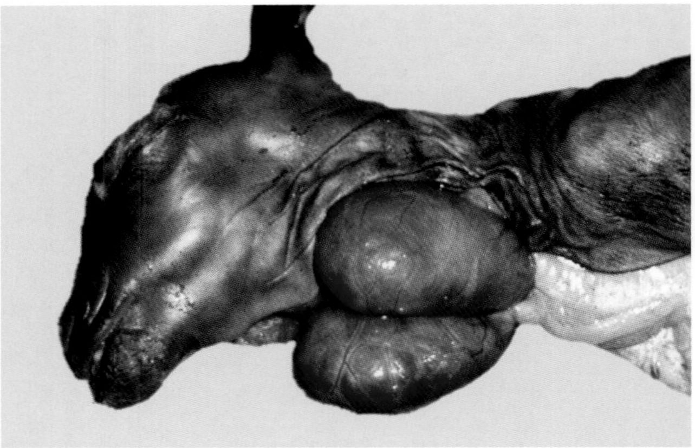

Fig. 12-37 **Hyperplasia, thyroid goiter, goat.**
Deficiency of maternal dietary iodine during pregnancy has resulted in bilateral hyperplasia (and hypertrophy) of thyroid follicular epithelial cells in this neonatal goat, which has resulted in a symmetric enlargement of the glands (goiter). (Courtesy Dr. O. Hedstrom, College of Veterinary Medicine, Oregon State University; and Noah's Arkive, College of Veterinary Medicine, The University of Georgia.)

cause of hyperthyroidism recurring several months to a year or more after surgical removal of a functional adenoma.

Hyperthyroidism in cats also occurs in association with bilateral multinodular adenomatous hyperplasia (goiter), which usually causes only slight enlargement of the affected lobe(s) (Fig. 12-36). In contrast to adenomas, areas of nodular hyperplasia are not encapsulated and the adjacent thyroid tissue is not compressed. Microscopically, hyperplastic nodules are composed of irregularly shaped, colloid-filled follicles lined by cuboidal follicular cells, and these nodules are considered a preneoplastic lesion as they can coalesce and form a thyroid follicular cell adenoma.

Cats with hyperthyroidism usually have notably increased serum T_4 and T_3 concentrations, but some euthyroid cats have histologic evidence of nodular disease. The serum T_4 concentrations in cats with hyperthyroidism range from 3.4 to 30 µg/dL (normal 1.5 to 5 µg/dL), and serum T_3 concentrations range from 179 to 470 ng/dL (normal 60 to 200 ng/dL). Moderately increased serum enzyme activities, including serum alanine aminotransferase (ALT, SGPT), serum aspartate aminotransferase (AST, SGOT), and especially alkaline phosphatase, occur in hyperthyroid cats.

Hyperthyroid cats often have disturbances of calcium homeostasis and a concomitant diffuse chief cell hyperplasia in the parathyroid glands. Blood ionized calcium and plasma creatinine concentrations are significantly decreased, whereas plasma phosphorus and intact PTH concentrations are increased. Hyperparathyroidism occurs in 77% of hyperthyroid cats, with PTH concentrations elevated up to 19 times that of the upper limit of the reference range. Hyperphosphatemia is present in approximately 40% of hyperthyroid cats. The mechanisms for the development of hyperphosphatemia in feline hyperthyroidism are uncertain but could be related in part to polyphagia, resulting in increased intestinal phosphorus absorption, increased catabolism of muscle proteins, release of phosphorus because of the gluconeogenic effects of the increased thyroid hormone concentrations, and increased bone resorption with release of phosphorus into the blood. Hyperparathyroidism and chief cell hyperplasia appear to be related to the reciprocal decline in amounts of circulating ionized calcium in response to the hyperphosphatemia. Increased blood phosphorus concentrations also could decrease renal 1α-hydroxylase activity and decrease the production of the active form of vitamin D, thereby reducing intestinal calcium absorption. However, circulating concentrations of 1,25-$(OH)_2$-dihydroxycholecalciferol were not decreased in a limited number of hyperthyroid cats evaluated.

Hyperplasia of Thyroid Follicular Cells (Goiter)

Goiter is a clinical term used to describe a nonneoplastic and noninflammatory enlargement of the thyroid gland (Fig. 12-37). It develops in all domestic mammals as a result of hyperplasia of follicular cells. Certain forms of thyroid hyperplasia, especially nodular, are difficult to differentiate from adenomas. The major pathogenetic mechanisms for the development of thyroid hyperplasia include iodine-deficient diets, goitrogenic compounds that interfere with thyroxinogenesis, excess dietary iodide, and genetically determined defects in the enzymes or thyroglobulin that are essential for the biosynthesis of thyroidal hormones. All of these result in inadequate thyroxine synthesis and decreased blood concentrations of T_4 and T_3, which are detected by the hypothalamus. This in turn stimulates the pituitary gland to increase the secretion of TSH, resulting in hypertrophy and hyperplasia of follicular cells.

Diffuse Hyperplastic and Colloid Goiter

Dietary iodine deficiency that resulted in diffuse hyperplastic goiter was common in many areas of the world before the widespread addition of iodized salt to animal diets. Iodine-deficient goiter still occurs worldwide in domestic animals, but cases are sporadic and few animals are affected. Marginally iodine-deficient diets that contain goitrogenic compounds can cause severe thyroid follicular cell hyperplasia and goiter. Goitrogenic substances include glucocorticoids, phenobarbital, sulfonamides, thiocyanate, perchlorate, and a number of plants of the family Brassicaceae. Offspring of females fed iodine-deficient diets are likely to develop severe thyroidal follicular cell hyperplasia and have clinical signs of hypothyroidism. Both lateral lobes of the thyroid gland are uniformly enlarged in young animals as a result of diffuse hypertrophy and hyperplasia of follicular cells (see Fig. 12-9). The enlargements, when extensive, result in palpable or visible swellings in the cranial ventral cervical area. The affected lobes are firm and dark red because an extensive interfollicular capillary network develops under the influence of long-term TSH stimulation.

Colloid goiter represents the involutionary phase of diffuse hyperplastic goiter in both young and adult animals. It develops either after sufficient amounts of iodide have been added to the diet or after the requirements for thyroid hormones have diminished as the animal ages. The notably hyperplastic follicular cells continue to produce colloid, but endocytosis of colloid from the lumen is decreased. This is a consequence of the diminished TSH concentrations produced in response to the return of blood T_4 and T_3 concentrations to normal. Both thyroid lobes are diffusely enlarged but are more translucent and lighter in color than in hyperplastic goiter. These differences in macroscopic appearances are the result of less vascularity in colloid goiter and development of macrofollicles distended with colloid. Follicles are progressively distended (see Fig. 12-10) with densely eosinophilic colloid because of diminished TSH-induced endocytosis. As a result, follicular cells lining the macrofollicles are flattened and atrophic. The interface between the colloid and luminal surface of the follicular cells is smooth, and the cells lack the endocytic vacuoles characteristic of actively secreting thyroid follicular cells. Some involuted follicles in colloid goiter have remnants of the papillary projections on follicular cells extending into their lumens.

The changes in diffuse hyperplastic and colloid goiters are uniform throughout the diffusely enlarged thyroid lobes. Follicles are irregular in size and shape in hyperplastic goiter because they contain varying amounts of colloid, which is lightly eosinophilic and vacuolated. Some follicles collapse because of the lack of colloid. The lining epithelial cells are columnar and have deeply eosinophilic cytoplasm and small hyperchromatic nuclei, which are often situated in the basilar portions of the cells. The follicles are lined by single or multiple layers of hyperplastic follicular cells that in some follicles form papillary projections into the lumens (Fig. 12-38). Similar proliferative changes are present in ectopic thyroid tissue in the neck and mediastinum.

Although seemingly paradoxic, an excess of iodide in the diet also can result in thyroid hyperplasia in animals. Foals of mares fed dry seaweed containing excessive iodide develop thyroid hyperplasia and clinically evident goiter. The thyroid glands of suckling animals are exposed to greater blood iodide concentrations than those of the dam because iodide is concentrated first by the placenta and then by the mammary gland. Increased blood iodide interferes with one or more steps of thyroidal hormone synthesis and secretion, leading to lowered blood T_4 and T_3 concentrations and resulting in a compensatory increase in pituitary TSH secretion. Excess iodine blocks the release of T_3 and T_4 by interfering with proteolysis of colloid by lysosomal enzymes in thyroid follicular cells.

Multifocal Nodular Hyperplasia

Multifocal nodular hyperplasia in thyroid glands occurs in old horses, cats, and dogs and appears as multiple, white-to-tan nodules of variable size (see Fig. 12-36), giving affected lobes a moderately enlarged and irregular contour. Multifocal nodular goiter in most animals except cats is endocrinologically inactive and is an incidental lesion at necropsy. However, functional thyroid adenomas often develop in the thyroid glands of aged cats with hyperthyroidism and multinodular hyperplasia of follicular cells. In contrast to thyroid adenomas, the areas of nodular hyperplasia are not encapsulated and cause minimal to no compression of adjacent parenchyma. Thus nodular goiter consists of multiple foci of hyperplastic follicular cells that are sharply demarcated but not encapsulated from the adjacent thyroid tissue.

The microscopic appearance of nodular hyperplasia often varies. Some hyperplastic follicular cells form small follicles with little or no colloid. Other nodules are composed of larger, irregularly shaped follicles lined by one or more layers of columnar cells that form papillary projections into the lumen. Some of the follicles have undergone colloid involution and are filled with densely eosinophilic colloid. These changes appear to be the result of alternating periods of hyperplasia and colloid involution in the thyroid glands of aged animals.

Epithelial Neoplasms of the Thyroid Gland

Follicular Cell Adenomas

Adenomas usually are white-to-tan, small, solid nodules that are well demarcated from the adjacent thyroid parenchyma (Fig. 12-39). The affected thyroid lobe is only moderately enlarged and distorted; usually only a single adenoma is present in a thyroid lobe. A distinct, white, fibrous connective tissue capsule of variable thickness separates the adenoma from the adjacent compressed parenchyma. Some thyroid adenomas are composed of thin-walled cysts filled with a yellow-red fluid. Their external surfaces are smooth and

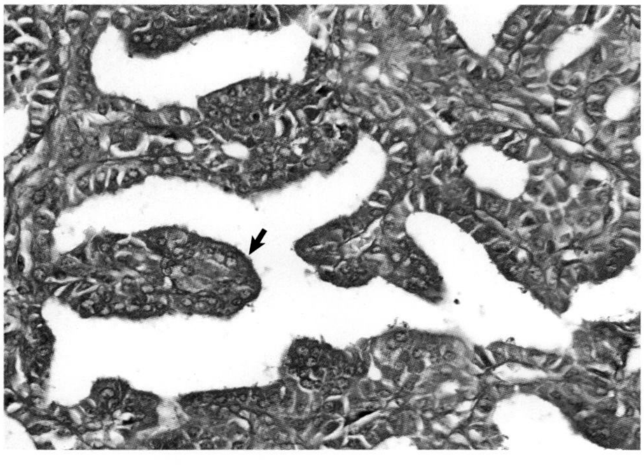

Fig. 12-38 Hyperplastic goiter, thyroid gland, dog.
Hyperplastic follicular epithelium forms a papillary projection *(arrow)*, which extends into the follicular lumen devoid of colloid. Note that the majority of follicular lumens are small and collapsed. Periodic acid–Schiff reaction. (Courtesy Dr. C. Capen, College of Veterinary Medicine, The Ohio State University.)

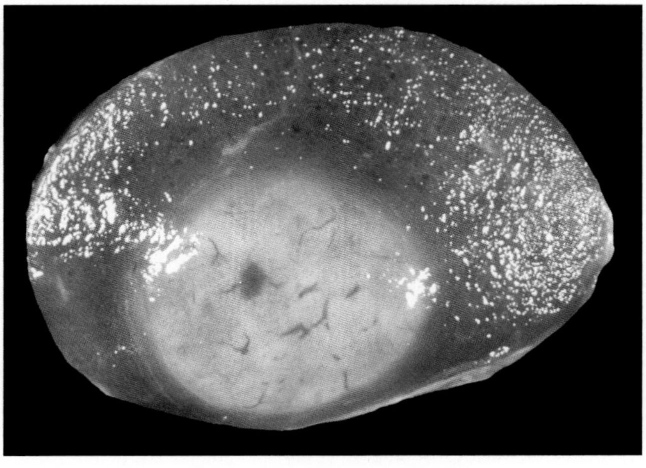

Fig. 12-39 Thyroid adenoma, thyroid gland, horse.
The thyroid gland contains an expansile, encapsulated, round, white-yellow mass that is well demarcated from normal thyroid gland. Note the prominent fibrous connective tissue capsule surrounding the adenoma. (Courtesy College of Veterinary Medicine, University of Illinois.)

covered by an extensive network of blood vessels. Small masses of neoplastic tissue remain in the wall and form rugose projections into the cyst. Adenomas are histologically classified as follicular and papillary types; the follicular type is more common in the thyroid gland of animals.

Follicular Cell Carcinomas

In dogs, thyroid carcinomas occur more often than adenomas, but in cats adenomas are more common. Boxers develop thyroid carcinomas more frequently than any other breed of dog, but beagles and golden retrievers have a higher risk of developing thyroid carcinomas. Approximately 60% of thyroid carcinomas in dogs are clinically detectable by palpation as a firm mass in the neck and by evidence of respiratory distress caused by tracheal compression. Carcinomas become fixed in position as a result of extensive local invasion of adjacent structures, whereas localized adenomas are freely movable under the skin. Neoplasms of thyroid origin also occur in accessory thyroidal tissue, located anywhere between the base of the tongue and the cranial mediastinum.

Thyroid carcinomas often grow rapidly and invade adjacent structures such as the trachea, esophagus, and larynx (Fig. 12-40). The earliest and most frequent site of metastasis is to lungs because thyroid carcinomas, early in the course of development, invade branches of the thyroid vein. The retropharyngeal and caudal cervical lymph nodes are infrequent sites of metastases.

Thyroid C (Ultimobranchial) Cell Neoplasms

Neoplasms derived from C cells of the thyroid gland occur most frequently in adult to aged bulls, occasionally in horses and dogs, and infrequently in other species. The incidence of C-cell neoplasms increases with advancing age in bulls that also typically have increased vertebral bone density. A high percentage of aged bulls fed calcium-rich diets develop C-cell neoplasms (30%) or hyperplasia of C cells and ultimobranchial derivatives (15% to 20%). The cause of C-cell neoplasms is unknown, but the chronic stimulation of C cells by large concentrations of calcium absorbed from the digestive tract can be responsible for their high incidence. A significant decline in the incidence of C-cell neoplasms occurs when the excessive calcium intake of bulls is reduced. Cows fed similar rations rarely develop proliferative lesions of C cells because of the greater physiologic requirements of pregnancy and lactation for calcium.

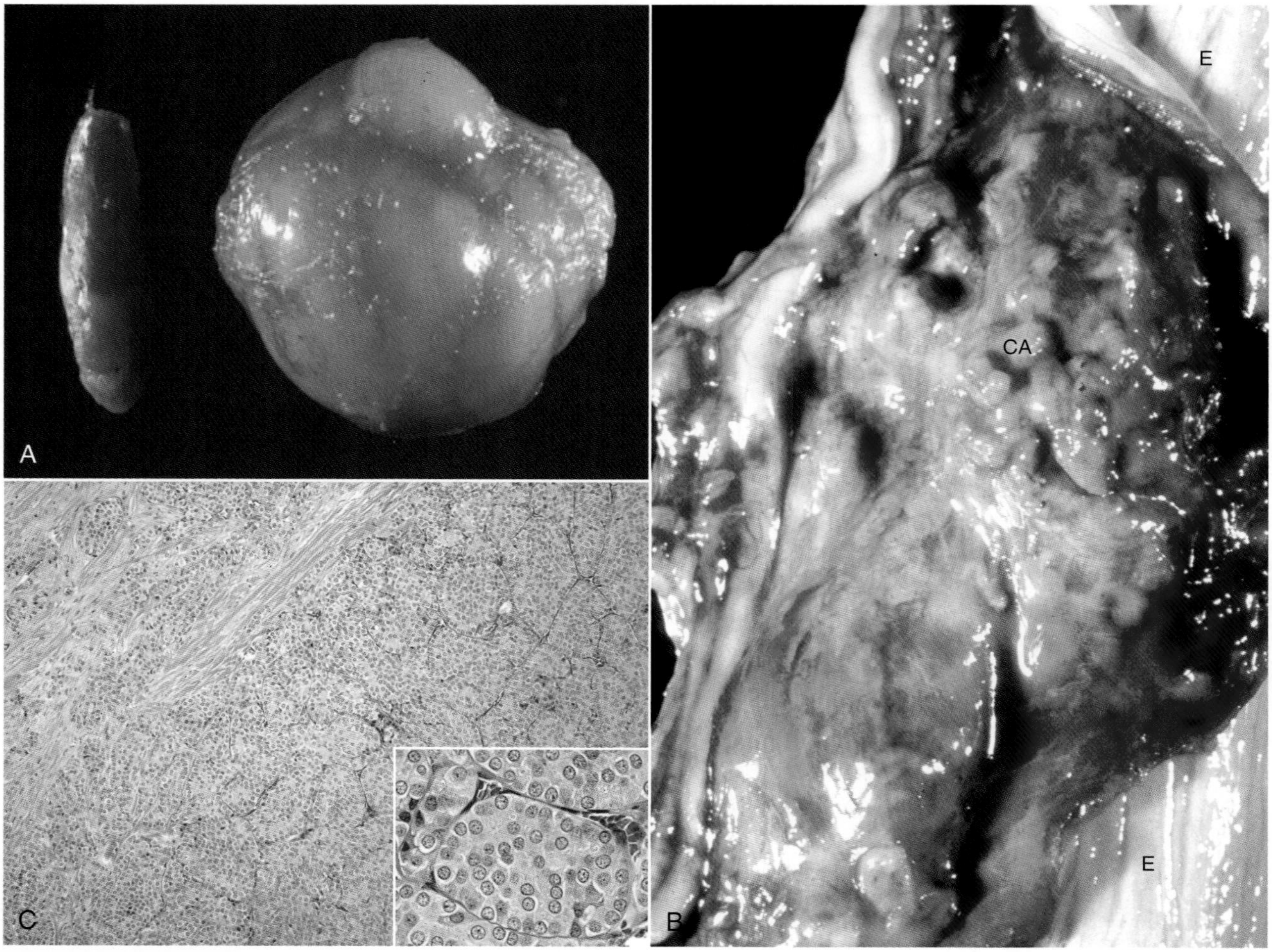

Fig. 12-40 Thyroid carcinoma, thyroid gland, dogs.

A, A large follicular carcinoma *(right side)* has obliterated the normal structure of the thyroid gland. A normal thyroid gland is shown on the left. **B,** The poorly demarcated and well-vascularized thyroid carcinoma *(CA)* is locally invasive and has extended into the wall of the esophagus. *E,* Esophageal mucosa. **C,** Neoplastic cells are haphazardly arranged into discrete islands. There is moderate variation in cellular and nuclear size and shape. Note the invasion of the tumor into the capsule of the thyroid gland *(upper left)*. *Inset,* Higher magnification of the cells in the thyroid carcinoma. H&E stain. (**A** courtesy Dr. W. Crowell, College of Veterinary Medicine, The University of Georgia and Noah's Arkive, College of Veterinary Medicine, The University of Georgia. **B** courtesy College of Veterinary Medicine, University of Illinois. **C** courtesy Dr. J.F. Zachary, College of Veterinary Medicine, University of Illinois.)

C-cell neoplasms in bulls are commonly found in association with other endocrine neoplasms, especially bilateral pheochromocytomas and occasionally pituitary adenomas. There are two distinct forms of the familial cancer syndrome known as *multiple endocrine neoplasia* (MEN) in humans. MEN1 is due to a disease-causing mutation in the MEN1 gene and is characterized by primary hyperparathyroidism, pancreatic islet cell tumors that are predominantly gastrinomas, and pituitary tumors that are predominantly prolactinomas. Other lesions that can be associated with MEN1 include duodenal gastrinomas, carcinoids, thyroid adenomas, adrenocortical tumors, and lipomas. Mutations in the receptor tyrosine kinase RET result in MEN2. There are two subtypes, MEN2A (also known as *Sipple's syndrome*) and MEN2B, both of which are associated with C-cell tumors, primary hyperparathyroidism, and pheochromocytomas. In addition, MEN2B patients frequently have mucosal neuromas and a marfanoid stature. There are increasing reports of MEN in veterinary medicine in cats, dogs, horses, and cattle. However, mutations in MEN1 or RET have never been documented in these cases.

Both C-cell adenomas and carcinomas can contain deposits of amyloid. The source of the localized amyloid deposits in the neoplasms is uncertain, but the amyloid appears to be produced by the neoplastic cells, as amyloid deposits are not present in other organs. Amyloid deposition is consistently documented with medullary thyroid carcinoma in humans, and amyloid has also been reported in certain other endocrine neoplasms. Amyloid in C-cell neoplasms is present between neoplastic cells, around vessels, and in the interstitium. Amyloid has been observed in bulls, horses, and dogs but in amounts varying (minimal to substantial) from case to case. Localized amyloid in C-cell tumors is derived from calcitonin.

Adenomas

C-cell adenomas occur as discrete, single, or multiple gray to tan nodules in one or both thyroid lobes. Adenomas are smaller (approximately 1 to 3 cm in diameter) than carcinomas and are separated from the adjacent thyroid gland parenchyma, which is compressed by a thin, fibrous connective tissue capsule. Larger C-cell adenomas replace most of the thyroid lobe, but a rim of dark, brown-red thyroid gland often is present on one side (Fig. 12-41). Histologically, thyroid C-cell adenomas are discrete, expansive masses composed of cells larger than a colloid-distended follicle. The adenoma is well-circumscribed or partially encapsulated, and adjacent follicles are compressed to varying degrees. The neoplastic C cells are well-differentiated and have abundant to clear, pale eosinophilic cytoplasm.

Carcinomas

Thyroid C-cell carcinomas result in extensive multinodular enlargements of one or both thyroid lobes and can replace an entire thyroid gland. Thyroid C-cell neoplasms in bulls and other animal species are firm, and in some areas, the stroma consists of dense bands of fibrous connective tissue. Multiple metastases occur in the cranial cervical lymph nodes (Fig. 12-42). These nodes are usually large and have areas of necrosis and hemorrhage. Pulmonary metastases appear as discrete tan nodules and occur infrequently. C-cell carcinomas are composed of neoplastic cells that are more pleomorphic than cells of adenomas. The carcinomatous cells are poorly differentiated, polyhedral to spindle-shaped, and have pale eosinophilic, finely granular, indistinct cytoplasm.

Ultimobranchial neoplasms in the thyroid glands of bulls often have a more complex histologic structure than the typical C-cell (medullary) carcinoma in dogs and horses. The neoplasm is composed of differentiated C cells arranged as focal accumulations of neoplastic cells with abundant pale eosinophilic cytoplasm, either within the wall of the thyroid and ultimobranchial follicles or present as larger solid nodules. Ultimobranchial thyroid neoplasms often are accompanied by multifocal hyperplasia of C cells in other parts of the thyroid. The neoplastic C cells often are embedded in an increased amount of hyalinized stroma, and there are deposits

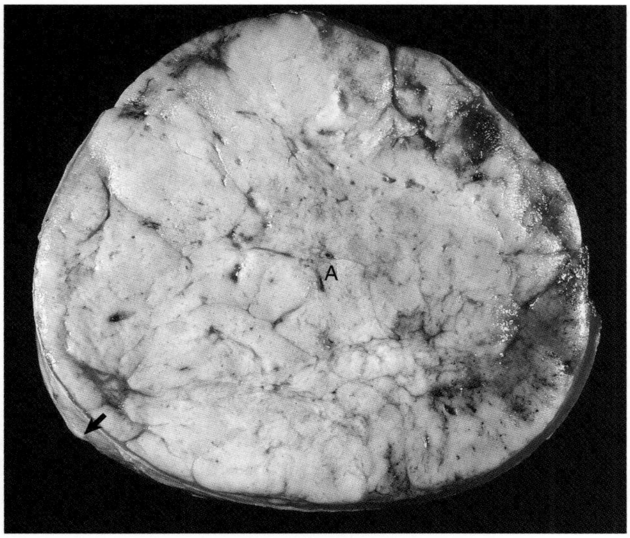

Fig. 12-41 C-cell adenoma, thyroid gland, horse.
The adenoma *(A)* is confined by the thyroid capsule and a rim of compressed thyroid gland *(arrow)* at the periphery of the mass. (Courtesy Dr. C. Capen, College of Veterinary Medicine, The Ohio State University.)

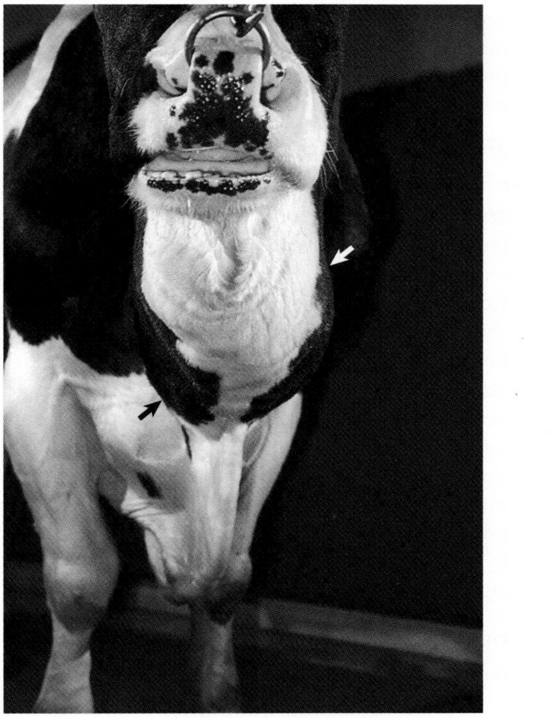

Fig. 12-42 C-cell carcinoma and metastases, thyroid and cervical lymph nodes, Holstein bull.
Note the swellings in the neck *(arrows)* as a result of metastases to the cervical lymph nodes. (Courtesy Dr. C. Capen, College of Veterinary Medicine, The Ohio State University.)

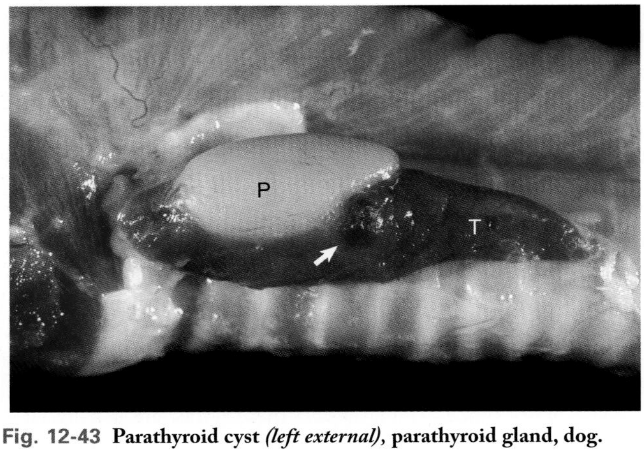

Fig. 12-43 Parathyroid cyst *(left external)*, parathyroid gland, dog. The parathyroid cyst *(arrow)* was formed from the persistent and distended embryonic duct that connects parathyroid-thymic primordia in the III and IV pharyngeal pouches (Kürsteiner's cyst). All parathyroid glands *(P)* were hyperplastic because of chronic renal failure. *T,* Thyroid gland. (Courtesy Dr. C. Capen, College of Veterinary Medicine, The Ohio State University.)

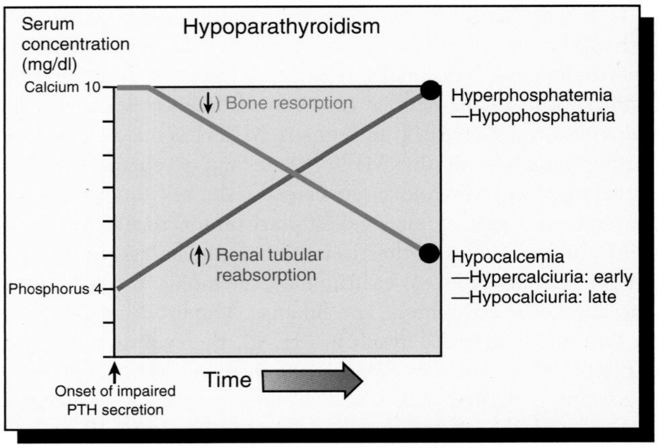

Fig. 12-44 Schematic diagram of the alterations in serum calcium and phosphorus concentrations in response to an inadequate secretion of parathyroid hormone *(PTH)*. A progressive increase in serum phosphorus concentration and a notable decline in the concentration of serum calcium resulted in increased neuromuscular excitability and tetany. (Redrawn with permission from Dr. C. Capen, College of Veterinary Medicine, The Ohio State University.)

of amyloid in some neoplasms. Portions of the thyroid neoplasm in bulls that are derived from less differentiated ultimobranchial remnants consist of follicle-like structures, cysts, and tubules composed of immature small basophilic cells. These neoplasms in bulls and other species closely resemble undifferentiated or stem cells of the normal ultimobranchial body that can differentiate into both C cells and follicular cells. Thyroid follicles and cribriform structures with colloid-like material formed by cells resembling differentiated follicular cells often are present in the neoplasms in close association with these more primitive ultimobranchial-derived structures. Histologically, the structure of ultimobranchial neoplasms in bulls is heterogeneous and resembles a variant of thyroid carcinoma in humans. This neoplasm, designated as an intermediate type of differentiated carcinoma, has structural and immunohistochemical characteristics of both C-cell (medullary) and follicular carcinomas.

DISORDERS OF THE PARATHYROID GLANDS

Developmental Disturbances

Parathyroid (Kürsteiner's) Cysts

Small cysts within the parenchyma of the parathyroid glands or in the immediate vicinity of the glands occur frequently in dogs but only occasionally in other animal species (Fig. 12-43). Parathyroid gland cysts are usually multiloculated, lined by a cuboidal to columnar, often ciliated epithelium, and filled with a densely eosinophilic proteinaceous material. Parathyroid gland cysts appear to develop from persistent and dilated remnants of the duct that connects the parathyroid and thymic primordia during embryonic development. Parathyroid gland cysts are distinct from midline cysts derived from remnants of the thyroglossal duct. The latter are lined by multilayered thyroidogenic epithelium that often has colloid-containing follicles and are usually located near the midline, from the base of the tongue to the mediastinum.

Hypoparathyroidism

In hypoparathyroidism, either the parathyroid glands secrete subnormal amounts of PTH or the hormone secreted is unable to interact with target cells. Hypoparathyroidism has been recognized in dogs, particularly in smaller breeds such as schnauzers and terriers, and infrequently in other animal species. Idiopathic hypoparathyroidism in adult dogs usually is caused by a diffuse lymphocytic parathyroiditis. Other infrequent causes of hypoparathyroidism include invasion and destruction of parathyroid glands by primary or metastatic neoplasms and trophic atrophy of parathyroid glands resulting from long-term hypercalcemia. In addition, the parathyroid glands are sometimes damaged or inadvertently removed during surgery involving the thyroid glands.

The functional disturbances and clinical manifestations of hypoparathyroidism primarily are the result of increased neuromuscular excitability and tetany. Because of the lack of PTH, bone resorption is decreased and blood calcium concentrations diminish progressively to 4 to 6 mg/dL (Fig. 12-44). Affected animals are restless, nervous, ataxic, and weak and have intermittent tremors of separate muscle groups. Tremors can progress to generalized tetany and convulsive seizures. Concurrently, blood phosphorus concentrations are increased because of increased renal tubular reabsorption.

Lymphocytic Parathyroiditis

Lymphocytic parathyroiditis is characterized by extensive degeneration of chief cells and replacement fibrosis. Mild lesions include infiltrates of lymphocytes and plasma cells and nodular hyperplasia of chief cells. Later, the parathyroid gland is completely replaced by lymphocytes, fibroblasts, and neocapillaries with few remaining viable chief cells (Web Fig. 12-7). Lymphocytic parathyroiditis develops by an immune-mediated mechanism, as evidenced by the production of a similar destruction of parathyroid gland parenchyma and lymphocytic infiltration in dogs injected with emulsions of parathyroid gland in adjuvant.

Hyperparathyroidism

Primary Hyperparathyroidism: Functional Chief Cell Neoplasms

Adenomas and carcinomas of parathyroid glands often secrete excessive amounts of PTH, resulting in a syndrome of primary hyperparathyroidism. Prolonged increased secretion of PTH accelerates osteolytic and osteoclastic bone resorption. Mineral is removed from the skeleton at an accelerated rate, and bone is replaced by immature fibrous connective tissue. The lesions of fibrous osteodystrophy are generalized throughout the skeleton but are accentuated in certain areas (e.g., maxilla, mandible, and subperiosteal areas of long bones).

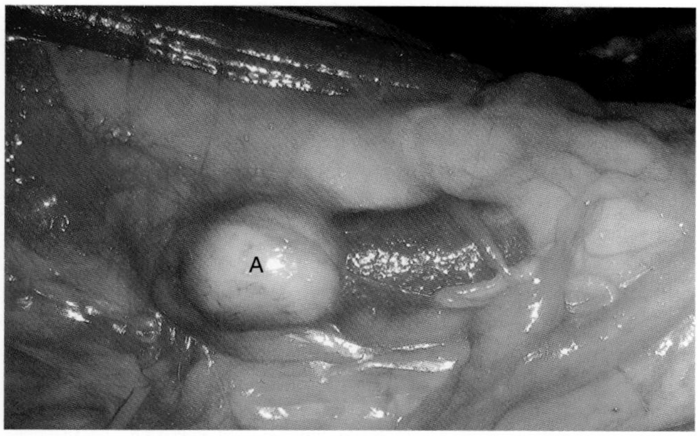

Fig. 12-45 Adenoma, parathyroid gland, dog.
Note the large parathyroid adenoma *(A),* well demarcated from the thyroid gland. (Courtesy College of Veterinary Medicine, University of Illinois.)

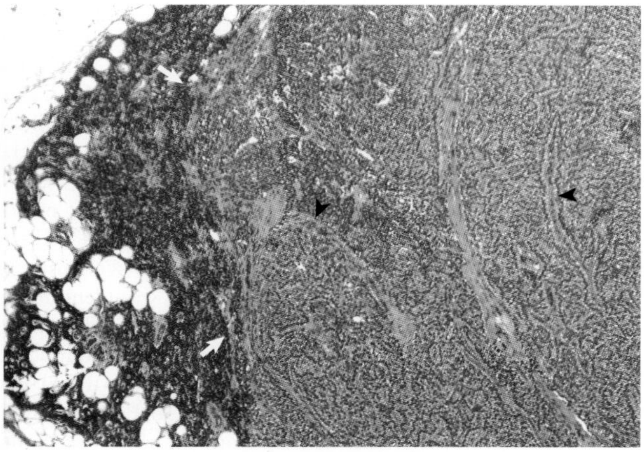

Fig. 12-46 Adenoma, parathyroid gland, dog.
The adenoma consists of closely packed chief cells arranged in small groups separated by fine fibrous septae containing capillaries *(arrowheads).* It is partially encapsulated and has compressed the adjacent, nonneoplastic parathyroid tissue *(arrows),* which has undergone trophic atrophy. H&E stain. (Courtesy Dr. C. Capen, College of Veterinary Medicine, The Ohio State University.)

Adenomas of parathyroid glands are encountered in older animals, particularly dogs, but parathyroid carcinomas are uncommon. Chief cell adenomas usually cause considerable enlargement of a single parathyroid gland. Parathyroid adenomas are encapsulated and sharply demarcated from the adjacent thyroid gland (Fig. 12-45).

Parathyroid gland adenomas are composed of small, closely packed groups of chief cells delineated by delicate vascular connective tissue septa that have many capillaries (Fig. 12-46). The neoplastic chief cells are round to polyhedral and have pale, expanded eosinophilic cytoplasm in which there are a few electron-dense secretory granules and prominent arrays of endoplasmic reticulum and Golgi complexes (Web Fig. 12-8).

The functional disturbances observed with endocrinologically active chief cell neoplasms are primarily the result of hypercalcemia and weakening of bones by excessive PTH-stimulated resorption of calcium. Cortical bone is thinned as a result of increased resorption by osteoclasts stimulated by the autonomous secretion of PTH (Fig. 12-47). Lameness can result from fractures of long bones that occur after relatively minor physical traumas. Compression fractures occur in vertebral bodies, resulting in pressure on the spinal cord and nerves that leads to motor and/or sensory dysfunction.

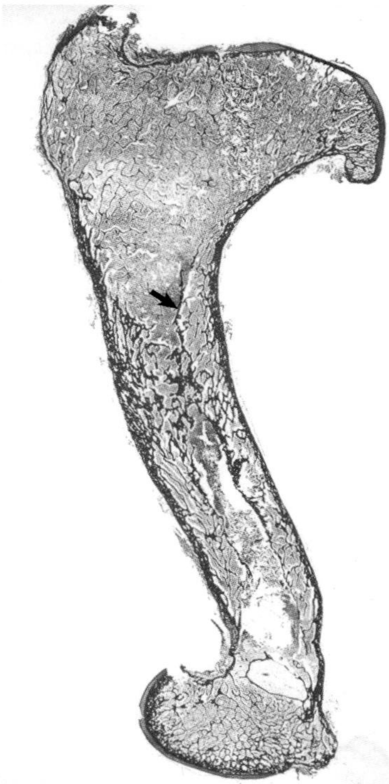

Fig. 12-47 Primary hyperparathyroidism, humerus, dog.
Severe thinning of cortical bone and large resorptive cavities *(arrow)* have resulted from localized resorption of bone by osteoclasts. (Courtesy Dr. C. Capen, College of Veterinary Medicine, The Ohio State University.)

Facial hyperostosis, caused by extensive osteoblastic proliferation and deposition of poorly mineralized osteoid and loosening or loss of teeth from alveolar sockets has been observed in dogs with primary hyperparathyroidism. Hypercalcemia results in anorexia, vomiting, constipation, depression, polyuria, polydipsia, and generalized muscular weakness because of decreased neuromuscular excitability.

The most practical laboratory test to aid in the diagnosis of primary hyperparathyroidism is quantification of the concentrations of total blood calcium, phosphorus, and circulating PTH (*N*-terminal or immunoradiometric [IRMA] assay). Dogs with primary hyperparathyroidism have greatly increased blood calcium concentrations (12 to 20 mg/dL or above). Blood phosphorus concentrations are low to normal (4 mg/dL or less) as a result of inhibition of renal tubular phosphorus reabsorption by the autonomous secretion of PTH. The urinary excretion of calcium and phosphorus is increased, which can predispose to the development of nephrocalcinosis and urolithiasis.

Secondary Hyperparathyroidism

Nutritional Imbalances

Nutritional hyperparathyroidism occurs commonly in cats, dogs, and horses. The increased secretion of PTH is a compensatory mechanism induced by nutritional imbalances. Such imbalances occur in diets low in calcium, diets with an excess of phosphorus, and diets with normal or low content of calcium and in New World primates housed indoors and fed diets with inadequate amounts of vitamin D_3. The significant result is hypocalcemia, which stimulates the parathyroid glands. Blood phosphorus concentrations, when elevated, contribute indirectly to parathyroid stimulation by decreasing blood calcium.

In response to the diet-induced hypocalcemia, chief cells undergo hypertrophy and hyperplasia with increased amounts of lightly eosinophilic or vacuolated cytoplasm. The organelles involved with protein synthesis (endoplasmic reticulum) and packaging of secretory products (Golgi apparatus) are well developed. Many chronically stimulated chief cells with well-developed secretory organelles accumulate glycogen after 5 to 14 weeks.

The most frequent nutritional imbalance causing hyperparathyroidism is the ingestion of excessive amounts of phosphorus. Hyperphosphatemia stimulates the parathyroid gland indirectly by lowering blood calcium. Horses that develop the disease usually have been fed grain diets with below-average-quality roughage. Evidence of excessive phosphorus intake might be difficult to determine, as the excess phosphorus could have been supplied as a bran supplement to the grain ration. The disease in horses is commonly referred to as "big head" because of the fact that the fibrous osteodystrophy is typically hyperostotic and most severe in the mandible and maxilla (see Fig. 16-55). The diet is usually palatable and nutritious, except for its excessive phosphorus and marginal or deficient calcium content. A diet deficient in calcium fails to supply the daily calcium requirement, and hypocalcemia develops, even though a greater proportion of calcium ingested is absorbed. Changes in concentrations of calcium and phosphorus in urine are more consistent and useful in the clinical diagnosis of nutritional secondary hyperparathyroidism in horses than changes in blood concentrations of these minerals. The increased secretion of PTH acts on normal kidneys to notably increase urinary phosphorus excretion and to decrease calcium loss in the urine.

Renal Disease

Hyperparathyroidism as a complication of chronic renal failure is characterized by excessive production of PTH in response to chronic hypocalcemia. When the renal disease is extensive enough to reduce the glomerular filtration rate, phosphorus is retained and hyperphosphatemia develops. The increased blood phosphorus concentration depresses ionized blood calcium concentration, resulting in parathyroid gland stimulation. Chronic renal disease also impairs the production of $1,25\text{-}(OH)_2D_3$ by the kidneys, thereby diminishing intestinal calcium transport and increasing mobilization of calcium from the skeleton. All parathyroid glands undergo notable chief cell hyperplasia, and the bones subsequently develop varying degrees of generalized fibrous osteodystrophy. The fibrous osteodystrophy that occurs with chronic renal failure is also most severe in the skull, but it is usually osteoporotic. Affected animals, especially dogs, have supple mandibles and/or maxillas known as "rubber jaws" (see Figs. 16-54 and 16-55).

Pseudohyperparathyroidism: Humoral Hypercalcemia of Malignancy

Hypercalcemia in animals is a common disorder with many causes. The most common form is cancer-associated hypercalcemia or humoral hypercalcemia of malignancy (HHM). Notable increases in serum calcium concentration resulting from an imbalance of calcium released from bones, excreted by the kidneys, or absorbed from the intestinal tract are reported with apocrine gland adenocarcinomas, metastases of solid neoplasms to bone, and hematologic malignancies such as lymphoma (lymphosarcoma).

The clinical signs of hypercalcemia are similar regardless of the underlying cause and depend on the rapidity of onset of increased concentrations of serum ionized calcium. Animals with total serum calcium values in excess of 16 mg/dL (4 mmol/L) generally have the most severe clinical signs. Exceptions to this rule occur, and some animals with severe hypercalcemia have only mild clinical signs. Horses and rabbits have normal total serum calcium concentrations greater than those found in other domestic animals, which should be considered before hypercalcemia is diagnosed in these species. Metabolic acidosis enhances the severity of clinical signs because it results in an increase in the ionized fraction of serum calcium. Increased serum ionized calcium induces clinical signs relating to the gastrointestinal, neuromuscular, cardiovascular, and renal systems.

The parathyroid glands in animals with HHM are small and difficult to locate or undetectable grossly. The parathyroid glands respond to the persistent cancer-associated hypercalcemia by trophic atrophy. Atrophic parathyroid glands in dogs are characterized by narrow cords of inactive chief cells with an abundant fibrous connective tissue stroma and widened perivascular spaces. Thyroid C cells undergo either diffuse or nodular hyperplasia in response to the persistent elevation in blood calcium.

Renal calcification has been detected microscopically in approximately 90% of dogs with HHM caused by anal sac apocrine gland adenocarcinomas, particularly when the calcium × phosphorus product is ≥50. Tubular calcification is most pronounced near the corticomedullary junction but is also present in cortical and inner medullary tubules, Bowman's capsule, and glomerular tufts. Calcification also occurs in the fundic gastric mucosa and endocardium.

Excessive secretion of biologically active PTHrP plays a central role in the pathogenesis of hypercalcemia in most forms of HHM; however, cytokines, such as interleukin-1 (IL-1), tumor necrosis factor-α (TNF-α), transforming growth factor-α (TGF-α) and TGF-β, or 1,25-dihydroxyvitamin D, can have synergistic or cooperative actions with PTHrP. Before PTHrP was identified, it was well understood that nonparathyroid neoplasms and humoral hypercalcemia of malignancy induced a syndrome that mimicked primary hyperparathyroidism because of secretion of a PTH-like factor that was antigenically unrelated to PTH. Purification of the substance with PTH-like activity from the adenocarcinoma derived from apocrine glands of the anal sac in dogs and multiple human neoplasms with documented HHM resulted in the discovery of PTHrP. PTHrP also can be demonstrated by immunohistochemical and biochemical analysis in a number of tissues, in which it appears to function primarily as a paracrine factor.

Apocrine Gland Adenocarcinoma

See the section on Disorders of Dogs for a discussion of apocrine gland adenocarcinoma.

Neoplasms Metastatic to Bone

Solid neoplasms that metastasize widely to bone and grow locally can produce hypercalcemia by inducing local bone resorption. This is not common in animals but is an important cause of HHM in humans, particularly patients with metastatic breast and lung carcinomas.

The pathogenesis of enhanced bone resorption is not well understood, but the two primary mechanisms include (1) secretion of cytokines or factors that stimulate local bone resorption and (2) indirect stimulation of bone resorption by tumor-induced cytokine secretion from local immune or bone cells. Cytokines or factors that are secreted by neoplastic cells and stimulate local bone resorption include PTHrP, TGF-α and TGF-β, and prostaglandins, especially prostaglandin E_2.

Lymphoma (Lymphosarcoma)

Lymphoma is the most common neoplasm associated with hypercalcemia in dogs and cats. Estimates of the prevalence of hypercalcemia in dogs with lymphoma vary from 20% to 40%.

Peripheral lymph node enlargement is present in some cases; cranial mediastinal or visceral nodes usually are involved. The hypercalcemia results from the production of humoral substances by neoplastic cells and/or from physical disruption of trabecular bone by lymphoma in bone marrow. Serum immunoreactive PTH concentrations are subnormal, and plasma prostaglandin E_2 concentrations are not different from those of controls.

Most dogs with lymphoma and HHM have significantly increased circulating PTHrP concentrations, but these concentrations are lower (2 to 15 pmol) than in dogs with carcinomas and HHM; there is no correlation with serum calcium concentration. The latter indicates that PTHrP is an important marker in dogs with HHM and lymphoma but is not the sole humoral factor responsible for the stimulation of osteoclasts and development of hypercalcemia. It is likely that cytokines, such as IL-1 or TNF, function synergistically with PTHrP to induce HHM in dogs with lymphoma. Some dogs with lymphoma and hypercalcemia have increased serum 1,25-dihydroxyvitamin D concentrations that could be responsible for or contribute to the induction of hypercalcemia. PTH (*N*-terminal) concentrations in dogs with lymphoma and hypercalcemia usually are in the normal range; however, a few dogs have concentrations that are increased slightly above the normal range.

Parturient Hypocalcemia

Parturient paresis in dairy cattle is a complex metabolic disease characterized by the development of severe hypocalcemia and hypophosphatemia near the time of parturition and the initiation of lactation. The serum calcium concentration decreases to less than 50% of normal in spite of an increased secretion of PTH by the cow's parathyroid glands. Bone resorption remains minimal, and few osteoclasts are present on bone surfaces. Biochemical and ultrastructural studies in cows indicate that the parathyroid glands are capable of responding to the acute hypocalcemia by increasing development of the cellular organelles responsible for hormonal synthesis and by increasing secretion of PTH.

The composition of the diet fed to dairy cows is a significant factor in the pathogenesis of parturient hypocalcemia. Diets with excessive calcium have been incriminated as significantly increasing the incidence of the disease. Conversely, diets low in calcium or diets supplemented with therapeutic doses of vitamin D reduce the incidence of parturient hypocalcemia. Calcium homeostasis in pregnant cows fed an excessive calcium diet appears to be maintained principally by intestinal calcium absorption (Fig. 12-48). This greater reliance on intestinal absorption rather than on PTH-stimulated bone resorption probably is a significant factor in the more frequent development of profound hypocalcemia near parturition in cows fed excessive calcium prepartal diets.

An increased prepartal secretion of calcitonin in cows that develop parturient hypocalcemia or milk fever, especially those fed excessive calcium diets, could be a factor contributing to the inability of increased PTH concentrations to mobilize calcium rapidly from skeletal reserves and to maintain blood calcium concentrations during the critical periparturient period. The thyroidal content of calcitonin is reduced, many C cells are degranulated, and plasma concentrations of calcitonin often are increased in cows before the development of profound hypocalcemia.

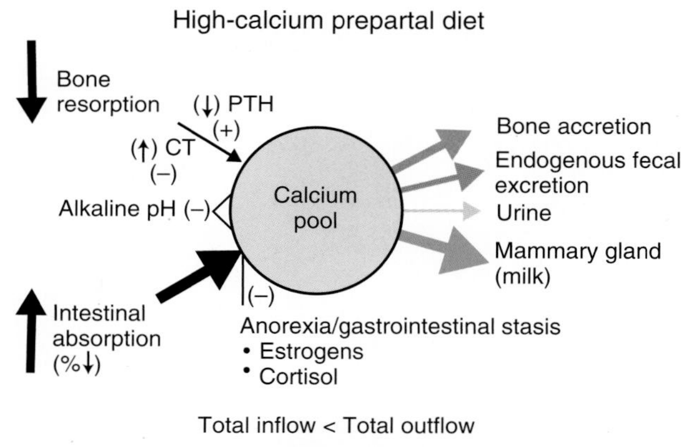

Fig. 12-48 Schematic diagram of calcium homeostasis in cows fed a high-calcium prepartal diet.
In this case, calcium homeostasis is primarily dependent on intestinal calcium absorption. The rate of bone resorption is low, and parathyroid glands are inactive. Anorexia and gastrointestinal stasis that often occur near parturition interrupt the major inflow of calcium into the extracellular fluid calcium pool. Outflow of calcium with the onset of lactation exceeds the rate of inflow into the calcium pool, and cows develop a progressive hypocalcemia and paresis. *CT,* Calcitonin; *PTH,* parathyroid hormone. (Redrawn with permission from Dr. C. Capen, College of Veterinary Medicine, The Ohio State University.)

DISORDERS OF PANCREATIC ISLET CELLS

Hypofunction of Pancreatic Islet Cells

Diabetes Mellitus

Diabetes mellitus is a metabolic disorder that results from a reduction of insulin available for normal function of many cells in the body. In some cases, increased concentrations of glucagon contribute to development of persistent hyperglycemia. Insulin unavailability could be due to degenerative changes in β cells of the pancreatic islets, reduced effectiveness of the hormone because of the formation of antiinsulin antibodies or inactive complexes, damage to β cells from immune-mediated islet cytotoxicity, or inappropriate secretion of hormones by neoplasms in other endocrine organs.

Diabetes mellitus is a common endocrinopathy in dogs and cats. Most cases of spontaneous diabetes occur in mature dogs and in females approximately twice as often as males. An increased incidence of diabetes mellitus has been observed in certain small breeds of dogs, such as miniature poodles, dachshunds, and terriers, but nearly all breeds of dogs can be affected.

Development of diabetes mellitus in young dogs is the result of idiopathic atrophy of the pancreas, acute pancreatitis with necrosis and hemorrhage, and aplasia of pancreatic islets; however, diabetes mellitus can also occur secondary to other endocrine disorders such as acromegaly, Cushing's syndrome, hyperaldosteronism, hyperthyroidism and various neoplasms. The pancreas with idiopathic atrophy is reduced to a third or less of its size. Hypoplasia of pancreatic islets in which the islets are absent but the pancreatic acini and ducts are present and functional has been a cause of diabetes mellitus in young dogs (2 to 3 months of age).

In the pathogenesis of diabetes mellitus, several factors are responsible for the decreased availability of insulin. Destruction of islets secondary to severe pancreatitis or the selective degeneration of islet cells are the most common causes in animals. In dogs, the pancreatic islets are often destroyed because of inflammation of the exocrine pancreas. Chronic relapsing pancreatitis with progressive loss of both exocrine and endocrine cells and replacement by fibrous connective tissue is a frequent cause of diabetes mellitus. In these dogs, the pancreas becomes firm, multinodular, and has scattered areas of hemorrhage and necrosis after a recent relapse (Fig. 12-49). Later in the course of the disease, all that remains of the pancreas is a thin fibrous band or nodule near the duodenum and stomach (Fig. 12-50).

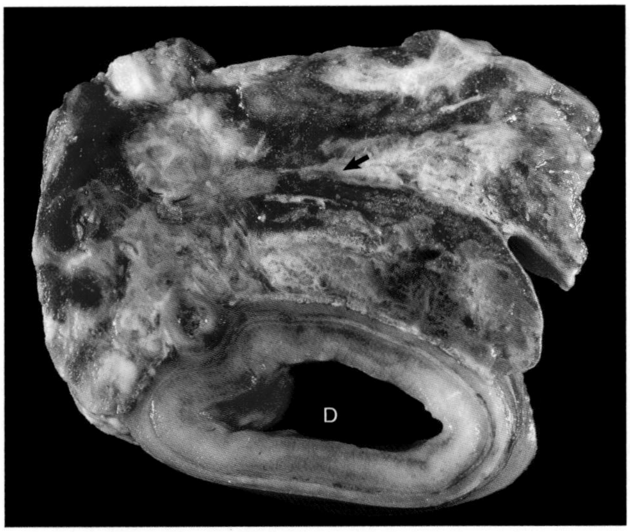

Fig. 12-49 Chronic relapsing pancreatitis, pancreas and duodenum, cross-section, dog.
The pancreas is multinodular and firm with areas of hemorrhage *(arrow)*, fibrosis, and necrosis. *D*, Duodenum. (Courtesy Dr. C. Capen, College of Veterinary Medicine, The Ohio State University.)

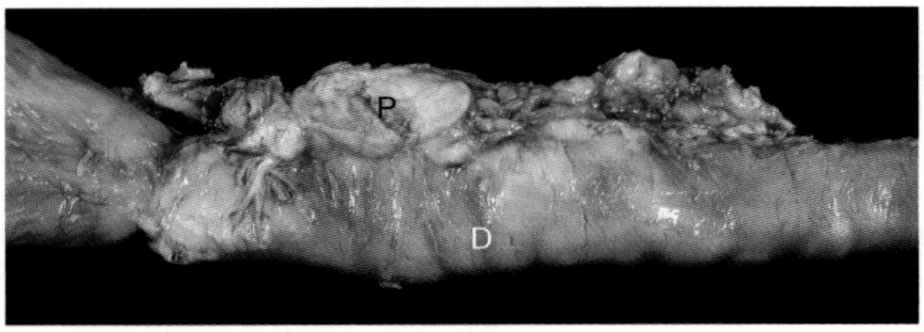

Fig. 12-50 Chronic pancreatitis, pancreas, dog.
The pancreas *(P)* is markedly atrophied and its parenchyma almost completely replaced by fibrous connective tissue in "end-stage" pancreatitis. *D*, Duodenum. (Courtesy Dr. C. Capen, College of Veterinary Medicine, The Ohio State University.)

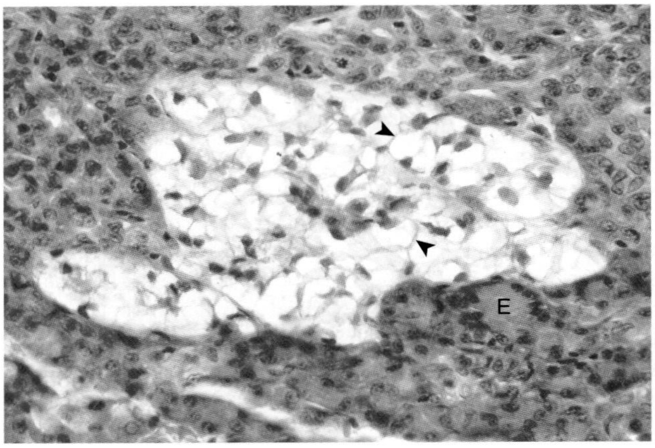

Fig. 12-51 Hydropic ("vacuolar") degeneration, pancreatic islet, cat.
Discrete vacuoles *(arrowheads)* are present in the cytoplasm of β cells. E, Exocrine pancreas. H&E stain. (Courtesy Dr. C. Capen, College of Veterinary Medicine, The Ohio State University.)

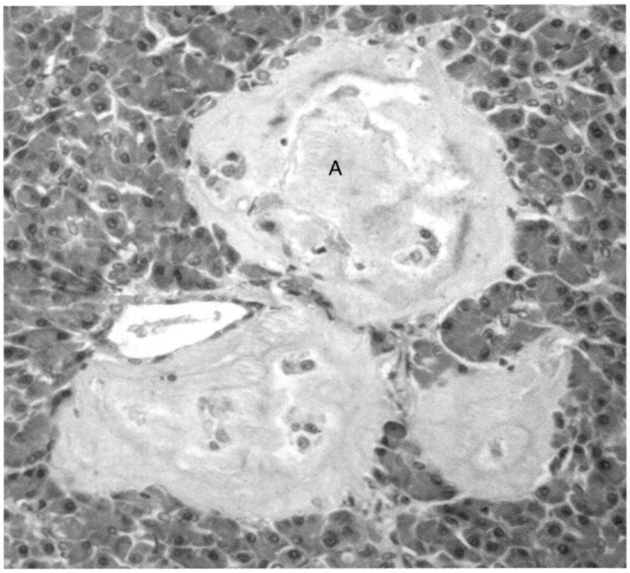

Fig. 12-52 Amyloidosis, pancreatic islets, cat.
Note the deposits of amyloid *(A)* and degeneration and loss of islet cells. H&E stain. (Courtesy College of Veterinary Medicine, University of Illinois.)

Histologically, β cells are reduced in number and remaining cells have vacuolated cytoplasm (Fig. 12-51). The cytoplasm of β cells is distended by massive amounts of glycogen particles (Web Fig. 12-9). Hydropic degeneration with glycogen accumulation, especially in cats, appears to develop in β cells in response to long-term overstimulation or exhaustion because of peripheral insulin resistance. When disease is chronic, the islets are difficult to find. Immune-mediated isletitis characterized by a progressive lymphoplasmacytic infiltration and selective destruction of β cells of the islets is another cause of diabetes mellitus (type 1) occasionally in dogs.

Another common pancreatic change in cats with diabetes is the selective deposition of amyloid in islets, resulting in degenerative changes in α cells and β cells (Fig. 12-52). Scattered amyloid deposits in pancreatic islets that increase progressively with age occur in the pancreatic islets of many cats without clinically apparent diabetes mellitus. Islet amyloid polypeptide (IAPP) (37 amino acids) and insulin are both secreted by β cells. The IAPP in cats has a unique amino acid sequence (amino acids 25 to 28: alanine, isoleucine, leucine, and serine), which is predisposed to polymerization and accumulation in pancreatic islets. As the insoluble amyloid fibers progressively accumulate in the islets, they disrupt β cells and surround islet capillaries, leading to the subsequent degeneration of islet cells.

Complete expression of the complex metabolic disturbances in diabetes mellitus appears to be the result of a bihormonal abnormality. Although a relative or absolute deficiency of insulin action in response to a rising extracellular glucose concentration has been long recognized as the sine qua non of diabetes mellitus, the importance of an absolute or relative increase of glucagon secretion in some forms of the disease in certain species has been appreciated only recently. Hyperglucagonemia in diabetic patients can be the result of increased secretion of pancreatic glucagon, enteroglucagon, or both. An increased blood glucagon concentration contributes to the severe endogenous hyperglycemia by mobilizing hepatic stores of glucose and to the development of ketoacidosis by increasing the oxidation of fatty acids by hepatocytes. The major glucoregulatory consequence of insulin deficiency is reduction in the movement of glucose into insulin-sensitive tissues (e.g., liver, adipose tissue, and muscle), with a corresponding increase in hepatic glucose production, resulting in notable endogenous hyperglycemia.

The onset of diabetes mellitus is insidious, and the clinical course is often chronic. Clinically, dogs with diabetes mellitus exhibit polydipsia, polyuria, weight loss in spite of polyphagia, bilateral cataracts, and weakness. The disturbances in water metabolism primarily have an osmotic basis. In dogs with persistent hyperglycemia and glycosuria, the renal tubular epithelium is unable to concentrate the urine effectively against the osmotic attraction of the glucose in the glomerular filtrate.

Diabetic animals have diminished resistance to bacterial and fungal infections, and diseases, such as suppurative cystitis, prostatitis, bronchopneumonia, and dermatitis, often become chronic or recurrent. This increased susceptibility to infection in patients with poorly controlled diabetes can be related in part to impaired chemotactic, phagocytic, and microbicidal functions and decreased adherence of polymorphonuclear leukocytes. The impaired microbicidal function of leukocytes can have a metabolic basis resulting from diminished production of cellular energy from glucose. Radiographic evidence of emphysematous cystitis is strongly suggestive of diabetes mellitus. Infections of the urinary bladder with glucose-fermenting organisms, such as *Proteus* sp., *Aerobacter aerogenes,* and *Escherichia coli* result in gas formation in the wall and lumen. Emphysema also develops in the wall of the gallbladder in some diabetic dogs.

Hepatomegaly occurs as a result of fatty degeneration (see Figs. 1-45 and 8-38). Lipids accumulate in the liver as the result of increased lipid mobilization, and hepatocytes injured by ketonemia have decreased usage of lipids. Individual hepatocytes are greatly enlarged by multiple droplets of lipid (Web Fig. 12-10). If the accumulation of lipids is extensive and long-standing, cirrhosis develops. The liver remains enlarged, and its surface becomes coarsely nodular because of extensive remodeling of hepatic parenchyma (Web Fig. 12-11; also see Fig. 8-21). Individual hepatocytes degenerate and are replaced by regenerative and hyperplastic nodules and interlobular fibrosis. Icterus and bilirubinuria often accompany severe cirrhosis.

Cataracts often develop in dogs with poorly controlled diabetes mellitus. They are stellate or asteroid in shape (Web Fig. 12-12; also see Fig. 20-95) and initially appear along the suture lines of lenticular fibers. Cataract formation in the diabetic patient is related to the unique sorbitol pathway by which glucose is metabolized in the lens. Glucose is first converted to sorbitol by the enzyme aldose reductase and subsequently to fructose by sorbitol dehydrogenase. These sugar alcohols accumulate within the lens and result in an intracellular accumulation of solute and hypertonicity. The initial structural change in the lens consists of swelling and hydropic degeneration of lenticular fibers. In long-standing cases of diabetes mellitus, swelling of lenticular fibers continues until the majority of lenticular fibers are affected. Later, macromolecular aggregation or precipitation of normally translucent lenticular proteins develops, accompanied by disruption of lenticular fibers and formation of interfibrillar clefts. The result is diffuse, often bilateral lens opacity observed in animals with chronic diabetes mellitus.

Other extrapancreatic lesions of diabetes mellitus, such as chronic renal disease, blindness, and gangrene, are the result of microangiopathy characterized by thickening of the capillary basement membrane. Dogs with long-standing, poorly controlled, spontaneous diabetes mellitus develop nodular or diffuse glomerulosclerosis characterized by PAS-positive fibrillar deposits of glycoprotein, which occasionally form spherical nodules in the glomerular capillary tufts. Other renal lesions include accumulation of glycogen within cells of the loop of Henle (intracytoplasmic) and distal convoluted tubule (intranuclear) (Web Fig. 12-13).

Hyperfunction of Pancreatic Islet Cells

β-Cell (Insulin-Secreting) Neoplasms (Insulinomas)

The neoplasms most frequently arising in pancreatic islets are adenomas and carcinomas derived from β cells. These neoplasms are often endocrinologically active and produce dramatic functional disturbances. Other pancreatic neoplasms appear to be derived from multipotential ductal epithelial cells that differentiate into one of several other cell types in the pancreatic islets. β-Cell neoplasms are seen most frequently in dogs 5 to 12 years of age (mean 9 years). These neoplasms also occur in older cattle and can cause periodic convulsions. Carcinomas of the pancreatic islets are more common than adenomas in dogs and are commonly found in the duodenal (right) lobe of the pancreas. Carcinomas of the pancreatic islets can be differentiated grossly from adenomas by their larger size, multilobular appearance, extensive invasion of adjacent parenchyma and lymph vessels, and metastases to extrapancreatic sites, such as regional lymph nodes (e.g., duodenal, mesenteric, hepatic, and splenic), liver, mesentery, and omentum.

The clinical alterations observed with functional β-cell neoplasms are the result of excessive insulin secretion and the development of severe hypoglycemia. The clinical signs are not specific for the hyperinsulinism produced by β-cell neoplasms. Initial signs include weakness, fatigue after vigorous exercise, generalized muscular twitching and weakness, ataxia, mental confusion, and changes in temperament. Dogs are easily agitated and have intermittent periods of excitability and restlessness. Periodic convulsive seizures of the tonic-clonic type occur later in the disease and increase progressively in frequency and intensity.

The predominance of clinical signs relating to the CNS demonstrates the primary dependence of the brain on glucose metabolism for energy. The failure to recognize dogs with functional islet cell neoplasms when they have clinical signs suggestive of primary disease of the nervous system has frequently led to the misdiagnoses of idiopathic epilepsy, brain neoplasm, or other organic neurologic disease. Repeated episodes of prolonged and severe hypoglycemia result in neuronal necrosis and permanent neurologic disability with terminal coma and eventually death.

Adenomas of the β cells of the pancreatic islets typically exist as single, yellow to dark red, small (1 to 3 cm), spherical nodules. The neoplasms are of similar consistency to or slightly firmer than that of the surrounding pancreas. Adenomas occur as a single nodule or less often as multiple nodules in one or both lobes and/or body of the pancreas. Islet cell adenomas are sharply delineated and surrounded by a thin capsule of fibrous connective tissue (Fig. 12-53). Small nests of acinar epithelial cells are sometimes present throughout the neoplasm but are more common at the periphery. Numerous connective tissue septa containing small capillaries radiate from the capsule into the neoplasm and subdivide the neoplasm into small lobules or packets. Well-differentiated neoplastic cells are round to polyhedral with distinct cell borders and pale eosinophilic, finely granular cytoplasm.

Islet cell carcinomas are consistently larger than adenomas, are multilobular, and invade into and through the fibrous capsule of the pancreas (Fig. 12-54). The dense bands of fibrous tissue that course through the neoplasm give rise to fine connective tissue septa containing capillaries that subdivide the neoplasm into small cords or lobules. Well-differentiated neoplastic cells in islet cell carcinomas are closely packed but are less uniform in size and shape than the cells in adenomas. They are round to polyhedral and have a granular eosinophilic cytoplasm. Mitotic figures are infrequent. Microscopic

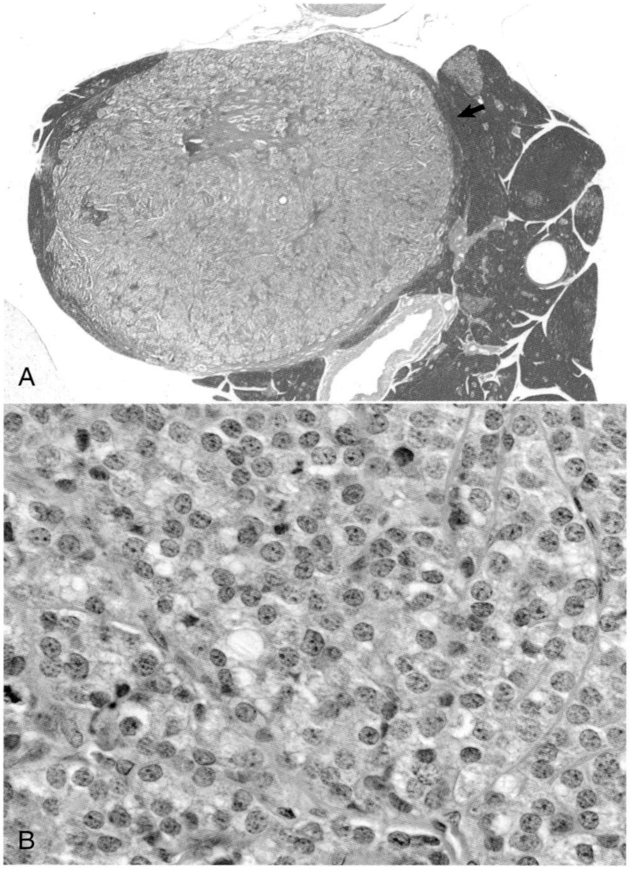

Fig. 12-53 β-Cell adenoma, pancreatic islet, dog.
A, A solid islet adenoma, surrounded by a fibrous capsule of variable thickness, has compressed the adjacent exocrine pancreas *(arrow)*. H&E stain. **B,** The neoplastic β-cells are arranged into packets and have abundant finely granular cytoplasm characteristic of neuroendocrine tumors. H&E stain. (**A** courtesy Dr. C. Capen, College of Veterinary Medicine, The Ohio State University. **B** courtesy Dr. J.F. Zachary, College of Veterinary Medicine, University of Illinois.)

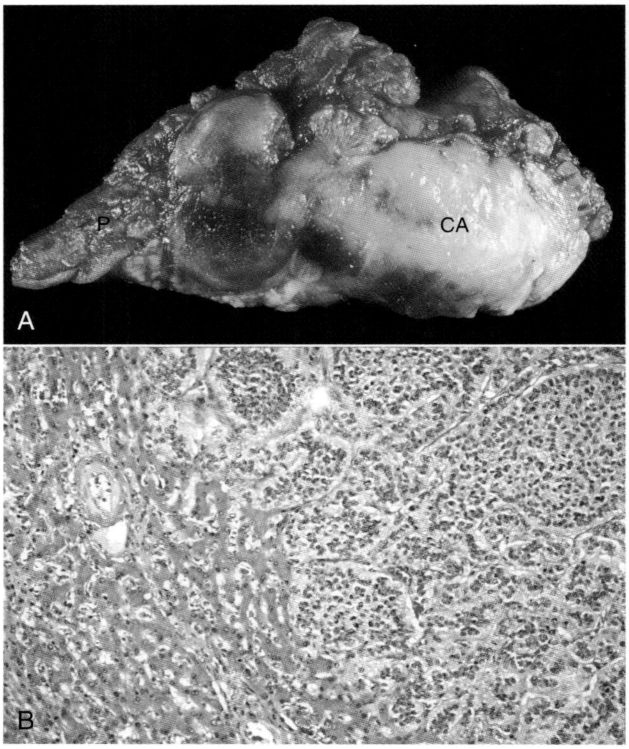

Fig. 12-54 β-cell carcinoma, pancreatic islet, dog.
A, The whitish-red carcinoma *(CA)* is well demarcated from the lobular exocrine pancreas *(P)*. **B,** The β-cell carcinoma *(right side of figure)* has metastasized to the liver and has expanded to compress adjacent hepatic parenchyma and invade sinusoids. H&E stain. (**A** courtesy Dr. C. Capen, College of Veterinary Medicine, The Ohio State University. **B** courtesy Dr. J.F. Zachary, College of Veterinary Medicine, University of Illinois.)

evidence of distinct local tissue invasion is the principal criterion for the diagnosis of islet cell carcinoma.

Cells composing functional islet cell neoplasms in dogs usually have histochemical and immunohistochemical characteristics of β cells. Ultrastructurally, the neoplastic β cells are electron dense because of numerous cytoplasmic organelles.

Non-β (Gastrin-Secreting) Islet Cell Neoplasms (Gastrinomas)

Gastrin-secreting, non-β islet cell neoplasms of the pancreas have been reported in dogs and cats. The hypersecretion of gastrin in humans results in the well-documented Zollinger-Ellison syndrome, consisting of hypersecretion of gastric acid and recurrent peptic ulceration in the gastrointestinal tract. The non-β islet cell neoplasms derived from ectopic amine precursor uptake decarboxylase (APUD) cells in the pancreas produce an excess of gastrin, which normally is secreted by cells of the antral and duodenal mucosa. The incidence of gastrin-secreting pancreatic neoplasms in dogs and cats is uncertain, but it appears to be uncommon compared with that of insulin-secreting β-cell neoplasms. In the comparatively few canine and feline cases studied, the clinical signs have included anorexia, vomiting of blood-tinged material, intermittent diarrhea, progressive weight loss, and dehydration, the result of the multiple ulcerations of the gastrointestinal mucosa because of gastrin-stimulated gastric acid hypersecretion (Zollinger-Ellison–like syndrome).

Animals with Zollinger-Ellison–like syndrome have single or multiple, variably sized neoplasms in the pancreas. These are firm, have increased amounts of fibrous connective tissue, and although partially encapsulated, the neoplasm usually extends into the surrounding pancreas.

Three histologic patterns of gastrin-secreting islet neoplasms in dogs are recognized: (1) the ribbon or trabecular pattern; (2) solid nests of cells with a delicate, highly vascularized stroma; and (3) an acinar pattern with cuboidal neoplastic cells arranged around a central lumen. The stroma is prominent and hyalinized in some gastrin-secreting neoplasms.

Canine gastrin-secreting islet cell neoplasms invade locally into the adjacent pancreas and often metastasize to regional lymph nodes and to the liver. These dogs have either single or multiple ulcerations of the gastric and/or duodenal mucosa and blood in the gut lumen.

Other non-β islet cell neoplasms reported in animals are those of glucagon-secreting α cells. Glucagonomas have been reported rarely in dogs and are associated with superficial necrolytic dermatitis.

DISORDERS OF THE PINEAL GLAND

Pinealitis

See the section on Disorders of Horses for a discussion of pinealitis.

Pineal Tumors

Pineal tumors are exceedingly rare in animals. The cases in domestic animals are isolated reports in a cow, goat, and horse. Tumors are classified as well-differentiated pinealocytomas, anaplastic pinealoblastomas, or mixed tumors. Immunoreactivity to synaptophysin has been shown to be the most consistent marker for pineal tumors.

DISORDERS OF THE CHEMORECEPTOR ORGANS

Neoplasms

Although chemoreceptor tissue appears to be widely distributed in the body, neoplasms develop principally in the aortic and carotid bodies. Aortic body chemodectomas are encountered more frequently in animals than those of the carotid body, but the reverse is true for humans. These neoplasms develop primarily in dogs and infrequently in cats and cattle. Brachycephalic breeds of dogs, such as the boxer and Boston terrier, are highly predisposed to develop neoplasms of the aortic and carotid bodies.

Neoplasms of the Aortic Body

Aortic body neoplasms appear most frequently as a single mass or as multiple nodules near the base of the heart (Fig. 12-55). They vary considerably in size (from 0.5 to 12.5 cm), with carcinomas larger than adenomas. Solitary small adenomas either are attached to the adventitia of the pulmonary artery and ascending aorta or are embedded in the adipose connective tissue between these major vessels. They have a smooth external surface and on cross-section are white and mottled with red-to-brown areas. Larger adenomas are multilobular and can compress and indent the wall of the atria, displace the trachea, and partially surround the major vessels at the base of the heart. Aortic body carcinomas are less frequent than adenomas in dogs. Carcinomas infiltrate the wall of the pulmonary artery and form papillary projections into its lumen or invade through the wall into the lumen of the atria. Although neoplastic cells often invade blood vessels, metastases to the lungs and liver occur infrequently in dogs.

Neoplasms of the aortic bodies in animals are not functional (i.e., they do not secrete excess hormone into the circulation), but as a space-occupying lesion they can produce a variety of functional disturbances. Larger aortic body adenomas and carcinomas put pressure on the atria, vena cava, or both and cause manifestations of cardiac decompensation. A higher percentage of aortic body neoplasms than carotid body neoplasms are benign. Aortic body carcinomas invade locally into the atria, pericardium, and adjacent vessels.

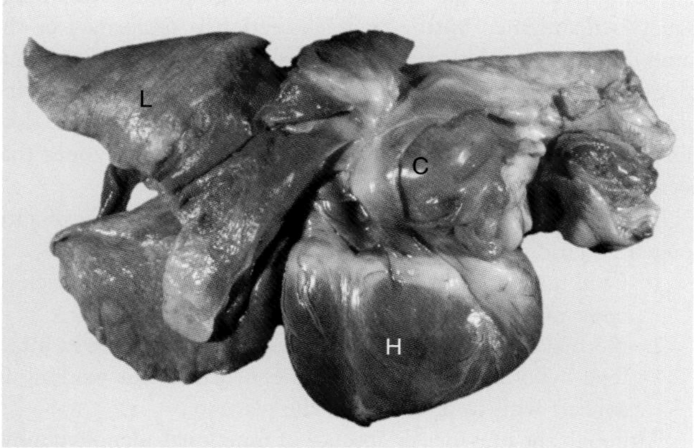

Fig. 12-55 Carcinoma, aortic body, dog.
Note the large mass *(C)* at the base of the heart *(H)*. Contiguous portions of the right-middle and diaphragmatic lung lobes are atelectatic. *L,* Lungs. (Courtesy College of Veterinary Medicine, University of Illinois.)

Neoplasms of the Carotid Body

Carotid body neoplasms arise near the bifurcation of the common carotid artery in the cranial cervical area. They are usually unilateral, only rarely bilateral, and are slow growing. Adenomas vary from approximately 1 to 4 cm in diameter, are well encapsulated, and have a smooth external surface. The bifurcation of the common carotid artery is incorporated in the mass, and neoplastic cells are firmly adhered to the tunica adventitia. Adenomas are firm, white with scattered areas of hemorrhage, and are extremely vascular.

Carotid body carcinomas are larger, more coarsely multinodular than adenomas, invade the capsule, and penetrate into the walls of adjacent blood and lymph vessels. The external jugular vein and some cranial nerves can be incorporated into the neoplasm. Metastases of carotid body carcinomas occur in approximately 30% of cases and have been found in the lungs, tracheobronchial and mediastinal lymph nodes, liver, pancreas, and kidneys. Multicentric neoplastic transformation of chemoreceptor tissue (aortic and carotid bodies) occurs frequently in brachycephalic breeds of dogs.

The microscopic features of chemoreceptor neoplasms ("chemodectomas") are essentially similar, whether they are derived from the carotid or the aortic body. The neoplasm is subdivided into lobules by prominent branching trabeculae of connective tissue, which originate from the fibrous capsule. Neoplasms are further subdivided into smaller nests by fine septa of collagenous and reticulin fibers and small capillaries. Neoplastic cells are commonly aligned along and around small capillaries and are discrete, round to polyhedral, and closely packed, with pale eosinophilic, finely granular, and often vacuolated cytoplasm.

Although the cause of carotid and aortic body neoplasms is unknown, a genetic predisposition aggravated by chronic hypoxia could account for the greater risk of development in certain brachycephalic breeds such as the boxer and Boston terrier. Carotid bodies of several mammalian species, including dogs, have developed hyperplastic foci when the animals were subjected to the chronic hypoxia of high altitude. Humans living at high altitudes have 10 times the frequency of chemodectomas as those residing at sea level.

Heart-Base Neoplasms Derived from Ectopic Thyroid Gland Tissue

Adenomas and carcinomas derived from ectopic thyroid gland account for approximately 5% to 10% of "heart base" neoplasms in dogs. They often compress or invade structures in the cranial mediastinum near the base of the heart (Fig. 12-56). Ectopic thyroid gland neoplasms have a compact cellular (solid) pattern that is difficult to distinguish histologically from that of aortic body neoplasms. Cells of ectopic thyroid gland neoplasms generally are smaller than those of aortic body neoplasms and have more hyperchromatic nuclei and an eosinophilic cytoplasm. Thyroidal neoplasms of follicular cells are not consistently subdivided into small packets by fine strands of connective tissue. Giant cells are infrequent in ectopic thyroid gland neoplasms, and the stroma is not prominent. Usually, primitive follicular structures or colloid-containing follicles can be demonstrated in ectopic thyroid gland neoplasms but not in aortic body neoplasms.

OBESITY

Obesity, defined as the accumulation of excessive amounts of adipose tissue in the body, is an increasing problem affecting

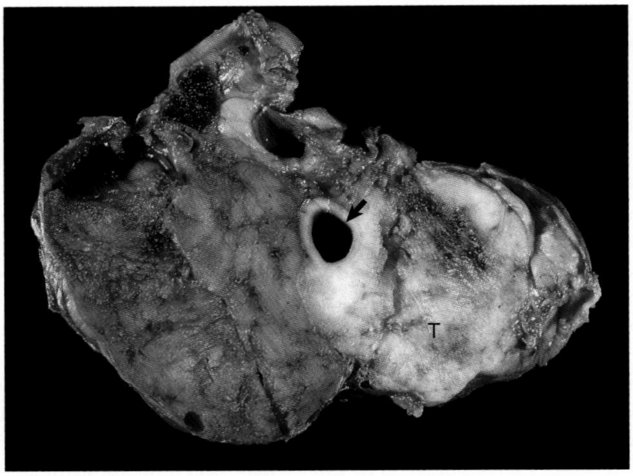

Fig. 12-56 Carcinoma, ectopic thyroid tissue, cranial mediastinum, cross-section, dog.
Neoplastic tissue *(T)* surrounds the trachea *(arrow)* and other structures in the cranial mediastinum. (Courtesy Dr. C. Capen, College of Veterinary Medicine, The Ohio State University.)

approximately 35% of dogs and cats. The primary cause is a positive energy balance, but there are many contributory factors, including breed predisposition, advancing age, sex, gonadal status, diet, and lifestyle. In addition, there is an unclear causal sequence between obesity and various endocrinopathies, including hyperadrenocorticism, hypothyroidism, and diabetes mellitus.

Adipose tissue is composed of unilocular white adipocytes and multilocular brown adipocytes; both store energy in the form of lipid, while brown adipocytes are also involved in thermogenesis. Preadipocytes and pluripotent stem cells are responsible for the expansion of adipose tissue in obesity. Adipose tissue is also recognized as an endocrine organ that synthesizes and secretes adipokines such as leptin and adiponectin. In fact, maintaining the balance between these opposing adipokines is essential for the prevention of obesity. Leptin is critical for appetite suppression and energy expenditure via thermogenesis but is also proinflammatory. Obesity ensues with leptin or leptin receptor deficiency, as well as decreased end-organ response to leptin in the hypothalamus. Interestingly, breed, glucocorticosteroid therapy, and neutering have been shown to impact leptin concentrations in dogs and/or cats. Adiponectin is essential for enhanced glucose uptake and metabolism and in contrast to leptin is antiinflammatory. Decreased circulating adiponectin levels have been reported in obese dogs and cats; however, altered proportions of high and low molecular weight adiponectin have not been examined as they have in humans. Monocytes and macrophages, the number and activity of which increase with expansion of adipose tissue, are also critical to the development of obesity. Together with white adipocytes, they produce procoagulant, acute phase reactant, and proinflammatory cytokines, particularly TNF-α and IL-6.

DISORDERS OF HORSES

PARS INTERMEDIA ADENOMAS

See the section on Disorders of the Adenohypophysis, Disorders of Domestic Animals for a discussion of hyperpituitarism and neoplasms of the adenohypophysis.

LYMPHOCYTIC (IMMUNE-MEDIATED) THYROIDITIS

See the section on Disorders of the Thyroid Gland, Disorders of Domestic Animals for a discussion of hypothyroidism.

NUTRITIONAL HYPERPARATHYROIDISM

See the section on Disorders of the Parathyroid Gland, Disorders of Domestic Animals for a discussion of hyperparathyroidism.

PINEALITIS

Pinealitis accompanying uveitis is well established in animal models of experimental autoimmune uveoretinitis after immunization with retinal antigens. Because the pineal gland is rarely, if ever, histologically examined during active uveitis in humans with autoimmune uveitis, there is no direct evidence of concurrent pineal pathology, but it is suspected. However, there are reports documenting lymphocytic and eosinophilic pinealitis in horses with recurrent uveitis.

DISORDERS OF RUMINANTS (CATTLE, SHEEP, AND GOATS)

APLASIA AND PROLONGED GESTATION

Subnormal function of the fetal endocrine system, seen especially in ruminants, can disrupt normal fetal development and result in prolonged gestation. In Guernsey and Jersey cattle, a genetically determined failure of development (aplasia) of the adenohypophysis has been described, but the neurohypophysis develops normally. This aplasia results in a lack of fetal pituitary trophic hormone secretion during the last trimester and hypoplasia of target endocrine organs, namely the adrenal cortex, gonads, and follicular cells of the thyroid gland. Fetal development is normal up to approximately 7 months of gestation, but then fetal growth ceases, irrespective of the length of time the viable fetus is retained in the uterus.

Prolongation of gestation occurs in ewes that ingest the plant *Veratrum californicum* between days 12 and 14 of gestation. *Veratrum californicum* contains potent alkaloids that inhibit neural tube development, resulting in cyclopia and extensive malformations of the CNS and hypothalamus in lambs. Arrhinencephalia and lack of development of nasal bones accompany the formation of a proboscis-like structure. Although the adenohypophysis may be present in some cases, it is unable to secrete normal amounts of trophic hormones (ACTH) because it lacks the necessary fine control derived from the hypothalamic-releasing hormones. Pregnancy is maintained until a cesarean section is performed or the lamb dies in utero. Although the lambs retained in utero continue to grow beyond the normal gestation period, target endocrine organs in the fetus are hypoplastic, and the adrenal cortex does not differentiate completely into the three distinctive zones that secrete corticosteroid hormones.

The following concepts have emerged from the study of prolonged gestation in cattle and sheep:

1. Fetal hormones are necessary for final growth and development of the fetus in certain animals.
2. Normal parturition at term in these species requires an intact fetal hypothalamic-pituitary-adrenocortical axis working in concert with trophoblasts of the placenta.

Although the presence or absence of functional adenohypophyseal tissue determines whether the fetus continues to grow in utero, the pathogenesis of prolonged gestation is similar in these two examples. The subnormal development of the fetal adrenal cortex in calves and lambs results in an inadequate secretion of cortisol and a failure to induce 17α-hydroxylase in the placenta, which converts precursor molecules, such as progesterone, to estrogen. Thus the dam's circulating progesterone is maintained near mid-gestational concentrations, and the notable increase in estrogens that normally occurs at term resulting in parturition is absent. The estrogen surge, when it occurs, stimulates prostaglandin synthesis in the uterus, which results in smooth muscle contractions and biochemical changes in collagen along the birth canal that normally permit delivery of the fetus.

CONGENITAL DYSHORMONOGENETIC GOITER

See the section on Disorders of the Thyroid Gland, Disorders of Domestic Animals for a discussion of hypothyroidism.

THYROID C-CELL (ULTIMOBRANCHIAL) NEOPLASMS

See the section on Disorders of the Thyroid Gland, Disorders of Domestic Animals for a discussion of epithelial neoplasms of the thyroid gland.

PARTURIENT HYPOCALCEMIA

See the section on Disorders of the Parathyroid Gland, Disorders of Domestic Animals for a discussion of hyperparathyroidism.

DISORDERS OF DOGS

PITUITARY CYSTS AND PITUITARY DWARFISM

Pituitary dwarfism in dogs is usually the result of a failure of the oropharyngeal ectoderm of Rathke's pouch to differentiate into trophic hormone–secreting cells of the pars distalis. This results in a progressively enlarging, multiloculated cyst and an absence of the adenohypophysis (Fig. 12-57). Other cysts originating in the craniopharyngeal duct or the pharyngeal hypophysis can also become large enough to induce clinical signs.

Juvenile panhypopituitarism occurs most frequently in German shepherd dogs, but it has been reported in Spitz, toy pinscher, and Karelian bear dogs. The dwarf pups appear normal from birth to about 2 months of age. Subsequently, the slower growth, retention of puppy hair coat, and lack of primary guard hairs gradually become evident (Fig. 12-58). A bilaterally symmetric alopecia develops gradually and often progresses to complete alopecia except for the head and tufts of hair on the legs. There is progressive hyperpigmentation of the skin until the skin is uniformly brownish-black over most of the body. Adult German shepherd dogs with panhypopituitarism vary in size from as small as 2 kg to nearly half normal size, depending on whether the failure of formation of the adenohypophysis is partial or complete.

The mode of inheritance is simple autosomal recessive. The activity of somatomedin, also known as *insulin-like growth factor* (a non–species-specific, cartilage growth-promoting peptide whose production in the liver and plasma activity is controlled by somatotropin) is low in dwarf dogs. Intermediate somatomedin activity is present in phenotypically normal ancestors suspected to be heterozygous carriers. Assays for somatomedin provide a useful indirect measurement of circulating growth hormone activity in dogs with suspected pituitary dwarfism if canine growth hormone assays are not available.

CRANIOPHARYNGIOMA

See the section on Disorders of the Adenohypophysis, Disorders of Domestic Animals for a discussion of hypopituitarism and neoplasms of the adenohypophysis.

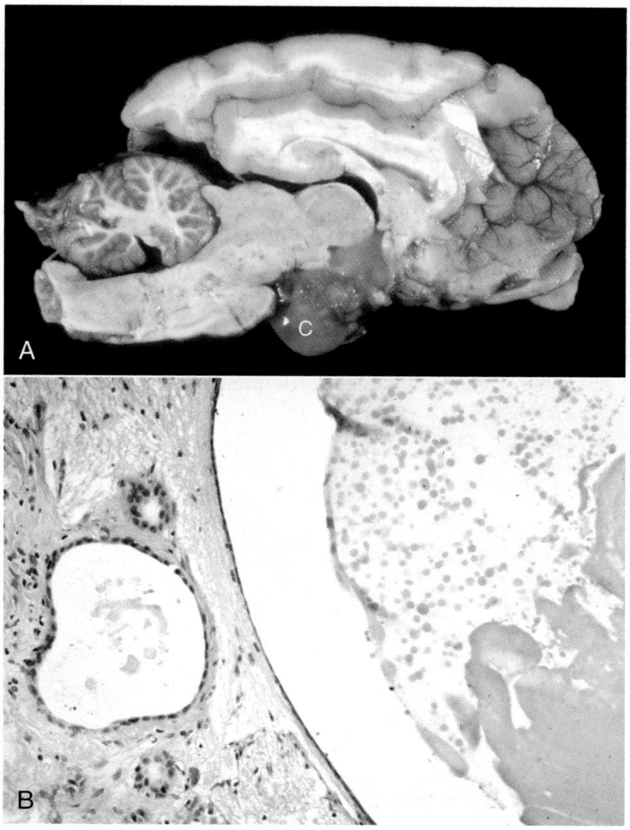

Fig. 12-57 Cystic Rathke's pouch, brain, sagittal section, dog.
A, A large, multiloculated cyst *(C)* is present on the ventral aspect of this brain where the adenohypophysis would normally be located. **B,** High magnification: the cyst is shown in the right half of the figure; the left half shows poorly organized and differentiated adenohypophysis. H&E stain. (Courtesy Dr. J.F. Zachary, College of Veterinary Medicine, University of Illinois.)

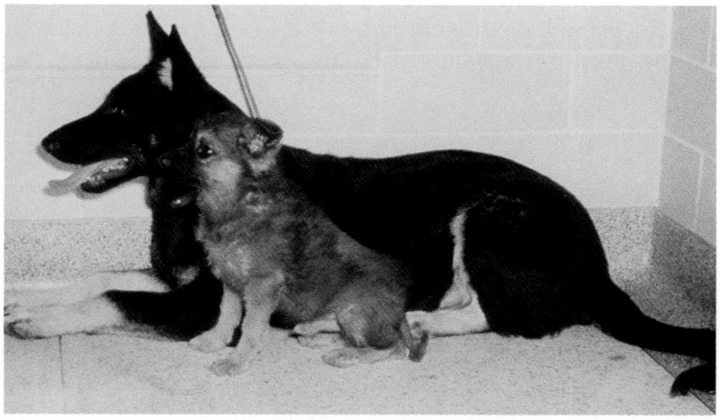

Fig. 12-58 Panhypopituitarism ("pituitary dwarfism"), 5-month-old German shepherd and littermate.
The unaffected littermate weighed 27.3 kg, whereas the dwarf puppy weighed only 4 kg. The pituitary dwarf has retained its puppy hair coat. (From Alexander JE: *Can Vet J* 3:83, 1962.)

PARS INTERMEDIA ADENOMAS

See the section on Disorders of the Adenohypophysis, Disorders of Domestic Animals for a discussion of hyperpituitarism and neoplasms of the adenohypophysis.

ACTH-SECRETING (CORTICOTROPH) ADENOMAS

See the section on Disorders of the Adenohypophysis, Disorders of Domestic Animals for a discussion of hyperpituitarism and neoplasms of the adenohypophysis.

PITUITARY APOPLEXY

Pituitary apoplexy is acute infarction or hemorrhage within a pituitary neoplasm or nonneoplastic pituitary gland. It has been reported in 5 dogs ranging in age from 4 to 12 years with no breed predisposition. Corticotroph adenomas of the pars distalis were present in 4/5 dogs. Although the exact pathogenesis of the hemorrhage and necrosis, particularly in nonneoplastic glands, has yet to be elucidated, they are hypothesized to be secondary to alterations in blood supply.

IDIOPATHIC ADRENOCORTICAL ATROPHY

Bilateral idiopathic adrenal cortical atrophy is an entity in young adult dogs that results in hypoadrenocorticism. The adrenal cortex is reduced to one-tenth or less of its normal thickness because of a marked reduction of all layers of the cortex. It consists primarily of the adrenal capsule (Fig. 12-59). Thus the adrenal medulla becomes relatively more prominent and along with the capsule, makes up the bulk of the remaining adrenal gland. The precise pathogenesis of idiopathic adrenal cortical atrophy is unknown, but the lesion is most likely immune-mediated. Early in the disease, multiple foci of lymphocytes and plasma cells are interspersed between the adrenal sinusoids and adrenal cortical cells. The capsule is thickened by condensation from the collapse of the adrenal cortex and fibroblastic proliferation. Pituitary gland lesions have not been observed in dogs with idiopathic adrenal cortical atrophy involving all three zones of the adrenal cortex, including the zona glomerulosa, which is not under ACTH control. By comparison, atrophy of the adrenal cortex caused by a destructive pituitary gland lesion that decreases ACTH secretion is characterized by severe atrophy only of the two inner cortical zones (zonae fasciculata and reticularis). The zona glomerulosa remains intact (see Fig. 12-16), and thus these animals do not have electrolyte abnormalities because the secretion of aldosterone remains within normal limits.

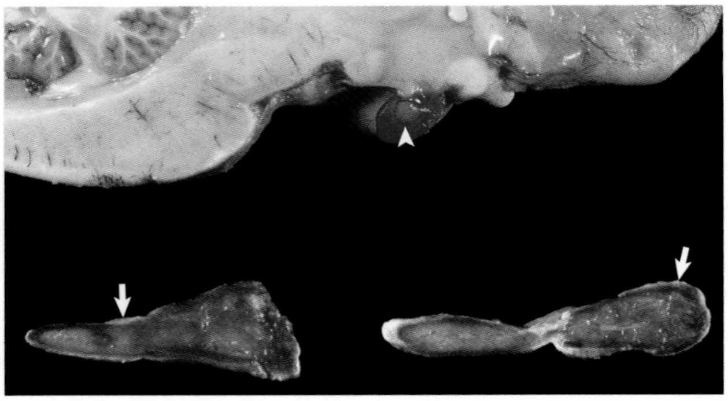

Fig. 12-59 Adrenal cortical atrophy, brainstem and pituitary gland, left and right adrenal glands, dog.

Note the marked bilateral atrophy of the cortices of the adrenal glands *(arrows)*. Atrophy of all three cortical layers is characteristic of hypoadrenocorticism. The pituitary gland *(arrowhead)* is grossly normal but had microscopic evidence of corticotroph hyperplasia. (Courtesy Dr. C. Capen, College of Veterinary Medicine, The Ohio State University.)

HYPOTHYROIDISM

See the section on Disorders of the Thyroid Gland, Disorders of Domestic Animals for a discussion of hypothyroidism.

RENAL HYPERPARATHYROIDISM

See the section of Disorders of the Parathyroid Gland, Disorders of Domestic Animals for a discussion on hyperparathyroidism.

APOCRINE GLAND ADENOCARCINOMA

A syndrome of HHM in aged, primarily female dogs with adenocarcinomas derived from apocrine glands of the anal sac has been characterized. Although a large case series of cats in the United Kingdom with apocrine gland adenocarcinoma was recently published, serum calcium was only measured in 5/64 cats with 1/5 having a marginal elevation and no clinical signs attributed to hypercalcemia. Dogs have persistent hypercalcemia (mean 16.2 mg/dL) and often mild hypophosphatemia, both of which return to normal after surgical excision of the neoplasm. The hypercalcemia persists after removal of the parathyroid glands, suggesting that the humoral factor produced by neoplastic cells does not stimulate an increased secretion of PTH. Increased circulating concentrations of PTHrP have been observed in hypercalcemic dogs with anal sac apocrine gland adenocarcinomas. The neoplasms are malignant, and most have metastasized to regional lumbar aortic lymph nodes at the time of initial presentation. Clinical signs include generalized muscular weakness, anorexia, vomiting, bradycardia, depression, polyuria, and polydipsia. These signs are primarily the result of severe hypercalcemia.

Apocrine gland adenocarcinomas develop as firm, usually unilateral masses, ventrolateral to the anus, and close to the anal sac but not attached to the overlying skin (Fig. 12-60). The neoplasm arises in the wall of the anal sac and projects as a variably-sized mass into the lumen (Fig. 12-61).

Histologically, apocrine gland adenocarcinomas are distinct from the more common perianal (circumanal) gland tumor, which arises in hepatoid glands. The majority of apocrine gland neoplasms histologically contain glandular and solid areas. Neoplastic cells form acini and papillary tufts that project into the acinar lumens Fig. 12-62; Web Fig. 12-14). The solid pattern is characterized by sheets, microlobules, and packets separated by a thin fibrovascular stroma. Pseudorosettes are common in solid areas adjacent to small blood vessels.

DIABETES MELLITUS

See the section on Disorders of Pancreatic Islet Cells, Disorders of Domestic Animals for a discussion of hypofunction of pancreatic islet cells.

DISORDERS OF CATS

ADRENOCORTICOTROPIC HORMONE-SECRETING (CORTICOTROPH) ADENOMAS

See the section on Disorders of the Adenohypophysis for a discussion of hyperpituitarism and neoplasms of the adenohypophysis.

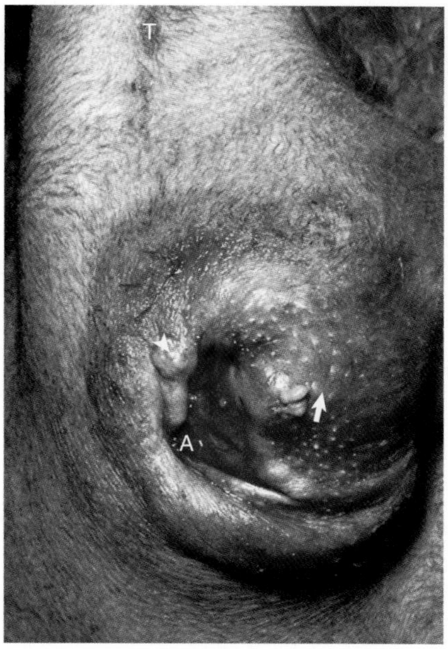

Fig. 12-60 Adenocarcinoma, apocrine glands of right anal sac, anus, dog.
The right perianal region is distended by an adenocarcinoma *(arrow)*, which has compressed the right side of the anus. It also projects as two nodules *(arrowhead)* on the dorsolateral margin of the anus. *T,* Tail; *A,* anus. (Courtesy Dr. C. Capen, College of Veterinary Medicine, The Ohio State University.)

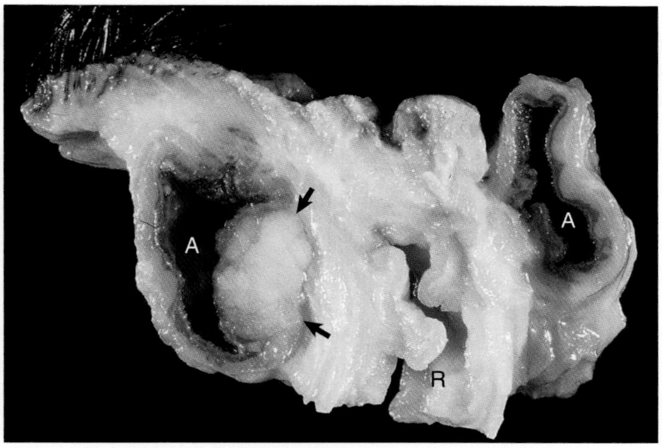

Fig. 12-61 Adenocarcinoma, apocrine glands, anal sac, dorsal plane, formalin-fixed specimen, dog.
A 1-cm diameter nodule *(arrows)* derived from apocrine glands of the wall of the right anal sac (glands of the perianal sinus) protrudes into the lumen of the right anal sac. Anal sacs *(A)* are present on both sides of the rectum *(R)*. (From Meuten DJ, Cooper BJ, Capen CC, et al: *Vet Pathol* 18:454-471, 1981.)

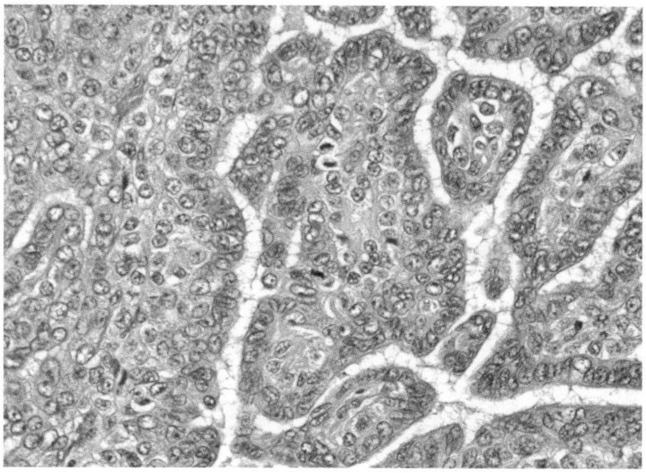

Fig. 12-62 Adenocarcinoma, apocrine glands, anal sac, dog.
Neoplastic cells form poorly arranged glands with papillary projections. There is moderate variation in cellular and nuclear size and shape as well as several mitoses, all characteristic of anaplasia. H&E. (Courtesy Dr. J.F. Zachary, College of Veterinary Medicine, University of Illinois.)

HYPERALDOSTERONISM

See the section on Disorders of the Adrenal Cortex, Disorders of Domestic Animals for a discussion of hyperaldosteronism.

HYPOTHYROIDISM

See the section on Disorders of the Thyroid Gland, Disorders of Domestic Animals for a discussion of hypothyroidism.

HYPERTHYROIDISM

See the section on Disorders of the Thyroid Gland, Disorders of Domestic Animals for a discussion of hyperthyroidism.

DIABETES MELLITUS

See the section on Disorders of Pancreatic Islet Cells, Disorders of Domestic Animals for a discussion of hypofunction of pancreatic islet cells.

SUGGESTED READINGS

Suggested Readings are available at evolve.elsevier.com/Zachary/McGavin/.

CHAPTER 13

Bone Marrow, Blood Cells, and the Lymphatic System*

Michael M. Fry[†] *and M. Donald McGavin*[‡]

BONE MARROW AND BLOOD CELLS

STRUCTURE AND FUNCTION

In adults, the bone marrow is the primary site of blood cell production, or *hematopoiesis,* which is a term is derived from *haima* (Gr., blood) and *poiein* (Gr., to make). Hematopoiesis may also occur elsewhere (extramedullary hematopoiesis), most commonly in the spleen. Hematopoiesis is also known as *hemopoiesis.*

Hematopoiesis is first seen as blood islands in the embryonic yolk sac. During gestation, the main site of hematopoiesis shifts from the yolk sac to the liver and spleen and eventually to the bone marrow. The composition of the marrow changes with age. The general pattern is that hematopoietic tissue (red marrow) regresses and is replaced with nonhematopoietic tissue, mainly fat (yellow marrow). Thus, in newborns and very young animals, the bone marrow consists largely of hematopoietically active tissue, with relatively little fat, whereas in geriatric individuals the marrow consists largely of fat. In adults, hematopoiesis occurs primarily in the pelvis, sternum, ribs, vertebrae, and the proximal ends of humeri and femora. Even within these areas of active hematopoiesis, fat may constitute a significant proportion of the marrow volume.

The marrow cavity is interlaced with venous sinuses composed of a luminal layer of specialized endothelial cells and an abluminal layer of specialized fibroblasts known as *adventitial reticular cells* (Figs. 13-1 and 13-2). Hematopoiesis takes place between these venous sinuses in the so-called hematopoietic spaces. Sinusoidal endothelial cells function as a barrier and regulate traffic of chemicals and particles between the intravascular and extravascular spaces. Reticular cells extend cytoplasmic processes into the hematopoietic spaces, forming a scaffold that supports the hematopoietic cells. Osteoblasts, osteoclasts, and elongated flat cells line the endosteum. Stromal cells, presumably of fibroblast origin, provide structural support and produce extracellular matrix components such as proteoglycans, glycosaminoglycans, collagen, fibronectin, and others. Adipocytes, macrophages, lymphocytes, and plasma cells are also components of the hematopoietic microenvironment.

Hematopoietic cells, supporting connective tissue cells, extracellular matrix components, and soluble factors form the bone marrow hematopoietic microenvironment. There is complex functional interplay among these components. Behavior of hematopoietic cells is influenced by direct cell-to-cell and cell-matrix interactions and by soluble mediators, such as cytokines and hormones, that interact with cells and with matrix proteins. Cells localize to specific niches within the hematopoietic microenvironment via adhesion molecules, such as integrins, immunoglobulins (Igs), lectins, and other receptors, that recognize ligands on other cells or matrix components. Cells also express receptors for soluble molecules such as chemokines (chemoattractant cytokines) and hormones that influence cell trafficking and metabolism.

The following basic concepts provide a framework for understanding the mechanisms of injury and diseases presented later in the chapter.

- Hematopoietic tissue is highly proliferative. Billions of cells per kilogram of body weight are produced each day.
- Pluripotent hematopoietic stem cells are a self-renewing population, giving rise to cells with committed differentiation programs, and are common ancestors of all blood cells. The process of hematopoietic differentiation is shown in Fig. 13-3.
- Hematopoietic cells undergo sequential divisions as they develop, so there are progressively higher numbers of cells as they mature. Cells also continue to mature after they have stopped dividing. Conceptually, it is helpful to consider cells in the bone marrow as belonging to mitotic and postmitotic compartments. Examples of developing hematopoietic cells are shown in Fig. 13-4.

*Dr. G.P. Searcy, Western College of Veterinary Medicine, University of Saskatchewan contributed to this chapter in the third edition.
[†]Contributor of the section on the bone marrow and blood cells.
[‡]Contributor of the section on the lymphatic system.

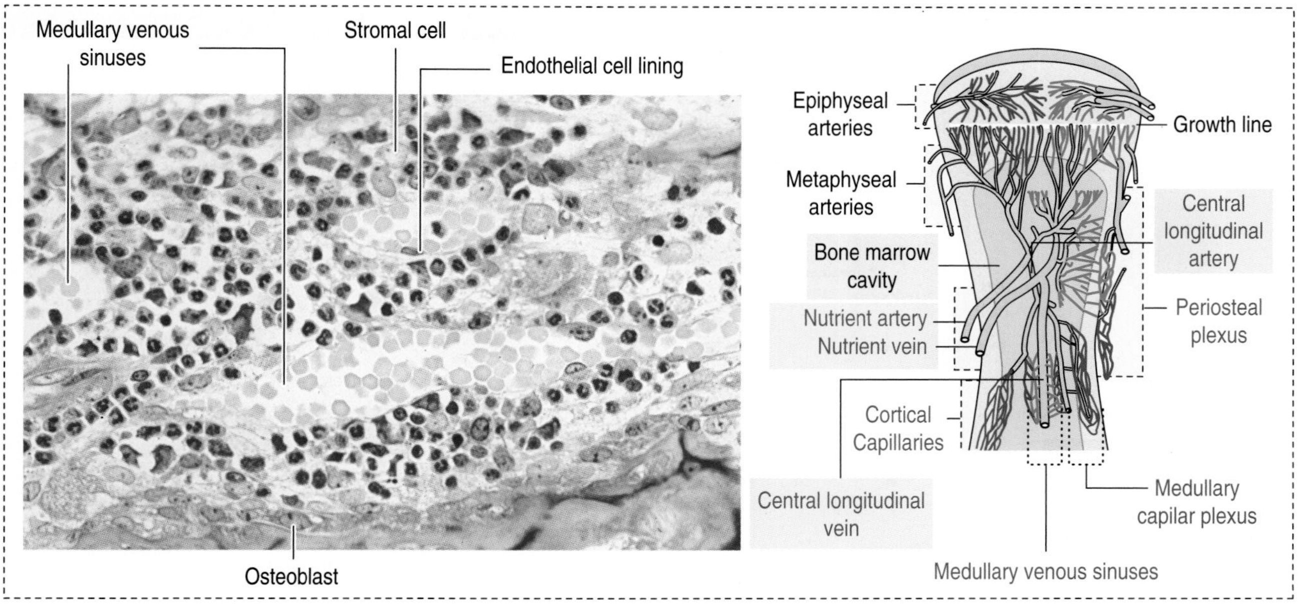

Fig. 13-1 Bone marrow: Structure and vascularization.
(From Kierszenbaum AL: *Histology and cell biology: an introduction to pathology*, ed 28, St Louis, 2007, Mosby.)

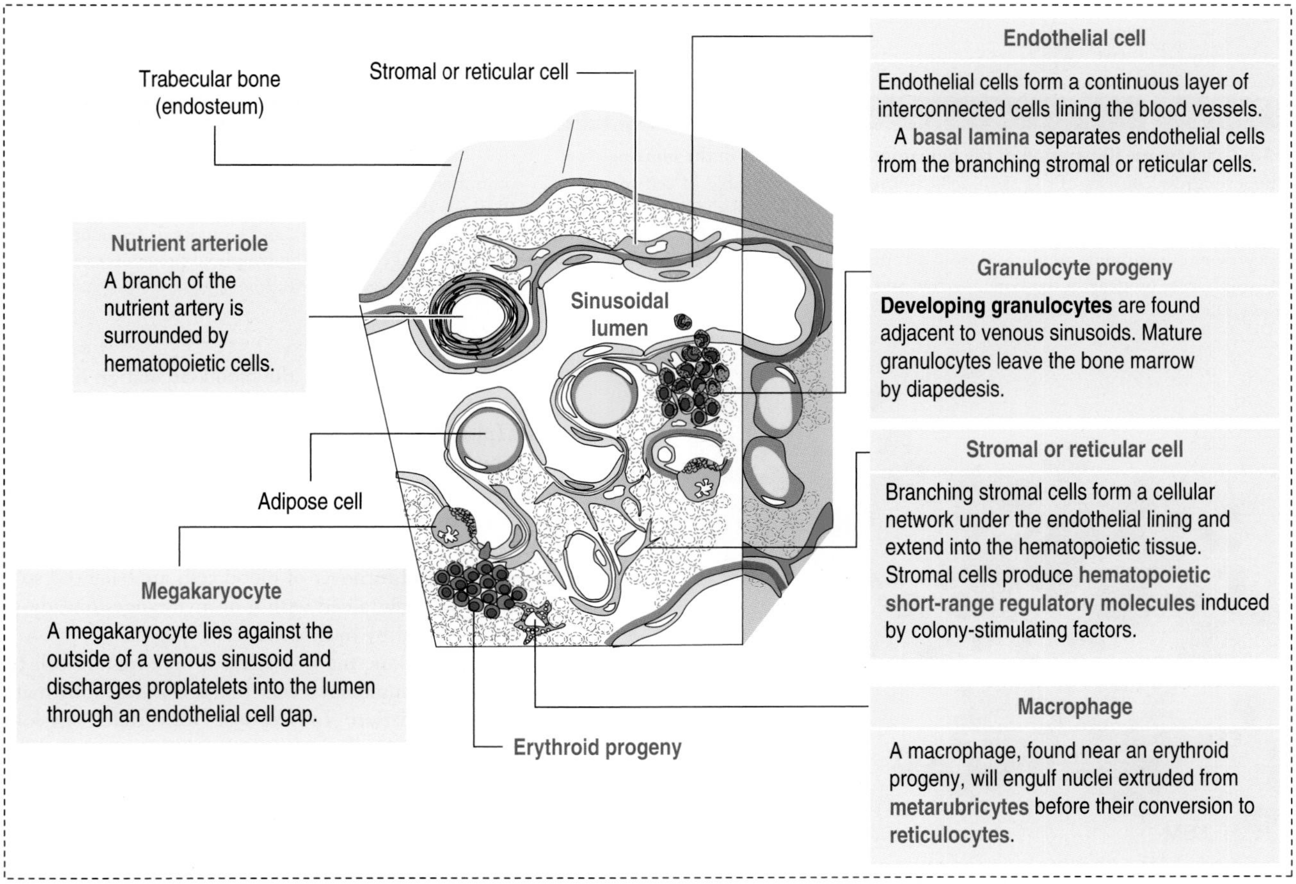

Fig. 13-2 Bone marrow: Structure.
(Adapted from Kierszenbaum AL: *Histology and cell biology: an introduction to pathology*, ed 2, St Louis, 2007, Mosby.)

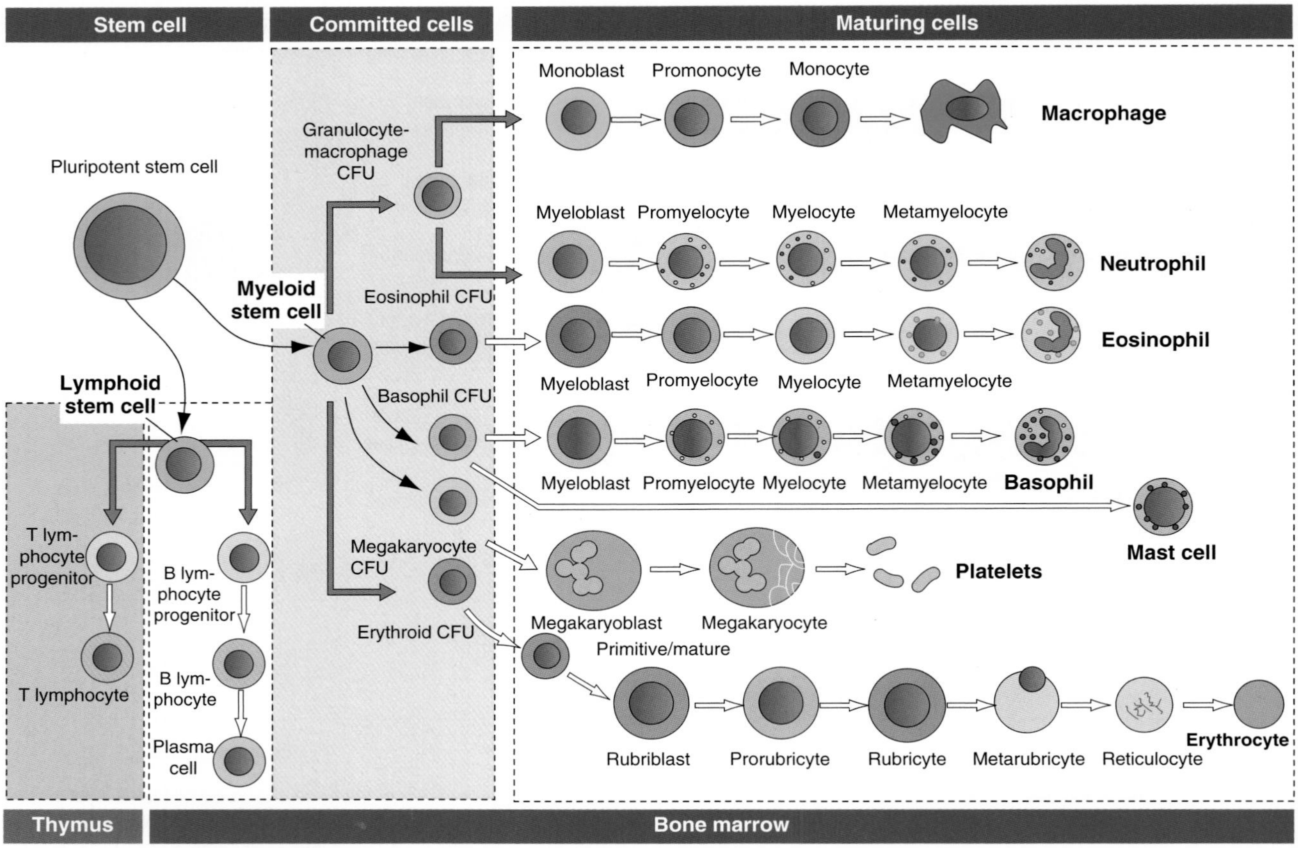

Fig. 13-3 Schematic illustration of the hematopoietic hierarchy in the bone marrow.
The bone marrow consists of (1) stem cells, pluripotent cells capable of self-renewal; (2) committed progenitor cells (myeloid and lymphoid progenitor cells); and (3) maturing cells. Maturing cells develop from cells called colony-forming units (CFUs). The myeloid stem cell gives rise to CFUs responsible for the regeneration of red blood cells (erythroid CFUs), platelets (megakaryocyte CFUs), basophils (basophil CFUs), and eosinophils (eosinophil CFUs). Monocytes and neutrophils are derived from a common committed progenitor cell (granulocyte-macrophage CFU). The lymphoid progenitor cell generates the B lymphocyte progeny in the bone marrow and T lymphocyte progeny in the thymus. (Adapted from Kierszenbaum AL: *Histology and cell biology: an introduction to pathology,* St Louis, 2002, Mosby.)

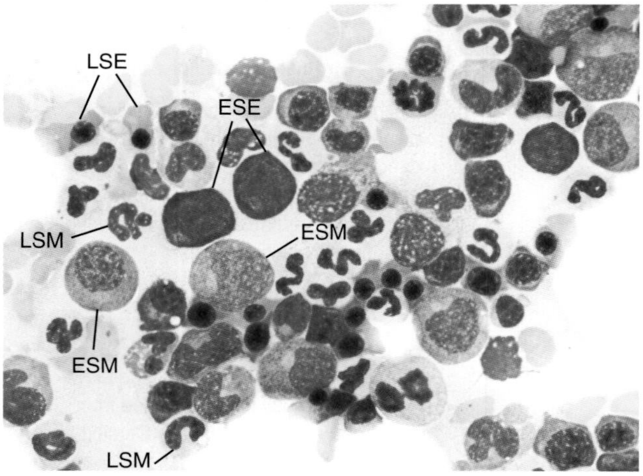

Fig. 13-4 Normal hematopoiesis, canine bone marrow aspirate.
Wright's stain. *ESE,* Early stage erythroid; *ESM,* early stage myeloid; *LSE,* late stage erythroid; *LSM,* late stage myeloid. (Courtesy Dr. M.M. Fry, College of Veterinary Medicine, University of Tennessee.)

- Mature cells released into the blood circulation have different normal lifespans, varying from hours (neutrophils), to days (platelets), to months (erythrocytes), and to years (some lymphocytes).
- The hematopoietic system is under exquisite local and systemic control and responds rapidly and predictably to various stimuli.
- Production and turnover of blood cells are balanced so that numbers are maintained within normal ranges (steady-state kinetics) in healthy individuals.
- Normally the bone marrow releases only mature cell types (and very low numbers of cells that are almost fully mature) into the circulation. In response to certain physiologic or pathologic stimuli, however, the bone marrow releases immature cells that are further back in the supply "pipeline."

REGULATION OF HEMATOPOIESIS

Control of hematopoiesis is complex, with many redundancies, feedback mechanisms, and pathways that overlap with other physiologic and pathologic processes. Many cytokines influence cells of different lineages and stages of differentiation. The aim of this section is not to explain these regulatory pathways in detail but rather to provide a broad overview and thus a basic framework for understanding mechanisms of disease involving the hematopoietic system.

ERYTHROPOIESIS

Erythropoiesis—from *erythros* (Gr., red)—refers to the production of red blood cells (RBCs), or erythrocytes, whose main function is gas (oxygen [O_2] and carbon dioxide [CO_2]) exchange. The dominant regulator of erythropoiesis is a glycoprotein aptly named erythropoietin (Epo). Epo acts on early erythroid progenitor cells in concert with other cytokines, including interleukins (IL-3, IL-4, and IL-9), granulocyte-macrophage colony-stimulating factor (GM-CSF), and insulin-like growth factor. Epo is synthesized primarily in the kidney, and exerts its effects by promoting proliferation and inhibiting apoptosis of developing erythroid cells that express Epo receptors. The stimulus for increased Epo production is hypoxia. Because erythrocytes are packed with hemoglobin, of which iron is an essential component, erythropoiesis requires adequate availability of iron. Physiologic systems exist to conserve and recycle iron, as discussed further later.

The earliest erythroid precursor identifiable by routine light microscopy is the rubriblast, which undergoes maturational division to produce 8 to 32 progeny cells. Late-stage erythroid precursors known as *metarubricytes* extrude their nuclei and become *reticulocytes*, which are the cells at the differentiation stage immediately preceding the mature erythrocyte. Reticulocytes start maturing in the bone marrow and finish maturing in the peripheral blood circulation and the spleen. (Horses are an exception in that they do not release reticulocytes into circulation, even in situations of increased demand.) The normal transit time from rubriblast to mature erythrocyte is approximately 1 week. Unlike mature erythrocytes, which lack organelles, reticulocytes still contain ribosomes and mitochondria, mainly to support completion of hemoglobin synthesis. These remaining organelles impart a bluish-purple cast (polychromasia) to reticulocytes on routine blood smear examination and when stained with dye, such as new methylene blue, precipitate to form irregular aggregates of dark-staining material (Fig. 13-5). Cats also have a more mature form of reticulocyte in circulation, the punctate reticulocyte, which has a much finer staining pattern when stained with new methylene blue and does not appear bluish-purple (polychromatophilic) on routine blood smear examination (see the section Anemia).

Mature erythrocytes circulate for a long time compared with other blood cells. The erythrocyte mean lifespan varies between species: approximately 150 days in horses and cattle, 100 days in dogs, and 70 days in cats. Erythrocytes therefore must be highly resilient cells capable of enduring continual mechanical and biochemical stresses. In most mammals, erythrocytes have a biconcave disk shape, sometimes called the *discocyte*. Species in which the discocyte is not the norm include goats (flat, irregularly shaped RBCs), camelids (oval RBCs), and some cervids (sickle-shaped RBCs). In dogs, some breeds (Akitas and Shibas) have smaller erythrocytes than others; erythrocytes in these breeds also have a high concentration of potassium, unlike erythrocytes in other dogs.

One of the key properties of erythrocytes is deformability; they change shape as they move through the microvasculature. This deformability is a function of interactions between the cell membrane, the cytoskeleton, and intracellular contents. Mature mammalian erythrocytes lack nuclei and organelles and are thus incapable of transcription, translation, and oxidative metabolism. However, they do require energy for various functions, including maintenance of shape and deformability, active transport, and prevention of oxidative damage, and they generate this energy entirely through glycolysis (also known as the *Embden-Meyerhof pathway*). Erythrocyte antioxidant biochemical pathways are discussed in more detail in the section on Defense Mechanisms.

The concentration of circulating erythrocytes typically decreases postnatally and remains below normal adult levels during the period of rapid body growth. The age at which erythrocyte numbers begin to increase and the age at which adult levels are reached vary among species. In dogs, adult values are usually reached between 4 and 6 months of age; in horses, this occurs at approximately 1 year of age. In most species, erythrocytes are larger at birth, and their mean volume decreases as fetal erythrocytes are replaced.

GRANULOPOIESIS AND MONOCYTOPOIESIS (MYELOPOIESIS)

Granulocytes (neutrophils, eosinophils, and basophils) and monocytes have key immunologic functions, including phagocytosis and microbicidal activity (neutrophils and monocyte-derived macrophages); parasiticidal activity and participation in allergic reactions (eosinophils and basophils); antigen processing and presentation; and cytokine production (macrophages). Inflammatory mediators, such as ILs and tumor necrosis factor α (TNF-α), stimulate fibroblasts, macrophages, and endothelial cells to produce cytokines, such as granulocyte colony-stimulating factor (G-CSF) and GM-CSF, that increase granulopoiesis and monocytopoiesis.

Granulocytic and monocytic cells are sometimes referred to collectively as *myeloid cells*. (NOTE: This terminology can be confusing because "myeloid" also has other meanings. In the most general sense, it refers to the bone marrow. In the context of hematology,

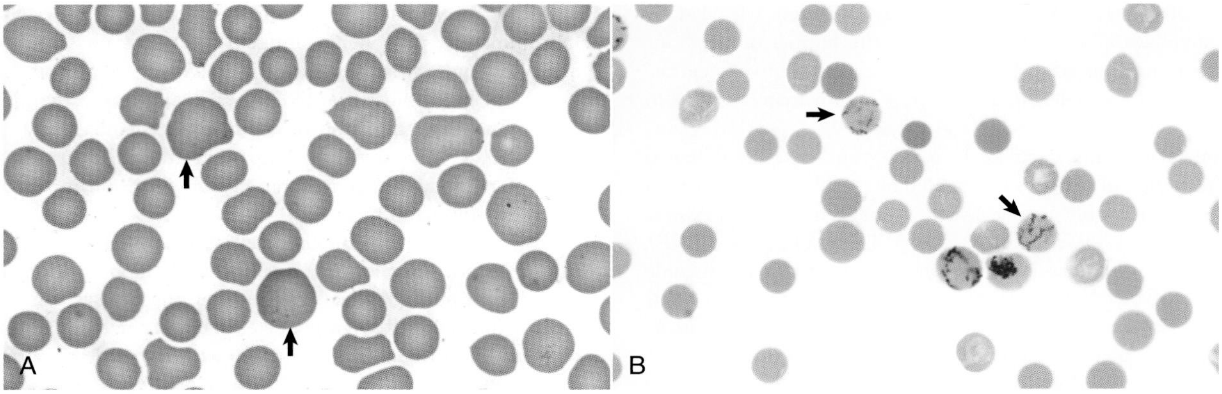

Fig. 13-5 Reticulocytosis, canine blood smears.
A, Reticulocytes *(arrows)* appear polychromatophilic with routine staining. Wright's stain. **B,** Reticulocytes. Precipitated aggregates of RNA are stained blue *(arrows)* with new methylene blue. (Courtesy Dr. M.M. Fry, College of Veterinary Medicine, University of Tennessee.)

"myeloid" is also sometimes used to mean a hematopoietic cell of nonlymphoid origin, a distinction reiterated in the classification of leukemias as discussed later in this chapter. In neuroanatomy, the prefixes "myelo-" or "myel-" can refer to the spinal cord or myelin.) The earliest granulocytic or monocytic precursor identifiable by routine light microscopy is the myeloblast, which undergoes maturational division to produce 16 to 32 progeny cells. The normal transit time from myeloblast to mature neutrophil is approximately 5 days. In addition, a reserve of fully mature neutrophils is maintained in the bone marrow. The size of this so-called storage pool is species-dependent. (Species differences and clinical significance of the storage pool are discussed in more detail in later sections.)

The concentration of granulocytes measured in the blood depends on the rate of production and release from the bone marrow, the proportions of cells circulating freely within the vasculature versus those transiently attached to the endothelial surface (marginated), and the rate of migration from the vasculature into tissues. Neutrophils normally are the predominant leukocyte type in blood of most domestic species. Neutrophils are only in circulation for a short time (less than 12 hours).

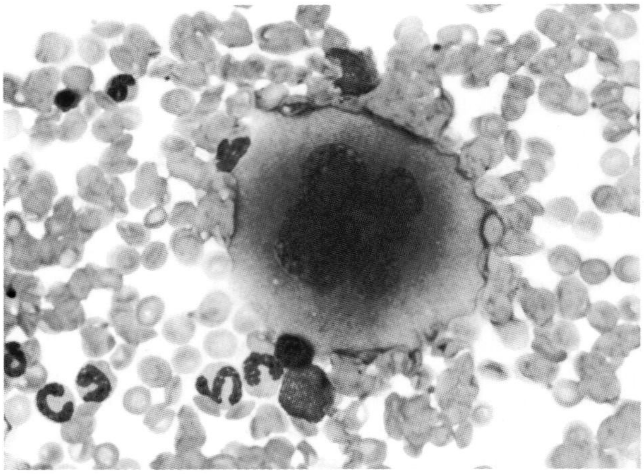

Fig. 13-6 Megakaryocyte, canine bone marrow aspirate. Note the cell's very large size, lobulated nucleus, and abundant granular cytoplasm. Wright's stain. (Courtesy Dr. M.M. Fry, College of Veterinary Medicine, University of Tennessee.)

THROMBOPOIESIS

Thrombopoiesis—from *thrombos* (Gr., clot)—refers to the production of platelets, which have a central role in primary hemostasis and also participate in coagulation and inflammatory pathways. Thrombopoietin (Tpo), synthesized primarily in the liver, is the dominant regulator of thrombopoiesis. Unlike Epo, which is upregulated in response to hypoxia, Tpo is produced at a relatively constant rate (constitutively). The mechanism regulating production is therefore different. Platelets and their precursors express the Tpo receptor, which binds Tpo in the plasma. When the platelet mass is decreased, less Tpo is bound to platelet receptors, and the increased concentration of Tpo free in the plasma stimulates thrombopoiesis.

Thrombopoiesis differs fundamentally from other forms of hematopoiesis. Platelets (sometimes called *thrombocytes*) are anucleate cells formed not by maturational division but by shedding of membrane-bound cytoplasmic fragments from precursor cells called *megakaryocytes.* (NOTE: Birds and reptiles produce thrombocytes in the manner of other blood cells and their thrombocytes and erythrocytes are nucleated.) As the name suggests, megakaryocytes are very large cells, much larger than any other hematopoietic cells (Fig. 13-6). Megakaryocytes arise from a progenitor cell and undergo endomitosis to become polyploid (usually 8N-32N). As they mature, megakaryocytes increase in size and their cytoplasm becomes more abundant. They change in staining pattern (Wright's stain of aspirates) from intensely basophilic to eosinophilic, and their nuclei change from round to highly lobulated. Megakaryocytes extend cytoplasmic processes into the lumina of the bone marrow venous sinusoids, where they shed platelets into circulation. The lifespan of a platelet in circulation is approximately 6 days in the dog.

Platelets normally circulate in a quiescent state, as flattened disks. Activation of platelets is triggered by soluble agonists, such as thrombin, or insoluble agonists, such as collagen. Platelets express surface receptors for fibrinogen, von Willebrand factor (vWF), collagen, and other ligands. Other key features of platelets include a network of membrane invaginations known as the *open canalicular system* (not present in cattle), which facilitates the expansion of surface area and release of granule contents in response to activation; specialized endoplasmic reticulum known as the *dense tubular system* that acts as a reservoir for calcium; and cytoskeletal components involved in mediating shape change, release of granule contents, receptor interactions, and clot retraction. When activated, platelets change to more spherical forms with pseudopodia and participate in a number of related processes at sites of vascular damage:

- Adhesion to exposed subendothelial collagen
- Secretion of bioactive granule contents (including calcium, adenosine diphosphate [ADP], fibrinogen, vWF, histamine, serotonin, and others)
- Aggregation with other platelets
- Eventual fusion with other platelets to form a platelet plug

Phospholipids (especially phosphatidylserine) expressed on the surface of activated platelets also help to localize coagulation (formation of an insoluble fibrin clot) to sites of vascular damage.

LYMPHOPOIESIS

Lymphopoiesis refers to the production of new lymphocytes. T lymphocytes and B lymphocytes are the key effectors of cell-mediated and humoral immunity, respectively. Lymphopoiesis is discussed in more detail in Chapter 5, but a brief overview is provided here. T lymphocytes originate in the bone marrow and migrate to the thymus, where they undergo differentiation, selection, and maturation processes before migrating to the peripheral lymphoid tissue as effector cells. B lymphocyte development occurs in two phases, first in an antigen-independent phase in the bone marrow and ileal Peyer's patches (the site of B lymphocyte development in ruminants), then in an antigen-dependent phase in peripheral lymphoid tissues (such as spleen, lymph nodes, and mucosa-associated lymphoid tissue [MALT]). Trafficking of lymphocytes occurs under the direction of chemokine (chemoattractant cytokine) signals. Once they have migrated to the peripheral lymphoid tissue, lymphocytes may undergo clonal expansion in response to antigenic stimulation.

Unlike other hematopoietic cells, which circulate only in the blood vessels, lymphocytes travel in both blood and lymphatic vessels, continually recirculating between the two systems. In most species, the majority of lymphocytes in blood circulation are T lymphocytes. According to conventional wisdom, cattle normally have higher numbers of lymphocytes than neutrophils in circulation. However, recent work suggests that is no longer the case, at least in mid-lactation Holstein cows, most likely because of changes in genetics and husbandry.

HEMOSTASIS (COAGULATION AND PLATELET FUNCTION)

Hemostasis—from *haima* (Gr., blood) and *stasis* (Gr., "a standing still")—refers to the cessation of bleeding. The main components responsible for hemostasis are platelets, blood vessels, and the coagulation system. Bleeding disorders may result if any of these systems are perturbed. Although coagulation factors are mainly synthesized in the liver, they are included in this chapter because of their inextricable link with the hematopoietic system.

Physiologic hemostasis involves coordinated processes: formation of a platelet plug at the site of vascular damage (primary hemostasis), development of a cross-linked network of insoluble fibrin that provides further clot stability (secondary hemostasis) and retraction and enzymatic degradation of the clot (tertiary hemostasis). The main components of these processes are summarized in Chapter 2 and Figs. 2-12 through 2-17. Signalment, history, and clinical signs are important in evaluating any patient with a suspected bleeding tendency, but laboratory testing is required to definitively identify specific defects in hemostasis. Routine assays for assessing hemostasis are summarized in Web Appendix 13-1.

Blood Vessels

Blood vessels have numerous functions in hemostasis. Endothelial cells produce and metabolize many molecules involved in promoting and regulating hemostasis (see Fig. 2-16). For example, they produce prothrombotic molecules, such as vWF and thromboxane A_2; antithrombotic molecules, such as prostacyclin (PGI_2), thrombomodulin, and nitric oxide; and fibrinolytic molecules, such as tissue plasminogen activator. When a blood vessel is damaged, a rapid, transient neuromechanical vasoconstriction occurs in response. Collagen underlying the damaged endothelium provides structural support for platelet adhesion and clot formation, and also acts as a key biochemical activator of platelets and the intrinsic pathway of the coagulation system (see next section).

Coagulation System

Stopping hemorrhage from a damaged blood vessel ultimately depends on the formation of a stable fibrin clot. This process depends on a number of plasma proteins, or clotting factors, that normally circulate in an inactive proenzyme state. These clotting factors, together with other molecules, including nonenzymatic proteins, calcium, and platelet phospholipids, are known collectively as the *coagulation system.* Activation of the coagulation system initiates a series of linked enzymatic reactions that result in the production of thrombin. Thrombin converts the soluble plasma protein fibrinogen to fibrin, which in turn is enzymatically cross-linked to form an insoluble clot. The coagulation system is conventionally considered to consist of three interrelated pathways for ease of understanding and interpretation of test results. These pathways—the intrinsic, extrinsic, and common pathways—are summarized in Fig. 2-13.

Anticoagulant and fibrinolytic pathways provide critical "checks and balances." These pathways are initiated simultaneously with activation of the coagulation system. Procoagulant and anticoagulant pathways are regulated at multiple levels and normally maintained in a balance that avoids hypercoagulable or hypocoagulable states. Some key regulators of hemostasis are listed in Web Box 13-1. Counterregulatory mechanisms are critical for the prevention of inappropriate or excessive clotting and the eventual dissolution of the clot (fibrinolysis) after it has formed. Fibrinolysis results from the action of plasmin on fibrin (see Figs. 2-14, 2-16, and 2-17). The inactive proenzyme plasminogen is converted to plasmin by several molecules, including tissue plasminogen activator, factor XII, and thrombin. Note that some of these molecules (e.g., factor XII and thrombin) have both procoagulant and anticoagulant effects. There are also regulators of fibrinolysis, including inhibitors of plasminogen and plasmin. Fibrinolysis results in production of fibrin degradation products (FDPs). D-dimer is a specific type of FDP that results from the degradation of insoluble cross-linked fibrin. Fibrinolytic products (FDPs and D-dimer) in the blood are often measured to detect inappropriate coagulation and are also of clinical importance because they can impair hemostasis by inhibiting fibrin polymerization and platelet function.

Platelets

The basics of platelet function are described in the previous section on Thrombopoiesis. Platelets normally circulate in a quiescent state, as flattened disks. Activation of platelets is triggered by soluble agonists, such as thrombin, or insoluble agonists, such as collagen. Platelets express surface receptors for fibrinogen, vWF, collagen, and other ligands. Other key features of platelets include a network of membrane invaginations known as the *open canalicular system* (not present in cattle), which facilitates the expansion of surface area and release of granule contents in response to activation; specialized endoplasmic reticulum known as the *dense tubular system* that acts as a reservoir for calcium; and cytoskeletal components involved in mediating shape change, release of granule contents, receptor interactions, and clot retraction. When activated, platelets change to more spherical forms with pseudopodia and participate in a number of related processes at sites of vascular damage:

- Adhesion to exposed subendothelial collagen
- Secretion of bioactive granule contents (including calcium, adenosine diphosphate [ADP], fibrinogen, vWF, histamine, serotonin, and others)
- Aggregation with other platelets
- Eventual fusion with other platelets (a process known as *viscous metamorphosis*) to form a platelet plug

Phospholipids (e.g., phosphatidylserine) expressed on the surface of activated platelets also help to localize the clot to sites of vascular damage.

PORTALS OF ENTRY

Invading cells or microorganism gain access to the bone marrow or blood circulation either hematogenously or by trauma. Trauma may be as obvious as a gaping wound or as subtle as the bite of an insect. Portals of entry for the bone marrow are summarized in Box 13-1.

DEFENSE MECHANISMS

The bone marrow is encased by a protective shell of cortical bone, and blood supply to the marrow provides access to systemic humoral and cellular defenses. Of course, leukocytes themselves function as an essential part of inflammation and immune function, as discussed briefly in the Granulopoiesis and Monocytopoiesis section and in greater detail in Chapters 3 and 5.

BOX 13-1 Portals of Entry into Bone Marrow

BONE MARROW
Hematogenously
Direct penetration (trauma)

Biochemical steps in the glycolytic pathway or linked to it generate antioxidant molecules that enable erythrocytes to withstand oxidative insults throughout their many days in circulation. In addition to producing energy in the form of adenosine triphosphate (ATP), glycolysis generates reduced nicotinamide adenine dinucleotide (NADH), which helps convert the oxidized, nonfunctional form of hemoglobin, known as *methemoglobin,* back to its active reduced state. Another antioxidant erythrocyte metabolic pathway, the pentose shunt or hexose monophosphate shunt pathway, generates reduced nicotinamide adenine dinucleotide phosphate (NADPH) to help maintain glutathione in the reduced state.

RESPONSES TO INJURY

The main mechanisms of disease in the bone marrow and blood cells are shown in Box 13-2, and are discussed in more detail here.

BONE MARROW

Bone marrow responses to injury include abnormal patterns of proliferation of normal hematopoietic cell types, proliferations of abnormal hematopoietic cell types (neoplastic or nonneoplastic), replacement of normal hematopoietic tissue by abnormal cells or fibrous tissue, necrosis, and inflammation. Each of these is discussed further; the relationship between altered hematopoiesis and concentrations of blood cells in circulation is discussed in more detail in the next section on Blood Cells.

The classic nomenclature for describing different types of abnormal cellular proliferations applies to the hematopoietic system, with some exceptions and modifications. Hyperplasia, an increase in cell number, may be an obviously appropriate response to a stimulus (e.g., erythroid hyperplasia in response to hypoxemia, or granulocytic hyperplasia in response to inflammatory stimuli). In other situations, hyperplasia is a secondary phenomenon for which the specific stimulus may not be clear—for example, a number of conditions (inflammation, neoplasia, iron deficiency, asplenia, and others) are associated with reactive thrombocytosis, in which an increased concentration of circulating platelets reflects megakaryocytic hyperplasia. Sometimes hyperplasia is idiopathic. For example, splenic nodular hyperplasia, which often includes a hematopoietic component, is frequently an incidental finding.

Hypertrophy, an increase in cell size, is not a conventional description for hematopoietic cells or for bone marrow as an organ. Abnormally large hematopoietic cells are considered evidence of dysplasia, or altered cell formation (alterations to shape or organization of cells are also evidence of dysplasia). Dysplasia of hematopoietic cells, indicating dyshematopoiesis, may be primary (idiopathic) or secondary to a number of conditions, including infection, nutritional imbalance, and toxicosis. Unfortunately, the terminology is sometimes confusing. For example, myelodysplastic syndromes are clonal hematopoietic stem cell disorders that are in fact neoplastic (see the section on Hematopoietic Neoplasia). Splenic hypertrophy is usually referred to as splenomegaly and may reflect processes other than hyperplasia or cellular hypertrophy (e.g., congestion). Similarly, lymph node enlargement is typically referred to as *lymphadenopathy* or *lymphadenomegaly* and may reflect lymphoid hyperplasia or other processes (e.g., neoplasia, inflammation, or edema).

Replacement of hematopoietic tissue in the bone marrow by abnormal tissue, usually fibrous tissue or malignant cells, is known as myelophthisis. The term *metaplasia,* describing the replacement of cells normally comprising a tissue with another well-differentiated cell type, is rarely used to describe hematopoietic tissues in veterinary medicine, although in humans, the terms *myeloid metaplasia* and *extramedullary hematopoiesis* are sometimes used interchangeably. Similarly, the term atrophy, which means a diminution in the size of a cell, tissue, organ, or part, is seldom used to describe bone marrow. Instead, a decrease in bone marrow hematopoietic tissue is typically referred to as *hypoplasia,* as discussed later in the section on cytopenias. The absence of bone marrow hematopoietic tissue of a particular lineage is typically referred to as *aplasia* or, if affecting all lineages, by the misleading term *aplastic anemia* (more aptly termed *aplastic pancytopenia*). An exception is "serous atrophy of fat," a condition associated with cachexia or starvation in which fat is catabolized and bone marrow reticular cells produce a mucoid ground substance (Web Fig. 13-1). However, neither hematopoietic cells nor fat is necessarily absent from the bone marrow in this condition, and other names, such as *gelatinous transformation,* have been suggested to describe it. Neoplasia of bone marrow or lymphoid organs may be primary or secondary (metastatic). Neoplasia may arise from any hematopoietic lineage. Specific types of hematopoietic neoplasia (leukemias, lymphomas, and others) are covered later in this chapter.

Bone marrow fibrosis (myelofibrosis) and necrosis are associated with many common underlying conditions, often occur in tandem, and are described most extensively in dogs. Conditions known or suspected to cause myelofibrosis and necrosis include sepsis, malignancy (especially hematopoietic malignancies), drug toxicity, and immune-mediated disease (especially nonregenerative immune-mediated hemolytic anemia [IMHA]).

Bone marrow inflammation can take different forms. Granulomatous inflammation in response to fungal infection (e.g., histoplasmosis) or mycobacteriosis may be evident histologically or as macrophage hyperplasia in cytologic preparations of aspirates. Phagocytosed organisms within macrophages are detectable with either type of sample. Dogs and cats with nonregenerative IMHA often have bone marrow inflammation, in addition to fibrosis and necrosis. The inflammation is evident as fibrin deposition, edema, and multifocal neutrophilic infiltrates; immune-mediated cytopenias are also associated with bone marrow lymphocytic and/or plasma cell hyperplasia.

BOX 13-2 Mechanisms of Disease in Bone Marrow and Blood Cells

BONE MARROW

Hypoplasia
Hyperplasia
Dysplasia
Aplasia
Neoplasia
Myelophthisis (fibrosis, metastatic neoplasia)
Necrosis
Inflammation

BLOOD CELLS

Increased destruction
Hemorrhage (especially erythrocytes)
Consumption (platelets)
Neoplasia
Altered distribution
Abnormal function

BLOOD CELLS

Responses of circulating blood cells to injury include decreased survival (destruction, consumption, or loss), altered distribution, and altered structure or function (or both). These responses are not mutually exclusive—for example, altered erythrocyte structure may lead to decreased survival. Often, but not always, these responses result in decreased concentrations of blood cells in circulation.

Abnormal Concentrations of Blood Cells

Cytopenia—from *kytos* (Gr., hollow vessel) and *penia* (Gr., poverty)—refers to a deficiency of blood cells in circulation, hence the terms *neutropenia, thrombocytopenia, lymphopenia,* and so on. Basic mechanisms causing cytopenias include decreased production (hypoplasia), increased destruction, blood loss, consumption, and altered anatomic distribution (e.g., shifts between marginated and circulating compartments in the blood, or between the spleen and the peripheral blood circulation). Most of these basic mechanisms may cause cytopenias of more than one lineage, and some processes affect multiple lineages simultaneously. Sustained decreased production of all three major bone marrow hematopoietic lineages results in pancytopenia (anemia, neutropenia, and thrombocytopenia). Pancytopenia may occur because of myelophthisis, in which normal bone marrow tissue is replaced by abnormal cells or tissue (as in the case of effacement by malignant cells or fibrous tissue) or because of an abnormality of hematopoietic cells themselves. Destruction of hematopoietic stem cells and progenitor cells causes a condition known as *aplastic anemia,* or *aplastic pancytopenia,* which is discussed further in the section on specific diseases.

The pattern of development of cytopenias is partly a function of normal blood cell kinetics. The lifespan of different blood cells in circulation varies markedly (neutrophils: hours, platelets: days, erythrocytes: months). Thus severe neutropenia typically develops within 1 week after cessation of granulopoiesis and after the bone marrow storage pool of neutrophils is depleted, whereas severe thrombocytopenia typically develops in the second week after cessation of thrombopoiesis. Anemia develops much more slowly after the cessation of erythropoiesis, if at all, depending in part on how rapidly the marrow recovers from the insult and on species variation in the erythrocyte lifespan.

Increases in the concentration of many blood cells are indicated by the suffix, *-osis* (erythrocytosis, lymphocytosis, monocytosis, and thrombocytosis). Increases in granulocytes are indicated by the suffix, *-philia* (neutrophilia, eosinophilia, and basophilia). Basic mechanisms causing increases in the concentration of blood cells vary considerably according to cell type and are discussed in more detail later. Neoplasia can result in increased or decreased numbers of blood cells. In many kinds of hematopoietic neoplasia, especially leukemias, there are readily detectable numbers of neoplastic cells in the blood. Specific types of hematopoietic neoplasia are discussed later in this chapter. Increased concentrations of blood cells can also occur secondary to many forms of neoplasia (i.e., as a paraneoplastic syndrome), including non-hematopoietic neoplasms, because of production of stimulatory cytokines by the tumor.

Veterinary laboratories typically provide species-specific hematology reference values based on a reference population of clinically normal adult animals. However, it is important to note that what is normal may vary not only between species but also as a function of other factors, such as age, breed, geographic location, and differences in laboratory methodology.

Mechanisms of disease causing cytopenias and abnormally increased concentrations of specific types blood cells are covered in more detail in the next section.

Anemia

Anemia refers to subnormal red blood cell mass or hemoglobin concentration. Anemia causes clinical signs referable to decreased oxygen-carrying capacity (pallor of mucous membranes, lethargy, weakness, exercise intolerance) and may also result in detectable abnormalities because of tissue hypoxia (e.g., increased liver enzyme activities as a result of hypoxia-induced damage to hepatocytes). Anemia also causes decreased viscosity of the blood, and in marked cases frequently causes heart murmurs as a result of a decrease in laminar blood flow.

Classifying anemia as regenerative or nonregenerative is clinically useful because it provides information about the mechanism of disease (Table 13-1). The hallmark of regenerative anemias, except in horses, is reticulocytosis (i.e., increased numbers of circulating reticulocytes [immature erythrocytes]), which is evident as polychromasia on a routinely stained blood smear. In ruminants, reticulocytosis is often accompanied by basophilic stippling (Fig. 13-7).

Reticulocytosis indicates increased bone marrow erythropoiesis (Fig. 13-8) and release of erythrocytes before they are fully mature (further back in the production "pipeline"). Reticulocytosis is an appropriate response to anemia. A strong regenerative response may produce an increased mean cell volume (MCV) and decreased mean cell hemoglobin concentration (MCHC) on the complete blood count (CBC), because reticulocytes are larger and have a lower hemoglobin concentration than mature erythrocytes. Horses are an exception to this classification scheme because they do not release reticulocytes into circulation even when their marrow is producing increased numbers of erythrocytes. Horses with a regenerative response may have an increased MCV and red cell distribution width (an index of variation in cell size). But definitive determination of regeneration in a horse requires either bone marrow examination, in which case the evidence of regeneration is erythroid hyperplasia, or sequential CBCs, in which case the evidence of regeneration is an increase in red cell mass over time. Punctate reticulocytes in cats are evident when blood is stained with new methylene blue, but they are not counted as reticulocytes on the CBC and have the same appearance as mature erythrocytes on routine blood smear examination.

Another finding that may accompany regeneration, in addition to reticulocytosis, is the presence of nucleated erythroid cells (nRBCs). However, the presence of circulating nRBCs is not in itself definitive evidence of regeneration and in fact may signify dyserythropoiesis (e.g., because of lead poisoning or bone marrow disease) or splenic dysfunction. When nRBCs are present as part of a regenerative response to anemia, they should be in low numbers relative to the numbers of reticulocytes.

Recall that the stimulus for increased erythropoiesis is increased secretion of Epo in response to hypoxemia. Although the action of Epo on erythropoiesis is rapid, evidence of a regenerative response is not immediately apparent in a blood sample. One of the main effects of Epo is to expand the pool of early stage erythroid precursors, and it takes time for these cells to differentiate to the point where they are released into circulation. In a case of acute blood loss, for example, it typically takes 3 to 4 days until reticulocytosis is evident on the CBC, and several more days until the regenerative response peaks. A similar lag occurs in cases of acute hemolysis. The term *preregenerative* is sometimes used to describe anemia with a regenerative response that is impending but not yet apparent on the CBC. Confirming a regenerative response in such cases requires either evidence of erythroid hyperplasia in the bone marrow or emergence of a reticulocytosis on subsequent days.

TABLE 13-1 Classification of Anemia

	Regenerative		Nonregenerative
CBC hallmarks	Reticulocytosis (except horses) Polychromasia, anisocytosis ±↑MCV, ↓MCHC		Absence of reticulocytosis ±↓MCV, ↓MCHC (iron deficiency*)
Causes	**Hemorrhage** Trauma Hemostasis defect Neoplasia GI ulceration Parasitism	**Hemolysis** Extravascular: immune-mediated, hemoparasitism, toxicity, PK, PFK deficiencies Intravascular: immune-mediated, hemoparasitism; toxicity, enzymatic (e.g., bacterial phospholipases), hypophosphatemia, PFK deficiency (with alkalemia)	Anemia of inflammation: ↓iron availability ↓RBC turnover Altered humoral signaling: ↓erythropoietin, endocrinopathies Ineffective erythropoiesis: immune-mediated; FeLV Primary production problem: toxicity, myelophthisis, pure red cell aplasia, pancytopenic disorders Iron deficiency*
Notes	Evaluate in concert with history, physical examination, other laboratory data. Fluid shift occurs within hours of hemorrhage. Regeneration takes approximately 3-4 days to become evident in blood, 7-10 days to reach maximum response.		Evaluate in concert with history, physical examination; other laboratory data may be indicated. Bone marrow evaluation may be indicated.

CBC, Complete blood count; *FeLV,* feline leukemia virus; *GI,* gastrointestinal; *MCHC,* mean cell hemoglobin concentration; *MCV,* mean cell volume; *PFK,* phosphofructokinase; *PK,* pyruvate kinase; *RBC,* red blood cell.
*Iron deficiency anemia is sometimes regenerative

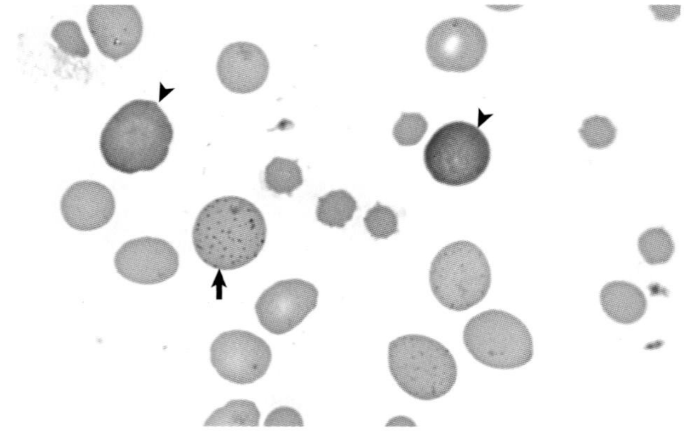

Fig. 13-7 Basophilic stippling and polychromasia, bovine blood smear. Erythrocytes from this cow with regenerative anemia include several cells with basophilic stippling *(arrow)* and two polychromatophilic cells (reticulocytes) *(arrowheads).* Wright's stain. (Courtesy Dr. M.M. Fry, College of Veterinary Medicine, University of Tennessee.)

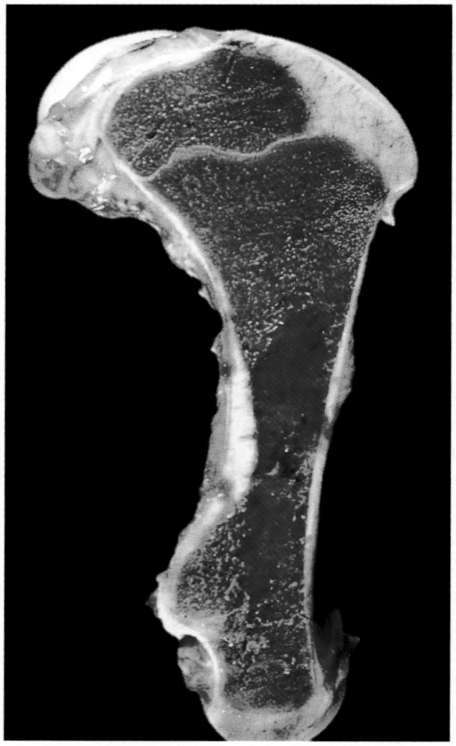

Fig. 13-8 Hemopoietically active bone marrow, femur, calf. Note that the bone marrow has a uniform consistency and is red to dark red. These responses are characteristic of hemopoietically active bone marrow. (Courtesy Dr. Ramos, Autonomous University of Barcelona; and Noah's Arkive, College of Veterinary Medicine, University of Georgia.)

Regenerative anemia occurs because of hemorrhage or hemolysis. Some find it useful to remember these as the "2 Hs" or alternatively, the "2 Ls" (loss or lysis). In the case of hemorrhage, erythrocytes and the other components of blood escape from the vasculature. Hemorrhage may be acute or chronic or internal or external. Causes of hemorrhage include trauma, abnormal hemostasis, certain forms of parasitism, ulceration, and neoplasia. Thus regenerative anemias usually occur not because of a problem with erythropoiesis but because of a process affecting erythrocytes that have already been released into the blood circulation. However, it is important to note that chronic hemorrhage can deplete the body's iron stores, leading to iron-deficiency anemia, which may be either regenerative or nonregenerative. A regenerative response may occur when the deficiency is resolving or temporarily compensated (e.g., when hemorrhage ceases, or when a patient suddenly gains access to increased dietary or parenteral iron). Nonregenerative anemias and iron-deficiency anemia specifically are discussed in more detail later in this chapter.

Hemolysis may be intravascular, in which case erythrocytes release their contents, mostly hemoglobin, directly into the blood, or extravascular, in which case macrophages phagocytose erythrocytes, and little or no hemoglobin is released into the blood. Both forms (mostly extravascular hemolysis) occur as part of normal homeostasis and involve pathways to conserve iron and other reusable components in hematopoiesis. However, some diseases are associated with increased destruction of erythrocytes by one, or both, of these mechanisms. The next sections discuss basic mechanisms of intravascular and extravascular hemolysis in health and disease in more detail.

Normal turnover of erythrocytes occurs mainly by extravascular hemolysis, in which senescent erythrocytes are phagocytosed by macrophages in the spleen and to a lesser extent in other organs such as liver (Kupffer cells) and bone marrow. The exact controls are not clear, but factors that likely play a role include the following:

- Exposure of membrane components normally sequestered on the inner leaflet of the cell membrane, particularly phosphatidylserine (this mechanism is also important in apoptosis of other cell types).
- Decreased deformability.
- Binding of IgG and/or complement.
- Oxidative damage.

Macrophages degrade erythrocytes into reusable constituents, such as iron and amino acids, and the waste product bilirubin. Intravascular hemolysis normally occurs at only extremely low levels. Hemoglobin is a tetramer that, when released from the erythrocyte into the blood, splits into dimers that bind to a plasma protein called *haptoglobin*. The hemoglobin-haptoglobin complex is taken up by hepatocytes and macrophages. This is the major pathway for handling free hemoglobin. However, free hemoglobin may also oxidize to form methemoglobin, which dissociates to form metheme and globin. Metheme binds to a plasma protein called *hemopexin,* which is taken up by hepatocytes and macrophages in a similar manner to hemoglobin-haptoglobin complexes. Free heme in the reduced form binds to albumin, from which it is taken up in the liver and converted into bilirubin.

In hemolytic anemia, erythrocytes are destroyed at an increased rate. Whether the mechanism is intravascular or extravascular, or a combination, depends on the specific disease process (specific diseases are discussed later in this chapter). A classic sequela of hemolytic anemias in general is hyperbilirubinemia, which is an increase in the plasma concentration of bilirubin. Bilirubin is a yellow pigment, which explains why hyperbilirubinemia, if severe enough, causes icterus—the grossly visible yellowing of serum or tissue (Fig. 13-9). Icterus of mucous membranes, skin, and other tissue is known as *jaundice.* Icterus is usually detectable when the plasma bilirubin concentration exceeds 2 mg/dL. Hemolysis is a cause of prehepatic hyperbilirubinemia, but it is important to note that hyperbilirubinemia can also occur as the result of hepatic or posthepatic conditions causing impaired bile flow (cholestasis).

Laboratory findings and clinical observations may point to a specific mechanism of hemolysis. In patients with extravascular hemolytic anemia, increased destruction of erythrocytes by splenic macrophages often results in splenomegaly (Fig. 13-10). Splenomegaly may also occur because of other conditions, as discussed elsewhere in this chapter. Intravascular hemolysis is grossly evident as hemoglobinemia (pink-tinged plasma or serum), if the concentration of extracellular hemoglobin is greater than approximately 50 mg/dL. Haptoglobin is saturated with dimeric hemoglobin at a concentration of approximately 150 mg/dL. When haptoglobin is saturated, any remaining free hemoglobin has a low enough molecular weight to pass through the renal glomerular filter into the urine (hemoglobinuria), imparting a pink or red discoloration to the urine. Thus extracellular hemoglobin can cause gross discoloration of the plasma, where it is bound to haptoglobin, before becoming grossly visible in urine. The half-life of haptoglobin is markedly decreased when bound to hemoglobin, so when

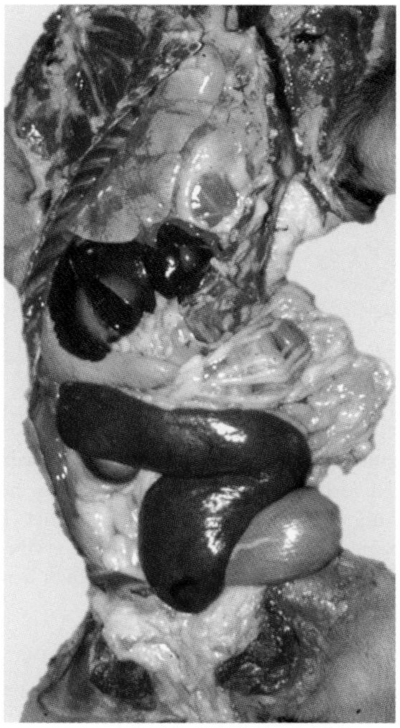

Fig. 13-9 Icterus, immune-mediated hemolytic anemia (IMHA), subcutaneous fat, splenomegaly, spleen, dog.
The marked yellow discoloration of tissues, most strikingly visible in the subcutaneous fat, is from high concentrations of serum bilirubin produced as a result of the hemolytic anemia. (Courtesy Dr. J.A. Ramos-Vara, College of Veterinary Medicine, Michigan State University; and Noah's Arkive, College of Veterinary Medicine, The University of Georgia.)

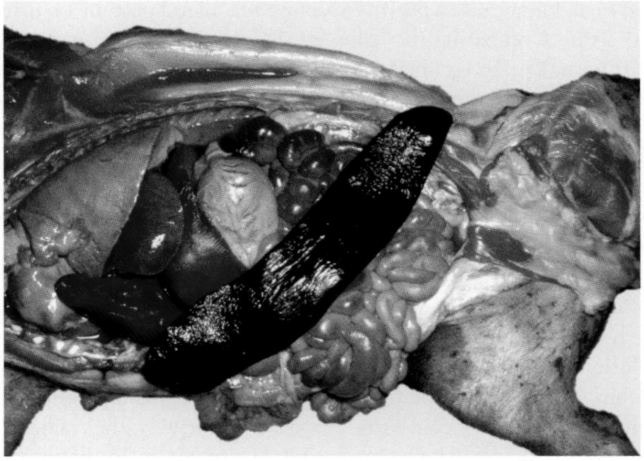

Fig. 13-10 Splenomegaly, fatal hemolytic anemia, *Mycoplasma suis,* pig.
The spleen is extremely enlarged, meaty, and congested. (Courtesy College of Veterinary Medicine, University of Illinois.)

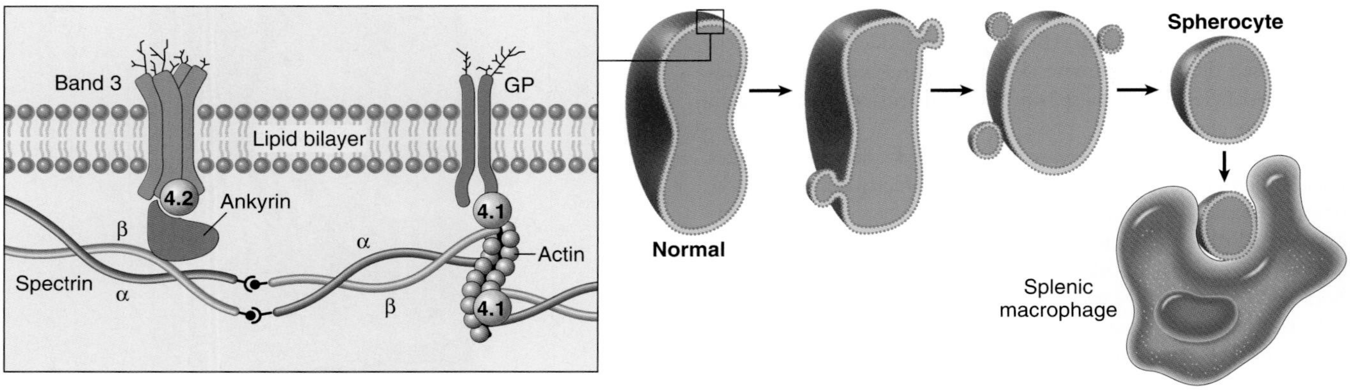

Fig. 13-11 Schematic representation of the mechanisms of spherocytosis and extravascular hemolysis (EVH). Hereditary spherocytosis occurs in humans (as shown here) because of mutations that weaken the connections between cytoskeletal and membrane proteins. In cases of immune-mediated hemolytic anemia (IMHA), the most frequent cause of spherocytes in animals, the underlying disease mechanism is different—spherocytes form when portions of the erythrocyte membrane bound with autoantibody are phagocytosed by macrophages—but the net result (spherocytosis and EVH) is similar to what is shown here. *GP,* Glycoprotein. (From Kumar V, Abbas AK, Fausto N, et al: *Robbins & Cotran pathologic basis of disease,* ed 8, Philadelphia, 2009, Saunders.)

large amounts of haptoglobin-hemoglobin complex are formed, the concentration of haptoglobin in the blood decreases and hemoglobin can pass through the glomerulus at even lower concentrations. Hemoglobinuria is a contributing factor in the renal tubular necrosis (hemoglobinuric nephrosis) that often occurs in cases of acute intravascular hemolysis (see Chapter 11). A similar lesion occurs in the kidneys of individuals with marked muscle damage and resulting myoglobinuria.

Hemoglobinuria cannot be distinguished grossly from hematuria (RBCs in the urine) or myoglobinuria, and both hemoglobin and myoglobin cause a positive reaction for "blood protein" on urine test strips. Comparing the colors of the plasma and the urine may be informative. In contrast to hemoglobin, myoglobin causes gross discoloration of the urine before the plasma is discolored. This is because myoglobin is a low-molecular-weight monomer, freely filtered by the glomerulus, and does not bind plasma proteins to a significant degree. Hematuria can be distinguished from hemoglobinuria on the basis of microscopic examination of urine sediment (RBCs are present in cases of hematuria).

CBC data are often useful in illuminating hemolytic mechanisms. Total hemoglobin concentration is conventionally measured by lysing all the erythrocytes and measuring the hemoglobin in solution spectrophotometrically. The value for mean cell hemoglobin (MCH) is calculated based on the total hemoglobin concentration and the concentration of erythrocytes. The value for MCHC is calculated based on the MCH and MCV. Thus although erythrocytes do not actually contain supranormal concentrations of hemoglobin, an excess of extracellular hemoglobin may cause an artifactual increase in the calculated MCH and MCHC. It is important to remember that similar increases may also occur artifactually because of positive interference with spectrophotometric measurement of hemoglobin such as occurs with lipemia.

Extravascular hemolysis also often produces characteristic CBC abnormalities that may reflect the mechanism of disease. For example, spherocytosis and autoagglutination are hallmarks of IMHA. Spherocytes form when macrophages (mainly in the spleen) phagocytose part of an erythrocyte plasma membrane bound with autoantibody (Fig. 13-11). The remaining portion of the RBC assumes a spherical shape, thus preserving maximal volume. This change in shape results in decreased deformability of the cells. Erythrocytes must be extremely pliable to traverse

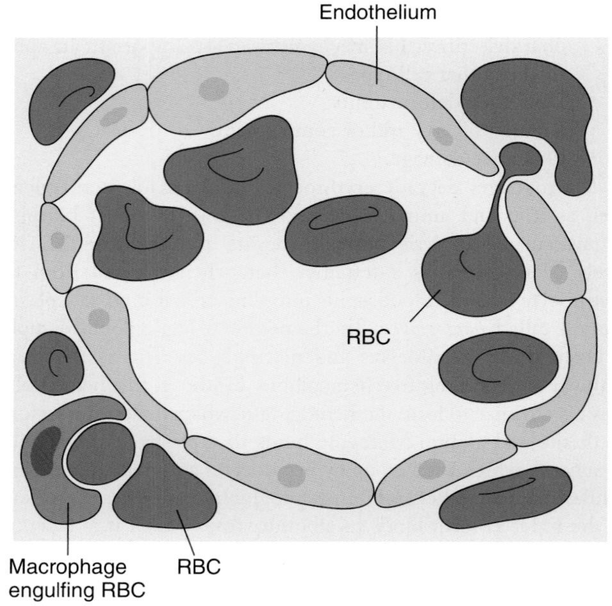

Fig. 13-12 Schematic representation of a splenic sinusoid. A red blood cell *(RBC)* is in the process of squeezing from the red pulp cords into the sinus lumen. Note the degree of deformability required for RBCs to pass through the wall of the sinus. (From Kumar V, Abbas AK, Fausto N: *Robbins & Cotran pathologic basis of disease,* ed 7, Philadelphia, 2005, Saunders.)

the splenic red pulp and sinusoidal walls (Fig. 13-12); spherocytes therefore tend to be retained in the spleen in close association with macrophages with risk of further injury and eventual destruction. In the dog, spherocytes appear smaller than normal and have uniform staining (Fig. 13-13, *A*), in contrast to normal RBCs, which have a region of central pallor imparted by their biconcave shape. This difference in staining between spherocytes and normal RBCs is not consistently discernible in many other domestic animals (including horses, cattle, and cats), whose erythrocytes differ from those of the dog in that they are smaller and have less pronounced biconcavity and therefore less pronounced central pallor. Autoagglutination occurs because of cross-linking of antibodies bound to erythrocytes. Autoagglutination is evident

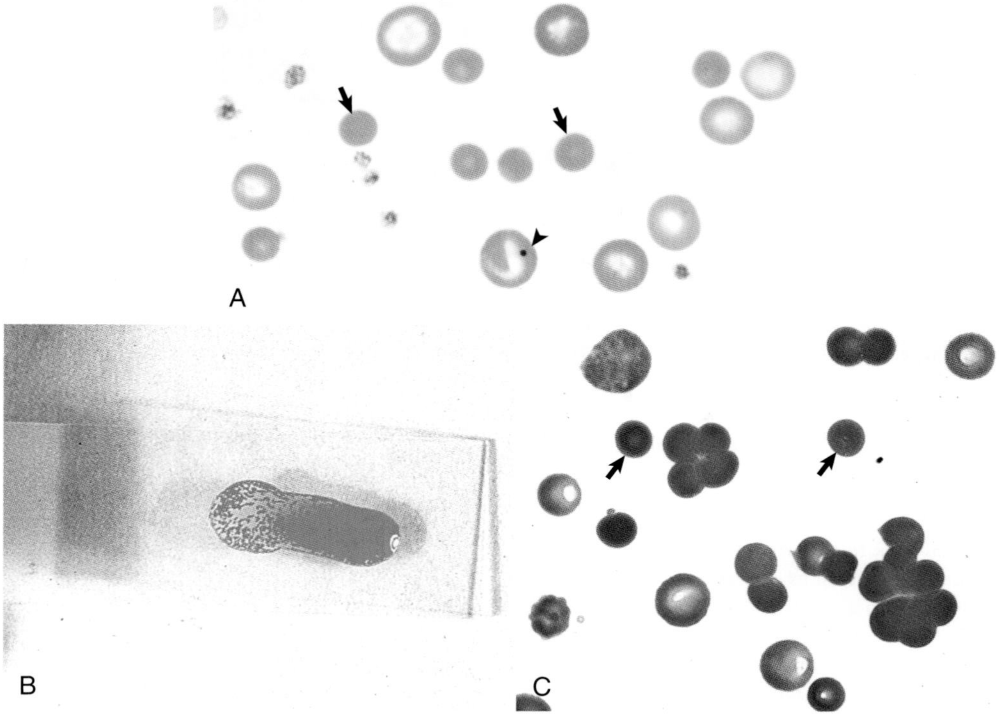

Fig. 13-13 Immune-mediated hemolytic anemia (IMHA), canine blood, dog.
A, Spherocytosis. Numerous spherocytes *(arrows)* and several polychromatophilic cells, one of which *(arrowhead)* contains a nuclear remnant known as a Howell-Jolly body, are visible. Wright's stain. **B,** Autoagglutination. Note the grossly visible agglutination. **C,** Spherocytosis and agglutination. Note the spherocytes *(arrows)* and microscopic agglutination of erythrocytes in a dog that received a blood transfusion. These abnormalities presumably indicate immune-mediated destruction of the donor erythrocytes. Wright's stain. (**A** courtesy Dr. M.M. Fry, College of Veterinary Medicine, University of Tennessee. **B** and **C** from Harvey JW: *Atlas of veterinary hematology: blood and bone marrow of domestic animals,* Philadelphia, 2001, Saunders.)

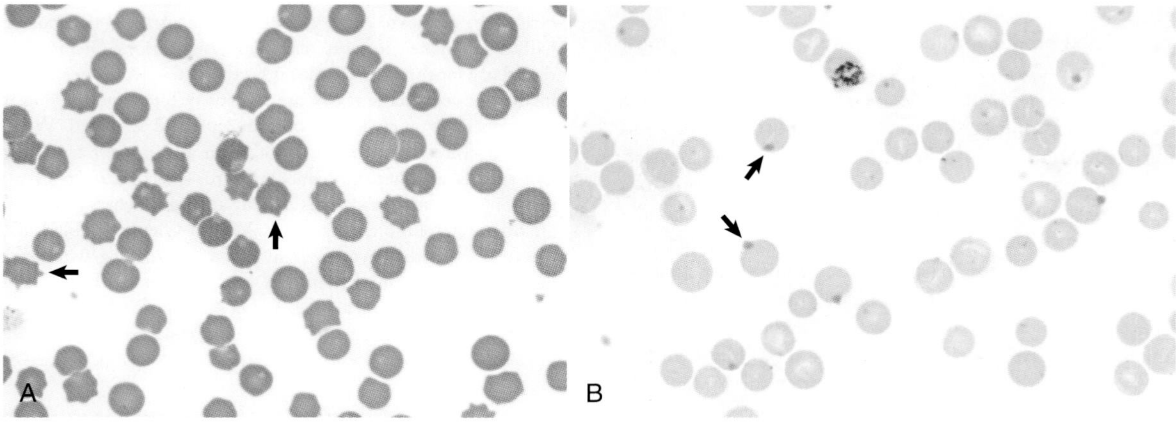

Fig. 13-14 Heinz bodies, blood smears.
A, Feline blood smear. With routine staining, Heinz bodies appear as pale circular intraerythrocytic inclusions that may protrude *(arrows)* from the margin of the cell. Wright's stain. **B,** Canine blood smear. Using a supravital stain, Heinz bodies are blue inclusions *(arrows)* and easier to see. New methylene blue stain. (Courtesy Dr. M.M. Fry, College of Veterinary Medicine, University of Tennessee.)

microscopically as clusters of erythrocytes, and macroscopically as blood with a grainy consistency (Fig. 13-13, *B*). Autoagglutination may also result in a falsely increased MCV and decreased RBC concentration when clustered cells are mistakenly counted as single cells by automated hematology analyzers.

Oxidative damage to erythrocytes occurs when normal antioxidative pathways that generate reducing agents (such as NADH, NADPH, and reduced glutathione) are compromised or overwhelmed and can result in hemolytic anemia, abnormal hemoglobin function, or both. Hemolysis caused by oxidative damage may be extravascular or intravascular, or a combination (predominant forms of hemolysis are discussed further in the section on specific diseases). Evidence of oxidative damage to erythrocytes may be apparent on examination of a blood smear, or even on gross physical examination. Heinz bodies are foci of denatured globin that interact with the erythrocyte membrane. They are usually subtly evident on routine Wright's-stained blood smears as pale circular inclusions or blunt, rounded protrusions of the cell margin and are readily discernible on smears stained with new methylene blue (Fig. 13-14). Cats are particularly susceptible to Heinz body formation and may have low numbers of small Heinz bodies normally. There is no unanimity of opinion, but some clinical pathologists believe that the presence of Heinz bodies in up to 10% of all RBCs in cats is within normal limits. This predisposition is believed to reflect unique features of the feline erythrocyte, whose hemoglobin has more sulfhydryl groups (preferential sites for oxidative damage) than do erythrocytes of other species and may also have lower intrinsic reducing capacity. It is also possible that the feline spleen, which is nonsinusoidal, does not have as efficient a "pitting" function as does a sinusoidal spleen, such as that of the dog (splenic structure and function are discussed in more detail later in this chapter). Eccentrocytes, evident as erythrocytes in which one side of the cell has increased pallor, are another manifestation of oxidative damage. They form because of cross-linking of membrane proteins, with adhesion of opposing areas of the cell's inner membrane leaflet, and displacement of most of the hemoglobin toward the other side (Fig. 13-15). Oxidative insult may also result in conversion of hemoglobin (iron in the Fe^{2+} state) to methemoglobin (iron in the Fe^{3+} state), which is incapable of binding oxygen. Methemoglobin is produced normally in small amounts but reduced back to oxyhemoglobin by the enzyme cytochrome-b5 reductase (also known as *methemoglobin reductase*). Methemoglobinemia results when methemoglobin is produced in excessive amounts (because of oxidative insult) or when the normal pathways for maintaining hemoglobin in the Fe^{2+} state are impaired (as in cytochrome-b_5 reductase deficiency). When present in sufficiently high concentration (approximately 10% of total hemoglobin), methemoglobin imparts a grossly discernible chocolate color to the blood.

Nonregenerative anemias are characterized by a lack of reticulocytosis on the CBC; however, reticulocytosis does not occur in horses even in the context of regeneration. Most often this is a result of decreased production in the marrow (i.e., erythroid hypoplasia). Erythrocytes circulate for a long time, so anemias caused by decreased production tend to develop slowly. The most common form of nonregenerative anemia is known as *anemia of inflammation* or *anemia of chronic disease.* In this form of anemia, RBCs are decreased in number but are typically normal in size and hemoglobin concentration (so-called normocytic, normochromic, anemia). It has long been known that patients with inflammatory or other chronic disease often become anemic and that this condition is associated with increased iron stores in the bone marrow. Sequestration of iron may be a bacteriostatic evolutionary adaptation because many bacteria require iron as a cofactor for growth. In recent years, investigators have begun to elucidate the molecular mechanisms underlying anemia of inflammation. Hepcidin, an acute phase protein synthesized in the liver that was first identified as an antimicrobial peptide, is a key mediator that acts by limiting iron availability. Hepcidin expression increases with inflammation, infection, or iron overload and decreases with anemia or hypoxia. Hepcidin exerts its effects by causing functional iron deficiency. It binds to and causes the degradation of the cell surface iron efflux molecule, ferroportin, thus inhibiting both absorption of dietary iron from the intestinal epithelium and export of iron from macrophages and hepatocytes into the plasma (Fig. 13-16).

Anemia of inflammation involves factors besides decreased iron availability. Inflammatory cytokines are likely to inhibit erythropoiesis by oxidative damage to and triggering apoptosis of developing erythroid cells, by decreasing expression of Epo and stem-cell factor, and by decreasing expression of Epo receptors. In addition, experimentally induced sterile inflammation in cats resulted in shortened erythrocyte survival, indicating that anemia of inflammation is likely also a function of increased erythrocyte destruction.

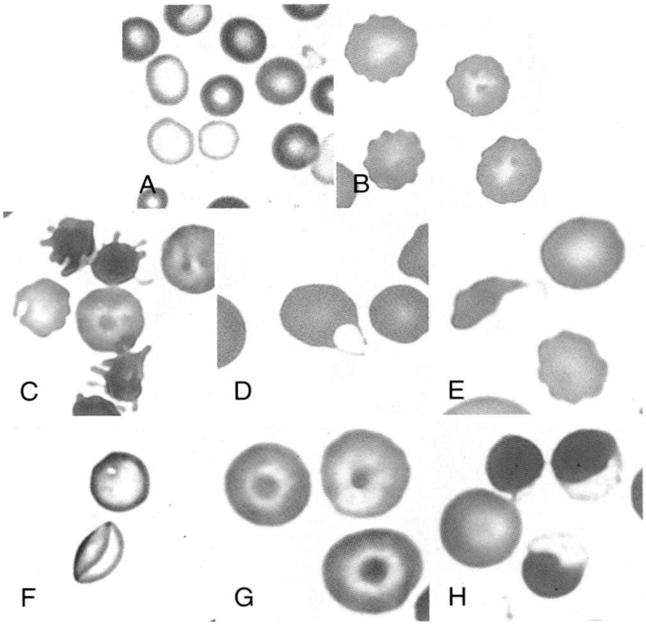

Fig. 13-15 Common erythrocyte morphologic abnormalities. **A,** Blood from a dog with a microcytic hypochromic iron-deficiency anemia was mixed with an equal volume of blood from a normal dog before blood smear was prepared. Because the hypochromic (pale-staining) cells are leptocytes shown in **F**, they have diameters similar to normal cells even though they are microcytic cells. Wright-Giemsa stain. **B,** Echinocytes appear as erythrocytes with scalloped borders; consequently, the old term "crenation" from Latin meaning "notched" is used. Wright-Giemsa stain. **C,** Three acanthocytes with irregularly spaced, variably sized spicules in blood from a dog with hemangiosarcoma. Wright-Giemsa stain. **D,** A keratocyte, exhibiting what appears to be a ruptured "vesicle" in blood from a cat with hepatic lipidosis. Wright-Giemsa stain. **E,** A schistocyte *(left),* discocyte *(top),* and echinocyte *(bottom)* in blood from a dog with disseminated intravascular hemolysis. Wright-Giemsa stain. **F,** Two thin flat hypochromic-appearing erythrocytes (leptocytes), with increased membrane-to-volume ratios, are present in blood from a dog with severe iron-deficiency anemia. The bottom leptocyte is folded. Wright-Giemsa stain. **G,** Three codocytes in blood from a Cairn terrier with a regenerative anemia and hepatic hemochromatosis secondary to pyruvate kinase deficiency. These erythrocytes exhibit a central density or "bull's-eye" and are often referred to as target cells. Wright-Giemsa stain. **H,** Three eccentrocytes and a discocyte *(left)* in blood from a dog with oxidant injury induced by the administration of acetaminophen. The cell at top center appears spherical with a small tag of cytoplasm and may be referred to as a pyknocyte. Wright-Giemsa stain. (From Harvey JW: *Atlas of veterinary hematology: blood and bone marrow of domestic animals,* Philadelphia, 2001, Saunders.)

True iron deficiency has long been recognized as a cause of anemia. In domestic animals, iron deficiency occurs most commonly because of chronic blood loss, and thus loss of iron in the form of hemoglobin, and less frequently because of nutritional deficiency. Although iron deficiency often results in nonregenerative anemia, it is not always so, especially when nutritional iron is not a limiting factor. Many underlying conditions can cause hemorrhage-induced iron deficiency anemia, including primary or secondary gastrointestinal (GI) disease (e.g., hookworms, neoplasia, ulceration) and marked ectoparasitism. The classic hematologic picture with iron deficiency is microcytic, hypochromic anemia. Microcytosis and hypochromasia are indicated on the CBC by abnormally low MCV and MCHC values, respectively. Microcytosis and hypochromasia may also be discernible on review of a

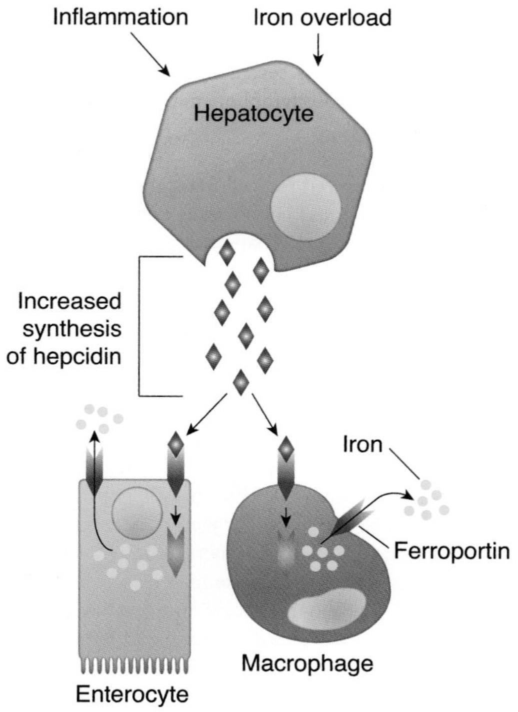

Fig. 13-16 Mechanism of action of hepcidin. Binding of hepcidin to ferroportin causes its internalization and degradation, thus inhibiting efflux of iron into the plasma. (Courtesy Dr. J.F. Zachary, College of Veterinary Medicine, University of Illinois.)

blood smear as RBCs that are abnormally small or paler-staining because of their subnormal hemoglobin concentration, respectively. However, microscopic examination is not a reliable means of detection, especially in the case of mild abnormalities. Low hemoglobin concentration is believed to contribute to microcytosis because one of the feedback mechanisms signaling erythroid cells to stop dividing is reaching a threshold hemoglobin concentration. Abnormally low hemoglobin concentration during erythropoiesis thus results in extra cell divisions and smaller erythrocytes. Microcytosis usually develops before hypochromasia.

Other causes of decreased erythropoiesis include the following:

- Decreased hormonal stimulation (e.g., chronic renal failure)
- Malnutrition
- Infection of erythropoietic cells
- Toxic insult to the bone marrow
- Other disease involving the bone marrow
- Immune-mediated destruction of erythroid precursors
- Inherited conditions

Specific examples of diseases causing nonregenerative anemia by these mechanisms are discussed later in this chapter. It is important to point out that nonregenerative anemia is not always caused by decreased erythropoiesis. For example, IMHA is typically strongly regenerative, but there are also nonregenerative forms of IMHA. Bone marrow findings in dogs with severe nonregenerative IMHA range from a complete absence of erythropoiesis, known as pure red cell aplasia, to erythroid hyperplasia in a majority of patients in one study. The latter situation is an example of ineffective hematopoiesis (in this case, ineffective erythropoiesis), in which cells are produced at abnormal or increased rate but are destroyed, presumably because of an immune-mediated mechanism, before they enter the circulation.

Neutropenia

Neutropenia refers to a decrease in the concentration of neutrophils in circulating blood. Neutropenia may be caused by decreased production, increased destruction, altered distribution, demand for neutrophils in inflamed tissue that exceeds the rate of granulopoiesis, or inherited disease. Decreased production is evident on bone marrow examination as granulocytic hypoplasia. This usually results from an insult that affects multiple hematopoietic lineages, such as chemical insult, radiation, neoplasia, infection, and fibrosis, but may also be caused by a process that preferentially targets granulopoiesis. Immune-mediated neutropenia is a rare but recognized condition in domestic animals. Bone marrow findings range from granulocytic aplasia or hypoplasia to hyperplasia, depending on where the cells under immune attack are in their differentiation programs. Neutropenia with no evidence of decreased production and in which other causes of neutropenia have been excluded may be a result of destruction of neutrophils before they leave the bone marrow, a condition known as *ineffective granulopoiesis.* Like other forms of ineffective hematopoiesis, this condition is often presumed to be immune mediated; in cats this condition may occur as a result of infection of hematopoietic cells with the feline leukemia virus (FeLV).

In marked contrast to erythrocytes, neutrophils have a very short lifespan in circulation. Once released from the bone marrow, a neutrophil is only in the bloodstream for hours before migrating into the tissues. The fate of neutrophils after they leave the bloodstream in normal conditions (i.e., not in the context of inflammation) is poorly understood. They migrate into the GI and respiratory tracts, liver, and spleen and may be lost through mucosal surfaces or undergo apoptosis and be phagocytosed by macrophages. When neutrophil production ceases, a reserve of mature neutrophils in the bone marrow (discussed in more detail later) may be adequate to maintain normal numbers of circulating neutrophils for a few days; however, after the bone marrow storage pool is depleted, neutropenia rapidly ensues.

Neutrophils within the blood vasculature are in two compartments: a *circulating pool,* consisting of those cells flowing freely in the blood, and a *marginated pool,* consisting of those cells transiently associated with the endothelial surface. (In reality, neutrophils are constantly shifting between these two pools, but the proportion of cells in either pool normally remains fairly constant in any given species.) Circulating neutrophils are part of the blood sample collected during routine venipuncture and are thus counted in the CBC, whereas marginated neutrophils are not. Pseudoneutropenia refers to the situation in which there are an increased proportion of neutrophils in the marginated pool. This may occur because of decreased blood flow or in response to stimuli, such as endotoxemia, that increase expression of molecules promoting interaction between neutrophils and endothelial cells.

Neutropenia may also result from increased demand for neutrophils in the tissue. How rapidly such a situation develops depends not only on the magnitude of the inflammatory stimulus but also on the reserve of postmitotic neutrophils in the bone marrow. The size of this reserve, or storage pool, is species dependent. In dogs, this pool contains the equivalent of 5 days normal production of neutrophils. Cattle represent the other extreme in that they have a small storage pool and thus are predisposed to becoming neutropenic more easily than are dogs. Horses and cats are somewhere between the two extremes, closer to cattle and dogs, respectively. It stands to reason that the clinical significance of neutropenia because of a supply and demand imbalance is also species dependent. In dogs, neutropenia as a result of inflammation is an alarming finding because it is evidence of a massive tissue demand for neutrophils that has exhausted the patient's storage pool and is exceeding the rate of granulopoiesis in the bone marrow, whereas in cows, neutropenia is commonly noted in a wide range of conditions involving acute inflammation and does not necessarily indicate an overwhelming demand.

Eosinopenia/Basopenia

In many laboratories, CBC reference values for eosinophils and basophils are as low as zero cells per microliter, precluding detection of eosinopenia or basopenia. When detectable, eosinopenia is often part of a stress (glucocorticoid-mediated) leukogram.

Thrombocytopenia

Thrombocytopenia refers to a decrease in the concentration of circulating platelets. Mechanisms of thrombocytopenia include decreased production, increased destruction, increased consumption, altered distribution, and hemorrhage. Decreased production may occur because of a condition affecting cells of multiple hematopoietic lineages, including platelets, or to one specifically depressing thrombopoiesis. In either case, decreased thrombopoiesis is evident on examination of a bone marrow sample as megakaryocytic hypoplasia. General causes of decreased hematopoiesis outlined earlier in the sections on anemia and neutropenia also apply to thrombocytopenia. Specific diseases causing thrombocytopenia are covered later in this chapter. Immune-mediated thrombocytopenia is a fairly common disease in dogs and may also occur in other species. Increased consumption of platelets is a hallmark of disseminated intravascular coagulation (DIC), a syndrome in which hypercoagulability leads to increased consumption of both platelets and coagulation factors in the plasma, with subsequent hypocoagulability and susceptibility to bleeding. The spleen normally contains a significant proportion of total platelet mass (up to one-third in some species), and abnormalities involving the spleen may result in changes in the number of circulating platelets. For example, splenic congestion may result in thrombocytopenia, and splenic contraction may result in thrombocytosis. Acute hemorrhage may result in mild to moderate thrombocytopenia. Potential mechanisms of thrombocytopenia caused by hemorrhage include loss and consumption. Of course, thrombocytopenia can also be a cause of hemorrhage. In the absence of other complicating factors, marked to severe thrombocytopenia (less than 50,000 platelets/μL) is more likely to be the cause of rather than the result of bleeding. Megakaryocytic hyperplasia on examination of a bone marrow sample is evidence of a regenerative thrombopoietic response, and an increase in the mean platelet volume (MPV) value on the CBC often accompanies such a response.

Lymphopenia

Lymphopenia refers to a decrease in the concentration of lymphocytes in blood circulation. It is a common CBC finding in sick animals. Usually the precise mechanism of lymphopenia is not clear. It is often presumed to be mediated at least in part by endogenous glucocorticoid excess. Lymphopenia may occur because of various mechanisms, including altered distribution of lymphocytes (increased trafficking of lymphocytes to, and decreased egress from, lymphoid tissues), lymphotoxicity (direct damage to lymphocytes or suppression of lymphopoiesis) of therapeutic or infectious agents, loss of lymphocyte-rich lymphatic fluid, or congenital disorders. Normal lymphocyte trafficking may be altered because of disruption of the normal architecture of lymphoid tissue (e.g., because of neoplasia or inflammation), or in response to cytokine signals. Glucocorticoid excess may cause lymphopenia via redistribution from the blood to lymphoid tissue, or via direct lymphotoxic effects. Anticancer treatments (chemotherapy or radiotherapy) and immunosuppressive drugs may also be lymphotoxic. Some hereditary immunodeficiencies (such as severe combined immunodeficiency or thymic aplasia) can cause lymphopenia.

Erythrocytosis

An increase in the measured red cell mass above the normal range (i.e., the opposite of anemia) is known as erythrocytosis. The term *polycythemia* is often used interchangeably with erythrocytosis, but technically and for the purposes of this chapter, polycythemia refers to a specific type of leukemia called *primary erythrocytosis* or *polycythemia vera*. Relative erythrocytosis occurs most frequently because of dehydration, when the decreased proportion of water in the blood results in hemoconcentration. A similar situation may occur as a result of epinephrine-mediated splenic contraction. Erythrocytosis caused by splenic contraction occurs to the most pronounced degree in the horse and may occur to a lesser extent in other species. In both of these cases, the total RBC mass is not in fact increased but appears to be so because of other factors. Secondary erythrocytosis refers to a true, Epo-mediated increase in red cell mass, either as an appropriate response to hypoxemia (such as may be seen in patients with cardiopulmonary disease and severely impaired oxygenation, or cardiovascular defects causing right-to-left shunting) or in rare cases an Epo-secreting tumor (inappropriate secondary erythrocytosis). Polycythemia vera is diagnosed based on a marked increase in red cell mass (hematocrit in normally hydrated dogs ranges from 65% to >80%), absence of hypoxemia, absence of other tumors, and normal or decreased concentration of plasma erythropoietin concentration. Absolute erythrocytosis, whether primary or secondary, causes increased viscosity of the blood and resulting impairment of blood flow and distention of the microvasculature. Affected individuals are at increased risk of tissue hypoxia and thrombosis or hemorrhage. Related clinical signs (hyperviscosity syndrome) may include erythematous mucous membranes (Fig. 13-17) and prolonged capillary refill time, prominent scleral vessels, evidence of thrombosis or hemorrhage, and secondary signs (e.g., neurologic and cardiovascular) related to specific organ systems affected.

Neutrophilia

Neutrophilia occurs in response to a number of different stimuli, which are not mutually exclusive. Major mechanisms of neutrophilia are shown in Fig. 13-18. Understanding the CBC findings characteristic of these responses is an important part of clinical veterinary medicine. Inflammation can result in neutropenia, as discussed earlier, or neutrophilia, as discussed next. However, before moving on to a discussion of inflammatory neutrophilia and the so-called left shift, it is important to mention two other common causes of neutrophilia.

Glucocorticoid excess, either because of endogenous production or exogenous administration, results in a CBC pattern known as the *stress leukogram,* characterized by mature neutrophilia (i.e., increased concentration of segmented neutrophils), lymphopenia, and, especially in dogs, monocytosis. Eosinopenia is another feature of the stress leukogram, although in many situations this is inapparent because the normal reference values for eosinophils are so low (in some laboratories, the lower reference value is zero). Mechanisms contributing to glucocorticoid-mediated neutrophilia include the following:

- Increased release of mature neutrophils from the bone marrow storage pool.
- Decreased margination of neutrophils within the vasculature, with a resulting increase in the circulating pool.

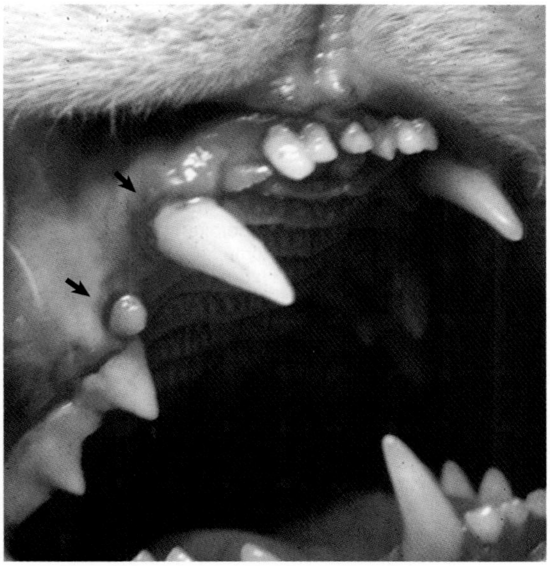

Fig. 13-17 Absolute erythrocytosis, hyperviscosity syndrome, erythematous mucous membranes, cat.
Erythema of mucous membranes is one of the signs associated with hyperviscosity syndrome. In this case, the oral mucous membranes are deeper red *(arrows)* than normal because of an abnormally high concentration of erythrocytes and associated sludging of blood. Hyperviscosity syndrome may also occur as the result of increased plasma immunoglobulin concentration. (Courtesy Dr. C. Patrick Ryan, Veterinary Public Health, Los Angeles Department of Health Services; and Noah's Arkive, College of Veterinary Medicine, University of Georgia.)

- Decreased migration of neutrophils from the bloodstream into tissues.

The magnitude of neutrophilia tends to be species dependent, with dogs having the most pronounced response (up to 35,000 cells/μL) and in decreasing order of responsiveness, cats (30,000 cells/μL), horses (20,000 cells/μL), and cows (15,000 cells/μL) less marked responses. With long-term glucocorticoid excess, neutrophil numbers tend to normalize, whereas lymphopenia persists.

Epinephrine release results in a different pattern, known as *physiologic leukocytosis,* characterized by mature neutrophilia (like the glucocorticoid response) and lymphocytosis (unlike the glucocorticoid response). This phenomenon is short lived (<1 hour). Neutrophilia occurs primarily because of a shift of cells from the marginated to the circulating pool. Physiologic leukocytosis is common in cats (especially when they are highly stressed during blood collection) and horses, less common in cattle, and uncommon in dogs.

Of course, neutrophilia may also indicate inflammation, and inflammatory stimuli of varying magnitude and duration produce different patterns of neutrophilia. A classic hematologic finding in patients with increased demand for neutrophils is the presence of immature forms in the blood, known as a "left shift." Not all inflammatory responses have a left shift, but the presence of a left shift almost always signifies active demand for neutrophils in the tissue. The magnitude of a left shift is assessed by the number of immature cells and their degree of immaturity. The mildest form is characterized by increased numbers of band neutrophils, the immediate predecessor to the segmented neutrophil normally found in circulation, with increasingly severe forms involving progressively immature predecessors. A left shift is considered orderly if the number of immature neutrophils in circulation decreases as they become progressively immature. The term *degenerative left shift* is sometimes used to describe cases where the number of immature forms exceeds the number of segmented neutrophils. As with glucocorticoid-mediated neutrophilia, the typical magnitude of neutrophilia caused by inflammation varies by species, with dogs having the most pronounced response.

Marked neutrophilia may also occur because of an inherited condition known as leukocyte adhesion deficiency (LAD), in which leukocytes lack normal expression of an adhesion molecule required for migration from the bloodstream into the tissue. This condition is described further in the section on specific diseases.

It might be useful to think of neutrophil kinetics in terms of a producer-consumer model in which the bone marrow is the factory, and the tissues (where the neutrophils eventually go) are the customers. The bone marrow storage pool is the factory inventory, and the neutrophils in the bloodstream are in delivery to the customer. Within the blood vessels, circulating neutrophils are on the highway, and marginated neutrophils are temporarily pulled off to the side of the road. During health, there is an even flow of neutrophils from the factory to the customer. Thus the system is in steady state, and neutrophil numbers remain relatively constant and within the normal range. However, disease states may perturb this system at multiple levels. Decreased granulopoiesis is analogous to a factory working below normal production level. Ineffective granulopoiesis is analogous to goods produced at a normal to increased rate but that are damaged during manufacturing and never leave the factory. A left shift is analogous to the factory meeting increased customer demand by shipping out unfinished goods. Cases of persistent, established inflammation are characterized by bone marrow granulocytic hyperplasia and mature neutrophilia, analogous to a factory that has had time to adjust to increased demand and is meeting it more efficiently by increasing its output.

Eosinophilia/Basophilia

Eosinophilia and, less commonly, basophilia (which, when present, often occurs concurrently with eosinophilia) may occur in response to parasitism, as part of an allergic response, as a paraneoplastic abnormality (because of production of cytokines by neoplastic cells or other inflammatory cells reacting to the neoplasm), as an atypical response to nonparasitic infectious disease, or in rare idiopathic conditions (e.g., hypereosinophilic syndrome).

Thrombocytosis

Thrombocytosis, or concentration of platelets in the blood above normal reference values, is a relatively common nonspecific finding in veterinary patients. In the vast majority of cases, thrombocytosis is reactive—a response to another, often apparently unrelated, disease process. Examples of conditions associated with reactive thrombocytosis include inflammatory and infectious diseases, iron deficiency, hemorrhage, endocrinopathies, and neoplasia. Factors that may contribute to reactive thrombocytosis include increased plasma concentration of thrombopoietin, inflammatory cytokines (e.g., IL-6), or catecholamines. Thrombocytosis may also occur as part of a regenerative response in patients recovering from thrombocytopenia, or as a result of redistribution because of splenic contraction (especially in horses) or splenectomy. In these cases, thrombocytosis is transient. In the case of splenectomy, thrombocytosis may be marked, but normalizes after several weeks. Because the body's total platelet mass regulates thrombopoiesis and a significant portion of the platelet mass is normally in the spleen, it makes sense that splenectomized animals develop thrombocytosis. However, the reason that the number of circulating platelets

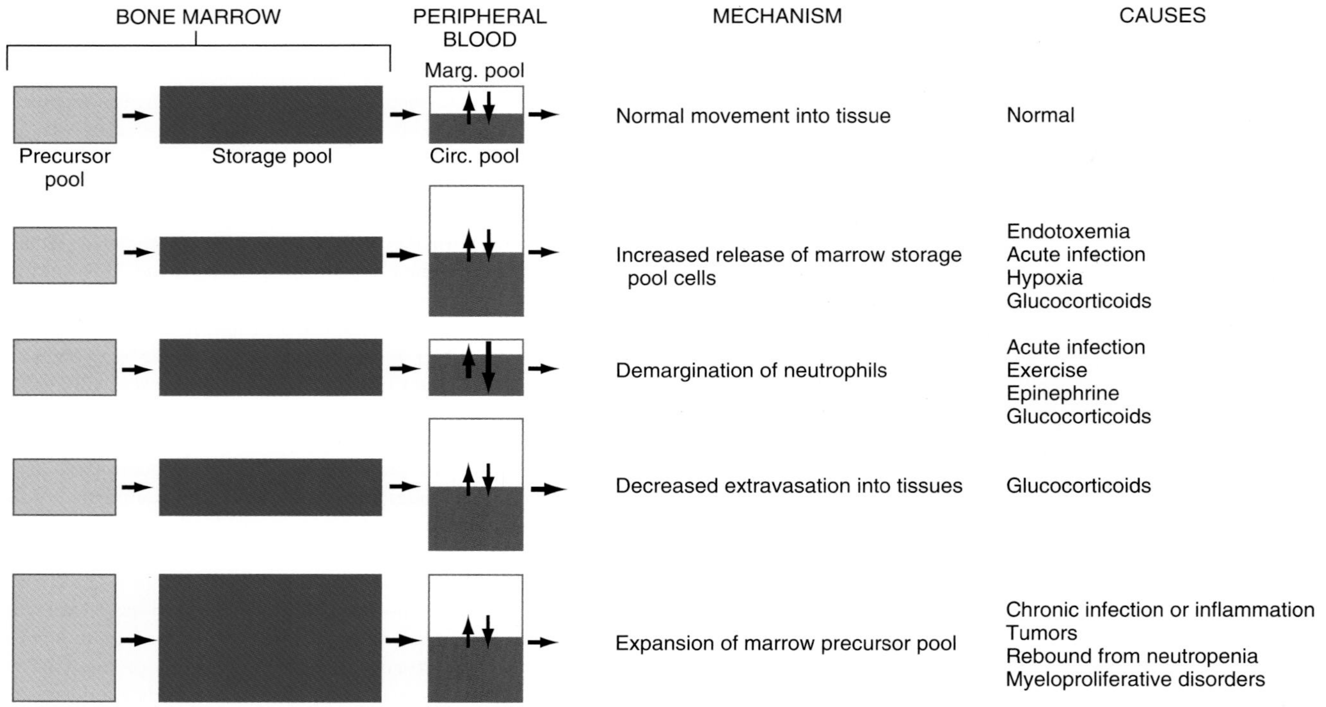

Fig. 13-18 Schematic illustration of the mechanisms of neutrophilic leukocytosis. Neutrophils and their precursors are distributed in five pools: a bone marrow precursor pool, which includes progenitor cells and more committed, mitotically active precursors; a bone marrow storage pool, consisting of mitotically inactive mature and slightly immature neutrophils (band forms); a peripheral blood marginating pool *(Marg. pool);* a peripheral blood circulating pool *(Circ. pool);* and a tissue pool. The relative size of each pool is represented by the size of its corresponding box. The peripheral blood neutrophil count measures only the circulating peripheral blood pool, which can be enlarged by increased release of cells from the marrow storage pool, increased demargination, diminished extravasation into tissue, or expansion of the marrow precursor cell pool. (Modified from Finch SC: *Hematology,* ed 3, New York, 1983, McGraw-Hill.)

normalize in these individuals in the weeks after splenectomy is not clear. There is also a rare form of leukemia known as *essential thrombocythemia,* which is characterized by marked thrombocytosis.

Lymphocytosis

Lymphocytosis refers to an increase in the concentration of lymphocytes in blood circulation. There are numerous causes of lymphocytosis. Young animals normally have higher concentrations of lymphocytes than older animals, and normal healthy young animals may have counts that exceed adult reference values. As discussed earlier in the section on neutrophilia, lymphocytosis is also a feature of epinephrine-mediated physiologic leukocytosis, resulting from redistribution of lymphocytes into the blood circulating pool. Epinephrine-mediated lymphocytosis may be more marked than neutrophilia, particularly in cats (lymphocyte counts of >20,000/μL are not uncommon). Antigenic stimulation may result in lymphocytosis, even in rare cases in marked lymphocytosis (up to approximately 30,000 cells/μL in dogs, and 40,000/μL in cats); however, this is not usually the case, even when there is clear evidence of increased immunologic activity in lymphoid tissues. In cases of antigenic stimulation, it is common for a minority of lymphocytes to have a "reactive" morphology—larger in size than small, mature lymphocytes, and with more abundant, deeply basophilic cytoplasm and incompletely condensed chromatin (Fig. 13-19). Just as glucocorticoid excess can cause lymphopenia, glucocorticoid

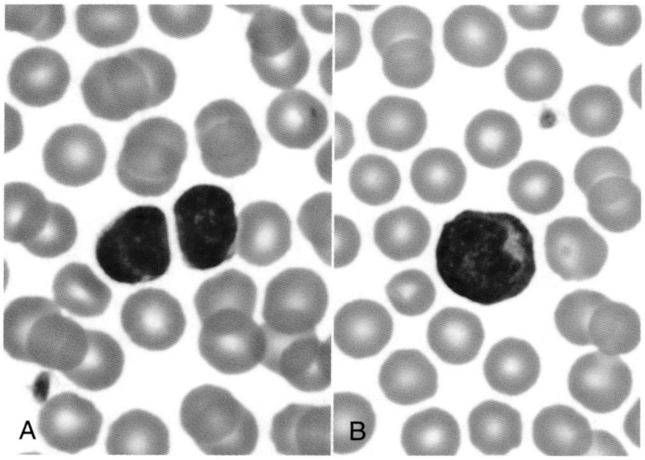

Fig. 13-19 Lymphocytosis (B), lymphocytes, canine blood smear. **A,** Small lymphocytes, the predominant type of lymphocyte in the blood under normal conditions. **B,** A reactive lymphocyte, characterized by mildly increased size and an increased amount of basophilic cytoplasm, from a recently vaccinated 16-week-old dog. Wright's stain. (Courtesy Dr. M.M. Fry, College of Veterinary Medicine, University of Tennessee.)

deficiency (hypoadrenocorticism) can cause lymphocytosis, or lack of lymphopenia under conditions of stress that typically result in glucocorticoid-mediated lymphopenia.

A condition known as *persistent lymphocytosis* (PL) occurs in approximately 30% of cattle infected with the bovine leukemia virus (BLV). The condition is defined as an increase in the blood concentration of lymphocytes above the reference interval for at least 3 months. This form of lymphocytosis is a nonneoplastic proliferation (hyperplasia) of B lymphocytes. In the absence of other disease, cattle with PL are asymptomatic. However, cattle infected with BLV, especially those animals with PL, are at increased risk to develop B lymphocyte lymphoma. (BLV and lymphoma in cattle are discussed in more detail later in this chapter in the section on Hematopoietic Neoplasia.) As in most other forms of benign lymphocytosis, the morphology of most lymphocytes is within normal limits in cattle with PL.

Secondary Abnormal Structure or Function of Blood Cells

The preceding section focused on abnormalities in the number of blood cells. There are also various acquired and congenital conditions involving abnormal structure or function of blood cells. This section briefly discusses abnormal blood cell structure or function occurring secondary to other underlying disease. Primary disorders of blood cells are discussed later in the chapter in the section on specific diseases,

Morphologic abnormalities detected on routine microscopic examination of blood smears may provide important clues about underlying disease processes. *Poikilocytosis* is a broad term referring to the presence of abnormally shaped erythrocytes in circulation. Web Table 13-1 lists conditions associated with and mechanisms involved in the formation of a number of specific types of erythrocyte morphologic abnormalities, and Fig. 13-15 shows some examples.

Similarly the acquired neutrophil morphologic abnormality known as *toxic change* (Fig. 13-20) reflects accelerated production of neutrophils as part of the inflammatory response. Features of toxic change include increased cytoplasmic basophilia, the presence of small blue-gray cytoplasmic inclusions known as Döhle bodies (often noted incidentally in cats) and in more severe cases, cytoplasmic vacuolation. Although not associated with impaired neutrophil function, toxic change occurs during granulopoiesis and thus is technically a form of dysplasia (e.g., Döhle bodies are foci of aggregated endoplasmic reticulum). Toxic change may accompany any inflammatory response, but in general the more marked the toxic change, the higher the index of suspicion for infection or endotoxemia. Other secondary changes to neutrophils may not be evident morphologically. For example, studies in humans and dogs have shown that individuals with cancer have abnormal neutrophil function (including phagocytic activity, killing capacity, and oxidative burst activity) before initiation of therapy. The clinical significance of this finding is not clear.

Platelet function disorders, also known as thrombopathies or thrombopathias, may be primary or secondary. Many conditions are known or suspected to cause secondary platelet dysfunction (hypofunction or hyperfunction) by altering platelet adhesion, aggregation, or by mechanisms that are not fully understood. Box 13-3 shows underlying conditions associated with secondary platelet dysfunction.

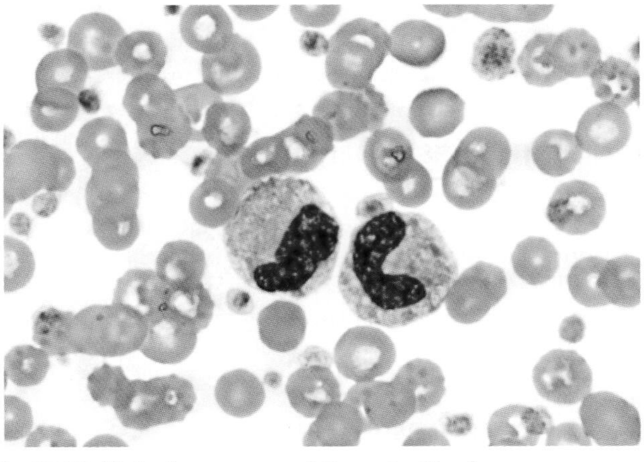

Fig. 13-20 Toxic change, neutrophils, canine blood smear. Two band neutrophils with basophilic, foamy cytoplasm indicate toxic change. This dog also has reactive thrombocytosis. Wright's stain. (Courtesy Dr. M.M. Fry, College of Veterinary Medicine, University of Tennessee.)

Methods for Gross and Microscopic Examination

Routine Tests

Routine diagnostic testing often provides great insight into disorders of the hematopoietic system. Information on this topic is available at evolve.elsevier.com/Zachary/McGavin/.

BOX 13-3 Conditions Known or Suspected to Cause Secondary Platelet Dysfunction in Animals

SECONDARY PLATELET HYPOFUNCTION

Underlying Disease

Uremia
Antiplatelet antibodies (also cause immune-mediated thrombocytopenia)
Infection (BVDV, FeLV)
Hyperglobulinemia
Increased fibrinolytic products
Hypoammonemia
Snake envenomation

Drugs or Other Exogenous Agents

Platelet inhibitors
NSAIDs—irreversible (aspirin) or reversible inhibition of cyclooxygenase
Colloidal plasma expanders (e.g., hydroxyethyl starch)
Other drugs and exogenous agents (many)

SECONDARY PLATELET HYPERFUNCTION

Underlying Disease

Infection (heartworm and RMSF in dogs, FIP, pasteurellosis in cattle)
Inflammation
Neoplasia
Taurine deficiency in cats
Nephrotic syndrome

BVDV, Bovine viral diarrhea virus; *FeLV,* feline leukemia virus; *FIP,* feline infectious peritonitis, *NSAIDs,* nonsteroidal antiinflammatory drugs; *RMSF,* Rocky Mountain spotted fever.

Additional Tests

Other tests that may help with evaluation of the hematopoietic system include bone marrow examination, aspiration cytology, direct antiglobulin test, immunophenotyping, and polymerase chain reaction and are discussed below. Information on this topic is available at evolve.elsevier.com/Zachary/McGavin/.

Hemostasis

Information on this topic is available at evolve.elsevier.com/Zachary/McGavin/.

DISORDERS OF DOMESTIC ANIMALS

APLASTIC ANEMIA (APLASTIC PANCYTOPENIA)

Aplastic anemia is a rare condition characterized by aplasia or severe hypoplasia of all hematopoietic lineages in the bone marrow and resulting cytopenias. The term is something of a misnomer because affected cells are not limited to the erythroid lineage (see the later discussion of pure red cell aplasia in the section on Immune-Mediated Disorders). Aplastic anemia is also known more accurately as *aplastic pancytopenia.* Destruction of hematopoietic stem cells or progenitor cells is recognized as a cause of the condition. Other proposed mechanisms include disruption of normal stem cell function because of mutation or perturbation of the hematopoietic microenvironment.

Many of the conditions reported to cause aplastic anemia in domestic animals do so only rarely, or idiosyncratically, and more frequently cause other hematologic or nonhematologic abnormalities. A partial list of reported causes of aplastic anemia in domestic animals includes the following:

- Chemical agents
  - Antimicrobial agents (dogs, cats)
  - Chemotherapeutic agents (dogs, cats)
  - Phenylbutazone (horses, dogs)
  - Bracken fern (cattle, sheep)
  - Estrogen (dogs)
  - Trichloroethylene (cattle, sheep)
  - Aflatoxin B_1 (horses, cattle, dogs, pigs)
- Infectious agents
  - Ehrlichiosis (dogs, cats)
  - Parvovirus (dogs, cats)
  - FeLV (cats)
  - Feline immunodeficiency virus (FIV; cats)
  - Equine infectious anemia (horses)
- Idiopathic (horses, cattle, dogs, cats)

Aplastic anemia occurs in both acute and chronic forms. Most of the chemical causes result in acute disease. As discussed in the earlier section on mechanisms of disease, severe neutropenia typically develops within 1 week of an acute insult to the bone marrow, after the bone marrow storage pool is depleted, and severe thrombocytopenia in the second week. The development of anemia is more variable, depending in part on how rapidly the marrow recovers from the insult, and on the RBC life span of the particular species. Severe neutropenia and thrombocytopenia predispose affected individuals to infection and hemorrhage, respectively. In addition to aplasia, pathologic bone marrow findings in animals with aplastic anemia may include evidence of necrosis, degeneration of hematopoietic cells, and an increase in phagocytic macrophages. Fig. 13-21 shows bone marrow aspirates from a dog with pancytopenia from acute 5-fluorouracil toxicosis, before and during recovery.

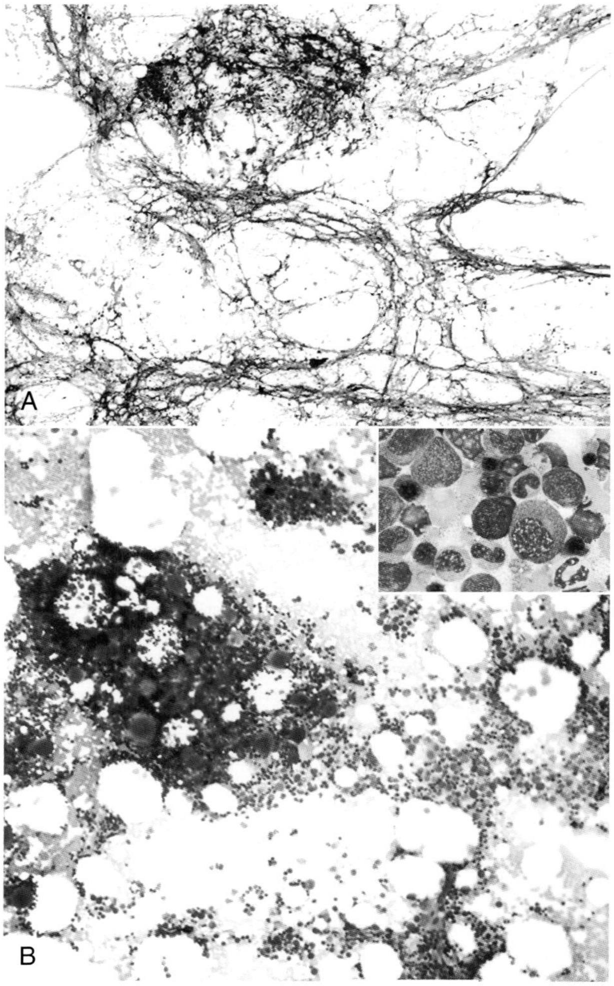

Fig. 13-21 Aplastic anemia, canine bone marrow aspirate. **A,** Bone marrow aspirate from a dog 8 days after ingestion of a toxic dose of 5-fluorouracil shows stromal cells but a lack of developing blood cells. **B,** Bone marrow aspirate from the same dog one week later, after resumption of hematopoiesis. *Inset,* Higher magnification of Fig. 13-22, *B* shows early- and late-stage erythroid and granulocytic precursors. Wright's stain. (Courtesy Dr. M.M. Fry, College of Veterinary Medicine, University of Tennessee.)

CONGENITAL DISORDERS

Many inherited or presumably inherited disorders of blood cells have been recognized in domestic animals, including rare or sporadic cases and conditions that are of questionable clinical relevance. This section and the later sections covering species-specific disorders are not comprehensive but instead focus on the more common, well-characterized, or recently reported conditions.

Erythropoietic Porphyrias

Porphyrias are inherited defects of enzymes involved in the synthesis of porphyrins, precursors of hemoglobin, and other heme proteins. Porphyrias result in accumulation of toxic porphyrin compounds. Congenital erythropoietic porphyria, transmitted as an autosomal recessive trait, occurs in Holstein and shorthorn cattle and is characterized by red-brown discoloration of teeth, bones, and urine caused by accumulation of porphyrins (see Fig. 1-75). Because of the circulation of the photodynamic porphyrins in blood, these animals have lesions of photosensitization of the nonpigmented skin and hemolytic anemia. All affected tissues, including erythrocytes, exhibit fluorescence with ultraviolet light. The premature destruction of developing and mature erythrocytes is caused by the accumulation within these cells of excess porphyrins. Bovine erythropoietic protoporphyria is an inherited disorder of heme synthetase, a terminal enzyme of the heme synthetic pathway, resulting in the accumulation of protoporphyrins in tissues and erythrocytes. It is inherited as an autosomal recessive trait and is confined to Limousin or Limousin-cross cattle. Photosensitivity is the only clinical manifestation of the disease; there is no anemia and no discoloration of teeth and bone. A congenital porphyria described in Siamese and domestic short-haired cats resembles congenital erythropoietic porphyria in cattle. These cats have brown teeth, photosensitization, and hemolytic anemia.

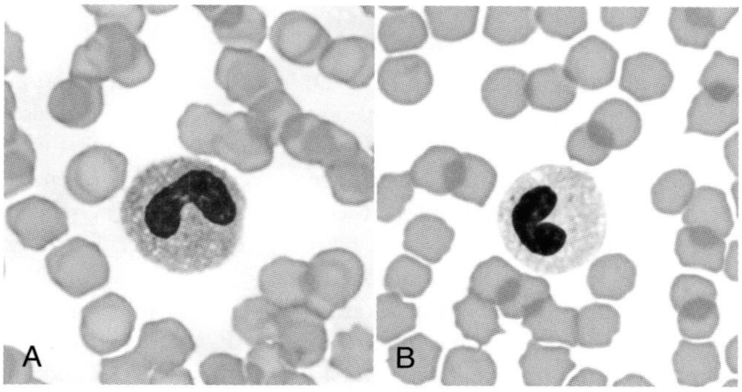

Fig. 13-22 Pelger-Huët anomaly, feline blood smear. Eosinophil **(A)** and neutrophil **(B)** have hyposegmented nuclei with mature, condensed chromatin. Wright's stain. (Courtesy Dr. M.M. Fry, College of Veterinary Medicine, University of Tennessee.)

Pyruvate Kinase Deficiency

Pyruvate kinase (PK) deficiency is an inherited autosomal recessive condition reported in many dog breeds and fewer cat breeds (Abyssinian, Somali, and domestic shorthair). The glycolytic isoenzyme that is deficient in erythrocytes of affected animals normally catalyzes the last ATP-generating reaction in glycolysis. Thus there is decreased production of ATP in PK-deficient individuals, which results in loss of normal membrane function and decreased erythrocyte lifespan. The disease is characterized by moderate to severe extravascular hemolytic anemia that is strongly regenerative. In dogs, PK deficiency typically also involves progressive iron overload, myelofibrosis, osteosclerosis, and cirrhosis. Dogs with PK deficiency usually die from complications of the disease between 1 and 5 years of age. In cats, PK deficiency is associated with milder hematologic abnormalities and is not associated with osteosclerosis; the prognosis is more favorable. Dogs with PK deficiency do not necessarily have the same genetic defect, so mutation-specific DNA-based assays are required. In contrast, a single DNA-based test is available to detect the common mutation affecting Abyssinian, Somali, and domestic shorthair cats.

Cytochrome b_5 Reductase Deficiency

Deficiency of cytochrome b_5 reductase (Cb_5R, also known as *methemoglobin reductase*), the enzyme that catalyzes the reduction of methemoglobin (Fe^{3+}) to hemoglobin (Fe^{2+}), has been recognized in many dog breeds and in domestic shorthair cats. It is probably an autosomal recessive trait. Affected animals may have cyanotic mucous membranes or exercise intolerance but are not anemic, usually lack clinical signs of disease, and have normal life expectancies.

Glucose-6-Phosphate Dehydrogenase Deficiency

Deficiency of the glycolytic enzyme glucose-6-phosphate dehydrogenase (G6PD), a common X-linked disease in people, has been reported in an American saddle bred colt with eccentrocytosis and persistent hemolytic anemia and in a partially deficient male dog without anemia or clinical signs.

Leukocyte Adhesion Deficiency

Information on this topic is available at evolve.elsevier.com/Zachary/McGavin/.

Pelger-Huët Anomaly

Pelger-Huët anomaly (PHA) is a condition characterized by lack of normal segmentation of the nuclei of mature granulocytes. This condition results in granulocyte morphology similar to that of band neutrophils in an inflammatory left shift; however, in the absence of any other disease process, animals with PHA should not have clinical signs or other laboratory findings indicating inflammation. PHA cells can be distinguished from immature forms of otherwise normal band forms on the basis of their mature chromatin pattern (Fig. 13-22). PHA has been described in dogs, cats, horses, and rabbits, as well as in humans. Prevalence is higher in certain dog breeds. In Australian shepherds, the mode of inheritance is autosomal dominant with incomplete penetrance. Most cases of PHA are the heterozygous form and probably of no clinical significance. In these cases, the shape of most granulocyte nuclei resembles those of band and metamyelocyte forms. A rare homozygous form of PHA has also been reported in rabbits and cats. It is associated with accompanying skeletal abnormalities and stillbirths or early mortality in these species (there are also rare reports of homozygous PHA in humans, without associated skeletal abnormalities or shortened lifespan). In homozygous PHA cells, granulocyte nuclei are round or oval. An acquired, reversible condition mimicking PHA, known as pseudo–PHA, is occasionally noted in animals with infectious disease, neoplasia, or in connection with drug administration.

Chédiak-Higashi Syndrome

Chédiak-Higashi syndrome (CHS) is a rare autosomal recessive condition characterized by recurrent pyogenic infections, bleeding tendencies, ocular and cutaneous hypopigmentation, and prominent cytoplasmic inclusions in blood cells. CHS has been described in several breeds of cattle and in Persian cats. The mutated gene encodes a protein called *beige* or *LYST* (lysosome trafficking regulator), the specific functions of which are still being investigated. Individuals with CHS have severely impaired cellular innate immunity because of neutropenia, impaired chemotaxis, and impaired killing by granulocytes and cytotoxic lymphocytes.

One of the classic features of CHS is a bleeding tendency caused by platelet dysfunction. Platelets in individuals with CHS lack the dense granules that normally contain key bioactive molecules involved in hemostasis, including platelet agonists, such as ADP and serotonin, and platelet aggregation in vitro in response to collagen, in particular, is severely impaired.

Glanzmann Thrombasthenia

Glanzmann thrombasthenia (GT) is an inherited platelet function defect caused by defective expression of the integrin $\alpha_{IIb}\beta_3$ (also known as GPIIb-IIIa). The $\alpha_{IIb}\beta_3$ molecule has multiple functions but is best known as a fibrinogen receptor that is essential for normal platelet aggregation. Bleeding tendencies vary widely between affected individuals, and bleeding tends to occur mainly on mucosal surfaces. The condition is characterized by an in vitro lack of response to all platelet agonists and severely impaired clot retraction. GT has been recognized in Great Pyrenees and Otterhound dogs and in a quarter horse, a thoroughbred-cross, and an Oldenburg filly. To date, all reported cases in animals have involved mutations to the IIb gene. Molecular testing is available to detect affected or carrier Great Pyrenees and Otterhound dogs and to detect the reported mutations in horses.

CalDAG-GEFI Thrombopathia

Conditions characterized by inability to relay signaling information in response to most platelet agonists have been described in basset hound, Eskimo spitz, and Landseer-ECT dogs and in Simmental cattle. The molecular basis involves mutations to the gene encoding the guanine nucleotide exchange factor, CalDAG-GEFI. Platelet receptor expression in affected animals is apparently normal. All reported mutations have been associated with a bleeding tendency.

TOXICOSES

Oxidative Agents

Rather than presenting an exhaustive list, this section describes some of the more commonly recognized oxidants that cause hemolytic anemia or impaired hemoglobin function in common domestic species. Oxidative insult may result in extravascular hemolysis because of phagocytosis of damaged erythrocytes by splenic macrophages, or in intravascular hemolysis if the damage is severe enough. In horses, red maple *(Acer rubrum)* toxicity is a well-characterized, potentially fatal cause of acute intravascular hemolytic anemia and methemoglobinemia. Ingestion of sufficient amounts of wilted or dried leaves or bark causes Heinz body formation, eccentrocytosis, severe intravascular hemolysis, and methemoglobinemia. Common postmortem findings include icterus, splenic hemosiderosis, splenomegaly, brown discoloration and swollen liver, and swollen kidneys that can be dark red to blue-black. Histologically, the kidneys have characteristic red-brown tubular casts (hemoglobinuric nephrosis).

Phenothiazine can cause Heinz body formation in horses. In ruminants, *Brassica* and rye grass are associated with Heinz body formation, and nitrite toxicity causes methemoglobinemia.

Copper toxicity is a well-known cause of acute intravascular hemolytic anemia in sheep and may also occur in goats and calves. The condition occurs in animals that have accumulated large amounts of copper in the liver. The copper is released under conditions of stress (e.g., shipping, starvation) and is believed to cause hemolysis as a result of direct interaction with membrane proteins, lipid peroxidation, formation of reactive oxygen species, and enzyme inhibition. Affected animals are often markedly icteric, and hemoglobinuric nephrosis is a classic postmortem lesion.

Onions and garlic are most commonly recognized as a cause of Heinz body hemolytic anemia in dogs and cats but can cause oxidative damage to erythrocytes in other domestic animals, including horses and cattle. Other causes of Heinz bodies in dogs include acetaminophen, benzocaine, naphthalene, phenylhydrazine, vitamins K_1 and K_3, and zinc toxicity. Other causes of Heinz bodies in cats include acetaminophen, benzocaine, methionine, naphthalene, propofol, and propylene glycol.

Snake Envenomation

Hemolytic anemia that results from snake envenomation has been reported in horses and dogs. Some venoms contain phospholipases that cause intravascular hemolysis; spherocytosis, consistent extravascular hemolysis, has also been reported.

NUTRITIONAL AND METABOLIC DISORDERS

Severe malnutrition is probably a cause of nonregenerative anemia in all species attributable to combined deficiencies of molecular building blocks, energy, and essential cofactors. By far the most commonly recognized specific deficiency that results in anemia is iron deficiency. Iron deficiency is usually not a primary nutritional deficiency but rather occurs secondary to depletion of iron stores via chronic hemorrhage. The most common route of loss is through the GI tract (e.g., a result of neoplasia, especially GI carcinoma or lymphoma, in older animals or hookworm infection in puppies). Chronic hemorrhage may also be caused by many other things, including marked ectoparasitism (e.g., pediculosis in cattle and massive flea burden in kittens and puppies), neoplasia in locations other than the GI tract, and bleeding diatheses. Rapidly growing nursing animals may be iron-deficient when compared with adults because milk is an iron-poor diet. In most cases, this has little clinical significance (and in fact is normal). An important exception is piglets with no access to iron, which may cause anemia, failure to thrive, and increased mortality. Neonatal piglets are routinely given parenteral iron (intramuscular injection of iron dextran) for this reason.

Other specific nutritional deficiencies causing anemia in animals are uncommon or rare. Copper deficiency can cause iron deficiency in ruminants, and may occur because of copper-deficient forage or impaired usage of copper by high dietary molybdenum or sulfate. It is believed that copper deficiency impairs production of ceruloplasmin, a copper-containing enzyme involved in GI iron absorption. Copper deficiency anemia, like iron deficiency anemia, is typically microcytic and hypochromic. Cobalamin (vitamin B_{12}) and folate deficiencies are recognized as causes of anemia in humans but are rare in animals.

INFECTIOUS DISEASES

This section covers infectious agents within the same genus that are recognized to cause disease in multiple species. Other infectious agents with more limited host specificity (for example, cytauxzoonosis in cats, feline and equine retroviruses) are covered in later sections on species-specific diseases. Throughout both sections, diseases are organized by taxonomy (protozoal, bacterial and rickettsial, and viral).

Babesiosis

Babesia spp. are intraerythrocytic protozoal organisms (piroplasmas) spread by arthropods (ticks, biting flies), transplacentally, and by blood transfusions. Evidence is accumulating that infection also is transmitted by dog fighting. *Babesia* spp. cause hemolytic anemia in horses, cattle, dogs, cats, and various nondomesticated animals. *Babesia* organisms are typically classified as large or small form, based on routine light microscopic morphology. Examples of large and small form organisms are shown in Fig. 13-23. *Babesia equi* and *B. caballi* infect horses and other equids in tropical and subtropical areas worldwide (*B. equi*, which also infects lymphocytes, is not considered a true *Babesia* but is phylogenetically more closely related to *Theileria* and *Cytauxzoon*). *B. bovis* and *B. bigemina* (small and large form organisms, respectively) are pathogenic *Babesia* spp. in cattle. These organisms have a worldwide distribution but have

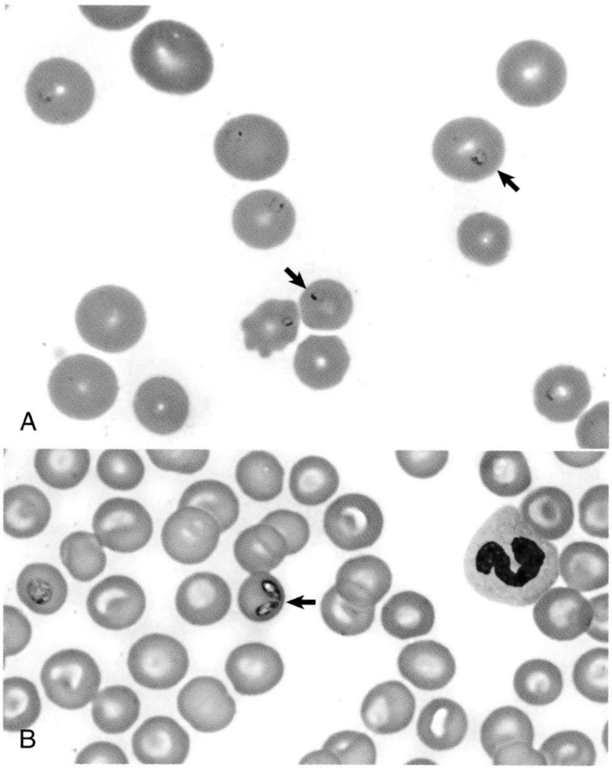

Fig. 13-23 Babesiosis, canine blood smear.
A, Small form *(arrows)* of *Babesia* (consistent with *Babesia gibsoni*). **B,** *Babesia canis (arrow)* organisms infecting erythrocytes. Wright's stain. (Courtesy Dr. M.M. Fry, College of Veterinary Medicine, University of Tennessee.)

been eradicated in North America. Other, less pathogenic *Babesia* spp. may also infect cattle. In dogs, large form and small form *Babesia* spp. infections are associated with hemolytic anemia. The predominant large form is *B. canis*, which has three subtypes (*canis, rossi,* and *vogeli*). *B. canis vogeli,* considered the least pathogenic strain, is the most common one in the United States (US). In some areas, particularly the southeastern US, the seroprevalence of *B. canis* is high, and many infected dogs are asymptomatic chronic carriers. There are also reports of dogs with other types of large form babesiosis, including one caused by an organism with highest molecular homology to *B. bovis*. Small form *Babesia* spp. in dogs include *B. gibsoni*, *B. conradae*, and a form known as the *Spanish isolate* (formerly *Theileria annae*). A number of *Babesia* spp. (*B. cati, B. felis, B. herpailuri, B. pantherae,* and others) have been reported in domestic and wild cats worldwide. Little is known about the epidemiology of feline babesiosis; the severity of disease ranges from asymptomatic to severe.

Babesiosis may cause both intravascular and extravascular hemolysis and is also associated with a wide range of other clinical signs. The wide variety of clinical signs is a result of variations in pathogenicity of the organisms and susceptibility of the host. Infection with highly virulent strains may cause severe multisystemic disease. In these cases, massive immunostimulation and cytokine release cause circulatory disturbances, which may result in shock, induction of the systemic inflammatory response, and multiple organ dysfunction syndromes. Mechanisms of hemolysis may include direct damage to the erythrocyte by protozoal proteases, immune-mediated destruction, and oxidative damage. In animals with acute disease, signs often include fever, lethargy, pallor, hemoglobinuria, splenomegaly, and icterus. Animals are often thrombocytopenic, presumably a result of immune-mediated destruction of platelets. They also may have lymphadenopathy. Less common signs include edema, ascites, signs of central nervous system dysfunction, renal failure, rhabdomyolysis, stomatitis, and gastroenteritis.

Babesia organisms can usually be detected on a routine blood smear in animals with acute disease. Infected erythrocytes may be more prevalent in capillary blood, so blood smears made from samples taken from the pinna of the ear or the nail bed may increase the likelihood of detecting organisms microscopically. Buffy coat smears also have an enriched population of infected RBCs. PCR testing is the most sensitive assay for detecting infection in animals with very low levels of parasitemia. At necropsy, animals dying of the acute disease have splenomegaly, jaundice, hemoglobinuria, swollen hemoglobin-stained kidneys, and subepicardial and subendocardial hemorrhages. The cut surface of the enlarged, congested spleen oozes blood. The gallbladder is usually distended with thick bile. A striking feature of *B. bovis* infections is congestion of gray matter throughout the brain, which is readily visible compared with the white matter. Parasitized erythrocytes are best visualized on impression smears of the kidney, brain, and skeletal muscle. Microscopic findings in the liver and kidney are typical of a hemolytic crisis and include anemia-induced degeneration, necrosis of periacinar hepatocytes and cholestasis, and hemoglobinuric nephrosis with degeneration of tubular epithelium. Erythroid hyperplasia is present in the bone marrow. In animals that survive the acute disease, there is hemosiderin accumulation in the liver, kidney, spleen, and bone marrow. In chronic cases, there is hyperplasia of macrophages in the red pulp of the spleen.

Theileriosis

Theileria spp. are tick-borne protozoal organisms that infect many domestic and wild artiodactyls worldwide. Infection is characterized by intralymphocytic schizonts and pleomorphic intraerythrocytic piroplasmas (merozoites and trophozoites). The latter stages closely resemble *Cytauxzoon* and small form *Babesia* spp. Recognized *Theileria* pathogens in cattle include *Theileria parva* (the cause of East Coast fever in Africa), *T. annulata* (the cause of tropical theileriosis in the Mediterranean regions, Middle East, and Asia), and *T. buffeli*, which has recently been documented as a cause of hemolytic anemia in the US. Possible mechanisms of anemia in theileriosis include invasion of erythroid precursors by merozoite stages and associated erythroid hypoplasia (as occurs with *T. parva* infection), immune-mediated hemolysis, mechanical fragmentation because of vasculitis or microthrombi, enzymatic destruction by proteases, and oxidative damage. Clinical signs in a severely anemic cow infected with *T. buffeli* included recumbency, fever, pallor, tachycardia, and lymphadenopathy. Necropsy findings included splenic hemosiderosis, edema of lymph nodes and the subcutis, thoracic and peritoneal effusions, and pneumonia.

Trypanosomiasis

Trypanosomes are flagellated protozoa that normally survive and are nonpathogenic in wildlife reservoir hosts. They are transmitted by arthropod vectors. Some *Trypanosoma* spp. are recognized as causing hemolytic anemia in animals in tropical and subtropical regions outside of North America. *Trypanosoma brucei* and *T. evansi* affect horses. *T. congolense* and *T. vivax* affect cattle. *Trypanosoma* spp. that cause anemia in other species include *T. simiae* in pigs and *T. brucei* in camels and horses. Trypanosomes also cause nonhemolytic disease (e.g., *T. cruzi*, the agent of Chagas' disease, or American trypanosomiasis) in many hosts, and nonpathogenic variants (e.g., *T. theileri* in cattle worldwide) are also recognized. Trypanosomal organisms do not infect erythrocytes

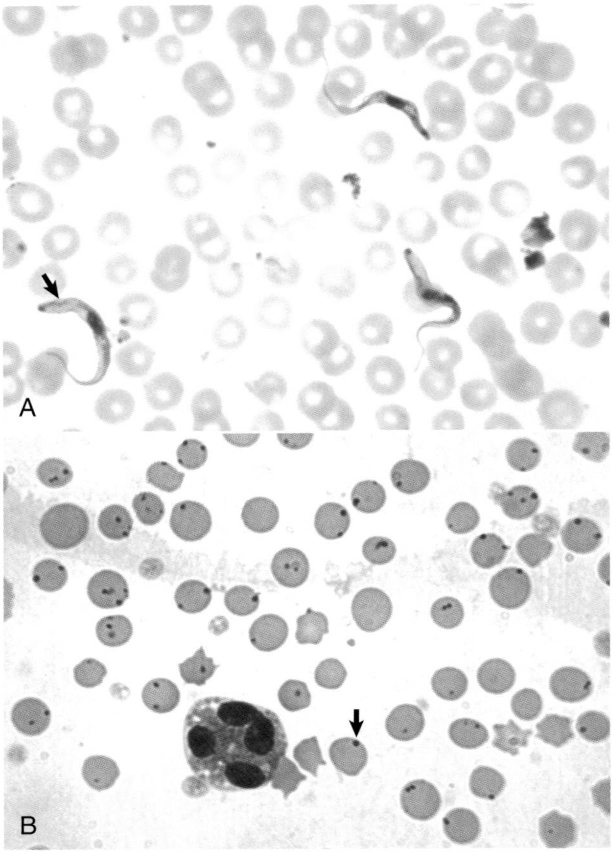

Fig. 13-24 Hemotropic parasites, bovine blood smear.
A, Trypanosomiasis. Trypanosomes are flagellated protozoa *(arrow)* characterized by an undulating membrane, kinetoplast, and nucleus. They may be identified in a wet mount made from the buffy coat portion of the packed cells. **B,** Anaplasmosis, *Anaplasma marginale.* Note the darkly stained organisms *(arrow)*, most of which are located on the edges of the erythrocytes. Anaplasmosis causes anemia mainly by immune-mediated extravascular hemolysis. (**A** courtesy Dr. M.D. McGavin, College of Veterinary Medicine, University of Tennessee. **B** courtesy Dr. J. Simon, College of Veterinary Medicine, University of Illinois.)

but rather exist as free trypomastigotes (flagellated forms with a characteristic undulating membrane) in the blood (Fig. 13-24, *A*) or as amastigotes in tissue. The mechanism of anemia is believed to be immune-mediated. Cattle with acute trypanosomiasis have significant anemia, which initially is regenerative, but less so with time. The extent of parasitemia is readily apparent with *T. vivax* and *T. theileri* infections because the organisms are present in large numbers in the blood. This is in contrast to *T. congolense*, which localizes within the vasculature of the brain and skeletal muscle. Cattle with *T. congolense* infections develop chronic debilitating disease; they have scruffy hair coats, appear "potbellied," and have fever, intermittent diarrhea, and exercise intolerance. Mortality is greater with *T. vivax* infections, usually because of intercurrent acute infectious diseases such as salmonellosis. Necropsy findings in cattle with trypanosomiasis include cachexia, generalized edema with increased fluid in body cavities, and generalized lymph node enlargement. Bronchopneumonia, a flabby heart, and serous atrophy of pericardial fat may be present. Liver and kidneys are symmetrically enlarged. Lymph nodes are enlarged up to four times normal size because of lymphoid hyperplasia, and most of the fatty bone marrow is replaced by red hematopoietic tissue. The spleen is enlarged because of lymphoid hyperplasia and is firm when incised.

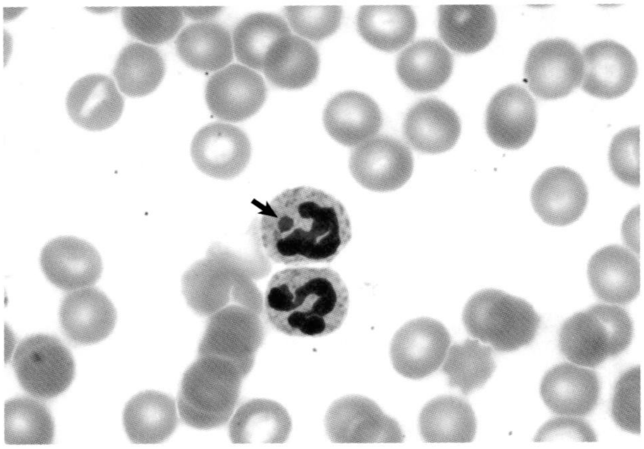

Fig. 13-25 Granulocytic ehrlichiosis, *Anaplasma phagocytophila*, canine blood smear.
The top neutrophil contains an inclusion *(arrow)* consistent with an *Anaplasma phagocytophila* morula. Wright's stain. (Courtesy Dr. M.M. Fry, College of Veterinary Medicine, University of Tennessee.)

Anaplasmosis and Ehrlichiosis

Anaplasma spp. are rickettsial organisms that may be transmitted by arthropod vectors (ticks, biting flies) or by blood-contaminated needles. Anaplasmosis is a cause of hemolytic anemia in cattle in tropical and subtropical areas of many parts of the world. *Anaplasma marginale*, considered the more pathogenic species, has a worldwide distribution. *A. centrale* is found in South America, Africa, and the Middle East. The genus names reflect the typical locations of the organisms when detected on examination of a blood smear, either on the periphery or more centrally within infected erythrocytes. A related species, *A. ovis*, affects sheep and goats in tropical and subtropical areas worldwide. Wild animals, such as deer, elk, and bison, may be latently infected and serve as reservoir hosts for *A. marginale*. Anaplasma organisms infect erythrocytes intracellularly.

Anaplasmosis causes anemia mainly by immune-mediated extravascular hemolysis. The severity of disease in infected animals varies with age. Infected calves under 1 year of age rarely develop clinical disease, whereas cattle 3 years of age or older are more likely to develop severe, potentially fatal, illness. The reason for this discrepancy is not clear. In clinically affected animals, common signs include lethargy or recumbency, pallor, and icterus. Animals dying of acute anaplasmosis have blood of low viscosity, pale to icteric tissue, an enlarged turgid spleen, and an icteric liver with a distended gallbladder. In animals with acute disease, it is usually easy to detect *A. marginale* organisms on routine blood smear evaluation (Fig. 13-24, *B*). However, in recovering animals, the organisms may be difficult to find. Surviving cattle become chronic carriers (and thus reservoirs for infection of other animals) and develop cyclic parasitemia, which is typically not detectable on blood smears. Splenectomy of carrier animals results in marked parasitemia and acute hemolysis. PCR testing is the most sensitive means of identifying animals with low levels of parasitemia.

Ehrlichiae are small, pleomorphic, Gram-negative, obligate intracellular bacteria that are transmitted by tick vectors. Some *Ehrlichia* spp. have a tropism for granulocytes, and morulae are sometimes found within the cytoplasm of neutrophils of affected animals (Fig. 13-25). Molecular analysis has shown that organisms previously considered to be distinct entities—*E. equi,* the agent of human granulocytic ehrlichiosis, and *E. phagocytophilum*—are genetically indistinguishable. All are now designated as *Anaplasma phagocytophilum*. Granulocytic ehrlichiosis occurs naturally in horses (*A. phagocytophilum*), dogs (*A. phagocytophilum* and *E. ewingii*), and cats (*A. phagocytophilum*). *A. phagocytophilum* survives within neutrophils by dysregulating key bactericidal functions, including the NADPH oxidase system, and delaying neutrophil apoptosis. Common clinical manifestations of infection include fever and signs referable to processes affecting cell or tissue types other than neutrophils (e.g., thrombocytopenia, anemia, immune-mediated polyarthritis). Neutropenia may occur in animals infected with *A. phagocytophilum*, but the mechanism is not clear. Judging from serologic evidence of exposure to *A. phagocytophilum*, most naturally infected dogs probably stay healthy.

Some Ehrlichieae have a tropism for mononuclear cells, but clinical manifestations are usually referable to other cell types or body systems. Morulae may be found in mononuclear cells of infected animals on routine examination of blood smears, and examination of buffy coat smears increases the probability of detecting the organism. In horses, *E. risticii*—the agent of Potomac horse fever (also known as equine monocytic ehrlichiosis)—infects monocytes and enterocytes and is primarily a diarrheal disease (see Chapter 7). In dogs, *E. canis*, the agent of canine monocytic ehrlichiosis, infects mononuclear cells. Infection with *E. chaffeensis*, the agent of human monocytic ehrlichiosis, has also been reported in dogs. Canine monocytic ehrlichiosis has acute and chronic forms. Acutely ill animals typically have a fever, lymph node enlargement, and splenomegaly. Thrombocytopenia and nonregenerative anemia are common findings. Untreated dogs recovering from acute disease develop a subclinical phase and may have persistent mild thrombocytopenia. A subset of these dogs develop chronic disease that may be debilitating and in some cases life threatening. Some studies indicate that German shepherd dogs with ehrlichiosis are predisposed to have particularly severe clinical disease. Severe cases are characterized by weight loss, lymph node enlargement, pyrexia, thrombocytopenia, and nonregenerative anemia. Thrombocytopenic animals may have severe bleeding tendencies. Some dogs with chronic disease develop pancytopenia. Necropsy findings vary with the stage of the disease. In the acute disease, there are widespread petechiae and ecchymoses, with splenomegaly and lymphadenomegaly. Chronically infected dogs are emaciated. The bone marrow is hyperplastic and red in the acute disease, but becomes hypoplastic and pale in animals with pancytopenia. Histologic findings include generalized perivascular plasma cell infiltration, which is most pronounced in animals with chronic disease. Multifocal, nonsuppurative meningoencephalitis, interstitial pneumonia, and glomerulonephritis are present in most dogs with the disease. *Ehrlichia* organisms are difficult to detect histologically; examination of Wright-Giemsa–stained impression smears of lung, liver, lymph nodes, and spleen is a more effective method for detecting the morulae in macrophages. Ehrlichiosis is often diagnosed on the basis of serologic testing, but PCR testing is more sensitive.

Anaplasma platys (previously called *Ehrlichia platys*) is a rickettsial organism that infects canine platelets, causing recurrent marked thrombocytopenia (the disease is also known as *infectious canine cyclic thrombocytopenia*). The disease is tick-borne and has been recognized worldwide. Evidence of megakaryocytic hyperplasia and organism-associated antigen within macrophages indicate that thrombocytopenia likely results from increased platelet destruction. Infection is generally considered to be asymptomatic, and morulae within platelets may be detected on blood smears incidentally, but there are rare reports describing more severe clinical signs in infected animals.

Clostridial Diseases

Certain *Clostridium* spp. may cause potentially fatal hemolytic anemias in animals. The mechanism of hemolysis involves a bacterial toxin (phospholipase C or lecithinase), which enzymatically degrades cell membranes, causing acute intravascular hemolysis. *C. haemolyticum* and *C. novyi* type D cause the disease in cattle known as *bacillary hemoglobinuria*. (The phrase "red water" has also been used for this disease and for hemolytic anemias in cattle caused by *Babesia* spp.) Similar naturally occurring disease has been reported in sheep and elk. In cattle, the disease is associated with liver fluke (*Fasciola hepatica*) migration in susceptible animals. Ingested clostridial spores may live in Kupffer cells of the liver for a long time without causing disease. However, when migrating flukes cause hepatic necrosis, the resulting anaerobic environment stimulates the clostridial organisms to proliferate and elaborate their hemolytic toxins, causing additional hepatic necrosis. Bacillary hemoglobinuria has also been associated with liver biopsy in calves. *C. perfringens* type A causes intravascular hemolytic anemia in lambs and calves—a condition known as *yellow lamb disease*, *yellows*, or *enterotoxemic jaundice* because of the characteristic jaundice. The organism is a normal inhabitant of the GI tract in these animals, but may proliferate abnormally in response to some diets. *C. perfringens* has also been associated with intravascular hemolytic anemia in horses with clostridial abscesses and in a ewe with clostridial mastitis.

Leptospirosis

Leptospirosis is recognized as a cause of hemolytic anemia in calves, lambs, pigs, and black rhinoceros. Specific leptospiral organisms associated with hemolytic disease include *Leptospira interrogans* serovars *pomona* and *ictohaemorrhagiae*. Proposed mechanisms of disease include immune-mediated (IgM cold agglutinin) extravascular hemolysis and enzymatic (phospholipase produced by the organism) intravascular hemolysis.

Leptospira organisms are ubiquitous in the environment. Infection occurs percutaneously and via mucosal surfaces and is followed by leptospiremia; organisms then localize preferentially in certain tissues (e.g., kidney, liver, and pregnant uterus). Leptospirosis can also cause many disease manifestations besides hemolysis (e.g., renal failure, liver failure, abortion, and other conditions) that are not discussed here.

In addition to anemia, common findings in animals with leptospirosis-induced hemolysis include hemoglobinuria and icterus. On necropsy, renal tubular necrosis, which occurs in part because of hemoglobinuria (hemoglobinuric nephrosis), may also be present.

Hemotropic Mycoplasmosis

The term *hemotropic mycoplasmas*, or *hemoplasmas*, encompasses a group of bacteria, formerly known as *Haemobartonella* or *Eperythrozoon* spp., that commonly infect RBCs of many domestic, laboratory, and wild animals. Hemotropic mycoplasmas affecting common domestic species are listed in Table 13-2. The mode of transmission is poorly understood but arthropods are believed to play a role; transmission in utero and through biting or fighting is also suspected. Effects of infection vary from subclinical to fatal anemia, depending on the specific organism, dose, and host susceptibility. Anemia occurs mainly because of extravascular hemolysis. Although the pathogenetic mechanisms are not completely understood, an immune-mediated component is highly probable. Hemotropic mycoplasmas (and nonhemotropic *Mycoplasma* spp.) induce cold agglutinins in infected individuals, although it is not clear whether these particular antibodies are important in

TABLE 13-2 Common Hemotropic Mycoplasmas in Domestic Animals

Host	Organism
Cattle	*Mycoplasma wenyonii* (formerly *Eperythrozoon wenyonii*)
Dog	*Mycoplasma haemocanis* (formerly *Haemobartonella canis*)
Cat	*Mycoplasma haemofelis* (formerly *Haemobartonella felis* large form or Ohio variant)
Cat	Candidatus *Mycoplasma haemominutum* (formerly *Haemobartonella felis* small form or California variant)
Cat	Candidatus *Mycoplasma turicensis* (to date, has only been identified by molecular methods)
Pig	*Mycoplasma suis* (formerly *Eperythrozoon suis*)
Alpaca	Candidatus *Mycoplasma haemolamae*

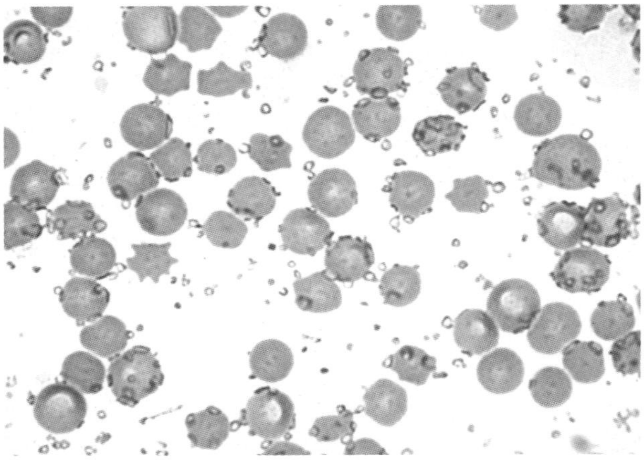

Fig. 13-26 Hemotropic mycoplasmosis, porcine blood smear.
Blood smear from a splenectomized pig infected with *Mycoplasma suis* (formerly *Eperythrozoon suis*). Note the small oval- to ring-shaped organisms attached to the surface of the erythrocytes and free in the protein of the blood smear. Wright's stain. (Courtesy Dr. J.F. Zachary, College of Veterinary Medicine, University of Illinois.)

the development of hemolytic anemia. Like other mycoplasmas, hemotropic mycoplasmas are small (0.3 to 3 μm in diameter), are Gram-negative, and lack a cell wall. They are epicellular parasites, residing in indentations and invaginations of the RBC surface. When detected on routine blood smear evaluation, the organisms are variably shaped (cocci, small rods, or ring forms) and sometimes arranged in short, branching chains (especially *M. haemocanis*). The organisms may also be noted extracellularly, in the background of the blood smear, especially if the smear is made after prolonged storage of the blood in an anticoagulant tube. A photomicrograph of hemotropic mycoplasma organisms in a peripheral blood smear are shown in Fig. 13-26.

Most hemotropic mycoplasma subspecies are more likely to cause acute illness in individuals that are immunocompromised or have concurrent disease. *M. haemofelis* infection is an exception, causing acute hemolytic anemia in immunocompetent cats. The disease in sheep and pigs has a seasonal incidence corresponding to the peak occurrence of biting insects. However, it can also occur at other times of the year as a recrudescence in a carrier animal secondary to another disease. In both sheep and pigs, unexpected death of one or two animals is often followed by anemia in other animals within the herd. *M. wenyonii* in cattle is less pathogenic than *M. ovis* and *M. suis* in sheep and pigs, respectively. Infection

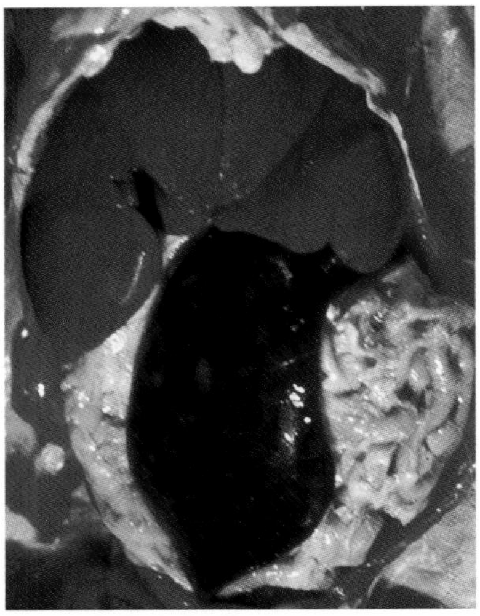

Fig. 13-27 *Mycoplasma haemofelis*, cat.
Note the splenomegaly, hepatomegaly, and icterus caused by infection of erythrocytes with this hemotropic parasite. Splenomegaly and icterus are the result of increased destruction (extravascular hemolysis) of infected erythrocytes. (Courtesy College of Veterinary Medicine, University of Illinois.)

with *M. wenyonii* appears to be widespread, but it rarely causes disease. Clinical signs in animals with acute disease include lethargy, fever, and pallor. Affected animals usually have mild to moderate hyperbilirubinemia and may be icteric. Animals probably remain chronically infected after recovery, even if treated with appropriate antibiotics. Chronically infected cattle, sheep, and pigs may have decreased production. Chronically infected dogs and cats are typically asymptomatic. In dogs, *M. haemocanis* infection is usually subclinical in immunocompetent animals but causes acute hemolytic anemia when infected animals receive a splenectomy. Two forms of hemoplasmas are known to infect cats. As mentioned earlier, *M. haemofelis*, the large form variant, causes acute hemolytic anemia in immunocompetent animals. Cats infected with the small form variant, which has the proposed name *M. haemominutum*, are typically asymptomatic or have only mild disease. Organisms are often but not always detected on routine blood smear examination in acutely ill animals. PCR testing is the most sensitive means of detecting infection in animals with low levels of parasitemia. In animals dying of hemotropic mycoplasma infection, the findings are typical of extravascular hemolysis, with pallor, icterus, and splenomegaly, and distended gallbladder (Fig. 13-27). Microscopic lesions in the spleen include congestion, erythrophagia, macrophage hyperplasia, extramedullary hematopoiesis, and increased numbers of plasma cells. Bone marrow has varying degrees of erythroid hyperplasia, depending on the duration of hemolysis.

IMMUNE-MEDIATED DISORDERS

Immune-Mediated Hemolytic Anemia

IMHA is a condition characterized by increased destruction of erythrocytes because of binding of immunoglobulin to cell surface antigens. It is a common, life-threatening condition in dogs and also has been described in horses, cattle, and cats. Although the clinical picture of IMHA is variable, it typically has an acute onset and causes severe anemia. Some studies have shown that certain dog breeds (cocker spaniels and others) are predisposed to develop IMHA, suggesting the possibility of a genetic component, and the disease is more common in young to middle-aged female dogs. In most cases the reactive antibody is IgG, and hemolysis is extravascular (i.e., RBCs with bound antibody are phagocytosed by macrophages, mainly in the spleen). IgM and/or complement proteins may also contribute to IMHA. Complement usually acts as an opsonin (C_3b) that promotes phagocytosis. However, formation of the complement membrane attack complex and resulting intravascular hemolysis is also a recognized mechanism and more likely to occur with IgM autoantibodies. Most immunoglobulins implicated in IMHA are reactive at body temperature (warm hemagglutinins). A smaller portion, usually IgM, are more reactive at lower temperatures and may lead to a condition known as *cold hemagglutinin disease*—ischemic necrosis at anatomic extremities (e.g., tips of the ears), where cooling of the circulation causes autoagglutination of erythrocytes and occlusion of the microvasculature. Typically, IMHA targets mature erythrocytes and is accompanied by a marked regenerative response. However, as discussed earlier in the chapter, immune-mediated destruction of immature erythroid cells in the bone marrow may also occur, resulting in nonregenerative anemia.

In veterinary medicine, IMHA is usually idiopathic (also called *primary IMHA* or *autoimmune hemolytic anemia*), and the specific trigger for the autoimmune reaction is not clear. Factors implicated in secondary IMHA include infection, drug administration, vaccination, neoplasia, and bee sting envenomation. Diagnosis of secondary IMHA is most often based on circumstantial evidence and exclusion of other known causes of hemolytic anemia, rather than on controlled experiments proving a direct causal relationship. Infectious agents affecting blood cells are discussed in more detail later. Drugs or chemicals associated with or suspected of causing IMHA in animals include antibiotics (cephalosporins, penicillin, and sulfonamides), levamisole, propylthiouracil, and the insecticide pirimicarb. Most drug-induced IMHA is believed to occur because of drug or drug metabolite interacting with the erythrocyte plasma membrane. Other proposed mechanisms include binding of drug-antibody immune complexes to the erythrocyte membrane, or induction of a true autoantibody directed against an erythrocyte antigen. A case of suspected vaccine-associated IMHA has been reported in a cow. Certain vaccines used in cows have been incriminated in the development of a specific form of IMHA in newborn calves: neonatal isoerythrolysis, which is discussed later. Retrospective studies investigating the relationship between vaccination history and development of IMHA in dogs have yielded conflicting results and are inconclusive.

Other common clinical findings in patients with IMHA include hyperbilirubinemia and splenomegaly (see Fig. 13-9), pyrexia, and inflammatory neutrophilia. These abnormalities vary in magnitude depending on the severity and duration of disease. Dogs with IMHA are also predisposed to develop hemostatic abnormalities (prolonged coagulation times, decreased plasma antithrombin [AT] concentration, increased plasma concentration of FDPs/D-dimer, thrombocytopenia, and DIC). The severity of postmortem lesions in dogs with IMHA, including ischemic necrosis within vital organs (liver, kidney, heart, and lung) and the spleen as a result of thromboembolic disease or hypoxia, has been shown to correlate with the severity of leukocytosis. Intravascular hemolysis (IVH) plays a relatively insignificant role in most cases of IMHA, but evidence of IVH (hemoglobinemia, hemoglobinuria) is noted occasionally, presumably in those cases in which IgM and complement are major mediators of hemolysis.

Neonatal Isoerythrolysis

A form of IMHA whose specific pathogenesis is well understood is neonatal isoerythrolysis (NI), a condition in which a newborn has colostrum-derived maternal antibodies, which react against its own erythrocytes. NI is common in horses (Fig. 13-28) and has been reported in cattle, cats, and some other domestic and wildlife species. In horses, this situation occurs as a result of immunosensitization of the dam from exposure to an incompatible blood type inherited from the stallion (e.g., transplacental exposure to fetal blood during pregnancy or mixing of maternal and fetal blood during parturition). A previously mismatched blood transfusion produces the same results. Some equine blood groups are more antigenic than others; in particular, types Aa and Qa are very immunogenic in mares. Severely affected foals become lethargic and weak as early as 8 to 10 hours after birth or at any time during the succeeding 4 to 5 days. They have pale, icteric mucous membranes and may have hemoglobinuria. Serum bilirubin concentrations are usually increased, and foals that die during a hemolytic crisis are notably icteric and have splenomegaly. In cattle, NI has been associated with vaccination with whole blood products or products containing erythrocyte membrane fragments. In cats, the recognized form of NI does not depend on prior maternal immunosensitization but on naturally occurring anti-A antibodies in queens with Type B blood. NI has been produced experimentally in dogs, but there are no reports of naturally occurring disease. NI can be prevented by typing the maternal and paternal blood and not allowing neonates from incompatible matings access to the mother's colostrum, or by not allowing animals with strongly incompatible blood types to breed.

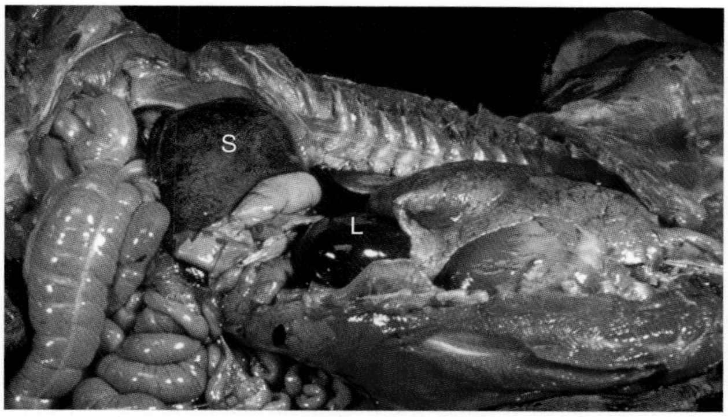

Fig. 13-28 Neonatal isoerythrolysis, foal.
Note the enlarged spleen *(S)* (also liver *[L]*) and icterus. The newborn foal had colostrum-derived maternal antibodies, which reacted against its own erythrocytes. Macrophages in the splenic red pulp remove erythrocytes whose membranes have bound antibody. (Courtesy College of Veterinary Medicine, University of Illinois.)

Pure Red Cell Aplasia

Pure red cell aplasia (PRCA) is a rare bone marrow disorder characterized by absence of erythropoiesis and severe nonregenerative anemia. Primary and secondary forms of PRCA have been described in dogs and cats. Primary PRCA is apparently caused by immune-mediated destruction of early erythroid progenitor cells, a presumption supported by the response of some patients to immunosuppressive therapy and by the detection of antibodies inhibiting erythroid colony formation in vitro in some dogs. Infection with FeLV subgroup C is associated with secondary erythroid aplasia in cats, probably because of infection of early stage erythroid precursors. Parvoviral infection has been suggested as a possible cause of secondary PRCA in dogs. Administration of recombinant human Epo (rhEpo) has been identified as a cause of secondary PRCA in dogs, cats, and horses, presumably caused by induction of antibodies against rhEpo that cross-react with endogenous Epo.

Experimentation with the use of species-specific recombinant Epo has produced mixed results. Dogs treated with recombinant canine Epo have not developed PRCA. However, in experiments reported thus far involving cats treated with recombinant feline Epo, at least some animals have developed PRCA.

Immune-Mediated Neutropenia

Immune-mediated neutropenia is a rare condition that has been reported in horses, dogs, and cats. The range of etiologies is presumably similar to that of the better characterized immune-mediated cytopenias (anemia and thrombocytopenia). The diagnosis may be supported by flow cytometric detection of immunoglobulin bound to neutrophils but is most often made on the basis of exclusion of other causes of neutropenia and response to immunosuppressive therapy.

Immune-Mediated Thrombocytopenia

Immune-mediated thrombocytopenia (IMT) is a condition characterized by immune-mediated destruction of platelets. There are numerous similarities between IMT and IMHA. IMT is a fairly common condition in dogs (it has also been described in horses and cats). It is more common in middle-aged animals, females, and perhaps some breeds of dogs. The disease is usually idiopathic and typically results in severe thrombocytopenia (often <10,000 platelets/μL), although less severe forms of the disease also occur. Affected animals have varying degrees of clinical bleeding tendencies. IMT also sometimes occurs together with IMHA, a condition known as *Evans syndrome.*

Underlying conditions associated with secondary IMT include infection (e.g., equine infectious anemia virus [EIAV] and ehrlichiosis), drug administration, neoplasia, and other immune-mediated diseases. Many types of infectious agents (viral, bacterial, fungal, and protozoal) have been associated with IMT, some of which may also cause thrombocytopenia by other mechanisms. Ehrlichiosis, for example, has been shown to elicit production of antibodies that are cross-reactive with platelet antigens in humans. Drugs suspected of causing IMT in animals include cephalosporins and sulfonamides.

Neonatal Alloimmune Thrombocytopenia

A form of immune-mediated thrombocytopenia, known as neonatal alloimmune thrombocytopenia, is recognized in neonatal pigs and foals. The pathogenesis of this disease is virtually identical to that of neonatal isoerythrolysis as a cause of anemia: a neonate inheriting paternal platelet antigens absorbs maternal antibodies against these antigens through the colostrum. In principle, a similar situation may occur after platelet-incompatible transfusion of blood or blood products containing platelets.

INFLAMMATORY DISORDERS

Hemophagocytic Syndrome

Hemophagocytic syndrome is a term used to describe proliferation of nonneoplastic (i.e., polyclonal), well-differentiated but highly erythrophagic macrophages. The condition is rare but has been recognized in dogs and cats. Unlike histiocytic sarcoma, which is neoplastic and in some forms also is characterized by highly erythrophagic macrophages, hemophagocytic syndrome is a secondary condition, occurring as a sequela of neoplasia, infection, or other underlying diseases. The macrophage proliferation and hyperactivation is a response to increased production of stimulatory cytokines occurring as part of the primary disease process. Macrophages are found in high numbers in the bone marrow and commonly in other tissues, including lymph nodes, spleen, and liver. Affected animals usually have cytopenias of two or more cell lines. Bone marrow findings reported in animals with hemophagocytic syndrome vary widely, ranging from hypoplasia to hyperplasia of cell lines with peripheral cytopenias, and may also include detection of macrophages containing phagocytosed hematopoietic precursor cells in addition to mature erythrocytes.

HEMATOPOIETIC NEOPLASIA

The term *hematopoietic neoplasia* encompasses a large, diverse group of clonal proliferative disorders of hematopoietic cells. This section is intended to help the student understand the basic biology (cell type, anatomic distribution, and biologic behavior) and diagnosis of hematopoietic neoplasia in veterinary medicine, with an emphasis on those forms that predominantly affect bone marrow, blood, and lymphoid tissue. Tumors of hematopoietic origin that predominantly affect other tissue, such as skin, are also mentioned briefly. Before listing specific diseases, it is worthwhile to consider the basic classification of hematopoietic neoplasia and mention some of the emerging diagnostic techniques used in veterinary medicine.

Hematopoietic neoplasia can be broadly classified as lymphoproliferative (lymphoid) or myeloproliferative (myeloid) disease, a distinction based on the fact that the earliest commitment of a pluripotent hematopoietic stem cell is to either a lymphoid or nonlymphoid lineage (see Fig. 13-3). Thus clonal proliferations of abnormal cells of lymphoid lineage are examples of lymphoid neoplasia, including the various forms of lymphoma (lymphosarcoma), lymphoid (lymphocytic) leukemia, and plasma cell tumors. Clonal proliferations of abnormal cells of nonlymphoid hematopoietic lineage (erythroid, granulocytic, monocytic and/or histiocytic, megakaryocytic), are considered myeloid neoplasms, including the various forms of myeloid (or myelogenous) leukemia, myelodysplastic syndrome, and histiocytic neoplasia. Mast cell tumors are not conventionally considered to be hematopoietic neoplasms, but in a technical sense they are also a form of myeloid neoplasia.

A number of techniques for diagnosing and classifying hematopoietic neoplasia are becoming increasingly available for routine use in veterinary medicine. For example, immunophenotyping refers to the use of antibodies recognizing specific molecules expressed on different cell types to determine the identity of a cell population of interest. Immunophenotyping on the basis of these lineage-specific or lineage-associated markers can be performed on histologic sections (immunohistochemistry), air-dried cytology smears (immunocytochemistry), or by laser analysis of cells in suspension in blood or buffer solutions (flow cytometry). Another emerging diagnostic technique is the clonality assay, a PCR test that can help identify neoplastic lymphoid proliferations on the basis of clonal rearrangements of genes encoding lymphocyte antigen receptors. In terms of practical application, the clonality assay is most useful in helping to distinguish lymphoid neoplasia from nonneoplastic lymphoid proliferations mimicking neoplasia.

In the last several decades, as new diagnostic techniques have become available, numerous systems for classifying hematopoietic neoplasia in humans have been proposed. These systems have been applied to veterinary medicine inconsistently but have helped to demonstrate the diversity of disease subtypes in animals. Some of these systems (the Rappaport and Kiel systems) did not attempt to correlate the classification of the neoplasm based on microscopic features with the clinical course of disease, whereas others (the Working Formulation for classification of lymphomas, sponsored by the National Cancer Institute) attempted to correlate survival data with morphologic criteria but did not take into account the cell of origin (i.e., B or T lymphocyte) of the tumor. A recently (2002) published system for classifying hematopoietic neoplasia in animals is an adaptation of the 2001 World Health Organization (WHO) system in humans. An effort is underway among a group of veterinary pathologists to coordinate the classification of hematopoietic neoplasia in humans and animals in a consistent, clinically relevant manner. The ultimate goal of this undertaking is to correlate pathologic findings (cell morphology, immunophenotype, tissue architecture, anatomic location) more precisely with clinical behavior of the neoplasm (prognosis, response to therapy).

The next section on hematopoietic neoplasia begins with leukemias and myelodysplastic syndromes, then covers the group of lymphoid malignancies known as lymphomas, and finishes by mentioning some other types of lymphoid and myeloid neoplasia.

Leukemia is an umbrella term referring to malignant hematopoietic neoplasms that originate in the bone marrow and typically have significant numbers of neoplastic cells in the blood. Hematopoietic neoplasms originating in the spleen, but primarily manifested in the blood, are also considered by some to be forms of primary leukemia. The term *leukemia* is also sometimes used to refer to other forms of neoplasia originating outside of the bone marrow or spleen, such as lymphoma, that progress to include significant bone marrow and blood involvement. For the purposes of this chapter, cases of secondary bone marrow or blood involvement are not considered leukemia but rather the "leukemic phase" of another primary neoplasm. Although primary leukemias usually have high numbers of neoplastic cells in circulation, this is not always the case. Some forms of leukemia (especially acute lymphoid leukemia in cats) have very low numbers of circulating neoplastic cells. This situation is sometimes known as *aleukemic leukemia,* although very close examination of blood smears usually reveals the underlying disease. The diagnosis may require confirmation by examination of the bone marrow, which in cases of leukemia contains disproportionately high numbers of neoplastic cells.

Leukemias are conventionally classified according to two criteria: as lymphocytic (lymphoid) or myelogenous (myeloid), based on the cell of origin, and as acute or chronic, based on the degree of differentiation of the neoplastic cells and their biologic behavior. This classification scheme is summarized in Table 13-3. Subcategories exist within each of these groups (e.g., lymphoid leukemias of B or T lymphocyte origin and myeloid leukemias of erythroid, granulocytic, monocytic, or megakaryocytic origin), as discussed further below.

Chronic leukemias are proliferations of well-differentiated cells and are typically indolent, slowly progressive diseases. Often the number of neoplastic cells in circulation is very high. It is not unusual for the concentration to be in the hundreds of thousands per microliter. Mild to moderate nonregenerative anemia is common, but other cytopenias are not usually present. With chronic leukemias, the lineage of the cells is easy to identify by examining a blood or bone marrow smear. The cells look normal, or relatively normal, under the microscope. However, this can pose a diagnostic challenge because it is often not easy to tell whether the cells are a malignant population (i.e., leukemia) or a benign, reactive population (as in the case of marked inflammatory neutrophilia, reactive lymphocytosis, or secondary erythrocytosis), particularly when the concentration of cells in the blood is consistent with either neoplastic or nonneoplastic disease. Diagnosis of chronic leukemia in veterinary species is thus typically one of exclusion. An exception is when the concentration of cells in the blood is so high as to reasonably exclude the possibility of nonneoplastic disease (e.g., the concentration of lymphocytes in cases of chronic lymphocytic leukemia often exceeds 100,000 cells/μL). Necropsy findings depend on the stage of disease. In advanced cases with marked organ infiltration with neoplastic cells, there is often uniform splenomegaly, hepatomegaly, and lymphadenopathy. The bone marrow is highly cellular (Fig. 13-29) and histologically is densely cellular with well-differentiated neoplastic cells. In lymph nodes, there may be follicular lymphoid hyperplasia and neoplastic cells in the sinuses and medullary cords. Similarly the spleen may have follicular lymphoid hyperplasia and accumulation of neoplastic cells in the red pulp. The liver may have accumulations of neoplastic cells in the sinusoids and periportal areas.

Chronic lymphoid leukemias (CLLs) are uncommon in veterinary species. The disease is rarely reported in horses and poorly characterized in cattle. In dogs, CLL is predominantly a disease of middle-aged to older dogs. Evidence indicates that most canine CLL cases are of T lymphocyte origin and that a subtype of granular T lymphocytes expressing CD8 (consistent with cytotoxic T lymphocyte lineage) is the most common form. Interestingly, most of these cases apparently originate in the spleen, with detectable bone marrow involvement occurring relatively late in the course of disease. In cats, evidence indicates that the majority of CLL cases have a T helper lymphocyte immunophenotype.

Chronic myeloid leukemias (CMLs) are rare in animals, with most reported cases occurring in dogs and cats. Types of CML reported in animals include chronic granulocytic leukemias of neutrophils, eosinophils, and basophils; chronic myelomonocytic

TABLE 13-3 Basic Classification of Leukemias

	Lymphoid	Myeloid
Chronic	CLL	CML
Acute	ALL	AML

ALL, Acute lymphoid leukemia; *AML,* acute myeloid leukemia; *CLL,* chronic lymphoid leukemia; *CML,* chronic myeloid leukemia.

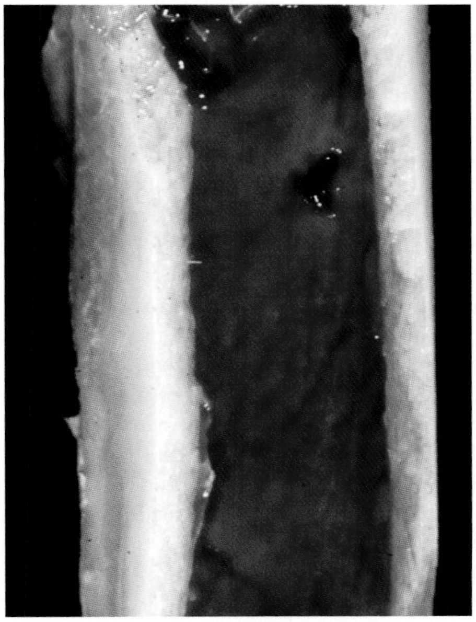

Fig. 13-29 Chronic leukemia, hypercellularity, bone marrow, dog. Grossly, the marrow consists entirely of hematopoietic tissue *(red)* and no fat *(yellow).* In this case, hypercellularity of the marrow is attributable to neoplastic proliferation, but hyperplasia may cause similar gross findings. (Courtesy Dr. B.C. Ward, College of Veterinary Medicine, University of Mississippi and Noah's Arkive, College of Veterinary Medicine, The University of Georgia.)

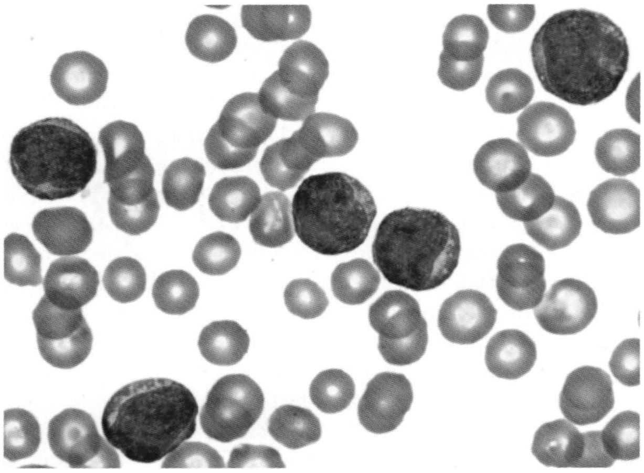

Fig. 13-30 Acute leukemia, canine blood smear. The specific lineage of the large, immature cells cannot be determined reliably based on routine staining. Wright's stain. (Courtesy Dr. M.M. Fry, College of Veterinary Medicine, University of Tennessee.)

leukemia; mast cell leukemia; essential thrombocythemia (CML of platelet lineage); and polycythemia vera (CML of erythrocyte lineage).

In contrast to chronic leukemias, acute leukemias are proliferations of poorly differentiated cells (Fig. 13-30) and typically have a rapid, aggressive clinical course. The distinction between chronic and acute leukemia is not always perfectly clear, either in terms of cell morphology or biologic behavior, and some cases fall "in the middle." Moreover, chronic leukemia may develop into a more acute form (presumably because of additional mutation), a situation sometimes referred to as "blast crisis." Acute leukemia has classically been defined by the presence of greater than 30% blast cells (large, immature cells) in the marrow or blood, although in human the threshold has been lowered to 20%. In general, the concentration of circulating neoplastic cells in acute leukemias does not tend to be as high as in chronic leukemias. Most animals with acute leukemia have cytopenias of two or more lineages, and pancytopenia (anemia, neutropenia, thrombocytopenia) is common. With acute leukemias, it is usually obvious from the presence of many large, immature cells in circulation that the patient has hematopoietic neoplasia. However, the cell of origin usually cannot be determined by routine microscopic examination because the cells are poorly differentiated. Identifying the specific cell type is best done by immunophenotyping and/or cytochemical staining. At necropsy, animals with acute leukemia have pale mucous membranes caused by anemia, and the bone marrow is highly cellular. Other findings depend on the degree to which neoplastic cells have infiltrated organs. There is often uniform splenomegaly, sometimes with infarcts. Histologically the bone marrow is densely cellular with poorly differentiated neoplastic cells. The splenic red pulp may be extensively infiltrated with neoplastic cells. The lymph nodes may have minor involvement of the medullary cords to diffuse involvement of the entire node.

Myelodysplastic syndrome (MDS) refers to a group of clonal myeloid proliferative disorders characterized by ineffective hematopoiesis. MDS does not meet the traditional definition of acute myeloid leukemia (AML) but is classically diagnosed based on these findings: less than 30% blasts in the bone marrow, cytopenias of more than one cell line, and morphologic evidence of dyshematopoiesis. Studies in people have shown that MDS also differs from AML on the molecular level (MDS is characterized by increased apoptosis compared with AML). MDS may lead to clinical illness and death as a result of the cytopenias and/or from transformation of the neoplasm into AML. MDS is rare in veterinary medicine, perhaps occurring most frequently in cats infected with FeLV.

The existing system for classification of AML and MDS in cats and dogs, an adaptation of the French-American-British (FAB) classification system in humans, was proposed by the Animal Leukemia Study Group (ALSG) in 1991 and generally has been accepted since then. However, the system does not include immunophenotyping or cytochemical staining characteristics, which have since become key aspects of classifying myeloid neoplasia in people.

The existing ALSG system in animals and the 2008 WHO classification system in humans are referenced in Web Box 13-2 and in the Suggested Readings list.

Acute lymphoid leukemia (ALL) is rarely recognized in horses and cattle. Cattle with lymphoid neoplasia caused by BLV infection often have high numbers of circulating neoplastic cells, but the disease is generally considered a form of lymphoma and is discussed next in the section on lymphoma. In a recent immunophenotypic study of 38 cases of ALL in dogs, 6 arose from B lymphocytes and 3 arose from $CD8^+$ granular T lymphocyte. Cats with ALL often have low numbers of neoplastic cells in circulation, and examination of the bone marrow may be necessary to make the diagnosis.

AML occurs most often in dogs and cats but has also been reported in other domestic and wild animals. In dogs, the majority of acute leukemias are of myeloid or probable myeloid origin (21 of 38 cases in one recent study). MDS is recognized most often in cats, especially in animals infected with FeLV, but has also been reported in dogs and horses.

Lymphoma (Lymphosarcoma)

The term *lymphoma* (also known as *lymphosarcoma* or *malignant lymphoma*) encompasses a diverse group of malignancies arising in lymphoid tissue(s) outside the bone marrow. There are many different forms, with notable variability in the following:

- Anatomic location—multicentric, alimentary, mediastinal/thymic, other
- Immunophenotype—B lymphocyte versus T lymphocyte versus non-B/non-T lymphocyte
- Cellular morphology—size, nuclear features, mitotic rate
- Histologic pattern—diffuse versus follicular
- Biologic behavior—from low-grade (indolent) to high-grade (aggressive) tumors

As mentioned previously, there is an ongoing effort to develop an updated system for classifying hematopoietic neoplasia animals. This effort includes a specific project focusing on classification of lymphoma in dogs. The principle underlying this effort is that each category should constitute a distinct disease entity based on cell morphology, immunophenotype, tissue architecture, anatomic distribution, patient signalment, and full clinical history. A critical component of this effort is to test interobserver and intraobserver variability of interpretation.

Lymphoma is often suspected on the basis of organomegaly (e.g., generalized lymph node enlargement) or abnormal ultrasound findings (e.g., thickened intestines with abnormal echogenicity). Initial diagnosis typically is made based on aspiration cytology, biopsy and/or histopathology, or both, of the affected organ(s). In both cytologic and histologic preparations, lymphoma is characterized by a monomorphic population of morphologically atypical lymphocytes. Histologically, lymphoma is also characterized by disruption of normal tissue architecture. In general, lymphomas of small, well-differentiated cells with low mitotic rates are low-grade (indolent, slowly progressive) diseases, whereas lymphomas of large, poorly differentiated cells with high mitotic rates are high-grade (aggressive, rapidly progressive) diseases (Fig. 13-31). The type of tumor and extent of disease may be characterized further by immunophenotyping and clinical staging, respectively. Immunophenotyping is done to determine whether a tumor is of B lymphocyte or T lymphocyte origin (this distinction cannot be made reliably based on routine staining) (see Fig. 13-31). It is not necessarily the case that B lymphocyte lymphomas have a more favorable prognosis than T lymphocyte lymphomas because lymphomas of both cell types occur in low-grade and high-grade forms. Clinical staging includes examination of aspirates of bone marrow and other enlarged organs (e.g., spleen, liver, and other lymph nodes).

In cases of advanced disease, there may be marked bone marrow and blood involvement and distinguishing lymphoma from lymphoid leukemia can occasionally be difficult. The distinction can often be made on the basis of immunophenotyping, especially for CD34, which typically is expressed by neoplastic cells in acute leukemias and not in lymphomas. Other laboratory findings with

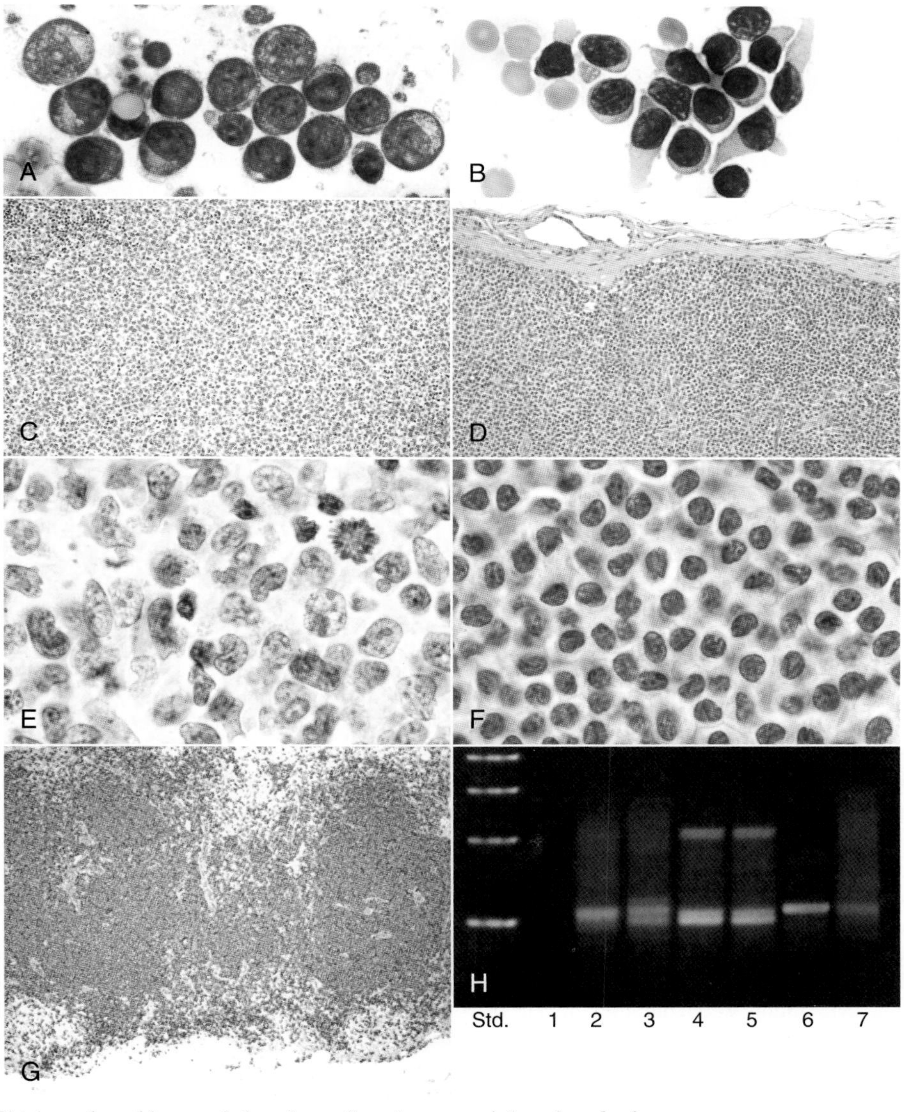

Fig. 13-31 Examples of high-grade and low-grade lymphoma (lymphosarcoma), lymph node, dog.
High-grade lymphoma: Fine-needle aspirate **(A)** and excisional biopsy (**C** and **E**) specimens. **C** and **E** are low- and high-magnification images, respectively, of the same specimen. Neoplastic lymphocytes are large and have large nuclei with dispersed chromatin and prominent nucleoli; a mitotic figure is evident at the top right of **C**. Low-grade lymphoma: Fine-needle aspirate **(B)** and excisional biopsy (**D, F,** and **G**) specimens, and results of polymerase chain reaction (PCR) testing of DNA extracted from the excisional biopsy. **D** and **F** are low- and high-magnification images, respectively, of the same specimen. In this sample, neoplastic lymphocytes are of small to intermediate size and have partially condensed chromatin; **G** shows a marked expansion of T lymphocytes. PCR results **(H)** confirm that these cells have a clonal T lymphocyte receptor gene rearrangement: Lane 1, negative control with no DNA; lanes 2 and 3, duplicates of a different case of T lymphocyte lymphoma; lanes 4 and 5, duplicates of this case; lane 6, positive control; lane 7, polyclonal control (i.e., normal). Wright's stain (**A** and **B**), H&E stain (**C-F**), immunostain for T lymphocyte marker CD3 **(G)**. (**A** courtesy Dr. M.M. Fry, College of Veterinary Medicine, University of Tennessee. **B** courtesy Dr. D.F. Edwards, College of Veterinary Medicine, University of Tennessee. **C-G** courtesy Dr. S.J. Newman, College of Veterinary Medicine, University of Tennessee. **H** courtesy Dr. W. Vernau, School of Veterinary Medicine, University of California, Davis.)

lymphoma are variable. Mild-to-moderate nonregenerative anemia is probably the most common hematologic abnormality. Lymphopenia is noted more frequently than lymphocytosis, presumably because of abnormal trafficking of normal, nonneoplastic lymphocytes. Hypercalcemia is often associated with lymphoma caused by production of parathyroid hormone-related peptide (PTHrP) by the neoplastic cells. Such paraneoplastic hypercalcemia (humoral hypercalcemia of malignancy) may lead to pathologic calcification and related complications (e.g., renal failure).

Necropsy findings in cases of multicentric lymphoma include enlarged lymph nodes that bulge on cut section and are gray-white to light tan or reddish (see Fig. 13-80). In advanced cases, the normal architectural distinction between the cortex and medulla is obliterated. Infiltration of spleen and liver can result in diffuse enlargement or nodules. In alimentary lymphoma, affected portions of the GI tract are thickened and may be nodular. The lesions may be ulcerated. Enlarged mesenteric nodes may coalesce to form large masses. The gross appearance of thymic lymphoma is a large, gray, soft mass in the cranial mediastinum (see Fig. 13-49). Renal lymphoma often affects both kidneys and is evident as bilateral diffuse renomegaly. Central nervous system and bone marrow involvement of lymphoma can be difficult to detect on necropsy because of the similar gross appearance of neoplastic and normal tissue. In any of the various forms of lymphoma, large masses may have areas of central necrosis.

Lymphoma is the most common hematopoietic malignancy in animals and has been reported in all the domestic species.

Lymphoma is uncommon in horses, representing 5% or less of all neoplasms. Multicentric lymphoma is the most common form, with lesions occurring more frequently in the abdominal and thoracic cavities than in peripheral lymph nodes. Cutaneous and other forms may also occur. Lymph nodes in different anatomic regions (e.g., superficial, mediastinal, and alimentary) are often similarly affected, and infiltration of liver and spleen is common. Reports of the frequency of concurrent blood involvement are highly variable. The alimentary form of equine lymphoma is a wasting syndrome, presumably because of involvement of the small intestine, resulting in malabsorption. Cutaneous lymphoma in horses, as in other species, is a chronic disease without blood or internal organ involvement. A recent report of 37 cases of equine lymphoma found T lymphocyte lymphoma to be more common than B lymphocyte lymphoma. Weight loss and ventral edema were the most common clinical signs. Laboratory abnormalities present in at least one-third of cases included hyperfibrinogenemia, hypoalbuminemia, hyperglobulinemia, anemia, thrombocytopenia, and neoplastic cells in circulation. In all tumors, normal nodal architecture was diffusely effaced. Extensive necrosis was common. Many of the tumors were composed of morphologically heterogeneous cells, and a smaller subset had marked infiltration with histiocytes and multinucleated giant cells. Most T lymphocyte tumors were composed of cells of small to medium size, and most B lymphocyte tumors were classified as T lymphocyte-rich B lymphocyte neoplasms.

In cattle, lymphoma is primarily a multicentric B lymphocyte disease of adults and is strongly associated with BLV infection and BLV-related persistent lymphocytosis. Approximately 30% of cattle infected with BLV develop nonneoplastic persistent lymphocytosis and of these, less than 5% develop lymphoma. The BLV-induced form of lymphoma is known as *bovine enzootic lymphoma.* BLV is a retrovirus that persists within lymphocytes for the life of the infected animal. Transmission of the virus is mostly horizontal caused by transmission of infected lymphocytes as opposed to free virus in secretions. Blood-sucking arthropods or other mechanical means of transferring small numbers of infected lymphocytes (such as contaminated needles) are the principal means of spread. BLV infection is more common in dairy cattle than in beef cattle, presumably because dairy cattle husbandry favors viral transmission. Incidence of infection varies widely between regions and between herds. Antibodies against viral antigen can be detected by an agarose gel immunodiffusion test, and some herds remain free of BLV by testing and culling infected animals. In addition to lymph nodes, lymphoma in cattle often involves other locations, such as abomasum, vertebral canal, kidney, heart, retro-orbital space, and uterus (see Fig. 13-86). Enlargement of superficial lymph nodes is common, and enlarged pelvic and abdominal lymph nodes are often found on rectal palpation. Involvement of the digestive tract and heart may cause vagal indigestion or diarrhea and congestive heart failure, respectively. Lymphoma of the central nervous system is most frequently manifested as posterior paresis or paralysis because of pressure by the extradural mass on the cauda equina or on the lumbar cord. Other sporadic forms of lymphoma not associated with BLV infection also occur in cattle, including thymic, multicentric, and cutaneous forms affecting young animals. The thymic form of sporadic bovine lymphoma is characterized by large cranial thoracic and lower cervical masses, respiratory distress, and weight loss in cattle less than 2 years of age. The sporadic multicentric form is characterized by disseminated disease in calves 3 to 6 months of age. Affected calves frequently have widespread lymph node enlargement in addition to hepatic, splenic, and renal involvement. Marked blood and bone marrow involvement may also occur. The cutaneous form is rare, occurs in young cattle, and consists of discrete cutaneous plaques or large scabby lesions.

In dogs, lymphoma is a common form of neoplasia, representing approximately 7% to 9% of all malignancies and the large majority of hematopoietic malignancies. No retroviral or other cause is known. Lymphoma is typically a disease of middle-aged to older dogs. Multicentric lymphoma with generalized lymph node enlargement is the most common form (80% to 85% of all cases of canine lymphoma), and the majority of these (approximately 80%) are intermediate- or high-grade tumors. Other less common forms of canine lymphoma include alimentary, thymic, and cutaneous forms, and sporadically occurring forms in virtually every conceivable location. Approximately 70% to 80% of canine lymphomas are of B lymphocyte origin. Although the remaining cases are mostly of T lymphocyte origin, "null" (non-B, non-T, possibly of natural killer cell origin) lymphomas also occur. Clinical signs may be referable to the specific organ systems affected but are usually absent or nonspecific when lymphoma is first diagnosed. Approximately 15% of dogs with lymphoma and approximately 40% of those with mediastinal lymphoma, are hypercalcemic. In the majority of canine lymphoma cases, significant blood or bone marrow involvement is not detected by routine methods on initial diagnosis but may be seen with advanced disease. Splenic and hepatic involvement is common in cases of canine multicentric lymphoma.

In cats, lymphoma is among the many hematopoietic abnormalities caused by FeLV, and the epidemiology of feline lymphoma has changed with the development of routine vaccination and testing for FeLV. Cats infected with FeLV are likely to develop lymphoma at a younger age, and are more likely to develop certain types of lymphoma, especially mediastinal and multicentric T lymphocyte forms, than FeLV-negative cats. These predispositions still apply, but the percentage of cats infected with FeLV has decreased dramatically. As a result, mediastinal (thymic) and multicentric forms of lymphoma, which used to represent the majority of cases, have become relatively uncommon. At present, approximately 80% to 90% of cats with lymphoma are FeLV-negative, and the majority of lymphoma cases are the alimentary form. Other less common locations in cats include mediastinal, multicentric, renal, and other extranodal sites. FeLV-positive cats with lymphoma still tend to be younger, and their tumors more often of T lymphocyte origin, than FeLV-negative cats. The large majority (>80%) of cats with mediastinal lymphoma, and approximately one-third of cats with multicentric lymphoma, are FeLV-positive. Mediastinal and multicentric forms, although less common now, are still more likely to occur in younger cats, whereas the alimentary form typically develops in older cats (>10 years of age). The neoplastic cell type also tends to vary by anatomic location. Alimentary lymphoma in cats is predominantly a B lymphocyte disease, whereas mediastinal lymphoma is predominantly a T lymphocyte disease (consistent with thymic origin). A subtype of intestinal lymphoma in cats, large granular lymphocyte (LGL) lymphoma, is predominantly a T lymphocyte disease with a highly aggressive biologic behavior. Unlike dogs, cats are usually clinically ill when lymphoma is first diagnosed. In addition to nonspecific signs, such as weight loss, anorexia, and poor grooming habits, cats often have signs referable to the affected organ systems. For example, animals with alimentary lymphoma often have chronic diarrhea and vomiting and may have palpable abdominal masses, whereas those with mediastinal lymphoma are often dyspneic.

Lymphoma is the most commonly reported malignancy in pigs and may be more likely to affect females than males. Multicentric lymphoma is the most common form of the disease in pigs. Lymph node enlargement is more common in visceral than peripheral nodes. Other commonly affected organs include spleen, liver, kidney, and bone marrow. Lymphoma often affects animals less than 1 year of age, and the mediastinal form of lymphoma tends to affect younger pigs more commonly than the multicentric form. A viral cause (C type viruses) for lymphoma in pigs has been suggested, but transmission studies are lacking. A form of hereditary multicentric lymphoma has also been reported in inbred herds.

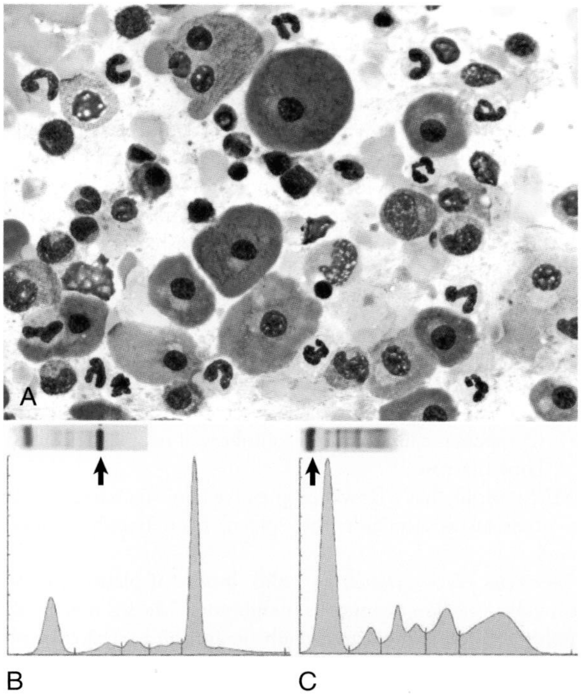

Fig. 13-32 Multiple myeloma and monoclonal gammopathy. **A,** Canine bone marrow aspirate. Many of the neoplastic plasma cells in the bone marrow aspirate have pink-tinged cytoplasm, the result of a high concentration of immunoglobulin. Wright's stain. **B,** Multiple myeloma, cat. Agarose gels and densitometry tracings showing results of serum electrophoresis. The serum has a high concentration of a monoclonal immunoglobulin (the dark band *[arrow]* on the right of the gel, corresponding to the tall peak on the right of the tracing). **C,** Normal cat. Agarose gels and densitometry tracings showing results of serum electrophoresis. The serum has a normal distribution of protein fractions, the most abundant being albumin (the dark band *[arrow]* on the left of the gel, corresponding to the tall peak on the left of the tracing). (**A** courtesy Dr. M.M. Fry, College of Veterinary Medicine, University of Tennessee. **B** and **C** courtesy Dr. S.A. Kania, College of Veterinary Medicine, University of Tennessee.)

Plasma Cell Neoplasia

There are two main forms of plasma cells tumors recognized in veterinary species: *multiple myeloma* (MM) and *plasmacytoma*.

MM is a malignant tumor of plasma cells that arises in the bone marrow and usually secretes large amounts of Ig. Blood involvement of the neoplastic cells is not a feature of the disease. MM is a rare disease in animals. Dogs are affected more frequently than other species, but MM has also been reported in horses, cattle, cats, and pigs. The hallmark laboratory finding in patients with MM is hyperglobulinemia, which occurs because of production of large amounts of Ig or Ig subunit by the neoplastic cells. This homogeneous protein fraction is often called paraprotein or M protein. Concentrations of other Igs are often decreased.

Diagnosis of MM is based on finding a minimum of two or three (opinions vary) of the following abnormalities:

- Markedly increased numbers of plasma cells in the bone marrow, especially in aggregates (Fig. 13-32, *A*). A threshold value of plasma cells constituting at least 30% of nucleated cells in the marrow has been proposed as a diagnostic criterion. The neoplastic cells composing the tumor may be well-differentiated plasma cells or poorly differentiated cells with increased anisocytosis and anisokaryosis, visible nucleoli, and multinucleation.
- Monoclonal gammopathy because of clonal production of Ig or Ig fragments by the neoplastic cells. Monoclonality is demonstrated by serum protein electrophoresis (Fig. 13-32, *B*) and can be characterized further using immunodiagnostic techniques (see later discussion). The term *gammopathy* is used because most Igs migrate in the γ-region of an electrophoresis gel, although some (especially IgA and IgM) may migrate in the β-region. Occasionally, biclonal or other atypical electrophoretic patterns may be seen with MM as a result of protein degradation, complex formation, or binding to other proteins, or when the tumor includes more than one clonal population. It is important to note that monoclonal gammopathy is not specific to MM but has also been reported in cases of B lymphocyte lymphoma and some nonneoplastic conditions such as canine ehrlichiosis or leishmaniasis. What appears to be a monoclonal pattern in the γ-region on routine serum electrophoresis may actually be oligoclonal (i.e., may include several Igs with a very similar migration pattern that are increased because of an immunologic response to antigenic stimulation). (This is unlikely to be the case with "spikes" in the β-region because nonneoplastic conditions typically do not result in high concentrations of IgA or IgM.) Definitively distinguishing monoclonal from oligoclonal patterns in the β-region requires immunoelectrophoresis or immunofixation using species-specific antibodies recognizing different Ig subclasses and subunits.
- Radiographic evidence of osteolysis. Work with human cell cultures has shown that osteoclasts support the growth of

myeloma cells and that direct contact between the two cell types increases the myeloma cell proliferation and promotes osteoclast survival.
- Light chain proteinuria. Free Ig light chains (Bence Jones proteins) are of low molecular weight and pass through the glomerular filter into the urine. These proteins do not react with urine dipstick protein indicators and are most specifically detected by electrophoresis and immunoprecipitation.

Other pathologic findings in patients with MM may include the following:
- Hypercalcemia, most likely caused by increased osteoclast activity
- Lesions associated with marked hyperglobulinemia (hemorrhage caused by secondary platelet dysfunction, renal amyloidosis, and hyperviscosity syndrome)
- Cytopenias caused by high numbers of neoplastic cells in the bone marrow

MM typically has a slowly progressive clinical course. Common sites of metastasis include the spleen, liver, lymph nodes, and kidneys.

Cutaneous plasmacytomas are solid tumors of plasma cell origin that involve the skin or mucous membranes. Masses may be single or multiple. These tumors are usually benign, and excision is usually curative, but more aggressive forms may occur. Cutaneous plasmacytoma is discussed in more detail in Chapter 17. The tumor type known as extramedullary plasmacytoma (EMP) is a malignant solid tissue tumor of plasma cells arising from sites other than the bone marrow. The tumor is rare in animals, occurring most often in dogs and also reported in horses and cats. In one study, there was a disproportionately high percentage of EMP cases in cocker spaniels. The tumors occur most frequently in the GI tract but may also occur in the trachea, spleen, kidney, uterus, central nervous system, and elsewhere. Grossly, the tumors may be multinodular or cause thickening of the intestinal wall. Metastasis to regional lymph nodes is common. As with MM, the neoplastic cells composing the tumor may be well-differentiated to poorly differentiated (Fig. 13-33). EMPs produce monoclonal immunoglobulins, and monoclonal gammopathy has been reported in some cases of EMP. If there is bone or bone marrow involvement of a malignant plasma cell tumor, it is considered to be MM. Amyloidosis is associated with EMP in many reports and may be useful in distinguishing extramedullary plasmacytoma from other tumors. The distinction between cutaneous plasmacytoma and extramedullary plasmacytoma is not always clear, and benign plasmacytomas of the skin have also been referred to as cutaneous extramedullary plasmacytomas.

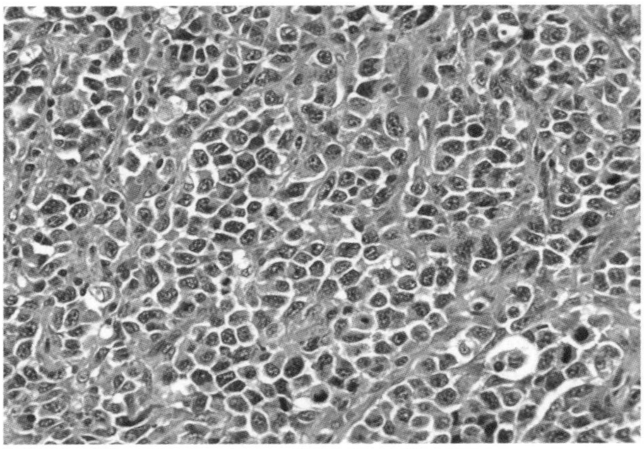

Fig. 13-33 Plasmacytoma, oral mucosa, dog. Note the moderately well-differentiated plasma cells arranged in small clusters separated by a fibrovascular stroma. H&E stain. (Courtesy College of Veterinary Medicine, University of Illinois.)

Histiocytic Neoplasia

Histiocytic sarcoma (HS) is an uncommon malignant neoplasm of histiocytic (macrophage or dendritic cell) origin. It occurs most frequently in the dog but has also been reported in the cat. There is a general belief that Rottweiler and Bernese mountain dogs are at increased risk for HS, although good epidemiologic data is thus far lacking. Some have called the disseminated form of this disease, with multiple organ involvement, by the name *malignant histiocytosis,* reserving the term *histiocytic sarcoma* for cases of single solid tumors, but there is an emerging consensus that the latter term encompasses both forms of the disease. The disseminated form of the disease has a rapid, aggressive clinical course. Sites commonly involved include the spleen, lung, lymph nodes, bone marrow, skin, and subcutis. Liver involvement occurs secondary to disease in the spleen. The solitary form of HS can occur at any of the aforementioned sites and also in joints (in close association with the subsynovium) or brain. Most cases of HS are of dendritic antigen-presenting cell origin, with a similar immunophenotype to (but dramatically different biologic behavior than) cutaneous histiocytoma. Fewer cases of HS are of macrophage cell origin. These malignant cells have an immunophenotype characteristic of resident macrophages in the splenic red pulp and the bone marrow, and frequently show marked phagocytosis of erythrocytes (hemophagocytosis). Dogs with this form of HS frequently have a hemophagocytic syndrome characterized by severe nonregenerative to mildly regenerative anemia (presumably a result largely of destruction of RBCs by the neoplastic cells), splenomegaly, hepatomegaly, and extramedullary hematopoiesis in the spleen and elsewhere. Microscopically, HS tumor cells are large, round-to-spindloid in shape and vary from relatively well-differentiated histiocytic morphology to cells with notable features of malignancy (Fig. 13-34).

Cutaneous histiocytosis (CH) and systemic histiocytosis (SH), nonneoplastic canine immunoregulatory disorders that share some clinical features of histiocytic malignancies, are covered in the section on canine immune-mediated diseases, and CH is discussed in more detail in Chapter 17.

Canine cutaneous histiocytoma, a benign neoplasm of epidermal Langerhans cell origin, and feline progressive histiocytosis, an initially indolent cutaneous neoplasm that is probably of dendritic cell origin, are discussed in detail in Chapter 17.

Mast Cell Neoplasia

Mast cell tumors (MCTs) of the skin and other organs are relatively common in animals, especially in dogs, and are covered in Chapter 6. Primary leukemia of mast cell origin is a rare form of myeloid leukemia. Mast cells normally are not present in circulation, but the finding of mast cells in the blood (mastocytemia) does not necessarily indicate myeloid neoplasia. In fact, one study found that severity of mastocytemia in dogs was frequently higher in animals without MCTs than those with MCTs and that random detection of mast cells in blood smears usually is not a result of underlying MCT.

Granulocytic Sarcoma

There are rare reports in animals of extramedullary solid tumors of granulocytic origin, known as *granulocytic* or *myeloid sarcomas.* These tumors are poorly characterized.

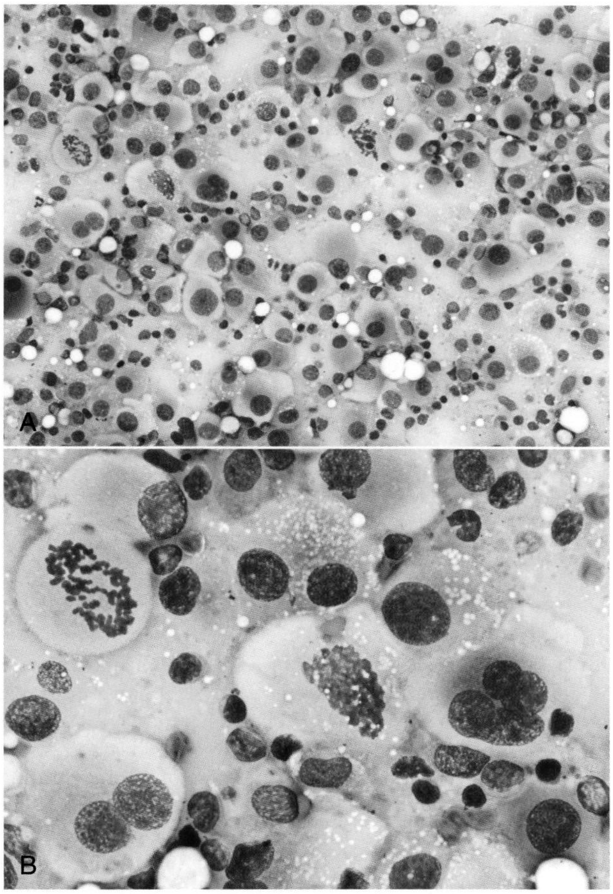

Fig. 13-34 Histiocytic sarcoma, canine mesenteric lymph node aspirate. The neoplastic cells are round cells with abundant gray-blue cytoplasm. Note the following features of malignancy: **A,** The low-magnification image shows notable variation in cell and nuclear sizes. **B,** The high-magnification image shows multinucleation, prominent nucleoli, and mitotic figures, as well as a background population of lymphocytes. Wright's stain. (Courtesy Dr. M.M. Fry, College of Veterinary Medicine, University of Tennessee.)

HEMOSTASIS

This section covers disorders of other components of hemostasis such as coagulation factors. Information on this topic is available at evolve.elsevier.com/Zachary/McGavin/. Platelet disorders are covered in the sections on disorders of bone marrow and blood cells.

CONGENITAL DISORDERS

Hemophilia

Information on this topic is available at evolve.elsevier.com/Zachary/McGavin/.

Other Inherited Factor Deficiencies

Information on this topic is available at evolve.elsevier.com/Zachary/McGavin/.

Other Inherited Coagulopathies

Information on this topic is available at evolve.elsevier.com/Zachary/McGavin/.

von Willebrand disease

Information on this topic is available at evolve.elsevier.com/Zachary/McGavin/.

TOXICOSES

Avitaminosis K

Information on this topic, including Web Fig. 13-2, is available at evolve.elsevier.com/Zachary/McGavin/.

DISSEMINATED INTRAVASCULAR COAGULATION (DIC)

DIC is a syndrome characterized by continuous activation of both coagulation and fibrinolytic pathways and is also known as consumptive coagulopathy. Information on this topic, including Web Fig. 13-3, is available at evolve.elsevier.com/Zachary/McGavin/ as well as in Chapter 2.

DISORDERS OF HORSES

CONGENITAL DISORDERS

Flavin Adenine Dinucleotide Deficiency

Flavin adenine dinucleotide (FAD) is a cofactor for cytochrome b_5 reductase, the enzyme that maintains hemoglobin in its functional reduced state, and for the glutathione reductase reaction that also helps protect erythrocytes from oxidative damage. Deficiency of erythrocyte FAD caused by abnormal erythrocyte riboflavin metabolism was recently reported in a Spanish mustang mare with methemoglobinemia and eccentrocytosis and has also been recognized in a Kentucky mountain saddle horse gelding.

INFECTIOUS DISEASES

Equine Infectious Anemia Virus

EIAV is a lentivirus that infects cells of the mononuclear phagocyte system in horses (also ponies, donkeys, and mules) throughout the world. Natural transmission is by arthropods, and the virus can also be transmitted transplacentally. Disease occurs in both an acute, potentially fatal form after initial infection, as well as a chronic intermittent form associated with recurrent viremia. Recurrent episodes happen mostly in the first year after infection, and tend to decrease in frequency and severity with time. Infection is lifelong and animals may become asymptomatic carriers. Viral antigen is found mainly within liver, spleen, and serum of infected animals, and also in bone marrow, lymph nodes, thymus, circulating mononuclear cells, and other tissues. EIAV causes anemia by both immune-mediated hemolysis and decreased erythropoiesis. Hemolysis is typically extravascular but may have an intravascular component during the acute phase. Decreased erythropoiesis may result from direct suppression of early-stage erythroid cells by the virus, as well as anemia of inflammation. Thrombocytopenia, likely caused by secondary immune-mediated destruction, is also a classic feature of acute EIAV infection and recurring febrile episodes. Clinical findings associated with viremic episodes include fever, depression, icterus, petechial hemorrhages, lymph node enlargement, and dependent edema. EIA infection is diagnosed on the basis of the Coggin's test, an agarose gel immunodiffusion test for the presence of the antibody against the virus.

Animals dying during hemolytic crises have icterus, anemia, and widespread hemorrhages. The spleen and liver are enlarged, dark and turgid, and they and other organs have superficial subcapsular hemorrhages. Petechiae are evident beneath the renal capsule and throughout the cortex and medulla. The bone marrow is dark red as a result of replacement of fat by hematopoietic tissue; the extent of replacement is an indication of the duration of the anemia. The severity of microscopic lesions is dependent on the chronicity of the disease, and they are most significant in the spleen, liver, and bone marrow. As would be anticipated, microscopic findings of the spleen are predominantly influenced by the number and activity of macrophages, which is a reflection of the duration of the disease and the frequency of hemolytic episodes. Hemosiderin-laden macrophages persist for months to years; therefore, large numbers are consistent with chronicity. Kupffer cell hyperplasia with hemosiderin stores and periportal infiltrates of lymphocytes are the most significant changes in the liver. Bone marrow histologic findings vary depending on the duration of the disease. In most animals, the marrow is cellular because of the replacement of fat by intense, orderly erythropoiesis. Granulocytes are relatively less numerous and plasma cells are increased. As in the spleen, hemosiderin-laden macrophages are present in large numbers in chronic cases. In more chronic cases, emaciated animals have serous atrophy of fat (see Web Fig. 13-1).

DISORDERS OF RUMINANTS (CATTLE, SHEEP, AND GOATS)

CONGENITAL DISORDERS

Congenital Dyserythropoiesis in Polled Herefords

A syndrome of congenital dyserythropoiesis and alopecia occurs in polled Hereford calves. The disease is often fatal. Hematologically, the condition is characterized by anemia that is nonregenerative to mildly regenerative (poorly regenerative given the degree of anemia). Bone marrow findings include marked erythroid predominance and morphologic abnormalities, consistent with ineffective erythropoiesis. The specific defect has not been identified.

Erythrocyte Band 3 Deficiency in Japanese Black Cattle

Japanese black cattle lacking band 3, an erythrocyte integral membrane protein that connects to the cytoskeleton, have moderate hemolytic anemia and retarded growth.

NUTRITIONAL AND METABOLIC DISORDERS

Hypophosphatemic Hemolytic Anemia

Marked hypophosphatemia is recognized as a cause of intravascular hemolytic anemia in postparturient dairy cows. Hypophosphatemia develops in these animals because of increased loss of phosphorus in their milk. Biochemical studies suggest that the mechanism of hemolysis involves decreased erythrocyte production of ATP, which may lead to compromised membrane and cytoskeletal integrity. An accompanying decrease in reducing capacity and increase in methemoglobin concentration have also been noted in experimental studies of hypophosphatemic hemolytic anemia in dairy cattle, suggesting that oxidative mechanisms may also contribute to anemia. Affected cows are anemic and hemoglobinuric. Gross postmortem findings include pallor, decreased viscosity of the blood, and discolored pale yellow and swollen liver and kidney. Renal tubular necrosis and hemoglobin pigment within the tubules is evident microscopically. Hemolysis has also been reported in association with hypophosphatemia in dogs and cats.

Water Intoxication

Calves with sporadic access to water sometimes drink excessively when water is available to the point where their plasma becomes hypotonic and osmotic intravascular hemolysis occurs. Hemoglobinuria is commonly observed in affected animals. The condition is rarely fatal.

INFECTIOUS DISEASES

Bovine Leukemia Virus

BLV is discussed in the earlier section on lymphoma.

Bovine Viral Diarrhea Virus

Thrombocytopenia, often severe, has been reported in association with acute bovine viral diarrhea virus (BVDV) infection in calves and adult cattle. Infection with type II BVDV has been specifically associated with a thrombocytopenic hemorrhagic syndrome. Calves infected with type II BVDV have also been shown to have impaired platelet function. Investigations of the mechanism of BVDV-induced thrombocytopenia have resulted in varying, sometimes conflicting, conclusions. More than one study has shown viral antigen associated both with bone marrow megakaryocytes and with circulating platelets. Evidence of impaired thrombopoiesis (megakaryocyte necrosis, megakaryocyte pyknosis, and degeneration) and increased thrombopoiesis (megakaryocytic hyperplasia, increased numbers of immature megakaryocytes) in the bone marrow has been reported in type II BVDV-infected animals, including concurrent megakaryocyte necrosis and hyperplasia in some experimental subjects. To our knowledge, antibody-mediated destruction of platelets has not been shown.

DISORDERS OF DOGS

CONGENITAL DISORDERS

Cyclic Hematopoiesis

Cyclic hematopoiesis is an inherited disorder of pluripotent hematopoietic stem cells, recognized in dogs and people. In dogs, the condition has an autosomal recessive inheritance pattern and is associated with dilute hair coat color. In dogs, cyclic hematopoiesis (also known as *lethal gray collie disease*) is characterized by predictable fluctuations in concentrations of blood cells that occur in 14-day cycles. The pattern is cyclic marked neutropenia and in a different phase, cyclic reticulocytosis, monocytosis, and thrombocytosis. Production of key cytokines involved in regulation of hematopoiesis is also cyclic. The specific lesion in cyclic hematopoiesis is believed to involve defective intracellular signaling but remains to be explained on the molecular level. Neutropenia predisposes affected animals to infection, and many die of infectious causes. Other related clinical manifestations include bleeding tendency, attributable at least in part to defective platelet function, and systemic amyloidosis, which occurs because of cyclic increases in concentration of acute phase proteins during phases of monocytosis.

Phosphofructokinase Deficiency

Inherited autosomal recessive deficiency of the erythrocyte glycolytic enzyme, phosphofructokinase (PFK), is described in English springer spaniel, American cocker spaniel, and mixed-breed dogs. The enzyme is also deficient in muscle tissue of affected dogs. Erythrocytes in PFK-deficient dogs have decreased ATP and 2,3-diphosphoglycerate production, and increased fragility under alkaline conditions. The disease is characterized by chronic, extravascular hemolysis with marked reticulocytosis. The marked regenerative response may compensate for the ongoing hemolysis, therefore affected animals are not necessarily anemic. However, acute intravascular hemolytic episodes may occur with hyperventilation and resulting alkalemia. There are three genes encoding PFK enzymes, designated M in muscle and erythrocytes, L in liver, and P in platelets. A point mutation in the gene coding for the M enzyme results in an unstable, truncated molecule. A single DNA-based test is available to detect the common mutation.

Erythrocyte Structural Abnormalities

A heterogeneous group of conditions, known as *hereditary stomatocytosis* because of the characteristic slit-shaped area of central pallor in RBCs on stained blood smears, has been described in several dog breeds. The clinical manifestations vary in affected animals, and the specific underlying defects have not been identified. In all cases, however, erythrocytes have increased osmotic fragility and decreased survival.

Other (presumably heritable) erythrocyte abnormalities in dogs that are not associated with clinical signs include elliptocytosis caused by band 4.1 deficiency or β-spectrin mutation, and familial macrocytosis and dyshematopoiesis in Poodles.

Scott-Like Syndrome

An inherited thrombopathy resembling Scott syndrome in humans, in which platelets lack normal procoagulant activity, has been recognized in a family of German shepherd dogs. Affected dogs have a mild to moderate clinical bleeding tendency characterized by epistaxis, hyphema, intramuscular hematoma formation, and increased hemorrhage associated with surgery. The specific defect in these dogs has not been identified on the molecular level, but involves impaired expression of phosphatidylserine on the platelet surface.

Breed-Related Platelet Abnormalities

Cavalier King Charles spaniels often have a lower than normal concentration of platelets, many of which are abnormally large (a condition known as macrothrombocytopenia). The molecular basis for this trait is a mutation in the gene encoding β1 tubulin. In general, affected dogs are asymptomatic. Cavalier King Charles spaniels have been shown to have abnormal platelet aggregation in vitro in some studies, although the clinical significance of these findings, including a possible causal relationship between platelet abnormalities and mitral valve disease in this breed, is not clear.

Greyhounds tend to have lower concentrations of circulating platelets than other dog breeds, although this is not of any known clinical significance. Other Greyhound traits include lower neutrophil and plasma protein concentrations and higher hematocrits than other dog breeds.

IMMUNE-MEDIATED DISORDERS

Cutaneous and Systemic Histiocytoses

CH, a rare immunoregulatory disorder caused by proliferation of activated dermal dendritic cells, is discussed in more detail in Chapter 17. SH is a familial disorder of Bernese mountain dogs (also found sporadically in other breeds) characterized by large, dense proliferations of activated interstitial dendritic cells in multiple tissues, including skin, peripheral lymph nodes, and ocular and nasal mucosa. The proliferating cells are immunophenotypically identical to those in CH, and the angiocentric skin lesions in SH are histologically identical to those in CH. Lesions of SH in locations other than skin are also angiocentric infiltrates consisting mostly of histiocytes and lymphocytes.

DISORDERS OF CATS

CONGENITAL DISORDERS

Increased Erythrocyte Osmotic Fragility

A condition characterized by increased erythrocyte osmotic fragility has been described in Abyssinian and Somali cats. The specific defect has not been identified, but pyruvate kinase deficiency (which has been reported in these breeds) was excluded as the cause. Affected cats have chronic intermittent severe hemolytic anemia and often have other lesions secondary to hemolytic anemia (e.g., splenomegaly and hyperbilirubinemia).

INFECTIOUS DISEASES

Cytauxzoonosis

Cytauxzoon felis is a protozoal organism causing severe, often fatal, disease in cats. Cytauxzoonosis in domestic cats is relatively common in the South Central United States, particularly during summer months. Bobcats (*Lynx rufus)*, and perhaps other wild felids, are believed to be the reservoir host. They are usually asymptomatic, with persistent parasitemia and transient schizogony. *Cytauxzoon felis* is transmitted by a tick vector, *Dermacentor variabilis*, which is probably essential for infectivity of the organism. Cytauxzoonosis has a schizogenous phase involving macrophages throughout the body (especially liver, spleen, lung, lymph nodes, and bone marrow) that causes systemic illness, and an erythrocytic phase that causes anemia of variable severity. Schizont-containing macrophages (Fig. 13-35) enlarge and accumulate within the walls of veins, eventually causing occlusion of the vessels. Merozoites are released and enter erythrocytes. Parasitemia develops relatively late in the course of infection. The signet ring–shaped erythrocytic inclusions (piroplasmas) of *Cytauxzoon felis* closely resemble small form *Babesia* (see Fig. 13-23, *A*) and some *Theileria* organisms. Affected cats typically become acutely ill with fever, pallor, and icterus and usually die within 2 to 3 days. For many years, cytauxzoonosis was considered to be almost always fatal. However, a recent report, in which numerous cats from a subregion of the endemic area in the United States survived infection with an organism with greater than 99% homology to *Cytauxzoon felis,* suggests the emergence of a less virulent strain. In affected cats, erythrophagocytosis is also often a prominent finding in tissue with the schizogenous phase.

Feline Leukemia Virus

FeLV is an oncogenic, immunosuppressive lentivirus associated with hematologic abnormalities of widely varying type and severity, including anemia in most infected cats. Manifestations of disease caused by FeLV infection vary depending on dose, viral genetics, and host factors, but normal hematopoiesis is probably suppressed to some degree in all cases. The virus infects hematopoietic precursor cells soon after the animal is exposed and continues to replicate in hematopoietic and lymphatic tissue of animals that remain persistently viremic. Persistently viremic cats are immunosuppressed

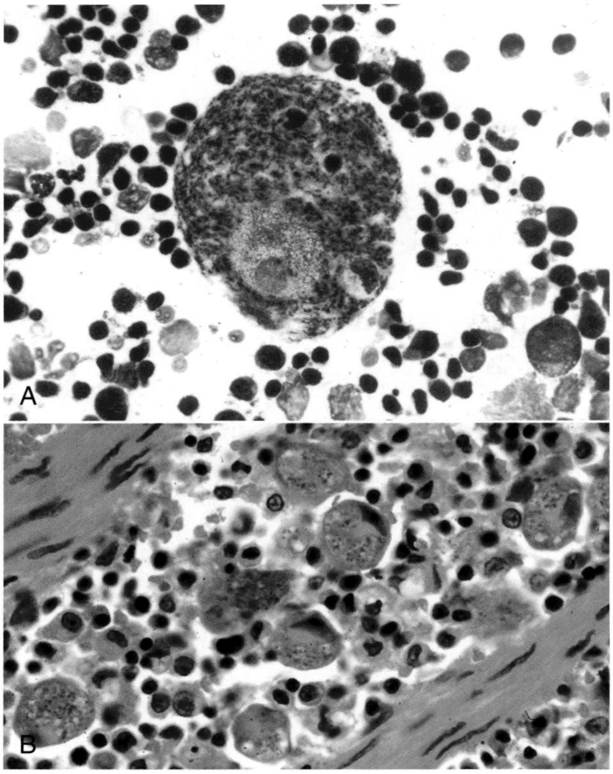

Fig. 13-35 Cytauxzoonosis, tissue aspirates, cat.
A, Lymph node aspirate. A large macrophage *(center of figure)* is laden with schizonts of *Cytauxzoon felis.* Wright's stain. **B,** Splenic macrophages are filled with *Cytauxzoon* organisms. H&E stain. (**A** courtesy Dr. D.F. Edwards, College of Veterinary Medicine, University of Tennessee. **B** courtesy Dr. A.R. Doster, University of Nebraska; and Noah's Arkive, College of Veterinary Medicine, The University of Georgia.)

and are prone to developing other diseases, including infectious diseases, bone marrow disorders, and lymphoma (lymphosarcoma).

FeLV-induced anemia is usually nonregenerative, presumably caused by direct effects of the virus on infected erythroid cells. However, macrocytosis and metarubricytosis (the presence of nucleated RBC precursors in circulation) are often noted in the absence of significant reticulocytosis—findings consistent with dyserythropoiesis, although the exact mechanism is not clear. Bone marrow of cats with FeLV-induced anemia often has evidence of arrested or disordered maturation of hematopoietic precursors. The relatively uncommon subgroup C viruses are associated with erythroid aplasia, probably because of infection of early stage erythroid precursors. Regenerative anemia may also occur with FeLV infection, often because of coinfection with *Mycoplasma haemofelis.*

FeLV infects hematopoietic cells and can produce a wide array of hematologic and other disease manifestations. FeLV may be detected in megakaryocytes and platelets in infected cats, and may result in platelet abnormalities, including thrombocytopenia, thrombocytosis, increased platelet size, and decreased function. Proposed mechanisms of FeLV-induced thrombocytopenia include direct cytopathic effects, myelophthisis, and immune-mediated destruction. Platelet life span and function have been shown to be decreased in FeLV-positive cats.

Feline Immunodeficiency Virus

FIV, another feline lentivirus, is associated with anemia in a minority of infected cats. Immunosuppressive effects of FIV from thymic depletion are discussed elsewhere. It is generally accepted that anemia does not result directly from FIV infection but instead develops because of concurrent disease such as co-infection with FeLV or hemotropic mycoplasma, other infection, or malignancy. The severity and type of anemia in FIV-infected cats depends on the other specific disease processes involved.

LYMPHATIC SYSTEM

The philosophy of this book is to describe the response of an organ or tissue to injury, based on its anatomic components and cell types. This approach works well with most organs and facilitates the reader's understanding of the pathologic processes. However, in the case of the lymphatic system, in which both the anatomic structures and immunologic functions are complex and interrelated, it is more difficult. Chapter 5 on the diseases of immunity describes some of these processes and to reduce repetition, the reader is referred to that chapter where appropriate. To understand the sequence of events in both normal and pathologic secondary lymphoid organs, it is desirable that the reader have an understanding of the three-dimensional anatomy of the spleen and lymph node, and particularly the pathways of the flow of blood, lymph, and lymphocytes through the lymph node and blood and lymphocytes through the spleen.

Under the classification of the *Nomina Anatomica Veterinaria,* the thymus, spleen, lymph nodes, and lymph nodules are part of the lymphatic system. They are also part of the immune system. Primary lymphoid organs are defined as the sites at which the component cells of the immune system (B and T lymphocytes) are formed. In most animals, there are two primary lymphoid organs (thymus and bone marrow), but in ruminants and birds, Peyer's patches (ileum) and the bursa of Fabricius, respectively, are sites of B lymphocyte production. The spleen, lymph nodes, and lymph nodules are secondary lymphoid organs and are responsible for the immune responses (i.e., production of antibody and cell-mediated immunity). Thus ruminant Peyer's patches are both primary and secondary lymphoid organs. However, because the spleen and lymph nodes contain numerous cells of the monocyte-macrophage system, they also have functions outside those of the immune system such as phagocytosis of particulate material (e.g., carbon, bacteria, and in the case of the spleen, senescent and altered erythrocytes).

The bone marrow is described in the first section of this chapter. The remaining primary lymphoid organ, the thymus, is described first in this section, followed by the secondary lymphoid organs: spleen, lymph nodes, and diffuse and nodular lymphatic tissues.

THYMUS

STRUCTURE AND FUNCTION

The thymus is essential for the development and function of the immune system, specifically for the differentiation, selection, and maturation of T lymphocytes. This is described in detail in Chapter 5, and the interrelationship of the T lymphocytes with the components of the thymus are described in this section. The shape and location of the thymus vary among young domestic animals. In ruminants and pigs, the thymus has two lobes: cervical and thoracic. The cervical lobe is large and extends along the lateral surfaces of the cervical trachea. The size of the cervical lobe varies in cats and horses but is usually small. Dogs do not have a cervical lobe. The thoracic lobe is present in all domestic animals and lies

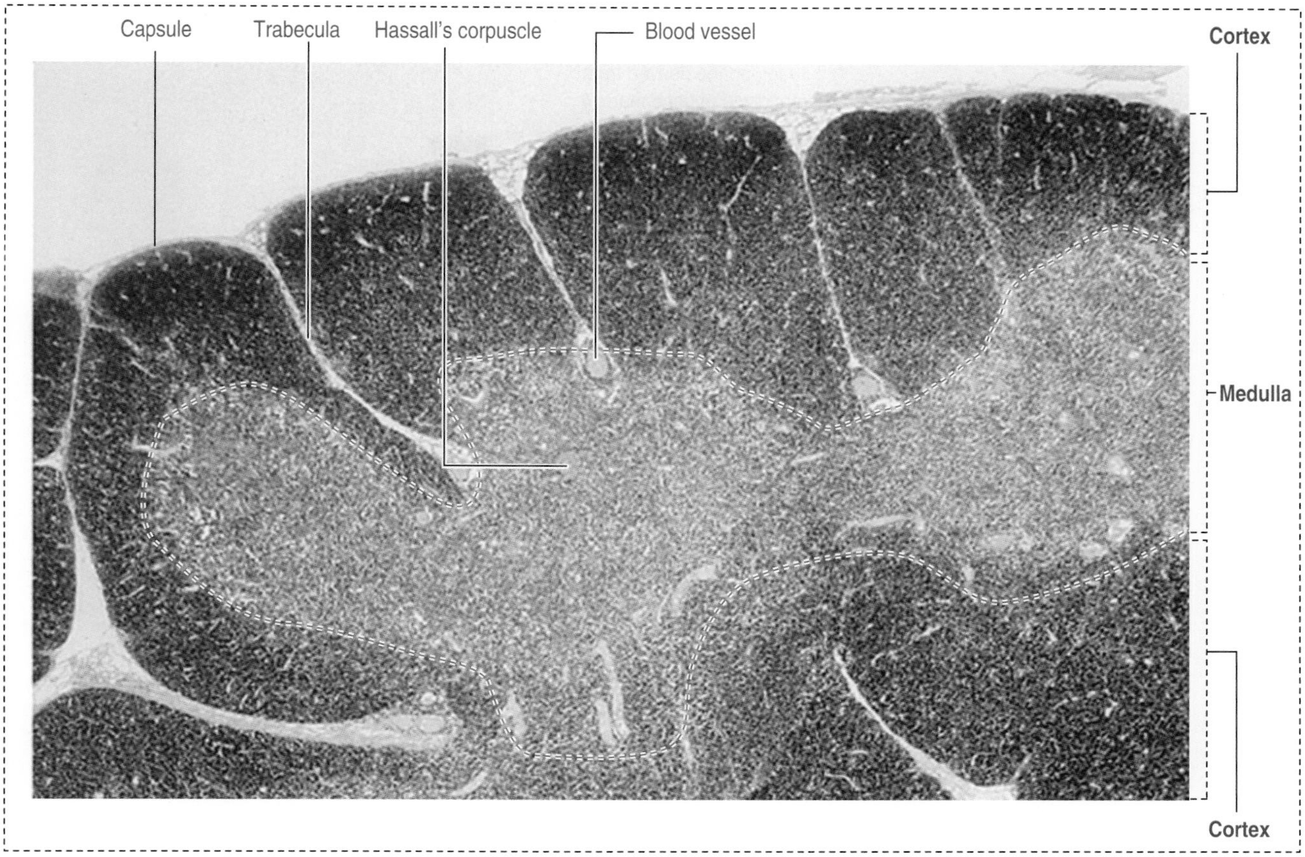

Fig. 13-36 Schematic illustration of the organization of the thymus.
The thymus consists of several incomplete lobules. Each lobule contains an independent outer cortical region, but the central medullary region is shared by adjacent lobules. Trabeculae, extensions of the capsule down to the corticomedullary region, form the boundary of each lobule. The cortex consists of stromal cells and developing T lymphocytes (thymocytes), macrophages, and cortical epithelial cells. Major histocompatibility complex class I and II molecules are present on the surface of the cortical epithelial cells. The characteristic deep blue nucleus staining of the cortex in histological preparation reflects the predominant population of T lymphocytes as compared with the less basophilic medulla, which contains a lower number of thymocytes. Hassall's corpuscles are a characteristic component of the medulla and are not seen in the cortex. (From Kierszenbaum AL: *Histology and cell biology: an introduction to pathology,* ed 2, St Louis, 2007, Mosby.)

in the cranial mediastinum, ventrally in the horse, pig, and dog and dorsally in ruminants.

The thymus has also been called a *lymphoepithelial organ* because besides lymphocytes it has an epithelial component. Histologically, it is divided into two portions, the stromal portion and the thymocyte portion (T lymphocytes at different stages of maturation and differentiation). All T lymphocytes in the thymus are derived from progenitor T lymphocytes in the bone marrow. The capsule, trabeculae, and blood vessels arise from the mesoderm of a branchial arch. Some stroma is designated "epithelial reticulum," reflecting its embryonic origin from branchial pouches and the third pharyngeal cleft. It produces no reticular fibers and thus is different from the reticulum composed of a meshwork of specialized fibroblast-like cells with long interdigitating filamentous projections (reticular cells), through which are dispersed macrophages and occasional myoid cells (smooth muscle-like).

The lymphoid component is composed of differentiating lymphocytes, which during gestation arise from hematopoietic progenitor cells, initially in the fetal liver, then spleen and later in the fetal bone marrow. The epithelial component consists of individual cells in the cortex and medulla and aggregates of epithelial cells in the medulla. The latter, called *Hassall's corpuscles,* are a characteristic histologic feature of the thymus. Cortical and medullary epithelial cells contribute to the microenvironment and are essential for differentiation, selection, and maturation of T lymphocytes in neonate and adult thymuses.

Microscopically, the thymus is divided into incomplete lobules, each of which has a cortex and a medulla, with the medullas being confluent centrally (Fig. 13-36). On the basis of functional and epithelial components, three zones are recognized: a subcapsular zone, a cortex, and a medulla. Bone marrow–derived T lymphocytes enter the circulation, travel to the thymus, and enter at the subcapsular zone (Fig. 13-37). Here, they begin differentiation and selection processes and develop into mature naïve T lymphocytes as they traverse the thymic cortex to the medulla. In the cortex, T lymphocytes that recognize self-molecules (i.e., major histocompatibility complex [MHC] molecules) but not self-antigens are permitted to mature by a process called *positive selection.* Cells that do not recognize MHC molecules are removed by apoptosis. Those T lymphocytes that recognize both MHC molecules and self-antigens are removed by macrophages at the corticomedullary junction, a process called *negative selection.* Because of the rigid differentiation requirements attributable to MHC restriction and tolerance (positive and negative selection, respectively) only a small fraction (<5%) of the developing T lymphocytes that arrive at the thymus from the bone marrow survive. Mature naïve T lymphocytes exit

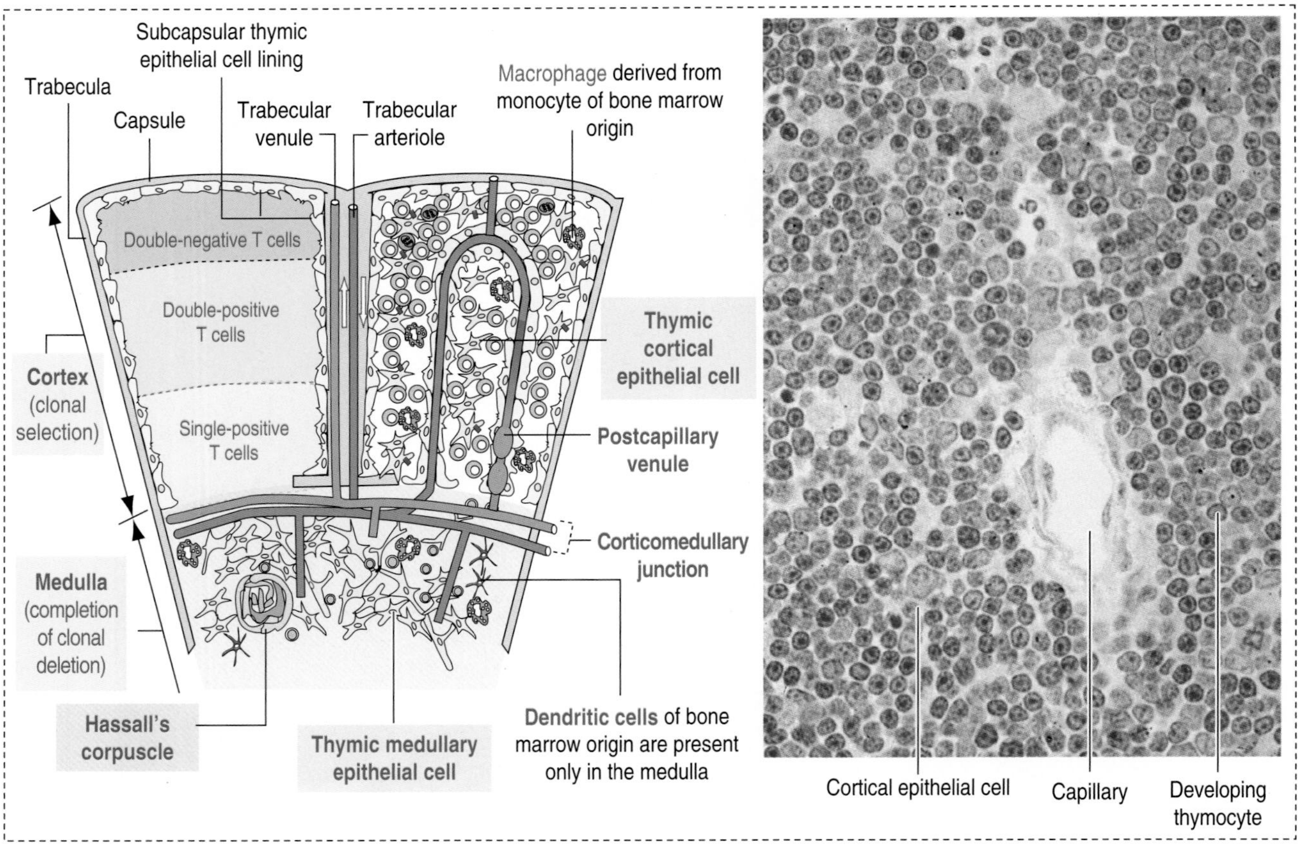

Fig. 13-37 Schematic illustration of the histology of the thymus.
The functional thymus consists of two cell populations: the stromal cells and the thymocytes. The stromal cells include *(1)* the subcapsular epithelial cells also lining the trabeculae and perivascular spaces; *(2)* the cortical epithelial cells of ectodermal origin; *(3)* the medullary epithelial cells of endodermal origin that give rise to Hassall's corpuscles; *(4)* macrophages present in both cortex and medulla, involved in the removal of apoptotic thymocytes eliminated during clonal selection; and *(5)* dendritic cells of bone marrow origin, confined to the medulla. *TCR,* T-cell receptor. (Adapted from Kierszenbaum AL: *Histology and cell biology: an introduction to pathology,* ed 2, St Louis, 2007, Mosby.)

the thymus through postcapillary venules in the corticomedullary region, enter the circulation, and recirculate through secondary lymphoid tissues in a highly regulated manner. The T lymphocyte regions of secondary lymphoid organs are specialized sites where these circulating mature naïve T lymphocytes (T lymphocytes that have not been exposed to their T lymphocyte receptor-specific antigen) are activated. On exposure to their specific antigens, they undergo additional phases of development and differentiate into effector and memory cells, some of which remain localized in lymph nodes and others migrate to sites of infection. The balance between the rates of production and distribution of T lymphocytes is critically important in maintaining immune homeostasis. In fact, immunodeficiency or autoimmunity may result from inadequate or overly zealous activity, respectively, of a particular subset of T lymphocytes.

The thymus attains its maximal mass relative to body weight at birth and involutes after sexual maturity. The lymphoid and epithelial components are gradually replaced by loose connective tissue and fat, although remnants remain histologically, even in aged animals.

RESPONSES TO INJURY

The responses of the thymus to injury are listed in Box 13-4, and the most common ones are lymphoid atrophy, inflammation, and neoplasia. The most common change is lymphoid atrophy caused by physical and physiologic stresses, toxins, drugs, and viral infections.

BOX 13-4 Response of the Thymus to Injury

Lymphoid atrophy
Inflammation—very rare
Hemorrhage and hematomas
Neoplasia

Atrophy

The causes of lymphoid atrophy are listed in Box 13-5. Because the thymus does not contain any lymphopoietic tissue, it depends on the bone marrow for the supply of T lymphocytes. Thus thymic lymphoid atrophy can be either the result of an inadequate supply of lymphocytes from the bone marrow or lysis of lymphocytes (lymphocytolysis) in the thymus.

Thymic atrophy must be differentiated from involution, which normally begins at sexual maturity. This distinction is difficult to make, unless the change is extreme or age-matched control animals are available. Viruses commonly cause injury to the thymus. Many viruses cause destruction of the lymphoid portion (e.g., from lymphocytolysis in equine herpesvirus-1 [EHV-1]) in aborted foals and feline panleukopenia virus in cats).

BOX 13-5 Causes of Lymphoid Atrophy

Lack of antigenic stimulus
Toxins
Chemotherapeutic agents
Infectious agents
  Viruses
  Bacteria
Ionizing radiation
Malnutrition
Cachexia
Aging

Inflammation

Inflammation of the thymus is rare. Inflammatory cells (neutrophils and sometimes macrophages) are often present within keratinized Hassall's corpuscles during involution, and this should not be mistaken for a true thymitis. A diffuse infiltration of inflammatory cells into the thymus has also been reported in salmon poisoning disease of dogs (see Chapter 7) and a diffuse infiltration of macrophages in epizootic bovine abortion (see Chapter 18). Porcine circovirus 2, the etiologic agent of postweaning multisystem wasting syndrome (PMWS) in pigs, is unusual in that it causes a granulomatous inflammation in lymphoid organs, which in the thymus affects chiefly the medulla (see the section on Disorders of Pigs).

Thymic Enlargement

Thymic enlargement is rare and occasionally is the result of hemorrhage, hematomas, or tumors and is discussed further in the section on Disorders of Domestic Animals.

Neoplasia

Primary malignant tumors of the thymus are chiefly thymomas and lymphomas and are discussed further in the section on Disorders of Domestic Animals. Thymomas are formed from the epithelial component of the thymus, and usually with a benign proliferating lymphoid component. They are encapsulated, grow slowly, and rarely metastasize. Thymic lymphomas have a malignant proliferating lymphoid component and are most frequent in young cattle, dogs and cats. Histologically, they are poorly encapsulated and usually have an increased mitotic rate. Metastases can be widely disseminated, but are rare.

SPLEEN

Understanding the relationships between anatomic structures and the different functions of the spleen is complicated. There are also anatomic differences among domestic animal species and a confused terminology. Most of the latter is the result of the complicated vascular structure of the spleen and changes in terminology over the years. For example, "sinus" and "sinusoid" have both been applied to the "splenic sinusoids," which in domestic animals are present only in the dog. Spleens, which have sinusoids, are often designated "sinusal" rather than "sinusoidal" and spleens without sinusoids as nonsinusal. Adding to the confusion, the word "sinus" has been used for the *red pulp vascular spaces*, which have also been called reticular spaces of the red pulp, interstices of the reticulum meshwork, and capillaries. Similarly, the white pulp has been termed splenic nodules, splenic follicles, and Malpighian corpuscles.

In this chapter, we use the following terms: *sinusoid, red pulp vascular space, marginal sinus, marginal zone, periarteriolar lymphoid sheath (PALS), periarteriolar macrophage sheath (PAMS), splenic or lymphoid follicles,* and *splenic cords.*

STRUCTURE

The spleen, suspended in the gastrosplenic ligament and covered by peritoneum, is located in the left cranial hypogastric region of the abdominal cavity between the diaphragm, stomach, and the body wall, except in domestic ruminants, where it is closely adhered to the left dorsolateral aspect of the rumen. The gross morphology (shape and size) of the spleen varies markedly among domestic animals, but generally it is a flattened, elongated organ. The spleen is covered by a thick fibromuscular capsule from which numerous intertwining fibromuscular trabeculae extend into the parenchyma and which along with the reticulum form the supporting stroma for the parenchymal components. The splenic parenchyma, unlike that of many organs, does not have a cortex and medulla but is divided into two distinct structural and functional components: the red pulp and white pulp. The red pulp consists of cells of the monocyte-macrophage system in the splenic cords and PAMS and red pulp vascular spaces and associated stroma (reticular cells and fibroblasts and myocytes in the trabeculae). The white pulp consists lymphocytes of the B lymphocyte regions (splenic follicles), T lymphocyte regions (PALS), and the marginal zone in which are macrophages, antigen-presenting cells, and trafficking B and T lymphocytes. There are minor differences in some of the splenic components of the domestic animals (e.g., the cat has a small marginal sinus but a well-developed PAMS).

The arterial and venous vasculature have minor differences among the domestic animals. The following account is correct for the canine spleen, and if the sinusoids, which are only in the canine spleen, are omitted, it applies in general to the nonsinusal spleens of the other domestic animals. The artery supplying the spleen is the splenic artery, a branch of the celiac artery, which is a major branch of the abdominal aorta. The splenic artery penetrates the splenic capsule at the hilus, branches, and enters the fibromuscular trabeculae as the trabecular artery (Fig. 13-38). As it leaves the trabecula, the trabecular artery becomes the central arteriole of the white pulp and is surrounded by a cuff of T lymphocytes (PALS). Adjacent to or eccentrically embedded in the PALS is a splenic follicle (B lymphocytes). A branch of the central artery goes to the marginal sinus, which surrounds the splenic follicle and carries blood-borne antigens and trafficking B and T lymphocytes into close contact with the follicle (Fig. 13-39). In the dog, the marginal sinus drains into the sinusoids, but in other domestic animals, it drains into the red pulp vascular spaces. It is significant that the first branch of the central artery goes to the marginal sinus. As a result, antigens, bacteria, particles, and other material are delivered to the marginal sinus first, before either the sinusoids (in the dog) or red pulp vascular spaces. After emerging from the PALS, the arteriole is surrounded by a sheath of macrophages known as PAMS. The PAMSs are very prominent in pigs. It then becomes the penicillary arteriole, and in horses, cattle, pigs, and cats, its terminal branches empty into the red pulp vascular space lined by reticular cells, which lie in and between the splenic cords. The term *red pulp vascular spaces* used here has the advantage of being descriptive and correct and clearly differentiates them from venous sinuses and sinusoids. In dogs and humans, branches of the central arteriole of the white pulp enter into venous sinusoids, which are lined by a discontinuous endothelium and these empty into splenic venules. The anatomic arrangement of arterioles opening into sinusoids is known as a *closed circulation* because the blood

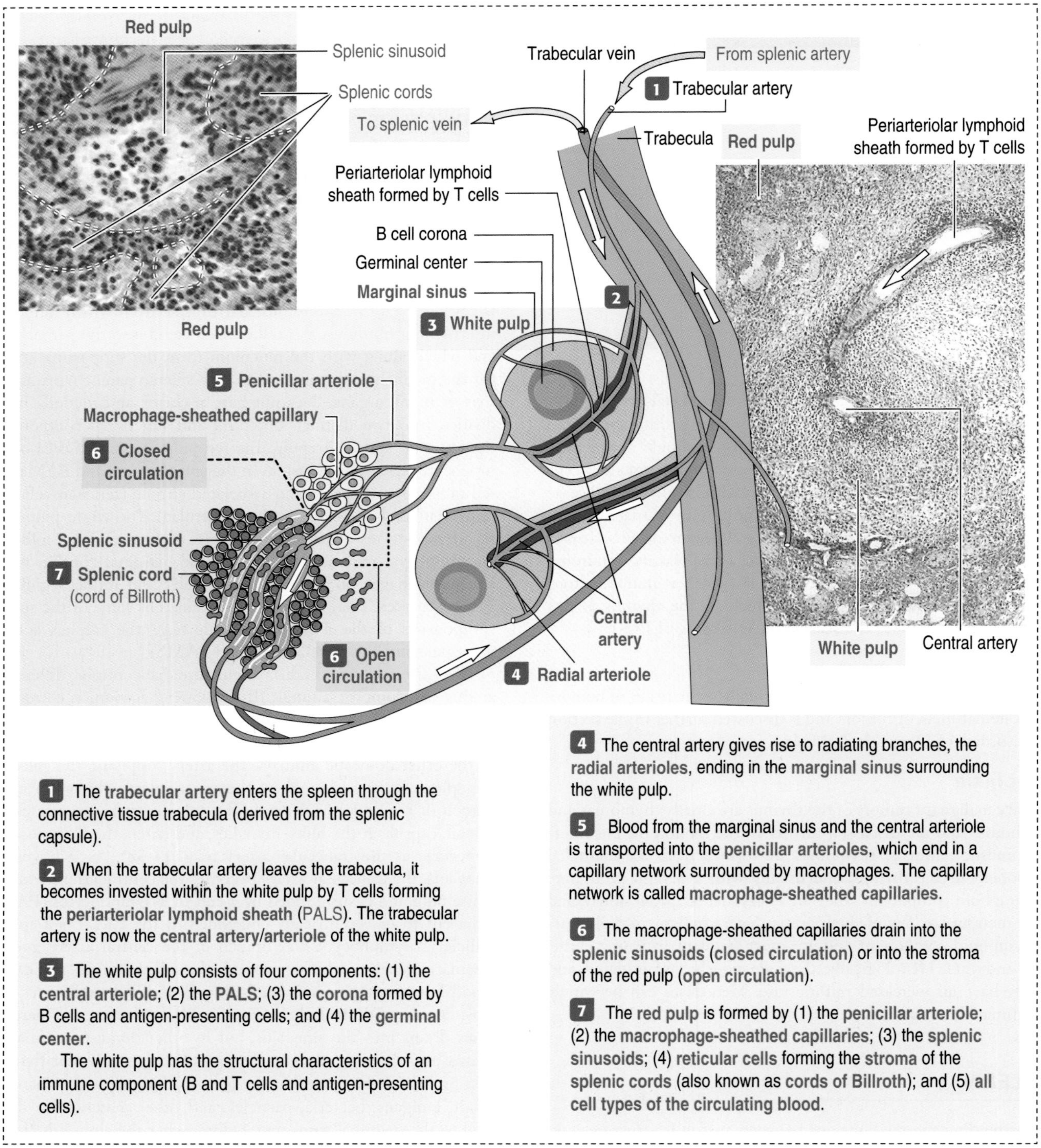

Fig. 13-38 Schematic representation of the human spleen.
The blood flow depicted is applicable in domestic animals only to the canine spleen, which has splenic sinusoids. The other domestic animals do not have splenic sinusoids. (Adapted from Kierszenbaum AL: *Histology and cell biology: an introduction to pathology,* ed 2, St Louis, 2007, Mosby.)

flow is through arterioles, capillaries, sinusoids, and venules, all of which are vessels lined by endothelium. The other route is through the red pulp vascular spaces, which are not lined by endothelium but by reticular cells and is designated an "open system" (see Fig. 13-38). Because the dog has sinusoids and red pulp vascular spaces, it has both open and closed splenic circulations. Blood flowing through either the sinusoids or red pulp vascular spaces is exposed to the surveillance of macrophages. These are located perivascularly around sinusoids, but their pseudopodia project into the sinusoidal lumen through the spaces in the discontinuous endothelium. In the red pulp, macrophages are present in the vascular spaces, attached to the reticular walls, and in the splenic cords. Blood then drains into the splenic venules, splenic veins, and ultimately the portal vein, which empties into the liver.

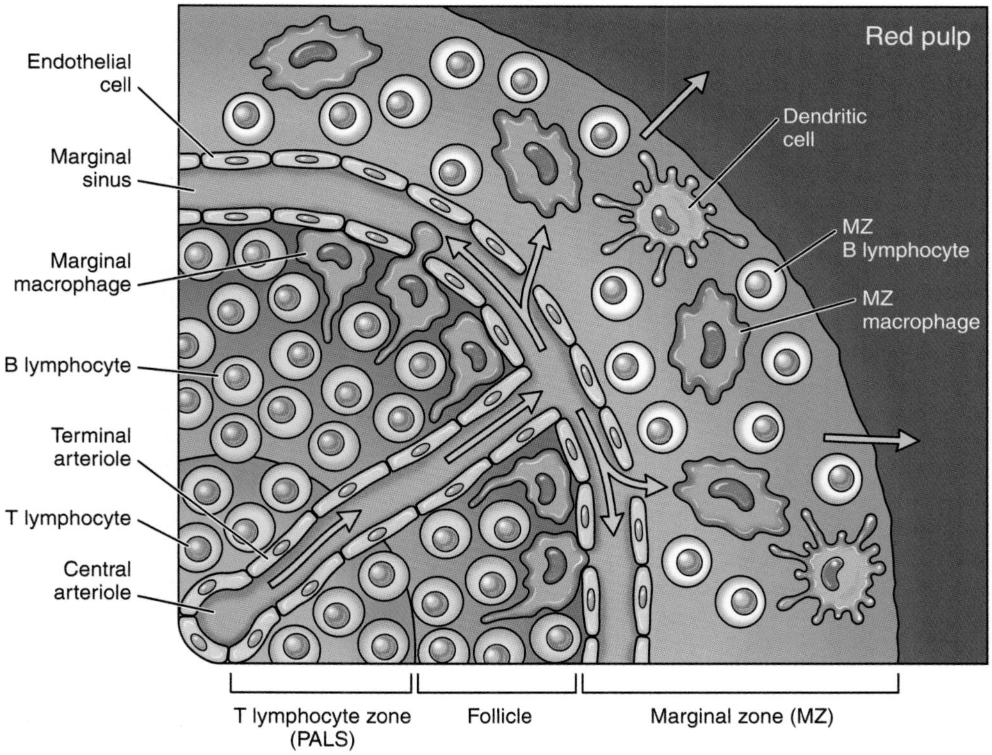

Fig. 13-39 **Structure of the marginal zone in the splenic follicle.**
Antigens from infections microorganisms enter the follicle via the central and terminal arterioles and reach the marginal sinus where they are phagocytosed by macrophages. Macrophages of the monocyte-macrophage system in the reticulum of the marginal zone, which is classified as part of the white pulp, form an important defense mechanism in the spleen through phagocytosis, antigen processing, and antigen presentation in splenic follicles to B lymphocytes resulting in the formation of immunoblasts that mature to plasma cells.

FUNCTION

The spleen filters blood and removes foreign particles, bacteria, and erythrocytes that are senescent, have structural membrane abnormalities, or are infected with hemotropic parasites. Its immunologic functions are those of a secondary lymphoid organ and include activation of macrophages to process and present antigen, B lymphocyte proliferation and production of antibody and biologic molecules, and the interaction of T lymphocytes and antigens. In some species, it stores significant quantities of blood (Box 13-6). These functions are best considered on the basis of the two grossly visible components of the splenic parenchyma: red and white pulp and the anatomic systems associated with them: (1) the monocyte-macrophage system, red pulp vascular spaces, and hematopoiesis within the red pulp and (2) the B and T lymphocyte systems within the white pulp.

Red Pulp

Monocyte-Macrophage System

Macrophages are located chiefly at two sites in the red pulp of the spleen: red pulp vascular spaces and splenic cords (and in the dog, perisinusoidally). Red pulp vascular spaces are supported by a reticular network, which is a fine meshwork of reticular fibers composed of type III collagen, in which macrophages are dispersed. These macrophages (and those in the reticulum of the marginal zone, which is classified as part of the white pulp) are responsible for phagocytosis of blood-borne foreign material (Fig. 13-40), bacteria, and senescent and/or damaged erythrocytes as in immune-mediated anemias and infections with hemotropic parasites. In the dog, sinusoidal macrophages remove entire erythrocytes

BOX 13-6 Functions of the Spleen

FILTRATION
1. Removal of erythrocytes
   a. Physiologic-senescent erythrocytes
   b. Pathologic
      - Removal of erythrocytes with abnormalities
      - Removal of erythrocytes with hemotropic parasites
2. Removal of particulate material–foreign material such as colloidal particles, bacteria, cell-associated viruses

IMMUNOLOGIC FUNCTIONS
1. Phagocytosis and processing of antigen
2. Homing of circulating lymphocytes in the blood
3. Lymphocyte transformation and proliferation
4. Production of antibody and lymphokines
5. Macrophage activation

STORAGE
1. Blood in storage spleens
2. Iron and its recycling

HEMATOPOIESIS
1. Extramedullary erythropoiesis in the case of severe demand
2. Production of B lymphocytes and some T lymphocytes and macrophages

Modified from Nieman RS, Attilo O: *Disorders of the spleen in major problem in pathology,* Philadelphia, 1999, WB Saunders.

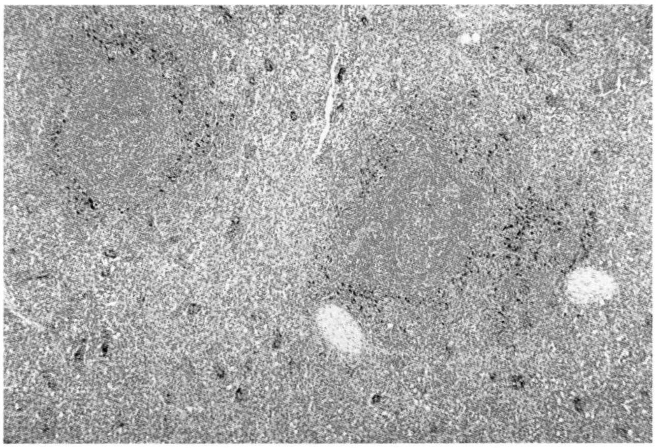

Fig. 13-40 Function of the marginal zone, splenic follicle, white pulp, spleen, calf injected intravenously with micronized carbon particles. Carbon particles *(black pigment)* are present in macrophages of the marginal zone. Macrophages of the monocyte-macrophage system phagocytose blood-borne foreign material, bacteria, viruses, and senescent and/or damaged erythrocytes as in immune-mediated anemias and infections with hemotropic parasites. Eosin counterstain. (Courtesy Dr. M.D. McGavin, College of Veterinary Medicine, University of Tennessee.)

(erythrophagocytosis), as well as portions of an erythrocyte's membrane and cytoplasmic inclusions, such as nuclear remnants like Heinz bodies, by a process called *pitting*. Indeed, the presence of large numbers of nuclear remnants in erythrocytes in canine blood smears may be indicative of splenic malfunction. The process of removal of senescent erythrocytes normally does not alter the size of the spleen, except when the spleen has to remove large numbers of defective erythrocytes, such as occurs in an acute hemolytic anemia, in which case, the spleen can be markedly enlarged. In nonsinusoidal spleens, macrophages of the splenic cords of the red pulp perform these functions, although the extent and location of the sites of pitting are unclear. The cat's spleen is deficient in pitting and thus in removal of Heinz bodies, presumably because it has no sinusoids. Also, there are no slits in the red pulp vascular spaces similar to the ones in the sinusoidal wall through which the erythrocytes have to squeeze to return to the circulation, or be either pitted or phagocytosed. Pitting takes place in the feline spleen, but the process is slow.

The sinusoidal, marginal sinus, and splenic cord macrophages are of bone marrow origin. They originate in the bone marrow, circulate in the blood as monocytes and migrate into the spleen. Fixed macrophages elsewhere in the body, in connective tissue, lymph nodes (sinus histiocytes), liver (Kupffer cells), lung (pulmonary intravascular macrophages and pulmonary alveolar macrophages), and brain (resident and perivascular microglial cells) are derived in a similar manner (see Chapters 5, 8, 9, and 14).

Red Pulp Vascular Spaces

Storage or Defense Spleens

Spleens are classified as either storage or defense spleens, based on whether or not they can store significant volumes of blood. The spleens of domestic animals have both storage and defense functions, but are classified as storage spleens. Their trabeculae and capsules contain smooth muscle, which allows them to expand and contract. Equine, canine, and feline spleens all have considerable capacity. It has been claimed that the canine spleen can store one-third of the dog's erythrocytes while the animal sleeps and the equine spleen holds one half of the animal's circulating red cell mass, which is considered an advantage as it reduces the viscosity of the circulating blood. The spleens of ruminants and the pig are intermediate in the amount of smooth muscle and have limited storage capacity. Spleens, whose capsules and trabeculae have a low percentage of smooth muscle and elastic fibers and thus cannot expand and contract (rabbit and human), are designated as defense spleens. Storage spleens expand and contract quickly under the influence of the autonomic nervous system (sympathetic and vagal fibers, which reach the reticular walls of the red pulp vascular spaces; catecholamines; "flight or fight") and other circulatory perturbations, such as in hypovolemic and/or cardiogenic shock (see the section on Small Spleens). Thus storage spleens may be either grossly enlarged and congested, or small with a wrinkled surface and a dry parenchyma (see the sections on Uniform Splenomegaly and Small Spleens). Also, the spleen responds to septicemia and acute hemotropic parasitic diseases by active hyperemia or acute passive congestion respectively, in the latter case the result of storing infected erythrocytes until they can be phagocytosed. Grossly congested spleens may be so enlarged that foci of white pulp are widely separated, making the white pulp look sparse and thus easily underestimated on gross examination.

Hematopoietic Tissue

Although the liver is the primary site of hematopoiesis in the developing fetus, the spleen also makes a minor contribution. Shortly before or after birth, depending on the species, hematopoiesis ceases in the liver and spleen and the bone marrow becomes the primary hematopoietic organ. However, often under conditions of severe demand, for example in a severe and prolonged anemia, this increased demand can be met partly through reactivation of splenic hematopoiesis. This outcome is called *extramedullary hematopoiesis* (EMH). It is also an incidental finding in splenic nodular hyperplasia (see the section on Nodular Spleens with Firm Consistency).

White Pulp

White pulp is grossly visible on the cut surface as distinct foci of grayish lymphoid tissue. Each focus consists of a periarteriolar lymphoid sheath and a splenic nodule surrounded by a marginal zone. There is considerable confusion regarding the terminology of splenic nodules or follicles. Histology books avoid the use of "lymphoid" as in "lymphoid nodule" or "lymphoid follicle". Terms used include "lymphoid-like follicle," "splenic follicle," "splenic nodule" and even just "white pulp." However, the pathology literature frequently uses the term "splenic lymphatic (or lymphoid) follicle". This chapter uses the terms *splenic nodule* and *splenic lymphoid follicle*.

Normally, foci of white pulp are small and may not be visible on gross examination of a cross section of spleen. However, if nodules are enlarged either by lymphoid hyperplasia or by a neoplastic process (e.g., lymphoma), these foci initially become visible on the cut surface, as 0.5- to 1.0-mm white dots scattered through the red pulp. Also, in animals with storage spleens, the distention of the red pulp from stored blood may separate white pulp, making it look sparse.

Splenic white pulp is organized around branches of the splenic artery, the central arteriole, in the form of PALS, which is populated primarily by T lymphocytes (see Fig. 13-38). Primary splenic follicles are located eccentrically in PALS and are primarily comprised of B lymphocytes. When exposed to antigen, the latter develop germinal centers characteristic of secondary lymphoid follicles (see the section on Lymph Nodes).

The marginal zone is the third component of the splenic white pulp. It is located at the interface of the white and red pulp and surrounds the marginal sinus, which is immediately adjacent to the follicle. The marginal sinus is supplied with blood by radial branches of the central artery, which drain into the marginal sinus (see Fig. 13-38) and is the portal of entry into the spleen for recirculating B and T lymphocytes. The marginal zone consists of macrophages, dendritic cells, and T and B lymphocytes and is an important transit area for B and T lymphocytes, which after they leave the circulation, enter the marginal zone. From here, T lymphocytes migrate to the PALS. Those B lymphocytes that recognize antigens for which they have been programmed are activated and enter the follicle and proliferate to form plasmablasts. Dendritic cells in the marginal zone capture blood-borne antigens, process them, and preset them to the follicular lymphocytes.

Macrophages in the white pulp or marginal zone are phenotypically distinct from those in the red pulp. The latter function primarily to actively phagocytose particles, senescent erythrocytes, erythrocytes containing hemotropic parasites (e.g., *Babesia* spp.), and pathogenic bacteria and fungi and thus are responsible for "filtering" the blood. Many of the marginal zone macrophages are involved in phagocytosis and processing of antigen. However, some marginal zone macrophages actively phagocytose particulate matter in the blood (see Fig. 13-40) and bacteria in septicemias.

RESPONSES TO INJURY

The responses of the spleen to injury (Box 13-7) include acute inflammation, hyperplasia of the monocyte-macrophage system, hyperplasia of lymphoid tissues, atrophy of lymphoid tissues, storage of blood or contraction to expel reserve blood, and neoplasia. These responses are reflections of the spleen's three chief anatomic components: (1) monocyte-macrophage system, (2) lymphoid (immune) system, and (3) vasculature, chiefly the red pulp vascular spaces and their supporting reticular stroma (reticulum). Because the spleen is examined on the basis of red and white pulp, this approach is used in the following description.

Red Pulp

Monocyte-Macrophage System

The distribution and function of macrophages in the spleen is described above under Structure and Function. These interactions are complex and their relationships to both innate and adaptive immunity, as well as cell turnover, are areas of intense study (see Chapter 5). The extent of phagocytosis by macrophages in the red pulp vascular spaces, which are attached to the reticulum forming the walls lining these spaces, splenic cords, and marginal sinuses, depends on the order in which they receive blood. In most species, the marginal sinus is the first, and consequently, particles and bacteria tend to be more concentrated here initially (see Fig. 13-40). However, again there are species differences, for example, in the cat, the marginal sinus is small and PAMS play a larger role in phagocytosis.

BOX 13-7 Response of the Spleen to Injury

- Acute inflammation—hyperemia, microabscesses, acute abscesses
- Monocyte-macrophage system hyperplasia—granulomatous diseases
- Lymphoid hyperplasia—production of plasma cells and antibody, cell-mediated immunity
- Lymphoid atrophy
- Storage of blood or contraction to expel reserve blood
- Neoplasia

The spleen is able to mount a very strong response to blood-borne pathogens. In immunized rabbits injected intravenously with pneumococci, the blood was cleared of 98% of those bacteria within 15 minutes and 100% of an inoculum of 1 billion bacteria was removed from the blood within an hour. Also, the rabbit spleen removed 10 times the number of bacteria per gram as the liver. When 1 billion pneumococci per pound of body weight were injected into the splenic artery of a dog over a 5-minute period, all bacteria were removed from the blood in 65 minutes. After splenectomy, blood-borne organisms multiply rapidly and are disseminated widely in the body and may cause "overwhelming post-splenectomy infection." It has also been shown that the phagocytic function of the spleen is critical in the control of plasmodium in humans with malaria and in cattle with babesiosis. To facilitate filtering, all of the blood in the body passes through the spleen at least once a day. In the dog, the blood flow and transit time depend on whether the spleen is contracted or distended. Blood flow is slower in the distended spleen, apparently because blood flows through the red pulp vascular spaces, rather than through the sinusoids as it does in the contracted canine spleen.

Sometimes in septicemias, the number of pathogenic bacteria arriving via the circulation can be so large that it exceeds the capacity of the splenic defenses to overcome them immediately. The result is acute splenic congestion and active hyperemia, followed by focal necrosis and or inflammation and a grossly enlarged and congested spleen. In the case of pyogenic bacteria, there may be neutrophils, other inflammatory cells, and bacteria throughout the red pulp. The marginal zone at the interface of the red and white pulp responds similarly to the red pulp vascular spaces and can be the initial site of response to blood-borne antigens and bacteria delivered by the radial branches of the central artery. As a result, it can be congested and in later stages (after only a few hours with highly pathogenic organisms) contain a diffuse spread or focal aggregates of neutrophils and macrophages. Histologically, the congestion forms a concentric ring, which may be incomplete, around the circumference of the splenic nodule (see the section on Anthrax).

Red pulp macrophages also proliferate in chronic hemolytic diseases in which there is a prolonged need to phagocytose erythrocytes and in chronic splenic congestion, which is usually a result of portal or splenic vein hypertension. The result is widened splenic cords. Unlike in humans, hepatic cirrhosis in animals does not cause chronic splenic congestion.

Macrophages in the red pulp (splenic cords and walls and lumens of red pulp vascular spaces) and marginal sinus also proliferate in response to fungi and facultative intracellular pathogens (e.g., *Mycobacterium bovis*) arriving hematogenously in the spleen. Their number may be augmented by monocytes recruited from the blood to form granulomatous inflammation. This inflammatory response can be diffuse (e.g. blastomycosis) or focal (tuberculosis).

Red Pulp Vascular Spaces

Red pulp vascular spaces respond to injury by congestion (see previous section).

White Pulp

The major system of the white pulp is the lymphoid system (PALS, splenic follicle), and the marginal zone, which lies at the junction of the red and white pulp but is not visible grossly.

The responses of the white pulp to injury are as follows:

- PALS (T lymphocyte areas)
  - Increase (hyperplasia) or decrease in size (atrophy)
- Splenic follicle

- Increase (hypertrophy) or decrease in the size (atrophy) and number (follicular hyperplasia)
- Germinal center
  - Activation or lymphocytolysis, necrosis, and reduction in size or disappearance (atrophy) of the follicle's germinal center. These are followed by atrophy of the splenic follicles and ultimately atrophy of the lymph node.
- Marginal zone.
  - Phagocytosis of antibody, particulate material and microorganisms, macrophage hyperplasia (see the section on Monocyte-Macrophage System).

Splenic follicular hyperplasia is a response to antigenic stimuli and results in the formation of secondary follicles and consequently an increase in the size of the white pulp, which may be visibly enlarged. Splenic lymphoid follicles, lymphoid follicles in lymph nodes, and diffuse and nodular lymphatic tissue have a well-established sequence of morphologic changes, chiefly in the germinal center, which are helpful in tracking the stage of the B lymphocyte response. These sequential changes are similar to those described later in the Lymph Nodes section on Responses to Injury.

Splenic follicular atrophy occurs in response to lack of antigenic stimulation or from regression after antigenic stimulation has ceased, and from the effects of toxins, antineoplastic chemotherapeutic agents, microorganisms such as viruses and bacteria, radiation, malnutrition, wasting/cachectic diseases, and aging (see Box 13-5). The follicles are depleted of lymphocytes and with time, germinal centers and follicles disappear. The amount of the total lymphoid tissue is reduced and the spleen may be smaller.

Monocyte-Macrophage System

The response of the monocyte-macrophage system in the marginal sinus and marginal zone to injury is phagocytosis and proliferation. Proliferation also occurs in the viral disease porcine PMWS where there is proliferation of both follicular macrophages and those in the deep cortex (see the section on Disorders of Pigs).

Capsule and Trabeculae

Apart from complete or partial rupture of the splenic capsule, usually from trauma or splenic distention, the capsule and trabeculae develop few lesions.

LYMPH NODES

STRUCTURE

The three dimensional structure of a lymph node is complex and difficult to fully appreciate in a two-dimensional histological slide or diagram. It is convenient from the point of view of understanding the pathological response of the lymph node to consider them based on its anatomic components (Fig. 13-41), which are as follows:

- Stroma: fibrous capsule and reticulum
- Cortex: outer cortex (B lymphocytes), deep cortex (paracortex; T lymphocytes)
- Medullary cords
- Vasculature: arteries, arterioles, high endothelium venules, efferent veins, lymphatic sinuses and vessels
- Cells of the monocyte-macrophage system

Stroma

The lymph node is almost completely enclosed by a fibrous capsule that is pierced by multiple afferent lymphatic vessels, which empty into the subcapsular sinus (see Fig. 13-41). Efferent lymphatic vessels and veins exit, and arteries enter at the hilus. The lymph node is supported by fibrous trabeculae and a reticulum of fibroblastic reticular cells. The reticulum also has an immunologic function of guiding lymphocytes and antigen-presenting cells to facilitate their interaction with B and T lymphocytes. Lymphocytes are such a predominant feature in lymph nodes that it is easy to overlook the fact that lymphocytes are transient cells, staying only a short time in the lymph node and that the lymph node itself is basically a fibrovascular structure within a dilated lymphatic.

Cortex

On gross examination of a cross-section of lymph nodes, two main areas are visible: cortex (outer) and medulla (inner) (see Fig. 13-41).

The outer cortex contains the lymphoid follicles. The morphologic and functional organization of the lymphoid follicle is similar to that of the splenic follicle, except there is no marginal zone. There are two types of lymphoid follicles, simply referred to as *primary* and *secondary.* Primary lymphoid follicles consist predominantly of densely packed resting B lymphocytes and follicular dendritic cells (see Chapter 5 for more complete discussion of dendritic cells). Mature naïve B lymphocytes expressing receptors for specific antigens exit primary lymphoid organs and circulate through the bloodstream, lymphatic vessels, and secondary lymphoid tissues. On their arrival at lymph nodes, B lymphocytes exit through high endothelial venules (HEVs) and home to the primary follicle. Those B lymphocytes that recognize the antigen for which they are expressing receptors are activated and proliferate to form secondary lymphoid follicles characterized by prominent germinal centers.

Germinal centers are areas with a specialized microenvironment that support the proliferation and further development of B lymphocytes to increase their antigen specificity (e.g., affinity maturation) and functional capacity (e.g., isotype switching). The germinal center has a "dark" zone, comprised of proliferating B lymphocytes, and an outer "light" zone comprised of nonproliferating B lymphocytes. Peripheral to that is the mantle zone that contains the inactive mature naïve B lymphocytes that have been displaced centrifugally as a result of the development and expansion of the germinal center. Plasma cell precursors (plasmablasts) formed in the germinal centers migrate from the cortex to the medullary cords.

The deep cortex (inner cortex, paracortex) consists of diffuse lymphoid tissue containing T lymphocytes and HEVs, through which T lymphocytes migrate from the blood into the deep cortex and B lymphocytes migrate to lymphoid follicles. Other T lymphocytes arrive via the afferent lymphatic vessels. T lymphocytes that are antigenically stimulated proliferate, but unless there is a marked increase in the number of T lymphocytes in the deep cortex, lymphoid hyperplasia here can be difficult to detect in H&E stained sections. Trabeculae, which are part of the stroma, are also in the cortex. They are collagenous bands extending radially inward from the capsule. They are often surrounded by trabecular (also called *paratrabecular*) sinuses, which are continuous with the subcapsular sinus and empty into the medullary sinuses (see Fig. 13-41).

Medullary Cords

The medulla consists of two major components: (1) medullary cords containing macrophages and lymphocytes—and in an immunologically stimulated lymph node, plasma cells actively secreting antibodies, which are released into the lymph in the medullary sinuses, and (2) the medullary sinuses lined by fibroblastic reticular cells. Macrophages (sinus histiocytes) cling to reticular fibers

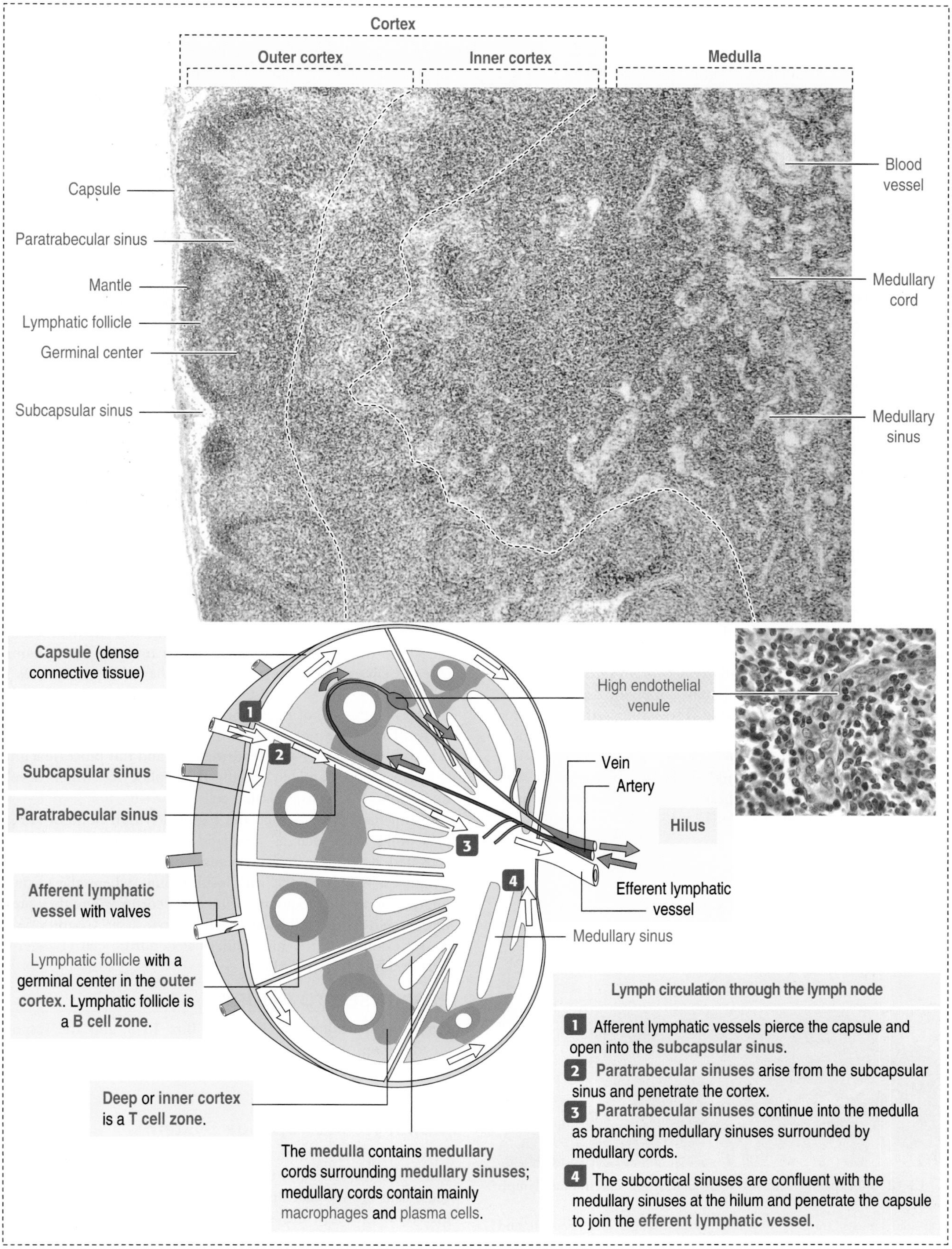

Fig. 13-41 Schematic illustration of the histology of the lymph node and lymph circulation.

(Adapted from Kierszenbaum AL: *Histology and cell biology: an introduction to pathology,* ed 2, St Louis, 2007, Mosby.)

crossing the lumen of the sinus and actively phagocytose foreign material, cellular debris, and bacteria in the incoming lymph.

The porcine lymph node has a different structure, but its immunologic functions are unchanged from those of other domestic animals. There is one afferent lymphatic vessel that enters at the hilus and discharges lymph into the center of the node, from where it flows to the subcapsular sinus and then drains into several efferent lymphatic vessels, which pierce the capsule. This reversal of flow is associated with an "inverted" structural organization, in which the lymphatic follicles present in the cortex of other domestic animals are located in the central region of the lymph node, and the medullary region is located peripherally. Consequently, any blood in the sinuses is also highly visible through the capsule.

Vasculature

The vasculature of the lymph node includes afferent lymphatic vessels, arteries, and veins and their branches including the HEVs and the sinuses—subcapsular, trabecular, and medullary through which lymph from the afferent lymphatic vessels flows to the efferent lymphatic vessels. Medullary sinuses are described with the medulla. Response of these vessels to injury is as for other vasculature (see Chapter 10). Afferent and efferent lymphatic vessels are part of the Cardiovascular System and are also discussed in Chapter 10.

All lymph nodes receive afferent lymphatic vessels from specific areas of the body. For example, peripheral lymph nodes such as the popliteal and superficial inguinal drain the hind leg. Central lymph nodes, such as the tracheobronchial and mesenteric lymph nodes (lymphocenters), drain the lungs and intestinal tract, respectively. The term *lymphocenter* is used in veterinary anatomy for a lymph node or a group of lymph nodes that occur constantly in the same region and receive lymphatic vessels from the same region in all species. Multiple afferent lymphatic vessels drain into the subcapsular sinus, but lymph from one afferent lymphatic drains into the adjacent portion of the lymph node. The result is that only this portion (lobule), particularly in lymph nodes from large domestic animals, may respond immunologically or with inflammation. Similarly, a neoplastic embolus initially lodges in that portion of the lymph node drained by the branch of the afferent lymphatic vessel arising in the neoplastic site (Fig. 13-42).

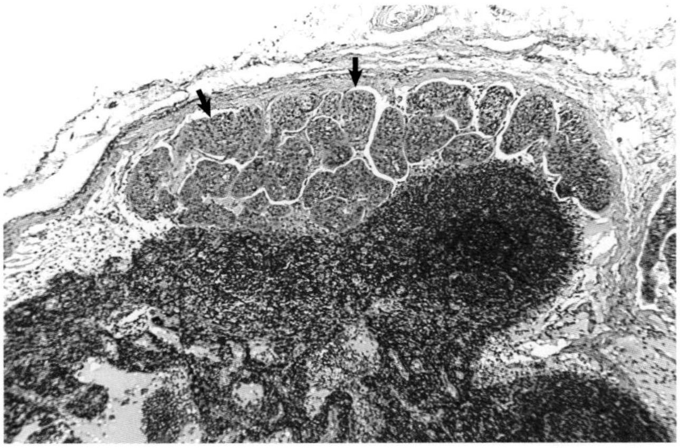

Fig. 13-42 Subcapsular sinuses with metastatic carcinoma, lymph node, dog.
Subcapsular sinuses are sites for embolization, lodgement, invasion, and growth of neoplastic emboli *(arrows)*, most commonly carcinomas. Emboli initially lodge in that portion of the lymph node drained by the branch of the afferent lymphatic vessel draining the primary carcinoma. H&E stain. (Courtesy Dr. M.D. McGavin, College of Veterinary Medicine, University of Tennessee.)

FUNCTION

The lymph nodes are one of the first lines of defense against lymph and blood borne infectious and non-infectious agents. The functions of the lymph node are to filter lymph of particulate matter and microorganisms, and to facilitate the surveillance of incoming antigens and their interaction with B and T lymphocytes and to produce B lymphocytes. It is helpful to consider the paths taken by particles, molecules, and cells arriving at a lymph node. This is accomplished via two possible routes: (1) via the arterial blood supply or (2) via lymphatic afferents. T lymphocytes arriving by the arterial route migrate out of the HEVs into the T lymphocyte areas adjacent to the follicle (interfollicular portion of the deep cortex) (see Chapter 3).

Material arriving in the lymph can be subdivided into the following three types:

- Particles and larger molecules
- Small molecules and free antigens
- Antigen in dendritic cells

Particles and molecules in the lymph arriving via the afferent lymphatic vessels enter the subcapsular sinus, which has been likened to a swamp. Hydrostatic pressure is low, particles tend to settle, and reticular fibers crossing the sinus impede the flow. All these factors facilitate phagocytosis by the sinus macrophages. Larger molecules and particles flow from the subcapsular into the trabecular sinuses and then into the medullary sinuses, where particles and bacteria are phagocytosed by the sinus histiocytes. This is well illustrated by the concentration of carbon in the medulla of the tracheobronchial lymph nodes of animals with anthracosis (see Fig. 13-40).

Smaller molecules, such as free antigens and chemokines, cytokines and other soluble products of the immune and inflammatory responses, penetrate the floor of the subcapsular sinus and are carried along reticular fibers to the outer cortex adjacent to the HEVs, the site of migration of B and T lymphocytes into the cortex. Thus these molecules are brought into close association with B and T lymphocytes and dendritic cells, and this process facilitates the activation of antigen specific B lymphocytes, which develops into antibody secreting plasma cells.

Antigens can also reach the regional lymph node in antigen-presenting cells such as dendritic cells. These cells have been activated by uptake and processing of antigen and migrate via lymphatic vessels to the subcapsular sinus where they exit and migrate along the reticulum to the outer cortex where they present the antigen to the follicular B lymphocytes (see Chapter 5). The classic example is the intraepidermal dendritic cell (Langerhans' cell) draining from the skin.

RESPONSES TO INJURY

Responses to injury are listed in Box 13-8, and the responses are discussed on the basis of the following systems: monocyte-macrophage system, outer cortex, inner cortex, medullary sinuses, and medullary cords.

Monocyte-Macrophage System

Like the spleen, lymph nodes contain cells of the monocyte-macrophage system and the lymphoid system (see Box 13-8), and these cells are the first line of defense against infectious and non-infectious agents in the incoming lymph. As most of these agents arrive in the afferent lymph, the sinus macrophages (histiocytes) are the first to respond. This is evidenced by an increase in their number (hyperplasia, so-called sinus histiocytosis) chiefly in the medullary sinuses (Fig. 13-43). Additional inflammatory cells, neutrophils

BOX 13-8 Response of the Lymph Node to Injury

HYPERPLASIA

Cells of the monocyte-macrophage system—sinus histiocytosis

Lymphoid tissue—outer cortex: follicular hyperplasia with the production of antibody; inner cortex: T lymphocyte hyperplasia

ATROPHY

Lymphoid atrophy

INFLAMMATION

Acute—microabscess and abscess formation

Chronic—abscesses, granulomas, and fibrosis

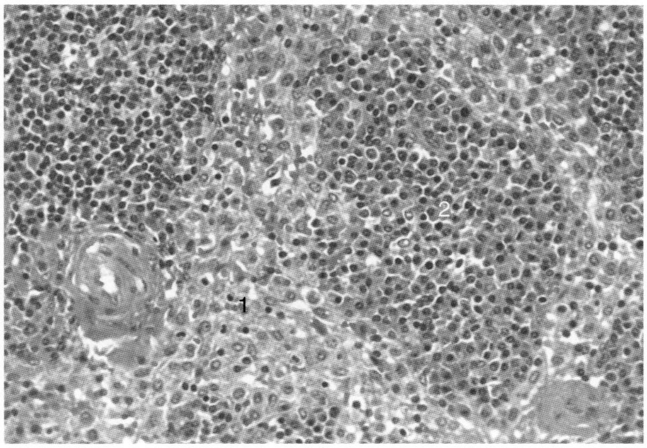

Fig. 13-43 Sinus histiocytosis, lymph node, medulla, dog.
The sinusoids *(1)* are filled with mostly macrophages and a few scattered neutrophils *(small dark nuclei).* Most of the macrophages are derived from the perisinusoidal macrophages, but some may arrive via the afferent lymphatics. The medullary cords *(2)* are filled with lymphocytes and plasma cells. Plasma cell precursors are formed in the germinal centers, mature into plasma cells, and migrate to the medullary cords. Thus the presence of large numbers of plasma cells in the medullary cords is indicative of ongoing production of antibody from an antigenic stimulus. (Courtesy Dr. M.D. McGavin, College of Veterinary Medicine, University of Tennessee.)

in acute lymphadenitis and monocytes in granulomatous lymphadenitis arrive in the blood and migrate into the parenchyma or the sinuses. Some of these leukocytes may contain viable intracellular pathogens (e.g., *Mycobacterium* spp. and fungi *[Blastomyces dermatitidis]*) or have cell-associated viruses (e.g., parvovirus) and infect the lymph node and then are disseminated throughout the lymphoid tissues of the body as a result of the normal trafficking of lymphocytes. Circovirus 2, the agent of porcine PMWS is unusual in that it causes an increase in macrophages in the lymphoid follicles and the deep cortex.

Outer Cortex: B Lymphocyte Areas

If the lymph tissue has not been antigenically stimulated, there may be no follicles or germinal centers visible, but within days of stimulation, a pale area, which is the site of a germinal center, appears (Fig. 13-44). It undergoes a predictable sequence of development, becomes larger, and contains mitotic figures, and lymphocytes proliferate. Because over 90% of these lymphocytes die by apoptosis in the germinal centers, nuclear debris is plentiful, and when this is phagocytosed by macrophages in the germinal center, these are named *tingible body macrophages. Tingible* is an old term meaning stainable, in this case referring to the phagocytosed nuclear debris. The immunoblasts formed here move to and mature in the medullary cords, which as a result are distended with plasma cells (medullary plasmacytosis). The concentration of medullary plasma cells correlates with the activity of the germinal centers. Thus an antigenically stimulated lymph node at the height of its response has numerous follicles (follicular hyperplasia) (Fig. 13-45), is enlarged, and has a tense capsule, and the cut surface may bulge. Histologically, there is follicular lymphoid hyperplasia and active germinal centers and medullary cord plasmacytosis. A subset of these B lymphocytes exit the lymph node and migrate to the bone marrow where they develop into fully differentiated plasma cells and secrete antibody. The majority of the serum antibody is secreted by plasma cells located in the bone marrow.

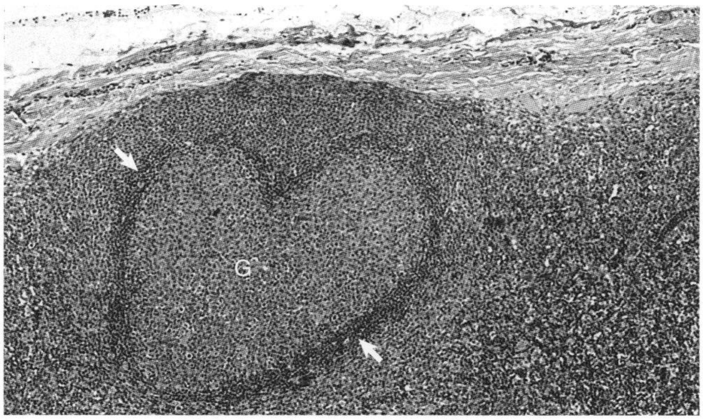

Fig. 13-44 Lymphoid hyperplasia, outer cortex: B lymphocyte areas, lymphoid follicles, lymph node, dog.
If the lymphoid follicle is antigenically stimulated by a bacterium for example, B lymphocyte areas undergo a predictable sequence of development and become larger and contain mitotic figures and B lymphocytes that proliferate. The central areas (germinal centers *[G]*) appear hypocellular as a result of rapid hypertrophy and hyperplasia of antigenically stimulated B lymphocytes followed by the death by apoptosis of more than 90% of these cells. The small numbers of immunoblasts formed in this proliferative response move to the mantle zone *(arrows)* of the follicle and then to the medullary cords, where they mature into plasma cells and secrete immunoglobulins. H&E stain. (Courtesy Dr. M.D. McGavin, College of Veterinary Medicine, University of Tennessee.)

As the immune response declines, mitoses in the germinal centers become less frequent and the concentration of cells in the germinal centers is reduced with the result that the follicular stroma (dendritic cells and macrophages) becomes visible. This stage is designated follicular lymphoid depletion (sometimes inappropriately referred to as *lymphoid exhaustion*). B lymphocyte areas (lymphatic follicles) can atrophy, and histologically, there are reduced numbers of lymphocytes in the outer cortex, smaller and reduced numbers of follicles. Causes of this are a failure of adequate numbers of B lymphocytes to arrive from the bone marrow as in myelofibrosis and destruction of lymphocytes in the bone marrow by viruses, radiation, and toxins. Disappearance of germinal centers is normal once antigenic stimulation has ceased.

Deep Cortex: T Lymphocyte Areas

T lymphocytes can also respond by a limited degree by proliferation. An increase in T lymphocytes has been reported in the deep and interfollicular cortices and in the PALS in malignant catarrhal fever (MCF) in cattle and in the deep cortex in pigs with porcine reproductive and respiratory syndrome. A diffuse proliferation of

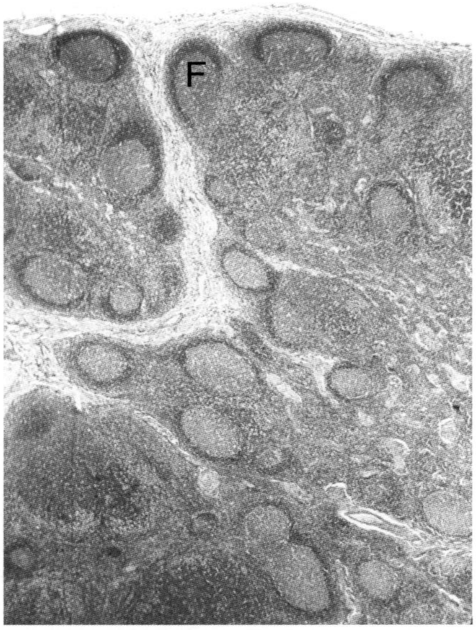

Fig. 13-45 Follicular lymphoid hyperplasia, chronic demodicosis, caudal cervical (prescapular) lymph node, dog.
The number of lymphoid follicles *(F)* has increased (hyperplasia), and all of these have germinal centers (secondary follicles) indicating active proliferation of B lymphocytes to form plasma cells in response to an antigenic stimulus. H&E stain. (Courtesy Dr. M.D. McGavin, College of Veterinary Medicine, University of Tennessee.)

macrophages occurs in the deep cortex in porcine circovirus 2 infection (PMWS).

Atrophy may indicate that there is a deficit in lymphocyte production in the bone marrow or in the differential selection in the thymus, or destruction by viruses, radiation, and toxins directly on the lymphocytes in the lymph node. Examination of H&E stained sections allows evaluation of follicular and germinal center activity and the concentration of plasma cells in the medullary cords and thus a reasonable estimate of B lymphocyte activity. However, because T lymphocytes cannot be differentiated from B lymphocytes in H&E stained sections, it is not possible to accurately evaluate their numbers in the deep cortex. For this, immunohistochemical staining of B and T lymphocytes is required. However, marked atrophy of the T lymphocyte areas can be detected histologically.

Medulla

Responses to injury of the medulla occur in the medullary sinuses and the medullary cords.

Medullary Sinuses

Responses to injury by the medullary sinuses are dilation and proliferation of the macrophages (histiocytes) in their lumens. Dilation can be caused by edema fluid draining from an edematous area (as in chronic cardiac failure), inflammatory edema fluid draining from an acutely inflamed area or inflammatory exudate in response to blood-borne bacterial emboli lodging in the lymph node. As the inflammation progresses (see the section on Acute Lymphadenitis), the sinuses become filled with inflammatory cells (neutrophils, macrophages) and hyperplastic sinus macrophages (see Fig. 13-43). Depending on the intensity of the inflammation, the adjacent parenchyma may be hyperemic and infiltrated with inflammatory cells. Sinus macrophages proliferate in response to a wide variety of particulate matter (see the section on Pigmentation), bacteria, and erythrocytes (erythrophagocytosis) draining from a hemorrhagic area.

Medullary Cords

As pointed out in the section on Structure and Function, after activation and proliferation of B lymphocytes in the follicle, the plasma cells produced migrate to and accumulate in the medullary cords, which at the height of the immune response are distended by plasma cells and some lymphocytes. As the immune response subsides, the number of plasma cells decreases and the medullary cords return to their resting state, populated by some lymphocytes and scattered plasma cells.

HEMAL NODES

STRUCTURE AND FUNCTION

Hemal nodes are prominent in ruminants, usually adjacent to lymph nodes. They are small dark red nodules whose architecture resembles that of lymph nodes. The sinuses are filled with blood and there are no afferent or efferent lymphatic vessels. Their function is unclear but erythrophagocytosis can be present. Further information on this topic, including Web Fig. 13-4, is available at evolve.elsevier.com/Zachary/McGavin/.

MUCOSA-ASSOCIATED LYMPHOID TISSUE

STRUCTURE

Histology books use the following terms: diffuse lymphatic tissue and solitary and aggregated lymphatic nodules to describe these forms of lymphatic tissue, but the immunology and pathology literature uses mucosa-associated lymphoid tissue (MALT). The importance of these three types of MALT is frequently overlooked because most of these tissues in the normal animal, apart from aggregated lymphatic tissue of the tonsil and Peyer's patches, are visible only microscopically. The actual mass is significant, and MALT is essential for mucosal immunity. It is a site where antigen is phagocytosed and from which immune cells and antigen flow via afferent lymphatic vessels to regional lymph nodes. MALT consists of three distinct morphologic types:

- **Diffuse lymphatic tissue** includes scattered lymphocytes surrounded by dendritic cells and connective tissue in the mucosa of many organs. In normal animals, it is most obvious in the mucosa of the alimentary tract. The lymphocytes secrete not only IgA, but also IgG and IgM.
- **Solitary lymph nodules,** also in the mucosa, are small unencapsulated clusters of lymphocytes, principally B lymphocytes that secrete various types of immunoglobulin. They are surrounded by small numbers of dendritic cells and lymphocytes. In the resting or antigenically unstimulated state, they are usually not visible grossly.
- **Aggregated lymphatic nodules** are unencapsulated and consist of groups of lymph nodules. There are considerable differences between the different domestic animals in their locations and whether they are present at birth. Because this tissue is antigen dependent and responds to antigenic

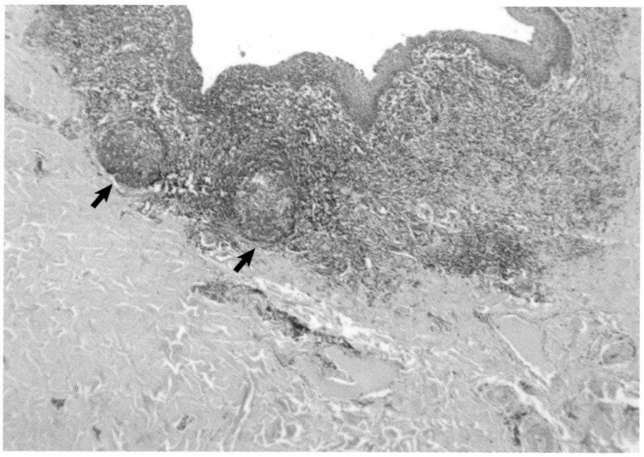

Fig. 13-46 Follicular lymphoid hyperplasia, conjunctiva, lymphoid nodules, cow.
The diffuse lymphoid tissue has increased in size, and there are two follicles with germinal centers *(arrows)*. This reaction is a frequent response to conjunctivitis from irritants and bacteria. H&E stain. (Courtesy Dr. M.D. McGavin, College of Veterinary Medicine, University of Tennessee.)

TABLE 13-4 Function of Mucosa-Associated Lymphoid Tissue (MALT) in Viral and Bacterial Diseases in Livestock

Function	Species	Microorganism
TONSILS		
Portal of entry	Sheep and goats	*Chlamydia psittaci*
Initial site of infection	Cattle	BVDV
Early site of infection	Cattle	BHV1
Site of replication	Pig	Porcine circovirus 2 PMWS infection
Carriers (reservoirs)	Horses	*Streptococcus zooepidemicus*
	Cattle	*Mannheimia haemolytica*
	Sheep	*Salmonella* spp.
		Pasteurella haemolytica
		Scrapie agent (PrPsc)
	Pigs	*Mycoplasma* spp.
		Streptococcus suis
		Salmonella spp.
		Yersinia pseudotuberculosis
GALT (PEYER'S PATCHES)		
Portal of entry	Cattle	*Brucella abortus*
		Mycobacterium avium spp. *paratuberculosis*
	Sheep and goats	*Yersinia tuberculosis*

Data from Liebler-Tenorio EM, Pabst R: *Vet Res* 37:257-280, 2006.
BVDV, Bovine virus diarrhea virus; *BHV-1,* bovine herpesvirus 1; *PMWS,* postweaning multisystem wasting syndrome.

BOX 13-9 Response of Mucosa-Associated Lymphoid Tissue (MALT; Lymph Nodule) to Injury

LYMPHOID ATROPHY
Viral infections
Malnutrition
Cachexia
Aging
Antineoplastic chemotherapeutic drugs
Toxins
Irradiation

LYMPHOID HYPERPLASIA
Antigenic stimulus

stimulus by hyperplasia, some of it is visible months or years after birth or infection.

The solitary lymph nodules and aggregated lymphatic tissues are classified by their anatomic locations and form the MALT. These lymphatic tissues include (1) the bronchus-associated lymphatic tissue (BALT), which is often at the bifurcation of the bronchi and bronchioles), (2) a ring of lymphoid tissue (pharyngeal and palatine tonsils [see below]) and lymph nodules (NALT, LALT, and ATALT [see below]) that surround the oral and nasal pharynges and encounter infectious microorganisms during ingestion and inhalation, and (3) the gut-associated lymphatic tissue (GALT), of which the most important and most obvious components are Peyer's patches and the pharyngeal and palatine tonsils. Lymph nodules can also be present in the mucosa of the conjunctiva-associated lymphatic tissue (CALT) (Fig. 13-46), mammary gland, urinary bladder mucosa, nose (NALT), larynx (LALT), auditory tube (ATALT), and genital tract.

FUNCTION

The primary function of MALT is to protect mucosal barriers and thus they are strategically placed to act as sentinels, but they can also become a portal of entry for bacteria and this is particularly true of the tonsils and Peyer's patches. Peyer's patches in the ileum are overlaid by a special epithelium known as the *follicle-associated epithelium* (FAE), in which there are numerous M cells. These M cells deliver macromolecules (including antigens), particles, pathogenic bacteria, and viruses across the epithelium to an area rich in dendritic cells, which are able to transport the material into the GALT. Table 13-4 lists the functions of the MALT with different microorganisms.

RESPONSES TO INJURY

The responses of MALT (diffuse lymphatic tissue and solitary and aggregated lymph nodules) to injury (Box 13-9) are similar to those of other lymphatic tissue: hyperplasia, atrophy, and inflammation.

Hyperplasia

After antigenic stimulation, activation of germinal centers, follicular hyperplasia (see Fig. 13-46), and increased production of plasma cell and antibodies occur. Lymph nodule hyperplasia can be marked in diseases, usually chronic diseases, for example, BALT in chronic *Dictyocaulus* spp. bronchitis or bronchiolitis in cattle, sheep, and goats; in *Metastrongylus* spp. bronchitis or bronchiolitis in pigs; and in some pneumonias. It is particularly marked in *Mycoplasma* spp. pneumonias of sheep and pigs and can be so extensive as to encircle bronchioles and bronchi and hence the designation of "cuffing pneumonia."

Hyperplastic lymph nodules can be so enlarged that they become grossly visible as white plaques or nodules. They can be seen in the conjunctiva of the eyelids and the third eyelid in chronic conjunctivitis (see Fig. 13-46), the pharyngeal mucosa in chronic pharyngitis, the gastric mucosa in chronic gastritis, and the urinary bladder in chronic cystitis (follicular cystitis). The normal fetus has no detectable BALT, but it may be present in fetuses aborted because of infections.

Atrophy

Atrophy of the diffuse lymphatic tissue and lymph nodules has the same causes as those affecting lymph nodes. These causes include lack of antigenic stimulation, cachexia, malnutrition, aging, and viral infections. The microscopic lesions of BVDV infection of Peyer's patches in ruminants (see Chapters 4 and 7) are distinctive and consist of lysis of cells of lymphoid follicles; in canine parvovirus infection, there is lymphoid necrosis of Peyer's patches and atrophy of these tissues can be a sequela.

Inflammation

Granulomas can form in Peyer's patches in paratuberculosis (Johne's disease) in goats (see the section on Disorders of Ruminants).

PORTALS OF ENTRY

Portals of entry used by microorganisms and other agents and substances to access the lymphatic system are summarized in Box 13-10. These portals include the blood vasculature (hematogenous) spread (cell-free or within leukocytes), direct penetration (trauma, wounds), afferent lymphatic vessels, or M cells and dendritic cells overlying MALT and tonsils.

THYMUS

Viruses and toxins, such as aflatoxins, enter the thymus hematogenously via the arteries.

SPLEEN

Infectious agents, such as bacteria, enter the spleen by two routes: via the blood vasculature or by direct penetration. The spleen has no afferent lymphatic vessels and efferent lymphatic vessels drain only the capsule and trabeculae. The splenic capsule is thick, and thus inflammation from an adjacent peritonitis is unlikely to penetrate it. Direct penetration is extremely rare, but foreign bodies occasionally do penetrate as a sequela to traumatic reticulitis in cattle. Contraction of the reticulum extrudes a foreign body, usually a nail or wire through the wall of the reticulum. Most of these objects travel cranially to penetrate the diaphragm and pericardium, causing traumatic reticulopericarditis. Less frequently, some enter the visceral surface of the ventral extremity of the spleen, often causing a splenic abscess. In horses, on rare occasions, splenic abscesses can develop secondary to perforation of the gastric wall. Also, small pieces of wire have been found in these splenic abscesses, presumably originating from the GI tract. Equine splenic abscesses can be secondary to gastric ulcers *(Gasterophilus intestinalis)* or by extension on the granulomatous inflammation around *Habronema* spp. in the wall of the stomach.

BOX 13-10 Portals of Entry into Lymphatic Organs

THYMUS
Hematogenously

SPLEEN
Hematogenously
Direct penetration (rare)

LYMPH NODE
Via afferent lymphatics
Hematogenously

MUCOSA-ASSOCIATED LYMPHOID TISSUE (MALT; LYMPH NODULE)
Hematogenously
In migrating macrophages and dendritic cells
Intestinal wall via M cells and dendritic cells to Peyer's patches

LYMPH NODES

Bacteria, viruses, and antigens enter the lymph node by two routes: afferent lymphatic vessels and via the blood vasculature (hematogenously).

Afferent Lymphatic Vessels

Infectious microorganisms, either cell free or within lymphocytes or monocytes, are transported in lymph to regional lymph nodes or lymphocenters. Here, some of these agents may escape removal by phagocytosis and are transported via the efferent lymphatic vessels to the next lymph node in the chain, where they can cause an inflammatory or immunologic response. This process can continue serially down a lymph node chain and if the agent is not removed it may eventually be transported via the lymphatic vessels to the circulating blood via the thoracic duct or truncus trachealis and disseminated throughout the body.

Blood Vasculature

Bacteria can arrive at lymph nodes hematogenously in septicemias and bacteremias. However, most pathogens arrive via afferent lymphatic vessels. B and T lymphocytes as part of their normal trafficking, arrive in the blood, enter the lymph node via the HEV and conduct surveillance for the specific antigens that they have been programmed to recognize. Macrophages containing microorganisms also arrive hematogenously (see Chapter 4).

Capsule

The lymph node is protected by a thick fibrous capsule, and thus direct penetration by inflammation, trauma, or neoplasms is rare. However, in sheep, in enzootic areas, during shearing, peripheral lymph nodes enlarged from caseous lymphadenitis (CLA) may be punctured by the comb of the shears, resulting in the shears becoming contaminated by pus. The infection may then transmit to other sheep through nicks and cuts in their skin.

LYMPH NODULES (MALT)

Lymph nodules do not have afferent lymphatic vessels and thus antigens arrive hematogenously, in migrating macrophages or across mucous membranes. M cells of Peyer's patches can transport infections agents. Live-attenuated *Salmonella* spp. bacteria induce dendritic cells in intestinal submucosal tissues to migrate to lymph follicles (B lymphocytes) and parafollicular (T lymphocytes) areas of Peyer's patches. Other pathogenic bacteria known or believed to enter via the M cells from the intestine include *Listeria monocytogenes, Mycobacterium avium* ssp. *paratuberculosis,* and *Yersinia pseudotuberculosis.* The scrapie agent also accumulates in Peyer's patches.

DEFENSE MECHANISMS

Defense mechanisms used by the lymphatic system to protect itself against microorganisms and other agents and substances are the innate and adaptive immune responses, which are discussed in Chapters 3 and 5. Viruses, bacteria, and particles arriving in the lymph and blood interact with cells of the monocyte-macrophage system through phagocytosis and antigen processing and presentation. Hyperplasia of the macrophages often occurs concurrently. Most of these macrophages are located in the medullary sinuses. If the material is antigenic, antigen processing and presentation are followed by an immune response resulting in proliferation of B lymphocytes and production of antibody and/or the proliferation of T lymphocytes. Other defense mechanisms are structural in nature and include the thick fibrous capsule of lymph nodes and the spleen, which protects them from external trauma.

METHODS OF GROSS AND MICROSCOPIC EXAMINATION

THYMUS

Information on this topic is available at evolve.elsevier.com/Zachary/McGavin/.

SPLEEN

Information on this topic is available at evolve.elsevier.com/Zachary/McGavin/.

LYMPH NODES

Information on this topic is available at evolve.elsevier.com/Zachary/McGavin/.

Microscopic Examination

Information on this topic is available at evolve.elsevier.com/Zachary/McGavin/.

Location of Affected Lymph Nodes

Enlarged lymph nodes can be distributed in several different patterns in the body. First, all lymph nodes throughout the body (systemic or generalized) may be enlarged (lymphadenomegaly). This pattern is generally attributed to systemic infectious, inflammatory, or neoplastic processes. If a regional lymph node (i.e., a lymph node draining a specific area such as one of the limbs or one side of the oral cavity) is enlarged, then the area drained by that node must be checked for infectious, inflammatory, or neoplastic processes. Finally, enlargement of the mesenteric lymph nodes or GALT suggests that the infectious, inflammatory, or neoplastic process originates within the gut, although they can be infected hematogenously. Normal mesenteric lymph nodes are continuously receiving and responding immunologically to barrages of antigens and bacteria received via their afferent lymphatic vessels from the intestinal tract. This role is reflected in their appearance. They are larger and have numerous well-developed lymphoid follicles (follicular lymphoid hyperplasia) with active germinal centers. Often the sinuses contain histiocytes (sinus histiocytosis), presumably in response to the need to phagocytose incoming material.

Multiple lymph nodes of a chain may be enlarged because infection or metastases spread via the lymphatic vessels, from one lymph node to the next in the chain. Thus it is important to know the area drained by specific lymph nodes; for example, all lymph from the head ultimately drains to the medial retropharyngeal lymph nodes, and lymph from the foreleg drains to either the axillary or superficial cervical (prescapular) lymph node. However, there are some surprises. Besides the thoracic cavity, the caudal sternal and caudal mediastinal lymph nodes drain the cranial abdomen and may be enlarged in the absence of thoracic lesions. Similarly, the celiac lymph nodes of dogs, pigs, and horses receive some afferent lymphatic vessels from thoracic organs and lesions in them do not necessarily mean that disease originated in the abdomen.

DISORDERS OF DOMESTIC ANIMALS: THYMUS

CONGENITAL DISORDERS

Congenital disorders of the thymus are discussed in detail in Chapter 5. Summaries of the gross and microscopic morphologic changes are described in the sections on Disorders of Horses and Disorders of Dogs.

Thymic cysts can be found within the developing and mature thymus and in thymic remnants in the cranial mediastinum. These cysts are often lined by ciliated epithelium and represent developmental remnants of branchial arch epithelium and are usually of no significance.

INFLAMMATORY AND DEGENERATIVE DISORDERS

Thymitis, an infrequent lesion, is seen in porcine circovirus 2 (PMWS) infection (see Disorders of Pigs and also Chapter 4), enzootic bovine abortion (EBA; see Chapter 18), and salmon poisoning disease of dogs (see Chapter 7). Variable degrees of acquired immunodeficiency may be caused by infectious agents (viruses), toxins, chemotherapeutic agents and radiation, malnutrition, aging, and neoplasia.

Infections that most commonly injure lymphoid tissues do so because they infect lymphocytes and destroy the lymphoid component of the thymus. Viruses, which can damage the lymphoid component of the thymus and are often found in other lymphoid tissues, include canine distemper virus, EHV-1 in aborted foals (Fig. 13-47), canine and feline parvovirus, FIV, BVDV, and hog cholera virus. In kittens infected with FIV, thymic lymphoid depletion is an early lesion, and in kittens with progressive FIV infection, ultimately there is complete loss of thymic architecture with only minimal thymic tissue remaining in the connective and adipose tissue of the mediastinum.

Environmental toxins, such as halogenated aromatic hydrocarbons (e.g., polychlorinated biphenyls and dibenzodioxins, lead, and mercury) have a suppressive effect on the immune system. Fumonisins B_1 and B_2, which are secondary fungal metabolites produced by members of the genus *Fusarium,* cause lymphocytolysis in the thymic cortex. In weaned and grower pigs, aflatoxin causes thymic atrophy because of lymphocyte depletion. In the case of the halogenated aromatic hydrocarbons, there is a genetic basis for susceptibility that is mediated through a complex composed of the aromatic hydrocarbon receptor and the aromatic receptor nuclear transporter. In general, the end result is that these chemicals cause severe atrophy of the primary and secondary lymphoid organs. Other environmental toxins, such as the metals lead and mercury, cause toxic effects through the interaction of the metal ion with enzyme systems, cell membranes, or organelles. Similarly, chemotherapeutic agents in general specifically target enzyme systems and cellular components essential for cell replication. Thus they can cause inhibition of a cellular function rather than cause a morphologic change.

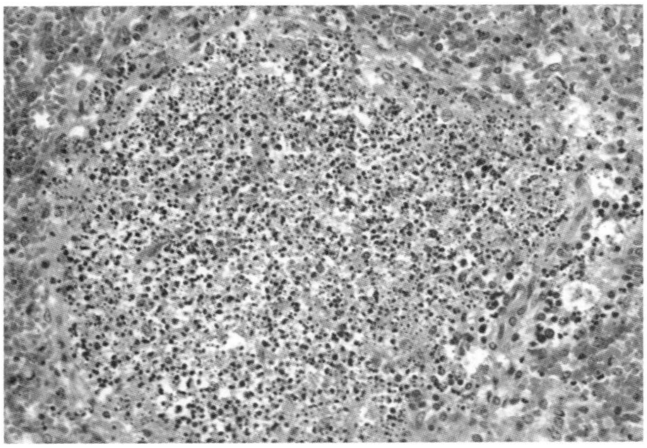

Fig. 13-47 Equine herpesvirus 1, spleen, aborted foal.
Most of the splenic follicle is occupied by nuclear debris, the result of lymphocytolysis. The splenic follicle is surrounded by red pulp. H&E stain. (Courtesy College of Veterinary Medicine, University of Illinois.)

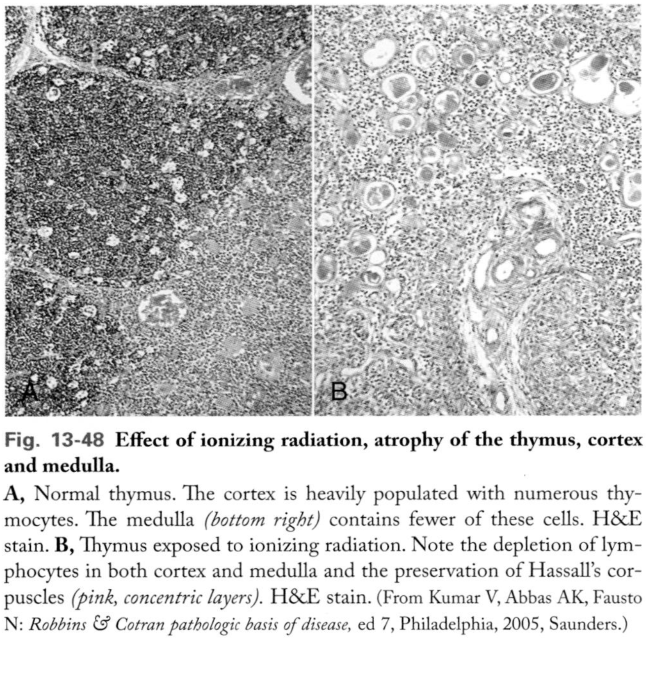

Fig. 13-48 Effect of ionizing radiation, atrophy of the thymus, cortex and medulla.
A, Normal thymus. The cortex is heavily populated with numerous thymocytes. The medulla *(bottom right)* contains fewer of these cells. H&E stain. **B,** Thymus exposed to ionizing radiation. Note the depletion of lymphocytes in both cortex and medulla and the preservation of Hassall's corpuscles *(pink, concentric layers).* H&E stain. (From Kumar V, Abbas AK, Fausto N: *Robbins & Cotran pathologic basis of disease,* ed 7, Philadelphia, 2005, Saunders.)

Anticancer drugs, radiomimetic anticancer drugs, or ionization radiation used in cancer therapy target dividing cells and destruction of lymphocytes can result in immunosuppression (Fig. 13-48). Lymphocytes are very sensitive to these agents. Most cytotoxic drugs used to treat cancer inhibit cell division by mechanisms that are centered on the function and activity of nucleic acids. Purine analogs (e.g., azathioprine) compete with purines in the synthesis of nucleic acids, whereas alkylating agents like cyclophosphamide cross-link DNA and inhibit the replication and activation of lymphocytes. Cyclosporin A specifically inhibits the T lymphocyte signaling pathway by interfering with the transcription of the IL-2 gene. Methotrexate, a folic acid antagonist, blocks the synthesis of thymidine and purine nucleotides. As chemotherapeutic drugs, they have the beneficial effect of targeting cancer cells and the detrimental effect of also targeting noncancerous immune cells, resulting in immunosuppression, the proverbial double-edged sword. Because of the desirable effect of these and other drugs, they

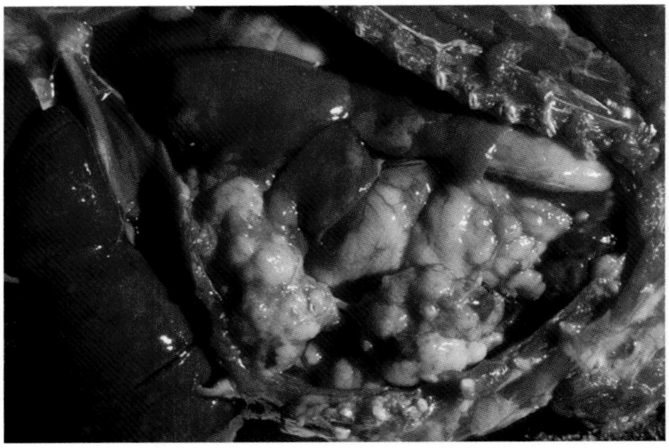

Fig. 13-49 Lymphoma (lymphosarcoma), thymus, dog.
The large pale mass in the cranial mediastinum is a thymic lymphosarcoma that has displaced the lungs caudad. (Courtesy Dr. M.D. McGavin, College of Veterinary Medicine, University of Tennessee.)

are also used to prevent allograft rejection after transplantation. Corticosteroids are considered to be immunosuppressive, although the degree of suppression is highly variable among species, and in general, humans and rodents are corticosteroid sensitive, whereas domestic species are considered corticosteroid resistant.

Ionizing radiation targets components of the cell's DNA and through nonlethal mechanisms such as the generation of highly reactive free radicals can damage and be lethal to lymphoid tissues and cells (see Fig. 13-48).

Malnutrition and cachexia impairs thymic function because they induce lymphoid deletion and resultant thymic atrophy, with resultant reduction in thymic hormone output. The result is a decrease in the number of circulating T lymphocytes in the blood, depletion of T lymphocytes from the secondary lymphoid organs, and impairment of T lymphocyte functions. Consequently, blood concentration of lymphocytes is decreased in starvation and immunosuppression. This effect of starvation is mediated by the hormone leptin, whose concentration in the blood is proportional to the mass of fat in the body.

AGING

Information on this topic is available at evolve.elsevier.com/Zachary/McGavin/.

NEOPLASIA

Because the thymus has both lymphoid and epithelial components, it is possible for either or both components to serve as cells of origin of neoplasm. Thymic lymphoma is a T lymphocyte neoplasm of young animals, particularly in cats and cattle and is less frequently seen in dogs (Fig. 13-49) (see the section on Hematopoietic Neoplasia). Clinical findings reflect the presence of a large mass in the cranial mediastinum. This mass can often be forced into the thoracic inlet with gentle compression of the cranial ribs. Thymomas are usually benign neoplasms that occupy the cranial mediastinum, usually of older animals. They are significantly less common than thymic lymphoma and are only distinguishable microscopically by the presence of neoplastic epithelial cells. Variable numbers of lymphocytes are present within thymomas but are not neoplastic. Nonneoplastic lymphocytes often outnumber the neoplastic epithelial cells. Thymomas have been associated with myasthenia gravis (which may be accompanied by megaesophagus) and polymyositis (immune-mediated) in dogs. A rare condition, thymic hyperplasia, which results from the formation of B lymphocyte follicles within the thymus, has also been reported in association with myasthenia gravis in dogs and cats.

MISCELLANEOUS DISORDERS

Thymic Hematomas

See the section on Disorders of Dogs.

DISORDERS OF DOMESTIC ANIMALS: SPLEEN

CONGENITAL DISORDERS

Asplenia or the failure of a spleen to develop in utero occurs occasionally in animals. This condition is usually incidental, because congenital asplenia is so rare, it has not been possible to be certain of the effect on the animal's immune status. Splenic aplasia is well known in certain strains of mice, but as these are usually maintained under either germ-free or specific pathogen–free (SPF) conditions the effect of asplenia cannot be evaluated. However, congenitally asplenic mice have a high mortality rate to experimental plasmodium infection. Splenectomy in the adult results in an increased susceptibility to pathogenic bacteria, particularly those with polysaccharide-rich capsular antigens such as pneumococci.

Congenital immunodeficiency diseases have been described in the discussions on the thymus in the sections on Disorders of Horses and Disorders of Dogs.

SPLENOMEGALY

The procedure for gross examination of the spleen is described in the discussion in the section on Methods of Gross and Microscopic Examinations; this examination involves deciding whether the spleen was enlarged (splenomegaly), normal, or small. Enlarged spleens are classified as congested and noncongested. The cut surface of severely congested spleens may be red to bluish-black and exude blood; these spleens are often termed *bloody* spleens. Enlarged spleens that are not congested but firm are often called *meaty* spleens because of their firmness and texture. Little blood oozes from their cut surfaces, and the color of this surface depends on how much of the normal red pulp has been replaced by inflammatory cells, stored materials, or neoplastic cells (see the section on Splenomegaly and Table 13-5). The spleen may be measured and weighed but because of the wide variation in the dimensions and weight of normal spleens and the amount of blood stored, these data can be difficult to interpret. The diseases and disorders associated with splenomegaly are discussed using the following categories:

- Uniform splenomegaly with a bloody consistency: bloody spleen (Fig. 13-50, *A*)
- Uniform splenomegaly with a firm consistency: meaty spleen (Fig. 13-50, *B*)
- Splenic nodules with a bloody consistency
- Splenic nodules with a firm consistency

Table 13-5 lists the common causes of uniform splenomegaly.

TABLE 13-5 Common Causes of Uniform Splenomegaly in Domestic Animals

Animal	Congestive (Bloody) Spleen	Firm (Meaty) Spleen
Horse	Septicemia Anthrax Salmonellosis (peracute) Hemolytic disease EIA (acute)	Septicemia Salmonellosis Hemolytic diseases EIA (chronic) IMHA Neoplasms Lymphoma Metastatic neoplasms
Cattle, sheep, and goat	Septicemias Anthrax Salmonellosis (acute) Hemolytic disease Babesiosis (acute)	Septicemia Salmonellosis Chronic hemolytic diseases Babesiosis (subacute) Anaplasmosis Trypanosomiasis Hemotropic mycoplasmosis Neoplasm Lymphoma
Pig	Septicemia Salmonellosis (peracute) Splenic torsion	Septicemias Salmonellosis Erysipelas Chronic hemolytic disease Hemotropic mycoplasmosis Neoplasm Lymphoma
Dog and cat	Barbiturate euthanasia or anesthesia Gastric torsion Neoplasms Hemangioma (nodular) Hemangiosarcoma (nodular)	Hemolytic disease IMHA Hematopoietic neoplasia Mast cell neoplasia (cat) Lymphoma Histiocytic sarcoma Granulomatous disease Histoplasmosis Amyloidosis

EIA, Equine infectious anemia; *IMHA*, immune-mediated hemolytic anemia.

Uniform Splenomegaly with a Bloody Consistency—"Bloody" Spleen

The common causes of a bloody spleen are (1) congestion (gastric volvulus with splenic entrapment, splenic volvulus, barbiturate euthanasia, anesthesia, and sedation), (2) acute hyperemia (inflammation, anthrax), and (3) acute hemolytic anemia (autoimmune disorder or hemotropic parasite).

Congestion

Splenic Volvulus and Gastric Volvulus with Splenic Entrapment

Volvulus of the spleen occurs mainly in pigs and dogs, and volvulus of the spleen and stomach together occurs in dogs (gastric volvulus), usually deep-chested ones (see Chapter 7).

In contrast to ruminants, in which the spleen is firmly attached to the rumen, the spleen of dogs and pigs is attached loosely to the stomach by the gastrosplenic ligament. It is the twisting of the spleen around this ligament that results initially in occlusion of the veins, causing splenic congestion, and later in occlusion of the artery, causing splenic infarction.

In dogs, the spleen is uniformly and markedly enlarged and may be blue-black from cyanosis (see Fig. 13-50, *A*). It is often folded back on itself (visceral surface to visceral surface) in the shape of the letter "C." Treatment for this condition is splenectomy, but removal of the spleen renders the animal susceptible to certain organisms (as discussed previously), such as hemotropic mycoplasma infections (previously known as *haemobartonellosis* and

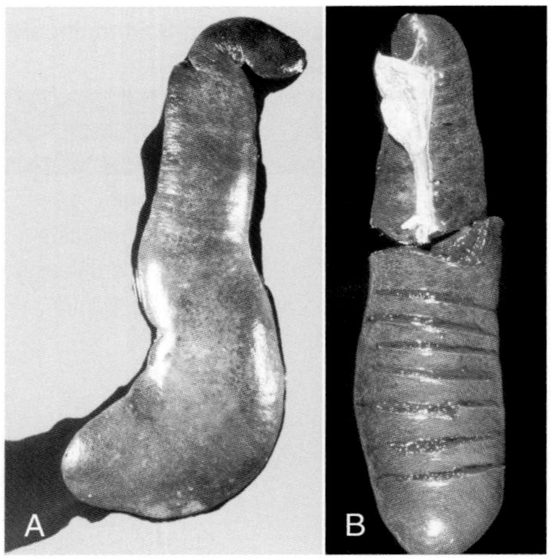

Fig. 13-50 Uniform splenomegaly.
A, Congested bloody spleen. This condition occurs secondary to compromises in vascular flow into and out of the spleen (e.g., vovulus), from intravenous barbiturates (e.g., euthanasia or anesthesia), and from acute hyperemia from septicemia. **B,** Meaty spleen. This condition most commonly results from proliferation of cells, most frequently macrophages in the red pulp and increased phagocytosis in, for example, septicemias, bacteremias, and hemolytic diseases. (Courtesy College of Veterinary Medicine, University of Illinois.)

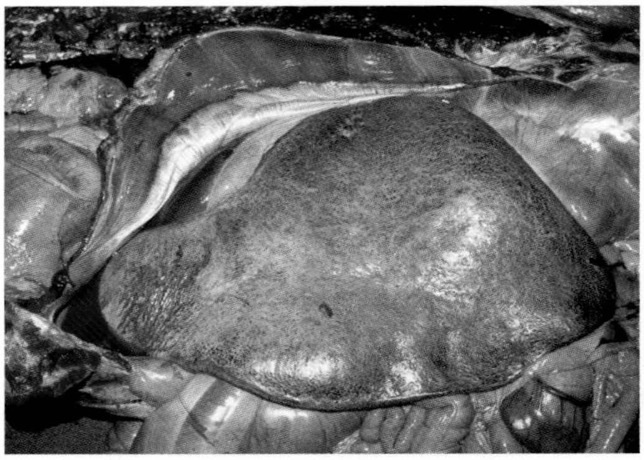

Fig. 13-51 Splenic congestion from barbiturate euthanasia, horse.
The spleen is enlarged and congested from storage of blood. (Courtesy Dr. M.D. McGavin, College of Veterinary Medicine, University of Tennessee.)

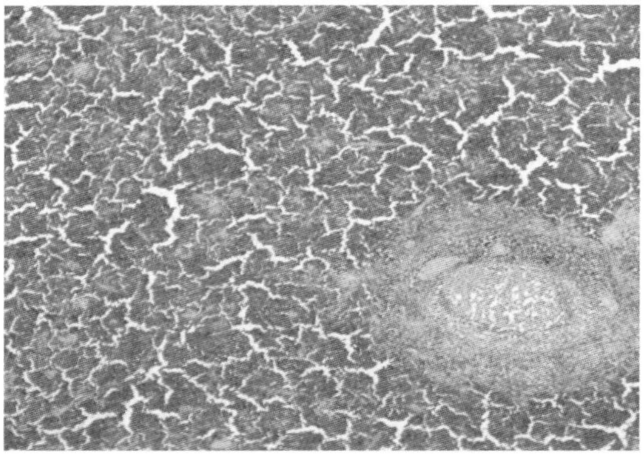

Fig. 13-52 Splenic congestion from barbiturate euthanasia, dog.
The red pulp vascular spaces are markedly distended by blood. One focus of white pulp—a splenic follicle with a pale germinal center—is present in the lower right. H&E stain. (Courtesy Dr. M.D. McGavin, College of Veterinary Medicine, University of Tennessee.)

eperythrozoonosis) in dogs and cattle, and babesiosis and theileriosis in cattle in endemic areas.

Barbiturate Euthanasia, Anesthesia, or Sedation

Acute passive congestion is seen most dramatically at necropsy in horses and dogs that have been euthanized or anesthetized by intravenous injection of barbiturate. The swollen spleen is thought to be the result of splenic relaxation of smooth muscle in the capsule and trabeculae, induced by the anesthetic When a dog under barbiturate anesthesia and with a markedly congested spleen from the anesthetic was injected with 1 mL of 1:1000 adrenaline into the splenic artery, the splenic volume was reduced by 75%.

Grossly, the spleen is extremely enlarged (Fig. 13-51), and the cut surface is notably congested and bulges and oozes blood. The splenic capsule can be fragile and easily ruptured. Histologically, as a result of the distention of the red pulp by blood, the normal architecture of the splenic parenchyma is almost obliterated by masses of blood cells, chiefly erythrocytes (Fig. 13-52). Because of the splenic distention, lymphoid tissues (periarteriolar lymphoid sheaths and splenic follicles) are widely separated and trabeculae and the capsule are thin.

Electric stunning of pigs at slaughter occasionally results in a large congested spleen, but the mechanism is unknown. It is important because it could be confused with a pathologically congested spleen. Splenic congestion in acute cardiac failure is rarely seen in animals.

Acute Hyperemia

Acute septicemias may cause acute hyperemia and concurrent acute congestion of marginal zones first and then the splenic cords. Microbes are transported hematogenously to these sites where they are rapidly phagocytosed by macrophages. Enormous numbers of intravenous bacteria can be cleared by the spleen from the blood in 20 to 30 minutes, but when this defensive mechanism is overwhelmed, the outcome is usually fatal. The response of the spleen depends on the duration of the disease. In acutely fatal cases, such as anthrax and fulminating salmonellosis, distention by blood may be the only finding. If the animal survives longer, as in swine erysipelas and the less virulent forms of salmonellosis, there may be time for neutrophils and macrophages to accumulate in the marginal zones and splenic cords (Fig. 13-53) and for macrophages to undergo hyperplasia.

In human medicine, it has been generally accepted that acute sepsis (septicemia) can cause acute splenitis, loosely defined as splenomegaly, which is the result of acute splenic congestion and neutrophilic infiltrates. A retrospective study in humans did not find splenitis, but rather there was little significant change in the spleen. However, in mice injected intraperitoneally with *Burkholderia mallei* (glanders bacillus), there was notable splenomegaly and histologically the spleen was infiltrated initially (within hours) with neutrophils and later (>24 hours) by pyogranulomatous inflammation. Although the Kupffer cells of the liver make up 80% to 90% of the body's macrophages in some animals, in these mice the greatest number of bacilli was present in the spleen.

Grossly in acute septicemias in domestic animals, the spleen is moderately enlarged and red from congestion, and the cut surface oozes blood. Microscopically, there is congestion of the marginal sinuses and red pulp vascular spaces, followed hours later infiltrations of neutrophils and a day or so later by granulomas in the marginal sinuses.

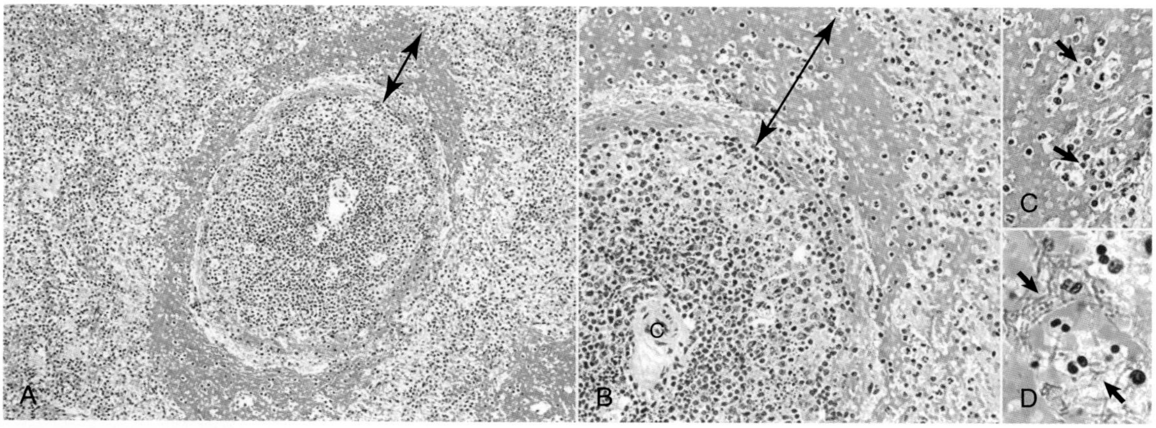

Fig. 13-53 Active hyperemia, anthrax, marginal zones, spleen, monkey.
Also see Fig. 13-40 for schematic illustration of the marginal zone. **A,** Acute septicemias may cause active hyperemia (inflammation) and concurrent acute congestion of the marginal zone *(double-headed line)* and then of the splenic cords (not shown). H&E stain. **B,** Higher magnification of **A.** Marginal zone *(double-headed line)*; central arteriole *(C)* of the follicle. H&E stain. **C,** Higher magnification of **B.** Note the small aggregates of neutrophils (active hyperemia) within the marginal zone *(arrows).* H&E stain. **D,** Higher magnification of **B.** Note the accumulation of the vegetative form *(arrows)* of anthrax (*light blue* and bacillus-shaped) within the marginal zone. This form produces anthrax toxins, which cause severe tissue injury resulting in inflammation and cell death. H&E stain. (Courtesy Dr. J.F. Zachary, College of Veterinary Medicine, University of Illinois. Photographed from slides provided by Toxicology Battelle Columbus to the Wednesday Slide Conference [2003-2004, Conference number 13, Case number 1], Armed Forces Institute of Pathology, Department of Veterinary Pathology.)

Anthrax

Anthrax is caused by *Bacillus anthracis* and is primarily a disease of ruminants, especially cattle and sheep (see Chapters 4, 7, 9, and 10). *Bacillus anthracis* is a Gram-positive, large rod-shaped, endospore-forming bacterium, which grows in aerobic to facultative anaerobic environments. If spores are ingested, they replicate locally in the intestinal tract, spread to regional lymph nodes, and then disseminate systemically, through the bloodstream, resulting in septicemia. *Bacillus anthracis* produces exotoxins, which degrade endothelial cell membranes and enzyme systems.

Grossly, the spleen is uniformly enlarged and dark red to bluish-black, and contains abundant unclotted blood. In peracute cases, the only histologic lesion may be marked congestion of the marginal sinuses and the splenic red pulp vascular spaces. At low magnification, congestion of the marginal sinus may appear as a circumferential red ring around the splenic follicle and there is marked lymphocytolysis of follicles and PALS. If the animal lives a little longer, neutrophils are scattered or in small foci in the marginal sinuses and red pulp vascular spaces (see Fig. 13-53). Bacilli are present intravascularly, presumably because death is so rapid from anthrax toxin that there is insufficient time for phagocytosis to take place. Impression smears of peripheral blood usually sampled at the ear vein or from blood exuding from their nostrils, oral cavity, or anus (see Chapters 4 and 7) can contain Gram-positive rod-shaped bacteria. Anthrax cases are not normally necropsied because exposure to air causes the bacteria to sporulate and anthrax spores are extremely resistant and contaminate the environment.

Acute Hemolytic Anemias

In hemolytic diseases, such as acute babesiosis, and during the hemolytic crises in equine infectious anemia, and some forms of immune mediated hemolytic anemia because of the need to remove large numbers of sequestered parasitized and altered erythrocytes from the circulation, the spleen is grossly enlarged and congested and the cut surface oozes blood. Histologically, there is dilation of the red pulp vascular spaces and erythrophagocytosis in the splenic cords. If the condition becomes chronic, hyperplasia of the red pulp macrophages takes place, and because of the decreased numbers of parasitized erythrocytes sequestered waiting to be phagocytosed, congestion is reduced.

Uniform Splenomegaly with a Firm Consistency—"Meaty" Spleen

The three basic mechanisms leading to uniform splenomegaly with a firm "meaty" consistency are as follows:

1. Phagocytosis
   a. Extensive removal of intravascular cells, cellular debris, or foreign agents
2. Proliferation of cells
   a. Hyperplasia of cells: such as lymphocytes producing biologic molecules like immunoglobulin, chemokines, and amyloid
   b. Inflammatory cells: macrophages
   c. Hemopoietic cells: in extramedullary hematopoiesis
   d. Diffuse primary neoplasms: primary splenic lymphoma, visceral mast cell tumor (cat)
   e. Diffuse metastatic neoplasms: lymphosarcoma, mast cell tumors, myeloid or erythroid tumors, plasma cell tumors
3. Storage of material: as in storage diseases and amyloidosis

The appearance of the cut surface of a "meaty" spleen varies with the extent of the change in the red and white pulp. In the early stages, red pulp has its normal color, but it becomes paler as lesions caused by any of these mechanisms become more extensive. The white pulp is not visible in normal spleens, but in cases of marked lymphoid hyperplasia, it may be visible on the cut surface as whitish foci, up to 1 to 2 mm in diameter, scattered through the red pulp. Moderately enlarged, firm spleens with visible white pulp are indicative of "reactive spleens," or lymphoma (lymphosarcoma).

Phagocytosis

Splenomegaly from an increased splenic phagocytosis could be considered a response to workload, a sort of "workload hyperplasia" of the macrophages in the splenic cords and red pulp vascular spaces to the need to phagocytose organisms in prolonged bacteremias or parasitemias from hemotropic organisms. While acute hemolytic anemias cause splenomegaly with congestion, the more chronic types of chronic hemolytic disease have less hemolysis and

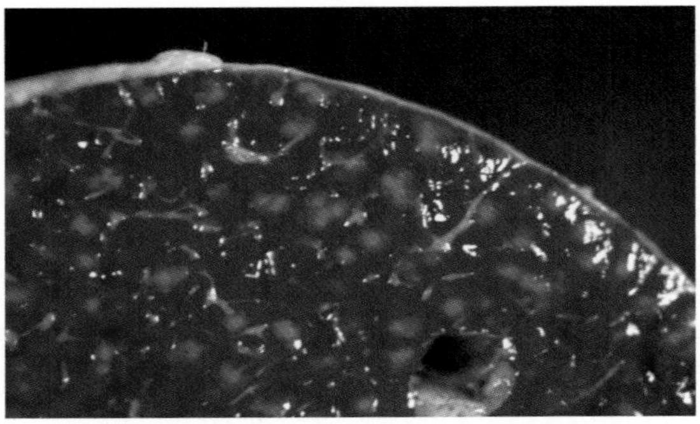

Fig. 13-54 Lymphoid hyperplasia, cross section of spleen, dog. Each of the 1- to 3-mm pale beige foci consists of hyperplastic periarteriolar lymphoid sheaths and splenic follicles. These structures are not visible in the normal spleen but become enlarged and visible from marked lymphoid hyperplasia or from lymphoma. (Courtesy Dr. S. Wolpert, USDA/FSIS; and Noah's Arkive, College of Veterinary Medicine, The University of Georgia.)

erythrophagocytosis and the spleen is firm (meaty) and red and not as congested. Because of the chronicity of the antigenic stimulus, there may be a concurrent hyperplasia of T and B lymphocyte areas. Equine infectious anemia has cyclical periods of viremia, immunologically mediated damage to erythrocytes and platelets, and phagocytosis to remove altered erythrocytes and platelets. These cycles result in proliferation of red pulp macrophages, hyperplasia of hematopoietic cells (EMH) to replace those lost, and hyperplasia of lymphocytes in T and B lymphocyte areas.

Proliferation of Cells

Cells Producing Biologic Molecules: Follicular Lymphoid Hyperplasia

Lymphoid hyperplasia has been described in detail in the section on Responses to Injury. The change in the splenic follicle is similar to that which occurs in the lymphoid follicle. Follicles become large and visible on gross examination (Fig. 13-54). Many of the chronic diseases previously listed above induce an immune response resulting in follicular lymphoid hyperplasia. In contrast to follicular lymphoid hyperplasia, in MCF in cattle there is T lymphocyte hyperplasia of the PALS.

Inflammatory Cells

Uniformly firm spleens resulting from infectious diseases are usually the result of chronic diseases. Splenitis caused by intracellular bacteria and fungi are commonly associated with uniformly enlarged firm spleens the result of macrophage hyperplasia and diffuse granulomatous disease and there may be some lymphoid hyperplasia.

Diffuse granulomatous diseases

These diseases occur (1) in response to bacteria that are intracellular facultative pathogens of macrophages, which include but are not limited to mycobacteria (*Mycobacterium bovis,* tuberculosis), *Brucella* spp. (brucellosis), and *Francisella tularensis* (tularemia) (see the section on Large Lymph Nodes); and (2) in systemic mycoses (see the section on Large Lymph Nodes), such as blastomycosis (*Blastomyces dermatitidis*). Some of these organisms may also produce nodular enlarged spleens with the formation of granulomas (see the section on Nodular Spleens with Firm Consistency). *Histoplasma capsulatum* causes a marked proliferation of cells of the monocyte-macrophage system, and the resultant accumulation of macrophages in the spleen may enlarge this organ to several times its normal size (Fig. 13-55, *A* and *B*). *Leishmania* spp. also cause

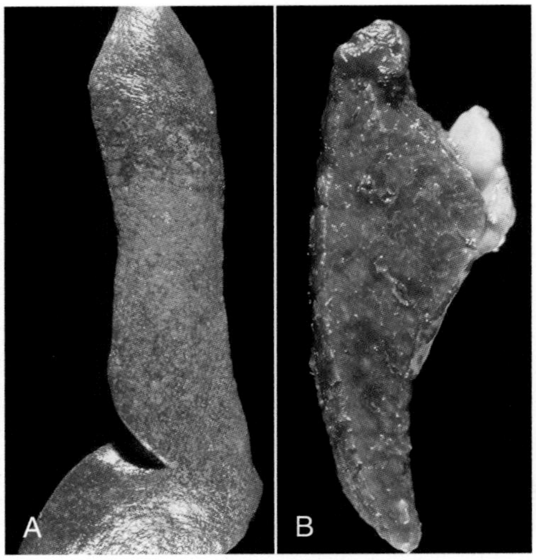

Fig. 13-55 Histoplasmosis, spleen, dog. **A,** There is uniform splenomegaly (meaty spleen) and the surface of the spleen is mottled from the diffuse granulomatous infiltrate. **B,** Cross-section of spleen. The red pulp has been almost completely replaced by diffuse noncaseous granulomatous inflammation. (Courtesy Department of Veterinary Biosciences, The Ohio State University; and Noah's Arkive, College of Veterinary Medicine, The University of Georgia.)

proliferation of macrophages, and large areas of the spleen may be replaced by macrophages. These cells also infiltrate the bone marrow and portal areas of the liver.

Extramedullary Hematopoiesis

Hormonal or physiologic signaling mechanisms within the spleen initiate the synthesis of progenitor cells from stem cells in an attempt to fulfill the cellular demands of the systemic circulation. However, splenic EMH is often found incidentally, and many consider its presence in the spleen to be within normal limits, at least in dogs. It usually involves cells of the erythroid, myeloid, and megakaryocytes lines, but one type usually predominates. Splenic enlargement from extramedullary hematopoiesis may be minimal, and EMH is often not detectable on gross examination. Extramedullary hematopoiesis may also occur in cases of chronic anemia and in conditions such as chronic respiratory disease or chronic cardiovascular disease, in which the circulation is not able to adequately maintain systemic partial pressure of oxygen (pO_2) concentrations. Extramedullary myelopoiesis may occur in suppurative bacterial diseases, such as canine pyometra, in which there is an excessive demand for neutrophils that exceeds the supply from the bone marrow. EMH is also present in splenic nodular hyperplasia.

Primary Neoplasms

Primary neoplastic diseases of the spleen arise from cell populations that normally exist in the spleen and include hematopoietic components, such as lymphocytes, mast cells and macrophages, and stromal cells, such as fibroblasts, smooth muscle, and endothelium. Primary splenic lymphoma, although rare, can produce a uniform splenomegaly (Fig. 13-56, *A*). Microscopically, the normal white pulp follicles are displaced, and the red pulp is occupied to varying degrees by neoplastic lymphocytes (Fig. 13-56, *B*). The different types of lymphoma in domestic animals are discussed in the section on Hematopoietic Neoplasia. In cats, visceral mast cell tumor typically presents as a uniform splenomegaly. In the advanced stages of disease, acute and chronic leukemias cause uniform splenomegaly. The splenic red pulp appears hypercellular from the extensive

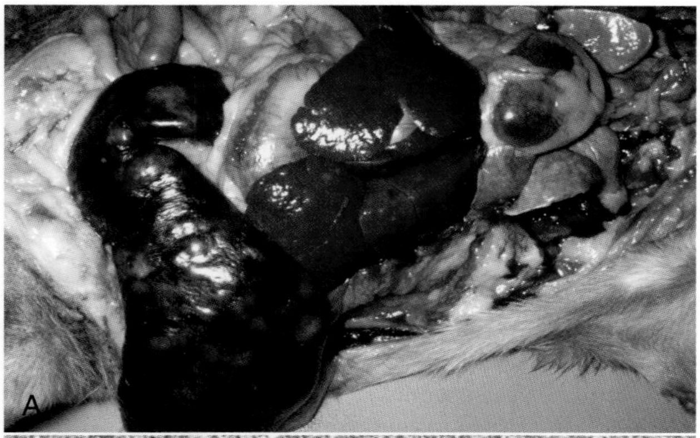

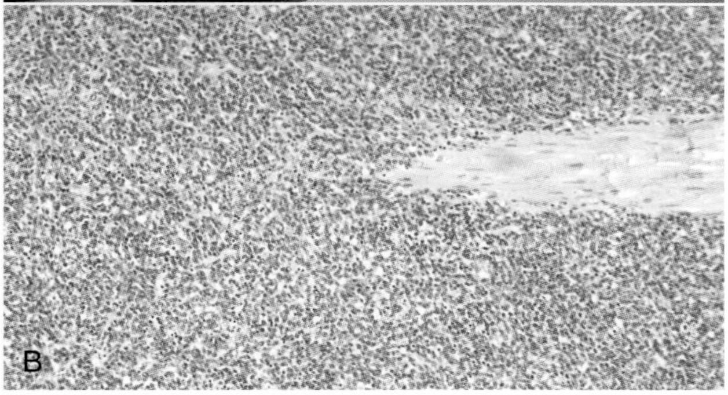

Fig. 13-56 Lymphoma (lymphosarcoma).
A, Spleen and liver, dog. The spleen is grossly enlarged with pale subcapsular nodules. The mottled appearance of the liver is caused by infiltration of malignant lymphocytes into the portal areas. **B,** Spleen, cow. The pale horizontal band on the upper right is a trabecula. The remainder of the spleen is diffusely infiltrated by malignant lymphocytes, which have completely obliterated all normal architecture. Note the absence of any normal red or white pulp. H&E stain. (**A** courtesy College of Veterinary Medicine, University of Illinois. **B** courtesy Dr. M.D. McGavin, College of Veterinary Medicine, University of Tennessee.)

infiltration of tumor cells. It should be appreciated that in some cases many of these different types of primary splenic neoplasms produce nodular lesions, which are discussed later.

Metastatic (Secondary) Neoplasms

The spleen is not a common site of metastatic neoplasia, but when it occurs, it generally causes nodules in the spleen—not a uniform splenomegaly. Metastatic neoplasms of the spleen, which cause uniform splenomegaly, can originate from the same hematopoietic cell populations as those that cause primary neoplastic disease, but the neoplastic cells metastasize to the spleen hematogenously. Lymphoma is the most common metastatic neoplasm of the spleen.

Storage of Material

Amyloid

The accumulation of amyloid in the spleen may occur with primary (AL) or secondary (AA) amyloidosis (see Chapters 1 and 5). Rarely can this accumulation be so severe as to cause uniform splenomegaly (Fig. 13-57), in which the spleen is firm, rubbery to waxy, and beige to orange. Microscopically, amyloid is usually in the splenic follicles. If these deposits are large enough, they are visible as approximately 2 mm gray nodules resembling sago pearls and the lesion has been called *sago spleen.* Sago is a starch extracted from the pith of sago palm stems and is processed into food in the form of gray or white opaque 2 mm diameter spherules. Splenic red pulp is rarely affected.

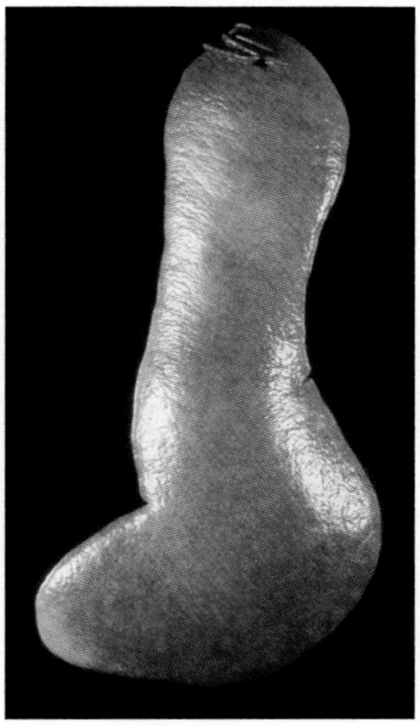

Fig. 13-57 Amyloid spleen, dog.
The spleen is pale beige, firm and waxy, and uniformly distended in this advanced case of amyloidosis. (Courtesy College of Veterinary Medicine, University of Illinois.)

Lysosomal Storage Diseases

Storage diseases constitute a large heterogeneous group of genetically determined and acquired disorders, which result from the lack of an enzyme required in the metabolism of a specific substrate. Storage diseases typically occur in animals less than 1 year of age. In general, these substrates are lipids and/or carbohydrates that accumulate in the cells, as the result of the lack of normal processing within lysosomes. Major categories of stored materials include mucopolysaccharides, sphingolipids, lipids, glycoproteins, glycogen, and mucolipids. Macrophages are the "cell of last resort" to phagocytose and degrade substances or microorganisms, but if the macrophages within the spleen are unable to degrade these substrates, they essentially serve to store them in an unprocessed form. Ultimately, the mass of this undigested substrate results in a uniformly enlarged firm spleen, which may be pale red, depending on the amount of unprocessed lipid or carbohydrate that has accumulated.

Splenic Nodules with a Bloody Consistency

The most common disorders of the spleen with bloody nodules are (1) hematomas, (2a) hematomas induced by hyperplastic lymphoid nodules, (2b) hematomas induced by splenic vascular neoplasms, (3) incompletely contracted areas of the spleen, (4) acute splenic infarcts, and (5) vascular neoplasms (hemangiosarcomas);. The term *nodule* has been applied rather loosely here. In some of these conditions, such as incompletely contracted areas of the spleen, the elevated area of the spleen is not as well defined as the term *nodule* would imply.

Hematomas

Bleeding into the red pulp, which is confined by the splenic capsule, produces a red to dark red soft bulging, usually solitary mass of varying size (2 to 15 cm in diameter) (Fig. 13-58). Resolution of a splenic hematoma progresses over days to weeks, through the stages of coagulation and breakdown of the blood into a dark red-brown soft mass (Fig. 13-59, *A*), infiltration by macrophages that phagocytose erythrocytes and break down hemoglobin to form bilirubin and hemosiderin (Fig. 13-59, *B*), and repair leading to tissue replacement by a scar. On occasions, the capsule (splenic capsule

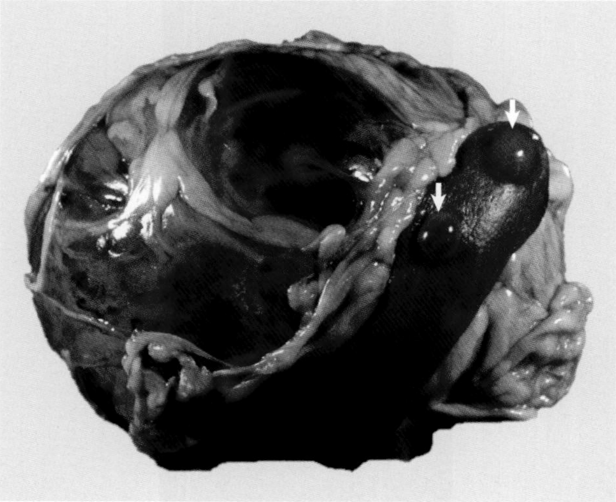

Fig. 13-58 Hematoma, spleen, dog.
The ventral extremity of the spleen has a large hematoma on its visceral surface. Note the two nodules *(arrows)* of splenic hyperplasia (dorsal extremity), a common site for hematomas to occur (see Fig. 13-63). (Courtesy College of Veterinary Medicine, University of Illinois.)

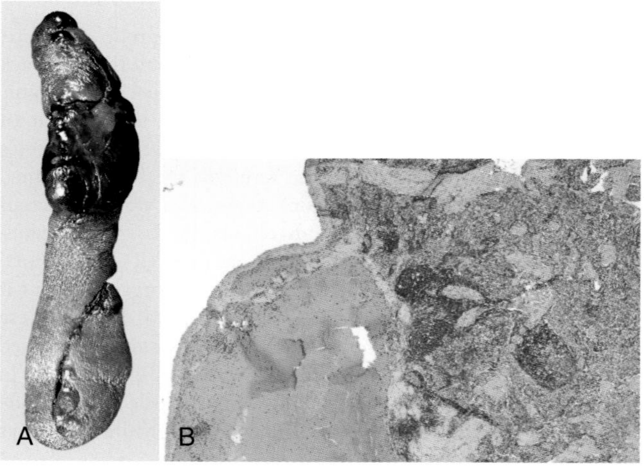

Fig. 13-59 Subcapsular hematoma, spleen, dog.
A, Note the separation of the splenic capsule from the underlying parenchyma by a mass of blood. **B,** The yellow material is bilirubin, resulting from the breakdown of erythrocytes in the subcapsular hemorrhage. H&E stain. (Courtesy Dr. M.D. McGavin, College of Veterinary Medicine, University of Tennessee.)

and visceral peritoneum) over the hematoma can rupture resulting in hemoperitoneum, hypovolemic shock, and death.

The origin or cause of many hematomas is unknown. Some are due to trauma, but two types are induced by (1) splenic hyperplastic lymphoid nodules and (2) splenic vascular neoplasms.

Hematomas Associated with Splenic Hyperplastic Nodules

Hematomas occur associated with these nodules, and it has been postulated that as the splenic follicles become hyperplastic they distort the adjacent marginal zone and marginal sinus, interfering with its drainage. The result is accumulation of pooled blood within and surrounding the hyperplastic nodule. Blood is unable to find its way into sinusoids or red pulp vascular spaces, and this leads to hypoxia and necrosis and hematoma formation.

Hematomas Induced by Splenic Vascular Neoplasms

Hematomas can also occur in the spleen secondary to the rupture of splenic neoplasms of primary or secondary vascular origin such as hemangiomas and hemangiosarcomas. Such tumors may arise from neoplastic transformation of endothelial cells in the spleen (primary tumors) or from metastases to the spleen (secondary tumors) from any location in the body, the more common sites include blood vessels of the right auricle, skin, and liver.

Incompletely Contracted Areas of the Spleen

Incompletely contracted areas of the spleen are areas that fail to empty during contraction induced by circulatory shock (hypovolemic, cardiogenic, or septic) or by a parasympathetic response, as in flight or fright situations. Also in the dog, microthrombi of disseminated intravascular coagulation (DIC) may block vascular flow in sinusoids and vascular spaces, resulting in incompletely contracted areas of the spleen. Acute splenic infarcts can be indistinguishable from areas of incompletely contracted splenic parenchyma. Incompletely contracted areas appear as numerous dark red to black, raised, soft, blood-filled areas of various sizes. These areas are usually at the margins of the spleen, and the intervening tissues are depressed and red. The latter areas are normal, contracted splenic red pulp devoid of blood. Incompletely contracted areas were previously confused with splenic infarcts and sometimes hematomas, but they are now recognized to be caused by failure of smooth muscle in some areas to contract, resulting in incomplete splenic evacuation of stored blood.

Acute Splenic Infarcts

Splenic infarcts occur principally in the subcapsular areas of the spleen, which are regarded as having poor perfusion and reduced venous return. In the dog, these areas are occupied by the splenic sinusoids. Infarcts are the result of splenic vein thrombosis in cattle with portal thrombosis, arterial thrombosis in bovine theileriosis, and hypercoagulable states such as those in immune hemolytic anemias. In classic swine fever, endothelial damage to the follicular artery is thought to be responsible for the infarction. Infarction from emboli is rare, and the cause for infarction may not be evident.

Acute splenic infarcts, which are initially hemorrhagic, are not always clearly visible in the early stages but appear as discrete, deeply congested areas with distention of the overlying capsule. As the lesion develops, it becomes somewhat wedge-shaped and gray-white with the base at the splenic capsule (Fig. 13-60). Later, a scar forms. Spleens distended with blood are prone to thrombosis and infarction.

Vascular Neoplasms

The most common causes of nodular spleens with a bloody consistency are benign and malignant neoplasms of vascular endothelial cell origin. Hemangiosarcomas (malignant) commonly occur, but hemangiomas (benign) are relatively uncommon. It may be differentiate between the two on gross examination.

Grossly, hemangiomas are usually solitary masses, dark red to bluish-purple, friable, and usually covered by a thin shiny serosa. Unlike hemangiosarcomas, there are no metastases to the liver or peritoneal mesothelium. Hemangiomas are composed of well-differentiated endothelial cells, which differentiate into relatively well-formed vascular spaces. Grossly, hemangiosarcomas can be difficult to differentiate from hemangiomas and hematomas. They are dark red to bluish-purple, friable, and usually covered by a thin serosa (Fig. 13-61), and they commonly occur as numerous large, discrete, and coalescing masses, scattered randomly throughout the spleen and effacing normal splenic architecture. The volume of

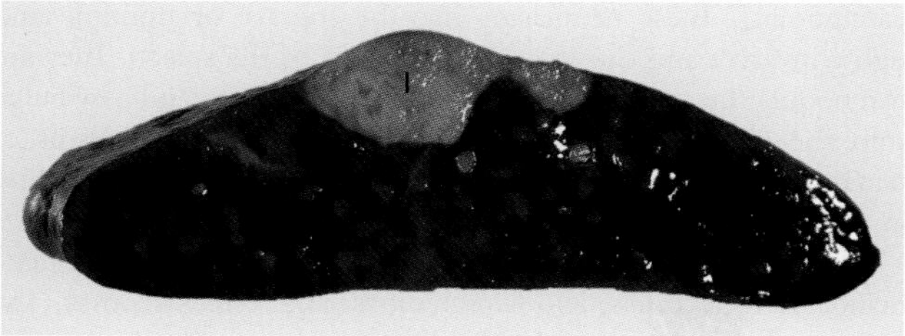

Fig. 13-60 Chronic splenic infarct, spleen, dog.
Note the characteristic pale beige, wedge-shaped area *(I),* with its base against the capsule of the spleen. (Courtesy Dr. M.D. McGavin, College of Veterinary Medicine, University of Tennessee.)

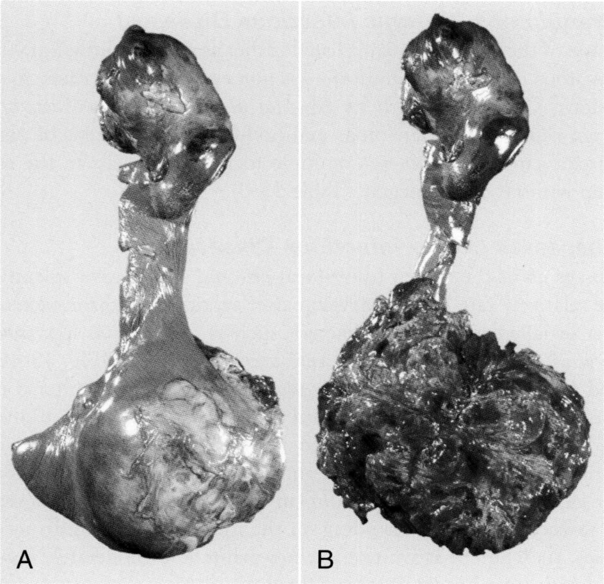

Fig. 13-61 Hemangiosarcoma, spleen, dog.
A, There are multiple nodules on the dorsal extremity and a large nodule on the ventral extremity of the spleen. **B,** The ventral mass has been incised to reveal the stroma of the hemangiosarcoma. (Courtesy Dr. M.D. McGavin, College of Veterinary Medicine, University of Tennessee.)

the actual tumor may be small when compared with that of the associated hemorrhage. They also may give rise to hepatic, pulmonary, and/or peritoneal transcoelomic metastases, the latter usually occurring by "seeding" of the peritoneal cavity. Hemangiosarcomas are composed of anaplastic endothelial cells, which form haphazardly arranged and poorly defined vascular spaces (Fig. 13-62) that most often contain liquid (unclotted) blood.

Splenic hemangiosarcomas can occur as primary masses that arise within the spleen or as metastases from distant sites, including skin or right atrium. Primary splenic hemangiosarcomas metastasize to the liver early and frequently; therefore evaluation of the abdomen must include a detailed examination of the entire abdominal cavity for hepatic and peritoneal metastases. Splenic hemangiosarcomas have a poor prognosis.

Splenic Nodules with a Firm Consistency

The most common disorders of the spleen with firm nodules are (1) splenic nodular hyperplasia, (2) fibrohistiocytic nodules, (3) primary neoplasms, (4) secondary (metastatic) neoplasms, (5) granulomas, and (6) abscesses.

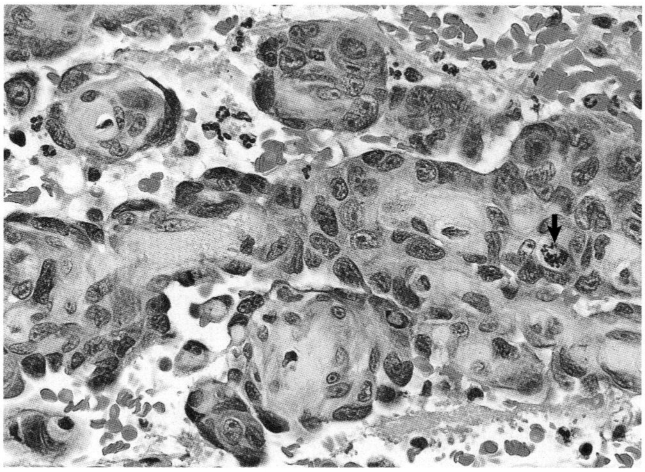

Fig. 13-62 Hemangiosarcoma, spleen, dog.
Note the haphazardly arranged vascular channels lined by anaplastic endothelial cells. Mitotic figure *(arrow).* H&E stain. (Courtesy Dr. J.F. Zachary, College of Veterinary Medicine, The University of Illinois.)

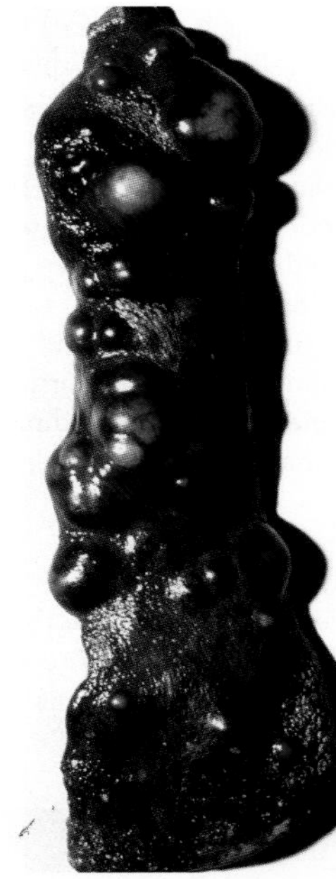

Fig. 13-63 Nodular hyperplasia, spleen, dog.
Several hemispherical 2- to 4-cm diameter nodules are protruding from the capsular surface. They are likely an aging change, formed by a mixture of hyperplastic extramedullary hemopoietic cells, and are prone to rupture from trauma, resulting in hemoabdomen and exsanguination. (Courtesy Dr. M.D. McGavin, College of Veterinary Medicine, University of Tennessee.)

Splenic Nodular Hyperplasia

Splenic nodular hyperplasia is most commonly seen in the spleen of older dogs and is often an incidental finding. Hyperplastic nodules are usually hemispherical and up to 2 cm or larger in diameter protruding from the surface (Fig. 13-63) and on cross-section have intermixed areas of red and white (Web Fig. 13-5). Nodules have no deleterious effect unless they result in a large hematoma, which can rupture and cause hemoperitoneum (see the section on Disorders of Dogs).

Fibrohistiocytic Nodules

See the section on Disorders of Dogs.

Primary Neoplasms

The primary neoplastic diseases of the spleen that result in nodular enlarged firm spleens commonly include lymphoma, histiocytic sarcoma, leiomyoma, leiomyosarcoma, and myelolipomas. These neoplasms may be solitary or multiple and are locally extensive. They are firm, are raised above the capsular surface, but usually confined by the capsular surface, and bulge from the cut surface. Because of the cell of origin (mesenchymal-spindle cells [fibroblasts, myocytes]), the cut surface of these spindle cell neoplasms may have a fibrillar appearance. Myxosarcomas have a distinctively mucinous or slimy character to the cut surface.

Malignant fibrous histiocytomas in canine spleens are considered a continuum of proliferations of fibrous and histiocytic cells (fibrohistiocytic nodule) normally found in the splenic reticular meshwork of the red pulp. They are most often seen as fibrous and histiocytic cellular proliferations in association with hyperplastic lymphoid cells. As the ratio of fibrohistiocytic cells to lymphoid cells increases, the malignant potential of the nodules also increases. Grossly, these tumors are often homogeneous and white and bulge from the cut surface of the spleen. To our knowledge, there is no evidence that malignant fibrous histiocytoma of the canine spleen is derived from the same cell of origin as the soft-tissue sarcoma of the same name (occasionally called *giant cell tumor of soft parts*) that occurs in dogs and cats.

Myelolipomas (neoplasms composed of approximately equal quantities of hematopoietic cells and adipose tissue) also may form nodules in the spleen, and these are softer than other mesenchymal-spindle cell neoplasms. Similarly, benign tumors of adipocytes (lipomas) can occur as a single neoplasm and cause splenomegaly.

In cats, the most common neoplasms (primary and secondary) forming nodules in the spleen are, in descending order of frequency, mast cell tumor, lymphoma (lymphosarcoma), myeloid neoplasms, and hemangiosarcomas.

Secondary (Metastatic) Neoplasms

Metastatic neoplastic diseases of the spleen that result in enlarged nodular firm spleens (Fig. 13-64) can arise from hematopoietic stem cells, from mesenchymal cells (sarcomas), or epithelial cells (carcinomas). These neoplasms may be solitary or multiple and highly invasive and can involve large areas of the spleen. They are firm nodular masses, usually confined by the capsule, and may bulge from the cut surface (see Fig. 13-64). Metastatic neoplasms of hematopoietic origin may be lymphoid or myeloid (see the section on Hematopoietic Neoplasia).

Metastatic neoplasms of mesenchymal origin (sarcomas) include fibrosarcomas, leiomyosarcomas, and osteosarcomas. The cut surface of mesenchymal neoplasms may have a fibrillar appearance, and they can be difficult to cut if osteoid and/or mineralized bone is present. Metastatic neoplasms of epithelial origin (carcinomas) include most of the common carcinomas (mammary, prostatic, lung, and endocrine). The cut surface of epithelial neoplasms may have a lobulated bulging appearance (see Fig. 13-64).

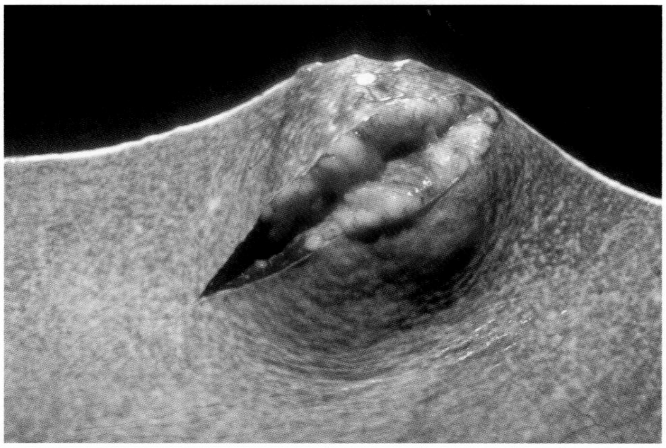

Fig. 13-64 Metastatic carcinoma, spleen, cow.
The white mass is an undifferentiated carcinoma, which has metastasized to the spleen. Note the lobular texture of the mass and how it bulges from the cut surface. (Courtesy Dr. M.D. McGavin, College of Veterinary Medicine, University of Tennessee.)

Granulomas (Chronic Infectious Diseases)

Some of the microorganisms listed earlier as causing diffuse granulomatous splenitis and uniform splenomegaly can also cause focal lesions. Organisms, such as *Brucella abortus* and *Mycobacterium bovis,* cause focal granulomas and nodules in the spleens of pigs. Porcine circovirus 2 causes multiple foci of giant cells in the red pulp without splenomegaly (Table 13-6).

Abscesses (Acute Infectious Diseases)

Abscesses in the spleen (multifocal chronic suppurative splenitis) are relatively rare but can develop after septicemia and/or bacteremia, usually from pyogenic bacteria such as *Streptococcus* spp., *Rhodococcus equi* (Fig. 13-65), *Arcanobacterium pyogenes* (Fig. 13-66), and *Corynebacterium pseudotuberculosis*. The bacteria are filtered by the monocyte-macrophage system in the spleen but are not killed and replicate within the splenic red pulp to form abscesses of various sizes, composition, and consistency. Abscesses bulge from the capsule of the spleen or from cut surfaces. The exudate can vary in texture and color depending on the inciting organism. In most cases, the content is white to yellow-white and moderately thick and with time becomes encapsulated.

Although there are a large number of diseases and conditions commonly associated with bacteremia, including navel ill, joint ill, chronic respiratory infections, bacterial endocarditis, chronic skin diseases, castration, tail docking, and ear trimming and/or notching, these rarely result in visible splenic abscesses. *Streptococcus equi*

TABLE 13-6 Granulomatous Diseases of the Spleen

Disorders	Agents
Noninfectious	Foreign bodies/particles
	Colloids (e.g., India ink)
Infectious	Bacteria: facultative pathogens
	Mycobacteriosis
	Tularemia
	Yersiniosis
	Brucellosis
	Fungi
	Blastomycosis
	Histoplasmosis
	Coccidioidosis
	Sporotrichosis
	Protozoa
	Toxoplasmosis
	Neosporosis

Modified from Nieman RS, Attilo O: *Disorders of the spleen in major problem in pathology,* Philadelphia, 1999, WB Saunders.

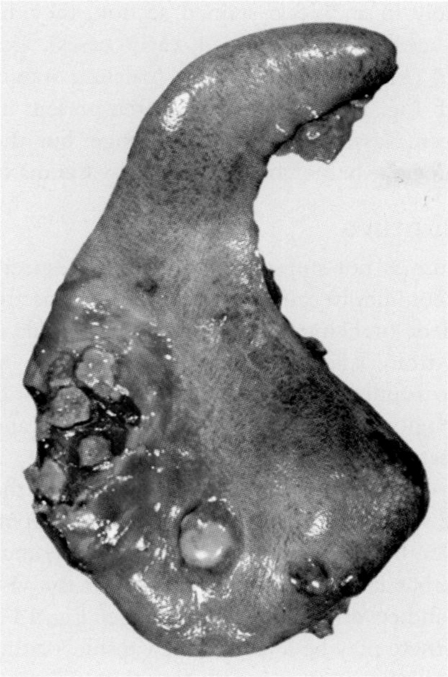

Fig. 13-65 Multiple subcapsular splenic abscesses, *Rhodococcus equi*, spleen, horse.
(Courtesy Dr. P. Carbonell, School of Veterinary Science, University of Melbourne.)

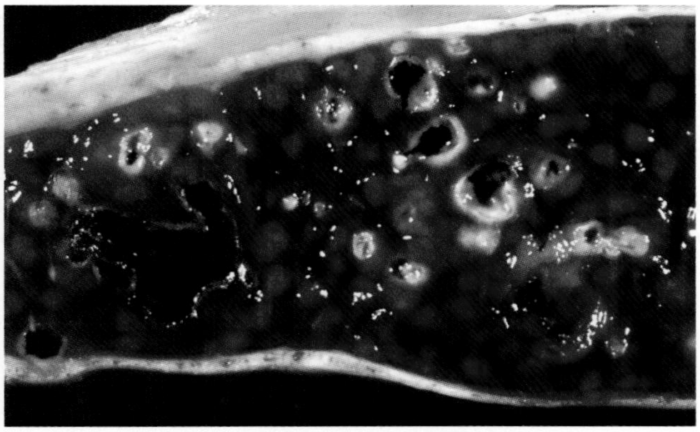

Fig. 13-66 Chronic multifocal suppurative splenitis, splenic abscesses, *Arcanobacterium pyogenes*, spleen, cow.
Multiple encapsulated abscesses are present throughout the parenchyma of the spleen, the result of a previous bacteremia. (Courtesy Department of Veterinary Biosciences, The Ohio State University; and Noah's Arkive, College of Veterinary Medicine, The University of Georgia.)

ssp. *equi,* the cause of equine strangles, is the prototypical bacterium of acute bacterial infections. The classic lesion of strangles is a nasopharyngitis with lymphadenitis of the regional lymph nodes, usually the mandibular and retropharyngeal. If the organism becomes bacteremic, it commonly causes abscesses in liver, kidney, synovial structures, mesenteric and mediastinal lymph nodes, and occasionally in the spleen. *Bastard strangles* is the term given to the form of the disease characterized by *Streptococcus equi* ssp. *equi* abscesses anywhere in the body other than the pharyngeal area.

In cattle, splenic abscesses can be the result of direct penetration by a foreign body from the reticulum (see the sections on Spleen and Portals of Entry). In horses, *Gasterophilus* and *Habronema* spp. have been reported causing perforating gastric ulcers and abscesses in the adjacent spleen. Splenic abscesses in horses have been found to contain short lengths of wire, which apparently have been ingested and migrated from the stomach.

SMALL SPLEENS (SPLENIC HYPOPLASIA AND ATROPHY)

The most common diseases or conditions associated with small spleens are (1) developmental anomalies, (2) aging changes, (3) wasting and/or cachectic diseases, (4) splenic contraction, (5) radiation of the spleen, and (6) splenic trauma.

Developmental Anomalies

Splenic Hypoplasia

Immunodeficiency diseases can result in small spleens (splenic hypoplasia), as well as small thymuses and lymph nodes. Small spleens occur most commonly with primary immunodeficiency diseases of young animals and involve defects in T or B lymphocytes or a combination. Severe combined immunodeficiency (SCID) in Arabian foals is a hereditary disease in which affected foals lack T and B lymphocytes and therefore is characterized by notable lymphoid hypoplasia of primary and secondary lymphoid tissues (see Fig. 13-81). Grossly, these spleens are exceptionally small, firm, and pale red. Spleens from affected animals lack lymphoid follicles and PALS, and there are few to no plasma cells. These diseases and their pathologic findings are discussed in Chapter 5.

Congenital Accessory Spleens

Accessory spleens can be either congenital or acquired (see the section on Splenic Trauma). Congenital accessory spleens are usually small and located in the gastrosplenic ligament.

Splenic Fissures

Fissures in the splenic capsule are elongated grooves whose axes run parallel to the borders of the spleen. This developmental defect is seen most commonly in horses but also occurs in other domestic animals. The surface of the fissure is smooth and covered by the normal splenic capsule.

Aging Changes

As part of the general aging change of cells as the body ages, there is reduction in the number of B and T lymphocytes in secondary lymphoid organs. This results in lymphoid atrophy and a sequela is a small spleen. Grossly, the organ is small and the capsule may be wrinkled. Microscopically, there is reduction in the white pulp; both PALS and splenic follicles may be undetectable, and if present, follicles lack germinal centers. Sinuses also lack blood, possibly because of anemia, and are collapsed, resulting in a condensation of their walls, which makes the red pulp appear fibrous.

Wasting/Cachectic Diseases

Any chronic disease, such as starvation, systemic neoplasia, and malabsorption syndrome, may produce cachexia. Starvation, although having a marked effect on the thymus with resultant atrophy of the T lymphocyte areas in the spleen and lymph nodes, has little or no effect on the B lymphocyte areas.

Splenic Contraction

Contraction of the spleen is a result of contraction of the smooth muscle in the capsule and trabeculae of storage and intermediate type spleens. It can be induced by the activation of the autonomic system and catecholamine release, which can occur in "fight or flight" situations, and in heart failure and cardiogenic, hypovolemic, and septic shock. It is also present in acute splenic rupture that has resulted in hemorrhage (hemoperitoneum). The contracted spleen is small, its surface is wrinkled, and the cut surface is dry.

Ionizing Radiation

There is atrophy of lymphoid tissue and with chronic radiation some red pulp fibrosis.

Splenic Trauma

Also see Miscellaneous Disorders of the Spleen-Splenic Rupture

Accessory Spleens Secondary to Splenic Trauma

Accessory spleens are the result of splenic rupture and seeding of the adjacent peritoneum with small implants of spleen (see the section on Disorders of Dogs).

MISCELLANEOUS DISORDERS OF THE SPLEEN

Hemosiderosis

Hemosiderin is a form of storage iron derived chiefly from the breakdown of erythrocytes, which normally occurs in the spleen. Thus some splenic hemosiderin is to be expected, and the amount varies with the species. It is most extensive in the horse. Excessive amounts of splenic hemosiderin are seen either from a reduced rate of erythropoiesis (less demand for iron) or from rapid destruction of erythrocytes, as in hemolytic anemias (increased stores of iron) such as those caused by immune hemolytic anemias or by hemotropic parasites. Excess hemosiderin may also occur in chronic heart failure and from the injection of iron dextran. Focal accumulations of hemosiderin in the capsule or parenchyma can be a sequela to hemorrhage, for example from trauma. Intraparenchymal deposits can also be sequelae to hematomas and infarcts. Hemosiderin is also present in siderotic plaques.

Siderotic Plaques

Siderotic plaques are also known as siderocalcific plaques and Gamna-Gandy bodies. Grossly, they are gray-white to yellowish, firm, dry encrustations on the splenic capsule. Usually, they are most extensive along the margins of the spleen but can be elsewhere on the capsule (Fig. 13-67) and sometimes in the parenchyma. Microscopically in an H&E-stained section, they are frequently multicolored: yellow (bilirubin in early cases), golden brown (hemosiderin) (Fig. 13-68), and blue (calcium stained by hematoxylin) (Web Fig. 13-6). As they are often present in older dogs, they have been classified as a senile change, but they are likely sequelae to previous hemorrhages induced by trauma of the spleen.

Splenic Rupture

Splenic rupture is not infrequent in animals, especially in dogs, and is most commonly caused by trauma, such as from an automobile accident or being kicked by other animals. Thinning of the capsule from splenomegaly can render the spleen more susceptible to rupture, and this occurs at sites of infarcts, hematomas, hemangiomas, hemangiosarcomas (dogs), and malignant lymphoma (cattle).

On gross examination, in acute cases when the capsule is ruptured, the spleen is markedly contracted in response to blood loss (Fig. 13-69). The rupture can be incomplete and involve just the red pulp, but leave the splenic capsule or the visceral peritoneum intact and covering the hematoma (see Fig. 13-59). In more severe cases, there may be a tear in the capsule, or the spleen may be broken into two or more pieces (see the section on Accessory Spleens). Small pieces of splenic parenchyma may be scattered on the peritoneum (sometimes called *splenosis* or *splattered spleen syndrome*) (Fig. 13-70). Clotted blood may adhere to the surface at the rupture site. If the rupture is not fatal, the spleen heals by scarring. There may be a capsular scar or two or more separate pieces of spleen adjacent to each other in the gastrosplenic ligament may be joined by a fibrous band. Exactly how functional the small accessory "spleens" are is questionable, although in human medicine, it is thought they may have some immune function and have a protective effect against postoperative infection. Because they have areas of erythrophagocytosis, it is presumed they are capable of removing senescent erythrocytes, but as most of them are supplied by small arteries and thus have a limited blood supply it is unlikely they are effective in filtering the body's blood. Also, it is generally considered that at least half of the original splenic mass is required for protection against blood-borne bacterial infections.

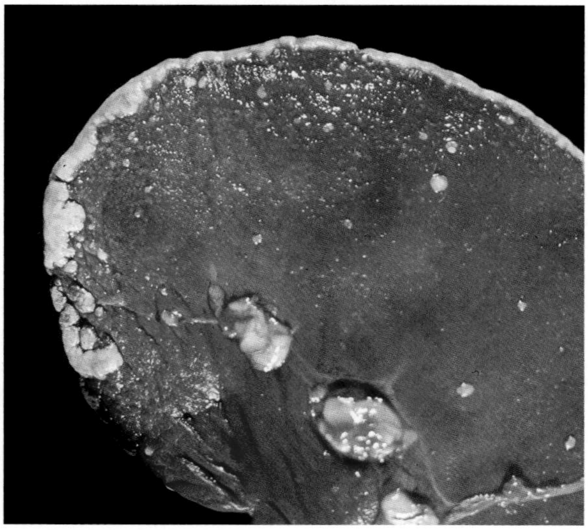

Fig. 13-67 Siderotic plaques, spleen, macroscopic view, dog. Note the yellow-white plaques on the capsular surface and along the border of the spleen. These plaques are likely the result of healing of sites of previous trauma and hemorrhage. The yellow color is attributable to hemosiderin and bilirubin, the white color to cacium and fibrosis. (Courtesy Dr. M.D. McGavin, College of Veterinary Medicine, University of Tennessee.)

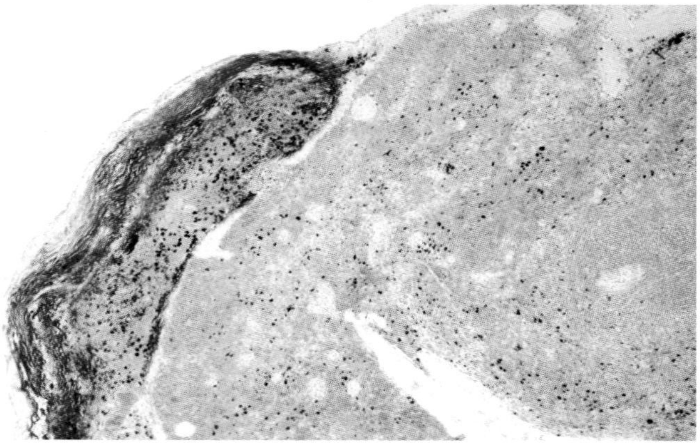

Fig. 13-68 Siderotic plaque, spleen, microscopic view, dog. The mass present on the capsular surface of the spleen on the right half of the illustration is a siderotic plaque formed by fibrous connective tissue of healing and hemosiderin pigment (*blue color* from stain reaction) and bilirubin pigment *(orange color)* from the breakdown of the heme molecule of hemoglobin from red blood hemorrhaged into the capsule from trauma. Prussian blue reaction. (Courtesy Dr. M.D. McGavin, College of Veterinary Medicine, University of Tennessee.)

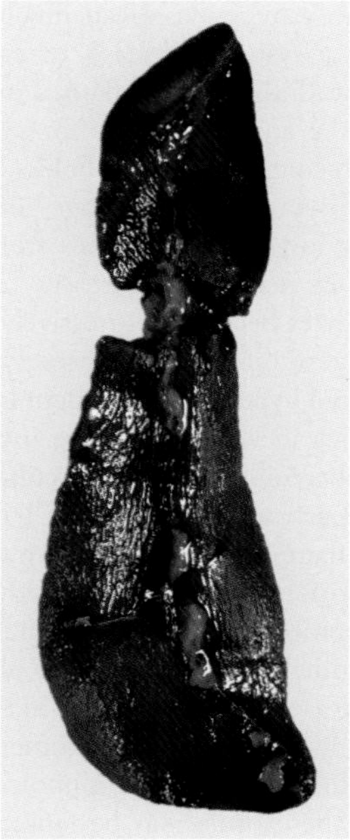

Fig. 13-69 Acute splenic rupture, spleen, dog.
The spleen has been almost transected by recent trauma. Because of the loss of blood, the spleen has contracted, the surface is crinkled, and the exposed surface of the parenchyma is dry. (Courtesy Dr. M.D. McGavin, College of Veterinary Medicine, University of Tennessee.)

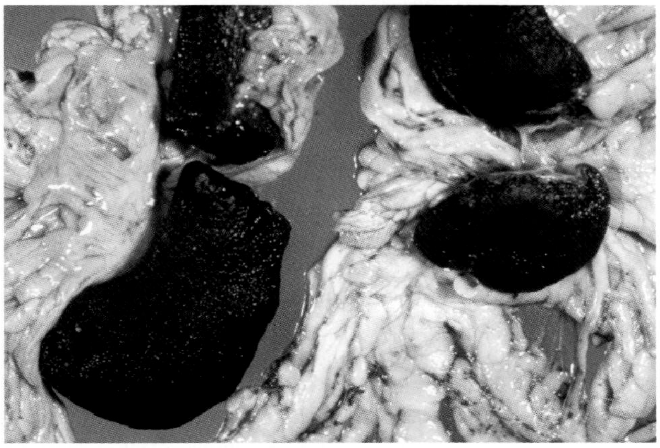

Fig. 13-70 Multiple "spleens," dog.
The spleen had been broken into several parts, and the rupture sites have healed by fibrosis. These small pieces of spleen on the gastrosplenic ligament, sometimes referred to as daughter or accessory spleens, are functional but not very effective in filtration because of their relatively paltry blood supply. (Courtesy Dr. H.B. Gelberg, College of Veterinary Medicine, Oregon State University.)

Consequently, if the ruptured spleen is removed, it is unlikely that these splenic implants are capable of the spleen's full function.

The bovine spleen has been reported to spontaneously rupture in acute septicemic anthrax.

Chronic Splenic Infarcts

In the early stage, splenic infarcts are hemorrhagic and may elevate the capsule (see the section on Nodular Spleens with a Bloody Consistency). However, as the lesions age, they diminish in size, become fibrotic, and may be depressed below the level of the surface of the adjacent capsule.

Parasitic Cysts

Occasionally, parasitic cystic nodules can be present within the spleen. These cysts are formed by intermediate stages of *Echinococcus granulosa* and *Cysticercus tenuicollis* and are seen most commonly in wild animal species.

LYMPH NODES

At necropsy the pathologist has to evaluate the size of lymph nodes, thus disorders are discussed on that basis.

Small Lymph Nodes

The most common diseases or conditions associated with small lymph nodes are as follows:

1. Developmental disorders
2. Lack of antigenic stimulation
3. Cachexia and malnutrition
4. Aging
5. Viral infections
6. Radiation

Developmental Disorders

Lymph Node Hypoplasia/Immunodeficiency Syndromes

Neonatal animals with primary immunodeficiency diseases of either B lymphocytes or T lymphocytes, or both, often have extremely small to undetectable lymph nodes. In dogs and horses with SCID, lymphoid tissues, including lymph nodes from affected animals, are characterized by an absence of lymphoid follicles and corticomedullary differentiation, and there are few to no lymphocytes and plasma cells (see Chapter 5).

Congenital Hereditary Lymphedema

Congenital hereditary lymphedema has been reported in certain breeds of cattle and dogs. Grossly, the most severely affected animals have generalized subcutaneous edema (see Fig. 2-11) and fluid in the serous cavities and are often stillborn. Histologically, in severe cases, lymphatic vessels are aplastic, and peripheral and central lymph nodes are hypoplastic.

Lack of Antigenic Stimulation

Size of the lymph node depend on whether it is "resting" or whether it is actively phagocytosing foreign material and/or responding to antigenic stimulation. In SPF animals, the lymph nodes are small because they have not been antigenically stimulated. Histologically, there is a small number of primary lymphoid follicles and few or no secondary follicles. This appearance can also be true of peripheral lymph nodes, such as the popliteal, of normal neonatal animals. However, those lymph nodes constantly receiving antigenic material and perhaps bacteria, such as lymph nodes draining the gut, are large, with active lymphoid follicles containing germinal centers. The number of follicles increases or decreases with changes in the intensity of the antigenic stimuli, and the germinal centers go through a cycle of activation, depletion, and rest as described previously. As the antigenic response wanes, germinal centers become depleted of lymphocytes and lymphoid and lymphoid follicles and lymph nodes become smaller.

Cachexia and Malnutrition

Any chronic disease, such as starvation, systemic neoplasia, or malabsorption syndrome, ultimately produces cachexia. As described in the sections on Inflammatory and Degenerative Disorders and

Wasting/Cachectic Diseases, starvation mainly reduces the production of T lymphocytes, resulting in atrophy of T lymphocyte areas but with little or no direct effect on B lymphocyte areas. This lymphoid atrophy can be the result of either lack of essential nutrients or physiological and emotional stress, which can be associated with the release of catecholamines and glucocorticoids. Thus cachexia and malnutrition have the potential to result in an immunosuppressed state.

Aging

Aging in the lymphoid system, as in aging of other organs results in reduced function and loss of cells followed by atrophy of all lymphatic tissues (see Chapter 1). Consequently, lymph nodes are small. The cortex is reduced, there is a loss of B lymphocytes and T lymphocytes, and lymphoid follicles may be absent.

Viral Infections

Many viral infections of animals target lymphocytes and cause the destruction of lymphoid tissue. In BVDV in the mesenteric lymph nodes, there is lymphocytolysis and necrosis of the germinal centers.

Canine distemper virus preferentially infects lymphoid, epithelial, and nervous cells. The distemper virus spreads from the tonsil and tracheobronchial lymph nodes to the spleen, bone marrow, and distant lymph nodes, where it causes lymphoid necrosis. The cortices of lymph nodes of dogs infected with canine distemper are depleted of lymphocytes 6 to 9 days after exposure. This loss of lymphocytes is also reflected hematologically by a profound lymphopenia. Although some viruses destroy lymphoid tissue, others can stimulate lymphoid tissue (e.g., Aleutian mink disease virus, maedi-visna virus, and MCF virus) or cause neoplasia (e.g., FeLV, BLV, and Marek's disease). Inclusion bodies, typical of porcine inclusion body rhinitis, are found in other epithelia and in lymph nodes.

Radiation

The response of lymphoid tissue to irradiation has been described in the section on Responses to Injury. After large doses of radiation and because of the susceptibility of lymphocytes and their rapid destruction, lymph nodes can quickly become smaller, but they can be restored to normal weeks later if the bone marrow can supply lymphocytes. With chronic radiation, besides the atrophy, there is fibrosis.

Large Lymph Nodes

Causes of large lymph nodes are as follows:

1. Lymphoid hyperplasia-follicular (B lymphocyte) and diffuse (T lymphocyte) lymphoid hyperplasia
2. Lymphadenitis—acute
3. Lymphadenitis—chronic, including encapsulated abscesses and granulomatous inflammation, either diffuse or focal
4. Primary neoplasms
5. Secondary (metastatic) neoplasms
6. Hyperplasia of the monocyte-macrophage system

Lymphoid Hyperplasia

Lymphoid hyperplasia may involve the follicles, deep cortex, or both. It is a common response after splenectomy of cattle with hemotropic parasite infections (babesiasis, theileriasis) and presumably is a compensatory response and results in marked generalized lymph node enlargement. Lymph nodes can be very large and have tense, distended capsules, and both cortex and medulla are hyperplastic.

Follicular lymphoid hyperplasia can involve large numbers of lymph nodes, as in a systemic disease, or can be localized to a regional lymph node draining an inflamed area. It is a common response, provided the animal survives for several days or longer after the initial antigenic stimulation. Follicular lymphoid hyperplasia can be present in the initial stages of a disease, but this may be followed by loss of lymphocytes from the follicles from lymphocytolysis as in many viral diseases (e.g., EHV-1). With time, the lymph follicles become progressively depleted and active proliferation in the germinal centers ceases.

Follicular lymphoid hyperplasia is evident in any regional lymph node draining an area in which there are inflammatory products or antigens (e.g., tuberculin from a tuberculin test or an injected vaccine). It is also particularly notable in lymph nodes draining areas of chronic inflammation (e.g., mammary lymph nodes in chronic bovine mastitis). Follicular lymphoid hyperplasia is characterized by proliferation of lymphoid follicles (see Fig. 13-45) and have active germinal centers to produce plasma cells to secrete antibody and an increase in T lymphocytes in the paracortical areas. In acute inflammation, these changes commence after a few days.

Grossly, when there is notable lymphoid hyperplasia, lymph nodes are enlarged, the capsule may be tense, and on incision the parenchyma bulges. The cortex may be increased in width.

Microscopically, lymph nodes are enlarged chiefly because of the expansion of the cortex by increased numbers of lymphoid follicles (follicular lymphoid hyperplasia), most of which have active germinal centers with numerous mitotic figures. Plasma cells precursors are generated here and then migrate to the medullary cords where they develop into antibody secreting plasma cells. After about 10 days or more, secondary lymphoid follicles can become depleted of mitotically active cells and lymphocytes. The result is pale germinal centers consisting primarily of stromal and precursor cells. Medullary cords originally densely packed with plasma cells also become depleted, approximately a couple of weeks after the antigenic stimulus ceases.

Diffuse (T lymphocyte) lymphoid hyperplasia. This is rarely detected in routine histologic examination but is seen in MCF of cattle, trypanosomiasis and a compensatory response in cattle after splenectomy, and in circovirus type 2 infections in pigs (see the section on Disorders of Pigs).

Acute Lymphadenitis

Acute lymphadenitis is usually the result of a regional lymph node draining an inflammatory site and becoming infected (e.g., the medial retropharyngeal lymph nodes in acute rhinitis, tracheobronchial lymph nodes in pneumonia [Fig. 13-71], and the supramammary [mammary] lymph node in acute mastitis). In cross-section, the affected lymph node is hyperemic and swollen with a tensed capsule (Fig. 13-72). In some instances, the afferent lymphatic vessels may also be inflamed (lymphangitis). The material draining to the regional lymph node may be bacteria, inflammatory products including mediators, a sterile irritant, or even parasites (such as *Demodex canis*). In septicemic diseases, such as bovine anthrax, the lymph nodes are grossly markedly congested, and histologically all lymphatic sinuses from the subcapsular to the medullary are filled with blood. Examination of these lymph nodes should include culturing for bacteria, examination of smears, and histologic sections for bacteria and fungi.

Grossly in acute lymphadenitis, lymph nodes are enlarged and may be soft or firm, depending on the amount of edema and exudate. The cut surface may be red, from hyperemia of local blood vessels, blood that has drained from an inflammatory site into the sinuses, or hemorrhage. Acute lymphadenitis should be

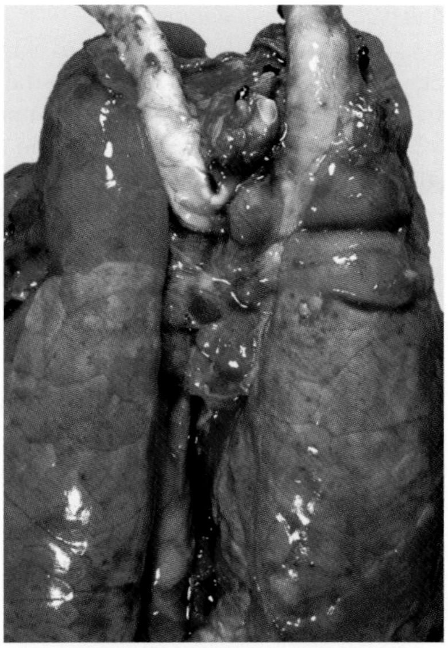

Fig. 13-71 Acute lymphadenitis, tracheobronchial lymph nodes, pig. The nodes are enlarged and reddened from draining the pneumonic cranial lung lobes. Because of the "reversed" anatomical arrangement in the porcine lymph node, the "medullary" sinuses filled with blood are obvious at the surface. Note the red consolidation of the dorsal portion of the cranial lung lobes. (Courtesy Dr. M.D. McGavin, College of Veterinary Medicine, University of Tennessee.)

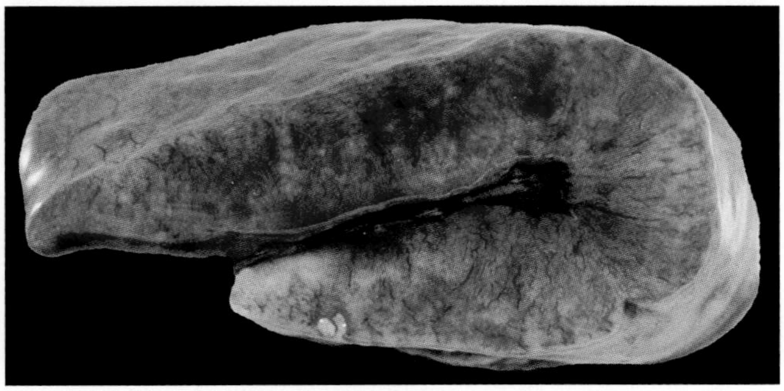

Fig. 13-72 Acute lymphadenitis, lymph node, dog. Acute lymphadenitis usually occurs when a regional lymph node drains an inflammatory site via afferent lymphatic vessels and becomes infected, most commonly with microorganisms. Note that this lymph node is firm, hyperemic (acute), and swollen with a tensed capsule. The cut surface bulges as the result of edema and the surface is wet with blood, lymph, and pus from acute inflammation. (Courtesy Dr. M.D. McGavin, College of Veterinary Medicine, University of Tennessee.)

differentiated from passive congestion of a lymph node diffusely reddened by congestion, from either post mortem (hydrostatic) congestion or from interference with the venous return, as occurs in the cervical tissues secondary to increased intrathoracic pressure in acute bovine bloat. When incised, the parenchyma may bulge, and the surface may be wet with blood, lymph, or pus (see Fig. 13-72). Suppuration is usually the result of pyogenic bacteria (e.g., *Streptococcus equi* ssp. *equi* in horses; *Streptococcus porcinus* in pig; and *Arcanobacterium pyogenes* in cattle and sheep). Microscopically, the lymph node is hyperemic. In the initial stages, neutrophils and usually erythrocytes are present in the sinuses, which are distended with lymph or exudate. After the passage of a day or so, numerous macrophages enter the sinuses (sinus histiocytosis), particularly the medullary sinuses (Fig. 13-73).

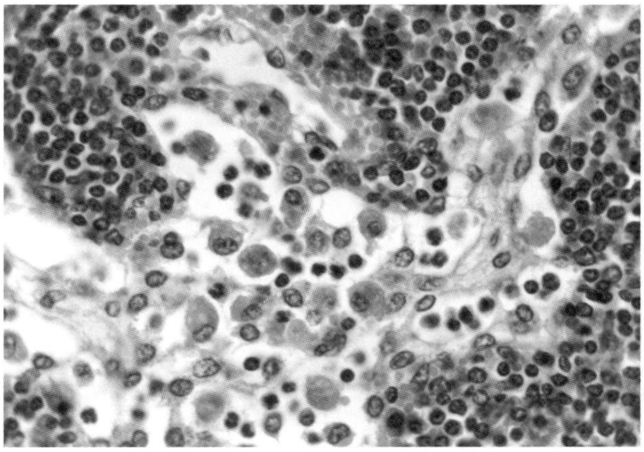

Fig. 13-73 Acute lymphadenitis (early), lymph node, medulla, dog. Medullary sinus with adjacent medullary cords. The lumen of the medullary sinus contains numerous macrophages (large cells, sinus histiocytosis) and a few neutrophils. This is the type of early response seen when a lymph node drains an inflamed area. The medullary cords are packed with lymphocytes and some plasma cells. H&E stain. (Courtesy Dr. M.D. McGavin, College of Veterinary Medicine, University of Tennessee.)

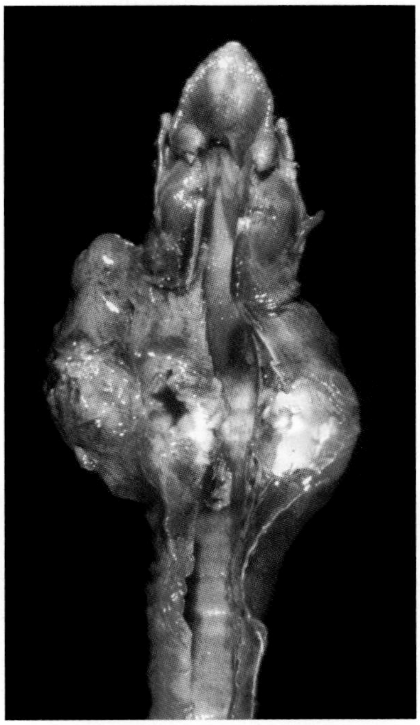

Fig. 13-74 Acute suppurative lymphadenitis, equine strangles (*Streptococcus equi* ssp. *equi*), dorsal view of larynx, left and right retropharyngeal lymph nodes, horse. The lymph nodes are grossly distended with pus. (Courtesy College of Veterinary Medicine, University of Illinois.)

In equine strangles caused by *Streptococcus equi* ssp. *equi*, the mandibular lymph nodes are the most often affected, but the retropharyngeal and parotid lymph nodes may be involved (Fig. 13-74). Multiple abscesses 1 to 10 cm in diameter may be present in the mandibular lymph nodes and may coalesce and rupture and discharge pus to the surface of the skin through a fistulous tract.

Focal areas of necrosis in lymph nodes are a common feature in many diseases, including toxoplasmosis, salmonellosis, tularemia, yersiniosis, Tyzzer's disease, and feline infectious peritonitis.

If inflammation in the lymph node continues for several days or longer, the lymph node is also enlarged by follicular hyperplasia and plasmacytosis of the medullary cords from the response of the immune system.

Chronic Lymphadenitis

Chronic lymphadenitis may be a chronic suppurative lymphadenitis with encapsulated abscesses as in ovine caseous lymphadenitis, granulomatous (diffuse or focal) or mixed (a mixture of microabscesses and fibrosis), follicular lymphoid hyperplasia, plasmacytosis and sinus histiocytosis. In chronic suppurative inflammation, abscesses range in size from small—causing no increase in the size of the lymph node—to large, even large enough to occupy the whole lymph node. In chronic recurrent lymphadenitis, as in the mammary (supramammary) lymph node draining a bovine udder with chronic mastitis, the lymph node is firm, and on cross-section, abscesses, chronic fibrosis, and follicular lymphoid hyperplasia are visible (see Web Fig. 13-5). Histologically, there are microabscesses or abscesses, fibrosis, follicular lymphoid hyperplasia, medullary cord plasmacytosis, and sinus histiocytosis.

Chronic Suppurative Lymphadenitis (Encapsulated Abscesses)

If an infection does not resolve then the result may be abscess formation. The classic example of chronic suppurative lymphadenitis is caseous lymphadenitis, a disease of sheep and goats caused by *Corynebacterium pseudotuberculosis* (Figs. 13-75 and 13-76) (see Disorders of Ruminants). It is also the cause of ulcerative lymphangitis in cattle and horses and pectoral abscesses in horses.

Granulomatous Lymphadenitis

Granulomatous lymphadenitis may be focal as in tuberculosis, focal coalescing as in blastomycosis and cryptococcosis, or diffuse as in histoplasmosis. Porcine circovirus 2 induces a diffuse granulomatous lymphadenitis with diffuse proliferation of macrophages in the lymphoid follicles and deep cortex.

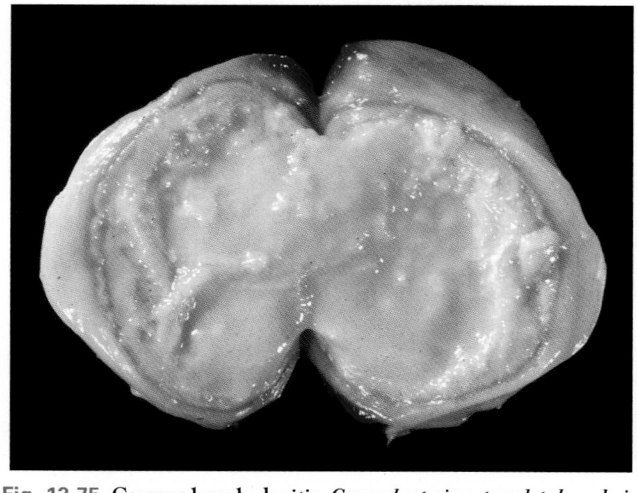

Fig. 13-75 Caseous lymphadenitis, *Corynebacterium pseudotuberculosis*, lymph node, sheep.
The whole lymph node has been replaced by an abscess containing mostly semifluid yellowish pus. This is an early stage of caseous lymphadenitis, before the pus has become inspissated and caseous. (Courtesy Dr. K. Read, College of Veterinary Medicine, Texas A&M University; and Noah's Arkive, College of Veterinary Medicine, The University of Georgia.)

Focal granulomatous lymphadenitis

The classic example of focal granulomatous lymphadenitis is tuberculosis caused by *Mycobacterium bovis,* but the more pathogenic members of the *Mycobacterium avium* complex can cause similar lesions in cattle and pigs. Initially, lesions in the lymphatic system are in the regional lymph nodes (e.g., the tracheobronchial lymph nodes in the case of pulmonary tuberculosis), but once tuberculosis is disseminated, for example, by trafficking macrophages, lymph nodes throughout the body will have lesions. *Mycobacterium bovis* lesions in lymph nodes are characterized by the formation of caseating granulomas. These are often multiple (Fig. 13-77) but can become coalescing and occupy the whole lymph node. Grossly, the lesions are pale, caseous, and often mineralized in cattle. Microscopically, the granulomas have central necrotic debris surrounded by a layer of epithelioid macrophages interspersed with scattered Langhans' giant cells and lymphocytes. Peripheral to this is a layer of lymphocytes, and in old lesions the granuloma may

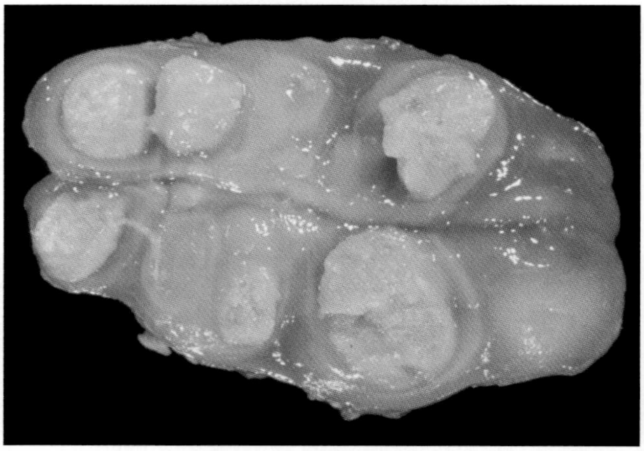

Fig. 13-76 Chronic caseous lymphadenitis, *Corynebacterium pseudotuberculosis,* lymph node, sheep.
The lymph node has been sliced longitudinally, exposing three chronic abscesses enclosed by thick fibrous capsules and containing yellowish caseous pus. (Courtesy Dr. W. Crowell, College of Veterinary Medicine, The University of Georgia; and Noah's Arkive, College of Veterinary Medicine, The University of Georgia.)

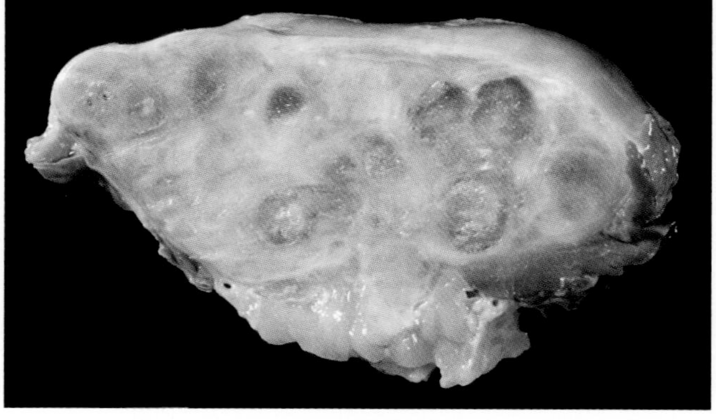

Fig. 13-77 Tuberculosis *(Mycobacterium bovis)*, lymph node, ox.
The normal architecture of the lymph node has been completely obliterated by multiple caseating granulomas, typical of *Mycobacterium bovis* lesions. (Courtesy Dr. M.D. McGavin, College of Veterinary Medicine, University of Tennessee.)

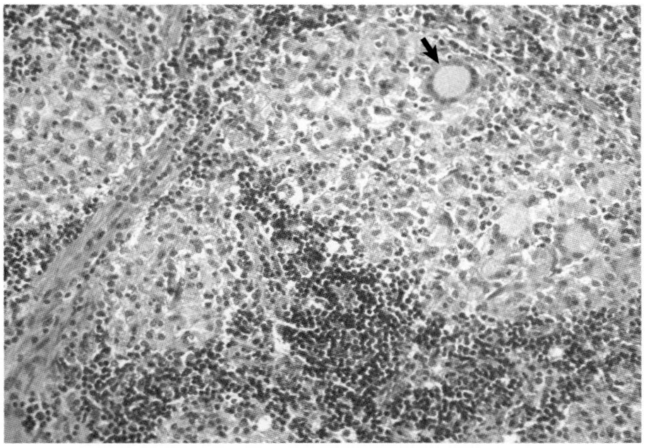

Fig. 13-78 Johne's disease (*Mycobacterium avium* ssp. *paratuberculosis*), lymph node, ox.

Several noncaseating granulomas *(pale areas)* have replaced the normal lymphoid tissue *(blue)*. Note the Langhans' giant cell *(arrow)*. H&E stain. (Courtesy College of Veterinary Medicine, University of Illinois.)

be surrounded by a fibrous capsule. Pigs ingesting one of the mycobacteria of the *Mycobacterium avium* complex may have caseous lesions confined to the retropharyngeal lymph nodes, and these lesions are self-limiting. In bovine Johne's disease, the mesenteric lymph nodes draining the infected intestine can have noncaseous granulomas (Fig. 13-78). Lesions may be seen in the spleen and Peyer's patches.

Chronic demodicosis is an unusual example of a focal granuloma. A foreign body granuloma develops around Demodex that have drained to a regional lymph node from an area of skin affected with chronic demodicosis. There is also marked follicular hyperplasia (see Fig. 13-45).

Diffuse granulomatous lymphadenitis

Blastomycosis and cryptococcosis are examples of focal coalescing granulomatous lymphadenitis. Both of these diseases frequently involve a regional lymph node draining an affected area (e.g., the tracheobronchial lymph nodes in the case of pulmonary infections). In advanced cases, the lymph node may be enlarged, the cut surface pale, and its normal architecture totally or almost completely obliterated (Web Fig. 13-7). In cryptococcosis in cats, there may be little or no inflammatory response (Web Fig. 13-8), and the enlargement of the lymph node is due mainly to a large mass of organisms *(Cryptococcus neoformans)*. For discussions of histoplasmosis and leishmaniasis, see the section on Disorders of Dogs. A diffuse granulomatous lymphadenitis characterized by diffuse proliferation of macrophages in the lymphoid follicles and deep cortex is seen in porcine PMWS (porcine circovirus 2; see the section on Disorders of Pigs).

Primary Neoplasms

Lymphosarcoma

Lymphoma can be primary or metastatic and both appear grossly similar. The different types of lymphoma are discussed in the section on hematopoietic neoplasia. The most common primary neoplasm is lymphoma (lymphosarcoma). Lymphoma can involve a wide range of organs and tissues, including alimentary (tonsils, stomach, and intestine), liver, respiratory (larynx and trachea), heart, kidneys, nerves, uterus, thymus, spleen, lymph nodes, and retrobulbar tissue. The actual incidence in any organ depends on the species of domestic animal and the type of lymphoma in that

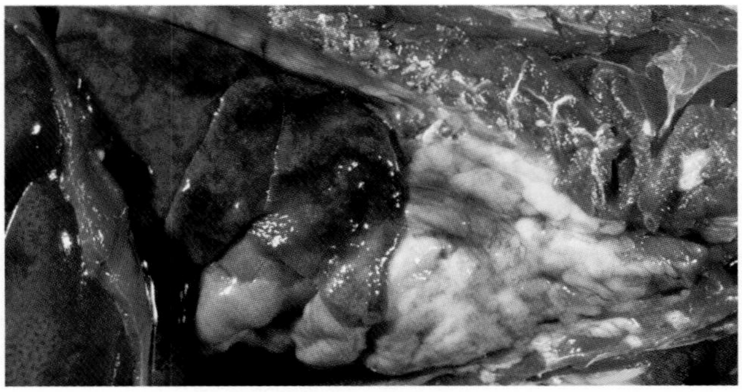

Fig. 13-79 Lymphoma (lymphosarcoma), cranial mediastinal lymph nodes, cat.

The cranial mediastinal lymph nodes are grossly enlarged, fill the cranial thoracic cavity, and have displaced the lungs and heart caudad. (Courtesy Dr. M.D. McGavin, College of Veterinary Medicine, University of Tennessee.)

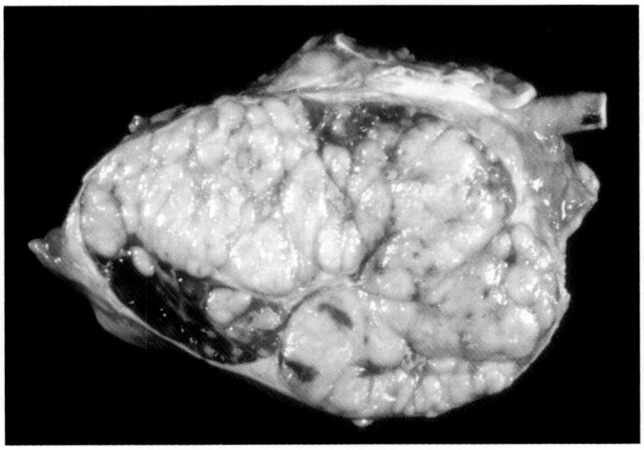

Fig. 13-80 Lymphoma (lymphosarcoma), bovine lymph node, cross section.

Normal architecture of lymph node has been completely obliterated by proliferating lobules of neoplastic tissue composed of malignant lymphocytes. (Courtesy College of Veterinary Medicine, University of Illinois.)

species. See appropriate chapters for each organ for the classification and distribution of lesions.

There is notable enlargement of lymph nodes (Figs. 13-79), and on cross-section the normal architecture (cortex and the medulla) may be obliterated by the malignant cells (Fig. 13-80). The cut surface is pale, is often homogeneous, and bulges (see the section on Hematopoietic Neoplasms).

Secondary (Metastatic) Neoplasms

Carcinomas typically metastasize to regional lymph nodes, at least initially. The hematogenous route is typical of metastasis of sarcomas but is often seen with carcinomas with systemic metastases. Thus metastatic carcinomas in regional lymph nodes are a common finding, and these lymph nodes may at least temporarily prevent further dissemination of the neoplasm. An incomplete list of metastatic tumors includes squamous cell carcinoma, mammary carcinoma, gastric carcinoma, pulmonary carcinoma, osteogenic sarcoma, malignant melanoma, and malignant mast cell tumor.

If the tumor has induced an inflammatory response at its primary site (e.g., from ulceration such as that caused by an ulcerating squamous cell carcinoma or a perforating gastric carcinoma), an acute lymphadenitis occurs in the regional lymph node.

Histologically, single cells or clusters of neoplastic cells travel via the afferent lymphatic vessels and are deposited in a sinus, usually the subcapsular sinus. Here, the cells proliferate and can ultimately occupy the whole lymph node. They can also send more malignant cells to the next lymph node in the chain via lymph drainage.

PIGMENTATION OF LYMPH NODES

Lymph nodes may have the following discolorations: red (blood in sinuses), black (carbon, tattoo ink), brown/yellow (melanin, parasitic hematin, hemosiderin), green (eosinophils, blue-green algae), and miscellaneous colors resulting from injected dyes and bilirubin from icterus. More information on this topic is available at evolve.elsevier.com/Zachary/McGavin/.

MISCELLANEOUS LYMPH NODE DISORDERS

Inclusion Bodies

Many viruses produce inclusion bodies, and some of these occur in lymph nodes. These viruses include EHV-1 in horses, bovine adenovirus, cytomegalic virus in inclusion body rhinitis and porcine circovirus 2 of pigs, herpesvirus of pseudorabies in pigs, parvovirus in dogs, and feline panleukopenia virus.

Emphysema

Emphysema in lymph nodes is a consequence of emphysema in their drainage fields and is seen most frequently in tracheobronchial lymph nodes in bovine interstitial emphysema and in porcine mesenteric lymph nodes in intestinal emphysema (see Chapter 7). The appearance of the lymph node varies with the extent of the emphysema. In severe cases, the lymph node is light, puffy, and filled with discrete gas bubbles, and the cut surface may be spongy. Histologically, the sinuses are distended with gas and their walls are lined by macrophages and giant cells. This change has been considered a foreign body reaction to the gas bubbles. Similar lesions are seen in afferent lymphatic vessels.

LYMPH NODULES (MALT)

MALT is involved in a variety of ways with bacteria and viruses, and these are summarized in Table 13-4. These interactions include being a portal of entry for pathogens, such as *Salmonella* spp., *Rhodococcus equi*, and BVDV; a site of replication for viruses (e.g., BVDV); occasionally a site infected hematogenously (panleukopenia virus and parvovirus); and a site of gross or microscopic lesions in some diseases caused by viruses. Bovine coronavirus, BVDV, Rinderpest virus, malignant catarrhal fever (MCF) virus, feline panleukopenia virus, and canine parvovirus all cause lymphocyte depletion. Bacteria such as *Salmonella* spp., *Rhodococcus equi, Yersinia pestis, Mycobacterium bovis, M. avium* ssp. *paratuberculosis* (goats), and *Listeria monocytogenes* infect Peyer's patches and cause disease.

DISORDERS OF HORSES

SEVERE COMBINED IMMUNODEFICIENCY (SCID)

SCID in Arabian foals is a hereditary disease in which affected foals lack T and B lymphocytes and therefore is characterized by notable lymphoid aplasia or hypoplasia of primary and secondary lymphoid tissues (Fig. 13-81). Reflecting the immunodeficiency, necropsy findings are often severe bronchopneumonia and a small thymus, spleen, and lymph nodes. The thymus may be difficult to identify or may consist of a few isolated lobules within the mediastinal fat and microscopically, it usually consists of a few islands of lymphocyte-like cells and Hassall's corpuscles. Grossly, spleens are exceptionally small, firm, and pale red. The spleen is smaller than normal because of a marked reduction in the white pulp owing to absence of germinal centers (see Fig. 13-81) and periarteriolar lymphoid sheaths. Microscopically, they lack lymphoid follicles and PALS, and there are few to no plasma cells. Grossly, peripheral lymph nodes and internal lymph nodes may be small and difficult to identify because of the absence of lymphocytes. Congenital immunodeficiency diseases are also discussed in detail in Chapter 5.

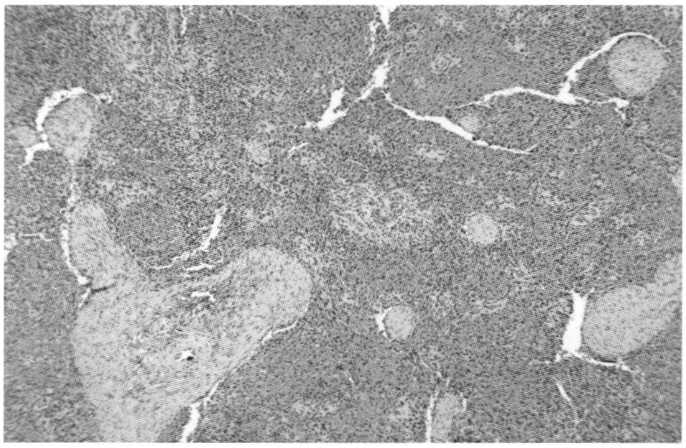

Fig. 13-81 Combined immunodeficiency disease, spleen, foal. The large pale pink areas are splenic trabeculae. Note the almost total absence of white pulp. H&E stain. (Courtesy Dr. M.D. McGavin, College of Veterinary Medicine, University of Tennessee.)

STRANGLES

Streptococcus equi ssp. *equi*, the etiologic agent of equine strangles, causes lesions typical of an acute bacterial infection. The classic lesion of strangles is a nasopharyngitis with lymphadenitis of the regional lymph nodes, usually the mandibular and retropharyngeal (see Fig. 13-74). This lymphadenitis can progress to the formation of abscesses and ultimately the abscesses may rupture and discharge pus through a sinus to the skin surface. If the organism becomes bacteremic, it commonly causes abscesses in liver, kidney, synovia, mesenteric and mediastinal lymph nodes, and occasionally in the spleen. Bastard strangles is the term given to the form of the disease characterized by *Streptococcus equi* ssp. *equi* abscesses anywhere in the body other than the pharyngeal area (see the discussion on acute infectious diseases in the section on Nodular Spleens with Firm Consistency).

RHODOCOCCUS EQUI INFECTION

The intestinal and pulmonary lesions have been described in Chapter 7 and 9, respectively. *Rhodococcus equi* enters the intestinal wall at Peyer's patches, causing a granulomatous inflammation and abscess formation and necrosis, which results in ulceration. The organisms drain to the regional lymph node (mesenteric, colonic, and cecal), causing a granulomatous lymphadenitis with granulomas and abscesses. Intestinal mucosal lesions are multiple and over sites of GALT. The diffuse lymphatic tissue in the lamina propria has increased numbers of macrophages and giant cells, many of which contain phagocytosed Gram-positive bacteria.

EQUINE LYMPHOMA

Equine lymphoma is divided into three anatomic types on the basis of the location of the majority of the lesions. These types are *alimentary,* which affects the rostral (upper) small intestine and its regional lymph nodes: abdominal with lesions in widespread lymph node involvement, large intestine and its regional lymph nodes, spleen, liver, peritoneum, and segmentally in the small intestine; *multicentric,* which can be a mediastinal mass that may extend into the heart and lungs and peripheral lymph nodes and abdominal cavity; and *cutaneously* (see Chapter 17).

DISORDERS OF RUMINANTS (CATTLE, SHEEP, AND GOATS)

JOHNE'S DISEASE

As the lesions of Johne's disease have been described in detail in Chapter 7, only those affecting the lymphatic system are mentioned here. Bovine Johne's disease is characterized by a chronic diffuse noncaseating (in contrast to sheep and goats) granulomatous enteritis affecting the submucosa and mucosa of the ileum, cecum, and colon. Secondary to this, there is a similar type of granulomatous lymphadenitis in the regional lymph node (see Web Fig. 13-7). Unlike bovine Johne's disease, which has a diffuse noncaseating (lepromatous) granulomatous inflammation in the intestine and lymph node, sheep and goats have caseous granulomas that may mineralize. Also, granulomas are scattered in other lymph nodes; in organs, such as the liver, lung, and spleen; and throughout the body.

ANTHRAX

Anthrax is caused by *Bacillus anthracis* and is primarily a disease of ruminants, especially cattle and sheep. It is discussed in the section on Uniform Splenomegaly of Bloody Consistency in this chapter and also in Chapter 4.

BOVINE VIRUS DIARRHEA

Lymphocytolysis and necrosis of the germinal centers of the mesenteric lymph nodes are found in the follicles of the GALT. Lesions are grossly striking in Peyer's patches where a fibrinonecrotic pseudomembrane covers the damaged GALT and outlines Peyer's patches (see Chapters 4 and 7).

BOVINE LYMPHOMA

The two forms of bovine lymphoma are a BLV-associated type and a sporadic type that is not associated with BLV (see the section on Bone Marrow), and the distribution of the lesions varies with the two types. In the BLV-associated type, lymphomas are located in the superficial, pelvic, and abdominal lymph nodes (see Fig. 13-80) and in the abdominal wall, extradurally in the vertebral canal, kidney, heart (right atrium), retrobulbar space, uterus, liver, and spleen (splenomegaly). The non-BLV lymphoma, designated *sporadic form,* is subdivided into thymic, cutaneous, multicentric, and calf form. The calf form affects calves at birth and up to 6 months of age and is rapidly progressive, with grossly visible infiltrations of neoplastic lymphocytes into all lymph nodes, liver, spleen, kidneys, and bone marrow. Bovine thymic lymphoma most often occurs in beef cattle 6 to 24 months of age and is characterized by massive thymic enlargement. The cause is unknown, and the occurrence of a concurrent leukemia is unusual. Microscopically, lymphomas are dominated by lymphocytes, which are homogeneous in size, shape, nuclear morphology, and nuclear-cytoplasmic ratio. The multicentric type has widespread symmetric lymph node enlargement and lesions in the liver spleen, kidneys (diffuse), and sometimes in skeletal muscle (see the section on Bone Marrow).

SPLENIC ABSCESSES

Splenic abscesses can be the result of direct penetration by a foreign body from the reticulum (see the sections on Spleen and Portals of Entry).

CASEOUS LYMPHADENITIS

Caseous lymphadenitis, a chronic suppurative lymphadenitis, is a disease of sheep and goats caused by *Corynebacterium pseudotuberculosis.* In sheep, the bacterium enters the skin through wounds, such as shearing cuts, and then drains to the regional lymph node. This node is usually either the superficial cervical (prescapular) or the subiliac (prefemoral) lymph node because the cuts are frequently on the legs, and these are a portal of entry for C. *pseudotuberculosis.* A suppurative lymphadenitis develops. Initially, there are multiple microabscesses with numerous eosinophils in the sinuses. These microabscesses coalesce and caseate and become encapsulated by fibrous tissue. However, they continue to enlarge, a process that results in the characteristic concentric laminations, which can often be seen on a cross-section of an old abscess. On gross examination, the pus in the abscess is initially greenish (because of the eosinophils) and semifluid (see Fig. 13-75), but it becomes caseous with age (see Fig. 13-76), loses its green color, and becomes inspissated. Old abscesses can reach a diameter of 4 to 5 cm. Similar abscesses may be found in the lungs, especially in older sheep. The abscesses in goats are usually more numerous and frequently involve lymph nodes of the head and neck.

DISORDERS OF PIGS

POSTWEANING MULTISYSTEM WASTING SYNDROME

PMWS, or porcine circovirus 2, is also discussed in Chapters 4 and 9. The major findings at necropsy are poor body condition, generalized lymphadenopathy, and interstitial pneumonia. In the lymphatic system, the disease is characterized by B and T lymphocyte depletion and a granulomatous response. The lymphocyte depletion affects all lymphatic tissues—spleen, lymph node, MALT (tonsil and Peyer's patches), and thymus. Microscopically, in the lymph node the characteristic lesions are granulomatous lymphadenitis and lymphocyte depletion. The increase in macrophages is chiefly in the follicles but also to a lesser degree diffusely throughout the deep cortex. The microscopic lesions in the follicles include depletion of lymphocytes, germinal center necrosis, and proliferation of macrophages with the formation of syncytial cells. Many of the macrophages contain inclusion bodies—intracytoplasmic, basophilic, round, and often multiple. Similar lesions are seen in the Peyer's patches. In the spleen, the T lymphocyte depletion affects the PALS and in the thymus there is a diffuse infiltration of macrophages.

PORCINE REPRODUCTIVE RESPIRATORY SYNDROME

Porcine reproductive respiratory syndrome (PRRS) is caused by a virus transmitted by contact with body fluids—saliva, mucus, serum, urine, and mammary secretions and from contact with semen during coitus. The virus infects macrophages at the site of contact. Infected macrophages migrate to lymphoid tissues (nasal or tonsillar in oral infections), infect and replicate in similar cells in these tissues, and then disseminate in macrophages throughout

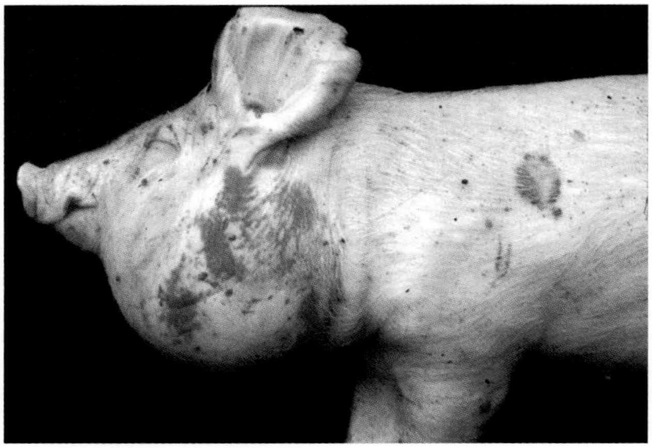

Fig. 13-82 Jowl abscess, pig.
The submandibular swelling is caused by marked enlargement of the mandibular lymph nodes from a suppurative lymphadenitis caused by *Streptococcus porcinus.* (Courtesy Dr. J.M. King, College of Veterinary Medicine, Cornell University.)

the body. The result is a reduction in the phagocytic and functional capacity of macrophages of the monocyte-macrophage system and as a consequence, reduction in resistance to common porcine bacterial and viral pathogens. The major lesions are interstitial pneumonia, generalized lymphadenopathy, and lymphocytic infiltrates into a wide variety of organs. Gross lesions are most likely in the tracheobronchial and mediastinal lymph nodes, which may be enlarged, pale, and firm. Microscopically, the lesions in the lymph nodes, tonsils, and spleens consist of follicular and deep cortical (T lymphocyte) hyperplasia, apoptosis of cells in the follicular germinal centers, and sometimes multinucleated macrophages.

PORCINE JOWL ABSCESS

In jowl abscess, *Streptococcus porcinus* colonizes the oral cavity, which results in infection of the tonsils and the regional lymph nodes. The mandibular lymph nodes are the most often affected, but the retropharyngeal and parotid lymph nodes may be involved (Fig. 13-82). Multiple abscesses 1 to 10 cm in diameter may be present in the lymph nodes.

LYMPHOMA

Lymphoma is a frequent tumor in pigs. There are two forms: multicentric in lymph nodes (more common in visceral lymph nodes) and in spleen, liver, kidney, and bone marrow and the mediastinal form, which tends to affect pigs less than one year of age.

DISORDERS OF DOGS

X-LINKED SEVERE COMBINED IMMUNODEFICIENCY

X-linked SCID (XSCID) has been reported in basset hounds, Jack Russell terrier, and Welsh corgi breeds of dogs. The thymus of these dogs is small and often obscured by mediastinal fat. Tonsils, lymph nodes, and Peyer's patches usually cannot be identified at necropsy. Microscopically, the thymic tissue consists of small dysplastic lobules with a variable number of Hassall's corpuscles. Congenital immunodeficiency diseases are also discussed in detail in Chapter 5.

THYMIC HEMATOMAS

Thymic hemorrhage and hematomas have been reported in dogs, especially young dogs. Many of these dogs die unexpectedly from hypovolemic shock as a result of massive thymic and mediastinal hemorrhage. A variety of causes have been implicated. These include rupture of dissecting aortic aneurysms, trauma from automobile accidents or excessive pulling on a collar, and ingestion of anticoagulant rodenticides (warfarin, dicumarol, diphacinone, and brodifacoum). In the last type, hemorrhage causes expansion of thymic lobules and interlobular septa and appears to originate in the medulla.

GASTROSPLENIC VOLVULUS

See the section on Uniform Splenomegaly with Bloody Consistency.

SPLENIC MYELOID METAPLASIA

Splenic myeloid metaplasia, with histiocytosis and hypersplenism, in the dog is characterized by severe, diffuse, and persistent splenomegaly, and the splenic capsule may be smooth or have multiple and confluent nodules. There is often random vascular thrombosis, producing grossly visible splenic infarcts. Microscopically, extramedullary hematopoiesis is present with interspersed foci of prominent macrophages (PAMS). The process effaces the splenic red pulp and is responsible for the splenic enlargement. This disease may be rather benign, not involving other organs, in which case splenectomy is generally curative. However, EMH may be systemic, involving bone marrow and liver, and this is indicative of a poor prognosis.

SPLENIC HEMATOMAS, HEMANGIOMAS AND HEMANGIOSARCOMAS, AND ACUTE SPLENIC INFARCTS

For more discussion on splenic hematomas induced by lymphoid hyperplastic nodules, splenic hematomas induced by splenic vascular neoplasms, splenic hematomas induced by lymphoid hyperplastic nodules, hemangiomas and hemangiosarcomas, and acute splenic infarcts, see the section on Nodular Spleens with Bloody Consistency.

SPLENIC NODULAR HYPERPLASIA

Splenic nodular hyperplasia is most commonly seen in the spleen of older dogs and is often an incidental finding. This lesion has also been called *canine nodular splenic hyperplasia and splenoma.* Nodules are formed by hyperplastic lymphoid cells or mixed accumulations of hyperplastic erythroid, myeloid, and megakaryocytic cells (EMH) with lymphoid cells. The nodules can be a single discrete nodule or multiple coalescing firm nodules protruding from the surface but covered by the splenic capsule. The capsular surfaces and cut surfaces often have a mottled red-white pattern because of the intermingling of erythrocytes and leukocytes. Hyperplastic nodules are usually hemispheric and up to 2 cm or larger in diameter (see Fig. 13-63) and on cross-section have intermixed areas of red and white (see Web Fig. 13-5). Nodules have no deleterious effect unless they interfere with the drainage of blood from the adjacent marginal sinus and cause a large hematoma, which can rupture and cause hemoperitoneum. Rupture is usually caused by trauma or even a misjudged jump from a couch. These masses must be distinguished from other types of nodules in the spleen, including those of hematoma, and fibrohistiocytic nodules, hemangioma, hemangiosarcoma, and primary or metastatic neoplasms.

FIBROHISTIOCYTIC NODULES

Fibrohistiocytic nodules are splenic masses in dogs that are typically solitary and spheric. They are composed of a mixed population of histiocytoid spindle cells, hematopoietic cells, plasma cells, and lymphocytes. These nodules likely represent a continuum between lymphoid nodular hyperplasia and malignant fibrous histiocytoma. A higher lymphoid-to-fibrohistiocytic cell ratio is associated with better long-term survival. Increased mitotic figures and fibrohistiocytic proportion are associated with metastasis and mortality, likely representing transformation into malignant fibrous histiocytoma.

MALIGNANT FIBROUS HISTIOCYTOMAS

Malignant fibrous histiocytomas in canine spleens are considered a continuum of proliferations of fibrous and histiocytic cells (fibrohistiocytic nodule) normally found in the splenic reticular meshwork of the red pulp (see Nodular Spleens with Firm Consistency.

ACCESSORY SPLEENS

Accessory spleens can be acquired after rupture of the spleen from traumatic injury in dogs (see Fig. 13-70). Fragments of spleen may be implanted onto peritoneal surfaces or embedded in the pancreas. Here, they become vascularized and functional. Implanted fragments grossly and histologically resemble normal splenic tissue. They have red and white pulp areas and a thick fibromuscular capsule. These features are important in differentiating accessory spleens from peritoneal implanted fragments (metastases) of hemangiosarcoma, which have a thin shiny serosal covering and a poor prognosis. It is thought that hyperplastic splenic nodules are more friable than normal spleen and thus are more likely to rupture and be a source of accessory spleens.

SIDEROCALCIFIC PLAQUES AND SPLENIC RUPTURE

See the discussion on miscellaneous disorders in the section on the Spleen.

HISTOPLASMOSIS

Histoplasmosis caused by *Histoplasma capsulatum* is a diffuse disease of the monocyte-macrophage system and causes a marked proliferation of macrophages in a wide variety of tissues including spleen, lymph nodes, liver, lungs, and intestine. The dimorphic fungus *Histoplasma capsulatum* grows as a mold in soil and as a yeast in animal tissue. The fungus is distributed throughout the world, in major river valleys, and in temperate and tropical climates; *Histoplasma capsulatum* grows especially well in soil enriched by bird feces. The greatest incidence of disease is in dogs; the incidence is lower in cats.

In most animals, the organism is inhaled and results in mild self-limiting infections in the lungs, but causes enlargement of tracheobronchial lymph nodes. Dogs and cats are usually asymptomatic. Because the fungus is confined to monocytes and macrophages, its spread beyond the respiratory tract is assumed to occur by hematogenous and lymphogenous dissemination of infected cells. Disseminated histoplasmosis in dogs and cats results in GI or hepatic disease of long duration.

Disseminated histoplasmosis is characterized by neutrophilia and monocytosis in some animals. Nonregenerative anemia is common because of the chronic inflammation. Nonspecific changes as a result of the damage to the liver are elevated serum alkaline phosphatase activity and hyperbilirubinemia. The total serum protein may be low, normal, or increased, depending on factors such as extent and duration of the diarrhea and emaciation.

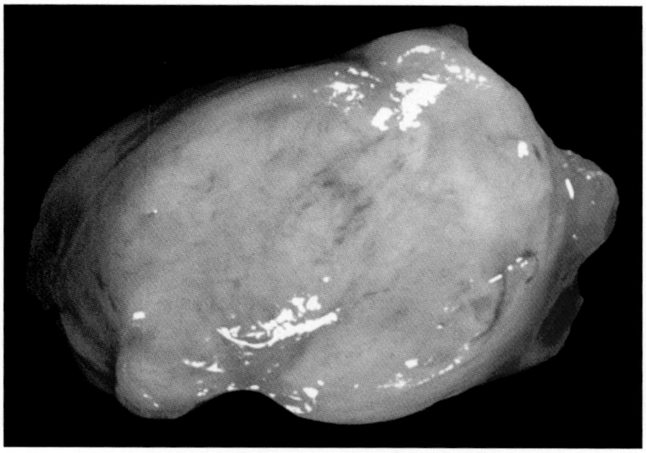

Fig. 13-83 Mesenteric lymph node, diffuse granulomatous lymphadenitis, histoplasmosis, dog.
Note that this lymph node is firm and swollen with a tensed capsule. The cut surface is grayish white and bulges from granulomatous inflammation (see Fig. 13-84). (Courtesy Dr. M.D. McGavin, College of Veterinary Medicine, University of Tennessee.)

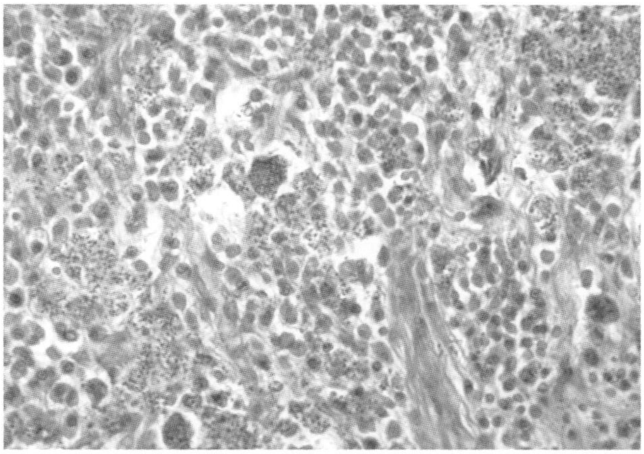

Fig. 13-84 Histoplasmosis, lymph node, dog.
Diffuse granulomatous lymphadenitis. Most of the field is occupied by macrophages, many of which have phagocytosed *Histoplasma capsulatum.* H&E stain. (Courtesy Dr. M.D. McGavin, College of Veterinary Medicine, University of Tennessee.)

Cytology is useful for the diagnosis of histoplasmosis. The least invasive procedures include examination of cells of body fluids, tracheal wash preparations, and aspirates of bone marrow and lymph nodes. The organisms are often visible in macrophages (Web Fig. 13-9).

Dogs dying of this disease are emaciated. The large bowel is thickened with mucosal corrugations caused by infiltration of the submucosa and lamina propria by macrophages, lymphocytes, and plasma cells. Lymph nodes are uniformly enlarged (Fig. 13-83), and normal architecture may be obscured (Fig. 13-84). In contrast to lymphoma, the nodes are firm when incised.

Histologically, in the lymph nodes, coalescing granulomas replace the normal cortical lymphoid tissue. Typical yeast organisms, which are 2- to 4-mm-wide hematoxylinophilic dots surrounded by a clear halo, are present in variable numbers in epithelioid macrophages (see Fig. 13-84). The spleen and liver are enlarged and firm, and the liver is diffusely gray. Affected organs can be imprinted on glass slides for cytologic evaluation.

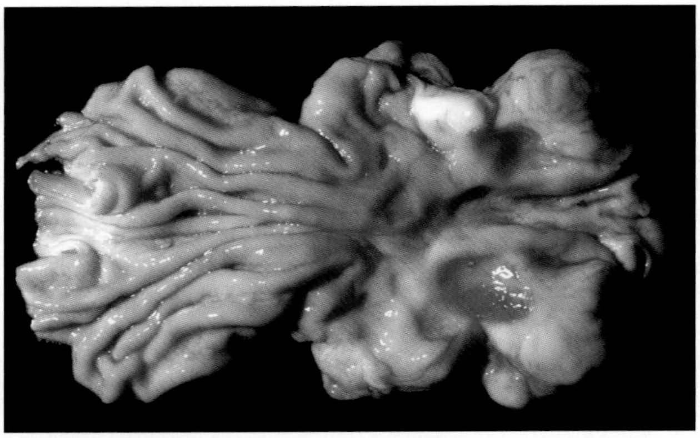

Fig. 13-85 Alimentary lymphoma (lymphosarcoma), stomach, cat. Note the notable thickening of the stomach, which occurred because of infiltration with neoplastic cells. Although uncommon, the mucosal epithelium is focally ulcerated. (Courtesy Dr. M.D. McGavin, College of Veterinary Medicine, University of Tennessee.)

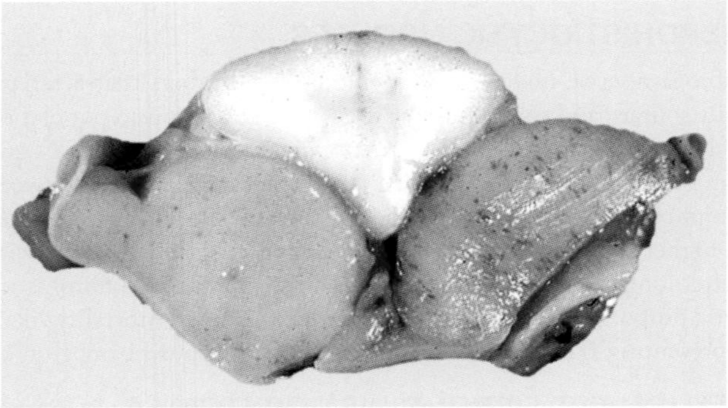

Fig. 13-86 Lymphoma (lymphosarcoma), vertebral canal, epidural space, cow. Bilateral ventrally located soft pink masses compress the spinal cord. In addition to lymph nodes, lymphoma in cattle often involves other locations such as abomasum, vertebral canal, kidney, heart, retroorbital space, and uterus. (Courtesy Dr. J.M. King, College of Veterinary Medicine, Cornell University.)

LEISHMANIASIS

Information on this topic, including Web Fig. 13-10, is available at evolve.elsevier.com/Zachary/McGavin/.

CANINE DISTEMPER

Canine distemper virus preferentially infects lymphoid, epithelial, and nervous cells (see Chapter 14). It spreads by aerosols of secretions, and the virus is phagocytosed and transported by macrophages to the adjacent lymphoid tissue—tonsil or tracheobronchial lymph nodes and disseminated to the spleen, bone marrow, and distant lymph nodes, where it causes lymphoid necrosis. The cortices of lymph nodes of dogs infected with canine distemper are depleted of lymphocytes 6 to 9 days after exposure. Accompanying this is a profound lymphopenia a result of the depression of lymphopoiesis in the bone marrow.

CANINE PARVOVIRUS

Parvovirus is cytolytic to dividing cells and attacks these in the bone marrow, liver, kidney, heart (myocytes) vessel, intestinal epithelium, and lung in neonatal dogs. The most striking lesions are in the dividing cells in the crypts of the small intestine. Hemorrhage from these drains to the regional lymph nodes. Because of a lack of supply of lymphocytes from the bone marrow, there is lymphoid depletion, followed by atrophy in the thymus and depletion of lymphocytes in the B and T lymphocyte areas in lymph nodes and MALT. Also in lymph nodes and MALT, follicular lymphocytes are lost from lymphocytolysis.

LYMPHOMAS

Lymphomas are common tumors in dogs, and there are five anatomic types: *multicentric* with generalized lymph node enlargement and often with splenic and hepatic involvement; *alimentary* (Fig. 13-85); *thymic* (see Fig. 13-49); *cutaneous;* and *epidural* (Fig. 13-86). The histologic appearance of the cell types is discussed in the section on Bone Marrow.

THYMOMAS

Thymomas are usually benign neoplasms that occupy the cranial mediastinum, usually of older animals. They are significantly less common than thymic lymphoma and are only distinguishable microscopically by the presence of neoplastic epithelial cells. Variable numbers of lymphocytes are present within thymomas but are not neoplastic, and these nonneoplastic lymphocytes often outnumber the neoplastic epithelial cells. Thymomas have been associated with myasthenia gravis (which may be accompanied by megaesophagus) and polymyositis (immune-mediated) in dogs. A rare condition, thymic hyperplasia, which results from the formation of B lymphocyte follicles within the thymus, has also been reported in association with myasthenia gravis in dogs and cats.

DISORDERS OF CATS

FELINE PANLEUKOPENIA (PARVOVIRUS)

Parvovirus causes lymphocytolysis of proliferating cells, including those in the bone marrow. As the thymus solely depends on bone marrow for the supply of lymphocytes, the result is thymic atrophy and collapse of the cortex. Similarly, in all secondary lymphatic organs such as spleen, lymph node and MALT (Peyer's patches), B lymphocyte (follicles) and T lymphocyte (inner cortex) areas become hypocellular. Also, follicular lymphocytes are destroyed by lymphocytolysis and microscopically only the pale staining stromal and stem cells remain.

PRIMARY AND SECONDARY NEOPLASMS

Lymphosarcoma

In cats, lymphoma is one of the manifestations of FeLV infections. Distribution of lesions varies widely but they are similar to those in canine lymphoma—mediastinal (thymic) (see Fig. 13-49) and multicentric and alimentary (see Figs. 7-79, 7-179, and 13-85). The thymus is an important site of lymphoma in cats. The tumors are large white or gray mediastinal masses that result in displacement of adjacent structures and in pleural fluid accumulation. In cats, the fluid is frequently chylous (see the discussion on lymph nodes in the section on Disorders of Domestic Animals).

In cats, the most common neoplasms (primary and secondary) forming nodules in the spleen are, in descending order of frequency, mast cell tumor, lymphoma (lymphosarcoma), myeloid neoplasms, and hemangiosarcomas. Splenic hyperplastic nodules and hematomas are less frequent than in the dog.

SUGGESTED READINGS

Information on this topic is available at evolve.elsevier.com/Zachary/McGavin/.

CHAPTER 14

Nervous System*

James F. Zachary

CENTRAL NERVOUS SYSTEM (CNS)

STRUCTURE AND FUNCTION

The CNS consists of neurons, glia, ependyma, endothelial cells and pericytes of blood vessels, and the meninges (Fig. 14-1 and Box 14-1). Neurons vary in size, shape, and function, and their cell bodies are organized into functional groups such as nuclei, gray columns, and cerebral lamina. Neuronal processes called axons and dendrites traverse through the brain and spinal cord, the former often as organized bundles (tracts, fasciculi) forming synapses on cell bodies, dendrites, and axons of other functionally related neurons. It is estimated that there are 1×10^{11} neurons in the human brain. Each neuron makes approximately 10,000 synapses with other neurons; therefore there are about 1×10^{15} synapses in the human brain.

Exactly which cells are classified as glia has varied over the last few decades. Originally, histologists included astrocytes (astroglia), oligodendrocytes (oligodendroglia), ependymal cells (ependymocytes), and microglia as glial cells; however, they currently recognize astrocytes, oligodendrocytes, and microglia as glial cells. Some classification schemes list astrocytes and oligodendrocytes as macroglia. Astrocytes, oligodendrocytes, and ependymal cells are derived from neuroectoderm; whereas microglia, part of the monocyte-macrophage system, are derived from mesoderm (bone marrow). In the mammalian CNS, glia outnumber neurons 10 to 1. Ependymal cells line the ventricular system, whereas choroid plexus epithelial cells form the outer covering of the choroid plexuses.

The CNS is arranged to form two basic parts: the gray and white matter (Figs. 14-2 and 14-3). In the CNS, gray matter is found in the cerebral cortex, in the cerebellar cortex and cerebellar roof nuclei, around the base of the cerebral hemispheres (basal nuclei [often called *basal ganglia*]: caudate nucleus, lentiform nucleus [putamen, globus pallidus], amygdaloid nucleus, claustrum), and throughout the brainstem, often in nuclei. The gray matter is typified by numerous neuronal cell bodies, plus a feltwork of intermingled thinly myelinated axons and dendrites, their synaptic junctions, and processes of oligodendroglia, astrocytes, and microglia. This network of processes and synapses in the gray matter is referred to as the *neuropil.* The white matter consists of well-myelinated axons that arise from neuronal cell bodies in the gray matter and terminate distally in synapses or myoneural junctions, plus oligodendroglia, astrocytes, and microglia. In the cerebral hemispheres, white matter is located centrally; whereas in the brainstem, white matter is intermingled with gray matter (nuclei). In the spinal cord, white matter is located peripherally surrounding the gray matter.

The exterior of the CNS is covered by the meninges. The meninges consist of three layers named, from outermost to inner most layers, the *dura mater, arachnoid,* and *pia mater.* The arachnoid and pia enclose the subarachnoid space.

Cells of the CNS

Neurons

The structure and basic cellular biology of neurons is similar to that of other cells (Fig. 14-4); however, there are, as discussed later, some notable differences. The neuron consists of three structural components: dendrites, a cell body, and a single axon. The length of the axon varies, depending on the function of the neuron. The length of axons of motor or sensory neurons can be 10,000 to 15,000 times the diameter of the neuronal cell body, which results in these axons being several meters in length. The axon terminates in synaptic processes or neuromuscular junctions.

Neuronal cell bodies vary considerably in size and shape, from the large neurons of the lateral vestibular nucleus, Purkinje cell layer of the cerebellum, and the ventral gray matter of the spinal cord to the very small lymphocyte-like granule cells of the cerebellar cortex (Fig. 14-5). Neuronal nuclei tend to be vesicular to spherical in shape, tend to be usually centrally located, and often, particularly in large neurons, tend to contain a prominent central nucleolus. Neurons contain focal arrays of rough endoplasmic reticulum and polysomes, termed *Nissl substance,* that are responsible for the synthesis of proteins involved in many of the neuron's vital cellular

*Dr. R.W. Storts, College of Veterinary Medicine, Texas A&M University, and Dr. D.L. Montgomery, Wyoming State Veterinary Laboratory, made contributions to this chapter in the third and fourth editions.

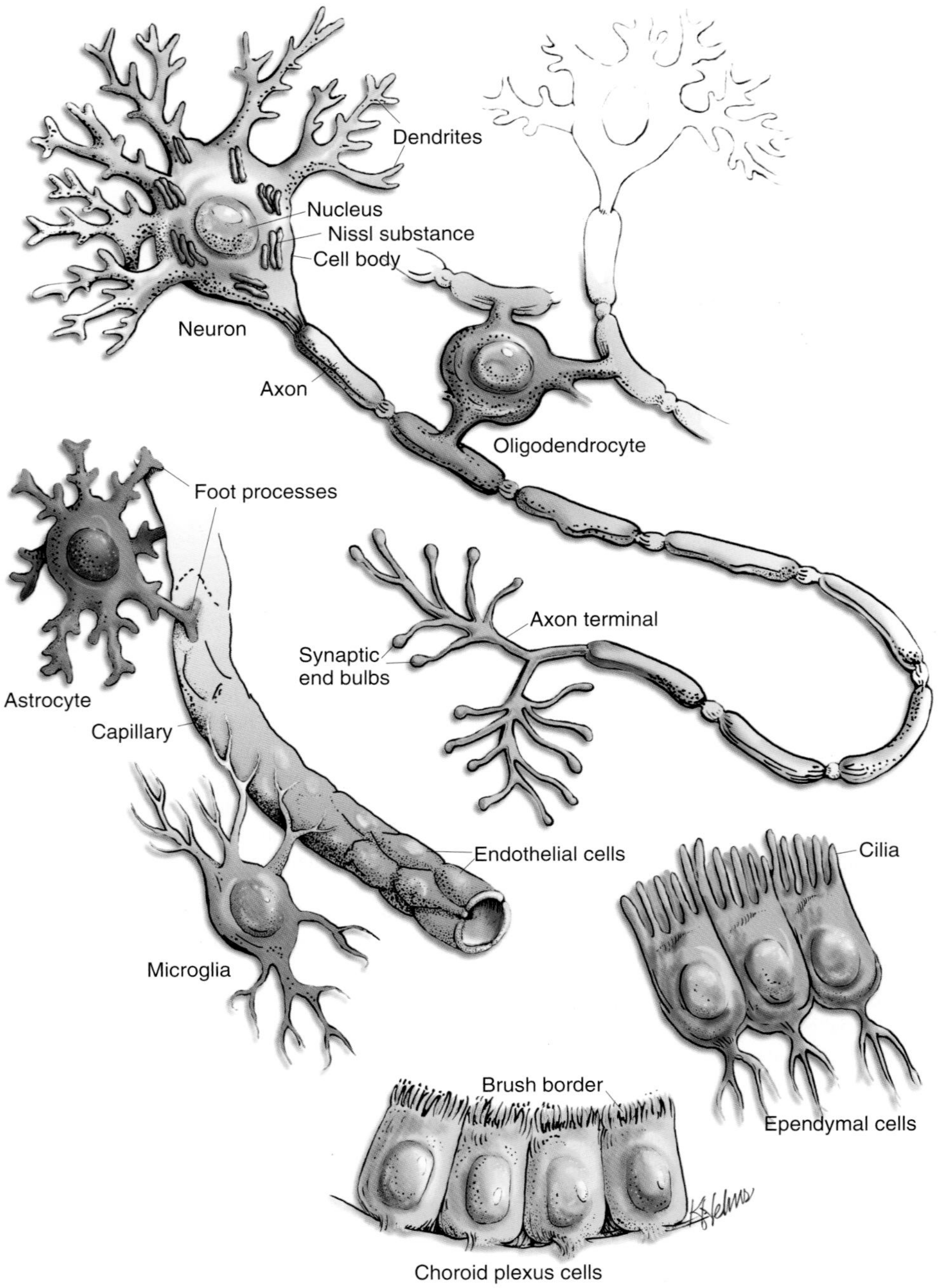

Fig. 14-1 Cell types in the CNS include neurons, astrocytes, oligodendroglia, microglia, ependymal cells, choroid plexus epithelial cells, and vascular endothelial cells.
(Courtesy Dr. J.F. Zachary, College of Veterinary Medicine, University of Illinois.)

processes such as axonal transport. Nissl substance is present in all neurons, regardless of the size of the cell body, but tends to be more prominent in those cells with voluminous cytoplasm such as motor neurons.

Axonal Transport

In most cells of the body, proteins and other molecules are distributed throughout the cell by simple diffusion. In neurons, simple diffusion alone is inefficient because synapses are a considerable distance away from the cell body of the neuron. As a result, molecules cannot diffuse the length of the axon; they must be transported the length of the axon to the synapse. In addition, there are no systems in axons or synapses to catabolize molecules resulting from normal metabolic processes in these structures. Thus these molecules need to be returned to the cell body for processing. These processes are facilitated in the axon by retrograde (toward the cell body) and anterograde (toward the synapse) axonal transport systems.

More information on this topic, including Web Fig. 14-1, is available at evolve.elsevier.com/Zachary/McGavin/.

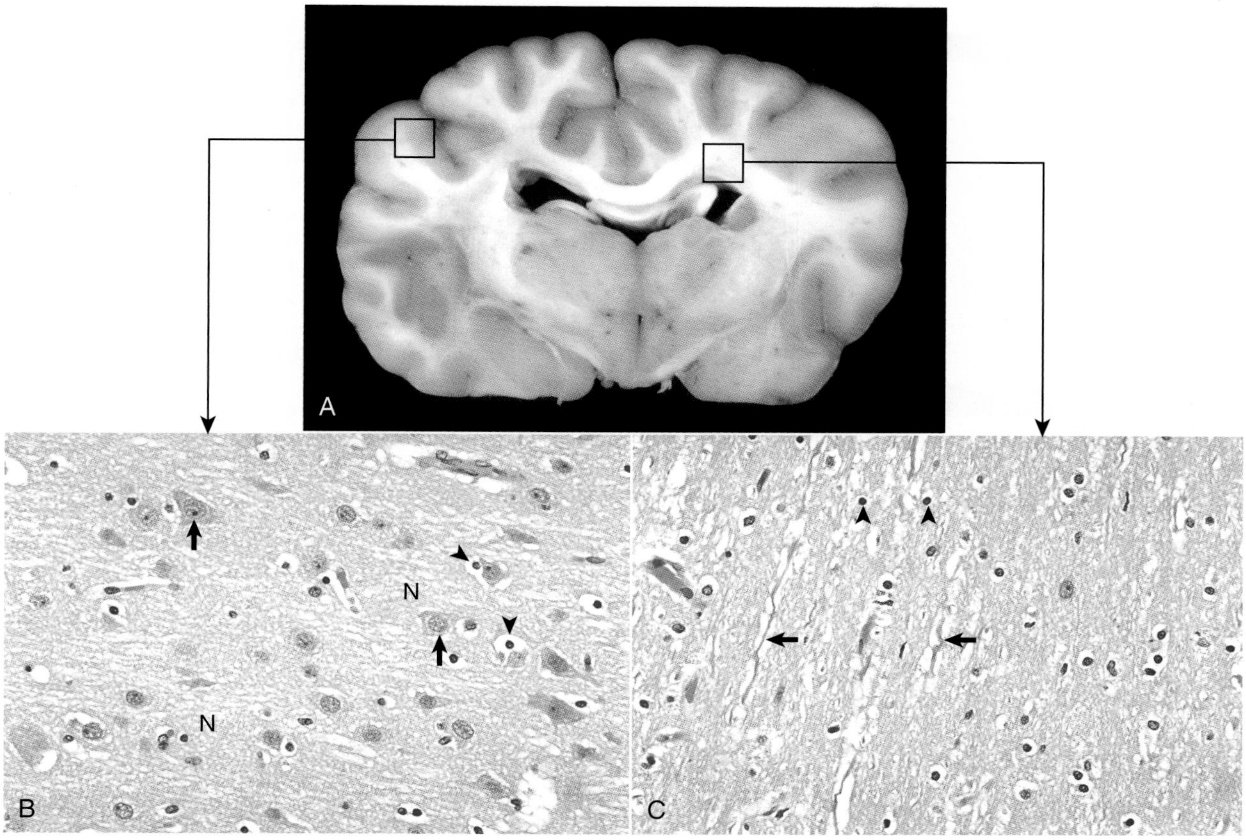

Fig. 14-2 Organization of the brain, gray matter, and white matter.
A, Transverse section at the level of the thalamus, dog. Gray matter *(darker areas)* of the cerebral cortex lies beneath the leptomeninges on the external surface of the brain, whereas in the thalamus there tends to be a mixture of gray and white matter. Major white matter areas *(light areas)* include corona radiata, centrum semiovale, and corpus callosum of the cerebrum, and internal capsule and optic tracts bordering the lateral and ventral surfaces of the thalamus, respectively. **B,** Gray matter consists primarily of the cell bodies of neurons *(arrows)* and a network of intermingled thinly myelinated axons, dendrites, and glial cell processes. This network is referred to as the neuropil *(N)*. Other components include oligodendroglia (perineuronal satellite cells) *(arrowheads)*, protoplasmic astrocytes, and microglia. H&E stain. **C,** White matter primarily consists of well-myelinated axons *(arrows)* plus oligodendroglia *(arrowheads)* and fibrous astrocytes. The clear spaces surrounding large axons are artifacts formed when the lipid components of myelin lamellae are dissolved away by solvents in the process of embedding tissue in paraffin for sectioning. H&E stain. (Courtesy Dr. J.F. Zachary, College of Veterinary Medicine, University of Illinois.)

BOX 14-1 Cells of the CNS and Their Primary Functions

NEURONS

Transmission of electric and chemical impulses
Spatial and temporal interpretation of impulses
Inhibitory and stimulatory regulation of impulses

ASTROGLIA (PROTOPLASMIC [TYPE I] AND FIBROUS [TYPE II])

Regulation of extracellular neurotransmitter concentrations and fluid/electrolyte imbalances
Repair of injury by proliferation of astrocytic cellular processes
Support and bundling of functionally related axons traversing through the CNS
Participation in barrier systems
- Glia limitans
- Blood-brain barrier

OLIGODENDROGLIA

Myelination of axons within the CNS
Proposed neuronal cell body homeostasis within the CNS

EPENDYMA

Movement of cerebrospinal fluid (CSF) through the ventricular system

CHOROID PLEXUS EPITHELIAL CELLS

Secretion of CSF
Barrier function (blood-CSF barrier)

MICROGLIA

Immunosurveillance, immunoregulation, phagocytosis
Monocyte-macrophage system

MENINGES

Arachnoid-CSF barrier
Subarachnoid CSF cushioning of head trauma

ENDOTHELIA

Barrier function (blood-brain barrier)
Selective molecule transport systems

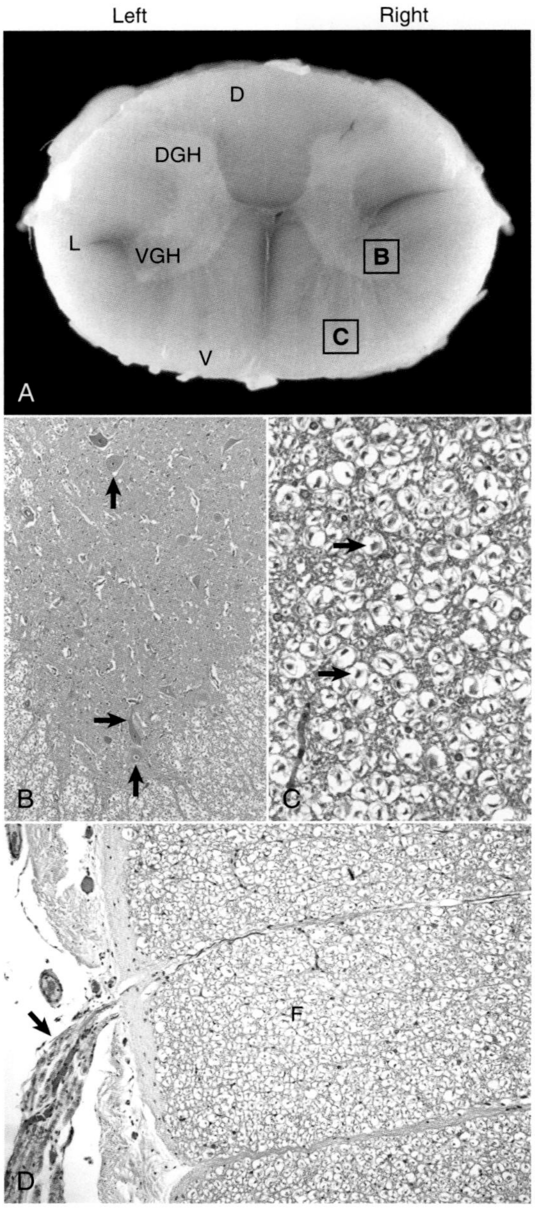

Fig. 14-3 Organization of the spinal cord, gray matter, and white matter. **A,** White matter in the spinal cord is located peripherally and divided into dorsal, lateral, and ventral funiculi. As a general rule, dorsal funiculi *(D)* consist of ascending sensory axons, lateral funiculi *(L)* have a mixture of sensory and motor axons, and ventral funiculi consist of descending motor axons *(V)*. *DGH,* Dorsal gray horn; *VGH,* ventral gray horn. Histologically, the right side is a mirror image of the left side. The areas labeled *B* and *C* and contained within the boxes correspond to the areas illustrated in **B** and **C. B,** Transverse section of spinal cord, ventral gray horn, horse. The cell bodies of large motor neurons *(arrows)* are those of lower motor neurons and their axons extend in peripheral nerves to myoneural junctions that innervate skeletal muscle. H&E stain. **C,** Transverse section of spinal cord, ventral funiculus, horse. Because most axons course up and down the length of the spinal cord, in a transverse section, axons *(arrows)* are cut in cross section. They are surrounded by myelin sheaths whose lipid components are dissolved out during the preparation of paraffin embedded sections, resulting in clear spaces that are an artifact. H&E stain. **D,** Efferent spinal nerve (longitudinal section shown here), transverse section of spinal cord, ventral funiculus, dog. Axons of lower motor neurons leave funiculi *(F)* and assemble as nerve rootlets *(arrow)* eventually forming peripheral nerves that innervate skeletal muscle. H&E stain. (Courtesy Dr. J.F. Zachary, College of Veterinary Medicine, University of Illinois.)

Diseases of the axon that result directly or indirectly from alterations in axonal transport systems are discussed later. The character of the histologic lesions affecting injured nerve fibers can often be related to alterations in specific transport systems. Neurofilament proteins are synthesized in the neuronal cell body and are assembled and transported into axons. If neurofilaments accumulate in neuronal cell bodies and proximal axons, this lesion is called an axonopathy and is characterized by alterations in slow transport systems, which results in axonal swelling or atrophy and perikaryal neurofibrillary accumulations. Axonal injury and alterations in neurofilament transport can also cause secondary demyelination.

Membrane Potentials and Transmitter/Receptor Systems

A fundamental activity of neurons is to modulate and effectively transmit chemical and electric signals from one neuron to another

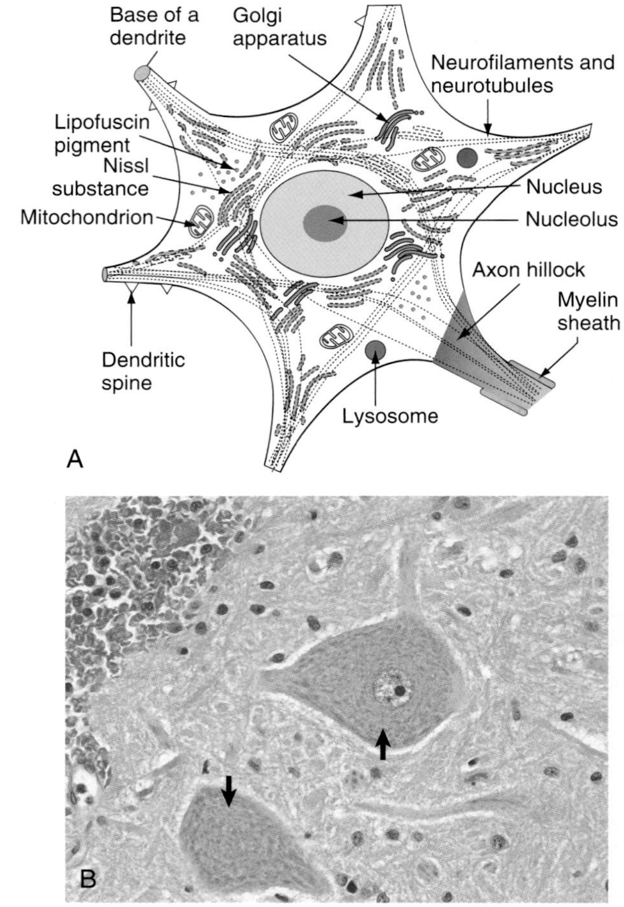

Fig. 14-4 Neuron structure.
A, Basic cell biology and structure of neurons are similar to other cells in the body. Additionally, neurons have dendritic arborizations and an axon, specializations for the initiation, propagation, and transmission of impulses that underlie the basic function of these cells. **B,** The cytoplasm of the neuronal cell body has blue (basophilic [H&E stain]) granular material (rough endoplasmic reticulum) called Nissl substance *(arrows)*. Nissl substance synthesizes proteins, including precursor neurotransmitter proteins and the structural proteins (neurofilaments), active in maintaining the integrity (length and diameter) of the axon. H&E stain. (**A** modified from Kierszenbaum AL: *Histology and cell biology,* St Louis, 2002, Mosby. **B** courtesy Dr. J.F. Zachary, College of Veterinary Medicine, University of Illinois.)

via synapses in the CNS or from one neuron to a muscle cell via junctional complexes, myoneural junctions, or motor end-plates in the PNS. The process of nerve impulse conduction is made possible by the establishment and maintenance of an electric potential across the cell membrane of the neuron/axon.

Information on this topic, including Web Fig. 14-2, is available at evolve.elsevier.com/Zachary/McGavin/.

Astrocytes

The functions of astrocytes in the CNS are regulation, repair, and support, as depicted in Fig. 14-6. Mature astrocytes differentiate from pluripotential progenitor cells during the development of the CNS. Astrocytes are the most numerous cell type in the CNS and have traditionally been classified into two types based on morphology. Protoplasmic astrocytes are located primarily in gray matter, whereas fibrous astrocytes occur chiefly in white matter. Microscopically, astrocytes have relatively large vesicular nuclei, indistinct or inapparent nucleoli, and no discernible cytoplasm with routine hematoxylin and eosin (H&E) staining (Fig. 14-7). With suitable histochemical stains, metallic impregnation, or immunohistochemical staining for glial fibrillary acidic protein (GFAP [the major intermediate filament in astrocytes]), the cell body and the extensive arborization and interconnections of astrocytic processes can be demonstrated. Processes vary from short and brushlike to long branching processes in protoplasmic and fibrous astrocytes, respectively (Fig. 14-8). These morphologic features and their corresponding histochemical and immunohistochemical staining reactions serve as important criteria for the classification of tumors of astrocyte origin.

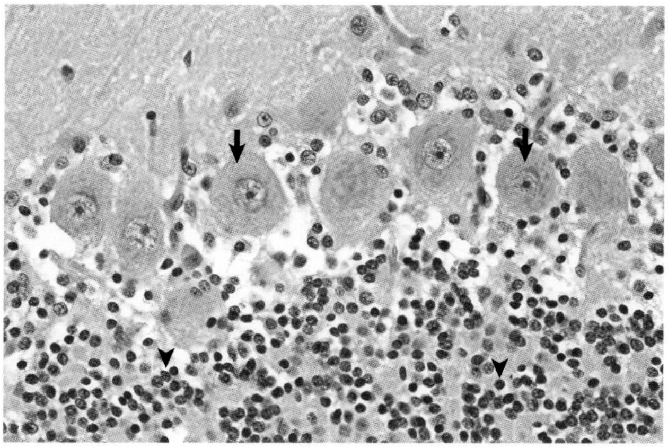

Fig. 14-5 Variations in neuronal morphology, cerebellum, granule cells, and Purkinje neurons, normal animal.
The granule cell neurons of the cerebellar cortex *(arrowheads)* are very small lymphocyte-like cells that have relatively little demonstrable Nissl substance when compared with Purkinje neurons *(arrows)* and large motor neurons (depicted in Fig. 14-4, *B*). H&E stain. (Courtesy Dr. J.F. Zachary, College of Veterinary Medicine, University of Illinois.)

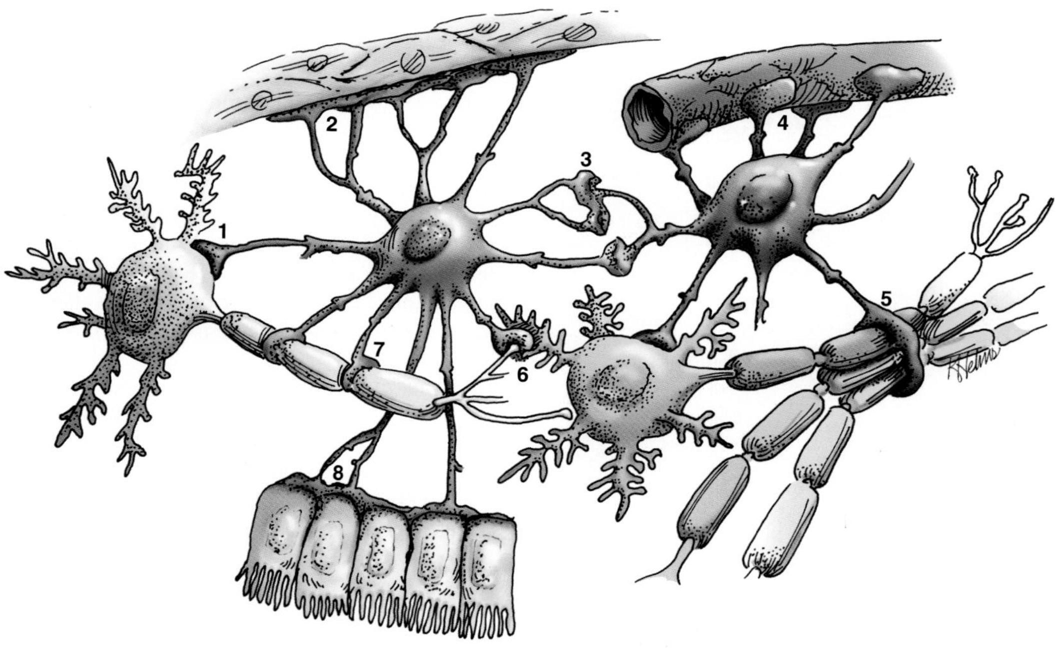

Fig. 14-6 Functions of astrocytes.
Astrocytes provide structural integrity and regulatory oversight, as depicted in this diagram. They: *1,* monitor and regulate fluid and electrolyte balances within neurons and surrounding extracellular space; *2,* form the glial limitans at the base of the pia mater; *3,* interconnect with other astrocytes to provide a system to monitor and regulate fluid and electrolyte balances throughout the CNS; *4,* possibly participate in the formation and functions of the blood-brain barrier; *5,* participate in the support of axon tracts of functionally related neurons; *6,* monitor for and remove excessive release of neurotransmitters in synapses; *7,* protect and insulate nodes of Ranvier; and *8,* participate in the cerebrospinal fluid–brain barrier. In addition, astrocytes are a reparative (healing) cell after CNS injury with loss of tissue because nervous tissue, per se, is devoid of fibroblasts. Fibroblasts exist in the pia mater and other meninges. Everywhere else, healing depends on the astrocyte, which responds by increased length, branching, and complexity of cellular processes (astrogliosis). The astrocyte has many functions in the nervous system; one of them is to act in healing to produce a scar in attempts to isolate cavities and abscesses. Fibroblasts may also contribute to the formation of a scar, if this cell type is present, as it is in the leptomeninges. (Courtesy Dr. J.F. Zachary, College of Veterinary Medicine, University of Illinois.)

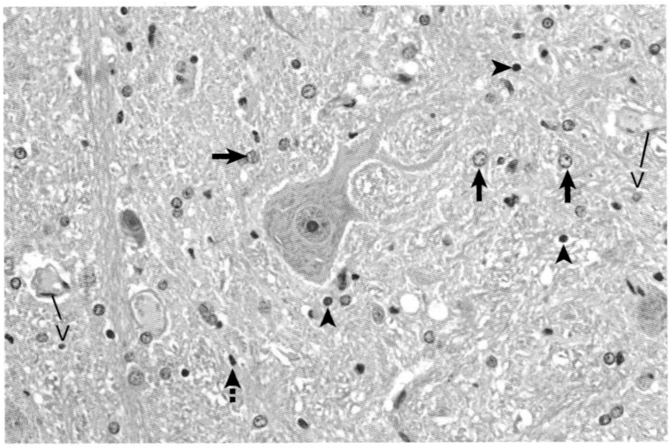

Fig. 14-7 Histologic features of glial cells, ventral gray horn, spinal cord, horse.
A neuronal cell body and its processes are in the center of the illustration. To the inexperienced, identifying specific types of glial cells in H&E stained histologic sections can be challenging. Astrocytes *(arrows)* have larger vesicular nuclei (dispersed chromatin) and the cell membrane and cytoplasm are rarely seen in nondiseased conditions. Thus these nuclei just seem to "sit" in the midst of the neuropil. The majority of nuclei in the neuropil here are astrocytic. Oligodendroglial cells *(arrowheads)* have smaller and dense round nuclei (condensed chromatin) often surrounded by a clear zone indicative of cell cytoplasm and a cell membrane. Oligodendroglial cells in gray matter are called perineuronal satellite cells; those in white matter are called interfascicular oligodendrocytes. Microglial cells are difficult to identify in H&E stained sections of the CNS, but they often appear as "rod cells," which have small, dense elongated nuclei *(dashed arrow)*. The light pink homogeneous tissue distributed in large quantities between these cell types is the neuropil. *V,* Blood vessels. H&E stain. (Courtesy Dr. J.F. Zachary, College of Veterinary Medicine, University of Illinois.)

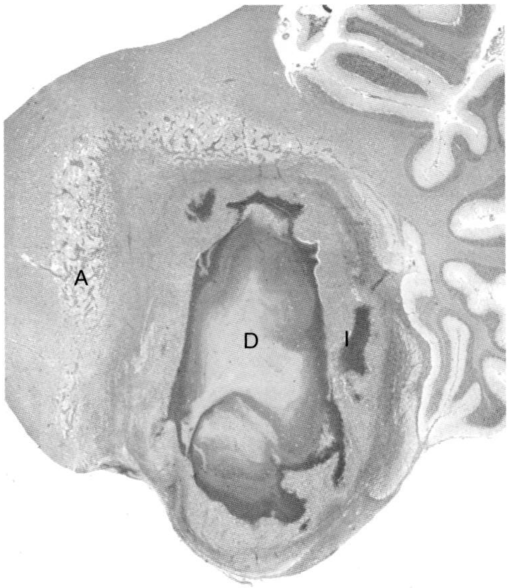

Fig. 14-9 Astrocytic repair, bacterial abscess, brainstem, sheep.
The abscess has a central core of necrotic debris *(D)* surrounded by a layer of inflammatory cells *(I)* and a less dense pink-staining zone representing an attempt by astrocytes and fibroblasts to form a capsule *(A)*. This capsule is formed by fibrous tissue on the ventral and right sides, those sides closest to the pia, which contains fibroblasts. A fibrous capsule is absent from the dorsal and left sides of the abscess, adjacent to brain parenchyma. Here, there is no population of resident fibroblasts and the capsule is formed by astrocytes and their processes, which are often delicate and do not form an effective capsule *(A)*. H&E stain. (Courtesy Dr. J.F. Zachary, College of Veterinary Medicine, University of Illinois.)

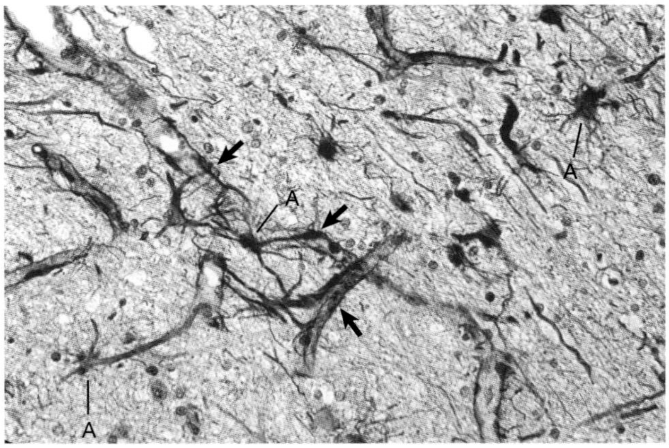

Fig. 14-8 Astrocytic processes, brain, cerebral cortex, normal animal.
Processes of astrocytes arborize extensively throughout the CNS (structures stained purple). Note that some of the processes are on the outside of blood capillaries (end feet) *(arrows)*. *A,* Cell body of astrocyte. Holzer's stain. (Courtesy Dr. M.D. McGavin, College of Veterinary Medicine, University of Tennessee.)

Functions of Astrocytes

Regulation of the microenvironment

The microenvironment of the CNS must be under strict control to maintain normal function. Astrocytes are involved in homeostasis of the CNS and regulate ionic and water balance, antioxidant concentrations, uptake and metabolism of neurotransmitters, and metabolism or sequestration of potential neurotoxins, including ammonia, heavy metals, and excitatory amino acid neurotransmitters such as glutamate and aspartate. Interactions between astrocytes, microglia, and neurons orchestrate immune reactions in the brain. In this regard, astrocytes can express major histocompatibility complex (MHC) class I and II antigens, a variety of cytokines and chemokines, and adhesion molecules that modulate inflammatory events in the CNS. Astrocytes also secrete growth factors and extracellular matrix molecules that play a role not only in development but also in repair of the CNS.

Repair of injured nervous tissue

In the CNS, reparative processes that occur after injury, such as inflammation and necrosis, are chiefly the responsibility of astrocytes. In these reparative processes, astrocytes are analogous to fibroblasts in the rest of the body. Astrocytes do not synthesize collagen fibers, as do fibroblasts. Instead, repair is accomplished by astrocytic swelling and division, and abundant proliferation of astrocytic cell processes containing intermediate filaments composed of GFAP, a process called *astrogliosis.* As an example, neuronal necrosis occurs in some viral diseases of the CNS. When neurons die, the spaces left by the loss of the neuronal cell bodies are filled and such spaces (<1 mm in diameter) are filled by processes of astrocytes. Larger spaces that form after injury, such as an infarct, are often too large to be filled and therefore exist in the CNS as fluid-filled spaces (cysts) surrounded by a capsule of astrocytic processes. Astrocytes will also attempt to wall off abscesses, but they are not as effective as fibroblasts and the capsule can be incomplete or weak (Fig. 14-9). In the case of direct extension of bacteria from the meninges or meningeal blood vessels, which contain or are surrounded by fibroblasts, respectively, fibroblasts play a larger role in isolating the inflammatory process.

Structural support of the CNS

Structurally, astrocytic processes provide support for other cellular elements and ensheathe and insulate synapses. Astrocytes also provide guidance and support of neuronal migration during development; thus, tracts and fasciculi of axons with similar functions are arranged and structurally supported by astrocytic processes. Processes of astrocytes (foot processes) also terminate on blood vessels throughout the CNS, forming a component of the blood-brain barrier. Astrocytes influence the induction of tight junctions between endothelial cells that serve as the structural basis for the blood-brain barrier. A dense meshwork of astrocytic processes also forms the glia limitans beneath the pia mater and is variably prominent in subependymal areas. During CNS development, cells termed *radial glia* provide a scaffold and guidance for migrating neurons. When development is completed, radial glia mature into astrocytes.

Oligodendroglia

There are two types of oligodendroglia: (1) interfascicular oligodendrocytes and (2) satellite oligodendrocytes (satellite cells). The function of interfascicular oligodendroglia is myelination of axons, whereas the function of satellite oligodendroglia is thought to be regulation of the perineuronal microenvironment. Oligodendroglia have been compared with neurons with regard to their total cell size in that their processes occupy much more space than the cell body. Neurons have very long axons, which account for their size; oligodendroglia have extensive myelin sheaths, which account for their size. In H&E stained sections, oligodendroglia are often confused with lymphocytes because of the similarity of the morphology of their nuclei and cytoplasmic volume. Interfascicular oligodendroglia and perineuronal satellite oligodendroglia are located primarily in white and gray matter of the CNS, respectively (Fig. 14-10); however, interfascicular oligodendroglia can also be found along axons that traverse through the gray matter. The mature, small oligodendrocyte has a spherical, hyperchromatic nucleus (see Figs. 14-7 and 14-10). As with astrocytes, the cell body and processes of this cell do not stain with conventional H&E staining methods and can only be demonstrated following special procedures that include metallic (silver) impregnation and immunohistochemical methods.

Most interfascicular oligodendroglia (see Fig. 14-10) are aligned in rows parallel to myelinated axons and are responsible for the formation and maintenance of segments (internodes) of myelin sheaths. One oligodendroglial cell can form as many as 50 different internodes of myelin, each of which can be located on many different axons (Fig. 14-11). Altered function of oligodendroglial cells, as occurs in infectious canine distemper virus (CDV) infection, can cause primary demyelination of these segments, resulting in severe neurologic dysfunction. Oligodendroglia also influence maturation and maintenance of axons and inhibit regeneration of established myelinated axons.

Perineuronal satellite oligodendroglia (see Fig. 14-10) are adjacent to neuronal cell bodies and are also located around blood vessels in the gray matter. They are thought by some investigators to regulate the perineuronal microenvironment and respond to perturbation by proliferation. When the perineuronal microenvironment is altered or neuron cells bodies are injured, perineuronal satellite oligodendroglia, in an attempt to regulate the environmental perturbation, hypertrophy and proliferate in a process referred to as *satellitosis*. Similarly, alterations in the microenvironment of gray and white matter away from areas surrounding neuron cell bodies results in hypertrophy of oligodendroglia (see Fig. 14-10). Finally, satellitosis can be quite prominent in normal CNS in various areas of the gray matter.

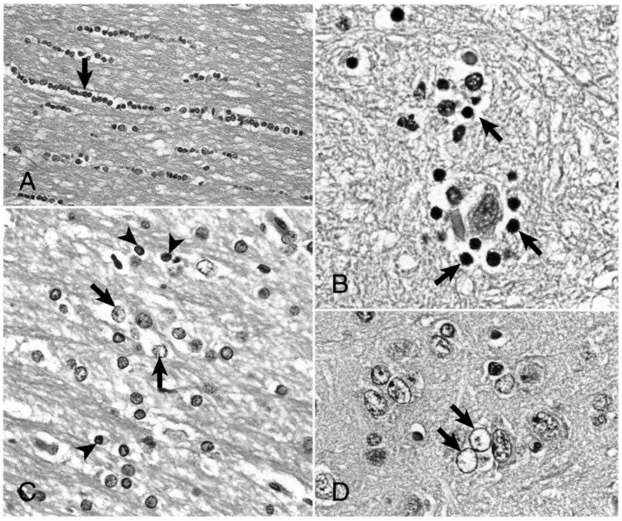

Fig. 14-10 Responses of glial cells to injury in H&E stained CNS sections.

A, White matter. In nondiseased states, oligodendroglia in white matter are often arranged linearly (interfascicular oligodendroglia) *(arrow)* and are responsible for the formation of myelin around axons. In gray matter (not shown; see Fig. 14-17), oligodendroglia are dispersed as individual cells around neuronal cell bodies as perineuronal satellite cells (Fig. 14-10, *B*). H&E stain. **B,** Gray matter. When neurons are injured or there exists some perturbation of the perineuronal microenvironment, a long-held belief was that oligodendroglia around neurons hypertrophy and proliferate in a process referred to as satellitosis. Currently, there is no uniform agreement that these cells respond to neuronal injury in this manner. Perineuronal satellite oligodendroglia *(arrows)* surround a small degenerate neuron with condensed chromatin and little cytoplasm. H&E stain. **C,** White matter. Astrocytes *(arrows)* and oligodendroglia *(arrowheads)* have a limited repertoire of responses to injury in the CNS. Astrocytic proliferation can occur but is very difficult to determine in sections stained with H&E. Here, astrocyte nuclei are somewhat enlarged and appear more numerous than expected. H&E stain. **D,** Gray matter. Astrocytes respond to injury in hyperammonemia, such as occurs with hepatic encephalopathy, by forming astrocytes with enlarged, markedly vesicular ("watery"), often elongated nuclei called Alzheimer's type II astrocytes *(arrows)*. This type of astrocyte may occur in pairs that are surrounded by a clear space indicative of cellular swelling. H&E stain. (**A** courtesy Dr. M.D. McGavin, College of Veterinary Medicine, University of Tennessee. **B** to **D** courtesy Dr. J.F. Zachary, College of Veterinary Medicine, University of Illinois.)

Microglia

The basic functions of microglia are immunosurveillance, immunoregulation, and reparative (phagocytic) activities after neural cell injury and death. The origin of microglia in the CNS has been debated for years. The current consensus is that the cells originate from circulating monocytes (mesoderm-derived) that enter and populate the CNS during embryonic development and early postnatal life, analogous to the formation of the monocyte-macrophage system in other organs. After entry into the CNS, the cells become amoeboid microglia, phagocytosing dead cells and cellular debris during remodeling and maturation of the CNS. Amoeboid cells then enter a quiescent stage and transform into ramified microglia. Ramified microglia constitute up to 20% of the glial cells and are present throughout the mature CNS, serving as sentinels of brain

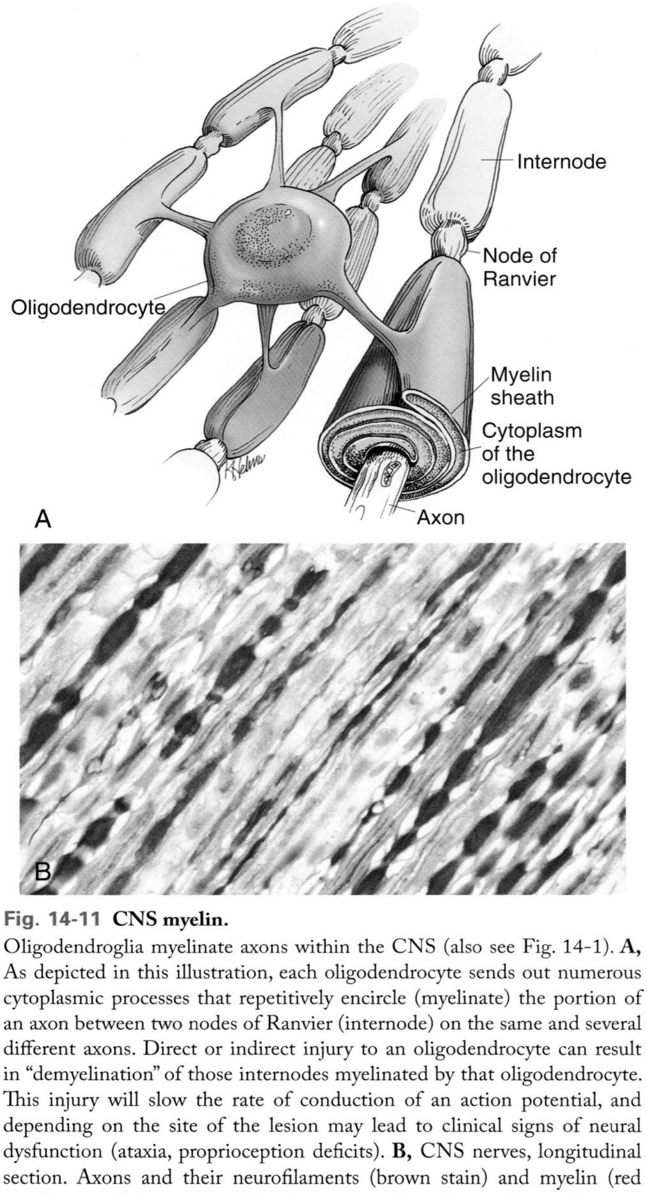

Fig. 14-11 CNS myelin.
Oligodendroglia myelinate axons within the CNS (also see Fig. 14-1). **A,** As depicted in this illustration, each oligodendrocyte sends out numerous cytoplasmic processes that repetitively encircle (myelinate) the portion of an axon between two nodes of Ranvier (internode) on the same and several different axons. Direct or indirect injury to an oligodendrocyte can result in "demyelination" of those internodes myelinated by that oligodendrocyte. This injury will slow the rate of conduction of an action potential, and depending on the site of the lesion may lead to clinical signs of neural dysfunction (ataxia, proprioception deficits). **B,** CNS nerves, longitudinal section. Axons and their neurofilaments (brown stain) and myelin (red stain) are well demonstrated by this immunohistochemical stain for neurofilaments and myelin basic protein. (Courtesy Dr. J.F. Zachary, College of Veterinary Medicine, University of Illinois.)

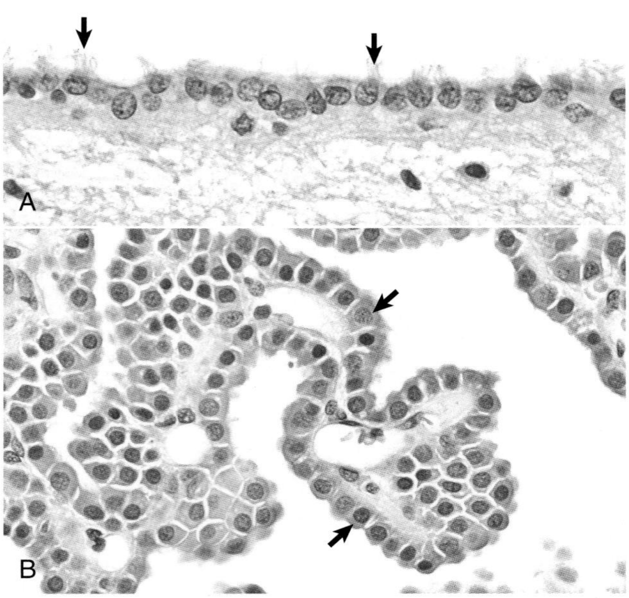

Fig. 14-12 Ependymal and choroid plexus epithelial cells.
A, Ependymal cells are ciliated *(arrows)* and assist with the flow of cerebrospinal fluid (CSF) through the ventricular system. H&E stain. **B,** Choroid plexus epithelial cells *(arrows)* secrete CSF from a brush-border (microvilli) on the luminal surface. The surface of the choroid plexus also has cilia that occur singly or more often in groups of three or more on a single cell. H&E stain. (Courtesy Dr. J.F. Zachary, College of Veterinary Medicine, University of Illinois.)

injury. Ramified microglia, also called *resting cells,* are most numerous in perineuronal and perivascular areas and in interfascicular locations in white matter. Evidence of pinocytosis in ramified cells suggests some role in maintaining the neural microenvironment. The principal function of microglia is phagocytosis, the initiation of and participation in the innate and adaptive immune responses, and in degenerative and inflammatory diseases of the CNS.

Microscopically, ramified microglia have small, hyperchromatic ovoid-, rod-, or comma-shaped nuclei and no appreciable cytoplasm with routine H&E staining, thus the term *rod cell* is sometimes used to describe them (see Fig. 14-7). With special labeling techniques or metallic impregnation, ramified cells have a few delicate branching processes. The small hyperchromatic nuclei and nuclear shape distinguish microglia from astrocytes and oligodendroglia. However, microglia are often difficult to identify in H&E stained sections without some expertise in neuropathology.

Activated microglial cells are not the major source of active macrophages in inflammation of the CNS. Blood monocytes recruited from the circulation account for up to 70% of the macrophages in inflammatory and degenerative diseases of the CNS. These macrophages differentiate from blood monocytes involved in normal "leukocytic trafficking" through the CNS and can be involved in immunologic and phagocytic responses (gitter cells) to disease processes and infectious organisms. They are found mainly in the leptomeninges, choroid plexus, and perivascular areas.

Ependyma (Including Choroid Plexus Epithelial Cells)

The basic functions of ependymal cells, which line the ventricular system, are to move cerebrospinal fluid (CSF) through the ventricular system via movement of their cilia and to regulate the flow of materials between the CNS and the CSF. The ependyma is a single-layered, cuboidal to columnar, epithelium that lines the ventricles and mesencephalic aqueduct of the brain, and central canal of the spinal cord (Fig. 14-12). This layer of cells is therefore situated between the CSF and nervous tissue. Ependymal cells have cilia that project into the CSF and beat in a coordinated manner in the direction of CSF flow. Other structures, referred to as *circumventricular organs,* which include the choroid plexuses, are covered by highly specialized ependymal cells. The surface of ependymal cells that form the choroid plexus have microvilli (microvillus border) and cilia that occur singly or more often in groups of three or more. The choroid plexus epithelial cells also have specialized tight junctions (zonulae occludentes) that are a functional part of the blood-CSF barrier. In contrast to the choroid plexus, junctions between the conventional ependymal cells include gap junctions (transmembrane proteins form a pore, allowing communication between adjacent cells) and zonulae and fasciae adherentes, which permit movement of materials, such as proteins from the CSF, into the extracellular space of the brain. This cellular lining, however, is not a static membrane in that it regulates several processes that involve interaction between the CSF and brain. The functions include regulation of fluid homeostasis between the ventricular cavities and the brain, secretion and absorption of CSF, endocytosis, phagocytosis, and metabolism of substances such as iron resulting from the lysis of erythrocytes after hemorrhage into the ventricular system. Finally, ependymal cells have the structural and enzymatic characteristics necessary for scavenging and detoxifying a wide variety of substances in the CSF.

During embryonic development, the medial wall of the lateral ventricle (choroid fissure), the roof of the third ventricle, and the rostral part of the roof of the fourth ventricle consist of a single layer of neuroectoderm that is adherent on its outer surface to the pia mater. This neuroectoderm-pia union forms the tela choroidea, providing an anchor for the choroid plexuses, which is formed by an invagination of this bilayer membrane into the ventricular spaces.

Choroid plexus epithelial cells are modified ependymal cells. The choroid plexus epithelium is a single-layered, cuboidal to columnar, epithelium with a microvillus border (see Fig. 14-12). CSF is secreted from the microvillus border. Choroid plexus epithelial cells, along with capillaries and the pia mater, form the choroid plexuses that project into the lateral, third, and fourth ventricles. The basic function of choroid plexuses is to produce the CSF that fills the ventricular system and the subarachnoid space. CSF has two important functions: (1) to act as a "shock absorber" to mitigate the effects of trauma to the brain and spinal cord and (2) to deliver nutrients to and remove wastes from the CNS.

The normal flow pattern of CSF is regulated by an intraventricular biologic pressure gradient in which the pressure created by secretion of CSF exceeds the pressure created by its absorption in arachnoid villi (arachnoid granulations). Arachnoid villi are focal extensions of the arachnoid and subarachnoid space that extend into the dorsal sagittal venous sinus of the brain. CSF is secreted by the choroid plexuses in the lateral, third, and fourth ventricles. It should be noted, however, that fluid from other sources, such as secretion by the ependyma, interstitial fluid of the brain, and ultrafiltrate of the blood, has also been reported to contribute to the formation of CSF. It moves from the lateral ventricles into the third ventricle, from the third ventricle through the mesencephalic aqueduct (aqueduct of Sylvius in humans), and then to the fourth ventricle. Once in the fourth ventricle, the CSF exits through the two lateral apertures of the fourth ventricle to enter the subarachnoid space. Lateral apertures are the two openings in the caudal medullary velum that forms the roof of the fourth ventricle into the subarachnoid space, one at each side of the cerebellopontine angle. Although the central canal of the spinal cord is connected to the ventricular system at the caudal end of the fourth ventricle, there apparently is little active movement of CSF within the central canal. CSF in the subarachnoid space is reabsorbed by the arachnoid villi in the brain. Recent evidence indicates that other routes of CSF drainage, in addition to arachnoid granulations, also exist and vary in different species. Venous sinuses, lymphatic drainage, and the cribriform plate appear to play important roles in CSF drainage and the maintenance of normal interventricular CSF pressure. In fact, experimental evidence suggests that the cribriform plate route may be the most important of the four. In humans, the entire volume of CSF is circulated approximately four times a day; however, with aging, the entire volume of CSF circulates less than two times a day.

Meninges

The meninges, which enclose the CNS, consist of three layers: the dura mater (outermost layer [pachymeninges]), the arachnoid membrane (mater), and the pia mater (innermost layer) (Fig. 14-13). Together, the arachnoid membrane and pia mater are frequently referred to as the *leptomeninges, pia-arachnoid layer,* or *pia-arachnoid.* The arachnoid membrane and pia mater are held together by bands of fibrous tissue called *arachnoid trabeculae.* This arrangement forms a compartment called the *subarachnoid space* in which CSF flows and which also contains blood vessels and nerves. There is also limited evidence based on studies in humans with neuro–acquired immunodeficiency syndrome that the brain has a primitive lymphatic system. The leptomeninges form a protective covering for the CNS and provide an external envelope filled with CSF that provides additional protection.

The dura mater, once referred to as the pachymeninx (thick meninges), is a strong and dense collagenous membrane (Fig. 14-14). In the cranium, the dura consists of two layers that are fused with each other. The outer layer serves as the periosteum of the cranial bone, except in the areas of the venous sinuses (surrounded by dura) and falx cerebri, which is the longitudinal layer that extends ventrally between the two cerebral hemispheres. At the level of the foramen magnum, the two layers become separated; the outer layer continues to function as the periosteum of the vertebral (spinal) canal, and the inner layer forms the free dural membrane that surrounds the spinal cord. The inner aspect of dura mater is lined by elongated, flattened mesothelial-like cells. Except in neonates, there is no epidural (extradural) space in the cranial vault as there is in the spinal cord. There can be a "potential" epidural or extradural space in mature animals from hemorrhage caused by trauma.

The arachnoid consists of both the multilayered membrane composed of cells that overlap one another and the trabeculae that join it to the pia. The arachnoid has tight junctions between its cells, although other junctions have also been described. It contains no blood vessels and has an outer smooth surface formed by mesothelial-like cells that abut similar cells in the dura mater. The mesothelium-like surfaces of the dura and arachnoid oppose and slide over each other, analogous to the parietal and visceral surfaces of other serous membranes.

The pia mater is closely adherent to the surface of the brain and spinal cord and is penetrated by a large number of blood vessels that supply the underlying nervous tissue (Fig. 14-15). The pia mater consists of flat, thin, overlapping connective tissue cells (fibroblasts) that are separated from the underlying neural tissue by variable amounts of loose collagen fibers and the glia limitans. In many areas the pia, which lacks a basal lamina, is only one-cell-layer thick and has fenestrations, so that the glia limitans is exposed directly to the subarachnoid space. Pial and arachnoid cells also ensheathe blood vessels, collagen bundles, and nerves that are within or cross the subarachnoid space and also are around arteries that penetrate into the CNS up to 1 to 2 mm in depth. Macrophages also are present throughout the leptomeninges.

Endothelium

The basic functions of endothelium in the CNS are to line luminal surfaces of blood vessels; form the blood-brain barrier; regulate thrombosis, thrombolysis, and platelet adherence; and maintain a nonthrombogenic boundary between coagulation cascade molecules and luminal surfaces of endothelial cells. Additionally, endothelial cells function as regulatory barriers to small and large molecules crossing the endothelium, and they control the adherence of leukocytes to their luminal surfaces. The endothelial cells

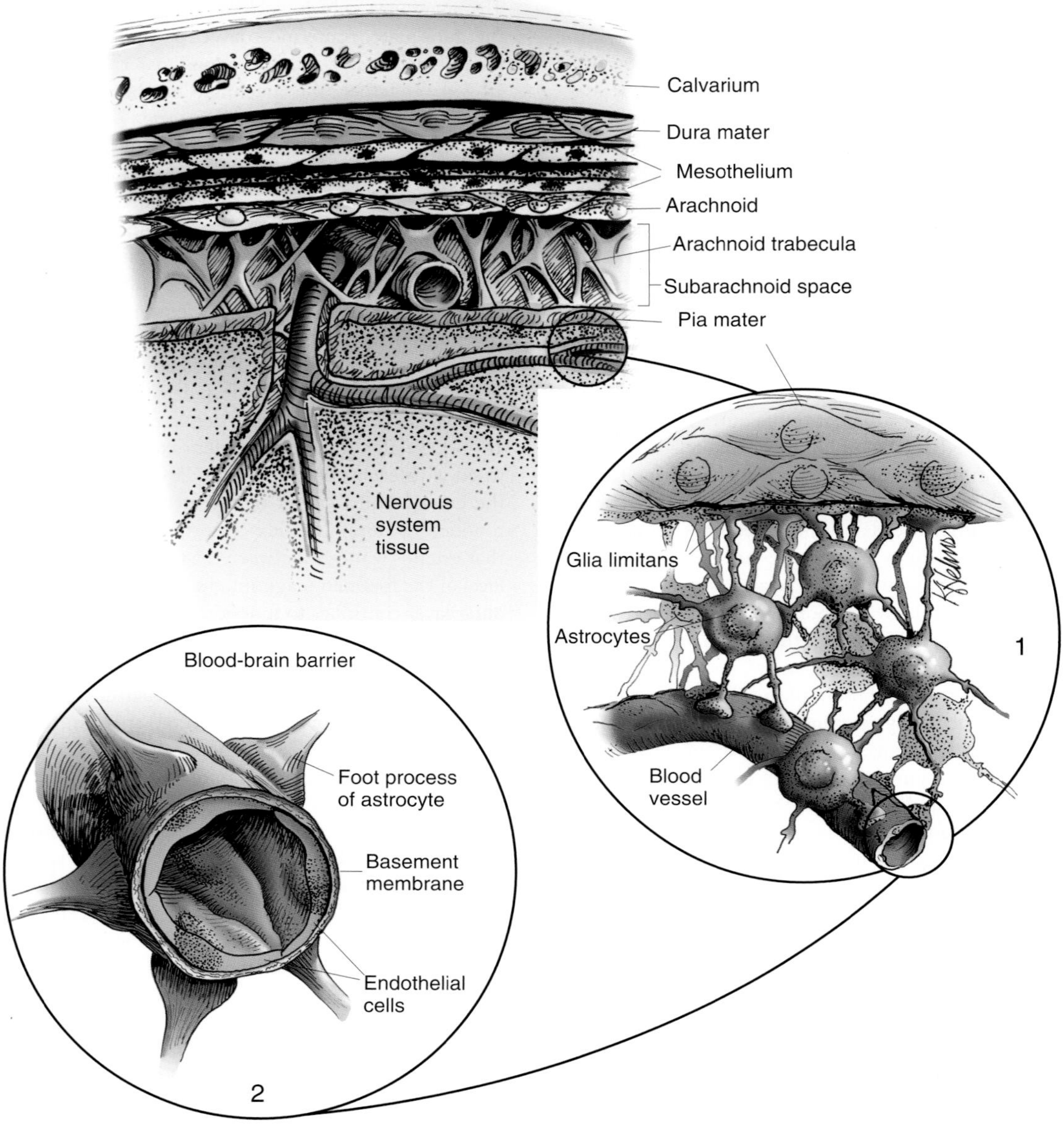

Fig. 14-13 Organization of the meninges.
The meninges, from outside to inside, are the dura mater, arachnoid mater, and pia mater as illustrated in the diagram. The arachnoid mater and the pia mater form the leptomeninges. These two layers of the leptomeninges also enclose the subarachnoid space, which contains the arteries, veins, and nerves and is filled with cerebrospinal fluid. The pia mater is attached to the surface of the CNS. Astrocytes and their foot processes underlie the pia mater and form the glia limitans *(inset 1)* and surround the endothelial cells that form the blood-brain barrier. As arterioles penetrate the cortex to supply the tissue with blood, they carry the pia and glia limitans with them for 1 to 3 mm until the arteriole structurally becomes a capillary. At this transition site within the cortex, the capillary penetrates the pia and is surrounded by the glia limitans, and the end feet of the astrocytes become part of the blood-brain barrier *(inset 2)*. Components of the blood-brain barrier are capillary endothelial cells, basement membrane, and astrocytic foot processes, but the barrier is formed structurally by tight junctions between endothelial cells and functionally by specialized transport systems in these cells. (Courtesy Dr. J.F. Zachary, College of Veterinary Medicine, University of Illinois.)

of the blood-brain barrier actively transport those molecules that the brain consumes rapidly and in large quantities such as glucose, amino acids, lactate, and ribonucleosides.

RESPONSES TO INJURY

Ground Rules for Understanding Injury in the CNS

Before the responses of the CNS to injury are discussed, some fundamental concepts are reviewed in Box 14-2.

Neurons

Neurons are the most vulnerable cells in the nervous system and probably within the body. They have large requirements for energy to maintain normal metabolism, transport systems, and the formation of cytoskeleton proteins in the axon, which can extend over long distances (>1 m), but neurons lack adequate intracellular glucose reserves. Therefore they are completely dependent for survival on an adequate blood supply to provide glucose. Additionally, neurons are vulnerable to free radical oxidative stresses and have a

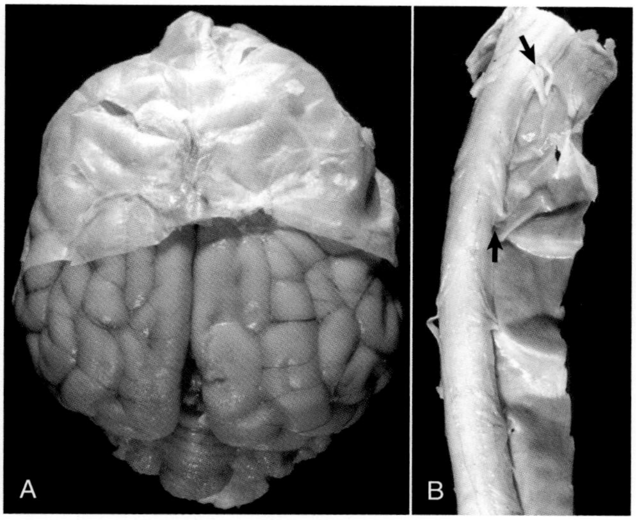

Fig. 14-14 Layers of the meninges.
A, Brain, dog. The dura matter is a thick opaque layer. Here it covers the rostral (cranial) half of the brain and has been dissected away from the caudal half of the brain to expose the underlying leptomeninges. In old animals, the dura mater often fuses with the periosteum of the calvarium, and at necropsy to expose the brain, it is usually removed attached to the calvarium. The leptomeninges are present, but because they are so transparent, in this photograph they are barely visible on the surface of the caudal half of the brain between gyri. **B,** Spinal cord, horse. The dura mater is the thick opaque layer dissected from and lying to the right of the spinal cord. The leptomeninges (pia-arachnoid layer) are present (but not readily visible in this photograph) on the exposed surface of the spinal cord. *Arrows* indicate spinal nerve roots. (Courtesy Dr. J.F. Zachary, College of Veterinary Medicine, University of Illinois.)

limited ability to buffer shifts of calcium ions into the cell, which can interfere with oxidative phosphorylation and ATP production, such as occurs with ischemia.

Neurons are especially sensitive to excessive stimulation with excitatory amino acid neurotransmitters called *excitotoxins* (e.g., glutamate and aspartate). These neurotransmitters are also released in a wide variety of neuronal injuries, especially in neuronal ischemia. Under normal conditions, astrocytic processes surrounding synapses have efficient uptake systems to remove excitotoxins, and neurons are not injured. In excessive quantities, persistent binding of excitotoxins to receptors can lead to neuronal degeneration and death.

The microscopic appearance of the neuronal cell body can vary according to the injury. Characteristic changes of the neuronal cell body are reviewed in Box 14-3.

Neuronal Cell Death

Neurons can die after injury as a result of one of two mechanisms: apoptotic cell death and necrotic cell death. These mechanisms are summarized next and discussed in greater detail in Chapter 1. Both apoptotic and necrotic neuronal cell death can occur concurrently or in temporal or spatial sequences within the nervous system. Although apoptotic and necrotic neuronal death represent different responses of neurons to injury, identical receptors, messenger systems, and mechanisms of cytotoxicity are likely involved in both apoptotic and necrotic cell death. Factors that determine whether the apoptotic or necrotic pathway is activated are unclear but appear to depend on the character on the initiating ligand or injury, type of cell membrane receptors activated, and caspases expressed in response to injury.

BOX 14-2 Concepts in Understanding Responses of the CNS to Injury

1. The cells of the CNS vary in their susceptibility to injury (neurons > oligodendroglia > astrocytes > microglia > blood vessels). Neurons are the most sensitive to injury, whereas glial and other cells are more resistant to injury.
2. Neurons have only small energy stores, therefore they depend on an intact blood flow to supply oxygen and nutrients, particularly glucose. Neurons with the highest metabolic rate, such as some neurons in the cerebral cortex, will die 6 to 10 minutes after the cessation of blood flow after cardiac arrest.
3. There is no regeneration of neurons. The neurons you have now are the ones you were born with; however, their metabolism is dynamic, and metabolites are continually turned over and replaced.
4. If nerve fibers in the CNS are cut by transection of the cord, no or little regeneration of nerve fibers results. Therefore if sufficient motor nerve fibers are cut, there is paralysis; if not, there is a neurologic deficit.
5. If fibers in the PNS are cut, they can regenerate under certain circumstances. This outcome depends on axoplasmic flow, alignment of the proximal and distal portions of the nerve, and the preservation and alignment of the proximal and distal portions of the endoneurial tube (the structure in which the axon lies).
6. Healing in the CNS is different than in the rest of the body. There are few fibroblasts in the CNS and they are principally found only in the leptomeninges and in the outer few millimeters of the CNS, where they are pulled into the cerebral cortex with blood vessels. Therefore wounds deep in the CNS heal by proliferation of astrocyte processes. Astrocytic processes fill small dead spaces of less than a few millimeters and encapsulate large dead spaces and abscesses. Superficial wounds or wounds that extend through the leptomeninges heal by synthesis and deposition of collagen by fibroblasts (fibrous connective tissue) and by proliferation of astrocytic processes. However, in contrast to the fibroblast, astrocytic processes produce a very poor capsule, which can break down easily.
7. The cranial cavity is nearly filled by the brain, its coverings, and fluids. Therefore many lesions, such as tumors, abscesses, hemorrhages, and hydrocephalus in the brain, produce clinical signs because they are space-occupying lesions, which in neuropathology implies that they cause atrophy or displacement of portions of the brain or cord, depending on the duration of the injury.
8. The blood-brain barrier can exert control over drugs and antibodies and prevent them from entering the intact brain. It is also a barrier to infection and is formed by the tight junctions of the endothelial cells, aided by basement membrane, and the end feet of the astrocytes, which lie on the outside of the capillary.
9. Although the CNS has the ability to resist infection and injury, once the CNS is infected, it has a low degree of resistance when compared with other tissues of the body. Microbes, such as *Cryptococcus neoformans,* which normally would be relatively nonpathogenic in other organs, may produce death if the CNS is infected. This outcome in part is attributable to the complexity of the CNS and the fact that it is the most vital organ in the body. Any disease process will often cause catastrophic results in the CNS, as opposed to tissues such as in the lung, liver, and kidney.

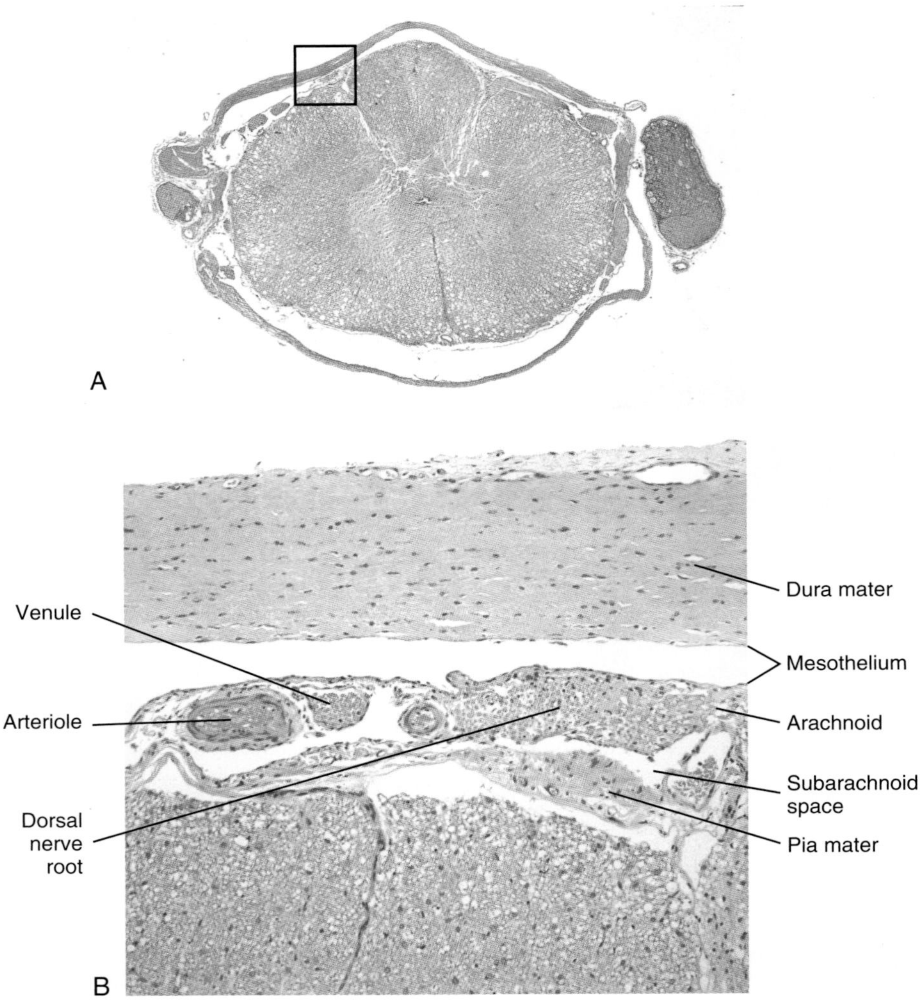

Fig. 14-15 Histologic section of spinal cord and meninges.
A, Low magnification of a cross-section of the spinal cord and meninges with spinal nerve rootlets and a dorsal root ganglion from which **B** was selected *(box).* H&E stain. **B,** The inner surface of the dura mater and the outer surface of the arachnoid mater are covered with mesothelial cells, and the space between them is the subdural space. Blood vessels and nerves of the dorsal and ventral roots traverse in the subarachnoid space. H&E stain. (Courtesy Dr. J.F. Zachary, College of Veterinary Medicine, University of Illinois.)

BOX 14-3 Microscopic Changes that Can Occur in the Neuronal Cell Body

1. Central chromatolysis after axonal injury
2. Ischemic cell change
3. Enlargement of the cell body in lysosomal storage diseases
4. Accumulation of lipofuscin pigment in aging
5. Accumulation of neurofilaments in certain neuronal degenerative diseases
6. Inclusion body formation in certain viral diseases
7. Cytoplasmic vacuolation in spongiform encephalopathies

Apoptotic Cell Death (Programmed Cell Death)

Apoptosis is a single cell-initiated, gene-directed cellular, and self-destructive regulatory mechanism that leads to "programmed" cell death. This mechanism is used (1) during the development of the nervous system to ensure proper migration and orientation of cell layers and removal of excess embryonic cells, (2) to remove "aged" cells (i.e., cell turnover) in organs, and (3) to maintain cell number homeostasis in organ systems that have regenerative capacity (endocrine glands).

Apoptotic neuronal death is characterized by a sequence of cellular degenerative steps that can be identified biochemically and morphologically. After appropriate signals are recognized and interpreted by cell membrane receptors (Fas, tumor necrosis factor [TNF] receptor-1, TNF-related apoptosis-inducing ligand receptors), a family of proteins known as caspases are activated. Caspases cleave cellular substrates that are required for cellular function and include cytoskeleton proteins and nuclear proteins such as DNA repair enzymes. Caspases also activate other degradative enzymes, such as DNAases, which cleave nuclear DNA.

The role of apoptotic neuronal death in specific neurologic diseases is discussed in greater detail in subsequent sections. As examples, some viral infections that occur in utero produce developmental anomalies by initiating apoptosis that leads to faulty differentiation of embryonic granule and Purkinje cell layers such as occurs in experimental Borna disease. Mild ischemia, excitotoxins, hormones, corticosteroids, and proinflammatory cytokines can induce apoptotic cell death. Rabies virus has been linked experimentally to apoptotic neuronal death.

Apoptosis results in characteristic morphologic changes in cells such as shrinkage, cytoplasmic condensation and blebbing, and chromatin clumping and fragmentation (see Figs. 1-30 through 1-34). As cells continue to shrink, nuclear chromatin is cleaved into smaller units and along with condensed cytoplasm is packaged for removal by macrophages. Inflammation is not induced by apoptotic cell death.

Necrotic Cell Death

Necrosis is a process that usually affects groups of cells in contrast to single isolated cells as observed in apoptosis. Necrosis is characterized by the following sequence: hydropic degeneration, swelling of mitochondria, pyknosis and fragmentation of the nucleus, and eventual cell lysis caused by cell membrane damage and the inability of the plasma membrane to control ion and fluid gradients (see Figs 1-11 through 1-17). Cellular debris associated with necrotic neuronal death elicits an inflammatory response in contrast to apoptotic neuronal death.

Acute neuronal necrosis (ischemic cell change)

Acute neuronal necrosis is a common response to a variety of CNS injuries, such as cerebral ischemia caused by blood loss and hypovolemic shock, vascular thrombosis, and cardiac failure; inflammatory mediators; bacterial toxins; thermal injury; heavy metals; and nutritional deficiencies, such as thiamine deficiency; and trauma. Additionally, conditions that reduce ATP generation through oxidative phosphorylation also lead to neuronal degeneration and death. Such conditions include (1) interference with cytochrome oxidase activity in mitochondria caused by cyanide poisoning, (2) competitive inhibition of oxygen uptake in carbon monoxide poisoning, and (3) inadequate availability of glucose for neuronal metabolism in hypoglycemia.

The susceptibility of cells and tissue structures of the CNS to ischemia in decreasing order of susceptibility are neurons, oligodendroglia, astrocytes, microglia, and blood vessels. However, within groups of neurons, some neurons are more sensitive to injury than others. This phenomenon is called *selective neuronal vulnerability.* Purkinje cells; some striatal neurons; neurons of the third, fifth, and sixth cerebral cortical lamina; and hippocampal pyramidal cells have the highest vulnerability. A regional vulnerability of neurons has also been reported (cerebral cortex and striatum > thalamus > brainstem > spinal cord). It is hypothesized that the most vulnerable neurons likely produce the most excitotoxins, such as glutamate, and are the most sensitive to them. Because of the microanatomic arrangement of the cerebral cortex, ischemic neurons often occur in a laminar pattern within the cerebrocortical gray matter. This microanatomic pattern accounts for the laminar lesions observed in thiamine deficiency–induced polioencephalomalacia in ruminants and in other diseases such as salt poisoning in pigs and lead poisoning in ruminants.

After the various types of CNS injury, there is an early increase in ATP-dependent release of normally sequestered intracellular calcium ions from altered mitochondria and endoplasmic reticulum. Also during this time, neuronal depolarization potentiates the release of the neuroexcitatory neurotransmitter glutamate. Persistent activation of glutamate receptors of target cells results in a disturbance referred to as excitotoxicity. This altered activity leads to a notable influx of extracellular calcium into cells, causing further impairment of mitochondrial function and the generation of reactive oxygen species, such as superoxide, hydrogen peroxide, hydroxyl radicals, and nitric oxide. These reactive oxygen species, exerting their effects especially on lipid-rich cell membranes, can enhance the existing excitotoxicity, cause further influx of calcium into cells as a result of membrane damage, and ultimately result in neuronal dysfunction and death. Additionally, reperfusion of ischemic tissue after the initial ischemic injury can enhance the generation of reactive oxygen metabolites, thus amplifying the tissue damage. Other influencing factors include the temperature of the brain at the time of ischemia, with lower temperatures (as little as 2° C decrease) having a sparing effect and elevated temperatures having an enhanced effect on neuronal injury following ischemia.

Neurons depend on a continuous supply of oxygen to remain viable, and if the supply is interrupted for several minutes, the vulnerable neurons as described previously degenerate. Ischemic cell change can also result from metabolic disturbances other than ischemia, such as in thiamine deficiency and cyanide toxicosis, which interferes with oxygen use. In H&E stained sections, the cytoplasm of the neuronal cell body is shrunken, deeply eosinophilic, and frequently sharply angular to triangular in shape (Fig. 14-16). The nucleus is reduced in size, is often triangular, and is pyknotic. The nucleolus and Nissl substance are usually not detectable. Ischemia neurons die and are removed either by a process called *neuronophagia,* which is phagocytosis by microglial cells and macrophages or

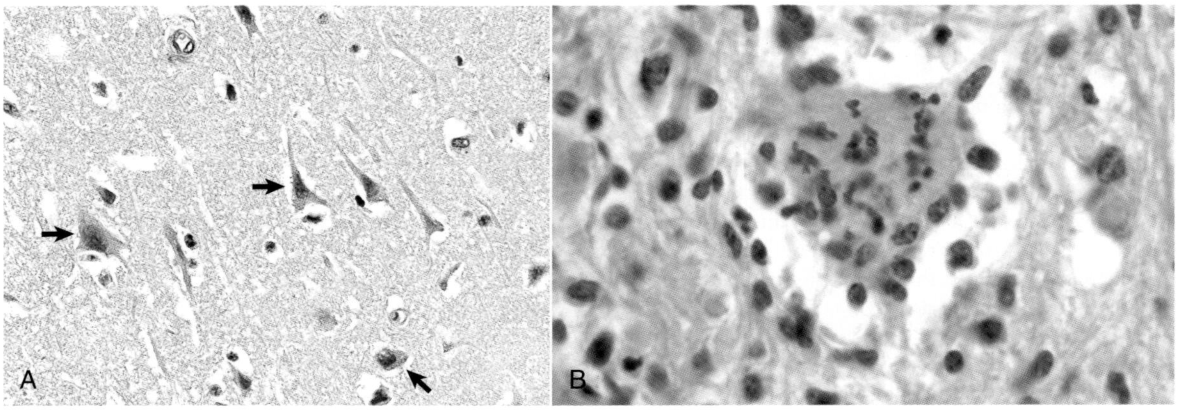

Fig. 14-16 Neuronal necrosis (acute), so-called ischemic cell change, cerebrum, dog.
A, Neuronal ischemia. Neuronal cell bodies of cerebral cortical laminae are red, angular, and shrunken *(arrows)* and their nuclei are contracted and dense. This lesion can be caused by neuronal ischemia. H&E stain. **B,** Neuronophagia. This necrotic neuron cell body *(center of figure)* is surrounded by macrophages that will phagocytose the cell debris. H&E stain. (**A** courtesy Dr. J. F. Zachary, College of Veterinary Medicine, University of Illinois. **B** courtesy Dr. M.D. McGavin, College of Veterinary Medicine, University of Tennessee.)

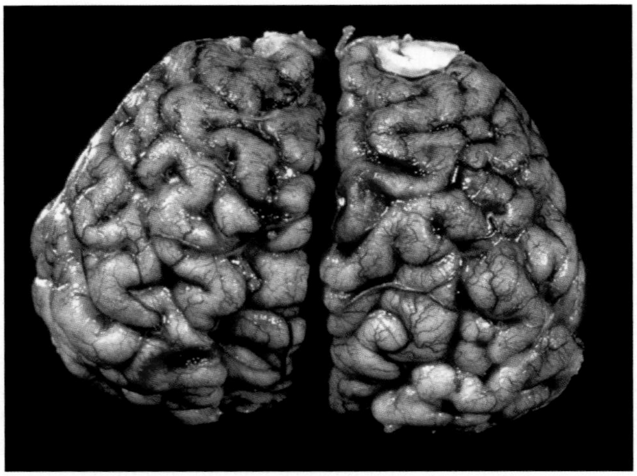

Fig. 14-17 Cerebral cortical atrophy, horse.
Atrophy is seen with a variety of slowly progressive neurologic diseases in which there is a progressive loss of neurons. These diseases include cerebral cortical atrophy of aging and ceroid-lipofuscinosis. The characteristic gross lesions are narrowing of the cerebral gyri with a consequent widening of the sulci. (Courtesy the Department of Veterinary Biosciences, The Ohio State University.)

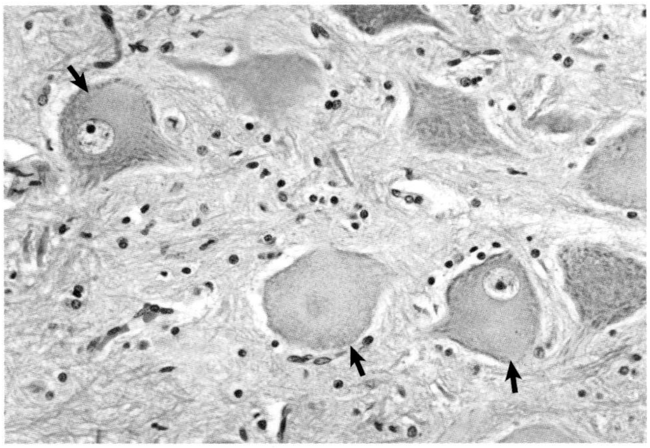

Fig. 14-18 Central chromatolysis, neuron cell body, dog.
Compare with Figs. 14-4, *B,* and 14-7. Affected neurons have eccentric nuclei and pale central cytoplasm with dispersed Nissl substance *(arrows).* (Courtesy Dr. M.D. McGavin, College of Veterinary Medicine, University of Tennessee.)

More information on this topic, including Web Fig. 14-3, is available at evolve.elsevier.com/Zachary/McGavin/.

by lysis (see Fig. 14-16). After neuronal necrosis, there is swelling of perineuronal and perivascular astrocytic processes.

Chronic neuronal necrosis (brain atrophy)

Neuronal death and loss of neurons can occur as a result of progressive disease processes of long duration in the CNS. This loss, termed *simple neuronal atrophy,* is seen with slowly progressive neurologic diseases, such as cerebral cortical atrophy of aging, ceroid-lipofuscinosis, and primary and multisystem and cerebellar neuronal degeneration. Gross lesions are usually not visible, but when cerebrocortical neurons die, there can be atrophy of cerebral gyri, which results in widening of the sulci (Fig. 14-17). Microscopic lesions indicative of an earlier loss of neurons are diminished numbers of neurons and astrogliosis and atrophy and loss of neurons in functionally related systems. Loss of neurons over time results in progressively worsening neurologic dysfunction.

Wallerian Degeneration and Central Chromatolysis

Injury to axons of the CNS and PNS can result from a variety of causes such as (1) traumatic transection leading to Wallerian degeneration, (2) compression and crushing, (3) therapeutic neurectomies, (4) nerve stretching injury, and (4) intoxication.

Wallerian Degeneration

In 1850, Dr. Augustus Volney Waller described the pattern of microscopic lesions (necrosis) in axons and myelin sheaths after transection. These changes are characteristic of Wallerian degeneration. Although Waller described this process in peripheral nerves, the term *Wallerian degeneration* is also used to describe necrosis that occurs in nerve fibers in the CNS after axons are injured (compressed or severed). These reactions include swelling of the neuronal cell body, dispersion of centrally located Nissl substance, and peripheral displacement of the nucleus termed *central chromatolysis* (Fig. 14-18) and swelling of the axon and myelin distal to the site of injury are to swell and break, and the rate is proportional to the diameter of the fiber (Fig. 14-19). Thus the larger the diameter of the axon, the faster the rate of Wallerian degeneration.

Macroglia

Astrocytes

Common astrocytic reactions in CNS injury are swelling, hypertrophy, division, and the laying down of intermediate filaments in cell processes. The term astrocytosis means that astrocytes have increased in size and number in response to injury, whereas the term *astrogliosis* (somewhat synonymous with hypertrophy) implies synthesis of intermediate filaments and an increased length, complexity, and branching of the astrocytic processes. The recognition of these differences is based on histopathologic evaluation.

Swelling is an acute response and is reversible, or it may progress with time to hypertrophy. Swollen astrocytes have clear-staining or vacuolated cytoplasm. Astrocytes swell after ischemia because of the increased uptake of sodium, chloride, and potassium ions and water in an effort to maintain homeostasis in the extracellular microenvironment. It is important to remember that such swelling depends on the astrocyte being viable and still having a semipermeable plasma membrane, even though its function may be altered. With progression and if the degree and duration of ischemia are sufficiently severe to result in cell death, the plasma membrane becomes fully permeable, and the cell does not swell but becomes shriveled or shrunken and undergoes disintegration, as described for the ischemic cell change of neurons.

If injury is severe, astrocytic processes fragment and disappear followed by lysis of the cell body. Hypertrophied astrocytes, often referred to as *reactive,* represent a response to a milder and more protracted injury to the CNS. Because of increases in intermediate filaments, mainly GFAP, the cytoplasm becomes apparent along with increased length and branching of the processes with H&E staining. The increase of intermediate filaments and consequently the intensity of GFAP immunohistochemical staining in these cells are so dramatic that some have defined reactive astrocytes on the basis of this change. In protracted degenerative conditions, astrocytes termed *gemistocytes* can be observed (Fig. 14-20). These cells have eccentric nuclei and abundant pink homogeneous cytoplasm, in contrast to the lack of visible cytoplasm in normal astrocytes, with routine H&E staining. Animals with hepatic encephalopathy

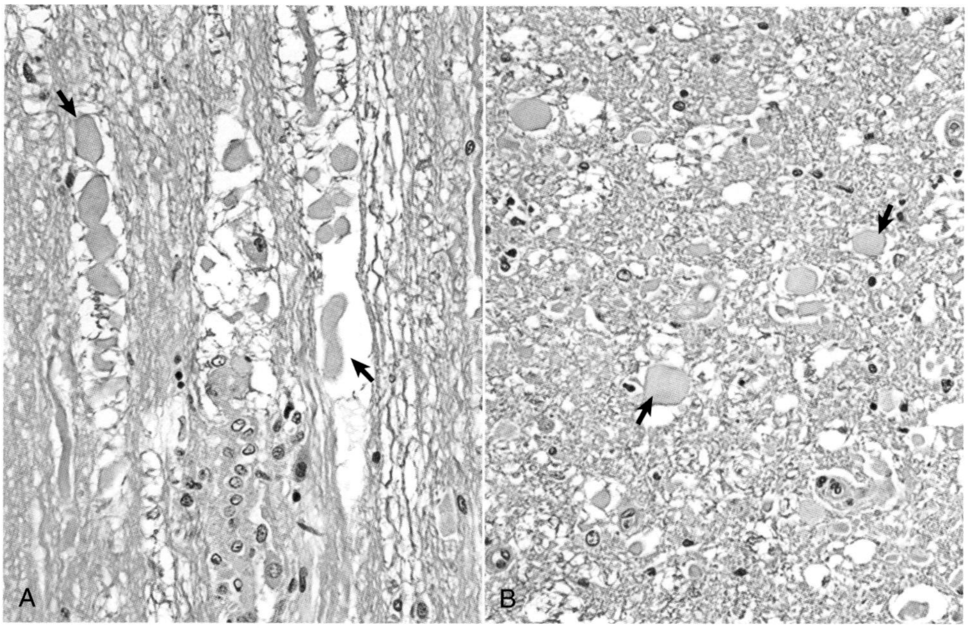

Fig. 14-19 Wallerian degeneration, transverse section of spinal cord, dog.
A, Longitudinal section. Arrows show swollen axons. H&E stain. **B,** Transverse section. H&E stain. Laceration and/or severe compression of myelinated nerves cause a specific sequence of structural and functional changes in the axon and the myelin (distal from the point of injury), referred to as Wallerian degeneration (see Web Fig. 14-3). Axons are initially swollen *(arrows)* and are eventually removed by phagocytosis to leave clear spaces, which were once the sites of nerve fibers. The cell bodies of affected neurons usually have central chromatolysis, but are metabolically active in an attempt to regenerate the lost portion of the axon (not shown; see Fig. 14-18). (Courtesy Dr. J.F. Zachary, College of Veterinary Medicine, University of Illinois.)

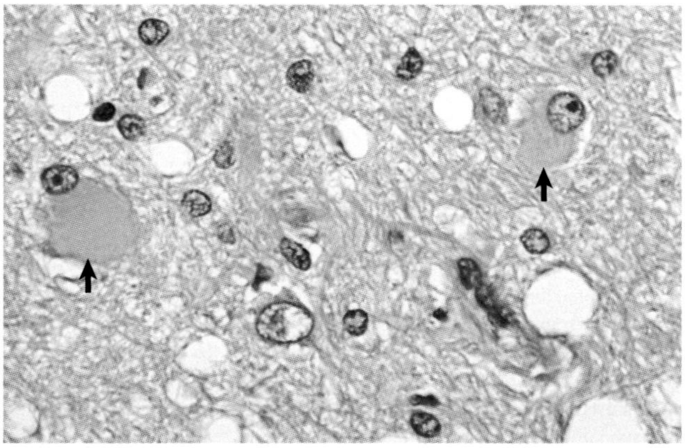

Fig. 14-20 Gemistocytes (gemistocytic astrocytes), cerebrum, dog. When astrocytes react to injury, initially by hypertrophy and later by the synthesis of increased glial filaments (astrogliosis), the nuclei enlarge and often the cell body, which is not normally visible in H&E stained sections, will become visible. These astrocytes are called gemistocytes (plump astrocytes) *(arrows)*. They occur in diseases in which there is alteration of intracellular and extracellular fluid balances or injury to the parenchyma, where healing will be by glial scarring (astrogliosis, e.g., to encapsulate a deep abscess or fill in a small area of dead space). H&E stain. (Courtesy Dr. J.F. Zachary, College of Veterinary Medicine, University of Illinois.)

can have a unique microscopic lesion in the brain affecting astrocytes of the cerebral cortices. Astrocytic nuclei tend to be in pairs occasionally with prominent central nucleoli and surrounded by a clear space, which is the edematous cytoplasm. They are called *Alzheimer's type II astrocytes* (see Fig. 14-10, *D*).

Astrocytic proliferation can occur in CNS injury, but in most instances, proliferative capacity is limited. When it occurs, the most dramatic examples are associated with attempts by reactive astrocytes (astrogliosis) to "wall off" abscesses and neoplasms or to fill in cavitated areas that result after lysis of necrotic neurons with the processes of astrocytes. This laying down of glial fibers is referred to as a *glial scar.* It is formed by a network of interlaced astrocytic processes and provides a loose barrier that separates the injured brain from the more normal adjacent tissue. This astroglia-fibroblast interface in injured CNS attempts to reform the glia limitans, restore the blood-brain barrier, and reestablish fluid and electrolyte balances.

Oligodendrocytes

Oligodendroglia react to injury by cell swelling, hypertrophy, and degeneration. Both perineuronal and interfascicular oligodendroglia can swell, hypertrophy, and degenerate; however, only oligodendroglia precursor cells can proliferate to replace degenerate cells. The role that perineuronal or satellite oligodendroglia play in normal neuronal function and neuronal injury has not been definitively clarified. Microscopically, these cells swell and hypertrophy around injured neurons; this response to injury has been called *satellitosis* (see Fig. 14-10, *B*).

Degeneration of interfascicular oligodendroglia caused by ischemia, certain viruses, lead toxicity, and autoimmunity can result in selective degeneration of myelin sheaths referred to as *primary demyelination.* Primary demyelination is the loss of myelin around an intact axon and results in the alteration of the conduction velocity of an action potential down the axon leading to clinical dysfunction (Fig. 14-21). Mechanisms of primary demyelination are summarized in Box 14-4. Protracted or repetitive injury to myelinating cells and their myelin sheaths can lead to irreversible neuronal atrophy. Oligodendroglia precursor cells located in the subventricular zone of the CNS can mature into interfascicular oligodendroglia and can also proliferate in response to

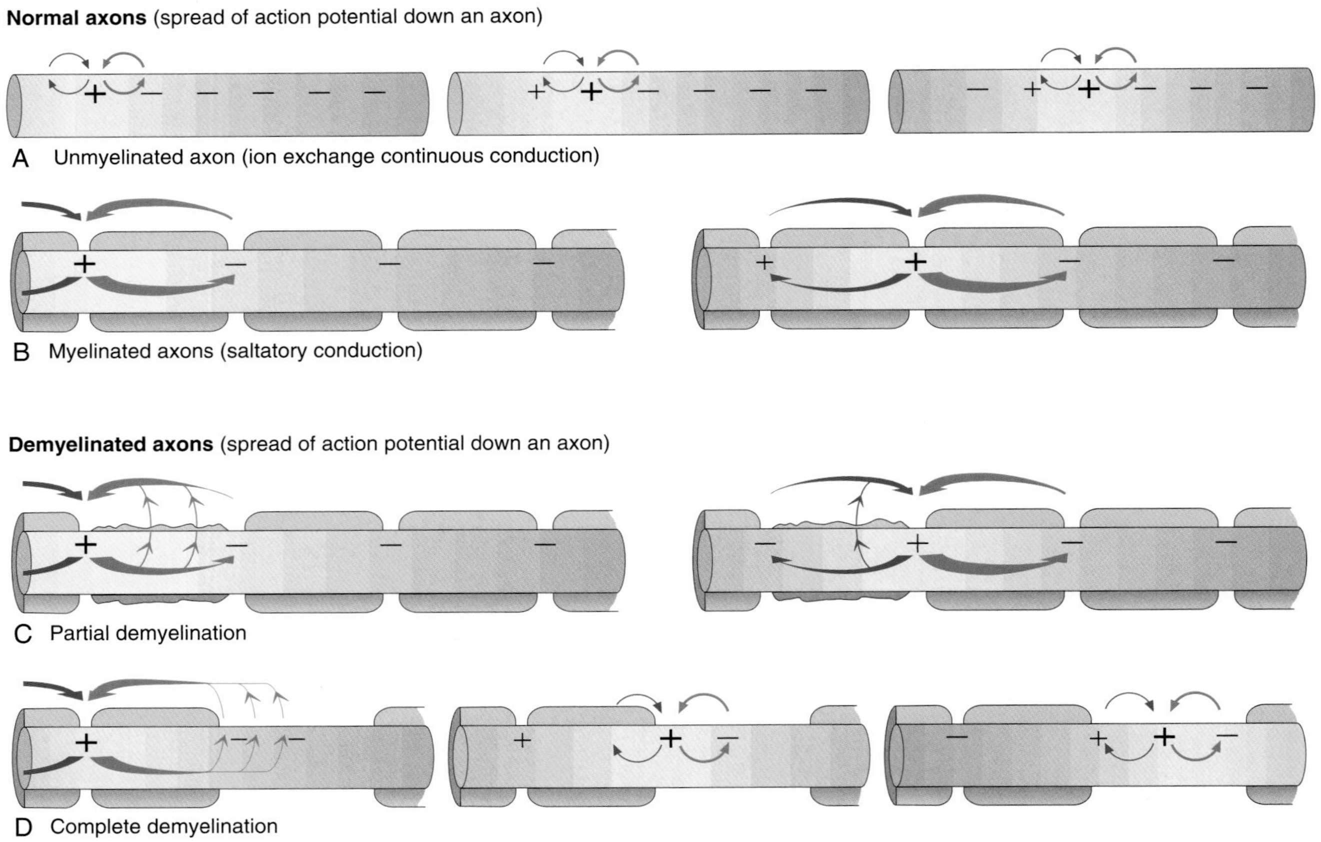

Fig. 14-21 Axonal action potential conduction and the effect of demyelination.
The speed of the conduction process is determined by the diameter of the axon and the degree of myelination. As axons increase in diameter, the resistance to ion flow decreases, allowing the action potential to flow faster. In addition, the degree of myelination is directly proportional to the diameter of the axon. Thus the concept that the more myelin the faster the speed of the impulse is true up to the point in which the myelin is normal in thickness. For an axon whose myelin is reduced, conduction of the action potential is slower. Under normal conditions, locomotion is a well-coordinated event that requires precise timing (speed) of impulse conduction to get coordinated movements. If the speed of the action potential is altered by disease, especially demyelination, then the conduction of the action potential will be delayed and what are normally coordinated movements become uncoordinated. **A,** In unmyelinated axons, action potentials are conducted at a relatively "slower" velocity by the process of ion exchange continuous conduction (Web Fig. 14-2). **B,** In myelinated axons, action potentials are conducted at a relatively "faster" velocity by a mechanism called saltatory conduction. Optimal function of saltatory conduction is dependent on having the proper degree of myelination of the axon (as determined by axonal diameter) throughout the full length of the axon. **C,** In axons that have lost some but not all of their myelin lamellae from one or more internodes so that there is a "thinner" covering of myelin, the speed of saltatory conduction is reduced because of leakage of the action potential across this thinner myelin sheath, resulting in clinical dysfunction of the nervous system. **D,** In axons that have lost all of their myelin from one or more internodes (complete primary demyelination of the internode), the speed of saltatory conduction is reduced because of the conversion from saltatory conduction to ion exchange continuous conduction in the areas where internodes have lost their myelin. Thus the speed and timing of the action potential is substantially reduced, leading to clinical dysfunction of the nervous system. (Courtesy Dr. J.F. Zachary, College of Veterinary Medicine, University of Illinois.)

noncytocidal injury and become involved in remyelination after primary demyelination.

CNS or PNS injury can also lead to loss of myelin secondary to injury of the axon and its cell body or to death of the neuron. When axons are injured, myelin lamellae forming the internodes are retracted and removed by phagocytosis. In some instances, oligodendroglia or Schwann cells, the myelin-forming cells in the PNS, also degenerate. This form of myelin degeneration is termed *secondary demyelination* and is secondary to axon degeneration or loss (resembles Wallerian degeneration).

Ependymal Cells

Ependymal and choroid plexus epithelial cell responses to injury include atrophy, degeneration, and necrosis. Atrophy usually occurs in response to enlargement of the ventricles as occurs with hydrocephalus. The cilia and microvilli of affected cells are reduced in number, and there is also a reduction in their cellular organelles such as endoplasmic reticulum and mitochondria. An additional lesion that accompanies ventricular enlargement is stretching and tearing of the ependymal lining. In such instances, the resulting areas of ependymal discontinuity result in the subependymal CNS

BOX 14-4 Mechanisms of Primary Demyelination

1. Inherited enzyme defects resulting in formation of abnormal myelin
   Leukodystrophies in man and animals
2. Impairment of myelin synthesis and maintenance
   Infection
   Mouse hepatitis virus in mice and progressive multifocal leukoencephalopathy in humans; in both cases oligodendrocytes are selectively destroyed by viral agents and myelin cannot be maintained.
   Nutritional
   Lack of maintenance of myelin is due to copper deficiency, malnutrition, vitamin B_{12} deficiency.
   Toxins
   Cyanide poisoning
   Cuprizone toxicity
3. Loss of myelin as a consequence of cytotoxic edema (status spongiosus)
   Hexachlorophene poisoning, usually prolonged edema
4. Destruction of myelin by detergent-like metabolites
   Lysolecithin, a metabolite of phospholipase A (normally present in the nervous system) may destroy myelin.
5. Immunologic destruction of myelin
   Cell mediated
   - Experimental allergic encephalitis (EAE)
   - Landry-Guillain-Barré (humans)
   - Coonhound paralysis
   - Marek's disease (chickens)
   - Various stages of multiple sclerosis in humans
   - Various stages of canine distemper

being directly exposed to the CSF. Unfortunately, mammalian ependymal cells do not regenerate and therefore do not repair the denuded areas. After 1 to 2 weeks, astrogliosis, which varies greatly in degree and uniformity, occurs in the exposed areas. Astrogliosis can extend into the ventricular space or be minimal in extent and confined to the periventricular area. Periventricular interstitial edema, myelin loss, and axon loss can ensue.

Inflammation of the ependyma, called *ependymitis,* can also occur, with infection being the most common cause. Microbes most commonly gain entrance to the ependyma via the circulation by lodging in the choroid plexuses, by direct contamination from a rupture of a cerebral abscess into the ventricular system, and by retrograde reflux through the lateral apertures of infected CSF from the subarachnoid space in cases of leptomeningitis. In the case of bacterial infection, the suppurative exudate that forms in the CSF can cause obstructive hydrocephalus, although the development of hydrocephalus cannot always be explained on the basis of obstruction.

Microglia

Microglia are often the first cells in the CNS to react to injury, and the magnitude of the response is graded to correlate with the severity of damage. The responses of microglia to injury include hypertrophy, hyperplasia, phagocytosis of cellular and myelin debris, and neuronophagia, which is the removal of dead neuron cell bodies. After injury, microglia progress through a stage of activation, becoming fully immunocompetent reactive cells. These reactive cells readily proliferate, either focally, forming glial nodules (Fig. 14-22), or more diffusely, depending on the nature of the injury.

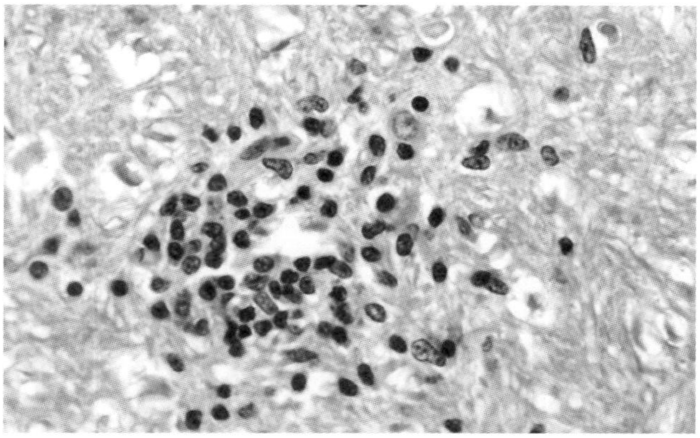

Fig. 14-22 Glial nodule, brainstem, dog.
These nodules *(center of figure),* formed by reactive microglial cells and macrophages, occur most frequently in viral encephalitides. H&E stain. (Courtesy Dr. M.D. McGavin, College of Veterinary Medicine, University of Tennessee.)

As mentioned, in concert with astrocytes and neurons, microglia help coordinate inflammatory events in the CNS. Resident microglia and blood-derived macrophages express MHC class I and II antigens, serve as antigen-presenting cells, and possess a broad armament of adhesion molecules, cytokines, and chemokines. Once activated, these cells can also produce nitric oxide, reactive oxygen intermediates, and other chemical mediators of inflammation that can damage the CNS if not under strict control. When tissue necrosis occurs, macrophages derived from blood monocytes phagocytose the lipid-laden debris of dead neurons and glia, and they become foamy macrophages termed *gitter cells* (Fig. 14-23) and accumulate in the damaged CNS.

Meninges

Pathologic processes that initially involve the meninges, most commonly the leptomeninges, can secondarily invade the CNS because of the close apposition between the two tissues. Conversely, processes that primarily affect the CNS can secondarily affect the meninges, most commonly the leptomeninges.

Meningitis refers to inflammation of the meninges. In common usage, the term generally refers to inflammation of the leptomeninges in contrast to inflammation of the dura mater, which is referred to as *pachymeningitis.* Leptomeningitis can be acute, subacute, or chronic and depending on the cause, suppurative, nonsuppurative, or granulomatous, and the exudate and inflammatory cells are chiefly in the subarachnoid space. Besides retrograde axonal transport, as occurs with, for example, *Listeria monocytogenes,* infectious agents spread to the meninges hematogenously by direct extension or by leukocytic trafficking.

Other meningeal lesions include (1) inflammation of the external periosteal dura after osteomyelitis, formation of extradural abscesses, and skull fracture and involve the inner dura as an extension of leptomeningitis and (2) proliferation of the inner dural mesothelial cells, arachnoid cells, fibroblasts, and cells of the pia mater in response to irritation. Additional lesions likely related to aging or degeneration include formation of cellular nests of mesothelial-like cells on the outer surface of the arachnoid membrane, mineralization of the arachnoid membrane in humans, and mineralization plus ossification of the dura mater of the spinal cord in both humans and dogs. Dural ossification in the dog, which tends to affect the ventral, cervical, and lumbar dura mater, is most commonly encountered in large breeds, although smaller breeds

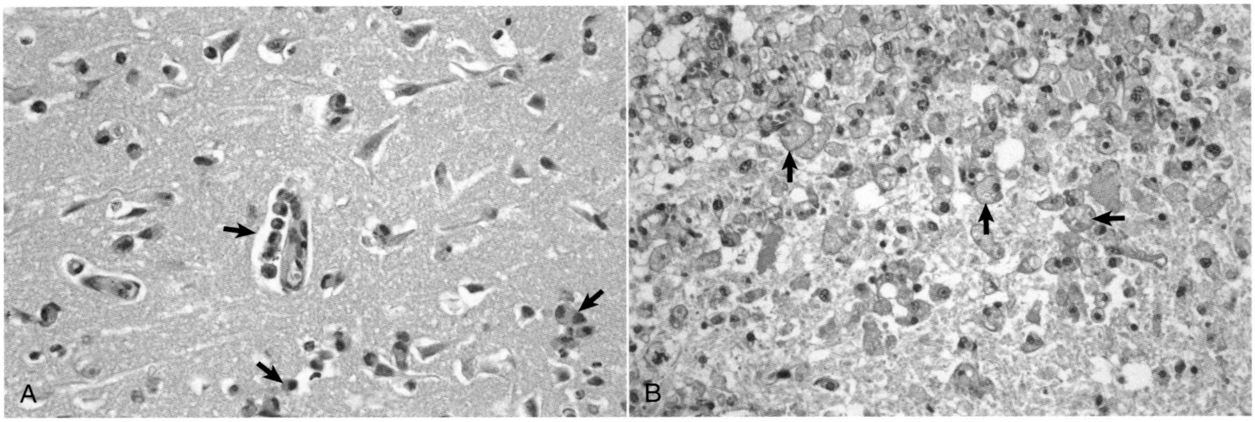

Fig. 14-23 Gitter cells, cerebrum.
A, Early polioencephalomalacia, cow. Note the angular, eosinophilic neurons with pyknotic nuclei (ischemic cell change). Monocytes *(arrows)* in the perivascular space have been recruited from the vasculature. These cells will become macrophages and phagocytose cellular debris from the necrotic neurons and the myelin from the nerve fibers undergoing degeneration after the death of their neurons. Microglia also participate in this phagocytic response. Macrophages, which have ingested degenerate myelin or other cellular debris, have foamy cytoplasm and are termed gitter cells. H&E stain. **B,** Old necrotic area, dog. The normal brain parenchyma has liquefied and the debris has been ingested by macrophages *(arrows)*, which has resulted in the cytoplasm of these cells becoming foamy. They are now designated as gitter cells or, simply, foamy macrophages. (Courtesy Dr. J.F. Zachary, College of Veterinary Medicine, University of Illinois.)

can be affected. The clinical significance of this lesion has been debated but not decided.

Circulatory System

Endothelial Cell (and Blood Vessel) Responses to Injury

Because many of the infectious and neoplastic disease processes demonstrated in this book are spread through the body via the circulatory system, endothelial cells lining blood vessels, especially capillaries, are subject to a variety of injuries. Bacterial hematogenous CNS diseases occur at the interface between the white and gray matter in the cerebral hemispheres. This phenomenon is thought to result from abrupt changes in vascular flow or luminal diameter of vessels at the interface. These changes may make endothelial cells more susceptible to injury, vasculitis, and thrombosis or predispose the vessels to entrapment of tumor or bacterial emboli.

Endothelial injury can be reversible or nonreversible, resulting in necrosis. Injury resulting in endothelial dysfunction can include the activation and release of vasoactive mediators, such as histamine, leading to local and/or systemic changes in vascular flow, pressure, and permeability. Bacterial products and elicited inflammatory cytokines can directly or indirectly cause vascular inflammation (vasculitis) leading to thrombosis and disseminated intravascular coagulation. Thrombotic meningoencephalitis of cattle caused by the bacterium *Histophilus somni* (formerly *Haemophilus somnus*) is an example of this type of injury (see Fig. 14-89). Certain herpesviruses and protozoa can also infect endothelial cells and cause endothelial necrosis with vasculitis, hemorrhage, and thrombosis. Finally, some pathogens, such as angioinvasive *Mucor* spp., directly invade blood vessels, resulting in necrosis of the endothelium. Vasculitis resulting in thrombosis can cause tissue ischemia, infarction, and vasogenic edema of the affected area of the CNS. A review of endothelial injury can be found in Chapter 2.

Infarction

Infarction means necrosis of a tissue after obstruction (ischemia) of its arterial blood supply. The rate at which ischemia occurs in the CNS determines the degree of injury that follows. The more rapid the onset of ischemia, the more severe the lesion. However,

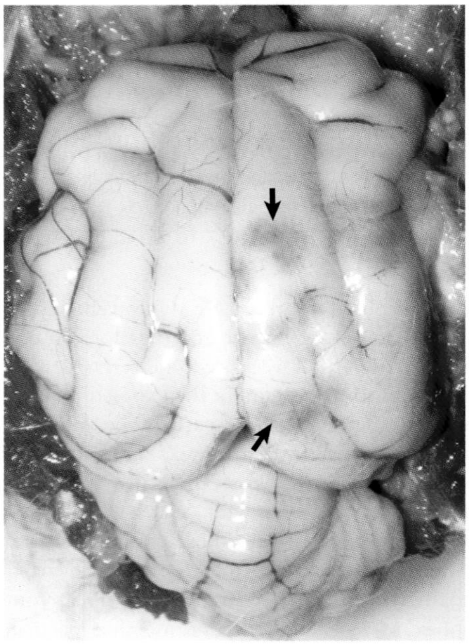

Fig. 14-24 Malacia, vascular occlusion, ischemia, infarction, cerebrum, cat.
Several red-pink foci *(arrows)* are areas of ischemic necrosis secondary to vascular occlusion caused by cerebral metastasis of a bronchoalveolar carcinoma. (Courtesy Drs. C.A. Lichtensteiger and R.A. Doty, College of Veterinary Medicine, University of Illinois.)

if the obstruction is sudden, as caused by an embolus formed as an example by tumor cells, many of the neurons can die within minutes and other components within hours (Fig. 14-24). This outcome also applies to compressive injuries to the CNS that produce a sudden reduction in blood flow, such as can happen with sudden compression in rapidly occurring Hansen type I disk herniation in the dog. If the blood flow through an artery is gradually reduced, for example, because of arteriosclerosis, there is often sufficient time for anastomotic vessels to dilate and compensate.

TABLE 14-1 Chronologic Sequence of Changes within Infarcted Tissue (in the Living Animal) after an Ischemic Event

Time Following Ischemic Event	Tissue Change
Immediate (seconds)	Cessation of blood flow (ischemia) and accumulation of waste products
Few minutes	Cellular injury and death; coagulation necrosis and edema; hemorrhage (especially in gray matter)
20 minutes	First microscopic evidence of neuronal injury (perfusion-fixation)
1-2 hours	First microscopic evidence of neuronal injury (immersion fixation)
2 hours	Pale staining of infarct microscopically (white matter); swelling of capillary endothelium; increase in size of astrocytic nuclei
3-5 hours	Ischemic cell change in most neurons; swelling of oligodendroglia and astroglia; beginning clasmatodendrosis of astrocytes
6-24 hours	Beginning neutrophilic infiltration; alteration of myelin (pale staining), 8-24 hours; degeneration and decrease of oligodendroglia, 8-24 hours; astrocytic swelling and retraction and fragmentation of processes (clasmatodendrosis), and degeneration*; cytoplasm of astrocytes visible, 8-24 hours*; vascular degeneration and fibrin deposition, 8-24 hours; thrombosis,† 6-24 hours; beginning endothelial proliferation at margin of infarct, 9 hours
8-24 (up to 48) hours	Initial gross detection of infarct unless hemorrhagic; infarct edematous (swollen), soft, pale, or hemorrhagic and demarcated
1-2 days	Swelling of axons and myelin sheaths; prominent neutrophilic infiltration
2 days	Prominent loss of neuroectodermal cells; continued proliferation of endothelial cells; reduced number of neutrophils; beginning increase in mononuclear cells (gitter cells)
3-5 days	Prominent number of mononuclear cells (gitter cells); disappearance of neutrophils; continued endothelial cell proliferation; number of capillaries appear increased; beginning of astrocytic proliferation (often at margin of infarct)
5-7 days	Grossly, swelling of infarct reaches maximum
8-10 days	Reduction in gross swelling of infarct; liquefaction necrosis; prominent number of mononuclear cells (gitter cells); continued endothelial cell proliferation; beginning fibroblastic activity with collagen formation, variable but most prominent in CNS tissue adjacent to the meninges; beginning increase of astroglial fiber production, 5-13 days
3 weeks-6 months	Mononuclear cells decreased; astroglial fiber density increased (especially at margin); astrocytic proliferation reduced; astrocytes return to original appearance; cystic stage of infarct, 2-4 months; vascular network may be present within cyst; endothelial cell proliferation reduced

*The degree of astrocytic injury depends on location (e.g., central or peripheral) of the cells within the infarct.

†Obviously, thrombosis may occur earlier than 6 hours. This is the time when it may initially be prominent.

Anastomoses of the arteries that penetrate from the ventral and cortical surfaces of the brain are insufficient to prevent infarction after sudden occlusion of one or more of these arteries. If the compression is slow—such as is caused by a slowly developing Hansen type II disk herniation in a dog or by a slowly growing neoplasm from the exterior, such as meningioma in a cat—adjacent neural tissue will atrophy to accommodate the mass.

Cerebral necrosis, comparable to infarction after vascular occlusion, can also result from other causes, including cessation of cerebral circulation caused by cardiac arrest, sudden hypotension caused by reduced cardiac output, and reduced or absent oxygen in inspired air. Additional causes include altered function of hemoglobin as a result of carbon monoxide poisoning, inhibition of tissue respiration after cyanide poisoning, ingesting toxic substances and poisons, and nutritional deficiencies.

When an artery supplying the CNS is suddenly occluded, blood supply to cells at the center of the infarcted area is rapidly stopped, and if maintained for a sufficient period, all cells die. Neurons at the border of this area continue to receive some blood from unobstructed vessels. It is proposed that the axonal terminals of degenerated ischemic neurons in the center of the infarct release excessive amounts of the neurotransmitter glutamate, causing injury to still-viable neurons in the borders, which increases the extent of the infarct. This process begins after the binding of the neurotransmitter glutamate to receptors on viable neurons in the borders, inducing an abnormal movement of calcium ions into the recipient cells followed by an increase in intracellular calcium ion concentration. This buildup of calcium ions contributes to a multifunctional cascade that leads to neuronal death. When there is hemorrhage with the infarct, the mechanical injury from the pressure, plus tissue displacement by the hemorrhage, can cause additional damage. See Table 14-1 for the reparative responses associated with the resolution of infarcts.

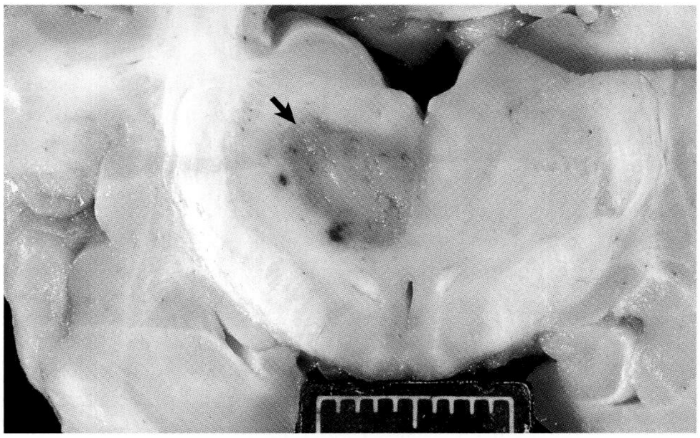

Fig. 14-25 CNS infarct, brain, thalamus, dog.
A focal, sharply demarcated area of yellow discoloration and malacia (softening) *(arrow)* in the left central thalamus is most likely an infarct. Scale bar = 2 cm. (Courtesy Dr. R. Storts, College of Veterinary Medicine, Texas A&M University.)

Although they occur through the same mechanisms, areas of cerebral infarction differ somewhat in gross appearance from infarcts in other tissues (Fig. 14-25). The abundance of lipids and enzymes, plus the relative lack of fibrous connective tissue stroma in the brain and spinal cord, results in the affected areas eventually becoming soft because of liquefaction necrosis. The gross

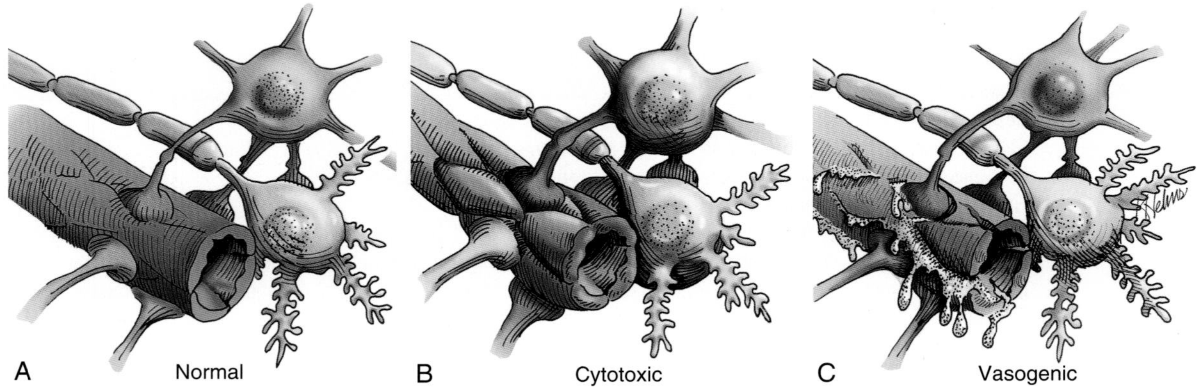

Fig. 14-26 Types of cerebral edema.
A, Normal blood-brain barrier. Endothelial cells are red; astrocytes are beige; neurons are light yellow. **B,** Cytotoxic edema. Cytotoxic edema is characterized by the accumulation of fluid intracellularly (in neurons, astrocytes, oligodendroglia, and endothelial cells) as a result of altered cellular metabolism, often caused by ischemia. The gray and white matter are both affected. The fluid taken up by swollen cells is primarily derived from the extracellular space, which becomes reduced in size and has an increased concentration of extracellular solutes. **C,** Vasogenic edema. This type of edema is seen in acute inflammation, and its basic mechanism is an increase in vascular permeability from the breakdown of the blood-brain barrier. This breakdown allows movement of plasma constituents such as water, ions, and plasma proteins into the extracellular space, particularly that of the white matter. (Courtesy Dr. J.F. Zachary, College of Veterinary Medicine, University of Illinois. Based on an illustration from Leech RW, Shuman RM: *Neuropathology: a summary for students,* Philadelphia, 1982, Harper & Row.)

appearance of infarction may also differ according to location. Lesions affecting the gray matter tend to be hemorrhagic, whereas infarction of the white matter is often pale. This difference is probably due in part to the less-dense capillary meshwork in the white matter and in part to the fact that the vessels supplying the white matter have fewer anastomoses than those of the gray matter. Infarcted tissue goes through a characteristic sequence of changes that can permit a relatively accurate determination of the age of the infarct. An outline of the chronologic events that occur after an ischemic episode that lasts more than 5 to 6 minutes and is followed by resuscitation of an animal is given in Table 14-1. As can be seen, the tissue changes listed in Table 14-1 take different periods of time to develop in the living resuscitated animal after ischemia occurs. Variation in the times that specific lesions occur depends on the extent and duration of the initial ischemic event. Following removal of cellular and myelin debris, the infarct is repaired by astrocytes. If the infarct is small (<1 mm), it is filled via astrogliosis; if the infarct is larger, it is encapsulated to form a cyst.

CNS Swelling and Edema

Congestive Brain Swelling

Congestive brain swelling, as distinguished from cerebral edema, is thought to represent, at least in part, an unregulated vasodilation after trauma, and it can cause serious brain damage (even more severe than the primary injury) if not properly controlled. This lesion therefore represents an enlargement of the brain resulting in elevated intracranial pressure caused by the increased diameter of the blood-containing vasculature, whereas edema results in an increased pressure following accumulation of fluid in the interstitium or intracellularly outside the circulation. Acute brain swelling can be localized (usually of lesser significance) when associated with focal lesions or generalized (often serious) when caused by diffuse brain injury. Although rarely seen in domestic animals, one exception to the importance of focal lesions is extracerebral hemorrhage (acute subdural hematoma in humans), which—though principally involving the surface of one hemisphere—can cause more mass effect (brain swelling) in the underlying cerebral hemisphere than the hematoma itself. In such circumstances (acute subdural hematoma), the small amount of blood in the subarachnoid space is not the sole reason for the patient's neurologic state. If the hematoma is removed, the acute brain swelling can progress so rapidly that the brain protrudes (herniates) through the craniotomy site.

The more serious forms of diffuse brain injury are associated with generalized acute brain swelling. It is sometimes difficult to determine the relative importance of swelling in affected individuals because initial acute swelling (detectable as soon as 30 minutes after injury in humans) can be followed after several hours to days by true cerebral edema (as a result of increased vascular permeability), which can be the actual deleterious lesion. Peroxidative injury to blood vessels has been one proposed cause of pathologic vasodilation in the posttraumatic CNS.

Cerebral Edema

The basis of our current understanding of cerebral edema was advanced by Klatzo in 1967 when he proposed two distinct types: (1) cytotoxic edema, or cell swelling, caused by increased intracellular fluid with normal vascular permeability and (2) vasogenic edema, or tissue swelling, caused by increased extracellular fluid resulting from increased vascular permeability (Fig. 14-26). Other types of cerebral edema have been identified as hydrostatic (or interstitial) edema associated with increased hydrostatic pressure of the CSF (resulting from obstructive internal hydrocephalus) and hypo-osmotic edema, which is dependent on development of an abnormal osmotic gradient between the blood and nervous tissue. The types of edema in the CNS are summarized in Table 14-2. It should be emphasized that, depending on the nature of the injury, multiple mechanisms can contribute to edema in the CNS and these distinctions are not always clearly defined or distinct. For continuity, spongiform change and status spongiosus will also be discussed in this section.

Vasogenic Edema

In animals, vasogenic edema is the most common type of edema in the CNS. It occurs following vascular injury often adjacent to inflammatory foci, hematomas, contusions, infarcts, cerebral hypertension, and neoplasms. The underlying mechanism of vasogenic cerebral edema is a breakdown of the blood-brain barrier that results in movement of plasma constituents, such as water, ions, and organic osmolytes, and proteins into the perivascular extracellular space, particularly that of the white matter (Fig. 14-27). In addition to extracellular accumulation of fluid, vasogenic edema can also be accompanied by some cellular swelling involving astrocytes. Vasogenic edema with the resulting accumulation of extracellular fluid can cause an increase in intracranial pressure within the CNS. This pressure can also be so severe as to cause neurologic dysfunction and caudal displacement of brain structures such as the parahippocampal gyri and cerebellar vermis (see Figs. 14-59 and 14-60).

Cytotoxic Edema

Cytotoxic edema is characterized by the accumulation of fluid intracellularly in neurons, astrocytes, oligodendroglia, and endothelial cells (called *hydropic degeneration* in other cells of the body) as a result of altered cellular metabolism, often caused by ischemia. Although not all of the cells listed previously may be involved in all cases of cytotoxic edema, affected cells swell within seconds of injury. The mechanism is thought to involve an energy deficit that interferes with normal function of the cell's Na^+/K^+-ATPase pump. Thus the cell cannot maintain homeostasis, which requires the secretion of intracellular sodium, and the elevated concentration of intracellular sodium and presumably other ions, as well as organic osmolytes, are followed by an increased influx of water. The gray and white matter of the brain are both affected, the brain swells, and the sulci and gyri become indistinct and flattened (Fig. 14-28), respectively. The fluid taken up by the swollen cells is primarily derived from the extracellular space, which becomes reduced in size and has an increased concentration of extracellular solutes.

However, for this lesion to be described accurately as cerebral edema, there must be additional fluid movement into the brain and not merely a change of existing fluid from extracellular to intracellular compartments. In practical terms, this is not always the case and can be difficult to determine. The term *cytotoxic edema* has been used rather loosely to refer simply to cellular swelling in many cases. Additional fluid may originate from the circulation by way of the transcapillary fluid exchange or possibly from the CSF, which has extensive diffusional communication with the extracellular fluid of the brain. The blood-brain barrier remains intact during development of this type of edema, so fluid does not enter the brain by a disturbance in vascular permeability. Specific causes of this lesion include hypoxia-ischemia, particularly in the early stages; intoxication with metabolic inhibitors, such as 2,4,dinitrophenol, 6-aminonicotinamide, and ouabain; and severe hypothermia.

TABLE 14-2 Types of Edema in the CNS

Type of Edema	Cause	Outcome
Cytotoxic	Altered cellular metabolism (often due to ischemia)	Intracellular accumulation of fluid (neurons, glial cells, endothelial cells)
Vasogenic	Vascular injury with breakdown of the blood-brain barrier	Extracellular accumulation of fluid (cerebrocortical white matter)
Hydrostatic (interstitial)	Elevated ventricular hydrostatic pressure (hydrocephalus)	Extracellular accumulation of fluid (periventricular white matter)
Hypo-osmotic	Osmotic imbalances (blood plasma versus extracellular and intracellular microenvironments of the CNS)	Extracellular and intracellular accumulation of fluid (cerebrocortical gray and white matter)

Interstitial (Hydrostatic) Edema

Interstitial edema is characterized by the accumulation of fluid in the extracellular space of the brain because of elevated ventricular hydrostatic pressure that accompanies hydrocephalus. Fluid moves across the ependyma of the ventricular wall and accumulates extracellularly in the periventricular white matter. Unlike the other forms of cerebral edema that cause swelling of affected CNS tissue, hydrostatic edema causes variable degeneration and loss of the periventricular white matter mostly through primary demyelination

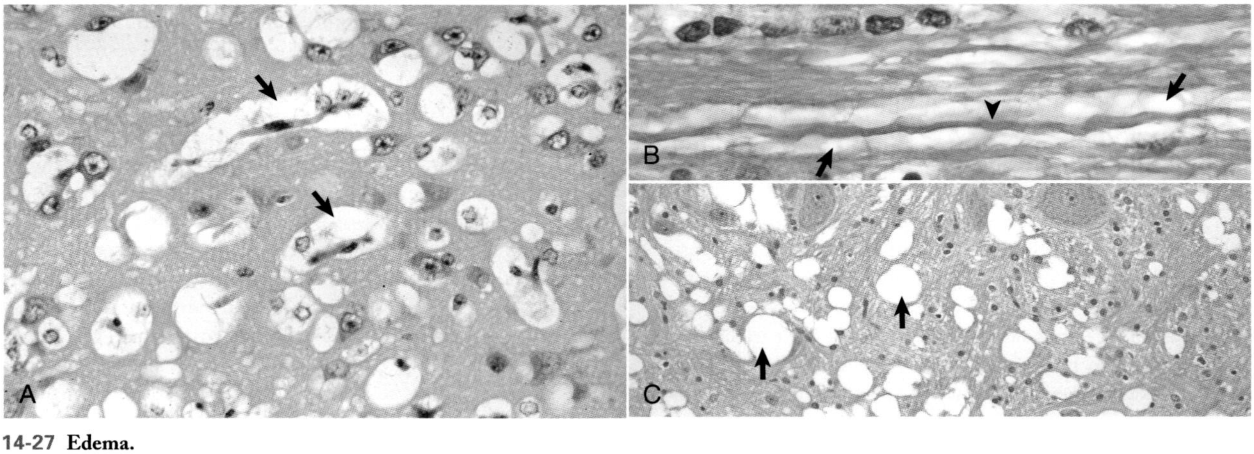

Fig. 14-27 Edema.
A, Vasogenic edema. The perivascular spaces are wide as a result of fluid leakage through the blood-brain barrier *(arrows)* (see Fig. 14-26). A similar change can be seen around neurons. These fluid-filled spaces are often very difficult to differentiate from artifactual spaces caused by shrinkage from fixation and dehydration in the preparation of the paraffin-embedded sections. H&E stain. **B,** Intramyelinic edema. Note the accumulation of edema fluid *(arrows)* between myelin lamellae that surrounds the axon *(arrowhead).* This lesion was caused by hexachlorophene added to a medicated shampoo. Such products are no longer available for use in veterinary practice. H&E stain. **C,** Edema (spongy change, status spongiosus), hepatic encephalopathy, dog. This lesion is characterized by variably sized fluid-filled spaces within the white matter *(arrows).* It can develop by several different mechanisms, which include splitting of myelin sheaths, accumulation of extracellular fluid, and swelling of astrocytic and neuronal cellular processes. Such changes can reflect osmotic imbalances as well as a direct toxic effect on cells (cytotoxic edema). H&E stain. (**A** and **C** courtesy Dr. J.F. Zachary, College of Veterinary Medicine, University of Illinois. **B** courtesy Dr. M.D. McGavin, College of Veterinary Medicine, University of Tennessee.)

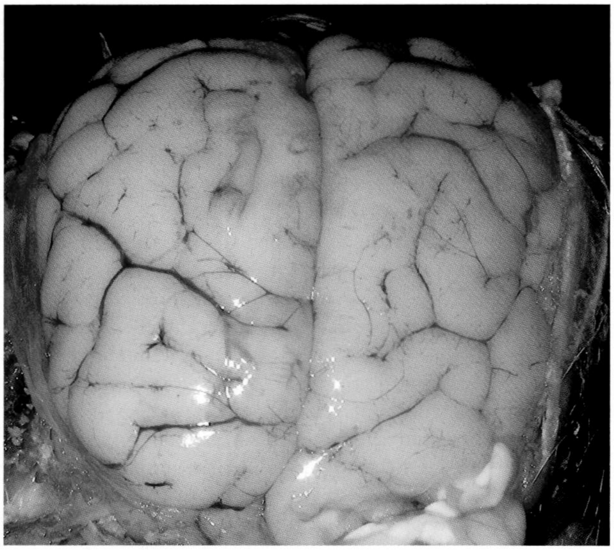

Fig. 14-28 Cerebral edema, dog.
On the dorsal surface, gyri are swollen and flattened and sulci have become less distinct. Accumulation of extracellular fluid has caused the brain to swell, and because space within the cranial vault is limited, the brain has been pressed against the calvarium. In extreme cases, notable brain swelling can cause caudal displacement of the vermis of the cerebellum and the parahippocampal gyri (see Figs. 14-59 and 14-60). (Courtesy Drs. C.A. Lichtensteiger and A. Gal, College of Veterinary Medicine, University of Illinois.)

accompanied by loss of axons. As the periventricular white matter is reduced in volume, the ventricle expands to fill the void by displacement, thereby exacerbating the hydrocephalus. The blood-brain barrier remains intact in hydrostatic edema.

Hypo-Osmotic Edema

Hypo-osmotic edema occurs after overconsumption of water (water intoxication), leading to dilution of the osmolality of the plasma. Under normal conditions the osmolality of CSF and extracellular fluid in the CNS is slightly greater than that of plasma. When the osmolality of plasma is further decreased, water moves from the vasculature into the brain after the osmotic gradient, resulting in osmotic edema. This form of edema accounts for the clinical signs and lesions in osmotic demyelination syndrome and salt poisoning, as discussed later.

Spongiform Change and Status Spongiosus

Spongiform change is a term whose exact meaning varies in different scientific disciplines and experimental situations. In this chapter, wherever possible, spongiform change is used to describe morphologic changes in H&E stained sections that occur primarily in gray matter. These changes are characterized by small clear vacuoles of varied sizes that form in the cytoplasm of neuron cell bodies and proximal dendrites in diseases such as the transmissible spongiform encephalopathies (TSEs) and rabies encephalitis and in the processes of astrocytes that are spatially related to the affected neurons.

Status spongiosus (spongy degeneration) is also a phrase whose exact meaning varies. It is defined as multiple fluid-filled clear spaces in the white matter of H&E stained sections of the CNS and may be extracellular or intracellular (see Fig. 14-27, *C*). This lesion results from the accumulation of edema fluid in the white matter secondary to a variety of causes, including cytotoxic edema, vasogenic edema, intramyelinic edema, Wallerian degeneration, and other hypoxic, toxic, and metabolic diseases.

In some instances, the term *spongy degeneration* or *spongy change* has been used in the veterinary literature to describe microscopic lesions in a group of diseases of young dogs, cats, and cows characterized by fluid accumulation in white matter. These diseases are discussed in later sections.

DEFENSE MECHANISMS

Barrier Systems

The CNS has several unique structural and functional barrier systems that serve to protect it from diseases affecting the vascular and ventricular systems and to actively facilitate transfer of necessary molecules, such as glucose, to cells within the CNS.

Blood-Brain Barrier

The blood-brain barrier, formed by vascular endothelial cells, endothelial-derived basement membrane, and foot processes of astrocytes, exists in the capillaries of the CNS (see Fig. 14-13). The most important structural component of the blood-brain barrier is the tight junctions between endothelial cells of cerebral capillaries. By means of the blood-brain barrier, the CNS can selectively regulate its extracellular compartment and isolate itself from sudden biochemical changes that may occur in the systemic circulation. In the majority of the CNS, endothelial cells are nonfenestrated and are held together by intercellular tight junctions. These tight junctions actively prevent the movement of protein, hydrophilic molecules, and ions from capillary lumina into the intercellular compartment of the CNS. Endothelial cells also have a transmembrane lipophilic pathway for the diffusion of small lipid molecules and numerous highly selective polarized receptor-mediated transport systems for molecules such as insulin, transferrin, glucose, purines, and amino acids. Finally, endothelial cells express a net negative charge on their abluminal side and at the basement membrane, providing an additional selective mechanism that impedes movement of anionic molecules such as chloride ions across the barrier. Foot processes of astrocytes cover more than 90% percent of the abluminal surface of capillary endothelial cells. Experimental evidence suggests that secretion of growth factors from astrocytes promotes the formation and maintenance of the blood-brain barrier.

Capillaries in the area postrema, median eminence, neurohypophysis, pineal body, subfornical organ, commissural organ, and supraoptic crest lack tight junctions and are fenestrated; thus the blood-brain barrier is absent at these sites.

Glia Limitans

The CNS is separated from the subarachnoid CSF by the pia mater and the glia limitans (see Fig. 14-13). The glia limitans, which covers the outer surface of the brain and spinal cord and is situated immediately subjacent to the pia mater, consists of astrocytic fibers with many foot processes that form a distinct layer that lies subjacent to the pia mater. In many areas the pia is only one-cell-layer thick and has fenestrations, so that the glia limitans is exposed directly to the subarachnoid space. As arterioles penetrate the cerebral cortex to supply the CNS with blood, they carry the pia mater and surrounding glia limitans with them until the arteriole structurally and functionally becomes a capillary. At the capillary level, the pia mater disappears, but the layer of pericapillary astrocytic foot processes remains and serves as a component of the blood-brain barrier. This transition zone occurs at a depth approximately 1 to 3 mm within the cerebral cortex.

Blood–Cerebrospinal Fluid Barrier

The blood-CSF barrier is formed by the choroid plexus and the arachnoid. This barrier is formed by tight junctions between apposing surfaces of choroid plexus epithelial cells that cover the choroid plexuses. As noted previously, blood vessels of the choroid plexus are fenestrated. The barrier formed by tight junctions between choroid plexus epithelial cells restricts the movement of molecules that leak from fenestrated capillaries into the extracellular compartment of the choroid plexus and then into the CSF. Similarly, the arachnoid membrane also has tight junctions that prevent the movement of molecules from the blood into the CSF. The arachnoid membrane is generally impermeable to hydrophilic molecules but lacks specialized transport systems, and its role in forming the blood-CSF barrier is largely passive.

Cerebrospinal Fluid–Brain Barrier (Ependymal Barrier)

The CNS is separated from ventricular CSF by ependymal epithelial cells and foot processes of astrocytes. Although the ependymal lining does form a cellular barrier of sorts, materials within the ventricular system can without too much difficulty penetrate into the brain. The CSF-brain barrier is far more permeable than the blood-brain barrier.

Innate and Adaptive Immune Responses

Although infectious agents have developed unique approaches to gain entry into the CNS, the body has also evolved a strong suite of defense mechanisms to protect the CNS against infectious pathogens and disease processes. The skin and mucous membranes of the alimentary, respiratory, and urinary systems provide structural and functional barriers against disease. The inflammatory response, immune system, and monocyte-macrophage system provide a strong local and systemic defense against pathogen replication and disease spread. Finally, barrier systems in the CNS, reviewed in an earlier section, represent structural and functional protection against a wide range of pathogens and toxic injuries. These defense mechanisms are summarized in Box 14-5.

BOX 14-5 Defense Mechanisms against Injury and Infectious Agents in the CNS

SKIN
Structural and functional (secretions) barrier

CALVARIUM, VERTEBRAE
Structural barrier

MENINGES, CEREBROSPINAL FLUID
Structural and functional (continuous flow of cerebrospinal fluid [CSF]) barrier

BARRIER SYSTEMS

Blood-Brain Barrier
Structural and functional barrier formed by vascular endothelium, basement membrane, and astrocytic foot processes. This barrier regulates the movement of agents from the blood to the CNS.

Blood-CSF Barrier
Structural and functional barrier formed by choroid plexuses cells and the arachnoid membrane. This barrier regulates movement of agents from the blood to the CSF.

Glia Limitans
Formed by astrocytic foot processes immediately subjacent to the pia mater. This structure may have some barrier function in preventing movement of microbes from CSF into the CNS through the pia mater.

MICROGLIA, TRAFFICKING MACROPHAGES
Resident and migrating cells that are part of the monocyte-macrophage system.

IMMUNOLOGIC RESPONSES
Innate and adaptive immunologic responses that form the body's overall immune system.

Inflammation of the CNS

Inflammation of the CNS is different from inflammation in other organs because of the presence of the blood-brain barrier. Under normal conditions, this barrier provides limited isolation of the CNS from circulating cellular and humoral elements of the immune system. Macrophages (monocytes) and T lymphocytes can penetrate an intact blood-brain barrier and enter the perivascular and subarachnoid spaces, transit these spaces, and return to the circulation in a role of protective immunologic surveillance of the CNS.

It is important to remember that inflammation in the CNS is regulated by a complex system of recognition and adhesion molecules, cytokines, chemokines, and their corresponding receptors (see Chapters 3 and 5). In particular within the CNS, chemokines and their receptors regulate physiologic and pathologic leukocyte trafficking and cellular migration events.

When pathogens use one of the four portals of entry to gain access to the CNS, the inflammatory process that ensues disrupts the blood-brain barrier. Thus, in addition to inflammation, edema and hemorrhage can result. Selectins and integrins in cooperation with chemokines are active in initiating and regulating the acute inflammatory response and the movement of neutrophils across the blood-brain barrier in response to a variety of pathogens. Migration of inflammatory cells within the CNS is poorly understood. Chemotactic gradients are likely established by chemokines that diffuse from sites of production within foci of inflammation. Activated glial cells, including astrocytes and resident microglia, form chemokine networks in areas of inflammation in response to cytokines produced by T lymphocytes that recognize foreign antigens.

Depending on the type of antigen and the pathogenicity of the infectious agent, the inflammatory response resolves (heals) or progresses to a chronic or granulomatous phase with attempts at resolution and clearance of the infectious agent. In the CNS, the type of inflammatory response can vary with the cause. A rather simplistic guideline, to which there are always exceptions, that compares the type of inflammation with different causal agents is as follows:

1. Serous to suppurative or purulent responses can be the result of several species of bacteria.
2. Eosinophil responses occur in salt poisoning of pigs and with parasitic larval migration.
3. Lymphocytic, monocytic/macrophage, nonsuppurative, lymphomonocytic, and lymphohistiocytic responses can be caused by viruses and certain protozoa.
4. Granulomatous response can be the result of fungi, certain protozoa, and some higher-order bacteria such as the *Mycobacterium* spp.

PORTALS OF ENTRY

Disease processes of the CNS enter the brain and spinal cord through one of four principal portals (Box 14-6). These portals

BOX 14-6 Portals of Entry into the CNS

DIRECT EXTENSION

Penetrating trauma through the calvarium or vertebral bodies

Extension of middle and/or inner ear infection

Extension of a nasal cavity/sinus infection through the cribriform plate or calvarium

Extension from osteomyelitis

HEMATOGENOUS

Localization within capillary beds of the meninges and parenchyma of the CNS

Localization within capillary beds of the choroid plexuses and extension into the cerebrospinal fluid

LEUKOCYTE TRAFFICKING

Macrophages or lymphocytes (containing microbes) during their migration through the CNS

RETROGRADE AXONAL TRANSPORT

Transported from the periphery into the CNS by neuronal retrograde axoplasmic flow

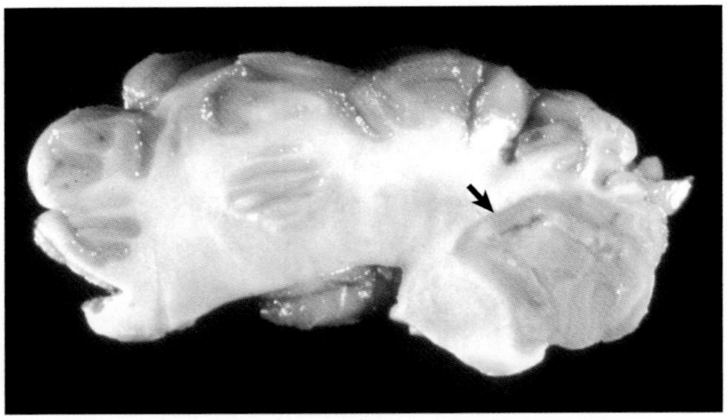

Fig. 14-29 Chronic bacterial abscess, leptomeninges of the cerebellum, sheep. The abscess *(arrow)* resulted from direct extension of infection from an inner ear infection and compresses and distorts the cerebellum. It is walled off from the adjacent cerebellum by a distinct fibrous capsule synthesized by fibroblasts from the adjacent leptomeninges. This abscess likely arose in the leptomeninges of the cerebellum and grew to compress adjacent cerebellum. (Courtesy College of Veterinary Medicine, University of Illinois.)

include (1) direct extension, (2) hematogenous entry, (3) leukocytic trafficking, and (4) retrograde axonal transport.

Direct Extension

Direct extension is a common portal of entry and includes a wide range of disease processes. Penetrating trauma through the calvarium or vertebrae as a result of a gunshot wound or other forms of trauma can provide a direct portal into the CNS. Disease processes can also extend into the brain and/or spinal cord as a result of (1) a middle and/or inner ear infection (Fig. 14-29), (2) nasal cavity/sinus infection or neoplasia through the cribriform plate or calvarium (Fig. 14-30), or (3) bacterial osteomyelitis or neoplasia of vertebral bodies with extension through the vertebrae into the vertebral canal.

Benign growths of the calvarium and vertebrae, such as osteomas, chondromas, and osteochondromas, often extend into and compress the brain and spinal cord. One specific neoplasm, the multilobular osteoma, has been described as originating from the periosteum of the canine skull. Also, malignant neoplasms adjacent to the cranium or spinal column can cause injury by direct invasion. Some examples include extracranial osteosarcoma and fibrosarcoma in the dog. Also, malignant melanoma of the soft palate in the dog and melanoma involving the paravertebral lymph nodes in the horse can invade adjacent CNS tissue. Other examples of direct extension include lymphosarcoma affecting the spinal cord in the bovine species and less frequently involving the spinal cord or brain in the dog and cat and carcinomas of the ethmoidal area and nasal cavity.

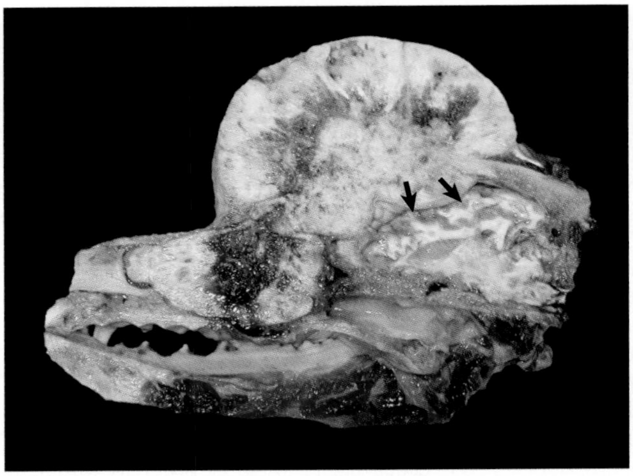

Fig. 14-30 Osteochondrosarcoma, calvarium, dog. The neoplasm has destroyed and penetrated the calvarium and compressed the cerebral hemispheres *(arrows)*. There is also invasion of frontal or nasal sinuses and nasal cavity. (Courtesy Dr. K. Bailey, College of Veterinary Medicine, University of Illinois.)

Hematogenous Entry

The most common portal of entry into the CNS is the bloodstream. In neonates, infectious agents, such as *Escherichia coli*, can enter the blood through the umbilical vein or through the venous system after surgical procedures such as castration. A CNS disease in cows called *thrombotic meningoencephalitis* is caused by *Histophilus somni* (formerly *Haemophilus somnus*) bacteremia with localization of bacteria in blood vessels of the brain, which leads to vasculitis, hemorrhage, and thrombosis (see Fig. 14-89). In adult animals, sites of chronic inflammation, such as abscesses, bacterial skin disease, and ear infections, can also serve as sustained sources of bacteria, which can enter the venous system and spread to distant sites through the bloodstream hematogenously.

Capillary beds of the meninges, neuropil, and choroid plexuses are common sites for localization of specific infectious agents. Such localization patterns may be attributable to receptor-mediated phenomena or vascular flow patterns related to the size of the infectious pathogen. Additionally the bloodstream is also a portal of entry into the CNS for metastasizing tumors such as hemangiosarcoma and a variety of carcinomas.

Leukocyte Trafficking

As part of the systemic immunologic surveillance system, macrophages (monocytes) and lymphoid cells continually move in and out of capillary beds in the CNS and thus serve as sentinel cells monitoring for the presence of disease processes within the brain and spinal cord (see Fig. 4-11). As examples, retroviruses, such as feline leukemia virus, and mycotic agents, such as *Blastomyces dermatitidis,* have stages of their life cycles within the cytoplasm of lymphocytes or macrophages. During the movement of lymphocytes and macrophages in and out of the CNS, cells infected with such agents are activated to release their infectious contents and infect cells of the CNS.

Retrograde Axonal Transport

Retrograde axonal transport provides a unique portal of entry for viruses such as rabies and the bacterium *Listeria monocytogenes.* These pathogens replicate in tissues richly innervated with receptors and motor end plates from sensory and motor neurons, respectively, which provide a connection between peripheral infection and the CNS. Retrograde axoplasmic flow is then used to gain entry into the CNS (see Web Fig. 14-1).

DISORDERS OF DOMESTIC ANIMALS

Disorders that occur in many or all animal species are discussed in this section. Disorders of individual animal species are discussed in later sections covering disorders unique to that species.

Malformations

Neural Tube Closure Defects (Dysraphia)

Dysraphia literally means an abnormal seam, and these anomalies appear to result from defective interaction of neuroepithelium with adjacent notochordal and mesenchymal cells during closure of the neural tube in the early stages of development. Neuroepithelium is the progenitor cell for neurons and astrocytes, oligodendrocytes, and ependymal cells.

Experimental studies of closure of the neural tube show that it occurs at four distinct locations called *closure initiation sites* in the embryo, and disruption of this process at these sites leads to site-specific dysraphic anomalies. Closure site I contributes to the posterior neuropore (the opening at the posterior end of the embryonic neural canal), whereas closure sites II to IV contribute to the anterior neuropore (the opening at the anterior end of the embryonic neural canal). Anencephaly is caused by a failure of closure sites II or IV; spina bifida is caused by a failure of closure site I. Genes possibly involved in neural tube closure defects include those of the folate metabolic pathway and folate transport.

Dysraphic anomalies, also called *neural tube closure defects,* in animals are typified by anencephaly and prosencephalic hypoplasia, cranium bifidum, and spina bifida.

Anencephaly and Prosencephalic Hypoplasia

Anencephaly literally means an absence of the brain, but in many instances of so-called anencephaly only the rostral part of the brain (cerebral hemispheres) is absent, or very rudimentary, and to varying degrees the brainstem is preserved. Thus this abnormality is best designated prosencephalic hypoplasia. Such anomalies result from an abnormal development of the rostral aspect of the neural tube. Although the cause for these anomalies is largely unknown, anencephaly has been reported to be associated with anomalies in other body systems in calves. Additionally, anencephaly—after initial cranium bifidum and exencephaly (protrusion of brain not covered by skin or meninges)—has been reported to occur in rat fetuses after exposure of the pregnant dam to excessive concentrations of vitamin A and cyclophosphamide.

Meningoencephalocele and Cranium Bifidum

Cranium bifidum is characterized by a dorsal midline cranial defect through which meningeal and brain tissue can protrude. The protruded material, which forms a sac (-cele), is covered by skin and

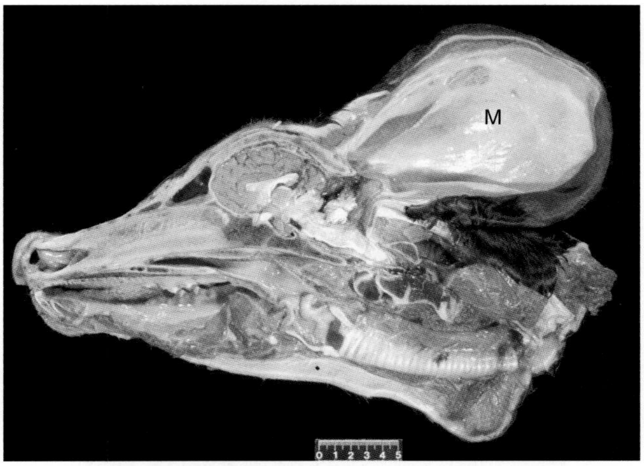

Fig. 14-31 Meningocele (M), brain, calf.
A defect in the caudodorsal portion of the skull has allowed the meninges to herniate into a large external pouch covered by skin. The pouch contains fluid and is lined by arachnoid and dura, which are continuous with those surrounding the brain. The cerebellum is small, and the occipital cortex truncated. Scale bar = 5 cm. (Courtesy Dr. R. Storts, College of Veterinary Medicine, Texas A&M University.)

can be lined by meninges (meningocele) or meninges accompanied by a part of the brain (meningoencephalocele) (Fig. 14-31). These malformations are hereditary in pigs and cats and are also caused by griseofulvin treatment in pregnant cats during the first week of gestation.

Meningomyelocele and Spina Bifida

Spina bifida is the vertebral counterpart of cranium bifidum. This lesion, which frequently tends to affect the caudal spine, is characterized by a dorsal defect in the closure of one to several vertebral arches that form the dorsal spinal column covering the spinal cord. The lesion results from a failure of the neural tube and developing vertebral arches to close properly, which may result in herniation of either meninges (meningocele) or meninges and spinal cord (meningomyelocele) through the defect, forming a sac covered with skin. In some cases there is no herniation of the meninges or spinal cord through the defect, and this variation is termed *spina bifida occulta* (Fig. 14-32). In this variation, there is an absence of skin over the affected vertebral arches, vertebral musculature is visible, and the dura mater and spinal cord can be seen in the spinal canal.

Spina bifida has been reported in several species, including horses, calves, sheep, dogs (especially English bulldogs), and cats, particularly the Manx breed, in which it is inherited as an autosomal dominant trait. An additional lesion, myeloschisis, is similar to spina bifida except in its severe form, it results from failure of the entire spinal neural tube to close. This lesion is therefore characterized by lack of development of the entire dorsal vertebral column.

Hydromyelia

Congenital hydromyelia is an abnormal dilation of the central canal of the spinal cord (Fig. 14-33) that leads to the formation of a cavity in which CSF may accumulate. In animals, this disorder likely results from infectious or genetic injury that results in damage to ependymal cells lining the canal and the subsequent disruption of the normal flow of CSF and the formation of abnormal CSF pressure gradients within the central canal. As CSF accumulates in the enlarging space, the increased pericanalicular pressure placed on the spinal cord compresses the white and gray

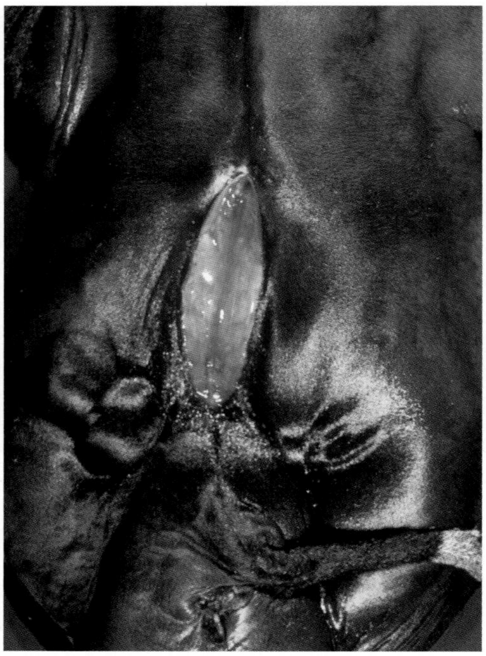

Fig. 14-32 Spina bifida occulta, calf.
There is a cleft in several vertebrae of the dorsal spinal column resulting from defective closure of the neural tube. Although not always the case, note the lack of herniation of the meninges or spinal cord through the defect. The spinal cord is not visible (i.e., occulta) because it is located in the vertebral canal at the deepest ventral extent of the cleft and is covered by edematous muscle. (Courtesy Dr. M.D. McGavin, College of Veterinary Medicine, University of Tennessee.)

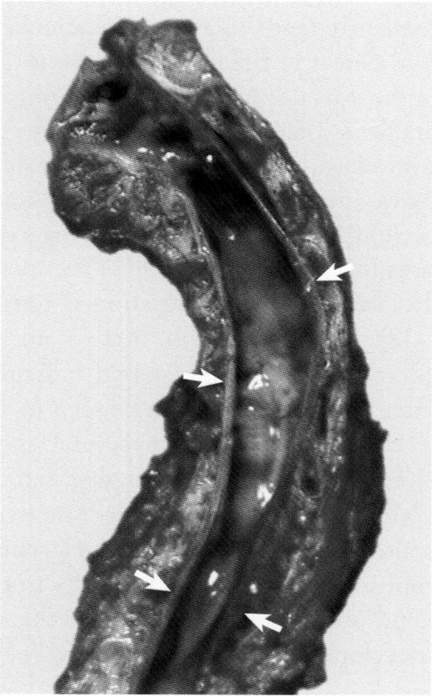

Fig. 14-33 End-stage hydromyelia, spinal cord, dog.
The white and gray matter of the spinal cord are missing as a result of compression atrophy from a space-occupying, fluid-filled central canal. The only recognizable remnants of nervous tissue is the dura *(arrows)*. In less severely affected animals, there would be variable dilatation of the central canal of the spinal cord with much less severe compression atrophy. (Courtesy College of Veterinary Medicine, University of Tennessee.)

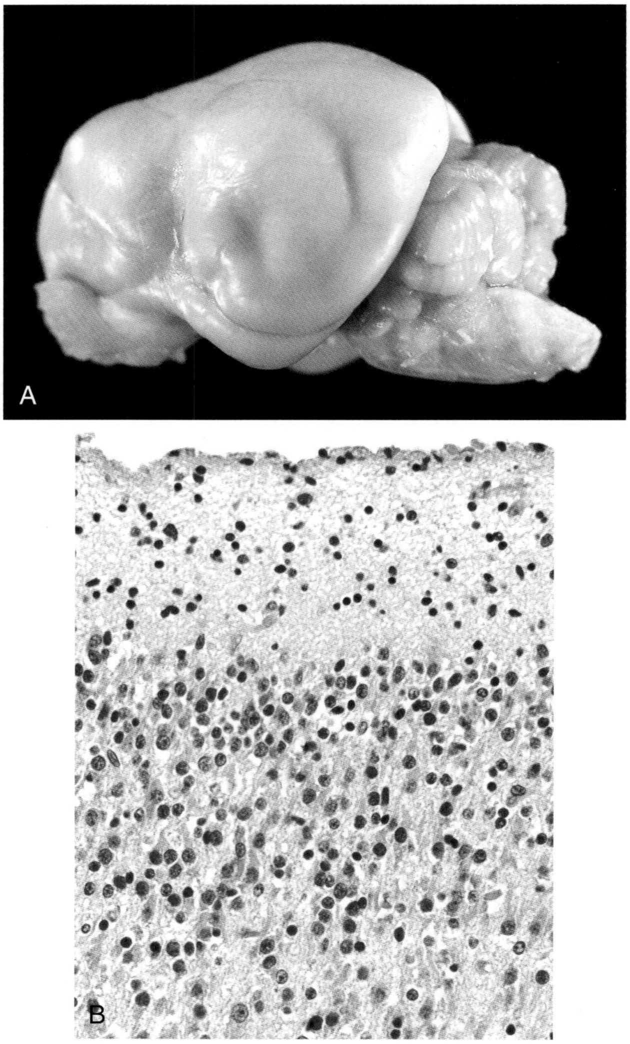

Fig. 14-34 Lissencephaly, brain, dog.
A, Note the smooth surfaces of the cerebral hemispheres, which are without gyri and sulci. Gyri and sulci fail to form, possibly from failure of neuronal development and migration. Lissencephaly is an abnormality in domestic animals, but is normal in mice, rats, rabbits, and birds. **B,** The development and migration of neurons have been disrupted such that the cortical gray matter lacks normal lamina formed by neuronal cell bodies. H&E stain. (**A** courtesy Dr. L. Roth, College of Veterinary Medicine, Cornell University. **B** courtesy Dr. R. Mantene, College of Veterinary Medicine, University of Illinois.)

matter, leading to loss of white matter and possibly neurons in gray matter. Acquired hydromyelia is rare and is caused by obstruction of the central canal CSF flow. Causes of obstruction include infection, inflammation, and neoplasia.

Clinical signs in young animals with congenital hydromyelia vary, depending on the location and size of the dilation of the central canal in the spinal cord. Signs may include ataxia, urinary incontinence, respiratory difficulty, muscle weakness in front and/or hind limbs, and abnormal proprioceptive reflexes.

Neuronal Migration Disorders

Lissencephaly

Lissencephaly (agyria) and a similar change called *pachygyria* (large gyria) are developmental anomalies that result in part of or the entire cerebrum having smooth surfaces lacking normal gyri and sulci (Fig. 14-34). The cortex is thicker than normal on a transverse section, and the normal laminar pattern of neurons is disrupted.

This lesion is thought to have a genetic basis and results from an arrest of or defect in neuronal migration during development. Recent experimental studies suggest that this migrational disorder is linked to mutations and/or deletions in the doublecortin, filamin-1, LIS1, and reelin genes. These genes control the spatial and temporal expression of proteins in the extracellular microenvironment that subsequently bind to receptors on migrating cells. Patterns of cell membrane binding signals are interpreted by migrating cells and are reflected in their movements by changes in intracellular cytoskeletal reorganization. This process allows cells to migrate to their final destinations within the CNS. Thus alterations in signaling pathways lead to abnormal neuronal migration and CNS anomalies.

The brains of some laboratory animals, such as rabbits, rats, and mice, lack gyri and sulci; therefore agyria is normal in these species and has no functional significance.

Encephaloclastic Defects

Porencephaly and Hydranencephaly

The formation of fluid-filled cavities in the brain, termed *porencephaly* (small cavities) and *hydranencephaly* (large cavities), usually occurs in utero during gestation. *Porencephaly* refers to a cleft or cyst in the wall of the cerebral hemisphere that typically communicates with the subarachnoid space, but it can also communicate with a lateral ventricle. The cavitation results from destruction of immature neuroblasts whose loss prevents normal development as a result of faulty or aberrant neuroblast migration. Hydranencephaly is considered a severe form of porencephaly and is characterized by cavitation in areas normally occupied by the white matter of the cerebral hemispheres and results from improper development of this part of the cerebrum. Hydranencephaly is often quite severe, with very little tissue present between the dilated lateral ventricles and the leptomeninges.

Type I and type II porencephaly have been described in human infants, and cases of porencephaly reported in animals can also be categorized using this scheme. Type I porencephaly is caused by vascular injury or vasculitis. Injury, resulting in infarction in the area of the subependymal germinal matrix, results in the formation of a cyst within the focus of dead cells and effete erythrocytes. The germinal matrix is very sensitive to ischemia because of sparse stroma, delicate vasculature, and high metabolism. The initial focus of hemorrhage can grow by centripetal expansion, depending on the severity of hemorrhage and hypoxia, into a cyst of considerable size. Type II porencephaly is caused by injury of neuroblasts in the germinal matrix and the failure of these neuroblasts to migrate within the matrix to form the cerebral cortex. A cyst results from the expansion of the subarachnoid space into the void left by the absence of the cortex.

Type II porencephaly appears to be the form of porencephaly that occurs in domestic animals. Viruses, such as those that cause Akabane disease, bovine virus diarrhea, blue tongue, border disease, Rift Valley fever, and Wesselsbron disease, infect and destroy differentiating neuroblasts and neuroglial cells in the developing fetus in utero. Although neuroblasts appear to be the primary target for viral infection in these diseases, additional experimental studies need to be conducted to clarify whether endothelial cells are also infected.

Grossly, porencephaly/hydranencephaly appears as thin-walled fluid-filled cysts of varied sizes in the cerebral hemispheres. Because of the lack of brain substance, the ventricles expand into this space (hydrocephalus ex vacuo), and the ependymal lining remains relatively preserved or may have scattered defects characterized by absent ependyma. The cranium and meninges are generally unaltered. In some cases, cerebellar hypoplasia (all or part of the cerebellum) and hypoplasia of the spinal cord may also occur. Microscopically, necrosis of undifferentiated cells, including potential neuroblasts and neuroglia, surrounding a fluid-filled cavity is present in the subventricular zone of the cerebral hemispheres. Degeneration and loss of motor neurons of the ventral horns of the spinal cord may also be observed. This lesion may result in denervation atrophy of limb muscles with a resultant lack of joint movement and arthrogryposis, a persistent congenital flexure or contraction of a joint. Nonsuppurative encephalitis, typified by the accumulation of macrophages, lymphocytes, and plasma cells, also occurs.

Malformations of the Cerebellum

Cerebellar Hypoplasia

In animals, the most common causes of cerebellar hypoplasia are parvoviruses (kittens: panleukopenia virus [Fig. 14-35] and puppies: canine parvovirus) and pestiviruses (calves: bovine viral diarrhea virus [Fig. 14-36] and piglets: classic swine fever virus). These viruses infect and destroy mitotic cells, primarily the cells of the external granular layer of the cerebellum that are still dividing during the late gestational and early neonatal periods. Necrosis of these cells means they are not available to migrate to form the internal granular layer, and thus the cerebellum is hypoplastic. In calves the cerebellar lesion (cerebellar hypoplasia/atrophy), which follows infection at 150 days of gestation (midtrimester), is considered to involve two processes. One process is typified by early necrosis of the undifferentiated cells in the external granular layer.

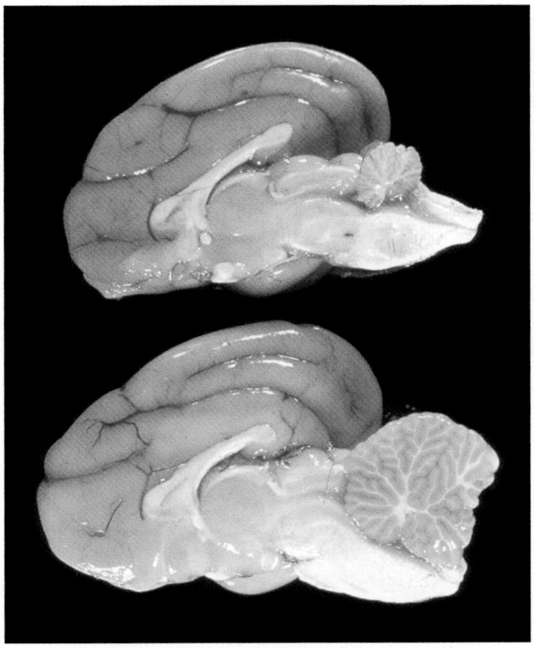

Fig. 14-35 Cerebellar hypoplasia, brain, cat.
In the cat, cerebellar hypoplasia (cerebellar hypoplasia, top specimen; normal cat, bottom specimen) most commonly is the result of in utero infection with feline panleukopenia virus (parvovirus). The virus infects and causes lysis of dividing cells in the external granular layer (on the outside of the cerebellum in the fetus). Because these cells are no longer available to migrate to form the (internal) granular layer, the cerebellum remains small. (Courtesy Dr. Y. Niyo, College of Veterinary Medicine, Iowa State University; and Noah's Arkive, College of Veterinary Medicine, The University of Georgia.)

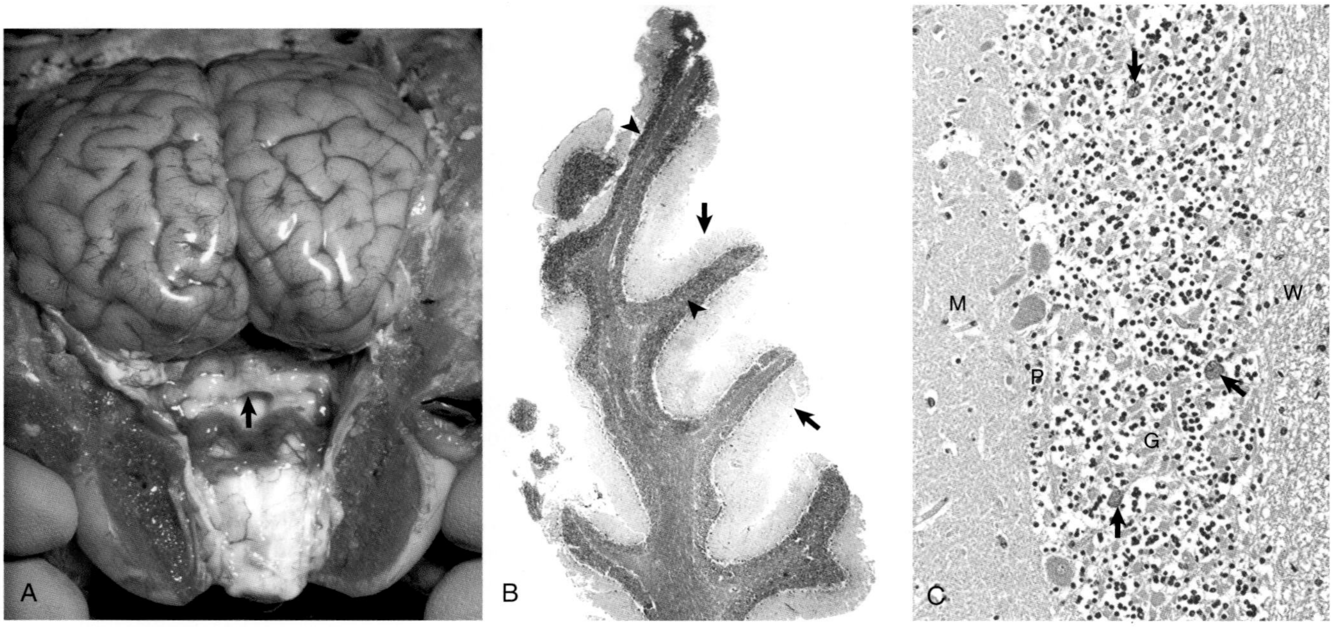

Fig. 14-36 Cerebellum, calf.
In the normal neonatal calf, cells of the external granular layer of the cerebellum migrate to form the (internal) granular layer (not shown). Bovine viral diarrhea virus infects and kills mitotic cells of the external granular layer of the cerebellum. These cells are still dividing during the late gestational and early neonatal periods in the cat and between 100 to 180 days of gestation in the calf. Necrosis of these cells means they are not available to migrate to form the internal granular layer, and thus the cerebellum does not obtain full size. Depending on the stage of gestation, injury can also alter development of cells in others ways including altered patterns of migration, resulting in various other lesions termed dysplasia. **A,** Cerebellar hypoplasia *(arrow).* In utero infection with bovine viral diarrhea virus (pestivirus) results in cytolysis of dividing germinal cells of the external granular layer and vascular impairment secondary to vasculitis of the cerebellum during organogenesis. The severity of the lesion involving the granule cells is at its greatest if dividing cells are infected during the earliest stages of cellular differentiation, and occurs between 100 to 180 days of gestation. **B,** Note the folia of the cerebellum are hypoplastic with a reduced thickness of the molecular layer *(arrows)* and haphazardly organized and thinned granular cell layer *(arrowheads).* **C.** The molecular layer *(M)* of the cerebellum is reduced in thickness and lacks the normal number of neuronal nuclei. The Purkinje cell layer *(P)* has large gaps between adjacent cells as the result of the loss of neuron cell bodies or the failure of neurons to migrate properly to form this layer. Note the retention of Purkinje cells *(arrows)* in the granular cell layer *(G).* The granular cell layer has significantly reduced numbers of neurons as shown by the lack of nuclei. White matter *(W).* H&E stain. (**A** courtesy Dr. M.D. McGavin, College of Veterinary Medicine, University of Tennessee. **B** and **C** courtesy Dr. J.F. Zachary, College of Veterinary Medicine, University of Illinois.)

A second process involves viral-induced vasculitis and ischemia of cerebellar folial white matter.

Grossly, the size of the cerebellum is reduced; the reduction in size varies in severity, depending on the age and developmental stage of the brain when the fetus or neonate is infected.

Microscopically, there is necrosis and loss of the external granular layer and degeneration and loss of Purkinje cells that are postmitotic but immature. Reasons for degeneration of Purkinje cells might include infection by the virus or lack of normal development of the cerebellar cortex. The Purkinje cells can also be malpositioned and located in the molecular layer as a result of the viral-induced alteration in development of the cerebellar cortex. In calves, edema of the folial white matter with focal hemorrhage in the cortex, followed by focal cavitation of the white matter and atrophy, may also be present. These latter lesions are due to ischemia resulting from vasculitis. Leptomeningitis, characterized by accumulation of lymphocytes and plasma cells and occasionally fibroplasia, may cause adhesions between adjacent cerebellar folia and focal obliteration of the subarachnoid space.

Malformations of the Spinal Cord

Syringomyelia

Syringomyelia (congenital and acquired forms) is a disorder in which a cyst forms in the spinal cord. The cyst, a tubular cavitation called a *syrinx,* is not lined by ependyma and is separate from the central canal. The syrinx can extend over several spinal cord segments. The lesion is well known in humans and has also been described in the dog (Weimaraner breed) and calves. The syrinx can communicate with the central canal but should not be confused with hydromyelia, which means dilatation of the central canal. The cavity contains fluid and is unlined, except for varying degrees of mural astrocytosis, which is usually very mild in the Weimaraner. Proposed causes include presence of an anomalous vascular pattern that results in low-grade ischemia, leading to infarction or failure of cells destined for this area to develop in utero trauma in humans or an infection that causes degeneration and cavitation. A rare acquired form of syringomyelia is similar to congenital syringomyelia; however, it occurs in older animals. Proposed causes include injury after trauma to the central canal or its vascular supply caused by trauma, infection, or neoplasia that result in degeneration and cavitation of the spinal cord.

Although the central canal of the spinal cord is connected to the ventricular system via the fourth ventricle, there apparently is little active movement of CSF within the central canal. Recently, it has been hypothesized that there may be alteration of "normal" CSF flow (see the discussion on ependyma in the section on Cells of the CNS) with redirection of the flow along a pressure gradient into the central canal and into the syrinx. It has also been suggested that pressure differences in the vertebral column cause CSF to continually move into the cyst, resulting in enlargement of the syrinx and additional compressive damage to the spinal cord.

Clinical signs in young dogs and calves with syringomyelia vary, depending on the location and size of the cyst in the spinal cord. Signs may include ataxia, urinary incontinence, respiratory difficulty, muscle weakness in front and/or hind limbs, and abnormal proprioceptive reflexes.

Hydrocephalus

The most common congenital malformations and developmental anomalies in veterinary medicine affecting cells that form the ependyma and choroid plexuses are hydrocephalus, hydromyelia, and syringomyelia. These anomalies are covered in greater detail later. Of these anomalies, hydrocephalus is the anomaly most likely to be caused by in utero injury following viral infection of the developing fetus. However, in some breeds (brachycephalic breeds), these disorders may have a genetic predisposition, but this mechanism of injury has not been as clearly established in domestic animals as it has in humans.

In laboratory animals, several neonatal in utero viral infections, including mumps virus, reovirus type I, and parainfluenza virus types I and II, can induce congenital hydrocephalus. Parainfluenza virus can also cause the lesion in the dog. Although there are some differences among the different viral infections, the basic lesion is stenosis of the mesencephalic duct (aqueduct of Sylvius in humans, mesencephalic aqueduct) that results in the development of noncommunicating hydrocephalus. In the dog, closure of the mesencephalic duct can be incomplete. The virus grows in and causes destruction of ependymal cells lining the ventricular system. The infection is initially accompanied by an inflammation that resolves within 2 weeks.

The notable lesion resulting from this injury to the ependyma of the mesencephalic duct is its occlusion. This end-stage lesion is not the result of an astroglial response or due to the presence of viral antigen. Instead, the original ependyma-lined aqueduct is replaced by focal aggregates of remaining ependymal cells that have separated from the adjacent tissue, which appears normal. The appearance of the final lesion is therefore more suggestive of an agenesis than a viral infection. Infection of adult laboratory animals (mice with influenza viral infection) also can induce mesencephalic duct stenosis resulting in hydrocephalus, but in contrast to neonatal infection, there is a persistent astroglial response in the area of stenosis.

Congenital Hydrocephalus

CSF can accumulate in the ventricular system, the subarachnoid space, or both. The type of hydrocephalus that develops depends on the site of blockage that disrupts normal flow of CSF.

Exactly which portions of the ventricular system will be dilatated in hydrocephalus depends on the site of the blockage:

1. Blockage of the interventricular foramen between a lateral and third ventricular leads to unilateral dilatation of that lateral ventricle.
2. Blockage of both interventricular foramina leads to bilateral dilatation of both lateral ventricles.
3. Blockage of the mesencephalic duct leads to bilateral dilatation of both lateral ventricles, the third ventricle, and the segment of the mesencephalic duct proximal to the blockage.
4. Blockage of the lateral apertures of the fourth ventricle leads to bilateral dilatation of lateral ventricles, the third ventricle, the mesencephalic duct, and the fourth ventricle.
5. Blockage of reabsorption leads to bilateral dilatation of lateral ventricles, the third ventricle, the mesencephalic duct, the fourth ventricle, and the subarachnoid space.

As an example, following blockage of the interventricular foramina, the pressure in the lateral ventricles increases; the ventricles dilate; the ependyma becomes atrophied and focally discontinuous; and because of the pressure gradient, CSF is forced into the periventricular white matter leading to hydrostatic edema. Hydrostatic edema results in degeneration and atrophy of myelin and axons, and this loss of tissue results in further expansion of the ventricles.

The forms of hydrocephalus are communicating and noncommunicating hydrocephalus. Communicating hydrocephalus, the least common of the two forms, occurs when there is communication of ventricular CSF with the subarachnoid space where the CSF can be in excess. Noncommunicating hydrocephalus results from obstruction within the ventricular system at, or rostral to, the lateral apertures of the fourth ventricle. An area of great vulnerability for obstruction is the mesencephalic aqueduct. Noncommunicating hydrocephalus can also occur without any evidence of obstruction to CSF flow as a result of failure of the reabsorption of CSF.

A recent hypothesis proposes that communicating hydrocephalus is caused by a decreased expansion of intracranial arteries during systole as a result of reduced compliance involving the arterial walls, or the subarachnoid space, and is referred to as *restricted arterial pulsation hydrocephalus*. Because the intracranial arteries cannot fully expand, a pressure gradient develops in which there is greater pressure within the brain tissue and the ventricles than outside the brain. Several causes have been advanced, including arteritis, subarachnoid hemorrhage, and meningitis.

A third type of hydrocephalus, referred to as *hydrocephalus ex vacuo* (or compensating hydrocephalus), is not usually a congenital abnormality but occurs secondary to absence or loss of cerebral tissue. This type of hydrocephalus can occur in utero from destruction and loss of cerebral tissue surrounding the lateral ventricles (e.g., in hydranencephaly). Hydrocephalus ex vacuo is discussed further in the next section on Acquired Hydrocephalus.

In domestic animals, congenital hydrocephalus can be caused by in utero viral infections leading to aqueductal stenosis (incomplete closure) in the dog that results in the development of noncommunicating hydrocephalus; however, a genetically programmed predisposition may occur in very small and brachycephalic breeds of dogs.

Gross lesions associated with communicating and noncommunicating congenital hydrocephalus include enlargement (doming) of the cranium if obstruction occurs before the sutures have fused (Fig. 14-37). The bones of the calvarium are extremely thin and the fontanelles are prominent (Fig. 14-38). In the brain there is prominent enlargement of the ventricular system proximal to the point of obstruction (Fig. 14-39). White matter adjacent to the dilated lateral ventricles is reduced in thickness, although the gray matter can retain a relatively normal appearance. As the hydrocephalus progresses, atrophy with fenestration of the interventricular septum (septum pellucidum), atrophy of the hippocampus in the floor of the lateral ventricles, and flattening of cortical gyri can occur. If the obstruction is abrupt and pressure builds rapidly, the cerebral hemispheres can be displaced caudally, causing herniation of the parahippocampal gyri under the tentorium cerebelli and of the vermis of the cerebellum through the foramen magnum. The resulting coning of the cerebellum can be accompanied by necrosis of cells in the cerebellar folia as a result of ischemia and infarction. Microscopically the ependyma can become atrophied and focally discontinuous, and there is loss of cells and cell processes in adjacent white matter and variably in the gray matter.

Clinically, congenital hydrocephalus occurs most frequently in brachycephalic or toy breeds such as the Chihuahua, Lhasa

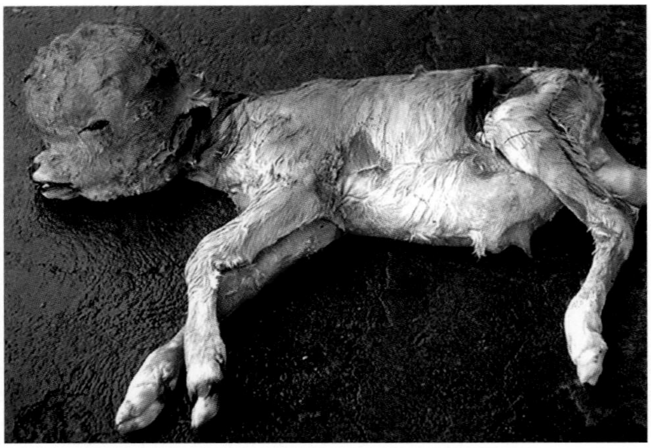

Fig. 14-37 Congenital hydrocephalus, brain, calf.
Note the symmetrically enlarged and dome-shaped calvarium. The bone of the calvarium is thinned and distorted from pressure from the expanding brain during gestation. (Courtesy Dr. J. King, College of Veterinary Medicine, Cornell University.)

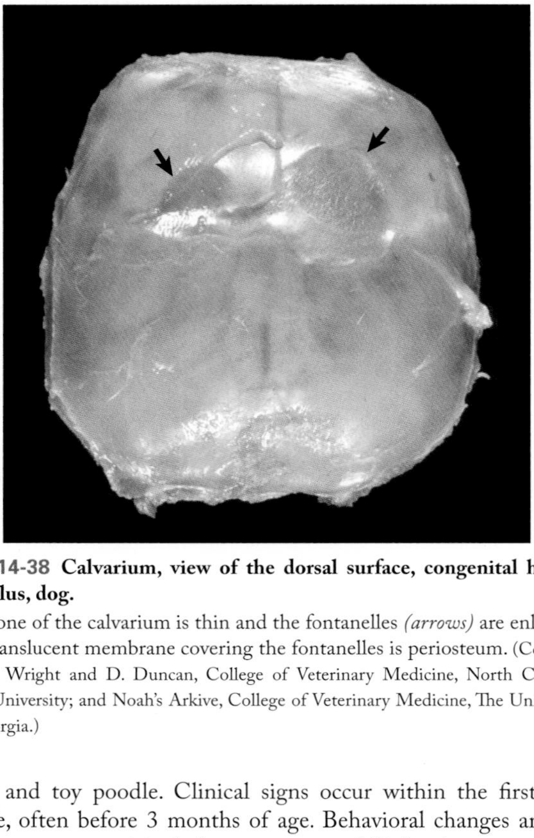

Fig. 14-38 Calvarium, view of the dorsal surface, congenital hydrocephalus, dog.
The bone of the calvarium is thin and the fontanelles *(arrows)* are enlarged. The translucent membrane covering the fontanelles is periosteum. (Courtesy Drs. J. Wright and D. Duncan, College of Veterinary Medicine, North Carolina State University; and Noah's Arkive, College of Veterinary Medicine, The University of Georgia.)

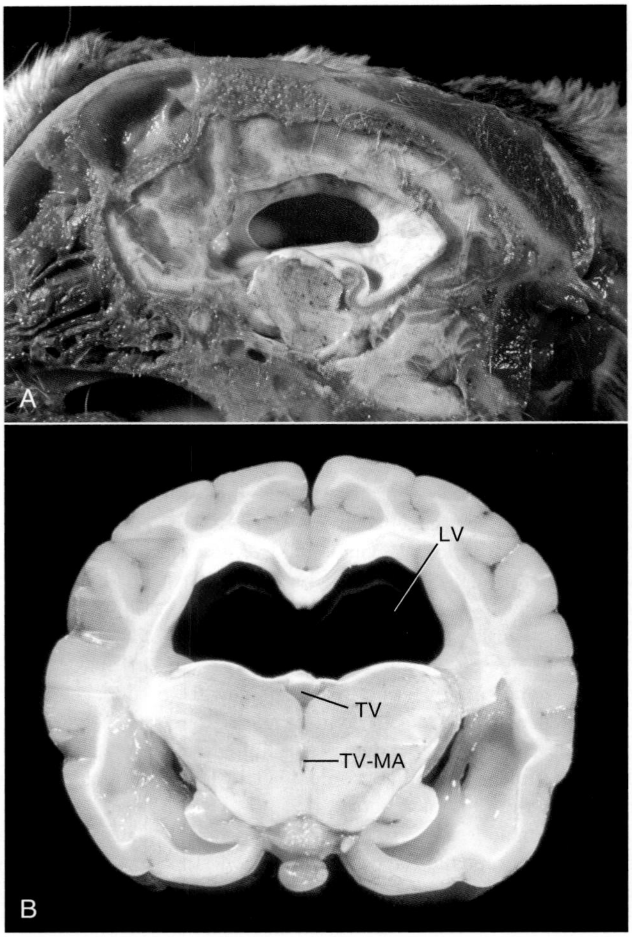

Fig. 14-39 Hydrocephalus, brain, dog.
A, Midsagittal section of the head, third ventricle. Note the dilated third and lateral ventricles and the absence of most of the septum pellucidum between the left and right lateral ventricles. **B,** Junction between parietal and occipital lobes, level of thalamus. Bilateral dilation of lateral ventricles dorsally *(LV),* and ventrolaterally. The fornix has separated and lies on the flattened floor of the ventricle. Note that the third ventricle *(TV)* and junctional area between the third ventricle and mesencephalic aqueduct *(TV-MA)* are not enlarged and are possibly even reduced in size, suggesting that the obstruction may be at, or rostral to, this plane of section. (**A** courtesy Dr. M.D. McGavin, College of Veterinary Medicine, University of Tennessee. **B** courtesy Dr. R. Storts, College of Veterinary Medicine, Texas A&M University.)

apso, and toy poodle. Clinical signs occur within the first year of life, often before 3 months of age. Behavioral changes are the most common and include poor motor skill development; delay in learned behavior, such as house training; somnolence; dullness; episodic confusion; circling; periodic aggression; and seizures.

Acquired Hydrocephalus

Noncommunicating acquired hydrocephalus has been associated with injury of the ependyma, resulting in obstruction of any of the following: the lateral apertures of the fourth ventricle, the cerebral aqueduct, or the interventricular foramen. Causes of obstruction include compression by cerebral abscesses and neoplasms, and blockages by infectious/inflammatory disease resulting in a ventriculitis and, uncommonly, by cholesteatomas in the choroid plexus of the lateral ventricles of the horse. Because the calvarium has now ceased to grow, unlike congenital hydrocephalus, it is of normal size and shape, and its bone is of normal thickness.

A second type of acquired hydrocephalus, referred to as hydrocephalus ex vacuo (or compensating hydrocephalus), usually occurs in the cerebral hemispheres secondary to loss of neural tissue. If there is loss of neurons in the cerebral cortex, as in bovine polioencephalomalacia or other types of laminar cortical necrosis, the axons of these neurons, which normally traverse the white matter of the cerebral hemispheres, will disappear by Wallerian degeneration, and there will be atrophy of the cortex from the loss of neuronal cell bodies and of the white matter from the loss of axons. The lateral ventricles will expand into the space once occupied by white matter. This dilatation of the lateral ventricles may be bilateral when there has been a loss of white and gray matter from both cerebral hemispheres, or it may be unilateral. If the loss of cortex is localized, as in an infarct, then dilatation of the lateral ventricle will not uniformly involve the whole lateral ventricle. Examples of disorders in which hydrocephalus ex vacuo occur include some storage diseases (ceroid-lipofuscinosis in sheep), aging, and postradiation exposure, all of which are associated with cerebral atrophy. There is no evidence of obstruction of the normal flow of CSF in this type of hydrocephalus.

Diseases Caused by Microbes

Bacteria

Brain Abscesses

Cerebral abscesses in animals are relatively uncommon but arise after entry of bacteria into the CNS. This may occur either from direct extension or hematogenously. With direct extension, abscesses occur following penetrating wounds, such as calvarial fractures, or from spread of infection from adjacent tissues, such as the leptomeninges, paranasal sinuses, and internal ear, and through the cribriform plate of the ethmoid (see Fig. 14-29). Diseases that cause bacteremia or septicemia result in infectious agents being trapped in vascular beds within the CNS and meninges. Abscesses usually arise within gray matter because it receives a disproportionate share of blood flow in the CNS, usually at the gray-white (cortex-subcortical white matter) junction. They exert effects in the CNS by disruption and destruction of tissue and by displacement as space-occupying lesions. If the abscess grows quickly, tissue is more likely to be disrupted and destroyed and in the worst case penetrate the wall of the lateral ventricle and cause a ventriculitis. Bacteria in the CSF may be carried into the subarachnoid space and cause a leptomeningitis. On the other hand, if growth is slow, tissue is more likely to be displaced. Chronic abscesses become encapsulated by either fibrous tissue if they are close to the leptomeninges or by astrocytes away from the meninges. The mechanism of tissue injury is likely a secondary bystander effect related to the actions of the mediators of inflammation and the toxins and other products elaborated from bacteria. Bacteria appear to localize in specific areas of the CNS based on receptor-mediated attachment or because of vascular flow patterns unique to the gray matter–white matter interface of the CNS that allows bacteria to attach to and move through the blood-brain barrier. This latter flow mechanism likely occurs because small blood vessels supplying the cerebrum fail to continue into the white matter and end with their horizontal branches running parallel to the surface of the gyrus within the gray matter at the interface with the white matter. Once within the CNS or meninges, bacteria replicate and elicit an inflammatory response. Lytic enzymes released from lysosomes of neutrophils and other inflammatory cytokines secreted by lymphocytes and macrophages destroy neurons and their processes and disrupt synapses, thus affecting neurotransmission.

Grossly, brain abscesses can be single or multiple, be discrete or coalescing, and have varied sizes (Fig. 14-40). Early in the process, abscesses consist of a white to gray to yellow, thick to granular exudate. The color of the exudate can be influenced by the exuberance of the pyogenic response elicited by the inciting bacteria and by any pigments produced by the bacteria. *Streptococcus* spp., *Staphylococcus* spp., and *Corynebacterium* spp. may produce a pale-yellow to yellow, watery-to-creamy exudate. Coliforms, such as *Escherichia coli* and *Klebsiella* spp., may produce a white to gray, watery to creamy exudate. *Pseudomonas* spp. may produce a green to bluish-green exudate. The borders of abscesses are often surrounded by a red zone of active hyperemia induced by inflammatory mediators acting on capillary beds. With chronicity, abscesses may be walled off by processes of astrocytes and fibrous connective tissue from the pia mater, especially when the abscess results from a penetrating wound.

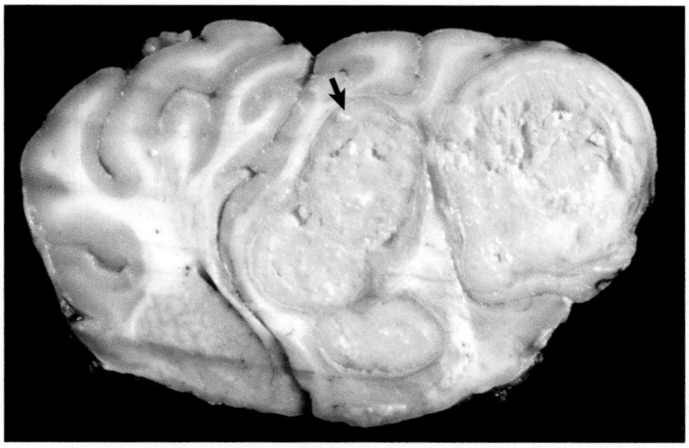

Fig. 14-40 Chronic cerebral abscesses, sheep. Abscesses with caseous centers *(arrow)* have replaced most of the right cerebral hemisphere, enlarged it, and displaced the midline to the left. The abscesses are encapsulated by a thick fibrous capsule generated by fibroblasts of the pia and perivascular spaces of the outer cortex. (Courtesy Dr. M.D. McGavin, College of Veterinary Medicine, University of Tennessee.)

Brain abscesses can arise in some food animal species from an extension of otitis interna (see Fig. 14-29). These animals often display evidence of facial nerve paralysis, such as a drooping ear. The cerebellopontine angle and adjacent structures are the common locations for such abscesses. In horses, *Streptococcus equi* (strangles) can cause brain abscesses via hematogenous spread from lymphoid tissues (Fig. 14-41). Direct penetration may also occur in small ruminants that lack frontal sinuses because of improper dehorning procedures. Brain abscesses are space-occupying lesions and as such can have a devastating effect on brain function. Depending on size and location, compression via mass effect (increased intracranial pressure) of vital structures (nuclei that regulate cardiac and respiratory rhythms) and brain displacements (cerebellar vermis, parahippocampal gyri) are two common sequelae to acute abscesses. Abscesses can occur in the spinal cord as a result of direct extension of bacterial vertebral osteomyelitis through the dura (Fig. 14-42), after tail docking in lambs, and occasionally from hematogenous spread.

Clinically, animals with brain abscesses can show abnormal mental behaviors, ataxia, head tilt, circling, and loss of vision.

Diffuse Encephalitis

Common bacteria have the potential to produce disease in the CNS by hematogenous spread and vasculitis (see the section on Neonatal Septicemia).

Ependymitis and Choroid Plexitis

Infectious agents, especially pus-forming bacteria, such as the coliform and *Streptococcus* spp., can enter the CNS hematogenously or via direct extension, invade the choroid plexuses, and be released into the CSF, gaining access to ependymal cells lining the ventricular system. Inflammation of the ependyma is called ependymitis, whereas inflammation of the choroid plexus is called choroid plexitis. Gross lesions usually consist of gray-white to yellow-green thick to gelatinous CSF within the ventricular system and choroid plexuses that are granular and gray-white, with areas of active hyperemia and hemorrhage. If the bacteria traverses through the lateral apertures of the fourth ventricle, they can enter and spread throughout the subarachnoid space, possibly inducing suppurative

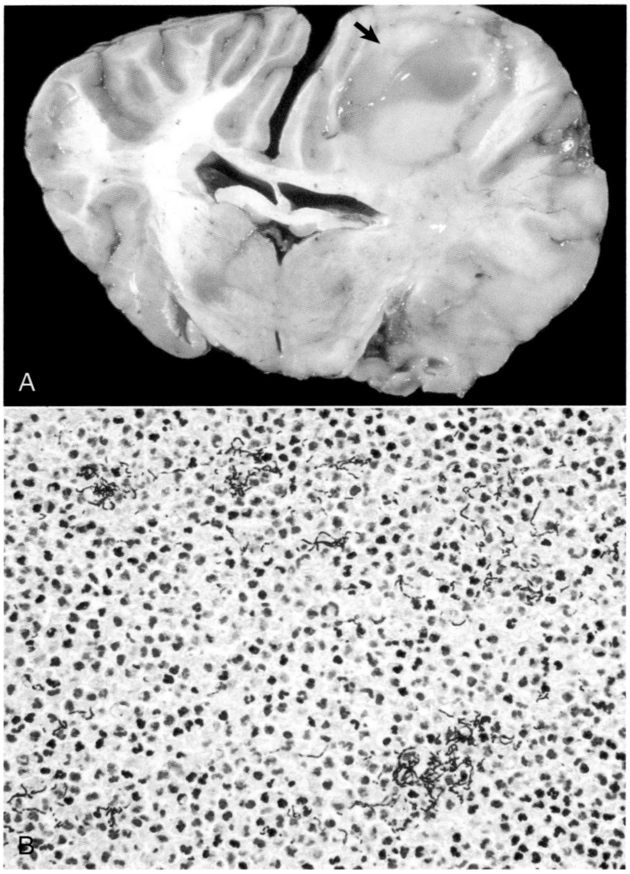

Fig. 14-41 Abscess, right cerebral hemisphere, horse.
A, The cerebral cortex contains an abscess *(arrow)* caused by *Streptococcus equi* entering the CNS via the blood (Strangles). A fibrous capsule is present on the lateral, medial, and dorsal sides of the abscess (most obvious on the lateral side as a gray band). There is no obvious capsule present on the ventral side (i.e., toward the right lateral ventricle). Microscopically, there is a thin glial capsule (astrogliosis). Note also the increased size of the right hemisphere with blurring of the distinction between gray and white matter, an indication of edema. **B,** Note the chains of Gram-positive (blue staining) cocci in the inflammatory exudate from an abscess caused by *Streptococcus zooepidemicus.* (**A** courtesy Dr. K. Read, College of Veterinary Medicine, Texas A&M University; and Noah's Arkive, College of Veterinary Medicine, The University of Georgia. **B** courtesy Dr. J.F. Zachary, College of Veterinary Medicine, University of Illinois.)

bacterial leptomeningitis. The exudate can also obstruct CSF flow, leading to noncommunicating hydrocephalus. Microscopically, inflammatory cells, especially neutrophils, mixed with fibrin, hemorrhage, and bacteria, can be seen in the exudate.

Meningitis

Meningitis refers to inflammation of the meninges (Fig. 14-43). In animals, meningitis is most commonly caused by bacteria such as *Escherichia coli* and *Streptococcus* spp. that traverse to the leptomeninges and subarachnoid space hematogenously. Bacteria can also spread to the meninges by direct extension and leukocytic trafficking. In common usage, the term meningitis generally refers to inflammation of the leptomeninges (the pia mater, subarachnoid space, and adjacent arachnoid mater) in contrast to inflammation of the dura mater, which is referred to as pachymeningitis. Leptomeningitis can be acute, subacute, or chronic and, depending on the cause, suppurative, eosinophilic, nonsuppurative, or granulomatous.

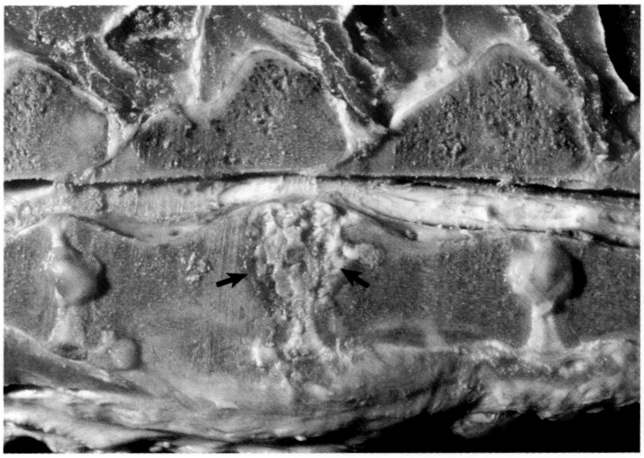

Fig. 14-42 Diskospondylitis, thoracic spinal cord, pig.
This type of abscess *(arrows)* is commonly caused by bacterial emboli that lodge in intervertebral disks or in the body of vertebrae causing osteomyelitis, which can extend into intervertebral disks. Large intervertebral abscesses can compress the spinal cord and cause Wallerian degeneration of nerves, mainly in the ventral funiculi but also in other funiculi. In this case, remodeling and proliferation of the vertebral bone secondary to the infection also contributed to the narrowing of the spinal canal and compression of the spinal cord. (Courtesy Dr. M.D. McGavin, College of Veterinary Medicine, University of Tennessee.)

Inflammation of specific parts of the dura mater of the cranial cavity can occur in the external periosteal dura after osteomyelitis, formation of extradural abscesses and pituitary abscesses, and skull fracture and involve the inner dura in association with leptomeningitis. Abscesses of the pituitary fossa occur with some frequency in cattle. Bacteria isolated from the cases include *Pasteurella multocida* and *Actinomyces pyogenes*. The abscess can result from spread of infection arising in the caudal nasal cavity or sinuses, possibly through direct extension or through the venous circulation. Incision of the pituitary fossa releases a thick viscous opaque tan to yellow exudate, which can elevate the dura mater surrounding the fossa. Infection can extend via the infundibular recess of the third ventricle into the ventricular system, resulting in ventriculitis, ependymitis, and empyema. Systemic bacterial infections in neonates are a common cause of acute meningitis (leptomeningitis), which are suppurative and fibrinous. In animals, leptomeningitis secondary to a selective viral infection only of the leptomeninges is very rare and is usually seen in combination with viral-induced encephalitides.

Neonatal Septicemia

Neonatal septicemia typically involves *Escherichia coli, Streptococcus* spp., *Salmonella* spp., *Pasteurella* spp., and *Haemophilus* spp. The release of endotoxins and bacterial cell wall components, such as lipopolysaccharide (LPS), teichoic acid, and proteoglycans, in the CNS vasculature leads to the secretion of cytokines (tumor necrosis factor [TNF], interleukin [IL], platelet-activating factor [PAF], prostaglandins, thromboxane, and leukotrienes) from the endothelium and trafficking CNS macrophages, followed by adhesion of neutrophils, injury to the endothelium and blood-brain barrier, and vasculitis resulting initially in brain swelling and brain edema and increased intracranial pressure.

Although there are differences in the diseases caused by these organisms, they tend to produce fibrinopurulent inflammation of membranous tissues (serosal surfaces) of the body. Leptomeninges, choroid plexus, and ependyma of the CNS—sites often preferentially involved in hematogenous spread of bacteria, synovium, uvea,

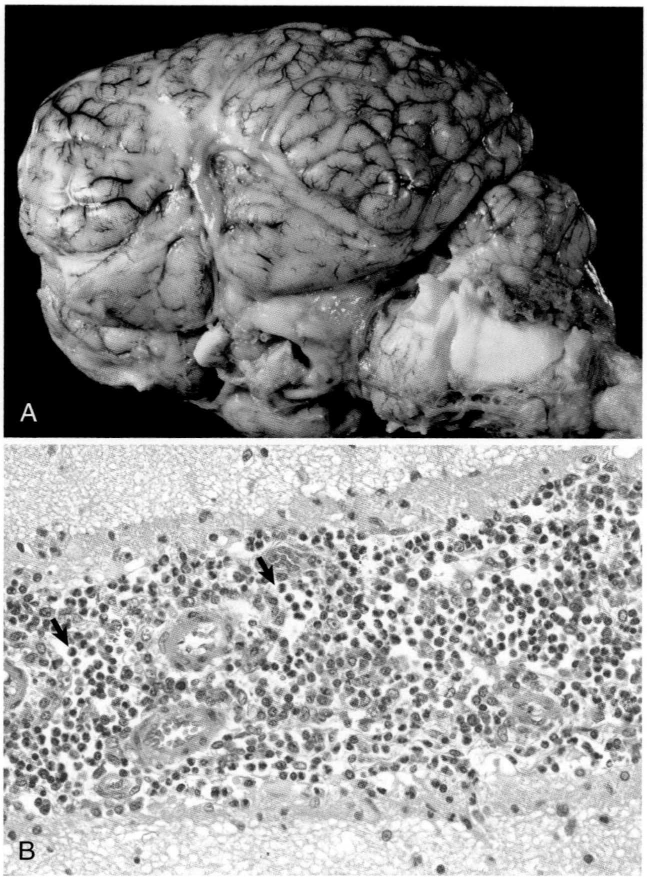

Fig. 14-43 **Suppurative bacterial meningitis, cerebral hemispheres, horse.**
A, Pale yellow-white thick exudate composed principally of neutrophils admixed with bacteria, cellular debris, edema fluid, and fibrin is present in the subarachnoid space on the lateral surface and also in the sulci. Overall the gyri are flattened, indicating brain swelling and compression. **B,** The arachnoid space of the leptomeninges in this sulcus contains a mixture of neutrophils *(arrows),* other mononuclear inflammatory cells, cellular debris, edema fluid, and fibrin. H&E stain. (**A** courtesy Dr. M.D. McGavin, College of Veterinary Medicine, University of Tennessee. **B** courtesy Dr. J.F. Zachary, College of Veterinary Medicine, University of Illinois.)

and the serosal lining of body cavities—can be affected in various combinations. Infections are often acquired perinatally, and onset is usually within a few days of birth up to 2 weeks (Box 14-7). The initial portal of entry can be oral; intrauterine; umbilical; or surgical, via postsurgical procedures such as castration and ear notching; or via the respiratory system, but the bacteria eventually spread to the CNS hematogenously.

Gross CNS lesions are commonly present and include congestion, hemorrhage, and diffuse to focal cloudiness or opacity in the leptomeninges, resulting in a leptomeningitis caused by accumulation of exudates (see Fig. 14-43). The ventricles contain fibrin, usually as a thin layer on the ependymal surface or as a pale coagulum in the CSF of the ventricular lumen, secondary to a choroid plexitis and/or ependymitis.

Microscopic lesions vary according to the organism. With the exception of *Salmonella* spp., the lesions consist of deposits of fibrin and an infiltration of mainly neutrophils in and around the blood vessels and capillaries of the leptomeninges, choroid plexus, and ependymal or subependymal areas of the brain. The epithelium of the choroid plexus and ependymal lining of the ventricles can be disrupted by cellular degeneration, disorganization, and necrosis, and this inflammation can extend into the adjacent CNS. A vasculitis with thrombosis and hemorrhage can be associated with lesions caused by *Escherichia coli.* Lesions caused by *Salmonella* spp. are not limited to the perinatal period. CNS involvement in salmonellosis is generally limited to foals and pigs and in contrast to the above infections, the leukocytic response tends to have a greater proportion of macrophages and lymphocytes, often to the extent that the inflammation is designated histiocytic or granulomatous. This difference presumably reflects the fact that *Salmonella* spp. can be facultative pathogens of the monocyte-macrophage system. As is true in other tissues, vasculitis, thrombosis, necrosis, and hemorrhage often accompany *Salmonella* infections of the CNS. *Haemophilus parasuis*, which causes Glasser's disease, is also a frequent cause of leptomeningitis, polyserositis, and polyarthritis in 8- to 16-week-old pigs. Again, lesions are as previously noted with fibrinopurulent inflammation involving the leptomeninges, serosal linings of body cavities, and joints.

Bacterial infection with CNS and visceral involvement occurs in neonatal pigs and through the weaning period. These diseases are deserving of special mention because of the incidence and stereotyped nature of the infections. Several strains of *Streptococcus suis* are capable of causing disease. Type 1 strains generally cause disease in suckling pigs ranging in age from 1 to 6 weeks, whereas type 2 strains affect older pigs 6 to 14 weeks old. Type 2 strains are recognized as one of the more important serotypes, causing meningitis not only in pigs but also in humans, particularly those working with pigs or handling porcine tissues. Other serotypes and untypable strains can also cause systemic disease that results in leptomeningitis, choroid plexitis, and ependymitis. Extension to involve cranial nerve roots or the central canal of the cervical spinal cord also occurs. The character of the inflammation is

BOX 14-7 CNS Bacterial Infections in Young Animals

CALF
Escherichia coli: leptomeningitis, choroiditis, ependymitis and ventriculitis, synovitis, ophthalmitis, and perioptic neuritis
Pasteurella/Mannheimia spp.: leptomeningitis, ependymitis and ventriculitis
Streptococcus spp.: leptomeningitis, synovitis, ophthalmitis

FOAL
Escherichia coli: leptomeningitis, ventriculitis, polyserositis, synovitis
Streptococcus spp.: leptomeningitis, polyserositis, synovitis
Salmonella typhimurium: leptomeningitis, ependymitis and ventriculitis, choroiditis, synovitis

LAMB
Escherichia coli: leptomeningitis, ependymitis and ventriculitis, peritonitis, synovitis
Pasteurella/Mannheimia spp.: leptomeningitis

PIG
Escherichia coli: leptomeningitis, ophthalmitis
Haemophilus parasuis: leptomeningitis, polyserositis, synovitis
Streptococcus suis type I and II: leptomeningitis, choroiditis, ependymitis, cranial neuritis, myelitis
Salmonella choleraesuis: leptomeningitis, ophthalmitis

TABLE 14-3 Viruses Causing CNS Disease in Domestic Animals

Virus Group	Disease	Type of Injury
Arbovirus	Equine encephalomyelitis	Encephalitis/myelitis/meningitis/vasculitis
	Japanese encephalitis	Encephalitis/myelitis/meningitis
	Louping ill	Encephalitis/myelitis/meningitis
	West Nile viral encephalomyelitis	Encephalitis/myelitis
	Wesselsbron virus	Malformations
Bunyavirus	Akabane disease	Malformations/encephalitis
	Arthrogryposis hydranencephaly complex (Cache Valley fever)	Malformations/encephalitis
	Rift Valley fever	Malformations/encephalitis
Coronavirus	Feline infectious peritonitis	Vasculitis/encephalitis/myelitis/meningitis
	Hemagglutinating encephalomyelitis	Encephalitis/myelitis/meningitis/ganglioneuritis
Enterovirus	Enterovirus-induced porcine polioencephalomyelitis	Encephalitis/myelitis
Herpesvirus	Equine herpesvirus 1 myeloencephalopathy	Encephalitis/myelitis/meningitis/vasculitis
	Bovine malignant catarrhal fever	Encephalitis/myelitis/meningitis/vasculitis
	Infectious bovine rhinotracheitis	Encephalitis
	Pseudorabies	Encephalitis/myelitis/meningitis
Lentivirus	Visna	Encephalitis/myelitis/demyelination
	Caprine leukoencephalomyelitis-arthritis	Encephalitis/myelitis/demyelination
Orbivirus	Blue tongue	Malformations/encephalitis
Paramyxovirus	Canine distemper	Demyelination/encephalitis/myelitis
	Old-dog encephalitis	Encephalitis/demyelination/meningitis/vasculitis
Parvovirus	Feline panleukopenia virus	Malformations/meningitis
Pestivirus	Classical swine fever	Malformations/hypomyelination/encephalitis/ meningitis/vasculitis
	Bovine viral diarrhea	Malformations/meningitis/dysmyelination
	Border disease	Malformations/hypomyelination
Polyomavirus	Progressive multifocal leukoencephalopathy	Demyelination
Rhabdovirus	Rabies	Encephalitis/myelitis/meningitis/vasculitis/ ganglioneuritis
Unassigned viruses	Borna disease	Encephalitis/myelitis

fibrinopurulent, and necrotic foci can be found in brainstem, cerebellum, and anterior spinal cord.

Clinically, affected animals are initially ataxic and then become laterally recumbent with rhythmic paddling of the limbs. As the disease progresses, they may become comatose and die.

Viruses

The viruses causing CNS disease in domestic animals are listed in Table 14-3.

Arboviruses

Japanese encephalitis

See Web Appendix 14-1.

Louping ill

See Web Appendix 14-1.

Herpesviruses

Encephalitic herpes viruses, members of the subfamily Alphaherpesvirinae, cause cell injury through (1) necrosis of infected neurons and glial cells, (2) necrosis of infected endothelial cells, and (3) secondary effects of inflammation, cytokines, and chemokines. Although necrosis appears to be the principal mechanism for cell injury, recent studies indicate that bovine herpesvirus–induced apoptotic cell death can occur.

Neurotropic herpes viruses enter the CNS principally by retrograde axonal transport; however, entry by hematogenous spread via viremia and leukocytic trafficking may occur. These viruses also have a unique survival mechanism that allows them to hide in a latent form in nervous tissue, for example, in trigeminal ganglion of pigs infected with pseudorabies virus. Stress or other factors can activate latent virus resulting in encephalitis.

Rhabdoviruses

Rabies encephalitis

Rabies virus (family Rhabdoviridae) is one of the most neurotropic of all viruses infecting mammals. It is generally transmitted by a bite from an infected animal; however, respiratory infection has also been uncommonly reported after exposure to virus in bat caves, accidental human laboratory exposure, and corneal transplants.

The proposed mechanism for spread of rabies virus from the inoculation site to the CNS is illustrated in Fig. 14-44. Rabies virus may first replicate locally at the site of inoculation. Infection of and replication in local skeletal muscle myocytes may be an important initiating event. The virus then enters peripheral nerve terminals by binding to nicotinic acetylcholine receptors at the neuromuscular junction. The probability is greater that the virus will be taken up by both axon terminals and myocytes after a large inoculation dose. If the virus directly enters peripheral nerve terminals, the incubation period will more likely be short, regardless of whether muscle cells are infected. With progressively lower doses of virus, however, there is a greater possibility that the virus will enter either nerve terminals or myocytes but not both. This situation can result in a short incubation period if the virus directly enters nerve terminals as described previously or could result in a more prolonged incubation period if there was initial infection

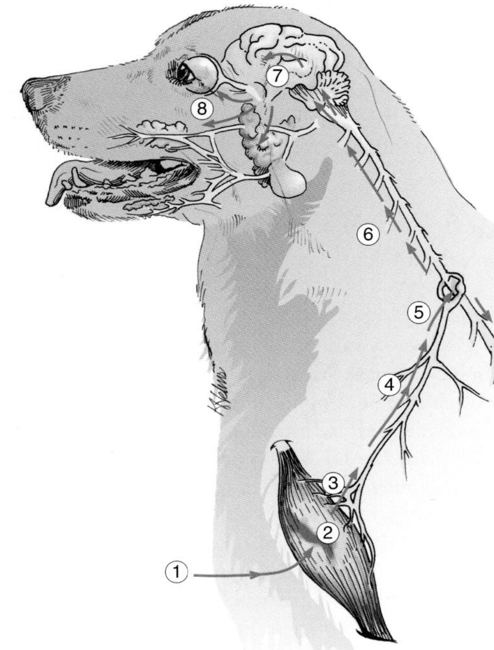

Fig. 14-44 Rabies pathogenesis.
After a bite wound, *1,* the rabies virus initially replicates in muscle (can enter peripheral nerves directly), *2,* enters, *3,* and ascends (retrograde axonal transport) the peripheral nerve *4,* to the dorsal root ganglion, *5,* enters the spinal cord *6,* and ascends *7,* to the brain via ascending and descending nerve fiber tracts, infects brain cells, spreads to salivary glands *8,* and the eye and is excreted in saliva. (Courtesy Dr. J.F. Zachary, College of Veterinary Medicine, University of Illinois. Based on an illustration from Robinson PA: Rabies virus. In Belshe RB, editor: *Textbook of human virology,* ed 2, St Louis, 1991, Mosby.)

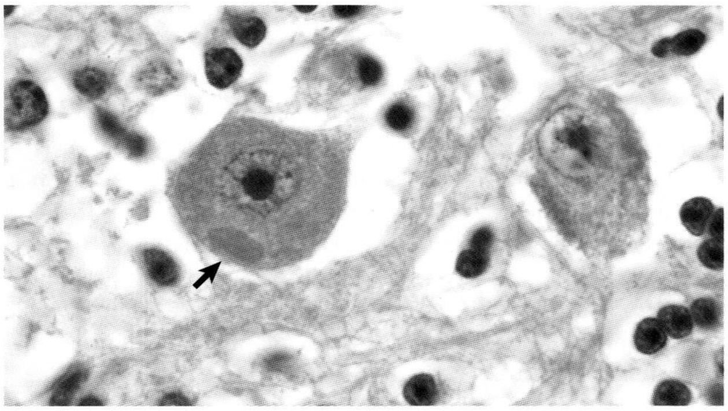

Fig. 14-45 Rabies, Negri body, cerebellum, Purkinje cell, cow.
A large pale red (eosinophilic) inclusion (Negri body) is present in the cytoplasm of the neuron cell body *(arrow).* In the cow, Negri bodies are seen in Purkinje cells and in other neurons, such as those of the red nucleus and cerebral cortex. H&E stain. (Courtesy Dr. M.D. McGavin, College of Veterinary Medicine, University of Tennessee.)

and retention of virus in myocytes before its release and uptake by nerve terminals.

The virus moves from the periphery to the CNS by fast retrograde axoplasmic transport, apparently via sensory or motor nerves, at a rate of 12 to 100 mm per day. Experimental data suggest that rabies virus phosphoprotein interacts with dynein LC8, a microtubule motor protein used in retrograde axonal transport. With sensory axons, the first cell bodies to be encountered after inoculation of a rear leg would be those of spinal ganglia, whose neuronal processes extend to the dorsal horn of the spinal cord. For motor axons, the cell bodies of the lower motor neurons in ventral horn gray matter or neuronal cell bodies of the autonomic ganglia are the ones initially infected. It is not known whether viral infection and replication in neurons of dorsal root ganglia are essential for infection of the CNS. The virus then moves into the spinal cord and ascends to the brain using both anterograde and retrograde axoplasmic flow. During the spread of the virus between neurons within the CNS, there is also simultaneous centrifugal movement via anterograde axonal transport of the virus peripherally from the CNS to axons of cranial nerves. This process results in infection of various tissues, including the oral cavity and salivary glands, permitting transmission of the disease in the saliva. An additionally important feature of rabies is that infection of nervous and nonnervous tissue, such as the salivary glands, occur at the same time, which permits affected animals to have the required aggressive behavior plus passage of the virus into the saliva to facilitate the transmission of the disease.

The results of recent experimental studies have helped clarify the mechanism by which the virus spreads within the CNS. After axoplasmic spread of the virus from an inoculated rear leg to neurons of the associated segments of the spinal cord, rapid spread of infection to the brain occurs via long ascending and descending fiber tracts, bypassing the gray matter of the rostral spinal cord. This early spread of the virus has been suggested to explain how induction of behavioral changes occurs before there is sufficiently severe injury to cause paralysis and allows dissemination of infection before there is time for a notable immune response. Spread of infection within neurons of the CNS recently has been proposed to occur via both anterograde and retrograde axoplasmic flow, with corresponding neuron-to-neuron spread by axosomatic-axodendritic and somatoaxonal-dendroaxonal transfer of virus. Transsynaptic spread can occur by budding of developing virions from the neuronal cytoplasm (cell body or dendrite) into a synapsing axon or in the form of bare viral nucleocapsid (ribonucleoprotein-transcriptase complexes) in the absence of a complete virion.

In vivo experimental studies using a laboratory strain of rabies virus showed that the virus caused a downregulation of about 90% of genes in the brain at more than fourfold lower levels. Affected genes were those involved in regulation of cell metabolism, protein synthesis, and growth and differentiation. Other experimental studies have shown increased quantities of nitric oxide in brains of rabies-infected animals, suggesting that nitric oxide neurotoxicity may mediate neuronal dysfunction. Finally, the rabies virus has been shown to induce apoptotic cell death of brain neurons in mouse models. The exact mechanism of rabies virus–induced neuronal injury in domestic and wildlife species remains to be fully determined.

Gross lesions of the infected central nervous tissue are often absent. Microscopic lesions of the CNS are typically lymphomonocytic (nonsuppurative) and include a variable leptomeningitis and perivascular cuffing with lymphocytes, macrophages, and plasma cells; microgliosis, which sometimes is prominent; variable, but often not severe, neuronal degeneration; and ganglioneuritis. Occasional and slight infection can also involve the leptomeninges, ependyma, oligodendroglia, and astrocytes. Emphasis should be given to the fact that infected neurons often are minimally altered morphologically. Neurons can also contain intracytoplasmic acidophilic (pale red to red) inclusions called Negri bodies (Fig. 14-45). Also, dogs are reported to have a tendency to develop a more severe inflammatory reaction than other species, such as the cow, in which little if any inflammation might occur. Nonneural lesions include variable nonsuppurative sialitis accompanied by necrosis and presence of Negri bodies in canine salivary epithelial cells.

Negri bodies, formed within neurons of the CNS and even in the cranial trigemina, spinal, and autonomic ganglia, have long been the hallmark of rabies infection, although they are not present in all cases. The inclusions are intracytoplasmic and initially develop as an aggregation of strands of viral nucleocapsid, which rather quickly transforms into an ill-defined granular matrix. Mature rabies virions, which bud from the nearby endoplasmic reticulum, can also be located around the periphery of the matrix. With time, the Negri body becomes larger and detectable by light microscopy. Classically, in H&E stained sections, the Negri body, which is eosinophilic, has one or more small, light clear areas called *inner bodies* that form as a result of invagination of cytoplasmic components (that include virions) in the matrix of the inclusion. Inclusions that do not possess "inner bodies" have been referred to as Lyssa bodies, but they are actually Negri bodies without cytoplasmic indentation. It should also be noted that both fixed viruses (adapted to the CNS by passage) and street viruses (that produce the naturally occurring disease) produce the same ultrastructural features, but fixed viral strains generally cause severe neuronal degeneration that precludes the development and thus the detection of Negri bodies. Negri bodies also tend to occur more frequently in large neurons such as the pyramidal neurons of the hippocampus, neurons of the medulla oblongata, and Purkinje cells of the cerebellum. Also, inclusions are frequently present in neurons not located in areas of inflammation. Therefore the preferred tissues for rabies examination by light microscopy and by florescent antibody technique for virus include hippocampus, cerebellum, medulla, and the trigeminal ganglion.

A spongiform lesion, indistinguishable qualitatively from the lesion characteristic for several of the spongiform encephalopathies, was described for the first time in 1984 by Charlton. This lesion was initially detected in experimental rabies in skunks and foxes and later in the naturally occurring disease in the skunk, fox, horse, cow, cat, and sheep. The lesion occurs in the neuropil of the gray matter, especially of the thalamus and cerebral cortex, initially as intracytoplasmic membrane-bound vacuoles in neuronal dendrites and less commonly in axons and astrocytes. The vacuoles enlarge, compress surrounding tissue, and ultimately rupture, forming a tissue space. Although the mechanism responsible for the development of this lesion has not been determined, it is thought to result from an indirect effect of the rabies virus on neural tissue (possibly involving an alteration of neurotransmitter metabolism).

The clinical signs in domestic animals are similar with some differences between species. The clinical disease in the dog has been divided into three phases: prodromal, excitatory, and paralytic. In the prodromal phase, which lasts 2 to 3 days, the animal can have a subtle change in temperament. *Furious rabies* refers to animals in which the excitatory phase is predominant, and *dumb rabies* refers to animals in which the excitatory phase is extremely short or absent and the disease progresses quickly to the paralytic phase. Cattle and carnivores generally have the furious form of rabies, and affected animals are restless and aggressive. Other somewhat unique signs of cattle with rabies include bellowing, general straining, tenesmus, and signs of sexual excitement followed by paralysis and death. Mules, sheep, and pigs usually have the excitatory form of rabies. Horses can have early signs that are atypical for a neurologic disease but terminally tend to have the excitatory form.

When conducting a necropsy on an animal suspected of having rabies, it is important to remember (1) to provide additional protection (double-gloves, mask, eye protection, and proper ventilation) for the prosector above those used for routine postmortem examination and (2) to collect the appropriate CNS tissues (hippocampus, cerebellum, and medulla and optionally the spinal cord) for examination by immunofluorescence and sometimes mouse inoculation. The remainder of the brain should be fixed by immersion in 10% neutral buffered formalin for histopathologic examination.

Bornaviruses

Borna disease

See Web Appendix 14-1.

Fungi and Algae

Infection of the CNS by a variety of fungi and algae has been reported in domestic animals. Most reported cases are isolated occurrences and often represent opportunistic infection in immunocompromised individuals. Rare infections have involved genera such as *Aspergillus, Candida,* and *Mucor*; dematiaceous fungi; and the blue-green algae, *Prototheca.* These infections do not have a predilection for the nervous system. Of the systemic fungi, CNS infections have occurred with *Coccidioides immitis, Blastomyces dermatitidis, Histoplasma capsulatum,* and *Cryptococcus neoformans*, but only *Cryptococcus neoformans* has a particular affinity for the CNS and is covered in a later section. These agents reach the CNS by leukocytic trafficking and hematogenous spread from primary sites of infection located in other areas (lung) of the body.

This group of pathogens usually elicits, as characterized by *Blastomyces dermatitidis,* a granulomatous to pyogranulomatous inflammatory response (Fig. 14-46). This response can be locally extensive, or distinct granulomas can form in the CNS and meninges. Grossly, CNS lesions consist of moderately well-demarcated expansile yellow-brown foci that displace and disrupt normal tissue (Fig. 14-47). Microscopically, the exudate consists of neutrophils, macrophages (epithelioid type), and multinucleated giant cells. The latter two cell types may contain organisms in their cytoplasm. *Blastomyces dermatitidis* organisms are broad-based, budding, spherical yeastlike organisms 8 to 25 mm in diameter (Fig. 14-48). The inflammatory response, including cells (granulomatous inflammatory cells) and cytokines, leads to the axonal, neuronal, and myelin disruption observed in these mycotic diseases.

CNS infections with *Coccidioides immitis* or *Histoplasma capsulatum* elicit an inflammatory response similar to that which occurs in *Blastomyces dermatitidis.* In coccidioidomycosis, the organisms

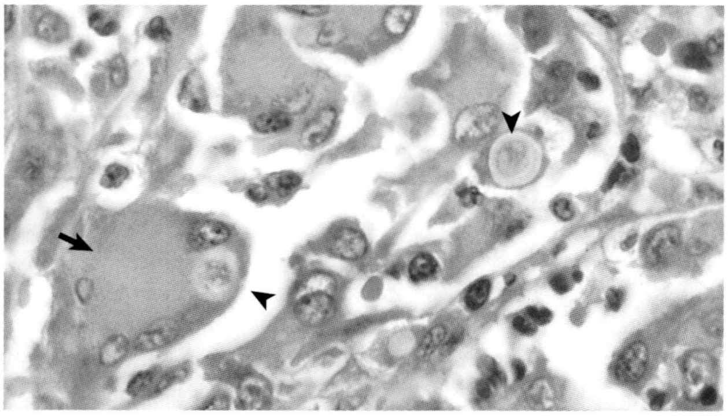

Fig. 14-46 Granulomatous encephalitis, blastomycosis, brain, dog. This inflammatory response, consisting of a mixture of macrophages, multinucleated giant cells *(arrow)*, lymphocytes, varying numbers of neutrophils, and occasional plasma cells, is typical of CNS infections by fungi and algae. *Blastomyces dermatitidis* organisms are present in the exudate and within macrophages and giant cells *(arrowheads)*. H&E stain. (Courtesy Dr. J.F. Zachary, College of Veterinary Medicine, University of Illinois.)

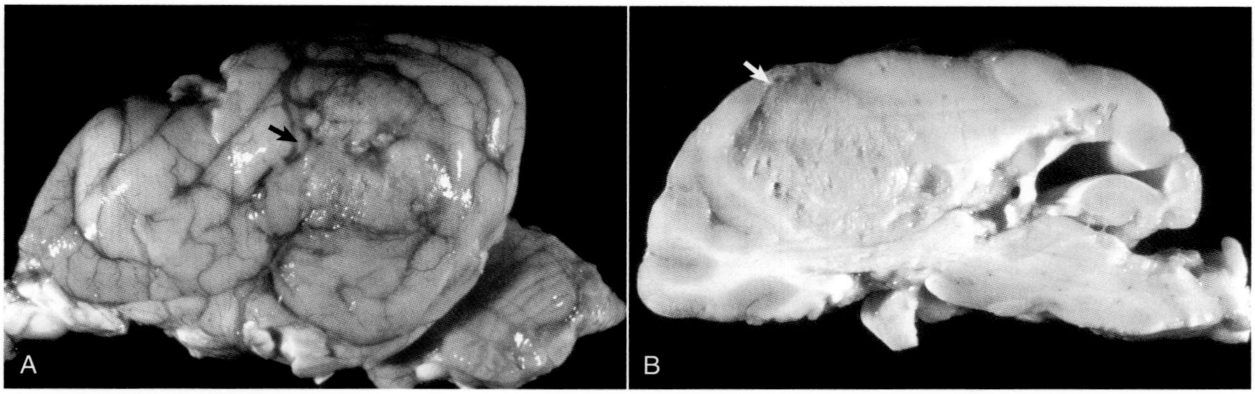

Fig. 14-47 Blastomycosis, cerebrum, dog.
A, The subarachnoid space (leptomeninges) of the left cerebral hemisphere (parietal-temporal lobes) contains a locally extensive focus (granuloma) of granulomatous inflammation caused by *Blastomyces dermatitidis (arrow)* with extension into subjacent cortex. **B,** A parasagittal section of a similar lesion from another dog shows a moderately well-demarcated granuloma in the white matter of the frontoparietal cortex *(arrow).* (Courtesy College of Veterinary Medicine, University of Illinois.)

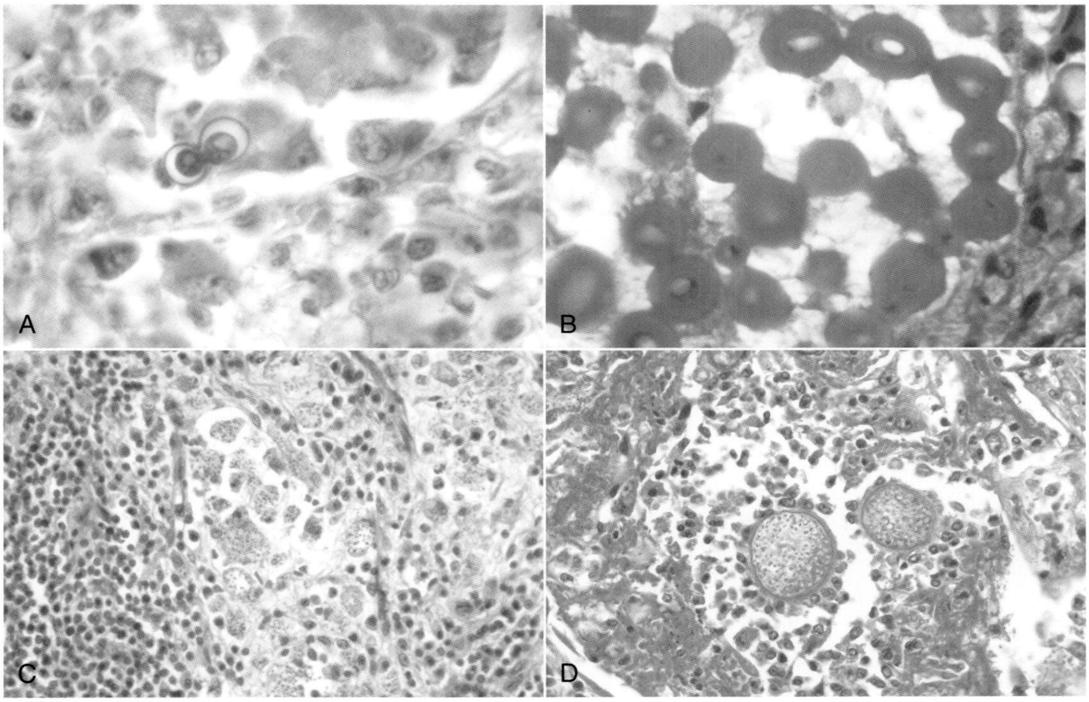

Fig. 14-48 Morphology of fungi that may infect the CNS.
A, *Blastomyces dermatitidis,* 8 to 25 mm in diameter, broad-based budding spherical yeastlike organisms, intracellular or extracellular location. H&E stain. **B,** *Cryptococcus neoformans.* In this illustration, the organism is surrounded by a mucinous capsule that is stained with Mayer's mucicarmine. The capsule varies in width, but can be so thick as to give the organism an overall diameter of 30 mm. The organism without its capsule is 5 to 20 mm in diameter. The capsule does not stain with H&E, thus causing the organism to appear to be surrounded by a clear halo (see Fig. 14-50, *A*). The organisms are oval to spherical, but may be crescentic or cup shaped in routine mucicarmine and H&E stained sections. Dehydration that occurs during processing of the tissue to embed it in paraffin causes this shrinkage and distortion. Mayer's mucicarmine stain, aqueous wet mount. **C,** *Histoplasma capsulatum,* located intracellularly, is spherical to elongated, 5 to 6 mm in diameter. H&E stain. **D,** *Coccidioides immitis,* spherules (20 to 30 mm in diameter) containing endospores (<5 mm in diameter), can be intracellular or extracellular. H&E stain. (Courtesy Dr. M.D. McGavin, College of Veterinary Medicine, University of Tennessee.)

are extracellular and/or intracellular spherules (20 to 30 mm in diameter) containing endospores (<5 μm in diameter), whereas in histoplasmosis, the organism principally is located intracellularly and is 5 to 6 mm in diameter. The microscopic features of these fungi are compared in Fig. 14-48.

Cryptococcus Neoformans

Cryptococcosis, most commonly occurring in cats, dogs, and horses, is caused by *Cryptococcus neoformans.* This pathogen enters the leptomeninges and subarachnoid space by direct extension through the cribriform plate after a nasal or sinus infection or hematogenously by leukocytic trafficking usually from a pulmonary infection. Leptomeningeal inflammation can also extend along the roots of cranial nerves. *Cryptococcus neoformans* secretes a thick mucopolysaccharide capsule that protects the organism from host defenses. The accumulation of the organism and its mucopolysaccharide capsule gives the leptomeninges a cloudy-to-viscous appearance. The leukocytic response can vary from sparse to granulomatous. In some infected cats, *Cryptococcus neoformans* may be present in large numbers without an inflammatory response. It is unclear whether this absence of inflammation is to the result of suppression of the immune response by the organism or a defect in the cat's immune and/or inflammatory responses to the pathogen.

Two virulence factors have been documented. First, a thick mucopolysaccharide capsule protects the organism from host defenses. Second, virulent organisms possess a biochemical pathway that can use catecholamines and that consists of a specific transport pathway and the enzyme phenoloxidase with production of a melanin or melanin-like compound through a series of oxidation-reduction reactions. This pathway can help protect the organism from oxidative damage in the brain. Both virulence factors are important for survival of the organism in the host. In addition, CSF lacks alternative pathway complement components that bind to the organism's carbohydrate capsule and facilitate phagocytosis and killing by neutrophils.

Grossly in CNS tissue and the leptomeninges, multiple small "cysts" with a viscous, gelatinous appearance can be seen (Fig. 14-49). Microscopically, leptomeningeal lesions have a loosely organized, lacy appearance with often myriad cryptococcal organisms and little or no inflammation. The leptomeningeal reaction can extend along the roots of cranial nerves. Spread of the CNS infection results in ventriculitis and choroiditis. In CNS tissue, in addition to the presence of the organism and its capsule, the response can vary from being sparse to a granulomatous inflammation.

The leukocytic response consists of neutrophils, eosinophils, macrophages, giant cells, and small mononuclear cells, depending on the immune status of the host. Animals with normal immune responses usually clear the infection from nasal cavities, sinuses, and the pulmonary system before its spreads systemically. Resistance to infection is provided by cell-mediated immunity. Immunosuppression of cell-mediated immunity caused by feline immunodeficiency virus (FIV) and feline leukemia virus (FeLV) in cats and by *Ehrlichia canis* or long-term glucocorticoid therapy in dogs appear to increase susceptibility to cryptococcosis.

The yeast is spherical (2 to 10 mm in diameter), crescentic, or "cup shaped," usually surrounded by a thick nonstaining (H&E stain) capsule (1 to 30 mm in diameter), and reproduces by narrow-based buds (Fig. 14-50, *A*). Special stains, such as periodic acid–Schiff (PAS) and Gomori's methenamine silver, demonstrate the organisms readily, and the capsule can be stained with mucicarmine and Alcian blue (Fig. 14-50, *B*).

Clinically, cryptococcosis with CNS infection occurs in cats, dogs, horses, and cattle. The character of neurologic signs varies with the location of the lesions but can include depression, ataxia, seizures, paresis, and blindness.

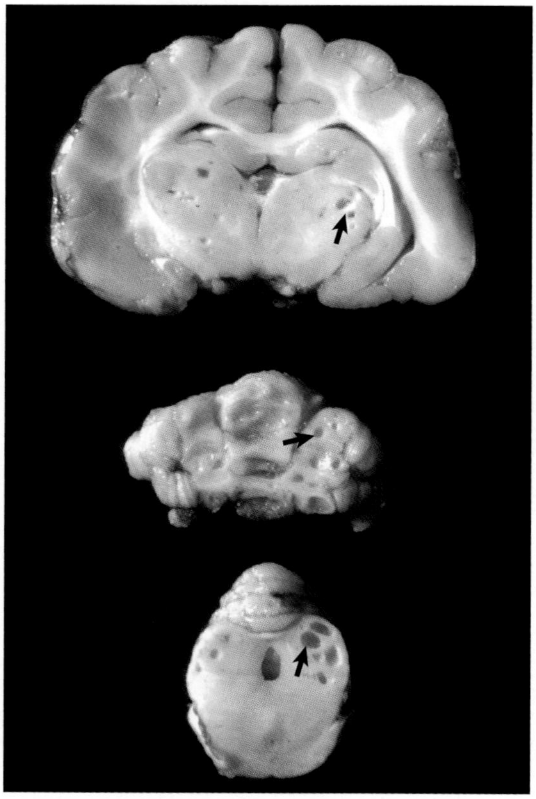

Fig. 14-49 Cryptococcosis, thalamus, cerebellum, and mesencephalon, transverse sections, cat.
Note the "cavitational" lesions caused by *Cryptococcus neoformans (arrows)*. Although the lesions look like cavities, they are filled with organisms, and the faint gray appearance is caused by the mucinous capsules of numerous cryptococci. *Cryptococcus neoformans* usually induces a granulomatous inflammation in most domestic animals, but in some animals, especially the cat, inflammation is minimal or absent. (Courtesy Dr. M.D. McGavin, College of Veterinary Medicine, University of Tennessee.)

Opportunistic Fungi

Opportunistic fungi, including those fungi in the Zygomycetes group, such as *Absidia corymbifera, Rhizomucor pusillus,* and *Rhizopus arrhizus,* and those fungi in the genus *Aspergillus,* such as *Aspergillus niger,* can invade blood vessels (angiotropic) and cause vascular thrombosis and infarcts in the CNS (Fig. 14-51). It must be noted that the term *opportunistic* implies that some form of tissue damage precedes fungal invasion. As an example, necrotizing enterocolitis caused by *Salmonella* spp. in the horse can provide an "open" vascular bed in the lamina propria of the intestinal mucosa that may be invaded by such fungi. Affected animals are often immunocompromised.

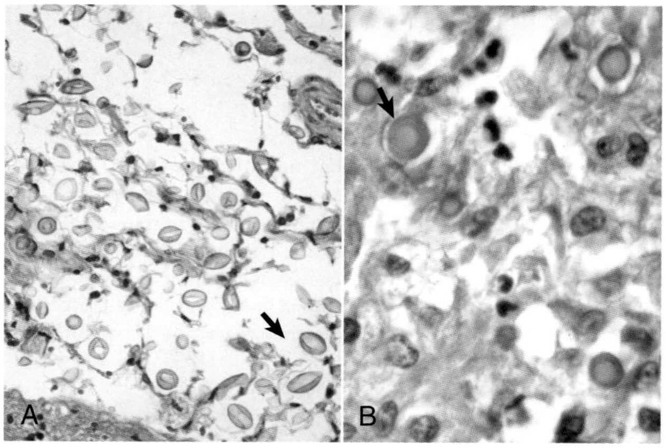

Fig. 14-50 Leptomeningeal cryptococcosis.
A, The thick unstained mucinous capsule surrounding the organism results in the formation of a clear space (halo) in H&E stained sections *(arrow)*. This feature is useful in identifying the organism in cytologic preparations and tissue sections. Also see Fig. 14-48, *B*. H&E stain. **B,** The mucinous capsule surrounding the organism also stains with mucicarmine, providing a simple method to identify the organism *(arrow)*. Mayer's mucicarmine stain. (Courtesy Dr. J.F. Zachary, College of Veterinary Medicine, University of Illinois.)

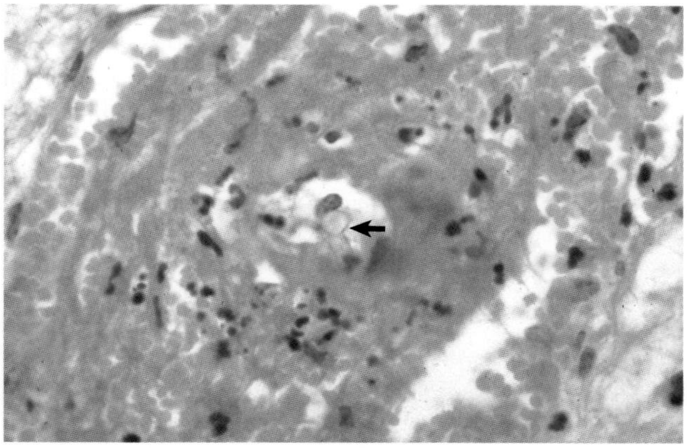

Fig. 14-51 Opportunistic angioinvasive fungi.
Fungi such as *Absidia corymbifera, Rhizomucor pusillus,* and *Rhizopus arrhizus* and fungi in the genus *Aspergillus,* such as *Aspergillus niger,* can invade blood vessels (angiotropic) and cause vascular necrosis and infarcts in the CNS. Note the vasculitis, hemorrhage, and disruption of the vessel and the fungal hyphae in the lumen *(arrow).* H&E stain. (Courtesy Dr. J.F. Zachary, College of Veterinary Medicine, University of Illinois.)

Protozoa

Neosporosis

Neosporosis, a naturally occurring or experimental disease caused by *Neospora caninum* or a Neospora-like coccidian, has been recognized in a variety of animals, including dogs, cats, cattle, sheep, and horses *(Neospora hughesi),* as well as laboratory rodents. First described in 1988 as a multisystemic infection in the dog, the organism has an affinity for the nervous system. The dog has recently been identified as the definitive host for the organism, but other hosts may exist. Some of the features of the organism are similar to those of *Toxoplasma gondii,* including division of tachyzoites by endodyogeny and having both proliferative (tachyzoites) and tissue cyst phases. However, *Neospora caninum* does not develop within a parasitophorous vacuole of a host cell, as does *Toxoplasma gondii.* This latter feature is evident only with the use of transmission electron microscopy.

Although there are morphologic differences between the organisms (*Neospora caninum* has a thicker cyst wall), differentiation by light microscopy is unreliable, and electron microscopic examination or immunohistochemistry is required. Apart from transplacental transmission proposed for a variety of species, the mechanism of infection is unknown. *Neospora caninum* can infect a variety of cell types, but outside of the CNS, it appears to have an affinity for cells of the monocyte-macrophage system. The most likely method of spread to the CNS is via leukocytic trafficking.

In the CNS, neurons and ependymal cells; mononuclear cells in the CSF; and cells of blood vessels, including endothelium, intimal connective tissue, and tunica media smooth muscle cells; can harbor organisms. Organisms have also been detected in spinal nerves. In all animals studied to date, the cyst form of *Neospora caninum* has been seen only in the CNS, whereas tachyzoites have been found in a variety of other tissue. Overall the morphologic pattern and character of lesions caused by *Neospora* spp. in the CNS are most consistent with endothelial tropism, vascular swelling and injury, tissue ischemia, and multifocal infarction.

Neurologic disease can be divided into two categories: that occurring during postnatal life and that associated with midterm to late-term abortions, the latter a notable problem in dairy cattle. Postnatal syndromes have been observed mainly in young and adult dogs, but horses are also affected. In young dogs, clinical signs are due to an ascending polyradiculoneuritis and polymyositis. In adult dogs, clinical signs are more referable to CNS lesions complicated by polymyositis, myocarditis, and dermatitis.

In horses, the pathogen causing neosporosis is *Neospora hughesi.* Clinical signs resemble those of protozoal myeloencephalitis caused by *Sarcocystis neurona.* Lesions in horses include meningoencephalomyelitis; variable vasculitis and necrosis with microgliosis; and perivascular cuffing by macrophages, multinucleated giant cells, lymphocytes, plasma cells, or neutrophils, most commonly in the gray and white matter of the spinal cord but also in the pons and medulla.

Gross lesions can involve the white and/or gray matter. Peracute gross lesions may include foci of hemorrhage and necrosis distributed in a vascular pattern. Acute lesions have the same pattern of distribution but are on cut surface granular in texture and yellow-brown to gray. In some cases the periventricular white matter may be more affected. Chronic lesions have larger areas of granular yellow-brown to gray discoloration, which often makes white matter indistinguishable from gray matter. Microscopically the lesions and their temporal occurrence are similar to those described for *Toxoplasma gondii,* including brain lesions that occur in aborted animals. *Neospora caninum* or Neospora-like organisms in lesions can be identified in tissue sections by H&E stain and immunohistochemical staining methods. Clinical signs are similar to those described for encephalitides induced by *Toxoplasma gondii.*

Toxoplasmosis

Toxoplasmosis is a disease in cats and other mammalian species caused by the obligate intracellular protozoan, *Toxoplasma gondii.* Domestic, feral, and wild cats are the definitive hosts of *Toxoplasma gondii.* Cats acquire *Toxoplasma gondii* by ingesting infective cysts, oocysts, or tachyzoites when eating infected prey, such as rodents or birds. Ingestion of one of these stages initiates the intraintestinal life cycle, which occurs only in members of the cat family. *Toxoplasma gondii* replicates and multiplies within epithelial cells of the small intestine and produces oocysts. Oocysts are released into the feces in large numbers for 2 to 3 weeks following initial ingestion of cysts, oocysts, or tachyzoites. When oocysts sporulate, usually within 5 days after passage in the feces, they become infectious for intermediate hosts. Sporulated oocysts are highly resistant and can survive in moist shaded soil or sand for months. Cats are unique in the biology of the organism, serving as both definitive (intraintestinal life cycle) and intermediate (extraintestinal life cycle) hosts.

Toxoplasma gondii can infect a wide variety of animals as intermediate hosts (extraintestinal life cycle), including fish, amphibians, reptiles, birds, humans, and many other mammals. New World monkeys and Australian marsupials are the most susceptible, whereas Old World monkeys, rats, cattle, and horses seem highly resistant.

Toxoplasma gondii can also parasitize a wide variety of cell types in the intermediate host and can cause lesions in such tissues as the lungs, lymphoid system, liver, heart, skeletal muscle, pancreas, intestine, eyes, and nervous system. After ingestion, bradyzoites from tissue cysts or sporozoites from oocysts enter intestinal epithelia and multiply. Evidence suggests active penetration of plasma membranes by organism-secreted lytic products, allowing a portal of entry rather than by uptake via phagocytosis. *Toxoplasma gondii* can then spread locally, free in lymph or intracellularly in lymphocytes, macrophages, or granulocytes to Peyer's patches and regional lymph nodes. Intracellularly, organisms multiply as tachyzoites within a parasitophorous vacuole by repeated cycles of endodyogeny during the early acute stages of infection. Dissemination to distant organs is via lymph and blood, either as free organisms or intracellularly in lymphocytes, macrophages, or granulocytes via leukocytic trafficking.

With chronicity and an increasing antibody response by the host, tachyzoites of *Toxoplasma gondii* transform into slow-growing bradyzoites that replicate in cysts within muscle. Infection of the CNS occurs hematogenously; neurons and astrocytes are the eventual target cells. The typical sequence of events in the pathogenesis of the characteristic lesion is similar to that in *Sarcocystis neurona* infection. In utero infections in animals and humans can result in CNS infection. In fetal brains, foci of necrosis are most common in the brainstem and induce the formation of microglial nodules. Additionally, foci of necrosis and mineralization occur in the cerebrocortical white matter and are caused by fetal hypoxia and ischemia resulting from severe placentitis, fetal myocardial damage, or initiation of a systemic inflammatory reaction in the fetus. In older more mature individuals, *Toxoplasma gondii* infections have been associated with immunosuppression such as occurs in concurrent CDV infection and toxoplasmosis. In some cases, this could represent activation of latent inactive *Toxoplasma gondii* cysts [bradyzoites] in neural tissues.

Immune-mediated mechanisms have been proposed to explain the vascular injury (type III hypersensitivity) and cellular or tissue necrosis (type IV hypersensitivity). Lysis of infected cells by primed cytotoxic, $CD8^+$ T lymphocytes also could potentially contribute to the tissue damage through the production of cytokines, such as interferon-γ (INF-γ), which can activate microglia and astrocytes to inhibit parasite replication and induce cytotoxic T lymphocytes to kill infected cells. This exuberant inflammatory response and the cytokine cascade that ensues to kill the organism also causes severe damage to cells in the area of inflammation, especially axons and neurons. Intracellular growth of tachyzoites also has been advanced as a cause of cellular necrosis. The organism does not produce a cytotoxin.

The blood-brain barrier of the CNS is breached when free organisms or those located intracellularly (leukocytic trafficking) infect endothelial cells of the CNS vasculature, especially capillaries. Gross lesions can involve any area of the CNS without predilection for gray or white matter, may also involve nerve rootlets, and may initially include foci of hemorrhage and necrosis and later, by granular, yellow-brown to gray foci. Peracute lesions initially include endothelial cell swelling as the result of infection by tachyzoites and vasculitis with hemorrhagic infarcts followed by vasogenic edema. If the edema is sufficiently severe to cause increased brain volume, the edema can lead to brain displacement and herniation.

Early microscopic lesions include infection of and proliferation within endothelial cells by *Toxoplasma gondii* tachyzoites. Endothelial injury results in endothelial cell swelling, endothelial cell degeneration, hemorrhage, capillary occlusion, ischemic necrosis, and edema of adjacent tissue. Subsequently, tachyzoites invade the CNS, inducing a prominent acute inflammatory response leading to necrosis and hemorrhage often striking in severity. With time, the inflammatory response consists of perivascular cuffing of blood vessels within the CNS and leptomeninges by lymphocytes and macrophages. CNS responses to injury consist of microgliosis and astrogliosis; however, these responses are often insufficient to replace the loss of tissue in the cerebral hemispheres, resulting in dilation of the lateral ventricles (hydrocephalus ex vacuo) and the formation of persistent cysts in the tissue. With chronicity and increasing inflammatory and immunologic responses by the host, tachyzoites change to slow-growing bradyzoites that replicate in and form tissue cysts. Organisms in lesions can often be identified with an H&E stain, but immunohistochemistry facilitates their detection and identification. As the infection is systemic, lesions can occur in several other tissues.

Occasionally, cysts (bradyzoites) can be observed in "normal" CNS tissue without an inflammatory or tissue lesion. These cysts are likely the result of a previous infection with *Toxoplasma gondii* that was successfully resolved. Experimental studies have confirmed that administration of corticosteroids and thus immunosuppression increases susceptibility or exacerbates the infection with *Toxoplasma gondii* or both or may contribute to the reactivation of tissue cysts.

Clinical signs can vary, depending on the age of the animal, species infected, and areas of the CNS involved and may include depression, weakness, incoordination, tremors, circling, paresis, and blindness.

Parasites

As a general concept, lesions resulting from parasitic infestation of the CNS vary in degree of severity and distribution, depending on the parasite and the host response to infection. Gross lesions of hemorrhage and malacia in parasite migratory tracts or space-occupying cysts occur with the various parasitic stages. Microscopically, there is necrosis, hemorrhage, and a leukocytic response, typically with a significant infiltrate of eosinophils. The extent of the host response is often dictated by the degree of trauma and disruption created by the parasite and the level of sensitivity of the host for parasite antigens. This section is not intended to be an extensive review of veterinary parasitology but will cover those parasites most commonly seen in veterinary practice.

Insect Larvae

Among the most common larvae are those of *Oestrus ovis* and *Hypoderma bovis*. The larvae of *Oestrus ovis* develop in the nasal cavity of sheep but can penetrate into the cranial vault through the ethmoid bone. Larvae of *Hypoderma bovis* can enter the spinal canal during their migration in the subcutis from the hoof to the dorsal midline in cattle and rarely as an aberrant parasite in the brain of horses. Damage in the CNS caused by *Hypoderma bovis* in cattle is typically the result of inflammation directed at the degenerating parasites after anthelmintic treatment. Larvae of *Cuterebra* spp., usually a parasite of rabbits and rodents, can invade the CNS of dogs and cats (see the section on Feline Ischemic Encephalopathy).

Cestodes

Coenurus cerebralis, the larval form of the dog tapeworm *Multiceps multiceps*, most commonly infests sheep and occasionally other ruminants. The larval forms presumably reach the CNS hematogenously and then cause damage during migration and encystation, forming space-occupying lesions. Another parasite for which humans are the definitive host is *Taenia solium*, with pigs being the intermediate host. The larval stage, *Cysticercus cellulosae*, generally develops in muscle of the pig but can also occur in the meninges and brain, resulting in a disease called "cysticercosis." Involvement of the CNS has been termed "neurocysticercosis."

Initially, viable cysticerci become "trapped" within capillaries of the CNS, but they do not apparently elicit an inflammatory response. At some point, the host responds immunologically and the cyst becomes denser, collapses inwardly, and disintegrates to eventually become calcified debris in a focus of inflammation. The inflammatory response has humoral and cellular components. Antibodies of the IgG family are directed against the cyst; however, cysts are likely killed by mediators released from eosinophils, which are attracted to the site by mediators released from lymphoid cells in the inflammatory exudate. For undetermined reasons, in "susceptible" animals viable cysts can become established and grow

TABLE 14-4 Nematodes Causing CNS Disease in Domestic Animals

Parasite	Normal Host	Aberrant Host
NEMATODE MIGRATION IN ABERRANT HOST		
Angiostrongylus cantonensis	Rat	Dog
Baylisascaris procyonis	Raccoon	Dog
Elaphostrongylus rangiferi	Reindeer	Sheep, goat
Parelaphostrongylus tenuis	Deer	Sheep, goat
Setaria digitata	Cattle	Sheep, goat, horse
ABERRANT NEMATODE MIGRATION IN NORMAL HOST		
Angiostrongylus vasorum	Dog (coyote)	
Dirofilaria immitis	Dog (cat)	
Stephanurus dentatus	Pig	
Strongylus spp.	Horse	

slowly for years. Viable cysticerci can cause asymptomatic infection by actively evading and suppressing the immune response of the host. These cysts cause vasogenic edema and increased intracranial pressure related to behavior as "space-occupying" masses.

Gross lesions are usually seen in the cerebral hemispheres, commonly at the interface of gray and white matter in a hematogenous pattern. Cysts can also be found in the cerebellum, medulla, ventricles, subarachnoid space, and the spinal cord. There are usually no gross changes in the CNS surrounding the cysts. Cysts are round to oval and of varied sizes and number, many of which can be large and visible up to centimeters in diameter. They have a translucent cyst wall and contain a thick, clear fluid. Within the fluid is a scolex, visible as a small 2- to 3-mm nodule. Microscopically, there is little or no inflammation or tissue injury surrounding the cysts, except for compression and edema.

Nematodes (Cerebrospinal Nematodiasis)

Aberrant migration of larval stages of nematode parasites into and through the CNS is called cerebrospinal nematodiasis. They gain access to the CNS hematogenously and actively enter the CNS by crossing the blood vessel wall through their locomotive processes. Nematodes cause damage in the cerebromedullary area of the brain and/or spinal cord either from aberrant migration in the definitive host or migration in an aberrant host (Table 14-4; Fig. 14-52). Larval stages of *Strongylus* spp. *and Baylisascaris procyonis*, for example, are typically involved, the exception being *Dirofilaria immitis,* where the adult parasite is found. Greater CNS damage is often created by the migration of the parasites in an aberrant host.

Macroscopic lesions of nematode larval migration often appear as linear or serpentine tracts of necrosis and/or hemorrhage in the tissue. Migration results in endothelial injury, vasculitis, and thrombosis, which may result in vascular occlusion and infarction. Larvae can often be found in histologic sections, and they induce a mononuclear cell inflammatory exudate, including abundant eosinophils (Fig. 14-53).

Halicephalobus (Micronema) deletrix is a free-living rhabditiform nematode that can infest the nasal cavity, CNS, and kidneys of the horse. The life cycle, pathogenesis, and route of infection of *Halicephalobus deletrix* are poorly understood. It has been proposed that the CNS is infected hematogenously in a manner similar to that described for cerebrospinal nematodiasis and that larvae penetrate skin and mucous membranes in recumbent horses with subsequent invasion of sinuses and/or blood vessels. In the CNS, microscopic lesions are prominently associated with blood vessels along which the parasite apparently migrates.

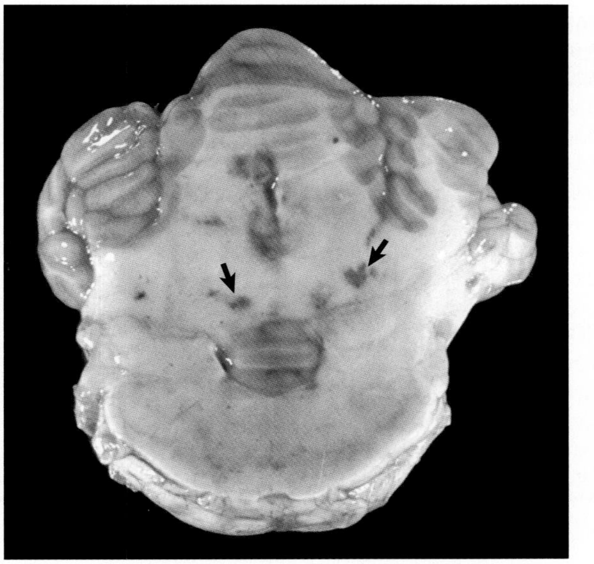

Fig. 14-52 Cerebrospinal nematodiasis, brain, cerebellum, and medulla at the level of the pons, horse.
Strongylus vulgaris migration. Several small foci of hemorrhage and necrosis in the cerebellar white matter are sites of larval migration *(arrows).* (Courtesy Dr. R. Storts, College of Veterinary Medicine, Texas A&M University.)

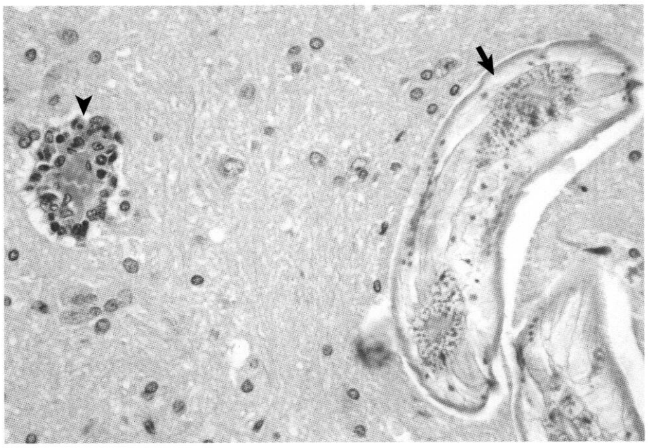

Fig. 14-53 Cerebrospinal nematodiasis, CNS, horse.
Migration of *Strongylus vulgaris* larvae *(arrow)* in the CNS elicits a perivascular lymphomonocytic inflammatory response mixed with eosinophils *(arrowhead)* and results in direct injury to blood vessels, axons, and dendrites. (Courtesy Dr. J.F. Zachary, College of Veterinary Medicine, University of Illinois.)

Prions

Transmissible Spongiform Encephalopathies

Ovine spongiform encephalopathy (scrapie), bovine spongiform encephalopathy (BSE), and human spongiform encephalopathies are classified within a group of diseases called *transmissible spongiform encephalopathies* (TSEs). Table 14-5 lists the known TSEs in animals and humans. These diseases are caused by proteinaceous infectious particles (prions) that (1) are composed of an abnormal isoform of a normal cellular protein, the prion protein (PrP^c [a 27- to 30-kD polypeptide]), designated PrP^{Sc} and (2) resist inactivation

TABLE 14-5 Transmissible Spongiform Encephalopathies (i.e., Prion Diseases)

Disease	Natural Host(s)	Prion	Pathogenic PrP Isoform
ANIMALS			
Ovine spongiform encephalopathy (scrapie)	Sheep, goats	Scrapie prion	$OvPrP^{Sc}$
Bovine spongiform encephalopathy (BSE)	Cows	BSE prion	$BoPrP^{Sc}$
Feline spongiform encephalopathy (FSE)	Cats	FSE prion	$FePrP^{Sc}$
Chronic wasting disease (CWD)	Mule deer, elk, black-tailed deer, white-tailed deer mink	CWD prion	$MdePrP^{Sc}$
Transmissible mink encephalopathy (TME)		TME prion	$MkPrP^{Sc}$
Exotic ungulate encephalopathy (EUE)	Nyala, greater kudu, oryx	EUE prion	$UngPrP^{Sc}$
HUMANS			
Kuru	Humans	Kuru prion	$HuPrP^{Sc}$
Creutzfeldt-Jakob disease (CJD)	Humans	CJD prion	$HuPrP^{Sc}$
Variant Creutzfeldt-Jakob disease (VCJD)	Humans	VCJD prion	$HuPrP^{Sc}$
Gerstmann-Sträussler-Scheinker syndrome (GSS)	Humans	GSS prion	$HuPrP^{Sc}$
Fatal familial insomnia (FFI)	Humans	FFI prion	$HuPrP^{Sc}$

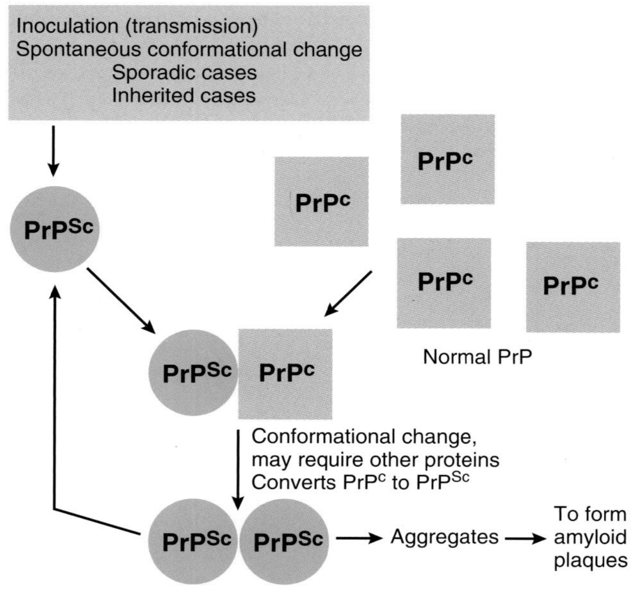

Fig. 14-54 Prion protein.
In prion diseases (spongiform encephalopathies), PrP (PrP^c), a normal neuronal protein, is converted to an abnormal β-pleated sheet isoform (PrP^{Sc}) through the interaction of PrP^{Sc} with PrP^c. (Modified from Cotran RS, Kumar V, Collins T, Robbins SL: *Robbins pathologic basis of disease,* ed 6, Philadelphia, 1999, Saunders.)

by procedures that degrade nucleic acids and proteins (i.e., heat, ultraviolet irradiation, and strong enzymes). PrP^c is expressed throughout the body and is the product of a highly conserved gene found in organisms as diverse as fruit flies and humans. The "Sc" superscript is derived from the word "scrapie" because scrapie is the prototype prion disease.

Although the mechanism by which PrP^{Sc} forms has not been completely explained, a posttranslational modification of PrP^c has been proposed (Fig. 14-54). This mechanism proposes that PrP^{Sc} acts as a template on which PrP^c undergoes a conformational change (is refolded) by a process facilitated by another protein (referred to as *protein X*), whereby the α-helical content of PrP^c diminishes and the amount of β-sheet increases, resulting in the formation of PrP^{Sc}. The features of a specific PrP^{Sc} is determined by the animal in which it is formed. When PrP^{Sc} of one species is inoculated into a different species, the recipient is less readily infected and generally has a prolonged incubation period. This resistance to infection is referred to as the *species barrier.* A review of prion biology and diseases can be found in Prusiner (2004) in the Suggested Readings on the Evolve site. Dr. Prusiner was awarded the Nobel Prize in Medicine in 1997 for his work on prion diseases.

Spongiform encephalopathies occur through horizontal transmission (scrapie-infected sheep offal fed to cows [BSE] has been proposed) and through an inherited mutation of the normal human prion gene (parent to child), resulting in the spontaneous formation of PrP^{Sc}. In animals, the primary route of infection appears to be through horizontal transmission. It has been proposed that prions ingested in infective feedstuffs enter the body through the intestine. The role of the rendering process in the pathogenesis of prion infectivity is also unclear. Prions are thought to cross the intestinal wall at Peyer's patches and are phagocytosed and transported to other lymph nodes by leukocytic trafficking. Prions replicate in lymphocytes and macrophages of the lymphoid system. Because these tissues are innervated, prions have been proposed to be transported by retrograde axonal transport to the brain; however, hematogenous spread via leukocytic trafficking may also be involved. In this example, scrapie infective ovine prions ($OvPrP^{Sc}$) accumulate in neurons and somehow result in the conversion of normal bovine prion proteins ($BoPrP^c$) in neurons to the disease-causing form, $BoPrP^{Sc}$, through a process in which a portion of the α-helical and coil structure of PrP^c is refolded into β-sheets (PrP^{Sc}). When neurons accumulate sufficient PrP^{Sc} to alter the normal function of neurons (it can take years), neurologic signs are observed.

Prion diseases are fatal. The adaptive immune system does not recognize prions as foreign; therefore no immunologic protection develops. How the accumulation of PrP^{Sc} causes neurodegeneration and neuron loss in prion diseases is not clear; however, astrocyte and microglial cell activation and apoptosis appear to be likely components of the pathway leading to neuronal injury.

No gross lesions of the nervous system are detectable in animals with spongiform encephalopathies. Microscopic lesions in scrapie-infected sheep and goats are limited to the CNS and are most commonly present in the diencephalon, brainstem, and cerebellum (cortex and deep nuclei), with variable lesions in the corpus striatum and spinal cord. Except for some minor changes, the cerebral cortex is essentially unaffected.

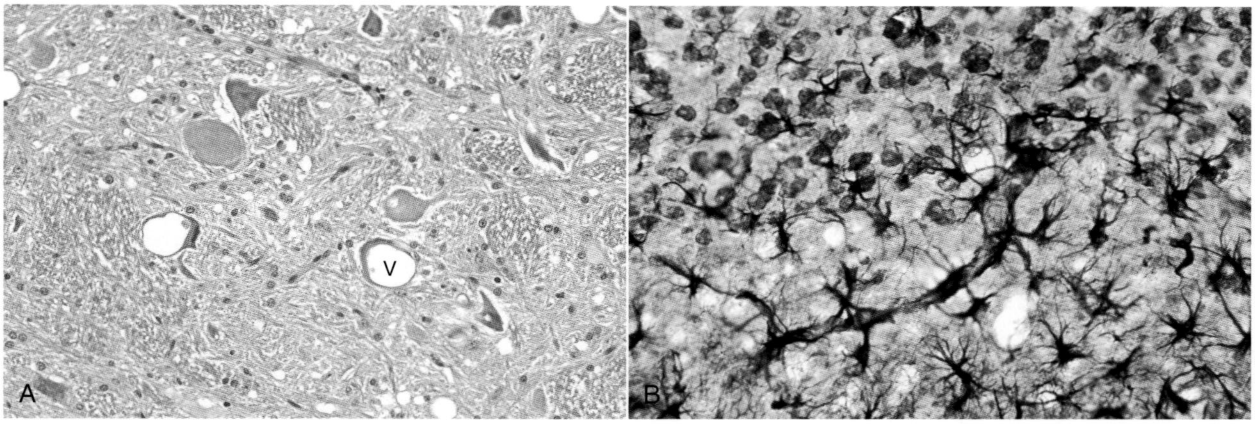

Fig. 14-55 Spongiform encephalopathy (scrapie), brain, motor neurons, sheep.
A, Neuronal cell bodies contain one or more discrete and/or coalescing clear vacuoles *(V)*. There are no inflammatory cells in this disease. Similar spongiosis is evident in the neuropil. H&E stain. **B,** Scrapie, experimental, brain, cerebellum, mouse. The cerebellar granule cells are at the top of the figure. There is notable hypertrophy and proliferation (astrocytosis) of astrocytes and their fibers (astrogliosis) *(black branching fibers)*. Some of the processes (running diagonally across the illustration) end, as is normal for astrocytes on the walls of capillaries. Cajal's gold sublimate stain for astrocytes. (**A** courtesy Dr. D. Gould, College of Veterinary Medicine and Biomedical Sciences, Colorado State University; and Dr. M. McAllister, College of Veterinary Medicine, University of Illinois. **B** courtesy Dr. W.J. Hadlow.)

The type of neuronal degeneration can vary and commonly is characterized by shrinkage with increased basophilia and cytoplasmic vacuolation (Fig. 14-55, *A*), although other changes, such as central chromatolysis and ischemic cell change, variably occur. Astrocytosis in affected areas of the brain, including the cerebellar cortex, can be severe (Fig. 14-55, *B*). There has been speculation whether the astrocytic reaction is a primary or a secondary response. An abnormal protein (prion amyloid protein) first accumulates in astroglial cells in the brain during scrapie infection, which could mean that this cell is the primary site of replication. The spongiform change tends to affect the gray matter, and greater severity of this lesion has been associated with long incubation periods. The lesion in the gray matter is the result of dilation of neuronal processes, but vacuolation of neuronal and astroglial perikarya, swelling of astrocytic processes, dilation of the periaxonal space, and splitting of myelin sheaths have also been reported. Finally, the disease is not accompanied by any notable inflammation within the CNS.

Degenerative Diseases

Metabolic

Aminoacidopathies

Two diseases characterized by errors of amino acid metabolism have been described in neonatal calves. One disease, maple syrup urine disease (MSUD), occurs in young polled Hereford and Hereford calves. The second disease, bovine citrullinemia, which was originally described in Australia, occurs in neonatal Friesian calves.

MSUD is caused by an inherited defect in branched chain ketoacid dehydrogenase enzyme complex necessary to metabolize the branched-chain amino acids leucine, isoleucine, and valine. These amino acids are essential and must be obtained from protein in the diet. After consumption, proteins are digested and the amino acids are released to be used to generate energy and for other metabolic processes. In MSUD there is a mutation in one or more of the genes that regulate this degradation process; therefore abnormal metabolites and ketoacids accumulate to toxic levels and cause disease. Urine has a sweet odor attributable to a derivative of isoleucine resembling maple syrup. In human infants, the disease is confirmed biochemically by finding elevated concentrations of leucine, isoleucine, and valine in the blood.

Gross lesions are not typically present. Microscopically, marked spongiosis, caused by vacuolation of myelin sheaths, is present throughout the neuraxis. The spongiosis affects both gray and white matter. Lesions are often most notable in areas, such as the brainstem, in which there is an intermingling of gray and white matter.

Affected calves may be normal at birth. Within a few days, depression, dullness, and weakness progress to recumbency and opisthotonus.

Bovine citrullinemia is a rare inborn error of metabolism of the urea cycle that results in a pronounced accumulation of citrulline and ammonia in the body fluids because of a failure of the normal synthesis of arginosuccinic acid by the enzyme arginosuccinate synthetase. In human infants, the disease is confirmed biochemically by finding elevated concentrations of citrulline in the blood. The cerebral lesions have also been suspected to result from the hyperammonemia or possibly some defect in excitatory neurotransmitter metabolism. However, the pathogenesis of the disease in calves remains unsettled.

Grossly, brains appear normal and have normal weights. Livers are pale yellow. Microscopically, there is fatty change in the liver. Lesions in the brain are characterized by mild-to-moderate diffuse astroglial swelling in the cerebral cortex.

Calves are normal at birth. Within a few days, a severe generalized CNS disorder develops characterized by apparent blindness, depression, and tremors that rapidly progress to seizures, coma, and death within a few hours.

Cerebral Cortical Atrophy

Brain atrophy caused by the loss of neurons in the cerebral cortex can occur in animal species but is observed most commonly in sheep with lipofuscinosis. Lipofuscin pigment, a "wear and tear" pigment associated with low-grade chronic membrane damage via lipid peroxidation, is often found in affected neurons. The cause of this lesion is unknown but thought to be related to long-term "wear and tear" on the CNS. Atrophy most frequently involves the cerebral hemispheres, especially the cortex. The cerebral hemispheres are increased in firmness and often have a tan color (lipofuscin), gyri are thinned, and the sulci widened. Microscopically, there is loss of neuron cell bodies in cortical laminae without inflammation. Astrogliosis in response to neuronal loss is also observed, as is an increased prominence of the adventitial layer of blood vessels.

Channelopathies

Channelopathies are a newly emerging group of inherited neuromuscular diseases of humans that affect the excitability of membranes of neurons and skeletal myocytes. These diseases result from mutations in genes encoding ion channel proteins that regulate calcium, sodium, and chloride channels and acetylcholine receptors. In humans, neurologic diseases, such as epilepsy and migraine headaches, have been attributed to channelopathies. In veterinary neurology, channelopathies will likely be shown in the future to be the underlying mechanism for epilepsy and other primary neuronal degenerations.

Degenerative Leukomyelopathies

Degenerative leukomyelopathies are a heterogeneous group of familial, likely inherited, and acquired diseases that have been described in dogs, cows, and horses. Although there is no universal agreement, the degenerative leukomyelopathies described here are best characterized as axonal degenerations with spheroid formation predominantly within spinal cord white matter and secondary changes in myelin sheaths and myelin loss. In dogs, familial or inherited diseases include degenerative axonopathy of Ibizan hounds, axonopathy in Labrador retrievers, and axonopathy in Jack Russell and smooth fox terriers. A disease in Rottweilers (see the section on Primary Cerebellar Neuronal Degenerations in Dogs and Cats) is another disorder with spinal cord white matter involvement that is familial and possibly inherited. An acquired disease, hound ataxia, has been described in the United Kingdom and Ireland in harrier, beagle, and foxhounds. Hound ataxia may represent a nutritional disorder in hunting dogs fed paunch (tripe). Degenerative leukomyelopathies in cattle can be inherited as an autosomal recessive trait or have a familial predisposition. Leukomyelopathies have been reported in Murray Grey, Holstein-Friesian, and in certain lines of Brown Swiss cattle. In horses, a degenerative leukomyelopathy is recognized that does not seem to have a well-defined familial or hereditary basis (see the section on Disorders of Horses).

Gross lesions are usually not observed. Microscopically, lesions in the white matter of the spinal cord are bilaterally symmetrical and consist of axonal degeneration with formation of spheroids, loss of axons, and secondary myelin degradation. Depending on the species or breed affected, lesions can involve any of the funiculi. Spinocerebellar tracts in the dorsolateral aspects of the lateral and septomarginal areas of ventral funiculi are commonly affected, as is the fasciculus gracilis in the dorsal funiculus. Severe involvement of the dorsal spinocerebellar tracts can extend into the caudal brainstem and via caudal cerebellar peduncles to the cerebellar cortex and Purkinje cells. In some species and breeds, there can also be involvement of additional specific brainstem structures.

Age of onset varies with the familial or inherited disorders. Paresis, ataxia, and dysmetria are the predominant clinical signs.

Epileptic Brain Damage

Brain damage caused by prolonged (usually >30 minutes) convulsive seizures (status epilepticus) is not widely recognized nor is its occurrence even accepted in domestic animals. In humans and experimental animals, brain damage resulting from status epilepticus is well documented. One study reported a relatively high incidence of brain lesions in dogs caused by status epilepticus. In this study, acute brain damage was widespread and corresponded well with areas of the brain prone to hypoxic-ischemic injury such as the cerebral cortex, pyriform cortex, basal nuclei, and hippocampus.

The cause of neuronal injury with prolonged convulsive seizures is debatable. It remains unclear if necrosis, apoptosis, or a combination of these two mechanisms causes neuronal injury in status epilepticus. During seizures, there is an increased metabolic demand for glucose and oxygen by neurons; however, cerebral blood flow increases during seizures so that the amount of glucose and oxygen available for neurons to generate energy remains adequate, at least during earlier stages. Acute neuronal necrosis still occurs even when cerebral blood flow, oxygenation, body temperature, and other metabolic parameters are maintained within normal limits in experimental animals with status epilepticus.

Excitotoxic injury caused by accumulation of neurotoxic amino acid neurotransmitters, such as glutamate during the extreme neuronal activity occurring in status epilepticus, is an attractive explanation for neuronal necrosis. Excitotoxicity would account for both the selective vulnerability of certain brain areas and the character of the lesions. Status epilepticus induced experimentally in rats with kainic acid, an excitatory amino acid receptor agonist, has been shown to cause primarily neuronal necrosis and some characteristics of apoptosis. Other experimental studies have suggested that astrocytes produce clusterin during status epilepticus. Clusterin (dimeric acidic glycoprotein), a sulfated glycoprotein, initiates apoptosis when expressed in cells in elevated concentrations. It is proposed that clusterin secreted by astrocytes during status epilepticus is actively endocytosed by hippocampal neurons, and these neurons die by an apoptotic mechanism. The exact mechanism of neuronal injury remains to be proved. There is some evidence that the mature brain is more prone to injury induced by status epilepticus than the immature brain.

Gross lesions, if present, usually consist of widened and flattened gyri and narrow indistinct sulci caused by cerebral edema. Acute neuronal ischemic cell change and astrocytic swelling are observed microscopically. In experimental animals with status epilepticus, neuronal degeneration is observed within 30 minutes and neuronal necrosis within 60 minutes.

Hepatic Encephalopathy

Acute and chronic liver failure, as well as hepatic atrophy associated with congenital or acquired vascular shunts, often results in hepatic encephalopathy and disordered neurotransmission because of the accumulation of toxic substances, principally ammonia, in the systemic circulation and thus the CNS. Ammonia is formed in the gastrointestinal tract by bacterial degradation of amines, amino acids, purines, and urea from proteins consumed in the diet. In healthy animals, ammonia is detoxified in the liver by conversion to urea by the ornithine citrulline arginine urea cycle. Urea is far less toxic than ammonia and is excreted in the urine. Ammonia has several neurotoxic effects such as (1) changing the transit of amino acids, water, and electrolytes across the neuronal cell membranes and (2) inhibiting the generation of both excitatory and inhibitory postsynaptic potentials in neurons. Ammonia and other toxic metabolites also appear to (1) cause increased permeability of the blood-brain barrier leading to vasogenic edema and (2) alter osmoregulation within the CNS. These mechanisms likely led to the spongy change (status spongiosus) characteristic of the disease microscopically. Because astrocytes play an important role in regulating fluid and electrolyte balances in the CNS and are the primary cell type having lesions (Alzheimer's type II astrocytes) in hepatic encephalopathy, it is not surprising that alterations in osmoregulation are a component of the pathogenesis of the disease. Ammonia and other toxic metabolites likely also affect oligodendroglia. Finally, it has been proposed that alterations in the blood-brain barrier may facilitate passage of neurotoxins such as

TABLE 14-6 Possible Mitochondrial Encephalopathies in Animals

Animal	Age of Onset (months)	Clinical Signs	Primary Lesions
Alaskan husky	6 to 9	Ataxia, other motor disturbances, anxiety, blindness, hypalgesia	Spongiosis and cavitation in thalamus caudal to medulla
Cattle dog	5 to 12	Seizures, behavioral abnormalities followed by locomotor signs	Spongiosis and cavitation in cerebellum, brainstem nuclei, and spinal gray matter
English springer spaniel	15 to 16	Ataxia, disorientation, visual deficits	Status spongiosus in accessory olivary nucleus; axon loss and gliosis in optic nerve and tracts
Jack Russell terrier (Parson)	2.5	Ataxia, hypermetria, and deafness	Neuronal degeneration and mineralization of the medulla oblongata, vestibulocochlear nerve, choroid plexus, and granule cell layer of the cerebellum
Limousin cattle	1 to 4	Locomotor signs, aggressive behavior, blindness	Spongiosis, cavitation in cerebral and cerebellar white matter, brainstem nuclei, optic chiasm
Simmental cattle	5 to 12	Ataxia, behavioral changes	Spongiosis and necrosis in internal capsule, caudate nucleus, putamen, brainstem nuclei, spinal gray matter

short-chain fatty acids, mercaptans, false (pseudo-) neurotransmitters (tyramine, octopamine, and β-phenylethanolamine), ammonia, and GABA into the CNS leading to neuronal dysfunction. A similar condition, termed renal encephalopathy, has been described in dogs, a horse, and a cow with renal failure. It is likely related to high concentrations of ammonia or ammonia-metabolites in the circulation because of inadequate renal clearance caused by severe glomerular or tubular injury.

In all species except the horse, lesions of hepatic encephalopathy are of two types: spongy change and formation of Alzheimer's type II astrocytes (see Fig. 14-10, *D*). Spongy change can be present throughout the neuraxis but typically involves areas of confluence or intermingling of gray and white. These areas include the deep cerebrocortical gray-white matter interface, basal nuclei and adjacent internal capsule, reticular areas throughout the brainstem, and deep cerebellar nuclei. The spongy change is due to intramyelinic edema, causing splitting and vacuolation of myelin sheaths. Spongy change can be produced experimentally by ammonia infusion and is reversible. Alzheimer's type II astrocytic change is a subtle alteration that has been reported in all domestic animals and is the only CNS change observed in horses with hepatic failure. Alzheimer's type II astrocytes are found in gray matter and have enlarged vesicular nuclei with peripheral chromatin, glycogen deposits, and demonstrable nucleoli or nucleolar-type bodies. Immunocytochemical staining for GFAP is typically weak or absent, possibly indicating a toxic effect on astrocytes.

Clinically, affected animals show CNS signs such as seizures, ataxia, depressed mentation, walking aimlessly, and head pressing.

Mitochondrial Encephalopathies

In humans, various encephalopathic and myopathic syndromes caused by point mutations in mitochondrial DNA affecting tRNA genes are grouped under the acronyms MELAS (mitochondrial encephalopathy, lactic acidosis, strokelike episodes) and MERRF (myoclonus epilepsy, ragged red fibers). The various human syndromes include Leigh's disease (subacute necrotizing encephalomyelopathy), Kearns-Sayre syndrome, and Leber's hereditary optic atrophy.

Diseases that might be classified as mitochondrial encephalopathies are not well characterized in animals. Despite this caveat, the diseases reported in the Alaskan husky, Australian cattle dogs, English springer spaniel dogs, and a Jack Russell terrier, as well as in Limousin and Simmental cattle and New Zealand South Hampshire sheep, could represent mitochondrial disorders. Table 14-6 summarizes the salient features of the diseases. Characteristics of these diseases in both humans and animals are symmetric bilateral involvement of the neuraxis and lesions typified by status spongiosus (edema of cerebral white matter) with variable progression to cavitation or necrosis. The CNS is highly dependent on oxidative metabolism and is therefore the most severely affected organ in mitochondrial disorders. Mitochondria isolated from affected human patients have impaired oxygen consumption and reduced respiratory chain enzyme complex activity. Recently, although quite controversial, it has been suggested that alterations in the function of genes in endothelial cells cause dysfunction of the blood-brain and CSF-blood barriers, which may play an important role in the underlying pathogenesis of mitochondrial encephalopathies.

Primary Neuronal Degeneration

Primary neuronal degeneration that occurs in many or all animal species is discussed in this section. Disorders of individual animal species are discussed in sections covering disorders unique to that species.

The term *primary neuronal degeneration* encompasses three groups of diseases affecting specific regions of the CNS in a temporally and spatially stereotyped manner and are characterized by degeneration, necrosis, and loss of specific populations of functionally linked neurons. Box 14-8 gives an overview of these diseases. The first group includes the multisystem neuronal degenerations, which are diseases that affect populations of functionally related neurons in the basal ganglia, brainstem, and cerebellum. The second group includes the primary cerebellar neuronal degenerations, which are diseases that affect populations of neurons restricted to the cerebellum and cerebellar roof nuclei. The third group includes primary spinal cord degenerations, which are diseases associated with axonal swellings (axonal spheroids) in the neuraxis termed neuraxonal dystrophies. Another term used to denote some of these diseases in the biomedical literature and veterinary textbooks is *abiotrophy*; this term was introduced by Gowers in 1902. The term literally means lack of ("a") a vital ("bios") nutrition ("trophy") required to sustain the life of a tissue. For discussion of the primary neuronal degeneration affecting individual animal species, see sections covering disorders specific for the species.

Multisystem Neuronal Degeneration

Multisystem neuronal degeneration is discussed in sections covering disorders unique to individual animal species.

BOX 14-8 Multisystem Neuronal Degenerations and Brainstem/Spinal Syndromes in Domestic Animals

MULTISYSTEM NEURONAL DEGENERATIONS
Canine: Kerry blue terrier, red-haired cocker spaniel, Cairn terrier

PRIMARY CEREBELLAR DEGENERATION
Neonatal Syndromes
Canine: beagle, Samoyed, Irish setter
Ovine: Welsh mountain, Corriedale
Bovine: Hereford, Hereford cross, Ayrshire

Postnatal Syndromes
Canine: Airedale, German shepherd, Gordon setter, rough-coated collie, border collie, Finnish terrier, Bernese mountain dog, Bern running dog, Labrador retriever, golden retriever, cocker spaniel, Cairn terrier, Great Dane
Bovine: Holstein-Friesian, Hereford cross, Angus
Equine: Arabian, Arabian cross, Gotland pony
Ovine: Merino
Porcine: Yorkshire

MITOCHONDRIAL ENCEPHALOPATHY (ENCEPHALOMYOPATHY)
Canine: English springer spaniel, Alaskan husky, Australian cattle dog, English setter dog, Jack Russell terrier
Bovine: Simmental, Limousin
Sheep: New Zealand South Hampshire

SPONGY DEGENERATION
Canine: Labrador retriever, Saluki, silky terrier, Samoyed
Bovine: Jersey, shorthorn, Angus-shorthorn, Hereford
Feline: Egyptian Mau

BRAINSTEM AND SPINAL SYNDROMES
Neuroaxonal Dystrophy
Canine: border collie, Chihuahua, Rottweiler
Feline: domestic
Equine: Morgan
Ovine: Suffolk

Motor Neuron Disease—Spinal Cord
Canine: Brittany spaniel, Swedish Lapland, English pointer, Rottweiler, German shepherd, sheepdog, collie, pug, dachshund, fox terrier
Feline: Siamese
Bovine: Brown Swiss, Hereford (shaker calf syndrome)
Equine: Various breeds (not believed hereditary)
Porcine: Hampshire, Yorkshire

Degenerative Leukomyelopathies (Spinal Cord—White Matter)
Canine: German shepherd, Afghan hound, Kooiker, Labrador retriever, Ibizan hound, harrier, beagle, foxhound, Rottweiler, smooth fox terrier, Jack Russell terrier
Bovine: Brown Swiss, Holstein-Friesian, Murray gray
Equine: Various breeds (see vitamin E deficiency)

Primary Cerebellar Neuronal Degeneration

Depending on the degree of maturation of the cerebellum and related systems at the time of birth in the various species, clinical signs in animals with the neonatal syndromes can be manifest in the immediate postnatal period (bovine, ovine) or can be delayed until the time of ambulation (canine). Hereditary transmission is known or suspected in some instances. Lesions vary among affected species and breeds but overall include degeneration or absence of Purkinje cells, proximal swelling of Purkinje cell axons, variable loss of granule cells, cortical astrogliosis, and degeneration of nuclei in the cerebellar medulla.

Animals with postnatal cerebellar syndromes are normal at birth or at the time of ambulation. Onset of ataxia with various other clinical signs referable to cerebellar disease begins weeks or months after a period of apparently normal development. Initial clinical signs are often subtle. Progression of the signs can be slow or rapid, relentless, or with static periods. Some individuals reach a stage without further progression of signs, but this is not typical of the syndrome in most animals.

Grossly, the cerebellum can be normal or reduced in size and atrophic. Microscopically, lesions are analogous to those that occur in the neonatal syndromes with loss of Purkinje cells, variable neuronal depletion in the granular layer, and astrogliosis in the molecular layer. Fusiform swellings of proximal Purkinje cell axons are found in the rough-coated collie and the Yorkshire pig. In the rough-coated collie and Merino sheep, lesions occur in other areas of the neuraxis. In these syndromes, degeneration and loss of neurons in the deep cerebellar and other nuclei are accompanied by axonal degeneration in the cerebellum, brainstem, and spinal cord. Loss of spinal ventral horn motor neurons has been noted in the rough-coated collie. An autosomal recessive mode of inheritance is suspected or documented in several of the diseases. For individual disorders, see sections covering disorders of individual animal species.

For discussion of the primary cerebellar neuronal degeneration affecting individual animal species, see sections covering disorders specific for the species.

Neuraxonal dystrophy

Diseases associated with axonal swellings (axonal spheroids) have been termed *neuraxonal dystrophy*. Diseases include those putatively associated with vitamin E deficiency or that have been interpreted as an aging change (see the section on Degenerative Diseases). Included here are diseases with a species and breed association and onset relatively early in life, generally before 1 year of age but varying between 4 weeks and 3 years. A hereditary basis is often suspected or proved. Neuraxonal dystrophies have been described in dogs, cats, horses, and sheep. Neuraxonal dystrophies of the horse are discussed in the section covering disorders unique to that species.

Dystrophy is defined as a disorder arising from defective or faulty nutrition of a cell, tissue, or organ, and the term is most commonly applied to muscle diseases. In this usage, it applies to neurons and their axons (neuraxonal). Lesions differ in severity and distribution but are characterized by prominent axonal swellings in various nuclei (often sensory) in the brainstem, cerebellum, and spinal cord. Loss of cerebellar Purkinje and granule cells have been reported in Rottweilers and cats and the loss of brainstem neurons in cats. In the Morgan horse, the axonal swellings are associated with vacuolation.

Neuroaxonal dystrophies are often characterized clinically by severe and often profound muscular weakness and widespread muscle atrophy. Sporadic cases in older adult animals also occur of unknown cause or suspected extraneous influence. Clinical signs vary but include gait abnormalities, dysmetria or hypermetria, proprioceptive disturbance, ataxia, or other cerebellar signs.

Motor neuron diseases

Motor neuron diseases have been described in dogs, cats, cows, horses, and pigs. Degeneration and loss of motor neurons in the ventral horns of the spinal cord and variable axonal degeneration in the ventral spinal nerve rootlets and peripheral nerves characterize the lesions in motor neuron diseases. In some of the motor neuron diseases, there is prominent swelling of ventral horn neuronal cells bodies or axons, or both, associated with marked accumulation of neurofilaments. This accumulation is presumably caused by posttranslational protein modification and impairment of neurofilament protein transport. Degeneration in some diseases is not strictly limited to motor neurons of the spinal cord or to motor neurons in general. Other sites of involvement are motor or sensory nuclei, or both, in the brainstem and white matter tracts in the spinal cord.

In horses, lesions in motor neurons are analogous to those already described. The disease affects various breeds, no definitive familial association or age predilections are known, and an inherited basis is not suspected. Generalized weakness, muscle atrophy, and weight loss progress over 1 to several months.

In calves, a disease known as *shaker calf syndrome* in horned Hereford calves can only be loosely termed a motor neuron disease. There is marked accumulation of neurofilaments within neurons of the central, peripheral, and autonomic nervous systems. All segments of the spinal cord are severely affected. Neurons and neuronal processes in ventral horns, intermediolateral nucleus, Clarke's column, and substantia gelatinosa are swollen and distended. Wallerian degeneration occurs in ventral nerve rootlets and white matter of the spinal cord. Brainstem lesions are less prominent. Swollen cerebellar Purkinje cells and neuronal degeneration in the lateral geniculate body and frontal cortex are reported. The disorder occurs in newborn calves and is characterized clinically by tremulous shaking of the head, body, and tail.

Nutritional

Vitamin B_1 (Thiamine) Deficiency

Thiamine diphosphate is the active form of thiamine. It is a critical cofactor for several thiamine-dependent enzymes involved in carbohydrate metabolism, and brain damage is thought to be related to a decline in thiamine-dependent enzymes, energy deprivation, and oxidative stress with the abnormal metabolism of free radicals in neurons. These enzymes are also important in the synthesis of several cell constituents, including neurotransmitters. Thiamine deficiency has been associated with neurologic disease in carnivores (Chastek paralysis), humans (Wernicke's encephalopathy), and ruminants. For discussion of nutritional diseases affecting individual animal species, see sections covering disorders specific for the species.

Vitamin A Deficiency

See the section on the PNS and Chapter 20.

Toxicoses

Space constraints do not allow a comprehensive discussion of all toxicities affecting the nervous system. Box 14-9 is a partial listing of poisons with the potential to cause CNS injury and neurologic illness. Some of these, such as mercury, have in the past caused high morbidity and mortality in isolated outbreaks. An example is the 1956 Minamata Bay incident in Japan of humans eating fish containing high concentrations of methylmercury. Methylmercury accumulates in the aquatic food chain, and thus the highest concentrations exist in predatory fish at the top of the food chain. In humans and animals with methylmercury toxicosis, neuronal cell bodies of the cerebral cortex and cerebellum die through a mechanism suggested to be apoptosis; however, microtubule dysfunction, oxidative stress, alterations of calcium homeostasis, and the potentiation of glutaminergic excitotoxicity may be involved. The potential remains for serious neurologic illnesses and death from these intoxications, and the interested reader is referred to more comprehensive reference sources. In this chapter, discussion of toxicities is limited to those conditions most likely to be encountered in veterinary practice.

BOX 14-9 Other Toxicities Involving the Nervous System

CHEMICALS

Heavy metals: cadmium, manganese, mercury, tin (trimethyltin), zinc
Hexacarbons: *n*-hexane, others
Pesticides: carbaryl, bromethalin, chlorinated hydrocarbons
Drugs: nitrofurazones, ivermectin, levamisole, metronidazole

PLANTS

Cycads, *Chrysocoma tenuifolia, Helichrysum* spp., *Solanum* spp. *(dimidiatum, fastigium, kwebense),* sorghum, *Stypandra* spp.

MYCOTOXINS

Acremonium, Aspergillus, Claviceps, Fumonisin, Penicillium

Chemicals

Chemically induced distal axonopathies have been classified by functional alterations affecting motor or sensory neurons, location of injury within the nerve (distal, proximal), or by the type of nerve affected (cranial or spinal). Because of the large number and wide use of chemicals in commerce, there exists an extensive list of experimental studies describing toxic axonopathies and neuropathies. Their complete discussion is outside the scope of this chapter.

Chemicals used in agricultural, industrial, and pharmaceutical commerce can injure nerves by interfering with axoplasmic flow. Such chemicals include acrylamide (polymerizing agent to strengthen paper), carbon disulfide (fat solvent, used for extraction of oil from oil-bearing fruit such as olives), triorthocresyl phosphate (high-performance lubricants in airplane engines), halomethane (refrigerants), methylene chloride (extraction agents, paint solvents, and degreasing agents), carbon tetrachloride (solvents), and butane (fuel source).

Acrylamide causes a unique distal axonopathy (dying-back axonopathy) primarily affecting axons of the PNS (less commonly the CNS) in which there is accumulation of neurofilaments within affected axons. Axonal spheroids are thought to be related to alteration of axonal transport resulting from phosphorylation of neurofilaments and their abnormal rearrangement within the axon. This "dying-back" axonopathy is microscopically characterized by degeneration of axons starting at or near synapses and proceeding toward the neuronal cell body. The most distal axonal projections are furthest from the cell body and thus cannot be maintained. Thus they are most vulnerable to functional alterations; however, it is unclear whether this degeneration is caused by energy deficits, lack of antioxidants, or physical obstruction of axoplasmic flow. Axonal degeneration is followed by secondary demyelination.

Certain types of toxic and biochemical injury to axons result in a stereotypic pattern of morphologic change that affects either distal or proximal segments of the axon and results in the formation of segmental axonal spheroids. Based on the location of the spheroids, such diseases are divided into one of two groups, either diseases affecting axons a distance away from their cell bodies (distal axonopathies) or diseases affecting axons near their cell bodies (proximal axonopathies).

It is hypothesized that axonal spheroid formation and subsequent axonal degeneration are caused by alterations in axoplasmic flow and by alterations of anterograde or retrograde flow, depending on the nature of the injury resulting in the accumulation and/or rearrangement of cytoskeletal proteins. The histologic lesion common to these two types of axonopathies is the formation of axonal spheroids with subsequent degeneration of the axon and secondary demyelination, which is a process that in many ways resembles the lesions described for Wallerian degeneration. Axonal spheroids are common to a variety of neuronal derangements; therefore distal and proximal axonopathies must be differentiated from other diseases that cause spheroids such as the compressive axonopathies.

Distal and proximal axonopathies have been further subdivided by some scientific disciplines into groups based on whether initial axonal lesions progress in an anterograde or retrograde direction. The terminology and classification schemes, although useful to some, are outside the scope of this chapter and are often confusing. The occurrence of secondary anterograde or retrograde lesions is discussed in the context of some of the diseases presented next.

Organophosphates

Organophosphates are divided into two groups according to their use, mode of action, and type of toxicity. The first group, organophosphate esters, used as pesticides (parathion, malathion, diazinon, carbaryl, or aldicarb), fungicides, herbicides, or rodenticides, cause acute toxicity by inhibiting cholinesterase either directly or indirectly and allowing acetylcholine to accumulate at synaptic (nerve-nerve junctions) or myoneural junctions (nerve-muscle junctions), resulting in persistent depolarization. In acute organophosphate toxicosis, clinical effects vary but are manifested in the following:

1. Parasympathetic nervous system, leading to salivation, lacrimation, urination, defecation, bradycardia, and pupillary constriction
2. Skeletal muscular system, resulting in muscle fasciculations followed by weakness and muscle paralysis (i.e., death is due primarily to respiratory failure)
3. CNS, leading to anxiety, restlessness, hyperactivity, anorexia, and generalized seizures (i.e., observed in dogs and cats but uncommon in cattle)

Gross and microscopic lesions in the nervous system are absent, and those in other tissues are nonspecific.

The second group causes chronic toxicosis and is the most common cause of chemically induced distal axonopathy in veterinary medicine. This group of organophosphates includes the cresyl and related compounds such as triorthocresyl phosphate used in hydraulic fluids, lubricants, flame-retardants, and plasticizers. The triaryl phosphate group of compounds used as high-temperature lubricants is toxic for several species of animals and humans.

Chronic exposure (delayed neuropathy) to certain organophosphate pesticides and herbicides (trichlorphon, merphos, triorthocresyl phosphate, leptophos, parathion, malathion, and diazinon) causes delayed neurotoxicity unrelated to cholinesterase inhibition as seen in acute organophosphate toxicosis. The type of axonal injury caused by these chemicals follows the stereotypic process of morphologic changes described previously and occurs approximately 10 to 14 days after exposure. Organophosphorus compounds causing delayed neurotoxicity inhibit the activity of an enzyme referred to as *neuropathy target esterase.* The function of the enzyme in the PNS and CNS is not fully understood.

Phosphorylation of the enzyme by the toxic compound is proposed to interfere with its normal function, resulting in axonal injury. Other studies have shown that organophosphates causing delayed neurotoxicity interact with Ca^{2+} or calmodulin kinase II, an enzyme responsible for phosphorylation of cytoskeletal proteins, such as microtubules, neurofilaments, and microtubule-associated protein-2, resulting in disassembly and accumulation of these proteins in the distal portions of axons, producing axonal swelling and degeneration.

No specific gross lesions are present in chemically induced distal axonopathies. Microscopically, there is retrograde degeneration beginning in the distal part of axons, especially those with a larger diameter. Affected areas in the spinal cord include dorsal funiculi, spinocerebellar tracts in lateral funiculi, and ventromedial aspects of the ventral funiculi. Central chromatolysis of cell bodies of affected nerves has occurred.

Clinically, signs of toxicity are usually delayed 1 to 2 weeks after exposure. Young animals, because of their ability to compensate for the neurologic deficits, tend to be less seriously affected, whereas recovery is slow and incomplete in adults. Susceptible animals include cats, domestic and exotic ruminants, chickens, pheasants, and ducks. Small laboratory animals, dogs, and some nonhuman primates are less sensitive. Clinical signs are those of combined sensory and motor neuropathy and spinal cord damage, such as proprioceptive deficits expected by damage to the spinocerebellar nucleus and tract, as well as the fasciculus gracilis.

Selenium

An acute paralytic syndrome termed *bilateral poliomyelomalacia* has been observed in feeder pigs associated with the inadvertent inclusion of toxic amounts of selenium (selenium-enriched yeast, sodium selenite, or sodium selenate) in pig rations. The pathogenesis of the lesions is not proved but could involve an induced nicotinamide or niacin deficiency. Experimentally, 6-aminonicotinamide, a gliotoxin and antagonist of the vitamin, causes lesions analogous to those seen in the natural porcine disease.

Grossly, bilateral (symmetric) areas of softening and yellow discoloration occur in the ventral spinal gray matter of the cervical and lumbar intumescences. Microscopically, acute lesions consist progressively of neuronal chromatolysis, neuronal necrosis, neuronal loss, microcavitation, and glial necrosis. As would be expected, these changes are subsequently followed by astrogliosis and the accumulation of gitter cells. Prominent capillaries are typical. Wallerian degeneration occurs in ventral spinal nerve rootlets of those cord segments whose ventral gray horn motor neurons have been destroyed. Identical lesions have been observed in the brainstem.

Clinically, affected pigs are alert, rest in sternal recumbency, and squeal loudly when disturbed. They eventually progress to quadriplegia with flaccid paralysis of the rear limbs. Cutaneous manifestations of the toxicity also occur and include rough hair coats, partial alopecia, and separation and sloughing of the hoofs. Historically, a similar ovine bilateral symmetric poliomyelomalacia has been reported from Africa, but an association with selenium toxicity was not made.

Sodium chloride

Sodium chloride toxicity, also known as *sodium ion toxicosis, water deprivation syndrome,* or *salt poisoning,* occurs primarily in pigs, poultry, and occasionally in ruminants, dogs, horses, and sheep. The disease occurs after overconsumption of sodium chloride in rations or supplements and can be complicated by limited availability of drinking water, resulting in severe dehydration. A similar sequence of events can occur with simple water restriction of sufficient duration to allow compensation by the brain's adaptive response to chronic hypernatremia (hyperosmolarity). Sodium chloride toxicity is due to hyperosmolarity (hypernatremia) caused by excessive intake of sodium salts or severe dehydration followed by rehydration and a "rapid" hypernatremic to normonatremic or hyponatremic shift.

During the initial hypernatremic phase, the brain "shrinks" because of the osmotic loss of water. An influx of sodium, potassium, and chloride ions into the brain, beginning within minutes after the osmotic loss of water, is an acute adaptive response to equalize the sodium imbalance. Maintenance of a normal ionic balance in the brain is critical, however, for normal function and although a new ionic equilibrium is established, this acute response alone cannot compensate for severe or prolonged hypernatremia.

A second, more delayed adaptive response of the brain is an influx or endogenous production of organic osmolytes, such as certain amino acids, polyols, and methylamines, to equalize the osmotic imbalance created by hypernatremia. This response requires hours or days to establish a new osmotic equilibrium. When animals are given free access to fresh water, an acute hypernatremic to hyponatremic shift occurs. Within minutes, the brain attempts to offset this osmotic imbalance by eliminating sodium, potassium, and chloride ions by actively transporting these ions into the vasculature. This early response cannot, however, offset the osmotic stress created by the increased organic osmolytes in the brain. As a result of the osmotic gradient created by the elevated organic osmolytes, water enters the brain with subsequent brain swelling.

Grossly, lesions are inconsistent but include cerebral and leptomeningeal congestion and edema. Zones of cerebrocortical laminar necrosis can be detected in transverse slices of fixed brain. Microscopically, cerebrocortical neuronal necrosis, often laminar, is accompanied by astrocytic swelling. In pigs, leptomeninges and perivascular spaces can have an infiltrate of eosinophils and with longer survival, an influx of macrophages occurs, depending on the extent of necrosis (Fig. 14-56). The leptomeningeal and perivascular infiltrate of eosinophils is an inconsistent finding. Pallor of subcortical white matter is indicative of edema, and prominence of small cortical blood vessels is due to congestion and swelling of endothelial cell nuclei. In ruminants, arteriolar degeneration with a transmural neutrophilic infiltrate, cerebellar Purkinje cell necrosis, and edema of basal nuclei, thalamus, and midbrain have been observed.

Clinical signs include inappetence and dehydration early followed by heading pressing, incoordination, blindness, circling, paddling, and convulsions. Animals are often found dead in their pasture or pen.

Metals

Arsenic

Toxicity caused by ingestion or cutaneous absorption can occur with inorganic and organic arsenicals and can affect multiple organs, including the nervous system. Inorganic compounds are predominantly herbicides or pesticides, whereas organic arsenicals (arsanilic acid, 3-nitro-4-phenylarsonic acid) have been used as feed additives in the pig and poultry industries as growth promoters and to control enteric diseases.

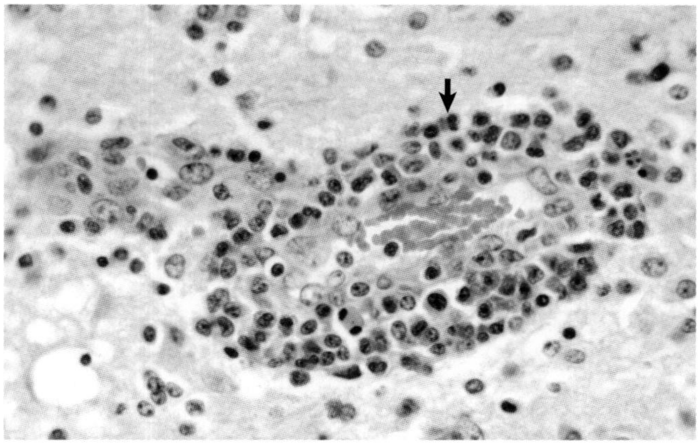

Fig. 14-56 Eosinophilic meningoencephalitis, cerebral cortex, gray matter, pig.
Note the accumulation of eosinophils *(arrow)* in the perivascular space. This response is characteristic of the lesions of hypo-osmotic edema caused by water deprivation or excessive consumption of sodium salts. The surrounding neuropil is edematous. H&E stain. (Courtesy Dr. M.D. McGavin, College of Veterinary Medicine, University of Tennessee.)

Poisoning with inorganic arsenicals is an acute enteric disease with hepatic and renal manifestations, but neurologic signs can occur. Probably because of the nature of the organic compounds and the manner of their use, there is greater potential for neurotoxicity. Arsanilic acid has a greater tendency to cause peripheral and optic nerve and tract damage, whereas 3-nitro compounds tend to affect the spinal cord more severely.

Gross lesions are not present. Microscopically, lesions in cranial and peripheral nerves and spinal cord consist of axonal degeneration and fragmentation of myelin sheaths. In the spinal cord after 3-nitro poisoning, lesions are found chronologically in the cervical and thoracic cord followed by lesions in the lumbar cord. Spinocerebellar tracts and dorsal funiculi are predominantly affected. The distribution of lesions suggests that the distal segments of long ascending fiber tracts can be preferentially injured. Inorganic arsenicals inhibit sulfhydryl enzyme systems and disrupt cellular metabolism. The exact mode of action of organic arsenicals is unknown.

In pigs, clinical signs include blindness resulting from damage to optic nerves and tracts and incoordination, paresis, and paralysis related to spinal cord and peripheral nerve lesions.

Lead

Lead poisoning has occurred in a variety of animals, but with the increased awareness of the potential for toxicity and environmental contamination and current regulations, such as reduced concentrations in paint and unleaded gasoline, poisoning is uncommon and if it occurs is most common in cattle. Potential sources include discarded car batteries and old flaking or peeling lead paint in barns and farm buildings.

Depending on the quantity absorbed, poisoning can be peracute with no gross or microscopic lesions, acute, subacute, or chronic. In peracute or acute cases, contents of the upper digestive tract, such as fragments of battery plates or flakes of paint, could indicate the possibility of lead poisoning. Lead poisoning can affect many tissues and organs, including CNS, PNS, liver, kidneys, gastrointestinal tract, bone marrow, blood vessels, and organs of the reproductive and endocrine systems. In horses grazing lead-contaminated pastures, a cranial neuropathy with laryngeal and facial paralysis has been described.

Lead poisoning in cattle and other species is via the oral route or less commonly, via the respiratory system or skin (inorganic lead). Lead can damage the brain through a variety of mechanisms. Direct toxic effects on neurons, astrocytes, and cerebral endothelial cells occur by disrupting metabolic pathways and altering the function of dopaminergic, cholinergic, and glutamatergic neurotransmitter systems. Lead crosses the blood-brain barrier rapidly using a cationic transporter, concentrates in the brain because of its ability to substitute for calcium ions in the pump, and enters astrocytes and neurons by voltage-sensitive cell membrane calcium channels. Lead disrupts calcium homeostasis, causing the accumulation of calcium in lead-exposed cells, and induces mitochondrial release of calcium, leading to apoptotic cell death. Astrocytes contain metallothionein and can sequester potentially toxic metals in the CNS, thus protecting more vulnerable neurons from the toxic effects of lead. However, astrocytes may also be sensitive to the toxic effects of lead, leading to functional deficits such as in the uptake, transport, and metabolism of neurotransmitters. Transplacental (humans and sheep) and neonatal lead exposure can result in delayed brain maturation and biochemical abnormalities.

Gross lesions in the CNS are usually absent. When present, they can resemble those present in polioencephalomalacia of cattle, but this is uncommon. In general, gross lesions, if present, are distributed in a laminar pattern and include meningeal and cerebrovascular congestion, brain swelling with flattening of gyri, or hemorrhage. With longer survival times, there may be foci of cerebrocortical malacia (softening), cavitation, and laminar necrosis followed by cerebral cortical atrophy, widened sulci, narrowed gyri, and loss of white matter.

Microscopically, lesions in peracute cases are absent. In acute cases, congestion, astrocytic swelling, status spongiosus, and microvascular prominence caused by endothelial hypertrophy are present, and often ischemic neuronal cell change is characteristically confined to the tips of cerebrocortical gyri. For most cases in cattle, only a few necrotic neurons at gyral tips and minimal astrocytic swelling, vascular prominence, and congestion can be found. With longer survival times, cerebrocortical lesions progress to laminar necrosis, accumulations of macrophages, or liquefactive necrosis, although the last is rare. Because of their similarities, lesions of lead encephalopathy in ruminants must be differentiated from those of thiamine deficiency-induced polioencephalomalacia and sulfur-related polioencephalomalacia.

Lesions in dogs resemble those in cattle, but vascular damage is more obvious and consistent. Vascular lesions can progress to mural hyalinization, necrosis, and thrombosis. Other lesions include neuronal necrosis in the cerebral cortex, hippocampus, and cerebellum (Purkinje cells), myelin destruction in cerebrocortical white matter, and a peripheral neuropathy.

Clinically, affected cows are often found down or dead in the pasture. If clinical signs are present, they range initially from depression, inappetence, and diarrhea to teeth grinding (bruxism), circling, head pressing, incoordination, and blindness later. In small animals, especially dogs, clinical signs include ataxia, tremors, clonic-tonic seizures, blindness, and deafness.

Organotins

Excessive exposure to organotins, such as triethyltin (stabilizer, catalyst, wood and textile preservative, fungicide, bactericide, and insecticide), causes cytotoxic edema principally affecting myelin sheaths of oligodendroglial cells in the white matter. Experimental studies have shown that triethyltin selectively damages myelin sheaths and causes a decrease in potassium concentrations in the white matter with a concurrent increase in intracellular water content. The blood-brain barrier is not affected. The mechanism of injury is thought to be uncoupling of oxidative phosphorylation and inhibition of mitochondrial ATPase activity within cell membranes. Loss of Na/K-dependent ATPase activity in cell membranes of myelin lamellae leads to the formation of intramyelinic edema.

Gross lesions, if present, consist of an enlarged brain and spinal cord. Because of compression against the cranium, an affected brain has flattened gyri and shallow indistinct sulci. Microscopically, fluid accumulates between myelin layers and leads to splitting of the myelin lamellae and the formation of intramyelinic spaces.

Microbial Toxins

Botulism

See the section on the PNS.

Tetanus

Tetanus is a spastic paralytic disease caused by the neurotoxin called *tetanospasmin* produced by *Clostridium tetani*. Similar to *Clostridium botulinum,* the bacterium is a ubiquitous Gram-positive spore-forming anaerobe commonly found in soil. Tetanospasmin is synthesized in anaerobic wounds and first binds at myoneural junctions and/or sensory receptors. It is transported via retrograde axoplasmic flow within the axon and across synaptic junctions until it reaches the CNS (see Fig. 4-28). In the CNS, the toxin is transferred across synapses until it becomes fixed to gangliosides in the presynaptic inhibitory motor neuron. Tetanospasmin blocks the release of inhibitory neurotransmitters such as glycine and GABA. Inhibitory neurotransmitters act to dampen the actions of excitatory nerve impulses from upper motor neurons that are imposed on lower motor neurons. If these impulses cannot be dampened by normal inhibitory mechanisms, the generalized muscular spasms characteristic of tetanus ensue. Tetanospasmin appears to act by selective cleavage of a protein component of synaptic vesicles, thus preventing the release of neurotransmitters by the cells. Once toxin is bound to synapses, the administration of antitoxin is useless.

This disease is most common in horses but may also occur in lambs castrated in areas contaminated with spores of *Clostridium tetani.* Tetanus also has been reported in cows, pigs, dogs, and cats. Except for the anaerobic wound, there are no macroscopic and microscopic tissue lesions in tetanus. Infected horses initially show signs of colic and muscle stiffness involving muscle groups of the lips, nostrils, ears, jaw (lockjaw), and tail. Horses are hyperesthetic and rapidly have a spastic and tetanic paralytic syndrome develop.

Plant Toxins

Astragalus, Oxytropis, *and* Swainsona *poisoning*

Astragalus, Oxytropis, and *Swainsona* represent three genera of plants with species that are toxic to livestock. As many as 300 species of *Astragalus* grow in North America, and the genus is the largest of any legume family in this part of the world. Three categories of toxicity can be observed with *Astragalus,* depending on the mechanism or manner of toxicity: nitro-containing, selenium-accumulating, and poisoning of the locoweed type. Only the last is discussed here. Locoweed poisoning, or locoism, is associated with ingestion of certain species of *Astragalus* and *Oxytropis* in North America and *Swainsona* in Australia. The toxic principles have been termed *locoine* and *swainsonine,* respectively.

The mechanism of toxicity has been clarified by the isolation of the indolizidine alkaloids swainsonine and swainsonine N-oxide from *Astragalus lentiginosus.* Both compounds inhibit lysosomal α-mannosidase, thus inducing an acquired α-mannosidosis that mimics the inherited storage disease mannosidosis. Mannosidases are glycoside-hydrolyzing enzymes that are found in the Golgi, lysosomes, and cytoplasm of all mammalian cells. Analyses of tissue from animals poisoned with swainsonine have shown that swainsonine is present in all tissue; however, neurons; epithelial cells in organ systems, such as the liver; and macrophages of the monocyte-macrophage system of the spleen and lymph nodes are commonly affected. Therefore, as occurs in the inherited storage disease (mannosidosis), acquired swainsonine-induced storage diseases affect similar cells throughout the body. Additionally, swainsonine interferes with normal synthesis of glycoproteins containing asparagine-linked complex oligosaccharides. Swainsonine also inhibits Golgi mannosidase II, an effect not recognized in the inherited disorder.

There are no specific gross lesions in acquired swainsonine-induced storage diseases. Microscopically, lesions involve neuronal cell bodies throughout the neuraxis and autonomic ganglia and are analogous to the inherited lysosomal storage diseases.

Microscopically, neuron cell bodies are swollen and nuclei are sometimes displaced to the periphery of the cell body. The cytoplasm appears foamy or finely vacuolated. The material that accumulates in the cytoplasm does not stain for lipid. Irregular fusiform enlargements, called *meganeurites,* occur in the proximal axon segment and aberrant synapses form. With time, lesions include distal axonal degeneration and neuronal necrosis with mineralization. The presence of cytoplasmic lesions in other cells of the CNS, such as astrocytes, depends on the degree to which α-mannosidase is expressed in individual cell populations. Astrocytes are hydropic or swollen, but their appearance is less dramatic and diagnostic when compared with changes in neurons. Macrophages recruited from the bloodstream to phagocytose debris and mannose released from dead neurons also are affected by swainsonine. Microgliosis and neuronophagia are present but inconspicuous.

Similar to the swelling and vacuolation of neurons, this process also occurs in cells throughout the body, including hepatocytes, exocrine pancreatic cells, renal tubular epithelium, endocrine organs (thyroid, parathyroid, and adrenal glands), circulating leukocytes, and cells of the monocyte-macrophage system in liver, spleen, and lymph nodes. Ingestion of the plants of these species by females during gestation can also result in abortion or birth of weak neonates that have similar lesions.

Cattle, sheep, and horses are generally affected. Toxicity is usually insidious, and clinical signs are not observed until after the plants have been grazed on for 14 to 60 days. Clinical signs include poor condition, depression, head pressing, incoordination, circling, blindness, recumbency, and paddling.

Miscellaneous Conditions

Meningeal Melanosis (Congenital)

The leptomeninges of animals and humans with heavily pigmented skin, especially black-faced sheep and black-skinned pigs, can have melanin (Fig. 14-57). The extent and degree of pigment deposition varies dramatically from animal to animal. Similar pigment deposits can be found in other areas of the body, including the lung, uterine caruncles, liver, and respiratory and alimentary systems' mucous membranes. Congenital meningeal melanosis produces no clinical impairment in affected animals.

Circulatory Disturbances

Many diseases of the CNS in veterinary medicine result from injury to the circulatory system and vascular endothelium. Vascular diseases of the CNS can result from inflammation/infection, either as a component of a systemic disease process or from extension of inflammatory meningeal or cerebral disease. The incidence of cerebrovascular diseases analogous to those in humans, including trauma, is low in animals, and neurologic manifestations associated with these diseases are uncommon. Arteriosclerosis ("hardening" of arteries) can be categorized as lipid (atherosclerosis) or nonlipid arteriosclerosis; the latter includes arterial fibrosis, mineralization, and amyloid deposition (see Chapter 10).

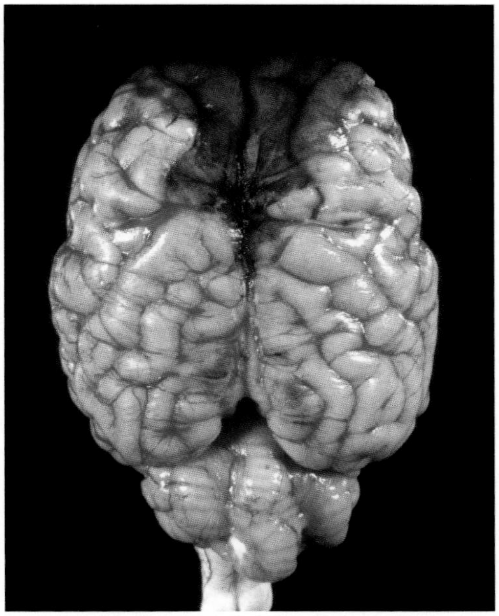

Fig. 14-57 Melanosis, leptomeninges (pia-arachnoid mater), sheep. Note the black pigmentation of the leptomeninges overlying the olfactory poles and dorsal aspect of the frontal lobe. Meningeal melanosis is a normal finding in black-faced sheep and other animals with heavily pigmented skin. (Courtesy Dr. D. Morton, College of Veterinary Medicine, University of Illinois.)

Atherosclerosis

Atherosclerosis is reported in a variety of animals, including nonhuman primates, pigs, dogs, and several avian species. Older pigs are most commonly and severely affected. Occasional older dogs with chronic hypothyroidism or diabetes mellitus can have severe atherosclerosis. The pathogenesis of atherosclerosis and atherosclerotic plaque formation is most well understood in humans, and the results of experimental studies may have some application to understanding atherosclerosis in domestic animals.

Atherosclerotic plaques arise from a complex and partially understood interaction among endothelium, smooth muscle cells, platelets, T lymphocytes, and monocytes. Endothelial injury induced by oxidized low-density lipoprotein [LDL] cholesterol results in vascular inflammation of the tunica intima. Monocytes migrate into the intima of the vessel wall to phagocytose LDL cholesterol. This process results in the formation of foam cells characteristic of early atherosclerosis (fatty streak). In addition, activated macrophages produce factors that also injure the endothelium. LDL cholesterol concentrations in foam cells and smooth muscle cells often exceed the antioxidant properties of normal endothelium. Oxidized LDL leads to additional metabolic changes that foster a procoagulant microenvironment and enhanced platelet-mediated thrombus formation, as well as initiates a cascade of events leading to the lesions associated with the development of mature atherosclerotic plaques (fibrous plaques with a cap [lipid-laden macrophages walled-off by connective tissue]). The location of atherosclerotic plaques in the circulatory system depends on fluid shear stresses and their interaction with injured vascular endothelium. Atherosclerotic plaques characteristically occur in areas of vessel branching or areas where blood undergoes a sudden change in velocity and/or direction of flow.

Although atherosclerotic plaques can reach sizes large enough to significantly reduce blood flow to regions of the brain, the stability of the plaques determines the seriousness of the disease. A stable plaque is characterized by an excess of smooth muscle cells with few lipid-containing macrophages. An unstable plaque is characterized by a large lipid-rich core with abundant lipid-containing macrophages, thin fibrous cap, and inflammation. Rupture of unstable plaques can lead to vascular thrombosis or thromboembolism and infarction of areas supplied by these vessels in the CNS.

Grossly, vessels that can be involved include the aorta and its major branches, extramural coronary arteries, renal arteries, and cerebral arteries. Affected arteries are rigid, irregularly thickened, and white to yellow-white (atheromatous plaques) (Fig. 14-58, *A*). Arterial lumina are narrowed or almost obliterated, but there is usually no appreciable ulceration, thrombosis, or hemorrhage (Fig. 14-58, *B*). Intimal thickening in intracranial arteries contain less lipid and have a greater tendency for fibrosclerosis than other vessels. In arteries within the brain, there is collagenous adventitial or transmural thickening. The arterial lesions can be associated with hemorrhage or infarcts involving basal nuclei, fornix, internal and external capsules, hippocampus, and thalamus.

In the dog, lesions involve cerebral, coronary, and renal arteries and vessels elsewhere in the body and are most severe in the intima and media. Hemorrhage, ischemia, and infarction of the cerebral cortex are uncommon but can occur.

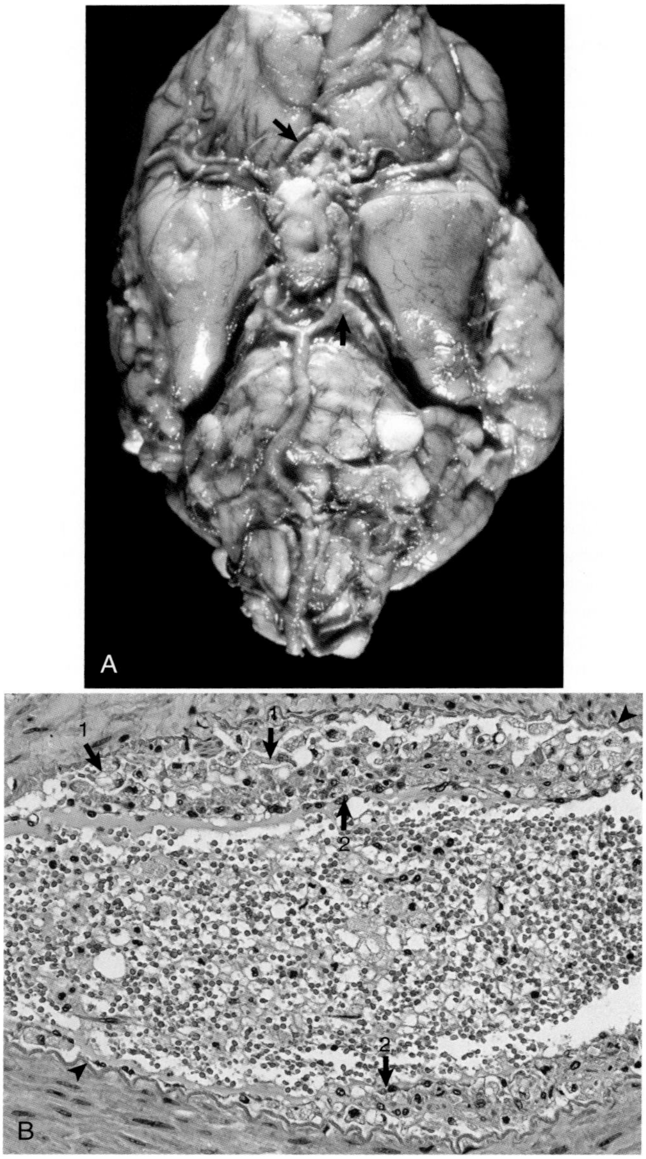

Fig. 14-58 Atherosclerosis, cerebral arteries, brain, ventral surface, dog. **A,** The basilar artery, the arteries of the circle of Willis, and the cerebral arteries are segmentally yellow, thickened, and beaded in appearance from atheroma *(arrows)*. This dog had long-standing hypothyroidism. **B,** The intima of this muscular artery with atherosclerosis contains numerous foamy (lipid laden) macrophages *(arrows 1)*. *Arrowheads* = internal elastic lamina; *arrows 2* = endothelium. H&E stain. (Courtesy Dr. J.F. Zachary, College of Veterinary Medicine, University of Illinois.)

Cerebral Edema (Permeability Changes)

The causes and mechanisms of cerebral edema are presented in the section on vasogenic, cytotoxic, and interstitial edema. Cerebral edema has also been associated with "water intoxication," which can result from an increased body hydration caused by (1) excessive, faulty intravenous hydration; (2) compulsive drinking caused by abnormal mental function; or (3) altered antidiuretic hormone secretion. The increased body hydration produces a hypotonic (hypo-osmolar) plasma, with subsequent development of an osmotic gradient between the hypotonic plasma and the relatively hypertonic state of the normal cerebral tissue. Fluid moves from the plasma into the brain. In this type of edema, the blood-brain barrier remains intact. If it did not, the change in plasma osmolarity would soon be transmitted to the brain tissue (through vascular leakage) and would abolish the necessary osmotic gradient. Fluid accumulation occurs primarily intracellularly but can also be present extracellularly. In addition, typically a pronounced increase occurs in the rate of formation of CSF originating from the choroid plexus and the extracellular fluid of the brain.

The gross lesions that accompany cerebral edema are the result of enlargement of an organ in an enclosed, limited space; the degree of swelling obviously determines the type and extent of lesions that develop. In evaluating lesions, it is particularly important initially to examine the brain and spinal cord in the fresh state and in situ.

Microscopically, in contrast to some other tissues, such as the lungs, the extracellular fluid associated with vasogenic edema fluid is often not detectable, except in instances of marked vascular injury. When the extracellular space-occupying fluid cannot be identified, only its effects (separation of the cells and their processes causing reduced staining intensity) can be recognized. Additionally, after prolonged vasogenic edema, the lesions include hypertrophy and hyperplasia of astrocytes, activation of microglia, and demyelination. Cytotoxic edema is characterized by cellular swelling, including swelling of astrocytes.

Because of compression against the cranium, an affected brain has flattened gyri and shallow sulci, and it can shift in position. If the edema is confined to one side, the displacement is unilateral, which can be associated with herniation of the cingulated gyrus under the falx cerebri; the extent of the unilateral intracerebral enlargement can be best appreciated after the examination of transverse sections. Diffuse swelling usually causes a caudal shifting that can result in herniation of the brain (parahippocampal gyri of temporal lobes) beneath the tentorium cerebelli (Fig. 14-59) or herniation of the cerebellar vermis through the foramen magnum, resulting in "coning" of the vermis (Fig. 14-60). On a cut surface, the white matter is most often affected (frequently with the vasogenic type of edema, which is the most common). It is swollen and soft, has a damp appearance, and is light yellow in the fresh, unfixed state.

Ischemic Myelopathy (Fibrocartilaginous Embolus Formation)

Ischemic myelopathy (necrotizing myelopathy) has been described in the dog, cat, horse, pig, lamb, and turkey. Herniation of degenerative disk material into the vasculature, forming occlusive emboli, is commonly accepted, but the route taken by fibrocartilaginous material into the spinal (or cerebral) vessels is unproved. It has been suggested that trauma to a metaplastic nucleus pulposus causes it to fragment and that the pressure of trauma forces small fragments into damaged veins, venous plexuses, or small arterioles.

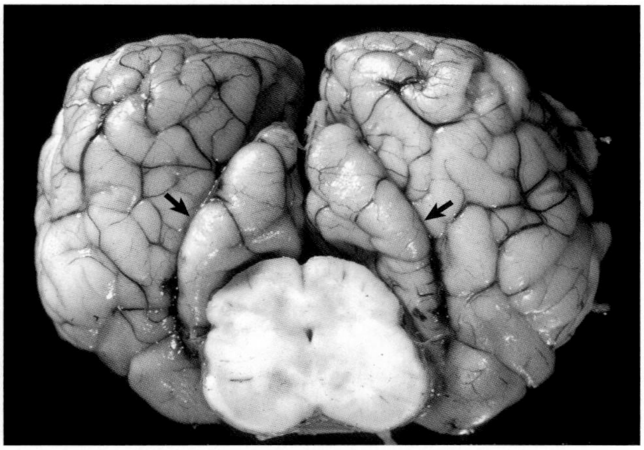

Fig. 14-59 Gyral herniation, parahippocampal gyri, brain, transverse section, caudal face, at level of the rostral colliculi and crus cerebri, horse. The caudal displacement of the parahippocampal gyri *(arrows)* was caused by a sudden swelling of the brain (increase in intracranial pressure) from severe cerebral blunt force trauma to the head. The other cerebral gyri are swollen and flattened and sulci are indistinct (cerebral edema). (Courtesy Dr. M.D. McGavin, College of Veterinary Medicine, University of Tennessee.)

The gross lesion is an acute focal infarct involving cervical or lumbar spinal cord most commonly, but any portion can be affected (Fig. 14-61). Microscopically, emboli histochemically identical to the fibrocartilage of the nucleus pulposus of intervertebral disks occlude meningeal or CNS arteries or veins, or both, in affected areas (Fig. 14-62). Clinically, there is a sudden onset of spinal cord deficits, sometimes with cerebral involvement, in certain species. In dogs, larger breeds are more commonly affected. The disease occurs in young and old animals. One study reported that 60% of confirmed cases of canine ischemic myelopathy had a history of trauma or exercise.

Nonlipid Arteriosclerosis

Arterial fibrosis occurs more frequently in older animals and has been described in dogs and horses. In the dog, fibrosis of the intima, media, or adventitia occurs with some frequency in cerebrospinal vessels of all types and caliber. Fibrous thickening of the adventitia of small meningeal and CNS arteries can be accompanied by variable degree of extension of fibrosis into other layers of the vessel wall. A preferential site is the choroid plexus. In old horses, a similar pattern of fibrosis occurs in vessels, and the adventitia may be preferentially affected. Amyloid deposits in meningeal and cerebral vessels are reported in older dogs and other animals. Mineralization (deposition of calcium or iron salts) of cerebral blood vessels occurs in the brains of several species but is especially common in adult horses. Vessels of the internal capsule, globus pallidus, cerebellar dentate nucleus, and infrequently the hippocampus are preferentially affected in horses, cattle, and less commonly, dogs. Meningeal vessels in old cats, old horses, and cattle and vessels of the choroid plexus in old cats are other sites of vascular mineralization. Overt ischemic damage is rarely associated with these nonlipomatous vascular lesions in any species, therefore clinical signs are not seen with this lesion.

Lysosomal Storage Diseases

Dysfunction of lysosome-mediated degradation of products (substrates) of normal cellular metabolism results in diseases referred to as *lysosomal storage diseases.* These substrates cannot be degraded by lysosomes, and the accumulated substrate eventually results in death of the affected cells.

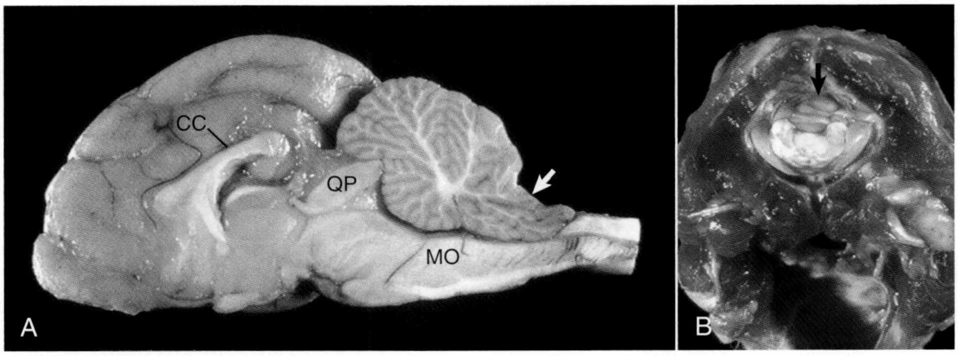

Fig. 14-60 Coning of the cerebellar vermis, brain, cat.

A, Sagittal section. Coning of the cerebellum. The caudal cerebellar vermis has been displaced caudally through the foramen magnum; note the notch on the dorsal surface *(arrow).* This result has compressed the medulla oblongata *(MO),* which can cause death from compression of the respiratory center. Note the elevation of the corpus callosum *(CC)* and focal compression of the rostral cerebellar vermis by the tectum (quadrigeminal plate) *(QP).* **B,** Coning of the cerebellum through the foramen magnum, caudal view through the foramen magnum. Note that in this case not only has the cerebellar vermis *(arrow)* been displaced caudally but also the medulla. The caudal cerebellar peduncles have been displaced caudally as far as the foramen magnum. (**A** courtesy Dr. D. Cho, College of Veterinary Medicine, Louisiana State University; and Noah's Arkive, College of Veterinary Medicine, The University of Georgia. **B** courtesy College of Veterinary Medicine, University of Illinois.)

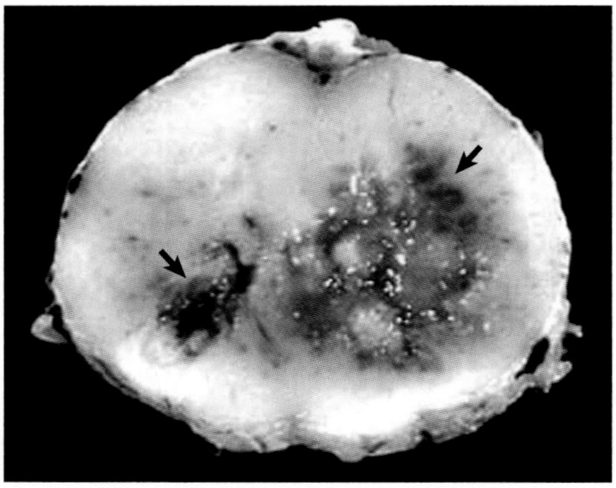

Fig. 14-61 Spinal cord infarction (ischemic necrosis), dog.
The yellow-brown region of necrosis *(arrows)* in the right lateral and ventral funiculi was the result of fibrocartilaginous emboli that occluded branches of the ventral spinal artery and obstructed blood flow. (Courtesy Dr. J. Edwards, College of Veterinary Medicine, Texas A&M University; and Dr. J. King, College of Veterinary Medicine, Cornell University.)

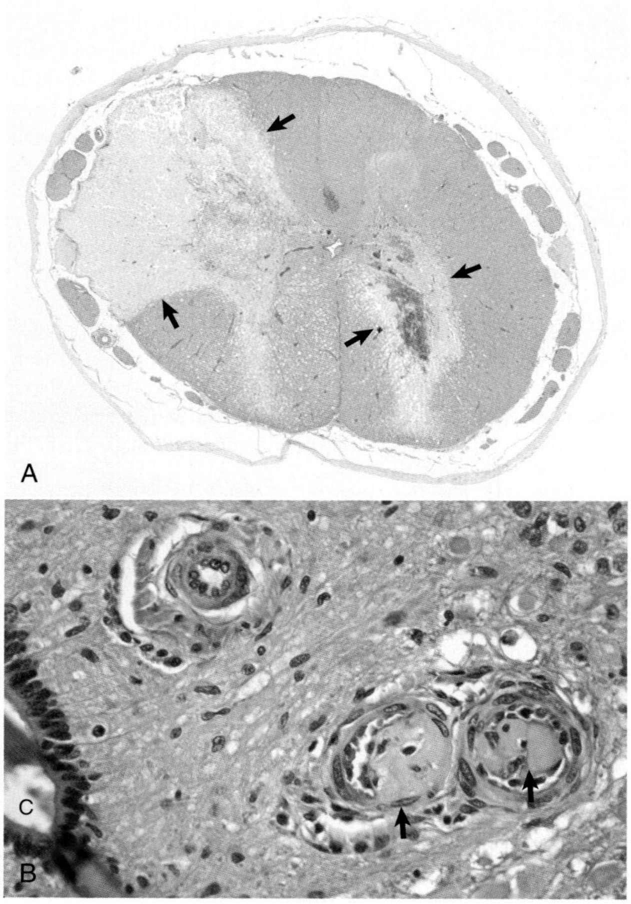

Fig. 14-62 Fibrocartilaginous embolus, spinal cord, dog.
A, Vascular occlusion and infraction. Fibrocartilaginous emboli have obstructed the dorsolateral artery *(top left)* and branches of the ventral spinal artery to the right ventral gray horn and adjacent white matter, causing infarction *(arrows)*. H&E stain. **B,** Fibrocartilaginous emboli in arterioles *(arrows)*. *C,* Central canal. H&E stain. (**A** courtesy Dr. M.D. McGavin, College of Veterinary Medicine, University of Tennessee. **B** courtesy Dr. J. Van Vleet, College of Veterinary Medicine, Purdue University.)

Cell death is the endpoint of a chronic and progressive process of substrate accumulation that interferes with cellular biochemical processes and transport systems. When neurons or myelinating cells die, they release their accumulated substrate into adjacent tissue. Macrophages are recruited from the bloodstream as monocytes, and they phagocytose cellular debris and unprocessed substrate released from dead cells. Macrophages, however, have the same genetic defect and thus also accumulate substrate in their lysosomes. Although less vulnerable to the effects of substrate accumulation, macrophages eventually die and their released substrate is phagocytosed by additional macrophages recruited from the blood.

Lipid storage diseases, such as globoid cell leukodystrophy, are covered in more detail later. Features of some selected lysosomal storage diseases of animals are provided in Table 14-7.

Lysosomal storage diseases were originally thought to develop exclusively because of mutations that result in a reduction in lysosomal enzyme synthesis. More recently, however, it has become clear that there are other defects such as the following:

1. Synthesis of catalytically inactive proteins that resemble normal active enzymes.
2. Defects in posttranslational processing (glycosylation, phosphorylation, addition of fatty acids in the Golgi) of the enzyme, which results in it being misdirected to sites (extracellular) other than to lysosomes.
3. Lack of enzyme activator (an enzyme that normally increases the rate of an enzyme-catalyzed reaction) or protector protein (facilitate repair and refolding of stress-damaged proteins).
4. Lack of substrate activator protein required to assist with the hydrolysis of substrate.
5. Lack of transport protein required for elimination of digested material from lysosomes.

Characterization of lysosomal disorders has therefore been broadened to include involvement of any protein that is essential for normal lysosomal function.

The best-known diseases are characterized by accumulation of the substrate or substrate precursors and sometimes even by the absence of a critical metabolic product for normal lysosomal function. As a general principle, cell swelling and cytoplasmic vacuolation occur because of the accumulation of unprocessed substrate in the lysosomes; therefore differences in the size and appearance of cells (neurons versus hepatocytes) depend on the availability of the substrate (carbohydrate or lipid) in the organ system. Many lipids and glycolipids are unique to the nervous system, thus, when there is a lysosomal defect, neural cells often accumulate in the substrate.

Examples of lysosomal storage diseases that affect humans and animals are the gangliosidoses. With few exceptions, these diseases are inherited in an autosomal recessive pattern. They are also often gene-dose dependent and correspondingly, recessive homozygotes manifest the disease, whereas heterozygotes are phenotypically and functionally normal, but the affected enzyme's activity is reduced by approximately 50% of normal. The age of onset of clinical signs and the severity of the disease process can vary among the different diseases because the deficiency of the involved enzyme is not always the same. If the gene defect is such that the mutant enzyme is not synthesized at all, there is an early onset of a severe disease. Conversely, if there is some residual synthesis of the deficient enzyme, later onset and a milder form of the disease result because partial catabolism of the accumulated substrate permits a longer period of time before the lysosomes are so distended with substrate that they cause loss of cell function.

Gross lesions of the CNS vary among the different types of lysosomal storage diseases. Brain atrophy occurs with globoid

TABLE 14-7 Classification of Selected Lysosomal Storage Diseases that Involve the CNS of Animals

Disease	Storage Product	Deficient Enzyme	Species	Breed
GM_1 gangliosidosis	GM_1 ganglioside	β-Galactosidase	Bovine	Holstein-Friesian
			Canine	Beagle, English springer spaniel, Portuguese water dog, Alaskan huskies
			Feline	Siamese, domestic shorthair
			Ovine	Suffolk, Coopworth-Romney
GM_2 gangliosidosis	GM_2 ganglioside	β-Hexosaminidase	Canine	German shorthair pointer, Japanese spaniel
			Feline	Domestic shorthair, Korat
			Porcine	Yorkshire
Globoid-cell leukodystrophy (Krabbe's-like disease)	Galactosylceramide (galactocerebroside) and galactosylsphingosine (psychosine)	Galactosylceramidase (galactocerebroside β-galactosidase)	Canine	West Highland terrier Cairn terrier, miniature poodle, blue tick hound, beagle, Pomeranian
			Feline	Domestic shorthair, domestic longhair
			Ovine	Polled Dorset
α-Mannosidosis	Mannose-containing oligosaccharide	α-Mannosidase	Bovine	Angus, Murray gray, Galloway
			Feline	Persian, domestic shorthair
β-Mannosidosis	Mannose-containing oligosaccharide	β-Mannosidase	Caprine	Nubian
			Bovine	Salers
Mucopolysaccharidosis	Different glycosaminoglycans	Several different enzyme deficiencies	Canine	Plott hound (type I, Hurler's disease), miniature pinscher (type VI, Maroteaux-Lamy disease) Breed? (type VII, Sly disease)
			Feline	Domestic shorthair (type I, Hurler's disease) Breed? (type VI, Maroteaux-Lamy disease) Domestic shorthair (type VII, Sly disease)
			Caprine	Nubian (type III, Sanfilippo's disease)
Ceroid-lipofuscinosis	Subunit c of mitochondrial ATPase	Prelysosomal defect?	Canine	English setter, border collie, Tibetan terrier
			Ovine	South Hampshire
			Bovine	Devon
	Sphingolipid	Palmitoyl protein thioesterase	Canine	Miniature schnauzer
	Activating proteins A and D		Ovine	Swedish Landrace
	Unknown	Unknown	Canine	Chihuahua, cocker spaniel, Saluki, terrier-cross, blue heeler, Yugoslavian shepherd, Dalmatian, Australian cattle dog, golden retriever, dachshund, corgi
			Ovine	Rambouillet
			Bovine	Beefmaster
			Feline	Siamese, domestic shorthair
Niemann-Pick type c disease	Primarily ganglioside in neurons	Unknown	Feline	Breed?
			Canine	Boxer

?, Unknown; *ATPase,* adenosine triphosphatase.

leukodystrophy in latter stages of the diseases because of the loss of myelin. Brain atrophy can also be seen with ceroid-lipofuscinosis but is not prominent in other lysosomal storage diseases, although brains of animals with gangliosidoses can have a firm, rubbery consistency. Microscopically, affected neurons often have a foamy, finely vacuolated, or granular cytoplasm, which is a reflection of the degree to which the stored material is removed during histologic processing (Fig. 14-63). The specific features of the stored material can be best appreciated by ultrastructural examination.

Ceroid-lipofuscinosis is a lysosomal storage disease characterized by abnormal sphingolipid (lipopigments) metabolism that occurs in cats, dogs, cattle, and sheep. Its lysosomal dysfunction has not been clearly identified, but experimental studies have shown alterations in the activity of palmitoyl-protein thioesterase and concentration of acid protease. The disease resembles other lysosomal storage diseases in that it can have a recessive mode of inheritance, but it is dissimilar in that it has no gene-dose effect. Brain atrophy occurs with ceroid-lipofuscinosis in later stages of the diseases (in sheep) (see Fig. 14-17). The atrophy, which most frequently involves the cerebral cortex but also sometimes the cerebellum, can result in a 50% reduction in brain weight. The cerebral hemispheres are increased in firmness and often have a tan color, whereas the gyri are thinned and the sulci widened, a clear indication of cerebrocortical atrophy. Microscopically, the cytoplasm of affected neurons has an eosinophilic granular material (with H&E staining) and a decrease in the number of neurons. Reactive astrogliosis is prominent, and microgliosis may also be observed.

Globoid Cell Leukodystrophy

As discussed previously, lysosomal storage generally refers to a cellular alteration in which an increased amount of substrate material, which normally is degraded, accumulates within lysosomes, often eventually resulting in cell death. These diseases have a hereditary basis, occur in young animals, and are transmitted in an autosomal recessive pattern. Features of some selected lysosomal storage diseases of animals are given in Table 14-7.

Globoid cell leukodystrophy, a sphingolipidosis, is a lysosomal storage disease; its principal lesion is primary demyelination

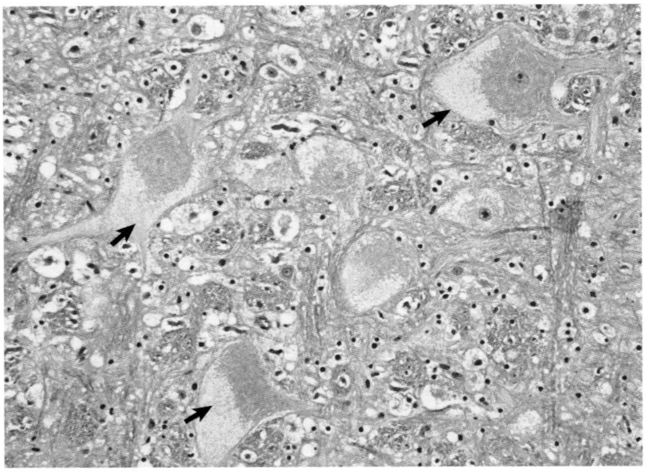

Fig. 14-63 Glycogen/carbohydrate (lysosomal) storage disease, brainstem, neuron cell bodies, cat.
Note the enlargement of the neuron cell bodies, displacement of nuclei, and accumulation of unprocessed substrate in the cytoplasm of the neuronal cell bodies *(arrows)* giving the appearance of "foamy" cytoplasm. H&E stain. (Courtesy Dr. J.F. Zachary, College of Veterinary Medicine, University of Illinois.)

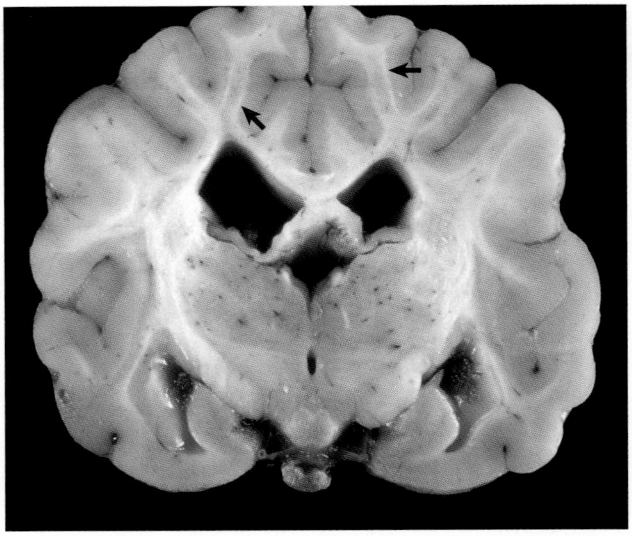

Fig. 14-64 Lipid storage disease, globoid cell leukodystrophy, brain, transverse section at the level of the mammillary body, dog.
The white matter, especially of the gyri, has an off-white to light gray appearance *(arrows)*. Macrophages (globoid cells) derived from blood monocytes (also enzymatically deficient in β-galactocerebrosidase) accumulate in white matter to phagocytose galactocerebroside and oligodendroglial debris secondary to the toxic effects of galactosylsphingosine (psychosine) on oligodendroglia (and in the PNS Schwann cells). There is also bilateral hydrocephalus of the lateral ventricles, presumably hydrocephalus ex vacuo, as a result of the loss of neurons and their axons. (Courtesy Dr. H.B. Gelberg, College of Veterinary Medicine, Oregon State University.)

involving oligodendrocytes of the CNS and Schwann cells of the PNS. The disease, which has an autosomal recessive inheritance in the Cairn and West Highland white terrier, is generally seen in younger animals, often younger than 1 year old. It has also been described in beagles, miniature poodles, basset hounds, Pomeranians, blue tick hounds, and domestic short- and long-haired cats.

Mechanistically, the proposed sequence of events in this disease includes (1) early "normal" myelination that progresses up to a certain stage; (2) disruption of normal myelin turnover because of deficient galactosylceramidase activity; (3) degeneration and necrosis of myelinating cells because of the accumulation of psychosine; (4) primary demyelination; (5) recruitment of phagocytes, both resident microglia and trafficking blood monocytes; and (6) infiltration of macrophages, which become globoid cells after phagocytosing myelin byproducts into the nervous tissue. The last-named changes occur in response to the demyelination and unmetabolized galactocerebroside.

Affected oligodendroglia and Schwann cells are deficient in the lysosomal hydrolase, galactosylceramide β-galactosidase (GALC), which is responsible for degradation of galactosylsphingosine (psychosine) and galactosylceramide (galactocerebroside). Psychosine is highly toxic and because it is not degraded, it has been hypothesized that it accumulates during the disease and causes direct injury to oligodendrocytes and Schwann cells, possibly through an apoptotic mechanism of cell death, in part, mediated by psychosine-induced production of cytokines and inducible nitric oxide synthase (iNOS).

In globoid cell leukodystrophy, the composition of myelin is not qualitatively abnormal. Galactosylceramide is highly concentrated in myelin but is nearly absent in systemic organs except for the kidney. Peak synthesis and turnover of galactosylceramide coincides with the peak period of myelin formation and turnover during the first year of life. GALC activity also increases in relation to the galactosylceramide peak. Myelination continues at a slower rate as animals mature, and in an adult myelin formation is stable with minimal turnover.

A deficiency in GALC activity results in the accumulation of galactosylceramide, especially during the early phase of myelin maturation and turnover, and in the formation of globoid cells discussed later. Psychosine also accumulates, leading to rapid and massive degeneration of oligodendroglia and Schwann cells, extensive myelinolysis, and reduction in myelination.

Gross lesions of the CNS are characterized by a gray discoloration of the white matter, especially of the centrum semiovale of the cerebral hemispheres and white matter of the spinal cord (Fig. 14-64). The lesion in the spinal cord tends to start in the peripheral white matter and spread inward. Microscopically, such areas have pronounced loss of myelin (Fig. 14-65, *A*) and prominent globoid cells containing galactocerebroside that can be demonstrated with a PAS stain (Fig. 14-65, *B*). Peripheral nerves are also affected and lesions are typified by primary demyelination and secondary axonal degeneration. Small sensory branches of peripheral nerves are useful sites to take biopsies to make diagnoses (see Fig. 14-112).

Clinically, affected animals are ataxic and have limb weakness and tremors that progress to paralysis and muscular atrophy. Poor vision or blindness may also occur.

Disease Processes Affecting Myelin Formation and Maintenance

Hypomyelination and Dysmyelination

Disorders of myelin formation include hypomyelinogenesis (hypomyelination) and dysmyelination. Hypomyelinogenesis is a process in which there is underdevelopment of myelin. Dysmyelination refers to the formation of biochemically defective myelin. Hypomyelinogenesis and dysmyelination most often occur in the early postnatal period and have similar clinical and pathologic features. There are some differences in the lesions and the mechanisms by which they develop. Some of these diseases in domestic animals are outlined in Table 14-8.

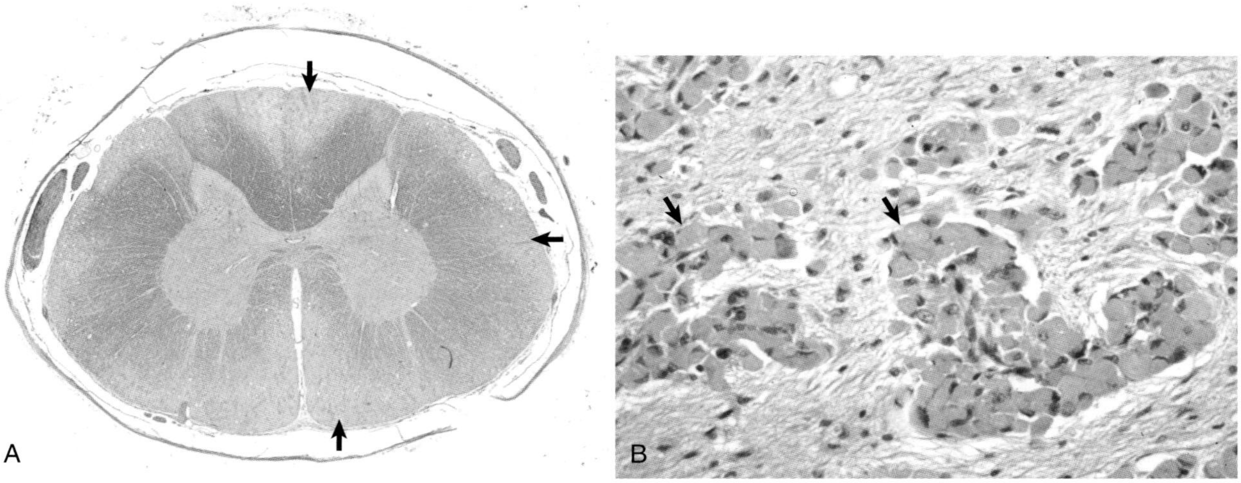

Fig. 14-65 Globoid cell leukodystrophy, dog.
A, Spinal cord. This section of spinal cord has been stained with Luxol fast blue, a histochemical reaction that stains myelin blue. Note the loss of myelin from the periphery of the cord, where axons are heavily myelinated *(arrows),* the first area to be affected. Luxol fast blue stain with a nuclear fast red counterstain. **B,** Cerebrum. Globoid cells deficient in β-galactocerebrosidase *(arrows),* usually located in the perivascular space, increase in size and number because they are unable to degrade galactocerebroside to a less complex substrate. H&E stain. (Courtesy Dr. M.D. McGavin, College of Veterinary Medicine, University of Tennessee.)

TABLE 14-8 Hypomyelinogenesis and Dysmyelination in Animals

Species	Breed	Disease Designation	Genetic Cause	Infectious Cause	Metabolic Cause
Bovine	All breeds	Bovine virus diarrhea (dysmyelination)		Bovine virus diarrhea (pestivirus)	
	Charolais	Progressive ataxia	Suspected		
Ovine	All breeds	Border disease (hypomyelinogenesis-dysmyelination)		Border disease virus (pestivirus)	
Porcine	Landrace	Congenital tremor (myelin agenesia)	Sex-linked recessive		
	Saddleback	Congenital tremor	Autosomal recessive		
	Chester-white	Myoclonia congenita	Autosomal recessive	Suspected	
	All breeds	Congenital tremor (dysmyelinogenesis and cerebellar hypoplasia)		Classical swine fever (pestivirus)	
	All breeds	Congenital tremor (dysmyelinogenesis)		Unknown virus suspected	
	All breeds	Congenital ataxia and tremor (hypomyelinogenesis and cerebellar hypoplasia)			Trichlorfon (acaricide)
Canine	Dalmatian	Hypomyelinogenesis			
	Chow Chow	Dysmyelination	Suspected		
	Springer spaniel	Shaking pups (hypomyelination)	Sex-linked recessive		
	Samoyed	Tremor (hypomyelination)	Suspected		
	Lurcher	Tremor syndrome (hypomyelination)			
	Weimaraner	Hypomyelination	Suspected		

Hypomyelinogenesis

Diseases caused by viruses

Classic swine fever (hog cholera) virus, a pestivirus, can be teratogenic in the porcine fetus. The best-known neural defects resulting from fetal infection are hypomyelinogenesis and cerebellar hypoplasia, although other lesions of the CNS, such as microencephaly and nonneural tissue, have been reported. The mechanism of lesion development has not been definitively determined, but a persistent infection that results in inhibition of cell division and function of selected tissues has been proposed.

Border disease viral infection (also a pestiviral infection) is capable of inducing maldevelopment in the CNS and nonneural tissues (skeleton) of lambs and goats after natural infection of the dam during pregnancy. One of the characteristic lesions in the CNS is hypomyelinogenesis, primarily affecting the white matter of the cerebrum and cerebellum. Grossly, it may be difficult to distinguish between white and gray matter in transverse sections of cerebrum and cerebellum. The brain and spinal cords from affected lambs may be smaller when compared with unaffected lambs. The PNS is unaffected. Hypomyelinogenesis may be related to a viral-induced decrease of myelin-associated glycoprotein, myelin basic protein, and activity of nucleotide phosphodiesterase in oligodendroglia. Other lesions detected in lambs include early inflammation, porencephaly-hydranencephaly, cerebellar malformation including hypoplasia, microencephaly, and reduction in diameter of the spinal cord.

Globoid Cell Leukodystrophy

See the previous section on Lysosomal Storage Diseases.

Spongy Degeneration (Status Spongiosus)

Spongy degeneration is a group of diseases of young animals characterized by a spongy lesion (referred to here as *status spongiosus*) that primarily occurs in the white matter of the CNS but also extends into the gray matter. Status spongiosus is a somewhat nonspecific term and can develop by several different mechanisms. It includes a variety of lesions, such as splitting of lamella forming myelin sheaths (characteristic of the diseases discussed here), accumulation of extracellular fluid (extracellular cerebral edema), swelling of cellular processes (astrocytic, neuronal), and Wallerian degeneration at a later stage when the necrotic myelin and axons have been phagocytosed and the spaces once occupied by these structures are empty.

Gross brain lesions reported for spongy degeneration range from no gross lesions to swelling, edema, and pallor of the white matter, and dilation of the ventricles. Microscopically, the lesion is characterized by variably sized empty spaces within the white matter. Ultrastructurally, with spongy degeneration and some other disease processes characterized by status spongiosus, there is splitting or separation of the myelin sheath at the intraperiod line with the formation of large intramyelinic spaces. In some cases, myelin formation is deficient.

Some species and breeds affected with spongy degeneration include the canine (Labrador retriever, Saluki, silky terrier, Samoyed), feline (Egyptian mau), and bovine (Jersey, shorthorn, Angus shorthorn, Hereford), and an autosomal recessive mode of transmission has been proposed for some forms of this disorder. A unique form of the spongy degeneration also occurs in a group of metabolic inherited diseases called *aminoacidopathies*.

The term *spongiform change* should not be confused with spongy degeneration. Spongiform change is characterized by small clear vacuoles of varied sizes that form in the cytoplasm of neuron cell bodies and proximal dendrites in diseases, such as the TSEs and rabies encephalitis, and in the processes of astrocytes that are spatially related to the affected neurons.

Demyelination

Demyelination, which means degeneration and loss of myelin already formed, can be divided into primary and secondary types. *Primary demyelination* refers to a disease process in which the myelin sheath is selectively affected, with the axon remaining essentially intact. *Secondary demyelination,* a designation criticized by some, refers to "secondary" degeneration of myelin after "primary" injury to and loss of the axon, as in Wallerian degeneration, and is not a selective injury of the myelin sheath.

Injury to oligodendroglia that results in myelin sheath breakdown or direct injury to myelin sheaths cause the release of lipids and other myelin components into the extracellular space. These materials readily activate microglial cells and attract blood monocytes, which phagocytose myelin debris.

Metabolic Causes

Osmotic demyelination syndrome

In humans, osmotic demyelination syndrome is termed *central* or *extrapontine myelinolysis.* The disorder was first reported in 1959, and the majority of cases were in severely malnourished alcoholics. Since then, the disorder has been observed in a variety of clinical disease states. A major risk factor is chronic hyponatremia treated in hospitals by the administration of intravenous saline solution. The disease has been experimentally reproduced in dogs and laboratory rodents by inducing hyponatremia, allowing a period of stabilization (3 to 4 days is sufficient), and then administering saline-containing fluids.

Two cases of osmotic demyelination syndrome have been reported in the veterinary literature, and one of the authors has observed a case. In all three, there has been a clinical diagnosis of Addison's disease. Treatment consisted of intravenous administration of fluids containing normal saline solution to correct the hyponatremia typical of hypoadrenocorticism. The reported rates of correction have been 22 mmol/L in 24 hours and 16.4 mmol/L in 24 hours. In the author's case, serum sodium increased by 42 mmol/L in 4 days. All of these rates of correction exceed the limits established for humans and are consistent with human cases of the syndrome.

The pathogenesis of osmotic demyelination syndrome is thought to be opposite to that occurring with salt poisoning (i.e., a hyponatremic to hypernatremic shift after saline administration). Lesions occur in areas of the brain in which there is a confluence or intermingling of gray and white matter. Rapid (within 24 to 48 hours) correction of chronic hyponatremia from an established equilibrium exceeds the adaptive responses of the brain, resulting in myelin destruction. The exact mechanism of demyelination is not known. It is proposed that osmotic imbalance and water shifts induce osmotic stress in the CNS that result in myelin destruction.

In contrast to humans, gross lesions in dogs are either not apparent or subtle. Slight softening and discoloration has been observed in affected brain regions. Microscopically, lesions can be limited to the reticular formation at the level of the pons or can be extensive, affecting cerebellar folia, midbrain, thalamus, basal nuclei, and at the interface of the corona radiata and cerebrocortical gray matter. In affected areas, the white matter is pale in routine H&E stained sections and is heavily infiltrated with foamy macrophages. Special stains (Luxol fast blue for myelin) confirm acute myelin destruction and accumulation of myelin debris in macrophages. As is typical of strictly demyelinating lesions, axons are well preserved.

Circulatory and Physical Disturbances

Physical compression of CNS tissue that results from various causes, usually chronic, can also induce demyelination. Some possible mechanisms include compression of myelin sheaths and oligodendroglia, interference with circulation resulting in CNS ischemia, and disease processes resulting in the accumulation of extracellular fluid.

It is well known that vasogenic and hydrostatic edema caused by inflammation, neoplasms, trauma, and obstructive hydrocephalus can cause degeneration of myelin sheaths. The underlying mechanisms for this injury are multiple and include creation of a hypoxic-anoxic environment, degeneration of oligodendroglia, and alteration in stability of the myelin sheath, permitting entrance of injurious proteolytic enzymes from the surrounding environment.

Diseases Caused by Microbes

Progressive multifocal leukoencephalopathy

See Web Appendix 14-1.

Immune-Mediated Diseases

In veterinary medicine, naturally occurring immune-mediated demyelination in domestic animals is rare, and other than canine polyradiculoneuritis (coonhound paralysis), it is usually only suspected rather than proved. These diseases are mostly known to occur in humans as sequelae to postinfectious and postvaccinal events. They result in primary demyelination of the CNS. Autoimmune diseases of the CNS are mechanistically either a type II hypersensitivity (antibody-mediated) or a type IV (cell-mediated) hypersensitivity, and T lymphocytes and macrophage-derived cytokines play contributory roles.

Autoimmune injury to oligodendroglia in the CNS arising from aberrant cellular and/or humoral immune responses can result from one of the following four proposed mechanisms:

1. Molecular mimicry: the CNS has antigens that are similar or identical to those expressed by certain pathogens (virus or bacterium). The normal inflammatory and immunologic responses to these pathogens result in the expression of antibodies that cross-react with "antigens" normally expressed by CNS cells.
2. Abrogation of immune tolerance: the CNS is an "immune privileged" organ (like the eye). The immune system therefore does not recognize CNS antigens as innate antigens, and if they are exposed to the immune system after inflammation or trauma, an autoimmune response can ensue. Injury, physical or otherwise, to blood vessels within the CNS can cause the release of "sequestered antigens" into the bloodstream, leading to an autoimmune response.
3. Genetic factors: Functions of the immune system that are strictly regulated genetically may be under the control of abnormal inherited genes or altered normal genes that regulate immune responses to CNS antigens and thus increase the susceptibility to autoimmune diseases.
4. Stress factors: Environmental stresses mediated through the CNS can depress the functions of the immune system, leading to the formation of autoantibodies.

The mechanism of myelin breakdown in immune-mediated demyelination is not clearly understood. The initial step is thought to be exposure of antigens in myelin basic protein of the major dense line of myelin lamellae after injury. Myelin proteins are substrates for calpain, a calcium-activated neutral proteinase. Calpain has been implicated in several autoimmune diseases and may play an important role in CNS demyelination. Exposed antigens are then recognized by the immune system, and experimental studies suggest that lesions result from a complex interaction between inflammatory cells and their mediators and lamellae of myelinating cells. T lymphocytes, some B lymphocytes, and activated macrophages (recruited monocytes) and microglia cells, adhesion molecules, cytokines, chemokines, and their receptors have been demonstrated in the lesions. This interaction results in primary demyelination.

Gross lesions are usually not present but can include a gray-to-yellow discoloration of white matter. Microscopically, lesions are best observed in white matter and are characterized by vacuolation of myelin and the presence of lymphocytes, macrophages, and plasma cells. Myelin sheaths degenerate from injury caused by (1) inflammatory mediators and (2) direct actions of macrophages on lamellae. Myelin lamellae separate as a result of intramyelinic edema, fragment, and are phagocytosed by macrophages.

The best-known model of immune-mediated demyelination is an experimental model referred to as *experimental allergic encephalomyelitis* (EAE). EAE is produced by inducing a hypersensitivity to myelin or more specifically, to myelin basic protein. If appropriate laboratory animals are inoculated with white matter or myelin basic protein (suspended in complete Freund's adjuvant), they become paralyzed after 2 to 3 weeks. Lesions are characterized by perivascular (perivenular) demyelination accompanied by accumulation of lymphocytes and macrophages.

A similar process, referred to as *postvaccinal encephalomyelitis,* occurred occasionally in humans when human rabies vaccine contained CNS tissue. The incidence decreased after 1957 when duck embryo rabies vaccine came into use. In some cases with mild clinical signs, recovery was complete and axons were remyelinated after immune-mediated demyelination.

A third situation in which this type of demyelination occurs follows infection with certain viruses in humans (rubeola virus) and animals (e.g., influenza virus). These diseases, which are rare and designated as postinfectious encephalomyelitis, are also characterized by development of lesions in the CNS comparable to those of EAE.

Traumatic Injury

Traumatic injury of the CNS is caused by physical insults such as compression, stretching, and/or laceration of neurons/axons. When the brain and spinal cord collide with the bony ridges lining the cranial vault and the bony wall of the vertebral canal, respectively, or when axial, rotational, and angular forces (Fig. 14-66) are applied to neurons and axons during trauma, the force of impact and sudden acceleration of neurons and axons, both within the CNS and in the adjacent cranial and spinal nerves, can cause them to compress, twist, stretch, and tear. Concurrently, the same type of forces can injure blood vessels in the CNS and leptomeninges and may result in small hemorrhages or hematomas within the parenchyma of the brain and in the leptomeninges (subarachnoid space) (Fig. 14-67).

Diffuse brain injury (often present in concussion) is caused by acceleration/deceleration forces applied to many areas of the CNS rather than in one specific location. Diffuse brain injury involves neuronal processes, cell bodies, transmitter mechanisms, and macroglial cells and blood vessels. The most severe injury to axons appears to be at the gray matter–white matter junction. A variant of diffuse brain injury is diffuse axonal injury in which axons of large myelinated nerve fibers are injured by shearing forces. In diffuse brain and axonal injury, mechanical deformation results in physical disruption of cell membranes and cytoskeleton and increased membrane permeability, resulting in major ionic fluxes in and out of the cell. Such changes can lead to excessive release of glutamate, excitotoxicity and cell death, free radical formation, apoptosis, and delayed inflammatory responses. The end result can be Wallerian degeneration.

In general, trauma of the CNS in animals occurs less frequently than in humans. Animals are not exposed as frequently to potentially trauma-causing situations (e.g., automobile travel) as are humans, and there are anatomic differences (see later), including a quadruped posture, which increases stability and helps protect the brains of animals.

Among animals, trauma to the brain is probably most frequently caused in dogs as a result of automobile-induced injury and in cats from falls from significant heights (high-rise apartment buildings, balconies, and roofs). Even after falling from considerable heights, cats often have remarkably minor injury to the CNS. Other examples include fracture of the spinal column or cranium of jumping horses and fractious animals, such as horses and ruminants, during excitement and restraint.

Predisposition to cerebral trauma is also influenced by anatomic differences. The percentage of brain mass in relation to skull size is much less in domestic animals than in primates, and in the bovine and porcine species, the cranial cavity is additionally protected dorsally by prominent frontal sinuses. Birth trauma, which can be important in humans, is essentially insignificant in animals because in the latter, the shoulders and particularly the pelvis, rather than the head, are likely to be compressed in the birth canal. Exceptions to this generalization include brachycephalic breeds of dogs. Several factors also influence the susceptibility of the spinal cord to trauma. The amount of space between the spinal cord and the wall

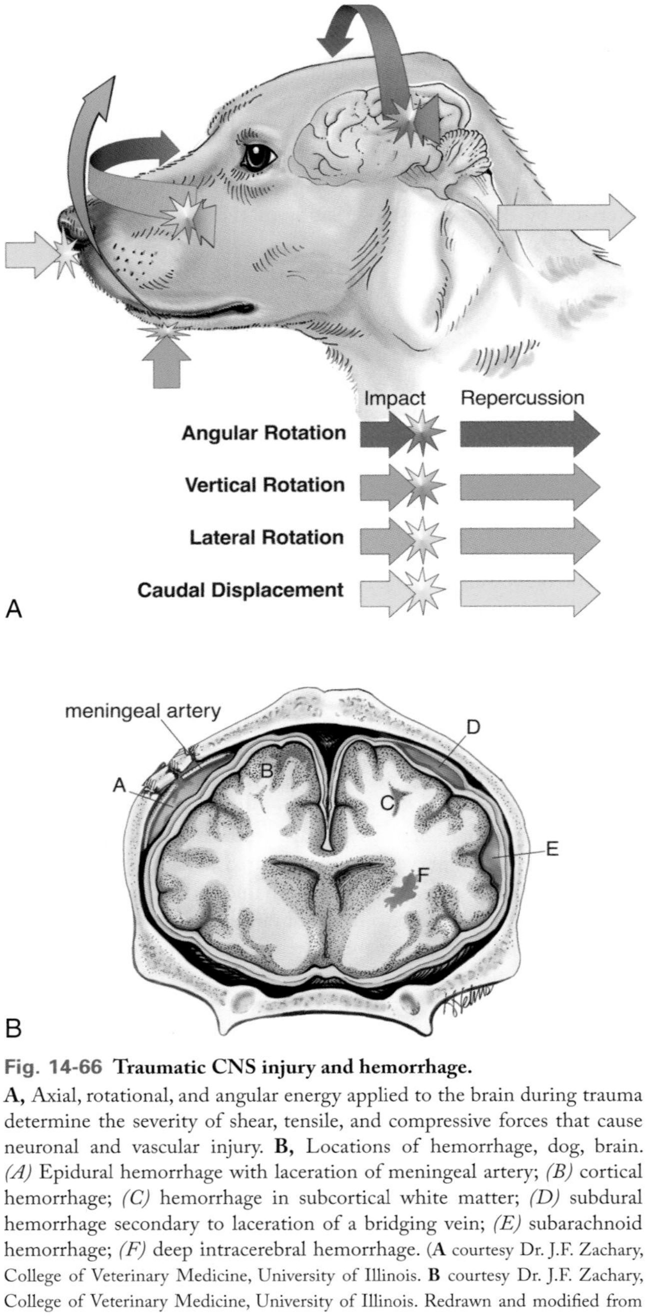

Fig. 14-66 Traumatic CNS injury and hemorrhage.
A, Axial, rotational, and angular energy applied to the brain during trauma determine the severity of shear, tensile, and compressive forces that cause neuronal and vascular injury. **B,** Locations of hemorrhage, dog, brain. *(A)* Epidural hemorrhage with laceration of meningeal artery; *(B)* cortical hemorrhage; *(C)* hemorrhage in subcortical white matter; *(D)* subdural hemorrhage secondary to laceration of a bridging vein; *(E)* subarachnoid hemorrhage; *(F)* deep intracerebral hemorrhage. (**A** courtesy Dr. J.F. Zachary, College of Veterinary Medicine, University of Illinois. **B** courtesy Dr. J.F. Zachary, College of Veterinary Medicine, University of Illinois. Redrawn and modified from Leech RW, Shuman RM: *Neuropathology: a summary for students,* Philadelphia, 1982, Harper & Row.)

of the vertebral canal is very important in determining the degree of injury after edema or compression with disk herniation. This space is greater in the cervical area of the dog than at the thoracolumbar level. Thus disk herniation at the latter area is more likely to result in severe spinal cord injury.

Functional factors also play an important role in brain injury. The brain of a freely movable head is much more susceptible to injury than one that is fixed in place. The increased susceptibility of the former has been attributed to the ability of the cranium (the bone) and its contents (the brain) to impact each other after nonpenetrating trauma. This interaction occurs because the brain does not completely fill the cranial cavity, thus resulting in a very short distance (or space) between brain and bone.

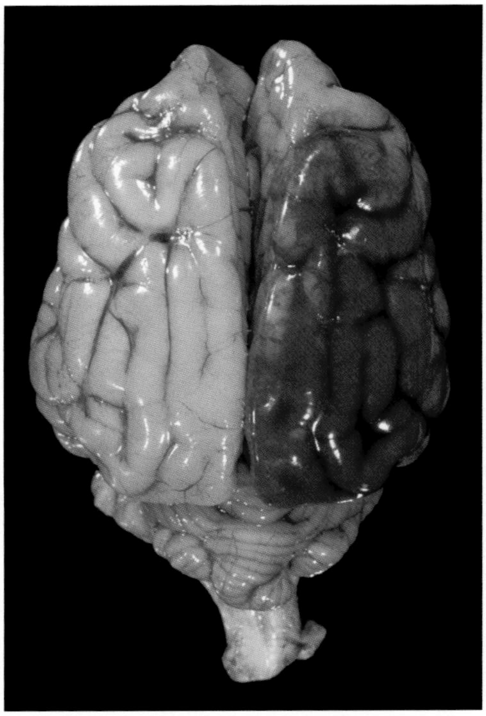

Fig. 14-67 Leptomeningeal (subarachnoid) hemorrhage, brain, right cerebral hemisphere, dog.
(Courtesy Dr. R. Storts, College of Veterinary Medicine, Texas A&M University.)

The type and location of the lesion (contusion and/or hemorrhage) depends on the location of the point of contact and the direction of the blow, relative to the head. If the blow is directly on the back or front of the head, the head and brain will move straightforward or backward, respectively (see Fig. 14-66, axial force). If the blow is horizontal to the top of the head or horizontal to the rostral portion, the head will rotate on the atlanto-occipital axis (angularly and rotationally, respectively). In the case of an axial blow to the back of the head (an animal falling onto the back of its head), the head and thus the cranial vault will accelerate faster than the brain, which will lag behind, and the caudal aspect of the vault may move forward and contact the caudal aspect of the cerebral hemispheres, usually the occipital cortex. In the case of an animal falling onto the back of its head, the head will accelerate abruptly and the momentum will carry the brain caudally, where it may strike the inside of the caudal brain in the cranial vault. A vertical blow delivered directly down onto the dorsal surface of the head will have the same type of result on the dorsal aspect of the cerebral hemispheres as the blow to the back of the head. It is more common, from the same blows described previously, to see hemorrhage, usually subarachnoid, on the opposite side of the point of impact with the brain. For example, a vertical blow to the top of the head causes hemorrhage of the ventral surface of the medulla and cerebral hemispheres. Thus, after an impact on a stationary, freely movable head, the bone of the cranial vault will move on the stationary brain and injure it (coup injury) and on the opposite side the nerves and blood vessels will be stretched, possibly resulting in nerve damage and hemorrhage (contrecoup injury). In addition, the mass and velocity of the object striking the head are important. Trauma after impact of a relatively large blunt object can create notable head movement and a large-impact injury, whereas a small object, such as a bullet moving at a high rate of speed, can cause less head movement and a smaller but deeper area of direct tissue damage. In summary, the basic concept is the transfer of kinetic energy by the striking object to the head. A large blunt object will cause the head to accelerate without deforming it; a smaller object, such as a bullet, will penetrate.

Factors involved in the protection of the brain include the rigidity of the cranium (depending on age), the round shape of the dorsum of the skull, the structure of the parietal, occipital, and temporal cranial bones (two layers of compact bone separated by spongy bone referred to as diploë), cranial sutures, sinuses, ridges in the floor of the cranial cavity, meninges, and CSF. The spinal cord is enclosed and protected by the vertebral column, which is surrounded by soft adipose tissue and muscle. Other structures that help protect the spinal cord by absorbing shock are the intervertebral disks and the cancellous bone of the vertebrae. Vertebral ligaments maintain the alignment of the vertebral column; denticulate ligaments support the spinal cord in the middle of the vertebral canal, and the meninges, particularly the CSF, cushions trauma.

Clinically, animals with CNS trauma have signs referable to the area injured, brain, or spinal cord. With brain trauma, signs can vary widely and range from unconsciousness lasting a few seconds followed by complete recovery and return to normal function to depression, abnormal behaviors such as disorientation and irritability, semiconsciousness with responsiveness only to noxious stimuli, and unconsciousness with no response to any stimulus. With spinal cord trauma, signs vary, depending on the severity of the injury and the rate of onset. Paralysis results from severance of the cord or ruptured disks. Paresis and ataxia result from less severe injury.

Concussion

Concussion is often thought of as a clinical designation of temporary loss of consciousness with recovery after head injury. As in humans, a movable head is much more susceptible to trauma than a fixed, supported one. Application of an appropriate concussive trauma to the mobile head of an animal results in a reversible cerebral dysfunction that lasts for a matter of seconds or at most, a few minutes and is usually reversible, with stronger blows causing more severe injury and even death.

Concussive injuries of the diffuse type also occur in animals, but there are some differences between animals and humans. For example, it is difficult to produce severe concussion in animals because the margin between the force of a stunning blow and one causing fatal injury is very small. The smaller the brain, the less vulnerable it is to rotational forces and the larger are the forces necessary to cause concussion. It should be noted, however, that concussion, particularly when there is rapid recovery from unconsciousness, can occur more frequently than appreciated in animals because the clinical signs may not be recognized.

Diffuse brain injury does not usually cause gross lesions. Microscopic lesions detected in animals include diffuse axonal injury characterized by axonal degeneration, and this may be followed by Wallerian degeneration. Damage to neurons ranges from central chromatolysis to death and neuronal loss. The more severe forms of diffuse brain injury can also have generalized acute brain swelling caused by unregulated vasodilation, which can be followed after some time by cerebral edema.

Spinal concussion is the term applied to the immediate and temporary loss of function that sometimes follows severe direct blows to the spinal column. Loss of function usually affects the long tracts/bundles of nerve fibers (funiculi), but usually there is no demonstrable external change in the vertebrae or spinal cord. As with cerebral concussion, there is often only a temporary functional disability of the cord after injury, but if the trauma is more severe, permanent neurologic deficits can result.

BOX 14-10 Pathogenesis of Coup-Contrecoup Contusion

CONDITIONS INVOLVED IN COUP-CONTRECOUP CONTUSION

1. Head freely movable.
2. Head accelerated rapidly (by being struck by a broad object, such as an automobile) or decelerated rapidly (head strikes pavement after a fall from a standing position).
3. Because the brain does not fill the cranial vault, it may lag behind the movement of the cranium when the head is accelerated or decelerated rapidly.
4. As a result, the inside of the cranial vault may strike the stationary brain at the point of impact (coup injury), or the lesion may occur on the opposite side (contrecoup), either from the stretching and tearing of vessels at that site or by the brain being struck by the inside of the cranial vault on the opposite side when there is reduced amount of cerebrospinal fluid buffer present.

Contusion

Contusion means bruising, which is generally associated with rupture of blood vessels, and in the cerebrum, this injury results in grossly detectable lesions, such as hemorrhage, which can, like concussion, result in unconsciousness and even death. The factors that cause concussion and contusion can occur together in the same animal. Lesions can be superficial (cerebral gyri) or more central (brainstem), and there can be concurrent skull fractures.

Although hemorrhage is the most common lesion, contusion of the brain can also result in tearing of CNS tissue. Tearing results in tissue necrosis and neuronal loss. Two designations are used to identify the location of contusive injury. A coup contusion is located at the impact site, and a contrecoup contusion at a location on the opposite side of the brain. When the two lesions occur together (coup-contrecoup or contrecoup-coup), the first term indicates the site of most severe injury. Box 14-10 summarizes the pathogenesis of coup-contrecoup contusion.

Many investigations have been made to determine the mechanisms involved in the development of contusive lesions, and the kinetics are complicated and still not completely resolved. Factors considered to be significant include the ability of the head to move freely, the occurrence of a rotational movement of the brain over rough surfaces on the inside of the cranial vault, and the development within the cranial cavity of positive and negative pressures and gravitational forces. The basic results of the different types of blows to the heads of animals have been discussed previously, and it is interesting to compare these with the lesions in humans. Several neuropathologic principles have been generally accepted regarding craniocerebral contusive trauma in humans, as follows:

1. A blow to the stationary (but freely movable) head produces a cerebrocortical coup contusion beneath the point of cranial impact, but with rare exceptions causes no cerebrocortical contrecoup contusion opposite the point of cranial impact. This outcome is not always true of animals, in which a blow to the dorsum of the head from a flat object, such as a spade, causes marked subarachnoid hemorrhage on the ventral surface (contrecoup).
2. An impact of a moving head (moving before impact, as in a fall from a standing position) against a firm or unyielding surface causes a cerebrocortical contrecoup contusion opposite the point of cranial collision (often at the poles and inferior surfaces of the frontal and temporal lobes), but with rare

exceptions there is no contusion beneath the point of impact. In contrast, horses that fall backward and land on their backs and strike the occiput often have subarachnoid hemorrhage over the occipital poles of the cerebral hemispheres.

3. Falls from great heights and crushing of the head between a strong external force and unyielding surface are generally not associated with the occurrence of contrecoup lesions.

Dawson and co-workers proposed a mechanism for both contrecoup and coup injury of the human brain that also addressed the specific deficiencies of mechanisms that have been advanced by others. An example explaining the mechanism of contrecoup injury states that when a person falls backward from a standing position because of loss of balance, the gravitational torque acting on the body causes downward acceleration of the head in excess of the acceleration as a result of gravity. Under these circumstances the brain lags toward the trailing anterior surface of the cranium before impact (causing displacement of the protective CSF layer between the brain and skull) and permits compressive stress to develop at this site, although impact occurs at the opposite side of the head. Because dissipation of the CSF at the anterior (contrecoup) site allows compressive stress to be focal at this contrecoup site and because of the shearing stress generated, injury occurs. In addition, a relative rotational gliding motion between the brain and skull is produced when the impact suddenly stops the skull's motion and rotation, thus creating an additive shearing stress because the fluid lubrication necessary to facilitate gliding of the brain over the cranial surface is reduced. The concentration of this rotational shearing stress is likely to occur beneath the frontal and temporal lobes because of the rough surface of the skull that exists in this location. In contrast to contrecoup injury, coup contusions occur infrequently in this type of fall. In such situations, the brain lags away from the impact site, which results in a thickening of the protective CSF layer between the brain and skull immediately beneath the point of impact, which helps explain the absence of coup injury in primates and humans in typical moving head trauma.

Coup injury in humans can occur when a stationary but freely movable head is impacted. In this type of trauma, there is neither brain lag nor disproportionate distribution of CSF before impact, which accounts for the typical absence of contrecoup contusions. With regard to falls from great heights, the dynamics involving rotation of the body about a fixed point of ground contact associated with a fall from a standing position do not occur. Because gravity produces no torque on a freely falling object, no angular acceleration of the body is produced, therefore such a fall is a true free-fall state that is associated with an absence of brain lag. For this reason, contrecoup lesions occur infrequently with this type of trauma. One point should be emphasized with regard to the evaluation of coup and contrecoup cortical contusions just described. Displacement of bone associated with skull fracture can contuse the subjacent brain, regardless of the resting or moving status of the head, and such fracture-contusions have nothing to do with the coup-contrecoup mechanisms described. Also, even though the basic mechanisms discussed earlier apply to humans, they should also be considered when evaluating cerebral contusions of domestic animals, but the situation in human brains is made far more complex because of the numerous wide bony ridges that project into the cranial vault.

Evaluation of spinal cord trauma should include examination not only of the spinal cord but also of the vertebral column and spinal nerve roots. Injuries to the spinal cord can involve concussion, contusion, hemorrhage, laceration, transection, and compression secondary to vertebral trauma and fracture. Contusion in the spinal cord is characterized by vascular tears, hemorrhage, and necrosis. Tears are generally focal and grossly visible. Contusion can occur without fracture of the vertebral column, with fracture, and with fracture plus dislocation of the spinal column. The latter combination can result in tearing and transection of the spinal cord.

CNS Hemorrhage

Although hemorrhage and hematomas in animal brains can be caused by a wide variety of injuries, trauma to the head is the most common cause. Box 14-11 lists common causes of brain hemorrhage)

After trauma to the head, hemorrhages can develop in the epidural, subdural, and subarachnoid space, under the pia mater (subpial), and in the brain (see Fig. 14-66, *B*). Hemorrhage can be diffuse (see Fig. 14-67) or focal (e.g., hematomas) (Fig. 14-68). Such hemorrhages can result from sliding of the brain over bony ridges (jugae) within the cranium, with resultant stretching and tearing of blood vessels and tissue, after the cutting and penetration of bone fragments from skull fracture. Cerebral epidural hemorrhage, which is not commonly described in animals, has been

BOX 14-11 Common Causes of Hemorrhage in Animal Brains

Vasculitis (such as *Histophilus somni* [formerly *Haemophilus somnus]* infection)
Damage to endothelium lining blood vessels (by the virus of canine infectious hepatitis, by septicemia or endotoxemia, by immune complexes, or by parasite larval migration)
Trauma
Contusion
- Coup lesion
- Contrecoup lesion

Penetrating wounds

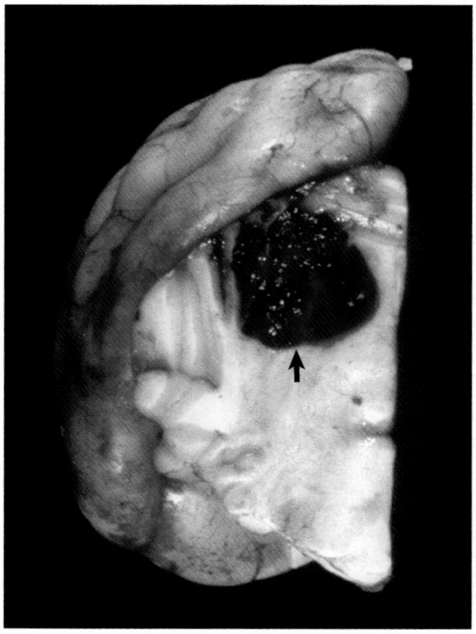

Fig. 14-68 Hematoma *(arrow)*, cerebellum, transverse section, dog. Traumatic injury to the head resulted in hemorrhage and the formation of a hematoma from shear, tensile, compressive axial, rotational, and angular forces. (Courtesy Dr. H.B. Gelberg, College of Veterinary Medicine, Oregon State University.)

reported in the horse, especially jumpers, resulting from falls while working. Epidural hemorrhage does not usually occur because the dura is tightly adhered to the inner surface of the calvarium and there is no epidural space. In trauma causing skull fractures, bleeding from local blood vessels can separate the dura from the calvarium, forming a hematoma in the epidural space.

Subdural hemorrhage, which is an extravasation of blood between the dura mater and arachnoid membrane, occurs in dogs and cats. It is rare and usually diffuse and does not form hematomas as seen in humans, where they can be life threatening from compression and herniation of the brain. Subarachnoid and intracerebral hemorrhages are most common in all species after head injury. Hemorrhage can result from injury to the brain with or without a fractured cranium by the mechanisms given previously and also from penetrating objects (bullets and stab wounds).

The same types of hemorrhage that affect the brain (epidural [rare], subdural [rare], leptomeningeal, and parenchymal) also occur in the spinal cord and its meninges. Causes are similar to those for the brain.

Hematomyelia (Hemorrhagic Myelomalacia)

Traumatic injury to the spinal cord can cause stretching and tearing of blood vessels, usually arterioles, within the gray matter, resulting in hematomyelia. Hematomyelia is also particularly associated with severe type I disk herniation. If larger vessels are torn, blood pressure can force blood into the gray matter. This outcome results in the formation of a dissecting blood-filled cavity ascending and/or descending initially within the gray matter of the spinal cord (Fig. 14-69). This lesion, which is characterized by a softening to semiliquefaction (myelomalacia) and hemorrhage of the tissue, can develop within 12 to 24 hours after injury and can progress both cranially and caudally from the original site of trauma. As the cavity extends cranially, the hemorrhage at the original site also extends into the white matter and can transect the spinal cord. If this lesion extends to the fifth cervical cord segment, the phrenic nerves to the diaphragm will be denervated and respiratory paralysis will result. Bleeding continues until pressure in the blood-filled cavity is equal to the vascular pressure or until bleeding ceases because of hemostasis in the vessel. Hemorrhage can also result from bleeding in arteriovenous malformations within the spinal cord. Hematomyelia is characterized by neurologic deficits consistent with a sudden onset of ascending or descending flaccid paralysis and sensory abnormalities.

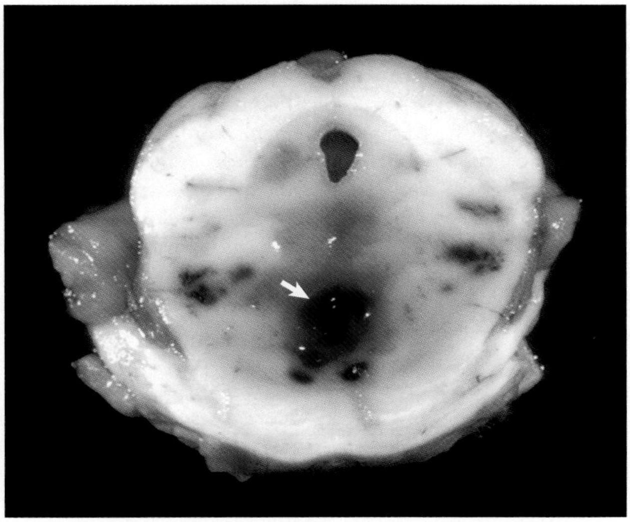

Fig. 14-69 "Duret" hemorrhages, brainstem, transverse section at the level of the pons.

Note the multiple hemorrhages in the periventricular white matter *(arrow)*. These hemorrhages are the result of twisting of the brainstem on a longitudinal axis from rotational and axial forces. (Courtesy Dr. M.D. McGavin, College of Veterinary Medicine, University of Tennessee.)

Compressive Injury

Diseases resulting in compressive injury can affect the brain, spinal cord, or both concurrently. In the brain, diseases, such as neoplasia, reticulosis, canine granulomatous meningoencephalitis, and chronic cerebral abscesses, can compress adjacent nervous tissue. In the spinal cord, compression can be intramedullary (within the spinal cord) or extramedullary (outside the spinal cord). Causes of intramedullary compression include hemorrhages, neoplasms such as nephroblastoma of the young dog, and chronic expansile inflammatory diseases. Extramedullary compression can be caused by intervertebral disk herniation in the dog; cervical stenotic myelopathy (wobbler syndrome) in the horse and dog; vertebral fracture and dislocation; neoplasms of the meninges, such as the meningioma; nerve rootlets, such as nerve sheath tumors; or tumor metastasis, such as lymphosarcoma. Finally, developmental anomalies of bone, such as atlanto-occipital malformation, and vertebral deformities with hemivertebrae, such as scoliosis, lordosis, and kyphosis (Fig. 14-70), can result in compression of the spinal cord.

Compression of CNS tissue causes neuronal dysfunction by impeding normal anterograde and retrograde axoplasmic flow in axons (see Web Fig. 14-1). In addition, compression of nerves may result in reduced blood flow to nerves and thus also contribute to neuronal dysfunction. Mild compression can result in partial blockage of slow axoplasmic flow and gradual accumulation of neurofilaments and microtubules, which results in mild enlargement of the axon proximal to the compression site and atrophy of the axon distal to the compression. Eventually, with a long period of time of complete blockage, the distal axon is lost.

Brain Displacements

See the discussion of cerebral edema (permeability changes) in the section on Circulatory Disturbances.

Cervical Stenotic Myelopathy

Cervical stenotic myelopathy, or wobbler syndrome, is characterized by stenosis of the cervical vertebral canal, which causes compressive trauma to the cervical spinal cord (Fig. 14-71). This disease occurs primarily in young rapidly growing large breeds of horses and dogs. Reports indicate that the disease is not caused by a straightforward mechanism but apparently involves several factors (multifactorial disease). For example, stallions that have a genetic predisposition for rapid growth and large body size are reported to be at greater risk of developing the disease. Oversupplementation with protein, vitamins, and minerals used to promote rapid growth may also be another environmental factor in developing cervical stenotic myelopathy.

Gross and microscopic lesions of the CNS in cervical stenotic myelopathy are similar to the lesions in intervertebral disk herniation. The severity depends on the speed and degree to which the compression is applied and the specific area of the cord that is involved. Central nervous tissue can tolerate a considerable degree of compression if it is applied slowly. Rapid compression can lead to quickly developing hypoxia-ischemia, necrosis, and direct damage to compressed axons. Lesions detected include a spectrum of changes characterized by axonal injury and disruption of myelin sheaths resulting in Wallerian degeneration and necrosis of the

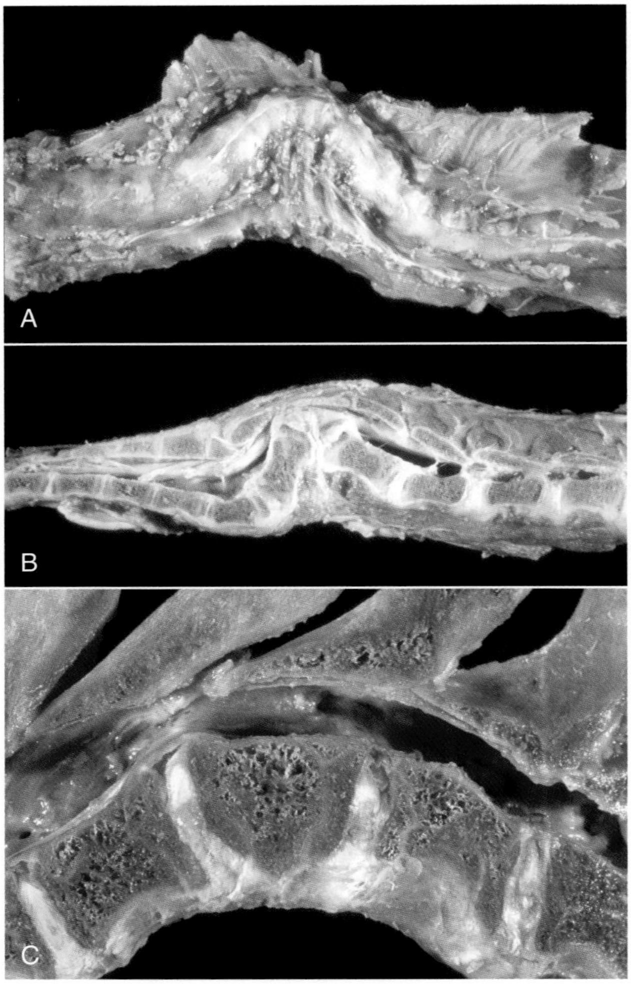

Fig. 14-70 Vertebral abnormalities, vertebral column.
A, Scoliosis, thoracic vertebrae, ventrodorsal view, sheep. Lateral deviation of the spinal column. **B,** Kyphosis, thoracolumbar vertebrae, lateral view, sheep. Dorsal deviation of several vertebrae and a wedge-shaped vertebra (hemivertebra; Fig. 14-70, *C*) have resulted in compression of the spinal cord. **C,** Hemivertebra, lumbar vertebrae, dog. Note that the craniodorsal portion of the body of the hemivertebra has protruded into the vertebral canal. (**A** and **B** courtesy College of Veterinary Medicine, University of Illinois. **C** courtesy Department of Veterinary Biosciences, The Ohio State University.)

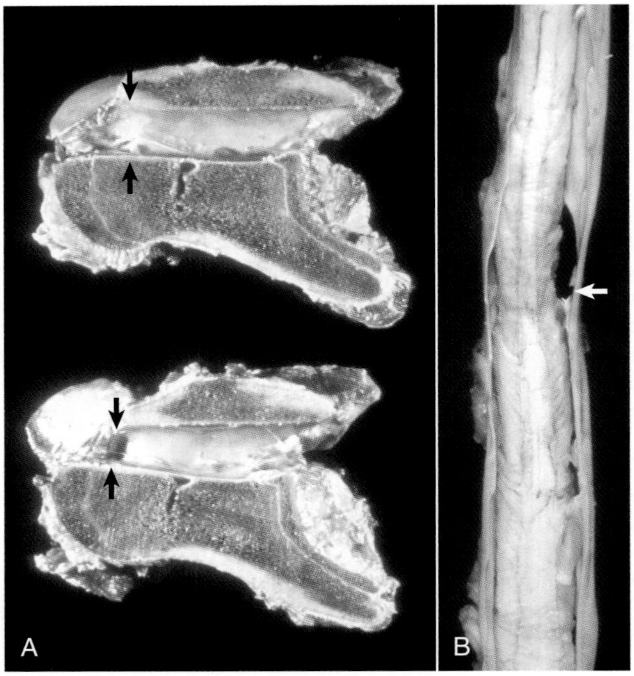

Fig. 14-71 Cervical stenotic myelopathy.
A, Cervical static stenosis, vertebral column, sagittal section, sixth cervical vertebra, horse. The vertebra on the bottom is stenotic *(arrows)* and will compress the spinal cord. The vertebra on the top is normal *(arrows)*. **B,** Cervical vertebral instability, spinal cord, fifth cervical segment, dog. Note the narrowing of the spinal cord at the site of compression *(arrow)*. (Courtesy College of Veterinary Medicine, University of Illinois.)

gray or white matter or of both. Lesions can be visible grossly from the exterior but are more commonly seen on cross-section of the spinal cord.

Microscopically, particularly at the site of injury, there is initial swelling of axons followed after several days by loss of architecture of the CNS as a result of necrosis and a beginning accumulation of gitter cells that have phagocytosed the lipid-rich tissue debris. Eventually the necrotic area is cleared and a cystic space is formed, which is surrounded by varying degrees of astrocytosis and astrogliosis, although not usually prominent unless there is severe destruction. Rostral and caudal to this location, the lesion is primarily one of Wallerian degeneration in the white matter, and the pattern of lesion development seen depends on the level of the spinal cord that is examined relative to the site of compression. At the site of injury, all parts of the white and gray matter of the spinal cord are affected and often necrotic, if the compressive force is sufficient. Rostral to this site, white matter degeneration is generally limited to the ascending tracts in the dorsal funiculi and the superficial portions of the dorsolateral part of the lateral funiculi. Caudal to the area of injury, degeneration is limited to the descending tracts in the ventral funiculi, and the more central portions of the lateral funiculi. It should also be noted that (1) a lesion may occur at the point of compression because of ischemia, but a lesion can also occur on the opposite side of the compression also because of ischemia that results from compression of the tissue against bone on that side, and (2) Wallerian degeneration can be observed in distal segments of affected axons far from the point of compression within the spinal cord. In the former case, compressive forces can be transferred through the spinal cord to axons and blood vessels away from the contact point, whereas in the latter example, degeneration of the distal axon segments can extend for a length of centimeters to meters away from the point of contact.

Cervical stenotic myelopathy has been known for many years to affect horses and more recently has been recognized in the large dog breeds. The disease in the horse has been referred to by several designations: the wobbler syndrome, wobbles, equine incoordination, and more recently, cervical stenotic myelopathy. The disease has been described in many horse breeds.

Cervical stenotic myelopathy in the horse has been divided into two syndromes: cervical static stenosis and cervical vertebral instability (dynamic stenosis). Cervical static stenosis commonly affects horses 1 to 4 years of age. The spinal cord is compressed at C5 through C7 as the result of an acquired dorsal or dorsolateral narrowing of the spinal canal (see Fig. 14-71). The stenosis is due to formation of bone that requires time to develop. The compressive effect with this type of stenosis is present regardless of head position. The second form of cervical stenotic myelopathy (cervical vertebral instability [dynamic stenosis]) occurs in horses ranging in age from 8 to 18 months and is characterized by a narrowing of the spinal canal during flexion of the neck, primarily at C3 through C5 vertebrae.

A disease process with many similarities to that in the horse also affects the dog. It has been known as wobbler syndrome, vertebral instability, vertebral subluxation, and cervical spondylolisthesis. The disease has been most frequently described in the Great Dane and Doberman pinscher breeds but has also been reported in the Saint Bernard, Irish setter, fox terrier, basset hound, Rhodesian ridgeback, and Old English sheepdog. Dogs can have signs develop between 8 months and 1 year of age, with a range of 1 month to 9 years. Great Danes tend to have lesions develop at a young age (8 months to 1 year), whereas Doberman pinschers are generally older, often more than 1 year of age. The vertebral and associated spinal cord lesions in the dog have been reported to most often involve the caudal cervical area from C5 through C7 vertebrae. An exception is the basset hound in which C3 is affected.

Tumors

In the brain, diseases, such as neoplasia, cause compression of adjacent nervous tissue. Compression of CNS tissue causes neuronal dysfunction by impeding normal anterograde and retrograde axoplasmic flow in axons (see the later discussion of specific types of CNS tumors).

Leptomeningeal Hemorrhage

Physical trauma to the CNS compresses, twists, and stretches blood vessels until they are torn. Such injury results in bleeding and leptomeningeal (subarachnoid) hemorrhage (see Fig. 14-67). In the spinal cord, laceration of a large artery or vein can result in prolonged bleeding that ascends or descends the leptomeninges, causing neurologic dysfunction on examination compatible with ascending or descending neurologic deficits in spinal nerve roots.

Tumors

Neoplasms of the CNS of animals are not as rare as was once believed. In fact, neoplasms occur with a frequency and variety, at least in the dog, similar to those in humans. The majority of the neoplasms described have been in the dog and cat, and a large portion of these tumors occur in the older population. The intention in discussing CNS neoplasms in this chapter is to present a brief overview of the more common or better-known neoplasms that occur in animals and is not meant to be all inclusive. The location and characteristics of the primary and common secondary (metastatic) tumors of the nervous system are summarized in Table 14-9.

Embryonal or Primitive Neoplasms

Considering the complexities of brain development and the fact that astrocytes and oligodendrocytes arise from common stem cells early in development, it should not be surprising that some neoplasms arising in the CNS have multiple lines of differentiation as indicated by immunohistochemistry. One such neoplasm is the rare primitive neuroectodermal tumor. This neoplasm has recently been recognized in a young calf. An additional report in a primate has been made. Peripheral neuroectodermal tumors are tumors composed of poorly differentiated embryonal cells, tend to occur in young age groups, and are aggressive. Immunohistochemical staining for specific markers confirms multiple lines of differentiation such as neuronal, astrocytic, and oligodendroglial. Typically, one cell type dominates, most commonly neuronal.

Another neoplasm of uncertain histogenesis is the rhabdoid tumor. In humans, this neoplasm most commonly arises in the kidneys and brain and is believed to develop from embryonal stem cells. As is true of other embryonal neoplasms, young individuals are commonly affected. A novel concept is the proposal that these neoplasms arise from primordial stem cells that adopt the phenotypic characteristics of cells in the tissue of origin.

Rhabdoid tumors arising in the brain have cell markers of neuronal or glial differentiation. Neoplasms in the kidneys typically lack these markers. Despite their primary location, cell morphology is similar. The cells are large and round to polyhedral, and cytoplasm is eosinophilic and abundant and contains large inclusions composed of skeins of intermediate filaments. A rhabdoid tumor has been reported in the brain of an 18-month-old dog. Immunohistochemical staining demonstrated that cells distributed throughout the tumor stained for vimentin; however, only scattered cells stained for neuron-specific enolase and GFAP. No cells in the tumor stained for S-100.

Medulloblastoma

Medulloblastoma has characteristics similar to the less frequently occurring neuroblastoma, and both are considered to arise from cells of the neuronal lineage. The cell of origin for the medulloblastoma has not been definitely determined, but it has been proposed that the neoplasm can arise from primitive cells originating in the neuroepithelial roof of the fourth ventricle that give rise to the external granular cell layer.

In animals, medulloblastomas have been reported in dogs, cats, cows, and pigs. There is a predilection for these tumors in young animals. The neoplasm chiefly occurs in the cerebellum of puppies and calves and sometimes also in adult dogs. The neoplasm is well circumscribed, soft, gray to pink, and usually does not have hemorrhages, cysts, or necrosis. The growth can compress the fourth ventricle and cause an obstructive hydrocephalus and can infiltrate adjacent structures, including the leptomeninges. It can metastasize through the CSF in the ventricles or subarachnoid space. Microscopically, the neoplasm is highly cellular and consists of round-to-elongated nuclei that have prominent chromatin in an ill-defined cytoplasm. The cells are arranged in sheets or broad bands and also can form pseudorosettes. Mitoses can be numerous.

Astrocytomas

Astrocytomas have been morphologically classified based on their degree of differentiation (histologic features in H&E stained sections) and include the following three types: diffuse astrocytomas, anaplastic astrocytomas, and glioblastoma multiforme. The degree of differentiation refers to how closely astrocytes forming the tumor resemble normal astrocytes within the CNS. Diffuse astrocytomas tend to have the most well-differentiated astrocytes, whereas glioblastoma multiforme has the most poorly differentiated astrocytes. All of these tumors are malignant; however, the degree of malignancy is often inversely related to the degree of differentiation.

Astrocytomas have been reported in dogs, cats, and cattle but are most frequently diagnosed in dogs (10% incidence) and uncommon in the cat. Brachycephalic breeds, such as Boston terriers and boxers, and dogs 5 to 11 years of age are most commonly affected. Common sites include the cerebral hemispheres, especially the temporal and pyriform lobes, thalamus-hypothalamus, midbrain, and less frequently, the cerebellum and spinal cord.

Astrocytomas often displace normal tissue; however, their gross appearance often depends on their rate of growth and degree of differentiation (Fig. 14-72). Slow-growing, well-differentiated astrocytomas (less malignant) are usually difficult to distinguish from normal tissue and are rather solid or firm and gray-white. Rapidly growing, poorly differentiated astrocytomas are more malignant

TABLE 14-9 Primary Tumors of the Nervous System

Cell of Origin	Tumor Type	Location	Species Affected	Gross Appearance
CNS				
Neuron	Medulloblastoma	Cerebellum (WM&GM)	Dog, cow, cat, pig (young animals)	Well-circumscribed, soft, gray to pink expansile mass (usually does not have hemorrhage, cysts, or necrosis).
Oligodendroglia	Oligodendroglioma	Cerebrum, brainstem, interventricular septum (WM&GM)	Dog, cat, cow	Well-demarcated, gray to pink-red, soft or gelatinous expansile mass, usually with areas of hemorrhage.
Astroglia	Astrocytoma	Pyriform lobe, cerebral hemispheres, thalamus-hypothalamus, midbrain, cerebellum, spinal cord (WM&GM)	Dog, cat, cow	Poorly demarcated, firm, gray-white when well differentiated; anaplastic neoplasms are moderately to well demarcated, soft and friable (usually with areas of necrosis, hemorrhage, edema, and cavitation).
Ependyma	Ependymoma	Ventricular system (lateral; less commonly, third and fourth), central canal of the spinal cord	Dog, cat, cow, horse	Poorly to moderately to well-demarcated, soft and gray-white, invasive, destructive gelatinous expansile mass (usually with areas of hemorrhage and cavitation).
Choroid plexus epithelium	Choroid plexus tumor	Ventricular system (fourth; less commonly, third and lateral)	Dog, horse, cow	Well-demarcated, granular to papillary, gray-white to red, expansile mass.
Microglia	Microgliomatosis (reticulosis)	Cerebrum, brainstem	Dog	Poorly demarcated, gray-white, infiltrative mass (may have perivascular pattern).
Endothelium	Hemangiosarcoma	Cerebrum, brainstem	Dog	Well-demarcated, invasive red to dark red, expansile mass.
Mesothelium (fibroblasts)	Meningioma	Meningeal surface of the CNS (basal cow, sheep areas, convexity and lateral surfaces of cerebral hemispheres, cerebellum-tentorium, falx cerebri, surface of the spinal cord)	Cat, dog, horse, cow, sheep	Well-demarcated, variable shapes, firm, encapsulated, and gray-white to soft, red-brown or gray, expansile masses (usually with areas of hemorrhage and necrosis).
PNS				
Schwann cells (other supportive cells)	Peripheral nerve sheath tumor*	Cranial nerves, spinal nerves (brachial plexus)	Dog, cow, cat	Firm or soft (gelatinous), white or gray, nodular masses.

WM&GM, White matter and gray matter.
*Other names for this tumor type include schwannoma, neurofibroma, and neurilemmoma.

and easier to discern because they have areas of necrosis, hemorrhage, cavitation, and edema.

Microscopically, the more well-differentiated diffuse astrocytomas consist of a rather uniform cell type loosely organized. Cell size varies, and distinct ramifying cytoplasmic processes can be observed. Nuclei vary in size and shape and contain more chromatin than normal astrocytes. Cells tend to be arranged around and along blood vessels. The boundary between neoplastic and normal tissue is indistinct. Anaplastic astrocytomas and glioblastoma multiforme have extreme cellular pleomorphism, often with giant cell formation.

Increasing usage of immunohistochemical markers for glial cells and indicators of cellular proliferation can undoubtedly enhance the specificity and prognostic significance of the diagnosis of different glial cell neoplasms in animals. The most reliable marker for astrocytomas is GFAP, although vimentin has proved useful in some cases.

Clinical signs in animals with astrocytomas vary, depending on the location of the tumor in the CNS but can include behavioral changes, ataxia, tetraparesis, seizures, circling, and abnormal cranial nerve and proprioceptive reflexes.

Choroid Plexus Papillomas and Carcinomas

Choroid plexus papilloma occurs most commonly in the dog but has been reported in the horse and in cattle. There is no breed predilection in dogs. In the dog, the neoplasm occurs most frequently in the fourth ventricle, but it also can be located in the third and lateral ventricles.

Grossly, the neoplasm is a well-defined, expansive, granular-to-papillary growth located within the ventricular system that is gray-white to red and compresses the adjacent nervous tissue (Fig. 14-73). Noncommunicating hydrocephalus may result from obstruction of CSF flow within the ventricular system. Microscopically, these neoplasms generally resemble the choroid plexus and are characterized by an arborizing vascular connective tissue stroma that is covered with a cuboidal to columnar epithelial layer. Mitoses are not present in the benign form. A more malignant variety, choroid plexus carcinoma, is characterized by invasiveness, presence of mitoses, additional occurrence of solid tumor growth, and a tendency to metastasize within the ventricular system or into the subarachnoid space (through the lateral apertures), where implantation in the ependyma or meninges, respectively, occurs. Currently, no reliable immunohistochemical markers for these tumors exist.

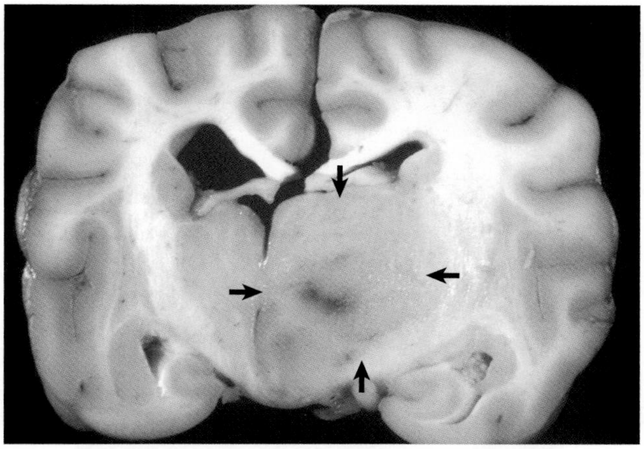

Fig. 14-72 Astrocytoma, brain, transverse section at the level of the thalamus, dog.
The deep ventromedial area (thalamus/hypothalamus) of the right hemisphere *(arrows)* contains a poorly demarcated, nonencapsulated, expansile mass, which is a space-occupying lesion that has displaced the midline to the left and compressed the right lateral ventricle. The left lateral ventricle is mildly dilated, most likely from compression of the interventricular foramen. (Courtesy Dr. M.D. McGavin, College of Veterinary Medicine, University of Tennessee.)

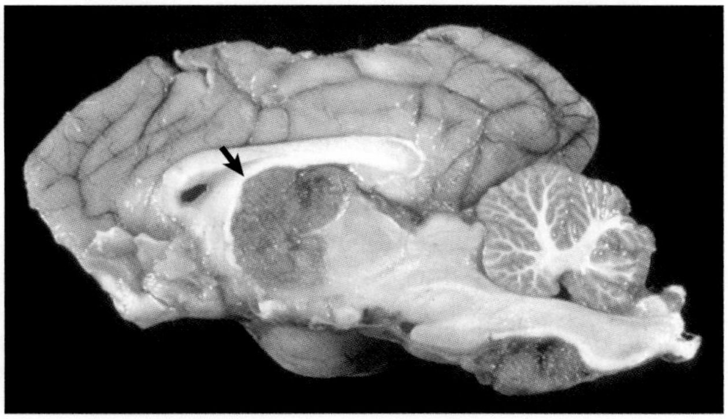

Fig. 14-73 Choroid plexus tumor (carcinoma), brain, sagittal section, dog.
The third ventricle contains an expansile mass *(arrow)* that has invaded the normal tissue ventral to it. The mass ventral to the medulla *(right)* may be a metastasis arising from tumor cells that entered the third ventricle and then spread in the cerebrospinal fluid caudally, through the mesencephalic duct, into the fourth ventricle, and out through a lateral aperture into the subarachnoid space. (Courtesy Dr. Y. Niyo, College of Veterinary Medicine, Iowa State University; and Noah's Arkive, College of Veterinary Medicine, The University of Georgia.)

The age range of dogs with choroid plexus tumors in one study was 5 to 13 years, except for one dog that was 2 years of age. Clinical signs in animals with choroid plexus tumors vary, depending on the location of the tumor in the CNS but can include behavioral changes, ataxia, paresis, seizures, circling, and abnormal cranial nerve and proprioceptive reflexes.

Ependymomas

Ependymomas are one of the less frequently occurring neoplasms in dogs, cats, cattle, and horses. Some reports on the dog indicate a higher frequency in brachycephalic breeds. Ependymomas usually involve the lateral or less commonly, third and fourth ventricles. They also occur in the central canal of the spinal cord. The neoplasm

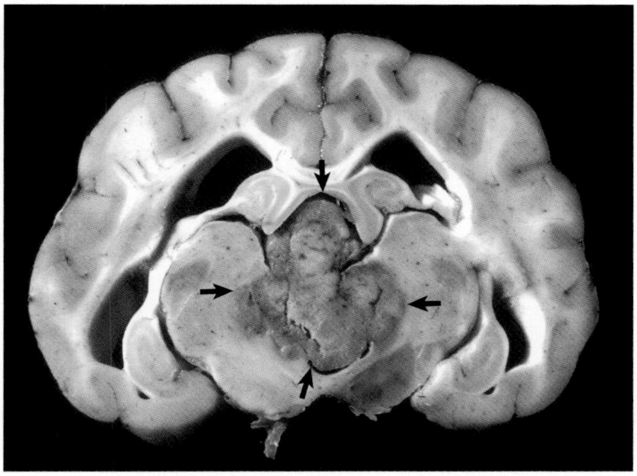

Fig. 14-74 Ependymoma, brain, transverse section at the level of the hippocampus, dog.
The third ventricle contains a moderately well-demarcated expansile mass *(arrows)* that has invaded normal tissue ventral to it. Moderate hydrocephalus is present in both lateral ventricles from blockage of the third ventricle. (Courtesy Dr. M.D. McGavin, College of Veterinary Medicine, University of Tennessee.)

can be observed within the ventricular system and subarachnoid space, likely attributable to local metastasis via the CSF. Noncommunicating hydrocephalus may result from obstruction of CSF flow within the ventricular system.

Grossly, ependymomas are usually large expansile intraventricular masses with generally well-demarcated margins (Fig. 14-74). The neoplasm is soft and gray-white to red, depending on blood content, and has a smooth cut surface in dogs. In cats, the cut surface can have a granular texture. In some ependymomas, the cut surface may have gelatinous consistency and be cavitated. More aggressive tumors show invasion into the normal tissue at its margins. Microscopically, ependymomas are highly cellular and well vascularized. Cells have hyperchromic, round-to-oval nuclei with scant or undetectable cytoplasm. Cells form perivascular rosettes (pseudorosettes) with nuclear polarity away from the vessel wall. Cells are also arranged in sheets and bands. The mitotic rate is variable. Hemorrhage, mucinous and cystic degeneration, and capillary proliferation occur. Malignancy is indicated by invasive growth, frequent mitoses, and anaplasia. Currently, no reliable immunohistochemical markers for ependymomas exist.

The average age of affected dogs ranges from 6 to 12 years. Occurrences in a cat as young as 18 months of age and in a calf 5 months of age have been reported. Clinical signs in animals with ependymomas vary, depending on the location of the tumor in the CNS but can include behavioral changes, ataxia, paresis, seizures, circling, and abnormal cranial nerve and proprioceptive reflexes.

Oligodendrogliomas

Neoplasms composed of oligodendrocytes occur most commonly in the dog, but cases have been reported in cats and cattle. The reported incidence varies; some reports indicate oligodendrogliomas as the most common neuroectodermal neoplasm (5% to 12% incidence), whereas others place it second to astroglial neoplasms. As with astrocytomas in dogs, there is a predilection for brachycephalic breeds (Boston terriers, boxers, and bulldogs), and the age range is the same as for astrocytomas (5 to 11 years of age). Neoplasms occur in all areas of the white matter of the cerebrum, brainstem, and interventricular septum (Fig. 14-75). Neoplasms

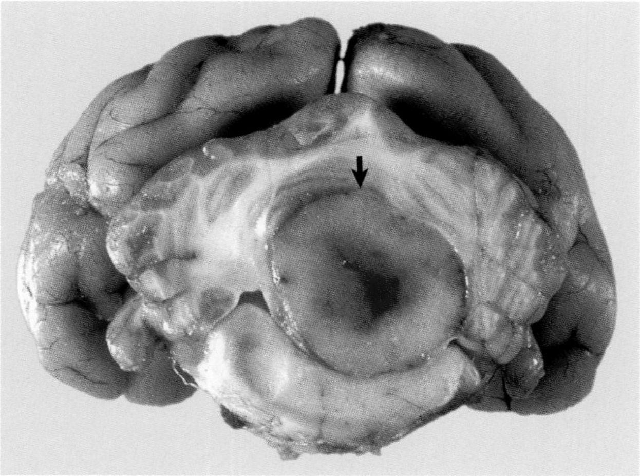

Fig. 14-75 Oligodendroglioma, brain, cerebellum, transverse section caudal to the pons, dog.
The tumor is relatively well demarcated from the surrounding cerebellum. Oligodendrogliomas may be well demarcated or merge with adjacent normal brain. They vary in size, are gray to pink-red, and are soft or gelatinous with areas of hemorrhage *(arrow)*. (Courtesy Dr. W. Crowell, College of Veterinary Medicine, University of Georgia; and Noah's Arkive, College of Veterinary Medicine, The University of Georgia.)

tend to extend to meningeal and ventricular surfaces, but dissemination in the CSF is uncommon.

Grossly, most oligodendrogliomas can be relatively well demarcated from surrounding tissue or their margins can be indistinct and blend in with adjacent normal white matter. The neoplasms vary in size, can grow quite large, are gray to pink-red, and are soft or gelatinous with areas of hemorrhage. In larger tumors, the central area may be cystic. Microscopically, the neoplasms are composed of densely packed cells. Nuclei are centrally located, hyperchromic, and surrounded by pale or nonstaining cytoplasm creating a perinuclear halo. Other patterns include cells arranged in rows, especially peripherally, or in semicircles. Mitoses are generally infrequent. Regressive changes include mucoid degeneration, edema, cavitation, and rarely mineralization. Extensive necrosis is uncommon. Currently, no reliable immunohistochemical markers for oligodendrogliomas exist.

Meningiomas

Meningioma is the most common mesodermal neoplasm of the CNS of animals, especially in cats. Sites of occurrence in the dog include the basal area of the brain, the area over the convexity of the cerebral hemispheres, the cerebellum-tentorium area, the lateral surface of the brain, the falx cerebri, and the surface of the spinal cord. Retrobulbar involvement (originating from the optic nerve sheath) also occurs. In the cat, the neoplasm uniquely occurs in the tela choroidea of the third ventricle but also occurs over the cerebral hemispheres, along the falx cerebri, over the cerebellum and tentorium, and rarely at the base of the brain. Occurrence in the meninges of the spinal cord is not common. Meningiomas have been reported to arise from arachnoid "cap cells," which are on the external surface of the arachnoid membrane. These cells cover the surface of the arachnoid layer that oppose the surface layer of the dura mater, and thus these tumors project into the subdural space and often into the CNS parenchyma.

Grossly, neoplasms in the dog are solitary and vary in size. The neoplasms are well defined, spherical, lobulated, lenticular, or plaquelike in shape; firm; encapsulated; and gray-white (Fig. 14-76). Sometimes on the cut surface there are soft, red, brown, or gray areas of hemorrhage and necrosis. Because these neoplasms grow slowly, they cause pressure atrophy of the adjacent nervous tissue. Meningiomas can be invasive, and sometimes there is hyperostosis of the overlying bone. In the cat, meningiomas vary in size from barely detectable to 2 cm in diameter. Cats and occasionally cattle can have more than one neoplasm. Other characteristics are comparable with those described in the dog.

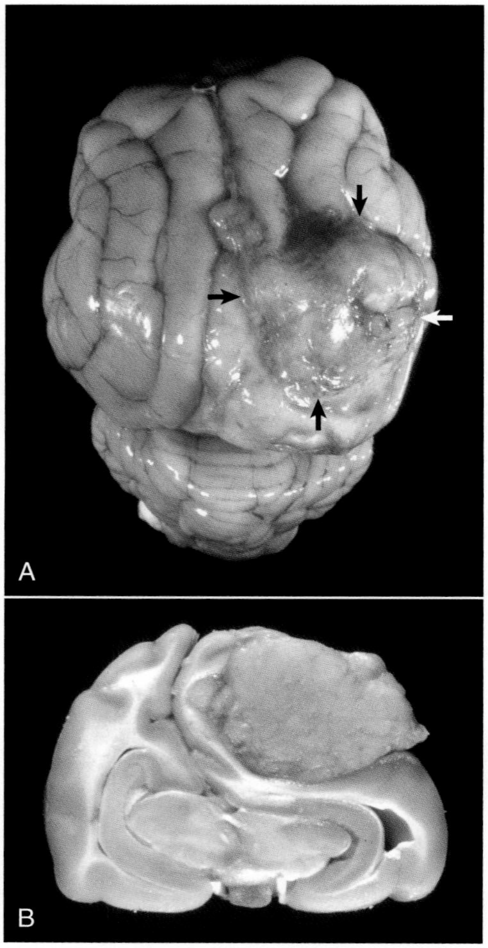

Fig. 14-76 Meningioma, brain, cat.
A, On the surface of the right parietal cortex is a mass *(arrows)* that has compressed and distorted the adjacent parenchyma. It is a space-occupying lesion that has displaced the midline (cerebral longitudinal fissure) to the left. **B,** Transverse section at the level of the hippocampus of the brain depicted in **A.** The tumor has compressed the right cerebral hemisphere and this has resulted in the midline being displaced to the left with compression of the left cerebral hemisphere. The meningioma does not invade the brain and can be "shelled" out at necropsy or surgery. (Courtesy College of Veterinary Medicine, University of Illinois.)

Microscopically, several patterns of neoplastic cells can occur, and more than one can be present in a given neoplasm. Based on their cytomorphologic features, these tumors are grouped into one of six categories: (1) epithelioid/meningotheliomatous; (2) fibroblastic; (3) transitional (features of both epithelioid and fibroblastic); (4) psammomatous; (5) angioblastic; and (6) anaplastic/malignant. Cytomorphologic features are beyond the scope of this chapter; however, the more common pattern is characterized by the formation of nests, islands, or laminated whorls of cells. The cells have large cell bodies with abundant cytoplasm, ill-defined cell boundaries, and elongated, oval, open nuclei with peripherally located chromatin. The number of cells making up a whorl can vary from a few to many, with mineralized material (referred to as psammoma bodies) in the center of such structures. A second pattern is characterized by strands or streams of elongated cells with a rather irregular or parallel orientation. Regressive changes include hemorrhage and cavernous vascular formations. Invasive growth occurs but is less common than growth by expansion. Currently, vimentin and pancytokeratin may be useful immunohistochemical markers for these tumors.

Meningiomas occur most frequently in the dog and cat but have been reported in other species of domestic animals, including horses, cattle, and sheep. In the dog, this neoplasm occurs in several breeds, with dolichocephalic animals being frequently represented. The majority of meningiomas are in dogs between 7 and 14 years of age and in cats 10 years old or older.

Other benign neoplasms of mesenchymal origin, such as neurofibromas of spinal cord nerve roots, occur in the meninges. Spindle cell sarcomas, such as neurofibrosarcomas and dural osteosarcomas, have also been reported in the meninges.

Microgliomatosis

Microgliomatosis, which has been classified as a proliferative neoplastic disease, has some features that are quite distinct from the inflammatory and neoplastic forms of reticulosis described in a later section (see the section on Reticulosis/Granulomatous Meningoencephalitis). Gross lesions are usually not present. The cells, which infiltrate the CNS without topographic perivascular arrangement, resemble microglia in that their nuclei, which vary in size and shape and have prominent chromatin, are the only visible cellular component after conventional staining. Also, mitoses can be common, and there is no accompanying reticulin fiber formation such as occurs in the inflammatory and neoplastic reticuloses. Microgliomatosis occurs in older dogs.

Hemangiosarcoma

Primary hemangiosarcoma of the CNS is a rare neoplasm arising from endothelial cells. The disease is most common in dogs but can occur in all domestic species. The neoplasm is a solitary expansile red-to-dark red mass within the cerebral cortex. Its color and bloody consistency are helpful in differentiating it from a primary or metastatic melanoma. Most hemangiosarcomas found in the CNS are from metastases.

Metastatic Tumors

Hematogenously metastasizing neoplasms occur and affect the brain more often than the spinal cord. The species in which metastasis has been most commonly reported is the dog; the next most frequent is the cat. Of the metastasizing carcinomas, mammary gland carcinoma in the dog has been reported to occur most frequently, although others have been described. Hemangiosarcoma of the heart, liver, and spleen is one of the most common metastasizing sarcomas in the dog; others are the mesenchymal component of the malignant mixed mammary gland tumor, lymphosarcoma, fibrosarcoma, and malignant melanoma. In the CNS, metastatic hemangiosarcomas appear to have predilection for the gray matter–white matter interface (Fig. 14-77). In the cat, the neoplasms that metastasize to the CNS include the mammary gland carcinoma (Fig. 14-78) and lymphosarcoma. Primary CNS lymphomas have been reported.

DISORDERS OF HORSES

Disorders that occur in many or all animal species are discussed in the section on Disorders of Domestic Animals.

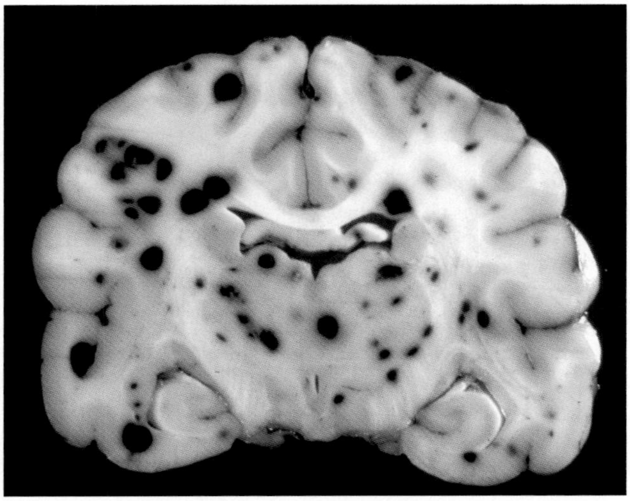

Fig. 14-77 Hemangiosarcoma, metastatic, brain, formalin-fixed, transverse section at the level of the thalamus, dog.
Note the prominent hematogenous metastases, which appear as black nodules of various sizes distributed throughout the brain, sometimes at the gray matter–white matter interface. In an unfixed (fresh) specimen, the nodules would be red to dark red from erythrocytes. Black nodules in a fresh specimen would be consistent with metastatic melanoma. (Courtesy Dr. M.D. McGavin, College of Veterinary Medicine, University of Tennessee.)

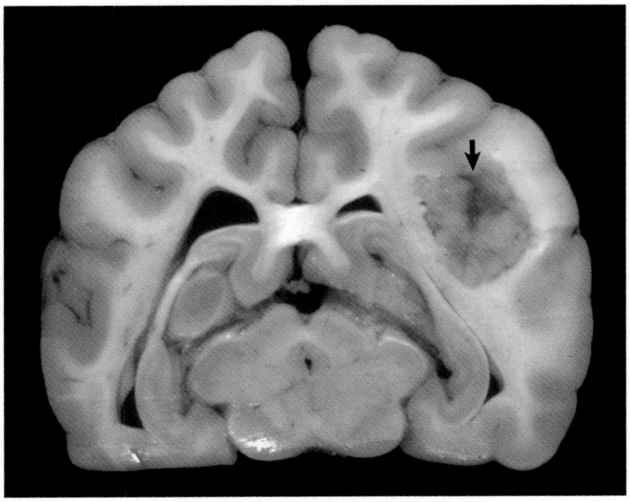

Fig. 14-78 Mammary carcinoma, metastatic, brain, transverse section at the level of the hippocampus, dog.
The right cerebral hemisphere contains a well-demarcated mass *(arrow)*, which has caused enlargement of the right cerebral hemisphere and compression of the right lateral ventricle. The left lateral ventricle is slightly dilated, probably because of pressure on the interventricular foramen. (Courtesy Dr. F. Moore and Dr. J. Carpenter, Angell Memorial Animal Hospital; and Noah's Arkive, College of Veterinary Medicine, The University of Georgia.)

Diseases Caused by Microbes

Viruses

Arboviruses

Equine encephalomyelitis

Eastern equine encephalomyelitis (EEE), western equine encephalomyelitis (WEE), or Venezuelan equine encephalomyelitis (VEE) viruses are members of the family Togaviridae, genus *Alphavirus*. The primary target cell for infection and injury is the neuron; however, these viruses can cause vasculitis followed by thrombosis. After inoculation (by mosquito), the hematogenously circulating virus initially infects several tissues, including bone marrow, lymphoreticular tissue, muscle, and connective tissue. In lymphoid tissue and bone marrow, this infection may cause cellular depletion, necrosis, or both. A second viremia results in hematogenous infection of the CNS. Experimental evidence suggests that the virus replicates in endothelial cells before entering the nervous system and infecting neurons, for which it has an affinity. There is also evidence that viruses of this group (VEE virus) can cause alterations in the metabolism of neurotransmitters in the CNS and that these alterations are responsible for some of the clinical signs.

Recent experimental evidence from in vivo and in vitro models of VEE suggests that the virus causes upregulation of multiple proinflammatory genes, including iNOS and TNF-α. This upregulation, occurring principally in astrocytes, affected other glial cells and influenced neuronal survival. In addition to these mediators of innate immune responses, apoptotic cell death was also described as contributing to neurodegeneration after virus infection.

In the CNS, all three viruses induce a polioencephalomyelitis that has similar characteristics, but there are some differences. Overall, gross lesions include cerebral hyperemia, edema, petechiation, focal necrosis, and increased CSF in the subarachnoid space. Gross lesions are usually found in gray matter, which is appreciated best in the spinal cord (Fig. 14-79). Microscopic lesions are most prominent in the gray matter of the brain and spinal cord and are characterized by perivascular cuffing with lymphocytes, macrophages, and neutrophils; variable neutrophilic infiltration of the gray matter; microgliosis; neuronal degeneration; focal cerebrocortical necrosis; perivascular edema and hemorrhage; necrotizing vasculitis; thrombosis; choroiditis; and leptomeningitis. Neutrophils are detectable during the early stages (2 days) of clinical EEE and VEE. Vasculitis, thrombosis, and cerebrocortical necrosis are particularly evident in VEE but also in EEE. No lesions are detected in the trigeminal ganglion.

Infection of horses with EEE, WEE, and VEE viruses produces a range of progressive clinical maladies, including fever, rapid heart rate, anorexia, depression, muscle weakness, and behavioral changes, such as dementia, aggression, head pressing, wall leaning, circling, blindness, and paralysis of facial muscles. EEE has also been reported in cattle and pigs.

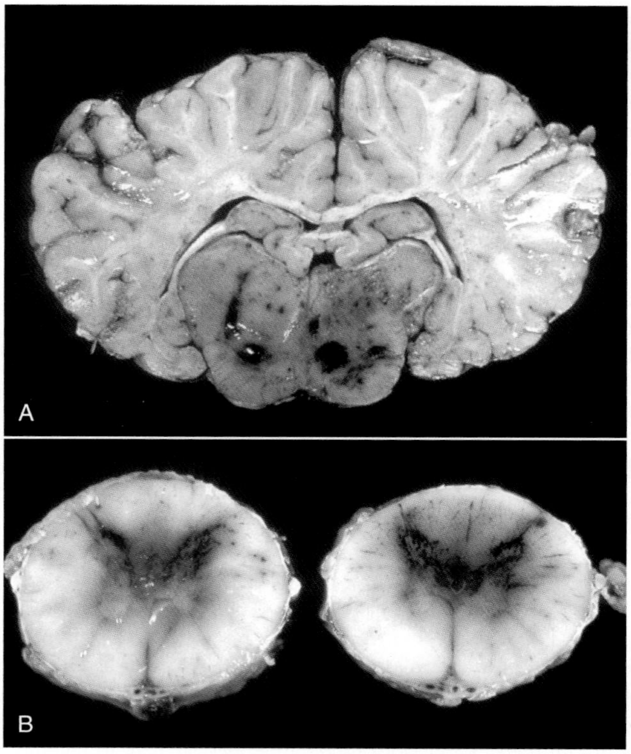

Fig. 14-79 Neuronal necrosis and vasculitis, eastern equine polioencephalomyelitis, brainstem and spinal cord, horse.
A, Brain, transverse section at the level of the hippocampus, horse. The gray matter of the brainstem has dark red-to-black discoloration as a result of congestion and hemorrhage. The lesion is the result of viral infection, which has an affinity for neurons; this virus also causes vascular necrosis followed by thrombosis, but this is not common. **B,** Spinal cord, horse. Note the red-to-brown discoloration of the gray matter in the dorsal and ventral horns (caused by congestion and hemorrhage). The lesion is the result of viral infection that has an affinity for neurons; however, this virus can also cause vascular necrosis followed by thrombosis. (Courtesy College of Veterinary Medicine, University of Florida; and Noah's Arkive, College of Veterinary Medicine, The University of Georgia.)

West Nile viral encephalomyelitis

West Nile virus, a mosquito-borne virus (family Flaviviridae, genus *Flavivirus*) that causes acute polioencephalomyelitis primarily in humans, birds, and horses, is most commonly transmitted via a bird-mosquito cycle. In 2002, West Nile virus infection was diagnosed in 47,000 horses in 40 states in the United States (US), and it was estimated that more than 4500 horses died after infection.

The pathogenesis of West Nile virus encephalomyelitis remains to be elucidated; however, it is likely to be similar to the mechanism described previously for equine encephalomyelitis viruses. The primary target cell for infection and injury appears to be the neuron; microglial cells are also affected. Experimental studies suggest that viral-induced apoptotic cell death is a mechanism possibly responsible for neuronal injury in experimental West Nile viral infections. Gross lesions of West Nile viral infection in horses usually involve the gray matter and include hyperemia and petechiation to prominent hemorrhage with prevalent involvement of the lower brainstem and ventral horns of the thoracolumbar spinal cord. Microscopic lesions in birds and horses that have died of the disease are characterized by a nonsuppurative (lymphocytic/histiocytic) polioencephalomyelitis and hemorrhage of the CNS that can vary in degree of severity. Clinical signs of the equine West Nile viral infection include variable fever, depression, ataxia, weakness to paralysis of the hind limbs, tetraplegia, convulsions, coma, and death.

Herpesviruses

Equine herpesvirus 1 myeloencephalopathy

Equine herpesvirus 1 (EHV-1) (an alpha-herpesvirus) is an important cause of equine abortion and perinatal foal infection and death, in addition to myeloencephalitis. EHV-1 can also cause rhinopneumonitis. EHV-1 does not appear to be neuronotropic, which is in contrast to some herpesvirus encephalitides of other species in which the virus replicates in neurons (herpes simplex viral infection in the human, infectious bovine rhinotracheitis viral infection in calves, and pseudorabies viral infection in pigs). In addition to vasculitis being the principal lesion, the infection in the horse also differs somewhat from most other herpetic infections of the CNS in being primarily a disease of the adult, although young animals can be affected.

Equine herpesvirus myeloencephalopathy begins with inhalation of the EHV-1. The virus infects epithelial cells of the nasopharynx and spreads to local lymphoreticular tissue, where it infects lymphocytes and macrophages (monocytes). Through leukocytic trafficking by macrophages (monocytes), EHV-1 is transferred to endothelial cells of the CNS.

The neurologic disease has been experimentally reproduced by intranasal inoculation of the virus (EHV-1, subtype 1), which can replicate in the epithelium of the respiratory or intestinal tracts after infection. Intranuclear inclusions occur in the nasal mucosa. Infection of mononuclear leukocytes (predominantly, but not exclusively, T lymphocytes and macrophages) then occurs and is followed by a cell-associated viremia. The virus, which is endotheliotropic, even though infection of neurons and astrocytes can occur, localizes in small arteries and capillaries of the CNS and some other tissues after direct spread from the circulating infected cells. Inflammation of endothelial cells then results in vasculitis leading to thrombosis and infarction of the neural tissue supplied by the thrombosed vessel. Latent infection of the trigeminal ganglion and lymphoid tissues can also occur.

The characteristic lesion in the CNS caused by EHV-1 infection is a vasculitis affecting endothelial cells of small blood vessels with thrombosis and resulting in focal CNS necrosis (infarction). Lesions occur in both the gray and white matter of the spinal cord, medulla oblongata, mesencephalon, diencephalon, and cerebral cortex (Fig. 14-80, *A*). The endothelium appears to be the initial site of involvement (Fig. 14-80, *B*), with the subsequent intimal and medial degeneration resulting in hemorrhage, thrombosis, extravasation of plasma proteins into the perivascular space, axonal swelling with ballooning of the myelin sheath and degeneration of the cell body, and variable mononuclear cellular cuffing. Other lesions include cerebrospinal ganglioneuritis and vasculitis in nonneural tissues, including the endometrium, nasal cavity, lungs, uvea of the eye, hypophysis, and skeletal muscle. Inclusion bodies are apparently not observed in CNS lesions.

The neurologic form of EHV-1 infection has a worldwide distribution and affects other Equidae, including zebras in addition to the horse, but appears to be relatively uncommon when compared with the incidence of abortion and upper respiratory tract disease caused by EHV-1. The neurologic disease may accompany or follow outbreaks of respiratory disease or abortion. An outbreak of epizootic acute encephalitis in Thomson's gazelle *(Gazella thomsoni)* was reported in 1997 from a zoologic garden in Japan. That disease resembled equine herpesvirus encephalitis, and the virus, named *gazelle herpesvirus 1* (GHV-1), was serologically related to EHV-1 and had a strong tropism for endothelium.

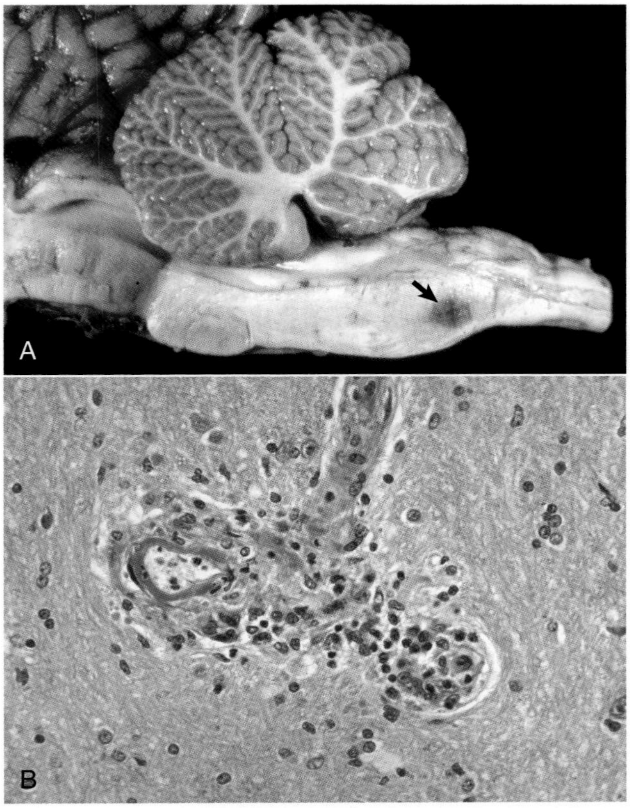

Fig. 14-80 Equine herpesvirus 1 myeloencephalopathy, brain, midsagittal section.
A, Hemorrhage, brainstem, horse. Focal or multifocal areas of hemorrhage and/or necrosis *(arrow)* are characteristic of equine herpesvirus encephalitis but also occur in equine arteritis virus encephalitis, cerebrospinal nematodiasis, and equine protozoal encephalomyelitis *(Sarcocystis neurona).* **B,** Chronic vasculitis and hemorrhage, brainstem, horse. Vasculitis is the primary lesion. The virus localizes in small arteries, venules, and capillaries of the CNS, resulting in vasculitis and fibrinoid necrosis, which at times leads to thrombosis and focal infarction of the brain and spinal cord. (**A** courtesy College of Veterinary Medicine, University of Illinois. **B** courtesy Dr. J. Simon, College of Veterinary Medicine, University of Illinois.)

Protozoa

Equine Protozoal Encephalomyelitis (Sarcocystosis)

Equine protozoal encephalomyelitis is a disease in horses caused by *Sarcocystis neurona*. The organism enters the body through ingestion of sporocysts, but how the parasite enters the CNS is unclear. Experimental studies suggest that ingested sporocysts multiply in visceral tissue, perhaps the intestine, and then are transported to the CNS probably via leukocytic trafficking. In the CNS, the typical sequence of events in the pathogenesis of the characteristic lesion is thought to be (1) leukocytic trafficking with focal parasitic activation and replication, (2) marked inflammation, (3) edema, and (4) pronounced tissue destruction affecting both white and gray matter.

Gross lesions can occur throughout the neuraxis but are more common in the spinal cord, particularly the cervical and lumbar intumescences, than in the brain. In the brain, lesions are most commonly seen in the brainstem. When gross lesions are present, they consist of discolored necrotic foci, often with hemorrhage of varied sizes (Fig. 14-81).

Microscopic lesions occur in both the white and gray matter and include necrosis, hemorrhage, and accumulations of lymphocytes, macrophages, neutrophils, eosinophils, and a few multinucleated giant cells in perivascular areas and the neuropil, or less commonly, the leptomeninges and the axonal swelling. Gemistocytic astrocytosis can be prominent. In lesions, *Sarcocystis neurona* is small and crescent-shaped to round, has a well-defined nucleus, and is often arranged in aggregates or rosettes (Fig. 14-82). Organisms can be difficult to detect but occur intracellularly in neurons, giant cells, neutrophils, or macrophages or occur extracellularly in cysts within the neuropil. *Sarcocystis neurona* is not typically seen in vascular endothelial cells, a common site for other members of this genus.

Sarcocystis neurona can be propagated in tissue culture where it develops in the host cell cytoplasm. It divides by endopolygeny, with development of schizonts containing merozoites arranged in rosettes around a prominent residual body. The schizont stage of the organism differs from those of the genera *Toxoplasma, Isospora, Eimeria, Besnoitia, Hammondia,* and *Neospora* because the merozoites lack rhoptries but resemble the schizont stage of other genera such as *Sarcocystis* spp. and *Frenkelia.* It is proposed that an opossum *coccidian, Sarcocystis falcatula,* and *Sarcocystis neurona* are

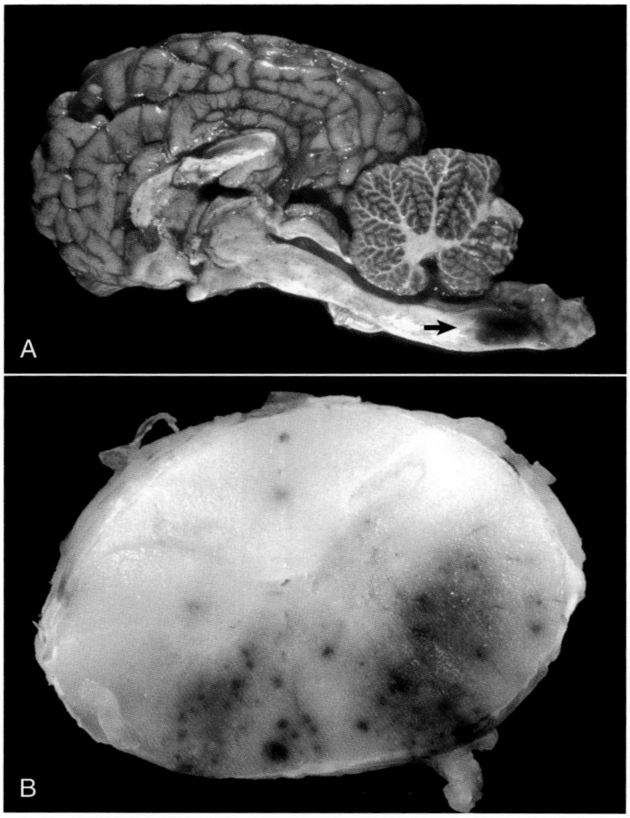

Fig. 14-81 Protozoal encephalomyelitis, brain, sagittal section, horse. **A,** Note the large focus of hemorrhage and necrosis *(arrow)* in the caudal medulla caused by *Sarcocystis neurona.* **B,** Lumbar spinal cord, transverse section. Myelitis due to *Sarcocystis neurona* infection. Prominent focal hemorrhage and necrosis are present in the right lateral funiculus and in the right and left ventral funiculi. (**A** courtesy College of Veterinary Medicine, University of Illinois. **B** courtesy Dr. R. Storts, College of Veterinary Medicine, Texas A&M University.)

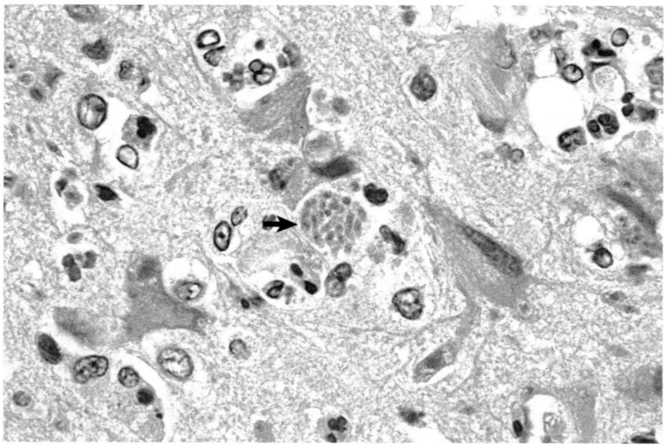

Fig. 14-82 *Sarcocystis neurona,* brain, horse. *Sarcocystis neurona* is a small, crescent-shaped to round protozoal organism found in neurons, endothelial cells, and microglial cells. They can be arranged in nonencysted aggregates *(arrow)* or rosettes intracellularly and in CNS tissue often with a mixed leukocytic cellular inflammatory response of varied severity. Organisms can be difficult to detect in histologic sections. H&E stain. (Courtesy Dr. J. Simon, College of Veterinary Medicine, University of Illinois.)

synonymous. Studies have suggested that the opossum represents the definitive host and avian species represent the intermediate host, providing a reservoir for infection of the horse.

Sarcocystis spp. infection in nonequine species involves organisms similar to *Sarcocystis neurona.* Such organisms have been associated with encephalomyelitis in cattle, sheep, and dogs, as well as raccoons, but such infections are sporadic. Lesions and organisms have additionally been seen in the CNS of infected bovine fetuses.

Clinical infection typically occurs in young adult horses, and signs depend on the area of the CNS parasitized. Signs can include depression, behavioral changes, seizures, gait abnormalities, ataxia, facial nerve paralysis, head tilt, paralysis of the tongue, urinary incontinence, dysphagia, atrophy of masseter and/or temporal muscles, and atrophy of the quadriceps and/or gluteal muscles.

Degenerative Diseases

Metabolic

Equine Degenerative Myeloencephalopathy

Equine degenerative myeloencephalopathy has been reported in a variety of pure and mixed breed horses. A similar disease has been reported in zebras. The specific cause of this disorder is unknown. Although a firm relationship does not currently exist, there is some evidence to suggest that vitamin E deficiency could play a role in this disease, as well as in a disorder in Morgan and Haflinger breeds termed *neuraxonal dystrophy.* Investigators have found low vitamin E levels in some horses and that vitamin E supplementation has resulted in clinical improvement or reduced the occurrence of the disease on some premises with a high incidence of degenerative myeloencephalopathy.

Vitamin E functions as an antioxidant, protecting cells from free radical–mediated injury. Vitamin E deficiency associated with abetalipoproteinemia and various fat malabsorption syndromes in humans, as well as experimentally induced deficiency, result in neurologic disorders with similarities to the equine diseases. A hereditary predisposition for equine degenerative myeloencephalopathy has not been excluded, but a specific mechanism has so far been elusive. Although this disease might be multifactorial or even represent entirely different syndromes with overlapping clinical presentations and lesions, they are grouped here because of similarities in clinical presentation and lesions.

In horses with degenerative myeloencephalopathy, lesions are microscopic. Axonal degeneration in the spinal cord is the most notable lesion, is bilateral, and can affect all funiculi, but the dorsal funiculus is least affected. Dorsal spinocerebellar tracts in lateral funiculi and septomarginal areas of the ventral funiculus are often severely affected. Myelin loss occurs secondary to the axonal degeneration. Depending on duration of clinical illness, astrogliosis occurs. Another less dramatic lesion in affected horses is the formation of eosinophilic spheroids (Fig. 14-83). In horses, spheroids have been described in the nucleus gracilis, medial and lateral cuneate nuclei of the terminal brainstem, and thoracic nucleus of the spinal cord. Spheroids represent a focal eosinophilic swelling in the course of an axon that can be somewhat homogeneous, laminated, or granular. The swellings are filled with amorphous debris, membranous profiles, and effete organelles.

Neuronal dystrophy is a clinically similar syndrome that occurs in Morgan and Haflinger horses. Lesions consist of eosinophilic spheroids in brainstem nuclei as previously noted, but the severe axonal degeneration does not occur in the spinal cord. The cause of axonal spheroids and dystrophic axons in equine degenerative myeloencephalopathy and neuraxonal dystrophy is unclear; however, alteration of axoplasmic flow is suspected. Immunohistochemical analyses have shown that spheroids and dystrophic

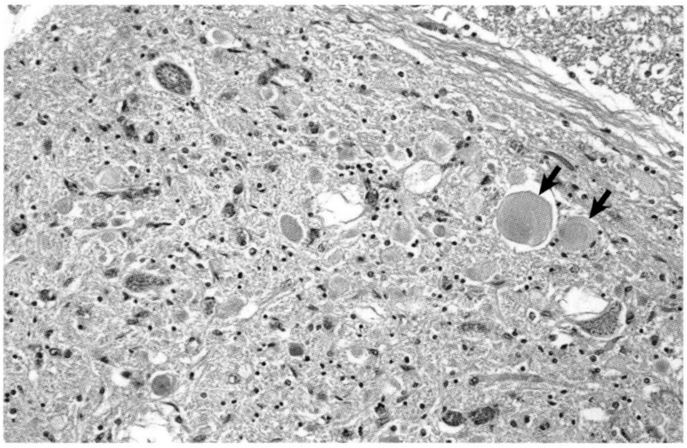

Fig. 14-83 Axonal spheroids and dystrophic axons, degenerative myeloencephalopathy, spinal cord, dorsal gray horn, horse. Axons of the thoracic nucleus are swollen, rounded, and pale pink (axonal spheroids, which are accumulations of neurofilaments and effete organelles) *(arrows)*. Although attributed to vitamin E deficiency, its role in CNS disease is not firmly established. Vitamin E functions as an antioxidant, protecting cells from free radical–mediated injury. H&E stain. (Courtesy Dr. J.F. Zachary, College of Veterinary Medicine, University of Illinois.)

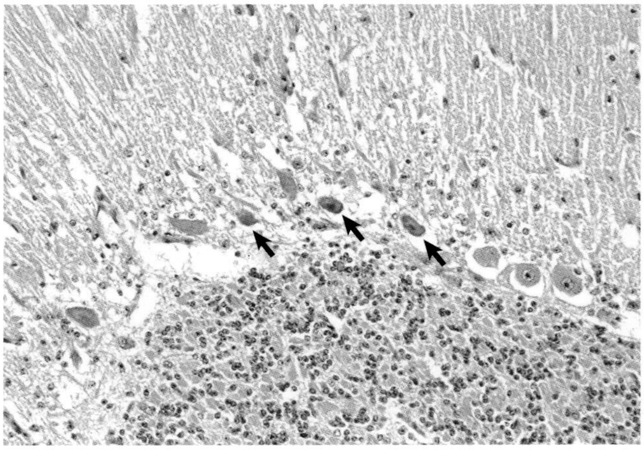

Fig. 14-84 Equine cerebellar degeneration, cerebellum, horse. Purkinje cells in the cerebellum show changes consistent with necrosis, such as shrunken cell bodies and nuclear pyknosis *(arrows)*. H&E stain. (Courtesy Dr. J.F. Zachary, College of Veterinary Medicine, University of Illinois.)

axons contain elevated quantities of proteins involved in movement, docking, and fusion of synaptic vesicles to plasma membranes. These findings suggest that disruption of axoplasmic flow plays a role in the pathogenesis of dystrophic axons in equine degenerative myeloencephalopathy and neuraxonal dystrophy.

Clinically, equine degenerative myeloencephalopathy and neuroaxonal dystrophies typically occur in young horses. The onset is insidious and clinical signs are symmetric with spasticity, ataxia, and paresis of the limbs.

Primary Neuronal Degeneration

Primary cerebellar neuronal degeneration

Equine cerebellar abiotrophy, a primary cerebellar neuronal degeneration, occurs in Arabian or part-Arabian foals and Swedish Gotland ponies. An autosomal recessive mode of inheritance is suspected, but the mechanism of injury is unclear. Although grossly the cerebellum may be slightly reduced in size, microscopically Purkinje cells and their proximal axons are swollen (Fig. 14-84). With time, there may be loss of Purkinje cells and neurons of the granular layer. Clinical signs appear between the time of birth and 9 months of age and include head tremors, ataxia, and spasticity.

Nutritional

Vitamin E Deficiency

See the previous section on Equine Degenerative Myeloencephalopathy.

Toxicoses

Microbial Toxins

Leukoencephalomalacia

Ingestion of moldy feed, mainly corn or corn by-products, contaminated with the fungus *Fusarium moniliforme* causes an acute fatal neurologic disease in horses called *leukoencephalomalacia.* The primary toxin isolated from *Fusarium moniliforme* has been named *fumonisin B1,* although other fumonisins have been extracted. The exact mechanism of injury has not been fully defined. Based on the character and progression of lesions, vascular damage has been inferred as the primary injury. Although unproved, the gross lesion is thought to be an infarct by some pathologists. Fumonisins disrupt cellular membranes, are associated with lipid peroxidation of cells and cellular membranes, inhibit synthesis of macromolecules and DNA, and may enhance production of TNF-α by macrophages. Also, fumonisins inhibit the enzyme ceramide synthase, interfering with the synthesis of sphingolipids. Sphingolipids are bioactive compounds that participate in the regulation of cell growth, cell differentiation, cell metabolic functions, and apoptotic cell death.

Gross lesions involve the white matter of the frontal and parietal lobes of the cerebral hemispheres most commonly, but cases with involvement of major white matter tracts in the brainstem and deep cerebellar white matter have occurred (Fig. 14-85). As a result of the white matter damage, including edema, brain swelling is marked with flattening of cerebrocortical gyri. The lesions are often bilateral but not symmetric, are unequal in severity, and can be quite extensive. The characteristic gross lesion at the time of death is yellow gelatinous malacia and liquefaction of the affected white matter due predominately to the breakdown of lipids accompanied by hemorrhage. The reason white matter, including subcortical white matter, is principally involved—whereas the cerebral cortical gray matter is spared—is thought to be related to a unique vulnerability of the blood vessels in the white matter. The mechanism for this selective vulnerability is unknown.

Microscopically, the affected white matter is coagulated or liquefied, and the neuropil is disrupted by accumulation of pink-staining proteinaceous fluid with scattered neutrophils and macrophages (Fig. 14-85, *C*). The border of the lesion is surrounded by diffuse or perivascular edema, perivascular hemorrhage, and blood vessels with small leukocytic cuffs. Blood vessel walls are degenerate or necrotic, and some are infiltrated with neutrophils, plasma cells, and eosinophils. Although not often detected, thrombosis occurs. Less characteristic changes include edema and perivascular cuffing in the leptomeninges and neuronal necrosis in deeper layers or the entire width of the overlying gray matter. Similar lesions have been reported in the spinal cord where gray matter is preferentially affected.

Leukoencephalomalacia can also be associated with hepatotoxicity, or hepatotoxicity can be the sole manifestation. Additionally, other animals, including pigs, ducks, and chickens, are susceptible, but clinical disease and lesions generally reflect pulmonary, hepatic, or renal injury. Clinical signs can include depression, somnolence,

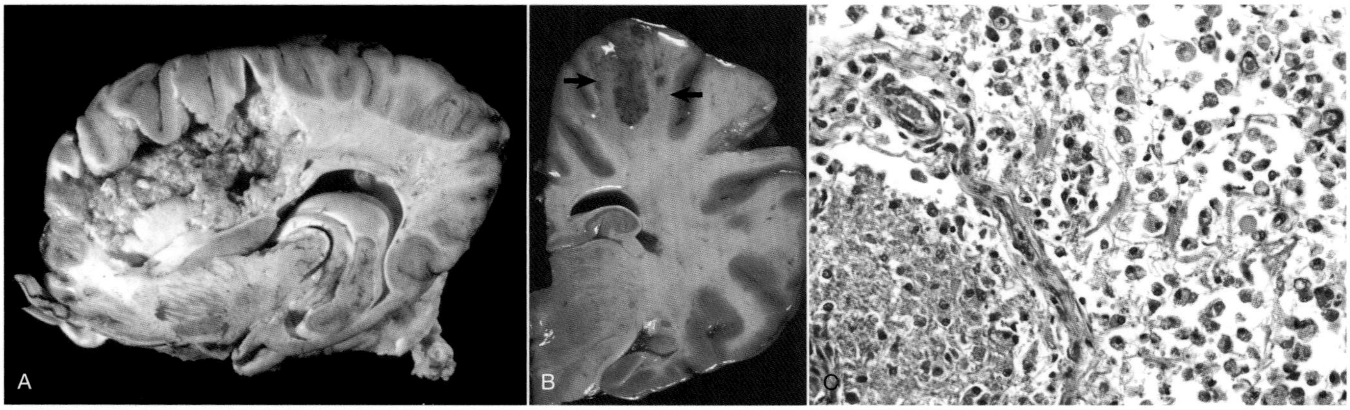

Fig. 14-85 Leukoencephalomalacia, brain, horse.
A, Sagittal section. The white matter of the frontal and parietal lobes is necrotic (malacia). The gray matter is not affected. This disease is caused by the toxin fumonisin B_1 produced by the fungus *Fusarium moniliforme* that grows in damaged feed grains. Note that this case demonstrates the extent and distribution of liquefactive necrosis in the white matter in this disease. A more typical presentation is shown in **B. B,** Transverse section. The white matter of the three cerebral gyri located at the top of the illustration has areas of yellow gelatinous softening *(arrows)* and hemorrhage. Because of the absence of cavitation (liquefactive necrosis), the age of this lesion is likely less than the lesion depicted in **C. C,** Note the severe injury of the white matter. Myelinated axons are fragmented, and myelin debris is abundant. Numerous macrophages are present in the space previously occupied by myelinated axons, and they are phagocytosing the cellular debris. H&E stain. (**A** courtesy Dr. J. Simon, College of Veterinary Medicine, University of Illinois. **B** courtesy Dr. W. Crowell, College of Veterinary Medicine, University of Georgia; and Noah's Arkive, College of Veterinary Medicine, The University of Georgia. **C** courtesy Dr. W. Haschek-Hock, College of Veterinary Medicine, University of Illinois.)

head pressing, aimless wandering, blindness, or seizures. Rapid progression of these clinical signs followed by death is typical ranging from 1 to 10 days after onset.

Plant Toxins

Centaurea spp. poisoning

Horses grazing *Centaurea solstitialis* (yellow star thistle) or *Centaurea repens* (Russian knapweed) develop a disorder known as *nigropallidal encephalomalacia.* This disease is similar to Parkinson's disease in humans and has been proposed as a model for experimental studies. The specific cause of the syndrome is not proved. A sesquiterpene lactone isolated from *Centaurea repens* termed *repin* could provide a basis for the neurotoxicity. Cytotoxicity in cell culture was associated with depletion of glutathione (a major antioxidant), an increase in reactive oxygen species, and evidence of membrane damage in PC12 cells (a pheochromocytoma cell line) and mouse astrocytes. High concentrations of monoamine oxidase involved in dopamine metabolism normally found in the dopaminergic striatonigral tract (i.e., striatum and substantia nigra [regulate balance and movement]) could render these areas of the brain more susceptible to oxidative damage caused by repin. The mechanism by which repin might cause an increased oxidative state with glutathione depletion, free radical production, and damage to cellular membranes is unknown. Repin is also reported to inhibit dopamine release in the rat striatum, potentially contributing to the clinical manifestations of the disorder. Other potential toxins isolated from *Centaurea solstitialis* include the excitotoxic amino acids aspartate and glutamate. It is unlikely that these amino acids are involved in the naturally occurring disease.

Gross brain lesions are sharply demarcated foci of yellow discoloration and malacia in the globus pallidus (pallidal) and substantia nigra (nigro) (Fig. 14-86). Lesions are usually bilateral and vary in severity; however, unilateral lesions also occur. Microscopically, necrosis with loss of neurons is the primary lesion; however, axons, glia, and blood vessels also are necrotic. The debris is phagocytosed by macrophages (monocytes) recruited into the lesion from the blood stream.

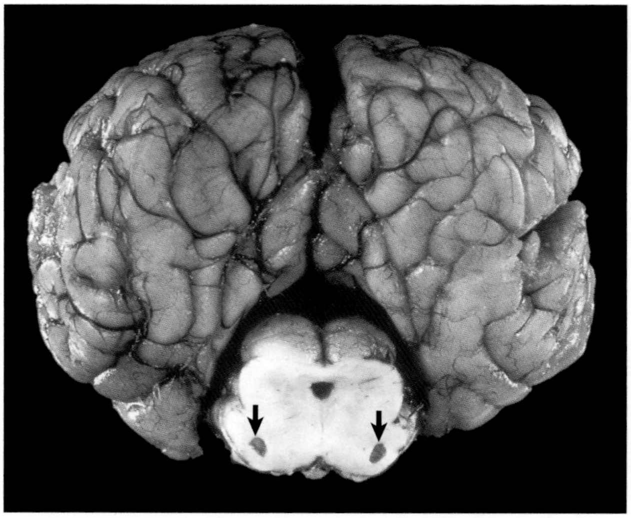

Fig. 14-86 Equine nigropallidal encephalomalacia, brain, transverse section through the midbrain at the level of the rostral colliculi, horse. This lesion is caused by yellow star thistle poisoning. Note the symmetrically cavitated (malacia) lesions in the substantia nigra *(arrows),* resulting from necrosis and phagocytosis by gitter cells. (Courtesy Dr. L. Lowenstine, School of Veterinary Medicine, University of California-Davis; and Noah's Arkive, College of Veterinary Medicine, The University of Georgia.)

Grazing the plants for 1 month or longer during the hot summer months when other forage is dried and unpalatable can cause clinical disease. Affected horses are somnolent, have persistent chewing movements, and have difficulty in prehension of feed and drinking water. Death generally is due to emaciation and starvation.

Miscellaneous Conditions

For discussion of miscellaneous conditions affecting individual animal species, see sections covering diseases specific for the species.

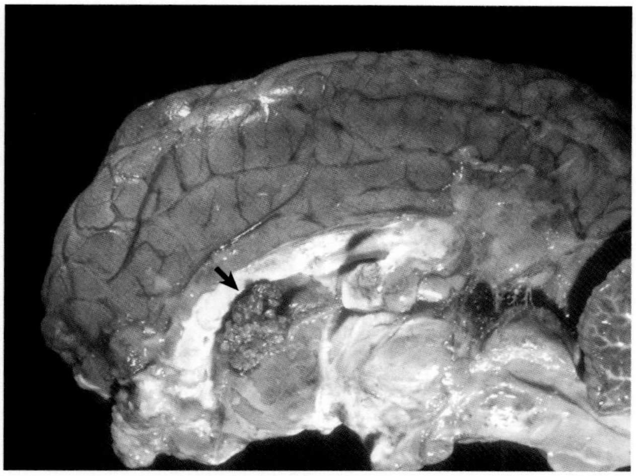

Fig. 14-87 **Cholesterol granuloma (cholesteatoma), brain, sagittal section, horse.**
The choroid plexus of the lateral ventricle contains an expansile mass consisting chiefly of cholesterol and a granulomatous inflammatory response *(arrow).* (Courtesy College of Veterinary Medicine, University of Illinois.)

Cholesteatomas

Cholesteatomas, also called *cholesterol granulomas,* form in choroid plexuses of the ventricles in horses as an aging change. These masses are usually incidental, but reports suggest that if they grow large enough and occlude the flow of CSF, acquired hydrocephalus can result. Cholesteatomas are tan to yellow-brown firm masses with a smooth to in some cases papilliform surface (Fig. 14-87). Occasionally the masses are mineralized. This lesion is thought to result from edema and minor but repeated hemorrhages within the choroid plexuses, which result in cholesterol deposits. These deposits elicit a foreign body inflammatory reaction (foreign body granuloma) in the choroid plexus.

Circulatory Disturbances

Peripartum Asphyxia Syndrome

Peripartum asphyxia syndrome (dummy foal, neonatal maladjustment syndrome, or barker foal) is attributed to impairment of normal umbilical blood flow between the mare and foal during parturition, resulting in decreased vascular flow to the brain. Causes usually are those related to interruption of umbilical blood flow, such as a twisted or pinched umbilical cord as occurs in a dystocia or premature separation of the placenta, possibly caused by endophyte fescue toxicity.

Gross lesions are laminar cortical necrosis and look similar to those described for bovine polioencephalomalacia. In the early stages of the disease, the cerebral gyri are edematous and swollen. The cortex may have a yellow-gray discoloration distributed in a laminar pattern several days after onset of the disease. If the animal survives for a longer period of time, there is cerebrocortical atrophy. Microscopically, initial lesions consist of laminar cortical edema and neuronal necrosis, followed by gitter cell accumulation and phagocytosis of cellular debris.

Clinical signs in foals with peripartum asphyxia syndrome include barking like dogs, seizures, aimless wandering, absence of a suckling reflex, and loss of affinity for the mare. Affected foals are usually normal for the first 12 to 24 hours and then decline rapidly as neuronal necrosis ensues.

DISORDERS OF RUMINANTS (CATTLE, SHEEP, AND GOATS)

Disorders that occur in many or all animal species are discussed in the section on Disorders of Domestic Animals.

Diseases Caused by Microbes

Bacteria

Listeriosis

Listeriosis, a bacterial disease with particular affinity for the CNS, is seen mainly in domestic ruminants. There is compelling evidence that *Listeria monocytogenes,* a facultative intracellular Gram-positive bacterium, invades through the mucosa of the oral cavity and into sensory and motor branches of the trigeminal nerve. Other cranial nerve branches that innervate the oral cavity and pharynx may also be involved. The bacteria migrate via sensory axons using retrograde axonal transport to the trigeminal ganglion and then into the brain (medulla) or via motor axons directly to the midbrain and medulla (motor neurons—nucleus of cranial nerve V). The infection can then spread rostrally and caudally to other areas of the brainstem. Lesions are occasionally found in the cerebellum and cranial cervical spinal cord. These sites are likely the result of direct extension of infection because *Listeria monocytogenes* is a motile bacterium that spreads from cell to cell in its replicative phase.

The mechanism of tissue injury is not completely defined; however, injury to neurons and axons is likely a secondary bystander effect related to inflammation. A correlation between the degree of cell-mediated immunity and severity of brain damage suggests that immunologic injury may occur. Recent studies in a murine model, however, indicate the T lymphocyte response is only slight in early stages of fatal listeriosis. Immunization before experimental infection enhances $CD4^+$ and $CD8^+$ T lymphocyte responses and provides greater survivability. Other studies have shown increased production of TNF-α and IL-10 in fatal murine infections. The former is capable of causing brain damage (apoptotic cell death) and augmenting other CNS immune responses; the latter has a suppressive effect on neuroimmunologic reactions. The organism also produces a hemolysin (listeriolysin) that is a virulence factor required for intracellular multiplication.

Once bacteria enter the CNS, recent experimental studies suggest that *Listeria monocytogenes* can directly infect neurons, microglia, choroid plexus epithelial cells, and macrophages recruited in the inflammatory exudate. The bacteria spread from cell to cell using a secreted phospholipase that cleaves a variety of phospholipids, including sphingomyelin (a component of myelin) and phospholipids in cell membranes (see Fig. 4-29). Axonal injury and neuronal death are likely attributable to inflammatory processes, especially to the action of listeriolysin and lipases.

Gross lesions are usually absent, but leptomeningeal opacity, foci of yellow-brown discoloration (0.1 to 0.2 mm in diameter in the area of the nuclei of cranial nerves V and VIII), hemorrhage, necrosis in the terminal brainstem, and cloudy CSF have been noted. Microscopically, a meningoencephalitis centered about the pons and medulla and involving both gray and white matter is characteristic (Fig. 14-88). The lesions, however, can extend from the diencephalon to the caudal medulla or cranial cervical spinal cord. Small, early lesions consist of loose clusters of microglial cells. With time, these lesions enlarge and contain variable numbers of neutrophils (Fig. 14-88, *B*) and later neutrophils dominate (microabscesses), but in some foci, macrophages can be the principal cell type. Necrosis and accumulation of gitter cells can be prominent in some cases. Numerous Gram-positive bacilli can be detected in some lesions (Fig. 14-88, *C*). Leptomeningitis is regularly present

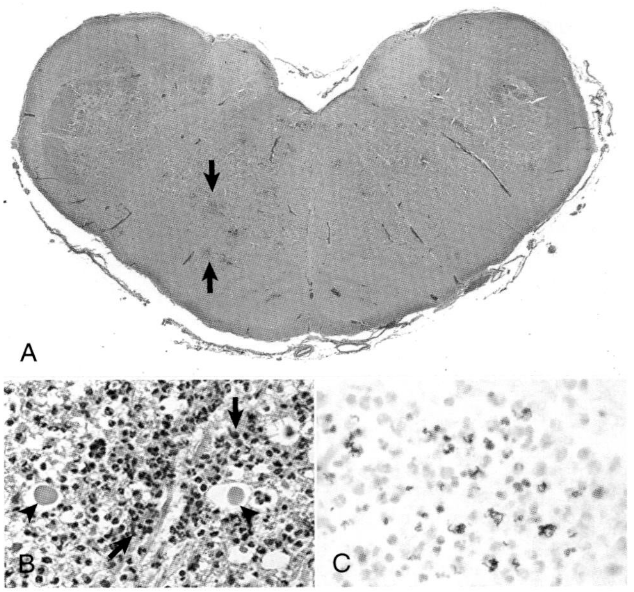

Fig. 14-88 Listeriosis, medulla, cow.
A, Microabscesses. Note the areas of faint blue discoloration in this subgross magnification of the medulla *(arrows).* The less well-defined blue areas are aggregates of neutrophils (microabscesses), and the blue linear lesions are perivascular cuffs. *Listeria monocytogenes,* the causative agent, uses retrograde axonal transport via the cranial nerves to enter the CNS and localize in the medulla (brainstem) and proximal cervical spinal cord. The lesion is rarely visible on gross observation. H&E stain. **B,** Early microabscesses *(arrows)* and inflammation are the result of inflammatory mediators that have injured axons *(arrowheads)* and will lead to Wallerian degeneration, seen here at the stage of swollen eosinophilic axons. H&E stain. **C,** *Listeria monocytogenes,* which is Gram-positive *(blue coccobacilli),* can sometimes be detected in microabscesses in a histologic section stained with a Gram stain. Gram stain. (Courtesy Dr. M.D. McGavin, College of Veterinary Medicine, University of Tennessee.)

and is often severe, and the exudate is composed of macrophages, lymphocytes, plasma cells, and fewer neutrophils. Cranial ganglioneuritis involving the trigeminal nerve and ganglion is often present.

Listeriosis presents in three disease forms: meningoencephalitis, abortion and stillbirth, and septicemia. The last commonly develops in young animals, possibly from an in utero infection. The encephalitic and genital forms of the disease rarely occur together in an individual animal or in the same flock or herd. Infections in humans also occur. Clinical signs in meningoencephalitic listeriosis are related to lesions in the brainstem and include dullness, torticollis, circling, unilateral facial paralysis, and drooling caused by pharyngeal paralysis. Signs of cranial nerve dysfunction occur because of inflammation in the medulla and pons. Death usually occurs within a few days after the initial signs and is preceded by recumbency and paddling of the limbs. Silage is the most common source of infection. If silage is contaminated with soil containing *Listeria monocytogenes* and is improperly prepared and stored (pH > 5.4), the organism can multiply.

Thrombotic Meningoencephalitis

Histophilus somni (formerly *Haemophilus somnus*), a small Gram-negative bacillus, causes a septicemic infection in cattle with variable clinical presentations, including pneumonia, polyarthritis, myocarditis, abortion, and meningoencephalitis. The disease is most prevalent in feedlot cattle but can occur in other situations. All manifestations, particularly meningoencephalitis, tend to be sporadic with single to multiple animals in a herd affected. The CNS form of the disease has been termed *thrombotic meningoencephalitis* (TME), previously referred to as *thromboembolic meningoencephalitis* (TEME). Mural thrombi from local vascular injury rather than thromboemboli from distal sites of vascular injury, such as the lungs, are the major type of thrombus in this disease.

The pathogenesis of *Histophilus somni* (formerly *Haemophilus somnus*) infection is not completely understood. Many cattle harbor the organism in the upper digestive tract without evidence of disease, but under some circumstances, it invades to cause severe clinical infection. The mechanism(s) of invasion into the bloodstream is not definitely known, but the respiratory tract is the initial site of bacterial replication followed by hematogenous spread to the CNS. Once the bacteria gain access to the circulation (bacterial emboli), emboli lodge at the interface of the gray and white matter in microvessels. Organisms adhere to endothelial cells, presumably via a receptor-mediated interaction, which results in endothelial cell contraction and desquamation. Subendothelial collagen is exposed, initiating a cascade of events culminating in vasculitis, thrombosis, and infarction. The bacteria within the infarct replicate and cause inflammation. Lipooligosaccharide, a toxic factor produced by *Histophilus somni* (formerly *Haemophilus somnus*), might protect the bacteria from host defenses. Bovine neutrophils, blood monocytes, and alveolar macrophages are incapable of killing the organism, allowing the infection to become established.

Gross lesions in the CNS are irregularly sized foci of hemorrhage and necrosis scattered randomly, and visible both externally and on cut surfaces (Fig. 14-89). Lesions are most frequent in the cerebrum, commonly at the cortical gray matter–white matter interface. The location of the lesion may reflect a change in the diameter and flow patterns of blood vessels, allowing bacteria to lodge, adhere, and replicate in these vessels. The spinal cord also has lesions. Other lesions include brain swelling caused by edema and leptomeningitis with cloudiness of the CSF.

Microscopic lesions in all organs, including the CNS, are initially marked vasculitis and vascular necrosis, which are followed by thrombosis and infarction. Septic vasculitis, the initial event, is followed by edema and an influx of neutrophils and macrophages in and around vessel walls and adjacent parenchyma. Colonies of small Gram-negative bacilli are frequent in thrombi, in and around affected vessels, and in areas of necrosis.

Clinically, affected cows are initially ataxic and circle, head-press, and appear blind. As the disease progresses, they may have convulsions, become comatose, and die.

Viruses

Herpesviruses

Bovine malignant catarrhal fever

Malignant catarrhal fever is usually a sporadic highly fatal disease of cattle and other ruminants, including deer, buffalo, and antelope, and can involve several animals in a herd. The disease has a worldwide distribution, and the clinicopathologic features do not differ significantly from one part of the world to another. The primary target tissues are the vasculature and lymphoid organs and epithelial tissue (particularly the respiratory and gastrointestinal tracts), but the kidneys, liver, eyes, joints, and CNS are also affected in some cattle. The virus appears to be transferred between lymphoid tissue/cells and endothelial cells via leukocytic trafficking in T lymphocytes. Two general types of the disease occur, the sheep-associated and wildebeest-derived forms. The causative agents involved belong to the herpesvirus subfamily Gammaherpesvirinae. The disease occurring outside Africa, caused by ovine

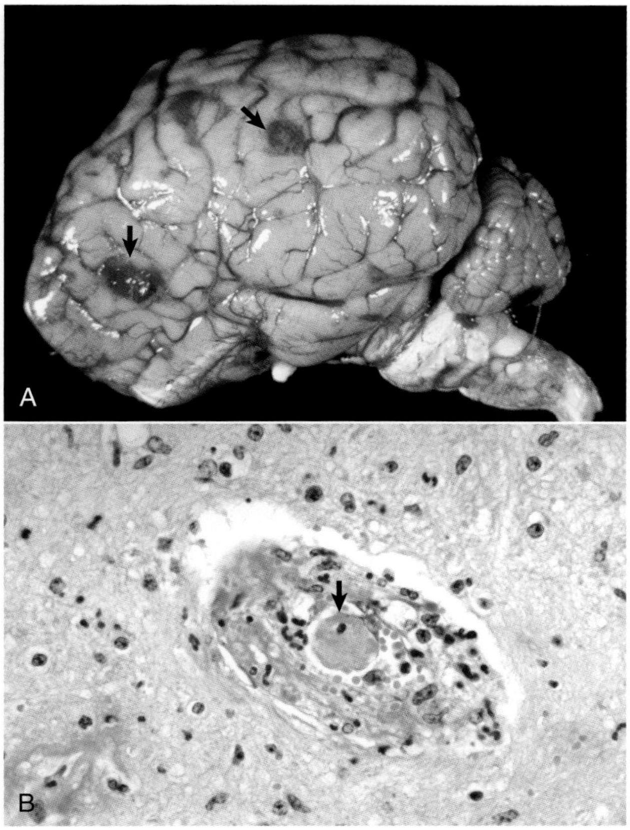

Fig. 14-89 Thrombotic meningoencephalitis (previously referred to as *thromboembolic meningoencephalitis*), cerebrum, steer.
A, On the surface of the cerebral cortex *(arrows)* are several red-brown lesions. These lesions are areas of necrosis, hemorrhage, and inflammation secondary to vasculitis and thrombosis caused by *Histophilus somni* (formerly *Haemophilus somnus*). Such septic infarcts are distributed randomly (hematogenous portal of entry) throughout the CNS, including the spinal cord. The lesions depicted here are unusually severe. **B,** A thrombus *(arrow)* is present in the vascular lumen. Note the acute inflammatory response, edema, fibrinogenesis, and hemorrhage in the vessel wall. H&E stain. (**A** courtesy Dr. H. Leipold, College of Veterinary Medicine, Kansas State University. **B** courtesy Dr. M.D. McGavin, College of Veterinary Medicine, University of Tennessee.)

herpesvirus 2 (OHV-2), often involves close contact of presumed "carrier" sheep with susceptible ruminants. The disease has recently been reported in muskox *(Ovibos moschatus),* Nubian ibex *(Capra nubiana),* and gemsbok *(Oryx gazella).* In Africa and occasionally in wildlife facilities outside the continent, the source of the infection (designated *Alcelaphine herpesvirus 1* [AHV-1]) is the wildebeest. Two other antigenically related viruses, which apparently do not cause natural disease, include Alcelaphine herpesvirus 2 (AHV-2) and Hippotragine herpesvirus 1 (HiHV-1), which have been isolated from African hartebeest and roan antelope, respectively. It is generally accepted that cattle and other susceptible ruminants contract the disease in nature after respiratory or oral infection during association with carrier sheep (presumed) and wildebeest, particularly at the time of parturition. A cell-mediated and cytotoxic lymphocytic process has been proposed as involved in the development of the necrotizing vasculitis.

Gross lesions of the CNS include active hyperemia and cloudiness of the leptomeninges caused by nonsuppurative meningoencephalomyelitis and vasculitis. Lymphocytic perivascular cuffing and varying degrees of necrotizing vasculitis occur in the leptomeninges and in all parts of the brain and occasionally in the spinal cord, with the white matter most consistently involved. Other lesions in the affected CNS include variable neuronal degeneration, microgliosis, choroiditis, necrosis of ependymal cells, and ganglioneuritis. Clinical signs referable to CNS infection may include trembling, shivering, ataxia, and nystagmus.

Infectious bovine rhinotracheitis

Although bovine herpesvirus 1 (BoHV-1) occasionally causes a nonsuppurative meningoencephalitis, primarily in young cattle, two variants of BoHV-1 isolated in Argentina and Australia (referred to as BoHV-1, subtypes 3a and 3b, respectively) and recently BoHV-5 (isolated in South America, mainly Argentina and Brazil) have a particular tropism for the CNS. Recent evidence suggests that BoHV-5 uses an intranasal route to infect and replicate in the nasal mucosa and then enters the CNS by retrograde axonal transport using the trigeminal and olfactory nerves.

Gross lesions are nonspecific and include meningeal congestion and petechiation in ventral areas of the brain. Microscopic lesions consist of lymphomonocytic meningoencephalitis (nonsuppurative) with the occasional presence of neutrophils. Other changes include neuronal degeneration, vasculitis, focal malacia, and presence of intranuclear acidophilic inclusions in neurons and astrocytes.

Clinically, outbreaks of disease occur in young cattle ranging in age from 5 to 18 months. Lesions can also involve the eyes (conjunctivitis) and tissues of the reproductive, alimentary, and integumentary systems in addition to the nervous system.

Lentiviruses

Visna

Visna, which means wasting, is a slowly progressive, transmissible disease of sheep. The disease is caused by a strain of the ovine maedi-visna virus (MVV) complex, one of the eight basic "lenti" (slow) viruses (family Retroviridae). A different strain of the same virus causes a lymphocytic interstitial pneumonia referred to as *maedi.*

In recent years, the understanding of the factors associated with infection, including the mechanism of lesion development, has improved. Visna is a persistent viral disease that probably results from the ability of the virus to form provirus and integrate into the host genome. The virus can also change its antigenic characteristics (antigenic drift), which enables it to escape the effects of the host's immune response. Although the visna virus and other lentiviruses can infect promonocytes and monocytes in the bone marrow and blood, viral replication is restricted in these cells, where it remains as provirus DNA until maturation and differentiation to macrophages. Primary viral replication occurs in cells of monocyte-macrophage-microglial lineage. Thus visna virus enters the CNS by way of leukocytic trafficking of virus-infected macrophages. Visna virus can also be present in oligodendrocytes and astrocytes located in foci of demyelination. It has been suggested that the virus gains access to these cells via close contact with infected monocytes. Recent studies suggest the virus can also infect and productively replicate in endothelial cells. This mechanism may provide an additional route for viral entry into the CNS and the potential for alterations of the blood-brain barrier.

Although gross lesions are not frequently observed, they may occur in areas of prominent inflammation where they appear as yellow-tan areas. Early microscopic lesions primarily affect the gray and white matter subjacent to the ependyma of the ventricular system of the brain and central canal of the spinal cord. These lesions are characterized by a nonsuppurative encephalomyelitis accompanied by pleocytosis, variable edema, CNS necrosis, astrocytosis, choroiditis, and nonsuppurative leptomeningitis. The inflammatory response is thought to be caused by the upregulation of expression of major histocompatibility complex class II genes that occurs in virus-infected macrophages. Degeneration of myelin sheaths also occurs at this time but is often accompanied by axonal degeneration, suggesting that it could be a secondary lesion, such as in Wallerian degeneration. Oligodendroglial and neuron injury and necrotic cell death are attributable to cytokines and other toxic factors secreted by inflammatory cells and glial cells. Recent in vitro studies suggest that caspase activation leading to apoptotic cell death may play a role in visna.

Neuronal cell bodies and oligodendroglia are normal (except in areas of necrosis) during this stage of the disease. The latter cells can become infected, however, which leads to later development of demyelination. Primary demyelination, particularly in the spinal cord, has been described in animals infected for prolonged periods (months to years). Such animals also have periventricular inflammation.

The primary demyelination that occurs during the late stages of the disease process (6 months to 8 years after infection) has been proposed to result from oligodendroglial cell infection. The main sources of excreted virus are the udder and lungs (as mainly cell-associated virus), and transmission occurs most readily between the dam and lamb via the milk and between confined individuals, probably via respiratory secretions. The MVV has also been detected in semen of infected rams. It is important to emphasize that no profound immune deficiency occurs with MVV infections, as is the case for immunodeficiency lentiviral infections that infect $CD4^+$ T lymphocytes. Nonetheless, secondary infections can still significantly accompany MVV infection.

In addition to pneumonia, MVVs can also cause mastitis, arthritis (uncommonly of the carpus or hind limb joints), and a mesangial glomerulitis. Irrespective of the target organ, the lesions are to be regarded as chronic and lymphoproliferative, in contrast to the well-known immunodeficiency infections caused by human immunodeficiency virus 1 (HIV-1), simian immunodeficiency virus (SIV), and FIV.

Viral strain differences and breed of sheep can influence the lesions that develop. For example, the visna form of the disease does not commonly occur in ovine breeds of North America, although some degree of visna-like lesions can be seen with maedi. Visna originally was described in Iceland, but sheep with similar lesions of the CNS have been detected in The Netherlands, Kenya, the US, and Canada. CNS signs include an abnormal hindlimb gait that progresses to incoordination and rear limb paresis over a period of weeks or months.

Caprine leukoencephalomyelitis arthritis

Caprine leukoencephalomyelitis arthritis was first described in the US and has since been recognized in other parts of the world. The infection can be readily transmitted by colostrum and milk after birth, or by direct contact. A close relationship exists between the MVVs of sheep and the caprine arthritis encephalitis (CAE) virus, but genomic differences between them can be demonstrated. As with MVV infection of sheep, CAE viral infection is also a lymphoproliferative disease with a tropism for the macrophage, which acts as a carrier for the virus.

Gross lesions in the nervous system include tan- to salmon-colored foci of necrosis and inflammation that can occasionally be detected in the brain (Fig. 14-90) and most prominently in the spinal cord. Microscopic lesions of the nervous system are similar to those of visna (nonsuppurative encephalomyelitis) but can be more severe with CAE. Nonneural lesions include interstitial pneumonia of moderate severity in some affected kids. Such lungs fail to collapse completely and are mottled red or blue. As discussed under visna, the mechanism of infection and cell death appear similar.

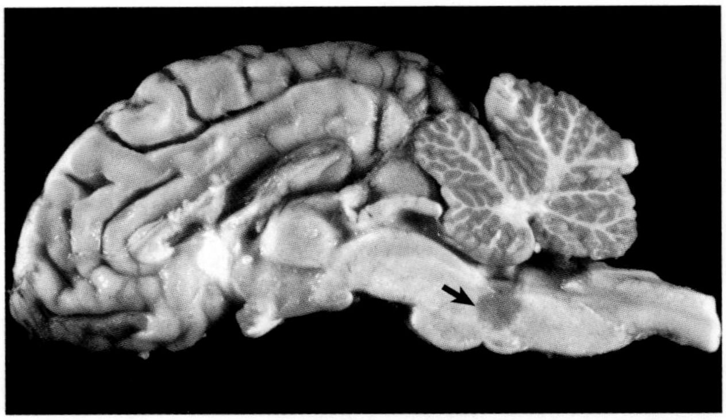

Fig. 14-90 **Leukoencephalitis, caprine retrovirus-induced encephalitis, brainstem, goat.**
A focal area of the brainstem *(arrow)* is yellow-brown and was found, microscopically, to be infiltrated by lymphocytes, plasma cells, and histiocytes. A similar lesion commonly occurs in the spinal cord. (Courtesy Dr. H.E. Whiteley, College of Veterinary Medicine, University of Illinois.)

The pattern of disease in CAE is age dependent. Neurologic manifestations are usually seen in young kids 2 to 4 months of age, but unlike visna in sheep, there is a more rapid progression and signs progressing to quadriplegia develop within weeks to months. As with visna, affected goats have pleocytosis. In adult goats, the primary target tissue is the synovium of the joints, and animals that survive the initial infection have lymphoproliferative synovitis and arthritis develop. Pneumonia, lymphocytic mastitis, and encephalomyelitis also occur in adult animals.

Chlamydia

Sporadic Bovine Encephalomyelitis

See Web Appendix 14-1.

Prions

See the section on Disorders of Domestic Animals for additional discussion of prions.

Bovine Spongiform Encephalopathy

BSE (mad cow disease) was originally identified in the United Kingdom in 1986 but likely existed there as early as April 1985. Through the end of 2003, more than 183,000 cows from more than 35,000 herds were reported with BSE. With regard to the origins of BSE, epidemiologic evidence strongly suggests that this disease was caused initially (during the early 1980s) by the feeding of rations containing meat and bone meal supplements that were contaminated with the scrapie agent. Countries that have reported cases of BSE or are considered to have a substantial risk to have animals with BSE include Albania, Austria, Belgium, Bosnia-Herzegovina, Bulgaria, Canada (confirmed May 2003), Croatia, Czech Republic, Denmark, Federal Republic of Yugoslavia, Finland, France, Germany, Greece, Hungary, Ireland, Israel, Italy, Liechtenstein, Luxembourg, former Yugoslavia Republic of Macedonia, The Netherlands, Norway, Oman, Poland, Portugal, Romania, Slovak Republic, Slovenia, Spain, Sweden, Switzerland, Japan, and United Kingdom (Great Britain, including Northern Ireland and the Falkland Islands).

In December 2003, BSE was confirmed in a single dairy cow from a herd in Washington state. This cow was apparently imported into the US 2 to 3 years earlier from a farm in northern Alberta,

Canada, which was the source of the positive BSE case in Canada confirmed in May 2003. In 2004, additional cases of BSE likely linked to a common source were reported in Washington state, Oregon, and Canada, and in June 2005 a cow tested positive for BSE in Texas.

Signs that accompany BSE include changes in behavior such as nervousness or aggressiveness, abnormal posture, abnormal gait, incoordination, difficulty in rising, decreased milk production, and loss of body weight despite continued appetite. Clinically affected cattle deteriorate until they either die or require euthanasia. This clinical period usually ranges from 2 weeks to 6 months. All cases of the disease in cattle have occurred in adult animals, with an age range of 3 to 11 years, but most animals have clinical signs develop between 3 and 5 years of age.

The National Veterinary Services Laboratory (Animal and Plant Health Inspection Service [APHIS]) of the US Department of Agriculture has developed and implemented through local and regional veterinary diagnostic laboratories procedures for sampling, preparing, and submitting brains for BSE analysis. Space limitations prevent describing these procedures. They can be obtained through APHIS or a diagnostic laboratory. Dead or sick animals that display neurologic signs and are suspected of being potential BSE candidates are tested using immunohistochemical analysis, Western blot analysis, or enzyme-linked immunosorbent assay (ELISA) to identify PrP^{Sc} in brain tissue. Genetically valuable animals that may be exported or have their embryos or DNA saved for future use and are from TSE risk groups can be tested for PrP^{Sc}. Immunohistochemical analysis for PrP^{Sc} of samples obtained (i.e., under anesthesia) from biopsies of tonsil and lymph follicles of the third eyelid from at-risk groups show promise as diagnostic tools.

Ovine Spongiform Encephalopathy (Scrapie)

Scrapie is best known as a degenerative disease that affects the CNS of sheep and was first recognized in Great Britain and other countries of Western Europe more than 250 years ago. The disease, which is currently reported throughout the world except for Australia and New Zealand, also occurs naturally in the domestic goat. The name is derived from the characteristic clinical signs of pruritus, which often results in loss of wool in sheep. The disease progresses inexorably with early signs of subtle change in behavior or temperament followed by scratching and rubbing against fixed objects because of the pruritus. Additional signs include incoordination, weight loss (despite retention of appetite), biting of the feet and limbs, lip smacking, gait abnormalities, trembling (when suddenly stressed), recumbency, and eventually death after 1 to 6 months or longer.

Much of our current understanding of the pathogenesis of the natural infection of scrapie in Suffolk sheep has been advanced by Dr. William Hadlow and co-workers. It should be noted that Dr. Hadlow is a veterinary pathologist and diplomate of the American College of Veterinary Pathologists, who first recognized and reported the similarity between scrapie and kuru of humans. This important contribution led to the current understanding of the TSEs and a Nobel Prize for the medical scientist (Dr. D. Gajdusek) who originally investigated kuru in the South Pacific.

Degenerative Diseases

Metabolic

Primary Neuronal Degeneration

Primary cerebellar neuronal degeneration

Primary cerebellar neuronal degeneration has also been reported to occur in Yorkshire piglets, Merino and Charolais lambs, Holstein Friesian calves, Angus calves, and a moose. An autosomal recessive mode of inheritance is suspected or documented in several of the diseases, but the mechanism of injury is unclear. Grossly, the cerebellum can be normal or reduced in size and atrophic. Microscopically, lesions may include loss of Purkinje cells, variable neuronal depletion in the granular layer, fusiform swellings of proximal Purkinje cell axons, and astrogliosis in the molecular layer.

Animals with postnatal primary cerebellar neuronal degeneration are normal at birth or at the time of ambulation. Onset of ataxia with various other clinical signs referable to cerebellar disease begins weeks or months after a period of apparently normal development. Initial clinical signs are often subtle. Progression of the signs can be slow or rapid, relentless, or with static periods. Some individuals reach a stage without further progression of signs, but this is not typical of the syndrome in most animals.

Nutritional

Vitamin B_1 (Thiamine) Deficiency

Thiamine deficiency in ruminants

Thiamine deficiency in cattle, sheep, and less commonly, goats, has been termed *polioencephalomalacia* or *cerebrocortical necrosis.* Rumen microbes are able to synthesize thiamine. Conclusive evidence of an absolute thiamine deficiency as the sole cause of polioencephalomalacia in ruminants has been elusive. Evidence or theories linking thiamine with the ruminant disorder include the following:

1. Clinical response to thiamine injection in some individuals
2. Decreases in ruminal thiamine, or overgrowth of thiaminase-producing microbes such as *Bacillus thiaminolyticus*
3. Ingestion of thiaminase-containing plants such as bracken fern
4. Production of inactive thiamine analogs
5. Decreased absorption or increased fecal excretion of thiamine

Gross lesions, if present, are limited primarily to the cerebral cortex. Initially, 2 days after onset, the surface of the brain can be swollen (cerebral edema) as indicated by flattening of cerebrocortical gyri and narrow sulci. In rare cases with more severe brain swelling, brain displacement with herniation of the parahippocampal gyri beneath the tentorium cerebelli and the vermis of the cerebellum into the foramen magnum can occur. By 4 days after onset, yellow discoloration of the cerebrocortical gray matter occurs (Fig. 14-91), and it is at this time that autofluorescence (see later for more detail) is seen when the brain is examined under

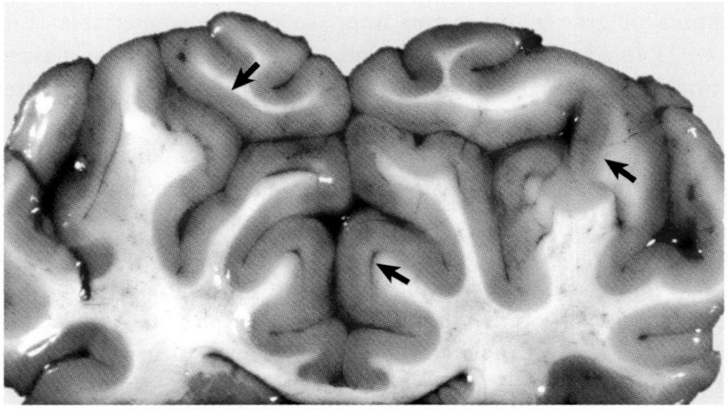

Fig. 14-91 Acute polioencephalomalacia, cerebral cortex, cross-sectional view, cow.
Cerebral cortical gyri are yellow and swollen *(arrows).* The cause of this yellow color is unknown but has been shown experimentally not to be caused by ceroid-lipofuscin pigments. Changes involving the sulci and gyri in acute polioencephalomalacia are shown in Fig. 14-93. (Courtesy Dr. L. Roth, College of Veterinary Medicine, Cornell University.)

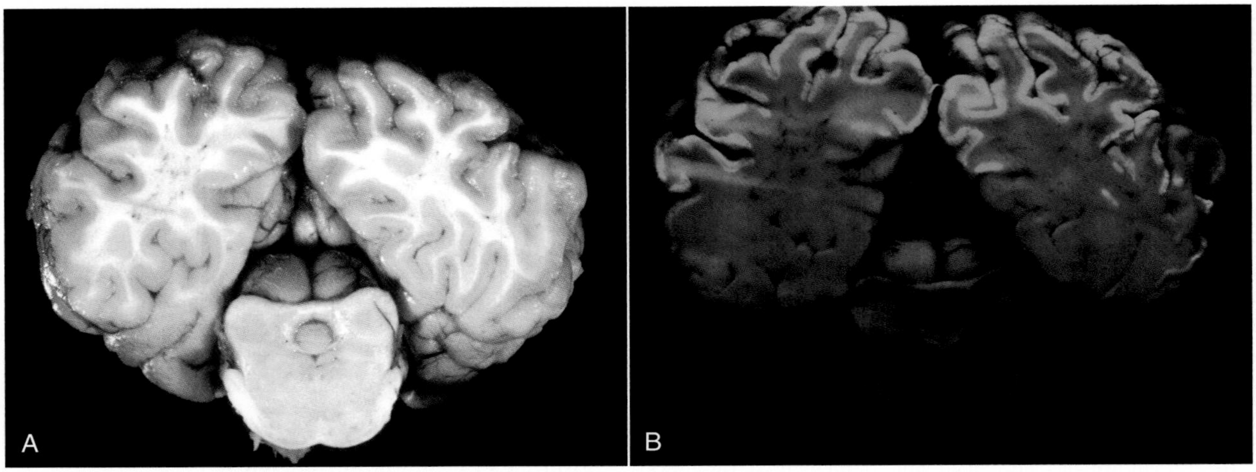

Fig. 14-92 Acute polioencephalomalacia, brain, cerebral hemispheres and midbrain, steer.
A, Compare the relative lack of gross lesions with those revealed by ultraviolet (UV) light in **B. B,** Bilaterally symmetric laminar pattern of apple-green autofluorescence (from mitochondrial derivatives) involving the full-thickness of the cortex indicates areas of necrosis in the gray matter. Although not shown here, the colliculi were also autofluorescent. The cerebrum is exposed to 365 nm ultraviolet (UV) light from a Wood's lamp. Similar results can be obtained with fixed (preserved) brain. (Courtesy Dr. P.N. Bochsler, School of Veterinary Medicine, University of Wisconsin-Madison.)

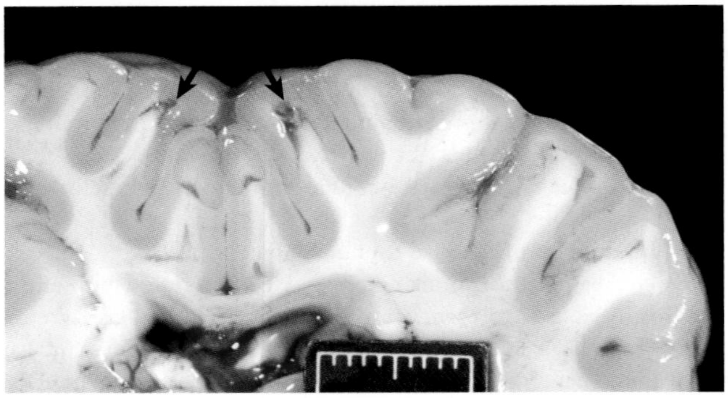

Fig. 14-93 Acute cerebrocortical polioencephalomalacia, thiamine deficiency, brain, parietal lobe, level of thalamus, goat.
Note the liquefactive necrosis with varying degrees of tissue separation *(arrows)* in the deep cortex. Scale bar = 2 cm. (Courtesy Dr. R. Storts, College of Veterinary Medicine, Texas A&M University.)

375 nm ultraviolet light (Fig. 14-92). Eight to 10 days after onset, edematous separation and necrosis involving the middle to deeper lamina or gray-white matter interface may be appreciable (Fig. 14-93). In advanced cases with prolonged survival, areas of marked atrophy of cerebral gyri with an attenuated or absent gray matter zone are covered by meninges (Fig. 14-94).

Microscopically, the earliest lesions are laminar cortical necrosis and astrocytic swelling. Laminar cortical necrosis is characterized by neuronal necrosis (ischemic change), with a laminar pattern of edema in the cerebral cortex. Neurons in the middle to deep lamina of the parietooccipital lobes of the cerebral cortex are preferentially affected (Fig. 14-95, *A*). In the early stages or in mild cases, lesions can be limited to the depths of cerebrocortical sulci, but generally there is involvement of entire gyri that may be confluent over extensive areas of the cortex. After 4 to 5 days, neuronal necrosis and edema are more severe, and there is an early influx of blood monocytes that mature into tissue macrophages and become gitter cells as they phagocytose necrotic debris. Macrophages and gitter cells are observed most commonly in perivascular and perineuronal spaces and in the pia arachnoid (see Fig. 14-23, *A*). After 8 to 10 days, necrosis and edema have resulted in laminar separation (at the

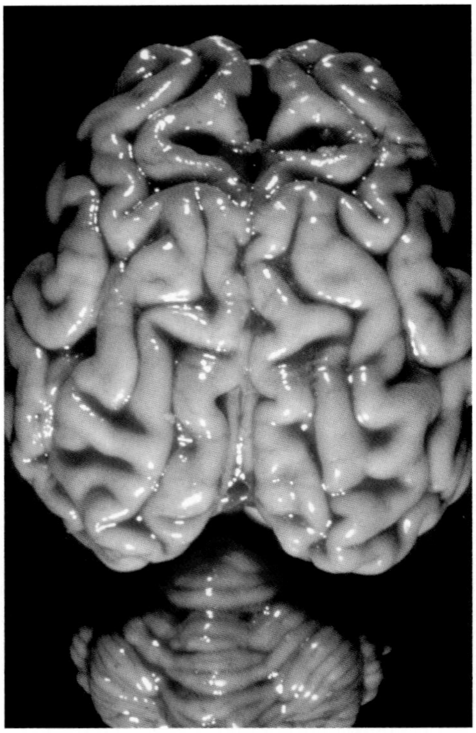

Fig. 14-94 Chronic cerebral cortical atrophy, brain, cow.
Cerebral cortical gyri are atrophic. Gyri are narrow, and as a result, the sulci are widened. In this case, the loss of cerebral cortex was caused by thiamine deficiency several years previously. (Courtesy College of Veterinary Medicine, University of Illinois.)

gray matter–white matter interface) in which there are prominent accumulations of macrophages (Fig. 14-95, *B*). Lesions that accompany the necrosis include vascular prominence caused by endothelial cell and perithelial cell hypertrophy and hyperplasia, congestion, and a minimal, if any, influx of neutrophils. Bilaterally symmetric focal lesions, similar to those seen in carnivores, occur in the thalamus and midbrain or colliculi and rarely in other brainstem structures. Animals that survive can have cerebral atrophy and develop

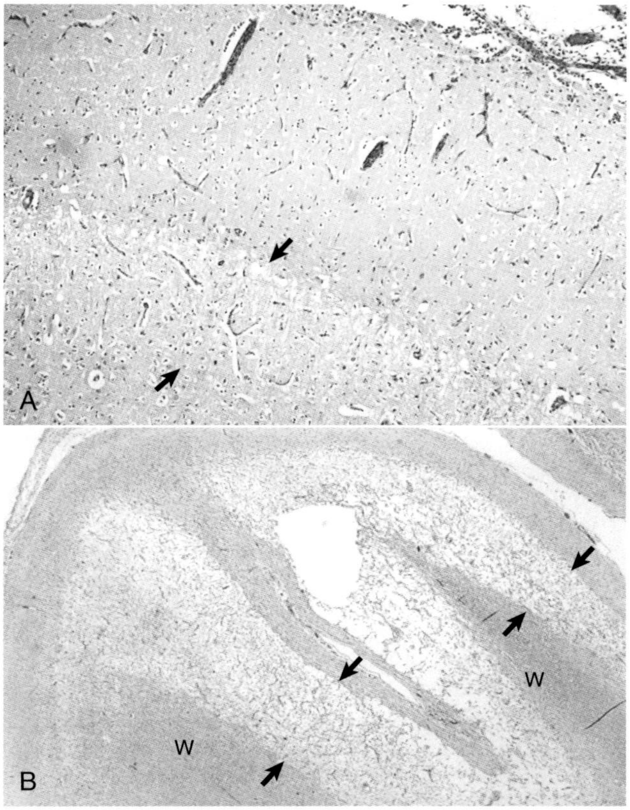

Fig. 14-95 Polioencephalomalacia, cerebral cortex, cross-sectional view, cow.

A, Acute stage. Note the zone of edema and acute neuronal necrosis affecting lamina 4-6 *(area between arrows)* of the cerebral cortex. Monocytes can be seen in the piarachnoid layer and subarachnoid space *(upper right)* in response to neuronal injury and the need to phagocytose cellular debris. Monocytes will also rapidly appear in perivascular spaces of blood vessels in the area of laminar edema and neuronal necrosis. H&E stain. **B,** Chronic stage. Areas of microcavitation in the deep cortical laminae next to the subcortical white matter are poorly stained *(area between arrows)* when compared with those of the normal superficial cortex *(left).* W, White matter. H&E stain. (**A** courtesy Dr. W. Haschek-Hock, College of Veterinary Medicine, University of Illinois. **B** courtesy Dr. J.F. Zachary, College of Veterinary Medicine, University of Illinois.)

hydrocephalus ex vacuo and have been known to live 1 to 2 years. It should be noted that laminar cortical necrosis can be caused by a variety of metabolic abnormalities. In ruminants, in addition to thiamine deficiency, water deprivation–sodium ion toxicosis, lead poisoning, and high sulfur intake can cause polioencephalomalacia and laminar cortical necrosis. Although autofluorescence at 365 nm ultraviolet light has been historically attributed to the accumulation of ceroid-lipofuscin in lipophages resulting from lipid degeneration in injured neuronal cell membranes, this supposition has recently been questioned. A recent study of cerebrocortical necrosis reported that autofluorescent substances in degenerating neurons occurred in structures resembling mitochondria and that ceroid-lipofuscin pigments were not demonstrated microscopically in damaged CNS. An association between mitochondria and autofluorescence has also been shown in the neuronal ceroid lipofuscinoses (Batten disease, ceroid-lipofuscin storage diseases). These diseases are characterized by the accumulation of an autofluorescent (365 nm ultraviolet light), intracytoplasmic storage material in CNS neurons composed mostly of subunit c of mitochondrial ATP synthase.

Clinically, the disease is seen most commonly in cattle 6 to 18 months of age fed concentrated rations. In sheep, most cases occur in younger age groups (2 to 7 months). Clinical signs in cattle and small ruminants may include depression, stupor, ataxia, head pressing, apparent cortical blindness, opisthotonos, convulsions, and recumbency with paddling and then death. If animals survive or respond to therapy, clinical signs can persist.

Polioencephalomalacia commonly occurs in cattle fed rations rich in carbohydrates with little roughage and is also associated with clinical or subclinical acidosis that may precipitate changes in rumen microflora. The disorder also occurs in association with other dietary factors, including cobalt deficiency, molasses- and urea-based diets, and diets high in elemental sulfur and sulfates and sulfides, some of which are not specifically associated with thiamine deficiency.

Recently, there has been considerable interest in the relationship of high dietary sulfur to polioencephalomalacia. All sources of sulfur, including formulated rations, plants rich in sulfur *(Kochia scoparia),* and high concentrations of sulfur in the drinking water, are additive. Total dietary intake should not exceed 0.3% to 0.4%. The exact mechanism to explain sulfur-induced polioencephalomalacia in ruminants has not been proved. Although deficiency or disordered metabolism of thiamine can be involved, it would seem not to be the sole cause or, in some instances, even a major factor in the disorder. Alternatively, polioencephalomalacia could represent a multifactorial metabolic disorder with multiple causes, all culminating in cerebrocortical necrosis. Any unifying hypothesis concerning the mechanism(s) of brain damage would have to reconcile all these variables.

Copper Deficiency

Swayback and enzootic ataxia are diseases caused by copper deficiency in lambs and kid goats. Swayback refers to the congenital form of the disease, whereas in enzootic ataxia, onset is delayed for up to 6 months after birth. Although copper deficiency is involved, the pathogenesis is poorly understood. Lesions occur in the cerebrum, brainstem, and spinal cord in the congenital form, but only in the brainstem and spinal cord in cases with a postnatal onset.

Additionally, deficiency of copper can affect wool, hair growth, and pigmentation; musculoskeletal development; and integrity of connective tissue. Copper deficiency can be primarily to the result of copper-deficient soils and inadequate intake from forage or secondary from defective absorption because of interactions between copper, molybdenum, zinc, cadmium, or inorganic sulfates. Copper is a component of several enzyme systems, including cytochrome and lysyl oxidases, such as mitochondrial cytochrome-c oxidase; dopamine β-monooxygenase; peptidyl α-amidating monooxygenase; tyrosinase; and superoxide dismutase and the protein ceruloplasmin. These enzyme systems are essential for energy generation by mitochondria in the brain, regulating oxidative stress, catecholamine synthesis, and the modification of peptide neurotransmitters.

The pathogenesis of the lesions that occur in swayback and enzootic ataxia is poorly understood. It has been suggested that cerebral lesions result from loss of embryonic cells at the same stage of brain development as occurs in porencephaly and hydranencephaly after in utero viral infection or dysgenesis caused by a biochemical disturbance. Biochemical disturbances could also account for the axonal/neuronal degeneration in the brainstem and spinal cord. Altered function of the mitochondrial enzyme cytochrome oxidase leading to energy failure could play a role in cerebral dysgenesis and axonal and ultimately neuronal degeneration.

More intriguing is the possible involvement of the enzyme copper-zinc superoxide dismutase. A mutation in this enzyme is present in approximately 20% of humans with familial amyotrophic lateral sclerosis (ALS) and in some individuals with the sporadic form of the disease. This human disorder, which is classified as a motor neuron disease, has a much later onset, and the mutation results in a "gain of function" of the enzyme rather than lack of function as might be present in copper deficiency. Neurofilament accumulation in brainstem and spinal ventral horn neurons and fiber tract degeneration (corticospinal in humans versus spinocerebellar in lambs and kids with copper deficiency) are similar. Drawing a relevant association between these diseases of humans and abnormal function of superoxide dismutase in swayback and enzootic ataxia in animals is premature at this time, however. It is also possible that the cortical white matter degeneration and brainstem or spinal lesions arise from different mechanisms.

Grossly, approximately 50% of congenitally affected lambs and rarely kids have bilateral cerebrocortical lesions. Externally the cerebral cortex can be focally soft and fluctuant or collapsed. These foci correspond to areas of rarefaction, which have either a gelatinous consistency or cystic cavities filled with clear serous fluid, in the white matter of the corona radiate and centrum semiovale. Microscopically, a variable astrogliosis is associated with the degeneration of white matter, but the cavities lack a capsule of glial fibers. Myelin degradation and an influx of macrophages are minimal. Delicate neuronal and astroglial processes traverse the cavities. Neuronal necrosis in cortical gray matter overlying these white matter lesions is sometimes observed.

Microscopic lesions in the brainstem and spinal cord in both the congenital (swayback) and delayed-onset (enzootic ataxia) forms of copper deficiency are similar in lambs and kids, and they affect both gray and white matter. Large multipolar neurons of the brainstem reticular formation, certain brainstem nuclei—such as the red and vestibular nuclei—and the ventral, lateral, and less commonly, dorsal horns of the spinal cord are affected. Neuronal cell bodies lack stainable Nissl's substance (chromatolysis). The cytoplasm is variably dense, pink, and homogeneous to fibrillar as a result of the accumulation of neurofilaments, and nuclei are often displaced to an eccentric position against the cell membrane. The extent of neuronal necrosis varies. Lesions in the white matter of the spinal cord consist of bilateral areas of pallor in the dorsolateral aspects of the lateral funiculi (corresponding roughly to the spinocerebellar tracts) and also in the ventral funiculi adjacent to the ventral median fissure. The pallor of the white matter is due to degeneration of myelinated axons. Involvement of the medial (septomarginal) aspect of the dorsal funiculi is infrequent. In the terminal brainstem, lesions are similar but have a somewhat scattered distribution. The spinocerebellar tracts extending into the middle cerebellar peduncles are affected. Astrogliosis is usually mild. Definitive microscopic lesions in the cerebellum and ventral spinal nerve rootlets and peripheral nerves are usually lacking in lambs but can be frequent in kids. Changes in Purkinje cells are analogous to those already noted in neurons in other areas. Additionally, ectopic Purkinje cells and thinning of the granular cell layer occur. Bergmann's glial cell processes in the molecular layer hypertrophy. Lesions in ventral spinal nerve rootlets and peripheral nerve are caused by axonal degeneration secondary to injury of motor neurons in the ventral gray horns.

Clinically, CNS disease as a result of copper deficiency in animals is mainly a disorder of sheep and goats and can be present at birth (swayback in lambs, rarely kids), or onset can be delayed up to 6 months (enzootic ataxia in lambs and kids). Swayback occurs in newborn lambs from ewes with inadequate dietary copper intake. Affected lambs can be born dead, weak, or unable to stand. If mobile, they are ataxic. Enzootic ataxia is characterized by ataxia.

Toxicoses

Microbial Toxins

Clostridium perfringens *type D encephalopathy (pulpy kidney disease, overeating disease)*

Clostridium perfringens type D enterotoxemia, associated with epsilon toxin production, is a disease of sheep, goats, and cattle, but only sheep commonly exhibit the neurologic manifestations of the disease. Brain damage is due to vascular injury and breakdown of the blood-brain barrier. Binding of epsilon toxin to endothelial cell surface receptors results in opening of tight junctions, disturbed transport processes, increased vascular permeability that results in vasogenic edema, swelling of astrocytic foot processes, and ultimately necrosis caused by hypoxic-ischemic mechanisms. Some of the effects of epsilon toxin can be mediated by an adenyl cyclase–cAMP system.

Gross lesions are absent in some peracute cases but when present, consist initially of bilaterally symmetric foci of malacia, leading to yellow-gray to red foci with malacia and cavitation (Fig. 14-96, *A*). Lesions can be found in the internal capsule, basal nuclei, thalamus, hippocampus, rostral colliculus and substantia nigra, pons, corona radiata of frontal cortex, and cerebellar peduncles, especially the middle peduncle. Lesions in other tissue consist of pulmonary congestion and edema, serous pericardial effusion, petechiation, and soft (pulpy) kidneys (see Fig. 11-49).

Microscopically, the CNS lesion in acute cases is vasogenic edema secondary to vascular injury. The fluid in perivascular spaces is frequently protein rich and eosinophilic. Walls of arterioles can be hyalinized, and endothelial cell nuclei swollen and vesicular (Fig. 14-96, *B*). Vasogenic edema, which is interstitial in location, gives a light or pink-staining, spongy appearance to the CNS parenchyma. Both gray matter and white matter are affected. Pericapillary hemorrhage and acute necrosis of neurons and macroglia occur. Other changes occur with longer survival and include axonal swelling, accumulation of neutrophils and foamy macrophages (Fig. 14-96, *B* and *C*), vascular prominence caused by perithelial-endothelial nuclear enlargement or swelling, lymphocytic perivascular cuffing, and liquefactive necrosis.

Sheep of all ages, except newborns, are susceptible; incidence peaks between 3 and 10 weeks of age and in feeder lambs shortly after arrival at a feedlot. Resistance of newborns can be related to lack in the gut of pancreatic proteolytic enzymes necessary for activation of the epsilon toxin, and to trypsin inhibitors in colostrum. Lambs are typically in good condition and are found dead.

DISORDERS OF PIGS

Disorders that occur in many or all animal species are discussed in the section on Disorders of Domestic Animals.

Diseases Caused by Microbes

Viruses

Enteroviruses

Enterovirus-induced porcine polioencephalomyelitis

See Web Appendix 14-1.

Coronaviruses

Hemagglutinating encephalomyelitis

See Web Appendix 14-1.

Herpesviruses

Pseudorabies

Pseudorabies virus (porcine herpesvirus 1), an alphaherpesvirus, causes encephalitis primarily in pigs; several species of domestic and wild animals are also susceptible. The disease is also known

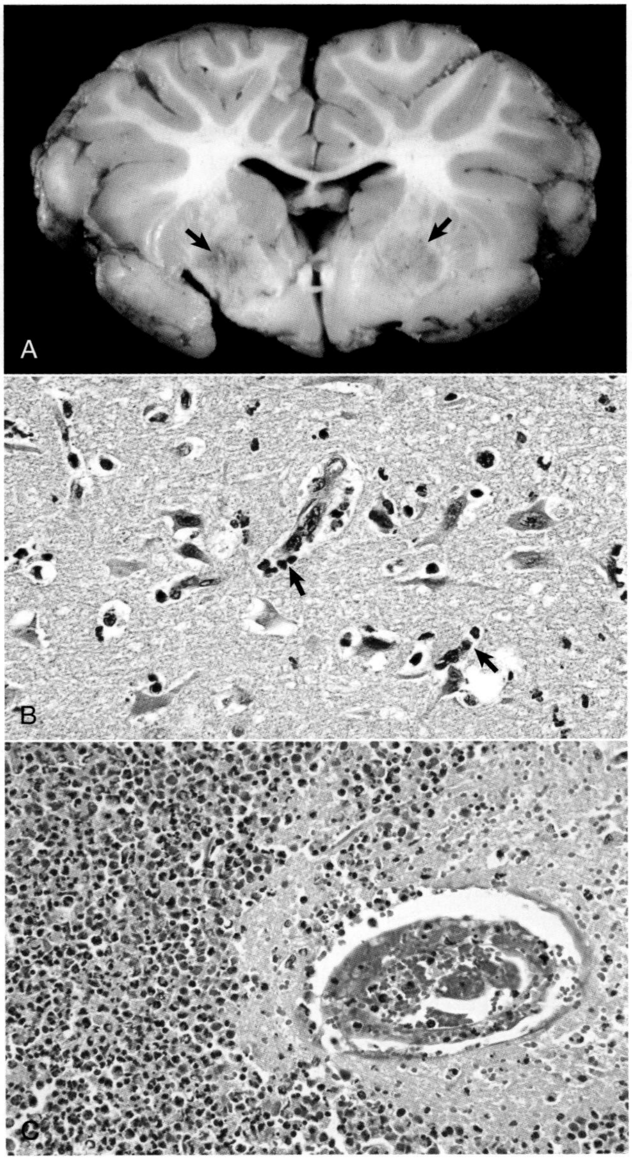

Fig. 14-96 Focal symmetric encephalomalacia, brain, transverse section at the level of the basal nuclei and rostral thalamus, sheep.
A, There are bilateral discoloration and malacia *(arrows)* in a portion of the basal nuclei. These lesions are caused by an enterotoxin produced by *Clostridium perfringens* type D. **B,** Early stage. Note the acute neuronal necrosis *(red neurons)* and perivascular and perineuronal edema. Inflammatory cells *(arrows),* including neutrophils and monocytes that will mature into macrophages, are beginning to appear in the perivascular space and will migrate to the necrotic neurons and phagocytose the debris. H&E stain. **C,** Later stage. Microscopically, the walls of arterioles can be hyalinized and endothelial cell nuclei swollen and vesicular (not shown here) with perivascular laking of proteinaceous fluid. Pericapillary hemorrhage and acute necrosis of neurons and macroglia can occur. With longer survival, as seen here, lesions include destruction of neuropil, accumulation of neutrophils and foamy macrophages (gitter cells *[left half of the figure]*), and lymphocytic perivascular cuffing. In this case, the inflammatory response is pronounced and would not be considered typical of this disease. H&E stain. (**A** courtesy Dr. D. Cho, College of Veterinary Medicine, Louisiana State University; and Noah's Arkive, College of Veterinary Medicine, The University of Georgia. **B,** Courtesy Dr. B.E. Walling, College of Veterinary Medicine, University of Illinois. **C,** Courtesy Dr. J. Simon, College of Veterinary Medicine, University of Illinois.)

as *Aujeszky's disease* and "mad itch." Pseudorabies is not related to rabies but was named because its clinical signs sometimes resemble those seen with rabies.

The route of natural infection in pigs is intranasal, pharyngeal, tonsillar, or pulmonary by direct contact or aerosolization, followed by reproduction of virus in epithelial cells of the upper respiratory tract. The virus then travels to the tonsil and local lymph nodes by way of the lymph vessels. After replication in the nasopharynx, virus invades sensory nerve endings and is then transported in axoplasm via the trigeminal ganglion and olfactory bulb to the brain. The virus has also been reported to be capable of spreading transsynaptically. Recent studies have additionally shown that some strains produce lesions in the gastrointestinal tract and myenteric plexuses, suggesting that infection might spread from the intestinal mucosa to the CNS via autonomic nerves. In latently infected pigs, the oronasal epithelium can be recurrently infected by virus spreading from the nervous system, followed by its excretion in oronasal fluid. The mechanisms that allow for latency and recrudescence are unclear, but neuronal apoptosis may play a role. The virus can also spread hematogenously, although in low titer, to other tissues of the body. Cellular attachment, entry, and cell-to-cell spread of the virus are mediated by glycoprotein projections that extend from the surface of the viral particle.

Gross lesions in pigs occur in several nonneural tissues, including organs of the respiratory system, lymphoid system, digestive tract, and reproductive tract. Focal tissue necrosis also occurs in the liver, spleen, and adrenal glands, particularly in young suckling pigs, and mortality can be high. The CNS is free of gross lesions except for leptomeningeal congestion. Microscopic lesions in pigs are characterized by a nonsuppurative meningoencephalomyelitis with trigeminal ganglioneuritis. Injury to CNS tissue can be marked, with neuronal degeneration and necrosis. Intranuclear eosinophilic inclusion bodies are not commonly detected in pigs but can be present in neurons, astrocytes, oligodendroglia, and endothelial cells. In cattle, sheep, dogs, and cats, the pathogenesis involving axonal spread to the CNS is comparable to that of pigs, with lesions that include nonsuppurative encephalomyelitis accompanied by ganglioneuritis. Intranuclear inclusion bodies, either eosinophilic or basophilic in their staining characteristics, have been described in neurons of the brain.

The disease in susceptible species other than pigs is generally fatal. Although pigs—particularly young, suckling piglets—can die from infection, most mature pigs remain persistently infected and act as latent carriers. Infection of secondary hosts, such as cattle, sheep, dogs, and cats, regularly involves direct or indirect contact with pigs. Secondary hosts acquire the virus through ingestion, inhalation, and wound infection. Dogs and cats often acquire the virus by ingesting organs from pigs that contain the pseudorabies virus.

Pestiviruses

Classic swine fever (hog cholera)

See Web Appendix 14-1 and Chapters 4 and 10.

Degenerative Diseases

Toxicoses

Microbial Toxins

Edema disease (enterotoxemic colibacillosis)

Edema disease is a disorder of rapidly growing, healthy feeder pigs being fed a high-energy ration. The disease is caused by strains of *Escherichia coli* producing a Shiga-like toxin, which is similar to toxins produced by *Shigella dysenteriae* and is designated Shiga-like toxin type IIe (SLT-IIe). This toxin causes necrosis of smooth muscle cells in small arteries and arterioles and a reduction focally in the degree of circulation to the CNS parenchyma, leading to infarction manifested grossly as malacia in the CNS. Glycolipid cell surface receptors on endothelial cells, globotriaosylceramide or globotetraosylceramide, are binding sites for the toxin, and their presence confers susceptibility to the disease. Binding of the toxin to these receptors can initiate a chain of inflammatory and immunologic reactions that lead to vascular damage.

The basic lesion is an angiopathy that leads to edematous and hypoxic-ischemic injury in a variety of tissue, including the brain. Grossly, edema is present in the subcutis often prominent in the palpebrae, cardiac region of the gastric submucosa, gallbladder, colonic mesentery, mesenteric lymph nodes, larynx, and lungs, and serous effusions occur in the thoracic cavity and pericardial sac (see Figs. 7-126 and 7-127). Congestion and sometimes hemorrhage also occur. The characteristic gross lesions in the brain are usually bilaterally symmetric foci of necrosis in the caudal medulla, but they can extend rostrally as far as the basal nuclei. The lesions are yellow-gray, soft, and slightly depressed.

The primary microscopic lesion, a degenerative angiopathy/vasculitis, is noted most frequently and is most severe in the caudal medulla to the diencephalon and in cerebral and cerebellar meninges (see Fig. 10-42). Cerebral, cerebellar, and spinal blood vessels are also affected. Initially, perivascular edema results from early vascular injury. Edema is followed by necrosis of medial smooth muscle cells, deposition of fibrinoid material, and accumulation of macrophages and lymphocytes in the adventitia. Although endothelial cells and their nuclei become swollen and vesicular, this layer generally remains intact, and consequently thrombosis is not a feature. Lesions associated with the angiopathy include pallor and spongiosis of the CNS parenchyma caused by vasogenic edema and necrosis of neurons and glia. An influx of macrophages into the necrotic lesions can be observed with longer survival times.

Pigs are usually 4 to 8 weeks of age, but younger and older pigs can be affected. Clinically, affected animals are initially ataxic and then become laterally recumbent with rhythmic paddling of the limbs. As the disease progresses, they may become comatose and die. Most pigs die within 24 hours; however, pigs that survive for several days typically develop CNS lesions (see Table 14-1).

DISORDERS OF DOGS

Disorders that occur in many or all animal species are discussed in the section on Disorders of Domestic Animals.

Diseases Caused by Microbes

Viruses

Morbillivirus

Canine distemper

Canine distemper is one of the most important diseases of the canine species. It is caused by a *Morbillivirus* (family Paramyxoviridae) and has a worldwide distribution. Morbilliviruses other than CDV include measles virus, rinderpest virus, peste des petits ruminants virus, phocine distemper virus of seals, equine *Morbillivirus,* and dolphin and porpoise Morbilliviruses. The virus is pantropic and has a particular affinity for lymphoid and epithelial tissues (lung, gastrointestinal tract, urinary tract, skin) and the CNS (including the optic nerve) and eye. In the CNS, there is demyelination without any substantial amount of inflammation.

Dr. Brian Summers (Cornell University, College of Veterinary Medicine) has commented on the sequence of events in CDV infection based on his studies of its pathogenesis. CDV is spread between dogs by aerosol transmission. The virus is trapped in the mucosa of the nasal turbinates (centrifugal turbulence), infects local macrophages, and is spread by macrophages (leukocytic trafficking) to regional lymph nodes (retropharyngeal). CDV replicates in these regional lymph nodes and replication is followed by a primary viremia that infects systemic lymph nodes, spleen, and the thymus approximately 48 hours after exposure. With infection of the lymphoid system, immunosuppression can occur, resulting in secondary bacterial infections, such as conjunctivitis, rhinitis, and bronchopneumonia, which are commonly seen in CDV infections.

Four to 6 days after the primary viremia, a secondary viremia occurs largely via leukocytic trafficking. CDV spreads from cells of the lymphoid system to infect the CNS and epithelial cells of the respiratory mucosa, urinary bladder mucosa, and gastrointestinal tract. In the CNS, trafficking leukocytes form perivascular cuffs, and from these cells CDV is disseminated throughout the CNS. It should be noted that the degree of inflammation in the CNS at this stage is minimal.

Under laboratory conditions, the severity of the disease and the cell populations and areas infected in the CNS depend on the (1) age of the dog, (2) strain of CDV, and (3) kinetics of the antiviral immune response. Virtually all cells of the CNS, including the meninges, choroid plexus, neurons, and glia, are susceptible to infection, but oligodendrocytes are novel in that the infection in these cells is usually defective (incomplete). In dogs infected experimentally with the A75-17 strain of CDV, isolated from a dog with CDV in 1975, approximately one-third of the dogs died from encephalomyelitis and the effects attributable to severe immunosuppression. One-third of infected dogs developed a timely systemic immune response, and the CNS disease was quickly resolved and they recovered. Finally, one-third of the dogs infected with CDV developed a subacute to chronic inflammatory/demyelinating disease of the white matter with some gray matter involvement because of a delayed and deficient immune response.

The encephalomyelitis of canine distemper is initiated after viral entry into the CNS, perhaps 1 week after exposure to CDV. Leukocytic trafficking spreads CDV to the gray and white matter of the CNS and to epithelial cells and macrophages of the choroid plexuses. The virus is shed from choroid plexus epithelial and ependymal cells into the CSF in infected macrophages. It is disseminated throughout the ventricular system, infects ependymal cells lining the ventricular system, and then spreads locally to infect astrocytes and microglia. Periventricular white matter lesions, especially those surrounding the fourth ventricle, are the result of this sequence of events.

By 25 days after exposure, CDV-infected leukocytes in the perivascular cuffs have disappeared; however, lesions in the white matter consist of periventricular foci of myelin degeneration and swollen astrocytes. CDV infects astrocytes, microglia, and other cells. Microglia and recruited blood monocytes phagocytose myelin fragments.

Inflammatory mediators released from lymphocytes, microglial cells, and trafficking macrophages result in expansion of the initial lesions. These inflammatory mediators may cause necrosis of cells and cell processes in the focus but do not result in a "selective" demyelinating process affecting axons. The characteristic white matter vacuolation (intramyelinic edema) seen in H&E stained sections of CDV-infected CNS is apparently caused by a direct effect of the virus on oligodendrocytes, as it appears in the earliest white matter lesions before they have acquired an "inflammatory" character—a dense infiltrate of lymphocytes, monocytes, and plasma cells.

Gross lesions characteristically occur in the cerebellum (medullary area, folial white matter, and subpial white matter) and cerebellar peduncles (with both white matter and sometimes gray matter

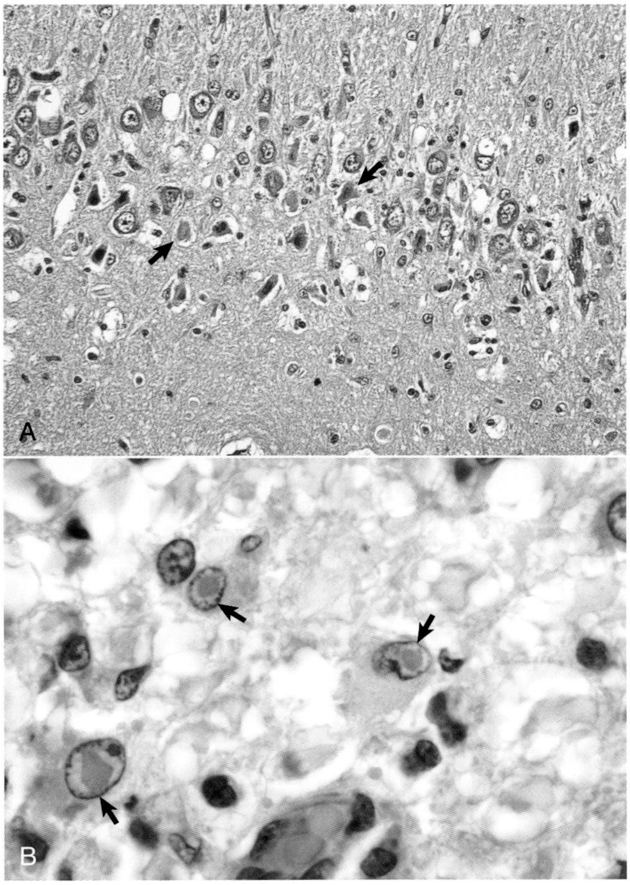

Fig. 14-97 **Canine distemper, dog.**
A, Acute polioencephalomyelitis. Hippocampal formation. Note the necrotic *(red [arrows])* neurons and edema of the dentate gyrus. Low numbers of mononuclear inflammatory cells are present. **B,** Inclusion bodies, brain, midbrain periventricular white matter, dog. Distinct acidophilic *(red)* intranuclear inclusion bodies *(arrows)* are present in astrocytes and some gemistocytes. Similar inclusions can be observed in the cytoplasm of epithelial cells throughout the body (bladder epithelium, respiratory epithelium, gastric epithelium). H&E stain. (**A** courtesy Dr. W. Haschek-Hock, College of Veterinary Medicine, University of Illinois. **B** courtesy Dr. M.D. McGavin, College of Veterinary Medicine, University of Tennessee.)

involvement of the pons). Lesions also occur in medulla oblongata (particularly in the subependymal area of the fourth ventricle), rostral medullary vellum, cerebrum (both white matter and gray matter), optic nerves, optic tracts, spinal cord, and meninges.

Microscopically, in addition to demyelination there is status spongiosus, astrocytic hypertrophy and hyperplasia with focal and variable syncytial cell formation, reduced numbers of oligodendroglia, and variable neuronal degeneration (Fig. 14-97, *A*). Inclusion bodies (cytoplasmic, nuclear, or both) are detectable, particularly in astrocytes, which are important target cells for the distemper virus, but also in ependymal cells and occasionally in neurons (Fig. 14-97, *B*). The earliest evidence of myelin injury is a ballooning change resulting from a split in the myelin sheath, or more degenerative changes including axonal swelling. This lesion is also variably associated with astroglial and microglial proliferation. This initial injury of the myelin sheath, which has been suggested to be a result of perturbed astrocytic function after viral infection, is followed by a progressive removal of compact myelin sheaths by phagocytic microglial cells that infiltrate the myelin lamellae and variable axonal necrosis.

A late stage of demyelination, which is a reflection of an affected animal's improved immune status, is more pronounced and is characterized by nonsuppurative inflammation (perivascular cuffing, leptomeningitis, and choroiditis) and also can be accompanied by tissue degeneration and accumulation of gitter cells.

In addition to the dog, animals of the families Ailuridae (red panda), Canidae (fox, wolf), Hyaenidae (hyena), Mustelidae (ferret, mink), Procyonidae (raccoon, panda), Ursidae (bear), Viverridae (civet, mongoose), and Felidae (exotic felids including lions, tigers, and leopards) are also reported to be susceptible to canine distemper viral infection. Additionally, canine distemper has recently been reported in javelinas (collared peccaries) of the family Tayassuidae in the US.

Neurologic signs in all affected species include convulsions, myoclonus, tremor, disturbances in voluntary movement, circling, hyperesthesia, paralysis, and blindness.

Old-dog encephalitis

Old-dog encephalitis is thought to arise from long-term persistent infection of the CNS with a defective form of CDV. This pathogenesis has been demonstrated in experimental infections with the CDV. Although the virus has the same general polypeptide composition and contains all of the major viral proteins as the one causing conventional distemper, some differences among peptides have been reported. The mechanisms involved in development of lesions are not known; however, they result in a proliferation of nonsuppurative inflammatory cells.

Lesions are primarily in the cerebral hemispheres and brainstem. Microscopic lesions are characterized primarily by demyelination with a disseminated, nonsuppurative encephalitis with variable, sometimes prominent, lymphoplasmacytic perivascular cuffing, microgliosis, astrogliosis, and variable leptomeningitis and neuronal degeneration. Nuclear and cytoplasmic inclusions, positive for distemper viral antigen, have been detected in neurons and astrocytes in the cerebral cortex, thalamus, and brainstem but in contrast to distemper, not in the cerebellum.

Old-dog encephalitis is a rare condition occurring in mature adult dogs. Clinical signs include depression, circling, head pressing, visual deficits, seizures, and muscle fasciculations.

Degenerative Diseases

Metabolic

Aging-Related Degenerative Myelopathy (German Shepherd Myelopathy)

A degenerative myelopathy is most commonly seen in the German shepherd, but a similar condition has been described in other large canine breeds (Belgium shepherd, Old English sheepdog, Rhodesian ridgeback, Weimaraner, and great Pyrenees). Based on its prevalence in German shepherds, it has been suggested that there is a genetic "aging" predisposition in this breed. Altered suppressor lymphocyte activity has been noted in affected dogs, but the relevance to the CNS disease is unknown. Some investigators have reported low vitamin E concentrations and suggested oxidative stress injury; others have found elevated concentrations of acetylcholinesterase in CSF. The cause of this disorder remains to be discovered.

Gross lesions in the CNS are not present in dogs with age-related degenerative myelopathy; however, atrophy of caudal axial and appendicular muscles occurs. Microscopic lesions are most notable in the thoracic spinal cord and can be diffuse or multifocal. Dorsal aspects of the lateral and ventromedial areas of ventral

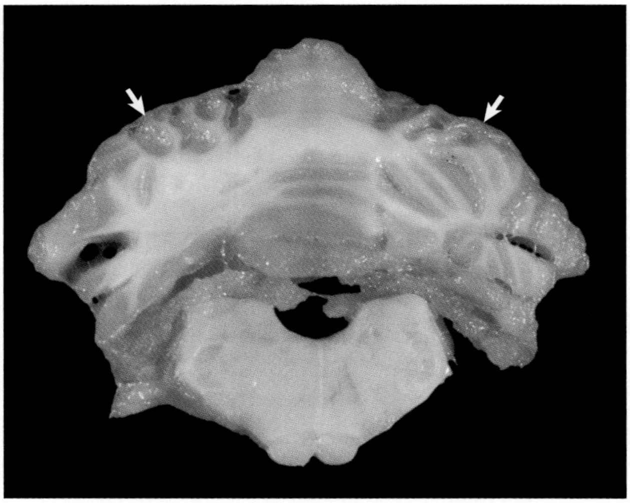

Fig. 14-98 Striatonigral and cerebello-olivary degeneration, brain, cerebellum, Kerry blue terrier.
Marked atrophy and thinning of folia of dorsal cerebellum *(arrows)* has resulted in increased width of sulci. (Courtesy Dr. D. Montgomery and Dr. R. Storts, College of Veterinary Medicine, Texas A&M University.)

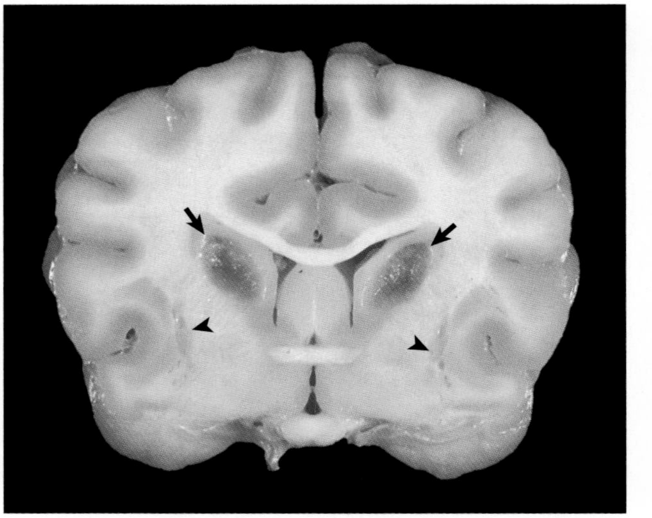

Fig. 14-99 Striatonigral and cerebello-olivary degeneration, brain, rostral parietal lobe, at level of optic chiasma, Kerry blue terrier.
Note malacia (softening), microscopically due to microcavitation and loss of neurons, in caudate nuclei *(arrows)* and putamen *(arrowheads)*. (Courtesy Dr. D. Montgomery and Dr. R. Storts, College of Veterinary Medicine, Texas A&M University; and *Vet Pathol* 20:143-159, 1983.)

funiculi can be more severely affected, but lesions can be diffuse in all funiculi. Lesions consist predominately of ballooning and degeneration of myelin sheaths and less prominently of axonal degeneration and loss. Degeneration of dorsal nerve rootlets and peripheral nerves and loss of neuron cell bodies in spinal gray matter occur as well.

Clinically, affected dogs are usually older than 8 years, but the disease has occurred as early as 5 years of age. They have progressive ataxia referable to the thoracolumbar spinal cord and muscle weakness.

Primary Neuronal Degeneration

Multisystem neuronal degeneration

Progressive neuronal abiotrophy of Kerry blue terriers. Progressive neuronal abiotrophy of Kerry blue terriers (cerebellar cortical and extrapyramidal nuclear abiotrophy of Kerry blue terriers, abiotrophy of Kerry blue terriers, or hereditary striatonigral and cerebello-olivary degeneration of Kerry blue terriers) is a well-characterized example of a disease with multisystem neuronal degeneration. The disease is inherited and affects connected neural systems, including basal nuclei and the substantia nigra (i.e., striatonigral) and the cerebellar cortex and caudal olivary nucleus (cerebello-olivary).

The pathogenesis is unknown, but an excitotoxic mechanism associated with abnormalities in the glutaminergic corticostriatal and in the granule–Purkinje cell neurotransmitter systems is proposed. The caudate nucleus and cerebellar cortex are believed to be the primary sites of involvement, whereas lesions in the olivary nucleus and substantia nigra represent transsynaptic degeneration.

Gross lesions are a slight reduction in size of the cerebellum and narrowing of cerebellar folia (Fig. 14-98). In more advanced stages, small foci of softening and discoloration occur in the caudal olivary nucleus and substantia nigra (Fig. 14-99). Lesions in the caudate nucleus initially consist of a vague area of pallor in the body of the nucleus that progresses to marked malacia and ultimately cavitation. There can be similar involvement of the putamen at this advanced stage. Microscopic lesions in chronologic order are degeneration and loss of cerebellar Purkinje and granule cells, followed by neuronal loss in the caudal olivary nucleus, caudate nucleus, putamen, and substantia nigra. Astrogliosis occurs in later stages and is especially prominent in the cerebellar molecular layer. The caudate nucleus and putamen are eventually reduced to microcystic cavities bisected by a few nerve and glial fibers.

In Kerry blue terriers, this hereditary disease, with onset from 5 weeks to 5½ months of age, is characterized clinically by rear limb ataxia, intention tremors, hypermetria of front and rear limbs, and atrophy of appendicular and epaxial muscles, presumably from disuse.

Multisystem neuronal degeneration of the red-coated English cocker spaniel. Multisystem neuronal degeneration of the red-coated English cocker spaniel is suspected of being inherited. The pathogenesis is unknown. Bilaterally symmetric diffuse nerve cell loss, astrogliosis, and axonal swellings occur in several nuclei, including septal nuclei, globus pallidus, subthalamic nuclei, substantia nigra, tectum, medial geniculate bodies, and cerebellar and vestibular nuclei. Central cerebellar white matter, corpus callosum, thalamic striae, and subcortical (particularly subcallosal gyri) white matter involvement also are noted. White matter lesions consist of axonal spheroids, intense astrogliosis, subtle myelin loss, and perivascular accumulation of macrophages. Clinical signs occur during the first year of life and consist of progressive ataxia and mental deterioration.

Multisystemic neuronal degeneration of the Cairn terrier. Multisystemic neuronal degeneration of the Cairn terrier has features of an inherited disorder. The pathogenesis is unknown. Widespread neuronal chromatolysis affecting multiple neuronal systems is observed in the CNS and PNS. Affected areas include brainstem sensory and motor nuclei, cerebellar roof nuclei, ventral and dorsal gray columns of the spinal cord, and spinal and autonomic ganglia. Other lesions include degeneration in lateral and ventral spinal funiculi, necrosis of substantia gelatinosa and adjacent white matter most notable in caudal thoracic and cranial lumbar segments, and degeneration in dorsal and ventral spinal nerve rootlets and peripheral nerves. Clinical signs occur between

2½ and 5 months of age, and there is onset of progressive cerebellar ataxia, spastic paresis, and collapse.

Primary cerebellar neuronal degeneration

Primary cerebellar neuronal degenerations, as described previously, have been reported to occur in many breeds of dogs and cats such as American Staffordshire terriers, Australian kelpie dogs, Italian hounds, border collies, Brittany dogs, beagle dogs, Portuguese podengo dogs, Scottish terriers, and domestic shorthair cats. This list is not inclusive and serves only to provide a few common examples. Although most common in young animals of the breeds listed, cerebellar degeneration in Brittany dogs occurs between 7 and 14 years of age. An autosomal recessive mode of inheritance is suspected or documented in several of the diseases. Grossly, the cerebellum can be normal or reduced in size and atrophic. Microscopically, the distribution and characteristics of lesions vary, depending on the breed and species of animal affected. A detailed discussion of the microscopic lesions for each breed and species is outside the scope of this chapter; however, lesions may include a combination of the following changes: loss of Purkinje cells and neurons of the granular layer, astrogliosis, fusiform swelling of proximal Purkinje cell axons, and axonal degeneration in the cerebellum, brainstem, and spinal cord.

Recently, neuronal vacuolation and spinocerebellar degeneration has been reported in young Rottweiler dogs. This breed variant of primary cerebellar neuronal degeneration raised biomedical concerns because of the similarities between the vacuolar lesions in neurons of this disease and those of the TSEs (scrapie, BSE). Analyses for protease-resistant scrapie prion protein were performed and were negative. The cause of this disease has not been determined but appears to have a hereditary basis. Apoptotic cell death is apparently not involved in neuronal degeneration. No gross lesions are observed in the brain, but atrophy of the dorsal cricoarytenoid muscles of the larynx has been reported. Microscopic lesions are characterized by spongiform change affecting neuron cell bodies and the neuropil. The cytoplasm of neurons of the cerebellar roof nuclei and nuclei of the extrapyramidal system contain one or more clear vacuoles (1 to 45 mm in diameter). Similar vacuoles are found in neurons in both dorsal nerve root ganglia, myenteric plexus, and other ganglia of the autonomic nervous system. Purkinje cells are also vacuolated, and in terminal stages of the disease there is degeneration with segmental Purkinje cell loss.

Clinical signs, seen as early as 6 weeks (commonly between 3 and 8 months of age in both sexes), include generalized weakness, ataxia, proprioceptive deficits, and paresis that progress in severity over the course of the disease.

Nutritional

Vitamin B_1 (Thiamine) Deficiency

Thiamine deficiency in carnivores

In monogastric carnivores and humans, the relationship between neurologic disease and thiamine deficiency per se is firmly established, and lesions in these species are similar. In carnivores (dog, cat, mink, and fox), there is an absolute dietary requirement for vitamin B_1. Dietary factors, such as the ingestion of fish containing thiaminase, deficient diets, or diets in which the vitamin has been destroyed by other means such as heating, can all lead to thiamine deficiency.

Gross and microscopic lesions are bilaterally symmetric and commonly involve brainstem nuclei, especially caudal colliculi and periventricular nuclei, but the cerebral cortex and cerebellum have also been affected (Fig. 14-100). Lesions consist of neuronal degeneration, neuronal necrosis, status spongiosus, myelin degeneration, and a secondary vascular endothelial and perithelial cell hypertrophy and hyperplasia. Necrotic neurons are those in the caudal colliculi (auditory nerves) that project via axons to the medial geniculate nucleus and those whose cell bodies are located in the periventricular nuclei of the hypothalamus that regulate the release of endocrine hormones from the anterior pituitary. Hemorrhage and an influx of macrophages also occurs in some cases.

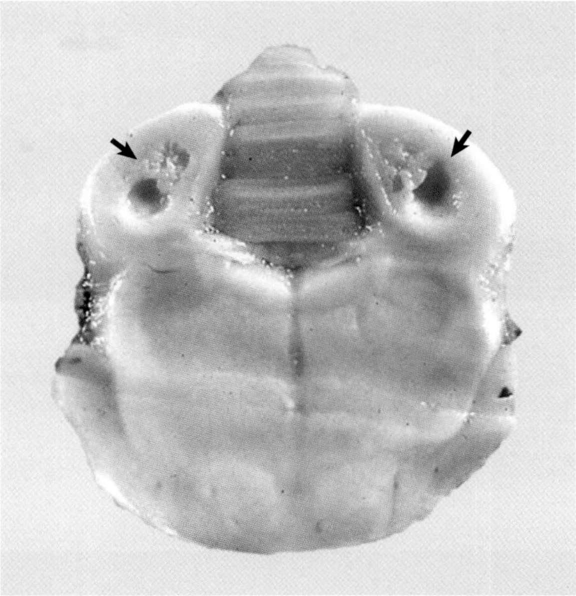

Fig. 14-100 Thiamine deficiency encephalopathy, midbrain, caudal colliculi, dog.
In the dog, lesions of thiamine deficiency encephalopathy are generally restricted to the brainstem. Note the symmetrically cavitated (malacic) lesions in the caudal colliculi *(arrows)* resulting from neuronal necrosis. (Courtesy Dr. J. Edwards, College of Veterinary Medicine, Texas A&M University; and Dr. J. King, College of Veterinary Medicine, Cornell University.)

Clinical signs in carnivores may include a combination of the following: anorexia, vomiting, depression, wide-based stance, ataxia, spastic paresis, circling, seizures, muscle weakness, recumbency, opisthotonus, coma, or death.

Miscellaneous Conditions

Dural Ossification

Dural ossification (ossifying pachymeningitis and dural metaplasia) is a metaplastic aging change in dogs, particularly the large breeds. The dura of the cervical and lumbar enlargements of the spinal cord, usually on the ventral and ventrolateral aspects, have well-differentiated bone that can form bone marrow, giving this bone a red color (Fig. 14-101). Thoracolumbar pain in affected dogs is thought to arise after flexion/extension of the spinal column as a result of compression of spinal roots as they penetrate the metaplastic dura.

Inherited Necrotizing Myelopathy of Afghan Hounds

Inherited necrotizing myelopathy of Afghan hounds seems to have an autosomal recessive inheritance. The lesions are similar to subacute combined degeneration of the spinal cord caused by vitamin B_{12} deficiency in humans and primates, but B vitamin status in affected dogs is considered normal. A similar disease has been reported in Dutch Kooiker dogs, but the relative degrees of axonal degeneration versus demyelination have not been adequately described.

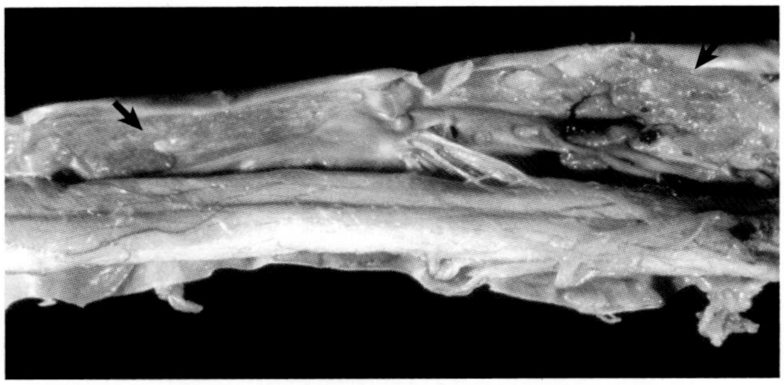

Fig. 14-101 Osseous metaplasia, dura mater, dog.
Also called *ossifying pachymeningitis* and *dural ossification,* the dura mater contains well-differentiated bone and bone marrow *(arrows).* With movement of the vertebrae, the metaplastic bone can impinge on nerve roots and cause pain in large breed dogs. (Courtesy College of Veterinary Medicine, University of Illinois.)

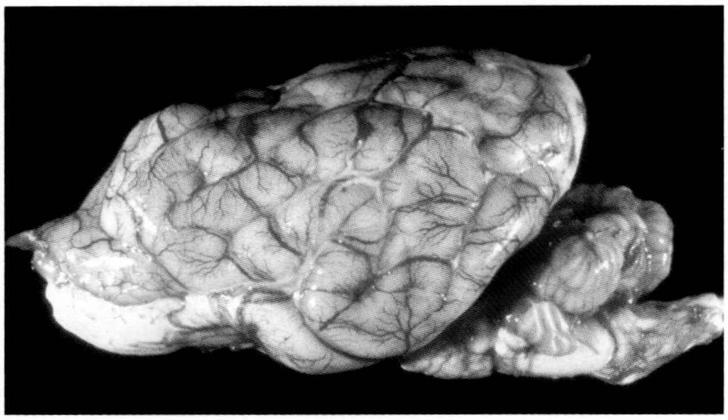

Fig. 14-102 Meningeal fibrosis, leptomeninges (pia-arachnoid mater), dog.
In old dogs, the leptomeninges can have areas of fibrosis *(white areas around blood vessels in sulci),* particularly in the sulci. This lesion must not be confused with acute leptomeningitis and accumulation of exudate in the leptomeninges and subarachnoid space. In the latter, the exudate extends into the sulci and also covers the gyri (see Fig. 14-43, *A*). (Courtesy College of Veterinary Medicine, University of Illinois.)

Topographically, gross lesions in the cervical cord are in ventral and less commonly dorsal funiculi, all funiculi in the thoracic cord, and ventral funiculi in lumbar areas. In well-developed lesions, there is severe destruction of the spinal white matter, with an influx of macrophages and myelin degradation that progresses to microcavitation. Neuronal cell bodies in spinal gray matter and ventral nerve rootlets are unaffected. Necrosis, perivascular accumulations of macrophages, and astrogliosis in the dorsal nucleus of the trapezoid body are variable.

Clinical signs begin between 3 and 13 months of age and progress rapidly to paraplegia or tetraplegia within 1 to 3 weeks.

Leptomeningeal Fibrosis

Aging dogs have varying degrees of leptomeningeal fibrosis involving the recesses of the cerebral sulci (Fig. 14-102). This lesion is not present in the leptomeninges covering the outermost surfaces of the gyri. This latter feature can be useful in differentiating meningeal fibrosis from suppurative meningitis. Except for mild meningitis, exudates also accumulate within the leptomeninges on the outermost surfaces of the gyri.

Reticulosis/Granulomatous Meningoencephalitis

Reticulosis has been reported to occur in several species but is most common in the dog. The term *reticulosis,* at best a somewhat imprecise designation, is used here to give a historic perspective. The spectrum of lesions originally included three disease processes: inflammatory (granulomatous meningoencephalitis) reticulosis, neoplastic reticulosis, and microgliomatosis (proliferation of microglia). Some pathologists have considered the inflammatory and neoplastic forms of reticulosis to represent two opposing ends of a spectrum, with intermediate or transitional forms falling in between. Microgliomatosis is considered to be distinct from the other two types. Recently, an additional designation, granulomatous meningoencephalomyelitis, has been used to describe a process that is considered to be analogous, at least in some instances, to the inflammatory form of reticulosis. Ophthalmic lesions also accompany this form and involve the optic nerve, optic disk, and retina.

When present, gross lesions of the three forms are rarely discrete. They frequently are gray-white to red, expansive areas within the brain, which result in a loss of structure (Fig. 14-103, *A*). However, lesions can have irregular, well-defined margins and a gelatinous or rubbery consistency or appear granular. Microscopically, the inflammatory form of reticulosis is characterized by perivascular accumulation of well-differentiated lymphocytes, monocytes, plasma cells, and epithelioid cells with occasional occurrence of neutrophils and giant cells, plus reticulin fibers and collagen (Fig. 14-103, *B*). Not infrequently, cells will be predominantly epithelioid. The inflammatory lesion has recently been characterized as consisting primarily of $CD3^+$ T lymphocytes and activated macrophages with strong MHC class II expression, which led to the suggestion that the underlying mechanism of the disease process was a T lymphocyte–mediated delayed-type hypersensitivity of an organ-specific autoimmune disease.

With the neoplastic form of reticulosis, cells are arranged around vessels and are also usually present in the tissue. The cells are less differentiated than in the inflammatory form of the disease, and mitotic figures are common. Also, prominent concentrically arranged reticulin fibers are present around vessels and around neurons and glial cells in the tissue.

Reticulosis, with clinical signs of ataxia and proprioceptive deficits, appears to occur more commonly in small breeds such as poodles and terriers. Age of affected dogs is variable and ranges from 9 months to 10 years. In three separate studies involving a total of 85 dogs with reticulosis (including all three forms), the sex distribution was 56 females and 29 males.

Traumatic Injury

Intervertebral Disk Disease

Although the anatomy of vertebrae and intervertebral disks is similar in dogs and humans, there are notable differences in the anatomy of the spinal cord and spinal nerve roots that result in differences between the two species in clinical signs caused by herniated disks. Disk herniations in humans commonly occur laterally, rather than dorsally as in dogs, contributing to the differences in clinical presentations (i.e., lateral herniations compress spinal nerve rootlets, whereas dorsal compression in dogs impinges on the spinal cord directly). In humans, the spinal cord terminates at the level of the second lumbar vertebra. Spinal nerve roots forming the cauda equina traverse in the remaining lumbar and sacral vertebrae before they exit the spinal canal to innervate structures. In dogs, the spinal cord terminates at the level of the sixth lumbar vertebra, and nerve roots forming the cauda equina traverse in the remaining lumbar, sacral, and coccygeal vertebrae before they

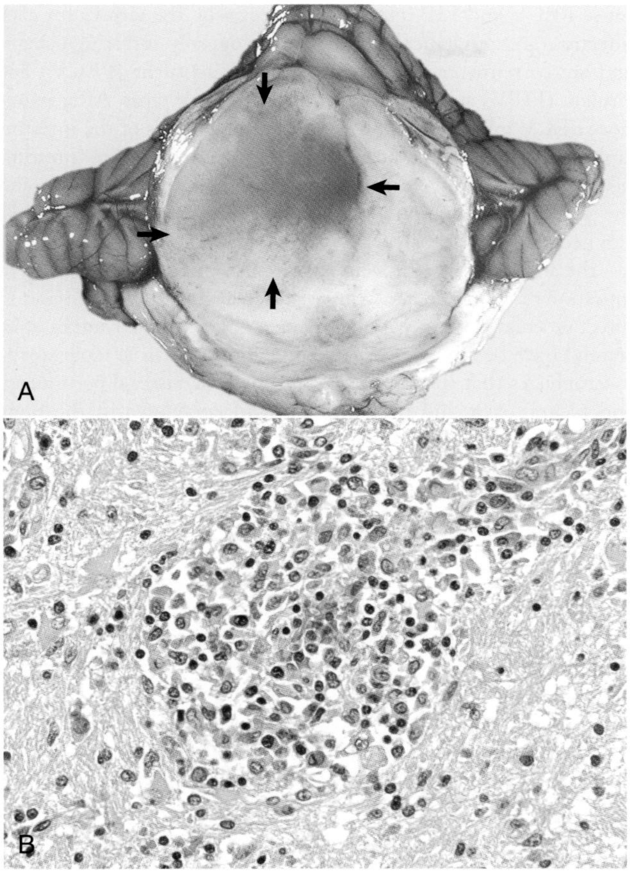

Fig. 14-103 **Granulomatous meningoencephalitis (GME), also termed *inflammatory reticulosis*, transverse section of midbrain just rostral to the pons, dog.**
A, The mesencephalon is swollen, discolored, markedly distorted, and soft as the result of extensive granulomatous inflammation *(arrows),* which has displaced the midline to the right. The mesencephalic aqueduct is also compressed and distorted. **B,** Note the accumulation of granulomatous inflammatory cells in the perivascular space. Such layers of cells expand over time and compress adjacent neural tissue, resulting in Wallerian-like degeneration of affected myelinated axons and atrophy of affected neuron cell bodies. H&E. (**A** courtesy Dr. J. Edwards, College of Veterinary Medicine, Texas A&M University; and Dr. J. King, College of Veterinary Medicine, Cornell University. **B** courtesy Dr. J.F. Zachary, College of Veterinary Medicine, University of Illinois.)

exit the spinal canal to innervate structures. Therefore in humans, disk disease involving the caudal lumbar vertebrae (caudal to L2) results in compression of spinal nerve roots that innervate limbs and are reflected clinically in a condition known as *sciatica* that is defined as referred pain in the sciatic nerve. In dogs, herniated disks in the lumbar vertebra primarily compress the spinal cord and under certain circumstances spinal nerves. Dogs thus present clinically with different neurologic signs.

Differences in clinical signs between dogs and humans caused by herniated disks arise not only from anatomic differences discussed previously but also from postural differences and the application of shear and stress forces applied to the vertebrae and intervertebral disks. Humans, with bipedal locomotion and erect posture, dissipate the forces of walking (also running) by transferring these forces from the legs up the vertebral column to the lumbar vertebrae (i.e., first in line to absorb and dissipate forces). In addition, lumbar vertebrae are not stabilized by the rib cage, and thus lumbar vertebrae must also absorb rotational forces (i.e., twisting forces) of motion. Therefore lumbar vertebrae are the primary sites for disk herniation in humans; however, because of the anatomy discussed earlier, herniated disks compress nerve roots and not the spinal cord. This arrangement results in pain but rarely leg paralysis.

Dogs, having quadrupedal locomotion and horizontal posture, normally dissipate the forces of walking by transferring these forces up the limbs at right angles to the vertebral column and spinal cord. However, when a dog jumps with downward motion, as an example, from a chair to the floor, the force is directed down the vertebral column and results in greater "end on" compression of disks and increased likelihood of herniation. Additionally, thoracic vertebrae are fixed in place by the ribs, and lumbar vertebrae can rotate freely around the axial skeleton. This arrangement directs the impact of stress and shear forces to the thoracolumbar vertebrae and is a primary site of disk herniation and spinal cord compression. In dogs, because the spinal cord is compressed, paralysis of the rear limbs results.

Intervertebral disk disease occurs in the canine species, particularly dogs of the chondrodystrophic breeds typified by the dachshund and Pekingese (Fig. 14-104). Contiguous vertebrae are held together by the annulus fibrosus of intervertebral disks and dorsal and ventral longitudinal ligaments. This anatomic arrangement results in the spinal canal being properly aligned in an axial plane, so the spinal cord can traverse through the space without compression. Extradural space surrounding the cervical, cranial thoracic, and caudal lumbar spinal cord is sufficient to allow for the accumulation of herniated disk material without substantial compression of the spinal cord. In contrast, there is little extradural space surrounding the thoracolumbar spinal cord; this is the site most likely to have clinically significant disk herniation. As a result in dogs, thoracolumbar disk herniation is often more debilitating then cervical disk herniation.

Degeneration of intervertebral disks in chondrodystrophic breeds of dogs is a genetically programmed metaplastic change of the nucleus pulposus, resulting in peripheral to central replacement of the nucleus pulposus with cartilage. It begins as early as 6 months of age, progresses rapidly, and results in the loss of elasticity of the nucleus pulposus. The loss of elasticity places additional mechanical stress forces on the annulus fibrosus, which itself is experiencing degenerative changes similar to those occurring in the nucleus pulposus. The annulus fibrosus is thinnest and thus weakest at its point of contact with the spinal canal. If the annulus fibrosus is ruptured after stress forces placed on the disk by movement, such as jumping downward from a chair, fragments of the nucleus pulposus can be released into the spinal canal (Hansen type I herniation). If the annulus fibrosus ruptures dorsally, fragments compress the ventral funiculi of the spinal cord. If the annulus fibrosus ruptures dorsolaterally to laterally, fragments compress the ventral funiculi, lateral funiculi, and/or spinal nerve roots. Degeneration of intervertebral disks in nonchondrodystrophic breeds of dogs is an aging change of the nucleus pulposus resulting from fibrous metaplasia. This change causes a gradual loss of elasticity of the nucleus pulposus, which may be noticed clinically by 8 to 10 years of age. The gradual loss of elasticity places mechanical stress forces on the annulus fibrosus and results in its protrusion into and compression of the spinal canal (Hansen type II herniation).

Disk herniation causes injury to the CNS by several mechanisms. As discussed previously, the primary injury is caused by the physical trauma of compression and the resulting Wallerian degeneration of affected axons. Additionally, disk material can compress the vascular supply to a spinal cord segment resulting in ischemia, neuronal excitotoxicity, and necrosis. Type I herniation causes the most severe spinal cord damage because there is insufficient time

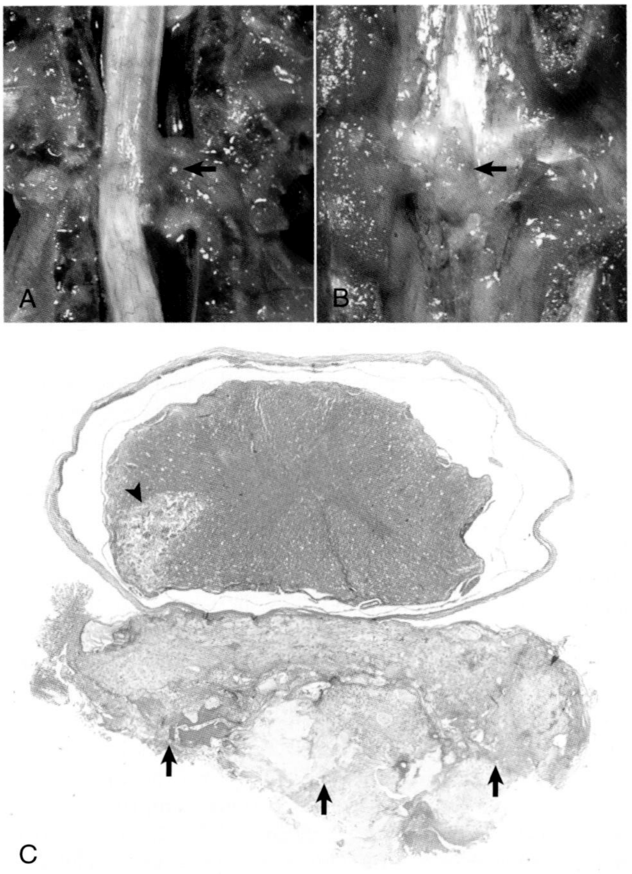

Fig. 14-104 Intervertebral disk disease, dog.
A, Disk rupture (herniated intervertebral disk), spinal cord compression. Disk material compresses the spinal cord *(arrow)* resulting in Wallerian degeneration. **B,** Vertebral column, lumbar vertebrae. Herniated intervertebral disk *(arrow)* protrudes into the vertebral canal. **C,** Herniated intervertebral disk, spinal cord. The disk material *(arrows)* lies in the epidural space, touches the dura mater, and compresses the overlying spinal cord. An area of necrosis, possibly caused by infarction is present in the ventral area of the left lateral funiculus *(arrowhead)*. The multiple small holes in all funiculi are the sites of lost nerves as the result of spinal cord compression, which caused Wallerian degeneration. (Courtesy Dr. M.D. McGavin, College of Veterinary Medicine, University of Tennessee.)

for the spinal cord to compensate and for collateral circulation to develop, as may occur in type II herniation.

DISORDERS OF CATS

Disorders that occur in many or all animal species are discussed in the section on Disorders of Domestic Animals.

Diseases Caused by Microbes

Viruses

Coronaviruses

Feline infectious peritonitis

Feline infectious peritonitis (FIP), which is caused by a coronavirus and has a worldwide distribution, is mainly a disease of domestic cats, although wild Felidae can be affected. There are two recognized feline coronaviruses (FCoV): feline enteric coronavirus (FECV) and feline infectious peritonitis virus (FIPV), which cause FECV and FIP infections, respectively. The viruses for each infection are antigenically and morphologically indistinguishable and are currently considered to represent avirulent (FECV) and virulent (FIPV) strains of the same basic FCoV virus. After ingestion, FECV infects and replicates in epithelial cells of the intestine and usually is an insignificant infection, although severe intestinal disease can occur. It has been proposed that when FECV gains the ability (by mutation) to replicate in macrophages, then FIP can occur.

The FIP virus (FIPV) enters the susceptible cat primarily by ingestion of contaminated saliva or feces, although transmission by direct inoculation (e.g., cat bites, licking open wounds) and in utero (rarely) have been reported. After infection, the virus replicates in macrophages that spread the virus to the liver, visceral peritoneum and pleura, uvea, and the meninges and ependyma of the brain and spinal cord.

After dissemination of the virus in the body, the development of disease depends on the type and degree of immunity that develops. Virus containment with resistance to disease occurs following development of a strong cell-mediated immunity. Humoral immunity by itself is not protective and can actually enhance development of the effusive form of FIP (wet form) by two proposed mechanisms. The first involves the development of virus-antibody-complement complexes that particularly accumulate in the same areas as infected macrophages around small blood vessels, resulting in inflammation and subsequent vascular injury (type III hypersensitivity) accompanied by effusion of large amounts of fluid. The second mechanism involves a process referred to as antibody-dependent enhancement (demonstrated to occur experimentally), which involves uptake of virus-antibody-complement complexes by macrophages followed by significant viral replication. The heavily infected macrophages, frequently perivascularly oriented, release cytokines that result in alteration of endothelial junctional complexes that leads to leakage of substantial amounts of fluid.

Noneffusive FIP (i.e., dry form), in comparison, is thought to occur when partial cell-mediated immunity (type IV hypersensitivity) develops and represents an intermediate stage between nonprotective humoral immunity alone and protective cellular immunity. Support for this mechanism is the fact that cats that develop the noneffusive form of FIP after experimental infection usually have a preceding and transient bout of effusive-type disease. In addition, there is evidence to support the theory that cats recovered from FIP are immune by a process of "infection immunity" or "premunition." Once these cats no longer retain such infections, they seem to also lose protective (cell-mediated) immunity and are, in fact, more sensitive to a subsequent challenge exposure because of the presence of humoral antibody.

The basic lesion in effusive and noneffusive FIP is a pyogranulomatous inflammation, leading to vasculitis followed by an inconsistent vascular necrosis resulting in infarction. The effusive form is typified by serositis, accumulation of fluid in the abdominal and thoracic cavities, with varying degrees of severity of inflammation. Lesions of the noneffusive form more frequently result in leptomeningitis, chorioependymitis, focal encephalomyelitis, and ophthalmitis, although involvement of the kidneys, hepatic and mesenteric lymph nodes, and less frequently, serosa and other abdominal viscera can occur. In the CNS, pyogranulomatous vasculitis tends to affect blood vessels of (1) the leptomeninges, especially in sulci and near their entrance into subjacent CNS tissue and around the circle of Willis (Fig. 14-105) and (2) the periventricular white matter, especially around the fourth ventricle (Fig. 14-106). The uvea, retina, and optic nerve sheath are also commonly involved in FIP.

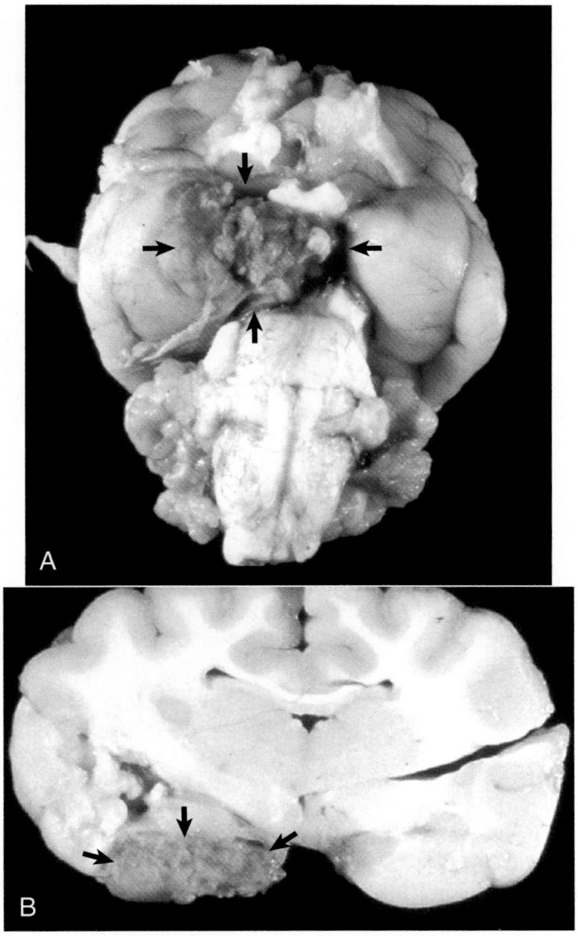

Fig. 14-105 Pyogranulomatous vasculitis, feline infectious peritonitis, cat.

A, Ventral brain, cerebral vasculature of the circle of Willis. A white-yellow pyogranulomatous inflammation distorts and obscures the blood vessels. Lesions are attributed to deposition of immune complexes (type III hypersensitivity), and in some cases possibly with a cell-mediated component, in the vessel walls that results in inflammation *(arrows)*. The character of the inflammatory response can vary from an exudate with accumulation of serous fluid and fibrin mixed with neutrophils and histiocytes to a reaction that is more pyogranulomatous, and in which commonly there are lymphocytes and plasma cells. The severity and magnitude of the lesion depicted here is much more dramatic than usual. **B,** A cross-sectional view of **A.** The pyogranuloma *(arrows)* is principally in the subarachnoid space and has compressed the adjacent cerebral cortex. (**A** and **B,** Courtesy Dr. J. Sundberg, College of Veterinary Medicine, University of Illinois.)

FIP generally occurs sporadically in cats of all ages, but it is most common in younger cats between the ages of 3 months and 3 years and can be clinically significant because it can result in death. The disease manifests itself in effusive (wet) or noneffusive (dry) forms. Clinical signs caused by involvement of blood vessels in the CNS can include behavioral changes, dullness, coma, paresis, ataxia, paralysis, and seizures.

Degenerative Diseases

Primary Neuronal Degeneration

Primary Cerebellar Neuronal Degeneration

A discussion of primary cerebellar neuronal degeneration in dogs and cats is in the previous section on Disorders of Dogs.

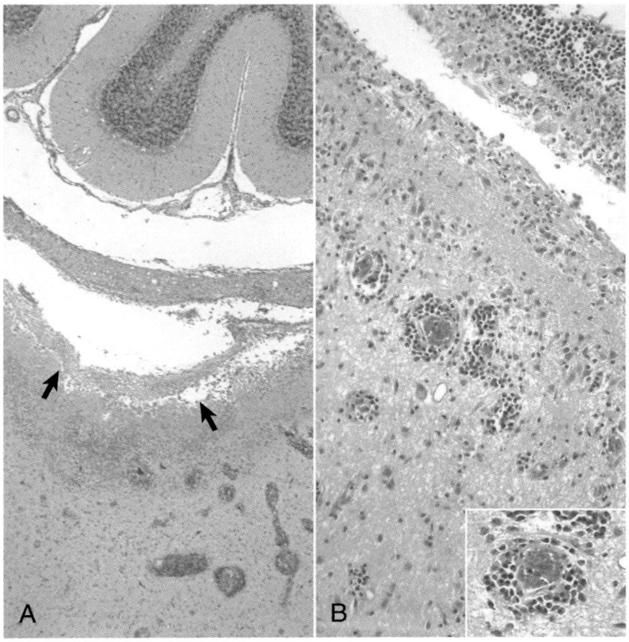

Fig. 14-106 Pyogranulomatous vasculitis, feline infectious peritonitis (FIP), cat.

A, Periventricular white matter *(arrows)* beneath the fourth ventricle (between the medullary velum and medulla). The type III hypersensitivity and pyogranulomatous inflammation that occur with FIP cause vascular and perivascular injury, vasogenic edema, and parenchymal disruption. H&E stain. **B,** A higher magnification of **A.** Ventriculitis and ependymitis are evident. Note the prominent perivascular cuffs of small mononuclear cells and macrophages. *Inset:* Higher magnification of **B.** H&E stain. (Courtesy Dr. J.F. Zachary, College of Veterinary Medicine, University of Illinois.)

Circulatory Disturbances

Feline Ischemic Encephalopathy

The cause of feline ischemic encephalopathy has not been definitively established. Although specific vascular lesions (thrombosis or vasculitis) have been found in only a few cases, an ischemic mechanism is suspected and is consistent with the character of the brain damage. Recent evidence strongly supports an aberrant cerebrospinal migration of *Cuterebra larva* after entry into the brain via the nasal cavity. A vascular-mediated vasospasm of the middle cerebral artery, resulting from hemorrhage or a toxin elaborated by the parasite, has also been proposed. Possible excitotoxic effects of a parasitic toxin have also been suggested.

The gross lesions are unilateral or uncommonly, bilateral necrosis (but not symmetric) of the white and gray matter of the cerebral hemispheres, usually in the area supplied by the middle cerebral artery (Fig. 14-107). The necrosis can be multifocal or involve up to two-thirds of one hemisphere. Hemorrhages can occur in the CNS or leptomeninges. In chronic cases, cerebral atrophy, most severe adjacent to the middle cerebral artery of the affected hemisphere, can occur. Microscopically, lesions include vasculitis, thrombosis, ischemia, and infarction, and the cerebral cortical lesions follow the sequence of changes in infarction listed in Table 14-1.

Feline ischemic encephalopathy has a peracute to acute onset and affects cats of any age. Clinical signs usually reflect unilateral cerebral involvement. The disease most often occurs in the summer months and is accompanied by signs that can include depression, mild ataxia, seizures, behavioral changes, and blindness.

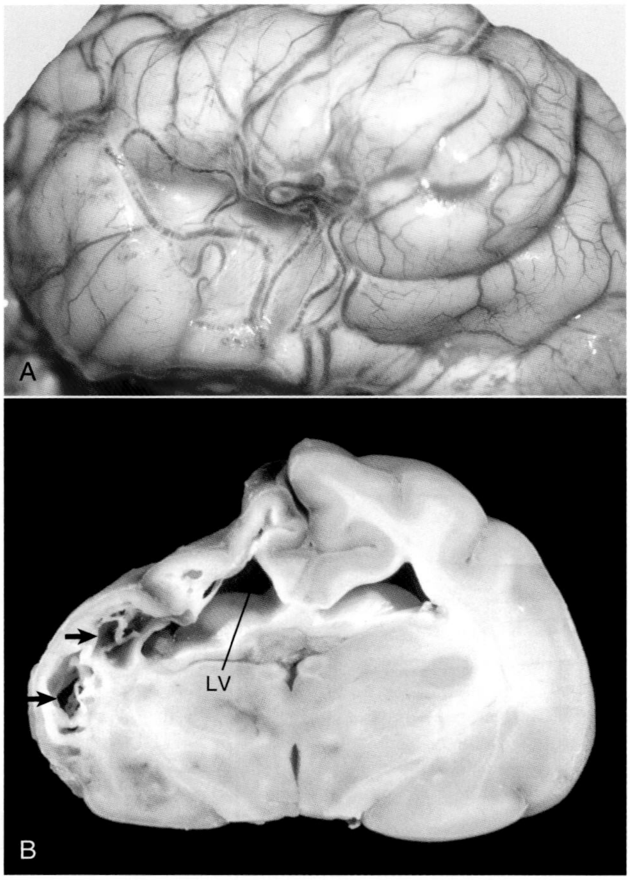

Fig. 14-107 Feline ischemic encephalopathy, brain.
A, Lateral view of a collapsed area of the cerebral cortex. Note the torturous pattern of the vascular supply, likely a component of the reparative response to ischemic injury. **B,** Transverse section at the junction between the left parietal and occipital lobes, level of thalamus, cat. Chronic feline ischemic encephalopathy with unilateral cerebral degeneration-atrophy. The dorsolateral aspect of the left cerebral hemisphere has undergone necrosis, followed by cyst formation and collapse after phagocytic removal of the necrotic debris. Cysts *(arrows)* have placed the previously existing parenchyma and the left lateral ventricle *(LV)* has expanded into the area of lost tissue (hydrocephalus ex vacuo). (**A** courtesy of Dr. V. Hsiao and Dr. A. Gillen, College of Veterinary Medicine, University of Illinois. **B** courtesy Dr. R. Storts, College of Veterinary Medicine, Texas A&M University.)

PERIPHERAL NERVOUS SYSTEM (PNS)

STRUCTURE AND FUNCTION

During the last few years, there have been important changes in the approach and terminology used to categorize diseases that involve that portion of the nervous system outside of the CNS. The traditional approach divided these diseases into those of the PNS and the autonomic nervous system (ANS). Advances in neuroscience have resulted in the PNS being divided into three divisions: the sensorimotor division (formerly the PNS), the autonomic division (formerly the ANS), and the enteric division (a newly labeled system). The sensorimotor division is formed by sensory neurons (afferent components of cranial and spinal nerves, sensory receptors, and cranial and spinal ganglia) and motor neurons (efferent components of cranial and spinal nerves, and lower motor neurons) that innervate skeletal muscle via myoneural junctions (Fig. 14-108). The autonomic and enteric divisions consist of networks of afferent and efferent nerves and their ganglia (Meissner's [submucosal] and Auerbach's [myenteric] plexuses) that regulate, as examples, the contractility and relaxation of smooth muscle of the vascular and alimentary (peristalsis) systems and glandular secretions via sympathetic and parasympathetic fibers. Afferent and efferent nerve fibers of the autonomic and enteric divisions are carried in the afferent and efferent branches of the sensorimotor division (cranial and spinal nerves).

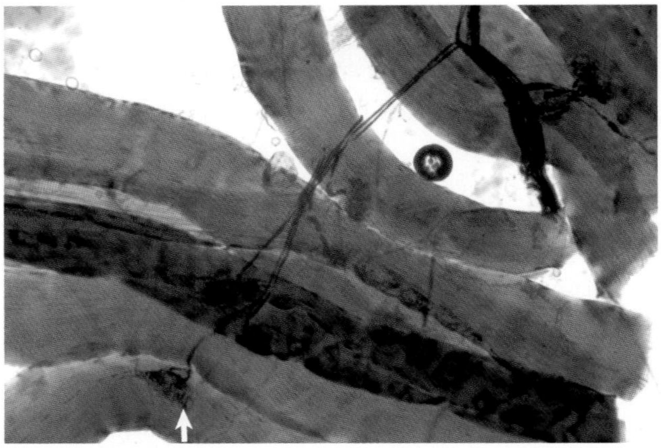

Fig. 14-108 Myoneural junctions.
Peripheral nerve with terminal axons ending at myoneural junctions on muscle fibers *(arrow)*. Dissected and glycerol-mounted muscle fibers. (Courtesy Dr. M.D. McGavin, College of Veterinary Medicine, University of Tennessee.)

Peripheral nerves are composed of groups of axons, both myelinated and nonmyelinated, and of varying caliber (Fig. 14-109). As with the CNS, conspicuous components of axons are neurofilaments and microtubules. Neurofilaments provide structural support; microtubules are intimately involved in bidirectional axoplasmic flow of structural components, nutrients, and trophic factors to and from the cell body required for maintenance of the axons and neuronal integrity. Transport from the neuron cell body to the distal axon (anterograde flow) occurs at fast (400 mm per day or about 0.25 mm per minute) and slow (1 to 4 mm per day) rates. Retrograde transport from the distal axon to the cell body progresses at a rate of 200 mm per day (about 0.125 mm per minute).

Supporting cells in the PNS include Schwann cells and fibroblasts of the endoneurium and the satellite cells (Schwann cell–like cells) of the dorsal root ganglion. Schwann cells surround both myelinated and nonmyelinated axons and are responsible for formation of the myelin sheaths (see Fig. 14-109). In contrast to the CNS, where one oligodendroglial cell can send out numerous processes to myelinate many different axonal internodes of several different axons, one Schwann cell myelinates one internode of one axon. As a result, the entire length of an axon in the PNS is myelinated by many individual Schwann cells.

Although Schwann cells do not appear to play a role in axon guidance during formation of the PNS, these cells are necessary for maintenance of axons and secrete neurotrophic factors that play a role in regeneration. Axons are grouped into fascicles along with surrounding loosely organized tissue fibrils and specialized endoneurial fibroblastic cells with phagocytic capabilities (see Fig. 14-109). When an axon is damaged so badly as to cause Wallerian degeneration, removal of the debris is by these putative endogenous phagocytic cells, augmented by an influx of blood monocytes. Mast cells and small blood vessels also are present among the nerve fibers.

Depending on species and anatomic location, endothelial cells of endoneurial blood vessels can be joined by tight junctions preventing free passage of some macromolecules and providing an

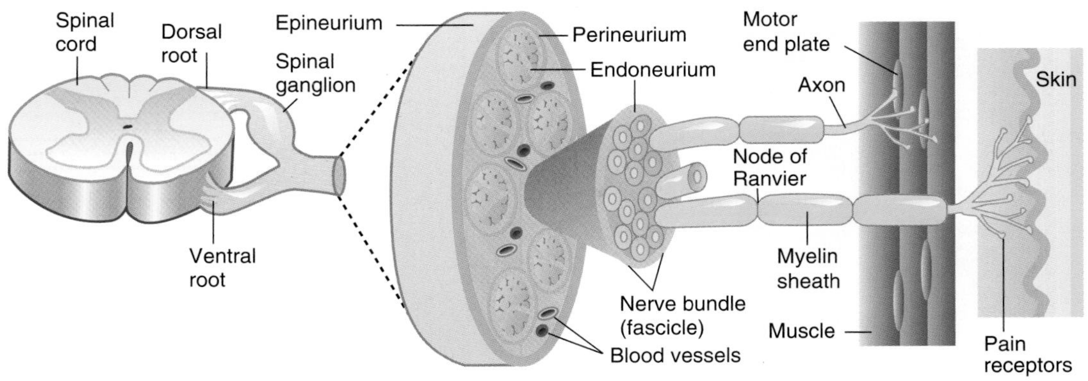

Fig. 14-109 Organization of a peripheral nerve, and sensory and motor branches and their coverings. In human (bipeds) neuroanatomy, spinal nerve rootlets are termed anterior and posterior rather than ventral and dorsal, respectively, in animals. (From McCance KL, Huether SE: *Pathophysiology: the biologic basis for disease in adults & children,* ed 4, St Louis, 2002, Mosby.)

incomplete blood-nerve barrier. Collagen bundles and modified fibroblastic cells, termed perineurial cells, form the perineurium that ensheathes individual nerve fascicles. The perineurium contributes some barrier properties by preventing the free diffusion of macromolecules into the nerve fascicles. The fibrous epineurium is continuous with the dura mater as a peripheral nerve joins the CNS and encloses groups of nerve fascicles. The epineurium contains fibroblasts, mast cells, and adipocytes, the latter probably providing some protection to the nerve. Satellite cells are found in dorsal root ganglia within the matrix formed by the endoneurium that envelops cell bodies of peripheral nerves. They function in a supportive, nonmyelinating role, much like perineuronal oligodendroglia in the CNS.

The autonomic and enteric divisions of the PNS function primarily to transmit impulses from the CNS to peripheral organs (efferent nerves) that regulate (involuntary control) the function of these organ systems (heart, vascular system, visceral smooth muscle, and exocrine and endocrine glands). These effects include but are not limited to the rate and force of contraction and relaxation in smooth (visceral organs and blood vessels) and striated muscle (heart). Afferent nerves, which transmit from the periphery to the CNS, mediate visceral sensation and vasomotor and respiratory reflexes through baroreceptors and chemoreceptors in the carotid sinus and aortic arch. Autonomic and enteric functions are regulated in the medulla, pons, and hypothalamus of the CNS.

The autonomic division has two structural and functional components: the sympathetic and parasympathetic systems. These systems usually have opposing effects on innervated organ systems. The parasympathetic system acts, for example, to lessen the effects of increased vasoconstriction (smooth muscle) and contractility (heart rate) exerted by the sympathetic system.

The enteric division of the PNS system exerts effects on digestive processes, such as motility, secretion, and absorption, and blood flow. The main components of the enteric nervous system are myenteric plexuses (Auerbach's plexuses), located between the longitudinal and circular layers of muscle, and submucosal plexuses (Meissner's plexuses) that innervate esophageal and intestinal smooth muscle. Injury to these plexuses can lead to dysautonomias, which are discussed in a later section.

DEFENSE MECHANISMS: BARRIER SYSTEMS

Blood-Nerve Barrier

The blood-nerve barrier regulates the free movement of certain substances from the blood to the endoneurium of peripheral nerves. Barrier properties are conferred by tight junctions between endothelial cells of the capillaries of the endoneurium and perineurium, and by selective transport systems in the endothelial cells.

RESPONSES OF THE AXON TO INJURY

See a discussion on wallerian degeneration and central chromatolysis in the section on Responses of Neurons to Injury in the section on the CNS.

DISORDERS OF DOMESTIC ANIMALS

Peripheral Neuronopathies and Myelinopathies

Many disorders affecting the CNS are also manifested in lesions in the PNS, either (1) because of damage to neuron cell bodies of lower motor neurons residing in the CNS or (2) because the PNS is equally vulnerable to the disease. An example in the first case is lysosomal storage diseases, in which substrate accumulates in cell bodies of lower motor neurons. Cell death and axonal degeneration of the PNS are the endpoints of a chronic and progressive process of substrate accumulation that interferes with cellular biochemical processes and transport systems. In the second case, substrate also accumulates in cell bodies of sensory neurons located in the dorsal root ganglion of the PNS, resulting in cell death and axonal degeneration. Despite this caveat, there are certain diseases that primarily affect the PNS. Depending on whether the lesion is in a sensory or motor nerve or both, diseases of the PNS can manifest clinically as motor disturbance, sensory deprivation, or a combination of motor and sensory alterations. Space constraints do not allow an exhaustive coverage of disorders of the PNS. Many of the reported disorders seem to represent isolated occurrences in a specific breed. This section covers the major types of PNS diseases with reference to specific disorders for illustrative purposes.

Congenital/Hereditary/Familial Diseases

Primary Sensory Neuropathies

Primary sensory neuropathies included here are the hereditary, familial, and breed- or species-associated syndromes reported in a variety of domestic animals that result in degeneration of PNS sensory neurons (dorsal root ganglion) or axons innervating the limbs. Two examples of primary sensory neuropathies have been described in English pointers and long-haired dachshunds. In pointer dogs, the onset is 2 to 12 months of age with signs of self-mutilation and insensitivity to pain resulting in neuropododermatitis or acral mutilation syndrome (Fig. 14-110). Additional signs can include ataxia, loss of conscious proprioception,

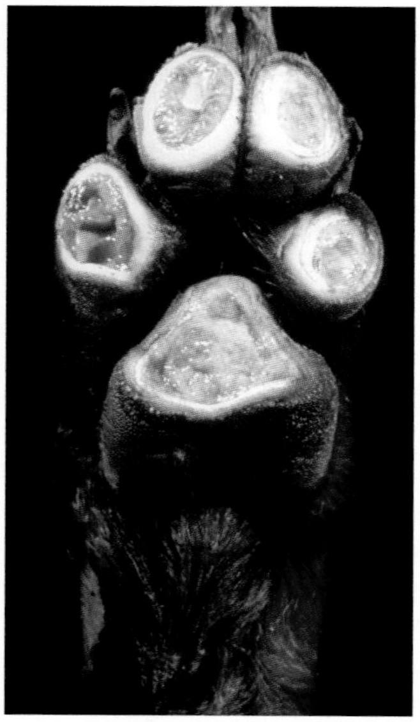

Fig. 14-110 Neuropododermatitis (acral mutilation syndrome), dog. This disorder, a primary sensory peripheral neuronopathy with self-mutilation and insensitivity to pain, is caused by the absence of (or small) dorsal root ganglia, reduction in size of dorsal nerve rootlets, and degeneration and loss of myelinated and nonmyelinated sensory axons. This dog wore off its footpads when placed on a concrete run. Satellite cell proliferation is commonly present in other large autonomic ganglia (i.e., celiac ganglion). (Courtesy College of Veterinary Medicine, University of Illinois.)

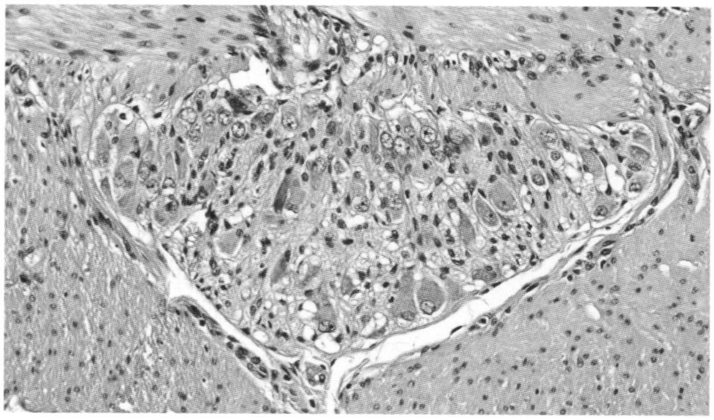

Fig. 14-111 Dysautonomia, submucosal (Auerbach's) plexus, dog. Neuronal central chromatolysis, nuclear pyknosis, and loss of neurons are the characteristic histologic features of enteric dysautonomia reported in dogs, cats, a llama, and horses. (Courtesy Dr. J.F. Zachary, College of Veterinary Medicine, University of Illinois.)

and patellar hyporeflexia. In dachshunds, a sensory neuropathy is manifested shortly after birth by ataxia and alterations in the function of the autonomic division of the PNS, such as urinary incontinence and digestive disturbances. Lesions in pointer dogs consist of small dorsal root ganglia with neuronal loss and replacement by satellite cells (nodules of Nageotte) and mild reduction in size of dorsal nerve rootlets because of degeneration and loss of myelinated and nonmyelinated axons with the presence of cell bands of Büngner (indicative of attempts at remyelination). In dachshunds, lesions are a distal axonopathy with loss of large myelinated and unmyelinated axons. Lesions can occur in the vagus nerve.

Other degenerative distal axonopathies of the PNS have also been reported in Birman cats and in dog breeds, including Bouvier des Flandres, Siberian huskies and crossbreeds, Boxer dogs (sensory axonopathy), Rottweilers (sensory axonopathy), dachshunds (sensory axonopathy), Dobermans (dancing Doberman disease is thought to be a primary myopathy), German shepherds (giant axonal neuropathy), and Dalmatians. They may have a genetic basis and be inherited.

Gross lesions in the PNS are inapparent; however, microscopically, depending on the breed involved, spheroids can be found in cranial and spinal nerves and brainstem nuclei. Affected animals are usually young (birth to 15 months of age) and show signs of ataxia, muscle weakness (paresis and tetraparesis) followed by muscle atrophy, proprioceptive deficits, urinary incontinence, and digestive disturbances (enteric division involvement).

Dysautonomias

Hereditary dysautonomias

Dysautonomia is a degeneration of neurons in the ganglia of the enteric division of the PNS that has been reported in dogs, cats (Key-Gaskell syndrome), a llama, sheep, and horses. The cause is unknown, and a hereditary basis is suspected in some cases. A toxic cause has been postulated in the cat. Lesions recently reported in sheep with abomasal emptying defect resemble those reported in dysautonomic diseases of humans and other animals.

Lesions are observed in peripheral and enteric (autonomic) ganglia and vary from neuronal chromatolysis and nuclear pyknosis in more acute cases to loss of neurons and proliferation of satellite cells in cases with longer duration (Fig. 14-111). Minimal-to-mild leukocytic infiltrates occur, but the lesions are not overtly inflammatory. In cats and dogs, clinical signs are varied and include gastrointestinal disturbances, urinary incontinence, mydriasis, unresponsive pupils, bradycardia, and other signs associated with autonomic dysfunction.

Acquired dysautonomias

Equine grass sickness (equine dysautonomia). Equine grass sickness (equine dysautonomia) is discussed in the later section on Disorders of Horses.

Peritonitis-induced dysautonomias

Degeneration of autonomic neurons in the myenteric and submucosal ganglion (plexuses) can occur in animals with peritonitis. The degree of neuronal degeneration appears to be related to the severity and type of inflammatory response in the peritoneal cavity and the ability of inflammatory mediators and other potentially toxic molecules to reach the ganglia by diffusion or hematogenously. Degeneration does not appear to progress to neuronal cell death if the peritonitis is resolved. Affected neurons have vesicular nuclei that are 2 to 3 times normal size (see Fig. 14-111). Nissl substance is also displaced (central chromatolysis). Nerve fiber bundles are edematous, and supporting cells can be remarkably hyperplastic and compress adjacent supporting stroma.

This lesion is thought to arise from inflammatory cytokine-mediated injury to autonomic neurons, and this may cause alterations of intestinal motility. It appears that the morphologic changes observed in autonomic and enteric neuron cell bodies are reversible with resolution of the peritonitis. Whether the neuronal lesion results from diffusion, hematogenous, or retrograde axonal transport of cytokines to the ganglion from the site of inflammation remains to be proved.

This lesion is likely the cause of paralytic ileus seen with peritonitis.

Hypomyelination/Dysmyelination Diseases

In contrast to the CNS, congenital and postnatal disorders of myelin formation are rare in the PNS but have been described in dogs, calves, and a cat. These disorders are thought to have a genetic predisposition and to be inherited. In dogs, hypomyelination has been described in golden retrievers with onset at approximately 7 weeks of age. Clinical signs include a peculiar hopping gait, depressed spinal reflexes, and circumduction of the limbs while walking. Lesions in peripheral nerves include thin myelin sheaths, increased numbers of Schwann cells, neurolemma cells with abnormally increased cytoplasmic volume, and no evidence of active demyelination or effective remyelination. The lesions are believed to involve a defect in Schwann cells or an abnormal axon–Schwann cell interaction.

In calves, a myelinopathic peripheral neuropathy has been described in Santa Gertrudis–Brahman cross-breeds. Microscopically, lesions were present in the vagus nerves, somatic peripheral nerves of the brachial plexuses, and the sciatic nerves. Dorsal and ventral spinal nerve roots also had similar lesions. There was "sausage-shaped" thickening of the myelin sheaths as a result of excess myelin arranged about the axons or as irregularly folded myelin sheaths not surrounding axons. Onset of clinical signs was at 6 to 10 months of age. Clinical signs were dysphagia, abnormal rumination with bloat, and a weak shuffling gait. Congenital hypomyelination has also been described in a 2-month-old Dorsett lamb with tremors and incoordination.

Demyelination Diseases

A variety of injuries similar to those described in the CNS can cause primary demyelination in the PNS. Specific demyelinating diseases are covered in the next sections. In response to injury, Schwann cells can proliferate to restore the myelin sheaths, often forming longitudinal columns along the course of a degenerated axon termed *cell bands of Büngner.* Remyelination results in internodes that are shorter than the internodes of adjacent normal myelinated axons, and this change is used microscopically to detect areas of remyelination in peripheral nerves. Another lesion that occurs with repeated episodes of demyelination is proliferation of Schwann cell processes forming concentric whirls, called *onion bulbs,* that surround the axon.

Coyotillosis

Another cause of primary demyelination is the shrub coyotillo *(Karwinskia humboldtiana)* affecting mainly small ruminants in the semidesert areas of the southwestern US. Seeds in the fruit contain polyphenolic compounds that are toxic when ingested. Four toxic compounds have been isolated, including a substance called *karwinol A* that induces primary demyelination of peripheral nerves.

Endocrine Diseases

Endocrine disorders, such as hypothyroidism, hyperadrenocorticism, and diabetes mellitus, can affect the PNS. The lesions of these neuropathies are not well characterized and can include evidence of primary demyelination, remyelination, and axonal degeneration. Distal portions of the axon are commonly affected. The extent to which demyelination or axonal degeneration is the primary lesion remains to be determined. From a clinical standpoint, it may be difficult to distinguish neurologic signs from those signs attributed to hormonal-influenced injury of myofibers. Clinical signs can be caused by sensory and motor deficits.

Nutritional Diseases

Vitamin A, Vitamin D, and Riboflavin Deficiencies

Nutritional axonopathies are relatively uncommon and are chiefly caused by vitamin A and some of the B vitamin deficiencies. Vitamin A deficiency results indirectly in peripheral neuropathy by affecting bone growth and remodeling. In neonatal calves, the neuropathy is due to narrowing of the optic foramina caused by continued bone deposition with decreased resorption resulting in compression of the optic nerves, Wallerian degeneration, and blindness. B vitamin deficiencies are primarily diseases of pigs and poultry. In pigs, deficiency of pantothenic acid (B-complex vitamin, vitamin B_5) causes a sensory neuropathy with axonal degeneration, demyelination, and chromatolysis and neuron loss in the dorsal root ganglia, resulting in proprioceptive deficits, goose stepping, and dysmetria. The exact sequence of events in pantothenic acid–deficiency neuropathy is controversial because one study in pigs described initial lesions in the axon, whereas a second study described initial lesions in the cell body. Riboflavin deficiency in poultry, named *curly toe paralysis,* is primarily a demyelinating neuropathy. Peripheral nerves are swollen because of endoneurial edema, and there is subsequent demyelination with mild axonal degeneration.

Vitamin E Deficiency

Equine motor neuron disease

Equine motor neuron disease is discussed in the later section on Disorders of Horses.

Toxic Diseases

Chemicals

Toxic diseases resulting from chemicals are discussed in greater detail in the section on the CNS. Examples of chemical toxins causing distal axonal degeneration are the vinca alkaloids, vincristine and colchicine, both causing disassembly of microtubules and inhibiting axoplasmic flow. Taxol, an alkaloid from the western yew *(Taxus brevifolia),* promotes the assembly of and stabilizes microtubules but also causes an axonopathy. An outbreak of distal polyneuropathy has been reported in cats fed commercial diets contaminated with the ionophore salinomycin, which is used as a coccidiostatic drug in poultry and growth promoter in cows. There was acute onset of lameness and paralysis affecting the hindlimbs that progressed to the forelimbs. Demyelination of peripheral nerves followed the axonal degeneration. Some toxins seem to cause different patterns of injury in the CNS and PNS. For example, in the CNS, lead is noted to cause neuronal necrosis, whereas in the PNS, demyelination, preferentially affecting Schwann cells, is prominent in some species.

Other Toxic Neuropathies

A number of toxins can affect the PNS, with or without damage in the CNS. The initial toxic effects can be at the level of the neuron cell body, the axon, or the myelin sheaths. Examples of toxins targeting neuronal cell bodies are organomercurial compounds such as methylmercury and the cancer chemotherapeutic agent doxorubicin. Methylmercury is particularly toxic because it directly alters biochemical reactions. Although methylmercury poisoning can result from ingestion of water or forage contaminated with industrial discharge, in animals the consumption of fish containing excessive concentrations of methylmercury is the most likely source of the toxin. Fish accumulate methylmercury in their muscle as a result of a "normal" environmental process called *biomethylation.* Biomethylation converts elemental mercury to methylmercury, which is ingested in the diet of fish. In mercury poisoning, sensory neuron cell bodies of the dorsal root ganglion are preferentially involved and the motor neurons are spared; whereas with doxorubicin, both dorsal root ganglion and autonomic cell bodies are affected. Experimental studies suggest that neuronal cell death is caused by apoptosis of neuronal cell bodies resulting in axonal and Wallerian degeneration.

Autoimmune Diseases

Neuromuscular Junction Diseases

Myasthenia gravis

Myasthenia gravis is a disorder of neuromuscular impulse transmission at myoneural junctions and results in flaccid paralysis of skeletal muscle. The disease can be caused by an autoimmune mechanism (acquired) or result from inherited genetic abnormalities (congenital). In autoimmune myasthenia gravis, the antibody binds to acetylcholine receptors (type II hypersensitivity) on postsynaptic muscle membranes. This interaction results in distortion of receptors and blocks binding of the receptors with acetylcholine. Acquired myasthenia gravis often occurs concurrently with thymic abnormalities such as thymoma and thymic hyperplasia. Because the thymus is responsible for immunologic self-tolerance, thymic abnormalities leading to induced alterations in tolerance have been suggested as the mechanism for developing an antibody response against acetylcholine receptors.

Congenital myasthenia gravis is caused by a genetically determined deficiency in the number of acetylcholine receptors expressed in motor end plates.

There are no gross or microscopic lesions in the PNS or CNS caused by myasthenia gravis. Clinical signs and lesions are the result of impairment of skeletal and esophageal muscles and muscle weakness followed by muscle atrophy.

Diseases Caused by Microbes

Bacteria

Botulism

Botulism is characterized by a flaccid paralysis caused by the neurotoxin of *Clostridium botulinum* type A, B, or C in North America and type D in South Africa. The bacterium is a ubiquitous Gram-positive spore-forming anaerobe commonly found in soil. This disease most commonly occurs in horses in North America and cows in South Africa. Different forms of botulism affect foals and adult horses. Toxicoinfectious botulism occurs in foals. Foals contract the disease by ingesting soil contaminated with clostridial spores. In past years, spores were thought to vegetate, replicate, and produce toxin in gastric or duodenal ulcers induced by stress or steroids and nonsteroidal antiinflammatory drugs (NSAIDs) passed in mares' milk. However, recent retrospective studies suggest that gastric or duodenal ulcers are not involved in the pathogenesis of toxicoinfectious botulism in foals. Currently, the site of bacterial colonization and toxicoinfection in foals is unknown. In human infants, the large intestine is thought to be the site of colonization and toxicoinfection.

In adult horses, poisoning after ingestion of toxin-contaminated forage and less commonly wound botulism occur. Adult horses contract the disease principally through the ingestion of preformed toxin in contaminated feeds, usually haylage that is prepared and stored improperly. Less commonly, adult horses contract the disease through tissue injury and an anaerobic environment, such as hoof abscesses and skin wounds. Spores of *Clostridium botulinum* are either carried into wounds by nails or other contaminated foreign objects or into gastric ulcers by ingestion of contaminated soil. In either case, the spores germinate only in necrotic tissue that has an anaerobic environment. The bacteria replicate and produce exotoxin, which is absorbed through the capillary endothelium and enters the bloodstream. In adult horses that ingest contaminated feeds, the toxin is absorbed from the alimentary system and enters the bloodstream.

Other than the wound where the bacteria replicates, the toxin of *Clostridium botulinum* causes no macroscopic and microscopic tissue lesions. Once botulinum toxin is in the bloodstream, it enters myoneural junctions and binds to receptors on presynaptic terminals of peripheral cholinergic synapses (see Fig. 4-27). The toxin is then internalized into vesicles, translocated to the cytosol, and then mediates the proteolysis of components of the calcium-induced exocytosis apparatus, thus interfering with acetylcholine release. Inhibition (blockage) of the release of acetylcholine results in flaccid paralysis of muscles innervated by cholinergic cranial and spinal nerves, but there is no impairment of adrenergic or sensory nerves.

Clinically, affected horses have progressive paralysis of the muscles of the limbs, mandible, larynx/pharynx, upper eyelid, tongue, and tail. Death is usually caused by flaccid paralysis of the diaphragm resulting in respiratory failure. Blockage of acetylcholine release at presynaptic cholinergic terminals is permanent. Improvement occurs only when axons develop (sprout) new terminals to replace those damaged by botulinum toxin.

Viruses and Protozoa

Inflammation of the PNS can occur in conjunction with viruses such as herpesvirus and rabies. Neuritis of the cauda equina in horses and dogs is primarily an inflammatory disorder with secondary demyelination. This neuritis could have an immune-mediated basis, and adenovirus type 1 has been isolated from affected horses, suggesting a previous viral infection. Polyradiculoneuritis and to a lesser extent ganglionitis occur in toxoplasmosis and neosporosis. The vomiting in pigs infected with hemagglutinating encephalomyelitis virus of pigs is presumed to result from altered function of the vagal nucleus and its ganglion and gastric intramural autonomic plexuses.

Lysosomal Storage Diseases

Globoid Cell Leukodystrophy

Peripheral nerves are also affected in globoid cell leukodystrophy and lesions are typified by primary demyelination followed by axonal degeneration. Small sensory branches of peripheral nerves are useful sites for biopsies to make the diagnoses (Fig. 14-112). Gross lesions are not evident; however, microscopically, such areas have pronounced loss of myelin and abundant globoid cells (activated blood monocytes).

Traumatic Injury

Trauma to peripheral nerves (lower motor or sensory) is relatively common in animals and can result from lacerations, violent stretching and tearing, or compression or contusion. Reaction patterns after PNS injury are analogous to those in the CNS, but peripheral nerves have a greater capacity for repair. Three patterns of lesions in the PNS have been described. Mild injury that leaves the axon intact (neurapraxia) can result in temporary conduction block, but total recovery of function is possible. More severe damage that destroys the axon but leaves the connective tissue framework intact (axonotmesis) results in Wallerian degeneration distal to the point of injury, but the potential for regeneration and reinnervation is good. Finally, severance of the nerve with destruction of the supporting framework (neurotmesis) results in Wallerian degeneration distal to the injury with the potential for regeneration but little chance of normal reinnervation. Destruction of the supporting framework results in fibrosis between the proximal and distal ends of the nerve and this gap may be large depending on the severity of the injury. Fibrous tissue can obstruct the regenerating proximal

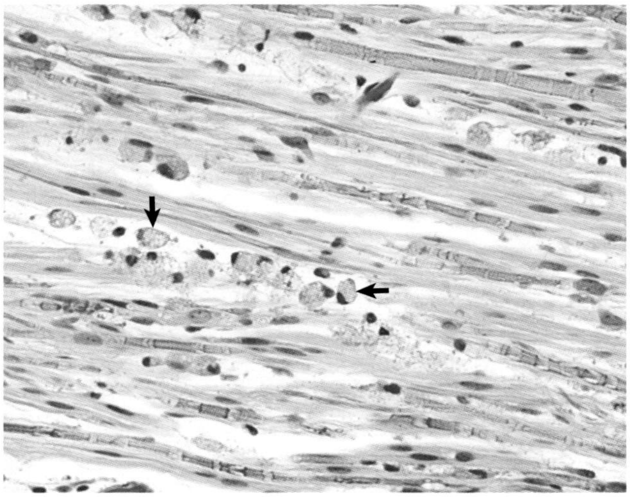

Fig. 14-112 Globoid cell leukodystrophy, small branch of a peripheral sensory nerve, dog.
Primary demyelination, secondary axonal degeneration, and globoid cells *(arrows)* between the nerve fibers. Also see Figs. 14-63 through 14-65. H&E stain. (Courtesy Dr. J.F. Zachary, College of Veterinary Medicine, University of Illinois.)

axon from reaching the distal supporting framework of the axon. If the regenerative response is exuberant but unproductive, a "potentially" palpable bulbous-like growth can form at the severed stump of the proximal axon called a "neuroma." The pattern of Wallerian degeneration and the reaction of the neuronal cell body to damage of its axon are described in an earlier section.

Recurrent Laryngeal Paralysis

Recurrent laryngeal paralysis is discussed in the later section on Disorders of Horses.

Neurogenic Cardiomyopathy (Brain-Heart Syndrome)

Neurogenic cardiomyopathy, or brain-heart syndrome, is discussed in the later section on Disorders of Dogs.

Neurogenic Shock

Neurogenic shock is caused by an alteration in the function of the ANS and its regulation of muscle tone in systemic blood vascular beds (Fig. 14-113). The onset of neurogenic shock usually coincides with traumatic injury to the CNS; however, the factors that determine whether it occurs are poorly understood. It is thought to be caused by massive discharge of the ANS. After trauma, there is immediate vasoconstriction of vascular smooth muscle. Vasoconstriction is shortly followed by vasodilatation, expanded circulatory volume, and a reduction in blood pressure leading to shock. Brain-heart syndrome in veterinary medicine is likely a manifestation of neurogenic shock and vasoconstriction of arterioles leading to myocardial necrosis.

Tumors

The objective of this section is to not be all encompassing regarding neoplasms of the PNS but to review one of the best-known examples of how neoplasia can involve this system. Terminology used for neoplasms considered to be of nerve origin in animals is quite confusing. For example, the terms *schwannoma, neurofibroma,* and *neurilemmoma* have all been used at various times by different pathologists to identify the same neoplasm. More recently, it has been accepted that the classification of such tumors in veterinary

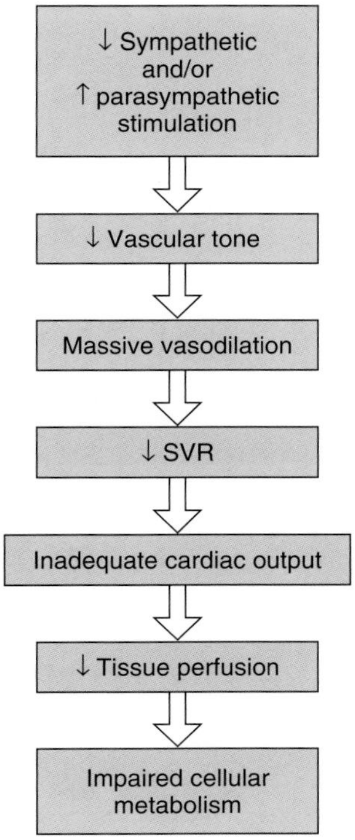

Fig. 14-113 Pathophysiologic mechanism of neurogenic shock. *SVR,* Systemic vascular resistance. (From Huether SE, McCance KL: *Understanding pathophysiology,* ed 2, St Louis, 2000, Mosby.)

pathology is somewhat arbitrary, therefore these tumors have been simply grouped as benign or malignant peripheral nerve sheath tumors. Malignant tumors show more anaplastic cytoarchitectural features and aggressive growth into adjacent normal tissue. Peripheral nerve sheath tumors occur in both cranial (Fig. 14-114) and spinal nerves (Fig. 14-115) of the PNS. Currently, there are no reliable immunohistochemical markers for these tumors.

Schwannomas of animals have been best recognized in the canine and bovine species and less commonly in the cat. In the dog, the neoplasm most commonly affects the cranial (fifth) or spinal nerve roots (posterior cervical-anterior thoracic roots of the brachial plexus and their extensions and roots at the thoracic and lumbar levels). Although schwannomas of the skin have been reported, there should always be careful consideration of other neoplasms, such as hemangiopericytoma and fibromas, that can have similar morphologic features. The bovine neoplasm occurs most commonly in mature animals, although the lesion has also been reported in young calves and involves the cranial eighth nerve, brachial plexus, and intercostal nerves. Additionally, autonomic nerves of the liver, heart, mediastinum, and thorax can be affected. The skin can be infrequently involved.

Grossly, schwannomas are nodular or varicose thickenings along nerve trunks or nerve roots. They can be firm or soft (gelatinous) and white or gray. Schwannomas of the spinal cord nerve roots can remain inside the dura mater or extend through the vertebral foramina to the exterior.

The main microscopic characteristics described for humans are also applicable for schwannomas of animals. In humans, the schwannoma is characterized by two morphologic features, known as *Antoni A and B tissue,* that occur in variable proportions within the neoplasm. Antoni A tissue is cellular and consists of monomorphic spindle-shaped Schwann cells. These cells have poorly defined eosinophilic cytoplasm and pointed basophilic nuclei and are present in a collagenous stroma of variable extent. The nuclei

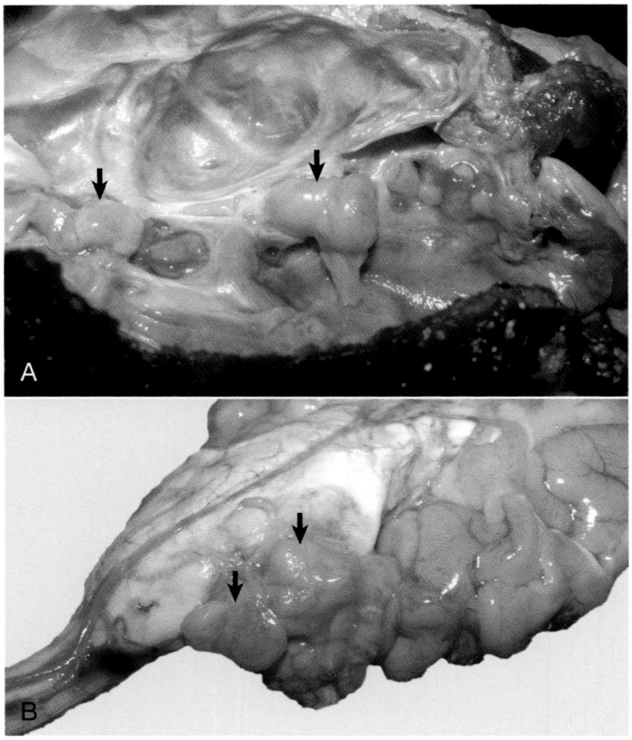

Fig. 14-114 Peripheral nerve sheath tumors.
A, Inner surface of the cranial vault, cranial nerves, dog. These tumors are usually lobulated, well-defined, tan, solitary to multiple masses that arise from the coverings of a cranial or spinal nerve *(arrows)*. In the CNS, the trigeminal nerve is usually affected, and the masseter and temporalis muscles innervated by them may atrophy. Tumors compress the nerves causing Wallerian degeneration. **B,** Brain from dog in **A.** Peripheral nerve sheath tumors *(arrows)*. (**A** and **B** courtesy Dr. J.F. Zachary, College of Veterinary Medicine, University of Illinois.)

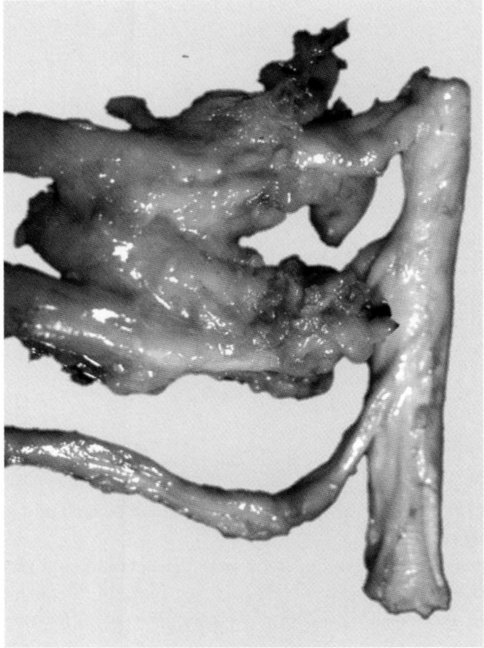

Fig. 14-115 Peripheral nerve sheath tumor, spinal nerve, cow.
These tumors are similar to those described in Fig. 14-114 and occur most commonly in cows and dogs. The terms *schwannoma, neurofibroma,* and *neurilemmoma* have been used by different pathologists to identify the same neoplasm. Although schwannoma has been proposed as the best term to classify these tumors, the term *peripheral nerve sheath tumor* groups all morphologic diagnoses under a common umbrella. (Courtesy College of Veterinary Medicine, University of Illinois.)

of these cells are commonly arranged in rows, between which are parallel arrays (stacks) of their cytoplasmic processes, and this arrangement is called a *Verocay body.* Antoni B areas are also composed of Schwann cells, but their cytoplasm is inconspicuous and their nuclei appear to be suspended in a copious myxoid, often microcystic, matrix. Also, schwannomas do not typically contain nerve fibers.

Schwannomas are differentiated from neurofibromas, which consist of Schwann cells, perineurial cells, and fibroblasts. Some microscopic features of the neurofibroma include elongated spindle cells with poorly defined pale eosinophilic, tapering wavy or buckled nuclei, and numerous small nerve fibers (that are not present in schwannomas). Presence of mast cells is also reported. These neoplastic components are situated in a variably prominent fibromyxoid to myxoid matrix (myxoid neurofibroma), although another variant of the neoplasm contains prominent collagen (collagenous neurofibroma).

DISORDERS OF HORSES

Peripheral Neuropathies

Congenital/Hereditary/Familial Diseases

Colonic Agangliosis

Colonic agangliosis (lethal white foal syndrome) is a disorder involving development of the enteric division of the PNS and is analogous to Hirschsprung's disease in infants. This disease occurs most commonly in foals of American Paint Horses with Overo markings. Affected foals have white or nearly white skin color. Specific information on these skin marking patterns can be obtained from the American Paint Horse Association. The gene, which results in the "colonic agangliosis" phenotype being expressed, is inherited as a homozygous dominant.

Recently, mutations in the endothelin-B receptor gene have been detected in affected horses and in some patients with Hirschsprung's disease. Both glial-derived neurotrophic factor (GDNF) and endothelin-3 (ET-3) are required for normal development of the enteric nervous system and enteric ganglia. It is proposed that GDNF is required for proliferation and differentiation of neuronal precursor cells destined to populate the gut. ET-3 might modulate these effects by inhibiting differentiation, thus allowing sufficient time for precursor cells to migrate and populate the intestinal wall in a cranial to caudal progression before they differentiate to form enteric ganglia.

There are no gross lesions in the intestine related to the enteric division of the PNS. Microscopically, the myenteric and submucosal enteric ganglia are absent and the areas affected vary but can extend anywhere between the ileum and distal large colon. Affected foals die soon after birth from functional blockage of the ileum and/or colon because of the lack of innervation and thus normal gut motility.

Toxic Diseases

Acquired Dysautonomias

Equine grass sickness (equine dysautonomia)

Equine dysautonomia has been suggested to be caused by ingestion of botulinum toxin–contaminated feeds principally affecting postganglionic sympathetic and parasympathetic neurons.

Brainstem cranial nerve nuclei have neuronal chromatolysis followed by degeneration and loss of lower motor neurons of the general visceral efferent nuclei of cranial nerves III and X and the general somatic efferent nuclei of cranial nerves III, V, VII, and XII. It has been suggested that equine dysautonomia should be classified as a multisystem disease. Clinically, injury of neurons results in dysphagia and gut stasis (colic).

Although the cause is unknown, oxidative stress, excitotoxicity, fungal toxins, and changes in weather have been proposed. Pasture grasses stressed by rapid growth or sudden cold weather can have reduced concentrations of antioxidants and increased concentrations of glutamate and aspartate (excitotoxic amino acids) and the neurotoxin malonate. It has been proposed that ingestion of high concentrations of these compounds either directly (excitotoxicity-apoptotic cell death) or indirectly (nitric oxide toxicity) induces neuronal injury within the ANS, resulting in alimentary system dysfunction. Because mycotoxins were suspected as a cause of equine grass sickness, studies conducted to investigate this hypothesis demonstrated six species of fungi in pastures from confirmed cases of grass sickness. The significance of these fungi in the pathogenesis of grass sickness is unclear. The similarity between neural lesions induced by *Clostridium botulinum* group III toxins and those in equine dysautonomia has been noted, but the role of such toxins in the disease remains unproved. A recent case report suggests that equine dysautonomia is caused by ingesting grass blades contaminated with botulinum neurotoxin; thus clinically, equine grass sickness has been referred to as a form of botulism.

There are no gross lesions in the PNS, except potentially for lesions related to paralytic ileus; however, microscopically and principally in the small intestine (ileum), the cell bodies of neurons in ganglia of the autonomic and enteric divisions of the PNS are chromatolytic, have displaced and pyknotic nuclei, are swollen and vacuolated, and with time there is neuronal loss and satellite cell proliferation in affected ganglia. Equine dysautonomia affects horses, ponies, and donkeys primarily between the ages of 2 and 7 years old. The disorder occurs principally between the months of April and July. Injury to enteric neurons results clinically in acute to chronic dysphagia and gut stasis (colic). The only way to diagnose equine grass sickness antemortem is by taking a biopsy of the small intestine during surgery.

Nutritional Diseases

Deficiencies

Equine motor neuron disease

Equine motor neuron disease (EMND) resembles amyotrophic lateral sclerosis (ALS) in humans. Because vitamin E concentrations are very low in affected horses, this and other dietary antioxidant deficiencies have been suggested as a possible factor in the mechanism of equine motor neuron disease. Thus dietary factors, especially the long-term absence (>1 year) of green feeds with high vitamin E concentrations, have been implicated in the pathogenesis of the disease. Vitamin E supplementation may be useful in treating this disease if detected and treated early in its course.

Neural injury in EMND involves the cell bodies and axons of lower motor neurons (ventral horn cells, cranial nerves). Microscopically, cell bodies are swollen, have chromatolysis, and contain spheroids. As the disease progresses, the cell bodies become shrunken and degenerate and are removed by neuronophagia. When the cell bodies are lost, the resulting empty neuronal space can be replaced by astrogliosis. The axons of affected lower motor neurons have lesions consistent with Wallerian degeneration.

The injury in lower motor neurons has been attributed to an oxidative stress mechanism because vitamin E is an antioxidant that offsets the harmful effects of free radicals and reactive oxygen species that can cause membrane lipid peroxidation. However, it is not linked to a mutation in the equine Cu/Zn superoxide dismutase gene. This gene regulates the production of the enzyme superoxide dismutase, whose function is to convert free radicals and reactive oxygen species (highly toxic to cells) to hydrogen peroxide (much less toxic to cells). The enzyme catalase is used to convert hydrogen peroxide to water and oxygen molecules. The muscle lesion in EMND is atrophy of type I myofibers secondary to loss of type 1 lower motor neurons.

Clinically, EMND is characterized by progressive degeneration and loss of lower motor neurons resulting in muscle atrophy, weight loss, difficulty standing, and muscle fasciculation

Vitamin E deficiency

Equine degenerative myeloencephalopathy. Equine degenerative myeloencephalopathy is discussed in the section on Disorders of Horses in the section on the CNS.

Traumatic Injury

Recurrent Laryngeal Paralysis

Laryngeal paralysis (roarer syndrome) is caused by axonal injury to the left recurrent laryngeal nerve, which results in atrophy of the left dorsal, lateral, and transverse cricoarytenoid muscles and consequently dysfunction of the larynx and laryngeal folds (see Fig. 15-18). The cricoarytenoid dorsalis muscle is the main abductor muscle of the larynx, which keeps the arytenoid cartilages in a lateral position. The cause of this axonopathy is unknown, and there may be different causes for different age groups of animals and different forms of the disease. Known causes include (1) transection of the axon by extension of inflammation from the guttural pouches because the nerve runs through the pouch within a connective tissue fold and (2) other trauma to the nerve. There is also some evidence that laryngeal paralysis may be inherited in younger horses. Currently a genetic age-onset abnormality of axoplasmic flow appears to be the most likely cause in horses in which trauma and inflammation can be excluded as causes.

Affected horses have disabilities of performance and a characteristic and diagnostic "roaring" sound with inspiration. Laryngeal hemiplegia can affect the right or left dorsal cricoarytenoid muscles; however, 95% of cases involve the left side. The cause of this specificity is unclear. Some have suggested it is related to the long course of the left recurrent laryngeal, which extends down into the chest and loops under the arch of the aorta to return to the larynx, but this hypothesis is weakened by the fact that the axonal injury is distal to where the nerve innervates the larynx.

Gross lesions can vary from being recognizable to being inapparent. Microscopically the lesion is Wallerian degeneration. Laryngeal hemiparesis is primarily a disease of large horse breeds between the ages 2 and 7 years old.

DISORDERS OF DOGS

Peripheral Neuropathies

Congenital/Hereditary/Familial Diseases

Dysautonomias

A discussion on hereditary dysautonomias can be found in the section on Disorders of Domestic Animals.

Miscellaneous neuropathies

Canine inherited hypertrophic polyneuropathy. Canine inherited hypertrophic polyneuropathy is a familial disorder in Tibetan mastiffs. The primary defect is in the Schwann cells, but the pathogenesis is undetermined. There are no gross lesions in the

PNS. Microscopic lesions consist of demyelination with onion bulb formation. The Schwann cell's cytoplasm is distended by accumulations of actin filaments. Axonal degeneration occurs but is mild. Clinical signs in canine inherited hypertrophic polyneuropathy begin at 7 to 10 weeks of age. They include pelvic limb muscle weakness, depressed spinal reflexes, and muscle atrophy that later progress to involve forelimbs and eventually cause recumbency. Neuropathies with primary developmental demyelination have also been reported in Alaskan malamutes and in beagle–basset hound crosses. A hypertrophic polyneuropathy has rarely been reported in unrelated domestic cats with onset at approximately 1 year of age.

Toxic Diseases

Dysautonomias

Acquired dysautonomias

Peritonitis-induced dysautonomias. Peritonitis-induced dysautonomias are discussed in the section on Disorders of Domestic Animals.

Miscellaneous Neuropathies

Acute Idiopathic Polyneuritis

Acute idiopathic polyneuritis (coonhound paralysis) is an acute, fulminating polyradiculoneuritis with ascending paralysis that occurs in dogs after the bite or scratch of a raccoon. By definition, polyradiculitis refers to disease or injury involving multiple cranial or spinal nerve roots, whereas polyradiculoneuritis refers to disease or injury involving multiple cranial or spinal nerve roots and their corresponding peripheral nerves.

Coonhound paralysis has been compared with Guillain-Barré syndrome. This human syndrome typically follows a viral illness, vaccination, or some other antecedent disease that results in an autoimmune response resulting in primary demyelination of cranial and spinal rootlets and nerves and delayed conduction of action potentials down the axon. Humoral and cell-mediated components are suspected to be involved in the autoimmune response.

Coonhound paralysis, like Guillain-Barré syndrome, is believed to represent an autoimmune primary demyelination. Despite the lack of close association of macrophages with the degenerating myelin and axons early in the development of the lesions, secretion of TNF-α by these cells could explain both the demyelination and axonal degeneration.

Acute idiopathic polyneuritis has been reported in dogs without an association with raccoons and also occurs rarely in cats, suggesting multiple factors might be involved in this type of nerve damage. Lesions in coonhound paralysis are most severe in ventral spinal nerve rootlets and progressively diminish distally in the peripheral nerve. Involvement of dorsal spinal nerve rootlets and ganglia is not constant and relatively minor. Lesions in the ventral nerve rootlets consist of segmental demyelination with a variable influx of neutrophils, depending on the acuteness and severity of clinical signs, along with lymphocytes, plasma cells, and macrophages (Fig. 14-116). Axonal degeneration is a common sequela. Evidence of remyelination with cell bands of Büngner and axonal sprouting occur during the recovery phase, but the effectiveness of the latter to establish continuity of the nerve rootlet and thus reinnervation of muscle is limited.

A chronic polyradiculoneuritis with infiltrations of lymphocytes, plasma cells, or macrophages; demyelination; and variable axonal degeneration in cranial and spinal nerve rootlets and cranial nerves is also reported in dogs and cats. With repeated episodes of demyelination, onion bulbs can be apparent. Both sensory and motor nerves can be involved with sensory disturbances and muscle atrophy.

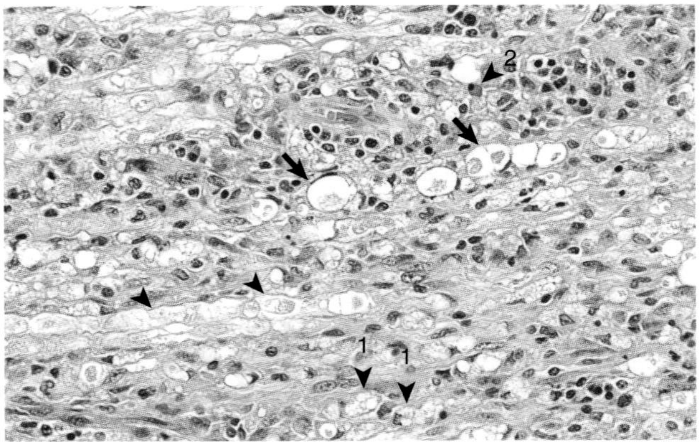

Fig. 14-116 Polyradiculoneuritis, coonhound paralysis, peripheral nerve, dog.
This disease is thought to result from an autoimmune response leading to primary demyelination of cranial and spinal rootlets and nerves. Myelin sheaths in this peripheral nerve are distended and fragmented along their length *(arrowheads)* and have been infiltrated by a mixed population of inflammatory cells consisting of lymphocytes, macrophages *(1)*, and plasma cells *(2)*. Enlarged spaces in the myelin sheath, termed *digestion chambers (arrows)*, which form in response to inflammatory and degradative processes, contain myelin debris and macrophages (not shown in this example). Axonal degeneration can occur secondary to primary demyelination. H&E stain. (Courtesy Drs. R.A. Doty, J.J. Andrews, and J.F. Zachary, College of Veterinary Medicine, University of Illinois.)

Clinically, affected dogs have signs of coonhound paralysis that develop 1 to 2 weeks after exposure to raccoon saliva. Initial signs of hyperesthesia, weakness, and ataxia are replaced in 1 to 2 days by tetraparesis and/or tetraparalysis that may last from weeks to months. Dogs can die from respiratory paralysis. Recovery is common, but the paralysis can be prolonged in dogs with extensive muscular atrophy.

Traumatic Injury

Neurogenic Cardiomyopathy (Brain-Heart Syndrome)

Neurogenic cardiomyopathy is a syndrome in dogs characterized by unexpected death 5 to 10 days after diffuse CNS injury (usually hit by car). Affected dogs die of cardiac arrhythmias caused by myocardial degeneration. Grossly the myocardium has numerous discrete and coalescing pale white streaks and/or poorly defined areas of necrosis. Neurogenic cardiomyopathy is thought to be caused by overstimulation of the heart by autonomic neurotransmitters and systemic catecholamines released at the time of trauma. It is unknown why there is a 5- to 10-day delay in the development of myocardial necrosis.

SUGGESTED READINGS

Suggested Readings are available at evolve.elsevier.com/Zachary/McGavin/.

CHAPTER 15

Skeletal Muscle

Beth A. Valentine and M. Donald McGavin

STRUCTURE

NORMAL SKELETAL MUSCLE

Understanding the normal structure and function of muscle, including gross, histologic, biochemical, physiologic, electrophysiologic, and ultrastructural features, is critical to understanding of muscle disease.

Structure of Myofibers

Structural and physiologic features of skeletal muscle determine much of its response to injury. Although muscle cells are frequently called muscle *fibers* or *myofibers,* they are in fact multinucleated cells of considerable length, which in some animals may approach 1 m. Myonuclei are located peripherally in the cylindrical myofiber (Fig. 15-1) and direct the physiologic processes of the cellular constituents in their area through a process known as *nuclear domains.* This anatomic arrangement allows segments of the cell to react independently of other portions of the cell. Myonuclei are considered terminally differentiated, with little or no capacity for mitosis and thus for regeneration.

Associated with myofibers are the satellite cells, also known as *resting myoblasts* (Web Fig. 15-1). These cells are distributed along the length of the myofiber, between the plasma membrane (sarcolemma) and the basal lamina. Satellite cells in skeletal muscle are very different from cells of the same name found within the peripheral nervous system. Muscle satellite cells are fully capable of dividing, fusing, and reforming mature myofibers. Thus, under favorable conditions, muscle cells (myofibers) are able to fully restore themselves after damage. Recent studies have found that pluripotent cells derived from bone marrow can also contribute to skeletal muscle repair, albeit only to a very small degree.

Each myofiber is surrounded by a basal lamina and outside of this by the endomysium, a thin layer of connective tissue containing capillaries. Myofibers are organized into fascicles surrounded by the perimysium, a slightly more robust layer of connective tissue (Web Fig. 15-2). Entire muscles are encased in the epimysium, a protective fascia that merges with the muscle tendon. This connective tissue framework is not inert, but in fact forms an integral part of the contractile function of muscle by storing and relaying force generated by myofiber contraction.

Ultrastructural examination reveals that skeletal muscle is a highly and rigidly organized tissue, with what are perhaps the most highly structured cells in the body. Each myofiber is composed of many closely packed myofibrils containing actin and myosin filaments. The striations visible with light microscopy (Fig. 15-2) represent the sarcomeric arrangement of muscle cells, in which actin and myosin filaments attached to transverse Z bands form the framework, and other organelles and intracytoplasmic materials are interspersed within this framework (Fig. 15-3). The endoplasmic reticulum of myofibers is called the *sarcoplasmic reticulum* and is modified to contain terminal cisternae that sequester the calcium ions necessary to initiate actin and myosin interaction and thus contraction. Sarcolemmal invaginations that traverse the cell, the T (for transverse) tubules, allow rapid dispersion of a sarcolemmal action potential to all portions of the myofiber. The terminal cisternae of two adjacent sarcomeres and the T tubule form what is called the *triad* (Fig. 15-3, *A*).

Neuromuscular junctions can only be visualized using electron microscopy or other specialized procedures (Fig. 15-4). Neuromuscular junctions occur only in specific zones within the muscle, usually forming an irregular circumferential "band" midway between myofiber origin and insertion.

Types of Myofibers

Mammalian muscles are composed of muscle fibers of different contractile properties. A common classification of these fibers is based on three major physiologic features: (1) rates of contraction (fast or slow), (2) rates of fatigue (fast or slow), and (3) types of metabolism (oxidative, glycolytic, or mixed). These physiologic differences form the basis of histochemical methods that demonstrate fiber types. There are several fiber-type classifications. Classification of fibers into type 1, type 2A, and type 2B (Table 15-1) has proved to have practical application in muscle pathology. It is the classification used in this text. Type 1 fibers are rich in mitochondria, rely heavily on oxidative metabolism, and are slow-contracting and

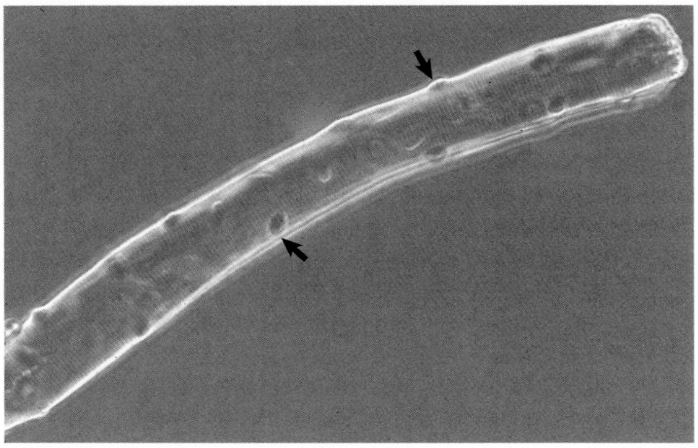

Fig. 15-1 Skeletal muscle, isolated intact myofiber.
Note the multiple peripherally located nuclei *(arrows)*. Phase contrast microscopy. (Courtesy Dr. B.A. Valentine, College of Veterinary Medicine, Oregon State University.)

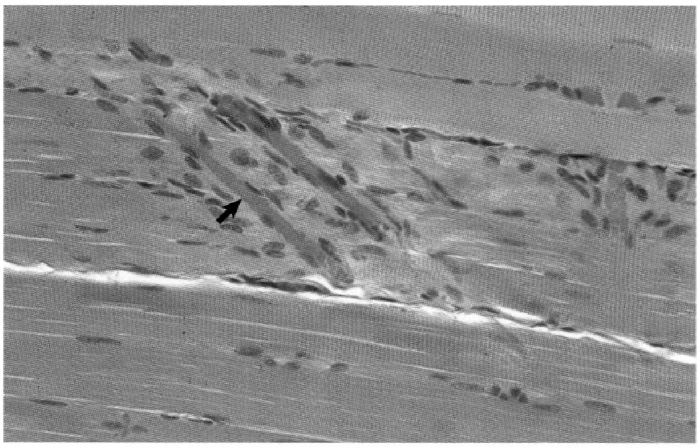

Fig. 15-2 Skeletal muscle, longitudinal section, normal mammalian muscle, cytoarchitectural characteristics.
Note the peripherally located myofiber nuclei and cross striations on the muscle fibers. The cross striations correspond to the A bands *(dark lines)* and I bands *(light lines)* in the transmission electron micrograph of Fig. 15-3, *B*. Myofibers are surrounded by an extensive capillary network *(arrow)*. Formalin fixation, H&E stain. (Courtesy Dr. M.D. McGavin, College of Veterinary Medicine, University of Tennessee.)

slow-fatiguing. Type 2 fibers have fewer mitochondria and are glycolytic, fast-contracting, and more easily fatigable. In most species, type 2 fibers can be subdivided into type 2A and type 2B. Type 2B fibers are the fast-contracting, fast-fatiguing, glycolytic fibers that depend on glycogen for their energy supply. Type 2A fibers are mixed oxidative-glycolytic and therefore, although fast-contracting, are also slow-fatiguing. Thus type 2A fibers are "intermediate" in the concentration of mitochondria, fat, and glycogen between type 1 and type 2B.

Most muscles contain both type 1 and type 2 fibers, and these can be demonstrated by the myosin adenosine triphosphatase (ATPase) reaction (Fig. 15-5, *A*). Notice that the different fiber types are normally intermingled, forming what is called a mosaic pattern of fiber types. In most mature muscles, the staining pattern of the ATPase reaction reverses when sections are preincubated in an acid rather than an alkaline solution. There are examples of both patterns in the illustrations in this section. Acid preincubation can also be used to distinguish type 2A and type 2B fibers (Fig. 15-5, *B*). Regenerating fibers, classified as type 2C fibers, stain darkly in both acid and alkaline preparations, which is a distinguishing feature. In most species, oxidative enzyme reactions to demonstrate mitochondria also demonstrate fiber types to some degree (Fig. 15-6, *A*). Fiber typing can also be done by utilizing immunohistochemical procedures to identify specific myosin isoforms.

The percentage of each fiber type varies from muscle to muscle (Fig. 15-7). Type 1 fibers (slow-contracting, slow-fatiguing, and oxidative) are plentiful in those muscles in which the main function is slow, prolonged activity, such as those that maintain posture. Type 1 predominant postural muscles are most often located deep in the limb. Within the same muscle, the percentage of type 1 fibers often increases in the deeper portions. Muscles that contract quickly and for short periods of time, such as those designed for sprinting, contain more type 2B fibers. Only rarely are muscles composed of only one fiber type (e.g., the ovine vastus intermedius is type 1). Athletic training causes some type 2B fibers to be converted to 2A. There are also variations within breeds and differences in the same muscle in different species. For example, the dog has no type 2B purely glycolytic fibers; all canine fibers have strong oxidative capacity (see Fig. 15-6, *B*).

Innervation and Motor Units

The axons of the peripheral nerve trunks contain terminal branches that innervate multiple myofibers. The terminal branches form synapses with the myofibers at the neuromuscular junction. The myofibers innervated by a single axon form a motor unit, all fibers of which will contract simultaneously after stimulation. Different muscles have different sized motor units that relate to their function. For example, extraocular muscle function does not call for forceful contraction, but rather for many fine movements to smoothly move the globe. Therefore these muscles have very small motor units, with only a small number of myofibers (1 to 4) innervated by each axon. In contrast, the quadriceps muscle is not designed for fine movement, but instead is designed for generation of force, therefore motor units are quite large, with many myofibers (100 to 150 or more) innervated by a single axon.

FUNCTION

Skeletal muscle has many functions in the body. Some obvious and major functions are maintaining posture and enabling movement, including locomotion. The rhythmic contraction of the respiratory muscles (the intercostal muscles and the diaphragm) is essential for life. In addition, muscles play a major role in whole body homeostasis and are involved in glucose metabolism and maintenance of body temperature. On a purely esthetic level, muscle contributes to pleasing body contours.

The function of skeletal muscle is intimately related to the function of the peripheral nervous system. The physiologic attributes of a muscle fiber—its rate of contraction and type of metabolism (oxidative, anaerobic, or mixed)—are determined not by the muscle cell itself but by the motor neuron responsible for its innervation (Fig. 15-8). This fact is significant in evaluating histologic changes in muscle fibers. It is possible to divide changes in muscle fibers into two major classes: neuropathic and myopathic. Neuropathic changes are those that are determined by the effect or the absence of the nerve supply (e.g., atrophy after denervation). The term *myopathy* should be reserved for those muscle diseases in which the primary change takes place in the muscle cell, not in the interstitial tissue and not secondary to effects from the nerve supply. The term *neuromuscular disease* encompasses disorders involving lower motor neurons, peripheral nerves, neuromuscular junctions, and muscles.

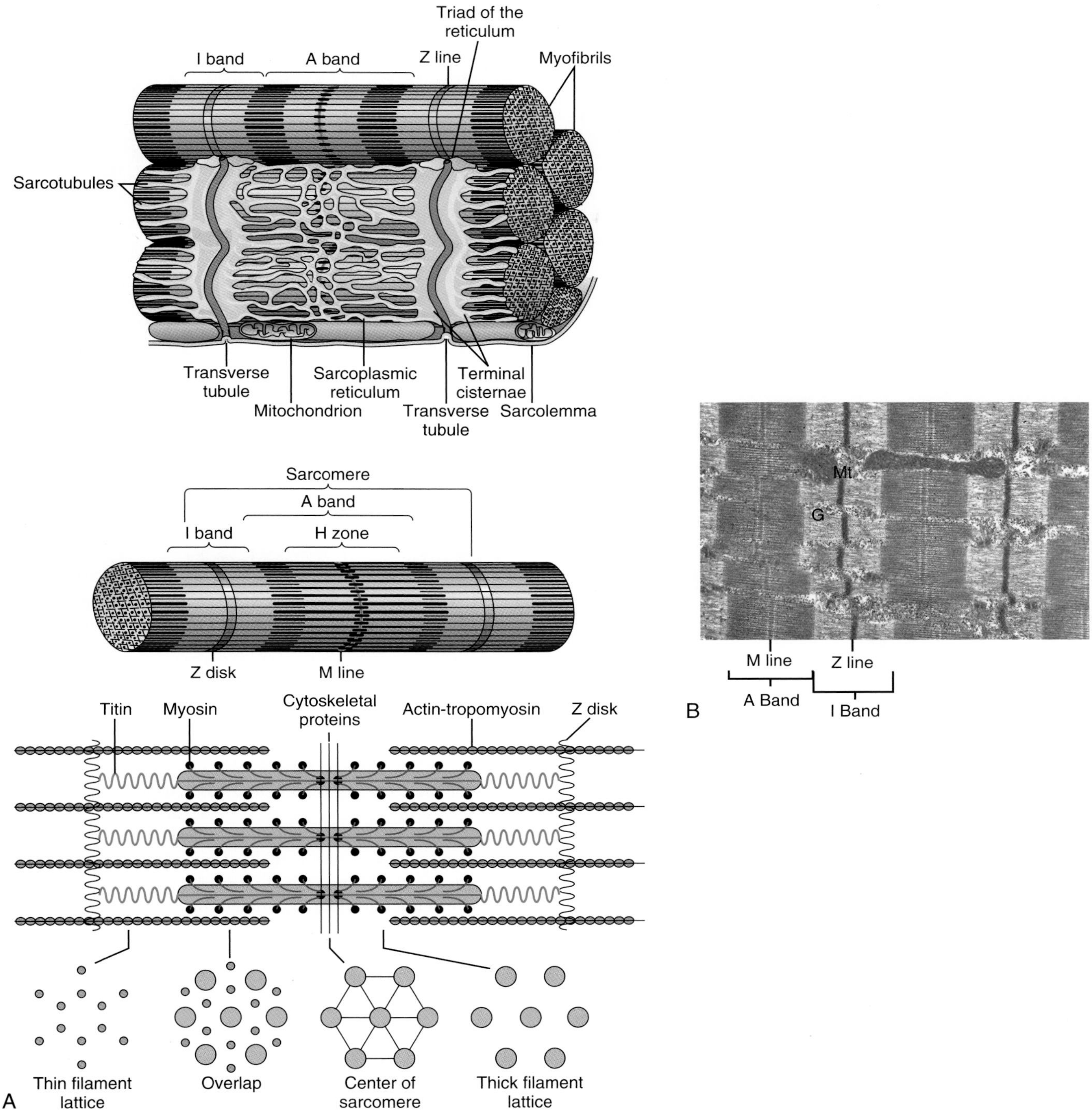

Fig. 15-3 Myofiber structure.

A, Schematic representation of myofiber orientation, secondary organelles, and ultrastructural arrangement of cytoskeletal proteins within sarcomeres. **B,** Skeletal muscle, longitudinal section, normal mammalian skeletal muscle. Sarcomeres are defined by Z lines, A bands composed of thick myosin filaments, and I bands composed of thin actin filaments. Dense M lines with adjacent clear H zones occur in the center of the A band. Mitochondria *(Mt)* and glycogen *(G)* are interspersed between the myofibrils. TEM. uranyl acetate and lead citrate stain. (**A** from Copstead-Kirkhorn LE, Banasik JL: *Pathophysiology: biological and behavioral perspective,* ed 3, St Louis, 2005, Saunders. **B** courtesy Dr. B.A. Valentine, College of Veterinary Medicine, Oregon State University.)

METABOLISM AND IONIC HOMEOSTASIS

Myofibers require a great deal of energy in the form of adenosine triphosphate (ATP) to generate force and movement. Type 1 oxidative and type 2A oxidative-glycolytic fibers use aerobic metabolism of glucose, stored in the muscle as glycogen, and fat. Type 2B glycolytic fibers rely primarily on anaerobic metabolism of glycogen for energy. Inherent or acquired metabolic defects that reduce skeletal muscle energy production can result in severe muscle dysfunction. A commonly encountered postmortem change, rigor mortis, illustrates the importance of ATP generation within skeletal muscle. The muscle contractile apparatus is still active immediately after death. ATP is necessary for the release of actin from

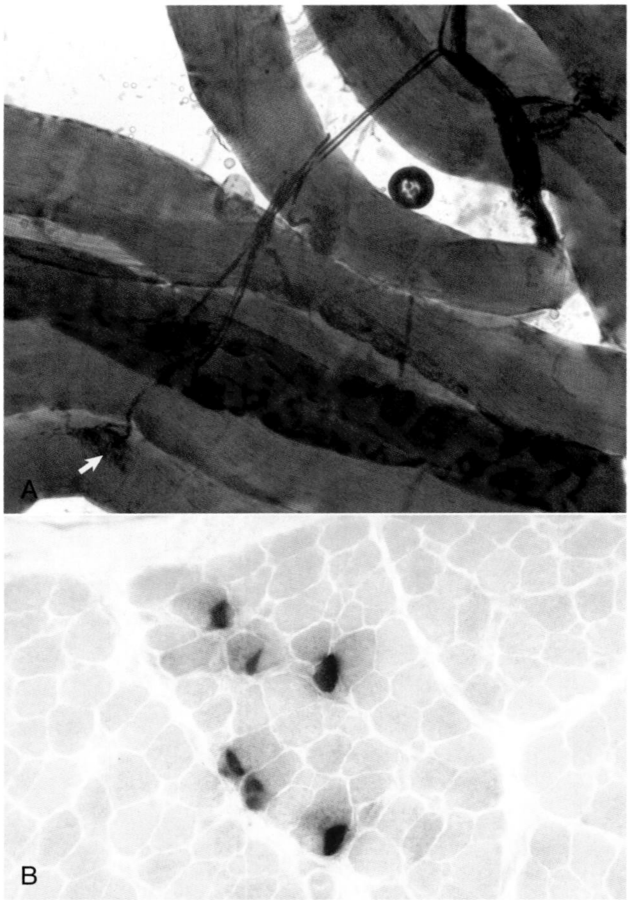

Fig. 15-4 Neuromuscular junctions.
A, An intramuscular nerve *(top right)* has given off axons, which terminate on a myofiber at a neuromuscular junction *(arrow)*. Teased preparation, silver impregnation method. **B,** Neuromuscular junctions, transverse section through the center region of normal mammalian muscle. The neuromuscular junctions *(red-brown stain)* form a cluster. Nonspecific esterase stain, frozen section. (**A** courtesy Dr. M.D. McGavin, College of Veterinary Medicine, University of Tennessee. **B** courtesy Dr. B.A. Valentine, College of Veterinary Medicine, Oregon State University.)

TABLE 15-1 Skeletal Muscle Fiber Types

Fiber Type	Physiologic Characteristics	Morphologic Characteristics
1	Slow twitch, oxidative, fatigue resistant, "red muscle," aerobic	High mitochondrial content, high fat content, low glycogen content
2A	Fast twitch, oxidative and glycolytic, fatigue resistant	Intermediate mitochondria, fat, and glycogen content
2B	Fast twitch, fatigue sensitive, glycolytic, "white muscle," anaerobic	Low mitochondrial and fat content, high glycogen content

myosin, the interaction that results in the sliding of myofilaments and contraction of muscle. After death, the absence of adequate ATP production causes the muscle fibers to undergo sustained contraction, which is known as *rigor mortis*. Rigor mortis eventually disappears because of muscle structural breakdown caused by autolysis or putrefaction (bacterial decomposition). The period of time for onset and release of rigor mortis varies, depending on physiologic (glycogen stores at the time of death) and environmental factors such as the environmental temperature (see Chapter 1).

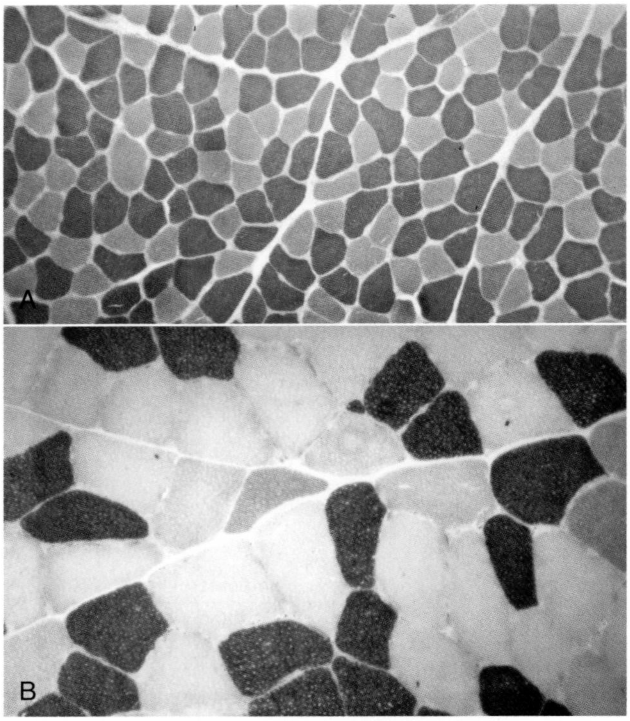

Fig. 15-5 Muscle fiber typing, myofibrillar adenosine triphosphatase (ATPase) reaction, normal skeletal muscle, transverse section.
A, Dog. Type 1 *(light)* and type 2 *(dark)* fibers are arranged in a mosaic pattern. Frozen section, ATPase pH 10.0. **B,** Horse. Acid preincubation allows differentiation of three fiber types, type 1 *(dark)*, type 2A *(light)*, and type 2B *(intermediate = gray)*. Frozen section, ATPase 4.35. (Courtesy Dr. B.A. Valentine, College of Veterinary Medicine, Oregon State University.)

Skeletal muscle is also excitable tissue, similar to that of the nervous system. Maintenance of proper ionic gradients across the sarcolemma is essential for initiation of the action potential. Internal ionic gradients, especially of calcium ions, are critical for initiation and termination of contraction. Alterations of ionic fluxes across the sarcolemma, or within the sarcoplasmic reticulum, can have a serious negative impact on myofiber function.

EXAMINATION OF MUSCLE: CLINICAL, GROSS, AND MICROSCOPIC

The decision to closely examine muscle, either by a biopsy or at necropsy, relies on recognition of indicators of neuromuscular dysfunction.

CLINICAL FINDINGS

Clinical signs of muscular disease are variable (Box 15-1). The most common manifestations are alteration in muscle size, muscle weakness, and abnormal gait. Depending on the nature of the disorder, clinical signs can be localized, multifocal, or generalized.

Alteration in muscle size is readily detected with careful physical examination. Unilateral atrophy is best appreciated by comparing muscles on both sides of the body. In cases of generalized atrophy, it is important to bear in mind the normal muscling of the breed. For example, the muscling of dairy cattle is less prominent

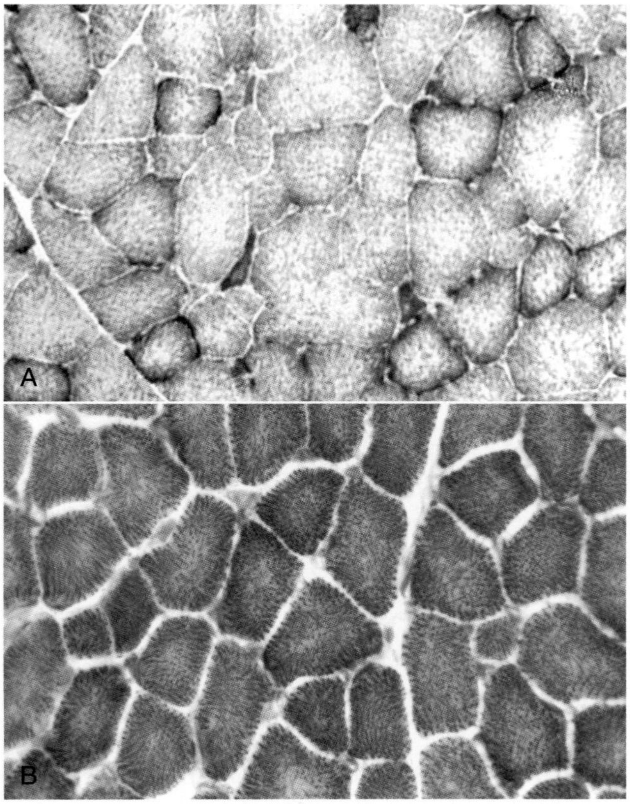

Fig. 15-6 **Mitochondria, NADH reaction *(blue stained)*, skeletal myocytes, normal skeletal muscle, transverse section.**
A, Horse. Type 1 fibers contain the most mitochondria, type 2B the least, and mitochondrial content of type 2A fibers is intermediate between type 1 and type 2B. Frozen section, NADH reaction. **B,** Dog. All fiber types have a similar mitochondrial content, therefore this reaction cannot be used to identify different types of myofibers in canine muscle. Frozen section, NADH reaction. (Courtesy Dr. B.A. Valentine, College of Veterinary Medicine, Oregon State University.)

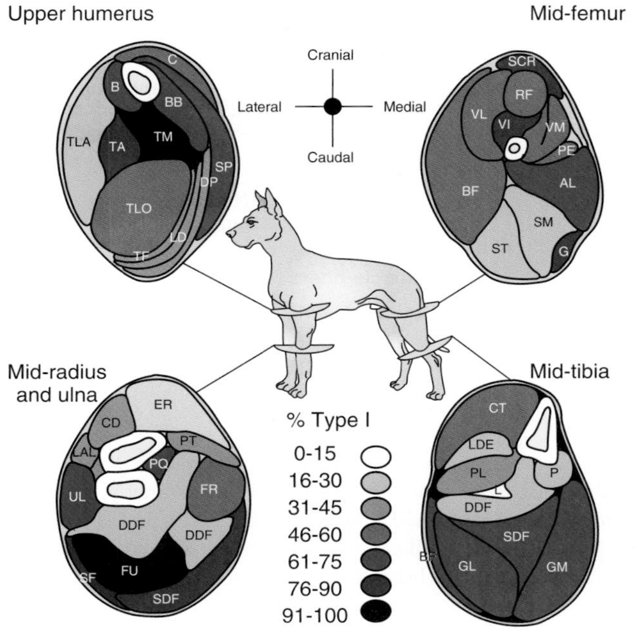

Fig. 15-7 **Schematic diagram of the percentage of type 1 and type 2 myofibers in limb muscles in the dog.**
There is a wide variation from muscle to muscle. Deeply located muscles have the most type 1 myofibers, indicative of their function in maintaining posture. (Redrawn from Armstrong RB, Sauber CW, Seeherman HJ, Taylor CR: *Am J Anat* 163:87-98, 1987.)

BOX 15-1 Clinical Signs of Muscle Disease

- Muscle atrophy
- Muscle hypertrophy
- Muscle swelling
- Weakness
- Muscle spasm
- Abnormal gait
- Esophageal dysfunction (dogs, cats, camelids)

than that of beef cattle, and mild generalized muscle atrophy in a draft horse breed is more difficult to detect than in a light horse breed.

Weakness can be obvious, as in an animal that is unable to rise or prefers to remain recumbent, or can be manifested primarily as exercise intolerance. Special attention should be paid to gait analysis. The gait of an animal with generalized weakness caused by muscle or peripheral nerve dysfunction will have a short stride and often be stiff, and all four legs are often positioned well under the body for support while standing. The abnormal gait of an animal with neuromuscular disease must be distinguished from a similar gait that can occur because of musculoskeletal disease (which is a misnomer, as these disorders affect bone and joint not muscle). Muscle or peripheral nerve dysfunction in the horse, with this species' unique biomechanics of the pelvic limb, can result in mechanical lameness that can be mistaken for neurologic disease. Odd equine hindlimb gaits designated with such terms as *shivers, stringhalt,* and *fibrotic myopathy* are caused by muscle or peripheral nerve disorders. A fibrotic myopathy-like condition also occurs less commonly in the dog and can involve the forelimb. Severe denervating or progressive myopathic conditions that begin in utero or at an early age can cause joint contractures and limb deviation (see Fig. 15-44).

Animals with myotonia often exhibit a stiff gait and develop episodic muscle spasms that can lead to collapse. Percussion of muscle groups can cause a persistent muscle contraction known as *dimpling.*

In dogs, horses, and ruminants, the esophagus contains a large percentage of skeletal muscle. In dogs and camelids, myopathic, neuropathic, and neuromuscular junction disorders can involve these muscles, causing esophageal dysfunction and megaesophagus. Denervation can also contribute to esophageal dysfunction in cattle with vagal indigestion.

As far as can be determined by clinical evaluation and extrapolation from similar conditions in other species, most neuromuscular disorders in animals are not associated with pain. Muscle cramps, caused by either primary myopathy or partial denervation, and muscle swelling are exceptions to this rule.

CLINICOPATHOLOGIC FINDINGS

If the plasma membrane of the myofiber is damaged or a segment of the myofiber becomes necrotic, some of the contents of the muscle cell will "leak out" and be taken up into the blood. The concentrations of some of these components in serum are used as an index of the extent of myofiber damage. The most commonly

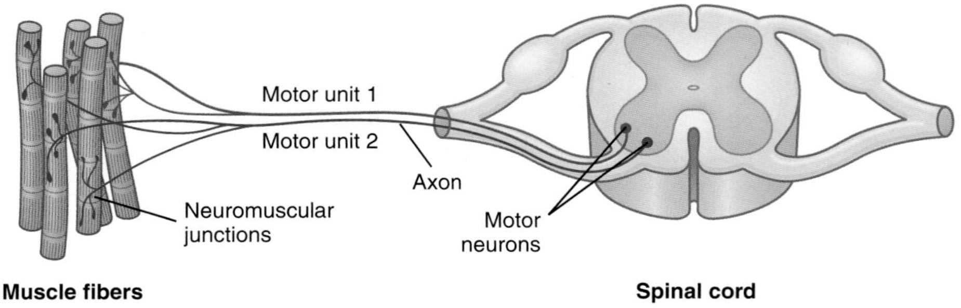

Fig. 15-8 Schematic diagram of motor units of a muscle.
Each motor unit consists of a motor neuron within the central nervous system and all the myofibers (muscle cells) supplied by the neuron and its axon branches. (From Huether SE, McCance KL: *Understanding pathophysiology,* ed 4, St Louis, 2008, Mosby.)

used is creatine kinase (CK), formerly called *creatine phosphokinase* (CPK). Aspartate aminotransferase (AST), formerly known as *serum glutamic-oxaloacetic transaminase* (SGOT), and lactic dehydrogenase (LDH) are also released but are not as specific an indicator of muscle damage because they are also present in other tissues. Because CK has a low renal threshold, it is quickly excreted in the urine. The half-life of circulating CK varies somewhat between species but is generally about 6 to 12 hours. The half-life of AST and LDH in the serum is much longer, and serum AST and LDH concentrations remain elevated for several days after muscle injury. Serum concentration of alanine aminotransferase (ALT) will also increase in all species from severe muscle cell necrosis. Other serum indicators of skeletal muscle injury include carbonic anhydrase III and fatty acid binding protein, but these latter proteins are not part of a routine serum chemistry panel. It has been speculated that the sarcolemma can become "leaky," leading to release of CK and other enzymes, without the affected segment becoming overtly necrotic. This possibility is very hard to prove or disprove.

Although the laboratory testing for CK and AST is relatively standardized, laboratory normal ranges may vary considerably within and among laboratories. Determining the normal range of blood values for animals is a difficult task. Normal serum CK concentration in animals is generally less than 500 U/L. Normal serum concentrations of AST, ALT, and LDH vary greatly between species. Tests included in chemistry panels also vary in different laboratories. Some laboratories do not include CK in small animal chemistry panels, which can result in a misdiagnosis of hepatic disease in a dog or cat with a persistent increase in serum AST and ALT concentrations because of degenerative muscle disease. For the purposes of discussion in this chapter, a mild increase in CK or AST is considered to be up to 2 to 3 times normal, a moderate increase is 4 to 10 times normal, and a severe increase is 10 times normal or more.

It should be emphasized that myofibers can be dysfunctional without undergoing necrosis. Myopathic and neuropathic conditions resulting in atrophy, weakness, spasm, stiffness, or myotonia rarely result in significant increase in serum muscle enzyme concentrations. At this time there is no biochemical parameter that will assess muscle fiber function; only morphologic or structural muscle fiber integrity can be assessed.

ELECTROMYOGRAPHY

Information on this topic is available at evolve.elsevier.com/Zachary/McGavin/.

METHODS OF GROSS AND MICROSCOPIC EXAMINATION OF MUSCLE

A variety of examination techniques are often necessary to best appreciate changes occurring in muscle.

Gross Pathology and Muscle Sampling

Gross examination includes evaluation of changes in size (atrophied, hypertrophied, or normal), color, and texture. The gross pathologic appearance of skeletal muscle can be quite deceiving. What appear to be mild changes in muscle on gross examination often can be severe on microscopic examination, and what appear to be severe changes on gross examination can turn out to be artefact. Subjective evaluation of size can be highly unreliable unless control muscles (e.g., from normal animals or from the opposite sides) are available for weighing and measuring.

Color changes are common. The intensity of the red color of muscle varies, depending on the type of muscle, the age and species of animal, and the extent of blood perfusion. Pale muscle can indicate necrosis (Fig. 15-9, *A* and *B*; see Figs. 15-26; 15-34, *A;* 15-36, *A;* and 15-40) or denervation (Fig. 15-9, *C;* see Fig. 15-37) but is also common in young animals and anemic animals. Pale streaking of muscle most often reflects myofiber necrosis and mineralization (see Fig. 15-9, *A* and *B*) or infiltration by collagen or fat (see Fig. 15-9, *C* and *D*), and is one of the more reliable indicators of gross pathologic changes. Muscle parasites can be grossly visible as discrete, round to oval, pale and slightly firm zones (see Figs. 15-41 and 15-42, *A*). Dark red mottling of skeletal muscle can indicate congestion, hemorrhage, hemorrhagic necrosis (see Figs. 15-32, *A,* and 15-38), inflammation, or myoglobin staining after massive muscle damage (see Fig. 15-36, *A*) or can simply reflect vascular stasis (hypostatic congestion) after death. Hemorrhagic streaks within the diaphragm often accompany death caused by acute exsanguination. A green discoloration can indicate either eosinophilic inflammation (Fig. 15-10) or severe putrefaction. Lipofuscin accumulation in old animals, especially cattle, can cause a tan-brown discoloration of muscle. Black discoloration of the fascia occurs in calves with melanosis as an incidental finding and in older gray horses with metastasis of dermal melanoma to muscle fascia.

Evaluation of texture is also important. Severely thickened and often calcified fascia occurs in cats with fibrodysplasia ossificans progressiva. Fat infiltration or necrosis can result in abnormally soft muscle. Decreased or increased muscle tone can be caused by denervation. Decreased tone can also occur as a result of a lack of muscle conditioning or postmortem autolysis.

Careful microscopic examination of multiple muscles is often required to detect lesions. In cases of suspected neuromuscular

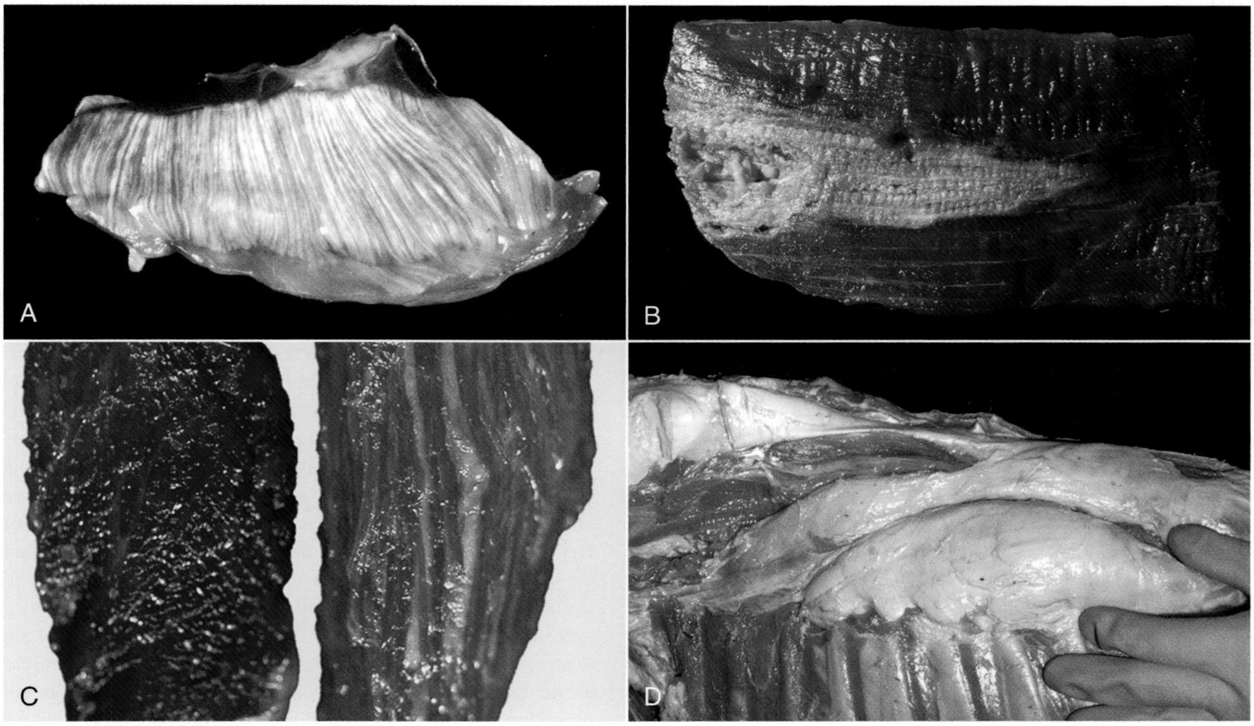

Fig. 15-9 Pathologic changes resulting in pale skeletal muscle.
A, Pale streaks, necrosis and mineralization, degenerative myopathy, canine X-linked muscular dystrophy, diaphragm *(left side),* dog. **B,** Localized pallor, necrosis, injection site of an irritant substance, semitendinosus muscle, cow. The irritant was injected just under the perimysium and caused necrosis and disruption of the myofibers. Some irritant seeped down between the fascicles to cause necrosis, but the fascicles of myofibers are still in place. **C,** Overall pale muscle with pale streaks from collagen and fat infiltration, denervation atrophy, equine motor neuron disease, horse. Equine motor neuron disease muscle *(right)* compared with normal muscle *(left).* **D,** Enlargement and pallor, steatosis, longissimus muscles, neonatal calf. The majority of the muscles have been replaced by fat. (**A** courtesy Dr. B.A. Valentine, College of Veterinary Medicine, Oregon State University. For histopathologic findings, see Fig. 15-45. **B** and **D** courtesy Dr. M.D. McGavin, College of Veterinary Medicine, University of Tennessee. For histopathologic findings, see Fig. 15-25. **C** courtesy Dr. A. de Lahunta, College of Veterinary Medicine, Cornell University. For histopathologic findings, see Figs. 15-19 and 15-37.)

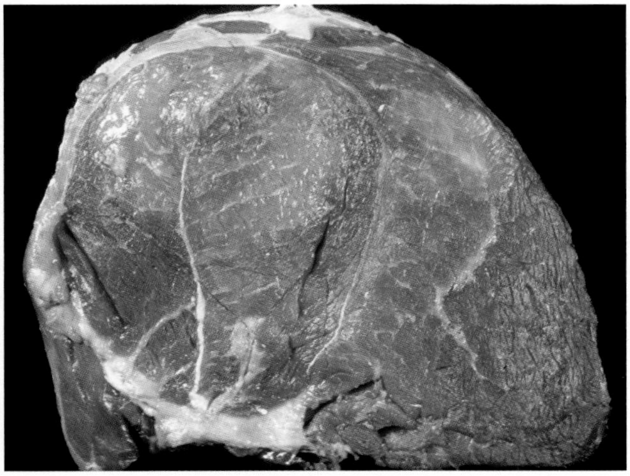

Fig. 15-10 Bovine eosinophilic myositis, gluteal muscles, cow.
Green discoloration of the muscle is due to inflammation that has abundant eosinophils. The inflammation is attributed to degenerating *Sarcocystis* spp. (Courtesy Dr. M.D. McGavin, College of Veterinary Medicine, University of Tennessee. For histopathologic findings, see Fig. 15-39.)

disease, multiple muscle samples should include active muscle (tongue, diaphragm, intercostals, and masticatory muscles), proximal muscle (lateral triceps, biceps femoris, semimembranosus, semitendinosus, and gluteal), and distal muscle (extensor carpi radialis, cranial tibial). For purposes of a biopsy, certain muscles (e.g., lateral triceps, biceps femoris, cranial tibial, semimembranosus, and semitendinosus) are easier to sample because of their parallel myofiber orientation. The ideal samples will also vary, depending on the suspected disorder, such as a type 1 predominant postural muscle for diagnosis of equine motor neuron disease; a type 2 predominant locomotory muscle for diagnosis of equine polysaccharide storage myopathy (EPSSM); and temporal or masseter muscle for diagnosis of masticatory myositis in dogs and masseter myopathy in horses. Short fibers, such as those in the intercostal muscle, are preferred for physiologic studies in which intact muscle fibers are necessary and for studies of neuromuscular junction zones.

To ensure proper fixation and orientation of sections prepared from fixed specimens, the sample should be a strip of muscle no more than 1 cm in diameter, with myofibers running lengthwise. Muscle maintains the ability to contract for some time after death, with the time varying, depending on the physiologic state.

Contraction of muscle after contact with fixative is the most common cause of an artefact called *contraction band artefact.* Contraction can be prevented or at least minimized by use of a specially designed muscle clamp (Web Fig. 15-3, *A*) or by placing the sample on a rigid surface, such as a portion of a tongue depressor, and fixing the ends with sutures, staples, or clamps before submersion in the fixative (Web Fig. 15-3, *B*).

Microscopic Examination

Frequently, lesions in muscles can be detected and evaluated only by microscopic examination. Proper microscopic examination requires evaluation of both transverse and longitudinal sections. Myofiber diameters, cytoarchitectural changes, and the percentage of abnormal myofibers are most reliably evaluated in transverse sections. Longitudinal sections reveal the length of changes such as segmental necrosis or regeneration or deposition of storage material. Improperly oriented samples, which result in sections that have obliquely oriented myofibers and thus neither longitudinal nor transverse myofibers, are difficult to evaluate. Use of a magnifying glass or dissecting microscope can aid in determining the orientation of myofibers during trimming of muscle before sectioning. Routine stains, such as hematoxylin and eosin (H&E), run the risk of offering the pathologist a "vast pink wasteland" for evaluation (Fig. 15-11, *A*) and are often inadequate for detecting subtle myopathic changes, lesions within intramuscular nerves, or presence of abnormal stored material. Various special stains, including reticulin, Masson trichrome, von Kossa, lipid (performed on frozen sections of fixed samples), and periodic acid–Schiff (PAS) for glycogen, are often invaluable in evaluation of routinely processed skeletal muscle (Web Table 15-1). Examples of many of these disorders can be found here in this chapter. Other valuable stains and reactions can only be performed on frozen sections of unfixed muscle samples (see Web Table 15-1).

For many decades, myofiber typing could be done only on frozen sections using the myosin ATPase reaction. Recently, immunohistochemical staining of myosin has been developed for demonstration of myofiber types in formalin-fixed muscle. This is a major advantage because fiber-type staining is often essential for the complete evaluation of muscle. It is most useful in demonstrating preferential involvement of a fiber type and alteration of the fiber-type pattern, the result of denervation and reinnervation.

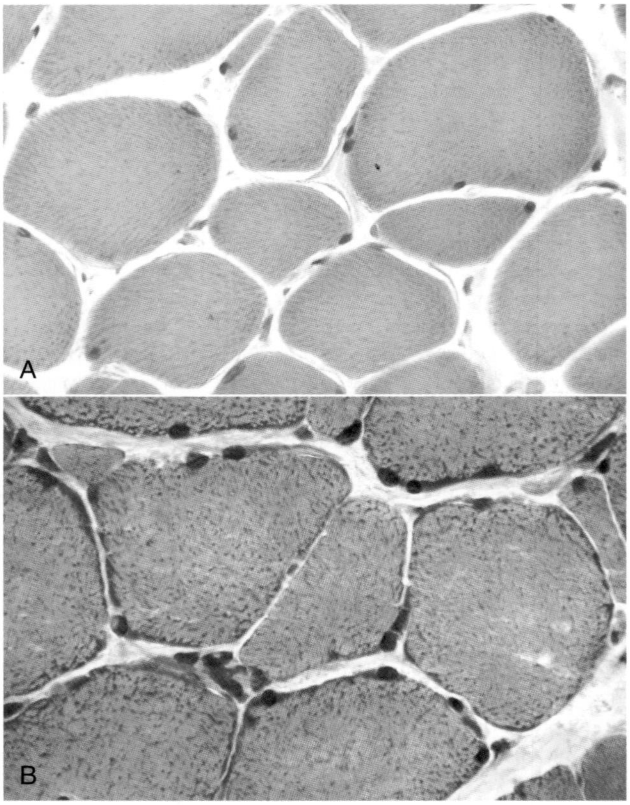

Fig. 15-11 Visibility of mitochondria, formalin-fixed vs. frozen sections, transverse sections of skeletal muscle.

A, Formalin-fixed, paraffin-embedded sample. Mitochondria stain faintly, and the myofibers lack detail when compared with **B.** H&E stain. **B,** Frozen section. Note the increased detail visible. Blue-stained mitochondria are seen throughout the cytoplasm and concentrated at the periphery of the myofibers. H&E stain. (Courtesy Dr. B.A. Valentine, College of Veterinary Medicine, Oregon State University.)

Enzyme Histochemistry and Immunohistochemistry

There is no question that frozen section histochemistry of unfixed muscle samples is the "gold standard" of muscle pathology. Skeletal muscle may be the one tissue in which the morphology of cells and cellular components is best appreciated in frozen sections (Fig. 15-11, *B*). Routine frozen section histochemistry on muscle includes a battery of stains applied to serial sections. Examples of many of these stains are illustrated in this chapter. Stains used include H&E, modified Gomori's trichrome, ATPase for fiber typing, nicotinamide adenine dinucleotide dehydrogenase (NADH), succinate dehydrogenase (SDH), cytochrome oxidase, and other mitochondrial enzyme stains, PAS for glycogen, alizarin red S for calcium, alkaline phosphatase and nonspecific esterase for macrophages and denervated fibers, and lipid stains. When indicated, frozen sections also allow for immunostaining for cytoskeletal proteins, such as dystrophin (see Fig. 15-46) and the dystrophin-associated proteins. Certain abnormal structures, such as nemaline rods formed by expansion of Z bands, as seen in nemaline rod myopathy, are not visible in routine sections but are readily identified in frozen sections stained with modified Gomori's trichrome.

The major disadvantage of frozen section histochemistry is that unless a neuromuscular disease laboratory is readily available to immediately process unfixed muscle samples, careful preparation for overnight shipping, on ice, in a moist but not overly wet environment, is necessary. Any delay in shipment or overwetting or overheating of the sample results in nondiagnostic samples. In addition, preparation of frozen sections is time and labor intensive, and in most cases only a single transverse section approximately 1 cm in diameter is examined. This can create a significant sampling error when evaluating a small sample of a large muscle in which lesions may not be evenly distributed.

Complete evaluation, which includes morphometric examination and calculation of the percentage and mean diameter of each fiber type, detects changes in the percentage of each fiber type and fiber atrophy or hypertrophy. But at this time, morphometric analysis is not routinely performed on samples submitted for diagnostic purposes.

Frozen section histochemistry is always a powerful tool for evaluation of muscle disease. But in many disorders, it is possible to obtain diagnostic sections from routinely processed muscle samples when appropriate sample selection, handling, and processing are performed, and sections are examined by a pathologist familiar with muscle pathology.

Electron Microscopy

Although much of what used to be determined by electron microscopy has been supplanted by newer immunohistochemical procedures, electron microscopic evaluation of muscle is still important. Various structural alterations, such as abnormalities of neuromuscular junctions, mitochondria, sarcomeric disarray, sarcotubular dilation, Z-line streaming, and cytoplasmic inclusions, may be best visualized, and in some cases only visualized, by this method. Sampling and handling methods to minimize contraction and other artefacts and to allow for precise transverse and longitudinal sections are imperative.

BOX 15-2 Portals of Entry into the Muscular System

DIRECT
Penetrating wounds
Intramuscular injections
Bone fracture causing trauma to adjacent muscle
External pressure causing crush injury

HEMATOGENOUS
Blood-borne pathogens, toxins, autoantibodies, and immune complexes
Cytotoxic lymphocytes causing immune-mediated damage
Other inflammatory cells

Other Methods of Evaluation

Physiologic testing of isolated intact myofibers in vitro forms the basis for diagnosis of malignant hyperthermia (MH). Short fibers, such as from samples of intercostal muscle, are preferred. While maintained in a physiologic solution, myofiber bundles are exposed to various agents, such as caffeine and halothane, to detect abnormal contractural sensitivity. Biochemical and molecular biologic analysis of muscle samples can evaluate levels of muscle enzymes and other proteins, and genetic analysis can be performed to detect specific gene defects. These latter tests require fresh muscle samples snap-frozen in liquid nitrogen and maintained at −70° C until analysis.

PORTALS OF ENTRY

Portals of entry are summarized in Box 15-2. Injury to muscle can occur secondary to trauma or infection. Muscle lying superficially can be damaged by penetrating wounds, including those created by intramuscular injections (Fig. 15-12; see also Fig. 15-9, *B*), which can also allow entry of infectious agents. Muscles located deeply are often injured after bone fracture. Crush injuries from external forces cause extensive muscle damage, and excessive tension can cause muscle tearing. Muscles are endowed with an extensive vascular network that can allow entry of blood-borne pathogens, immune complexes, antibodies and toxins, and inflammatory cells.

Other routes by which muscle can become dysfunctional are summarized in Box 15-3. Some muscular disorders are genetically determined. Inherited or acquired dysfunction of motor neurons or nerves causes muscle injury in the form of atrophy. Toxins or an altered endocrine or electrolyte status can affect muscle, and physiologic damage can be caused by exhaustive or overexuberant exercise.

DEFENSE MECHANISMS

Defense mechanisms are summarized in Box 15-4. The thick encircling fascia (epimysium) of many muscles provides some protection from penetrating injuries and from extension of adjacent infection. This fascia can, however, also contribute to injury under circumstances that lead to increased intramuscular pressure causing hypoxia (compartment syndrome). Tissue macrophages are not typically found in normal muscle but are recruited rapidly from circulating monocytes in the vasculature. Macrophages can cross even an intact basal lamina and effectively clear debris from damaged portions of myofibers, allowing for rapid restoration of the myocyte through satellite cell activation. Neutrophils and other inflammatory cells are also recruited from the bloodstream in response to injury or infection. The extensive vascular network of muscle includes extensive collateral circulatory pathways that render muscle relatively resistant to ischemic damage caused by thrombosis or thromboembolism. Despite the high vascular density of muscle, metastasis of neoplasms to muscle is quite rare. There is some evidence to suggest that the capillary endothelium of skeletal muscle is inherently resistant to neoplastic cell adhesion and invasion.

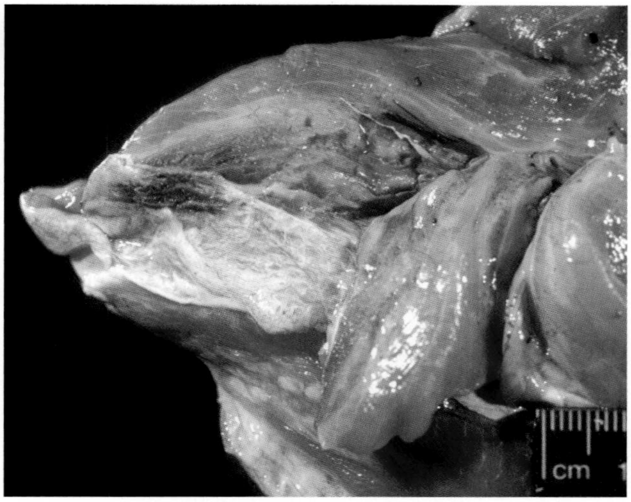

Fig. 15-12 **Inflammation and myofiber necrosis, injection site, muscles, lateral thigh, cow.**
Necrotic muscle has been stained green by the injected material, which has spread distally down the fascial plane between the two muscles from the original injection site *(top right)*. (Courtesy Dr. M.D. McGavin, College of Veterinary Medicine, University of Tennessee.)

BOX 15-3 Other Causes of Muscle Dysfunction

PHYSIOLOGIC
Excessive muscle tension causing muscle rupture
Exercise-induced damage to myofibers
Loss of innervation
Loss of blood supply
Endocrine and electrolyte abnormalities

GENETIC
Inborn errors of metabolism
Genetic defects of myofiber structural components
Developmental defects

NUTRITIONAL/TOXIC
Deficiency of selenium and/or vitamin E
Toxic plants or plant products
Feed additives (ionophores)
Other toxins (e.g., some snake venoms)

BOX 15-4 Defense Mechanisms of Skeletal Muscle

SKIN, SUBCUTIS, AND FASCIA
Form structural barriers to protect against external injury

VASCULATURE
Collateral circulation to protect against ischemia
Recruitment of monocytes that become tissue macrophages
Recruitment of neutrophils and other inflammatory cells
Capillary endothelium resistant to tumor metastasis

IMMUNOLOGIC RESPONSES
Innate humoral and cellular immunologic responses

OTHER
Adequate tissue antioxidant concentrations
Physiologic adaptation (e.g., hypertrophy, fiber type alteration)
Regenerative capacity of myofibers

RESPONSES TO INJURY

It is often said that the range of response of muscle to injury is limited, consisting primarily of necrosis and regeneration. Actually, muscle is a remarkably adaptive tissue, with a wide range of response to physiologic and pathologic conditions. Myofibers can add or delete sarcomeres to cause elongation or shortening of the entire muscle. In addition to necrosis and regeneration, myofibers can atrophy and hypertrophy, they can split, they can undergo a variety of cytoarchitectural alterations, and they can completely alter their physiologic functions when undergoing fiber-type conversion. To describe muscle response to injury as stereotypical does not do justice to this inherent plasticity. What is true, though, is that it is frequently not possible to determine the cause of muscle injury based on gross or histologic lesions alone. Supplementary tests and clinical histories are often essential.

NECROSIS AND REGENERATION

Myofiber necrosis can accompany a variety of disorders. Because of their multinucleate nature, myofibers often undergo segmental necrosis, with involvement of only one or several contiguous segments within the cell. Global necrosis of the entire length of the myofiber occurs only under severe duress, such as extreme pressure to the entire muscle causing crush injury, or widespread ischemia because of pressure on, or thromboembolism of, a large artery.

Necrotic portions of myofibers have several different histologic appearances. The earliest change is often segmental hypercontraction, resulting in segments of slightly larger diameter that are slightly darker staining ("large dark fibers") that are best seen on transverse sections (Fig. 15-13, *A*). On longitudinal sections, "twisting" or "curling" of affected fibers is often seen. But similar changes occur as an artifactual change in improperly handled samples. The cytoplasm of fully necrotic portions of the fiber is often homogeneously eosinophilic and pale (hyaline degeneration), with loss of the normal cytoplasmic striations and the adjacent muscle nucleus. The affected cytoplasm then becomes floccular or granular as that portion of the myofiber starts to fragment (Fig. 15-13, *B*; see Fig. 15-15, *B*).

Increased intracellular calcium is a common trigger of necrosis in all cells, and myofibers contain a high level of calcium ions stored in the sarcoplasmic reticulum. Therefore myofibers may be particularly sensitive to calcium-induced necrosis, either as a result of damage to the sarcolemma, causing influx of extracellular calcium, or from damage to the sarcoplasmic reticulum, releasing intracellular stores of calcium. Small wonder then that necrotic myofibers are often prone to overt mineralization. Overtly mineralized myofibers appear as chalky white streaks on gross examination (see Fig. 15-9, *A*) and as basophilic granular to crystalline material within myofibers on histologic examination. Large deposits of mineral can induce a foreign body granulomatous response. Although the presence or absence of myofiber mineralization has sometimes been used as a diagnostic aid, the circumstances under which a necrotic myofiber segment can become mineralized are so diverse that myofiber mineralization must be considered a nonspecific response, indicative only of myofiber necrosis. Myofiber mineralization can be confirmed with histochemical stains, such as alizarin red S and von Kossa. Histochemical staining for calcium in frozen sections also detects increased intracytoplasmic calcium in damaged myofibers that are not overtly necrotic or mineralized (Fig. 15-14, *A*).

Provided there is still an adequate blood supply, macrophages derived from transformation of blood monocytes rapidly infiltrate areas of myofiber necrosis (Fig. 15-14, *B*). Macrophages are able to traverse the basal lamina and rapidly clear cytoplasmic debris (Fig.

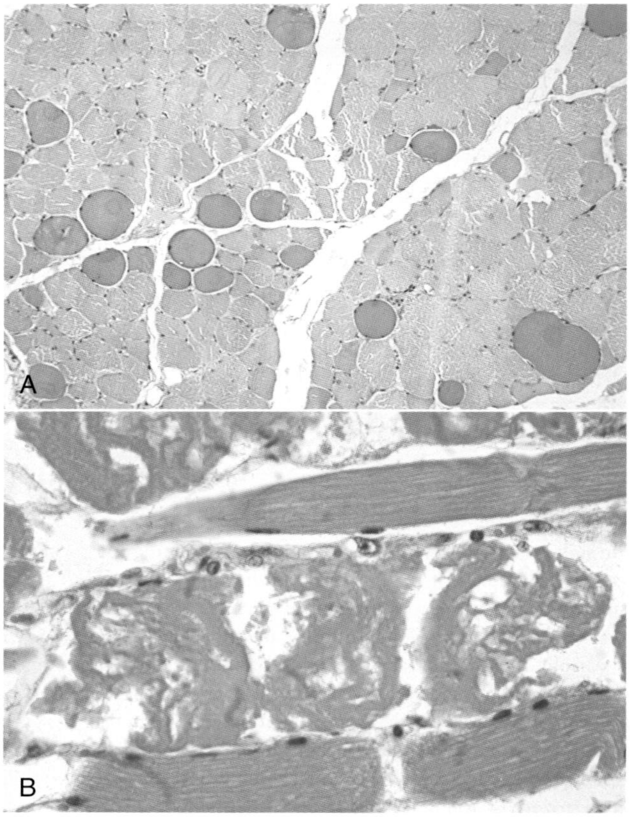

Fig. 15-13 Myofiber necrosis, skeletal muscle.
A, Hypercontraction, transverse section. Large, deeply stained fibers ("large dark red fibers") are hypercontracted segments of a myofiber, the initial stage of necrosis. Note the rounded outline of these myofibers compared with the polygonal outlines of normal myofibers. Formalin fixation, H&E stain. **B,** Segmental necrosis, monensin toxicosis, longitudinal section, horse. Segments of the myofibers have undergone hypercontraction *(center of figure)*, and the remaining cytoplasm is fragmented. Formalin fixation, H&E stain. (Courtesy Dr. M.D. McGavin, College of Veterinary Medicine, University of Tennessee.)

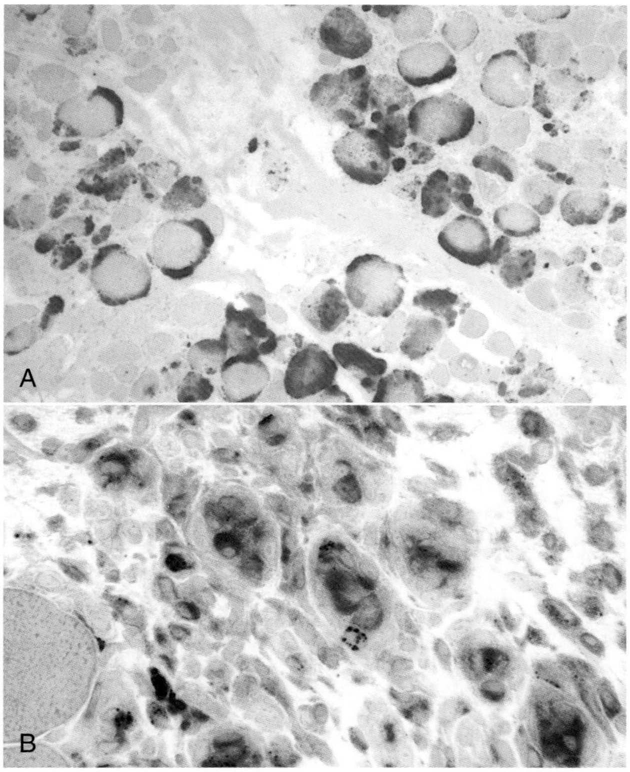

Fig. 15-14 Myofiber necrosis, skeletal muscle, transverse section. **A,** There has been a massive influx of calcium *(stained orange)* into acutely necrotic fibers. Frozen section, alizarin red S stain. **B,** Macrophages with red-brown staining cytoplasm invading necrotic myofibers. Portions of intact fibers are in the lower left. Frozen section, nonspecific esterase stain. (**A** courtesy Dr. B.A. Valentine, College of Veterinary Medicine, Oregon State University. **B** courtesy Dr. B.J. Cooper, College of Veterinary Medicine, Oregon State University.)

15-15, *A*). Other leukocytes, including neutrophils, eosinophils, and lymphocytes, can also be recruited to sites of extensive myonecrosis, presumably because of various cytokines released from damaged muscle. The infiltration of macrophages and other cells into areas of damaged muscle to clear away necrotic myofibers does not in any way constitute a form of myositis.

Because myonuclei are unable to divide, regeneration of muscle relies on satellite cell activation. Muscle satellite cells are resistant to many of the insults that result in myofiber necrosis, and activation of satellite cells is triggered by necrosis of adjacent segments of that myofiber. Therefore, as macrophages are clearing cytoplasmic debris, satellite cells are becoming activated and begin to divide in preparation for regeneration of the affected myofiber segment. If the myofiber basal lamina is still intact, it will leave an empty cylindrical space known as a *sarcolemmal tube.* This name is clearly a misnomer, dating from the days when the term *sarcolemma* was applied to the tube formed by the basal lamina that remains after segmental myofiber necrosis. Clearly what is now termed the sarcolemma (plasmalemma) of necrotic fiber segments is lost, but this is a misnomer that is firmly entrenched. The important concept to remember is that, if intact, the basal lamina forms a cylindrical scaffold to guide proliferating myoblasts and to keep fibroblasts out. Satellite cells may be seen undergoing mitosis, at which stage they are known as *activated myoblasts,* on the inner surface of this tube (see Fig. 15-15, *A*). Within hours, proliferating myoblasts will fuse end-to-end to form myotubes (Fig. 15-15, *B* and *C*), and within

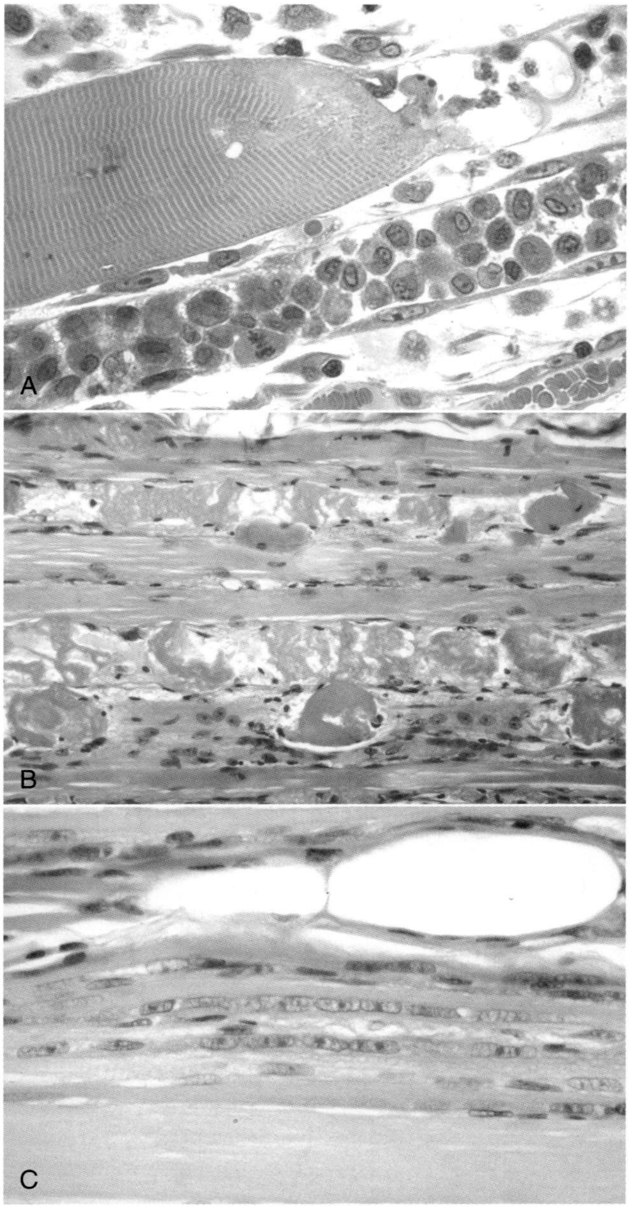

Fig. 15-15 Segmental necrosis and regeneration. **A,** Monophasic segmental coagulation necrosis, skeletal muscle, longitudinal section of two myofibers. A segment of the upper fiber *(right)* and all the visible portion of the lower fiber have undergone necrosis, and macrophages have invaded through the intact basal lamina and cleared the cytoplasmic debris. Satellite cells on the inner surface of the basal lamina of the lower fiber are activated, and one *(lower left side)* is in mitosis. One-mm plastic-embedded section, H&E stain. **B,** Polyphasic injury, segmental coagulation necrosis and regeneration of myofibers, muscle, longitudinal section. Between each of the foci of coagulation necrosis in the lowest myofiber is a segment of small-diameter faintly basophilic cytoplasm lacking cross striations, in which there is an internal chain of euchromatic nuclei. This is a late stage of regeneration. Formalin fixation, H&E stain. **C,** Monophasic injury, late stage regeneration, skeletal muscle, longitudinal section. The regenerating segment of the myofiber consists of myotubes, which have small diameters, with slightly basophilic cytoplasm and internal rows of large euchromatic nuclei. Formalin fixation, H&E stain. (**A** courtesy Dr. A. Kelly, University of Pennsylvania. **B** courtesy Dr. B.A. Valentine, College of Veterinary Medicine, Oregon State University. **C** courtesy Dr. B.J. Cooper, College of Veterinary Medicine, Oregon State University.)

days the myotube produces thick and thin filaments and undergoes maturation to a myofiber, reestablishing myofiber integrity. If the basal lamina is ruptured, myotubes are said to be able to bridge gaps of 2 to 4 mm and larger ones heal by fibrosis (see later discussion). The process of myofiber regeneration recapitulates embryologic development of skeletal muscle and is depicted schematically in Fig. 15-16. A percentage of dividing satellite cells do not fuse with the forming myotube but instead become new satellite cells capable of future regeneration.

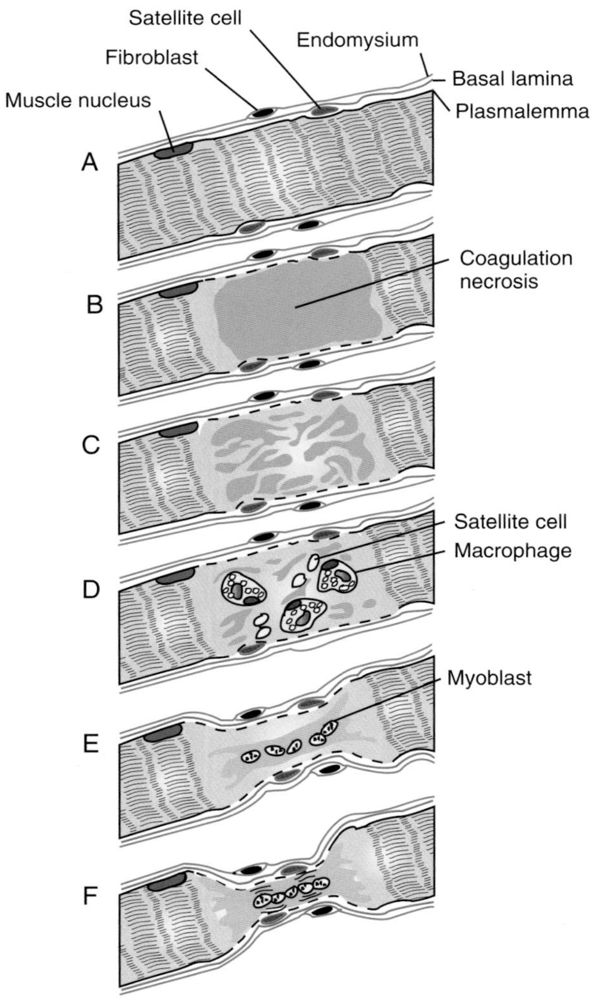

Fig. 15-16 Schematic diagram of segmental myofiber necrosis and regeneration.

A, Myofiber, longitudinal section. **B,** Segmental coagulation necrosis. **C,** The necrotic segment of the myofiber has become floccular and detached from the adjacent viable portion of the myofiber. The satellite cells are enlarging. **D,** The necrotic segment of the myofiber has been invaded by macrophages, and satellite cells are migrating to the center. The latter will develop into myoblasts. The plasmalemma of the necrotic segment has disappeared. **E,** Myoblasts have formed a myotube, which has produced sarcoplasm. This extends out to meet the viable ends of the myofiber. The integrity of the myofiber is maintained by the sarcolemmal tube formed by the basal lamina and endomysium. **F,** Regenerating myofiber. There is a reduction in myofiber diameter with central rowing of nuclei. There is early formation of sarcomeres (cross striations), and the plasmalemma has re-formed. Such fibers stain basophilically with H&E. (Redrawn with permission from Dr. M.D. McGavin, College of Veterinary Medicine, University of Tennessee.)

In summary, the success of muscle regeneration depends on (1) the presence of an intact basal lamina and (2) the availability of viable satellite cells. The stages of successful muscle regeneration are summarized in Box 15-5.

Thus myofibers undergoing segmental necrosis in which the basal lamina is preserved, as in metabolic, nutritional, and toxic myopathies, regenerate very successfully. However, when large areas of satellite cells are killed (e.g., by heat, intense inflammation, or infarction), the situation is very different. In this case, a return to normal is not possible, and healing is chiefly by fibrosis.

If the insult to the muscle is sufficient to disrupt the myofiber basal lamina but not enough to damage the satellite cells, regeneration attempts are ineffective. Because the basal lamina is not intact, there is no tube to guide the myoblasts proliferating from each end. Myoblast proliferation under these conditions results in formation of so-called muscle giant cells (Fig. 15-17). Thus the presence of muscle giant cells indicates that conditions for regeneration have not been optimal and occurs after destructive lesions, such as those caused by trauma that transects myofibers, infarction, and intramuscular bacterial infection or injection of irritants. Muscle giant

BOX 15-5 Stages of Muscle Regeneration under Optimal Conditions

1. Muscle nuclei disappear from the necrotic segment and the sarcoplasm becomes hyalinized (eosinophilic, amorphous, and homogeneous) because of the loss of normal myofibrillar structure (see Fig. 15-16, *B*). The necrotic portion may separate from the adjacent viable myofiber (see Fig. 15-13, *B;* Fig. 15-15, *A* and *B;* and Fig. 15-16, *C*).
2. Within 24 to 48 hours, monocytes emigrate from capillaries, become macrophages, and enter the necrotic portion of the myofiber (see Fig. 15-14, *B;* Fig. 15-15, *A;* and Fig. 15-16, *D*). Concurrently, the satellite cells, located between the basal lamina and the sarcolemma, begin to enlarge (see Fig. 15-15, *A,* and Fig. 15-16, *C* and *D*), become vesicular with prominent nucleoli, and then undergo mitosis to become myoblasts.
3. Myoblasts migrate from the periphery to the center of the sarcolemmal tube, admixed with macrophages (see Fig. 15-16, *D*).
4. Macrophages lyse and phagocytose necrotic debris and form a clear space in the sarcolemmal tube, and the shape and integrity of the sarcolemmal tube is maintained by the basal lamina (see Fig. 15-15, *A*).
5. Myoblasts fuse with one another to form myotubes, which are thin, elongated muscle cells with a row of central, closely spaced nuclei. Developing myotubes send out cytoplasmic processes in both directions within the sarcolemmal tube (see Fig. 15-16, *E*). When the processes contact each other or a viable portion of the original muscle fiber, they fuse. The regenerating fiber is characterized by (1) basophilia as a result of increased RNA content; (2) internal nuclei, often in rows, that have differentiated to myonuclei; (3) a lack of striations; and (4) a smaller-than-normal diameter (see Fig. 15-15, *B* and *C,* and Fig. 15-16, *F*).
6. The fiber grows and differentiates. Its diameter increases, the sarcoplasm loses its basophilia, and longitudinal and cross striations appear, indicating the formation of sarcomeres.
7. In most species, within several days, the muscle nuclei of regenerating fibers move to their normal position at the periphery of the fiber, just under the sarcolemma.

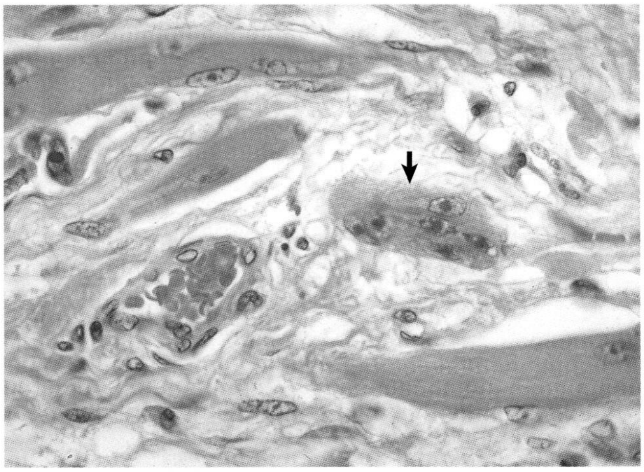

Fig. 15-17 Ineffectual regeneration.
Large, bizarre multinucleate muscle giant cells *(arrow)* are indicative of regeneration in an area in which the myofiber's basal lamina has been damaged. Because the wall of the "myotube" of basal lamina is not intact, regenerating sarcoplasm exudes through the defect and in cross section this appears as a "muscle giant cell." Formalin fixation, H&E stain. (Courtesy Dr. M.D. McGavin, College of Veterinary Medicine, University of Tennessee; and Noah's Arkive, College of Veterinary Medicine, The University of Georgia.)

cells are often accompanied by fibrosis, which will unite the ends of the damaged myofibers. This also occurs in muscle damaged by invasive or metastatic sclerosing carcinomas. Cytokines released from damaged muscle fibers contribute to the signaling pathways that initiate macrophage infiltration and regeneration, but they also contribute to interstitial fibroblast activation. Collagen is inelastic, and thus large areas of fibrosis inevitably reduce the ability of the muscle to contract and to stretch. Fibrosis within locomotory muscles often results in obvious alteration of the gait.

Because segmental necrosis and regeneration are such a common result of a wide variety of insults (e.g., overexertion, selenium deficiency, and toxic injury), a histologic diagnosis of segmental necrosis is often not helpful in determining the cause of the disease. Pathologic classification of lesions according to distribution (i.e., focal, multifocal, locally extensive, and diffuse) and duration (i.e., acute, subacute, chronic) has proven to be extremely useful in determining the possible causes of segmental muscle necrosis. Pathologic classification of degenerative myopathies has been further enhanced by Dr. Byron Kakulas, who introduced the terms *monophasic necrosis* and *polyphasic necrosis.* Monophasic lesions are of the same duration, indicative of a single insult. Polyphasic lesions indicate an ongoing degenerative process. Thus a focal monophasic lesion could be the result of a single traumatic incident such as an intramuscular injection (see Fig. 15-9, *B*). A multifocal monophasic lesion could represent a single episode of overly strenuous exercise (exertional myopathy) or a toxin being ingested on one occasion (e.g., a horse eating one dose of monensin; see Figs. 15-13, *B,* and 15-34, *B*). However, if the insult is repeated or ongoing, such as occurs in muscular dystrophy (see Fig. 15-45), selenium deficiency, or continuous feeding of a toxin, then new lesions (segmental necrosis) will form at the same time that regeneration is taking place; in other words, it will be a multifocal and polyphasic disease (see Fig. 15-15, *B*). Using this approach, it is sometimes possible to rule out a diagnosis (e.g., muscular dystrophy and selenium deficiency myopathy are typically polyphasic), but this is not an invariable rule. For example, in livestock with borderline concentrations of selenium, a sudden stress can cause a monophasic necrosis.

BOX 15-6 Findings Associated with Chronic Myopathic Change

- Excessive fiber-size (diameter) variation
- Internal nuclei
- Fiber splitting
- Other cytoarchitectural changes
- Fibrosis
- Fat infiltration

The term *rhabdomyolysis* is often encountered, particularly in the clinical arena, and especially in association with exercise-induced muscle injury (exertional rhabdomyolysis) in humans, horses, and dogs. Technically, *rhabdomyolysis* simply means necrosis (lysis) of striated muscle. This term was coined years ago to replace the term *myoglobinuria* as a description for the clinical entity of severe muscle injury associated with myoglobin release causing dark red discoloration of the urine. Thus rhabdomyolysis generally indicates the presence of a severe degenerative myopathy with a large degree of myofiber necrosis (see Fig. 15-36). In horses, the term *exertional rhabdomyolysis* has become firmly entrenched as a clinical entity in which exercise-induced muscle injury is the presenting sign. The term *recurrent exertional rhabdomyolysis* is often employed in cases in which repeated bouts of exercise-induced muscle damage have been documented.

ALTERATION IN MYOFIBER SIZE

The normal myofiber diameter will vary, depending on fiber type, the muscle examined, the species, and the age of the animal. In some species (e.g., horse, cat, and humans), there are three distinct populations based on diameter: Type 1 fibers are the smallest, type 2B fibers the largest, and type 2A fibers are intermediate in size. Different sizes in diameters are in part a reflection of the oxidative needs of the fibers; oxygen diffuses more readily into the interior of small-diameter fibers. In the dog, all fiber types are oxidative, and fiber-type diameter is much more uniform. A histogram generated from morphometric analysis of fiber diameters will reveal the characteristics of individual muscles in various species. Not surprisingly, this type of detailed information is more readily available for human patients than for animals. Even without morphometric analysis, however, a pathologist experienced in examination of muscle can often determine whether there is a normal fiber-size distribution (based on fiber diameter in transverse section), or whether there is an increase in fiber-size variation. The finding of increased fiber-size variation suggests that something is wrong but in itself does not give any indication of cause. Increased fiber-size variation can be a result of fiber atrophy, fiber hypertrophy, or both and is considered part of the spectrum of changes included in the term *chronic myopathic change* (Box 15-6).

Atrophy

The term *atrophy* is used to imply either a reduction in the volume of the muscle as a whole or in the diameter of a myofiber. In the early stages of atrophy, it may be difficult or impossible to detect loss of muscle mass by gross observation, and morphometric evaluation of myofiber diameters may be required. Several cellular physiologic processes can be activated to result in muscle atrophy. These include induction of lysosomal action to result in autophagy of cytoplasmic components, apoptosis (programmed cell death), and

BOX 15-7 Fiber Types Affected in Different Types of Muscle Atrophy

1. Denervation: Type 1 and type 2 fibers; reinnervation leads to altered fiber-type patterns (fiber-type grouping)
2. Disuse: Predominantly type 2 fibers; may vary, depending on the species and cause
3. Endocrine disease: Predominantly type 2 fibers; associated with hypothyroidism and hypercortisolism
4. Malnutrition, cachexia, and senility: Predominantly type 2 fibers
5. Congenital myopathy: Often predominantly type 1 fibers

activation of the cytoplasmic ubiquitin-proteosomal machinery. Lysosomal activation is prominent in denervation atrophy and is the basis for the positive reaction of denervated fibers in alkaline phosphatase and nonspecific esterase preparations. The causes of muscle fiber atrophy include physiologic and metabolic processes and denervation. In most instances, muscle atrophy is reversible provided the cause is corrected. The type of fiber undergoing atrophy varies, depending on the cause, therefore fiber typing is often required for a definitive diagnosis. Interestingly, type 2 fibers are the most likely to atrophy under a variety of circumstances (Box 15-7). Signalling molecules involved in muscle atrophy include tumor necrosis factor α (TNF-α) and interleukin (IL)-1 and IL-6.

Physiologic Muscle Atrophy

Decrease in myofiber diameter and therefore in the overall muscle mass is a physiologic response to lack of use (disuse atrophy), cachexia, and aging. Type 2 fibers are preferentially affected (Web Fig. 15-4). Disuse atrophy occurs relatively slowly, and only in muscles not undergoing normal contraction, as is caused by severe lameness or in muscles of a limb that is splinted or enclosed in a cast. The degree of disuse atrophy will be variable, but typically is not as severe as the atrophy of cachexia or denervation (see later discussion). Disuse atrophy is often asymmetric. Muscle atrophy caused by cachexia can be profound, especially in cases of cancer cachexia in which increased circulating levels of TNF alter the muscle metabolism, favoring catabolic processes rather than anabolic processes. Cachexia also develops relatively slowly and causes symmetric muscle atrophy. Muscle atrophy caused by aging can be considered a milder form of cachexia. Starvation, malnutrition, and chronic renal and cardiac diseases can also result in cachexia.

Atrophy Caused by Endocrine Disease

Preferential atrophy of type 2 fibers causing symmetric muscle atrophy also occurs because of various endocrine disorders. The most common are hypothyroidism and hypercortisolism in dogs. Aging horses with pituitary dysfunction or tumors (leading to equine Cushing's syndrome) often develop type 2 muscle fiber atrophy. Myofibers contain a high concentration of surface receptors for several hormones, and atrophy caused by endocrine disease reflects the intimate interrelationship between the endocrine and the muscular systems.

Denervation Atrophy

Denervation atrophy, also known by the misnomer *neurogenic atrophy,* is not uncommon in veterinary medicine. Maintenance of normal myofiber diameter depends on trophic factors generated by an intact associated nerve. Loss of neural input results in rapid muscle atrophy, and more than half the muscle mass of a completely denervated muscle can be lost in a few weeks. This trophic effect

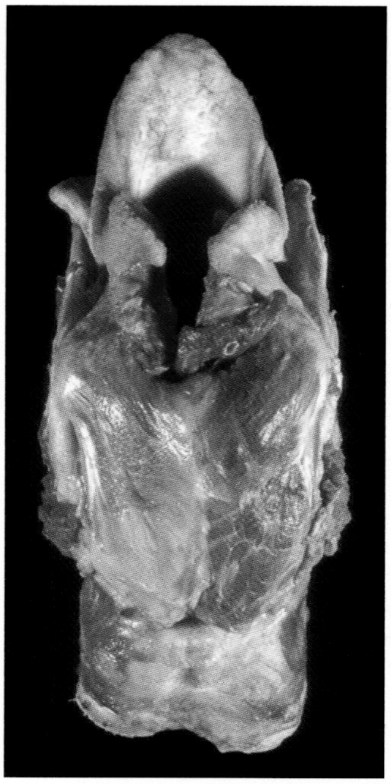

Fig. 15-18 Denervation muscle atrophy, left cricoarytenoideus dorsalis muscle, larynx, dorsal surface, horse.
Note the unilateral *(left side)* atrophy and pale gray-to-white discoloration of the muscle. This horse had a peripheral neuropathy, which led to laryngeal hemiplegia. (Courtesy College of Veterinary Medicine, University of Illinois.)

is not dependent on contractile activity because denervation atrophy is not a feature of neuromuscular junction disorders such as botulism and myasthenia gravis. In these disorders, there is a failure of neuromuscular transmission, but the nerve to the muscle is intact; therefore the muscle is technically still innervated. Generalized neuropathies or neuronopathies, such as equine motor neuron disease, result in widespread and symmetric muscle atrophy. More commonly, however, only select nerve damage is present, resulting in asymmetric muscle atrophy. One example is equine laryngeal hemiplegia (roaring) secondary to damage to the left recurrent laryngeal nerve (Fig. 15-18). It should be pointed out that purely demyelinating disorders of peripheral nerves can cause profound neuromuscular dysfunction, but axons are still intact. Associated myofibers are not technically denervated and therefore do not undergo denervation atrophy.

After denervation, fibers become progressively smaller in diameter as peripheral myofibrils disintegrate. If an atrophic fiber is surrounded by normal fibers, it will be pressed into an angular shape, called an angular atrophied fiber. The angular atrophied fibers of denervation atrophy most often occur either singly or in small contiguous groups (small group atrophy) (Fig. 15-19, *A*). In more severe denervating conditions, in which many fibers within muscle fascicles are undergoing denervation atrophy, there are no normal fibers to cause compression and angularity, and affected fibers occur as larger groups of small-diameter, rounded fibers (large group atrophy; Fig. 15-19, *B*). Although myofibrils disappear rapidly, muscle nuclei do not do so at the same rate, and therefore denervation atrophy is often associated with a notably increased concentration of myonuclei. The breakdown of glycogen in the myofiber is an early change in denervation atrophy, and therefore denervated fibers stain faintly or not at all with the PAS reaction.

A histologic diagnosis of denervation atrophy may be suspected, based on the characteristic features of routinely processed muscles,

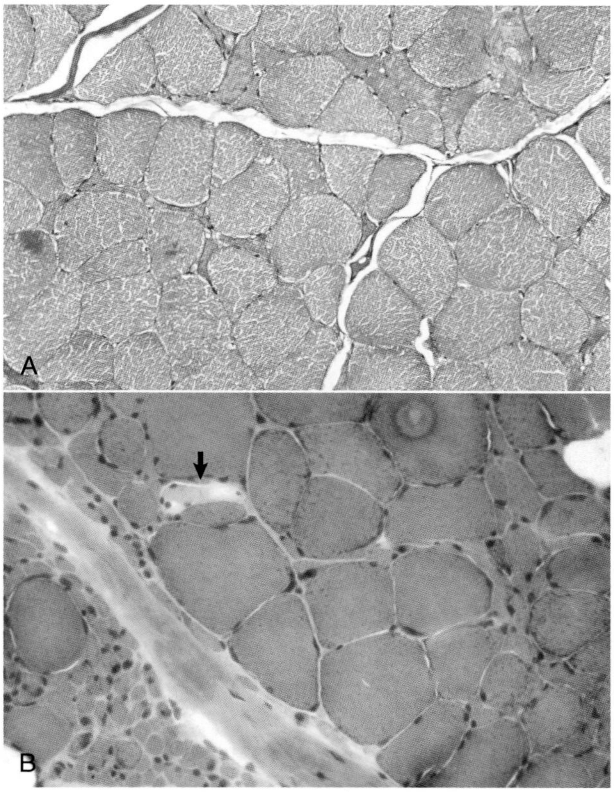

Fig. 15-19 Denervation atrophy, transverse sections.
Both sections are from horses with equine motor neuron disease. **A,** In relatively mild denervation, severely atrophied and angular fibers form small contiguous clusters indicative of small group atrophy. Formalin fixation, Masson trichrome stain. **B,** In severe denervation, entire fascicles of fibers undergo rounded atrophy characteristic of large group atrophy *(lower left).* Small group atrophy and admixed fiber hypertrophy are also present. A single pale stained fiber *(arrow)* is undergoing acute necrosis. There is also mild endomysial and perimysial fibrosis and mild fat infiltration *(empty vacuoles in the upper right and lower left).* Frozen section, modified Gomori's trichrome stain. (Courtesy Dr. B.A. Valentine, College of Veterinary Medicine, Oregon State University.)

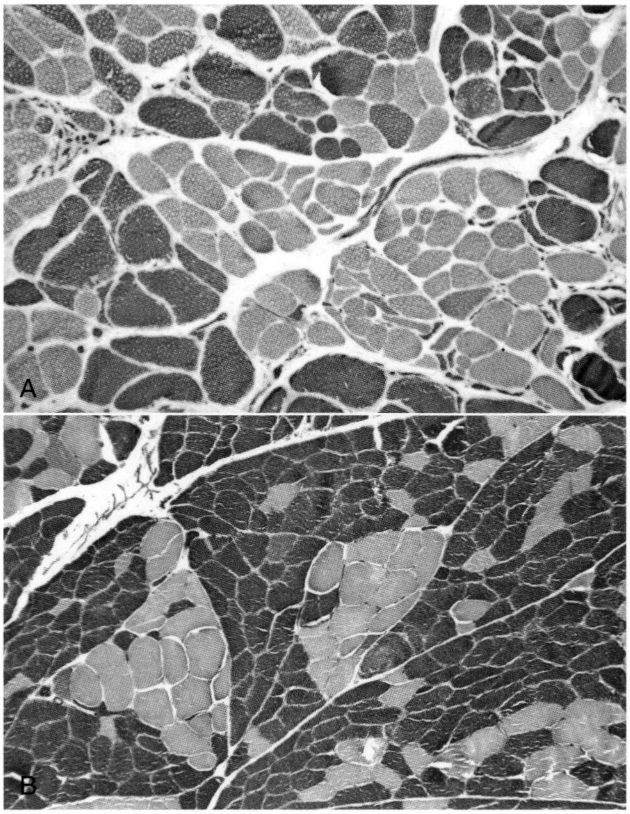

Fig. 15-20 Denervation atrophy and reinnervation, skeletal muscle, transverse sections.
A, Fiber typing reveals angular atrophy of both type 1 *(light)* and type 2 *(dark)* fibers, characteristic of denervation atrophy. In this case, there is also a loss of the normal mosaic pattern of fiber types, with groups of type 1 and of type 2 fibers indicative of reinnervation. This section is from a horse with laryngeal hemiplegia. Frozen section, ATPase pH 10.0. **B,** Fiber-type grouping in a dog indicative of denervation and reinnervation secondary to corticosteroid therapy. There is a loss of the normal mosaic pattern of fiber types, with grouping of type 1 *(light)* and type 2 *(dark)* fibers. The lack of angular atrophied fibers indicates that active denervation is not occurring at this time. Frozen section, ATPase pH 9.8. (**A** courtesy Dr. B.A. Valentine, College of Veterinary Medicine, Oregon State University. **B** courtesy Dr. M.D. McGavin, College of Veterinary Medicine, University of Tennessee.)

but is most reliably documented with histochemistry or immunohistochemistry to detect fiber types. The loss of a nerve fiber to a muscle results in atrophy of all myofibers innervated by that nerve. Because of the intermingling of motor units forming a mosaic pattern of fiber types, myofibers undergoing denervation atrophy are scattered in a section of muscle. Because the motor neuron determines the histochemical myofiber type and because denervating diseases typically involve both type 1 and type 2 neurons or nerves, atrophy of both type 1 and type 2 myofibers in muscle fasciculi is the hallmark of denervation atrophy (Fig. 15-20, *A*).

In denervation atrophy, histologic examination of the intramuscular nerves is warranted because it may reveal axonal degeneration or loss of myelinated fibers. Masson trichrome stain can be useful here because it will differentiate myelin (red) from collagen (blue). If the nerve damage does not incapacitate the animal and the muscle can still be used (e.g., in locomotion), the remaining innervated myofibers often undergo notable hypertrophy because of increased workload. Often, the hypertrophied fibers in chronic denervation are type 1. Even without fiber typing, a pattern of severe small or large group atrophy (see Fig. 15-19, *A*), especially if associated with notable fiber hypertrophy (see Fig. 15-19, *B*), is strongly suggestive of denervation atrophy. A finding of damage in an associated peripheral nerve is definitive.

Under many circumstances, denervated muscle fibers can be reinnervated by subterminal sprouting of axons from adjacent normal nerves. Reinnervation results in return to normal myofiber diameter, but reinnervation is often from sprouts of a different type of nerve. Because muscle fiber type is a function of the motor neuron, the newly innervated myofiber takes on the fiber type determined by that neuron. This process results in a loss of the normal arrangement of type 1 and 2 myofibers and the formation of groups of the same fiber type adjacent to each other, called *fiber-type grouping* (see Fig. 15-20). Thus fiber-type grouping is the hallmark of denervation followed by reinnervation. What appears to be fiber-type grouping can also occur because of fiber-type conversion (most often to type 1 fibers) in chronic myopathic conditions. Careful evaluation of the structure and function of peripheral nerves helps distinguish neuropathic from myopathic changes. If previously reinnervated fibers are denervated again, the pattern includes large groups of atrophied fibers of a single fiber

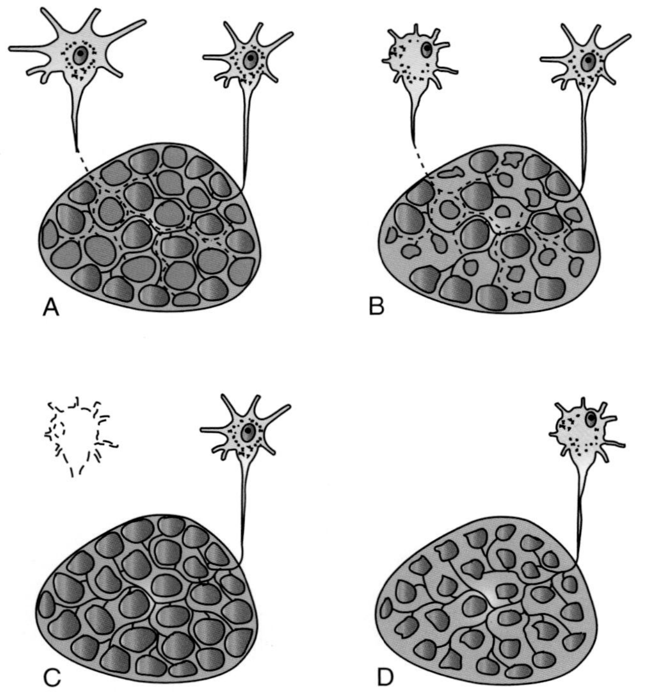

Fig. 15-21 **Schematic diagram of motor units undergoing denervation and reinnervation.**

A, Terminal axon branches innervate multiple myofibers, and myofiber type is determined by the electrical activity of the type of neuron innervating the myofiber. Normally the terminal axons of the motor units are intermingled, with the result that the differently stained myofiber types form a mosaic pattern. **B,** If a neuron (or axon) is damaged, the axon will undergo Wallerian degeneration, and the myofibers in that motor unit will undergo denervation atrophy. Small group atrophy is illustrated here. **C,** Axonal sprouts from a healthy neuron can reinnervate affected fibers and cause restoration of their normal diameter. The myofibers will assume the fiber type of the new motor unit, which often causes fiber-type conversion, leading to fiber-type grouping. **D,** If neuronal (or axonal) damage is progressive, denervation atrophy of large groups of fibers of a single type can occur, known as type-specific group atrophy. This type of atrophy is less common in animals than in humans. (Redrawn with permission from Dr. B.A. Valentine, College of Veterinary Medicine, Oregon State University.)

type, a process known as *type-specific group atrophy.* Type-specific group atrophy is far less common in animals than in humans. Fiber-type grouping and type-specific group atrophy can only be detected by methods that distinguish fiber types. Changes occurring as a result of denervation and reinnervation are illustrated in Fig. 15-21.

Atrophy Caused by Congenital Myopathy

Congenital myopathy in children is often associated with selective type 1 fiber atrophy. This finding is less common in the congenital myopathies identified thus far in animals. Selective type 1 atrophy is, however, a feature of feline nemaline myopathy, an animal model of congenital nemaline myopathy in children.

Hypertrophy

Myofibers increase in diameter by the addition of myofilaments. Physiologic hypertrophy is the normal process of myofiber enlargement that occurs with exercise conditioning. Compensatory hypertrophy occurs because of pathologic conditions that (1) decrease the number of functional myofibers and therefore increase the load on remaining fibers or (2) interfere with normal cellular metabolic or other physiologic processes. Compensatory myofiber hypertrophy is therefore considered a relatively nonspecific response to a variety of insults. Fibers undergoing compensatory hypertrophy can enlarge to more than 100 μm in diameter (normal is less than approximately 60 to 70 μm). Fiber hypertrophy often accompanies fiber atrophy, which contributes to increased fiber-size variation in various myopathic and neuropathic conditions.

Compensatory hypertrophy can occur because of a decrease in the number of functional myofibers. Thus, in a partially denervated muscle, the remaining innervated fibers hypertrophy (see Fig. 15-19, *B*), presumably as a result of increased workload. Pathologically hypertrophied fibers have less oxygen diffusion from interstitial capillaries to internal portions of the myofiber because of the increase in the distance from the capillary to the internal portions of the myofibers, which can lead to myofiber damage. Mechanical overloading of hypertrophied muscle fibers is also possible. For example, overloading of hypertrophied fibers can result in segmental necrosis of the hypertrophied fibers (see Fig. 15-19, *B*), or fibers can undergo longitudinal fiber splitting to generate one or more smaller-diameter "fibers," all contained within the same basal lamina (Fig. 15-22). Serial sections of areas of fiber splitting generally reveals that splits do not extend the entire length of the myofiber. Fiber splitting is considered a form of cytoarchitectural alteration (see later discussion). Insulin-like growth factor 1 (IGF-1) is an important molecular signal involved in skeletal muscle hypertrophy. Genetic inactivation of the regulatory gene myostatin results in muscle hypertrophy caused by an increase in the number of myofibers.

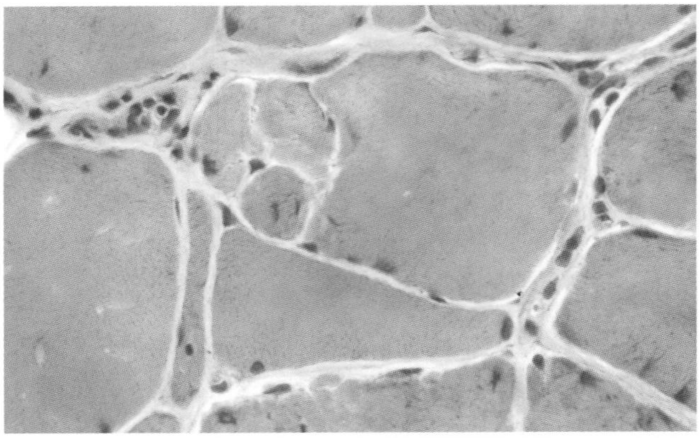

Fig. 15-22 **Fiber type splitting of hypertrophied myofibers, nemaline myopathy, skeletal muscle, transverse section, cat.**

Sarcolemmal ingrowth into the myofiber has resulted in multiple partitions with the formation of four myofibers; however, all myofibers are enclosed by one basal lamina. Frozen section, modified Gomori's trichrome stain. (Courtesy Dr. B.A. Valentine, College of Veterinary Medicine, Oregon State University.)

CYTOARCHITECTURAL CHANGES

In addition to fiber splitting, a variety of other cytoarchitectural changes can occur within myofibers. Some are degenerative, the result of an insult that damages the myofiber but does not culminate in myofiber necrosis. Others reflect underlying ultrastructural alterations that may be either pathologic or compensatory in nature. The functional significance of many of the myofiber cytoarchitectural changes is not known.

Vacuolar Change

Vacuolar change is a common cytoplasmic alteration. In formalin-fixed paraffin-embedded sections or in any sample subjected to less than ideal handling, true vacuolar change can be very difficult to distinguish from artifacts. Vacuoles can be an early manifestation of processes leading to necrosis, they can reflect underlying sarcotubular dilation as occurs in many myotonic conditions (see later discussion), and they can be caused by abnormal storage of carbohydrate or lipid, or they can reflect underlying myofibrillar abnormalities. Additional studies are often necessary to determine the nature of the vacuoles. When severe, such as in glycogen storage diseases, the term *vacuolar myopathy* is often employed.

Internal Nuclei

Myonuclei of mature myofibers in domestic animals are normally found peripherally, just beneath the sarcolemma. Nuclei located one nuclear diameter or more from the sarcolemma are known as *internal nuclei.* (NOTE: The previously used term *central nuclei* is considered incorrect because few abnormally placed nuclei are exactly centrally located.) Internal nuclei are rare in normal mammalian muscle, but a small percentage can be found normally in avian and reptilian species. Rows of internal nuclei in small-diameter, slightly basophilic myofibers are characteristic of the myotubular stage of regeneration (see Fig. 15-15, *B* and *C*). In most species, myonuclei return to the normal peripheral location early in regeneration, within days of myotube formation. Rodents are the exception. In rodents, internal nuclei are retained after regeneration, which, in these species, provides a handy marker for identification of fibers that have undergone necrosis and regeneration. In other mammalian species, the presence of internal nuclei in normal or hypertrophied fibers is a nonspecific finding indicative of chronic myopathic change (Fig. 15-23; see Box 15-6). In hypertrophied fibers, the migration of myonuclei to the internal portion of the myofiber can precede the sarcolemmal infolding that creates longitudinal fiber splitting.

Whorled and Ring Fibers

The cytoarchitectural rearrangements resulting in whorled and ring fibers are best appreciated in transverse sections. Whorled fibers contain spirals of cytoplasm with internally located nuclei. Whorled fibers can be seen in areas of chronic denervation, and also in areas in which myofiber necrosis with incomplete regeneration has occurred. Ring fibers (also known as *ringbinden*) contain a peripheral rim of sarcomeres oriented perpendicular to their normal orientation, resulting in peripheral radiating striations. Ring fibers are visible with many stains, both in frozen sections and in routinely processed sections. In either frozen or routine sections, they are best visualized in sections stained with PAS (Fig. 15-24, *A*) or iron hematoxylin. In humans, ring fibers are common in a specific form of inherited muscular dystrophy known as *myotonic dystrophy,* but they are also seen in other myopathic and in neuropathic conditions and therefore are not specific for myotonic dystrophy. Similarly,

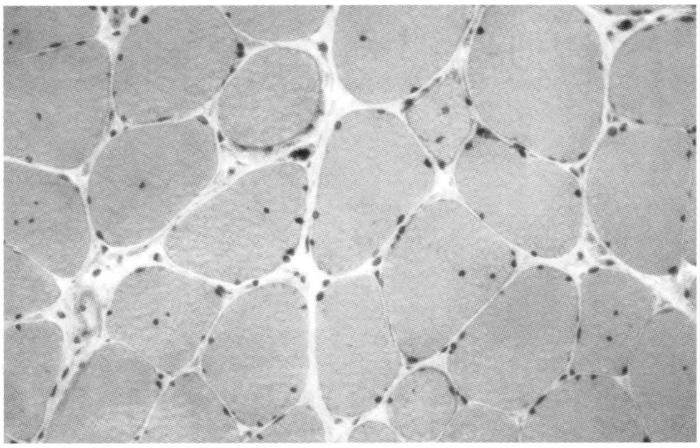

Fig. 15-23 Chronic myopathic change, medial triceps muscle, horse.
The variation in myofiber diameter and the presence of one or more internal nuclei in most myofibers are indicative of a chronic myopathic change. Frozen section, H&E stain. (Courtesy Dr. B.A. Valentine, College of Veterinary Medicine, Oregon State University.)

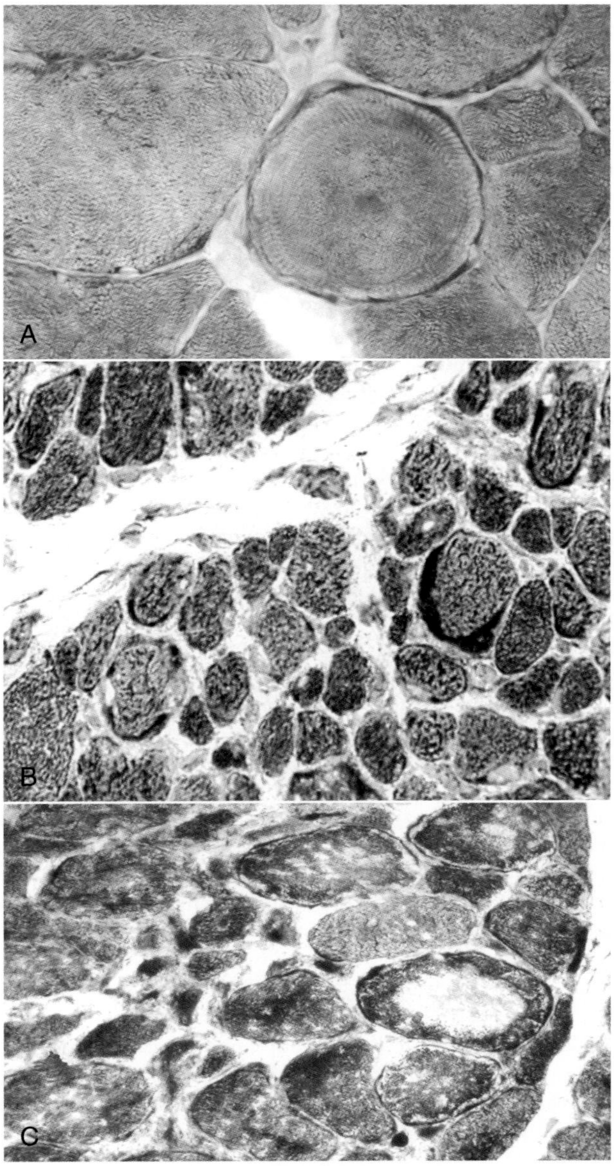

Fig. 15-24 Cytoarchitectural changes, skeletal muscle, transverse sections.
A, Ring fiber, extensor carpi radialis muscle, horse. A ring fiber is characterized by a peripheral rim of sarcomeres, arranged circumferentially around a myofiber and with their length at right angles to the long axis of the myofiber. Frozen section, PAS reaction. **B,** Irregular mitochondrial distribution with peripheral aggregates of mitochondria, Labrador centronuclear myopathy, temporalis muscle, dog. Frozen section, NADH reaction. **C,** Irregularity of mitochondrial distribution and "moth-eaten" fibers, polyneuropathy, dog. Fibers containing pale zones are characteristic of moth-eaten fibers. Frozen section, NADH reaction. (Courtesy Dr. B.A. Valentine, College of Veterinary Medicine, Oregon State University.)

there is no animal disorder in which ring fibers are specific, and these fibers can be seen in a variety of myopathic and neuropathic conditions such as ovine congenital muscular dystrophy. The presence of ring fibers can only be considered a chronic myopathic change. For example, numerous ring fibers were found in muscle from the contralateral weight-bearing limb from a horse with long-standing, non–weight-bearing foreleg lameness.

Other Cytoarchitectural Changes

Many other cytoarchitectural changes reflect alterations in mitochondrial density or integrity and are best appreciated on examination of frozen sections, in which mitochondria can be visualized, or on ultrastructural examination. The presence of peripheral aggregates of mitochondria, which stain red with modified Gomori's trichrome stain, form the basis of "ragged red" fibers. Ragged red fibers are a hallmark of mitochondrial myopathy in humans. In animals, however, ragged red fibers are common in various myopathic conditions and also occur in normal dog and horse muscle. Mitochondrial abnormalities are also detected by oxidative enzyme reactions such as NADH (Fig. 15-24, *B* and *C*) and SDH in frozen sections. Nemaline rods, formed by expansions of the Z-line material, stain purple to red with modified Gomori's trichrome stain in frozen sections. These rods can also be seen in animals with other myopathic conditions. Moth-eaten fibers contain multiple pale zones because of loss of mitochondrial oxidative enzyme activity on frozen sections and occur in denervating disorders and in myopathic conditions (Fig. 15-24, *C*). Sarcoplasmic masses are pale-staining zones usually at the periphery of myofibers, but occasionally central. These can be seen in H&E-stained muscle sections and appear as light blue areas with few or no myofibrils. Ultrastructurally they often contain disarrayed myofilaments with or without degenerate mitochondria. Other less commonly encountered alterations in animal muscle are pale central cores visible with mitochondrial stains, tubular aggregates composed of sarcotubular membranes, and target fibers in which mitochondrial oxidative enzyme reactions reveal central clear zones surrounded by a thin rim of highly reactive cytoplasm. Other less commonly encountered alterations in H&E-stained sections of animal muscle are pale central cores. As demonstrated in sections stained by mitochondrial oxidative enzyme reaction (e.g., SDH) these are of three types: (1) cores rich in mitochondria and similar to the peripheral sarcoplasmic masses described above; (2) target fibers so designated because of a pale center surrounded by a rim of densely staining mitochondria; and (3) aggregates of sarcotubular membranes that do not stain with mitochondrial stains.

CHRONIC MYOPATHIC CHANGE

Evaluation of abnormal skeletal muscle often reveals chronic myopathic change, which includes alterations in myofiber diameter, cytoarchitectural alterations, and interstitial fibrosis and fat infiltration (see Box 15-6). Chronic myopathic change accompanies a variety of myopathic and neuropathic conditions. In particularly severe cases, a definitive cause may not be identified. Chronic inflammation or denervation and chronic degenerative myopathy resulting in repeated bouts of myonecrosis and regeneration often cause diffuse endomysial and perimysial fibrosis (see Figs. 15-19, *B*, and 15-48, *B*). Interstitial infiltration of muscle by mature adipocytes is less common than fibrosis and occurs most commonly in chronically denervated muscle (see Fig. 15-19, *B*), particularly neonatal muscle that lacks appropriate innervation (Fig. 15-25). Fat infiltration can also occur because of severe chronic degenerative myopathy. A chronically damaged or denervated muscle that develops profound fibrosis and/or fat infiltration can be grossly

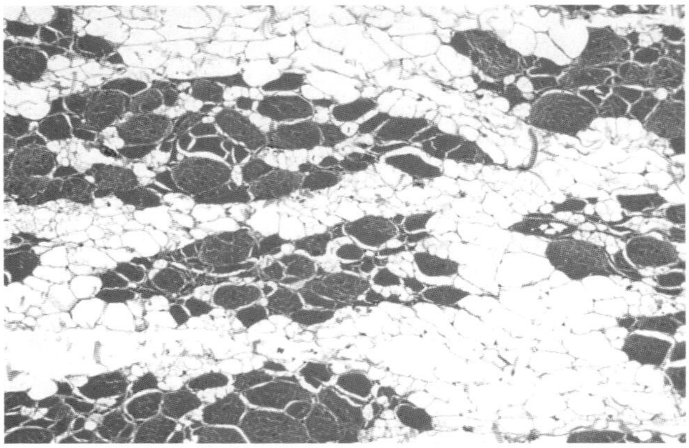

Fig. 15-25 Lipomatosis (steatosis), calf.
Lost myocytes have been replaced by mature adipocytes *(clear [nonstaining] areas)*. Islands of remaining myofibers have groups of angular atrophied fibers admixed with hypertrophied fibers, suggestive of denervation atrophy. Formalin fixation, H&E stain. (Courtesy Dr. M.D. McGavin, College of Veterinary Medicine, University of Tennessee.)

enlarged, despite atrophy or loss of myofibers—a condition known as *pseudohypertrophy* (see Fig. 15-9, *D*).

DISORDERS OF DOMESTIC ANIMALS

TYPES OF MUSCLE DISEASE

Classification of muscle diseases based on lesions alone is not very satisfactory, and many classifications are based on cause (e.g., toxic myopathy or nutritional myopathy). An example of such a classification is given in Table 15-2. Myopathic conditions can be inherited or acquired. Inherited disorders can affect muscle metabolism or myofiber structure. Acquired muscle disease in livestock is often associated with nutritional deficiency or with ingestion of myotoxins, whereas acquired muscle disease in the dog is most often caused by immune-mediated inflammatory conditions. Other causes of acquired myopathies include ischemia, infectious agents, hormonal or electrolyte abnormalities, and trauma. There are also many neuropathic conditions that result in denervation atrophy (see peripheral nerve discussion). More information on most of the disorders described in this section can also be found under the appropriate species heading or in Web Appendix 15-1.

Degenerative

Degenerative myopathies are those resulting in segmental or global myofiber necrosis in which inflammatory cells are not the cause of the myofiber damage.

Disturbance of Circulation

Given the numerous capillary anastomosis and rich collateral circulation of skeletal muscle, only disorders that result in occlusion of a major artery or that cause widespread intramuscular vascular damage will result in myofiber necrosis (Box 15-8). Vascular occlusion of a major artery, most often aortoiliac thrombosis, occurs most commonly in cats (thromboembolism) and horses (mural thrombosis). Intramuscular vascular damage occurs in many species, and there are a variety of causes.

The basic factor in determining the effect of ischemia on muscle is the differential susceptibility of the various cells forming the muscle as a whole. Myofibers are the most sensitive, satellite cells less sensitive, and fibroblasts the least sensitive to anoxia. Thus

TABLE 15-2 Classification of Muscle Disease

Classification	Cause or Type of Disorder
Degenerative	Ischemia Nutritional Toxic Exertional Traumatic
Inflammatory	Bacterial Viral Parasitic Immune-mediated
Congenital and/or inherited	Anatomic defects Muscular dystrophy Congenital myopathy Myotonia Metabolic Malignant hyperthermia
Endocrine	Hypothyroidism Hypercortisolism
Electrolyte	Hypokalemia Hypernatremia Other electrolyte imbalances
Neuropathic	Peripheral neuropathy Motor neuronopathy
Neuromuscular junction disorders	Myasthenia gravis Botulism Tick paralysis
Neoplasia	Primary tumors (rhabdomyoma, rhabdomyosarcoma) Secondary tumors (hemangiosarcoma, fibrosarcoma, infiltrative lipoma, other tumor phenotypes) Metastatic tumors

BOX 15-8 Causes of Muscle Ischemia

1. Occlusion of a major blood vessel
2. External pressure on a muscle
3. Swelling of a muscle in a nonexpandable compartment ("compartment syndrome")
4. Vasculitis/vasculopathy

obstruction of the blood supply to an area of muscle leads first to myofiber necrosis, then to death of satellite cells, and finally to the death of all cells, including the stromal cells. The size of skeletal muscle infarcts depends on the size of the vessel obstructed and the duration of blockage. Because of the numerous anastomoses, blockage of capillaries causes less severe ischemia but can result in segmental myofiber necrosis, which is usually multifocal and if the cause is ongoing, polyphasic, with regenerating and necrotic myofibers. However, when larger arteries are blocked, whole areas of muscle, including the satellite cells, are killed, resulting in a monophasic necrosis and healing by fibrosis. Ischemia can also cause peripheral nerve damage and neuropathy, leading to denervation atrophy of intact myofibers.

Increased intramuscular pressure can occur in a recumbent animal of sufficient weight after a prolonged period of recumbency, either because of disease or general anesthesia. Myofiber necrosis caused by recumbency can occur because of (1) decreased blood flow as a result of compression of major arteries, (2) reperfusion injury causing massive calcium influx into muscle cells when the animal moves or is moved and the compression relieved, (3) increased intramuscular pressure causing compartment syndrome (see later definition), or (4) any combination of these factors. Localized myonecrosis caused by recumbency is common in horses, cattle, and pigs; occurs only in large breeds of dogs; and is virtually unheard of in cats. In downer cows, the weight of the body of the animal in sternal recumbency can cause ischemia of the pectoral muscles and of any muscles of the forelimbs or hindlimbs that are tucked under the body. Ewes in advanced pregnancy with twins or triplets can develop an ischemic necrosis of the internal abdominal oblique muscle, which can lead to muscle rupture. Plaster casts or bandages that are too tight can put external pressure on muscles, leading to ischemia. The duration of ischemia determines the severity of necrosis and the success of regeneration (see the section on Necrosis and Regeneration). Postanesthetic myopathy is a monophasic, multifocal necrosis. In the downer cow, the lesions are multifocal to locally extensive (Fig. 15-26) and, depending on the duration since the onset of recumbency, can be either monophasic or polyphasic.

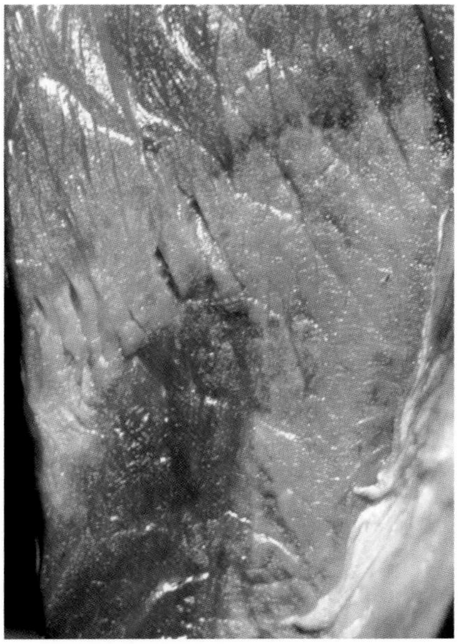

Fig. 15-26 Ischemic necrosis, downer cow syndrome, pectoral muscle, cow.
Increased intramuscular pressure during prolonged periods of recumbency has resulted in localized muscle pallor (lighter-colored areas of muscle) from myofiber necrosis secondary to decreased blood flow caused by compression of arteries. (Courtesy Dr. M.D. McGavin, College of Veterinary Medicine, University of Tennessee.)

Any severe insult, whether it be ischemia caused by recumbency or another myodegenerative disorder that causes myonecrosis within a muscle covered by a tight and nonexpansible fascia, can result in ischemic injury because early in the necrosis, there is increased intramuscular pressure. The resulting compromise of blood circulation leads to ischemic myodegeneration, which is known as *compartment syndrome.* The phenomenon of compartment syndrome is best illustrated in the anterior tibial muscle of humans after strenuous exercise. This condition is believed to be a consequence of swelling of the anterior tibial muscle, which is surrounded anteriorly by the inelastic anterior fascial sheath and posteriorly by the tibia. Swelling impedes blood supply, resulting in ischemia. A similar phenomenon occurs in muscles surrounded by tight fascia in animals, particularly horses. Horses that are recumbent because of general anesthesia can develop compartment syndrome affecting gluteal or lateral triceps muscles. Horses can also develop compartment syndrome in gluteal muscles because of exertional rhabdomyolysis and in temporal and masseter muscles because of selenium deficiency. Compartment syndrome is also possible in the temporal and masseter muscles of dogs with masticatory myositis.

Damage to intramuscular blood vessels will also cause myofiber necrosis. Vasculitis can cause areas of muscle damage (e.g., in horses with immune-mediated purpura hemorrhagica because of *Streptococcus equi* infection [see Fig. 15-33] and in pigs with erysipelas). Viral diseases that target blood vessels of many organs, such as bluetongue in sheep, can also affect muscle. Exotoxins produced by clostridial organisms cause myositis and severe localized vascular damage, leading to hemorrhage and myofiber necrosis (Table 15-3). The familial myopathy of Gelbvieh cattle is characterized by fibrinoid necrosis of intramuscular blood vessels and associated myonecrosis.

Nutritional Deficiency

Myofibers are particularly sensitive to nutritional deficiencies that result in the loss of antioxidant defense mechanisms. Nutritional myopathies are most common in livestock, including cattle, horses, sheep, and goats (Table 15-4). Although nutritional myopathy of livestock is often referred to as *selenium/vitamin E deficiency,* in the vast majority of cases, it is deficiency of selenium that is the cause of myofiber degeneration. The trace mineral selenium is a vital component of the glutathione peroxidase system, which helps to protect cells from oxidative injury. The high oxygen requirement combined with contractile activity makes striated muscle, both skeletal and cardiac, particularly sensitive to oxidative injury. Neonatal animals, which rely on stores of selenium accumulated during gestation, are most frequently affected. Affected muscle is pale as a result of necrosis (see Fig. 15-40); thus the common name *white muscle disease.* As should be evident from the previous discussion, a gross observation of pale muscle is not specific for necrosis caused by nutritional deficiency; therefore the term *nutritional myopathy* is much preferred.

TABLE 15-3 Clostridial Toxins Causing Muscle Damage

Toxin	Type	Action
α-Toxin	Calcium-dependent phospholipase	Hydrolyzes membrane phospholipids
θ-Toxin	Oxygen-labile cytotoxin (perfringolysin-O)	RBC and WBC lysis Induces platelet- activating factor leading to leukostasis and decreased tissue perfusion
κ-Toxin	Collagenase	Contributes to tissue lysis
μ-Toxin, γ- toxin	Hyaluronidases	Disruption of muscle integrity
ε-Toxin	Lipase	Lipid membrane lysis

RBC, Red blood cell; *WBC,* white blood cell.

TABLE 15-4 Nutritional and Toxic Myopathies

Disorder	Species Affected	Cause
Nutritional myopathy	Horses, cattle, sheep, goats, camelids, pigs	Selenium or (less commonly) vitamin E deficiency
Ionophore toxicity	Horses, cattle, sheep, goats, pigs	Monensin, other ionophores used as feed additives
Plant toxicity	Horses, cattle, sheep, goats, pigs	*Cassia occidentalis,* other toxic plants; gossypol in cottonseed products
Pasture-associated myopathy (United Kingdom, midwestern United States)	Horses	Unknown—possible clostridial or fungal toxin

Toxic Myopathies

Livestock are the animals most prone to develop a degenerative myopathy from the ingestion of a toxin (see Table 15-4). Myotoxins can be present in plants in pastures or hay and in plants or plant products in processed feed. Examples of toxic plants and plant products include *Cassia* (coffee senna), *Karwinskia* (coyotillo), *Eupatorium* (white snakeroot), *Thermopsis* spp., and gossypol present in cottonseed. Clinical signs are weakness, often leading to recumbency, and are accompanied by a moderate-to-severe increase in serum muscle enzyme concentrations. Gross and histologic findings of multifocal necrosis that can be either monophasic or polyphasic are typical. Diagnosis is based on identification of causative plants within feed, pasture, or stomach contents or when available, detection of toxic compounds in stomach content or liver.

Ionophore antibiotics, such as monensin, lasalocid, maduramicin, and narasin, are often added to ruminant feeds to enhance growth. Ionophores form lipid soluble dipolar reversible complexes with cations and allow movement of cations across cell membranes, often against the concentration gradient. This causes a disruption of ionic equilibrium that can be detrimental, especially to excitable tissue such as the nervous system, heart, and skeletal muscle. Ionophore toxicity results in calcium overload and death of skeletal (see Figs. 15-13, *B,* and 15-34) and cardiac muscle. Most domestic ruminants are quite tolerant of moderate ionophore levels, but toxicity occurs at very high levels. Most cases of ionophore toxicity involve the ingestion of monensin. The LD_{50} (the dose at which 50% of animals die) of monensin in cattle is 50 to 80 mg/kg, and the LD_{50} for sheep and goats is 12 to 24 mg/kg. Horses are exquisitely sensitive to ionophores and even very low levels are toxic, with an LD_{50} for monensin of only 2 to 3 mg/kg of body weight.

Exertional Myopathies

The ionic and physical events associated with myofiber contraction can under certain circumstances predispose a myofiber to necrosis. Exercise-induced myonecrosis, which can be massive, can occur because of simple overexertion. This outcome is well known in the capture and restraint of nondomesticated species, a syndrome known as *capture myopathy.* More often, however, exercise-induced myofiber damage occurs in animals with preexisting conditions such as selenium deficiency, muscular dystrophy, severe electrolyte depletion, or glycogen storage disease. The term *exertional rhabdomyolysis* (also known as *exertional myopathy, azoturia, setfast, blackwater, Monday morning disease,* and *tying up*) has long been applied to a syndrome recognized in horses (see Fig. 15-36). Only recently have underlying myopathic conditions been identified as the most common predisposing cause of equine exertional rhabdomyolysis (see the section on Muscular Disorders of the Horse). A similar disorder affects working dogs such as racing sled dogs and greyhounds, the cause of which is still unclear.

Trauma

External trauma to muscle includes crush injury, lacerations and surgical incisions, tearing caused by excessive stretching or exercise, burns, gunshot and arrow wounds, and certain injections. Some of these result in complete or partial rupture of a large muscle. The diaphragm is the most common muscle to rupture and in dogs and cats is most often the result of a sudden increase in intraabdominal pressure such as from being hit by a car. In horses, diaphragmatic rupture is thought to occur most often during falls in which the pressure of the abdominal viscera causes diaphragmatic damage. A partial rupture of a muscle results in a tear in the fascial sheath, through which the muscle can herniate during contraction. In racing greyhounds, spontaneous rupture of muscles, such as the longissimus, quadriceps, biceps femoris, gracilis, triceps brachii, and gastrocnemius, can occur during strenuous exercise. In horses, damage to the origin of the gastrocnemius muscle has been linked to overexertion during exercise or while struggling to rise. Tearing of muscle fibers occurs in the adductor muscles of the hind limbs of cattle doing the "splits" (sudden bilateral abduction) on a slippery floor. Because there is often extensive disruption of the myofibers' basal laminae, most of the healing is accomplished by fibrosis. If muscle trauma is accompanied by fractures of bones and the animal moves the limb, further trauma by laceration by sharp bone fragments can result.

An abnormal response to localized muscle trauma is thought to be a possible underlying cause of two uncommon reactions of muscle: myositis ossificans and musculoaponeurotic fibromatosis. The term *myositis ossificans* is a misnomer, as the lesion does not involve inflammation, but it has attained the status of acceptance by common usage. Myositis ossificans is a focal lesion usually confined to a single muscle and has been seen in horses, dogs, and humans. The lesion is essentially a focal zone of fibrosis with osseous metaplasia, often with a zonal pattern. The central zone contains proliferating undifferentiated cells and fibroblasts; the middle one, osteoblasts depositing osteoid and immature bone; and the outer one, trabecular bone, which may be being remodeled by osteoclasts. These lesions can cause pain and lameness, which are often cured by surgical excision. A connective tissue disorder in cats, fibrodysplasia ossificans progressiva, has been inappropriately called *myositis ossificans.* Musculoaponeurotic fibromatosis has so far been described only in horses and humans. It is a progressive intramuscular fibromatosis that has also been called a *desmoid tumor.* Musculoaponeurotic fibromatosis is not, however, considered to be a true neoplastic process. Progressive dissecting intramuscular fibrosis accompanied by myofiber atrophy are the characteristic features. In most cases, the extent of intramuscular involvement makes surgical excision impossible, although wide excision of early lesions has proved to be curative.

Inflammatory Myopathies (Myositis, Myositides [Plural])

In addition to the misnomer "myositis ossificans," the term *myositis* has been inappropriately applied to various other veterinary disorders, such as exertional and nutritional myopathy, in the horse. These two disorders are degenerative myopathies not inflammatory myopathies. It is vitally important to distinguish between a true myositis and a degenerative myopathy in which there is a secondary inflammatory response. In the normal response to the myofiber necrosis, the necrotic segment is infiltrated by macrophages recruited from the circulating monocyte population (see Figs. 15-14, *B,* and 15-15, *A*), which phagocytose the cellular debris. Severe acute necrotizing myopathy can also be accompanied by a certain degree of infiltrating lymphocytes, plasma cells, neutrophils, and eosinophils. Cytokines released from damaged muscle fibers are likely to recruit a variety of inflammatory cells under various circumstances, but these cells are not involved in causing the muscle cell damage. True myositis occurs only when inflammatory cells are directly responsible for initiating and maintaining myofiber injury and when inflammation is directed at the myofibers and not at the stroma. In some cases, it may take careful evaluation of the overall tissue changes, an understanding of the probable underlying cause, and years of experience with muscle pathology to differentiate a florid cellular response with macrophages on a "clean-up" mission from true inflammation. Lymphocytic myositis must also be distinguished from lymphoma involving skeletal muscle (see the section on Neoplasia).

TABLE 15-5 Bacterial Myopathies

Infectious Agent	Species Affected
Clostridium spp. causing myositis *(e.g. Cl. septicum, Cl. chauvoei,*	Horses, cattle, sheep, goats, pigs
Clostridium botulinum	Horses, cattle, sheep, goats, dogs
Pyogenic bacteria *(e.g., Arcanobacterium pyogenes, Corynebacterium pseudotuberculosis)*	Horses, cattle, sheep, goats, pigs, cats
Bacteria causing fibrosing and granulomatous lesions *(e.g., Actinomyces bovis, Actinobacillus lignieresii)*	Cattle, sheep, goats, pigs

Bacterial

Bacterial infections of muscle are not uncommon, particularly in livestock. Bacteria can cause suppurative and necrotizing, suppurative and fibrosing, hemorrhagic, or granulomatous lesions (Table 15-5). Bacterial infection can be introduced by direct penetration (wounds or injections), hematogenously, or by spread from an adjacent cellulitis, fasciitis, tendonitis, arthritis, or osteomyelitis (see the section on Portals of Entry).

Various clostridial species, particularly *Clostridium perfringens, Clostridium chauvoei, Clostridium septicum,* and *Clostridium novyi,* can elaborate toxins (see Table 15-3) that damage myofibers and intramuscular vasculature, resulting in hemorrhagic myonecrosis (see Figs. 15-32 and 15-38). Toxemia is typical and often lethal. *Clostridial myositis* is most common in cattle and horses. *Clostridial myositis* has also been called *gas gangrene* and *malignant edema* in horses and *blackleg* in cattle.

Pyogenic bacteria introduced into a muscle usually cause localized suppuration and myofiber necrosis. This may resolve completely or become localized to form an abscess. In some cases, the infection can spread down the fascial planes (see Fig. 15-12). For example, a nonsterile intramuscular injection into the gluteal muscles of cattle can cause an infection that extends down the fascial planes of the muscles of the femur and tibia and erupts to the surface through a sinus proximal to the tarsus. Although the majority of inflammation involves fascial planes, some bacteria extend into and cause necrosis of adjacent muscle fasciculi. *Streptococcus zooepidemicus* (horses), *Arcanobacterium pyogenes* (cattle and sheep), and *Corynebacterium pseudotuberculosis* (horses, sheep, and goats) are common causes of muscle abscesses. After bite wounds from other cats, cats can develop cellulitis caused by *Pasteurella multocida* that extends into the adjacent muscle.

Bacteria causing single or multiple granulomas (focal or multifocal granulomatous myositis) are relatively uncommon. Most such lesions are caused by *Mycobacterium bovis* (tuberculosis), usually in cattle and pigs, but this disease is rare in North America.

Chronic fibrosing nodular myositis of the tongue musculature in cattle is the result of infection with *Actinobacillus lignieresii* (wooden tongue) or *Actinomyces bovis* (the agent causing lumpy jaw). A similar lesion caused by *Staphylococcus aureus* is known as *botryomycosis* and is most commonly seen in horses and pigs. It is most often wound related and can occur at a variety of sites. Histologically, actinobacillosis, actinomycosis, and botryomycosis are similar in that the lesions are encapsulated inflammatory lesions containing a central focus of "radiating clubs" of amorphous eosinophilic material associated with bacteria and neutrophils (Splendore-Hoeppli reaction). Neutrophils admixed with macrophages (pyogranulomatous inflammation) can also be seen. Gram-stained tissue can be used to differentiate between the clusters of Gram-positive cocci in *Staphylococcus* infection, the Gram-positive bacilli causing actinomycosis *(Actinomyces bovis),* and the Gram-negative bacilli causing actinobacillosis *(Actinobacillus lignieresii).*

Viral

Relatively few of these are recognized in veterinary medicine. Spontaneous ones are listed in Table 15-6. Gross lesions may or may not be visible and if present, are small, poorly defined foci or streaks. Muscle lesions induced by viruses are either infarcts secondary to a vasculitis, as seen in bluetongue in sheep, or multifocal necrosis, presumably because of a direct effect of the virus on the myofibers.

Parasitic

Parasitic infections of the skeletal muscles of domestic animals are not uncommon and include protozoal organisms and nematodes. The most important ones are listed in Table 15-7 and are discussed under the appropriate species heading. Most parasitic diseases have little pathologic or economic importance, with the exceptions of *Neospora caninum, Hepatozoon americanum,* and *Trypanosoma cruzi* in dogs and *Trichinella spiralis* in pigs.

TABLE 15-6 Viral Myopathies

	RNA VIRUSES	
Disease	**Family**	**Causal Agent**
Porcine encephalomyelitis	Picornaviridae	Enterovirus
Foot-and-mouth disease	Picornaviridae	Aphthovirus
Bluetongue	Reoviridae	Orbivirus
Akabane disease	Bunyaviridae	Akabane virus

TABLE 15-7 Parasitic Myopathies

Infectious Agent	Type of agent	Species Affected
Sarcocystis spp.	Protozoan	Horses, cattle, sheep, goats, camelids, pigs
Trichinella spiralis	Nematode	Pigs
Neospora caninum	Protozoan	Dogs, fetal cattle
Trypanosoma cruzi	Protozoan	Dogs
Cysticercus spp.	Cestode (larval form)	Cattle, sheep, goats, pigs
Nematode larval migrans	Nematode	Dogs
Hepatozoon americanum	Protozoan	Dogs

As the name *Sarcocystis* suggests, intramyofiber protozoal cysts caused by *Sarcocystis* spp. are a common finding. This protozoal organism is a stage in the life cycle of an intestinal coccidium of carnivores that uses birds, reptiles, rodents, pigs, and herbivores as an intermediate host. Ingestion of oocysts by an intermediate host releases sporozoites that penetrate through the intestinal wall, enter blood vessels, and are hematogenously disseminated and invade tissue, including muscle. This parasite rarely causes clinical disease and is therefore most often considered an incidental finding. *Sarcocystis* infection of muscle is seen most often in horses, cattle, and small ruminants and occasionally in cats. Because they are intracellular, cysts are protected from the host's defense mechanisms; thus there is no inflammatory response (Fig. 15-27).

Immune-Mediated

Immunologically induced myositis, not associated with vascular injury, has been recognized primarily in the dog. Rarely, immune-mediated myositis occurs in cats and horses. Infiltrating lymphocytes, most often cytotoxic T lymphocytes, are the cause of myofiber injury. Although cytotoxic T lymphocytes are the effector cells causing myofiber damage, the inflammatory infiltrate is a mixture of lymphocyte types. The characteristic histologic pattern of immune-mediated myositis is an interstitial and perivascular lymphocytic infiltration (Fig. 15-28, *A,* see also Fig. 15-48), often with invasion of intact myofibers by lymphocytes (Fig. 15-28, *B*). A variety of forms of immune-mediated myositis occur in the dog and can be localized to specific muscles, presumably because of unique myosin isoforms within those muscles. These are listed in Table 15-8. Acquired myasthenia gravis is also an immune-mediated disease and is included in this table for completeness, but this is a disorder causing damage to the neuromuscular junction rather than to myofibers. In cats, feline immunodeficiency virus infection is a cause of immune-mediated myositis. In horses, lesions consistent with immune-mediated myositis are occasionally found after exposure to *Streptococcus equi* ssp. *equi* or infection with equine influenza virus. It should be pointed out that small perivascular and interstitial infiltrates of lymphocytes, with no apparent myofiber damage, are a frequent incidental finding in equine muscle.

Immune-mediated vasculitis resulting in muscle injury occurs in horses and is known as *purpura hemorrhagica.* Purpura hemorrhagica has been classically associated with *Streptococcus equi* ssp. *equi*, but other bacteria, such as *Corynebacterium pseudotuberculosis,* can also cause purpura hemorrhagica.

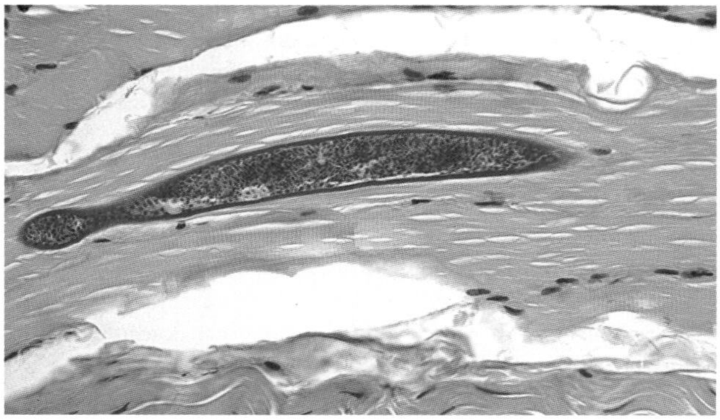

Fig. 15-27 Sarcocystosis, skeletal muscle, longitudinal section, cow. The elongate encysted intramyofiber protozoan is characteristic of *Sarcocystis* spp. There is no associated inflammation. These parasites are common in the muscles of many species of domestic animals and are usually an incidental finding. Formalin fixation, H&E stain. (Courtesy Dr. M.D. McGavin, College of Veterinary Medicine, University of Tennessee.)

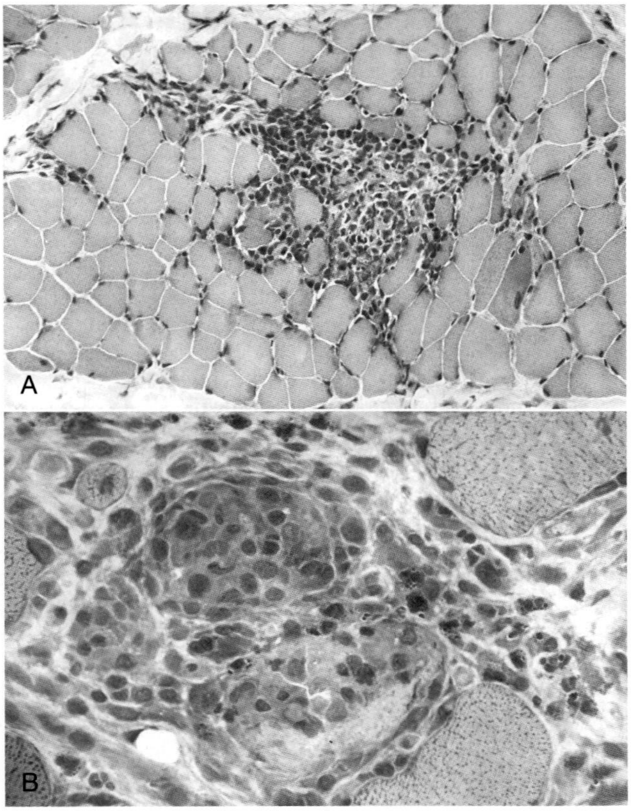

Fig. 15-28 Immune-mediated myositis, canine polymyositis, skeletal muscle, transverse sections, dog.
A, There is a dense interstitial infiltrate of primarily mononuclear inflammatory cells. Formalin fixation, H&E stain. **B,** Note the interstitial infiltrate of mononuclear inflammatory cells and mononuclear cells that have invaded intact myofibers causing myofiber necrosis. Frozen section, modified Gomori's trichrome stain. (**A** courtesy Dr. M.D. McGavin, College of Veterinary Medicine, University of Tennessee. **B** courtesy Dr. B.J. Cooper, College of Veterinary Medicine, Oregon State University.)

TABLE 15-8 Immune-Mediated Muscle Disorders

Disorder	Species Affected
Purpura hemorrhagica	Horses
Viral-associated	Horses, cats
Polymyositis	Dogs, horses (rare)
Masticatory myositis	Dogs
Extraocular muscle myositis	Dogs
Acquired myasthenia gravis	Dogs, cats

Congenital and Inherited Disorders

Muscle is subject to numerous hereditary, congenital, and neonatal defects (Web Table 15-2). Muscular disorders that are apparent at birth are congenital, but they may or may not be inherited. Inherited disorders can manifest at birth or soon thereafter, or they may not be apparent for many years. Molecular biologic studies and development of molecular genetic tests have greatly enhanced our understanding of several muscular disorders of animals and the ability to detect affected and carrier animals.

Anatomic Defects

Anatomic defects in skeletal muscle are apparent at birth or soon thereafter. These defects can be either genetic or acquired and result from either abnormal in utero muscle development or abnormal innervation.

Innervation Defects

Congenital defects in the lower motor neuron system, involving motor neurons or peripheral nerves, result in severe alteration of myofiber development. Denervation occurring in fetal and neonatal animals can result in very complex muscle lesions because of the importance of innervation in myofiber development and maturation. Depending on the nature of the nervous system defect, muscular lesions can reflect failure of innervation, denervation of previously innervated fibers, or a combination of both. The most common example of this is arthrogryposis in cattle and sheep in which in utero infection or toxin ingestion causes nervous system lesions that lead to failure of innervation or to denervation of skeletal muscle. Additionally, a disorder thought to have a genetic basis has been reported in black Angus cattle and results in failure of innervation of skeletal muscle. Failure of innervation or severe denervation injury in utero most often result in failure of the myofibers to develop and their subsequent replacement by adipose tissue (fatty infiltration). This outcome can be severe in affected muscle and may be the basis for some cases of congenital muscular steatosis in livestock (see Figs. 15-9, *D,* and 15-25).

Genetic Defects

Congenital muscular hyperplasia (double muscling) is a genetic disease causing a congenital anatomic skeletal muscle defect (increased number of myofibers) in cattle, dogs, and children. This disorder is caused by defects in the myostatin gene, which controls in utero muscle development. There is more information on this disease in Web Appendix 15-1. With continued selective breeding and advancement in molecular biologic techniques, it is likely that other genetic defects affecting muscle structure may occur or be recognized.

Failure of Normal Development

In addition to failure of myofiber maturation caused by innervation defects, inherent myofibrillar developmental defects can occur. This is exemplified by myofibrillar hypoplasia causing splay leg in neonatal pigs. A similar condition has been reported in a calf.

Congenital defects in the diaphragmatic muscle (diaphragmatic hernia) can occur in all species but are most well documented in dogs and rabbits. A genetic basis with a multifactorial inheritance is suspected. Clinical signs of respiratory distress caused by herniation of abdominal viscera into the thoracic cavity generally occur at or shortly after birth. Defects in the left dorsolateral and central portions of the diaphragm because of failure of closure of the left pleuroperitoneal canal are most common.

Muscular Dystrophy

The term *muscular dystrophy* has been grossly misused in the veterinary literature. In the 1930s, the term *nutritional muscular dystrophy* was applied to a disease more appropriately classified as nutritional myopathy, and the misuse of this term has been a source of confusion for years as to exactly what is meant by muscular dystrophy. Using the definition applied to humans, muscular dystrophy is an inherited, progressive, degenerative primary disease of the myofiber characterized histologically by ongoing myofiber necrosis and regeneration (polyphasic necrosis). Several types of muscular dystrophy occur in humans and animals. The enormous recent advances in genetic and molecular characterization of muscle diseases have resulted in defining their exact genetic defects, such as those in the dystrophin gene responsible for Duchenne's muscular dystrophy and trinucleotide repeat sequences in myotonic dystrophy, and in the reclassification of others. Similarly, reevaluation of some inherited disorders previously classified as muscular dystrophy, such as muscular dystrophy in sheep and cattle, suggests that they would be better classified as progressive congenital myopathies.

Congenital Myopathies

Those inherited disorders of muscle that do not qualify as anatomic defects, muscular dystrophy, myotonia, or a metabolic myopathy (see later discussion) are classified as congenital myopathies. These include structural defects leading to abnormal myofiber cytoarchitecture. In some cases, the defective gene is known, whereas the cause of others remains undetermined.

Myotonia (Channelopathies)

Myotonia is defined as the inability of skeletal muscle fibers to relax, resulting in spasmodic contraction. Various inherited myotonic conditions have been recognized in humans and animals for many years. Only recently has the basis for many of these myopathies been determined. Most have been found to be related to inherited defects resulting in abnormal ion channel function. Maintenance of ionic equilibrium and control of the ionic fluxes of excitable tissue, such as muscle, are critical to normal muscle functioning. A variety of sarcolemmal ion channels exist that control fluxes of ions such as sodium, potassium, chloride, and calcium. Defective sodium or chloride channels most often result in myotonia.

Metabolic Myopathies

Inherited disorders of muscle metabolism (see Web Table 15-2) are characterized by reduced muscle cell energy production. Clinical signs include exercise intolerance, exercise-induced muscle cramps, and rhabdomyolysis (acute segmental myofiber necrosis). Metabolic defects can involve glycogen metabolism, fatty acid metabolism, or mitochondrial function. Metabolic disorders often cause increased blood lactate after exercise. Inheritance patterns vary. Glycolytic, glycogenolytic, and nonmitochondrial DNA–encoded enzyme defects are generally inherited in an autosomal recessive manner. Defects involving mitochondrial DNA–encoded enzymes are inherited through the dam because all mitochondria are contributed by the oocyte.

The pathways of glycolysis and glycogenolysis are complex, involving a cascade of enzymatic reactions. Deficiency of a glycolytic or glycogenolytic enzyme leads to accumulation of glycogen and in some cases glycogen-related proteoglycans. There are many different types of glycogen storage diseases and their categorization is dependent on which enzyme is deficient. Of the types of glycogenoses recognized in humans, five types (II, III, IV, V, and VII) cause glycogen accumulation in muscle. Of the glycogenoses affecting muscle, only types II (acid maltase deficiency), IV (glycogen branching enzyme deficiency), V (myophosphorylase deficiency), and VII (phosphofructokinase deficiency) have so far been recognized in animals. Storage diseases in which glycogen accumulates in muscle have been described in horses, cattle, sheep, dogs, and cats.

Inherited lipid storage myopathies have not yet been described in animals, although dogs appear to have a predilection for development of neuromuscular weakness because of acquired lipid storage myopathy with concurrent reduction in skeletal muscle carnitine activity. Mitochondrial myopathies are rarely recognized in animals, perhaps because of the difficulty in confirming mitochondrial defects. A few such disorders have been described in dogs, and a mitochondrial myopathy has been reported in one Arabian horse. Mitochondrial disorders may affect only muscle, or muscle involvement may be part of an encephalomyopathic condition.

Malignant Hyperthermia (MH)

MH is a condition characterized by unregulated release of calcium from the sarcoplasmic reticulum, leading to excessive myofiber contraction that generates heat, resulting in a severe increase in body temperature. MH is often fatal. In humans, pigs, horses, and dogs, a congenital defect in the sarcoplasmic reticulum calcium-release channel, the ryanodine receptor, causes dysregulation of excitation-contraction coupling leading to MH. Episodes in affected individuals can be triggered by general anesthetic agents, especially halothane, or by stress, thus the name *porcine stress syndrome* for the disorder in pigs (see Fig. 15-43).

A MH-like condition can also occur because of other myopathic conditions, especially those that result in uncoupling of mitochondrial oxidative phosphorylation from the electron transport chain. Inherently uncoupled mitochondria within brown fat are the physiologic basis for production of heat during breakdown of this fat in neonates, and pathologically uncoupled or loosely coupled mitochondria in muscle as a result of an underlying myopathy release energy as heat.

Gross and microscopic lesions are described in the discussion on the disorder in the section on Disorders of Pigs.

Endocrine and Electrolyte Abnormalities

Various endocrinologic abnormalities can result in myopathic conditions (Table 15-9). The most common are hypercortisolism and hypothyroidism in dogs. In horses, pituitary hyperfunction resulting in Cushing's disease also causes muscle disease. In most cases of endocrine myopathy, the end result is myofiber atrophy, particularly of type 2 fibers. A unique syndrome of muscle hypertrophy and pseudomyotonia occurs in dogs associated with hypercortisolism. Endocrine myopathies can also be complicated by the fact that endocrinopathy can also cause pathologic changes in peripheral nerves, leading to a mixture of myopathic (type 2 fiber atrophy) and neuropathic changes (denervation atrophy and alteration in fiber-type pattern) within muscle. Denervation followed by reinnervation leading to fiber-type grouping can be seen in dogs with chronic hypercortisolism (see Fig. 15-20, *B*) and hypothyroidism.

Normal electrolyte status is vital to normal skeletal muscle function. Hypocalcemia, hypokalemia, hypernatremia, and hypophosphatemia can cause profound skeletal muscle weakness, sometimes associated with myofiber necrosis, in various species.

TABLE 15-9 Myopathies Caused by Endocrine and Electrolyte Abnormalities

Disorder	Species Affected
Hypothyroidism	Dogs
Hypercortisolism	Dogs
Hypokalemia	Cattle, cats
Hypophosphatemia	Cattle
Hypernatremia	Cats
Hypocalcemia	Cattle
Hypothalamic/pituitary dysfunction	Horses

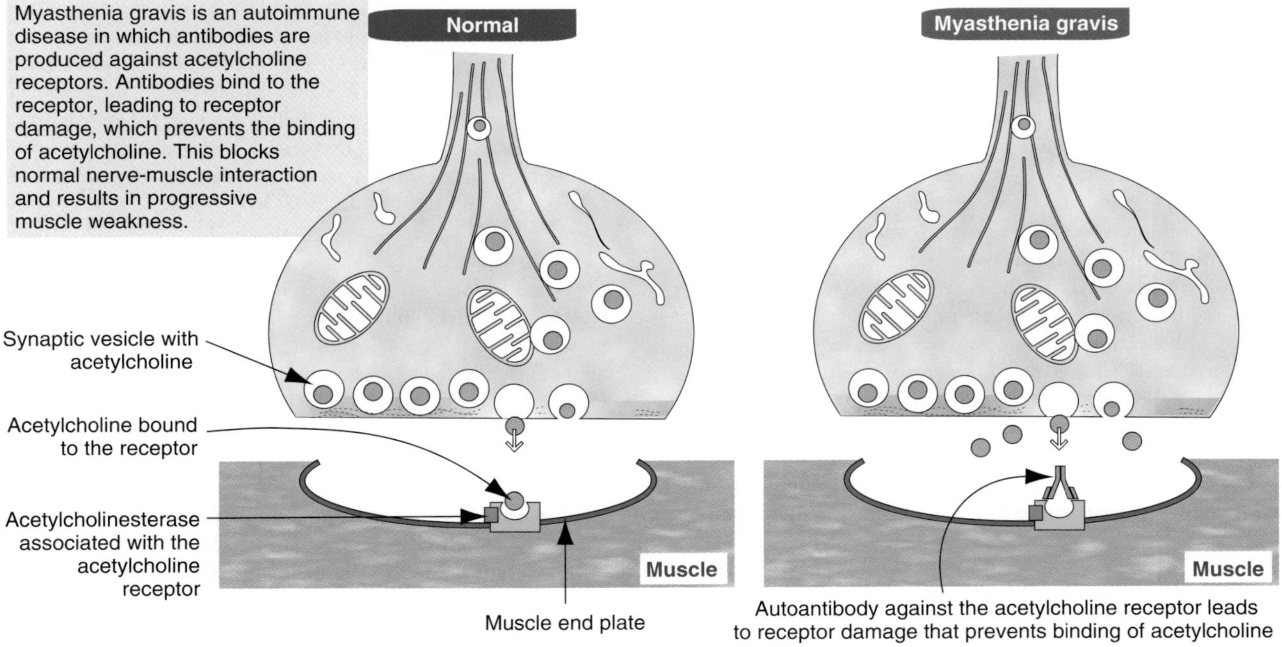

Fig. 15-29 Schematic diagram of the pathogenesis of acquired (autoimmune) myasthenia gravis. (Modified from Kierszenbaum AL: *Histology and cell biology: an introduction to pathology,* ed 2, St Louis, 2006, Mosby.)

Neuropathic and Neuromuscular Junction Disorders

Dysfunction of the lower motor neurons, peripheral nerves, or neuromuscular junction can have profound effects on muscle function.

Neuropathic Disorders

There are many peripheral nerve disorders and a few motor neuron disorders that can lead to denervation atrophy of muscle in animals. These can be inherited or acquired. Long nerves, such as the sciatic and left recurrent laryngeal nerves, appear to be particularly sensitive to development of acquired neuropathy. Many of the peripheral nerve disorders of animals are discussed in Chapter 14. Characteristic features of denervation atrophy are described in the section on Responses of Muscle to Injury.

Neuromuscular Junction Disorders

The neuromuscular junction is a modification of the postsynaptic myofiber membrane. At the neuromuscular junction, the membrane is folded to increase surface area and is studded with specialized ion channels known as *acetylcholine receptors.* After arrival of an action potential at the distal end of a motor nerve, the terminal axons release acetylcholine, which diffuses across the synaptic space to bind to the acetylcholine receptors. Binding opens these channels, leading to sodium influx, which initiates the skeletal muscle action potential that culminates in muscle contraction. Acetylcholine is rapidly degraded by acetylcholinesterase released from the postsynaptic membrane, which prevents continued stimulation and thus contraction of the muscle fiber.

Disorders that impair the ability of nerve impulses to travel across the neuromuscular junction have profound effects on skeletal muscle function. Technically, however, the myofibers are still innervated, so denervation atrophy does not occur and no light microscopic abnormalities in the muscle or nerve are present. Various neurotoxins (i.e., in snake and spider venom and in curare-containing plants) and drugs can affect the neuromuscular junction, but the most common neuromuscular junction disorders affecting animals are myasthenia gravis, botulism, and tick paralysis.

Myasthenia Gravis

Myasthenia gravis can be either acquired or congenital. Acquired myasthenia gravis is an immune-mediated disorder caused by circulating autoantibodies against skeletal muscle acetylcholine receptors (Fig. 15-29). Binding of these antibodies to the acetylcholine receptor on the postsynaptic membrane leads to a severe decrease in the number of functional receptors. The mechanisms by which antibodies damage these receptors are (1) direct damage to the neuromuscular junction, which may be visible with electron microscopy as simplification of the folding of the membrane, and (2) formation of cross-linked antibodies leading to receptor internalization. Sufficient functional acetylcholine receptors are present to initially allow normal neuromuscular transmission, but if there is sustained muscular activity the decrease in the number of available receptors leads to progressive weakness and collapse. Therefore acquired myasthenia gravis results in episodic collapse, and repetitive nerve stimulation causes a characteristic rapid decrease in amplitude of the muscle compound motor action potential. Diagnosis of myasthenia gravis can also be made after intravenous injection of cholinesterase inhibitors such as edrophonium chloride (Tensilon, ICN Pharmaceuticals, Costa Mesa, CA) in collapsed animals. The reduction in cholinesterase activity leads to more active acetylcholine being available within the synapse and rapid, although transient, restoration of skeletal muscle contraction. Detection of autoantibodies to acetylcholine receptors in the blood confirms the diagnosis of acquired myasthenia gravis.

The origin of the autoantibodies causing myasthenia gravis is not always known, but there is a strong link between thymic abnormalities and development of myasthenia gravis in both humans and animals. Specialized cells within the thymic medulla, known as *myoid cells,* express skeletal muscle proteins, including those of the acetylcholine receptor. It is thought that these cells participate in development of self-tolerance. Abnormalities of the thymus, most commonly thymoma in animals and thymic follicular hyperplasia in humans, can lead to loss of self-tolerance to acetylcholine receptors. In such cases, removal of the abnormal thymus can result in restoration of normal neuromuscular junction activity. When thymic abnormalities are not present, treatment with long-acting anticholinesterase agents and in some cases immunosuppressive agents, such as corticosteroids, is necessary.

Congenital myasthenia gravis is an inherited disorder that is much less common than acquired myasthenia gravis. To date it has been described only in humans, dogs, and cats. Animals with congenital myasthenia gravis are born with defective neuromuscular junctions that often have a decreased membrane surface area, best visualized with electron microscopy, and as a consequence an inherently reduced acetylcholine receptor density. Such animals may be normal at birth because there are sufficient functional acetylcholine receptors to support muscle contraction in a neonate. But, with rapid postnatal growth, clinical signs of profound, sustained, and progressive weakness occur as a consequence of insufficient functional receptors to support the function of growing muscles.

Botulism

Botulism is a neuromuscular disorder caused by the exotoxin of the bacterium *Clostridium botulinum.* Botulinum toxin is considered one of the deadliest of the known toxins. Botulism is characterized by profound generalized flaccid paralysis. Seven serologically distinct but structurally similar forms of botulinum toxin are designated A, B, C, D, E, F, and G. Sensitivity to these toxin types varies among different species. Dogs are most sensitive to type C toxin, ruminants to types C and D, and horses to types B and C.

Botulinum toxin consists of a light chain and a heavy chain linked by a disulfide bond. Binding of botulinum toxin to receptors on the presynaptic terminals of peripheral nerves is followed by endocytosis of the toxin. Within the endocytotic vesicle of the terminal nerve, the disulfide bond is cleaved, and the released light chain is translocated into the axonal cytoplasm (see Fig. 4-27). Botulinum toxin light chains are metalloproteinases. Numerous proteins are involved in the release of acetylcholine from presynaptic vesicles, and botulinum toxin blocks release of acetylcholine by irreversible enzymatic cleavage of one or more of these proteins. Different forms of botulinum toxin affect different proteins, but the end result is the same. Active neuromuscular junctions are the most sensitive, which has led to the use of low concentrations of locally injected botulinum toxin as a treatment for localized muscular disorders resulting in spasm.

Clostridium botulinum spores are commonly present in the gastrointestinal tract of animals and in the soil. Under favorable anaerobic and alkalinic conditions, these spores become active, with resultant toxin production. Botulism can occur because of ingestion of preformed toxin, such as in feed contaminated by dead rodents or soil-borne organisms, or from toxin produced by *Clostridium botulinum* organisms within the gastrointestinal tract or superficial wounds (Box 15-9). Dogs and cats are the species most likely to ingest dead rodents containing botulinum toxin and are quite resistant to developing botulism. In veterinary medicine, horses are the most sensitive to botulinum toxin. Death of horses, most often the result of respiratory muscle paralysis, can result from exposure to only very small amounts of botulinum toxin. The damage to presynaptic axon terminals is irreversible, and recovery from botulism occurs only after terminal axon sprouting and reestablishment of new functioning synapses.

BOX 15-9 Portals of Entry—Equine Botulism

Gastrointestinal colonization of ingesta: Foals up to 6 months of age
Ingestion of preformed botulinum toxin: Adults, usually from rodent carcasses in hay or concentrated feed, or environmental contamination
Wound contamination: Adults, deep wounds, uncommon

Tick Paralysis

Dermacentor and *Ixodes* ticks can elaborate a toxin that also blocks release of acetylcholine from axon terminals. Tick paralysis is seen most often in dogs and children. Recovery after tick removal can be rapid (within 24 to 48 hours), indicating that the mechanism of toxin action in tick paralysis does not result in irreversible presynaptic damage and thus is different from that of botulinum toxin.

Neoplasia

Neoplasms involving skeletal muscle are most often those that arise within the muscle or its supporting structures or that invade muscle from adjacent tissue. Neoplasms metastatic to muscle are rare.

Primary Muscle Tumors

Tumors with striated muscle differentiation are thought to arise from intramuscular pluripotential stem cells rather than from satellite cells. These tumors are uncommon and are either benign (rhabdomyoma) or malignant (rhabdomyosarcoma [Fig. 15-30]). Primary intramuscular tumors can also arise from fibrous tissue, vasculature, or neural elements. The most common tumor to arise from muscle-supporting structures is hemangiosarcoma.

Rhabdomyoma and Rhabdomyosarcoma

Tumors of striated muscle that occur at sites other than within muscle are rhabdomyomas of the heart or lung and botryoid rhabdomyosarcomas of the urinary bladder; these are not discussed in this section. Rhabdomyoma and rhabdomyosarcoma arising within skeletal muscle are most common in the dog, followed by the horse and cat. Morphologic variants include round cell, spindle cell, and mixed round and spindle cell, reflecting the developmental stages of skeletal muscle. Historically, diagnosis of tumors of skeletal muscle has relied on identification of cross striations indicative of sarcomeric differentiation. Cross striations are most often seen in elongated multinucleate cells known as *strap cells* (Fig. 15-30, *C*) and in ovoid cells known as *racquet cells.* They are most easily recognized after staining with phosphotungstic acid hematoxylin (PTAH) stain, but the search for cross striations can be extremely frustrating and often unrewarding. These days the diagnosis of tumors of skeletal muscle origin relies primarily on results of immunohistochemical examination using antibodies for muscle-specific proteins. Muscle actin and desmin are expressed by smooth and skeletal muscle tumors, but myoglobin, sarcomeric actin, myogenin, and MyoD1 are specific for skeletal muscle. Evidence of muscle differentiation, such as primitive myofilaments and Z-band structures, can also be detected by electron microscopy.

Rhabdomyoma is most often a round cell tumor and occurs most commonly in the larynx of adult dogs. The youngest reported age is 2 years. Tumors are generally smooth and nodular, pink, and unencapsulated. Histologic features are closely packed plump round cells that have central euchromatic nuclei, generally with a single prominent nucleus, and abundant vacuolated to granular eosinophilic cytoplasm. A small number of multinucleate and elongate strap cells can also be seen. Mitoses are rare, and evidence of invasion is uncommon.

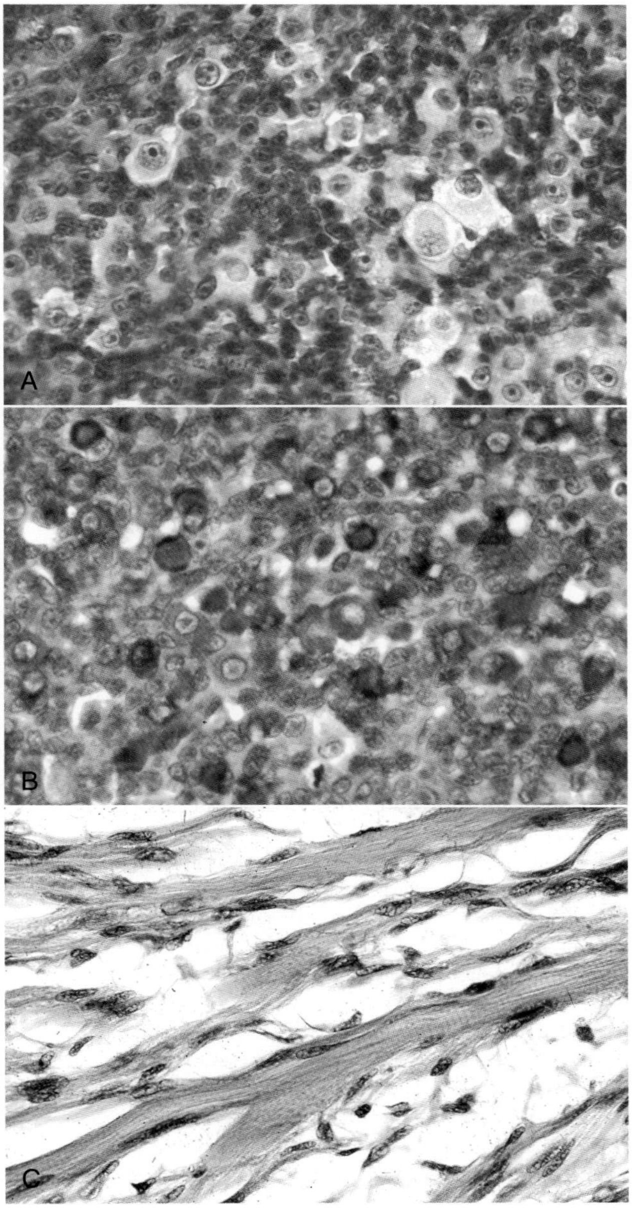

Fig. 15-30 Rhabdomyosarcoma.
A, Skeletal muscle, cat. An admixture of small round basophilic cells with a lesser number of larger round cells with prominent eosinophilic cytoplasm is characteristic of embryonal rhabdomyosarcoma. Nuclei are central and euchromatic, most often with a single large nucleolus. H&E stain. **B,** Immunostaining reaction of the same rhabdomyosarcoma as depicted in **A,** showing intense cytoplasmic expression of desmin in many tumor cells, indicative of muscle origin (skeletal, cardiac, or smooth). These cells also express myoglobin and sarcomeric actin (not shown), which differentiates skeletal muscle tumors from smooth muscle tumors. Immunoperoxidase reaction for desmin. **C,** Botryoid rhabdomyosarcoma, urinary bladder, large breed dog. Cross-striations, characteristic of a well-differentiated rhabdomyosarcoma, are present in the elongated multinucleate tumor cells. H&E stain. (**A** and **B** courtesy College of Veterinary Medicine, Cornell University. **C** courtesy Dr. B.A. Valentine, College of Veterinary Medicine, Oregon State University.)

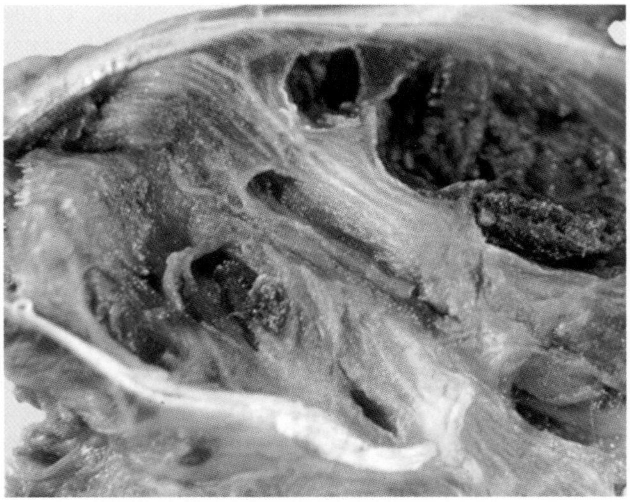

Fig. 15-31 Intramuscular hemangiosarcoma, cervical skeletal muscle, horse.
Multiple irregular zones of cavitated *(upper right)* to solid tumor with hemorrhage have replaced normal muscle. Formalin-fixed specimen. (Courtesy Dr. A. de Lahunta, College of Veterinary Medicine, Cornell University.)

Similar to the situation in humans, rhabdomyosarcomas in animals most often occur at a young age and are most common in the neck or oral cavity, especially in the tongue. These tumors are pink and fleshy, and they often have prominent local invasion. The most common and most distinctive form of rhabdomyosarcoma in animals is embryonal rhabdomyosarcoma, composed of primitive round cells with prominent euchromatic nuclei, a single prominent nucleolus, and either indistinct or prominent eosinophilic cytoplasm ("rhabdomyoblasts"; see Fig. 15-30, *A* and *B*). Rhabdomyosarcoma can also contain elongate multinucleate strap cells (see Fig. 15-30, *C*) and ovoid racquet cells. Cellular and nuclear pleomorphism is common, as is mitotic activity. These tumors are locally invasive and frequently metastasize, although too few cases have been studied to document any pattern of metastasis.

Hemangiosarcoma

Malignant vascular neoplasms (hemangiosarcoma) arising within muscle are most common in the horse and dog (Fig. 15-31). Clinical signs include swelling within a muscle, often with associated lameness. Cytologic preparations frequently reveal only peripheral blood, which is suggestive of a hematoma. Pathologic diagnosis can be difficult if multiple sites within the lesion are not sampled, as the amount of hemorrhage often far exceeds the area composed of proliferating neoplastic endothelial cells. Intramuscular hemangiosarcoma has a high incidence of metastasis, often to the lungs.

Other Tumors Involving Skeletal Muscle

A variant of lipoma, known as infiltrative lipoma, is often located in skeletal muscle. Characteristic gross pathologic and histopathologic findings are mature adipocytes invading skeletal muscle. This tumor is most common in the dog but has also been reported in young horses. Wide excision is the treatment of choice because this tumor recurs as a result of local invasion, but it does not metastasize.

Infiltration of skeletal muscle by neoplastic lymphocytes is not uncommon. Neoplastic lymphocytic infiltrates surround myofibers and can cause myofiber atrophy. These cells do not invade myofibers, however, and myonecrosis is rare. This helps to distinguish intramuscular lymphoma from lymphocytic myositis. Careful examination of infiltrating neoplastic cells typically reveals a relatively monomorphic population of lymphocytes, which may be atypical in appearance. Immunohistochemistry to confirm a single infiltrating cell type is also useful.

Vaccine-associated sarcoma in the muscle of the cat can arise within an intramuscular vaccination site or extend into underlying skeletal muscle from a subcutaneous injection site. Occasionally, mast cell tumors and carcinomas exhibit prominent skeletal muscle invasion. Melanoma arising in the skin of older gray horses often metastasizes to muscle fascia and may exhibit some extension into the muscle itself. Intramuscular metastasis of tumors is rare (see the section on Defense Mechanisms). Intramuscular metastasis of carcinoma, particularly prostatic, can occur in dogs. When carcinomas with areas of sclerosis involve muscle, either by extension or by metastasis, the muscle basement membrane of adjacent myofibers is typically destroyed, often resulting in bizarre multinucleate cells representing attempts at muscle regeneration (see Fig. 15-17). These bizarre cells should not be misidentified as tumor cells.

DISORDERS OF DOMESTIC ANIMALS BY SPECIES

Adequate muscle function is essential for the survival of any species. Many domestic animals have been selectively bred for improved musculature for meat production, performance, or appearance. Therefore muscle disease in animals can have a significant economic impact. In some cases, it is selection pressure imposed by humans that has resulted in development and perpetuation of various myopathic conditions in animals. It is likely that continued selection for what appears to be a phenotypically desirable trait will lead to the recognition of new genetic mutations and myopathic conditions in the future.

It is interesting to compare the effects of muscular disorders that affect humans and animals. The four-footed stance of animals allows for greater stability, which can allow an animal to remain ambulatory for some time, when a similarly affected person would be confined to a wheelchair. However, disorders that result in recumbency, even if it is transitory, can be devastating in livestock. It is much more difficult to nurse a large animal through a period of recumbency than it would be for a hospitalized human or small animal.

The most common and important muscle disorders of animals are discussed by species because this is the way diseases are considered clinically. The same disease may occur in different species. Details of less common muscle disorders are presented in Web Appendix 15-1.

DISORDERS OF HORSES

There is perhaps no other domestic animal species for which optimal muscle development and function is so critical as the horse. Selective breeding for better muscling has occurred in virtually all horse and pony breeds. The ability of such selection pressure to perpetuate equine muscle mutations is exemplified by the relatively recent occurrence of hyperkalemic periodic paralysis (HYPP), in which a muscle mutation results in visually appealing increased muscle bulk and definition. Unfortunately, as you will see in the discussion of HYPP later, such mutations do not often result in improved muscle function.

Bacterial and Parasitic Myopathies

Infection by various bacterial organisms and clostridial toxins can cause myopathy in the horse. Protozoa (*Sarcocystis* spp.) are common incidental findings in equine muscle, but *Sarcocystis*-induced muscle damage resulting in clinical signs of muscle disease is rare.

Clostridial Myositis (Malignant Edema; Gas Gangrene)

Clostridial myositis in the horse is an often fatal disorder caused by infection by various toxin-producing clostridial species, which are large Gram-positive anaerobic bacilli. *Clostridium septicum* is the most common cause of clostridial myositis in horses, but *Clostridium perfringens* types A to E, *Clostridium chauvoei, Clostridium novyi, and Clostridium fallax* can also cause infection. Infection can involve more than one clostridial species. *Clostridium* spp. are ubiquitous organisms that form spores within the soil and within the gastrointestinal tract. Unlike cattle, in which nonpenetrating trauma can cause muscle bruising and anaerobic conditions that activate clostridial spores already in the muscle, clostridial myositis in horses is virtually always secondary to a penetrating wound. Most often, this is an injection site of a nonantibiotic substance, but infection of sites of puncture wounds and of perivascular leakage of irritants in intravenously administered compounds are also possible. It is also possible that clostridial bacteria entering the blood from an injured gastrointestinal tract can colonize damaged muscle. This is one possible explanation for the frequent occurrence of signs of colic before development of clostridial myositis at the site of intramuscular injection of medications such as flunixin meglumine that cause localized muscle damage. Under anaerobic conditions, clostridia proliferate and produce toxins that damage blood vessels, resulting in hemorrhage and edema, and cause necrosis of adjacent muscle fibers (see Table 15-3).

Clinical signs are acute onset of heat, swelling, and pain within a muscle group and adjacent fascia, with concurrent fever, depression, dehydration, and anorexia. If sufficient muscle necrosis is present, serum CK and AST concentrations may be mildly to moderately increased. Death from toxemia and/or septicemia often occurs within 48 hours. Affected muscle and adjacent fascia are swollen and often hemorrhagic, with edema, suppurative inflammation, and necrosis; gas may also be present (Fig. 15-32). Vasculitis is not seen. Gram-positive bacilli characteristic of *Clostridium* spp. are generally demonstrable within affected tissue.

The diagnosis can be made with reasonable certainty based on typical historic, gross pathologic, cytologic, and histopathologic findings. *Clostridium* spp. can also be identified by culture under anaerobic conditions or by a fluorescent antibody test. Treatment must be initiated rapidly and includes surgical incisions into affected muscle to allow drainage and oxygenation, antibiotic therapy, and supportive care.

Botulism

Technically, this disease is a neuromuscular junction disorder and is included in this section for convenience. Botulism is caused by *Clostridium botulinum* toxin and is often not associated with *Clostridium botulinum* infection. The portals of entry of botulinum toxin in horses are summarized in Box 15-9. *Clostridium botulinum* bacteria are found as spores within the gastrointestinal tract of many mammals, and spores are common in the soil. Preformed toxin within contaminated feed or soil is the most common cause of botulism in adult horses. However, in foals, usually between 1 week and 6 months of age, ingestion of *Clostridium botulinum* spores can lead to proliferation of toxin-producing *Clostridium botulinum* within the intestinal tract, resulting in toxicoinfectious botulism (shaker foals). Wound infection is an uncommon cause of botulism in horses.

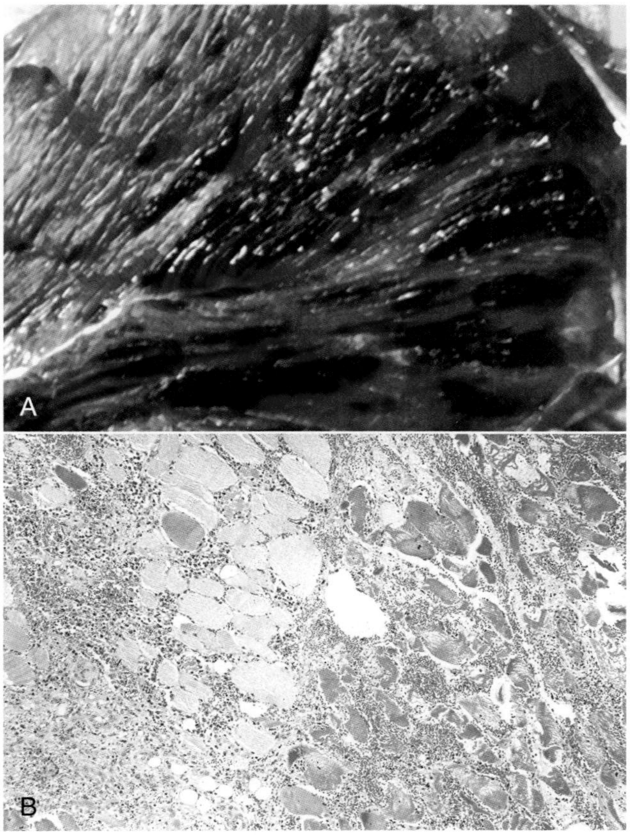

Fig. 15-32 Clostridial myositis, malignant edema, horse. **A,** *Clostridium septicum* is the most common cause of clostridial myositis in horses. Affected muscle *(shown here)* and adjacent fascia *(not shown here)* are swollen and often hemorrhagic. **B,** Interstitial edema, hemorrhage, and inflammatory cells surround numerous swollen and fragmented necrotic myofibers. Formalin fixation, H&E stain. (**A** courtesy College of Veterinary Medicine, Cornell University. **B** courtesy Dr. B.A. Valentine, College of Veterinary Medicine, Oregon State University.)

The pathogenesis of botulism has been previously discussed in the section on Neuropathic and Neuromuscular Junction Disorders). Irreversible binding of toxin to presynaptic nerve terminals and blockage of acetylcholine release lead to the profound generalized flaccid paralysis that is the hallmark of botulism. Clinical signs are acute and progress rapidly, generally resulting in recumbency. Dysphagia and tongue weakness are common findings that help to distinguish botulism from other neuromuscular diseases causing recumbency. Serum concentrations of CK and AST are within normal limits (indicating the absence of damage to myofibers) or are possibly slightly increased as a result of ischemic myopathy secondary to recumbency (see later discussion).

No specific gross or histopathologic lesions are present in horses dying with botulism, although aspiration pneumonia caused by dysphagia can occur. Muscle fibers are intact unless recumbency has compromised their blood supply, causing ischemia and localized myofiber necrosis.

Evaluation of stomach contents or contaminated feed may reveal the presence of toxin. However, horses are exquisitely sensitive to botulinum toxin, and since only a small concentration of the toxin may be present in an affected horse, available tests may not detect such a low concentration of toxin. In most equine cases, the diagnosis is made based on the clinical history after elimination of other possible causes of profound muscular weakness. Affected animals should be treated with polyvalent botulinum antitoxin to prevent further binding of toxin. Recovery occurs after terminal axon sprouting and reestablishment of functional neuromuscular junctions. Vaccination with botulinum toxoid is an effective preventive measure.

Corynebacterium pseudotuberculosis *(Pigeon Fever)*

Intramuscular abscesses caused by *Corynebacterium pseudotuberculosis* occur almost exclusively in horses in arid regions of the western United States and Brazil. *Corynebacterium pseudotuberculosis* is a Gram-positive pleomorphic facultative anaerobic bacillus present within the soil. It can enter muscle via penetrating wounds, including injection sites. The biotype most common in horses is different from that which affects sheep and goats because it is unable to reduce nitrates to nitrites. The high lipid content of the bacterial cell wall contributes to the survival of *C. pseudotuberculosis* within macrophages. Bacterial exotoxins, such as phospholipase D, contribute to vascular damage and inhibition of neutrophil function. Equine infections occur most frequently during the fall and early winter, and a higher incidence of the disease is often seen after rainy winters. Infections are most common in the pectoral musculature, but other locations are possible. Affected muscles are swollen and edematous and contain variably sized zones of localized suppurative inflammation. Fever is common. The causative agent is readily isolated from affected tissue and can be seen in aspirates from intramuscular abscesses. Treatment is generally curative and includes antibiotic therapy and establishment of drainage of abscesses. Rarely, infection with *Corynebacterium pseudotuberculosis* in horses leads to immune-mediated vasculitis (purpura hemorrhagica; see next section).

Streptococcal-Associated Myopathies

Two distinct degenerative myopathies are associated with infection or exposure of the horse to *Streptococcus equi* ssp. *equi.* One, known as *purpura hemorrhagica,* has been recognized for many years. The other, known as *streptococcal-associated rhabdomyolysis and muscle atrophy,* has only recently been recognized.

Purpura Hemorrhagica

In this disease, muscle damage is not caused by the direct infection of the muscles but rather by an immune response to the bacterial pathogen. *Streptococcus equi* is the most common cause of purpura hemorrhagica in horses, but *Corynebacterium pseudotuberculosis* and possibly other bacteria can also cause purpura hemorrhagica. In cases caused by *Streptococcus equi*, circulating immune complexes composed of immunoglobulin A (IgA) antibodies and streptococcal M antigen deposit in the walls of small vessels. This leads to vasculitis and vascular wall necrosis (Fig. 15-33), with resultant hemorrhage and infarction of myofibers. It is also possible that antibodies to streptococcal M protein cross-react with skeletal and cardiac muscle myosins to cause direct injury.

Signs of myopathy often accompany systemic signs of post-streptococcal purpura in horses (i.e., depression, fever, dependent edema, petechiae or ecchymoses, leukocytosis, increased serum fibrinogen, and anemia), but myopathy can also be the primary presenting disease process. Affected horses are weak, may have a short-strided gait, and can become recumbent. Myoglobinuria and very high increases in serum concentrations of CK and AST are common.

Multiple muscles are involved (as opposed to the locally extensive lesion of clostridial myositis), and affected muscles contain multifocal to locally extensive hemorrhage and edema that dissects between necrotic muscle fibers and muscle fasciculi. Gross

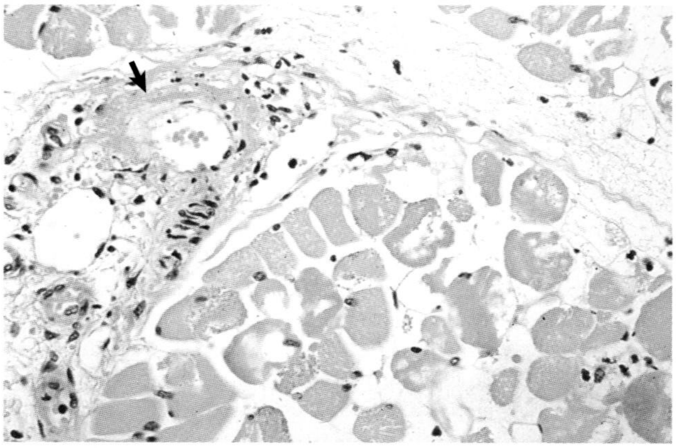

Fig. 15-33 Intramuscular vasculitis, purpura hemorrhagica, skeletal muscle, transverse section, horse.
In the wall of the blood vessel *(arrow)* is a band of circumferential fibrinoid necrosis containing nuclear debris. Many of the adjacent myofibers are necrotic *(center to lower right areas)*. Some of these myofibers are fragmented, and a small number contain fine basophilic deposits of mineral. Formalin fixation, H&E stain. (Courtesy Dr. B.A. Valentine, College of Veterinary Medicine, Oregon State University.)

pathologic findings are similar to those seen in clostridial myositis (see Fig. 15-32, *A*), but lesions do not contain gas bubbles. Vascular injury (leukocytoclastic vasculitis and fibrinoid necrosis of blood vessels; see Fig. 15-33) is seen on microscopic examination and is the diagnostic feature.

Diagnosis is based on a history of exposure of the horse to *Streptococcus equi* and the typical clinical, clinicopathologic, and histopathologic findings. Because this is an immune-complex disorder, histopathology, cytology, and bacterial cultures of affected muscle do not reveal *Streptococcus equi*. This bacterium or other causative bacteria may be cultured from other affected tissues, especially lymph nodes or guttural pouch. A high serum titer to *Streptococcus equi* M protein is strongly supportive of a diagnosis of streptococcal-associated purpura hemorrhagica. Treatment includes corticosteroid therapy and supportive care, but horses frequently succumb to other sequelae of systemic vasculitis, such as gastrointestinal infarcts.

Streptococcal-Associated Rhabdomyolysis and Muscle Atrophy

A syndrome of severe acute rhabdomyolysis resulting in profound rapidly progressive generalized loss of muscle mass has also been seen in horses with clinical infection by *Streptococcus equi* or in horses that have been exposed to this bacterium but that did not develop obvious clinical signs of infection. This syndrome occurs most frequently in young to young adult quarter horses, but young horses of other breeds can also be affected. Clinically recognizable muscle atrophy is often most evident in paraspinal and gluteal muscles. Some cases have microscopic evidence of concurrent EPSSM (see the section on Inherited or Congenital Myopathies), which may be a predisposing factor. In others, nonsuppurative perivascular and interstitial inflammation has been detected, and the proposed mechanism is immune-mediated damage caused by cross-reaction of streptococcal antibodies with muscle proteins. Affected horses do not show typical signs of purpura hemorrhagica but often have very high serum concentrations of CK (often greater than 100,000 units per liter) and AST (often greater than 10,000 units per liter). Affected horses may respond to corticosteroid therapy. Most will recover, but recurrence after subsequent exposure to *Streptococcus equi* is possible.

Protozoal Myopathy

Protozoa (*Sarcocystis* spp.) are common incidental findings in equine skeletal and cardiac muscles. As the protozoa are in cysts within the myofiber itself and thus are protected from the body's surveillance, there is no inflammatory response. Massive infection by *Sarcocystis fayeri* is suspected of causing a degenerative myopathy in horses, but this is rare. Rarely, localized thickening of the tongue has been found in horses with granulomatous myositis, the result of sarcocystis organisms within tongue musculature. The cause of the intense inflammation apparently incited by protozoa in these rare cases is unknown.

Ear Tick–Associated Muscle Spasms

Episodic muscle spasms of various muscle groups can occur in horses with ear ticks *(Otobius megnini)*. The mechanism is not known. Dimpling of affected muscles after percussion can be seen, but myotonic discharges are not found with electromyography. Treatment for ear ticks results in rapid recovery.

Nutritional and Toxic Myopathies

Nutritional deficiency, most often of selenium, and various toxins are relatively common causes of degenerative myopathy in the horse.

Nutritional Myopathy

Foals (most commonly up to 2 weeks of age) and young adult horses are most susceptible to nutritional myopathy because of a deficiency of the antioxidants selenium or (less commonly) vitamin E. In severely selenium-deficient areas, such as the Pacific Northwest, selenium deficiency myopathy can occur in horses of any age. Normally the selenium present in the soil is taken up by growing plants. In many areas, the soil is selenium deficient, and selenium supplements to the animal's ration must be provided. Vitamin E deficiency occurs in horses that eat marginal- to poor-quality grass hay and have little or no access to pasture and no supplemental vitamin E. Oxidative injury to actively contracting muscle fibers occurs as a result of a lack of antioxidant activity.

Affected foals are most likely to be those born to selenium-deficient mares. Foals have generalized weakness, which may be present at birth or become apparent soon after birth. Affected foals may become recumbent but are generally bright and alert. They often continue to suckle if bottle fed, but weakness of the tongue and pharyngeal muscles can lead to weak suckling.

Affected adult horses are most often stabled horses fed only selenium-deficient hay, with clinical disease being seen most commonly in the late winter or early spring. In the Pacific Northwest, selenium deficiency myopathy can occur in adult horses fed only pasture or hay, and it can occur at any time of year. Affected adult horses often show preferential involvement of the temporal and masseter muscles (the condition is sometimes inappropriately termed *maxillary myositis* or *masseter myositis*) with swelling and stiffness of these muscles and impaired mastication. Involvement of pharyngeal muscle results in dysphagia and involvement of the tongue results in impaired prehension of food, which can be mistaken for botulism. In more chronic cases, bilaterally symmetric atrophy of the masseter muscles may be evident, which can be mistaken for atrophy secondary to protozoal myeloencephalitis. Careful examination of these horses often reveals generalized weakness, evident as a stiff, short-strided gait. Severely affected horses can have an acute onset of recumbency that mimics neurologic disease.

Serum concentrations of CK and AST are generally mildly to moderately increased, although extremely high concentrations can be seen in severely affected foals and horses. Concentric needle EMG of affected muscles results in abnormal spontaneous activity (positive sharp waves, fibrillations, and myotonic bursts).

Muscles of affected horses appear pale (hence the common name white muscle disease), often in a patchy distribution (see Fig. 15-40). The most severely affected muscles are those that have the highest workload (e.g., cervical muscles in foals used during suckling and "bumping" the udder, proximal limb muscles, tongue, and masticatory muscles). The gross appearance depends on the extent of the necrosis and the stage. In early stages, yellow and white streaks are present, and later pale, chalk white streaks often appear. Horses with impaired swallowing can have cranioventral aspiration pneumonia. Severely selenium-deficient foals and horses also have pale areas of necrosis within the myocardium, especially the left ventricular wall and septum, which are areas that have a high workload. The stage of the necrosis depends on the age of the lesions. In foals with severe, acute myopathy leading to death or euthanasia, lesions are at the stage of massive muscle necrosis and mineralization with minimal macrophage infiltration (monophasic). In animals that have lived longer (i.e., subacute cases), the lesions are polyphasic, and active necrosis, macrophage infiltration, and regeneration are present. Although type 1 fibers may be more likely to develop necrosis because of nutritional myopathy, in severely affected muscles almost all fiber types are affected. In cases with myocardial involvement, myocardiocyte necrosis and mineralization are present. If the animal survives, the necrotic myocardiocytes are replaced by fibrovascular connective tissue that matures to form a scar.

A provisional diagnosis of nutritional myopathy is based on typical history, increases in serum concentrations of CK and AST, and characteristic gross and histopathologic findings. The diagnosis is confirmed by detecting deficient concentrations of selenium or vitamin E in blood of live animals or in liver samples obtained at necropsy. If horses live long enough, myofiber regeneration can restore the muscles to normal. This disorder in foals can be prevented by supplementing the ration of mares with selenium during gestation. Foals born in selenium-deficient areas can also be given injectable vitamin E and selenium soon after birth. Young adult horses should be given sufficient dietary vitamin E and selenium. Treatment with selenium and vitamin E after the onset of clinical signs is far less effective than prevention.

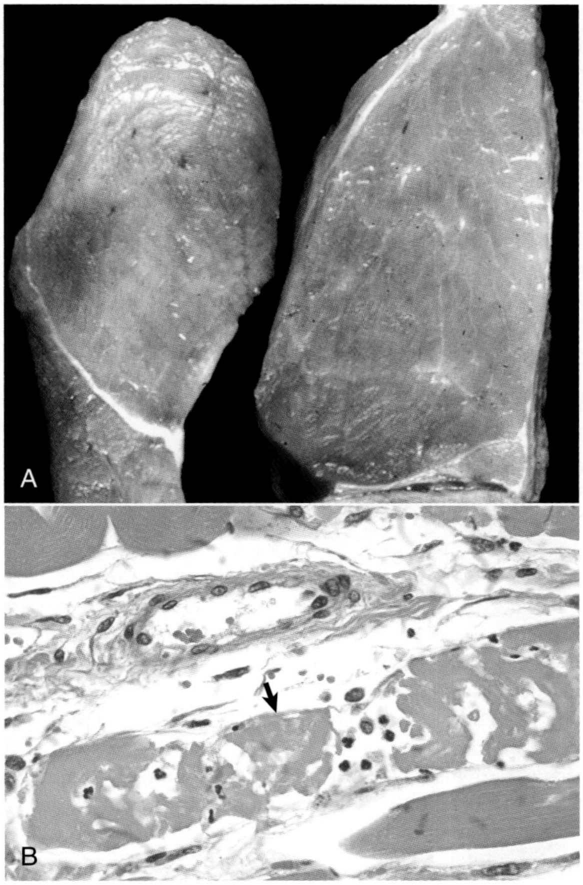

Fig. 15-34 Ionophore toxicity, monensin, skeletal muscle.
A, Necrosis. The pale white to gray foci are areas of necrotic myofibers. Myocardium will often contain similar lesions. **B,** Segmental myofiber necrosis (2 days old), longitudinal section, horse. The segment of myofiber *(arrow)* visible here is necrotic, fragmented, and infiltrated by macrophages and neutrophils. Note the intact basal lamina and endomysium on both sides of the myofiber, which will contain the regenerating myofiber and thus facilitate resolution. Ionophore toxicity results in calcium overload and death of skeletal (also cardiac) myocytes. Formalin fixation, H&E stain. (**A** courtesy Dr. J. Wright, College of Veterinary Medicine, North Carolina State University; and Noah's Arkive, College of Veterinary Medicine, The University of Georgia. **B** courtesy Dr. M.D. McGavin, College of Veterinary Medicine, University of Tennessee.)

Ionophore Toxicity

The pathogenesis of ionophore toxicity is discussed in the section on Toxic Myopathies. Horses are exquisitely sensitive to ionophores and succumb to very small doses. Ionophores may be present as contaminants within horse feed, or the horse may be accidentally fed ionophore-containing feeds intended for other domestic animals.

Most of the available literature relates to monensin toxicity, but the effects of other ionophores should be similar. In acute monensin toxicity, death occurs because of shock and cardiovascular collapse, and no specific lesions are seen on postmortem examination within the first 48 hours, although these may be stained diffusely pink by myoglobin. If the horse survives 3 to 4 days, affected skeletal and cardiac muscles often contain pale streaks (Fig. 15-34, *A*) and, microscopically, cardiac muscle necrosis and segmental necrosis of skeletal muscle is present (Fig. 15-34, *B*; see Fig. 15-13, *B*), with concurrent increases in serum concentrations of CK and AST, which may be severe. Given the profound sensitivity of horses to ionophores, ionophore toxicity in horses is typically the result of a single dose and thus the lesion is a monophasic multifocal process. This helps to differentiate ionophore toxicity from nutritional myopathy, which is often polyphasic. Both type 1 and type 2 fibers are affected. If the horse survives, necrosis is followed by myofiber regeneration, which can restore the muscles to normal, but necrotic myocardiocytes are replaced by fibrosis because of the lack of significant regeneration by myocardiocytes. Horses dying at 14 days after ionophore exposure often have normal skeletal muscles and extensive myocardial fibrosis. Acute cardiac failure and death because of myocardial scarring can occur months to years after apparent clinical recovery from ionophore exposure.

Diagnosis is based on a history that includes both ingestion of ionophores and the presence of the characteristic gross or histopathologic findings. Analysis of feed or stomach contents for ionophores is definitive. Treatment for ionophore-intoxicated horses is supportive, as there is no specific therapy.

Plant Toxicities

A number of toxic plants are known to cause muscle necrosis in horses (see also Toxic Myopathies). These include *Cassia occidentalis* (coffee senna) and *Thermopsis* spp. Most plant-associated toxicities in horses are associated with plants growing in pastures or in baled hay. Necrosis is most often polyphasic indicating a prolonged period of ingestion. Cardiac myonecrosis may or may not also be present. In the United Kingdom and less commonly in the midwestern United States, a syndrome of pasture-associated myonecrosis has been documented in horses. The cause of this disorder, also known as *atypical myoglobinurium,* is still unknown. Clostridial toxins (specifically *Clostridium sordellii* and *Clostridium bifermentans*) and environmental mycotoxins are considered possible causes.

Inherited or Congenital Myopathies and Myotonic Disorders

Hyperkalemic Periodic Paralysis

Hyperkalemic periodic paralysis (HYPP) is a myotonic disorder that affects horses whose ancestry traces back to a quarter-horse stallion named *Impressive.* Affected horses generally have remarkably well-defined muscle groups, which has led to their popularity for showing in halter. The disease is inherited as an autosomal dominant disease; therefore affected horses can be either heterozygotes or homozygotes. Homozygous foals often have a distinctive laryngeal muscle dysfunction that results in laryngospasm and labored breathing. Most homozygous horses do not survive; if they do, they are invalids.

The underlying defect in HYPP is a point mutation in the gene encoding the α subunit of the skeletal muscle sodium channel. This defect causes abnormal (delayed) inactivation of sodium channel activity, resulting in membrane instability and continuous muscle fiber electrical activity, which is reflected in EMG findings (see later discussion). The pathogenesis of clinical signs of HYPP is complex and not entirely understood, either in horses or in humans with a similar disorder. Affected heterozygotes have a mosaic of abnormal and normal sodium channels, and resting muscle membrane potentials are typically lower than normal. This leads to an increased likelihood of electrical generation of a prolonged muscle action potential, resulting in transient myotonia. When abnormal sodium channels are activated, the response to the resulting abnormally increased intracellular sodium is release of potassium into the extracellular space and bloodstream, resulting in hyperkalemia. Hyperkalemia is not, however, a consistent finding. Feeding of high potassium feeds, such as alfalfa products or feeds with added molasses, can precipitate clinical signs of HYPP, possibly by activating abnormal sodium channels. Another potential consequence of prolonged activation of abnormal sodium channels is inactivation of normal sodium channels, resulting in flaccid paralysis and collapse. This result would explain the typical signs seen during episodes, which include transient muscle spasm (myotonia), with protrusion of the third eyelid, followed by generalized flaccid paralysis. Decreased muscle temperature, as can occur as a result of a chilling rain, can precipitate episodic collapse in HYPP horses, possibly by decreasing the activity of the muscle sodium-potassium exchanger (the Na-K ATPase), an important means by which affected muscle compensates for abnormal sodium channel activity. Postanesthetic recumbency and anesthesia-associated hyperthermia have also been seen in HYPP horses. Affected horses can appear normal for many years, can have multiple episodes of collapse, or can die acutely. Serum concentrations of CK and AST are generally normal. Abnormal ionic fluxes occur at all times in affected horses, and concentric needle EMG between paralytic episodes reveals characteristic persistent myotonic bursts.

There are no gross pathologic findings in HYPP horses other than gross prominent muscling. Skeletal muscle dysfunction in HYPP horses is due to abnormal ionic fluxes that can lead to spasms and weakness, therefore affected skeletal muscle is generally histologically normal. In some cases, scattered intracytoplasmic vacuoles (vacuolar myopathy) can be present in type 2 fibers. The characteristic pathologic finding of HYPP is only evident at the ultrastructural level, where dilated terminal cisternae of the sarcoplasmic reticulum are found.

Diagnosis can be made with reasonable certainty based on characteristic clinical signs (muscle spasms often leading to flaccid paralysis) and clinicopathologic findings (hyperkalemia) in a horse of Impressive line breeding. Myotonic bursts with concentric needle EMG are also diagnostic. The simplest and most reliable test, however, is a DNA-based test performed on peripheral white blood cells or, as described more recently, on cells obtained from the base of pulled mane or tail hairs. Treatment consists of feeding a low-potassium diet, which means avoiding alfalfa products and molasses. A low-potassium diet can be successful in controlling signs in many cases. More severe cases can be treated with the diuretic acetazolamide, which causes increased urinary excretion of potassium. Acute episodes can be treated with intravenous dextrose or insulin or oral sugar solutions such as sugar syrup. Administration of glucose to stimulate insulin secretion, or of insulin itself, aids in alleviating signs by helping drive the intracellular movement of potassium along with glucose.

Equine Polysaccharide Storage Myopathy (EPSSM)

EPSSM is a myopathy most commonly recognized in quarter horse, warm blood, Arabian, Morgan, pony of the Americas, and draft-related breeds. It also occurs in many other horse and pony breeds, including miniature horses. Surveys of equine muscle samples have revealed an astonishingly high incidence of approximately 66% in all draft-related horses and approximately 30% in all light horses. Not all affected horses exhibit obvious clinical signs of muscle dysfunction. This disorder is inherited as an autosomal dominant trait.

In contrast to other glycogenoses affecting skeletal muscle, to date no abnormality in the glycolytic or glycogenolytic pathways in skeletal muscle has been identified, making this equine disorder unique, but an underlying carbohydrate metabolic disorder is still suspected. Affected horses appear to have a more rapid intramuscular uptake of blood glucose than controls, although the exact mechanism for this phenomenon is still unknown. A point mutation in the skeletal muscle glycogen synthase 1 (GYS1) gene has recently been associated with some, but not all, cases of EPSSM. A DNA test for this mutation is available. Abnormal accumulation of intracytoplasmic glycogen (confirmed by being PAS-positive, amylase-sensitive) within type 2 fibers is the histologic finding. In severe cases, aggregates of abnormal glycogen are eventually ubiquitinated, resulting in amylase-resistant inclusions composed of glycogen and filamentous protein. Certain breeds, such as quarter horse and draft-related breeds, seem to be most prone to the development of amylase-resistant inclusions, whereas glycogen aggregates are more common in other breeds. The explanation for this difference is as yet unknown, although breeds prone to developing amylase-resistant inclusions are also those breeds most likely to have the GYS1 mutation.

Clinical signs are variable, but all are thought to be caused by insufficient energy production by affected muscle fibers. Abnormal myofiber function caused by architectural alteration secondary to intramyofiber deposition of complex polysaccharide is also a possible mechanism, but the excellent response to therapy, even in horses with severe intramyofiber inclusions of accumulated polysaccharide, suggests that this is less significant than is altered energy metabolism. Recurrent exertional rhabdomyolysis (see later discussion) is a commonly recognized sign, but unexplained pelvic limb lameness is even more common than clinical rhabdomyolysis. Affected horses can also have a stiff gait, symmetric muscle atrophy, back soreness, muscle-cramping resulting in abnormal hindlimb flexion characteristic of shivers, and bilateral pelvic limb or generalized weakness. In draft horses, sudden onset of spontaneous recumbency or postanesthetic recumbency because of myopathy can occur. Serum concentrations of CK and AST are markedly increased after episodes of exertional rhabdomyolysis but may be only mildly to moderately increased in affected horses after exercise or onset of recumbency. Normal serum concentrations of CK and AST in affected horses are thought to indicate that the muscle dysfunction is not accompanied by overt myonecrosis. Concentric needle EMG may reveal abnormal spontaneous activity (scattered positive sharp waves and fibrillations).

In severe cases, in which horses have died or been euthanatized because of rhabdomyolysis or recumbency, muscles may be pale pink or diffusely red-tinged (myoglobin staining), which can be mistaken for autolysis. Multifocal pale zones may be present (see Fig. 15-36, *A*). In draft horses and sporadically in horses of other breeds, chronic myopathy can result in overall reduction in muscle mass. Muscles in severely affected draft horses can also be of normal size but may contain pale streaks where myofibers have been replaced by fat. The most severely affected muscles are those of the proximal hind limb (especially gluteal, semimembranosus, and semitendinosus muscles) and epaxial muscles of the back (e.g., longissimus), although any of the large "power" muscle groups, including pectoral and shoulder girdle muscles, can be affected. Swollen, dark kidneys (pigmentary nephrosis) caused by myoglobinuria can be seen in horses dying with severe rhabdomyolysis. The extent of overt myofiber necrosis is extremely variable; massive necrosis or regeneration can be seen after severe rhabdomyolysis, whereas only minimal scattered necrotic fibers may be seen in recumbent horses. Lesions are monophasic if there has been only a single bout of exertional rhabdomyolysis, or polyphasic if there have been repeated bouts of less severe exercise-induced injury. Abnormal polysaccharide is always present, but fiber necrosis is uncommon in muscle biopsy samples taken from affected horses while they are clinically normal.

The characteristic histologic finding is aggregates of intracytoplasmic material that stain positively with the PAS reaction for glycogen (Fig. 15-35, *A*). In severe cases, multiple pale intracytoplasmic inclusions are also present in H&E stained sections (Fig. 15-35, *B*). These inclusions are PAS-positive (Fig. 15-35, *C*) and resist digestion by amylase and are thus not glycogen. Terms used to describe this amylase-resistant material include *amylopectin, polyglucosan,* and *complex polysaccharide.* In chronic cases, myofibers also have chronic myopathic change (atrophy, hypertrophy, or internal nuclei), and fat replacement of myofibers after myofiber loss can occur in severely affected cases.

At this time, the detection of the GYS1 mutation provides a definitive diagnosis of EPSSM, but this test is not very sensitive. The most sensitive test for diagnosis of EPSSM depends on finding characteristic histopathologic changes in muscle samples of horses with appropriate clinical signs. Gluteal, semimembranosus, or semitendinosus muscle samples are preferred, although changes in longissimus muscle are also found, especially in horses with back pain. A presumptive diagnosis of EPSSM can be made based on characteristic clinical findings in a predisposed breed. Treatment has relied on altering the diet to minimize starch and sugar intake (less than 15% of total daily calories) and maximize fat intake (at least 20% to 25% of total daily calories from fat). Grains and sweet feeds are replaced by high-fiber, low-starch, low-sugar feeds, with added fat in the form of vegetable oil, powdered fat, or high-fat rice bran supplements. Providing the horse with regular exercise and as much time as possible in a pasture or paddock are also important. Treatment is very successful in most cases.

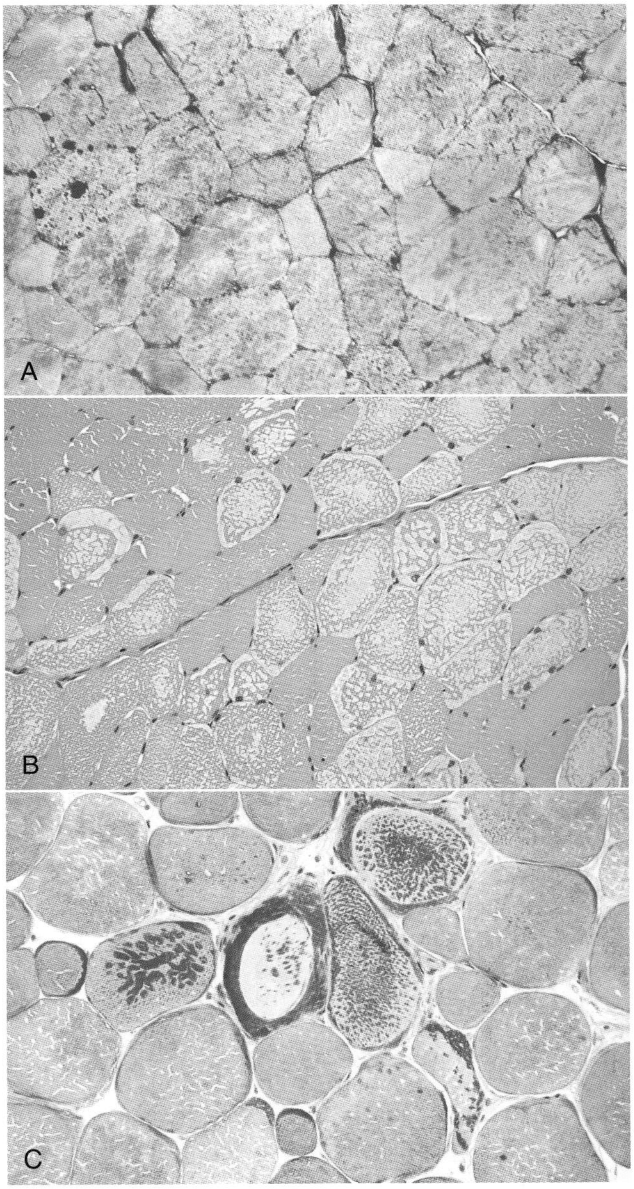

Fig. 15-35 Equine polysaccharide storage myopathy, semimembranosus muscle, transverse sections, horse.
A, Note the increased amount of and irregularly distributed dark-pink staining glycogen. Abnormal aggregates are present both beneath the sarcolemma and within the cytoplasm. Formalin fixation, PAS reaction. **B,** Severe form. Numerous myofibers contain multiple pale *(very light pink)* subsarcolemmal and intracytoplasmic inclusions of stored polysaccharide. Formalin fixation, H&E stain. **C,** These inclusions shown in **B** stain intensely with PAS but are not digested by amylase *(not shown)* and are characteristic of what is called *complex polysaccharide, amylopectin,* or *polyglucosan.* Formalin fixation, PAS reaction. (Courtesy Dr. B.J. Cooper, College of Veterinary Medicine, Oregon State University.)

Glycogen Brancher Enzyme Deficiency

Glycogen brancher enzyme (GBE) deficiency, or glycogenosis type IV, is a disorder caused by a congenital lack of a glycogenic enzyme, GBE, and is an emerging disease in quarter horses and American paint horses. It is inherited as an autosomal recessive trait. Affected foals may be aborted, stillborn, or weak at birth or can have contracted tendons, rhabdomyolysis, or cardiac failure at an early age. The consequence of GBE deficiency is the accumulation of long unbranched chains of glucose within cells that leads to abnormal glycogen formation and intramyofiber deposits. These molecules would normally be converted into glycogen in the presence of GBE in the final step in the formation of glycogen. There are no specific gross pathologic findings. Pulmonary edema may be found in foals that die from cardiac failure. Characteristic histologic findings are round hyaline inclusions resembling amylopectin (polyglucosan bodies) within skeletal and cardiac myocytes, especially Purkinje fibers, and to a lesser degree within hepatocytes. Unlike glycogen, inclusions are PAS-positive and resistant to amylase digestion. As with other carbohydrate metabolic defects, a lack of energy production by affected fibers is thought to underlie cellular dysfunction. Disruption of cytoarchitecture caused by amylopectin deposition may also contribute. Analysis of peripheral blood or skeletal muscle for GBE activity identifies affected animals with severely reduced GBE activity and carriers in which GBE activity is moderately reduced. A DNA test to detect carriers and affected horses using pulled mane or tail hairs is now available. There is no treatment for this disorder.

Myotonia and Mitochondrial Myopathy

A myotonic disorder occurs occasionally in horses, and a mitochondrial myopathy has been described in an Arabian horse. These disorders are discussed in more detail in Web Appendix 15-1.

Other Equine Myopathies

Exertional Rhabdomyolysis

Equine exertional rhabdomyolysis (tying up, azoturia, Monday morning disease, setfast, blackwater) is characterized clinically by sudden onset of stiff gait, reluctance to move, swelling of affected muscle groups (especially gluteal), sweating, and other signs of pain and discomfort. Serum concentrations of CK and AST are often markedly increased. Signs may appear during or immediately after exercise, but only rarely is exertional rhabdomyolysis associated with exhaustive exercise. In severely affected horses, even minimal exercise, such as walking out of a stall, can cause clinical signs. High grain feeding and lack of regular exercise have been recognized to be factors leading to exercise-induced muscle injury for many years. Previous theories regarding the pathogenesis of equine exertional rhabdomyolysis include development of muscle lactic acidosis, vitamin E and/or selenium deficiency, hypothyroidism, and systemic electrolyte abnormalities. It is only recently that studies have concluded that lactic acidosis is not a finding in horses with exertional rhabdomyolysis, that hypothyroid horses show no signs of degenerative myopathy, and that electrolyte abnormalities as a primary cause of equine exertional rhabdomyolysis are rare. It is still thought that vitamin E or selenium deficiency can exacerbate signs of exertional rhabdomyolysis in predisposed horses, but neither vitamin E nor selenium deficiency is considered a primary cause. Recent studies have found that affected horses typically have an underlying myopathy, most often EPSSM. There is some evidence to suggest that recurrent exertional rhabdomyolysis in thoroughbreds is the result of abnormal calcium homeostasis within skeletal muscle, although some affected thoroughbreds have been found to have EPSSM. As muscle necrosis per se is not painful and does not cause muscle swelling, it is suspected that other factors play a role in this disorder in the horse. These factors include oxidative injury to muscle membranes occurring secondary to segmental necrosis and the subsequent production of oxygen-derived free radical compounds and vascular compromise resulting in ischemia (i.e., compartment syndrome when muscle damage occurs in a muscle with a tight and relatively nonexpandable fascia such as the gluteal and longissimus muscles). Oxidative injury may explain the perceived benefit of supplemental vitamin E and selenium to affected horses.

Gross findings are similar to those described for EPSSM (i.e., initially areas of muscle that are pale pink or diffusely red-tinged; Fig. 15-36, *A*). Histologic findings are localized or widespread muscle fiber necrosis (Fig. 15-36, *B*), followed by the usual sequence of events: macrophage infiltration and regeneration. Affected fibers are primarily type 2 fibers. Lesions can be either monophasic or polyphasic.

Diagnosis is based on typical clinical signs and clinicopathologic evidence of muscle injury (increased activity of CK or AST). Treatment for an acute episode includes nonsteroidal

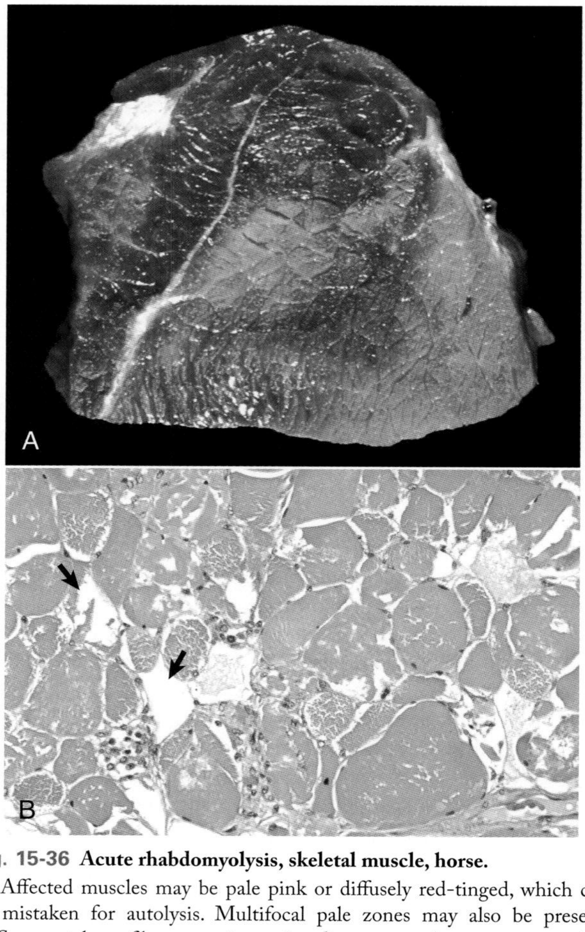

Fig. 15-36 Acute rhabdomyolysis, skeletal muscle, horse. **A,** Affected muscles may be pale pink or diffusely red-tinged, which can be mistaken for autolysis. Multifocal pale zones may also be present. **B,** Segmental myofiber necrosis, semitendinosus muscle, transverse section. Most of the myocytes are necrotic and at the stage of coagulation necrosis. In a few myofibers, necrosis is at a later stage and the necrotic sarcoplasm has lysed, leaving empty sarcolemmal tubes *(arrows)*. A couple of necrotic myofibers are at an even later stage and contain a small number of macrophages. Formalin fixation, H&E stain. (**A** courtesy Dr. W. Crowell, College of Veterinary Medicine, University of Georgia; and Noah's Arkive, College of Veterinary Medicine, The University of Georgia. **B** courtesy Dr. B.J. Cooper, College of Veterinary Medicine, Oregon State University.)

antiinflammatory agents, acepromazine, and rest. Careful evaluation of the patient for evidence of renal damage ([pigmentary] myoglobinuric nephrosis) because of myoglobin released from damaged muscle is indicated. Long-term treatment and prevention include correction of any concurrent electrolyte, mineral, or vitamin deficiencies and most importantly, a change in diet to one that is high in fat and fiber and low in starch and sugar, as described for horses with EPSSM (see the section on Inherited or Congenital Myopathies). Thoroughbreds with recurrent exertional rhabdomyolysis caused by suspected underlying skeletal muscle calcium-handling abnormalities also respond well to this type of diet.

Malignant Hyperthermia

In horses, malignant hyperthermia (MH) can occur during general anesthesia. Hyperthermia can also occur during recovery from anesthesia, which is sometimes called *hypermetabolism* to distinguish it from true MH. A genetic defect in the skeletal muscle ryanodine receptor, similar to that in MH in humans, dogs, and pigs, has been identified in some horses with MH triggered by anesthetic agents. A genetic test for the MH mutation is available. Some horses affected with a hyperthermia-like syndrome during anesthesia or during recovery from anesthesia have HYPP or EPSSM, but in some cases the exact cause of the hyperthermia is not clear. It is likely that, as is similar to hyperthermia in humans, a variety of underlying myopathies, especially those that result in uncoupling of mitochondria within skeletal myocytes (see the section on Malignant Hyperthermia), can predispose animals to anesthesia-associated hyperthermia. Studies of muscle from horses with exertional rhabdomyolysis have detected loosely coupled mitochondria, which could predispose them to MH–like episodes. The extent of overt muscle fiber necrosis caused by hyperthermia varies but is often severe.

Ischemic Myopathy

In addition to vascular damage resulting from clostridial toxins or immune-mediated vasculitis, ischemic myopathy of pectoral and limb muscle can be seen in recumbent horses as the result of pressure interfering with vascular perfusion. Once the horse is moved or is standing, reperfusion injury can occur. Development of compartment syndrome can contribute to ischemic injury (see the section on Disturbance of Circulation). Ischemic myopathy of the abdominal muscles can be seen after prolonged pressure from being supported in a sling. In these cases, affected muscles generally show degenerative or regenerative changes that are all at about the same stage (monophasic necrosis). Concurrent necrosis and regeneration (polyphasic necrosis) can also be seen in horses that are in a sling or recumbent for an extended period of time such as for several days. Recovery depends on the extent of the ischemic area and the ability of the muscle to regenerate (i.e., depending on whether the basal lamina is intact and whether satellite cells have become necrotic from ischemia).

Transient pelvic limb muscle ischemia as the result of aortoiliac mural thrombosis occurs in horses. The cause of the thrombosis is unknown, although it has been attributed to migration of strongyle larvae through the aortic wall, damaging the intima. Typically the thrombus is not occlusive, and clinical signs of pelvic limb dysfunction occur only during or after strenuous exercise, such as racing. A short-stride gait and a decreased surface temperature of the distal portion of the affected limb during episodes are characteristic. Because the ischemia is transient, pathologic studies are few. But overt myofiber necrosis is thought to be minimal, and recovery is typically rapid. Surgery to remove the thrombus can be curative.

Postanesthetic Myopathy

Degenerative myopathy can occur in horses undergoing prolonged recumbency during general anesthesia. In some cases, muscle damage may be the result of ischemia from systemic hypotension leading to muscle hypoxia or from pressure caused by the weight of large muscle masses during recumbency, especially when adequate padding has not been provided. Underlying myopathy of various types also predisposes to postanesthetic myopathy. In ischemic damage, the location of the lesions depends on the position of the horse during anesthesia. In dorsal recumbency, the gluteal and the longissimus muscles are ischemic; in lateral recumbency, the triceps brachii, pectoralis, deltoideus, and brachiocephalicus muscles of the leg under the body become ischemic. The basic mechanism is that the pressure in the muscle exceeds the perfusion pressure in the capillaries. The use of adequate padding under the recumbent horse and the maintenance of normal blood pressure during anesthesia have greatly reduced the incidence of postanesthetic myopathy from muscle ischemia in horses. These days, underlying myopathy, particularly EPSSM, appears to be the most common cause of postanesthetic myopathy in horses.

Endocrine Myopathies

Although hypothyroidism is often suggested to be a cause of muscle dysfunction in the horse, studies of experimentally thyroidectomized horses have failed to support hypothyroidism as a cause of equine myopathy. Pituitary hyperfunction caused by adenoma or hyperplasia in older horses, causing equine Cushing's disease, is the most common equine endocrine disorder causing muscle atrophy (preferentially of type 2 fibers) and weakness. The characteristic pot-bellied appearance of affected horses is thought to be secondary to abdominal muscle weakness.

Denervating Diseases

Localized or generalized muscle dysfunction can be caused by disorders affecting motor neurons or peripheral nerves. Several syndromes of peripheral nerve dysfunction are recognized in the horse.

Peripheral Neuropathy

Injury to the motor nerves in a peripheral nerve results in localized muscle atrophy and dysfunction of those myofibers innervated by those nerves. Damage to the suprascapular nerve results in unilateral scapular muscle (supraspinatus and infraspinatus) atrophy, and the clinical condition is known as sweeney. In working draft horses, this nerve can be compressed by a poorly fitted harness collar. In nonharness horses, trauma is the most common cause. Traumatic injury to the radial nerve or axillary plexus is also relatively common in horses.

Stringhalt is a sporadic pelvic limb neuropathy characterized by an exaggerated flexion of one or both hindlimbs. It can be caused by trauma to the hind leg, ingestion of plant toxins, or can be of unknown cause. Outbreaks of stringhalt in pastured horses in Australia and New Zealand are the result of ingestion of *Hypochoeris radicata* and related species, also known as flatweed, false dandelion, and hairy cat's ear. Lesions of denervation atrophy are found in the distal lateral digital extensor muscle, and surgical removal of this muscle is one method of correction. *Hypochoeris radicata* grows prolifically in the Pacific Northwest, and a similar syndrome of plant-induced stringhalt is said to occur there, but evidence to support this hypothesis has been hard to find. Feeding trials at Oregon State University have failed to reproduce the syndrome.

Fibrotic myopathy is a condition most often attributed to hamstring (semitendinosus, semimembranosus, and biceps femoris) muscle trauma, but pelvic limb neuropathy as a result of trauma or unknown causes can also cause fibrotic myopathy. Fibrotic myopathy causes a restriction of the forward swing of the affected pelvic limb. Gross examination often reveals pale, firm muscle caused by collagen deposition. When fibrotic myopathy is actually the result of neuropathy, affected muscle shows characteristic microscopic lesions of chronic denervation atrophy.

Laryngeal hemiplegia is a well-documented condition in horses in which degeneration of nerve fibers within the left recurrent laryngeal nerve results in unilateral laryngeal muscle denervation atrophy (see Fig. 15-18) and laryngeal dysfunction. Affected horses often make a characteristic respiratory noise during exercise, hence the name *roaring*. There are many possible causes of injury to the left recurrent laryngeal nerve, including extension of infections from the guttural pouches or tumors in that area, lead toxicity, and direct trauma. Most cases, however, are considered idiopathic. Although the exact cause of idiopathic laryngeal hemiplegia in horses is not known, the fact that it occurs only in tall, long-necked horses, and virtually never in ponies, suggests that whatever the mechanism of injury, very long nerves (particularly the very long left recurrent laryngeal nerve of tall long-necked horses) are predisposed.

Lead intoxication can also cause generalized peripheral neuropathy resulting in muscle atrophy and weakness mimicking equine motor neuron disease (see later discussion). Polyneuritis equi (neuritis of the cauda equina) and peripheral nerve lymphoma also cause denervation atrophy in horses. Polyneuritis equi most often involves the caudal nerve roots and facial nerves, and lymphoma has been found affecting multiple nerve roots or selectively involving the facial nerve.

Motor Neuronopathy

Damage to motor neurons in the nuclei of the brainstem or in the ventral horns of the spinal cord will result in Wallerian degeneration of peripheral nerves. In the horse, protozoal myeloencephalitis caused by *Sarcocystis neurona* is a common cause of unilateral denervation atrophy, usually of facial or gluteal musculature because of preferential damage to cranial nerve nuclei in the brainstem or motor neurons of the lumbosacral intumescence. Affected horses often also have Wallerian degeneration in spinal cord white matter and exhibit ataxia and proprioceptive deficits.

Equine motor neuron disease occurs as the result of severe and prolonged vitamin E deficiency, which leads to motor neuron degeneration. Clinical signs are sudden onset of rapid muscle wasting, weakness, trembling, and increased time spent in recumbency. Type 1 motor neurons and muscles are preferentially affected, supporting the proposed pathogenesis of oxidative injury to motor neurons secondary to vitamin E deficiency. The severe denervation atrophy occurring in postural muscles (medial head of the triceps, vastus intermedius, and sacrocaudalis dorsalis medialis) in horses with motor neuron disease often results in a remarkable pale yellow-tan color (Fig. 15-37, see Fig. 15-9, *C*) and gelatinous texture of the affected muscle. Severely affected horses may become persistently recumbent, leading to death or euthanasia. In some cases, high-dose vitamin E supplementation (10,000 IU or more per day) can halt the progression of the disorder, and affected horses on vitamin E therapy can even develop some compensatory muscle hypertrophy and regain muscle mass. There is little or no evidence of reinnervation in this disorder, and affected horses are considered disabled for life.

DISORDERS OF CATTLE

Although cattle have not been selected for muscle performance, many breeds have been selected for meat quality. This process has led to selection for at least one genetic disorder. Disorders affecting muscle can have a profound economic effect on the cattle industry.

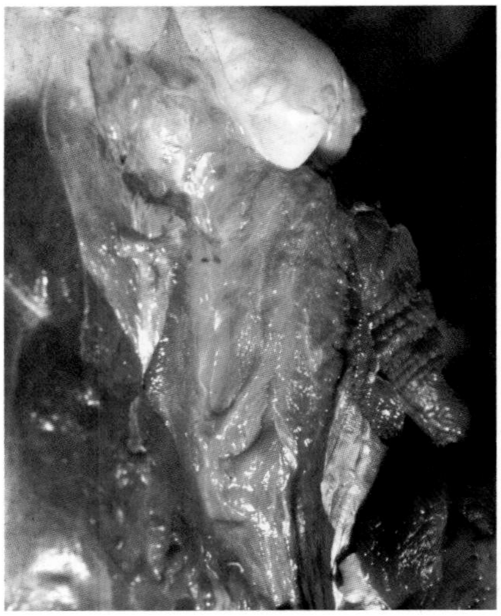

Fig. 15-37 **Denervation atrophy, equine motor neuron disease, medial triceps muscle, horse.**
The medial triceps muscle *(center, top to bottom)*, a type 1 predominant postural muscle deep in the foreleg, is diffusely pale tan and gelatinous in appearance because of severe denervation atrophy. The adjacent muscles (*left* and *right*) have a normal appearance. (Courtesy College of Veterinary Medicine, Cornell University. For histopathologic findings, see Fig. 15-19.)

Bacterial and Parasitic Myopathies

Clostridial Myositis (Blackleg)

Clostridial myositis (blackleg), due to *Clostridium chauvoei*, is an extremely economically important disease that is most common in beef cattle. It can also occur in dairy cattle, especially those housed in free-stall barns where jostling and muscle bruising are possible. *Clostridium chauvoei* is a spore-forming, Gram-positive anaerobic bacillus. Its spores are ubiquitous in the soil, and after ingestion they are capable of crossing the intestinal mucosa, entering the bloodstream, and being carried to skeletal muscles. The spores lie dormant until localized trauma to the muscle, which in cattle is most often caused by bruising during handling in a chute or from trauma in a crowded feedlot, results in muscle damage and localized hypoxia and anoxia. The resultant anaerobic conditions allow the spores to activate and the bacteria to proliferate and produce toxins (see Table 15-3) that cause capillary damage with resultant hemorrhage, edema, and necrosis of adjacent myofibers.

The most common presentation is acute death. Signs before death are referable to toxemia; to the heat, swelling, crepitus, and dysfunction of the affected muscle group; and to fever. Serum concentrations of CK and AST are typically increased. Locally extensive hemorrhage and edema, often with crepitus caused by gas bubbles, are seen in affected muscles and in overlying fascia and subcutaneous tissue. Necrotic muscle fibers appear dark red to red-black. Lesions are either wet and exudative (early lesions) or dry (later lesions) (Fig. 15-38, *A*). A characteristic odor of rancid butter from butyric acid is typical. Cardiac muscle can also be involved. In other parts of the body, hemorrhages and edema can occur from the toxemia. Affected carcasses autolyze rapidly, likely because of the effects of clostridial toxins on tissue and of high body temperature before death. Histologically, locally extensive areas of muscle fibers undergoing coagulation necrosis and fragmentation, and

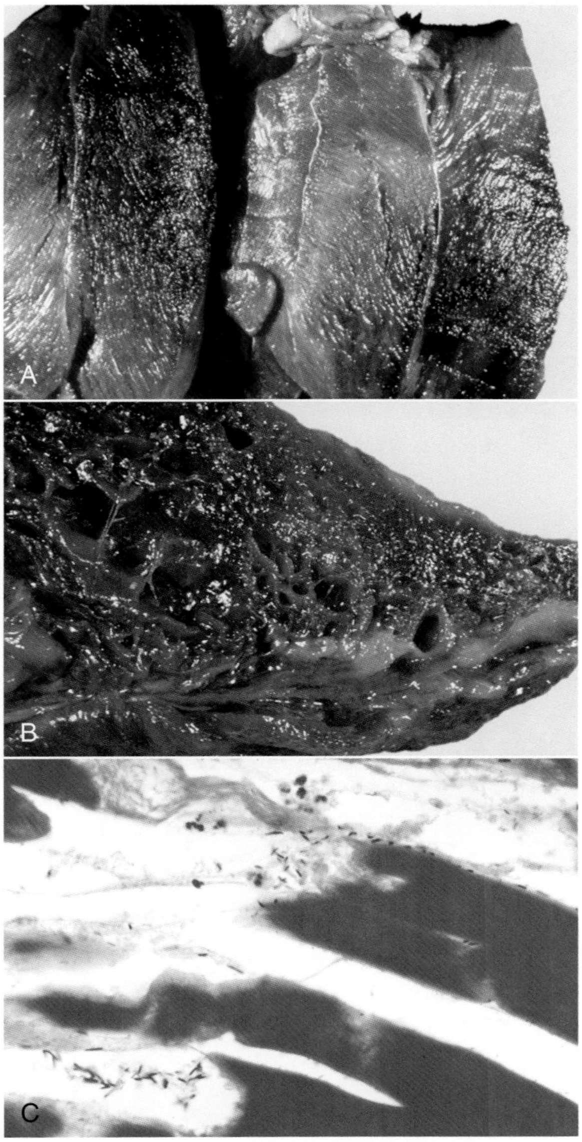

Fig. 15-38 **Blackleg, hemorrhagic-necrotizing myositis *(Clostridium chauvoei)*, thigh muscle, cow.**
A, The dark red areas are caused by hemorrhagic necrosis of the affected muscle. These lesions are characteristic of blackleg. **B,** *Clostridium chauvoei* can also produce substantial quantities of gas within infected tissues as shown here by the numerous ("pseudocystic") spaces within hemorrhagic and necrotic muscle. **C,** Gram-positive bacilli are present in the serous exudate. Formalin fixation, Gram stain. (**A** courtesy College of Veterinary Medicine, Cornell University. **B** and **C** courtesy Dr. M.D. McGavin, College of Veterinary Medicine, University of Tennessee.)

interstitial edema and hemorrhage are seen. Overt vasculitis is not seen. Gas bubbles are typical. Gram-positive bacilli whose appearance is compatible with that of *Clostridium chauvoei* may be demonstrable within affected muscle (Fig. 15-38, *C*).

Isolation of *Clostridium chauvoei* on anaerobic media or visualization by fluorescent antibody techniques are useful for the diagnosis of blackleg but are confirmatory only if typical gross and histopathologic lesions are present because dormant spores of *Clostridium chauvoei* can be found in normal muscle. The vaccination history and evaluation of husbandry practices are also important; unvaccinated or inadequately vaccinated (i.e., vaccinations not up-to-date) animals in situations in which muscle trauma is possible are most at risk. There is generally no effective treatment for cattle with blackleg, and death occurs rapidly. Prevention is the best approach. Vaccination against clostridial toxins and maintenance of a safe environment are critical.

Botulism

Botulism caused by ingestion of *Clostridium botulinum* toxin from contaminated feed or soil occurs in cattle, and clinical signs of flaccid paralysis and pathogenesis are similar to those in the adult horse. Cattle are most susceptible to type C and D botulinum toxins, and herd outbreaks are possible. Cattle, however, are much more resistant to botulism than are horses. Botulinum toxin, most often from animal cadavers such as mice or rats, within silage, haylage, or hay is the most common cause of outbreaks of botulism in cattle. Abnormal eating habits (pica) can result in ingestion of *Clostridium botulinum* toxin from the soil or carrion. Botulism in cattle is usually fatal.

Pyogenic Bacteria

Cattle are prone to develop abscesses and cellulitis (fasciitis) from infections with pyogenic bacteria, most commonly *Arcanobacterium pyogenes*. Abscesses in muscle occur most commonly in the hindleg. Swelling and lameness of the affected limb caused by widespread necrotizing cellulitis and myositis are seen.

Arcanobacterium pyogenes is a ubiquitous bacterium that can infect muscle by two routes: by direct contamination of wounds and injection sites and hematogenously. The bacterium can be found within the reproductive tract of cows and within the rumen wall, and it has been speculated that *Arcanobacterium pyogenes* from a transient bacteremia after parturition or from disruption of the rumen wall can result in colonization of damaged muscle. Lesions vary, depending on the virulence of the bacteria and the age of the lesions. They vary in extent from encapsulated intramuscular abscesses adjacent to the site of injection to a diffuse purulent cellulitis extending down the tissue and fascial planes. The cellulitis may be so severe as to involve much of the musculature of the affected limb. When abscesses are present, the gross appearance is of an encapsulated mass filled with thick, yellow-green, foul-smelling pus. In cases of cellulitis, pus dissects along fascial planes outside the muscle and between perimysial sheaths within muscles. Inflammation extends into the adjacent myofibers, resulting in myonecrosis and subsequent replacement by fibrous tissue. The greenish color of the exudate is distinctive, and small Gram-positive pleomorphic bacteria are often seen within tissue sections or cytologic preparations. *Arcanobacterium pyogenes* is readily isolated on aerobic culture.

Actinobacillus lignieresii (Wooden Tongue)

Infection of oral tissue, particularly of the tongue musculature (see Figs. 7-26 and 7-27), by *Actinobacillus lignieresii* results in a severe chronic granulomatous to pyogranulomatous and fibrosing myositis. Infection occurs through oral wounds or by penetrating plant fragments. Affected cattle have difficulty prehending and swallowing and often have excessive salivation. Histologic features include marked fibrosis caused by tissue destruction and chronicity and foci of inflammation containing eosinophilic material ("radiating clubs") and characteristic Gram-negative bacilli. Aggressive antibiotic therapy can be curative.

Actinomyces bovis (Lumpy Jaw)

Actinomyces bovis frequently involves bones of the jaw, causing chronic granulomatous to pyogranulomatous and fibrosing osteomyelitis (see Fig. 16-58). Occasionally *Actinomyces bovis* involves the musculature of the tongue, causing gross and histologic lesions similar to those caused by *Actinobacillus lignieresii*. Gram stain reveals Gram-positive bacilli, which distinguishes this lesion from the Gram-negative *Actinobacillus lignieresii* infection.

Protozoal Myopathies

Sarcocystis spp. forming intracytoplasmic cysts (see Fig. 15-27) is a common incidental finding that may even be grossly visible as nodules within skeletal and cardiac myofibers of cattle (see Fig. 15-41). Massive infection may result in fever, anorexia, and progressive wasting, but this is uncommon. More often, *Sarcocystis* infection is diagnosed as an incidental finding at necropsy or during meat inspection at slaughter. If the cyst wall breaks down, a focus of myofiber necrosis and later granulomatous inflammation result.

Eosinophilic myositis is a disease of cattle thought to be a relatively uncommon manifestation of *Sarcocystis* infection that may involve hypersensitivity. There is overt green discoloration (see Fig. 15-10) of affected muscles caused by the massive infiltration of eosinophils (Fig. 15-39, *A* and *B*). This is accompanied by myofiber necrosis and, in chronic cases, fibrosis. Fragments of degenerating intralesional protozoa can sometimes be found (Fig. 15-39, *C*).

Neospora caninum can also infect cattle. Adults have no clinical disease, but infection of the fetus can cause multifocal nonsuppurative inflammation of skeletal muscle and heart and brain.

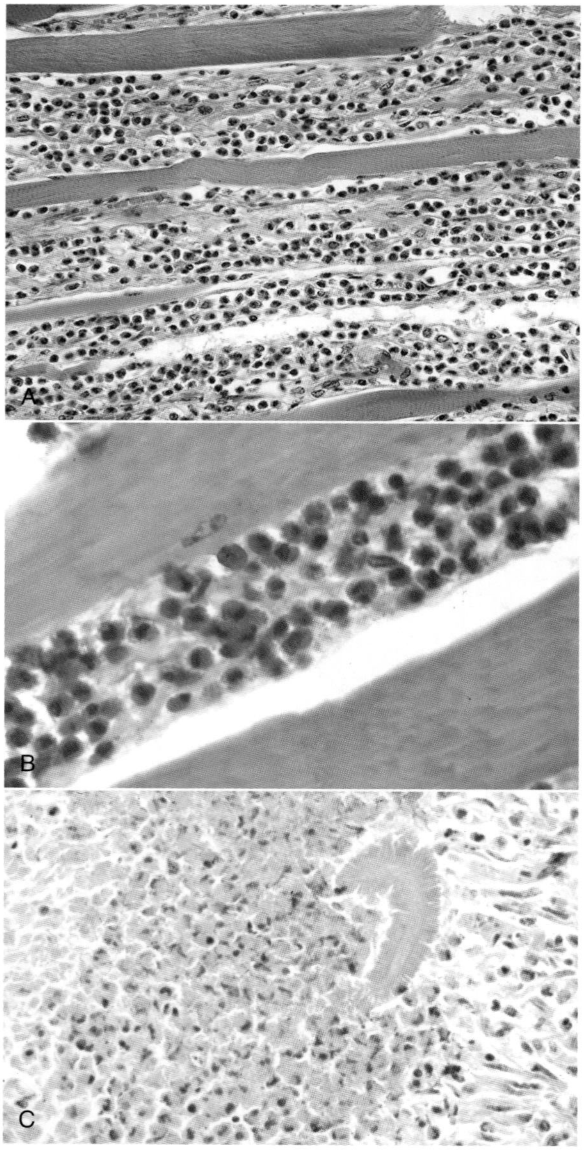

Fig. 15-39 Bovine eosinophilic myositis, skeletal muscle, longitudinal section, cow.

A, Dense interstitial infiltrate of eosinophils has separated the muscle fibers, some of which are atrophic. Formalin fixation, H&E stain. **B,** Higher magnification demonstrating the large population of eosinophils in the inflammatory exudate. Formalin fixation, H&E stain. **C,** Degenerate *Sarcocystis* organism surrounded by degenerate eosinophils. Formalin fixation, H&E stain. (**A** courtesy Dr. M.D. McGavin, College of Veterinary Medicine, University of Tennessee; and Noah's Arkive, College of Veterinary Medicine, The University of Georgia. **B** courtesy Dr. M.D. McGavin, College of Veterinary Medicine, University of Tennessee. **C** courtesy Dr. R. Bildfell, College of Veterinary Medicine, Oregon State University.)

Nutritional and Toxic Myopathies

Nutritional Myopathy

Similar to horses, calves and young cattle are susceptible to nutritional myopathy caused by a selenium or (less commonly) vitamin E deficiency. But the profound involvement of temporal and masseter muscles ("maxillary myositis") that can occur in horses is not seen in cattle. In the latter species, the postural muscles and muscles of locomotion are most commonly affected. Muscles of affected calves appear pale pink to white, often in a patchy distribution and in cervical muscles used during suckling and "bumping" the udder. The gross appearance depends on the extent of the necrosis and the stage of the lesion. In early stages, yellow and white streaks are present, and later pale, chalk white streaks from calcification often appear, thus the common name *white muscle disease* (Fig. 15-40). Confirmation of the diagnosis is based on blood or liver analysis for selenium and vitamin E.

Plant Toxicities

Cassia occidentalis (coffee senna, coffee weed) is the most common cause of degenerative myopathy in cattle as the result of plant toxicity. This plant grows throughout the southeastern United States. Pale areas within skeletal muscle, with lesser involvement of cardiac muscle, are caused by myofiber necrosis, generally with minimal to no mineralization. Other plant toxicities are discussed in the toxic myopathies section.

Ionophore Toxicity

The pathogenesis of ionophore toxicity is discussed in the toxic myopathy section. Ionophore toxicity in cattle is seen only with overdoses because of improper feed mixing. Anorexia, diarrhea, and weakness are the primary clinical signs. Serum concentrations of CK and AST are often extremely high (e.g., CK greater than 50,000 U/L and AST greater than 5000 U/L). Pale areas within skeletal and cardiac muscle are due to myofiber necrosis. In animals that survive, regeneration will restore the skeletal muscle completely, but cardiac lesions heal by fibrosis.

Congenital or Inherited Disorders

Steatosis

Steatosis in cattle, sometimes called *lipomatosis,* is most often recognized as an incidental finding at necropsy or at slaughter. This disorder is thought to be the result of defective in utero muscle development, in which large areas of myofibers are replaced by adipocytes. An inherited basis has not been established. Lesions can be symmetric or asymmetric, with the most severely affected

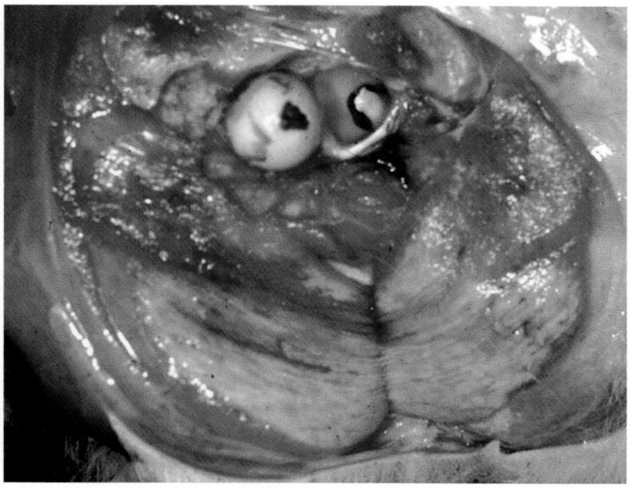

Fig. 15-40 Nutritional myopathy (white muscle disease), skeletal muscles of the caudal thigh, sagittal section, calf.
In this early stage, affected muscles have yellow and white streaks, often in a patchy distribution. These streaks are areas of necrotic myofibers. Later as the necrotic myofibers calcify, white streaks (chalky texture, mineralization) are visible grossly. (Courtesy Dr. G.K. Saunders, Virginia-Maryland Regional College of Veterinary Medicine; and Noah's Arkive, College of Veterinary Medicine, The University of Georgia.)

muscles being those of the back and loin (longissimus muscles; see Fig. 15-9, *D*). The most severely affected muscles are composed entirely of fat, whereas less severely affected muscles appear streaked because of partial replacement by fat. Histologically, the space normally occupied by myofibers is filled with mature adipocytes. In utero denervation or failure of innervation results in a similar muscle lesion (see Fig. 15-25), and careful evaluation of the peripheral nerves and spinal cord is indicated.

Diagnosis is readily made on gross examination and can be confirmed by histologic examination, specifically in frozen sections stained with oil-red-O or Sudan black for fat. Because this condition is usually not diagnosed during life and the loss of myofibers is irreversible, treatment is neither necessary nor possible.

Other Bovine Congenital or Inherited Myopathies and Neuronopathies

Congenital muscular hyperplasia ("double muscling") resulting from defects in the myostatin gene occurs in a variety of cattle breeds. An unusual multisystemic disease with characteristic necrotizing vasculopathy occurs in young Gelbvieh cattle. Glycogenosis type II (acid maltase deficiency) has been recognized in shorthorn and Brahman cattle, and glycogenosis type V (myophosphorylase deficiency) occurs in Charolais cattle. An inherited motor neuron degenerative disease occurs in Brown Swiss cattle. These disorders are discussed in more detail in Web Appendix 15-1.

Electrolyte Abnormalities

Hypokalemic Myopathy

Decreased potassium interferes with normal muscle cell function and can lead to muscle weakness and myofiber necrosis. Type 2 fibers are preferentially affected. The pathogenesis of hypokalemic myopathy is not clear, but myofiber necrosis may be the end result of either decreased myofiber energy production or of focal ischemia secondary to vasoconstriction. Hypokalemia can also interfere with normal cardiac conduction, and atrial fibrillation is common. Hypokalemia in cattle can be the result of anorexia. A history of ketosis occurring within a month of parturition is common. Glucocorticoids with high mineralocorticoid activity, such as isoflupredone acetate used to treat ketosis, are a recognized cause of hypokalemic myopathy in cattle. Activation of glucose transport into cells by intravenously administered glucose or insulin also causes intracellular movement of potassium and can result in hypokalemia. No specific findings are present at postmortem examination, although ischemic necrosis secondary to recumbency can be seen in muscles of the hindlimbs (see later discussion). Lesions of multifocal polyphasic myofiber necrosis and vacuolated myofibers (vacuolar degeneration) are present in all muscles, including those not involved in weight-bearing, and are indicative of myodegeneration as a direct effect of hypokalemia.

Affected cows are profoundly weak and become recumbent and unable to support the weight of their heads. Serum concentration of potassium is below normal (<2.3 mEq/L), and CK and AST levels are moderately high (CK up to approximately 25,000 U/L, AST up to approximately 2000 U/L). The diagnosis is based on typical historic and clinical findings and a low serum potassium concentration. Intravenous and oral supplementation with potassium salts and supportive therapy may result in recovery in some cases, but this disorder is often fatal.

Other Electrolyte Abnormalities

Both hypocalcemia and hypophosphatemia can result in profound muscle weakness and recumbency in cattle. In hypocalcemia, weakness is primarily the result of disruption of neuromuscular transmission. Significant changes are not seen in affected muscles, although ischemic necrosis can occur secondary to recumbency (see later discussion). Diagnosis relies on clinical findings and identification of abnormally low serum calcium or phosphorus concentrations. Treatment includes correction of the electrolyte defect by intravenous administration of the appropriate electrolyte-containing fluids, supportive care, and correction of any dietary abnormalities that may predispose to electrolyte problems.

Ischemic Myopathy

Ischemic muscle necrosis caused by recumbency is common in cattle. The muscular lesion is similar to that seen in other species, but in cattle, prolonged sternal recumbency is more common than lateral recumbency, and pectoral muscles and muscles of limbs tucked under the body or splayed out limbs are most prone to injury (see Fig. 15-26).

DISORDERS OF SHEEP AND GOATS

Selection pressures and economic consequences of muscle disorders similar to those in beef cattle exist in small ruminants raised for meat. In goats, selection for an interesting mutant has resulted in perpetuation of myotonia.

Bacterial and Parasitic Myopathies

Clostridial Myositis (Blackleg)

Clostridial myositis (blackleg) occurs occasionally in sheep and goats and is similar to the disease in cattle.

Botulism

Botulism can occur in small ruminants, but, as in cattle, it is rare.

Protozoal Myopathy

Intracytoplasmic cysts of *Sarcocystis* spp. are commonly found within skeletal and cardiac muscle fibers of sheep and goats as an incidental finding, similar to findings in muscle and heart of cattle. Eosinophilic myositis as a result of sarcocystosis is rare in sheep

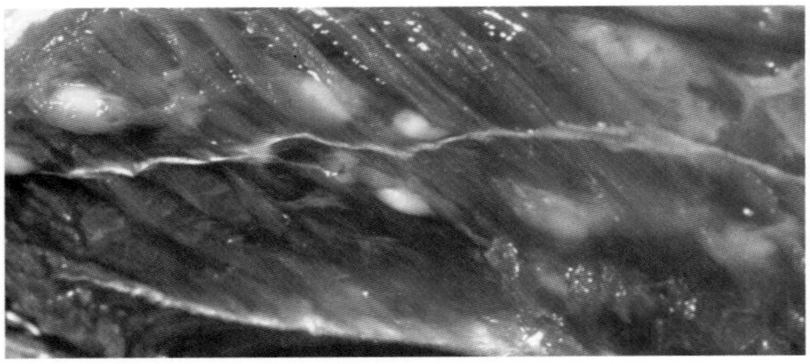

Fig. 15-41 Sarcocystosis, skeletal muscle, alpaca. Multiple pale gray-white nodules within the muscle indicate the location of *Sarcocystis* cysts. (Courtesy College of Veterinary Medicine, Cornell University.)

and is not recognized in goats. In camelids, massive infection with *Sarcocystis* can occur (Fig. 15-41), especially in animals imported from South America where sarcocystosis is common. In rare cases, *Sarcocystis* infection in camelids is associated with widespread eosinophilic myositis.

Nutritional and Toxic Myopathies

Degenerative myopathy caused by nutritional deficiency or toxin ingestion is relatively common in many small ruminant species. The nonselective eating habits of goats make them particularly likely to ingest poisonous plants.

Nutritional Myopathy

Young goats and sheep are susceptible to degenerative myopathy associated with selenium or, less commonly, vitamin E deficiency. A similar disorder occurs rarely in young camelids. The disease in these species is similar to the disease in young cattle.

Toxic Myopathies

Sheep and goats are susceptible to plant and ionophore toxicities, similar to those in cattle. In goats, ingestion of honey mesquite *(Prosopis glandulosa)* causes degeneration of the motor nucleus of the trigeminal nerve, resulting in denervation atrophy of the muscles of mastication, and consequent inability to adequately chew feed, leading to progressive emaciation.

Congenital or Inherited Myopathies

Myotonia in Goats

Myotonia in the goat is inherited as an autosomal dominant trait, and the variable clinical severity is attributable to increased severity in homozygotes compared with heterozygotes. The genetic defect affects the skeletal muscle chloride channel, resulting in decreased chloride conductance and associated ionic instability of the sarcolemma. Starting at about 2 weeks of age, affected goats develop severe muscle spasms in response to sudden voluntary effort, for example, when startled by the blowing of a locomotive's horn, Episodes of myotonia can last from 5 to 20 seconds and are characterized by generalized stiffness and adoption of a "sawhorse" stance. Goats often fall over. Sustained dimpling of muscle occurs after percussion. Serum concentrations of CK and AST are normal. Concentric needle EMG reveals the characteristic waxing and waning ("dive bomber") spontaneous activity of myotonia. There are no gross pathologic findings. Histologically, muscle fibers in affected goats may show moderate hypertrophy. But characteristic abnormalities are revealed only with ultrastructural examination in which dilated and proliferated T tubules and terminal cisternae of sarcoplasmic reticulum are seen. Diagnosis is based on characteristic clinical signs and EMG findings. There is no treatment for this disorder, and it is rarely fatal. Affected animals are actually prized by collectors of so-called fainting goats. If nothing else, housing for these animals is simplified, as fencing need not be nearly as high as that required for normal goats.

Other Inherited Myopathies

An inherited myopathy (ovine muscular dystrophy) in Merino sheep and an inherited glycogen storage myopathy have been identified in sheep in Australia. These disorders are discussed in more detail in Web Appendix 15-1.

Megaesophagus in Camelids

The tunica muscularis of the esophagus of camelids contains a large amount of skeletal muscle, and adult llamas and alpacas are prone to develop abnormal motility and dilation of the esophagus (megaesophagus). Affected animals often lose body condition and exhibit abnormal rumination of feed boluses. Histopathologic findings of angular atrophy of type 1 and type 2 fibers in the esophagus of affected older llamas suggest that this disorder is an acquired denervating disease, but further studies are necessary. Megaesophagus in alpacas occurs in young animals and to date no diagnostic muscular lesions have been detected.

DISORDERS OF PIGS

The economic impact of muscle disease in pigs is profound. The high percentage of pigs with the genetic defect that predisposes to malignant hyperthermia is another example of selection pressure leading to skeletal muscle genetic mutations.

Bacterial and Parasitic Myopathies

Clostridial Myositis (Malignant Edema)

Pigs occasionally develop clostridial myositis (usually *Clostridium septicum*), particularly at sites of intramuscular injection. The resulting disease is similar to that seen in cattle, sheep, and goats, although heart involvement appears to be rare.

Pyogenic Bacteria

Abscesses within muscles and their fascia as a result of infection by pyogenic bacteria, such as *Arcanobacterium pyogenes*, are common in pigs and are similar to those in cattle.

Trichinosis

Infection of pigs by the nematode parasite *Trichinella spiralis* is of major economic importance to the porcine industry and poses a serious health hazard to humans. Pigs infected with *Trichinella spiralis* show no clinical signs.

The adult nematode resides in the mucosa of the small intestine. Larvae penetrate the intestinal mucosa and enter the bloodstream, through which they gain access to the muscle. Larvae invade and encyst within myocytes. Encysted larvae are typically not visible on gross examination, although dead larvae can calcify and be visible as 0.5- to 1-mm white nodules (Fig. 15-42, *A*). Active muscles, such as the tongue, masseter, diaphragm, and intercostal, laryngeal, and extraocular muscles, are preferentially affected. Focal inflammation consisting of eosinophils, neutrophils, and lymphocytes occurs associated with invasion of the muscle by *Trichinella* larvae. After cyst formation, the larvae are protected from the host's immune response and inflammation is minimal to absent (Fig. 15-42, *B*).

Diagnosis is based on identification of the characteristic nematode larvae encysted within muscle fibers. In those cases in which the larvae have died and calcified, a presumptive diagnosis of trichinosis can still be made.

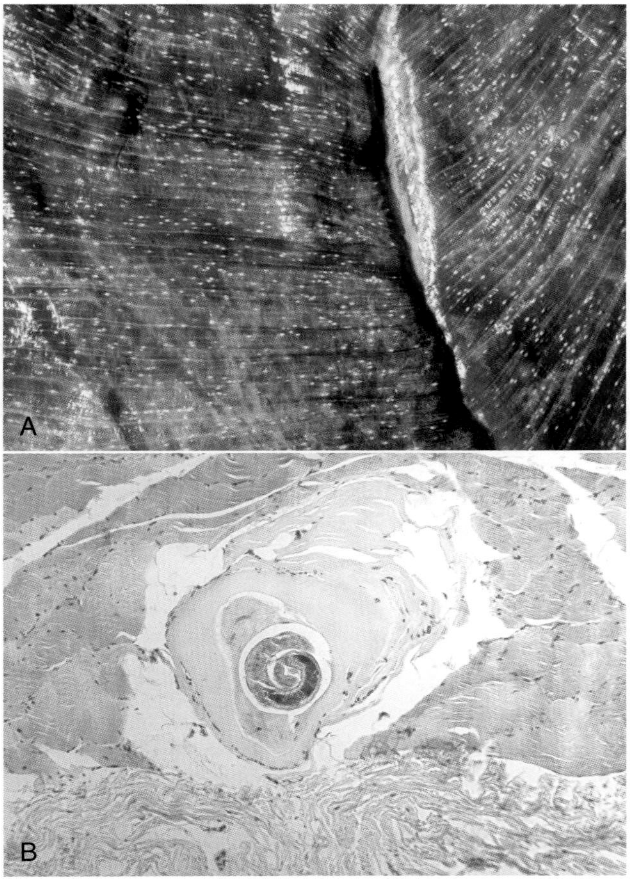

Fig. 15-42 **Trichinosis, encysted larvae, diaphragm, bear.** **A,** Encysted larvae of *Trichinella spiralis* appear as pale elongated gray-white foci in the muscle. **B,** Encysted larvae *(center)* of *Trichinella spiralis* incite minimal inflammation until they die. Formalin fixation, H&E stain. (Courtesy Dr. M.D. McGavin, College of Veterinary Medicine, University of Tennessee.)

Protozoal Myopathies

Intracytoplasmic cysts of *Sarcocystis* spp. are not common in pigs but can occasionally be found in the skeletal and cardiac muscle fibers as an incidental finding. Eosinophilic myocarditis has been reported after experimental infection.

Nutritional and Toxic Myopathies

Nutritional Myopathy

Young pigs are susceptible to degenerative myopathy caused by selenium or vitamin E deficiency, and the pathologic changes are similar to those seen in calves. A distinctive clinical disorder seen in very young Vietnamese pot-bellied pigs, in which affected piglets have a short, stilted gait and tend to stand on their toes, is thought to be related to selenium or vitamin E deficiency. Histologically, there is multifocal polyphasic myofiber necrosis. Affected piglets appear to recover spontaneously.

Toxic Myopathies

Pigs are susceptible to poisoning by *Cassia occidentalis* and develop segmental necrosis of myofibers, especially in the diaphragm. Monensin toxicity results in segmental necrosis of skeletal muscle and necrosis of cardiac muscle, particularly of the atria. The pathogenesis of ionophore toxicity is discussed in the earlier section on Toxic Myopathies. Gossypol present in cottonseed products is toxic to pigs when these products are fed at 10% or more of the ration and causes skeletal and cardiac muscle necrosis, as well as lesions in the liver and lung.

Congenital and Inherited Myopathies

Myofibrillar Hypoplasia (Splay Leg)

Myofibrillar hypoplasia (splay leg) is a congenital disorder that affects young piglets and results in splaying of the limbs laterally (abduction). Affected animals propel themselves by pushing against the ground with the pelvic limbs. This posture results in progressive flattening of the sternum. Although delayed myofibril development has been suggested, the histopathologic findings are inconclusive because similarly poorly developed myofibers can be seen in normal littermates. Affected piglets can recover with treatment, which includes the use of a harness that partially supports their bodies, holds their legs under their bodies, and encourages locomotion. Providing affected pigs with a nonslip floor is also important.

Steatosis

Pigs can have large areas of muscle replaced by mature adipose tissue, similar to that described in cattle.

Malignant Hyperthermia (Porcine Stress Syndrome; Pale Soft Exudative Pork)

MH (porcine stress syndrome, pale soft exudative pork) affects several strains of pigs, most commonly those with unpigmented hair coats. A similar syndrome occurs in Vietnamese pot-bellied pigs. Incidence varies but can be very high within certain herds. The disease in pigs is an accurate animal model of the disease in humans and is an important cause of economic losses in the pig industry. Susceptibility to MH is inherited as an autosomal recessive trait. The genetic defect results in abnormal activity of the skeletal muscle ryanodine receptor. The ryanodine receptor is a calcium release channel located in the sarcoplasmic reticulum terminal cisternal membrane that links the T tubule to the sarcoplasmic reticulum during excitation-contraction coupling. Uncontrolled intracytoplasmic calcium release because of abnormal ryanodine receptor activity leads to excessive contraction with resultant heat production. Clinical disease occurs only in pigs homozygous for the defect, although human heterozygotes can also be susceptible to hyperthermic episodes after halothane anesthesia. It is suspected that this defect originated more than 50 years ago in a foundation animal and resulted in offspring with increased muscling and reduced body fat. Affected pigs are clinically normal until an episode of hyperthermia is triggered by a precipitating factor such as halothane anesthesia or stress. Episodes consist of severe muscle rigidity and dramatically increased body temperature. Severe cases progress rapidly to death. Serum concentrations of CK and AST are markedly increased during episodes.

In animals dying during a hyperthermic episode, affected muscles are pale, moist, and swollen and appear "cooked" (Fig. 15-43), thus the common name "pale, soft, exudative pork." Muscles of the shoulder, back, and thigh are preferentially affected. Affected fibers are either hypercontracted or if the animal has survived for some hours, are undergoing coagulation necrosis. Histopathologic findings in susceptible pigs sampled during clinically normal periods include chronic myopathic change (fiber-size variation, internal nuclei) and rare necrotic fibers.

This disorder is most commonly diagnosed in pigs dying acutely and is made based on the clinical history of a precipitating stress and on the characteristic gross and histopathologic findings. Given that the precise defect is known, genetic testing allows for identification of carrier and affected animals. Avoidance of precipitating stress factors in susceptible pigs and removal of carrier and affected

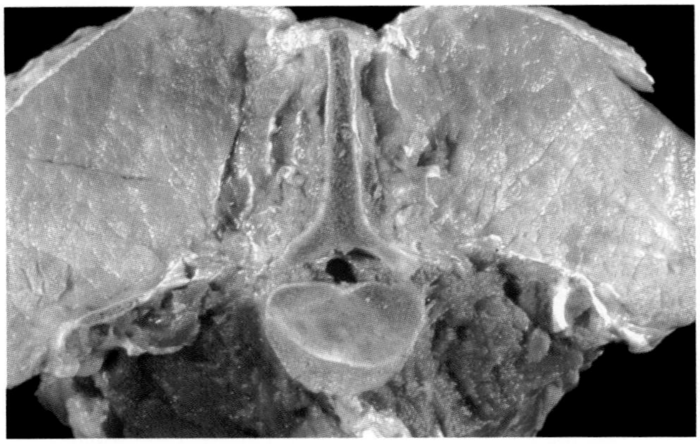

Fig. 15-43 Malignant hyperthermia (porcine stress syndrome, pale soft exudative pork), lumbar epispinal muscles, transverse section, pig. The affected muscles are pale pink, moist, and swollen and have a "cooked" pork appearance ("parboiled"). (Courtesy Dr. J. Wright, College of Veterinary Medicine, North Carolina State University; and Noah's Arkive, College of Veterinary Medicine, The University of Georgia.)

animals from the breeding stock reduces the incidence of this disorder.

Ischemic Myopathy

Large pigs are susceptible to ischemic myopathy secondary to recumbency, resulting in ischemic necrosis similar to that seen in horses and cattle. The proximal limb muscles are most susceptible.

DISORDERS OF DOGS

Selection pressures for a certain type of muscular development are far less frequent in dogs than in livestock. A few disorders, such as myotonia, have been suggested to occur more often in dogs originally bred for meat, but this is pure speculation. The canine genome may have genes prone to new mutations, similar to humans, leading to genetic disorders, such as X-linked muscular dystrophy. In general, the impact of muscular disorders in dogs is much less than in livestock. Dogs with muscular weakness can still make good house pets.

Parasitic Myopathies

Protozoal Myopathy

The parasitic diseases affecting skeletal muscle in the dog are primarily caused by protozoal organisms, of which *Neospora caninum* is the most important. It is now suspected that early reports of myositis and radiculoneuritis attributed to *Toxoplasma gondii* in young dogs were actually the result of *Neospora caninum* infections. *Neospora caninum* is often transmitted in utero, and evidence suggests that affected bitches are chronic carriers of the organism. Both the peripheral nervous system and the skeletal muscle are invaded by organisms. Ventral spinal roots are preferentially involved, and damage results in denervation atrophy of muscles. Signs of progressive neuromuscular weakness, most profound in the pelvic limbs, begin in affected pups several weeks of age. Marked muscle atrophy of the pelvic limb muscles occurs rapidly, and fixation of pelvic limb joints occurs as a result of denervation of muscle in an actively growing limb. Serum concentrations of CK and AST may be slightly increased. Concentric needle EMG reveals dense, sustained spontaneous activity (fibrillations and positive sharp waves) consistent with denervation.

Pelvic limb muscles are severely atrophied, firm, and pale. Fixation of the pelvic limb joints persists after anesthesia or death. Scattered foci of mixed inflammation with associated segmental myofiber necrosis are often seen within skeletal muscle, and characteristic intracytoplasmic protozoal cysts may be present.

Neospora caninum infection should be suspected based on characteristic progressive neuromuscular dysfunction in a young growing pup. Infection of older dogs is also possible but is uncommon. The finding of a mixed inflammatory-neuropathic lesion within affected skeletal muscle should prompt a search for protozoa, although these are often present in small numbers and may not be seen. Serologic tests can detect antibodies to *Neospora caninum,* and antibodies are available for immunohistochemical studies of paraffin-embedded, formalin-fixed tissue. Antiprotozoal treatment may kill the organisms, but denervation atrophy and pelvic limb fixation will persist.

Hepatozoon americanum and *Trypanosoma cruzi* are other protozoal organisms that can affect canine skeletal muscle. These parasitic diseases are discussed in more detail in Web Appendix 15-1.

Other Parasites

Rarely, cysts of *Trichinella spiralis* are found as an incidental finding in canine muscle.

Congenital or Inherited Myopathies

X-Linked Muscular Dystrophy (Duchenne's Type)

X-linked muscular dystrophy (Duchenne's type) has been confirmed or suspected in several breeds of dogs, including Irish terrier, golden retriever, Labrador retriever, miniature schnauzer, Rottweiler, Dalmatian, Shetland sheepdog, Samoyed, Pembroke Welsh corgi, Japanese spitz, and Alaskan malamute. This canine disorder is homologous to Duchenne's muscular dystrophy of humans and involves defects in the dystrophin gene, which codes for a membrane-associated cytoskeletal protein present in skeletal and cardiac muscle. The absence of dystrophin renders skeletal muscle fibers susceptible to repeated bouts of necrosis and regeneration. Necrosis of cardiac myocytes also occurs and is followed by replacement with connective tissue, resulting in a progressive cardiomyopathy. This disorder is inherited as an X-linked recessive trait, affecting approximately 50% of males born to a female carrier. Experimentally, affected females have been produced from breeding of an affected male to a carrier female. It is suspected that new mutations in the canine dystrophin gene may be relatively common, as is the case in humans. Therefore this disorder could occur in any breed, including crossbreeds. There is variable severity of clinical disease even within littermates, and small breed dogs are often less severely affected than are large breed dogs.

Severely affected pups develop a rapidly progressive weakness and die within the first few days of life. In less severely affected dogs, clinical signs are a stiff, short-strided gait and exercise intolerance beginning at 8 to 12 weeks of age, followed by progressive weakness and muscle atrophy. Development of a degree of joint contracture and splaying of the distal limbs is typical (Fig. 15-44). Weakness of the tongue, jaw, and pharyngeal muscles results in difficulty with prehension and swallowing of food, and affected dogs often drool excessively. Involvement of skeletal muscle within the esophagus can result in megaesophagus, which can cause regurgitation, and aspiration pneumonia. Markedly increased concentrations of serum CK, AST, and ALT are characteristic, even before the onset of obvious clinical disease. Concentric needle EMG reveals remarkable spontaneous activity in the form of pseudomyotonic bursts. Muscles do not dimple with percussion.

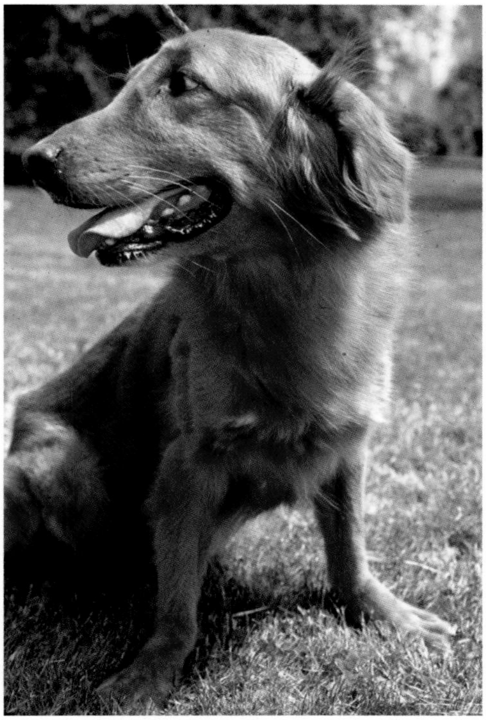

Fig. 15-44 Canine muscular dystrophy, X-linked muscular dystrophy, adult golden retriever.
Note the diffuse muscle wasting and splaying (outward rotation) of the forelimbs. (Courtesy Dr. B.A. Valentine, College of Veterinary Medicine, Oregon State University.)

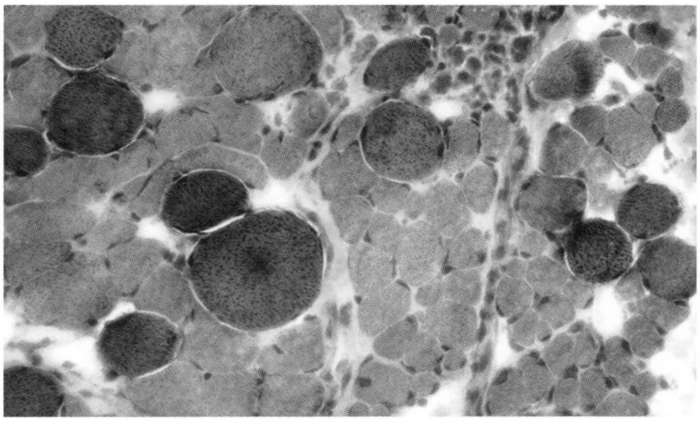

Fig. 15-45 Canine muscular dystrophy, X-linked muscular dystrophy, biceps femoris muscle, transverse section, dog.
The numerous large dark fibers *(left)* are undergoing acute necrosis, and the cluster of small-diameter fibers with large prominent nuclei *(top right)* are regenerating. The presence of both necrotic and regenerating fibers is indicative of polyphasic necrosis. Frozen section, modified Gomori's trichrome stain. (Courtesy Dr. B.A. Valentine, College of Veterinary Medicine, Oregon State University.)

In pups dying within the first few days of life, the thin superficial muscles of the shoulder, neck, and pelvic limbs (trapezius, brachiocephalicus, deltoid, and sartorius), and the diaphragm have pale yellow-to-white streaks throughout (see Fig. 15-9, *A*). Death in these cases is thought to be caused by respiratory failure related to severe diaphragmatic myonecrosis. In animals with clinical disease beginning at 8 to 12 weeks, pale streaks within muscle are much less evident, although affected muscles often appear diffusely pale and may be fibrotic. All skeletal muscles, with the exception of the extraocular muscles, appear to be affected to varying degrees. Overt myofiber necrosis is most severe in earlier stages of the disorder and typically affects small clusters of contiguous myofibers. Scattered large, darkly stained myofibers ("large dark fibers") in the early stages of hypercontraction and segmental necrosis are common (see Fig. 15-13, *A*) Regeneration of affected segments occurs rapidly, and characteristically both myofiber necrosis and fiber regeneration are present within the same section (i.e., the lesion is a multifocal polyphasic necrosis) (Fig. 15-45). Scattered mineralized fibers can also be found. With time, ongoing necrosis and regeneration are less common, and endomysial fibrosis occurs. Chronically affected muscles can have remarkable fibrosis, infiltration by adipocytes, and other chronic myopathic changes. Fiber-type conversion can also be seen as a chronic myopathic change.

In all dogs 6 months of age or older, multifocal pale yellow-to-white zones will be present within the heart, predominantly involving the subepicardial region of the left ventricular wall, the papillary muscles, and the ventricular septum. Histologically, necrosis, mineralization, and progressive dissecting myocardial fibrosis are found. Death in older animals is the result of either aspiration pneumonia secondary to dysphagia or to progressive cardiac failure, although affected dogs may survive for many years.

The diagnosis should be suspected based on characteristic clinical findings in a young male dog but must be confirmed by muscle biopsy and analysis of muscle for dystrophin. The absence of dystrophin in muscle fibers of affected dogs can be confirmed using immunohistochemical staining on frozen sections (Fig. 15-46) or by Western blot analysis. There is no treatment for this disorder.

Carrier females show no clinical signs, but scattered necrotic and regenerating fibers and moderate increases in serum CK and AST are common in young carriers. At birth, dystrophin in carriers is expressed as a mosaic pattern in individual cardiac and skeletal myofibers (Fig. 15-46, *C*). Because they are multinucleate, skeletal myofibers are able to eventually upregulate and translocate dystrophin to restore this protein to those segments where it is missing throughout the entire myofiber. Fiber necrosis is therefore rare in older carriers. Cardiac muscle, however, remains mosaic for life. Foci of necrosis and development of fibrosis occurs in the cardiac muscle of carrier females, but to date, none have developed overt cardiac failure. Any female dog producing affected pups is a carrier, and approximately half of all of her female offspring will also be carriers. Carrier females can also be identified either by dystrophin or DNA analysis and should be spayed.

Other Canine Muscular Dystrophies

Dystrophin has been found to be associated with a series of dystrophin-associated proteins, forming a membrane complex. The genes for many of these proteins are autosomally inherited; therefore not all canine muscular dystrophies are X-linked disorders. Autosomal recessive inheritance of dystrophin-associated gene defects leading to muscular dystrophy is common in humans, and defects in dystrophin complex proteins leading to non-Duchenne's type muscular dystrophy have also been identified in various breeds of dogs. These are discussed in more detail in Web Appendix 15-1.

Labrador Retriever Centronuclear Myopathy

Labrador retriever centronuclear myopathy is inherited as an autosomal recessive trait. Affected dogs occur within the working or sporting breed lines rather than the show dog lines. Studies suggest similarity to inherited centronuclear myopathy of humans and a genetic test to detect carrier and affected dogs has been developed. Affected Labrador retrievers develop signs of neuromuscular

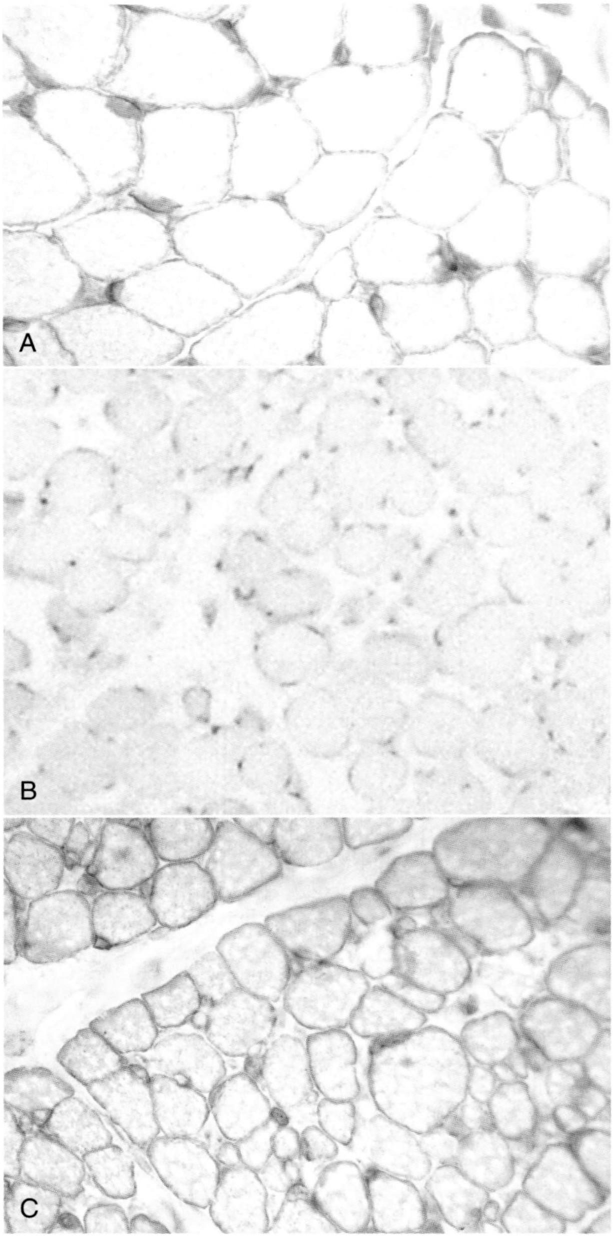

Fig. 15-46 Dystrophin localization in transverse sections of canine muscle, immunostain for dystrophin, skeletal muscle.

A, Normal dog. Note that the dystrophin is localized at the sarcolemma. Frozen section, immunoperoxidase reaction for dystrophin. **B,** X-linked muscular dystrophy, dog. Dystrophin is completely absent. Frozen section, immunoperoxidase reaction for dystrophin. **C,** X-linked muscular dystrophy carrier, young carrier female dog. Note the mosaic pattern in which some fibers contain normal dystrophin and others completely lack dystrophin. Frozen section, immunoperoxidase reaction for dystrophin. (Courtesy Dr. B.J. Cooper, College of Veterinary Medicine, Oregon State University.)

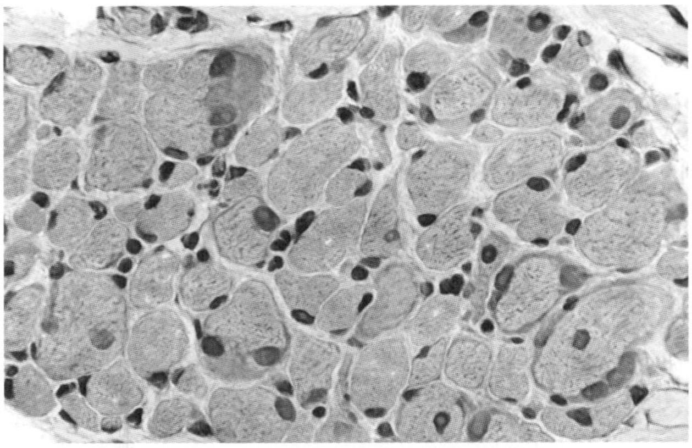

Fig. 15-47 Labrador retriever centronuclear myopathy, skeletal muscle, transverse section, Labrador retriever dog.

There is excessive fiber-size variation, and some fibers contain one or rarely two internal nuclei. Nuclei are abnormally large. Frozen section, H&E stain. (Courtesy Dr. B.A. Valentine, College of Veterinary Medicine, Oregon State University.)

weakness within the first 6 months of life. Exercise intolerance leads to collapse during prolonged exercise, and episodes of collapse can also be elicited by exposure to cold. Loss of triceps and patellar reflexes is characteristic. Affected dogs usually do not develop normal muscle mass. Concentric needle EMG reveals intense and abnormal spontaneous activity with normal motor nerve conduction velocities. Serum concentrations of CK and AST are often normal, although they can be mildly to moderately increased. Megaesophagus can be present.

The only specific abnormalities seen at necropsy are generalized poor muscling and possibly megaesophagus. On histologic examination, affected dogs have remarkable myopathic changes characterized by clusters of atrophic myofibers, myofiber hypertrophy, and internal nuclei (Fig. 15-47). Abnormal mitochondrial distribution, often with peripheral mitochondrial aggregates (identified as ragged red fibers in frozen sections stained with modified Gomori's trichrome stain), can also be seen (see Fig. 15-24, *B*). Segmental necrosis and regeneration are rare, therefore this disorder does not qualify as a muscular dystrophy. Although the initial reports described this disorder as a type 2 deficiency myopathy, further studies have shown that fiber-type proportions vary remarkably between muscles and between dogs, although an increase in type 1 fibers (type 1 fiber predominance) is often seen. Alteration of the normal mosaic pattern of myofiber types is also seen. There is fiber-type grouping, usually considered a neuropathic change, despite the absence of peripheral nerve lesions. These changes are thought to reflect fiber-type conversion unassociated with denervation.

Based on the clinical findings, the diagnosis may be suspected but should be confirmed by genetic testing. There is no treatment for the disorder, although the disease is nonprogressive after 6 months to 1 year of age, and affected animals can still be kept as pets. Dogs producing affected pups should not be rebred.

Congenital Myotonia

Myotonia is seen most commonly in the Chow Chow dog, miniature schnauzer, and Staffordshire terrier. Autosomal recessive inheritance has been confirmed in the miniature schnauzer, and available evidence supports similar inheritance in the Chow Chow. The underlying cellular defect in miniature schnauzers is decreased chloride conduction, and a similar defect is suspected in Chow Chow dogs. Affected pups can begin to show signs of a stiff gait as early as 6 weeks of age. The signs progress for several months and then stabilize with variable severity. Affected dogs move with splayed, stiff thoracic limbs and often a "bunny hop" gait in the pelvic limbs. Signs are most severe on initiation of movement and improve with continued exercise. But affected dogs are never clinically normal. During severe episodes, dogs can fall over, and laryngospasm can result in transient dyspnea and even cyanosis. The musculature becomes remarkably hypertrophied, and sustained muscle dimpling occurs after percussion. Characteristic waxing and waning ("dive bomber") myotonic bursts are found with concentric needle EMG. Serum concentrations of CK and AST are normal or mildly increased.

Overall muscle hypertrophy, with prominently defined muscle groups, is the only finding on postmortem examination. In early stages of the disease, muscle appears relatively normal on histologic examination. With time, myofiber hypertrophy and myofiber atrophy of both type 1 and type 2 fibers and rare scattered segmental necrosis or regeneration are seen. Fibrosis is mild to inapparent.

Diagnosis is based on clinical signs and can be confirmed by concentric needle EMG or by examination of a muscle biopsy. Molecular testing is available to detect carrier and affected miniature schnauzers. Therapeutic agents that act to stabilize excitable cell membranes, such as quinidine, procainamide, and phenytoin, can relieve some of the signs of myotonia.

Swimmer Pups

Swimmer pups are clinically similar to piglets with splay leg. Affected pups cannot adduct the limbs beneath their bodies and develop a characteristic "swimming" gait and, because of the weight of the body, progressive dorsoventral flattening of the sternum and thoracic wall. Although this syndrome can occur in pups with neuromuscular disease of any sort that leads to weakness, it is more commonly associated with overfeeding leading to excess body weight. Affected overfed pups often recover completely after reduction in total daily milk intake, provision of a nonslippery floor surface, and development of harnesses and physical therapy to encourage them to bring their legs underneath their bodies and walk. In pups that die or are euthanized, sternal flattening and abnormal lateral deviation of the limbs are consistent necropsy findings. Histopathologic abnormalities in muscle vary, depending on the cause (e.g., myofiber necrosis and regeneration in pups with muscular dystrophy, denervation atrophy in denervating disease) and are absent in pups in which this disorder simply reflects overfeeding.

Endocrine Myopathies

Hypothyroidism

Because of its role in muscle metabolism, decreased thyroid hormone often results in skeletal myofiber weakness and atrophy. Hypothyroidism can also cause a peripheral neuropathy, and damage to motor nerves can cause denervation atrophy and contribute to the neuromuscular weakness. Signs of neuromuscular dysfunction caused by hypothyroidism are extremely varied and include generalized weakness, muscle atrophy, laryngeal paralysis, and megaesophagus. EMG studies are often normal; abnormal spontaneous activity and decreased motor nerve conduction velocities can be found if there is concurrent peripheral neuropathy. Serum concentrations of CK and AST are generally normal. Other systemic manifestations of hypothyroidism may or may not be present.

At necropsy, overall muscle atrophy can be seen. Thyroid glands are often bilaterally atrophied, and megaesophagus can be present. Symmetric alopecia (endocrine dermatopathy) can also be seen. Type 2 myofibers are preferentially atrophied. Axonal degeneration can occur in peripheral nerves and because of denervation, can lead to angular atrophy of both type 1 and type 2 fibers and to fiber-type grouping as a result of reinnervation.

Diagnosis is suspected on the basis of clinical findings and selective type 2 atrophy or evidence of denervation or reinnervation in affected muscles, but should be confirmed by evaluation of thyroid function. In many cases, replacement thyroid hormone improves the signs of neuromuscular weakness.

Hypercortisolism

Hypercortisolism can occur because of either increased adrenocortical cortisol production or administration of exogenous corticosteroids. Clinical findings of neuromuscular weakness can be very similar to those in hypothyroidism. A unique manifestation of hypercortisolism in some dogs is development of a remarkably stiff, stilted pelvic limb gait, with increased bulk and tone of proximal thigh muscles (Cushingoid pseudomyotonia). The cause of Cushingoid pseudomyotonia is not known, although induction of sarcolemmal ionic instability is postulated. Concentric needle EMG of these muscles reveals myotonic bursts that do not wax and wane (pseudomyotonic activity). Muscles do not dimple after percussion. Other systemic signs of hypercortisolism, such as symmetric muscle atrophy and alopecia, can also be present. Serum concentrations of CK and AST are normal. Adrenal glands have bilateral cortical atrophy caused by exogenous corticosteroid administration or bilateral hypertrophy caused by stimulation secondary to pituitary neoplasia. Adrenal cortical neoplasia causes enlargement of the affected gland and atrophy of the contralateral gland. Findings in affected muscle and peripheral nerves are similar to those seen in hypothyroid myopathy (i.e., selective type 2 fiber atrophy) and evidence of axonal degeneration in peripheral nerves, type 1 and type 2 fiber atrophy indicative of denervation atrophy, and fiber-type grouping reflecting reinnervation are possible (see Fig. 15-20, *B*).

Diagnosis is suspected on the basis of clinical and histopathologic findings but should be confirmed by evaluation of adrenocortical function and total serum cortisol. Cessation of exogenous corticosteroids, removal of adrenal neoplasms, or chemical destruction of hyperplastic adrenal cortical tissue results in improvement in muscle mass and strength, although signs of pseudomyotonia may persist.

Immune-Mediated Myopathies (see Table 15-8)

Polymyositis

Polymyositis is the result of immune-mediated inflammation that attacks components of the skeletal myofibers and results in myofiber necrosis (see Fig. 15-28). The immunologic injury can be directed against skeletal muscle only or can be part of a more generalized immune-mediated disease such as systemic lupus erythematosus. Polymyositis can also occur in dogs with thymoma. This inflammatory myopathy can have an acute and rapidly progressive course or an insidious onset of muscle atrophy and generalized weakness. Muscles throughout the body are affected, but atrophy of temporal and masseter muscles may be most obvious, mimicking the appearance of dogs with masticatory myositis (see later discussion). Esophageal muscle involvement can lead to esophageal fibrosis and esophageal dysfunction, including megaesophagus. Respiratory muscle involvement can occur and if severe, will cause respiratory distress. Pain on palpation of muscles is rare. Serum concentrations of CK, AST, and ALT can be increased, but in chronic cases these concentrations can also be within normal limits. Concentric needle EMG often reveals scattered foci of abnormal spontaneous activity, and motor nerve conduction velocities are normal.

At necropsy, overall muscle atrophy may be the only finding. Aspiration pneumonia can occur secondary to megaesophagus. Histologic findings within affected muscles are extremely variable. In acute, fulminating cases, the muscle sections are filled with inflammatory cells, predominantly lymphocytes (Fig. 15-48, *A*), although interstitial eosinophils and neutrophils can also be

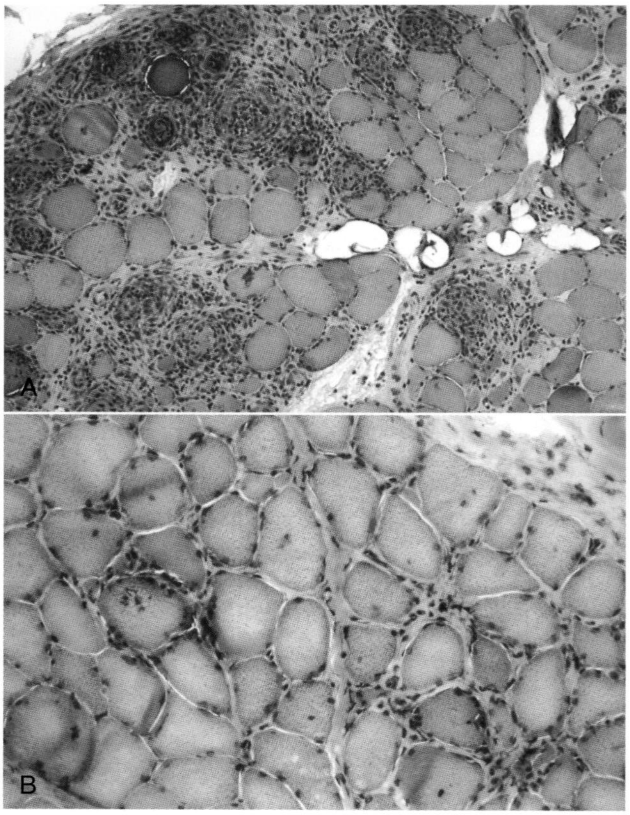

Fig. 15-48 Canine polymyositis, skeletal muscle, transverse section, dog.
A, Acute polymyositis. Dense interstitial and intramyofiber mononuclear inflammatory cell infiltrates are associated with myofiber necrosis. Frozen section, H&E stain. **B,** Chronic polymyositis. At this stage, there are only scattered interstitial mononuclear inflammatory cell infiltrates, scattered degenerate fibers, and chronic myopathic change (excessive fiber-size variation, internal nuclei, endomysial fibrosis). Frozen section, H&E stain. (**A** courtesy Dr. L. Fuhrer, Clinic Vétérinaire de St. Avertin, France. **B** courtesy Dr. B.A. Valentine, College of Veterinary Medicine, Oregon State University.)

present. The degree of myofiber necrosis is variable. Necrotic fibers in early stages are surrounded by lymphocytes that can be seen to invade intact myofibers (see Fig. 15-28, *B*). Similar to human polymyositis, $CD8^+$ cytotoxic/suppressor T lymphocytes are the primary infiltrating cells. Necrosis is followed by regeneration, but basal lamina damage is common and results in some degree of healing by fibrosis. In more chronic and insidious cases, the only lesion consists of scattered lymphocytes in the interstitial tissue adjacent to myofibers, with a variable degree of fibrosis and chronic myopathic change (Fig. 15-48, *B*). Sampling multiple muscles for histopathologic examination is recommended.

Polymyositis should be suspected based on the clinical findings, but identification of characteristic changes within muscle sections is often necessary to confirm the diagnosis. A positive circulating antinuclear antibody titer (ANA) is useful but is not always present. Treatment with immunosuppressive drugs, such as corticosteroids, can be curative, but affected animals may require lifelong therapy.

Masticatory Myositis (Eosinophilic Myositis; Atrophic Myositis)

The type 2 myofibers in the masticatory muscles of the dog contain a unique myosin isoform (type 2M myosin). On occasions, antibodies to this myosin form, and the result is an inflammatory

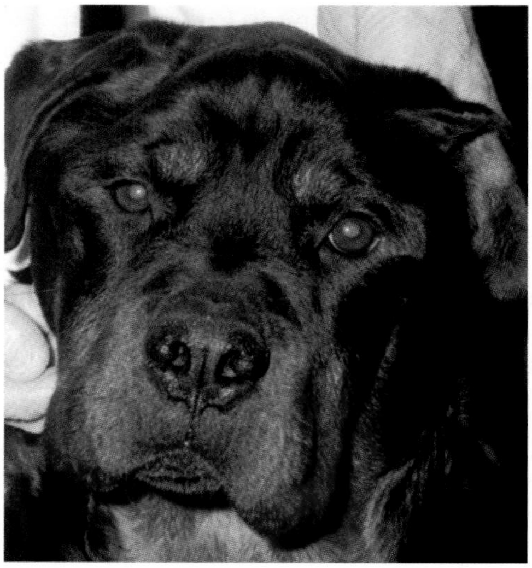

Fig. 15-49 Chronic masticatory myositis, skeletal muscle, dog. Note the severe atrophy of the temporalis and masseter muscles. (Courtesy Dr. W. Hornbuckle, College of Veterinary Medicine, Cornell University.)

myopathy confined to the temporalis and masseter muscles. Severe, acute cases display bilaterally symmetric swelling of, and pain in, those muscles, and an inability to fully open the jaw. Affected dogs can have difficulty prehending food. More chronic or insidious cases have bilaterally symmetric atrophy of the temporal and masseter muscles (Fig. 15-49) and decreased jaw mobility. Pain may or may not be evident at this stage. Concentric needle EMG often reveals foci of spontaneous activity in active cases but can be normal in more chronic cases. Serum concentrations of CK and AST are normal or only mildly increased.

Severely atrophied muscles often contain pale streaks. The degree and nature of the inflammation are variable. In acute cases, infiltrates of lymphocytes and plasma cells, similar to those in polymyositis, are present. But, in contrast to canine polymyositis, the infiltrating cells in masticatory myositis are primarily B lymphocytes. There can also be numerous eosinophils, and these can be the predominant cell type. Neutrophils are much less common. Inflammation is associated with myofiber necrosis. Regeneration can restore myofibers, but because the basal lamina is often damaged, healing by fibrosis is common. The presence of fibrosis is an important prognostic indicator because fibrosis is an irreversible change.

The diagnosis is suggested on the basis of characteristic clinical findings. Masticatory myositis must be differentiated from polymyositis, which can also have severe involvement of the temporal and masseter muscles. Serologic testing to detect anti–type 2M myosin antibodies specific to masticatory muscle myositis is available, and serum from affected dogs will bind to type 2M fibers (Fig. 15-50). EMG and histopathologic evaluation of multiple muscles can also help to differentiate these two disorders. Treatment with immunosuppressive doses of corticosteroids generally alleviates pain and results in increased mobility of the jaw and an increase in muscle mass. Some degree of atrophy and loss of complete jaw mobility can persist. A single course of corticosteroids can be curative; however, some cases require extended therapy.

Extraocular Muscle Myositis

An immune-mediated attack directed specifically at extraocular muscles is the suspected cause of this disorder. Acute onset of bilateral exophthalmos is seen. Affected dogs are usually less than

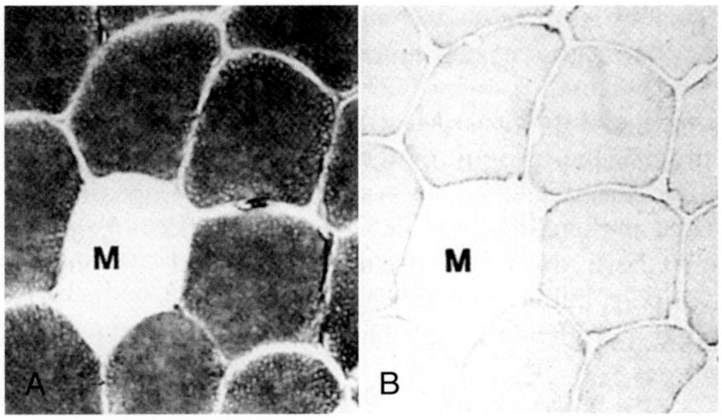

Fig. 15-50 Canine masticatory myositis, skeletal muscle, temporalis muscle, transverse sections, normal dog.
A, A single type 1 fiber *(light staining, M)* surrounded by type 2 fibers *(dark staining).* Frozen section, ATPase pH 9.8. **B,** After incubation with serum from a dog with masticatory myositis, type 2 fibers stain positively because of binding of anti–type 2M myosin antibodies from the affected dog. Notice that the type 1 fiber *(M)* is unstained. Frozen section, staphylococcal protein A-peroxidase. (Courtesy Dr. G.D. Shelton, University of California, San Diego.)

2 years of age, and golden retriever dogs appear to be predisposed. Serum concentrations of CK and AST are generally normal.

The extraocular muscles, with the exception of the retractor bulbi muscle, are swollen and pale yellow. A predominantly lymphocytic inflammation resulting in myofiber necrosis and regeneration is seen. Because it is difficult to obtain a biopsy sample of the extraocular muscles, diagnosis is generally based on typical clinical findings. Corticosteroid therapy is effective, but episodes can recur.

Disorders of the Neuromuscular Junction

Myasthenia Gravis

The pathogenesis of myasthenia gravis is discussed in the section on neuropathic and neuromuscular junction disorders (see Fig. 15-29). In most cases, myasthenia gravis is an acquired disease, with circulating antibodies directed at the acetylcholine receptors of the neuromuscular junction. An inherited predisposition to development of acquired myasthenia gravis has been reported in Newfoundland dogs. In some cases, onset of myasthenia gravis occurs because of thymoma or less commonly, thymic hyperplasia. Myasthenia gravis associated with hypothyroidism also occurs in dogs but is rare. Congenital myasthenia gravis is due to abnormal development of the neuromuscular junction and is inherited as an autosomal recessive trait in Jack Russell terriers, smooth fox terriers, and Springer spaniels. Congenital myasthenia gravis also occurs in smooth-haired miniature dachshunds. Typical signs of acquired disease are episodic collapse in an adult dog, with normal gait and strength after rest. Clinical signs can, however, be variable. The canine esophagus contains a large percentage of skeletal muscle throughout the length of the tunica muscularis; therefore megaesophagus is common in dogs with myasthenia gravis and may be the only presenting sign. This differs from humans, in which only the proximal one-third of the esophageal muscularis is completely skeletal muscle and the lower third is completely smooth muscle. In some cases, mild weakness persists between episodes. Clinical signs of congenital myasthenia gravis appear at an early age (6 to 8 weeks of age) and in most affected breeds are progressive and typically quite severe. Affected dachshunds, however, appear to recover by 6 months of age. Repetitive motor nerve stimulation reveals an initial sharp decremental response, followed by relatively uniform amplitude potentials. Serum concentrations of CK and AST are normal.

No findings are evident at postmortem examination unless megaesophagus, thymic abnormalities, or thyroid abnormalities are present, and no abnormalities in muscle are seen on light microscopic examination. Ultrastructural abnormalities of the neuromuscular junctions (simplification of the postsynaptic membrane) may be present.

Diagnosis is suspected on the basis of typical clinical findings and results of repetitive nerve stimulation. In patients with acquired myasthenia gravis, dramatic transient improvement in muscle strength after administration of intravenous acetylcholinesterase inhibitors such as edrophonium (Tensilon) is seen, and the diagnosis is confirmed by identification of circulating antibodies to skeletal muscle acetylcholine receptors. In cases of acquired myasthenia gravis, the presence of a thymic abnormality should be determined, because removal of a thymoma or of a hyperplastic thymus results in resolution of clinical signs. In other cases, long-acting acetylcholinesterase inhibitor therapy, sometimes combined with corticosteroid therapy, is often beneficial. There is no effective treatment for congenital myasthenia gravis.

Tick Paralysis

In a dog with flaccid tetraparesis, a diagnosis of tick paralysis should be considered along with polyradiculoneuritis (coonhound paralysis; see Chapter 14) and botulism. Clinical signs of tick paralysis appear 5 to 7 days after infestation with causative *Dermacentor* or *Ixodes* ticks. Initial clinical signs are pelvic limb weakness, with progression to recumbency within 48 to 72 hours. Cranial nerve function is normal. Clinical signs of tick paralysis are very similar to those of coonhound paralysis (see Chapter 14). Treatment for tick infestation can result in recovery within a few days, although death from respiratory muscle paralysis is still possible.

Botulism

Botulism occurs in dogs, resulting in rapid onset of flaccid tetraparesis, but is rare. Reported cases of canine botulism are most often the result of types C and D of *Clostridium botulinum* neurotoxins. Diagnosis is often presumptive, based on a failure to identify other causes of diffuse neuromuscular weakness and with luck, a history of consumption of a rotted carcass. Recovery has been reported in dogs with botulism, although many cases are fatal.

Other Canine Myopathies

Exertional Rhabdomyolysis

Massive acute rhabdomyolysis associated with exertion occurs in racing greyhounds and sled dogs. Muscles of the back (longissimus) and thigh (gluteal) are most often affected and may be severely swollen. Predisposing factors are not clear, but in sled dogs a change to a very high-fat diet has resulted in a decrease in exercise-induced muscle injury.

Malignant Hyperthermia (MH)

MH occurs sporadically in dogs, and breeding studies indicate an autosomal dominant inheritance. The cause has been determined to be a genetic defect in the muscle ryanodine receptor, which is also the cause of MH in pigs and humans. MH-like episodes can also occur in any dog after ingestion of hops used for brewing beer.

Other Breed-Specific Myopathies

A number of breed-specific myopathies have been reported in the dog, and include dermatomyositis in collies and Shetland sheepdogs, mitochondrial myopathy in Old English sheepdogs and other breeds, central core myopathy in Great Danes, exercise-induced collapse in Labrador retrievers, and myopathy of Bouvier des Flandres dogs, English Springer spaniels, and Rottweilers. Myoclonus and intramuscular Lafora-like bodies occur in wirehaired miniature dachshunds. These are discussed in more detail in Web Appendix 15-1.

Idiopathic Masticatory Muscle Atrophy

Dogs can develop a progressive atrophy of temporal and masseter muscles that is not associated with pain or difficulty opening the jaw or prehending food. Examination of affected muscle from these dogs reveals mild generalized atrophy of myofibers, but there is no evidence of inflammation, degeneration, fibrosis, or denervation. The cause is not known, and there is no treatment.

Denervating Diseases

There are numerous causes of inherited and acquired peripheral nerve disorders causing axonal damage and resultant denervation in dogs (see Chapter 14). Motor neuron disease is most often inherited, as in the Brittany spaniel and Rottweiler. Such disorders cause symmetric atrophy of affected muscles. Neoplasms arising in peripheral nerves (nerve sheath neoplasms) cause compression of the nerve resulting in Wallerian degeneration, leading to progressive gait abnormalities and ultimately denervation atrophy of muscles of the affected limb.

DISORDERS OF CATS

Relatively few muscular disorders have thus far been identified in cats. This may in part be the result of low performance expectations of the average house cat. It is entirely possible that there are many cats lying around with muscular disorders that have as yet gone unrecognized.

Inherited or Congenital Myopathies

X-Linked Muscular Dystrophy (Duchenne's Type)

Dystrophic cats lack the muscle cytoskeletal protein dystrophin, which is also the cause of Duchenne's dystrophy in boys and X-linked muscle dystrophy in the dog. Affected cats develop a progressive, persistent, stiff gait associated with marked muscular hypertrophy. The cause of the remarkable muscular hypertrophy seen in affected cats, as opposed to the muscle atrophy seen in the dog and in humans, and the pseudohypertrophy as a result of fat infiltration into affected muscle that can occur in humans, is not known. Age of onset is from a few months to 21 months of age. Affected cats have difficulty grooming, jumping, and lying down. Concentric needle EMG reveals dense and sustained abnormal spontaneous activity, similar to findings in the dystrophic dog. Serum concentrations of creatine kinase (CK), AST, and ALT are elevated, typically to very high levels. Affected cats can die under anesthesia or after restraint or sedation because of a MH-like syndrome.

At necropsy, all muscles are severely hypertrophied and may contain pale areas. Focal pale or chalky areas within the myocardium are typically found. Histologically, muscles show a range of changes. Concurrent segmental myonecrosis and myofiber regeneration (polyphasic necrosis) are characteristic. Chronic myopathic changes, found in older animals, include severe myofiber hypertrophy, myofiber atrophy, internal nuclei, and mild-to-moderate endomysial fibrosis. Myocardial lesions consist of multifocal necrosis and mineralization of cardiac myofibers and fibrosis, primarily in the left ventricular free wall, papillary muscles, and septum. Affected cats may have a relatively normal lifespan, although unexpected death during anesthesia or forced restraint is common. The exact cause of this is unclear.

The diagnosis is suspected on the basis of characteristic clinical, clinicopathologic, and histopathologic findings in a young male cat. Confirmation relies on assay of muscle samples for dystrophin or on immunohistochemical staining for dystrophin in frozen sections.

Other Feline Inherited or Congenital Myopathies

A form of autosomal recessively inherited muscular dystrophy due to deficiency of the dystrophin complex protein α-dystroglycan occurs in Sphinx and Devon Rex cats. Glycogenosis type IV (GBE defect) affecting skeletal muscle is seen as an inherited disorder in Norwegian Forest cats. A histologically similar condition occurs occasionally in other breeds. Feline nemaline myopathy is a rare congenital myopathy in the cat. These disorders are discussed in more detail in Web Appendix 15-1.

Myopathies Caused by Electrolyte Abnormalities (Hypokalemia and Hypernatremia)

Similar to cattle, cats with severe electrolyte abnormalities can show signs of neuromuscular weakness that can be caused by degenerative myopathy. Although degenerative myopathy has been reported secondary to increased blood sodium concentrations (hypernatremia), hypokalemic myopathy occurs far more frequently.

The cause of the weakness and myofiber necrosis associated with electrolyte abnormalities is complex and involves abnormal skeletal muscle energy metabolism and possible ischemia because of vasoconstriction. Hypokalemia (serum potassium concentration less than 3.5 mEq/L) can occur because of decreased dietary intake or increased urinary excretion of potassium. In cats, hypokalemia is often a consequence of chronic renal disease. It can also occur secondary to gastrointestinal disease or inappropriate fluid therapy. Hyperthyroidism has been associated with development of hypokalemic myopathy in cats. Hypernatremic myopathy is less common but has been reported in a 7-month-old cat with hydrocephalus and transient hypopituitarism.

Affected cats show severe generalized weakness, with notable ventroflexion of the neck. Concentric needle EMG often demonstrates foci of abnormal spontaneous activity. Serum concentrations of CK, AST, and ALT are often increased, sometimes severely. Clinically diagnosed cases of hypokalemia and hypernatremia can be confirmed by determining if the serum potassium is low or the serum sodium is high, respectively.

No specific gross pathologic findings are present except in cats with hypokalemia as a result of chronic renal disease, in which the kidneys are small and fibrotic. In hypokalemic myopathy, myofiber necrosis and regeneration of variable severity are present concurrently (polyphasic necrosis). Chronic renal disease is commonly due to chronic interstitial nephritis. No abnormalities were detected in a muscle biopsy from a cat with hypernatremic myopathy, although the mildly increased serum concentration of CK and the abnormal EMG suggest mild and perhaps transient myofiber necrosis and regeneration.

Diagnosis is based on characteristic clinical findings of weakness and concurrent hypokalemia or hypernatremia. Treatment of affected cats has been very successful. Immediate fluid therapy is used to correct the electrolyte abnormality, followed by diet change to maintain normal electrolyte concentrations. If there is an underlying hyperthyroidism, this should also be treated.

Immune-Mediated Disorders

An immune-mediated myositis has been described in cats infected with feline immunodeficiency virus. Serum concentration of CK is moderately increased, but clinical signs of muscle dysfunction are not apparent. Infiltration of muscle by $CD8^+$ lymphocytes, similar to human immunodeficiency virus (HIV)-associated polymyositis is characteristic.

Disorders of the Neuromuscular Junction

Myasthenia Gravis

Feline acquired and congenital myasthenia gravis are similar to these disorders in the dog but occur less commonly.

Botulism

Although theoretically possible, we are not aware of any confirmed or highly suspicious cases of botulism in cats. This likely reflects both an inherent resistance to botulinum toxin and the typical feline fastidious appetite.

Denervating Diseases

Disorders affecting peripheral motor nerves are much less common in cats as compared with dogs. A chronic relapsing polyneuritis primarily affecting ventral spinal roots has been seen in young adult cats, which can cause denervation atrophy in affected muscles. Diabetes mellitus can also result in peripheral neuropathy in cats.

SUGGESTED READINGS

Information on this topic is available at evolve.elsevier.com/Zachary/McGavin/.

CHAPTER 16

Bones, Joints, Tendons, and Ligaments

Cathy S. Carlson and Steven E. Weisbrode

The skeleton consists of bones and joints and their supporting structures and is responsible for supporting and protecting the body and enabling movement initiated by the nervous system and facilitated by muscles. The skeleton can be divided into axial skeleton (head, vertebrae, ribs, and sternum) and appendicular skeleton (thoracic and pelvic limbs). Information on the methods for postmortem examination and evaluation of the skeleton is available in Web Appendix 16-1, which can be found at evolve.elsevier.com/Zachary/McGavin/.

STRUCTURE AND FUNCTION OF BONE

BONE AT THE CELLULAR LEVEL

Structure and function can be discussed at the organ, tissue, and cellular levels. In this section, normal structure and function are briefly reviewed, beginning at the cellular level and including bone matrix and mineral. Cells directly involved with the structural integrity of bone include osteoblasts, osteocytes, and osteoclasts (Box 16-1).

Osteoblasts are cells on any bone surface (periosteal, endosteal, trabecular, intracortical) that produce bone matrix (osteoid), initiate the mineralization of this matrix (deposition of hydroxyapatite), and seemingly paradoxically initiate the resorption of this matrix by osteoclasts. Osteoblasts are derived from mesenchymal stem cells. Active osteoblasts are plump (Fig. 16-1), with abundant basophilic cytoplasm that is rich in rough endoplasmic reticulum and contains prominent Golgi apparatus and numerous mitochondria (Web Fig. 16-1). Inactive osteoblasts are disk-shaped with little cytoplasm because fewer organelles are needed for matrix synthesis and secretion (Fig. 16-2 and Web Fig. 16-2). Osteoblasts likely interact with osteocytes to assist in fine control of calcium homeostasis and detection of mechanical use and microscopic damage to bone, as discussed later. Indirect measurements of osteoblast activity are reflected in blood concentrations of the bone-specific isoform of alkaline phosphatase, an enzyme on the cell membrane of osteoblasts, and the noncollagenous protein, osteocalcin, that is secreted by osteoblasts and is present in bone matrix. Both are thought to have roles in mineralization and calcium ion homeostasis.

Osteocytes are osteoblasts that have been surrounded by mineralized bone matrix (Web Fig. 16-3) and are the most numerous and longest living of the bone cell types. They occupy small spaces in the bone called *lacunae* (singular: lacuna) and make contact with osteoblasts and other osteocytes by means of long cytoplasmic processes that pass through thin tunnels in the bone called *canaliculi* (singular: canaliculus). Under conditions of extreme stress to calcium homeostasis, osteocytes might have the ability to resorb perilacunar mineral and matrix, thus enlarging the lacuna (osteocytic osteolysis). This process apparently is rare and likely does not contribute significantly to development of osseous lesions. Osteocytes also retain a limited capacity to form bone and are exquisitely sensitive to mechanical strain in the form of shear stress. Other functions of osteocytes are somewhat speculative and are presented later in osteoblast-osteocyte interactions.

Osteoclasts are multinucleated cells that are derived from hematopoietic stem cells of the granulocyte-monocyte series and are responsible for bone resorption (Fig. 16-3). They have abundant eosinophilic cytoplasm and a specialized brush border along the margin of the cell that is adjacent to the bone surface that is being resorbed (Web Fig. 16-4). For osteoclasts to resorb bone, they must gain access to the bone surface that is usually covered by osteoblasts, and they must attach to the mineralized surface by transmembrane receptors in their sealing zones. These receptors bind to specific ligands in the matrix, likely residing in noncollagenous proteins. Osteoclasts are not able to bind to unmineralized bone matrix even though it contains these same ligands. Once bound to the matrix, the osteoclast resorbs bone in two stages. First, the mineral is dissolved by secretion of hydrogen ions through a proton pump located in the brush border. These hydrogen ions are derived from carbonic acid produced within the osteoclast from water and carbon dioxide by the enzyme carbonic anhydrase. Second, the collagen of the matrix is cleaved into polypeptide fragments by cysteine and metalloproteinases and cathepsins, particularly cathepsin K, released from the numerous lysosomes in the osteoclast and secreted through the brush border. The concavity in the bone created by the resorbed bone matrix is called a *Howship's lacuna,* or a resorption lacuna. Physiologically, osteoclast activation is controlled by osteoblasts and bone marrow stromal cells (see

BOX 16-1 Bone Cell Function

Osteoblasts: Cells of stromal stem cell origin that reside on the surface of bone and form bone matrix, initiate bone mineralization, and initiate bone resorption (by signaling to osteoclasts) in response to physiologic stimuli

Osteocytes: Osteoblasts that have become encased in bone matrix. These cells detect changes in stress (force applied to the bone) and strain (structural deformation in response to the force) in the bone and signal these changes to osteoblasts to either form bone or initiate resorption; may mobilize calcium from the bone through osteocytic osteolysis

Osteoclasts: Cells formed by the fusion of cells of the monocyte-macrophage cell line; function is to resorb mineralized bone matrix

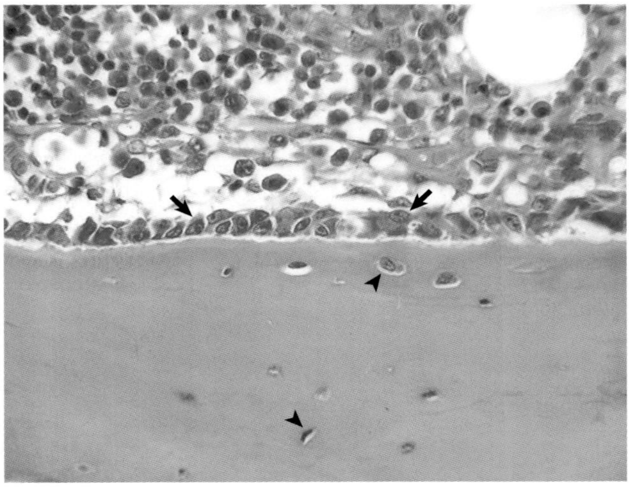

Fig. 16-1 **Osteoblasts and osteocytes, long bone, young dog.** Prominent cuboidal osteoblasts *(arrows)* line the endosteal surface. Hematopoietic marrow is present *(above the endosteal surface)*. More mature (older) osteocytes are present deeper in the cortex *(below the endosteal surface)* and are recognizable as small elliptical cells *(arrowheads)* residing in lacunae. The more recently embedded (younger) osteocytes are in larger lacunae closer to the endosteal surface. H&E stain. (Courtesy Dr. S.E. Weisbrode, College of Veterinary Medicine, The Ohio State University.)

later discussion of interactions). Calcitonin is a systemic inhibitor of osteoclasts. Osteoclasts have receptors for calcitonin and respond to this hormone by involuting their brush border and detaching from the bone surface. The activity of osteoclasts can be indirectly measured by determining serum concentrations of collagen degradation products (pyridinoline and deoxypyridinoline cross-links) or tartrate-resistant acid phosphatase (TRAP) activity. TRAP is a glycosylated monomeric metalloenzyme that is highly expressed by osteoclasts. TRAP staining also may be used as a cytochemical marker of osteoclasts in histologic sections (Web Fig. 16-5).

Osteoblast-osteocyte interactions are apparent from their connections to each other by thin, tortuous, cytoplasmic processes. This network of osteoblasts and osteocytes forms a functional membrane that separates the extracellular fluid bathing bone surfaces from the general extracellular fluid and can regulate the flow of calcium and phosphate ions to and from the bone fluid compartment (Fig. 16-4). Because of the large surface area of perilacunar and canalicular bone available for rapid ion exchange, significant amounts of calcium can be shifted from the bone fluid compartment to the extracellular fluid compartment without structural changes within

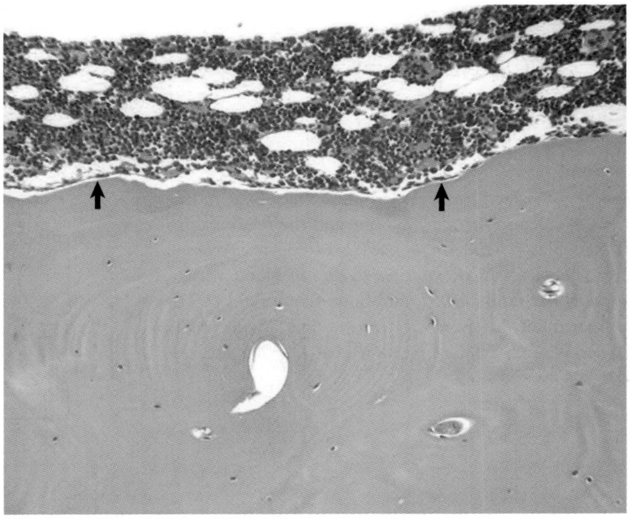

Fig. 16-2 **Osteoblasts, vertebra, adult dog.** Quiescent osteoblasts *(arrows)* on the endosteal surface of adult bone are fusiform with little cytoplasm and form an inconspicuous layer between the cortical bone *(below the endosteal surface)* and active hematopoietic marrow *(above the endosteal surface)* of the adult axial skeleton. H&E stain. (Courtesy Dr. S.E. Weisbrode, College of Veterinary Medicine, The Ohio State University.)

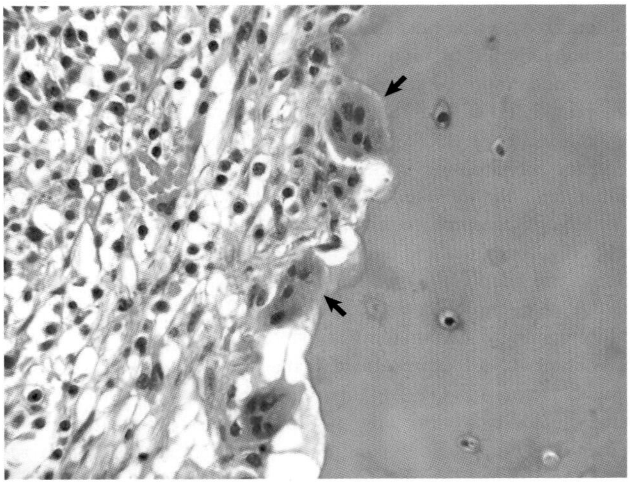

Fig. 16-3 **Osteoclasts, long bone, young dog.** Several multinucleated cells (osteoclasts) *(arrows)* are resorbing endocortical bone and creating a scalloped endosteal surface. These scalloped cavities of resorbed bone are called *Howship's* (or erosion) *lacunae.* H&E stain. (Courtesy Dr. S.E. Weisbrode, College of Veterinary Medicine, The Ohio State University.)

the bone. In addition, this network allows osteocytes to detect alternations in the fluid flow within the bone extracellular fluid compartment. It is thought that such flow contributes to electric currents called *streaming potentials.* Changes in these streaming potentials caused by altered stress and strain on the bone or disruption of these potentials by microcracks (minuscule fractures within the bone visible only microscopically) might be detected by osteocytes with subsequent signaling to the overlying osteoblasts to initiate bone formation or resorption.

Osteoclast-osteoblast/stromal cell interactions are required for physiologic resorption of bone. The bone surface is protected from osteoclastic resorption by a continuous layer of osteoblasts and also by a very thin layer of unmineralized bone matrix normally

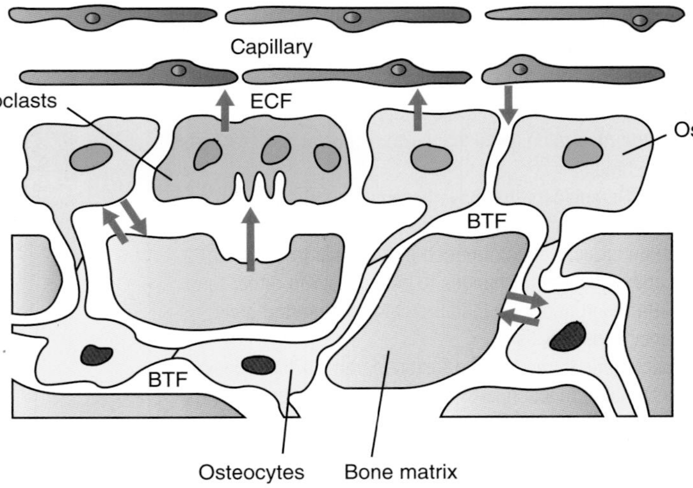

Fig. 16-4 Schematic diagram of the movement of calcium.
The hypothesized intracellular and extracellular movement of calcium *(arrows)* in bone and the relationships of osteoblasts *(blue, single nuclei),* osteocytes *(yellow),* and osteoclasts *(blue, multiple nuclei)* to blood vessels, extracellular fluid *(ECF),* and bone tissue fluid *(BTF)* compartment is shown. (Redrawn from Matthews JL, Vander Wiel C, Talmage RV: *Adv Exp Med Biol* 103:456, 1978.)

present beneath resting osteoblasts (lamina limitans) (see Web Fig. 16-2). Osteoclasts are not able to bind to unmineralized bone matrix. For parathyroid hormone (PTH) to initiate bone resorption, receptors on the osteoblast bind PTH (osteoclasts do not usually express receptors for PTH). The binding of PTH to osteoblasts signals them to retract and secrete collagenases, which erode the unmineralized layer of matrix and allow osteoclasts access to a mineralized bone surface. In addition, osteoblasts and stromal cells that are activated by binding PTH and in response to a variety of other bone-resorbing stimuli (1, 25 dihydroxyvitamin D_3; interleukin [IL]-1, IL-6, and IL-11; tumor necrosis factor-α [TNF-α]; prostaglandin E_2 [PGE_2]; and glucocorticoids) express or secrete receptor activator for nuclear factor κ B ligand (RANKL), also called *osteoclast differentiation factor* (ODF). RANKL binds to the RANK receptor on osteoclasts and activates the resorption process. Osteoblasts and bone marrow stromal cells also can secrete osteoprotegerin (OPG), a RANK homolog that works by binding to RANKL, thus blocking the RANK-RANKL interaction and inhibiting the differentiation of osteoclast precursors into mature osteoclasts. OPG expression can be stimulated by transforming growth factor-β (TGF-β). Therefore osteoblasts and stromal cells have the ability to both up- and down-regulate osteoclastic bone resorption (Fig. 16-5). In conditions of inflammation and necrosis, inflammatory mediators, such as IL-1 and TNF-α, can stimulate osteoclasts directly, causing bone resorption independent of the presence of viable osteoblasts.

BONE AT THE ORGANIC MATRIX AND MINERAL LEVEL

The mineralized matrix of bone provides the organ's strength. Bone organic matrix consists of type I collagen and "ground substance" (the noncollagenous extracellular matrix: water, proteoglycans, glycosaminoglycans, noncollagenous proteins, and lipids, which are discussed later). Type I collagen polymers are secreted by osteoblasts and assembled into fibrils that are embedded in the ground substance and then mineralized. The type I collagen molecule is composed of three intertwined amino acid chains, unique to which is the hydroxylated form of the amino acid proline (hydroxyproline). Type I collagen molecules have extensive cross-linkages among the amino acid chains within the molecule and between adjacent molecules. Collagen molecules are deposited in rows with a gap between each molecule and with the rows staggered so that the molecules overlap by one-quarter of their length. This specific packing of the collagen molecules and the cross-linkages contribute

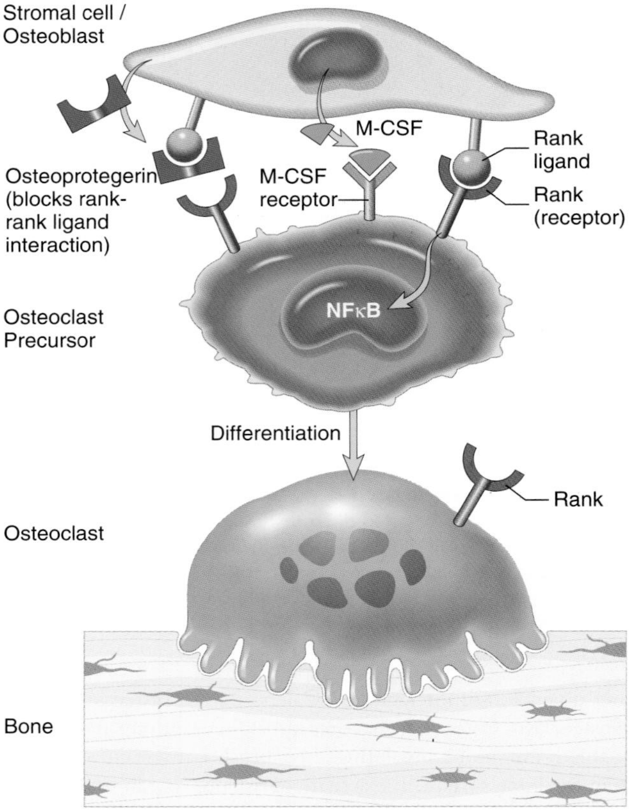

Fig. 16-5 Schematic diagram showing interaction between stromal cells/osteoblasts and osteoclast/osteoclast precursors.
Stromal cells and osteoblasts produce "rank ligand," which binds to the "rank" receptor on the osteoclast and its precursors; this binding stimulates osteoclasis. Conversely, osteoblasts and stromal cells can inhibit the activation of osteoclasts by secreting osteoprotegerin, which can bind to "rank ligand" and block its binding to "rank receptor." *M-CSF,* Macrophage colony-stimulating factor; *NFκB,* nuclear factor κ B. (From Kumar V, Abbas AK, Fausto N, et al: *Robbins & Cotran pathologic basis of disease,* ed 8, Philadelphia, 2009, Saunders.)

to the strength and insolubility of the fibrous component of the bone matrix. Other than in rapidly deposited bone (woven bone found in primary trabeculae, bone of early fetal development, and pathologic conditions such as fracture repair), collagen fibers are arranged in parallel lamellae (singular: lamella) and the tissue is called *lamellar bone*. In cortical (compact) bone, lamellae are arranged concentrically (Fig. 16-6). In trabecular bone, the lamellae usually are arranged parallel with the bone surface. The collagen content of bone and its lamellar arrangement give bone its strength and flexibility. The ground substance of bone, which also is synthesized by osteoblasts, consists of noncollagenous proteins, proteoglycans, and lipids. Many of the noncollagenous proteins are cytokines that are capable of influencing bone cell activity. These cytokines, such as TGF-β, may play pivotal roles in controlling the extent of bone formation and resorption in normal remodeling and in disease (Fig. 16-7). Also, among the noncollagenous proteins are enzymes that can function in the degradation of collagen (e.g., matrix metalloproteinases) and can destroy inhibitors of mineralization (e.g., pyrophosphatases). Other noncollagenous proteins in the matrix can function as adhesion molecules and help bind cells to cells, cells to matrix, and mineral to matrix. Examples of these are osteonectin and osteocalcin. The role of proteoglycans in bone matrix is uncertain; however, there is some evidence that they influence bone cell differentiation and proliferative activity. Lipids may assist in binding calcium to cell membranes and in promoting calcification.

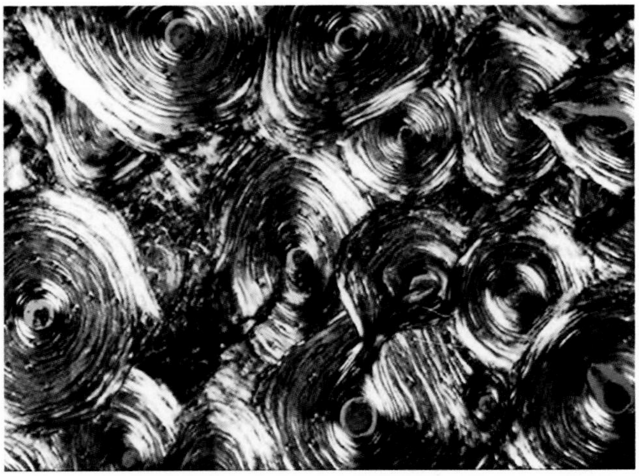

Fig. 16-6 Osteonal remodeling, cortical bone. Endocortical surface of bone has undergone extensive osteonal remodeling.
Collagen fibers are birefringent when viewed in appropriate plane with polarized light; alternate lamellae polarize when viewed in the same plane. This alternating pattern of birefringence demonstrates the parallel arrangement of collagen layers in lamellar bone. Much of the cortex has been remodeled into osteonal bone (concentric layers with central channel for vessels and nerves), but there are a few small areas of cortex that remain unosteonized (unremodeled). Unstained and fully mineralized. Polarized light micrograph. (Courtesy Dr. L. P. Krook, College of Veterinary Medicine, Cornell University.)

Bone mineral is in the form of a crystal called *hydroxyapatite*. Fully mineralized bone composes approximately 65% of the bone by weight and consists in part of calcium, phosphorus, carbonate, magnesium, sodium, manganese, zinc, copper, and fluoride. The mineral content gives bone its hardness. The production of osteoid (unmineralized organic matrix) by osteoblasts is followed by a period of maturation, after which mineral is deposited in exchange for water. Mineralization in woven bone is initiated within cytoplasmic blebs (matrix vesicles) of osteoblasts in the osteoid (see Web Fig. 16-1). Initiation of mineralization involves concentrating calcium, phosphorus, and other elements in these matrix vesicles to a level that causes precipitation of the mineral in the form of amorphous (not yet crystalline) hydroxyapatite. Matrix vesicles contain phospholipids and enzymes such as alkaline phosphatase and adenosine triphosphatase in their membranes. It is speculated that the membrane phospholipids attract calcium and phosphorus to the surface of the vesicle and that the alkaline phosphatase and adenosine triphosphatase enzymes might function

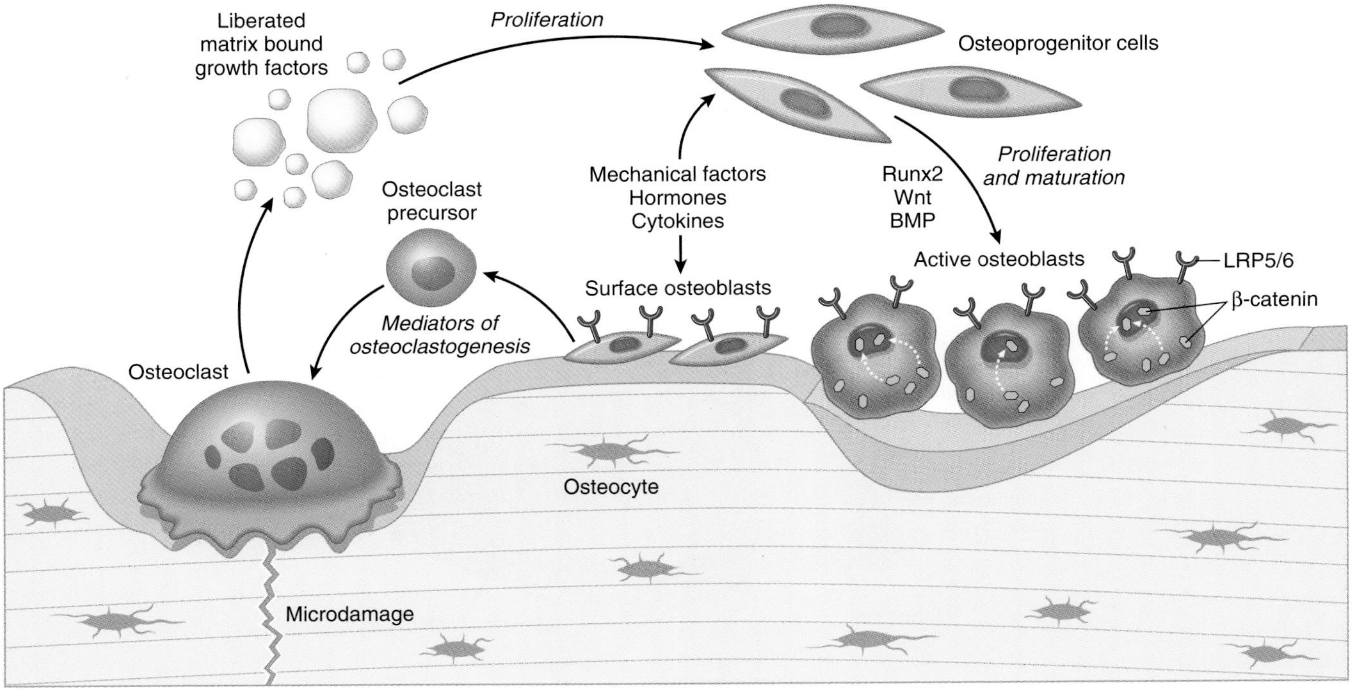

Fig. 16-7 Schematic diagram of the relationship between osteoclasts, osteoblasts, and growth factors.
Osteoclasts are able to liberate and activate growth factors from the matrix that are stimulatory to osteoblast progenitor cells and "couple" the process of osteoclastic bone lysis with subsequent bone formation. (From Kumar V, Abbas AK, Fausto N et al: *Robbins & Cotran pathologic basis of disease*, ed 8, Philadelphia, 2009, Saunders.)

in the pumping of these ions into the cell against a concentration gradient.

On reaching a critical mass, the amorphous mineral becomes crystalline. The crystalline hydroxyapatite pierces the lipid membrane of the matrix vesicle and extends to the gaps (holes) between collagen molecules. It is within these holes that the mineral crystals are first deposited in collagen. For the mineralization to spread beyond these gaps between the tropocollagen molecules, it is necessary for naturally occurring inhibitors of mineralization, such as inorganic pyrophosphate, in the matrix to be destroyed. Inorganic pyrophosphates are normal by-products of cellular metabolism and are deposited in unmineralized matrix by osteoblasts. The phosphatase enzymes described previously on the matrix vesicles have the ability to cleave these inorganic pyrophosphates and in doing so, destroy these inhibitors. Once the gaps are filled with mineral and the inhibitors of mineralization are destroyed, the process continues so that eventually the surfaces of collagen fibers, as well as spaces between collagen fibers, are mineralized. Initiation of mineralization in lamellar bone might not require matrix vesicles because glycoproteins, such as sialoprotein and osteonectin, can act as the nidus for the mineralization process.

BONE AS A TISSUE

In the cortex and subjacent to articular cartilage (subchondral bone), bone is organized into osteons (also called *Haversian systems*), which are cylinders of concentric layers of lamellae that are oriented parallel to the longitudinal axis of the bone and contain centrally located vessels and nerves (Fig. 16-8; see also Fig. 16-6). The bone between the osteons is called *interstitial lamellae.* Layers of bone oriented parallel to the internal and external circumference of the bone (beneath the endosteal and periosteal surfaces) are called *circumferential lamellae.* The osteonal system provides channels for the vascular supply to the cortex and also acts as tightly bound cables, giving the cortical bone strength and limited flexibility.

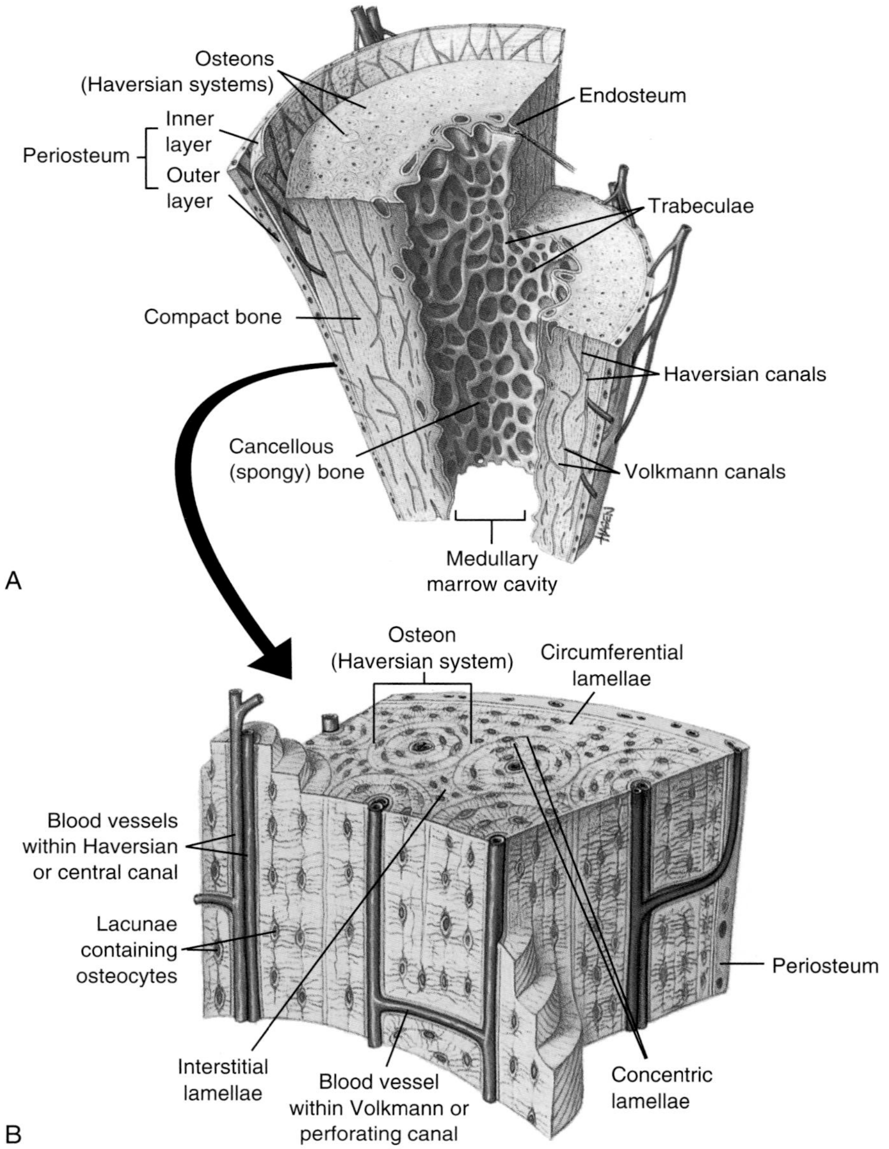

Fig. 16-8 Schematic diagram of the structure of compact and cancellous bone.
A, Longitudinal section of a long bone showing both cancellous and compact bone. **B,** Magnified view of compact bone.

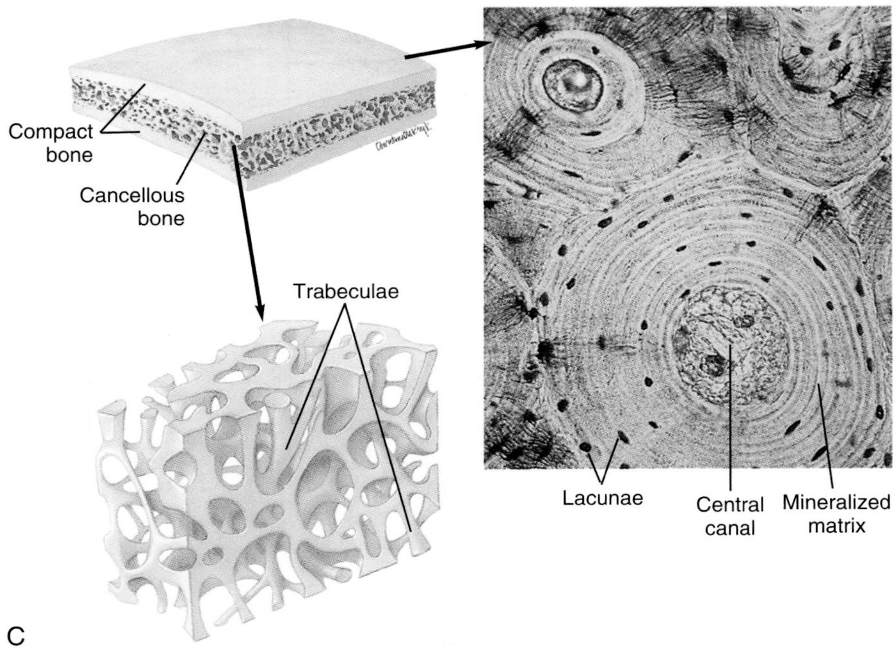

Fig. 16-8, cont'd **C,** Section of a flat bone. Outer layers of compact bone surround centrally located cancellous bone. Fine structure of compact and cancellous bone is shown at a higher magnification. (From Thibodeau GA, Patton KT: *Anatomy and physiology,* ed 6, St Louis, 2007, Mosby.)

This osteonal system also might be important in limiting propagation of microcracks in bone by diverting cracks along cement lines, which are collagen-poor, proteoglycan-rich seams between adjacent remodeling or modeling units (see later discussion). In H&E-stained histologic sections of decalcified bone, cement lines appear as basophilic lines.

In contrast to the dense compact bone of the cortex and the subchondral bone plates, the bone in the medullary cavity is in the form of anastomosing plates or rods and is called *cancellous, trabecular,* or *spongy bone* (see Figs. 16-8 and 16-10). The orientation of the trabeculae usually reflects adaptation (modeling) to mechanical stresses applied to the bone. This is readily apparent when examining the trabeculae in the femoral neck, which are oriented in lines and arcs that are perpendicular to the stress applied and are thicker and more numerous on the ventral aspect (side of compression) compared with the dorsal aspect (side of tension). The lamellae within a trabecula usually are arranged parallel to the surface of the trabecula and are not arranged into tubes or osteons, as they are in cortical bone.

In most species, bone undergoes a low but constant replacement called *remodeling:* old bone is resorbed and replaced by new bone. The basal level of this remodeling activity (number of sites in the skeleton being remodeled at any one time) is likely "programmed" for each species. The number of active remodeling sites, however, can be markedly increased or decreased in response to altered mechanical use (see later discussion). This turnover of old bone to new bone allows for the repair of accumulated microscopic injury in the bone (microfractures). In normal bone remodeling, slightly less bone is replaced than removed, leaving a small negative net change in bone mass with each remodeling cycle and explaining in part the reduced bone mass in aged animals. Furthermore, in disease states, such as hyperparathyroidism, resorption is often increased and formation decreased, leaving a significant net negative bone balance. Interestingly, in small, short-lived animals, such as the mouse and rat, cortical bone is not remodeled. In addition, not all areas of bone in larger species undergo remodeling.

The remodeling unit of cortical bone is called the *osteon,* whereas the remodeling unit of trabecular bone is called the *basic structural unit.* The shape of the osteon is cylindric; however, the basic structural unit has the contour of a shallow trench filled with parallel lamellae. The time required from initiation to completion of these remodeling units (from initiation of bone removal by osteoclasts to complete filling of the defect by osteoblasts), regardless of the type of bone, is estimated to be 3 to 4 months in humans. Basophilic cement lines that mark the limit of previous resorptive activity are usually somewhat scalloped, following the contours of the Howship's lacunae created by osteoclasts, and are called *reversal lines* (where resorption stopped and the process was reversed by formation) (Fig. 16-9). Cement lines also can occur when osteoblast formation ceases and subsequently resumes, and these are called "resting lines" and are usually smooth, following the contour of the overlying surface.

The term *modeling* is used to describe change of the shape or contour of a bone in response to normal growth, altered mechanical use, or disease. In modeling, bone surfaces (periosteal, endosteal, intracortical, and trabecular) can go directly from resting to either formation or resorption, depending on the stimulus. This process allows the shape or size of bone to change, enables the medullary cavity to enlarge, and allows the overall shape of the bone to be maintained while it is growing. Modeling is in contrast to remodeling, in which resorption must precede formation to keep bone mass and shape constant.

BONE AS AN ORGAN

Individual bones of the skeleton vary in their manner of formation, growth, structure, and function. Flat bones of the skull develop by the process of intramembranous ossification, in which mesenchymal cells differentiate into osteoblasts and produce bone directly, in the absence of a preexisting cartilage model. In contrast, most bones develop from cartilaginous models by the process of endochondral ossification, in which cartilage is invaded by vessels, undergoes mineralization, and forms primary (diaphyseal) and

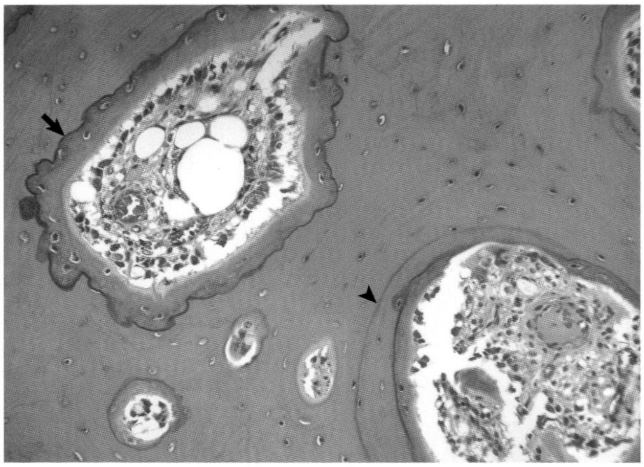

Fig. 16-9 Remodeling in compact subchondral bone adjacent to a joint with bacterial infection, bone, horse.

Resting cement lines appear as basophilic smooth lines indicating where formation has temporarily stopped *(arrowhead)*. Reversal lines are scalloped basophilic lines *(arrow)* indicating where bone resorption stopped and was followed by formation. H&E stain. (Courtesy Dr. S.E. Weisbrode, College of Veterinary Medicine, The Ohio State University.)

secondary (epiphyseal) centers of ossification. Bones forming by endochondral ossification, such as the long bones of the appendicular skeleton and the vertebral bodies, are divided anatomically into epiphyses, metaphyseal growth plates (physes), metaphyses, and diaphyses (Fig. 16-10).

BLOOD SUPPLY TO BONE

Arterial blood from the systemic circulation enters bones through nutrient, metaphyseal, periosteal, and epiphyseal arteries (Fig. 16-11). Nutrient arteries penetrate the diaphyseal cortex through a nutrient foramen covered by strong, protective fascial attachments; once within the medulla, these arteries divide into proximal and distal intramedullary branches. Other arteries penetrating the cortex are the proximal and distal metaphyseal arteries, which are smaller and more numerous than the nutrient arteries. They penetrate the cortex and anastomose with the terminal branches of the nutrient arteries in the medullary cavity, protecting against infarction in case of obstruction of a nutrient artery.

Small periosteal arteries also pass through the diaphyseal cortex at sites of fascial attachment and can supply one quarter to one third of the outer cortex. The remainder of the cortex is supplied by the nutrient artery and its anastomotic branches. This blood flow is centrifugal (from medulla to periosteum) because of greater pressures in the intramedullary vessels. The chondrocytes of the physis nearest the epiphysis are supplied by epiphyseal arteries, whereas the chondrocytes of the physis nearest the metaphysis are supplied by branches of metaphyseal and nutrient arteries. As capillaries from these vessels approach the metaphyseal side of the physis, they make abrupt turns (loops), which are sites of predisposition to bacterial embolization in neonatal sepsis, sometimes resulting in osteomyelitis.

BONE GROWTH

Bone grows in length by interstitial growth within the metaphyseal growth plates (physes) (Fig. 16-12). The mineralized longitudinal septa of the growth plates serve as struts on which bone is deposited, a process called *endochondral ossification.* The metaphyseal growth plate is primarily responsible for lengthening the bone and

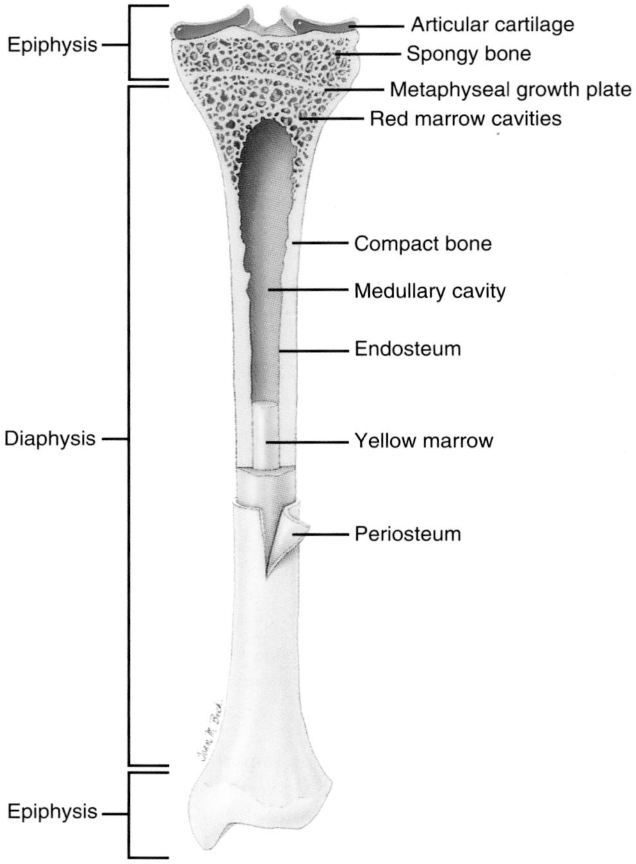

Fig. 16-10 Schematic diagram of a longitudinal section of long bone (tibia) showing spongy (cancellous) and compact bone and names of the regions of bone.

(From Thibodeau GA, Patton KT: *Anatomy and physiology,* ed 6, St Louis, 2007, Mosby.)

is divided into a reserve or resting zone, a proliferative zone, and a hypertrophic zone (Fig. 16-13). The hypertrophic zone is sometimes further subdivided into zones of maturation, degeneration, and calcification. The resting or reserve zone serves as a source of cells for the proliferating zone in which cells multiply, accumulate glycogen, produce matrix, and become arranged in longitudinal columns. In the hypertrophic zone, chondrocytes secrete macromolecules that modify the matrix to allow capillary invasion and initiate matrix mineralization. The hypertrophic zone chondrocytes eventually die. The overall lengthening of the bone is due both to chondrocyte proliferation and hypertrophy. Calcification begins in the longitudinal septa of cartilaginous matrix between columns of chondrocytes. Matrix vesicles derived from chondrocytes (analogous to those described previously for mineralization of bone) form in the hypertrophic zone and initiate the mineralization process. The processes of mineralization and vascular invasion of the growth plate are codependent events. To supply salts for the mineralization, a nearby blood supply is necessary, and vascular invasion, a critical step in endochondral ossification, does not take place in mammalian growth plates unless there is mineralization of the longitudinal septum. Blood vessels from the metaphysis invade into the advancing growth plate, providing an entryway for osteoblasts that form bone on the cartilage spicules (see Fig. 16-13). The chondro-osseous junction in the metaphysis is a fragile lattice of bone-covered spicules of calcified cartilage (primary trabeculae).

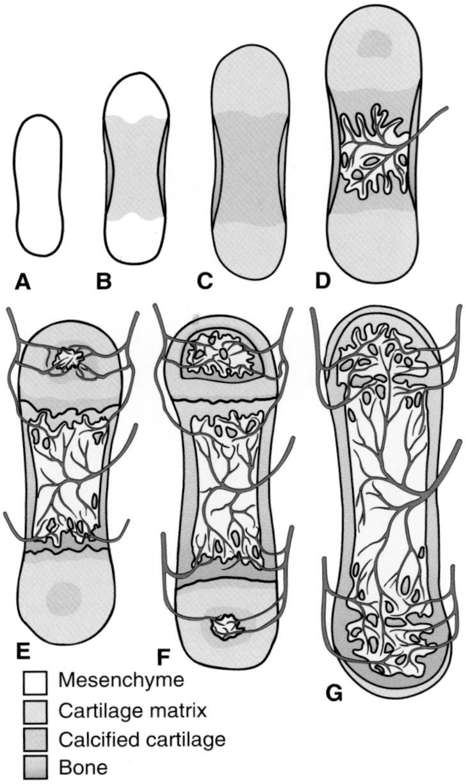

Fig. 16-11 Correlation of long bone development and vascularization. The primitive mesenchyme that makes up the skeletal primordia contains no blood vessels **(A).** This mesenchyme condenses and undergoes central mineralization; a bony collar forms in the periosteum of the diaphysis (**B** and **C**). The nutrient artery enters the mineralized cartilaginous tissue in the diaphysis, bringing osteogenic and osteoclast precursors and enabling endochondral ossification to occur (primary center of ossification) **(D).** Similarly, the epiphyseal arteries bring these cells to the secondary centers of ossification in the epiphyses **(E).** Extensive anastomoses develop as the bone continues to develop and as the growth plates close (**F** and **G**). (Redrawn from Banks WJ: *Applied veterinary histology,* ed 3, St Louis, 1993, Mosby.)

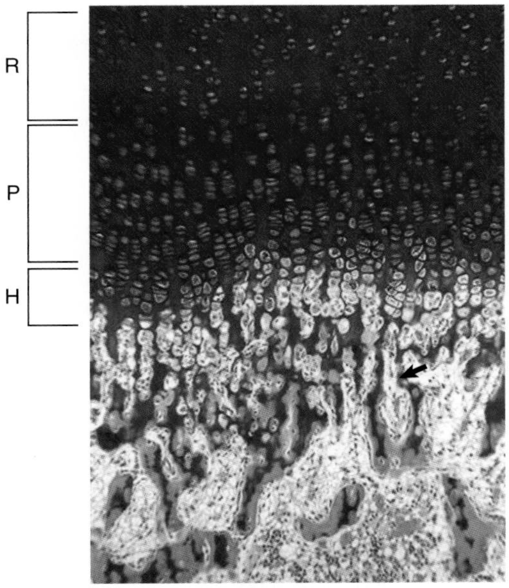

Fig. 16-12 Growth plate, long bone, dog. Resting *(R),* proliferating *(P),* and hypertrophic *(H)* zones of the growth plate are visible. Apoptotic chondrocytes are released from their lacunae by invading vessels and chondroclasts leaving only the longitudinal septa *(arrow)* as a template on which bone will be deposited to form a primary trabeculae. H&E stain. (Courtesy Dr. S.E. Weisbrode, College of Veterinary Medicine, The Ohio State University.)

As the growth plate advances and elongates the metaphysis, the more mature trabeculae deeper in the metaphysis become fewer and thicker (secondary and tertiary trabeculae) and often contain residual fragments of cartilage.

Growth plates are thickest when growth is most rapid; as growth slows, the plate becomes thin and "closes" (becomes replaced by bone) at skeletal maturity. The age at which a growth plate closes varies, depending on site, species, and gender. For example, the physes of vertebrae usually remain open longer than the physes of the long bones. Androgens and estrogens play a major role in determining the time of growth plate closure, and early castration results in delayed growth plate closure with subsequent increased length of bones compared with intact individuals.

Growth of the epiphysis contributes both to the overall length of the bone and to the shape of the ends of the bone. This is accomplished by endochondral ossification at the articular-epiphyseal complex (AEC). The AEC is composed of permanent articular cartilage, as well as a subjacent temporary growth/epiphyseal cartilage that is vascularized and contains the same zones as the growth plate (Fig. 16-14). In the mature individual, endochondral ossification no longer occurs at the AEC. Although the articular cartilage remains throughout life, the epiphyseal cartilage is completely replaced by bone once growth has ceased (Fig. 16-15). Bone grows in width by intramembranous bone formation. Except for articular surfaces (including the ends of the vertebral bodies), the surfaces of bones are covered by periosteum. This covering is a thin membrane that is loosely attached to underlying bone except at heavy fascial attachments on bony prominences and at tendon insertions, where its attachments are strong and are associated with large vessels penetrating the underlying bone. Microscopically, the periosteum is composed of an outer fibrous layer that provides structural support and an inner osteogenic or cambium layer, capable of forming normal lamellar appositional bone on the cortex of growing bones and of forming abnormal woven bone formation in response to injury (Fig. 16-16). The periosteum is well supplied with lymph vessels and with fine myelinated and nonmyelinated nerve fibers that account for the intense pain that occurs with periosteal injury.

The periosteum covering the physis is called the *perichondrial ring.* The perichondrial ring adds new cartilage to the periphery of the physis, enabling it to expand in width as the animal grows. The metaphyseal cortex immediately adjacent to the perichondrial ring is normally very thin in the growing bone because its surfaces are the sites of very active osteoclastic bone resorption. Structurally, this area is the weakest part of the bone.

STRUCTURE AND FUNCTION OF JOINTS

Joints (articulations) join skeletal structures, provide for movement, and in some cases have shock-absorbing functions. This section of the chapter is primarily devoted to synovial joints, also called *movable* or *diarthrodial joints.*

Synovial joints occur in both the axial and appendicular skeleton. These joints allow for a variable degree of movement, and anatomically, they are composed of two bone ends joined together by a fibrous capsule and ligaments. The inner surface of the articular

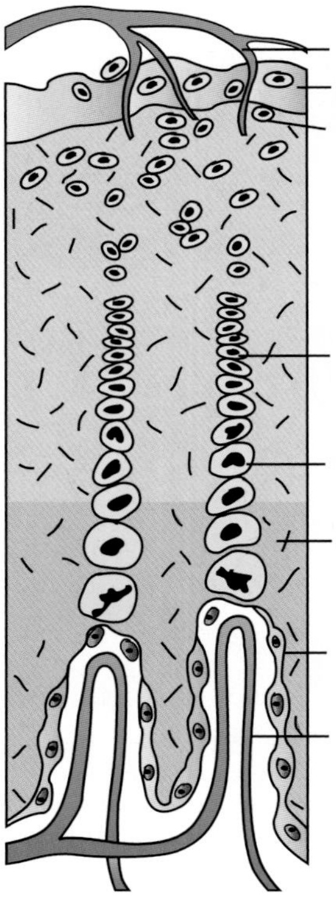

Fig. 16-13 Schematic diagram of the major blood supply to the physis. Branches of the epiphyseal artery supply the resting zones of the growth plate. Branches of the metaphyseal artery form capillary loops at the metaphyseal side of the physis where endochondral ossification is occurring. (Redrawn from Banks WJ: *Applied veterinary histology,* ed 3, St Louis, 1993, Mosby.)

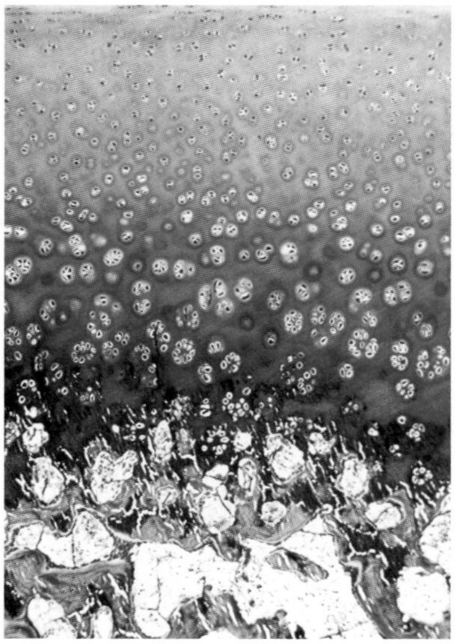

Fig. 16-14 Articular-epiphyseal complex *(AEC)*, bone, immature pig. The AEC is composed of a layer of articular cartilage *(AC)* and a subjacent layer of growth (epiphyseal) cartilage *(EC)*. The growth cartilage is present only in immature individuals, and its structure and function is similar to that of the physis. Compare with Fig. 16-15. Toluidine blue stain. (Courtesy Dr. C.S. Carlson, College of Veterinary Medicine, University of Minnesota).

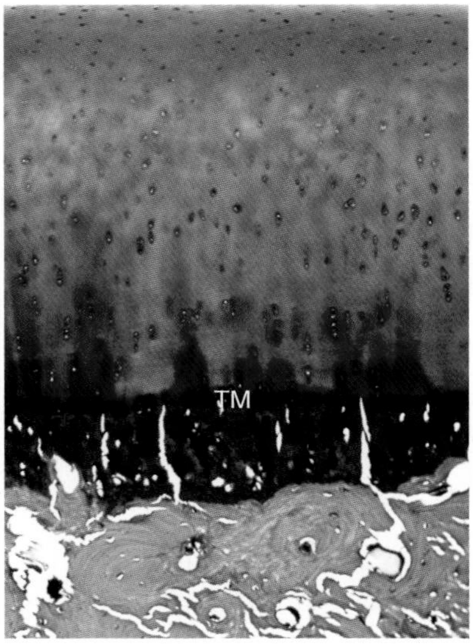

Fig. 16-15 Articular cartilage, bone, adult dog. The articular cartilage is present throughout life; however, the epiphyseal cartilage is absent in adults. In adults, endochondral ossification has ceased and the tidemark *(TM)* delimits the boundary between the uncalcified articular cartilage *(AC)* and the calcified cartilage *(CC)*. Compare with Fig. 16-14. Toluidine blue stain. (Courtesy Dr. C.S. Carlson, College of Veterinary Medicine, University of Minnesota.)

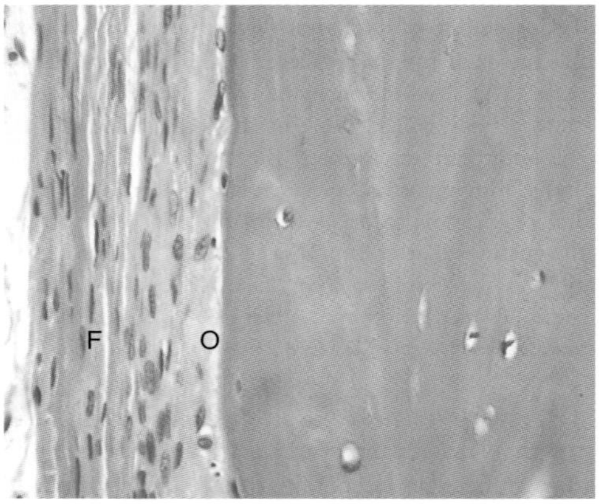

Fig. 16-16 Periosteum, bone, dog. The outer fibrous layer *(F)* and inner osteogenic layer *(O)* line the periosteal surface. The osteogenic layer is able to rapidly deposit woven bone as a nonspecific response to injury. H&E stain. (Courtesy Dr. S.E. Weisbrode, College of Veterinary Medicine, The Ohio State University.)

capsule is lined by a synovial membrane, and the bone ends are covered by articular cartilage. The joint space contains synovial fluid, and fibrocartilaginous menisci or disks are present at some sites (e.g., femorotibial and temporomandibular joints). Synovial joints operate with very low coefficients of friction and are self-lubricating. Articular cartilage serves as the bearing substance and subchondral bone as the supporting material. Articular cartilage functions to minimize friction created by movement to transmit mechanical forces to underlying bone and to maximize the contact area of the joint under load. Joints receive and absorb energy of impact. Both articular cartilage and subchondral bone deform under pressure, but it is the subchondral bone that has the most significant force-attenuating properties.

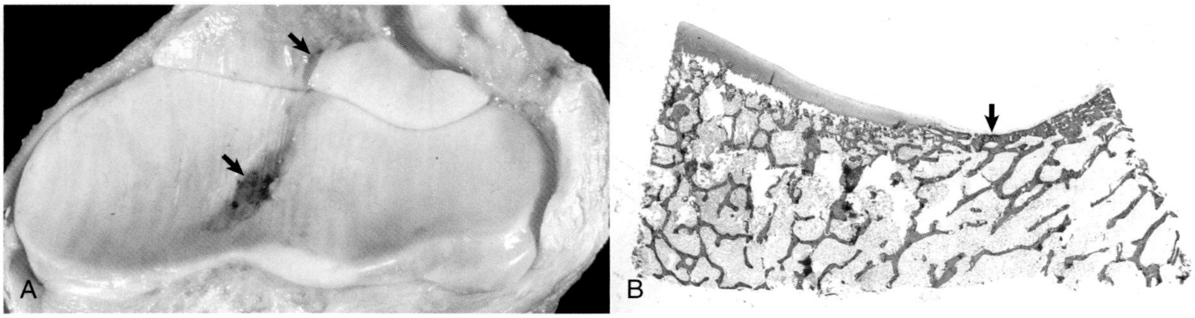

Fig. 16-17 Synovial fossa, joint, radius and ulna, bone, proximal end, adult horse.
A, Synovial fossae are depressions in the cartilage on the non–weight-bearing surfaces of the sagittal ridge of the radius and in the semilunar notch of the ulna *(arrows)*. The parallel linear grooves apparent on the weight-bearing surface (articular cartilage) of the radius are the result of degenerative joint disease. **B,** Histologically, the surface of the synovial fossae is covered by a thin fibrous membrane *(arrow)* rather than articular cartilage. H&E stain. (Courtesy Dr. S.E. Weisbrode, College of Veterinary Medicine, The Ohio State University.)

ARTICULAR CARTILAGE

Articular (hyaline) cartilage is normally a white to blue-white material with a smooth, moist surface. Cartilage thickness is greatest in the young and at sites of maximal weight bearing. Thinning and yellow discoloration occur in old age. At its margins, articular cartilage merges with a periosteal surface that is lined by fibrous tissue contiguous with the synovial membrane. Synovial fossae are normal depressions on non–weight-bearing articular cartilage surfaces (Fig. 16-17) that develop bilaterally in the larger appendicular joints of the horse, pig, and ruminant. These fossae are not present at birth but are fully formed by skeletal maturity. The function of synovial fossae is not known; however, they are significant because they are often mistaken for lesions. Adult articular cartilage contains no nerves or blood or lymph vessels, and its nutrients are obtained by diffusion from synovial fluid and to a lesser extent from subchondral vessels. In the immature skeleton, articular cartilage overlies the temporary growth cartilage of the epiphysis (epiphyseal cartilage). The epiphyseal cartilage is highly dependent on a network of blood vessels that originate from the perichondrium and the subchondral bone. Similar to the physis, it undergoes endochondral ossification and thereby contributes to the growth/development of the epiphysis. At skeletal maturity, the epiphyseal cartilage has been entirely replaced by bone, and the only joint cartilage remaining is the adult articular cartilage, which includes a thin subjacent zone of mineralized cartilage. In skeletally mature individuals, the junction between the unmineralized articular cartilage and the deeper mineralized cartilage forms a thin basophilic line in H&E stained sections called the *tidemark* (see Fig. 16-15). As animals age, multiple tidemarks can be formed, indicating an advance (thickening) of the mineralized layer of articular cartilage and thinning of the overlying nonmineralized articular cartilage. The mineralized cartilage serves to anchor articular cartilage to subchondral bone and limits the diffusion of substances between bone and cartilage.

Articular cartilage is 70% to 80% water by weight. It is a viscoelastic, hydrated fiber-reinforced gel that contains chondrocytes, collagen fibers (mostly type II), noncollagenous proteins, and proteoglycan aggregates. The largest proteoglycan in articular cartilage is aggrecan, which is composed of the immensely long, nonpolysulfated glycosaminoglycan, hyaluronan, to which core proteins are attached in a perpendicular arrangement like bristles on a brush. Similarly, smaller, negatively charged polysulfated glycosaminoglycans (chondroitin sulfate and keratan sulfate) are attached to the core proteins. The large content of negatively charged polysaccharide chains in the aggrecan aggregate is responsible for the extremely high osmotic swelling pressure of cartilage. The swelling pressure provided by aggrecan is counteracted by the resistance of the intact type II collagen fibers, giving cartilage its characteristic properties of being able to resist compressive forces and having a high tensile strength. Collagen fibers are arranged in arcades so that the tops of the arcades are parallel to the articular surface, and the sides are perpendicular to the surface and parallel with the radial or intermediate zone of chondrocytes. Functionally, the superficial zone of articular cartilage resists shearing forces, the middle zone functions in shock absorption, and the mineralized deep zone of cartilage serves to attach articular cartilage to the subchondral bone by its irregular (and therefore interlocking) interfaces. By scanning electron microscopy, the surface of articular cartilage is not smooth, but rather contains numerous depressions that can serve as reservoirs for synovial fluid.

Articular cartilage contains a single population of cells called *chondrocytes* that are responsible for the production, maintenance, and turnover of intercellular substances. In routine histologic sections, chondrocytes appear to be present within lacunae. However, although the lacunae within which osteocytes reside contain fluid spaces, the apparent lacunae of chondrocytes have been clearly demonstrated to be the result of shrinkage artifact. In fact, the chondrocyte cell membrane is in direct contact with the pericellular matrix and contains surface receptors for matrix components (e.g., hyaluronan).

Normal matrix turnover is enzymatic and this process is balanced by enzyme inhibitors. Proteases capable of degrading aggrecans are called *aggrecanases* and are members of the ADAM (A Disintegrin And Metalloprotease) protein family, whereas proteases capable of breaking the peptide bonds in collagen are called *collagenases*. Disease occurs if there is increased destruction or decreased synthesis of matrix components. It is important to remember that compared with bone that normally renews itself by remodeling, articular cartilage has extremely poor regenerative capabilities. Although there is evidence for proteoglycan synthesis in normal articular cartilage, the turnover of cells and type II collagen occurs at an extremely low rate. Correspondingly, the cellularity of articular cartilage declines with age.

ARTICULAR CAPSULE/SYNOVIUM/SYNOVIAL FLUID

The articular capsule consists of outer fibrous and inner synovial tissue layers. The outer layer is a heavy sheath that contributes to joint stability and at its insertion, attaches to bone at the margins of the joint, thereby enclosing a segment of bone of variable length

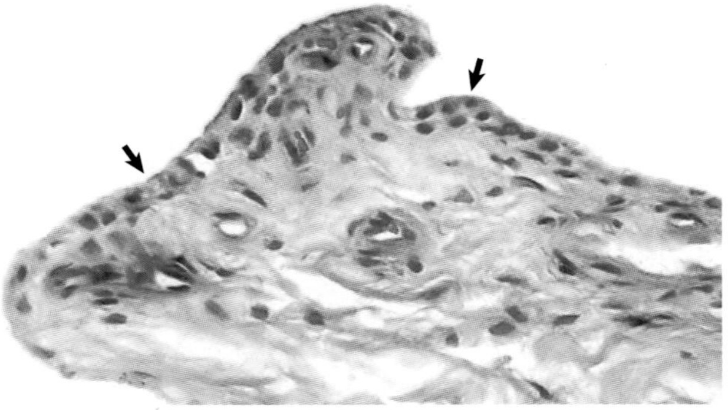

Fig. 16-18 Synovial membrane, joint, dog.
The normal synovial membrane *(arrows)* consists of an incomplete layer of histiocytes (phagocytic cells) and fibrocytes with subjacent loose fibrous and/or fibrofatty tissue. The joint lumen is at the top of the figure. H&E stain. (Courtesy Dr. S.E. Weisbrode, College of Veterinary Medicine, The Ohio State University.)

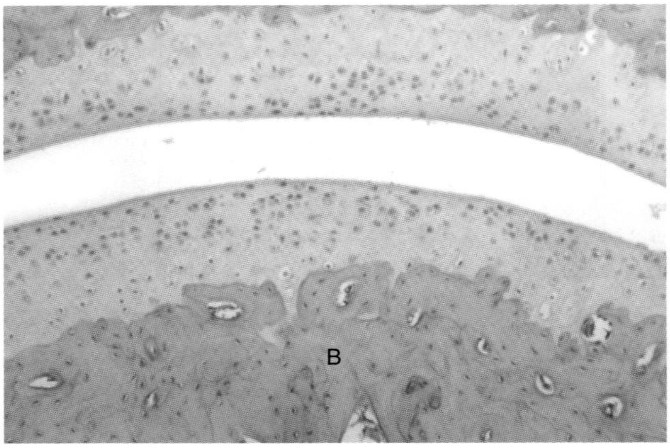

Fig. 16-19 Rat.
Compact bone *(B)* supports the articular cartilage in the adult animal when there is no longer endochondral ossification occurring at the articular epiphyseal complex. H&E stain. (Courtesy Dr. S.E. Weisbrode, College of Veterinary Medicine, The Ohio State University.)

within the joint cavity. It is well supplied with blood vessels and nerve endings. The inner synovial tissue layer is called the *synovial membrane* and covers all the inner surfaces of the joints except for the surface of the articular cartilage. The synovial membrane is normally very thin, lacks a basement membrane, and is barely visible grossly. In fact, collection of normal synovial membrane for histologic evaluation is best done immediately after opening the joint because otherwise, it will retract and become difficult to locate. The inner surface of the synovial membrane may be flat or may contain tiny projections (villi). Synovial intimal or lining cells, one to four cells thick, form a discontinuous surface layer and include two cell types: (1) A cells, which are macrophages that are responsible for the removal of microbes and the debris resulting from normal wear and tear in the joint (Fig. 16-18) and (2) B cells, which are fibroblast-like cells that produce synovial fluid. Normal synovial fluid contains hyaluronic acid, lubricin (a water-soluble glycoprotein), proteinases, and collagenase and is clear, colorless to pale yellow, and viscous. In addition to lubricating the joint surfaces, it supplies oxygen and nutrients to and removes carbon dioxide and metabolic wastes from the chondrocytes in articular cartilage. The synovial subintima can be classified according to the type of tissue that predominates (areolar, adipose, or fibrous), and contains blood and lymph vessels that supply and drain the intraarticular structures. Adipose tissue sometimes accumulates in the deep layers of the synovium, forming fat pads that serve as soft cushions in joint cavities (e.g., the infrapatellar fat body of the stifle joint).

Joint lubrication depends on the microscopic roughness, elasticity, and hydration of articular cartilage and on the presence of hyaluronic acid and lubricin in synovial fluid. The lubricating properties of lubricin depend on its ability to bind to articular cartilage, where it retains a protective layer of water molecules. In contrast, hyaluronic acid, the molecule that makes synovial fluid viscous, has largely been excluded as a lubricant of the cartilage-on-cartilage bearing and instead, lubricates the site of surface contact between synovium and cartilage. When pressure is applied to the joint, such as during weight bearing, the articular surface is supplied with pressurized fluid that carries most of the load. This fluid is synovial fluid admixed with water that is released from the underlying cartilage, subsequent to pressure of weight bearing. When the load is removed, the water returns to the cartilage because of the hydrophilic properties of proteoglycans. This flushing of fluid in and out of the articular cartilage enables nutrients to enter cartilage from the synovial fluid and waste products to be removed.

SUBCHONDRAL BONE

The subchondral bone acts to support the overlying cartilage and dissipate concussive forces to the peripheral cortical bone (Fig. 16-19). The thickness of the subchondral bone plate varies in proportion to the degree of weight bearing. Increased subchondral bone thickness is a common pathological finding in osteoarthritis. In larger animals (nonrodent species), subchondral bone often is composed of compact osteonal bone rather than trabecular bone.

STRUCTURE AND FUNCTION OF TENDONS AND LIGAMENTS

A tendon is a unit of musculoskeletal tissue that transmits force from muscle to bone. Morphologically, tendons are similar to ligaments and fascia; however, ligaments join bone to bone and fascia connects muscle to muscle. The musculotendinous unit is composed predominately of parallel arrays of closely packed collagen fibers and rod- or spindle-shaped fibroblast-like cells (tenocytes) within a well-ordered extracellular matrix (Fig. 16-20). Collagen fibrils are bundled into large fibers that are evident throughout the tendon and are visible under light microscopy as a crimped or a sinusoidal pattern that facilitates a 1% to 3% elongation of the tendon. This elongation of the individual fibers serves to buffer the tendon from sudden mechanical loading. Water represents approximately 55% of the weight of tendon, is present mainly in the extracellular matrix, and is believed to reduce friction, facilitating the gliding of fibrils in response to mechanical loading. The major fibrillar component of tendon is type I collagen, which constitutes approximately 80% of the dry weight, whereas type III collagen is present in the endotenon and epitenon. The remainder of the tendon components include elastin, proteoglycans, and inorganic components. Collagen is synthesized by the tenocytes and constitutes the basic structural unit of tendon. The collagen polypeptides form a triple helix, which self-assembles into collagen fibrils with intermolecular cross-links that form between adjacent helixes. The collagen polypeptides and the ensuing triple helix are synthesized inside the cell, secreted into the extracellular matrix, and assembled into the microfibrillar

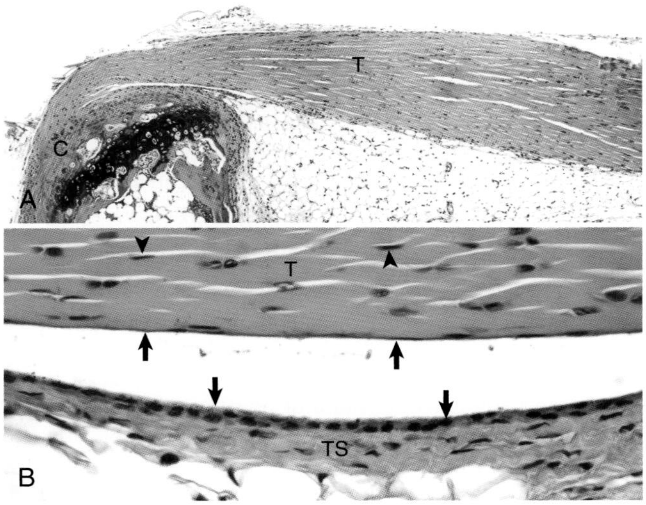

Fig. 16-20 Tendon, joint, mouse.
A, Gastrocnemius tendon *(T)*. The tendon is composed of parallel arrays of closely packed collagen fibers and low numbers of fibroblast-like cells called *tenocytes* (see higher magnification in **B**; *arrowheads*). The tendon is covered by flattened synoviocytes (see higher magnification in **B**), so it may glide smoothly over the synoviocytes of the tendon sheath. *C,* Calcaneus insertion. H&E stain. **B,** Higher magnification of tendon sheath. The enveloping structure enclosing the tendon is the tendon sheath *(TS)*, and it is lined by synoviocytes *(arrows)*. *T,* Gastrocnemius tendon. H&E stain. (Courtesy Dr. J.F. Zachary, College of Veterinary Medicine, University of Illinois.)

units that constitute the collagen fibers. This step is promoted by a specialized enzyme called *lysyl oxidase,* which promotes crosslink formation—a process involving placement of stable crosslinks within and between the molecules. Crosslink formation is the critical step that gives collagen fibers their strength. Tendon is stronger per unit area than muscle, and its tensile strength equals that of bone, although it is flexible and slightly extensible. The parallel arrangement of tendon collagen fibers resists tension so that contractile energy is not lost during transmission from muscle to bone. The mechanical properties of tendons depend on the collagen fiber diameter and orientation; however, the proteoglycan components of tendons also are important to the mechanical properties. While the collagen fibrils allow tendons to resist tensile stress, the proteoglycans allow them to resist compressive stress.

Skeletal ligaments are defined as dense bands of collagenous tissue that span a joint and then become anchored to the bone at either end. They vary in size, shape, orientation, and location. Their bony attachments are called *insertions.* Biochemically, ligaments are approximately two-thirds water and one-third solid. Type I collagen accounts for 85% of the collagen (other collagen types include III, VI, V, XI, and XIV) and the collagens account for approximately 75% of the dry weight, with the balance being made up by proteoglycans, elastin, and other proteins. While the ligament appears as a single structure, during joint movement some fibers appear to tighten or loosen depending on the bone positions and the forces that are applied, confirming the complexity of these structures. Histologically, ligaments are composed of fibroblasts that are surrounded by matrix. The cells are responsible for matrix synthesis and are relatively few in number, representing a small percentage of the total ligament volume. Recent studies have indicated that normal ligament cells may communicate by means of prominent cytoplasmic extensions that extend for long distances and connect to cytoplasmic extensions from adjacent cells, thus forming an elaborate three-dimensional architecture. Gap junctions have also been detected in association with these cell connections, raising the possibility of cell-to-cell communication and the potential to coordinate cellular and metabolic responses throughout the tissue. Ligament microstructure reveals collagen bundles aligned along the long axis of the ligament and displaying an underlying "waviness" or crimp along the length, similar to that present in tendon. Crimp is thought to play a biomechanical role, possibly relating to the ligament's loading state with increased loading likely resulting in some areas of the ligament uncrimping, allowing the ligament to elongate without sustaining damage.

One of the main functions of ligaments is mechanical as they passively stabilize joints and help guide those joints through their normal range of motion when a tensile load is applied. Another function of ligaments relates to their viscoelastic behavior in helping provide joint homeostasis. Ligaments "load relax," which means that loads/stresses decrease within the ligament if they are pulled to constant deformations. A third function of ligaments is their role in joint proprioception. In joints such as the knee, proprioception is provided principally by joint, muscle, and cutaneous receptors. When ligaments are strained, they invoke neurologic feedback signals that then activate muscular contraction, which appears to play a role in joint position sense.

Tendons and ligaments attach to bone in a similar manner, through osteotendinous or osteoligamentous junctions, respectively. These junctions are known as *entheses* and are distinguished as fibrous and fibrocartilaginous according to the type of tissue present at the attachment site. At fibrous entheses, the tendon or ligament attaches either directly to the bone or indirectly to it via the periosteum. Fibrocartilaginous entheses are sites in which chondrogenesis has occurred and commonly contain four tissue types: dense fibrous connective tissue, uncalcified fibrocartilage, calcified fibrocartilage, and bone.

RESPONSES OF BONE TO INJURY

Mechanical forces that can affect bone are both internal and external. Internal forces associated with extremes in work or exercise can influence modeling or remodeling (see previous discussion) and occasionally cause fracture (failure of the bone). External forces (trauma) are more commonly associated with damage to the periosteal surface or fracture of the cortex and/or trabecular bone.

Hormonal agents, particularly calcitriol and PTH, enter the bone by the bloodstream as described previously. Infectious agents are discussed later in the section on Inflammation of Bone.

Defense against mechanical forces includes the structure of the bone and the bone's ability to model and remodel to adapt to chronic changes in forces applied to it. The dense bone of the cortex enables the bone to resist most external forces. The formation of osteons and cement lines in the cortex (primary remodeling) facilitates dissipation of microcracks and bending of the bone in response to stress.

Defense against hormonal agents that are capable of resorbing bone include the protective covering on mineralized surfaces by the lamina limitans and osteoblasts. In addition, hormonal signaling to resorb bone is done through the osteoblast, which has the ability to modulate the resorption signal. Defense against infectious agents is discussed later in the section on Inflammation of Bone.

The hard tissue of bone can be likened to the rings in a tree that leave clues to the history embedded in its hard structure. Interpreting these clues requires understanding the ways in which bone uniquely responds to injury (Box 16-2).

BOX 16-2 Bone-Specific Reactions to Injury

1. Disruption of endochondral ossification affects metaphyseal trabeculae.
2. Bone changes its shape to adapt to damage and abnormal use.
3. Bone alters its mass in response to systemic disease and altered use.
4. Bone deposited rapidly is woven rather than lamellar.
5. Injured periosteum often responds by forming bone.

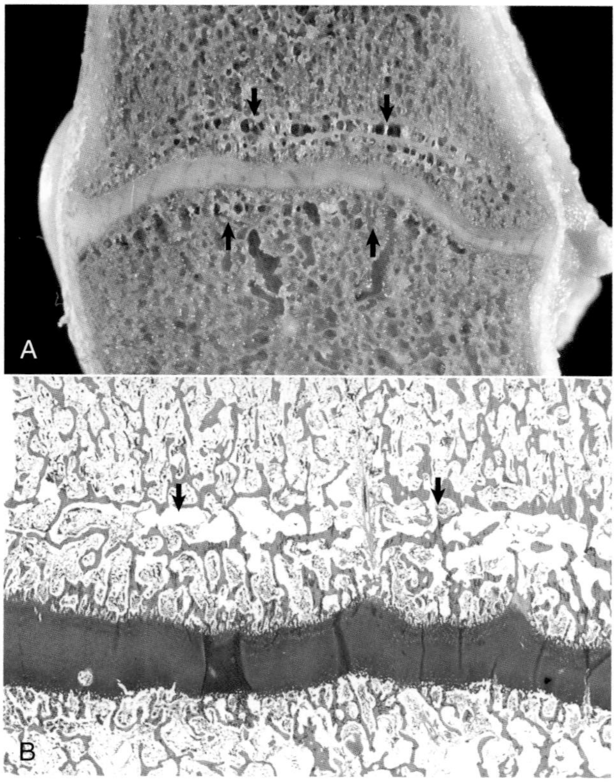

Fig. 16-21 Growth arrest lines, long bone, metaphysis, young zebra. Gross **(A)** and microscopic **(B)** appearance of growth arrest lines. The zebra was ill from a bacterial renal infection and became anorexic. The animal made a brief clinical recovery before euthanasia. The period of inappetence is responsible for the parallel horizontal lines of bone in the metaphysis (growth arrest lines; *arrows*). These lines are the result of transverse (horizontal) orientation of the trabeculae during the period of slowed growth. H&E stain. (Courtesy Dr. S.E. Weisbrode, College of Veterinary Medicine, The Ohio State University.)

Disruption of endochondral ossification can alter the appearance of the primary trabeculae. Examples of this are growth retardation lattice and growth arrest lines. Growth arrest lines can be seen in cases in which multiple nutrient deficiencies are present such as occur in debilitating disease or general malnutrition. The growth plate becomes narrow (growth is impaired), and the metaphyseal face of the plate can be sealed by a layer of bone as a result of transverse trabeculation (trabecular bone forming parallel versus perpendicular, immediately subjacent to the growth plate). If endochondral ossification resumes, this layer of bone becomes separated from the physis and becomes located more distally in the metaphysis (Fig. 16-21, *A* and *B*). The resulting bony trabeculae parallel to the growth plate that also can be seen grossly and radiographically are called *growth arrest lines.*

A growth retardation lattice results from acquired impairment of osteoclastic resorption of bone within the primary trabeculae, resulting in retention of primary trabeculae. These trabeculae elongate because of continued endochondral ossification. The retention of the primary trabeculae results in a dense band of vertically oriented trabecular bone subjacent to the growth plate called a *growth retardation lattice* (Fig. 16-22). The band is apparent because the normal modeling process that resorbs many primary trabeculae completely and molds the remaining ones into progressively fewer but thicker secondary and tertiary trabeculae is impaired. Diseases that cause growth retardation lattices include canine distemper and bovine viral diarrhea, in which viral infection of osteoclasts results in defects in cell function. Similarly, toxic damage to osteoclasts, such as in lead poisoning, can cause a growth retardation lattice ("lead line"). Abnormal retention of primary trabeculae also can be seen with congenital defects in the function of osteoclasts (see later discussion of osteopetrosis). The phrase *growth retardation lattice* is perpetuated here because it is in common use; however, it is important to understand that the lesion is caused by a failure in modeling of the trabeculae rather than by a reduction in longitudinal growth. Weakening or destruction of the matrix of the physeal cartilage, such as occurs in animals with hypervitaminosis A and with manganese deficiency, can lead to premature closure of growth plates. If the entire plate is affected, no further longitudinal growth is possible. If closure is focal, such as can be seen subsequent to localized inflammation or traumatic damage to vessels, the remainder of the growth plate continues to undergo endochondral ossification, resulting in an angular limb deformity.

Osteochondrosis is an important example of a disease caused by disruption of endochondral ossification and is discussed later under disorders of endochondral ossification.

The ability of bone to change its shape and size (modeling) to accommodate altered mechanical use is called *Wolff's Law* (see example in Fig. 16-23). Tension and compression are important mechanical factors that affect bone modeling with formation favored at sites of compression and resorption favored at sites of tension. In addition, trabecular bone aligns along lines of stress. The ways in which bone cells detect altered mechanical use are not precisely known but likely include input from a variety of signals, including stretch receptors on bone cells, streaming potentials, and piezoelectrical activity. Streaming potentials are electrical currents in bone that are detected by the osteocyte-osteoblast network and are caused by fluid fluxes through canalicular spaces. Piezoelectrical activity refers to the production of electrical currents in bone as a result of deformation of collagen fibers and mineral crystals. Electrical currents can affect cell function (bone formation and resorption) and thus influence bone modeling. In fact, several types of portable devices that are designed to produce an electrical current are available for use in humans to promote fracture healing.

Bone mass can be altered to accommodate mechanical use. Normal mechanical use suppresses programmed bone resorptive activity and is required for maintenance of bone mass. Decreased mechanical use reduces this inhibition (allowing resorption to proceed) and also suppresses bone formation. The net effect of decreased mechanical use therefore is a reduced amount of bone as a result of increased resorption and decreased formation (Fig. 16-24). In contrast, increased mechanical use suppresses bone resorption and allows bone mass to increase (Fig. 16-25). Chronic suppression of remodeling, however, could result in retention of aged bone and lead to accumulated microcracks, which in turn could override the suppression and stimulate remodeling in these regions.

Woven bone is newly-formed, hypercellular bone that is deposited in reaction to injury. Although woven bone is normally present

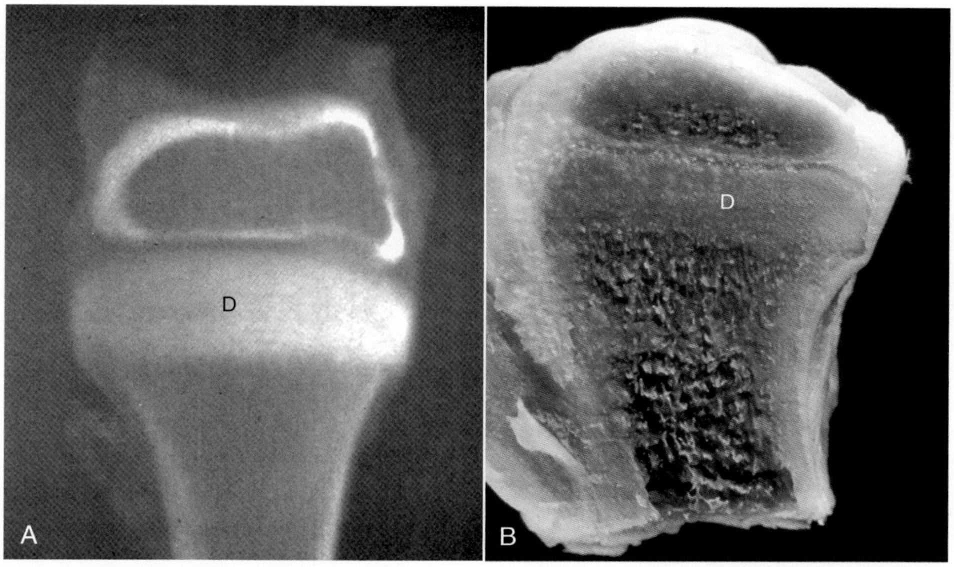

Fig. 16-22 Growth retardation lattice, bone, radius, distal end, dog. Radiograph **(A)** and longitudinal section **(B)** of a growth retardation lattice. The increased bone density *(D)* of the metaphysis represents failure of osteoclasts to resorb unnecessary primary trabeculae. In this case, the failure of osteoclastic resorption was caused by canine distemper virus infection of osteoclasts. (Courtesy Dr. S.E. Weisbrode, College of Veterinary Medicine, The Ohio State University.)

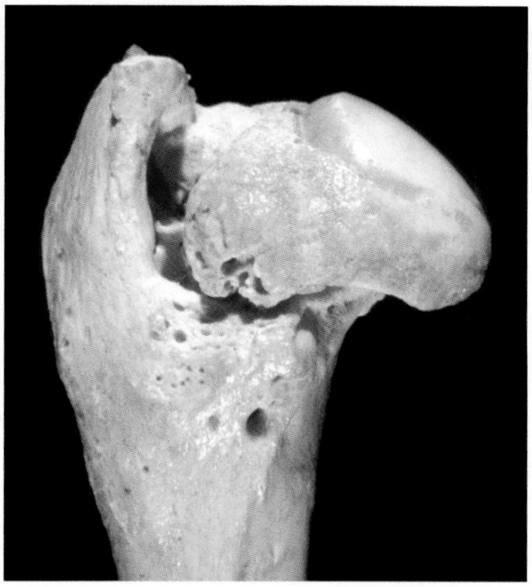

Fig. 16-23 Hip dysplasia, bone, femoral head and neck, dog. The femoral head is severely flattened and periosteal new bone and coalescing osteophytes have formed a massively thickened femoral neck. Macerated and bleached specimen. (Courtesy Dr. S.E. Weisbrode, College of Veterinary Medicine, The Ohio State University.)

in immature individuals, the presence of woven bone in the adult skeleton is considered to be pathologic. The collagen fibers in woven bone are irregularly/randomly arranged rather than being oriented in a lamellar pattern, a change that is best appreciated using polarized light microscopy (Fig. 16-26). In addition, osteocytes are larger and more numerous per unit area than in lamellar bone, and there is no preferred orientation to their lacunae versus in lamellar bone in which the alignment of the elliptical lacunae is parallel to the lamellae. Over time, woven bone remodels into lamellar bone.

The periosteum is programmed to respond to injury by producing woven bone, which usually is oriented perpendicularly to the long axis of the cortex. Although nodular periosteal new bone is sometimes referred to as *osteophytes,* the use of this term should be restricted to periarticular new bone that occurs in response to joint injury/instability. Reactive periosteal woven bone may be admixed with hyaline cartilage and sometimes is composed predominantly of cartilage. The extent to which cartilage is produced by the periosteum is thought to be a result of the available oxygen. When oxygen tension is low, cartilage proliferation may predominate; however, when oxygen tension is normal, there may be no cartilage present. Cartilage produced in such circumstances can eventually undergo endochondral ossification. In addition, woven bone produced by the periosteum may be remodeled to lamellar bone or may be removed by osteoclastic resorption. In addition to producing woven bone in response to injury, the periosteum also is capable of producing lamellar bone during slower stages of appositional growth of the diaphysis, and this bone also is subject to osteoclastic resorption. During growth, the regions of the cut-back zone of the metaphysis, in which the bone diameter is reduced from a larger diameter at the physis to the narrower diameter of the diaphysis, exhibit marked osteoclastic bone resorption at the periosteal bone surface. Infectious inflammation of the periosteum also can lead to marked osteoclastic bone resorption at the periosteal bone surface.

RESPONSES OF JOINTS TO INJURY

ARTICULAR CARTILAGE

Although articular cartilage contains metabolically active cells, it has a limited response to injury and minimal capacity for repair that is a result in large part to its lack of a blood supply. Superficial cartilage defects (cartilage erosions) that do not penetrate into subchondral bone persist for long periods with few or no histologic changes. Clusters or clones of chondrocytes (evidence of local chondrocyte replication in response to injury) may be present, particularly along the margins of the defect, but are ineffective

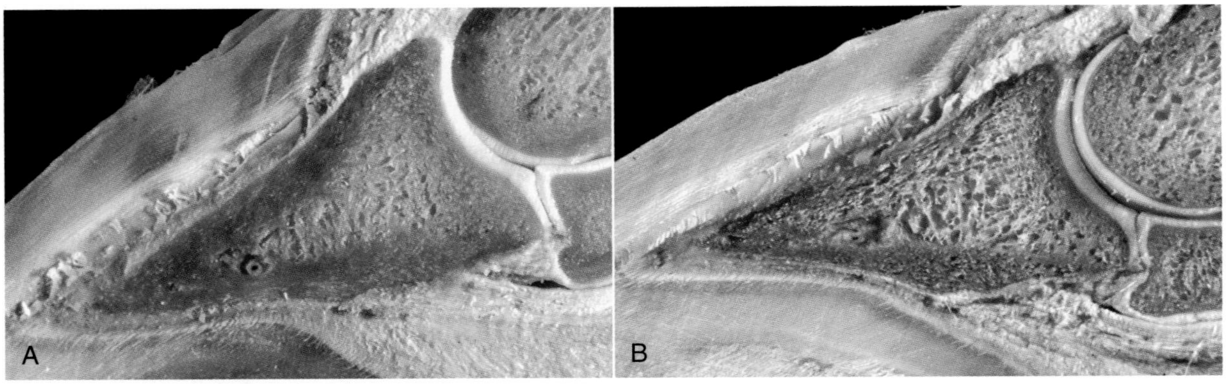

Fig. 16-24 Bone, third phalanx, left rear leg, foal.
The leg was in a cast for 2 months to repair an avulsion of gluteal muscles from their insertions. **A,** Normal right third phalanx. **B,** Left third phalanx. There is pronounced disuse osteopenia (atrophy) compared with the right third phalanx shown in **A.** The increase in resorption and decrease in formation associated with disuse has resulted in marked porosity of the cortical and subchondral bone. The cortex now has the appearance of trabecular bone (trabeculation of the cortex). (Courtesy Dr. S.E. Weisbrode, College of Veterinary Medicine, The Ohio State University.)

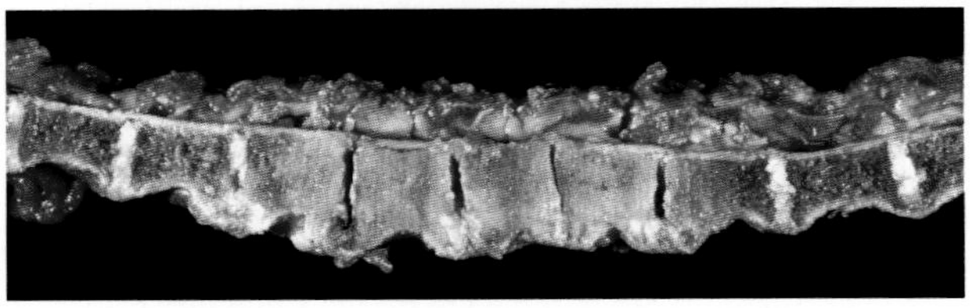

Fig. 16-25 Osteosclerosis, bone, vertebrae, dog.
Osteosclerosis (increased bone per unit of area) is evident in the four vertebrae in the center of the vertebral column. The cancellous bone of the medullary cavities has been obliterated by newly formed compact bone. The osteosclerosis is in response to increased mechanical stress in the bodies of the vertebrae as a result of degeneration and loss of the intervertebral disks between these vertebrae. (Courtesy Dr. S.E. Weisbrode, College of Veterinary Medicine, The Ohio State University.)

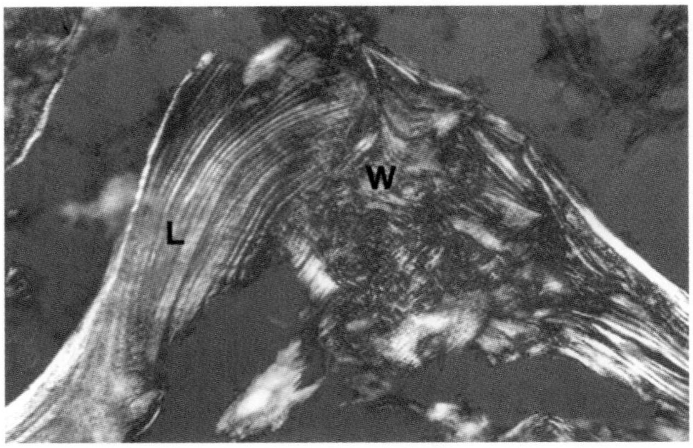

Fig. 16-26 Cancellous and woven bone, polarized microscopy.
A spicule of bone composed of areas of lamellar *(L)* and woven *(W)* bone. The woven bone , which may represent the site of a healing fracture, exhibits a disorganized orientation of collagen fibers compared with the adjacent lamellar bone, in which the collagen fibers are arranged in parallel layers. Unstained and fully mineralized. Polarized light micrograph. (From Burkitt HG, Young B, Heath JW: *Wheater's functional histology: a text and color atlas,* ed 3, New York, 1993, Churchill Livingstone.)

in filling it. Progression of the lesion, with matrix degeneration and eventual loss of the remaining articular cartilage, may occur over time, particularly if thickened (sclerotic) subchondral bone is present subjacent to the defect. In contrast, if a cartilaginous defect extends into subchondral bone (cartilage ulceration), allowing mesenchymal cells access to the defect, it is quickly filled with vascular fibrous tissue that often undergoes metaplasia to fibrocartilage but rarely, if ever, to hyaline cartilage. Formation of fibrocartilage can be hastened in full-thickness cartilaginous defects by exercise or prolonged passive motion. Injury to articular cartilage is not painful unless the synovium or subchondral bone is involved. Having no blood supply of its own, articular cartilage does not participate directly in the inflammatory response but is very much affected by inflammation in the synovium, subchondral bone, or subarticular growth (vascularized) cartilage of the epiphysis in young animals. Given that alternating compression and release of normal weight bearing facilitates the diffusion of fluid with nutrients into the articular cartilage and fluid with metabolic waste products out of articular cartilage, it follows that constant compression or lack of weight bearing leads to atrophy (thinning) of articular cartilage.

Sterile injury to cartilage can be a consequence of trauma, joint instability, or lubrication failure because of changes in synovial fluid, synovial membrane, or incongruity in joint surfaces. Destruction of articular cartilage in response to sterile injury and infectious inflammation is mediated by a combination of enzymatic digestion of matrix and failure of matrix production when chondrocytes become degenerate or necrotic. These changes can be initiated by damage to the cartilage directly or may occur indirectly, secondary to lesions in the synovium.

Matrix metalloproteinases are enzymes capable of matrix digestion; they are normal constituents of the matrix, but are present in an inactive form. Matrix metalloproteinases can be broadly categorized as gelatinases, collagenases, and stromelysins. Collagenases are most capable of digestion of collagen fibers; gelatinases digest type I collagen and basement membrane collagens but are less effective against type II collagen of cartilage. Stromelysins destroy noncollagenous proteins. Matrix metalloproteinases can be activated by products of degenerating or reactive chondrocytes and inflammatory cells. In addition, tissue inhibitors of metalloproteinases (TIMPs) are present in the matrix, acting as a control on the destructive effects of activated metalloproteinases. As mentioned earlier, proteases capable of degrading aggrecans are called aggrecanases and are members of the ADAM protein family. The loss of proteoglycans from cartilage alters the hydraulic permeability of the cartilage, thereby interfering with joint lubrication and leading to further mechanically induced injury to the cartilage. The loss of proteoglycans, with subsequent inadequate lubrication of the

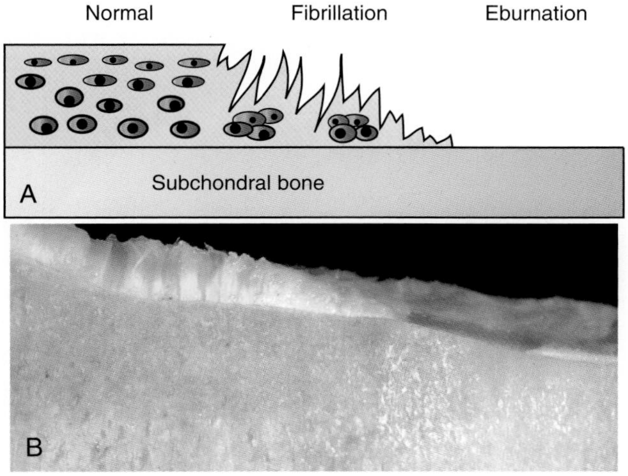

Fig. 16-27 Fibrillation.
A, Schematic diagram showing the structural changes that characterize fibrillation and loss of articular cartilage and adjacent eburnated subchondral bone. In the area of eburnation, the cartilage is missing, and the exposed subchondral bone has increased density. **B,** Fibrillation and ulceration, degenerative joint disease, tibia, proximal articular cartilage, sagittal section, bull. To the left, the cartilage is frayed (fibrillation) and its surface has the appearance of a shag rug. To the right of the fibrillated region is an ulcer (full-thickness loss of articular cartilage). The cartilage to the right of the ulcer is very thin, indicating erosion. (**B** courtesy Dr. S.E. Weisbrode, College of Veterinary Medicine, The Ohio State University.)

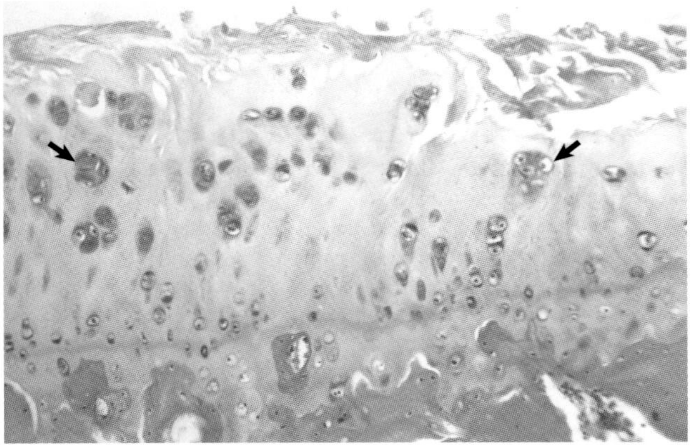

Fig. 16-28 Degenerative joint disease, hip dysplasia, femoral head, articular cartilage, dog.
The superficial cartilage is fibrillated and hypocellular (necrosis) with clusters of chondrocytes *(arrows)* representing ineffectual attempts at repair. H&E stain. (Courtesy Dr. S.E. Weisbrode, College of Veterinary Medicine, The Ohio State University.)

articular surface, leads to disruption of collagen fibers on the surface of articular cartilage. Grossly, the surfaces of affected areas of cartilage are yellow-brown and have a dull, slightly roughened appearance. As more proteoglycans are lost, the collagen fibers condense and fray (fibrillation) with multiple clefts and/or fissures forming along the vertical axis of the arcades of collagen fibers (Figs. 16-27 and 16-28). The vertical axis of the collagen fibers in these arcades is perpendicular to the plane of movement of the joint. Fibrillation is accompanied by loss of surface cartilage (erosion) and eventual thinning of the articular cartilage. Subsequent to fibrillation and erosion, necrosis of individual chondrocytes occurs in the radial zone, resulting in hypocellularity of the remaining cartilage. In

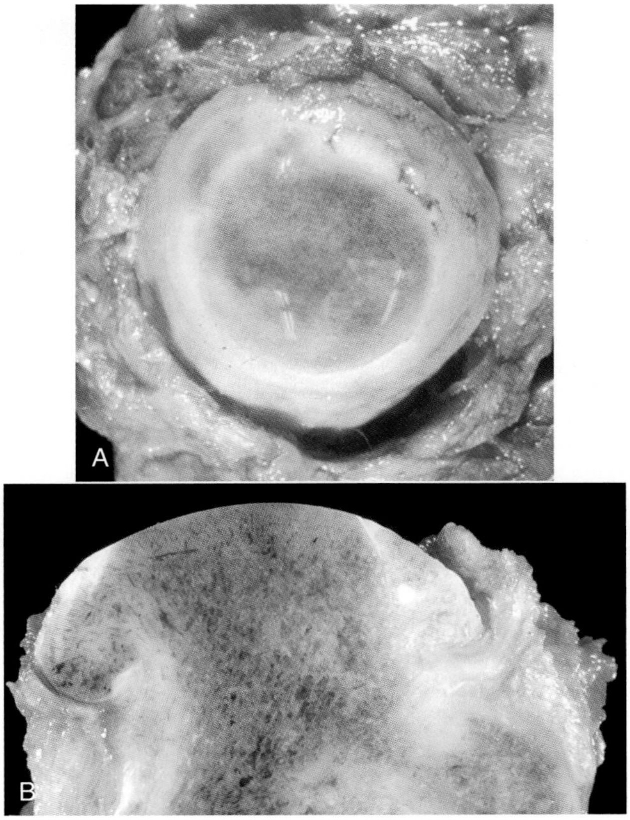

Fig. 16-29 Degenerative joint disease, hip dysplasia, bone, femoral head with eburnation, dog.
The femoral head viewed from the medial aspect **(A)** and in a sagittal plane **(B).** The head is flattened and ulcerated. The ulcerated region appears darker because of congestion of blood vessels in the marrow spaces of the subchondral bone. The zone of attachment of the round ligament to the head of the femur has been destroyed. Note in **A** how the subchondral bone has become smooth and shiny (eburnation). (Courtesy Dr. S.E. Weisbrode, College of Veterinary Medicine, The Ohio State University).

response to the fibrillation, erosion, and necrosis of chondrocytes, remaining chondrocytes can undergo regenerative hyperplasia (cluster or clone formation), but the ability of chondrocytes in the adult to divide is limited and the regenerative attempt is almost always ineffective. Loss of articular cartilage can become complete, resulting in exposure of subchondral bone (ulceration), which typically is eburnated (thickened/sclerotic) (Fig. 16-29).

ARTICULAR CAPSULE/SYNOVIUM/SYNOVIAL FLUID

Intraarticular prostaglandins, nitric oxide, TNF-α, IL-1, and neurotransmitters—such as substance P, among other cytokines and chemokines—are increased in degenerative and inflammatory joint disease. Prostaglandins and nitric oxide inhibit proteoglycan synthesis in synovium and chondrocytes; this reduction in proteoglycan content can lead to degeneration and loss of the cartilage (see previous discussion). IL-1 and TNF-α are cytokines secreted by activated macrophages (synovial type A cells or subintimal macrophages); they promote secretion of prostaglandins, nitric oxide, and neutral proteases from synovial fibroblasts and chondrocytes. Increasing concentrations of these agents decreases matrix synthesis and increases matrix destruction. Cytokines and growth factors that can be anabolic to cartilage include IL-6, TGF-β, and insulin-like growth factor (IGF).

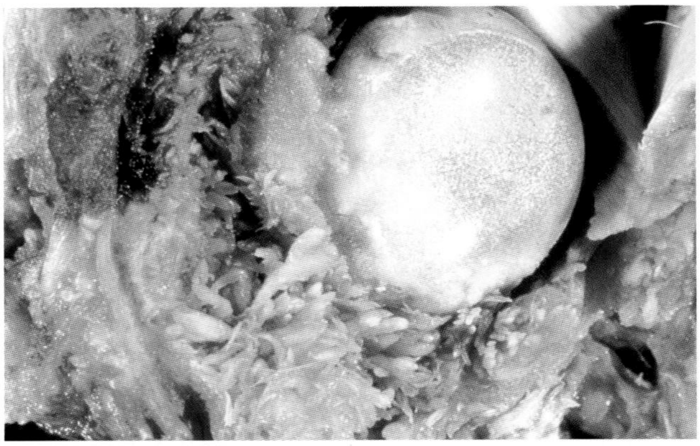

Fig. 16-30 Synovial villous hyperplasia, hip dysplasia, coxofemoral joint, articular capsule, and femoral head, dog.
There is marked villous synovial hyperplasia. The extent of the proliferation is unusually severe for hip dysplasia. Microscopically, villous synovial hyperplasia is routinely accompanied by variable lymphoplasmacytic inflammation that is independent of the cause of the articular damage. (Courtesy Dr. S.E. Weisbrode, College of Veterinary Medicine, The Ohio State University.)

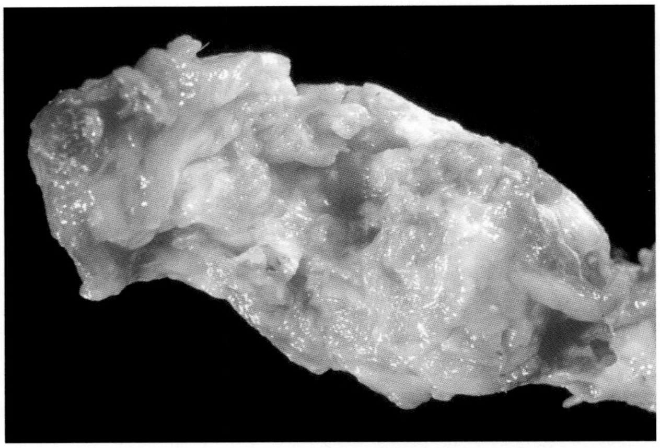

Fig. 16-31 Pannus, rheumatoid-like arthritis, proximal radius and ulna, dog.
Fibrovascular tissue (pannus) covers all articular surfaces. (Courtesy Dr. S.E. Weisbrode, College of Veterinary Medicine, The Ohio State University.)

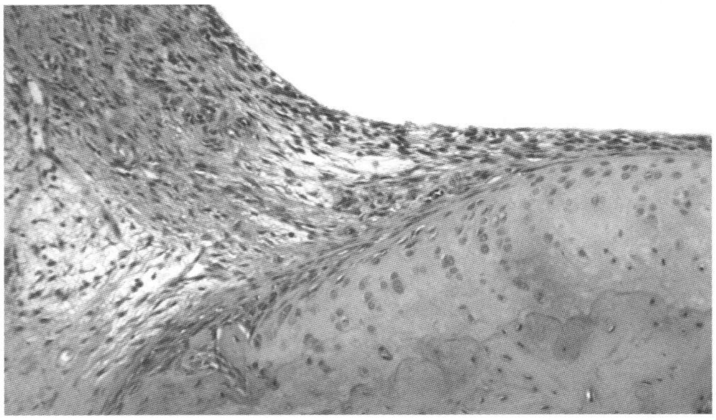

Fig. 16-32 Pannus, rheumatoid-like arthritis (experimentally induced), distal articular cartilage, tibia, rat.
The experimentally induced rheumatoid-like arthritis was produced by injecting Freund's adjuvant and *Mycobacterium butyricum* into the subcutis at the base of the tail. The pathogenesis of "adjuvant arthritis" is uncertain, other than it appears to be T lymphocyte mediated. Here, fibrovascular repair tissue (pannus) is seen arising from the synovium *(left)* and growing onto the surface of the articular cartilage, which is relatively undamaged at this stage of the disease. H&E stain. (Courtesy Dr. S.E. Weisbrode, College of Veterinary Medicine, The Ohio State University.)

Lysosomal enzymes (collagenase, cathepsins, elastase, and arylsulfatase) and neutral proteases, which are capable of degrading proteoglycans or collagen, can be derived from inflammatory cells, synovial lining cells, and chondrocytes.

The synovial membrane commonly responds to injury by villous hypertrophy and hyperplasia (Fig. 16-30), hypertrophy and hyperplasia of synoviocytes, and pannus formation (see later discussion). Villous hypertrophy occurs with or without synovitis. The proportions of A (macrophages) and B (fibroblast-like) cells in the synovium also can change in various disease processes. Fragments of articular cartilage can adhere to the synovium, where they are surrounded by macrophages and giant cells. Larger pieces of detached cartilage (as in osteochondrosis) can float free and survive as chondral or osteochondral fragments ("joint mice") that continue to remain viable through nutrient supply from synovial fluid.

Inflammatory cell infiltrates (see the discussion on infectious and noninfectious arthritis in the section on Inflammatory Lesions) in the synovial membrane can impair fluid drainage from the joint and can cause joint fluid to lose some of its lubricating properties as the result of degradation of hyaluronic acid by the superoxide-generating systems of neutrophils.

Pannus can develop in association with chronic infectious fibrinous synovitis and with some immune-mediated diseases; the classic example is rheumatoid arthritis. Pannus is a fibrovascular and histiocytic tissue (also called an *inflammatory granulation tissue*) that arises from the synovial membrane and spreads as a membrane over articular cartilage (Figs. 16-31 and 16-32). In the pannus, tissue histiocytes and monocytes of bone marrow origin transform into macrophages and they, along with the collagenases from fibroblasts, cause lysis and destruction of the underlying cartilage (Fig. 16-33). In time, if both opposing cartilaginous surfaces are involved, the fibrous tissue can unite the surfaces, causing fibrous ankylosis (fusion of the joint). In some cases of immune-mediated arthritis, pannus is present in the subchondral bone marrow (bone marrow pannus), as well as in the synovium, and may penetrate into the overlying articular cartilage.

Sterile degenerative changes in articular cartilage are often accompanied by the formation of periarticular osteophytes (Fig. 16-34) and by some degree of secondary synovial inflammation and hyperplasia. The synovitis is characterized by the presence of variable numbers of plasma cells, lymphocytes, and macrophages in the synovial subintima (beneath the layers of synoviocytes) and by hyperplasia and hypertrophy of synovial lining cells. The pathogenesis of this synovitis is not known but is suspected to be the result in part of the presence of degenerate cartilage debris within the joint. The pathogenesis of osteophytes also is unclear. They can arise from mesenchymal cells with chondro-osseous potential within the synovial membrane at the junction of the synovial membrane with the perichondrium/periosteum, just peripheral to the articular cartilage, or on the surface of the bone where the articular capsule and the periosteum merge. Osteophytes do not grow continuously, but once formed, they persist as multiple periarticular spurs of bone. These spurs can be confined within the joint cavity if they arise from the perichondrium or can be protrusions from the periosteal surface of the bone if they arise from the insertion site of the joint capsule with the periosteum. Osteophytes can result from mechanical instability within the joint, causing stretching or tearing of the insertions of the articular capsule or ligaments, or they can form

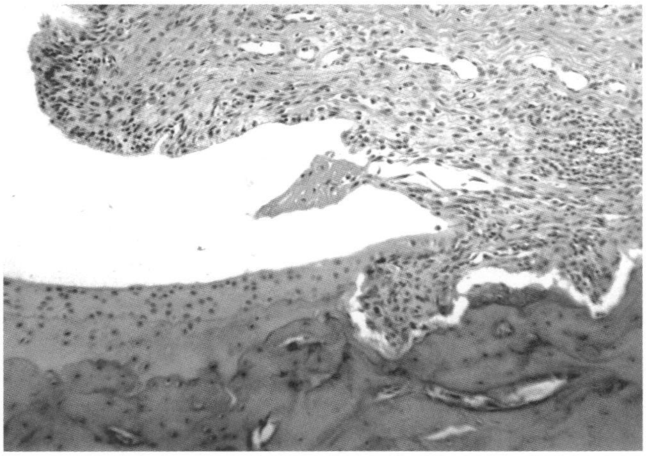

Fig. 16-33 **Pannus, rheumatoid-like arthritis (experimentally induced), articular cartilage, distal tibia, rat.**
Pannus originating from the synovium *(right)* is invading and destroying the articular cartilage and subchondral bone. H&E stain. (Courtesy Dr. S.E. Weisbrode, College of Veterinary Medicine, The Ohio State University.)

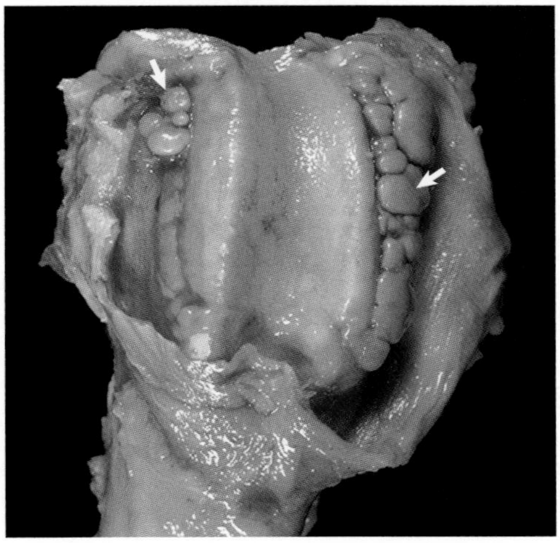

Fig. 16-34 **Osteophytes, degenerative joint disease, distal femur, dog.**
Note the large number of osteophytes *(arrows)* along the lateral and medial margins of the trochlear ridges. (Courtesy Dr. H. Leipold, College of Veterinary Medicine, Kansas State University; and Noah's Arkive, College of Veterinary Medicine, The University of Georgia.)

from stimulation by cytokines such as TGF-β that are released from reactive or degenerating mesenchymal cells within the joint.

Because of their antiinflammatory effects, glucocorticoids often are therapeutically injected into joints. Although the usual result is decreased pain and inflammation, glucocorticoid injection sometimes is followed by a rapid progression of degenerative changes within the joint that is designated "steroid arthropathy." These degenerative changes relate to the antianabolic effects of glucocorticoids on chondrocytes, in which synthesis of cartilaginous matrix is reduced, proteoglycans are depleted, repair is retarded, and the mechanical strength of cartilage is reduced.

SUBCHONDRAL BONE

With the loss of matrix proteoglycans in degenerate articular cartilage, a greater component of concussive forces is transmitted to the subchondral bone. The bone responds to the increased mechanical use by decreasing resorption and increasing formation, resulting in a net increase in amount of bone per unit area (increased subchondral bone density or subchondral sclerosis). If the cartilage ulcerates to the level of the bone and the joint is still being used, the surface of the dense subchondral bone can become smooth and shiny (eburnation) (see Fig. 16-29, *A*). There is interest in the possible role subchondral bone might play in initiating cartilage damage in degenerative joint disease, as some studies have reported an increase in subchondral bone thickness/density before the development of articular cartilage lesions. Some believe that this dense bone is less effective in dissipating normal concussive forces and causes some of the impact to be deflected back into the articular cartilage, causing injury to the chondrocytes.

RESPONSES OF TENDONS AND LIGAMENTS TO INJURY

The site where ligament or tendon attaches to bone is known as an *enthesis* but is also called an *insertion site* or an *osteotendinous* or *osteoligamentous junction.* Entheses are vulnerable to acute or overuse injuries in sports as the result of stress concentration at the hard-soft tissue interface. Osteophytes located in these regions are termed *enthesophytes.*

The initial stage of repair of tendons and ligaments involves formation of scar tissue to provide continuity at the injury site. For tendons in particular, mobility must be maintained during healing to prevent or at least decrease the formation of adhesions and to increase strength. The sequence of repair includes three phases: (1) tissue inflammation, (2) cell and matrix proliferation, and (3) remodeling and maturation. The inflammatory stage usually involves the formation of a hematoma, which activates the release of chemotactic factors, including TGF-β, IGF-1, platelet-derived growth factor (PDGF), and basic fibroblast growth factor (bFGF). Inflammatory cells are attracted from the surrounding tissues to engulf and resorb the clot, cellular debris, and foreign material. Fibroblasts are recruited to the site to begin to synthesize components of the extracellular matrix and angiogenic factors that are released during this phase initiate the formation of a vascular network. During the cell proliferation phase, recruitment and proliferation of fibroblasts continues because these cells are responsible for the synthesis of collagens, proteoglycans, and other extracellular matrix components, which initially are arranged randomly. At this point in the repair process, the extracellular matrix is composed largely of type III collagen. At the end of the proliferative stage, the repair tissue is highly cellular and contains relatively large amounts of water and an abundance of extracellular matrix components. The remodeling stage begins 6 to 8 weeks after injury and is characterized by a decrease in cellularity, reduced matrix synthesis, a decrease in type III collagen, and an increase in type I collagen synthesis. The type I collagen fibers are organized longitudinally along the tendon axis and are responsible for the mechanical strength of the regenerating tissue. Despite multiple ongoing phases of remodeling, the repair tissue never achieves the characteristics of normal tendon.

PORTALS OF ENTRY INTO BONE

Infectious agents can enter bone directly through the periosteum and cortex or through the vasculature. Agents can gain access through the periosteum by means of trauma that may or may not break the bone or by extension from adjacent inflammation, as in periodontal tissue (e.g., periodontitis progressing to mandibular or maxillary osteomyelitis) or the middle ear (otitis media extending into the bone, resulting in osteomyelitis of the tympanic bulla).

Blood vessels gain access to the marrow cavity of the diaphysis and metaphysis through the nutrient foramen. The primary blood supply of the epiphysis in young animals is the epiphyseal artery, multiple branches of which arborize into the growth plate, providing vascularization of the proliferative zone. Blood-borne bacterial infection of bone in the perinatal animal may originate from the umbilicus or more commonly, by the oral-pharyngeal route. In theory, hematogenous osteomyelitis can begin in any capillary bed in bone in which viable bacteria localize. In practice, it occurs most commonly in young animals and is localized typically at the zone of vascular invasion on the metaphyseal side of the growth plate (Fig. 16-35) or immediately subjacent to the AEC (Fig. 16-36) where capillaries in both sites make sharp bends to join medullary veins (Fig. 16-37). In these locations, bacterial localization is apparently facilitated by slow flow and turbulence of blood, a lower phagocytic capacity, and a discontinuous endothelial lining. In addition, no vascular anastomoses are located in this region, therefore thrombosis of these capillaries results in bone infarction that is a predisposing factor for bacterial localization. From this nidus, the inflammation can extend into other structures, including the overlying joint cavity for AEC lesions (see Fig. 16-36) and the epiphysis, periosteum, or joint cavity for physeal lesions (Fig. 16-38; see also Fig. 16-37).

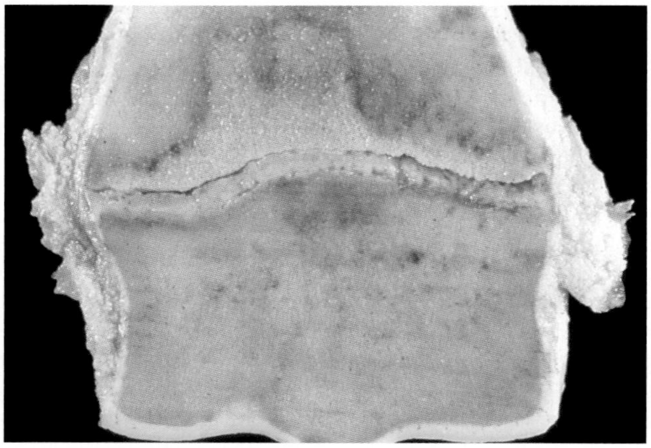

Fig. 16-35 Embolic (suppurative) osteomyelitis and physitis, bone, distal radius, foal.
The pale region in the metaphysis extending upward to the top middle border of the illustration represents suppurative inflammation and necrosis. It is bordered by a red rim of active hyperemia. A fissure (the linear space along the metaphyseal margin of the growth plate) and the porosity *(darker regions within the growth plate, right)* are the result of bone lysis (primary trabeculae) caused by the infection. (Courtesy Dr. S.E. Weisbrode, College of Veterinary Medicine, The Ohio State University.)

PORTALS OF ENTRY INTO JOINTS

Microbial and other agents enter the joints via hematogenous spread (Fig. 16-39). For example, neonatal bacteremia secondary to omphalitis or oral-intestinal entry commonly leads to polyarthritis. Bacteria can also reach the joint by direct inoculation, as in a puncture wound, by extension from adjacent periarticular soft tissues, or by extension from adjacent bone.

PORTALS OF ENTRY INTO TENDONS/LIGAMENTS

Infection of tendons and ligaments usually requires a laceration or puncture wound because of the dense connective tissue covering of the tendon (epitenon) or ligament (epiligamentum). Less commonly, there may be extension of infection from infected skin or from an adjacent joint. The sequelae of bacterial infection of tendons and ligaments most often include adhesions and accompanying loss of function.

DEFENSE MECHANISMS OF BONE

The defense against infectious agents is no different in bone than in other tissues. However, the consequences of an inflammatory

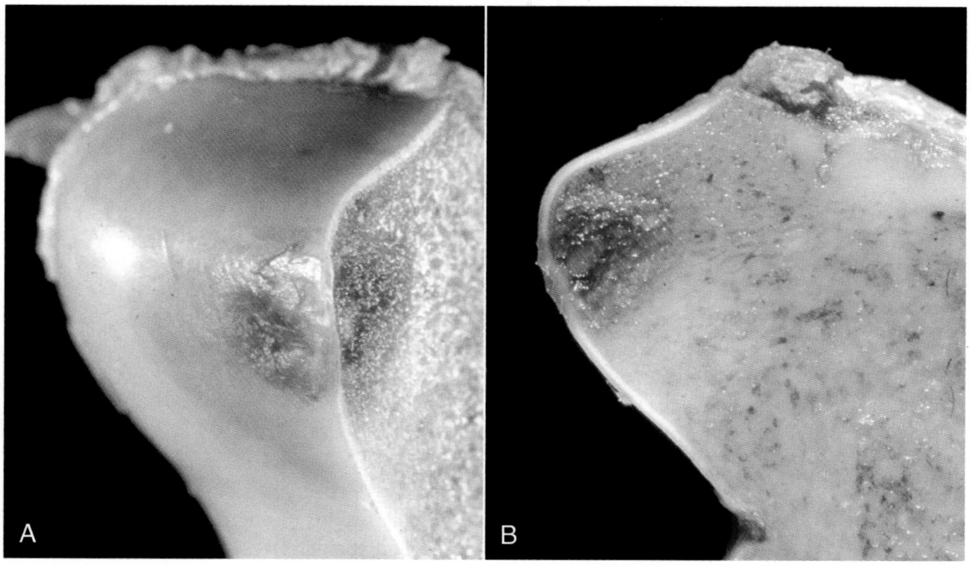

Fig. 16-36 Embolic (suppurative) osteomyelitis, bone, distal femur, medial trochlear ridge, transverse section, horse.
A, Oblique view of articular cartilage and transverse section. **B,** The suppurative osteomyelitis has extended from its site of origin in the cancellous bone into the articular-epiphyseal complex, with resulting collapse and fragmentation of the articular cartilage. (Courtesy Dr. S.E. Weisbrode, College of Veterinary Medicine, The Ohio State University.)

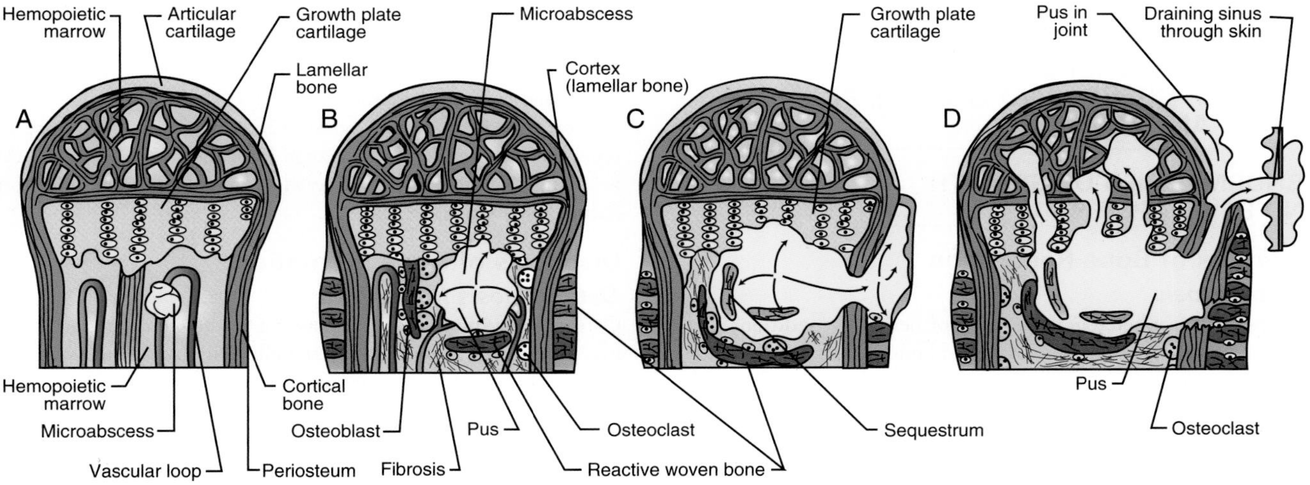

Fig. 16-37 Schematic diagram showing patterns of spread of embolic osteomyelitis from the physis.
The septic embolus lodges in capillary loops at the metaphyseal side of the physis **(A)**. The inflammation causes lysis of metaphyseal bone and growth plate cartilage which can cause mechanical instability, to which the periosteum responds by producing reactive bone **(B)**. The exudates can lyse the cortex at its thinnest point (the metaphyseal cut back zone) and extend into the periosteum (periostitis) or into the joint (arthritis) (**C** and **D**). (Redrawn from Rubin E: *Essential pathology*, ed 3, 2001, Lippincott Williams & Wilkins).

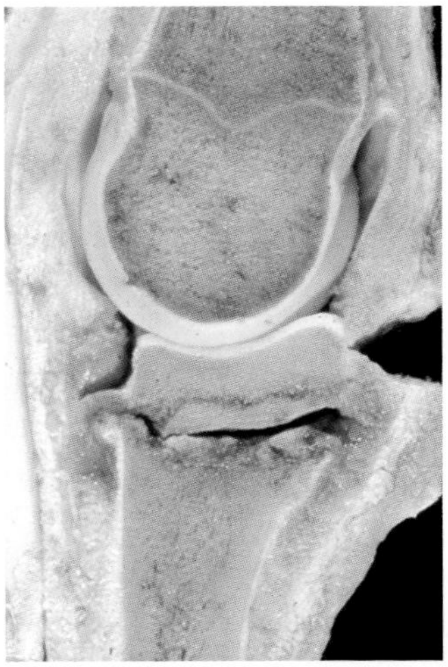

Fig. 16-38 Embolic bacterial physitis, osteomyelitis, periostitis, proximal first phalanx and arthritis, metacarpal-phalangeal joint, horse.
Bacterial inflammation has destroyed the physis and has extended into the periosteum and joint cavity *(left)*. (Courtesy Dr. S.E. Weisbrode, College of Veterinary Medicine, The Ohio State University.)

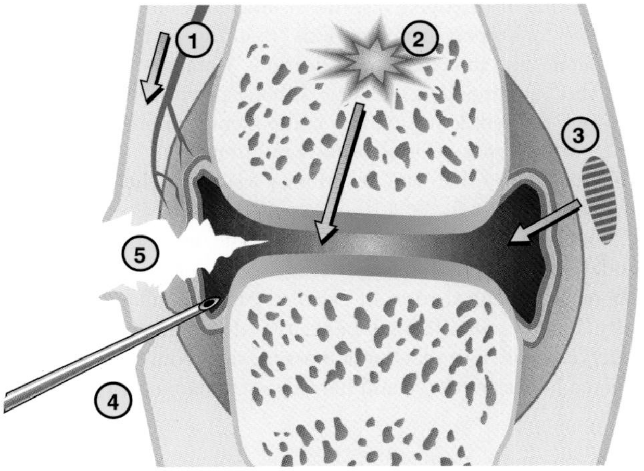

Fig. 16-39 Schematic diagram of the routes of infection for a joint in an adult.
1, The hematogenous route. *2,* Extension from osteomyelitis. *3,* Spread from an adjacent soft tissue infection. *4,* Diagnostic or therapeutic procedures. *5,* Penetrating damage from puncture or cutting. (From Huether SE, McCance KL: *Understanding pathophysiology,* ed 4, St Louis, 2008, Mosby.)

response can greatly affect the structure and function of bone. Many soluble inflammatory mediators can increase both bone formation and resorption, resulting in varying degrees of reactive bone formation and bone lysis. The exudate associated with some acute infections in the medullary cavity can increase the pressure in this region and cause compression of the nutrient artery, resulting in ischemic necrosis. If resorbed cortical bone is replaced by fibrous repair tissue, the bone can become unstable.

DEFENSE MECHANISMS OF JOINTS

The cellular and humoral defenses against infectious agents are no different in the joint from those in other tissues. However, because articular cartilage has such limited ability to regenerate, the consequence of inflammation that destroys the ability of synovium to provide nutrients and synovial fluid to the cartilage or that destroys areas of the cartilage could be the subsequent progression to degenerative joint disease.

DEFENSE MECHANISMS OF TENDONS/LIGAMENTS

The cellular and humoral defenses against infectious agents are no different in tendons and ligaments from those in other tissues.

DISORDERS OF BONE IN DOMESTIC ANIMALS (HORSES, RUMINANTS [CATTLE, SHEEP, AND GOATS], PIGS, DOGS, AND CATS)

ABNORMALITIES OF GROWTH AND DEVELOPMENT

Disorders of Bone Resorption

Osteopetrosis

Osteopetrosis is a heterogenous group of heritable conditions that result in diffuse osteosclerosis (increased bone matter per unit area) caused by a defect in bone resorption by osteoclasts. Although bone mineral density is increased, the bones can be more fragile. Pathologic fractures are reported in animals that survive birth. The cause of the fragility is not certain but is likely related to failure of normal bone modeling in both cortex and medulla. The disease occurs in humans and in multiple animal species, including dogs, sheep, horses (Peruvian Paso breed), cattle (Angus and Herefords), rats, and several strains of mice. Specific immune regulators and growth factors that influence osteoclast ontogeny and/or activation have been implicated in the pathogenesis of some of the naturally occurring mutations associated with osteopetrosis in animals. In severe forms of osteopetrosis, the insufficient bone marrow cavity is unable to support hematopoiesis, resulting in thrombocytopenia, anemia, and infectious complications. Because osteoclasts arise from the hematopoietic precursors, bone marrow transplantation (in which normal donor marrow components are injected) is curative for some types of osteopetrosis in humans.

Growth plate: There are no primary lesions in the growth plate in osteopetrosis.

Trabecular bone: Osteoclasts are unable to resorb and shape (model) the primary trabeculae (Fig. 16-40). As a result, spicules of bone with central cores of calcified cartilage fill the medullary cavity. This process affects all bones that develop in a cartilaginous model (elongate by endochondral ossification from a growth plate). Affected bones are dense and have no medullary cavity. The defect in Angus cattle is inherited as an autosomal recessive trait. Affected calves are typically stillborn a few weeks premature and also have brachygnathia inferior, impacted molar teeth, and deformed cranial vaults that compress the brain.

Cortical bone: Cortical bone lesions in osteopetrosis are not reported consistently but can range from the cortex being too thin to it being inadequately compacted in animals that have plexiform (laminar) cortical bone growth.

Disorders of Bone Formation

Osteogenesis Imperfecta

Osteogenesis imperfecta is a hereditary osteopenic (reduced bone mass) disease that is characterized clinically by multiple fractures, joint laxity, and defective dentin. It is the most common heritable connective disorder in humans and has been described in the veterinary literature in calves, lambs, kittens, and puppies. The tissues involved include bone, dentin, tendons, and sclera, and clinical signs include bone fractures, joint laxity, dental abnormalities, and blue sclerae. In humans, the disease is most commonly caused by mutations in one or both of the genes that code for type I collagen, and this also has been reported in animals. Genes coding for enzymes responsible for posttranslational modification of collagen are mutated less commonly. Mild forms of the disease, caused by inactivation of an allele of one the genes, result in reduced amounts of normal collagen. Conversely, mutations causing substitutions in critical amino acids necessary for collagen helix formation and cross-linking can result in production of normal amounts of structurally inferior collagen. Interestingly, the clinical manifestations of these mutations are usually limited to the bone, teeth, and eyes, even though type I collagen is also the major structural collagen in skin. A mutation in the *SERPINH1* gene has been reported in osteogenesis imperfecta in dachshund dogs. *SERPINH1* is present in high concentration in the endoplasmic reticulum and specifically binds to and stabilizes the triple helices of nascent collagens.

Growth plate: Growth plates are not affected in osteogenesis imperfecta (primary collagen of hyaline cartilage is type II collagen).

Trabecular bone: In severe cases, there is greatly reduced trabecular bone without evidence of marked osteoclasis or proliferation of

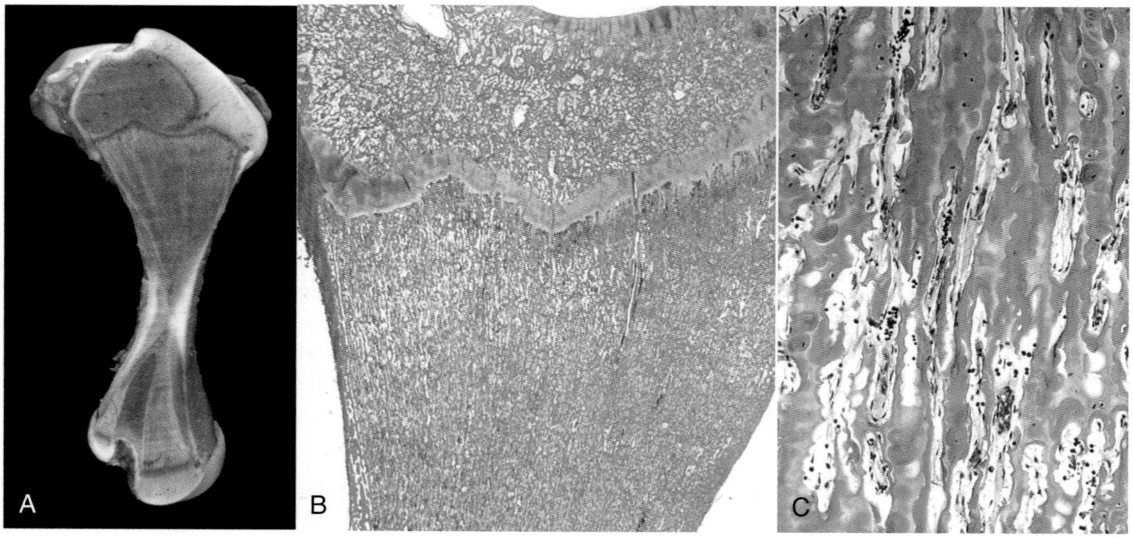

Fig. 16-40 Osteopetrosis, bone, femur, calf (Aberdeen Angus).
A, The primary trabeculae are retained and fill the entire medullary cavity. **B** and **C,** Retained straight unremodeled trabeculae containing cartilaginous cores fill the medullary cavity. H&E stain. (**A** courtesy Dr. H. Leipold, College of Veterinary Medicine, Kansas State University. **B** and **C** courtesy Dr. S.E. Weisbrode, College of Veterinary Medicine, The Ohio State University.)

fibrous tissue, as would be expected in severe cases of fibrous osteodystrophy (see later discussion). Osteoblasts may appear normal or small. In some cases, the amount of bone and its microscopic appearance are normal, but there is evidence of fractures. These fractures may occur in utero and are recognized at birth by callus formation. Bone fragility in cases in which bone morphology and mass are normal is likely to be caused by errors in helix formation or cross-linking of tropocollagen molecules. These individuals may become osteopenic with age, possibly the result of decreased mechanical use because of bone pain from fractures.

Cortical bone: There is a delay in the compaction of cortical bone. During normal development, species-dependent spaces of varying size and contour remain between laminae of woven bone in the developing cortex. The filling of these spaces by bone to solidify the cortex is called *compaction*. The cortices in osteogenesis imperfecta may be composed of woven bone containing large vascular spaces that remain empty. If the animal survives, these vascular spaces may eventually fill in with bone to form compact cortical bone.

Teeth: In some cases, bones may be structurally normal at birth other than the presence of fractures; therefore examination of teeth can be important in reaching a diagnosis of osteogenesis imperfecta. Grossly, teeth in cases of osteogenesis imperfecta may be pink because of visibility of the dental pulp through the thin crown. Dental fractures also may be present. Histologically, the dental tubules are short, tortuous, and sometimes absent. The disorganization of the dentin is a qualitative change that allows confirmation of the diagnosis without requiring an age-matched control animal.

Disorders of Bone Modeling

Congenital Cortical Hyperostosis

Congenital cortical hyperostosis is an autosomal recessive hereditary disease of newborn pigs that is characterized by abnormal periosteal bone formation involving the major long bones. Lesions may be a consequence of disorganization of the perichondral ossification groove (the chondrogenic membrane surrounding the growth plate that enables the growth plate to expand in diameter), and one or several limbs may be affected. Piglets are stillborn or die shortly after birth because of other defects; the pathophysiology of the bone lesions is not understood.

Growth plate: Growth plates are not involved.

Trabecular bone: Trabecular bone is not involved.

Cortical bone: The underlying cortex is normal; however, trabeculae of woven bone, oriented perpendicularly to the long axis of the cortex, radiate outward from its periphery. These trabeculae arise from the cambium layer of the periosteum and other than extent of the change, are typical of the nonspecific reaction of the periosteum to injury described previously.

Craniomandibular Osteopathy

Craniomandibular osteopathy, also known as *lion jaw*, typically occurs as an autosomal recessive condition in West Highland white terriers; however, similar lesions have been reported as isolated occurrences in other breeds and also have been associated with a leukocyte adhesion molecule deficiency in a colony of Irish setter pups that had concurrent metaphyseal osteopathy (see the discussion of noninfectious inflammation in the section on Inflammation of Bone). Lesions are bilaterally symmetric, resulting in diffuse, irregular thickening of the mandibles, occipital and temporal bones, and occasionally, other bones of the skull (Fig. 16-41). The tympanic bullae are often severely affected. Less commonly the disease can affect the appendicular skeleton. The disease often becomes apparent at 4 to 7 months of age and can regress. For affected dogs, mastication is painful and difficult, and the muscles of the skull

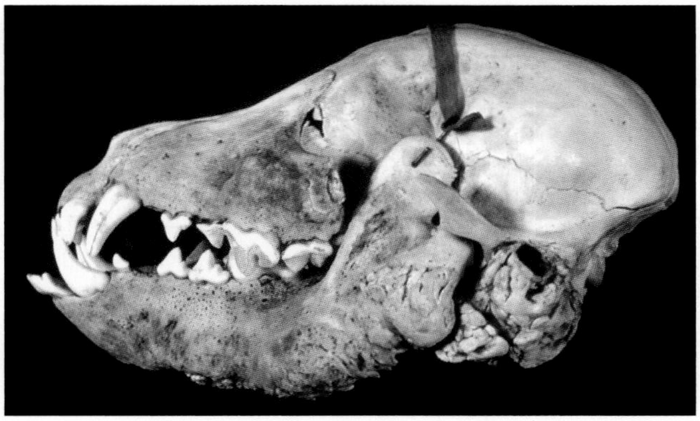

Fig. 16-41 Craniomandibular osteopathy, bone, skull, dog (West Highland white terrier).
Extensive periosteal new bone formation on the lateral surfaces of the body and ramus of the mandible, caudolateral maxilla, bulla tympanica, and occipital condyle. Macerated and bleached specimen. (Courtesy Dr. H. Leipold, College of Veterinary Medicine, Kansas State University.)

become atrophic from disuse. The etiopathogenesis of this disease is unknown. A similar self-limiting disease has recently been reported in the calvaria of young Bullmastiff dogs.

Growth plate: Growth plates are not involved.

Trabecular bone: In the medullary cavities of the bones of the skull and jaw, trabeculae become osteosclerotic (increased bone density per unit area) because of proliferation of woven bone by the osteoblasts of the endosteum with subsequent modeling and remodeling (see next discussion on cortical bone).

Cortical bone: In the skull and jaw, the cortices are thickened because of proliferation of woven bone by the periosteum. Characteristic of the disease is rapid disorganized modeling and remodeling, causing a mosaic of reversal cement lines with regions of lamellar bone adjacent to regions of woven bone.

Disorders of Endochondral Ossification

Chondrodysplasias

Chondrodysplasias (also called *chondrodystrophies*) are hereditary disorders of bone growth that occur as a result of primary lesions in growth cartilage. Growth cartilage is present in the physis (responsible for longitudinal bone growth) and the epiphyseal cartilage of the AEC (growth cartilage at the ends of growing long bones; responsible for development of epiphysis), both of which are replaced by bone in the adult individual. Chondrodysplasias can result in disproportionate dwarfism. Affected animals usually are short-legged with normal-sized heads because the bones of the calvarium (but not the maxilla and mandible) arise from intramembranous, rather than by endochondral, ossification. Primordial dwarfism, in which the limbs are proportional to body length, may occur secondary to underlying endocrine disease (pituitary dwarfism) or malnutrition but also may be genetically determined. Both types of dwarfism are represented by distinct breeds. For example, dachshund, Pekingese, and Bassett hounds are examples of chondrodysplastic dwarfs and miniature poodles, miniature schnauzers, and miniature pinschers are examples of primordial dwarfs.

The mechanisms of chondrodysplasias in animals are becoming better understood through genetic studies and often involve inherited errors in genes that control chondrogenesis. In humans, the most common dwarfism is called *achondroplasia* (a misnomer because growth cartilage is present). The condition is inherited as an autosomal dominant trait caused by a single point mutation in the fibroblast growth factor receptor 3 (FGFR3) gene, which is a

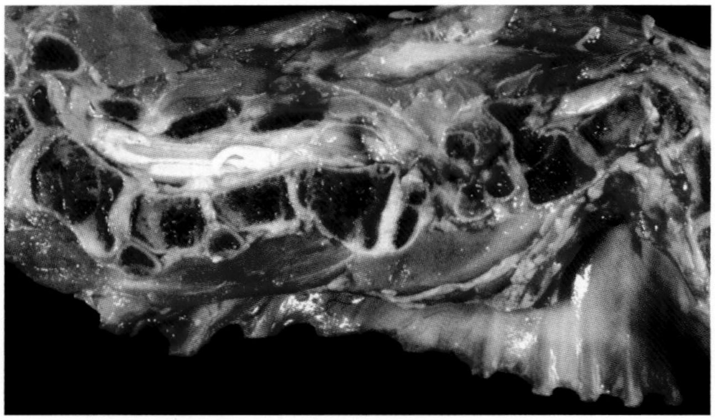

Fig. 16-42 Spider lamb chondrodysplasia, spine, longitudinal section, Suffolk lamb.
The vertebral column has multiple, disorganized ossification centers resulting in variation of the size, shape, and orientation of the vertebrae. (Courtesy Dr. Cathy Carlson, College of Veterinary Medicine, University of Minnesota.)

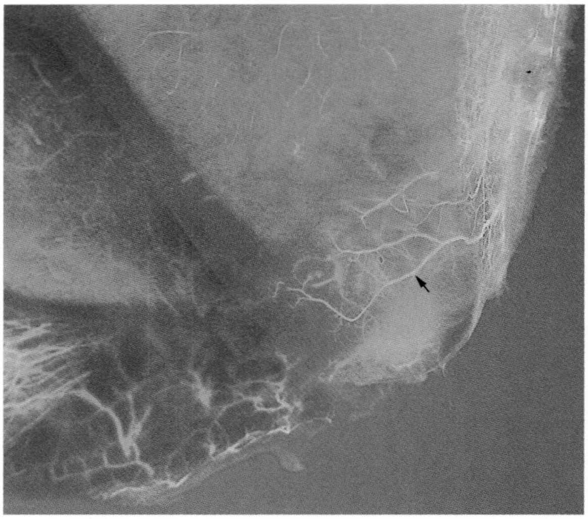

Fig. 16-43 Vascular supply to cranial aspect of distal intermediate ridge, tibia, 14-day-old Standardbred foal.
The arteries have been perfused with micronized barium and the tissues cleared by the modified Spälteholz technique. The cartilage has become translucent, and the subchondral bone is reddish-brown. The image shows a perfused vessel coursing distally on the cranial aspect of the tibia before turning, branching, and continuing within the cartilage on the articular aspect of the distal tibia *(arrow)*. (Courtesy Dr. Kristin Olstad, Norwegian College of Veterinary Medicine, Oslo, Norway.)

negative regulator of bone growth. This mutation results in constant activation of this receptor causing downregulation of chondrocyte proliferation. Conversely, spider lamb chondrodysplasia, which occurs in Suffolk and Hampshire sheep, is the result of a single-base change in the tyrosine kinase II domain of FGFR3, which removes the FGFR3-induced inhibition of chondrocyte proliferation and results in elongation of the limbs and the presence of multiple secondary centers of ossification in the epiphyses (Fig. 16-42). Recently, the genetic mutation for the chondrodysplasia typifying the commonly recognized chondrodysplastic canine breeds, including dachshunds, Pekingese, and Bassett hounds has been identified as a conserved fibroblast growth factor 4 (*fgf4*) retrogene on canine chromosome 18 that likely arose before the division of early dogs into modern breeds Atypical expression of the FGF4 transcript in the chondrocytes may cause inappropriate activation of one or more of the FGF receptors, such as FGFR3.

Skeletal dysplasias have also been reported in animals with inherited lysosomal storage diseases such as mucopolysaccharidosis and gangliosidosis. In these individuals, chondrocytes may be vacuolated due to cytoplasmic retention of glycosaminoglycans and lipid.

Growth plate: Growth plate widths can be normal or reduced depending on the disease. Likewise, chondrocytes can be arranged in normal columns or markedly disorganized. The cartilage matrix also may have a normal appearance or may be rarefied (less compact or dense, characterized by reduced staining intensity).

Trabecular bone: Trabeculae in the primary and secondary spongiosa may be thickened and irregular and may exhibit lateral bridging between trabeculae. Cartilage cores may be larger than normal and may be retained in the secondary spongiosa. These changes may vary greatly, depending on the type of chondrodysplasia.

Cortical bone: Lesions in cortical bone are greatly variable and are reflected primarily by grossly apparent abnormalities in shape or size. Histologically, this tissue usually has a normal appearance.

Osteochondrosis Latens and Manifesta

The osteochondroses consist of a heterogeneous group of lesions in growth cartilage of young animals and are characterized by focal or multifocal failure (or delay) of endochondral ossification. The sites where these lesions occur are the metaphyseal growth plate and the epiphyseal cartilage of the AEC. The lesions are common, often occur in bilaterally symmetric sites and represent an important orthopedic entity that has a number of different clinical manifestations in pigs, dogs, horses, cattle, and poultry. The hallmark of the uncomplicated gross lesions of osteochondrosis is focal retention of growth cartilage because of its failure to become mineralized and replaced by bone (a failure of endochondral ossification). In the growth plate, this is the result of an accumulation of viable hypertrophic chondrocytes, whereas in the AEC, it results from an area of necrosis of epiphyseal cartilage.

The etiology of osteochondrosis appears to be multifactorial, with genetics, rapid growth rate, vascular factors, and trauma all being implicated. Trauma is the most widely proposed etiology in both humans and animals; however, its most likely role is as a final insult to compromised epiphyseal cartilage rather than as an initiating factor in the development of early lesions. Rapid growth and nutritional factors also are cited. Although osteochondrosis occurs during the period of rapid growth and is most common in species that grow rapidly, most experimental work has failed to document rapid growth as a cause of the disease. In addition, little evidence is available to indicate that the lesions of osteochondrosis result from a specific nutritional deficiency. Copper deficiency, perhaps induced by excess dietary zinc, produces lysis of the AEC and formation of thin flaps of cartilage in thoroughbred suckling foals; however, the distribution of these lesions and their extent and severity distinguish them from the multifocal failure of endochondral ossification that is the hallmark of osteochondrosis.

Recent experimental work in pigs and horses has demonstrated that a defect (unknown cause) in vascular supply to growth cartilage, resulting in localized areas of ischemic necrosis, is important in the initiation of preclinical lesions. Although articular cartilage is avascular throughout life, subarticular epiphyseal cartilage of the AEC and growth plate cartilage both are highly vascularized tissues and depend on a vascular supply for viability (Fig. 16-43). The blood vessels supplying growth cartilage run in channels that are termed *cartilage canals.* Both growth plate and epiphyseal (growth) cartilage are temporary, by definition. During growth,

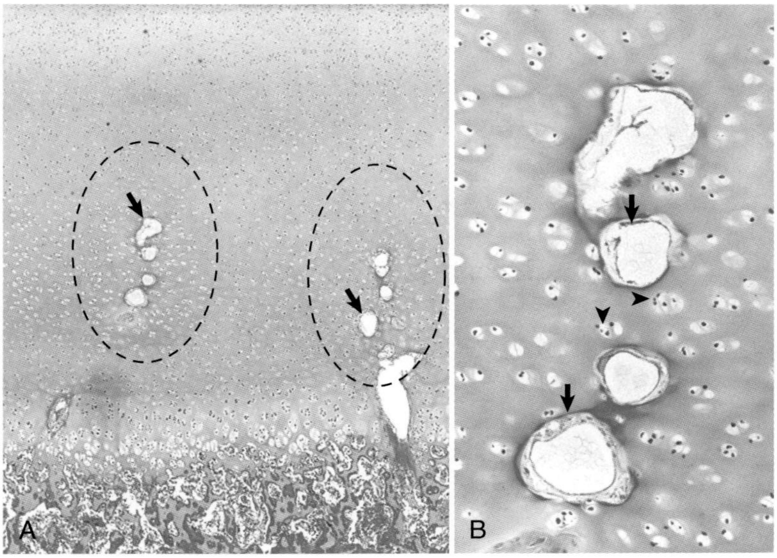

Fig. 16-44 Osteochondrosis latens, lateral femoral condyle, 12-week-old pig.
A, Locally extensive area of chondronecrosis (within ellipses) within the epiphyseal cartilage of the articular-epiphyseal complex (AEC), centered on necrotic cartilage canal blood vessels *(arrows)*. Neither the overlying articular cartilage or the subjacent subchondral bone are involved at this stage of the disease. H&E stain. **B,** Higher magnification of **A** showing necrotic cartilage canal blood vessels *(arrows)* and necrotic chondrocytes *(arrowheads)*. H&E stain. (Courtesy Dr. Cathy Carlson, College of Veterinary Medicine, University of Minnesota.)

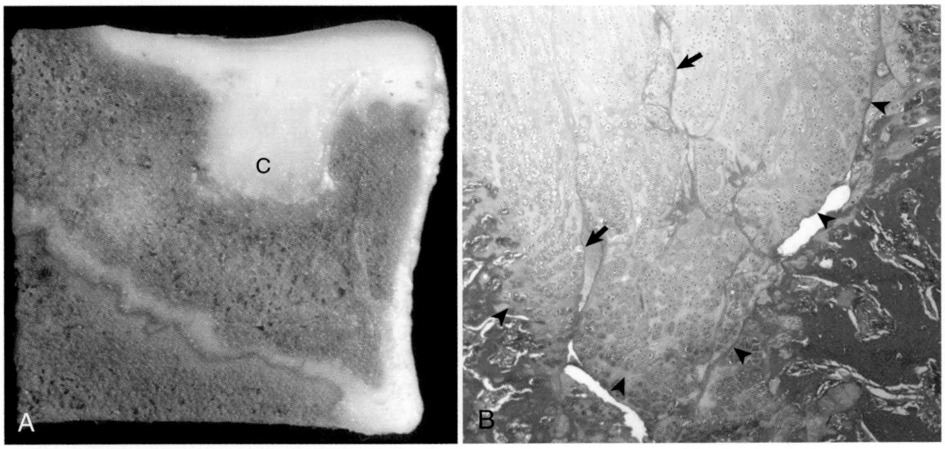

Fig. 16-45 Osteochondrosis manifesta, bone, distal femur, lateral trochlear ridge, horse.
A, The cartilage *(C)* extending into the epiphysis is composed of necrotic epiphyseal cartilage that has failed to undergo endochondral ossification and been retained, whereas the remainder of the epiphysial cartilage has been converted to bone. The retained cartilage has a yellowish appearance compared with the overlying articular cartilage due to degeneration/necrosis of the retained cartilage. **B,** Histologically, there is evidence of a marked cartilage repair process that is characterized by chondrocyte proliferation. The chondro-osseous junction *(arrowheads)* contains a thin margin of acellular, eosinophilic matrix that is associated with several small clefts and is interpreted as necrotic cartilage; eosinophilic streaks *(arrows)* within the retained cartilage may represent collapsed, necrotic vascular channels. H&E stain. (Courtesy Dr. S.E. Weisbrode, College of Veterinary Medicine, The Ohio State University).

the epiphyseal cartilage gradually becomes reduced in volume (until it disappears at maturity) and requires the nutritional support of fewer vascular channels, until it becomes entirely avascular and eventually is completely replaced by bone. It is during the time frame in which the epiphyseal cartilage is supplied by blood vessels that subclinical lesions of osteochondrosis occur. This time frame varies, based on site, age, and species, which likely explains, along with biomechanical factors, why different species have different lesion predilection sites for the development of osteochondrosis. Detailed studies in pigs and horses have revealed that these subclinical lesions occur at a much younger age in horses than in pigs. The finding of extensive areas of necrosis of epiphyseal cartilage in 2-week-old foals suggests that the underlying lesion may, in some cases, even occur in utero or shortly after birth. Although the nature of the insult to the vessel(s) is unclear, the result is a well-demarcated area of necrosis of epiphyseal cartilage that is centered on necrotic blood vessels, is visible only microscopically, and is termed *osteochondrosis latens* (Fig. 16-44). When the ossification front of the secondary center of ossification reaches the area of necrosis, failure of endochondral ossification occurs, resulting in an area of retained necrotic epiphyseal cartilage that is visible grossly (Fig. 16-45). The lesion at this stage is termed *osteochondrosis manifesta*. This lesion is highly vulnerable to traumatic clefting through the area of necrosis, termed *osteochondrosis dissecans,* even with physiologic pressure. Once clefting occurs and subchondral bone is exposed, the lesion is highly painful and results in clinical signs

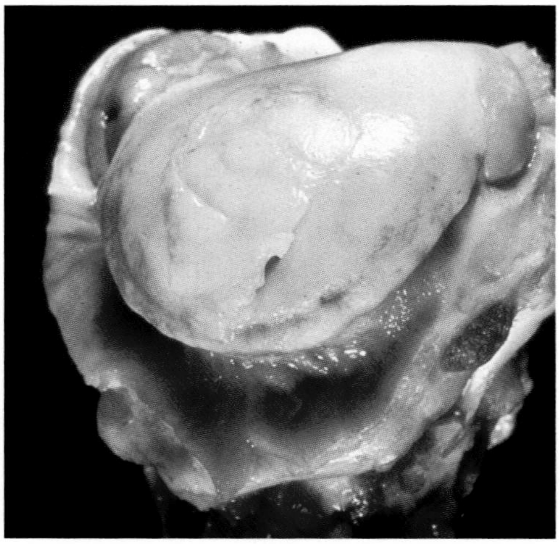

Fig. 16-46 Osteochondrosis dissecans, bone, articular cartilage, humerus, proximal end, dog.
A flap of thickened cartilage has detached from the underlying bone. The synovium is hyperemic and hyperplastic. (Courtesy Dr. S.E. Weisbrode, College of Veterinary Medicine, The Ohio State University.)

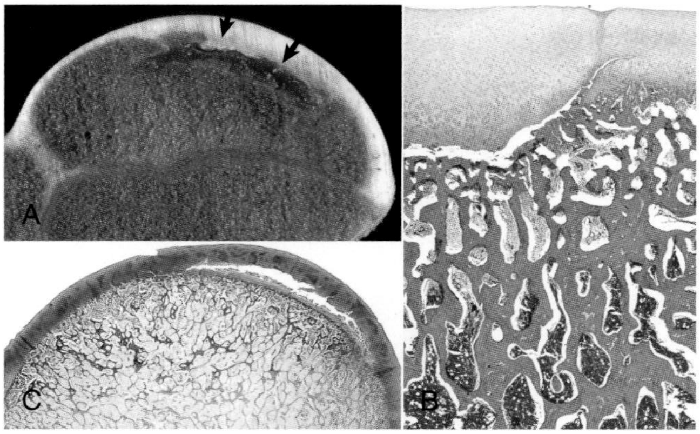

Fig. 16-47 Osteochondrosis of the articular-epiphyseal complex (AEC), bone.
A, Humerus, pig. The retained cartilage has separated from the subchondral bone *(arrows)* but a fissure extending to the articular surface (osteochondrosis dissecans) has not formed. **B,** AEC, distal femur, horse. A linear fissure between the thickened epiphyseal cartilage and subjacent underlying (subchondral) bone is extending into adjacent normal *(right)* articular cartilage. H&E stain. **C,** Humerus, horse. Note the linear fissure within the epiphyseal cartilage of the AE complex, which likely occurred secondary to ischemic necrosis of cartilage before the occurrence of a failure of endochondral ossification. H&E stain. (**A** and **B** courtesy Dr. S.E. Weisbrode, College of Veterinary Medicine, The Ohio State University. **C** courtesy Dr. C. Bridges, College of Veterinary Medicine, Texas A&M University; and Dr. J. King, College of Veterinary Medicine, Cornell University.)

of lameness. Cleft formation most commonly does not occur, and in most cases, the necrotic epiphyseal cartilage becomes surrounded by subchondral bone, gradually diminishes in size, and eventually becomes completely replaced by bone. In horses, particularly in the medial femoral condyle (weight-bearing location), some of these early lesions of osteochondrosis have been hypothesized to develop into subchondral bone cysts.

Physeal lesions of osteochondrosis also are likely have a vascular etiology but are characterized by multifocal areas of retained, viable, hypertrophic cartilage. If these involve an extensive area of the growth plate, the growth plate may fracture, either partially or completely, resulting in a variety of clinical sequelae.

Growth plate and AEC: Lesions of osteochondrosis are not recognized grossly until they result in a focal failure of endochondral ossification, at which time they are composed of a well-demarcated wedge of retained cartilage involving the epiphyseal cartilage at the AEC (osteochondrosis manifesta) or physis (physeal osteochondrosis) (Fig. 16-46). Hemorrhage and mineralized debris may be present at the junction of the retained cartilage and the underlying bone. Small lesions that have not undergone clefting produce no clinical signs and are much more common than those causing clinical disease. Predilection sites for both clinical and subclinical lesions include the AEC of the distal femur (especially the medial femoral condyle) and humerus (condyles and head) of pigs; the distal femur (medial condyle and both trochlear ridges), distal tibia (cranial intermediate ridge and medial malleolus), talus (trochlear ridges), and articular processes of the cervical vertebrae of horses; the humerus (humeral head and medial humeral condyle), distal femur (both condyles) and tibiotarsal bone (medial trochlear ridge) of dogs; the distal talus (medial and lateral trochlear ridges), distal femur (medial and lateral trochlear ridges) of cattle; and the proximal tibia of rapidly growing birds.

Osteochondrosis latens lesions are only recognized histologically in the AEC and occur as well-demarcated areas of necrosis of epiphyseal cartilage, usually adjacent to or surrounding one or more necrotic cartilage canal blood vessels (see Fig. 16-44). The overlying articular cartilage and subjacent subchondral bone are not affected at this stage of the disease. Osteochondrosis manifesta lesions also are composed of necrotic epiphyseal cartilage, but at this point of the disease, the ossification front has reached and partially surrounded the area of necrosis so that it is grossly visible (see Fig. 16-45). Lesions of physeal osteochondrosis, in contrast to those occurring in the AEC, are composed of columns of retained, viable, hypertrophic chondrocytes without evidence of mineralization or vascular invasion.

Trabecular bone: In lesions of osteochondrosis latens, trabecular bone is normal. Osteochondrosis manifesta lesions, however, include direct contact of the subchondral bone with an area of necrotic cartilage. Marked myelofibrosis and bony remodeling, with formation of locally extensive areas of woven bone, are nearly always present; however, inflammatory cells are rarely a feature of the lesion. A closely similar bony reaction is seen in lesions of physeal osteochondrosis. In both sites, cleft formation may occur at the junction of the retained cartilage and the underlying bone (see Figs. 16-46 and 16-47, *A* and *B*).

Cortical bone: Lesions in cortical bone are not expected at any stage of osteochondrosis of the AE complex or physis.

Osteochondrosis Dissecans

Osteochondrosis dissecans (OCD) is the name given to osteochondrosis at the AEC that forms clefts in the necrotic cartilage with subsequent fracture of the overlying articular cartilage (Fig. 16-47). The result is a cartilaginous or osteochondral flap, depending on whether bone is present with the cartilage. This may change with the duration of the lesion because cartilaginous flaps that have a blood supply may ossify over time. Should this flap fracture off and become free in the joint space, it is sometimes referred to as a *joint mouse.* OCD can be accompanied by pain, joint effusion, and nonspecific secondary lymphoplasmacytic synovitis. Free-floating chondral or osteochondral fragments ("joint mice") occasionally interfere with mechanical movement of the joint. The lesions of OCD develop in various synovial joints, including those of the facets of the vertebral column. Common sites of OCD are the same as those of osteochondrosis manifesta (see previous section). The disease is extremely common in young breeding pigs and is a significant cause of lameness in this species. Although less common in horses and dogs, it remains an important cause of lameness in these species. The articular cartilage defect in OCD has poor healing capabilities, and such joints commonly develop some degree of degenerative joint disease. Surgical removal of the flap reduces the long-term clinical consequences; however, the defect repairs by the formation of fibrocartilage, which provides suboptimal biomechanical properties to the joint surface compared with articular cartilage.

For the development of OCD, clefts must develop in the epiphyseal cartilage of the AEC, usually at the stage of osteochondrosis manifesta (see Fig. 16-45). Cleft formation can cause mechanical instability and lead to separations within cartilage or between cartilage and the underlying bone. "Trauma" (most commonly normal physiologic activity) can cause the cleft to extend through the overlying articular cartilage, resulting in the formation of a flap. At this stage of the disease, the affected animal has acute pain.

Cartilage flap formation involving extensive areas of multiple joints can develop in horses without predisposing lesions of osteochondrosis latens or manifesta. In these cases, articular cartilage of normal thickness can be peeled from the subjacent bone because of fissuring in the deeper layers of the AEC. Such lesions have been seen in foals that have licked fences with zinc-based white paint. The pathogenesis of the lesion is thought to involve copper deficiency induced by the zinc excess. Copper is a required cofactor for enzymes that facilitate cross-linkages between tropocollagen molecules; however, these foals do not appear to have a generalized collagen dysplasia. The extensive distribution of the articular lesions distinguishes them from OCD, which occurs multifocally in species-dependent predilection sites.

Growth plate and AEC: The growth plate is not involved in OCD. The lesion in the AEC includes a locally extensive area of fibroplasia, neovascularization, and bony remodeling at the chondro-osseous junction. Even in the most chronic lesions, variably sized areas of necrosis of epiphyseal cartilage often can be identified at the chondro-osseous junction or along the deep surface of the articular cartilage. The superficial zones of the articular cartilage may be normal, other than the presence of a fissure that extends from the necrotic zone of epiphyseal cartilage to the articular surface. In cases in which the cartilage fragment has been displaced, all or part of the AEC is replaced by an area of cartilage ulceration overlying reactive and fibrotic subchondral bone.

Trabecular bone: The severity of changes in trabecular bone of the epiphysis reflects the extent of the cleft formation and depends on whether the flap has detached. Marked fibrosis and formation of reactive woven bone is expected at the base of the flap.

Cortical bone: Lesions in cortical bone are not expected with OCD.

Epiphysiolysis

Epiphysiolysis is the separation of the epiphysis from the metaphysis as the result of the formation of a horizontal fissure through an abnormal physis. The condition is most common in pigs and dogs. In market-weight pigs and in young gilts, the femoral head may be involved, whereas, in sows, separation of the ischial tuberosity (site of insertion of semimembranosus, semitendinosus, and biceps femoris muscles) at its growth plate (often bilaterally) is a common cause of caudal weakness and inability to stand and often occurs at parturition. In dogs, the process of epiphysiolysis can affect the anconeal process of the ulna, resulting in a condition known as *ununited anconeal process.* This may occur as one aspect of a condition known as the *elbow dysplasia syndrome,* which includes one or more of the following: OCD of the medial humeral condyle, fragmentation of the coronoid process, ununited anconeal process, and elbow incongruity (shortening of the ulna relative to the radius secondary to lesions in the distal ulnar growth plate). Because these lesions have primarily been studied in their chronic stages, the nature of the initial lesion is unclear; however, it is strongly suspected that they occur secondary to an extensive area, or to multifocal coalescing areas, of physeal osteochondrosis. A somewhat similar disease, known as *diffuse physeal dysplasia with slipped capital femoral epiphysis,* is described in heavy young adult castrated male cats. The growth plates in these cats appear to remain open longer than expected, are widened, and histologically, have a disorganized appearance in which chondrocytes are present in clusters, rather than columns, and are separated by variable amounts of matrix. It has been hypothesized that this dysplastic lesion may be present in all growth plates in affected animals, but fractures occur only in sites (e.g., femoral head) where shear forces occur during weight bearing. Osteochondrosis is rarely reported in cats, and the histologic changes in affected and contralateral growth plates are more characteristic of a physeal dysplasia (diffuse process) than of osteochondrosis (focal to multifocal process) in this species.

Several types of underlying conditions may result in partial closure of the physis, causing an angular limb deformity in the affected limb. This condition is most common in horses, where it usually occurs secondary to lesions of physeal osteochondrosis. Other causes include trauma and inflammation of the growth plate and/or primary trabeculae.

Growth plate: Grossly there is a horizontal fissure/fracture through the physis with complete or partial separation of the epiphysis from the metaphysis. In cats, the remaining physeal cartilage is dysplastic, as described above (disorganized arrangement of chondrocytes with separation by variable amounts of matrix). In pigs and dogs, the remaining physeal cartilage contains areas of delayed endochondral ossification. The chronicity of the lesions (with accompanying secondary changes) complicates their interpretation.

Trabecular bone: The response to trabecular bone in epiphysiolysis is characteristic of reaction to trauma and fracture and includes myelofibrosis, proliferation of reactive woven bone, and variable hemorrhage.

Cortical bone: There are no primary changes in cortical bone with this condition; any lesions that develop would be secondary to altered mechanical use.

Cervical Vertebral Myelopathy

Cervical vertebral stenotic myelopathy (CVSM) is a neurologic disease of horses and dogs (usually giant breeds) that occurs secondary to static or dynamic compression of the spinal cord by abnormally developed cervical vertebrae. This compression can be constant as the result of an anatomic stenosis of the canal termed *cervical vertebral static stenosis* (CVS), or may occur only during movement (usually flexion), which is termed *cervical vertebral instability* (CVI). CVS involves the less mobile caudal cervical vertebrae, mainly C5-C6 and C6-C7, and most commonly affects older horses (usually 1 to 4 years old). In contrast, the spinal cord lesions of CVI are centered on the more mobile cranial cervical vertebrae, primarily at C3-C4 and C4-C5, in younger horses (6 to 15 months of age). In both syndromes, anatomic localization of the lesion by neurologic examination, myelography, or computed tomography is very helpful to the pathologist. In thoroughbred and standardbred horses and in dogs, the static compression is usually the result of a grossly appreciable narrowing of the spinal canal from caudal to cranial within a single vertebral body that likely occurs during development (Fig. 16-48). In adult quarter horses, localized hyperplasia and fibrocartilaginous metaplasia of the ligamentum flavum (the ligament between the dorsal lamina), likely secondary to chronic mechanical irritation and/or trauma, can protrude into the spinal canal causing static compression of the spinal cord and closely similar clinical signs.

The lesions associated with dynamic compression of the cord are more variable and less definitive because identical lesions often occur in asymptomatic animals. In horses, the most common lesions are those of osteochondrosis (see previous discussion) of the cervical facets. Osteochondrosis can cause abnormal and asymmetric development of the facets or abnormally large cranial vertebral epiphyses. With either lesion, the dorsal aspect of the vertebral body may compress the ventral aspect of the cord during flexion, causing transient ischemia. Such compression may initially cause functional deficits without lesions in the spinal cord but also may progress to produce notable Wallerian degeneration. The frequency of osteochondrosis of the cervical vertebrae in clinically normal horses is the same as in horses with clinical signs of dynamic cervical vertebral myelopathy; however, the severity is worse in the latter cases. In addition, the frequency and severity of osteochondrosis lesions in the appendicular skeleton are greater in horses with clinical signs, further supporting the hypothesis that osteochondrosis may be an important underlying cause for this condition. The diameter of the vertebral canal is smaller in horses in which there is dynamic compression of the cord, suggesting that this change contributes to the development of clinical signs.

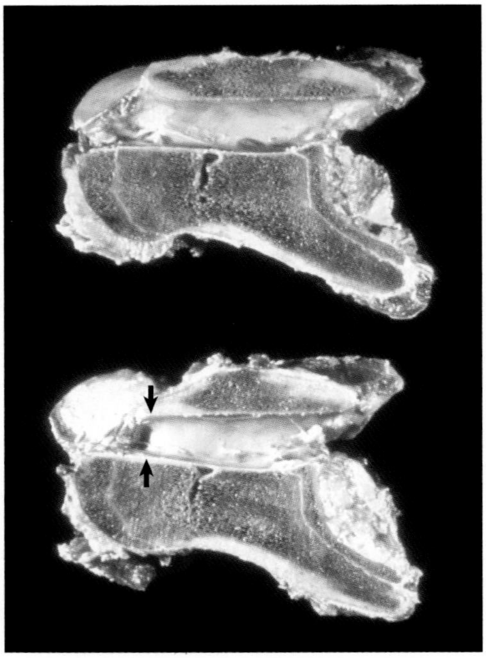

Fig. 16-48 Static stenosis, bone, cervical vertebra, sagittal section, horse.
Static stenosis (narrowing) of the vertebral canal caused by malformation of the vertebra *(bottom vertebra, arrows)*. The top vertebra is normal. (Courtesy College of Veterinary Medicine University of Illinois.)

METABOLIC BONE DISEASES

Metabolic bone diseases are systemic skeletal diseases that are generally of nutritional, endocrine, or toxic origin (Table 16-1 and Web Table 16-1) and occur in both growing and adult skeletons. Metabolic bone diseases are often called *osteodystrophies,* which is a general term that implies defective bone formation. The classic metabolic osteodystrophies are osteoporosis, fibrous osteodystrophy, rickets, and osteomalacia. These terms imply specific pathologic changes but do not necessarily imply specific causes. For example, osteoporosis can be the result of a calcium deficiency, glucocorticoid therapy, or physical inactivity. In addition, different osteodystrophies can coexist in the same skeleton. For example, the skeleton of an animal with a severe calcium deficiency accompanied by excess dietary phosphorus might have features of both osteoporosis and fibrous osteodystrophy. In practice, most nutritional deficiencies in domestic animals do not involve a single element. More often, deficiencies are multiple, relatively mild, and do not produce the "classic" lesions that occur under experimental conditions.

Osteoporosis

Osteoporosis is a disease in which bone fractures occur secondary to a reduction in bone density or mass (Fig. 16-49). The bone present, although reduced in amount, is normally mineralized. When there is reduced bone mass but no clinical disease (fractures), the term osteopenia is more appropriate; however, once fractures occur, the disease is called *osteoporosis.* In senile osteoporosis in humans, in addition to decreased bone density, the turnover rate is

TABLE 16-1 Metabolic Bone Disease

Disease	Characteristics	Causes
Osteoporosis	Reduced bone mass: porous, thin, and fragile bones	Protein calorie malnutrition, immobilization, dietary calcium deficiency, glucocorticoid excess, estrogen or androgen deficiency and advanced age
Osteomalacia (adult animals)	Decreased bone mineralization (accumulation of osteoid): soft bones	Vitamin D deficiency, phosphorus deficiency
Rickets (growing animals)	Decreased bone mineralization (accumulation of osteoid): soft bones; thickened hypertrophic zone of growth plate (failure of endochondral ossification)	Vitamin D deficiency, phosphorus deficiency
Fibrous osteodystrophy	Decreased bone mass and increased pliability of bone due to resorption and replacement by fibro-osseous tissue	Hyperparathyroidism 1. Primary: functional chief cell adenoma of parathyroid gland 2. Paraneoplastic: parathyroid hormone–related protein secreted from neoplasms such as adenocarcinoma of apocrine glands of anal sac 3. Secondary nutritional: from diets low in calcium and high in phosphorus 4. Secondary renal: from failure of the kidney to secrete phosphorus and reduced synthesis of 1,25-dihydroxyvitamin D

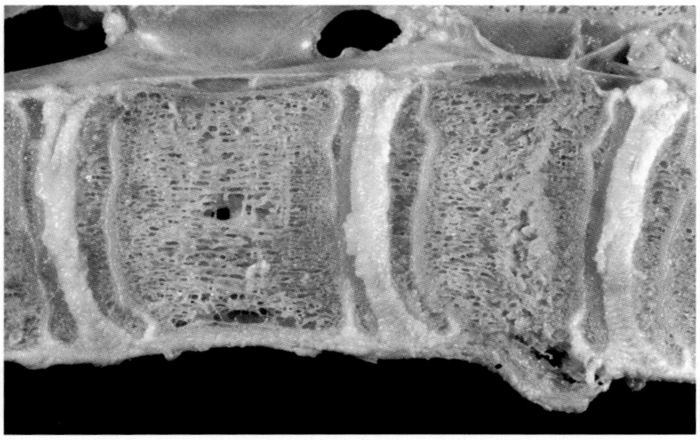

Fig. 16-49 Osteoporosis, bone, cervical vertebrae, sagittal section, horse.
Note the markedly thin cortices, particularly dorsally. The thickness of trabeculae also has been reduced, but this is difficult to appreciate grossly. The vertebra to the right has a compression fracture, causing shortening of the length of the vertebral body between the growth plates and fracture of the ventral cortex. The marrow has been flushed from the specimen in order to illustrate the bone changes. (Courtesy Dr. S.E. Weisbrode, College of Veterinary Medicine, The Ohio State University.)

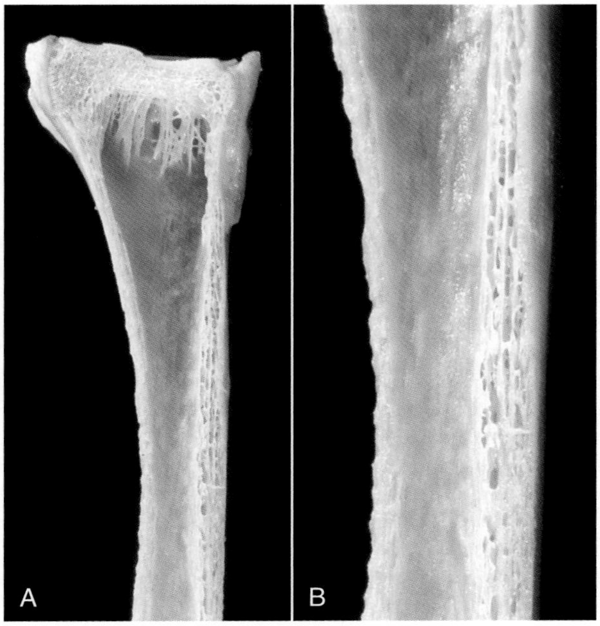

Fig. 16-50 Osteopenia, bone, metatarsal, sheep.
A, There is marked reduction in the number and length of metaphyseal trabeculae. **B,** The cranial cortex *(right)* is markedly porous (trabeculated), and the caudal cortex *(left)* is thin. The marrow has been flushed from the specimen. (Courtesy Dr. S.E. Weisbrode, College of Veterinary Medicine, The Ohio State University.)

reduced, allowing microcracks (small cracks in the bone visible only microscopically) to accumulate. These microcracks, superimposed on the reduced bone mass, make bones more brittle than would be predicted from the reduced mass alone. In growing animals, osteoporosis is potentially reversible. In adults, however, loss of trabecular bone is generally considered to be permanent. Although osteoporosis affects both cortical and trabecular bone, the loss of trabecular bone occurs earlier because of its higher surface area. Although the thickness and density of cortical bone generally determines bone strength, trabecular bone contributes significantly to bone strength in some locations, including the femoral neck, vertebral bodies, and distal radius. This explains why osteoporotic fractures in humans occur most commonly in these locations. Some causes of osteopenia include calcium deficiency, starvation, physical inactivity, hypogonadism, and chronic glucocorticoid administration. A calcium deficiency can result in hypocalcemia, which is compensated for by increased PTH output and increased bone resorption. Starvation and malnutrition can result in arrested growth and osteoporosis, largely because of reduced bone formation resulting from deficiencies of protein and mineral. Reduced physical activity (disuse or immobilization osteoporosis) causes increased bone resorption and decreased bone formation. This loss of bone from disuse might be mediated through changes in piezoelectrical activity, streaming potentials, and stretch receptors that are able to detect decreased mechanical use of the skeleton. Loss of bone mass associated with long-term paralysis or immobilization is not necessarily progressive; rather, the skeleton stabilizes at a new (reduced) level. Postmenopausal osteoporosis is a common and important disease in women, often resulting in vertebral deformity or collapse and pathologic fractures of the femoral neck and distal radius (wrist). Declining concentrations of estrogens, physical inactivity, reduced muscle tone, and inadequate calcium intake are factors that can be responsible for causing osteopenia to progress to osteoporosis; however, in postmenopausal women, estrogen deficiency is the most important. Estrogen generally potentiates bone formation and inhibits bone resorption, likely by altering cytokine production from osteoblasts and monocytes. Estrogens promote secretion of TGF-β (an anabolic cytokine) and decrease production of IL-1, IL-6, and TNF-α (cytokines that promote osteoclasis). The loss of estrogen after menopause has the opposite effect. For example, IL-6 knockout mice do not develop osteopenia after ovariohysterectomy, confirming the critical role of cytokines in this process. Interestingly, ovariohysterectomy in the bitch is associated with only a transient osteopenia that does not develop into clinical osteoporosis. Thus dogs are not particularly useful as an animal model of this disease. Osteopenia associated with reduced estrogens from ovarian atrophy or ovariectomy appears to be greatest in animals with estrous cycles that extend throughout the year (e.g., rat, pig, and primate), rather than being seasonal.

Growth plate: Lesions in the growth plate are not expected in osteoporosis unless the disease is related to pituitary dysfunction or protein calorie malnutrition, in which case the plate would be thin.

Trabecular bone: Trabeculae become thinner, decrease in number, and develop perforations (loss of continuity) within the plates. With time the normal structure of trabecular bone (anastomosing plates) is replaced by strut or rodlike bone. The loss of these anastomoses results in reduced ability of the trabeculae to withstand stress. In most long bones of adults, trabeculae extend from the epiphysis to the metaphyseal-diaphyseal junction. The degree to which the trabeculae fail to reach this distance is an indication of the severity of the osteopenia (Fig. 16-50, *A*).

Cortical bone: Cortical bone becomes thin because of osteoclastic resorption on the endosteal surface, with corresponding enlargement of the medullary cavity. The porosity of the cortex also increases because of increased osteoclastic resorption within the cortical vascular spaces and Haversian systems and/or decreased osteoblastic activity and may more closely resemble trabecular bone than cortical bone (Fig. 16-50, *B*). In severe cases, loss of cortical bone results in an increased susceptibility to fracture.

Rickets and Osteomalacia

Failure of mineralization with subsequent bone deformities and fractures is called rickets in the growing skeleton and osteomalacia (soft bone) in the adult. Rickets is a disease of bone and epiphyseal (growth) cartilage in immature animals, whereas osteomalacia is a disease where the lesions are confined to bone and only occurs in adults. Affected animals have bone pain, pathologic fractures, and deformities such as kyphosis and scoliosis.

The most common causes of rickets and osteomalacia are deficiencies of vitamin D or phosphorus. However, both diseases can occur in chronic renal disease and in chronic fluorosis. Dietary phosphorus deficiency is not common but can occur in herbivores grazing on phosphorus-deficient pastures. Phosphorus-deficient animals often have reduced feed intake, are unthrifty, and have impaired reproductive performance. Vitamin D deficiency is rare because of the common addition of this vitamin to commercial feed. In addition, animals exposed to adequate sunlight should be able to synthesize vitamin D if their kidneys are normal. Although calcium deficiency is not commonly considered to be a cause of rickets in animals, studies in humans provide evidence that some cases of rickets may be attributable to extremely low dietary calcium intakes in the presence of adequate vitamin D intake, particularly in infants and younger children (versus adolescents). In addition, low dietary calcium is known to exacerbate the development of vitamin D deficiency rickets in children. The mechanisms of this phenomenon are not known; however, it has been shown that knockout mice with no receptors for vitamin D develop rickets that can be corrected by feeding a high-calcium diet.

Growth plate: The growth plates in rickets are diffusely but irregularly thickened because of failure of cartilage matrix mineralization and endochondral ossification (Fig. 16-51). This lesion may be evident in the costal-chondral junctions as prominent, nodular thickenings that historically have been called *rachitic rosary* due to its resemblance to a string of prayer beads. This thickening is apparent grossly as retained epiphyseal cartilage. Microscopically, the columns of chondrocytes in the plate are somewhat disorganized, and in mammals, there is a marked increase in the number of chondrocytes in the zone of hypertrophy compared with normal. It is uncertain if the disorganization of chondrocytes in vitamin D-deficiency rickets is caused by a primary effect of a lack of vitamin D metabolites (specifically, 24,25-dihydroxyvitamin D) or to a mechanical consequence of the failure of endochondral ossification. Because of the inadequate absorption of calcium, the rickETic growth plate does not undergo mineralization. In mammals, when mineralization of the cartilage matrix does not occur, blood vessels with accompanying chondroclasts do not invade the physis and the process of endochondral ossification does not proceed.

Trabecular bone: Grossly and radiographically, the metaphyses are "flared" in rickets because of failure of bone and cartilage removal in the cutback zones (see Fig. 16-51). Poorly mineralized matrices cannot be resorbed because osteoclasts cannot bind to an unmineralized matrix (see previous discussion). Microscopically, the surfaces of trabecular bone in rickets and osteomalacia contain excessive amounts of osteoid (unmineralized matrix) (Fig. 16-52). Because osteoclasts are not able to adhere to or resorb osteoid, bone modeling and remodeling is impaired. Hypocalcemia can develop concurrently with vitamin D deficiency, and lesions of secondary hyperparathyroidism (fibrous osteodystrophy [see later discussion]) also can develop.

Cortical bone: Grossly, cortical bone can appear normal or the softened bone can be deformed by weight bearing. In severe cases, the bones are so soft that they can be cut with a knife. Microscopically, endocortical and trabecular surfaces in the cortex can have numerous wide seams of unmineralized osteoid. Osteomalacic bone is susceptible to accumulation of microcracks because of the impaired remodeling and modeling secondary to the failure of osteoclasts to bind to osteoid surfaces.

Fibrous Osteodystrophy

Fibrous osteodystrophy is the name given to the skeletal lesions that result from primary hyperparathyroidism, secondary hyperparathyroidism, and pseudohyperparathyroidism. These disorders are characterized by increased, widespread osteoclastic resorption

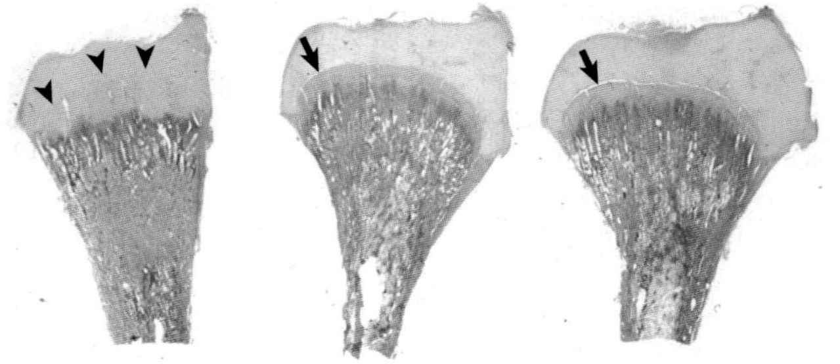

Fig. 16-51 Vitamin D deficiency (experimental), bone, tibia, chicken. Left specimen: rachitic tibia; middle and right specimens: normal chicken and a chicken fed a vitamin D–deficient diet supplemented with calcitriol. The latter two specimens appear normal and are indistinguishable from each other. The growth plate in the rachitic bird is thickened. The arrowheads indicate the junction between the growth plate and the epiphyseal cartilage. The metaphysis has not undergone modeling ("cutback"). In the normal-appearing bones, notice the tapering of the metaphysis ("cutback" zone) and the thickness of the growth plate. In these normal chickens, the cleft *(arrows)* separating the growth plate from the epiphyseal cartilage is an artifact. There is no ossification center present in the epiphysis, which is normal for young broilers. H&E stain. (Courtesy Dr. L. Nagode.)

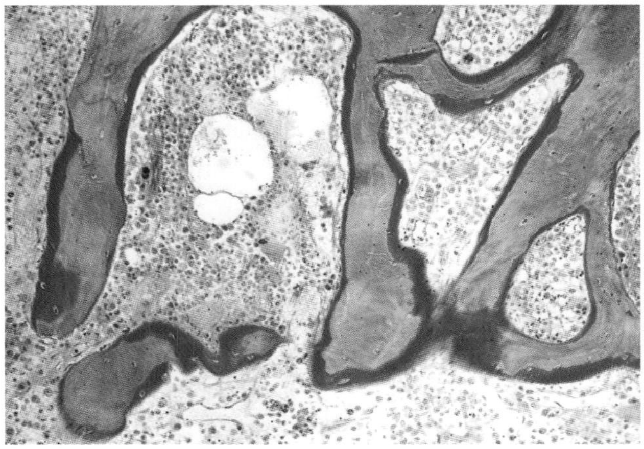

Fig. 16-52 Osteomalacia, bone, cross-section, metaphysis, trabeculae, human. This person had osteomalacia secondary to malabsorption of fat soluble vitamins (including vitamin D) associated with gastrectomy. This section was not demineralized and was stained to show the difference between osteoid *(red)* and fully mineralized bone *(blue-green)*. Normally, no more than 10% of trabecular surfaces should be covered by osteoid seams; however, in this case almost all surfaces are covered by osteoid. Goldner's trichrome stain. (Courtesy Dr. S.E. Weisbrode, College of Veterinary Medicine, The Ohio State University.)

of bone and replacement by primitive fibro-osseous tissue, which results in a weakened bone structure. Sequelae include lameness, pathologic fractures, and deformities. As described previously, osteoblasts—but not osteoclasts—have receptors for PTH and respond by upregulating production of RANKL and downregulating secretion of OPG. Bone marrow stromal cells also have receptors for PTH, and when the hormone is expressed constantly at high levels, these cells differentiate into fibroblasts. Paradoxically, intermittent dosing of PTH has the opposite effect on bone and is used clinically in humans for the treatment of osteoporosis.

In domestic animals, primary hyperparathyroidism, which includes functional parathyroid adenoma, parathyroid carcinoma, and idiopathic bilateral parathyroid hyperplasia, is rare. Secondary hyperparathyroidism is more common and can be either nutritional or renal in origin. Nutritional hyperparathyroidism is caused by dietary factors that tend to decrease the concentration of serum ionized calcium, to which the parathyroid glands respond by increasing output of PTH. Nutritional hyperparathyroidism is most common in young, growing animals that are fed rations that are deficient in calcium and have a relative excess of phosphorus. Unsupplemented cereal grain rations fed to pigs, all-meat diets fed to dogs and cats, and bran fed to horses are examples of low-calcium, high-phosphorus diets that can cause secondary nutritional hyperparathyroidism and eventually, fibrous osteodystrophy. Increased concentrations of dietary phosphorus are important in the evolution of fibrous osteodystrophy, perhaps by interfering with the intestinal absorption of calcium. Pseudohyperparathyroidism is also known as humeral hypercalcemia of malignancy and is discussed in Chapter 12.

Growth plate: No lesions are expected in the growth plate or AEC.

Trabecular bone: Trabeculae are replaced by irregular spicules of woven bone that are separated by variable amounts of fibrous connective tissue and are accompanied by numerous osteoclasts. Osteoblastic proliferation can be marked but ineffectual in that little osteoid is produced. Proliferation of fibrous tissue in the marrow space is usually marked but may be subtle in early stages, consisting of only two or three layers of fibroblasts between the bone lining cells and the marrow space (Fig. 16-53). In severe cases, the marrow cavity is filled with fibrous tissue.

Cortical bone: Bone resorption and replacement by fibrous tissue can be so extensive that the bone becomes pliable (Fig. 16-54). Clinically and at postmortem examination, severely affected bones can be bent at a right angle without fracture. Osteoclastic resorption begins on the endocortical bone surface, but any vascular spaces within the wall of the bone can undergo marked enlargement by osteoclastic resorption and replacement by fibrous tissue. In advanced disease, the entire width of the cortex may be replaced by reactive woven bone and fibrous tissue. Sometimes the proliferation of fibrous tissue is so exuberant that the external dimension of the bone is increased (Fig. 16-55). This process is most common in the maxilla and mandible and may reflect the response of the weakened bone to the intense mechanical stress of mastication.

Renal Osteodystrophy

Renal osteodystrophy is a general term that refers to the skeletal lesions that develop secondary to chronic, severe renal disease. In humans, this can include osteomalacia and fibrous osteodystrophy, either as separate diseases or in combination. Similarly, although fibrous osteodystrophy is the most common consequence of chronic renal disease, particularly in dogs, this sometimes is complicated by osteomalacia. Clinical signs of the disease include bone pain (lameness) and loss of teeth and deformity of the maxilla or mandible as the result of osteoclastic resorption of bone and replacement by fibro-osseous tissue. Renal osteodystrophy has a complex pathogenesis that likely varies, depending on the extent and nature of the renal disease and the availability of dietary vitamin D. Loss of glomerular function, inability to excrete phosphate, inadequate renal production of 1,25-dihydroxyvitamin D (calcitriol), and acidosis are central to its development. As the glomerular filtration rate falls in chronic renal disease, hyperphosphatemia develops, stimulating PTH synthesis and secretion. Hyperphosphatemia also suppresses the renal hydroxylation of inactive 25-hydroxyvitamin D to 1,25-dihydroxyvitamin D (calcitriol). Hypocalcemia develops primarily from decreased intestinal calcium absorption because of low serum calcitriol levels. Low serum calcitriol levels, hypocalcemia, and hyperphosphatemia have all been demonstrated to independently promote PTH synthesis and secretion. If serum levels of PTH remain elevated, fibrous osteodystrophy develops. The reduced production of 1,25-dihydroxyvitamin D by the diseased kidneys, together with impaired mineralization because of the acidosis of uremia, explain the development of osteomalacia.

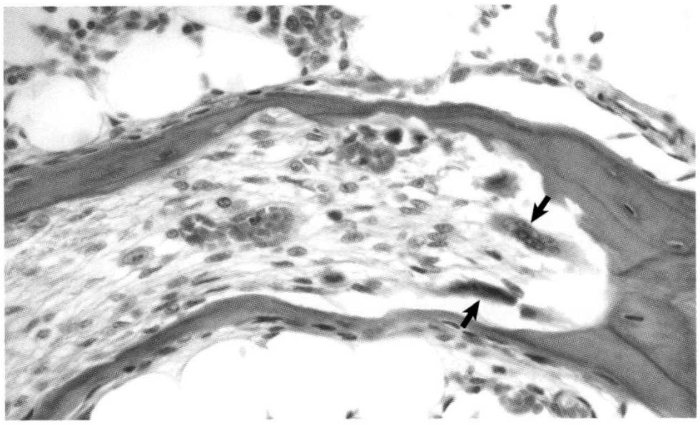

Fig. 16-53 Tunneling resorption (within a trabecula), fibrous osteodystrophy, bone, longitudinal section, dog.

Osteoclasts *(arrows)* have resorbed the central portion of the trabecula, and this tissue is being replaced by fibrous tissue rather than bone. H&E stain. (Courtesy Dr. S.E. Weisbrode, College of Veterinary Medicine, The Ohio State University.)

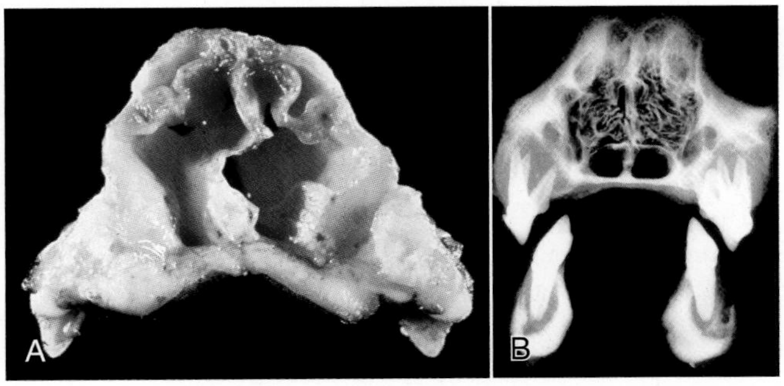

Fig. 16-54 Fibrous osteodystrophy, bone, maxillae and mandible, transverse section, dogs.

A, The pliable nature of the bone can be seen by the collapsed and folded (not fractured) appearance of the nasal septum and maxilla. **B,** Radiograph. There is marked loss of bone density around the teeth in both maxillae and mandibles. (Courtesy Dr. S.E. Weisbrode, College of Veterinary Medicine, The Ohio State University.)

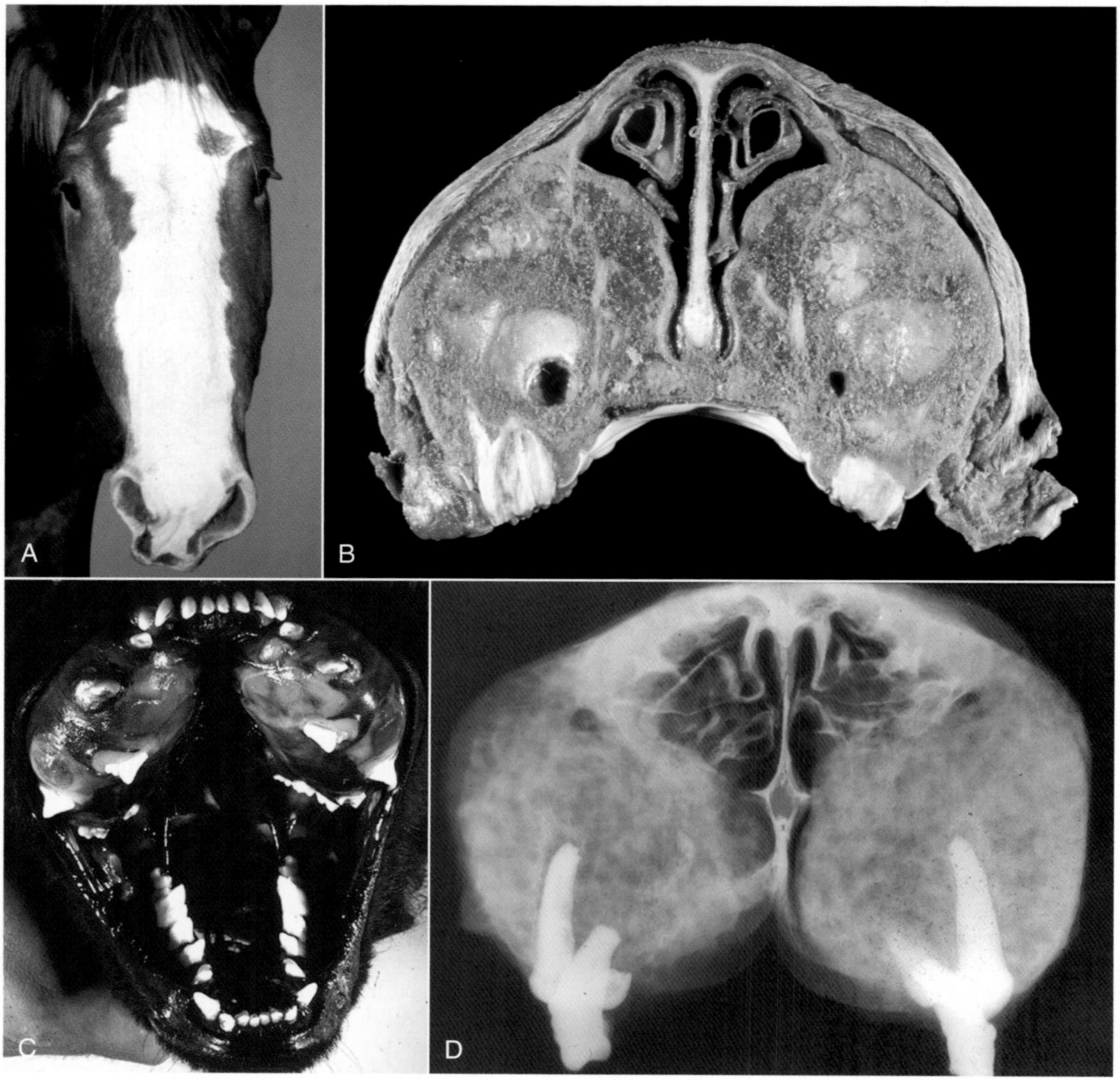

Fig. 16-55 Fibrous osteodystrophy, bone, maxillae and mandibles.
A, Nutritional fibrous osteodystrophy, horse. Note the swelling of the facial crest. **B,** Maxillae, cross-section, horse. Proliferating and poorly organized fibroosseous tissue in the maxillae has distorted and extended their contours laterally and compressed the nasal cavity medially. Note the absence of normal bone. **C,** Renal fibrous osteodystrophy, dog. Exuberant poorly mineralized woven bone and fibrous tissue has caused the maxillary bones to expand and distort the positioning of the teeth. Similar changes affect the mandible, and the teeth at this site are also malpositioned. **D,** Radiograph, renal fibrous osteodystrophy, dog. Note the reduced bone density (radiodensity) of the proliferative woven bone and fibrous tissue that has replaced the preexisting maxillary bones and the absence of normal radiodense bone. Postmortem transverse slab section. (**A** and **D** courtesy Dr. S.E. Weisbrode, College of Veterinary Medicine, The Ohio State University. **B** courtesy Dr. W. Crowell, College of Veterinary Medicine, The University of Georgia; and Noah's Arkive, College of Veterinary Medicine, The University of Georgia. **C** courtesy Department of Veterinary Biosciences, The Ohio State University; and Noah's Arkive, College of Veterinary Medicine, The University of Georgia.)

INFLAMMATION OF BONE

Infectious Inflammation of Bone

Inflammation of bone is termed *osteitis*. *Periostitis* occurs if the periosteum is involved, and *osteomyelitis* is the appropriate term if the medullary cavity of the bone is involved (Table 16-2). These conditions generally occur together and may be life threatening, requiring early diagnosis and vigorous treatment. They often involve the simultaneous necrosis and removal of bone and the compensatory production of new bone, occurring over a prolonged period. Infectious inflammation of bone in animals is usually caused by bacteria. Hematogenous bacterial osteomyelitis is uncommon in dogs and cats, but it is common in neonatal foals and animals used for food and fiber production. A wide range of Gram-positive and Gram-negative bacteria is responsible for hematogenous osteomyelitis in calves and foals. *Arcanobacterium pyogenes* and other pyogenic bacteria (e.g., *Streptococcus* spp., *Staphylococcus* spp.) and *Salmonella* spp., *Escherichia coli,* and other coliforms are among the most common microbes that cause hematogenous osteomyelitis. *Staphylococcus intermedius* is the most common cause of hematogenous osteomyelitis in dogs.

Fungi, viruses, and protozoa also can cause bony lesions. Mycotic agents, such as *Coccidioides immitis* and *Blastomyces dermatitidis,* frequently spread hematogenously to bone to produce granulomatous or pyogranulomatous osteomyelitis, with bone lysis and irregular new bone formation. The viruses of hog cholera and infectious canine hepatitis can cause endothelial damage, resulting in metaphyseal hemorrhage, necrosis, and acute inflammation.

TABLE 16-2 Lesions of Inflammatory Joint Disease

	Synovial Fluid	Synovial Membrane	Articular Cartilage
TIME/EXUDATE			
Acute suppurative	Reduced viscosity Neutrophils	Hyperemia Edema	No lesions
Subacute suppurative	Reduced viscosity Neutrophils	Hyperplasia Lymphoplasmacytic inflammation	Usually no lesions
Chronic suppurative	Reduced viscosity Neutrophils	Hyperplasia Lymphoplasmacytic inflammation Fibrosis	Erosion Ulceration
Acute fibrinous	Reduced viscosity Fibrin	Hyperemia Edema	No lesions
Subacute fibrinous	Reduced viscosity Fibrin	Hyperplasia Lymphoplasmacytic Inflammation	Usually no lesions
Chronic fibrinous	Reduced viscosity Fibrin	Hyperemia Lymphoplasmacytic Fibrin Pannus	Erosion Ulceration Pannus

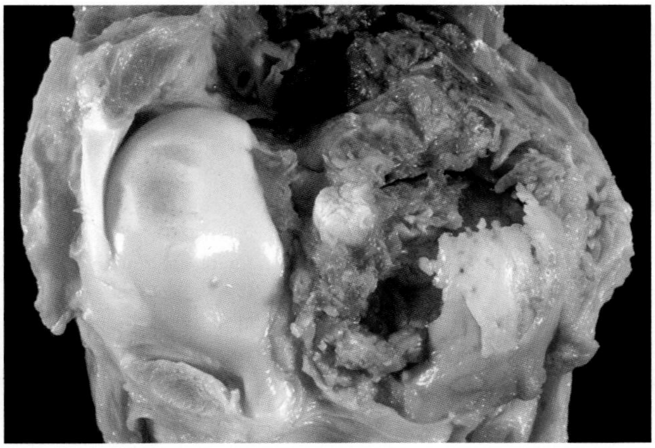

Fig. 16-56 Emboli (suppurative) epiphysitis, bone, distal femur, foal. Bacterial emboli in the articular-epiphyseal complex (AEC) have produced suppurative inflammation that has destroyed both the subchondral bone and overlying articular cartilage of the condyle *(right).* (Courtesy Dr. S.E. Weisbrode, College of Veterinary Medicine, The Ohio State University.)

Osseous localization of the distemper virus injures osteoclasts, disrupting metaphyseal modeling and producing a growth retardation lattice (described earlier), and a variant of the feline leukemia virus (FeLV) has been associated with myelosclerosis (increased density of medullary bone) in cats; however, these latter two viruses do not cause inflammation of bone.

Growth plate: Epiphyseal cartilage (Fig. 16-56) (cartilage of the epiphysis that has yet to undergo endochondral ossification) and physeal cartilage can be eroded by invasion of inflammation from adjacent bone or may undergo direct bacterial embolization via cartilage canal blood vessels or in the blind-loop vessels at sites of endochondral ossification (see the section on Portals of Entry of Bone). Growth cartilage may appear thickened secondary to osteomyelitis because of disruption of endochondral ossification by the inflammatory process and the resulting failure to replace cartilage with bone (see Fig. 16-35). In growing animals, articular cartilage can undergo lysis by extension of osteomyelitis from the subjacent AEC, a lesion that may be mistaken for primary arthritis (see Fig. 16-36).

Trabecular bone: The composition of the exudate in metaphyseal osteomyelitis is determined by the infectious agent and typically is purulent in bacterial infections in domestic animals. Exudate in the medullary cavity increases the intramedullary pressure and can cause compression of vessels resulting in thrombosis and infarction of intramedullary fat, hematopoietic marrow, and bone. In areas of inflammation, bone resorption is mediated primarily by osteoclasts that are stimulated by prostaglandins and cytokines released by local tissue and inflammatory cells. Reduced blood flow through large vessels also promotes osteoclastic bone resorption, possibly by altering electrostatic charges in bone. Proteolytic enzymes released by inflammatory cells and activation of matrix metalloproteinases by the acid environment of inflammation also assist in resorbing matrix. Lack of drainage and persistence of the offending agent in areas of necrotic bone account for the chronicity of the process, which may continue for years. Inflammation in the medullary cavity also may penetrate into and through cortical bone and undermine the periosteum, where it can further disrupt the blood supply to the bone at the nutrient foramen and nutrient canal.

Cortical bone: The lesions involving cortical bone that occur with infectious osteomyelitis may vary based on the route of entry of the organism and the nature of the exudates (Fig. 16-57). Bone lysis is expected with suppurative inflammation and is subperiosteal for bacteria induced traumatically via the periosteum and endosteal in cases of embolic osteomyelitis. Lysis within the cortex begins within existing vascular channels and can occur with either route of entry. Periostitis can develop by direct inoculation from trauma (e.g., puncture wounds) or by centripetal spread of inflammation from the marrow cavity and through the cortex. Chronic bacterial periostitis is characterized by multiple coalescing pockets of exudate and areas of irregular periosteal new bone formation and cortical lysis (Fig. 16-58). Additional sequelae of osteomyelitis include extension of inflammation to adjacent bone, hematogenous spread to other bones and to soft tissues, pathologic fractures, and development of sinus tracts that penetrate cortical bone and drain to the exterior. Occasionally, fragments of dead bone become isolated from their blood supply and surrounded by exudate (bone sequestrum). Sequestra can form when bone fragments are contaminated at the site of a compound fracture, when the fragments at a fracture site become infected hematogenously, or when fragments of necrotic bone become isolated (and thus avascular) in osteomyelitis (Fig. 16-59). These sequestra and associated exudates can become surrounded by a dense collar of reactive bone, which is termed the *involucrum.* Extracellular matrix is not living tissue; therefore it cannot be resorbed in an area in which the cells (bone or marrow) are dead. For this reason, relatively large sequestra can persist for long periods and may interfere with repair. Grossly, they often become pale and chalky and lack the glistening appearance of normal bone.

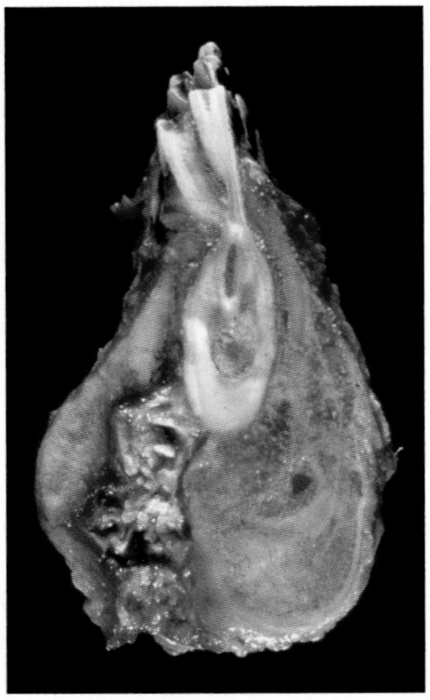

Fig. 16-57 Chronic (suppurative) osteomyelitis, bone, mandible, transverse section, sheep.
Chronic suppurative osteomyelitis has caused a fistulous tract that penetrates through the full dorsoventral thickness of the mandible. This lesion likely began as a periodontal bacterial infection. (Courtesy Dr. S.E. Weisbrode, College of Veterinary Medicine, The Ohio State University.)

Noninfectious Inflammation of Bone

Metaphyseal Osteopathy

Metaphyseal osteopathy, previously termed *hypertrophic osteodystrophy,* is a disease of young (usually 3 to 6 months of age), growing dogs of the large and giant breeds. Both names, unfortunately, are misleading, since the initial lesion is a suppurative and fibrinous osteomyelitis of the trabecular bone of the metaphysis, which is replaced in the chronic stages of the disease by the formation of abundant periosteal new bone. Remissions/exacerbations may occur over weeks to months, but most cases resolve completely. The cause and pathogenesis are unknown; infectious agents have not been isolated. There are reports of metaphyseal osteopathy in litters of Weimaraners, in which granulocytopathies have been suspected, and in littermates of Irish setters, in which canine leukocyte adhesion deficiency was confirmed. The lack of CD18 expression on the neutrophil surface in the affected Irish setters results in the failure of neutrophils to marginate or extravasate, as well as a failure of these cells to phagocytose by CD18. Affected dogs have an underlying genetic defect that is expressed clinically to various degrees, ranging from normal to the development of severe, repeated infections. Interestingly, 75% to 85% of these dogs develop metaphyseal osteopathy by 10 to 12 weeks of age, and hematopoietic stem cell transplants lead to resolution of all lesions. Based on these findings, it is possible that neutrophil entrapment at the chondro-osseous junction in the metaphysis (same location that is predisposed to the development of osteomyelitis in young animals; see section on Portals of Entry into Bone) results in autoinflammation and necrosis, with the periosteal proliferation occurring as a secondary event. Clinically, metaphyseal osteopathy is characterized by lameness, fever, and swollen, painful metaphyses in multiple long bones.

Growth plate: Lesions in the growth plate are not expected in metaphyseal osteopathy.

Trabecular bone: Lesions are usually bilaterally symmetric. Radiographically, alternating metaphyseal zones of increased lucency and increased density are present parallel to the physes (Fig. 16-60,

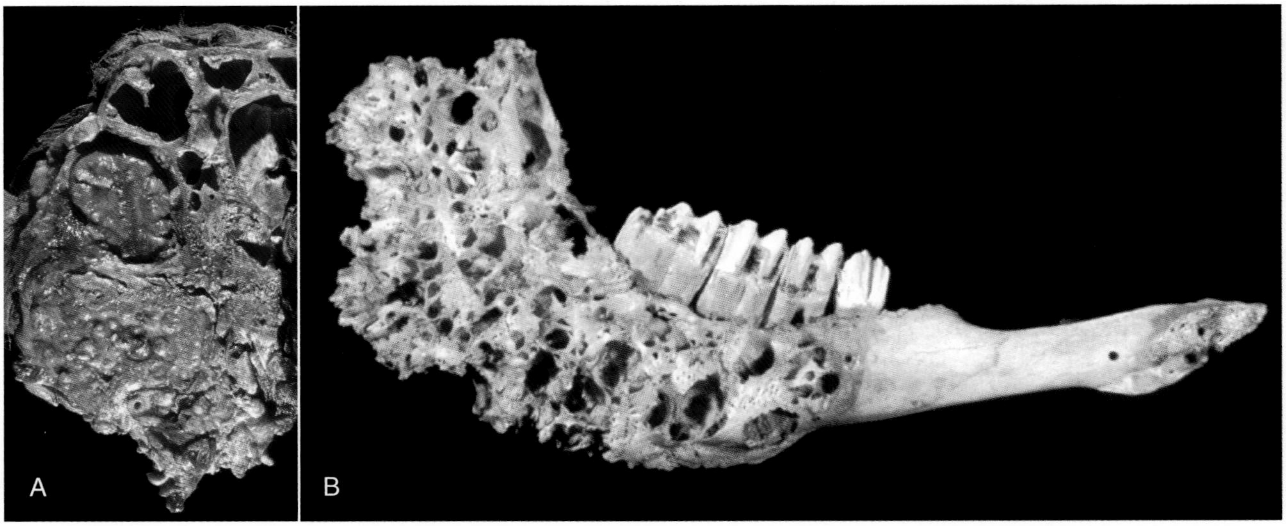

Fig. 16-58 Chronic (pyogranulomatous) osteomyelitis and sinusitis, actinomycosis *(Actinomyces bovis)*, maxillary sinus, cow.
A, Transverse section of the maxillae. The nodules apparent within the masses in the sinuses and maxilla represent pockets of pyogranulomatous inflammation that are surrounded by fibrous tissue and woven bone. **B,** Macerated and bleached specimen of the mandible. Note the spicules of woven bone radiating from the mandible. Within the spaces formed by this reactive bone were nodules of pyogranulomatous inflammation and colonies of *Actinomyces bovis.* (Courtesy Dr. S.E. Weisbrode, College of Veterinary Medicine, The Ohio State University.)

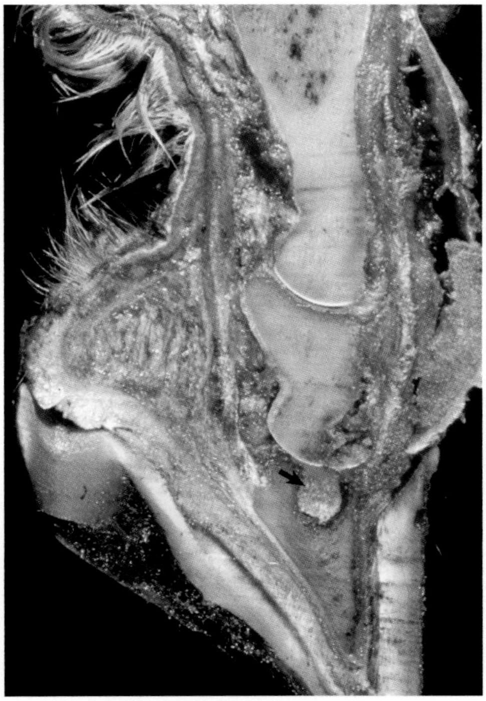

Fig. 16-59 Suppurative periostitis and osteomyelitis, phalanges, horse. Trauma to the dorsal aspect of the hoof inoculated bacteria into the subcutis, causing suppurative cellulitis and periostitis and, subsequently, cortical osteolysis of the dorsal aspect of the distal first phalanx and the entire dorsal surface of the second phalanx. From there, the infection spread to the distal interphalangeal joint and then to the third phalanx, where it caused suppurative osteomyelitis, loss of articular cartilage, and formation of a sequestrum in the proximal portion of the third phalanx *(arrow)*. The viable tissue immediately adjacent to the sequestrum is not different from that which is more distant, implying that in this case an involucrum (reactive bone surrounding the exudate around a sequestrum) was not formed. (Courtesy Dr. S.E. Weisbrode, College of Veterinary Medicine, The Ohio State University.)

A and *B*). Microscopically, the lucent areas represent suppurative and fibrinous inflammation and necrosis of the metaphyseal marrow and bone (Fig. 16-60, C). The death of osteoblasts results in primary trabeculae that are not reinforced by apposition of bone matrix. These trabeculae collapse and fracture without external distortion of the bone (infractions) and appear radiographically as relatively dense regions.

Cortical bone: The inflammation can extend from the medulla through the cutback zone into the periosteum. This periosteal inflammation, along with mechanical instability caused by the metaphyseal infractions, can cause notable new metaphyseal periosteal bone formation in chronic cases.

Eosinophilic Panosteitis

Eosinophilic panosteitis is another canine bone disease with an unfortunate name, since the lesion is neither inflammatory nor eosinophilic. The cause is unknown, and the disease is almost always self-limiting. It occurs in growing (commonly large-breed) dogs, usually at 5 to 12 months of age, and is painful. German shepherd dogs appear to be predisposed. Morphologic studies are few because the disease is easily recognized clinically and resolves spontaneously so that biopsy evaluation is rarely necessary. Radiographically, the lesions are recognized as increased densities in the medullary cavity in the diaphysis, usually beginning near the nutrient foramen. Increased densities can also be present in the periosteum. These densities are the result of proliferation of well-differentiated woven bone and fibrous tissue. No inflammation is present. The cause of the lameness is presumed to be pressure on nerves by the proliferating woven bone both within the medullary cavity and on the periosteum.

ASEPTIC NECROSIS OF BONE

Aseptic necrosis of bone in humans occurs in a variety of clinical conditions, including occlusive vascular disease (bone infarction), hyperadrenocorticism, fat embolism, nitrogenous embolism, sickle cell anemia, and intramedullary neoplasms, all of which likely result in arterial or venous infarction of the bone (Table 16-3). In domestic animals, aseptic necrosis of bone has been associated with intramedullary neoplasms and various nonneoplastic lesions, which likely result in decreased venous outflow from the bone and

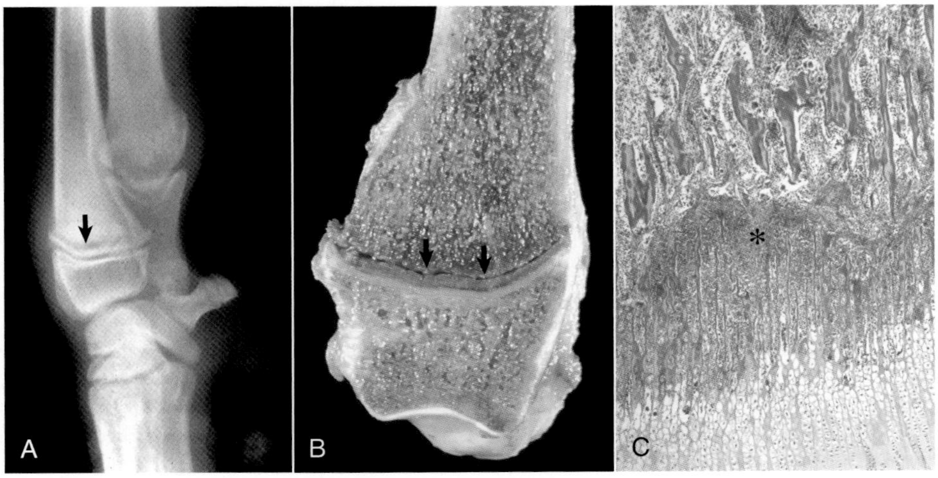

Fig. 16-60 Metaphyseal osteopathy, bone, distal radius, dog.
A, Radiograph. The radiolucent line in the metaphysis *(arrow)*, parallel with growth plate, is characteristic of metaphyseal osteopathy. **B,** Grossly, this line appears to be a fracture *(arrows)* within the metaphysis. **C,** Histologically, this line is a hypercellular band *(asterisk)* of neutrophils between the primary and secondary trabeculae. (Courtesy Dr. S.E. Weisbrode, College of Veterinary Medicine, The Ohio State University.)

TABLE 16-3 Necrosis of Bone

Cause/Duration of Necrosis	Lesion	Clinical Significance
Acute aseptic (ischemic) necrosis	Death of bone cells and marrow; bone structure intact.	Can be clinically silent.
Chronic aseptic (ischemic) necrosis	1. If no revascularization, dead bone can remain intact structurally for a long time but will accumulate microcracks. 2. If revascularization takes place, dead bone can be resorbed slowly and replaced by new bone. 3. If revascularization takes place, dead bone may be resorbed slowly and NOT be replaced by bone but by fibrous tissue.	1. Can remain clinically silent, but risk of microcrack progressing to complete clinical fracture increases with time and mechanical use. 2. Can remain clinically silent from initiation of lesion to completion of repair. 3. Can cause structural failure and collapse of the bone (e.g., chronic idiopathic necrosis of the femoral head).
Acute septic necrosis	Exudate, usually suppurative, forms at junction of dead bone and viable tissue with subsequent bone lysis and reactive bone formation.	Pain caused by cytokines from the inflammation and pressure in marrow cavity and periosteum.
Chronic septic necrosis	1. If the focus of dead bone is relatively small, it can be completely resorbed by the inflammatory process and osteoclastic bone lysis; there can be marked modeling of bone, usually with resorption predominating and replacement by fibrous tissue; in some cases excess formation can occur. 2. If the focus of dead bone is relatively large, it can be sequestered (sequestrum) by a peripheral wall of reactive fibrous tissue or reactive bone (involucrum).	Pain caused by cytokines and pressure in marrow cavity and periosteum; draining tracts can form; strength of the bone can be weakened because of resorption or its function can be affected by exuberant new bone formation.

increased bone marrow pressure. Although the long-term use of steroids in humans has been associated with necrosis of the femoral head in adults, steroids do not appear to induce osteonecrosis in domestic animals.

The gross appearance of necrotic bone varies with the extent of the affected area and the response of the body to it. Microscopically, the hallmark of bone necrosis is cell death and loss of osteocytes from their lacunae.

After an episode of ischemia leading to infarction, the cellular elements of the marrow lose their differential staining, and circular spaces (pooled lipid) develop within a few days. If the region of dead bone remains avascular, the coagulated tissue and mineralized matrix can persist for some time. Dead osteocytes elicit little reaction; their nuclei become pyknotic, but their disappearance from lacunae is slow and might not be complete for 2 to 4 weeks.

Reaction to and repair of necrotic bone requires revascularization that is associated with infiltration of macrophages and invasion by fibrous tissue that advances from the margins of the lesion. The bone marrow might eventually regenerate entirely, or a scar might form and remain. The necrotic matrix remains fully mineralized and might even "hypermineralize" because of calcification of the dead osteocytes and their lacunae. This mineralization is only possible if there is vascularization that brings additional calcium to the region. Dead bone is slowly removed by osteoclasts. The resorption of necrotic bone with simultaneous replacement by new bone is termed *creeping substitution.* The process is slow and often incomplete. Small areas of bone necrosis might not be detected clinically or radiographically.

Growth plate: Ischemic necrosis of metaphyseal bone and bone marrow can result in retained growth cartilage. The metaphyseal necrosis would not directly affect the zones of proliferating and hypertrophying chondrocytes; however, the physeal thickness would increase because the conversion of epiphyseal cartilage to bone by endochondral ossification at the chondro-osseous junction would be impaired. Ischemic necrosis of the epiphysis could result in premature closure of the growth plate because of the death of the proliferating chondrocytes, which depend on the epiphyseal blood vessels. Endochondral ossification would continue normally if the metaphyseal blood supply was not affected, and the plate would close because of failure to generate new proliferating zone chondrocytes.

Trabecular bone: In the femoral heads of young, small, and miniature breed dogs, aseptic necrosis of the femoral head is associated with clinical signs because of the collapse of the articular cartilage as a result of resorption of the necrotic subchondral bone (Legg-Calvé-Perthes disease) that occurs late in the course of the disease. Apparently the initial infarction is asymptomatic (Fig. 16-61). The cause of the infarction is usually not determined but might be caused by venous compression or increased pressure within the articular cavity. This pressure can result in increased intraosseous pressure and bone necrosis. In clinical cases of aseptic necrosis, the dead bone is not replaced by creeping substitution but is ultimately resorbed and replaced by fibrous tissue. The fibrous tissue does not provide adequate support for the articular cartilage, and the femoral head collapses. In stages preceding complete resorption, it is common, in revascularized necrotic medullary bone, for reactive new bone to be deposited on trabeculae of necrotic bone (Fig. 16-62). This sandwich of central dead bone covered by viable reactive woven bone can persist for months and may give (along with osteocyte mineralization described previously) the affected region a radiodense appearance. Ultimately, in clinical cases of aseptic necrosis of the femoral head, even these foci of new bone formed over dead bone are resorbed and replaced by fibrous tissue.

Cortical bone: Large areas of necrotic cortical bone have a dry, chalky gross appearance and the periosteum can be removed easily. These areas can remain as a subclinical lesion for years. The formation of sequestra almost always requires inflammation; sequestra formation after sterile necrosis of bone is unlikely.

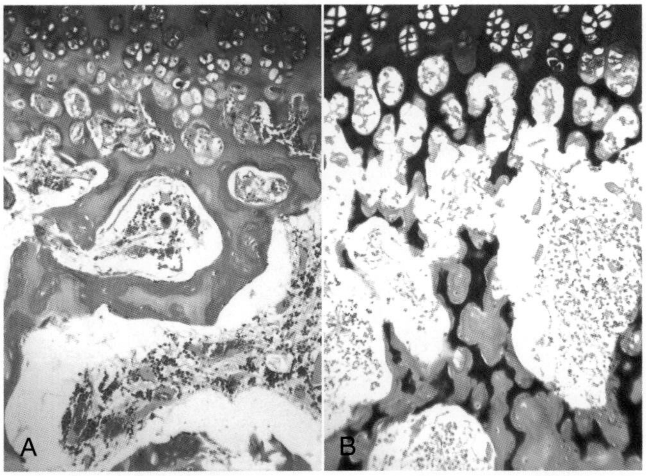

Fig. 16-61 Femoral head, necrosis (experimental), bone, femur, pig. Necrosis was produced experimentally by a ligature placed around the femoral neck. Several days after the procedure, the only difference between the control **(A)** and the infarcted bones **(B)** is the coagulation necrosis of the marrow and bone cells. The hard tissue of the cartilage and bone remains unaffected. H&E stain. (Courtesy Dr. S.E. Weisbrode, College of Veterinary Medicine, The Ohio State University.)

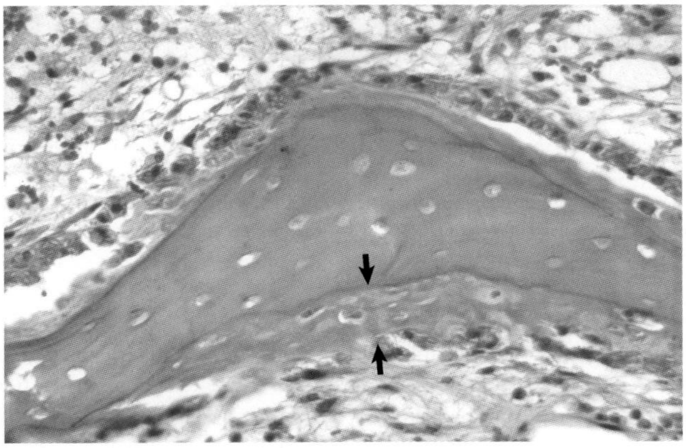

Fig. 16-62 Revascularization, ischemic necrosis (experimentally induced), 1-month duration, femoral head, epiphyseal (cancellous) bone, pig.
Reactive woven bone *(between arrows)* has been deposited on the surface of the necrotic bone, which contains empty lacunae and karyolytic nuclei. Fibrovascular repair tissue in the marrow surrounds the bone. H&E stain. (Courtesy Dr. S.E. Weisbrode, College of Veterinary Medicine, The Ohio State University.)

PROLIFERATIVE AND NEOPLASTIC LESIONS

Surprisingly, bone, as a tissue, offers little resistance to an expanding or invading neoplasm, and many skeletal neoplasms are accompanied by bone resorption as well as new bone formation (Fig. 16-63). Pain, hypercalcemia, increased serum alkaline phosphatase activity, pathologic fracture, and distant metastases are other possible manifestations of a skeletal neoplasm. New bone formation occurs, at least in part, in response to mechanical stress on a weakened cortex and is prominent in neoplasms that have a marked fibrous stroma. Neoplasms with little stroma, such as plasma cell myeloma and lymphosarcoma, have minimal reactive bone formation, even though bone may be destroyed by marked bone lysis. Tumor-associated bone destruction is largely accomplished by osteoclasts, but prostaglandins, cytokines, acid metabolic by-products, and lytic enzymes released by inflammatory or neoplastic cells can also be responsible for local bone resorption and formation. Hypercalcemia, a result in part of bone resorption induced by release of bone-resorbing factors from extraskeletal neoplasms, is well documented and is termed *humoral hypercalcemia* of malignancy. The best-known examples in animals occur in dogs secondary to adenocarcinoma of the apocrine glands of the anal sac and T lymphocyte lymphoma, in which the neoplastic cells produce PTH-related protein.

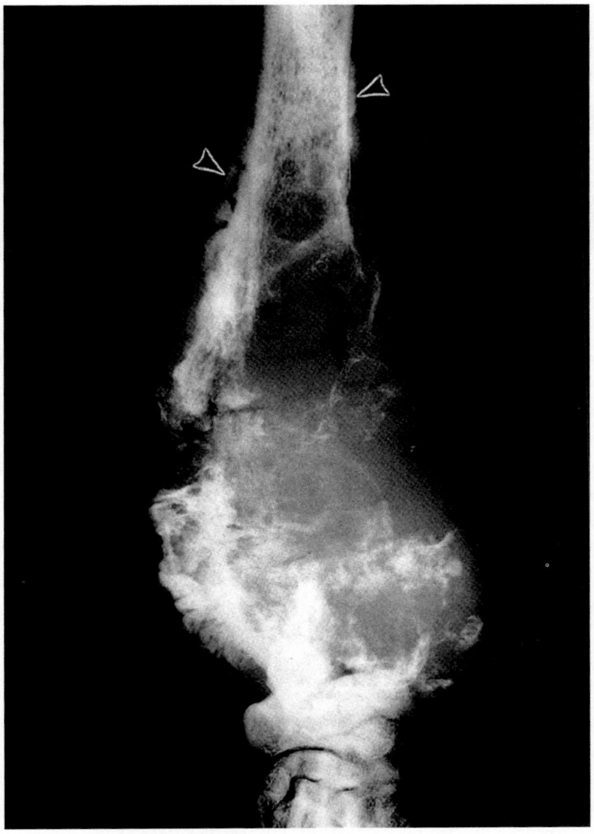

Fig. 16-63 Osteosarcoma, bone, distal radius, dog.
Radiograph of osteosarcoma with extensive destruction of preexisting bone; small areas of new bone formation on the periosteal surface *(arrowheads)*. (Courtesy Dr. S.E. Weisbrode, College of Veterinary Medicine, The Ohio State University.)

NONNEOPLASTIC PROLIFERATIVE AND CYSTIC LESIONS

The nonneoplastic proliferative and cystic lesions considered here vary widely in their cause, structure, and ultimate effect on the host. Reactive bone formation, sometimes exuberant, can occur in fracture repair, chronic osteomyelitis, and degenerative joint disease in the form of periarticular osteophytes. An exostosis is a nodular, benign, bony growth projecting outward from the surface of a bone. An osteophyte is a similar growth that occurs at the margins of a diarthrodial (movable) joint. An enthesophyte is the calcification of a tendon or ligament at the point of its insertion into the bone. In addition to bone, these proliferations may include variable amounts of cartilage. The bone component can be woven and/or lamellar, depending on rate of growth and duration of lesion. Hyperostosis usually is used to indicate that the diameter of the bone has increased and implies more uniform thickening on the periosteal surface rather than the nodular appearance of an osteophyte or exostosis. An enostosis is a bony growth within the

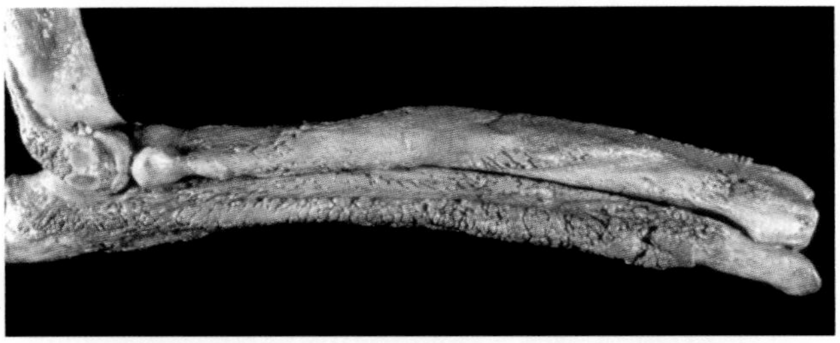

Fig. 16-64 Hypertrophic osteopathy, bone, radius and ulna, dog. Marked periosteal proliferation of woven bone has resulted in the surfaces of both bones, but particularly the ulna, being irregularly roughened/thickened. Macerated and bleached specimen. (Courtesy Dr. S.E. Weisbrode, College of Veterinary Medicine, The Ohio State University.)

medullary cavity, usually originating from the cortical-endosteal surface, and can result in obliteration of the medullary cavity. These lesions are nonneoplastic proliferative lesions in which growth is seldom continuous. Some exostoses can remodel (e.g., an osteophyte may become indistinguishable from the preexisting bone over time, and its presence is only recognizable by a change in shape of the affected area) and some regress. Nonneoplastic proliferative lesions can be mistaken for skeletal neoplasia, particularly in small biopsy specimens. Conversely, a malignancy may be missed when small superficial biopsies contain only nonneoplastic reactive bone that is present adjacent to the tumor. These statements serve to highlight the problem of making a morphologic diagnosis from a small biopsy specimen, without the benefit of a clinical history, radiographic findings, and other laboratory data. One must also remember that more than one process might be active at any one site (e.g., osteosarcoma might be complicated by fracture repair or by osteomyelitis).

Hypertrophic Osteopathy (Hypertrophic Pulmonary Osteopathy)

Hypertrophic osteopathy (hypertrophic pulmonary osteopathy) occurs in humans and domestic animals; dogs are the most commonly affected species. The disease is characterized by progressive, bilateral, periosteal, new bone formation in the diaphyseal regions, particularly of the distal limbs, that occurs as a secondary reaction to a primary lesion (Fig. 16-64). The word "pulmonary" is sometimes included because most cases occur in association with intrathoracic neoplasms or inflammation. Other, less commonly associated lesions or agents include endocarditis, heartworms, rhabdomyosarcoma of the urinary bladder in young giant-breed dogs, and ovarian neoplasms in the horse. Although the association between the pulmonary lesions and the proliferation of new periosteal bone on the extremities is not clear, it has been postulated that pulmonary lesions lead to reflex vasomotor changes (mediated by the vagus nerve) and to increased blood flow to the extremities. Evidence to support this theory includes the observation that the bony lesions regress after the primary lesion is removed, as well as after vagotomy. In addition, lesions similar to hypertrophic osteopathy can be reproduced in dogs by creating shunts that allow blood to bypass the pulmonary circulation, thereby increasing the stroke volume of the left side of the heart, leading to increased blood flow to peripheral tissues. Increased arterial pressure, hyperemia, and edema of the periosteum lead to thickening first by fibrous tissue and later by new bone formation. Similar periosteal woven bone deposition can occur in the metaphysis, but in hypertrophic osteopathy (as opposed to metaphyseal osteopathy) the lesions are usually less severe and less frequent in the metaphysis than in the diaphysis.

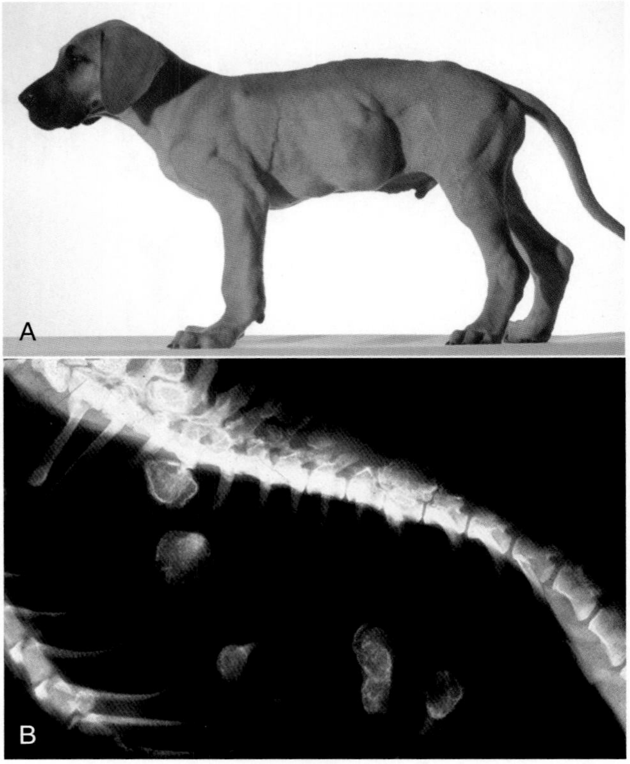

Fig. 16-65 Osteochondromas, young dog.
A, Multiple osteochondromas (cartilaginous exostoses) are present as single and coalescing masses on the ribs. **B,** Radiograph. The cartilaginous exostoses have the density of bone and appear in this case as exophytic nodules on the ribs and the dorsal spinous processes of the vertebrae. (Courtesy Dr. S.E. Weisbrode, College of Veterinary Medicine, The Ohio State University.)

Osteochondromas

Osteochondromas (multiple cartilaginous exostoses) reflect a defect in skeletal development (lesions appear shortly after birth) rather than being true neoplasms and are confirmed to have a hereditary etiology in humans and horses. A hereditary basis has been suggested in dogs as well. Osteochondromas project from bony surfaces as eccentric masses that are located adjacent to physes. They arise from long bones, ribs, vertebrae, scapulas, and bones of the pelvis, and they may be numerous (Figs. 16-65 and 16-66). Microscopically, they have an outer cap of hyaline cartilage that undergoes orderly endochondral ossification to give rise to trabecular bone that forms the base of the lesion (Fig. 16-66, *C*). The medullary cavity of the osteochondroma usually communicates with the medullary cavity of the underlying bone because the cortex of the underlying bone at this site has not completely developed. Normally, growth ceases at skeletal maturity when the cartilage cap is replaced by bone. Although the origin of osteochondromas is not clear, some arise secondary to a defect in the perichondral ring as peripheral areas of physeal cartilage that are separated and removed from the growth plate during longitudinal growth. Clinically, their importance is threefold: they might interfere mechanically with the action of tendons or ligaments; they can act as space-occupying masses that protrude into the vertebral canal and cause spinal cord compression; and they can undergo malignant transformation and give rise to chondrosarcomas. Osteochondromas in cats are different in that they develop in mature animals, less commonly affect long bones, do not have orderly endochondral ossification, and might be of viral origin; however, like those in horses and

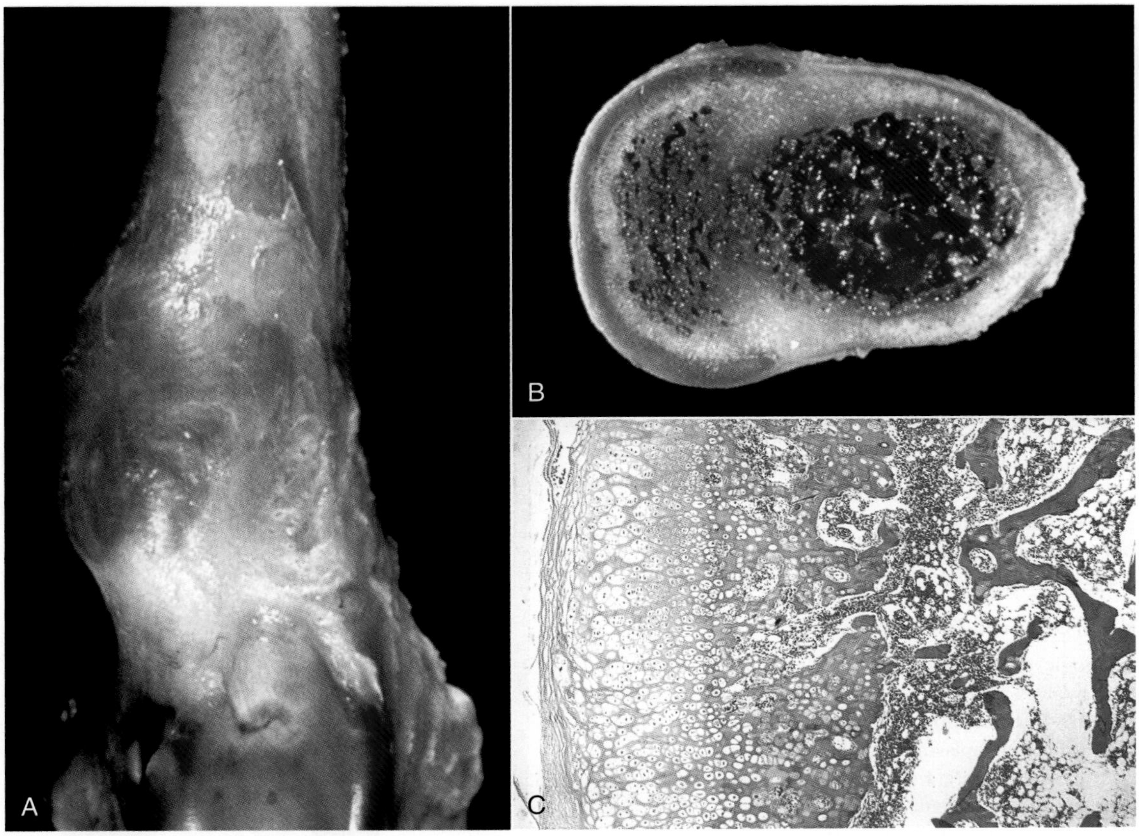

Fig. 16-66 Osteochondroma (cartilaginous exostosis), bone, distal femoral metaphysis, dog. **A,** A plateaulike mass *(left)* protrudes from the metaphyseal cortex. **B,** On cross-section, the mass *(left)* has a cartilage cap. **C,** Histologically, the cartilage cap is undergoing endochondral ossification, similar to that which occurs in an articular-epiphyseal complex. H&E stain. (Courtesy Dr. S.E. Weisbrode, College of Veterinary Medicine, The Ohio State University.)

dogs, osteochondromas in cats may undergo malignant neoplastic transformation. The term *osteochondroma* is not recommended for cartilaginous osteophytes that have undergone central endochondral ossification. As will be discussed regarding callus formation in the section on Fracture Repair, the osteogenic tissue (cambium layer) of the periosteum can form hyaline cartilage instead of bone when the oxygen tension of the tissue is low.

Fibrous Dysplasia

Fibrous dysplasia is an uncommon focal to multifocal, lytic, intraosseous lesion that has been found at various sites (skull, mandible, and long bones) in young animals and may be a developmental defect. Typically, preexisting bone is replaced by an expanding mass of fibro-osseous tissue that can weaken the cortex and enlarge the external contour of the bone. The lesion is firm, often contains mineralized areas, and may contain multiple cysts filled with sanguinous fluid. Microscopically, the lesion is composed of well-differentiated fibrous tissue containing trabeculae of woven bone that are relatively regularly spaced and sized. Osteoblasts are not recognizable on trabecular surfaces, which is a feature that helps to distinguish this lesion from ossifying fibroma.

Bone Cysts

Bone cysts are classified as subchondral, simple, or aneurysmal. Radiographically, all appear as well-demarcated lucent areas without evidence of aggressive growth. Subchondral cysts are sequelae to osteochondrosis and degenerative joint disease. Subchondral bone cysts caused by osteochondrosis represent failure of endochondral ossification with subsequent necrosis and cavitation of retained growth cartilage and are most common in the medial femoral condyle in young horses (1 to 3 years of age). Although less commonly, these lesions also may occur in older horses. Subchondral cysts secondary to degenerative joint disease represent herniation of synovial fluid into the subchondral bone through fissures in degenerated articular cartilage. These herniations become lined by a synovial–like membrane, and the lysis of bone occurs by osteoclasis, secondary either to pressure or to cytokines released from the expanding cyst. Trauma to intact articular cartilage also is proposed as an etiology because cystic lesions have been reproduced experimentally by lacerating the articular cartilage to the level of the subchondral bone.

Simple bone cysts can contain clear, colorless, serum-like fluid or serosanguineous fluid. The wall of the cyst is composed of variably dense fibrous tissue and woven to lamellar bone. The bone located peripheral to the cyst undergoes modeling to accommodate the expansile growth of the cyst. Simple bone cysts may be difficult to distinguish from fibrous dysplasias, depending on the biopsy sample and radiographic and clinical information that is available.

Aneurysmal bone cysts contain spaces, filled with blood or serosanguineous fluid, that are not usually lined by endothelium. Tissue adjacent to the spaces can vary from well-differentiated fibrous or fibro-osseous tissue to pronounced proliferation of undifferentiated mesenchymal cells admixed with osteoclast-like multinucleated giant cells. Hemorrhage and hemosiderosis are frequent. The

TABLE 16-4 Primary Skeletal Neoplasms of the Dog

Name	Cell of Origin	Incidence	Primary Site	Biologic Behavior
Osteoma	Osteoblast	Rare	Flat bones	Benign
Osteosarcoma	Osteoblast	Common	Predominantly metaphyses of larger appendicular bones	Highly malignant with metastases early in clinical course
Chondroma	Chondroblast/chondrocyte	Rare	Flat bones	Benign
Chondrosarcoma	Chondroblast/chondrocyte	Relatively rare	Ribs, sternum, nasal cavity	Metastases not common and late in clinical course
Fibroma	Fibroblast			Not commonly recognized as a primary tumor of bone
Fibrosarcoma	Fibroblast	Relatively rare	Diaphysis of bones of appendicular skeleton	Metastasizes relatively late in clinical course

cause of simple and aneurysmal bone cysts is unknown; however, they could be consequences of ischemic necrosis, hemorrhage, or congenital or acquired vascular malformations. Caution should be exercised in the interpretation of microscopic lesions in biopsy specimens of cysts, and these lesions should be correlated with the radiographic appearance to rule out cystic cavitation in a neoplasm.

PRIMARY NEOPLASMS OF BONE

The histopathologic diagnosis of skeletal neoplasia in domestic animals often involves evaluation of needle, trephine, or wedge biopsies (Table 16-4). Bone biopsy samples usually are small relative to the size of the neoplasm, and the most easily accessible tissue often is reactive periosteal tissue that is located exterior to the neoplasm, therefore it is important that the pathologist incorporate the radiographic and clinical findings in the interpretation of the sample. Cases in which there are radiographically aggressive lesions that have an effect on bone mass are usually associated with malignancy or inflammation; therefore, if the microscopic findings from these cases indicate the presence of a benign lesion and/or provide no explanation for the radiographic changes, it may be necessary to examine additional tissue to reconcile these differences.

Ossifying fibromas are uncommon masses in the maxillae and mandibles of horses and cattle. In their early stages, these are intramedullary neoplasms; however, although considered benign, they destroy adjacent cortical and trabecular bone by expansile growth. Microscopically, they are composed of well-differentiated fibrous tissue with scattered spicules of woven bone covered by osteoblasts.

Fibrosarcomas are malignancies of fibroblasts that produce collagenous connective tissue but not bone or cartilage. Microscopically the matrix of fibrosarcomas should not mineralize or entrap cells in lacunae as occurs in normal and neoplastic bone and cartilage, and the cells may be arranged in a whirling or interlacing pattern. Central fibrosarcomas arise from fibrous tissue within the medullary cavity, whereas periosteal fibrosarcomas arise from periosteal connective tissue. Central fibrosarcomas must be distinguished grossly and microscopically from osteosarcoma. In general, central fibrosarcomas grow more slowly, are accompanied by less formation of reactive new bone, are slower to metastasize, and produce a smaller tissue mass than osteosarcomas. Grossly, fibrosarcomas are gray-white, fill part of the medullary cavity, and replace cancellous and cortical bone.

Chondromas are benign neoplasms of hyaline cartilage. They are very rare neoplasms of dogs, cats, and sheep and often arise from flat bones; those arising in the medullary cavity are termed *enchondromas.* Cartilaginous neoplasms in the skeleton do not arise from articular cartilage, most likely because of its low mitotic potential and avascularity. Because they usually occur in adult animals, which do not possess growth cartilage, the cell of origin is presumed to be

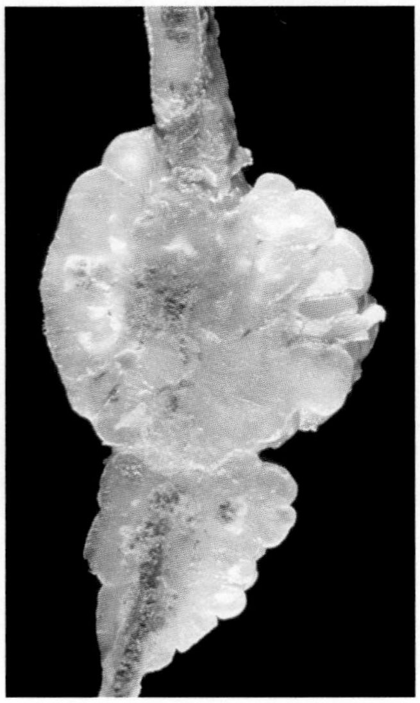

Fig. 16-67 Chondrosarcoma, bone, rib, cat.
A chondrosarcoma arising in a rib has destroyed and replaced the normal bone structure. (Courtesy Dr. S.E. Weisbrode, College of Veterinary Medicine, The Ohio State University.)

a stromal cell with chondrogenic potential. Chondromas are multilobulated and have a blue-white appearance on cut surface. They tend to enlarge slowly, but progressively, and can cause thinning of underlying bone. Microscopically, they are composed of multiple lobules of well-differentiated hyaline cartilage that may include areas of endochondral ossification. Chondromas may be very difficult to distinguish from low-grade, well-differentiated chondrosarcomas; distinguishing between these two tumor types may require clinical information. Chondrosarcomas are malignant neoplasms in which the neoplastic cells produce cartilaginous matrix but not osteoid or bone. Chondrosarcomas arise most frequently in the flat bones of the skeleton and occur most commonly in mature, large-breed dogs and in sheep (Figs. 16-67 and 16-68). In dogs, the major sites of origin are the nasal bones, ribs, and pelvis; in sheep, they arise from the ribs and sternum. Most chondrosarcomas arise in the medullary cavity and destroy preexisting bone. Given time, they become large, lobulated neoplasms with a gray or blue-white cut surface. Grossly, some neoplasms are gelatinous, and some contain large areas of hemorrhage and necrosis. Microscopically (Fig. 16-69), the range of differentiation of neoplastic cells is wide: Some neoplasms are well differentiated, lack mitotic figures, and are difficult to distinguish from chondroma (grade I

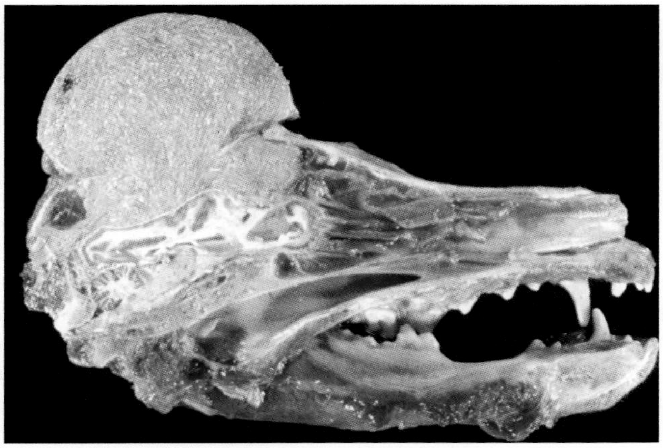

Fig. 16-68 Chondrosarcoma, bone, calvarium, dog.
A chondrosarcoma protrudes from the skull, compresses the underlying brain, and has invaded the frontal sinus. The widespread white foci within the mass represent areas of mineralization. (Courtesy Dr. K. Read, College of Veterinary Medicine, Texas A&M University; and Noah's Arkive, College of Veterinary Medicine, The University of Georgia.)

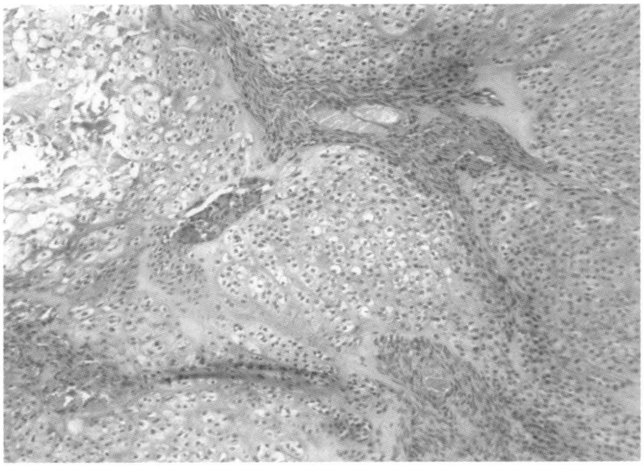

Fig. 16-69 Chondrosarcoma, bone, dog.
Chondrocyte lacunae are prominent in well-differentiated regions *(left)* but are less apparent in the more poorly-differentiated regions *(lower right).* (Courtesy Dr. S.E. Weisbrode, College of Veterinary Medicine, The Ohio State University.)

chondrosarcomas). Grade II chondrosarcomas are composed of pleomorphic chondrocytes, contain low-to-moderate numbers of mitotic figures, and contain no undifferentiated areas. Grade III chondrosarcomas exhibit marked nuclear pleomorphisms, numerous mitotic figures, and contain areas of undifferentiated sarcoma. Some chondrosarcomas are composed primarily of primitive mesenchyma tissue and contain abundant basophilic interstitial mucin and rare foci of chondroid differentiation (mesenchymal chondrosarcoma). Nonneoplastic bone can be present as the result of endochondral ossification of the malignant cartilage; however, the presence of malignant osteoblasts in close association with foci/areas of osteoid supports a diagnosis of osteosarcoma, even in tumors in which the majority of the tissue present is cartilaginous. Chondrosarcomas have a longer clinical course, grow more slowly, and develop metastases later than osteosarcomas. Metastases are usually pulmonary via the venous system, without metastasis to the regional or bronchial lymph nodes. Osteomas are uncommon

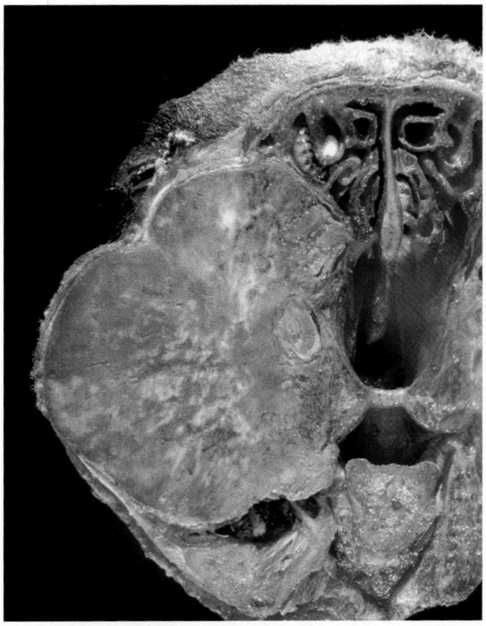

Fig. 16-70 Osteoma, bone, maxilla and maxillary sinus, sheep.
The osteoma has proliferated and formed a dome-shaped mass above the normal contour of the maxilla and has compressed the maxillary sinus. Grossly, this mass was diffusely hard; histologically, it was composed of closely spaced trabeculae lined by well-differentiated osteoblasts. An *Oestrus ovis* larva is present in the nasal cavity. (Courtesy Dr. S.E. Weisbrode, College of Veterinary Medicine, The Ohio State University.)

benign neoplasms that usually arise from bones of the head as a single, dense mass that projects from the surface of the bone (Fig. 16-70). They do not invade or destroy adjacent bone; their growth is slow and progressive but not necessarily continuous. Microscopically, osteomas are covered by periosteum and are composed of cancellous bone; trabeculae are lined by well-differentiated osteoblasts and osteoclasts. The intertrabecular spaces contain delicate fibrous tissue, adipocytes, and hemopoietic tissue.

Osteosarcomas are malignant neoplasms in which neoplastic cells form bone, osteoid, or both. These tumors are common neoplasms in dogs and cats, in which they comprise approximately 80% and 50%, respectively, of all the primary bone neoplasms; however, they are rare in other domestic animals. Osteosarcomas typically occur in mature dogs of the large and giant breeds and arise most commonly in the metaphyses. The distal radius, distal tibia, and proximal humerus are the usual sites (Fig. 16-71); however, osteosarcomas can occur in ribs, vertebrae, bones of the head, and various other parts of the skeleton (Fig. 16-72). Rarely, they arise in soft tissue (extraskeletal osteosarcoma). Growth of the neoplasm is often rapid, aggressively locally invasive, and painful. Except for those arising in the axial skeleton and in particular, the head, early hematogenous pulmonary metastasis is common. Metastasis also may be widespread, involving soft tissues, as well as other bones.

Osteosarcomas can be classified as simple (bone formed in a collagenous matrix), compound (both bone and cartilage are present) or pleomorphic (anaplastic, with only small islands of osteoid present). Classification has also been based on cell type and activity (osteoblastic, chondroblastic, or fibroblastic), radiographic appearance (lytic, sclerotic, or mixed), or site of origin (central/intraosseous, juxtacortical, or periosteal). An uncommon form of osteosarcoma is the telangiectatic type that grossly resembles hemangiosarcoma and is composed of osteoblasts, osteoid, and large cystic, blood-filled cavities lined by malignant osteoblasts. Because there may be a great deal of heterogeneity within an individual tumor, classifying osteosarcomas may be difficult and is not recommended when the diagnosis is based solely on a small biopsy sample.

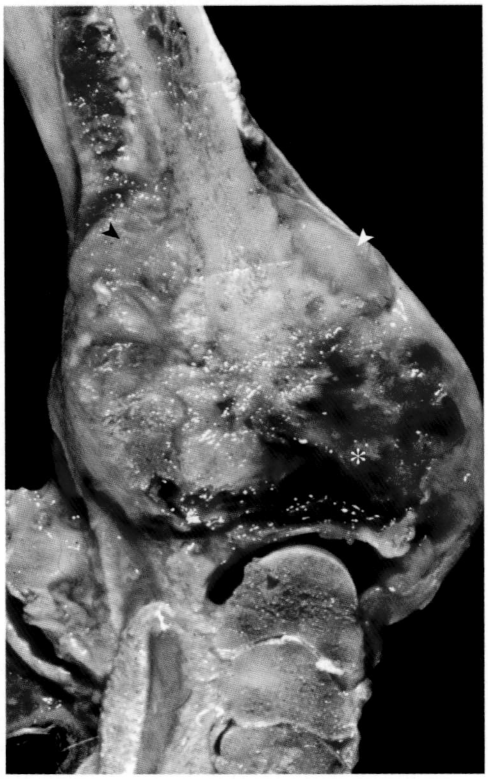

Fig. 16-71 Osteosarcoma, bone, distal radius, dog.
Osteosarcoma has lysed and replaced normal bone. There is reactive periosteal new bone formation *(arrowheads)* and a large area of hemorrhage and necrosis *(asterisk)*. (Courtesy Department of Veterinary Biosciences, The Ohio State University; and Noah's Arkive, College of Veterinary Medicine, The University of Georgia.)

Central (intraosseous) osteosarcomas have a gray-white gross appearance and contain variable amounts of mineralized bone. Large, pale areas surrounded by zones of hemorrhage (areas of infarction) and irregular, randomly located areas of hemorrhage are common in rapidly growing intramedullary neoplasms. Neoplastic tissue tends to fill the medullary cavity locally and can extend proximally and distally but typically does not penetrate articular cartilage and therefore does not invade the joint space. Cortical bone is usually destroyed, and neoplastic cells penetrate and undermine the periosteum and can extend outwardly as an irregular lobulated mass. Destruction of cortical bone is accompanied by varying amounts of reactive (nonneoplastic) periosteal bone, which may be differentiated from tumor bone microscopically by its regular appearance and well-differentiated lining osteoblasts. Variable amounts of woven bone or osteoid are produced by the neoplastic osteoblasts; in fact, bone/osteoid production by the tumor cells is the hallmark lesion of this neoplasm (Fig. 16-73). Bone formation by the malignant cells can be abundant and widespread, or it can be minimal, as in anaplastic or fibroblastic osteosarcomas that are composed of sheets of poorly differentiated mesenchymal cells or fibroblastic tissue.

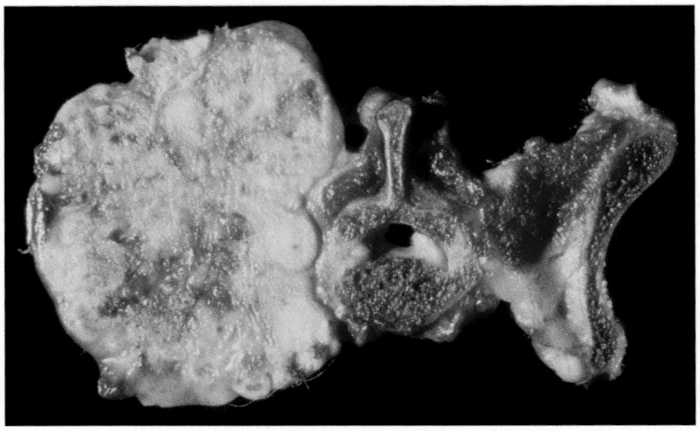

Fig. 16-72 Osteosarcoma, bone, wing of ilium, dog.
Although the mass appears to be growing primarily by expansion into the adjacent soft tissues, there is evidence of invasion and lysis of the underlying ilium and focal invasion of the lumbar vertebra. (Courtesy Dr. S.E. Weisbrode, College of Veterinary Medicine, The Ohio State University.)

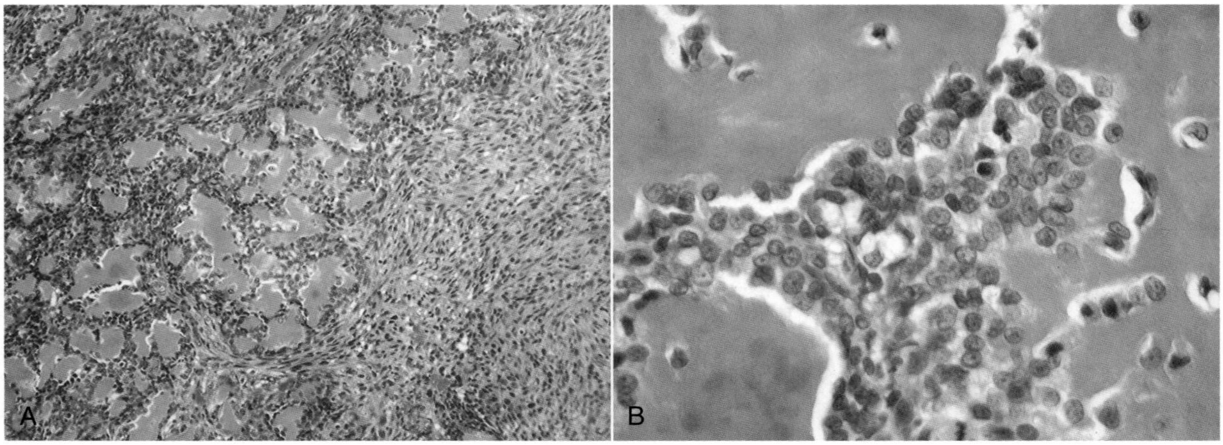

Fig. 16-73 Osteosarcoma, bone, dog.
A, Islands of eosinophilic osteoid are being produced by sheets of malignant osteoblasts. **B,** At higher magnification, malignant osteoblasts surround and invest (malignant osteocyte formation) the osteoid. Mineralization is not apparent in this decalcified section. H&E stain. (Courtesy Dr. J. Sagartz, College of Veterinary Medicine, The Ohio State University; and Noah's Arkive, College of Veterinary Medicine, The University of Georgia.)

Periosteal osteosarcomas also have an aggressive behavior and invade into the medullary cavity from the periphery. As with central or intraosseous osteosarcomas, periosteal osteosarcomas cause bone lysis and reactive bone formation in addition to production of neoplastic bone. At the time of presentation, it is often impossible to determine if the osteosarcoma originated from the periosteum or the medullary cavity. Rarely, osteosarcomas are also juxtacortical (parosteal) in origin. These neoplasms arise within the periosteum and form an expansive mass that adheres to and surrounds but does not invade the underlying cortex. Invasion of the shaft and metastasis can occur with parosteal osteosarcomas but is a late event; therefore early en bloc excision might effect a cure. Although parosteal osteosarcomas are very rare, it is important to distinguish them from periosteal osteosarcomas because of their more favorable prognosis.

Multiple skeletal osteosarcomas occur in humans and dogs, and these may represent a primary neoplasm that has metastasized to bone or may have a multicentric origin. The lesions have a random distribution, and pulmonary metastases are likely to be present. Although the cause of naturally occurring osteosarcomas is largely unknown, in both humans and domestic animals, it is known that osteosarcomas can develop in association with or subsequent to other conditions at the same bony site, including infarction, fracture, and the presence of metallic fixation devices. Osteosarcomas of viral origin are reported in mice.

A unique form of skeletal malignancy occurs in the skull of the dog and is awkwardly called a *multilobular tumor of bone* (referred to as *chondroma rodens* in the older literature). These tumors are single, nodular, smooth-contoured, immovable masses on the flat bones of the skull (bones of membranous origin) and the hard palate. Neoplastic tissue is firm and the cut surface is composed of multiple, gray, partially mineralized lobules separated by fibrous tissue. These neoplasms are slow growing and locally invasive and may compress and invade the brain. They metastasize to the lungs late in the clinical course; however, the metastases are frequently small and clinically silent. Histologically, these tumors consist of multiple lobules, each having centrally located cartilage or bone, that are surrounded by plump mesenchymal cells that blend into well-differentiated interlobular fibrous tissue.

Various other neoplasms, such as liposarcomas, giant cell tumors, and hemangiosarcomas, can arise in bone, and neoplasms, such as lymphosarcomas and plasma cell myeloma, can involve the bone marrow and surrounding bone. Most cases of tumor metastases to bone involve carcinomas, with the most common primary sites being mammary gland, liver, lung, and prostate gland.

SECONDARY NEOPLASMS OF BONE

At autopsy, 60% of human cancer patients have skeletal metastases. These metastases are predominantly in red bone marrow, in which the vascular sinusoidal system is apparently predisposed to trap circulating malignant cells. The true incidence of skeletal metastasis in animals is unknown and estimates might be artificially low because early euthanasia shortens the course of the disease and because bone scanning and other types of clinical imaging techniques are done less often than in humans. Metastatic neoplasms in bone can be associated with pain, hypercalcemia, lysis of bone, pathologic fracture, and reactive new bone formation. Rib shafts, vertebral bodies, and humeral and femoral metaphyses (proximal appendicular skeleton) are common sites of metastatic neoplasms in dogs, and these most commonly involve carcinomas. The most common primary sites are the same as those in humans (mammary gland, liver, lung, and prostate gland). In cats, skeletal metastases are rare but, when present, appear to involve the distal appendicular skeleton. Clinically silent pulmonary carcinomas in cats are reported to metastasize to the digits, particularly the third phalanx, causing destruction of the nail bed epithelium and sloughing of the claw.

In about 50% of the carcinomas that are identified in the proximal appendicular skeleton in the dog, there is no clinical evidence of a primary tumor nor is one located at postmortem, raising the possibility that these are primary intraosseous carcinomas. Primary intraosseous carcinomas are reported in the mandible and maxilla of humans but are uncommon and are nearly always diagnosed as squamous cell carcinomas, some of which have features indicating an odontogenic origin.

FRACTURE REPAIR

Broken bones are a common occurrence, therefore it is important to understand how and why fractures heal and more importantly, why in some cases they do not heal. Fractures can be classified as traumatic (normal bone broken by excessive force) or pathologic (an abnormal bone broken by minimal trauma or by normal weight bearing). Osteoporosis, osteomyelitis, and bone neoplasia are examples of lesions that can weaken a bone and predispose it to pathologic fracture.

Growth plate: The Salter-Harris classification of growth plate fractures has been widely accepted and can be readily found in texts on clinical orthopedics. Growth plate fractures that involve only the hypertrophied layers of cartilage and/or the primary bone trabeculae (Salter-Harris I and II) usually heal with few or no complications. Fractures that cross the growth plate (III and IV) or crush the plate (V and VI) have the potential to heal with secondary growth abnormalities. Fractures that crush or cross the growth plate could irreversibly injure chondrocytes of the reserve (resting) cell layer of the growth plate or damage the branch of the epiphyseal artery that nourishes these cells. Loss of reserve cells can result in premature closure of the growth plate in these regions.

Trabecular bone: Fractures of trabeculae without external deformation of the cortex are called *infractions.* Inflammation and/or necrosis of bone often are predisposing factors.

Cortical bone: Fractures of cortical bone can be classified in many other ways: closed or simple, if the skin is unbroken; open or compound, if the skin is broken and the bone is exposed to the external environment; comminuted, if the bone has been shattered into several small fragments; avulsed, if the fracture was caused by the traction of a ligament at its insertion onto bone; greenstick, if one cortex of the bone is broken and the other cortex is only bent so that there is no separation or displacement of the fracture site; and transverse or spiral, depending on the orientation of the fracture line.

Stable fracture repair means that the fracture ends have been immobilized to give relative clinical stability (not necessarily weight-bearing ability) but have not been rigidly fixed surgically (Table 16-5). The events that normally occur in the healing of

TABLE 16-5 Stable Fracture Repair

Time	Tissue at Repair Site	Stability
Immediate	Hematoma	Unstable
24-48 hr	Undifferentiated mesenchymal cells and neovascularization	Unstable
36 hr	Earliest woven bone	Unstable
4-6 wk	Primary callus of woven bone and possibly hyaline cartilage	Stable
Months to years	Modeling of woven bone into lamellar bone	Stable

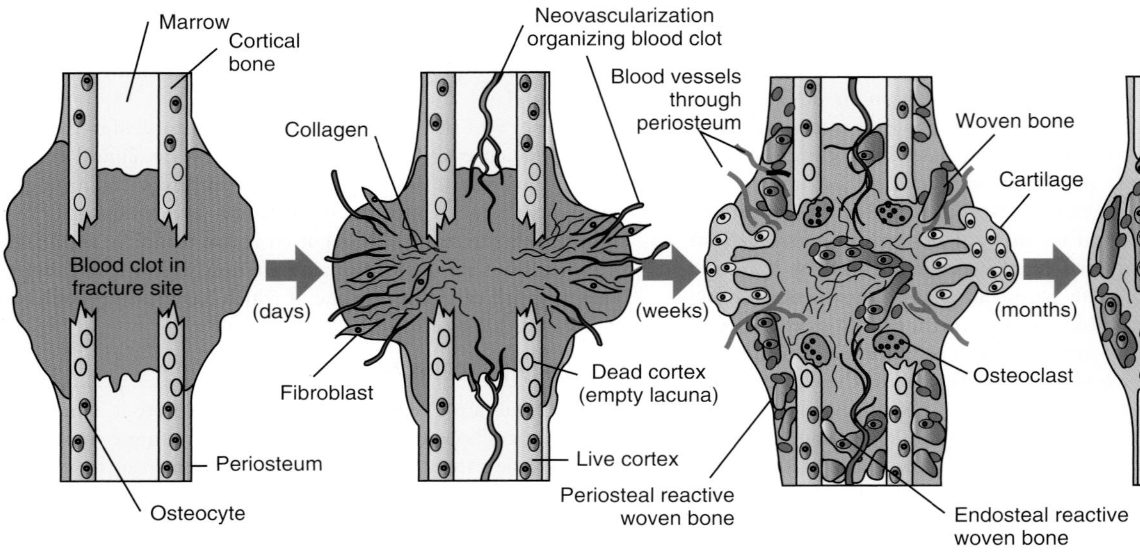

Fig. 16-74 Schematic diagram of the temporal course of callus formation and fracture repair. (Redrawn from Rubin E: *Essential pathology,* ed 3, Baltimore, 2001, Lippincott Williams & Wilkins.)

a closed stable fracture of cortical bone are summarized below; however, the reader should understand that this description represents a summary of a complex process that is subject to a great deal of variation. At the time of fracture, the periosteum is torn, bone fragments are displaced, soft tissue is traumatized, and bleeding occurs to form a hematoma (Fig. 16-74). Because of impaired blood flow and the presence of isolated bone fragments, bone and marrow tissue adjacent to the fracture sites can (and often does, at least to some extent) undergo necrosis. The hematoma and tissue necrosis can be important in subsequent callus formation. Growth factors are released by macrophages and platelets in the blood clot and the proliferating osteogenic tissue and even from the dead bone through the lysis and acidification of the matrix. These growth factors (bone morphogenetic proteins, TGF-β, and PDGFs among others) are important in stimulating proliferation of repair tissue (woven bone). Undifferentiated mesenchymal cells having osteogenic potential, along with proliferating blood vessels, begin to penetrate the hematoma from the periphery in 24 to 48 hours. The mesenchymal cells are derived from the periosteum, endosteum, stem cells in the medullary cavity, and possibly from metaplasia of endothelial cells. These mesenchymal cells proliferate in the hematoma to form a loose collagenous tissue that, combined with neovascularization, has been called *granulation tissue;* however, this is misleading because the ultimate outcome of granulation tissue is fibrous tissue, whereas the mesenchymal cells in the early stages of fracture healing have the potential to undergo metaplasia to cartilage and bone. Woven bone is visible microscopically as early as 36 hours, and regenerating nerve fibers are visible in the hematoma as early as 3 days, after the fracture has occurred.

The term *callus* refers to a disorganized meshwork of woven bone that forms after a fracture. It can be external (formed by the periosteum) or internal (formed between the ends of the fragments and in the medullary cavity or endosteum). This "primary" callus should bridge the gap, encircle the fracture site, and stabilize the area (Fig. 16-75). In time, woven bone at the fracture site is replaced by stronger, mature lamellar bone (secondary callus). Depending on the mechanical forces acting at the site, the callus can eventually be reduced in size by osteoclasts until the normal shape of the bone is restored. This process, however, might take years to complete.

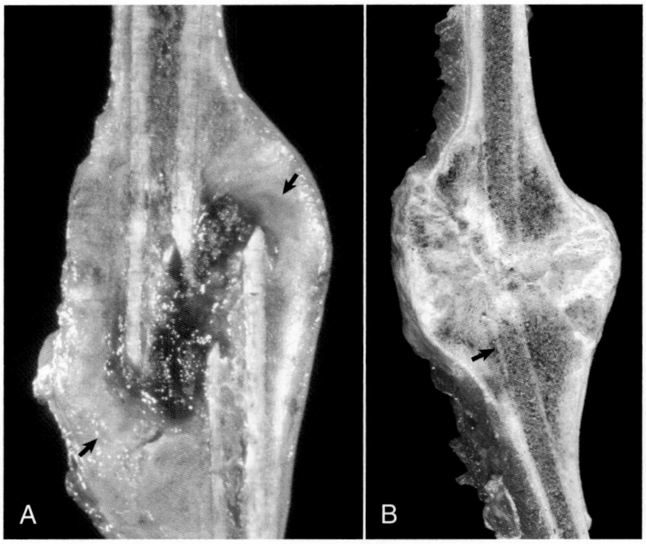

Fig. 16-75 Fractures, stable and unstable, bone, rib. **A,** Unstable fracture. The fractured edges of the rib are improperly aligned, and there is abundant external callus composed of cartilage and bone *(arrows);* also present are areas of fibrous tissue admixed with hemorrhage. Fibrous tissue is produced in regions of tension in an unstable fracture. **B,** Stable fracture. The fractured edges of the rib are adequately aligned, and the fracture is stabilized by abundant cartilaginous callus that is being replaced by new bone. Note the location of the original cortex (*arrow* indicates original periosteal surface). (**A** courtesy College of Veterinary Medicine, University of Illinois. **B** courtesy Dr. F. A. Leighton, College of Veterinary Medicine, University of Saskatchewan; and Noah's Arkive, College of Veterinary Medicine, The University of Georgia.)

A callus often contains hyaline cartilage, the amount of which reflects the adequacy of the blood supply, as less than optimal oxygen supply promotes mesenchymal stem cells to differentiate into chondroblasts rather than osteoblasts. Cartilage does not provide as strong a callus as woven bone; however, it will eventually undergo endochondral ossification and therefore ultimately contribute to the formation of the bony callus.

Rigid fracture repair is usually a result of surgical intervention that involves the application of devices to keep the bone ends in contact or in very close proximity for fracture stability during the repair process. Ideally (but rarely achieved across an entire fracture), contact healing, in which the fractured ends are touching each other and there is no instability, occurs. In such conditions, healing is by direct osteonal bridging of the fracture site (Web Fig. 16-6). Osteoclasts forming channels for new osteons will "jump" the fracture line and the new osteons will "knit" the bone ends together without formation of a callus. If a gap less than 1 mm is present between the bone ends, bone cells will migrate from the fracture ends and form lamellar bone at a right angle to the fracture line. This will eventually model into osteonal bone parallel to the long axis of the bone. In rigid fractures with gaps greater than 1 mm, woven bone fills the gap and must be modeled into osteonal bone (Web Fig. 16-7).

The most common complications of fracture healing are inadequate blood supply, instability, and infection. If the blood supply is less than optimal, hyaline cartilage will form; if blood supply is disrupted to the point of anoxia, necrosis will occur. Mechanical tension and compression at the fracture site also influence the reparative process because excessive movement and tension favor the development of fibrous tissue. Mature fibrous tissue is not desirable; it does not stabilize the fracture and unlike cartilage, does not act as a template for bone formation. Excessive fibrous tissue between bone ends in a fracture might result in a nonunion. With time, the bony ends of the nonunion can become smooth and move in a pocket of fibrous tissue and cartilage to form a false joint or pseudoarthrosis. Other factors that can interfere with the normal repair process include malnutrition and the interposition of large fragments of necrotic bone, muscle, or other soft tissue that might lead to delayed union or nonunion. Fractures heal more slowly in aged animals likely because of decreased red marrow and its constituent stromal stem cells.

There are several complications of fracture repair specifically associated with metallic implants used in fracture stabilization. Metallic devices that are too large deprive the bone of normal mechanical forces (stress shielding) and result in bone loss (disuse atrophy). Intramedullary fixation devices have the potential to damage the blood supply. Implanted material (metal, plastics, and bone cement) often is separated from the surrounding bone by a thin layer of fibrous tissue, sometimes with metaplastic cartilage that forms in response to operative trauma, implant mobility, or corrosion of the implant. In addition, the implant surface can be a nidus for bacterial growth, and the admixture of bacteria with amorphous host fluid can form a biofilm that is resistant to antibiotics and host inflammatory cells. Microscopic particulate debris from implanted fixation materials ("wear debris") can elicit a macrophage or multinucleated giant cell response. These inflammatory cells can release cytokines and growth factors that result in bone resorption and deterioration at the bone-implant surface, causing loosening and failure of the implant. Neoplasia thought to be induced by metallic fracture fixation devices has been reported rarely in human and veterinary literature and is usually secondary to chronic osteomyelitis. The mechanism by which chronic osteomyelitis could be a predisposing factor for development of osteosarcoma is not known for certain. Generally, it is believed that any lesion that causes cell proliferation (as would be expected in chronic osteomyelitis) can increase the chance of cancer-causing spontaneous DNA damage by, for example, free radicals and solar radiation.

Pulmonary embolization of marrow fat from the trauma of the fracture or from trauma associated with repair of the fracture can cause severe clinical disease in humans. It appears that the frequency of fat embolization secondary to trauma to the bone marrow is relatively common in humans and dogs, but that clinical consequences of such embolization are relatively rare. Experimentally, fat embolization can be created readily in dogs by reaming the medullary cavity, followed by pressurization. Interestingly, fat released from the marrow cavity in dogs by reaming is greater from intact bones than from fractured bones because of decompression of the marrow cavity by the fracture in the latter.

DISORDERS OF THE JOINTS IN DOMESTIC ANIMALS (HORSES, RUMINANTS [CATTLE, SHEEP, AND GOATS], PIGS, DOGS, AND CATS)

The joints, or junctions between the bones, can be classified as those that allow essentially no movement (fibrous joints or synarthrosis [e.g., sutures between the bones of the skull]), those that allow limited movement (cartilaginous joint or amphiarthrosis [e.g., intervertebral joints]), and joints that are freely movable (synovial joint or diarthrosis [e.g., stifle joint]). The guide for postmortem examination of the joints is presented in Web Appendix 16-1.

ABNORMALITIES OF GROWTH AND DEVELOPMENT

Arthrogryposis

Arthrogryposis refers to the congenital contracture of a joint, a condition that usually occurs with bilateral symmetry. The cause of arthrogryposis is often not established when it occurs sporadically. However, the pathogenesis is well established in outbreaks involving damage to the fetal central nervous system (CNS) with intrauterine viral infections (Akabane virus and bluetongue virus) in cattle and sheep. In some cases, the CNS lesions are clearly hereditary, with significant numbers of offspring affected after introduction of a new sire. The CNS lesions result in degeneration or atrophy of muscle groups with subsequent contraction of the distal limb. Alternatively, maternal intoxication with certain alkaloids (coniine in poison hemlock) and lupine plants (anagyrine) is believed to result in fetal paralysis. Lack of fetal motion during a critical window of development results in arthrogryposis, and this has been well documented experimentally. In arthrogryposis occurring secondary to lack of fetal motion in utero, there is no primary problem in the joint. Usually, on sectioning the tendons or the articular capsule, these contractures can be relieved and the joint can be straightened. In rare circumstances, there is congenital articular malformation resulting in incongruous joint surfaces.

Articular cartilage: Articular cartilage is usually normal, but subtle malformations can be present.

Articular capsule/synovium/synovial fluid: Articular capsule/synovium/synovial fluid is without gross lesions other than the lack of flexibility.

Subchondral bone: Subchondral bone is usually normal other than subtle malformation.

Hip Dysplasia

Hip dysplasia of the dog is a major orthopedic problem and is most common in large and giant breeds. It is inherited as a complex polygenic trait, and gene expression in individuals may be modified by environmental factors, including weight and exercise. Dogs on restricted caloric intake have a significantly delayed time of onset of both hip dysplasia and degenerative joint disease. Many different theories regarding the etiopathogenesis have been advanced, but most agree that it is a biomechanical disease in which joint laxity of the hip (instability) is one of the essential early findings, eventually resulting in chronic subluxation and severe secondary degenerative joint disease with marked modeling of the acetabulum and femoral head and neck. The lesions are not present at birth but can be well advanced by 1 year of age. The earliest radiographic lesion is delayed ossification of the craniodorsal acetabular rim, which may be identified as early as 7 weeks of age in severely affected individuals.

Hip dysplasia also occurs as an inherited disease (recessive, sex-limited) in bulls of certain beef breeds, including Herefords. Affected animals have shallow acetabula and joint laxity and instability, which lead to degenerative joint disease early in life.

Articular cartilage: In the advanced disease, there is notable erosion and ulceration of articular cartilage of both the femoral head and acetabulum.

Articular capsule/synovium/synovial fluid: In advanced disease, the articular capsule is distended and thickened, sometimes containing areas of osseous and cartilaginous metaplasia, and synovial fluid is increased in amount. The round ligament of the femoral head may be ruptured. It has been reported that the earliest detectable microscopic lesion in hip dysplasia is a mild lymphoplasmacytic synovitis, which probably occurs secondary to early cartilage breakdown.

Subchondral bone: In advanced disease, the dorsal rim of the acetabulum flattens and becomes shallow and wide. Subsequent to ulceration of cartilage of the femoral head, there is eburnation of underlying bone and formation of periarticular osteophytes on both the femur and the acetabulum.

INFLAMMATORY LESIONS

The term *synovitis* is restricted to inflammation of the synovium, whereas the term *arthritis* implies that lesions also are present in articular cartilage. Although arthritis is characterized by the presence of inflammatory cells in the synovial membrane, the nature of the inflammatory process is often reflected best in the volume and character of the exudate in the joint fluid. In general, it is useful to classify joint diseases as inflammatory (e.g., rheumatoid arthritis) or noninflammatory (e.g., osteoarthritis), although some degree of inflammation may be present in noninflammatory joint disease. Arthritis also can be classified by cause (bacterial, viral, sterile immune-mediated, or urate deposits of gout), duration (acute, subacute, or chronic), or the nature of the exudate produced (serous, fibrinous, purulent, or lymphoplasmacytic). The term *arthropathy* is all-encompassing and refers to any joint disease. Like osteomyelitis, arthritis can be a serious threat to the well-being of an animal by causing pain and leading to permanent deformity. Chronicity can be the result of an inability of the animal to remove the causative agent or substance, repeated trauma, persistence of bacterial cell wall material, or ongoing autoimmune-mediated inflammation. If there is irreversible damage to cartilage or synovium, even if the cause of the primary inflammation is cleared, the joint could progress to degenerative joint disease. In fact, end-stage rheumatoid arthritis in humans (the prototype of inflammatory arthritis) may be indistinguishable from end-stage osteoarthritis (considered by most to be a noninflammatory condition). Injury to intraarticular structures can be the result of the offending agent or substance, to the inflammatory process, to proteolytic enzymes released from cells of cartilage or synovial tissues, to activation of latent matrix metalloproteinases, or to failure of degenerating or necrotic chondrocytes to maintain the proteoglycan content of the matrix. Mediators of inflammation that contribute to joint injury include prostaglandins, cytokines, leukotrienes, lysosomal enzymes, free radicals, nitric oxide, neuropeptides, and products of the activated coagulation, kinin, complement, and fibrinolytic systems in synovial fluid.

Infectious Arthritis

Neonatal bacteremia secondary to omphalitis or oral-intestinal entry commonly leads to polyarthritis in lambs, calves, piglets, and foals. Bacteria can also reach the joint by direct inoculation, as in a puncture wound, by direct extension from periarticular soft tissue, or by extension from adjacent bone, although these routes are less common. Bacterial osteomyelitis can extend through the cortex at the metaphysis (see Figs. 16-37 to 16-39) (especially in young animals in which this cortex is thin or incomplete) into the joint, or epiphyseal osteomyelitis can lyse directly through articular cartilage (see Fig. 16-56). Bacterial arthritis is not common in dogs or cats. In a retrospective study in a university veterinary hospital, most cases of bacterial arthritis in dogs involved the stifle and occurred as complications from surgery on this joint.

The lesions of infectious arthritis may be very similar regardless of the agent; therefore the lesions in the next section are presented by time frame and whether the initial exudates are/were mostly neutrophilic (suppurative arthritis) or fibrinous (fibrinous arthritis) (see Table 16-2).

Articular cartilage: The response of cartilage to inflammation with time depends on the nature and severity of the exudates. In acute inflammation, independent of the nature of the initial exudate, the articular cartilage is normal grossly and microscopically. In subacute suppurative or fibrinous arthritis, there can be thinning of the cartilage because of lysis and erosion (see previous discussion) of collagenous matrix by the enzymes in the exudates, activation of matrix metalloproteinases, and collapse of the cartilage as a result of a loss and failure to replace the water-binding proteoglycans by the degenerate or necrotic chondrocytes. In chronic suppurative arthritis, extensive cartilage erosion and ulceration is expected (Fig. 16-76). In chronic fibrinous arthritis, cartilage ulceration may occur but not as consistently as with chronic suppurative arthritis. Pannus formation also may occur in chronic fibrinous arthritis but is unusual with chronic suppurative arthritis. As described previously, cartilage erosion and ulceration is expected subsequent to pannus formation. In chronic infectious arthritis in which there was no acute exudate in the joint, cartilage loss might be quite slow and occur secondary to low grade lymphoplasmacytic synovitis (see later discussion).

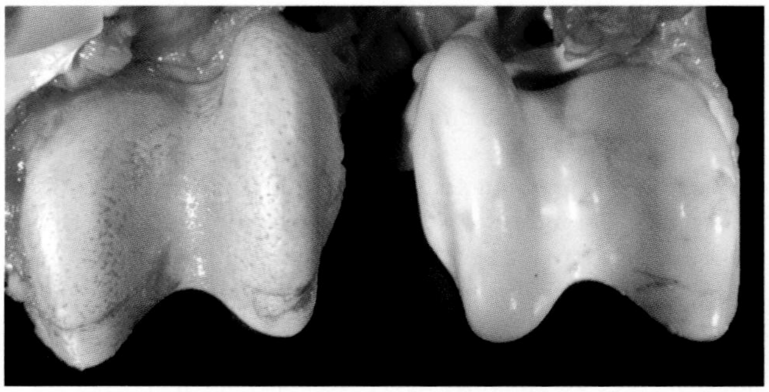

Fig. 16-76 **Chronic suppurative (active) arthritis, tibial-tarsal bone, articular surface, hock, horse *(left)* and normal contralateral bone *(right)*.** The suppurative inflammation has caused widespread erosions (lysis) of the articular cartilage that appear as darkened pitted areas on the articular surface *(left)*. The reddish discoloration of these areas is due to the subchondral (vascularized) bone marrow, which is now visible subjacent to the thinned areas of cartilage. Normal left tibial-tarsal bone is on the right. (Courtesy Dr. S.E. Weisbrode, College of Veterinary Medicine, The Ohio State University.)

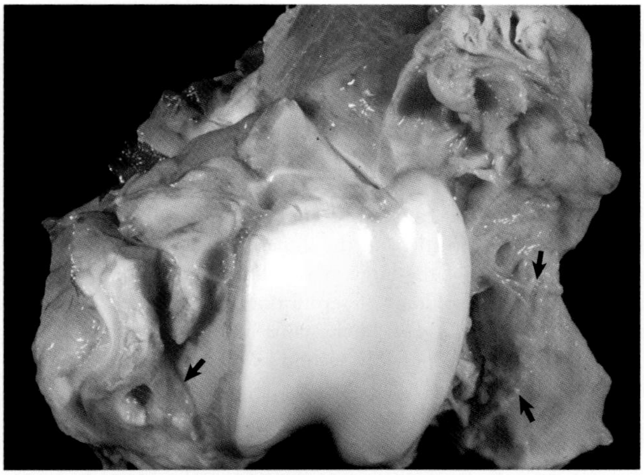

Fig. 16-77 Acute fibrinous arthritis, bone, tibial-tarsal joint (hock), calf.
The joint space is distended by layers of yellowish-brown fibrin that coat the synovial surface *(arrows)* of the joint capsule. (Courtesy Dr. C.S. Patton, College of Veterinary Medicine, University of Tennessee.)

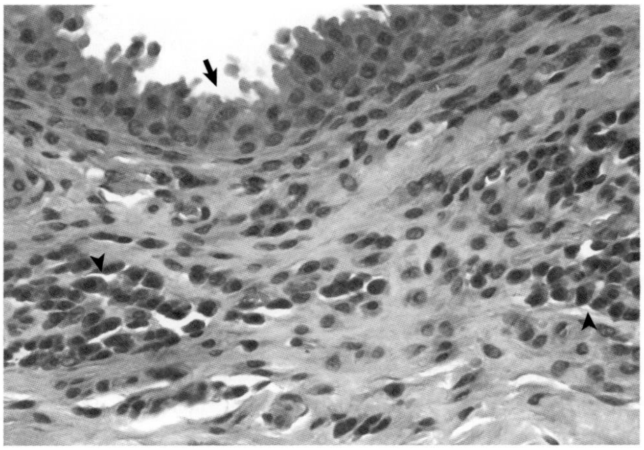

Fig. 16-78 Subacute synovitis, joint capsule, dog.
There is marked synovial cell hyperplasia *(arrow)* and infiltration of lymphocytes and plasma cells into the synovial subintima *(arrowheads)*. H&E stain. (Courtesy Dr. S.E. Weisbrode, College of Veterinary Medicine, The Ohio State University.)

Articular capsule/synovium/synovial fluid: In acute suppurative and fibrinous arthritis, the synovial fluid is usually reduced in viscosity because of a combination of enzymatic digestion of the glycosaminoglycans and dilution of the synovial fluid with edema. The fluid may be turbid because of the presence of neutrophils and strands of fibrin and may be reddened because of mild hemorrhage. Exudate in the synovial fluid can be extensive in acute lesions (Fig. 16-77), whereas the synovial membrane can appear only slightly hyperemic and edematous even microscopically. Therefore, in acute arthritis, evaluation of synovial fluid may be much more informative than evaluation of synovial membrane. Reports in the horse suggest that culturing for bacteria in synovial fluid is more sensitive than either culturing synovial membrane or examining synovial membrane histologically using special stains to identify bacteria. In contrast, in the dog, culturing the synovial membrane has been reported to be more sensitive than culturing synovial fluid. Given these discrepancies, it may be prudent to culture both tissues. In acute fibrinous or suppurative bacterial arthritis that has been treated effectively with antibiotics, the lesions can resolve without residual defects.

In subacute suppurative and fibrinous arthritis and subacute infectious arthritis in which there was no acute exudation into the joint, the synovium is expected to contain lymphoplasmacytic inflammation and exhibit variable hyperplasia of synovial lining cells, regardless of the cause (Fig. 16-78). The lymphoplasmacytic inflammation reflects the immunogenicity of the infectious agent. The synovial hyperplasia is a nonspecific response but presumably is an attempt to increase production of synovial fluid. In subacute (and chronic) suppurative and fibrinous arthritis, it is uncommon to find significant numbers of neutrophils and fibrin deposits, respectively, in the synovial membrane since they are expected to exude from the membrane and enter the joint space.

In chronic suppurative arthritis, granulation tissue with pronounced lymphoplasmacytic inflammation can replace the synovial membrane and there can be notable fibrosis of the articular capsule. In chronic fibrinous arthritis, if deposits of fibrin are extensive, they can be invaded and replaced by fibrous tissue, leading to restricted articular movement. Chronic fibrinous arthritis (e.g., erysipelas and mycoplasmosis [see later discussion]) of long duration is often accompanied by pronounced villous hypertrophy, lymphoplasmacytic synovitis and pannus formation, and progressive destruction of cartilage (Fig. 16-79). In both chronic fibrinous arthritis and chronic suppurative arthritis, fibrin and pus (suppurative exudate) continue to be produced and are present in the joint space in active (bacteria is still present) lesions. Fibrous ankylosis of joints can occur in extreme cases of either fibrinous or suppurative arthritis.

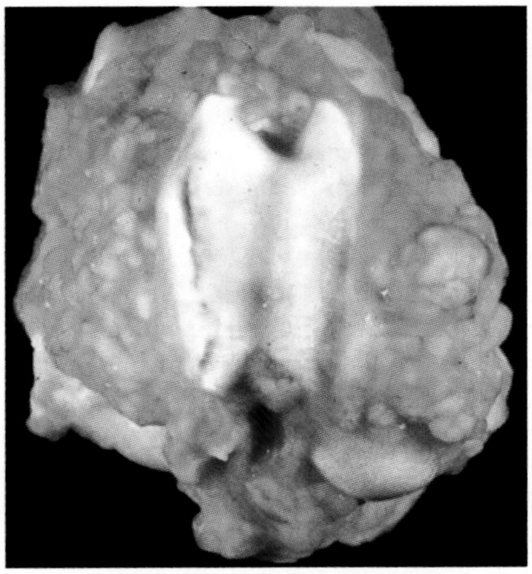

Fig. 16-79 Chronic fibrinous (active) synovitis, erysipelas, stifle joint, pig.
A chronic arthritis from *Erysipelothrix rhusiopathiae* has resulted in villous hypertrophy of the synovial membrane. The tips of some villi are hemorrhagic and necrotic. (Courtesy Dr. D. Harrington, College of Veterinary Medicine, Purdue University; and Noah's Arkive, College of Veterinary Medicine, The University of Georgia.)

Subchondral bone: Subchondral bone is affected only secondarily in infectious arthritis. In chronic purulent arthritis, the exudates can erode the overlying cartilage and extend into the subchondral bone plate (Fig. 16-80). If there is severe chronic lameness, the subchondral bone can undergo disuse atrophy and appear osteopenic.

Bacterial Arthritis

Many different bacteria cause arthritis in animals. The duration of bacterial arthritis is variable; some organisms are rapidly removed

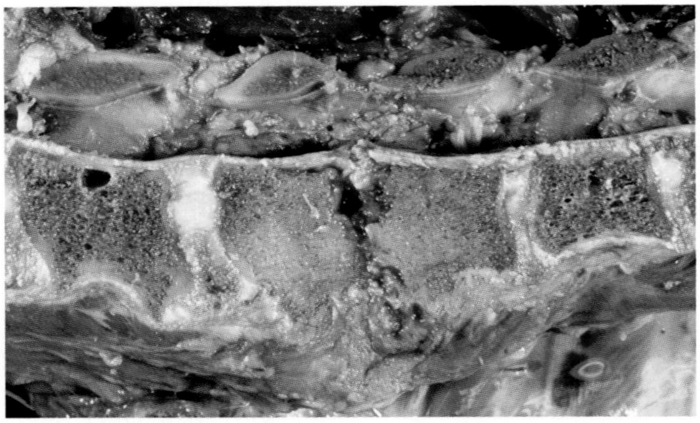

Fig. 16-80 Suppurative discospondylitis, joint, intervertebral disk, dog. Chronic marked suppurative discospondylitis (inflammation of the intervertebral disc and adjacent vertebrae) with marked lysis of the disk and cortices, epiphyses, and metaphyses of the adjacent vertebrae. (Courtesy Dr. S.E. Weisbrode, College of Veterinary Medicine, The Ohio State University.)

and synovitis is short-lived. In other instances, bacteria can persist, and the inflammatory process can become chronic but remain active. The extent and mechanism of cartilaginous destruction differ somewhat, depending on the nature of the exudates. In turn, the nature of the exudates can depend on the infectious agent involved. Generally, fibrinous inflammation is expected more often with Gram-negative bacteria, whereas suppurative arthritis is expected more often with Gram-positive bacteria. The exudates in the joint in acute stages of infection with Gram-positive bacteria, however, can be primarily fibrinous but become purulent with time. An example of chronic fibrinous arthritis is that caused in pigs by *Erysipelothrix rhusiopathiae* septicemia, which is an exception to the previous generality about fibrinous inflammation being caused by Gram-negative bacteria. *Erysipelothrix rhusiopathiae*, a Gram-positive bacteria, causes a fibrinous arthritis that does not become purulent with time. Survivors may have lesions secondary to localization of *Erysipelothrix rhusiopathiae* in the skin, synovial joints, valvular endocardium, or intervertebral disks. Chronic painful polyarthritis is a common sequela. *Arcanobacterium pyogenes* is a common cause of suppurative arthritis in cattle and pigs. *Escherichia coli* and streptococci initially cause septicemia in neonatal calves and piglets and then localize in joints, meninges, and, sometimes, serosal surfaces. The synovitis often is acutely serofibrinous, becoming more purulent with time. *Haemophilus parasuis* causes Glasser's disease in pigs 8 to 16 weeks of age. Lesions consist of fibrinous polyserositis, polyarthritis, and meningitis. Acute serofibrinous polyarthritis is seen frequently in cattle dying of thrombotic meningoencephalitis caused by *Haemophilus somnus.*

Borrelia burgdorferi, a spirochete, is the tick-borne cause of Lyme disease (borreliosis). Arthritis occurs with Lyme disease in dogs, cattle, and horses and affects single or multiple joints. In experimental studies in dogs, lameness developed in about half of the infected animals 2 months or longer after infection. In the acute stages of the disease, the exudate is a combination of fibrinous and suppurative (fibrinopurulent) inflammation. In the chronic stages, pannus (usually a sequela to fibrinous arthritis) and chronic suppurative inflammation can be seen.

Mycoplasma Arthritis

Generally, the lesions of mycoplasma arthritis are similar to those described previously for bacteria causing fibrinous arthritis. Multiple joints usually are involved, indicative of a hematogenous route of infection. *Mycoplasma hyorhinis* causes fibrinous polyarthritis and polyserositis in weanling pigs, and *Mycoplasma hyosynoviae* causes fibrinous polyarthritis in pigs older than 3 months of age. It is not certain how these mycoplasma gain access to the circulation and ultimately, the joints; however, it is likely an oral-pharyngeal/pulmonary route secondary to stress or concurrent respiratory disease, as both agents are commonly isolated from nasal and pharyngeal regions in asymptomatic individuals.

Mycoplasma bovis causes fibrinous to pyogranulomatous polyarthritis in feedlot cattle, and the disease is characterized by lameness and swelling of the large synovial joints of the limbs, which can contain large volumes of serofibrinous to frankly suppurative exudate. *Mycoplasma bovis* likely gains access to joints through a hematogenous route, possibly secondary to mycoplasma pneumonia or mastitis.

Viral Arthritis

Reoviral arthritis in chickens was the first viral arthritis to be discovered. At the time, there was great hope that idiopathic arthritides (such as rheumatoid arthritis) would also be shown to have a viral etiology; however, other than in goats, viral arthritis does not appear to be a significant, or even recognized, disease in domestic mammals. The caprine arthritis-encephalitis virus (a retrovirus) causes chronic fibrinous arthritis in older goats. The disease is characterized by debilitating lameness, carpal hygromas, and distention of the larger synovial joints. Chronic cases exhibit lymphoplasmacytic synovitis, synovial villous hyperplasia, and pannus formation typical of chronic fibrinous arthritis. An additional lesion that is peculiar to chronic cases of this disease is necrosis and mineralization of synovial villi that may give the membrane a chalky white appearance.

Noninfectious Arthritis

Noninfectious arthritis includes specific joint diseases that have inflammation as the initiating event but are known to be sterile. These disorders are often classified as erosive or nonerosive, depending on the effect of the disease on articular cartilage. Three examples of sterile erosive arthritis follow. These diseases often are chronic, sometimes lasting for months, as they can be very difficult to control with medication.

Rheumatoid Arthritis

Rheumatoid arthritis in dogs is an uncommon, chronic, sterile, erosive polyarthritis that resembles the disease in humans. The cause is unknown in both species, although it is clear that the process is immune mediated (humoral and cell-mediated immunity). Antibodies (rheumatoid factor) of the immunoglobulin (Ig) G (IgG) or IgM classes are produced in response to an unknown stimulus. Factors that may be involved include alterations in the stearic configuration of IgG, persistent bacterial cell wall components that cross-react with normal proteoglycans, anticollagen antibodies, and defective suppressor T lymphocyte activity. Neutrophils that are activated by ingestion of immune complexes release lysosomal enzymes, which sustain the inflammatory reaction and injure intraarticular structures. In addition to inflammatory mediators and their effects on synovium and cartilage, rheumatoid arthritis characteristically includes exuberant pannus formation (see Figs. 16-31 and 16-32). Fibroblasts in pannus can enzymatically degrade cartilage, and pannus may additionally act as a physical barrier between the synovial fluid and the cartilage to prevent nutrition of the chondrocytes. Antibodies against normal and altered articular cartilage collagen are present in human cases of rheumatoid arthritis and might be important mediators of the ongoing joint inflammation and injury that occur in this disease. In dogs, rheumatoid arthritis is characterized clinically by progressive lameness involving primarily the distal joints of the limbs (carpal, tarsal, and phalangeal joints).

Reactive Arthritis

Reactive arthritis is the name given to a sterile erosive oligoarthritis of uncertain pathogenesis. This condition is rarely reported in domestic animals but is a recognized problem in primate research colonies as occurring subsequent to diarrheal disease and is likely to be underdiagnosed in other species. Reactive arthritis is defined clinically as sterile inflammation in joints that occurs subsequent to infectious inflammation in other organ systems—usually intestinal and urogenital in humans and usually caused by bacteria such as *Yersinia, Salmonella, Campylobacter, and Shigella.* Several hypotheses have been presented that are not mutually exclusive, including cross-reactivity (molecular mimicry) between bacterial heat-shock proteins and articular glycosaminoglycans, inexplicable homing of sensitized gut lymphocytes to joints, and inexplicable localization of antigenic bacterial peptidoglycans in joints.

Postinfectious Sterile Arthritis

Postinfectious sterile arthritis is suspected to represent the immune reaction to antigenic breakdown products of bacterial cell walls that can remain sequestered in a joint after a confirmed bacterial infection within the joint. A description of the lesions occurring in all three types of erosive, noninfectious arthritis follows.

Articular cartilage: Cartilage erosion that is clearly related to the presence of pannus is expected at the subacute phases of disease and is later followed by ulceration that may be extensive.

Articular capsule/synovium/synovial fluid: Grossly, the lesions in advanced cases consist of marked villous hypertrophy of the synovial membrane, pannus formation that may appear as a velvet-like layer overlying the subchondral bone, periarticular osteophytes, and in some cases, fibrous ankylosis of affected joints. Microscopically, the alterations in the joint include hyperplasia of synovial lining cells and infiltration of the synovium by large numbers of plasma cells and lymphocytes. Additionally, necrotic foci, fibrinous exudate, and infiltrating neutrophils may be present. The synovial fluid contains large numbers of neutrophils.

Subchondral bone: Particularly in cases of active disease in which there is pannus formation, subchondral bone exhibits lytic changes. Secondary osteoarthritis may be present in chronic disease and may result in subchondral bone sclerosis.

Nonerosive Noninfectious Arthritis

Nonerosive noninfectious arthritis has been best described in the dog. Most cases are idiopathic symmetric oligoarthritides, but they can be associated with concurrent sterile immune-mediated diseases such as steroid responsive meningitis/arteritis, neoplasia, infectious inflammation in other organ systems (nonerosive reactive arthritis), and systemic lupus erythematosus (SLE). Dogs with SLE may also have dermatitis, anemia, thrombocytopenia, polymyositis, and glomerulonephritis. It is not clear why nonerosive noninfectious arthritis, which is thought to be mediated by synoviotrophic immune complexes, does not result in articular destruction, as occurs in rheumatoid arthritis.

Articular cartilage: Articular cartilage lesions are not expected in nonerosive arthritis even in chronic cases.

Articular capsule/synovium/synovial fluid: Villous hypertrophy can be minimal to marked, with variable neutrophilic and lymphoplasmacytic synovitis. Pannus formation does not occur; the exudate in the synovial fluid in chronic nonerosive arthritis is neutrophilic.

Subchondral bone: Subchondral bone lesions are not expected in nonerosive arthritis.

In sterile inflammatory joint disease, a definitive diagnosis is often not possible. It should be remembered that response to antibiotics does not confirm that a process was a result of infectious agents. Antibiotics that reduce Gram-positive bacteria in the intestine may allow coliform overgrowth and increased lipopolysaccharide production. Increased intestinal absorption of lipopolysaccharide is associated with decreased clinical signs in autoimmune arthritis, possibly by downregulation of the immune system or by establishing a more rigorous recognition of self.

Crystal Deposition Disease

Crystal deposition disease is characterized by deposits of minerals, such as urates, calcium phosphates, and calcium pyrophosphates, in articular cartilage and/or the soft tissue of joints. Clinical disease caused by crystal deposition is rare in domestic mammals. Species that lack the enzyme uricase (primates, birds, and reptiles), an enzyme that promotes the oxidation of uric acid to allantoin, may experience excessive accumulation of uric acid in the bloodstream. Crystal-induced synovitis with secondary degeneration of articular cartilage occurs when urate crystals are deposited in and around joints, a condition known as *gout.* Deposits of urate, called *tophi,* incite an acute to chronic granulomatous inflammation and can appear grossly as white caseous material. Joint disease involving one or multiple joints also has been reported in young dogs resulting from deposition of calcium and phosphorus in different forms (calcium pyrophosphate deposition disease, pseudogout, and calcium phosphate deposition disease) in the soft tissue of the synovium, articular capsule, and adjacent ligaments. Underlying metabolic disease in this condition is not recognized. Intraarticular crystal deposition disease is perhaps the most common of the crystal deposition diseases but usually is clinical silent. This condition is usually caused by calcium pyrophosphate deposition and may occur in locations in horses and dogs that are subjected to increased mechanical use (scapulohumeral joint of racing dogs and metacarpophalangeal and metatarsophalangeal joints of horses). The deposition is initiated around the chondrocytes and can be seen grossly as bright white foci. The significance of the deposition is uncertain, but it might play a role in the progression of degenerative joint disease.

DEGENERATIVE JOINT DISEASE

Degenerative joint disease (osteoarthritis, osteoarthrosis), recognized since antiquity, is a destructive disease of synovial joints that occurs in all animals with a bony skeleton (Table 16-6). It can be monoarticular or polyarticular, can occur in immature or mature animals, and can be symptomatic or clinically silent. Affected animals have variable degrees of joint enlargement and deformity, pain, and articular malfunction. The etiopathogenesis of degenerative joint disease is incompletely understood, and it is likely that the term encompasses a variety of diseases that have a common end-stage (Fig. 16-81). Initial changes can be the result of traumatic injury to articular cartilage; inflammation of the synovium; increased stiffness of the subchondral bone; or abnormalities in conformation, joint stability, and congruence of joint surfaces (Fig. 16-82). The number one risk factor for degenerative joint disease in humans is age, although the disease is not considered to be an inevitable consequence of aging. Most cases in humans are primary (no identifiable cause); however, most cases in animals appear to be secondary, with osteochondrosis being an important predisposing factor in those species having a high prevalence of this disease.

TABLE 16-6 Degenerative Joint Disease

Name of Stage	Gross Appearance	Microscopic Lesion
Early degeneration	Normal; articular cartilage may be somewhat softened on palpation	Mild increase in thickness of articular cartilage; decreased proteoglycan content apparent with histochemical stains for sulfated polysaccharides (e.g., toluidine blue, safranin O)
Mild	May appear normal; articular cartilage may contain superficial erosions and may have normal or reduced thickness	Degenerative changes involving superficial articular cartilage, including chondrocyte degeneration/death and superficial fibrillation
Moderate	Articular cartilage contains locally extensive areas of fibrillation (frayed appearance)	Loss of articular cartilage integrity, with fibrillation and loss of tissue extending into tangential and radial zones; this change may be accompanied by a mild synovitis, locally extensive increased thickness of subchondral bone, and the presence of periarticular osteophytes
Chronic	Full thickness loss of articular cartilage with exposure of the subchondral bone, which is thickened; the surface of the thickened subchondral bone may be smooth (eburnation); osteophytes may be grossly visible and joint capsule is thickened	Loss of cartilage to the level of the subchondral bone; subchondral bone may be severely thickened; periarticular osteophytes are often present; subchondral cysts may be present; synovium exhibits chronic inflammation and fibrosis

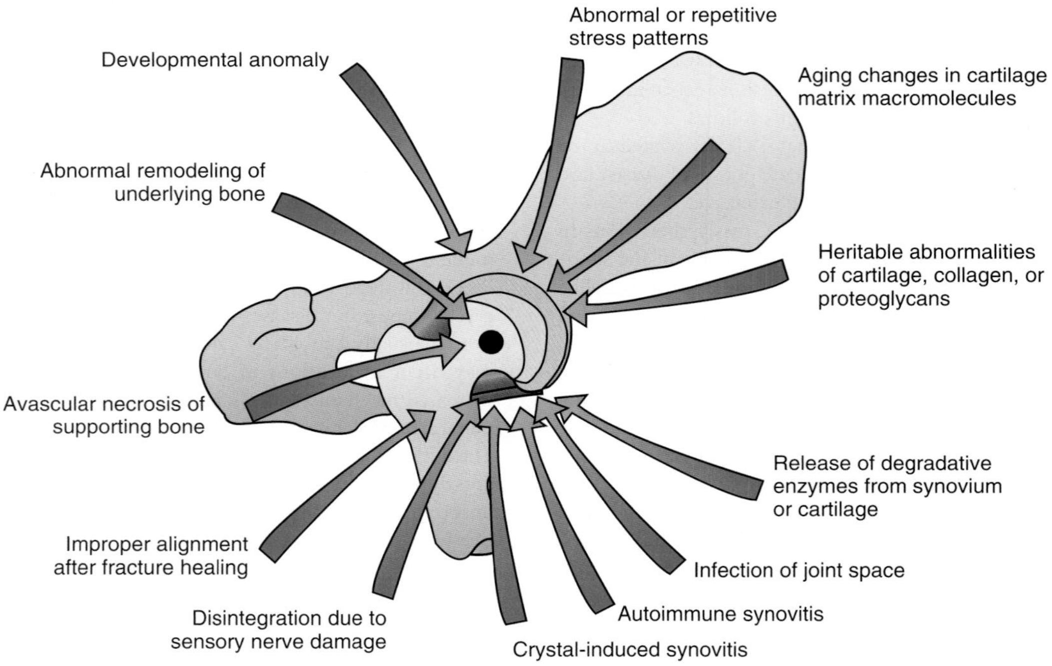

Fig. 16-81 Schematic diagram illustrating degenerative joint disease of the coxofemoral joint. (Redrawn from Damjanov I, Linder J: *Anderson's pathology,* ed 10, St Louis, 1996, Mosby.)

The initial biochemical change in articular cartilage in degenerative joint disease is loss of proteoglycan aggregates. In the early stages of degeneration, this loss of proteoglycans is associated with an increase in water content in the cartilage matrix that causes swelling of the tissue. This may seem contradictory because proteoglycans in normal cartilage play a critical role in binding water. The explanation is not clear; however, the increased water in the matrix in early degenerative joint disease is not bound normally to the proteoglycans and does not contribute to the normal lubrication and flushing of nutrients and waste products. In addition, core proteins of proteoglycan aggregates are susceptible to the action of neutral proteoglycanases, which are increased in early degenerative joint disease. In electron micrographs, the findings in early degenerative joint disease include focal loss of the amorphous layer covering the surface of the articular cartilage and fraying of the superficial collagen fibers. Continued proteoglycan loss interferes with joint lubrication and allows collagen fibers to collapse along lines perpendicular to the joint surface because of the loss of the hydrated gel of proteoglycans and water that normally keeps the fibers separated.

Synovitis in degenerative joint disease is generally mild and occurs secondary to release of inflammatory mediators by injured chondrocytes and from synovial macrophages that have phagocytosed cartilaginous breakdown products.

Articular cartilage: Lesions often are topographically variable within a joint. The loss of proteoglycans and improper binding of water (actual increase in water content) causes the articular cartilage to become soft (chondromalacia). In hinge-type joints, linear

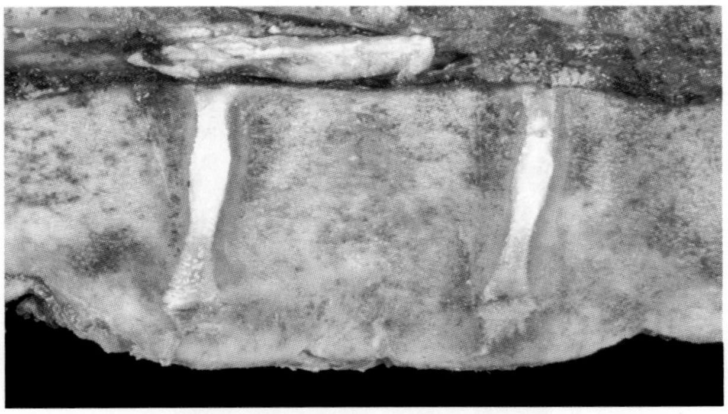

Fig. 16-82 Ankylosing spondylosis, joints, intervertebral, bull. The bony proliferation (ventrally) has bridged the intervertebral space between the adjacent vertebrae and caused fusion (ankylosis) of several joints. Periosteal new bone formation on the ventral and lateral periosteal surfaces of the vertebrae is called spondylosis and may result from mechanical instability or excess mechanical stress on the intervertebral joints. (Courtesy Dr. S.E. Weisbrode, College of Veterinary Medicine, The Ohio State University.)

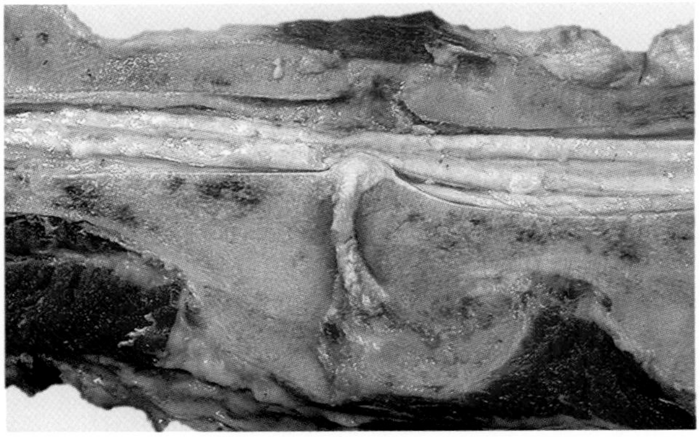

Fig. 16-83 Intervertebral disc disease, degenerate intervertebral disc, prolapsed disc, ankylosing spondylosis, intervertebral joint, dog. Dorsal protrusion of a degenerate nucleus pulposus has compressed the spinal cord. Marked ventral ankylosis (coalescing periarticular osteophyte formation) is secondary to the instability of the joint. (Courtesy J. King, College of Veterinary Medicine, Cornell University.)

grooves often are present, particularly in horses (see Fig. 16-17). Histologically, these represent linear depressions in the cartilage associated with scattered necrotic chondrocytes and localized loss of proteoglycan. The pathogenesis of these grooves is uncertain, but they might represent sequelae to jetties of synovial fluid secondary to incongruities of the joint surfaces. Alternatively, these may appear on an opposite joint surface to a lesion such as a chip fracture, in which case direct mechanical injury is more likely. Chondromalacia is followed by abnormal wearing of the cartilage and loss of superficial articular cartilage (early erosion). As the lesions progress, erosions becomes deeper (cartilage becomes thinner) and grossly apparent fraying of collagen fibers along their radial arrangement can be seen (fibrillation [see Figs. 16-27 and 16-28]). This outcome can be appreciated grossly as a roughened, opaque articular surface, often with discoloration of the cartilage to yellow or brown. Advanced lesions can have notable loss of cartilage down to the mineralized layer and subchondral bone (ulceration [see Fig. 16-29]).

Articular capsule/synovium/synovial fluid: Synovitis characterized by villous hypertrophy, hyperplasia of synoviocytes, and infiltration of lymphocytes, plasma cells, and macrophages is usually present in chronic cases. The synovial fluid does not contain exudates and is clear and colorless but might have reduced viscosity because of increased plasma filtrate relative to glycosaminoglycans in the synovial fluid and increased degradation of glycosaminoglycans by enzymes released by the inflamed synovium. Fibrosis of the articular capsule caused by instability or release of cytokines, such as TGF-β, might contribute, along with osteophytosis and joint incongruity, to the joint stiffness and limited range of motion seen in advanced degenerative joint disease.

Subchondral bone: In advanced disease, sclerosis of subchondral bone, which may be severe, is a consistent finding. Some investigators consider a mild increase in subchondral bone thickness to be an early lesion of degenerative joint disease, possibly preceding articular cartilage damage. If the articular cartilage is ulcerated and the joint remains in use, the exposed subchondral bone may develop a smooth, polished appearance (eburnation). Marginal (periarticular) osteophytes form, particularly with joint instability, and there can be pronounced modeling of the epiphyseal and metaphyseal bone because of altered mechanical use. Joint fusion, caused by a combination of bony or fibrous bridging (ankylosis) of the joint space may occur. Subchondral bone cysts, cavities in the subchondral bone with a synovial-like lining and peripheral osteoclastic bone lysis and fibrosis, may be present, particularly in severe cases. Presumably, these cysts arise secondary to fissures in the overlying cartilage or eburnated bone that allow synovial fluid to be forced into the subchondral bone. These cysts appear to be more common in humans than domestic animals, possibly the result of the longer duration of the disease in humans. The Hartley guinea pig spontaneously develops degenerative joint disease in the stifles before 1 year of age. Subchondral cysts are present in the proximal tibial articular surface and in this model, they appear to be invaginations of synovial membranes surrounding the cruciate ligaments as they insert into the subchondral bone.

DEGENERATION OF INTERVERTEBRAL DISKS

Degeneration of the intervertebral disks is an age-related phenomenon in many species. In general, loss of water and proteoglycans, reduced cellularity, and an increase in collagen content of the nucleus pulposus occur, so that the distinction between the nucleus pulposus and the annulus fibrosus is obscured. Grossly, the central part of the degenerated disk is yellow-brown and is composed of friable fibrocartilaginous material (Fig. 16-83). These degenerative changes are likely caused by various metabolic and mechanical insults that lead to a breakdown of proteoglycan aggregates in the nucleus pulposus and to degenerative changes in the annulus fibrosus. Both rotational and compressive types of movement may further injure the annulus fibrosus. Changes in structure of the nucleus pulposus, together with a weakened annulus, often lead to concentric and radial tears or fissures in the annulus that allow bulging or herniation of the nucleus pulposus material (Fig. 16-84). Herniation usually occurs dorsally in domestic animals. In humans (rarely in domestic animals), disk material can be extruded through the end-plate into the vertebral body, producing a lesion known as *Schmorl's node.*

In chondrodystrophic breeds of dogs, such as the dachshund, chondroid metaplasia of the nucleus pulposus is followed by calcification during the first year of life. These alterations can result in disk prolapse, with total rupture of the annulus fibrosus and extrusion of disk material into the vertebral canal at sites of mechanical stress such as the cervical and thoracolumbar vertebrae.

Senile degenerative disk disease is independent of breed in the dog and also occurs in humans, pigs, and horses. These lesions

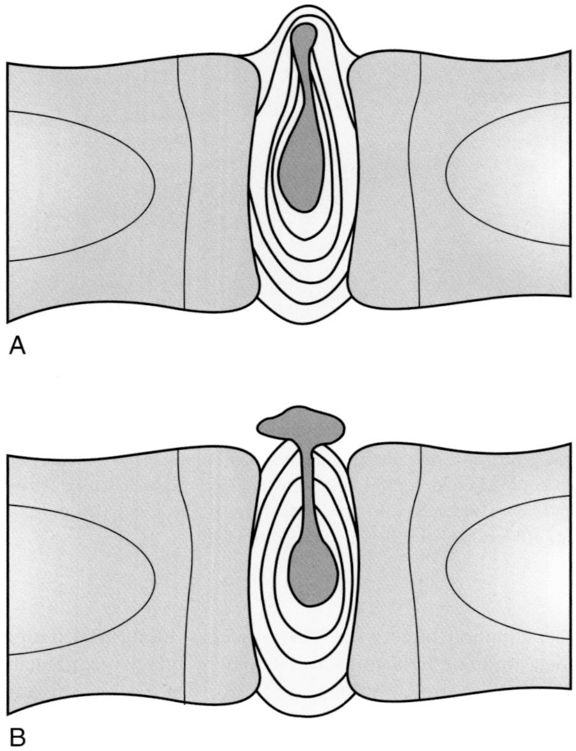

Fig. 16-84 Schematic diagram illustrating stages of prolapse of the nucleus pulposus in intervertebral disc disease.
A, Prolapse of the nucleus pulposus may be secondary to partial rupture of the annulus fibrosus. **B,** Complete rupture of the annulus fibrosus allows extrusion of the nucleus pulposus into the vertebral canal.

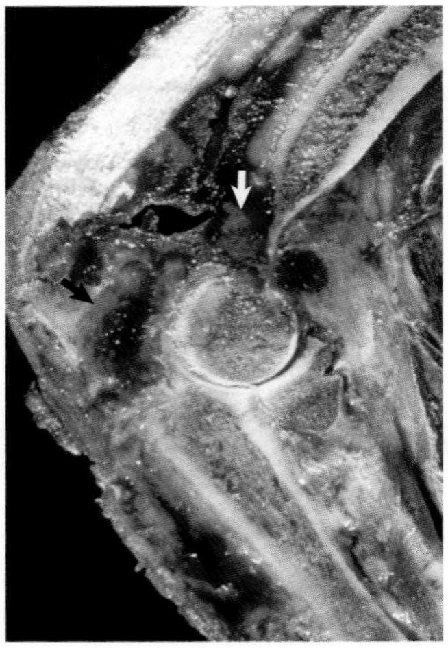

Fig. 16-85 Synovial cell sarcoma, joint, elbow, dog.
Synovial cell sarcoma presenting as a tan and hemorrhagic mass within the joint has invaded into the distal humeral condyle *(white arrow)* and caused pronounced lysis of the proximal ulna *(black arrow)*. (Courtesy Dr. S.E. Weisbrode, College of Veterinary Medicine, The Ohio State University.)

are characterized by progressive dehydration and collagenization of the nucleus pulposus and degeneration of the annulus fibrosus. The lesions develop slowly, and calcification is rare. Prolapse of the disk is secondary to partial rupture of the annulus fibrosus and is characterized by bulging of the dorsal surface of the disk into the vertebral canal. An important consequence of degeneration of intervertebral disks is prolapse of the disk. Prolapse or herniation can be dorsal (spinal cord compression) or lateral (spinal nerve compression and entrapment). Because each intervertebral joint is a three-joint complex (intervertebral joint and two facet joints), the reduced disk thickness that follows degeneration and dehydration allows overriding of articular facets and some degree of joint instability. These changes contribute to the development of degenerative disease and enlargement of articular facets, which may cause impingement on spinal nerves and even compression of the spinal canal because the medial aspect of these facets is adjacent to the intervertebral foramen. Degeneration of intervertebral disks and the ensuing intervertebral joint instability can result in the development of osteophytes at the margins of the vertebral bodies around or adjacent to the disk (spondylosis) in many species, including dogs, cattle, pigs, and horses (see Figs. 16-82 and 16-83). Vertebral osteophytes are usually located ventrally and laterally; if present dorsally, they may cause stenosis of the vertebral canal.

NEOPLASMS OF JOINTS

Primary neoplasms within joints arise from the synovial membrane and are considered to be malignant, but vary notably in their metastatic potential. These tumors are uncommon in dogs and very rare in other species. Two different malignancies of the synovium are recognized. One is derived from histiocytes and is called a *histiocytic sarcoma.* As the name implies, these cells have a histiocytic phenotype; atypia is sometimes extreme with bizarre mitotic figures and pronounced pleomorphism. Histiocytic sarcomas have a high probability of distant metastasis.

Synovial cell sarcoma is the term given to a malignancy of synovial fibrocyte origin (Fig. 16-85). These tumors are more common in joints but may also occur in synovia of tendon sheaths. The malignant cells composing synovial cell sarcoma are negative for histiocytic cell markers, positive for mesenchymal markers (vimentin); inexplicably, a small percentage are positive for epithelial markers (cytokeratins). Such epithelial cell expression is not found in the synovia of normal joints. In humans, there is a characteristic gene translocation that occurs in synovial cell sarcomas. Synovial cell sarcomas have a moderate-to-low chance of distant metastasis. Some fibrocytic cell tumors in the synovium have notable myxomatous metaplasia and have been called *myxomas.* These tumors appear not to have metastatic potential. However, because of their ability to invade bone, these should also be considered low-grade malignancies. The following lesions are characteristic of fibrocytic synovial cell sarcoma and not histiocytic sarcoma.

Articular cartilage: Articular cartilage is usually not affected other than secondarily as a result of a loss of subchondral bone support caused by invasion by the tumor.

Articular capsule/synovium/synovial fluid: Synovium can be markedly and asymmetrically thickened by the presence of a gray-to-tan mass that contains variable hemorrhage. The tumor tissue can be firm to gelatinous (myxoid matrix produced by the neoplastic cells) and usually is relatively confined to the region of the joint. Microscopically, the mass has the appearance of a moderate- to low-grade fibrosarcoma, with little collagen production. Myxomatous metaplasia of the malignant cells can be seen in some cases, causing the tumor to resemble a myxosarcoma.

Subchondral bone: Radiographically, there is evidence of invasion into subchondral and periosteal bone, usually on both sides of the joint space and ranging from minimal to extensive. However, this bone invasion can be subtle and often is not apparent on gross examination.

DISORDERS OF TENDONS AND LIGAMENTS IN DOMESTIC ANIMALS (HORSES, RUMINANTS [CATTLE, SHEEP, AND GOATS], PIGS, DOGS, AND CATS)

Of the 33 million musculoskeletal injuries reported in the United States in humans each year, roughly 50% involve injuries to the soft tissue, including tendons and ligaments. These injuries also are common in veterinary medicine, particularly in dogs and horses. Traumatic injuries may result in either partial or complete ligament or tendon discontinuities. Aging changes that occur in tendons/ligaments, including cartilaginous metaplasia, ischemia, and local fibroblastic proliferations, may make them more susceptible to traumatic injury, although these changes often are present in animals with intact tendons/ligaments.

Degeneration and rupture of the cranial cruciate ligament is a common cause of lameness in some large breed dogs. The clinical disease is known as *cranial cruciate ligament deficiency* and can lead to severe degenerative joint disease. The pathogenesis is not well understood but appears to require the presence of synovial inflammation and is likely complicated by genetic and conformational factors. It is uncertain if the synovitis associated with the disease is the same or different from the pathogenesis of the synovitis seen in degenerative joint disease (see previous section) of other causes. The degenerative changes in the ruptured ligament consist of variable coagulation necrosis and loss of fibroblasts, chondroid metaplasia of some of the remaining fibroblasts, and loss of the normal crimp of the collagen fibers (see previous section).

NEOPLASMS OF TENDONS AND LIGAMENTS

A lesion termed *localized nodular tenosynovitis* has been diagnosed occasionally in dogs and may actually be better characterized as a benign neoplasm. Histologically, the lesion has cleft-like spaces lined by synoviocytes and proliferating fibrous connective tissue. Variable numbers of multinucleated giant cells, hemosiderin-laden macrophages, and mononuclear inflammatory cells also are present. Some nodules contain a spindle cell population, resembling fibroma. Lesions containing increased numbers of multinucleated giant cells may fall under the category of benign giant cell tumor but may just be a variant of localized nodular tenosynovitis. Similarly, fibromas arising from the mesenchyme of the paratenon have been described in horses, but these may actually be sclerotic variants of localized nodular tenosynovitis. Regardless of the histologic subtype, these lesions are slow growing, lack malignant change, and are not reported to metastasize. Malignant tumors originating in tendons and ligaments are rare.

SUGGESTED READINGS

Suggested Readings are available at evolve.elsevier.com/Zachary/McGavin/.

CHAPTER 17

The Integument

Ann M. Hargis and Pamela Eve Ginn

STRUCTURE

The skin is the largest organ in the body and has haired and hairless portions (Figs. 17-1 and 17-2). The skin consists of epidermis, dermis, subcutis, and adnexa (hair follicles and sebaceous, sweat, and other glands). The histologic structure varies greatly by anatomical site and among different species of animals. The haired skin is thickest over the dorsal aspect of the body and on the lateral aspect of the limbs and is thinnest on the ventral aspect of the body and the medial aspect of the thighs. Haired skin has a thinner epidermis, whereas nonhaired skin of the nose and pawpads has a thicker epidermis (see Figs. 17-1 and 17-2). The skin of large animals is generally thicker than the skin of small animals. The subcutis, consisting of lobules of adipose tissue and fascia, connects the more superficial layers (epidermis and dermis) with the underlying fascia and musculature.

EPIDERMIS

The epidermis is divided into layers based on the morphology of the keratinocyte, the major cell type of the epidermis. The epidermis of haired skin consists of four basic layers: stratum corneum, stratum granulosum, stratum spinosum, and stratum basale (Fig. 17-3). The epidermis of hairless skin consists of five layers; the fifth layer is the stratum lucidum, which is located between the stratum granulosum and stratum corneum. Keratinocytes originate from germinal cells in the stratum basale of the epidermis, ascend through the layers of the epidermis, changing in appearance and other characteristics in each layer until they reach the stratum corneum as fully keratinized, dead corneocytes. Keratinocytes are continuously shed from the stratum corneum. The transit time for a keratinocyte from the stratum basale to shed in the stratum corneum is approximately 1 month, although this time can be accelerated in some disorders such as primary seborrhea characterized clinically by scaling.

The outermost layer of the epidermis is the stratum corneum, which consists of many sheets of flattened, keratinized cells termed corneocytes. Keratin is an intracellular fibrous protein that is in part responsible for the toughness of the epidermis, enabling the epidermis to form a protective barrier. The next layer is the stratum granulosum, which consists of effete cells with basophilic keratohyalin granules. In nonhaired skin, the stratum corneum and stratum granulosum are separated by an additional layer of compacted, fully keratinized cells, the stratum lucidum, best seen in the pawpad. Deep to the stratum granulosum is the stratum spinosum, a layer of polyhedral-shaped cells attached to one another by desmosomes. During fixation and processing for microscopic examination, the cells of the stratum spinosum contract, except for the desmosomal attachments. These attachment sites create the appearance of "spines" or intercellular bridges, leading to the name of this layer. The visibility of the intercellular bridges is enhanced when there is intercellular edema of the epidermis. The stratum spinosum in haired areas is thinner in dogs and cats and is thicker in horses, cattle, and pigs. The innermost layer of the epidermis is the germinal layer or stratum basale, which consists of a single layer of cuboidal cells resting on a basement membrane. Intermixed within the basal cell layer are melanocytes, Langerhans' cells, and Merkel cells.

Melanocytes, embryologically derived from neural crest cells, are also present in lower layers of the stratum spinosum and produce melanin pigment, giving skin and hair their color. Melanocytic granules are transferred to and distributed in keratinocytes as a caplike cluster of granules between the nucleus and the external surface of the skin to help protect the nucleus from UV light–induced injury. Langerhans' cells are bone marrow–derived cells of monocyte-macrophage lineage that process and present antigen to sensitized T lymphocytes, thereby modulating immunologic responses of the skin. Langerhans' cells are present in the basal, spinous, and granular layers of the epidermis but have a preference for a suprabasal position. Merkel cells are located in the basal layer and join with keratinocytes via desmosomal junctions. Merkel cells are located in haired and hairless skin, particularly in regions of the body with high tactile sensitivity (digits and lips), and in the outer portion of hair follicles. When Merkel cells are associated with an axon, they form a Merkel cell–neurite complex and function as a slowly adapting mechanoreceptor. The specialized areas of the skin containing these Merkel cell–neurite complexes are known as *tylotrich pads* (hair discs, tactile pads). The axon associated with the Merkel cell is myelinated but near the epidermis, the myelin sheath is lost, and the nerve fibers terminate at the basal

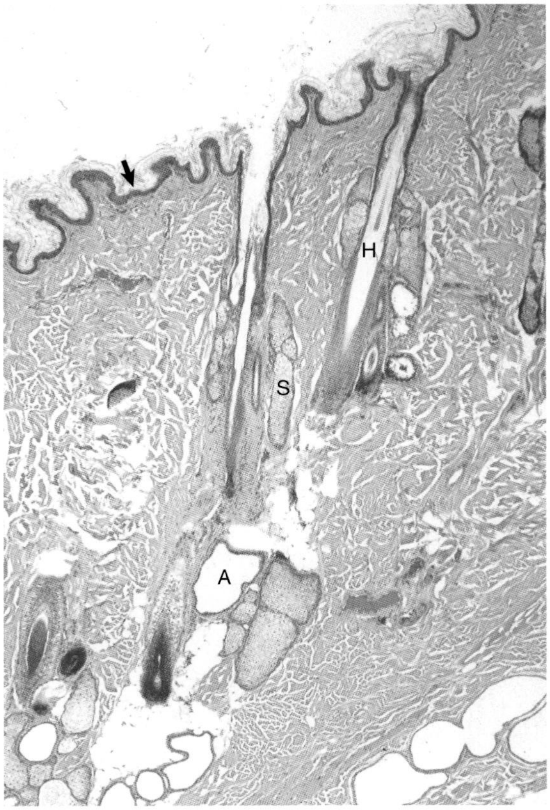

Fig. 17-1 Normal skin, haired, thorax, dog.
The epidermis *(arrow)* in haired skin has an undulating surface but lacks rete ridges. The epidermis in haired skin has fewer nucleated cell layers than the epidermis in nonhaired (hairless) skin such as that on the nose and pawpads (see Fig. 17-2); thus it is referred to as "thin" skin. Hair follicles *(H)*, apocrine glands *(A)*, and sebaceous glands *(S)* are present. The haired skin is thickest over the dorsal aspect of the body and on the lateral aspect of the limbs, and it is thinnest on the ventral aspect of the body and the medial aspect of the thighs. H&E stain. (Courtesy Dr. Ann M. Hargis, DermatoDiagnostics.)

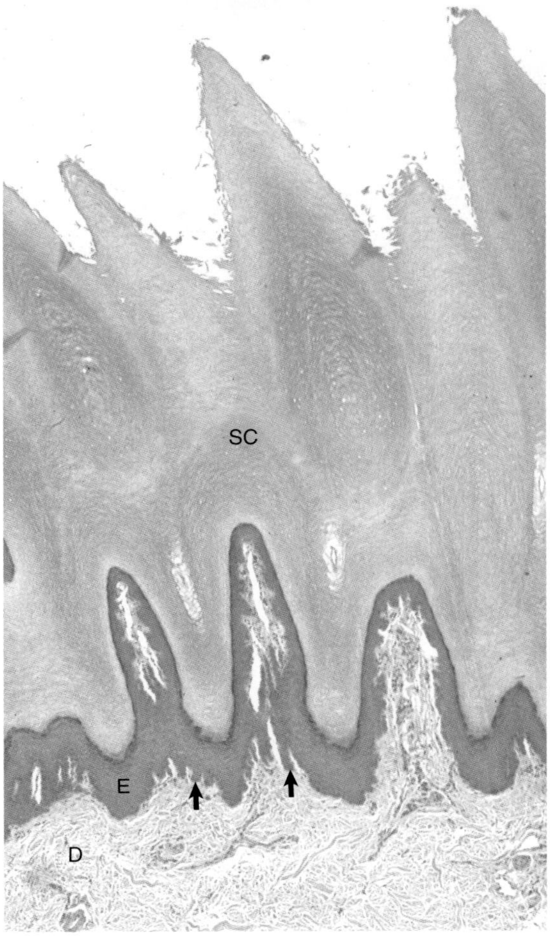

Fig. 17-2 Normal skin, hairless, pawpad, dog.
The epidermis *(E)* in hairless (nonhaired) skin has more numerous nucleated cell layers and more abundant stratum corneum than the epidermis in haired skin; thus it is referred to as "thick" skin. Note the dense zone of compact stratum corneum *(SC)* over the surface. The epidermis and dermal papillae in the superficial dermis *(D)* interdigitate to form rete ridges *(arrows)*. The rete ridges strengthen the attachment between the epidermis and dermis. In the dog, the contour of the epidermal surface follows the epidermal ridges and thus is papillated. H&E stain. (Courtesy Dr. Ann M. Hargis, DermatoDiagnostics.)

aspect of the Merkel cell. Merkel cells have granules that contain chemical mediators (met-enkephalin, vasoactive intestinal peptide, chromogranin A, acetylcholine, calcitonin gene-related peptide, neuron-specific enolase, and synaptophysin). The specific role or pathophysiologic mechanism that these chemical mediators have in nerve transduction or in paracrine influence of keratinocytes or hair follicle epithelial cells remains unknown. The origin of Merkel cells also remains unknown.

BASEMENT MEMBRANE ZONE

The epidermis and dermis are separated by a basement membrane. In hairless areas, such as the pawpads and nasal planum, this junction is irregular because of epidermal projections that interdigitate with dermal papillae (e.g., rete ridges/also known as rete pegs), thus strengthening the epidermal-dermal attachment by providing resistance to shearing. In densely haired areas, the junction is smoother and has an undulating appearance as the epidermal-dermal attachment is strengthened by the hair follicles. The more sparsely haired skin of pigs has more epidermal-dermal interdigitations (rete ridges) and fewer hair follicles. The basement membrane zone is composed of hemidesmosomes of basal cells (i.e., keratin intermediate filaments and attachment plaques), the lamina lucida (plasma membrane, subdesmosomal dense plate, and anchoring filaments), and the lamina densa (i.e., type IV collagen), which also serve to anchor the epidermis to dermis (Fig. 17-4). The importance of the basement membrane in anchoring function is noted in some immune-mediated diseases in which antibodies target, bind, and ultimately damage a component in the basement membrane and result in the formation of bullae (see the discussion on reactions characterized grossly by vesicles or bullae as the primary lesion and histologically by vesicles or bullae within the basement membrane [bullous dermatoses] section on Selected Autoimmune Reactions). The basement membrane zone also serves as a scaffold for migration of epidermal cells in wound healing and as an initial barrier to invasion of the dermis by neoplastic keratinocytes.

DERMIS

The dermis (corium), consisting of collagen and elastic fibers in a glycosaminoglycan ground substance, supports hair follicles, glands, vessels, and nerves. By convention, the dermis is generally

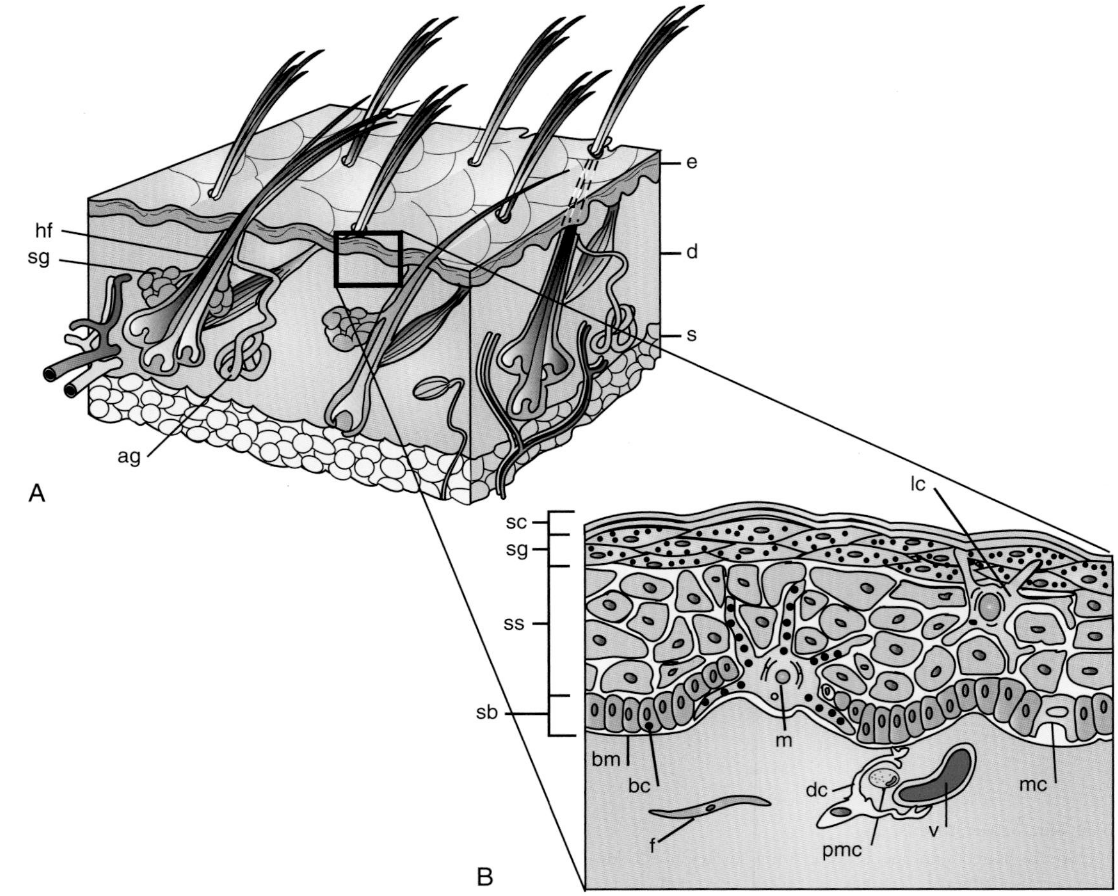

Fig. 17-3 Schematic diagram of the structure of the skin.
A, The skin is composed of epidermis *(e)*, dermis *(d)*, and subcutis *(s)*, with adnexa consisting of hair follicles *(hf)*, sebaceous glands *(sg)*, and apocrine glands *(ag)*. **B,** This projection of the epidermis demonstrates the progressive upward maturation of basal cells *(bc)* in the stratum basale *(sb)* through the stratum spinosum *(ss)*, stratum granulosum *(sg)* into the cornified squamous epithelial cells of the stratum corneum *(sc)*. Melanocytes *(m)*, midepidermal dendritic Langerhans' cells *(lc)*, and Merkel cells *(mc)* are also present. The subjacent dermis contains small vessels *(v)*, fibroblasts *(f)*, perivascular mast cells *(pmc)*, and dendrocytes *(dc)*, potentially important in dermal immunity and repair. (Adapted from Kumar V, Abbas AK, Fausto N, et al: *Robbins & Cotran pathologic basis of disease,* ed 8, Philadelphia, 2009, Saunders; Gawkrodger DJ: *Dermatology: an illustrated colour text,* ed 2, New York, 1997, Churchill Livingstone.)

subdivided into superficial and deep layers that blend together without a clear line of demarcation. The superficial dermis conforms to the contour of the epidermis and generally supports the upper portion of the hair follicle and sebaceous glands. It is composed of fine collagen fibers and is wider in the skin of cattle and horses than in the skin of dogs and cats. The deep dermis supports the lower portion of the hair follicle and apocrine glands and is composed of collagen bundles larger than those in the superficial dermis. Smooth muscle fibers of the arrector pili muscle attach the connective tissue sheath of the hair follicle to the epidermis and are responsible for causing the hair to stand erect. Skeletal muscle fibers from the cutaneous muscle extend into the lower dermis and are responsible for voluntary skin movement. Mast cells, lymphocytes, plasma cells, macrophages, and rarely eosinophils and neutrophils can be found in normal dermis. These cells are bone marrow derived–cells and arrive via the blood vascular system, thus they are typically concentrated around small superficial blood vessels.

VESSELS AND NERVES

Cutaneous arteries give rise to three vascular plexuses: deep, middle, and superficial. The deep plexus supplies the subcutis and deep portions of follicles and apocrine glands; the middle plexus supplies the sebaceous glands, midportion of follicles, and arrector pili muscles; and the superficial plexus supplies the superficial portions of follicles and epidermis. Lymph capillaries arise in the superficial dermis and connect with a subcutaneous plexus. The lymph vessels then converge to form larger channels that eventually reach peripheral lymph nodes.

The skin is an important sensory organ containing millions of microscopic nerve endings that perceive itch, pain, temperature, pressure, and touch (Fig. 17-5). The nerve endings consist of Meissner's corpuscles, pacinian corpuscles (Pacini's corpuscles), free sensory nerve endings, and mucocutaneous end organs (similar to Meissner's corpuscles but located in mucocutaneous skin). These nerve endings are minute, and the free sensory nerve endings are so delicate that they require special staining techniques, such as silver impregnation, to be visualized microscopically. The sensations of itch, pain, touch, temperature, and displacement of body hair are detected by the free sensory nerve endings. Itching, a form of mild pain that promotes the desire to scratch, is one of the most common reasons animals are presented to veterinarians. The sensations of touch and pressure are detected by Meissner's and Pacini's corpuscles. Sensations detected by free sensory nerve endings and by the corpuscles are transmitted to the spinal cord via the dorsal

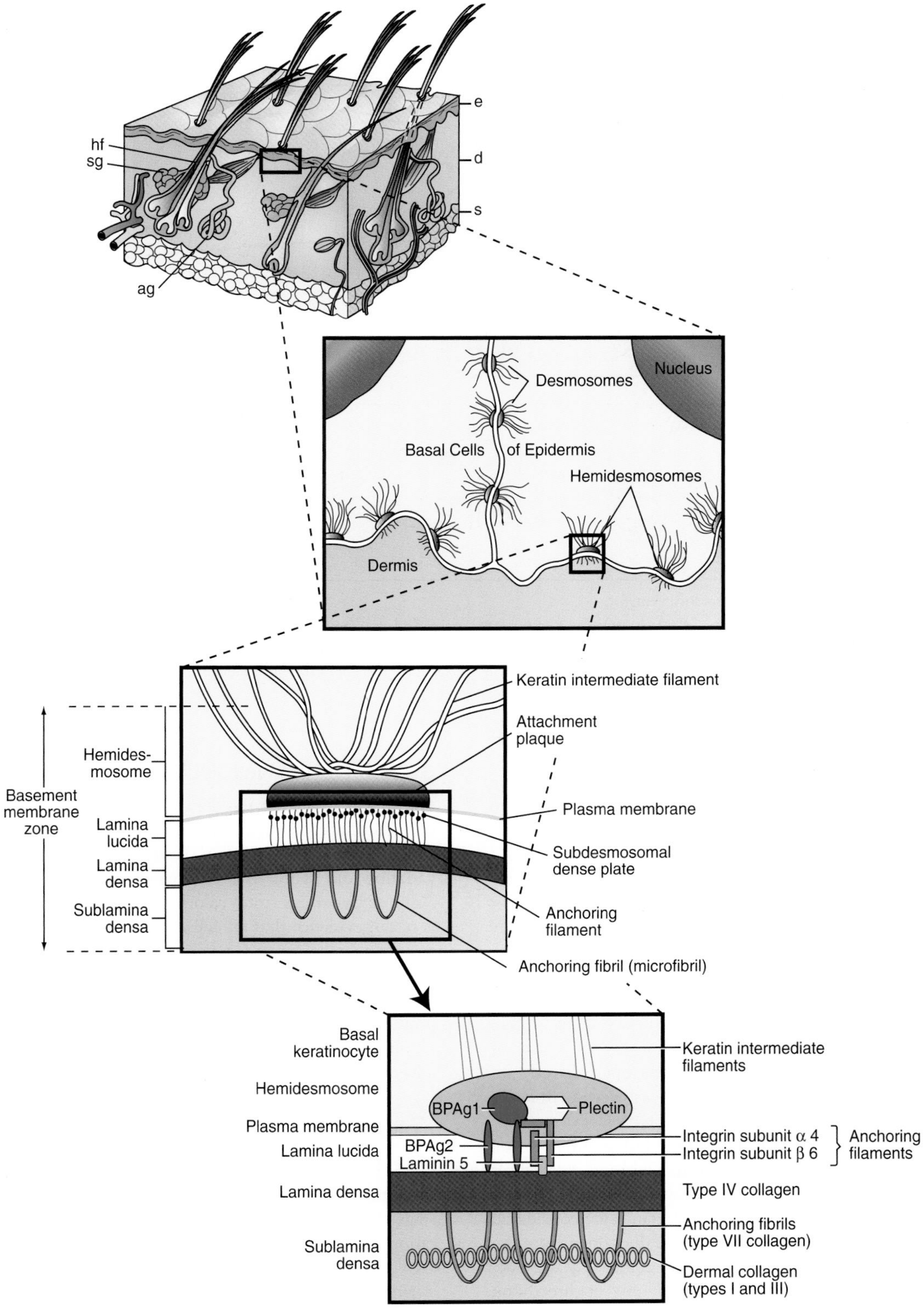

Fig. 17-4 Schematic diagram of basement membrane structure of the skin.
Keratinocytes attach to each other via desmosomes and to the basement membrane via hemidesmosomes. The projection of the basement membrane zone illustrates the multiple, interconnecting layers of this zone. The most superficial layer consists of the basal layer hemidesmosomes (keratin intermediate filaments and attachment plaques). The next layer, the lamina lucida, is an electron-lucent zone composed of the plasma membrane, subdesmosomal dense plate, and anchoring filaments. The deepest layer is the lamina densa, an electron-dense zone that consists of type IV collagen. Anchoring fibrils (type VII collagen), serve to attach the lamina densa and epidermis to the papillary dermis. The interconnecting layers of the basement membrane zone provide an important function in epidermal-dermal adherence, are the site of immune reactant deposition in cutaneous disease (see Table 17-11), and serve as a barrier to invasion by malignant epidermal tumors. *ag,* Apocrine glands; *d,* dermis; *e,* epidermis; *hf,* hair follicles; *s,* subcutis; *sg,* sebaceous glands. (Adapted from Kumar V, Abbas AK, Fausto N, et al: *Robbins & Cotran pathologic basis of disease,* ed 8, Philadelphia, 2009, Saunders; Rubin E, Farber JL: *Pathology,* ed 3, Philadelphia, 1999, Lippincott-Raven; and Elder DE: *Lever's histopathology of the skin,* ed 10, Philadelphia, 2009, Lippincott Williams & Wilkins.)

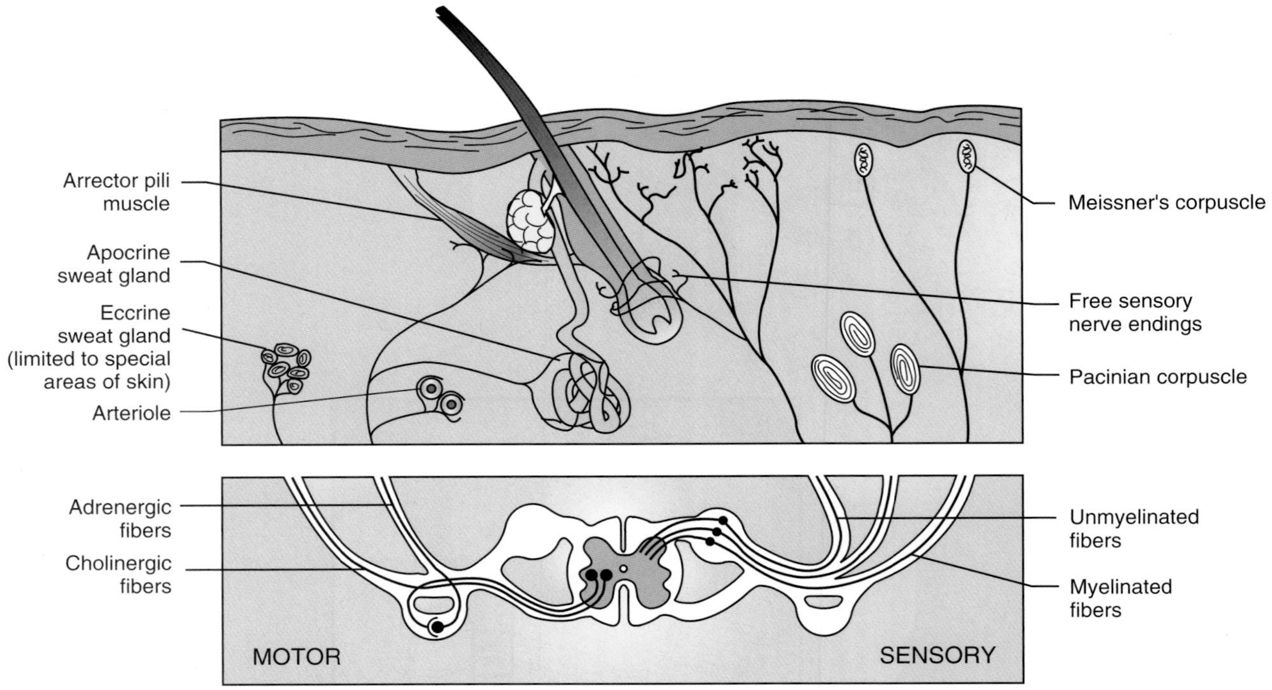

Fig. 17-5 Schematic diagram of cutaneous innervation.
Cutaneous nerve endings transmit sensations of touch, pressure, temperature, pain, and itch (pruritus) via dorsal root ganglia to the central nervous system. Motor fibers in skin are supplied by the autonomic nervous system. Adrenergic fibers activate arterioles, arrector pili muscles, and apocrine glands; cholinergic fibers stimulate eccrine glands. (Adapted from Ackerman AB: *Histologic diagnosis of inflammatory skin diseases,* Philadelphia, 1978, Lea and Febiger.)

root ganglia. Sensory fibers to the facial area are supplied by the trigeminal nerve. Motor fibers (adrenergic and cholinergic) are supplied by the sympathetic component of the autonomic nervous system (see Fig. 17-5). Adrenergic fibers travel from the spinal cord through postganglionic fibers in peripheral nerves and arborize into plexuses that innervate blood vessels, arrector pili muscles, and apocrine sweat glands. Stimulation by these adrenergic fibers causes vasoconstriction and piloerection (raising of the hair shafts). Cholinergic fibers travel from the spinal cord and arborize into plexuses that innervate the eccrine sweat glands. Stimulation of these fibers in humans causes widespread eccrine sweating, important in thermoregulation and recognized clinically as "beads of sweat" on the skin. Because the eccrine ducts open directly on the surface of the skin, the secretion is more easily seen clinically. This phenomenon does not occur in dogs or cats because they lack eccrine glands in haired skin. However, cholinergic and to a lesser degree adrenergic fiber stimulation in dogs and cats causes sweating of the eccrine glands of pawpads at times of excitement or agitation. In the haired skin, equine sweat glands are considered to be the epitrichial (apocrine) type, where the duct opens into the follicular canal near the skin surface, but less commonly the duct may open in a depression near the follicle opening or directly on the skin surface. As in humans, sweating in the horse is important in thermoregulation. However, the precise mechanisms that control sweating in the horse are unknown. The horse has a rich supply of vessels and nerves around sweat glands. It appears that equine sweat gland secretion is controlled by an interaction among neural, humoral, and paracrine factors. The only other domestic animal in which apocrine gland secretion is thought to play a thermoregulatory role is cattle, but sweating is not typically clinically visible except in horses.

SUBCUTIS (PANNICULUS, HYPODERMIS)

The subcutis attaches the dermis to subjacent muscle or bone and consists of adipose tissue and collagenous and elastic fibers, which provide flexibility. Adipose tissue insulates against temperature variation and in the case of pawpads, serves in shock absorption. Adipose tissue also stores calories as triglycerides. In addition, there is recent evidence that fat cells secrete via autocrine, paracrine, and endocrine mechanisms a variety of cytokines, chemokines, and hormone-like factors such as adiponectin, leptin, resistin, tumor necrosis factor-α (TNF-α), interleukin-6 (IL-6), and acute-phase proteins. These factors have been called *adipokines* and are thought to play a role in metabolism, and some may also contribute to adverse events associated with obesity.

ADNEXA

Hair Follicles

The growth of hair occurs within hair follicles in a sequence of stages (Fig. 17-6). These stages include hair genesis, growth, maturation, and loss. In the anagen stage of the hair cycle, mitotic activity and growth occur. The catagen stage is a transitional phase during which cellular proliferation ceases. The follicle then enters a resting stage, telogen, after which mitotic activity and new hair production resumes. The exogen stage is the phase in which the old hair is shed. In many animals hair follicle growth occurs in cycles, resulting in periodic loss or shedding of the hair coat. The reason the hair growth occurs in cycles is not clear. Some hypotheses include that the cycle provides the ability to: (1) shed fur to cleanse the body surface, (2) adapt and change body cover in response to changing environment (winter to summer) or social conditions, or (3) protect against malignant transformation that might occur in

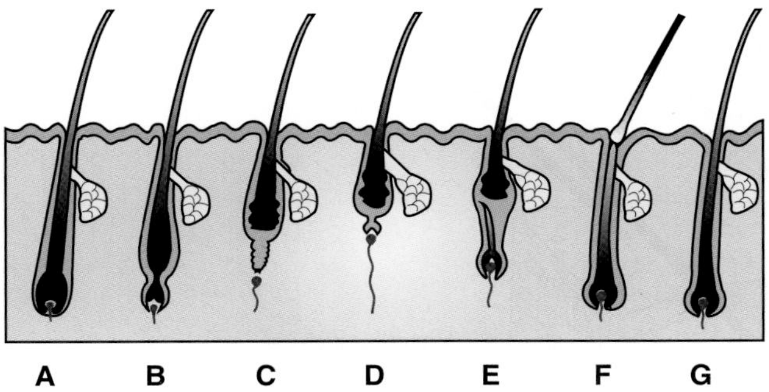

Fig. 17-6 Schematic diagram of the hair cycle.
A, Anagen. During this growing stage, hair is produced by mitosis in epithelial cells covering the apex of the follicular papilla (dermal papilla), which is enveloped by hair matrix cells at the hair bulb. **B,** Early catagen. In this transitional stage, a constriction occurs at the hair bulb, and the hair shaft above this becomes a "club hair." **C,** Catagen. The distal follicle becomes thick and corrugated and pushes the hair outward. **D,** Telogen. This is the resting stage in which the follicular papilla separates and an epithelial strand shortens to form a secondary germ. **E,** Early anagen. The secondary germ grows down to enclose the follicular papilla, and a new hair bulb forms. **F,** Exogen. This refers to the shedding of the old hair shaft. **G,** Anagen. The hair elongates as growth continues. Note that the anagen hair bulbs are located deeper in the dermis than the catagen and telogen hair bulbs. (Adapted from Scott DW, Miller WH Jr, Griffin CE: *Muller and Kirk's small animal dermatology,* ed 6, Philadelphia, 2001, Saunders.)

a rapidly dividing tissue. The regulation of hair cycling is exceedingly complex and incompletely understood. Factors that play a role include genetics, photoperiod, temperature, nutrition, hormones, health status, and neural mechanisms. Genetic factors determine the hair shaft length (e.g., short-haired versus long-haired breeds of dogs). The exact signals that control the hair cycle have not been identified; however, growth factors, such as epidermal growth factor, fibroblast growth factor (FGF), hepatocyte growth factor, platelet-derived growth factor (PDGF), transforming growth factor-β (TGF-β), and insulin-like growth factor (ILGF), have been localized to the skin and hair follicles. These growth factors probably play a crucial role in regulation of the hair cycle and follicle growth.

Photoperiod acts via the hypothalamus, pituitary, and pineal glands, which secrete tropic hormones, such as melatonin and the gonadal, thyroid, and adrenal hormones, that also influence hair growth. Some hormones, such as thyroid and growth hormone, stimulate hair growth, whereas excessive levels of estrogen or glucocorticoids suppress hair growth. The cells in the follicular papilla (sometimes called *dermal papilla*) regulate epithelial growth and are probably the target of the tropic hormones. Nutrition and health status have a significant influence on hair growth and quality. Hair is largely composed of protein. Thus diets low in protein or disease states associated with severe protein loss result in poor quality hair coat. Animals in poor health have larger numbers of hair follicles in telogen, and because telogen hairs are more easily shed than anagen hairs, animals in poor health tend to shed more heavily than healthy animals. Also, in disease states, cuticle formation can be defective, resulting in a dull or dry hair coat. It is also thought that the hair cycle is influenced by the nervous system. Evidence of such is implied by the abundant nerve supply of the hair follicle, the high density of Merkel cells in the hair follicle epithelium, and facts that keratinocytes express several neurotransmitter and neuropeptide receptors whose stimulation can alter keratinocyte proliferation and differentiation. Indirect influence by autonomic nerves could also be mediated by alteration of hair follicle blood flow and thus of oxygen and nutrient supply.

Forms of hair follicles vary in different animals (Fig. 17-7). Horses and cattle have evenly distributed simple follicles with one large (i.e., primary) follicle, usually with sebaceous and apocrine glands and arrector pili muscles. Pigs have simple follicles grouped in clusters. Goats, dogs, and cats have compound follicles that consist of primary follicles and smaller secondary follicles. Sheep have simple follicles in hair-growing areas and compound follicles in wool-growing areas. Primary follicles have the hair bulb rooted more deeply in the dermis than secondary follicles. The depth of the hair bulbs varies with species. In dogs and cats, the anagen hair bulbs of primary follicles are at the dermal-subcutaneous junction, whereas in horses and cattle the anagen hair bulbs are in the mid-dermis. In all species, the bases of telogen follicles are more superficially located than the bases of anagen follicles. Typically, primary and secondary hair shafts emerge through a common follicular opening. Tactile hairs include sinus and tylotrich hairs. Sinus hairs, also termed *vibrissae,* arise in simple follicles with a blood-filled sinus located between the inner and outer layers of the dermal sheath. Sinus hairs generally occur on the nose, above the eyes, on the lips and throat, and on the palmar aspect of the carpus of cats. Sinus hairs function as mechanoreceptors (i.e., touch receptors). Tylotrich hairs also function as mechanoreceptors and are scattered among the regular body hairs. The arrector pili muscles extend from the connective tissue sheath of the hair follicles at the junction of the middle and inferior portion of the follicle and attach to the superficial dermis. The arrector pili smooth muscles are oriented almost perpendicularly to the wall of the follicle and are well developed on the back of animals, especially dogs. Muscle contraction causes erection of hairs and expression of the contents of sebaceous glands.

Sweat Glands

There are two basic types of sweat glands: apocrine glands and eccrine glands. Apocrine glands are located throughout haired areas of skin in domestic animals and are tubular- or saccular-coiled glands (see Fig. 17-7). The ducts of the apocrine glands open in the superficial portion of the hair follicle; thus these glands are also called *epitrichial glands.* The glands are lined by secretory cuboidal to low columnar epithelium surrounded by contractile myoepithelial cells. Other apocrine glands include the interdigital glands of small ruminants, glands of the external ear canal and eyelids of domestic animals, anal sac glands of dogs and cats, and the mental organ of pigs. Eccrine glands are merocrine in secretion and in contrast to ducts of apocrine glands, the ducts open directly onto the surface of the epidermis. Thus eccrine glands are also called *atrichial glands.* They are tubular glands lined by cuboidal epithelium surrounded by myoepithelium and are confined mainly to pawpads of dogs and cats, frog region of ungulates, carpus of pigs, and nasolabial region of ruminants and pigs.

Sebaceous Glands

Sebaceous glands are simple, branched, or compound alveolar glands that undergo holocrine secretion, with ducts opening into hair follicles except at some mucocutaneous junctions where the glands open on the surface of the skin (e.g., meibomian gland/also known as tarsal gland). Well-developed sebaceous glands are found in the supracaudal gland of dogs and cats; infraorbital, inguinal, and interdigital regions of sheep; the base of the horn of goats; the anal sac glands of cats; the preputial glands of horses; and the submental organ of cats.

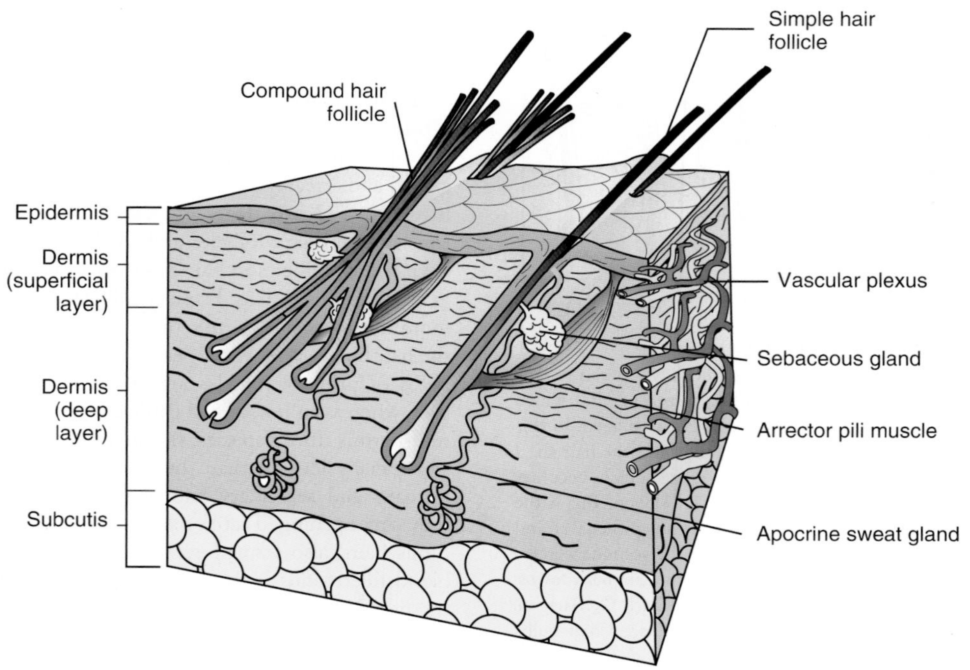

Fig. 17-7 Schematic diagram of the skin and simple and compound hair follicles.
For the purpose of simplification, the vascular supply is illustrated on one face only. Note the simple hair follicle *(right)* and the compound hair follicle *(left)*. Simple follicles consist of one large primary follicle with the hair bulb in the dermis or subcutis (depth varies with species), and with sebaceous and apocrine glands, and arrector pili muscles. Compound follicles consist of a large primary follicle and smaller secondary follicles. The hair bulbs of secondary follicles are located more superficially in the dermis than the hair bulbs of primary follicles. Secondary follicles may have sebaceous glands but lack apocrine glands and arrector pili muscles. (From Dellman DH, Brown EM: *Textbook of veterinary histology,* ed 3, Philadelphia, 1987, Lea and Febiger.)

Specialized Structures

Anal sacs are specialized cutaneous structures that are especially prone to develop lesions. Anal sacs are bilateral diverticula located between internal and external anal sphincter muscles in dogs and cats and have ducts that open onto the anus at the level of the anocutaneous junction. Ducts and sacs are lined by stratified squamous epithelium. In cats, the sac wall has sebaceous and apocrine glands, but in dogs, the wall has only apocrine glands. The anal sacs can become distended with secretory products, rupture after trauma, and cause bacterial infection and chronic inflammation (foreign body reaction) in contiguous tissues. Carcinomas of the apocrine gland of the anal sac in dogs are often associated with tumor cell production of parathyroid hormone-related protein (PTHrP) and humoral hypercalcemia of malignancy.

Hepatoid (i.e., circumanal or perianal) glands occur most commonly in the skin around the anus and are also present in skin near the prepuce, tail, flank, and groin. These glands are modified sebaceous gland that have nonpatent ducts and are composed of peripheral reserve cells that surround lobules of differentiated cells resembling hepatocytes, resulting in the name "hepatoid" glands. Adenomas of the perianal glands in male dogs are often testosterone dependent.

The claws of dogs and cats shield the third phalanx and consist of a wall (i.e., dorsal and lateral sides) and sole (i.e., ventral side), both of which are stratified squamous keratinizing epithelium. The wall consists of hard keratin and the sole of softer keratin. The dermis of the claw consists of dense collagen, elastic tissue, and blood vessels that can bleed profusely if the claw is trimmed too short. The claw fold is a fold of skin that covers the wall laterally and dorsally for a short distance. Hooves consist of the wall, sole, and frog in solipeds; and a wall, sole, and prominent bulb in ruminants and pigs. The hoof wall comprises three structurally distinct layers (i.e., stratum externum, stratum medium, and stratum internum), which are formed by the proliferation and downward movement of epidermal cells arising from a specialized junction of the epidermis and dermis, a region known as the *coronary band* or *coronet.* The stratum internum of the inner hoof wall interdigitates with the dermal lamina of the corium, thereby anchoring the inner hoof wall to the dermis that covers the third phalanx. If the attachment of the stratum internum to the dermal lamina fails, the shearing forces of body weight and movement lead to vascular damage in this region and ultimate damage to the corium of the sole and coronet. The separation of the third phalanx from the inner hoof wall is the primary pathologic process leading to the painful condition of laminitis most often seen in horses and cattle.

The digital pads of dogs and cats have a thick epidermis composed of all layers, including the stratum lucidum. The surface is covered by compacted layers of stratum corneum and is smooth in the cat; however, in the dog, the surface is covered by conical papillae that conform to the outline of the epidermal surface (see Fig. 17-2). The epidermis and dermis interdigitate via rete ridges and dermal papillae, thus providing resistance to shear forces. Eccrine (atrichial) glands are present in the dermis and the adipose tissue. Lobules of adipose tissue that act as a cushion are subdivided by collagenous stroma and elastic tissue.

The chestnuts and ergots of the horse are considered to be vestiges of the first, second, and fourth digits. Chestnuts are located in the supracarpal and tarsal area on the medial surface of the limbs, and the ergot is located at the flexion of the fetlocks

BOX 17-1 Functions of the Skin

Provides a protective barrier against fluid loss, microbiologic agents, chemicals, and physical injury
Regulates temperature and blood pressure
Produces vitamin D
Acts as sensory organ
Stores nutrients
Absorptive surface
Participates in innate and adaptive immunity and inflammation and repair

(metacarpophalangeal articulation). Chestnuts and ergots are histologically similar and consist of compact stratum corneum covering thick cellular layers of the epidermis. The rete ridges are long and interdigitate with long dermal papillae.

FUNCTION

The skin is not only the largest organ in the body, but one of the most important. Without the skin, terrestrial mammalian life could not exist. The skin has numerous functions, which are listed in Box 17-1. The skin prevents significant loss of fluid and electrolytes (e.g., the stratum corneum barrier), protects against physical and chemical injury (e.g., the stratum corneum barrier, keratin filaments, desmosomal and hemidesmosomal junctions, collagen, and elastic fibers), participates in temperature and blood pressure regulation (e.g., the hair coat, sweat glands, and vascular supply), produces vitamin D (e.g., ultraviolet [UV] light photolysis of dehydrocholesterol), serves as a sensory organ (e.g., tactile hairs, Merkel cells, and nerves), and stores fat, water, vitamins, carbohydrates, protein, and other nutrients (e.g., subcutaneous fat). Absorption, although not a primary function, also occurs. In addition, the keratinocyte, a major source of cytokines and antimicrobial peptides, is now considered to be an integral part of the innate and adaptive immune systems protecting against microbial injury and participating in inflammation and tissue repair.

PORTALS OF ENTRY

Normal intact skin has many natural defenses and barriers that render it impenetrable to most organisms and protect the body from a variety of other types of insults that include pressure, friction, mild mechanical trauma, temperature extremes, UV light exposure, and chemical absorption.

The route by which an infectious agent gains entry into the body is called the *portal of entry* (Box 17-2). Many pathogens can only cause disease when entering the body via their specific portal of entry. A few pathogens, such as hookworm larvae, are able to penetrate intact normally functioning skin. Dermatophytes are able to colonize the cornified structures (hair, claws) and the stratum corneum and cause disease without ever entering living tissue. Clinical disease in a dermatophyte infection is the result of the host's reaction to the organism and its by-products. The skin only becomes an efficient portal of entry for microorganisms when the barrier is damaged by trauma, excessive moisture, heat or cold, or by disruption of the normal flora of the integument. A number of microorganisms (e.g., *Staphylococcus intermedius, Streptococcus* sp., *Corynebacterium pseudotuberculosis, Pasteurella* sp., *Proteus* sp., *Pseudomonas* sp., and *Escherichia coli*) gain entrance to the body by either entering through natural pores, such as hair follicles or glands with ducts that traverse the epidermis, or by the parenteral route, which includes all types of breaks in the skin, including injections, insect bites, and other types of wounds. Organisms that are able to inhabit hair follicles, such as mites or bacteria, gain entry to the body when the wall of the follicle is ruptured, leading to emptying of follicular contents into the dermis. Similarly, rupture of glands or ducts can lead to entry of microorganisms. From here, infectious agents can stimulate a robust host immune response or possibly spread to other areas of the body by gaining entry to the bloodstream or traveling to regional and distant lymph nodes via lymph flow.

BOX 17-2 Portals of Entry into the Skin

EPIDERMIS
Absorption through stratum corneum and epidermis
Penetrating trauma, including injection from exterior
Penetration of ultraviolet or γ-radiation
Direct contact with heat, cold, irritants, caustic substances, and microbiologic agents

ADNEXA
Penetration through follicular openings
Rupture of follicle, gland, or other structure (anal sac)

DERMIS AND PANNICULUS
Vessels (Hematogenous)
Drugs or toxins
Localization within capillary beds
Embolism
Leukocyte trafficking

Nerves
Migration from ganglion along sensory nerves via axonal flow to epithelial cells

SUPPORT STRUCTURES
Penetrating trauma from bone fracture
Extension of tumor or infection from adjacent lymph node, gland, muscle, or bone

Intact skin with its waterproof barrier provides some protection against weak acids and alkali substances and water-soluble compounds, but certain lipid-soluble compounds can be absorbed directly through intact skin as can some artificially engineered gases developed for chemical warfare. UV radiation (UVR) can damage the skin by direct exposure if the body's natural defenses, such as the hair coat and melanin pigments, are not present or are inadequate. The lesions of solar (actinic) dermatitis (see the section on Disorders of Physical, Radiation, or Chemical Injury: Solar (Actinic) Dermatosis, Keratosis, and Neoplasia) typify the effects of chronic exposure to UVR. In addition to solar dermatitis, squamous cell carcinomas, hemangiomas, and hemangiosarcomas have an increased tendency to develop in skin chronically damaged by UVR.

The dermal capillaries can be a portal of entry to the skin via the hematogenous route. Embolization of infectious agents, such as bacteria (*Erysipelothrix rhusiopathiae* [diamond skin disease]) or fungi (systemic infection with *Blastomyces dermatitidis*) can damage the skin via this route during hematogenous dissemination. Tumor cells (hemangiosarcoma) can also embolize to the skin and lead to metastatic tumor foci or possible cutaneous infarction. The hematogenous route is also most often the delivery system for drugs (adverse cutaneous reactions to the administration of trimethoprim-potentiated sulfonamides; photosensitization dermatitis that occurs with phenothiazine ingestion) and toxins (gangrenous ergotism caused by the mycotoxin of *Claviceps purpurea*) to reach the skin.

Rarely, an infectious agent that is neurotropic can migrate from a ganglion along sensory nerves via axonal flow to the skin (reactivation of feline herpesvirus 1 (FHV-1) infection in cats resulting in ulcerative facial dermatitis). The skin can also be secondarily infected or traumatized or damaged by extension of pathologic processes affecting adjacent support structures such as bone, muscle, lymph nodes, or glands (locally invasive mammary gland carcinoma resulting in cutaneous ulceration).

DEFENSE MECHANISMS

The skin is a complex organ composed of many integrated components structurally and functionally designed to protect the host. Host defenses against injury principally consist of three broad mechanisms: (1) physical defense, (2) immunologic defense, and (3) repair mechanisms. The most critical defense is the barrier derived from the more superficial layers of the skin, which include the stratum corneum, epidermis, basement membrane, and superficial dermis. Without these outer layers of the skin, animals cannot survive (consider, for example, the deleterious effects of extensive burns and immune-mediated diseases such as pemphigus vulgaris). One of the most important cells in the skin is the keratinocyte. The keratinocytes terminally differentiate to form the stratum corneum, the outermost barrier of the skin. The keratinocytes produce keratin filaments, desmosomes, and hemidesmosomes, providing structural integrity to the cytoplasm and an interconnecting network that anchors the keratinocytes to each other and the basement membrane. Keratinocytes produce cytokines (including IL-1, IL-6, IL-8, IL-3, TNF-α, colony-stimulating factors) and growth factors (including TGF-α, TGF-β, PDGF, FGF), thus participating in innate and adaptive immunity and in the communication between the two. Keratinocytes also dissolve desmosomes and hemidesmosomes and form actin filaments so they can migrate to cover skin wounds and then proliferate to regenerate the wounded skin. Keratinocytes thus not only orchestrate the activities of the skin but also serve as many members of the orchestra.

PHYSICAL DEFENSE MECHANISMS

Barrier Functions

Barriers of the skin against physical injury are listed in Box 17-3. The hair coat, particularly the long dense hair coat of some dogs and cats, serves as a physical barrier to temperature extremes, UVR, and minor trauma. The hair coat also sheds water as a result of the lipids provided by sebaceous gland secretion. Vibrissae, or tactile hairs, and sensory neurons provide awareness of the physical environment, allowing the animal to make appropriate reactions for survival such as reflex responses to heat and other noxious stimuli. Claws, especially on cats, serve as a quite effective barrier against predators by providing traction for climbing and serve as weapons to be used against aggressors. Horns of cattle, sheep, and goats also provide some physical defense capabilities.

The stratum corneum is an exceedingly important component of the barrier, imparting protection from the exterior and preventing water loss from the interior. The stratum corneum is composed largely of keratins, a family of proteins called *intermediate filaments.* Keratin proteins are the major structural proteins of the skin, hair, and claws. The stratum corneum is considered to be the "bricks and mortar" of the barrier. The bricks are the flattened cornified cells (corneocytes) with their resistant cell envelopes and keratin microfibrils, and the mortar consists of intercorneocyte lipids.

The bricks are formed at the level of the stratum granulosum when the keratinocytes are transformed into the flattened corneocytes. The transformation occurs when (1) the nucleus is digested, (2) the keratin intermediate filaments aggregate into microfibrils oriented parallel to the skin surface, (3) the lipids are released into the intercellular space, and (4) the cell membrane is replaced by a resilient cell envelope consisting of cross-linked protein with lipids covalently bound to its surface. Filaggrin (which is an acronym for filament-aggregating protein) from the keratohyalin granules in the stratum granulosum plays a significant role in formation of the bricks by participating in the aggregation of keratin filaments into tight bundles. The keratin intermediate filaments and filaggrin compose 80% to 90% of the protein mass of the epidermis. Later, filaggrin is digested by proteolytic enzymes to produce components of amino acids that form the "natural moisturizing factor" of the stratum corneum, which serves to help maintain hydration, flexibility, and proper desquamation. Concurrent with the aggregation of the keratin filaments, the resistant cornified envelope is transformed from the water-permeable phospholipid cell membrane of the keratinocyte when the membrane-bound enzymes (e.g., transglutaminases), cross-link proteins from the keratohyalin granules (e.g., loricrin) and the cytoplasm (e.g., involucrin) in isopeptide bonds. Other proteins (including trichohyalin and small proline-rich proteins) are similarly cross-linked and eventually the entire

BOX 17-3 Host Defense Mechanisms Against Injury: Physical Defense Mechanisms

BARRIER FUNCTIONS

Hair follicles: Physical and thermal
Tactile hairs and neurons: Sensory
Claws and horns: Physical defense
Stratum corneum: Barrier function
Adnexal glandular secretions: Barrier function
Apocrine glands horses and cattle: Defense against excessive heat
Melanin: Defense against ultraviolet radiation
Basement membrane zone: Filter to macromolecules, and barrier to invasion of neoplastic epidermal cells
Panniculus: Barrier against temperature extremes

RESISTANCE TO MECHANICAL FORCES

Hair follicles and epidermal-dermal interdigitations: Anchor epidermis to dermis
Stratum corneum: Corneocyte, corneocyte envelope, and intercellular lipid adhesion
Desmosomes and hemidesmosomes: Intercellular and basement membrane adhesion
Basement membrane: Anchors epidermis to dermis
Collagen and elastic tissue: Resilience, strength, and support of adnexa
Panniculus: Shock absorption, facilitates movement, anchors dermis to fascia

cell membrane consists of cross-linked proteins. The proteins of the cornified envelope compose 7% to 10% of the protein mass of the epidermis. The corneocytes are joined together by desmosomes that are modified from those joining keratinocytes in lower layers of the epidermis by the addition of a protein called corneodesmosine. These stratum corneum desmosomes are referred to as *corneodesmosomes.*

The mortar is formed when lipids, from the lamellar bodies in the stratum granulosum, are released into the intercellular space. These intercorneocyte lipids (glycosyl ceramides, cholesterol, cholesterol esters, and long-chain fatty acids) are hydrophobic and prevent transepidermal water loss. Lamellar bodies have other important functions: (1) they provide enzymes that generate ceramides and free fatty acids that are incorporated into the lipid membranes; (2) they provide proteases and antiproteases that regulate digestion of corneodesmosomes and shedding of cornified cells to the exterior; and (3) they secrete antimicrobial peptides including defensins into the intercellular compartment of the stratum corneum. The lipid component of the stratum corneum surrounds the protein component to which it is covalently bound and provides adhesion of the cornified cells (i.e., bricks) to the intercellular lipids (i.e., mortar). Layers of the corneocytes and their corneocyte envelope (i.e., bricks), and intercellular lipids (i.e., mortar) form a tough and resilient protective barrier. The waterproofing and repellency of the stratum corneum is in part provided by the keratinocyte and sebum-derived lipids.

Other barrier functions of the skin include defense against antioxidant injury provided by vitamin E in sebaceous gland secretion and defense against UV light provided by the hair coat and also by melanin pigment in keratinocytes. The cap of melanin pigment over the nucleus helps protect the nucleus (and its nucleic acid) against UV light–induced injury by scattering and absorbing UV light rays. The basement membrane zone serves as an initial barrier to invasion of the dermis by neoplastic epidermal cells. The panniculus through its insulating properties serves as a barrier against cold temperatures. Secretion from apocrine glands in cattle and horses provides defense against excessive heat.

Resistance to Mechanical Forces

Anatomic features of the skin that provide resistance to physical injury are listed in Box 17-3. Hair follicles help anchor the epidermis to the dermis, as do epidermal-dermal interdigitations, thus these interdigitations are most numerous in nasal planum and pawpad where hair follicles are absent and resistance to shearing force is necessary. Host defense against mechanical injury is also provided by the tightly bundled keratin filaments of the corneocyte, the resilience of the cornified envelope, the adhesion of the cornified envelope and intercellular lipids, and the corneodesmosomes. In addition, the keratinocytes contain keratin filaments and form desmosomal junctions with adjacent cells (see Fig. 17-4). The keratin filaments perform a structural role (i.e., cytoskeletal) in the cells, and the desmosomes promote adhesion of epidermal cells and resistance to mechanical stresses. The basement membrane anchors the epidermis to the dermis via hemidesmosomes providing structural integrity against trauma. Dermal collagen and elastic tissue provide resilience and strength to the skin and support for the vessels, nerves, and adnexa. The panniculus protects against surface trauma by providing some shock absorption (e.g., pawpads), by facilitating movement, and by anchoring the dermis to fascia. Thus the various components of the epidermis, dermis, adnexa, and panniculus provide a flexible interconnecting framework to protect the host against mechanical injury.

IMMUNOLOGIC DEFENSE MECHANISMS

Innate Immunity

Information on this topic, including Web Table 17-1 and Web Fig. 17-1, is available at evolve.elsevier.com/Zachary/McGavin/.

Acquired (Adaptive) Immunity

Information on this topic, including Web Table 17-2, is available at evolve.elsevier.com/Zachary/McGavin/.

Disease Example of Barrier Dysfunction

Information on this topic, including Web Figs. 17-2 and 17-3, is available at evolve.elsevier.com/Zachary/McGavin/.

REGENERATION AND REPAIR

Information on this topic, including Web Box 17-1 and Web Fig. 17-4, is available at evolve.elsevier.com/Zachary/McGavin/.

Healing of Wounds with Opposed Edges

Information on this topic is available at evolve.elsevier.com/Zachary/McGavin/.

Healing of Wounds with Separated Edges

Information on this topic is available at evolve.elsevier.com/Zachary/McGavin/.

RESPONSES TO INJURY

A PRIMER TO HISTOLOGIC PATTERNS

A number of "new" terms commonly used to classify diseases of the skin are used throughout this chapter. For convenience and to provide quick reference, these terms are listed online in Web Glossary 17-1. Although there are many new terms to learn, it should be realized that the system used to form these terms is similar to that used for other anatomic systems. Basically, prefixes and suffixes are added to word roots to create specific terms that define the pathology of the skin. For example, the prefix "epi" (meaning on or above) combined with the word root "dermat(o)" (referring to skin) creates the word "epidermis," which simply means the portion of the skin above the dermis. Likewise, the term *hypodermis* refers to the portion of the skin below the dermis, also called the *subcutis* or *panniculus.* Suffixes are used in the same way. For example, the suffix "itis" (meaning inflammation) combined with the word root "dermat(o)" forms the word "dermatitis," which simply means inflammation of the skin. Similarly, terms referring to inflammation predominantly within the epidermis, follicles, or the panniculus are epidermitis, folliculitis, and panniculitis, respectively. The suffix "osis" refers to a disease process, often noninflammatory. Thus combining dermat(o) and osis forms the word "dermatosis," which means any disease of the skin, especially one not characterized by inflammation. Dermatoses are the plural of dermatosis and thus mean noninflammatory skin diseases.

Numerous endogenous and exogenous factors can potentially cause injury of the skin (Fig. 17-8). Determining a definitive diagnosis of a skin disorder depends on obtaining a complete history, including age, breed, and sex of the animal; conducting a thorough physical examination, paying particular attention to the distribution of skin lesions; and performing additional diagnostic tests, such as skin scrapings, surface cytology, a complete blood count, serum chemistry panel, skin biopsy sampling, and microbiologic cultures. Results from cutaneous biopsy sampling are often useful and can be necessary to establish a definitive diagnosis for skin diseases. Although the skin has a limited range of responses to injury, the distribution and types of inflammatory cells in the lesion often represent a recognizable pattern that can be used to (1) formulate a list of specific etiologic agents that could cause the lesion or (2) suggest categories of disease with similar lesions and a common pathogenesis. Algorithms (i.e., a set of directions for accomplishing some task that has a recognizable endpoint) have been developed for the recognition of histopathologic patterns in veterinary dermatopathology (Table 17-1). Recognition of patterns, both clinically and histologically, can facilitate differential diagnoses of skin disease (Table 17-2). Patterns of responses to injury are illustrated by changes in the epidermis, dermis, adnexa, and panniculus and are discussed in the next sections.

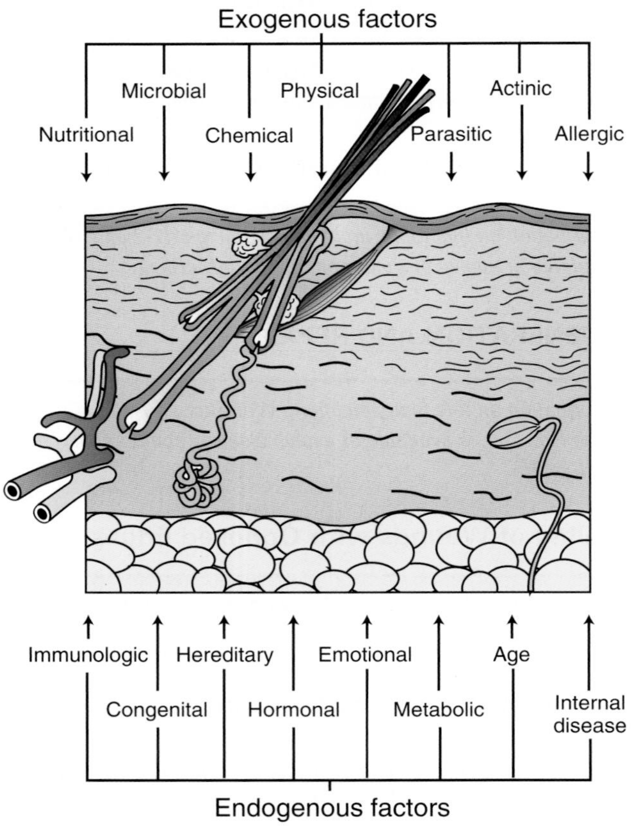

Fig. 17-8 Schematic diagram of the exogenous and endogenous factors that influence the skin.

A myriad of exogenous and endogenous factors influence the gross and microscopic appearance of the skin. Because the skin can respond to these factors in a limited number of ways, different skin disorders may have a similar appearance. Identification of the cause of a skin disorder therefore often requires not only histopathologic evaluation but also clinical history, including clinical lesion distribution and appearance. (Redrawn from Dr. Ann M. Hargis, DermatoDiagnostics.)

Responses of the Epidermis to Injury

Alterations in Epidermal Growth or Differentiation

The basal cells (i.e., basal keratinocytes) in their postmitotic state migrate outward from the basal layer, eventually forming the cornified layers (stratum corneum) of the epidermis. In the normal epidermis, balance is established between the rate of proliferation of the basal cells (germinal cells) and the rate of loss of differentiated cells (squamous epithelial cells) from the surface, resulting in the constant thickness of the epidermis and each of the layers. The orderly proliferation, differentiation, and cornification of epidermal cells is regulated by cytokines (e.g., epidermal growth factor, FGFs, ILGFs, ILs, and TNF), hormones (e.g., cortisol and vitamin D_3), and nutritional factors such as protein, zinc, copper, fatty acids, and vitamin A and B vitamins. The cytokines that regulate keratinocyte growth and differentiation are produced by a variety of cell types in the skin, including endothelial cells, leukocytes, fibroblasts, and keratinocytes. Thus keratinocytes also have a self-regulatory role (i.e., autocrine) in their growth and differentiation, and inflammatory cells, among others, can influence keratinocyte growth and differentiation.

Disorders of Cornification

Disorders of cornification (i.e., alterations in the formation of the stratum corneum) can be primary, such as in primary seborrhea, but more often are secondary to a variety of factors such as inflammation, trauma, or metabolic or nutritional disorders. A disorder

TABLE 17-1 Examples of Pattern Diagnosis in the Skin

Component of Skin	Reaction to Injury	Pattern	Disease Examples
Epidermis	Prominent hyperkeratosis	Hyperkeratotic diseases of the epidermis	Primary seborrhea Ichthyosis Vitamin A deficiency Callus
Dermis	Interface inflammation	Interface dermatitis	Lupus erythematosus Dermatomyositis
Follicle	Inflammation of the follicular lumen	Luminal folliculitis	Infection with staphylococci, dermatophytes
Panniculus	Predominantly neutrophilic inflammation	Neutrophilic panniculitis	Abscess Feline pansteatitis (early)

A pattern consists of two parts: a component of the skin (e.g., epidermis) + a histologic reaction of that component to injury (e.g., hyperkeratosis) = pattern (hyperkeratotic diseases of the epidermis).

TABLE 17-2 Differential Diagnoses of Selected Patterns that Can Be Recognized Clinically and Histologically

Pustules Crusts (epidermal)	Vesicles Bullae (epidermal to subepidermal)	Necrosis or ulceration (epidermal)	Scaling or other hyperkeratotic lesions* (epidermal)	Nodules ± draining tracts (dermal and pannicular)	Alopecia (adnexal)	Hypopigmentation or depigmentation (epidermal)
DISORDERS						
Superficial bacterial infection	Pemphigus vulgaris	Vasculitis/infarction	Primary seborrhea	Masses caused by deep infections with bacteria, fungi, algae, *Pythium,* migratory parasites (e.g., abscesses, actinomycosis, feline leprosy, mycetoma, blastomycosis, pythiosis, habronemiasis)	Folliculitis: infectious/noninfectious	Vitiligo
Pemphigus foliaceous and panepidermal pustular pemphigus	Paraneoplastic pemphigus	Chemical and thermal burns	Ichthyosis	"Sterile" nodular inflammation (e.g., foreign body reactions, histiocytosis, sterile pyogranuloma, xanthoma, venomous bites, injection site reactions, eosinophilic granulomas)	Postinflammatory and posttraumatic	Uveodermatologic syndrome
Dermatophilosis	Lupus erythematosus	Superficial necrolytic dermatitis	Zinc responsive dermatosis	Panniculitis/steatitis	Endocrine alopecia	Lupus erythematosus
Exudative epidermitis	Dermatomyositis	Erythema multiforme	Sebaceous adenitis	Neoplasms	Idiopathic flank alopecia	Copper deficiency
Subcorneal pustular dermatosis	Subepidermal bullous dermatoses	Stevens-Johnson syndrome	Ear margin seborrhea		Telogen effluvium	Alopecia areata (healing stage)
Pawpads*	Drug reactions	Toxic epidermal necrolysis	Vitamin A responsive dermatosis		Anagen effluvium	Inherited disorders (Chédiak-Higashi syndrome, Maltese and other coat color dilutions)
Pemphigus foliaceous	Chemical and thermal burns	Ergot/fescue grass toxicity	Feline exfoliative dermatosis and thymoma		Postclipping alopecia	Waardenburg-like syndrome
Superficial necrolytic dermatitis	Photosensitization	Frostbite	Callus		Follicular dysplasia	Piebaldism
Lupus erythematosus	Viral diseases	Feline indolent ulcer	Cutaneous horn		Congenital alopecia and hypotrichosis	Albinism
		Feline ulcerative dermatosis syndrome	Solar (actinic) dermatitis		Feline psychogenic alopecia	Cyclic hematopoiesis
		Vesicular cutaneous lupus erythematosus			Poor nutrition with protein deficiency	Contact with rubber
		Self-trauma			Feline paraneoplastic alopecia	
		Epitheliogenesis imperfecta				

Some of these disorders could be placed in different patterns. For instance, disorders characterized by vesicles or bullae may develop into an ulcerative pattern after the vesicles or bullae rupture.
*Hyperkeratotic disorders may also affect the nasal planum and pawpads; see Box 17-11.

of cornification called *hyperkeratosis* is characterized by an increase in the thickness of the stratum corneum and occurs in two forms: orthokeratotic and parakeratotic hyperkeratosis. In orthokeratotic hyperkeratosis (also referred to as hyperkeratosis), squamous epithelial cells are anuclear, and in parakeratotic hyperkeratosis (also referred to as parakeratosis), the squamous epithelial cells have nuclei. Subtypes of hyperkeratosis include basket weave (exaggerated undulating pattern of layers of the normal stratum corneum), compact (compacted layers of basket weave stratum corneum), and laminated (layers of stratum corneum that are more linear and less undulating). Both parakeratosis and hyperkeratosis are common nonspecific responses to chronic stimuli (e.g., superficial trauma, inflammation, or sun exposure) and also occur as primary lesions. For example, hyperkeratosis is a feature of the cornification disorder, primary seborrhea, of the cocker spaniel (Fig. 17-9), ichthyosis, and vitamin A deficiency. Diffuse parakeratosis is a feature of zinc-responsive dermatosis and superficial necrolytic dermatopathy (hepatocutaneous syndrome) (Fig. 17-10). Hyperkeratosis and parakeratosis can be accompanied by alterations in the thickness of the granular cell layer (stratum granulosum). Generally, hyperkeratosis is associated with an increased thickness of the granular cell layer (hypergranulosis), and parakeratosis is associated with a decreased thickness of the granular cell layer (hypogranulosis).

Epidermal Hyperplasia

Epidermal hyperplasia is an alteration in epidermal growth or differentiation characterized by an increase in the number of cells within the epidermis, most often within the stratum spinosum, and is also referred to as *acanthosis.* Hyperplasia is a response common to a variety of stimuli, often chronic, and occurs in a variety of types, including regular, irregular, papillated, and pseudocarcinomatous (pseudoepitheliomatous) (Fig. 17-11). Some forms of epidermal hyperplasia (regular, irregular, and pseudocarcinomatous) can develop in sequence. In early stages of epidermal hyperplasia, the epidermal dermal interface is mildly undulating, but as the hyperplasia progresses, there often is an elongation of the rete ridges (ridges that extend into the dermis and interdigitate with dermal papillae) that can be regular or irregular. In regular epidermal

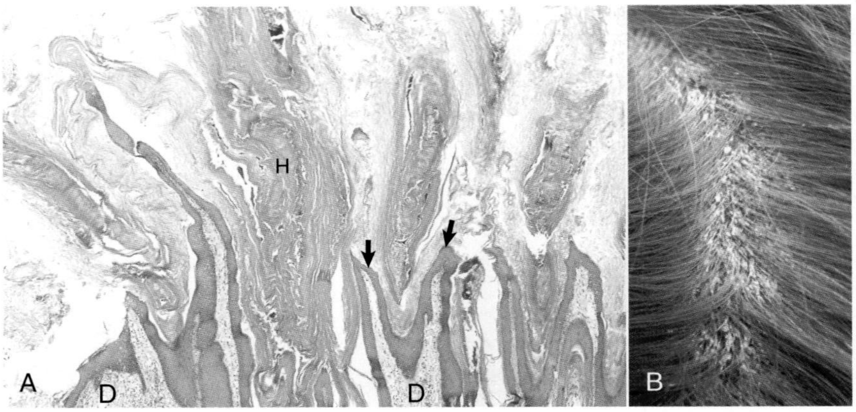

Fig. 17-9 Primary idiopathic seborrhea, skin, haired, dog.
A, Note the marked orthokeratotic hyperkeratosis *(H)*. The stratum corneum within the hair follicles is increased in quantity, extends through the follicular opening to the external skin surface, and distends follicular openings *(arrows)*, creating a papillomatous appearance in the epidermis. *D,* Dermis. H&E stain. **B,** Hair is parted to reveal excessive scaling, the result of orthokeratotic hyperkeratosis. (Courtesy Dr. Ann M. Hargis, DermatoDiagnostics.)

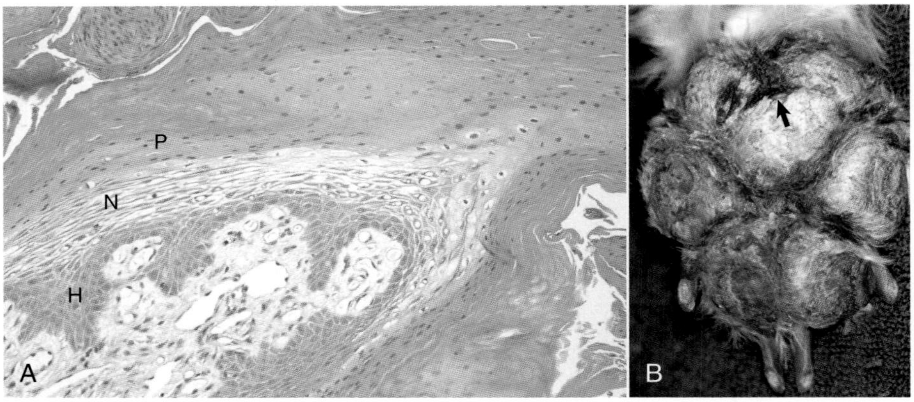

Fig. 17-10 Superficial necrolytic dermatitis, skin, dog.
A, Nuclei of the thickened stratum corneum have been retained (parakeratotic hyperkeratosis [parakeratosis]). The epidermis has a trilaminar pattern (red, white, and blue) created by three layers: (1) parakeratotic layer *(P)*, (2) subparakeratotic edema/necrolytic layer *(N)*, and (3) deep epidermal hyperplastic layer *(H)*. The pathogenesis of superficial necrolytic dermatitis is not completely understood but is speculated in most cases to be the result of an underlying systemic disease (such as severe liver disease or diabetes mellitus) that interferes with the normal nutrient metabolism needed to form a healthy epidermis. H&E stain. **B,** Pawpad. Note the fissure *(arrow)* and crusts. The crusting is largely a result of the parakeratosis. Secondary infections by bacteria, yeast, and fungi can also contribute to the formation of crusts by causing fluid, leukocytes, and other cellular debris to accumulate on the surface. (Courtesy Dr. Ann M. Hargis, DermatoDiagnostics.)

hyperplasia, the rete ridges are approximately evenly sized and shaped, whereas in irregular epidermal hyperplasia, the rete ridges are less uniform. Pseudocarcinomatous hyperplasia is a chronic and late stage of epidermal hyperplasia that develops after milder forms (regular or irregular). It refers to marked hyperplasia of the epidermis, resulting in many branching and anastomosing epidermal ridges that deeply interdigitate with dermal collagen fibers. Mitotic figures can be numerous in proliferating basal cells, but in contrast to squamous cell carcinoma, the keratinocytes maintain normal polarity, are not atypical, and do not penetrate the basement membrane. Pseudocarcinomatous hyperplasia develops after chronic injury, as seen with chronic dermal suppurative or granulomatous inflammation or at the edges of persistent, nonhealing ulcers. Psoriasiform epidermal hyperplasia is an exaggerated type of regular epidermal hyperplasia in which the epidermis forms elongated rete ridges that are of similar length and width and that interdigitate with similarly elongated dermal papillae. This type of hyperplasia has very regular or uniform histologic appearance and is a feature of certain disease syndromes, such as psoriasiform lichenoid dermatitis of the Springer spaniel and porcine juvenile pustular psoriasiform dermatitis (pityriasis rosea). Papillated epidermal hyperplasia is a unique form of epidermal hyperplasia in which fingerlike (papillary) projections of epidermis develop above the skin surface; it is a feature of some papillomas, hamartomas, and calluses.

Dyskeratosis

Dyskeratosis is an alteration in epidermal differentiation characterized by premature keratinization of cells in the viable layers of the epidermis. Dyskeratotic keratinocytes are shrunken, are separated from adjacent keratinocytes, and have a pyknotic nucleus and brightly eosinophilic cytoplasm because of the accumulation of keratin filaments. Dyskeratosis occurs when epidermal maturation is deranged such as in zinc-responsive dermatosis. Dyskeratosis is also a feature of epidermal dysplasia, which is a premalignant change in solar (actinic) keratoses.

Apoptosis

Apoptosis refers to programmed cell death. Apoptotic keratinocytes have the morphologic features of dyskeratotic cells. However,

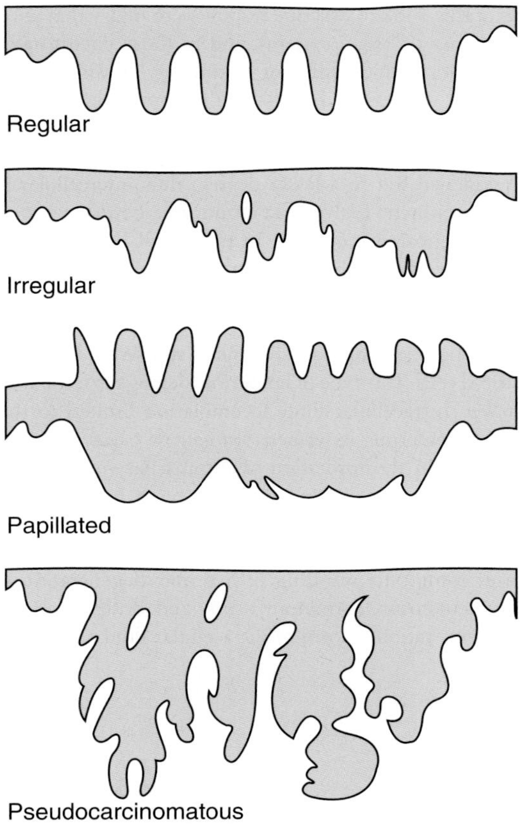

Fig. 17-11 Schematic diagram of the patterns of epidermal hyperplasia. Exaggerated regular epidermal hyperplasia is also called *psoriasiform* epidermal hyperplasia, named after the human condition *psoriasis,* which is characterized by this type of epidermal hyperplasia. (Adapted from Ackerman AB, Boer A, Bennin B, et al, eds: *Histologic diagnosis of inflammatory skin diseases,* ed 3, New York, 2005, Ardor Scribendi.)

in apoptosis, the cytoplasmic eosinophilia is caused by condensation of cytoplasmic organelles. Apoptotic cells are phagocytosed by adjacent keratinocytes. Phagocytosis before cellular disintegration prevents the development of an acute inflammatory response that would be elicited by the liberated cellular constituents. Thus the process of apoptosis is significantly different from that of necrosis, in which cell lysis releases cellular contents into the extracellular space and causes an inflammatory response. Apoptosis is seen with diseases such as lupus erythematosus and erythema multiforme (Fig. 17-12).

Necrosis

Necrosis refers to the death of cells and is characterized by nuclear pyknosis (shrunken and dense nucleus), karyorrhexis (nuclear membrane rupture with fragmentation and release of contents), or karyolysis (complete dissolution of the nucleus with loss of chromatin material), organelle swelling, plasma membrane rupture, and release of cytoplasmic elements into the extracellular space accompanied by an acute inflammatory response. Causes of epidermal necrosis include physical injury (lacerations, thermal burns), chemical injury (irritant contact dermatitis), and injury as a result of ischemia and infarction (vasculitis, thromboembolism). Necrosis of the epidermis can result in erosion (loss of a superficial portion of the epidermis) or ulceration (loss of an area of the entire epidermis and portion of the dermis).

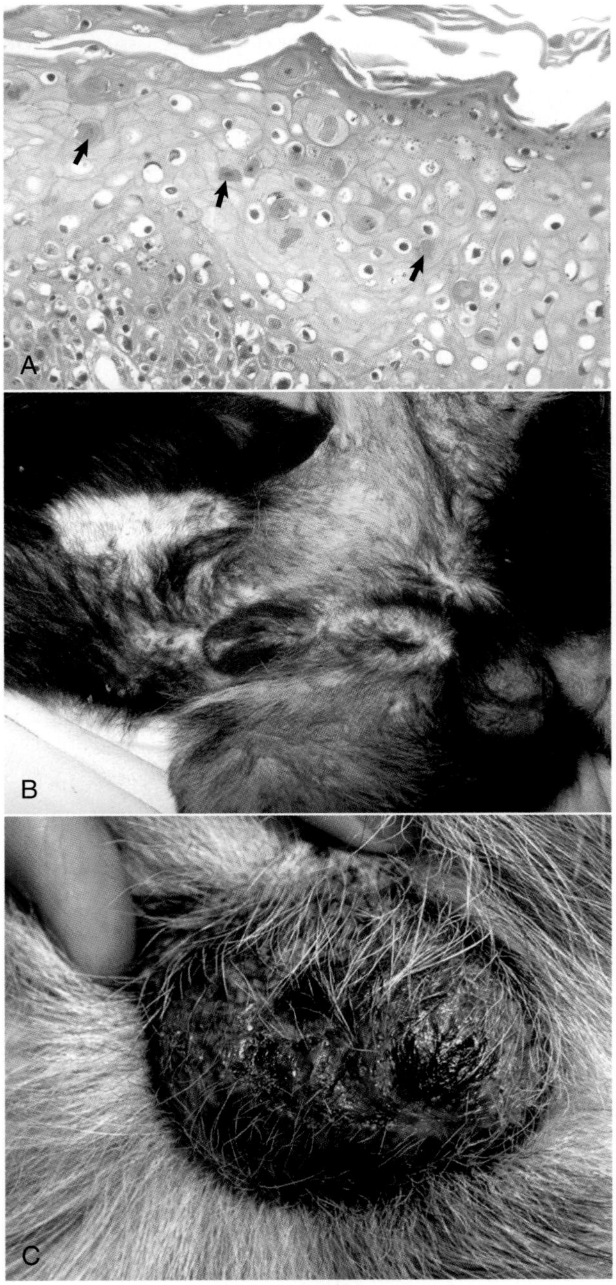

Fig. 17-12 Erythema multiforme, skin, dog. **A,** Apoptotic keratinocytes *(arrows)* are present in the cellular layers of the epidermis. The increased staining intensity of apoptotic keratinocytes is a result of condensation of cytoplasmic organelles and nuclei. H&E stain. **B,** Skin of abdomen, inguinal region, and scrotum. Note the circular and linear erosions. The clinical lesions resulting from apoptotic keratinocytes depend on the prevalence and location of the apoptotic cells in the epidermal strata. Numerous deeply located apoptotic keratinocytes can lead to loss of part of the epidermis, resulting in erosions that develop into ulcers. **C,** Scrotum, erythema, ulceration, and crusting are present. Crusts form because the ulceration (injury) results in the release of inflammatory mediators, leading to the accumulations of fluid and cellular exudate that cover and dry on the ulcerated surface. (**A** courtesy Dr. Ann M. Hargis, DermatoDiagnostics. **B** courtesy Clinical Dermatology Service, College of Veterinary Medicine, University of Florida. **C** courtesy Dr. Alexander Werner, Valley Veterinary Specialty Service.)

Dysplasia

Dysplasia is defined as abnormal development. Classically, it refers to alteration in size, shape, and organization of adult cells (keratinocytes). Dysplasia is a stage of abnormal development that precedes the formation of a noninvasive (in situ) carcinoma. This is the stage of carcinoma that occurs before the abnormal epidermal cells penetrate the basement membrane. The histologic features include irregular stratification of keratinocytes, variation in cell and nuclear size, increase in number of mitoses, dyskeratosis, and large hyperchromatic nuclei.

Epidermal Atrophy

Atrophy is a decrease in the number and size of the cells within the epidermis and occurs as a consequence of sublethal cell injury. Cutaneous atrophy can affect the epidermis, follicles, sebaceous glands, and dermal collagen and occurs in response to hormonal imbalances, such as hyperadrenocorticism in dogs and cats, partial ischemia, and in severe malnutrition.

Alterations in Epidermal Fluid Balance and Cellular Adhesion

Edema and Intracellular Fluid Accumulation

Edema refers to fluid accumulation between cells. Intercellular edema of the epidermis is called *spongiosis* because as the intercellular space expands with fluid, the epidermis develops a "spongy" appearance (Fig. 17-13). The term "spongiosis" is used in other chapters of this book to describe responses to injury that are unique to other tissues or organ systems, and in those circumstances the term "spongiosis" has different meanings. Severe intercellular edema of the epidermis results in the formation of spongiotic vesicles, which are variably sized vesicular spaces in the epidermis. The spongiotic vesicles often blend with intercellular spaces that are also widened but to a lesser degree; thus intercellular bridges are often prominent between keratinocytes bordering spongiotic vesicles. Spongiosis is common in epidermal inflammation (epidermitis) caused by staphylococci or *Malassezia* sp.

Intracellular fluid accumulation results in cytoplasmic swelling of keratinocytes, and if the swelling is severe, the swollen keratinocytes can burst, forming microvesicles supported by the walls of the ruptured cells. This type of epidermal damage is termed *reticular degeneration.* Intracellular fluid accumulation limited to the basal layer of the epidermis is termed *hydropic* or *vacuolar degeneration* and can result in the formation of intrabasilar vesicles. Hydropic degeneration is a consequence of damage to basal keratinocytes when the basal keratinocytes cannot maintain normal homeostasis, and fluid accumulates within the cells (Fig. 17-14). Examples of diseases commonly resulting in hydropic degeneration include lupus erythematosus, dermatomyositis, and drug eruptions. Ballooning degeneration, a form of intracellular fluid accumulation of

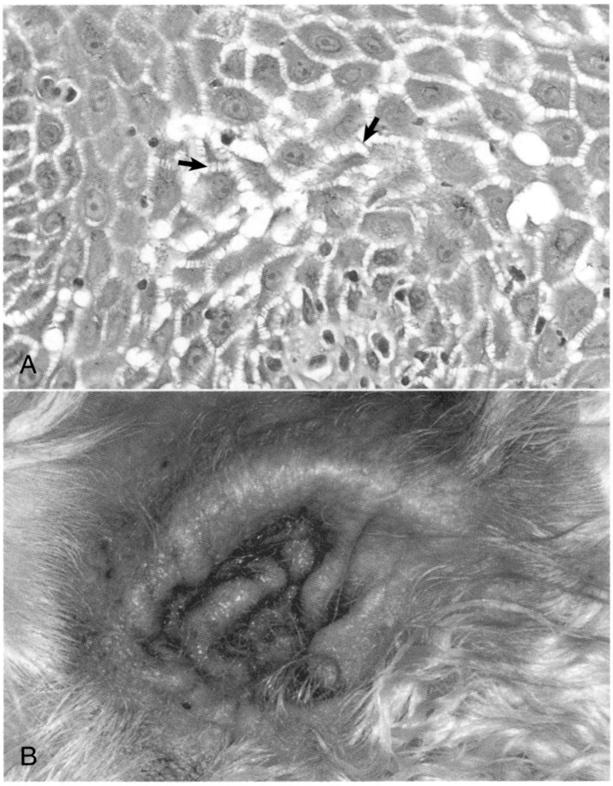

Fig. 17-13 Edema, skin, dog.
A, Intercellular epidermal edema. Note the appearance of "spines" between keratinocytes *(arrows)* of the stratum spinosum caused by widening of the intercellular spaces by edema. The keratinocytes remain connected to each other via desmosomal attachment sites (see Fig. 17-4). H&E stain. **B,** Acute allergic otitis, ear. Note erythema from dermal congestion (hyperemia) and the moist glistening surface of the skin from dermal and epidermal edema. (**A** courtesy Dr. Ann M. Hargis, DermatoDiagnostics. **B** courtesy Dr. David Duclos, Animal Skin and Allergy Clinic.)

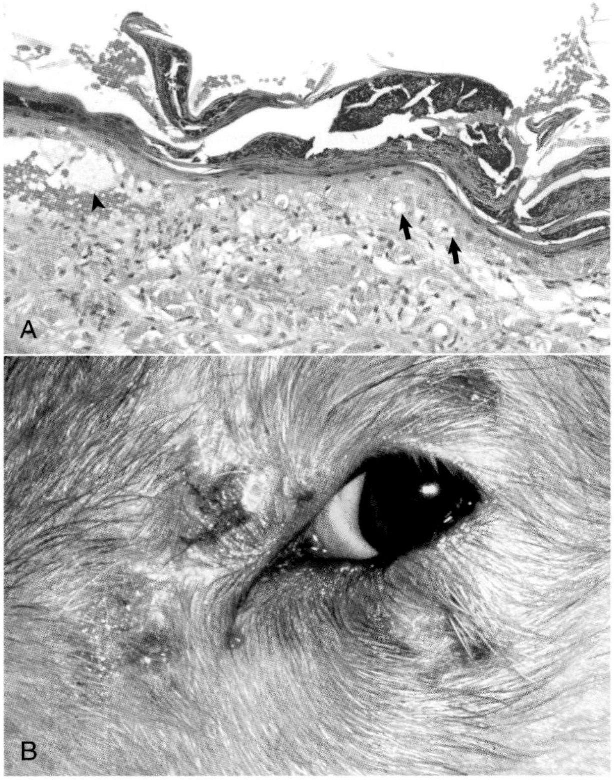

Fig. 17-14 Hydropic degeneration, skin, dog.
A, Note vacuolization of the cells of the basal layer *(arrows).* The vacuolated basal cells have resulted in a cleft *(arrowhead)* between the epidermis and dermis. A few lymphocytes are also present in the superficial dermis and lower layers of the epidermis. H&E stain. **B,** Dermatomyositis, periocular. Erythema, depigmentation, erosion, and crusting are the result of injury to basal cells. The vacuolar degeneration of basal cells weakens the epidermal dermal attachment and results in formation of vesicles, erosions, and ulcers. In addition, inflammatory mediators are released, resulting in fluid and cellular exudate, which dry on the surface and form crusts. (Courtesy Dr. Ann M. Hargis, DermatoDiagnostics.)

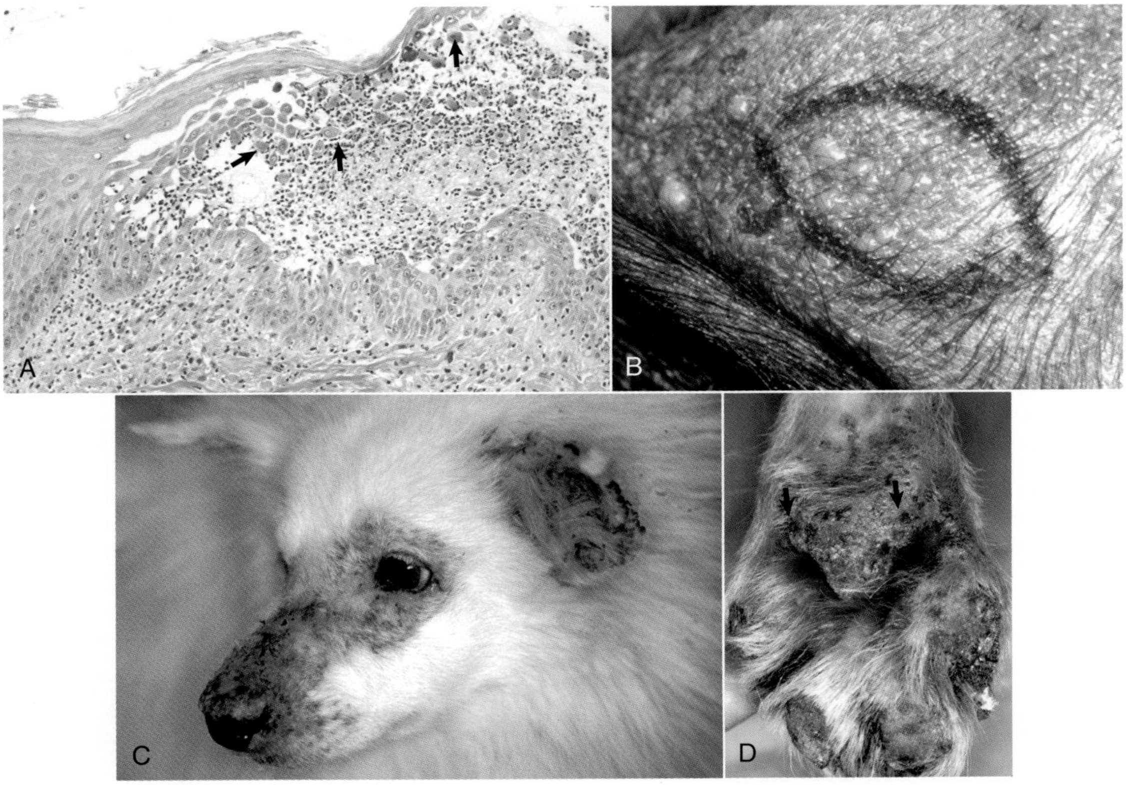

Fig. 17-15 Pemphigus foliaceous, skin.
A, Horse. The subcorneal pustule contains neutrophils and acantholytic cells *(arrows),* which are epidermal cells separated from each other as a result of the loss of desmosomal attachments. In pemphigus foliaceous, the pustule is located in the superficial epidermis, resulting in clinical lesions that are superficial (pustules that can rupture to form erosions and crusts). The roof of the pustule is the stratum corneum, and the base of the pustule is the stratum spinosum. Forceful clipping or scrubbing the surface of the pustule can lead to rupture and thus can make the sample nondiagnostic. H&E stain. **B,** Inguinal region, dog. Multiple pustules (circumscribed accumulations of pus in the epidermis visible as irregularly ovoid, slightly elevated tan areas) are present in the sparsely haired skin of the inguinal region. The skin within the black ellipse has been injected with local anesthetic in preparation for biopsy sampling. **C,** Face, dog. Erythema, alopecia, focal erosion, crusting, and depigmentation are present on medial surface of the pinnae, periocular skin, and dorsum of the muzzle and the nasal planum. Crusts develop as the result of upward growth of the epidermis and disruption of pustules. Erosions develop as the result of loss of stratum corneum and pustular exudate, which exposes the stratum spinosum. Depigmentation can result from inflammation and damage to pigment containing epidermal cells. **D,** Pawpad, dog (same dog as in **C**). Erosions *(arrows),* depigmentation, and crusts are present. (**A** courtesy Dr. Pamela E. Ginn, College of Veterinary Medicine, University of Florida. **B** courtesy Dr. David Duclos, Animal Skin and Allergy Clinic. **C** and **D** courtesy Dr. Ann M. Hargis, DermatoDiagnostics.)

keratinocytes in more superficial layers of the epidermis, such as the stratum spinosum, is characterized by swollen cells losing their intercellular attachments. This type of degeneration can result in the formation of a fluid-filled vesicle. Viruses that infect cells of the epidermis, such as the pox and parapox viruses, can cause lysis of cytoplasmic keratin and a buildup of excessive fluid, resulting in ballooning degeneration (see the section on Pathologic Reactions of the Entire Cutaneous Unit).

Acantholysis

Acantholysis is the disruption of intercellular junctions (desmosomes) between keratinocytes of the epidermis. The process is initiated by damage to transmembrane glycoproteins belonging to the cadherin family of adhesion molecules and leads to splitting of the extracellular core of the desmosomes. Subsequently, the desmosomal plaques dissolve and intermediate filaments retract to the perinuclear region of the keratinocytes. Acantholysis occurs with immune-mediated injury, as seen in pemphigus (type II cytotoxic hypersensitivity) or with neutrophilic enzymatic destruction, as seen in superficial pyoderma or uncommonly with some *Trichophyton* sp. infections. The microscopic lesions vary with the location of acantholysis within the various layers of the epidermis. In pemphigus foliaceous, acantholysis occurs in the subcorneal epidermis, resulting in release of free-floating keratinocytes in subcorneal vesicles and pustules (Fig. 17-15). In pemphigus vulgaris, acantholysis occurs in the epidermis, just above the basal layer, resulting in the separation of the upper epidermis from the basal cells (which are often referred to as *a row of tombstones*) attached to the basal lamina (Fig. 17-16). Fluid accumulating between the separated layers of the epidermis forms vesicles of varied sizes and shapes.

Vesicles

Vesicles are fluid-filled cavities within or beneath the epidermis (Web Fig. 17-5). If the cavity is less than 1 cm in diameter, it is called a *vesicle;* if it is greater than 1 cm in diameter, it is called a *bulla* (pl. bullae). Vesicles can develop in any layer of the epidermis or beneath the epidermis and can form as the result of acantholysis, epidermal or dermal edema, degeneration of basal cells and keratinocytes, or other processes, such as immune mediated targeting of components of the basement membrane, or frictional trauma and burns that damage proteins and lead to a lack of cohesion between the epidermal cells or between the epidermis and dermis, resulting in the accumulation of fluid within a cavity. The location of vesicles

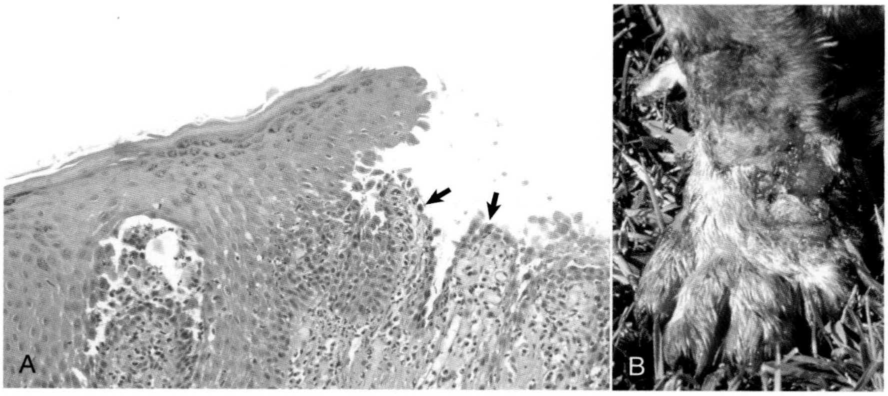

Fig. 17-16 Pemphigus vulgaris, skin, dog.
A, Suprabasilar clefting has left a row of basal cells *(arrows)* attached to the dermis. The single row of basal cells is fragile and easily damaged leading to formation of ulcers, with subsequent fluid loss and secondary bacterial infection. H&E stain. **B,** Leg. Note the erythema and large confluent areas of ulceration. In contrast to pemphigus foliaceous (more commonly characterized by erosions and crusts), pemphigus vulgaris is characterized by larger more confluent ulcers because the acantholysis in pemphigus vulgaris occurs deeper in the epidermis (in the cells of the lower epidermis). Vesicles are not frequently seen as they rapidly progress to ulcers, the more common clinical lesion. (**A** courtesy Dr. Ann M. Hargis, DermatoDiagnostics. **B** courtesy Dr. Alan Mundell, Animal Dermatology Service.)

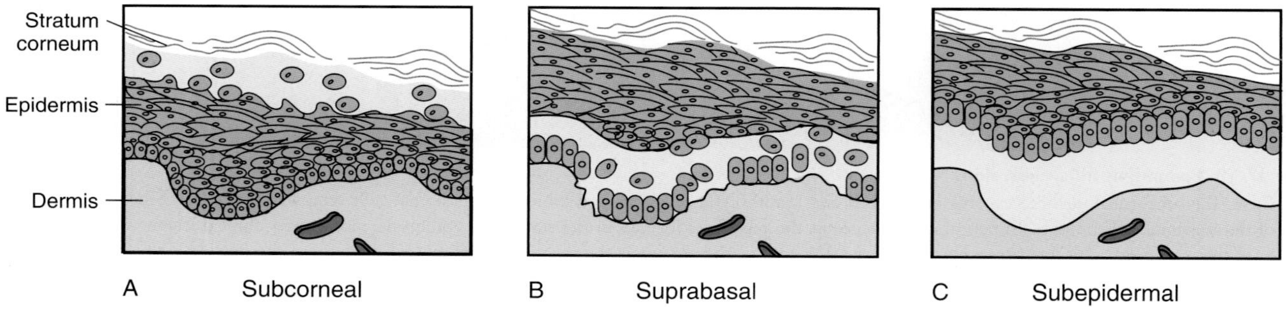

Fig. 17-17 Schematic diagram of the sites of vesicle formation in the skin.
A, In a subcorneal vesicle, the stratum corneum forms the roof of the vesicle (as in impetigo or pemphigus foliaceous). **B,** In a suprabasal vesicle, a portion of the epidermis (stratum spinosum) forms the roof (as in pemphigus vulgaris). **C,** In a subepidermal vesicle, the entire epidermis separates from the dermis and forms the roof (as in bullous pemphigoid). (From Kumar V, Abbas AK, Fausto N, et al: *Robbins & Cotran pathologic basis of disease,* ed 8, Philadelphia, 2009, Saunders.)

or bullae within the layers of the epidermis is suggestive of certain diseases. For instance, intraepidermal vesicles can occur in viral infections, subcorneal vesicles in pemphigus foliaceous, suprabasilar vesicles in pemphigus vulgaris (see Fig. 17-16), and subepidermal vesicles in bullous pemphigoid or thermal burns (Fig. 17-17).

Inflammatory Lesions of the Epidermis

Acute inflammation of the epidermis actually begins in the dermis with active hyperemia, edema, and migration of leukocytes, often neutrophils (see inflammatory disorders of the dermis section). The edema fluid arises from dilated venules and can move intercellularly through the epidermis, widening the intercellular spaces and causing spongiosis. In thermal burns of the skin, larger quantities of fluid accumulate within or below the epidermis forming vesicles; the fluid reaching the epidermal surface dries to form a largely acellular crust. The leukocytes (often neutrophils in acute inflammation) migrate from the superficial dermal vessels, through the superficial dermis, and into the intercellular spaces of the deep and then superficial layers of the epidermis. The aggregation of migrating leukocytes in the epidermis is termed *exocytosis.* Exocytosis of leukocytes is common in inflammation and is usually accompanied by spongiosis. If the inflammation progresses, the migrating leukocytes form pustules within the epidermis or the stratum corneum. Pustules usually dry rapidly and become crusts (Fig. 17-18). The type of leukocyte recruited into the epidermis is influenced by complex interactions of cytokines involved in the pathogenesis of the disease and can be useful in classifying and ultimately diagnosing the disease. For instance, intraepidermal eosinophils can be seen in association with ectoparasite bites. Lymphocytic infiltrates into the epidermis are often seen with immune-mediated diseases such as lupus erythematosus. Malignant lymphoma affecting the epidermis is also characterized by intraepidermal lymphocytes. Erythrocytes can also be present in the epidermis, usually associated with trauma, or circulatory disturbances, such as marked vasodilation and vasculitis.

Pustules

Pustules (microabscesses) are accumulations of inflammatory cells (pus) within the epidermis (see Fig. 17-15). Epidermal pustules vary in inflammatory cell content and location in the epidermis, depending on the pathogenesis of the disease. The pustules of superficial bacterial infections generally contain degenerate neutrophils and coccoid bacteria and are often located beneath the stratum corneum (subcorneal). In ectoparasitic hypersensitivity, pemphigus foliaceous, and feline eosinophilic plaque, the pustules can be filled with eosinophils. Small pustules containing neoplastic lymphocytes (Pautrier's microabscesses) are present in epitheliotropic lymphoma.

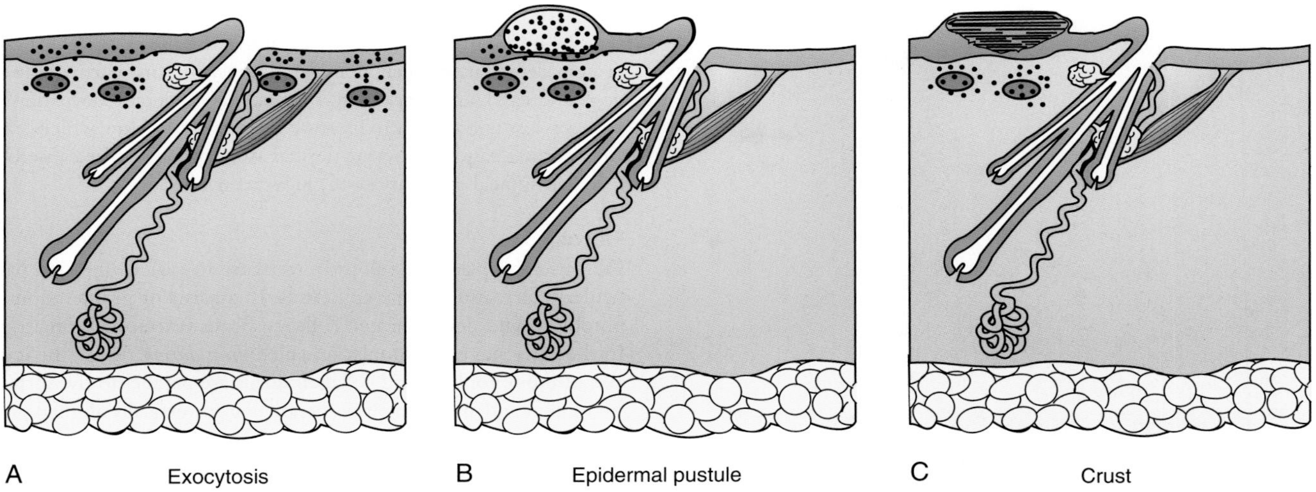

Fig. 17-18 Schematic diagram of the inflammatory patterns of the epidermis.
A, Leukocytes *(black dots)* migrate from the perivascular dermis into the epidermis, a process called exocytosis. **B,** Leukocytes migrate into the epidermis and accumulate to form a pustule. **C,** The pustule dries to form a crust. (Redrawn from Dr. Ann M. Hargis, DermatoDiagnostics; and Dr. Pamela E. Ginn, College of Veterinary Medicine, University of Florida.)

Crusts

Crusts are composed of dried fluid and cellular debris (i.e., dried exudates) located on the epidermal surface; thus crusts are indicative of a previous exudative process. Crusts are not specifically diagnostic but can hold the key to diagnosis in some diseases. For example, in dermatophilosis, the most diagnostic portion of the skin sample is the crust, which is multilaminated and contains the Gram-positive, branching coccoid organism *Dermatophilus congolensis*. Similarly, crusts formed through aging of pustules in pemphigus foliaceous are multilaminated and frequently contain numerous acantholytic cells. Crusts can also contain hair shafts infected with spores and hyphae of dermatophytes.

Alterations in Epidermal Pigmentation

Pigmentary alterations include hyperpigmentation, hypopigmentation, and pigmentary incontinence. Melanin is produced by melanocytes located in the basal and lower spinous layers of the epidermis, in the external root sheath and hair matrix of follicles, and perivascularly in the dermis. Melanocytes have surface receptors for hormones, such as melanocyte-stimulating hormone, and these hormones regulate melanogenesis. Other factors that influence the amount of melanin pigment in skin and hair are genes, age, temperature, and inflammation.

Hyperpigmentation

Hyperpigmentation results from an increased production of melanin from existing melanocytes or an increase in the number of melanocytes. An example of hyperpigmentation caused by an increased number of melanocytes is a lentigo, a rare localized non-neoplastic proliferation of melanocytes confined to the epidermis and resulting in formation of a black macular circumscribed lesion that is usually less than 1 cm in diameter. Most hyperpigmentation of the epidermis results from increased production of melanin from existing melanocytes. Possible mechanisms of increased melanin production include increases in the rate of production of melanosomes (i.e., granules within melanocytes that contain tyrosinase and synthesize melanin), in melanosome size, in rates of melanosome transfer to keratinocytes and increased survival of melanosomes in keratinocytes. Examples of epidermal hyperpigmentation by increased production of melanin include chronic inflammatory diseases (most common cause), such as chronic allergic dermatitis, and endocrine dermatoses, such as hyperadrenocorticism. Hyperpigmentation secondary to inflammation is thought to result from release of melanocyte-stimulating factors from keratinocytes. It is thought that these factors are present in normal epidermis, but that their level or activity is increased in response to stimulation or keratinocyte stress.

Hypopigmentation

Hypopigmentation can be congenital or hereditary and develops because of a lack of melanocytes, failure of melanocytes to produce melanin, or failure of transfer of melanin to epidermal cells. Hypopigmentation can also be acquired via a loss of existing melanin or melanocytes (depigmentation). Because copper is a component of tyrosinase, production of melanin pigment depends on copper, and copper deficiency can result in reduced pigmentation.

Pigmentary Incontinence

Pigmentary incontinence refers to the loss of melanin pigment from the basal layer of the epidermis or outer root sheath or bulb of the hair follicles caused by damage to the cells of the basal layer or of the follicular components and the accumulation of the pigment in macrophages in the upper dermis or perifollicular regions, respectively. Basal layer pigmentary incontinence can be a nonspecific lesion associated with inflammation; however, it is also seen with diseases that specifically damage basal cells or melanocytes such as lupus erythematosus or vitiligo. Perifollicular pigmentary incontinence occurs in diseases in which inflammation targets the follicular wall, such as demodicosis, or there is abnormal growth or development of hair follicles, such as in some types of follicular dysplasia. Leukotrichia and leukoderma (Fig. 17-19) refer to decreased pigmentation of hair and skin, respectively.

Responses of the Dermis to Injury

Alterations in Growth, Development, or Tissue Maintenance

Dermal Atrophy

Dermal atrophy results from a decrease in the quantity of collagen fibrils and fibroblasts in the dermis and leads to a decrease in the thickness of the dermis noted clinically by thin, translucent

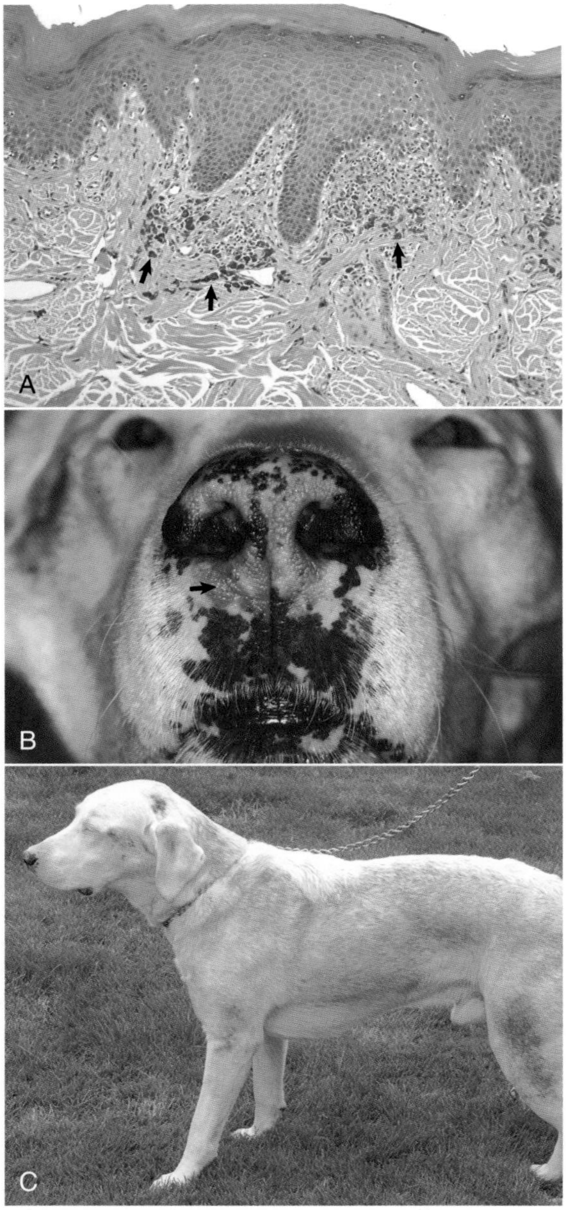

Fig. 17-19 Leukoderma, skin, dog.

A, Injury to the epidermal pigment containing cells (predominantly melanocytes) has caused loss of melanin pigment in the epidermis (leukoderma). The pigment from the damaged melanocytes has been phagocytosed by dermal macrophages (pigmentary incontinence) *(arrows).* Mild to moderate lymphocytic inflammation is present along the epidermal dermal interface. H&E stain. **B,** Nose and lips. Areas of the normally black skin of the planum nasale and lips have been partially *(bluish-gray)* or totally *(pink)* depigmented. The bluish-gray areas are in the process of becoming depigmented. Biopsy samples should be collected from the bluish-gray areas *(arrow)* to identify active inflammation and diagnostic lesions. Biopsy samples from black skin or from already totally depigmented skin will likely only show normal appearing black or nonpigmented skin, respectively, with no evidence of inflammation. **C,** Leukotrichia, body. This dog is the same one depicted in **B.** He was a black Labrador retriever mix. More than 90% of the black hair coat became white (leukotrichia). Biopsy samples from white-haired areas may be normal because the inflammatory event that caused the pigment loss is likely gone by the time nonpigmented hair shafts emerge from the hair follicles. (**A** courtesy Dr. Ann M. Hargis, DermatoDiagnostics. **B** and **C** courtesy Dr. David Duclos, Animal Skin and Allergy Clinic.)

skin with more visible vasculature. The principal causes of dermal atrophy in domestic animals are catabolic diseases associated with protein degradation, such as hyperadrenocorticism (particularly in dogs and cats), and starvation. In cats with hyperadrenocorticism, collagen loss is sufficient to increase fragility of the skin, which tears with normal handling. Severe dermal atrophy can also be caused by repeated topical application of glucocorticoids.

Fibrosis

Fibrosis (fibroplasia) develops in response to various injuries, particularly ulceration of the epidermis. It consists of proliferation of fibroblasts and newly formed collagen fibrils (extracellular matrix). In the early stage of fibroplasia (called *granulation tissue*), the long axis of the fibroblasts and collagen fibrils are parallel to the surface of the skin and are oriented perpendicular to vertically aligned proliferative vessels. Clinically, the capillaries are seen on the surface as minute red dots that create a "granular" appearance, thus the name "granulation tissue." Microscopically, the orientation pattern provides a "lattice-work" appearance to the tissue (Fig. 17-20). Fibrosis refers to the gradual deposition and maturation of collagen to form a scar. During fibrosis, collagen production increases and fibroblast and capillary numbers decrease, resulting in less cellular dense collagen oriented in thick hyaline bundles in parallel arrangement (e.g., a scar), which grossly appear white and glistening.

Collagen Dysplasia

Collagen dysplasia is generally an inherited abnormality of collagen that results in decreased tensile strength and an increased ability of the skin to stretch beyond normal limits. Because the tensile strength is reduced, even minor trauma can cause the skin to tear. Healing results in formation of scars. Microscopic features vary among the different types of collagen dysplasia disorders, and in some the skin has no microscopic alterations. Collagen bundles can vary in size and shape and consist of tangled fibers with an abnormal organizational pattern.

Solar Elastosis

Solar elastosis is caused by chronic exposure of the skin to the UV spectrum of sunlight. Sunlight consists of visible, UV, and infrared light rays. The portion of the UV light most damaging to the skin is ultraviolet B (UVB) and is in the range of 290 to 320 nm. The amount of light reaching the skin is dependent on a variety of environmental and host factors that can greatly influence the geographic incidence and anatomic locations of solar damage. Environmental factors include quantity of ozone, smog, and cloud cover that tend to absorb and scatter some of the UV rays. Altitude and latitude are also very important. The atmosphere at high altitude is thinner, so there is less oxygen and particulate matter to absorb and scatter the UV rays. Latitude is also critically important. It has been estimated that the incidence of sunlight-induced cancer in humans doubles for every 265 miles closer to the equator that humans reside. At high latitudes, the path of sunlight through the ozone layer is longer than at lower latitudes, so the ozone absorbs more of the harmful UV light. The path of sunlight through the ozone layer is also one of the reasons that sunlight has more damaging UV rays in summer months and at midday. Increased wind velocity has also been shown to have an enhancing influence on damaging effects of UV light on the skin. Local environmental factors can influence the quantity of UV light reaching an animal's skin. Such factors include availability of shelter from sunlight in the form of trees, shade panels, or indoor housing, and color of the ground material (lightly colored sand) that can increase exposure to UV light through reflection. Host factors include quantity of hair,

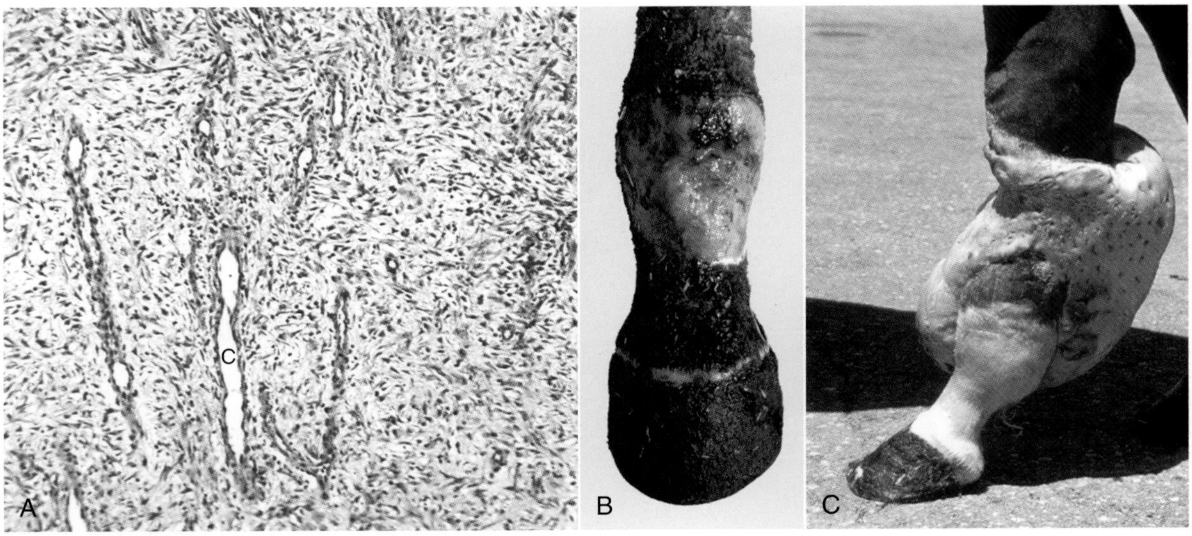

Fig. 17-20 **Granulation tissue, skin, horse.**
A, Note vertically oriented capillaries *(C)* and horizontally oriented fibroblasts and a few collagen fibers providing a "lattice-work" appearance to the granulation tissue. **B,** Leg. Note ulcerated area filled with granulation tissue. **C,** Exuberant granulation tissue, leg. Granulation tissue is a normal component of wound healing. However, excessive or exuberant granulation tissue can develop as a pathologic process. This condition occurs especially in horses, when an ulcer fails to become reepithelialized. Although this process is commonly called "exuberant granulation tissue," at the stage depicted in this photograph, most of the granulation tissue has been converted to fibrous connective tissue. (Courtesy Dr. M.D. McGavin, College of Veterinary Medicine, University of Tennessee.)

degree of pigmentation, thickness of stratum corneum, and other difficult to define genetic factors. Therefore solar damage is more prevalent in high altitude, low latitude parts of the world and in animals residing outside for long periods of time. Lesions generally develop in poorly haired and lightly pigmented sites. Solar elastosis develops in the superficial dermis of chronically sun-exposed skin, and consists of increased numbers of thick, interwoven, basophilic fibers with the staining characteristics of elastin (thus the name, "solar elastosis"). In the nonpigmented abdominal skin of dogs, solar elastosis may develop intermixed with or below a linear band of scarring parallel to the epidermal surface (laminar fibrosis). The pathogenesis of the development of solar elastosis is complex and not fully understood and may vary with species. Current evidence involving studies in humans and mouse models supports the view that a majority of the elastotic material (elastin, fibrillin, and glycosaminoglycans) is newly formed as the result of altered function of sun-damaged fibroblasts, but that degradation of preexisting dermal matrix proteins, including elastin and also most likely collagen, seems to be involved as well. Solar elastosis is less prominent in the skin of domestic animals than in humans but is often prominent in lightly pigmented, poorly haired sun-exposed skin and eyelids of horses and in the lower eyelids of Hereford cattle residing in sunny locations.

Degenerative Collagen Disorders of the Dermis

The term *collagen degeneration* has been used to refer to an altered histologic appearance of collagen fibers in hematoxylin and eosin (H&E) stained sections, whereby there is brightly eosinophilic granular to amorphous material bordering the fibers and somewhat obscuring the fiber detail. The collagen fibers and bordering eosinophilic material have also been referred to as *flame figures,* a result in part to the irregular, sometimes radiating edges and brightly eosinophilic staining intensity. Electron microscopic studies in cats and humans indicate that the collagen fibers can be disrupted, but they are not "degenerate." Instead, the brightly eosinophilic granular and amorphous material consists of aggregates of many eosinophils and eosinophil granules that border slightly disrupted but otherwise normal collagen fibers. These flame figures are seen in conditions in which eosinophils are prominent, including in reactions to insect bites, mast cell tumors, and eosinophilic granulomas (collagenolytic granulomas) (Fig. 17-21). Collagen lysis refers to dissolution of collagen fibrils morphologically consisting of amorphous, lightly eosinophilic material lacking fibrillar detail. Collagen lysis is likely a secondary event caused by proteolytic enzymes released by a variety of cells, including eosinophils (collagenase) and neutrophils (collagenolytic proteinase, collagenase).

Disorders Characterized by Abnormal Deposits in the Dermis

Amyloid

Amyloid is an abnormal proteinaceous substance that can be deposited in a localized site in the body (organ limited) or can be "systemic" where multiple organs are involved. In the systemic form, amyloid deposition can be the result of a primary abnormality of plasma cells (primary amyloidosis), in which case the amyloid is derived from components of immunoglobulin light chains (AL amyloid), or as a result of chronic inflammatory conditions (secondary amyloidosis), in which case the amyloid is derived from serum amyloid-associated protein (SAA protein), an acute-phase reactant produced by the body in response to inflammation. Cutaneous amyloid deposition can occur in association with systemic amyloidosis, but visceral involvement is more common and clinically important. Cutaneous deposition of amyloid is rare but is seen in horses, dogs, and cats. In horses, it can occur in association with secondary systemic amyloidosis or in a localized (organ-limited) form. In organ-limited amyloidosis, the skin and/or upper respiratory tract are typically involved, the condition is not associated with recognized triggering causes, and the amyloid is produced from immunoglobulin light chains (AL amyloid). Clinical lesions vary from papules and plaques to nodules that usually are covered by a normal hair coat. Similar nodules can also develop in the respiratory mucosa and regional lymph nodes. Histologic lesions include nodular to diffuse granulomatous dermatitis and panniculitis with deposition of amyloid, an eosinophilic hyaline material. Cutaneous

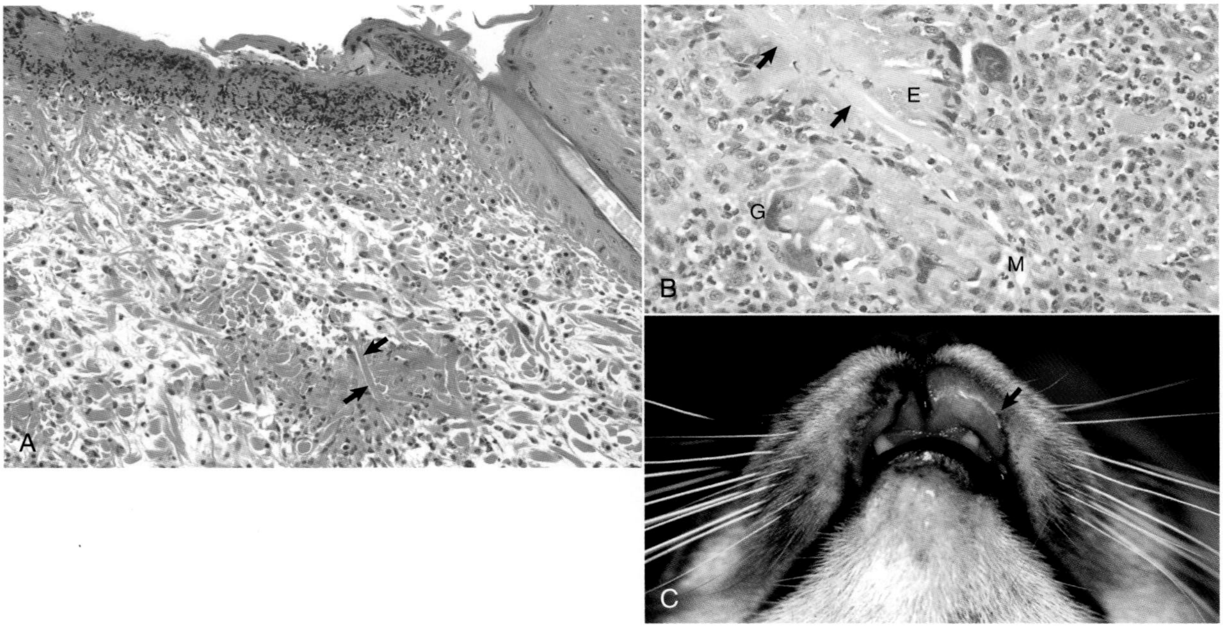

Fig. 17-21 Eosinophilic granuloma, skin, cat.
A, Ulcerated skin *(left)* with fragmented collagen *(arrows)* is bordered by degranulated eosinophils. H&E stain. **B,** Fragmented collagen *(arrows)* is bordered by a row of macrophages *(M),* multinucleated giant cells *(G),* and degranulated eosinophils *(E),* somewhat resembling a flame ("flame figure"). H&E stain. **C,** Upper lip. Bilateral ulcers are present on the upper lips, but the ulcer on the right side of the photograph is more extensive *(arrow).* (Courtesy Dr. Ann M. Hargis, DermatoDiagnostics.)

deposition of amyloid in dogs and cats is usually the localized type, and is seen in association with extramedullary plasma cell tumors (AL amyloid). However, cutaneous deposition of amyloid in dogs also can be triggered by a monoclonal gammopathy (AL amyloid). Clinical and histologic lesions reflect the triggering disease.

Mucin

Mucin (glycosaminoglycan [GAG]), a normal component of the ground substance of the dermis, consists of protein bound to hyaluronic acid and can be deposited in increased quantity in focal areas or diffusely. Because hyaluronic acid has a great affinity for binding water, the skin in cases of mucin deposition (mucinosis) has a thick, puffy appearance. In cases of severe mucinosis, the skin, when pricked with a needle, can exude mucin (a stringy fluid material). In histologic sections, much of the water is lost and mucin appears as fine amphophilic granules or fibrils that separate dermal collagen. Examples of disorders with dermal mucin deposition are termed *myxedema* in hypothyroidism and *mucinosis* in the Chinese Shar-Pei dog.

Calcium Deposits

Mineralization is a general term for the deposition of insoluble, inorganic minerals in the cutaneous tissue and usually consists of calcium in combination with phosphate or carbonate. Because the mineral most often deposited is calcium, the terms *mineralization* and *calcification* are often used interchangeably. Mineralization can occur in four basic forms: (1) dystrophic, (2) metastatic, (3) idiopathic, and (4) iatrogenic. Mineralization can also occur in tissues that have been traumatized, which may encompass more than one of these pathogenic mechanisms. Dystrophic mineralization occurs as a result of injury or degeneration of cellular and extracellular components of the skin, with normal serum calcium levels, and without abnormalities in calcium metabolism. Examples include deposition of mineral in granulomas and calcinosis cutis seen in some cases of hyperadrenocorticism. In metastatic mineralization, the calcium deposits develop without preceding tissue injury or degeneration and in association with hypercalcemia, usually the result of abnormal metabolism of calcium, phosphorus, or vitamin D. Examples include deposition of calcium salts in soft tissues in chronic renal disease and in poisoning with cholecalciferol (vitamin D_3). Mitochondria have a high affinity for calcium and phosphate, and participate in both dystrophic and metastatic calcification by concentrating intracellular calcium and phosphate to levels that allow crystallization. Mechanisms leading to calcium deposition in dystrophic mineralization involve reduced pH of injured tissue, the influx of calcium into injured cells, and then into mitochondria. Metastatic calcification may be the result of increased extracellular calcium levels and the failure of the cell's normal ability to strictly regulate intracellular calcium with resultant accumulation within mitochondria. Mineralization can affect individual or groups of collagen fibers, resulting in increased basophilia and fragmentation of fibers in H&E-stained sections. The causes of idiopathic mineralization are not known; it occurs in the absence of tissue injury or abnormalities in calcium or phosphorus metabolism. Calcinosis circumscripta is a form of tissue mineralization in which calcium is deposited as amorphous nodular aggregates in the soft tissues of the tongue and in the subcutis of the pawpads of dogs. The pathogenesis is not defined, but some cases are considered idiopathic, whereas others may be the result of tissue trauma. Calcium deposits can elicit a granulomatous inflammatory response, a foreign-body reaction to the deposits. Iatrogenic mineralization develops via direct exposure to calcium salts such as occurs with topical exposure to calcium chloride deicing solutions.

Inflammatory Disorders of the Dermis

Dermatitis is inflammation of the dermis. Acute dermatitis begins with active hyperemia (increased blood flow), edema, and migration of leukocytes and results from release of cytokines and other mediators of acute inflammation (see Chapter 3). Active hyperemia is caused by vasodilation of arterioles, which causes increased blood flow at reduced velocity to capillary beds and postcapillary venules. Edema is caused by increased vascular permeability. Fluid leaves vessels mostly through widened interendothelial cell junctions. With a mild increase in vascular permeability, the edema fluid is clear (serous) because there are very few plasma proteins in the fluid. With increasing vascular permeability or endothelial cell injury, larger protein molecules, such as fibrinogen, escape from vessels, and the edema fluid becomes more eosinophilic and amorphous to fibrillar (fibrinous). The next step in acute dermatitis is migration of leukocytes from vessels into the perivascular dermis. The slowing of the blood flow and the endothelial cell expression of adhesion molecules that bind circulating leukocytes permit the migration of leukocytes in acute inflammation. The slowing of the blood flow allows leukocytes to move from the center of the vessel, where blood flow is fastest, to the margin, where they contact and attach to the activated endothelial cells.

After attaching to activated endothelial cells, leukocytes migrate between the endothelial cells into the perivascular dermis. The type of leukocyte that migrates and the sequence of cellular influx depend on activation of different adhesion molecules and chemotactic factors in the different phases of inflammation. In many types of acute inflammation, neutrophils are one of the first cells to arrive. Neutrophils predominate in the first 6 to 24 hours of injury and are generally replaced by macrophages in 24 to 48 hours. This sequence of cellular exudation can vary. For example, in reactions mediated by IgE cross-linking, such as type I hypersensitivity responses, mast cells (located in the perivascular dermis) are stimulated to release contents of granules (occurs in seconds) and synthesize and release inflammatory mediators (prostaglandins, leukotrienes, and cytokines), resulting in the influx of eosinophils, basophils, $CD4^+$ T_H2 lymphocytes, and macrophages. Mast cell degranulation and T_H2 lymphocyte activation cause eosinophils to accumulate in large numbers. Thus eosinophils often comprise the majority of leukocytes in inflammatory reactions against parasites and other allergic reactions.

Acute dermatitis typically results in one of four outcomes. First, there can be complete resolution, which occurs when the inciting stimulus has short duration and there is little tissue damage that is completely repaired. Second, an abscess can form, which occurs with pus-producing (pyogenic) bacterial infections. Third, healing occurs by replacement of the injured area by fibrous connective tissue (e.g., scarring), which occurs when there is significant tissue destruction (such as a deep burn) in which the parenchymal tissues are lost and thus cannot regenerate. Fourth, there is progression of acute dermatitis to chronic dermatitis.

Chronic dermatitis is inflammation of the skin that lasts weeks or months. Histologic features of chronic dermatitis include accumulation of macrophages, lymphocytes, and plasma cells; tissue destruction in part caused by the inflammatory cells; and a reparative host response of fibrosis and angiogenesis. Chronic dermatitis is usually caused by persistent infections often associated with delayed hypersensitivity and the formation of granulomas (e.g., *Mycobacteria* sp.), presence of foreign material in the skin (e.g., embedded suture), or autoimmune reactions in which self-antigens provoke an ongoing immunologic inflammatory response against host tissue (e.g., lupus erythematosus). Macrophages are a key cell in chronic dermatitis. They arise from monocytes in the peripheral blood and mature to macrophages whose primary function is phagocytosis. Macrophages also become activated by a variety of chemical mediators, including the cytokine IFN-γ secreted by sensitized T lymphocytes. When activated, macrophages also secrete many mediators of tissue injury (toxic oxygen metabolites, proteases, and coagulation factors) that contribute to chronic inflammation and fibrosis (growth factors, angiogenesis factors, and collagenases). The presence of lymphocytes and plasma cells in chronic inflammation is indicative of a host immune response.

The inflammatory milieu in the progression of acute and chronic dermatitis can be further complicated by other superimposed factors, notably physical injury from self-trauma, secondary bacterial infection of traumatized surface, injury from insect bites attracted by odor or exudate, and moderation by the host immune response or therapy. Thus dermal inflammatory responses to different stimuli often have overlapping histologic features, providing a diagnostic challenge for the dermatopathologist. Even so, the distribution of leukocytes often evolves into recognizable patterns that, when combined with the inflammatory cell type and other morphologic changes, suggest a group of differential diagnoses or the cause or pathogenesis of a specific disease (see Tables 17-1 and 17-2). Dermal patterns of inflammation that have been used in histologic diagnosis include perivascular dermatitis, interface dermatitis (inflammation affecting the basilar epidermis and superficial dermis that often obscures the epidermal dermal interface), nodular to diffuse dermatitis with infectious agents, and nodular to diffuse dermatitis without infectious agents (Fig. 17-22). For example, perivascular dermatitis with eosinophils is suggestive of hypersensitivity associated with parasites or other antigens; interface dermatitis with lymphocytes is suggestive of an immune response directed toward epidermal cells, such as lupus erythematosus or erythema multiforme; and nodular dermatitis with macrophages (granulomatous dermatitis) indicates a persistent stimulus, such as infection with acid-fast bacteria or fungi. Thus patterns of inflammation combined with cellular composition of infiltrates are useful in microscopic diagnosis.

Responses of the Adnexa to Injury

The term *adnexa* refers to appendages or adjunct parts, which in the skin includes hair follicles and glands. The major clinical and histologic changes involve the hair follicles, and thus follicular lesions are emphasized in the next discussion.

Alterations in Maintenance, Growth, and Development

Atrophy

Atrophy refers to gradual reduction (involution) in size and can be physiologic or pathologic. Physiologic atrophy is related to the normal progression of the hair follicle cycle (i.e., the hair cycle stages of growth [anagen], transition [catagen], rest [telogen], and shed [exogen]). Pathologic atrophy occurs when the degree of atrophy is greater than that expected for a given stage of the hair cycle. Causes of follicular atrophy include hormonal abnormalities, nutritional abnormalities, inadequacy of blood supply, inflammation, and general state of health, including stressful events or systemic illness. Some types of pathologic atrophy can be reversed when the underlying cause is corrected. Damage to germinal epithelium can result in destruction or total loss of the adnexa with replacement by a scar. Examples include extensive inflammation and disruption of the follicle (folliculitis and furunculosis) and bordering glands and dermis that destroy a significant portion of the adnexal germinal epithelium, thermal burns sufficiently deep to involve the adnexa and dermal vessels, thrombosis causing infarction (i.e., diamond skin disease in pigs), and severe physical trauma such as lacerations that remove components of the skin, including adnexa.

Hypertrophy

Hypertrophy is an increase in the unit size of a structure or an individual cell. Follicular hypertrophy, which results in follicles

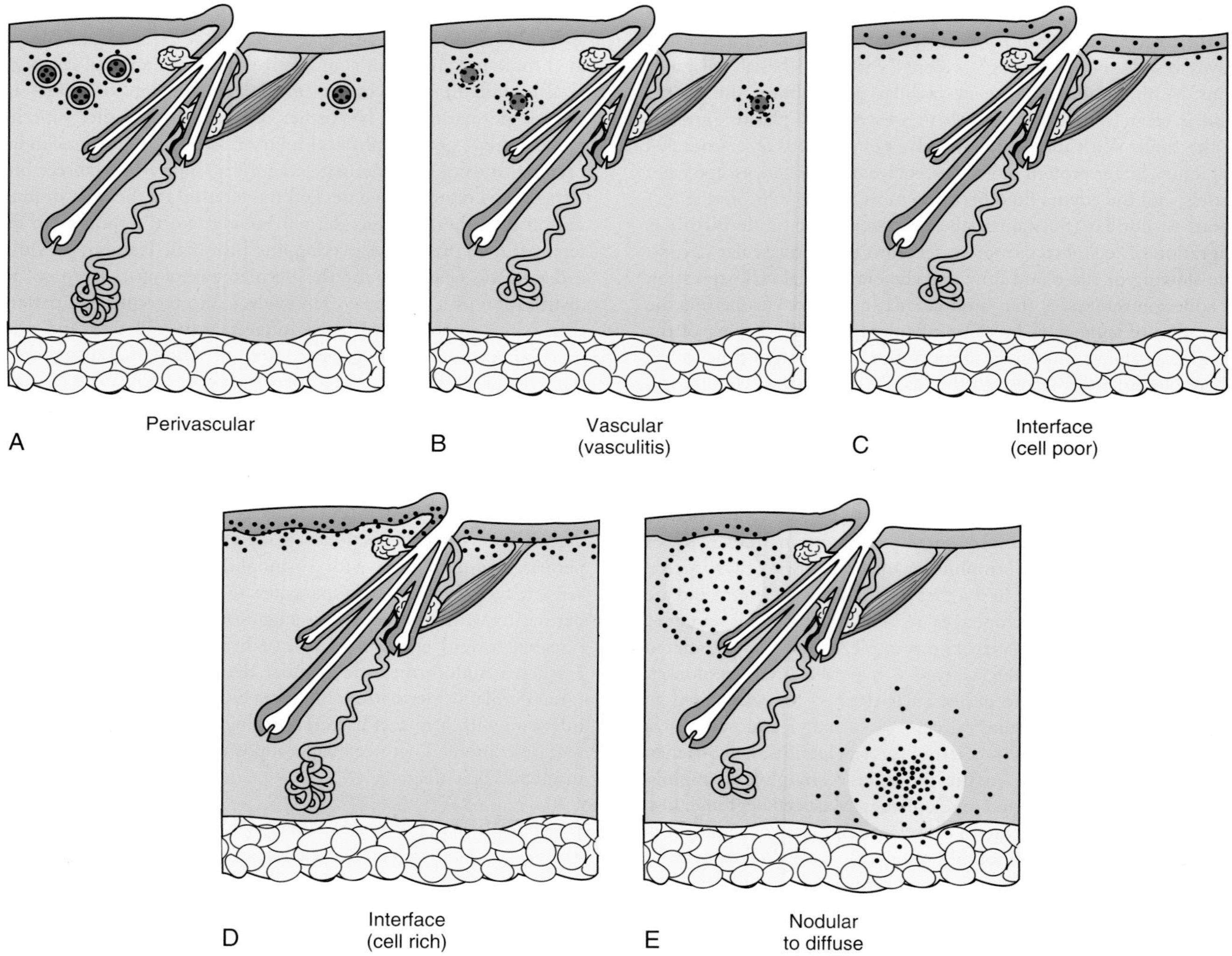

Fig. 17-22 Schematic diagram of the inflammatory patterns of the dermis.
A, Perivascular: Leukocytes *(black dots)* migrate from the dermal vessels into the perivascular dermis. This is the least specific pattern because all inflammatory patterns are at one stage, perivascular. **B,** Vascular (vasculitis): Leukocytes target the vessel wall, resulting in necrosis, inflammation, leakage of fibrin and red blood cells, and if severe, thrombosis and infarction. **C,** Interface, cell poor: Mild, often lymphocytic, inflammation located along the epidermal dermal interface with vacuolar or apoptotic degeneration of basal cells. **D,** Interface, cell rich: Dense band of inflammation along the epidermal dermal interface, obscuring the basilar layer of the epidermis, and with vacuolar or apoptotic degeneration of basal cells. **E,** Nodular to diffuse with or without microorganisms. Inflammation, typically granulomatous to pyogranulomatous, which partially effaces the architecture of the dermis may be associated with infectious agents or may be sterile. (Redrawn from Dr. Ann M. Hargis, DermatoDiagnostics; and Dr. Pamela E. Ginn, College of Veterinary Medicine, University of Florida.)

that are longer and wider than normal for the site, develops secondary to repeated surface trauma such as in acral lick dermatitis. Hyperplasia is an increase in the number of cells in a structure. Enlargement of adnexa, a common response to injury, usually involves both hypertrophy and hyperplasia and is observed in follicles and sebaceous and apocrine glands associated with chronic allergic dermatitis.

Abnormalities of Hair Cycle Stages

Abnormalities of hair cycle stages occur when there is disruption in the normal progression from the anagen, catagen, telogen, and exogen stages of the hair cycle (see Fig. 17-6). Clinical and histologic lesions are diverse. Some animals have failure of hair to regrow after clipping (hypothyroidism, postclipping alopecia). Other animals have sudden shedding of hair coat (synchronous change of many follicles from telogen into anagen, resulting in loss of old telogen hair shafts as new hair shafts emerge, termed *telogen effluvium*). Yet other animals have gradual but progressive loss of hair shafts associated with endocrine disease such as hyperadrenocorticism.

Follicular Dysplasia

Follicular dysplasia refers to incomplete or abnormal development of follicles and hair shafts and is usually an inherited abnormality of the hair follicles in which there is failure of hair growth, production of defective hair shafts, or failure to maintain hair within follicles. The conditions may be congenital or tardive (late occurring). Different types of follicular dysplasia syndromes are described, but most are poorly characterized. Microscopic features vary but include abnormal keratinocytes in the hair matrix or abnormally formed follicles, which produce abnormal hair shafts, resulting clinically in a reduced or absent hair coat. The lesions of follicular dysplasia that are most easily recognized microscopically are color associated and include color mutant alopecia (color

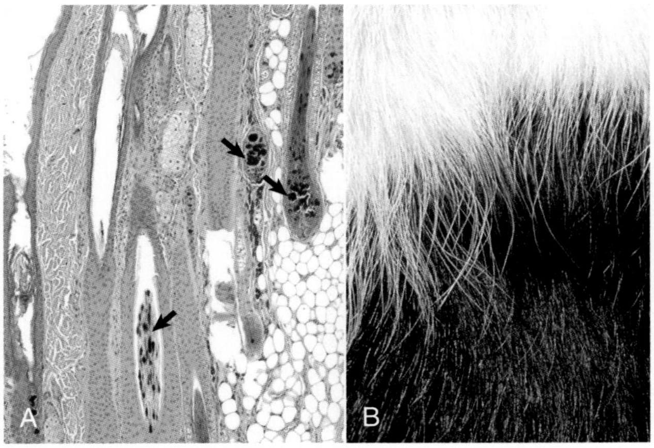

Fig. 17-23 Black hair follicular dysplasia, skin, dog. **A,** Large and variably sized and shaped melanin pigment granules are present in hair shafts and hair matrix cells *(arrows)*. Macrophages that have phagocytosed melanin pigment are present in the dermis, most prominently near hair bulbs. The melanin presumably comes from damaged hair matrix cells. H&E stain. **B,** Note alopecia in black-haired area and normal hair coat in white-haired area. The skin in the black-haired area is pigmented; thus alopecia is not easily recognized from a distance. (**A** courtesy Dr. Ann M. Hargis, DermatoDiagnostics. **B** courtesy Blackwell Publishing.)

dilution follicular dysplasia) and black hair follicular dysplasia (Fig. 17-23), in which melanin pigment abnormalities serve as a marker for the dysplasia. These pigment abnormalities include abnormally clumped melanin pigment granules in melanocytes in the epidermis and follicular hair matrix cells; irregularly sized, shaped, and distributed melanin pigment clumps in hair shafts; and macrophages containing melanin pigment and located in the perifollicular dermis. The pathogenesis of the abnormal hair coat appears to involve breakage of hair shafts in areas of large pigment clumps, an abnormality of development of the cuticle, and also possibly an abnormality of hair shaft development caused by damaged hair matrix cells.

Sebaceous Gland Dysplasia

Abnormal development of sebaceous glands is rare, is presumed to be genetic in origin, and has been reported in dogs and cats. The pathogenesis is unknown. Histologically, in early stages, there are increased numbers of small epithelial reserve cells compared with mature sebaceous gland cells. The number of mature sebaceous gland cells may be reduced, cytoplasmic vacuolization may be irregular, and the orderly differentiation of reserve cells to mature cells is missing. In the late stage, there is subtotal atrophy, where only a few reserve cells and a few mature sebaceous gland cells remain. Clinical lesions consist of adherent scales, poor hair coat, and progressive alopecia. The poor hair coat and alopecia are presumed to be the result of follicular atrophy and dysplasia that develop after or secondary to the sebaceous gland lesions.

Adnexal Inflammatory Disorders

Folliculitis

Folliculitis is inflammation of a hair follicle. Folliculitis can be histologically classified according to the anatomic segment of the hair follicle affected and the type of leukocytes present in the inflammatory infiltrate (Fig. 17-24). The types of follicular inflammation include perifolliculitis, mural folliculitis, luminal folliculitis, and inflammation of the hair bulb (bulbitis). The inflammation of hair follicles begins in the perifollicular blood vessels with the same hemodynamic, permeability, and leukocytic changes that comprise dermal inflammation. Leukocytes migrate from perifollicular blood vessels to the dermis, resulting in perifolliculitis (inflammation around but not involving the hair follicle). Perifolliculitis is not specific for any category of disease but is an initial event in the development of folliculitis. Perifolliculitis also often coincides with folliculitis of a variety of causes. The perifollicular inflammatory cells then migrate into the follicular wall, resulting in mural folliculitis (inflammation limited to the wall of the follicle). Depending on the cause of the inflammatory process, the leukocytes can remain localized to the follicular wall or can progress into the follicular lumen.

Mural

In mural folliculitis, leukocytes remain largely confined to the follicular wall. Mural folliculitis is further subdivided by the location, type, or severity of involvement of the follicular wall such as interface (outer aspect of the follicular wall), infiltrative (more infiltration into the follicular wall), pustular (presence of pustules in the follicular wall), or necrotizing (necrosis and disruption of the follicular wall). The subtype of mural folliculitis can provide insight into the pathogenesis of folliculitis (e.g., disease process). For example, pustular mural folliculitis is a feature of pemphigus foliaceous, and interface mural folliculitis is a feature of demodicosis (Fig. 17-25).

Bulbitis

Bulbitis refers to inflammation directed at the deepest portion of the follicle, the hair bulb. Alopecia areata is a specific example of bulbitis. It develops in horses, cattle, dogs, and cats; is characterized by lymphocytic infiltrates around and in growing hair bulbs; and results in alopecia. In horses and dogs, antifollicular cell-mediated immunity and humoral immunity participate. Cellular infiltrates of the hair bulb are mostly cytotoxic $CD8^+$ lymphocytes and $CD1^+$ dendritic antigen-presenting cells, whereas $CD8^+$ and $CD4^+$ lymphocytes predominate in the peribulbar infiltrate. Autoantibodies target trichohyalin, hair keratins, and other components of the hair follicle. The damage to hair matrix cells within the hair bulb results in formation of dystrophic (abnormal) hair shafts. Alopecia areata can spontaneously resolve, but the newly growing hairs can be white instead of pigmented, probably as a result of damage to melanocytes in the hair bulb.

Luminal

Luminal folliculitis refers to inflammation involving the lumen of the follicle and usually the wall of the follicle (Fig. 17-26). Luminal folliculitis develops when the leukocytes in the follicular wall migrate into the lumen, usually as a result of a stimulus in the follicular lumen, such as a follicular infection with bacteria (staphylococci) or dermatophytes *(Microsporum, Trichophyton)*, or infestation with parasites *(Demodex, Pelodera)*. The inflammation can weaken the follicular wall leading to rupture, known as *furunculosis* (Fig. 17-27), and release of follicular contents into the dermis. There are other causes of furunculosis, including trauma to the surface of the skin resulting in epidermal hyperplasia at the opening of the follicle, plugging of the follicle by stratum corneum, and accumulation of follicular contents including glandular secretions (comedo formation). The gradual accumulation of this luminal material can cause distention of the follicle and thinning of the follicular wall, leading to rupture. Regardless of the cause of furunculosis, the presence of hair fragments, keratin proteins, sebum, and possible infectious agents in the dermis leads to a suppurative inflammatory response that progresses to more

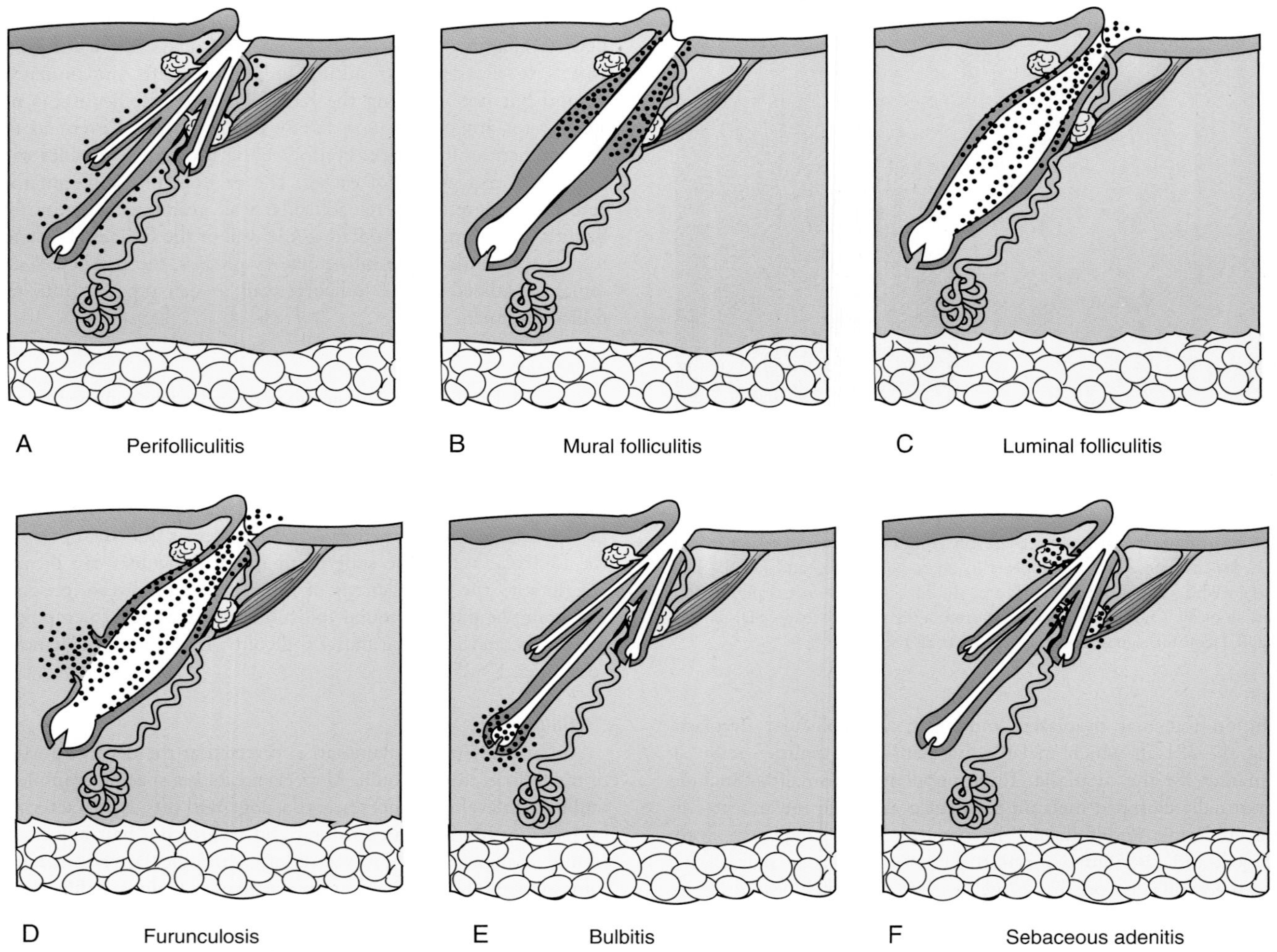

Fig. 17-24 Schematic diagram of the inflammatory patterns of the adnexa.
A, Perifollicular: Leukocytes *(black dots)* migrate from the dermal vessels near follicles into the perifollicular dermis. **B,** Mural folliculitis: Inflammation targets the follicular wall. There are subtypes of mural folliculitis that vary with level of involvement (superficial versus inferior), type of the inflammation (pustular versus necrotizing), and the degree or severity of penetration into the follicular wall (interface versus infiltrative). **C,** Luminal folliculitis: Inflammatory exudate is present in the follicular lumen, and inflammation also usually involves the wall, often a response to follicular infection. **D,** Furunculosis: Disruption of the follicular wall resulting in release of luminal contents into the bordering dermis. **E,** Bulbitis: Inflammation targeting the inferior segment of the hair follicle, also called the *hair bulb.* **F,** Sebaceous adenitis: inflammation targeting the sebaceous glands. For purposes of simplification, a simple hair follicle is illustrated in parts **B, C,** and **D.** (Redrawn from Dr. Ann M. Hargis, DermatoDiagnostics; and Dr. Pamela E. Ginn, College of Veterinary Medicine, University of Florida.)

long-standing chronic pyogranulomatous inflammation and scarring. Perifolliculitis, luminal folliculitis, and furunculosis often follow in sequence (Fig. 17-28). The inflammation can resolve with appropriate therapy, can extend into the deep dermis and panniculus, and/or can form sinuses that drain to the surface of the skin and are difficult to resolve. Severe inflammation can lead to complete destruction of adnexal units and replacement by scar tissue.

Sebaceous Adenitis

Sebaceous adenitis is a specific inflammatory reaction that targets sebaceous glands; it is largely a disease of dogs (Fig. 17-29), but rarely is seen in cats and horses. Early histologic lesions are characterized by accumulations of lymphocytes around sebaceous ducts. Fully developed lesions consist of lymphocytes, neutrophils, and macrophages that efface sebaceous glands. Chronic lesions have total loss of sebaceous glands (atrophy), scarring, and epidermal and follicular hyperkeratosis. Sebaceous gland inflammation also can occur secondary to folliculitis, demodicosis, uveodermatologic syndrome, or leishmaniasis, in which the inflammation targets other areas of the skin (follicles, epidermal cells, or dermis) and involves the neighboring sebaceous glands because of their proximity to the inflammation.

Hidradenitis

Hidradenitis, which is inflammation of apocrine glands, has rarely been studied in detail in domestic animals. Suppurative hidradenitis has been described in dogs in which most cases developed in conjunction with staphylococcal folliculitis and furunculosis, either affecting the same or other follicular units. It is speculated, because of the physical connection between the apocrine gland and hair follicle in dogs, that suppurative hidradenitis is most often an extension of hair follicle infection and is the result of the bacteria that cause the folliculitis. There are no clinical signs that are unique to or suggest the presence of hidradenitis other than the association with follicular bacterial infection. Histologically, dogs with hidradenitis associated with bacterial folliculitis and

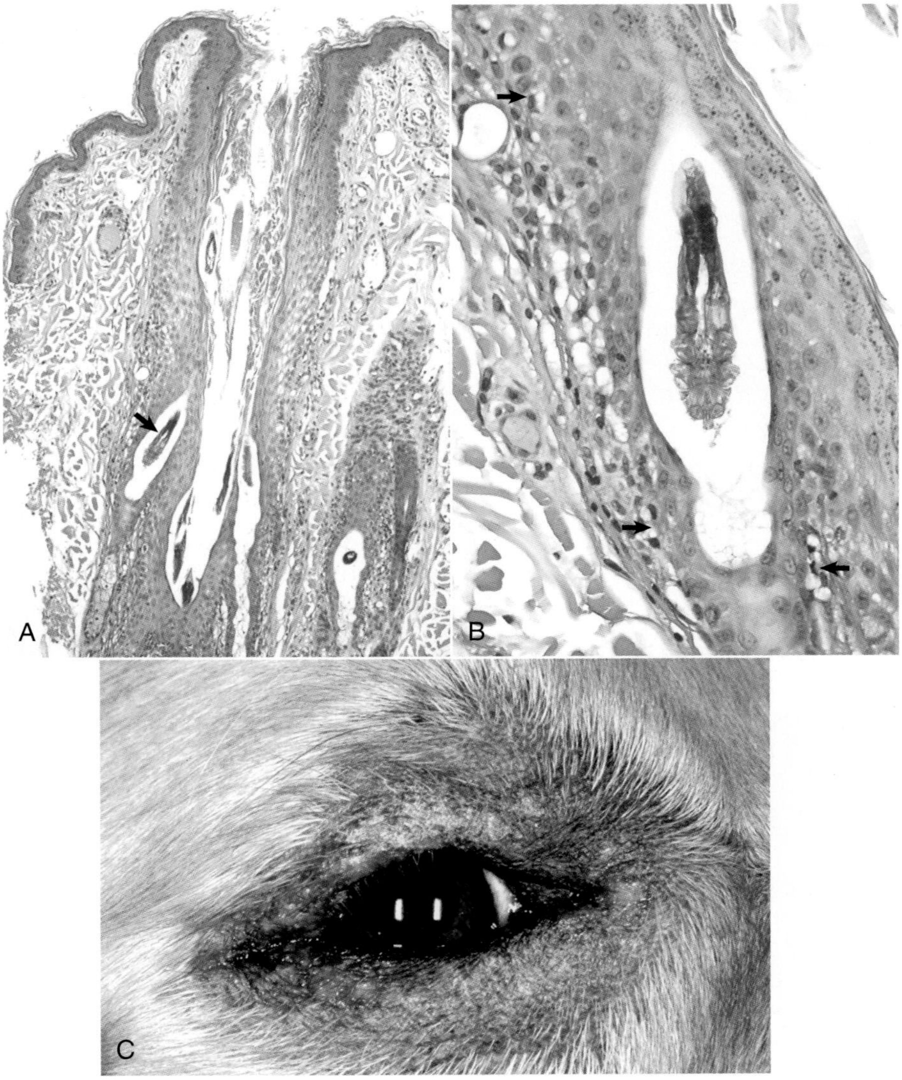

Fig. 17-25 Demodicosis, skin, dog.
A, Note mites deep in the lumens of follicles *(arrow)* and also inflammation in the outer wall of the follicle (interface mural folliculitis) and in the perifollicular dermis (perifolliculitis). H&E stain. **B,** Note the mite in the follicular lumen. There are a few lymphocytes bordering the follicular wall and mild vacuolar degeneration of basal cells *(arrows)* (lymphocytic interface mural folliculitis) of the follicular wall. H&E stain. **C,** Localized demodicosis, periocular. Skin is alopecic, lichenified, and hyperpigmented. Alopecia is likely caused by inflammation, initiated by an immune response to mite infestation and possibly secondary bacterial infection, that results in damage and sometimes disruption of the follicular wall (furunculosis). (Courtesy Dr. Ann M. Hargis, DermatoDiagnostics.)

furunculosis have suppurative inflammation of the apocrine gland and surrounding dermis.

Responses of the Vessels to Injury

Vasculitis, inflammation of vessels (see Fig. 17-22, *B*) in which the vessels are the primary target of injury, can be the result of infection by microbes, immunologic injury, toxins, photodynamic chemicals, or disseminated intravascular coagulation (DIC) or can be idiopathic. The species most commonly presenting with vasculitis are the horse and the dog, and most cases are idiopathic in that a specific cause cannot be determined. Histologic diagnosis of vasculitis is often challenging because it is difficult to differentiate between vessels taking part in inflammation simply by providing a conduit for inflammatory cells to reach a site of injury in the epidermis or dermis from those vessels that are actually the target of injury. Also, the type of inflammatory cell that participates in the inflammatory process can vary more with the age of the vascular lesion than with the type of disease process. Histologic lesions in vasculitis include damage to the vessel wall such as the presence of few necrotic cells or foci of fibrinoid necrosis, mural infiltrates of leukocytes, and intramural or perivascular edema, hemorrhage, or fibrin exudation. Vascular injury leads to the clinical lesions of edema and hemorrhage and if severe, can include ischemic necrosis and infarction. Ulceration with or without sloughing of the skin can occur. Partial ischemia can lead to atrophic changes in the components of the skin. Classic examples include immune-complex deposition in vessel walls (systemic lupus erythematosus and equine purpura hemorrhagica), rabies vaccination–associated vasculitis and ischemic dermatopathy, infection with an endotheliotropic organism *(Rickettsia rickettsii),* and septicemia with bacterial embolism and infarction in pigs *(Erysipelothrix rhusiopathiae).*

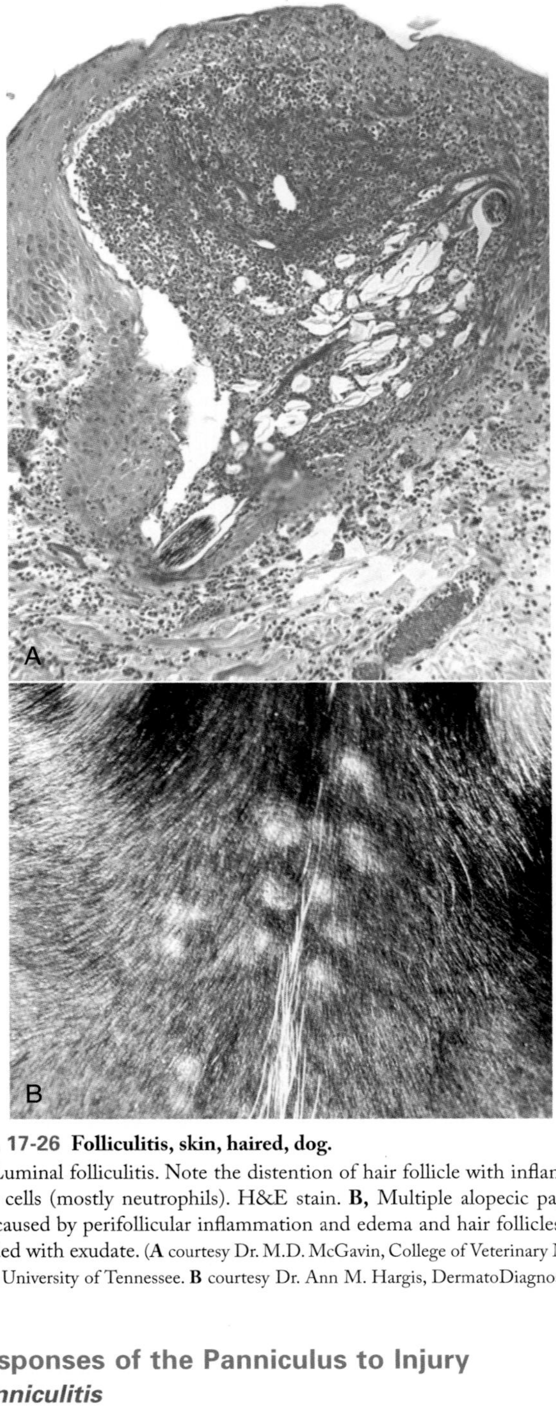

Fig. 17-26 Folliculitis, skin, haired, dog.
A, Luminal folliculitis. Note the distention of hair follicle with inflammatory cells (mostly neutrophils). H&E stain. **B,** Multiple alopecic papules are caused by perifollicular inflammation and edema and hair follicles distended with exudate. (**A** courtesy Dr. M.D. McGavin, College of Veterinary Medicine, University of Tennessee. **B** courtesy Dr. Ann M. Hargis, DermatoDiagnostics.)

Responses of the Panniculus to Injury

Panniculitis

Panniculitis, which is inflammation of the subcutaneous adipose tissue, can be caused by infectious agents (bacteria, fungi), immune-mediated disorders (systemic lupus erythematosus), physical injury (trauma, injection of irritant material, foreign bodies), nutritional disorders (vitamin E deficiency), or pancreatic disease (pancreatitis, pancreatic carcinoma) or can be of undetermined cause (idiopathic). Panniculitis can be primary or secondary. In primary panniculitis, the subcutaneous adipose tissue is the target of the disease process (Fig. 17-30). An example of primary panniculitis is feline pansteatitis, which occurs in cats fed diets high in polyunsaturated fats and low in antioxidants, such as vitamin E. Lack of vitamin E leads to oxidation of lipids (free radical–induced membrane lipid peroxidation) of the subcutaneous adipose tissue, inciting a pyogranulomatous inflammatory response. In secondary panniculitis, the subcutis is affected by inflammation primarily involving the contiguous dermis; the inflammation extends down into the subcutis. For example, deep bacterial folliculitis with furunculosis can lead to a secondary panniculitis, as can a penetrating wound contaminated with microbial agents or a foreign body. Animals with panniculitis clinically have palpable nodules that can ulcerate and drain an oily or hemorrhagic material. Lesions are most often on the trunk and proximal limbs and can be solitary or multifocal. Solitary lesions may be cured by excision, whereas multiple lesions may resolve with specific therapy or result in scar formation. In animals, panniculitis is subdivided based on cell type and presence or absence of microorganisms into the following basic categories: predominantly neutrophilic, predominantly lymphocytic, predominantly granulomatous to pyogranulomatous with infectious agents, predominantly granulomatous to pyogranulomatous without infectious agents, and fibrosing.

Pathologic Reactions of the Entire Cutaneous Unit

Disease processes involving the skin uncommonly affect just one component of the skin (i.e., only the epidermis or only the lumens of hair follicles). More often, multiple components of the skin are involved in the disease process. In addition, lesions evolve through different stages; some lesions can resolve, and there can be secondary lesions, such as self-induced trauma, complicating the initial lesions. Therefore multiple biopsy samples collected from different areas of the skin are often necessary to help illustrate the range of lesions necessary to reach a diagnosis. Multiple biopsy samples provide a more representative picture of the disease process than could a single biopsy sample. Even so, evaluation of multiple biopsy samples does not always lead to a specific diagnosis, but the pattern of lesions identified often suggests categories of disease and rules out other differential diagnoses.

The involvement of the multiple components of the skin in a disease process can be illustrated by a poxvirus infection (Fig. 17-31). When a poxvirus invades the epidermis, the virus replicates in the cells of the stratum spinosum and causes cytoplasmic swelling (ballooning degeneration) and rupture (reticular degeneration) of some of the epidermal cells. Cytoplasmic viral inclusions form in some cells. Cellular constituents released from damaged epidermal cells act as chemical mediators of the acute inflammatory response and are chemotactic for leukocytes. These chemical mediators and chemotactic factors (1) increase blood flow to the site of viral invasion by dilation of arterioles, (2) cause margination of leukocytes in capillaries and postcapillary venules in the dermis, (3) increase vascular permeability (dermal edema), and (4) cause migration of leukocytes out of vessels into the tissue, creating the formation of macular lesions. The epidermal degeneration, dermal edema, and perivascular inflammation can progress to exudative lesions. Ballooning and reticular degeneration of keratinocytes result in the formation of intraepidermal vesicles. Leukocytes in perivascular sites under the influence of inflammatory mediators from the epidermis migrate to the epidermis and enter the vesicle to form pustules. Some poxviruses also cause epidermal hyperplasia by stimulating host cell DNA synthesis, presumably by a viral gene product similar to epidermal growth factor, resulting in pseudocarcinomatous hyperplasia. The pustule enlarges and eventually ruptures, releasing the exudates onto the skin surface. The exudates dry and form a crust (scab). The primary lesions of vesicles and pustules are fragile and often transient, lasting only hours, and so are difficult to identify and collect in biopsy samples. The secondary

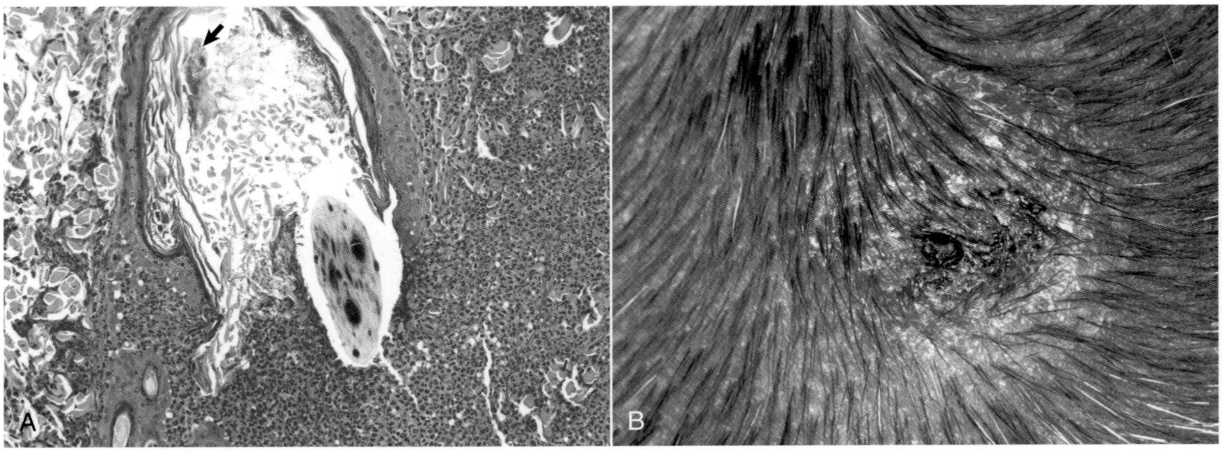

Fig. 17-27 Folliculitis and furunculosis, skin, haired, dog.
A, The wall of the follicle has become disrupted, resulting in the release of follicular contents (a hair shaft, stratum corneum of the follicle, and exudate) into the dermis. The follicular lumen also contains numerous coccoid bacteria *(arrow)*. The hair shaft has variably sized and shaped melanin pigment granules, indicating that this dog also has coat color dilution. H&E stain. **B,** A circular area of erythema, scaling, and crusting is caused by follicular inflammation and rupture (furunculosis). The inflammation in the perifollicular dermis has extended into the surrounding dermis and formed a draining sinus to the epidermal surface. The exudate on the surface has dried to form a crust. (Courtesy Dr. Ann M. Hargis, DermatoDiagnostics.)

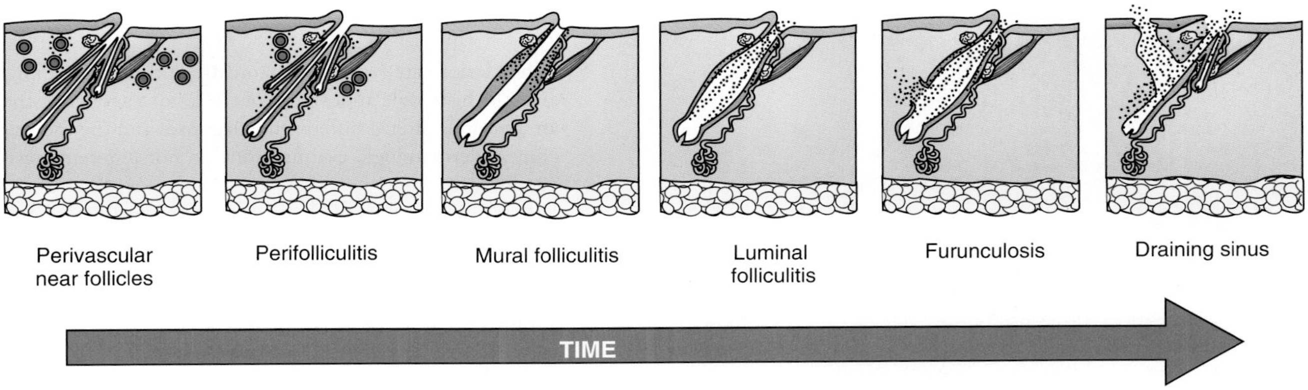

Fig. 17-28 Schematic diagram of the progression of folliculitis.
Inflammation begins with migration of leukocytes *(black dots)* from perifollicular dermal vessels into the perifollicular dermis (perifolliculitis). Inflammation progresses to involve the follicular wall (mural folliculitis) and then the lumen (luminal folliculitis). If the inflammation continues, the follicular wall is weakened, ruptures, and follicular contents are released into the dermis. The inflammation can extend into the deep dermis and panniculus, and/or form sinuses that drain to the surface of the skin. For purposes of simplification, a simple hair follicle is illustrated in some frames. (Redrawn from Dr. Ann M. Hargis, DermatoDiagnostics; and Dr. Pamela E. Ginn, College of Veterinary Medicine, University of Florida.)

lesions of crusting and scarring are more long-standing. In this way, multiple components of the skin participate in the development of the lesions and are responsible for the clinical stages of macule, papule, vesicle, pustule, crust, and scar.

DEFINITIONS OF CLINICAL TERMS

Knowledge of the clinical appearance of skin lesions, distribution of lesions, and correlation between the gross and histologic lesions is often critical in formulating differential and final diagnoses. In skin diseases, the clinical lesions represent the gross lesions and are typically examined by a practitioner, not the pathologist; thus the practitioner essentially serves as the eyes for the pathologist. It is therefore important for the practitioner to develop the ability to accurately recognize clinical lesion morphology and translate that information to the pathologist. To facilitate this process, Table 17-3 is provided to illustrate the morphology of the various clinical lesions and provide examples of the disease processes in which those lesions occur.

TECHNIQUES FOR SKIN BIOPSY SAMPLING

Important tips for biopsy sampling of the skin are listed in Table 17-4. Biopsy do's and don'ts are listed in Boxes 17-4 and 17-5, respectively.

When to Collect Biopsy Samples

Knowing when to collect biopsy samples helps obtain the most diagnostic samples; facilitates obtaining samples early so acute, serious, or neoplastic disorders are diagnosed quickly; and prevents the frustration and economic loss when samples are inappropriately collected, such as when concurrent therapy might alter diagnostic lesions, when lesions are in a quiescent stage and might not be diagnostic, and when clinical dermatologic evaluation would have been a better method of achieving a diagnosis. Biopsy sampling is recommended when the following are present:

1. The therapy for the skin disorder is associated with significant side effects (to confirm the clinical diagnosis before starting therapy).

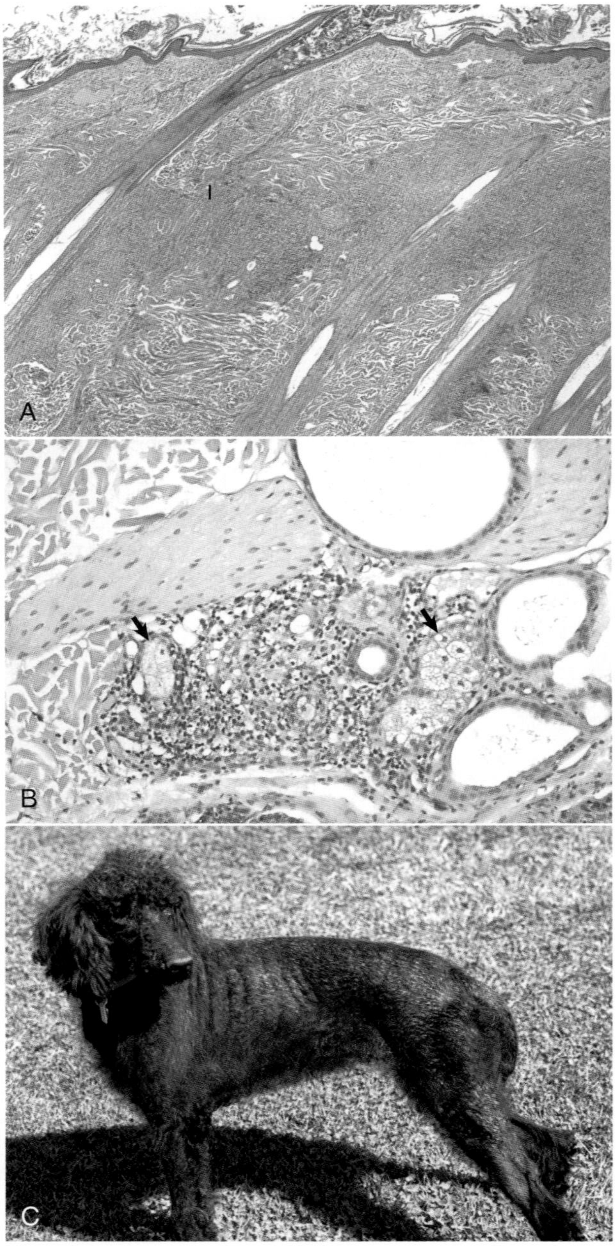

Fig. 17-29 Sebaceous adenitis, skin, haired, dog.
A, Note the inflammation (I) concentrated in and around sebaceous glands. The inflammation forms a band of inflammatory cells parallel to the epidermis at the level of the sebaceous glands. H&E stain. **B,** Inflammation is beginning to efface the sebaceous glands. A few sebaceous glands *(arrows)* are visible within the area of inflammation. H&E stain. **C,** Alopecia and scaling are evident. The pathogenesis of sebaceous adenitis and the alopecia and scaling is incompletely understood. (Courtesy Dr. Ann M. Hargis, DermatoDiagnostics.)

2. A nodular lesion, ulcer, or nonhealing wound might represent a tumor (so that surgical excision of the tumor can be performed as early as possible).
3. Lesions develop suddenly, are severe, or are unusual (to help identify a serious disease so that therapy can be instituted early).
4. Lesions develop during the course of therapy (to identify a potential adverse reaction to drug therapy).

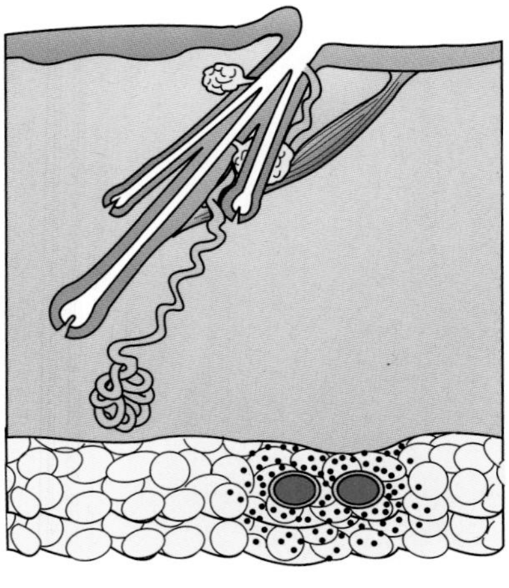

Fig. 17-30 Schematic diagram of inflammation in the panniculus. Note the leukocytic inflammation *(black dots)* in the subcutaneous adipose tissue (panniculitis). In addition to spreading locally, the inflammation can form a sinus through the dermis and epidermis to the surface. The exudate can have an oily composition as a result of the fat content of the panniculus. (Redrawn from Dr. Ann M. Hargis, DermatoDiagnostics; and Dr. Pamela E. Ginn, College of Veterinary Medicine, University of Florida.)

5. When lesions are active and before use of therapy that might alter the histologic appearance of the lesions and when there are multiple clinical differential diagnoses and the thorough clinical dermatologic examinations do not differentiate the conditions.
6. When a skin disorder fails to respond to apparently appropriate therapy or when the disorder responds to therapy but recurs when therapy is stopped (to establish the correct diagnosis, or evaluate for predisposing factors). Recall that antiinflammatory therapy can alter lesions.

Site Selection

Multiple cutaneous sites representative of the range of lesions should be selected for biopsy. Fully developed nontreated primary lesions, such as macules, papules, pustules, nodules, neoplasms, vesicles, and wheals, are often the most useful for diagnosis (see Table 17-3). However, primary lesions may not be present at the time the animal is examined, so secondary lesions, such as scales, crusts, ulcers, comedones, or scars then need to be sampled and evaluated (see Table 17-3). These secondary lesions can be diagnostic or contribute substantially to the diagnosis when multiple cutaneous sites are selected for biopsy. One of the most useful secondary lesions is the crust because acantholytic cells from drying pustules in pemphigus foliaceous and organisms, such as *Dermatophilus congolensis* or dermatophytes, may be identified in crusts, providing the information necessary for diagnosis. Also, the margin of a chronic ulcer may represent a squamous cell carcinoma, or the scale at the edge of an epidermal collarette (i.e., peripherally expanding ring of epidermal scales) may represent superficial spreading pyoderma, thus providing the key to diagnosis.

Methods

Excisional biopsy samples (entire lesions) are recommended for large pustules or vesicles that can be damaged by use of a smaller punch biopsy instrument. Deeper excisional biopsy samples are generally necessary for diagnosis of lesions, such as panniculitis, that are deep to the epidermis and dermis. Digital amputation

Text continued on p. 1006

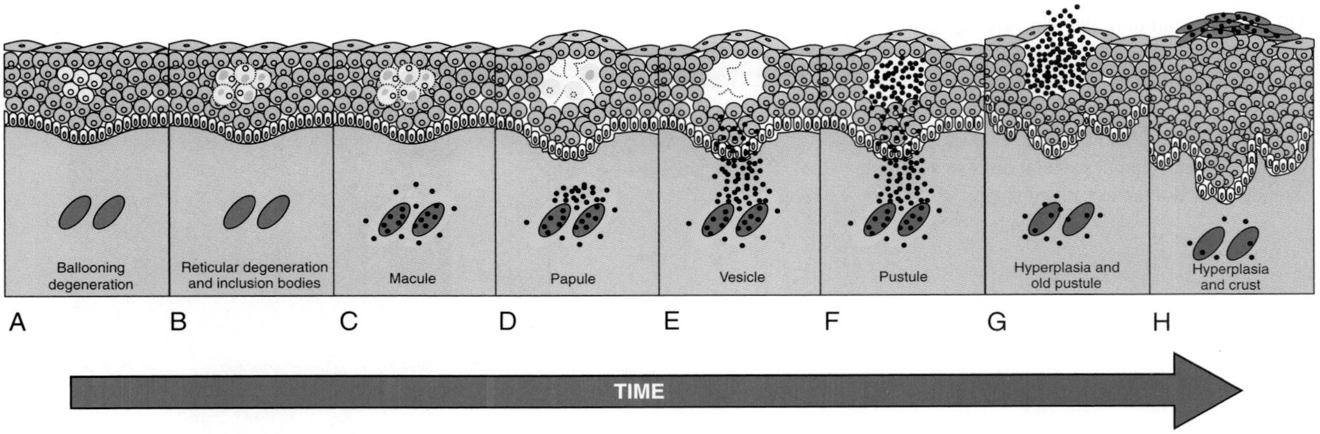

Fig. 17-31 Schematic diagram of the development of a poxvirus lesion over time.
A, Ballooning degeneration. **B,** Reticular degeneration with cytoplasmic inclusion bodies of keratinocytes. Both **A** and **B** are subclinical stages. **C,** Congestion, edema, margination, and migration of leukocytes *(black dots)* form the macule stage. **D,** Continued epidermal reticular degeneration, epidermal hyperplasia (acanthosis), dermal edema, and perivascular inflammation form the papule stage. **E,** The vesicle stage develops by coalescing of areas of reticular degeneration (disruption of swollen keratinocytes). **F,** Inflammatory cells migrate from the dermal vessels into the vesicle and accumulate in the vesicle to form the pustule stage. **G,** The epidermis begins to proliferate and becomes more acanthotic, and the old pustule is moved toward the epidermal surface. **H,** Epidermal hyperplasia progresses with the formation of elongated epidermal dermal interdigitations, and the old pustule ruptures to form a crust. Larger pustules can be umbilicated, involve the dermis, and result in scarring. (Redrawn from Dr. Ann M. Hargis, DermatoDiagnostics; and Dr. Pamela E. Ginn, College of Veterinary Medicine, University of Florida.)

TABLE 17-3 Definition and Morphology of Primary and Secondary Skin Lesions

Lesion Definition	Drawing	Clinical Photograph
CALLUS* Thick, hard, hairless plaque with increased skin creases Example: Trauma over bony prominence such as elbow or sternum	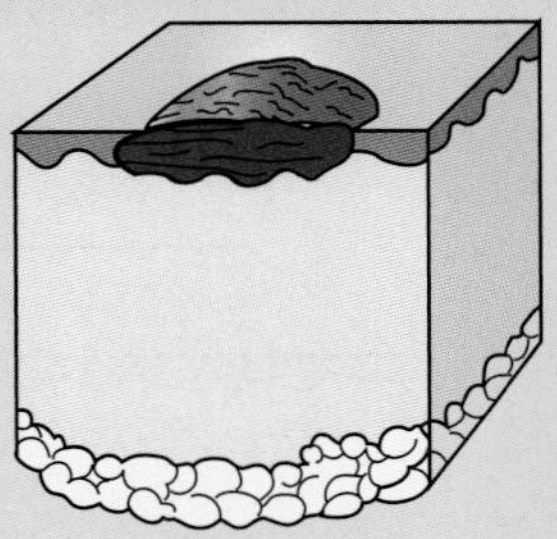	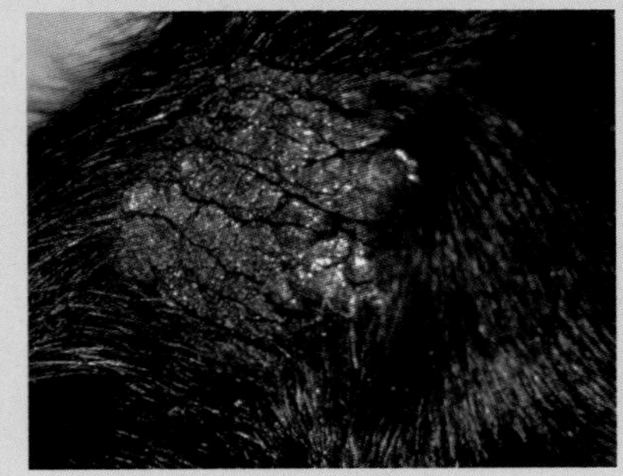
COMEDO Plug of stratum corneum and sebum *(arrows)* within the lumen of a hair follicle Examples: Canine solar (actinic) dermatosis, chin acne, Schnauzer comedo syndrome, hyperadrenocorticism	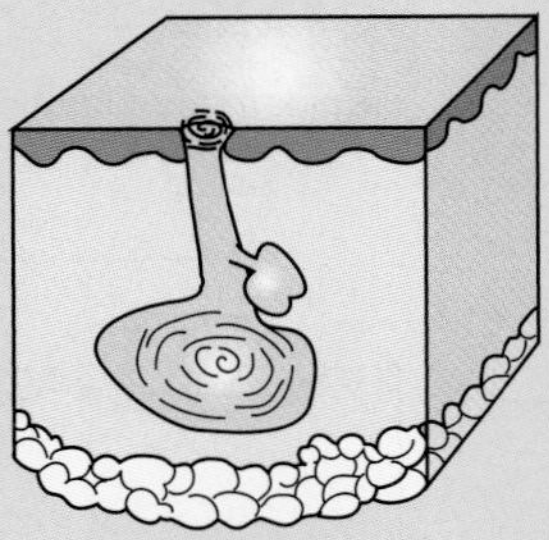	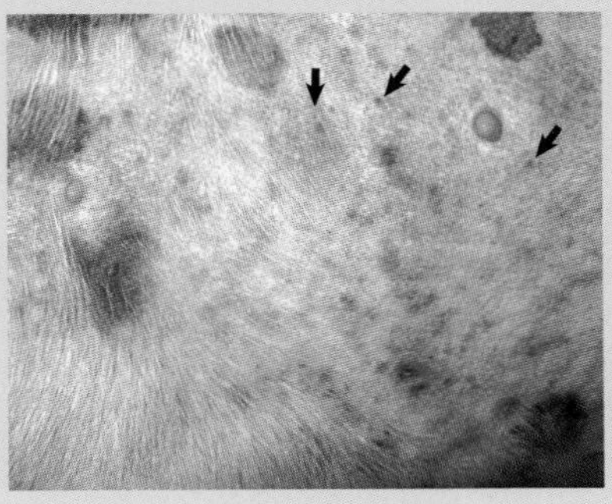

Continued

TABLE 17-3 Definition and Morphology of Primary and Secondary Skin Lesions—cont'd

Lesion Definition	Drawing	Clinical Photograph
CRUST Dried exudate on the skin surface Example: Chronic stage of pustular disease such as staphylococcal infection or pemphigus foliaceous	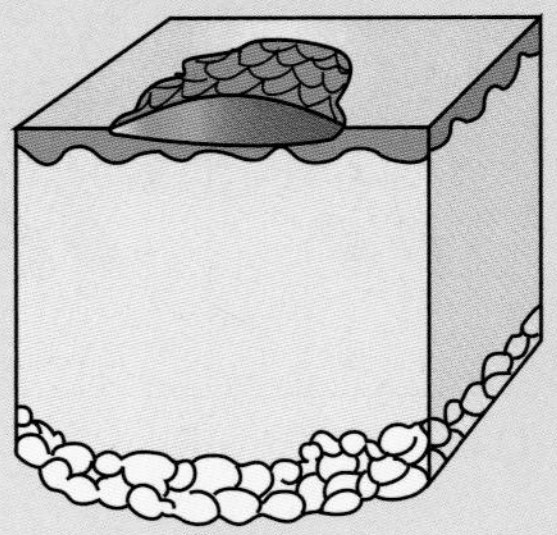 Crust	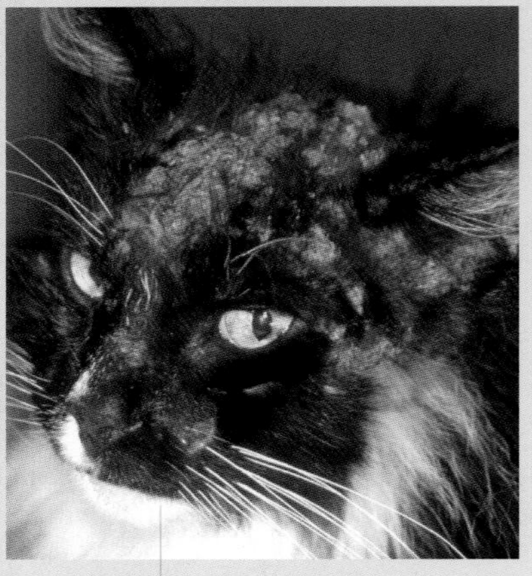
CYST Cavity lined by epithelium and filled with liquid or semisolid material and located in the dermis or subcutis Examples: Follicular cyst, dermoid cyst, apocrine gland cyst	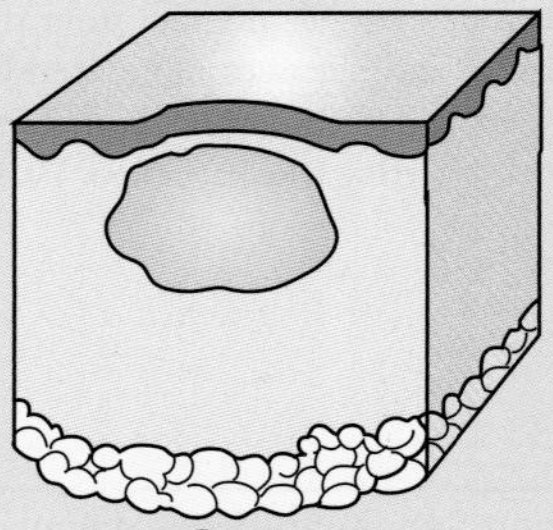 Cyst	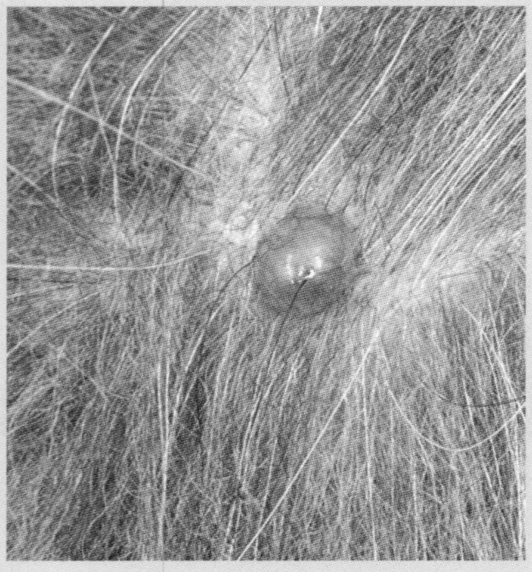
EPIDERMAL COLLARETTE Flat to minimally elevated ring *(arrows)* of scale that enlarges peripherally Examples: Superficial bacterial infection, insect bite, fungal infection	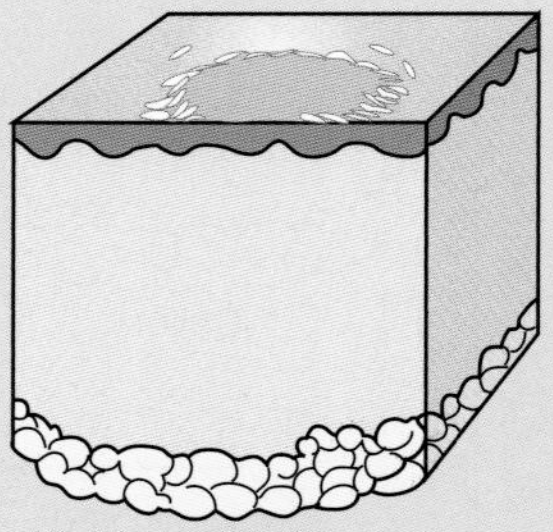 Epidermal collarette	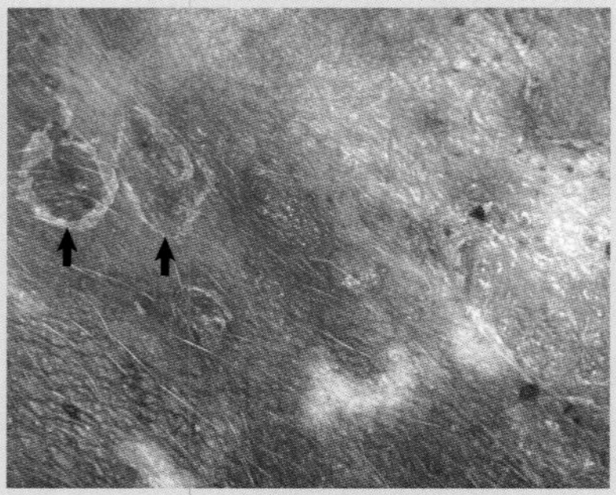
EROSION Loss of part of the epidermis; depressed, moist, glistening *(arrows)* Examples: Secondary to vesicle or pustule rupture or secondary to surface trauma	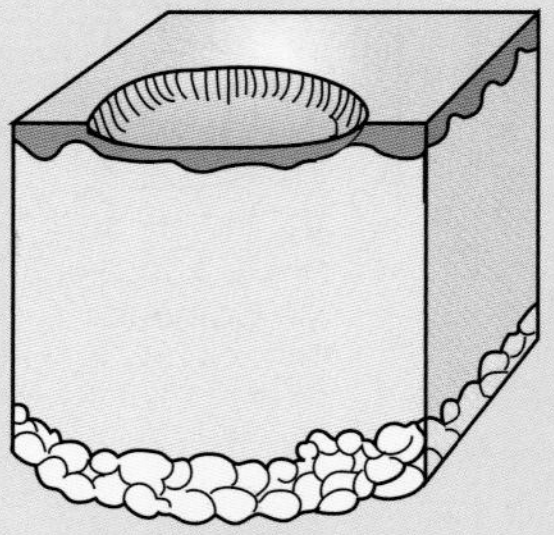 Erosion	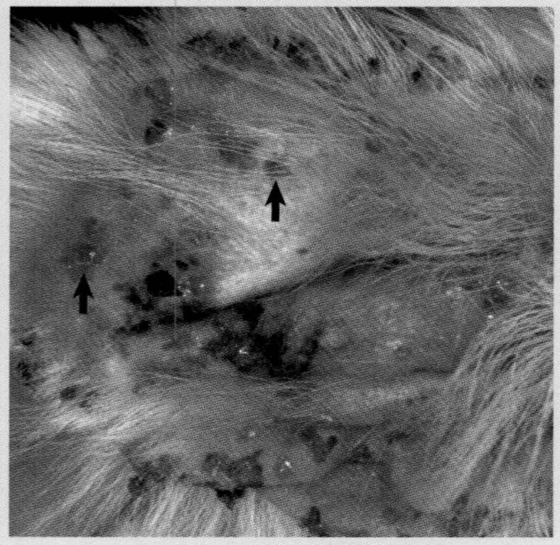

TABLE 17-3 Definition and Morphology of Primary and Secondary Skin Lesions—cont'd

Lesion Definition	Drawing	Clinical Photograph
EXCORIATION[†] Linear loss of epidermis *(arrows)* Example: Abrasion or scratch	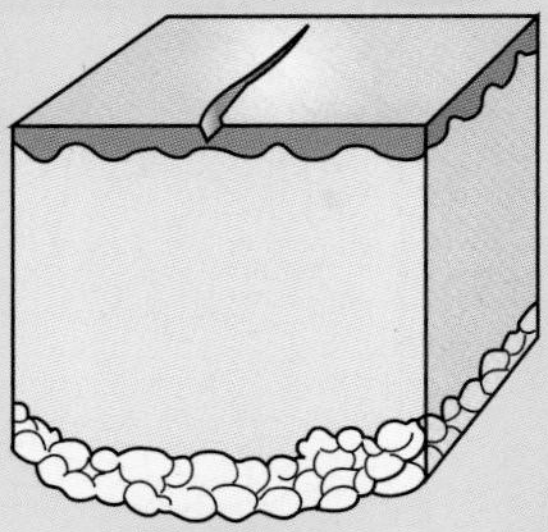 Excoriation	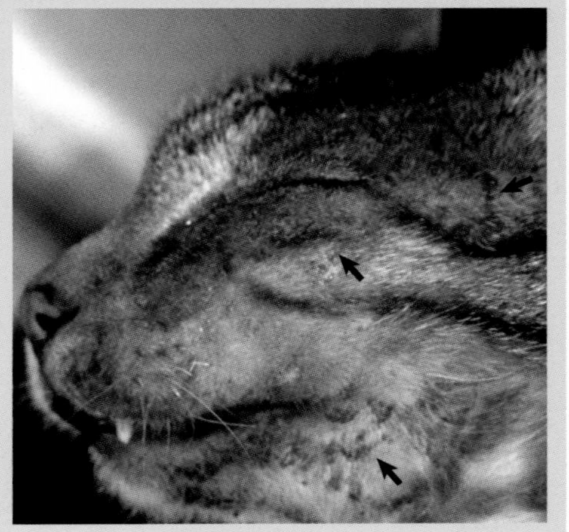
FISSURE Linear crack or break *(arrow)* from the epidermis to the dermis Examples: Pawpad fissure seen in pemphigus foliaceous, superficial necrolytic dermatitis, or digital hyperkeratosis	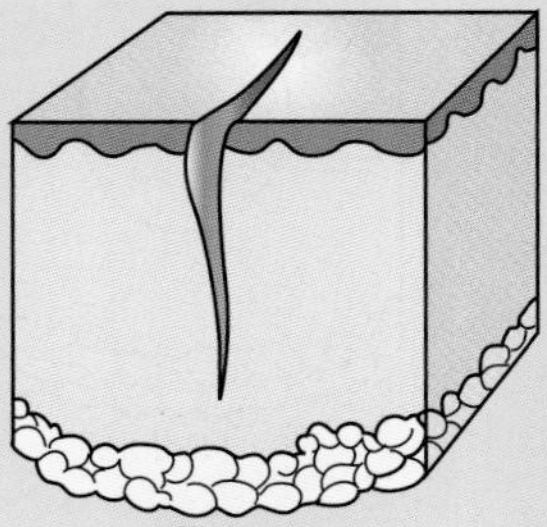 Fissure	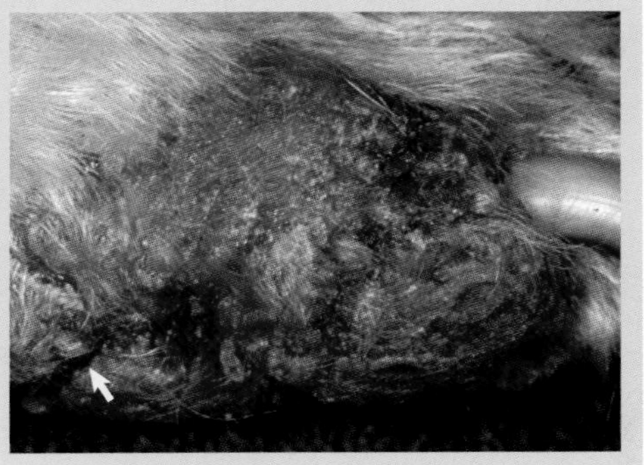
LICHENIFICATION[‡] Rough, thickened epidermis secondary to persistent rubbing, scratching, or irritation Example: Chronic dermatitis	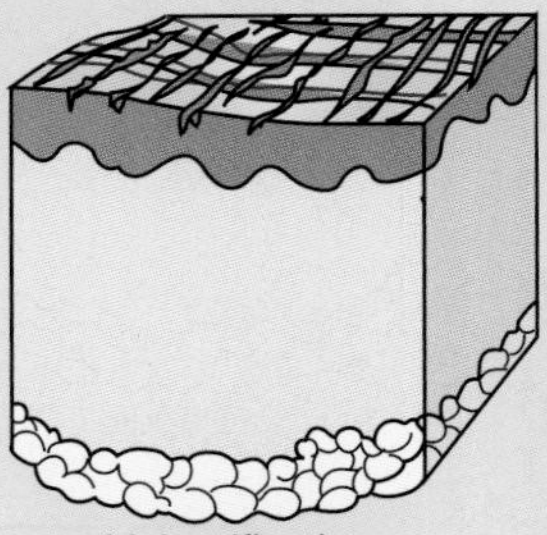 Lichenification	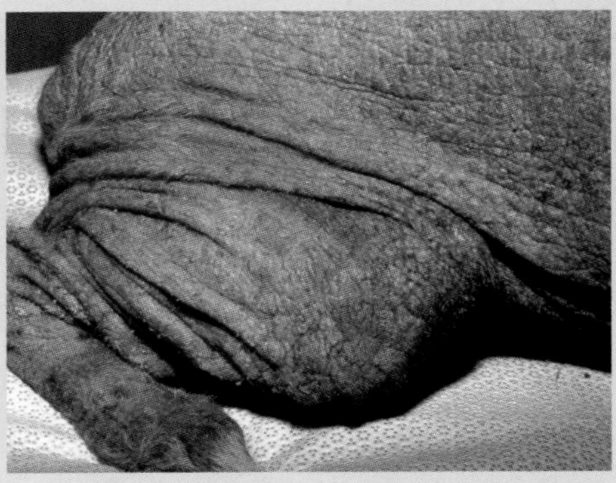
MACULE Flat, circumscribed area that is a change in the color of the skin, <1 cm in diameter Examples: Hemorrhage, lentigo, vitiligo	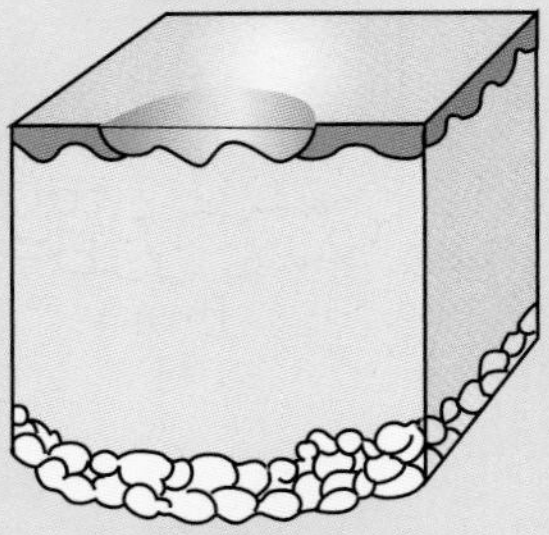 Macule	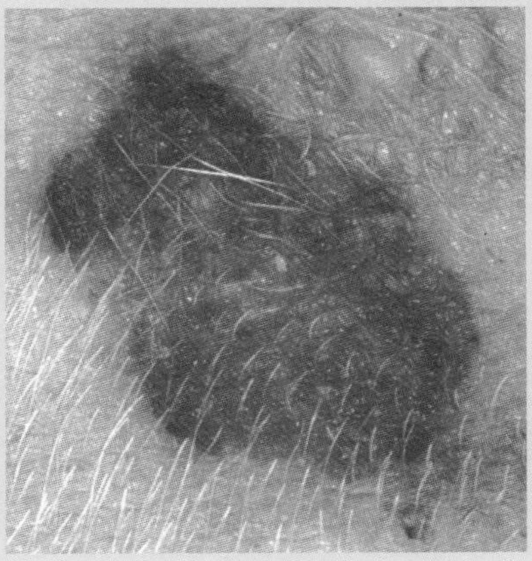

Continued

TABLE 17-3 Definition and Morphology of Primary and Secondary Skin Lesions—cont'd

Lesion Definition	Drawing	Clinical Photograph
NEOPLASM[§] "An abnormal mass of tissue, the growth of which exceeds and is uncoordinated with that of normal tissue and persists in the same excessive manner after cessation of the stimuli, which evoked the change[¶]" Examples: Lipoma, mast cell tumor, squamous cell carcinoma	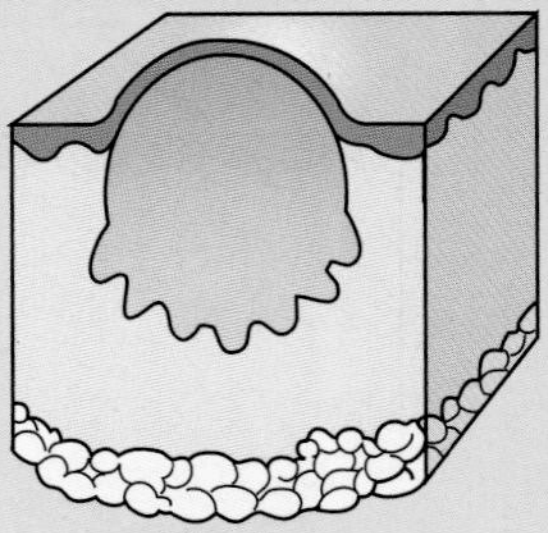 Neoplasm	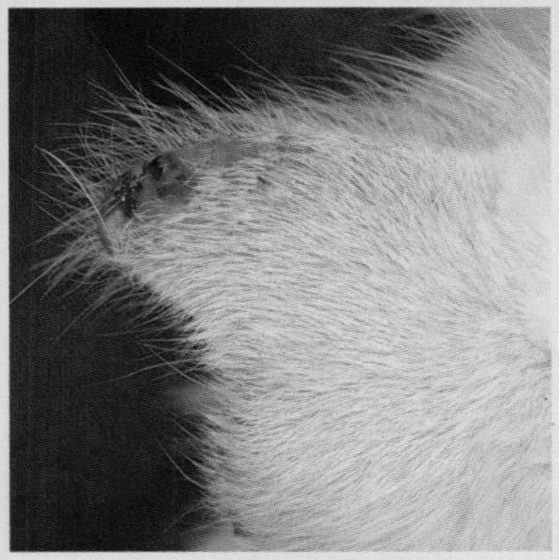
NODULE[¶] Elevated, firm, circumscribed lesion ≥1 cm in diameter Examples: Bacterial or fungal infection, infectious or sterile granuloma	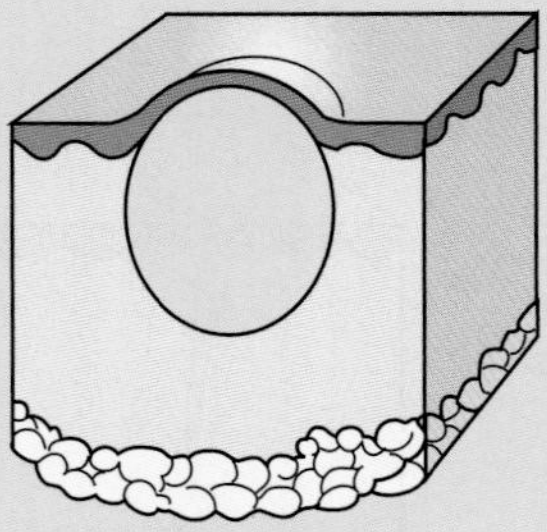 Nodule	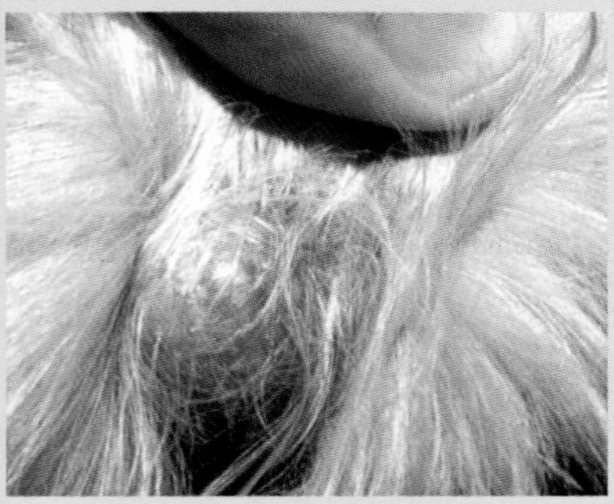
PAPULE Elevated, firm, circumscribed area <1 cm in diameter *(arrows)* Examples: Insect bite, papilloma, superficial folliculitis	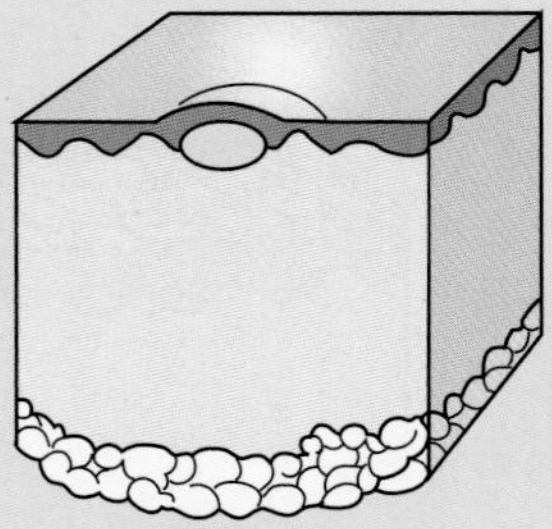 Papule	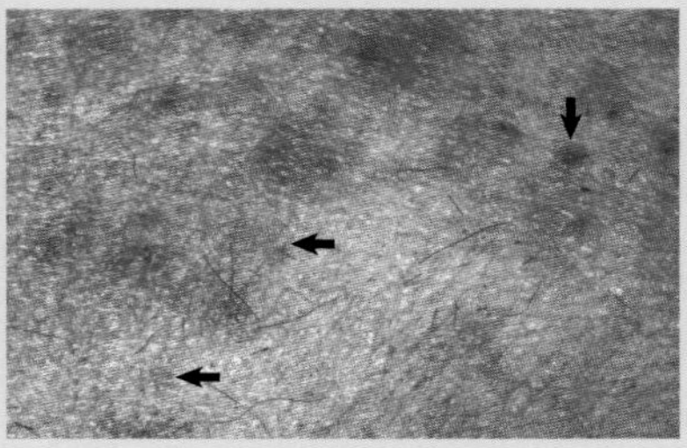
PLAQUE Elevated, firm lesion with a flat top surface ≥1 cm in diameter Examples: Calcinosis cutis, reactive histiocytosis, eosinophilic plaque	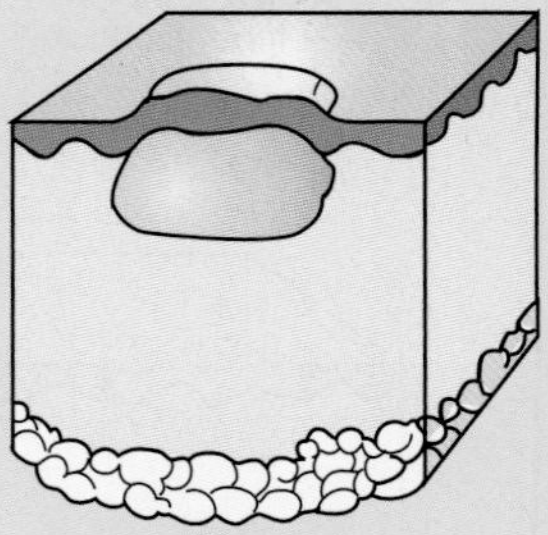 Plaque	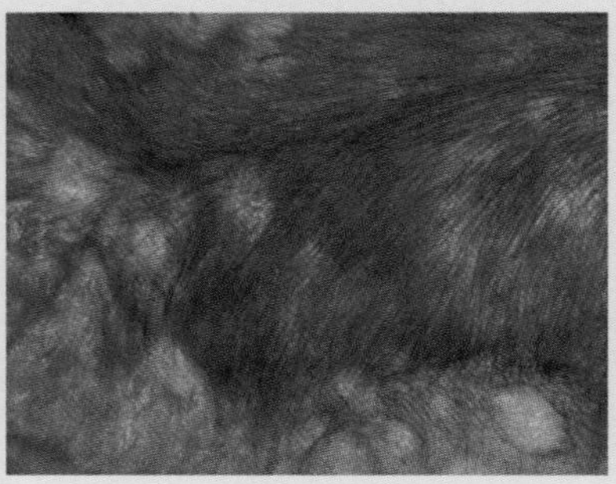

TABLE 17-3 Definition and Morphology of Primary and Secondary Skin Lesions—cont'd

Lesion Definition	Drawing	Clinical Photograph
PUSTULE, EPIDERMAL[†] Elevated superficial accumulation of purulent fluid within the epidermis *(arrow)* Examples: Bacterial infection, pemphigus foliaceous	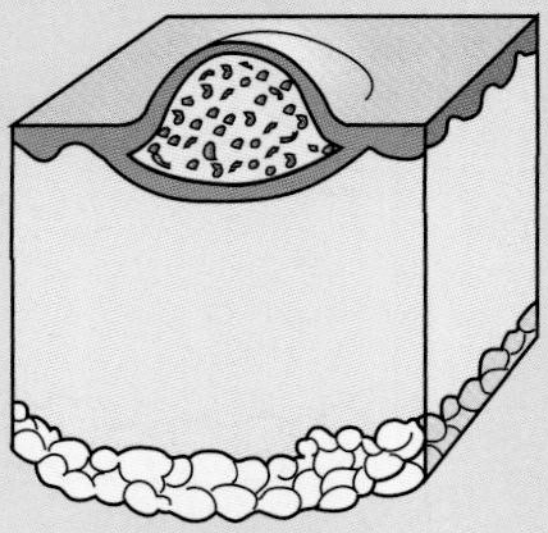 Pustule	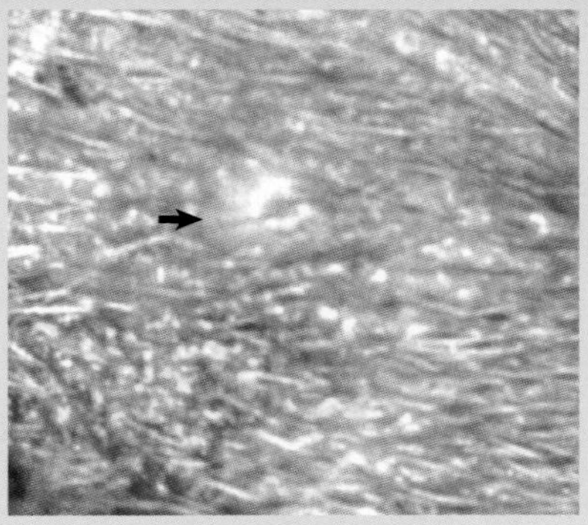
SCALE Fragmented, keratinized cells, flaky skin, irregular, thick or thin, dry or oily Examples: Cornification disorders, sebaceous adenitis, ichthyosis	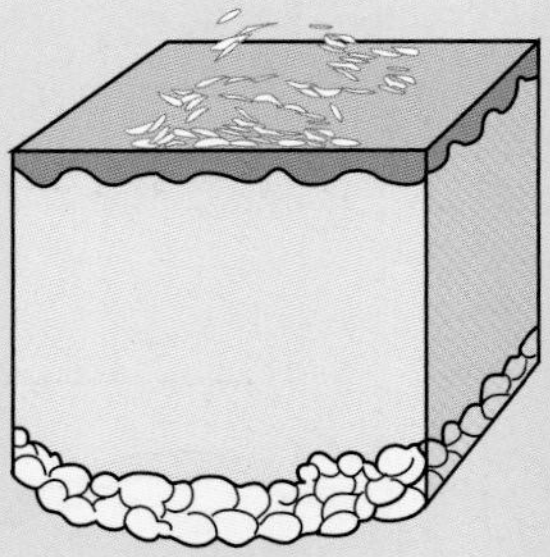 Scale	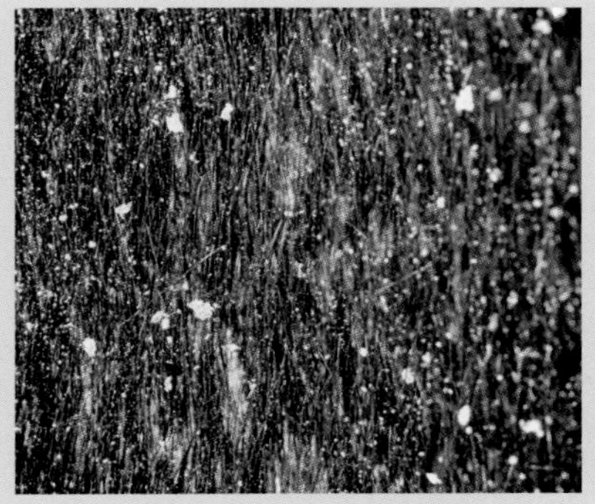
SCAR Thin to thick fibrous tissue that replaces normal skin following injury or laceration to the dermis Examples: Healed wound, surgical scar	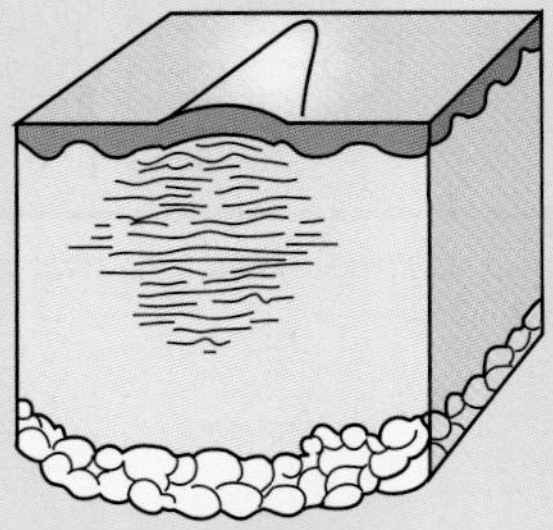 Scar	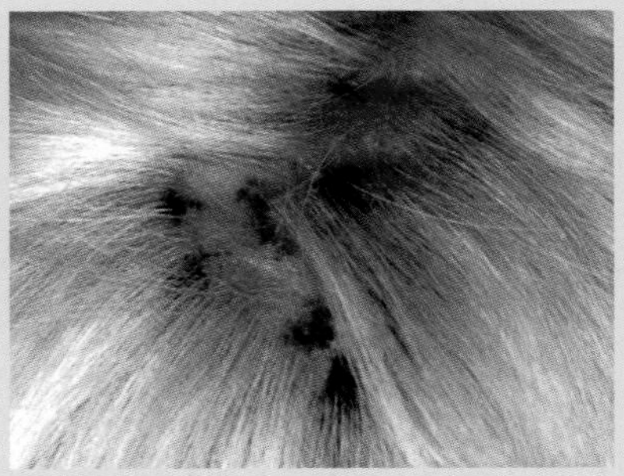
ULCER[†] Loss of epidermis and basement membrane with exposure of dermis, concave Examples: Ischemic lesions resulting from vasculitis, indolent ulcer, feline herpesvirus infection, feline ulcerative dermatosis syndrome	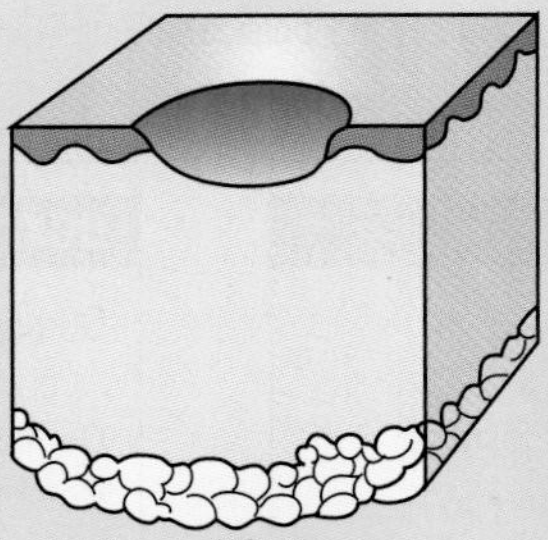 Ulcer	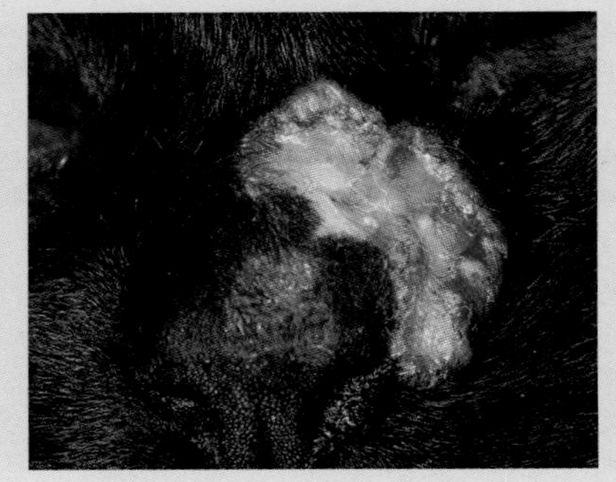

Continued

TABLE 17-3 Definition and Morphology of Primary and Secondary Skin Lesions—cont'd

Lesion Definition	Drawing	Clinical Photograph
VESICLE AND BULLA** Vesicle: Elevated, circumscribed, fluid-filled lesion <1 cm in diameter Bulla: A large vesicular lesion ≥1 cm in diameter *(arrows)* Examples: Burn, viral infection, immune- mediated diseases such as bullous pemphigoid	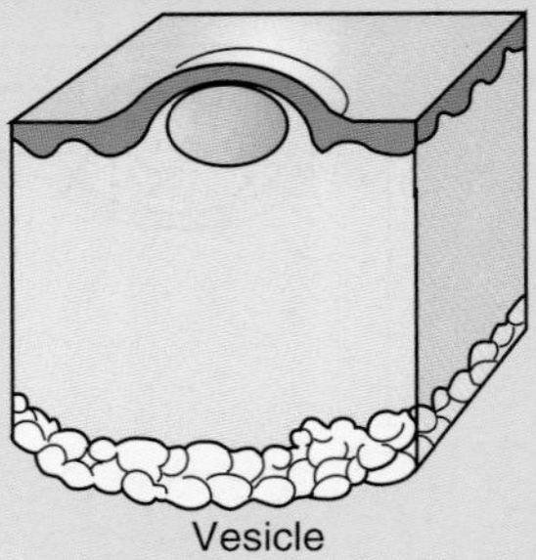	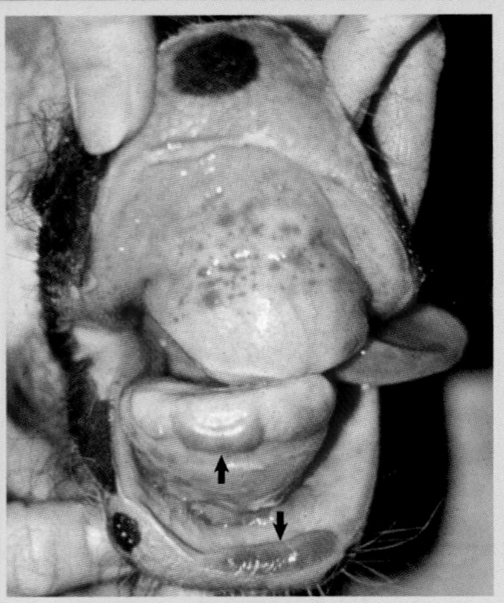
WHEAL† Elevated, irregular-shaped area of cutaneous edema; solid, transient *(arrows)* Examples: Insect bites, urticaria, allergic reaction	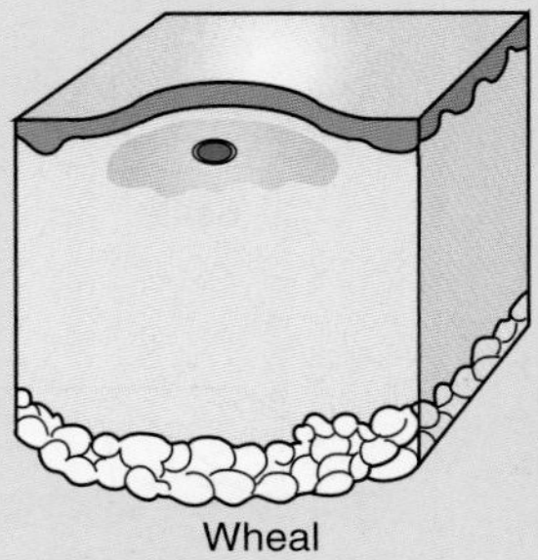	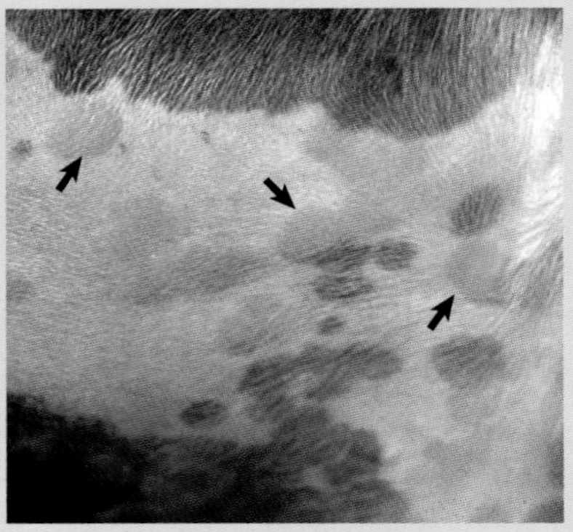

All drawings modified from Copstead LC, Banasik JL: *Pathophysiology: biological and behavioral perspectives,* ed 3, Philadelphia, 2005, Saunders. All clinical photographs courtesy Dr. Ann M. Hargis, DermatoDiagnostics, unless otherwise noted.
*Courtesy Washington Animal Disease Diagnostic Laboratory.
†Courtesy Dr. David Duclos, Animal Skin and Allergy Clinic.
‡Courtesy Dr. Helen Power, Dermatology for Animals
§Courtesy Dr. David Duclos, Animal Skin and Allergy Clinic.
¶From Willis RA: *Pathology of tumors,* Philadelphia, 1948, FA Davis.
¶Courtesy Dr. Alan Mundell, Animal Dermatology Service.
**Courtesy Dr. Pamela E. Ginn, College of Veterinary Medicine, University of Florida; and Ginn PE, Hillier A, Lester GD: *Vet Dermatol* 9:249-256, 1998.

BOX 17-4 Biopsy Sampling Do's

Be gentle
Biopsy early
Collect multiple samples representative of the range of lesions
Include crusts
Biopsy before using antiinflammatory therapy
Use the correct biopsy procedure for the type of lesion
Label samples from different areas
Prevent samples from freezing

BOX 17-5 Biopsy Sampling Don'ts

Do not surgically prepare the site if lesions are in the epidermis or dermis
Do not use electrocautery or laser for small biopsy samples
Do not grasp the punch biopsy samples or lesion areas of larger samples with a tissue forceps
Do not use a biopsy instrument that is too small (4 mm is the minimum useful diameter)
Do not forget to collect multiple samples
Do not forget to submit a history

can be required, particularly in dogs, for the diagnosis of claw bed lesions. Electrocautery or laser should not be used for small biopsy samples because the samples can be damaged and rendered nondiagnostic. Tissue forceps (small toothed) should grasp, if at all, only one nonaffected margin, preferably in the subcutis.

Site Preparation

Generally, the skin at a punch biopsy site should not be surgically prepared because the procedure may remove a diagnostic portion of the sample. Gentle clipping of hair is acceptable, and surgical preparation of the skin is acceptable for an excisional biopsy of

TABLE 17-4 Biopsy Sampling Tips

Preparation	Very gently clip or scissor if necessary. Do not surgically prepare the site if sampling lesions in epidermis or dermis. Caveat: Can surgically prepare site for excision of lesions deep in the subcutis or to remove large nodular mass such as a neoplasm.
Lesions	Collect multiple samples representative of the range of lesions. If crusting is significant, collect crust, wrap in lens paper, and place in formalin. For alopecic conditions: Collect samples from the most alopecic areas; draw a line on the sample in the direction of the hair coat. For ulcers or depigmenting lesions (junction important): Use incisional or excisional method or use an 8-mm biopsy punch instrument, and draw a line on the sample perpendicular to the junction between lesion and normal skin.
Punch samples	Use 6- or 8-mm punch instruments for haired skin. Use 4-mm punch for periocular skin, pawpads, or nasal planum.
Incisional and excisional samples	Use incisional or excisional methods if smaller punch would damage large pustule or vesicle. Gently place thin incisional or excisional samples, subcutis side down, on a piece of cardboard; let adhere for about 30 seconds, then place in formalin (prevents warping). NOTE: Do not let sample dehydrate. For lesions in the panniculus, use incisional or excisional method to ensure that the sample is of sufficient size and depth for diagnosis.
Fixation	Fix samples in 10% buffered formalin with 10 times the volume of formalin for the volume of samples. For diagnosis of autoimmune skin disease or tumors, begin with standard histopathology; selected immunohistochemical stains can usually be done later on the formalin-fixed samples if desired.
Important finale	Submit a history with differential diagnoses.

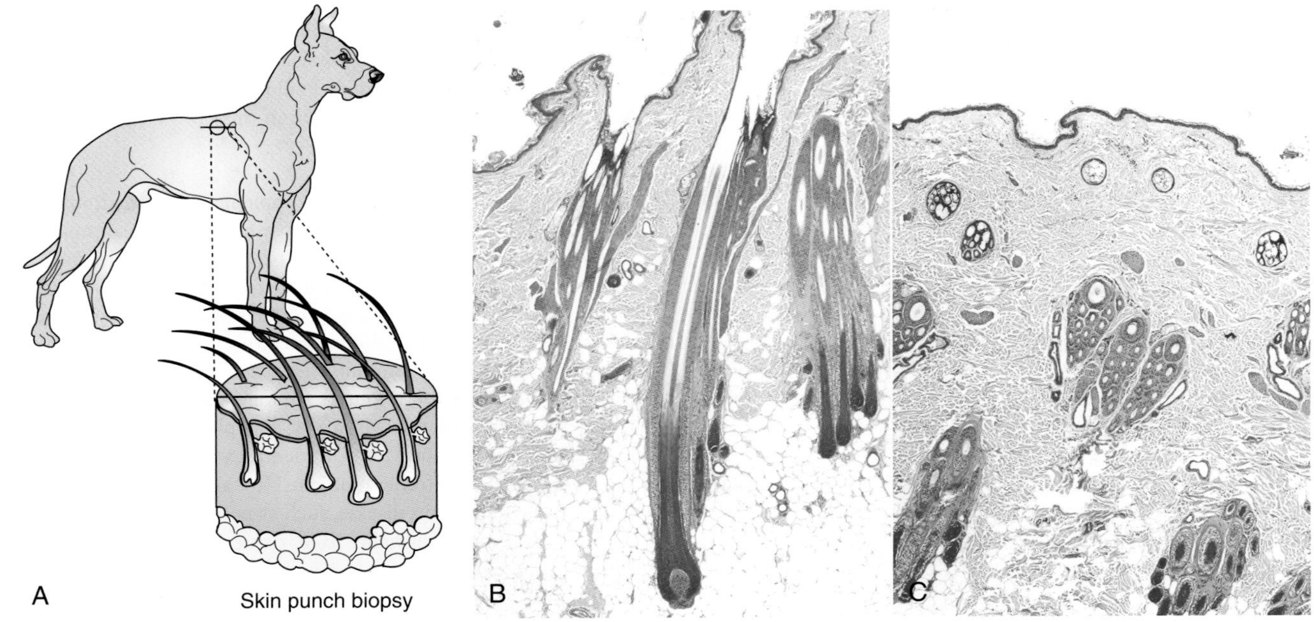

Fig. 17-32 Sampling of the skin for histopathologic evaluation, haired, dog.
A, Schematic diagram of the line drawn (with fine tipped permanent marking pen) on the skin in the direction of the hair coat. The line directs laboratory personnel to cut and embed the sample parallel to the hair follicles. Cutting the sample parallel to the hair follicles allows visualization of the entire length of the follicles during microscopic examination, which facilitates evaluation for causes of alopecia. For simplicity, simple follicles are used in this illustration. **B,** Section of skin trimmed parallel to the hair follicles. Note that the hair follicles are cut longitudinally and that the full length of the hair follicle is present. H&E stain. **C,** Section of skin trimmed in cross-section to the hair follicles. Note that the hair follicles are cut tangentially and that only portions of each follicle are present for examination, which reduces the ability to evaluate follicular morphology. H&E stain. (**B** and **C** courtesy Dr. Ann M. Hargis, DermatoDiagnostics.)

lesions deep to the epidermis. For collection of biopsy samples in areas of alopecia, drawing a line with a fine-tipped permanent marking pen in the direction of the hair coat helps laboratory personnel orient the sample (Fig. 17-32, *A*). In the laboratory, the sample is cut along the line so that the hair follicles are oriented longitudinally (Fig. 17-32, *B*). If the line is not drawn on the sample, the sample might be cut so that the follicles are in cross or tangential section rather than longitudinal section (Fig. 17-32, *C*), which reduces histologic value of the sample when evaluating for follicular disease. For collection of ulcers, depigmented lesions, or other lesions where the interface between normal and affected skin is critical to diagnosis, use of incisional or excisional samples collected from affected skin and contiguous normal skin is often preferable. However, a large (8 mm) biopsy punch instrument can be used to collect the junction between normal and affected skin, if a line with a fine-tipped permanent marking pen is drawn perpendicular to the junction between the normal and affected tissue before sample collection (Fig. 17-33). The line instructs laboratory personnel how to trim the sample to ensure that the critical areas are present for dermatopathologic evaluation. For lesions suspected

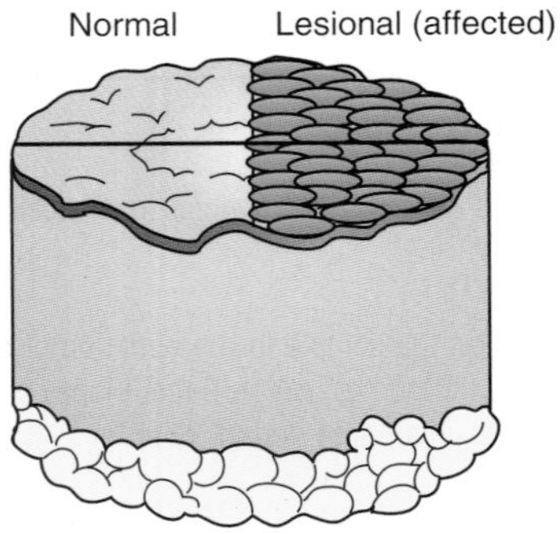

Fig. 17-33 Schematic diagram of collecting the margin of a lesion and normal skin using a large punch biopsy instrument (8 mm).
It is necessary to draw a line on the sample from normal into affected skin to direct laboratory personnel to cut and embed the sample so that the interface between the normal and affected skin is present for microscopic examination. Without this line, the sample could be cut at a right angle to the desired line and thus miss the interface between normal and affected skin essential for histologic examination of the area most likely to have diagnostic changes.

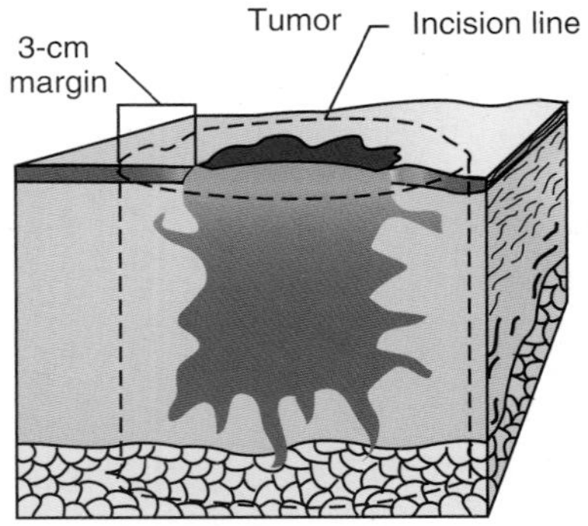

Fig. 17-34 Schematic diagram of excisional sampling.
If possible, 3-cm margins should be collected if the nodule is suspected of being an invasive neoplasm. This facilitates examination of the margins for completeness of excision.

of being invasive tumors, complete excision of the mass, including a 3-cm margin of clinically normal skin around all borders, is recommended (Fig. 17-34).

Fixation

Punch biopsy specimens should be placed in 10 times the volume of 10% neutral buffered formalin (NBF). To prevent warping in the fixative, thin excisional biopsy specimens should be gently attached to a flat object, such as a piece of cardboard or tongue depressor, and permitted to dry for 20 to 30 seconds. Twenty to 30 seconds is all that is necessary for the sample to adhere to the flat object. The specimen and flat object are then immediately immersed in formalin. Care should be taken not to let the sample become dehydrated (i.e., remain unfixed for longer than 20 to 30 seconds), which could damage the morphology of small samples and the lesions. In cold climates during winter months, adding 1 part alcohol to 9 parts 10% NBF reduces the chance of freezing of specimens during transport.

History

Accurate histopathologic diagnosis and interpretation require knowledge of the gross features of the lesions. Therefore it is essential to include with biopsy samples the following information: (1) age, breed, and sex of the animal; (2) location, gross appearance, and duration of the lesions; (3) presence or absence of lesion symmetry; and (4) presence or absence of pruritus affecting the animal (Box 17-6). Clinical information, including results of laboratory evaluations (i.e., hemograms, serum biochemical analyses), results of skin cultures, scrapings, or cytology, current medications, and response to therapy, should be included along with a list of clinical differential diagnoses. History can be critical to reaching a diagnosis. For example, presence of luminal and mural folliculitis with no apparent follicular infectious agents in H&E-stained sections in conjunction with the history of lack of response to appropriate antibiotic therapy would suggest to the pathologist that a fungal stain to evaluate for occult dermatophyte infection should be performed. Without the history of lack of response to appropriate antibiotic therapy, the folliculitis could easily be presumed to be of bacterial origin, and a fungal infection missed.

BOX 17-6 What Constitutes a History?

Age, breed, sex
Lesion distribution
Lesion appearance and severity
Lesion duration
Influence of specific and/or recent therapy that could change lesions
Other clinical problems
Laboratory analyte abnormalities
Differential diagnoses (important)

Ancillary Procedures

Other diagnostic procedures can supplement information gained from histologic examination of biopsy samples. These procedures include aspiration of pustule contents for cytologic evaluation, performing touch imprints of the cut surface of suspected neoplastic or infectious lesions for cytologic evaluation, aseptically collecting a tissue sample for microbiologic culture, and collecting biopsy samples of suspected immune-mediated diseases or poorly differentiated tumors for immunostaining. Use of immunostaining for identification of cell surface or cytoplasmic proteins (to aid in diagnosis of tumors) or for identification of immunoglobulin, complement, or other antigens (to aid in the diagnosis of immune-mediated skin disease, such as pemphigus) can be helpful in some cases. The formalin-fixed tissue submitted for histopathology also can be used for most routine immunohistochemical procedures, since most employ immunoperoxidase staining rather than immunofluorescence.

Unfortunately, immunostaining techniques for immune-mediated skin diseases can give false-positive or false-negative results, thus they must be done in conjunction with standard histopathology. For autoimmune diseases, if immunofluorescence evaluation is desired, specimens can be fixed in Michel's medium, which preserves immunoglobulin and complement. If immunohistochemistry (immunoperoxidase) staining is desired, formalin-fixed samples are used; however, for best results, samples should not remain in formalin longer than 48 hours. Prolonged fixation in formalin results in cross-linking of proteins and false-negative results. For autoimmune disease, newer techniques that detect more specific antigens, such as desmoglein (transmembrane glycoproteins found in desmosomes that provide physical connections between keratinocytes), use of "salt-split" skin sections (a technique used in immunostaining of the skin where sodium chloride splits the epidermis from the dermis through the lamina lucida, allowing better differentiation of subepidermal bullous diseases), use of better substrates for indirect immunostaining, and use of immunoblotting

TABLE 17-5 Examples of Antibodies to Cell Surface or Cytoplasmic Proteins that May Differentiate Tumors with Similar Histologic Appearance

Tumor Type	Antibodies	
	VIMENTIN	**PAN CYTOKERATIN**
Carcinoma	–	+
Sarcoma	+	–
	CYTOKERATIN 5/6	**CYTOKERATIN 8**
Squamous cell carcinoma	+	–
Sweat gland carcinoma	–	+
	α-SMOOTH-MUSCLE ACTIN	**GFAP**
Neurofibrosarcoma	–	+
Leiomyosarcoma	+	–
	CYTOKERATIN	**FACTOR VIII**
Carcinoma	+	–
Epithelioid hemangiosarcoma	–	+
	CD3	**CD79A**
B cell lymphoma	–	+
T cell lymphoma	+	–

GFAP, Glial fibrillary acidic protein; *CD,* cluster of differentiation.

and enzyme-linked immunosorbent assay (ELISA) techniques may improve diagnostic accuracy of immune-mediated skin diseases in the future.

Identification of cell surface or cytoplasmic proteins can help identify the cell type in poorly differentiated tumors (Table 17-5). However, there can be anomalous expression of proteins in some tumors (e.g., anomalous expression of cytokeratin in melanoma); thus evaluation of a series (panel) of antibodies is preferred because the pattern of staining with a panel of antibodies is more reliable than staining with one or two antibodies. Formalin-fixed specimens are acceptable for most procedures, but for others, fresh or frozen specimens are better. Discussion with a pathologist is recommended regarding when to use immunostaining procedures.

DISORDERS OF DOMESTIC ANIMALS

CONGENITAL AND HEREDITARY DISORDERS

The terms *congenital* and *hereditary* are not synonymous. Congenital lesions develop in the fetus (in utero), are present at birth, and have a variety of causes. An example is hypotrichosis in the fetus associated with maternal dietary iodine deficiency. Inherited conditions are transmitted genetically and are not always manifested phenotypically in utero or at birth but may develop later in life. An example is sebaceous adenitis, which may not develop until 1 to 2 years of age or later. Web Box 17-2 lists selected cutaneous inherited diseases in animals. There are many other diseases (e.g., cutaneous and renal glomerular vasculopathy in greyhounds, atopic dermatitis in selected breeds) that may also be inherited, but the mode of inheritance has not been documented.

Congenital Alopecia and Hypotrichosis

Congenital alopecia or atrichia (absence of hair from skin where hair is usually present) and hypotrichosis (less than the normal amount of hair) have been reported in most species of domestic animals. In most instances, congenital hypotrichosis is a hereditary condition caused by spontaneous genetic mutations affecting genes responsible for or influencing the normal development and/or maintenance of hair follicles or other components of the skin. In most cases, the exact mutation has not been identified. In some of these animals, the alopecia or hypotrichosis has been recognized as standard for the breed (e.g., Mexican hairless pig, Chinese crested dog, Mexican hairless dog, and Sphinx cat), and the mutation is purposefully propagated. The congenital alopecia and hypotrichosis syndromes have been considered to be forms of congenital follicular dysplasia because there is an abnormal development of the hair follicles. Animals with congenital hereditary hypotrichosis can have defects in other body systems, including brachygnathism (abnormal smallness of the mandible), and dental, thymic, and genital abnormalities. When the condition involves the hair follicles plus adnexal glands and teeth, which all arise from the ectoderm, the condition is also termed *ectodermal dysplasia.* In addition to health problems created by oral, dental, or thymic defects (inability to efficiently chew or graze and immune deficiency that can lead to death), animals with hypotrichosis are more susceptible to sunburn, temperature extremes, and bacterial and fungal infections. The degree, location, and age of onset of hairlessness vary. Hair that is present is usually abnormally coarse or fine and easily broken or epilated. Morphologic changes in the skin and hair follicles vary from species to species, most likely representing differences in mutations. A useful example is congenital hypotrichosis with anodontia in German Holstein calves (Fig. 17-35). In this condition, hypotrichosis, lack of most teeth, and complete absence of eccrine nasolabial glands is inherited as a monogenic X-linked recessive trait. Because the condition affects the hair follicles, some adnexal glands, and teeth, it is also classified as an ectodermal dysplasia. The condition varies in severity, with some calves more affected than others. Affected calves have reduced numbers of hairs per surface area in various anatomic locations (especially head, pinnae, neck, back, and tail), and also have reduced length and numbers of eyelashes and vibrissae. The alopecia and hypotrichosis are most severe in newborn calves because the presence of fine hairs increases with age. There are no defects in the horns, endocrine glands, genital organs, or other internal organs. Histologically, hair follicles and adnexal glands are absent in the skin on the back of the ears. Hair follicle density is often reduced in other areas. When present, hair bulbs are small and poorly developed. In some areas, the apocrine glands are reduced in quantity, and eccrine nasolabial glands are absent.

Especially for purposes of herd health management and disease prevention, it is important to differentiate the congenital inherited alopecia and hypotrichosis disorders from the nongenetic congenital alopecic disorders. The latter includes congenital hypotrichosis caused by maternal iodine deficiency in pigs, calves, lambs, and foals; in utero infection with bovine virus diarrhea or hog cholera virus; and defects in other systems such as adenohypophyseal hypoplasia in some breeds of cattle (Table 17-6).

Collagen Dysplasia and Mucinosis

Collagen dysplasia (hyperelastosis cutis, dermatosparaxis, and cutaneous asthenia) occurs in most domestic animals and comprises a clinically, genetically, and biochemically heterogeneous group of diseases that are rare. In each, skin tears easily, is hyperextensible,

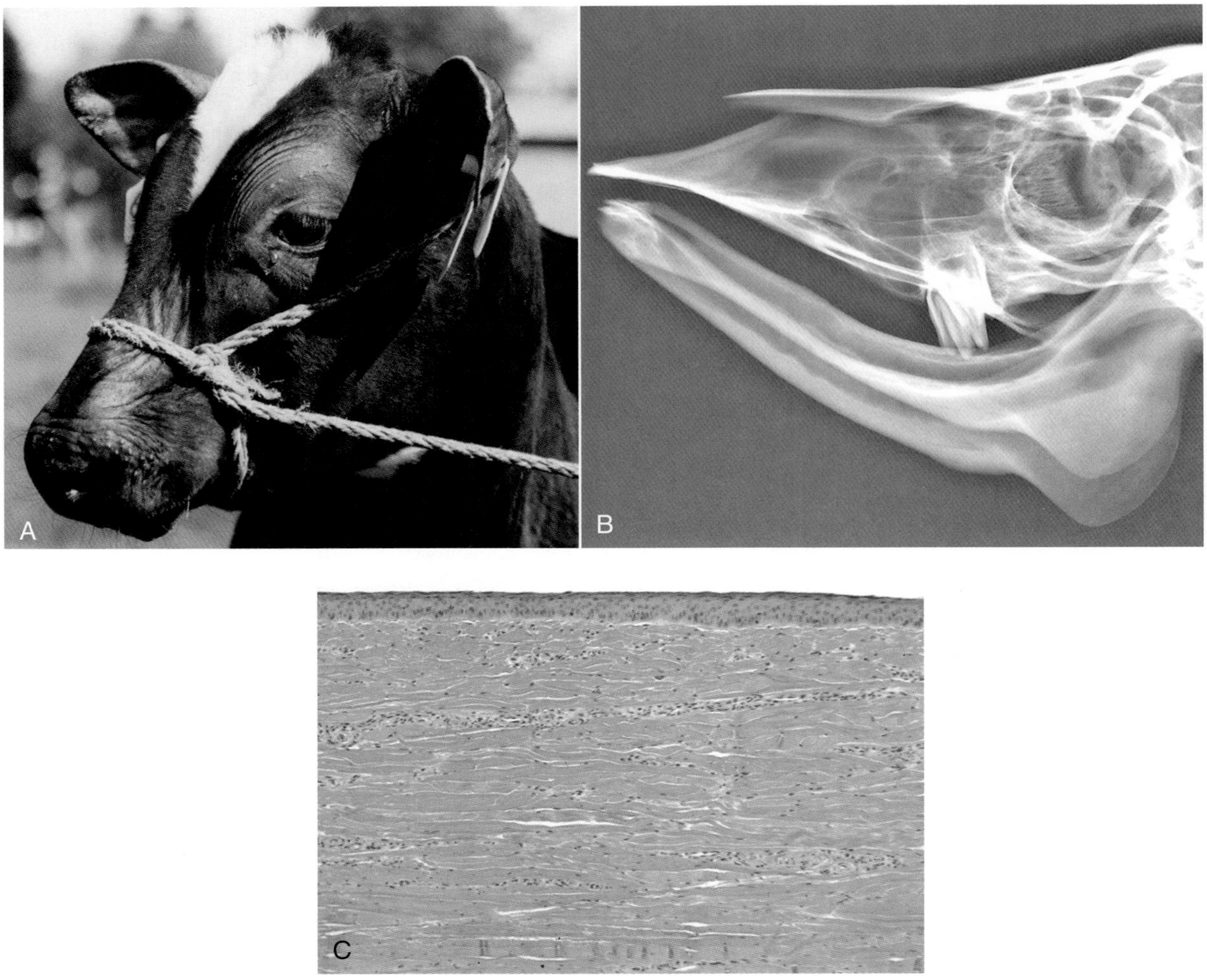

Fig. 17-35 Congenital hypotrichosis with anodontia, calf.
A, The hair coat is sparse and short. Eyelashes and tactile hairs are also sparse and very short. The tail switch (not in this photograph) was about one-third the normal length. **B,** Radiograph, skull. Note that most of the teeth are missing. When congenital hypotrichosis involves the hair follicles plus adnexal glands and teeth, which all arise from the ectoderm, the condition is also termed *ectodermal dysplasia.* **C,** Affected skin. Note the lack of hair follicles. Animals with hypotrichosis are susceptible to extremes of temperature, and the skin is more likely to sustain traumatic injury and secondary infection because of the lack of the protective hair coat. H&E stain. (**A** courtesy Professor Tosso Leeb, Institute of Animal Breeding, School of Veterinary Medicine Hannover; Drogemuller C, Kuiper H, Peters M, et al: *Vet Dermatol* 13:6;307-313, 2002. **B** courtesy Professor Tosso Leeb, Institute of Animal Breeding, School of Veterinary Medicine Hannover; and Tierarztl Prax. **C** courtesy Dr. Frank Seeliger, Department of Pathology, Tieraerztliche Hochschule Hannover.)

and loose, but the severity of these lesions varies among species. Specific enzyme defects affecting collagen synthesis or processing are the cause of some collagen dysplasia syndromes. Abnormal synthesis or processing of collagen leads to structurally abnormal dermal collagen that has decreased tensile strength. The causes of other collagen dysplasia syndromes have not been established. Gross lesions consist of cutaneous hyperextensibility and laxity (Fig. 17-36), frequent skin wounds that result even from normal handling and activity, and numerous scars, which are the result of previous tearing of the dermal connective tissues. Microscopic features vary among the different types of collagen dysplasia syndromes, and in some, the skin is histologically normal. If microscopic lesions are present, the collagen bundles can vary in size and shape, can be separated by wide spaces, have laminar splits in various levels of the dermis, or have a haphazard arrangement. Electron microscopy or biochemical analyses are sometimes required to make a definitive diagnosis.

Mucinosis (mucin deposition in the dermis) occurs as an inherited dermal connective tissue disorder in the Chinese Shar-Pei dog where the presence of dermal mucin causes the thick, wrinkly skin that typifies this breed. However, in some Shar-Pei dogs, the mucin deposition is excessive, and "lakes" or pools of mucin develop. In these areas of mucin accumulation, there is a concomitant reduction in dermal collagen fibers and lymphatic channels may be dilated. These areas of the skin are fragile, and if traumatized, thick, stringy mucin exudes from the dermis. Mucin deposition may also develop in association with myxedema of hypothyroidism.

Epidermolysis Bullosa (Red Foot Disease)

Epidermolysis bullosa refers to a group of mechanobullous diseases, resulting in development of cutaneous blisters (bullae) in response to minor mechanical trauma. Blisters develop as a result of poor cohesion of the epidermis and dermis as a result of structural defects at the basement membrane zone. The structural defects are the result of mutations in genes responsible for the synthesis of a variety of structural components of this anatomic region of the skin and include abnormalities in keratin intermediate filaments, hemidesmosome-associated proteins, and anchoring fibrils such as

TABLE 17-6 Categories, Causes, and Age of Onset of Hypotrichosis and Alopecia

Category	Cause	Age of Onset	Species
Congenital hypotrichosis or alopecia	Usually inherited, may be accompanied by odontogenic, thymic, genital, or other defects that influence neonatal viability. Can be classified as congenital follicular dysplasia syndromes.	Usually present at birth or within the first month of life	Mostly calves; less often piglets, puppies, kittens; rarely foals
	Maternal dietary influences (e.g., iodine deficiency)	Present at birth	Calves, piglets, lambs, foals
	Secondary to other defects (adenohypophyseal hypoplasia)	Present at birth	Guernsey and Jersey calves
	In utero infection with bovine virus diarrhea or hog cholera virus	Present at birth	Calves, pigs
Tardive follicular dysplasia	Usually inherited	Months to years after birth	Dogs, cattle, horses
Endocrine disorders*	Abnormal function of pituitary, thyroid, adrenal or pineal glands, or gonads; or iatrogenic administration of hormones	Develops in young adults to aged	Predominantly dogs
Nonendocrine hair cycle abnormalities	Nonendocrine factors that influence hair growth such as therapy with antimitotic drugs, stress, fever, illness (telogen effluvium), or clipping plush-coated breeds of dogs (postclipping alopecia)	Typically adults	Any species, often dogs
Neoplasia	Paraneoplastic: internal malignancy, often of pancreas or liver	Aged	Cats
	Direct involvement of epidermis, dermis, or adnexa (example: epitheliotropic lymphoma)	Usually adult to aged	Dogs, cats
Inflammatory conditions or trauma	Follicular infection Posttraumatic and inflammatory Sebaceous adenitis Alopecia areata Traction alopecia	Any age	Any species; dogs most frequently affected with follicular infection and sebaceous adenitis
Excessive grooming	Hypersensitivity reactions or psychogenic causes	Any age	Most often affects cats
Nutrition	Severe protein or protein-calorie nutrition	Any age, especially young or pregnant	Any species
Alopecia X	Undetermined	Usually 1 or 2 years of age	Plush-coated breeds of dogs

*Endocrine:
1. Clinically manifested endocrine disease in cats is usually caused by hyperadrenocorticism where marked dermal atrophy leads to tearing of the skin with normal handling procedures. Alopecia can be a feature, but skin fragility is a more significant problem.
2. Clinically manifested endocrine disease in horses is usually caused by hyperadrenocorticism and is typified paradoxically by hypertrichosis rather than alopecia (possibly because of production of adrenal androgens, other hormones, or pressure of the pituitary on thermoregulatory areas of the hypothalamus).

type VII collagen. The diseases vary in mode of inheritance, clinical manifestations, and anatomic location of the blisters. Animals affected with the diseases usually die because of their inability to obtain nourishment, loss of fluid and protein, and secondary infection leading to bacteremia. Epidermolysis bullosa has been reported in horses, cattle, sheep, dogs, and cats. Lesions can be present at birth or develop shortly thereafter and are located where epithelial surfaces are subjected to minor mechanical trauma, such as oral mucosa, lips, and extremities, and can include sloughing of claws, hooves, or pawpads. Shearing forces that normally cause no problem are sufficient to cause injury in these animals. Microscopic lesions are those of an epidermal vesicular disease in which vesicles form in different locations (subepidermal, epidermal-dermal junction, or intraepidermal), depending on the specific disease. The vesicles progress to ulcers or if secondarily infected, become pustules. As healing occurs, the reepithelization causes sloughing of the dried exudates over the ulcer, and the pustules dry to form crusts.

Epitheliogenesis Imperfecta (Aplasia Cutis)

Epitheliogenesis imperfecta results from the failure of the stratified squamous epithelium of skin, adnexa, and/or oral mucosa to develop completely. The disease varies in severity and has been reported in most domestic species. It is the result of inherited genetic mutations in some species, but inheritance is not proved in other species. Additional information regarding the pathogenesis is not known. Without the protective covering of the stratified squamous epithelium, the underlying tissue is easily traumatized, can become infected, and bacteremia can develop. Grossly, lesions consist of sharply demarcated areas devoid of the epidermis and adnexa or mucosa, exposing the underlying red, moist dermis or submucosa. Lesions are located most often on the face, extremities, or mucous membranes and can be small (1 cm) or involve extensive regions such as the entire distal limb (Fig. 17-37). Small lesions can heal with scarring and not interfere with life. With extensive involvement, the entire skin can be affected, including hooves, ears, lips, and eyelids, and may result in abortion of the affected fetus. Animals born alive with extensive lesions usually die from infection or dehydration and electrolyte abnormalities from extensive fluid loss through nonepithelialized surfaces.

Congenital Hypertrichosis

Congenital hypertrichosis refers to excessive growth of hair, which can be congenital or hereditary. Congenital hypertrichosis has developed in fetal lambs secondary to hyperthermia in pregnant ewes living in areas of high environmental temperature. In addition

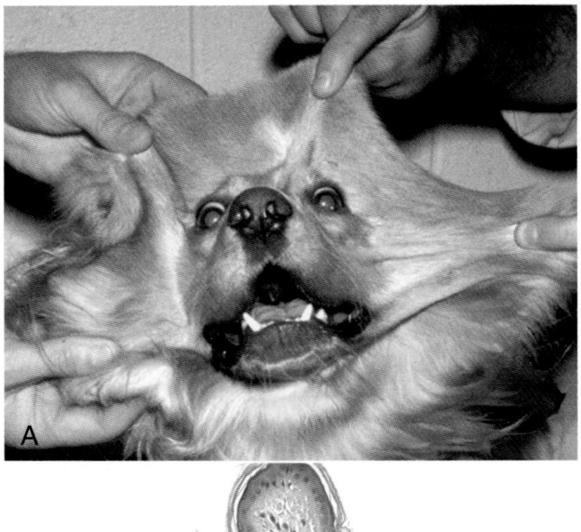

Fig. 17-36 Collagen dysplasia, skin, dog.
A, The skin is hyperextensible. In this dog, the skin can be stretched more than the skin of a normal dog. **B,** The collagen bundles are irregular in size and shape and are arranged haphazardly. The abnormally formed collagen is responsible for the hyperextensibility of the skin, which predisposes to tearing with normal handling and activity. H&E stain. **C,** Deeper level of the sample shown in **B.** Collagen bundles are stained blue. The variation in diameter and shape of the collagen bundles and their haphazard arrangement is accentuated with this stain. Masson's trichrome stain. (**A** courtesy Dr. Ben Baker, Washington State University. **B** and **C** courtesy Dr. Ann M. Hargis, DermatoDiagnostics.)

to the hypertrichosis, the lambs are small and few survive the first 2 months of life.

In utero border disease virus infection of fetal lambs results in an abnormally hairy fleece at birth, muscle tremors, defective myelination of the brain and spinal cord, abnormalities of body conformation, poor growth, and reduced viability. The fleece abnormalities and the muscle tremors result in the name *hairy shaker disease.* Fleece abnormalities are only noted in fine- and medium-wooled (smooth-coated) breeds. Fetal infection before 80 days of gestation results in an initial phase of retardation of follicular growth, followed by an extended period of rapid growth of primary follicles. The altered growth rate of follicles results in production of larger, more heavily medullated primary wool fibers, and the clinical appearance of the "hairy" fleece. The exact mechanism controlling the exaggerated growth of primary follicles is unknown. It has been speculated that reduction in number of the later developing secondary fibers could be the result of impaired nutrition because of placentitis. Microscopically, primary follicles and wool fibers are enlarged and the number of the secondary follicles and wool fibers is reduced (see the discussion on hair follicles in the section on Morphology of the Skin and also Fig. 17-7).

Dermatosis Vegetans

Dermatosis vegetans is an inherited disorder of young pigs characterized by vegetating skin lesions, hoof malformation, and giant cell pneumonia. The condition is a simple autosomal recessive trait of Landrace pigs. The pathogenesis of lesion formation is unknown. Skin lesions can be present at birth but might not develop until 2 to 3 months of age. Lesions begin as erythematous papules on the ventral abdomen and medial aspect of the thighs and possibly the sides and back. The papules enlarge peripherally to form plaques with a depressed center filled with gray to brown-black granular brittle material. Each crusty plaque is sharply demarcated from normal skin by a hyperemic raised border. As lesions spread peripherally, they coalesce to form extensive horny, papilloma-like areas covered by black crusts. Hoof lesions, if they occur, are always present at birth. Usually all digits, including accessory digits, on more than one limb are affected. The coronary region is markedly swollen and erythematous, and a yellow-brown greasy material covers the skin. The wall of the hoof is thickened by ridges and furrows parallel to the coronary band. Histologically, fully developed cutaneous lesions have marked orthokeratotic and parakeratotic hyperkeratosis, prominent irregular epidermal hyperplasia, intercellular edema, and intraepidermal pustules and microabscesses containing eosinophils and neutrophils. Affected piglets frequently die of secondary infection when skin lesions reach the typical papilloma-like stage (5 to 8 weeks of age) either from entrance of bacteria from skin lesions or a bacterial pneumonia complicating the giant cell pneumonia characteristic of this disease. Skin lesions begin to resolve if the pig survives.

DISORDERS OF PHYSICAL, RADIATION, OR CHEMICAL INJURY

Solar (Actinic) Injury

Sunlight is composed of visible (400 to 700 nm), UV (100 to 400 nm), and infrared (700 to 20,000 nm) light rays. The portion of the UV light most damaging to the skin is UVB and is in the range of 290- to 320-nm wavelength. However, photodynamic chemicals, if present in the skin, can chemically react with longer wavelengths, thus releasing energy and leading to the formation of reactive oxygen intermediates that initiate a chain of reactions resulting in cutaneous damage (photosensitization, phototoxicity). The amount of light reaching the skin depends on a variety of environmental and host factors, such as quantity of ozone, smog, and cloud cover (tend to absorb and scatter some of the UV rays), and the amount of pigment and hair, which reflect or otherwise block UV rays from reaching the skin. Solar damage is more prevalent at high altitudes and at latitudes close to the equator, in areas with a high number of cloudless days, in animals spending most of their time outdoors, and in older animals that have had more exposure to the sun. The susceptibility of animal skin to solar injury depends on the density of hair, degree of pigmentation, and thickness of the

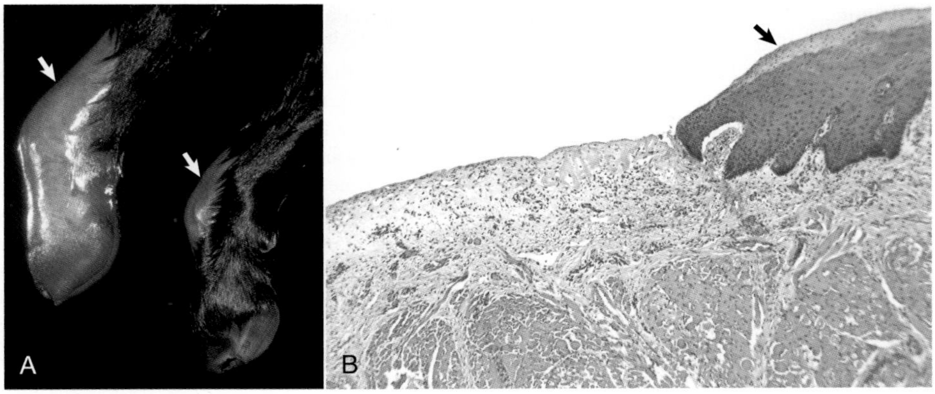

Fig. 17-37 Epitheliogenesis imperfecta, calf.
A, Skin. Areas of epidermis over the extremities are missing *(arrows)*. This condition is the result of inherited genetic mutations in some species, but inheritance is not proven in other species. **B,** Oral mucosa. Junction of normal and affected mucous membrane. Epithelium is present on the right (normal area) *(arrow)* but is abruptly missing on the left. The lack of germinal epithelium results in the failure of the epidermis, adnexa, or mucosal epithelium to develop completely. Skin, adnexa, and oral mucosa can be affected in this disease. (Courtesy Dr. M.D. McGavin, College of Veterinary Medicine, University of Tennessee.)

stratum corneum. Lesions generally develop in poorly haired and lightly pigmented skin.

Solar (Actinic) Dermatosis, Keratosis, and Neoplasia

The damage to skin by UV light can be acute (sunburn) or chronic (solar dermatosis, neoplasia). An early transient erythema may be caused by the heating effect of the light rays and possibly to photochemical changes. The later developing erythema is called "sunburn erythema," and the skin is warm, tender, and swollen. The pathogenesis of sunburn erythema may involve diffusion of inflammatory mediators, such as cytokines, from radiation-damaged keratinocytes, or from direct damage to endothelial cells of superficial dermal capillaries by UV light. Chronic sun exposure, particularly to UVB, causes damage primarily in the epidermis leading to the development of neoplasia. The damage occurs in three broad categories, as follows:

1. One of the most detrimental changes occurs when UVB radiation contacts the nucleus and causes the formation of "photoproducts," which are abnormal covalent or single bonds between two adjacent pyrimidine bases in a strand of DNA. The two major UVB-induced photoproducts are pyrimidine dimers (covalent bonds between two thymine or two cytosine bases) and 6-4 photoproducts (single-bond bridging carbon 4 in one cytosine and carbon 6, either in a cytosine or a thymine). These photoproducts form in keratinocyte DNA (and also in DNA of Langerhans' cells and dermal dendritic cells). The damage can be easily and accurately repaired before the cell undergoes mitosis by the nucleotide excision repair enzyme system that removes the damaged area and synthesizes a new strand of DNA. However, if the cell undergoes mitosis before the damage is repaired, a gap in the DNA strand is left at the location of the photoproduct. The gap is repaired by a postreplication repair method that is thought to be error-prone and may lead to mutations and the development of neoplasms. Factors that irritate the skin and increase the rate of cell division increase the number of cells repaired by the postreplication repair method and therefore can enhance development of neoplasms.
2. Chronic exposure to UVB radiation also causes damage to DNA in the form of mutations to tumor-suppressor genes, in particular to the p53 gene. Normally, UVR–induced DNA damage causes keratinocyte induction of the p53 gene, which leads to cell cycle arrest, thus allowing the UVR–caused DNA damage to be corrected by the nucleotide excision repair system before the cell undergoes mitosis, and a functional p53 gene also facilitates apoptosis (programmed cell death) of cells with excessive unrepaired damaged DNA so that those defective cells are removed. The p53 gene mutations develop when UVR–induced photoproducts are not repaired before keratinocyte mitosis. The photoproducts form small structural abnormalities in the DNA strand that can result in faulty base paring (i.e., mutations) during replication. The mutations are characterized by the replacement of a cytosine with a thymine (C to T) or double-base changes in which a cytosine dimer is replaced by two non-dimerized thymine bases (CC to TT). Although p53 gene mutations occur in a variety of tumors, those mutations caused by UVR (the C to T or CC to TT mutations) are unique and do not occur with other types of DNA damage or in non–UVR-associated tumors, thus are termed *signature mutations*.
3. UVB causes immunosuppression by depressing host cell-mediated immune reactions that normally serve to eliminate or destroy mutated proliferating cells. A variety of mechanisms contribute and involve UVB-damaged keratinocytes, Langerhans' cells, dendritic cells, and others. Mechanisms include release of immunosuppressive cytokines such as IL-10 and IL-4, reduction in the number of Langerhans' cells (antigen-presenting cells), a switch in Langerhans' cell antigen presentation from T_H1 lymphocytes (involved in immune response against tumors) to T_H2 lymphocytes (release immunosuppressive cytokines), induction of suppressor T lymphocytes, and release of cytokines and other biologic response modifiers that downregulate the immune response.

Other factors may also contribute. For example, papillomaviruses recently have been identified in mucosal and cutaneous in situ and invasive squamous cell carcinomas, including invasive squamous cell carcinomas arising in sun exposed skin in cats. However, it is currently not known if the papillomavirus identified within the tumor is merely infecting the tumor or if the virus could have a role in tumor induction. Some papilloma viral gene products have been shown to bind p53 tumor-suppressor gene protein products in cervical squamous cell carcinomas in women leading to disruption of the cell cycle regulation.

The lesions of sun-induced injury occur in all domestic animals. In horses, lesions occur on the eyelids and nose and around the prepuce. The eyelids of Hereford cattle are also prone to development of lesions. In lightly colored dairy goats, lesions can develop on the lateral aspects of the udder and teats. Lightly pigmented young pigs are also susceptible to more acute solar injury, and the pinnae and tip of the tail can slough if injury is severe. In dogs, lesions develop most commonly in nonpigmented, sparsely haired skin of the ventral abdominal, inguinal, and perianal areas (Fig. 17-38). In cats, gross lesions occur where there is little or no hair and little pigment, particularly on external ear tips, eyelids, nose and lips, and are most severe in white cats. Grossly, lesions begin as erythema, scaling, and crusting. After years of exposure, the skin becomes wrinkled and thickened secondary to epidermal hyperplasia, hyperkeratosis, fibrosis, and in some species, elastosis. One or more papular or plaquelike foci covered with thick scale (hyperkeratosis) known as *solar (actinic) keratoses* may develop, some of which progress to invasive squamous cell carcinoma. Occasionally the hyperkeratosis is dense and compact, and resembles a "horn" (Fig. 17-38, *B*). Hemangiomas and hemangiosarcomas have developed in the nonpigmented conjunctiva of dogs and horses and in the dermis of sparsely pigmented and sparsely haired skin of dogs, cats, and a few goats. The cutaneous hemangiomas and hemangiosarcomas are often seen on the abdomen and flanks of dogs that spend time resting in the sun. The difference in type of neoplasm can be a result in part to thickness of the epidermis, which influences the depth of penetration of the UV rays. UV light may also play a role in the development of melanomas in goats.

Microscopically, in early UV-induced injury, the number of apoptotic cells (sunburn cells) scattered in the epidermis can be so numerous as to form a band of these cells along with intercellular edema, vacuolation of keratinocytes, and loss of granular cell layer. By 72 hours, hyperkeratosis, parakeratosis, and acanthosis are present along with dermal lesions of hyperemia, edema, perivascular mononuclear infiltrates, capillary endothelial cell swelling, and hemorrhage. Hyperkeratosis, parakeratosis, and acanthosis can persist. Comedones (hair follicles dilated with a plug of follicular stratum corneum and sebum) develop in some dogs (Fig. 17-38, *C*).

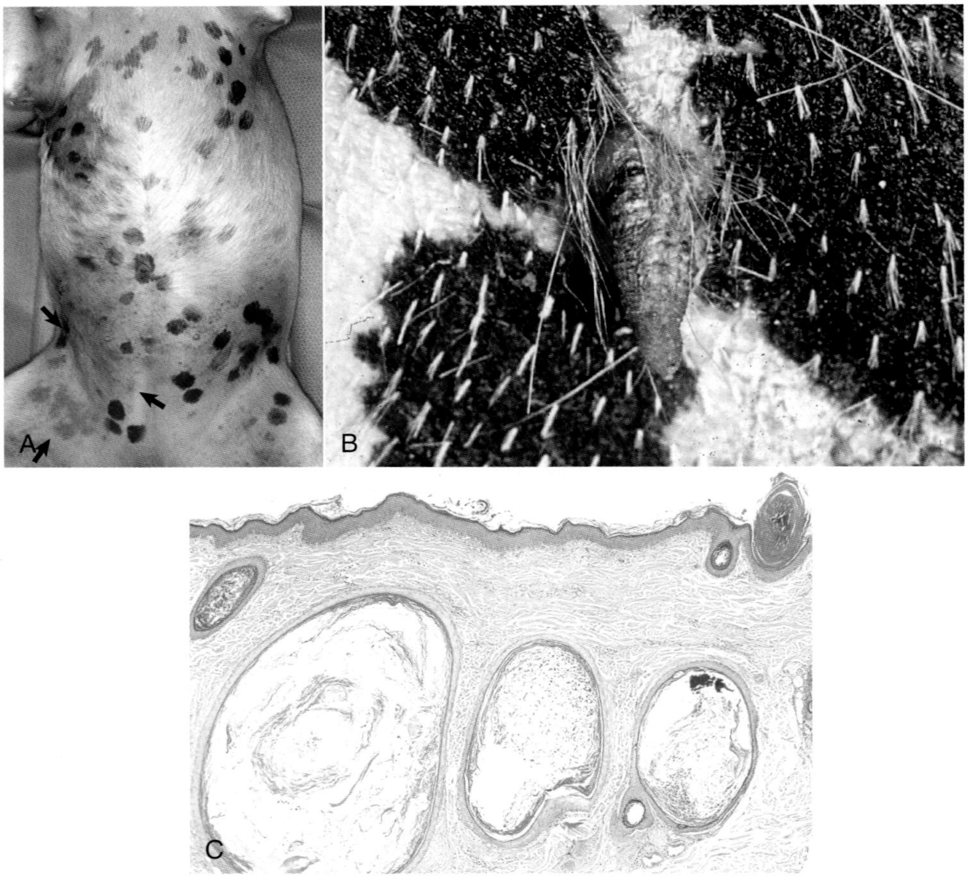

Fig. 17-38 Solar dermatitis, skin, dog.
A, Ventral abdomen and thorax. The nonpigmented and sparsely haired skin is erythematous, has comedones and crusts, and is palpably thickened *(arrows)*. The densely pigmented black spots are clinically unaffected, but lightly pigmented spots are affected. Comedones can rupture (furunculosis), releasing follicular contents that cause a foreign body inflammatory response and secondary bacterial infection. Clinically, the inflammation is prominent (erythema and furuncles) and can be misinterpreted as primary. Clinically, the distribution pattern of affected nonpigmented sparsely haired skin and unaffected haired or pigmented skin is supportive of the diagnosis of solar dermatitis. **B,** Ventral abdomen. Solar dermatitis with a solar (actinic) keratosis that has formed a cutaneous horn. Cutaneous horns are keratoses formed from multiple layers of compacted stratum corneum. They may arise from benign or malignant lesions in the epidermis (solar actinic keratosis, squamous cell carcinoma) or adnexa (infundibular keratinizing acanthoma). **C,** The epidermis is thickened by acanthosis, and three comedones (follicular distention and hyperkeratosis) are present. If comedones rupture, a large amount of endogenous foreign material (stratum corneum, hair shafts, and sebum) is released into the dermis, causing a foreign-body inflammatory response. Bacteria are also released and cause a secondary bacterial infection. H&E stain. (Courtesy Dr. Ann M. Hargis, DermatoDiagnostics.)

Affected follicles are often surrounded by a thin layer of fibrosis. In dogs, superficial dermal vessels may have hyalinized or sclerotic walls, and endothelial cells may be missing (solar vasculopathy). In some animals and in some anatomic locations, elastic tissue and collagen are damaged by solar radiation, and the dermis may be thickened by a zone of fibrosis parallel to the epidermal surface (laminar dermal fibrosis). Solar elastosis characterized by deposits of wavy basophilic elastin fibers in the superficial dermis is often present in horses and sometimes dogs. With continued UV exposure, solar keratoses develop. The epidermal surface is thickened by compact hyperkeratosis or parakeratosis. The acanthotic epidermis has atypical keratinocytes starting in the basal layer and progressing into the spinous layer. Keratinocytes are irregularly stratified and irregularly sized and shaped. Nuclei are large and often vary in size. Nucleoli may be large. There may be increased mitoses and premature cornification. The keratinocytes may form downward proliferations, usually as short buds, but occasionally as branching and anastomosing epidermal ridges. However, in solar keratoses, the basement membrane remains intact. Invasive squamous cell carcinoma can develop in the site of solar keratoses when atypical keratinocytes breach the basement membrane and invade into the contiguous dermis and, less often, subcutis. In some instances the atypical keratinocytes invade lymphatic channels, and can metastasize to lymph nodes, lungs, and can more widely disseminate.

Photosensitization

Photosensitization is a disorder caused by long-wavelength UV, or less frequently visible light, absorbed by a photodynamic chemical in the skin, or by a complex of photodynamic molecule and a biologic substrate, which results in a release of energy that produces reactive oxygen molecules, including free radicals. Generation of reactive oxygen molecules leads to mast cell degranulation and the production of inflammatory mediators, which causes damage to cell membranes, nucleic acids, proteins, and organelles. The photodynamic agent usually enters the dermis via the systemic circulation. However, direct contact and absorption of some photodynamic agents can result in localized contact photosensitization.

Photosensitization can occur in several forms. Type I or primary photosensitization, is often caused by ingestion of preformed photodynamic substances contained in a variety of plants; thus herbivores are most commonly affected. The plants causing photosensitization usually contain helianthrone or furocoumarin pigments. The helianthrone pigments are red fluorescent pigments such as hypericin (found in *Hypericum perforatum* [St. John's wort]) and fagopyrin (found in *Fagopyrum esculentum* [buckwheat]). Photosensitization attributed to furocoumarin pigments is caused by the presence of psoralens, photodynamic agents found in a variety of plants, including *Cymopterus watsonii* (spring parsley), *Ammi majus* (bishop's weed), and *Thamnosma texana* (Dutchman's breeches). Furocoumarin pigments also form phytoalexins, a group of compounds formed in plants in response to fungal infection or other injury and that inhibit or destroy the invading agent. The phytoalexins formed in fungus-infected parsnips and celery have caused phytophotocontact dermatitis when they are absorbed into the skin and react with UV light.

Primary photosensitization can also occur with the administration of drugs such as phenothiazine, which is converted to a photoreactive metabolite in the intestinal tract. This metabolite is usually converted to a nonphotoreactive compound in the liver by mixed function oxidases, but occasionally, either the reactive metabolite bypasses the liver or mixed function oxidase activity in the liver is compromised or insufficient and the reactive metabolite reaches the skin.

Type II photosensitization develops because of abnormal porphyrin metabolism, leading to the blood and tissue accumulation of photodynamic agents. These diseases usually are inherited as an enzyme deficiency, resulting in abnormal synthesis of photodynamic agents, including uroporphyrin and coproporphyrin. Examples include bovine congenital porphyria and bovine erythropoietic (hematopoietic) protoporphyria. Photosensitization caused by abnormal porphyrin metabolism has also been reported in pigs and cats.

Type III or hepatogenous photosensitization is caused by impaired capacity of the liver to excrete phylloerythrin, which is formed in the alimentary tract from the breakdown of chlorophyll. This is the most common type of photosensitization and occurs most commonly in herbivores, but any animal with generalized hepatic disease on a chlorophyll-rich diet that is exposed to sufficient solar radiation can develop hepatogenous photosensitization. Hepatogenous photosensitization occurs secondary to primary hepatocellular damage, inherited hepatic defects, or bile duct obstruction. Toxic plants, including but not limited to *Lantana camara* (lantana) and *Tribulis terrestris* (puncture vine), and mycotoxins, such as sporidesmin, are the most common cause of this type of photosensitization. Other plants that cause hepatic damage (such as those that contain pyrrolizidine alkaloids) can also contribute to the development of hepatogenous photosensitization.

Grossly, in photosensitization, lesions are located on areas of the body with nonpigmented skin and hair, and on parts of the body exposed to the sun such as the face, nose, and distal extremities in horses. In cattle, lesions occur in white-haired areas and on the teats, udder, perineum, and nose. In sheep with heavy fleeces, lesions occur on the pinnae, eyelids, face, nose, and coronary band, but in shorn sheep, lesions can occur on the back. Sheep can have extensive edema of the head, prompting terms that are synonyms: "swelled head" and "facial eczema." Onset of lesions may take only hours and initially include erythema and edema, followed by blisters, exudation, necrosis, and sloughing of necrotic tissue. The microscopic lesions consist of coagulative necrosis of the epidermis and possibly follicular epithelium, adnexal glands, and superficial dermis. Subepidermal vesiculation can occur. Endothelial cells of the superficial, middle, and deep dermal vessels are swollen and necrotic, and fibrinoid degeneration and thrombosis can result in edema; infarction; sloughing of the epidermis, dermis, and adnexa; and secondary bacterial infection.

Ionizing Radiation Injury

Advances in the treatment of cancer in companion animals have made the possibility of radiation-induced skin injury more likely. Ionizing radiation consists of electromagnetic radiation (x-rays, γ-rays) and particulate radiation (e.g., electrons, neutrons, protons) and is most damaging to highly proliferative cells, such as those of the anagen hair matrix, but epidermal basal cells and vascular endothelial cells are also affected. Available radiation modalities offer differing degrees of tissue penetration and thus differing potential for tissue injury. Some forms of radiotherapy penetrate deeper tissues while sparing the skin, and others are more concentrated in the superficial tissues or are preferentially absorbed by specific tissues. The type of radiation therapy and the source, dose, intensity, and duration of exposure dictate the range of possible side effects. Ionizing photons disrupt chemical bonds in cells, leading to injury or cell death. Some cells are not lethally damaged, but sustain DNA damage to the extent that replication and/or replacement are not possible. The effects of radiation damage can be divided into acute and chronic forms.

Acute radiation injury to the skin is a result of damage to rapidly dividing cells. Damage is self-limiting, and recovery is associated with rapid cell turnover. Clinical lesions of radiation dermatitis appear 2 to 4 weeks after exposure. Initially, there is erythema, pain, edema, and heat, followed several weeks later by dry or moist desquamation depending on the degree of injury. Histologically, the lesions resemble a second-degree burn, with suprabasilar or subepidermal bullae formation, dermal edema with fibrin exudation, and a marked leukocytic infiltrate. Reepithelialization occurs over a period of 10 to 60 days. The damage sustained to germinal epithelium of hair follicles and sebaceous glands leads to alopecia within 2 to 4 weeks after exposure. Hair regrowth follows over the next several months, but damage to sebaceous glands is not reversible and leads to permanent scaling manifesting histologically as hyperkeratosis. The chronic lesions of radiation injury are evident months to years after treatment and are primarily the result of damage to the microvasculature. Chronic changes include pigmentary alterations (hyperpigmentation with lower doses and hypopigmentation with higher doses), leukotrichia (depigmentation of hair shafts because of loss of follicular melanocytes), dermal scarring, epidermal atrophy, and ulceration. The epidermis is thin, friable, and in some areas, hyperplastic and can become neoplastic. Squamous cell carcinomas can develop in some sites of severe radiation damage because of sublethal DNA damage. Chronic nonhealing exudative ulcers can develop, but granulation tissue does not form. The dermis is fibrotic with atypical fibroblasts, telangiectasia, and possibly deep arteriolar changes. Endothelial swelling, necrosis, and thrombosis lead to occlusion and excessive endothelial proliferation, which, when combined with the effects of vascular leakage, leads to vascular collapse. This condition of progressive vessel abnormalities is referred to as *obliterative endoarteritis* and is known to form a "histohematic" (tissue-blood) barrier to surrounding tissue, leading to continued anoxia and nutrient shortage.

Chemical Injury

Chemical injuries to the skin can result from local application directly onto the skin or from absorption of chemicals via the gastrointestinal tract and subsequent distribution to the skin. For a chemical to cause injury via local application, it must penetrate the hair and protective epidermal layers. Penetration is enhanced by physical damage to the stratum corneum, especially that caused by excessive moisture. Chemical injuries of the skin include contact irritant dermatitis (local application), systemically distributed chemicals, such as arsenic, mercury, thallium, iodine, and organochlorines and organobromines, and poisonings by fungal-contaminated plants and plants containing selenium, mimosine, and trichothecenes. Externally applied agents that produce irritant contact dermatitis induce cutaneous damage by altering the water-holding capacity of the epidermis or by penetrating the epidermis and directly damaging cells. Systemically absorbed and distributed chemical agents cause lesions by a wide variety of mechanisms, some of which are not known. An example is toxicity caused by systemic absorption of some organochlorine and organobromine compounds, such as highly chlorinated naphthalenes, which were used as additives in lubricants for farm machinery such as feed pelleting equipment. As a result, highly chlorinated naphthalenes were frequent feed contaminants. Toxicosis occurred most commonly in cattle, the most susceptible species, and was known as X-disease or bovine hyperkeratosis. Fortunately, this toxicosis is largely historically interesting, as highly chlorinated naphthalenes have not been used in lubricants since the 1950s. Lesions of chlorinated naphthalene toxicity are the result of the interference of the conversion of carotene to vitamin A and result in vitamin A deficiency. Vitamin A is necessary for normal differentiation of stratified squamous epithelium. Clinical lesions consist of alopecia and lichenified, fissured plaques of scale that spare only the legs. Histologic lesions consist of marked hyperkeratosis of the epidermis and follicles. Squamous metaplasia of the epithelial lining of the glands and ducts of the liver, pancreas, kidneys, and reproductive tract also develop.

Irritant Contact Dermatitis

There are two forms of contact dermatitis, one is immunologically mediated (see the discussion on allergic contact dermatitis in the section on Selected Hypersensitivity Reactions), and the other is caused by direct damage by irritant substances. Allergic contact dermatitis (immunologically mediated) requires prior sensitization to the offending agent. Most cases of contact dermatitis are nonimmunologic and are caused by direct contact with substances, such as body or wound secretions; application of drugs; or exposure to acids, alkalies, soaps, detergents, or irritant plants. These substances overwhelm the protective mechanisms of the skin and directly injure cells. It is important to realize that the two types of contact dermatitis can produce very similar histologic lesions, thus differentiation between immune-mediated and irritant contact dermatitis largely depends on history, clinical signs, and anatomic distribution of the lesions. Horses develop lesions on the nose, ventrum, lower limbs, and where riding tack contacts the body, and on the perineum and caudal aspect of the rear legs. In dogs and cats, lesions of irritant contact dermatitis develop on the glabrous (sparsely haired) skin of the abdomen, axillae, flanks, interdigital spaces, perianal area, ventral tail, ventral chest, legs, eyelids, and feet. Grossly, erythematous patches, papules, and rarely, vesicles develop, but self-inflicted trauma can lead to ulcers and crusts. Microscopically, lesions consist of spongiotic dermatitis, neutrophilic vesicopustules, and superficial dermal perivascular neutrophilic inflammation. Chronic lesions consist of epidermal hyperplasia, hyperkeratosis, sometimes confluent parakeratosis, and superficial perivascular inflammation. Lesions can be obscured by self-inflicted trauma, making histologic diagnosis difficult. Corrosive substances (strong acids or alkalies) can cause epidermal necrosis.

Injection Site Reactions

Injections of vaccines or therapeutic drugs into the subcutis can result in granulomatous nodules. Injected materials, such as adjuvant and other vaccine components, are highly antigenic and can incite a local and persistent immunologic response resulting in a palpable subcutaneous nodule. Histologic descriptions of the acute or subacute reactions to similar injected materials are not reported in the literature. Histologic changes represented by the palpable nodules at the site of previous vaccination consist of a localized area of deep dermal or subcutaneous necrosis containing foreign material thought to be adjuvant or vaccine components. The central zone of foreign and necrotic material is bordered by macrophages and multinucleated giant cells with a peripheral zone of lymphocytes and variable numbers of plasma cells and eosinophils (foreign body granuloma). Macrophages usually contain amphophilic granular foreign material. Lymphoid follicular development at the margins of these lesions can be extensive. Although many injection site lesions heal without serious consequences, in cats there is a causal relationship between postvaccination inflammation and development of fibrosarcomas, myxosarcomas, osteosarcomas, rhabdomyosarcomas, chondrosarcomas, and histiocytic sarcomas. The antigen load and degree of persistent inflammation and eventual fibroblastic proliferation caused by subcutaneous vaccine administration are thought to be important factors predisposing cats to tumor development. It is speculated that during tissue repair, fibroblasts

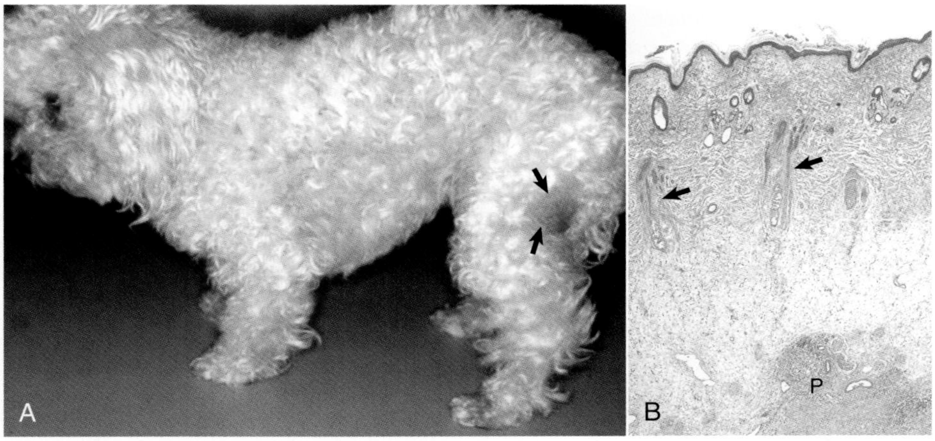

Fig. 17-39 Rabies vaccine–associated alopecia, skin, haired, dog.
A, This type of alopecia *(arrows)* generally develops 3 to 6 months after vaccination and is the result of partial ischemia. **B,** Note panniculitis *(P)* with lymphocytes, plasma cells, and histiocytes that has resulted from subcutaneous injection of killed rabies vaccine. Small, atrophic hair follicles *(arrows)* are in the dermis. H&E stain. (**A** courtesy Dr. Lynn Schmeitzel, College of Veterinary Medicine, University of Tennessee. **B** courtesy Dr. Ann M. Hargis, DermatoDiagnostics.)

or myofibroblasts are stimulated by the immunogenic substances in the vaccine reaction site and this, in combination with other factors such as oncogene alterations or unidentified carcinogens, leads to malignant transformation of cells. Tumor development can take months to years, with eventual neoplastic transformation of mesenchymal cells.

In small, often soft-coated, breeds of dogs, especially poodles, injection of killed rabies vaccine can result in localized lymphoplasmacytic panniculitis, subtle vasculitis, and localized ischemia leading to severe follicular atrophy in overlying dermis (Fig. 17-39) that is clinically apparent as a focal area of alopecia and hyperpigmentation. Immunofluorescence staining has identified rabies antigen in the vessels and epithelium of the hair follicles. A low-grade, immune-mediated vasculitis with resultant tissue hypoxia leading to the atrophic changes in the adnexa has been suggested as the pathogenesis. Vascular lesions are characterized by hyalinization of the vessel wall, lack of endothelial cells, intramural karyorrhectic debris, and perivascular lymphocytic infiltrates. Rarely, small numbers of lymphocytes are found within the walls of affected vessels.

Injection site eosinophilic granulomas with necrotic centers have been reported to occur in horses 1 to 3 days after injections of various substances using silicone-coated needles. The reaction is suspected to be a form of delayed hypersensitivity.

Snake and Spider Bites (Envenomations)

The families Elapidae (coral snake) and Viperidae (rattlesnake, water moccasin, and copperhead) contain the majority of the poisonous snakes in the United States (US). The genera *Latrodectus* (e.g., black widow) and *Loxosceles* (e.g., brown recluse) are the most common venomous spiders causing cutaneous injury. Effects depend on composition of the venom, individual victim response, anatomic location of the envenomation, and specific characteristics of the offending snake or spider, which can be influenced by season of the year, geographic location, time since last inflicted bite or sting, depth of injury, and so forth. Different species of animals respond differently to the same venom.

Spider bites occur most often on the face and legs. The brown recluse spider (*Loxosceles reclusa*) is the spider most known to induce dermal necrosis, although there are a number of others. Brown recluse venom contains hyaluronidase and sphingomyelinase-D, which degrade tissue. A blister with a surrounding pale halo and more peripheral erythema characterizes initial reactions documented in humans and some experimental animals. Necrosis and eschar formation occur within 5 to 7 days. Ulceration can be extensive. Histologically, there is hemorrhage and edema, neutrophilic vasculitis, and arterial wall necrosis. The epidermis and dermis undergo infarction, which can extend into the subcutis and underlying muscle. Panniculitis can be present. Eventually, there is dermal scarring and replacement of the subcutis and muscle by hypocellular connective tissue. Brown recluse spider bites in humans can also lead to massive hemolysis. Differentials include other venomous bites, vasculitis, slough caused by iatrogenic injection of irritating substances, thermal burns, necrotizing fasciitis or other cutaneous infection, septic embolization, or trauma. Some putative spider bites (and possibly wasp and bee stings) in the dog develop as acute, painful, swollen areas on the dorsal or lateral nose that histologically consist of severe eosinophilic folliculitis and furunculosis (see the discussion on nasal eosinophilic folliculitis and furunculosis in dogs in the section on Miscellaneous Skin Disorders,), leading to the theory that these lesions are probably caused by hypersensitivity reactions to injected venom.

Snakebites are common in the horse and dog and to a lesser degree in cats and most often inflicted on the head or legs. Snake venom contains various enzymes, proteins, peptides, and kinins. Of the five genera of venomous snakes in the US, crotaline venom (rattlesnake, copperhead, cottonmouth, and others) contains the highest concentration of proteolytic enzymes. Snakebite envenomation produces pain, edema, and erythema that, if severe, are followed by necrosis and sloughing of tissue, and sometimes death of the animal. Variable systemic effects occur, including paralysis, coagulation disturbances, shock, increased capillary permeability, myocardial damage, rhabdomyolysis, and renal failure.

Ergot

Ergot poisoning is caused by the ingestion of toxic alkaloids produced by the fungus *Claviceps purpurea.* This fungus infects the seed heads of grasses and grains. The alkaloids, particularly ergotamine, cause direct stimulation of adrenergic nerves supplying arteriolar smooth muscle, resulting in marked peripheral arteriolar vasoconstriction and damage to capillary endothelium. Arteriolar spasm and damage to capillary endothelium lead to thrombosis and ischemic necrosis (infarction) of tissue. Cold temperatures increase the severity of the lesions. The species most commonly poisoned are cattle fed contaminated grain or cattle grazing pastures infected with the alkaloid-producing fungus. Lesions develop after about 1 week of consumption and begin as swelling and redness of the extremities, particularly the hindlegs. Lesions begin at the coronary bands and extend to the fetlocks (metatarsophalangeal joints). The feet may become necrotic, with viable and nonviable tissue separated by a distinct line (dry gangrene). The front feet and tips of ears, teats, and tail can be affected and in severe cases can slough.

Tall Fescue Grass

Lesions identical to those of ergot poisoning occur after the ingestion of tall fescue grass, a common pasture plant, infected by the endophytic fungus *Neotyphodium coenophialum* (formerly *Acremonium coenophialum*). Lesions develop about 2 weeks after ingestion of the toxic plant and consist of necrosis (dry gangrene) of distal extremities. The ergot alkaloids, particularly ergovaline, are responsible for toxicity and act as peripheral vasoconstrictors.

Selenium

Selenium poisoning is caused by ingestion of plants that have accumulated toxic concentrations of selenium, or to an overdose of a selenium supplement. Some plants selectively accumulate selenium, regardless of soil selenium content. These selective accumulators (obligate accumulators; e.g., *Astragalus, Stanleya*) require selenium for growth, generally are not palatable, and are eaten only when other plants are unavailable. Many other plants (facultative accumulators; e.g., *Aster, Atriplex*) do not require selenium for growth but will accumulate toxic concentrations of selenium if grown in soil with high selenium levels. These facultative accumulator plants are commonly eaten by livestock and more often are the cause of poisoning. The mechanism by which selenium is thought to exert its effects on the integument and appendages is through its competitive replacement of sulfur, which modifies the structure of keratin, a sulfur-containing molecule. Replacement of sulfur by selenium in other molecules can also contribute to toxicity. Acute or chronic selenium poisoning has developed in most domestic animals, although susceptibility to selenium poisoning varies with species, dosage, diet, rate of consumption, chemical form, and other factors. In acute poisonings, signs relate to involvement of multiple organ systems. Chronic selenium toxicity usually develops in livestock (horses, cattle, and sheep) consuming seleniferous forages. It occurs worldwide but is more frequent in Nebraska, Wyoming, and the Dakotas in the US and in portions of Western Canada. Animals with chronic selenium intoxication are emaciated, have poor quality hair coat, and have partial alopecia. Horses lose the long hair of the mane and tail, develop hoof deformities, and shed the hooves.

Vetch Toxicosis and Vetch-Like Diseases

Vetch toxicosis is most commonly seen as a syndrome characterized by dermatitis, conjunctivitis, diarrhea, and granulomatous inflammation of many organs. It occurs in cattle and to a lesser extent in horses after consumption of vetch-containing pastures. Hairy vetch (*Vicia villosa* Roth) is a cultivated legume used as pasture, hay, and silage in most of the US and other countries. Toxicity from vetch seeds is known to be a result of the presence of prussic acid. The cause of the granulomatous inflammation in this syndrome remains unclear. One proposed pathogenesis is that ingestion of vetch or another substance leads to antigen formation in the form of a hapten or a complete antigen that sensitizes lymphocytes and evokes the cell-mediated immune response upon repeat exposure.

Initial lesions in cattle consist of a rough coat with papules and crusts affecting the skin of the udder, teats, escutcheon (back of udder and perineum), and neck, followed by involvement of the trunk, face, and limbs. The skin becomes less pliable, alopecic, and lichenified. Marked pruritus leads to excoriations from self-induced trauma. The dermis has perivascular to diffuse infiltrates of monocytes, lymphocytes, plasma cells, multinucleated giant cells, and eosinophils. There is marked hyperkeratosis and dermal and epidermal edema.

The clinical syndrome begins 2 or more weeks after consumption and consists of pruritic dermatitis, diarrhea (possibly bloody), and wasting. Morbidity is low and mortality is high. Holstein and Angus cattle and cattle 3 years or older are more often affected. Death in cattle occurs approximately 10 to 20 days after illness begins. At necropsy, yellow nodular infiltrates of mononuclear leukocytes are seen that disrupt the architecture of a wide range of organs but are most severe in myocardium, kidney, lymph nodes, thyroid, and adrenal glands. In cattle, other species of *Vicia* and additional compounds are capable of inducing disease indistinguishable from vetch toxicity. These include feed additives such as di-ureido isobutane and citrus pulp.

Hairy vetch toxicosis in horses resembles that in cattle, except for the infrequent finding of eosinophils in the infiltrate and lack of heart involvement. Conditions very similar to vetch toxicosis have been reported in horses with no vetch exposure. These cases have been variably referred to as *idiopathic granulomatous disease involving the skin, systemic granulomatous disease, generalized granulomatous disease,* or *equine sarcoidosis.* Organ involvement is variable. Skin lesions include scaling, crusting, and alopecia on the face or limbs that progress to a generalized exfoliative dermatitis. Histologically, the skin has multifocal, sometimes perifollicular, to deep dermal nodules of granulomatous inflammation. These idiopathic conditions in the horse are fairly indistinguishable and should be considered "vetch-like disease" until more information is available.

The diagnosis of vetch toxicity or vetch-like disease is a diagnosis by exclusion. It is made after review of the herd history and of character and distribution of the lesions. The combination of lesions is fairly distinctive.

Physical Injury

Acral Lick Dermatitis

Acral lick dermatitis (lick granuloma, neurodermatitis) is a relatively common psychogenic dermatitis usually developing on an extremity (acral = extremity or apex) in dogs and is caused by persistent licking or chewing. The cause is not known, but a mild sensory polyneuropathy that incites a sensation of pruritus or pain may be associated with lesion development. Boredom can also play a role. The constant licking and chewing of the skin is a form of repeated trauma that leads to the gross and histologic changes. Usually a single lesion develops in carpal, metacarpal, metatarsal, tibial, or radial areas. Grossly, lesions are circumscribed, hairless, and sometimes, ulcerated (Fig. 17-40). Microscopically, there is compact hyperkeratosis and acanthosis of the epidermis and follicular epithelium. Ulcers are occasionally seen, the result of chronic irritation from licking. The dermis is thickened by fibrosis. Capillaries and some collagen fibers are oriented parallel to hair follicles, called *vertical streaking.* Sebaceous glands and hair follicles are hypertrophic, and there is perivascular and periadnexal plasmacytic dermatitis. Some lesions are complicated by secondary bacterial folliculitis and furunculosis.

Pyotraumatic Dermatitis (Acute Moist Dermatitis, "Hot Spots")

Pyotraumatic dermatitis, especially common in dogs, is secondary to irritation and principally the result of self-inflicted trauma from

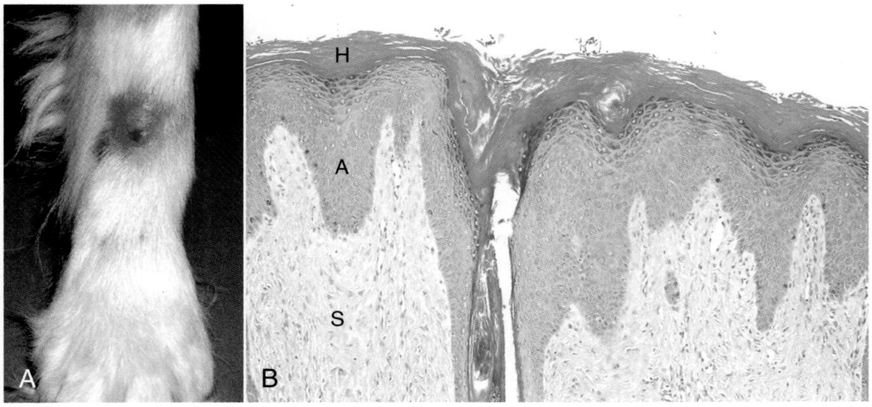

Fig. 17-40 Acral lick dermatitis, skin, leg, dog. **A,** Chronic licking has resulted in an area of alopecia and a small dark ulcer in the alopecic area. Alopecia can be caused by mechanical removal of the hair or breakage of hair from licking, and in cases with secondary folliculitis, alopecia can also be caused by follicular inflammation (folliculitis) and sometimes follicular rupture (furunculosis). Ulceration also can be caused by mechanical trauma to the skin surface. **B,** The epidermis is thickened by compact hyperkeratosis *(H)* and acanthosis *(A)*, and the dermis is thickened by granulation tissue and fibrosis (scarring *[S]*). H&E stain. (Courtesy Dr. Ann M. Hargis, DermatoDiagnostics.)

biting or scratching because of pain or itching caused by allergies, parasites, matted hair, or irritant chemicals. Dogs with long hair and dense undercoats are predisposed, and lesions develop more commonly in hot humid weather. Flea bite dermatitis is a common predisposing cause, and lesions can coalesce to involve large portions of dorsal lumbar and thigh skin. Type I hypersensitivity reaction to flea bites leads to severe pruritus and self-trauma. Excoriated, moist skin is conducive to bacterial colonization. Grossly the lesions are hairless, red, exude fluid, and have circumscribed edges. Microscopically, affected dogs have either superficial erosive to ulcerative exudative dermatitis or a deeper suppurative folliculitis (pyotraumatic folliculitis, deep pyoderma). The pyotraumatic folliculitis lesions are considered to represent a deep pyoderma and develop more commonly on the cheek and neck of young golden retrievers, Saint Bernard, Labrador retriever, and Newfoundland dogs. Biopsy is required to differentiate the more superficial pyotraumatic dermatitis from the deeper suppurative folliculitis.

Feline Ulcerative Dermatitis Syndrome

Feline ulcerative dermatitis syndrome is an uncommon disorder that may have more than one underlying cause. Previous injections and hypersensitivity are thought to initiate the syndrome in some but not all cats. The pathogenesis is not known, but self-trauma appears to significantly contribute to and perpetuate lesions. Lesions develop most commonly in the skin of the dorsal neck or interscapular regions, and grossly consist of a nonhealing ulcer with serocellular exudate that can mat the adjacent hair. Microscopic lesions consist of an ulcer covered by fibrinonecrotic crust. The dermis subjacent to the ulcer contains components of necrotic epidermis and adnexa intermixed with degenerate neutrophils. Adnexal effacement by fibrosis is seen in severe cases. Inflammation in adjacent and deeper dermis is variable but often scant and consists of a few neutrophils, eosinophils, and mixed mononuclear cells. Chronic lesions consist of acanthosis of bordering epidermis with a linear band of fibrosis beneath and parallel to the adjacent intact epidermis. In those cases attributed to previous vaccination, nodular lymphoplasmacytic to histiocytic panniculitis is present.

Callus

A callus is a raised, irregular, patch of thickened skin that develops because of friction, usually over pressure points on bony prominences or on the sternum (see Table 17-3). Callosities can develop in all domestic animals but are particularly common in giant breed dogs and in pigs kept on concrete or other hard flooring without adequate bedding. Secondary folliculitis, furunculosis, and ulceration can develop. Microscopically the epidermis and follicular epithelium are thickened by hyperkeratosis and acanthosis. Regular epidermal hyperplasia (rete ridge and papillary dermal interdigitation) also occurs. Comedones are present in some lesions. The follicular openings can be widened by excessive keratin. Dilated follicles can rupture (furunculosis), releasing bacteria, keratin proteins, and sebum, resulting in secondary pyoderma and a foreign body inflammatory response (callus pyoderma).

Intertrigo (Skin Fold Dermatitis)

Intertrigo is superficial dermatitis occurring on apposed skin surfaces. It occurs in cows with large pendulous udders and develops between the udder and the medial thigh (udder-thigh dermatitis). Intertrigo also occurs in dogs in the skin of the facial fold (brachycephalic breeds), lip fold (breeds with large lips such as the Saint Bernard), body fold (Shar-Pei breed), vulvar fold (obese female dogs with a small vulva), and tail fold (dogs with corkscrew tails such as English bulldogs) (Fig. 17-41). The cause and pathogenesis involve the presence of closely apposed skin surfaces, frictional trauma between the skin surfaces, accumulated moisture (from tears, saliva, cutaneous glandular secretions, or urine), and bacterial infection. The moisture and frictional trauma predispose to bacterial growth and subsequent infection. Early gross lesions of intertriginous dermatitis typically consist initially of erythema and edema. Later, pustules, ulcers, and crusts can develop. Late lesions in cows can be severe, with occasional sloughing of skin and subcutis. Microscopically, in early stages there is congestion and edema with early perivascular inflammation that progresses to a more diffuse band of inflammation in the superficial dermis, parallel to the epidermis, but often sparing the epidermal-dermal junction. Inflammatory cells include plasma cells, fewer lymphocytes, neutrophils, and macrophages. In more severe cases, there can be exocytosis of neutrophils into the epidermis, epidermal pustules, crusts, ulcers, and, in cows, necrosis that leads to sloughing of tissue. If the cause is corrected, early and mild chronic lesions heal without scarring (most cases). However, when there is ulceration or necrosis and sloughing of tissue (minority of cases), lesions heal by second intention with the formation of granulation tissue, wound contraction, and scarring.

Temperature Extremes

Information on this topic is available at evolve.elsevier.com/Zachary/McGavin/.

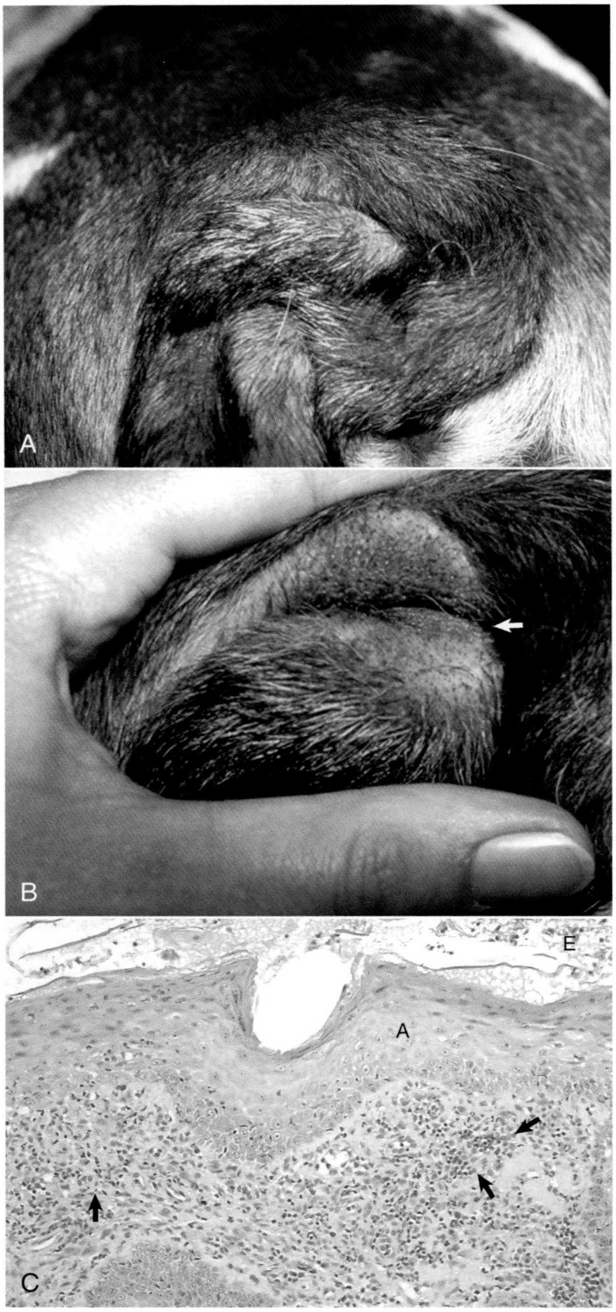

Fig. 17-41 Intertriginous inflammation (screw tail), skin, tail, dog. **A,** "Screw tail," English bulldog. Excessive skin folds around the tail cause friction and moisture accumulation, predisposing to bacterial growth. **B,** Intertriginous pyoderma, English bulldog. The skin fold *(arrow)* of the dog depicted in **A** has been opened to expose the erythema, hyperpigmentation, and lichenification. **C,** Intertriginous dermatitis. The epidermis is acanthotic *(A)* and partially covered by fluid and cellular exudate *(E)*, and there is inflammation composed of numerous plasma cells and fewer lymphocytes and neutrophils in the dermis *(arrows)*. H&E stain. (**A** and **B** courtesy Dr. Alexander Werner, Valley Veterinary Specialty Service. **C** courtesy Dr. Ann M. Hargis, DermatoDiagnostics.)

MICROBIAL AND PARASITIC DISORDERS

Cutaneous infections develop when there is disruption in the defense mechanisms of the skin (see the section on Host Defense Mechanisms Against Injury). Predisposing factors to skin infections involve compromised epidermal barrier integrity caused by friction, trauma, excessive moisture, dirt, matted hair, chemical irritants, freezing or burning, irradiation, and parasitic infestation. Suppressed immune function resulting from inadequate nutrition, therapy with glucocorticoids, and other acquired or inherited immunologic abnormalities can also contribute to increased susceptibility to microbial and parasitic infections. Infectious agents enter the body via their specific portal of entry (see the section on Portals of Entry into the Skin), which includes traversing the epidermal surface, entering via hair follicles or the ducts of glands, and migrating via nerves or sometimes via the hematogenous route.

Viral Infections

Poxviruses

Poxviruses are DNA epitheliotropic viruses that infect most domestic, wild, and laboratory animals and birds (Table 17-7). Dogs and cats are rarely infected with poxviruses, although infection with contagious ecthyma (parapoxvirus) has been reported in dogs, and cutaneous infection caused by a poxvirus of the orthopoxvirus genus (cowpox) has been reported in cats in Europe. There are rare anecdotal reports of poxvirus infection in the skin of cats in North America, but, with the exception of one case, the poxvirus or viruses involved have not been characterized. In the single case in which the virus was identified, polymerase chain reaction (PCR) and gene sequencing identified raccoonpox, an orthopoxvirus, in the skin lesions. There are major differences between different poxviruses and in the range of species they infect; some are species-specific and others are zoonotic. Many poxviruses of animals, such as the contagious ecthyma parapoxvirus, can cause skin lesions in humans. Poxviruses induce lesions by a variety of mechanisms. Lesions develop secondary to poxviral invasion of epithelium, by ischemic necrosis caused by vascular injury, and by stimulation of host cell DNA, resulting in epidermal hyperplasia. Hyperplasia may be explained by a gene, present in several poxviruses, including molluscum contagiosum, whose product has significant homology with epidermal growth factor. Poxviruses also encode for functions that may counteract host defenses. These include genes related to those encoding the serpins (a superfamily of related proteins important in regulating serine protease enzymes that mediate kinin, complement, fibrinolytic, and coagulation pathways) and genes encoding antiinterferon activities. The severity of poxviral infection varies, depending on whether the infection is localized (cutaneous) or systemic and whether there are secondary infections. The sequence of the cutaneous lesions are macule, papule, vesicle (varies in severity), umbilicated pustule, crust, and scar (see Fig. 17-31). Histologically, pox lesions begin as keratinocyte cytoplasmic swelling and vacuolation, usually first affecting the cells of the outer stratum spinosum. Rupture of the damaged keratinocytes produces multiloculated vesicles, so-called reticular degeneration. The early dermal lesions include edema, vascular dilation, a perivascular mononuclear cell infiltrate, and a variable neutrophilic infiltrate. Neutrophils migrate into the epidermis and aggregate in vesicles to form microabscesses. Large intraepidermal pustules can form and sometimes extend into the superficial dermis. There is usually marked epithelial hyperplasia and sometimes pseudocarcinomatous hyperplasia of the adjacent epithelium. This contributes to the raised border of the umbilicated pustule. Rupture or drying of the pustule produces a crust, often colonized on its surface by

TABLE 17-7 Viral Infections of the Skin

Virus	Diseases	Species Affected	Distribution
Parapoxvirus	Contagious pustular dermatitis	Sheep, goats, cattle; rarely dogs	Cutaneous
	Papular stomatitis	Cattle	
	Pseudocowpox	Milking cows; zoonotic	
Orthopoxvirus	Cowpox	Many species, including cats in Europe	Cutaneous
Molluscipoxvirus	Molluscum contagiosum	Horses, rarely dogs	Cutaneous
Capripoxvirus	Sheeppox	Most are species specific	Systemic
	Goatpox		
	Lumpy skin disease	Cattle	
Suipoxvirus	Swine pox	Pigs	Cutaneous
Unclassified poxvirus	Ulcerative dermatosis of sheep	Sheep	Cutaneous
Bovine herpesvirus 2 (dermatotropic)	Bovine ulcerative mammillitis (bovine herpes mammillitis)	Cattle	Cutaneous
	Pseudo–lumpy skin disease		
Bovine herpesvirus 4 (dermatotropic)	Bovine herpes mammary pustular dermatitis	Cattle	Cutaneous
Feline herpesvirus 1	Feline facial dermatitis and stomatitis	Cats	Cutaneous, oral, ocular, upper respiratory
Ovine herpesvirus 2* (in United States)	Malignant catarrhal fever	Cattle	Cutaneous, oral, systemic
Papillomavirus	Papilloma, wart	All species	Cutaneous, oral, mucocutaneous
Papillomavirus	Epidermal viral plaques	Dog, cat	Cutaneous
Papillomavirus	Bowenoid disease	Cat, less in dog	Cutaneous
	Multicentric carcinoma in situ		
Papillomavirus	Fibropapilloma	Cattle	Cutaneous, genital
Papillomavirus	Sarcoid (fibropapilloma)	Horse, cat	Cutaneous
Picornavirus	Foot-and-mouth disease	Ruminants, pigs	Oral, cutaneous
Picornavirus	Swine vesicular disease	Pigs	Oral, cutaneous
Rhabdovirus	Vesicular stomatitis	Horses, cattle, pigs	Oral, cutaneous
Calicivirus	Vesicular exanthema	Pigs	Oral, cutaneous
Calicivirus	Feline calicivirus	Cats	Oral, cutaneous, systemic
Parvovirus	Porcine parvovirus	Piglets	Oral, cutaneous
Retrovirus	Feline leukemia virus	Cats	Secondary skin infections; cutaneous horns with feline leukemia virus
	Feline immunodeficiency virus		

*Indirect evidence of viral involvement.

bacteria. Poxvirus lesions often contain characteristic intracytoplasmic eosinophilic inclusion bodies. These are single or multiple and of varying size and duration. The inclusions are primarily comprised of proteins. Sheeppox and goatpox are the most pathogenic poxviruses, and infection causes significant mortality, especially in young animals as a result of systemic disease. Sheeppox and goatpox do not occur in the US or Canada.

Molluscum Contagiosum

Information on this topic is available at evolve.elsevier.com/Zachary/McGavin/.

Cowpox

Cowpox virus infections occur rarely in cattle in the United Kingdom and other areas of Europe. There is increasing evidence that small wild rodents (i.e., mice, squirrels, voles) serve as a reservoir for infection and that cattle, cats, and rarely other mammals become infected through contact with the wild rodents. Cutaneous infections in cattle usually develop on the teats and udder of cows and on the muzzle of suckling calves. Lesions follow the typical sequence of cutaneous poxviral infections. In cats, poxvirus infection is uncommon and usually occurs in outdoor cats living in rural areas, presumably because these cats hunt and have contact with rodents harboring the poxvirus. Primary cutaneous lesions typically develop on the face, neck, or forelegs and consist of an ulcerated or crusted macule or plaque. Lesions can develop into deep ulcers that heal with granulation tissue or less commonly develop into abscesses or cellulitis. Rarely, oral or mucocutaneous junctional areas are affected. Additional secondary cutaneous lesions can develop within about 2 weeks after viremic distribution to other cutaneous sites and less commonly to the upper or lower respiratory tract. The microscopic lesions are sharply demarcated, often deep ulcers covered by fibrinonecrotic exudate. Intracytoplasmic inclusion bodies in keratinocytes or follicular or sebaceous glandular epithelial cells help establish the diagnosis.

Bovine Papular Stomatitis

Bovine papular stomatitis virus is distributed worldwide, and although it causes disease more commonly in cattle more than 2 years old, it can occur at any age and in any breed. Lesions occur on the muzzle, nostrils, lips, and mouth, and cows with suckling calves can develop teat and udder lesions. The development and appearance of the lesions are similar to pseudocowpox, with resolution of lesions in days to weeks. A chronic form has been described in which exudative necrotic dermatitis involves the trunk, as well as the mouth, and in which the animals died in 4 to 6 weeks. Transmission to humans induces lesions identical to "milker's nodule" caused by *Pseudocowpox virus* infection. The histologic appearance of lesions is typical of other poxviral infections.

Capripoxviral Diseases

Capripoxviruses are the cause of sheeppox and goatpox. These viruses cause significant economic losses in countries where they are endemic, and the geographic distribution of these viruses is expanding. Sheeppox and goatpox are present in Africa, Asia, the Middle East, and most of the Indian subcontinent where, despite attempts at vaccination, capripoxvirus is responsible for cycles of epidemic disease followed by periods of endemic maintenance with low morbidity. The disease is exotic to the Americas, Australia, and New Zealand. Although eradication measures eliminated the disease from Britain in the mid-nineteenth century, they have only recently been successful in Eastern European countries. The diseases they cause lead to constraints on international trade of livestock and related products and can prevent the importation of new breeds of sheep or goats into endemic areas because fatality rates can be very high in nonindigenous breeds. Capripoxviruses are highly contagious and spread by the respiratory tract in times of close contact and mechanically by insect vectors and fomites. Virus is shed in saliva, conjunctival secretions, milk, urine, and feces, as well as in skin lesions and scabs. Vaccination of susceptible animals for sheeppox and goatpox provides lifelong immunity. The viruses share a high percentage of homology at the nucleotide and amino acid levels but are distinguishable phylogenetically using PCR-RFLP techniques. These viruses are also considered potential agents of agroterrorism.

Sheeppox

Sheeppox is caused by the sheeppox virus and is the most serious of the pox diseases of domestic animals. Sheeppox causes extensive economic loss through high mortality, reduced meat, milk or wool yields, commercial inhibitions from quarantine requirements, and the cost of disease prevention programs.

Transmission of infection is by direct contact with diseased sheep or indirect contact via contaminated environment. Sheeppox virus is resistant to desiccation and remains viable for up to 2 months on wool or 6 months in dried crust. There are breed differences in disease susceptibility. Fine-wooled Merino sheep are particularly sensitive, whereas breeds native to endemic areas, such as Algerian sheep, are comparatively resistant. Sheeppox occurs in all ages of sheep with a high morbidity and a mortality as high as 50%; but the disease is most severe in lambs, with mortality reaching 80% to 100%. A high level of background immunity, such as occurs in endemic areas of Kenya, is associated with low mortality, even in the young.

Sheeppox is a systemic disease. Infection is usually by the respiratory route but may occur through skin abrasions. The incubation period varies from 4 to 21 days and is followed by a leukocyte-associated viremia. The virus localizes in many organs, including the skin where the virus concentration is highest 10 to 14 days postinfection. The initial clinical signs are fever, lacrimation, drooling, serous nasal discharge, and hyperesthesia. Skin lesions develop in 1 to 2 days and have a predilection for the sparsely-wooled areas and typically involve eyelids, cheeks, nostrils, vulva, udder, scrotum, prepuce, ventral surface of the tail, and medial thigh. There is usually a concurrent superficial lymphadenopathy.

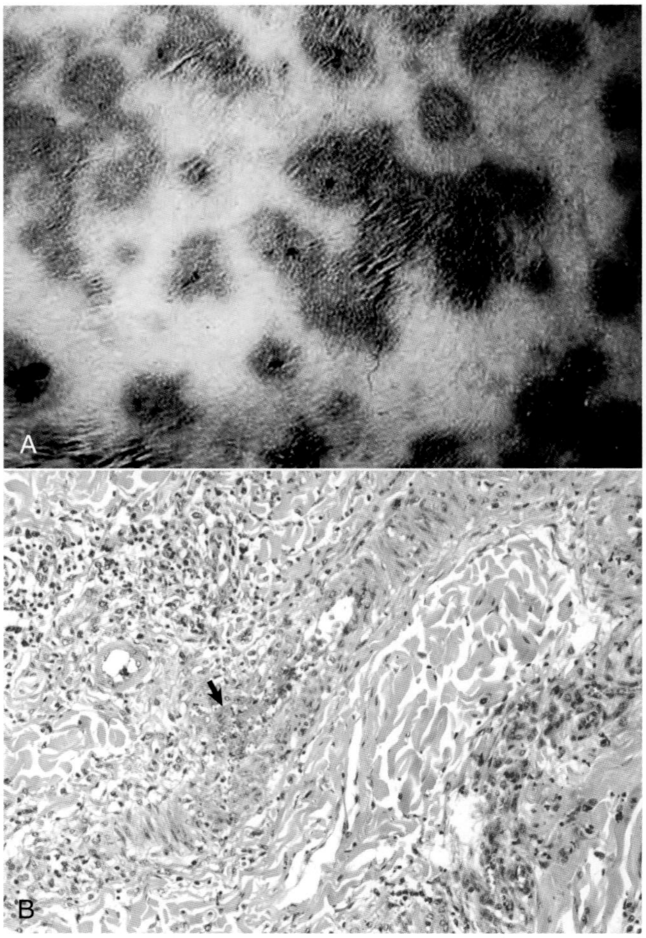

Fig. 17-42 **Capripoxvirus, skin, lamb.**
A, The clinical lesions are multifocal coalescing macules and plaques that are indurated, hemorrhagic, and necrotic likely a result of vasculitis. **B,** Note necrosis of vessel wall with fibrin deposition, red blood cells, and neutrophils and lymphocytes in the bordering dermis (vasculitis) *(arrow).* H&E stain. (**A** courtesy of *Foreign animal diseases*, ed 7, 2008, United States Animal Health Association. **B** courtesy Dr. A.M. Hargis, DermatoDiagnostics. Photographed from slides provided by Division of Animal Medicine, Animal Technology Institute Taiwan. From AFIP WSC October 8, 2008, Conference 5, Case III.)

The macroscopic lesions follow the typical pattern for pox infections. Erythematous macules progress to papules, which may be firm. Sheeppox lesions have a variably prominent vesicular stage. The pustule stage is characterized by the formation of a thin crust. In severely affected animals, the lesions coalesce and form areas of edema, hemorrhage, necrosis, and induration, involving all layers of the skin and subcutis (Fig. 17-42). These areas correspond to the development of vasculitis described later with microscopic lesions (Fig. 17-42, *B*). Highly susceptible animals often develop hemorrhagic mucosal papules early in the course of the disease, and ulcerative lesions in the gastrointestinal and respiratory tracts develop later. Approximately one-third of animals develop multiple pulmonary lesions that comprise foci of pulmonary consolidation. The kidneys have multifocal, circular, and fleshy nodules throughout the renal cortices.

Healing of the skin lesions is slow, taking up to 6 weeks, and a scar may remain. In the milder form of the disease, seen in endemic areas, the full range of pox lesions does not develop. Instead, epidermal proliferation produces papules covered by scale-crust, which

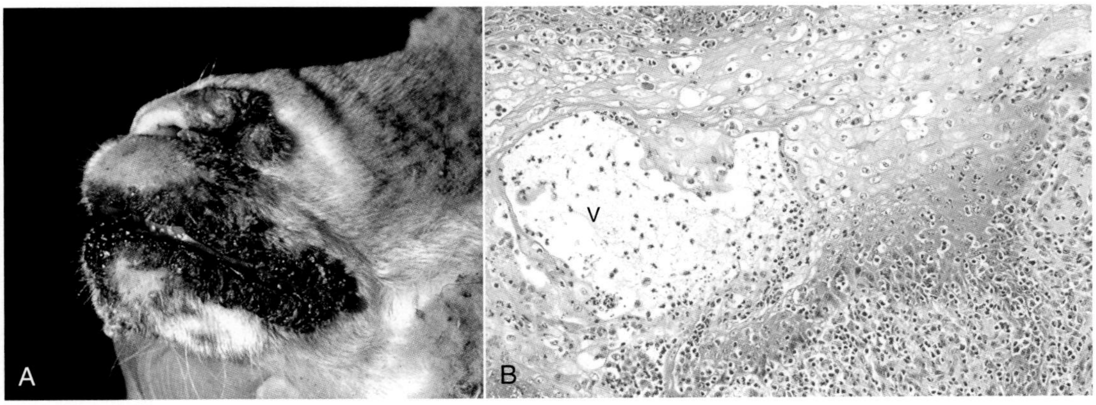

Fig. 17-43 Contagious ecthyma, skin, lamb.
A, Note crusts around nose and lips. These lesions are the late stage of the disease, are formed after rupture of vesicles and pustules, and are responsible for the common name *scabby mouth.* **B,** Note the epidermal hyperplasia (acanthosis), ballooning degeneration, vesicle *(V),* and neutrophils accumulating in the vesicle, which subsequently results in the formation of a pustule. Epidermal hyperplasia, upward movement of the pustule, and rupture of the vesicle or pustule contribute to crust formation as seen in **A.** H&E stain. (**A** courtesy Dr. M.D. McGavin, College of Veterinary Medicine, University of Tennessee. **B** courtesy Dr. Ann M. Hargis, DermatoDiagnostics.)

heal with desquamation in a few days. Such lesions often occur on the ventral surface of the tail.

Sheeppox lesions have the typical microscopic poxviral epithelial lesions, including intracytoplasmic inclusion bodies. The lesions affect both surface epithelium and that of the hair follicles. There are also marked dermal lesions reflecting the systemic route of cutaneous involvement and possibly implicating immune-mediated lesions in addition to those caused by direct viral damage. The initial dermal lesions, corresponding to the macroscopic erythematous macule, are marked edema, hyperemia, and neutrophilic exocytosis. During the papular stage, large numbers of mononuclear cells accumulate in the increasingly edematous dermis. These mononuclear cells are called *sheeppox cells* and are characteristic of the disease. The nuclei of sheeppox cells are vacuolated and have marginated chromatin. The vacuolated cytoplasm contains single, occasionally multiple, eosinophilic intracytoplasmic inclusion bodies. Sheeppox cells are virus-infected monocytes, macrophages, and fibroblasts, but not endothelial cells. Approximately 10 days postinfection and corresponding with the most prominent epithelial lesions and peak of skin infectivity, severe necrotizing vasculitis develops in arterioles and post-capillary venules (Fig. 17-42, *B*). Virus particles have not been identified in endothelial cells, and the vasculitis may be the result of immune-complex deposition. Ischemic necrosis of the dermis and overlying epidermis follows. The pulmonary lesions are proliferative alveolitis and bronchiolitis with focal areas of caseous necrosis. Alveolar septal cells contain intracytoplasmic inclusion bodies. Additional histologic lesions, characterized by the accumulation of sheeppox cells, may involve heart, kidney, liver, adrenal gland, thyroid gland, and pancreas.

The course and outcome of sheeppox depend not only on the usual host-virus relationship but also on the nature and location of secondary infections. The virus itself may cause death during the febrile, eruptive phase of the disease. Secondary bacterial infection and even septicemia and pneumonia can be the cause of death because animals are susceptible to fly strike and while the skin lesions are in the healing stage.

Goatpox

Goatpox, caused by goatpox virus, occurs in the previously described geographic distribution, and a benign form of goatpox occurs in California and Sweden. The clinical signs of goatpox vary in different geographic areas. The disease is generally milder than sheeppox with a low mortality rate (5%), although generalized eruption with mortality rates approaching 100% may occur, with a course of disease similar to that of sheeppox infections in sheep. The cutaneous lesions have a predilection for the same areas as for sheeppox. In nursing kids, lesions may appear on the buccal mucosa or anterior nares. In animals with higher levels of resistance, the lesions may be confined to the udder, teats, inner aspects of thighs, or ventral surface of the tail.

Contagious Ecthyma

Contagious ecthyma (contagious pustular dermatitis, orf, sore mouth) is a common localized infection of young sheep and goats caused by a parapoxvirus with worldwide distribution. Less commonly, humans, cattle, wild ungulates, and dogs are infected. Morbidity in lambs is usually great, and although mortality is usually low, it can approach 15% in lambs. Lesions are initiated by abrasions from pasture grasses or forage, begin at the commissures of the mouth, and spread to the lips (Fig. 17-43), oral mucosa, eyelids, and feet. Lambs can transfer the virus to the teats of ewes, and the lesions can spread to the skin of the udder. Contagious ecthyma is economically important as the result of weight loss in lambs that are reluctant to eat because of the pain associated with oral and perioral lesions. Pathogenesis of lesion formation and gross and microscopic features are consistent with the typical poxvirus lesions (see previous discussion and Fig. 17-31), except that the vesicle stage is very brief, the ulcer and crust stage persists and is clinically prominent, and the epidermis is markedly hyperplastic. Inclusion bodies are only briefly detectable histologically at the vesicular stage.

Swinepox

Pox lesions in pigs are caused by the host-specific poxvirus *Suipoxvirus* (swinepox). Normally, swinepox is transmitted by contact, although transplacental infection has not been ruled out. The sucking louse *Haematopinus suis* often acts as a mechanical vector and assists infection by causing skin trauma. The virus persists in dried crusts from infected animals. The pathogenesis of lesion formation and morphology of the gross and histologic lesions are consistent with the typical pox infection. The gross lesions typically affect the ventral and lateral abdomen, lateral thorax, and

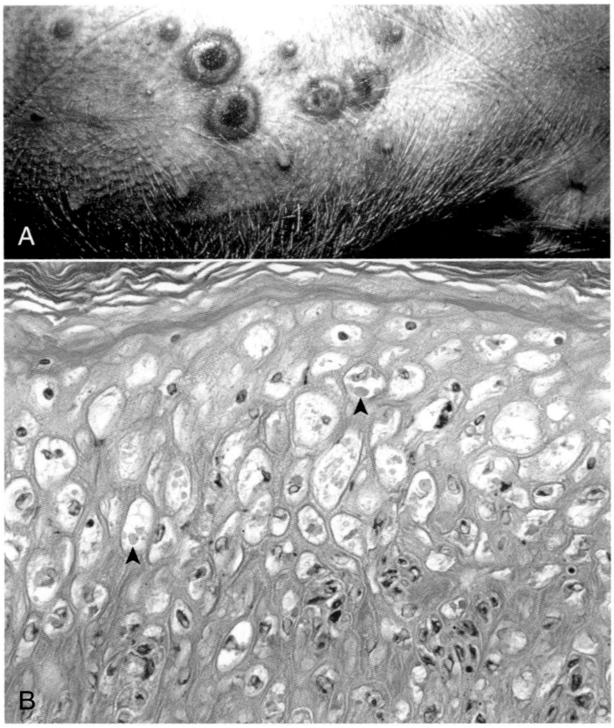

Fig. 17-44 **Swinepox, skin, piglet.**
A, Note the four umbilicated pustules in the abdominal skin. **B,** Note keratinocytes with ballooning degeneration and eosinophilic cytoplasmic inclusion bodies *(arrowheads).* Ballooning degeneration develops before vesicle formation. H&E stain. (**A** courtesy Dr. M.D. McGavin, College of Veterinary Medicine, University of Tennessee. **B** courtesy Dr. A.M. Hargis, DermatoDiagnostics. Photographed from slides provided by Department of Veterinary Pathology, Western College of Veterinary Medicine, University of Saskatchewan. From AFIP WSC January 21, 1998, Conference 15, Case IV.)

medial foreleg and thigh. Occasionally, lesions on the dorsum predominate. Lesions can be generalized and rarely involve the oral mucosa, pharynx, esophagus, stomach, trachea, and bronchi. The erythematous papules usually transform into umbilicated pustules without a significant vesicular stage (Fig. 17-44). The inflammatory crust eventually sheds to leave a white scar. The disease occurs worldwide and is endemic to areas of intensive swine production. The disease affects young, growing piglets and is mild with very low mortality.

Herpesviruses

Herpesviruses are DNA viruses that only occasionally produce cutaneous lesions (see Table 17-7). Cutaneous lesions have rarely been reported in nondermatotropic herpesvirus infections, such as infectious bovine rhinotracheitis (bovine herpesvirus 1) and equine coital exanthema (equine herpesvirus 3), and in cats with FHV-1 infection. Two dermatotropic herpesvirus infections with economic importance are bovine herpesvirus 2 and bovine herpesvirus 4. Herpesviruses can be latent, with inactive virus persisting in tissue such as the trigeminal nerve ganglia. It is speculated that up to 80% of adult cats recovered from FHV-1 infection as kittens or young cats have latent herpesvirus 1 infections. During times of stress, the virus is reactivated and lesions can recur. Herpesviruses infect epithelial cells and replicate in the nucleus, leading to lysis of nuclear contents. As immature viral particles enter the cytoplasm, there is degeneration of cytoplasmic organelles, accumulation of cytoplasmic lipid, and precipitation of protein. Death of keratinocytes leads to spread of virus to neighboring cells, leading to rapid necrosis of focally extensive areas of the epidermis. Gross lesions consist of vesicles that rupture to form ulcers that are then covered by crusts. Microscopic lesions in herpesvirus infections depend on the stage, but early degenerative changes include ballooning and reticular degeneration, the sequelae of degeneration of epidermal cells and acantholysis. Syncytial cells may be seen. Intranuclear inclusions develop, but because of rapidly developing necrosis may not be found except at the margins of ulcers. The appearance of the viral inclusions varies with the specific herpesvirus. Some herpesviruses produce large, hyaline amphophilic inclusions that fill the nucleus (FHV-1), whereas others (bovine herpes mammillitis) produce typical Cowdry type A inclusions, which are also intranuclear but smaller and eosinophilic.

Bovine Herpesvirus 2

Bovine herpesvirus 2, a dermatotropic virus (Allerton virus), can cause generalized disease (pseudo–lumpy skin disease) or as seen in the US, localized infection of the teat called *bovine ulcerative mammillitis* (bovine herpes mammillitis). Mammillitis is inflammation of the teat or nipple. Localized infection occurs more commonly in lactating dairy cows but can develop in beef cows, pregnant heifers, and suckling calves. Trauma is implicated in the pathogenesis because normal skin is resistant to viral penetration. The pathogenesis of lesion formation was discussed earlier. Bovine ulcerative mammillitis is economically important because of decreased milk production and secondary bacterial mastitis. Lesions develop on the teats and skin of the nearby udder or occasionally the perineum. Suckling calves develop lesions on the muzzle (nose).

Bovine Herpesvirus 4

Bovine herpesvirus 4 (bovine herpes mammary pustular dermatitis) causes a similar but milder disease than the localized form of bovine herpesvirus 2.

Feline Ulcerative Facial Dermatitis and Stomatitis

Feline herpesvirus 1 is an uncommon cause of ulcerative, often persistent, facial dermatitis or stomatitis in cats of various ages and sexes. Glucocorticoid therapy or stresses, such as overcrowding, are thought to play a role in lesion development. Most lesions develop under circumstances suggesting reactivation of latent herpesvirus infection. The pathogenesis is typical of that described for herpesviruses in the previous section. Gross lesions are ulcerative and crusted (see Table 17-3). Histologically, there is extensive necrosis of the epidermal, follicular, and sometimes sebaceous gland epithelium accompanied by prominent mixed dermal inflammation that frequently includes numerous eosinophils. Follicular epithelium can be destroyed, and free keratin in the dermis is associated with eosinophils and foci of eosinophil degranulation bordering collagen fibers and collagen degeneration. Large amphophilic or hyaline intranuclear inclusions are present in the surface and adnexal epithelium. Inclusion bodies are often easily overlooked, variable in number, and sometimes present in small rafts of epithelial cells surrounded by necrotic debris. The lesions are different from those previously reported in domestic cats in that they persist and are limited to the skin of the face or oral mucosa and often have significant eosinophilic inflammation. The inflammation in feline herpesvirus dermatitis overlaps with that of the hypersensitivity reactions, including mosquito bite hypersensitivity, and also with that of eosinophilic ulcers, thus warranting close scrutiny of eosinophilic necrotizing cutaneous lesions for intranuclear inclusion bodies.

Papillomaviruses

Papillomaviruses are typically species- and site-specific pathogens that infect the squamous epithelium and cause benign proliferative masses and less commonly malignant tumors. As more precise methods of papillomavirus identification have been developed, including in situ hybridization, PCR, and DNA sequencing, increasing numbers of papillomaviruses have been identified. Papillomaviruses reproduce exclusively in keratinocyte nuclei. They gain access through defects in the epithelium and enter the basal layer epithelial cells. Once in the cell, there are three possible outcomes: (1) the virus can remain within the basal cell nucleus outside of the chromosomes in a circular DNA episome where the virus replicates synchronously with the host cell causing a latent infection without morphologic changes in keratinocytes; (2) as the basal cells mature, the virus can convert from latent to productive infection with the formation of complete infectious virions and with morphologic changes recognized as viral cytopathology, including epithelial hyperplasia, keratinocytes with clear cytoplasm and pyknotic nuclei, and sometimes with cytoplasmic or intranuclear inclusion bodies; or (3) the virus can become integrated into the genome of the host cell, resulting in malignant transformation and the morphologic changes of neoplasia. Malignant transformation occurs because the viral genes that remain after integration into the host cell are those associated with cellular regulation. These viral genes promote keratinocyte cell growth by inactivating tumor-suppressor proteins such as p53 and pRb. These events lead to uncontrolled cell proliferation, inability to repair DNA damage, and eventual malignant transformation.

All domestic animals are affected by one or more papillomaviruses (see Table 17-7), and some cross-species infections have been detected, particularly with the bovine papillomaviruses. Recently, a papillomavirus in an exophytic papilloma on the dorsal surface of the nose of a cat had 98% similarity to human papillomavirus type 9. The specific type or types of papillomaviruses involved in some infections have yet to be determined. Papillomavirus infections cause diverse clinical and histologic lesions ranging from papillomas, epidermal pigmented plaques, and fibropapillomas, including sarcoids. Papillomavirus DNA has also been identified within in situ and invasive squamous cell carcinomas in animals, but further work is necessary to prove a cause and effect relationship.

A common type of cutaneous papillomavirus infection (papilloma, wart, cutaneous papillomatosis) consists of clinical lesions that may be exophytic (proliferating to the exterior) (Fig. 17-45) or endophytic (inverted) papilliferous benign masses. Other papillomas may be flat, plaque-like lesions that lack the prominent papilliferous projections. Histologically, stratified squamous epithelium is covered by thickened orthokeratotic or parakeratotic keratin, is acanthotic, and in the exophytic and endophytic papillomas, has elongated epidermal-dermal interdigitations that project outwardly or inwardly, depending on the type. In some papillomas, keratinocytes, especially of the upper stratum spinosum, are swollen, have clear cytoplasm or a perinuclear halo, and a pyknotic nucleus; these

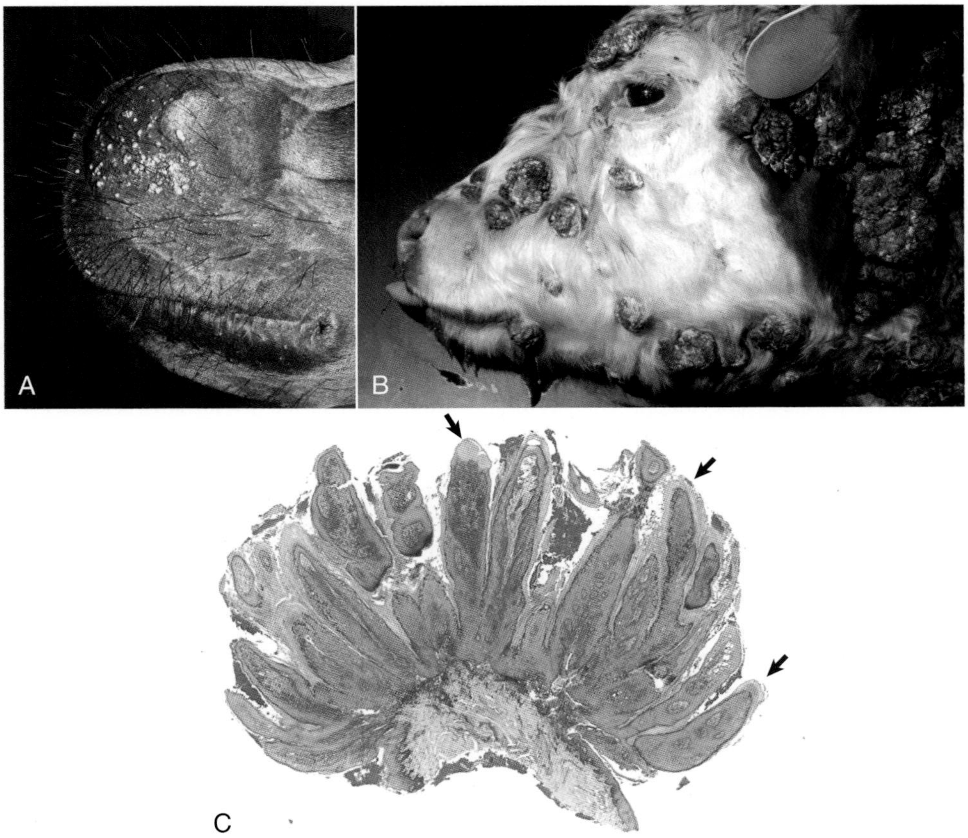

Fig. 17-45 Cutaneous papillomas, skin.

A, Chin, horse. Note multiple, small, verrucous masses arising in the skin. **B,** Head, cow. Note multiple, irregular, alopecic, verrucous papillomas. **C,** The papillary projections *(arrows),* often called fronds, are composed of hyperkeratotic epidermis covering a collagenous core. H&E stain. (**A** courtesy Dr. David Duclos, Animal Skin and Allergy Clinic. **B** and **C** courtesy Dr. M.D. McGavin, College of Veterinary Medicine, University of Tennessee.)

keratinocytes are termed *koilocytes* (meaning hollow or concave). Keratohyalin granules are irregular. Also, pale basophilic intranuclear inclusion bodies, located in degenerating cells in the outer layers of the stratum spinosum and granulosum in which virion production is taking place, occur in some but not all papillomas. Many papillomas spontaneously regress, and in regressing stages, there is reduced epidermal hyperplasia, increased proliferation of fibroblasts, deposition of collagen, and infiltration of T lymphocytes at the epidermal dermal interface and in the epithelium. Some papillomas, such as those on the ears of horses and some affecting the teats of cattle, often do not regress.

Viral plaques have been described in dogs and cats. Canine pigmented viral plaques are associated with papillomavirus infection in certain breeds of dogs (miniature schnauzers, pugs, and Shar-Peis) or in other breeds of dogs that are immunosuppressed. Novel papillomaviruses have been detected in some of these plaques. Clinical lesions occur most commonly on the ventral abdomen, groin, ventral thorax, or neck and consist of variably irregular, pigmented macules, or plaques. Histologically, the lesions are sharply demarcated, hyperkeratotic foci, or plaques with pigmented, acanthotic epidermis, and large keratohyalin granules. These pigmented epidermal plaques do not regress, are slowly progressive, and occasionally develop into a squamous cell carcinoma. Feline viral plaques are usually multiple, ovoid, slightly raised pigmented or nonpigmented, and slightly scaly and rough plaques less than 8 mm in greatest dimension. Papillomavirus has been detected in the lesions but not specifically identified to type. Histologically, there is an abrupt transition between normal epithelium and the plaque, which consists of epidermis thickened by hyperkeratosis, hypergranulosis, and acanthosis. Keratohyalin granules may be enlarged, and koilocytes (keratinocytes with clear cytoplasm and pyknotic nuclei), and cytoplasmic pseudoinclusions may be present. Malignant transformation commonly occurs; lesions resemble the in situ bowenoid carcinoma (see next paragraph).

Papillomavirus infection also has been implicated in the development of another syndrome in cats and less often in dogs termed *multicentric squamous cell carcinoma in situ* (Bowen's-like disease, in situ bowenoid carcinoma). Although not all the factors contributing to lesion formation have been documented, papillomavirus DNA has been identified in these lesions in cats, suggesting a nonproductive infection promotes the epithelial hyperplasia characteristic of this disease. The papillomaviruses identified in some of these lesions have homology with human papillomaviruses. Multicentric squamous cell carcinoma in situ clinically consists of sharply demarcated single, or more often multiple, scaly verrucous or irregular plaque-like lesions 0.5 to 3.0 cm in diameter. Histologically, the epidermis and follicular infundibular epithelium are thickened by proliferation of basal keratinocytes that tend to stream together, providing a "windblown" appearance to the epidermis. Nuclei are often varied in size with hyperchromatic nuclei, large nucleoli, and numerous mitoses, some of which are located above the basal layer. The basement membrane, at the time of histologic examination, is intact. Most lesions remain as "in situ" carcinomas indefinitely, but an occasional lesion has progressed to invasive basal cell carcinoma or invasive squamous cell carcinoma.

Some types of papillomaviruses, particularly bovine papillomaviruses 1 and 2, can infect fibroblasts and cause fibropapillomas, flat, verrucous, or nodular masses in which the proliferation of dermal fibroblasts is the prominent feature, often surpassing that of the epidermal hyperplasia (Fig. 17-46). Fibropapillomas occur in horses, mules, donkeys, cattle, sheep, and cats. These lesions in horses are called *sarcoids,* which are thought to represent a nonproductive infection by distinct variants of bovine papillomavirus.

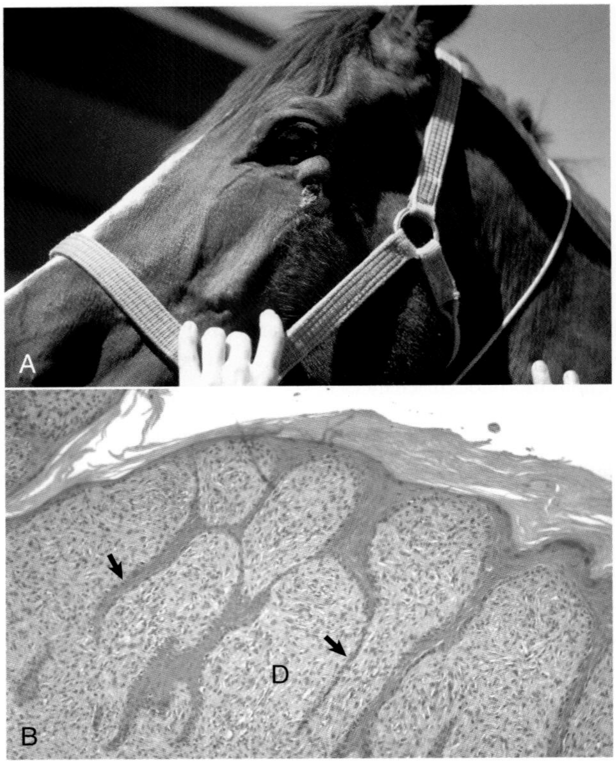

Fig. 17-46 Sarcoid, skin, horse.
A, Equine sarcoid, face. The irregular multinodular mass is present on the ventrolateral periocular skin, especially below the eye. **B,** Sarcoid. The sarcoid consists of an epidermal and dermal component. The hyperplastic epidermis has thin rete pegs that extend into the dermis *(arrows)*. The dermis *(D)* is thickened by proliferating fibroblasts and collagen. H&E stain. (**A** courtesy Dr. Helen Power, Dermatology for Animals. **B** courtesy Dr. Pamela E. Ginn, College of Veterinary Medicine, University of Florida.)

Equine sarcoids are locally aggressive, nonmetastatic fibroblastic skin tumors of horses, mules, and donkeys. They are the most common skin tumor of horses, accounting for up to 30% of tumors, and occur in any breed, sex, or age. Young adult horses 3 to 6 years of age are most commonly affected. Sarcoids frequently develop in areas subjected to trauma or at sites of wounds 6 to 8 months after wound healing and develop anywhere but are most common on the head, legs, and ventral trunk. They can be single or multiple. The tumors are classified according to their gross appearance as verrucous, fibroblastic, mixed, or occult. The verrucous type is a small wartlike growth, usually measuring less than 6 cm in diameter, with a dry, rough surface and variable alopecia. The fibroblastic type of sarcoid is more variable in appearance and can range from a well-circumscribed firm nodule with intact surface to a large mass, greater than 25 cm in diameter, with an ulcerated surface prone to hemorrhage, and resembling exuberant granulation tissue. The mixed type is a transitional form in which a verrucous sarcoid becomes a fibroblastic type as a result of trauma or biopsy. The occult form consists of a slow-growing, slightly thickened area of skin with slight surface roughening and alopecia that remains static for a long period.

Histologically, sarcoids are typically biphasic tumors composed of both epidermal and dermal components; however, the epidermal component may be minimal or absent in some tumors, especially those with extensive ulceration. When the epidermis is intact, hyperkeratosis, parakeratosis, and acanthosis with thin rete pegs extending deep into the dermis are common features. The dermal component consists of fibroblasts and collagen in various proportions. The fibroblasts have plump nuclei, and nucleoli may be prominent. The mitotic index is usually low. Fibroblasts at the dermal-epidermal junction are frequently oriented perpendicular to the basement membrane in a "picket fence" pattern, which is a distinctive histologic feature seen in most sarcoids. The cells are arranged in whorls, interlacing bundles, or haphazard arrays of variable density. Tumor margins are typically indistinct and adequacy of excision is frequently difficult to determine. Spontaneous remission can occur after several years in up to 30% of cases. The tumors are characterized by a high rate of recurrence, up to 50%, after surgical excision. Feline fibropapillomas (also called *sarcoids*) are similar morphologically to the equine lesion, and also likely represent a nonproductive infection with papillomavirus with similarities to bovine, ovine, deer, and European elk papillomaviruses. Affected cats often live in rural areas and have had exposure to cattle. Bovine fibropapillomas are caused by bovine papilloma virus 1 (teats, penis) or bovine papillomavirus 2 (head, neck, shoulder, legs, and teats) and occur in young animals. The lesions generally spontaneously regress within 1 to 12 months.

Papillomaviruses, some as yet to be identified by type, have been found in canine and feline invasive squamous cell carcinoma. However, the presence of the virus in the tumors does not allow differentiation between actual induction of the tumor and mere infection of the tumor. Further work to characterize the types of papillomaviruses and the role the viruses play in epidermal hyperplasia and neoplasia is necessary.

Other Viruses

Information on this topic is available at evolve.elsevier.com/Zachary/McGavin/.

Bacterial Infections

The portals for entry of bacteria into the skin include pores (follicular openings), hematogenous spread, or direct entry through damaged skin. Cutaneous bacterial infections vary in location (e.g., epidermis, dermis, subcutis, adnexa, or systemic), morphology (e.g., pyogenic, granulomatous, or necrotizing), distribution (e.g., focal, multifocal, regional, mucocutaneous, haired skin, or interdigital), and severity (e.g., mild and asymptomatic to severe with systemic signs). The variation is caused by the specific organism involved, predisposing or coexisting factors, and host-immune response. The so-called superficial and deep bacterial infections are frequently pus-producing infections (pyogenic) and are thus referred to as pyodermas. In contrast, bacterial granulomas are characterized by an abundance of macrophages and are usually caused by traumatic implantation of bacteria that generally are saprophytes of low virulence. Systemic bacterial infections or localized infection with toxin-producing bacteria are often most severe because of vascular damage or the presence of endotoxins or exotoxins that have systemic consequences. The most common bacterial infections of the skin are listed in Box 17-7.

Bacterial skin disease is seen much more frequently in dogs than other domestic species, possibly the result of the thin stratum corneum with small amount of lipids, lack of a protective lipid seal at opening of the canine hair follicles, and the relatively high pH of canine skin. Until recently, *Staphylococcus intermedius* has been considered the cause of most cases of pyoderma in dogs. However, recent molecular studies involving multilocus gene sequencing have revealed that bacterial isolates phenotypically consistent with *Staphylococcus intermedius* consist of three separate species (considered to be the *Staphylococcus intermedius* group), which include *S. intermedius*, *Staphylococcus pseudintermedius*, and *Staphylococcus delphini*. *Staphylococcus pseudintermedius* is now considered to be responsible for most cases of pyoderma in dogs. Coagulase-positive staphylococci are also the most common bacteria isolated from pyoderma in horses (*S. aureus*, *S. intermedius*), in cattle and sheep (*S. aureus*), and in goats (*S. aureus*). Molecular studies will likely be required to identify the species involved in some of these infections, particularly those of the *Staphylococcus intermedius* group. *Staphylococcus hyicus* causes exudative epidermitis in piglets and has been associated with superficial pyoderma in several other species. Many other bacteria can cause skin infections. *Dermatophilus congolensis* is responsible for superficial pyoderma in many species. Many Gram-negative bacteria are opportunistic pathogens that can invade already diseased or compromised skin.

BOX 17-7 Cutaneous Bacterial Infections

SUPERFICIAL PYODERMAS

Superficial pustular dermatitis (impetigo)
Exudative epidermitis
Canine superficial pyoderma (superficial spreading pyoderma)
Mucocutaneous pyoderma
Dermatophilosis
Ovine fleece rot
Superficial folliculitis (see bacterial folliculitis and furunculosis below)

DEEP PYODERMAS

Bacterial folliculitis and furunculosis
Abscesses

BACTERIAL GRANULOMATOUS DERMATITIS

Mycobacterial granulomas
Granulomas caused by nonfilamentous bacteria
- *Staphylococcus* spp.
- *Streptococcus* spp.
- *Pseudomonas aeruginosa*
- *Actinobacillus lignieresii*
- *Proteus* spp.

Filamentous bacterial granulomas
- *Nocardia* spp.
- *Actinomyces* spp.
- *Streptomyces* spp.
- *Actinomadura* spp.

SYSTEMIC OR TOXIC REACTIONS

Erysipelothrix rhusiopathiae
Systemic salmonellosis, pasteurellosis, *Escherichia coli* infection
Canine toxic shock syndrome
Clostridial dermatitis

BACTERIAL DIGITAL INFECTIONS OF HORSES AND RUMINANTS

Proliferative pododermatitis (horse)
Necrotizing pododermatitis (horse)
Papillomatous digital dermatitis (cattle)
Necrobacillosis of the foot (cattle and sheep)
Contagious foot rot (cattle and sheep)
Contagious ovine digital dermatitis (sheep)

Superficial Bacterial Infections (Superficial Pyodermas)

Superficial bacterial infections (superficial pyodermas) involve the epidermis and the upper infundibulum of hair follicles, usually heal without scarring, and usually do not involve the regional lymph nodes. Gross lesions include erythema, alopecia, papules, pustules, crusts, and peripheral expanding rings of scale also called "epidermal collarettes" (see Table 17-3). The early microscopic feature of superficial bacterial infection that involves the epidermis is intraepidermal pustular dermatitis. The intraepidermal pustules are fragile and can rupture, leading to crust and superficial scale formation. The major microscopic feature of superficial bacterial infection that involves the follicles is superficial suppurative luminal folliculitis. The cellular infiltrate in and around hair follicles plus dermal congestion and edema correspond to the clinically evident papules and follicularly oriented pustules. Follicular injury leads to alopecia. Although Gram-positive cocci, such as *Staphylococcus* sp., are usually the cause of the superficial bacterial infections, the bacteria are not always microscopically demonstrable. Predisposing factors, such as allergy, seborrhea, and immune deficiency, and other causes of follicular inflammation or dysfunction often play a role.

Superficial Pustular Dermatitis

Superficial pustular dermatitis, typically caused by staphylococci, encompasses several syndromes including impetigo in a variety of animal species, exudative epidermitis in pigs, and superficial pyoderma in dogs. Pathogenicity may correlate with various proteins and toxins produced by the bacteria and thought to act as virulence factors. One of the factors that has come under recent scrutiny includes the exfoliative toxins. These toxins have been isolated from strains of *Staphylococcus aureus* in humans with impetigo, an acute contagious superficial bacterial skin infection that usually affects children and is characterized by vesicles and pustules that form yellowish crusts. In addition, similar exfoliative toxins have been identified as a source of another skin condition usually affecting infants and children, termed *staphylococcal scalded-skin syndrome.* In impetigo and staphylococcal scalded-skin syndrome, it has been shown that virulent forms of *S. aureus* produce exfoliative toxins that cause the loss of adhesion of keratinocytes in the superficial epidermis. These toxins are glutamate-specific serine proteases that cleave a single peptide bond in desmoglein 1, present in the extracellular protein core of the desmosome. The separation of these superficial keratinocytes results in intraepidermal splitting and initiation of lesion development in these infections. In impetigo, the *S. aureus* that produce exfoliative toxins can be isolated from the intact pustules. In contrast, in staphylococcal scalded-skin syndrome, there are generalized blisters and superficial exfoliation of the stratum corneum, but cultures from intact vesicles usually are negative for exotoxin producing *S. aureus*. It appears that the exfoliative toxins are produced in a distant area of infection and reach the skin via the bloodstream (a process called *toxemia*) where they cause the vesicular and exfoliative lesions. Investigative studies in two domestic species (pigs and dogs) suggest that a similar pathogenic mechanism involving exfoliative toxins may play a role in development of superficial pustular dermatitis caused by staphylococci. For example, it has been shown that *Staphylococcus hyicus*, which causes exudative epidermitis in piglets, produces an exfoliative toxin that can cleave swine desmoglein 1, and produce cutaneous exfoliation similar to that in pigs with exudative epidermitis. Similarly, an exfoliative toxin isolated from strains of *Staphylococcus intermedius (pseudintermedius)* from dogs with pyoderma has caused cutaneous exfoliation when injected into the skin of dogs. In addition, the exfoliative toxin gene has been identified in *Staphylococcus intermedius* and *Staphylococcus pseudintermedius* isolated from skin, wound, and ear infections in dogs suggesting a role for the toxin in pathogenicity. Although the exfoliative toxins in canine pyoderma have not been fully characterized, these findings suggest that some strains of *Staphylococcus* sp. in dogs and *Staphylococcus hyicus* in pigs may cause superficial bacterial infections via a pathologic mechanism involving exfoliative toxins. Further studies are necessary to determine if exfoliative toxins or other virulence factors contribute to the development of superficial pyoderma in other species.

Impetigo

Impetigo is observed most commonly in cows, ewes, does, and dogs and is usually caused by coagulase-positive *Staphylococcus* sp. Predisposing factors, such as cutaneous abrasions, viral infections, increased moisture, and poor nutrition, may contribute. Lesions of impetigo in cows, does, and ewes, occur predominantly on the ventral abdomen, perineum, medial thigh, vulva, ventral tail, teats, and udder. In dogs, lesions are largely in nonhaired ventral skin. Prepubescent puppies are usually healthy otherwise, but older dogs with impetigo often have underlying disease, including immunosuppression associated with hyperadrenocorticism. Gross lesions consist of nonfollicular pustules that develop into crusts. The microscopic lesion is a nonfollicular neutrophilic subcorneal pustule. In bullous impetigo, a more severe condition occurring in older dogs with underlying disease, the lesions are large interfollicular flaccid pustules (bullae) that when ruptured lead to more extensive loss of the superficial epidermis. Acantholytic cells may be present in the pustules, probably the result of the cleavage of desmoglein 1 by the exfoliative toxin, thus requiring differentiation between impetigo and pemphigus foliaceous (see Fig. 17-15). The presence of coccoid bacteria within intact pustules can help provide support for a bacterial origin of the lesions. Perivascular to interstitial neutrophilic to mixed mononuclear dermal inflammation is present.

Exudative Epidermitis of Pigs (Greasy Pig Disease)

Exudative epidermitis, usually caused by *Staphylococcus hyicus*, is an acute, often fatal, dermatitis of neonatal piglets, but a mild disease in older piglets. Predisposing factors include cutaneous lacerations and poor nutrition. In piglets, brownish exudates develop around the eyes, pinnae, snout, chin, and medial legs and spread to the ventral thorax and abdomen, giving the animal an overall "greasy" appearance (Fig. 17-47). The lesions rapidly coalesce and become generalized, resulting in greasy, malodorous exudates covering an erythematous skin. If piglets survive, the exudate hardens, cracks, and forms fissures. Subacute disease develops gradually in older piglets, and lesions are generally localized to the skin of the face, pinnae, and periocular regions. Grossly, the epidermis is thickened with scaling. The early histopathologic lesion is subcorneal pustular dermatitis, which extends to the hair follicle, resulting in superficial suppurative folliculitis. In the fully developed lesion, the epidermis is hyperplastic and has thick crusts of keratin, microabscesses, and cocci. The term *exudative epidermitis* is descriptive of this condition as the inflammatory changes largely involve the epidermis, and there is an accumulation of exudates on the surface. The dermis is congested and edematous. In the early stages, the dermatitis is superficial and perivascular with neutrophils and eosinophils, and in the later stages is perivascular and mononuclear.

Canine Superficial Pyoderma (Superficial Spreading Pyoderma)

Superficial spreading pyoderma is a common, often pruritic, superficial bacterial infection in dogs caused by *Staphylococcus pseudintermedius.* Clinical lesions are most frequently recognized in the

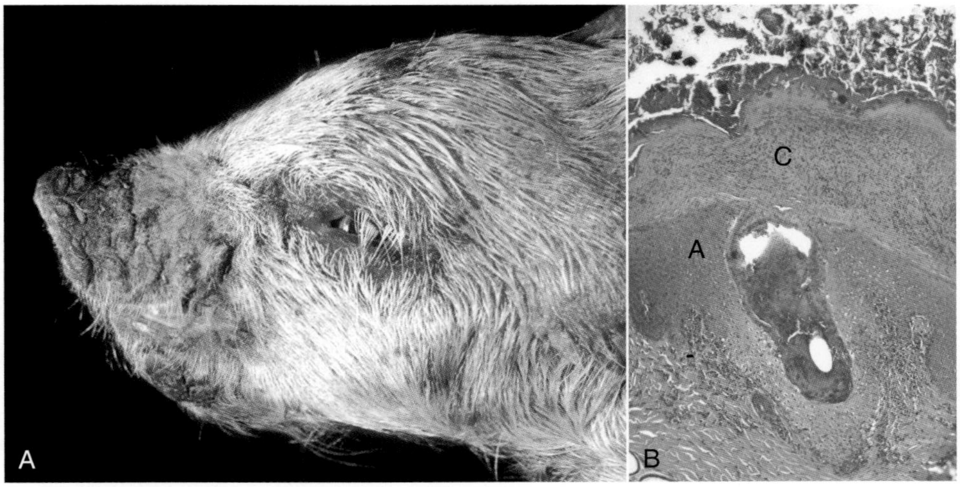

Fig. 17-47 **Exudative epidermitis, *Staphylococcus hyicus (hyos)*, skin, piglet.**
A, Head. Exudative epidermitis is also called greasy pig disease. The skin in this pig is lichenified and has fissures. Greasy exudate focally has adhered to the hair and the surface of the skin. **B,** Note the epidermal hyperplasia (acanthosis *[A]*) and suppurative exudate within the lumen of a hair follicle and on the surface of the epidermis. The exudate has dried to form a crust *(C)* that is fragmenting superficially. H&E stain. (**A** courtesy Dr. M.D. McGavin, College of Veterinary Medicine, University of Tennessee. **B** courtesy Dr. Pamela E. Ginn, College of Veterinary Medicine, University of Florida.)

glabrous ventral thoracic and abdominal skin but can affect the haired skin of the dorsal and lateral trunk as well. Early clinical lesions include erythematous macules, papules, and transient pustules. Older clinical lesions include epidermal collarettes, crusts, alopecia, and hyperpigmentation. Early microscopic lesions are superficial, spongiotic epidermal pustules that rapidly crust and form basophilic debris, often with cocci, on the surface of the epidermis. This basophilic debris can dissect peripherally (laterally) between the epidermis and stratum corneum and is thought to form the rim of scale that clinically represents the epidermal collarette. In this way, the lesions "spread" outwardly from the initial lesion. Occasionally, superficial spreading pyoderma can originate from superficial folliculitis where follicular pustular formation is minor and epidermal collarette formation more prominent. Dermal lesions include superficial perivascular to interstitial accumulations of neutrophils, eosinophils, and mixed mononuclear cells. Some dogs have neutrophilic vasculitis involving superficial venules possibly caused by immune-complex deposition, a feature suggesting a hypersensitivity response to bacterial antigens. Dermal congestion and edema are usually present.

Mucocutaneous Pyoderma

Mucocutaneous pyoderma is a putative bacterial infection of mucocutaneous junctional skin in dogs. Antibiotic responsiveness suggests that bacteria contribute, however, the etiology is likely more complex and may involve immunologic factors as well. A variety of breeds are affected, but the German shepherd breed is thought to be predisposed. The pathogenesis is unknown. Lesions consist of erythema, swelling, and crusting, and in severe cases, ulceration. Depigmentation may develop in chronic cases. Lesions are most common on mucocutaneous skin of the lips, but mucocutaneous skin of prepuce, vulva, and anus can be affected. Histologic lesions include a dense band of lymphoplasmacytic inflammation with variable numbers of neutrophils at the epidermal dermal junction (lichenoid inflammation), typically without basal cell degeneration. Other features include spongiosis and cellular exocytosis into the epidermis, neutrophilic pustular crusts, and folliculitis of adjacent follicles. Over time, pigmentary incontinence develops. Although classic cases are said not to have basal cell degeneration, apoptotic keratinocytes above the basal layer can be present. In addition, there can be interface inflammation obscuring the epidermal-dermal interface. These features prevent definitive histologic differentiation from discoid lupus erythematosus.

Dermatophilosis (Streptothrichosis)

Dermatophilosis, caused by *Dermatophilus congolensis,* is characterized by crusty cutaneous lesions (Fig. 17-48) and occurs in horses, cattle, and sheep more often than goats, pigs, dogs, or cats. The bacterium is transmitted by carrier animals and is more common in tropical and subtropical climates and during wet weather, thus the layman's term *rain rot.* Lesions tend to develop on the dorsum of the back and distal extremities and after epidermal irritation from ectoparasites, trauma, or prolonged wetting of the skin, hair, or wool, which allows penetration of the damaged epidermis by the *Dermatophilus* "zoospore."

The bacterium grows in the outer root sheath of the hair follicle and superficial epidermis and produces Gram-positive filamentous branches that subdivide longitudinally and transversely (see Fig. 17-48). These bacteria stimulate an acute inflammatory response in which neutrophils migrate from superficial vessels into the dermis and through the epidermis to form intraepidermal microabscesses. The inflammation inhibits further penetration of the bacterium. However, residual bacterial organisms subsequently invade the newly regenerated epidermis. Thus repeated cycles of bacterial growth, inflammation, and epidermal regeneration result in the formation of the multilaminated pustular crusts. Grossly, lesions consist of papules, pustules, and thick crusts that can coalesce and mat the hair or wool (see Fig. 17-48). The microscopic lesions consist of hyperplastic superficial perivascular dermatitis with multilaminated crusts of alternating layers of keratin and neutrophils covering the skin surface. Samples of crusts obtained by biopsy are necessary to identify organisms and make a definitive diagnosis.

Ovine Fleece Rot

Ovine fleece rot is a superficial bacterial dermatitis usually caused by excessive moisture (usually in the form of rain) that penetrates the fleece (wool), wets the skin, and causes proliferation of *Pseudomonas* spp. Approximately 1 week of continual wetting is usually

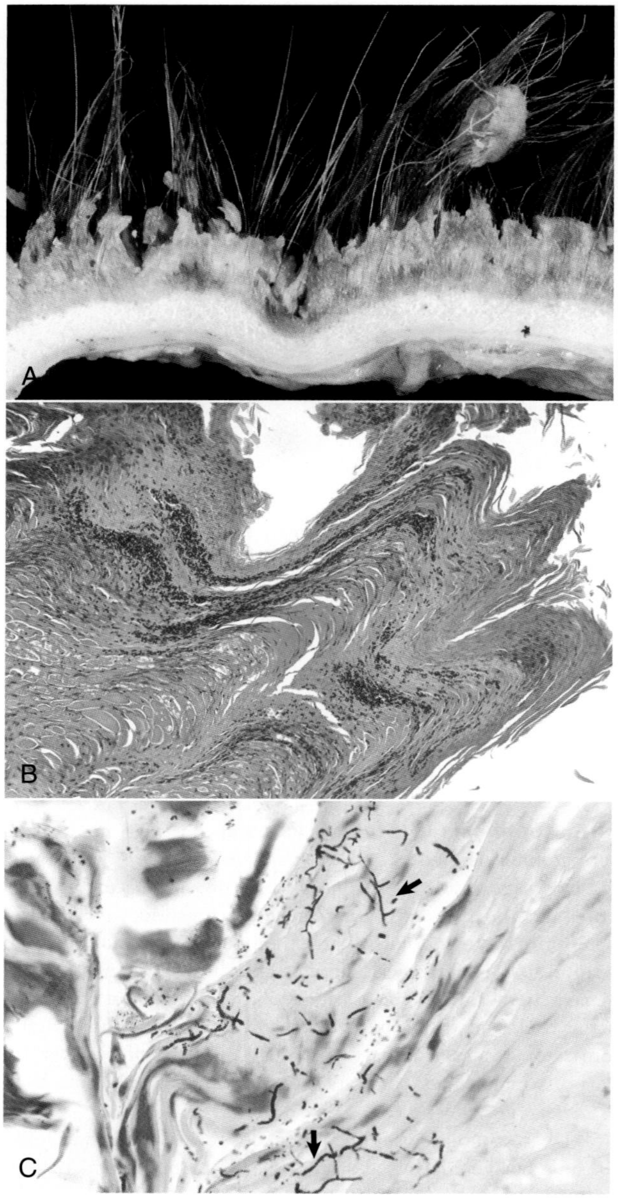

Fig. 17-48 ***Dermatophilus congolensis*** **infection, skin, haired, cow.** **A,** The hair is matted by a crust composed of dried exudate, stratum corneum, and bacteria. **B,** Note thick laminated crust formed of alternating layers of hyperkeratotic/parakeratotic stratum corneum and degenerate neutrophils. H&E stain. **C,** The stratum corneum contains filamentous bacteria *(arrows)*. These bacteria subdivide longitudinally and transversely and can result in a "railroad track" appearance (not evident here). Brown and Brenn stain. (**A** courtesy Dr. F. Lozano-Alarcon. **B** courtesy Dr. M.D. McGavin, College of Veterinary Medicine, University of Tennessee. **C** courtesy Dr. Ann M. Hargis, DermatoDiagnostics.)

sufficient to cause marked proliferation of the bacteria on the skin and in the fleece. This is followed by an acute inflammatory response with serum exudation and matting of the fleece. The fleece is also discolored because of production of pigments (chromogens) by the *Pseudomonas* bacteria and has a rotten odor. Microscopic lesions include epidermal pustular dermatitis and superficial folliculitis. Ovine fleece rot is important economically because the malodor attracts flies, predisposing to myiasis (infestation of tissue by the larvae of dipterous flies), and the value of the affected wool is reduced.

Superficial Bacterial Folliculitis

Staphylococcal folliculitis and furunculosis are discussed with deep bacterial infections in the next section.

Deep Bacterial Infections (Deep Pyodermas)

Deep pyodermas are bacterial infections of the hair follicle, dermis, and/or subcutis. They are caused by a variety of bacteria, including *Staphylococcus* sp., *Streptococcus* sp., *Corynebacterium pseudotuberculosis, Pasteurella* sp., *Proteus* sp., *Pseudomonas* sp., *and Escherichia coli. Staphylococcus pseudintermedius* is the primary pathogen of canine skin. Organisms typically enter the skin via natural pores such as hair follicles or any form of wound, including direct penetration of the skin. Deep bacterial infections of hair follicles often have predisposing causes, such as immune suppression, demodicosis (dogs), or disorders associated with follicular hyperkeratosis (callus or comedo formation), and also originate as a sequela to superficial bacterial folliculitis. Deep bacterial infections are less common than superficial infections and develop most frequently in dogs.

Bacterial Folliculitis and Furunculosis (Table 17-8)

Infection of the hair follicle can be superficial or deep. Superficial infections involve the follicular infundibulum but can spread to involve the deeper portions of the follicle (the infundibulum and below). Mild-to-moderate folliculitis without furunculosis can resolve completely with appropriate antibiotic therapy. However, untreated or severe folliculitis can progress to involve deeper aspects of the follicle and result in follicular distention with rupture (furunculosis) and release of follicular contents (hair, follicular stratum corneum, and bacteria) into the dermis and sometimes subcutis. The bacteria proliferate in the deep dermis and subcutis and can reach draining lymph nodes. Draining tracts often develop as a foreign body response to extruded follicular contents (e.g., hair and follicular stratum corneum). Thus the infection and severe inflammation spread into the surrounding dermis and subcutis, resulting in the need for intensive long-term treatment and increasing the potential for systemic infection and local scarring.

Numerous bacteria can cause folliculitis and furunculosis, but staphylococcal bacteria are the most commonly involved. Staphylococcal folliculitis and furunculosis develop most commonly in the dog (see Figs. 17-26 and 17-27), frequently affect the horse, sheep, and goat but are uncommon in the cow, pig, and cat.

In horses, lesions develop most commonly in association with tack, especially on the skin of the saddle area, the tail, or the caudal aspect of the pastern (proximal interphalangeal articulation) or fetlock (metacarpophalangeal articulation). When the skin of the pastern or fetlock is involved, the condition is called equine pastern folliculitis (also known as grease heel, scratches). Equine pastern folliculitis is a complex disorder in which secondary staphylococcal folliculitis plays a role. Predisposing factors are numerous and include excessive moisture, trauma, and contact dermatitis. Also, many other conditions affect the pastern skin in horses, including immune-mediated diseases (pemphigus foliaceous, vasculitis, or photosensitization), other infections (dermatophilosis, dermatophytosis), and mite infestation (*Chorioptes* sp.), necessitating an early thorough clinical evaluation and sometimes microbiologic or histopathologic evaluation to differentiate staphylococcal folliculitis of the skin of the pastern from these other disease processes. In severe chronic lesions, initiating causes may no longer be identifiable.

TABLE 17-8 Bacterial Folliculitis and Furunculosis

Organisms	Predisposing Causes	Portal of Entry	Clinical Lesions	Histologic Lesions	Anatomic Locations	Species
Staphylococcus sp. are most frequently involved. Others: *Streptococcus* sp., *Corynebacterium pseudotuberculosis,* *Pasteurella* sp., *Proteus* sp., *Pseudomonas* sp., and *Escherichia coli*	**Superficial folliculitis:** Allergy Seborrhea Parasitic infestations Hormonal factors Local irritants Matted hair coats **Deep folliculitis:** Sequel to superficial bacterial folliculitis Immune suppression Stresses (large animals) Demodicosis (dogs) Follicular hyperkeratosis (callus or comedones) Irritation from tack (horses) Increased environmental temperature and moisture (horse) **Pastern folliculitis (horses):** Excessive moisture, trauma, contact dermatitis, mite infestation	Hair follicle openings	**Superficial folliculitis:** Papules, crusted papules, pustules, epidermal collarettes, and alopecia **Deep folliculitis:** Same as superficial folliculitis plus hemorrhagic bullae, nodules, and draining tracts	**Superficial:** Superficial luminal folliculitis **Deep:** Superficial and deep suppurative luminal folliculitis with follicular distention often in conjunction with furunculosis Pyogranulomatous dermatitis in response to release of follicular contents Tracts that drain to the surface Scarring with loss of adnexa and permanent alopecia localized to affected skin	Dorsal nose, pressure points, interdigital areas, chin, and can be generalized	Dog; common
					Area covered by tack, especially the skin of the saddle area, the tail, or on the caudal aspect of the pastern* or fetlock†	Horse; frequent
					Face, pinnae, distal limbs, and glabrous areas of the udder, ventral abdomen, medial thighs, and perineum	Goat; frequent
					Adult sheep: face, especially around the eyes, ears, base of horns, limbs, or teats Lambs: mild lesions most commonly on the lips and perineum; usually spontaneously regress	Sheep; frequent
					Tail, perineum; less often scrotum and face	Cattle, more in young bulls; uncommon
					Piglets younger than 8 weeks: generalized body hindquarters, abdomen, chest Young growing piglets: facial lesions related to sharp canine teeth	Piglets; uncommon
					Crusted papular eruption indistinguishable from miliary dermatitis, anywhere, including head and neck	Cat; rare

*Pastern (proximal interphalangeal articulation).
†Fetlock (metacarpophalangeal articulation).

In adult sheep, lesions develop on the face, especially around the eyes, or on the limbs or teats. In otherwise healthy lambs, mild lesions develop most commonly on the lips and perineum and usually spontaneously regress. In goats, the face, pinnae, distal limbs, and glabrous areas of the udder, ventral abdomen, medial thighs, and perineum are most commonly affected.

In dogs, lesions are localized or generalized and develop on the dorsal nose, pressure points, interdigital areas, and chin. Other cutaneous areas can also be affected, especially if predisposing conditions (e.g., follicular dysplasia, cornification disorders, or demodicosis) are present. Deep pyoderma of adult German shepherd dogs (German shepherd folliculitis, furunculosis, and cellulitis) is a unique deep pyoderma with an apparent genetic predisposition. Lesions are located on the dorsal lumbosacral, ventral abdominal, and thigh areas. Hypersensitivity to the bites of fleas or alterations in immune or neutrophil function have been proposed as predisposing causes, but most of these potential causes have been discounted. Deep folliculitis and furunculosis, especially on the cheek area or neck of some large-breed dogs (golden and Labrador retriever, Saint Bernard, and Newfoundland), can clinically resemble superficial pyotraumatic dermatitis (acute moist dermatitis), belying the deep nature of the lesions.

Postgrooming furunculosis is an uncommon but acute, severe, and painful form of furunculosis in the dog that is believed to be associated with grooming. A variety of bacteria have been cultured from lesions, including *Staphylococcus intermedius (pseudintermedius), Pseudomonas aeruginosa, Escherichia coli,* and *Proteus* sp.

Grossly the lesions of superficial folliculitis include papules, crusted papules, pustules, epidermal collarettes, and alopecia. Deep folliculitis can have similar lesions plus hemorrhagic bullae, nodules, and draining tracts. The microscopic patterns include superficial or deep luminal folliculitis, pyogranulomatous furunculosis, draining sinuses, and occasionally, panniculitis. Microscopic lesions include suppurative luminal folliculitis with follicular distention often in conjunction with furunculosis. Pyogranulomatous dermatitis in response to release of follicular contents is often severe, may efface the dermal architecture, extend into the deep dermis and panniculus, and form tracts that drain to the surface. Scarring can lead to loss of adnexal structures and permanent alopecia localized to affected skin.

Subcutaneous Abscesses

Subcutaneous abscesses are localized collections of purulent exudate located within the dermis and subcutis. Abscesses are common in cats because of the frequency of bacterial contamination of puncture wounds. Abscesses also are common in large animals. In addition to puncture wounds, other predisposing causes include foreign bodies, injections, and shearing and clipping wounds. Granulation tissue or mature fibrous connective tissue borders the exudate. Subcutaneous abscesses frequently rupture and drain spontaneously, and heal by scarring. A wide variety of bacteria can cause subcutaneous abscesses. Commonly isolated bacteria include *Pasteurella multocida* (dog and cat bite wounds), *Corynebacterium pseudotuberculosis* (horses, sheep, and goats), and *Arcanobacterium pyogenes* (sheep, goats, cattle, pigs). Other frequently isolated bacteria include β-hemolytic streptococci, *Fusobacterium* sp., *Peptostreptococcus* sp., *Bacteroides* sp., *Staphylococcus* sp., *and Clostridium* sp.

Cellulitis

Cellulitis, in contrast to an abscess, is a poorly defined suppurative bacterial infection of the dermis and subcutis that dissects and spreads through surrounding soft tissues. The affected skin is often swollen, erythematous, and warm and may become devitalized and slough. The bacteria can cause a foul odor and some, such as *Clostridium* sp., can produce subcutaneous gas bubbles (subcutaneous emphysema). Cellulitis may be accompanied by fever and enlargement of regional lymph nodes. Histologic lesions consist of poorly defined areas of purulent to pyogranulomatous inflammation that may include hemorrhage, necrosis, and thrombosis. Bacteria may be visible histologically. As with subcutaneous abscesses, the source of the infection is usually a penetrating wound in the area of infection. A variety of bacteria, including those found in subcutaneous abscesses, can cause cellulitis. A rare but particularly severe subtype of cellulitis, termed *necrotizing fasciitis* has been described most commonly in dogs with *Streptococcus canis* infection (see later discussion of infection with toxin-producing bacteria).

Bacterial Granulomatous Dermatitis (Bacterial Granulomas)

Bacterial granulomatous dermatitis is usually caused by traumatic implantation of bacteria, which are generally saprophytes of low virulence. Causative organisms usually stimulate a strong cell mediated-immune response by persisting as an antigen in the tissue. Grossly, lesions are slowly progressive, nodular or diffuse, and can ulcerate and drain through the surface of the skin via fistulas. Microscopic lesions consist of mixed populations of inflammatory cells, especially macrophages, thus lesions are granulomatous to pyogranulomatous. Multinucleated giant cells and caseous necrosis are present in some lesions. Causal agents can be present in macrophages, exudate, or in clear spaces or fat vacuoles within tissue but are often in such low numbers that they are difficult to identify in histologic sections.

Mycobacterial Granulomas

Mycobacterial organisms produce granulomatous to pyogranulomatous dermatitis and panniculitis in many species of animals, particularly cats and less frequently dogs and cattle. The majority of mycobacteria are intracellular pathogens that are able to persist in tissue by entering macrophages. Many are able to survive and replicate within the macrophages by inhibiting fusion with lysosomes. Tissue destruction results from persistence of antigen in the tissue and a cell-mediated inflammatory response. Infection occurs with obligate pathogens that require a vertebrate host to multiply and saprophytes in the environment that occasionally cause opportunistic infections. Infection occurs with the tuberculosis group considered to be obligate pathogens *(Mycobacterium tuberculosis, Mycobacterium bovis),* the leprosy group considered to be obligate pathogens *(Mycobacterium lepraemurium),* and the opportunistic group considered to be saprophytes or facultative pathogens (subdivided based on growth rate and pigment production). Rapid-growing opportunistic organisms (*Mycobacterium fortuitum, Mycobacterium smegmatis, Mycobacterium chelonae, Mycobacterium abscessus,* and *Mycobacterium thermoresistible*) and slow-growing opportunistic organisms (*Mycobacterium avium-intracellulare* complex, *Mycobacterium kansasii,* and *Mycobacterium ulcerans*) are inhabitants of soil, water, and decomposing vegetation, and infection tends to occur via wound contamination or traumatic implantation. To avoid confusion in terminology, by convention, infections caused by *Mycobacterium tuberculosis* and *Mycobacterium bovis* are referred to as *tuberculosis.* In contrast, infections caused by other mycobacterial agents are referred to as *mycobacteriosis,* which is sometimes further defined by the group of agents involved (e.g., atypical, opportunistic, or avian).

Mycobacterial infection is more common with the rapidly growing opportunistic mycobacteria (also called *atypical mycobacteria*), and infections are more common in cats, in which lesions

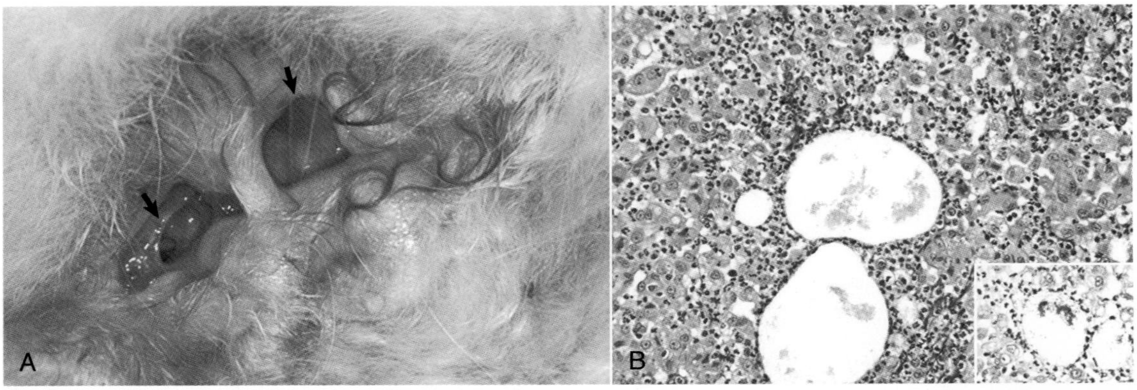

Fig. 17-49 Atypical mycobacteriosis (opportunistic mycobacterial infection), rapidly growing *Mycobacterium* sp., pyogranulomatous panniculitis, skin, abdomen, cat.
A, Note the draining sinuses *(arrows)* that overlie areas of nodular pyogranulomatous inflammation in the dermis and panniculus. **B,** Note pyogranulomatous inflammation (neutrophils and macrophages) surrounding a vacuole containing bacteria. In atypical *Mycobacterium* sp. infections of this type, the mycobacterial organisms are extracellular. H&E stain. *Inset,* Pyogranulomatous inflammation with a vacuole containing acid-fast bacilli that are stained red. Fite's method for acid-fast organisms. (**A** courtesy Dr. David Duclos, Animal Skin and Allergy Clinic. **B** and **Inset** courtesy Dr. Pamela E. Ginn, College of Veterinary Medicine, University of Florida.)

are characterized by recurrent nodules, with draining sinuses frequently located in the dermis and subcutis of the inguinal area. The microscopic lesions are characterized by pyogranulomatous inflammation. Organisms are more often found extracellularly in clear spaces sometimes lined by neutrophils (Fig. 17-49). Infections with the slow-growing, opportunistic mycobacteria are more commonly disseminated (not limited to the skin) and resemble those caused by *Mycobacterium tuberculosis.*

In cattle, cutaneous infections with opportunistic mycobacterial organisms, historically called *skin tuberculosis,* occur as single or multiple nodules 1 to 8 cm in diameter in the dermis and subcutis, particularly of the lower legs. But lesions can spread to the thighs, proximal forelimbs, shoulders, and abdomen through skin lymphatics. The skin of the udder is sometimes involved. The lymph nodes are unaffected. The causative organisms are thought to be saprophytic atypical mycobacteria that probably enter through cutaneous abrasions. In most of these infections, the specific mycobacteria have not been identified by culture, but *Mycobacterium kansasii* has been identified in a few cases. A more appropriate name for this condition is *bovine cutaneous opportunistic mycobacteriosis.* Clinical lesions are either firm or fluctuant nodules connected by thin cords of tissue that represent inflamed lymphatic channels (lymphangitis). The firm nodules consist of pyogranulomatous inflammation with fibrosis and sometimes mineralization. The fluctuant nodules are thick-walled abscesses that can ulcerate, rupture, and drain thick, tan exudate. Small lesions can spontaneously resolve, but larger lesions are persistent. This disease became apparent during the time of intense tuberculosis eradication efforts because infection with these opportunistic mycobacterial organisms can cause false-positive reactions to bovine tuberculin tests. Bovine cutaneous opportunistic mycobacteriosis is much less commonly identified in current times, partly because the prevalence of and thus testing for bovine tuberculosis has been reduced.

Feline leprosy, caused by *Mycobacterium lepraemurium* and probably other mycobacterial organisms (see later discussion) develops in cats living in cold, wet areas of the world, including the northwestern US and Canada. Mode of transmission is not known, but bites of cats or rodents, soil contamination of cutaneous wounds, or possible transmission via biting insect vectors may be involved. *Mycobacterium lepraemurium* does not grow in culture using standard techniques but has been identified by PCR with DNA sequencing. These molecular techniques have resulted in the identification of other, potentially causative, mycobacterial agents (i.e., *Mycobacterium visibilis*) in cutaneous lesions clinically consistent with feline leprosy. Additional mycobacterial species will likely be identified in lesional tissue in the future. Lesions develop most commonly on the head, neck, and limbs but can occur anywhere (Fig. 17-50). Histologically, two distinct morphologic patterns of inflammation are present. In one, there is diffuse granulomatous inflammation without necrosis and with large numbers of intracellular acid-fast bacilli; some of these infections have been caused by *Mycobacterium visibilis.* In the other pattern, there are granulomas with central necrosis surrounded by a zone of lymphocytes. Few to moderate numbers of acid-fast bacilli are generally limited to the areas of necrosis. Some of these infections have been caused by *Mycobacterium lepraemurium.*

Rarely, a nodular granulomatous dermatitis caused by acid-fast bacilli develops on the head, dorsal pinnae, or other distal extremities in dogs, often with short-hair coats (canine leproid granuloma syndrome). Saprophytic mycobacterial organisms transmitted via the bites of flies are thought to be the cause of the syndrome. The dogs are healthy otherwise, and cultures are negative.

Cutaneous infections caused by *Mycobacterium tuberculosis* and *Mycobacterium bovis* are rare; alimentary and pulmonary infections are more common, but skin infections can develop alone or in combination with disseminated infection. Tentative diagnosis of mycobacterial infections is made by considering the animal species affected, clinical lesion appearance and location, and cytologic or histopathologic detection of acid-fast bacilli. In the past, culture was required for definitive identification of the organism involved. The acid-fast bacilli can be rare in tissue sections, especially with the saprophytic opportunistic agents, and some organisms, such as those in feline leprosy and canine leproid granuloma syndrome, are exceedingly difficult to grow on culture media; thus diagnosis is challenging. Fortunately the need for cultural identification is being reduced by use of immunohistochemistry and PCR techniques that can identify the organisms or their genetic material in tissue and can be completed within a few days. The use of genetic techniques is enhancing studies of mycobacterial diseases in humans and animals. It is likely that taxonomy of mycobacterial diseases will be refined, based on the use of the genetic techniques.

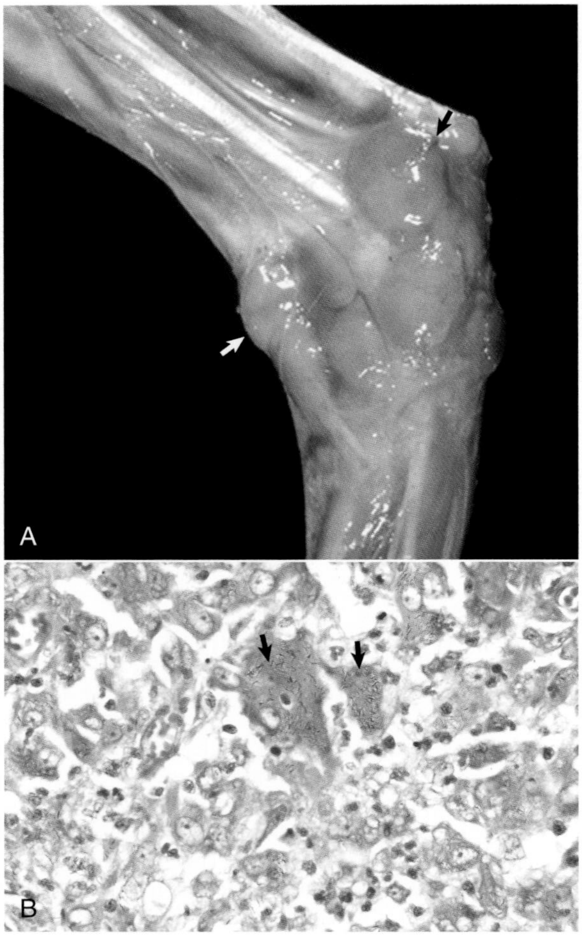

Fig. 17-50 Feline leprosy syndrome, *Mycobacterium lepraemurium* (and sometimes other *Mycobacterium* sp. such as *Mycobacterium visibilis*), nodular granulomatous panniculitis, subcutis, cat.

A, Leg. Note multiple grouped nodules *(arrows)* consisting of granulomatous inflammation. In feline leprosy, slowly growing nodules are present in the skin or subcutis, especially of the face, forelegs, or trunk. **B,** Macrophages contain numerous mycobacteria that are stained red *(arrows)*. Ziehl-Neelsen stain. (**A** courtesy Dr. Charles Leathers, Washington State University. **B** courtesy Dr. Ann M. Hargis, DermatoDiagnostics, Edmonds, Washington.)

Bacterial Granulomatous Dermatitis Caused by Other Bacteria

Botryomycosis is a term for a granulomatous dermatitis caused by nonfilamentous bacteria, typically *Staphylococcus* spp., *Streptococcus* spp., *Pseudomonas aeruginosa, Actinobacillus lignieresii*, and *Proteus* spp. In botryomycosis, these bacteria form small yellow "sulfur" granules, which consist of centrally located bacterial colonies surrounded by radiating club-shaped bodies of homogeneous eosinophilic material termed *Splendore-Hoeppli material.* This material is considered to be antigen-antibody complexes. Clinically, the lesions are progressive nodular masses located in cutaneous or subcutaneous areas that are composed of granulomatous inflammation with the embedded bacterial colonies bordered by the Splendore-Hoeppli material. Histologic differential diagnoses of botryomycosis include infections with filamentous bacteria that cause similar nodular masses (actinomycotic mycetomas) and nodular masses caused by fungi (eumycotic mycetomas).

Filamentous bacteria also cause bacterial granulomatous dermatitis with granules bordered by Splendore-Hoeppli material and are differentiated from botryomycosis by Gram staining and culture. The bacteria are introduced through traumatic injury; are Gram-positive, filamentous, and branching; and include various species of *Nocardia* and *Actinomyces.* Other actinomycetes (e.g., *Actinomadura, Streptomyces*) can also contribute. The granules contain mycelial filaments that are 1 μm or less in diameter. *Nocardia* spp. have a limited tendency to clump together; thus they typically do not form granules. The clinical lesions are progressive nodular cutaneous and subcutaneous masses, often with draining sinuses, which can extend into and involve underlying bone. These nodular masses are called *actinomycotic mycetomas.* Histologic lesions are nodular areas of granulomatous inflammation with abundant fibrosis and embedded bacterial colonies bordered by Splendore-Hoeppli material. Histologic differential diagnoses include botryomycosis and mycetomas caused by fungi (see the discussion of eumycotic mycetomas in the section on Subcutaneous Mycoses). A classic example of actinomycotic mycetoma in cattle is the so-called lumpy jaw, wherein the infection begins via traumatic implantation of *Actinomyces bovis* into the mandibular mucosa (rather than skin), which progresses to involve mandibular bone (see Chapter 16).

Dermal Lesions Secondary to Systemic Bacterial Infections or Infection with Toxin-Producing Bacteria

Systemic bacterial infections can cause skin lesions in animals by bacterial embolization to the skin during sepsis, toxin production, direct infection of vascular endothelial cells, or precipitation of immune-complex disease. In some infections, more than one mechanism is involved. Lesions often reflect vascular damage, specifically vasculitis and thrombosis.

Cutaneous lesions caused by *Erysipelothrix rhusiopathiae* (erysipelas) in pigs are a result of bacterial embolization to the skin during sepsis. Lesions consist of square to rhomboidal, firm, raised, pink to dark purple areas (Fig. 17-51) and are caused by vasculitis, thrombosis, and ischemia (infarction). The rhomboidal shape likely represents the area of skin supplied by the thrombosed vessel.

Septicemic salmonellosis causes cyanosis of the external ears and abdomen because of capillary dilation, congestion, and thrombosis. The thrombosis leads to necrosis of distal extremities. The mechanism of vascular damage involves endotoxin-induced venous thrombosis. Systemic infection with *Pasteurella multocida* can cause similar lesions in pigs. *Escherichia coli* production of Shiga toxin 2e (verotoxin 2e) causes edema disease of pigs. The Shiga toxin damages the endothelium and tunica media of small arteries and arterioles in various areas of the body, causing vascular degeneration, necrosis, and edema. Gross lesions of the skin in edema disease consist of accumulation of clear fluid (edema) in the subcutis of the snout, eyelids, submandibular area, ventral abdomen, and inguinal areas. Histologically, the subcutis is edematous, and sometimes, edema, hemorrhage, smooth muscle necrosis, and hyaline degeneration of the tunica media of vessels may be evident in the skin and other areas of the body.

Recently, conditions that resemble toxic shock syndrome in humans have been described rarely in dogs and more rarely in other domestic species. In humans, toxic shock syndrome is an acute febrile illness that results in hypotension, shock, an extensive cutaneous rash, and involvement of three or more visceral organ systems. The pathogenesis involves the release of bacterial exotoxins (e.g., toxic shock syndrome toxin-1 and enterotoxins) produced by certain strains of *Staphylococcus aureus* that usually cause minor or occult infections. The exotoxins act as superantigens, thus do not need to be processed by antigen-presenting cells to cause T lymphocyte activation and result in activation of large numbers

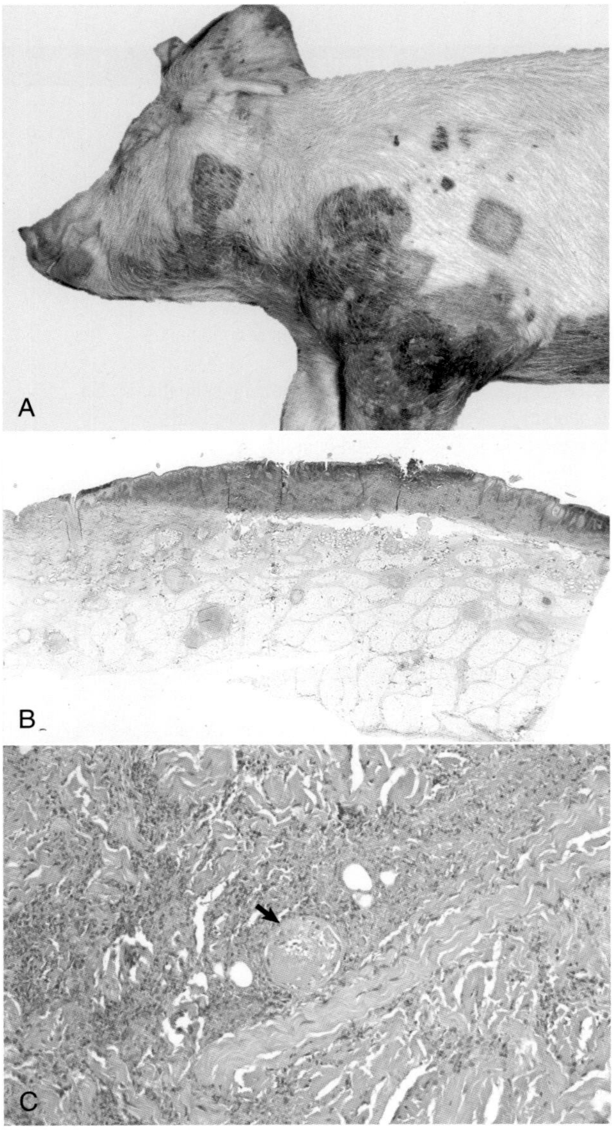

Fig. 17-51 ***Erysipelothrix rhusiopathiae*** **infection, skin, haired, pig.** **A,** The reddish rhomboidal lesions in the skin are infarcts secondary to thrombosis, from the embolization of septic emboli. **B,** The epidermis and dermis are necrotic from infarction. The only normal dermis and epidermis are at the extreme left. H&E stain. **C,** Note the thrombosis of the vessel *(arrow).* H&E stain. (**A** and **B** courtesy Dr. M.D. McGavin, College of Veterinary Medicine, University of Tennessee. **C** courtesy Dr. Pamela E. Ginn, College of Veterinary Medicine, University of Florida.)

of T lymphocytes in a short period of time. The T lymphocytes are stimulated to produce cytokines, including TNF-α, IL-1, and interferon, which are thought to cause the tissue damage and signs of toxic shock syndrome. Less commonly, group A streptococci are the cause of toxic shock syndrome. However, in contrast to the minor or occult infections associated with *Staphylococcus aureus* toxic shock syndrome, the streptococcal toxic shock syndrome is usually associated with bacteremia and severe necrotizing fasciitis (inflammation of the subcutaneous fat and fascial planes). The involved streptococci produce pyrogenic exotoxin A that has similarities to toxic shock syndrome toxin-1 and is thought to contribute to the development of the syndrome.

As in humans, two types of toxic shock–like syndrome occur in dogs. In one, *Streptococcus canis* is usually the cause of a severe localized infection in the skin or another site (e.g., lung or urogenital tract) with presumed release of bacterial toxins that cause severe secondary systemic shock. Clinically, the skin lesion, termed *necrotizing fasciitis,* is painful, hot, and swollen. The subcutaneous fat, fascia, and overlying skin can become necrotic and can slough. The swelling is caused by necrosis of fat and exudate accumulating between the fascial planes (fasciitis and/or cellulitis). Histologic lesions include edema, hemorrhage, necrosis, suppurative inflammation, and thrombosis. Occasionally, vasculitis and colonies of cocci are seen. The condition can rapidly lead to sepsis, multiorgan failure, and death if not treated early and aggressively. Fever or shock-like symptoms are present. With the exception of the area with necrotizing fasciitis, the skin is not otherwise affected.

The second type of toxic shock–like syndrome has been described in dogs without necrotizing fasciitis. This syndrome has distinct clinical and histologic similarities to the staphylococcal toxic shock syndrome in humans, but the site of infection and production of exotoxin have not yet been documented. The dogs are depressed, febrile, and anorectic. The clinical skin lesions include generalized macular erythema predominantly involving the trunk and legs. Some dogs also have edema of the limbs. Vesicles or pustules are seen in some dogs and can progress to crusts. Ulcers may be seen in advanced lesions. The histologic lesions are identical to those seen in the human staphylococcal toxic shock syndrome. The dogs have superficial to mid-dermal perivascular to periadnexal and interstitial neutrophilic to mixed cellular dermatitis with dermal congestion, edema, and sometimes hemorrhage. A unique feature is the presence of apoptotic keratinocytes in the epidermis and superficial follicular epithelium bordered by neutrophils or occasional eosinophils. Superficial epidermal pustules and crusts may be seen. Apoptosis may become confluent, resulting in full-thickness necrosis and ulceration of the epidermis. The lesions can be fatal without early therapy with appropriate antibiotics.

Bacterial infections can also develop from direct extension of bacterial infections of deeper tissue, such as clostridial myositis and cellulitis. *Clostridium novyi* can cause severe cellulitis, toxemia, and death in young rams whose heads have been traumatized by butting during the breeding season. Spores in the soil gain entrance through cutaneous lacerations at the base of the horns, germinate, produce toxins, and result in cellulitis and toxemia. Swelling of the head and neck result in the common term *big head* or *swelled head. C. chauvoei* is a secondary invader of wounds, where spores can germinate, proliferate, and produce necrotizing and hemolytic exotoxins leading to extensive necrosis of the skin and underlying tissue (gas gangrene).

Rocky Mountain spotted fever, the most important rickettsial disease associated with cutaneous lesions, is caused by *Rickettsia rickettsii*, an organism that infects endothelial cells. This organism is transmitted by ticks, mainly *Dermacentor andersoni* and *Dermacentor variabilis.* The disease is seasonal, corresponding with the increased activity of ticks and contact with ticks. In addition to systemic signs, affected dogs have cutaneous, ocular, genital, and oral erythema with petechiae, edema, necrosis, and ulceration as a result of the direct endothelial cell damage and vasculitis caused by the rickettsia.

Digital Infections of Horses and Ruminants (Bacterial Pododermatitis) (Table 17-9)

Proliferative Pododermatitis (Canker)

Proliferative pododermatitis in horses, also known as canker, is a painful, proliferative, and inflammatory condition of the hoof. The

TABLE 17-9 Digital Infections of Horses and Ruminants

Species	Disorder	Predisposing Factors	Bacteria Involved	Severity	Contagious
Horse	Proliferative pododermatitis (canker)	Moisture, unclean environment	*Bacteroides* sp., *Fusobacterium necrophorum*, possible spirochetes	Lameness, can be severe	No
Horse	Necrotizing pododermatitis (thrush)	Moisture, impacted manure, mud, hoof conformation	*Fusobacterium necrophorum*	Severe lameness, foul discharge, loss and deformity of frog, infection of deeper tissues	No
Cattle	Papillomatous digital dermatitis (foot warts; hairy heel warts)	Prolonged wet conditions	Probably *Treponema* sp. spirochete	Moderate to severe lameness	Yes
Cattle	Necrobacillosis of the foot (foul-in the-foot)	Trauma	*Fusobacterium necrophorum* *Bacteroides melaninogenicus*	Can be severe with cellulitis involving tendons, joints, and bone	No
Cattle	Contagious foot rot	Trauma and moisture	*Dichelobacter nodosus* *Fusobacterium necrophorum* Other bacteria	Mild; similar to benign foot rot in sheep	Yes
Sheep	Contagious foot rot, virulent form	Moisture and trauma	*Dichelobacter nodosus* plus *Fusobacterium necrophorum* and other bacteria	Severe; virulent strains of *Dichelobacter nodosus* produce more proteolytic enzymes	Yes
	Contagious foot rot, benign form (foot scald)	Moisture and trauma	*Dichelobacter nodosus* *Fusobacterium necrophorum*	Mild; less virulent strains of *Dichelobacter nodosus* produce fewer proteolytic enzymes and are less pathogenic	Yes
	Necrobacillosis of the foot I. Ovine interdigital dermatitis		*Fusobacterium necrophorum* Other bacteria but no *Dichelobacter nodosus*	Clinically similar to benign foot rot	No
	II. Foot abscesses A. Heel abscesses (infective bulbar necrosis) B. Toe abscesses (lamellar abscesses)	Wet seasons Heavy adult sheep	*Fusobacterium necrophorum* *Arcanobacterium pyogenes*	Can cause severe lameness with permanent foot deformity	No
Sheep	Contagious ovine digital dermatitis (CODD)	Moisture and trauma	Probably *Dichelobacter nodosus* and *Treponema* sp. spirochete	Severe lameness, pain, with possible sloughing of hoof wall	Yes

cause of proliferative pododermatitis in the horse is unknown, but the disease appears to be polymicrobial in nature. The condition has been associated with the presence of a variety of Gram-positive and Gram-negative bacteria and, in some cases, with tissue colonization by an as-of-yet unidentified species of spirochetes. *Bacteroides* sp. and *Fusobacterium necrophorum* have been isolated in some cases. The pathogenesis of lesion formation is not yet known but moisture and unclean environments often predispose to the condition. It most often affects the rear feet of draft horses but can affect any foot or multiple feet of any breed of horse and even those kept in dry, clean environments. Initial lesions consist of a focal raised pink lesion resembling granulation tissue that bleeds easily and is surrounded by a gray or brown zone located in the frog. This lesion will progress to excessive, soft, white filiform papillomatous-like proliferations emanating from the frog, bars, sole, and sometimes hoof wall of the affected foot. Some cases will be foul smelling and have surface collections of caseous white exudate. Microscopically, areas of marked papillary epidermal hyperplasia associated with hyperkeratosis and neutrophilic infiltrates of the epidermis are present. The outer stratum spinosum may have areas of marked ballooning degeneration. The dermis contains superficial neutrophilic to lymphoplasmacytic infiltrates. A mixed population of Gram-positive and Gram-negative bacteria can be identified on the surface epithelium, but the organisms are not consistently associated with the areas of inflammation. In some cases, spirochetes have been identified within the proliferative epidermis.

Necrotizing Pododermatitis (Thrush)

Necrotizing pododermatitis of the horse, commonly known as thrush, is a painful, necrotizing condition of the frog and central and lateral sulci of the hoof. It is caused by the anaerobic bacterium, *Fusobacterium necrophorum*. Trapping of moist and bacterial-ridden materials such as manure and mud lead to softening of the tissue of the frog and allow colonization by the bacterium. The condition most often affects the hind feet but can affect all hooves. Initial lesions consist of black discoloration and softening of the frog accompanied by a very foul odor. Over time, the black discoloring and softening spread to involve deeper tissues and more areas of the frog. The lesions consist of foul-smelling black exudate and loss of frog tissue. In chronic severe cases, the distal limb can be swollen and the frog becomes spongy and ragged, easily shreds, and can bleed. There can be long-term atrophy of the frog as tissue disintegration occurs. Gross characteristics are usually diagnostic, but microscopic lesions consist of degeneration, necrosis, and suppurative inflammation of the frog epithelium and sometimes of deeper tissues. Bacterial colonization of the tissues is usually present.

Papillomatous Digital Dermatitis

Papillomatous digital dermatitis, also known as *foot warts* or *hairy heel warts,* is a painful, contagious dermatitis of the feet of cattle. It occurs worldwide. The cause of papillomatous digital dermatitis is unknown, but the disease appears to be polymicrobial, with spirochetes belonging to the genus *Treponema* playing a predominant role. The condition is also usually associated with management conditions in which the feet of cattle remain wet for prolonged periods. The pathogenesis of lesion formation is not yet known. Papillomatous digital dermatitis most commonly affects the skin proximal and adjacent to the interdigital space at the caudal (plantar) aspect of the hind feet. Early gross lesions are well-circumscribed, round-to-oval, red plaques up to 6 cm in diameter with a moist granular surface prone to bleeding and with a very strong, pungent odor. Lesions are partially to completely alopecic and can be bordered by hypertrophied hairs two to three times longer than normal. Microscopically, this corresponds to areas of mild epidermal hyperplasia with foci of erosion, necrosis, ballooning degeneration, and microabscesses. The dermis contains minimal perivascular inflammation. Mixed bacteria can be present in the outer necrotic debris, but only spirochetes are present in the deeper viable epidermis. The lesions become progressively more proliferative and less painful with time. Mature lesions are irregular wartlike growths or filamentous papillae that measure 0.5 to 1.0 mm in diameter and 1 mm to 3 cm in length and are pale yellow, gray, or brown. Histologically the older lesions are composed of frondlike projections or plaques of markedly hyperplastic epidermis with parakeratosis and hyperkeratosis. Foci of necrosis and hemorrhage, ballooning degeneration, and aggregates of neutrophils are scattered throughout the hyperplastic epidermis (Fig. 17-52). At this later stage, inflammation is more intense in the dermis and plasma cells can be numerous. Lesions are painful, forcing the animal to shift its weight to the toe of the affected foot, which results in a smooth contour to the toe (clubbing) and atrophy of the bulbs of the heels.

Papillomatous digital dermatitis is economically important because it frequently causes moderate to severe lameness that results in weight loss, decreased milk production, and poor reproductive performance. The vast majority of cases are in dairy cows, but the infection has also been reported in beef cattle. Although the disease occurs in cattle of all ages, the highest incidence appears to be in replacement dairy heifers.

Necrobacillosis of Cattle

Necrobacillosis (foul-in-the-foot) of cattle occurs secondary to trauma to the interdigital skin and is caused by *Fusobacterium necrophorum* and *Bacteroides melaninogenicus.* There is lameness with an interdigital dermatitis and cellulitis with fissures and necrosis that may extend into the deeper structures of the foot such as the distal phalanx, distal sesamoid bone, distal interphalangeal joint, and tendons.

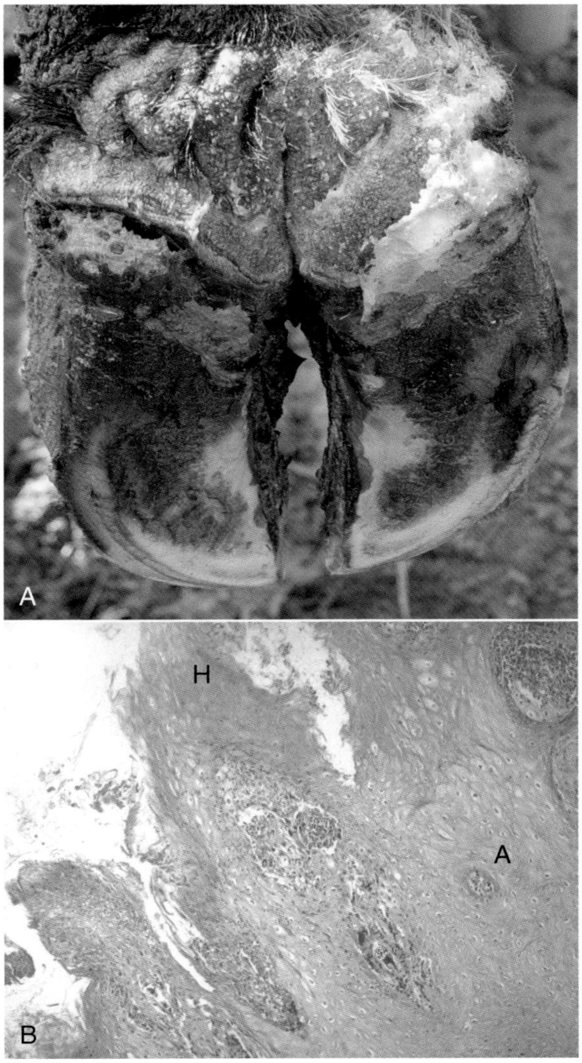

Fig. 17-52 Papillomatous digital dermatitis, skin, cow.
A, Note the moist, irregular, and reddened alopecic areas on the bulbs of the heel. The lesions are of several weeks to a few months duration. **B,** Note the papillated epidermal hyperplasia (also see Fig. 17-11). The epidermis is thickened by hyperkeratosis *(H)* and acanthosis *(A)*. Most of the acanthotic cells have ballooning degeneration. The hyperplastic epidermis covers dermal papillae, which contain congested vessels and foci of mixed inflammatory cells. H&E stain. (**A** courtesy Dr. Jan Shearer, College of Veterinary Medicine, University of Florida. **B** courtesy Dr. Pamela E. Ginn, College of Veterinary Medicine, University of Florida.)

Contagious Foot Rot

Contagious foot rot in cattle and sheep develops when predisposing factors, such as moisture and trauma, damage the interdigital epidermis and allow colonization by a variety of microorganisms, including *Fusobacterium necrophorum* from skin or feces. If the obligate anaerobic bacteria *Dichelobacter nodosus* is present in interdigital skin, foot rot will develop. Contagious foot rot is a synergistic bacterial infection principally involving *D. nodosus* (elaborates proteases and growth-enhancing factors, which aid bacterial penetration of the epidermis and bacterial growth) and *F. necrophorum* (responsible for most of the necrosis and inflammation). Contagious foot rot in sheep occurs in virulent and benign forms, whereas foot rot in cattle occurs in a benign form. The virulent form of foot rot in sheep is caused by more virulent *D. nodosus* that produces significantly more proteolytic enzymes (proteases including elastase), allowing more bacterial penetration of the epidermis. The proteases in the virulent form also tend to be more heat stable. Virulent foot rot is more persistent (and can last for more than 1 year if not treated), affects a high percentage of sheep, affects more than one foot, and can result in death of sheep because of emaciation as a result of severe pain and reluctance to graze. Early lesions of virulent foot rot begin in the interdigital axial (inner) bulbar notch, affect both digits, and consist of red, moist, and swollen eroded skin. The infection spreads around the bulb of the heel to the epidermal matrix of the hoof and results in a malodorous exudate that separates the horn from the interdigital skin. Lesions progress to the bulb and sole and finally to the axial and abaxial (outer) surfaces of the hoof wall. The germinal epithelium is not destroyed and regeneration is attempted, but the new horn is destroyed. In chronic infections, hooves can become long and misshapen. Benign foot rot in sheep (foot scald) and benign foot rot in cattle are mild, confined to interdigital skin, and can have slight separation of the horn of the heel; also the hoof can overgrow.

Necrobacillosis of Sheep

Necrobacillosis of the foot in sheep includes ovine interdigital dermatitis and foot abscesses. Ovine interdigital dermatitis is an acute necrotizing dermatitis that clinically is similar to benign foot rot. Ovine interdigital dermatitis is differentiated from foot rot by the failure to demonstrate *Dichelobacter nodosus* in smears or cultures of exudate. Foot abscesses include heel abscesses (infective bulbar necrosis) and toe abscesses (lamellar abscesses). Foot abscesses are more common in wet seasons and in heavy adult sheep. In addition to *Fusobacterium necrophorum, Arcanobacterium pyogenes (Actinomyces pyogenes)* may be isolated from the lesions.

Contagious Ovine Digital Dermatitis

Contagious ovine digital dermatitis (CODD) is a newly documented and severe infection of the ovine hoof reported in the United Kingdom and rarely in Ireland. The disease is of major animal welfare concern. The cause of this form of digital dermatitis in sheep is not yet completely defined but thought to be polymicrobial, with *Dichelobacter nodosus* and possible spirochetes belonging to the genus *Treponema* playing a role. The condition differs from typical contagious foot rot in sheep in that the lesions have an acute onset, are more severe, and are characterized by ulcerative lesions of the coronary band and hoof wall in some cases (contagious foot rot lesions affect the heel and interdigital region). CODD also fails to respond to conventional treatment and is not preventable by vaccines. The pathogenesis of lesion formation is not yet known. Early gross lesions consist of ulcers at the coronary band and progress to loosening, and possible shedding, of the hoof wall. Interdigital lesions are not reported. Microscopic lesions have not been described.

Fungal (Mycotic) Infections

Mycotic infections have been classified into four basic categories: superficial, cutaneous, subcutaneous, and systemic (Box 17-8). Ability to mount an inflammatory response is paramount to clearing the infection. Mycotic infections tend to occur more often in animals with compromised resistance because of debilitating systemic diseases, such as diabetes mellitus or neoplasia, or in animals treated with glucocorticoids or other immunosuppressive agents or with long-term, broad-spectrum antibiotics.

BOX 17-8 Cutaneous Fungal Infections

SUPERFICIAL (LIMITED TO HAIR OR STRATUM CORNEUM)

Piedra
- *Trichosporon beigelii*

CUTANEOUS (LIMITED TO HAIR, STRATUM CORNEUM, CLAWS)

Dermatophytes
- *Microsporum canis*
- *Microsporum gypseum*
- *Trichophyton mentagrophytes*

Candida spp.
Malassezia spp.

SUBCUTANEOUS (USUALLY LIMITED TO CUTANEOUS AND SUBCUTANEOUS TISSUE, SOMETIMES LYMPHATICS)

Eumycotic mycetoma
- *Curvularia geniculata*
- *Madurella* spp.
- *Acremonium* spp.
- *Pseudoallescheria* spp.
- *Phaeococcus* spp.

Dermatophyte pseudomycetoma
Phaeohyphomycosis
Hyalohyphomycosis
Sporotrichosis
Entomophthoromycosis (zygomycosis)
Oomycosis (pythiosis and lagenidiosis)

SYSTEMIC (USUALLY PULMONARY PORTAL OF ENTRY, BUT CAN AFFECT DERMIS AND SUBCUTIS)

Blastomycosis
Coccidioidomycosis
Cryptococcosis
Histoplasmosis

Superficial Mycoses

Superficial mycoses are infections restricted to the stratum corneum or hair with minimal or no dermal reaction. Piedra is a rare superficial mycosis caused by *Trichosporon beigelii* and has been reported in horses and dogs. Lesions consist of minute swellings restricted to the extrafollicular portion of the hair shaft.

Cutaneous Mycoses

Cutaneous mycoses (also included as superficial mycoses by some authors) are infections of keratinized tissue, including hair, claws, and epidermis. The fungi are usually restricted to the cornified layers and only very rarely are found in the dermis or subcutis, but tissue destruction and host response can be extensive. Infections in animals include dermatophytosis, cutaneous candidiasis, and *Malassezia* dermatitis.

Dermatophytoses

Dermatophytoses are fungal infections of the skin, hair, and claws of animals caused by taxonomically related fungi known as dermatophytes. Pathogenic genera include *Epidermophyton, Microsporum,* and *Trichophyton*. Dermatophytosis occurs worldwide, is the most important cutaneous (superficial) mycosis, and is common

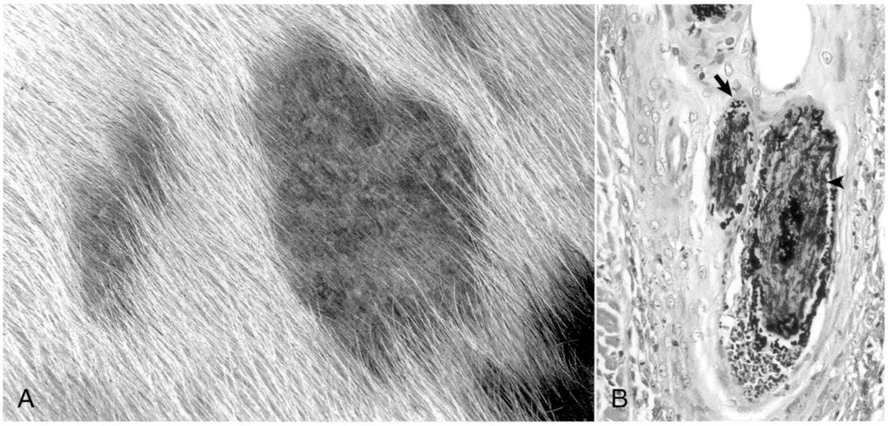

Fig. 17-53 Dermatophytosis, luminal folliculitis, skin, haired.
A, Dermatophytosis, presumed to be *Trichophyton verrucosum,* cow. Note irregularly ovoid, hairless dark brown areas with mild surface crusting. **B,** Dermatophyte infection presumed to be *Microsporum canis,* involving hair follicle, dog. Note spores *(arrow)* along periphery and hyphae *(arrowhead)* within hair shaft. The hair loss is caused by breakage of hair shafts and mural and luminal folliculitis, which interfere with production of new hairs and cause increased loss of old hairs. Gomori's methenamine silver nitrate–H&E counter stain. (**A** courtesy Dr. H. Denny Liggitt, University of Washington. **B** courtesy Dr. Ann M. Hargis, DermatoDiagnostics.)

in humans and animals, especially cats. Superficial and cutaneous mycoses (dermatophytosis) are acquired by contact with infected animals or by contact with scales shed from infected animals. Dermatophytes are able to colonize the cornified structures (hair, claws) and the stratum corneum and cause disease without ever entering living tissue. Clinical disease in a dermatophyte infection is the result of the host's reaction to the organism and its by-products. Dermatophytes are more contagious than other fungal infections, are more common in hot, humid environments, and young animals are more susceptible than adults. Animals kept in overcrowded, dirty, or damp areas and those with inadequate nutrition are also more susceptible. Fungal species that more commonly infect domestic animals are included in the genera *Microsporum* and *Trichophyton. Epidermophyton* is adapted to humans (anthropophilic) and rarely infects animals. Zoophilic dermatophytes (e.g., *Microsporum canis*) are primary animal pathogens but can infect humans. *Microsporum canis* is so well adapted, especially in long-haired, purebred cats that inapparent infections occur. Geophilic dermatophytes (e.g., *Microsporum gypseum*) occur in soil as saprophytes, but under favorable conditions can infect humans and animals if the integrity of the skin is broken or the host immune system is compromised.

Dermatophytes invade cornified tissues (stratum corneum, hair shafts, and claws) by producing proteolytic enzymes, which help them penetrate the surface lipid coat. The fungal hyphae invade the cornified tissue, and the hyphae break into chains of arthrospores. The products elaborated by the dermatophytes cause dermal irritation and damage to the epidermis. The fungal products and cytokines released from damaged keratinocytes result in epidermal hyperplasia (hyperkeratosis, parakeratosis, and acanthosis) and dermal inflammation. Inflammatory cells arrive via the superficial vessels (superficial perivascular dermatitis) and, subsequently, migrate through the epidermal layers (exocytosis) to the invaded keratinized layers, forming intracorneal microabscesses. Exocytosis of inflammatory cells into follicular walls and lumens results in mural and luminal folliculitis and, if the follicular wall is destroyed, in furunculosis. Bacterial infection increases the severity of the folliculitis and furunculosis. Gross and microscopic lesions are highly variable and range from an asymptomatic infection to an eruptive nodular mass (kerion), to deep granulomatous nodular dermal and pannicular masses containing distorted fungal hyphae (pseudomycetoma), to discolored, malformed, friable, broken, or sloughed claws (onychomycosis).

Gross lesions in haired skin are often circular or irregularly shaped, scaly to crusty patches of alopecia (Fig. 17-53), which can coalesce to involve large portions of the body. Fungi tend to die in areas of inflammation in the center of lesions but are viable at the periphery, thus giving rise to the peripheral red ring and the term *ringworm.* Hair loss is caused by breakage of hair shafts and loss of hair shafts from inflamed follicles. Follicular papules and pustules can be present. In animals with severe furunculosis, the inflammation can extend into the deep dermis and subcutis leading to draining tracts. Microscopic patterns include perifolliculitis, luminal folliculitis, or furunculosis, and epidermal hyperplasia with intracorneal microabscesses. In many lesions, septate hyphae or spores are present in hair shafts and in the stratum corneum of the epidermis or follicles (Fig. 17-53, *B*).

Candidiasis

Candidiasis is a yeast infection caused by *Candida* sp., normal inhabitants of the skin and gastrointestinal tract (see Figs. 7-28 and 7-29). Infection occurs when host resistance is compromised. Infections with *Candida* sp. are rare in domestic animals and usually occur on mucous membranes and at mucocutaneous junctions. Gross lesions consist of exudative and pustular to ulcerative inflammation of the lips (cheilitis), oral mucosa (stomatitis), and external ear canal (otitis externa). Microscopic lesions consist of spongiotic neutrophilic pustular inflammation, parakeratosis, and ulceration with exudation. The yeast organisms are present in the superficial exudates.

Malassezia Dermatitis

Malassezia dermatitis is caused by *Malassezia pachydermatis (Pityrosporum canis),* a lipophilic yeast isolated from the normal external ear canal and skin. This yeast proliferates and causes clinical disease when the microclimate or host defenses are altered. Lesions can be regional (interdigital, otic, perianal, or intertriginous) or more generalized (Fig. 17-54). Grossly the lesions are erythematous, often hyperpigmented, lichenified, alopecic, and scaly. Microscopic lesions consist of hyperkeratosis, focal parakeratosis, variable spongiotic pustular dermatitis, acanthosis, and the presence of *Malassezia*

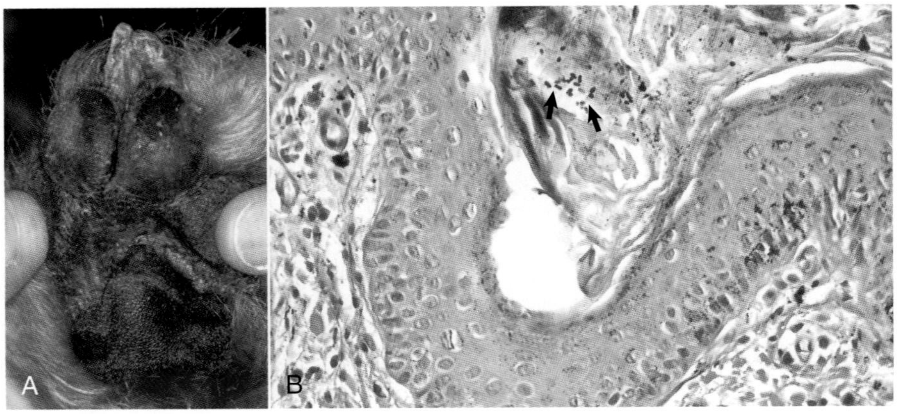

Fig. 17-54 Interdigital dermatitis *(Malassezia pachydermatis)*, skin, dog.
A, In this dog with atopic dermatitis, the interdigital skin is erythematous, moist, and mildly lichenified indicating chronicity. **B,** Haired skin. Stratum corneum contains numerous *Malassezia pachydermatis* yeast *(arrows),* which are bilobed ("peanut"-shaped). The dermis is mildly edematous—note the mild separation of the collagen bundles by nonstaining to lightly amphophilic extracellular fluid. Gomori's methenamine silver stain–H&E counter stain. (**A** courtesy Dr. David Duclos, Animal Skin and Allergy Clinic. **B** courtesy Dr. Ann M. Hargis, DermatoDiagnostics.)

pachydermatis within the surface keratin. Because *Malassezia* organisms can be lost during tissue processing, cytology is often a more reliable method of assessing the number of yeast present. Low numbers in histologic sections with lesions compatible with *Malassezia* dermatitis are often considered significant, especially with concurrent characteristic gross lesions (see Fig. 17-54).

Subcutaneous Mycoses

Subcutaneous mycoses are caused by fungi that, after traumatic implantation, invade cutaneous and subcutaneous tissue. Some infections remain localized, but others spread to the lymph vessels. Diseases in this category include eumycotic mycetomas, dermatophyte pseudomycetoma, subcutaneous phaeohyphomycosis, subcutaneous hyalohyphomycosis, sporotrichosis, subcutaneous entomophthoromycosis, and oomycosis (pythiosis and lagenidiosis, not true fungi). The gross appearance of subcutaneous mycoses and deep granulomatous infections caused by bacteria are similar, usually one or more ulcerative nodules, sometimes with draining sinuses. Microscopically the lesions of subcutaneous mycoses consist of nodular to coalescing, suppurative, pyogranulomatous, or granulomatous inflammation.

Eumycotic Mycetomas

Eumycotic mycetomas develop most often in horses and dogs and are rare fungal infections resulting in progressive cutaneous and subcutaneous nodular enlargements of granulomatous inflammation that can have draining sinuses and that resemble botryomycosis and actinomycotic mycetomas. The portal of entry is through traumatic injury into the dermis or subcutis, and most of the fungi involved in these infections are saprophytes. *Curvularia geniculata* is the most commonly isolated fungus in animals; other fungal genera include *Madurella, Acremonium, Pseudoallescheria,* and *Phaeococcus.* Histologic lesions are nodular masses of granulomatous inflammation with fibrosis and exudate in which there are embedded granules composed of masses of septate, branching fungal hyphae measuring 2 to 4 µm in diameter. The granules vary in size, shape, color, and texture and are bordered by Splendore-Hoeppli material. Culture identifies the organism involved.

Dermatophytic Pseudomycetoma

Dermatophytic pseudomycetoma is a rare, deep dermal and subcutaneous infection, usually caused by *Microsporum canis,* that develops predominantly in Persian cats, suggesting the possibility of a specific genetic deficit in innate or adaptive immunity in this breed. It is presumed that follicles rupture, releasing dermatophytes into the subfollicular dermis. Gross lesions are similar to other subcutaneous mycoses. Microscopic lesions are in the subfollicular dermis or subcutis and consist of a granulomatous inflammatory response and intermixed aggregates of fungal hyphae with irregular dilations. Hair shafts within adjacent follicles contain *Microsporum hyphae* and spores.

Phaeohyphomycosis

Phaeohyphomycosis is a mycotic infection caused by species of pigmented fungi (dematiaceous) of a variety of genera that have dark-walled, septate hyphae. Genera include *Alternaria, Drechslera, Exophiala, Phialophora,* and others. These fungi are plant pathogens, soil saprophytes, or in some instances, normal flora that enter the skin at sites of trauma. Most of these infections remain localized to the skin and subcutaneous tissue, but they can spread to other tissue via lymphatic drainage in immunocompromised hosts. Grossly, lesions consist of alopecic or haired cutaneous nodules that can ulcerate and drain (Fig. 17-55). Microscopically, lesions consist of foci of granulomatous, pyogranulomatous, or lymphocyte-rich granulomatous inflammation containing pigmented fungal organisms. Culture is necessary for specific identification of the fungus involved. Subcutaneous phaeohyphomycosis occurs in horses, cattle, cats, and rarely dogs. Hyalohyphomycosis (paecilomycosis) is similar to phaeohyphomycosis except that the fungal hyphae in tissue are nonpigmented (nondematiaceous). Organisms include *Pseudoallescheria* sp., *Acremonium* sp., *Fusarium* sp., *Paecilomyces* sp., and *Geotrichum* sp.

Sporotrichosis

Sporotrichosis, caused by *Sporothrix schenckii,* is an uncommon mycosis that occurs in cutaneous, cutaneolymphatic, and disseminated forms in horses, mules, cattle, cats, and dogs. *Sporothrix schenckii* is a saprophytic dimorphic fungus found in moist organic debris, and entry into the body is by traumatic implantation. Ulcerated cutaneous nodules and fistulas develop at the site of inoculation and along lymph vessels (lymphangitis), but visceral dissemination is uncommon. Deep dermal to subcutaneous pyogranulomatous inflammation develops. Organisms are ovoid to elongate (cigar-shaped) bodies, which are often sparsely distributed and difficult to find in histologic sections. Immunohistochemistry or culture or both may be required to document infection. The exudate containing organisms is infectious to humans if introduced into cutaneous wounds.

Oomycosis (Pythiosis and Lagenidiosis)

Oomycosis refers to dermal and subcutaneous infection by *Pythium insidiosum* or *Lagenidium* sp., which are both aquatic dimorphic

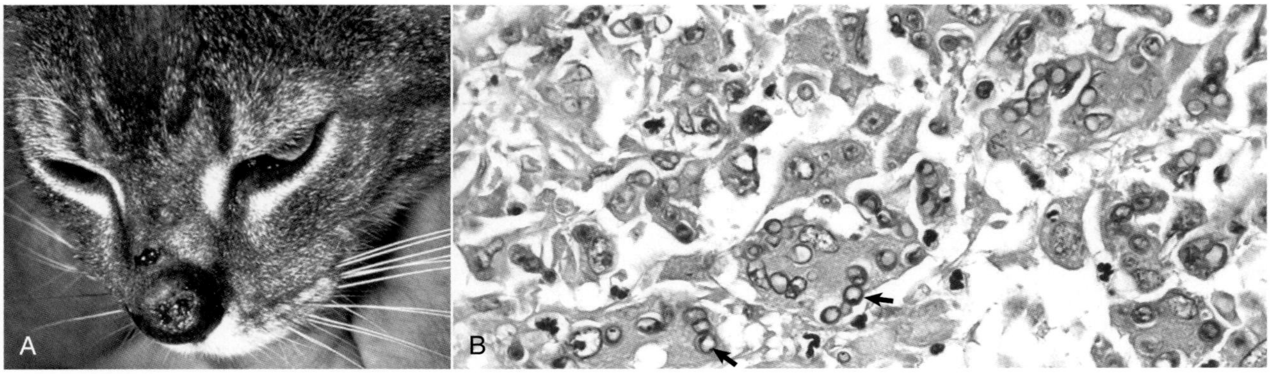

Fig. 17-55 **Cutaneous opportunistic fungal infection, phaeohyphomycosis, granulomatous dermatitis, skin, cat.**
A, Infection of nasal planum and dorsum of muzzle. There is nodular ulcerative and granulomatous dermatitis primarily on the planum nasale. An ulcer is on the dorsum of the muzzle. **B,** Granulomatous dermatitis. Note macrophages containing yeastlike pigmented (dematiaceous) fungi *(arrows)*. The presence of the pigmented fungi indicate that the condition is phaeohyphomycosis. The specific fungal organism was not cultured. H&E stain. (**A** courtesy Dr. Alexander Werner, Valley Veterinary Specialty Service. **B** courtesy Dr. Ann M. Hargis, DermatoDiagnostics.)

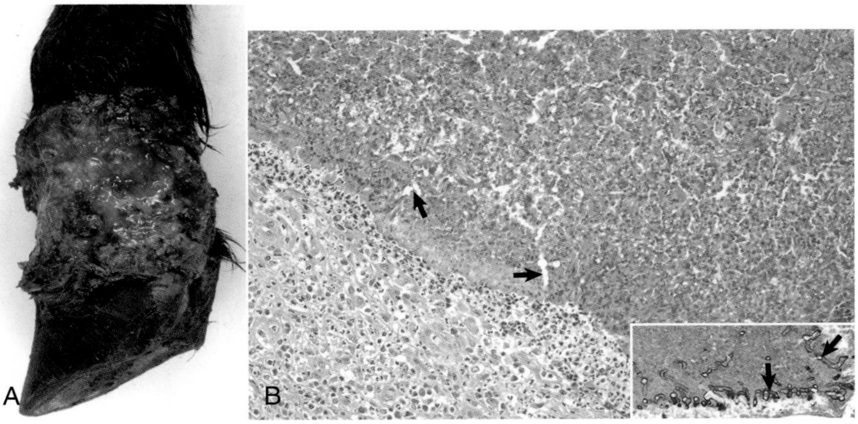

Fig. 17-56 **Cutaneous pythiosis, *Pythium insidiosum* skin, horse.**
A, Distal leg. Note the extensive ulcer with multinodular coalescing granulomatous and exudative dermatitis. Infection with *Pythium insidiosum* results in extensive inflammation and tissue damage. Necrotic tissue and inflammatory debris exude from the ulcerated surface. **B,** Note margin of necrotic debris *(top right half of figure)* and granulomatous and eosinophilic dermatitis *(bottom left corner of figure)*. Hyphal-like structures of *Pythium insidiosum* do not stain well with H&E but may be visible as irregular clear hyphal-like spaces embedded within the necrotic debris *(arrows)*. H&E stain. *Inset,* Numerous *Pythium insidiosum* organisms stained black *(arrows)*. Gomori's methenamine silver stain. (**A** courtesy University of Florida Clinical Dermatology Service. **B** and **Inset** courtesy Dr. Pamela E. Ginn, College of Veterinary Medicine, University of Florida.)

water molds and members of the Oomycetes in the kingdom Stramenopila. Pythiosis most often affects the skin of the limbs and trunk of horses, cattle, dogs, and cats. Lagenidiosis has only been reported in dogs. Many infections develop in conjunction with exposure to freestanding water. Contamination of minor skin wounds is thought to be necessary for infection to occur. Infections are more common in tropical or subtropical climates, including the Gulf Coast of the US, and are characterized clinically by erythematous, sometimes necrotizing, nodular lesions that ulcerate and drain (Fig. 17-56). There can be extensive tissue destruction by inflammation and necrosis. A unique gross feature of pythiosis in the horse are yellow, friable fragments of necrotic tissue and hyphae, which can be dislodged from the lesions. Pythiosis in the dog is a rapidly progressive, debilitating, and often fatal disease seen most often in young, large-breed dogs. Although cutaneous pythiosis is most common, gastric pythiosis also occurs in dogs of this same signalment. Lagenidiosis in the dog is also a very aggressive disease, and dogs may have lesions in organs other than the skin and lymph nodes. Histologically, hyphae or hyphal-like structures are in areas of eosinophilic to pyogranulomatous dermal or subcutaneous inflammation. Organisms may not be readily visible in H&E-stained sections; thus special stains, such as Gomori's methenamine silver stain, may be required to identify the organisms. Pythiosis, lagenidiosis, and entomophthoromycosis (see next discussion) cannot be reliably differentiated from one another via examination of histologic sections. PCR assays to detect oomycotic DNA and immunoblot analyses are required to differentiate these diseases from one another. Special collection and culture techniques are also necessary.

Entomophthoromycosis (Zygomycosis)

Entomophthoromycosis refers to dermal and subcutaneous infections caused by *Basidiobolus* sp. *and Conidiobolus* sp., which are saprophytic fungi that gain entry to the body by inhalation or traumatic implantation by wounds or insects. Most *Basidiobolus* sp. infections have been seen in the horse. Infections with *Conidiobolus* sp. have been seen in horses, llamas, sheep, and dogs. Systemic dissemination of *Conidiobolus* sp. has developed in the sheep and dog. As in oomycosis, infections are more common in tropical or subtropical climates. Clinical and histologic features are similar to those of oomycosis. Differentiation between entomophthoromycosis and oomycosis requires culture and other techniques, such as PCR assays and immunoblot analyses, and is therapeutically important because infections with Zygomycetes (true fungi) can be responsive to antifungal treatment, whereas infections with Oomycetes are not.

Systemic Mycoses

The respiratory tract, especially the lung, is almost invariably the primary portal of entry and infection in the systemic mycoses, but cutaneous and subcutaneous infections can occur as part of the disseminated disease or by direct implantation of fungi by trauma. Systemic mycoses include *Blastomyces dermatitidis, Coccidioides immitis, Cryptococcus neoformans,* and *Histoplasma capsulatum.* Infections with these fungi can occur in animals with apparently normal immune function but are more extensive in immunocompromised animals. Grossly, one or more nodular areas in the skin can ulcerate and have draining sinuses. Histopathologically, there are nodular areas of granulomatous or pyogranulomatous inflammation in the dermis and possibly subcutis. *Cryptococcus neoformans* can cause a granulomatous response, but generally the inflammation is less severe than with the other fungi. The cryptococcal organisms have a mucinous capsule that does not stain with H&E. When inflammation is mild, the capsules of the numerous organisms in a lesion give the tissues a multicystic appearance microscopically. Cytology or microscopy is required for diagnosis. The morphologic features of the organisms (including mucicarmine-positive capsule) are sufficient for diagnosis.

Algal Infections

Information on this topic is available at evolve.elsevier.com/Zachary/McGavin/.

Parasitic Infections

Ectoparasites include mites and ticks (which have eight legs), and lice, fleas, and flies (which have six legs) (Box 17-9). The presence of these ectoparasites is called an *infestation.* Endoparasites causing cutaneous lesions include nematodes, trematodes, and protozoa, and their presence is called an *infection.* Parasites cause a number of untoward effects including damage to hides and predisposition to secondary infection. Arthropod parasites (jointed limbs) also serve as vectors of bacterial, spirochetal, helminthic, rickettsial, protozoal, and viral infections. The cutaneous reaction to parasites varies with parasite number, location, feeding habits, and host immune response. The cutaneous reaction is often mediated in part by immune mechanisms (hypersensitivity).

BOX 17-9 Cutaneous Parasitic Infestations

MITES
Demodex sp.
Sarcoptes sp.
Notoedres sp.
Otodectes sp.
Psoroptes sp.
Chorioptes sp.
Cheyletiella sp.
Psorergates sp.
Neotrombicula and *Eutrombicula* spp.

TICKS
Argasid (soft)
Ixodid (hard)

LICE
Mallophaga (biting)
Anoplura (blood sucking)

FLEAS
Ctenocephalides felis and *Ctenocephalides canis*

FLIES
Adult fly bites
Horn fly, stable fly, horse fly, deer fly, black fly, biting gnats, mosquitoes
Myiasis
Calliphoridae, Sarcophagidae, *Cuterebra* sp., *Hypoderma* sp., screwworm, *Dermatobia* sp.

HELMINTHS
Larvae
Hookworms, *Habronema* sp., *Pelodera* sp., *Necator* sp., *Strongyloides* sp., *Gnathostoma* sp., *Bunostomum* sp.

Filarial
Onchocerca sp., *Stephanofilaria* sp., *Elaeophora* sp., *Parafilaria* sp., *Suifilaria* sp., *Dirofilaria* sp., *Acanthocheilonema* sp.

PROTOZOA
Leishmania sp.
Rarely other genera

Mites

Mite infestations can cause serious cutaneous lesions in domestic animals and economic loss in food animals. Sheep in the US are free of mite infestation except for *Demodex* sp. Cattle, however, can be infested with a variety of mites, including *Sarcoptes, Psoroptes,* and *Chorioptes* genera, which are reportable diseases. Mite infestations are rare in horses, except for *Chorioptes* sp., which produce dermatitis of distal limbs in heavy breeds. Mite infestations can also cause serious cutaneous diseases in dogs (*Demodex canis, Sarcoptes scabiei, Otodectes cynotis*), cats (*Demodex cati, Demodex gatoi, Otodectes cynotis, Notoedres cati*), and pigs (*Sarcoptes scabiei*). In *Sarcoptes scabiei* infestation, mites can be difficult to find, except for infestation of the skin of the external ears of pigs.

Most species of *Demodex* mites live their entire life cycle in the lumens of hair follicles or sebaceous glands as part of the normal fauna of the skin of most mammals. It is only when the normal equilibrium between the host and the parasite is changed to favor proliferation of the mite that skin lesions of demodectic mange are produced. Thus identification of large numbers of adult mites or an increased number of immature mites in skin scrapings or biopsy samples is required for diagnosis of demodicosis. Demodicosis is caused by host-specific mites; it is a major problem in dogs but is uncommon in other animals.

Demodicosis

Demodectic mange is rare in the horse. *Demodex caballi* is commonly present in pilosebaceous units of eyelids and nose, generally without producing lesions. In contrast, *Demodex equi* is distributed over the body. Clinical lesions are rare, but when present, develop on the face, neck, shoulders, or forelimbs, and consist of localized to diffuse alopecia and scaling or of papules, nodules, and pustules.

Demodicosis in cattle (*Demodex bovis, Demodex tauri,* and *Demodex ghanaensis*) and goats (*Demodex caprae*) is of little clinical significance, but extensive infection can damage hides by development of multifocal nodules in the skin of shoulders, neck, and face or in a more generalized distribution. Nodules correspond to follicular cysts that are filled with mites and keratinaceous material. Rupture of the cysts leads to severe granulomatous dermatitis and damage to the hide.

Sheep have two species of mites. *Demodex ovis* is located in hair follicles or sebaceous glands distributed over the body and can cause alopecia, erythema, scaling, pustules, and matted fleece. Lesions develop on the face, neck, shoulders, and back, but the ears, limbs, and coronary bands can also be affected. *Demodex aries* is located in sebaceous glands of the vulva, prepuce, and nostrils and can cause papular, rarely pustular, or nodular lesions.

Demodex phylloides of pigs causes scale-covered papules progressing to nodules that are filled with keratinaceous debris and mites and that damage the hide. Lesions develop in the ventral body skin, eyelids, and snout.

Demodicosis is one of the most common skin disorders of dogs in North America. Several different demodectic mites have been identified in dogs, *Demodex canis* (most common), *Demodex injai* (rare), and *Demodex cornei* (rare), a short-bodied mite. *Demodex canis* and *Demodex injai* live in hair follicles and can be found in sebaceous glands. *Demodex cornei* is found on the skin surface. Mixed infections with *Demodex canis* and *Demodex injai* and *Demodex canis* and *Demodex cornei* have been reported. *Demodex injai* has been associated with generalized demodicosis and a clinically greasy hair coat. *Demodex cornei* has been associated with generalized and localized demodicosis. Most cases of canine demodicosis are caused by *Demodex canis,* and occur in two clinical forms, localized and generalized, both of which are more common in juvenile dogs. Transmission from mother to offspring occurs via close skin contact, as occurs during suckling. Purebred dogs of many breeds are predisposed to infestation, suggesting an inherited basis for the disease related to a primary deficit in cell-mediated immunity. Research studies suggest the defect is one of T lymphocyte helper dysfunction, resulting in damage by cytotoxic T lymphocytes. Active lesions of demodicosis result in lymphocytic mural folliculitis with lymphocyte-mediated damage to the keratinocytes of the follicular wall. It is speculated that follicular keratinocytes express altered self-antigens or *Demodex* antigens, which leads to immune-mediated destruction of the follicular wall. Secondary immunodeficiency, caused by T lymphocyte suppression, is also associated with demodicosis, particularly if a secondary *Staphylococcus intermedius (pseudintermedius)* infection is present. The secondary immunodeficiency improves as the demodicosis resolves. Results of studies conflict as to whether the secondary immunodeficiency is caused by the accompanying bacterial infection or the mite infestation. Demodicosis occurs in adult dogs with underlying metabolic disorders (hypothyroidism, hyperadrenocorticism) or that are given drugs (glucocorticoids or cytotoxic drugs) that can compromise the immune system. Idiopathic cases also occur.

Gross lesions of localized demodicosis in the dog consist of one to several small scaly, erythematous, alopecic, areas on the face or forelegs (see Fig. 17-25). Canine generalized demodicosis usually involves large areas of the body; lesions consist of larger coalescing patches of erythema, alopecia, comedones, scales, and crusts. The early microscopic lesions include epidermal hyperkeratosis, perifolliculitis, and lymphocytic interface mural folliculitis, including mild degeneration of follicular basal cells, follicular pigmentary incontinence, and intraluminal mites (see Fig. 17-25). Follicles can become plugged with large numbers of mites, keratin, and sebum. Secondary bacterial infection leads to neutrophilic folliculitis that in conjunction with mite proliferation and follicular hyperkeratosis, progresses to follicular rupture. Mites, bacteria, keratin, and sebum spill into the dermis, stimulating a granulomatous to pyogranulomatous dermatitis. Perifollicular granulomas with portions of mites are often seen. Gross lesions in dogs with severe secondary bacterial infection include papules, pustules, edema, and draining tracts. In severe demodicosis, inflammation and organisms spread into the subcutis, and lymphadenitis and septicemia can develop. Severe chronic lesions consist of dermal fibrosis with effacement of adnexal structures.

In cats, demodicosis is rare and is caused by two species of mites, one (*Demodex cati*) lives in follicles and sebaceous glands, and the other (*Demodex gatoi*) resides on the skin surface within the stratum corneum. Unless the immune response is compromised, lesions associated with *Demodex cati* are usually localized to the chin, eyelids, head, or neck. When the immune response is compromised, as in feline retroviral infections, generalized lesions of erythema, scaling, alopecia, pustules, and crusts develop. Histologically, cats with *Demodex cati* have epidermal and follicular hyperkeratosis and follicular atrophy. Inflammation is minimal. The most common sign associated with the presence of *Demodex gatoi* is pruritus, resulting in excessive grooming and symmetric alopecia. *Demodex gatoi* is contagious between cats, and there is an asymptomatic carrier state.

Scabies

Scabies is caused by *Sarcoptes scabiei.* This highly contagious and zoonotic mite is the most important ectoparasite of pigs, is common in dogs, and is uncommon to rare in horses, cattle, sheep, goats, and cats. The mites burrow in tunnels in the stratum corneum and cause intense pruritus principally as a result of hypersensitivity reactions, although irritation from secretions also plays a role. Lesions begin on the external ears, head, and neck and can become generalized. Early gross lesions include erythematous macules, papules, crusts, and excoriations. Chronic lesions are scaly, lichenified, and hairless (Fig. 17-57). Microscopically, early lesions consist of superficial perivascular dermatitis with eosinophils, mast cells, and lymphocytes. Mild focal spongiosis can be seen. Small parakeratotic crusts can develop as spongiotic lesions age. Chronic lesions are associated with epidermal acanthosis with marked rete ridge formation, compact hyperkeratosis, parakeratosis, crusting, and perivascular dermatitis with eosinophils, mast cells, and lymphocytes. In areas of excoriation, neutrophils—and with time, dermal scarring—may be evident. Mites, mite eggs, or feces may be found in tunnels in the stratum corneum (see Fig. 17-57, *B*) but are not commonly seen in tissue sections because of small numbers of mites.

Notoedric Mites

Notoedric mite infestation is caused by *Notoedres cati.* This mite infests cats, rabbits, and occasionally foxes, dogs, and humans. It is a rare but highly contagious pruritic disease characterized initially by an erythematous papular rash followed by scales, crusts, and alopecia, and when chronic, with lichenification. Lesions begin on the neck and pinnae and extend to the head, face, and paw and can become generalized. Microscopic lesions consist of a hyperplastic, perivascular eosinophilic dermatitis with mild spongiosis and crusts. In cats, mites are readily found in the stratum corneum in tissue sections or in skin scrapings.

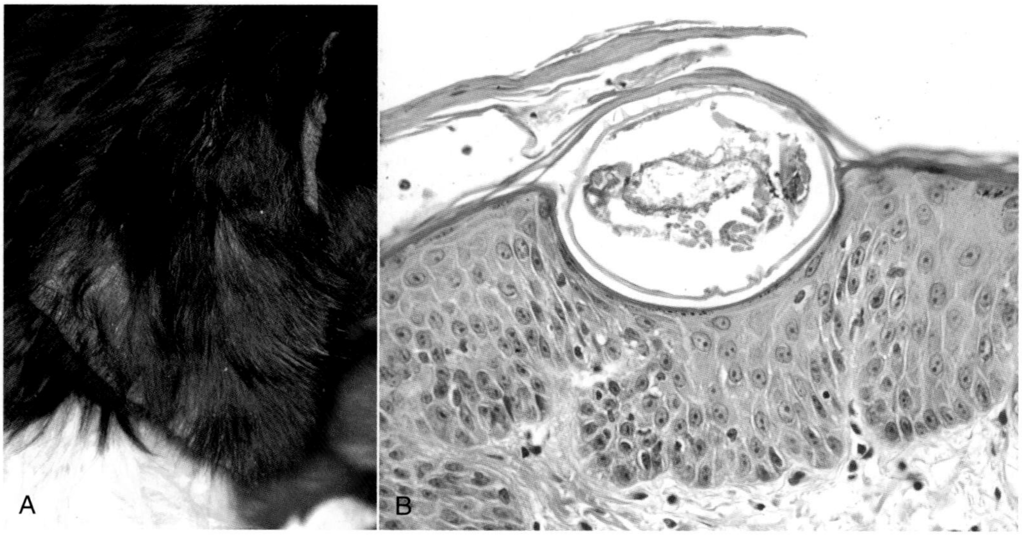

Fig. 17-57 ***Sarcoptes scabiei* infestation, skin, dog.**
A, Ear. Note the alopecia, erythema, and scaling along the margin of the ear. **B,** Note the section of a mite in the stratum corneum. The epidermal hyperkeratosis, acanthosis, and rete ridge formation are in response to both the mite itself and also to self-trauma caused by intense pruritus. H&E stain. (**A** courtesy Dr. Ann M. Hargis, DermatoDiagnostics. **B** courtesy Dr. M.D. McGavin, College of Veterinary Medicine, University of Tennessee.)

Otodectic Mites

Otodectic mite infestation caused by *Otodectes cynotis* occurs in the external ear canals of dogs and cats and occasionally can be present on other parts of the body. The mite lives on the skin surface and can be seen by direct visualization. Because *Otodectes* can be present in areas of the body other than ears, it is important to differentiate it from *Sarcoptes* and *Notoedres* mites, which can be identified in microscopically examined skin scrapings or sometimes in tissue sections.

Psoroptic Mites

Psoroptic mite infestation in horses, cattle, sheep, goats, rabbits, and other animals is caused by several species of host-specific mites. *Psoroptes cuniculi* live on the surface of the skin, feeding on lipids and later on serous and hemorrhagic crusts that exude from the traumatized skin. It infests the external ear canals of horses, sheep, goats, and rabbits. *Psoroptes equi* infests the base of the mane and tail, and skin under the forelock of horses. *Psoroptes ovis* causes serious disease in cattle and sheep, producing parasitic lesions of thickened skin and dry scales and crusts that begin on the withers and spread because of persistent self-inflicted trauma. In sheep, psoroptic mite infestation is called *sheep scab.* Lesions develop on the withers and sides. The wooled areas are chiefly involved with crusts that become adherent to the matted fleece and in time expand and coalesce. Damage is the result of self-inflicted trauma, caused by the pruritus associated with irritation and hypersensitivity reactions. The microscopic lesion is a spongiotic, hyperplastic, hyperkeratotic, or exudative superficial perivascular dermatitis with eosinophils. Self-trauma leads to erosions, ulcers, and exudation of serum and leukocytes. No cases of *Psoroptes ovis* have been reported in sheep in the US since 1970.

Chorioptic Mange

Chorioptic mange, caused by *Chorioptes bovis*, affects horses, cattle, goats, and in some countries, sheep. The mite is not host specific. Mites on the skin surface cause irritation and pruritus leading to self-trauma and the gross lesions of erythematous, papular, crusted, scaly, hairless, thickened skin on the lower limbs and tail of horses; lower hind limbs, scrotum, tail, perineum, udder, and thigh of cattle; scrotum and lower hind limbs of sheep; and lower limbs, hindquarters, and the abdomen of goats. Microscopic lesions are similar to those seen in other surface-dwelling mite infestations.

Cheyletiellosis

Information on this topic is available at evolve.elsevier.com/Zachary/McGavin/.

Psorergatic (Psorobic) Mites

Information on this topic is available at evolve.elsevier.com/Zachary/McGavin/.

Trombiculiasis

Information on this topic is available at evolve.elsevier.com/Zachary/McGavin/.

Ticks

Ticks comprise two families, Ixodidae (hard ticks that contain a scutum, a hard chitinous plate on the anterior dorsal surface) and Argasidae (soft ticks that lack the scutum). Most of the pathogenic ticks are in the family Ixodidae. An exception is *Otobius megnini,* the spinose ear tick, which is parasitic to all domestic animals and causes severe otitis externa. Heavy tick infestations, particularly by adult argasid ticks that engorge repeatedly, can cause anemia. As obligate bloodsucking ectoparasites, ticks also serve as vectors for many potentially severe blood-borne diseases such as *Rickettsia rickettsii* (Rocky Mountain spotted fever), *Borrelia burgdorferi* (Lyme disease), *Anaplasma marginale* (anaplasmosis), and African swine fever. Tick bites also cause direct damage to the skin at the site of attachment, which predisposes to secondary bacterial infection leading to abscesses or septicemia and to myiasis. Adverse reactions to ticks depend in part on the content of salivary secretions. Tick saliva has been shown to contain factors that are antihemostatic, antiinflammatory, and immunosuppressive. These factors are thought to facilitate feeding and the transmission of tick-borne diseases. In addition, salivary secretions of several species of ixodid ticks (e.g., *Dermacentor andersoni* and *Dermacentor variabilis* in North America) contain neurotoxins that can cause an acute ascending lower motor neuron paralysis of the host. If the tick is removed, symptoms disappear rapidly.

The severity of local cutaneous reactions varies not only with salivary secretions but also with host resistance. In experimental studies, it has been shown that in nonsensitized hosts, the inflammatory response to tick mouth parts embedded deeply in the dermis develops in the immediate site of the bite, is composed largely of neutrophils, and is minor even about 2 days after the tick attaches. In contrast, previously sensitized hosts develop more rapid and intense local reactions (as early as 1 hour postattachment). Cutaneous lesions are present a greater distance from the site of attachment, and basophils, eosinophils, and neutrophils are present in the epidermis and dermis. Cutaneous basophil hypersensitivity, a form of delayed-type hypersensitivity, plays an important role in immunity to ticks.

In naturally occurring cases, gross lesions include red papules that progress to circular erythematous areas up to 2 cm in diameter. Lesions progress to foci of necrosis, erosions, ulcers, crusts, and in some animals, nodules. Lesions heal with scarring and alopecia. Histologic lesions include congestion, edema, and sometimes hemorrhage with an intradermal cavity below which the tick mouthparts may be present. Inflammation consists of perivascular to diffuse accumulations of neutrophils, eosinophils, and basophils. Later-developing lesions include epidermal and dermal necrosis, the granulocytic leukocytes of more acute lesions plus accumulations of lymphocytes and macrophages at the margin of the necrotic dermis. In a vertical section of skin (from epidermis to panniculus), these lesions can be triangular with the apex at the panniculus. Some lesions comprise granulomas (arthropod bite granulomas) in which the inflammatory cells efface the tissue architecture and lymphoid follicles form.

Lice

Pediculosis is infestation with lice and is caused by two orders of lice: Mallophaga (biting lice) and Anoplura (blood-sucking lice). Infestations are relatively host specific, are spread by direct contact, and are relatively easy to control because the life cycle takes place entirely on the host. Pediculosis occurs more commonly in winter when temperatures are cooler, the wool or hair coat is longer, animals are congregated, and the plane of nutrition is lower. Thus heavy infestations are usually an indication for underlying problems, such as overcrowding, poor sanitation, or poor nutrition. Generally, pediculosis is not a significant threat to the host, and animals with low infestations may not have clinical signs or lesions. Most problems are related to skin irritation and resultant pruritus. However, the Anoplura have piercing mouth parts and suck blood, thus heavy infestations can cause anemia. In addition, *Haematopinus suis,* a sucking louse that parasitizes pigs, is economically important because the lice transmit *Eperythrozoon suis* and the viruses of swinepox and African swine fever. The Mallophaga cause less severe signs as they feed on epithelial cellular debris. Primary lesions caused by lice are few, and most are secondary to scratching, rubbing, or biting. The cause of the pruritus is not known, but is thought to be a result of more than mechanical irritation alone. Gross lesions consist of papules, crusts, excoriations, and self-induced damage to hair and wool. Lice and eggs are visible on hair or wool. Animals infested with sucking lice can be anemic. Weight loss and reduced production of milk can result from the constant irritation associated with some infestations.

Fleas

Flea infestation is principally a problem in dogs and cats. *Ctenocephalides felis* is the most common flea causing infestation, and it also transmits *Dipylidium caninum*. Infestation can occur with *Ctenocephalides canis* and less commonly with fleas that parasitize other mammals and birds. Fleas can cause severe skin irritation because of frequent biting and release of enzymes, anticoagulants, and histamine-like substances; hypersensitivity reactions to saliva; and secondary host-inflicted trauma from scratching and biting. Severe infestations can cause blood loss (anemia), especially in puppies, kittens, or small debilitated adults. Lesions occur over the dorsal lumbosacral region (Fig. 17-58), caudomedial thighs, ventral

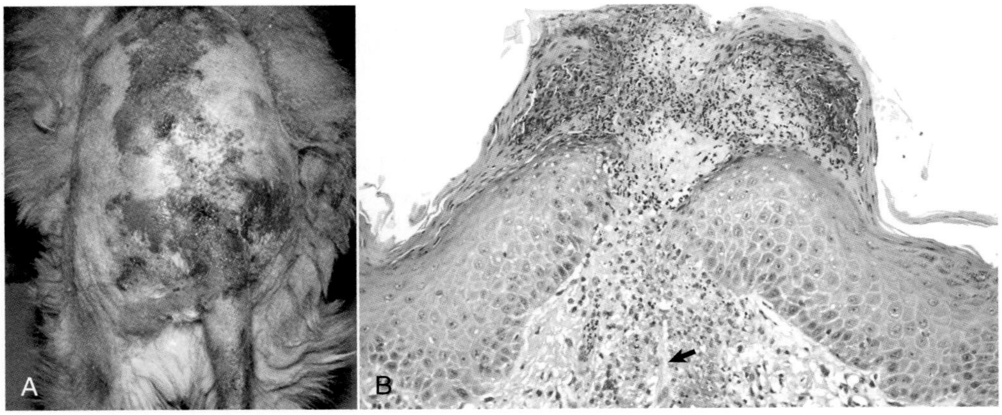

Fig. 17-58 Insect bite hypersensitivity, skin, acute moist dermatitis (pyotraumatic dermatitis), dog.

A, Flea bite hypersensitivity. The hair has been clipped to allow better visualization of the lesions. Self-inflicted trauma is largely the source of the erosion, moist exudation, and crusting in the skin of this dog with flea bite hypersensitivity. **B,** Insect bite. The serocellular crust on the epidermal surface covers a defect in epidermis, beneath which in the dermis is a vertical zone of necrosis infiltrated by eosinophils *(arrow)*. Hypersensitivity reactions to insect bites can be pruritic and initiate scratching and result in acute moist dermatitis. H&E stain. (**A** courtesy Dr. Ben Baker, Washington State University. **B** courtesy Dr. Ann M. Hargis, DermatoDiagnostics.)

abdomen, flanks, and the neck area in cats and consist of multiple red papules and secondary excoriations (see the section on Insect Bite Hypersensitivity).

Flies

Information on this topic, including Web Fig. 17-6, is available at evolve.elsevier.com/Zachary/McGavin/.

Helminths

Cutaneous infections with helminths are generally not life threatening but can be unsightly and irritating in companion animals and cause hide damage in food animals. Infections are caused by migration of helminth larvae, which live in noncutaneous sites as adults, or by filarial infections (filarial dermatitis), in which adults or microfilaria spend some time in the skin or subcutis.

Helminth Larval Migrans

Cutaneous habronemiasis

Cutaneous habronemiasis (summer sores) occurs in horses and is caused by infection with the larvae of *Habronema* sp. *or Draschia* sp. deposited on the skin by house or stable flies. Larval deposition and lesions occur on parts of the body where the skin is either traumatized, such as the legs, or moist and soft, such as the prepuce and medial canthus of the eye (Fig. 17-59). Larvae are unable to penetrate normal skin, but fly bites cause sufficient damage to allow larval penetration. Grossly, single or multiple, proliferative, ulcerated red to brown, nodular masses are present that on section have small, yellow to white, gritty foci. The microscopic lesion is a nodular dermatitis with eosinophils, epithelioid macrophages, and sometimes, giant cells bordering larvae or necrotic debris (Fig. 17-59, *B*). Granulation tissue infiltrated by neutrophils is present on the ulcerated surface.

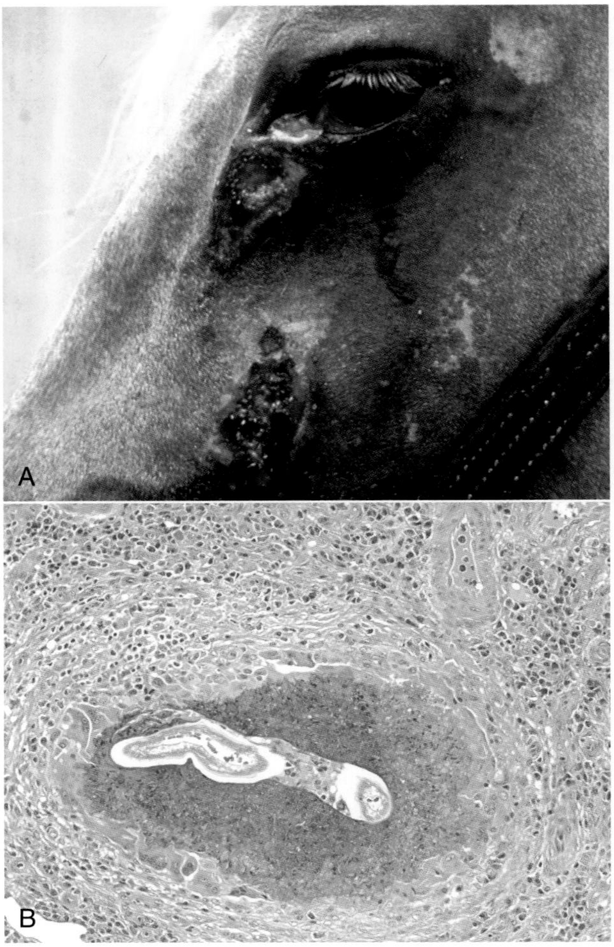

Fig. 17-59 Cutaneous habronemiasis, *Habronema* sp., skin, horse. **A,** Face. Multiple coalescing nodular granulomatous and ulcerated areas are present on the skin of the medial canthus, skin immediately ventral to the eye, and the skin of the lateral surface of the face. Lesions of cutaneous habronemiasis develop in areas of the skin that are traumatized (often the legs) or in soft moist skin (around the genitalia or eyes). In this case, moisture from ocular secretion (tears) may have predisposed to bites of house or stable flies, with subsequent emergence and migration of *Habronema* sp. larvae into the dermis. **B,** Note sections of larvae within necrotic debris bordered by macrophages and mixed inflammation including eosinophils. H&E stain. (**A** courtesy Dr. Valerie Fadok, College of Veterinary Medicine, University of Florida. **B** courtesy Dr. Pamela E. Ginn, College of Veterinary Medicine, University of Florida.)

Hookworm dermatitis

Hookworm dermatitis is caused by cutaneous migration of the larvae of *Ancylostoma* or *Uncinaria* sp. Red papules that coalesce and develop into lichenified alopecic areas occur on the feet of dogs and less frequently, on other areas in contact with an unsanitary environment contaminated by hookworm larvae. Pawpads can become soft, the keratinized portion can separate, and secondary bacterial dermatitis and paronychia can develop. Hyperplastic spongiotic perivascular dermatitis with eosinophils, serocellular crusts, and migration tracks are the microscopic lesions. Parasitologic evaluation of fresh tissue may allow larval identification.

Other helminth parasites associated with cutaneous larval migration include *Pelodera, Necator, Strongyloides, Gnathostoma,* and *Bunostomum.* Schistosome cercariae, especially of birds, can cause similar lesions.

Filarial dermatitis

Onchocerciasis is a filarial dermatitis principally affecting horses. Adult parasites are located in nodules in connective tissue and can be asymptomatic. Microfilariae are located in the dermis, particularly of the ventral midline, and are the source of the major lesions. Intermediate hosts, such as the Simuliidae (black flies, gnats) and Ceratopogonidae (biting midges), transmit the microfilariae. Not all horses with microfilariae have clinical signs or lesions. In those horses with cutaneous inflammation attributed to microfilariae, dead or dying microfilariae induce the most intense inflammation, and inflammation can be enhanced by microfilaricidal therapy. Differences in lesion severity between horses may reflect different degrees of hypersensitivity to microfilariae, different degrees of hypersensitivity to the bites of intermediate hosts, or possibly other factors. Recent evidence in human filarial disease has revealed that the acute inflammatory response in two important diseases, elephantiasis and river blindness, may largely be a result of the endosymbiotic bacteria *(Wolbachia)* harbored within the filarial parasites and released into the blood by living parasites or following death or damage of the adults or microfilariae. The inflammatory stimulus is thought to be induced by proinflammatory and chemotactic cytokines and depends on pattern recognition receptors known to contribute to innate immunity. *Wolbachia* have been identified in a number of filarial parasites in animals, including *Onchocerca gutturosa, Onchocerca lienalis, Onchocerca cervicalis, Dirofilaria immitis,* and *Dirofilaria repens.* However, further research is needed to determine the role of these bacteria in filarial parasitic diseases in animals. In equine onchocerciasis, clinical lesions related to microfilariae develop on the head, neck, medial forelimbs, ventral thorax, and abdomen and consist of patchy to diffuse alopecia, erythema, scaling, crusting, and pigmentary changes. Some horses have a characteristic, variably pigmented, circular area of dermatitis on the forehead. Keratitis, conjunctivitis, and uveitis are observed in some horses. Microscopic cutaneous lesions vary from none to superficial and deep perivascular to interstitial dermatitis with eosinophils, lymphocytes, and microfilariae. Fibrosis is seen in older lesions.

Stephanofilariasis, a filarial dermatitis of cattle, buffalo, and goats, is transmitted by flies and caused by six species of parasites of the genus *Stephanofilaria.* Each species of *Stephanofilaria* causes lesions in a different body location. Cutaneous lesions are caused by a reaction to the parasites free in the dermis, to the bites of the flies serving as the vector, and self-inflicted trauma. *Stephanofilaria stilesi* occurs in cattle in the US and causes lesions along the ventral midline that consist initially of small (1 cm) circular patches with moist erect hairs, foci of epidermal hemorrhage, and serum exudation. Such foci expand and coalesce into a large area covered by crusts, which, on healing, consist of thickened hairless plaques as large as 25 cm in diameter (Fig. 17-60). Microscopic lesions consist of superficial and deep perivascular dermatitis with eosinophils, epidermal hyperkeratosis, parakeratosis, acanthosis with spongiosis, eosinophilic microabscesses, and crusts. Adult parasites and microfilaria can be seen. Other causes of filarial dermatitis include *Elaeophora* sp., *Parafilaria* sp., *Suifilaria* sp., and rarely *Dirofilaria* sp. or *Acanthocheilonema* sp.

Protozoa

Information on this topic is available at evolve.elsevier.com/Zachary/McGavin/.

IMMUNOLOGIC SKIN DISEASES

Immunologic diseases are classified as either hypersensitivity (allergic) or autoimmune. Hypersensitivity is a mild-to-severe reaction that develops in response to normally harmless foreign compounds, including antiserum, pollen, and insect venoms. In contrast, autoimmune diseases develop when antibodies or T lymphocytes react against self-antigens, rather than against foreign antigens. *Autoimmune disease* in this section is a general term referring to a spectrum of diseases in which autoimmune mechanisms appear to participate in lesion production. Four basic immune reactions, types I, II, III, and IV, mediate the tissue damage in both hypersensitivity and autoimmune diseases (Table 17-10). Most cutaneous hypersensitivity reactions are mediated either by type I or type IV reactions, or by a combination of one or more of the four reactions. Autoimmune mechanisms tend to be mediated by type II or III reactions, although more than one mechanism can be involved. Hypersensitivity reactions are common in dogs and horses, less common in cats, and are uncommon in food animals. Autoimmune diseases with cutaneous manifestations are uncommon in domestic animals, accounting for 1% to 2% of dermatoses in most species. Of the cutaneous autoimmune disorders, pemphigus foliaceous is the most prevalent, followed in incidence by discoid and systemic lupus erythematosus. In domestic animals, certain breeds of dogs, horses, and cats seem to be predisposed to develop particular autoimmune diseases.

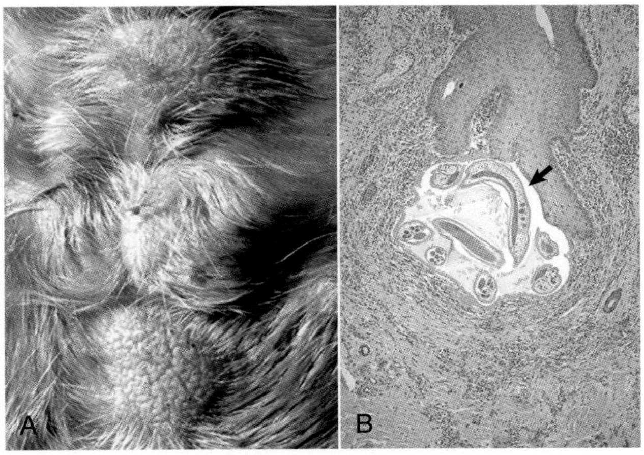

Fig. 17-60 *Stephanofilaria* dermatitis, *Stephanofilaria stilesi*, skin, cow. **A,** Ventral abdomen. Note the thickened plaque-like area of alopecia and lichenification. **B,** Note longitudinal and cross sections of adult parasite. The adult parasites usually live in a cystlike space at the base of a hair follicle *(arrow)* and can destroy follicles. Note the marked infiltrate of mixed mononuclear cells around the cystic space and base of the follicle (perifolliculitis). H&E stain. (**A** courtesy Dr. M.D. McGavin, College of Veterinary Medicine, University of Tennessee. **B** courtesy Dr. Pamela E. Ginn, College of Veterinary Medicine, University of Florida.)

Mechanisms of Tissue Damage in Hypersensitivity Reactions

Type I Hypersensitivity Reactions

Type I hypersensitivity reactions are mediated by preformed or newly synthesized pharmacologically active substances released by mast cells and basophils after reaction between foreign antigen and specific antibody (usually IgE) bound to high affinity IgE receptors on the membrane of the mast cells or basophils (see Table 17-10). Preformed substances released from mast cells include histamine, factors chemotactic for eosinophils and neutrophils, prostaglandins, serine esterases, and TNF-α. Substances synthesized on mast cell stimulation include leukotrienes, cytokines, and platelet-activating factor. Type I hypersensitivity can be systemic (anaphylaxis), localized to the skin, or both. In the skin, the reaction results clinically in pruritic, circumscribed wheals with raised, erythematous borders. The reaction occurs in two phases, immediate (15 to 30 minutes) and late (6 to 12 hours), and is generally referred to as an *immediate hypersensitivity reaction.* The eosinophil products, major basic protein and eosinophil cationic protein, are toxic to epithelial cells and contribute to tissue damage in the late-phase reaction. The production of IgE is genetically controlled, and therefore inherited predispositions to type I hypersensitivity occur. Cutaneous type I hypersensitivity reactions include atopic dermatitis (most common), urticaria, angioedema, hypersensitivity resulting from bites of flies such as *Culicoides* sp. and mites such as *Sarcoptes* sp., the presence of gastrointestinal parasites, and ingested dietary components (e.g., proteins, grains, preservatives). This type of reaction is characterized microscopically by mast cell degranulation, capillary dilation, edema, and infiltrates of eosinophils.

Type II Hypersensitivity Reactions

Type II hypersensitivity reactions, also called *cytotoxic reactions,* depend on IgG antibodies formed against either normal or altered cell membrane antigens. The reaction engages Fc receptor and complement-mediated effector mechanisms. Cell damage occurs by either complement-mediated lysis, antibody-dependent cell-mediated cytotoxicity, or antibody-directed cellular dysfunction (see Table 17-10). The first two mechanisms are most common in type II reactions affecting the skin. Examples include deposition of

TABLE 17-10 Mechanisms of Tissue Damage in Hypersensitivity or Autoimmune Diseases

There are four types of hypersensitivity reactions (type I, II, III, IV) that cause tissue damage by immunologic mechanisms. Types I, II, and III are mediated by antibodies and are distinguished by the type of antigen and class of antibody involved. Type I responses are mediated by IgE bound to the high-affinity IgE receptor on the surface of mast cells. Binding of foreign (exogenous) antigen to IgE cross-links these receptors, inducing mast-cell activation. Type II responses are mediated by IgG or IgM directed to antigens bound to the surface of the cell or part of cell membrane. The reaction can engage Fc receptor and complement-mediated effector mechanisms. Type III responses are mediated by IgG or IgM directed against soluble antigens, and the tissue damage is caused by responses triggered by immune complexes. Type IV hypersensitivity reactions are mediated by T lymphocytes and can be subdivided into three groups. In the first group, tissue damage is caused by $CD4^+$ T_H1 lymphocytes directed to soluble antigen bound to MHC II and that release cytokines including IFN-γ, resulting in an inflammatory response via macrophage activation. In the second, damage is caused by activation by $CD4^+$ T_H2 (helper) lymphocytes directed to soluble antigen bound to MHC II and that release IL-4 and IL-5, resulting in an inflammatory response in which eosinophils predominate. In the third, damage is caused by cytotoxic T lymphocytes ($CD8^+$) directed to cell-associated antigen bound to MHC I.

	Type I	Type II	Type III	Type IV		
Immune reactant	IgE	IgG or IgM	IgG or IgM	$CD4^+$ lymphocyte, T_H1 type	$CD4^+$ lymphocyte, T_H2 type (T-helper)	$CD8^+$ cytotoxic lymphocyte
Time frame	15-30 min	Minutes to hours	3-10 hr	48-72 hr	48-72 hr	48-72 hr
Antigen	Exogenous antigen	Antigen is bound to surface of cell or is a part of the cell membrane	Soluble antigen, endogenous or exogenous	Soluble antigen bound to MHC II—injected into skin	Soluble antigen bound to MHC II	Cell-associated antigen bound to MHC I
(Examples)	(pollens, molds, insect salivary antigens)	(desmosomal or hemidesmosomal proteins)	(DNA, histones, ribosomes) *(Streptococcus equi)*	(tuberculin)	(atopic dermatitis: mites, pollens)	(contact antigen or self-antigen)
Effector Mechanism	Mast cell activation	FcR^+ cells (macrophages, NK cells) complement	FcR^+ cells complement	Macrophage activation	Eosinophil activation	Cytotoxicity
	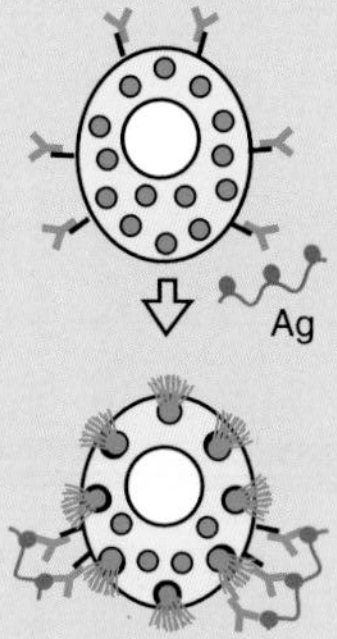	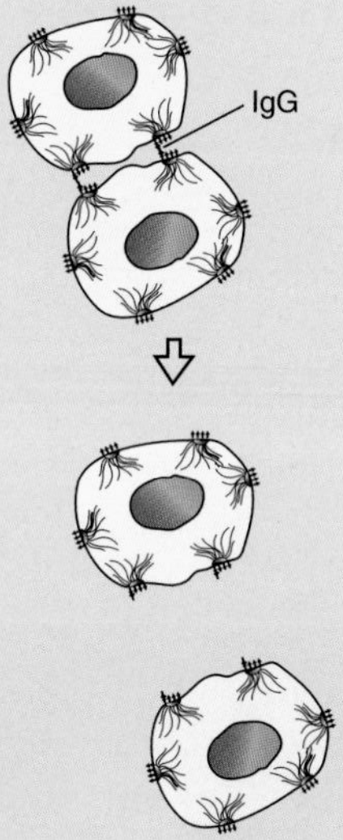	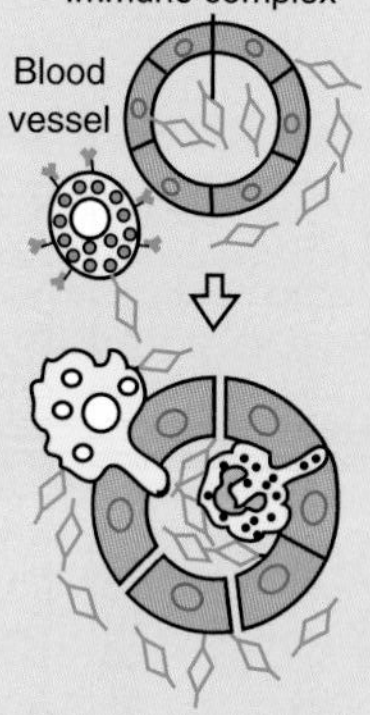	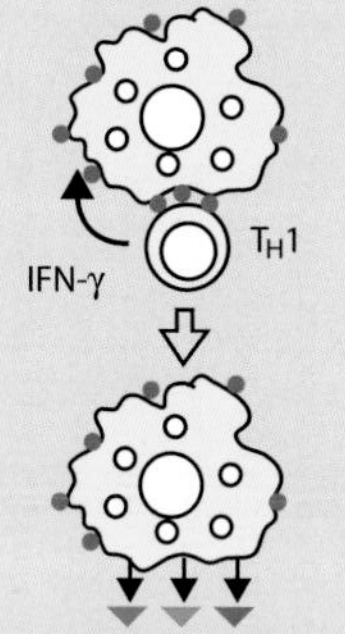	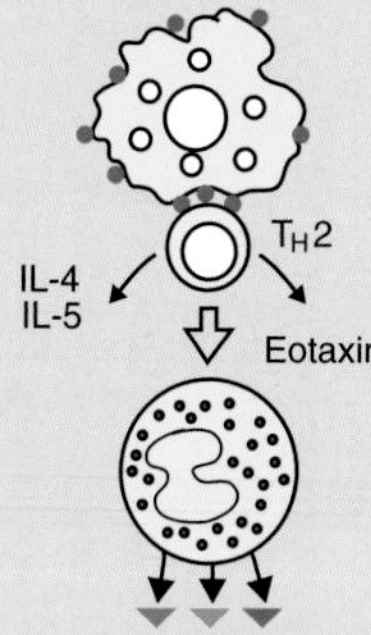	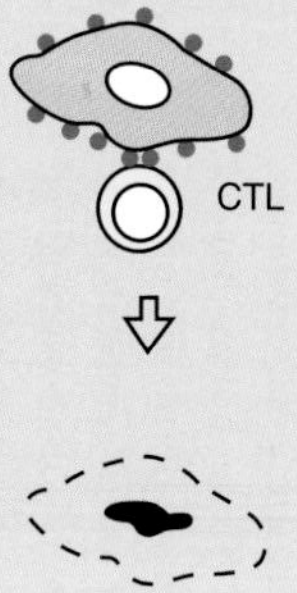
Examples of hypersensitivity	Atopic dermatitis, urticaria, anaphylaxis	Pemphigus, pemphigoid	Systemic lupus erythematosus Purpura in *Streptococcus equi* infection	Diagnosis of infections by *Mycobacteria* spp. and systemic fungal infections	Atopic dermatitis	Contact hypersensitivity Graft-versus-host disease

Adapted from Janeway CA, Travers P, Walport M et al: *Immunobiology: the immune system in health and disease,* ed 5, New York, 2001, Garland Publishing.

IFN-γ, Interferon-γ; *Ig,* immunoglobulin; *IL,* interleukin; *MHC,* major histocompatibility complex; *NK,* natural killer.

autoantibody to desmoglein 1 and desmoglein 3, transmembrane proteins found in desmosomes that provide physical connections between keratinocytes and are present in pemphigus (uncommon), and autoantibody to bullous pemphigoid antigen 2, a 180 kD hemidesmosomal transmembrane molecule in bullous pemphigoid (rare). The lesions vary with the location of the target antigen. In pemphigus foliaceous, desmosomal damage leads to formation of superficial epidermal vesicles that rapidly become pustules and crusts, whereas in bullous pemphigoid the deeper hemidesmosomal damage leads to formation of subepidermal vesicles that rapidly become ulcers.

Type III Hypersensitivity Reactions

Type III reactions are mediated by soluble immune complexes mostly of the IgG class formed in the circulation or in tissues. The antigen can be exogenous (e.g., bacterial) or endogenous (organ specific as in systemic lupus erythematosus). Immune complexes are often deposited in vessel walls and result in complement fixation and in the generation of cytokines and leukotactic factors, leading to vasculitis (see Table 17-10). Tissue damage results from lysosomal enzymes released from neutrophils, activation of complement and coagulation systems, platelet aggregation, and free oxygen radicals. Immune-complex vasculitis is believed responsible for the purpura seen in infections in horses with *Streptococcus equi* and is responsible for some of the lesions of systemic lupus erythematosus. Clinical lesions associated with immune-complex vascular damage include hemorrhages and edema with serum exudation. In severe cases, vascular damage leads to ischemic necrosis and ulceration of the skin. Microscopic lesions consist of the vascular wall disrupted by neutrophils (neutrophilic vasculitis), perivascular edema, hemorrhage, and fibrin exudation.

Type IV Hypersensitivity Reactions (T Lymphocyte–Mediated Hypersensitivity Reactions)

Type IV reactions are mediated by antigen-specific effector T lymphocytes. These include sensitized $CD4^+$ lymphocytes (T_H1 or T_H2), or $CD8^+$ lymphocytes (cytotoxic T lymphocytes) (see Table 17-10). The reaction mediated by sensitized $CD4^+$ T_H1 lymphocytes develops after contact with a specific persistent or nondegradable antigen (such as tuberculin), causing the release of cytokines and recruitment of other lymphocytes and macrophages. The reaction largely depends on IFN-γ or other cytokines, including IL-2. IFN-γ activates macrophages that work to eliminate the targeted antigen. In reactions mediated by $CD4^+$ T_H2 lymphocytes (T-helper lymphocytes), contact with soluble antigen bound to MHC II results in inflammatory responses in which eosinophils predominate. This type of reaction is believed to participate in the pathogenesis of atopic dermatitis. In the cytotoxic reaction, the $CD8^+$ T lymphocytes kill the targeted host cell directly. This is the mechanism of damage associated with allergic contact dermatitis associated with antigens such as poison ivy and can also participate in graft-versus-host disease. Type IV reactions take many hours to develop and are initiated by antigens bound to host cell major histocompatibility molecules. Type IV reactions mediated by $CD4^+$ T_H1 lymphocytes are used in the diagnosis of diseases such as tuberculosis, histoplasmosis, and coccidioidomycosis. The skin reaction typically develops 24 to 48 hours after exposure to the specific antigen and consists of perivascular mononuclear cell accumulations and dermal edema.

Combination Hypersensitivity Reactions

The strict categorization of hypersensitivity reactions is an oversimplification. Categories and lesions can overlap, and there are species differences. Hypersensitivity to fleas, ticks, *Staphylococcus* sp., hormones, and drugs are mediated by a combination of types I, II, III, or IV reactions. Therefore histopathologic examination may provide the general category of inflammatory reaction pattern and rule out other disease processes but may not lead to a diagnosis of the specific type of hypersensitivity present.

Selected Hypersensitivity Reactions

Urticaria and Angioedema

Urticaria (hives) and angioedema occur most commonly in horses and dogs, and consist of multifocal or localized areas of edema. In urticaria, the edema involves the superficial dermis, whereas in angioedema, the edema involves the deep dermis and subcutis. There are immunologic (foods, drugs, antisera, and insect stings) and nonimmunologic (heat, exercise, and stress) stimuli. Immunologic mechanisms involve type I and type III hypersensitivity reactions. A unique form of urticaria has been described in Jersey and Guernsey cattle because of a type I hypersensitivity reaction to casein in their milk. Urticarial lesions are wheals that typically arise suddenly and remain a few hours, although chronic urticaria (lasting weeks or longer) has been described. In some animals, serum oozes from the wheals matting the hair coat. Angioedema is a localized or generalized area of extensive deep dermal and subcutaneous edema. Histologic lesions in urticaria and angioedema are subtle and consist of vascular dilation and edema with or without perivascular eosinophilic to mixed mononuclear dermatitis. Occasionally, the intercellular epidermal edema (spongiosis) progresses to epidermal vesicles, serum exudation, and serous crusting.

Atopic Dermatitis (Atopy, Allergic Inhalant Dermatitis)

Atopic dermatitis is defined as a genetically predisposed inflammatory and pruritic allergic skin disease with characteristic clinical features associated most commonly with IgE antibodies to environmental allergens. It is an example of a type I hypersensitivity reaction, although type IV mechanisms also participate. The skin is the major target organ in horses, dogs, and cats. There is increasing evidence that the major route of allergen exposure is percutaneous and that epidermal barrier dysfunction contributes to the development of atopic dermatitis. A discussion of the pathogenesis of atopic dermatitis can be found in the section on Host Defense Mechanisms Against Injury, disease example of barrier dysfunction.

The predominant clinical sign of atopy is pruritus. Horses can have pruritus of the head, pinnae, ventrum, legs, and tail head, or recurrent urticaria. Pruritus causes horses to bite themselves, rub against objects, stomp their feet, and switch their tails. In dogs, pruritus is often manifested as face rubbing (see Web Fig. 17-2) and paw licking. Severely affected dogs may be restless and may not be able to sleep because of frequent scratching. Pruritus may affect the face, distal extremities, ears, and ventrum or may be generalized. Pruritus of the distal extremities and otitis externa are frequent features of dogs with atopic dermatitis. Clinical signs of feline atopy vary and include pruritus of the face, neck, or ears, or generalized pruritus manifested as self-induced trauma or alopecia. Miliary dermatitis, eosinophilic granuloma complex, and symmetric alopecia are often features of feline atopic dermatitis. Primary clinical lesions are rare, and most lesions are the result of self-inflicted trauma such as excoriations, erythema, and alopecia. More chronic lesions include lichenification and hyperpigmentation. Microscopic lesions collected from nontraumatized skin in atopic dermatitis consist of superficial perivascular accumulations of lymphocytes, mast cells, variable numbers of eosinophils, and cells with a histiocytic morphologic appearance. Immunohistochemistry of atopic dog skin has revealed that the lymphocytes are T lymphocytes and the cells with the histiocytic appearance are dendritic antigen-presenting cells. Some animals, particularly horses, have deep perivascular inflammation as well. Eosinophils are seen less frequently in dogs than other species but are the predominant inflammatory cell in horses and cats, which can also develop eosinophilic folliculitis. The epidermis in atopic dermatitis is hyperplastic, and sometimes epidermal intercellular edema (spongiosis) progresses to small foci of parakeratosis (see Web Fig. 17-2, *B*). In dogs, epitheliotropic mononuclear cells identified as T lymphocytes and Langerhans' antigen-presenting cells are present. Langerhans' cells can occur in clusters. Uncommonly, intraepidermal eosinophils and subcorneal eosinophil microabscesses have been observed in dogs. Lesions of self-trauma, such as excoriations, and secondary infections with staphylococci and *Malassezia* sp. with the accompanying perivascular inflammation and exocytosis of leukocytes into the epidermis sometimes associated with epidermal or follicular pustules, can mask mild lesions of atopic dermatitis. Diagnosis of atopy is based on clinical signs, physical examination, intradermal skin testing, and the use of the radioallergosorbent test (RAST) and the ELISA for elevated allergen-specific IgE.

Insect Bite Hypersensitivity

Culicoides Hypersensitivity

Culicoides hypersensitivity in horses is a common worldwide pruritic dermatitis, caused principally by type I and type IV hypersensitivity reactions to salivary antigens from bites of *Culicoides* sp. Signs can be seasonal or nonseasonal depending on climate and thus the prevalence of *Culicoides.* Signs usually develop in horses more than 2 years of age and in the geographic areas in which *Culicoides* live. Gross lesions depend on the stage of disease and severity of pruritus. Initial lesions are papules. Later-developing lesions are pustules and nodules. Self-trauma can cause excoriations, erosions, and sometimes ulcers, crusts, alopecia, and lichenification. Common sites are the tail base, withers, and head. Microscopic lesions include superficial and usually deep perivascular dermatitis with numerous eosinophils. Some horses also have eosinophilic folliculitis, intraepidermal pustules, crusts, erosions or ulcers, and eosinophilic granulomas. Older lesions have epidermal hyperplasia, hyperkeratosis, cellular crusts, and dermal fibrosis, usually the result of ulceration or folliculitis and furunculosis.

Flea Bite Hypersensitivity

Flea bite hypersensitivity is the most common hypersensitivity dermatitis in dogs and cats. It is mediated by type I and type IV reactions, including cutaneous basophil hypersensitivity. Flea bite hypersensitivity is pruritic. In dogs, cutaneous lesions occur principally along the dorsal lumbosacral area (see Fig. 17-58), ventral abdomen, caudomedial aspects of the thighs, and flanks. In cats, lesions occur around the neck but can be generalized, especially in highly sensitive animals. Secondary lesions are caused by self-inflicted trauma. Grossly, there is a papular dermatitis with secondary excoriations. Chronic lesions include lichenification (see Table 17-3), and some dogs develop multiple firm alopecic nodules (fibropruritic nodules) in the dorsal lumbosacral area. Microscopically, flea bite hypersensitivity in dogs consists of superficial perivascular dermal accumulations of mast cells, basophils, eosinophils, lymphocytes, and histiocytes. Occasionally, small foci of epidermal necrosis and eosinophils called nibbles are seen, which strongly suggest flea bite hypersensitivity. Fibropruritic nodules consist of a core of coarse thick collagen bundles covered by a hyperplastic epidermis; the end result of chronic inflammation associated with flea bites. In cats, the inflammatory lesions are in the superficial and deep perivascular dermis, and eosinophilic folliculitis and furunculosis also can be a feature. The overlying epidermis is acanthotic.

Mosquito Bite Hypersensitivity in Cats

Mosquito bite hypersensitivity develops in cats hypersensitive to mosquito antigens, presumably present within the injected mosquito saliva. Experimental studies using intradermal skin tests and Prausnitz-Kustner tests in cats indicate that these lesions are initiated by a type I hypersensitivity reaction. A delayed hypersensitivity reaction also may occur but has not been fully characterized. Mosquito bite hypersensitivity develops primarily on the haired skin of the nose, but lesions can involve nasal planum, periocular skin, pinnae, and less commonly the flexor surface of the carpi and margins of pawpads. Lesions begin as erythematous papules and progress to crusts, erosions, ulcers, and alopecia (Fig. 17-61). Inactive lesions can be hypopigmented or hyperpigmented, presumably from damage to or regenerative hyperplasia of melanin-containing cells in the epidermis. Histologic lesions include extensive superficial and deep, perivascular and interstitial eosinophilic to mixed dermatitis, occasionally with foci of degranulated eosinophils (flame figures) and eosinophilic folliculitis and furunculosis. The epidermis is acanthotic with foci of erosion, ulceration, and cellular crusting (see Fig. 17-61).

Allergic Contact Dermatitis

Allergic contact dermatitis, an example of a type IV hypersensitivity reaction, is primarily the result of contact with chemicals such as aniline dyes in carpets, plant resins, chemicals in shampoo, and historically to plastics in food dishes. These chemical substances contain low molecular weight haptens that require binding to cell-associated proteins before they are recognized by cytotoxic T lymphocytes ($CD8^+$). Lesions develop on reexposure to the antigen. The lesions are pruritic, result in self-inflicted trauma, vary in severity, and are located in regions in contact with the antigen, typically in areas of glabrous (smooth and bare or hairless) skin unless the antigen is a liquid or aerosol. Grossly, lesions consist of erythema, papules with or without vesicles, and exudates that develop into crusts. Chronic lesions consist of lichenification, hyperpigmentation, and alopecia. Early microscopic lesions are spongiotic superficial perivascular dermatitis with lymphocytes, macrophages, and usually, infrequent eosinophils. However, some lesions have many perivascular eosinophils and eosinophilic epidermal pustules. More chronic lesions, often those identified in biopsy samples, have acanthosis and foci of parakeratotic cellular crusts. Lesions associated with self-induced trauma can also be seen.

Hypersensitivity Reactions to Drugs

Hypersensitivity reactions to drugs are uncommon in dogs and cats, are rare in other domestic animals, and can result from any of the four types of hypersensitivity reactions. The drugs most commonly associated with hypersensitivity reactions include penicillins and trimethoprim-potentiated sulfonamides, but many drugs can cause a hypersensitivity reaction. Gross and microscopic lesions vary greatly. Microscopic lesions have different histopathologic patterns and include perivascular dermatitis, interface dermatitis, epidermal necrosis, vasculitis, vesiculopustular dermatitis, necrotizing dermatitis, perforating folliculitis (i.e., furunculosis), or panniculitis.

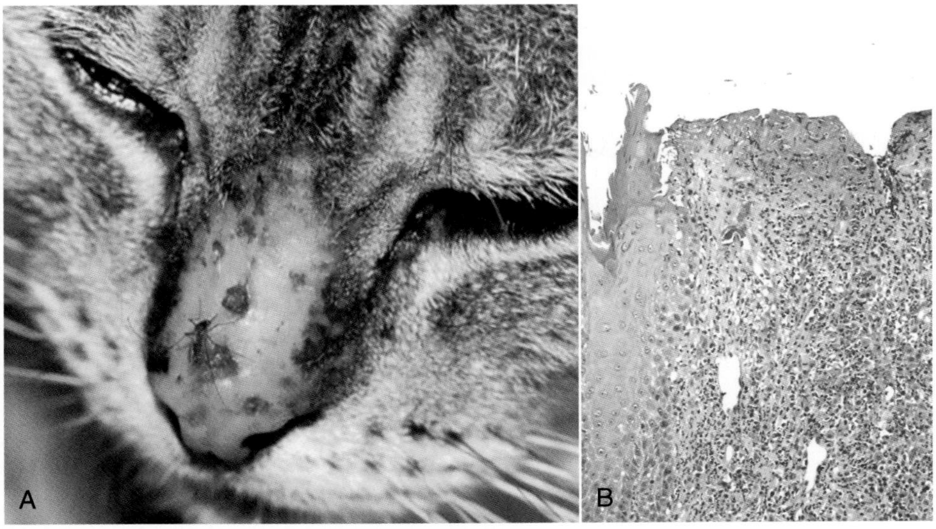

Fig. 17-61 Resolving mosquito bite hypersensitivity dermatitis, skin, face, cat.
A, Alopecia, erythema, and erosions are present. Note the mosquito that is biting the skin. The two red depressions nearest the mosquito are healing biopsy sites collected previously during a more active stage of the disease. Mosquitoes have been kept away from this cat for one week, allowing the active lesions of hemorrhagic crusting to resolve. **B,** The dermis under the ulcer is heavily infiltrated with eosinophils, lymphocytes, and plasma cells. H&E stain. (**A** courtesy of Dr. Kenneth V. Mason, Animal Allergy and Dermatology Service, Springwood, Queensland, Australia. **B** courtesy Dr. Ann M. Hargis, DermatoDiagnostics.)

Selected Autoimmune Reactions

Reactions Characterized Grossly by Vesicles or Bullae as the Primary Lesion and Histologically by Acantholysis

Pemphigus represents a group of diseases clinically characterized by transient vesicles or bullae and histologically by acantholysis (Table 17-11). This group of diseases is caused by a type II response and involves autoantibodies produced against proteins responsible for keratinocyte cell-to-cell adhesion (desmosomes, in particular desmoglein-1 and desmoglein-3). Desmosomes are the sites where cells of the stratum spinosum attach to each other, and during fixation and processing for microscopic examination, the cells of the stratum spinosum contract, except for the desmosomal attachments, which provide the appearance of "spines" or intercellular bridges (see the discussion on epidermis in the section on Morphology of the Skin). These desmosomal protein antigens are found in various stratified squamous epithelia, including skin, mucocutaneous junctions, oral mucosa, esophagus, and vagina. Damage to desmosomes results in acantholysis, which leads to the formation of vesicles or bullae within varying levels of the epidermis according to the location of the target antigen. The pathogenesis of acantholysis is not fully understood and is an active area of investigation. However, the autoantibodies themselves induce acantholysis and thus are considered pathogenic. The pathogenesis of acantholysis may differ between the superficial form of the disease (pemphigus foliaceous) versus the deeper form (pemphigus vulgaris). For both pemphigus foliaceous and pemphigus vulgaris, accumulating experimental evidence suggests that antibody binding to specific desmoglein proteins initiate acantholysis by triggering intracellular signaling pathways, which indirectly results in loss of desmoglein-mediated binding. The signaling pathways involve p38MAPK (mitogen-activated protein kinase) and RhoA (a small protein known to regulate the actin cytoskeleton). In pemphigus vulgaris, plakoglobin (a protein in the desmosomal plaque that is thought to be part of a receptor complex required to transfer the signal from autoantibody-bound desmoglein-3 into the cell) also contributes. In addition, in pemphigus vulgaris direct inhibition of desmoglein-3 binding and desmoglein-3 depletion from desmosomes, as well as activation of other signaling pathways (involving the transcription factor c-Myc, phospholipase C, protein kinase C, and others) appear to contribute to the pathogenesis of acantholysis, but their role in pemphigus foliaceous is uncertain. Other factors, such as desmoglein proteolysis, mechanical stress, and secondary changes such as altered extracellular calcium concentration, may also play a role in acantholysis.

The severity of clinical disease is in part related to the depth of the formation of the vesicles. The more severe signs are caused by separations deep within the epidermis and or oral mucosa, and the more mild signs are caused by separations in the subcorneal epidermis. The reasons that blisters develop in the superficial versus deeper epithelium are controversial. One theory, the compensation theory, suggests that different histologic sites of blister formation in superficial versus deep forms of pemphigus are the result of different distribution patterns of desmoglein-1 and desmoglein-3 within the skin and mucous membranes and the ability of these desmoglein proteins to compensate for the loss of each other in regard to the adhesion of keratinocytes. However, other studies using mouse models and in vitro systems have suggested that this compensation theory does not fully explain the difference in depth of blister formation and that various signaling pathways required for the maintenance of desmosomal adhesion in the specific epidermal layers may play a role, but these pathways have not been fully elucidated.

Pemphigus Foliaceous

Pemphigus foliaceous (PF) is the most common and milder form of pemphigus and in domestic animals has been reported in the horse, goat, dog, and cat. The disease develops spontaneously and in dogs and cats, as an adverse reaction to drug therapy. In humans, PF autoantibodies recognize the desmosomal protein, desmoglein-1, which is expressed predominantly in the upper layers of the epidermis. This expression pattern of desmoglein-1 in conjunction with expression patterns of other intercellular adhesion molecules and signaling pathways appear to play a role in location of the vesicles and the anatomic distribution pattern of lesions. Antibodies

TABLE 17-11 Immune-Mediated Dermatoses in Which Bullae Form within or below the Epidermis

Disorder	Species	Relative Prevalence	Clinical Distribution	Target	Location of Bullae
Pemphigus foliaceous (PF)	Dog Cat Horse Goat	Common, but rare in goat	Skin	Dogs: Dsg 1 in <10% of dogs (minor antigen). Unknown antigen in most dogs and other species.	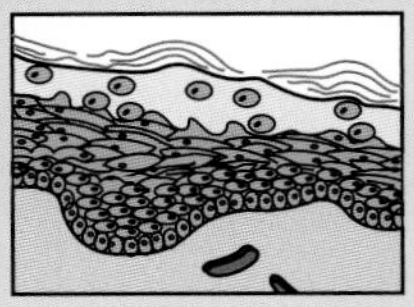
Pemphigus foliaceous subtype (panepidermal pustular pemphigus [PPP])	Dog	Uncommon	Skin, largely facial	Not defined immunologically, probably variant of PF	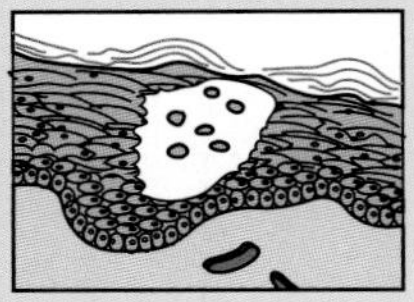
Pemphigus vulgaris (PV)	Dog Cat	Rare	Mucosal or mucocutaneous types	Dog: Dsg 3 (mucosal) Dsg 3 + Dsg 1 (mucocutaneous)	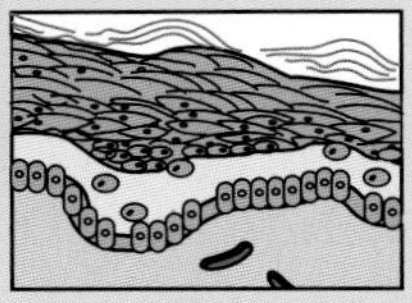
Paraneoplastic pemphigus (PNP)	Dog	Rare	Oral, mucocutaneous, skin	Dsg 3, envoplakin, periplakin	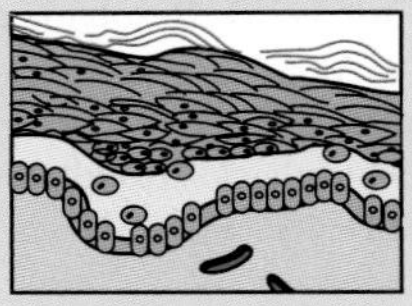
Bullous pemphigoid (BP)	Dog Cat Horse Pig	Rare, but one of the more frequently seen subepidermal bullous dermatoses in multiple species	Skin, mucocutaneous, mucosal epithelium Pigs: skin only	BPAG2-NC16A domain (collagen XVII and the NC16A noncollagenous extracellular domain)	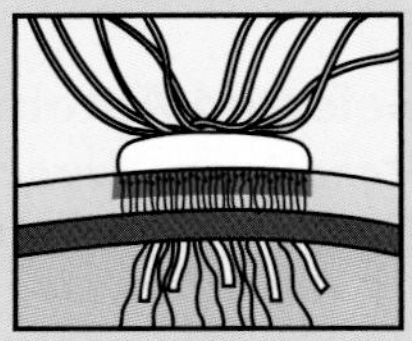
Epidermolysis bullosa acquisita (EBA)	Dog	Rare, but one of the most frequently seen subepidermal bullous dermatoses of dogs	Oral, mucocutaneous junctions, skin, areas of trauma	Type VII collagen-NC1, anchoring fibrils in sublamina densa	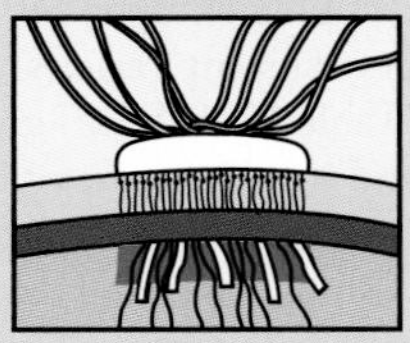
Linear IgA dermatosis	Dog	Rare	Oral, ocular conjunctiva, skin of face and extremities	LAD-1 (processed extracellular segment of type XVII collagen in upper lamina lucida)	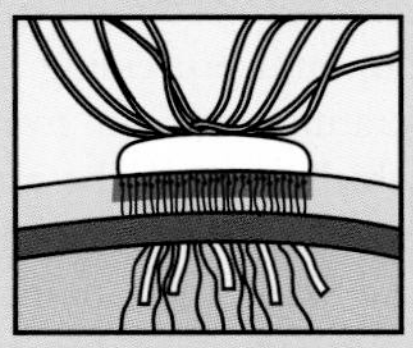
Mucous membrane pemphigoid (MMP)	Dog Cat	Rare, but one of the more common subepidermal bullous dermatoses in dogs	Predominantly mucous membranes and mucocutaneous junctions	Different antigens are targets: Laminin-5 Collagen XVII Integrin alpha-6 beta-4	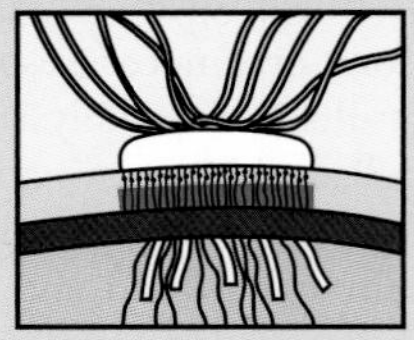
Lupus erythematosus* (systemic and cutaneous forms)	Dog Cat Horse	Uncommon Bullous SLE subtype, rare, dog	Oral Skin Systemic form	Many membrane and solid antigens including DNA, RNA, nucleoprotein, histone-related antigens, and in bullous SLE subtype, type VII collagen	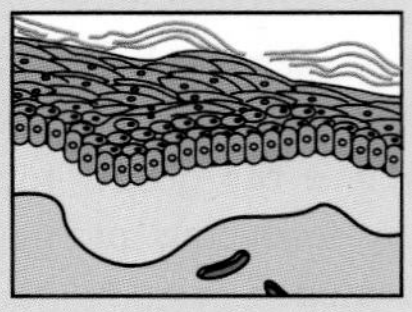

*The level of bulla formation depends on subtype of lupus erythematosus and antigen targeted, typically subepidermal with basal cell degeneration. Bullous SLE subtype is similar to EBA.

BPAG, Bullous pemphigoid antigen; *Dsg,* desmoglein; *IgA,* immunoglobulin A; *LAD-1,* leukocyte adhesion deficiency-1; *SLE,* systemic lupus erythematosus.

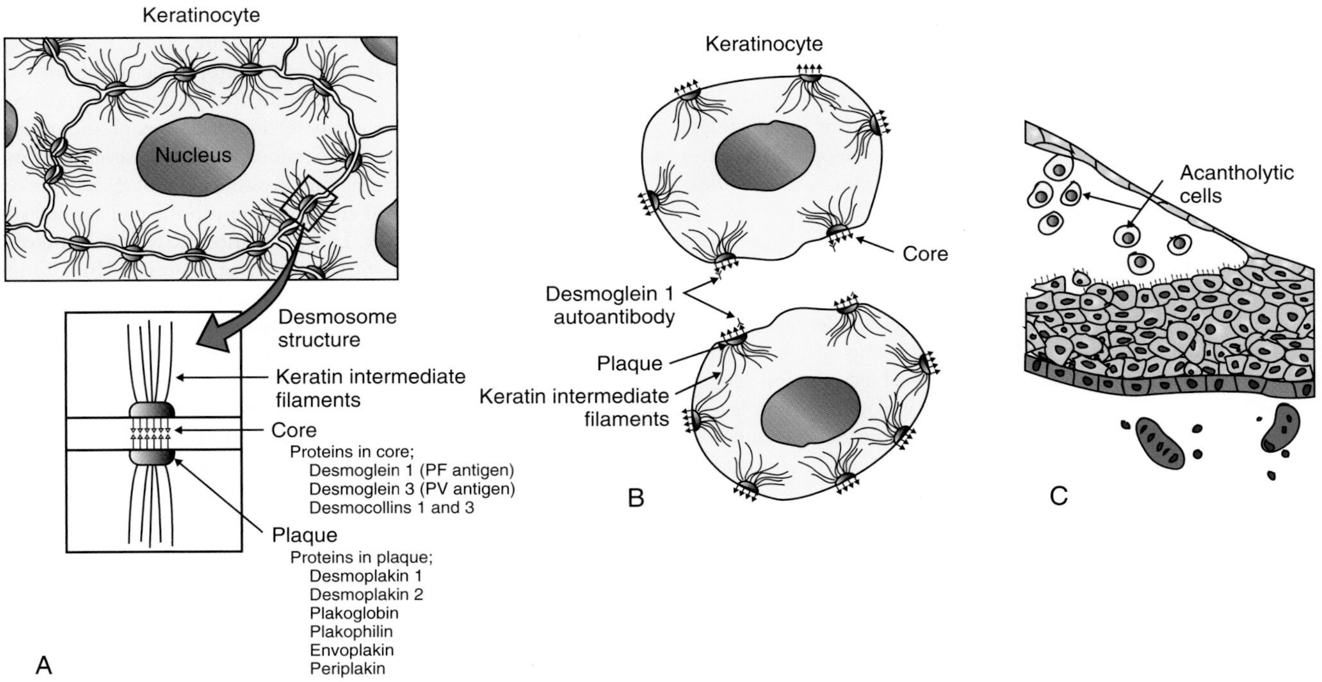

Fig. 17-62 Schematic diagram of the development of acantholysis in pemphigus foliaceous.
In humans and about 6% of dogs with pemphigus foliaceous, acantholysis develops when autoantibodies bind to desmoglein-1, a glycoprotein within the extracellular core of the desmosome. **A,** Desmosomes provide physical connections between keratinocytes and consist of keratin intermediate filaments, an intracytoplasmic plaque region in which the intermediate filaments insert, and an extracellular core region. Proteins in the plaque region consist of desmoplakins, plakoglobin, and others. Proteins in the core region consist of desmogleins-1 and -3 and desmocollins-1 and -3. **B,** Autoantibody attaches to desmoglein-1, which is located predominantly in desmosomes of the upper layers of the epidermis. Simple binding of the autoantibody to desmoglein-1 induces keratinocyte detachment. Experimental evidence suggests that antibody binding to desmoglein-1 initiates acantholysis by triggering intracellular signaling pathways, which indirectly result in loss of desmoglein-mediated binding. Other factors, such as desmoglein proteolysis, mechanical stress, and secondary changes, including altered extracellular calcium concentration, may also play a role in acantholysis. **C,** An intraepidermal vesicle containing acantholytic keratinocytes is the result of loss of desmosomes between keratinocytes in the upper layers of the epidermis. *PF,* Pemphigus foliaceous; *PV,* pemphigus vulgaris. (Adapted from Rubin E, Farber JL: *Pathology,* ed 3, Philadelphia, 1999, Lippincott-Raven; and Lin MS, Mascaro JM Jr, Liu Z et al: *Clin Exp Immunol* 107 suppl 1:9-15, 1997.)

targeting desmoglein-1 cause cutaneous, rather than oral lesions, and the acantholytic process occurs at a superficial level in the epidermis, producing clinical lesions that are typically exfoliative (Fig. 17-62). PF in animals is thought to be similar to that in humans. In fact, autoantibodies to desmoglein-1 have been identified in the serum of a small percentage of dogs with PF. In addition, serum autoantibodies, largely of the IgG4 isotype, that target intercellular autoantigen(s) in the stratum granulosum or less commonly autoantibodies that bind cytoplasmic basal antigen(s) have been identified in dogs with PF. Other studies have revealed IgG autoantibodies directed against intracellular keratinocyte antigens in various layers of the epidermis, nuclear epidermal antigens, and rarely basement membrane antigens. It also has been shown using immunoprecipitation-immunoblotting that serum autoantibodies of canine PF target desmosomal proteins, including desmoglein-1 and other as yet to be identified proteins localized to desmosomes. Thus it appears that PF is immunologically heterogeneous and that autoantibodies, including those directed toward desmosomal proteins, contribute to the pathogenesis of canine PF. Autoantibodies involved in the development of PF have not been studied in horses, goats, or cats.

The gross lesions are similar in all species. The primary lesions consist of transient vesicles that rapidly become pustules, which can be localized to specific areas of the skin (nose, pinnae, periocular skin, pawpads, claw beds, and coronary bands), or can be more generalized and symmetric. The pustules are in the superficial epidermis, covered by only a small amount of stratum corneum or a few epidermal cells. Because the pustules are fragile, they quickly rupture from minor mechanical pressure on the surface, and this leads to secondary crusts, scales, alopecia, and superficial erosions (see Fig. 17-15). In horses, lesions often begin on the face or distal extremities or can be localized to the coronary bands. Most horses have multifocal to generalized crusting, scaling, and alopecia of the face, neck, trunk, and extremities. Some horses have been depressed and lethargic. In goats, pustules, crusts, scales, and alopecia develop on the face, abdomen, limbs, perineum, and tail, and in females, udder and teats. In most dogs, lesions are bilateral and symmetric and appear first on the dorsal muzzle, planum nasale, periocular skin, and ears. Pawpads are frequently involved, and claws may be affected and may slough. In more than half the cases, lesions become generalized. Mucosal lesions are rarely seen in dogs with PF. Pruritus is present in about one-fourth of affected dogs. Systemic signs (anorexia, depression, fever, and weight loss) usually are seen in dogs with more generalized and erosive lesions. In the cat, lesions are similar to those in the dog and occur on the face, ears, and feet and consist of erosions and crusts, as pustules are exceptionally transient. Skin around the nipples may be affected. Pustular exudate and crusting may be seen in the skin of the claw folds. In any species, the lesions can become generalized.

Microscopically, lesions in all species are similar. Subcorneal and intragranular acantholysis result in the formation of very transient "vesicles" (in animals the vesicle stage is not a major clinical feature as it is in humans because the vesicle stage in animals very rapidly progresses to the pustular stage). Pustules contain neutrophils, less often eosinophils, and acantholytic keratinocytes. The acantholytic keratinocytes may "cling" to the roof of the pustules and occur in clusters. In dogs, cells resembling apoptotic keratinocytes have been noted, but significance is unknown. Pustules are often large and bridge multiple follicles. The pustules may affect the follicular infundibular epithelium. Pustules progress to crusts. In the horse, subcorneal or intragranular pustules are observed, but in the dog, pustules may occur in the stratum spinosum. Crusts should be included in the biopsy sample, especially if well-developed pustules are no longer present because laminated crusts with acantholytic cells can help establish the histologic diagnosis. The laminated crusts are composed of multiple layers of dried pustules, one on top of the other. The dermis contains perivascular to interstitial accumulations of mixed inflammatory cells. Eosinophils are the predominant inflammatory cell in about one-third of the canine and equine cases. Deposition of IgG at intercellular bridges in all layers of the suprabasilar epidermis or in the superficial epidermis demonstrated by immunofluorescence (IF) or immunohistochemistry (IHC) is a feature of PF but is not specific for PF. With immunostaining, there are frequent false negative results (poor lesion selection or prior glucocorticoid or immunosuppressive therapy) and false positive results (chronic skin lesions with plasma cells and secondary immunoglobulin diffusion into the epidermis), thus immunostaining must be interpreted carefully and in conjunction with clinical and histologic findings. Newer techniques that detect more specific antigens, such as desmoglein, and use of better substrates for indirect immunostaining may improve diagnostic accuracy of superficial forms of pemphigus in the future.

Pemphigus Vulgaris

Pemphigus vulgaris (PV) is a very severe form of pemphigus and has been reported in the dog and cat (see Table 17-11). In the dog, autoantibodies are formed against desmoglein-3, one of the prominent desmosomal proteins involved in adhesion of basal cells of the epidermis and mucosal epithelium. In addition, autoantibodies to other proteins involved in intercellular adhesion have been reported in some dogs with PV, including desmoglein-1. It is thought that the distribution patterns of desmoglein-3 in conjunction with desmoglein-1 in skin and oral mucosa in combination with antibodies to other proteins involved in intercellular adhesion result in vesicular lesions deep in the epidermis, oral mucosa, or both. Thus some forms of PV largely affect the oral mucosa (mucosal-dominant PV) whereas others affect the skin and oral mucosa (mucocutaneous PV). The deep vesicular lesions lead to formation of vesicles or secondary erosions and ulcers in the oral mucosa, at mucocutaneous junctions, and or skin subject to mechanical stress such as in the axilla or groin. Animals can be febrile, depressed, and anorectic and have leukocytosis. Drooling is often a presenting complaint, as involvement of the oral mucosa is almost always present. Microscopic lesions consist of separation of keratinocytes of the lower epidermis owing to loss of intercellular attachments. However, basal cell keratinocytes remain attached to the basement membrane, resulting in a suprabasilar vesicle leaving a row of basal cells attached to the basement membrane ("row of tombstones") (see Fig. 17-16). There usually is accompanying superficial perivascular to interface mixed inflammation. Direct IF or IHC reveal immunoglobulin and sometimes complement in the intercellular epidermis. Indirect IF has revealed circulating antikeratinocyte antibodies, typically toward desmoglein-3.

Paraneoplastic Pemphigus

Paraneoplastic pemphigus (PNP) is a rare, aggressive form of pemphigus associated with solid or hematopoietic neoplasms (see Table 17-11). PNP has been documented in humans and dogs. Cutaneous lesions can precede detection of the neoplastic process, and are resistant to treatment. Lesions consist of severe mucosal and mucocutaneous blistering and erosions. Histologically, lesions have a pattern of combined erythema multiforme and suprabasilar acantholysis resembling PV. Lymphohistiocytic cell–rich interface dermatitis with apoptosis of keratinocytes is present. In addition, lymphocytes border apoptotic keratinocytes (this is often called *lymphocytic satellitosis*). Labeling of intercellular bridges is detected by IHC or IF. In humans, immunoprecipitation reveals a typical set of five protein bands with molecular weights of 250, 230, 210, 190, and 170 kD. These protein bands have been identified as desmoplakin I and II, bullous pemphigoid antigen 1, envoplakin and periplakin. In dogs, immunoprecipitation has revealed the main antigen targets are 210 kD (envoplakin), 190 kD (periplakin), and a 130 kD protein that likely represents desmoglein-3. In addition, in one dog, immunoprecipitation also revealed other proteins, including 250 kD (desmoplakin-I), 210 kD (desmoplakin-II, a superposition of envoplakin), and 230 kD (bullous pemphigoid antigen I), whereas in another dog, immunoprecipitation revealed a 170 kD transmembrane molecule. Thus PNP in dogs is similar to that in humans.

Pemphigus Subtypes

Subtypes of pemphigus include pemphigus erythematosus, pemphigus vegetans, and "facially prominent" PF. Pemphigus erythematosus occurs in dogs and cats and is considered to be a variant of PF with a facial lesion distribution. Currently, there is insufficient clinical, histologic, immunologic, or prognostic evidence to clearly separate pemphigus erythematosus from facially predominant PF.

Pemphigus vegetans has very rarely been reported in dogs. Original designations of pemphigus vegetans in dogs were based on similarities to pemphigus vegetans in humans, a mucocutaneous condition in which pustules evolve into hyperplastic verrucous (vegetating) cutaneous lesions in conjunction with mucosal suprabasilar acantholysis as seen in PV. Antibodies to desmoglein-3 are identified in human patients, and sometimes, circulating autoantibodies to other proteins involved in intercellular adhesion have been identified. Some of the dogs diagnosed with pemphigus vegetans have not had oral lesions. In another dog with lesions suggestive of pemphigus vegetans antibodies to desmoglein-1 rather than desmoglein-3 were identified, thus the rare cases of pemphigus vegetans diagnosed in dogs to date are not directly comparable to those in the human.

Panepidermal pustular pemphigus (PPP) refers to a form of pemphigus in the dog that has some of the features of PF, pemphigus vegetans, and pemphigus erythematosus. It appears to represent a variant of PF. The term was originally developed when a facially predominant form of PF was identified in Akitas, Chows, and a few other breeds of dogs, and there appeared to be a need to reconsider the classification of pemphigus subtypes. The principal diagnostic feature used to distinguish dogs with PPP from those with PF is based solely on histopathology: the presence of acantholytic cell–containing pustules located in all layers of the epidermis and the follicular infundibular outer root sheath (e.g., pustules located in deeper epidermis than typical for PF). An explanation for the difference in pustule depth may simply reflect the regional variation in various antigens targeted by autoantibodies in different anatomic locations of canine skin. For example, it has been shown that desmoglein-1 can be identified on keratinocytes in all layers of the epidermis in skin from the dorsal muzzle, pinna, and pawpads, whereas desmoglein-1 is only detected in the upper layers of the epidermis in skin from the shoulder, groin, or abdomen. Thus the difference in desmoglein expression could influence pustule location. Further classification of subtypes of pemphigus require in-depth studies, including immunopathology, as well as the results of therapeutic trials.

Reactions Characterized Grossly by Vesicles or Bullae as the Primary Lesion and Histologically by Vesicles or Bullae within the Basement Membrane (Bullous Dermatoses)

Bullous dermatoses are a rare group of disorders caused by autoantibodies directed toward one or more antigens within the basement membrane zone (see the discussion on the basement membrane zone in the section on Morphology of the Skin and Table 17-11) and characterized clinically and histologically by vesicles and bullae. The disorders include bullous pemphigoid (autoantibodies against bullous pemphigoid antigen 2 [BPAG2; BP180], which is type XVII collagen, a hemidesmosomal transmembrane molecule), epidermolysis bullosa acquisita (autoantibodies against type VII collagen in the anchoring fibrils), linear IgA bullous dermatosis (autoantibodies against the 120-kD linear IgA bullous dermatosis antigen [LAD-1] in the upper lamina lucida), mucous membrane pemphigoid (laminin-5, collagen XVII, and integrin alpha-6 beta-4), and bullous systemic lupus erythematosus (autoantibodies against the noncollagenous amino terminus of type VII collagen) reported in one dog. Bullous pemphigoid is described as it affects the greatest number of species. Basic features of the other subepidermal bullous dermatosis are listed in Table 17-11.

Bullous Pemphigoid

Bullous pemphigoid (BP) is caused by autoantibodies directed against hemidesmosomal proteins. In humans, the autoantibodies are directed toward BPAG1, a 230-kD intercellular antigen, and BPAG2, also called type XVII collagen, a 180-kD hemidesmosomal transmembrane molecule. In animals, only BPAG2 has been identified. BP has been reported in the horse, Yucatan minipig, dog, and cat. Clinical lesions are similar between species and consist of vesicles, erosions, ulcers, and crusts. The location and severity of clinical lesions vary. In horses, lesions are severe and associated with systemic signs; involve the oral mucosa, the squamous lining of the esophagus, and the stomach in some cases; and are generalized in the skin (Fig. 17-63). In Yucatan minipigs, lesions are usually limited to the skin of the back and rump. Dogs are usually mildly affected and have cutaneous lesions in the skin of the abdomen and axillae, concave pinnae, or mucocutaneous junctions. Oral lesions occur in about half the dogs. Cats usually have few lesions limited to the face and oral mucosa. Separation of the hemidesmosomes of the basal layer cells from the upper lamina lucida of the basement membrane leads to the microscopic lesions of vesicles and bullae, often with eosinophils and neutrophils in the superficial dermis or within the subepidermal vesicles. Lesions in dogs and pigs have more inflammatory cells than those in horses and cats. Direct immunofluorescence staining most commonly reveals IgG and in some dogs, complement linearly distributed at the dermoepidermal junction. Evaluation of salt-split epithelial substrates with indirect IF reveals staining on the epithelial side of the artificial split, helping to differentiate BP from epidermolysis bullosa acquisita and mucous membrane pemphigoid that are located in the sublamina densa or lower lamina lucida, respectively. The presence of eosinophils is considered to be suggestive of bullous pemphigoid.

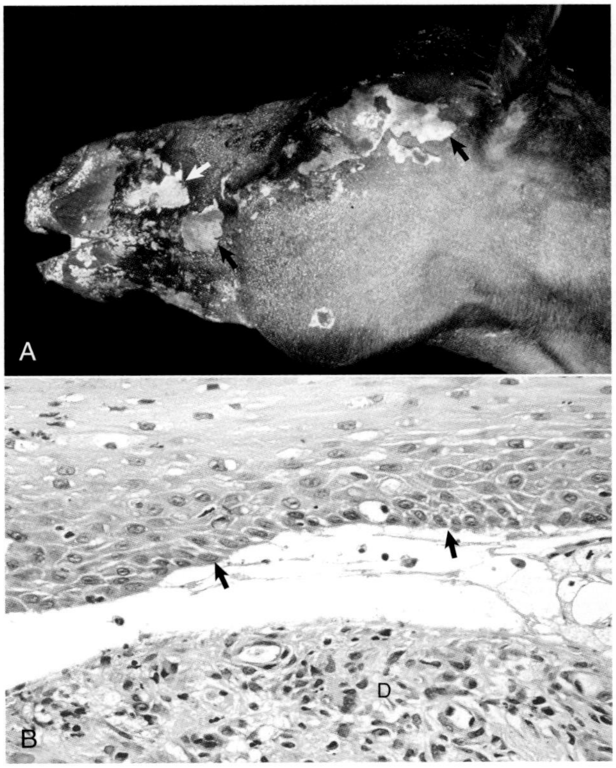

Fig. 17-63 **Bullous pemphigoid-like dermatitis, skin.**
A, Bullous pemphigoid-like dermatitis, face, horse. Severe ulceration and hemorrhage are present in the skin, especially lateral to and above the eye, on the nose, and on the chin. Both cutaneous and mucocutaneous sites of the body lined by stratified squamous epithelium were affected. The epidermis had separated easily from the underlying dermis, leading to the formation of vesicles, bullae, and areas of ulceration *(arrows)*. **B,** Subepidermal bullous dermatosis, dog. Note subepidermal vesicle formed when the intact epidermis, including the stratum basale *(arrows)* separated from the dermis *(D)*. H&E stain. (**A** courtesy Dr. S. Terrell, College of Veterinary Medicine, University of Florida. **B** courtesy Dr. Ann M. Hargis, DermatoDiagnostics.)

Reactions Characterized Grossly by Depigmentation, Pleomorphic Papular to Macular Eruptions, or Ulceration and Histologically by Basal Cell or Keratinocyte Degeneration

Systemic Lupus Erythematosus

Systemic lupus erythematosus (SLE) is a multiorgan disease of dogs and rarely cats and horses. Factors involved in development include genetic predisposition, viral infections, hormones, and UV light. SLE is a disease of immune dysregulation, with abnormalities in both cellular and humoral immunity, including defective T lymphocyte suppressor function and cytokine dysregulation. The defective T lymphocyte suppression function may be caused by anti–T lymphocyte antibodies or a primary suppressor T lymphocyte deficiency. The defective T lymphocyte suppression function results in B lymphocyte hyperactivity and in the formation of autoantibodies to a variety of membrane and soluble antigens, including nucleic acids. Antibodies are also directed to organ-specific antigens, clotting factors, and cells (e.g., erythrocytes, leukocytes, and platelets). The antinuclear antibody titer should be positive. Although the autoantibodies can damage tissue, the principal mechanism of injury in SLE occurs via antigen-antibody binding (i.e., immune-complex formation), and deposition of the antigen-antibody complexes in a variety of tissues, including skin.

The deposition of these immune complexes, which in the skin occurs at the basement membrane and in the walls of dermal blood vessels, results in a type III hypersensitivity response. Lesions are intensified by exposure to UV light. The enhanced damage may occur via UV-induced expression of nuclear antigens on the keratinocyte surface, autoantibody binding to the newly expressed antigens with resultant keratinocyte damage, and release of keratinocyte cytokines (e.g., IL-1, IL-6, and TNF-α). UV light may also act by inducing the expression of adhesion molecules, thus facilitating trafficking of leukocytes to the epidermis. Systemic signs are variable but can include polyarthritis, fever, anemia, proteinuria (from glomerulonephritis), and thrombocytopenia.

Cutaneous lesions are highly variable, can be localized or generalized, but commonly involve the face, pinnae, and distal extremities. Lesions consist of erythema, depigmentation, alopecia, scaling, crusting, and ulceration. Stomatitis or panniculitis can be present. Microscopic lesions include lymphohistiocytic interface dermatitis with basal cell apoptosis, pigmentary incontinence, and the presence of subepidermal vacuolization. The basal cell degeneration and subepidermal vacuolization can lead to formation of subepidermal vesicles, which can rapidly ulcerate and crust. Basement membrane thickening caused by accumulation of immune complexes, and immune-complex vasculitis of small dermal vessels can also be seen.

Discoid lupus erythematosus (DLE), also called *localized cutaneous lupus erythematosus* and *photosensitive nasal dermatitis,* is seen most commonly in the dog but is rare in the horse. Historically, DLE has been considered to be a mild variant of SLE in which there is no involvement of other organ systems and the antinuclear antibody titer is negative. However, with the recent recognition of another disease, "mucocutaneous pyoderma" (see the section on Superficial Bacterial Infections), and the clinical and histologic overlap between localized cutaneous lupus erythematosus and mucocutaneous pyoderma, the classification of DLE as a distinct entity is being revisited. Investigative studies are needed to better define these two conditions. Clinical lesions of DLE consist of depigmentation, erythema, scaling, erosion, ulceration, and crusting, and generally occur in the skin of the nasal planum, dorsal surface of the nose, and less commonly, the pinnae, lips, periocular region, and rarely in the oral mucosa. The nasal planum may lose the normal surface architecture and become atrophic, scarred, and bleed easily when traumatized. DLE can be exacerbated by sunlight. Microscopic lesions include accumulations of lymphocytes and plasma cells at the epidermal dermal interface. In early cases the infiltrate can be sparse, but in some cases the lymphocytes and plasma cells are arranged in a dense bandlike pattern that obscures the epidermal-dermal interface. In addition, there are apoptotic basal cells resulting in loss of epidermal pigment that is phagocytosed by dermal macrophages (pigmentary incontinence). As with SLE, the basal cell degeneration can, in more severe cases, lead to subepidermal vesicles, loss of the epidermis, and ulceration and crusting. Other forms of lupus erythematosus also uncommonly occur in dogs.

Exfoliative cutaneous lupus erythematosus is formerly known as *lupoid dermatosis of the German shorthair pointer.* Lesions develop in German shorthair pointers between 3 months and 3 years of age. Clinical lesions consist of scaling and crusting first seen on the face, ears, and back. Lesions then become generalized. The lesions persist but wax and wane. Fever and lymphadenopathy can be present. Rarely, there is a positive antinuclear antibody titer. Histologic lesions consist of lymphocytic interface dermatitis with hydropic degeneration of basal cells and apoptosis of keratinocytes. Interface inflammation also affects the basilar epithelium of follicles and sebaceous glands, resulting in sebaceous gland atrophy.

Vesicular cutaneous lupus erythematosus is a disorder formerly known as *ulcerative dermatosis of the collie and Shetland sheepdog.* Lesions develop in middle age to older dogs. The Shetland sheepdog and collie appear predisposed to lesion development. Dogs with this form of lupus have a negative antinuclear antibody titer, but some have antibodies to extractable (soluble) nuclear antigens (e.g., Ro/SSA and La/SSB). Clinical lesions develop most commonly in the groin and axillary areas but may also occur in the mucocutaneous junctions around eyes, mouth, external genitalia, and anus. Lesions consist of vesicles and bullae that progress to ulcers. Lesions can be cyclic, and worsen in association with estrus. Lesions also tend to occur in spring and summer; season plus location in less-haired areas has suggested a possible role for sunlight in the pathogenesis of lesions. Histologic lesions include interface lymphocytic dermatitis with hydropic degeneration of basal cells, keratinocyte apoptosis, and extensive vesicles and bullae at the epidermal-dermal junction that progress to ulcers. Mixed inflammation is present in ulcerated lesions and subepidermal fibrosis may be extensive.

Lupus panniculitis is a rare manifestation of lupus erythematosus and is seen in dogs. Clinical lesions consist of nodules occurring predominantly in the subcutis of the trunk and proximal aspects of the legs. Histologic lesions consist of nodular masses of lymphoplasmacytic and histiocytic inflammation often with fat necrosis. Vasculitis can also be present. In addition, there may be apoptotic basal cell degeneration, pigmentary incontinence, and thickening of the basement membrane.

Immunostaining in cases of lupus erythematosus may reveal the presence immunoglobulin and sometimes complement or both at the basement membrane zone.

Erythema Multiforme, Stevens-Johnson Syndrome, and Toxic Epidermal Necrolysis

Erythema multiforme (EM), Stevens-Johnson syndrome (SJS), and toxic epidermal necrolysis (TEN) are uncommon to rare conditions affecting the skin and sometimes mucous membranes. They have been reported in humans, horses, cattle, dogs, and cats. They have been studied most extensively in the human and less so in the dog. Until recently, the conditions were considered to represent different ends of a spectrum of disease from mild (EM) to severe (TEN). However, in-depth studies scrutinizing the character and extent of clinical and histologic lesions in correlation with the clinical history have prompted a modification. Currently, EM in humans is considered to be a separate entity usually associated with infection, particularly with herpesviruses. Stevens-Johnson syndrome and TEN most often represent adverse reactions to drug therapy. Classification of EM, SJS, and TEN in animals is controversial. The results of a multicenter study aimed at better defining these conditions in animals suggested SJS and TEN were more likely to be associated with drug exposure, whereas EM was unlikely to be associated with drug exposure, but the cause or causes of EM in animals remains unclear. A variety of causes for EM (bacterial infection, diet, drugs, and neoplasia) have been proposed, but usually not proved. One dog with EM-like lesions had parvovirus infection. Drugs (sulfonamides, cephalexin, levamisole, and others) appear to be the main cause of SJS and TEN in animals, but drug causation is not usually proved because of the unwillingness to purposely reexpose a patient to the suspected offending drug. The pathogenesis in EM is thought to involve a cell-mediated (type IV) immune response directed against antigens (foreign peptides that are components of infectious agents, drugs, or others) expressed on the surface of keratinocytes. A main effector cell is the cytotoxic T lymphocyte ($CD8^+$ lymphocyte) that recognizes and binds to the foreign peptide-MHC I complex on the surface of keratinocytes (see Table 17-10) resulting in apoptosis. In EM the apoptosis of keratinocytes is patchy, whereas in SJS and TEN, it is more extensive to confluent. The pathogenesis for the more extensive apoptosis in SJS and TEN is unclear, but in humans, it is thought to involve the binding of a transmembrane receptor (called *FasL*) to its corresponding receptor (Fas) expressed on the surface of keratinocytes. Soluble FasL is increased in serum of patients with TEN, and the binding of FasL to Fas causes keratinocyte apoptosis via activation of an intracellular enzyme cascade. The inability to remove the drug metabolites probably also contributes.

In animals, EM has been studied most extensively in dogs and is characterized clinically initially by polymorphous, coalescing circular areas of erythema. The erythema disappears from the center of the lesions, producing targetlike lesions that are most common on the trunk, axillae, and groin. Papules, vesicles, ulcers, erosions, and serpiginous erythematous lesions also can be seen (see Fig. 17-12). EM can occur in minor or major forms, depending on the extent of clinical involvement. In EM minor, mucosal surfaces are usually not involved or mucosal involvement is restricted to one site. In contrast, more extensive mucous membrane and cutaneous involvement are seen in EM major, referred to as *Stevens-Johnson syndrome* (SJS) by some pathologists. Histologically, individual keratinocytes in all layers of the epidermis undergo apoptosis (see Fig. 17-12) and are surrounded by lymphocytes (lymphocytic satellitosis). Apoptotic keratinocytes can coalesce, leading to the clinically visible erosions and possibly ulcers. There are perivascular mononuclear cells in the dermis with minor obscuring of the epidermal dermal interface.

In animals, TEN is seen principally in dogs and cats, is a much more serious condition than EM, and may overlap in the spectrum of gross and histologic lesions with SJS. TEN is a life-threatening, severe ulcerative disorder of the skin and oral mucous membranes that begins clinically as widespread erythematous macules that coalesce. Later there is full-thickness epidermal detachment that results in large subepidermal bullae and widespread ulceration as the confluently apoptotic (necrotic) epidermis is sloughed. Lesions are often present on the face, mucocutaneous junctions, and pawpads, but can be more widespread. Histologically there is full-thickness coagulative necrosis of the epidermis, with separation of the epidermis from the dermis forming bullae, which detach and leave the dermis denuded. Dermal inflammation in the acute lesions is minimal. The lesions in acute TEN are distinguished from thermal burns, by the lack of dermal necrosis in TEN. The diagnosis of EM and SJS requires both clinical, as well as histologic, findings because it is not possible to distinguish these conditions by histopathology alone. The extent of clinical involvement including presence of absence of mucosal lesions is paramount.

Reactions Characterized Grossly by Hemorrhage, Edema, Necrosis, Ulceration, Infarction, or by Alopecia and Scarring and Histologically by Vasculitis or Thrombosis

The diagnosis of cutaneous vasculitis is challenging because it can be difficult to distinguish between inflammatory cells targeting a vessel from inflammatory cells simply migrating through a vessel physiologically to reach an area of inflammation elsewhere in the epidermis or dermis. Disproportionate numbers of inflammatory cells in the vessel wall in comparison to the surrounding dermis suggest the vessel is a target of the inflammation. Vasculitis can be primary or secondary to systemic processes such as drug ingestion (e.g., sulfonamides), connective tissue disease (e.g., SLE), infections (e.g., *Rickettsia rickettsii*, *Erysipelothrix rhusiopathiae*), or it may be incidental to a local process such as ulceration or a thermal burn. In many instances, the cause of the vasculitis is unknown (idiopathic). Two principal mechanisms are thought to contribute to the pathogenesis of vasculitis; these include direct invasion of vessels by infectious agents (e.g., *Rickettsia*, herpesvirus) and immune-mediated mechanisms (e.g., allergic, antibody-mediated cytotoxic, immune complex, or cell mediated). The type of inflammatory cell may suggest the pathogenesis. For example, eosinophils may predominate in allergic reactions (arthropod bites or collagenolytic granulomas), neutrophils may predominate in immunologic reactions associated with immune complex deposition (lupus erythematosus, some drug reactions), and lymphocytes may predominate in cell-mediated immune responses (malignant catarrhal fever). However, the cell type may simply reflect stage of disease rather than the mechanism. In animals, type III hypersensitivity reactions (immune complex–mediated processes) are thought to contribute to many cases of immunologic vasculitis, but it is likely that multiple immunologic mechanisms contribute. Evidence for the role of immune-complex deposition is derived from experimental studies (Arthus phenomenon and serum sickness) and from identification of immune complexes in serum and tissues in patients with vasculitis caused by infectious agents and hypersensitivity reactions to drugs. Thus infectious agents can contribute to immune complex–mediated vasculitis. The immune complexes can form in the circulation, in the vessel wall, or both.

Small arterioles, capillaries, and postcapillary venules are most the most commonly affected vessels. Involvement of the deep vascular plexuses suggests a systemic component is contributing to the vasculitis. Clinical lesions include edema and hemorrhage and in severe cases in which thrombosis can develop, ischemic necrosis and infarction. Ulceration and sometimes sloughing of the skin can occur. In some cases, partial ischemia leading to alopecia and scarring are the main features. Histologic lesions may include the presence of variable numbers of intramural inflammatory cells, intramural or perivascular edema, hemorrhage, or fibrin exudation. Necrosis and fibrin exudation (fibrinoid necrosis) can occur but are rarely seen in small animals. Thrombosis may develop. There is often significant overlap in the clinical and histologic lesions of vasculitis, depending on the severity and stage of disease at the time lesions are examined. Vasculitis is most common in horses and dogs and is rare in cattle, sheep, pigs, and cats.

Vasculitis in Horses

Purpura hemorrhagica

Purpura (from the Latin meaning purple) are red or purple macules or patches caused by hemorrhage in the skin or mucous membranes. Purpura hemorrhagica in the horse occasionally develops as a sequela to *Streptococcus equi* infection and more rarely is seen after other infections or vaccinations. The clinical lesions of subcutaneous edema and petechial and sometimes ecchymotic hemorrhages of the skin and mucous membranes develop as a consequence of immune-complex vasculitis. There may be serum exudation of distal extremities. Severely edematous areas may ooze serum and become necrotic and slough. Microscopic lesions consist of vascular wall disruption by neutrophils (neutrophilic vasculitis), perivascular edema, hemorrhage, and fibrin exudation.

Pastern leukocytoclastic vasculitis

Pastern leukocytoclastic vasculitis may represent a photoenhanced dermatosis; however, the cause and pathogenesis are unknown. Sun exposure appears to trigger lesion development in some horses, but lesions do not always resolve with removal from sun exposure. The disease is not considered a form of photosensitization because liver function is normal and exposure to photosensitizing chemicals has not been documented. Lesions typically develop in the white-haired legs, but rarely, similar lesions occur in legs covered with dark hair. Lesions initially consist of well-demarcated erythematous, moist, and crusted areas. More chronic lesions consist of plaques of epidermal acanthosis, hyperkeratosis, and crusting. Microscopically, lesions occur in small, thin-walled vessels of superficial dermal papillae. Early changes include vessel wall degeneration or necrosis and thrombosis. There is controversy regarding the presence of inflammation and true vasculitis. Although leukocytoclasia of neutrophils is described, the failure to demonstrate active vasculitis in many cases leads some veterinary dermatologists and pathologists to the preference of the term *vasculopathy.* Chronic changes include thickening and hyalinization of vessel walls. Epidermal changes include degeneration and hyperplasia, depending on stage of the disease. There may be mixed perivascular inflammation.

Vasculitis in Ruminants

Vasculitis is rare in cattle. It is seen with malignant catarrhal fever (see Chapters 4 and 7). Capripoxvirus causing lumpy skin disease in cattle causes damage to endothelial cells resulting in vasculitis that is central to the pathogenesis of lesions in this condition. Systemic infection with *Salmonella dublin* can also cause gangrene of the distal extremities, tail, and pinnae as a result of endotoxin-associated venous thrombosis.

Vasculitis in sheep and goats is also rare and is seen as part of systemic capripoxvirus infections (see the section on Viral Infections).

Vasculitis in Pigs

Vasculitis is uncommon to rare in pigs, and usually is seen in association with bacterial infection such as *Erysipelothrix rhusiopathiae,* and Gram-negative septicemias caused by *Salmonella, Pasteurella,* or *Escherichia coli* (discussed in the section on Bacterial Infections).

In addition, a condition called *porcine dermatitis and nephropathy syndrome,* predominantly affecting the vessels in the skin and kidneys, has been described. The incidence is usually low (less than 1%); however, epizootics where the incidence reaches 10% to 20% or higher have been described. Mortality is high (80% to 90%). The cause and pathogenesis are unknown, but the condition may be associated with infection with porcine circovirus 2, porcine reproductive and respiratory syndrome (PRRS) virus, or *Pasteurella multocida.* Immune complex deposition is thought to play a role. Immunoglobulin and complement have been detected in cutaneous vessel walls and glomeruli. Clinical lesions consist of cutaneous erythematous to hemorrhagic papules, macules, and plaques that are most severe on the hind limbs, ventral abdomen, flanks, and perineum. Necrosis and ulceration may develop. Histologic lesions are necrotizing vasculitis with hemorrhage, edema, and fibrin deposition affecting small and medium-sized arteries of the skin, kidney and other tissues.

Vasculitis in Dogs

Dermatomyositis and similar disorders with cutaneous and vascular lesions (ischemic dermatopathy)

Dermatomyositis is an inherited disease with variable expressivity that occurs in juvenile and adult onset forms in collies and Shetland sheepdogs (Fig. 17-64). Other breeds are occasionally affected. The pathogenesis involves vasculitis of skin, muscle, and sometimes other tissues. The vascular lesions are subtle and include mild thickening of the vessel wall, occasionally pyknotic cells in the vessel wall, and occasionally lymphocytes within the wall; these changes are termed *cell-poor vasculitis.* Circulating immune complexes have been identified and likely play a role. Dermatomyositis develops in puppies as early as 8 weeks of age. Early lesions include vesicular dermatitis of face, lips, and external ears, which progresses to involve the distal extremities, especially over bony prominences and the tip of the tail. Myositis and atrophy of muscles of mastication, distal extremities, and sometimes, of the esophagus develop after

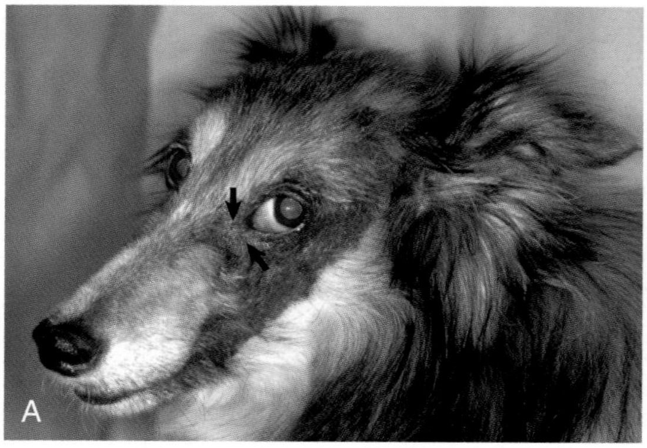

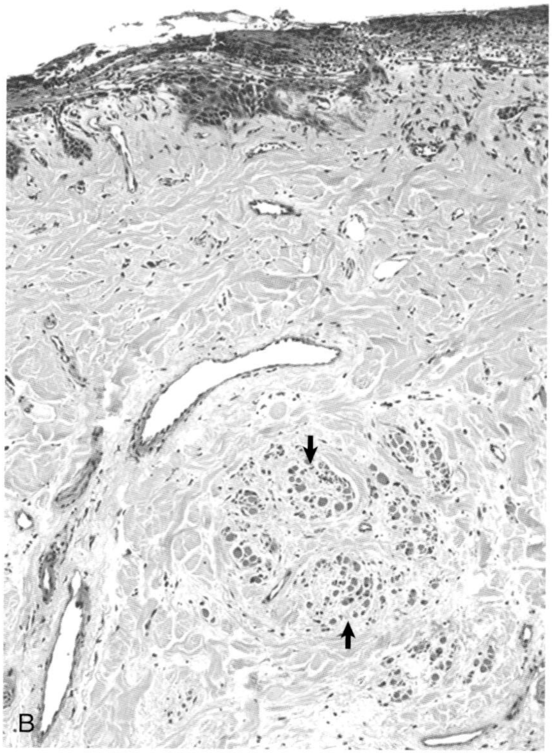

Fig. 17-64 Dermatomyositis, skin, dog.
A, Face. Chronic lesions of hair loss, hyperpigmentation, and scarring are present in the skin around the eye and on the lateral side of the face. Interface dermatitis, myositis, and vasculitis have resulted in ischemic follicular atrophy, muscle atrophy, and scarring. The scarring and possibly also some muscle atrophy have contributed to the contraction of the skin of the eyelid and the inability to close the eyelids fully at the medial canthus *(arrows).* **B,** Lip. Erosion is present on the surface of the lip skin at the far right. Atrophy of the adnexa, not present here, and dermis can predispose to injury of the epidermis and superficial dermis by minor trauma. Muscle atrophy *(arrows)* and scarring around the muscle fibers are present. If muscle is present in skin biopsy samples with features of dermatomyositis and if muscle atrophy or myositis are seen, the diagnosis of dermatomyositis is strengthened. H&E stain. (Courtesy Dr. Ann M. Hargis, DermatoDiagnostics.)

the dermatitis (see Fig. 17-64). The myositis is variably severe and multifocal, but more prevalent in peripheral anatomic locations. The muscle inflammation consists of lymphocytes, plasma cells, histiocytes, and fewer neutrophils or eosinophils. Perifascicular myofiber atrophy (atrophy at the periphery of muscle fascicles) occurs occasionally. The rostral and most superficial portion of the temporalis muscle is the biopsy site of choice to confirm the myositis. Dermatomyositis varies in severity. Mild skin lesions heal without scarring, but moderate skin lesions heal with permanent foci of alopecia, hyperpigmentation, and scarring. Hypopigmentation can also develop from damage to melanin-containing cells in the basal layer of the epidermis. Skin and muscle lesions in dogs with severe disease are progressive and disfiguring, the result of severe scarring of the skin and atrophy of muscle. Microscopic skin lesions include interface dermatitis with basal cell degeneration of the epidermis and follicular wall, variable epidermal vesicles and pustules, follicular atrophy, and dermal scarring. Cell-poor vasculitis, a major feature contributing to the lesions in dermatomyositis, is not always identified in small biopsy samples. The combination of interface dermatitis and mural folliculitis with follicular atrophy and cell-poor vasculitis has been considered to represent ischemic lesions, and is referred to as *ischemic dermatopathy.*

Skin and vessel lesions indistinguishable from those in dermatomyositis (e.g., ischemic dermatopathy) have developed in other ages and breeds of dogs sometimes in association with vaccination and have been organized into the following groups: (1) juvenile dogs other than collies and Shetland sheepdogs without known breed predilection to dermatomyositis, and sometimes with temporal association with vaccination; (2) dogs with localized reactions to subcutaneous injection of killed rabies and sometimes other killed vaccines; (3) dogs with more generalized postrabies vaccine–associated disease, and (4) dogs with generalized ischemic dermatopathy in which correlation with previous vaccination cannot be documented.

Rabies vaccine–induced ischemic dermatitis develops as a localized form limited to the site of vaccination and as a more widespread form, both developing in the months after rabies vaccination. Poodles, Yorkshire and Silky terriers, and other soft-coated breeds of dogs are predisposed to the localized form but it can occur in any breed. In the localized form, an alopecic, hyperpigmented patch of atrophic skin appears at the site of vaccination. Microscopically, in addition to lesions of *ischemic dermatopathy*, mild chronic lymphocytic cell-poor vasculitis, a mild diffuse increase in mononuclear cells throughout the dermis, and lymphocytic panniculitis are present. Rabies antigen has been detected in follicular epithelial cells and in vessels in affected skin. In the widespread form, lesions are present at the site of vaccination, ear margins, periocular skin, and skin over bony prominences, tip of tail, and pawpads. Lingual erosions and ulcers also occur. In addition, some dogs develop perifascicular muscle atrophy and perimysial fibrosis, with C5b-9 in the microvasculature. The microscopic lesions are similar to the localized form with the addition of possible muscle lesions. The development of lesions after vaccination and the identification of rabies-virus antigen in the vessels and follicular epithelial cells in dogs with the localized form of rabies vaccine–induced dermatitis have resulted in the speculation that lesions might be a result of an immunologic reaction to viral antigen in these sites in genetically predisposed dogs.

Familial vasculopathy of German shepherd dogs

Familial vasculopathy of German shepherd dogs appears to have a genetic basis, but the underlying cause and pathogenesis are unknown. Cutaneous and vascular lesions have similarities to ischemic dermatopathy. Puppies, about 1 to 2 months of age, are affected, and some puppies develop lesions after vaccination. The major clinical lesion is swelling of pawpads, and some puppies develop ulcers on the pawpads, ear margins, tail tip, and nasal planum with depigmentation of the nasal planum or nasal commissures. Histologically, early vessel lesions include neutrophil infiltration of small venules and arterioles, but more commonly, vascular lesions are subtle and consist of cell-poor vasculitis (mild thickening of the vessel wall with occasional pyknotic cells and lymphocytes within the wall). In addition, cutaneous lesions consist of mild interface dermatitis with pigmentary incontinence. The nodular lesions in pawpads are in the dermis and subcutis, and early lesions consist of focal collagen degeneration bordered by neutrophils and mononuclear cells. Chronic lesions have dermal and subcutaneous fibrosis sometimes accompanied by degeneration and fibrosis of skeletal muscle bundles.

Cutaneous and renal glomerular vasculopathy of the greyhound

Greyhounds with cutaneous and renal glomerular vasculopathy are typically from race track environments. The cause and pathogenesis are unknown; however, there is speculation that the disorder is similar to hemolytic-uremic syndrome in humans in which a verotoxin (Shiga-like toxin) damages vascular endothelium. Most racing greyhounds eat raw meats, which could contain the *Escherichia coli*–producing toxin. Clinical lesions include hemorrhagic macules that progress to deep ulcers of the tarsus, stifle, or inner thigh. Occasionally, lesions develop on the front legs, groin, or trunk. Lesions heal slowly (usually over 1 to 2 months) by fibrosis. Histologically, capillaries, venules, and arterioles in the dermis and occasionally the subcutis have degenerate walls with pyknotic or karyorrhectic nuclei, as well as occasional fibrinoid necrosis. Fibrin thrombi can result in cutaneous infarction. About 25% of the affected greyhounds also have systemic signs of renal failure because of glomerular arteriolar inflammation, necrosis, and thrombosis.

Cold Agglutinin Disease

Information on this topic is available at evolve.elsevier.com/Zachary/McGavin/.

Vasculitis in Cats

Information on this topic is available at evolve.elsevier.com/Zachary/McGavin/.

DISORDERS WITH ALOPECIA OR HYPOTRICHOSIS

Cutaneous endocrine disorders are due to imbalances in hormones and generally are manifested as nonpruritic, bilaterally symmetric alopecia or hypotrichosis (Box 17-10). The remainder of the hair coat is dull, dry, easily epilated, and fails to regrow after clipping. The epidermis is often hyperpigmented. These lesions are referred to as *endocrine alopecia.* In disorders associated with alterations in sex hormones, the alopecia often begins in the perineal and genital areas and can extend cranially. However, it is not uncommon for a cutaneous endocrine disorder to have asymmetric alopecia and epidermal hyperpigmentation along with secondary pyoderma or seborrhea. Microscopically, uncomplicated endocrine disorders of the skin consist of hyperkeratosis of superficial epidermis and of hair

BOX 17-10 Conditions with Prominent Alopecia or Hypotrichosis

ENDOCRINE DISORDERS
Hypothyroidism
Hyperadrenocorticism
Hyperestrogenism
Hypersomatotropism
Hyposomatotropism
Cyclical flank alopecia (pineal gland)

NONENDOCRINE HAIR CYCLE ABNORMALITIES
Postclipping alopecia
Telogen effluvium
Chemotherapy-associated alopecia

DISORDERS ASSOCIATED WITH EXCESSIVE GROOMING
Feline psychogenic alopecia
Feline hypersensitivity reaction

FOLLICULAR DYSPLASIA
OTHER CONDITIONS ASSOCIATED WITH ALOPECIA
Alopecia X*
Acquired pattern alopecia
Trauma-associated alopecia

*Alopecia X (synonyms: adrenal sex hormone alopecia, castration responsive dermatosis, growth hormone responsive dermatosis) is a poorly understood syndrome. Hormonal association has not been proved.

follicles; normal, atrophic, or hyperplastic epithelium; dilated follicles from hyperkeratosis; increased numbers of catagen or telogen hair follicles; lack of hair shafts in follicles; and increased epidermal pigmentation. These general features support the diagnosis of an endocrine disease but often are not sufficiently specific to be diagnostic for an individual endocrine disorder. Also, inflammation caused by secondary seborrhea or pyoderma frequently complicates the diagnosis. Selected clinical and histologic features of individual endocrine disorders (e.g., clinical evidence of cutaneous and muscle atrophy and histologic evidence of mineral deposition in the case of hyperglucocorticoidism) in conjunction with clinical testing are used to establish a more definitive diagnosis. Cutaneous endocrine disorders are more common in dogs than in cats, food animals, or horses.

Cutaneous Endocrine Disorders

Hypothyroidism

Deficiency of thyroid hormone develops most commonly in dogs and usually is caused by idiopathic thyroid atrophy and lymphocytic thyroiditis. Thyroid hormones play an essential role in normal growth and development of many organs, including the skin, and can result in a variety of systemic and cutaneous signs and lesions. In dogs, the hair follicle is considered to be an important target for thyroid hormones, where the hormones are thought to be necessary for the initiation of the anagen stage of the hair cycle. Clinical lesions of thyroid deficiency consist of a dull, dry, easily epilated hair coat that fails to regrow after clipping. Alopecia develops in areas of wear, including the tail, elbows, hips, around the neck (wear from the collar), and on the dorsal surface of the nose. Symmetric truncal alopecia is not as common as once thought. Microscopically, in areas of advanced alopecia, hair follicles are usually in the telogen stage of the hair cycle, generally without hair shafts (hairless telogen follicles). Follicular infundibular hyperkeratosis with plugging of the follicular opening is also present. Other histologic changes seen in some dogs with hypothyroidism include acanthosis of epidermis and follicular infundibular epithelium. Myxedema, an increase in dermal mucin resulting in dermal thickening, is a rare manifestation of canine hypothyroidism. Secondary staphylococcal infection can develop.

Hypothyroidism can also be the result of congenital iodine deficiency. Iodine deficiency develops in fetuses because of maternal ingestion of diets deficient in iodine or containing substances that interfere with production of thyroid hormones (goitrogens). These factors result in insufficient synthesis of thyroxine and reduced blood levels of thyroxine and triiodothyronine. The reduced levels of these hormones are detected by the hypothalamus and pituitary gland, stimulating secretion of thyrotropin and resulting in hyperplasia of the thyroid follicular cells. Regions of North America that are deficient in iodine include the Great Lakes Basin, the Rocky Mountains, the Northern Great Plains, the upper Mississippi Valley, and the Pacific Coast region. Paradoxically, maternal diets high in iodine can also result in congenital hypothyroidism. High blood iodine also interferes with one or more steps of thyroid hormone production, leading to low blood thyroxine levels, hypothalamic and pituitary stimulation, and secretion of thyrotropin. Congenital iodine deficiency can occur in any domestic animal but usually is seen in large animals; it is associated with the birth of dead fetuses or weak neonates. These neonates can have alopecia, and thyroid glands are usually enlarged because of the follicular cell hyperplasia.

Hyperadrenocorticism

Hyperadrenocorticism results in cutaneous lesions principally in dogs, less often in cats, and rarely in other domestic animals. It is usually caused by bilateral adrenal cortical hyperplasia secondary to a functional pituitary neoplasm, and less often by a functional adrenal cortical neoplasm or a functional nodule of cortical hyperplasia. Particularly in dogs, the administration of exogenous glucocorticoids is also a cause. In dogs, cutaneous lesions include endocrine alopecia that generally spares the head and extremities, thinning of the skin, comedones, increased bruising, poor wound healing, and increased susceptibility to infection (Fig. 17-65). Dystrophic calcification of the dermis of the dorsal cervical region, inguinal, and axillary areas can occur in dogs, particularly in iatrogenic hyperadrenocorticism (calcinosis cutis) (Fig. 17-66). Grossly, lesions of calcinosis cutis are firm, thickened, sometimes gritty, often ulcerated and alopecic crusted plaques or nodules (see Fig. 17-66). In cats, the dermal collagen fibers can be markedly thin and atrophic, resulting in extremely fragile skin that can tear with normal handling. Microscopically, the lesions of hyperadrenocorticism include epidermal, dermal, and follicular atrophy (see Fig. 17-65), and follicular hyperkeratosis. Hair follicles are in the telogen stage of the hair cycle and have lost their hair shafts (hairless telogen). In cats, the atrophic hair follicles often have brightly eosinophilic keratin (trichilemmal keratin) in the lumens, a feature considered highly suggestive of hyperadrenocorticism. Calcinosis cutis may develop in dogs (see Fig. 17-66). A foreign body reaction (granulomatous inflammation) and draining sinuses can develop in association with the calcium deposits.

Pituitary Dysfunction in the Horse

Tumors of the pars intermedia of the pituitary gland occur in older horses and can reach a large size, destroy the pituitary gland, and cause hypopituitarism and diabetes insipidus. The clinical signs in

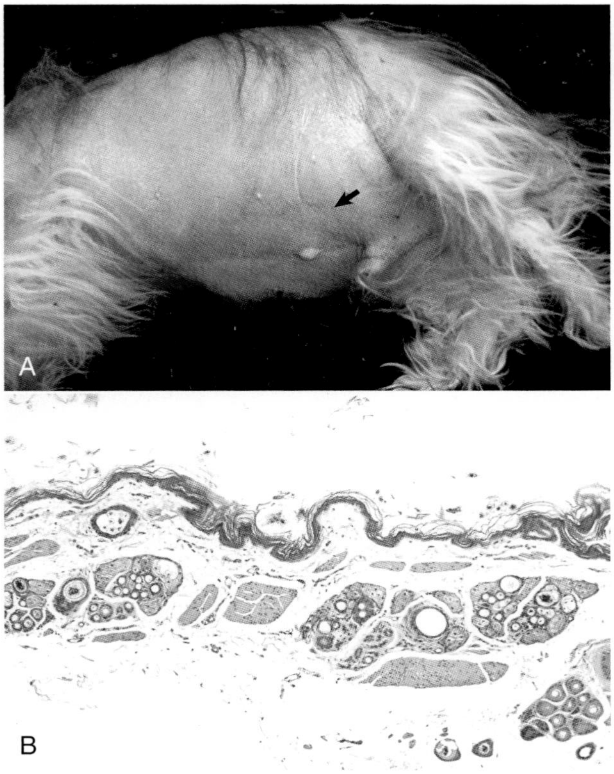

Fig. 17-65 Truncal alopecia, hyperadrenocorticism, skin, dog. **A,** Note the alopecia, distended abdomen, and thin skin in which blood vessels are faintly visible *(arrow)*. The distended abdomen and visibility of blood vessels are a result of protein catabolism and loss of muscle and dermal collagen, respectively. The distended abdomen and thin skin with greater visibility of blood vessels in conjunction with symmetric alopecia suggest that a catabolic endocrine disease, such as hyperadrenocorticism, is likely. **B,** Atrophy of dermal collagen fibers is so severe that the collagen has almost disappeared, leaving the adnexa and arrector pili muscles readily visible. Hair follicles are in the telogen (resting) stage of the hair cycle. H&E stain. (**A** courtesy Dr. Alan Mundell, Animal Dermatology Service. **B** courtesy Dr. Ann M. Hargis, DermatoDiagnostics.)

horses with pars intermedia pituitary tumors (polyphagia, polydipsia, polyuria, increased sweating, and an excessively long and thick hair coat) are largely mediated through dysfunction of the hypothalamus or neurohypophysis caused by an underlying expanding pituitary tumor. The long hair coat, also called *hypertrichosis* or *hirsutism,* is the result of failure to seasonally shed; cyclic shedding is mediated through the hypothalamus. Some tumors of the pars intermedia are functional and result in production of proopiomelanocortin (POMC), which is processed into high levels of various pars intermedia–derived peptides, including corticotropin-like intermediate lobe peptide, melanocyte-stimulating hormone, and beta endorphin, and much smaller levels of adrenocorticotropin. The combination of hypothalamic dysfunction and differential expression of pars intermedia–derived peptides over that of adrenocorticotropin result in a unique syndrome of hyperpituitarism in horses that differs from functional pituitary tumors in dogs and cats, which usually are associated with high levels of adrenocorticotropin. Some horses with large pituitary tumors also develop insulin-resistant hyperglycemia, which may be the result of downregulation of insulin receptors secondary to chronic polyphagia and hyperinsulinemia. Insulin resistance is associated with an increased prevalence of laminitis.

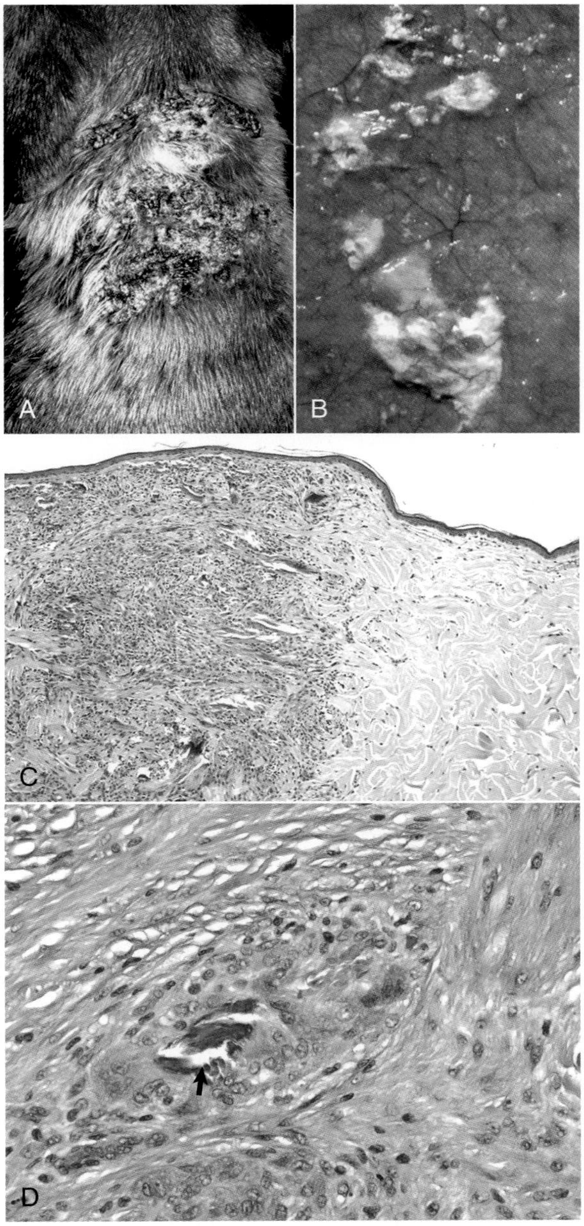

Fig. 17-66 Calcinosis cutis, hyperadrenocorticism, skin, dog. **A,** Dorsal neck. The skin is partially alopecic, ulcerated, and crusted. It is also palpably thickened. **B,** Subcutis. Mineral deposits are visible as white nodular foci. **C,** Skin at the margin of a plaque is thickened by dermal mineralization and granulomatous inflammation *(left half)*. H&E stain. **D,** Higher magnification of dermal mineralization *(arrow)* and granulomatous inflammation. H&E stain. (**A** courtesy Dr. Alan Mundell, Animal Dermatology Service. **B** courtesy Dr. M.D. McGavin, College of Veterinary Medicine, University of Tennessee. **C** and **D** courtesy Dr. Ann M. Hargis, DermatoDiagnostics.)

Hyperestrogenism

Hyperestrogenism can develop in male and female dogs. In females, the estrogen originates from ovarian cysts, rarely an ovarian neoplasm, or from estrogen administration. In males, elevated serum concentrations of estrogen are usually derived from a functional testicular Sertoli cell tumor. Iatrogenic estrogen administration has also caused hyperestrogenism in male dogs (Fig. 17-67). In addition to endocrine alopecia, female dogs have an enlarged vulva and abnormalities of the estrus cycle. Male dogs can develop

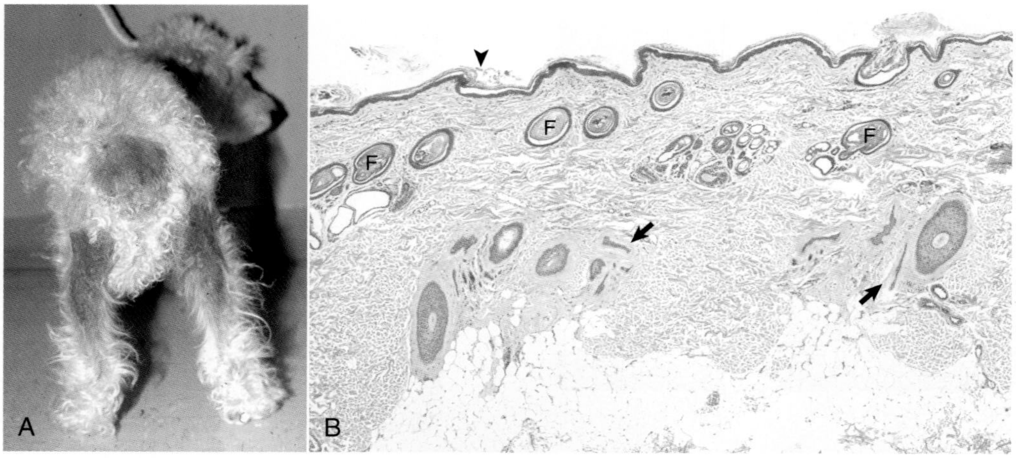

Fig. 17-67 **Symmetric alopecia and hyperpigmentation, hyperestrogenism (iatrogenic from diethylstilbestrol therapy), skin, dog.** **A,** Note the symmetric alopecia and hyperpigmentation over the caudal dorsal trunk and caudolateral hind legs. In male dogs, the symmetric alopecia in conjunction with enlargement of nipples, pendulous prepuce, and attraction of other male dogs suggest the possibility of hyperestrogenism. **B,** Note epidermal orthokeratotic hyperkeratosis *(arrowhead),* follicles dilated with keratin *(F),* and small atrophic follicles *(arrows)* in the telogen (resting) stage of the hair cycle. H&E stain. (Courtesy Dr. Ann M. Hargis, DermatoDiagnostics.)

gynecomastia, pendulous prepuce, or an enlarged prostate because of squamous metaplasia of prostatic ducts. Cutaneous microscopic lesions include orthokeratotic hyperkeratosis, follicular hyperkeratosis, and telogen follicles without hair shafts (hairless telogen) (see Fig. 17-67).

Hypersomatotropism

Hypersomatotropism rarely occurs in adult dogs and is a result of excess levels of growth hormone (somatotropin). The excess growth hormone can arise from acidophil tumors of the anterior pituitary gland, injection of pituitary gland extracts, administration of progestins, or with the metestrus (luteal) phase of the estrous cycle in intact female dogs. Elevated levels of growth hormone result in increased production of connective tissue, bone, and viscera. Clinical lesions consist of acromegaly (enlargement of parts of the skeleton, especially distal extremities) and thick, folded myxedematous skin over the head, neck, and extremities. The hair coat can be long and thick, and the claws can be thick and hard. Histologic lesions include thickened dermis caused by increased production of glycosaminoglycans and collagen by dermal fibroblasts. Myxedema is present in about a third of cases.

Hyposomatotropism

Deficiency of growth hormone in dogs younger than 3 months of age is usually the result of failure of the normal development of the pituitary gland leading to cyst formation. Deficiencies of thyroid, adrenal, and gonadal hormones are frequent accompanying problems. Pituitary deficiency results in failure to grow, retention of the puppy hair coat, and development of endocrine alopecia. Microscopically, the features are consistent with endocrine alopecia (e.g., hyperkeratosis of superficial epidermis and of hair follicles; normal or atrophic epithelium; follicular dilation from hyperkeratosis; increased numbers of telogen hair follicles; lack of hair shafts in follicles; and increased epidermal pigmentation). The numbers of dermal elastic fibers are reduced in the skin of some dogs.

Cyclical or Seasonal Flank Alopecia (Idiopathic Flank Alopecia)

Cyclical or seasonal flank alopecia develops more commonly in dogs living in northern latitudes. The cause of cyclical flank alopecia is not known, but changes in the photoperiod and thus melatonin released from the pineal gland might play a role. Many breeds are affected, but English bulldogs, boxers, and Airedale terriers are among the more commonly affected breeds. Alopecia develops seasonally or cyclically in the skin of the flank, usually bilaterally (Fig. 17-68). Histologically, follicles are in the telogen stage of the hair cycle, generally without hair shafts (hairless telogen), and primary follicles are markedly dilated and distorted by follicular hyperkeratosis. The follicular hyperkeratosis also distends the openings of secondary follicles as they enter the primary follicle, giving the follicles the distorted appearance of an upside-down "footprint" (see Fig. 17-68, *B*). The condition, as the name suggests, is often transient but can be recurrent.

Cutaneous Nonendocrine Disorders Associated with Hair Cycle Abnormalities

Postclipping Alopecia

Postclipping alopecia is a failure of the hair to regrow in apparently normal dogs after close clipping. The condition usually occurs in long-haired or heavily coated (plush-coated) breeds of dogs such as the Chow Chow. It is thought that heavily coated breeds of dogs have a prolonged telogen stage of the hair cycle, possibly to conserve energy by avoiding frequent cycles of shedding. Thus clipping when the hair coat is in a prolonged inactive stage of the hair cycle would result in lack of quick regrowth of the hair coat. The hair coat may not regrow until there is another significant growth phase, which may take 6 to 12 months. Most affected dogs regrow hair coat after they go through a cycle of heavy shedding. Histologic lesions consist of normal epidermis, dermis, and sebaceous glands and hair follicles in the telogen stage of the hair cycle, with prominent trichilemmal keratin resembling flame follicles but in which the hair shafts are retained.

Telogen Effluvium

Telogen effluvium develops when an animal is systemically ill or is severely stressed such as occurs with high fever, pregnancy and lactation, or anesthesia and surgery. The illness or stressful event triggers a sudden termination of the growth stage of follicles. This causes a majority of the hair follicles to synchronously enter the catagen and then telogen stages of the hair cycle. Gross lesions do

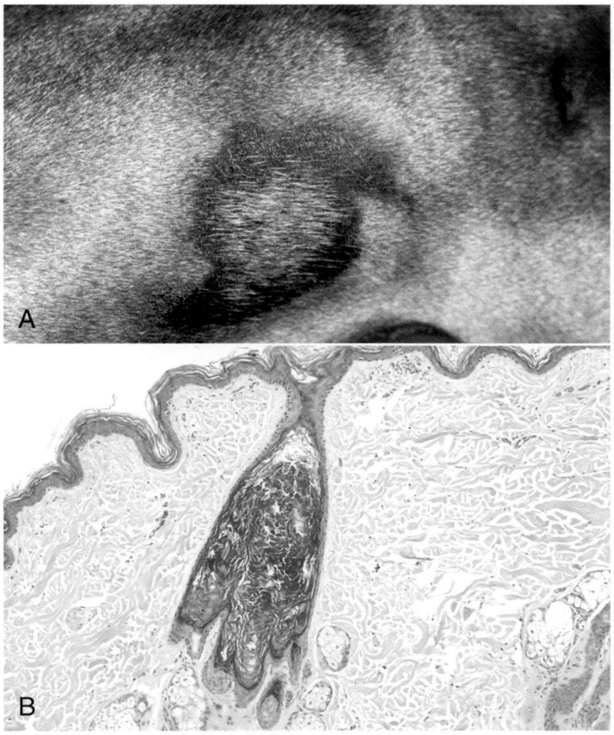

Fig. 17-68 Cyclical flank alopecia (seasonal flank alopecia), skin, dog. **A,** Alopecia and hyperpigmentation are present in the skin of the flank of a boxer dog. The breed of dog, location of the alopecia, and often cyclic nature of the condition suggest that cyclical flank alopecia is a likely diagnosis. Hair is regrowing in the central area of alopecia *(brown area within hyperpigmented zone),* indicating that lesions are resolving. **B,** Note the distorted follicle with dilations at the base. The follicle resembles an upside-down "footprint." This histologic feature, in conjunction with clinical history of cyclical flank lesions in the predisposed breeds, supports the diagnosis of this condition. H&E stain. (**A** courtesy Dr. David Duclos, Animal Skin and Allergy Clinic. **B** courtesy Dr. Ann M. Hargis, DermatoDiagnostics.)

not develop until about 1 to 3 months after the systemic illness or stress resolves, and the telogen (or inactive) follicles synchronously enter into the anagen stage of the hair cycle. When the new anagen hair shafts emerge from the follicle, the old telogen hair shafts are suddenly shed. The alopecia resolves as the new hair shafts emerge from the follicles, and the new hair coat becomes visible. Histologic changes vary with the time of biopsy sampling. In late stages (during the stage of excessive shedding), the skin and follicles are essentially normal and consist of the majority of follicles in the anagen stage of the hair cycle. In early stages (before shedding), telogen follicles predominate.

Chemotherapy-Associated Alopecia

Chemotherapy-associated alopecia is best documented in humans and occurs when there is a severe injury to the anagen (or growing) hair bulbs, and is thus called *anagen effluvium*. It is usually diagnosed clinically by examination of pulled hairs, so scalp biopsy sampling is rarely performed. It is the result of an injury that interrupts the mitotic activity of the epithelial cells in the hair bulb, which have the greatest proliferative activity. The abrupt cessation of mitotic activity is thought to lead to weakening of the partially keratinized proximal portion of the anagen hair shaft, which subsequently breaks at its narrowest point within the hair canal. The consequence of anagen effluvium is hair shedding that usually begins within a week or two after initiation of chemotherapy and is complete by 1 to 2 months after therapy. Because about 90% of human scalp hair is in the anagen phase, the hair loss is usually significant and alopecia obvious. Diagnosis can be made early in the course of hair loss by gently pulling out the damaged anagen hairs, which have narrow or pointed ends when examined microscopically. Diagnosis can also be made late in the course of hair loss after anagen hairs have been lost. Because telogen hair follicles are immune to this injury, they remain intact. Thus examination of hairs pulled during the late stage of hair loss reveals a vast majority of telogen hairs, essentially confirming the presence of anagen effluvium. Chemotherapy-associated alopecia also occurs in dogs and cats, but has not been well studied. In dogs, it has been reported most commonly with doxorubicin therapy and occurs in longer coated breeds such as poodles and old English sheepdogs, and also in some terrier breeds. The prolonged anagen hair phase in some of the longer haired breeds may explain why they are predisposed. The degree of hair loss varies substantially and depends on drug, dose, method of administration, and treatment schedule, as well as animal variables (dogs with long versus short anagen hair cycle phases). Hair loss may begin within 7 to 10 days, and is usually apparent within 1 to 2 months. The hair loss may be complete or partial (generalized thinning of the hair coat or loss of primary versus secondary hairs) and can affect different regions of the body (head and site of intravenous injection of the drug; skin of ventral trunk and medial legs; somewhat symmetrical involvement of facial skin). Hair loss can include vibrissae in both dogs and cats. With doxorubicin therapy, cutaneous hyperpigmentation is also present. Hair growth resumes after therapy is terminated, but the color or texture of the haircoat may be altered. Diagnosis is based on clinical history, physical examination, and examination of pulled hairs. Histopathologic examination has rarely been done and is not considered to be diagnostic. It has revealed a prominence of telogen follicles, which is more consistent with an early stage of telogen effluvium. The reason for this discrepancy is unknown, but may reflect stage of hair loss at time of biopsy sampling (late in the course of hair loss) or differences in hair follicle cycling, response to chemical injury, or regenerative capabilities between dogs and humans.

Alopecic Disorders Associated with Normal Follicles

Excessive grooming, particularly in cats, can result in symmetric alopecia or hypotrichosis that clinically resembles endocrine dermatoses. Excessive grooming can be the result of pruritus (usually associated with cutaneous hypersensitivity reactions) or allegedly from psychogenic problems such as boredom or stress (feline psychogenic alopecia). Thus it is important to determine if the alopecia or hypotrichosis is the result of excessive grooming, and if so, what the underlying stimulus is.

Feline Psychogenic Alopecia

Psychogenic alopecia occurs in cats of the more emotional breeds, including Siamese and Abyssinian, and possibly others. A partial alopecia is the result of the breaking of hairs from gentle but persistent licking. Linear or symmetric areas of alopecia are found along the caudal dorsal midline or in the perineal, genital, caudomedial thigh, or abdominal areas. Microscopically, the skin is generally normal, but there may be trichomalacia (twisted or broken hair shafts within hair follicles). The principal differential diagnosis is alopecia resulting from hypersensitivity (see next discussion). Endocrine-associated alopecia is rare in the cat.

Alopecia Caused by Hypersensitivity Reactions in the Cat

Clinical signs of alopecia caused by hypersensitivity reactions are often identical to those of feline psychogenic alopecia. Pruritus typically is the result of hypersensitivity reactions of a variety of causes (food allergy, parasitism, or atopy). Histologically, there is perivascular dermatitis, usually with eosinophils, mast cells, and lymphocytes. The inflammation helps to distinguish alopecia associated with hypersensitivity from that of feline psychogenic alopecia.

Disorders Associated with Dysplastic Follicles

Follicular Dysplasia Syndromes

Follicular dysplasia syndromes, defined as incomplete or abnormal development of follicles and hair shafts, comprise a group of generally poorly characterized disorders recognized most commonly in dogs but occasionally in horses, cattle, and cats. Clinical lesions are alopecia or hypotrichosis, and consequently, there is clinical resemblance to the endocrine disorders. Some of the more common follicular dysplasia syndromes are associated with coat color dilution (color dilution follicular dysplasia, color mutant alopecia) or occur in black versus white haired areas (black hair follicle dysplasia) (see Fig. 17-23). Microscopic features of follicular dysplasia vary with the syndrome. The conditions associated with coat color dilution or those that occur in black-haired areas have densely clumped melanin pigment in the hair bulb, hair shafts, and also in the basal layer of the epidermis (see Fig. 17-23). Lesions in other conditions include lipid distention of hair matrix cells, abnormally formed follicles or hair bulbs, and abnormal hair shafts. The microscopic features help to differentiate syndromes of follicular dysplasia from the endocrine dermatosis.

Other Conditions Associated with Alopecia

Alopecia X

Alopecia X (adrenal sex hormone alopecia, castration responsive dermatosis, growth hormone responsive dermatosis) is seen most often in breeds of dogs with plush hair coats (e.g., Pomeranian, Chow Chow, Samoyed, Keeshond, and Alaskan malamute). Toy and miniature poodles and sporadically other breeds of dogs are also affected. Dogs with this condition (or conditions) are grouped together by having in common (1) plush hair coats in the normal state (e.g., when not affected with this condition), (2) alopecia-sparing head and distal extremities, (3) normal thyroid and glucocorticoid levels, and (4) skin biopsy samples with telogen follicles that retain their hair shafts (haired telogen), and often prominent flame follicles (follicles with prominent trichilemmal keratin that forms spikes into the follicular stratum spinosum). The alopecia often develops at 1 or 2 years of age in otherwise healthy dogs of either sex. The alopecia is symmetric and involves the perineum, caudal thighs, ventral abdomen and thorax, neck, and trunk. The head and distal extremities are spared. Hyperpigmentation is usually present (Fig. 17-69). Thyroid function testing, adrenocorticotropic hormone (ACTH) response test, low-dose dexamethasone suppression test, and serum chemistry results are normal. Although abnormalities in a number of hormones have been detected, the cause of this condition remains unknown. Microscopic lesions include haired telogen follicles and prominent and diffuse formation of flame follicles (Fig. 17-69, *B*). Prominent diffuse flame follicle formation is suggestive of alopecia X, but flame follicles can be seen in other endocrine dermatoses (hyperestrogenism and hyperadrenocorticism, particularly in plush-coated breeds), and in follicular dysplasia of the Siberian husky. Follicles similar to flame follicles but with less exaggerated trichilemmal keratin spikes and with hair shafts retained are seen in normal plush-coated breeds of dogs and in post clipping alopecia. Epidermal hyperpigmentation and dermal atrophy are variable.

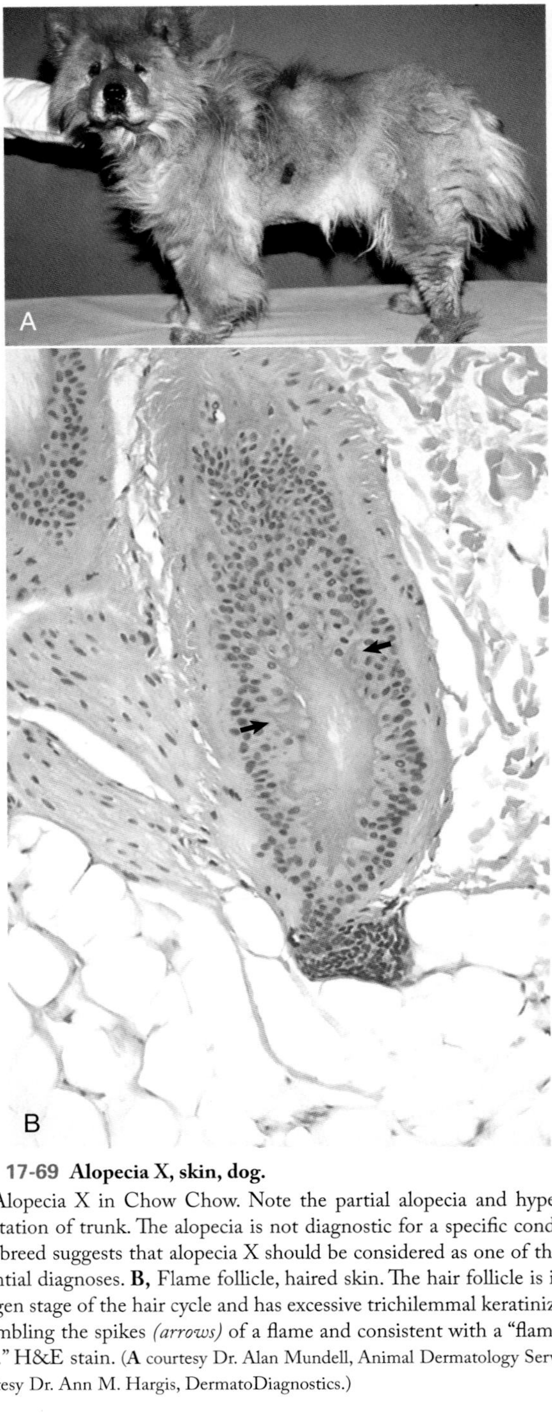

Fig. 17-69 Alopecia X, skin, dog.
A, Alopecia X in Chow Chow. Note the partial alopecia and hyperpigmentation of trunk. The alopecia is not diagnostic for a specific condition. The breed suggests that alopecia X should be considered as one of the differential diagnoses. **B,** Flame follicle, haired skin. The hair follicle is in the telogen stage of the hair cycle and has excessive trichilemmal keratinization resembling the spikes *(arrows)* of a flame and consistent with a "flame follicle." H&E stain. (**A** courtesy Dr. Alan Mundell, Animal Dermatology Service. **B** courtesy Dr. Ann M. Hargis, DermatoDiagnostics.)

Acquired Pattern Alopecia (Pattern Baldness)

Pattern alopecia develops in selected toy breeds of dogs (Dachshund, Boston terrier, Chihuahua, Italian greyhound, and Whippet). Breed predilections suggest a genetic basis. Generally, before 1 year of age, these dogs gradually develop a bilaterally symmetric thin hair coat in specific areas of the body such as the pinnae, skin caudal to the pinna, caudal thighs, perineal skin, or ventral neck, chest, and abdomen. The dogs are otherwise healthy. Histologic findings reveal miniaturized hair follicles and small (vellus) hair shafts.

Trauma-Associated Alopecia

Traction alopecia in dogs and posttraumatic alopecia in cats are presumed a result of interference with the local blood supply to follicles and adjacent skin. Traction alopecia develops in long-haired breeds of dogs in which rubber bands or other devices are used chronically to apply tension to the hair. Lesions usually occur on the top of the head or on the ears, the location where the traction devices are usually applied. Posttraumatic alopecia has been reported in cats that have suffered traumatic pelvic fracture. Alopecic lesions develop in the lower back several weeks after the fracture. The gross lesion in both conditions is alopecia, which is long term and generally permanent. Histologically, in both traction alopecia and posttraumatic alopecia, follicles are in hairless telogen, are atrophic, and may be partially or completely replaced by dermal fibrosis. Adnexal glands are also usually atrophic and may be absent. In traction alopecia some follicles may contain damaged hair shafts (malacic hairs) or melanin pigment debris indicating previous traction and fracture of hairs. In posttraumatic alopecia, the shearing force is severe and abrupt and results in degeneration of pannicular adipose tissue and more extensive dermal and superficial subcutaneous scarring.

DISORDERS RELATED TO NUTRIENT IMBALANCES, DEFICIENCIES, OR ALTERED METABOLISM

Malnutrition

Information on this topic is available at evolve.elsevier.com/Zachary/McGavin/.

Protein-Calorie Malnutrition

Information on this topic is available at evolve.elsevier.com/Zachary/McGavin/.

Zinc Deficiency

Zinc deficiency occurs chiefly in pigs and dogs and is of less importance in ruminants. It results from diets containing high concentration of phytic acid (binds zinc), low concentration of zinc, or high concentration of calcium (reduces absorption of zinc), or from inherited defective absorption or metabolism.

Dietary Zinc Deficiency in Ruminants

Information on this topic is available at evolve.elsevier.com/Zachary/McGavin/.

Hereditary Zinc Deficiency in Calves

Information on this topic is available at evolve.elsevier.com/Zachary/McGavin/.

Zinc Deficiency in Pigs

Information on this topic is available at evolve.elsevier.com/Zachary/McGavin/.

Canine Zinc-Responsive Dermatosis

Canine zinc-responsive dermatosis occurs in two forms. One form occurs principally in Siberian huskies and Alaskan malamutes, but other large-breed dogs can be affected. Alaskan malamutes have an inherited reduced ability to absorb zinc from the intestine. Scaling and crusting develop in the skin around the mouth, chin, eyes (Fig. 17-70), external ears, pressure points, and pawpads. The second form of zinc deficiency occurs in rapidly growing pups of large-breed dogs fed diets low in zinc or high in calcium or phytates, which can interfere with zinc absorption. Clinically dogs with this form have scaly plaques located on those areas of the skin subjected

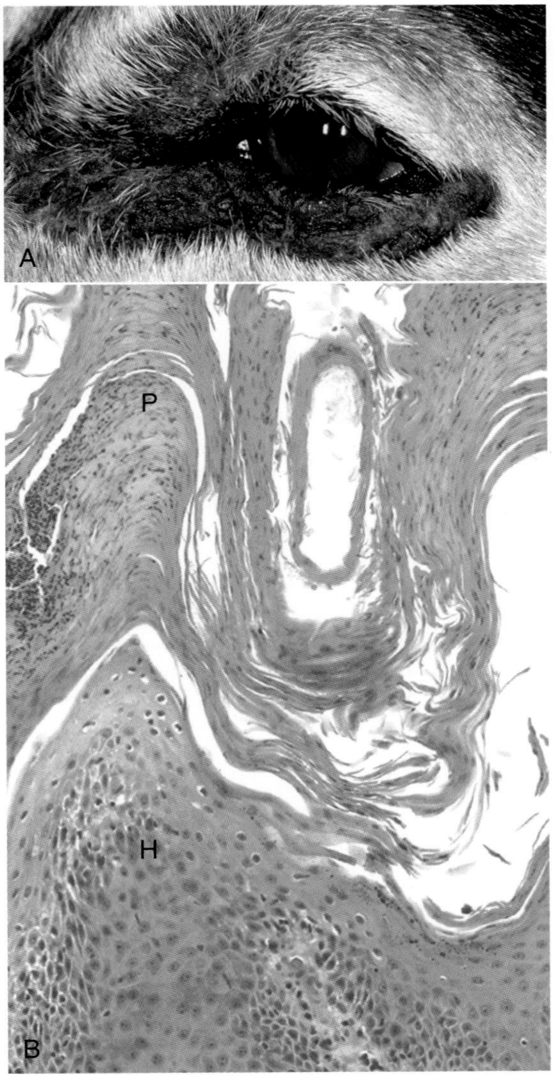

Fig. 17-70 **Zinc-responsive dermatosis, skin, dog.**
A, Siberian husky. Periocular skin is thickened, alopecic, pigmented, and covered by tightly adherent scale. In Siberian huskies and Alaskan malamutes in particular, scaling and crusting develop in the skin around the mouth, chin, eyes, external ears, pressure points, and pawpads. **B,** Note the papillary epidermal hyperplasia *(H)* with marked parakeratosis *(P)*. The parakeratotic hyperkeratosis and acanthosis form the thickened adherent scale. Although epidermal hyperplasia and parakeratosis are features of zinc-responsive dermatosis, they also occur in other conditions (such as superficial necrolytic dermatitis, chronic surface trauma, and nasal parakeratosis). Therefore breed, lesion distribution, and other features in the clinical history or clinical chemistry analysis are important in differential diagnosis. H&E stain. (Courtesy Dr. Ann M. Hargis, DermatoDiagnostics.)

to repeated trauma (e.g., elbows and hocks), the pawpads, and planum nasale. Microscopically, there is marked diffuse parakeratosis (see Fig. 17-70, *B*) that extends into the hair follicles, and an accompanying superficial perivascular lymphocytic and sometimes eosinophilic dermatitis. Another disorder, generic dog food dermatosis, a largely historic disease that occurred in the 1980s in dogs fed generic dog foods, has clinical and histologic lesions similar to those of canine zinc-responsive dermatosis. However, dogs with generic dog food dermatosis had a more rapid onset of lesions and also had systemic signs such as fever, depression, lymphadenopathy, and pitting edema of the dependent areas. The acute onset and systemic signs suggested that more than zinc deficiency played a role in generic dog food dermatosis.

Lethal Acrodermatitis of Bull Terriers

Lethal acrodermatitis is an autosomal recessive inherited disease of defective zinc metabolism in white bull terriers. The exact cause or pathogenesis of the disorder is not known. Although defective zinc metabolism and/or absorption are thought to play a role, affected dogs do not respond to oral or parenteral zinc supplementation. The concentrations of serum zinc and copper are low in affected bull terriers compared with those of control dogs, suggesting that copper deficiency might contribute. Lesions generally begin between 6 and 10 weeks of age. Most affected dogs are dead by 15 months of age, usually because of bronchopneumonia. The thymus is small or absent, and T lymphocytes are deficient in lymphoid tissues, likely contributing to immunodeficiency and increasing the potential of infection. Cutaneous lesions begin between the digits and on pawpads and progress to involve mucocutaneous areas, especially of the face. Severe interdigital pyoderma, paronychia (inflammation of the skin around the claws), and villous thickening and fissuring of pawpad keratin ensue. Exfoliative dermatitis can also develop on pinnae, external nose, elbows, hocks, and in some dogs, can become more generalized, with crusting, ulceration, and secondary pyoderma. Microscopically, the principal lesions are extensive diffuse parakeratotic hyperkeratosis, responsible for the exfoliative dermatitis, and accompanying acanthosis. Lesions of secondary infection consist of epidermal pustular dermatitis and folliculitis.

Copper Deficiency

Information on this topic is available at evolve.elsevier.com/Zachary/McGavin/.

Vitamin E Deficiency

Cats fed diets containing an excess of dietary fatty acids, such as canned red tuna, can develop inflammation of the subcutaneous and abdominal fat (steatitis). This condition develops when the diet is high in fat and when food processing or oxidation inactivate vitamin E. Vitamin E has a number of functions that contribute to its role as an antioxidant that stabilizes lysosomes. Grossly, the subcutaneous fat contains firm, nodular, yellow to orange masses. Microscopic lesions consist of fat necrosis that stimulates a lobular to diffuse neutrophilia followed by granulomatous inflammatory response. Macrophages and multinucleated giant cells contain ceroid pigment, which is responsible for the yellow to orange color of the affected fat.

Vitamin A–Responsive Dermatosis

Vitamin A–responsive dermatosis is a rare disorder primarily occurring in cocker spaniels, although a few other breeds of dogs have been affected. Because lesions respond to vitamin A therapy and relapse when treatment is withdrawn, vitamin A plays a role in the pathogenesis. However, vitamin A deficiency is not the cause of the lesions, as plasma concentrations of vitamin A are within the normal range. Vitamin A might contribute to lesion resolution by influencing epithelial differentiation. Gross lesions consist of generalized scaling, dry hair coat, and hyperkeratotic plaques with large "fronds" of stratum corneum extending from distended follicular openings (large open comedones). The plaques are most prominent in the ventral and lateral thorax and abdominal skin but can also occur on the face and neck. Microscopic lesions consist of mild orthokeratotic hyperkeratosis, mild irregular epidermal hyperplasia, and follicles markedly distended by hyperkeratosis.

DISORDERS OF EPIDERMAL GROWTH OR DIFFERENTIATION

Predominant Epidermal Hyperkeratosis (Scale)

Primary Idiopathic Seborrhea

Primary idiopathic seborrhea is a disorder of epidermal hyperproliferation that results in increased production of corneocytes and visible scale. It occurs most commonly in dogs and less commonly in horses and cats. Most experimental work has been performed in cocker spaniels. The pathogenesis of the disease involves hyperproliferation of the epidermis, hair follicle infundibulum, and sebaceous glands. The basal cell labeling indices are 3 or 4 times higher in cocker spaniels with seborrhea than in normal dogs. The hyperproliferation results in reduction in the epidermal turnover time to about one third (e.g., from 22 days to 8 days in the cocker spaniel). In the cocker spaniel the disorder appears to be the result of a primary cellular defect in the keratinocyte, as the epidermal cells remain hyperproliferative when grown in culture and after being grafted onto the dermis of normal dogs. However, the molecular basis of the defect has not been studied. In seborrhea, quantitative studies on sebum production have not been performed, but it is known that there is a relative increase in free fatty acids and a relative decrease in diester waxes on the surface of the seborrheic skin of various breeds. In addition, there is a change from nonpathogenic resident bacteria to pathogenic, coagulase-positive staphylococci. Clinically, two forms of seborrhea have been described, a dry form (seborrhea sicca), with dry skin and white-to-gray scales that exfoliate (see Fig. 17-9), and a greasy form (seborrhea oleosa), with scaling and excessive brown to yellow lipids that adhere to the surface of the skin and hair. An animal can have seborrhea sicca in some areas of the body and seborrhea oleosa in others. Microscopic lesions include marked hyperkeratosis of the epidermis and follicular epithelium. The epidermis has a papillary appearance caused by widening of follicular ostia by the follicular hyperkeratosis (see Fig. 17-9). Comedones (follicles dilated with a plug of follicular stratum corneum and sebum) are present in some animals. At the edges of follicular ostia, foci of parakeratosis form over a spongiotic epidermis containing a few scattered leukocytes. The superficial dermis is congested and edematous.

Ichthyosis

The ichthyoses are a heterogeneous group of inherited skin disorders seen principally in cattle and dogs. In severe forms of ichthyosis, the skin is thickened by marked scaling and can crack into plates resembling fish scales, thus the disease is named "ichthys" from the Greek word meaning fish. Recently, advances in molecular diagnosis have improved the understanding of the defects in some of these disorders. In humans, most of the ichthyoses are associated with defects in the epidermal barrier, including the intercellular lipid layers, cornified envelope, and keratin proteins. These defects

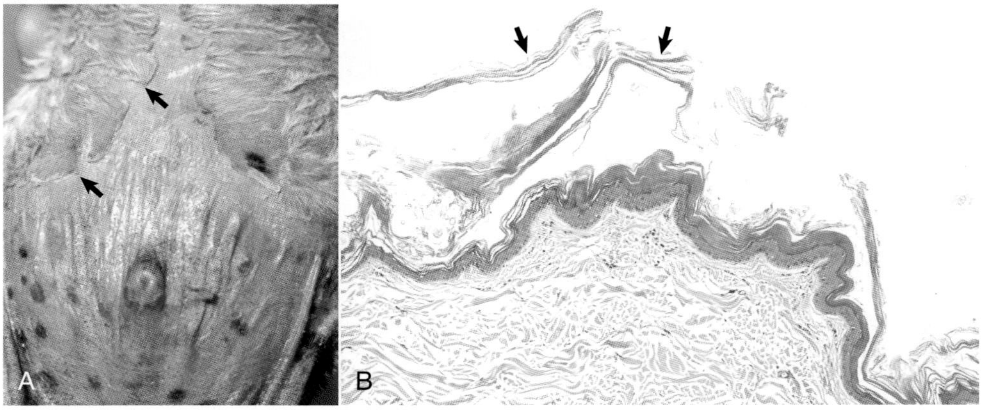

Fig. 17-71 Ichthyosis, skin, dog.
A, Abdomen. The skin is covered with adherent plates of scale *(arrows),* and the skin surface is wrinkled. **B,** Compact hyperkeratosis is present. Plates of stratum corneum are separating from each other and are lifting off the surface *(arrows).* H&E stain. (**A** courtesy Dr. Diane Lewis, College of Veterinary Medicine. University of Florida. **B** courtesy Dr. Ann M. Hargis, DermatoDiagnostics.)

result in increased production of stratum corneum (scaling) characteristic of the disease and can result in an increased prevalence of secondary infections. Recently, molecular defects similar to those in the human ichthyoses have been identified as a cause of some forms of ichthyoses in cattle and dogs.

In cattle, two forms of the disease have been described; both are thought to have an autosomal recessive mode of inheritance. One (ichthyosis fetalis) is lethal, and most calves are stillborn or die within days of birth. Ichthyosis fetalis markedly resembles harlequin ichthyosis in human infants. Defects in a gene (ABCA12, a member of the adenosine triphosphate [ATP]-binding cassette family) have been identified as a cause of harlequin ichthyosis. The ABCA12 gene is involved in the production of a protein necessary for lipid transfer in lamellar granules, a process required for formation of intercellular lipid layers and epidermal barrier structure and function. Because of barrier dysfunction, infants with harlequin ichthyosis develop excessive loss of fluids (dehydration) and life-threatening infections in the first few weeks of life. A loss of functional ABCA12 protein disrupts the normal development of the epidermis, resulting in the hard, thick scales characteristic of harlequin ichthyosis. Recently, a mutation in ABCA12 has been identified in Chianina cattle, one of the breeds of cattle known to develop ichthyosis fetalis, confirming the similarity of the genetic defect for the disease in cattle and humans. Grossly, the skin in affected calves is covered by thick cornified plaques separated by fissures. Fissuring of the skin can lead to exudation of protein, and secondary bacterial and fungal infections that often lead to death or euthanasia. The ears may be small, and there may be eversion of the eyelids, lips, and other mucocutaneous junctional areas. Microscopically, the epidermis is thickened by marked compact hyperkeratosis with variable parakeratosis. Follicular infundibular epithelium is also affected, and stratum corneum surrounds entrapped hairs. In the less severe form of ichthyosis in cattle (ichthyosis congenita), the defect has not been identified molecularly. Lesions may be mild at birth and progress with age. The skin becomes thickened, folded, and covered by platelike scales separated by shallow fissures and in which hairs are entrapped. More severe lesions are seen where hair is shorter, particularly on the limbs, abdomen, and nose. Microscopically, the epidermal surface is wrinkled, variably thickened by acanthosis, and covered by prominent laminated orthokeratotic hyperkeratosis.

Ichthyosis in dogs is usually divided into two basic subtypes, epidermolytic and nonepidermolytic, based on the presence or absence of vacuolization of the keratinocytes of the superficial stratum spinosum and granulosum in conjunction with hyperkeratosis. The molecular basis of canine ichthyosis rarely has been investigated; however, recently, transglutaminase 1-deficient recessive lamellar ichthyosis, an autosomal recessive inherited disorder in Jack Russell terrier dogs, has been described. The disease is nonepidermolytic and resembles lamellar ichthyosis in humans, which is associated with defects in the cornified cell envelope and is caused by mutations in the transglutaminase 1 gene. Transglutaminases catalyze cross-linking of proteins that form the cornified envelope. Clinical lesions in the Jack Russell terriers include generalized adherent and loosely attached scales, as well as large, adherent white or tan scales in sparsely haired skin (Fig. 17-71). Pawpads are moderately hyperkeratotic, and claws are soft. Secondary infection with coccoid bacteria and yeast are common, likely the result of the epidermal barrier defect. Histologic lesions consist of laminated to compact hyperkeratosis of the epidermis and follicular infundibulum without epidermolysis. Secondary infections result in inflammation. Ultrastructurally, many layers of corneocytes are present. Corneocytes have irregular margins and linear or oval lamellar inclusions and in comparison to control animals, thin or less prominent cornified envelopes.

Perhaps the most common form of nonepidermolytic hyperkeratosis in dogs occurs in young, otherwise healthy Golden retrievers. The mode of inheritance is uncertain, but an autosomal recessive mode of inheritance is suspected. Clinical lesions vary in severity and consist of large flat scales on the surface of the skin and within the haircoat. Pawpads and nasal planum are not affected. Histologic lesions consist of mild-to-moderate compact orthokeratotic hyperkeratosis without epidermal acanthosis, epidermolysis, or dermal inflammation. Ultrastructurally, affected dogs have more cohesive corneocytes and more numerous corneodesmosomes, suggesting that the disorder may be caused by delayed degradation of corneodesmosomes.

The molecular basis of an autosomal recessive inherited form of epidermolytic hyperkeratosis recently has been described in Norfolk terrier dogs that have a mutation in the gene that encodes for keratin 10 (KRT10). Similar histologic lesions have been seen in a few other breeds of dogs (Fig. 17-72). This condition is similar to epidermolytic hyperkeratosis in humans, caused by defects in keratin proteins 1 and 10. Keratin intermediate filaments are important structural proteins in the epidermis, and defects can be associated with irregular keratin filament aggregation and loss

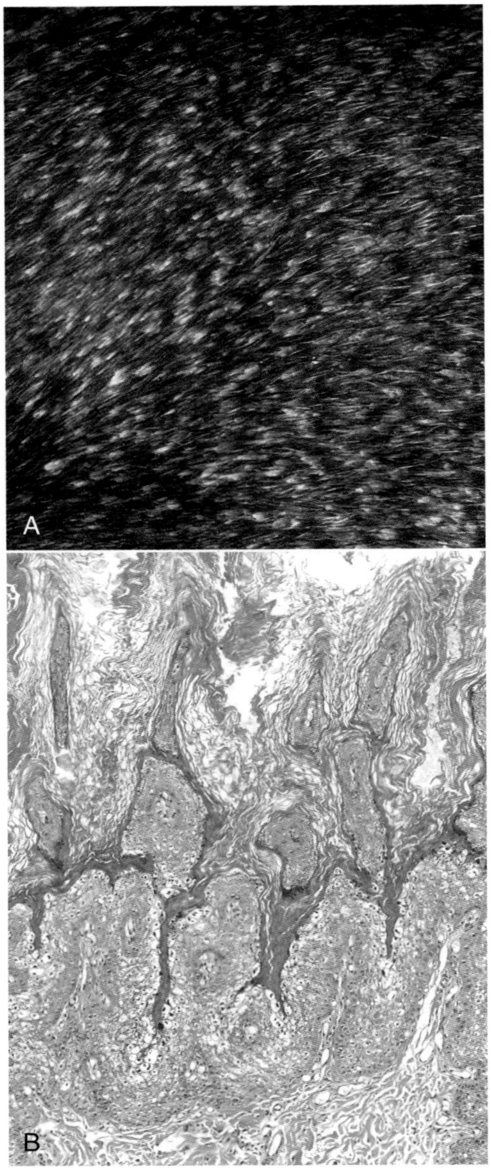

Fig. 17-72 Epidermolytic hyperkeratosis, skin, dog.
A, Lateral thorax of Rhodesian ridgeback. There are fronds of keratin adherent to hairs. **B,** Papillary epidermal hyperplasia with disruption and clefting of the granular layer and large keratohyalin granules. The papillary hyperplasia and hyperkeratosis contribute to the accumulation of keratin on the hairs in this breed of dog. H&E stain. (Courtesy of Dr. Ann M. Hargis, DermatoDiagnostics.)

of strength, resulting in disruption of keratinocytes, especially in association with trauma. In Norfolk terrier dogs, the clinical lesions include scaling and epidermal fragility, and the superficial epidermis can slough after mild mechanical trauma. Pigmented scaling, especially in intertriginous areas, is present. Pawpads, claws, and hair are normal. Histologically, there is papillary epidermal hyperplasia with minimal-to-moderate hyperkeratosis, large keratohyalin granules, and disruption (epidermolysis) and clefting of granular cell keratinocytes (see Fig. 17-72). Ultrastructurally, keratinocytes in the upper stratum spinosum and granulosum have a reduction of tonofilaments and abnormal filament aggregation.

BOX 17-11 Hyperkeratosis of the Nasal Planum or Pawpads in Dogs

IMMUNE MEDIATED
Pemphigus foliaceous
Lupus erythematosus
Drug reaction

INFECTIOUS
Canine distemper
Leishmaniasis

METABOLIC
Superficial necrolytic dermatitis
Zinc-responsive dermatosis

INHERITED
Familial pawpad hyperkeratosis (may be a form of ichthyosis)
Ichthyosis
Nasal parakeratosis of the Labrador retriever
Acrodermatitis of bull terriers

IDIOPATHIC
Idiopathic seborrhea
Idiopathic nasodigital hyperkeratosis

NEOPLASTIC
Cutaneous lymphoma

Sebaceous Adenitis

Sebaceous adenitis, inflammation of sebaceous glands, occurs most commonly in dogs and rarely is seen in cats and horses. The cause and pathogenesis are uncertain, but an inherited component of the disease is proposed for two breeds of dogs (Standard poodle and Akita) in which the disease has been studied more extensively. Clinical lesions are variable between breeds of dogs. In general, there is multifocal to coalescing or diffuse alopecia and scaling with fronds of keratin adherent to hair shafts. Similar lesions are reported in cats. Progressive patches of nonpruritic scaling, crusting, alopecia, and leukoderma are reported in the horse. The reason scaling and alopecia develop in association with loss of sebaceous glands is speculative. Microscopic lesions include lymphocytes, neutrophils, and macrophages that efface sebaceous glands (see Fig. 17-29), and in some dogs, extensive orthokeratotic hyperkeratosis. Chronically affected dogs have no remaining sebaceous glands, but mild residual inflammation and fibrosis are present in the perifollicular dermis near the isthmus (site normally occupied by sebaceous glands).

Hyperkeratosis of Nasal Planum or Pawpads in Dogs

Nasal and/or digital hyperkeratoses have a variety of underlying causes, including infectious disease (e.g., canine distemper [see Chapter 14], leishmaniasis), immune-mediated disorders (e.g., PF and lupus erythematosus), familial or inherited disorders (e.g., idiopathic seborrhea, familial pawpad hyperkeratosis of Irish terriers and Dogue de Bordeaux, ichthyosis, nasal parakeratosis of the Labrador retriever, and acrodermatitis of bull terriers), metabolic or nutritional disease (e.g., superficial necrolytic dermatitis, zinc-responsive dermatosis), adverse reaction to drug therapy, and neoplasia (e.g., cutaneous lymphoma) (Box 17-11). In some cases, an underlying cause is not determined, thus the condition is considered to be idiopathic (occurs most commonly in old dogs). Some of the disorders in which nasal or digital hyperkeratosis is a feature also have skin lesions in other sites, and systemic disease can be present. Gross lesions on the pawpads or nasal planum include a dry, thick, irregular and rough surface in which crusts, fissures, or erosions can develop (see Figs. 17-10 and 17-15). The edges of the pawpads and non–weight-bearing pads are more severely affected because friction on weight-bearing surfaces wears through some of the excessively thick stratum corneum. Histologic lesions of nasal and/or digital hyperkeratoses may reflect the underlying cause (e.g., infectious, immune mediated, metabolic, or neoplastic). In the idiopathic nasodigital hyperkeratosis of old dogs, irregular epidermal hyperplasia with marked orthokeratotic to parakeratotic hyperkeratosis is present. In familial nasal parakeratosis of Labrador retrievers, there is variable parakeratotic hyperkeratosis with intraepidermal serum and leukocytic exocytosis. The dermis has perivascular to interface or interstitial mixed inflammation. In familial pawpad hyperkeratosis, there is moderate-to-extensive epidermal acanthosis and marked diffuse orthokeratotic hyperkeratosis in which the surface stratum corneum forms many papillary projections.

Predominant Follicular Hyperkeratosis (Comedones)

Comedones (see Table 17-3) occur in numerous skin disorders, including those associated with surface trauma (callus, solar dermatosis), endocrine dermatosis (especially hyperadrenocorticism), nutritional or inherited disorders of cornification (primary seborrhea, vitamin A responsive dermatosis), and in some disorders associated with follicular infection (especially demodicosis). In addition, comedones are prominent in two conditions wherein the comedones are considered a major feature of the disease.

Schnauzer Comedo Syndrome

Schnauzer comedo syndrome affects some miniature schnauzers and probably has an inherited basis. Gross lesions develop on the dorsum of the back and consist of comedones, papules, and crusts. Histologic lesions consist of follicles distended with a plug of follicular stratum corneum and sebum (comedones). Because the follicular opening is connected to the epidermis, the dilated follicles can contain coccoid bacteria. The dilated follicles can rupture (furunculosis) and release contents into the dermis, resulting in a foreign body response and bacterial infection.

Acne

Feline acne develops in the skin of the chin, lower lip, and less commonly upper lip. Cats of a variety of ages, sexes, and coat lengths are affected. The cause and pathogenesis are unclear, but defects in follicular cornification and poor grooming habits have been suggested. Gross lesions consist of comedones that can progress to papules, crusts, nodules, and diffuse swelling. Histologic lesions begin as mild follicular hyperkeratosis and progress to comedones, which can become secondarily infected by bacteria, result in folliculitis, follicular rupture (furunculosis), and localized to diffuse dermatitis, panniculitis, and cellulitis.

Canine acne is a chronic disorder that develops in the skin of the chin and lips of young dogs, usually with short hair coats. The cause of the disorder is not known, but a follicular cornification disorder has not been definitively documented. Early lesions consist of follicular papules and comedones that with time enlarge to nodules that can ulcerate and drain. Histologically, early lesions consist of moderate-to-marked follicular hyperkeratosis (the papules and comedones) and later of folliculitis, furunculosis, and draining sinuses (the nodular, ulcerated, and draining lesions).

Predominant Epidermal Hyperplasia (Lichenification or Crusts)

Equine Coronary Band Dystrophy

Equine coronary band dystrophy is a condition of unknown etiology and pathogenesis. Clinically, the coronary band (coronary border of hoof) is thickened, crusty, and scaly. Cracks and fissures can lead to lameness. The chestnuts and ergots (cornified protuberances considered to be vestiges of the first, second, and fourth digits) are similarly affected and can be ulcerated. Usually all four limbs are affected; however, the lesion may not involve the entire coronary band. Histologically, the epidermis of affected areas has marked papillary epidermal hyperplasia (see Fig. 17-11) and marked orthohyperkeratosis to parakeratotic hyperkeratosis. In some areas, there is ballooning degeneration of keratinocytes. Dermal inflammation is minimal unless secondary infection is present. The diagnosis is made by ruling out the various differential diagnoses, including PF, hepatocutaneous syndrome, bacterial or fungal infection, selenium toxicosis, mite infestation, and eosinophilic exfoliative dermatitis. The condition is chronic and treatment palliative. Although the condition affects adult horses of any breed, draft breeds are considered predisposed.

Porcine Juvenile Pustular Psoriasiform Dermatitis (Pityriasis Rosea)

Porcine juvenile pustular psoriasiform dermatitis (pityriasis rosea) develops in suckling and young pigs (3 to 14 weeks of age), usually resolves spontaneously by 4 weeks of onset, and is thought to be inherited. A few piglets in the litter or entire litters can be affected. Lesions are symmetric and develop on the abdomen, groin, and medial thigh and begin as small papules covered by brown crusts. The lesions coalesce and spread and develop into umbilicated plaques with white centers and erythematous, scaly borders that can progress into mosaic patterns (Fig. 17-73). These clinical lesions resemble those of dermatophytosis, swinepox, and dermatosis vegetans, from which they need to be differentiated, but otherwise the clinical lesions are of no significance. Microscopically, the early histologic lesions are superficial and deep perivascular neutrophilic, eosinophilic, and mixed mononuclear dermatitis. Epidermal spongiosis and leukocytic exocytosis result in spongiform pustules. Later, lesions consist of marked psoriasiform epidermal hyperplasia (regular epidermal hyperplasia with epidermal ridges of uniform length and width) and parakeratotic cellular crust.

Secondary Seborrhea

Secondary seborrhea is not a primary disorder of cornification; however, it clinically resembles the primary cornification disorders (dry exfoliative or greasy adherent scales) and thus needs to be differentiated from them. Secondary seborrhea is common and is caused by a variety of unrelated cutaneous disorders such as allergy, ectoparasitism, fungal infection, dietary deficiency, endocrine disease, and internal diseases. The lesions of secondary seborrhea resolve completely if the underlying disease is eliminated. Microscopic changes include epidermal and follicular hyperkeratosis with or without parakeratosis plus the lesions associated with the underlying disease.

DISORDERS OF PIGMENTATION

Melanin pigments are responsible for the coloration of the hair, skin, and eyes and also play an important role in photoprotection. Melanin is synthesized by melanocytes, which are dendritic

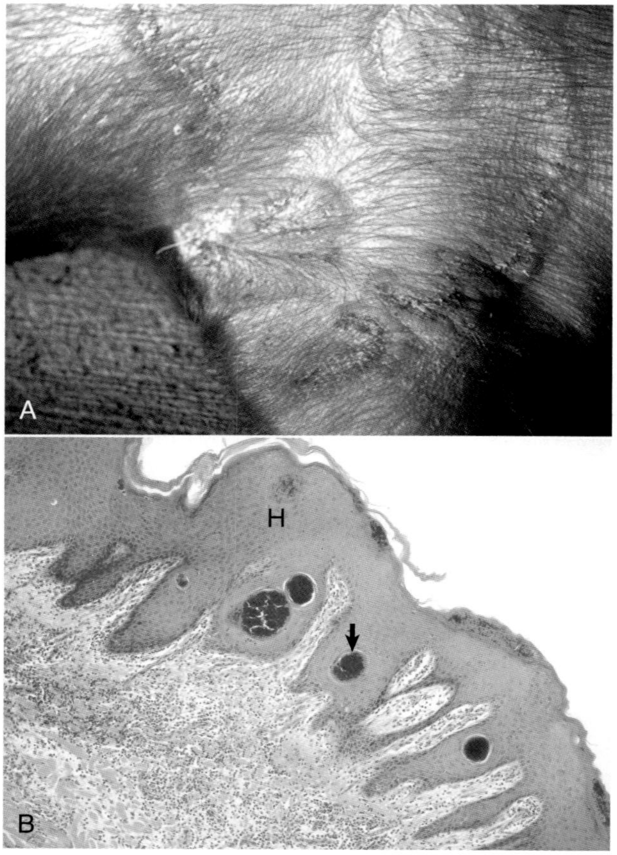

Fig. 17-73 Porcine juvenile pustular psoriasiform dermatitis (pityriasis rosea), skin, pig.
A, Abdomen. Note the circular to serpiginous (wavy) lesions with distinct raised and reddened border and the adjacent scale. These lesions need to be differentiated from those of dermatophytosis, swinepox, and dermatosis vegetans. **B,** Note the epidermal hyperplasia (acanthosis with elongated rete ridges) *(H)* and intraepidermal pustules *(arrow)*. The dermis contains diffuse accumulations of neutrophils and mixed mononuclear inflammatory cells. The disease receives its name from the juvenile age of onset, the formation of epidermal pustules, and the exaggerated regular epidermal hyperplasia (psoriasiform hyperplasia). H&E stain. (**A** courtesy Dr. M.D. McGavin, College of Veterinary Medicine, University of Tennessee. **B** courtesy Dr. Pamela E. Ginn, College of Veterinary Medicine, University of Florida.)

cells originating as melanoblasts in the neural crest. Melanoblasts develop in the neural crest and migrate to peripheral sites, including the basal and lower spinous layers of the epidermis, hair follicles, and dermis. Melanoblasts differentiate into melanocytes and synthesize melanosomes and melanin. Tyrosinase, a copper-containing enzyme, plays a critical role in the synthesis of melanin. Genetic mutations affecting any of the steps in the formation of melanin can lead to hereditary hypopigmentation. Many types of exogenous influences, such as inflammation, UVR, endocrinopathies, autoimmune diseases, and nutritional status, can affect melanocytes in the skin, resulting in acquired hypopigmentation or hyperpigmentation. Examples of some of the disorders include Chédiak-Higashi syndrome, color mutant (dilution) alopecia, the Maltese dilution of cats, leukoderma and/or leukotrichia of Doberman pinschers and Rottweilers, periocular leukotrichia in Siamese cats, and Arabian fading syndrome. Immune-mediated disorders associated with depigmentation include discoid lupus erythematosus and uveodermatologic syndrome (Vogt-Koyanagi-Harada [VKH]–like disease).

Hypopigmentation

Disorders associated with reduced pigment can (1) be inherited or acquired, (2) involve skin or hair, (3) be generalized or localized, or (4) be idiopathic or linked with other diseases. Reduction in pigmentation of the skin is leukoderma and of the hair is leukotrichia. Leukoderma and leukotrichia can occur independently. They can result from a decrease in melanin (hypomelanosis), a complete absence of melanin (amelanosis), or from a loss of existing melanin (depigmentation). These events result from either an absence of the pigment-synthesizing melanocytes or from a failure of melanocytes to produce normal amounts of melanin or to transfer it to adjacent keratinocytes. Because copper is a component of tyrosinase, production of melanin pigment depends on copper, thus copper deficiency can result in reduced pigmentation.

Inherited Hypopigmentation

Hereditary hypopigmentation can be divided into melanocytopenic hypomelanosis, characterized by the absence of melanocytes in affected areas, and melanopenic hypomelanosis, in which melanocytes are present but defective. Hypopigmentation can be localized, focally extensive, or generalized.

Syndromes analogous to the human Waardenburg-Klein syndrome have been reported in horses, dogs, and cats. In this melanocytopenic hypomelanosis, there is failure of melanoblasts to migrate from the neural crest into the skin or failure to survive in the skin. Affected animals typically have white coats and blue or heterochromatic irides and are deaf. In dogs, this syndrome has been described in breeds such as the Dalmatian, bull terrier, Sealyham terrier, collie, and Great Dane. In horses and dogs, the condition is inherited as an autosomal dominant trait with incomplete penetrance. In the cat, the inheritance is autosomal dominant with complete penetrance for the loss of pigmentation and an incomplete penetrance for the inner ear degeneration.

Overo lethal white foal syndrome, analogous to human Waardenburg type-4 (Hirschsprung's disease), has been reported in American Paint horses in which white foals from the breeding of two Overo spotted paint horses are born with aganglionic colons. The condition has autosomal recessive inheritance and is the result of a genetic mutation in the endothelin signaling pathway, which is critical for correct development and migration of neural crest cells. Neural crest cells give rise to melanocytes and enteric neurons. These foals develop colic from greatly distended colons and die shortly after birth.

Piebaldism is also a form of genetic melanocytopenic hypomelanosis resulting in multifocal white patches in which there is an absence of melanocytes because of either a congenital failure of melanoblasts to migrate from the neural crest to the skin, or by their inability to survive and proliferate in the skin. Piebaldism has been seen in many species, including horses, cattle, dogs such as the Dalmatian, and cats.

The various forms of albinism are examples of melanopenic hypomelanosis. In albino animals and humans, melanocytes are present and normally distributed but are defective in function and fail to synthesize melanin. The extent of the biochemical defect varies, so that albinism covers a spectrum from amelanosis, oculocutaneous albinism, through graded pigmentary dilution. Oculocutaneous albinisms and pigment dilutions are inherited as autosomal recessive traits. In albino animals with white hair and skin and translucent irides, there is a mutation in the tyrosinase gene resulting in no residual enzyme activity.

Chédiak-Higashi syndrome in humans; Hereford, Brangus, and Japanese Black cattle; Persian cats; and various other animal species is an example of partial albinism and is inherited as an autosomal recessive trait. While melanin is produced, there is a mutation of the beige gene, which plays a major role in generating cellular organelles. This results in a membrane defect leading to the formation of giant melanosomes that are transferred with difficulty to the keratinocytes. The clumping of these giant melanosomes produces the color dilution effect. Chédiak-Higashi syndrome is discussed with the hematopoietic system (see Chapter 13).

Cyclic hematopoiesis (cyclic neutropenia), a lethal hereditary disease of collie dogs, is caused by an autosomal recessive gene with a pleiotropic effect on coat color dilution. Affected dogs are silver-gray. The abnormal hair pigmentation results from the diminished formation of melanin from its precursor tyrosine rather than from pigment clumping. The normal collie coat color is partially restored in animals receiving bone marrow transplants to correct cyclic hematopoiesis. The hematologic aspects of this disease are considered in the discussion on the hematopoietic system in Chapter 13.

Coat color dilution has been reported in many species. It occurs in many breeds of horses, cattle, dogs, and cats but is particularly common in Siamese cats. The pale coat coloration is caused by clumping of large melanin granules in hair shafts, hair matrix cells, and sometimes in the epidermis. In cats, dilute coat color is thought to be a result of an autosomal recessive trait (Maltese dilution).

Acquired Hypopigmentation

Acquired hypopigmentation follows damage to the epidermal melanin unit by various insults, including trauma, inflammation, radiation, contactants, endocrinopathies, infections, nutritional deficiencies, and neoplasia. In general, the severity of the injury determines whether an insult will result in hypopigmentation or hyperpigmentation. Mild injury results in pigmentary incontinence and epidermal hypopigmentation from death of melanin-containing keratinocytes. However, hyperpigmentation can occur, possibly from release of melanocyte-stimulating factors from surviving keratinocytes and subsequent increase in production of melanosomes. It is thought that these factors are preset in normal epidermis, but their level or activity is increased in response to stimulation or keratinocyte stress. In contrast, severe injury results in the death of melanocytes, which do not regenerate, and thus there is no repigmentation.

Vitiligo is a melanocytopenic hypomelanosis of humans and animals, which is characterized by gradually expanding pale macules that are often symmetric or segmental in distribution. The immediate cause of vitiligo is the destruction of melanocytes. Theories regarding the pathogenesis of this disease include autoimmune destruction of melanocytes, a neurogenic theory involving release of a neurochemical from peripheral nerves that inhibits melanogenesis, a self-destruction theory that involves failure of protection of melanocytes against the toxic effects of melanin precursors, or a combination of factors. Vitiligo has been described in horses, cattle, dogs, and cats. The condition is best characterized in Belgian Tervuren dogs. The depigmentation in this breed occurs chiefly on the pigmented skin and mucous membranes of the face and mouth in young adult dogs. Histologic examination of affected skin shows an epithelium devoid of both pigment granules and DOPA-positive cells. Electron microscopy confirms the lack of melanocytes in the lesions, their place being taken by Langerhans' or indeterminate dendritic cells.

Uveodermatologic syndrome (Vogt-Koyanagi-Harada[VKH]–like syndrome) is a rare syndrome of histiocytic interface dermatitis and granulomatous uveitis in dogs, particularly Akitas, Chow Chows, Samoyeds, Alaskan malamutes, and Siberian huskies. The strong breed associations suggest there is an inherited basis for this disease. In fact, in the Akita, specific DLA class II gene alleles appear to predispose to the development of this disease. The pathogenesis is thought to involve an immune-mediated attack against melanin or melanocytes, but there are conflicting results regarding the role of humeral versus cell-mediated immune responses. Ocular lesions usually develop before cutaneous lesions. Clinical lesions consist of symmetrical patchy to diffuse depigmentation of the skin of the nose, lips, eyelids, scrotum or vulva, anal skin, ears, and pawpads. Lesions are occasionally more widespread. Leukotrichia of adjacent hair can be present. Uncommonly, lesions are more severe and consist of erosion, ulceration, and crusting. Fully developed histologic lesions are cell-rich interface inflammation, primarily of histiocytic cells containing melanin pigment (pigmentary incontinence). The inflammation occurs parallel to the epidermal surface but usually does not obscure the interface and may extend around adnexa. Basal cell degeneration is uncommon.

Cutaneous depigmentation in horses and dogs can result from contact with rubber. The monobenzene ether of hydroquinone, a common ingredient in rubber, inhibits melanogenesis. In horses, lesions result from contact with equipment such as rubber bit guards, crupper straps, or with feed buckets (lips, buttocks, and face). In dogs, lesions result from contact with rubber dishes or toys (lips or nose).

In dogs, hypopigmentation can occur in immune-mediated diseases targeting the epidermal-dermal interface, such as lupus erythematosus and dermatomyositis, and in association with neoplastic conditions, such as epitheliotropic lymphoma (mycosis fungoides). The hypopigmentation develops from injury and subsequent loss of the melanin-containing keratinocytes or melanocytes. Leukotrichia (depigmentation of hair) can be seen in the healing stage of alopecia areata, an immune-mediated condition characterized clinically by alopecia, and microscopically by lymphocytic inflammation of the hair bulb.

Hyperpigmentation

Secondary Hyperpigmentation

Hyperpigmentation can result from inflammation, irritation, and metabolic disorders. Consequently, hyperpigmentation is seen in all species with epidermal melanin pigment. Hypermelanosis results from an increased rate of melanosome production, an increase in melanosome size, or an increase in the degree of melanization of the melanosome. It is usually associated with an accelerated melanocyte turnover with an increased number of melanosomes, as occurs after trauma.

Acanthosis Nigricans

Primary idiopathic acanthosis nigricans is considered a genodermatosis (genetically determined skin disorder) of young dachshunds. The disease is manifested by bilateral axillary hyperpigmentation, lichenification, and alopecia, which can involve large areas and include secondary seborrhea and pyoderma. Histologic examination reveals hyperplastic dermatitis with orthokeratotic and parakeratotic hyperkeratosis, acanthosis, and rete ridge formation. All layers of the epidermis are heavily melanized. Spongiosis, neutrophilic exocytosis, and serous crusts can also be present. The dermal inflammatory reaction is mild, pleomorphic in cell type, and superficial perivascular in location. The term *acanthosis nigricans* has also been used to encompass a variety of chronic inflammatory and pruritic disorders that in their chronic form are manifested by axillary or more diffuse lichenification, alopecia, and hyperpigmentation. Consequently, the diagnosis of primary acanthosis nigricans requires clinical correlation together with the histologic findings

BOX 17-12 Disorders Characterized by Infiltrates of Eosinophils or Plasma Cells

- Eosinophilic plaques
- Eosinophilic granulomas
- Nasal eosinophilic folliculitis and furunculosis in dogs
- Hypereosinophilia syndromes with systemic signs or lesions
  - Multisystemic eosinophilic epitheliotropic disease in the horse
  - Feline hypereosinophilic syndrome
  - Eosinophilic dermatitis with edema in the dog
- Feline plasma cell pododermatitis
- Hypersensitivity and parasitic dermatitis (see the section on Mechanisms of Tissue Damage in Hypersensitivity Reactions)
- Feline herpesvirus facial dermatitis (see the section on Herpesvirus)

to support the diagnosis in a young dachshund with compatible lesion distribution.

MISCELLANEOUS SKIN DISORDERS

Disorders Characterized by Infiltrates of Eosinophils or Plasma Cells

Disorders characterized by infiltrates of eosinophils or plasma cells are listed in Box 17-12. In addition to the syndromes discussed herein, eosinophils are often a prominent feature of hypersensitivity or parasitic dermatoses, especially in cats and horses, and are also often a feature in feline herpesvirus facial dermatitis.

Eosinophilic Plaques

Eosinophilic plaques are common lesions of the skin of cats that occur on the abdomen and medial thigh and are thought to be associated with hypersensitivity reactions. Lesions consist of raised, variably sized erythematous, pruritic, and eroded to ulcerated plaques. Microscopically, epidermal lesions include acanthosis, variable spongiosis, erosion, and ulceration, accompanied by superficial and deep, perivascular to diffuse, predominantly eosinophilic dermatitis.

Eosinophilic Granulomas (Collagenolytic Granulomas)

Eosinophilic and granulomatous lesions with brightly eosinophilic, granular to amorphous material bordering collagen fibers and somewhat obscuring the fiber detail (flame figures) occur in horses, dogs, and cats. The causes of these syndromes are poorly understood. The tinctorial change can develop in any lesion with large numbers of eosinophils such as reactions to parasites, foreign bodies (including hair), or in mast cell tumors. Eosinophils congregate and degranulate near collagen bundles causing the tinctorial change. Eosinophil degranulation results in release of a wide range of toxic granule proteins (e.g., major basic protein), enzymes (peroxidase, collagenase), cytokines (IL-3, IL-5, granulocyte macrophage colony-stimulating factor [GM-CSF]), chemokines (IL-8), and lipid mediators (leukotrienes and platelet-activating factor) augmenting an inflammatory response. Gross lesions include papules, nodules, plaques (sometimes linear), and ulcers in the skin (see Fig. 17-21). Nodular or ulcerated lesions can also develop in the oral mucosa of dogs and cats and in the pawpads of cats. Microscopically, nodular dermatitis (or stomatitis) consists of an inflammatory response with a prominence of eosinophils, flame figures, and macrophages, some of which are multinucleated (see Fig. 17-21). Collagen lysis develops in some lesions, likely a secondary event caused by the proteolytic enzymes (e.g., collagenase). Some indolent ulcers on the upper lip of cats have areas of flame figures and granulomatous inflammation and are considered to be eosinophilic granulomas.

Nasal Eosinophilic Folliculitis and Furunculosis in Dogs

Nasal eosinophilic folliculitis and furunculosis develops primarily on the dorsal and lateral surfaces of the nose of young dogs and is thought to be a result of arthropod bites (bees, wasps, spiders). Lesions develop acutely and are often painful swollen areas that rapidly ulcerate and can drain bloody fluid. Lesions can progress to involve the periocular, pinnal, and sometimes the glabrous ventral abdominal skin. Because lesions develop rapidly and appear clinically severe, biopsy samples are typically collected early in the course of the disease. At this time, microscopic lesions consist of ulceration, superficial and deep interstitial eosinophilic to mixed inflammation with eosinophilic folliculitis and furunculosis.

Hypereosinophilic Syndromes with Systemic Signs or Lesions

Multisystemic Eosinophilic Epitheliotropic Disease in the Horse

Multisystemic eosinophilic epitheliotropic disease is a generalized, exfoliative dermatitis of horses that is of unknown etiology; however, one case report documents the coexistence of an intestinal T cell lymphoma and postulates a role for tumor cell overproduction of IL-5, a powerful eosinophilopoietin. Initial cutaneous lesions include dry scales and serous exudates of the epithelium of the skin of the head, coronary bands, and oral mucosa. The lesions progress to generalized excoriations with ulceration and alopecia. Secondary infections are common. Histologically, there is superficial and deep, perivascular to interstitial, eosinophilic lymphoplasmacytic, and sometimes granulomatous dermatitis with irregular epidermal hyperplasia and orthokeratotic and parakeratotic hyperkeratosis. Eosinophils, lymphocytes, and apoptotic keratinocytes can be prominent in the epidermis, and eosinophilic folliculitis, furunculosis, and flame figures are occasionally seen. The dermatitis is accompanied by a similar inflammatory response with fibrosis in other organs, including the alimentary tract, pancreas, liver, uterus, and bronchial epithelium. Clinically, the horses lose weight and become progressively debilitated.

Feline Hypereosinophilic Syndrome

Feline hypereosinophilic syndrome is a rare multisystemic disorder of unknown cause that is associated with moderate-to-marked peripheral eosinophilia and infiltrates of mature eosinophils in multiple organ systems, sometimes including the skin. Middle-aged female cats are more often affected. Gross lesions of the skin include erythema and excoriations associated with severe pruritus. Histologically, there is superficial and deep, perivascular dermatitis with prominent eosinophils. Clinical signs include anorexia, diarrhea, weight loss, and vomiting.

Eosinophilic Dermatitis with Edema in the Dog

Eosinophilic dermatitis with edema is a newly described condition affecting adult dogs of a variety of breeds, although Labrador retrievers may be overrepresented. The cause is not known, but a hypersensitivity reaction to medications, arthropod bites, or other antigens is suspected. Gross lesions consist of extremely erythematous macules that progress and coalesce into arciform and serpiginous plaques. Facial or generalized pitting edema is often seen. Lesions involve the pinnae, ventral abdomen and thorax, and less often the extremities. Histologic lesions consist of diffuse, predominantly eosinophilic dermatitis, vascular dilation, and edema.

Eosinophil aggregation and degranulation are seen in some lesions. Depression, hypoproteinemia, and pyrexia are present in some dogs.

Plasma Cell Pododermatitis

Feline plasma cell pododermatitis is an uncommon condition of undetermined cause or pathogenesis. Immunohistochemical staining with a polyclonal anti-*Mycobacterium bovis* antibody cross reactive to a broad spectrum of bacteria and fungi, and PCR for a variety of potential feline pathogens, including *Bartonella* spp., *Ehrlichia* spp., *Anaplasma phagocytophilum, Chlamydophila felis, Mycoplasma* spp., *Toxoplasma gondii,* and feline herpesvirus 1 (FHV-1) have been negative. However, some cats have tested positive for FIV. Affected cats have hypergammaglobulinemia and a response to immunomodulating therapy leading to the hypothesis that feline plasma cell pododermatitis is an idiopathic immune-mediated disease. It is characterized clinically by soft, painless swelling of multiple pawpads that can lead to collapse of the pawpad and ulceration, hemorrhage, and lameness. Histologically, the skin of the pawpad is heavily infiltrated by plasma cells with variable numbers of Russell body plasma cells, neutrophils, and lymphocytes. This condition is sometimes accompanied by plasmacytic stomatitis, immune-mediated glomerulonephritis, or renal amyloidosis.

Nodular Granulomatous Inflammatory Disorders without Microorganisms

Nodular granulomatous inflammatory disorders without microorganisms are listed in Box 17-13. The diseases in this category have traditionally been considered to be sterile because no microorganisms have been identified by microscopic examination, including with special stains for organisms, by electron microscopic examination, by cultures, or by cytologic evaluation for organisms. However, newer techniques, including the PCR that detects minute amounts of DNA, suggest the potential for microbial participation in the pathogenesis of some of these seemingly sterile inflammatory disorders, especially in humans. It is possible, for instance, for an abnormal immune response to an as yet unidentified microbial antigen to initiate a macrophage-dominated inflammatory response. Defective downregulation of the immune response to the organism could lead to a persistent granulomatous inflammatory process. Currently, this issue remains unresolved, but as more of these lesions are probed for microbial agents, a better understanding of these so-called "sterile" inflammatory disorders will hopefully develop.

BOX 17-13 Nodular Granulomatous Inflammatory Disorders without Microorganisms

- Juvenile sterile granulomatous dermatitis and lymphadenitis
- Sterile pyogranuloma syndrome (idiopathic sterile granuloma and pyogranuloma)
- Canine reactive histiocytosis
- Canine Langerhans' cell histiocytosis
- Feline dendritic cell histiocytosis
- Idiopathic sterile nodular panniculitis
- Xanthoma (xanthogranuloma)
- Equine generalized granulomatous disease (see the section on Vetch Toxicosis and Vetch-Like Diseases)
- Feline nutritional pansteatitis (see the section on Vitamin E Deficiency)

Juvenile Sterile Granulomatous Dermatitis and Lymphadenitis (Juvenile Cellulitis, Juvenile Pyoderma, Puppy Strangles)

Juvenile sterile granulomatous dermatitis and lymphadenitis, also known as juvenile cellulitis, juvenile pyoderma, or puppy strangles, is a disorder of unknown cause that occurs in pups younger than 4 months (Fig. 17-74), with one or more of the pups of a litter developing pustular and nodular dermatitis and edema of the face, ears, and mucocutaneous junctions. The pustular and nodular lesions tend to rupture, drain, and crust. Microscopically, early lesions consist of multifocal granulomatous or pyogranulomatous perifolliculitis and dermatitis (see Fig. 17-74). Early lesions are adjacent to but do not involve follicles; however, lesions typically progress to folliculitis, furunculosis, panniculitis, cellulitis, and granulomatous to pyogranulomatous lymphadenitis. The lesions initially are considered to be sterile, but secondary bacterial infections develop and can lead to sepsis if not treated. About half of the puppies are lethargic, and anorexia, fever, and joint pain can also occur. This condition occasionally has been reported in adult dogs.

Idiopathic Sterile Granuloma and Pyogranuloma (Sterile Pyogranuloma Syndrome)

Idiopathic sterile granuloma and pyogranuloma, or sterile pyogranuloma syndrome, are seen most commonly in dogs and rarely horses and cats, are of unknown cause, and are characterized grossly by single or multifocal papules, plaques, or nodules most commonly in the skin of the head and extremities. Early microscopic lesions include periadnexal to coalescing nodular accumulations of leukocytes predominantly consisting of macrophages (histiocytes), neutrophils, and lymphocytes. Organized granulomas and pyogranulomas are present. Older lesions can efface adnexa and extend into the subcutis. Neither microorganisms nor foreign material are found microscopically, and cultures and cytology for organisms are negative. The lesions must be differentiated from those of the infectious granulomatous disorders and reactive histiocytosis in dogs.

Canine Reactive Histiocytosis

Canine reactive histiocytosis is a poorly understood disorder that occurs in cutaneous and systemic forms in dogs of a variety of ages and breeds. Cultures and special stains fail to reveal causative agents, and the disorder is thought to be the result of immune dysregulation. The disorder typically has a slowly progressive, waxing and waning course but can respond favorably, at least for a time, to immunomodulatory therapy. The lesions require long-term management and often lead to death, particularly if there is systemic involvement. The cutaneous form consists of single or multifocal, nonpainful plaques or nodules composed of histiocytic cells that are immunophenotypically identified as dermal perivascular activated dendritic antigen-presenting cells ($CD1^+$, $CD4^+$, $CD11c^+$, MHC II^+, and $CD90^+$). Also intermixed with the histiocytic cells are $CD3^+$, $CD8^+$, $TCR\alpha\beta^+$ T lymphocytes, and $CD11b^+$ neutrophils. The systemic form is identical immunophenotypically but can also involve the nasal mucosa, eyelids, sclera, lung, spleen, liver, bone marrow, and multiple lymph nodes in addition to the skin. Gross lesions in the cutaneous form are restricted to the skin and subcutis, can be alopecic or haired, and are most often on the head, neck, perineum, scrotum, and extremities. Histologically, there are single or multifocal infiltrates of large, round-to-oval histiocytes mixed with lymphocytes and neutrophils that, in early lesions, are periadnexal to elongate and are oriented vertically. Later, the infiltrates coalesce into larger deep dermal and subcutaneous masses. Vessels are often surrounded

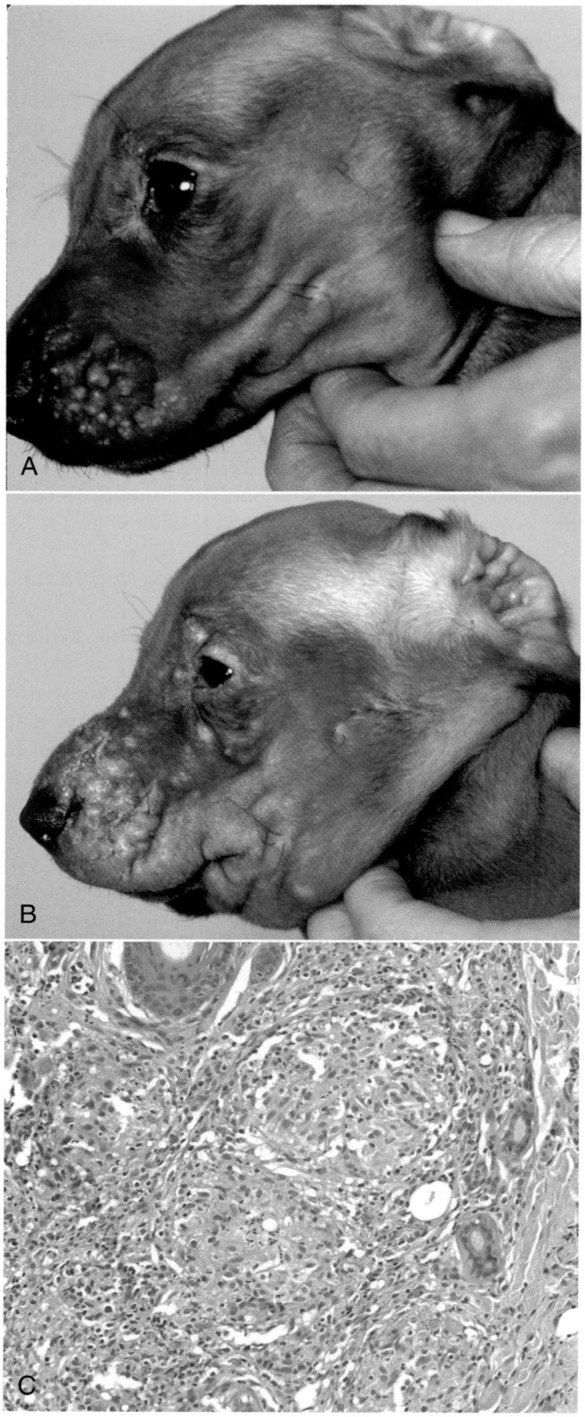

Fig. 17-74 Granulomatous dermatitis, skin, dog.
A, Juvenile sterile granulomatous dermatitis and lymphadenitis (juvenile pyoderma), dachshund puppy. The pustules on the muzzle are of 1-day duration. The mandibular lymph node (held between thumb and index finger) is enlarged. **B,** Juvenile sterile granulomatous dermatitis and lymphadenitis (juvenile pyoderma), dachshund puppy (same as in **A**). The lesions, of 12-days duration, have progressed to include alopecia, thickening of the skin from edema, and crusting. The mandibular lymph node (held between thumb and index finger) has at least doubled in size. **C,** Note the periadnexal mixture of macrophages and fewer lymphocytes, plasma cells, and neutrophils in the dermis. No microorganisms are present. H&E stain. (**A** and **B** courtesy Dr. David Prieur, College of Veterinary Medicine, Washington State University. **C** courtesy Dr. Ann M. Hargis, DermatoDiagnostics.)

and invaded by the infiltrates, which can result in thrombosis and infarction.

Canine Langerhans' Cell Histiocytosis

Canine Langerhans' cell histiocytosis is a rare condition in dogs resulting from progression of single or multiple persistent or recurrent canine cutaneous histiocytomas that spread to regional lymph nodes and subsequently to internal organs. The cell of origin is the Langerhans' cell, a cell immunophenotypically identified as the intraepithelial dendritic Langerhans' antigen-presenting cell ($CD1^+$, $CD11c^+$, $CD90^-$, $CD4^-$, MHC II^+, and ICAM-1^+, and usually E-cadherin$^+$). Expression of E-cadherin may diminish as the Langerhans' cells lose their connections with epidermal and follicular epithelial cells. The lesions begin with the development of one or more nodular, dome shaped often hairless masses (histiocytomas). In contrast to the majority of histiocytomas, the lesions fail to regress and become persistent or they may recur after excision. The masses extend more deeply into the subcutis. There is enlargement of regional lymph nodes, the result of spread of Langerhans' cells to the nodes. With time, infiltrative nodular masses of Langerhans' cells develop in internal organs.

Histologically, the initial lesion consists of one or more circumscribed but nonencapsulated dermal-to-superficial panicular masses that are broader at the surface than at the base. The masses consist of cords and sheets of round to polyhedral cells with a rounded sometimes indented or folded nucleus (Langerhans' cells). The epidermis may be acanthotic with exaggerated epidermal dermal interdigitations. Langerhans' cells are often present in the epidermis. Ulceration and secondary bacterial infection can develop. In the persistent lesions, the cellular infiltrates extend more deeply into subcutis, become less well-differentiated, have increased mitotic index, and lack peripheral T lymphocyte infiltrates and foci of necrosis (features of regression of typical more common cutaneous histiocytomas). In addition, clusters of Langerhans' cells are located within dermal lymphatic channels. These cells spread to efface architecture of regional nodes and form infiltrative nodular masses in internal organs. The condition has a poor prognosis. Immunomodulatory therapy is not effective and not recommended in cases of Langerhans' cell histiocytosis.

Feline Dendritic Cell Histiocytosis

Feline dendritic cell histiocytosis is a rare condition in cats resulting in development of histiocytic masses. The cell of origin is immunophenotypically identified as a dendritic cell (CD 18, $CD1^+$, MHC II^+), but variable expression of E-cadherin in different cases prevents further identification as to whether this cell normally functions as an intraepithelial or dermal dendritic antigen-presenting cell. Gross lesions begin with the development of one or more dermal masses that may subsequently enlarge and coalesce into larger plaque-like areas that may remain limited to the skin. In some cases, there may be spread to regional lymph nodes. In addition, some masses may become poorly differentiated and develop invasive features of histiocytic neoplasia with spread to one or more internal organs.

Histologic lesions consist of circumscribed, but nonencapsulated masses in the dermis and panniculus that are broader at the surface than the base. The masses consist of large rounded to polyhedral cells with a large central vesicular nucleus. Mixed inflammatory cells, including numerous vacuolated macrophages, may be present. In some masses, the histiocytic cells are also present in the epidermis.

Idiopathic Sterile Nodular Panniculitis

Idiopathic sterile nodular panniculitis develops in dogs, cats, and rarely horses. These lesions are of unknown cause and are characterized grossly by single or multifocal plaques or nodules in the subcutis and occasionally deep dermis of any anatomic site. Lesions can rupture and drain, thus they involve the dermis secondarily. Microscopic lesions consist of discrete, coalescing, or diffuse accumulations of macrophages (histiocytes), neutrophils, lymphocytes, and occasionally other leukocytes. The lesions must be differentiated from those of the infectious granulomatous disorders, sterile pyogranuloma syndrome, and reactive histiocytosis in dogs.

Xanthomas (Xanthogranulomas)

Xanthomas are rare, usually multifocal, light tan to yellow papules, plaques, or nodules located in the skin of cats and more rarely horses and dogs. The lesions take their name from the Greek "xanthos" meaning yellow. Some xanthomas are associated with abnormalities in triglyceride or cholesterol metabolism and are thus seen in animals with hereditary defects in lipid metabolism or with metabolic disorders such as diabetes mellitus, hypothyroidism, or hyperadrenocorticism. Histologically, xanthomas associated with abnormalities in triglyceride or cholesterol metabolism consist of sheets of macrophages filled with foamy cytoplasm, scattered giant cells, and interstitial areas of granular to amorphous lipid material and cholesterol clefts. The lipids in the lesions impart a yellow to tan color to the clinical lesions, which is responsible for the name. Rarely, xanthogranulomas also have developed in apparently healthy cats and dogs.

Other syndromes, including equine generalized granulomatous disease (see the section on Vetch Toxicosis and Vetch-Like Diseases), and nutritional pansteatitis (see the section on Vitamin E Deficiency), are also categorized as sterile granulomatous disorders.

Disorders of the Claw Bed and Lupoid Onychodystrophy

Onychodystrophy refers to abnormal formation of the claw (nail), onychomadesis to sloughing of claws, and paronychia to inflammation of the skin of the claw fold. These conditions are rare. Onychodystrophy and paronychia of multiple claws on multiple feet have a variety of causes, including infections (e.g., bacterial, fungal), immune-mediated disorders (e.g., pemphigus, lupus erythematosus), systemic disease (e.g., hyperadrenocorticism, disseminated intravascular coagulation), and disorders of unknown cause (e.g., lupoid onychodystrophy, idiopathic onychodystrophy). Diagnosis can require amputation of the third phalanx and the adjacent skin proximal to the claw fold for histopathologic evaluation. Lupoid onychodystrophy is probably the most common cause of onychomadesis that leads to onychodystrophy of multiple claws involving multiple feet in dogs. The condition affects many breeds of dogs of varying ages; the dogs are healthy otherwise. History includes sudden loss of claws, eventually involving all claws on all feet. There is partial regrowth of misshapen, friable claws that continue to slough. Paronychia is usually absent. Histologic lesions are more prominent on the dorsal aspect of the claw and claw bed skin and include interface lymphoplasmacytic inflammation with basal cell vacuolation and apoptosis and pigmentary incontinence. Secondary bacterial infection and osteomyelitis can develop.

CUTANEOUS MANIFESTATIONS OF SYSTEMIC DISORDERS

Laminitis

The term *laminitis* refers to inflammation of the laminar structures of the hoof, but laminitis is a complex disease in which inflammation is only a part of the disease process. Laminitis occurs when there is failure of the basal epithelial cells of the epidermal laminae (attached to the inner hoof wall) to adhere to the basement membrane and underlying dermal laminae (attached to the third phalanx), which results in loss of support of the distal phalanx within the hoof. In the severe form of the disease, the loss of support leads to a devastating, crippling disease. Laminitis can be seen in any hoofed animal but is of greatest importance in horses and cattle. Laminitis occurs in three phases (developmental or preclinical, acute, and chronic). By definition, chronic laminitis (also called *founder*) refers to the stage of laminitis associated with radiographic or physical evidence of rotational or vertical displacement of the third phalanx relative to the hoof wall. In severe laminitis, rotation can occur as early as 24 hours after the appearance of lameness. Laminitis develops as a consequence of three broad types of disease processes. These include systemic disease (e.g., carbohydrate overload, endotoxemia or septicemia, metritis, enterocolitis, or contact with black walnut shavings), metabolic disease (e.g., hyperadrenocorticism, insulin resistance, obesity, or glucocorticoid administration), and trauma (excessive contusion, excessive weight bearing on a single limb). The pathogenesis of laminitis is complex, not completely understood, and controversial. Various theories have been developed to explain how the hoof's lamellar structure is initially damaged in laminitis. The vascular theory suggests that there are abnormalities in the hoof blood flow, including increased capillary pressure, flow in arteriovenous anastomoses, and venoconstriction, which deprive the laminae of oxygen/nutrients and can lead to ischemia. The enzymatic theory suggests that increased digital blood flow delivers cytokines or other laminitis-triggering factors to the digit where they activate matrix metalloproteinases, which are enzymes shown to contribute to the separation of the laminar epithelial cells from the basement membrane. Matrix metalloproteinases are present in the laminar tissue because these enzymes are important in hoof remodeling. The inflammatory theory suggests that in the early stages of laminitis local digital cytokine (IL-1-beta, IL-6, and IL-8) and adhesion molecule (ICAM-1 and E-selectin) gene expression is associated with infiltration of leukocytes (neutrophils) into laminar tissue, creating inflammation and tissue damage. Another theory, the metabolic theory, was developed because it was discovered that horses and ponies with metabolic disease, including obesity, insulin resistance, hyperinsulinemia, and hypertriglyceridemia, are at increased risk for developing laminitis. The reasons for this are unclear, but it has been shown that laminitis can be induced in healthy ponies by maintaining superphysiologic circulating concentrations of insulin. Thus it has been hypothesized that laminitis can be triggered in an insulin-resistant horse or pony by conditions that increase insulin resistance or hyperinsulinemia (e.g., diets high in carbohydrates, overfeeding, administration of glucocorticoids, or episodes of endotoxemia). Recent research suggests that there are interconnecting links between these various theories, so they probably are not mutually exclusive. Further research is necessary to unravel the sequences of events leading to laminar failure. Gross findings of the external foot in acute laminitis can be minimal. Swelling or edema of the coronary band can be seen. Extravasation of serum through the skin above the coronary band is indicative of severe laminitis. Chronic lesions are highly variable, ranging from minimal gross changes to a totally gangrenous foot. Common gross lesions include parallel circumferential hoof rings (ridges, founder rings), altered foot shape, separation of the wall from the epidermis at the coronet, depression of the coronary band, a flattened sole, and in some cases, penetration of the third phalanx through the sole.

The principal clinical sign of laminitis is pain manifested as lameness, abnormal stance, or reluctance to move. Diagnosis of laminitis is based principally on clinical, radiographic, and gross findings. Histopathology is used to facilitate understanding of the pathogenesis of laminitis. Regardless of the initial stimulus, the lesions of acute laminitis include degeneration and necrosis of epithelial cells of the laminae, separation of epithelial cells from the basement membrane, and loss of the basement membrane. If the epithelial and basement membrane damage is minor and patchy, regeneration of the damaged cells and basement membrane occurs, preserving structural integrity of the epithelial laminae and hoof, and the animal does not enter into the chronic stage of laminitis. If the epithelial and basement membrane damage is more severe and confluent, the stability created by the interdigitating epithelial laminae attaching the hoof wall to the dermis and third phalanx is disrupted and the structural integrity of the foot is weakened. In addition, the epithelial necrosis causes release of inflammatory mediators, such as cytokines, which result in congestion, edema, and an influx of a small-to-moderate number of neutrophils and mixed mononuclear cells. The edema adds to the soft tissue swelling and in the confines of the rigid hoof wall, further compromises digital perfusion. If the tissue damage is subtotal, remaining epithelial cells regenerate. The hyperplasia and increased cornification of epithelial cells of the primary and secondary laminae cause broadening and fusion of the laminae, which reduces the surface area of the laminae and weakens the structural support of the hoof wall. The weakened structure of the epithelial laminae and basement membrane as a result of degeneration, necrosis, and subsequent epithelial hyperplasia, combined with the weight of the animal on the hoof and pulling force of the digital flexor tendon, contribute to displacement of the third phalanx, the hallmark of chronic laminitis, and to the altered shape of the foot in chronic laminitis (Fig. 17-75). For example, the circumferential hoof rings develop because the heel growth exceeds that of the dorsal wall. The unequal growth rate of the heels compared with the dorsal wall plus the mechanical forces on the wall also lead to abnormal hoof shape, such as the concave profile of the dorsal hoof, often accompanied by long under-run heels. Depression of the coronary band and flattened or dropped sole are a result of displacement of the distal phalanx relative to the hoof wall, thus are an indication that collapse of the foot has occurred.

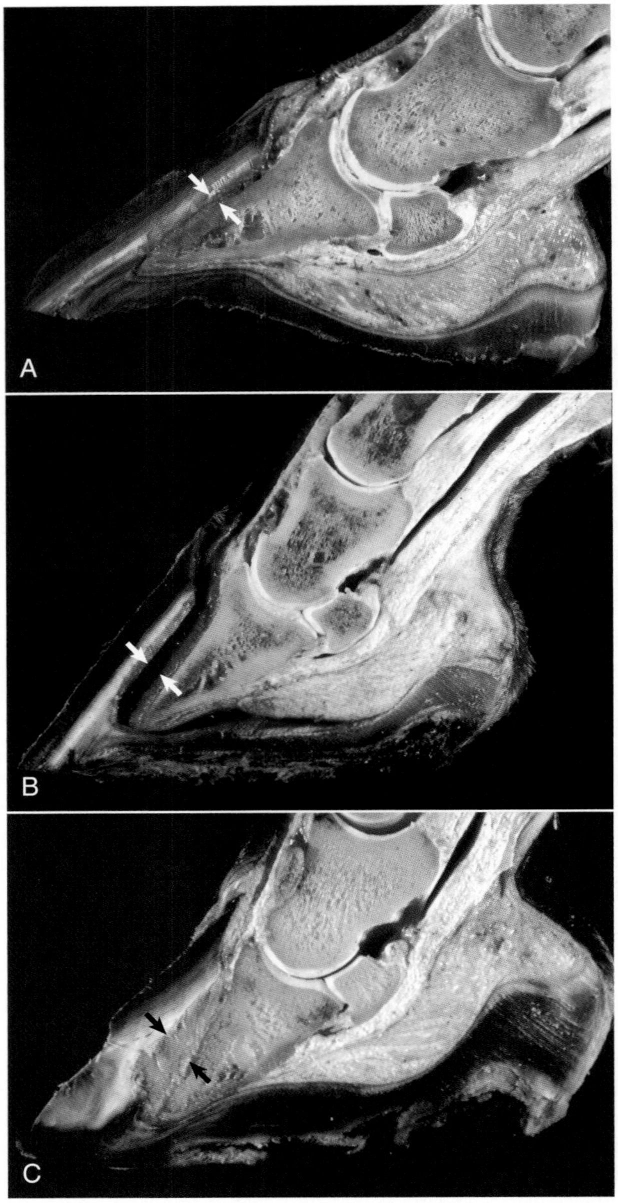

Fig. 17-75 Laminitis, hoof, horse.
A, Normal hoof, midsagittal section. Note that the dorsal surface of the third phalanx is parallel to the epidermal laminae of the inner surface of the hoof wall *(arrows)*. No space is visible at this junction or at the junction of the ventral surface of the third phalanx and the internal (weight-bearing) surface of the hoof. **B,** Acute laminitis. Note that the dorsal surface of the third phalanx has separated from the epidermal laminae of the inner surface of the hoof wall *(arrows)*, leaving a large gap. The tip of the third phalanx has rotated ventrally slightly, resulting in a space between the ventral aspect of the third phalanx and the internal surface of the horny sole (weight-bearing surface of the hoof). **C,** Severe chronic laminitis. The dorsal surface of the third phalanx is widely separated from the epidermal laminae of the inner surface of the hoof wall, and the tip of the third phalanx has rotated ventrally. This space is filled with proliferated epithelium, connective tissue, and areas of inflammation *(arrows)*. The shape of the entire weight-bearing surface of the hoof, the external surface of the horny sole, has been altered, leading to turning up and irregular wear of the toe region and thickening of the heel of the horny sole. (**A** courtesy Dr. Pamela E. Ginn, College of Veterinary Medicine, University of Florida. **B** courtesy College of Veterinary Medicine, University of Illinois. **C** courtesy Dr. T. Boosinger, College of Veterinary Medicine, Auburn University; and Noah's Arkive, College of Veterinary Medicine, The University of Georgia.)

Cutaneous Paraneoplastic Syndromes

Cutaneous paraneoplastic syndromes are rare dermatoses that occur in association with internal malignancies (Box 17-14). Confirmation of a dermatosis as a paraneoplastic syndrome requires strict adherence to established clinical, histopathologic, and in some instances, immunologic criteria. Conditions meeting these criteria currently recognized in animals include PNP (discussed in the section on Selected Autoimmune Reactions); paraneoplastic alopecia and internal malignancies in the cat; exfoliative dermatosis and thymoma in the cat, dog, and rabbit; and superficial necrolytic dermatopathy in the dog and cat. Dermatofibrosis in the dog, pancreatic panniculitis, and multisystemic eosinophilic epitheliotropic disease in the horse (see the section on Disorders Characterized by Infiltrates of Eosinophils or Plasma Cells) have also been associated with underlying neoplasia; however, they have not yet been proved to be true paraneoplastic syndromes. This list is exclusive of the endocrine dermatoses associated with functional tumors of endocrine organs. Many other syndromes are documented in humans, and it is likely more will be documented in animals in the future. The refractory nature of these syndromes and their

BOX 17-14 Principal Cutaneous Paraneoplastic Syndromes

Paraneoplastic alopecia and internal malignancies in the cat
Exfoliative dermatitis and thymoma
Superficial necrolytic dermatitis
Pancreatic panniculitis (necrotizing panniculitis)
Nodular dermatofibrosis and renal or uterine tumors in dogs
Paraneoplastic pemphigus (see the section on Selected Autoimmune Diseases)

significance as an indicator of systemic disease underscores the importance of their recognition.

Paraneoplastic Alopecia Associated with Internal Malignancies in the Cat (Pancreatic Paraneoplastic Syndrome)

Paraneoplastic alopecia associated with internal malignancies in the cat (pancreatic paraneoplastic syndrome) is a rapidly progressive, largely ventrally distributed, symmetric alopecia that develops in older cats with metastatic pancreatic or biliary carcinomas. The pathogenesis of this condition is not known. The alopecia typically affects the ventral abdomen, thorax, and legs. The ears and periocular skin are less frequently involved. Alopecic skin is smooth, soft, and often has a shiny or glistening appearance. The pawpads are dry with circular rings of scale. Histologically, affected skin has small inactive hair follicles with a reduction or absence of the stratum corneum. Some cats groom excessively, and it has been suggested that the smooth shiny appearance of the skin is caused by the absence of the stratum corneum. In other areas of the skin, there is variable orthokeratotic and parakeratotic hyperkeratosis in which *Malassezia pachydermatis* is sometimes identified. In addition to the alopecia, the cats have systemic signs of anorexia, weight loss, and lethargy.

Exfoliative Dermatitis and Thymoma

A generalized exfoliative dermatitis has been documented as a paraneoplastic syndrome of older cats with thymomas. More recently, the condition has been recognized in dogs and rabbits. T lymphocyte immune dysregulation probably plays a role in lesion development. Rarely, identical cutaneous lesions are recognized in cats without evidence of underlying neoplasia or internal disease, suggesting that the histologic lesions in this disease syndrome may represent a cutaneous reaction pattern associated with T lymphocyte immune dysfunction. Gross lesions begin as scaling and erythema of the head, neck, and ears and progress to generalized alopecia with scales, crusts, and ulcers. Histologically, the lesions include basal cell hydropic degeneration, lymphocyte exocytosis, and lymphocyte clustering around apoptotic keratinocytes of the epidermis and outer follicular root sheath. Sebaceous glands may be absent. The lesions are compatible with the diagnosis of erythema multiforme or a graft-versus-host-type reaction. *Malassezia pachydermatis* is sometimes identified. Cats with this syndrome may have clinical signs referable to an intrathoracic mass resulting in dyspnea.

Superficial Necrolytic Dermatitis (Diabetic Dermatopathy, Hepatocutaneous Syndrome, Necrolytic Migratory Erythema, Metabolic Epidermal Necrosis)

Superficial necrolytic dermatitis (also known as diabetic dermatopathy, hepatocutaneous syndrome, necrolytic migratory erythema, metabolic epidermal necrosis) is an uncommon disorder reported primarily in older dogs with deranged nutrient metabolism associated with hepatic dysfunction, diabetes mellitus, or less commonly with a glucagon-secreting tumor usually within the pancreatic islets. Long-term anticonvulsant therapy and the rare ingestion of mycotoxins also have preceded the development of superficial necrolytic dermatitis. The disorder is rare in cats, and has been associated in some instances with pancreatic carcinoma and/or hepatopathy, but other conditions also have been present, including thymic amyloidosis and intestinal lymphoma. The pathogenesis of superficial necrolytic dermatitis is not completely understood and may vary with the underlying defect. When glucagon is elevated, persistent gluconeogenesis is thought to result in a negative nitrogen balance with protein degradation, including proteins in the epidermis. However, when glucagon is not elevated, as occurs in humans with some types of hepatic or malabsorptive disease and in dogs with diabetes and multinodular vacuolar hepatopathy, it is thought that deficiencies of certain essential fatty acids, zinc, and amino acids play a role. In dogs, clinical lesions of scales, thick adherent crusts, erythema, alopecia, erosions, and ulcers develop on the mucocutaneous junctions, genitalia, pinnae, skin subjected to trauma (elbows, hocks), and ventral thorax. Pawpad lesions consist of crusting and fissuring or ulceration (see Fig. 17-10) and result in lameness. In cats, alopecia and scaling of trunk and limbs have been seen; another cat had alopecia of the ventral trunk and medial thighs and ulceration and crusting of the oral mucocutaneous and interdigital regions. Microscopic lesions, when fully developed, are considered diagnostic and consist of trilaminar thickening of the epidermis in which the stratum corneum has marked parakeratosis, the upper stratum spinosum is pale with reticular degeneration, and the lower spinous and basal cell layers are hyperplastic (see Fig. 17-10). Secondary infections with bacteria or yeast frequently complicate lesions, and secondary infection with dermatophytes also has been seen.

Pancreatic Panniculitis (Necrotizing Panniculitis)

Pancreatic panniculitis (necrotizing panniculitis) is an acute rare disorder that has developed in dogs with pancreatic neoplasia and pancreatitis. It is seen less frequently in cats in which it has been associated with pancreatitis. The lesions are thought to be a result of the release of pancreatic enzymes (e.g., lipases) either from damaged pancreatic exocrine cells or from neoplastic exocrine cells. The lipases enter the systemic circulation and subsequently locate in the panniculus. Gross lesions are mostly truncal and consist of multiple, frequently ulcerated and hemorrhagic nodules or poorly defined swellings within the subcutis. Lesions may drain purulent, oily material. Histologically, there is necrosis of adipose tissue (caused by the lipases) with fine basophilic granularity (caused by mineralization of the necrotic fatty tissue). Suppurative to pyogranulomatous inflammation occurs at the periphery of the necrotic foci. Hemorrhage and fibrin exudation may be evident, and lesions may extend into the dermis and rupture through the epidermis.

Nodular Dermatofibrosis and Renal Disease in the Dog

In nodular dermatofibrosis, multiple cutaneous nodules composed of excessive collagen coexist with renal cystadenomas, cystadenocarcinomas, hyperplastic epithelial cysts, or uterine smooth muscle tumors. Renal lesions are often bilateral and may not be detectable clinically for months or years after the appearance of the cutaneous nodules. The syndrome has been described most commonly in the German shepherd but has been seen in a few other purebred dog breeds and mixed-breed dogs and is thought to have an autosomal dominant mode of inheritance in the German shepherd. Whether the condition is a true paraneoplastic syndrome with the renal neoplasm inducing dermal fibrosis or the simultaneous occurrence of two independent conditions with a common hereditary linkage is undetermined. Gross lesions consist of firm dermal and subcutaneous nodules on legs, head, or ears. Histologic lesions consist of nodular dermal and subcutaneous aggregates of poorly cellular, mature dermal collagen bundles that are slightly thickened. In the dermis, the collagen bundles blend often imperceptibly with bordering collagen, but in the subcutis, the nodules are usually circumscribed. Adnexa are normal or hyperplastic. The cutaneous nodules are benign but serve as a marker for the more serious renal lesions.

Paraneoplastic Pemphigus

See the discussion on paraneoplastic pemphigus (PNP) in the section on Selected Autoimmune Reactions.

CUTANEOUS NEOPLASIA

The skin is a common site of neoplastic growth in most animals; the neoplasms are of ectodermal, mesodermal, and melanocytic origin (Box 17-15). Ectodermal neoplasms of the epidermis and adnexa are most often benign with the exception of the neoplasms of the apocrine sweat glands, apocrine glands of the anal sac, and neoplasms of the surface epithelium (squamous cell carcinomas).

Benign neoplasms do not metastasize or invade adjacent tissue. In general, benign neoplasms are circumscribed, grow by expansion, and are composed of well-differentiated cells that closely resemble the cells or tissue of origin (see Box 17-15). Malignant neoplasms are locally invasive and often metastasize. They are more often composed of anaplastic cells with a high mitotic index that no longer resemble the cells of origin. Anaplastic cells are pleomorphic (vary in cell size and shape) and have a large, vesicular nucleus with increased size and number of nucleoli (see Box 17-15). Malignant cells develop surface alterations such as altered antigenicity, decreased numbers or altered location of receptors for adjacent cells, and increased receptors for components of the extracellular matrix. Changes such as these allow malignant cells to detach from the primary site of tumor growth, move through tissues, and in some cases escape detection by the host's immune system. A specific example is the loss of E-cadherins (proteins responsible for epithelial cell-to-cell attachment) by some types of carcinomas. E-cadherins are partially responsible for the "contact inhibition" that leads to density control and inhibits uncontrolled proliferation of epithelial cells.

Neoplasms of the skin develop secondary to the same basic molecular changes, leading to the development of neoplasms of any tissue. The neoplastic transformation of a cell is the end result of a series of events causing damage to the cellular DNA. Most agents that are known to be carcinogenic target and damage DNA. Solar radiation, x-radiation, viral infections, and continued trauma are important contributors to neoplastic transformation of components of the skin. Continued trauma contributes to tumor development by increasing cell turnover, which in turn increases the chance of mutations. Not all factors contributing to the development of cutaneous neoplasms are known.

Four categories of genes encode for a large number of proteins responsible for regulation of cellular proliferation and differentiation. These categories are the tumor-suppressor genes, the protooncogenes, genes that regulate apoptosis, and genes that regulate DNA repair. Damage to these genes results in deranged cellular proliferation by the abnormal expression or function of proteins such as growth factors, growth factor receptors, signal-transducing proteins, cell cycle regulators, and nuclear transcription factors. The majority of malignant neoplasms have evidence of damage (mutation) of multiple genes within these categories. Mutations are often collected by cells in a stepwise manner that imparts increasing degrees of malignant potential. These molecular changes are known to correlate with morphologic changes and the clinical behavior of some neoplasms. For example, it is known that squamous cell

Text continued on p. 1084

BOX 17-15 Examples of Tumors of the Skin

ECTODERMAL TUMORS

Trichoblastoma

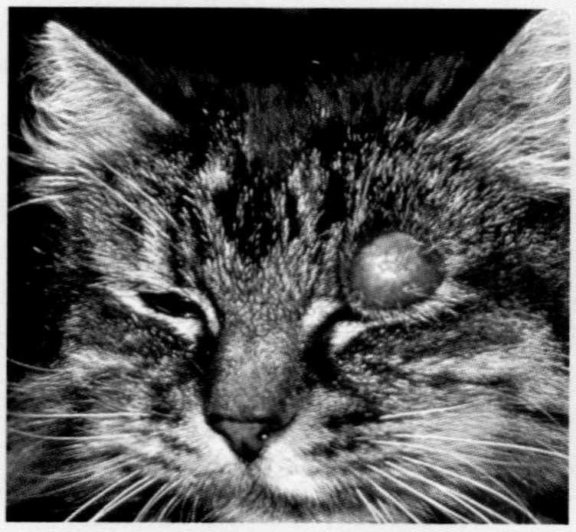

Trichoblastoma, skin, upper eyelid and dorsal to eye, cat. The tumor is circumscribed, raised, and sparsely haired. The tumor and bordering skin can be easily moved from side to side above the deeper tissue because the tumor has not invaded into underlying tissue.*

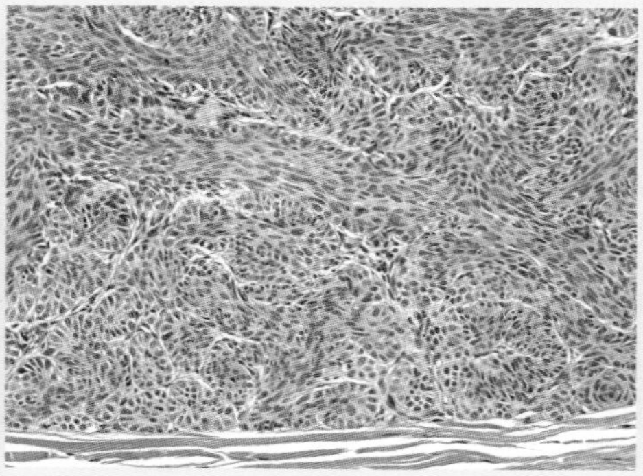

Trichoblastoma, skin, cat. H&E stain. A circumscribed tumor of basaloid epithelial cells (trichoblasts) arranged in irregular aggregates. Some of the trichoblasts are elongate (spindle-shaped), a feature of some trichoblastomas in cats. H&E stain.†

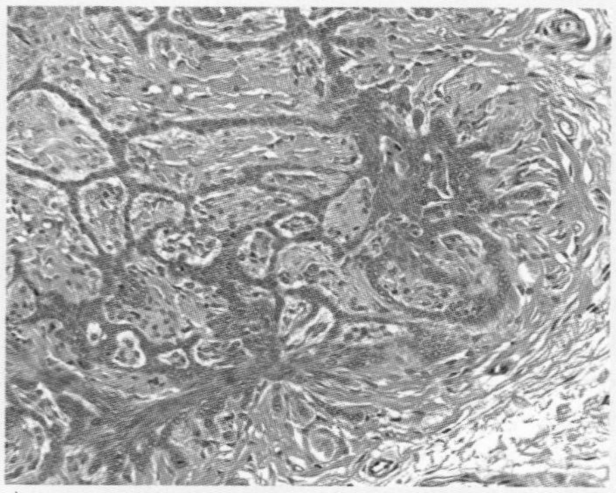

Trichoblastoma skin, dog. Note ribbon (medusoid) pattern produced by the proliferating basal cells. This pattern is one of several patterns (ribbon, trabecular, granular cell, spindle cell) typical of trichoblastomas in dogs. H&E stain.‡

BOX 17-15 Examples of Tumors of the Skin—cont'd

Infundibular Keratinizing Acanthoma

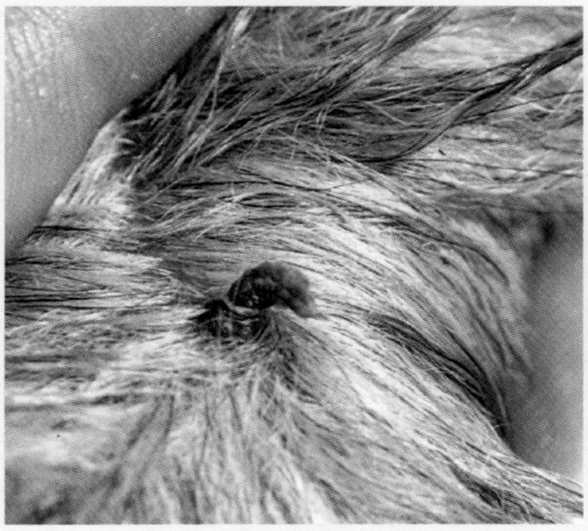

Infundibular keratinizing acanthoma (intracutaneous cornifying epithelioma, keratoacanthoma), skin, dog. Note horny growth (cutaneous horn) projecting from surface of the tumor. Cutaneous horns can arise from a variety of benign or malignant epidermal lesions (solar keratosis; Fig. 17-38, *B,* squamous cell carcinoma) or adnexal lesions, especially infundibular keratinizing acanthomas.[§]

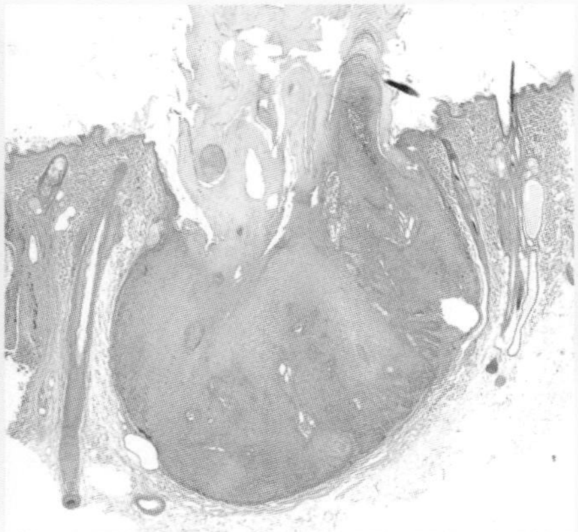

Infundibular keratinizing acanthoma, skin, dog. Note the circumscribed tumor located in the dermis and subcutis. The tumor consists of irregularly sized lobules of stratified squamous cornifying epithelium supported by a small quantity of collagenous stroma. The tumor is often "cystic" and contains laminations of stratum corneum, which can extend through the epidermal surface and form a "cutaneous horn." The epithelium forming the lobules of the tumor blends with the overlying epidermis. H&E stain.

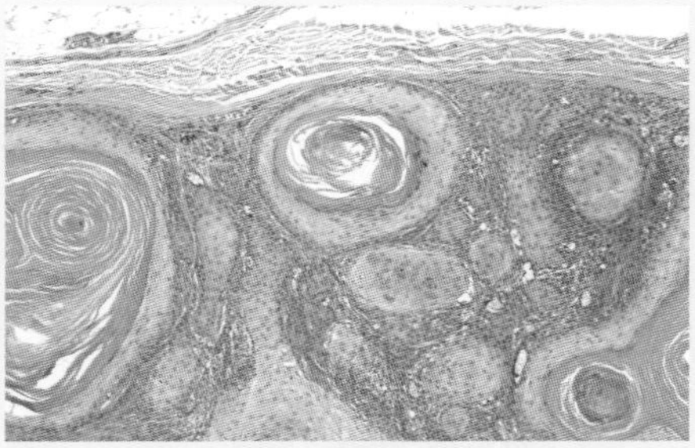

Infundibular keratinizing acanthoma, skin, dog. Infundibular keratinizing acanthoma, skin, Higher magnification of wall of the tumor. The lobules border concentric laminations of stratum corneum and are supported by scant mucinous stroma. These tumors resemble squamous cell carcinoma but have a circumscribed, noninvasive border. H&E stain.

Sebaceous Gland Adenoma

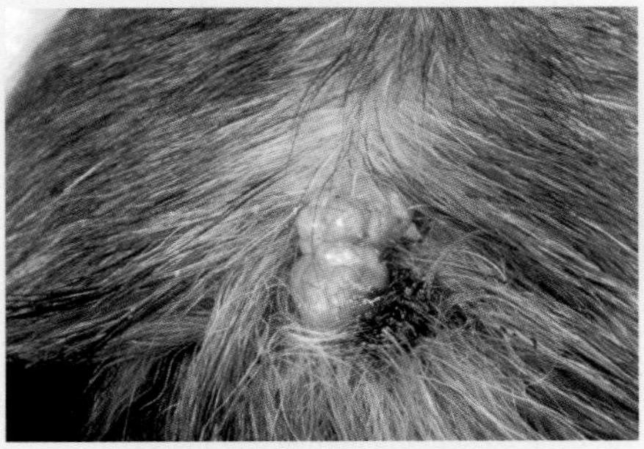

Sebaceous gland adenoma, skin, dog. This common tumor of sebaceous glands often protrudes above the epidermal surface. The tumors are hairless and greasy because of sebaceous gland secretion.

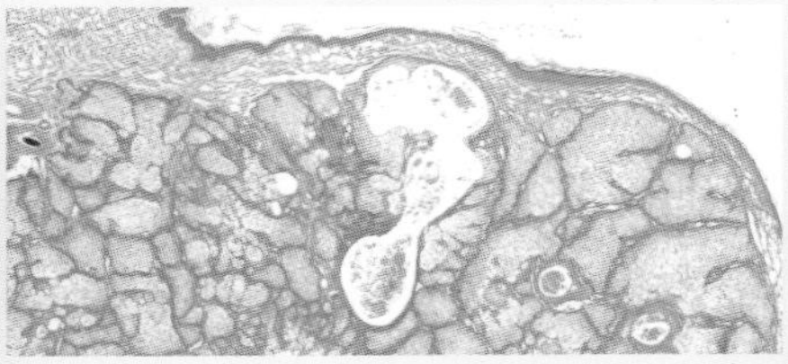

Sebaceous gland adenoma, skin, dog. Lobules of well-differentiated sebaceous glands are present in the dermis and cause polypoid elevation of the overlying epidermis. A duct with sebaceous secretion is also present. Ducts connect via follicular epithelium to the epidermis providing the sebaceous (greasy) secretion to the surface. H&E stain.

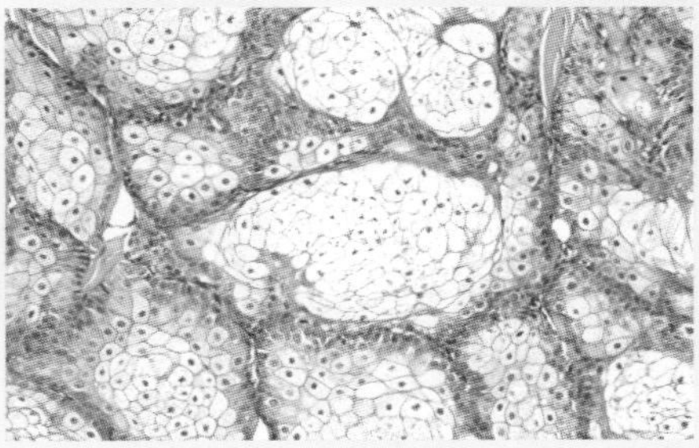

Sebaceous gland adenoma, skin, dog. Note the close resemblance of the lobules of tumor cells to those of nonneoplastic sebaceous glands, a feature suggesting benign behavior. H&E stain.

Continued

BOX 17-15 Examples of Tumors of the Skin—cont'd

Squamous Cell Carcinoma

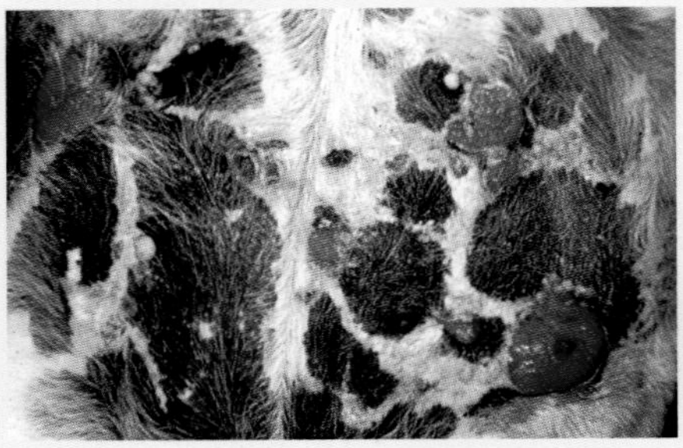

Squamous cell carcinomas, skin, abdomen, dog. Note multiple ulcerated squamous cell carcinomas in nonpigmented, sparsely haired abdominal skin. These are solar induced squamous cell carcinomas that developed in a beagle dog living outdoors at a high altitude region where the level of UV light is increased.

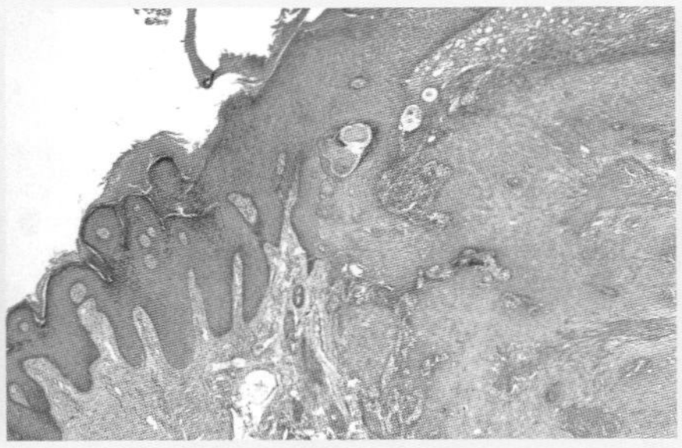

Squamous cell carcinoma, skin, dog. The dermis is invaded by neoplastic squamous epithelial cells that have arisen from the basal cells of the epidermis *(above center)* and that have differentiated to form irregular islands of squamous epithelium. H&E stain.†

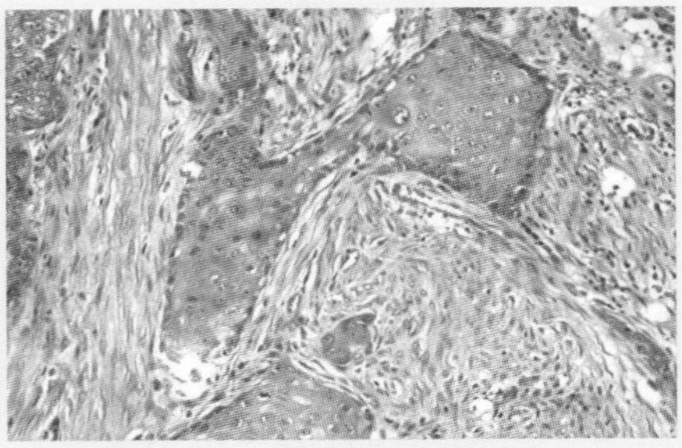

Squamous cell carcinoma, skin, dog. Islands of neoplastic epithelial cells with squamous differentiation have invaded the dermis and are surrounded by proliferating fibroblasts and collagen (desmoplasia). H&E stain.†

MESODERMAL TUMORS

Cutaneous Histiocytoma

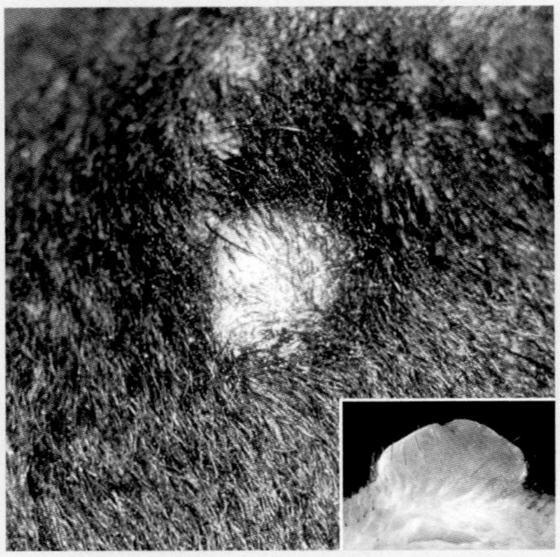

Cutaneous histiocytoma, skin, nose, dog. Circular raised alopecic tan nodule is present. Cutaneous histiocytomas frequently spontaneously regress.

Inset, section of cutaneous histiocytoma illustrating the nonencapsulated, solid dermal mass protruding above the epidermal surface.

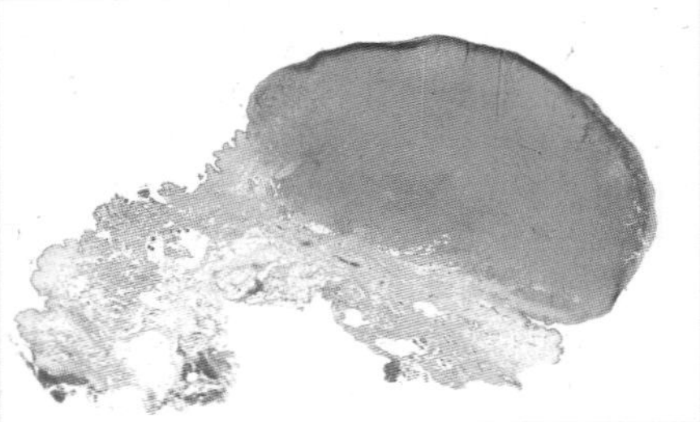

Histiocytoma, skin, dog. The histiocytoma elevates the epidermal surface, and consists of a solid mass of histiocytic cells. H&E stain.†

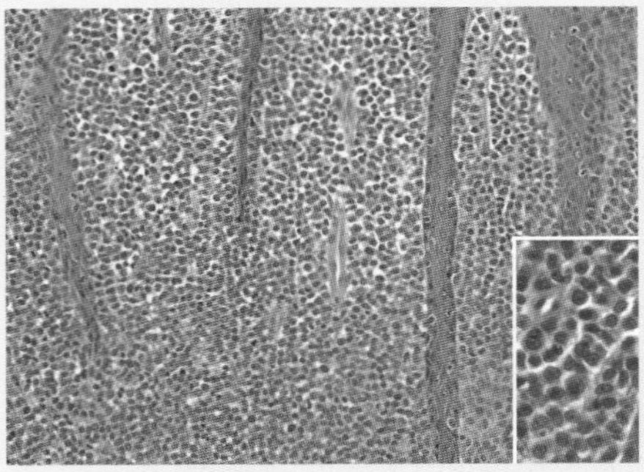

Histiocytoma, skin, dog. Note the polyhedral to round cells in the dermis and the down-growth of epidermis (rete ridges) into the histiocytoma (a common feature of these tumors). Inset: Higher magnification of the histiocytic cells. H&E stain.

BOX 17-15 Examples of Tumors of the Skin—cont'd

Cutaneous Lymphoma

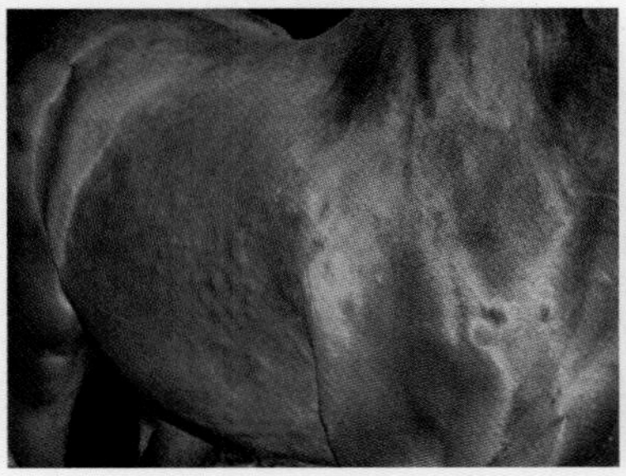

Cutaneous lymphoma, skin, neck and lateral thorax, horse. Note the nodules that are masses of neoplastic lymphocytes and infiltrating nonneoplastic lymphocytes in the dermis, causing elevation of overlying epidermis.¶

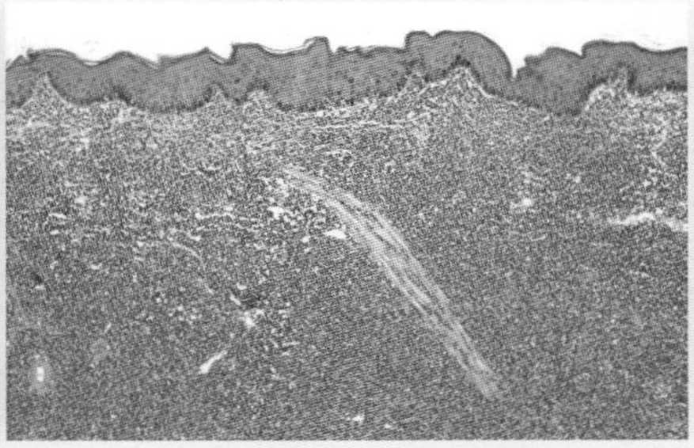

Cutaneous lymphoma, skin, horse. Sheets of neoplastic lymphocytes and infiltrating nonneoplastic lymphocytes have obliterated the normal dermal architecture except for an arrector pili muscle *(center)*. The overlying epidermis is normal. H&E stain.

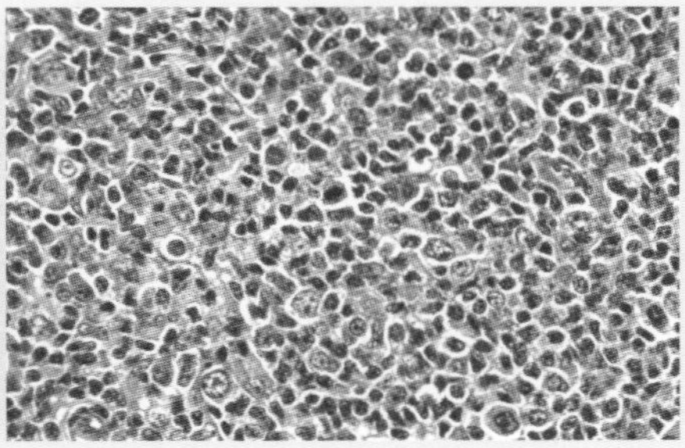

Cutaneous lymphoma, skin, horse. Note the population of different appearing lymphoid cells. Some resemble normal lymphocytes and are small and well differentiated, whereas others are large and pleomorphic with vesicular nuclei and prominent nucleoli. Immunohistochemical and genetic studies of many cases of cutaneous lymphoma in the horse have demonstrated that the small well-differentiated lymphocytes are nonneoplastic T lymphocytes, whereas the large pleomorphic lymphocytes are neoplastic B lymphocytes. It is speculated that the neoplastic B lymphocytes produce cytokines that lead to infiltrates of nonneoplastic T lymphocytes and sometimes other leukocytes. Cutaneous lymphoma in the horse with this morphology and immunophenotype is referred to as a T lymphocyte–rich B cell lymphoma subtype. H&E stain.

Epitheliotropic Lymphoma

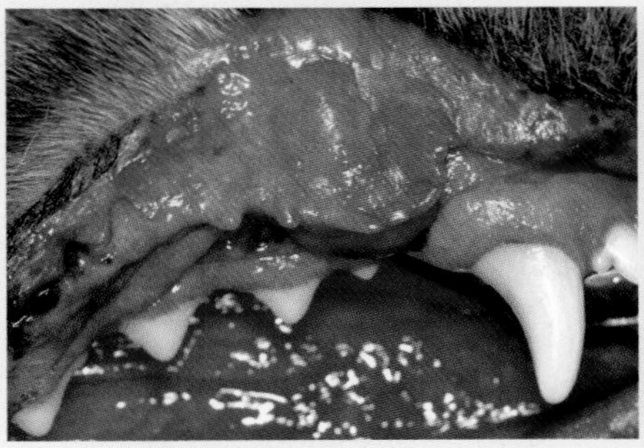

Epitheliotropic lymphoma, skin of lip and oral mucosa, dog. Note swelling, erythema, and depigmentation. Lymphocytes invade the epithelium and can cause depigmentation by displacing and damaging pigment containing epithelial cells and resident melanocytes of the basal region of the epidermis. Because of the involvement of the oral mucosa and mucocutaneous junctions and the presence of depigmentation and sometimes erosions, epitheliotropic lymphoma can be clinically confused with immune-mediated diseases such as SLE.

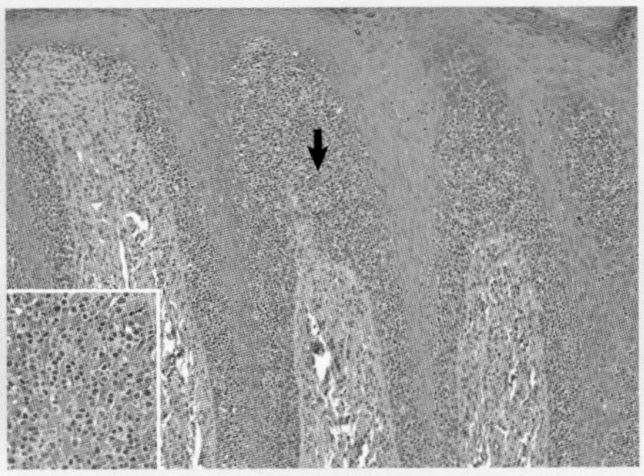

Epitheliotropic lymphoma, skin, pawpad, dog. Neoplastic lymphocytes are located predominantly in the lower layers of the epidermis *(arrow)*. *Inset,* Higher magnification of the neoplastic lymphocytes in the epidermis. Some of the lymphocytes are clustered together, forming microabscesses (Pautrier's microabscesses). H&E stain.

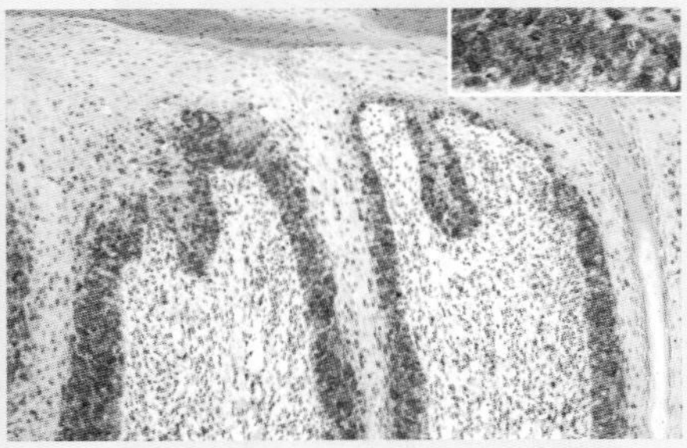

Epitheliotropic lymphoma, skin, pawpad, dog. Neoplastic lymphocytes are located predominantly in the lower layers of the epidermis and are labeled for CD3, indicating that they are T lymphocytes. *Inset,* Higher magnification of the malignant lymphocytes in the epidermis. Immunohistochemical stain for $CD3^+$ lymphocytes.

Continued

BOX 17-15 Examples of Tumors of the Skin—cont'd

Mast Cell Tumor

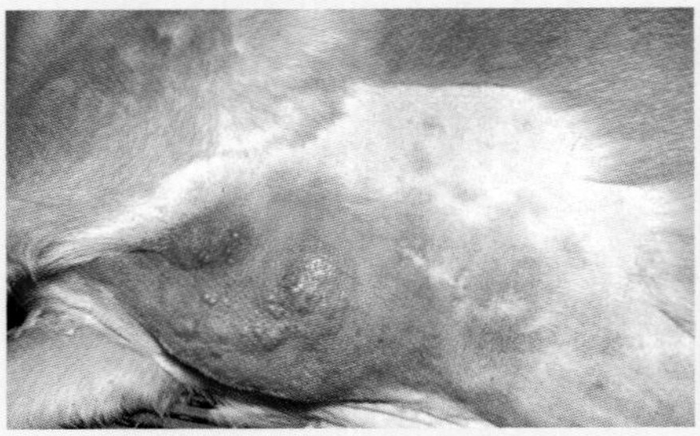

Mast cell tumor, skin, ventral thorax, dog. Note the irregular nodular and erythematous masses. Mast cell tumors in dogs can clinically resemble areas of inflammation because mast cells can degranulate and release inflammatory mediators (e.g., histamine, factors chemotactic for eosinophils and neutrophils, prostaglandins, serine esterases, and TNF-α) causing the inflammatory response.[¶]

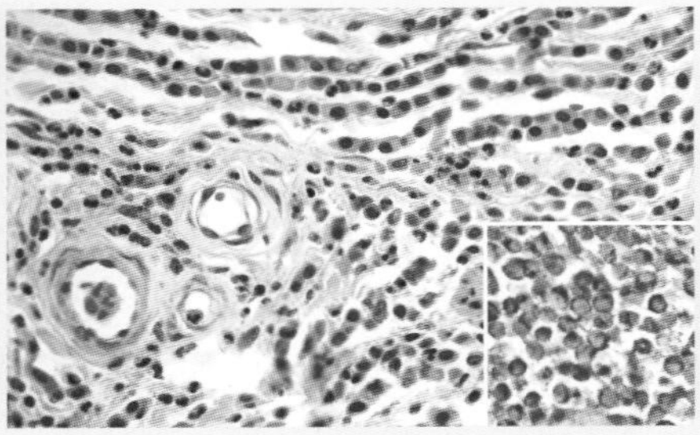

Mast cell tumor, skin, dog. The dermis is infiltrated by well-differentiated neoplastic mast cells with abundant gray to blue, finely granular cytoplasm and centrally located nuclei. H&E stain. *Inset,* Mast cells stained to illustrate metachromatic granules. In some cases, it can be difficult to differentiate round cell tumors such as histiocytomas, lymphomas, and mast cell tumors from each other. Demonstration of metachromatic cytoplasmic granules is an indicator of the presence of mast cells. Metachromasia means that the tissue or cellular component stains a color different from that of the staining dye because of a chemical reaction between the dye and the tissue component. For example, mast cell granules stain purple with the blue dye, toluidine blue. Toluidine blue stain.[†]

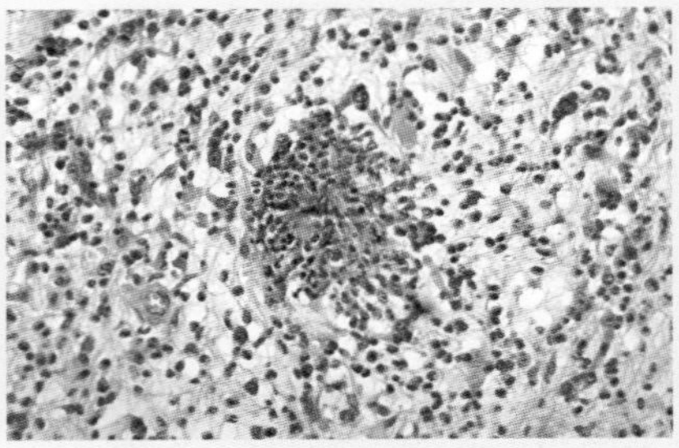

Mast cell tumor, skin, dog. Mast cell tumor with degranulated eosinophils that border a collagen fiber. The collagen fibers and bordering eosinophilic material have been referred to as *flame figures* in part because of their irregular, sometimes radiating, edges and brightly eosinophilic staining intensity. H&E stain.[†]

Fibrosarcoma

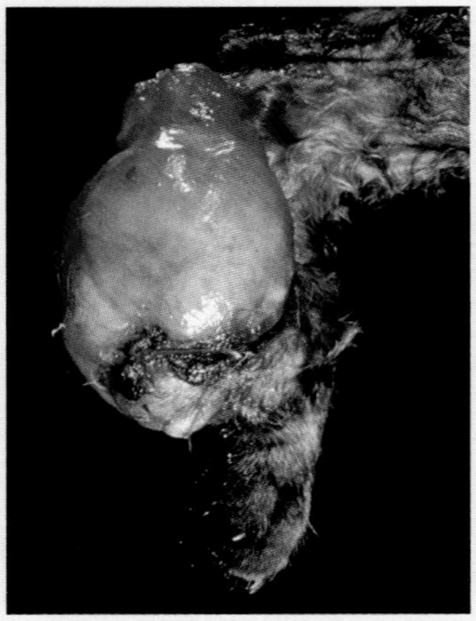

Fibrosarcoma, skin, leg, cat. The tumor has enlarged to such a degree that it has caused ulceration of the epidermis. Fibrosarcomas are locally invasive and difficult to excise completely. Amputation is an option for fibrosarcomas located on distal extremities.

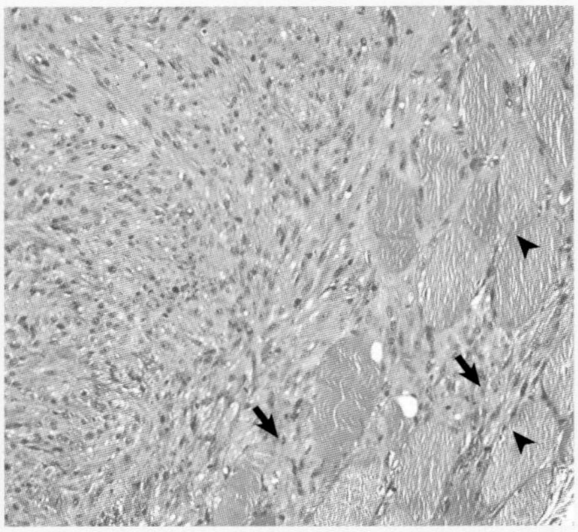

Fibrosarcoma, skin, cat. Cells of the fibrosarcoma *(arrows)* have infiltrated between skeletal muscle fibers *(arrowheads).* H&E stain.

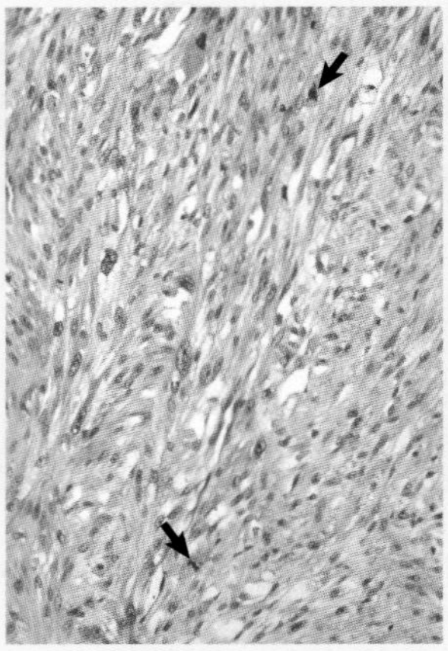

Fibrosarcoma, skin, cat. Note haphazardly arranged intersecting bundles of anaplastic spindle-shaped neoplastic cells within a collagenous stroma. Anaplastic cells are pleomorphic in that they vary in cell size and shape and have a large, vesicular nucleus with increased size and number of nucleoli. Numerous mitotic figures are also present *(arrows).* H&E stain.[†]

BOX 17-15 Examples of Tumors of the Skin—cont'd

Hemangioma

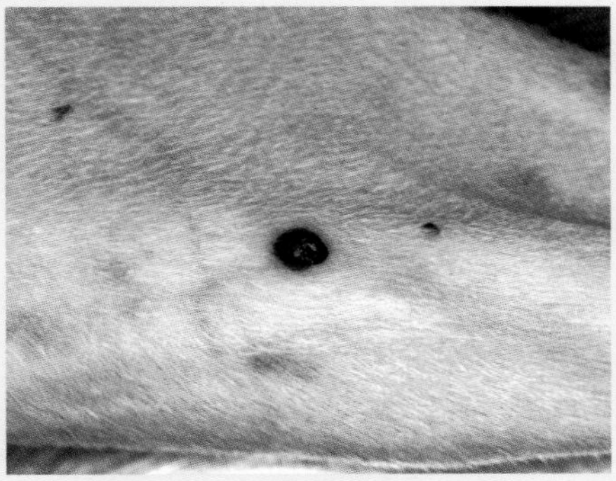

Hemangioma, skin, hind leg, dog. Note raised red to dark red circumscribed mass in nonpigmented and sparsely haired skin.

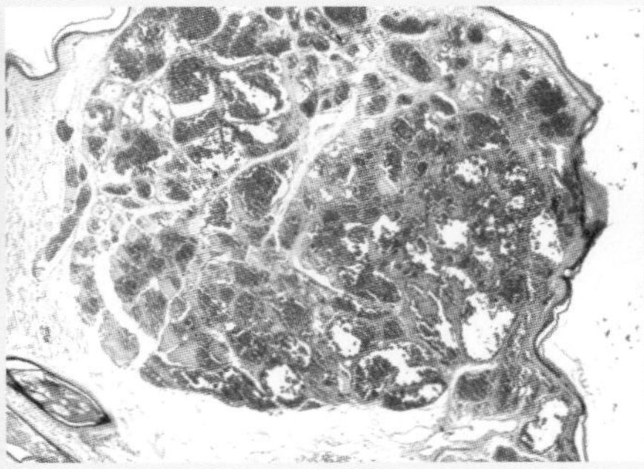

Hemangioma, skin, dog. Well-defined mass of proliferative, blood-filled, vascular channels in the dermis has elevated the epidermis. H&E stain.

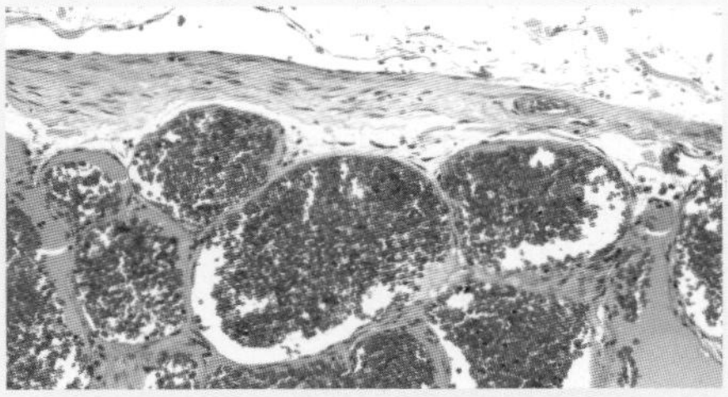

Hemangioma, skin, dog. The dermis is expanded by a circumscribed mass of blood-filled vascular channels lined by well-differentiated endothelial cells. The flattened well-differentiated endothelial cells form a single uniform layer. H&E stain.†

Hemangiosarcomas

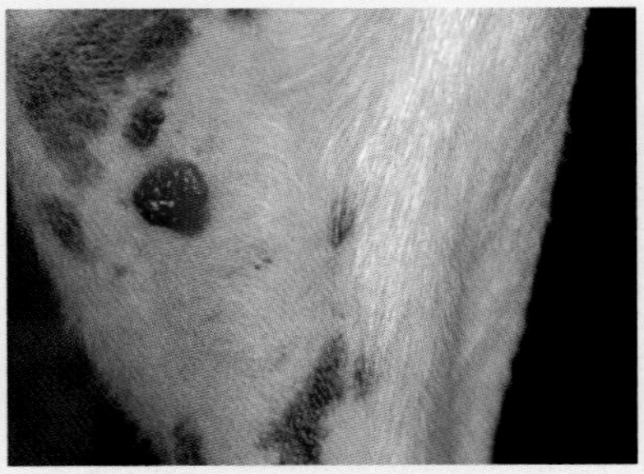

Hemangiosarcoma, skin, dog. Note multiple raised red masses in nonpigmented and sparsely haired skin of whippet.

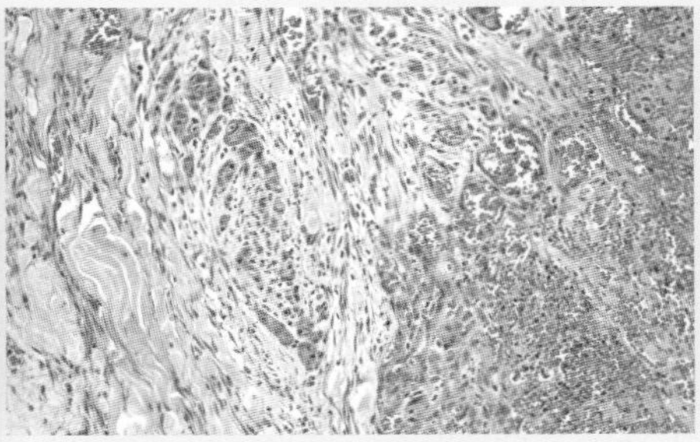

Hemangiosarcoma, skin, dog. Note poorly demarcated margin between tumor (mostly on the *right*) and normal tissue (mostly on the *left*). H&E stain.

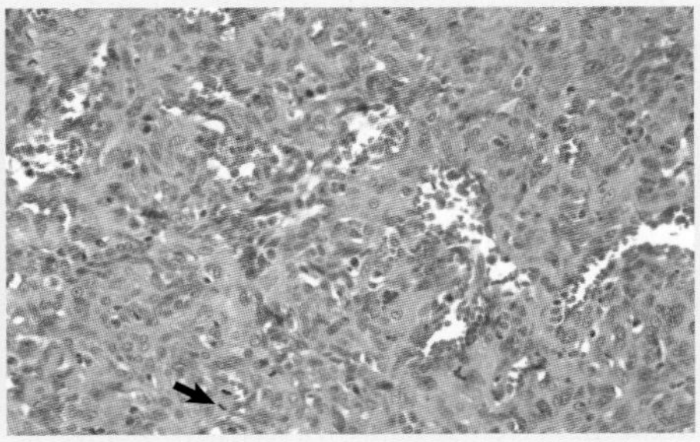

Hemangiosarcoma, skin, dog. The dermis is effaced by highly irregular vascular channels lined by plump, hyperchromatic endothelial cells with numerous mitotic figures *(arrow)*. H&E stain.†

Continued

BOX 17-15 Examples of Tumors of the Skin—cont'd

MELANOCYTIC TUMORS

Melanocytoma and Melanoma

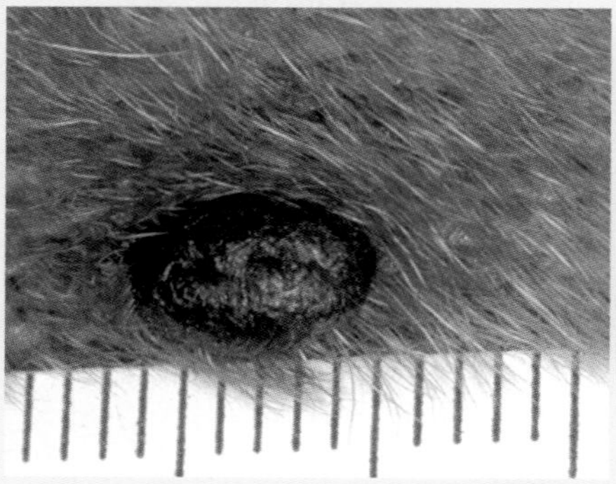

Melanocytoma, skin, dog. Note raised pigmented brown to black hairless mass.[¶]

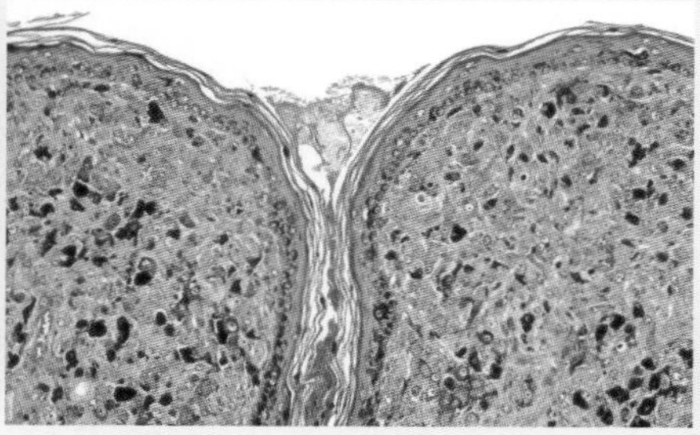

Melanocytoma, skin, dog. The dermis is diffusely infiltrated by sheets of variably pigmented melanocytes, which have prominent nucleoli and moderate variation in the size of cells and nuclei. H&E stain.[†]

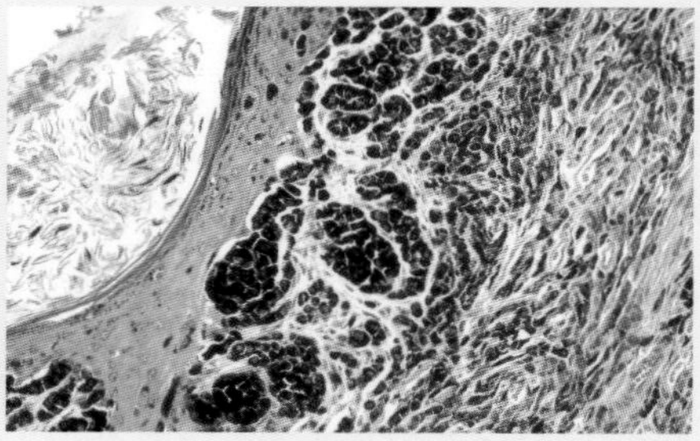

Melanoma, skin, dog. Note clusters of pigmented melanocytes within the epidermis. This is called *junctional activity* and is a feature of melanocytic tumors. H&E stain.[†]

All photographs courtesy Dr. Ann M. Hargis, DermatoDiagnostics, unless otherwise noted.
SLE, Systemic lupus erythematosus; *UV*, ultraviolet; *TNF-α*, tumor necrosis factor-α.
*Courtesy Dr. Peter Ihrke, College of Veterinary Medicine, University of California-Davis.
†Courtesy Dr. Pamela E. Ginn, College of Veterinary Medicine, University of Florida.
‡Courtesy Dr. M. Donald McGavin, College of Veterinary Medicine, University of Tennessee.
§Courtesy Dr. Helen Power, Dermatology for Animals.
¶Courtesy Dr. David Duclos, Animal Skin and Allergy Clinic.

carcinomas often develop in a stepwise manner and progress through several recognizable stages: hyperplasia (increased number of cells; no cellular atypia or tissue disorganization) → dysplasia (increased mitoses, cellular atypia, and tissue disorganization consisting of loss of polarity) → carcinoma in situ (increased tissue disorganization, mitoses, anaplastic nuclei, but no invasion of underlying basement membrane) → invasive squamous cell carcinoma (disruption of the basement membrane with dermal invasion by anaplastic carcinoma cells).

The progression of the disease from mere hyperplasia to an invasive carcinoma represents a series of molecular events whereby the population of cells harbors an increasing number of damaged genes belonging to the four categories of genes listed. This series of changes takes place over long periods of time, often years, before a tumor reaches full malignant potential. The process may be halted in the early stages if the agents causing continued genetic damage can be removed (e.g., exposure to UVR).

Most cutaneous neoplasms are primary because the skin is an uncommon to rare site for metastasis; however, the skin can be the site of secondary tumor growth. Examples include mammary gland neoplasms that invade into adjacent skin, feline pulmonary bronchogenic carcinomas that metastasize to multiple digits of the feet, and canine visceral hemangiosarcomas that can metastasize to the skin. Web Tables 17-3 to 17-6 provide a listing of the salient features of the common neoplastic-like lesions and neoplastic lesions in domestic animals.

SUGGESTED READINGS

Information on this topic is available at evolve.elsevier.com/Zachary/McGavin/.

CHAPTER 18

Female Reproductive System and Mammary Gland*

Robert A. Foster

The reproductive system is arguably the most important system for the survival of a species. In production animals, reproduction is essential for the continued supply of product, whether it is meat, fiber, milk, or any of the many other by-products. Diseases of the reproductive system have not changed much in the last few decades, but our understanding of many of the processes has progressed dramatically and many of the accepted "dogmas" were challenged and/or modified. In addition, the traditional approach to diseases of the reproductive system focused on specific diseases for which information is known, rather than taking into consideration the overall significance in a clinical setting. In this chapter, each anatomic component or region is examined, and the relative importance of specific diseases or processes is emphasized. The traditional approach also concentrated on bovine and to a lesser extent equine reproductive diseases. In this chapter, diseases of all species, including companion animals, is included in more detail.

STRUCTURE

FEMALE REPRODUCTIVE SYSTEM

The female reproductive systems of domesticated animals, although diverse in anatomy, share many similarities in structure and function. Embryologic development of the female reproductive tract was thought to be the default when the male reproductive tract did not form, but now we know many unique genes and subsequent processes control it.

Genes initiate the pathways of ovarian differentiation and development. *Dax1* is one gene that both promotes ovarian development and inhibits testicular development. In the development of the ovary, the germ cells undergo meiosis and the supporting cells surround the oocytes to become the granulosa and theca cells of the follicles. The differentiation of a female phenotype occurs with the development of the paramesonephric (Müllerian) ducts to form the uterine tube, uterus, and cranial vagina and for the urogenital sinus to develop into the caudal vagina and vulva.

The structural arrangement of the ovary is similar in all species except in the mare. The ovary itself has an outer layer of epithelium, which is of mesothelial origin. The cortex of the ovary contains follicles, stromal connective tissue, and blood vessels. The medulla has large blood vessels, lymphatic vessels, nerves, and loosely arranged connective tissue. Remnants of the mesonephric tubules, called the *rete ovarii,* are present in this region.

The follicles are where the ova develop and are named according to their stage of development: primordial, primary, secondary, and tertiary types. Each developing follicle has multiple layers of granulosa cells and peripheral theca cells. Ovulation occurs when the follicle ruptures, releasing the ovum and allowing the space to fill with blood and then with luteal cells to form the corpus hemorrhagicum and corpus luteum, respectively. Follicles that do not ovulate become atretic. In addition to these various ovarian structures, cats have interstitial glands that are cells of an endocrine type. The canine ovary has small ingrowths of the ovarian surface that are called *subsurface epithelial structures* and structures called *granulosa cell rests* that are aggregates of granulosa cells in a tubular arrangement.

Oogenesis is usually completed by birth. In most species, ovulation occurs through the outer surface of the ovary and the ovum is collected by the infundibulum.

The ovary of the mare differs from the other species in several ways. Equine fetal gonads undergo hypertrophy wherein interstitial endocrine cells, stimulated by equine chorionic gonadotropin (formerly called pregnant mare serum gonadotropin), expand in number and produce an extremely large gonad. These atrophy and disappear before birth. The ovary of the mare has a kidney shape with a depression called the *ovulation fossa.* The ovum is released from this depression. The follicles in the mare can attain a large size—up to 7 cm. Mares can therefore form a large corpus hemorrhagicum. On occasion, a corpus hemorrhagicum and a corpus luteum can be visible externally as structures that extend outward through the ovulation fossa.

*Dr. Helen M. Acland made contributions to this chapter in the third edition.

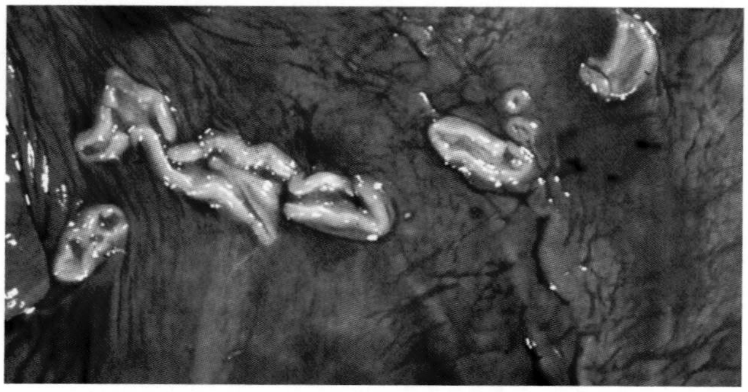

Fig. 18-1 Endometrial cups, uterus, mare.
Endometrial cups are plaque-like structures in the endometrium that form when trophoblasts invade the endometrium early in pregnancy. They are present between 37 and 150 days of pregnancy and secrete equine chorionic gonadotropin. The chorionic surface opposite each cup is called the chorioallantoic pouch and is avillous. (Courtesy Dr. K. Read, College of Veterinary Medicine, Texas A&M University; and Noah's Arkive, College of Veterinary Medicine, The University of Georgia.)

The uterine tube has four regions—the infundibulum, ampulla, isthmus, and uterotubal junction. It is supported by a mesosalpinx. The mesosalpinx of the dog completely surrounds the ovary to form the bursa and has a large amount of fat; a small hole connects the interior aspect to the abdominal cavity. The infundibulum surrounds the ovary of each species, except in the horse where it only covers the ovulation fossa. The uterine tube is where fertilization occurs, and the conceptus then moves into the uterus.

All species have a bicornuate uterus with uterine horns and a uterine body. The uterus of the mare has longitudinal folds. Endometrial cups are present in the endometrium between 37 and 150 days of gestation and are the site of production of equine chorionic gonadotropin, formerly pregnant mare serum gonadotropin (Fig. 18-1). These typically form around the pregnant horn at the bifurcation. Their disappearance is an immune-mediated event. The placenta of the horse is diffuse and microcotyledonary. In ruminants, each uterine horn contains four rows of protuberances that become the caruncles. These may be pigmented in sheep. The placenta of ruminants is cotyledonary. The placenta of the pig is diffuse with small ridges. Dogs and cats have a zonary placenta with marginal hematomas.

The cervix is the structure that separates the external genitalia from the uterus and is an effective barrier from the external environment. Cervical mucus is viscous except during estrus when it becomes more plentiful and thinner. The cervix in the mare, dog, and cat does not have transverse folds as it does in the ruminants and sows. The cervix of the dog and cat opens on the dorsal aspect of the cranial vagina.

Cell Types

In general terms, much of the reproductive system has a barrier between the external environment and the internal environment that is based on epithelium and on an active mucosal immune system. Superimposed on this arrangement are the modifications that occur with the estrous cycle and with pregnancy.

The cell types of the ovary include the epithelium (surface epithelium, subsurface epithelial structures of the bitch, and the rete ovarii), the stroma, germ cells, and follicular cells. Lymphoid cells are usually absent. Control of ovarian function is from the hypothalamus and pituitary through release of gonadotropin-releasing hormone (GnRH), as well as follicle-stimulating hormone (FSH) and luteinizing hormone (LH) (see Fig. 12-3).

The uterus is a unique environment that is separated from the external environment by the cervix. Because it is designed to protect and nourish the fetus, there are some unique features of the endometrium. The endometrium has an epithelial lining of columnar and sometimes ciliated cells. There is also a stromal component of the endometrium. Inflammatory and immune cells are present, particularly during estrus, when the uterus is open to the external environment and to spermatozoa or semen (horses and pigs have intrauterine insemination). Mild inflammation is a "normal" part of the estrous cycle, especially in mares after breeding.

The "external" component of the female reproductive tract, which is the vulva, vagina, and part of the cervix, is lined by a stratified squamous epithelium that varies with the stage of cycle. This is best illustrated in the bitch and queen, in which vaginal cytology is a practical guide to determine the stage of cycle. During anestrus, the epithelium is predominantly of a basal type, with a large nucleus and a small amount of cytoplasm. With the progressive approach of estrus (i.e., during proestrus), the epithelium becomes more mature so that at estrus the majority of cells are superficial epithelial cells with either pyknotic nuclei or no nuclei. Lymphoid follicles beneath the epithelium are a normal part of the distal vagina.

Pregnancy brings about a world of change to the reproductive system. The maintenance of pregnancy and the exchange of nutrients between mother and fetus and the exchange of other products from fetus to mother depend on the interactions of the trophoblasts with the endometrium. During pregnancy, the trophoblasts are directly opposed to and in contact with the endometrial epithelium. In cattle, the maintenance of pregnancy depends on the inhibition of prostaglandin $F_{2\alpha}$ ($PGF_{2\alpha}$) production in the endometrium so luteolysis does not occur. The trophoblast must avoid rejection by the mother and maintain a barrier yet provide a system for the exchange of nutrients and waste products. There is much to be learned about the enigma that is pregnancy.

Some of the cells that we would ordinarily consider "inflammatory" have specific and individual functions separate from their usual roles. Thus uterine macrophages, natural killer cells, and in some cases, neutrophils have separate and distinct functions. For example, macrophages are important in maintaining the size and shape of bovine caruncles, $CD2^+$ T lymphocytes and natural killer–like cells are important in early pregnancy in pigs, and neutrophils are involved in cervical relaxation at parturition in sheep. Thus the usual function of inflammatory cells can be modified or used by the reproductive tract for specific but otherwise unexpected purposes that result in the maintenance of pregnancy.

MAMMARY GLANDS

Mammary Development, Lactation, and Involution

The ventrolateral ectoderm of the embryo becomes the mammary ridge and then the mammary complex. In development, mammary buds push into mesenchyme with their number equaling the number of mammae: mares 2, cows 4, ewes and does 2, sows 14, bitches 10, and queens 8. Sprouts form from each mammary bud, and the number equals the number of papillary ducts (and therefore mammary glands) per mamma: mares 2; cows, ewes, and does 1; sows 2; bitches 8 to 14; and queens 3 to 7. Mammae develop in male embryos, but in domesticated species, they only regress fully in the stallion.

As puberty approaches, there is branching of ducts mediated by prolactin, growth hormone, insulin-like growth factors, and many other factors. There is an intimate interaction between the mesenchyme and epithelium in the formation of ducts and alveoli. Mammary development is maximal at the onset of lactation. Milk flows from alveoli through the lactiferous ducts to a lactiferous sinus (in large animals) and with suckling, through the papillary duct or ducts.

There is variation between the species in the amount of regression that occurs when milking ceases. All species reduce the area of secretary epithelium and increase the relative amount of stroma of the gland. When secretion ceases completely, mammary fluid is resorbed. Bovine mammary glands do not regress as much as in other species, and they complete involution in about 2 weeks. Ewes take about 4 weeks to involute. Leukocytes, especially macrophages, infiltrate the involuting gland.

Cell Types

The mammary glands are sequestered from the outside world by the gatekeeper functions of the sphincter of the mammary papilla (teat) and the papillary duct and at least in the ruminant, its lining of keratinized squamous epithelium. The lactiferous sinus and ducts are lined by columnar epithelial cells, and the alveoli have the secretory epithelium. Secretion of milk components occurs in the alveoli. Mammary epithelial cells, specifically the alveolar cells, have receptors for immunoglobulin G (IgG); they are present for about 1 week before parturition, but the receptors disappear during lactation. Epithelial cells also allow for the transfer of IgA, which is produced locally in subepithelial plasma cells, into the alveolar lumens.

Lymphoid cells in the normal glands are derived from blood, and there is also homing of lymphocytes from the intestine (the enteromammary link) as part of the common mucosal immune system. Lymphocytes of the cellular immune system are present also but in low numbers.

FUNCTION

FEMALE REPRODUCTIVE SYSTEM

The overall function of the female reproductive tract is to provide a location for the conception, development, and eventual release of viable offspring. One offspring is sufficient for dairy cows, but the largest number possible is required for other production animals. Each anatomic site has its own particular function.

The function of the ovary is to develop and release an ovum or ova and to produce hormones, such as estrogen and progesterone, that influence animal behavior and affect other organs and tissue to maintain pregnancy.

The uterine tube acts as a transport system and storage site for spermatozoa. It also collects and transports the ovum or ova and provides a location for fertilization. The conceptus is nourished and eventually transported to the uterus for subsequent development.

The uterus provides a sterile and inert environment for the development of the conceptus. Exchange of nutrients and trophic factors, immunologic components such as immunoglobulin molecules, and waste products is a major function. This is achieved via placental attachment sites that increase the surface area of the interface between maternal and fetal tissue. At the appropriate time, the muscles of the uterus contribute to the release and birth of the developing individual.

The cervix functions as a gatekeeper by holding the products of conception within the uterus until the appointed time. It also provides a seal that prevents organisms and substances from entering the cranial vagina. Its dilation is an important part of parturition.

The vagina and vulva provide a passageway that allows semen to be deposited within an internal site, which protects the spermatozoa from desiccation and excessive contamination with organisms and materials that would excessively irritate or infect the uterus and uterine tube. The vagina also reduces contamination of the cervix, especially during pregnancy. It is also a portal for the fetus at parturition.

MAMMARY GLANDS

The mammary glands provide immunity and nutrients to neonates. Milk is the source of many defenses, including antimicrobial, anti-inflammatory, and immune-modulating molecules and substances. In the immediate neonatal period, passive transfer of immunoglobulin via colostrum is an important means of providing immediate immunity to offspring of all domestic species. Most domestic species rely on colostrum ingested in the first 24 hours as the sole source of serum immunoglobulin. Dogs and cats are exceptions because there is some transplacental transfer. Components of the cellular immune system, such as lymphocytes and cytokines, are also transferred in milk. After the immediate postnatal period, substances in ingested milk (including immunoglobulin) provide some local protection against intestinal and respiratory pathogens.

The mammary glands of the modern dairy animal are expected to provide much more milk than is necessary for these functions, and the high-producing dairy cow is a special creature, developed to provide a product of good quality with a long shelf-life and modifications to the components of milk to suit consumers. This includes high production with a low somatic cell count.

RESPONSES TO INJURY

FEMALE REPRODUCTIVE SYSTEM

Little is known about the response of the ovary to infection or insults. Observations of neutrophilic and in viral infections, lymphocytic inflammation indicates that the ovary is capable of inflammatory and immune responses as one would expect with other parts of the body. Hyperplasia of the surface epithelium is a common response, just as it is with mesothelium elsewhere.

The uterine tube is such a narrow structure that its function is altered readily with edema, inflammation, and scarring. Exocytosis of neutrophils from blood vessels via the interstitium can be rapid. In sufficient numbers, pus is formed. Local immune responses can develop and result in the presence of lymphocytes, plasma cells, and in some instances, lymphoid follicles. Granulation tissue formation in severe inflammatory conditions leads to scarring, and subsequent obstruction of the tube is followed by an accumulation of fluid (hydrosalpinx) or pus (pyosalpinx).

There are many studies of the response of the uterus to infection. Inflammation varies from mild, in postmating endometritis, to severe, in bacterial metritis and pyometra. In mild acute inflammation of the endometrium (endometritis) of species—apart from the dog and cat—neutrophils and macrophages migrate through the epithelium into the lumen, and the stratum compactum is edematous. This becomes more florid with an increased severity. Neutrophils and necrotic debris accumulate in the uterus until pyometra forms. Lymphocytes and plasma cells accumulate in the stroma of the endometrium. With chronicity and in severe situations, the epithelium becomes squamous, thus squamous metaplasia develops. Necrosis and erosion of the epithelium results in the formation of granulation tissue, and varying degrees of fibrosis are commonplace in severe infectious or inflammatory disease.

The canine endometrium in particular, as well as the feline endometrium, responds with cystic endometrial hyperplasia. Any injury or insult, whether inert foreign material or pathogenic infectious agents, stimulates this response, which occurs in diestrus. The luminal epithelium becomes papillated and can resemble a placental site.

In the vulva and vagina, inflammation and infection of the external part of the reproductive tract results in hyperplasia and keratinization of the stratified squamous epithelium. Exocytosis of inflammatory cells does occur, predominantly with neutrophils. These inflammatory cells do so with some difficulty because of the intercellular junctions between epithelial cells. The inflammatory response is typically lymphocytic and plasmacytic, and these cells can form a thick band of cells beneath the epithelium. Lymphoid follicles often form and give the affected region of the vagina a granular macroscopic appearance.

Reactions of the placenta are stereotyped and rely heavily on the maternal and to a lesser extent, the fetal immune systems. Some species variability is related to the types of placenta and the usual route of infection. The response of the fetus and placenta tends to be relatively rudimentary. Trophoblasts are phagocytic, and they will take up debris, blood, and infectious agents. Reactions of fluid exudation and connective tissue with granulation and fibrosis occur as elsewhere. The reactions of fetal macrophages and neutrophils are less obvious than is seen where maternal leukocytes are readily accessible. Placentitis occurs when there is sufficient time for a response; fetal loss can be rapid with fetal distress, and there can be insufficient time to mount an effective response. Chronic lesions are much more obvious and especially occur in ruminants. The cotyledonary placenta means that attachment of the placenta to the endometrium is restricted to a relatively small area in relation to what may appear to be the total placental area, but the extensive papillation of the components of the placentome produces a very large surface area. The intercotyledonary area is a potential space that can accumulate a large volume of exudate. Chronic inflammation in ruminants is common and identified by fibrosis of the placenta. The neutrophils are probably of maternal origin. Lymphoid follicles and plasma cells are a lesser component of the reaction, but lymphocytes do accumulate beneath the layer of trophoblasts and around blood vessels. In the equine placenta, placentitis involves a small area, usually around the cervical star. There is no potential space because of the diffuse microcotyledonary type of placenta, thus exudates and suppuration are much less prominent; chronic placentitis is rare. The inflammatory reaction in the pig, dog, and cat placenta is mild, and chronic placentitis is rare.

MAMMARY GLANDS

The mammary glands are usually sterile but can respond rapidly to infection or other irritants. The responses are stereotyped, however. The columnar epithelial cells can become hyperplastic, but the cells are not able to withstand injury to the same extent as stratified squamous epithelium, thus squamous metaplasia is a frequent occurrence when irritants, such as infection or intramammary preparations, are introduced. Necrosis of the epithelium is common in infectious disease, and granulation and scarring of the lining of the ducts and sinus are frequent.

Although the immune system of the normal mammary glands is quiescent, injury quickly results in recruitment of the various elements. Neutrophils and macrophages are rapidly recruited. Humoral and cellular immunity is typically seen in infectious conditions. The presence of large numbers of plasma cells with the development of a local immune system is an invariable component of the immune response in infection. Edema and subsequent fibrosis are part of the reaction to injury. The flow of milk is often halted by injury and exudates, thus the normal involutionary processes that result in resorption of secretion (macrophage and epithelial uptake) also operate.

BOX 18-1 Portals of Entry into the Female Reproductive System, Especially the Uterus

Ascending infection through cervix
- At insemination
- Excessive vaginal contamination
- Postpartum and with retained fetal membranes

Hematogenous
- Localization in maternoplacental interface

Descending from ovary via uterine tube

Transneural with recrudescence of herpesvirus infection

PORTALS OF ENTRY

FEMALE REPRODUCTIVE SYSTEM

It is critical that infectious organisms are excluded from the uterus, otherwise fertility or pregnancy can be jeopardized. Portals of entry are listed in Box 18-1. Organisms that cause inflammation of the uterus can enter through the vulva (ascending infection) or can arrive via the blood (hematogenous infection). Reinfection of the external genitalia from nerves is a unique feature of infection with some herpesviruses.

Ascending infections occur at estrus, breeding, and parturition. At estrus, the cervix is open to admit spermatozoa. Contamination of the cranial vagina is very important in determining whether infection of the uterus occurs or not. Conformational and structural changes in the vulva and vagina are also important determinants of infection. These are discussed in more detail later. A subcategory of ascending infection is infection of semen by infectious agents. There are many agents, including bacteria, viruses, protozoa, and *Ureaplasma* and *Mycoplasma* spp. , which can be acquired in this fashion. These are discussed further in the discussion on disorders of the uterus in the section on disorders of the Female Reproductive System. Ascending infection is the major portal by which the equine placenta becomes infected with bacteria or fungi. The cervix in the mare is "loose," attains a much larger diameter, and can be readily opened with digital pressure. It is virtually impossible to penetrate the cervix of other species with a probe without creating severe trauma. Infection of the uterus and/or placenta by the ascending route with *Streptococcus zooepidemicus* is common in the mare, but most ascending infections in other species include a mixture of bacteria. This is particularly the case with postpartum infection.

Hematogenous infections are less common and are usually involved in specific infections, such as in brucellosis, salmonellosis, pestivirus, and herpesvirus infections, and they usually occur during pregnancy. Many of the fungal infections of the placenta occur via the hematogenous route.

There are some instances in which infections appear to descend from the ovary through the uterine tube. Some viral, chlamydial, and *Ureaplasma* infections can be descending.

Transaxonal infection of the distal reproductive tract occurs with some herpesviruses, where stressful events, such as parturition, cause a recrudescence. Neonates can be exposed and infected via this route, but clinical disease in the mother is unusual.

MAMMARY GLANDS

Portals of entry are listed in Box 18-2. Most infectious agents and foreign material (intramammary preparations) enter the gland in an ascending fashion via the papillary duct. Small (bacteria) and large (leaches) pathogens can enter the gland via this route. There are some instances in which organisms home to the mammary glands from systemic infection, but their number is small. Viruses, such as the retroviruses of caprine arthritis and encephalitis, ovine maedi-visna, and *Mycoplasma* spp., are good examples. Penetrating injury is rare.

DEFENSE MECHANISMS

FEMALE REPRODUCTIVE SYSTEM

Innate, nonimmune, or physical factors are very important in the defense of the reproductive system. An adaptive immune system occurs after these have failed. In many instances, failure of the physical factors that result in infection of the tract is too late for the fetus, and infertility and failure of pregnancy occurs. Defense mechanisms are listed in Box 18-3.

Innate Immunity

The reproductive tract requires a defense system that provides a sterile environment for the fetus but allows entry of antigenic and infectious materials (semen). It does this by providing specialized epithelium in the "contaminated" environment of the vulva and vagina, and then has a specialized structure, the cervix, to exclude most agents from the upper "sterile" regions. Vaginal epithelium has intercellular tight junctions that inhibit the transepithelial migration of agents and molecules, and it has molecules that detect pathogen-associated molecular patterns. These pattern recognition receptors, including Toll-like receptors and defensins, exclude or direct actions against many pathogens.

The anatomy and integrity of the cervix is very important in the exclusion of infectious agents from the uterus. Contamination of the cranial vagina is an additional factor, and conformation of the external genitalia is the physical factor that has received the most attention in relation to uterine infections. In older multiparous mares, the vulva is frequently higher than the floor of the pelvic canal and tends to become horizontal; air and contaminants, including feces, are sucked in or allowed entry into the vagina or even into the uterus. Urine can pool in the vagina of mares with defective function of the vestibule and vulval muscles. When contamination and pooling of urine occur, the vestibule and vagina become inflamed. Subsequently, the cervix and uterus also become affected, either from direct contact with environmental organisms or from local spread of the inflammation.

Muscular contractions of the uterus and gravitational drainage of secretions (mucus, lochia) from the uterus and vagina are physical factors that can flush out infectious organisms. Congenital malformations and anomalies, such as persistent hymen, can reduce outflow and increase pooling in the vagina and uterus. The altered environment of the vagina in spayed, obese bitches can predispose the vagina and vulva to infection.

After infection or irritation from semen, changes include hyperemia and edema of the uterine wall and lumen. These have the theoretical effect of diluting infectious or irritant substances. Recruitment of neutrophils from the blood occurs in response to chemotactic substances released by bacteria, complement, and inflammatory mediators from endometrium and leukocytes. Attracted neutrophils infiltrate the endometrium, enter the uterine lumen, and contribute additional amounts of inflammatory mediators, providing additional chemotactic stimuli. Complement activation, directly by bacteria via the alternate pathway or by specific antibody via the classical pathway, can eliminate bacteria, either by lysis after attack on their membranes or by phagocytosis enhanced by opsonization.

Adaptive Immunity

The reproductive tract is a unique environment because it must respond adequately to challenge from pathogens, yet tolerate the allogeneic spermatozoa and fetus. Adaptive immune responses, whether humoral or cellular, have to be carefully controlled. Control is achieved by differing cytokine expression of epithelial cells and their effects on regulatory T lymphocytes that make "decisions" as to the type and extent of the response. There is likely to be variation in the response, depending on the location. The response in the "sterile" compartments of the uterus and uterine tube are different from that of the "nonsterile" vagina and ectocervix.

Although the upper reproductive tract is part of the common mucosal immune system, it differs from intestinal and bronchial tissues because it does not have mucosal-associated lymphoid tissue (MALT) analogous to Peyer's patches. This difference occurs because of the lack of continuous antigenic stimulation. Lymphoid follicles, however, are present in the vulva and distal vagina. The uterus also has the added potential influence of hormones to modify responses.

T lymphocytes are critical in determining whether the appropriate response is predominantly humoral or cell mediated. $CD8^+$ T lymphocytes are the most common lymphocytes of the luminal endometrial epithelium and stroma (stratum compactum

BOX 18-2 Portals of Entry into the Mammary Glands

Ascending ductular route
- Bacteria, fungi, parasites
- Teat lesions
- Therapeutic agents

Systemic infection and localization
- Systemic fungi, viruses, mycoplasmas, mycobacteria

Direct penetration
- Penetrating injury

BOX 18-3 Defenses of the Female Reproductive System

Innate defenses
- Vaginal epithelium
- Cervical barrier
- Conformation
- Myometrial tone and contraction
- Drainage of secretions
- Neutrophils
- Macrophages
- Complement
- Cytokines
- Microbial recognition molecules

Adaptive defenses
- Humoral immunity including common mucosal immune system
- Cellular immunity

especially), although there is variation, depending on the location in the uterus. For example, $CD4^+$ lymphocytes are more common in the horns of the uterus of mares, whereas $CD8^+$ lymphocytes are more numerous in the body.

Little is known of the T lymphocyte and cell-mediated immune system of the reproductive tract; much more is known about its humoral immune system. It is generally believed that locally produced antibodies are more important in those diseases that are acquired by ascending infection, for example, *Tritrichomonas foetus* in cattle, whereas systemic immunity is more important in systemically or hematogenously acquired infections, such as *Brucella* sp. infection. The immunoglobulin isotype (IgA or IgG) and subisotype (IgG_1 or IgG_2) that is found in an individual infection is unique to that infection. The generalization that IgA is the main mucosal antibody is not always the case. The response to specific infectious agents is not uniform, and there are differing responses between species. Protection against *Tritrichomonas foetus* in cattle, for example, is mostly by IgG_1. Local transfer of immunoglobulin occurs at all levels of the tract.

Leakage of serum into the uterine lumen from an inflamed endometrium also contributes to the antibody content of the uterine fluid. Opsonization of bacteria by antibodies, especially IgG, promotes more efficient phagocytosis by neutrophils and macrophages; thus they enhance the innate cellular response by phagocytes.

The influence of the estrous cycle on antibodies in the uterus is controversial, but data suggest that concentrations of luminal immunoglobulins and immunoglobulin-containing cells in the endometrium are not influenced by the stage of the estrous cycle.

Locally produced IgA interferes with attachment of bacteria to mucosal surfaces and can activate complement via the alternate pathway. It is not directly bactericidal and acts neither as an opsonin nor as a macrophage activator. Variations occur among species on the position in the tract where the concentration of IgA is greatest, but the sites correspond to the site of semen deposition (uterus in mares, vagina in cows).

Hormonal Influences on Innate and Adaptive Immunity

Infections of the uterus are more easily overcome at estrus than at other stages of the cycle. This increased response at estrus is probably a result at least in part to better drainage through an open cervix. Both estrogen and progesterone affect neutrophil and lymphocyte function, but there is variation in results obtained when the effects of hormones were studied. In some species, such as the mouse, estrogen induces an influx of neutrophils and macrophages (at estrus). Estrogen can also be involved in the upregulation of subsets of T lymphocytes. There is variation in the numbers of lymphocytes in the reproductive tract during the estrous cycle. Even so, there is evidence that $CD4^+$ lymphocytes increase in number with increases in estrogen concentration. Progesterone, which dominates during the luteal phase and pregnancy, antagonizes the "proinflammatory" activity of estrogen. Studies in cattle and sheep indicate an upregulation of T and B lymphocyte responses during the follicular phase of the estrous cycle when estrogen dominates. Major histocompatibility complex II (MHC II) expression is enhanced at estrus in direct relationship with rising estrogen concentration. The influence of the estrous cycle on antibodies in the uterus is controversial, but data suggest that concentrations of luminal immunoglobulins and immunoglobulin-containing cells in the endometrium are not influenced by the stage of the estrous cycle. Generally, the uterus is more susceptible to infection during the progestational or luteal phase of the estrous cycle and during pregnancy. The nonpregnant uterus is highly resistant to infection. The mechanisms involved in the effect of sex hormones on neutrophils are unknown, and receptors for sex hormones have not been demonstrated in them.

Prostaglandins are normally produced by the epithelium of the endometrium. In most species (excluding the dog, cat, and primates), prostaglandins are responsible for lysis of the corpus luteum. In acute inflammation, prostaglandin production by the endometrium is increased, and lysis of the corpus luteum occurs. When there is epithelial and mucosal surface loss, production of prostaglandins is decreased, the corpus luteum persists, and the more susceptible progestational uterine environment is maintained.

MAMMARY GLANDS

As with the body in general, the mammary glands have a full range of mechanisms to prevent and control infectious disease. It relies heavily on isolation. The structure and function of the papillary duct of the teat and the keratin that accumulates there to form a plug prevent many potential pathogens from entering the gland. Secretions of the gland contain antimicrobial, antiinflammatory, and immune-modulating substances. Within the gland, there also are humoral and cellular defenses. Innate defense mechanisms are listed in Box 18-4.

Innate Immunity

Physical factors are very important in the resistance to infection. The teat orifice, with its sphincter, and the papillary duct offer mechanical resistance to the entry of organisms. The keratin and waxy nature of the inner aspect of the papillary duct can be protective by having bactericidal fatty acids, by adsorbing bacteria and desquamating when coated with bacteria, and by desiccating. Delays in the formation of the keratin plug at drying off or cracks in the teat ends increase the risk of intramammary infection. Regular milking of the lactating mammary glands probably is a natural defense mechanism because of the flushing of organisms and products of inflammation from the gland.

Soluble factors are numerous and contribute to resistance to infection. Lactoferrin, the major iron-binding protein of saliva and milk, is a nonspecific natural protective factor in milk. Mammary epithelial cells produce the bulk of lactoferrin in milk. Lactoferrin concentration is increased in acute mastitis and in the involuting gland. The binding of iron withholds this essential nutrient from pathogenic bacteria and thus has a bacteriostatic effect. The lactoperoxidase-thiocyanate-H_2O_2 system temporarily inhibits some streptococci and coliforms and *Staphylococcus aureus*.

BOX 18-4 Innate or Nonspecific Defenses of the Mammary Glands

Physical factors
- Sphincter and keratin of teat orifice
- Flushing action of milk

Soluble factors
- Lactoferrin
- Lysozyme
- Complement
- Cytokines

Cellular factors
- Macrophages
- Neutrophils
- Natural killer cells

Lactoperoxidase is synthesized by mammary epithelium, thiocyanate is derived from certain green feeds, and H_2O_2 is produced by enzymic constituents of milk by streptococci or from an exogenous source. Hypothiocyanite produced by the lactoperoxidase system damages the inner bacterial membrane, killing the bacteria. Lysozyme, synthesized locally or from blood, destroys bacteria by lysis of cell wall peptidoglycan. Complement activated in mastitis by the alternate pathway in response to the presence of bacterial endotoxin can be important in bactericidal activity, opsonization, and promoting inflammation. Normal milk is antiinflammatory. Cytokines have a broad range of immunomodulation. Molecules of this general group include the interleukins (IL-2, especially), colony-stimulating factors (CSF), interferons (IFN), and tumor necrosis factor (TNF).

Cells that are not part of the adaptive or acquired immune system include macrophages, neutrophils, and natural killer cells. Macrophages are usually the most numerous leukocyte in mammary secretions. They phagocytose bacteria and act as antigen-presenting cells. Macrophages can be found free in the alveoli and the interstitium, as well as in the lamina propria of the lactiferous sinus and interlobular and intralobular lactiferous ducts. In a lactating cow, at least 500,000 phagocytes per milliliter of milk are necessary for defense of the mammary glands against invading bacteria. In uninfected bovine mammary glands, 50,000 to 200,000 neutrophils and macrophages per milliliter of milk are present, with the macrophages predominating. Lymphocytes represent about 10% of the leukocytes in lactation. Neutrophils are present only in low numbers unless there is bacterial infection or injury, when their influx can be dramatic. Neutrophils play an extremely important role in antibacterial action by phagocytosis and the release of antibacterial substances. Their function is inhibited in the periparturient period. Recruitment can be so rapid that neutrophils are the dominant cells as soon as 2 hours after infection. Cell counts in milk can average 700,000 per milliliter in subclinically infected quarters, and millions of neutrophils per milliliter are common in clinical infections.

Although neutrophils recruited from the blood are important in fighting infection in the mammary glands, they do not kill bacteria as well in milk as they do in blood. Milk seems to be a poor medium for the functioning of neutrophils. Some possible reasons include the absence of glucose in milk for the glycolytic metabolism of neutrophils, decreased amounts of glycogen in milk neutrophils, deficiency of opsonins and complement in milk, coating of the surface of neutrophils with casein, loss of neutrophil pseudopodia caused by phagocytosis of fat, and a decrease of hydrolytic enzymes within neutrophils after phagocytosis of casein and fat.

In experimental staphylococcal mastitis, the numbers of inflammatory cells (mostly neutrophils) in milk cycle up and down every several days, with a corresponding inverse cycling of the number of viable bacteria. When cell counts are at a peak, phagocytosis is optimal and bactericidal activity per cell is most efficient, by as much as 10,000-fold higher. The frequency and periodicity of the cycle, as well as the amplitude of the cell and bacterial counts, are independent for each infected quarter. The likely source of reinfection of the mammary glands is neutrophils that are inefficient at killing phagocytosed bacteria at the time of low cell count. As these cells undergo necrosis and lysis, their previously protected intracellular viable bacteria are released to multiply, and the inverse cycling of neutrophils and bacterial numbers continues.

In the first week after parturition, when neutrophils are most needed to deal with mammary infections, bovine blood neutrophils already are defective before they pass into the mammary glands. They have significantly impaired chemokinesis and decreased superoxide anion production, antibody-dependent cell-mediated cytotoxicity, and phagocytosis of bacteria. The causes are probably some combination of the effects of stress, energy, and protein demands of early lactation and the hormonal fluxes of this stage of the reproductive cycle. In the parturient period, the concentration of glucocorticoids is increased. This means that leukocyte function is less effective, because expression of L-selectin and CD18 on neutrophils are downregulated by glucocorticoids. This downregulates adhesion between neutrophils and vascular endothelium and transendothelial migration of neutrophils. Neutrophils are also important in creating bystander injury when the products of neutrophil granules, such as superoxide anions and enzymes, are released during phagocytosis and with neutrophil destruction.

Natural killer cells use perforin to kill bacteria in a major histocompatibility complex (MHC) independent way and is part of the nonspecific defenses of the gland.

Adaptive Immunity

The humoral immune system operates in the mammary glands in several ways apart from the transfer of immunoglobulin in colostrum and during lactation. Antibody concentration in normal bovine milk is small, about 1 mg/mL, and includes IgA, IgM, IgG_1, and IgG_2. IgA and IgM are synthesized locally in the stromal tissue of the acini of the mammary glands and may be part of the enteromammary link of the mucosal immune system, whereby lymphocytes from gut-associated lymphoid tissue (GALT) home to the gland. Most IgG is serum derived; IgG_1 is selectively transferred into mammary secretion and is the major immunoglobulin class in milk obtained from healthy mammary glands. IgG_2 is both serum derived and locally produced by resident plasma cells, especially in inflammation.

Particulate antigens, such as bacteria, stimulate an antibody response in the mammary glands of the cow, whereas soluble antigens do not. In colostrum and in milk from inflamed mammary glands, antibody concentration approaches 50 mg/mL. Early in inflammation, IgG_1 and IgG_2 opsonize bacteria to enhance phagocytosis by macrophages, but later the importance of IgG_2 as an opsonin increases as neutrophils enter the gland. Neutrophils can transport IgG_2 to the mammary glands as they move to the site of inflammation. IgM also functions as an opsonin. IgA does not opsonize but could prevent bacterial adherence to epithelium, inhibit bacterial multiplication, neutralize leukocyte-inhibiting bacterial toxins, and agglutinate bacteria. Concentrations of immunoglobulin are reduced in the periparturient period and may contribute to the increased susceptibility of the gland to infection.

Cell-mediated immunity in the gland is stimulated in infectious disease. Interleukins from mammary macrophages stimulate the immune system by activating T and B lymphocytes. Only a few B lymphocytes are present in the normal mammary glands and milk. T lymphocytes in normal mammary tissue and milk of cows and pigs are mostly $CD8^+$ α/β T lymphocytes. The $CD4^+/CD8^+$ ratio is <1, which is reversed from the ratio in blood. The mammary glands thus have selective lymphocyte trafficking, favoring $CD8^+$ lymphocytes, which have either cytotoxic or suppressor function. T lymphocytes that activate B lymphocytes, T lymphocytes, and macrophages are underrepresented in normal mammary tissue and milk. $CD8^+$ T lymphocytes are found in the lactiferous duct and alveolar epithelium, whereas the lesser numbers of $CD4^+$ lymphocytes and B lymphocytes are in clusters in the connective tissues. In early lactation, the $CD8^+$ lymphocytes in milk function more as suppressor lymphocytes than cytotoxic lymphocytes, but the situation is reversed in mid and late lactation. Suppressor T lymphocytes control, modulate, or suppress the immune response, and cytotoxic T lymphocytes can act as scavengers, removing damaged mammary cells. $CD4^+$ (T helper [T_H]) lymphocytes predominate in goat mammary glands and in mastitis. In response to bacterial infection, an influx of $CD4^+$ T lymphocytes occurs in milk, and these lymphocytes eventually outnumber $CD8^+$ T lymphocytes. During the periparturient period, T_H2 lymphocytes (cell-mediated response) secreting IL-4 and IL-10 predominate over T_H1 lymphocytes (humoral-mediated response) secreting IL-2 and INF-γ. T lymphocytes may be cytotoxic, and they preferentially migrate to epithelial surfaces and can destroy altered epithelial cells. γ/δ T lymphocytes are present in greater numbers in mammary secretions and parenchyma when compared with blood. The percentage of γ/δ T lymphocytes of mammary parenchymal lymphocytes decreases in the postpartum period, a time of increased susceptibility of the mammary glands to disease, which suggests that γ/δ T lymphocytes can be important in defense against infection.

DISORDERS OF DOMESTIC ANIMALS (HORSES, RUMINANTS [CATTLE, SHEEP, AND GOATS], PIGS, DOGS, AND CATS)

FEMALE REPRODUCTIVE SYSTEM

Disorders of Sexual Development

An understanding of the development of the reproductive tract of domesticated animals is from studies in multiple species, including humans, laboratory rodents, and pigs. Sequencing of the genomes of animals now makes identification of genes and processes responsible for sexual development easier. Developmental anomalies and neoplasia are better understood, too. There is a pragmatic reason for examining embryology: it is easier to learn the mechanisms of how anomalies occur and to determine their significance rather than memorize every possible disorder.

Normal Sexual Development

Sexual development occurs in three sequential processes: (1) chromosomal sex is established at conception, (2) gonadal sex occurs early in fetal development, and (3) phenotypic sex soon follows. Germ cells migrate from the yolk sac to the genital ridge, and without germ cells the ovaries do not develop, and dysgenesis is the result. The undifferentiated and bipotential gonad acquires germ cells, mesenchymal cells, coelomic epithelial cells, and mesonephric epithelial cells. These form the major cell types in the developed gonad: germ cells; supporting, steroid-producing cells and unspecialized mesenchyme; and epithelium. Before differentiation into male and female, the embryo has a double set of ducts: the mesonephric (Wolffian) ducts and tubules and the paramesonephric (Müllerian) duct (Fig. 18-2). In individuals with a chromosomal sex of XX (female), without the sex-determining region of the Y chromosome (*SRY* negative), there is activation of genes and gene products so that a normal ovary develops. Development of a testis is inhibited. The tubular genitalia of the female develop from the paramesonephric ducts, and the mesonephric ducts disappear. The paramesonephric ducts are paired and join the urogenital sinus. They fuse to form the cranial vagina and the uterine body. The urogenital sinus forms the vulva and posterior part of the vagina. The external genital tubercle forms the clitoris. All stages of the development of the genitalia are under the control of genes and gene products; the female reproductive system is not a "default" system.

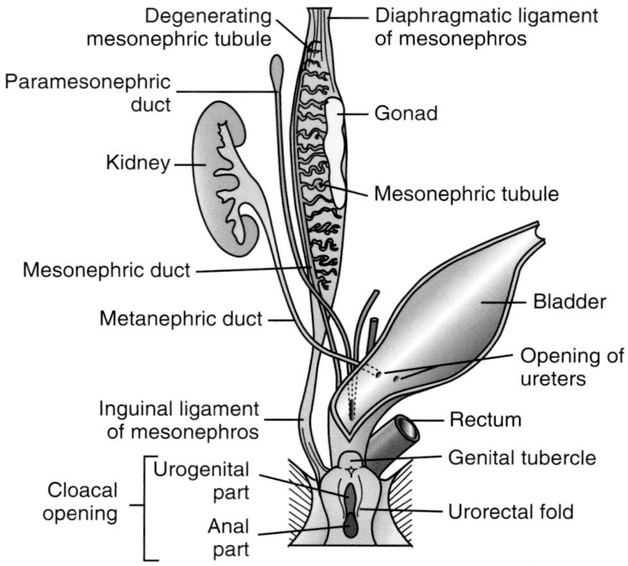

Fig. 18-2 Schematic diagram of the normal components of the female reproductive system and the embryonic structures, especially the paramesonephric (Müllerian) duct and urogenital sinus and tubercle from which they were derived.
The paired paramesonephric ducts fuse to form the body of the uterus, cervix, and cranial vagina. The mesonephric tubules remain as the microscopic rete ovarii, but the mesonephric ducts usually regress completely.

Major Anomalies

Major anomalies are those that result in dramatic abnormalities in sexual phenotype and usually result in infertility. Affected animals are phenotypically male, female, or ambiguous or altered. The exact defect cannot be reliably determined from phenotypic characteristics alone. There are a large number of individual steps involved in sexual development and differentiation, and missing or changing one step can have major effects on subsequent differentiation. Common disorders of sexual development (DSD) are listed in Table 18-1.

Abnormal location and size of the external genitalia creating phenotypic ambiguity is often an indication of a major underlying anomaly. A basic definition of syndromes and identifying the underlying defect and pathogenesis requires an assessment of the sex chromosomes, presence or absence of genes like *SRY*, gonadal type, and phenotype.

Sex chromosome DSD are those with an abnormal number and/or mixture of sex chromosomes, including XXY (Klinefelter syndrome), X_ (Turner syndrome), and XX/XY (chimerism). XY disorders of sexual development are those with disorders of testicular development, disorders of androgen synthesis or action, and miscellaneous conditions (see Chapter 19). XX DSD includes disorders of ovarian development, androgen excess, or miscellaneous disorders. The greater availability of tests for the *SRY* gene means a greater ability to define the underlying anomaly. XX disorders are now defined as XX *SRY* positive and XX *SRY* negative, and XY disorders are subdivided into XY *SRY*-positive and XY *SRY*-negative genotypes.

Gonadal anomalies are found at surgery or necropsy. Histologic assessment is necessary to differentiate between rudimentary gonads (gonadal dysgenesis), testis, ovary, and ovotestis or a combination of both male and female gonadal structures in a single gonad. In phenotypic females, the lack of an estrous cycle, an enlarged clitoris, and/or an increased distance from the anus to

TABLE 18-1 Common Syndromes of Disorders of Sexual Development (DSD)

Category of DSD	Syndrome	Species	Comments
Chromosomal DSD	Freemartinism	Bovine, ovine	Chimerism in twinning
XX DSD, *SRY* negative with testis	XX sex reversal	American cocker spaniels	Autosomal recessive inheritance
XX DSD, *SRY* negative with testis	XX sex reversal	Polled goats	Associated with the poll gene
XY DSD, *SRY* positive with testis	Male feminization syndrome	Equine, canine	Lack of testosterone receptors
XY DSD, *SRY* positive with testis	Müllerian remnant syndrome	Miniature schnauzer	Complete internal female tubular genitalia
XY DSD, *SRY* positive with testis	Failure of testicular descent	All species	Discussed under male genital system
XX DSD, *SRY* negative with ovary or	Segmental aplasia	All species	Rare anomaly often missed at clinical examination
XY DSD, *SRY* positive with testis	Gonadal hypoplasia	All species	Males especially

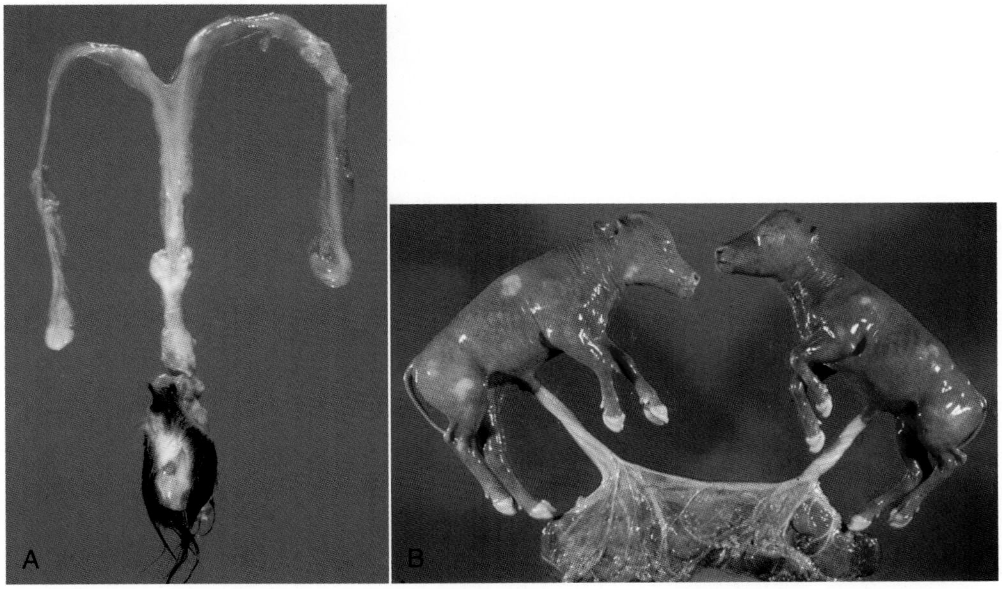

Fig. 18-3 Chromosomal disorder of sexual development, bovine freemartinism, cow.
A, Phenotypically female, reproductive tract, cow. The freemartin is the female of a set of male and female twins. Freemartins are chimeras. There is a vulva and vagina with a prominent clitoris. The internal genitalia consist of bulbourethral and vesicular glands, deferent duct, and short incomplete segments of uterus. The gonads are testis with epididymides attached. This major anomaly renders the cow infertile. **B,** Placenta, twin fetuses. Placental vascular anastomosis, which allows exchange of blood between fetuses, is a requirement for freemartinism. These anastomoses occur most often in the bovine species. (Courtesy Dr. R.A. Foster, Ontario Veterinary College, University of Guelph.)

vulva may indicate an abnormality. Sex reversal, hermaphroditism, pseudohermaphroditism, and feminization are examples of clinical terms used to describe an abnormality. Descriptions of the phenotypic and gonadal anomalies are often done without the benefit of genotype, but it is preferable to describe the disorder completely as outlined next.

Sex Chromosome Disorders of Sexual Development

True chromosomal DSD is very rare. Cases of X_ (Turner syndrome) and XXY (Klinefelter syndrome) are reported. They usually have gonadal dysgenesis and a feminine phenotype.

Chimerism is more common. Chimeras and mosaics have two or more somatic cell types, each with a different chromosomal constitution. Chimeras have two genetically distinct cell types that come from different individuals, whereas mosaicism is a different chromosomal constitution from altered mitosis. The most common chimera in domestic animals is the freemartin calf (Fig. 18-3). Vessels of the placentas from two different fetuses fuse and exchange blood between fetuses. Each fetus becomes a hematopoietic chimera. Anastomosis of placental vessels occurs most often in bovine species and less frequently in other ruminants and pigs. The freemartin is the female of a set of male and female twins. Gene products from the cells of the male fetus induce fetal Sertoli cells and seminiferous cordlike structures in the ovaries of the female twin. The ovaries are small and can have reduced number of or no germ cells or organs partially converted to testes. The paramesonephric (Müllerian) duct derivatives vary from almost normal to cordlike structures, but their lumens do not communication with the vagina. The vagina, vestibule, and vulva are hypoplastic. Vesicular glands are always present; other mesonephric (Wolffian) structures are present to varying degrees. Externally, the animal has a female phenotype, but the vestibule and vagina are short, the vulva is hypoplastic, and the clitoris is enlarged. The male twin is minimally affected.

XY Disorders of Sexual Development

XY DSD has a normal male chromosomal component (XY) and a female phenotype. They have abnormal gonadal development that drives phenotypic abnormalities, abnormal androgen synthesis, or lack androgen receptors. They are described according to the presence or absence of the *SRY* gene and the gonadal type. The most extreme example is XY DSD, *SRY*-positive with testes and female

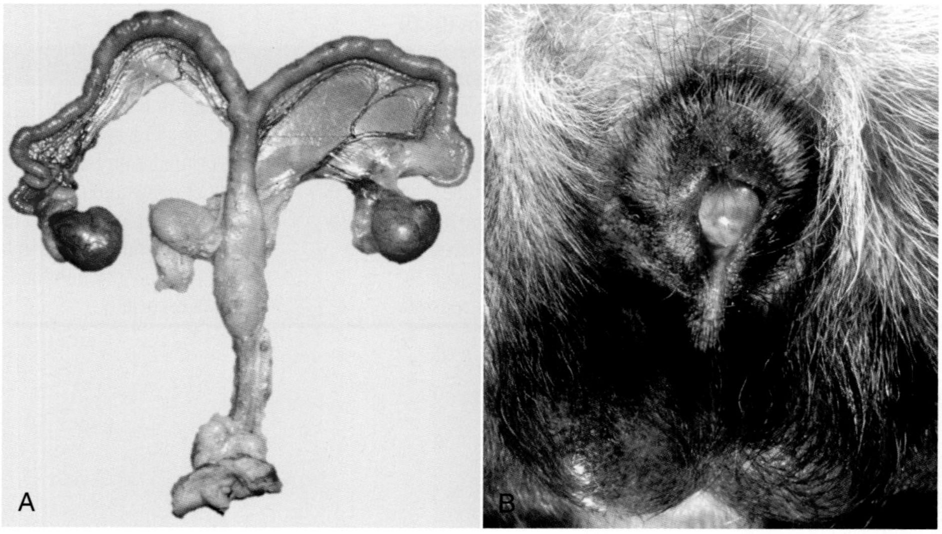

Fig. 18-4 Disorder of sexual development with testis, male pseudohermaphrodite, reproductive tract.
A, Pig. A testis and epididymis are present on each side. Note the well-developed uterus, cervix, and vagina. No ovarian tissue is present. **B,** Clitoral enlargement, dog. The clitoris protrudes between the labia of the vulva and is visible on the ventral floor of the vulva. Note the formation of a bifid scrotum ventral to the vulva. (Courtesy Dr. K. McEntee, Reproductive Pathology Collection, University of Illinois.)

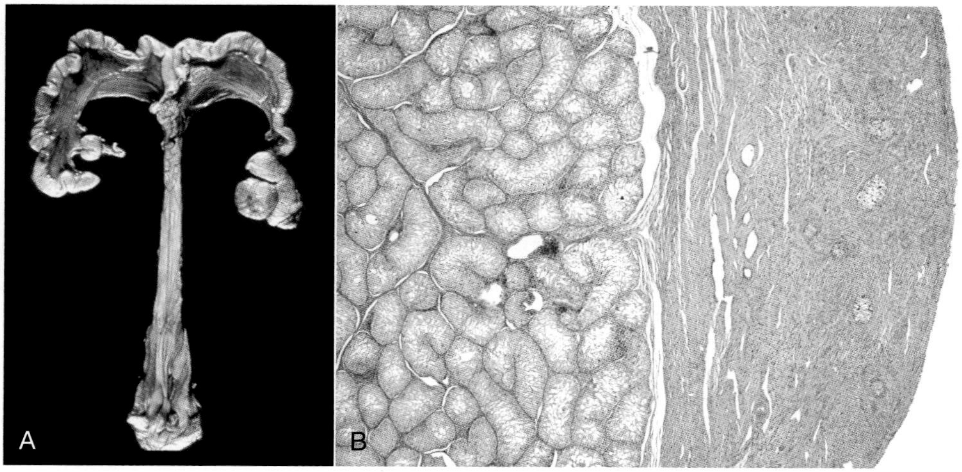

Fig. 18-5 Disorder of sexual development with ovotestis, true hermaphrodite, reproductive tract.
A, Gilt, an ovotestis is on the left and a testis on the right. Note the well-developed uterus, cervix, and vagina. **B,** Dog, ovotestis, at the periphery *(right half of image)* is the ovarian component with capsule and stroma. No active follicles are visible. The testicular component contains seminiferous tubules lined by Sertoli cells *(left half of image)*. There is no spermatogenesis in these tubules. H&E stain. (**A** courtesy Dr. K. McEntee, Reproductive Pathology Collection, University of Illinois. **B** courtesy Dr. J.F. Zachary, College of Veterinary Medicine, University of Illinois.)

phenotype. These were called *male pseudohermaphrodites, testicular feminization,* or *XY sex reversal* (Fig. 18-4). They usually lack androgen receptors. Serum testosterone is present, but the genitalia are female. A mild form occurs in Miniature schnauzers with persistent Müllerian duct syndrome. They are XY males with a complete paramesonephric system, including uterine tube, uterus, and cranial portion of the vagina. They lack the anti-Müllerian hormone (AMH, previously called Müllerian inhibitory substance) or its receptor. XY DSD, *SRY* negative with gonadal dysgenesis and female phenotype is another category and is found in horses and other species. They have hypoplastic or undifferentiated gonads and a female phenotype.

XX Disorders of Sexual Development

The only category of XX DSD reported in animals is XX DSD, *SRY* negative. Most are XX DSD, *SRY* negative with ovotestes and a female but ambiguous phenotype. They are usually true hermaphrodites with both male and female gonads (Fig. 18-5). They are phenotypically female, with masculinization, for example, an enlarged clitoris. American cocker spaniels and some other breeds of dog have this autosomal recessive trait. In goats, it is associated with the polled gene. Confirmation of this syndrome requires genotyping because in the case of goats, the presence of mammary development in bucks is not always an indication of an XX DSD.

Anomalies with Normal Sexual Development

There are many different anomalies found in individuals with normal genotypic, gonadal, and phenotypic sex. They include failure of the normal maturation, hypoplasia, or aplasia of parts of the internal or external genitalia. Because normal development requires such intricate timing of events, including regression of some parts, the joining of tubes and tubules, migration of components from

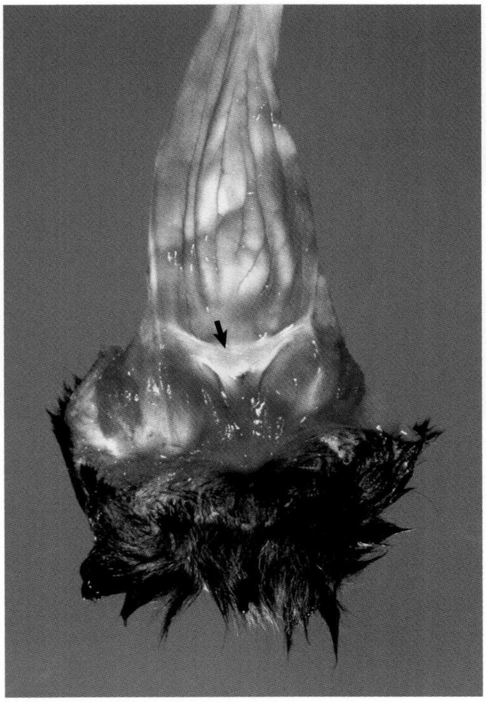

Fig. 18-6 Persistent hymen, vagina, and vulva, bitch.
The membrane *(arrow)* partially separates the vestibule from the vagina and is just cranial to the urethral opening. This minor anomaly is of little consequence and does not interfere with coitus or parturition. (Courtesy Dr. R.A. Foster, Ontario Veterinary College, University of Guelph.)

one site to another, the interaction of genes, and hormones and local factors, it is no wonder there are myriad anomalies.

Segmental aplasia of the paramesonephric duct can affect any part and little is known of its pathogenesis. A genetic basis is implicated in shorthorn cattle, in which it is linked to the recessive gene for white coat color. The simplest form is failure of the paramesonephric duct to make a proper connection with the urogenital sinus, leaving a persistent hymen, a membrane at the site where the two precursor tissues join (Fig. 18-6). A perforated hymen sometimes persists and is not clinically significant. If the hymen is complete and there is no drainage of fluid from the uterus, the upstream portion of the vagina, cervix, and uterus distend with normal secretions. In the more severe forms of segmental aplasia, one or more segments of the vagina, cervix, uterine body, and uterine horns are absent or rudimentary. Aplasia of a segment of the uterus (Fig. 18-7) occurs in cattle. Prostaglandin can be synthesized and released from the blind ending uterine horn, just as is produced by a normally connected uterine horn. In those with a local utero-ovarian pathway for luteolysis, such as the cow, the absence of a segment of the uterus could result in insufficient $PGF_{2\alpha}$ to cause regression of the corpus luteum. In the pig, where systemic transmission of $PGF_{2\alpha}$ from the endometrium to the corpus luteum is important, prostaglandins from the blind uterine horn can have a lytic effect on the corpora lutea of pregnancy in the contralateral ovary. In the dog and cat, the uterus does not play a role in the regression of the corpus luteum.

Imperfect lateral fusion of the paired paramesonephric ducts results in anomalies. Normally the two ducts unite first at the cloacal end to form the vagina. The fusion moves cranially to form the cervix and the uterine body. Malformations caused by imperfect fusion are most common in and adjacent to the cervix. They range

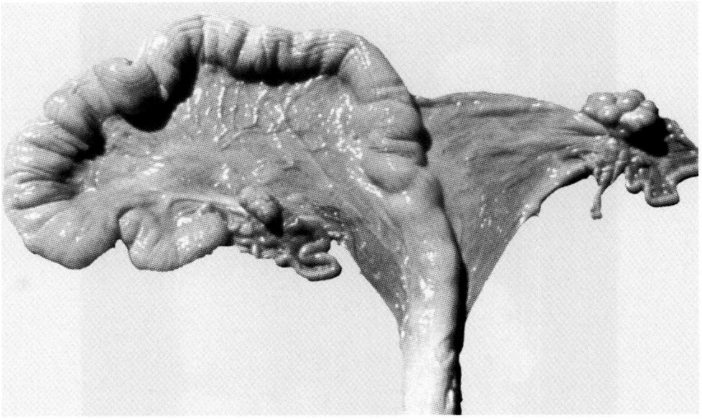

Fig. 18-7 Segmental aplasia of a uterine horn, uterus, pig.
The right uterine horn is completely missing. (Courtesy Dr. K. McEntee, Reproductive Pathology Collection, University of Illinois.)

from a dorsoventral fibrous band in the cranial vagina, failure of fusion of the caudal cervix with bifurcation of the cervical canal, to complete duplication of the cervix and body of the uterus (uterus didelphys).

Hypoplasia (and its extreme, aplasia) of a portion of the reproductive tract apart from the tubular genitalia comes in many different degrees. Gonadal hypoplasia is common, especially in males, and these are discussed in the relevant sections.

Minor Anomalies

Minor or incidental anomalies are myriad in the reproductive tract. The same factors influencing the development of major anomalies in animals with normal sexual differentiation also operate here. Minor anomalies are incidental and not clinically significant apart from potentially being mistaken for lesions that do cause infertility, subfertility, or are life threatening. Foremost of these are the numerous cysts and tubular remnants. Periovarian cysts are extremely common and can be confused with cystic neoplasms. They can be derived from paramesonephric ducts, mesonephric ducts, and mesonephric tubules. Web Table 18-1 lists the location and names of common incidental cystic anomalies. They are discussed in more detail later.

Inclusion cysts of the reproductive tract are isolated cysts not derived from embryonic elements. The serosal inclusion cyst of the uterus in bitches is a common type (Fig. 18-8). It arises from a small group of mesothelial cells trapped beneath the serosal surface during involution of the uterus. These grapelike clusters of semitransparent thin-walled cysts are located on the serosal surface of the uterus. Subsequent distention and enlargement result in numerous cysts developing.

Common Syndromes

Many of the commonly seen syndromes of sexual development are listed in Table 18-1.

Ovary

Developmental Anomalies

Agenesis, a total lack of ovarian tissue, can involve one or both ovaries. The entire reproductive tract also can be absent. In cases of bilateral agenesis, the tubular genitalia remain infantile.

Duplication of an ovary is a rare anomaly that arises by two different mechanisms: originating separately or splitting of an already developing ovary. The latter type is close to the normally located organ and may be connected to it. This anomaly is an

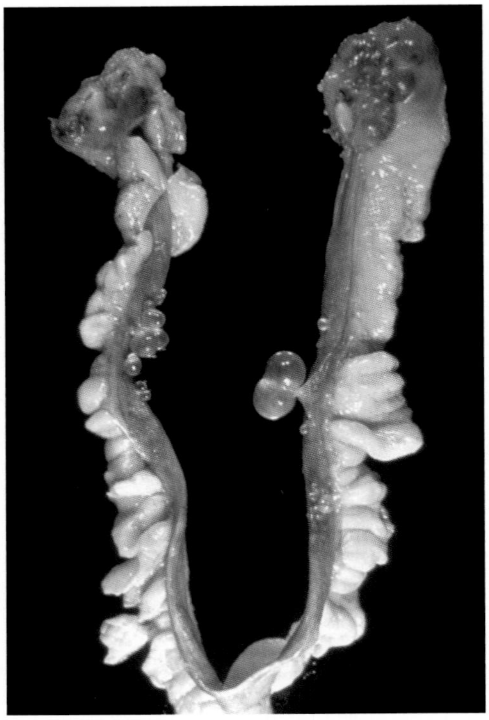

Fig. 18-8 Uterine serosal inclusion cysts, reproductive tract, bitch. The cysts projecting from the serosal surface of the uterus are believed to arise from mesothelial cells trapped within serosal connective tissue. These cysts are an incidental finding at ovariohysterectomy. Note that there are also multiple thin-walled cysts around the right ovary. These cysts are remnants of embryonal ducts and are called periovarian cysts. (Courtesy Dr. K. McEntee, Reproductive Pathology Collection, University of Illinois.)

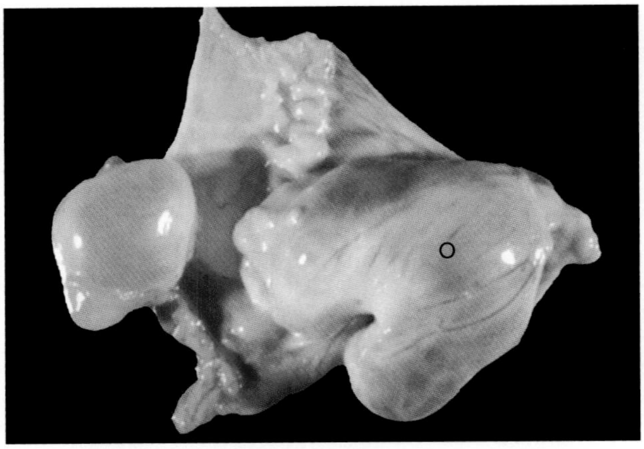

Fig. 18-9 Hydatid of Morgagni, ovary, mare. This cystic structure is located in the fimbria, adjacent to the ovary *(O)*. They are very common in mares and are cystic remnants of paramesonephric ducts. (Courtesy Ontario Veterinary College, University of Guelph.)

uncommon cause of ovarian remnant syndrome, in which previously but incompletely spayed cats and dogs come into heat (estrus) again.

Hypoplasia of the ovaries occurs most commonly in cows. It occurs in Swedish Highland cattle as an autosomal recessive trait with incomplete penetrance. It is either unilateral or bilateral. The number of primordial follicles and the proportion of Graafian follicles are fewer than normal. Ovarian hypoplasia occurs with chromosomal DSD such as XXX and X_ chromosomes in mares and XXX DSD in cows. It is usually bilateral but not symmetric. The affected ovaries are small and lack follicles or surface scars from ovulation. Microscopically, cortical stroma and ova are absent or poorly developed. The tubular genitalia remain infantile after the expected time of puberty. Other causes of an infantile reproductive tract are malnutrition or other forms of debility. Ovaries in these animals, however, have numerous primordial follicles and can respond to gonadotropic hormones after removal of the debilitating factor.

Vascular hamartomas of the ovary are incidental findings in the mare, cow, and sow. They appear as a dark red mass on the surface of the ovary and consist of connective tissue and vascular channels lined by mature endothelial cells.

Cysts In and Around the Ovary

Periovarian (paraovarian) cysts are cysts that are external to the ovary. They are common findings in dogs and cats during ovariohysterectomy (see Web Table 18-1). Intraovarian cysts are the cysts within the ovary. These should be differentiated from cystic neoplasms (see next section).

Periovarian cysts

Periovarian cysts are usually cystic remnants of embryonic structures, either paramesonephric ducts or mesonephric tubules or ducts. Location of the cyst helps differentiate them. Cystic remnants of the paramesonephric ducts include the fimbrial cyst and the cystic accessory uterine tube. This is common in the mare and called the *hydatid of Morgagni* (Fig. 18-9). Hydatid of Morgagni measure up to several centimeters in diameter and are cranial to the ovary in the mesovarium. Cystic accessory uterine tubes are in the mesosalphynx. Histologically, they resemble the normal uterus and have a thin coat of muscle. There are cysts that arise from mesonephric remnants, either ducts or tubules. Cysts of the mesonephric duct are in the cranial or caudal mesovarium and histologically have a thick smooth muscle coat.

Intraovarian cysts

Intraovarian cysts are numerous and common. Many are derived from Graafian follicles but others are epithelial cysts from the surface epithelium or from the intraovarian rete ovarii, embryonic structures of mesonephric tubular origin. The most common in the mare is an epithelial inclusion cyst, and the most common in the dog and cat is the cystic rete ovarii (Fig. 18-10).

Epithelial inclusion cysts in mares can cause infertility (see Web Table 18-1). They are located in the ovary around the ovulation fossa. Epithelium from the surface of the ovary becomes pinched off and embedded in the stroma during ovulation. This epithelium produces fluid that causes the structure to enlarge and eventually reach several centimeters in diameter. They are identical in appearance to large follicles, but they do not appear and disappear as follicles should; histologic assessment is necessary for diagnosis. Their size and number may block ovulation. Epithelial inclusion cysts in other species, or cysts of subsurface epithelial structures in bitches form in a similar manner, but they are in the capsule of the ovary and are small and incidental.

Cystic ovarian (Graafian) follicles, or follicular cysts, are defined as follicles that are larger than normal. They are especially important in cows and sows. The disease in cows is called *cystic ovarian degeneration* (COD). Bovine cystic follicles are 2.5 cm or more in diameter (Fig. 18-11) and persist for 10 or more days without the formation of a corpus luteum. The prolongation of the postpartum interval to first estrus (so called *days-open*) is the main consequence of cystic follicles. Ovulation does not occur. These cysts probably

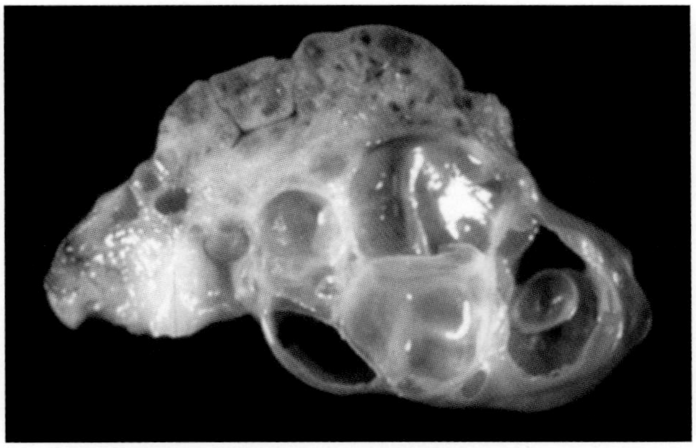

Fig. 18-10 Multiple cystic rete ovarii, ovary, bitch.
Note the multiple cysts *(lower right half of image)* within the ovary at the hilus. They are incidental findings in bitches and are of little consequence. They develop from the rete (mesonephric tubules) of the ovary and become cystically distended. In cats, they can be unilocular and very large and cause pressure atrophy of the ovary. They must be differentiated from cystadenomas and cystadenocarcinomas, histologically. (Courtesy Dr. R.A. Foster, Ontario Veterinary College, University of Guelph.)

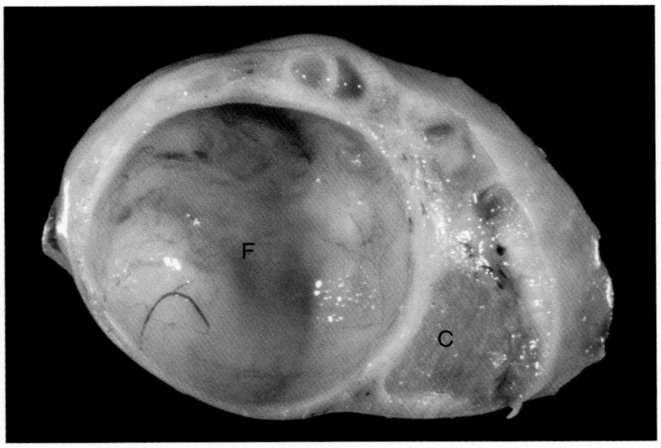

Fig. 18-11 Cystic Graafian follicle, ovary, cow (also called follicular cysts).
Follicular cysts *(F)* are larger than normal follicles and usually greater than 2.5 cm in diameter. They are the macroscopic lesions of cystic ovarian disease in the cow. They arise when ovulation of a normal follicle does not occur. *C,* Corpus luteum. (Courtesy Dr. R.B. Miller, Ontario Veterinary College, University of Guelph.)

develop because of an abnormality of the hypothalamo-hypophyseal-ovarian axis that causes a deficiency of LH or of the LH receptor in the ovary, although the mechanism is not confirmed. Cystic ovarian degeneration is treated with GnRH, which causes release of LH in the pituitary, and with chorionic gonadotropin (high in LH). Evidence suggests that stress is involved wherein adrenocorticotropic hormone (ACTH) or cortisol inhibits GnRH release from the hypothalamus and prevents upregulation of LH receptors in the ovary. Higher concentrations of progesterone can have a similar effect. The end result is an inadequate LH surge and failure of ovulation. In a similar way, postpartum uterine infection can cause cystic follicles. *Escherichia coli* infection of the uterus increases concentrations of serum $PGF_{2\alpha}$ metabolites and cortisol. It was proposed that bacterial endotoxins, or the prostaglandins produced because of damage caused by endotoxins, stimulate the adrenal cortical secretion of cortisol; cortisol excess suppresses the preovulatory release of LH, resulting in the development of cysts.

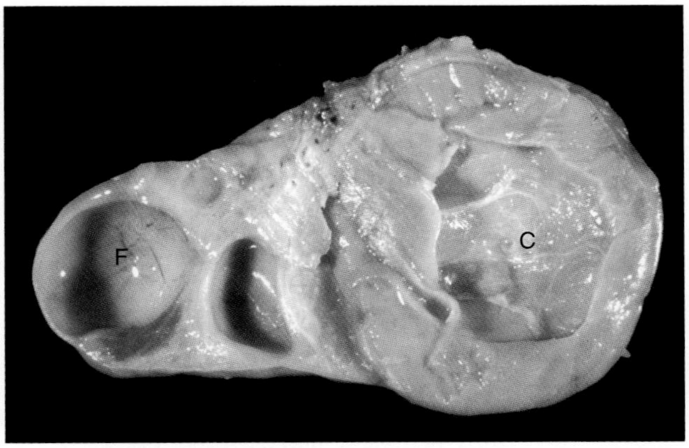

Fig. 18-12 Cystic corpus luteum, ovary, cow.
A cystic corpus luteum *(C)* is a normal corpus luteum complete with an ovulation papilla and a prominent cystic center. There is also a normal Graafian follicle *(F)* present. (Courtesy Dr. R.B. Miller, Ontario Veterinary College, University of Guelph.)

Luteinized cysts are anovulatory luteinized follicular cysts. They develop from follicular cysts by delayed or insufficient release of LH and are therefore part of COD (see Web Table 18-1). It therefore occurs in cows and sows more often than in other species. Luteinized cells line the cystic cavity. Cystic follicles and luteinized cysts can occur in the same ovary.

Cystic corpus luteum is a corpus luteum with a cystic center. It is unknown why a follicle fails to luteinize fully. The cystic center is larger than the normal small central cavity that occurs normally in some corpora lutea. Ovulation occurs in a normal follicle, but a large irregular cystic center develops (Fig. 18-12). The length of the estrous cycle is not affected, and most cysts are incidental.

Inflammation of the Ovary

Oophoritis, or inflammation of the ovary, is rare in domestic animals. Infectious bovine rhinotracheitis virus (bovine herpesvirus 1 [BoHV-1]) viremia in experimental studies can induce necrotizing oophoritis in the postestrus cow. A cloudy fibrinous fluid fills some follicles. Microscopically, the lesions in the corpus luteum range from focal necrosis and the presence of mononuclear cells to diffuse hemorrhage and necrosis. Most affected ovaries also have necrotic follicles and mononuclear cells in the stroma. Bovine viral diarrhea (BVD) virus, a vertically and horizontally transmitted virus responsible for mild-to-fatal enteric disease and reproductive failure, can localize in bovine oocytes and cumulus cells and cause chronic oophoritis. Infection of ovarian oocytes with BVD virus is one of several possible routes of transmission of the virus from cow to fetus. Bacterial oophoritis occasionally is found in cats and dogs. In cats, it must be differentiated from feline infectious peritonitis (FIP). The inflammation is around the ovary and within the uterine tube, suggesting that the causative bacteria ascended from the uterus.

Miscellaneous Diseases of the Ovary

Supernumerary follicles occur in bovine ovaries when FSH is used in doses to cause superovulation in preparation for embryo transfer. There may be more than a dozen well-developed ovarian follicles or corpora lutea.

Adhesions between infundibulum and ovary vary from thin bands to large sheets of fibrous tissue binding the walls together.

The lesion is often bilateral in cows and results from ascending infection after postpartum metritis. Physical trauma from rectal palpation and manipulation of the ovary is another possible cause; infundibular adhesions are common in beef heifers. Adhesions can obstruct or cause retention of fluids and result in a cystic infundibulum.

A small amount of hemorrhage is normal at the time of ovulation in all species. The mare is an exception because the follicles are large and the cavity of the ovulated follicle fills with blood to form a large corpus hemorrhagicum. In rare cases, the hemorrhage can be extensive enough to form an ovarian hematoma or even hemoperitoneum. If the hematoma extends through the ovulation fossa, the corpus luteum develops external to the ovarian capsule. In the mare and cow, a focal area of serositis is detectable at the point of ovulation. Progression through a fibrinous to a fibrous stage is rapid, and an "ovulation tag" is formed. The manual expression of a persistent corpus luteum in the cow sometimes results in severe periovarian hemorrhage. Organization of the hematoma results in adhesions between the ovary and adjacent structures, such as infundibulum of the uterine tube, and causes infertility. Excessive hemorrhage into follicles is sometimes present in calves, and hemorrhage into cystic follicles occurs occasionally in the bitch.

Atretic follicles are those that become arrested at any stage of development and then regress. In any estrous cycle, only one or a small number of follicles is destined to mature, whereas the others undergo atresia at various stages of maturation. A similar process occurs in seasonal anestrus and in all domestic species during pregnancy, except for the mare. Follicular atresia is considered abnormal when it is a part of any disease process that interferes with the release of or the pituitary response to GnRH. Development of the follicle can be arrested at any stage, and after an undetermined amount of time, it degenerates. The ovum undergoes apoptosis first; then the granulosa cells become pyknotic, vacuolated, and desquamate. The follicle either persists as a cyst with a partial thin lining of granulosa cells or is replaced by macrophages, theca cells, and fibrous connective tissue, eventually becoming a small scar.

Neoplasms

There are three main groups of primary ovarian neoplasms in domesticated animals: germ cell, sex cord stromal, and epithelial neoplasms. Little is known of ovarian carcinogenesis. Neoplasms rarely metastasize to the ovary of domestic mammals.

Germ cell neoplasms

Neoplasms arising from germ cells can differentiate along either embryonic or extraembryonic lines and are benign or malignant. The majority of neoplasms of germ cells are benign and undifferentiated (dysgerminoma) or benign with somatic differentiation (teratoma).

Dysgerminoma is a rare neoplasm of all species. It is usually a white solid friable lobulated mass with areas of hemorrhage and necrosis. It is composed of large round cells with a high nuclear to cytoplasmic ratio and many mitoses. This neoplasm is identical to seminoma in the testis. Metastases are rare.

Ovarian teratomas are rare and usually well differentiated and benign. They have disorganized elements of at least two of the three embryonic germ layers: ectoderm, including neuroepithelium; mesoderm; and endoderm. Skin with hair is often present (Fig. 18-13). Bone, cartilage, nervous tissue, fat, and respiratory epithelium are frequently seen. Malignant teratomas occur less often, and they are usually poorly differentiated with primitive tissue types.

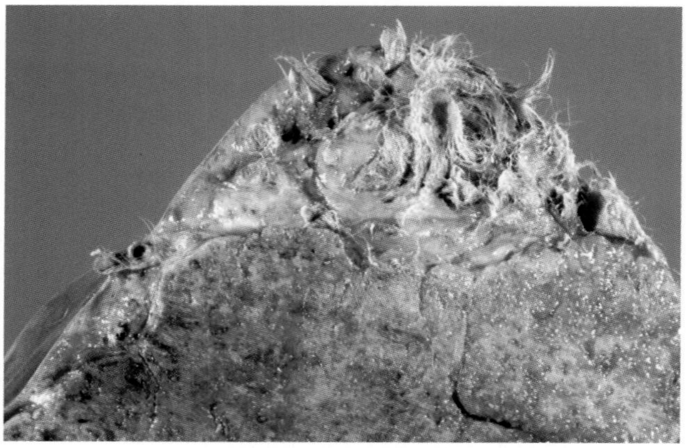

Fig. 18-13 Ovarian teratoma, ovary, bitch.
These tumors have cells that represent all three germ cell lines: ectodermal (epithelium, including neuroepithelium), mesodermal (mesenchymal tissue), and endodermal (intestine and respiratory tissues). The most common tissues seen macroscopically include hair, cartilage, and bone. This teratoma was 30 cm in diameter and surrounded by a bursa, but residual ovarian tissue was not found. Hair *(top half of image)* and bone are the main structures visible. (Courtesy Dr. R.A. Foster, Ontario Veterinary College, University of Guelph.)

Sex cord stromal neoplasms

Sex cord stromal neoplasms have a phenotype that resembles the tissues derived from the sex cords and/follicles. Most have regions with any combination of granulosa cell, theca cell, luteal cell, Sertoli cell, or interstitial endocrine cell phenotypes. Granulosa cell phenotype usually predominates, thus most are called *granulosa cell tumors.* Most produce estrogens, androgens, and/or inhibin. The mare can have signs of anestrus (inhibin-producing), nymphomania (estrogen-producing), or stallion-like behavior (androgen-producing); the bitch is likely to have prolonged estrus and may develop pyometra.

Granulosa cell tumors. Granulosa cell tumors are the most common ovarian neoplasms reported in large animals. They are unilateral, smooth surfaced, and round and can be 20 to 30 cm in diameter. They can be solid, cystic, or polycystic (Fig. 18-14, *A* and *B*). The cysts can vary from microscopic size to several centimeters in diameter. Often, the fluid within the cysts is red-brown. Microscopically, the neoplastic cells resemble normal granulosa cells and often are arranged as they would be in normal Graafian follicles: in single or multiple rows of round to columnar cells lining fluid-filled spaces (Fig. 18-14, *C*). In less differentiated areas, the neoplastic cells are arranged in sheets. Sometimes, especially in queens, Call-Exner bodies are present. These are rosettes of granulosa cells around a central space. The stroma can be sparse or plentiful. Granulosa cell tumors in the mare and cow are usually benign, are sometimes malignant in the bitch, and are often malignant in the queen; prognostic criteria are not well established.

Pure thecomas are sex cord stromal tumors with predominantly thecal differentiation. The cytoplasm of cells in a thecoma can contains lipid droplets, as do the cells of the internal theca. Areas of luteinization in sex cord stromal neoplasms occur, but pure luteomas, neoplasms with a uniform population of luteinized cells, are rare. Sertoli cell, Leydig cell, and interstitial cell tumors are also reported.

Epithelial neoplasms

The ovaries are covered by coelomic epithelium, the same layer of tissue that invaginates in early fetal life to form the lining of the internal tubular genitalia. Neoplasms of the ovarian surface

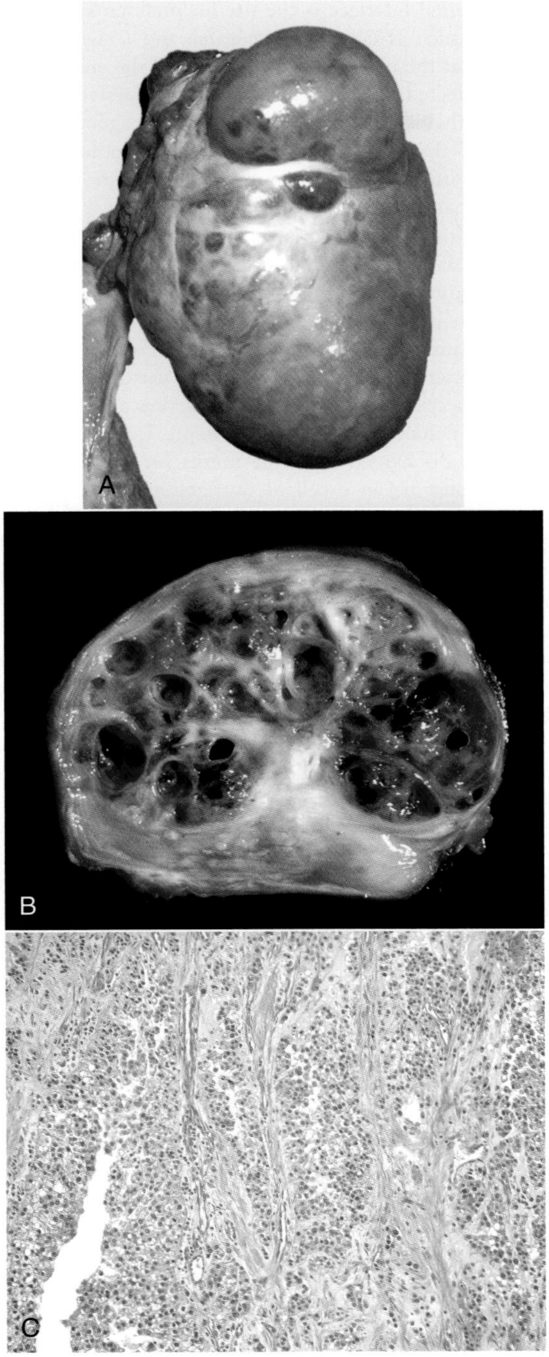

Fig. 18-14 Sex cord stromal neoplasm, granulosa cell tumor, ovary, cow. **A,** This large, lobulated neoplasm has obliterated the normal structure of the ovary. They can be solid (as in this case) or multicystic. **B,** Multiple fluid-filled cysts and solid areas have caused the dramatic ovarian enlargement. Granulosa cell tumors are part of the group of neoplasms known as sex cord stromal tumors. **C,** This granulosa cell tumor has solid and cystic regions. The cysts are lined by cells that resemble granulosa cells of the follicle. H&E stain. (**A** courtesy College of Veterinary Medicine, University of Illinois. **B** and **C** courtesy Dr. R.A. Foster, Ontario Veterinary College, University of Guelph.)

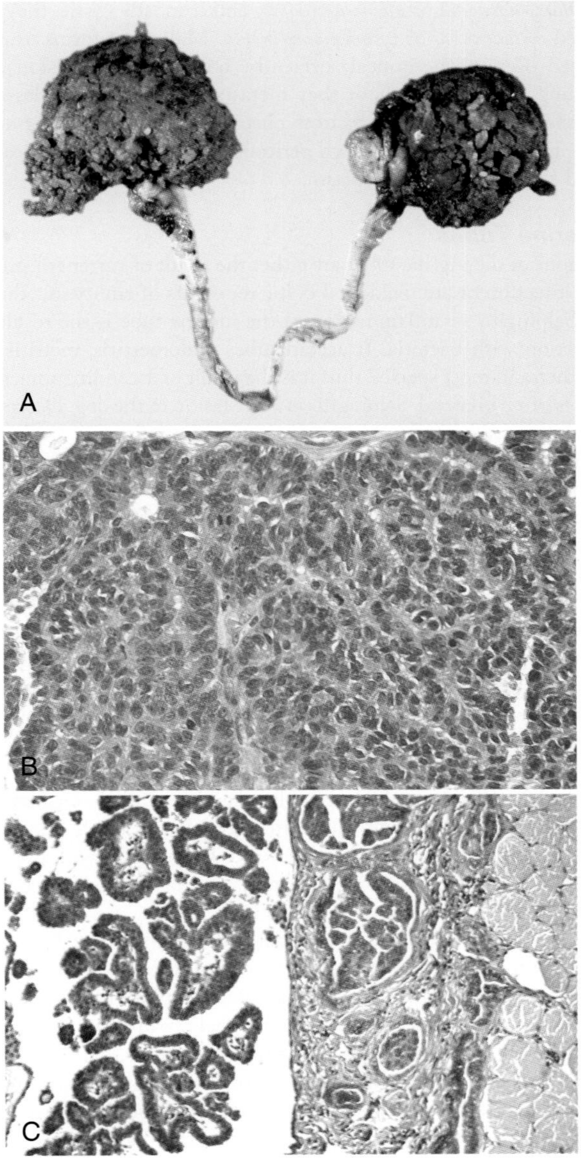

Fig. 18-15 Papillary ovarian carcinoma, ovary, bitch. **A,** Both ovaries are enlarged by neoplastic epithelium that has formed papillary structures that give the masses a shaggy outer surface. These neoplasms are often malignant and bilateral, and they seed the abdomen, producing carcinomatosis. **B,** Neoplastic epithelial cells are arranged in cords and papillae, are pleomorphic, and have many mitoses. H&E stain. **C,** This papillary carcinoma has seeded the abdominal cavity, implanted on the peritoneum, invaded into the muscle of the diaphragm, and is in subserosal lymphatic vessels adjacent to the diaphragmatic skeletal muscle *(right)*. H&E stain. (**A** courtesy Dr R.B. Miller, Ontario Veterinary College, University of Guelph. **B** courtesy Dr. M.D. McGavin, College of Veterinary Medicine, University of Tennessee. **C** courtesy Dr. K. McEntee, Reproductive Pathology Collection, University of Illinois.)

epithelium can thus resemble the several neoplastic types of the endometrium. The cells overlying the ovaries, while contiguous with the mesothelium, are called *ovarian epithelium.* Neoplasms of the ovarian epithelium are adenoma and carcinoma, and these occur commonly in the bitch (Fig. 18-15, *A*). In dogs, they originate from the subsurface epithelial structures that are invaginations of the epithelium into the capsule of the ovary. Neoplasms also arise in the rete ovarii of the ovarian hilus but only very rarely. They are often multifocal, not from metastasis but instead from multiple de novo development. They also may be bilateral. Macroscopically, the affected ovary is large and multinodular and has a cystic or shaggy appearance. Histologically, they have a combination of papillary and cystic regions. When predominantly papillary, they are called *papillary adenoma* or *adenocarcinoma,* and if mostly cystic, they are called *cystadenoma* or *cystadenocarcinoma.* Malignant forms usually spread over the peritoneal surface by both lateral extension and seeding (Fig. 18-15, *C*), or they metastasize to lymph nodes and other organs. Ascites results from obstruction of the diaphragmatic lymph vessels, which reabsorb peritoneal fluid, and/or from excess fluid secretion by the neoplasm.

Uterine Tubes

Lesions of the uterine tubes are either the result of current or previous infection or are incidental cystic remnants of embryonic ducts.

Salpingitis or inflammation of the uterine tube is the result of infection with bacteria. It accompanies endometritis, metritis, or pyometra in most species, thus it is the result of ascending infection and is often bilateral. Salpingitis is a rare lesion in the dog. Descending infection from the ovary may occur with viral infection. Direct hematogenous infection is possible. Macroscopic lesions are minimal. There may be hyperemia, thickening of the mucosa, and small amounts of luminal exudate. Inflammation of the infundibulum of the uterine tube accompanies perioophoritis. Microscopically, the inflammation ranges from mild to severe and from acute to chronic. Early mild lesions are loss of cilia and desquamation of epithelial cells at the tips of the mucosal folds. When severe, salpingitis involves other parts of the mucosa and sometimes the muscle layer. Exudate is present in the lumen. When adhesions form between the erosions and adjacent mucosa, the tube becomes cystic, reepithelializes, or is replaced by granulation tissue. Obstruction of the uterine tube combined with suppurative inflammation results in pyosalpinx, which is a dilated and pus-filled uterine tube. Neutrophils predominate and form large lakes in the lumen or in mucosal cysts derived from the glands of the tube. As with pyometra, the epithelium is missing or hyperplastic or develops squamous metaplasia.

Hydrosalpinx is a dilated and fluid-filled uterine tube. Obstruction of the uterine tube prevents normal fluid from exiting to the uterus. Obstruction results from previous salpingitis and scaring, from trauma in cattle after aggressive rectal palpation or manual expression of a corpus luteum, ovarian hematoma, or from cystic dilation of embryonic remnants or segmental aplasia. Macroscopically, there is dilation of the tube with clear fluid so that it becomes thin-walled, tortuous and appears to be longer than normal.

Lesions commonly encountered in dogs and cats are duct remnants in the mesosalpinx, more often of the mesonephric duct (simple tubular structures lined by low columnar to cuboidal cells) than paramesonephric duct (lined by a folded mucosa similar to the uterine tube mucosa) origin. Mesonephric and paramesonephric duct remnants are described in the discussion on periovarian cysts in the section on the Ovary.

Ectopic pregnancy of humans occurs when the conceptus develops in the Fallopian (uterine) tube. This is not reported in domesticated mammals. Ectopic pregnancy in dogs and cats occurs with traumatic rupture of the pregnant uterus and release of the fetus into the abdomen.

Uterus

Inflammation

Uterine disease is a significant cause of infertility and mortality in some cases. Foremost of these are inflammatory diseases, usually the result of contamination of the uterus with bacteria.

Most uterine infections are the result of ascending infection that arises when the cervix is open—at estrus, parturition, or the postpartum period. Infection can descend from the ovary and uterine tube or via the hematogenous route, particularly in pregnancy when the uteroplacental interface is the site for preferential localization of organisms such as *Coxiella, Chlamydia,* and *Ureaplasma* spp. It is assumed that the placenta is the target and the endometrium is secondarily affected, but the interface of the two systems is a unique environment that is suitable for many infectious agents to multiply. Resistance of the uterus to infection is influenced by physical factors, the hormonal environment, and the innate and acquired immune mechanisms as discussed previously.

Endometritis is inflammation of the endometrium, usually to seminal fluid and bacterial infection in nonpregnant animals. In cows, herpesvirus infections are also a cause. In pregnancy, organisms that cause placentitis, fetal infection, and failure of pregnancy also cause inflammation of the endometrium. Postpartum endometritis occurs after a normal pregnancy and parturition, but endometritis is especially common and more severe after an abnormal parturition or failure of the uterus to involute. Lochia, the fluid and debris that is discharged from the uterus for a short time after parturition, must be an excellent nutrient medium for bacterial growth.

Mild cases of acute endometritis are not detectible grossly. In more severe cases of acute endometritis, the mucosa is swollen and has a corrugated surface, often with adherent fibrin and necrotic debris. At microscopic examination, neutrophils are found in the endometrial stroma and glands, with a range of surface changes from desquamation of a few surface epithelial cells to severe necrosis of the entire endometrium. Mild lesions resolve completely or incompletely with residual changes of cystic glands and periglandular fibrosis. Severe acute endometritis often becomes chronic, and necrotic endometrium is replaced by granulation tissue and subsequently fibrous tissue. Release of $PGF_{2\alpha}$ in acute endometritis in large animals with 4 or 5 days of progesterone priming causes premature regression of the corpus luteum and shortening of the estrous cycle. The loss of endometrium (which produces $PGF_{2\alpha}$) in chronic endometritis decreases the amount of $PGF_{2\alpha}$, especially in the mare and the cow, and results in a persistent corpus luteum.

Persistent mating-induced endometritis is recognized in mares. Affected animals are unable to resolve acute endometritis that follows mating. It is normal for inflammation, presumably because of the local effects of seminal fluid, to last 24 to 36 hours in mares. Those mares with reduced uterine contractility fail to clear this inflammation and accumulate uterine and seminal fluid in the uterus and develop persistent edema. Reduced uterine contractility, which is the result of an intrinsic dysfunction or release of nitric oxide in the endometrium, is proposed as the cause. Greater susceptibility occurs with repeated pregnancies, loss of body condition, and genetics. The position of the uterus also plays a role, and normal mares have a more horizontal uterus that allows better drainage of fluid than the more drooped or vertical orientation of susceptible mares.

In the mare, endometrial biopsy is a breeding management tool because the severity of endometritis is correlated directly with the inability of the uterus to carry a fetus to term. To give a prognosis based on the features of the endometrium, the stage of cycle, number and presence of inflammatory cells, contents of the glands, and frequency and severity of periglandular fibrosis are scored (Fig. 18-16). The endometrium of individual mares is categorized as predicted high, reduced, or low likelihood of the birth of a live foal.

Metritis is inflammation of all layers of the uterine wall (Fig. 18-17). It is a more severe and advanced form of endometritis. In its acute stage, the serosa is dull, finely granular, and has petechial hemorrhages and fine adhering strands of fibrin. Microscopically, there is edema and neutrophils in the endometrium, muscle layers, and the serosa.

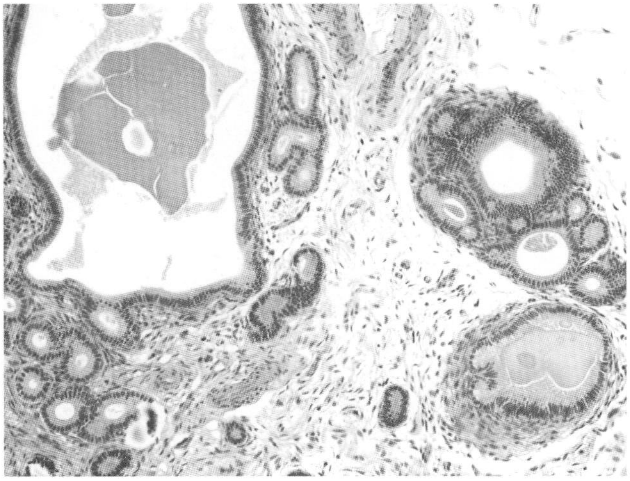

Fig. 18-16 Endometrial fibrosis, endometrial biopsy, mare.
Fibrosis from endometrial inflammation and edema results in endometrial glands forming nests *(right)* and cysts *(left)*. This fibrosis results in reduced fertility due to a lack of attachment of the conceptus, or a failure of formation of normal microcotyledons and a reduced placental area. H&E stain. (Courtesy Dr. R.A. Foster, Ontario Veterinary College, University of Guelph.)

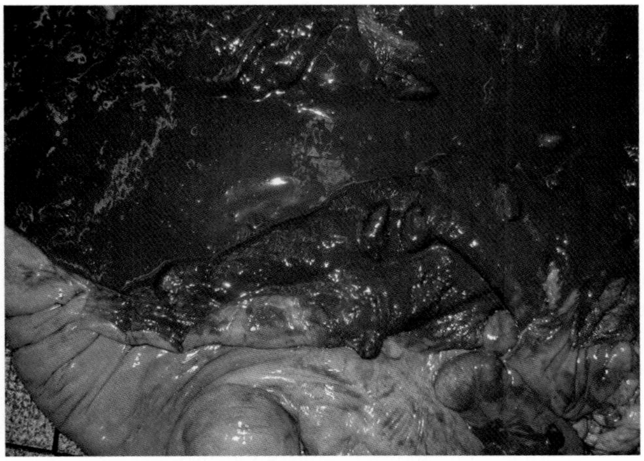

Fig. 18-17 Postpartum metritis, uterus, cow.
The uterus is distended and filled with foul-smelling dark brown fluid. The endometrium was red-black and dull, indicating an endometritis secondary to bacterial infection. This cow developed a severe metritis immediately after calving. (Courtesy Dr. R.A. Foster, Ontario Veterinary College, University of Guelph.)

Pyometra (accumulation of pus in the uterine lumen) occurs as a sequel to endometritis or metritis. It is an acute or chronic infection of the uterus with dilation and accumulation of pus in the lumen (Fig. 18-18). The closure of the cervix is not always complete, and if not, exudate is discharged into the vagina. In cows, endometritis and pyometra prevent prostaglandin release and the corpus luteum is retained thus mimicking pregnancy. In the bitch and queen, pyometra follows endometritis, which requires a corpus luteum for its development (see the discussion on cystic endometrial hyperplasia later in this chapter) (see Fig. 18-18, *A* and *B*). The color and consistency of the exudates vary with the infecting bacteria. Exudate is viscid and brown with *Escherichia coli* infection and creamy yellow with streptococcal infection. The uterus can be greatly distended but not necessarily uniformly. Macroscopically, necrotic, ulcerated, and hemorrhagic areas are present in the endometrium, with dry, white, thickened, finely cystic areas. Microscopically, the dry white areas have hyperplasia and squamous metaplasia, a common occurrence in chronic inflammation of any mucous membrane. The cystic areas are cystic endometrial hyperplasia (Fig. 18-19). Lesions outside the genital tract secondary to pyometra include widespread extramedullary hematopoiesis and immune complex glomerulopathy and are common in the bitch.

Noninflammatory Diseases

Torsion of the uterus occurs in pregnant animals and most frequently in the cow. It occurs rarely in the pregnant bitch and queen (Fig. 18-20) but can occur when the uterus is enlarged by pyometra or mucometra (accumulation of mucus in the uterine lumen). The rotation is around the mesometrium and occurs at the level of the cervix in the cow and mare and at the junction of the uterine horn and body in the bitch and queen. Torsion results in circulatory compromise and venous infarction. The veins, which have a lower pressure and are thinner walled, are compressed and occluded before the arteries. The uterine wall and placenta become congested and edematous. The fetus dies and mummifies or if the cervix is open enough to allow the entrance of bacteria or fungi, putrefies. The uterine wall is friable and prone to rupture.

Rupture of the uterus occurs as a sequel to torsion, in severe dystocia and during treatment of uterine diseases by infusion of drugs and fluids. The torsion and dystocia-related ruptures are likely to be in the caudal part of the uterus and are often fatal because of hemorrhage or infection. The rupture that follows overvigorous infusion of medications into the uterus occurs at the lesser curvature of an infused horn, dissects beneath the serosa and into

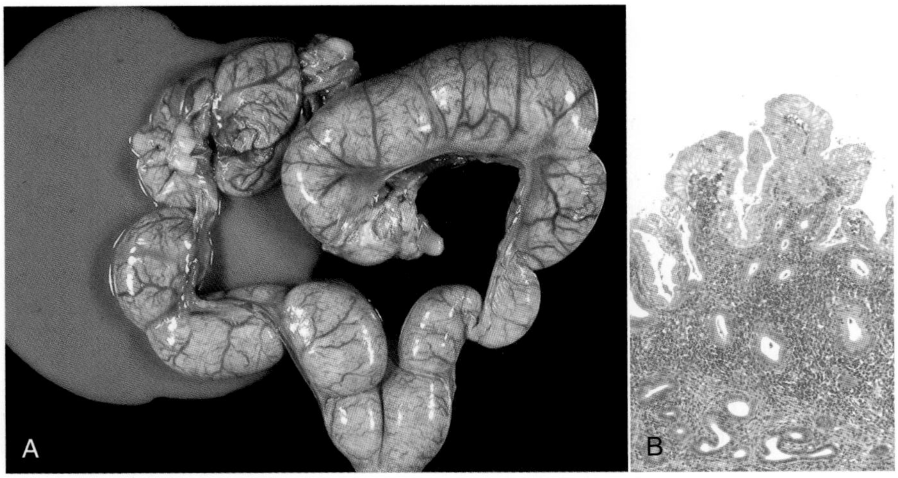

Fig. 18-18 Metritis-pyometra-endometrial hyperplasia, uterus, bitch.
A, Pyometra occurs several weeks after estrus. Bacteria grow in the uterus and induce a suppurative response. The uterus fills with pus and is distended. **B,** Endometritis and pyometra. There are large numbers of lymphocytes and plasma cells in the endometrial stroma. The surface epithelium is hyperplastic and papillary. The luminal epithelial cells are highly vacuolated. Pus in the lumen of the uterus was removed during processing of the histologic section. H&E stain. (**A** courtesy Dr. J. Wright, College of Veterinary Medicine, North Carolina State University; and Noah's Arkive, College of Veterinary Medicine, The University of Georgia. **B** courtesy Dr. R.A. Foster, Ontario Veterinary College, University of Guelph.)

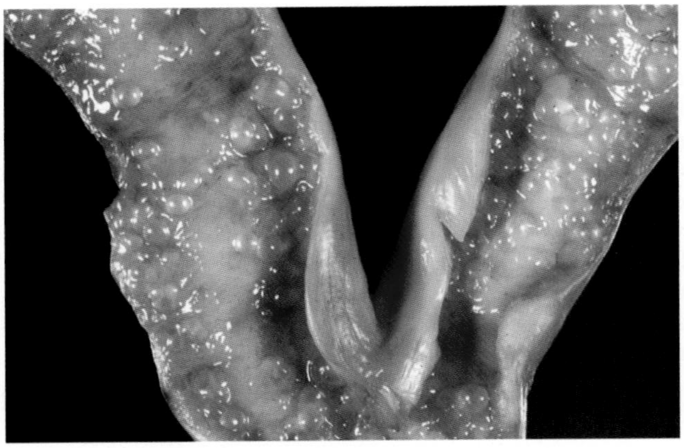

Fig. 18-19 Cystic endometrial hyperplasia, uterus, bitch.
Note the cysts in the mucosa of the endometrium. This change occurs under the influence of progesterone after estrus. Cystic hyperplasia may provide a suitable environment for bacteria to grow and cause pyometra, or alternatively, cystic hyperplasia may be secondary to uterine infection and endometritis. (Courtesy Dr. W. Crowell, College of Veterinary Medicine, The University of Georgia; and Noah's Arkive, College of Veterinary Medicine, The University of Georgia.)

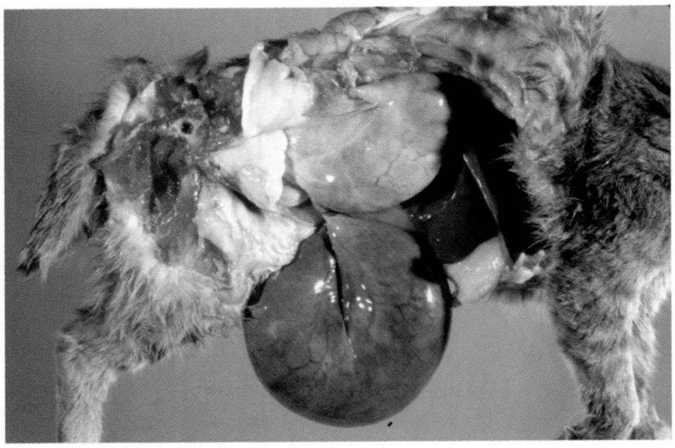

Fig. 18-20 Uterine torsion, cat.
The dark red black structure *(bottom center)* is a twisted uterine horn that contains a fetus. Its color is the result of venous infarction. (Courtesy Dr. R.A. Foster, Ontario Veterinary College, University of Guelph.)

the mesometrium, and results in inflammation around the uterus (perimetritis).

Prolapse of the uterus after parturition is important in the cow, ewe, and sow. A flaccid uterus and excessive straining are predisposing conditions. Factors that cause uterine inertia, such as prolonged dystocia, hypocalcemia, and ingestion of estrogenic plants, usually contribute to prolapse of the uterus. The anatomic structures that are prolapsed can be restricted to the previously pregnant horn, cervix, or vagina or can include all of the uterus, the bladder, and sometimes some of the small intestine. As the structures prolapse, there is vascular compromise, and congestion and edema result (Fig. 18-21). Constriction by the vaginal and vulval tissues exacerbates this by further compressing blood vessels, and as edema develops, the tissues exposed to the outside environment continue to swell, hang down further, dry, and become traumatized. This further exacerbates the swelling. Continued straining and the effects of gravity on the prolapsed tissues continue to contribute to stretching of internal structures, including ligaments and blood

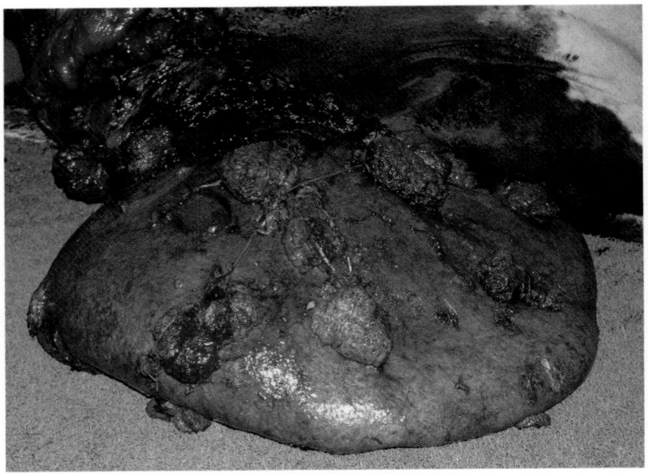

Fig. 18-21 Uterine prolapse, vulva, cow.
The uterus, cervix, and part of the vagina have prolapsed. The uterus has become swollen from dependent edema and from reduced venous outflow. The mucosae of the uterus and uterine caruncles are exteriorized and exposed to the environment, and thus they have become dehydrated and traumatized. (Courtesy Dr. R.A. Foster, Ontario Veterinary College, University of Guelph.)

vessels. Hemorrhage and shock can cause death even if the uterus is manually returned to its normal anatomic position in the abdominal cavity. If the animal survives, the intervening drying, trauma, venous infarction, and infection that occur may prevent future fertility.

Retention of fetal membranes for longer than normal after parturition is common, especially in the cow. In cows, membranes are considered retained if not expelled by 24 hours postpartum and by 3 hours in the mare. In cattle, where this is studied the most, there are many processes and mechanisms thought to operate to cause the fetomaternal interface (cotyledon and endometrium) to separate. These include the following:

1. The effects of increasing relaxin and decreasing progesterone concentrations in increasing collagenase activity to favor enzymatic breakdown of collagen linkages.
2. Increased expression of MHC-1 by trophoblasts and a maternal immune response to allow leukocytes (especially neutrophils) and cytokines to promote separation.
3. Mechanical effects of uterine contraction induced by prostaglandin and estrogen upregulation of oxytocin receptors.
4. A turnover of maternal epithelial cells of the caruncle in normal pregnancy, where as parturition approaches, there is a gradual loss and flattening of the cells.

Trophoblasts compensate by hyperplasia. Normal separation of cotyledon from caruncle involves reduced cell proliferation and increased apoptosis of placental tissue. Parturition before there is complete "maturation" of the epithelium is believed to result in retention of placental membranes. Retention is common in cases in which cesarean section is medically necessary before the time of normal parturition because there may be insufficient time for complete maturation to occur. Infectious, nutritional, hormonal, circulatory, hereditary, and weather factors may inhibit the "maturation" process. Retained membranes can act as a nutrient medium for growth of contaminant bacteria and for the development of severe endometritis from the transient mild postparturient endometritis. Bacterial endometritis can even cause systemic disease, such as toxemia, septicemia, or disseminated intravascular coagulation (DIC).

Subinvolution of placental sites is a disease unique to the bitch. It is the longer than normal persistence of placental sites in the uterus after parturition beyond the normal 12 weeks. In the normal canine placenta, trophoblasts are found in the endometrium and around the blood vessels of the myometrium, but they rapidly degenerate in the postpartum period. Subinvolution of placental sites is identified clinically by an excessive bloody vaginal discharge that lasts for weeks or months after delivery instead of the normal 1 to 6 weeks. Grossly, subinvoluted placental sites are about twice as wide as normal sites for the same time after parturition, but their appearance is identical to normal except that fibrin adherent to the site is more prominent (Fig. 18-22). As such, multiple segmental thickenings of the walls of the uterine horns are visible from the serosal surface. The luminal surface of each site is a raised, rough, ragged, gray-to-brown plaque of hemorrhage and fibrin. Microscopically, the luminal part of the plaque consists of cell debris, hematoma, thrombus, and regenerating endometrium. In the deeper part of the site, the changes are an abundance of an eosinophilic matrix, hemorrhage, distention, and decreased density of endometrial glands. Trophoblasts appear to be more numerous in subinvolution sites than in normally involuting placental sites and are abundant at the deepest portion of the eosinophilic matrix; these cells can invade the myometrium and penetrate the full thickness of and perforate the wall of the uterus. Affected animals have a prolonged bloody discharge and can become anemic, and those dogs with coagulation disorders, such as von Willebrand's disease, can exsanguinate. The uterus is prone to develop ascending infection, endometritis, and open pyometra.

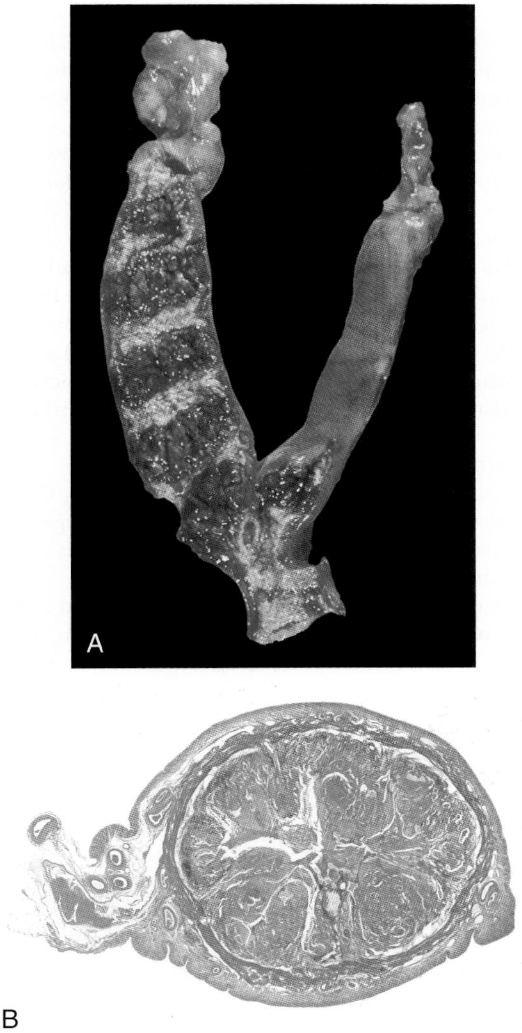

Fig. 18-22 Subinvolution of placental sites, uterus, bitch.
A, Incompletely involuted placental sites. The red transverse stripes are placental sites with hemorrhage, fibrin, and necrotic debris. They are larger than normal sites for the same stage after parturition and remain long after normal sites would have disappeared (12 to 15 weeks postpartum). **B,** Transverse section of the uterus at a subinvoluted placental site. The two pink outer layers are normal myometrium and underlying endometrial stroma. Most of the distended lumen is filled with large irregularly sized clots of blood, fibrin, and necrotic debris around which are endometrial epithelium and trophoblasts. H&E stain. (Courtesy Dr. M.D. McGavin, College of Veterinary Medicine, University of Tennessee.)

Pseudopregnancy is an exaggerated form of a normal physiologic process. Every nonovariectomized female dog has a prolonged luteal phase of estrus, and this is called *covert pseudopregnancy* or *physiologic pseudopregnancy*. Some dogs, especially of the toy breeds, develop an exaggerated reaction. The mechanism is poorly understood, but prolactin or its receptors play a role. The presence of progesterone is necessary for the changes to occur. Overtly pseudopregnant dogs either have an increased concentration of prolactin, or they have increased sensitivity to prolactin. This can occur with a more rapid than usual decline in progesterone when dogs are spayed during diestrus. Hyperprolactinemia that occurs in response to visual stimuli of the presence of surrogate neonates results in the mammary development, lactation, maternal behavior, and other clinically apparent changes of pseudopregnancy. Uterine changes in pseudopregnancy can include the formation of structures that resemble placental sites (now called *localized endometrial hyperplasia of pseudopregnancy* or *pseudoplacentation endometrial hyperplasia*) and mucometra; obviously there are no fetuses.

Endometrial atrophy is usually the result of loss of ovarian function. It occurs (1) at anestrus, (2) with a debility such as malnutrition or cachexia, and (3) in DSD. Focal endometrial atrophy of unknown cause sometimes occurs in the mare. Atrophic endometrium is macroscopically thin. In the mare, the longitudinal folds are indistinct, and in the cow, the caruncles are flat. The uterus of the mare is the most studied microscopically because data from uterine biopsies is frequently used for the management of breeding. The endometrium of the uterus of the anestrous mare has cuboidal luminal and glandular epithelium, with short, straight glands.

Endometrial polyps are common lesions in older bitches and queens. The cause is unknown, but they usually occur with cystic endometrial hyperplasia. They are localized and often pedunculated hyperplastic nodules of endometrial stroma and glands that vary from microscopic up to several centimeters long (Fig. 18-23). They can cause obstruction of the uterine lumen and mucometra.

Endometrial hyperplasia can be localized or generalized; is an important lesion in the ewe, bitch, and queen; and is rare in the mare. Cystic follicles, granulosa cell tumors, and estrogens from plants are causes of endometrial hyperplasia in the cow. In ewes, it is caused by prolonged hyperestrogenism. Ingested estrogenic clover, such as subterranean (*Trifolium subterraneum*), and red (*Trifolium pratense*) clover is the most likely source of estrogen. In ewes, endometrial hyperplasia results in reduced fertility, dystocia, and uterine prolapse because of uterine hypotonicity. Glands of the endometrial type can develop in the cervical mucosa. Even when nonpregnant, ewes have mammary gland enlargement. Endometrial cysts develop beside and beneath the caruncles, and they are about 1 cm in diameter and are filled with clear fluid. The mycotoxin zearalenone obtained from moldy feed causes endometrial cysts in the sow. In the bitch and presumably the queen, cystic endometrial hyperplasia (CEH) is a common response of the uterus (see Fig. 18-19) that occurs in diestrus. The disease can be reproduced by estrogen priming of dogs followed by progesterone administration, but this may not be the physiologic mechanism. Bacteria are almost always present in the uterus of dogs with CEH and are probably the cause. Increased concentration of progesterone in late estrus or early diestrus and aberrant hormonal function may alter hormonal receptor expression. This may prime the uterus so that inflammation or irritation by bacteria (or other substances, such as suture material and oil) stimulates the uterus to undergo hyperplasia and the type of change seen in early pregnancy (the so-called *decidual reaction*).

Simple endometrial hyperplasia can be overlooked or recognizable macroscopically when the endometrium has patchy or diffuse thickening. When it is cystic, the lesion is readily recognized at surgery or at necropsy. Microscopically, the main component of endometrial hyperplasia is an increase in the size and number of glands with no change in the stroma except for edema. The glandular epithelium is progestational in appearance (i.e., the cells are columnar, hypertrophic, and hyperplastic and have a clear vacuolated cytoplasm) (see Fig. 18-18, *B*). As the glands become cystic with increased pressure of retained secretion the epithelium of the glands becomes flattened and simple squamous in type (compression atrophy). Mucometra and hydrometra are the accumulation of mucus and clear fluid, respectively, in the uterine lumen (Fig. 18-24, *A* and *B*). The cause is congenital or acquired obstruction of the outflow of the fluid and/or mucus that is produced by the endometrium and released when the cervix opens. However, hydrometra and mucometra can develop with excessive production in hyperestrogenism. Hydrometra and mucometra occur in pseudopregnancy, where it resolves spontaneously.

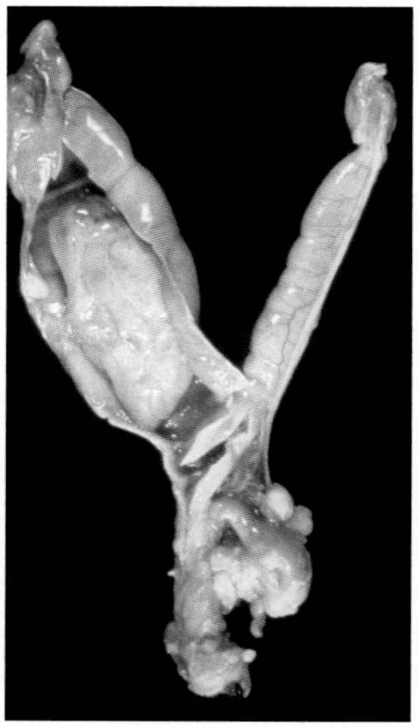

Fig. 18-23 Endometrial polyp, cat.
The uterine horn on the left is distended by a solid cylindrical polyp that is connected to the endometrium by a narrow stalk. (Courtesy Dr. G. Foley, Pfizer Inc.)

Adenomyosis is the presence of endometrium within the myometrium, and the effect generally is negligible in domestic animals, which do not menstruate. Adenomyosis is found in the cow, bitch, and queen. It is thought that endometrium is either forced into the myometrium by pressure of pregnancy or pyometra, or that the epithelium "migrates." In primates, adenomyosis is considered part of *endometriosis,* which is a general term in which endometrium is found in ectopic locations. Endometriosis, in which endometrium is found on serosal surfaces, around the ovary, or in the chest, is not reported in domestic species. Macroscopic changes in adenomyosis are primarily localized thickening of the myometrium. In dramatic cases, there are cysts formed in the myometrium. Sometimes, in bitches the uterus undergoes diffuse symmetric or focal asymmetric enlargement near the cervix (Fig. 18-25). Microscopically, endometrial glands, stroma, or both are within the myometrium.

Neoplasms

Uterine neoplasms are uncommon in domestic animals. Carcinoma in the cow and leiomyoma in the bitch are the most frequently seen. Lymphoma, which affects multiples sites of the body, is a common neoplasm in the cow.

Endometrial carcinoma is well known in cattle and is found at the time of meat inspection. The cause is unknown. The early microscopic lesion is most often in the depths of the endometrial

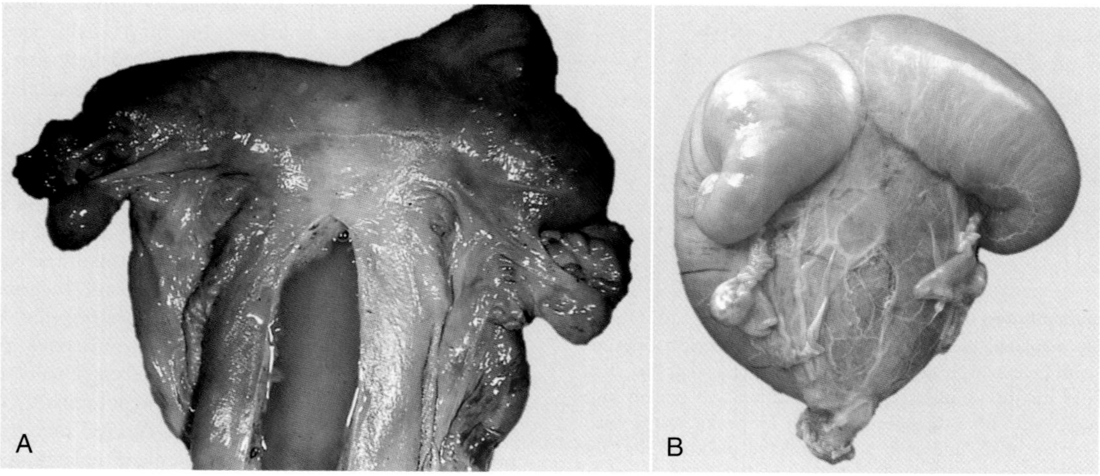

Fig. 18-24 Mucometra and hydrometra, uterus.
A, Mucometra, mare. Note the accumulation of mucus within the opened body of the distended uterus. **B,** Hydrometra, goat. The uterine horns and body are filled with clear watery fluid. (**A** courtesy Dr. K. McEntee, Reproductive Pathology Collection, University of Illinois; and Dr. J. King, College of Veterinary Medicine, Cornell University. **B** courtesy Dr. P. W. Ladds, James Cook University of North Queensland.)

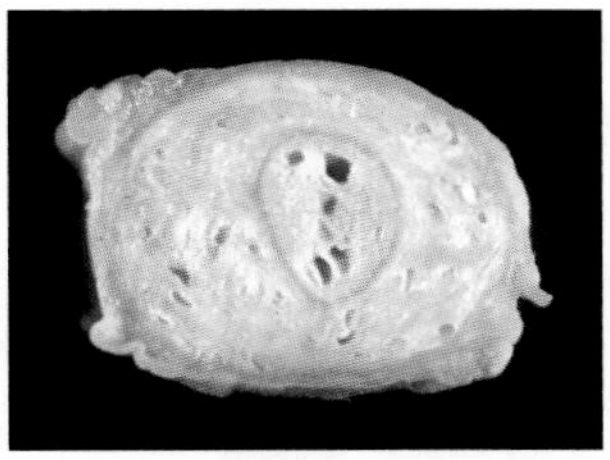

Fig. 18-25 Adenomyosis, uterine body, bitch. Formalin fixed specimen. The myometrium *(outer portion)* is infiltrated and expanded by multiple cysts of endometrial stroma and glands. Many of these glands are filled with pus, and the endometrium is expanded as a result of inflammation secondary to bacterial infection. (Courtesy Dr. R.B. Miller, Ontario Veterinary College, University of Guelph.)

glands of the horns and less often in the body of the uterus. As it increases in size, the neoplasm thickens the uterine wall without altering the luminal epithelium. A scirrhous response, the deposition of large amounts of fibrous tissue, is a characteristic lesion and this makes the neoplasm firm and tough, and causes localized constriction bands on the serosal surface. The neoplasms can be small and annular or involve a large area of the uterine wall. Microscopically, the neoplasm is readily distinguished from normal endometrium by the increased size, pleomorphism, and disarray of the glandular epithelial cells and the accompanying scirrhous reaction. Metastases occur to the regional (iliac) lymph nodes and lungs, and they seed the serosal surfaces of the abdomen.

Lymphosarcoma in the cow in the enzootic form is caused by the bovine leukemia retrovirus and commonly affects a triad of organs, namely the heart, abomasum, and uterus, as well as the lymph nodes. In the uterus, as in other locations, the neoplastic cells can be focal, multifocal, or multifocally coalescing and up to 3 cm thick (Fig. 18-26). Affected areas are light yellow, slightly friable, and sometimes centrally necrotic and thicken or replace any or all layers of the uterine wall. An extensively involved uterus can support pregnancy, even to an advanced stage.

Uterine leiomyomas in the bitch are often multiple neoplasms and can occur in the cervix and vagina (Fig. 18-27, *A* and *B*). Estrogens likely have a role in provoking and maintaining these neoplasms. In other domestic species, however, these neoplasms are rare and tend to be solitary. They are well demarcated, unencapsulated, spheric, and vary in size. If they are small, they are confined within the wall of the vagina, cervix, or uterus or can protrude into the lumen or project to the serosal surface of the uterus or into the pelvic canal. Some luminal neoplasms, especially those in the vagina, are pedunculated, making them liable to trauma or torsion. They are usually firm, pink or white, and occasionally calcified or edematous. The color is related to the amount of fibrous tissue present along with the whorled smooth muscle cells; in the macroscopically white neoplasms, fibrous tissue is the dominant component.

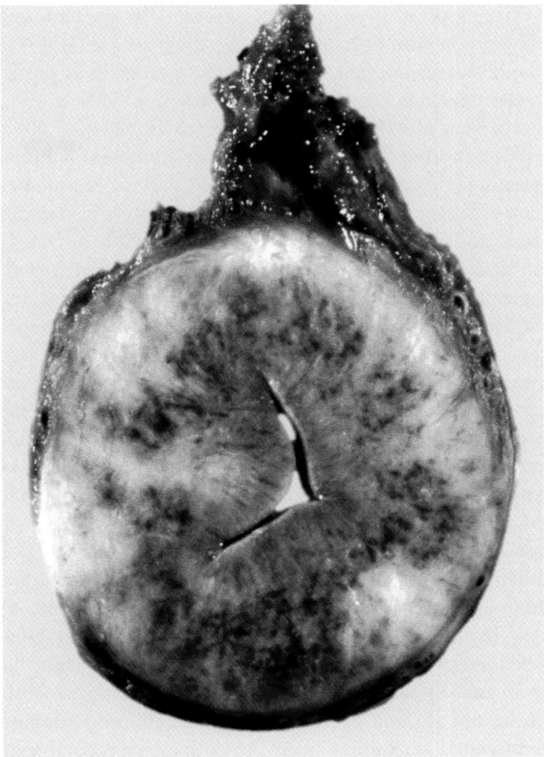

Fig. 18-26 Lymphoma (lymphosarcoma), uterus, cross-section, cow. The mucosa, lamina propria, and myometrium are expanded by neoplastic lymphocytes. The dark-red to brown regions are areas of necrosis and hemorrhage. (Courtesy Dr. R.A. Foster, Ontario Veterinary College, University of Guelph.)

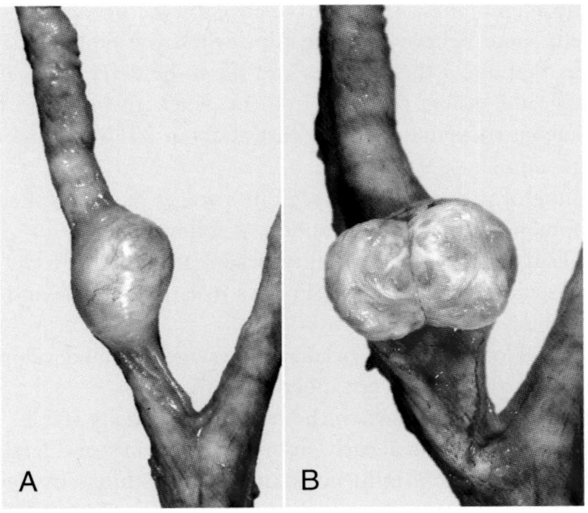

Fig. 18-27 Leiomyoma, uterus, bitch. **A,** Note the well-circumscribed, firm mass in the left uterine horn. **B,** The cut section of the leiomyoma reveals gelatinous content and bands of smooth muscle and connective tissue. This mass is within and arising from the myometrium. (Courtesy Dr. D.D. Harrington, College of Veterinary Medicine, Purdue University; and Noah's Arkive, College of Veterinary Medicine, The University of Georgia.)

Placenta and Fetus

Failure of Pregnancy

Maintenance of pregnancy is one of those miraculous events that defy logic, and there is probably more that is not known than is known about pregnancy and embryonic and fetal development. The fetus is allogeneic and therefore foreign to the mother. Yet it survives, even though both fetus and mother could mount an immune response to each other. Tolerance or suppression of the maternal immune system is required, but the mechanisms are incompletely understood, and there is little agreement about how this actually occurs. Mechanisms in rodents and primates are studied in detail and involve several potential processes, including:

- An active role of systems like the Fas/Fas ligand system in which active immune cells undergo apoptosis when they contact trophoblasts expressing the Fas ligand.

- The suppression of material immunity in the endometrium by production of indolamine 2,3 dioxygenase (IDO), which inhibits tryptophan, an amino acid necessary in the growth and development of T lymphocytes.
- The lack of MHC expression on trophoblasts.
- Alteration of the balance of T_H and suppressor lymphocytes.

Immunologic considerations are only part of maintenance of pregnancy. There are hormonal influences, especially maintenance of serum and uterine progesterone concentration by the corpus luteum and placenta. Stressors and systemic cytokines, such as prostaglandin, can cause luteolysis of the corpus luteum and terminate pregnancy during the time when pregnancy is dependent on the corpus luteum (all of pregnancy in cattle, goats, pigs and dogs, and up to 50 days of gestation in horses, sheep, and cats).

It is generally believed that fetuses initiate their own parturition. Disease conditions mimic normal parturition so that in conditions of fetal stress, such as maternal or fetal illness, hyperthermia, and hypoxia, the fetal pituitary secretes ACTH that results in glucocorticoid production by the fetal adrenal gland. Corticosteroids increase the synthesis of estrogens in the placenta, which causes upregulation of oxytocin receptors in the myometrium and the synthesis and release of $PGF_{2\alpha}$ from the endometrium. $PGF_{2\alpha}$ initiates myometrial contraction and causes luteolysis and a decreased progesterone production. Lysis of the corpus luteum results in relaxin secretion and a further decline in progesterone concentration. Relaxin secretion and reduced progesterone promotes placental separation from the endometrium by promoting collagenase activity. Initiation of birth by this process should result in a fresh (nonautolyzed) fetus, whereas rapid fetal death results in loss of pregnancy by other mechanisms, and the fetus, having spent additional time at body temperature, will be autolyzed.

The conceptus is the product of conception, and it is composed of the embryo, that part of the conceptus that gives rise to the adult, and the membranes. The time when embryos become fetuses is debated; some believe it is the time when the embryo develops features that allow their species and sex to be determined phenotypically and others consider it to be when the embryo begins spontaneous movement. This occurs at about 35 to 45 days of age in large animals.

Failure of pregnancy is divided into stages based on the fetus's development and potential viability, as follows:

- Early embryonic mortality occurs at the embryonic stage, usually less than 35 to 45 days in large animals and about 20 days in dogs and cats.
- Fetal loss (abortion) occurs at the stage of fetal development, when the fetus is not independently viable.
- Stillbirth occurs when the fetus is potentially viable.

The exact outcome of early embryonic mortality and fetal death is unpredictable and is influenced, among other things, by the cause of the failure of pregnancy, species, stage of gestation, and number of fetuses. The main outcomes are the following:

1. Embryonic death and return to estrus at the normal interval
2. Embryonic death and delayed return to service
3. Fetal loss with no autolysis
4. Fetal loss with autolysis
5. Mummification
6. Maceration
7. Stillbirth

Embryonic mortality occurs in all species, and the causes are outlined in the next section. Fetal loss with no autolysis is the norm in horses, sheep, and goats. In the bitch and queen, the lifespan of the corpus luteum is long in the nonpregnant animal and similar to pregnancy. When embryonic or fetal death occurs, the corpus luteum and products of conception may be retained until approximately the normal time of parturition. Fetal autolysis is therefore usual.

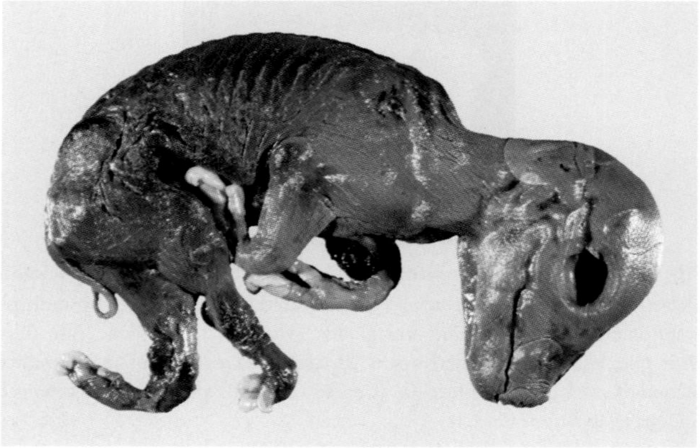

Fig. 18-28 Failure of pregnancy, mummified fetus, pig. This fetus died in utero, and the fluids were resorbed. Dehydration of a fetus in utero following death of the fetus usually takes longer than 1 week to occur. (Courtesy Ontario Veterinary College, University of Guelph.)

Mummification is one of the possible outcomes of fetal death. Rather than being expelled soon after death, the fetus is retained and progressively dehydrates to become a firm, dry mass, which is discolored by degraded hemoglobin to brown or black, and consists of leathery skin enclosing the other dehydrated organs (Fig. 18-28). The cause of death can be infectious or noninfectious, and organisms that promote lysis of dead tissue must be absent and the cervix must be closed to prevent the entry of putrefactive organisms. The situations in which mummification most commonly occurs are listed in Table 18-2. In twin pregnancy in the mare, the mummified fetus and the longer surviving fetus abort together before term. In parvovirus infection in the sow, mummified fetuses are retained and born at term along with live fetuses. In any species with a single fetus pregnancy, the mummified fetus can be expelled at any time or retained indefinitely.

Maceration is when the fetus becomes liquefied (Fig. 18-29). This requires bacteria in the uterus, and these could be those that caused the fetal death or they could be putrefactive organisms that entered the uterus via the cervix. In addition to disintegration of the fetus (see Fig. 18-29), the uterus has lesions also. Endometritis or pyometra is present; the type of lesion depends on whether the cervix remains open or closed. Endometritis and pyometra tend to become severe and chronic. Emphysema occurs when the bacteria are gas forming, such as clostridia. Maternal toxemia and death are likely if the bacteria produce potent exotoxins. Fetal bones resist maceration, and if the uterus eventually regains some muscular tone, the bones can cause perforation.

The general diagnostic rate published by veterinary diagnostic laboratories for determination of the cause of sporadic failure of pregnancy is about 50%. Identifying the cause of embryonic loss is very low because there are seldom embryonic or placental tissues to examine. The embryo is thought to dissolve, but the conceptus is so small that it may not be found. There are recognized infectious causes of early embryonic mortality, and the infection often occurs at or near the time of coitus or conception. Agents such as *Campylobacter, Tritrichomonas, Ureaplasma,* and nonspecific endometrial infections are among the common examples. It appears that chromosomal abnormalities account for the majority of noninfectious causes.

TABLE 18-2 Failure of Pregnancy

GUIDE TO FETAL AUTOLYSIS*	
Time Since Death	**Change**
12 hr	Cornea cloudy, amnionic fluid blood tinged
24 hr	Fluid in body cavities
36 hr	Gelatinous fluid in subcutis
72 hr	Eyes dehydrated
144 hr	Carcass dehydrated, no abomasal contents
COMMON CAUSES OF FETAL MUMMIFICATION	
Mare	Twinning
Cow	BVD virus infection, trichomoniasis
Bitch	Canine herpesvirus
Queen	Torsion of a uterine horn
Sow	Parvoviral infection

ABORTOGENIC AGENTS COMMON TO ALL SPECIES

Brucella sp.
Campylobacter sp.
Chlamydophila abortus
Coxiella burnetii
Herpesviruses
Leptospira interrogans
Listeria monocytogenes
Mycoplasma and *Ureaplasma* spp.
Neospora caninum
Salmonella sp.
Toxoplasma gondii

BVD, Bovine viral diarrhea.
*Data from Dillman RC, Dennis SM: *Am J Vet Res* 37: 403-407, 1976.

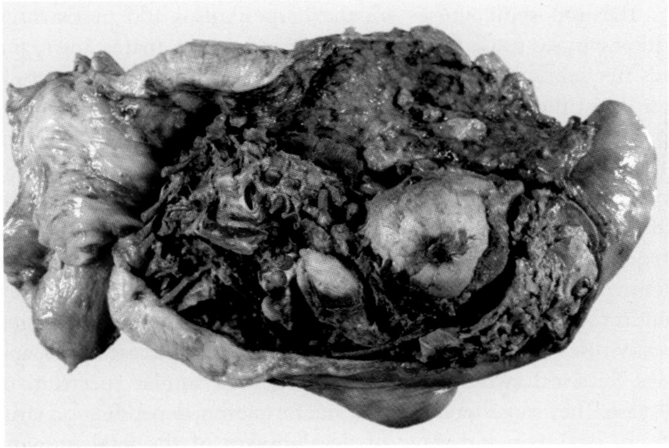

Fig. 18-29 Failure of pregnancy, macerated fetus, lamb. Fetal bones, hair, and brown pasty material fill the uterus. The ewe was infertile. (Courtesy Dr. R.A. Foster, Ontario Veterinary College, University of Guelph.)

Although the overall diagnostic success rate in sporadic fetal loss (abortion) is about 50%, the success rate is greater in outbreaks. Many of the recognized causes are infectious because infections are usually easy to diagnose (Table 18-3). This has led to the general approach of determining if the loss of pregnancy is infectious or not.

TABLE 18-3 Occurrence of Causes of Sporadic Failure of Pregnancy in Various Domesticated Species

Cause	Equine (%)	Bovine	Ovine	Caprine	Porcine
No diagnosis	40	60	60	52	53
Noninfectious	26*	3	5	10	1
Infectious	34	37	35	38	46
Placentitis	12	5	9	3	7
Viral	9	3	0	0	20
Bacterial	10	16	25	31	32
Protozoal	0	16	10	7	0

*See Box 18-5.

TABLE 18-4 Specific or Regionally Important Diseases that Cause Failure of Pregnancy

Species	Cause
Equine	Insufficient serum progesterone
	Equine herpesvirus 1
	Fescue toxicosis *(Neotyphodium coenophialum)*
	Thyroid hyperplasia/musculoskeletal syndrome
Bovine	*Brucella abortus*
	Foothills abortion
	Ponderosa pine abortion
	Campylobacter fetus
	Tritrichomonas foetus
Ovine	*Listeria monocytogenes*
	Brucella ovis
	Wesselsbron disease
	Rift Valley fever
	Cache Valley virus
	Salmonella sp.
	Iodine deficiency
Caprine	*Brucella melitensis*
	Iodine deficiency
Porcine	Leptospirosis

These are not the most common in all areas. Common causes are listed in Table 18-3.

Examination of fetus and placenta

Regardless of which species is involved, investigating failure of pregnancy requires a keen sense of what can be achieved. Depending on the situation, the investigation may have an economic impact, a zoonotic impact, or it may appeal to scientific curiosity. Maternal, fetal, and placental factors should be considered. There are infectious causes common to all species (see Table 18-2), causes that are species specific, and those that are geographically important (Table 18-4).

Examination of the fetus and placenta and sampling of tissue are primarily to answer the question: Are there any fetal or placental abnormalities to explain the failure of pregnancy? Some of the lack of success in determining the cause is the failure to submit the appropriate specimens. Where feasible, send the whole fetus and membranes to the laboratory. When this is not feasible, success in ruling out fetal or placental factors depends on submission of the correct specimens, and this in part depends on knowing what specimens to send. Each diagnostic laboratory has a recommended list of samples to maximize diagnostic success.

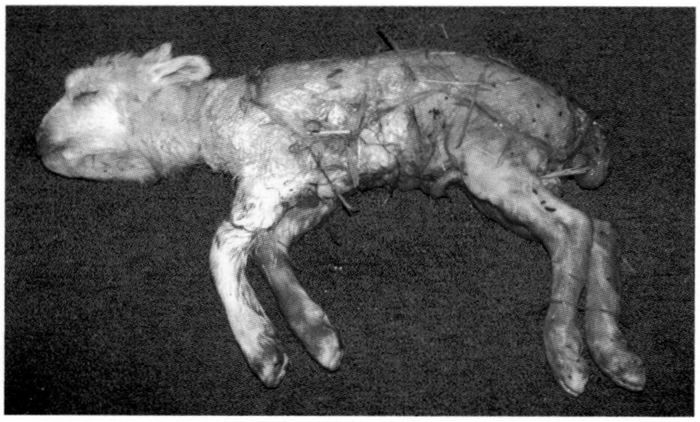

Fig. 18-30 Dystocia, lamb.
This large lamb died during parturition. It was trapped in the birth canal by the shoulders and right foreleg, which has flexed (folded back). The lamb became hypoxic and defecated meconium, visible as a yellow deposit on the skin of the body caudal to the shoulder. The head and left foreleg became swollen and the skin dry. The skin of the rest of the body is moist from amniotic fluid (and meconium), indicating that this portion of the body was in the vagina and uterus. (Courtesy Dr. R.A. Foster, Ontario Veterinary College, University of Guelph.)

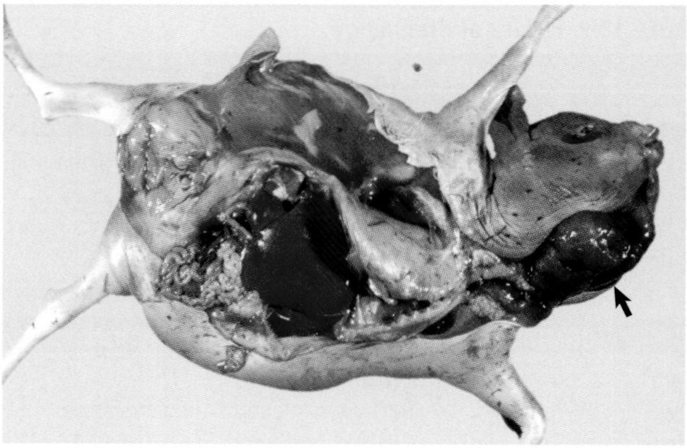

Fig. 18-31 Iodine deficiency, goiter, goat fetus.
This fetus has bilaterally extremely enlarged thyroid glands, alopecia *(arrow)*, and myxedema evident subcutaneously over the thorax and abdomen, which are the classic lesions of severe hypothyroidism. (Courtesy Dr. R.A. Foster, Ontario Veterinary College, University of Guelph.)

Each species and breed of animal has an expected rate of development and an average size at birth. Variation from this normal development indicates an abnormality to explain. Fetal and placenta weight, fetal size including crown-rump length, and degree of development for gestation length are basic parameters and changes may indicate increased or inadequate maternal nutrition, concurrent disease, or placental sufficiency.

The degree of fetal autolysis and evidence of fetal distress provide useful information. When distressed and hypoxic, a fetus gasps and aspirates amniotic contents, and meconium is released into the amniotic fluid. Meconium staining of the skin can be seen grossly (Fig. 18-30). Keratin squames and meconium from the amniotic fluid are found in the lungs on histologic examination. A fetus caught in the birth canal for a sufficient period of time develops localized swellings such as a swollen tongue and face (see Fig. 18-30). Pressure from the birth canal restricts venous and lymphatic flow, and any fetal part trapped exterior to the birth canal is edematous. Fetal autolysis was studied in sheep and gives an approximation of the time of fetal death before expulsion. It is generally believed that an autolyzed fetus dies too quickly for it to initiate its own parturition, as would occur with septicemia or viremia. A fetus without autolysis initiated its own parturition.

The fetus is similar to an adult in the general response to diseases (Fig. 18-31), particularly near parturition, but many of the responses are rudimentary, depending on the stage of gestation. The fetus is in a sterile environment and has no flora or fauna. Exposure to environmental or pathogenic agents occurs from contact with the external environment or with maternal infection. Many of the pathogens have an affinity for the reproductive tract and may infect and/or initiate failure of pregnancy in many species. Agents common to all species are listed in Table 18-2. Some of them are discussed next.

Failure of Pregnancy in Domestic Animals

Each species has common and known causes and profile of lesions and conditions that result in the failure of the pregnancy. Table 18-3 lists the likely laboratory diagnostic success and the types of diseases and conditions to expect.

In most species, the known causes of failure of pregnancy are infectious diseases and therefore one of the initial diagnostic processes is to separate the causes into infectious and noninfectious. Noninfectious causes affect the fetus or placenta, or both. Knowing the normal anatomy is therefore essential, and some of the unique structures of each species are listed next. Noninfectious fetal lesions are relatively uniform across the species. Anomalies affect the fetus primarily, unless they are sufficiently severe or large to cause dystocia and subsequent maternal death. Examples are hydrocephalus, hydrops fetus, and arthrogryposis. These are found sporadically in all species.

Many of the known causes of failure of pregnancy are infectious, and some of these infectious agents affect all species (see Table 18-2). Microorganisms of the same genus produce similar lesions in different species.

Viral diseases

The important viruses are the herpesviruses and pestiviruses. Herpesviruses cause failure of pregnancy in cows, mares, sows, and less frequently, other domestic species. Generally, the macroscopic lesions in the fetuses are multiple randomly distributed pale gray to white foci of acute necrosis, most commonly seen in the liver (Fig. 18-32, *A*). Often, the fetal liver is enlarged, and the necrotic foci are large enough to be visible as 1- to 2-mm white areas (Fig. 18-32, *B*). Foci can be red from hemorrhage. Similar lesions less frequently occur in other organs, including the lungs, kidneys, brain, or virtually any other organ. The placenta can be edematous, but in the majority of domestic species, there are no other changes. Pestiviruses in cattle (BVD virus), sheep (border disease virus), and pigs (classical swine fever virus) produce a similar spectrum of disease. They cause fetal death or malformation, depending on virus strain, fetal age, and stage of development of the fetal immune system. Placental and fetal lesions either are absent or are restricted to microscopic lymphocytic infiltrates in the heart and brain. Fetal malformations caused by these are discussed in the next section and in other chapters, especially of the nervous system.

Bacterial diseases

Bacterial species causing inflammation of the placenta and fetal sepsis are numerous. Almost any organism that causes bacteremia and septicemia can infect the pregnant uterus; common examples are the *Brucella, Salmonella, Listeria,* and *Campylobacter* spp. Entry into the body is often after fecal-oral transmission and then hematogenous spread. Some gain entry by venereal transmission. The

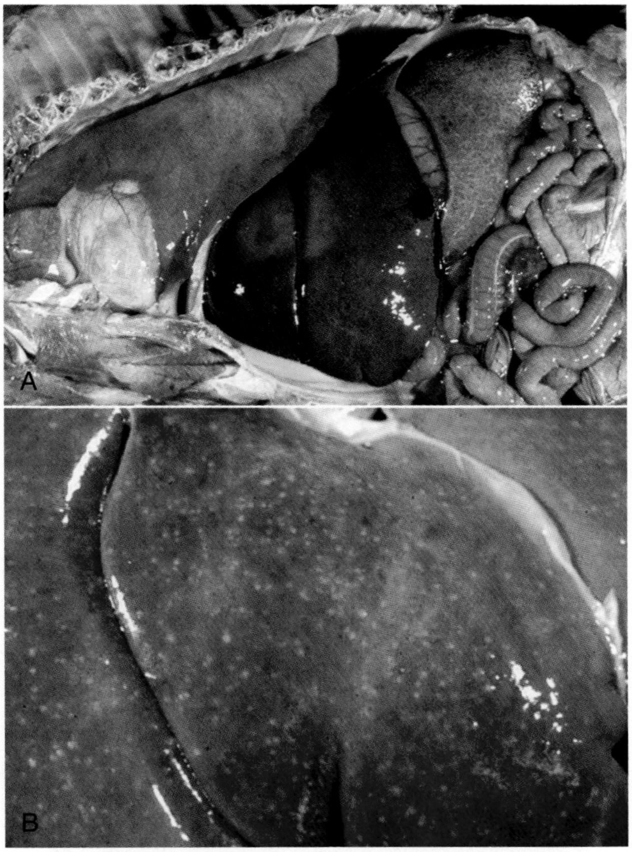

Fig. 18-32 Equine herpesvirus 1 infection, aborted equine fetus. **A,** The changes typical of herpesvirus abortion include solid rubbery lungs and multiple foci of necrosis in the liver. **B,** Randomly distributed multiple 1-mm white foci in the liver are characteristic of necrosis caused by herpesvirus infection. This case is more florid than most. (**A** courtesy Dr. R.B. Miller, Ontario Veterinary College, University of Guelph. **B** courtesy Dr. J. King, College of Veterinary Medicine, Cornell University.)

important genera are listed in Table 18-2. In all species of domestic animals, *Salmonella, Campylobacter,* and *Listeria* sp. cause intestinal disease, and if bacteremic, can cause placental and fetal infection. Some bacteria have a particular affinity for the reproductive tract, and there are genera that infect virtually every domestic animal species. *Brucella, Leptospira, Chlamydophila,* and *Coxiella* spp. are particularly important. Common or important bacterial causes of failure of pregnancy are outlined for those species in which they are especially important.

Protozoal diseases

The protozoa of importance are *Toxoplasma gondii* and *Neospora caninum. Toxoplasma gondii* can cause failure of pregnancy in virtually every species except cattle. Likewise, the list of domestic animals affected by *Neospora caninum* is growing. There are sporadic cases of *Sarcocystis* sp. abortion also. The lesions seen with these protozoa include multifocal placental necrosis and microscopic foci of necrosis and inflammation in many fetal organs, especially the brain.

Failure of Pregnancy in Horses

Noninfectious failure of pregnancy

Any failure of pregnancy without an infectious cause is placed into the noninfectious failure of pregnancy category. The potential list is very long, and specific conditions vary with the domestic species. All domestic species have sporadic fetal anomalies, thyroidal hyperplasia and goiter, and dystocia.

Horses are unique in that they have a large number of noninfectious causes of failure of pregnancy (Box 18-5), related in some instances to the apparent lack of placental reserve and their microcotyledonary placentation.

BOX 18-5 Noninfectious Causes of Failure of Equine Pregnancy

Twinning
Umbilical cord anomalies
- Excessive length
- Torsion
- Too short

Inadequate villus development
- Endometrial fibrosis

Thyroid hyperplasia and musculoskeletal disease
Premature placental separation
Body pregnancy

Fetal anomalies are usually rare and sporadic in horses. In some regions, especially where feed quality during winter is inadequate, foals are lost because of thyroid hyperplasia and musculoskeletal disease (TH-MSD). The thyroid lesion is a microscopic hyperplasia, but there is no macroscopic enlargement of the glands. Routine histologic examination of the thyroid is therefore necessary to make this diagnosis. Musculoskeletal diseases seen in this syndrome include prognathia, flexural deformity, joint laxity, and tendon ruptures, presumably from hypothyroidism.

Examination of the placenta for lesions requires knowledge of normal anatomy, and there are many features and structures that are normal but have the appearance of being a lesion (Box 18-6). It is important to assess the equine placenta for the following:

BOX 18-6 Normal Structures of the Equine Placenta Confused with Lesions

Amniotic plaques
Avillous regions of:
- Chorioallantoic pouches
- Large vessels
- Insertion of cord
- Location of uterine tube
- Cervical star

Hippomane
Allantoic pouches
Yolk sac remnant

- Anything that reduces placental area, such as avillous regions
- Lesions of the cervical star (Fig. 18-33)
- Excessive length (normal is 36 to 83 cm) and torsion (Fig. 18-34) of the umbilical cord
- Lesions of the amnion (amniotic plaques [Fig. 18-35, *A*])

Normally, chorionic villi develop where contact is made between the endometrium and the chorion. Small and insignificant regions of avillous placenta occur in the following:

- At the contact area between chorion and endocervix (cervical star).
- At sites of the endometrial cups (chorioallantoic pouches).

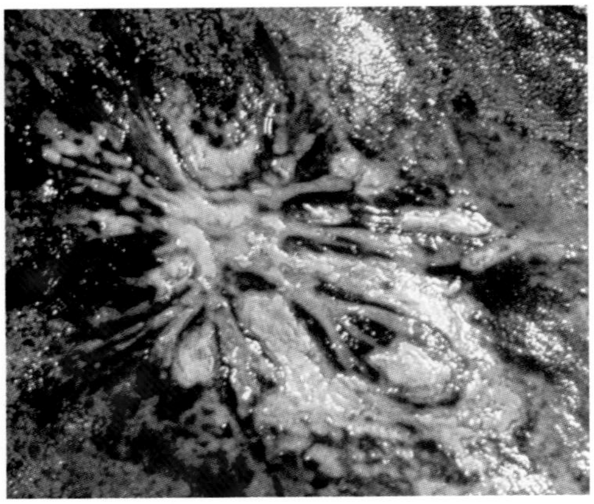

Fig. 18-33 Bacterial placentitis, cervical star, mare.
The chorion at the cervical star is thickened by edema, and there is fibrin, necrotic debris, and suppurative exudate on the surface. (Courtesy Dr. K. McEntee, Reproductive Pathology Collection, University of Illinois.)

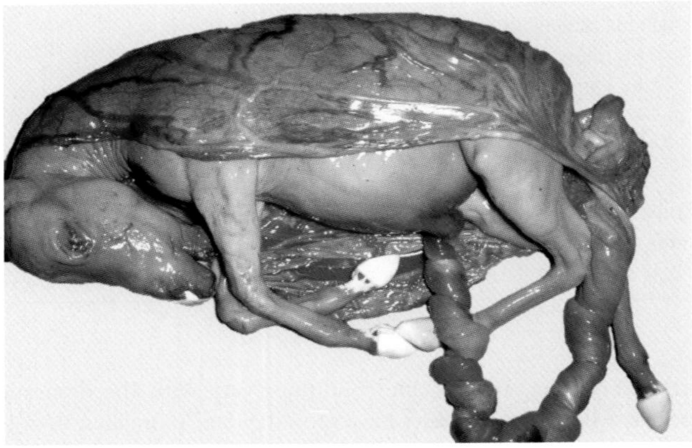

Fig. 18-34 Umbilical cord torsion, equine fetus.
This aborted fetus, wrapped in its amnion, has a very long and twisted umbilical cord. Twisted cords are often longer than 83 cm, a risk factor for torsion of the cord. (Courtesy College of Veterinary Medicine, University of Illinois.)

- Where there are folds of the chorion.
- Over large vessels in the chorioallantois.
- At the site of insertion of the umbilical cord.

Two structures that often cause confusion are the hippomane and the yolk sac remnant. Almost all equine placentas have a hippomane in the allantoic cavity. These are rubbery concrements of allantoic precipitates that vary in color from white to tan to red (Fig. 18-35, *B*). The yolk sac remnant is the remaining tissue of the yolk sac that is a circular cystic structure found in the allantoic portion of the umbilical cord from its junction with the amnion to the chorioallantois. It may be surrounded by the umbilical vessels or extend from the cord with a stalk (Fig. 18-35, *C*). This remnant is often mineralized and has a fluid-filled center and an ossified wall. The outer surface is smooth, but the inner surface has a pattern that resembles the inner surface of the calvarium. It is sometimes mistaken for the skull of a twin or an amorphous globosus (see the section on Failure of Pregnancy in Ruminants; Fig. 18-36). The final common normal finding is allantoic pouches. These are outpouches of the allantois into the allantoic cavity to form a small polyp. Sometimes these have a long stalk.

Twinning is a common noninfectious cause of abortion in mares. Chorionic villi do not develop over the contact area between

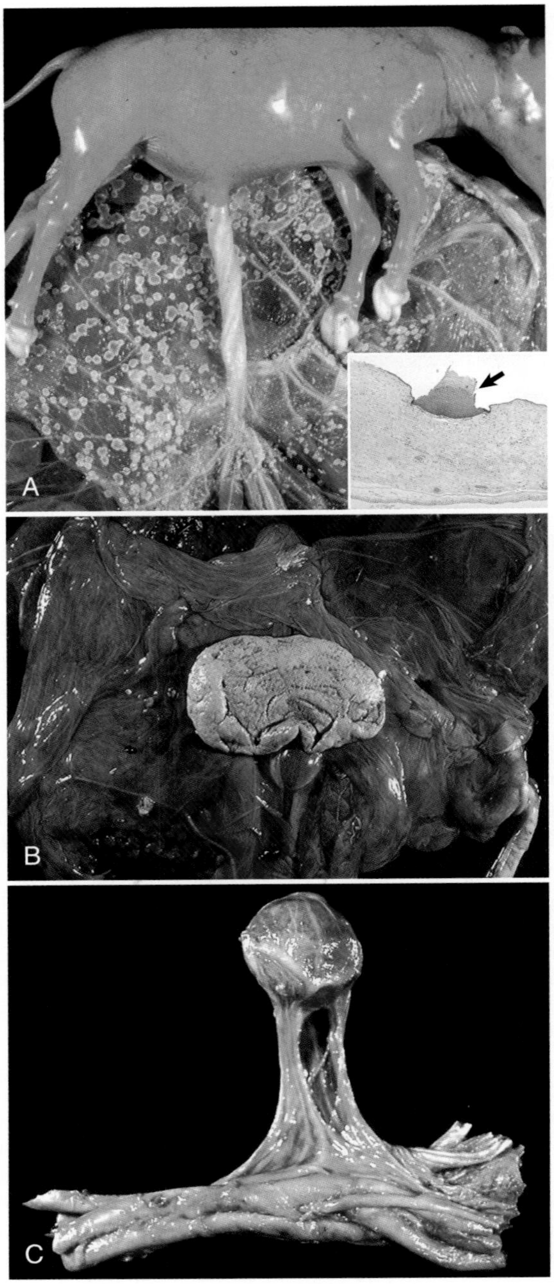

Fig. 18-35 Incidental structures, placentas.
A, Amniotic plaques, bovine fetus and placenta. Multiple white, raised circular plaques up to 1.5 cm in diameter are present on the fetal side of the amnion. They are normal incidental structures composed of stratified squamous keratinizing epithelium. *Inset,* An amniotic plaque *(arrow).* H&E stain. **B,** Hippomane, allantois, equine placenta. These rubbery flattened discs up to 10 cm in diameter are the end result of aggregation of sediments of allantoic fluid in the horse and other equids. They are incidental findings. **C,** Mineralized yolk sac remnant, umbilical cord, equine fetus. Yolk sac remnants seen on the allantoic portion of the umbilical cord are incidental structures. Note that in this case the yolk sac is connected by a stalk containing blood vessels and is located at the junction of the umbilical cord and the allantois. (**A** courtesy Department of Veterinary Biosciences, The Ohio State University; and Noah's Arkive, College of Veterinary Medicine, The University of Georgia. **Inset** courtesy Dr. M.D. McGavin, College of Veterinary Medicine, University of Tennessee. **B** courtesy Dr. M. McCracken, College of Veterinary Medicine, University of Tennessee; and Noah's Arkive, College of Veterinary Medicine, The University of Georgia. **C** courtesy Dr. J. King, College of Veterinary Medicine, Cornell University.)

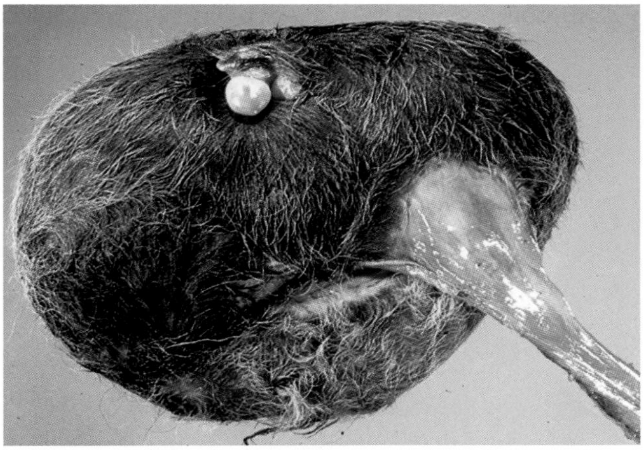

Fig. 18-36 Acardiac monster (bovine amorphous globosus). This structure, covered with hair, is the remnant of a twin fetus and is attached to the placenta of the normal twin by a stalk. It is a rare finding in cattle and is usually of little consequence. (Courtesy Dr. J. Edwards, College of Veterinary Medicine, Texas A&M University; and Dr. J. King, College of Veterinary Medicine, Cornell University.)

the two placentas. The combined functional area of the chorions of both twins is only slightly larger than that for a normal nontwin foal. Twin fetuses often have growth retardation. Aborted twin equine fetuses often appear to have died at different times. Death is thought to be from placental insufficiency. When the available space in the uterus is divided evenly, which is approximately 80% of cases, both twins usually die and are aborted in midgestation. In cases in which great disparity exists in the apportioning of space, the favored twin has a chance of survival, whereas the other dies and mummifies.

There are several abnormalities of the equine umbilical cord, inadequate or excessive length, and torsion. In torsion of the umbilical cord, the cord is usually longer than normal and excessively twisted (more than three complete turns). For a twisted cord to qualify as being functionally significant, there must be compromise of the umbilical vessels and urachus. The wall of the urachus is thinner and more pliable than the umbilical arteries or vein and thus is more easily constricted. Local distentions of the urachus occur between the twists and anywhere along its course in the cord from the umbilicus to the allantoic cavity. The cord is edematous and hemorrhagic, and red distended segments alternate with pale constricted twisted segments (see Fig. 18-34). Fibrin is sometimes present on the outer surface of affected areas of the cord.

In the mare, endometrial fibrosis, often the result of a previous endometritis, reduces the area of the endometrium available for the formation of the maternofetal interface (see Fig. 18-16). Chorionic villi–microcotyledons do not develop where there are no endometrium with glands. Thus in large areas of endometrial fibrosis, the chorion does not develop microcotyledons and their villi. Severely affected mares may become pregnant but do not carry the fetus to term because the functional area of the placenta is too small.

Premature placental separation in the mare has been described in two forms. One form occurs around the time of parturition, causing the chorioallantois to appear at the vulva with the cervical star intact. This is known as a "red bag" delivery because the exposed chorion is a bright red color. Although the caudal part of the chorioallantois is detached from the uterus, the cranial part remains in place, and there is tearing of the chorioallantois across the body of the placenta rather than at the cervical star. The other form occurs any time before parturition. Prematurely detached areas become brown and dehydrated.

Another equine placental disease is called *body pregnancy.* Fetal death and abortion occur as a result of placental insufficiency and fetal malnutrition. The initial site of fetal embryonic attachment is in the body of the uterus rather than at the bifurcation of the uterine horns. The fetus occupies the uterine body only rather than the body and horns, and the placenta is underdeveloped in the horns. Some fetuses expand in size so that the placenta extends through the cervix, where it is avillous and becomes infected with vaginal organisms.

Infectious failure of pregnancy

Viruses. Equine herpesvirus 1 (EHV-1) is one of the most important causes of failure of pregnancy in mares. EHV-1 infects respiratory epithelium, but after lymph nodal involvement, the virus is transported to the uterus (and other tissues) in leukocytes where infection of uterine arteriolar endothelial cells occurs. Virus is also located between the maternofetal interface and in microcotyledons. The resultant microvascular damage leads to thrombosis, edema, hemorrhage, and infarction of microcotyledons. The endometrium has perivascular lymphocytes, neutrophils, and histiocytes. Fluid that escapes through the damaged endometrium separates the maternal and fetal layers, thus allowing virus from the endometrium to enter the placenta and then fetus. Fetal endothelial cells and the cells of most organs are then infected with the virus. The classic lesion, as with most herpesviruses, is focal hepatic necrosis. Focal necrosis occurs microscopically in many other organs also. Bronchiolar epithelial death and fibrin exudation produces a diffuse pneumonia. Fibrin casts in the trachea are formed in some cases, and this is a characteristic lesion. EHV-3 (equine coital exanthema) and EHV-4 produce a similar lesion but much less frequently.

Equine viral arteritis virus (an Arterivirus) in the mare causes failure of pregnancy, but in the majority of cases, there are no lesions in the fetus. The mechanism is probably fetal anoxia caused by compression of uterine blood vessels by virus-induced myometritis, although a few cases of arteritis in the chorion and myocardium of aborted fetuses are described.

Bacteria. In the mare, most bacterial pathogens enter the pregnant uterus through the cervix (see Fig. 18-33), and several bacteria are involved. These include hemolytic streptococci, especially *Streptococcus zooepidemicus* (frequently cultured from fetal organs, placentas, and uterine discharges), *Escherichia coli,* and other Gram-negative bacteria. Inflammation of the chorioallantois is most severe at the cervical star, opposite the cervix. Fetal expulsion and death occur because of a reduction in placental area caused by placentitis and/or fetal sepsis, which is probably more important. Because many cases have only a small area of placenta affected, the cervical star must be examined carefully for placentitis. Affected parts of the placenta are edematous and brown and covered by small amounts of fibrinonecrotic exudate. Macroscopic fetal lesions attributable to the infection are rare. Microscopically, the lesions include neutrophils in debris on the surface of affected microcotyledons, and severe inflammation of the stroma of microcotyledons and desquamation of trophoblasts. Microscopic fetal lesions are rare, despite the ease with which bacteria are recovered from many fetal organs.

Failure of Pregnancy in Ruminants (Cattle, Sheep, and Goats)

The diagnostic process to determine the failure of pregnancy in ruminants is similar to that of other species. There are many

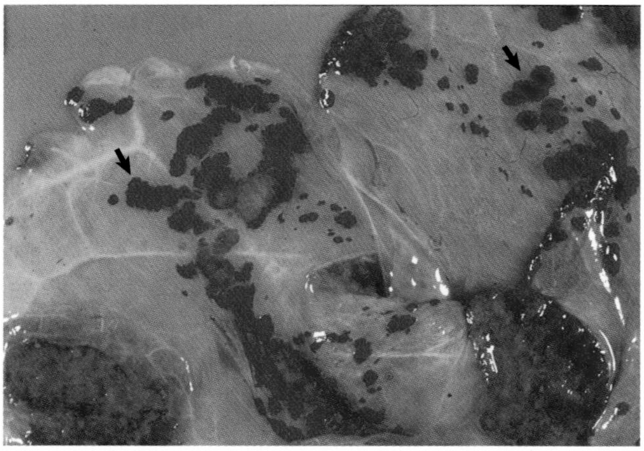

Fig. 18-37 Adventitial placentation, placenta, chorion, cow.
Additional sites of placentation are visible in the intercotyledonary chorion. They appear as red plaques *(arrows)*, sometimes with villi, that extend from cotyledons. There is a corresponding change on the endometrium. (Courtesy Drs. W. Crowell and Tyler, College of Veterinary Medicine, University of Georgia; and Noah's Arkive, College of Veterinary Medicine, University of Georgia.)

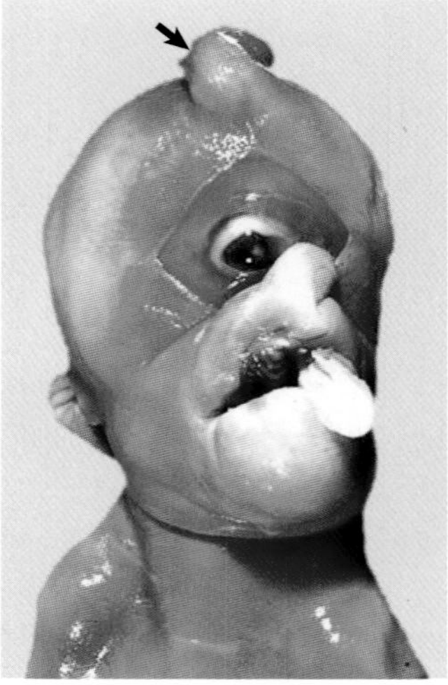

Fig. 18-38 Cyclopia, porcine fetus.
A defect of ocular and cranial development has resulted in fusion of the eyes (cyclops) and a proboscis *(arrow)* above the eye. Cyclopia can occur in the lambs of ewes that ingest the plant *Veratrum californicum* on the fourteenth day of gestation. (Courtesy Dr. J. King, College of Veterinary Medicine, Cornell University.)

similarities in the pathogenesis and morphology of the lesions of failure of pregnancy among ruminants because they all have a cotyledonary placenta. There are only several anatomically normal structures that are mistaken for lesions. These are adventitial placentation, mineralization of the membranes, and amniotic plaques.

Adventitial placentation in cattle is the formation of additional placentome (Fig. 18-37). More is seen in cows with a higher parity. It is also considered to be a hyperplastic response to inadequacy of existing placentome surface area. A reduction in the area of placentomes from the loss of caruncles can occur because of endometritis, removal of cotyledons during aggressive manipulations, removal of retained placental membranes, and chronic placentitis. Compensation for a reduced placentome area is also achieved by enlargement of the existing functional maternal caruncles. Adventitial placentation is also seen in hydroallantois and when fetuses are the result of cloning. These adventitious areas initially form near the normal placentomes but can expand to involve much of the chorionic surface.

All species have amniotic plaques (see Fig. 18-35, *A*). They are small raised plaques of epidermal tissue, and some may have hair growing from them. In ruminants, they are up to 2 cm in diameter and are only on the amnion, thus on the same side as the fetus. In particular, ruminants normally have mineralization of the placenta, which appears as a white lacy change, especially to the chorion.

Because the placentation of ruminants is cotyledonary, there is a large potential space between the placentomes in which exudates and agents can accumulate. Chronic placentitis involving the pericotyledonary areas and the intercotyledonary portions of the chorion is common. The lesions are stereotyped and include the following:

1. Placental edema and fibrosis
2. Cupping of the cotyledon
3. Exudate on the chorionic surface
4. Cotyledonary necrosis

Most agents cause a similar change and the etiologic diagnosis depends on microbiologic examination. The list of possible infectious agents is long, although there are species of bacteria and fungi that are more prevalent in some geographic locations and in some ruminant species (see next).

Amorphous globosus is a rare and incidental finding, especially in bovine placentas. It is a type of acardiac monster and is a severely anomalous second fetus. Macroscopically, it is usually spheric, covered in hair, and attached to the placenta by a cord (see Fig. 18-36). Various organs can be identified within the structure, histologically.

Noninfectious failure of pregnancy

There is considerable geographic variation in the types of noninfectious failure of pregnancy. Fetal anomalies not related to infectious agents can take innumerable forms. Anomalies, such as aplasia or hypoplasia of the adrenal glands, or anomalies of the anterior pituitary cause prolonged gestation by altering the pituitary-adrenal axis. One classic example is prolonged gestation in ewes that ingest the plant *Veratrum californicum* on the fourteenth day of gestation. Along with cyclopia (Fig. 18-38) and holoprosencephaly, the pituitary may be absent.

Hydramnios and hydroallantois refer to the excessive accumulation of fluid in the amniotic and allantoic sacs, respectively. These lesions occur mostly in the cow but could occur in any species. The volume and composition of placental fluids is mostly regulated by the membranes (amnion and allantois), and the nature of the dysregulation in hydramnios and hydroallantois is not known. Hydramnios also occurs with some fetal facial muscle and skeletal abnormalities in which impairment of the fetal drinking reflex reduces amniotic fluid removal by the fetus. Allantoic fluid is formed in part from fetal urine received through the urachus, thus excessive urination is implicated. In the cow, hydroallantois occurs in conjunction with adventitial placentation and in some twin pregnancies. The allantoic fluid composition changes from normal to that closely resembling maternal or fetal extracellular fluid. When these membranes are retained after delivery of a fetus, fluid sometimes continues to be produced.

Infectious failure of pregnancy

Diseases of cattle. In cattle, *Neospora caninum* and bacteria are among the most common causes of failure of pregnancy, according to the results from diagnostic laboratories worldwide.

Bacterial diseases. *Brucella abortus* is eradicated from some countries but is a classic disease that is still important. Cattle are infected by exposure to infected placental fluids by several routes but most often through the alimentary tract. Infection via conjunctiva or inhalation are both possibilities. After exposure, the bacterium is found in macrophages in the draining lymph nodes. Bacteremia ensues, and systemic infection and localization in the pregnant uterus, testes (in bulls) and mammary gland occur. The trophism of *Brucella abortus* to the pregnant uterus is related to erythritol and steroid hormones. Bacteria enter the erythrophagocytic trophoblasts of the hemophagic organ of the placentome, at the base of the chorionic villi. They replicate in the rough endoplasmic reticulum of the periplacentomal and interplacentomal trophoblasts, a unique mechanism of intracellular parasitism. Macroscopic lesions of the placenta are those of a typical chronic placentitis and include thickening and edema of the intercotyledonary chorioallantois, a fibrinonecrotic coating of the intercotyledonary chorion, and cupping of the cotyledon. There are no unique lesions, but histologically, large numbers of bacteria are in trophoblasts and there is a vasculitis in both maternal and fetal tissues, a lesion that could be a response to endotoxin released from the *Brucella* organisms. Most fetuses develop pneumonia that ranges from minimal to severe. Microscopically, the pneumonia is either a chronic bronchopneumonia with numerous macrophages and lymphocytes and some neutrophils or a fibrinous pneumonia. Microscopic granulomas that include multinucleate giant cells occur in organs such as the lung, liver, spleen, and lymph nodes.

Other bacterial causes of placentitis produce similar and often identical lesions. *Bacillus licheniformis* is a common example. The pathogenesis of *Bacillus licheniformis*, based on experimental studies, suggests there is localization in the placentomes after bacteremia. Cotyledonary necrosis and suppurative inflammation occurs, with fetal infection from fetal bacteremia or by ingestion of contaminated amniotic fluid. Campylobacteriosis is a sporadic disease unless it is newly introduced into a herd. *Campylobacter fetus* var. *venerealis* can be a long-term inhabitant of the preputial cavity of bulls. It is transmitted venereally and can survive on the vaginal mucosa, but the cow must become pregnant for it to establish itself in the uterus. Early embryonic death is the most likely manifestation of campylobacteriosis and often the only clinical abnormalities are an irregular estrous cycle or the return to estrus of an animal thought to be pregnant. Much less frequently, abortion occurs at a later stage of pregnancy. Cows become resistant to subsequent infections by the bacterium. Gross and microscopic lesions in placentas are similar to those described in brucellosis (edema of the intercotyledonary chorioallantois and necrosis of cotyledons with microscopic inflammation of both) but are less severe and with fewer bacteria in the desquamated trophoblasts.

Leptospirosis is another disease where failure of pregnancy is a common outcome. Results of serologic studies indicate that a large percentage of cattle are infected, but most do not have clinical signs. Several different serovars are associated with abortion, especially *Leptospira interrogans* serovar Hardjo. In adult animals, the bacteria localize in the kidneys after the bacteremic phase. Pregnant cows abort weeks after the bacteremic phase, usually in the last trimester. Placental lesions are usually limited to edema, where fetal lesions often are mild and obscured by autolysis. Some dead fetuses expelled near term have the gross lesions of ascites and fibrinous peritonitis. Microscopic fetal lesions include interstitial nephritis and necrotizing hepatitis. Leptospires can be demonstrated in peritoneal or pleural cavity fluid by dark-field microscopic examination and in renal tubular lumens by silver stains or by immunohistochemical techniques. Measurement of the leptospiral antibody in fetal fluids (serum, cavity fluids) is a common method for diagnosis.

Epizootic bovine abortion (EBA), also known as *foothill abortion,* occurs in California and adjacent states. The causative agent, known as *the agent of EBA,* is carried by the tick *Ornithodoros coriaceus.* A novel Deltaproteobacterium is the suspected agent. The fetal disease is chronic with notable microscopic lesions 50 days after exposure of the dam to ticks. The lesions are sufficiently specific for a diagnosis in fetuses whose gestational age is greater than 100 days. Gross lesions include petechial hemorrhages of the conjunctiva and oral cavity, an enlarged nodular liver and ascites (both presumably from heart failure secondary to myocarditis), and enlarged lymph nodes and spleen. Lymphoid follicles are hyperplastic and have large numbers of histiocytes. The thymus is atrophic because of the loss of cortical lymphocytes. The thymic parenchyma and interstitium contain many histiocytes. Foci of acute necrosis are present in several organs, especially the lymph nodes and spleen. These foci frequently develop into pyogranulomas. Vasculitis occurs in several organs. Deposits of IgG and IgM are present in the vascular lesions.

Ureaplasma diversum causes failure of pregnancy at different times of gestation in cattle. The characteristic lesion in abortions is amnionitis, a change only occasionally seen in other bacterial or fungal infections. There is focal or diffuse reddening of the amnion especially and also the chorioallantois. There is thickening and yellow discoloration of the amnion (Fig. 18-39). The lesions are chronic and ongoing with fibrosis, edema, inflammation, and necrosis of the amnion occurring together with focal inflammation and necrosis of the cotyledons and the intercotyledonary chorioallantois. Many fetuses have a chronic bronchopneumonia with large lymphoid follicles near bronchi.

Any bacterium with a bacteremic phase in cows could cause lesions in the placenta and fetus. *Salmonella*, *Mannheimia*, and *Pasteurella* spp. and *Histophilus somni* are therefore potential causes of placentitis, fetal pneumonia, hepatitis or other lesions, and failure of pregnancy.

Protozoal diseases. *Neospora caninum* is now recognized as a major cause of abortion in cows. Fetuses are 3 to 9 months' gestational age and have no gross lesions, except in rare cases in which there is fetal heart failure from myocarditis. There are no macroscopic placental lesions. In the fetal brain, multiple foci of necrosis or groups of microglial cells are often adjacent to capillaries. Groups of *Neospora caninum* zoites in or around these foci are either extracellular or occur in glial or endothelial cells. In the heart, the lesions include multifocal epicarditis, myocarditis, endocarditis, and protozoal organisms in either myofibers or endothelial cells. Lymphocytic portal hepatitis, multifocal hepatocellular necrosis, and fibrin thrombi in hepatic sinusoids are also seen. Foci of lymphocytes are present in additional organs, including the placenta.

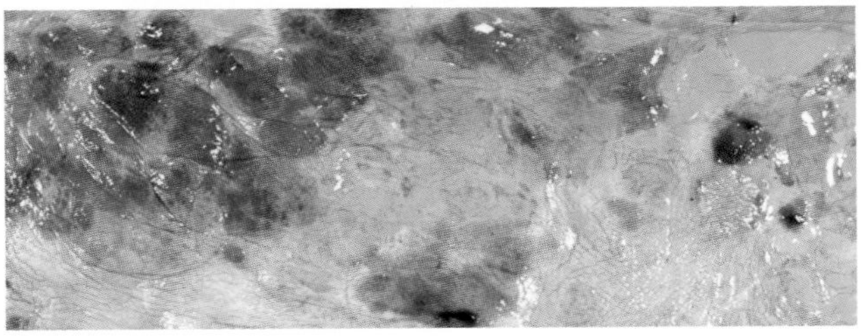

Fig. 18-39 Amnionitis, *Ureaplasma diversum* infection, cow.
The amnion has large, opaque, red and white areas of granulation tissue and fibrous tissue, respectively *(left half of image)*. Amnionitis without placentitis in cattle is a good indicator of *Ureaplasma* sp. infection. (Courtesy Dr. R.B. Miller, Ontario Veterinary College, University of Guelph.)

Tritrichomonas foetus causes transient vaginitis, cervicitis, and endometritis and therefore infertility. It can cause early embryonic mortality but only occasionally causes abortion. Macroscopic lesions are usually absent. Microscopically, there is placental edema and a mild lymphocytic and histiocytic chorionitis and focal necrosis of trophoblasts. Large numbers of trichomonads are present. Fetal pneumonia with intrabronchiolar neutrophils, macrophages, and some multinucleated giant cells may occur in one-half of cases. The diagnosis is confirmed when trichomonads are seen in the contents of the fetal abomasum or in fetal and placental tissues. Endometritis can be severe and result in pyometra.

Fungal diseases. Fungal abortion caused by *Aspergillus* spp. and the Zygomycetes (*Absidia, Mortierella, Rhizopus,* and *Mucor*) in cattle is a major cause in some geographic locales but is sporadic in most places. The fungi spread to the placenta hematogenously because the placentomes are involved first and there is multifocal involvement. In some cases, lesions occur in the placenta in the tip of the horn with the degree of fibrosis suggesting movement caudally; this suggests descending intrauterine spread. The placental changes are those of chronic necrotic placentitis as the cotyledons become enlarged, brown, and friable and the intercotyledonary chorioallantois becomes leathery and covered with a brown exudate (Fig. 18-40 and 18-41). In a small number of cases, the amnion may be thick, white, or yellow with leathery areas resembling the lesions caused by *Ureaplasma diversum.* Fetal dermatitis may be present wherein small, white, raised plaques are present on the skin of the fetus, often over the neck and shoulder. Microscopically, the lesions include large numbers of neutrophils, macrophages and lymphocytes in the amnion (if affected) and chorioallantois, and necrosis and desquamation of trophoblasts. The vessels at the base of the cotyledons have vasculitis and fungal vascular invasion. Lesions in the fetus may include a superficial perivascular and hyperkeratotic dermatitis and bronchopneumonia. Fungal hyphae, septate in *Aspergillus* and nonseptate in the Zygomycetes, are abundant in lesions of the placenta. Fungi can also be recovered from the fetal stomach, presumably from swallowed amniotic fluid.

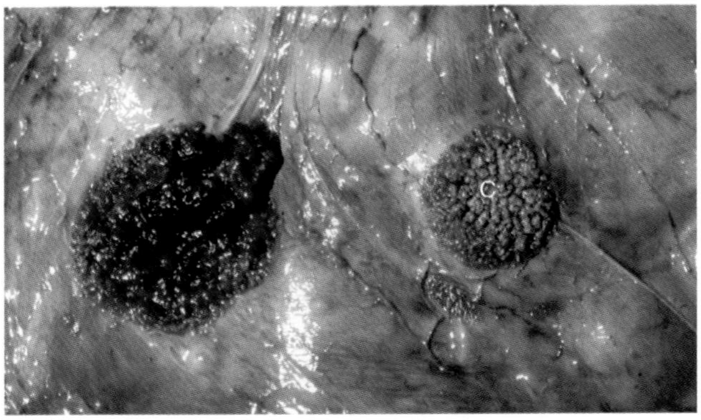

Fig. 18-40 Mycotic intercotyledonary placentitis, cow.
Marked edema, fibrosis, and thickening of the intercotyledonary placenta has caused it to be opaque. The cotyledon *(C)* on the right is necrotic. (Courtesy Dr. R.A. Foster, Ontario Veterinary College, University of Guelph.)

Viral diseases. The frequency of viral causes of failure of pregnancy in cattle is probably underreported, especially those caused by BVD virus. There are seldom macroscopic or microscopic lesions of BVD virus infection in the fetus and placenta, and the virus may not be found. The pathogenesis of BVD is outlined in Chapters 4 and 7.

Bovine herpesvirus 1 (BoHV-1) is a sporadic cause of bovine abortion. Fetal autolysis is usually present because of rapid death of the fetus. Fetal lesions are typical of herpesvirus infection in other species with multifocal necrosis and hemorrhage (see previous discussion). There are usually no macroscopic or microscopic placental lesions, although vascular endothelial necrosis and villous necrosis with neutrophils in the necrotic tissue occurs in experimental infection. In addition, BoHV-1 produces an acute necrotizing endometritis in the uterine body or caudal parts of the uterine horns of the cow, particularly in the postpartum period. Microscopically, the lesions range from mild focal lymphocytic endometritis to severe diffuse necrotizing metritis.

Bunyaviruses, such as Akabane virus, and the bluetongue viruses cause fetal infection and abortion and produce a range of lesions in the developing fetal central nervous system, including hydranencephaly, microencephaly, cerebellar hypoplasia, and a lack of spinal cord ventral horn neurons. The loss of ventral horn neurons causes denervation muscle atrophy that leads to arthrogryposis (fixation of limb joints) and skeletal deformities such as torticollis and scoliosis.

Diseases of sheep

Bacterial diseases. In sheep, many cases of failure of pregnancy are caused by bacteria, including *Chlamydophila abortus, Campylobacter fetus,* and *Brucella ovis.*

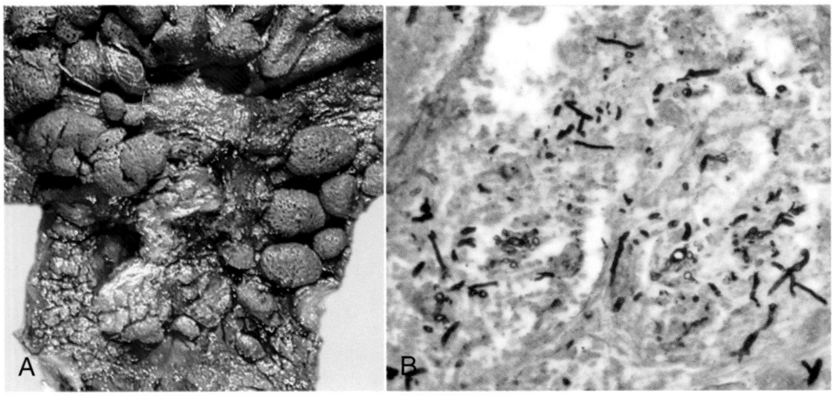

Fig. 18-41 Mycotic endometritis, postpartum uterus, cow.
A, The endometrial surface of the middle and lower portion of this uterus is irregularly thickened and corrugated. Caruncles are small or missing. **B,** The placenta is necrotic, and the numerous fungal hyphae *(black)* are irregular in diameter, do not have regular septation, and branch at odd angles, all features typical of the *Aspergillus* spp. and Zygomycetes. Gomori's methenamine silver stain. (**A** courtesy Dr. J. King, College of Veterinary Medicine, Cornell University. **B** courtesy Dr. K. McEntee, Reproductive Pathology Collection, University of Illinois.)

Enzootic abortion of ewes is caused by *Chlamydophila abortus* and is one of the most common abortifacient agents in sheep. It occurs in all sheep-producing countries, producing late-term abortion. It occurs in two forms: outbreaks when first introduced into susceptible flocks or as an enzootic condition of ewe lambs. Infection is from placentas and fluids to the oral cavity, and ewes are immune to reinfection after the first abortion, but they may remain carriers. Ewes infected before 5 or 6 weeks of gestation abort in late gestation, but ewes infected after 5 or 6 weeks of gestation abort in the subsequent pregnancy. The pathogenesis of failure of pregnancy involves infection of susceptible animals and persistence of *Chlamydophila abortus* in an unknown site of the body. After about day 90 of pregnancy, there is proliferation of the *Chlamydophila abortus* in the placentome and then in trophoblasts in the intercotyledonary placenta. This leads to a cytokine and chemokine cascade, with inflammation and thrombosis of placental vessels and subsequent abortion. The placentitis is similar to that described in general terms in placentitis of cattle (see the discussion on bacterial disease in the section on Diseases of Cattle). *Coxiella burnetii* (see the section on Disease of Goats) and *Brucella ovis* infection induce an identical placentitis. The organisms distend the trophoblasts and are obvious with such special stains as modified Ziehl-Neelsen or Gimenez stains. In the fetus, foci of lymphocytes and macrophages may be present in the liver, lungs, and muscle.

Sheep develop coxiellosis, but it is more common in goats and is described in the section on Diseases of Goats.

Brucella ovis in sheep is probably transmitted venereally from a ram with epididymitis shedding large numbers of bacteria in the semen. Gross placental lesions are similar to those produced by *Brucella abortus* in cattle. There are no specific fetal lesions. Calcified plaques on the hooves are reported, but this is not a specific change. Microscopically, as with *Brucella* sp. infections in other species, large numbers of coccobacilli are found in trophoblasts and are free in the chorionic mesenchyme. There is a vasculitis that involves the larger chorionic vessels. Lesions in the fetus when present are bronchopneumonia, lymphadenitis, interstitial nephritis, and pericholangitis. In younger fetuses, the cells are monocytes and macrophages, whereas older fetuses have well-formed nodules of lymphocytes and plasma cells.

Campylobacter fetus ssp. *fetus* and *Campylobacter jejuni* are primarily intestinal inhabitants. These bacteria are transmitted fecal-orally or from infected placentas or fluid to the oral cavity. Failure of pregnancy occurs in outbreaks and continues throughout the flock as organisms spread from an aborting to an uninfected ewe. Infection of the pregnant uterus results in late-term abortion or the birth of live but sick lambs. Ewes become immune after the first infection. The placentitis results in an edematous intercotyledonary chorioallantois and friable, yellow cotyledons, as is seen in other cases of acute placentitis. At necropsy, about 25% of the fetuses have multiple, well-circumscribed, up to 20 mm in diameter yellow hepatic foci with red depressed centers, which are areas of necrosis. Microscopically, the lesions are those of an acute neutrophilic and necrotic placentitis, as occurs with other bacteria, including *Brucella ovis*. The chorioallantois and especially the cotyledon have necrotic neutrophils and trophoblasts along the surface. *Campylobacter* organisms are abundant among the inflammatory cells, within trophoblasts, and there may be dense emboli of bacteria in the capillaries of the chorionic villi. The hepatic lesion is a multifocal necrotizing hepatitis with abundant intralesional bacteria. *Flexispira rappini* causes an identical lesion in the ovine placenta and fetal liver, but infections are less common and sporadic.

Listeriosis caused by *Listeria monocytogenes* is a cause of sporadic abortions in many species, including cattle, sheep, and goats and of outbreaks of abortion in sheep. Although both nervous disease and reproductive disease occur in the same flock or herd, this is rare. Listerial abortions occur in the last trimester of pregnancy. Some aborting dams are septicemic and also have endometritis. The placental lesion, as with other bacterial placentitis, is severe diffuse necrotizing and suppurative placentitis of both the cotyledons and the intercotyledonary areas. There are multiple 1-mm yellow or white foci in many organs, but they are readily seen in large numbers in the liver. These foci are areas of acute multifocal necrotizing hepatitis in which the Gram-positive *Listeria* organisms are numerous. The microscopic lesions in the placenta are identical to those of campylobacteriosis and brucellosis, except that the trophoblasts, especially in the intercotyledonary areas, are filled with Gram-positive listerial bacilli.

Viral diseases. Bluetongue, border disease, Cache valley, and Akabane viruses are important causes of failure of pregnancy in some geographic regions. Bluetongue virus *(Orbivirus)* is an important viral infection of the ovine fetus in those areas in which bluetongue occurs. Fetal lambs with this infection can develop hydranencephaly. They have viral antigen in immature neural cells in areas of necrosis in the periventricular zone of the cerebral hemispheres. Bluetongue is discussed elsewhere. The pestivirus of sheep is border disease virus (BDV), and it produces a disease in pregnant sheep identical to that of BVD virus in pregnant cattle (see the section on Diseases of Cattle). Cache valley virus and Akabane virus produce an identical disease; Akabane viral disease is described in the section on Diseases of Cattle.

Protozoal diseases. *Toxoplasma gondii* is an important cause of abortion in ewes. Susceptible ewes eat food contaminated by cat feces that contain oocysts. Macroscopic lesions in the placenta are the characteristic white 1- to 2-mm foci of necrosis in the cotyledons (Fig. 18-42). There may be edema of the intercotyledonary chorioallantois. Microscopically, the cotyledonary lesions are distinctive and consist of multiple foci of necrosis with rare groups of *Toxoplasma* organisms within trophoblasts. Immunohistochemistry is often needed to detect them. A small percentage of fetuses aborted because of toxoplasmosis have cerebral leukoencephalomalacia, a nonspecific effect of fetal anoxia secondary to placentitis.

Diseases of goats. *Coxiella burnetii* infection is extremely important in goats especially but also in sheep and potentially in all species. *Coxiella burnetii*, the cause of Q fever in humans, causes abortion or the birth of dead or weak lambs or kids. Abortion occurs in newly exposed animals and repeat infection resulting in abortion is possible. *Coxiella* is acquired by ingestion or by

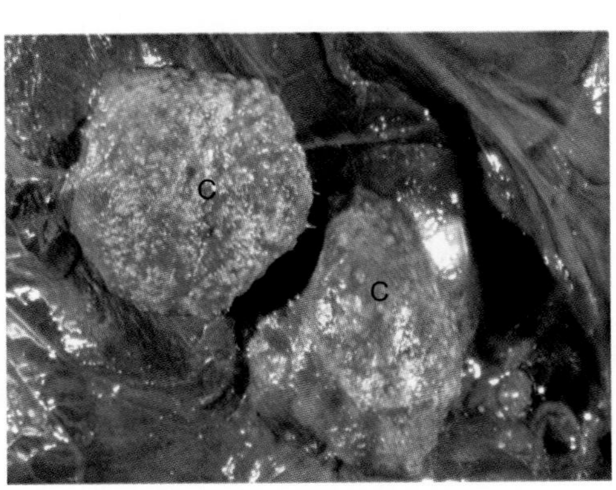

Fig. 18-42 Ovine protozoal placentitis, toxoplasmosis, abortion, placenta, sheep.
The cotyledons *(C)* have hundreds of white foci of necrosis, a lesion that is characteristic of *Toxoplasma gondii*–induced abortion in sheep and goats. (Courtesy Ontario Veterinary College, University of Guelph.)

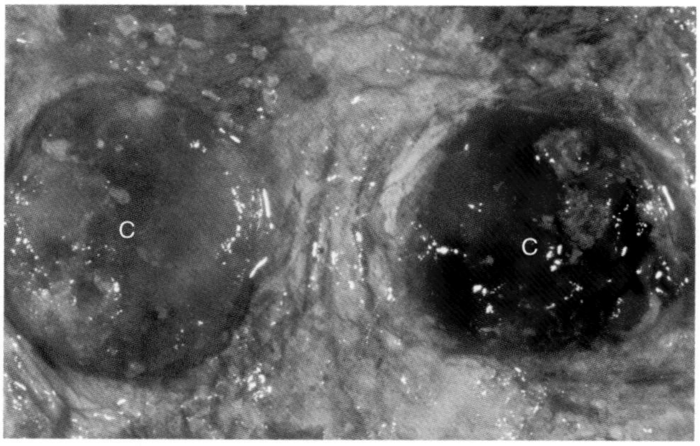

Fig. 18-43 Intercotyledonary placentitis *(Coxiella burnetii)*, goat. Note the opacity of the intercotyledonary placenta caused by thickening from inflammation and fibrosis. The cotyledons *(C)* have variable areas of gray discoloration, indicating necrosis and inflammatory exudates. The gross appearance of the lesions of placentitis tends to be similar, regardless of the etiologic agent identified by microbiological examination. (Courtesy Dr. R.A. Foster, Ontario Veterinary College, University of Guelph.)

inhalation. It is shed in vaginal discharges at parturition and in the milk. In affected placentas the intercotyledonary chorioallantois is thick, leathery, yellow, and covered with surface exudate (Fig. 18-43). There are no macroscopic fetal lesions. Microscopically, the placental lesions are most severe in the intercotyledonary areas where there is necrotic inflammatory debris on the chorionic surface and neutrophils, macrophages, and lymphocytes in the chorionic stroma. Hypertrophic trophoblasts contain myriad *Coxiella* organisms. Fetal lesions, if present, consist of peribronchiolar, renal medullary, and hepatic portal lymphocytic aggregates.

Goats also develop chlamydophilosis and campylobacteriosis as described for sheep. *Brucella melitensis* infection in goats (and sheep) occurs mainly in Mediterranean countries. There is an initial bacteremic phase, and subsequently, inflammation is localized to the mammary glands and pregnant uterus. Goats develop a more severe febrile disease and more severe mastitis than do sheep. The lesions are similar to those caused by *Brucella abortus* in cattle and *Brucella ovis* in sheep. Toxoplasmosis of goats is common but less so than in sheep.

Failure of Pregnancy in Pigs

The principles of diagnosis used in other species apply to pigs (disease of mother, fetus, or placenta; infectious and noninfectious disease); however, the approach in intensive pig production is different and more epidemiologic in nature. Strict biosecurity has eliminated many potential diseases.

For the majority of causes, there are no fetal or placental lesions and the testing for infectious agents is more microbiologic and molecular (i.e., polymerase chain reaction [PCR]) in nature.

Noninfectious failure of pregnancy

There are many potential noninfectious causes of failure of pregnancy. Fetal anomalies and goiter are readily identified, but most others are not. There are often no lesions in the mother, placenta, or fetus. Seasonal infertility wherein there is failure of pregnancy at a regular time each year is very common in large production units. It may be in the summer, when heat is implicated, or in the fall or with the onset of cold weather. This diagnosis is based on the appropriate history and a failure to identify other causes.

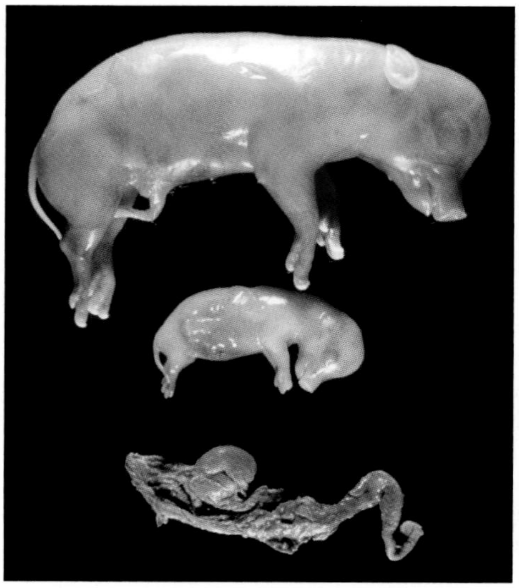

Fig. 18-44 Stillbirth, mummification, embryonic death and infertility (SMEDI), abortion, pig fetus. Viruses, such as porcine parvovirus and porcine enteroviruses, induce SMEDI. These viruses affect the fetuses to differing degrees and at different stages of gestation. Those fetuses that die early in gestation are usually mummified *(bottom fetus)* or resorbed. (Courtesy College of Veterinary Medicine, University of Illinois.)

Infectious failure of pregnancy

Viruses. Viral diseases are the most important infectious causes of reproductive failure in pigs. Porcine reproductive and respiratory syndrome (PRRS) virus, porcine parvovirus (PPV), pseudorabies virus (PRV), and porcine circovirus 2 (PCV-2) are the most important.

PRRS virus, an Arterivirus, is transmitted horizontally through body fluids and vertically to the fetuses of those sows without immunity. Transplacental infection of pig fetuses causes abortion, usually in the later stages of pregnancy, but there are seldom macroscopic and microscopic lesions in the fetuses or placentas. The diagnosis is based on evidence of herd exposure, maternal serology, and virus isolation. Lesions, when present, are segmental or diffuse hemorrhage in the umbilical cord as a result of necrotizing umbilical arteritis. Ascites, hydrothorax, and edema of perirenal tissue, splenic ligament, and mesentery are seen in some fetuses. Microscopically, a segmental arteritis occurs in the umbilicus and fetal lungs, heart, and kidneys. Alveolar septa in the lungs are thickened by lymphocytes and histiocytes, and proliferation of type 2 pneumocytes. Aggregates of lymphocytes, plasma cells, and macrophages are present in blood vessels in the heart, portal tracts, and cerebellar white matter. Endometritis and myometritis also occur with edema and lymphocytes and histiocytes in the interstitium and around uterine vessels.

PPV is an important cause of embryonic and fetal loss and causes death and mummification of affected fetal pigs (Fig. 18-44). Sows usually are not ill, but fetuses are infected and die at varying stages—all in the one pregnancy. This suggests fetus-to-fetus transmission within the uterus. The characteristic findings in fetuses therefore are some fresh fetuses, and then varying stages of autolysis and mummification, with the most mummified fetuses being the smallest. This indicates fetal death occurred at different stages of gestation. Microscopically, fetuses that were infected after immunocompetence had developed have widespread lymphocytes and plasma cells in the liver, lungs, kidneys, and cerebellum.

PCV-2 is capable of causing reproductive failure at any stage of gestation. The virus crosses the placenta and replicates in lymphoid tissues. Death of the fetus and expulsion occurs without macroscopic or microscopic lesions. Some affected litters have fresh, autolyzed, and mummified fetuses. Interstitial edema of the heart, a lymphocytic interstitial myocarditis, and ascites and hepatic congestion of heart failure may occur.

Porcine herpesvirus (PHV) is eradicated from many jurisdictions. Although it can cause typical herpesviral lesions in fetuses, it is one of the few where typical inclusion bodies are seen in the chorion.

Bacteria. Numerous bacteria are implicated in causing reproductive failure. Any bacteria that become bacteremic could localize in the placenta and cause failure of pregnancy; they are listed in Table 18-2. The bacteria that are especially important are *Brucella suis* and *Leptospira* sp.

Brucella suis causes failure of pregnancy, but the disease in pigs differs in several respects from brucellosis in ruminants. Suppurative endometritis, focal granulomas, and multiple hyperplastic lymphoid nodules may occur in the endometrium of nonpregnant sows. Endometrial glands become distended with neutrophils, and the luminal epithelium is eroded and focally has squamous metaplasia. In pregnancy, the lumen of the uterus between placentas has mucopurulent exudate in which trophoblasts contain intracellular bacteria. The chorioallantois has edema and some focal hemorrhage. Microscopically, there are many neutrophils in the tissue, necrotic debris on the chorionic surface, and loss of trophoblasts.

Leptospirosis is an important cause of pregnancy failure. The pathogenesis is similar to that of cattle and is discussed in Chapters 4 and 11. *Leptospira interrogans* serovar *pomona* is commonly isolated. Sows abort after a bacteremic phase, and there are no placental lesions. Fetuses become septicemic, die, and are autolytic. Some develop nephritis and/or neutrophils may be found in the peritoneal serosa.

Failure of Pregnancy in Dogs

Much less is written about failure of pregnancy in dogs than with production animals, in which the economic importance of pregnancy failure provides an incentive to identify the cause and prevent further disease. The following includes some traditional causes.

Infectious failure of pregnancy

Viruses. Canine herpesvirus is capable of causing failure of pregnancy, although it is far more likely to cause mortality of puppies up to 8 weeks of age. The lesions of herpesvirus infection of pups are similar to the stereotypical changes of herpesviruses discussed in other species. In pups, infection is acquired in the perinatal period from recrudescence of the virus in the bitch. Chilling of the puppies and the subsequent lower body temperature facilitates viral replication and viremic spread. Multifocal hemorrhage of the kidney is a characteristic change, and microscopically, there is widespread focal necrosis and hemorrhage with typical intranuclear herpesviral inclusion bodies.

Bacteria. *Brucella canis,* as with other brucella, is acquired by the dog either through ingestion or venereally. Dogs acquiring the bacterium by ingestion initially develop lymphadenitis of the head and neck and bacteremia. Epididymitis and testicular degeneration are the lesions in male dogs, and pregnant females develop placentitis and fetal endocarditis, pneumonia, and hepatitis. Microscopically, trophoblasts of the marginal hematoma and zonary placenta are packed with *Brucella* organisms and there may be neutrophils within the chorion. Other possible fetal lesions include renal hemorrhage, inflammation of the pelvic connective tissue, and lymphadenitis.

There are reports of *Salmonella* sp., *Campylobacter jejuni, Streptococcus canis,* and *Leptospira* serovars causing abortion in dogs. Maternal illness and bacteremia results in infection of the placenta, but the lesions are mild and often are limited to a neutrophilic placentitis.

Protozoa. *Toxoplasma gondii* and *Neospora caninum* both cause failure of pregnancy, although it is uncommon. Macroscopic lesions in fetuses are absent, and microscopically, there may be focal necrosis of all tissues, but often there are protozoa that can only be found by immunohistochemistry.

Leishmania infantum is a reported cause of failure of pregnancy. Placental lesions are large numbers of amastigotes within trophoblasts of the zonary portion of the placenta. No lesions occur in other tissues.

Failure of Pregnancy in Cats

The causes of failure of pregnancy of cats include many of the important general diseases of cats, and little is known of the mechanisms of action. Lesions are seldom seen or reported unless there are obvious fetal anomalies. Feline herpesvirus, feline leukemia virus (FeLV), feline panleukopenia virus, and FIP virus are all implicated, either directly or epidemiologically, in pregnancy failure. Cases are from maternal illness rather than from placental or fetal lesions. Bacteria implicated in disease are those that cause failure of pregnancy in a wide range of species, including *Coxiella burnetii, Salmonella,* and *Mycoplasma.*

Cervix

Diseases involving only the cervix are rare in domestic mammals because most are extensions of uterine disease. There is considerable variation between species in the anatomy of the cervix, and this has an impact on uterine and placental health. The equine cervix is relatively loose, whereas the cervix of cattle and dogs is not. The responses are identical to those of the uterus because the cervix is a part of the uterus. Anatomic features and responses to injury are detailed earlier in this chapter. Humans and some primates develop papillomavirus infection and subsequently cervical carcinoma; domesticated species do not.

Noninflammatory Disease

Anomalies are rare, except in the cow where there can be hypertrophy or hypoplasia of the whole structure, aplasia of one or more of the usual five rugae, tortuosity, and dilation or diverticulum formation of the cervical canal. Two entire cervices or a single bifurcated cervix is recognized. This can occur as the only lesion or it is part of a more extensive failure of proper fusion of the paired paramesonephric ducts and can be found with a divided vagina and two compete uteri.

Ewes exposed to estrogenic substances in subterranean and red clover develop a permanent infertility because of alteration of the cervix. Affected animals have a cervix that has fused cervical folds and uterine-like glands that produce less viscous mucus. Alteration of cervical mucus affects spermatozoal migration and results in reduced fertility.

Neoplastic disease of the cervix of domestic animals is very rare and unlike humans, in which cervical dysplasia and neoplasia linked to human papillomavirus types is well recognized.

Inflammatory Disease

Cervicitis usually occurs as a minor lesion concurrently with more severe endometritis or vaginitis. This is observed in specific infectious diseases, such as contagious equine metritis caused by *Taylorella equigenitalis,* and in nonspecific postparturient endometritis, metritis, cervicitis, and vaginitis. Inflammation restricted to the cervix can result from poorly performed traumatic artificial insemination. In cows with acute cervicitis, the caudal rugae are edematous and prolapse into the vagina. Inflammatory exudate covers the cervical simple cuboidal epithelium and collects in the vagina. The cervical mucosa is thin with epithelium and a small amount of stroma, and the underlying fibromuscular tissue is relatively impervious to infection; thus most cases of cervicitis resolve readily. Those infections that follow traumatic dystocia are likely to involve the muscle layer from the onset and can produce severe lesions, including paracervical abscesses, local peritonitis with granulating tracts into the connective tissue of the pelvic canal, stenosis with adhesions across the lumen of the cervix in areas denuded of epithelium, or cervical glandular cysts filled with mucus or neutrophils.

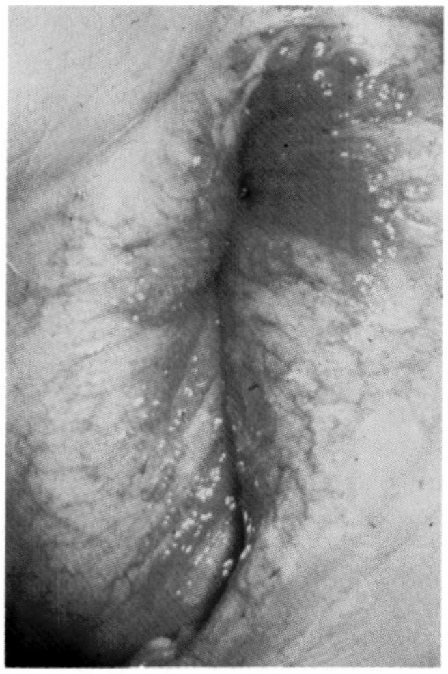

Fig. 18-45 Granular vulvitis, vulva, cow.
Granular vulvitis is a nonspecific condition resulting from development and hyperplasia of subepithelial lymphoid follicles of the vulva and vestibule. Inflammation of the vulva, in the initial stages, causes hyperemia. There is subsequent hyperplasia of lymphoid tissue, visible as 1 to 2 mm raised white nodules on the vulval mucosa. It is commonly seen in cows with infection of the vulva or vagina with *Ureaplasma diversum* and results in a granular appearance of the mucosa. (Courtesy Dr. R.B. Miller, Ontario Veterinary College, University of Guelph.)

Vulva and Vagina

There are few diseases that are unique to or commonly affect one domesticated species, and these are indicated next. For the majority of diseases, lesions occur sporadically and the disease in one species is similar in appearance to that of a different species. The two main categories of disease of the vagina and vulva are (1) infectious (and inflammatory) disease and (2) noninflammatory conditions, including anomalies, hyperplasia, and neoplasia.

Disorders of Domestic Animals

Inflammatory diseases

Postparturient vulvitis and vaginitis occur when they are lacerated during dystocia and become infected. Trauma unrelated to parturition, such as during coitus, artificial insemination, embryo transfer or other human intervention, also could progress similarly. Inflammation of the cervix and cranial vagina after dystocia can have a more serious outcome because of local spread of infection into and through the wall into the peritoneal cavity.

Granular vulvitis describes the clinical appearance of the vulva and vagina in inflammatory diseases. Inflammation causes red coloration (hyperemia) and exudates, and the granular appearance is usually the result of development and hyperplasia of lymphoid follicles (Fig. 18-45). Thus any infectious agent can be a cause if there is sufficient time for cell-mediated or humoral immunity.

Genital herpesvirus infection occurs in most species. The virus is venereally spread and causes multifocal epithelial necrosis and apoptosis and erosion at the first exposure. As with the general pathogenesis of herpesvirus infection, the virus enters the nerves and remains in neuronal cell bodies and ganglia in a latent state until there is recrudescence and shedding. Macroscopic lesions begin as 1 to 2 mm white, raised foci that soon erode (Fig. 18-46). Vesicle formation is unusual. In some species, the lesions will coalesce to form large ulcers, up to several centimeters diameter (Fig. 18-47). Affected pigmented skin loses pigmentation and remains as white regions of depigmentation (Fig. 18-48).

Noninflammatory disease

Swelling of the vulva is normal during estrus. Excessive or persistent swelling is abnormal and occurs commonly in dogs (see below). It also occurs in hyperestrogenism, such as with estrogen-producing ovarian neoplasms or exposure to estrogenic substances (Fig. 18-49). The vaginal mucosa also swells with edema and protrudes through the vulva, exposing the mucosa.

Vaginal polyps occur in most species, but they are particularly common in dogs (Fig. 18-50, also see Disorders of Dogs). They begin as local edema because their stroma is either normal vaginal stroma swollen with edema fluid or there is diffuse fibrosis from longstanding edema. They may protrude from the vulva and frequently ulcerate.

Cysts in the vaginal wall arise from remnants of the mesonephric ducts (Gartner's ducts) or vestibular (Bartholin's) glands. Causes of cyst formation include inflammation of the lining of the duct or gland and hyperestrogenism, in which edema caused by estrogen stimulation is prolonged. The mesonephric ducts do not normally open into the vagina. When they become cystic, they form single or multiple cysts or a tortuous tube in the lateral floor of the vagina between the cervix and near the urethral opening. Major vestibular glands are found on the ventral and lateral walls of the vestibule and become cystic when edema, inflammation, or scar tissue obstructs their openings. Other anomalies of the vagina and vestibule include persistent hymen and vaginal septum (double vagina). Stricture or stenosis of the vagina or vestibule occurs as a congenital anomaly or follows traumatic injury at parturition.

The most common neoplasm of the vagina and vulva is the squamous cell carcinoma of the vulva. Leiomyoma and carcinoma of the vagina occur sporadically in all species but are most common in dogs. They are discussed later.

Squamous cell carcinoma of the vulva occurs in all species but especially in the cow, ewe, and mare (Fig. 18-51). Exposure to sunlight is a known cause. Ewes subjected to the Mules operation (surgery of the perineum and inguinal areas intended to prevent urine wetting the wool) and to short tail docking have a greater sun exposure of the vulva and a greater incidence of squamous cell carcinoma of the vulva. The lack of pigmentation of the vulva is an additional risk factor. Squamous cell carcinoma originates on the hairless and less pigmented skin of the vulva and has the appearance and biologic behavior of squamous cell carcinomas of the eye and conjunctiva, skin, and other sites. The neoplasm metastasizes late in the course of the disease to the iliac lymph nodes.

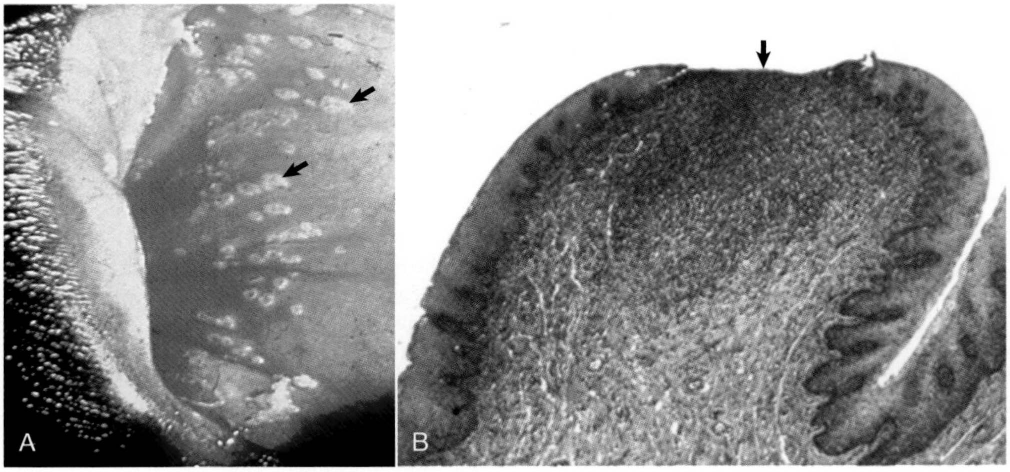

Fig. 18-46 Infectious pustular vulvovaginitis, bovine herpesvirus 1 infection, cow.
A, Focal ulceration of mucosa of the vestibule. The multiple white regions *(arrows)* are areas of necrotic epithelium and ulceration. **B,** Ulceration of mucosa of the vestibule. Note the ulcer *(arrow)* with loss of the epithelium over an aggregate of lymphocytes. H&E stain. (Courtesy Dr. K. McEntee, Reproductive Pathology Collection, University of Illinois.)

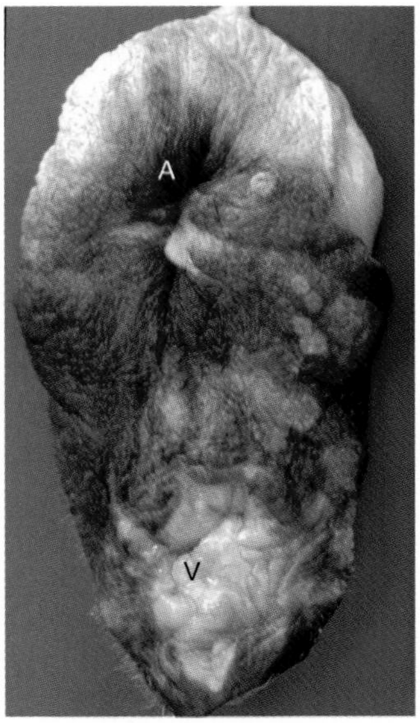

Fig. 18-47 Ulcerative vulvitis, caprine herpesvirus infection, goat.
The vulva *(V)* has numerous vesicles on the mucosa. The skin of the perineal region around the anus *(A)* and vulva has multiple circular regions of epithelial necrosis and erosion. Herpesviral infection of the genital tract has the classic lesions of vesicles that rupture to form ulcers, which are irregularly distributed on the affected areas. (Courtesy Dr. P.W. Ladds, James Cook University of North Queensland.)

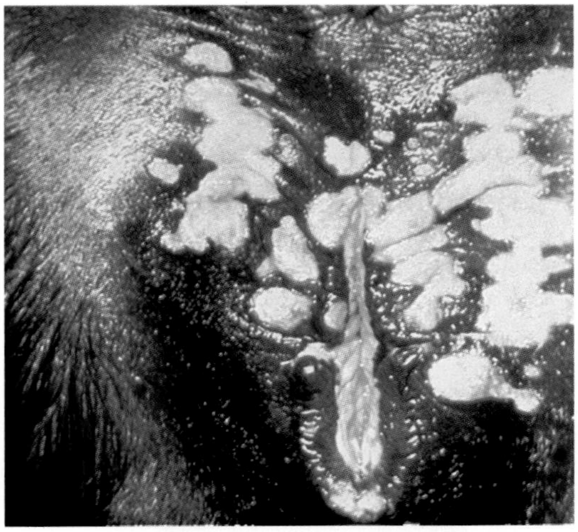

Fig. 18-48 Coital exanthema, ulcerative vulvitis, mare.
Large full-thickness ulcers around the perineum and on the vulvar skin heal with depigmented regions. (Courtesy Dr. K. McEntee, Reproductive Pathology Collection, University of Illinois.)

Disorders of Horses

Equine herpesvirus 3 (EHV-3) is the cause of equine coital exanthema. It is a typical genital herpesviral disease of the vulva, and the virus is spread venereally, results in transient vesicles and erosions of the external genitalia of both mares and stallions (see Fig. 18-48). Depigmentation of pigmented skin of the vulva occurs.

Disorders of Ruminants (Cattle, Sheep, and Goats)

Granular vulvitis in cattle occurs with many different agents, and it is not a specific diagnosis. It simply indicates a local immune reaction to antigen. It can begin as an acute vulvitis or as a subclinical disease. *Ureaplasma diversum* is a classic cause of granular vulvitis. In the acute stage, there is a purulent vulvar discharge and a hyperemic vulvar mucosa with 2-mm raised granules (see Fig. 18-45). The disease can become chronic, and lesions resolve within 3 months. In about 10% of infected cows, discrete, raised, white nodules of follicular lymphoid hyperplasia, 2 to 5 mm in diameter,

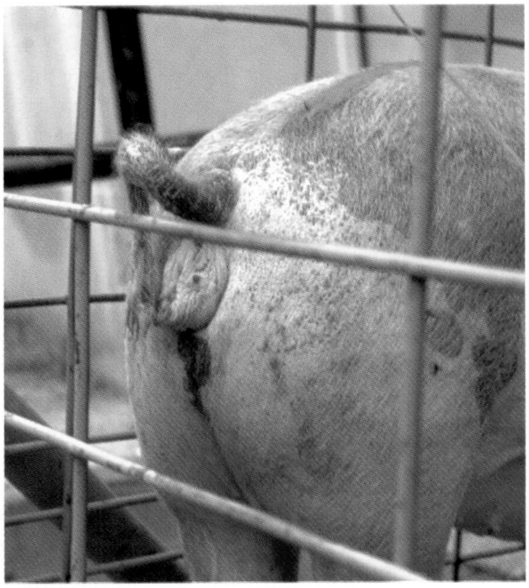

Fig. 18-49 Vulva hypertrophy and edema, estrogenic effect, sow.
The vulva of this sow is swollen with edema. This swelling is typical of hyperestrogenism secondary to mycotoxicosis. (Courtesy Dr. J. Simon, College of Veterinary Medicine, University of Illinois.)

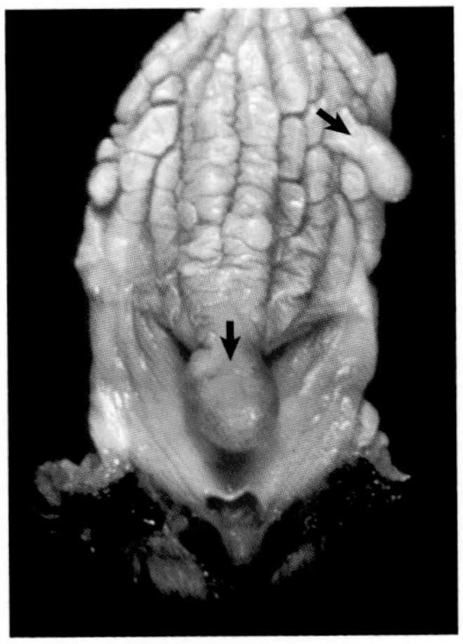

Fig. 18-50 Polyps, vagina, bitch.
There are several vaginal polyps *(arrows)* arising from the wall of the vagina. The larger caudal polyp adjacent to the urethra protrudes caudally through the labia of the vulva and is ulcerated. (Courtesy Dr. K. McEntee, Reproductive Pathology Collection, University of Illinois.)

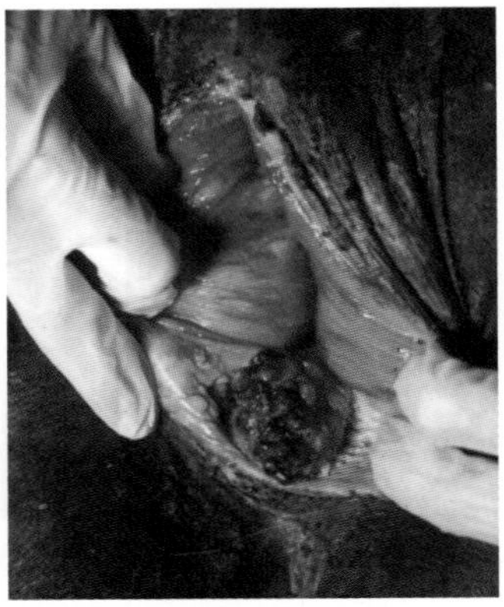

Fig. 18-51 Squamous cell carcinoma, vulva, mare.
The clitoris has been replaced by a multinodular and ulcerated tumor. (Courtesy Dr. J. King, College of Veterinary Medicine, Cornell University.)

occur in rows or clusters on the dorsolateral wall of the vulva. Infection is usually self-limiting, but herds can have a persistent infection. The prepuce of bulls and their semen can remain infected and spread the infection during mating or artificial insemination. Reduced fertility with return to service or abortion occurs with pathogenic strains of the organism as a sequel to infection of the embryo or placenta.

Infectious pustular vulvovaginitis of cattle is caused by BoHV-1, which is similar to the BoHV-1 that is the cause of infectious bovine rhinotracheitis (IBR). The two diseases behave as separate entities, but their occurrence can overlap in a herd or in an individual animal. Vulvovaginitis is transmitted by coitus, artificial insemination, and possibly nose-to-vulva contact. The first evidence of the disease includes hyperemia and edema of the vagina and vulva; this is followed by petechial hemorrhages and slight nodularity of the mucosal surfaces because of edema within epithelial cells. A rapidly coalescing multifocal erosion of the mucosa follows (see Fig. 18-46). Microscopically, changes are detected in the epithelium, the lamina propria, and the lymphoid nodules. The epithelium develops eosinophilic intranuclear inclusions and undergoes ballooning degeneration or apoptosis, followed by desquamation, but usually without discrete stages of vesicle or pustule formation. The lamina propria is hyperemic and edematous. The subepithelial lymphoid nodules become prominent and hyperplastic. Resolution of the disease is rapid and by 7 and 10 days, the lesions are a slightly thickened epithelium and hyperplastic lymphoid nodules. Lesions are similar on the penis of affected bulls. An identical disease occurs in goats and rarely in sheep. Caprine herpesvirus 1 causes lesions in goats similar to those of bovine vulvovaginitis (see Fig. 18-47).

Disorders of Pigs

Toxicosis of pigs by the mycotoxin zearalenone found in *Fusarium* sp.–infected grain and corn is a cause of vaginal and vulval hypertrophy, particularly in prepubertal gilts (see Fig. 18-49). The toxin is a nonsteroidal estrogen that binds to the estrogen receptor. The vaginal and vulval lesions are stromal edema. Other effects of the mycotoxin are altered time of first estrus, both early and late, reduced numbers of live embryos, endometrial hyperplasia, and precocious mammary development.

Disorders of Dogs

In bitches, so-called nonspecific vaginitis or vulvitis is common. The lesions range from acute vaginitis to chronic granular vulvitis (see previous section).

Vaginal hyperplasia, hypertrophy, and/or prolapse of bitches are common diseases seen during the follicular stage (proestrus) of the first to third estrus periods in young animals, particularly of the brachiocephalic breeds. An increased sensitivity to estrogen is assumed, and there is excessive edema of the submucosal tissues of the vagina. The vaginal mucosa swells and interferes with coitus. Dramatic swelling can, if severe, result in vaginal tissue protruding from the vulva that becomes excoriated and ulcerated. Spontaneous regression during diestrus is the norm.

Vaginal polyps are relatively common in older bitches (see Fig. 18-50). They are often solitary, up to several centimeters in diameter, and have a thin stalk of attachment to the vaginal wall. Most are located on the ventral floor of the vagina. They are indistinguishable from leiomyomas macroscopically. Excision is usually curative.

Canine transmissible venereal tumor (CTVT) of dogs is transmitted at coitus by the transfer of intact neoplastic cells. CTVT cells have 59 chromosomes compared with the normal canine number of 78. Immunohistochemical evaluation suggests that these tumors have a histiocytic origin. Both sexes are affected. The neoplasm begins as a nodule beneath the vaginal or vestibular mucosa and when enlarged, breaks through the overlying mucosa. The lesion often begins in the dorsal wall of the vagina at the junction with the vestibule. It bulges into the lumen of the vagina and can protrude through the vulva as an ulcerated, friable mass (Fig. 18-52, *A*). Microscopically the neoplastic cells are large, round or oval, and uniform in size (Fig. 18-52, *B*) but with occasional large, bizarre nuclei. The cytoplasm is pale staining and may have peripheral vacuoles. This neoplasm can develop multifocal necrosis and spontaneously regress. Lymphocyte-mediated cytotoxicity occurs in some and results in regression of tumors. This neoplasm is particularly sensitive to vincristine. In countries with stray dogs and dogs in poor health, metastases to other sites, especially the skin, are relatively common.

Carcinoma of the vagina in bitches is a recognized entity. Some clearly arise from the urethra, especially when they extend from the urethral orifice. Others arise from vaginal epithelium, but little is known of their cause. They are phenotypically similar to transitional cell carcinomas. The long-term prognosis is poor, but the prevalence of metastatic disease varies and urethral obstruction often is the complication that is difficult to control.

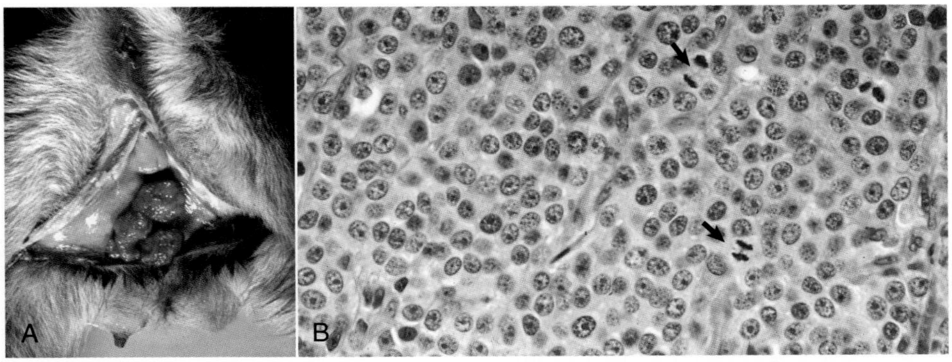

Fig. 18-52 Canine transmissible venereal tumor (CTVT), vulva and vagina, bitch.
A, The multinodular tumors markedly distend the lumens of the vagina and vestibule and are grossly characteristic of CTVT. **B,** Neoplastic cells are round and often divided into packets by a fine fibrous stroma. Mitoses are frequent *(arrows)*. H&E stain. (**A** courtesy Dr. J. King, College of Veterinary Medicine, Cornell University. **B** courtesy Dr. M. J. Abdy, College of Veterinary Medicine, The University of Georgia; and Noah's Arkive, College of Veterinary Medicine, The University of Georgia.)

Bitches develop single or multiple leiomyomas of the vagina. These usually only occur in entire bitches, so a hormonal link is proposed. Ovariohysterectomy may be curative, further supporting a hormonal dependence. The common differential diagnosis of leiomyoma is vaginal polyps (see previous discussion). These have a similar macroscopic appearance, and histologic examination is usually required to differentiate them because each is a well-circumscribed nodule up to several centimeters in diameter arising from the vaginal wall (see Fig. 18-50).

MAMMARY GLANDS

Mastitis and mammary neoplasia are the major diseases of the mammary glands. Mastitis is inflammation of mammary glands. Most cases of mastitis begin with galactophoritis, which is inflammation of the mammary ducts. Mastitis is the most economically important disease of the mammary glands, and although it occurs in all species, it is a particular problem in animals used for milk production.

Galactostasis is milk retention, and there is no systemic illness, even though the glands become engorged, hot, and painful. It occurs after weaning or in pseudopregnancy and is thought to result from inadequate oxytocin release because of fear, stress, or lack of mammary stimulation.

Agalactia is a failure of milk production and is rare. It is one of the manifestations of caprine arthritis and encephalitis virus (CAEV) infection in goats and maedi-visna virus infection of ewes. The udders are hard, thus it is called *hard udder* and no milk is produced. There is usually microscopic interstitial inflammation present.

Galactorrhea (also called *inappropriate lactation* and *precocious lactation*) is also unusual. It is seen in male goats of high milk production lines. In bitches, it is part of pseudopregnancy and occurs at the termination of diestrus when there is a prolactin surge in response to a reduction in progesterone concentration. It also occasionally occurs after ovariohysterectomy during diestrus.

Disorders of Horses

Mammary disease is sporadic in mares, although the full gamut of changes of other species does occur. Mastitis is the more prevalent disease of those reported. It is assumed that the pathogenesis of mastitis in mares is similar to that of other species, especially as the agents are similar, at least in type. *Streptococcus zooepidemicus* is the most prevalent, with Gram-negative species second. Early weaning of foals and seasonal insect feeding is implicated in predisposing a mare to mastitis. Mastitis occurs at any stage of lactation, is usually unilateral, and may just affect one mammary gland (mares have two or three per mamma), and results in local pain, swelling, and pyrexia in about 50% of cases.

Mammary carcinoma is also sporadic and very rare. No cause is known. Case reports indicate they are often metastatic.

Disorders of Ruminants (Cattle, Sheep, and Goats)

Disorders of Cattle

Mastitis in dairy cattle is an extremely important disease. Most of the organisms responsible for mastitis are bacteria, and the number and range of lesions they cause is large. The majority of cases are caused by *Staphylococcus aureus* and are of subclinical or moderate clinical forms.

Mammary pathogens can be divided into groups based on the source of infection. In one group are those organisms, such as *Streptococcus agalactiae, Staphylococcus aureus*, and *Mycoplasma* sp., for which the mammary glands are the principal site of persistence or reservoir. Coliform organisms are in the group acquired from the external environment, such as fecal matter, soil, water, or bedding. An overlap group has members, such as *Streptococcus uberis* and *Streptococcus dysgalactiae*, capable of persisting in either location. Cow-to-cow transmission is important for the mammary reservoir group, whereas contamination of the teat end is important for disease caused by the environmental group. The rates of new mammary gland infections in dairy cows caused by environmental pathogens are greatest during the first and the last 2 weeks of a 60-day nonlactating period. Coliform and streptococcal infections that are established during the nonlactating period with organisms from the environment are present at the time of parturition and cause clinical mastitis soon afterward.

Another way to group the pathogenic organisms is by the disease they cause. The three main groups, based on their virulence and effects, including systemic disease, are the Gram-negative pathogens, Gram-positive pathogens that cause acute severe necrotizing disease, and Gram-positive pathogens that cause chronic suppurative mastitis. Gram-negative organisms, particularly *Escherichia coli*, can cause severe mastitis and systemic effects because of endotoxin release. Gram-positive pathogens cause disease that ranges from subclinical mastitis to gangrenous mastitis. Many induce a chronic suppurative disease.

Gram-negative bacteria gain access to the glands and release endotoxins, and cytokine release results in necrosis and severe

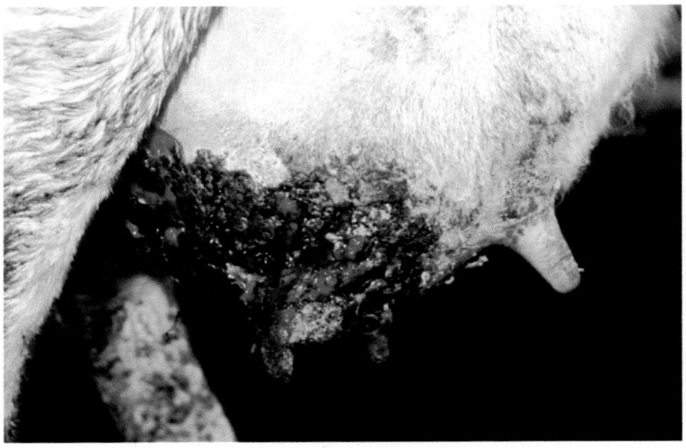

Fig. 18-53 Severe necrotic mastitis, coliform mastitis, mammary gland, cow.
Serum oozes through the dead skin of the affected right rear quarter. (Courtesy Dr. M.D. McGavin, College of Veterinary Medicine, University of Tennessee.)

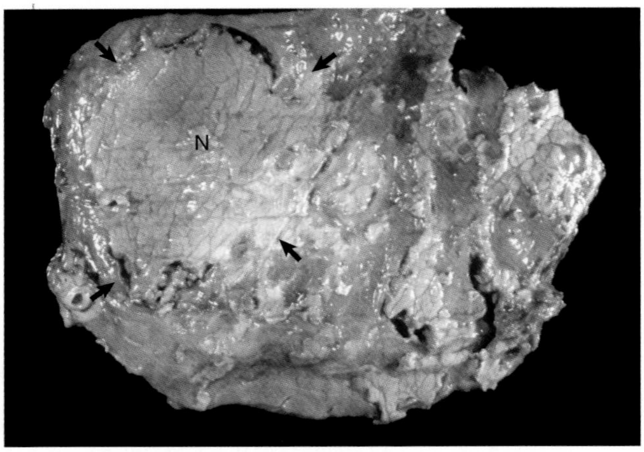

Fig. 18-54 Necrotizing mastitis, coliform mastitis, mammary gland, transverse section of quarter, cow.
Note the dry and pale gray-white area, typical of coagulative necrosis, to the left of center (delineated by *arrows*). The necrotic tissue *(N)* is partially surrounded by a zone of edema and by a thin light-gray band of fibrous tissue. Encapsulated necrotic tissue is designated a "sequestrum." (Courtesy College of Veterinary Medicine, University of Illinois.)

vascular leakage (Fig. 18-53). A systemic acute-phase reaction induced by endotoxins and cytokines causes fever, anorexia, leukopenia, hyperfibrinogenemia, and hypocalcemia. This latter feature can be mistaken for primary milk fever. Edema of the mamma and surrounding areas is often prominent. Local changes include death and sequestration of glandular tissue, wherein regions of the gland become dry, friable, and surrounded by a red border of hyperemia and hemorrhage (Fig. 18-54). The massive outpouring of edema fluid causes the gland to be dramatically swollen and hard and the "milk" to be watery and/or contain fibrin. Fibrin can obstruct the ducts and sinuses. Not only is this type of mastitis potentially life threatening because of endotoxemia, but also the severe effects on the gland often lead to reduced defenses to other pathogens so that secondary, pus-forming pathogens also proliferate.

Severe acute mastitis is caused when necrotizing Gram-positive bacteria, including virulent *Staphylococcus aureus* and streptococci, gain entry to the glands. With severe staphylococcal mastitis, neutrophils enter the tissue within minutes to hours, and the products of neutrophils contribute to the death of the glandular tissue. Cell

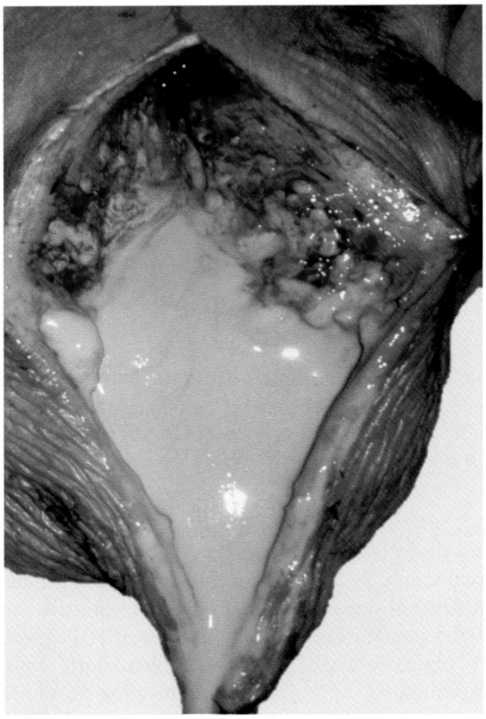

Fig. 18-55 Suppurative mastitis, mammary quarter, cow.
The lactiferous sinus and ducts are filled with viscous yellow pus. (Courtesy College of Veterinary Medicine, University of Illinois.)

surface–associated (adhesions, protein A, and capsular polysaccharides) and extracellular secretory products (leukotoxins, extracellular enzymes, and coagulase) of these organisms contribute to the damaging effect of these bacteria. The combined result is hemorrhage and death of the gland, with the result that the gland or part of the gland becomes gangrenous, hard, dry, and red-black. When severe, systemic effects of the acute-phase response caused by systemic cytokines induce fever, anorexia, weight loss, leukopenia, and hyperfibrinogenemia.

Chronic suppurative mastitis occurs when pus-forming bacteria do not induce the degree of necrosis, vascular effects, or systemic effects of the first two groups. These bacteria invoke a neutrophilic response that dominates the lesion and results in a buildup of necrotic leukocytic debris that typifies the suppurative response. The lesions they induce are centered on lactiferous ducts and sinus, and filling these with suppurative exudate (Fig. 18-55). *Arcanobacterium pyogenes, Mycoplasma bovis, Streptococcus dysgalactiae,* and various aerobes and anaerobes are prime candidates. Nocardial mastitis can be included in this group as well. Infection with these organisms, especially *Arcanobacterium pyogenes,* can occur with long-acting intramammary preparations used in the nonlactating or dry cow period. The occurrence in dry cows, initially recognized in the summer months, led to the name "summer mastitis." Careful culture reveals up to five or six different species of the *Arcanobacterium, Streptococcus, Bacteroides, Peptostreptococcus*, and *Fusobacterium* genera. Because these are found in other pyogenic infections, it is assumed that they are environmental contaminates. Dry cows are not usually closely monitored, so the mastitis is typically chronic, with thick intramammary exudates and fibrosis. *Arcanobacterium pyogenes* causes mastitis in lactating, nonlactating, and even immature bovine mammary glands with abscesses in the small and large lactiferous ducts. Abscesses range from those microscopic in size to those grossly visible. Fistulas from the abscesses can form at the base of the teat. Fibrosis of the abscess walls can result in loss of small unaffected ducts and involution and fibrosis of the parenchyma they drain.

Streptococcal Mastitis

Streptococcus agalactiae was the most important pathogen of the bovine mammae in the era before adequate mamma hygiene and efficient antibacterial drugs. Resistance of cows to mastitis caused by this organism is subject to great individual variation; in general, resistance decreases with age. The mamma is the only organ affected by this organism. *Streptococcus agalactiae* does not persist long in the environment. Once a cow is infected, however, the organism persists in the lactiferous sinus, with periodic waves of multiplication, increase in virulence, and tissue invasion. The initial response to invasion of *Streptococcus agalactiae* is interstitial edema and an influx of neutrophils into the interstitium and alveoli. The alveolar epithelium undergoes either brief hyperplasia or vacuolation and then desquamates. Macrophages quickly become a component of the cell population of infected alveoli, and fibrosis rapidly obliterates the lumen of these alveoli. Edema, cellular infiltration, and fibrosis are lesions found in infected and adjacent alveoli, so that pressure is increased within the lobule and within adjacent lobules. The increased pressure causes stagnation of milk flow, thereby initiating premature involution of a portion of the gland. After the acute phase, periductal fibrosis occurs and granulation tissue replaces part of the normal cuboidal to columnar epithelium of smaller ducts. Fibrous polyps can completely obstruct milk flow. Regeneration of ductal epithelium can occur after the granulation tissue has matured and contracted. The lactiferous ducts and sinuses, with their normally two-layered columnar epithelium, are similarly but less severely affected, often going through a phase of squamous metaplasia of the epithelium.

The macroscopic appearance depends on the stage of the disease; different stages occur in different areas. Usually more than one mamma is involved. In the acute stage, there is hyperemia of the lactiferous sinus. Milk quality is altered, and strands or clumps of debris are present in the milk, or the milk is transformed into pus. The areas of parenchymal edema and cellular infiltration are gray and turgid. Groups of alveoli, in which the secretion is retained because of obstruction of the duct by granulation tissue, resemble small abscesses. Involuting parenchyma and fibrotic parenchyma appear similar to one another and can be difficult to differentiate grossly. The lactiferous sinus becomes granular and thickened because of underlying projecting areas of granulation tissue and surrounding fibrosis.

Staphylococcal Mastitis

Staphylococcus aureus has a greater propensity than *Streptococcus agalactiae* to invade the interstitial tissue between alveoli, and thus can induce a more severe disease. Isolates of *Staphylococcus aureus* obtained from bovine mammary glands range from nonpathogenic to highly pathogenic. The severest form of staphylococcal mastitis is the gangrenous form (Fig. 18-56), usually seen shortly after parturition and involving a variable proportion of the udder. Severe acute inflammation, with classic heat, redness, swelling, and pain, progresses to coldness of the affected area, a blue-black color, and fluid exudation, indicating tissue death. Microscopically, during the first 48 hours after infection with toxigenic *Staphylococcus aureus,* the tissue has severe interstitial edema that increases the interalveolar stromal area. Progressive swelling, vacuolation, and focal erosion of epithelial cells occur throughout the ducts and are prominent near the junction of stratified squamous epithelium and columnar

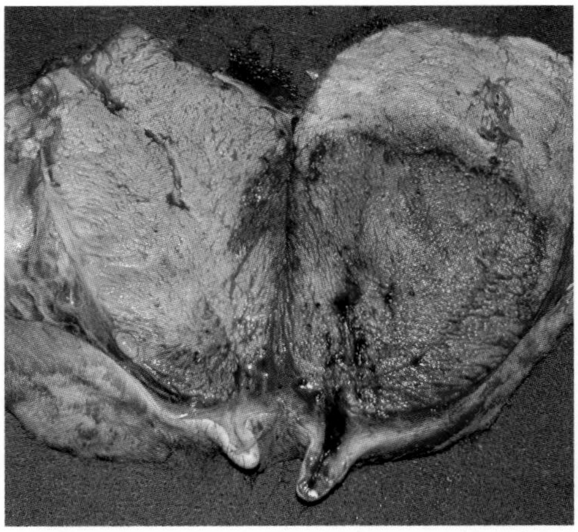

Fig. 18-56 Gangrenous mastitis (*Clostridium* sp.), mammary gland, transverse section of udder, cow.
Most of the right quarter and some of the adjacent left quarter are dark red with hemorrhage. A well-demarcated hyperemic (darker red) border has formed at its junction with the adjacent normal gland *(right udder).* There is also marked subcutaneous edema between the gland and the skin. (Courtesy Dr. R.A. Foster, Ontario Veterinary College, University of Guelph.)

epithelium of the papillary duct. The bacteria attach to epithelial cells, cause focal damage, and later can be seen on, within, and below ductal and alveolar epithelia The cellular phase of the inflammatory response is rapid, with neutrophils initially in the subepithelial tissues of the duct system, then within the epithelium, and later in the lumen of alveoli.

The less severe form follows a course similar to that of streptococcal mastitis. Initially, damage occurs to the epithelium of the lactiferous sinus and larger lactiferous ducts. Bacteria expand rapidly along the ducts and produce acute inflammation in groups of adjacent terminal alveoli. In chronically infected quarters, macrophages are the principal cell type in the epithelial lining, in lumens, and especially in the glandular interstitium. Lymphocytes increase in number, but some investigators have reported a lack of increase in plasma cells. These observations suggest that mammary lymphocytes could become hyporesponsive to antigenic stimulation in chronically infected mammary glands. Some data indicate that mammary lymphocyte function is compromised; blastogenesis is depressed in lymphocytes recovered from infected mammary glands. Studies have documented that plasma cells are prevalent in the stroma of mammary glands with chronic *Staphylococcus aureus* mastitis; more cells produce IgA than IgG antibody, and IgA-containing cells increase in number as the disease progresses. The extent of regeneration is uncertain; it is unclear whether damaged alveoli redevelop secretory tissue or remaining healthy tissue undergoes compensatory hypertrophy, or whether both processes occur.

In chronic suppurative staphylococcal mastitis, abscess formation follows acute disease. Abscesses, scattered and often coalescing, vary in size from those that are microscopic to those grossly visible. Sometimes staphylococcal bacteria are surrounded by rosettes of club-shaped material (the term *botryomycosis* was applied to such lesions). An equally important and parallel set of events occurs in the lobules not invaded by bacteria as the obstruction of milk flow by granulation tissue and pressure from surrounding fibrosis result in involution. Multiple, small, soft cream to pink nodules, some containing pus, are separated by bands of fibrous tissue. Disease caused by less pathogenic strains of staphylococci, such as nonhemolytic coagulase-negative strains, progresses less dramatically and

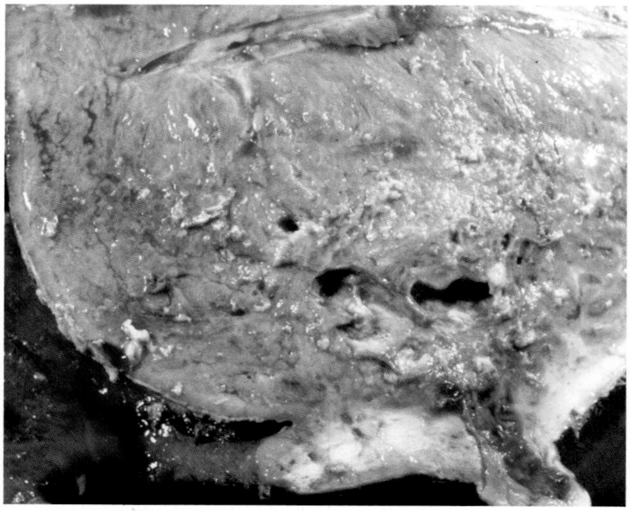

Fig. 18-57 Coliform mastitis, mammary glands, cow.
There is marked thickening of the walls of the lactiferous ducts. White to yellow fibrin and pus have collected in the lactiferous ducts and the upper portion of the lactiferous sinus. (Courtesy College of Veterinary Medicine, University of Illinois.)

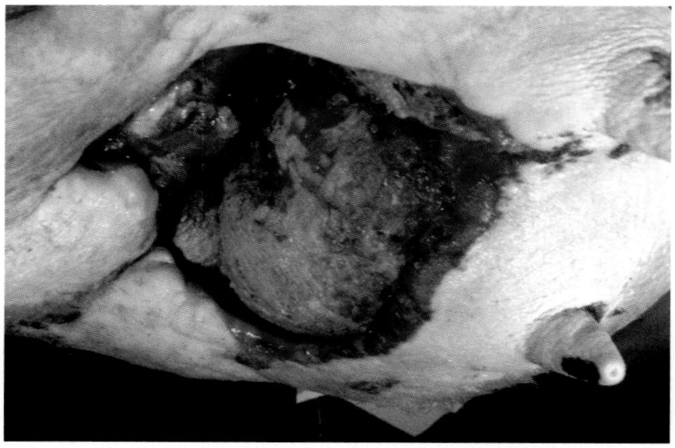

Fig. 18-58 Sloughed quarter, mammary gland, necrotizing mastitis, cow.
The necrotic right rear quarter has recently sloughed, leaving a large ulcerated area covered by a thin gray layer of exudate. The surface of the ulcer is finely granular, indicating the formation of granulation tissue. (Courtesy College of Veterinary Medicine, University of Illinois.)

not necessarily with obvious abscess formation. However, the same components of granulation tissue and fibrosis are present, causing obstruction and pressure, which in turn cause atrophy of adjacent lobules.

Coliform Mastitis

Coliform mastitis occurs when bacteria from the environment contaminate the opening of the papillary duct and ascend. The most common bacteria are *Escherichia coli, Enterobacter aerogenes,* and *Klebsiella pneumoniae.* Coliform bacteria probably exert their damaging effect via endotoxin acting on the vasculature. In the acute form of the disease, the lesions are hyperemia, hemorrhage, and edema of the affected areas centered on the lactiferous ducts. The fluid in the lactiferous sinus is cloudy and blood stained and has clumps of fibrin (Fig. 18-57). Microscopically, interlobular septa are edematous and fibrin thrombi are in lymph vessels. Epithelium of ducts and alveoli is necrotic, and only low numbers of inflammatory cells are within them. Coliform bacteria are numerous within both the alveoli and the epithelium. The severity of the disease in postparturient cows is attributed to a delay in the influx of neutrophils. The cow's response to endotoxin is influenced by the stage of the reproductive cycle. The nonlactating mammary glands are much less sensitive to the effects of endotoxin than are the lactating ones.

If the cow survives endotoxemia, the necrotic mammary tissue, which can be a large portion of a mamma, separates from the viable tissue and is sequestered or eventually sloughs (Fig. 18-58). Cows in early lactation with less severe coliform mastitis often develop chronic mastitis that has alterations of hyperplasia, disorganization, and filiform processes of the epithelial lining of the papillary duct and lactiferous sinus.

Mycoplasmal Mastitis

Mycoplasma mastitis in cows occurs as individual sporadic cases or in outbreaks. Several mycoplasmas are capable of causing bovine mastitis, but *Mycoplasma bovis* is the most prevalent. The disease caused by *Mycoplasma bovis* can affect one or all mammae; mycoplasmas inoculated into one mamma often spread to all. Hematogenous spread and contamination of the teat are therefore routes by which the gland becomes infected. Affected quarters initially are enlarged, firm, and light brown and have a nodular parenchyma. The nodules are abscesses that can be up to 10 cm in diameter. Large numbers of neutrophils are found in the lobular interstitium and alveoli in the early stages. This changes with chronicity to include lymphocytes and macrophages. Early vacuolation and degeneration of alveolar epithelium is followed by hyperplasia and then by metaplasia to a relatively undifferentiated multilayered epithelial lining. Focal erosions of ductal epithelium are replaced by granulation tissue. Aggregates of lymphocytes occur in the lobular interstitium and around ducts. Interstitial fibrosis and lobular atrophy occur in the late stages. Spread of the organism to calves and resultant otitis, arthritis, and pneumonia can occur.

Granulomatous Mastitis

Granulomatous mastitis in the cow occurs when drugs for the treatment or prevention of mastitis are introduced through the teat and are contaminated with *Nocardia asteroides, Cryptococcus neoformans,* atypical *Mycobacterium* sp. (other than *Mycobacterium bovis*), or *Candida* spp. These infectious agents can also cause spontaneous mammary disease. Nocardial mastitis is the best known of these diseases because it occurs in outbreaks. Severely affected cows develop pyrexia that may last for several weeks. Cows become lethargic and lose weight, as would be expected with systemic cytokine release. The glands are hot and swollen and may have multiple abscesses or granulomas. Small white particles may be found in the exudate. Lesions in the mammary glands are centered on the lactiferous ducts and sinuses because galactophoritis is the prominent finding. Because the infection is chronic and ascending, lobules are affected to a varying degree. Granulomas and pyogranulomas predominate microscopically. These are usually surrounded by fibrous tissue, and extensive involvement results in the gland being replaced by a framework of fibrous tissue surrounding pockets of inflammatory cells and central necrotic debris (Fig. 18-59). An udder affected with cryptococcal mastitis has the same yellow gelatinous material that is typical of cryptococcal lesions elsewhere.

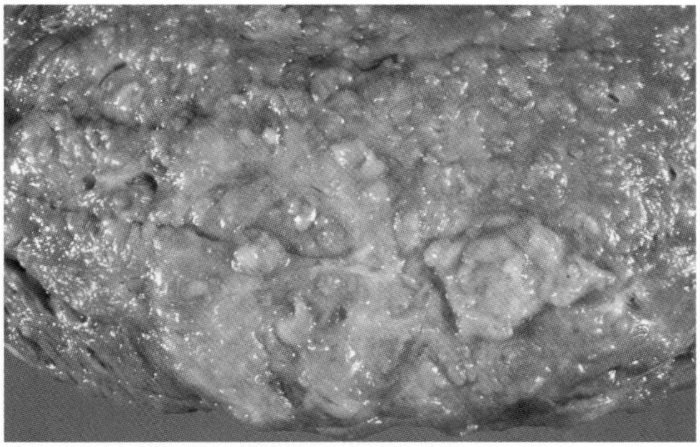

Fig. 18-59 Chronic mastitis and galactophoritis (*Nocardia* spp.), mammary glands, transverse section, cow.
Chronic inflammation of the lactiferous ducts and adjacent mammary glands has resulted in the replacement of most of this gland by pyogranulomas and abscesses containing yellow pus. The adjacent normal glandular tissue has involuted. This cow was infected when the dry cow medication was contaminated by *Nocardia* spp. (Courtesy Dr. R.A. Foster, Ontario Veterinary College, University of Guelph.)

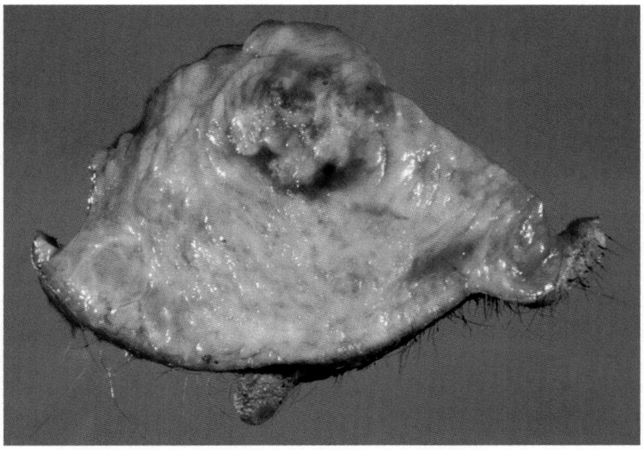

Fig. 18-60 Mammary carcinoma, mammary gland, bitch.
This mammary carcinoma has infiltrated and replaced normal mammary glands and contiguous soft tissue. The upper nodule is the neoplasm, and the lower and surrounding white tissues are composed of infiltrating neoplastic cells and fibrous tissue, the result of a desmoplastic response. (Courtesy Dr. R.A. Foster, Ontario Veterinary College, University of Guelph.)

Disorders of Sheep and Goats

There are two main agents recovered from the mammary glands of sheep: *Mannheimia haemolytica* and *Staphylococcus aureus*. In many sheep flocks, the main manifestation of infection with these agents is unexpected death because these bacteria are responsible for an acute necrotizing or gangrenous mastitis. It is difficult to be certain, but the morbidity can be about 5% and mortality 20%. Mastitis in goats is similar, and as with the disease in sheep, is assumed to have a similar pathogenesis to the disease in cattle. For mycoplasmal mastitis, *Mycoplasma agalactiae* or *Mycoplasma mycoides* ssp. *mycoides* are usually the causative agents.

Goats infected with CAEV can develop a "hard udder." The udder is hard, and little milk can be expressed from the teat. Recovery occurs, but milk production is reduced. Histologically, there are large numbers of lymphocytes and lymphoid follicles in the interstitium between the glands. The virus grows in mammary epithelium and is present in milk. The newborn is infected through infected milk. A similar disease in sheep is seen with infection with maedi-visna virus. The pathogenesis is provided in more detail in the chapter of respiratory disease; briefly the virus is spread through respiratory secretions rather than milk, the virus replicates in macrophages and results in slowly progressive lesions with large numbers of lymphocytes and plasma cells in many organs, the mammary glands being one.

Disorders of Dogs

Neoplasia of the mammary glands is common in the dog, and it has the highest incidence of all domesticated species (Fig. 18-60). Most canine mammary tumors are clinically benign. There has been much interest in canine mammary neoplasia both from the viewpoint of prognosis and treatment, from a logical pathogenetic viewpoint, and as a tool in comparative oncogenesis. Although the phenomenon of mammary neoplasia is well recognized, the cause is not. Ovariohysterectomy after the second estrus dramatically increases the prevalence of this disease. The "window of susceptibility" is up to 2 years of age. A high-protein diet decreases susceptibility, whereas treatment with medroxyprogesterone acetate and being a purebred increases it.

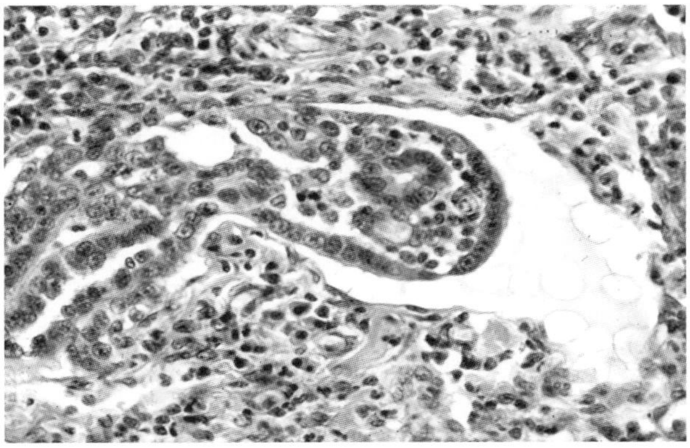

Fig. 18-61 Adenocarcinoma, invasion into lymphatic vessels, bitch.
Note the neoplastic cells infiltrating through the wall of the lymphatic *(above left)*. Microscopic invasion by mammary carcinoma into a lymphatic, as depicted here, is an indicator of a poor prognosis. In this case, there are lymphocytes and plasma cells in the perilymphatic tissues. H&E stain. (Courtesy Dr. M. Domingo, Autonomous University of Barcelona; and Noah's Arkive, College of Veterinary Medicine, The University of Georgia.)

Mammary neoplasms are a diverse group that are dominated by epithelial and combined epithelial and myoepithelial tumors. Sarcomas, such as fibrosarcoma and osteosarcoma, are much less common but are particularly aggressive and metastatic. The embryology of the mammary glands involves a close association between the epithelium and mesenchyme, so it is not surprising that tumors are often combinations of stroma and epithelium with the so-called complex adenomas and carcinomas, with a mixture of epithelial and myoepithelial components, and the mixed mammary tumor with those elements plus cartilage and bone.

The development of mammary epithelial neoplasia can proceed from ductal or lobular hyperplasia to dysplasia and on to neoplasia and subsequent progression from benign adenoma to noninvasive carcinoma and to invasive forms (Fig. 18-61). Once progression begins, an individual will often continue to develop neoplasia, and the development of multiple mammary masses is likely. The prognosis for each subsequent mass is not dependent on the previous one, so that many different types of neoplasia can be found in one animal.

Predicting behavior of mammary neoplasms is an inexact science. From a pragmatic and simplistic view, invasion is an indicator of a poor prognosis. It is the reason that excisional biopsy is the best procedure for diagnosis in dogs; cytology can be useful in identifying inflammation and sarcomas but can give a false impression of malignancy in epithelial tumors. The neoplasms that arise are variable in their phenotypes and as such, there are many different classification schemes.

General principles of neoplasia apply, and in dogs, those that are locally invasive are more likely to be life threatening. The threat increases with the lack of differentiation, and there is an increasing risk of metastasis with tubulopapillary, solid, and anaplastic carcinomas, respectively. Those with metastasis to the local lymph node have an especially poor prognosis. Because there is a potential for progression from benign to malignant, neoplasms (either because of rapid growth or having additional time to develop) larger than 5 cm in diameter have a poorer prognosis.

In dogs, mastitis caused by bacteria or *Mycoplasma* sp. occurs early in lactation or pseudopregnancy. Staphylococci, streptococci, and *Escherichia coli* are major isolates. It is assumed that the pathogenetic pathways of mastitis in dogs are the same as for dairy cows. Infection of fissures in nipples and adjacent skin spreads via the lactiferous ducts into the gland and results in suppurative inflammation and/or abscesses. The glands become swollen, large, firm, and edematous because the toxins and tissue destruction by the agents or the cytokine and contents of inflammatory cell granules cause acute inflammation. It may be superimposed on mammary hyperplasia or mammary neoplasia, especially on tumors of ducts. Systemic illness is often seen.

Disorders of Cats

Fibroadenomatous hyperplasia (mammary hypertrophy) is highly prevalent and is the most common disease; it occurs in young intact female cats. Those less than 2 years old are most likely to develop mammary enlargement, which usually occurs in the spring and with the first several estrous cycles. Much of what is known about this disease is based on its coinciding with the luteal phase of estrus, early in pregnancy, or after progestin therapy. High concentrations of progesterone or progesterone-like substances are the common link. As expected, megestrol acetate treatment of an old neutered male or female can induce this also. What is difficult to explain is the distribution of the lesion, as all mammary glands, only one mamma, or parts of one mammary gland may be as well. The lesion is proliferation of mammary ducts and adjacent stroma (Fig. 18-62). This overstimulation of an otherwise normal process is likely to be the result of a local dysregulation of tissue growth with the stimulation of receptors by progesterone. Some have theorized an exaggerated response to prolactin as well. Hemorrhages, coagulative necrosis, and/or ulceration of affected areas can occur. In young females, resolution is spontaneous or ovariohysterectomy is effective. Older neutered animals on progestin require drug withdrawal and sometimes mastectomy.

Mammary neoplasia in cats is relatively uncommon, so studies of causal factors are limited. There is not the same relationship with early desexing as there is with dogs. Progression from focal hyperplasia to adenoma to carcinoma is recognized, but this progression is presumably rapid, as many of the carcinomas are small.

The majority of neoplasms in cats are carcinomas and they metastasize. They are usually single and occur in the tissue adjacent to the nipple; 75% to 96% are adenocarcinomas and show rapid growth (Fig. 18-63). They metastasize to regional lymph nodes (axillary or the superficial inguinal nodes), lungs, or other mammary glands. The average age of affected animals is 11 years, and there is a 7- to 9-year-old risk plateau. Intact animals are at a slightly greater risk, but there is no beneficial effect of early spaying. The poorest prognosis is in older cats with neoplasms that are greater than 3 cm in diameter, with the presence of regional lymph node involvement, with increased number of mitoses, and with the presence of necrosis. Well-differentiated tumors have a better prognosis. The interval between diagnosis and death is often short, less than 1 year, but the range is wide. There is no or only a weak correlation between histologic features, including proliferation indices and prognosis, except perhaps size.

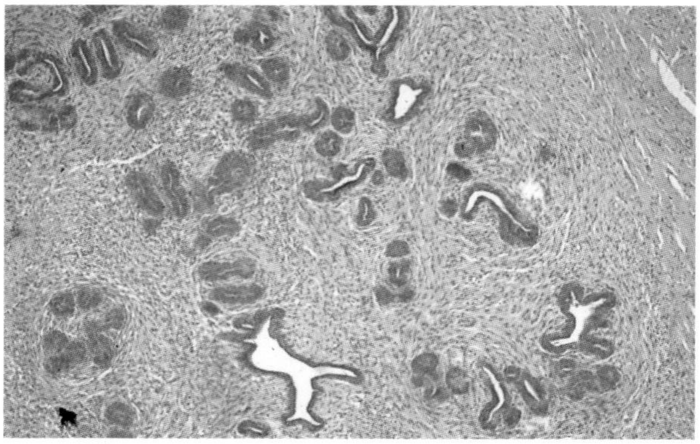

Fig. 18-62 Mammary hypertrophy (fibroadenomatous hyperplasia), mammary gland, cat.
Mammary ducts have proliferated and are surrounded by abundant loosely arranged stromal tissues. Typically, cats with mammary hypertrophy are young and develop enlargement of one or several mammary glands in the spring. H&E stain. (Courtesy Dr. W. Crowell, College of Veterinary Medicine, The University of Georgia; and Noah's Arkive, College of Veterinary Medicine, The University of Georgia.)

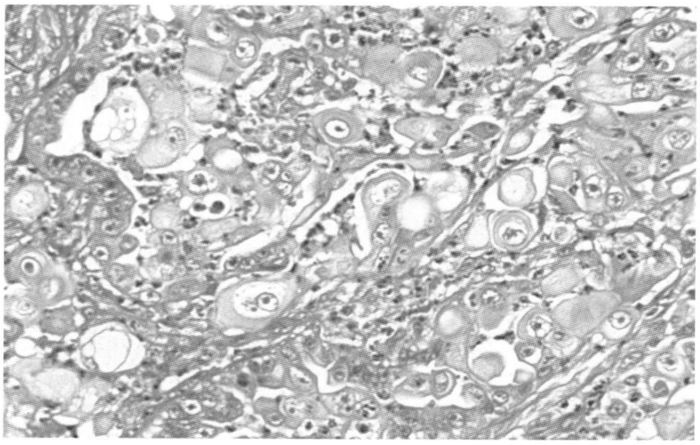

Fig. 18-63 Mammary carcinoma, mammary gland, cat.
The cells of this anaplastic neoplasm do not resemble those of normal epithelium but are large and round. They are arranged either in clusters or as individual cells within a fibrous stroma. Inflammatory cells, including neutrophils and lymphocytes, are also present. H&E stain. (Courtesy College of Veterinary Medicine, University of Illinois.)

SUGGESTED READINGS

Information on this topic is available at evolve.elsevier.com/Zachary/McGavin/.

CHAPTER 19

Male Reproductive System

Robert A. Foster

The reproductive system is arguably the most important in terms of survival of a species. In production animals, reproduction is essential for the continued supply of product, be it meat, fiber, milk, or many other products. Most production animals rely on a small number of males as breeding stock, so in addition to being 50% of the reproductive team, an infertile male or one carrying an undesirable trait has a major impact.

The male reproductive system usually receives little attention and time; with some exceptions, replacement of a breeding male is often more effective than diagnosis and treatment. Infertility in the male is difficult to reverse unless the cause can be readily found and corrected. This is where knowledge of the disease processes, responses to injury, and prognosis are so important.

Companion animals are not given the same amount of study as production animals, especially the bull and ram. The aim here is to emphasize the disorders of all species and highlight the mechanisms and reactions of the male reproductive tract by examining the disorders of each anatomic location.

STRUCTURE

The male reproductive tract can be divided into three major areas based not only on anatomic location but also on functional characteristics and important disease processes. These are the scrotum and its contents, the accessory genital glands, and the penis and prepuce.

THE SCROTUM AND CONTENTS

The purpose of the scrotum and its contents is to supply spermatozoa for transportation to the female. Although the general focus is on the testis and its germinal cells contained in the seminiferous tubules, other parts have important functional characteristics that allow this to happen. Testicular development is quiescent until puberty when spermatogenesis begins. The testes therefore are small until puberty, when they increase to their adult size. The testes are covered by a capsule (once called the *tunica albuginea*), which is relatively nonexpansile and usually maintains the testicular contents under slight pressure. Within the testis are the interstitial and intratubular regions. Within the interstitium are the interstitial endocrine (Leydig) cells, blood vessels, lymphatics, and macrophages, dendritic cells, mast cells, and T lymphocytes. Each seminiferous tubule has a lining of myoid cells and a limiting membrane. There is a basement membrane between these structures. The arrangement of the seminiferous tubules varies from species to species, but the end result is the formation of spermatozoa. After spermatogenesis, spermatozoa are transported through rete tubules into the efferent ductules and then into the epididymis, a single and extremely long duct. In doing so, the spermatozoa mature and are concentrated. The pathway out of the scrotal area is through the deferent duct.

The purpose of the scrotum, vaginal tunics, and spermatic cord (deferent duct, pampiniform plexus, and cremaster muscle) is to protect and maintain spermatogenesis at a temperature slightly lower than body temperature. The testes are raised or lowered, according to ambient temperature, by the cremaster muscle. There is a counter current vascular system that allows the testes to be at a lower temperature than body temperature; the pampiniform plexus assists this process. The pulsatile nature of arterial blood flow is altered to form a continuous and lower pressure system. In addition, the scrotal skin, which is thin, often hairless, and in most species has abundant apocrine sweat glands, helps to maintain a lower testicular and epididymal temperature. The vaginal tunic, which is an outpouching of the peritoneum, allows for free movement of the testes within the scrotal sac. The scrotum is composed of skin, dartos muscle, and scrotal fascia. It is fused with the parietal layer of the vaginal tunic.

Cell Types

The functions of the male reproductive system are the production of testosterone and the production and transportation of spermatozoa. Spermatozoa are formed from germ (stem) cells by a process of spermatogenesis. Spermatogenesis occurs in three stages: the proliferative, meiotic, and spermatogenic stages. The proliferative phase involves the mitotically active spermatogonia. They are present at the periphery of the seminiferous tubules on the basement membrane. The second phase is the meiotic phase, in which

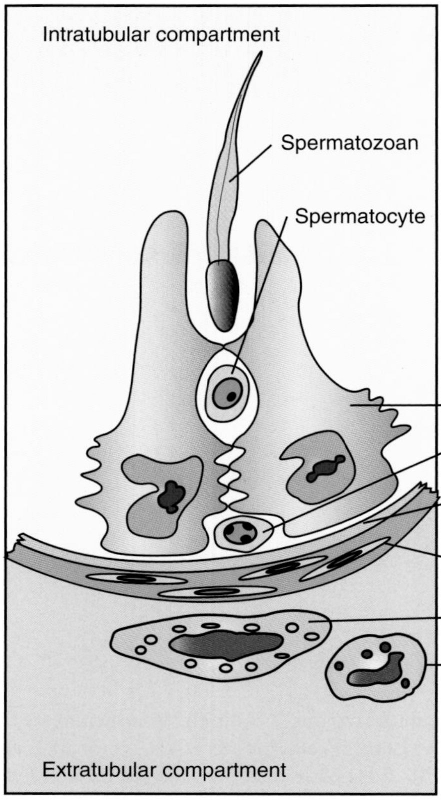

Fig. 19-1 Schematic diagram of the normal components of the testis. The Sertoli cells, germ cells, and interstitial endocrine cells are closely integrated, and considerable messaging occurs between them. The blood-testis barrier is at the level of the Sertoli cells, with contributions from the myoid cells and basement membrane. Spermatogonia are on the interstitial side of the blood-testis barrier.

spermatocytes are formed. In the spermatogenic phase, spermatids and finally spermatozoa are formed. Spermatozoa have a head, body, and tail. The head contains the nucleus and an acrosome, which contains enzymes required for the penetration of the zona pellucida. The body or midpiece contains mitochondria, and the tail is a flagellum.

Sertoli cells provide support, nutrients, hormones, and cytokines to permit spermatogenesis. During spermatogenesis, the cells pass into a region that is separated from and external to the immune system of the body. The barrier is called the *blood-testis barrier*, and it is maintained by the Sertoli cells (Fig. 19-1). Control of spermatogenesis is achieved through a combination of both central (luteinizing hormone [LH] on the interstitial endocrine cells and follicle-stimulating hormone [FSH] on Sertoli cells) and local (paracrine and autocrine molecules, including testosterone) factors, and there is considerable crosstalk between germ cells, Sertoli cells, and interstitial endocrine cells. Local modification of spermatogenesis is achieved through increased or decreased apoptosis at any stage of development. Many of the disorders and conditions that affect spermatogenesis increase or decrease the apoptotic rate.

The cells lining the various ducts, including the rete tubules, efferent ductules, and epididymides, are epithelial cells that have a variety of functions, in addition to being a barrier. Absorption, phagocytosis, and secretion are all part of their physiologic role. Movement of spermatozoa along these ducts and tubules is achieved through smooth muscle contraction and the cilia.

In the accessory genital glands, storage of spermatozoa (particularly in the ampulla, where present) and secretion of various substances are the major roles for the epithelium of these glands. From the pelvic urethra and through the penile urethra, the lining cells are urothelial in type.

THE ACCESSORY GENITAL GLANDS

The purpose of the accessory glands is to provide nutrition and a transport medium for spermatozoa. There are four main accessory glands: the ampullae, vesicular glands, prostate, and bulbourethral glands. There is considerable species variation in the size, type, and number of these accessory glands. Horses and ruminants have all four glands, although the prostate of ruminants is either very small (bull) or is disbursed within the pelvic urethra (ram and buck). Pigs lack ampullae, dogs have only a prostate, and cats have a small prostate and bulbourethral glands. The secretion of the vesicular gland and prostate is serous, but the bulbourethral gland typically has a viscous mucoid product.

THE PENIS AND PREPUCE

There is considerable structural difference between the penis and prepuce of the various species. In prepubertal animals, the prepuce is attached to the penis, but they become separated at sexual maturity. The penis of the horse is erectile and is located within a prepuce that produces a thick, waxy material called *smegma*. Ruminants and pigs have a long fibrous penis that has some erectile tissue. To accommodate a penis of sufficient length, there is a series of bends called the *sigmoid flexure*, and there is a retractor muscle to hold the penis in the prepuce. There is an extension of the urethra in small ruminants that is called the *vermiform appendage* or the *urethral process*. During ejaculation, this appendage spins and sprays semen onto the cervix. The glans of the penis of the boar has a corkscrew shape that allows it to insert into the cervix. The penis of dogs and to a lesser extent cats is erectile and has an os penis. The cat has projections of penile epithelium called *spines* or *barbs* on its penis, and they are testosterone dependent.

FUNCTION

The overall function of the male reproductive system is to provide genetic material to the female for combination with female genetic material to produce an offspring with a combined and hopefully better genetic makeup. This is achieved by several separate areas—the scrotum and contents, accessory genital glands, and the penis and prepuce.

THE SCROTUM AND CONTENTS

The testes are the location of preparation of genetic material for transfer to the female. One-half of the chromosomes are produced by the process of meiosis in the seminiferous tubules in the process of spermatogenesis (see the section on cells of the male reproductive system). The testes also produce the hormone testosterone to ensure development of male phenotypic and behavioral characteristics. It also provides the signals that stimulate females to come into heat and become receptive. The testis also produces other substances for the regulation of spermatogenesis. Spermatozoa leave the testis in a high volume of fluid—the rete testis fluid—and enter the epididymis. The epididymis has the function of supporting and directing spermatozoal maturation and concentrating the spermatozoa for ejaculation. The function of the testis and epididymis depends on unique requirements, including maintenance of a temperature below body temperature, and a continuous nonpulsatile blood flow. The scrotum provides support and with the cremaster muscle in concert with the dartos muscle of the scrotal wall, thermoregulation by raising the testis and epididymis closer to the body wall. The pampiniform plexus is a countercurrent system that assists in maintaining a lower temperature, and the long and tortuous testicular artery removes the pulses of the arterial supply. The deferent duct is the conduit for taking the concentrated spermatozoa to the accessory genital glands.

THE ACCESSORY GENITAL GLANDS

The function of the accessory glands is to produce ejaculatory fluid to support, nourish, and protect spermatozoa as they are transferred to the female. The energy source of spermatozoa includes fructose produced by the accessory glands, usually the vesicular glands. Accessory genital glands also provide the fluid for territorial scent marking. The domestic species have a differing size and arrangement of accessory glands to do this. The amount and type of fluid varies according to the unique arrangements and mating behavior of the species. Coitus in ruminants is a rapid event, and they produce a small and highly concentrated ejaculate that is deposited around the external os of the cervix. On the other end of the scale are pigs, where coitus takes about 20 minutes, insemination is intrauterine, and the ejaculate is high volume (up to 500 mL). Pigs have large vesicular glands that produce a watery fluid and large bulbourethral glands that produce a viscous mucoid product. The prostate of the dog is the only gland, and it provides all the seminal fluid. All species except the dog and pig have ampullae of the deferent ducts; these provide secretion and a storage site for spermatozoa.

THE PENIS AND PREPUCE

The penis is designed to enter the vagina of the female and to deposit the ejaculate in a location unique to each species. Pigs and horses are intrauterine inseminators, whereas the others deposit semen around the cervix and proximal vagina. This ensures protection of spermatozoa, including the prevention of desiccation. There are also adaptations and functions that ensure the spermatozoa of the dominant male are the ones that fertilize the ova. This may explain why pigs and dogs have prolonged coitus. The penis of the cat has barbs that stimulate the vagina of the queen and induce ovulation. Small ruminants have a urethral process that sprays spermatozoa around the cervix, and the pig has a preputial diverticulum for scent production.

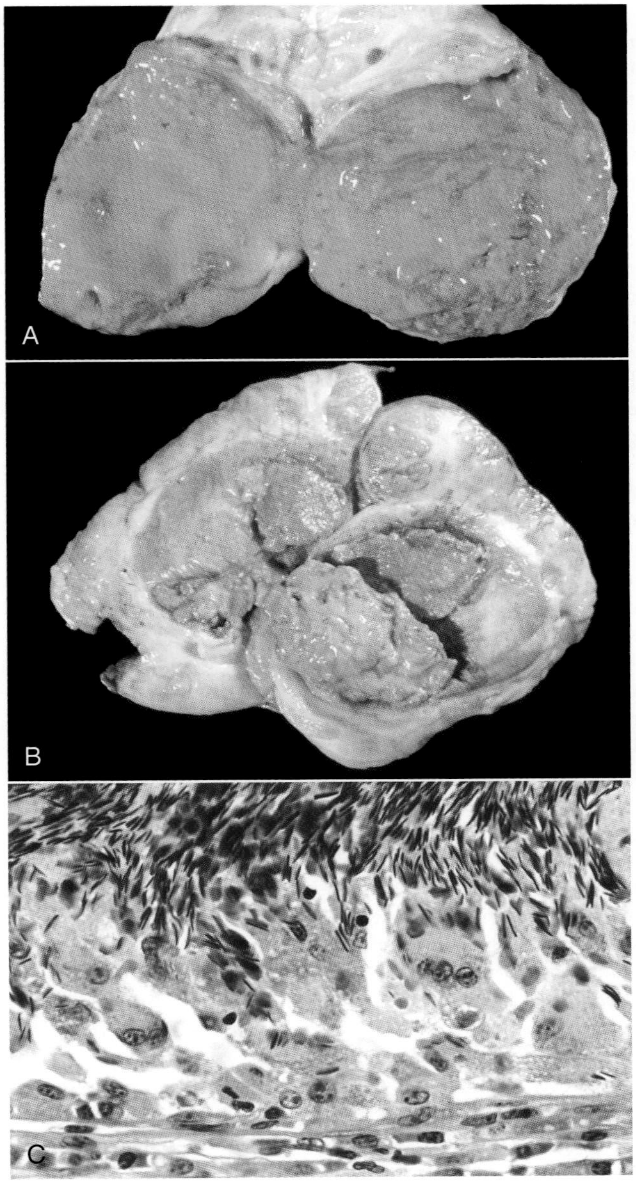

Fig. 19-2 Spermatic granulomas, tail of the epididymis, ram. **A**, Most of the tail of the epididymis (bisected and reflected) has been replaced by a yellow-tan, semiliquid spermatic granuloma. These granulomas are any color from white to red. They are frequently and incorrectly called abscesses. **B**, Multiple encapsulated (chronic) spermatic granulomas with white caseous centers. **C**, A mass of spermatozoa free in the interstitium *(upper half of image)* is surrounded by epithelioid macrophages and multinucleated giant cells, some of which have phagocytosed spermatozoa. Lymphocytes, plasma cells, and fibrous connective tissue surround these granulomas *(lower half of image)*. H&E stain. (**A** and **B** courtesy Drs. P. W. Ladds and R. A. Foster, James Cook University of North Queensland. **C** courtesy Dr. R. A. Foster, Ontario Veterinary College, University of Guelph.)

RESPONSES TO INJURY

Injury to the male reproductive system comes in many different forms, and there are many potential targets, including the pituitary and endocrine control, interstitial endocrine cells, Sertoli cells, spermatogenic germ cells, and the various ducts. Apart from the obvious redundancy of having bilateral systems, the male reproductive tract has very little functional reserve and cannot undergo compensatory change to any significant degree. Some testicular compensatory hypertrophy is possible and is discussed later in this chapter.

The formation of spermatic granulomas (Fig. 19-2) is one of the most dramatic and important responses of the male reproductive system to injury. Spermatic granulomas occur with rupture of a duct; spermiostasis and spermatocele are the usual preliminary stages. Spermatozoa are "foreign" to the body. Immunity to spermatozoa with the formation of antisperm antibody is a well-recognized phenomenon. The cell wall constituents and the high chromatin content make them resistant to degradation. Any injury that exposes spermatozoa to the tissue of the body results in severe inflammation, mostly of a granulomatous type. This can be a foreign body type response, an immunologic response, or both. The inflammation produced is usually chronic and results in severe scarring, which further obstructs tubules and ducts, leading to even more inflammation so that it becomes self-perpetuating. It is therefore critical to prevent such injury.

Injury to the testis can be the result of a primary attack on a target cell or may be secondary to interruption of hormonal regulation, whether systemic or local. The endpoint of an injury can therefore be far reaching. Regardless of the primary target, most injurious events result in germ cell degeneration and depletion. Germ cells are sensitive, but Sertoli cells are relatively resistant to injury. As a result, severe injury often results in seminiferous tubules containing only spermatogonia and Sertoli cells. As Sertoli cells degenerate, they become vacuolated and swollen. Exfoliation of normal germ cells can also occur. The spermatogenic epithelium responds to injury by increasing or decreasing apoptosis, resulting in spermatogenic arrest or a complete failure of spermatogenesis. As long as spermatogonia remain, spermatogenesis can restart. Failure of release of spermatozoa is an early indication of degeneration. The formation of multinucleated spermatid giant cells and phagocytosis of spermatozoa by Sertoli cells occur.

A major effect of injury to interstitial endocrine cells is the failure of the release of testosterone. This can effectively stop spermatogenesis by increasing apoptosis and by inhibiting maturation of spermatids. Direct damage to spermatozoa can affect motility and fertilizing capability. Recovery from injury, while taking time, is achieved by restarting spermatogenesis from the relatively resistant spermatogonia.

The testis is a specialized immunologic environment and has a reduced immune responsiveness, no doubt because of the importance of not developing an immunologic response to germ cells. Unfortunately, if an inflammatory response does occur within the testis, it is likely to be sustained.

Injury to the epididymis can have permanent and devastating effects. Injury affects not only the functions of the epididymides—including maturation and storage of spermatozoa, resorption of fluid, and secretion of materials—but severe injury also results in inflammation. Any constriction of the epididymal duct results in spermiostasis, potential rupture, and the formation of spermatic granulomas. Because the epididymis is very limited in its responses, alteration to the structure and function of the epididymis is often permanent and affects fertility in a dramatic fashion.

Injury to the accessory genital glands is not common, and they can recover, often with a reduced function. Functional reserve is often sufficient to maintain fertility.

The peritesticular tissues, in particular the vaginal tunics, are also prone to injury from peritoneal reactions secondary to epididymal disease or from a direct penetrating injury. The reaction of these tissues is identical to that of the peritoneum, and as such, fibrosis and adhesion are a common response. Adhesion can limit the movement of the testes and alter its ability to thermoregulate.

PORTALS OF ENTRY

There are four main portals of entry of infectious and injurious agents to the male reproductive tract (Box 19-1). They include direct penetration and injury, ascending infection, hematogenous localization, and peritoneal spread.

BOX 19-1 Portals of Entry

Direct penetration
Ascending infection
Hematogenous localization
Peritoneal spread

The external location of the penis, prepuce, and scrotum makes them prone to direct penetrating injury and to blunt force trauma. Surprisingly, this is a relatively rare occurrence.

Ascending infection is relatively common. It occurs sporadically in adults but curiously is particularly a problem in pubertal animals when hormonal changes make the system more prone to infection from bacteria. This pubertal change was shown for *Actinobacillus seminis* and *Histophilus somni*, which are resident flora of the prepuce of sheep. The accessory genital glands in particular are targets, but there can be further ascension to the epididymis. It is exceedingly rare, because of the long length of the epididymis, for the testis to be involved in ascending infection. The male reproductive tract is also a target of pathogens that are spread by sexual activity. Spread from females or in some circumstances from other males is well recognized.

Hematogenous localization is a recognized portal of entry by specific pathogens, such as the various *Brucella*. The epididymis and the accessory genital glands are the main targets.

The vaginal tunic is an outpouching of the peritoneal cavity and any process affecting the peritoneum, whether infectious or neoplastic, affects the peritesticular tissues.

DEFENSE MECHANISMS

The male reproductive tract, and in particular the internal genitalia, is so exquisitely sensitive to injury that it is extremely important to prevent rather than respond to injury. The combined effect of the high antigenicity of spermatozoa and the exceedingly long and very narrow duct system means that there is little tolerance for inflammation, necrosis, or other injurious situations. Much of the reproductive system relies on isolation for protection and the prevention of infection or injury.

INNATE IMMUNITY

There are multiple factors that prevent infection and injury to the vulnerable tissues. The testes and epididymides are hidden from the external environment by their intrascrotal location and by the extremely long and narrow tube that connects them to the outside world. The thin luminal diameter and extreme length of the deferent duct makes ascending infection unlikely. There is almost continuous flow of fluid along the deferent duct and the epididymis, thus the flushing action is protective. Even the accessory genital glands are protected by the flushing action of urine and by the long length of the urethra in species, such as ruminants, and the pig.

Testicular and epididymal fluid has antibacterial properties. The high chlorine content may be partially responsible. Antimicrobial proteins in seminal plasma are numerous and include bovine seminal plasmin, lactoferrin, β-defensins, and the antibacterial CXC chemokine granulocyte chemotactic protein-2/CXCL6. Some of these are acquired in the epididymis, where they are bound to spermatozoa. There are also numerous cytokines normally produced in the tract. Epithelial cells of the reproductive tract have physical barrier proteins, including mucin, that prevent infection, and Toll-like receptors to stimulate inflammation.

Nonspecific cellular defenses are relatively few. Neutrophils are not normally present in seminal plasma but can infiltrate rapidly if required. Macrophages are present within tissue and particularly within the testes, where they are recruited and maintained by the interstitial endocrine cells. Their presence inhibits the immune response; the cell-mediated responses, such as natural killer cells, lymphocyte-activated killer cells, and cytotoxic T lymphocytes, are inhibited as part of immune privilege and tolerance.

ADAPTIVE IMMUNITY

Much of the reproductive tract can produce an adaptive immune response if called on to do so. Where it is important is in the more distal portions of the tract, particularly the accessory genital glands and the prepuce. Unfortunately, development of an adaptive response in the testis and the epididymis is often "too little, too late." Also, development of adaptive responses in the testis is inhibited by local immunosuppressive factors. This does not, however, prevent adaptive immunity from developing in the testis. The epididymis and deferent duct do not have a developed mucosal immune system, but there is evidence that such a system exists in the accessory genital glands, particularly the ampulla and bulbourethral glands. When infection occurs, local immunity and transfer of serum immunoglobulin is present. Preputial immunity is also mediated by local humoral and cellular mechanisms. Immunoglobulin G (IgG)- and IgA-based systems are present. Much less is known of cell-mediated immune mechanisms in the male reproductive tract.

Using local immunity to protect against infectious disease, particularly those important sexually transmitted diseases, has had little success. Response to vaccination has been variable with some individuals having protective immunity, particularly with *Campylobacter fetus* infection in bulls. Systemic immunity to reproductive disease has also been of variable effectiveness. Although protecting against systemic infection, challenge to the reproductive tract has in some instances increased the response to the infection and caused more damage than would normally occur.

INFLAMMATION

In general terms, inflammation of the male reproductive tract is similar to that of other systems. What is unique about the male genital tract is inflammation to spermatozoa. Spermatozoa and germ cells outside the blood-testis barrier are antigenic. There are also antigenic components within seminal fluid. Spermatozoa have antigens that attract immune cells and also nonspecifically bind immunoglobulin. These reactions can have a minimal effect on the tissues directly and act by agglutinating spermatozoa or by opsonization. In some instances, the effect is much more dramatic and immunization against spermatozoa can result in a severe inflammatory response. This inflammation can be local or spermatozoa can be "attacked" in those areas in which the tissue-spermatozoal barrier is the weakest. In many species, this is the region of the efferent ductules and the epididymis. This so-called autoimmune reaction to spermatozoa can be experimentally created, but a clinical correlate is infrequent. Local effects, however, are much more recognized. Direct damage to testicular parenchyma can result in granulomatous inflammation centered on the seminiferous tubules, the so-called intratubular orchitis. Where spermatozoa are exposed to the tissues of the body, the reaction is that of granulomatous inflammation. Macrophages and multinucleate giant cells are found adjacent to spermatozoa (see Fig. 19-2, *C*). Initially at least, $CD4^+$ T lymphocytes are abundant. Immunoglobulin-producing cells, particularly IgG-containing cells, are found. Granulomas are formed with the characteristic appearance of layers of epithelioid macrophages with multinucleate giant cells and then lymphocytes and plasma cells with a surrounding of fibrous tissue. In advanced cases, inspissated spermatozoa are found within a fibrous capsule. The production of a fibrous capsule and resultant contraction leads to further obstruction to the various adjacent ducts and tubules, with the result that additional spermiostasis, spermatocele, and spermatic granuloma formation continues. This inflammation therefore has devastating effects on fertility. Further complications occur if spermatozoa are released into the cavity of the vaginal tunics because a severe periorchitis develops and results in fibrosis and the lack of ability to adequately thermoregulate the testes.

DISORDERS OF DOMESTIC ANIMALS (HORSES, RUMINANTS [CATTLE, SHEEP, AND GOATS], PIGS, DOGS, AND CATS)

There are many different ways to approach disorders of the male reproductive system (see Appendix 19-1). Each approach has its own advantages and disadvantages. Some of the disorders affect more than one region, yet there are many disorders that have a primary manifestation in one anatomic location. Approaching disorders from a pathogenetic viewpoint is logical; however, it does not always account for clinical relevance or assist in the correlation between clinical signs and prognosis. Disorders are approached based on their anatomic location: scrotal contents, accessory genital glands, and the penis and prepuce—this approach is more clinically relevant. Before doing so, it is prudent to examine disorders of sexual development (DSD) because they fall in a distinct category.

DISORDERS OF SEXUAL DEVELOPMENT

There are a large number of anomalies of the male reproductive system (Box 19-2). Some have clinical relevance and others do not. Differentiating between these is very important. Some of the anomalies represent the most common disease of a particular species. Where this is the case, the disease is discussed under disorders of a particular anatomic location because this is the most clinically relevant place. We have attempted to divide the various anomalies into those that are major and minor based on effects on fertility and on the future breeding potential of the animal. Some anomalies have a genetic basis and such individuals should not be used as a stud animal, even though the animal may still be fertile.

Male Embryology

Normal males have an XY chromosomal sex. The differentiation of the bipotential fetal gonad to a testis depends on the presence of a gene—the sex-determining region of the Y chromosome *(SRY)*

BOX 19-2 Selected Congenital Anomalies

MAJOR ANOMALIES

Cryptorchidism
Testicular hypoplasia
Spermatic granuloma of the epididymal head
Ambiguous genitalia
- Tricolor cat (chimera)
- Persistent Müllerian duct syndrome
- Testicular feminization syndrome

Ciliary dyskinesia (immotile cilia syndrome)
Segmental aplasia of mesonephric duct

MINOR ANOMALIES

Inclusion cysts
Remnants of mesonephric ducts
- Internal and external paradidymis

Remnants of paramesonephric (Müllerian) ducts
- Appendix testis
- Cystic uterus masculinus

Hypospadias
Retained preputial band

that codes for the testis-determining factor and on other genes that cause the germ cells to go into mitotic arrest. Supporting cells become the Sertoli cells, the steroid-producing cells become the interstitial endocrine cells (Leydig cells), and the mesenchyme develops the appearance of a testis. Further development requires the activation of many other genes that are not on the Y chromosome. The expression of *SRY* occurs briefly in the somatic cells of the indifferent gonads (or genital ridges). Because expression ceases shortly before Sertoli cells can be recognized, it is proposed that the functional gene product of *SRY* influences other genes, such as *SOX9,* that ensure the differentiation and maintenance of Sertoli cells. *SOX9* is upregulated in XY individuals just before gonadal differentiation. Sertoli cells signal the other supporting cell precursor lines to differentiate along the male pathway. Early in sex differentiation, the embryo has a double set of ducts. The paramesonephric (Müllerian) ducts are female precursors, arising by invagination of the celomic cavity. The mesonephric (Wolffian) tubules and ducts are male precursors, arising from the primitive kidney, the mesonephros. The rete testis and efferent ductules are derived from mesonephric tubules. There are about 20 efferent ductules, although the number varies with species. The epididymis is derived from the part of the mesonephric duct within the mesonephros. The deferent duct, ampulla, and vesicular gland are derived from the distal part of the mesonephric duct, outside the mesonephros (Fig. 19-3).

After germ cells migrate from the yolk sac and the testes develop in the tissue of the genital ridge, the testes produce two hormones. Sertoli cells secrete the polypeptide hormone anti-Müllerian hormone (AMH, previously called Müllerian inhibitory substance) during embryonic development and at lower concentrations postnatally. AMH causes regression of the ipsilateral paramesonephric duct, indirectly through action on mesenchymal tissue. Sertoli cells stimulate differentiation of interstitial endocrine cells from the cells of the interstitium. Interstitial endocrine cells secrete the steroid hormone testosterone, which causes persistence and differentiation of the mesonephric ducts. Testosterone is likely transported down the mesonephric ducts rather than moving by simple diffusion. A third hormone, dihydrotestosterone, which is a metabolite of testosterone, is required for formation of the prostate gland, the closing of the urethral folds, and the formation of the penis and scrotum. The enzyme steroid 5α-reductase is produced by cells in the urogenital sinus, genital tubercle, and genital swellings and reduces testosterone to dihydrotestosterone. Functional androgen receptors on target tissues are necessary for androgen-dependent differentiation and growth. Species differences exist in whether the production of testosterone by interstitial endocrine cells is under the control of gonadotropin produced by the fetal pituitary gland or the placenta. Fetal interstitial endocrine cells are replaced by postnatal interstitial endocrine cells, which are relatively quiescent until puberty. The production of testosterone is regulated by luteinizing hormone (LH), which is under the control of gonadotropin-releasing hormone (GnRH) from the hypothalamus. Also, follicle-stimulating hormone (FSH) is controlled by GnRH; FSH is produced by the anterior pituitary gland. FSH regulates the activity of Sertoli cells and can thus influence AMH production. Sertoli cells stimulated by FSH produce a glycoprotein, androgen-binding protein, which fosters high testosterone concentration around the germ cells for the progression of spermatogenesis.

The external genitalia form when the genital tubercle is masculinized by the presence of androgens. Elongation of the tubercle forms the phallus; opposing urethral folds form the penile urethra; and the genital swellings fuse to form the scrotum.

Testicular Descent

The testes and epididymides undergo descent from their original location to the scrotum. There are three main phases in testicular descent: the abdominal translocation, the transinguinal migration and the inguinoscrotal migration. The developing gonads are held in place by cranial and caudal suspensory ligaments. The caudal ligament, the primitive gubernaculum testis, attaches the developing testis to the site of the inguinal canal. It develops into an intraabdominal and extraabdominal part that protrudes into the scrotum. Evagination of the peritoneum forms the inguinal canal and the vaginal tunic.

With the abdominal translocation phase particularly, stimulation of gubernaculum mesenchymal cells is controlled in rodents by the insulin-like peptide (INSL) hormone, INSL3. The receptor for INSL appears to be GREAT/LGR8. Other molecules are likely involved. The subsequent enlargement of the gubernaculum and progressive weakening of the cranial suspensory ligament anchors the testis so that with fetal growth, the testis retains its position near the inguinal canal.

Little is known of the transinguinal phase, apart from the lack of involvement of testosterone or INSL3. Dilation of the inguinal canal by the gubernaculum and then intraabdominal pressure is involved with movement of the testis through the inguinal canal to bring the testis and epididymis into a subcutaneous location. The third and inguinoscrotal phase of testicular descent is mediated by the hypothalamopituitary-induced production of gonadal androgens. Having said this, domestic animals with failure of testicular

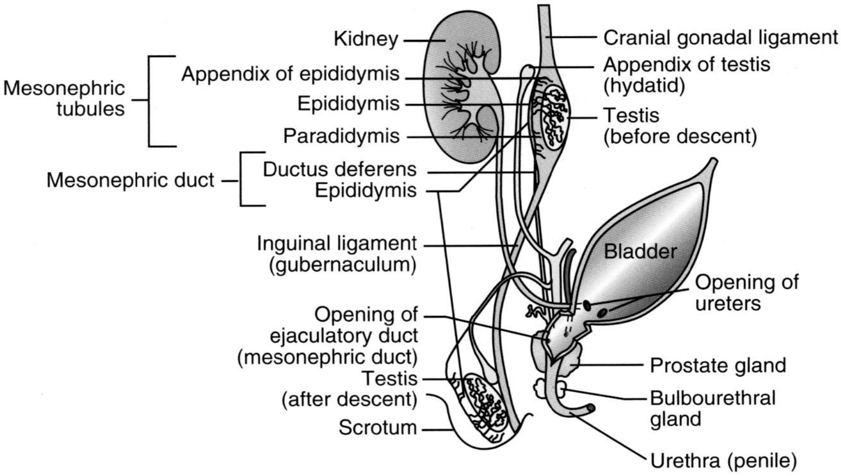

Fig. 19-3 Schematic diagram of the normal components of the male reproductive system and the embryonic structures, especially the mesonephric (Wolffian) duct and urogenital sinus and tubercle, from which they were derived.

The rete tubules and efferent ductules are formed from the mesonephric ductules; the epididymis, deferent duct, ampullae, and vesicular glands form from the mesonephric duct; the prostate and bulbourethral glands form from the urogenital sinus; and the penis, prepuce, and scrotum form from the genital tubercle and swellings.

descent into the scrotum seldom have a deficiency of testosterone or a lack of the androgen receptor. The genitofemoral nerve and calcitonin gene–related proteins or binding sites are involved in rodents.

Major Anomalies

The most common and important major anomaly of the male reproductive system is failure of testicular descent or cryptorchidism. Testicular hypoplasia and segmental aplasia of the epididymis are a close second. These disorders and conditions are discussed further in the section on Disorders of the Scrotum and Contents. Much less common, but nevertheless important, are other DSD.

Disorders of Sexual Development

Errors of chromosomal, gonadal, or phenotypic sex are usually manifested by abnormalities in sexual dimorphism. Many of the abnormalities result in a female phenotype and are mentioned in more detail in Chapter 18. The concentration here is on those disorders that involve animals that have male gonads or are predominantly phenotypic males. One cannot always tell the underlying cause of sexual ambiguity by examining phenotype or even identifying the gonadal type. Complete definition of a DSD requires knowledge of all three components: chromosomal, gonadal, and phenotypic types.

Chromosomal Disorders of Sexual Development

Sex chromosomes can be abnormal in structure or number. Two examples of abnormal structure of the Y chromosome are deletion of the short arm and isochromosome formation (duplication of one arm and loss of the other). Affected individuals have a female phenotype and extremely hypoplastic gonads. A few cattle have been identified with an isochromosome Y. With duplication of one of the sex chromosomes in an individual with a Y chromosome (XYY or XXY), or a mosaic (as occurs with the calico or tricolor male cats), the external genitalia are male in character. Klinefelter syndrome (XXY) is discussed in the section on Testicular Hypoplasia. Chimeras, such as XX/XY, are phenotypically sexually ambiguous, and the degree depends on the relative amounts of each chromosome. Freemartins are chimeras and are discussed in Chapter 18.

XX Disorders of Sexual Development

Animals with an XX genotype, testicular tissue, and a male phenotype are called XX sex reversal individuals. They may be *SRY* positive or *SRY* negative. XX *SRY*-negative DSD is reported in many breeds of dogs, in goats, and in horses. Affected individuals have an ovotestis or testis. Those with ovotestes or a testis and an ovary are called *hermaphrodites.* Some ovotestes have an end-to-end arrangement of ovarian and testicular tissue, with clear demarcation between the two. Others have central testicular tissue with a periphery of ovarian structures. Bilateral hermaphrodites have an ovotestis on each side; unilateral hermaphrodites have an ovotestis on one side; and lateral hermaphrodites have a testis on one side and an ovary on the other. The genital tract in hermaphrodites is ambiguous and can be phenotypic male, female, or various combinations of the two, depending on the amount of hormones, including testosterone and AMH. It is assumed that XX *SRY*-negative individuals have a testis-determining region on another chromosome. XX *SRY*-positive DSD is not reported in domestic mammals.

XY Disorders of Sexual Development

There are three classifications of XY disorders of sexual development; those with disorders of gonadal development (gonadal dysgenesis, ovotestes, or aplasia), disorders of androgen synthesis or action, and miscellaneous types. They can be either XY *SRY*-positive or XY *SRY*-negative. XY DSD are identified in many species, including dogs and horses.

XY *SRY*-negative individuals usually have primitive and undifferentiated gonads, called *gonadal dysgenesis,* and a female phenotype. Their classification is therefore XY *SRY*-negative, gonadal dysgenesis DSD. XY *SRY*-positive individuals with a female phenotype usually have testes and are called *male pseudohermaphrodites* (Figs. 19-4 and 19-5). The differentiation of the genital tract can be slightly or greatly abnormal. In many cases, the mechanism for the abnormal differentiation is unknown, but there are well-recognized

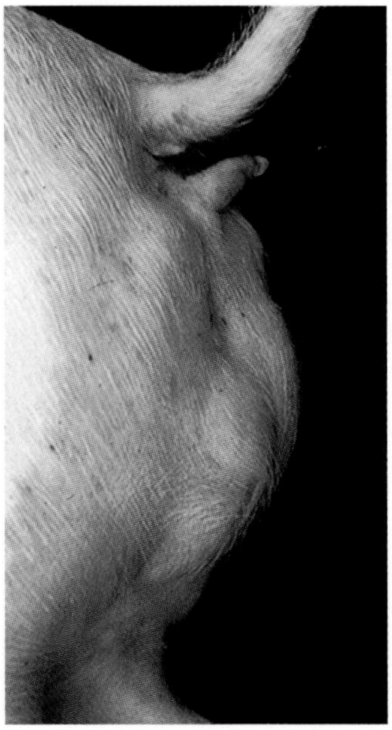

Fig. 19-4 XY disorder of sexual development, male pseudohermaphrodite, external genitalia, boar.
This pig has a scrotum and intrascrotal testes, but the penis is small and clitoris-like and has a terminal urethral opening (ventral to the tail). (Courtesy Dr. D. Dodd; and Noah's Arkive, College of Veterinary Medicine, The University of Georgia.)

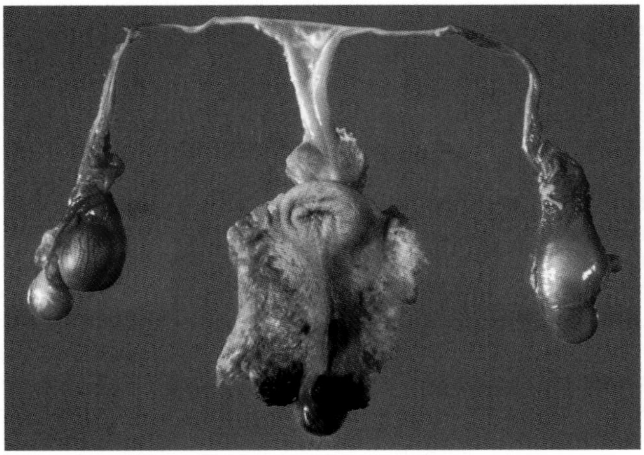

Fig. 19-5 XY disorder of sexual development, male pseudohermaphrodite (male feminization syndrome), reproductive tract, ram.
This sheep has testes, deferent ducts, and accessory genital glands but also a vulva and a prominent clitoris. An androgen receptor defect would explain these anomalies. (Courtesy RA Foster, Ontario Veterinary College, University of Guelph.)

syndromes in which the underlying pathogenesis is known. Three such syndromes are persistent Müllerian duct syndrome (PMDS), androgen insensitivity, and steroid 5α-reductase deficiency.

PMDS is a rare disorder of AMH production or function. AMH can be absent or present in affected humans; the syndrome can be a result of either a mutation in the *AMH* gene or the AMH receptor. In animals, the syndrome is described in miniature schnauzer dogs and basset hounds with an autosomal recessive mode of inheritance and in a goat with an unknown mode of inheritance. Affected dogs have XY (or XXY) chromosomes and externally are normal males, with the common exception of unilateral or bilateral cryptorchidism. The testes, however, are attached to the cranial ends of uterine horns. When a testis has descended into the scrotum, the uterine horn passes through the inguinal ring. The deferent duct can be found microscopically within the myometrium. The cranial vagina and the prostate gland are often present. AMH is present in the testes of normal male dogs up to 143 days of age. AMH is present in the testes of young affected dogs also and is bioactive. A mutation in the structural gene for the AMH receptor results in AMH resistance in PMDS-affected dogs. Dogs with unilateral or bilateral scrotal testes can be fertile. Affected dogs may develop Sertoli cell tumor, hydrometra, and pyometra. Testicular abnormalities in PMDS, such as reduced spermatogenesis and tubular sclerosis, could be attributable to cryptorchidism. Cryptorchidism could be the result of interference with the MIS-controlled first phase of the function of the gubernaculums, the phase in which the testis migrates to the inguinal area.

Deficiency of 5α-reductase type 2, inherited as an autosomal recessive trait in humans, has not yet been documented in animals, but in all likelihood, it does exist. The enzyme converts testosterone to dihydrotestosterone, which is required for the masculinization of the urogenital sinus, tubercle, and genital swellings. Without dihydrotestosterone, these structures become caudal vagina, vestibule, clitoris, and vulva. Internally, mesonephric structures (deferent duct, epididymis) develop. The testes are likely to be retained.

Androgen receptor disorders are becoming increasingly recognized. Most cases are caused by a mutation in the androgen receptor gene, which is located on the X chromosome and thus in a single copy. Hundreds of mutations have been identified in other species, and the effects range from complete androgen insensitivity with female external genitalia (testicular feminization) (see Fig. 19-5) to mild male pseudohermaphroditism. The testes produce testosterone, but the stimulation of the mesonephric system is not normal because of defective androgen receptors. The normal androgen receptor has a hormone-binding and a DNA-binding domain; once activated by androgen, the domain changes shape and is able to bind to specific DNA sequences and regulate the transcription of other specific genes, leading to normal male differentiation. In humans with androgen insensitivity, the gene is rarely deleted, but numerous point mutations in the receptor gene have been identified, mostly in the hormone-binding and DNA-binding domains. Whether the result is partial or complete androgen insensitivity depends on the location of the mutation and the change in function of the receptor. Dihydrotestosterone binds to the androgen receptor with greater affinity than that of testosterone, and the receptor, when it acts as a transcriptional factor, might interact with different genes other than the testosterone-bound receptor. In domestic animals, complete androgen insensitivity is described in the equine, bovine, and feline species. The testes are often cryptorchid and are in the inguinal area. The first and second phases of testicular migration is normal. The inguinoscrotal third phase, which is under the control of androgens, does not occur. AMH produced by the testes causes regression of the paramesonephric ducts. External genitalia are female in complete androgen insensitivity, with a cranial blind end to the vagina, and neither the paramesonephric nor mesonephric ductal system is present.

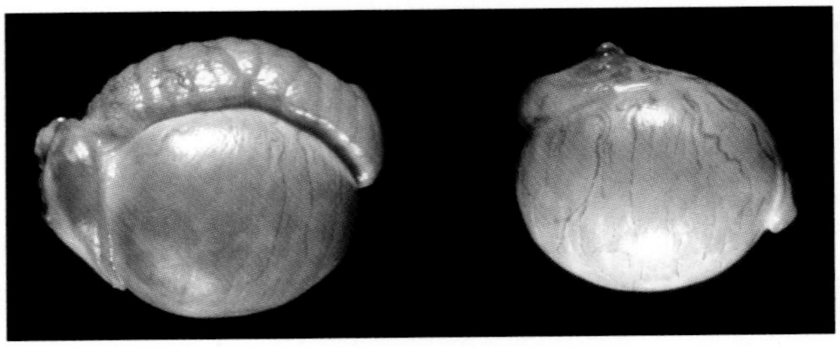

Fig. 19-6 Segmental aplasia, epididymis, dog.
There is no tail of the epididymis of the right testis. This portion of the mesonephric duct did not develop. The left testis is normal. (Courtesy College of Veterinary Medicine, University of Illinois.)

Cryptorchidism is an XY *SRY*-positive DSD but is examined in detail as a separate entity in the discussion of the testis in the section on Disorders of the Scrotum and Contents.

Segmental Aplasia of Mesonephric Duct Derivatives

Segmental aplasia of the structures of mesonephric ductal origin (epididymis, deferent duct, ampulla, or vesicular gland) can involve any of the structures, but it most commonly involves the epididymis alone (Fig. 19-6) and less commonly other structures. Segmental aplasia is reported mainly in the bull and most commonly involves the body and tail of the epididymis and is unilateral. Its inheritance is thought to be autosomal recessive. Spermatozoa become impacted because the epididymal duct is blind ending; local dilation or rupture occurs secondarily, allowing escape of spermatozoa and formation of spermatic granulomas.

Ciliary Dyskinesia (Immotile Cilia Syndrome)

One or more of several defects in the axoneme of cilia throughout the body and of the flagellum of spermatozoa causes ciliary dyskinesia, a rare disease identified in humans, dogs, pigs, mice, and rats. An autosomal recessive mode of inheritance is proposed. In dogs, heterogeneity of ultrastructural abnormalities of microtubule doublets and their dynein arms or central microtubules is reported. The effect on the reproductive system is immotile or hypomotile spermatozoa caused by flagellar lesions or to oligospermia (a subnormal concentration of spermatozoa) or azoospermia (no spermatozoa), presumably because of defective cilia in the epididymis and deferent duct. Because of defective cilia in the nasal mucosa, bronchial and bronchiolar mucosa, and ependyma, commonly associated lesions are rhinitis, bronchopneumonia, bronchiectasis, and hydrocephalus. Also associated is situs inversus, but the pathogenesis of the reversal of the normal left and right orientation of organs is unclear. Female infertility is related to defective function of cilia of the uterine tube.

Minor Anomalies

There are myriad minor anomalies that are of little consequence except when they are confused with other conditions that do affect fertility. Foremost of the minor anomalies are the various cysts that occur as a result of duplication or failure of regression of embryonic ducts and tubules.

Cysts of the Male Tract

It is often difficult to identify the origin of an individual cyst or group of cysts. In many instances, anatomic location is the

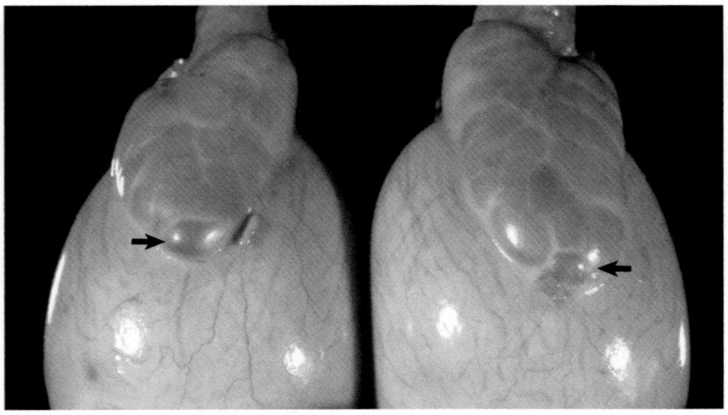

Fig. 19-7 Congenital inclusion cysts, testis and epididymis, ram. These 7-mm cysts *(arrows)* in the tissue between the head of the epididymis and testis are incidental findings and are not significant. (Courtesy Drs. P. W. Ladds and R. A. Foster, James Cook University of North Queensland.)

determining factor. Many of the cysts are simply called *inclusion cysts* (Fig. 19-7). These have a wall of compressed collagen, a thin inner lining of flattened cells, and a clear fluid content. They are found where mesothelial cells are trapped adjacent to a serosal surface. Inclusion cysts attached to the head of the epididymis are good examples.

The testis is derived from gonadal cords that form between the gonadal ridge on the medial side of the mesonephros and remnants of mesonephric tubules. The rete testis and efferent ductules are derived from mesonephric tubules. Within the mesonephros, many mesonephric tubules enter the single mesonephric duct. It is from the mesonephric part of the duct that the epididymis is derived. The deferent duct, ampulla, and vesicular gland are derived from the more caudal part of the mesonephric duct, outside the mesonephros. In the developed testis, about 20 efferent ductules are found, but the number varies with the species. Efferent ductules normally link in the head of the epididymis. Blind efferent ductules result when there is no connection to the epididymis and can be resorbed or persist and enlarge to form cysts or rupture. Blind-ending efferent ductules can be present in sufficient numbers to cause spermiostasis, spermatocele, and spermatic granulomas. The condition known as *spermatic granuloma of the epididymal head* (SGEH) is thus formed (see the section on Spermatic Granulomas and Epididymitis).

Unconnected with the lumen of the epididymal duct and efferent ductules, remnants of tubules of the mesonephros can form cysts adjacent to the head of the epididymis (external paradidymis) or within the head of the epididymis (internal paradidymis). Cysts, both connected and unconnected with the ductular system, are lined by ciliated columnar epithelium. They are clinically significant if they become large enough to cause stasis of spermatozoa in adjacent structures, or if they rupture and liberate spermatozoa into the surrounding tissue. The remnant of the paramesonephric duct, called the appendix testis, is not clinically significant and located on the cranial or cranioventral surface (depending on the species orientation of the testes) of the testis near the head of the epididymis. Sometimes, this small nodule of tissue can appear cystic. A similar cystic structure is found in the band of tissue between the ampullae. It is called the *cystic uterus masculinus* (Fig. 19-8). Some prostatic cysts of dogs have a similar origin.

DISORDERS OF THE SCROTUM AND CONTENTS

Disease of the scrotal contents is based on a clinical approach in which the scrotal skin, vaginal tunics, testis and the epididymis are examined in turn. The most economically important disorders are those that affect the testis and epididymis, although the importance of disorders of the scrotal skin and tunics should not be forgotten. They directly affect thermoregulation and can be confused with disorders of the testis, epididymis, or spermatic cord.

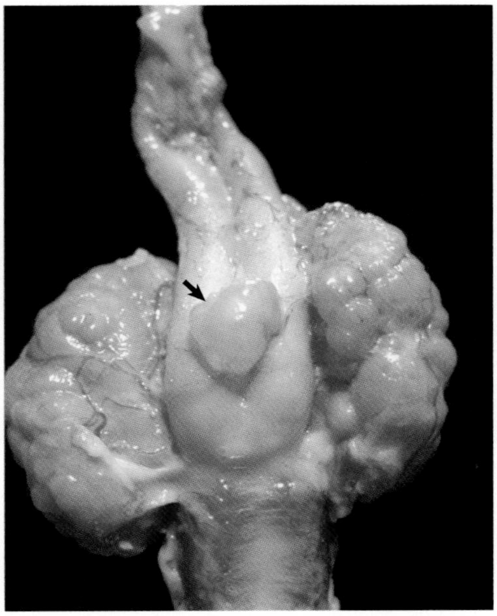

Fig. 19-8 Cystic uterus masculinus, accessory genital glands, ram. This sheep has a 1-cm thin-walled cyst in the tissue between the ampullae of the deferent ducts *(arrow)*. (Courtesy Drs. P. W. Ladds and R. A. Foster, James Cook University of North Queensland.)

The Scrotum

The fusion of the paired primordia of scrotal skin depends on androgens produced by cells of the gonad after it has differentiated into a testis. Altered androgen concentration or a lack of androgen receptors can lead to defects in the scrotum such as failure of fusion, cleft formation, or bifurcation. Defects can be local, confined to the scrotum and penis, or part of a wider range of defects in DSD. Hypospadias, in which the urethra opens on the ventral side of the penis, can be part of these anomalies.

Dermatitis of the scrotal skin is common. Often, it is nonspecific or involved in generalized dermatopathies. Dermatitis restricted to the scrotum can be the result of trauma, frostbite (Fig. 19-9), or exposure to environmental irritants such as cement dust. Some pathogens have the scrotum as a predilection site. These include *Dermatophilus congolensis* and *Besnoitia besnoiti* in the bull and *Chorioptes bovis* in the ram (Fig. 19-10). The heat generated in scrotal dermatitis can interfere with the thermoregulatory function of the scrotum, leading to testicular degeneration.

Neoplasms of any of the types that occur in the skin can occur in the scrotum but are much less common in the scrotal skin. Neoplasms occasionally encountered are papillomas in the boar and mast cell tumors and hemangiosarcomas in the dog. Testicular tumors, especially Sertoli cell tumors and interstitial cell tumors, occur in the scrotum of previously castrated male dogs and cats, respectively, presumably from cells inadvertently transplanted at surgery. Vascular abnormalities, often called *hemangiomas* and which are probably hamartomas, occur on the scrotum of the boar and dog. The scrotal veins of bulls sometimes become varicose.

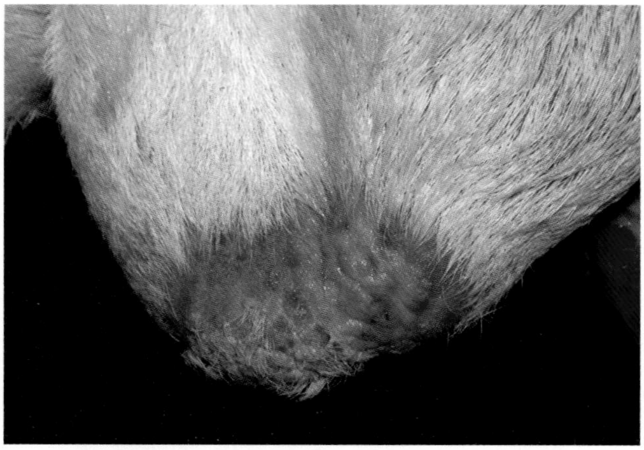

Fig. 19-9 Frostbite, scrotum, ram.
The skin of the lower portion of the scrotal sac has sloughed. The ventral scrotal skin is alopecic or covered by crusts from previous frostbite. (Courtesy Dr. R. A. Foster, Ontario Veterinary College, University of Guelph.)

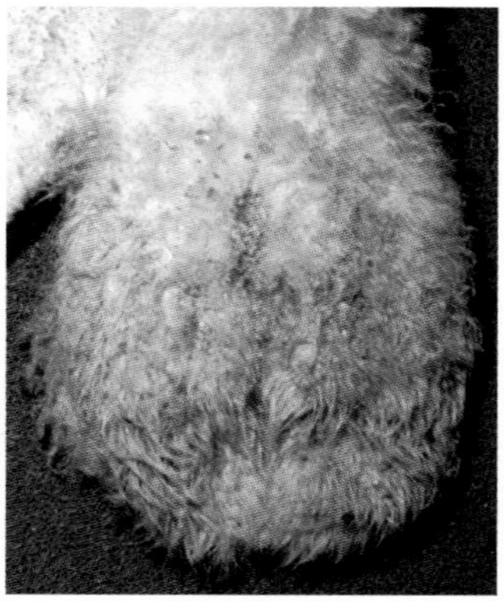

Fig. 19-10 Scrotal dermatitis *(Chorioptes bovis)*, scrotum, ram.
There is extensive crusting and exudation of the skin in response to the chronic irritation and inflammation caused by the mites. (Courtesy Dr. R. A. Foster, Ontario Veterinary College, University of Guelph.)

Vaginal Tunic

The vaginal tunics are the extension of the peritoneum that lines the scrotal sac as the parietal layer and covers the testis, epididymis, and spermatic cord as the visceral layer. The cavity between the two layers is continuous with the peritoneal cavity. The tunics and the cavity thus are subject to all the disorders of the peritoneum and peritoneal cavity. Ascites therefore results in hydrocele or fluid accumulating within the tunics around the scrotal contents. Polyserositis in pigs especially and feline infectious peritonitis (FIP) in cats causes inflammation of the tunics and periorchitis. Neoplasia is uncommon; mesothelioma and peritoneal carcinomatosis are the most frequently encountered. Parasitic disease, especially the cysts of *Cysticercus tenuicollis* in rams, occurs periodically and can be confused with cysts or spermatic granulomas.

Inflammation of the vaginal tunics without initial inflammation of the abdominal peritoneum can be the result of trauma or local infection. The latter is likely to be an extension from orchitis or epididymitis. Especially well-known causes are trypanosomiasis in bulls, rams, and bucks, and *Brucella ovis* and *Actinobacillus seminis* in rams. Adhesions between the parietal and visceral vaginal tunic are fibrinous at first and later fibrous.

BOX 19-3 Intrascrotal Disorder–Based Differences in Size of the Testis and/or Epididymis

DECREASED SIZE
Cryptorchidism
Hypoplasia
Segmental aplasia
Testicular atrophy/degeneration

INCREASED SIZE (INCLUDING MASSES)
Spermatic granuloma of epididymal head
Epididymitis
Orchitis
Periorchitis
Testicular neoplasia
- Seminoma, teratoma
- Sertoli cell tumor
- Interstitial cell tumor

Congenital cysts
Varicocele
Torsion
Inguinal hernia
Scrotal lymphadenopathy

Testis and Epididymis

The testis and epididymis are inseparable, and disease of one usually results in disease of the other. Scrotal palpation is the main clinical method to identify abnormalities of this region, and the changes in size are the most obvious. We therefore use a size approach, beginning with those that cause small scrotal contents, then with those that result in enlargement of one or more of the intrascrotal structures (Box 19-3).

Reduced Testicular and Epididymal Size

Missing or aplastic components are rare. Segmental aplasia of the mesonephric duct, usually aplasia of the epididymal tail (see Fig. 19-6), is one example. It is described earlier under major anomalies. If one complete side of the scrotal contents is missing, either unilateral castration was performed or the affected animal was a unilateral cryptorchid. Sometimes, the undescended testis and epididymis subsequently descend, or the castration operator may have missed a testis and epididymis. Affected sheep, for example, often have the scrotum removed, and the testis is located beneath the underlying skin. A lack of both sides of the scrotal contents can represent castration or bilateral cryptorchidism and requires additional investigation, including measurements of hormonal concentrations, especially after treatment with GnRH, or surgical exploration. A search for secondary characteristics that are testosterone dependent, such as the barbs on the penis of the cat and the presence of a prostate in dogs, can assist in separating behavioral characteristics from similar behaviors in incompletely castrated males.

A small testicular size is of great importance, especially to production animals, as daily sperm output is correlated to testicular volume and weight. A small size indicates hypoplasia or atrophy. It can be extremely difficult to differentiate unless there is a history of size change. Hypoplasia is a congenital condition in which the testis does not increase to its full size at puberty. It is often seen as part of other syndromes, most commonly cryptorchidism.

Cryptorchidism

Cryptorchidism occurs when there is incomplete descent of the testis (normal testicular descent is discussed earlier). In most mammalian species, the testis normally descends into the scrotum by the time of birth. Cryptorchidism is more often unilateral than bilateral, with the side being somewhat species dependent. Many undescended testes are on the right side. In the horse, the distribution is equal left to right, and in the bull, the left side is usually affected. The undescended testis can be anywhere along its path from caudal to the kidney (Figs. 19-11 and 19-12, *A*) to the scrotum but is commonly within the abdomen near the internal inguinal ring, within the inguinal canal or in a subcutaneous location just outside the external inguinal ring. Epididymal development is coordinated with testicular development and consequently is slowed in cryptorchidism.

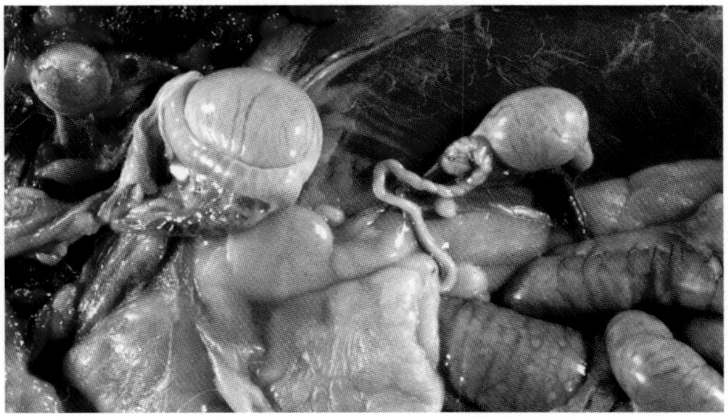

Fig. 19-11 Cryptorchid testis, intraabdominal, dog.
The retained testis and epididymis *(right)* are hypoplastic. The other descended testis *(left)* is normal. Intestines are below the right testis. (Courtesy Dr. Y. Niyo, College of Veterinary Medicine, Iowa State University; and Noah's Arkive, College of Veterinary Medicine, The University of Georgia.)

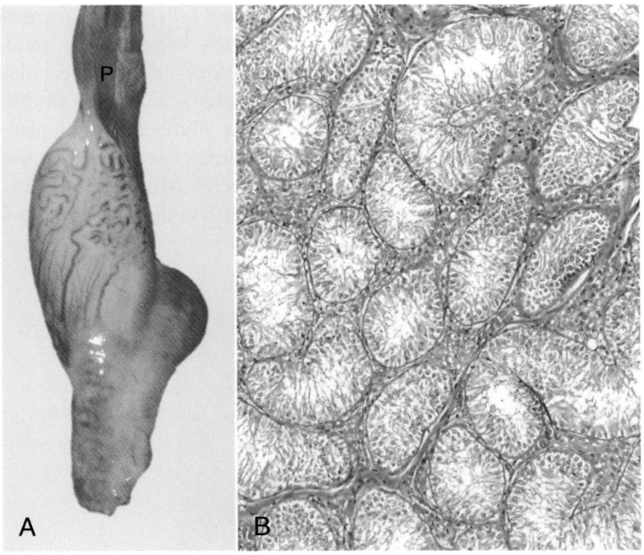

Fig. 19-12 Cryptorchid testis.
A, Cryptorchid testis and epididymis, bull calf. The testis and epididymis are hypoplastic and are barely larger than the pampiniform plexus above *(P)*. There are no attachments to the vaginal tunic. **B**, Cryptorchid testis, dog. There is complete absence of spermatogenesis; however, the Sertoli cells are normal. H&E stain. (**A** courtesy Dr. R.A. Foster, Ontario Veterinary College, University of Guelph. **B** courtesy Dr. J.A. Ramos-Vara, College of Veterinary Medicine, Michigan State University; and Noah's Arkive, College of Veterinary Medicine, The University of Georgia.)

Cryptorchidism is the most common disorder of sexual development (DSD). Most are XY *SRY*-positive with testes but with a disorder of phenotypic sex. It has a polygenetic basis and a reasonable working hypothesis is a sex-limited autosomal recessive mode of inheritance. It can be the result of a failure of normal production or regulation by one or more genes for the production of testosterone, androgen receptor, INSL3, INSL3 receptor, and/or calcitonin gene–related protein. Descriptions of cryptorchidism should include whether it is unilateral or bilateral and which stage of descent is abnormal (abdominal translocation, transinguinal migration, and inguinoscrotal migration).

In the horse, left and right testicular retention are almost equal in occurrence and the left retained testis is more likely to be abdominal than inguinal in location. Three breeds (Percheron, American saddle horse, and American quarter horse), ponies, and crossbred horses were significantly overrepresented in a large hospital-based study of cryptorchidism.

Abnormalities in the gubernaculum could cause cryptorchidism by its failure to develop, improper positioning, excessive growth, or failure to regress. In humans, some other predisposing or contributing factors for cryptorchidism include testicular hypoplasia, estrogen exposure in pregnancy, breech labor compromising blood supply to the testes, and late closing of the umbilicus, delaying the ability to increase abdominal pressure.

A cryptorchid testis remains small at puberty, probably because of its higher than optimal temperature. Superimposed atrophy occurs in the cryptorchid testis after puberty. The testis is small and fibrotic and has interstitial collagen deposition, hyaline thickening of the tubular basement membranes, and degeneration of germinal epithelium so that only a few spermatogonia remain with the normal complement of Sertoli cells (Fig. 19-12, *B*).

Cryptorchid testes are much more prone to develop neoplasia than scrotally placed ones. In the dog, Sertoli cell tumors are more likely to occur in the testes present in the abdomen (Fig. 19-13), whereas seminomas tend to develop more commonly in inguinally placed testes. The contralateral testis is also at increased risk for

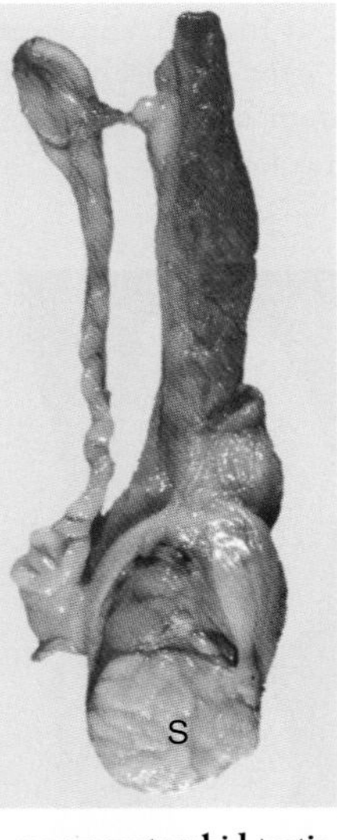

Fig. 19-13 Sertoli cell tumor, cryptorchid testis, dog.
The testicular parenchyma has been replaced by a white multilobular Sertoli cell tumor *(S)*. The texture is firm, indicating fibrosis. This dog had bilaterally retained testes and epididymides and bilateral Sertoli cell tumors. (Courtesy Dr. R. A. Foster, Ontario Veterinary College, University of Guelph.)

developing a neoplasm, even if that testis is located in the scrotum. A retained testis, especially if enlarged by a neoplasm, is prone to torsion.

Cryptorchidism is a phenotypic DSD. Many animals with other DSD have cryptorchidism, and genetic testing can identify these disorders. Some of these individuals have ovotestes. The greater the ratio of testicular to ovarian tissue, the more likely an ovotestis has descended into the scrotum. A testis most often lies in the scrotum, and an ovary is in its normal position. The ovary or ovarian portion of an ovotestis is histologically normal, but the seminiferous tubules of a testis or ovotestis are abnormal because of a combination of cryptorchidism and the effects of estrogen produced by the ovarian tissue.

Testicular Hypoplasia

Hypoplasia of the testes is a common condition in which the testis is smaller than normal for the age of the animal, and it is often present in disorders such as cryptorchidism and other DSD. Hypoplasia of the testis and epididymis in an otherwise normal male is the specific focus here.

It is difficult to distinguish hypoplasia from testicular atrophy by using morphologic features. Both testicular hypoplasia and atrophy can occur alone, with no apparent contributing or influencing factors; either can also be associated with, secondary to, or part of some other lesion. Testicular and epididymal hypoplasia (Fig. 19-14, *A* and *B*) has been causally linked to poor general nutrition, zinc deficiency, specific genes in the Swedish red and white breed of cattle, and endocrine and cytogenetic abnormalities. Endocrine disturbances causing testicular hypoplasia are those that reduce production of either luteinizing hormone by the pituitary gland, which in turn influences testosterone production by the interstitial endocrine cells, or FSH by the pituitary gland, which stimulates the nurturing function of the Sertoli cells.

A wide range of cytogenetic abnormalities, from translocations and mosaics to nondisjunctions causing polysomies of sex chromosomes, result in testicular hypoplasia. The best known example of polysomy is the XXY karyotype of Klinefelter syndrome seen in stallions, bulls, boars, dogs, and tricolor cats. In cats, the syndrome is recognized in males with the tricolor, tortoise shell, or calico coat types. These cats can be XXY, XX/XXY, or more complex chimeras or mosaics with two or more X chromosomes and one or more Y chromosomes. The gene for black and the gene for orange are carried one per X chromosome, and so a normal male cat should not have hair of both colors.

Hypoplasia of the testis can theoretically occur when the number or length of seminiferous tubules is reduced, or when there are no or insufficient germ cells. Usually before puberty, the seminiferous tubules have only Sertoli cells and spermatogonia (see Fig. 19-14, *B*). At puberty, the tubules of hypoplastic testes undergo an irregular progressive sclerosis and become collagenous, presumably from concurrent degeneration. Interstitial endocrine cells appear to be more numerous and clustered.

Hypoplasia of the testes is not apparent until after puberty. Unilateral hypoplasia is more common than bilateral hypoplasia, but this difference in prevalence could be a reflection of the relative ease of recognizing a size abnormality when the normal contralateral testis is available for ready comparison. Unilateral hypoplasia is difficult to explain because most of the causes seem to act systemically and therefore should produce a bilateral effect.

The size range of a hypoplastic testis generally is from a prepubertal size (see Fig. 19-14, *A*) to almost normal. The consistency of a hypoplastic testis is near to normal. The severity of the hypoplasia can be graded histologically by the proportion of hypoplastic tubules scattered through the organ. Hypoplastic tubules have a small diameter and are lined only by Sertoli cells and sometimes a few spermatogonia. Interstitial endocrine cells appear proportionally more numerous, but this is only because the tubular area is reduced and the relative amount of interstitium is increased. In severe testicular hypoplasia, most or all of the tubules are abnormal; the tubules have a small diameter and a uniform microscopic appearance with only infrequent vacuolation of Sertoli cells and without a thickened basement membrane. In moderate hypoplasia, fewer tubules are small, those of normal size have some differentiation of the seminiferous epithelium, and a few tubules have complete spermatogenesis. In most tubules, however, when the stage of spermatocyte formation is reached, the spermatocytes undergo apoptosis or degeneration, leaving tubules lined by Sertoli cells with a vacuolated cytoplasm. The lumen of such tubules can contain cellular debris and multinucleate cells that are formed when dividing cells fail to separate. When hypoplasia is mild, only a few small tubules are lined only by Sertoli cells; most tubules have normal spermatogenesis. Mild hypoplasia is difficult to distinguish from testicular degeneration. The number of hypoplastic tubules would not be expected to increase with age because hypoplastic tubules do not arise after puberty. Mild hypoplasia is detected when scrotal circumference is just less than the accepted minimum.

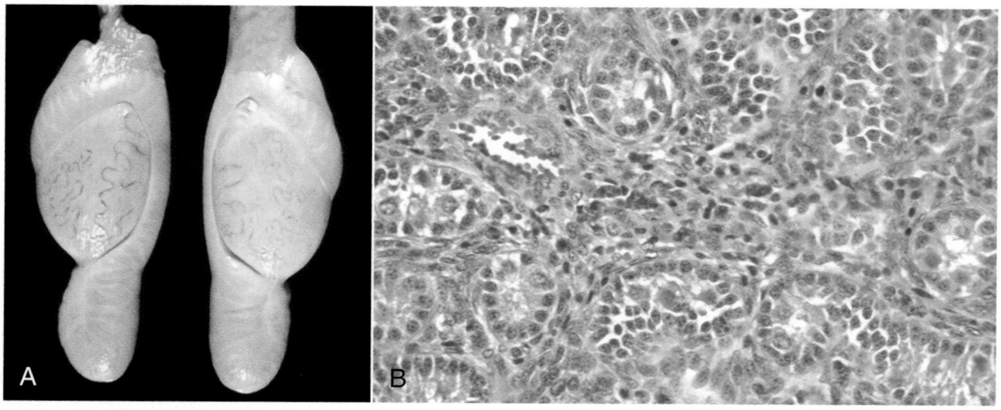

Fig. 19-14 Bilateral hypoplasia, testes, yearling ram.
A, Both testes and epididymides from this yearling ram are very small compared with normal age-matched controls. **B**, The seminiferous tubules are lined only by Sertoli cells, and there is no spermatogenesis. H&E stain. (Courtesy Dr. R. A. Foster, Ontario Veterinary College, University of Guelph.)

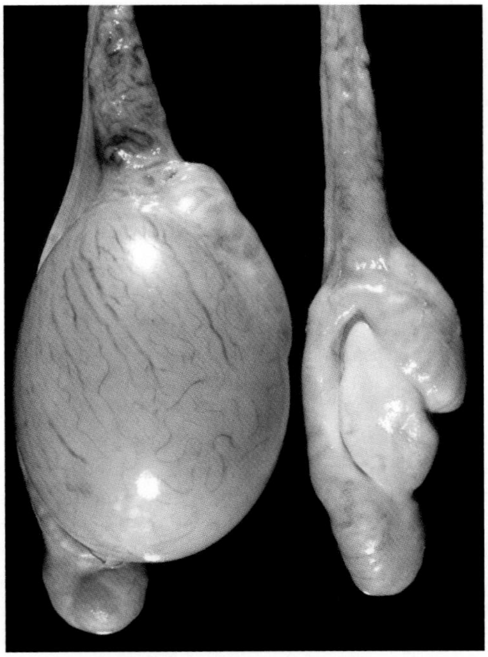

Fig. 19-15 Unilateral testicular atrophy and epididymitis, testis and epididymis, ram.
The affected testis *(right)* is small, and testicular veins are not visible on the capsule of the testis because of fibrosis and contraction of the connective tissue. The other testis *(left)* is bulbous, indicating hypertrophy. (Courtesy Drs. P. W. Ladds and R. A. Foster, James Cook University of North Queensland.)

Testicular Atrophy and Degeneration

Testes that reduce in size after puberty are macroscopically atrophic, and the microscopic change is degeneration of the seminiferous tubules. Testicular atrophy is a common lesion. Mild testicular degeneration can be detected only microscopically, but when it is severe and chronic, the testis is small and firm (Fig. 19-15). The causes are many, and in a particular individual, the specific cause is often unknown. Degeneration can be unilateral or bilateral, depending on whether the cause is local or systemic. In young growing males, the distinction between testicular degeneration and hypoplasia is often difficult to make using morphologic features. Both lesions are often present together because hypoplastic testes are prone to degeneration. Inflammation also can be superimposed on degeneration when there is obstruction, leading to back pressure, rupture of seminiferous tubules, and spermatic granuloma formation. Recovery of a testis with degeneration back to a normal testis is possible if the injurious agent is eliminated and damage is not too severe.

Specific causes of testicular degeneration are numerous (Box 19-4). Increased apoptosis of germ cells is a common endpoint of many causes, regardless of whether the initial effect is on the hypothalamo-pituitary-gonadal endocrine axis or on the Sertoli cell–interstitial cell–germ cell axis. Fever or local heat from inflammation of the scrotal skin is a classic cause of degeneration. Obstruction of flow of spermatozoa causes testicular degeneration. Obstruction can be the result of developmental anomalies such as segmental aplasia of mesonephric duct derivatives, local injury, or inflammation of the epididymis. Vascular events, such as impairment from aging, torsion, or severe crushing of the spermatic cord, cause degeneration. Systemic injurious factors include nutritional deficiency, hormonal aberrations, toxins, irradiation, and oxidative stress. Hypovitaminosis A and zinc deficiency are specific nutritional deficiencies; general malnutrition also causes testicular degeneration. Interference with GnRH, LH and its control of androgen production by interstitial endocrine cells, or FSH and its effect on the production of androgen-binding protein by Sertoli cells can have a deleterious effect on the seminiferous epithelium. Such interference could happen, for example, when a neoplasm of the pituitary gland causes local compression of the pituitary gland, the hypothalamus, or both. Estrogen produced by Sertoli cell tumors induces testicular degeneration. Environmentally acquired endocrine disruptors are also implicated. Some therapeutic drugs, such as amphotericin B, gentamicin, and chemotherapy compounds, cause testicular degeneration.

Many toxins are capable of causing testicular degeneration, and most damage the spermatogonia and dividing primary spermatocytes, but some damage later stages and spermatocytes and spermatids or injure Sertoli cells.

BOX 19-4 Some of the Known Causes of Testicular Atrophy/Degeneration in Mammals, Including Rodents

Advancing age
Chlorinated naphthalenes
Epididymitis
Chemicals
- Chemotherapy
- Halogenated compounds, including hexachlorophene
- Nitrogen-containing compounds, including benzimidazoles and nitrofurans

Heat
Hormones
- Dexamethasone
- Estrogen
- Testosterone
- Zeranolone

Metal compound toxicosis
Neoplasia
- Pituitary tumors
- Sertoli cell tumors

Nutritional disorders
- Negative energy balance
- Fatty acid deficiency
- Hypovitaminosis A
- Hypervitaminosis A
- Hypovitaminosis B
- Hypovitaminosis E
- Hypovitaminosis C
- Oxidative stress
- Protein and amino acid deficiency
- Zinc deficiency

Plants
- Locoweed (*Astragalus*)
- Lysine seeds

Radiation
Scrotal disease
Stress/corticosteroid therapy
Trauma
Ultrasound
Viral infection
- Distemper virus
- PRRS (porcine reproductive and respiratory syndrome) virus

A testis undergoing degeneration initially is softer than normal, and as the degeneration progresses, the testis becomes smaller. The cut surface of the normal testis and the acutely degenerated testis bulges slightly. After the acute phase, the testis becomes firmer and has small flecks or large areas of mineralization, especially in ruminants. Degeneration can be either generalized or regional, occurring in the ventral portion of the testis of bulls or in the dorsal part of the testis (near the head of the epididymis) in rams. If the degeneration is caused by ischemia after a vascular accident in the spermatic cord, small islands of parenchyma beneath the testicular capsule can survive the infarction because of diffusion of oxygen from vessels of the epididymis and capsule of the testis. Degeneration can occur locally around a lesion, such as a neoplasm, that expands and causes compression.

Microscopically, the initial change is spermatogenic arrest at one or more stages of the spermatogenic cycle. The seminiferous tubules have a smaller diameter. With further degeneration, there is a thickened basement membrane, decreased numbers of germinal cells, vacuolated Sertoli cells, intratubular multinucleated spermatids, and interstitial fibrosis (Fig. 19-16, *A* and *B*). A key lesion in the differentiation of testicular degeneration from testicular hypoplasia is the wavy basement membrane found in testicular degeneration because affected tubules had at some stage reached full size and then subsequently collapsed. At the end stage of testicular degeneration, Sertoli cells are the only lining cells remaining, but with time, these also disappear, leaving only the basement membranes. Mineralization can involve intratubular cellular debris, tubular basement membranes, or the interstitium.

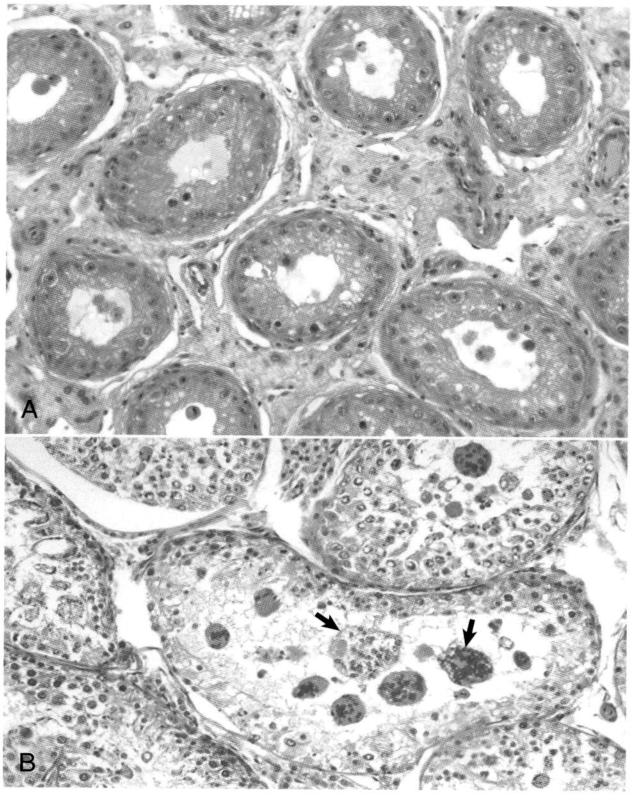

Fig. 19-16 Testicular degeneration, testis.
A, Ram. There is interstitial fibrosis that separates the seminiferous tubules. Spermatogenic arrest at the spermatocyte stage, vacuolation of Sertoli cells, and a wavy basement membrane caused by a reduction in tubular diameter are present. H&E stain. **B**, Dog. In addition to reduced spermatogenesis, there is formation of multinucleated spermatids *(arrows)* as a result of failure of spermatids to separate. This is a common change in testicular degeneration. (Courtesy Dr. R. A. Foster, Ontario Veterinary College, University of Guelph.)

Degeneration of the epididymis is less well studied but does occur. In degenerative conditions, the epididymis is much less likely to be reduced in size. This lack of reduction in size can be helpful in differentiating testicular atrophy from hypoplasia macroscopically. In the former, the epididymis approximates adult size, whereas in hypoplasia the epididymis is small in size.

Testicular and Epididymal Enlargement

There are several disorders that result in testicular and epididymal enlargement. Foremost is inflammation, especially epididymitis and orchitis. Testicular neoplasia is a common cause in dogs.

Spermatic Granulomas and Epididymitis

Spermatic granuloma of the epididymal head is a unique congenital disease of most species. It is not an infectious condition, but inflammation dominates as a response to extravasated spermatozoa. It affects the efferent ductule region first, and then spreads to involve the head of the epididymis (Fig. 19-17, *A*). All efferent ductules should connect to the single epididymal duct in the head of the epididymis, but some are blind-ended. At puberty, the blind-ending ductules fill with spermatozoa and the resultant spermiostasis proceeds to spermatocele and then spermatic granulomas (Fig. 19-17, *B*). These progress over time and result in infertility because of obstruction of the epididymal duct. The back pressure produced by the spermatic granulomas causes dilation of the mediastinum of the testis and testicular atrophy.

Epididymitis is very important in rams (Fig. 19-18) and dogs (Fig. 19-19) and is rare in other species. The tail of the epididymis is almost always affected, allowing the majority of cases to be differentiated from spermatic granuloma of the epididymal head. Because the epididymis is only a single coiled duct, any lesion along its length has the potential to cause obstruction of spermatozoal flow and the formation of spermatic granulomas. Thus epididymitis is frequently accompanied by spermatic granulomas and also periorchitis. Epididymitis is most frequently encountered as a unilateral, chronic lesion of the tail of the epididymis and thus can be recognized by comparing the size and shape of the abnormal organ with the normal one. In acute inflammation, the epididymis is swollen and soft. In chronic inflammation, it is enlarged and firm because of abundant fibrous tissue and the presence of spermatic granulomas. Epididymitis is one of the causes of testicular degeneration, and macroscopically, the testis is atrophic. Focal fibrinous or fibrous adhesions occur between the visceral and parietal vaginal tunics over the epididymis (see Fig. 19-18). If a spermatic granuloma ruptures into the cavity of the vaginal tunic, diffuse inflammation can result (Fig. 19-20), followed by adhesions across the cavity. In some cases, fistulas discharge through the scrotum.

Microscopically, the early lesions of epididymitis begin when bacteria are within the lumen of the duct. Neutrophils infiltrate, and their products combined with bacterial products, such as exotoxin and endotoxin, cause ductal and stromal necrosis, fibrin exudation, and edema. Spermatozoa extravasate, and spermatic granulomas form. With time, there will be neutrophils and macrophages within the tubules, epithelial hyperplasia, metaplasia, intraepithelial cavities, or lumina, and many lymphocytes and plasma cells within the interstitium. (Fig. 19-21).

Noninfectious causes of epididymitis are exceedingly rare, and frequently, cases that have no recoverable agent have spermatic granulomas that remain after a previous infection is otherwise controlled.

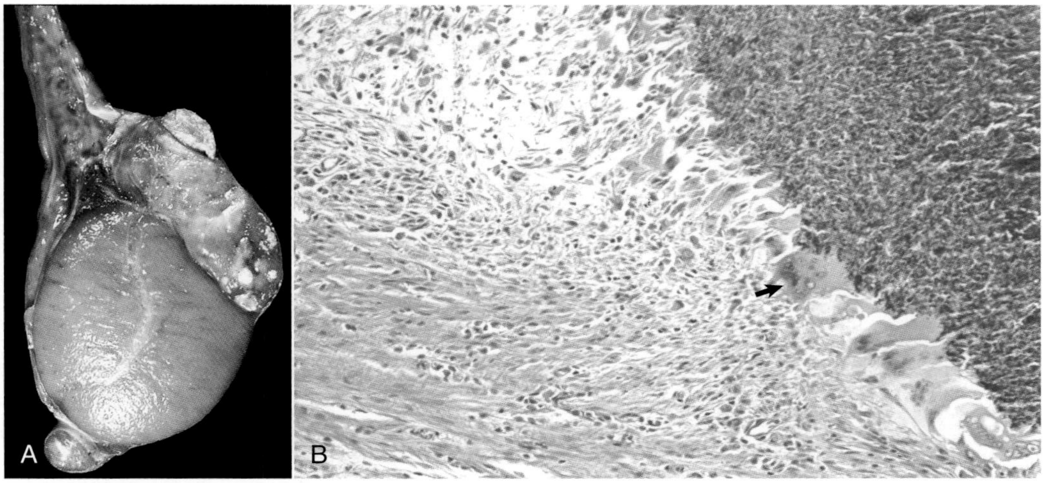

Fig. 19-17 Spermatic granuloma, head of the epididymis, dog.
A, The head of the epididymis is tremendously enlarged because of spermatic granulomas *(white-yellow masses)*. The body and tail of the epididymis (ventral) are small, as the spermatic granulomas have obstructed the flow of spermatozoa from the testis to the epididymis. **B**, The mass of spermatozoa *(right)* in the interstitial connective tissue of the epididymis is surrounded by macrophages and multinucleated giant cells *(arrow)*. H&E stain. (**A** courtesy College of Veterinary Medicine, University of Illinois. **B** courtesy Dr. K. McEntee, Reproductive Pathology Collection, University of Illinois; and Dr. J. King, College of Veterinary Medicine, Cornell University.)

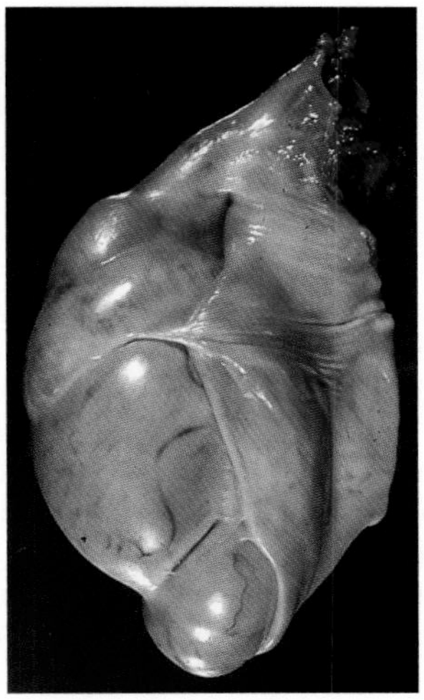

Fig. 19-18 Epididymitis *(Brucella ovis)*, tunic adhesions, epididymis, ram.
Note the dramatic enlargement of the epididymis *(left half of the image)* and the adhesion of the parietal vaginal tunic to the visceral vaginal tunic around the affected epididymis. (Courtesy Dr. K. McEntee, Reproductive Pathology Collection, University of Illinois; and Dr. J. King, College of Veterinary Medicine, Cornell University.)

Orchitis

True orchitis (inflammation of the testis) is much less common than epididymitis, probably because the testis is much further "upstream" than the epididymis and possibly because of its altered immunologic environment, which is antiinflammatory. Orchitis is, unfortunately, the clinical term for inflammation of the scrotal contents, even though most cases are epididymitis. Orchitis is usually accompanied by epididymitis; it may be an extension of epididymitis. Primary orchitis is usually hematogenous, with examples, including *Brucella abortus* in bulls, *Corynebacterium pseudotuberculosis* in rams, and *Brucella suis* in boars. It happens in several forms. Intratubular orchitis is centered on the seminiferous tubules, so it is assumed the agent and the inflammatory reaction begin there. Intratubular orchitis appears grossly as poorly defined, up

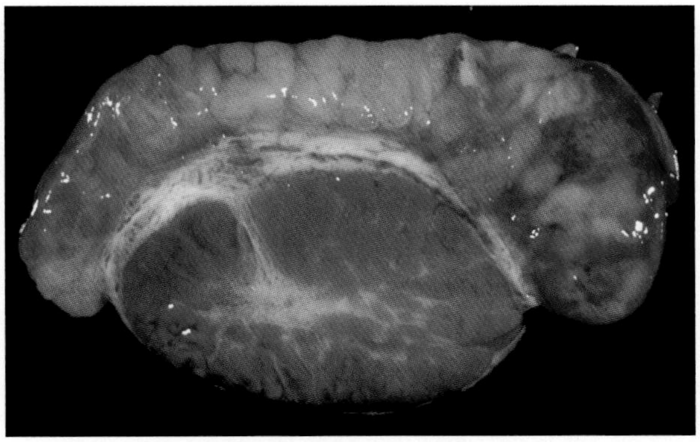

Fig. 19-19 Acute epididymitis, epididymis, dog.
The head *(left)* and tail *(right)* of the epididymis are grossly hyperemic and contain pale foci of suppurative exudate and spermatozoa. (Courtesy Dr. K. McEntee, Reproductive Pathology Collection, University of Illinois; and Dr. J. King, College of Veterinary Medicine, Cornell University.)

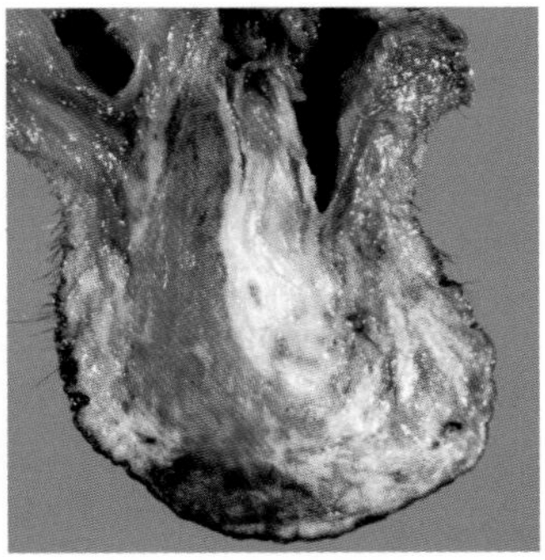

Fig. 19-20 Scrotal cellulitis and periorchitis, scrotum (testis has been removed), dog.
The vaginal tunic is thickened by inflammatory exudate, granulation tissue, and fibrous tissue. The inflammation extends into the skin. There is an ulcer in the ventral skin from self-mutilation. (Courtesy Dr. R. A. Foster, Ontario Veterinary College, University of Guelph.)

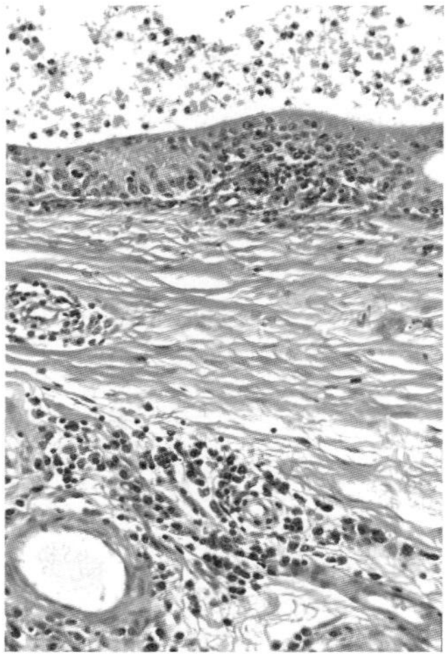

Fig. 19-21 Chronic epididymitis, epididymis, ram.
Note the intertubular fibrosis and large numbers of lymphocytes and plasma cells in the interstitium *(lower half of image)*. The epithelium of the epididymal duct *(top)* is hyperplastic, and the lumen contains neutrophils and spermatozoa. H&E stain. (Courtesy Dr. R. A. Foster, Ontario Veterinary College, University of Guelph.)

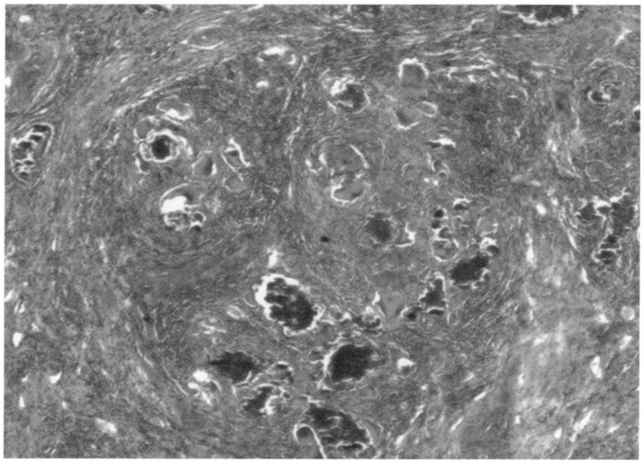

Fig. 19-22 Granulomatous interstitial orchitis, testis, ram.
There is granulomatous inflammation surrounding aggregates of spermatozoa and mineral that replaced the seminiferous tubules after they were destroyed. Lymphocytes and plasma cells predominate in the surrounding interstitium. H&E stain. (Courtesy Dr. R. A. Foster, Ontario Veterinary College, University of Guelph.)

to 1-cm yellow foci that become firm and white as the lesions become chronic. Initially, the affected tubules have acute inflammatory debris. The lining of the tubules is lost, but the tubular outlines remain. Spermatic granulomas frequently form. In the center of these granulomas, spermatozoa are free within the tissue and within macrophages. Macrophages and lymphocytes surround the spermatozoa and with time, collagen is formed at the edge of the lesion. When the lesion is predominantly in the interstitium, it is called *interstitial orchitis* (Fig. 19-22).

Necrotizing orchitis, such as is caused by *Brucella abortus* and *Brucella suis,* is the most severe form of orchitis. It is a more severe form of intratubular or interstitial orchitis, but in some cases the affected areas are so severely inflamed and the necrosis is so extensive that the original structures form a caseous mass. Gray-brown, initially soft and later firm, necrotic debris replaces an irregular

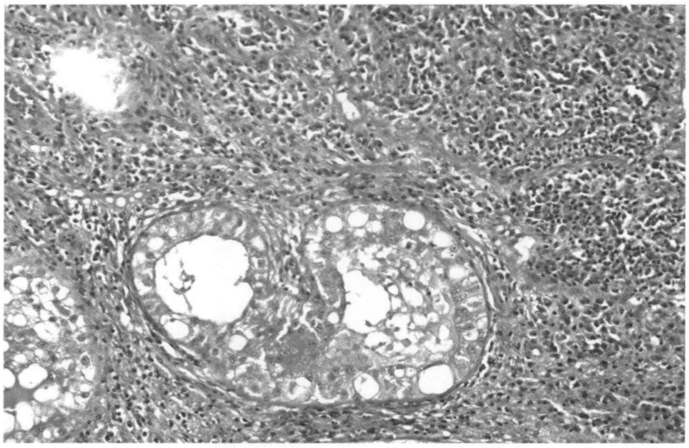

Fig. 19-23 Severe fibrinous interstitial orchitis, feline infectious peritonitis (FIP), testis, cat.
Note the severe orchitis with a mixture of fibrin and plasma cells in the interstitium. The tubules are degenerate and not directly involved. The testicular lesion was the first manifestation of FIP in this cat. H&E stain. (Courtesy Dr. R. A. Foster, Ontario Veterinary College, University of Guelph.)

but large portion of the testis. In a few extremely severe cases, a fistula develops through the scrotum. One manifestation of FIP is a fibrinous and necrotic orchitis (Fig. 19-23).

Granulomatous orchitis, especially tuberculous orchitis, is now very rare as countries eradicate *Mycobacterium bovis.* Mycotic orchitis caused by *Blastomyces dermatitidis* occurs sporadically in dogs in endemic areas.

Neoplasia

Testicular neoplasms are common in older dogs, much less frequent in horses, and rare in other species. They usually arise from germ cells, Sertoli cells, or interstitial endocrine cells. Occasionally, neoplasms of testicular mesenchymal structures or metastatic neoplasms are found. The three common primary testicular neoplasms are seminoma, Sertoli cell tumor and interstitial cell tumor; they occur singly or in combination. These primary neoplasms are almost always benign, and there are no features that indicate the likelihood of metastasis. Metastasis, when it does occur, is identified by nodules in the spermatic cord, scrotal lymph node, or beyond.

Germ cell neoplasms are seminoma, teratoma, and other less common types such as embryonal carcinoma. Seminomas are the most common testicular neoplasm in the aged stallion and the second most common canine testicular neoplasm (Fig. 19-24, *A*). They are more prevalent in cryptorchid testes than in descended testes. Multicentric origin within the testis and local invasiveness are characteristic, but metastasis is rare. The neoplasm is homogenous, white or pink-gray, and firm; bulges when cut; and has fine fibrous trabeculae. Microscopically, seminomas are either intratubular or diffuse, and the neoplastic cells are large round cells with scant cytoplasm and a large nucleus with a prominent nucleolus. Anisokaryosis is up to sixfold, but most cells are large and uniform in size. The mitotic rate is usually high. Giant cells, with either a single nucleus or multiple nuclei, are sometimes present (Fig. 19-24, *B*). Aggregates of $CD8^+$ T lymphocytes are often present around blood vessels in seminomas and are a useful diagnostic feature, since they are not seen in other testicular neoplasms. Teratomas arise from totipotential primordial germ cells. They are uncommon but are best known in the young horse, especially in a cryptorchid testis. The neoplasms can be large, cystic, or polycystic and can contain recognizable hair, mucus, bone, or even teeth. Microscopically, derivatives of two of the three embryonic germ

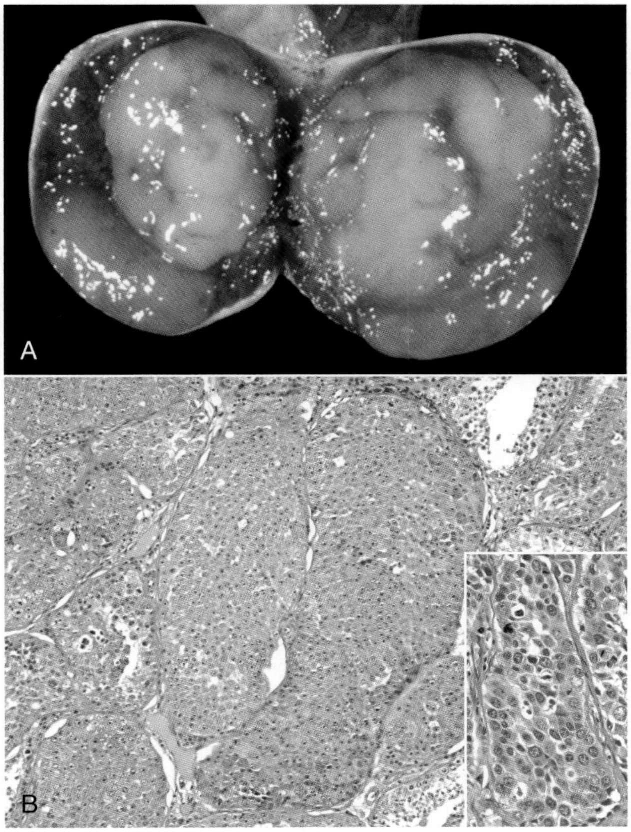

Fig. 19-24 Seminoma, testis, bisected and reflected section, dog.
A, Note the pale pink to beige circumscribed homogeneous mass. The cut surface has a gelatinous texture and has bulged slightly on incision. The contralateral testis was atrophic. **B**, Seminomas consist of round germinal cells with a high nuclear-to-cytoplasmic ratio and frequent mitoses *(not shown here)*. Note how the cells have filled and expanded the seminiferous tubules. *Inset:* Higher magnification of the neoplastic cells. Note the mitoses. Despite this "malignant" appearance, most are behaviorally benign. H&E stain. (**A** courtesy Dr. K. Read, College of Veterinary Medicine, Texas A&M University; and Noah's Arkive, College of Veterinary Medicine, The University of Georgia. **B** courtesy College of Veterinary Medicine, University of Illinois. **Inset** courtesy Dr. R.A. Foster, Ontario Veterinary College, University of Guelph.)

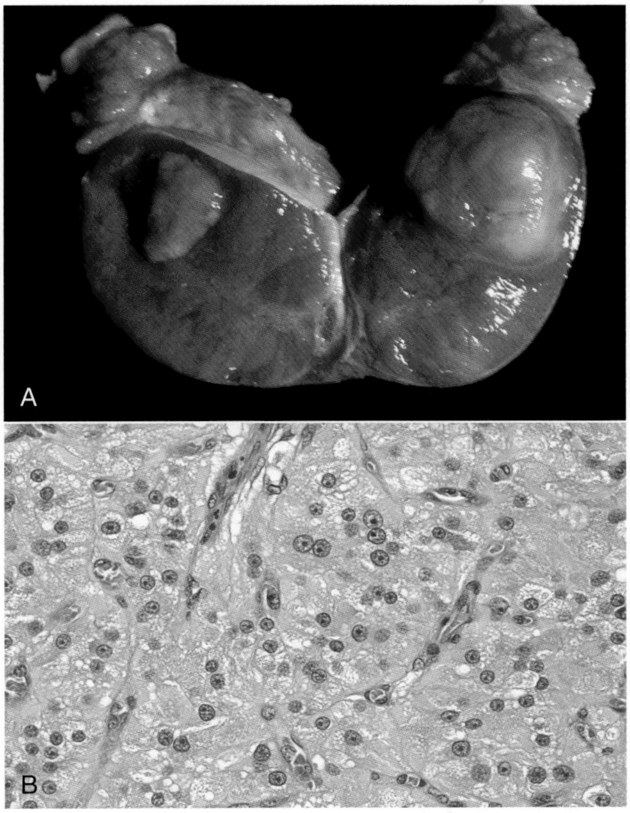

Fig. 19-25 Interstitial cell tumor, testis, bisected and reflected section, dog.
A, Note the well-demarcated, yellow-tan mass, which has bulged on incision. Such masses become hemorrhagic when they become large. Atrophy of an affected testis as the result of pressure is common when the tumor is large. **B**, Cells are arranged in packets surrounded by a fine fibrous stroma typical of endocrine cells. Their cytoplasm is pale, eosinophilic, and abundant and often has fine vacuoles. Mitoses are rare. H&E stain. (**A** courtesy Dr. M.D. McGavin, College of Veterinary Medicine, University of Tennessee. **B** courtesy Dr. W. Crowell, College of Veterinary Medicine, The University of Georgia; and Noah's Arkive, College of Veterinary Medicine, The University of Georgia.)

layers (ectoderm, mesoderm, and endoderm) are present. Most teratomas have well-differentiated tissue and are benign.

Interstitial cell tumor is the most common testicular neoplasm of the bull, dog, and cat. These neoplasms are almost always benign. They likely begin as regions of nodular hyperplasia. Some cases produce hormones, including estrogenic substances. They are readily identifiable grossly because they are spherical and well demarcated (Fig. 19-25, *A*), a tan-to-orange color, often with regions of hemorrhage. Microscopically, they are noninvasive and finely encapsulated. The neoplastic cells are arranged in solid sheets or packed into small groups by a fine fibrous stroma (Fig. 19-25, *B*). The cells of the bovine neoplasms vary little, but in the dog, the cells can be large, round, and polyhedral or spindle shaped. The cells have abundant cytoplasm that is often finely vacuolated and often has brown lipofuscin pigment. Nuclei are round, and anisokaryosis is usually minimal. Hemorrhage and necrosis is common.

Sertoli cell tumor is the third most common testicular neoplasm of the dog. It is rare in other species. In the dog, more than 50% of Sertoli cell tumors are located in retained testes. The neoplasm is well circumscribed, expansile, firm, white, and lobulated by fibrous bands and can cause dramatic enlargement of the affected testis (Fig. 19-26, *A*). Metastasis is rare but when present, is in the spermatic cord and occasionally spreads to the superficial inguinal (scrotal) lymph node. Metastases beyond the regional lymph node are reported but are very rare. Microscopically, the abundant fibrous tissue in Sertoli cell tumors distinguishes them from the other two common types of testicular neoplasm. Neoplastic Sertoli cells have an intratubular or a diffuse arrangement and tend to palisade along the fibrous stroma or form tubular structures (Fig. 19-26, *B*). They either resemble normal Sertoli cells or are pleomorphic. In addition to the effects of pressure and local invasion, about a third of Sertoli cell tumors produce a feminizing effect, causing gynecomastia (enlargement of the mammary glands), alopecia, hyperplasia, or squamous metaplasia of the acini of the prostate gland (Fig. 19-26, *C*). The amount of hormone produced is generally proportional to the size of the neoplasm. Although some produce estrogen, many produce inhibin, which inhibits GnRH secretion and subsequently LH and FSH release. This alters the balance between estrogen

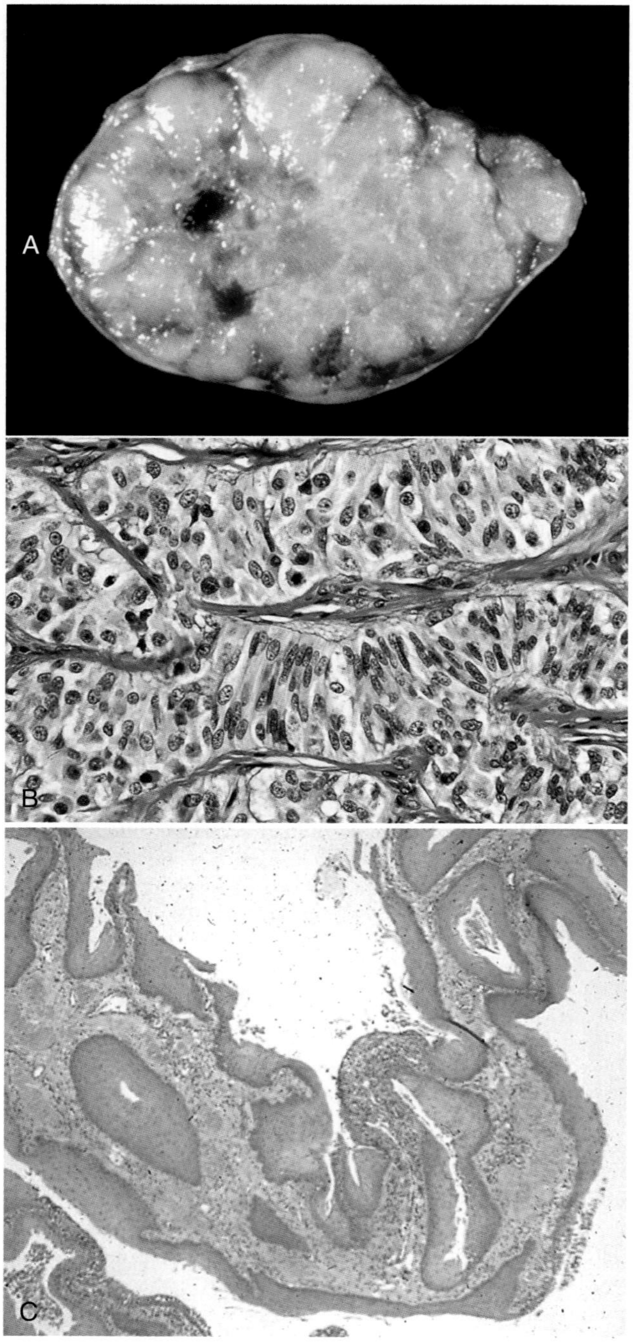

Fig. 19-26 Sertoli cell tumor, testis, dog.
A, Sertoli cell tumors are firm, white, and often lobulated, and the lobules are surrounded by fibrous bands. **B**, Histologically, Sertoli cell tumors have tubular structures lined by cells that resemble Sertoli cells and are supported by fine septa of fibrous tissue. H&E stain. **C**, Prostate, squamous metaplasia. Functional Sertoli cell tumors that secrete estrogen can induce hyperplasia and/or squamous metaplasia of the prostate gland. Normal epithelium of the prostatic ducts (transitional) and glandular acini (columnar) is replaced by stratified squamous keratinizing epithelium. H&E stain. (**A** courtesy Dr. K. McEntee, Reproductive Pathology Collection, University of Illinois. **B** courtesy Dr. R. A. Foster, Ontario Veterinary College, University of Guelph. **C**, Courtesy Dr. W. Crowell, College of Veterinary Medicine, The University of Georgia; and Noah's Arkive, College of Veterinary Medicine, The University of Georgia.)

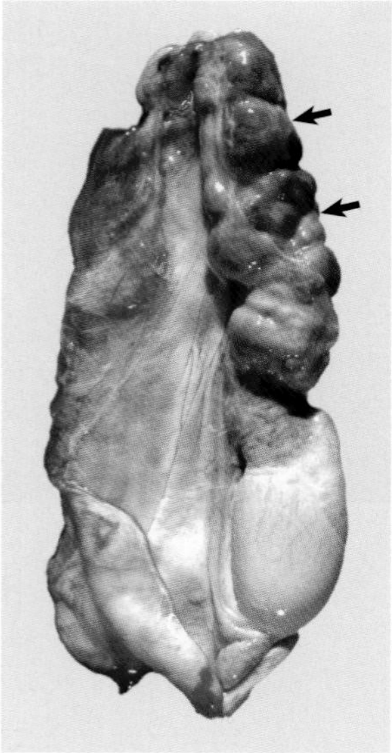

Fig. 19-27 Varicocele, pampiniform plexus, ram.
This extremely large varicocele *(arrows)* is larger than the testis. It is multinodular from large thromboses filling the dilated veins. (Courtesy Dr. P. W. Ladds, James Cook University of North Queensland.)

and testosterone production. A possibly life-threatening effect of hyperestrogenism is myelotoxicity, resulting in a poorly regenerative anemia, granulocytopenia, and thrombocytopenia.

Mixed germ cell–stromal neoplasms are described also. The neoplasm-bearing testis is large and often cryptorchid. The testis is partially or completely replaced by a firm, gray-white to tan, single multilobed mass that is almost identical in appearance to the Sertoli cell tumor. Microscopically, germ cells intermingle with Sertoli cells in tubular structures of various sizes, thus it is a mixture of seminoma and Sertoli cell tumor.

Spermatic Cord

The spermatic cord is composed of the deferent duct, pampiniform plexus, and cremaster muscle. The scrotal lymph node and the inguinal canal are adjacent structures. The most common disease is varicocele or varicose dilation of veins of the pampiniform plexus (Fig. 19-27). This is seen most commonly in older rams and is described in the section on Disorders of Ruminants. It can be found in any species.

Torsion of the spermatic cord is seen in retained testes, especially when there is a testicular neoplasm present. Torsion also occurs periodically in the stallion and is a cause of colic. Torsion causes venous occlusion with a resultant venous infarction of the testis especially and also of the epididymis.

Inflammation of the spermatic cord (funisitis, scirrhous cord) occurs after the contamination of a castration wound. Sometimes the lesion is neutrophilic and necrotizing, but more often it is chronic and a scirrhous cord is encountered. Great enlargement of the distal part of the cord is caused by exuberant granulation tissue in which numerous small pockets of pus are scattered. Staphylococci are the bacteria frequently recovered from the pus in the horse. The term *botryomycosis* was used for these staphylococcal pyogranulomas. Radiating club-shaped eosinophilic deposits (Splendore-Hoeppli reaction) are present around the central clusters of bacteria. This is surrounded in turn by neutrophils and multinucleated giant cells and then by granulation and fibrous tissue.

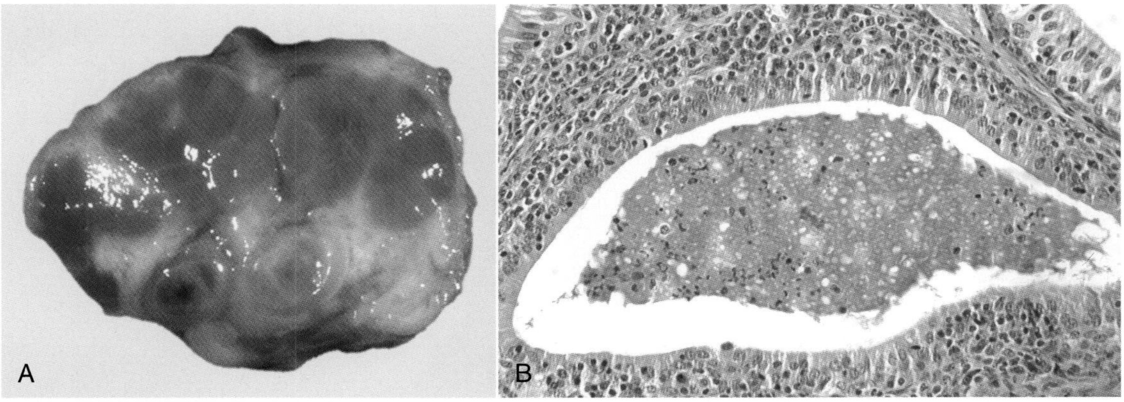

Fig. 19-28 Chronic vesicular adenitis, vesicular gland, cut surface, ram.
A, The normal lobulation of the vesicular gland is distorted by white-gray fibrous tissue that surrounds the glandular tissue. **B**, Chronic vesicular adenitis *(Brucella ovis)*. Glandular acini are filled with degenerating neutrophils and debris, and neutrophils are migrating through the acinar epithelium. The interstitium is heavily infiltrated by plasma cells and lymphocytes. H&E stain. (Courtesy Dr. R. A. Foster, Ontario Veterinary College, University of Guelph.)

Inguinal hernia is a differential diagnosis for masses or swellings in the region of the spermatic cord and scrotum. Stallions, older rams, and some Pietrain strains of pigs are particularly prone to inguinal hernia. It is an important cause of scrotal enlargement and colic in stallions. Little is known about the cause of inguinal hernia in domesticated animals. The herniated structures are usually a part of the intestine, and they can be free within the vaginal tunics or encased in a second fold of peritoneum. In stallions, the entrapped intestine undergoes venous infarction, causing life-threatening colic. In other species, intestinal infarcts are unusual.

Scrotal lymphadenopathy is another cause of swelling in the region of the spermatic cord. Caseous lymphadenitis in rams and lymphoma in dogs are causes of enlargement of the scrotal lymph nodes.

DISORDERS OF THE ACCESSORY GENITAL GLANDS

The accessory genital glands include the ampullae, vesicular glands, prostate, and bulbourethral glands. The ampullae and vesicular glands are derived from the mesonephric duct, and the prostate and bulbourethral glands are derived from the urogenital sinus. Their hidden location within the pelvis means they are not routinely examined.

Ampulla

Disease of the ampullae is unusual, and the majority are microscopic. Bulls have variation in the patterns of insertion of ampullae at the seminal colliculus. The ampullae can be above or below the vesicular glands. The membrane between the ampullae is the location for the remnants of the paramesonephric duct—the cystic uterus masculinus—in bulls and rams especially. Hyperestrogenism can cause these to become greatly enlarged.

Ampullitis is a feature of infection with agents that cause epididymitis and vesicular adenitis, including but not restricted to *Brucella abortus, Brucella ovis, Actinobacillus seminis, Histophilus somni,* and many other agents. It may precede epididymitis as part of an ascending infection or occur when organisms and inflammatory products pass through the deferent duct from an infected epididymis.

Vesicular Glands

The major disease of the vesicular glands (seminal vesicles) is inflammation of the gland, and often, it is clinically silent, except in the bull where it is an important disease (see the section on Disorders of Ruminants).

Vesicular adenitis is occasionally seen in stallions and can be a part of lesions caused by *Burkholderia pseudomallei* in boars and the many *Brucella* species, especially *Brucella ovis* in sheep (Fig. 19-28).

Prostate Gland

The prostate gland is derived from the urogenital sinus. Both estrogens and androgens are trophic to the prostate gland.

The only animal with any frequency of prostatic disease is the dog. There are three main disorders and their prevalence is, in descending order: hyperplasia (Fig. 19-29), neoplasia (Fig. 19-30), and prostatitis (Fig. 19-31). These disorders are discussed in the section on Disorders of Dogs and Cats.

Bulbourethral Glands

The bulbourethral gland, as with the prostate, is derived from the urogenital sinus. There are few lesions of the bulbourethral glands, no doubt because of their dense structure and lack of lumina to allow bacterial growth and persistence. The major disease of this gland is seen in castrated male sheep grazing clover pasture with a high estrogen content. The glands of these wethers become so large that they cause perineal swellings. The glands have massive hypertrophy, squamous metaplasia, and cyst formation.

DISORDERS OF THE PENIS AND PREPUCE

Disorders of the penis and prepuce are relatively rare, yet infection is common and extremely important for food-producing animals. Many of the venereally transmitted organisms, such as *Tritrichomonas foetus, Campylobacter fetus,* herpesviruses, and papillomaviruses, are present in the prepuce and do not cause severe disease or have a mild and self-limiting course. The penis is protected from trauma and drying by the prepuce and this environment is permissive of many infections. Only some induce an immune reaction and/or inflammation.

Phimosis is the inability to extrude the penis, paraphimosis is the inability to retract the penis into the prepuce, and priapism is a persistent erection; all are seen occasionally.

Developmental Anomalies

Persistent frenulum is a band of tissue between the ventral raphe of the penis and the prepuce. The raphe of the penis and prepuce

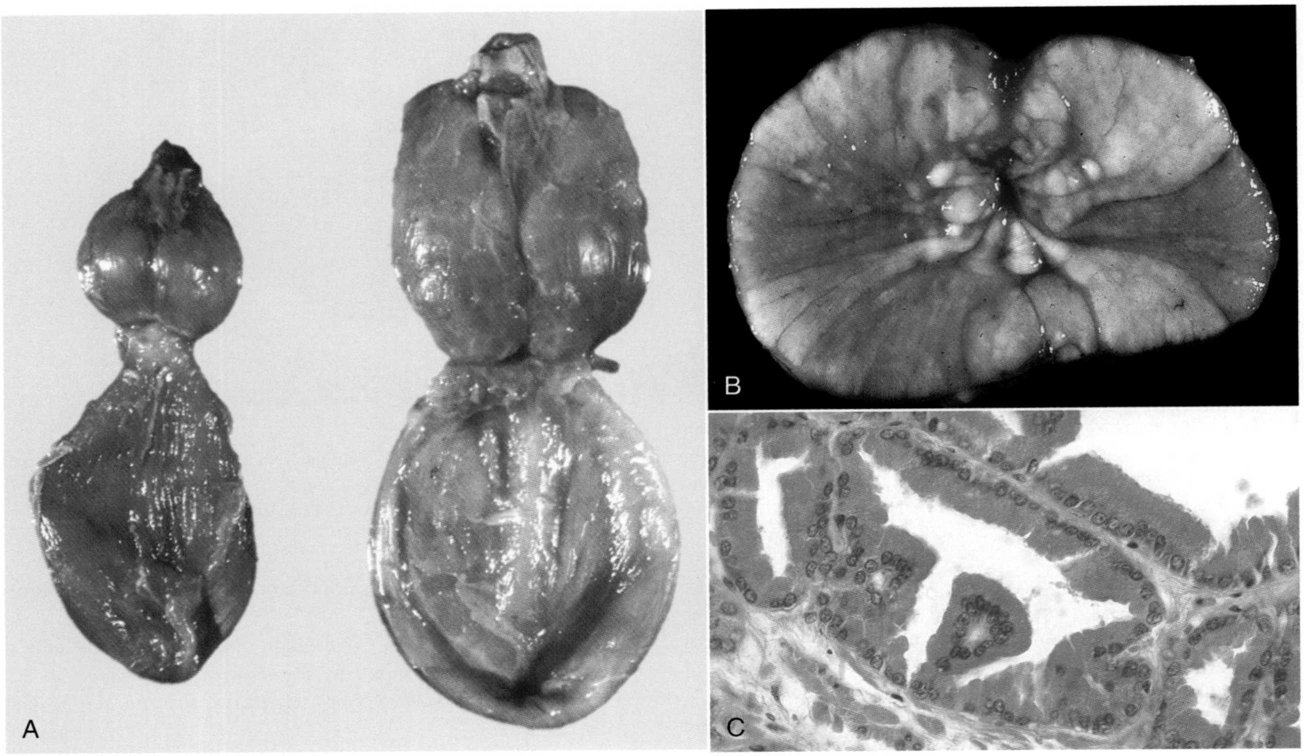

Fig. 19-29 Prostatic hyperplasia, prostate, dog.
A, Prostates of two dogs of different ages (oldest on the right [age-related growth]). Both prostates are bilaterally and symmetrically larger than normal postpubertal prostates. **B**, The lighter white tissues that in some areas bulge from the cut surface are areas of hyperplasia. A hyperplastic prostate is symmetrically enlarged and detectable on rectal palpation, ultrasonography, or by gross examination at necropsy. **C**, The prostatic acini are larger than normal, as the epithelium is hyperplastic and the cells enlarged (hypertrophy). Note the abundant granular apical cytoplasm and the uniform size and shape of the cells. Mitotic activity is very low. H&E stain. (**A** courtesy Dr. R. A. Foster, Ontario Veterinary College, University of Guelph. **B** courtesy Department of Veterinary Biosciences, The Ohio State University; and Noah's Arkive, College of Veterinary Medicine, The University of Georgia. **C** courtesy Dr. R.K. Myers, College of Veterinary Medicine, Iowa State University.)

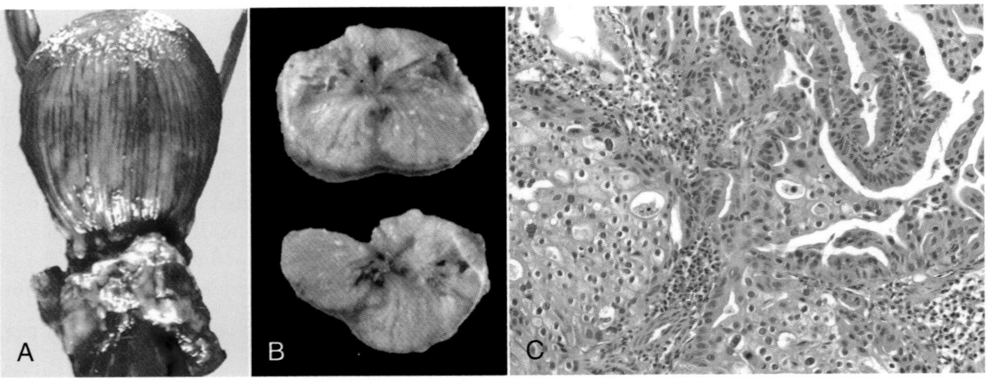

Fig. 19-30 Carcinoma, prostate, dog.
A, The adjacent pelvic tissues of this dog contain many coalescing nodules of metastatic carcinoma that have spread from the prostate, which is barely recognizable beneath the bladder *(opened, upper half of image)*. Prostatic carcinomas are usually asymmetric and lobulated white-to-gray masses that expand the size of the gland and may compress the urethra (dysuria) and the colon (difficulty defecating, ribbon stools). **B**, Cross-section. Note the asymmetric enlargement. The focal white areas are regions of necrosis within a gland that is enlarged by neoplastic epithelial cells that induce the abundant fibrous tissue that is also present. **C**, Note the anaplastic prostatic epithelial cells arranged in acini *(upper right)* and solid lobules *(lower left)*. Mitoses can be frequent in some cases. There also may be stromal or lymphatic invasion and desmoplasia (scirrhous response). H&E stain. (**A** courtesy Dr. M. Howard, College of Veterinary Medicine, Iowa State University; and Noah's Arkive, College of Veterinary Medicine, The University of Georgia. **B** courtesy Dr. J. A. Ramos-Vara, College of Veterinary Medicine, Michigan State University; and Noah's Arkive, College of Veterinary Medicine, The University of Georgia. **C** courtesy Dr. R.A. Foster, Ontario Veterinary College, University of Guelph.)

are remnants of the frenulum, a thin membrane ventral to the penis that normally ruptures at puberty, probably as the result of simple mechanical forces. Balanopreputial bands are similar but are located elsewhere on the penis. They are relatively common and minor anatomic abnormalities rather than serious defects, but they can have an important deleterious effect in limiting the extent to which the penis can be protruded from the sheath and in causing the erect penis to be curved instead of straight (Fig. 19-32). Persistent frenulum is important in bulls and boars. Judging by the frequent occurrence of large flaps and tags of tissue on the ventral raphe

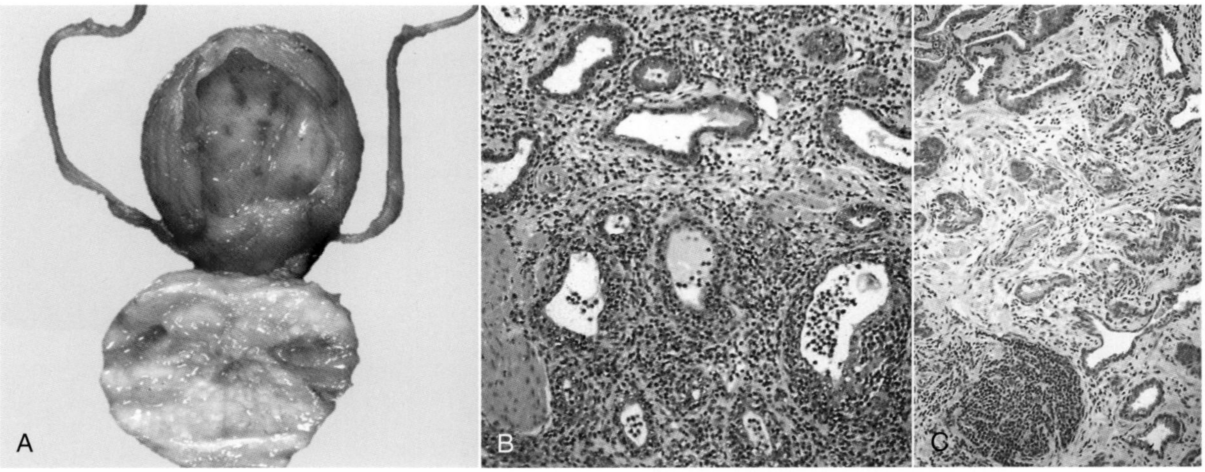

Fig. 19-31 Prostatitis, prostate, dog.
A, Acute prostatitis, cut surface. The prostate is enlarged with edema, and there are many white foci of inflammatory cells instead of the usually smooth red surface. Clinically, this condition is usually painful. **B,** Acute prostatitis. Note that the glands and interstitium contain large numbers of neutrophils. Most of these infections are of bacterial origin and develop after bacteria ascend the urethra. H&E stain. **C,** Chronic prostatitis. Note that the glands and interstitium contain large numbers of lymphocytes and macrophages and a large lymphoid nodule *(bottom half of image).* Follicular lymphoid hyperplasia is a common finding in chronically infected tissue. The abundant interstitial stroma is from fibroplasia and chronic inflammation. Most cases of chronic prostatitis have a bacterial origin. H&E stain. (Courtesy Dr. W. Crowell, College of Veterinary Medicine, The University of Georgia; and Noah's Arkive, College of Veterinary Medicine, The University of Georgia.)

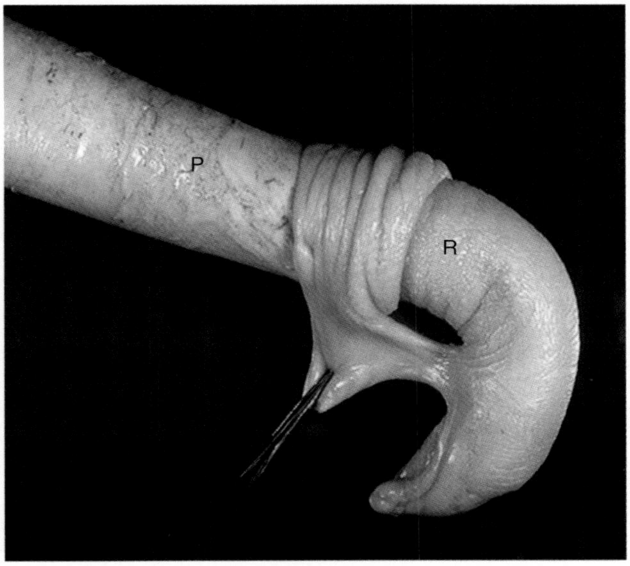

Fig. 19-32 Persistent frenulum, penis, bull.
A tag of tissue *(forceps),* a frenulum remnant, connects the ventral surface of the penis to the prepuce *(R)* at its reflection from the penis and has caused the penis *(P)* to grow curved ventrally as the animal has matured, thus making intromission impossible. (Courtesy Dr. W. Crowell, College of Veterinary Medicine, The University of Georgia; and Noah's Arkive, College of Veterinary Medicine, The University of Georgia.)

of the penis, transitory persistence of the frenulum is quite common.

The penis is subject to many abnormalities of size and form, such as congenital absence, hypoplasia, duplication, directional deviations, and in ruminants, absence of the sigmoid flexure and abnormal locations of the insertions of the retractor penis muscles. None of these lesions is common.

Hypospadias and epispadias are malformations of the urethral canal that create abnormal openings of the urethra on the ventral surface of the penis (hypospadias) or on the dorsal surface (epispadias). In hypospadias, the urinary opening is anywhere from the head to the shaft of the penis, penoscrotal junction, or the perineum. Their importance is in the potential for causing urinary obstruction and in interference with normal insemination.

Hemorrhage and Penile Hematoma

The penis is a highly vascular structure, and the presence of erectile tissue and high pressures during erection and coitus make the potential for severe or even fatal hemorrhage high (Fig. 19-33). Trauma to the penis is usually responsible; cuts, lacerations, and surgical incisions bleed profusely. Forced deviation of the penis in ruminants causes rupture and hemorrhage (see later) that can be fatal.

Inflammation

Inflammation of the penis is phallitis, of the head (glans) of the penis is balanitis, and of the prepuce is posthitis. Inflammation of the penis and prepuce (phaloposthitis or balanoposthitis) occurs mostly in castrated animals. This could be the result of alterations to structure because of a lack of testosterone and/or normal development and the tendency of these animals to urinate within their prepuce. Retention of urine in the preputial cavity creates an environment for the overgrowth of bacteria. Those that produce urease split urea to ammonia, a toxic molecule that damages the preputial epithelium, causing erosion and ulceration. Ovine posthitis (see later) is a classic disease.

Nonspecific posthitis occurs in all species and in the gelding, is believed to occur because of a lack of extrusion of the penis with a resultant buildup of the waxy smegma and bacterial overgrowth. A foul-smelling prepuce and posthitis is the result. Dogs commonly develop a nonspecific and purulent discharge of the prepuce.

Herpesviruses cause a multifocal phaloposthitis in several species. Equine herpesvirus 3 is the cause of equine coital exanthema, a disease of stallions and mares with a similarly short clinical course, but with larger (15 mm) ulcers with a predilection for the body rather than the head of the penis. Bovine herpesvirus 1 (BoHV-1) causes a phaloposthitis in the bull, progressing over the course of a few days from hyperemia and swelling to vesicles and

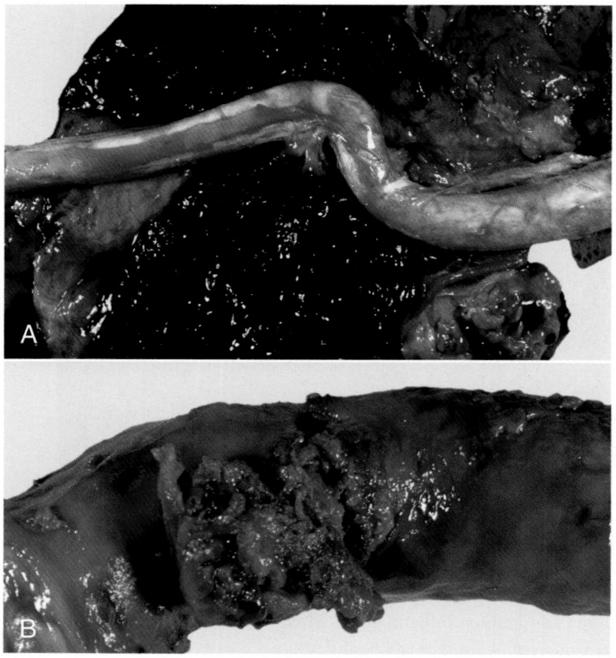

Fig. 19-33 Penile hematoma, penis, bull.
A, The large hemorrhage around the penis at the sigmoid flexure is a hematoma from rupture of the penis during forced deviation. **B**, Illustrated is the site of rupture of the penis with a blood clot filling the rupture site. (Courtesy Dr. M.D. McGavin, College of Veterinary Medicine, University of Tennessee.)

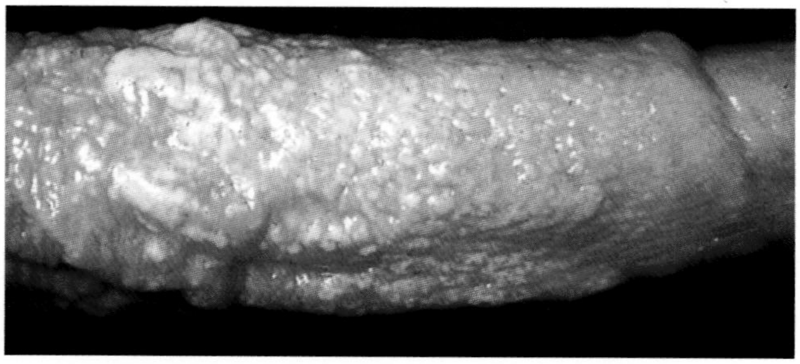

Fig. 19-34 Phaloposthitis, bovine herpesvirus 1, penis (free part), bull.
Note the vesicles and pustules of the mucosa. Bovine herpesvirus 1 causes hyperemia, swelling, vesicles, pustules, and 1- to 2-mm ulcers, especially of the prepuce. Intranuclear inclusion bodies are present microscopically, briefly in epithelial cells of the penis and prepuce during the vesiculopustular stage. (Courtesy Dr. K. McEntee, Reproductive Pathology Collection, University of Illinois; and Dr. J. King, College of Veterinary Medicine, Cornell University.)

pustules and then 1- to 2-mm ulcers, especially of the head of the penis (Fig. 19-34). In the vesiculopustular stage, intranuclear inclusion bodies are present briefly in epithelial cells of the penis and prepuce. Ulcerative balanoposthitis with acidophilic intranuclear inclusions has been observed in goats and is considered a result of caprine herpesvirus infection. Canine herpesvirus reportedly causes inflammation at the base of the penis and the reflection of the prepuce but does not cause the formation of pustules or ulcers. Resolution of these lesions in the affected species is rapid, leaving only hyperplastic mucosal lymphoid nodules and small areas of depigmented mucosa (see Chapter 18 for a detailed description). BoHV-1, suid herpesvirus 1 (pseudorabies virus) in pigs, caprine herpesvirus 1, and canine herpesvirus can persist in a latent state, capable of becoming reactivated by stress or treatment with corticosteroids.

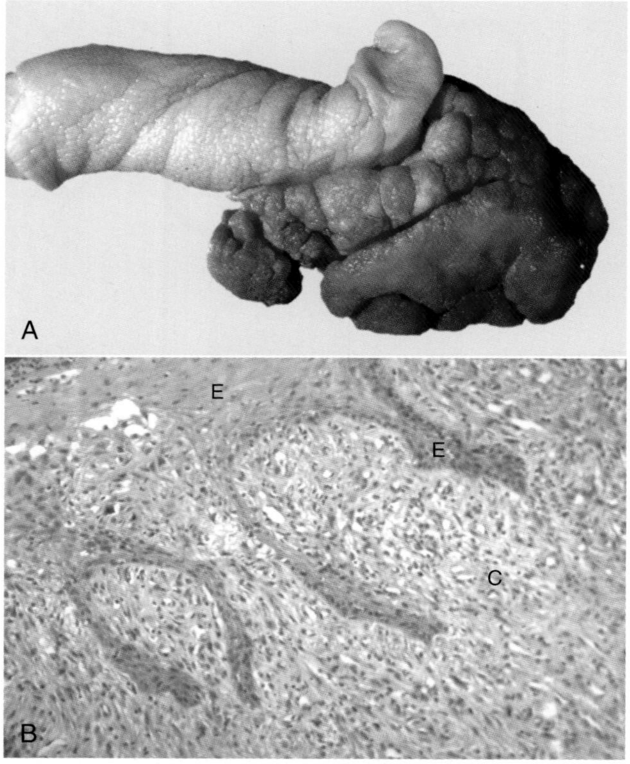

Fig. 19-35 Penile fibropapilloma, glans penis, bull.
A, There is a large exophytic papillary mass protruding from the penile epithelium. This large proliferative lesion on the penis is typical of a fibropapilloma. **B**, Note the abundant connective tissue *(C)* covered by hyperplastic stratified squamous epithelium *(E)* that is thickened and has elongated epidermal-dermal interdigitations that penetrate deeply into the connective tissue. H&E stain. (**A** courtesy Dr. R. A. Foster, Ontario Veterinary College, University of Guelph. **B** courtesy Dr. J. Simon, College of Veterinary Medicine, University of Illinois.)

Other organisms are capable of causing phaloposthitis. These include the larvae of *Habronema* spp. in the horse and *Strongyloides papillosus* in the bull. The well-known bovine venereally transmitted diseases of campylobacteriosis and trichomoniasis cause no lesions or minimal nonspecific lesions of the penis and prepuce, even though they reside there.

Foreign material sometimes is found in the prepuce; bulls, rams, bucks, and tomcats can have matted hair around their penis to form a constricting ring (colloquially called *hair ring*). This "ring" can cause a posthitis or even avascular penile necrosis. It is assumed the deposition of hair in this location is, at least in ruminants, the result of homosexual activity and the rubbing of the penis on the posterior of other animals. Dogs, especially those of the chondrodystrophic breeds with short legs, impact their prepuce with sand.

All species can have traumatic wounds of a variety of types and severity, resulting from mating injuries. Mating or attempting to mate through fences can cause lacerations of varying severities. Owners attempting to "untie" mating dogs can cause degloving injuries to the penis. Horses with penile laceration can develop exuberant granulation tissue ("proud flesh") of the penis.

Many species develop preputial prolapse, but it is well known in the bull and is discussed later.

Papillomaviruses affect the penis of many species. Typical "warts" are produced in the dog, sarcoids are seen in horses, and the bull develops fibropapilloma (Fig. 19-35, *A* and *B*). The bovine disease is discussed in the section on Disorders of Ruminants.

Obstruction of the penile urethra, especially at the sigmoid flexure of all ruminants and the urethral process of small ruminants, is common with urolithiasis (see Chapter 11). The narrowest part of the urethra is the urethral process, and small uroliths that pass through the rest of the urethra become lodged near the tip. Depending on the degree of obstruction, necrosis, and rupture, penile and preputial necrosis can occur. Many animals die of bladder rupture before necrosis of the urethral process or penis occurs.

Neoplasms

Primary neoplasms of the penis and prepuce are mostly restricted to a limited number of types and species affected. Metastatic or multicentric neoplasms affect these tissues rarely. Dogs develop the xenotransplanted canine transmissible venereal tumor (CTVT; see the section on Disorders of Dogs and Cats). Papilloma and squamous cell carcinoma occur in the horse, bull, and dog. Horses develop sarcoids of the penis. The equine disease is described in more detail later.

DISORDERS OF HORSES

The most common disorders of horses are listed in Appendix 19-1. The common and important disorders of the scrotum and contents are cryptorchidism (as previously described), testicular and epididymal torsion, scirrhous cord, and inguinal hernia. Disorders of the accessory genital glands are rare. In the penis and prepuce, nonspecific posthitis in geldings, squamous cell carcinoma, habronemiasis, exuberant granulation tissue, and equine sarcoid are common. The disorders of the scrotum and contents and accessory genital glands are as previously described. Disorders of the penis and prepuce are described next.

PENILE SQUAMOUS CELL CARCINOMA

Both stallions and geldings develop squamous cell carcinomas of the glans penis (Fig. 19-36, *A*). Although exophytic masses do occur, the usual growth habit is infiltrative. These carcinomas induce abundant fibrous tissue, which results in an enlarged firm penis with focal ulcers. Microscopically, the neoplasm is well differentiated with the classic appearance of invasive nests, cords, and nodules of neoplastic epithelium with differentiation toward the stratum spinosum, often with well-developed keratin pearls (Fig. 19-36, *B*) or keratin squames mixed with neutrophils. The neoplastic cells are surrounded by fibrous tissue, as well as lymphocytes and plasma cells. Metastasis is to the superficial inguinal (scrotal), deep inguinal, and medial iliac lymph nodes. The prepuce often becomes edematous because of lymphatic obstruction, and the preputial cavity becomes distended by retained smegma, inflammatory debris, and urine.

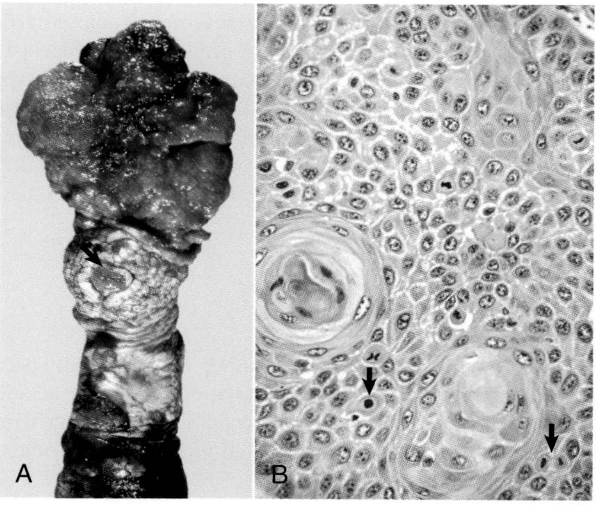

Fig. 19-36 Squamous cell carcinoma, penis, ventral surface, horse (gelding).
A, A very large ulcerated mass protrudes from the glans penis. The urethral opening is visible *(arrow)*. **B**, Neoplastic squamous epithelial cells are often arranged around "keratin pearls." Mitoses are frequent *(arrows)*. H&E stain. (**A** courtesy Dr. R. A. Foster, Ontario Veterinary College, University of Guelph. **B** courtesy Dr. M. J. Abdy, College of Veterinary Medicine, The University of Georgia; and Noah's Arkive, College of Veterinary Medicine, The University of Georgia.)

PENILE HABRONEMIASIS

Habronemiasis is the lesion caused by aberrant migration of the larvae of *Habronema muscae* and *Draschia megastoma,* which are deposited by infected flies on wounds on the penis or prepuce of horses. The gross lesion is an ulcerated, often exophytic mass on the penis or prepuce. It has the same appearance as exuberant granulation tissue or equine sarcoid. Microscopically, however, the lesions are multiple distinct nodules and tracts containing larvae and/or are filled with debris and eosinophils. Granulation and fibrous tissue surround the nodules and tracts.

Equine sarcoids and exuberant granulation tissue of the penis or prepuce are identical to their dermal counterparts (see Chapter 17). As with habronemiasis, these form ulcerated proliferative lesions on the penis and prepuce. Histologic evaluation is necessary to separate them.

DISORDERS OF RUMINANTS (CATTLE, SHEEP, AND GOATS)

Disorders of the scrotum and contents are very similar between the bull, ram, and buck. All commonly develop cryptorchidism, testicular hypoplasia, and testicular atrophy/degeneration (described previously). Rams develop epididymitis commonly and varicocele (see next section). For the disorders of the accessory genital glands, vesicular adenitis is especially important in bulls. The disorders of the penis and prepuce of importance in the bull are penile-forced deviation and hematoma and in the ram, ovine posthitis and urolithiasis.

EPIDIDYMITIS

Infectious epididymitis is most common and important in rams. It occurs in two main ways in rams: hematogenously by *Brucella ovis* and by ascending infection with bacteria such as *Actinobacillus seminis, Histophilus somni*, and *Escherichia coli.* Regardless of the causative agent, the lesion is similar and is dominated grossly and microscopically by swelling and the formation of spermatic granulomas. Macroscopically, the lesions are usually restricted to the tail of the epididymis, regardless of the causative bacterium. The tail of the epididymis is enlarged up to tenfold and is largest when spermatic granulomas form. Microscopically, the duct lumina contain a mixture of spermatozoa, neutrophils, and macrophages and multinucleate foreign body–type giant cells. The epithelium changes from simple columnar and ciliated to pseudostratified columnar and cuboidal with focal hyperplasia. These regions often develop a secondary lumen or intraepithelial lumina. Some of the epithelium becomes stratified squamous in type (squamous metaplasia). The smooth muscle wall of the duct and the interstitium contain many lymphocytes and plasma cells, plus edema and fibrin initially.

Fibrous tissue rapidly develops with granulation tissue and eventually mature fibrous tissue (see Fig. 19-21). Interstitial abscesses and spermatic granulomas develop after either death of the tissue or rupture of the duct and development of a spermatocele. These often rupture into the cavity of the vaginal tunics and produce a periorchitis. With time and severity, the tunics become thickened with edema and fibrin deposition, followed by granulation tissue and finally fibrosis.

VARICOCELE

Varicocele is the local dilation of the spermatic vein in the pampiniform plexus. Older rams are most commonly affected, but the underlying defect is unknown. About half the cases are bilateral, and the unilateral cases are evenly divided between the left and right side. Thrombosis of affected vessels is common. The dilated veins are located near the inguinal ring; the complex distal part of the pampiniform plexus is not affected (see Fig. 19-27). The thrombosed and dilated vessels are up to 10 cm diameter and are so large that they interfere with thermoregulation, either by their sheer size or by interfering with the countercurrent system. Venous flow from the testis could theoretically be restricted and this could subsequently alter testicular oxygen tension and create oxidative stress, thus causing testicular degeneration, poor spermatozoal motility, and immature spermatozoa in the semen.

VESICULAR ADENITIS

Vesicular adenitis (seminal vesiculitis) is a significant disease because it reduces fertility, particularly in young bulls. Inflammation in the vesicular glands contributes inflammatory cells and mediators to the semen. It also reduces the ability of spermatozoa to survive freezing. Young bulls, in their first breeding season, are especially affected. The cause is most likely infectious; various organisms, including viruses, protozoa, *Chlamydophila* sp., *Ureaplasma diversum, Mycoplasma* sp., *Brucella abortus,* and other bacteria, have been investigated over the years. The pathogenesis is uncertain, but hypotheses include ascending infection, descending infection, hematogenous spread, congenital malformation preventing excretion of fluid and spermatozoa, and reflux of spermatozoa or urine into the glands.

The common form of vesicular adenitis is a chronic interstitial inflammation (see Fig. 19-28, *A* and *B*). It begins with an acute form where the glands are swollen with edema, and they are painful on palpation. Microscopically, neutrophils enter the lumen of glands and there is edema and fibrin in the interstitium. In the more chronic and interstitial form, the glands are enlarged and firm and have loss of lobulation. Glandular lumina contain neutrophils and debris, but there are many lymphocytes and plasma cells in the interstitium, and collagen is deposited between the acini (see Fig. 19-28, *B*). Metaplasia of glandular epithelium to a stratified squamous type is common.

PENILE FORCED DEVIATION AND HEMATOMA

Penile hematoma (penile deviation; broken penis) after forced deviation is an important disease in bulls. A similar disease in the ram is reported. During mating, the penis probes for the vulva, and when appropriate, the copulatory thrust and ejaculation is done with great force. If the penis deviates from its intended target, lateral pressure is applied to the region of the sigmoid flexure and insertion of the retractor penis muscles, resulting in rupture and hemorrhage (see Fig. 19-33). The swelling of the hematoma is just cranial to the scrotum, and can be up to 50 cm diameter. In severe cases, hemorrhagic shock occurs. Small hematomas heal without complications, but depending on the extent of the injury and hematoma, granulation and scar tissue is formed and prevents extension of the penis (phimosis). Some hematomas become infected and result in a penile abscess.

PENILE FIBROPAPILLOMA

Fibropapilloma occurs on the glans penis of young bulls (see Fig. 19-35, *A* and *B*). It is caused by bovine papillomavirus type 1 infection, but the pathogenesis is incompletely understood. Affected animals are young, usually in their first breeding season, and the lesions are self-limiting. Larger neoplasms can interfere with breeding by causing pain or by their physical size. Affected bulls can develop an aversion to mating. Macroscopically, the single or multiple warty masses have a papillary epithelial covering and a fibrous core. Surface ulceration is often extensive. They are histologically typical of fibropapillomas elsewhere, with epithelial and stromal hyperplasia and long projections of epithelium into the fibrous tissue. Intranuclear inclusion bodies are seen in some. The proportions of epithelial and fibrous tissue vary greatly from case to case.

PREPUTIAL PROLAPSE

Trauma is part of the pathogenesis of preputial prolapse in bulls. Bulls of the *Bos indicus* type have a pendulous prepuce, and many have a small or absent preputial retractor muscle. Temporary eversion of the prepuce for urination is common in bulls, but affected bulls have inadequate muscular control. The everted preputial mucosa is injured and becomes swollen with edema and inflammation. The prepuce remains everted (prolapsed), swells further, dries, and is further lacerated, leading to a cycle of injury and inflammation that is permanent. Affected bulls are unable to mate.

OVINE POSTHITIS

Ovine posthitis (pizzle rot) is a disease of wethers mostly and is caused by urease-producing *Corynebacterium renale.* When the diet is high in protein and the urine has a high concentration of urea, *Corynebacterium renale* cause the urea to be broken down to ammonia, which is cytotoxic. This produces ulceration of the prepuce near the orifice. Lack of testosterone (from castration) is also involved because the disease can be prevented by administration of androgens to wethers. If the preputial orifice becomes blocked by swelling, the disease becomes much more severe, spreading beyond the initial small ulcer on the hairless skin of the prepuce to diffusely involve the mucosa, with ulceration of the head of the penis and loss of the urethral process. Scarring and phimosis can result. In severe cases, the preputial orifice becomes blocked and the animals die from urinary retention.

DISORDERS OF PIGS

Boars develop the full range of disorders that affect all species, especially cryptorchidism and testicular atrophy and degeneration. They do have a short list of unique conditions, including scrotal hemangiomas (described previously) and preputial diverticulitis.

PREPUTIAL DIVERTICULITIS

Boars are the only domesticated animal with a preputial diverticulum; it is located dorsal to the preputial orifice. Inflammation of the preputial diverticulum, preputial diverticulitis, has an unknown pathogenesis. Deflection of the penis into the diverticulum because of malformation or masturbation is suspected, and local infection occurs. Macroscopically, there is swelling above the preputial orifice and foul-smelling fluid and exudate can be expressed instead of the normal clear fluid. Histologically, the epithelium is eroded and covered with fibrin, debris, and neutrophils. Lymphocytes and plasma cells and granulation tissue are located in the wall. The diverticulum is also a location for papillomas to develop.

DISORDERS OF DOGS AND CATS

Dogs and cats have reproductive disorders that are common to all species, including cryptorchidism and testicular atrophy/degeneration. Dogs have a high prevalence of testicular neoplasia (described previously). The only accessory genital gland in the dog is the prostate, and dogs develop all of the disorders seen in humans, including prostatic hyperplasia, prostatic and paraprostatic cysts, prostatitis, and prostatic carcinoma. Of the many disorders of the penis and prepuce, canine transmissible venereal tumor is unique and outlined later.

ORCHITIS AND EPIDIDYMITIS

Infectious orchitis and epididymitis occur most commonly in mature dogs, and not just at puberty. The reason for this is unknown. Most cases are caused by Gram-negative bacteria such as *Escherichia coli,* and presumably by ascending infection. Orchitis is surprisingly common too, and hematogenous or local spread are both possible. In severe disease, dogs have a large painful and doughy scrotum plus endotoxemia and the systemic response to infection with anorexia, lethargy, and fever. The tail of the epididymis and vaginal tunics are usually affected, but in some cases, a severe necrotizing orchitis also occurs. Dogs will lick and chew at the affected scrotum and create a fistula to the scrotal contents (see Fig. 19-20). *Brucella canis* infection also causes epididymitis but by the hematogenous route. The lesions in the testis and epididymis (see Fig. 19-18) are identical to those described previously in the discussion of epididymitis in the section on Disorders of Ruminants. Testicular atrophy and degeneration is an invariable consequence of epididymitis, and many dogs also have prostatitis.

PROSTATE GLAND (PROSTATIC) HYPERPLASIA

The dog is the only domestic animal species to spontaneously develop prostatic hyperplasia with age (see Fig. 19-29, *A* and *B*). The clinical consequence of prostatic enlargement includes constipation from the "ball valve" effect of a large prostate forced into the pelvis during attempted defecation. Although obstruction of the urethra is a feature of prostatic hyperplasia in humans, stenosis of the urethra only occasionally occurs in the canine disease. Enlargement of the prostate is hormone related, but the precise mechanisms are unknown. Enlargement of the gland does not occur in castrated dogs, and removal of androgens by castration of affected dogs causes atrophy. Administration of estrogens causes enlargement of the gland because estrogen and testosterone operate in concert. Estrogen is responsible for the fibromuscular hyperplasia and testosterone is mostly responsible for the epithelial hyperplasia (see Fig. 19-29, *C*). Enlargement of the gland is usually uniform. On occasion, the hyperplasia is cystic, and in extreme cases, a large single cyst or multiple small cysts are found. Microscopically, there is hyperplasia of the acinar epithelium and individual epithelial cells are larger than normal and their apical cytoplasm is expanded and filled with eosinophilic globules. Stromal hyperplasia causes a larger amount of the interlobular and to a lesser extent the intralobular fibromuscular stroma. Some acini are distended with fluid and have a flattened epithelium.

Estrogen-induced hypertrophy of the canine prostate gland is most often seen with a testicular Sertoli cell tumor. Hyperestrogenism also causes squamous metaplasia of acinar epithelium, ducts, prostatic urethra, and any uterus masculinus (see Fig. 19-26, *C*). Flattened keratinized epithelial cells are desquamated into the acini, and neutrophils and other inflammatory cells are present. Squamous metaplasia of the prostate gland in dogs is not preneoplastic.

PROSTATIC AND PARAPROSTATIC CYSTS

Prostatic and paraprostatic cysts occur periodically in dogs, and their origin is debated. Intraprostatic cysts occur in prostatic hyperplasia, squamous metaplasia, and prostatitis. Paraprostatic cysts are outside the capsule of the prostate. Some are an enlarged cystic uterus masculinus (see Cysts of the Male Tract) and some are serosal inclusion cysts or pseudocysts that do not have an epithelial lining. Many are probably hyperplastic cysts formed when cystic acini extrude through the incomplete muscular layer of the prostatic capsule, in a manner similar to adenomyosis of the uterus. Paraprostatic cysts can attain giant proportions, as large as 30 cm in diameter. Some become infected and abscessed. They have a thin wall, and some have mineralization and ossification of the collagen in the capsule. Microscopically, they have an inner lining of either flattened cuboidal epithelium, cells resembling mesothelium, or granulation and fibrous tissue. They have a thin fibrous capsule. Those with mineralization and ossification have normal woven or lamellar bone within the capsule. Most have no inflammation.

CARCINOMA OF THE PROSTATE GLAND

Canine prostatic carcinoma is the only prostatic neoplasm of importance in domestic animals (see Fig. 19-30, *A*). A similar disease is exceedingly rare in the cat. The cause is not known, and castration is not protective. Prostatic hyperplasia and metaplasia appear not to precede neoplasia, although hyperplasia and carcinoma are found together in intact dogs. Prostatic intraepithelial neoplasia (PIN) is only found in a high-grade form in prostates that already have carcinoma—there is no recognized low and intermediate grade PIN to suggest progression from one to the next. Some of the clinical signs of carcinoma of the prostate are similar to those of prostatic hyperplasia because of the enlargement of the organ. Carcinoma and its metastases cause cachexia and locomotor abnormalities through pressure and invasion of nearby structures, including the bones of the spine and pelvis. Macroscopically, there are two general appearances. The most obvious is the type that causes asymmetric extreme enlargement (see Fig. 19-30, *B*). The prostate gland becomes very large and attached to other pelvic structures. The second type is mostly periurethral, with a necrotic and cystic cavity within the prostatic capsule. It causes minimal enlargement of the gland, but urinary obstruction and metastatic disease are present. Castrated dogs are usually affected with this latter form.

Much has been written and said about the prevalence of different types of neoplasia of the prostate. Some authors have divided them into adenocarcinoma and transitional cell carcinoma; the latter presumably arise from the pelvic urethra or from prostatic ducts. There is also an intermediate category of mixed glandular and transitional types. Attempts to accurately phenotype carcinomas by histochemical, immunohistochemical, and molecular methods are unsuccessful because there are no specific markers to separate acinar from urothelial types. This is probably because of the common origin of prostatic ducts and glands and for urothelium in general. Because of this, the term *carcinoma of the prostate* is a general term used to refer to adenocarcinoma, mixed carcinoma, squamous cell carcinoma, and transitional cell carcinoma when the histologic type is purely glandular, mixed, squamous, or urothelial. The appearance of a carcinoma reflects attempted differentiation toward glandular, urothelial, or epidermal tissues, or mixtures of two or more (see Fig. 19-30, *C*). There are varying degrees of stroma between the neoplastic epithelial cells. Some also contain sarcomatous tissue.

The prognosis for carcinoma of the prostate is generally poor. About 80% of affected dogs have metastases to a lymph node and/or lung at the time of diagnosis, and 20% of these have metastasized to bone.

PROSTATITIS

Prostatitis is seen periodically and can be clinically significant if toxemia accompanies the infection or if there is urinary obstruction. Prostatitis is found in older animals, often together with hyperplasia, or in young animals without hyperplasia. Although increased concentrations of zinc in prostatic fluid is associated with antimicrobial properties in humans and dogs, resistance to infection and resolution of infection are not correlated with zinc concentrations in prostatic tissue in the dog. Prostatitis can usefully be divided into acute, chronic, abscess formation, and specific *(Brucella canis)* forms. Organisms, such as *Escherichia coli, Proteus vulgaris*, and others, invade from the urethra. The affected organ can be diffusely or focally involved, swollen, red, and edematous (see Fig. 19-31, *A*). The early microscopic lesion is neutrophilic, and acini contain neutrophils and debris. The degree of necrosis varies and is extensive in some cases. Abscesses can form (see Fig. 19-31, *B*). The abscesses can persist or be replaced by fibrous tissue. With continued inflammation, lymphocytes and plasma cells are present in the interstitium in large numbers. Usually, fibrosis is an accompanying change (see Fig. 19-31, *C*). Prostatitis is part of the spectrum of lesions caused by *Brucella canis* in the dog, and the prostate can be the site of persistence of the bacterium.

CANINE TRANSMISSIBLE VENEREAL TUMOR

Canine transmissible venereal tumor (CTVT) is a type of xenotransplantation. Based on immunologic, cytogenetic, and nucleotide sequence studies, the neoplasm is thought to arise from a specific genetic alteration of canine histiocytes, followed by the transmission of abnormal cells from dog to dog via direct contact with the tumor (see Fig. 18-52). The primary neoplasm is usually on the external genitalia, but extragenital primaries and metastases also occur, particularly in stray dogs and those in poor health. The neoplasm is found on the penis, more often on the proximal parts, and not often on the prepuce (Fig. 19-37, *A*). The neoplasm can be single or multiple and up to 10 cm in diameter, with a red, ulcerated, multinodular surface. Microscopically, the neoplastic cells form a diffuse sheet with minimal stroma. They are large, round or oval, and uniform in size, thus resembling lymphocytes (Fig. 19-37, *B*). The cytoplasm is pale staining and may have peripheral vacuoles that are readily identified on cytologic preparations. This neoplasm can develop multifocal necrosis and spontaneously regress because of lymphocyte-mediated cytotoxicity.

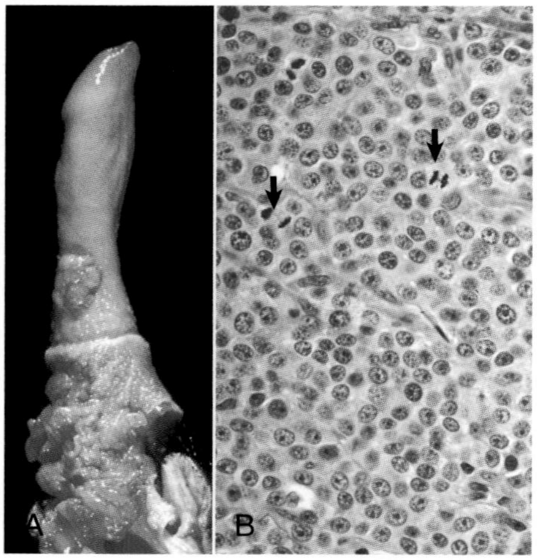

Fig. 19-37 Transmissible venereal tumor, penis, dog. **A,** There is a large multinodular mass involving the penis and the prepuce at its reflection from the penis. **B,** Neoplastic cells are round, uniform in size, and often divided into packets by a fine fibrous stroma. Mitoses are frequent *(arrows)*. H&E stain. (**A** courtesy Dr. M.D. McGavin, College of Veterinary Medicine, University of Tennessee. **B** courtesy Dr. M. J. Abdy, College of Veterinary Medicine, The University of Georgia; and Noah's Arkive, College of Veterinary Medicine, The University of Georgia.)

SUGGESTED READINGS

Information on this topic is available at evolve.elsevier.com/Zachary/McGavin/.

CHAPTER 20

The Ear and Eye*

Bradley L. Njaa† *and Brian P. Wilcock*‡

EAR

The ear is a specialized sense organ formed by a highly organized mixture of cutaneous, nasopharyngeal, osseous, and neurologic tissues. Within the ear are several air- and fluid-filled interfaces involved in the transduction of sound and pressure waves to action potentials that are conducted by the nervous system to the brain for interpretation and appropriate motor and cognitive responses.

In the context of interacting with animals, hearing is often considered of secondary or tertiary importance when compared to vision or olfaction. For many years, specific breeds predisposed to auditory dysfunction were maintained in colonies to facilitate investigation as animal models of human disease. More recently, throughout the world, deaf and hearing-impaired people are greatly benefiting from professionally trained hearing dogs. In addition, animal trainers, pet owners, and producers rely on a fully functioning auditory system to train, address, keep safe, or herd their animals. Therefore a much better understanding of conditions affecting this special sense is needed.

Many current textbooks focus on one species or one aspect of the ear. The focus of this chapter is to (1) clarify the anatomy of the ear by comparing and contrasting anatomic features of the domestic animal species, (2) address the responses to injury and the defense mechanisms protecting against injury, and (3) delineate various otic diseases that either affect many different species or are more unique to certain species.

STRUCTURE AND FUNCTION

EXTERNAL EAR

The external ear comprises the auricle (also known as pinna) and external acoustic meatus terminating medially at the tympanic membrane. Developmentally, the external ear arises from tissue elevations called *auricular hillocks,* three from the first branchial or pharyngeal arch and three from the second branchial or pharyngeal arch. The first pharyngeal groove or cleft between the two arches forms the external acoustic meatus. As they come into apposition early in development, the auricle and external acoustic meatus form. The auricle is a highly mobile and flexible, cartilaginous structure that is covered by haired skin with adnexa more dense on the convex than concave surface. The structural characteristics of auricles are closely tied to breed specifications. Among the species and breeds covered in this chapter, auricles can be erect, semi-erect, lop-eared, pendulous, microtic, or folded.

The auricle functions to collect, focus, and direct sound down the funnel-shaped external acoustic meatus to the tympanic membrane (Fig. 20-1). Because the rostroauricular and caudoauricular muscles are innervated by motor branches of the facial nerve, the flexible (cartilaginous) auricle is able to move rostrally, laterally, and caudally about a central auricular axis. The position of the auricle can signal an animal's behavior or emotion. Fearful cats often flatten their ears in a defensive posture, whereas angry horses often completely flatten their ears caudally as an initial warning before they strike. Alternatively, a dog may flatten its ears when content or when it is being verbally scolded.

The external acoustic meatus (ear canal) is a conical opening made up of elastic cartilage and bone (Fig. 20-2). The more lateral portions are composed of auricular cartilage that narrows and overlaps with annular cartilage. Dense fibrous connective tissue forms a bridge between the annular cartilage ring and the osseus portion of the external acoustic meatus. In cats and dogs, the osseous portion (1) is a very narrow rim of bone and (2) is a broad opening exposing the tympanic membrane that is readily visible during otic examination. In horses, ruminants, and pigs, the osseous portion of the external acoustic meatus is an elongate cylinder of bone with a narrow lumen (Fig. 20-3). In horses, the junction between the cartilaginous and osseous portions of the external acoustic meatus is grossly identified by an abrupt change from pigmented to non-pigmented epithelium. Visualization of the deeper portions of the external acoustic meatus in livestock species requires specialized equipment and heavy sedation.

Although there are wide species variations, the cartilaginous and osseous portions of the external acoustic meatus are lined by

*Dr. W.W. Carlton, College of Veterinary Medicine, Purdue University, and Dr. J.A. Render, North American Science Associates, contributed to the section on the eye and ear in the third edition.
†Contributor of the section on the ear.
‡Contributor of the section on the eye.

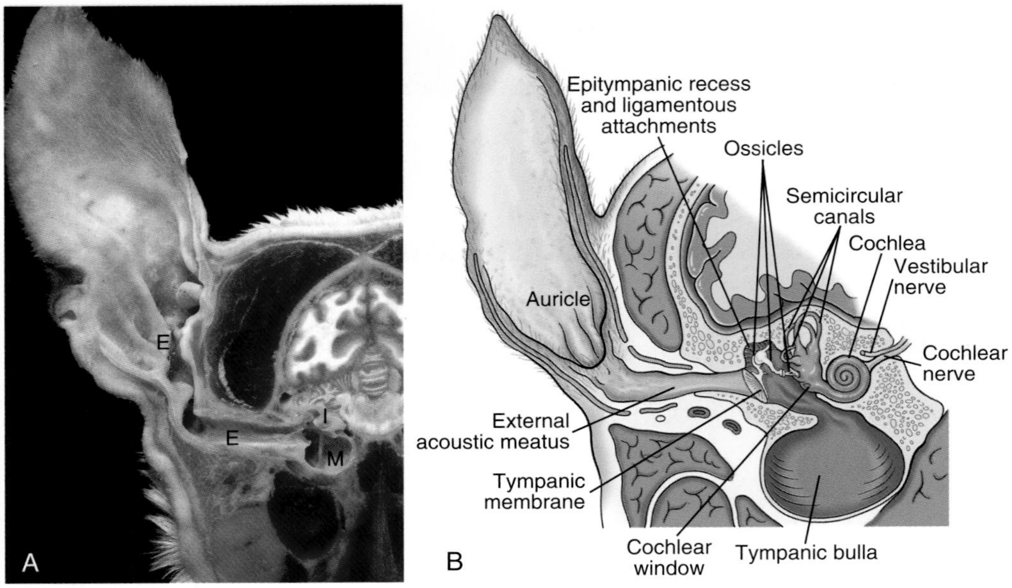

Fig. 20-1 Major regions of the ear.
A, Cross-section, head through the right ear, rostral surface, dog. External *(E),* middle *(M),* and inner *(I)* ear are illustrated. The tympanic membrane has been removed in this section. The external ear consists of the auricle and external acoustic meatus; the middle ear consists of the ossicles, tympanic cavity, and bulla; and the inner ear consists of the cochlea and semicircular canals. **B,** Schematic diagram depicting a cross-section through the external, middle, and inner ear of a dog. (**A** courtesy Dr. B.L. Njaa, Center for Veterinary Health Sciences, Oklahoma State University.)

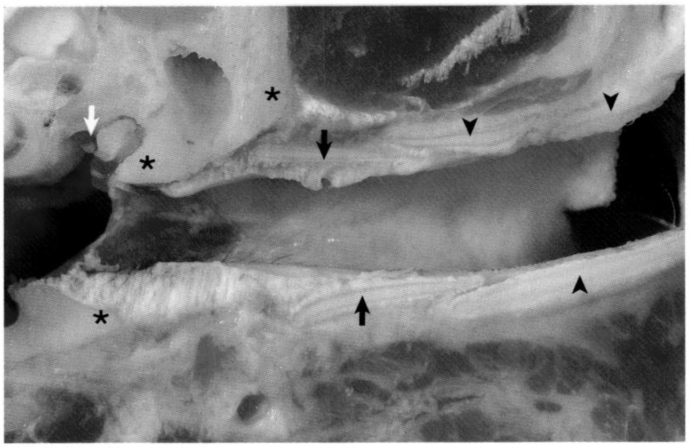

Fig. 20-2 External acoustic meatus, osseous and cartilaginous portions, cross-section through the left ear, dog.
Annular *(black arrows)* and auricular cartilage *(black arrowheads)* form the structure of the cartilaginous portion of the external acoustic meatus. Dense, white, fibrous connective tissue attaches the annular cartilage to the osseous rim of the external acoustic meatus *(asterisks).* The incudostapedius joint is visible in this image *(white arrow).* The tympanic membrane is removed in this section. (Courtesy Dr. B.L. Njaa, Center for Veterinary Health Sciences, Oklahoma State University.)

a thin epidermis formed by stratified squamous epithelium and a thin dermis that contains a relatively uniform allotment of sebaceous glands, fewer hair follicles, and greater ceruminous glands when comparing medial to lateral portions (Fig. 20-4). Sebaceous glands are composed of 6 to 10 club-shaped acini surrounded by thin fibrous tissue with ducts opening into associated hair follicles. Relative to ceruminous glands, they tend to be located in the more superficial dermis. Ceruminous glands are simple, coiled, tubular glands that resemble apocrine sweat glands. Their ducts open either into hair follicles or directly to the epidermal surface.

Although motor innervation of muscles of the external acoustic meatus is provided by the facial cranial nerve, sensory innervation is more complex. Branches of the trigeminal, facial, and vagal cranial nerves and branches of the second cervical spinal nerve innervate the skin. Sensory innervation to the mucosa of the external acoustic meatus is provided by the mandibular branch of trigeminal and auriculotemporal cranial nerves. The primary blood supply to the ear is through the caudal auricular artery, which branches into the lateral, intermediate, deep, and medial auricular arteries. The caudal auricular artery is a main branch of the external carotid artery.

MIDDLE EAR

Tympanic Membrane (Tympanum)

The tympanic membrane, also known as the tympanum, is an extremely thin, three-layered, semitransparent membrane peripherally suspended from the tympanic ring by a fibrocartilaginous ring. The tympanic membrane is formed when the endoderm of the first pharyngeal pouch comes into close contact with the ectoderm of the first pharyngeal cleft or groove. Most of the tympanic membrane is held under tension so it can be deformed by and responsive to sound waves (Fig. 20-5). It covers the medial extremity of external acoustic meatus, demarcating the junction between the external ear and middle ear. Both surfaces of the tympanic membrane have an air interface.

In most species, the tympanum is an oval-to-round structure, whereas in ruminants, it is shaped more like a broad triangle (Fig. 20-6). Embedded in the tympanum is the manubrium of the malleus. The placement of the manubrium in the tympanic membrane is highly variable between species. It is more centrally located in horses versus a more rostromedial location in ruminants and pigs.

The tympanum is divided into two sections, the *pars tensa* and the *pars flaccida.* The majority of the tympanic membrane is made up of the pars tensa, which is a very thin, translucent, and taut membrane that bulges convexly into the tympanic cavity (Fig. 20-6,

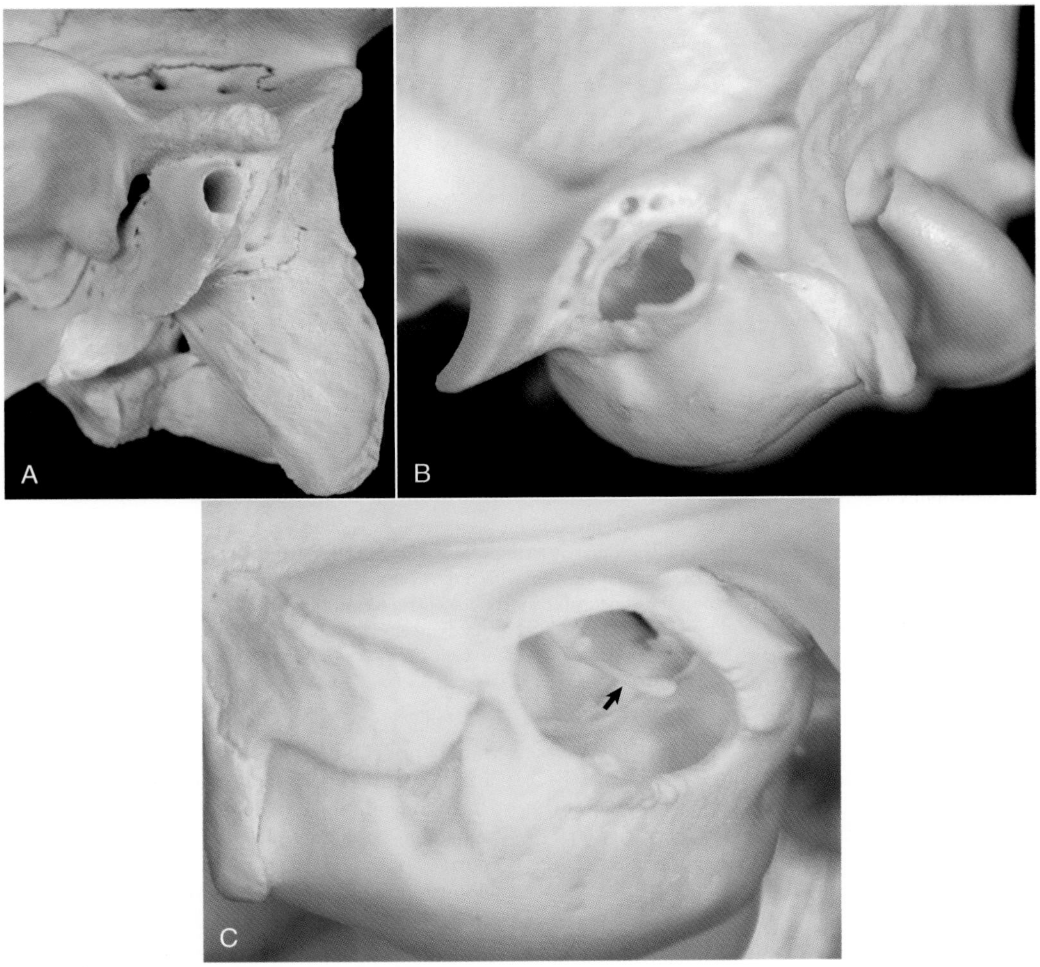

Fig. 20-3 Osseous external acoustic meatus, macerated specimens.
A, Ox. The bony external acoustic meatus in most livestock is much longer and narrower when compared to dogs and cats. Visualization of the middle ear is obscured by the elongate osseous external acoustic meatus. **B,** Dog. The osseous portion of the external acoustic meatus is a thin rim of bone allowing easy visualization of the middle ear. **C,** Cat. The osseous portion of the external acoustic meatus is very thin and the opening is very large, allowing easy visualization of the middle ear and malleus *(arrow)*. (Courtesy Dr. B.L. Njaa, Center for Veterinary Health Sciences, Oklahoma State University.)

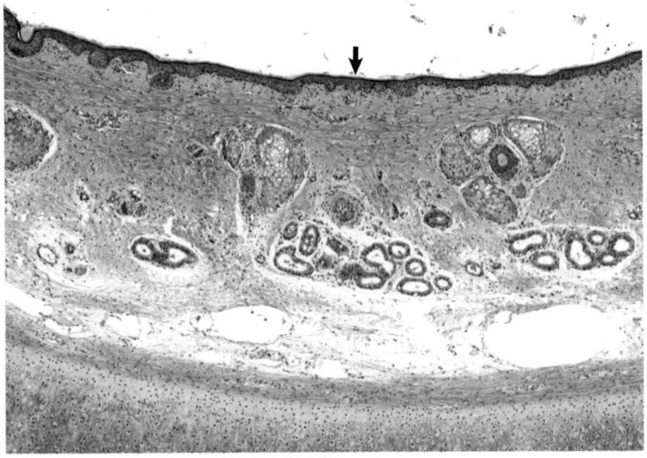

Fig. 20-4 External acoustic meatus epithelium and adnexa, pig.
Stratified squamous epithelium *(arrow)* lines the external acoustic meatus. Adnexa present are mixtures of sebaceous glands, most often flanking hair follicles, and deeper eccrine glands referred to as *ceruminous glands.* Auricular cartilage is present along the lower edge of the image. H&E stain. (Courtesy Dr. B.L. Njaa, Center for Veterinary Health Sciences, Oklahoma State University.)

E). The pars tensa is made up of three layers: (1) outer layer of keratinizing squamous epithelium derived from ectoderm of the first pharyngeal groove; (2) middle layer of thin, variably vascularized fibrous connective tissue originating from the pharyngeal wall; and (3) inner layer of very low cuboidal to nonkeratinizing squamous epithelium, which is of pharyngeal pouch origin.

The dorsal most portion of the tympanic membrane is the pars flaccida, which is roughly triangular, thicker, more vascular, and flaccid when compared to the pars tensa (see Fig. 20-6, *E*). Overlain by keratinized epithelium, the underlying stroma of the pars flaccida in dogs is made of loosely arranged collagen, rare mast cells, and few elastin fibers. This latter feature is in direct contrast to humans in which there are abundant elastin fibers. Visualized from the external acoustic meatus, this portion of the tympanic membrane may bulge into or away from the middle ear.

The tympanic membrane is placed roughly at a 45-degree angle relative to the central axis of horizontal portion of the external acoustic meatus (Fig. 20-7, *A*). However, commonly, the actual placement of the tympanic membrane is more variable with the external, concave surface of the tympanic membrane angled more rostrally (Fig. 20-7, *B* and *C*). Cats have a similar orientation to their tympanum (Fig. 20-8). Interestingly, the surface area of the

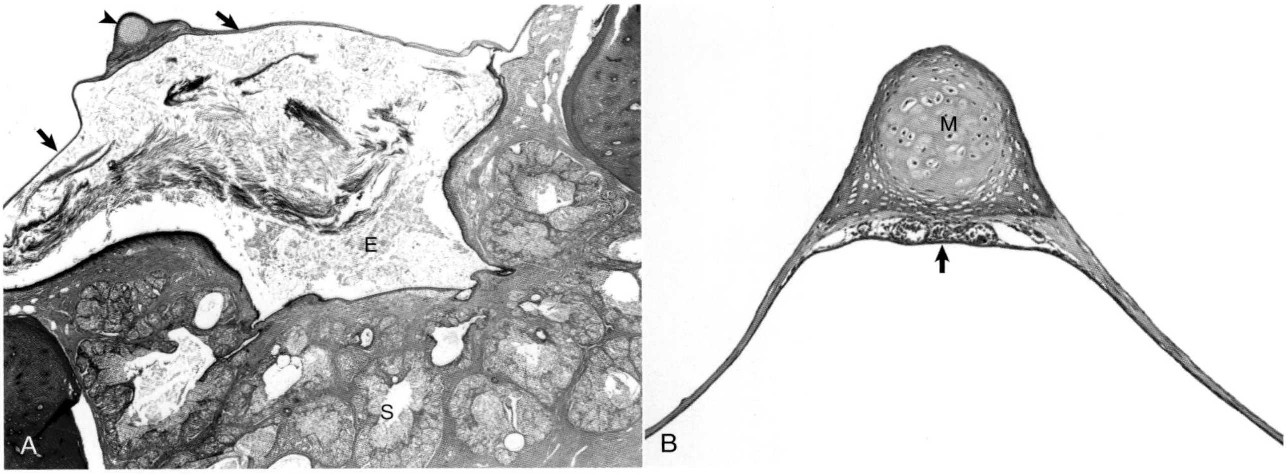

Fig. 20-5 Tympanic membrane.
A, Cat. Cross-section through the tympanic membrane *(arrows)*, manubrium of the malleus *(arrowhead)*, and external acoustic meatus *(E)*. An intact tympanic membrane at the level of the pars tensa is very thin. It is lined by a single layer of cornified squamous epithelial cells externally, and low cuboidal to noncornified squamous epithelium line the inner surface. The abundant keratin within the external acoustic meatus is not uncommon. The prominent, multiple, branching sebaceous glands *(S)* are common in the deepest portions of the external acoustic meatus. H&E stain. **B,** Higher magnification of the tympanic membrane and malleus, pig. The manubrium *(M)* of the malleus is embedded in the tympanic membrane. Numerous blood vessels are present beneath the manubrium *(arrow)* and are located in the middle layer of the tympanic membrane beneath the external concave surface, which corresponds with the region of germinative epithelium. H&E stain. (Courtesy Dr. B.L. Njaa, Center for Veterinary Health Sciences, Oklahoma State University.)

tympanic membrane from an approximately 550-kg horse is larger than the tympanic membrane of a Maltese dog but is approximately 15% smaller than the surface area of the tympanic membrane of a German shepherd dog. Additionally, the tympanum of the fetal goat is approximately 20% larger than that of large dog breeds.

Tympanic Cavity

The tympanic cavity is an air-filled compartment surrounded by bone that is separated from the external ear by a thin tympanic membrane (tympanum) and is in direct communication with the pharynx via the auditory tube (also known as the eustachian or pharyngotympanic tube). Both the tympanic cavity and the auditory tube are derived from the endoderm of the first pharyngeal pouch. The epitympanic recess is the dorsal extremity of the tympanic cavity within which lies the head of the malleus and short curs of the incus. Ligaments stabilize and anchor the incudomallearis joint and the short crus of the incus within this recess (Fig. 20-9).

In many species, there is a bulbous, ventral portion of the tympanic cavity called the *tympanic bulla* (see Fig. 20-3, *B* and *C*). Within the bulla of the dog and cat is a bony septum referred to as the *septum bulla.* In the cat, the septum bulla abuts the petrous portion of the temporal bone and separates the tympanic cavity into two compartments: the dorsolateral epitympanic cavity and the ventromedial tympanic cavity (see Fig. 20-8). This separation is incomplete, which allows communication between the two compartments through a narrow opening between the septum bulla and petrous portion of the temporal bone and a larger opening at its caudal edge. In the dog, this septum is a much smaller, incomplete bony ridge that only makes contact with the petrous portion of the temporal bone rostrally and often has tiny, elongate bony spicules with bulbous ends (see Fig. 20-7, *B*). The mucosal surfaces of the tympanic bullae of cats and dogs are lined by an epithelium that varies, depending on location. Dorsally, close to the auditory tube opening, the mucosa is composed mostly of ciliated columnar cells mixed with goblet cells and basal cells similar to the cells in the nasopharyngeal mucosae (Fig. 20-10 and see Fig. 20-20). Ventrally, the number of ciliated cells and goblet cells decreases and the number of cuboidal, less differentiated cells increases. The surfaces of the petrous portion of the temporal bone, auditory ossicles, and tympanic membrane are lined by cuboidal to noncornifying squamous epithelium. In ruminants, camelids, and pigs, the ventral portion of the tympanic cavity or bulla is made of more numerous bony compartments lined by noncornifying squamous epithelium (Fig. 20-11). In cattle and pigs, these compartments are air-filled with direct communication with the tympanic cavity. In camelids and small ruminants, the tympanic cavity does not appear to directly communicate with the bullae. Horses do not have readily identifiable tympanic bullae.

Auditory Ossicles

A chain of three bones or auditory ossicles forms the mechanical transduction system of hearing: the malleus, incus, and stapes (Figs. 20-12 and 20-13). The malleus and the incus, as well as the tensor tympani, are derived from the mesenchyme of the first branchial or pharyngeal arch. The stapes and the stapedius muscle originate from the mesenchyme of the second branchial or pharyngeal arch.

Malleus

The largest of the ossicles is the malleus. The manubrium of the malleus is embedded in the tympanic membrane (see Fig. 20-5). The most ventromedial convexity of the malleus is the "umbo" (see Figs. 20-6, *F,* and 20-12). The muscular process of the manubrium near the neck of the malleus is the attachment site of a thin tendinous portion of the tensor tympani muscle. Various ligaments stabilize the malleus in the epitympanic cavity by anchoring the long, thin rostral process, the neck, and the head of the malleus. The head of the malleus articulates with the articular surface of the body of the incus forming the incudomallearis joint (see Figs. 20-9, 20-12, and 20-13). In the horse and cow and in aged dogs and cats, the incudomallearis joint capsule is a narrow but thick ligament that makes disarticulation difficult and gives the external appearance of a falsely fused joint. In younger dogs and cats, the incudomallearis ligament is not nearly as tenacious and disarticulation is much less difficult.

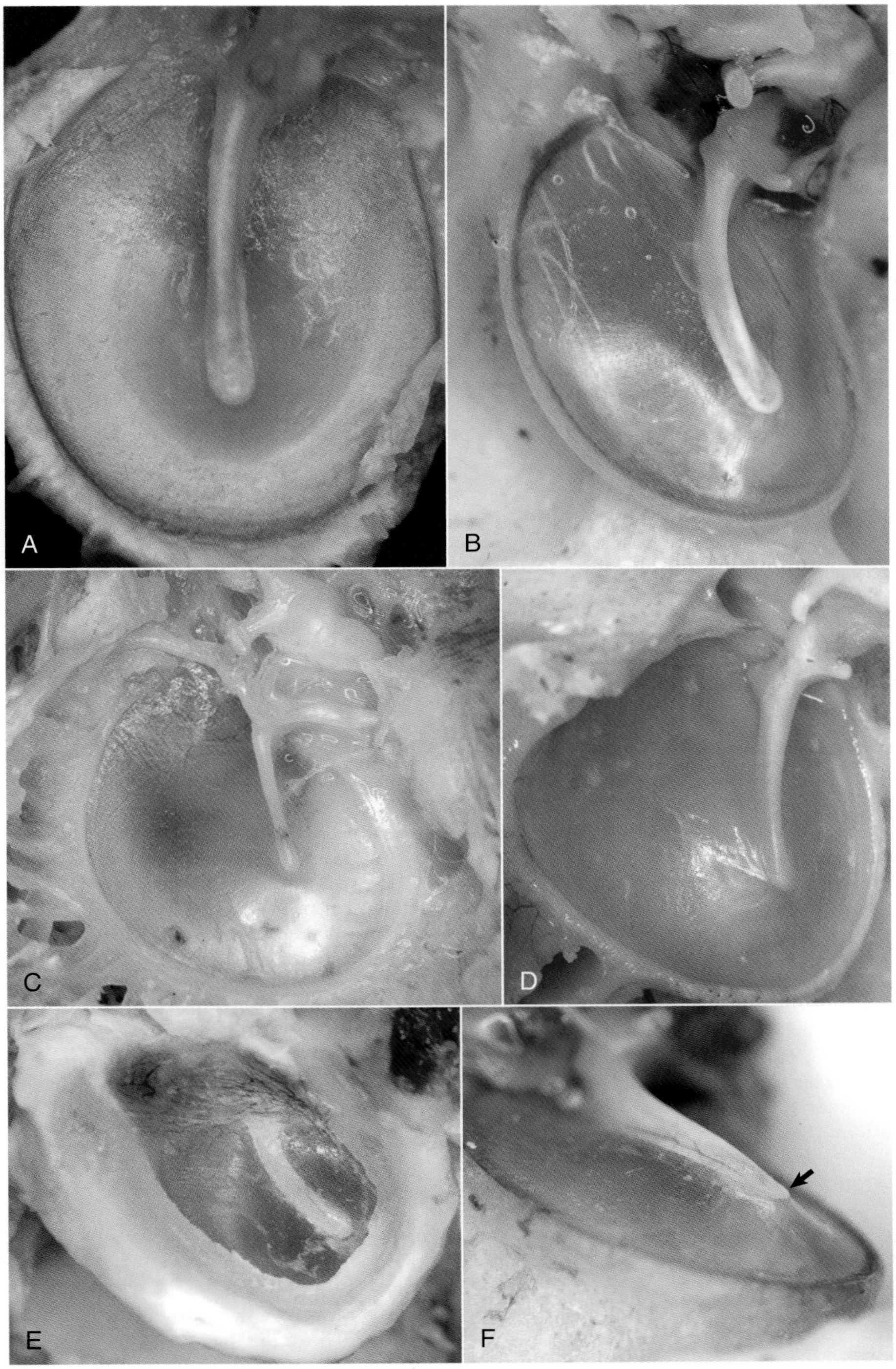

Fig. 20-6 **Tympanic membrane.**
A, Horse. In the horse, the tympanic membrane (tympanum) is more round than other species. The manubrium of the malleus forms a very shallow arc and is centrally located in the tympanum. **B,** Dog. The tympanum is oval to comma-shaped in dogs, and the manubrium of the malleus is C-shaped. **C,** Pig. The shape of the tympanic membrane is similar to that of the dog, but the manubrium of the malleus is shorter and straighter. **D,** Goat. Ruminants tend to have a more triangular-shaped tympanic membrane. In both pigs and ruminants, the manubrium of the malleus is more rostral and medial than in other species. **E,** Dog. Lateral view of tympanic membrane. The transparent portion of the tympanic membrane held under tension and associated with the manubrium of the malleus is the pars tensa. The highlights depict the radial striations of the normal pars tensa. Dorsally, the tympanic membrane is thicker, highly vascular and is under much less tension, and is designated as the pars flaccida. **F,** Dog. The tympanic membrane is convex on its medial surface in the tympanic cavity. The ventromedial extremity of the manubrium is called the umbo *(arrow)*. (Courtesy Dr. B.L. Njaa, Center for Veterinary Health Sciences, Oklahoma State University.)

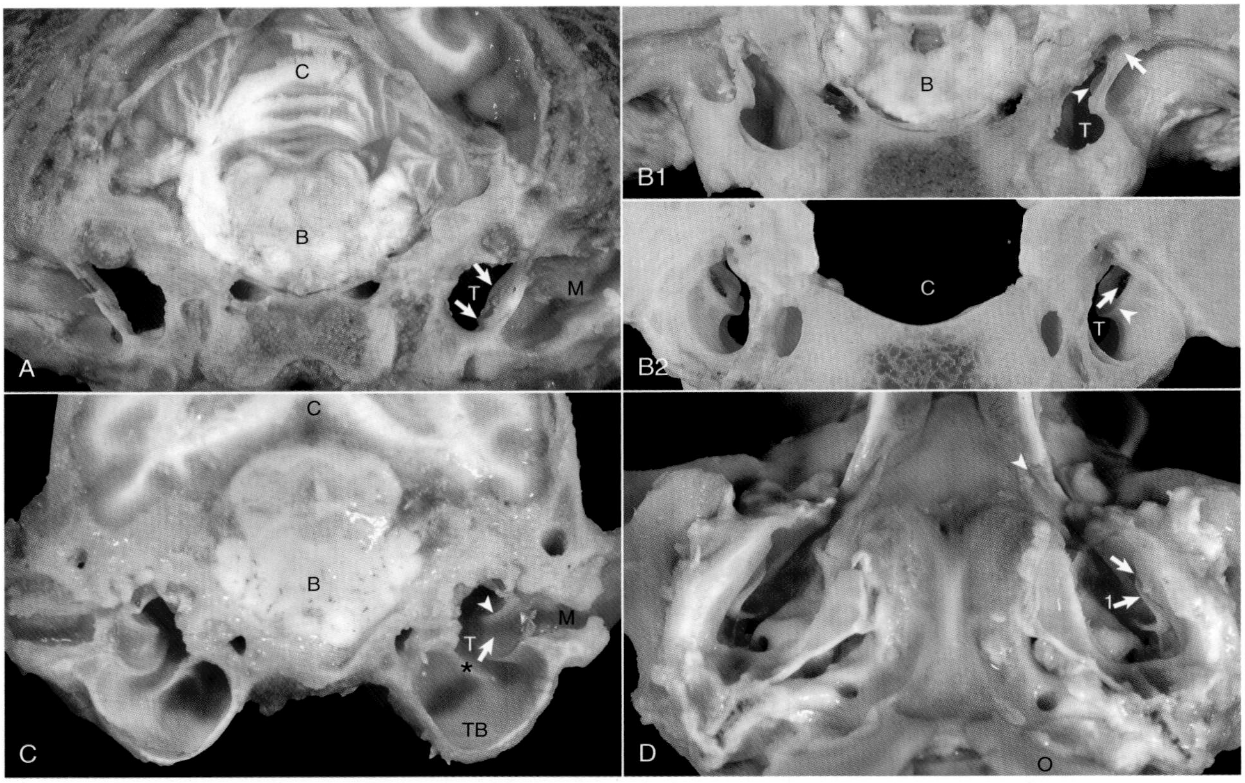

Fig. 20-7 External acoustic meatus, tympanic membrane, tympanic cavity. Compare unlabeled contralateral side with labeled side for more structural detail.

A, Transverse section, rostral surface, dog. The tympanic membrane *(arrows)* extends medially towards the tympanic cavity *(T)* at an approximate 45-degree angle from dorsal to ventral, in relation to the central axis of the horizontal part of the external acoustic meatus *(M).* Portions of the rostral edge of the tympanic ring have been inadvertently removed during sample preparation. Brainstem *(B);* cerebellum *(C).* **B,** Transverse section, rostral (1) and caudal (2) surfaces, goat. The tympanic cavity *(T)* has been opened bilaterally. In the cranial view *(1),* the tympanic membrane is not visualized because it is hidden by the tympanic ring *(arrows),* which surround the membrane. The manubrium of the malleus *(arrowheads)* is minimally visible. However, from the caudal view *(2),* the tympanic membrane *(arrows)* is clearly visible and is positioned so that the concave or external surface is tilted rostrally. Brainstem *(B);* calvarium where brainstem would be positioned *(C);* tympanic ring *(arrowheads).* **C,** Transverse section, caudal surface, dog. The external or concave surface of the tympanic membrane *(arrow)* is angled almost fully rostral rather than lateral. Note that the septum bullae *(asterisk)* are short and incomplete in the dog when compared with a cat (see Fig. 20-10). Brainstem *(B);* Cerebellum *(C);* Tympanic cavity *(T);* Manubrium of the malleus *(arrowheads);* External acoustic meatus *(M),* Tympanic bullae *(TB).* **D,** Ventral-dorsal view, opened bullae. Bilaterally, the concave surface of the tympanic membranes *(arrow)* are tilted rostrally. Occipital condyles *(O)* appear at the bottom of the image. Extending rostrally and medially from the tympanic cavity are the auditory tubes *(arrowhead),* which provide direct communication between the tympanic cavity and nasopharynx. Manubrium of the malleus *(arrow 1).* (Courtesy Dr. B.L. Njaa, Center for Veterinary Health Sciences, Oklahoma State University.)

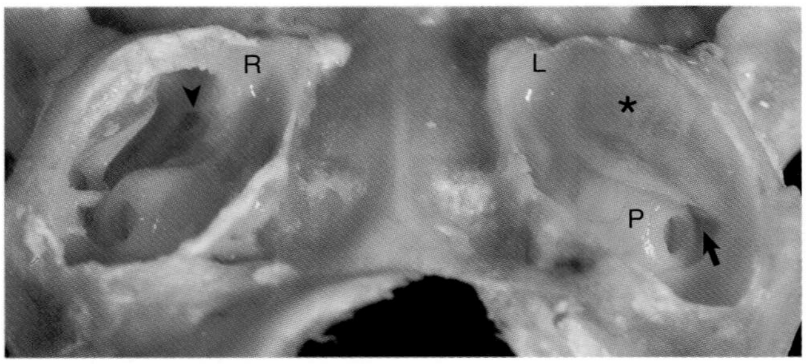

Fig. 20-8 Tympanic bullae, cat.

Caudoventral section, with both tympanic bullae opened ventrally. The septum bulla *(asterisk)* is intact in the left bulla *(L)* and opened ventrally in the right bulla *(R).* From rostral to caudal, the septum bulla dorsally abuts the petrous portion of the temporal bone. At its caudal extreme is an opening that allows communication between the two cavities *(arrow).* The auditory tube opening into the tympanic cavity is observed in the dorsal, rostral extremity of the right epitympanic cavity *(arrowhead).* The large bulge rostral to the round window corresponds to the start of the cochlea and is called the promontory *(P).* In both specimens the tympanic membrane is tilted rostrally. (Courtesy Dr. B.L. Njaa, Center for Veterinary Health Sciences, Oklahoma State University.)

Incus

The incus is a bicuspid-shaped bone that lies caudal and dorsal to the malleus. It has two crura, one designated as the short crus, which is anchored in the epitympanic recess along with the body of the incus by a band of narrow connective tissue, and the other designated as the long crus, which transmits vibrations to the stapes. The lenticular process is at the end of the long crus (see Fig. 20-13), and in young animals, the lenticular process is a separate bone. In older animals, it fuses with the distal end of the long crus of the incus and articulates with the head of the stapes. Regardless of age, the incudostapedius joint capsular ligament is more translucent than the incudomallearis joint capsule and there is inherently more joint laxity.

Stapes

The stapes, named for its close resemblance to stirrups of a saddle, is often considered the smallest bone in the body.* However, its size

*This categorization depends on the age of the animal. In young animals, the unfused lenticular process of the long crus of the incus is the smallest bone in the body.

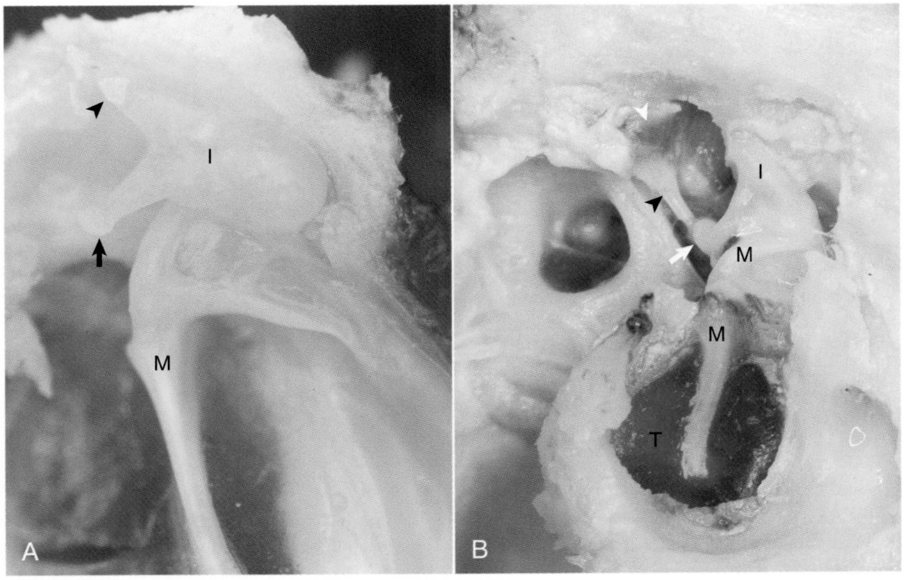

Fig. 20-9 Malleus, incus, incudomallearis joint, epitympanic recess.
A, Cat. Medial view. Seated in the epitympanic recess is the rounded head of the malleus *(M)* and the incus *(I)*; together they are articulated to form the incudomallearis joint. The smaller crus of the incus *(arrowhead)* and the head of the malleus are anchored to the epitympanic recess by ligaments (see Fig. 20-1). At the end of the longer crus of the incus is the lenticular process *(arrow)*. **B,** Giraffe. Lateral view, right ear. The tympanic membrane is intact *(T)*. The small crus of the incus *(I)* along with the head of the malleus *(M)* are firmly anchored in the epitympanic recess by ligamentous attachments. The lenticular process of the long crus articulates with the head of the stapes seated in the oval window to form the incudostapedius joint *(white arrow)*. The facial nerve has been removed in order to expose the stapedius muscle *(white arrowhead)*, which is firmly attached to the stapes via its tendon *(black arrowhead)*. (Courtesy Dr. B.L. Njaa, The Center for Veterinary Health Sciences, Oklahoma State University.)

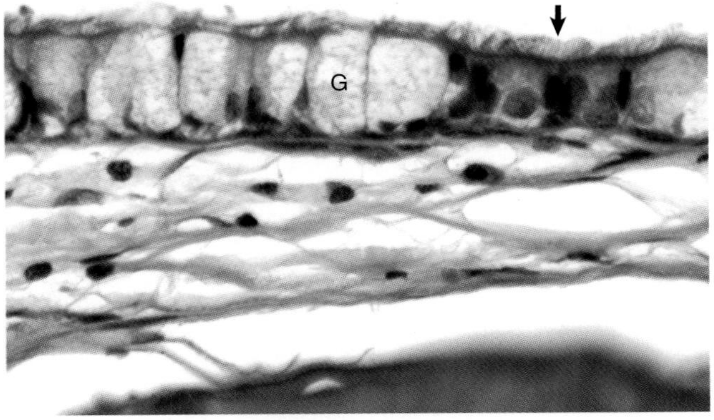

Fig. 20-10 Tympanic cavity mucosa, cat.
The mucosa of the tympanic cavity is not uniform. In cats and dogs, the mucosal epithelium in the more dorsal portions of the bullae morphologically mirrors mucosae of the nasopharynx. Included are ciliated columnar epithelial cells *(arrow)* and goblet cells *(G)* mixed with fewer nonciliated columnar epithelial cells. H&E stain. (Courtesy Dr. B.L. Njaa, Center for Veterinary Health Sciences, Oklahoma State University.)

and shape is somewhat variable, depending on species (Fig. 20-14). Its base or footplate is convex and firmly seated in the oval or vestibular window of the petrous portion of the temporal bone and anchored by the annular ligament of the stapes. This arrangement forms a syndesmosis between the stapes base and cartilage of the oval window (Fig. 20-15). The stapedius muscle, fittingly referred to as the smallest muscle in the body, is attached to the muscular process of the shorter caudal crus close to the head of the stapes. Vibrations of the tympanic membrane are linearly transduced to stapes vibrations that lead to fluid waves of the perilymph of the internal ear.

MIDDLE EAR MUSCLES AND NERVES

The middle ear has two muscles associated with the auditory ossicles that help modulate auditory transduction and a third muscle that controls patency of the auditory tube. The tensor tympani muscle originates rostrally and medially from the bony recess in the petrous portion of the temporal bone and makes its tendinous insertion onto the muscular process of the neck of the malleus (Fig. 20-16; see Fig. 20-13, *A*). It receives its innervation via a motor branch of the trigeminal nerve. Contraction of the tensor tympani muscle pulls the tympanic membrane medially and rostrally, placing greater tension on the auditory ossicle chain, which results in an increased resonant frequency of the auditory sound conduction system.

The stapedius muscle originates in the stapedius muscular fossa located dorsomedial to and obscured by the facial nerve as it courses through the facial groove of the temporal bone (Fig. 20-17). The stapedial branch of the facial nerve innervates this muscle as it converges into a thin tendon that inserts onto the muscular process of the short crus of the incus close to the head of the stapes. In the cat, the displacement variance of the stapes in its vestibular window is approximately 0.2 μm, whereas the maximal contraction of the stapedius muscle leads to dorsal and caudal stapedial bone displacement of between 40 and 60 μm. This displacement, which is perpendicular to the normal movement of the stapes, maximally attenuates sound transmission up to 30 decibels. Contraction of the stapedius muscle is an integral part of what is termed the *acoustic reflex,* defined as consensual, reflexive contraction of the muscle in response to stimuli (frequently sound) that leads to attenuated acoustic transmission.

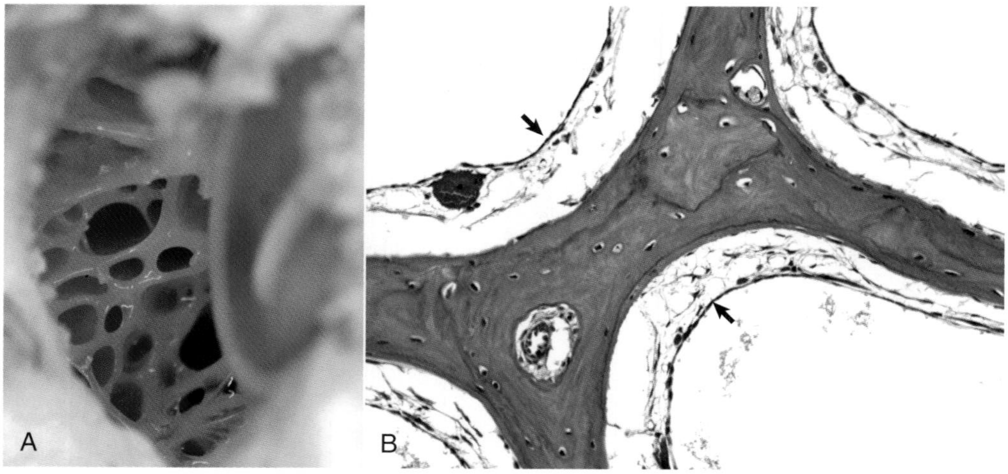

Fig. 20-11 Tympanic cavity and bulla.
A, Dorsal view into the middle ear, ox. Ruminants and pigs have small tympanic cavities but much larger tympanic bullae. The bullae are made of multiple, arborizing air-filled channels with numerous bony septa as shown here. **B,** Histologic section of tympanic bulla, pig. Bony septa are lined by low cuboidal to nonkeratinizing squamous epithelial cells *(arrows)*. H&E stain. (Courtesy Dr. B.L. Njaa, Center for Veterinary Health Sciences, Oklahoma State University.)

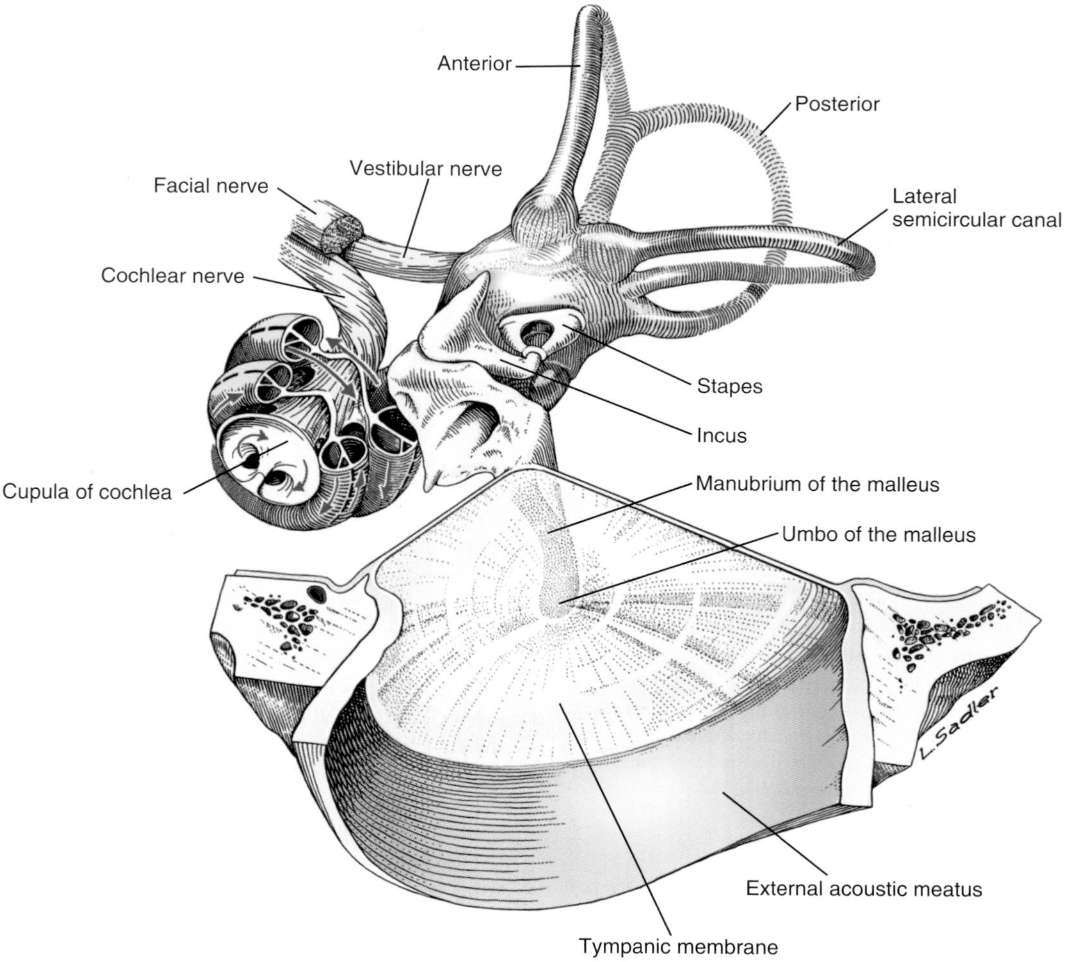

Fig. 20-12 Schematic diagram of the middle and inner ear, dog.
Tympanic membrane, auditory ossicles, and membranous labyrinth. The bony labyrinth has been removed to demonstrate the orientation of the cochlea and semicircular canals relative to the auditory ossicles and tympanic membrane. The facial nerve and vestibulocochlear nerve enter the ear together through the internal acoustic meatus.

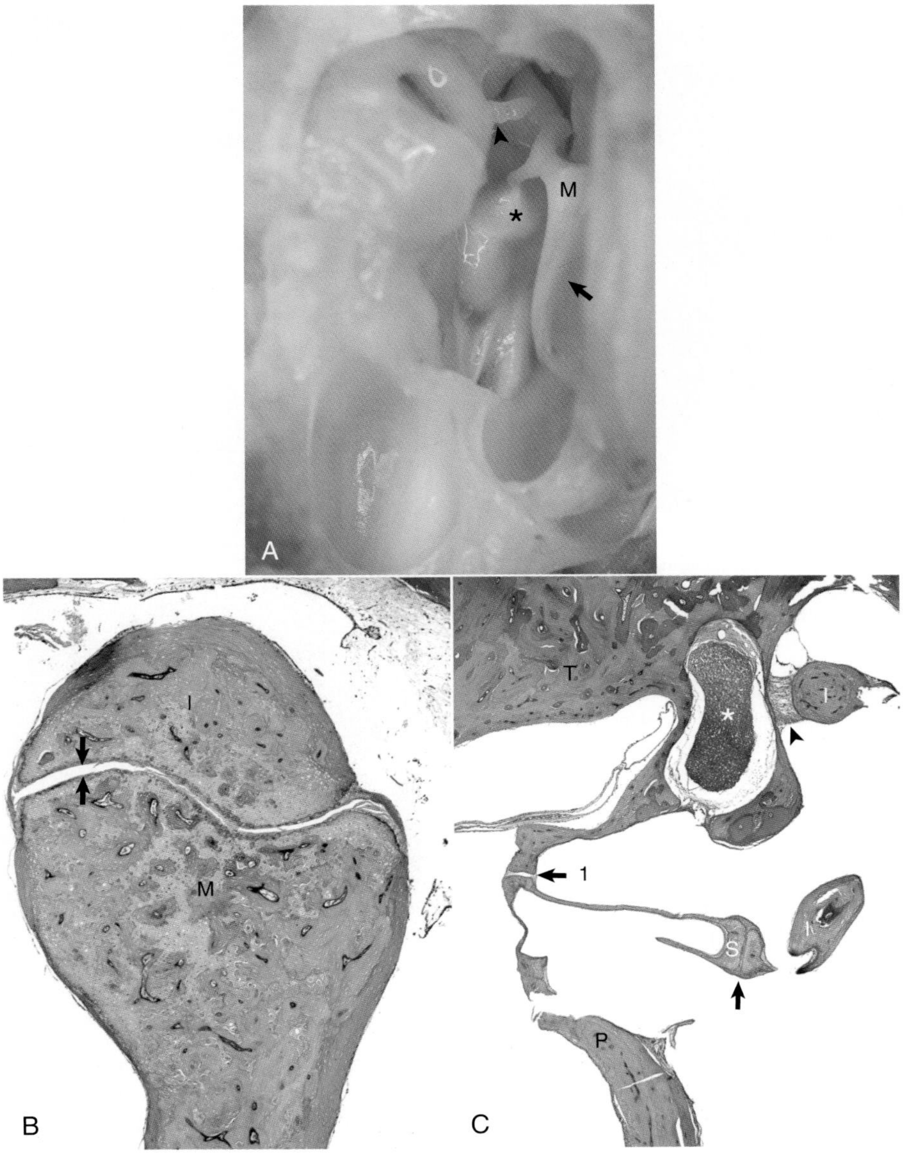

Fig. 20-13 **Auditory ossicles and ossicular joints, cat.**
A, Tympanic cavity, tympanic membrane, auditory ossicles, petrous portion of the temporal bone, auditory muscles, ventral view. The manubrium of the malleus is embedded in the tympanic membrane. The head of the malleus and incus are anchored in the epitympanic recess and form the incudomallearis joint. The long crus of the incus is shown articulating with the stapes to form the incudostapedius joint *(arrowhead).* Attached to the muscular process of the malleus *(M)* is the tensor tympani muscle *(asterisk).* Tympanic membrane *(arrow).* **B,** Histologic section of the incudomallearis joint *(between the arrows),* normal. The articulation of the malleus *(M)* and incus *(I)* is shown in the epitympanic recess. Similar to the petrous portion of the temporal bone, these ossicular bones lack a medulla. **C,** Histologic section of the incudostapedius joint. Positioned in the oval window is the stapes *(S),* held in place by a syndesmosis *(arrow 1).* The more ventral edge of the stapes has artifactually fractured. Articulating with the head of the stapes is the lenticular process of the long crus of the incus *(I)* to form the incudostapedius joint *(arrow).* The lenticular process of the incus is to the right of the incudostapedius joint. A portion of the short crus is positioned in the epitympanic recess and anchored by a ligamentous attachment *(arrowhead).* The facial nerve is present coursing through the facial groove *(asterisk).* Note the lack of complete bony encasement allowing communication with the tympanic cavity. Promontory *(P),* petrous portion of the temporal bone *(T).* H&E stain. (**A** and **B** courtesy Dr. B.L. Njaa, Center for Veterinary Health Sciences, Oklahoma State University.)

The tensor veli palatine muscle arises from a groove in the petrous portion of the temporal bone medial and ventral to the tensor tympani muscle. Along with its nerve, the tensor veli palatine nerve, a branch of the trigeminal nerve, this long, slender muscle extends rostrally from the tympanic cavity parallel to the auditory tube. In concert with the levator veli palatine muscle, which is innervated by the facial nerve, coordinated contraction of these muscles open the pharyngeal orifice of the auditory tube.

Two cranial nerves provide motor branches to the muscles of the middle ear. Branches of the trigeminal nerve named for their respective muscles innervate the tensor tympani and tensor veli palatine muscles within the tympanic cavity. The facial nerve initially leaves the cranial cavity through the internal acoustic meatus (see Fig. 20-17), along with the vestibulocochlear cranial nerve, and then courses through the facial groove of the petrous portion of the temporal bone in close proximity to the oval window

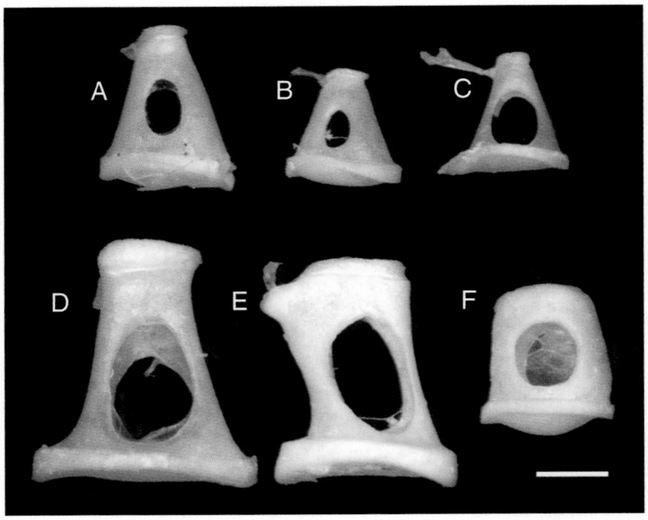

Fig. 20-14 Stapes, species variations.
Stapes are highly variable in size and shape, depending on the species. The first two stapes, beginning from the top row left are from different sized dogs. The larger stapes is from a 20 kg mixed breed dog **(A).** The smaller stapes is from a Maltese dog **(B).** The third stapes of the upper row is from a cat **(C).** The lower row depicts stapes from a horse **(D),** cow **(E),** and slaughter-age pig **(F).** In all cases, the lower plate of the stapes is convex. Also, in each case, the tendinous attachment of the stapedius muscle is affixed to the shorter crus or limb of the stapes. Scale bar = 1 mm. (Courtesy Dr. B.L. Njaa, Center for Veterinary Health Sciences, Oklahoma State University.)

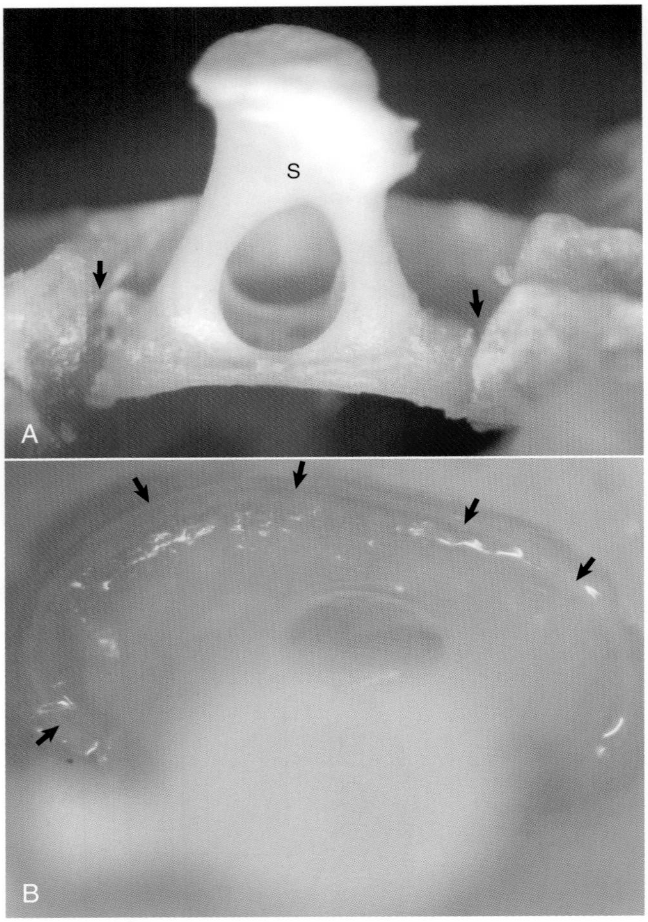

Fig. 20-15 Stapes in situ, horse.
A, Partially opened oval window. The stapes *(S)* is seated in the oval window connected to the petrous portion of the temporal bone by the annular ligament *(arrows).* **B,** Ventrolateral view of the stapes, in situ. A thin rim of annular cartilage is visible denoting the syndesmosis formed between the stapes and cartilage of the oval window of the petrous portion of the temporal bone *(arrows).* (Courtesy Dr. B.L. Njaa, Center for Veterinary Health Sciences, Oklahoma State University.)

(Fig. 20-18). Several millimeters medial and lateral to the tendon of the stapedius muscle, the bony casing of the facial groove is incomplete, which allows direct communication between the epineurial connective tissue of the facial nerve and the tympanic cavity (see Fig. 20-18). This proximity and exposure of the facial nerve to the tympanic cavity explains why middle ear disease can manifest as facial nerve dysfunction. The facial nerve emerges from the middle ear through the stylomastoid foramen immediately caudal to the external acoustic meatus.

AUDITORY TUBE (EUSTACHIAN OR PHARYNGOTYMPANIC TUBE)

In most mammalian species, the middle ear communicates with the pharynx through the auditory tube, which originates from the first pharyngeal pouch (Fig. 20-19). In the middle ear, the auditory tube opens into the most rostral and dorsal portion of the tympanic cavity called the *epitympanic cavity.* In the pharynx, the auditory tube originates from a narrow slit-like opening in the nasopharyngeal cavity and is lined by epithelium that is contiguous with the nasopharynx, namely ciliated, columnar pseudostratified epithelium mixed with goblet cells (Fig. 20-20). In many species, flanking the auditory tube are clusters of lymphocytes referred to as the tubal tonsil.

Infectious organisms can migrate via the auditory tube between the nasopharynx and the middle ear, thus serving as a portal of entry for each area. Additionally, the auditory tube is an important route for clearance of an infectious organism from the middle ear via the nasopharynx to the alimentary system.

Unique to the horse and other Equidae, guttural pouches (see Chapters 9 and 17) are enlarged diverticula of the auditory tubes that extend further rostrally, medially, and ventrally when compared to auditory tubes of other mammalian species. Although the precise function of guttural pouches remains controversial, their proximity to internal carotid arteries and their ability to inflate during vigorous exercise makes the idea of an extracalvarial brain cooling apparatus a provocative hypothesis.

INTERNAL EAR

The internal ear is confined to a single bone, the petrous portion of the temporal bone. In most mammalian species, it is a triangular, wedge-shaped bone that forms the dorsomedial margin of the tympanic cavity. Often referred to as the hardest bone of the body, it is frequently slightly more yellow than surrounding bone and lacks the cancellous bony arrangement or medullary cavities present in other portions of the temporal bone. The internal ear is derived from a focal area of ectoderm referred to as the *otic placode.* This eventually forms an otic vesicle and through interaction with surrounding embryonic tissues, differentiates into this highly specialized tissue.

The internal ear is essentially made up of several membranous compartments, collectively known as the *membranous labyrinth,* derived from ectoderm, that contain *endolymph.* The membranous labyrinthine compartments include the cochlea, sacculus, utricle,

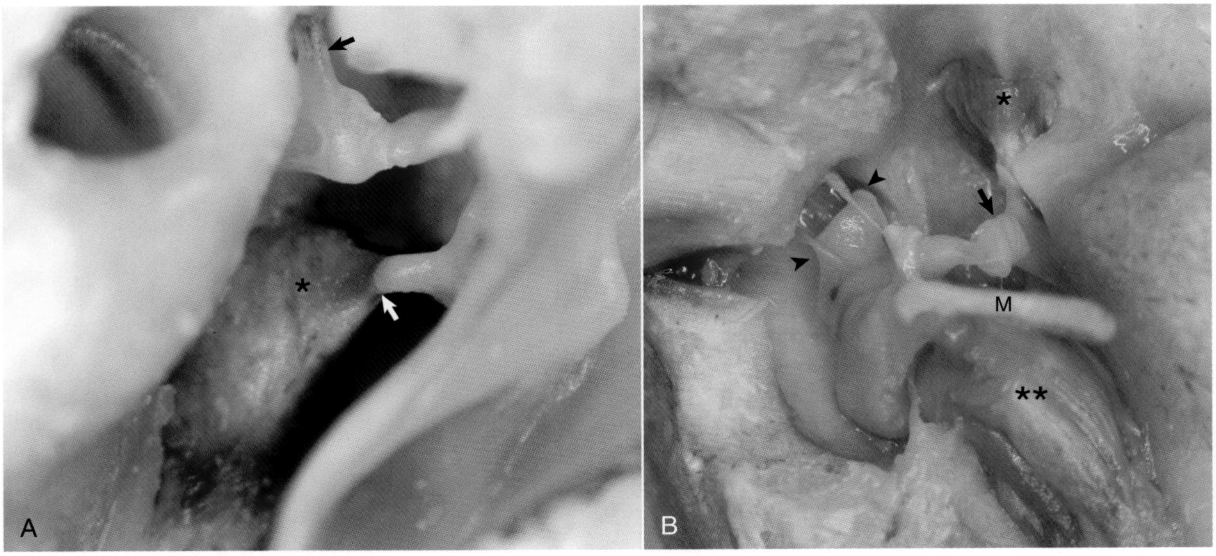

Fig. 20-16 Auditory ossicular muscles.
A, Middle ear, caudal view, ox. The external acoustic meatus is to the right on this image with the caudal edge of the tympanic membrane removed. The tensor tympani muscle *(asterisk)* is attached via its tendon to the muscular process of the malleus *(arrow)*. The tendon of the stapedius muscle *(arrowhead)* is attached to the stapes bone near the head of the stapes. **B,** Middle ear, ventral view, horse. The bony external acoustic meatus, tympanic membrane, and associated connective tissue have been removed. The articulated incus and malleus form the incudomalleolar joint and are anchored in the epitympanic recess *(arrowheads)*. The incudostapedius joint is opened *(arrow)*. The facial nerve and some of the surrounding bone have been removed to expose the stapedius muscle *(asterisk)* attached to the stapes seated in the oval window. The muscular process of the malleus is obscured by the position of the manubrium *(M)* of the malleus, which is attached to the tensor tympani muscle *(two asterisks)*. (Courtesy Dr. B.L. Njaa, Center for Veterinary Health Sciences, Oklahoma State University.)

and each semicircular canal with associated ampullae (Fig. 20-21). Surrounding the membranous labyrinth is a protective bony shell, derived from mesoderm, known as the *osseous labyrinth* (i.e., petrous portion of the temporal bone). The membranous labyrinth is classically a rostrally coiled tube or cochlea with an intermediate compartment or vestibule and a caudal semicircular canal region. However, the shape of the petrous portion of the temporal bone is very different. The beginning of the cochlea is denoted by the prominent bulge in the petrous portion of the temporal bone known as the *promontory*. Caudally, portions of this bone give the appearance of the tubular membranous labyrinth that likely represent the semicircular canals. Within the membranous labyrinth are biologic mechanosensory hair cells (see later) responsible for hearing (the auditory compartment) and for assessing head position, acceleration, and balance (the vestibular compartment).

Cochlea

The cochlea is the most complex portion of the membranous labyrinth comprising two closed-end tubular structures that are highly coiled (see Fig. 20-21). The central core of bony labyrinth around which the cochlea spirals nearly three times is the modiolus. Sound waves vibrate the tympanic membrane and are converted by coordinated movements of the malleus, incus, and stapes to fluid waves within the perilymph by vibrations of the vestibular or oval window. Fluid waves travel through the scala vestibuli toward the cupula, reaching the helicotrema, and then returning within the scala tympani toward the round (also known as cochlear) window. Positioned between the scala vestibuli and the scala tympani is the second closed compartment known as the *cochlear duct* or *scala media*. The cochlear duct is separated from the scala vestibuli by the vestibular membrane (also known as Reissner's membrane), which transmits fluid waves of perilymph in the scala vestibuli into fluid waves of endolymph in the cochlear duct. Within the cochlear duct is a ribbonlike strip of extracellular matrix called the *tectorial membrane*. It is composed of several genetically distinct types of collagen (collagen types II, IX, and XI) and three distinct noncollagenous glycoproteins (α-tectorin, β-tectorin, and otogelin). The tectorial membrane rests on and is affixed to tips of hair cells that make up the mechanosensory portion of the organ of Corti that lies on the basilar membrane (Fig. 20-22). There are a series of three rows of outer hair cells and a single row of inner hair cells (see Fig. 20-21). Fluid waves in the cochlear duct result in movement of the tectorial membrane, which distorts inner and outer hair cells (neural-like cells), resulting in their depolarization and afferent transmission of action potentials via the cochlear branch of the vestibulocochlear cranial nerve to the vestibular nucleus.

Vestibular System

The vestibular system is made of several endolymph-filled compartments located in the caudal third to half of the petrous portion of the temporal bone. It represents a major sensory system that (1) maintains balance in concert with general proprioception and visual systems, (2) coordinates body posture, and (3) helps maintain ocular position in relation to the position or motion of the head. Included in the vestibular system are the semicircular canals, utricle, saccule, vestibular ganglia, vestibular portion of cranial nerve VIII (vestibulocochlear nerve), vestibular nuclei, and vestibular lobules of the cerebellum.

There are three semicircular canals oriented at right angles relative to each other occupying three planes. Each canal has a terminal dilation or ampulla that contains a specialized surface sensory organ called the *crista*. In aggregate, the sensory portion is referred to as *crista ampullaris*. Each crista is lined by specialized sensory hair cells that send continuous tonic neural signals to the vestibular nucleus. Deflection of these sensory hair cells during acceleration, deceleration, or rotation results in variation of the tonic signals sent

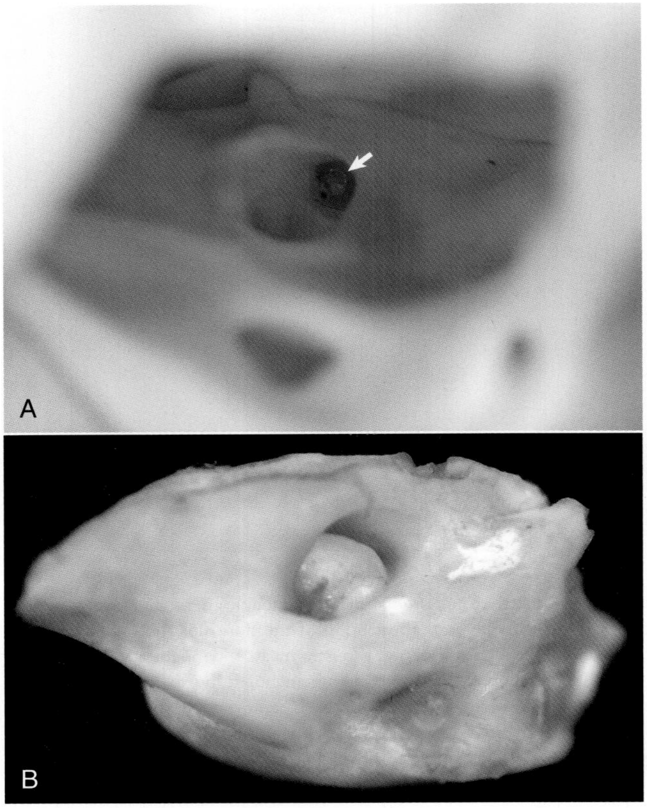

Fig. 20-17 Internal acoustic meatus, cat.
A, Right internal acoustic meatus. Viewed through the open left external acoustic meatus, the right internal acoustic meatus *(arrow)* represents the bony opening into the petrous portion of the temporal bone, through which the vestibulocochlear nerve and facial nerve exit the cranial cavity. **B,** Petrous portion of the temporal bone, cat. The yellow hue is very typical of this bone in all species. The large central opening is the internal acoustic meatus within which lie the vestibular and cochlear nerves. (Courtesy Dr. B.L. Njaa, Center for Veterinary Health Sciences, Oklahoma State University.)

to the vestibular nucleus. However, the hair cells are not activated during constant velocity.

Maculae are receptors located within the membranous utricle and saccule of the vestibule. The saccular macula is oriented in the vertical plane, whereas the macula of the utriculus is oriented in the horizontal plane. Surface lining neuroepithelial hair cells of the macula project into an otolithic membrane. Movement of the otolithic membrane causes deflection of the hair cells and triggers action potential. As in the case of the crista ampullaris, macular receptors provide a continuous tonic nervous input, with a net effect of maintaining static head positioning relative to gravity.

On stimulation of sensory nerve endings, action potentials are transmitted through bipolar cells whose cell bodies are located in the vestibular ganglia of the vestibular branch of the vestibulocochlear nerve. Signals travel to the vestibular nuclei in the medulla. From the vestibular nuclei, connections are made with the oculomotor, trochlear, and abducent nuclei of the rostral brainstem via the medial longitudinal fasciculus, the vestibulocerebellum by the caudal cerebellar peduncle, and the spinal cord via the vestibulospinal tract located in the ventral funiculus.

Histologic Evaluation of the Internal Ear

See Web Appendix 20-1.

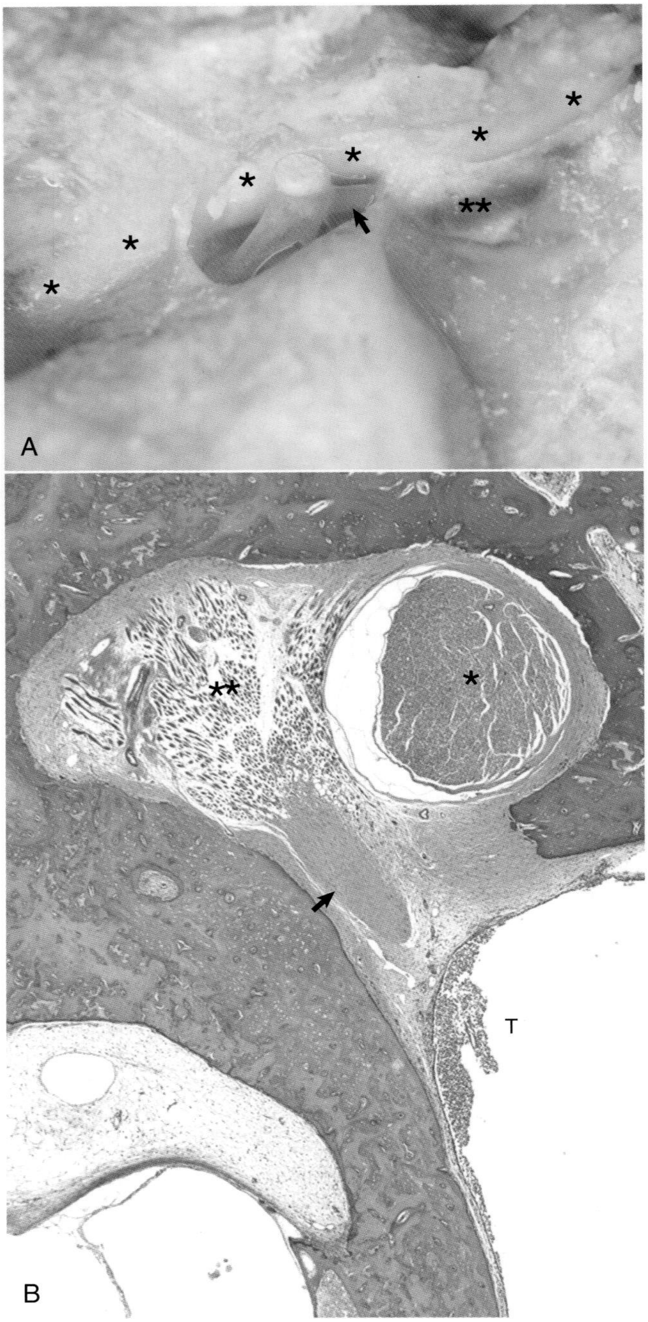

Fig. 20-18 Stapedius muscle and its proximity to the facial nerve.
A, Horse. The facial nerve *(asterisks)* courses through the facial groove in close proximity to the stapes and partially obscures the stapedius muscle *(two asterisks)*. The tendon of the stapedius muscle *(arrow)* is shown attached to the short arm of the stapes, near the head of the stapes. **B,** Dog. Histology of facial nerve and stapedius muscle. The facial nerve *(asterisk)* is present within the facial groove partially obscuring the stapedius muscle *(two asterisks)* anchored in its stapedius muscular fossa. The tendon of the stapedius muscle *(arrow)* is observed in oblique, transverse section, but the stapes is not in this plane of section. Within the tympanic cavity *(T)* are moderate numbers of neutrophils, indicative of suppurative otitis media. H&E stain. (Courtesy Dr. B.L. Njaa, Center for Veterinary Health Sciences, Oklahoma State University.)

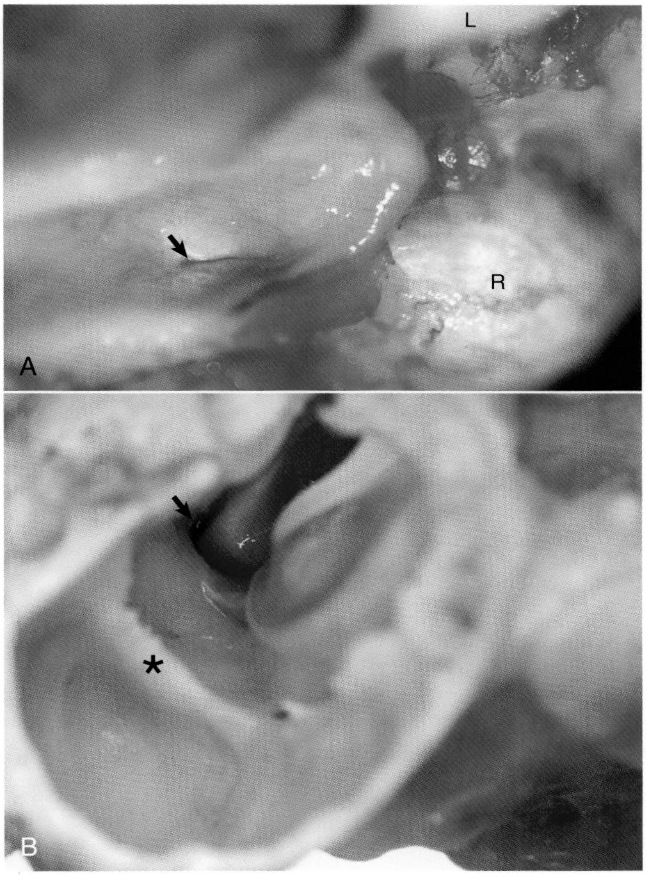

Fig. 20-19 Auditory tube.
A, Nasopharynx, cat. A thin slit-like opening, normally maintained in a closed position, represents the opening of the right auditory tube into the nasopharynx *(arrow)*. *L,* Left occipital condyle; *R,* right occipital condyle. **B,** Middle ear, tympanic bulla, right ear, caudal, oblique view, dog. The auditory tube *(arrow)* is located dorsal, medial, and rostral to the tympanic ring of the tympanic membrane just to the left of the tympanic membrane and manubrium of the malleus. The septum bulla *(asterisk)* is short and incomplete when compared to the cat. (Courtesy Dr. B.L. Njaa, Center for Veterinary Health Sciences, Oklahoma State University.)

PORTALS OF ENTRY

Portals of entry into the ear are listed in Box 20-1.

BOX 20-1 Portals of Entry into the Ear

EXTERNAL EAR
Extension from the external environment (acoustic meatus)
Hematogenous spread
Extension from the middle ear

MIDDLE EAR
Extension through perforation of the tympanic membrane
Ascension of the auditory tube
Extension via degeneration of the temporohyoid joint
Extension via erosion through the tympanic bulla
Migration along vascular or neural pathways

INTERNAL EAR
Extension from the middle ear
Hematogenous spread
Migration along vascular or neural pathways

EXTERNAL EAR

Extension from the External Environment

Extension from the external environment is a common portal of entry into the external ear. It is a specialized invagination of the skin that terminates medially at the tympanic membrane of the middle ear. As the external acoustic meatus gradually narrows, its funnel shape is conducive in directing foreign materials, fomites, parasites, and/or infectious microorganisms into the external ear and toward the tympanic membrane of the middle ear. Additionally, its moist environment favors colonization of skin and/or mucosa by pathogenic microorganisms (Table 20-1). Although dermatitides can affect any part of the dermis, including the external ear, occasionally, involvement of the ear is an important feature used to arrive at a definitive diagnosis.

Hematogenous Spread

Hematogenous spread is a portal of entry into the external ear. Septicemias and/or specific types of viremias are thought to contribute to the development of external ear disease. Otitis externa and possibly deafness have been attributed to canine distemper virus, but it is unclear if the virus is a primary cause or one of several factors leading to otic disease. In an animal with septicemia, circulating bacteria have the potential to adhere to the endothelium of the capillary beds of the external ear, colonize the endothelium, and spread into adjacent tissues (see Chapter 4).

Extension from the Middle Ear

Extension from the middle ear is another portal of entry into the external ear, especially in cavalier King Charles spaniels with primary secretory otitis media. In primary secretory otitis media, the external ear is typically unaffected unless the tympanic membrane is ruptured and mucoid debris is spread into the external acoustic meatus. However, it has been suggested that this breed may have underlying failure of mucosae of the middle ear predisposing these spaniels to auditory tube dysfunction and thus otitis media leading to rupture of the tympanic membrane.

MIDDLE EAR

Extension through Perforation of the Tympanic Membrane

Extension from the external ear through a perforated tympanic membrane is a portal of entry into the middle ear (Fig. 20-23). In dogs with chronic otitis externa, secondary otitis media may occur in as many as 80% of affected dogs. At the time of clinical diagnosis, the tympanic membrane is most often intact, although some studies report perforations in over 40% of cases with otitis externa and concurrent otitis media. Based on the results of bacteriologic studies, it has been shown that a majority of dogs with concurrent otitis externa and otitis media have different bacteria isolated from each compartment. Thus it is unclear if the portal of entry in otitis media involves perforation of the tympanic membrane and spread of otitis externa into the middle ear with subsequent healing of the tympanic membrane or if otitis media results from bacteria ascending a poorly functioning auditory tube. Multiple studies implicate the latter mechanism (see later).

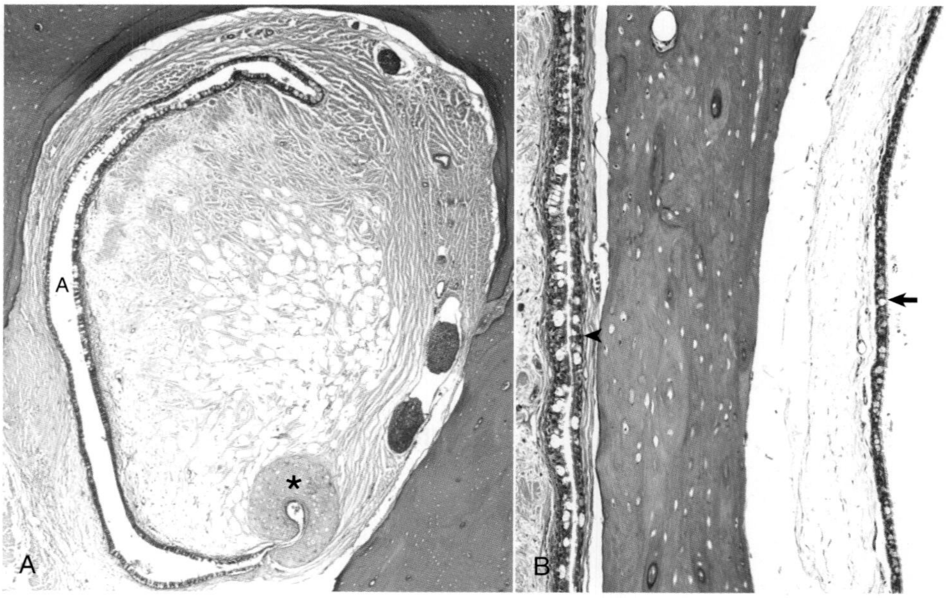

Fig. 20-20 Histology of the auditory tube mucosa, cat.
A, Rostral opening of the auditory tube. The auditory tube *(A)* in cross-section is typically C-shaped. Comma-shaped cartilage *(asterisk)* provides structural support to portions of the auditory tube. The mucosal lining is composed of ciliated, pseudostratified, columnar epithelium mixed with goblet cells and nonciliated epithelial cells. H&E stain. **B,** Cross-section through tympanic bulla and auditory tube. The mucosae of the tympanic bulla *(arrow)* and the lining of the auditory tube *(arrowhead)* are composed of pseudostratified, ciliated columnar epithelial cells mixed with goblet cells and basal cells. This mucosa is virtually identical to the nasopharyngeal mucosa. H&E stain. (Courtesy Dr. B.L. Njaa, Center for Veterinary Health Sciences, Oklahoma State University.)

Ascension of the Auditory Tube

Ascension up the auditory tube is a portal of entry into the middle ear. It appears that dysfunction of the auditory tube is a necessary precursor for development of otitis media and likely leads to impaired clearance of middle ear effusions and prolonged periods of negative pressure within the tympanic cavity. Dysfunction may be related to impairment of the opening of the auditory tube into the pharynx during swallowing when pressure equalization takes place or it could be related to alterations of mucociliary clearance facilitated by epithelial cells lining the tube. Via either mechanism, it appears that microorganisms can use this portal to reach the middle ear.

Extension Via Degeneration of the Temporohyoid Joint

Direct extension into the middle ear can occur from degeneration of the temporohyoid joint and release of microorganisms. See the discussion on temporohyoid osteoarthropathy in the section on Disorders of Horses.

Extension Via Erosion through the Tympanic Bulla

Erosion through the tympanic bullae is a rare portal of entry into the middle ear. Neoplastic processes, such as oral squamous cell carcinomas, regional lymphosarcoma, or local compression by an abscess, can lead to bone remodeling, as well as bone lysis, with subsequent spread into the middle ear.

Migration along Vascular or Neural Pathways

Branches of the caudal auricular artery and the facial nerve traverse within the middle ear and have the potential to serve as pathways for spread of microorganisms and neoplasms from the brain to the middle ear. This migratory process likely occurs via the extracellular matrix of arteries and nerves (see Chapters 3, 10, and 14) and via anterograde axonal transport in nerves (see Chapter 14). As an example, cranial nerve sheath tumors (see Chapter 14) in the brain have been reported to migrate along branches of the facial nerve and vestibulocochlear nerves and enter the ear via the internal acoustic meatus.

INTERNAL EAR

Extension from the Middle Ear

Extension from the middle ear is a portal of entry into the internal ear, thus otitis interna or labyrinthitis is most commonly thought of as occurring by direct extension from an infection of the middle ear. The most likely portal is the round or cochlear window. Based on studies in cats, the permeability of the round window is increased for elements (sodium) and macromolecules (tritiated albumin) during mild cases of experimentally induced otitis media. Penetration through the oval or vestibular window is less likely because of the annular syndesmosis that is formed between the petrous portion of the temporal bone and the stapes (Fig. 20-24). Although otitis media may be diagnosed in isolation, otitis interna is rarely diagnosed without concurrent otitis media.

Hematogenous Spread

Entry through hematogenous spread occurs in the internal ear (see the previous discussion on the middle ear in the section on Portals of Entry for details).

Migration along Vascular or Neural Pathways

Migration along vascular or neural pathways as a portal of entry occurs in the internal ear (see the previous discussion on the middle ear in the section on Portals of Entry for details).

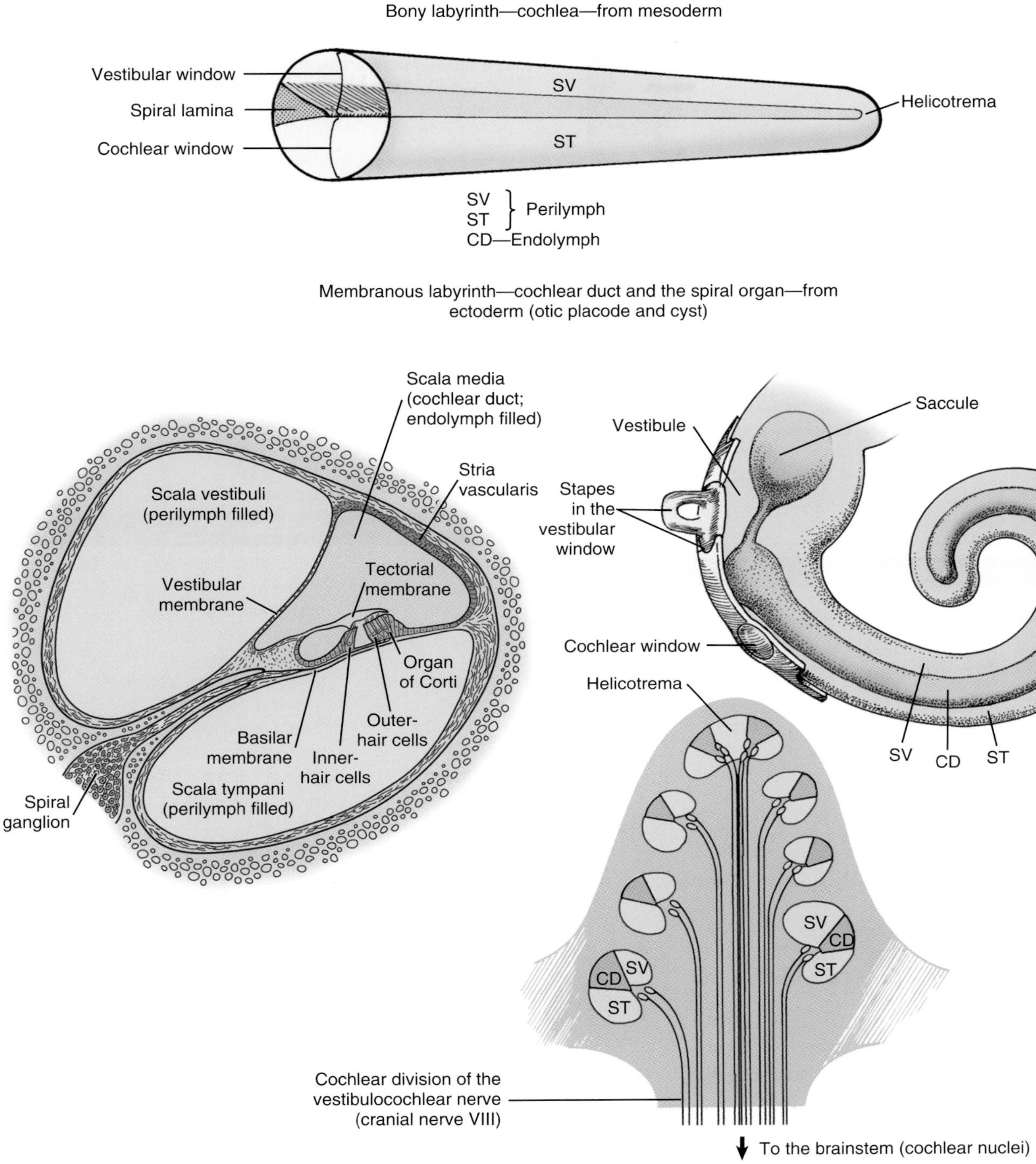

Fig. 20-21 Schematic diagram of the structure of the cochlea, cochlear duct, and spiral organ.
(Modified from de Lahunta A, Glass E: *Veterinary neuroanatomy and clinical neurology*, ed 3, St Louis, 2009, W.B. Saunders.)

RESPONSES TO INJURY

The ear's responses to injury are listed in Box 20-2.

EXTERNAL EAR

The external ear is an extension of the integument, and it responds to inflammatory stimuli similarly. All of the hallmarks of inflammation occur in otitis externa. Initially, there is reddening and warmth of the affected auricle associated with otitis externa caused by vascular dilatation and hyperemia. Transudation of fluid out of leaky vessels leads to edema affecting both the auricle (see Fig. 17-13) and external acoustic meatus. Edema within the tissues results in swelling of the tissues and discomfort when the tissues are touched. As the inflammatory response progresses, the transudate becomes an exudate, infiltrating the dermis of the external ear. Epithelial and adnexal changes, described later, result in further expansion of the external ear dermis. Eventually, the lumen of the external acoustic meatus may become so stenotic that hearing function becomes impaired.

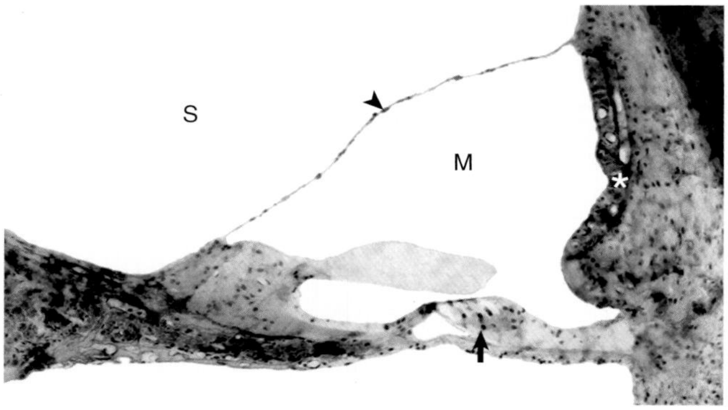

Fig. 20-22 Cochlear duct, cat.
The tectorial membrane is positioned over the inner and outer hair cells of the organ of Corti *(arrow)*. The intact vestibular membrane *(arrowhead)* becomes distorted when auditory ossicular movements create fluid waves in the perilymph of the scala vestibuli *(S)*. The stria vascularis *(asterisk)* is the source of endolymph production and maintenance. See Fig. 20-21 for a diagram of the structure. *M,* Scala media. Thick tissue section, toluidine blue stain. (Courtesy Dr. D.A. Ryugo; from Ryugo DA, Cahill HB, Rose LS, et al: *Hear Res* 181:73-84, 2003.)

BOX 20-2 Responses to Injury of the Ear

EXTERNAL EAR
Inflammation, acute and chronic
Epithelial and adnexal hyperplasia
Fibrosis
Osseous metaplasia
Neoplasia (occasionally)

MIDDLE EAR
Inflammation (myringitis)
Healing of the tympanic membrane
Goblet cell metaplasia
Impaired mucociliary clearance (likely atrophy of ciliated epithelial cells)
Osteosclerosis of the tympanic bulla
Formation of inflammatory polyps
Horner's syndrome/Pourfour du Petit syndrome

INTERNAL EAR
Sensory cell degeneration/death
Inflammation: Auditory ossicular chain damage (osteolysis/osteonecrosis)

As has already been described, the external acoustic meatus and auricle are lined by haired skin. Large, abundant, multiple, branching, and actively secreting sebaceous glands are most prominent in the deeper portions of the external acoustic meatus associated with hair follicles (see Fig. 20-5, *A*). Smaller, tubular, eccrine sweat glands, referred to as *ceruminous glands,* are located in the deeper layers of dermis. The epidermis, which is best studied in dogs, in response to inflammation, becomes hyperplastic and hyperkeratotic, although in some conditions it becomes ulcerated. Glandular changes include smaller, less abundant, less active sebaceous glands and more numerous, typically large, dilated ceruminous glands. Neutrophils, lymphocytes, and macrophages typically infiltrate the dermis, as well as the ectatic ceruminous glands (Fig. 20-25). Aggregates of lymphocytes form when the process is chronic. With

TABLE 20-1 Predisposing Factors and Primary Causes of Otitis Externa

Predisposing Factors	Outcomes
Conformation	Stenotic external acoustic meatus Hairs within the external meatus Pendulous pinnae
Excessive moisture	Swimmer's ear High-humidity climate
Excessive cerumen production	Overactive glands
Treatment effects	Trauma from treatment swabs Irritation from topic products Altering normal microflora
Obstructive ear disease	Neoplasms Polyps Granulomas
Systemic disease	Immune suppression Viral disease Debilitation Catabolic states
Primary Causes	**Outcomes**
Parasites	Ticks, mites, nematodes (see Table 20-2)
Hypersensitivity reactions	Atopy Food hypersensitivity Contact hypersensitivity Drug reactions
Keratinization disorders	Primary idiopathic seborrhea Hypothyroidism Sex hormone imbalances Lipid-related conditions
Foreign bodies	Plants (especially foxtails) Hair Sand, dirt Hardened secretions, medications
Glandular disorders	Ceruminal gland hyperplasia Sebaceous gland hyperplasia or hypoplasia Altered secretion rate Altered type of secretions
Autoimmune diseases	Lupus erythematosus Pemphigus foliaceous Pemphigus vulgaris Pemphigus erythematosus
Vascular diseases	Cold agglutinin disease Solar dermatitis Frostbite Vasculitis Juvenile cellulitis Aural chondritis
Secondary Causes	**Outcomes**
Bacteria	*Staphylococcus intermedius* *Proteus* spp. *Pseudomonas* spp. *Escherichia coli* *Klebsiella* spp.
Yeast	*Malassezia pachydermatis* *Candida albicans*

Modified from Griffin CE, Kwochka KW, MacDonald JM: Otitis externa and media. In *Current veterinary dermatology: The art and science of therapy,* St. Louis, 1993, Mosby; and Scott DW, Miller WH, Griffin CE: *Muller & Kirk's small animal dermatology,* ed 6, Philadelphia, 2001, WB Saunders.

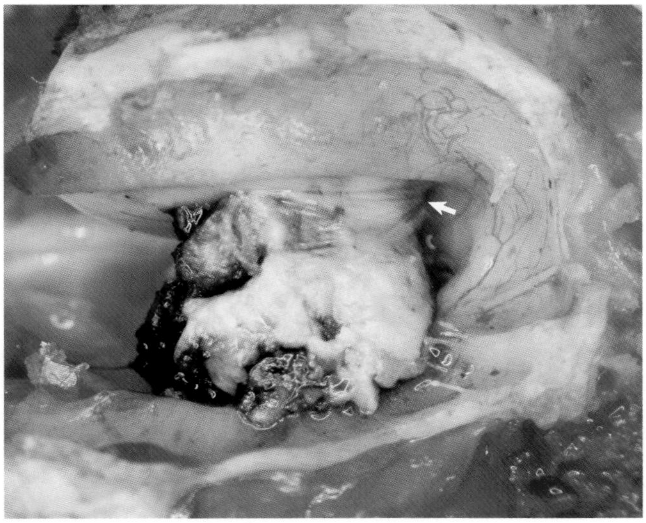

Fig. 20-23 Ruptured tympanic membrane, dog.
A large aggregate of cerumen bulges through a tear in the caudal portion of the pars tensa between the manubrium of the malleus and the caudal bony tympanic ring into the tympanic cavity. The wrinkled flap of the torn pars tensa can be seen *(arrow)*. There was no evidence of otitis media and likely the tear was acute. A ceruminous gland adenoma was identified in the horizontal portion of the external acoustic meatus unassociated with the tympanic membrane causing complete obstruction. (Courtesy Dr. B.L. Njaa, Center for Veterinary Health Sciences, Oklahoma State University.)

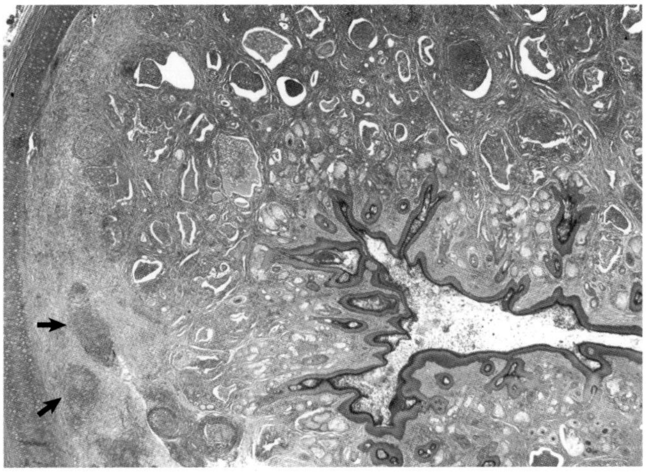

Fig. 20-25 Otitis externa, external acoustic meatus, dog.
In this histologic section, the dermis contains increased numbers of ceruminous glands that are dilated and filled with inflammatory cells, typically neutrophils, macrophages, lymphocytes, and plasma cells. These inflammatory cells are also present in the periadnexal dermis. Lymphoid aggregates form nodules *(arrows)* in the deep dermis near the cartilaginous rings of the external acoustic meatus. The overlying epidermis is mildly to moderately thickened (acanthosis). The luminal diameter has been markedly reduced, which can further exacerbate the problem of otitis externa. H&E stain. (Courtesy Dr. B.L. Njaa, Center for Veterinary Health Sciences, Oklahoma State University.)

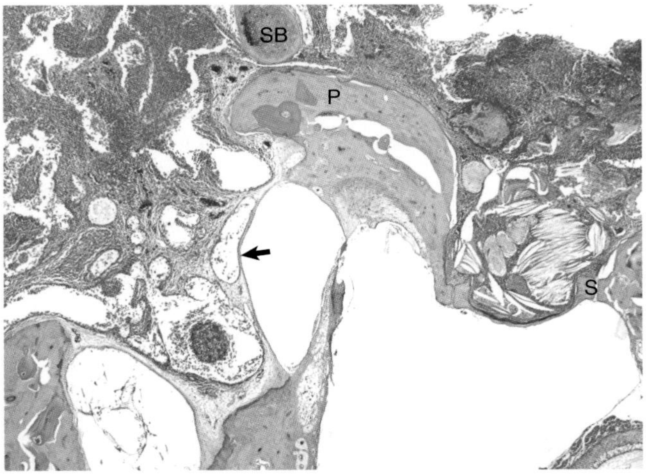

Fig. 20-24 Chronic otitis media, cat.
Histologic section of middle ear, petrous portion of the temporal bone through the round and oval window with the stapes in situ. The syndesmosis formed between the bone of the oval or vestibular window of the petrous portion of the temporal bone seems to prevent otitis media from spreading into the inner ear. Conversely, the membranous covering of the round or cochlear window is infiltrated by inflammatory cells. During episodes of otitis media, the permeability of this membrane is increased. Otitis interna was diagnosed in this cat (not depicted in this image). At the top of the image is the edge of the septum bulla abutting the petrous portion of the temporal bone, anatomic indication that this is from a cat. Edge of stapes *(S)*; round window membrane *(arrow)*; promontory *(P)*; septum bulla *(SB)*. H&E stain. (Courtesy Dr. B. L. Njaa, Center for Veterinary Health Sciences, Oklahoma State University.)

increased chronicity, there is greater infiltration by fibroblasts and collagen, which can lead to more permanent stenotic changes. Finally, soft tissues, such as the dermis or auricular cartilage, may become ossified through metaplasia in the most chronically inflamed ears.

Auricles of lightly pigmented cats chronically exposed to ultraviolet (UV) light are prone to developing squamous cell carcinoma (described later in the chapter; also see Chapter 17). UVB light leads to cellular transformation of the epithelial cells leading to a clonal population of neoplastic squamous epithelial cells.

MIDDLE EAR

Myringitis

Inflammation of the tympanic membrane is called *myringitis* and is most commonly caused by bacterial infection of the external or middle ear (see Fig. 20-39, *B*). Macroscopically, the tympanic membrane may be congested, hemorrhagic, or thickened, resulting in opacity. Microscopically, the tympanic membrane has all of the characteristics of acute inflammation and if the inciting cause is unresolved results in chronic inflammation (see Chapter 3). Prolonged and severe myringitis may lead to perforation of the tympanic membrane and prevent its healing.

Healing of the Tympanic Membrane

The tympanic membrane is a regionally well-vascularized membrane that has an air-interface along each surface. It can be perforated by traumatic injury, sudden exposures to high pressures, degradative enzymes and pressures from acute and chronic inflammation, chronic mite infestations, and neoplasms. Unique to the tympanic membrane, and likely related to its function, is its inherent ability to heal rapidly while maintaining its thin structure during healing through a process called *epithelial migration*. Unlike most other tissues, in which granulation tissue forms and bridges the defect followed by reepithelialization, the tympanic membrane closes the defect, first with migrating epithelial cells followed by a granulation tissue response that closes the mesenchymal portion of the tympanic membrane.

Within minutes to hours of the initial perforation, injured tissue at the edge of the perforation initiates an acute inflammatory response. Within hours, epithelial cells proliferate initially along the annulus and along the margin of the manubrium, corresponding to areas in which the blood supply is most prominent and epithelial stem cells of the tympanum are thought to reside. Proliferating epithelium advances toward the perforation using keratin as a scaffolding to initially bridge and reepithelialize the defect. As this epithelium is migrating across the defect, granulation tissue forms on the inner edge of the perforated membrane. Anchored to the epithelium that initially closes the perforation, the middle, mesenchymal layer of the tympanic membrane is repaired by this advancing granulation tissue. As granulation tissue remodels to its normal thin layer, the inner epithelial layer finally bridges the defect to complete the healing process. In an experimental animal model, 2.5-mm perforations were completely healed by 9 days after injury.

Goblet Cell Metaplasia and Impaired Mucociliary Clearance

An important defense mechanism of the middle ear is the mucociliary apparatus of the auditory tube and contiguous tympanic cavity. Chronic otitis media causes a decrease in the number of ciliated cells (ciliary atrophy) in the mucosa of the auditory tube. Studies in cats determined that neutrophil lysate (likely consisting of degradative enzymes) or lipopolysaccharide did not significantly reduce the number of ciliated cells in the auditory tube, but auditory tube obstruction and likely increased pressure in the middle ear resulted in a dramatic decrease in the number of ciliated epithelial cells. In the same study, there was a marked increase in the total number of goblet cells lining the tympanic cavity and bulla. It was hypothesized that obstruction of the auditory tube elevated partial pressure of carbon dioxide (pCO_2) in the mucus layer of the mucosa, triggering mucosal stem cells to differentiate toward goblet cells rather than ciliated cells. The viscoelasticity of the mucus produced by these goblet cells was greater than normal and resulted in a marked decrease of mucociliary clearance of the middle ear, probably further contributing to auditory tube obstruction, increased pressure in the middle era, and metaplasia of ciliated cells to goblet cells.

Osteosclerosis of the Tympanic Bulla

In infections of the middle ear caused by microorganisms, mediators of acute and chronic inflammation, such as cytokines and degradative enzymes, may lead to excessive periosteal proliferation of new bone and osteosclerosis (thickening) of the wall of the tympanic bulla (Fig. 20-26; see Chapter 16). The bulla may become grossly distorted, and the lumen volume typically decreases. Inflammation also can contribute to bone lysis.

Formation of Inflammatory Polyps

Inflammatory polyps are discussed later but are thought to represent both inflammatory and hyperplastic responses to injury induced by otitis media. Inflammation of the middle ear results in the formation of polypoid masses by an undetermined mechanism. These masses then result in clinical disease referable to where they exert their greatest effect. Polyps that involve the auditory tube and the nasopharynx can result in dysphagia and dyspnea, whereas those involving the tympanic membrane and external acoustic meatus lead to signs of otitis externa.

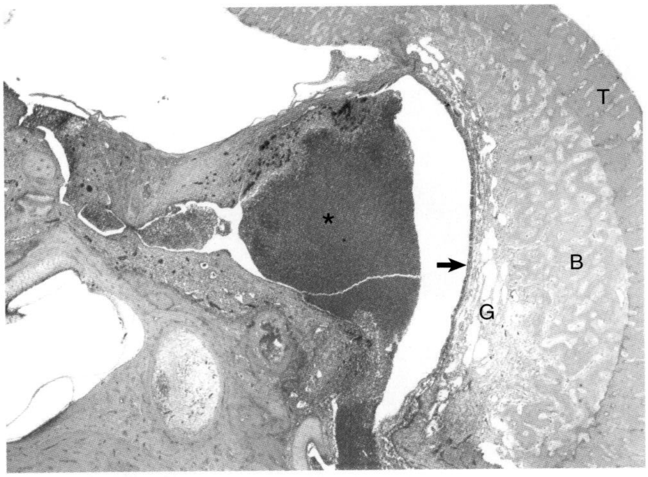

Fig. 20-26 Chronic otitis media with osteosclerosis, guinea pig. The tympanic cavity is partially filled with a suppurative exudate (*asterisk,* center of the image). The inner surface of the tympanic bulla is lined by a thickened hyperplastic mucosa *(arrow)*. Below the mucosa is an area of granulation tissue *(G)* that overlies the formation newly remodeled bone *(B)*, a reparative or healing response to injury. Tinctorially, the tympanic bulla *(T)* is the darker blue area along the right margin of the image. H&E stain. (Courtesy Dr. B.L. Njaa, Center for Veterinary Health Sciences, Oklahoma State University.)

Horner's Syndrome/Pourfour Du Petit Syndrome

Postganglionic sympathetic fibers that innervate the eye course through the middle ear with branches of the internal carotid artery via the tympano-occipital fissure. Smooth muscle that lifts the upper eye, retractor muscles of the third eyelid, smooth muscle that tonically pulls the eyes rostrally, and dilator muscles of the pupil are all innervated by these fibers. Thus, in otitis media, cells and mediators of inflammation can act on postganglionic sympathetic fibers that innervate the eye as they traverse through the middle ear, leading to primary demyelination and axonal injury.

Most commonly, injury resulting in partial paralysis of postganglionic sympathetic fibers causes Horner's syndrome. This syndrome has the following clinical signs: miosis, enophthalmos, ptosis, a narrowed palpebral aperture, protrusion of the third eyelid, and peripheral vasodilation of the skin of the face. Resolution of signs typically follows clearance of the cause.

Injury to the postganglionic sympathetic fibers can much less commonly result in hyperexcitability or hyperirritability. This is most commonly reported in cats that have had their ears examined, sampled, and flushed while under anesthesia. Clinical signs include mydriasis, exophthalmos, widening of the palpebral aperture and cool skin over the face. In all cases reported, clinical signs resolved spontaneously. This hyperirritability syndrome is the opposite of Horner's syndrome and is referred to by some as the *Pourfour du Petit syndrome.*

INTERNAL EAR

Sensory Cell Degeneration/Death

Within the organ of Corti are the outer and inner sensory hair cells, as well as spiral ganglion neurons. The sensory hair cells are the most vulnerable to injury. Damage to the sensory cells or ganglion cells results in impaired function that is often permanent. Whether the cause is labyrinthitis, noise-induced hearing loss (85 dB sound pressure level or higher), chemical ototoxins, or the poorly understood disorder called *presbycusis* (i.e., age-related hearing loss), sensory hair cells are targeted and undergo degeneration or death leading to hearing impairment or hearing loss. Bursts of intense noise are thought to result in disarrangement or breakage to the stereocilia, whereas continuous exposure to damaging noise leads to death of the hair cells.

Auditory Ossicular Chain Damage

Chronic otitis media can potentially lead to conductive hearing loss by damaging the auditory ossicles. Chronic exposure to infection, bacterial or fungal toxins, and degradative enzymes from inflammation can result in bony lysis. Excessively lytic bones may develop pathologic fractures. Additionally, chronic inflammation can result in fibrosis, which may restrict the movement of the ossicles. Finally, chronic inflammation can damage the articulations of the ossicles, thus impairing transmission of vibrations.

DEFENSE MECHANISMS

Defense mechanisms of the ear are listed in Box 20-3.

EXTERNAL EAR

Integumentary Defenses

Defense mechanisms of the skin are discussed in Chapters 3 and 17.

Epithelial Migration

Migration of cornified epithelial cells to the periphery of the tympanic membrane and onto the external acoustic meatus continuously replaces the effete epidermal layer of the tympanic membrane. Epithelial migration is thus an important means of maintaining tympanic membrane thickness, clearance of debris and likely microorganisms and parasites from the tympanic membrane and external acoustic meatus, and retaining vibratory sensitivity. Alterations in this epithelial migratory pattern can lead to or may be the cause of disease of the external or middle ear. As discussed previously, epithelial migration is also the method by which perforations of the tympanic membrane are repaired.

BOX 20-3 Defense Mechanisms of the Ear

EXTERNAL EAR
Integumentary defenses
Epithelial migration
Cerumen barrier and acidity
Cerumen immunoglobulins
Commensal organisms
Structural defense from the osseous external acoustic meatus

MIDDLE EAR
Mucociliary apparatus
Surfactant
Auditory tube–associated lymphoid tissue (ATALT)
Commensal microorganisms

INTERNAL EAR
Structural defense from the petrous portion of the temporal bone
Acoustic reflex

Adnexa and Cerumen

Cerumen is an oily emulsion that coats and protects the integument of the external acoustic meatus. Its naturally hydrophobic properties make it an important barrier to the entry of excessive moisture into the epidermal cells or underlying dermis. In normal ears of dogs, cerumen is made of sloughed superficial squamous cells mixed with ceruminous and sebaceous gland secretions. There is a high lipid content in cerumen made up of neutral lipids. In otitic ears, the cerumen changes because ceruminous glands are typically more numerous and active during periods of inflammation and thus contribute more to the content of cerumen (see Fig. 20-25). One consequence is a decrease in the lipid content, a decrease in hydrophobicity, and impairment of a natural barrier.

Cerumen in otitic ears becomes more acidic than normal, which is believed to impair bacterial growth. This outcome is due to greater contribution by ceruminous glands during periods of external ear inflammation. The pH of the external acoustic meatus is variable in dogs, ranging from 4.6 to 7.2. During periods of inflammation, the mean pH in acute otitis externa may decrease, whereas the mean pH in chronic otitis externa tends to increase. The mechanistic consequences of these changes are poorly understood.

Immunoglobulins IgA, IgG, and IgM have been identified in canine cerumen; however, the predominant immunoglobulin is IgG. This high level of IgG is believed to be related to transudation of serum in the inflamed external ear. Lysozyme and interleukins have also been identified in cerumen and provide an antimicrobial function.

Commensal Organisms

A mixture of bacteria and yeast normally populates the external acoustic meatus. Various species of "potentially pathogenic" microorganisms have been cultured from external ears of dogs with no evidence of disease. They include *Bacillus* spp., *Corynebacterium* spp., *Escherichia coli*, *Micrococcus* spp., *Staphylococcus* spp., *Streptococcus* spp., and yeast organisms, most commonly *Malassezia* spp. Rarely, *Pseudomonas* spp. and *Proteus* spp. have been isolated. Based on a single study of horses, *Corynebacterium* spp. and *Staphylococcus intermedius* were isolated from normal ears. Presumably, these organisms live symbiotically and defense mechanisms limit or prevent proliferation of a monoculture. However, the spectrum of microorganisms cultured from diseased external ears closely mirrors this list.

Osseous External Acoustic Meatus

The length and diameter of the osseous portion of the external acoustic meatus are highly variable among species and provide a unique structural defense mechanism. Animals with longer and narrower osseous portions have tympanic cavities and tympanic membranes that are better protected than those with shorter osseous portions.

MIDDLE EAR

Mucociliary Apparatus

Various portions of the middle ear are lined by epithelium similar to that found in the nasopharynx. A combination of goblet cells and ciliated columnar epithelial cells extend through the auditory tube into the tympanic cavity. See Chapters 4 and 9 for discussion of the mucociliary apparatus.

Surfactant

Surfactant in the lung has long been recognized for its central role in reducing surface tension in alveoli, allowing them to expand

and collapse normally during inspiration and expiration, respectively (see Chapter 9). However, recently, it has been shown that surfactant has other roles, especially in the function of the auditory tube. Surfactant is a complex mixture made up of 90% lipid and phospholipid and 10% surfactant proteins, designated surfactant protein-A (SP-A), SP-B, SP-C, and SP-D. Cuboidal epithelial cells lining the auditory tube are the source of surfactant and contain apical secretory granules analogous to what are seen in type II pneumocytes of the lung. One major difference between pulmonary surfactant and auditory tube surfactant is the ratio of phosphatidylcholine to sphingomyelin. Pulmonary surfactant has a ratio of 67 to 1, whereas auditory tube surfactant has a ratio of 2 to 1. This dramatic difference in auditory tube surfactant phospholipid content is reflected in a reduced ability to modify surface tension.

The most abundant surfactant protein in lung surfactant is SP-B, a strongly hydrophobic protein with high surface activity. However, auditory tube surfactant has a paucity of SP-B and relative abundance of SP-A and SP-D, two highly hydrophilic surfactant proteins. This difference may indicate a different function for auditory tube surfactant, namely, acting as a release agent and antiadhesive rather than a surface tension modifying substance. Antiadhesive properties would facilitate opening of the auditory tube.

Surfactant proteins are collectins that have two domains: (1) a lectin moiety that binds to the surface of foreign substances and organisms and (2) a collagenous domain that functions as a ligand for phagocytosis and complement activation (see Chapter 3). Finally, surfactant is believed to play a protective role against free radicals by early termination of free radical propagation, and protecting against oxidative injury. A lipid-binding pocket in surfactant proteins may prevent free radicals from propagating.

Auditory Tube–Associated Lymphoid Tissue (ATALT)

Dorsal to the opening of the auditory tube is an aggregate of lymphoid tissue. In humans and rodents, this aggregate is referred to as the *tubal tonsil.* Based on a limited number of dissections of presumed normal auditory tubes, lymphoid aggregates have not commonly been identified in the species covered in this text; however, it is reasonable to assume that they exist in this location (see Chapters 4 and 9) and should be thought of as a component of MALT. Lymphoid tissue in the nasopharynx may proliferate and become locally prominent in response to inflammation or infection.

Commensal Microorganisms

Resident microflora in the middle ear are similar to microbes found in the nasopharynx and the external ear. They include aerobic and anaerobic bacteria and yeast in small numbers. *Staphylococcus* spp., *Streptococcus* spp., *E. coli*, *Branhamella* spp., *Bordetella bronchiseptica*, *Enterococcus* spp., and *Bacillus* spp. have been isolated from the middle ear of normal dogs. *Clostridium perfringens* has also been isolated from tympanic cavities of normal dogs.

INTERNAL EAR

Petrous Portion of the Temporal Bone

Referred to as the hardest bone in the body, the petrous portion of the temporal bone is the bony labyrinth that encases and protects the membranous labyrinth held within. The thick and extremely dense bony labyrinth ensures maximal protection to the sensory portions of the internal ear. In addition, its dorsomedial location in the body deep to the external acoustic meatus provides one of the most protected sites in the body.

Acoustic Reflex

Reflexive contraction of the tensor tympani and stapedius muscles in response to loud and injurious noise functions to protect the internal ear by dampening sound conductance. Contraction of the tensor tympani pulls the malleus rostrally and applies tension to the tympanic membrane. The stapedius muscle applies tension to the stapes in a dorsocaudal direction, relative to the tensor tympani muscle; parallel to the long axis of the oval window and perpendicular to the direction the stapes oscillates in the oval window. Thus the delicate structures of the internal ear are protected.

DISORDERS OF DOMESTIC ANIMALS

DEVELOPMENTAL ANOMALIES OF THE EXTERNAL EAR

Auricular Agenesis/Aplasia

Auricular agenesis/aplasia (also known as anotia) has been reported in sheep, cattle, and a dog. Auricular hillocks or ridges of the first and second branchial (pharyngeal) arches, which normally interact to form the auricle and the first groove or cleft that normally forms between the two arches, which becomes the external acoustic meatus, fail to interact properly during embryologic development. This failure to develop normally results in anotia and a lack of an external acoustic meatus. It can manifest as a unilateral or bilateral lesion. In sheep, auricular agenesis has been associated with deafness, as well as other congenital anomalies.

Auricular Hypoplasia

Auricular hypoplasia (also known as microtia) is a normal feature of certain animal breeds. Auricles are what distinguish the La Mancha breed from other goat breeds. Ear length in goats is inherited as an incompletely dominant trait. Two auricular phenotypes exist in the breed: "gopher ears" and "elf ears." Goats with gopher ears have microtic ears that possess little or no auricular cartilage and either fold dorsally or ventrally. La Mancha goats with elf ears have microtic auricles that are larger than gopher ears, up to 5 cm in length with folded, distorted auricular cartilage (Fig. 20-27, *A*) that either folds upward or downward.

Scottish fold cats have slightly microtic ears with a characteristic forward or rostrally folded auricular cartilage. Cats with this simple autosomal dominant inherited trait have unaffected auricles at birth, but the fold of the auricle begins to develop at 3 to 4 weeks of age. Defective cartilage is believed to be the primary problem in these cats, whereby the auricular cartilage either develops abnormally or lacks resiliency succumbing to gravitational forces. Presumably, present-day Scottish fold cats are descendants of a single Scottish female cat that had a spontaneous mutation of the folded ear allele (Fd). It is believed that all Scottish fold cats with the folded-ear phenotype, whether homozygous or heterozygous, suffer with mild or severe, respectively, forms of osteochondrodysplasia of their distal limbs and tails. The mode of inheritance for this skeletal abnormality is also believed to be incomplete dominant.

Unilateral microtia was first reported in a 1950s report involving six slaughter-age pigs in Denmark. Affected auricles were one-third their normal size, and there was atresia of both the bony and cartilaginous portions of the external meatus. In addition, the tympanic cavity was poorly developed with complete absence of tympanic membranes and auditory ossicles. Specimens were never examined histologically. Other species, such as dogs, may be affected sporadically (Fig. 20-27, *B*).

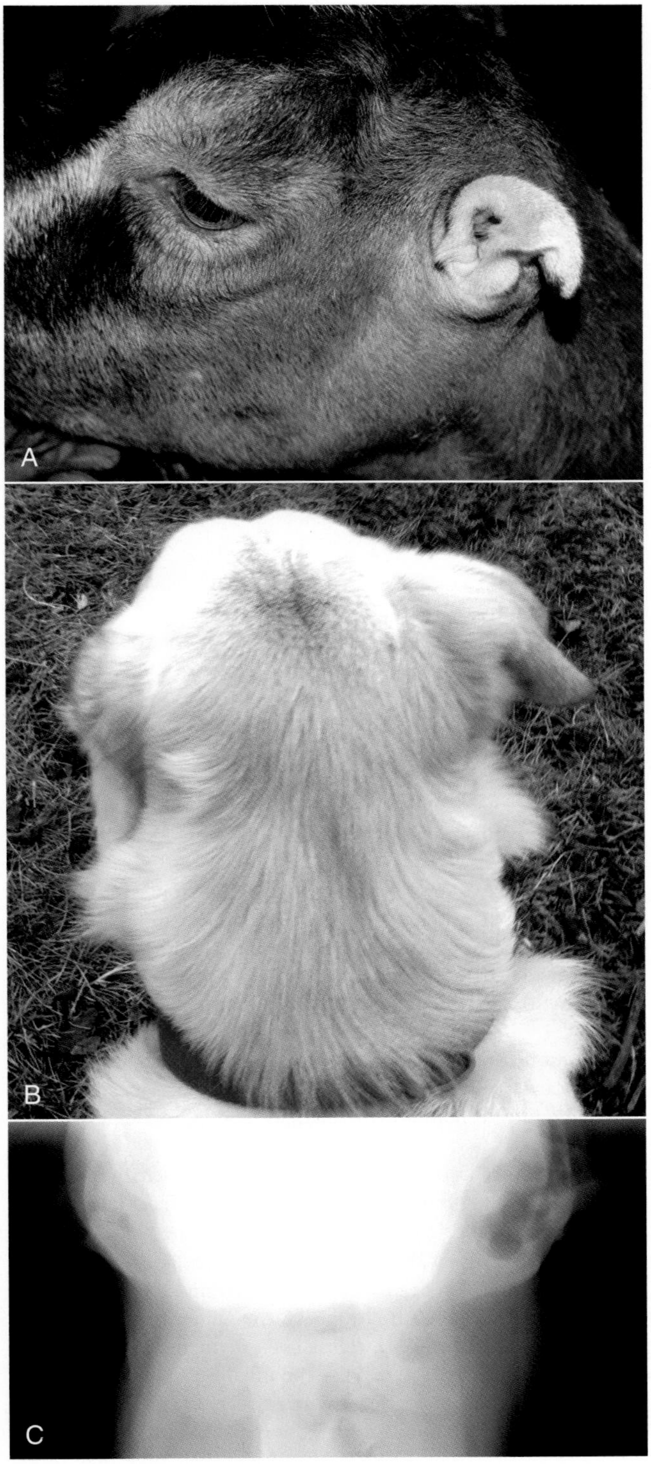

Fig. 20-27 Microtic and distorted ears, goat and cat.
A, La Mancha doe. Elf ears are one of two breed-standard auricle phenotypes accepted for La Mancha goat registry. **B,** Labrador retriever dog. The left auricle is smaller than the right and has always been. The dog is deaf as a result of impaired development of the ear. **C,** Radiograph of the same dog in **B.** The left external acoustic meatus, middle ear, and bulla are very small and underdeveloped when compared to the right side. (**A** courtesy Dr. M. Smith, College of Veterinary Medicine, Cornell University; **B** and **C** courtesy Dr. T. Lykins, Pet Pro, and Ms. T. Maxey, owner.)

Auricular Agenesis/Aplasia

Preauricular malformations (tags, cysts, pits, fissures, and sinuses) are a group of developmentally related disorders of soft tissues that occur rostral to the auricle (Web Fig. 20-1). Preauricular tags are pedunculated outgrowths of skin that contain no bony, cartilaginous, or cystic components and do not communicate with the external or middle ear. The remaining malformations often have an opening rostral to the auricle that is contiguous with a sinus tract that travels under the skin following alongside the cartilage of the external acoustic meatus. These latter malformations are lined by squamous epithelial cells, which may lead to the formation of cysts filled by squamous cell debris or if infected with microorganisms can result in abscesses and with rupture cellulitis.

Preauricular malformations should be differentiated from branchial cysts that arise developmentally from the first branchial cleft. Cleft malformations are closely linked with other structures that may develop normally from the clefts and arches such as the external acoustic meatus, tympanic membrane, and facial nerve. Animals with preauricular or cleft malformations should be examined for congenital anomalies affecting other organ systems.

Cropped or Notched Ears

Cropped or notched ears was a deformity identified in a group of Highland cattle, affecting 45 of 46 progeny from one breeding sire. The inheritance was determined to be incomplete dominance of a single autosomal gene. Other auricular anomalies that have been reported, primarily in sheep, include polyotia (presence of more than one auricle), macrotia (enlarged auricles), synotia (fusion of auricles), and misplaced auricles (heterotopic otia). A single case report of a Friesian cross calf with epitheliogenesis imperfecta had one ear deformed from rolling of its lateral margins followed by fusion of the surfaces after being brought into close proximity.

Atresia of the External Acoustic Meatus

The external acoustic meatus is normally atretic or stenotic for the first days of life in altricial animals but is open at birth in precocial animals.* For example, beyond this initial neonatal period, atresia of the external acoustic meatus is reported as congenital or secondary to trauma (Fig. 20-28). When congenital, it occurs in animals as a lone defect or with other congenital abnormalities such as anotia, microtia, middle ear hypoplasia, auditory ossicular malformation or agenesis, agenesis of ossicular musculature, abnormal positioning of the facial nerve, hydrocephalus, and soft palate hypoplasia. The external acoustic meatus arises from the first branchial cleft or groove and disturbances of its embryonic development result in congenital atresia. Atresia has been described in all species typically covered in this text.

Stenosis of the External Acoustic Meatus (Congenital Hypothyroidism)

Stenotic external acoustic meatuses can occur in toy fox terriers that develop goiter caused by a fully penetrant, autosomal recessive nonsense mutation of the thyroid peroxidase gene resulting in dyshormonogenesis and congenital hypothyroidism. Clinically, puppies are lethargic, do not walk, and are able to hear normally.

A congenital hypothyroidism and dysmaturity syndrome with multiple congenital musculoskeletal abnormalities has been

*Altricial refers to animals that are helpless at birth and require greater parental care (i.e., puppies, kittens). Precocial refers to animals that are active very shortly after birth (i.e., calves, lambs, kids, foals, and piglets).

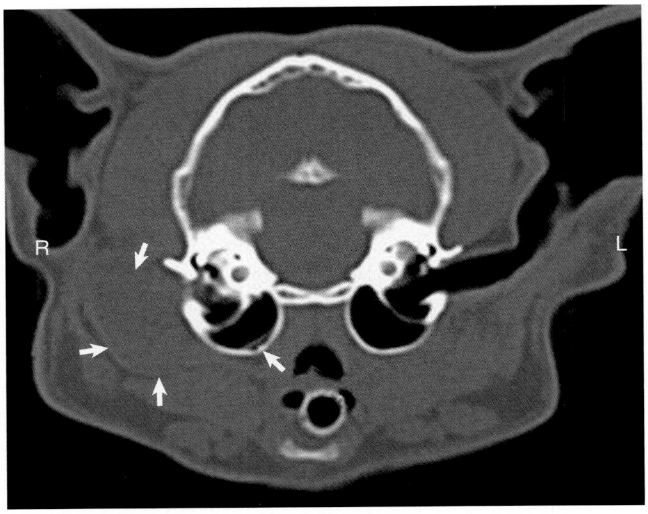

Fig. 20-28 **Congenital, unilateral external acoustic meatus atresia, right ear, cat.**
Axial computed tomography (CT) scan of the head of the cat demonstrating replacement of the right horizontal canal by a hypodense round, well-marginated fluid attenuating material located immediately lateral to the right tympanic bulla, outlined by the solid white arrows. The open white arrow illustrates the soft-tissue material accumulating in the dependent portion of the bulla. *R,* Right side; *L,* left side. (With permission of *J Feline Med Surg* 11:864-868, 2009.)

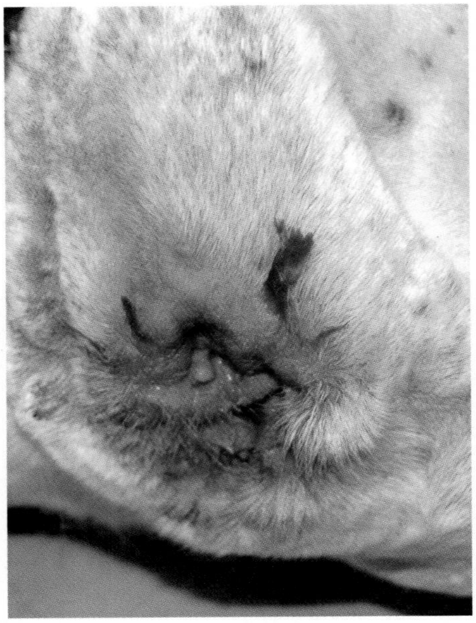

Fig. 20-29 **Otitis externa, dog.**
The auricle is thickened, reddened, and painful (otalgia) with obvious otorrhea and presumed otiasma. (Courtesy Dr. W.H. Miller, College of Veterinary Medicine, Cornell University).

described in foals in western Canada. In addition to tendon laxity and bony changes, some foals have floppy ears that likely are caused by congenital defects in the formation of auricular cartilage. External acoustic meatus, middle ear, or internal ear abnormalities have never been investigated in foals affected by this syndrome.

Otognathia

Otognathia, a rudimentary accessory mouth found at the base of the ear, is an unusual condition reported in sheep and cattle. This accessory orifice is either blind or continuous with the pharynx, lined by a mucous membrane, and may contain rudimentary teeth, mandible-like bones, and lateral extensions of the tongue. Both unilateral and bilateral otognathia have been reported. Embryologically, the first branchial pouch (endodermal origin) makes contact with the first branchial cleft (ectodermal origin), eventually thinning to form a membrane, which normally becomes the tympanic membrane. In otognathia, during development, this membrane between the developing first pharyngeal cleft and first pharyngeal pouch ruptures and forms persistent fistulae. Dentigerous cysts, most commonly reported in horses and described later, may have a similar embryologic origin.

INFLAMMATION OF THE EXTERNAL EAR

Otitis Externa

Otitis externa is rarely a primary condition but arises from the interaction of predisposing factors, primary causes, and secondary causes (see Table 20-1). Predisposing factors, such as conformation, auricular phenotype, breed, and external ear moisture, act as inherent risk factors for the development of otitis externa but are not directly causative. Primary causes, such as ectoparasites, keratinization defects, foreign bodies, hypersensitivity reactions, and systemic immune-mediated disorders that affect the integument, may initiate inflammation of the external acoustic meatus. Secondary factors, such as bacterial and fungal infections, tend to intensify the inflammatory reaction and subsequent severity of otitis externa.

Dogs are most severely affected and therefore examined the most. The most common primary causes appear to be atopic dermatitis, adverse food reactions, ectoparasites, and foreign bodies. It is estimated that the prevalence range of otitis externa in dogs is 15% to 20.4%, which is much higher than the estimated prevalence of 4% in cats. In addition, long-standing chronic external ear infections that have excessive healing responses with extensive fibrosis, cartilage remodeling, and osseous metaplasia can make an eventual return to normal structure and function difficult or nearly impossible.

Macroscopically, otitis externa may include discharge from the ear (also known as otorrhea), hemorrhage from the ear (also known as otorrhagia), and pain elicited when palpating the ear (also known as otodynia or otalgia). The auricles tend to be red, warm, and edematous (see Fig. 17-13) due to increased congestion of dermal blood vessels (Fig. 20-29). With chronicity, the epidermis may become thickened and bosselated, as well as hyperpigmented. The normally pliable auricular cartilage may be modified by fibrosis or osseous metaplasia and become stiffer. The most severely affected ears may develop acquired stenosis of the external acoustic meatus. This feature is an important perpetuating factor that promotes recurrent episodes of otitis externa and prevents satisfactory resolution.

Microscopically, many of the changes have already been discussed. The dermis thickens initially because of edema followed by exudation and infiltration by inflammatory cells. Initially, neutrophils predominate but later, with more chronic inflammation, macrophages are prominent, mixed with lymphocytes and plasma cells. The formation of multiple lymphoid aggregates is not uncommon (see Fig. 20-25). The adnexa transforms from an initially dominant sebaceous gland population to an overabundance of ceruminous glands that tend to be large, ectatic, and infiltrated by inflammatory cells. The overlying epidermis is typically both hyperplastic and hyperkeratotic, although it may be multifocally eroded or ulcerated in acute episodes. All of this thickening in aggregate leads to a reduction in the luminal diameter of the external acoustic meatus.

In chronically affected ears, thick bands of dense fibrous connective tissue replace dermal adnexa. The lack of ceruminous and sebaceous glands results in a lack of cerumen production. Without this natural, typically hydrophobic barrier, the epidermal surface is perpetually hyperplastic and hyperkeratotic. The reduced hydrophobicity results in an increased amount of moisture, superficially resulting in more intercellular edema (see Fig. 17-13) of the epidermis. Cartilage may undergo metaplastic change, resulting in the formation of cartilaginous nodules or more commonly undergo osseous metaplasia. The net affect is a permanent, severe reduction in the luminal diameter of the external acoustic meatus.

Clinically, affected animals have an increased tendency to scratch their ears or shake their heads incessantly. Otitis externa is frequently associated with a malodorous aural discharge or otiasma.* In general, animals have a reluctance to allow examination of affected ears. For those animals that are chronically affected, signs of middle and internal ear disease may develop.

VASCULAR INJURY OF THE EXTERNAL EAR

Infarction

Vascular injury to the auricle occurs in all domestic animal species and results in responses ranging from ear tip necrosis to sloughing of the entire auricle. Various causes, such as bacterial septicemia, immune-mediated vasculitis, frostbite, and toxins, injure and activate endothelium, platelets, and clotting cascades often resulting in vascular thrombosis.

- In pigs, septicemic salmonellosis and its endotoxins can injure vascular endothelium leading to thrombosis of small vessel and tissue infarction of the ear tip and tail (see Chapter 3 for mechanistic details). Ears initially are dark red to purple-black and painful and then become dry (dry gangrene) and scabbed and eventually slough.
- In cats with feline infectious peritonitis (FIP) and also hypothesized in German shepherd dogs with familial vasculopathy (autosomal recessive inheritance pattern), immune complex–mediated vasculitis (type III hypersensitivity) has the potential to cause systemic or cutaneous vasculitides of extremities such as the ears, tails, and potentially feet.
- Severe drops in ambient temperature in newborn animals or animals that are poorly sheltered can result in frostbite. In these cases, blood is shunted away from the extremities to preserve the core body temperature and the poorly perfused extremities, such as ears, tails, feet, and nose, are compromised. Affected tissues demonstrate a clear line of demarcation between tissue that has died or has become infarcted as the result of inadequate circulation and the tissue that retained adequate circulation. The dead tissue darkens, is cool to the touch, and becomes dry from dry gangrene (Fig. 20-30).
- Ingested preformed toxins, such as ergot alkaloids, cause vasoconstriction leading to vascular compromise, infarction, and sloughing of extremities.

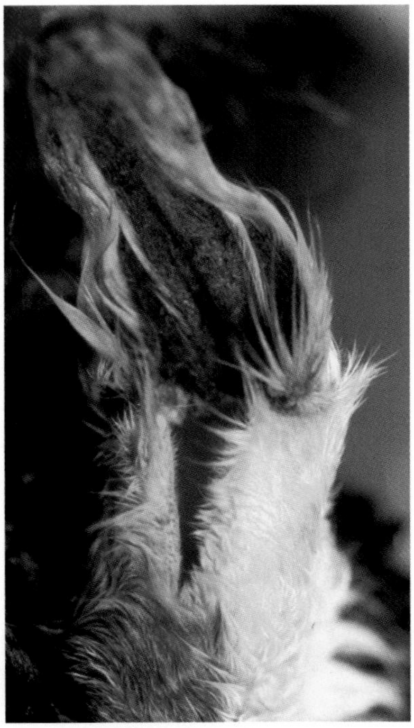

Fig. 20-30 Auricular infarction, frostbite, goat. Note that the distal *(upper)* half of the ear has dry gangrene from frostbite. (Courtesy Dr. B.L. Njaa, Center for Veterinary Health Sciences, Oklahoma State University.)

Hematomas

Animals with chronic external or middle ear disease often respond clinically to discomfort by continuously and vigorously shaking their heads. This action applies severe centrifugal shearing forces (trauma) to blood vessels and auricular cartilage at the sides and tips of the auricles. Since auricular cartilage is elastic and the blood vessels pass through perforations, repeated trauma results in fractures of auricular cartilage, most likely at these areas of perforation. Presumably, the sharp edges of the fracture cartilage and the shearing forces lead to laceration of associated blood vessels. Hemorrhage from these ruptured auricular blood vessels is the genesis of aural hematomas with blood collecting either intrachondrially or subparachondrially.

Aural hematomas are most common in dogs, pigs, and cats but have been reported in sheep, goats, a cow, and a foal. Affected auricles are markedly swollen, most obvious on the concave surface, and are warm, hyperemic, painful, and heavy and tend to droop (Fig. 20-31, *A*). Large breed dogs, in particular golden retrievers and Labrador retrievers, and middle-aged to older dogs with ear disease are prone to develop aural hematomas. If untreated, hematomas eventually heal by fibrosis resulting in a very firm to hard, thickened, and permanently malformed auricle. When opened, the cavity that forms is filled with clotted blood and a meshwork of fibrin (Fig. 20-31, *B*). Microscopic changes typically include cartilage fractures and splitting, cartilage erosion, and granulation tissue formation.

PARASITIC DISEASES OF THE EXTERNAL EAR

Numerous ectoparasites parasitize or infest domestic and wild animals, including mites, ticks, and nematodes (Table 20-2). Most affect their hosts by infesting various parts of the integumentary system (see Chapter 17). A small proportion of these organisms preferentially infest the ear. Reactions vary from minimal irritation to gross deformity. External ear infections may be isolated or extend to the middle and internal ears. The clinical signs are prototypic,

**Otiasma* is a proposed term for foul-smelling otorrhea, derived from two root words: *oto* for ear and *miasma* for noxious odors from putrid organic matter.

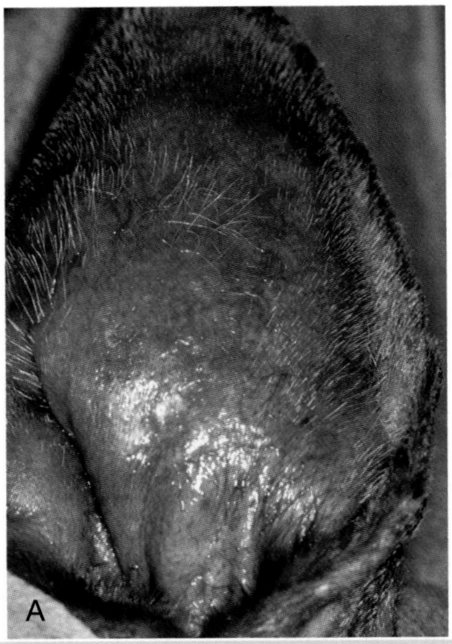

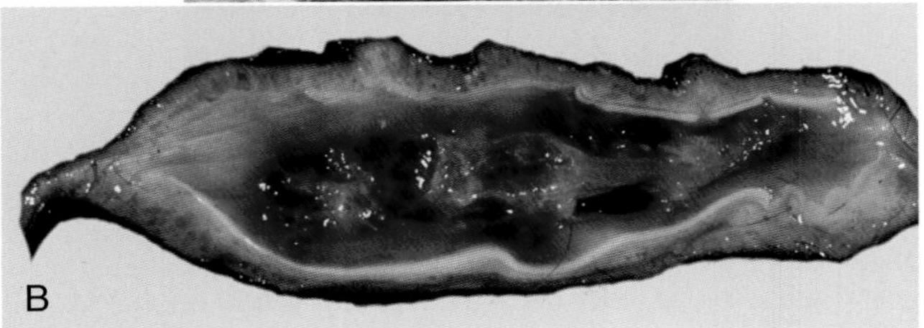

Fig. 20-31 Aural hematoma, dog.
A, Left auricle. The concave aural surface has become convex due to expansion of the underlying connective tissue by mixtures of blood and fibrin. **B,** Auricle, cross-section. Portions of the auricular cartilage are present on both sides of the cavity. Within the cavity are abundant strands of lighter, eosinophilic fibrin strands mixed with thicker, larger dark red blood clots. (**A** courtesy Dr. M.C. Rochat, Center for Veterinary Health Sciences, Oklahoma State University; **B** courtesy Dr. D.D. Harrington, School of Veterinary Medicine, Purdue University; and Noah's Arkive, College of Veterinary Medicine, The University of Georgia.)

TABLE 20-2 Ticks, Mites, and Nematodes Affecting the External or Middle Ears of Animals

Name	Type	Host
Notoedres cati	s, e, m	Cat. Rabbits, dogs
Sarcoptes scabiei	s, m	Dog, pig
Otodectes cynotis	e, m	Cat, dog, other carnivores
Psoroptes cuniculi	e, m	Rabbit, sheep, goat, horse, deer
Raillietina species	e, m	Cattle, buffalo, goat, others
Otobius megnini	e, t	Dog, cat, horse, ruminants, swine
Otobius lagophilus	e, t	Rabbits
Rhipicephalus species	s, e, t	Dog, horse, ruminants, others
Amblyomma species	s, t	Dog, horse, ruminants
Amblyomma maculatum	e, t	Ruminants, others
Amblyomma americanum	s, e, t	Ruminants, others
Boophilus species	s, t	Ruminants, horse
Dermacentor nitens	s. t	Horse, ruminants
Haemaphysalis leporispalustris	s, t	Horse, ruminants
Ixodes ricinus	s, t	Dog, horse, ruminant
Rhabditis spp.	e, n	Cattle
Mammomonogamus auris	e, n	Cat (otitis media)

s, Skin; *e,* ear; *n,* nematode; *m,* mite; *t,* tick,
Modified from Thomson RG: *Special veterinary pathology,* Toronto, 1988, BC Decker.

including head shaking, repeated ear twitching, excessive ear itching, and traumatization of the auricle and base of the ear.

Ear Mite Infestations (Otoacariasis)

Mites are categorized as burrowing or nonburrowing. Many species, such as *Sarcoptes* spp. (see Fig. 17-57) and *Demodex* spp., can cause more generalized lesions with possible involvement of the ear. However, there are few mites that spend much or all of their life cycle within the concave portion of the auricle or in the external acoustic meatus.

Otodectes Cynotis

Otodectes cynotis infest the external acoustic meatus of domestic and wild cats, dogs, and occasionally ruminants. The main route of infestation is from dam to offspring. Other routes of spread include contaminated combs, brushes, bedding, or other grooming accessories. They are nonburrowing and feed on the cerumen, keratin, and lipids. These mites are a prominent primary cause of otitis externa with up to 50% of cats and 10% of dogs developing otitis externa. They cause intense irritation by mechanisms not well understood. Copious cerumen production ensues until a thick, waxy, dark brown exudate obstructs the external acoustic meatus. Auricles are often alopecic and have "scratching" wounds from trauma that form in response to intense pruritus. These areas may also become infected secondarily with bacteria. The mucosa becomes hyperkeratotic with acanthosis and parakeratotic hyperkeratosis with crusts that contain mites and mite detritus mixed with cerumen. Small-to-moderate numbers of lymphocytes and macrophages infiltrate the dermis and subcutis. Ceruminous glands are typically hypertrophied and hyperplastic.

While a majority of cats are infested, a minority manifest clinical disease possibly owing to early exposure as kittens and the development of Arthus- and immediate-type hypersensitivity reactions.

Notoedres Cati

Notoedres cati is primarily a cat pathogen but can infest dogs, foxes, rabbits, and rarely people. Usually, infestations are restricted to the auricles, head, face, neck, and shoulders. Infestation produces alopecia, pruritus, thick crusting, and excoriation of the rostral pinnae as the female mite burrows in the stratum corneum and occasionally penetrates hair follicles and sebaceous glands. Microscopic lesions include epidermal hyperplasia and spongiosis with perivascular eosinophilic dermatitis and crusting.

Raillietina *Species*

Raillietina spp. of mites occur most commonly in cattle, buffalo, and goats of nearly every continent. Cattle are most commonly parasitized by *Raillietina auris,* whereas the mite infesting goat ears is *Raillietina caprae. Raillietina flechtmanni* is found in buffalo and cattle ears. These mites often go undetected because of their small size and their tendency to reside deep in the external acoustic meatus adjacent to the tympanic membrane, and they do not commonly cause clinical disease. When clinically apparent, there is often a thick plug of cerumen and debris, with variable suppuration, behind which the mites reside. Additionally, the external acoustic meatus may be ulcerated. Affected animals rarely may develop central nervous system (CNS) signs related to heavy infestations that penetrate the middle and internal ear. Otitis externa is more severe with concurrent bacterial infections or if the host is additionally infected with *Rhabditis* spp. of nematodes. In goats, there are often concurrent infections with *Raillietina caprae* and pathogenic *Mycoplasma* spp.

Psoroptes cuniculi

Psoroptic otoacariasis is most commonly caused by *Psoroptes cuniculi,* infesting sheep, goats, deer, horses, donkeys, mules, and antelope. Although capable of feeding on any part of the animal, it prefers the ear in goats, sheep, and horses. They live on the surface feeding on lipids, keratin, crusts, and cerumen. Pruritus can be intense and is related to surface irritation by infesting mites and hypersensitivity reactions leading to self-trauma to the auricle and periauricular skin. As described (see Chapter 17), histologic lesions include eosinophilic perivascular dermatitis that can be spongiotic, hyperplastic, hyperkeratotic, or exudative. In affected goats, care must be taken to check that the infestation is not complicated by *Raillietina* spp.

Ticks

Ticks and tick-borne diseases rank as some of the most important health constraints of livestock in many parts of the world. Ticks serve as vectors for the spread of disease, affect production parameters such as weight gain or milk production, can lead to significant anemia, may impair individual or herd immunity, and can be a source of aggravation or irritation. Sites of attachment and feeding may occur in multiple locations, but many species of ticks have preferred sites. What follows is a discussion of a few species of mites that preferentially feed in the ears.

Rhipicephalus *Species*

The brown ear tick, *Rhipicephalus appendiculatus,* is found most commonly in southern and southeastern African countries. Adults primarily attach to the ears of domestic and wild ruminants whilst larvae and nymphs attach to ears, head, and neck of most ruminant species, as well as equids, carnivores, and hares. *Bos indicus* cattle become fairly resistant to tick infestations, but exotic *Bos taurus* cattle can have severe production losses and very significant ear damage. *R. appendiculatus* secrete proteins in their saliva, some of which react with the host animal enzymes to form a hard feeding cone and others have inherent enzymatic activity. The protein that forms the cone is called *cement,* and it provides an anchor for feeding ticks and may interfere with a robust inflammatory reaction by the host animal. Affected ears can range from minimally injured to very deformed and sometimes can appear shredded. Microscopically, at the feeding sites, neutrophils predominate in the dermis immediately surrounding the cement layer and are also mixed with macrophages and variable numbers of eosinophils. Brown ear tick toxicosis is a poorly understood condition that occurs in susceptible cattle, presumably the result of tick saliva toxins. Some saliva-derived toxins have an immunosuppressive effect, although the exact mechanism is not understood. These animals may have suppression of adaptive immune responses and lose protection against other environmental pathogens that they have encountered and resisted. In some instances, tick toxicosis can be fatal.

Gulf Coast Ear Tick

Another tick that preferentially infests the ear is variably named the Gulf coast tick or Gulf coast ear tick. *Amblyomma maculatum* is native to North, Central, and South America. In North American, this tick can be found all along the Gulf coast, extending as far inland as Oklahoma, Kansas, and Arkansas and along the southern Atlantic coast. Adult ticks preferentially feed on cattle, sheep, horses, and mules by attaching to the external ears but can also infest deer, cats, foxes, dogs, and pigs. Heavy infestations cause intense auricular inflammation and swelling and may even cause the destruction of the auricular cartilage resulting in a droopy ear sometimes referred to as "gotch ear"* (Fig. 20-32). *A. maculatum* is an experimental vector for transmitting *Cowdria ruminantium*, the causative agent for heartwater disease, but it has not been implicated in field outbreaks in North America. It has also been shown that the Gulf coast ear tick in Florida, Georgia, Kentucky, Mississippi, Oklahoma, and South Carolina may serve as a reservoir for *Rickettsia parkeri.*

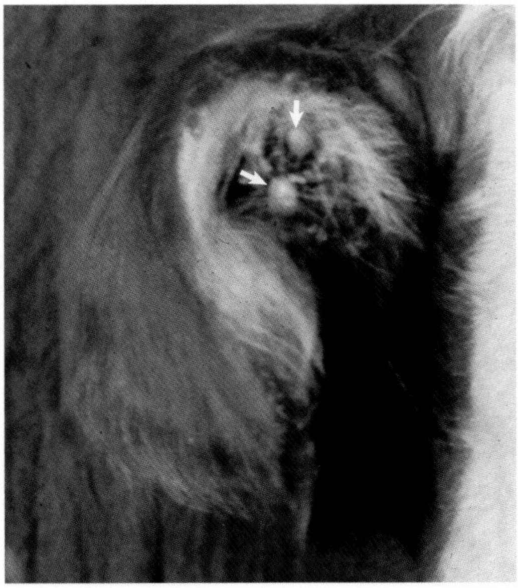

Fig. 20-32 **Gotch ear, bovine.** The left ear of a Hereford cow is severely deformed because of infestation by numerous Gulf coast ear ticks, *Amblyomma maculatum.* The bodies of several ticks *(arrows)* are attached to the concave surface of the medially, ventrally, and rostrally deviated auricle. (Courtesy Dr. J.A. Hair, Oklahoma State University.)

Spinose Ear Tick

Otobius megnini, the "spinose ear tick," has a broad host range, including ungulates, sheep, goats, cattle, horses, dogs, and humans. Adults are free living and nonparasitic, but nymph and larval stages are parasitic. Newly hatched larvae remain in the environment until they climb onto a suitable host. Owing to their small size and propensity for living very deep in the external acoustic meatus, larvae are rarely identified in host ears. As these ticks moult and mature, some can be found attached to and blood feeding in the more shallow portions of the external acoustic meatus or attached to the auricular skin (Fig. 20-33). After several months of feeding in or on host ears, nymphs drop off the host, seeking dry, sheltered places where they moult into adults. Lesions are attributable to blood feeding, which results in local irritation and secondary otitis externa. As has already been described, local reactions to the feeding sites include perivascular to interstitial dermatitis laden with neutrophils and eosinophils. Infested animals may develop clinical symptoms such as head shaking and pruritus related to nymph feeding on blood and lymph of the skin of the external acoustic meatus.

*"Gotch ear" is a colloquial term with Spanish roots coined by cowboys and defined as a type of earmark used to identify cattle that resulted in severe rostral, medial, and ventral flexion of the auricle.

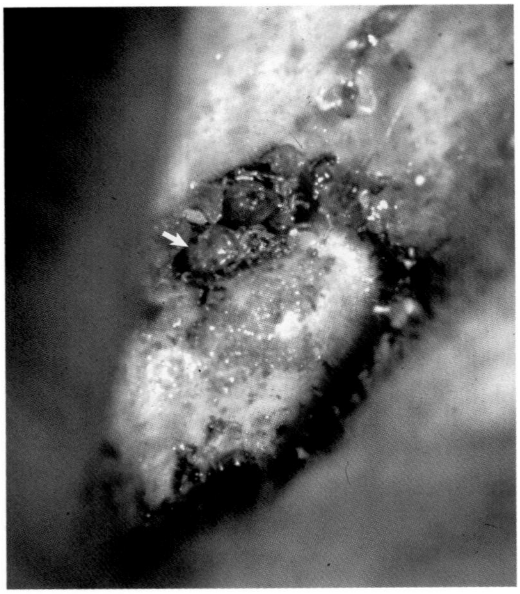

Fig. 20-33 Spinose ear tick, bovine.
Deep within the concave surface of the auricle are numerous *Otobius megnini,* or spinose ear tick *(arrow).* Associated with these ticks is an increased amount of brown ceruminous exudate. (Courtesy Dr. J.A. Hair, Oklahoma State University.)

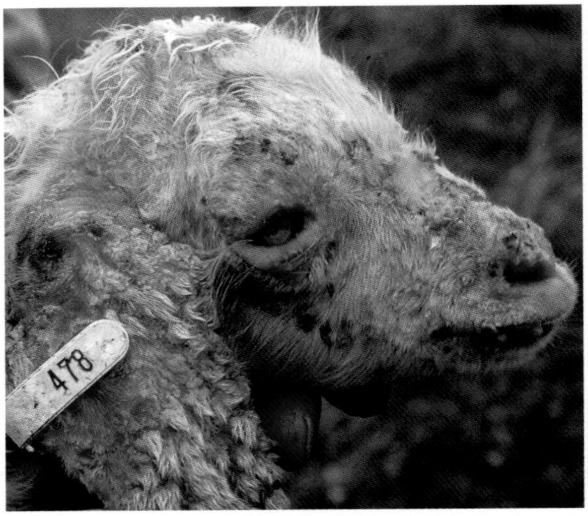

Fig. 20-34 Cutaneous dermatophilosis, goat.
The auricular skin, as well as skin of the muzzle, face, and periocular region, is matted from a severely exudative dermatitis caused by *Dermatophilus congolensis.* (Courtesy Dr. K.G. Thompson, Institute of Veterinary, Animal, and Biomedical Science, Massey University.)

BACTERIAL DISEASES OF THE EXTERNAL EAR

Dermatophilosis (Streptothrichosis)

Dermatophilosis (also known as streptothrichosis) is caused by *Dermatophilus congolensis* and is a zoonotic bacterium of the skin and mucosae of the nose, commissures of the lips, distal or proximal limbs, and ears but may proliferate virtually anywhere on the body. The bacterium prefers moist areas and requires the integrity (i.e., barrier) of the skin to be impaired. Thus damaged skin with scabs and crusts on the face and ears are sites of colonization by *D. congolensis* in younger animals. *D. congolensis* is transferred during nursing from damp and traumatized skin of the inguinal region of lactating dams to the ears of nursing kids (Fig. 20-34). Colonization begins by invasion of flagellated zoospores that penetrate the epidermis and reach the level of the basement membrane in which they transform to a filamentous morphology. They also penetrate into the dermis and follicular adnexa, inciting a prominent neutrophilic response. This acute inflammation halts further invasion. However, residual bacteria colonies are able to invade nascent, regenerated epidermis. This cycle of bacterial growth, inflammation, and epidermal regeneration leads to the multi-laminated pustular crusts so typical of dermatophilosis. Damage to the cutaneous barrier system can also be caused by other invasive bacteria, fungi, or ectoparasites such as mites and ticks. Macroscopically, lesions are characterized by a crusting and exudative dermatitis (see Chapter 17) with thick crusts covering an epidermis that is ulcerated and hemorrhagic. Microscopically, crusts are made of alternating layers of markedly parakeratotic hyperkeratosis, degenerate neutrophils, and coagulative necrosis all laden with *Dermatophilus congolensis.* It can be identified by its filamentous morphology with longitudinal and transverse septa (see Fig. 17-48).

NEOPLASMS OF THE EXTERNAL EAR

Most frequently, aural neoplasia is a unilateral disease; bilateral involvement is rare. Sebaceous gland tumors, histiocytomas, plasmacytomas, and mast cell tumors (see Chapter 6) are the most common types of aural neoplasms in dogs. Sebaceous gland tumors are most often benign, but diagnoses of aural masses resembling sebaceous glands include sebaceous gland hyperplasia, sebaceous adenoma, sebaceous epithelioma, and sebaceous adenocarcinoma. Differentiating between histiocytomas, plasmacytomas, and mast cell tumors requires a surgical biopsy (see Chapter 17) and histologic examination.

In cats, basal cell tumors, vascular tumors, and squamous cell carcinomas are the most common types of aural neoplasms. Vascular neoplasms and squamous cell carcinomas arise on lightly pigmented pinna of outdoor cats exposed to the sun for prolonger periods of time as a result of UVB light-induced neoplastic transformation (see Chapter 6). With squamous cell carcinomas, the margins at the base and tips of the ears are most often affected (Fig. 20-35; also see Table 17-3). However, they can also arise within the external acoustic meatus and the tympanic cavity and bulla. Macroscopically, they are raised, ulcerated, and hemorrhagic neoplasms. Growth is often a combination of local stromal invasion and concurrent vascular invasion with metastasis via regional lymphatic vessels. Initially, these tumors can be misdiagnosed as exudative dermatitic lesions.

Neoplasms of the external acoustic meatus in the dog or cat are infrequently diagnosed but the most common types include ceruminous gland tumors, sebaceous tumors, and epithelial neoplasms of undetermined origin. In fact, the majority (85%) of feline aural neoplasms are malignant compared to 60% of canine aural neoplasms being malignant. Of these, ceruminous gland adenocarcinomas are the most common neoplasm diagnosed in the external acoustic meatus of both dogs and cats. Typically, middle-aged to older animals are affected.

Canine ceruminous gland adenomas are more commonly diagnosed than adenocarcinomas. By comparison, adenomas are multiple, small, pedunculate, irregular, and firm masses. These masses may develop secondarily to recurrent bouts of chronic otitis externa. Some speculate that the chemical mediators of chronic inflammation and products of cerumen decomposition are carcinogenic and contribute to dysplasia and neoplastic transformation. Ceruminous

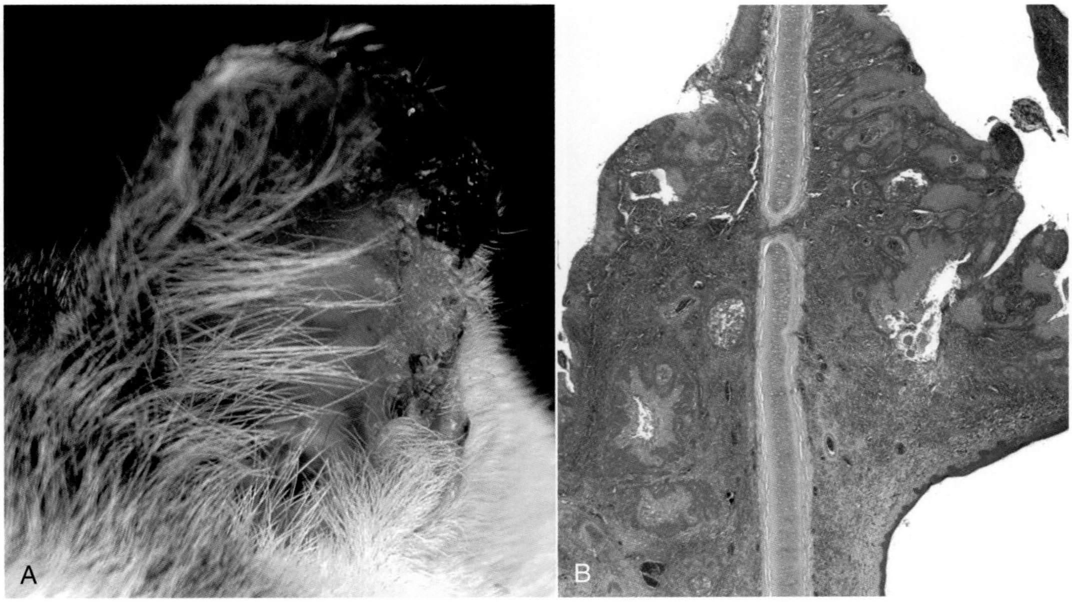

Fig. 20-35 **Aural squamous cell carcinoma, cat.**
A, Lateral view. The lateral margin and tip of the left auricle are ulcerated and covered by a serohemorrhagic crust caused by an underlying squamous cell carcinoma. **B,** Histologic section of aural squamous cell carcinoma. Note the cords and islands of anaplastic squamous epithelial cells that have infiltrated the dermis. The tumor may penetrate through the auricular cartilage as it grows. H&E stain. (**A** courtesy Dr. W.H. Miller, College of Veterinary Medicine, Cornell University; **B** courtesy Dr. B.L. Njaa, Center for Veterinary Health Sciences, Oklahoma State University.)

gland adenocarcinomas tend to be locally invasive and expansile (Fig. 20-36, *A*). There is a tendency for metastasis to regional lymph nodes, lungs, and systemic viscera.

By contrast, ceruminous gland adenocarcinomas are much more frequently diagnosed in cats than adenomas and account for up to 2% of all feline neoplasms. They tend to be locally invasive and up to 50% are reported to metastasize to regional lymph nodes, lungs, or systemic viscera. There is a greater tendency for adenocarcinomas to be diagnosed in aged male cats.

These neoplasms are readily capable of growing between overlapping areas of auricular cartilage extending into the periauricular dermis and subcutis (Fig. 20-36, *B*). Histologically, the neoplastic cells tend to form acini, small ducts, irregular tubular structures, or small clusters (Fig. 20-36, *C*). Neoplastic cells are typically basaloid to low columnar with intensely basophilic cytoplasm. Variation in nuclear and cytoplasmic size is variable, but neoplastic cells may be quite uniform. The occurrence and number of mitotic figures are highly variable. There tends to be a very prominent desmoplastic response to the surrounding tissue. Large areas of necrosis are not uncommon.

MISCELLANEOUS DISORDERS OF THE EXTERNAL EAR

Pinnal Alopecia

Pinnal alopecia occurs as a congenital disease in cattle or an acquired disease in dogs and cats. In Polled Hereford calves, this congenital disease begins at birth as an alopecic disease of the muzzle, auricular margins, and base of the ears. Pedigree analysis suggests this disorder is an inherited disease but the mode of inheritance remains undermined. A detailed analysis of this condition consistently found evidence of epidermal maturation and keratinization defects. At birth, the hair coat was wiry and tightly curled; it epilated easily. Alopecia and hyperkeratosis became generalized by 3 months of age. Marked wrinkling of the skin developed over the face and neck as the cattle aged. Microscopically, the density of hair follicles was normal, but a higher proportion of these follicles were in telogen phase. Additionally, there was premature keratinization and degeneration of the internal root sheath of the follicle, sebaceous gland atrophy, and dilated sweat glands that were lined with a thinned epithelium. This process resulted in easy epilation of hair. In older affected calves, the hyperkeratotic skin was also inflamed with a mild, superficial, perivascular, lymphocytic perivascular dermatitis. Interestingly, hyperkeratotic lesions also affected the rumen mucosa. Clinically, the anemia was characterized as nonregenerative, normocytic to macrocytic, and normochromic.

Acquired pinnal alopecia occurs primarily in dogs and cats (Box 20-4). The condition in dogs primarily affects dachshunds, but has also been reported in Chihuahuas, Boston terriers, whippets, and Italian greyhounds. Siamese cats are more commonly diagnosed with acquired pinnal alopecia that is patchy to complete but unlike the dog spontaneously resolves. In dogs, it is often symmetrical, and auricular hair of the convex surface becomes miniaturized. Then gradually over time, auricles become alopecic (Fig. 20-37). Rarely, the auricle becomes completely alopecic; however, the remainder of the body hair coat is typically unaffected. Biopsies show affected anagen hair follicles that are smaller diameter or shorter.

DEVELOPMENTAL ANOMALIES OF THE MIDDLE EAR

Primary Ciliary Dyskinesia (Immotile Cilia Syndrome)

Described most completely in the dog, primary ciliary dyskinesia (also known as immotile cilia syndrome) has also been suspected or confirmed in horses, ruminants, pigs, and cats. Typically, affected animals are under a year of age, have a persistent cough and nasal discharge related to chronic rhinitis, and have chronic recurrent respiratory disease related to impaired or ineffective mucociliary clearance without evidence of immunologic impairment.

In dogs, the most common ciliary defects include dynein arm deficiency, abnormal microtubular patterns, random orientation of

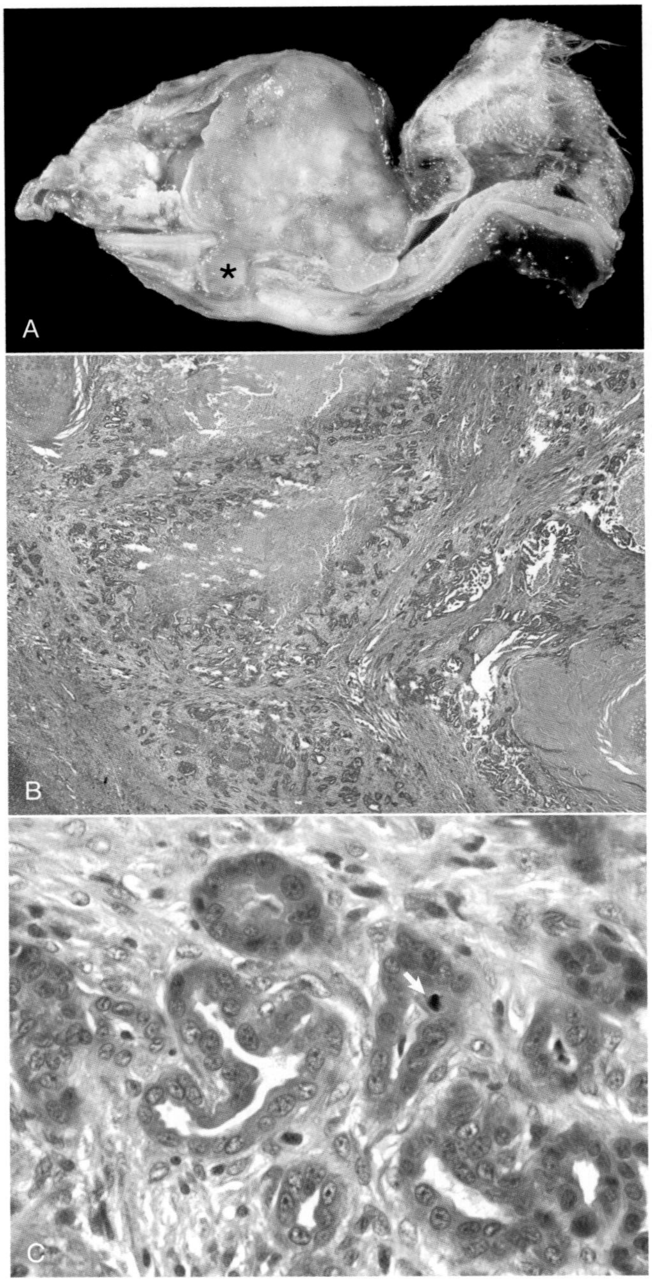

Fig. 20-36 Ceruminous gland adenocarcinoma.
A, Cross-section of external acoustic meatus. This ceruminous gland adenocarcinoma fills the external acoustic meatus and expands its luminal diameter. Ventrally, there is a small extension of the neoplasm *(asterisk)* either through or between overlapping layers of auricular and annular cartilage. **B,** Histology of ceruminous gland carcinoma. Neoplastic ceruminous glands induce a prominent desmoplastic response and are shown invading through the cartilage *(bottom center of image)*. H&E stain. **C,** Higher magnification of **B.** The neoplasm has haphazardly arranged and formed tubules and acini with evidence of anaplastic and mitotically active cells *(arrow)*. It is shown growing through the auricular cartilage. H&E stain. (**A** courtesy Dr. W.N. Evering, Pfizer Global Research; **B** and **C** courtesy Dr. B.L. Njaa, Center for Veterinary Health Sciences, Oklahoma State University.)

BOX 20-4 Causes of Pinnal Alopecia

Adverse drug reactions
Alopecia areata
Atopy
Canine hypothyroidism
Canine pinnal alopecia
Color dilution alopecia
Congenital anemia, dyskeratosis, and progressive alopecia of Polled Herefords
Congenital hypotrichosis
Demodicosis
Dermatophytosis
Epitheliotropic T lymphocyte lymphoma
Estrogen-responsive dermatosis
Feline hypothyroidism
Feline pinnal alopecia
Food allergy
Hyperadrenocorticism
Leishmaniasis
Pattern baldness
Topical steroid-induced alopecia
Vasculitis/ischemic dermatitis

the microtubules, and electron-dense inclusions in the basal body that anchors the cilium to the cell. In horses, the total number of cilia may be decreased and the vast majority have central microtubule pair defects. The middle ear relies in part on fully functioning ciliated epithelial cells and mucus-producing goblet cells for clearance of fluid and debris through the auditory tube. Thus abnormal cilia equates to abnormal auditory tube clearance.

Macroscopic lesions include bilateral mucopurulent rhinitis, sinusitis, and chronic tracheitis. There is frequently unilateral or bilateral otitis media evident with mucopurulent exudate or with sterile, gelatinous material filling the tympanic cavity. Tympanic bullae may be thickened or sclerotic. Microscopically, the tympanic cavity contains proteinaceous material mixed with variable numbers of inflammatory cells, typically neutrophils and macrophages with variable aggregates of lymphocytes and plasma cells.

Clinically, animals present with a chronic cough and persistent nasal discharge, and the symptoms are unresponsive to antibiotics. Typically, middle or internal ear signs are not evident clinically. Frequently, animals are neutrophilic, likely caused by persistent secondary bacterial infections of the upper respiratory tract. Affected males are frequently infertile.

INFLAMMATION OF THE MIDDLE EAR

Otitis Media

Infections of the middle ear affect all domestic animal species but vary in prevalence and which pathogens are isolated. Ruminants and pigs are most severely affected, whereas cats are less commonly affected.

Otitis media in pigs occurs naturally as a result of nasopharyngeal ascent of bacteria through the auditory tubes. *Pasteurella multocida, Arcanobacterium pyogenes,* and *Mycoplasma hyorhinis* are likely pathogens, separately or concurrently, that first colonize the nasopharynx and ascend the auditory tube to gain entry and cause otitis media. Studies of the pathogenesis of otitis media in young piglets suggest that dysfunction of the auditory tube is an initial contributing factor. Dysfunction is linked to acute inflammation, goblet cell hyperplasia of mucosae and occasional acute inflammation of

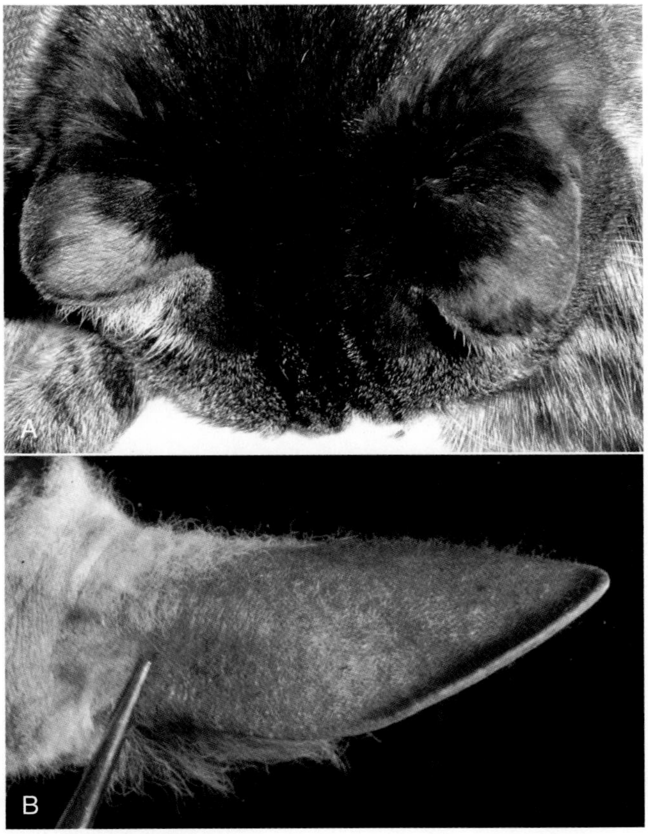

Fig. 20-37 Pinnal alopecia.
A, Dorsal view, cat. Alopecia is present as bilaterally symmetric lesions most severely affecting the convex surface of the auricles of the distal half of each ear *(light pink areas)*. In the dog, this lesion tends to be permanent, whereas in the cat, typically Siamese breeds, this often spontaneously resolves. **B,** Auricle, convex surface, calf. Note the absence of hair on the convex surface of the ear. This case is an example of congenital pinnal alopecia in Polled Hereford calves. (**A** courtesy Dr. W.H. Miller, College of Veterinary Medicine, Cornell University. **B** courtesy Drs. W. Crowell and D.E. Tyler, College of Veterinary Medicine, The University of Georgia; and Noah's Arkive, College of Veterinary Medicine, The University of Georgia.)

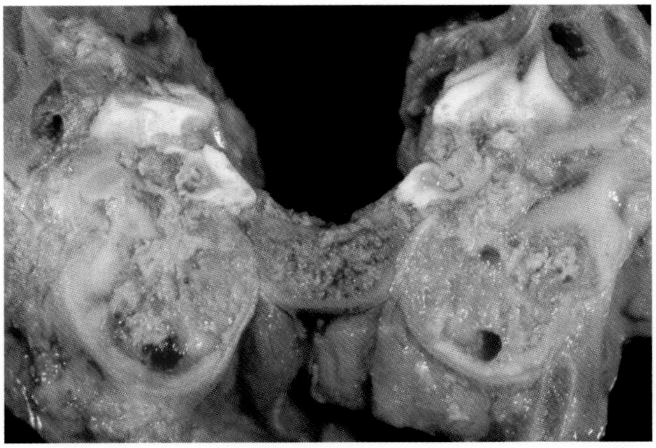

Fig. 20-38 Suppurative otitis media, rostral view, cow.
Bilaterally, tympanic cavities and bullae are filled with suppurative exudate. (Courtesy Dr. B.L. Njaa, College of Veterinary Medicine, Cornell University.)

the tympanic cavity. In older pigs, otitis media was more severe and suppurative and auditory tube lesions were more severe and characterized by interepithelial infiltration by neutrophils, intraluminal exudation of neutrophils and fibrin, marked goblet cell hyperplasia, mucosal erosion to ulceration, and infiltration of the propria submucosa by lymphocytes and macrophages. Bacterial colonies of *Pasteurella multocida* and *Arcanobacterium pyogenes* were present in the exudate. Colonization of the tympanic cavity resulted in lysis of bone of the wall and of the osseous septa of tympanic bullae. In severe cases, lesions spread and caused otitis interna and acute fibrinous inflammation of the cochlea and vestibule, as well as extension into the leptomeninges and neuropil of the brain. Pigs older than 4 months more commonly had severe, chronic otitis media with extensive expansion as described above.

In ruminants, *Histophilus somni*, *Pasteurella multocida*, *Arcanobacterium pyogenes*, *Mycoplasma bovis*, and *Streptococcus* spp. have been isolated from animals with otitis media. Various mites (see previous discussion) and nematodes may also contribute to the occurrence and severity of disease. As in pigs, otitis media occurs as a result of nasopharyngeal ascent of bacteria through the auditory tubes. In natural infections, potential routes of initial exposure to these bacteria include congenital infection, ingestion of colostrum, ingestion of contaminated milk, exposure to infected vaginal secretions, or ingestion or inhalation of respiratory secretions leading to nasopharyngeal colonization. Other factors include concurrent bacterial or viral infections, nutritional status of the herd, level of contamination in the environment, and host immune status.

Macroscopically, lesions may be unilateral or bilateral. Mucosae lining tympanic bullae are congested and edematous (see Fig. 17-13). Bullae can be filled with fibrinopurulent to caseous exudate and the underlying mucosa is often ulcerated (Fig. 20-38). There may be remodeling of bony septa of the bullae or osteolysis, as well as osteolysis of auditory ossicles. With chronicity, the mucosa of the tympanic cavity and bullae becomes markedly thickened by fibrosis and granulation tissue. In severely affected animals, tympanic membranes and auditory ossicles are missing. Microscopic lesions reflect what is seen grossly, namely bony lysis of bullae septa, infiltration by mixtures of neutrophils and macrophages, abundant cellular debris, and variable numbers of bacteria. When examined, auditory ossicles have superficial erosion of bone. The epithelium of the tympanic cavity is highly variable, with areas lined by squamous epithelium, whereas others are lined by ciliated, pseudostratified columnar epithelium mixed with goblet cells. The latter mucosae often form small cystic cavities surrounded by exudate. The propria submucosa is infiltrated by variable numbers of lymphocytes, plasma cells, macrophages, and neutrophils.

Clinical signs frequently include facial nerve paralysis, head tilt, drooping ears, epiphora, and mucopurulent nasal discharge. Severe otitis media can result in tympanic membrane rupture leading to purulent otorrhea and otiasma. Rarely, infections spread to cause meningitis.

Otitis media is an uncommon disease in cats. Numerous bacteria have been isolated including *E. coli*, *Enterobacter* spp., *Enterococcus* spp., *Streptococcus* spp., β-hemolytic *Streptococcus* spp., *Staphylococcus* spp., *Proteus* spp., and *Clostridium* spp. Although more frequently a unilateral disease, bilateral disease is reported. Grossly, any tympanic bulla that contains fluid of any kind should be suspected as being otitis media. Tympanic cavity effusions may be translucent, gray mucoid, yellow-green, red-tinged, or hemorrhagic (Fig. 20-39, *A*). Flushing the effusion may allow visualization of ruptured tympanic membranes, bony proliferation of the tympanic bulla, or

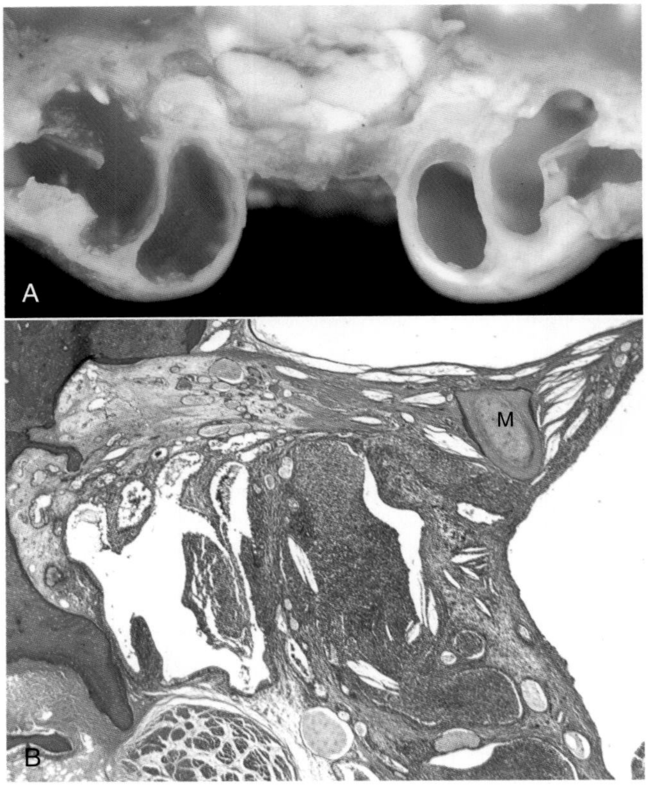

Fig. 20-39 Otitis media, cat.
A, Rostral view. Red-tinged, viscous fluid fills the tympanic compartments of the left ear. The right ear is normal with no luminal exudate. The septum bulla is complete and separates the tympanic cavity into the dorsolateral epitympanic cavity and the ventromedial tympanic cavity. **B,** Histologic section of middle ear. The tympanic cavity contains abundant suppurative exudate *(center)* mixed with numerous cholesterol clefts. The propria submucosa of the tympanic cavity is thickened by edematous fibrous connective tissue. Throughout are numerous cystic cavities lined by mucosa. The manubrium *(M)* of the malleus is embedded in a tympanic membrane that is thickened as a result of chronic inflammation (myringitis) with fibrosis and cholesterol cleft formation. (Courtesy Dr. B.L. Njaa, Center for Veterinary Health Sciences, Oklahoma State University.)

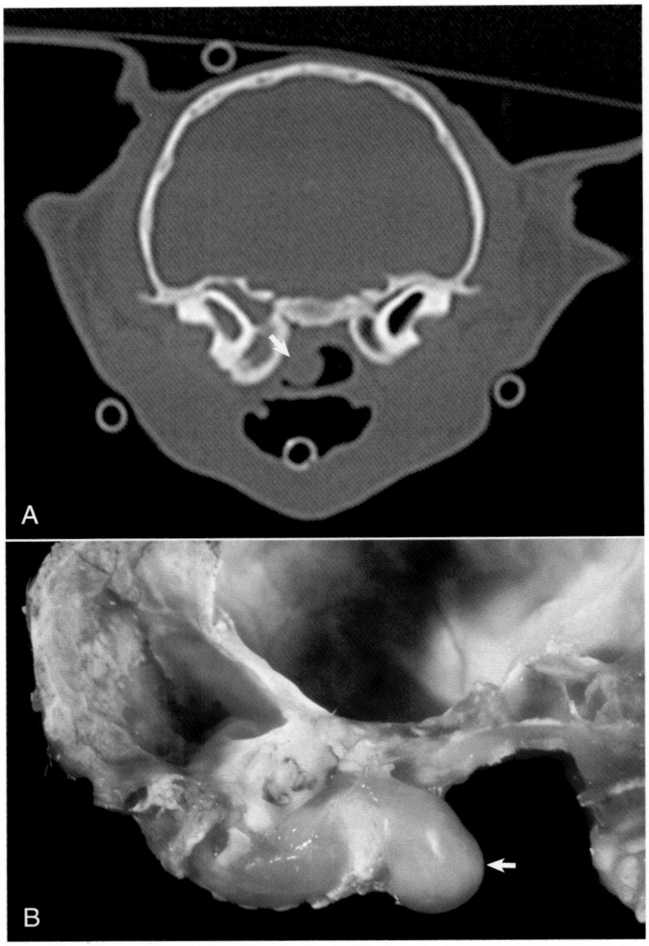

Fig. 20-40 Nasopharyngeal polyp, cat.
A, Computed tomography (CT) of tympanic bullae and pharynx. A small, central bulge of hypoechoic tissue *(arrow)* extends from the left tympanic cavity into the nasopharynx, presumably through the auditory tube. **B,** Cross-section through the left tympanic bulla and nasopharynx. A nasopharyngeal polyp *(arrow)* fills the tympanic bulla and extends through the auditory tube into the nasopharynx. The smooth, shiny surface indicates it is covered by epithelium. The inner ear is opened in this view, and the rostral, ventral spiral turns of the cochlea are present. (**A** courtesy Dr. N. Dykes, College of Veterinary Medicine, Cornell University; **B** courtesy Dr. J. Render, North American Science Associates.)

deformities to the auditory ossicles, when examined with the use of a dissecting microscope. Microscopically, there are abundant neutrophils, typically degenerate, mixed with macrophages, and variable numbers of lymphocytes and plasma cells (Fig. 20-39, *B*). Often, the pseudostratified, ciliated columnar epithelium of the tympanic bulla is undermined by the infiltrate and frequently forms smaller, gland-like structures. Areas of cholesterol cleft formation are common as are areas of hemorrhage. The amount of fibrosis within the tympanic cavity is variable and relates to the chronicity of the otitis media. Osseous proliferation of the tympanic bulla is seen more often than bony erosions. The earliest necropsy survey of cats submitted for routine postmortem examinations found that 9.1% had evidence of middle ear inflammation. A recent *Journal of the American Veterinary Medical Association* (JAVMA) study suggests a much lower prevalence; however, more importantly, the study confirmed that clinical disease caused by otitis media is rare when compared to the number of cats with gross evidence of disease. Therefore both bullae should be routinely opened when performing postmortem examinations of cats.

Nasopharyngeal Polyps (Inflammatory Polyps)

Nasopharyngeal polyps are the most common, nonneoplastic, inflammatory masses affecting cats often under 2 years of age. They also occur much less frequently in dogs and have been reported once in a horse. A confirmed cause has not yet been determined, but proposed etiologies include chronic upper respiratory tract infections, otitis media, ascending middle ear infections via the auditory tube, or congenital defects such as aberrant growths from remnants of the branchial arches. As their name suggests, inflammatory polyps are pedunculated and polypoid, often with a smooth surface (Fig. 20-40). They may be confined to the middle ear, protrude through the auditory tube into the nasopharynx, or penetrate through a ruptured tympanic membrane into the external acoustic meatus. Histologically, inflammatory polyps have a fibrovascular core that is infiltrated with lymphocytes, plasma cells, and macrophages of varying numbers and are covered by epithelium. The

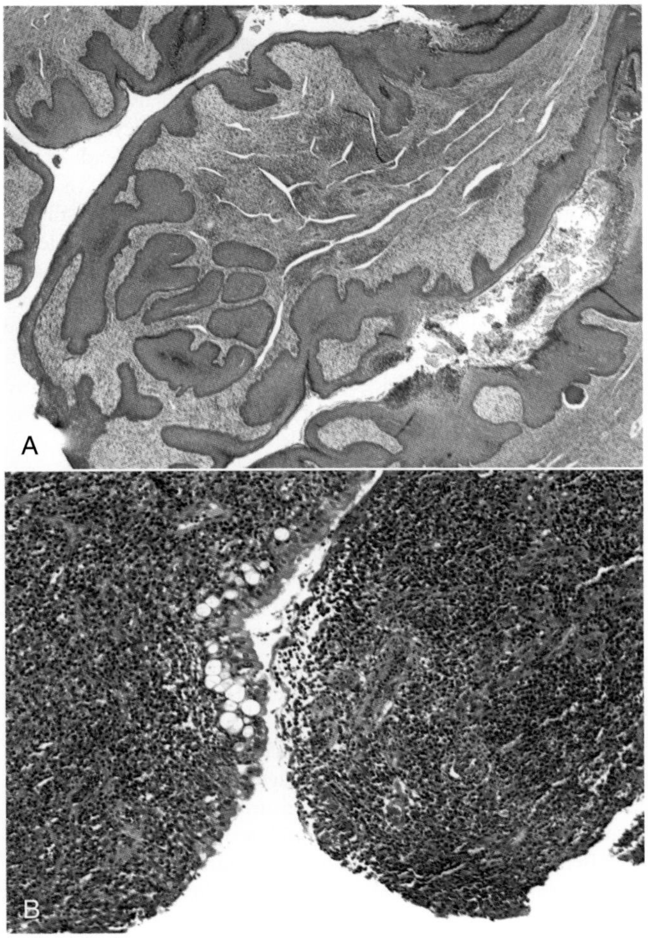

Fig. 20-41 Nasopharyngeal inflammatory polyps, cats.
A, Histologic section of the polyp depicted in Fig. 20-40, *A*. The mucosa covering the surface of this polyp is primarily hyperplastic stratified squamous epithelium but in some cases polyps may also by covered by ciliated columnar epithelium mixed with goblet cells. The lamina propria contains abundant chronic inflammatory cells. H&E stain. **B,** The lamina propria of this polyp is partially obscured by dense infiltrates of lymphocytes, plasma cells, and macrophages. The mucosa is composed of ciliated, columnar, pseudostratified epithelial cells mixed with goblet cells and is focally eroded or ulcerated. H&E stain. (**A** courtesy Dr. D. Schafer, College of Veterinary Medicine, Cornell University; **B** courtesy Dr. B.L. Njaa, Center for Veterinary Health Sciences, Oklahoma State University.)

overlying epithelium reflects the tissue of origin whether arising from the nasopharynx, auditory tube, tympanic bulla, or other portions of the tympanic cavity and varies from stratified squamous epithelium to pseudostratified ciliated columnar epithelium mixed with goblet cells (Fig. 20-41). Signs of disease vary, depending on the location of the polyps. Signs of otitis externa or otitis media may commonly indicate the presence of polyps. Other symptoms include nasal, otic, or ocular discharge; sneezing; dyspnea; stridor; voice change; dysphagia; head tilt; Horner's syndrome; nystagmus; and ataxia. Much less commonly, obstructing polyps may lead to cyanosis and syncope.

Inflammatory polyps reported in dogs and horses occur much less frequently. Based on published accounts, the age of onset is typically much older. In the few reports of inflammatory polyps in dogs, they primarily occur in male dogs. Macroscopic and histologic features as well as clinical signs are virtually identical to what has been described in cats.

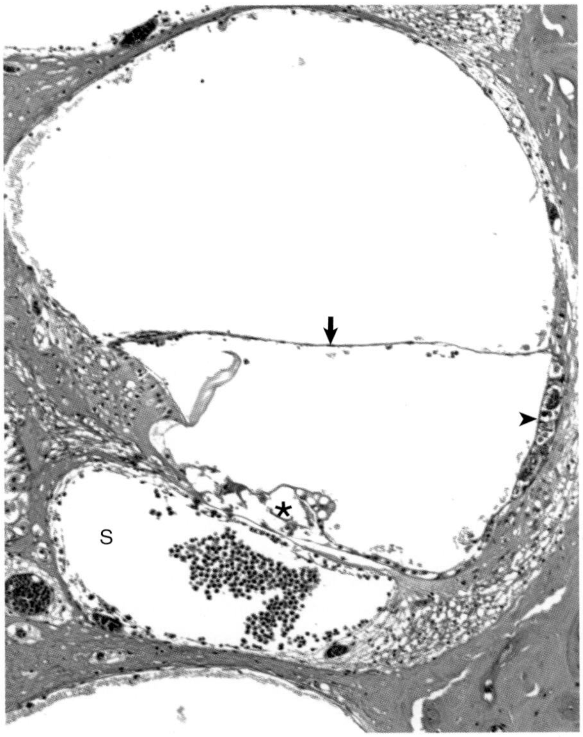

Fig. 20-42 Otitis interna, guinea pig.
The ventral compartment known as the scala tympani *(S)* contains a large luminal aggregate of inflammatory cells, mainly heterophils (neutrophils). Fewer inflammatory cells are present in the cochlear duct and scala vestibuli. The vestibular membrane *(arrow)* is intact. The tectorial membrane is artifactually separated from the organ of Corti that is also presumably artifactually distorted *(asterisk)*. Stria vascularis *(arrowhead)*. See Fig. 20-21 for a diagram of the structure. H&E stain. (Courtesy Dr. B.L. Njaa, Center for Veterinary Health Sciences, Oklahoma State University).

NEOPLASMS OF THE MIDDLE EAR

Neoplasms occur rarely in the middle ear. Squamous cell carcinomas have been diagnosed most frequently in dogs and cats. Neoplasms may originate within the middle ear or arise in the external ear canal and penetrate through the tympanic membrane into the tympanic cavity. Neoplastic growth tends to be expansile and infiltrative with evidence of bony lysis of bullae, lysis of the petrous portion of the temporal bone, or intracranial invasion. Local damage to the facial nerve or vestibulocochlear nerve may lead to vestibular signs, facial nerve paralysis, or Horner's syndrome. In both dogs and cats, pain on opening the mouth is very common.

INFLAMMATION OF THE INTERNAL EAR

Otitis Interna (Labyrinthitis)

Otitis interna results from extension of otitis media. It may occur with or without osteomyelitis of the petrous portion of the temporal bone. With time and severity, lesions progress retrograde through the internal acoustic meatus into the cranial cavity, resulting in meningitis, ventriculitis, and encephalitis. Macroscopically, there is typically a middle ear exudate that varies from serosanguineous to suppurative to granulomatous. Microscopically, the inflammatory infiltrate affecting the middle ear is typically composed of neutrophils, macrophages, lymphocytes, and plasma cells. Within the membranous labyrinth, smaller numbers of neutrophils mixed with fibrin can be found in the perilymph (Fig. 20-42). Fewer lymphocytes and plasma cells may infiltrate the lamina propria of the internal ear mucosa. The most plausible portal of entry is through the membranous covering of the round or cochlear window (see Fig. 20-21).

VESTIBULAR DISEASE OF THE INTERNAL EAR

Injury to any portion of the vestibular system (see the previous section on the Vestibular System) leads to a condition collectively referred to as *vestibular disease.* Although the lesion may be located peripherally (internal ear sensory receptors, vestibular ganglia, or peripheral axons of cranial nerve [CN] VIII) or centrally (vestibular nuclei of the medulla, vestibular projections to the rostral brainstem, cerebellum, or spinal cord), affected animals typically exhibit a head tilt, nystagmus, asymmetric ataxia, circling, and variable facial paralysis.

Congenital vestibular disease has been reported to occur in certain breeds of dogs (Doberman pinschers, German shepherd dogs, Cocker Spaniels, Beagles, or Akitas) and more commonly in oriental breeds of cats (Siamese, Tonkinese, or Burmese). The cause of this disease is not well understood largely because most affected animals recover spontaneously or compensate within the first few weeks of life. Gross lesions are typically absent. As a result of the clinical course, histologic lesions are usually not reported. However in one report, a small number of Doberman pinscher puppies had evidence of intense lymphocytic infiltration of the middle and internal ear propria submucosa. The most common clinical sign is a head tilt with varying degrees of ataxia. Nystagmus is reported but a less prominent feature. Deafness has been reported in some cases.

Concurrent otitis media and otitis interna is the most common cause of peripheral vestibular disease. Otitis media in isolation will not result in vestibular disease, but if deficits are detected that are compatible with peripheral vestibular disease, concurrent internal ear involvement is confirmed. Causes include (1) viral infections such as those caused by canine distemper virus and feline infectious peritonitis virus and (2) various bacterial, rickettsial (Rocky Mountain spotted fever, ehrlichiosis, bartonellosis), protozoal (toxoplasmosis, neosporosis), and mycotic (cryptococcosis, blastomycosis, histoplasmosis, coccidiomycosis) infections. A small group of affected horses had concurrent facial nerve paralysis as well. Refer to previous discussions of gross and histologic features of otitis media and otitis interna.

Idiopathic peripheral vestibular disease is considered the second most common form of this disease diagnosed in dogs and cats. Dogs are typically geriatric at the time of diagnosis. In cats, age is less important, but most cases are diagnosed in the summer and fall months in the northeastern and mid-Atlantic regions of the United States. A cause has not been determined and specific lesions have not been identified. One key clinical feature in making this diagnosis is the presence of peripheral vestibular disease signs in the absence of concurrent facial nerve paralysis or Horner's syndrome.

Aural or intracranial neoplasia may arise within, compress on, or infiltrate into the labyrinthine or neural portions of the vestibular system. Vestibular neurofibromas or schwannomas may primarily arise within the vestibulocochlear nerve (see Figs. 14-114 and 14-115. Compression or invasion of soft tissues of the head and ear, the skull, brainstem, or cerebellum can result in significant vestibular deficits. Based on diagnostic imaging, lytic lesions of the tympanic bullae or petrous portions of the temporal bone are more often associated with aural neoplasia than with otitis media or otitis interna. Signs associated with intracranial neoplasia depend more on the location of the neoplasm versus the kind of neoplasm. Grossly, the neoplasm may arise within or infiltrate a portion of the central vestibular system. Alternatively, the mass may cause obstructive hydrocephalus or brain herniation, resulting in more widespread neurologic deficits.

Various therapeutic agents can cause vestibular disease. Ototoxic agents, such as aminoglycoside antimicrobials, furosemide, platinum-containing antineoplastic agents, and salicylates, are a few categories of chemicals that cause injury to or death of the neurosensory hair cells of the membranous labyrinth. In most instances, deafness that develops is permanent, whereas vestibular disease from other nontoxic causes may improve or completely resolve with time. Metronidazole is an antimicrobial agent capable of causing neurotoxicity with resultant vestibular disease. The exact mechanism is not fully known but theorized to be modulated by γ-aminobutyric acid (GABA) receptors in the vestibulocerebellum and may result in axonal degeneration. The signs typically resolve on cessation of therapy. There is very little published documenting lesions associated with metronidazole therapy.

Hearing Loss and Deafness

Hearing loss and deafness can be congenital or acquired, and each type further categorized as conduction or neurosensory deafness. Deafness in animals with a patent external acoustic meatus is likely congenital in origin. Audiometrics first detect sound perception in kittens 5 days old and puppies 14 days old. Animals that are known to hear normally that subsequently undergo hearing loss have acquired deafness. A patent external acoustic meatus, intact tympanic membrane, functioning auditory ossicles, and normal perilymph and endolymph of the cochlea define the conduction portion of hearing and thus any damage or loss of these structures leads to conduction deafness. The neurosensory contribution to hearing includes the membranes and neurosensory cells of the membranous labyrinth and associated neural connections. Any interference with the neural pathways or injury to the mechanosensory hair cells leads to neurosensory deafness.

Causes of conduction hearing loss include (1) external acoustic meatus stenosis that may be congenital or acquired secondary to otitis externa, (2) chronic otitis externa leading to narrowing of the external acoustic meatus or tympanic membrane rupture and impaired sound transmission, (3) auditory ossicle damage or tympanic membrane injury from otitis media, and (4) damage from neoplasms affecting any portion of the conduction system. Repair or removal of the cause of the conduction deafness can result in return to normal function and hearing.

Congenital inherited sensorineural deafness is a common disorder, especially in dogs and cats. Alterations in the function of microphthalmia-associated transcription factor (MITF) occurs in Dalmatian dogs with congenital sensorineural deafness and blue iris color. The merle color pattern is a pigment dilution related to variable expression of the merle allele of the pigment locus mouse *Silver* pigment locus homolog *(SILV).* Dogs homozygous for the dominant merle allele are significantly more likely to be deaf than heterozygotes. The piebald gene, which results in a coat color that alternates between white and darkly pigmented, also has been linked with deafness. Both the piebald and merle genes cause the blue eye phenotype by suppressing melanocytes in the iris and deafness by suppressing melanocytes in the stria vascularis of the cochlear duct.

Congenital sensorineural deafness has been classified into two major categories based on mechanism: albinotic and abiotrophic. The albinotic form or Scheibe deformity is also known as *cochleosaccular degeneration.* It is associated with hypopigmentation and stria vascularis dysfunction. Deafness due to stria vascularis dysfunction is related to lack of melanocytes. Endolymph is produced and maintained by the stria vascularis, but in the absence

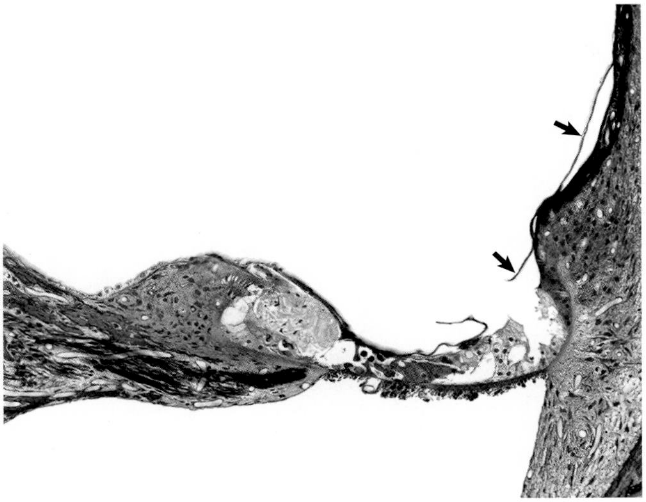

Fig. 20-43 **Albinotic or Scheibe-type deafness, cat.**
The vestibular membrane *(arrows)* is ruptured and collapsed onto the organ of Corti *(asterisk)* and the tectorial membrane is difficult to discern in the section. The scala media or cochlear duct is obliterated. See Fig. 20-21 for a diagram of the structure. Thick tissue section, toluidine blue stain. (Courtesy Dr. D.A. Ryugo; from Ryugo DA, Cahill HB, Rose LS, et al: *Hear Res* 181:73-84, 2003.)

of melanocytes, this function is inhibited. Abnormal endolymph leads to degeneration of hair cells of the cochlea characterized by atrophy of stria vascularis, collapse of the cochlear duct, degeneration of the organ of Corti, abnormal tectorial membrane, delayed spiral ganglion degeneration, and collapse of the saccules (Fig. 20-43). Deafness may be unilateral or bilateral with up to 50% of white-coated, blue-eyed cats affected. Dalmatian dogs have a 30% incidence of the albinotic form, which is inherited as an autosomal dominant gene.

The abiotrophic form is caused by abiotrophy of sensory hair cells (neuroepithelial) with subsequent atrophy of the organ of Corti, yet the cochlear duct and stria vascularis are normal. Typically a bilateral condition, hair cells of the vestibular system and cochlear system are affected. This form of deafness is a progressive condition, most often recognized at a later age. This mechanism may be the cause of deafness in cavalier King Charles spaniels, which typically is not recognized until 3 to 4 years of age. Although much is known clinically and functionally about this disease, because of the need for rapid fixation and decalcification of affected tissues, little is known about the pathogenesis or histopathology of this form.

Acquired sensorineural deafness most commonly occurs secondary to otitis media. Inflammation extends through the round or cochlear window into the membranous labyrinth. Inflammation causes damage to the sensorineural hair cells resulting in both vestibular signs and deafness. Less commonly, neoplasia involving the petrous portion of the temporal bone and associated nerves can cause deafness via compression.

Presbycusis refers to age-associated deafness that occurs as an animal ages. The pathogenesis of presbycusis may relate to arthrosis of the auditory ossicle articulations or more likely to a late form of abiotrophy of the sensory hair cells of the cochlea. Thus it represents an acquired form of deafness that may be the result of conduction or neurosensory abnormalities. Histologic studies have demonstrated profound hair cell loss and neuronal loss, most prominent in the basal coils of the cochlea. This is comparable with presbycusis in people.

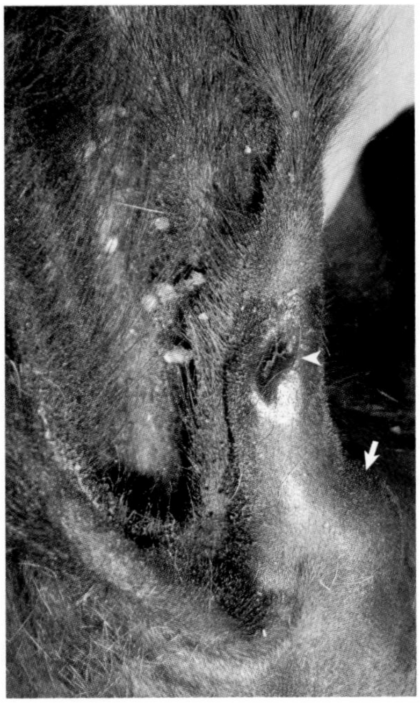

Fig. 20-44 **Dentigerous cyst, right auricle, horse.**
Within the craniomedial edge of the right auricle is a firm mass that represents a dentigerous cyst *(arrow)*. Along the craniodorsal edge of this mass is an external opening to a fistulous tract *(arrowhead)*. Scattered over the concave surface of the auricle are several pale, aural plaques (see Fig. 20-46). (Courtesy Dr. P. Fretz, The Western College of Veterinary Medicine, University of Saskatchewan.)

Acoustic noise trauma is a leading cause of deafness in people. The injury is primarily focused on the organ of Corti. Tears form in the supporting structures of the organ of Corti, causing release of hair cells into the endolymph and vascular injury resulting in bleeding into the compartments of the cochlea. Several weeks after the initial injury, the organ of Corti is completely degenerated caused initially by outer hair cell loss followed by inner hair cell loss. There is also a retrograde degeneration of the associated nerve tracts.

Ototoxicity is another means of acquired deafness. Many compounds are known to be ototoxic, including aminoglycoside antimicrobials, platinum-containing chemotherapeutic agents, furosemide, salicylates, and otic cleansers. To exert toxicity, ototoxins much reach the internal ear. This process may occur via hematogenous spread, enhanced diffusion through a tympanic membrane under the influence of otitis media, or through a perforated tympanic membrane. Once in the tympanic cavity, ototoxic compounds gain access to the internal ear by diffusing through the round window. The target of ototoxicity is the hair cells. As has already been discussed, hair cells of the vestibular and cochlear systems succumb and become injured or die from apoptosis. Deafness tends to be permanent, whereas vestibular disease is more transient.

DISORDERS OF HORSES

DEVELOPMENTAL ANOMALIES

Dentigerous Cysts (Temporal Odontomatas, Periauricular Cysts)

Dentigerous cysts (also known as temporal odontomatas, temporal teratomas, temporal cysts, ear or aural fistulas, ear teeth, and heterotopic polydontia) are rare, nonheritable, congenital cysts that occur rostral and ventral to the base of the ear pinna (Fig. 20-44). They also occur in the forehead, paranasal sinuses, and petrous portion of the temporal bone. Typically flask-shaped due to a long narrow fistula that drains to the surface, dentigerous cysts are most often unilateral arising in the temporal region as the result of malpositioned tooth stem cells from the first branchial arch that are displaced within the first branchial cleft. Microscopically, the fistula and cavity are lined by stratified squamous epithelium and teeth of varied stages of differentiation composed of dentin, cementum, and enamel. Teeth are loosely or firmly attached to underlying temporal or parietal bones of the skull. Salivary gland tissue may also be present. When dentigerous cysts do not contain teeth or dental structures, they are called *dermoid cysts.* In sheep, dentigerous cysts occur in the mandibular incisor region and are called *ovine odontogenic cysts.*

MISCELLANEOUS DISORDERS

Auricular Chondrosis

Auricular chondrosis is a condition in horses with similarities to auricular chondritis (see the section on Disorders of Dogs and Disorders of Cats) but with one main difference and that is a lack of inflammation and chondritis. A cause for this condition has not been determined. The lack of inflammation and lack of response to corticosteroids in the lone case report indicate the pathogenesis is likely distinct from auricular chondritis. Macroscopically, lesions were characterized by nodular thickenings of both pinnae that ranged from 3 to 8 mm in diameter palpable below the surface with no apparent involvement of the overlying epidermis. With the exception of mild parakeratotic hyperkeratosis, microscopic lesions were primarily confined to the auricular cartilage. Cartilage plates were markedly thickened with central areas that lacked chondrocytes and had areas of degeneration and necrosis. Other regions contained adipocytes and were invaded by small blood vessels. Along the margins of the damaged cartilage were areas of nascent cartilage formation with macrocytic chondrocytes and deeply basophilic matrix present at the interface. However, there was no evidence of infiltration of the cartilage or peripheral soft tissue by inflammatory cells. In the lone reported case, nodules were nonpainful and persistent.

Temporohyoid Osteoarthropathy

The temporohyoid joint is a permanent synchondrosis connecting the proximal stylohyoid bone to the petrous portion of the temporal bone via tympanohyoid cartilage. This articulation is in very close proximity to the middle and inner ear. A complete understanding of normal joint movement is lacking but the temporohyoid joint is believed to function by dampening movement of the hyoid apparatus during tongue movement. Temporohyoid osteoarthropathy is a bony proliferative disease of the temporohyoid articulation that may result from (1) infectious agents inciting the disease by local extension of otitis media/interna, hematogenous spread, ascending infection from the respiratory tract, or extension from guttural pouch disease or (2) premature degenerative joint disease of the temporohyoid joint.

Infectious Microorganisms

Otitis media causes ventral osteitis of the tympanic cavity and because of proximity to the temporohyoid joint, osteoarthritis of the joint ensues by extension of inflammation. Osteomyelitis and periosteal proliferation of bone results in ankylosis of the temporohyoid joint and fusion of the stylohyoid bone to the petrous portion of the temporal bone (Fig. 20-45). Additionally, the bony portion of the external acoustic meatus is also in close apposition and may become narrowed as a result of exostosis and osteoarthritis. Infectious agents may also affect this region via other routes leading to similar lesions.

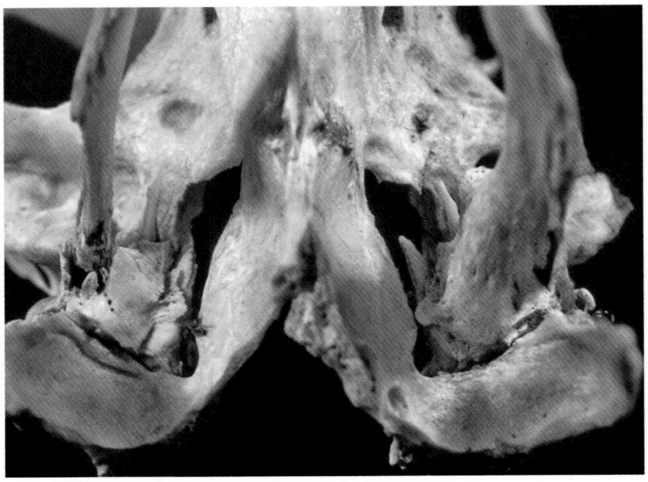

Fig. 20-45 Temporohyoid arthropathy, horse. The left stylohyoid bone from this mature thoroughbred mare is thickened and fused with the temporal bone. (Courtesy Dr. R. Peters, Cummings School of Veterinary Medicine, Tufts University.)

Premature Degenerative Joint Disease

Thickening of the proximal stylohyoid and ankylosis of the temporohyoid joint can result from degenerative joint disease. In a recent study, age-related, bony remodeling changes were documented in the temporohyoid joint, including (1) club-shaped development to the proximal stylohyoid bone; (2) rounding of the synostosis with the petrous portion of the temporal bone; and (3) extension of osteophytes from the petrous portion of the temporal bone, typically enveloping the stylohyoid head and in some cases bridging the joint. These proliferative changes were typically observed bilaterally but were never as severe as is seen in temporohyoid osteoarthropathy. Histologic changes were most pronounced in the oldest horses in the study. There was marked disorganization of the joint with marked irregularity in the depth of the joint fibrocartilage, a variation of lipping to fragmentation of the petrous portion of the temporal bone along the joint margin, markedly irregular chondro-osseous junctions, extensive fibrous replacement of periarticular bone, marked periosteal thickening, and marked clustering of chondrocytes with heterogeneity of the surrounding and intervening matrix. There were no areas of active inflammation in any of the examined sections.

Clinical disease is often categorized into two syndromes. In the first scenario, horses demonstrate abnormal behavior, such as shaking their heads, ear rubbing, and problems chewing, and resent having a bit in their mouths. The second syndrome is related to a fracture through the ankylosed joint leading to signs attributable to acute vestibular or facial nerve injury. Rarely, affected horses may develop meningitis.

Aural Plaques (Aural Papillomatosis)

Aural plaques (also known as equine ear papillomas, papillary acanthoma, hyperplastic dermatitis of the ear, or "ear fungus") occur in horses over 1 year of age and are thought to be caused by papilloma virus spread between horses by fly bites. Macroscopically, lesions are characterized as raised, well-demarcated, hypopigmented, hyperkeratotic plaques arising from the inner concave surface of the

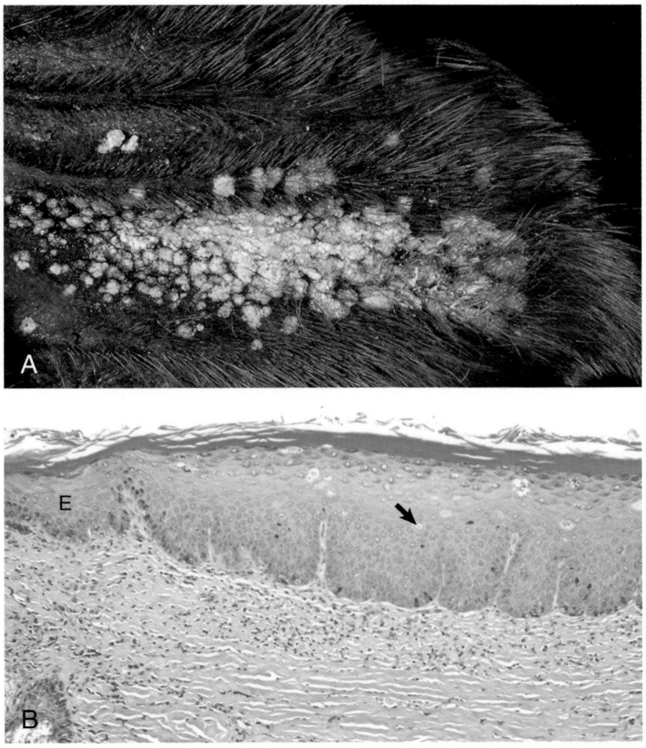

Fig. 20-46 Aural plaques, horse.
A, Concave surface of right auricle. Multiple, hypopigmented, exophytic gray-to-white masses cover the central portion of the auricle. Often, these plaques coalesce to form a large mass. **B,** Histologic section of an aural plaque. The stratified squamous epithelium is hyperplastic. When compared to the adjacent more normal and basally pigmented epithelium *(E)*, the basal epithelial cells are hypopigmented. Scattered through the sessile mass are koilocytes *(arrow)*. H&E stain. (**A** courtesy Dr. Rob Fairley, The Western College of Veterinary Medicine, University of Saskatchewan; **B** courtesy Dr. Rob Bildfell, College of Veterinary Medicine, Oregon State University.)

auricle (Fig. 20-46, *A*). Plaques are typically 1 to 3 mm in diameter but can overlap to involve larger areas. Microscopically, the epidermis is moderately hyperplastic with a stratum corneum that is variably hyperkeratotic. The granulosis layer tends to be quite prominent. Scattered through the affected epidermis are singlets or clusters of koilocytes. Basal epithelial cells tend to be more poorly pigmented when compared to peripheral, more normal epidermis (Fig. 20-46, *B*). Various molecular techniques have been used to demonstrate papillomavirus in the epidermis of the plaques. Clinically, aural plaques rarely resolve spontaneously, but they are usually of little clinical significance unless infected by bacteria secondary to trauma.

Guttural Pouch Disease

See Chapters 9 and 17.

DISORDERS OF RUMINANTS (CATTLE, SHEEP, AND GOATS)

DEVELOPMENTAL ANOMALIES

β-Mannosidosis of Cattle and Goats

β-Mannosidosis is an autosomal recessive lysosomal storage disease caused by a deficiency of glucohydrolase β-D-mannosidase leading to the accumulation of oligosaccharide substrates of β-mannosidase in lysosomes of multiple cell types located in nervous, renal, thyroid, and lymphoid tissues. This disease was first described in Nubian kids and has subsequently been reported in Salers calves. Newborn animals were unable to rise and had dome-shaped heads, intention tremors, nystagmus, and bilateral Horner's syndrome. Macroscopically, affected animals have bilaterally kinked and folded auricles that are most severe in Nubian kids but less severe in Salers calves. Additionally, Nubian kids have sensorineural deafness, Salers calves have normal auditory function. In both species, there is narrowing of the cartilaginous portions of the external acoustic meatus. Tympanic bullae are normal in the goats but smaller in the calves. Mucosa of the middle ear of the goats forms prominent polypoid projections, thus reducing the volume of the tympanic cavity.

Microscopically in both species, prominent intracytoplasmic vacuoles (lysosomes, see Chapter 14) are present in cells of the cochlear duct, including cochlear hair cells, supportive cells of the organ of Corti, cells of the stria vascularis, mesothelial cells covering the scala tympani, neurons of the spiral ganglion, cells of Reissner's membrane, endothelial cells, and fibroblasts.

PARASITIC DISEASES

Stephanofilarial Otitis

Stephanofilarial otitis, commonly referred to as *ear-sore,* occurs in cattle and buffalo and is caused by *Stephanofilaria zaheeri.* Biting flies have been implicated in the transmission of the parasite to the auricle and infestation is painful. Macroscopic lesions are most evident on the concave surface of the auricle and vary from congestion to inflammation with hemorrhage, to severe crusting (parakeratosis) if chronic, and to alopecia with depigmentation. Microscopically, microfilaria are present in the auricular epidermis and dermis along with lymphocytes, macrophages, hyperplastic or degenerate sebaceous glands, and hemorrhage. Microfilaria in the dermis are usually dead and located in areas that are infiltrated by macrophages, eosinophils, and plasma cells. It has been hypothesized that this lesion may represent a form of immune-mediated response. Chronic cases of "ear-sore" can result in dysplastic or neoplastic transformation of cells of the epidermis likely linked to excessive cellular mitoses and mutations of genes that arise in rapidly dividing somatic cells (see Chapters 1 and 6).

Rhabditis Species Otitis

A free-living, saprophytic, rhabditiform-nematode of the genus *Rhabditis* is a cause of otitis externa in cattle. Concurrent infections with the ear mite *Raillietina auris* and the yeast *Malassezia* spp. are also common. *Rhabditis* spp. occur in tropical and subtropical climate zones that occur in Africa and some regions of Brazil. *Rhabditis* spp. infect and proliferate in the external acoustic meatus. Infested cattle may be asymptomatic or may have depression, otorrhea, otitis media and interna, cranial nerve paralysis, meningitis, circling, recumbency, and death. Elevated environmental temperature and high humidity are primary risk factors that contribute to the occurrence of this disease; additional risk factors include the breed, presence of horns, irritation or injury of the auricular skin caused by certain types of insecticide dips, and age. Examples of risk factors are (1) purebred and crossbred *Bos indicus* cattle, such as Gyr, have long, pendulous auricles that provide a more favorable environment for infection; (2) in *Bos indicus* cattle breeds, horns are thought to compress the external acoustic meatus and thus increase their susceptibility to infection; (3) cattle "dip-treated" with an acaricide had greater infestations with *Rhabditis* spp. compared to cattle treated by a spray method; and (4) because older cattle

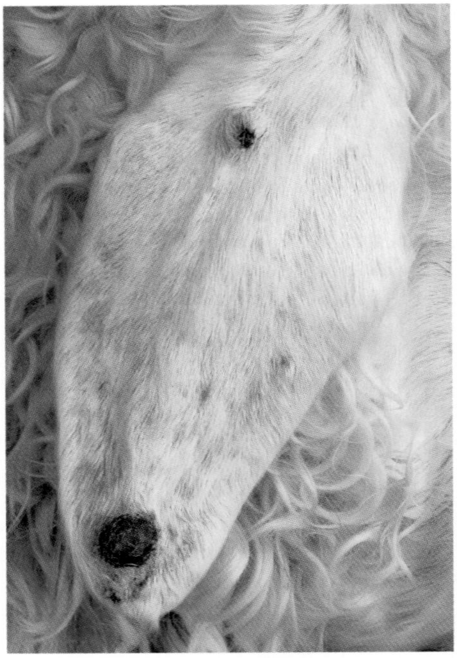

Fig. 20-47 Auricular melanomas, white Angora goat. Two large exophytic, dark black, ulcerated melanomas are growing from the convex surface of the auricle. Closer inspection reveals several smaller melanomas. These neoplasms are highly malignant and are believed to be caused by ultraviolet (UV) irradiation. (Courtesy Dr. K.G. Thompson, Institute of Veterinary, Animal & Biomedical Sciences, Massey University.)

accumulate more organic matter in their external acoustic meatuses, it is thought that this outcome provides a better environment for infestation with *Rhabditis* spp.

NEOPLASMS

Aural Melanomas of Angora Goats

UV radiation (see Chapter 6) plays a significant role in the induction of malignant melanomas on the dorsal surface of the auricle of Angora goats (Fig. 20-47); a less common site is the base of the horns and coronary band of the hooves. Macroscopically, this neoplasm is characterized by single or multiple black nodules either superficially or subcutaneously. Aural melanomas are highly aggressive and spread initially by local invasion to areas, such as the frontal sinuses, followed by rapid and widely disseminated metastases to regional lymph nodes and other organ systems, such as the liver. Microscopically, these neoplastic cells are polygonal to spindle shaped, typically heavily pigmented, and moderately pleomorphic. Mitotic figures can be numerous. Typically, neoplastic cells stain strongly for melanin A. One report determined strong expression of p53 in neoplastic cells but its significance remains undetermined (see Chapter 6).

DISORDERS OF PIGS

MISCELLANEOUS DISORDERS

Aural Chewing (Ear Chewing or Ear Cannibalism)

Aural chewing (also known as ear chewing or ear cannibalism) appears to be linked to the practice of intensified confinement rearing systems and docking of tails. High population density, heightened competition for food, low protein or inadequate nutrition, boredom, and inadequate microclimatic conditions probably increase the stress on and irritability of piglets, resulting in restlessness and aberrant behaviors. It is likely that tail docking simply redirects the focus of such behavior to the ears, as they represent two protruding and readily assessable objects. Eventually, piglets begin to suck or chew the ears of penmates until they become reddened and ulcerated. The appearance of these lesions and the taste of the serum and blood likely attract additional piglets to suck or chew the ears, thus worsening the lesions. At this stage, the affected piglets experience intense pain. Macroscopically, lesions are typically bilateral most often affecting the ventral portions of the ears and are characterized by torn and traumatized auricular edges with crusting. The remainder of the auricle is typically red and thickened. Repeated trauma may lead to localized intradermal or intrachondral abscess formation. It may also represent a nidus of infection that disseminates systemically as a septicemia such as *Streptococcus* spp. Microscopically, lesions are consistent with those tissue changes described in acute inflammation (see Chapter 3).

Ear Necrosis (Necrotic Ear Syndrome and Ulcerative Spirochetosis of the Ear)

Ear necrosis, which is also known as necrotic ear syndrome and ulcerative spirochetosis of the ear, occurs in 6- to 9-week-old piglets and is thought to be caused by a spirochetal bacterium of the genus *Treponema* that is transmitted between animals through broken skin caused by biting of ears. Macroscopically, lesions appear as ulcerated, hemorrhagic, and crusted areas along the lower margin of the auricle near the base of the ear. When severe, the entire ear margin may be affected. The dermis and subcutis beneath the crusts are typically thickened due to edema and active hyperemia and vary in color from gray-black to red. Microscopically, thick serocellular crusts often containing cocci or coccobacilli cover the ulcerated epidermis that also contains large numbers of neutrophils mixed with cellular debris (acute inflammation). Vasculitis is evident in both arterioles and venules of the deeper dermis with fibrinoid degeneration, medial hyperplasia, and thrombosis. Adjacent, nonulcerated epidermis is hyperplastic with prominent, deeply invaginating epidermal pegs (reparative response). The Warthin-Starry stain (silver impregnation methodology) has been used to identify spirochetes in the junction between necrotic and healing tissues, as well as in the deeper dermis that has vasculitis, edema, and hemorrhage.

DISORDERS OF DOGS

PARASITIC DISEASES

Auricular Parasitic Dermatitis: *Stomoxys calcitrans*

The adult stable fly, *Stomoxys calcitrans,* is responsible for a hemorrhagic, crusting dermatitis in dogs. Although infestations may also affect the face, these stable flies have a tendency to feed at the ear tips of dogs with erect ears or along ear margins of pendulous ears. Affected ears are typically red and alopecic with dark red, crusted hemorrhage over the surface. Chronically, ears may become very thickened and firm owing to a granulomatous inflammatory response. Histologically, there is an intense perivascular to interstitial dermatitis with areas of necrosis and infiltration by numerous eosinophils, plasma cells, and macrophages. The overlying epidermis is irregularly acanthotic with compact orthokeratotic or parakeratotic hyperkeratosis. Chronically affected ears tend to have more dense infiltrates of macrophages mixed with lymphocytes, mast cells, eosinophils, and plasma cells that obscure normal adnexal architecture. There may be prominent lymphoid aggregates. Discrete granulomas may be present. Dogs typically experience intense pruritus and pain.

INFLAMMATION

Otitis Externa, Media, and Interna

See the section on Disorders of Domestic Animals.

Canine Leproid Granuloma

Canine leproid granuloma is an uncommon mycobacterial disease affecting the subcutis and dermis of dogs. A causative agent has never been cultured but through molecular techniques the cause of canine leproid granuloma is a novel, slow-growing mycobacterium of the *Mycobacterium simiae*–related group. Thought to be an environmental saprophytic organism, lesions form as a result of dermal inoculation through traumatic wounds or arthropod vectors. Single to multiple, firm, painless nodules most frequently arise on the dorsal surface of the auricle at its base but may affect the auricular tip, the head, or distal forelimbs. The largest lesions, upward of 5 cm in diameter, are alopecic and frequently ulcerated.

Histologically, a multinodular to diffuse, pyogranulomatous infiltrate extends from the dermis into the subcutis (Fig. 20-48). Macrophages may be large with abundant cytoplasm and may form multinucleated giant cells. Neutrophils are intermixed with the macrophages or may aggregate into focal clusters. The occurrence and number of lymphocytes and plasma cells are highly variable, often scattered throughout, and more prominent along the deep edge of the mass. The morphology of the mycobacteria is not uniform and includes filamentous to bacilliform morphologies with or without beading, to coccoid. In contrast to rapidly growing mycobacteria of the Runyon group IV, which typically have discrete pyogranulomas centered on clear spaces that contain acid-fast positive bacteria, this morphology is absent in leproid granulomas. In addition, caseous exudation and mineralization are not features typical of leproid granulomas. This condition is a self-limiting disease that typically resolves spontaneously within 6 months of the initial diagnosis. Neither regional lymph node involvement nor systemic disease has ever been reported. Shorthaired dog breeds are predisposed to developing canine leproid granulomas with no sex predilection. Based on Australian studies, more than half of the cases were described in Boxers and Boxer crossbred dogs. In a much smaller North American study, German Shepherd dogs were overrepresented.

Cholesterol Granulomas

Cholesterol granulomas are an uncommon condition of dogs and cats that develop in the middle ear. Predisposing factors include hemorrhage into the middle ear, impairment of auditory tube drainage, and diminished or obstructed ventilation of the middle ear. These benign, expansile masses develop most often in association with concurrent otitis media or some other middle ear disease (Fig. 20-49). A prominent microscopic feature for which these masses are named are scattered and clustered acicular clefts (cholesterol clefts), derived from red cell membranes in areas of hemorrhage. Surrounding these clefts are mixtures of macrophages, plasma cells, lymphocytes, and variable numbers of neutrophils, depending on the duration and type of otitis media. In addition to fibroplasia, there may be areas of necrosis and other regions of mineralization.

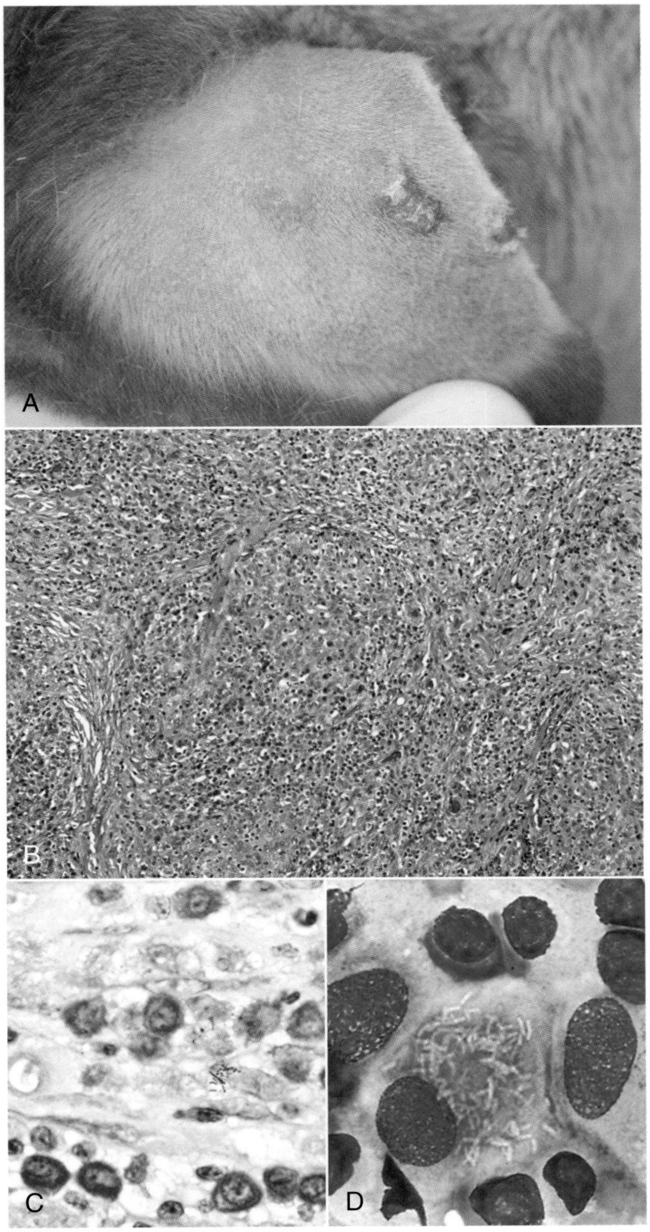

Fig. 20-48 Canine leproid (lepromatous) granulomas, auricle, dog. **A,** Several pyogranulomas are present in the subcutis of the convex surface of the external ear. Overlying skin is eroded or ulcerated; the leftmost ulcer has healed. **B,** The granulomas contain numerous large macrophages, many lymphocytes, and fewer plasma cells and neutrophils. H&E stain. **C,** Higher magnification of **B.** Short to long acid-fast bacilli *(red color),* some with a beaded morphology, are present in the granulomatous exudate. Acid-fast stain. **D,** Fine needle aspirate of a mass. In this cytologic preparation, there is a large macrophage that contains numerous bacilli consistent with a diagnosis of a canine leproid granuloma. Aqueous Romanowsky stain. (**A** courtesy Dr. D. Crow, Animal Dermatology Clinic, Dallas, TX; **B** courtesy Dr. B.L. Njaa, The Center for Veterinary Health Sciences, Oklahoma State University; **C** and **D** courtesy Dr. R.W. Allison, The Center for Veterinary Health Sciences, Oklahoma State University.)

MISCELLANEOUS DISORDERS

Aural Cholesteatoma (Aural Epidermal Cyst)

Aural cholesteatomas are masses most commonly found in the middle ear of middle-aged to aged dogs, possibly more commonly in cocker spaniels (see Fig. 20-49). Although aural cholesteatomas

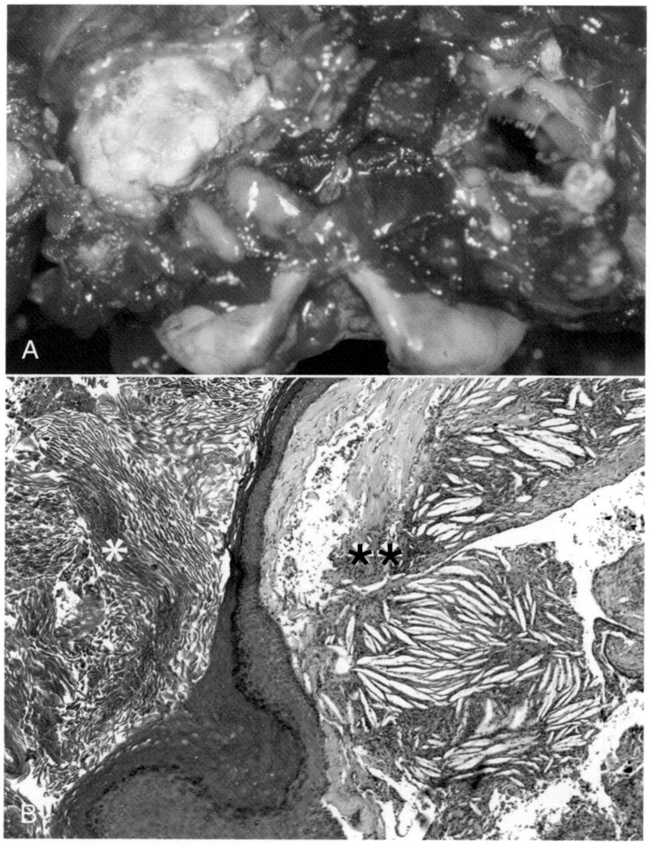

Fig. 20-49 Aural cholesteatoma with middle ear cholesterol granuloma, dog.
A, Ventral-dorsal view. The right tympanic cavity is filled with thick white cholesterol-laden material that obliterates its lumen. The left tympanic cavity is considered within normal limits. Note the fine spicules of bone with bulbous ends that represent a typical septum bulla in dogs. **B,** Histologic section of the tympanic cavity depicted in **A.** The left half of the figure shows an epithelial lined cyst filled with keratin flakes. This is a cholesteatoma *(asterisk).* The right half of the figure shows a mass composed of fibrous connective tissue mixed with numerous acicular spaces representing cholesterol clefts. This mass is a cholesterol granuloma *(two asterisks).* In this case, both a cholesteatoma and cholesterol granuloma are present in the same middle ear. H&E stain. (**A** courtesy Dr. M. Rozmanec, College of Veterinary Medicine, Cornell University; **B** courtesy Ms. J.M. Cramer and Dr. A. Alcaraz, College of Veterinary Medicine, Cornell University.)

are benign cysts, by virtue of their location, concurrent otitis, and expansile growth, they can be locally destructive and rarely lead by extension to meningitis.

Two main theories exist that account for the origin of these epithelial cysts. The first and least popular is the congenital theory in which embryonic epithelial rests are the genesis for their formation. However, the precedent of otitis media and otitis externa in all canine cases strongly supports cyst formation as an acquired change. The more likely pathogenesis is a combination of otitis media and otitis externa resulting in prolonged negative pressure within the middle ear leading to deformity of and likely perforation or invagination of a portion of the tympanic membrane into the middle ear forming a cyst lined by cornifying, stratified squamous epithelium. Because of the inherent epidermal migration of the external surface of the tympanic membrane, these cysts continue to expand as a result of continuous keratin production. In addition, chronic otitis externa can lead to external acoustic meatal stenosis or obstruction preventing the normal flow of keratin from the external tympanic membrane out the external acoustic meatus. Membrane rupture may ensue (see Fig. 20-23) and a cholesteatoma may develop.

Macroscopically, although the name implies something very different, cholesteatomas are not true neoplasms, but expansile cysts lined by keratinizing stratified squamous epithelium and filled with abundant laminated keratin. Thus more appropriate nomenclature for this entity is aural epidermal cyst or epidermal cyst of the middle and external ear. Expansion of the cyst within the middle ear can result in enlargement of the tympanic bulla, as well as bony lysis of bullae. Lysis of the petrous portion of the temporal bone may occur and is always associated with neurologic signs. Sclerosis or periosteal reactions of the ipsilateral temporomandibular joint is a common sequela.

Microscopically, aural cholesteatomas resemble epidermal cysts commonly diagnosed elsewhere in the skin. The lumen contains abundant layers of keratin flakes. A band of well-vascularized fibrous connective tissue that may contain neutrophils, lymphocytes, and macrophages forms the wall of the cyst. Outside of the wall is mature granulation tissue, most likely a reparative response to chronic, recurrent otitis media. Cholesterol granulomas may develop in concert with cholesteatomas. Depending on the duration, severity of otitis media, and size of the cholesteatoma, the tympanic bulla may be osteosclerotic or osteolytic.

Clinical signs are referable to concurrent otitis externa and otitis media and may include facial nerve palsy, head tilt, ataxia, nystagmus, and circling. Lesions are most typically unilateral. Hearing may be impaired from damage to the tympanic membrane or ossicular chain. Temporomandibular joint involvement often results in pain when opening the mouth.

Craniomandibular Osteopathy

Craniomandibular osteopathy is a proliferative, non-neoplastic lesion affecting bones of the head, in particular of the tympanic bullae (see Chapter 16 for more detail). It is an autosomal recessive disorder of terrier breeds, especially West Highland white terriers. Macroscopically, tympanic bullae are markedly enlarged and filled with new bone. Typically a bilateral lesion, affected bullae fuse with the adjacent mandible, restricting movement of the mandible. Microscopically, normal lamellar bone undergoes osteoclastic resorption and is replaced by a primitive, coarse type of bone that expands beyond the normal confines of the periosteum. Lymphocytes, plasma cells, and neutrophils invade the periphery of the affected bone. Presumably, filling of tympanic bullae with new bone impairs hearing by interfering with auditory ossicular function; however, there is a paucity of confirmatory reports.

DISORDERS OF CATS

DEVELOPMENTAL ANOMALIES

Feline Lysosomal Storage–Induced Microtia

Mucopolysaccharidosis (MPS) VI is a lysosomal storage disease reported most commonly in cats (see Chapter 14). Affected cats have mutations in their 4-sulfatase gene that leads to the accumulation of dermatan and chondroitin sulphate in lysosomes of cells. This accumulation is thought to lead to inhibition of other lysosomal enzymes and possibly the accumulation of other glycolipids. Aside from other features of facial dysmorphism, one characteristic of MPS VI is microtia or small auricles that are typically set lower on their heads (Fig. 20-50). The gross lesions

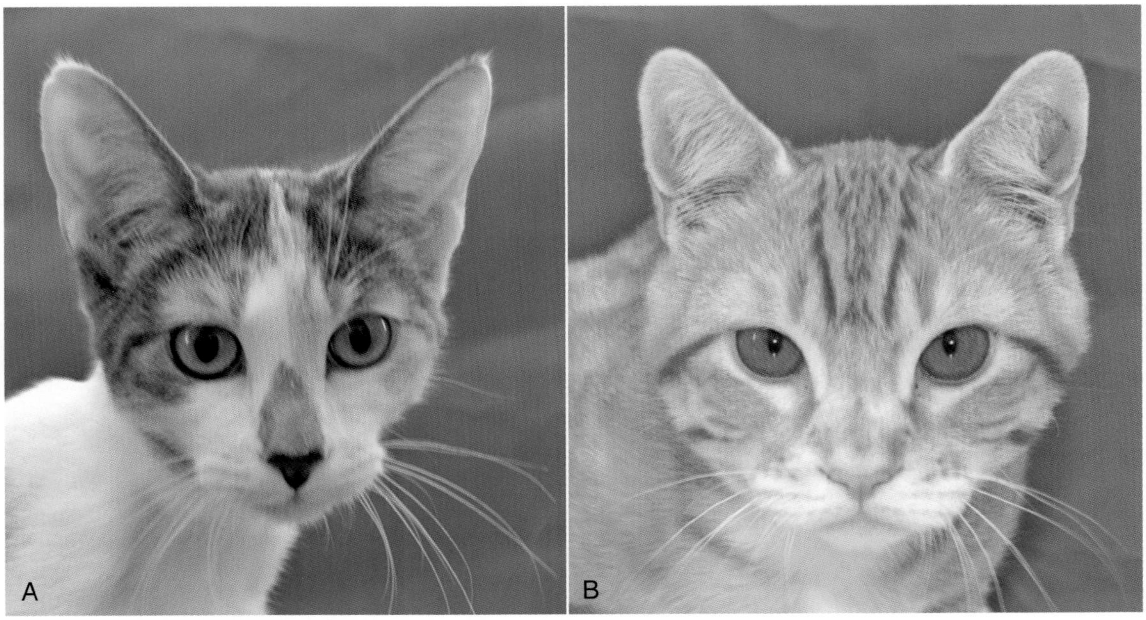

Fig. 20-50 **Mucopolysaccharidosis (MPS) VI, cat.**
A, Normal cat. **B,** Cat with MPS VI. The auricles in the cat with MPS VI are smaller than the normal cat. The bridge of the nose is also broader in the cat with MPS VI when compared with the normal cat. (Courtesy Dr. M.E. Haskins, School of Veterinary Medicine, University of Pennsylvania.)

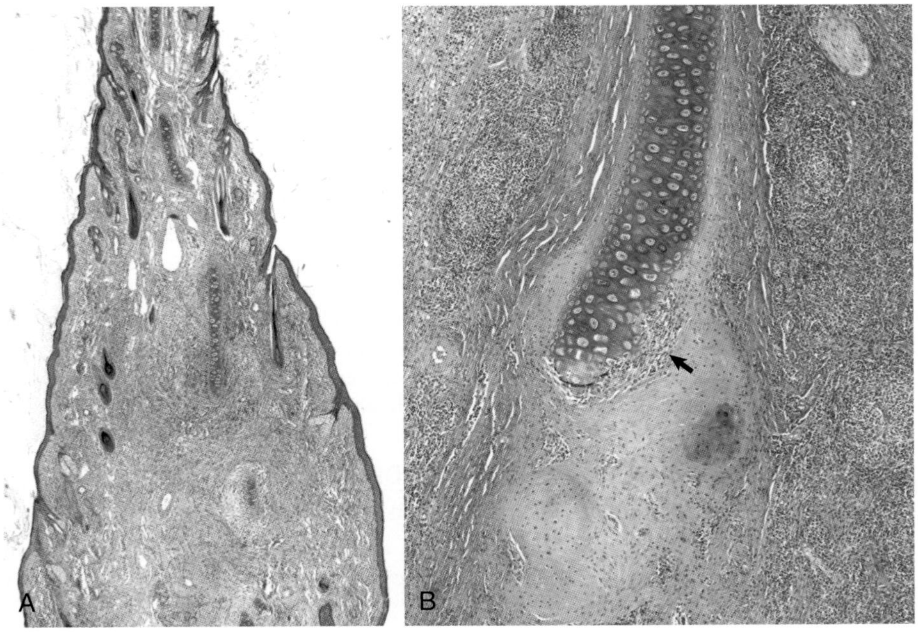

Fig. 20-51 **Auricular chondritis, cat.**
A, Histologic section of an auricle. The auricle is thickened and expanded by a chronic inflammatory exudate containing lymphocytes and fewer numbers of macrophages. The auricular cartilage is incomplete and made of individual cords surrounded by inflammatory cells and nascent cartilage. H&E stain. **B,** Higher magnification of **A.** Abundant lymphocytes have migrated into the dermis of the auricle. There is both calcified and uncalcified cartilage present adjacent to the preexisting auricular cartilage. A thick layer of neutrophils *(arrow)* are shown invading and destroying the preexisting auricular cartilage. H&E stain. (Courtesy Ms. J.M. Cramer, College of Veterinary Medicine, Cornell University.)

can be extremely subtle unless a direct comparison is made to age-matched, unaffected cats. There are no histologic features specific to the auricles. Clinical disease is referable to neurologic symptoms (see Chapter 14).

INFLAMMATION

Otitis Externa, Media, and Interna

See Disorders of Domestic Animals.

Auricular Chondritis (Relapsing Polychondritis)

Auricular chondritis (also known as relapsing polychondritis) is a rare inflammatory condition in cats (and dogs) affecting cartilage. It is thought to be caused by an immune-mediated response to type II collagen in cartilage. Macroscopically, lesions are characterized by a bilateral auricular chondritis and rarely by concurrent nonerosive polyarthritis, tracheal and laryngeal chondritis, nasal chondritis, ocular inflammation, and audiovestibular damage. Auricles are swollen, erythematous, painful, pruritic, variably alopecic, and curled. Over time, they become permanently deformed, thickened, and firm. Microscopically, auricular cartilage is distorted and wrinkled rather than being a typical straight band caused by cartilage degeneration (Fig. 20-51). Inflammation characterized by infiltration with lymphocytes, plasma cells, macrophages, multinucleated giant cells, and neutrophils is observed. Distinct lymphoid follicles are typically seen peripheral to the damaged cartilage. In the

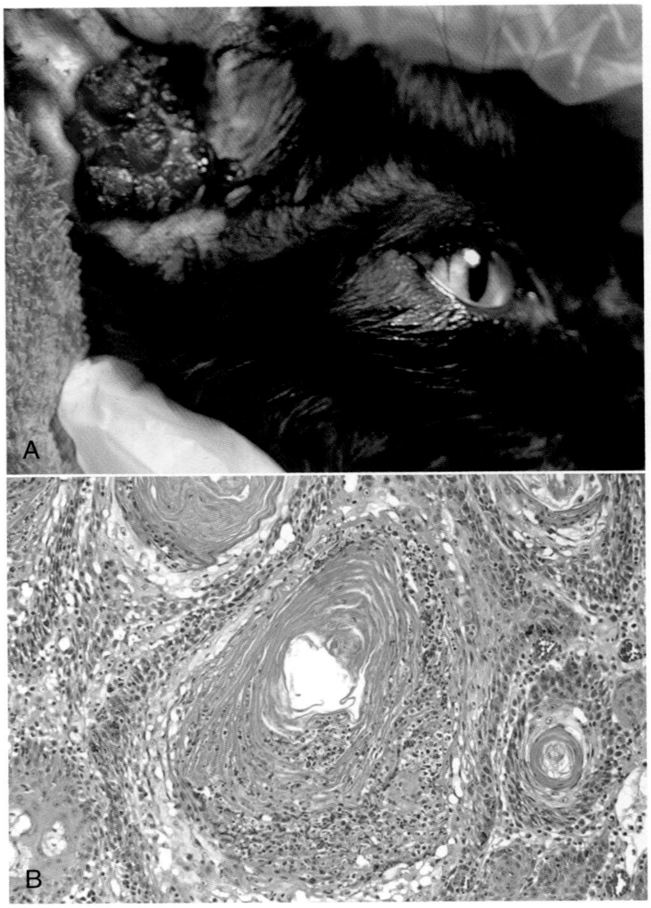

Fig. 20-52 Proliferative, necrotizing otitis externa, cat. **A,** A large, thick proliferative mass grows from the inner, concave surface of the auricle and extends into the external acoustic meatus. **B,** The epithelium of the hair follicle is markedly hyperplastic and hyperkeratotic with luminal folliculitis. Numerous necrotic keratinocytes are present within the follicular lumen mixed with necrotic inflammatory cells and cellular debris. H&E stain. (Courtesy Dr. E.A. Mauldin, School of Veterinary Medicine, University of Pennsylvania.)

severe chronic cases, cartilage is necrotic with areas of regenerative or dysplastic chondroid nodule formation, neovascularization, and extensive fibrosis throughout the auricle.

Proliferative, Necrotizing Otitis Externa

Otitis externa is an uncommon condition in cats. A rare, unique condition of unknown etiology is proliferative necrotizing otitis externa that affects cats. Large, well-demarcated erythematous plaques develop over the concave auricular surface and are covered by thick, tan-to-brown keratinous debris (Fig. 20-52, *A*). These lesions may extend into and partially occlude the external acoustic meatus. Microscopically, these plaques are sharply demarcated from the adjacent normal skin. The key diagnostic features include (1) superficial acanthosis with pronounced hair follicle outer root sheath hyperplasia, (2) marked neutrophilic luminal folliculitis, (3) mild to moderate follicular hyperkeratosis, and (4) scattered individually necrotic keratinocytes of the outer root sheath of hair follicles (Fig. 20-52, *B*). Cats may range from 2 months to 5 years of age. Lesions may cause no discomfort or mild pruritus and pain. Lesions typically resolve spontaneously.

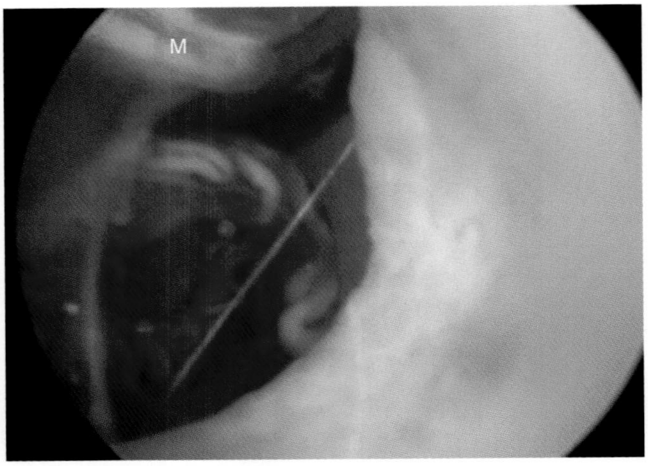

Fig. 20-53 *Mammomonogamus auris*, middle ear, cat. *Mammomonogamus auris* is shown through the intact tympanic membrane using video-otoscopy. Manubrium of the malleus *(M)*. (With permission from Tudor EG, Lee ACY, Armato DG, et al: *J Feline Med Surg* 10:501-504, 2008.)

PARASITIC DISEASES

Mammomonogamus auris

Mammomonogamus auris, a strongyloid nematode, is a rare and regionally distinct cause of otitis media in cats of the Asian pacific region. It is unknown how the adult nematode infects and spreads to and in the middle ears of affected cats. The tympanic membrane is not considered a portal of entry because it is always intact at the time of diagnosis. The need for an intermediate host has been speculated but as of yet has not been identified. However, after infection, some nematodes mature in the trachea, larynx, nasal sinuses, or middle ear and can readily pass in and out of these locations via the auditory tube, nasopharynx, and laryngopharynx. Frequently, a unilateral infection with a single worm pair is observed, although bilateral infections occur and up to eight pairs have been recovered from middle ears of affected cats (Fig. 20-53). Samples of the middle ear have never been collected for microscopic or microbiologic examination. Most cats infected with *M. auris* are asymptomatic, although head shaking can be a feature of this disease.

MISCELLANEOUS DISORDERS

Acquired Folding of the Auricle

Acquired folding of the auricle is a disease of sudden onset in adult cats. In nearly all cases, affected cats have a prolonged history of treatment with otic preparations containing glucocorticoids. Affected cats typically have biochemical evidence of iatrogenic adrenocortical insufficiency. The lesion consists of bilateral rostral and lateral folding of the distal or apical third of the auricles. They are cool and thin and appear to lack palpably normal cartilage. Histologic features have not been reported.

Feline Ceruminous Cystomatosis

The cause of feline ceruminous cystomatosis is unknown. It is characterized by benign, cystic, non-neoplastic proliferation of ceruminous glands on the medial surface of the auricle, the base of the auricle, and extending to variable depths into the external acoustic meatus. These glands are markedly dilated, clustered, and filled with brown, inspissated ceruminous secretion and are dark blue to black. As a result, they may be misdiagnosed as melanocytic or vascular neoplasms (Fig. 20-54). Microscopically, cysts are

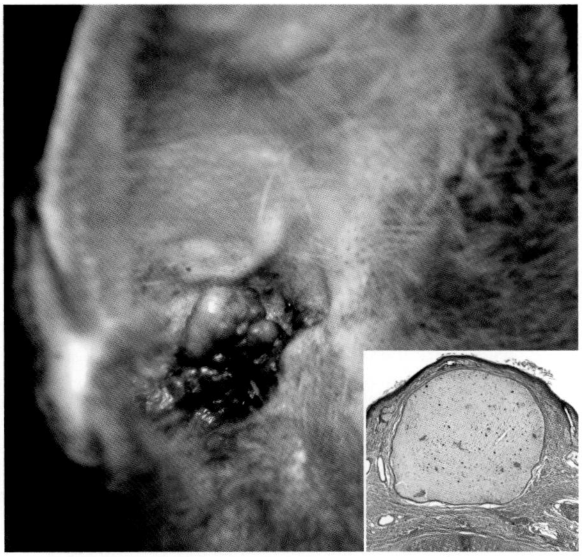

Fig. 20-54 **Feline ceruminous cystomatosis, auricle, Abyssinian cat.** **A,** Multiple, dark grey to blue to black nodules extend from the concave surface of the auricle and are characteristic of feline ceruminous cystomatosis, a cystic dilatation and hyperplasia of ceruminous glands. **B,** Flattened, squamous epithelial cells line the surface of the cyst. The lumen is filled with gray cerumen. H&E stain. (**A** courtesy B. Moyes and Dr. B. Milleson, Briarglen Veterinary Clinic, Tulsa, OK; **B** courtesy Dr. B.L. Njaa, Center for Veterinary Health Sciences, Oklahoma State University.)

massively dilated, cerumen-filled glands surrounded by minimal to moderate, mononuclear inflammation. Typically, affected cats exhibit no signs attributable to these nodules.

EYE

Because of its superficial anatomic location and the transparency of its anterior pole, the globe is the only organ that can be directly examined in great detail by the clinician. As a result, the evaluation of the gross lesions of the eye is really the realm of the clinical practitioner and especially the clinical ophthalmologist. The terminology of ophthalmic pathology is identical to the terminology of clinical ophthalmology, which unfortunately is complex and seemingly designed to intimidate anyone other than the most determined.

Examining a globe is really a miniature postmortem in itself. The embryologic development, general reactions to injury, and specific diseases are as different among the cornea, uvea, and retina as they are among the lung, liver, and kidney. Therefore it is traditional to consider the diseases of the eye as a series of relatively separate topics defined by the anatomic portion of the eye under consideration. There are certainly some diseases affecting the eye as a whole, but they are actually in the minority.

All adult mammalian globes have similar general anatomy, depicted in Fig. 20-55. The globe is a spherical biologic camera with an elaborate autofocus lens derived from surface ectoderm and a light-absorbing film plate (retina) created by an outgrowth of specialized neurons from the brain. All other structures within

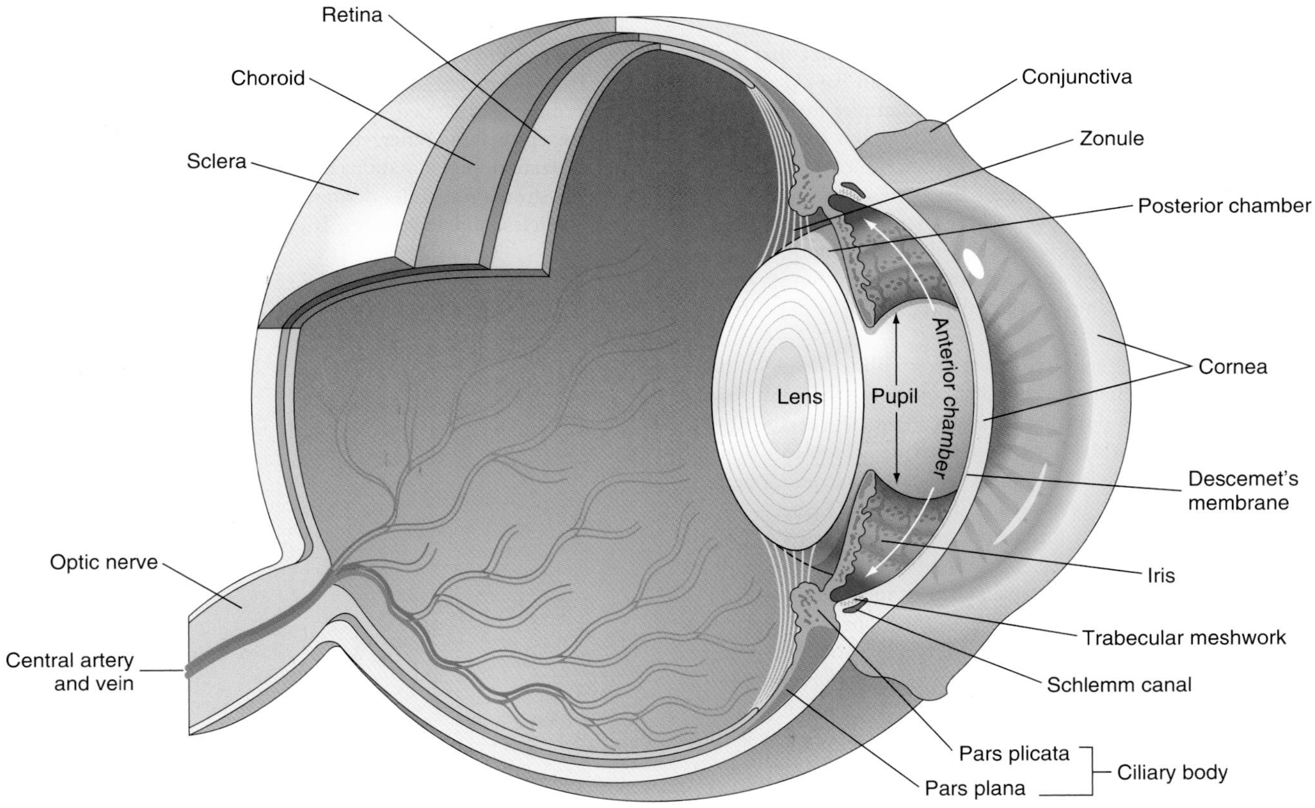

Fig. 20-55 **Schematic diagram of the anatomy of the eye.**
(Modified from Kumar V, Abbas AK, Fausto N: *Robbins & Cotran pathologic basis of disease*, ed 7, Philadelphia, 2005, Saunders; and Slatter D: *Fundamentals of veterinary ophthalmology*, ed 3, Philadelphia, 2001, Saunders.)

and surrounding the globe are simply there to ensure the optimal function of the cornea, lens, and retina.

The eye develops as a tentacle of brain tissue that reaches out to just under the skin surface of the developing embryo. The eye's purpose is to gather sensory information in the form of photons of light, which are absorbed by neurons specifically adapted to convert light into electrical energy. To facilitate access by those photons to the light-sensitive neurons of the retina, the surface ectoderm, which would normally form ordinary skin, undergoes specialized differentiation into the cornea and lens as the tentacle of the brain comes into proximity with it. Details of embryogenesis are discussed in later sections of this chapter.

The details of ocular anatomy can be found in any histology text, but there are some specific features that are particularly relevant to ocular pathology. A few of the most important features are emphasized in the following:

1. The globe is a sealed, fluid-filled sphere, which is protected from noxious influences by a bony orbit, mobile eyelids, a thick fibrous outer shell of cornea and sclera, and a series of vascular and epithelial tight junctions within the uvea and retina referred to as the *blood-eye barrier.*
2. Although the anatomy and physiology of the globe serve to protect it from many injuries affecting other parts of the body, the same unique features make it extremely susceptible to the propagation of injury once those defenses have been overcome. The fluid media within the globe allows diffusion of infectious agents and chemical mediators of inflammation throughout the globe. The same defenses that prevent entry of various types of chemical or biologic agents also prevent drainage of dangerous by-products of tissue injury and inflammation.
3. Proper visual function requires that very precise anatomic relationships be maintained among the constituent parts of the globe. Minor changes in those relationships that would be insignificant in most other tissues can have devastating results within the globe. Common examples include blindness resulting from minor accumulations of serous exudate behind the retina (serous retinal detachment), or accumulation of edema fluid within the cornea that significantly alters corneal clarity even to the point of blindness. Many of the critical tissues within the globe are unforgiving even of minor changes associated with inflammation or wound healing that in most other tissue would be regarded as insignificant.
4. Most of the visually critical tissues within the globe have negligible regenerative capacity. Some, like the adult retina, are essentially postmitotic and cannot regenerate at all. Others, such as the lens and cornea, are capable of limited regeneration, but the regeneration never recreates a perfect structural or functional replica of the original tissue. Many of the most significant intraocular lesions are related to events of wound healing (epithelial proliferation, angiogenesis, and fibrosis), which are desirable events in most tissue but cause serious functional impairments in the globe.
5. Unlike most other tissue, the eye has essentially no reserve capacity. In many tissues, we struggle to determine whether a lesion is or is not "functionally significant." There is probably no such thing as a functionally insignificant lesion within the globe. Every single focus of necrosis, inflammation, or scarring probably has a visual consequence even if the degree of impairment is not easily measured.
6. Vision requires that the cornea, lens, and fluid media within the globe remain optically clear. This means that accumulation of exudates, or changes in refractive properties related to conditions such as edema and fibrosis, are extremely damaging even though these reactions to injury may be beneficial to the survival of the globe itself. There is not much point in having a globe that has survived but has forfeited vision.
7. Ocular bystander injury occurs when injury to one component of the globe "spills over" and affects other parts of the globe. Examples include the following:
   - Inflammatory effusion from choroiditis, which can cause retinal detachment
   - Alteration in aqueous composition and flow, which can lead to cataracts
   - Organization of intraocular exudates, which can cause tractional retinal detachment or glaucoma secondary to pupillary block or peripheral anterior synechia
   - Chemical mediators of wound healing in chronic uveitis that stimulate preiridal fibrovascular membranes and corneal stromal vascularization

STRUCTURE AND FUNCTION

CORNEA

The cornea is the anterior third of the fibrous tunic that provides structural support for the retinal and uvea. It is a three-layered sandwich about 1 mm thick. It has a thick center of densely compacted collagen fibrils covered on its anterior surface by stratified squamous epithelium derived from fetal surface ectoderm. On its inner (posterior) surface, it is covered by a single layer of cuboidal epithelial cells, known as the *corneal endothelium,* which is derived from periocular mesenchyme (Fig. 20-56). The corneal epithelium is 6 to 10 cells thick and has a turnover time of 5 to 7 days. The adult corneal endothelium of most domestic mammals does not replicate.

The cornea is an adaptation of skin. These adaptations to the epidermis are designed specifically to render it transparent. The surface epithelium differs from that of skin in that there is no keratinization, pigmentation, hair follicles, or adnexal glands. The corneal stroma resembles dermis, except that it lacks blood vessels, hair follicles, and leukocytes. It has relatively few fibroblast-like

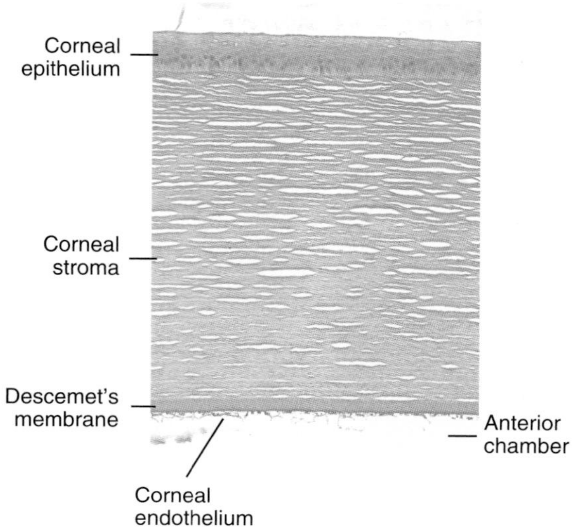

Fig. 20-56 Normal cornea, dog.
H&E stain. (Courtesy Dr. B. Wilcock, Ontario Veterinary College.)

cells (keratocytes) and a highly regimented organization of its collagen fibrils. These fibrils are arranged in compact lamellae with a space between them that matches the wavelength of visible light. Thus the cornea allows the passage of light without any scattering. To further facilitate the unimpaired passage of light, the corneal stroma is maintained in a dehydrated state compared with that of most other tissue. That dehydrated state is maintained passively by intercellular junctions within the corneal epithelium and endothelium, which exclude water from the tear film and anterior chamber, respectively. It is further maintained by the active removal of electrolytes (and thus water) by energy-dependent membrane pumps within the corneal endothelium and to a much lesser degree the overlying epithelium. The avascular cornea is permitted to exist in this highly privileged anatomic and physiologic state only as long as its "support system" is working properly. It must be protected from desiccation and irritation by properly functioning eyelids and lacrimal secretion, nourished by a tear film that is biochemically normal and delivered in adequate amounts, and replenished by germinal cells resident in the adjacent conjunctiva and sclera. The failure of any of these support systems results in corneal decompensation, seen clinically either as necrosis or as reversion of the cornea to a skinlike state, which although much more durable is unfortunately also opaque.

UVEA

The uvea is the nourishing vascular tunic of the globe. It is made up of the iris, ciliary body, and choroid. It includes the pigmented stroma and muscles of the iris and ciliary body and the light-reflecting mirror known as the *tapetum,* which is buried within the dorsal choroid of all domestic species except the pig. It borders the fluid-filled cavities of the globe: the anterior chamber, posterior chamber, and vitreous. The uvea is surrounded exteriorly by the sclera.

The uvea is formed in part by neuroectoderm from the primary optic vesicle, and in part by periocular mesenchyme. Its primary function is to provide nutrients to the avascular lens and to the outer half of the retina. In its general structure, it is similar to the lamina propria of the various tubular organs such as the intestine or reproductive tract. It is rich in fibrous tissue, nerves, blood vessels, and melanocytes. In contrast to the lamina propria of other tissue, however, it contains virtually no resident lymphocytes or plasma cells. Although the vasculature of the uvea is in free communication with systemic vasculature, access by infectious agents or tumor cells from the blood into the globe via the uvea is normally prevented by a series of strategically located tight junctions, which are collectively referred to as the blood-eye barrier (see later discussion in the section on Defense Mechanisms).

LENS

The lens is a biconvex, avascular, transparent accumulation of elongated epithelial cells, suspended within the pupillary aperture. Its shape and elasticity vary greatly by species and with age. It is surrounded by the lens capsule, which is a thick basement membrane (predominantly type IV collagen) produced throughout life by the lens epithelium. Germinal epithelium forms a single layer of cuboidal epithelial cells just below the capsule along the anterior surface of the lens. The epithelium is absent from the posterior surface of the lens. Near the equator of the lens, these epithelial cells migrate inwardly and elongate to become lens fibers. As they elongate, the cells also lose most of their cytoplasmic organelles and eventually lose their nuclei. They develop complex "ball and socket" interdigitations of their plasma membranes and many gap junctions that allow each lens fiber to adhere tightly to all of its adjacent fibers.

New lens fibers are recruited from the germinal cells of the lens epithelium throughout life, so the lens continues to grow. Its net growth is partially counterbalanced by a progressive increase in the density of the center of the lens (the lens nucleus), which is formed by the oldest lens fibers. Gradually the increasing number of aged fibers within the progressively expanding lens nucleus makes the lens less transparent (so-called nuclear sclerosis) and less flexible, so that at least in some species, there is a loss of focusing ability (accommodation) with age.

The purpose of the lens is to further refract light that has passed through the cornea and to focus that light onto the retina. To accomplish this, the lens obviously must remain transparent and in its proper location within the pupillary aperture. Its transparency depends on its highly regimented structure, the paucity of cytoplasmic organelles, the very precise molecular character of its intracellular crystalline proteins, and on its maintenance of a critical state of dehydration. This dehydration is maintained primarily by excretion of electrolytes through an active sodium-potassium–dependent adenosinetriphosphatase pump, located mostly in the anterior lens epithelium.

The location of the lens within the pupillary aperture (with the iris resting on its anterior surface and its posterior surface embedded in a depression in the anterior surface of the vitreous) is maintained by a ring of transparent elastin-like fibers (the lens zonules or zonular fibers) stretching from the lens capsule to the nonpigmented ciliary epithelium. The exact arrangement of these fibers varies greatly by species. Contraction and relaxation of the ciliary muscles alters tension on these fibers and allows the lens to change shape or position, and thus to focus.

The health of the lens almost totally depends on the aqueous humor delivering nutrients and removing its waste products. Lens metabolism is primarily via anaerobic glycolysis. Glucose is delivered via the aqueous humor and is absorbed across the lens capsule, which is impermeable to most other substances. This metabolic peculiarity of the lens is vital in understanding the development of diabetic cataracts (see later discussion).

RETINA AND VITREOUS

The retina is the raison d'être for the entire globe. The cornea, lens, uveal tract, and sclera are simply a "supporting cast" to allow the retina to do its job of converting photons of visible light into electrical impulses, which are transmitted to the visual cortex of the brain. It is the most fascinating of the ocular tissues, yet at the same time the one that we can influence the least. It is one of the sad realities of ocular disease that we are often powerless spectators, able to view the evidence of active or previous retinal disease, yet with virtually no ability to influence it. Most frequently, at the time of clinical examination, the eye is already blind from retinal detachment, inherited photoreceptor disease, or the devastating effects of glaucoma.

The retina is literally an outpouching of brain tissue. It is formed from the neuroectoderm of the anterior half of the primitive optic vesicle. As the optic vesicle invaginates to form the optic cup, the presumptive retinal neuroectoderm is pushed into apposition with the neuroectoderm from the posterior half of the optic vesicle, which will form the retinal pigment epithelium (RPE). The proper development of the retina requires that proximity to the retinal pigment epithelium. This dependence of retina on the retinal pigment epithelium continues throughout life. It is impossible to review all significant features of the very complex retinal structure and function here, but those features that are most important in understanding the retinal diseases are as follows:

1. Macroscopically the retina resembles a slightly opaque vascularized membrane, resembling tissue paper, held against the RPE, choroid, and sclera by the gel-like vitreous. It is not actually attached to that RPE and/or choroid except at the optic disc and at its very periphery, where it becomes continuous with the epithelium of the pars plana of the ciliary body (the site of transition is known as the ora ciliaris retinae).
2. The retina consists of three layers of neurons (ganglion cells, inner nuclear layer, and outer nuclear layer) separated by cell-free layers created by the intermingling of the axons and dendrites of those neurons. The innermost layer, adjacent to the vitreous, is the nerve fiber layer. It is made up of the ganglion cell axons that, as they exit the globe, become the optic nerve. The RPE is usually listed as the outermost layer of the retina, but it is derived from the posterior half of the optic vesicle and is not directly involved in vision. Anatomically and functionally, the RPE is more appropriately considered a part of the choroid. The combination of retina, RPE, choroid, and tapetum that is responsible for the ophthalmoscopic appearance of the posterior pole of the globe is known as the *ocular fundus* (Fig. 20-57).
3. The outer nuclear layer is formed by the cell bodies of the photoreceptors, which are specialized cilia containing photoactivated pigments that are responsible for converting light into electrical impulses. These photoreceptors are embedded into crevices within the surface of the adjacent RPE, but there are no actual cellular junctions. This intimate contact is essential to allow the RPE to deliver nutrients to and remove waste products from the metabolically demanding photoreceptors. The potential space between the photoreceptors and the RPE is the remnant of the lumen of the primary optic vesicle. It is in this space that hemorrhage, edema fluid, and inflammatory exudate accumulate, resulting in exudative retinal detachment.
4. The inner (vitreal) half of the retina in most species is supplied by blood vessels entering the globe through the optic nerve. In contrast, the outer nuclear layer, photoreceptors, and RPE are totally dependent on diffusion of nutrients from the adjacent choroid. Separation of the retina from the RPE results in rapid ischemic degeneration of photoreceptors, and eventually of the outer nuclear layer. In the horse, in which retinal blood vessels are almost absent, the assumption is that the retina relies almost completely on choroidal diffusion to obtain nutrients, and the consequences of retinal detachment should therefore be even more devastating.
5. The optic nerve is the continuation of the nerve fiber layer of ganglion cell axons into the brain and uses the preexistent tube formed by the embryonic optic stalk. Ganglion cell axons exit the globe through a series of perforations, known as the *lamina cribrosa,* in the sclera at the posterior pole of the globe. In most species, axons become myelinated at about the level of the lamina cribrosa, as they leave the globe. The combination of axons, myelin, and supporting glia on the vitreal side of that lamina cribrosa forms the optic disc. The amount of myelin and how far the myelinated fibers extend into the retina are responsible for the ophthalmoscopic appearance of the optic disc, which varies among species (Fig. 20-58). In dogs, the myelin extends several millimeters internal (anterior) to the lamina cribrosa and this extension is responsible for the prominence of the optic disc in that species. Because the optic nerve is a tract of the brain rather than a true peripheral nerve, the myelin is laid down by oligodendrocytes instead of Schwann cells (see Chapter 14).
6. Vision requires that the light gathered and refracted by the cornea is focused by the lens onto the photoreceptors. Light passes through the minimally absorptive inner two-thirds of the retina so that most of it can be absorbed by the pigments within the photoreceptors. The electrical signal generated by activation of the photopigment is transmitted in a stepwise fashion from the outer nuclear layer to the neurons of the inner nuclear layer, then to the ganglion cells, and finally via the nerve fiber layer to the optic nerve and brain. The number of photoreceptors "feeding" to a single ganglion cell varies greatly among species and is one of the variables determining visual acuity and the efficacy of dim-light vision. In all domestic animals except the pig, photons not absorbed on the initial pass through the photoreceptors are then reflected back by the cytoplasmic crystals embedded within the tapetum to stimulate the photoreceptors a second time. The tapetum is therefore assumed to be a choroidal adaptation to increase the efficiency of vision in dim light.

The vitreous is an optically clear, gelatinous mass that fills the interior of the globe from the back of the lens to the retina. It is about 99% water, with collagen and hyaluronic acid making up most of the remaining 1%. Little is known about the production and turnover of the vitreous humor. It is thought to be made mostly by secretion from nonneuronal cells of the retina and the nonpigmented epithelium of the ciliary body. The vitreous contains only a scattering of histiocyte-like cells, known as *hyalocytes,* and a few fibroblasts. Along the anterior surface of the vitreous is a shallow depression known as the *hyaloid fossa,* in which lies the posterior surface of the lens. The anterior surface of the vitreous undergoes condensation to form the anterior hyaloid membrane, which separates the vitreous from the aqueous humor. The vitreous seems to function mainly to maintain the shape of the globe and to help support the retina in its normal position against the RPE and choroid.

EYELIDS, CONJUNCTIVA, AND ORBIT

The central theme in ophthalmology is the degree to which proper ocular function rests on the ability of the critical visual tissues, such as the retina and lens, to function thanks to a carefully controlled, protected environment. Thus the eye depends entirely on a long list of factors in a "supporting cast" to protect the sensitive visual tissues against the external environment. The first line of defense is the eyelids, conjunctiva, and bones of the orbit that create a wall around the globe. This protective wall is designed to let in light and nutrients but to exclude the many elements of the external environment that might injure this very sensitive organ.

From the perspective of a pathologist, the diseases of the eyelids, conjunctiva, and orbit are much less intriguing than those of the globe itself. From a clinical perspective, however, the diseases of the eyelid and conjunctiva form a major part of what the primary care veterinarian is likely to diagnose and treat.

Eyelids

The epithelium of the eyelids develops from the surface ectoderm adjacent to the cornea. After separation of the lens vesicle, the surface ectoderm regains continuity to form the cornea. Ectoderm at the periphery of the cornea then migrates over the surface of the embryonic cornea, accompanied by some underlying periocular mesenchyme to form the eyelids. The ectoderm forms the surface epithelium and glands; the accompanying periocular mesenchyme forms the deeper dermis and the eyelid muscles. These ingrowing

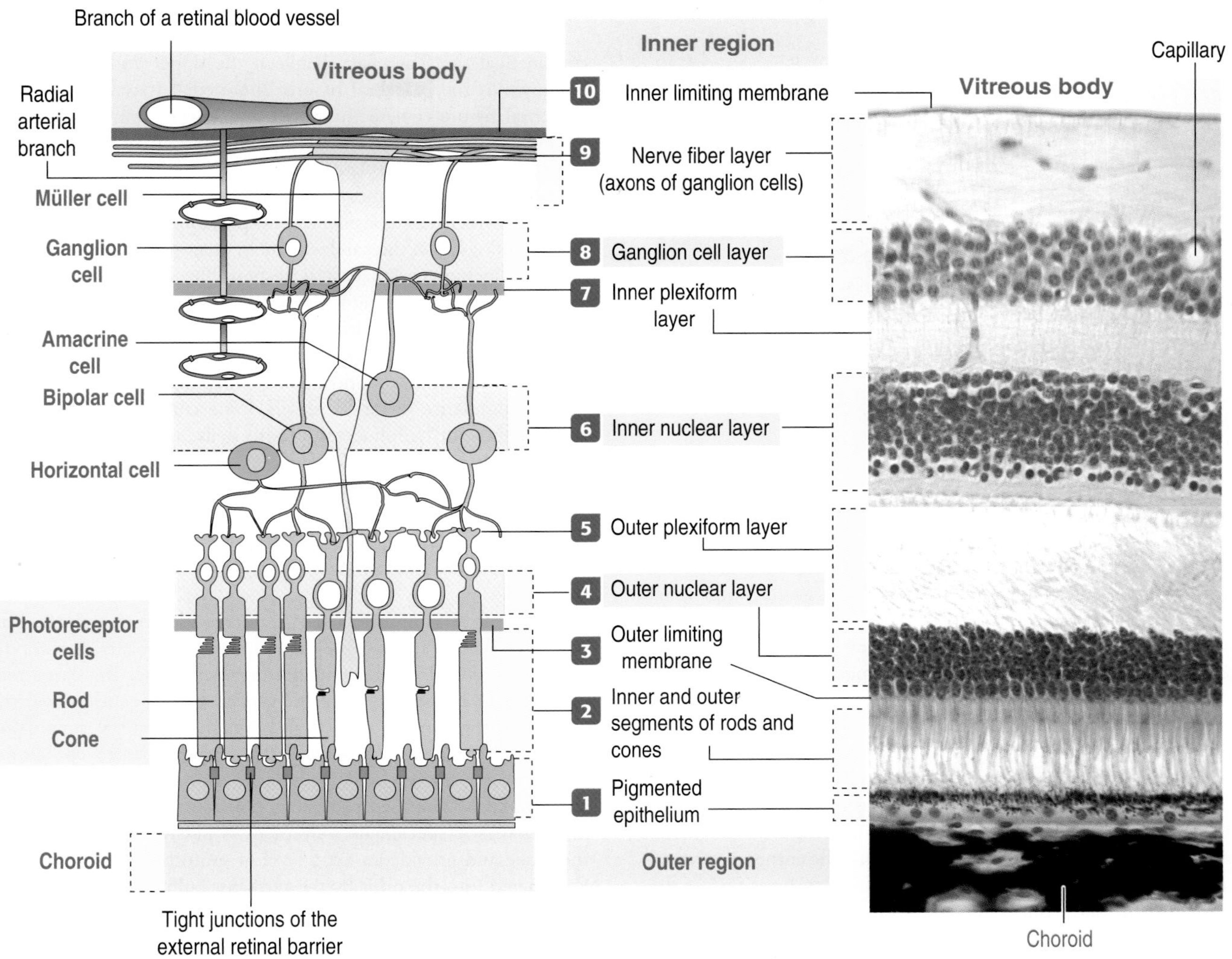

Light passes through several layers of the retina before activating the rod and cone photoreceptor cells. The layers of the retina observed in the photomicrograph are represented in the adjacent diagram. The synapses between the cells of each layer of the retina are also illustrated.

Radial branches from blood vessels (arteries and veins)—located on the retinal surface—are interconnected by capillary beds present in the inner layers of the retina. Retinal capillary beds are lined by endothelial cells linked by tight junctions creating an internal blood-retinal barrier. An external retinal barrier is formed by tight junctions linking the cells of the pigmented epithelium.

Note that the neclei of rods and cones are present in the outer nuclear layer.

The axons of the cones and rods project into the outer plexiform layer and synapse with dendrites of the bipolar cells.

Nuclei of the bipolar cells contribute to the inner nuclear layer.

Axons of the bipolar cells synapse with dendrites of the ganglion cells in the inner plexiform layer.

Axons of the ganglion cells become part of the optic nerve.

Müller cells span most of the retina. The inner limiting membrane represents their basal lamina. Their nuclei form part of the inner nuclear layer.

The outer limiting membrane corresponds to junctional complexes (zonula adherens) between rods, cones, and Müller cells.

Horizontal cells synapse with several rods and cones.

Amacrine cells synapse with axons of bipolar cells and dendrites of ganglion cells.

Fig. 20-57 Normal mammalian retina.

(From Kierszenbaum AL: *Histology and cell biology: an introduction to pathology*, St Louis, 2002, Mosby.)

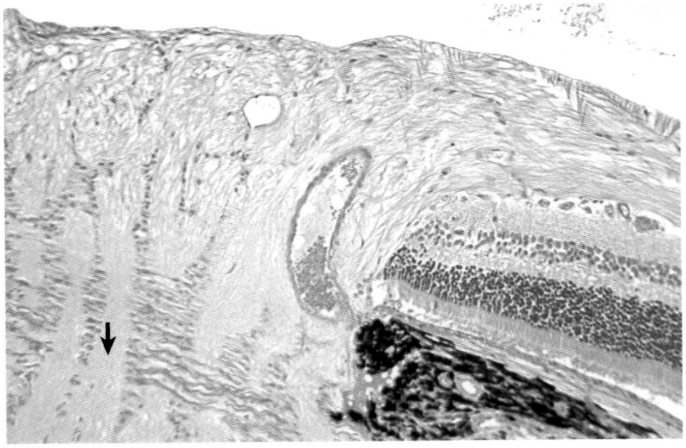

Fig. 20-58 Normal optic disc, dog.
The dense fibrous tunic of the sclera becomes fenestrated to permit the exit of the nerve, creating the lamina cribrosa *(arrow)*. H&E stain. (Courtesy Dr. B. Wilcock, Ontario Veterinary College.)

lid buds fuse with each other over the central cornea. How long this fusion persists varies with the species. In dogs and cats, it persists until about 2 weeks after birth and provides the immature cornea with a secure, sterile environment in which to complete its embryologic development.

The mature eyelids are movable folds of skin that slide across the surface of the cornea on a film of mucus and fluid known as the tear film. This blinking movement serves to help distribute the protective tear film across the corneal surface and to remove unwanted particulate debris from the corneal surface. Each eyelid has an anterior surface of haired skin, with all of the adnexal glands as seen in skin anywhere else. The dermis is modified by the addition of striated muscle (orbicularis oculi and levator muscles). The inner surface of the eyelid, which rests against the cornea, is covered by a mucous membrane known as the *palpebral conjunctiva* (see the next section on the Conjunctiva). The site of transformation from eyelid skin to palpebral conjunctiva at the eyelid margin is characterized by the presence of a row of very large modified sebaceous glands known as *Meibomian glands* and by the emergence of several rows of large modified hairs that are the eyelid cilia (eyelashes). The Meibomian glands contribute a lipid component to the tear film, which aids in the dispersal of the aqueous component of the tear film and helps prevent evaporation. The cilia are largest and most numerous along the margin of the upper eyelid; they may be infrequent or absent along the lower eyelid.

Conjunctiva

The conjunctiva is a mucous membrane extending from the palpebral margin of the eyelid to the periphery of the cornea. The portion of conjunctiva that covers the posterior surface of the eyelid is the palpebral conjunctiva, and the portion attached to the surface of the globe and continuous with the peripheral cornea at the limbus is the bulbar conjunctiva.

The palpebral conjunctiva consists of stratified squamous nonkeratinized epithelium near its origin at the eyelid margin but quickly becomes stratified columnar epithelium with numerous goblet cells. At the base of the eyelid, it is reflected back onto the surface of the sclera. Now named the bulbar conjunctiva, it extends over the eyeball as far as the periphery of the cornea. The epithelium of the bulbar conjunctiva lacks goblet cells. It becomes continuous with the corneal epithelium at the limbus. At the junction between bulbar conjunctiva and corneal epithelium, there is a population of germinal cells that are the permanent replicative cells of the corneal epithelium. They are the source of replacement corneal epithelial cells in cases of persistent corneal ulceration.

The space between the palpebral and bulbar conjunctiva is the conjunctival sac. The space between the upper and lower eyelid is known as the palpebral fissure. The medial (nasal) limit of the palpebral fissure (where the upper and lower eyelids join) is the medial canthus. The lateral (temporal) margin of the palpebral fissure is known as the lateral canthus. It is the palpebral fissure that determines what most people would regard as the "shape of the eye," which has considerable importance in the breeding of purebred dogs. It is the careless genetic manipulation of the shape of the palpebral fissure that is responsible for the frequency of some of the most common eyelid diseases (see later discussion of entropion and ectropion in the section on Diseases of the Eyelid).

The lamina propria of both the palpebral and bulbar conjunctiva resembles the lamina propria of any other mucous membrane. It has an abundance of blood vessels, loose connective tissue, variable numbers of lymphocytes, plasma cells, and diffuse lymphoid tissue and lymphoid nodules (mucosa-associated lymphoid tissue [MALT]). The MALT responds immunologically to the microbial flora within the conjunctival sac. In patients with chronic conjunctivitis, the lymphoid nodules are often grossly visible, indicating the intensity and duration of the response of the MALT to antigenic stimuli.

The ventral conjunctiva, as it transforms from palpebral to bulbar conjunctiva, undergoes an additional specialization in the form of the third eyelid or nictitating membrane. This large fold of conjunctiva protrudes from the ventral-medial canthus over the anterior surface of the cornea and contains a central supporting plate of cartilage and a stroma of dense fibrous tissue, containing an accessory lacrimal gland. Both its anterior and posterior surfaces are covered by stratified squamous nonkeratinized epithelium. In most domestic species, its movement is passive, serving to cover the globe and provide an extra level of protection when the globe is retracted into the orbit by the retractor bulbi muscle.

Orbit

The orbit is the bony fossa that surrounds most of the globe, except the cornea, and separates the globe from the brain. Along its posterior border are numerous foramina through which blood vessels and nerves reach or leave the globe. The orbit is formed by the fusion of five to seven bones, depending on the species. It is a complete bony shell, except in dogs, cats, and pigs, in which the dorsal roof of the orbit is formed only by the supraorbital ligament that extends from the frontal bone to the zygomatic bone, leaving the dorsal orbit incomplete. The orbit contains the globe itself but also the extraocular muscles, abundant fat, lacrimal gland, zygomatic salivary gland, and all the muscles and nerves that support these structures.

The lacrimal gland is a specialized serous salivary gland located in the orbit, dorsolateral to the eyeball. Along with the histologically similar gland of the third eyelid, it is responsible for the production of the serous component of tears. It empties through 15 to 20 small excretory ducts at the lateral part of the fornix of the superior conjunctival sac.

It is unclear how much interdependence there is between the ocular and orbital embryologic development. On one hand, animals with severe microphthalmia often have a relatively normal orbit, but usually there is some reduction in size and distortion of shape. It may be that the critical issue is the stage of embryogenesis at which the developing globe is injured and subsequently atrophies (remember that most microphthalmia in domestic animals

BOX 20-5 Portals of Entry for Corneal Injury

DESTRUCTION OF CORNEAL EPITHELIUM
Desiccation
Trauma
Chemical injury

PENETRATION OF THE CORNEAL STROMA

DIFFUSION INTO STROMA FROM LIMBAL BLOOD VESSELS

INJURY TO CORNEAL ENDOTHELIUM
Glaucoma
Lens luxation
Leukocyte-mediated injury

BOX 20-6 Portals of Entry for Uveal Injury

HEMATOGENOUS
Toxins
Infectious agents
Neoplastic emboli

PENETRATING INJURY INTO ONE OR MORE OF THE OCULAR CHAMBERS VIA AQUEOUS OR VITREOUS
Diffusion of chemical mediators of inflammation

is "secondary" and is the result of in utero atrophy rather than true hypoplasia).

PORTALS OF ENTRY

CORNEA

Portals of entry into the cornea are listed in Box 20-5. Injury to the cornea may arise from altered homeostasis of the corneal surface, by penetrating injury through the surface epithelium, secondary to injury to corneal endothelium, or rarely by migration into the cornea from the blood vessels at the limbus. Regardless of the route of entry, virtually all significant corneal diseases reflect stromal injury, whether this stromal injury was the primary lesion or simply a consequence of injury to the surface epithelium or to the endothelium of the cornea.

UVEA

Portals of entry into the uvea are listed in Box 20-6. Microbes and other injurious agents enter the uvea via the bloodstream (hematogenous), penetrating injury, or aqueous or vitreous. Hematogenous entry is used by toxins, infectious agents, and metastatic neoplasia. Injury to the blood vessels themselves (thrombosis, occlusion by neoplastic emboli) may cause ischemic damage. Penetrating injury provides infectious agents entry into one or more of the ocular chambers, causing uveal injury either by production of toxins or (more often) by stimulating a uveal inflammatory response. Injury that causes lens rupture can initiate a phacoclastic uveitis (see later discussion). Chemical mediators of inflammation released from an injured cornea, lens, or retina diffuse into and throughout the aqueous or vitreous, thus providing the opportunity for additional injury in contiguous tissues.

BOX 20-7 Portals of Entry into the Lens

RADIATION
Light
Therapy (x-rays, cancer treatment)
Incidental or accidental exposure

PERFORATION
Through the cornea
Through the sclera
By lens-adapted organisms

BLUNT TRAUMA
Rupture of lens capsule
Dislocation of lens

VIA AQUEOUS HUMOR
Altered chemical composition
Altered volume and/or flow
Toxins
- Inflammatory mediators
- Chemicals
- Biotoxins

LENS

Portals of entry into the lens are listed in Box 20-7. Although the lens is occasionally injured by a direct perforating injury (see later discussion on phacoclastic uveitis in the section on Lens-Induced Uveitis) or becomes displaced by blunt trauma (lens luxation), the vast majority of injuries to the lens are related to defective lens nutrition. This involves either inadequate delivery of nutrients because of defective flow of aqueous humor or chemically abnormal aqueous humor. The aqueous humor may contain by-products of intraocular necrosis or inflammation, or excessive/deficient levels of specific chemicals. Common examples include cataracts caused by excessive glucose levels in animals with diabetes mellitus and cataracts associated with systemic hypocalcemia. Degenerative changes in the lens are also seen in dogs with inherited photoreceptor disorders (so-called progressive retinal atrophy), probably caused by diffusion of toxic by-products of photoreceptor degeneration. Inherited cataracts in dogs are the single most frequent type of cataract seen in veterinary practice, but virtually nothing is known about the specific biochemical pathogenesis.

Among the more exotic causes of lens injury are injury from therapeutic radiation; electrical shock, including lightning strike; and penetrating intralenticular metallic foreign bodies. Dietary imbalances, excessive sunlight exposure, and parasitic migration are common causes of cataracts in some nonmammalian species (especially fish) but have rarely been reported in domestic mammals. Cataracts have been reported in puppies and wolf cubs fed a commercial milk replacer, and in kittens fed feline milk replacer. Cataract development was attributed to a dietary deficiency of arginine, although the precise nature of the dietary deficiency was not identified in every instance.

Because the lens is avascular and surrounded by a dense collagenous capsule, it is relatively impervious to the entry of infectious agents from elsewhere in the globe. The one rare exception in domestic mammals is the seemingly specific targeting of the lens capsule by systemic aspergillosis and presumably by other species of hyphal fungi occurring as a sequela to mycotic abomasitis in calves or opportunistic mycoses in dogs immunosuppressed by cancer chemotherapy. These fungi exhibit a tropism for basement membranes throughout the body, including the lens capsule. In rabbits, the lens capsule is frequently penetrated by the protozoon *Encephalitozoon cuniculi,* which causes spontaneous lens rupture. In fish, cataracts induced by the selective intralenticular penetration by fluke larvae are exceedingly prevalent. Several viral diseases, notably bovine viral diarrhea, are occasionally associated with congenital cataracts as a consequence of generalized systemic infection in utero before the establishment of the blood-eye barrier.

RETINA AND VITREOUS

It has been said that anything in notable excess or deficiency is harmful. This statement is particularly applicable to the retina, which, despite its sheltered intraocular niche, probably is injured by a wider range of noxious stimuli arriving by a wider variety of routes than any other tissue in the body.

Portals of entry into the retina are listed in Box 20-8. The retina can be injured by light and other types of radiation arriving through the cornea and lens, by hematogenous dissemination of chemical or infectious agents, by objects penetrating through the cornea or through the sclera, and by microorganisms arriving via the optic nerve. Because the retina is part of the brain, it is susceptible to most of the infectious, degenerative, and metabolic diseases of the brain, including the storage diseases. Exactly how frequently the retina is involved in diseases affecting primarily the brain is unknown, but the risk appears to be quite low.

The retina is sensitive to injury from chemical mediators of inflammation and toxic products of infectious agents within the vitreous and is particularly sensitive to increased intraocular pressure. Especially in purebred dogs, there is also a huge list of inherited defects in photoreceptor metabolism, which result in progressive destruction of photoreceptors and their nuclei.

The most important and most frequent causes of injury are those related to retinal detachment (see later discussion), increased intraocular pressure, vascular hypertension, and genetically determined photoreceptor diseases. It is important to view this list in perspective. Despite the long list of potentially injurious stimuli and the innumerable routes by which such stimuli can impact the retina, retinal disease is actually quite infrequent.

BOX 20-8 Portals of Entry into the Retina

HEMATOGENOUS
Infectious
Toxic
Vascular hypertension
Thrombosis/thromboembolism
Metastasis

TRAUMATIC
Perforation
Blunt trauma

TRANSCORNEAL
Light
Therapeutic radiation

VITREOUS
By-products of endophthalmitis
Traction detachment
Liquefaction
Glaucoma

CHOROID
Exudative detachment

RETINAL PIGMENT EPITHELIUM (RPE)
RPE disease (Vogt-Koyanagi-Harada syndrome, central progressive retinal atrophy)

OPTIC NERVE
Dieback retinopathy
Retrograde infection
Retrograde malignancy

GENETIC
Canine progressive retinal atrophy syndromes
- Primary retinal dysplasia

EYELIDS, CONJUNCTIVA, AND ORBIT

Eyelids

The outer surface of the eyelid is skin and therefore is susceptible to the same diseases as the skin elsewhere on the body. For palpebral skin, the portals of entry are the same as for skin at other sites, as follows:

1. Through the skin's surface or through adnexal glands by colonization of niche-adapted infectious agents
2. Penetrating injury
3. Hematogenous localization

Conjunctiva

The conjunctiva is a mucous membrane similar in structure to other mucous membranes and is therefore susceptible to injury from the same range of physical and chemical injuries affecting any other mucous membrane. The routes of entry are predictable and as follows:

1. Colonization of the epithelial surface by niche-adapted infectious agents
2. Absorption of injurious antigenic stimuli across an intact epithelium
3. Implantation via penetrating injury
4. Direct physical or chemical injury to the epithelial surface, allowing opportunistic infection
5. Hematogenous localization

Orbit

Portals of entry into the orbit are as follows:

1. Orbital fractures from external trauma
2. Extension of inflammatory or neoplastic disease originating within the gingiva or the nasal cavity
3. Extension of intraocular inflammatory or neoplastic disease through the sclera
4. Direct extension of inflammatory or neoplastic foci from the conjunctiva or eyelid
5. Penetrating injuries through the skin or upwardly through the mouth, or migrating foreign bodies implanting infectious agents
6. Hematogenous localization of microorganisms, neoplasms, and influx of antibodies in immune-mediated diseases (muscle, lacrimal gland)

BOX 20-9 Corneal Defenses Against Infection

Intact corneal epithelium
- Constant washing of the corneal surface
- Tears rich in antimicrobial substances (e.g., immunoglobulin A, lysozyme, and lactoferrin)
- Surface mucus inhibits bacterial colonization

Leukocytes
- Present in small numbers within the tear film
- Rapid recruitment from the capillaries at the limbus

7. Extension from the cranial vault via the optic nerve or through one of the other foramina; this is rare

Of these portals of entry, infectious orbital cellulitis resulting from penetrating foreign body or migration from tooth root cellulitis is the most common. In dogs and cats, spread of osteolytic nasal carcinoma, oral squamous cell carcinoma, or malignant melanoma into the orbit is relatively frequent. In cattle, the orbit is a frequent location for metastatic malignant lymphoma in those animals that survive long enough with the disease.

DEFENSE MECHANISMS

CORNEA

The cornea is defended against injury by its protected anatomic location, by several reflexes, and by the tear film (Box 20-9). Passive (anatomic) protection is provided by the eyelids, the eyelashes, and the bony orbit. Various reflexes are activated by mechanical stimulation of eyelids, eyelashes, or the cornea itself. The blink reflex causes the eyelids to close when the eyelids or eyelashes are stimulated by contact with any solid material or even strong air currents. The menace reflex causes the eyelids to blink when there is visual perception of a threat to the globe. The corneal reflex causes the eyelids to close when the cornea itself is irritated by external stimuli. Reflex retraction of the globe into the orbit, with subsequent passive sliding of the third eyelid to cover the cornea, occurs in response to corneal trauma.

The tear film is a serous secretion produced by the lacrimal gland and by the gland of the third eyelid, with contributions from goblet cells in the conjunctiva and several accessory glands within the conjunctival lamina propria. It not only provides the majority of the nourishment for the avascular cornea but also provides a mucus coat to prevent evaporation of the protective fluid, soluble antibacterial chemicals, and a flushing action to protect the cornea against colonization by bacteria and fungi that live in the conjunctival sac.

UVEA

The uveal tract, like any other lamina propria, is in free communication with peripheral blood and is therefore not protected against any noxious agents in circulation. It is protected from physical injury (as are most other parts of the globe) by the thick fibrous tunic of the sclera and by the bony orbit.

Direct uveal injury, however, seems to be less important to the globe than the spread of the uveal disease to other parts of the eye that are less able to resist an insult or regenerate (particularly the lens and retina). The protection of other portions of the globe from inflammation in the uvea rests on two main mechanisms: the blood-ocular barrier and the unique immunologic phenomenon known as *anterior chamber immune deviation.*

The blood-ocular barrier is created by tight junctions between endothelial cells of the iris and retinal blood vessels and tight junctions between adjacent epithelial cells of the inner nonpigmented ciliary epithelium and the retinal pigment epithelium. Unless the damage to the uvea itself is so severe as to disrupt these tight junctions, they prevent most chemical and infectious agents from gaining access to vulnerable intraocular tissues such as the lens and retina.

The location of this barrier is important in understanding the different reactions to injury by different parts of the uveal tract. For example, the presence of tight junctions between the RPE cells is extremely important in preventing exudate from within the choroid gaining access to the subretinal space. Subretinal fluid accumulation can cause vision-threatening retinal detachment, so the blood-eye barrier at that site provides important protection.

In the anterior chamber, however, the situation is quite different. Here the barrier is at the level of the endothelial cells of the iris. During any substantial inflammation, this barrier is broken as part of the increased vascular permeability inherent in any acute inflammation. This allows infectious agents, inflammatory mediators, and leukocytes to flood into the stroma of the iris. Because the iris has no "barrier" along its anterior surface, these agents, cells, and chemicals then quickly diffuse into aqueous humor of the anterior chamber. From here, they may disperse throughout the globe and damage the lens or even the retina.

Anterior chamber-associated immune deviation (ACAID) is a specialized immune response by which infectious agents and many other antigens introduced into the anterior chamber cause only a highly controlled immune response that effectively eliminates the provoking antigen, while producing minimal bystander tissue injury that would threaten nearby ocular tissue. ACAID protects the eye from antigen-specific, immune-mediated injury from delayed-type hypersensitivity (DTH). The eye contains no lymphoid tissue. To initiate an immune response, antigens within the anterior chamber must first be captured by intraocular antigen presenting cells, exit the globe through the normal aqueous outflow pathways, and reach the marginal zones of the spleen. Here antigen-specific T lymphocytes are activated to differentiate into regulatory cells that interfere with the induction of DTH, thus muting DTH and sparing the eye from inflammation induced by DTH.

LENS

The defenses of the lens against injury are almost purely passive. They are the fibrous tunic of the cornea and sclera, the bony orbit, the eyelids, and a thick collagenous resilient lens capsule.

RETINA AND VITREOUS

The retina and vitreous, like the lens, rely mostly on their protected intraocular niche, and like the lens, their active defense mechanisms are negligible. They are protected from most physical and chemical injury by the bony orbit, the fibrous shell of cornea and sclera, and by the uvea and from infectious (and to some extent, from toxic and metabolic) diseases by the blood-eye barrier created by tight junctions between RPE cells and by the tight junctions of the retinal vascular endothelium. The retina has essentially no defense against infectious agents, radiation, or noxious chemicals arriving through the vitreous. Ischemic injury is a major threat to retinal viability. It is protected by having an autoregulated vascular system that allows retinal perfusion to remain relatively normal despite wide fluctuations in systemic blood pressure. The injured retina also produces angiogenic growth factors and has a powerful system of scavengers to counteract the damaging effects of excitatory neurotoxins, nitric oxide, and other potentially damaging by-products of ischemia. The retina and vitreous have no resident phagocytes or other cellular components of the immune system.

EYELIDS, CONJUNCTIVA, AND ORBIT

Eyelids

Like skin anywhere else, the defenses of eyelid against injury include both structural and cellular defenses, including hair, keratin, epithelial tight junctions, and a potent intraepithelial and superficial dermal immune system (see discussion on skin). Like skin, it becomes susceptible to infectious disease when those defenses are compromised by excessive moisture, metabolic disease, or mechanical injury. The eyelid is susceptible to all of the same infectious, nutritional, and immune diseases as skin in any other location.

Conjunctiva

The conjunctiva is protected from most physical and chemical injuries by the eyelids and by the tear film. It has tight junctions between the epithelial cells to prevent easy access by infectious or chemical agents into the underlying lamina propria. It is capable of rapid replication in the event of injury and readily undergoes squamous metaplasia as an adaptive survival mechanism in response to chronic low-grade irritation of any type. The resident mucosal immune system (MALT) functions similarly to immune systems in other mucosal sites, such as the upper respiratory tract, lungs (bronchus-associated lymphoid tissue [BALT]), and gastrointestinal tract (gut-associated lymphoid tissue [GALT]) (see Chapter 13).

RESPONSES TO INJURY

CORNEA

Injury to the corneal epithelium occurs from chemical or physical injury, from deficiency in the quantity or quality of the tear film, or by colonization of the corneal epithelium by infectious agents specifically adapted to that environmental niche. Common examples of such damage include abrasion from misdirected eyelashes or improperly structured eyelids, irritating plant or other foreign bodies within the conjunctival sac, or lacerations inflicted in the course of fighting or running through heavy brush. The cornea is also very susceptible to changes in the quality or quantity of the tear film that may result from primary disease of the lacrimal gland or from desiccation caused by enlargement of the globe or impaired closure of the eyelids.

The corneal endothelium may be injured by increased intraocular pressure (glaucoma), mechanical damage from an anteriorly displaced lens, or from injury mediated by leukocytes (so-called corneal endothelialitis).

The corneal stroma is most frequently injured as a sequela to epithelial damage. It may also be directly injured by lacerations and penetrating injury, implantation of infectious agents subsequent to penetrating injury, or rarely by percolation of chemical or infectious agents into the corneal stroma from the blood vessels at the limbus. Injury to the corneal endothelium will also affect the stroma, allowing the dehydrated but strongly hydrophilic stroma to absorb fluid from the aqueous humor. This results in corneal edema and substantial visual impairment (Box 20-10).

The great majority of corneal lesions encountered in clinical practice result from epithelial injury as a result of trauma or desiccation. Almost all corneal diseases listed in clinical textbooks reflect one or more of only three pathologic processes: adaptive cutaneous metaplasia in response to mild irritation, epithelial and/or stromal necrosis, and repair (wound healing) (Box 20-11). The varied clinical manifestations of these three fundamental processes are often given specific clinical names that serve to confuse rather than clarify.

BOX 20-10 Causes of Corneal Edema

Injury to corneal epithelium
- Resulting in osmotic absorption of water from the tear film

Injury to corneal endothelium from:
- Anterior lens luxation
- Increased intraocular pressure (glaucoma)
- Primary corneal endothelial dystrophy
- Immune-mediated inflammatory destruction

Inflammation of the cornea
- Corneal stromal ingrowth of new, leaky blood vessels

BOX 20-11 Corneal Responses to Surface Injury

ADAPTIVE METAPLASIA

Keratinization
Rete ridge formation
Epithelial and stromal pigmentation
Superficial stromal fibrosis and vascularization from the limbus

SHALLOW ULCERATION

Edema
Return to normal via epithelial regeneration

DEEP ULCERATION

Edema
Inflammation (primarily neutrophilic)
Neutrophil-mediated stromal lysis
Stromal repair via ingrowth of fibroblasts and blood vessels from the limbus
Return to nearly normal via epithelial regeneration following stromal rebuilding

Adaptive Cutaneous Metaplasia to Mild Persistent Irritation

The usual response of the cornea to persistent mild irritation is cutaneous metaplasia, which is a combination of keratinization, epithelial hyperplasia, epithelial pigmentation, subepithelial fibrosis, and vascularization (Figs. 20-59 and 20-60). In short, a cornea that is challenged to adapt to mild persistent irritation does so by recalling its genetic heritage as skin and comes to resemble skin in every way except for the acquisition of hair follicles. Not all examples of cutaneous metaplasia involve the entire range of adaptive changes; it is possible, for example, to have keratinization without pigmentation or epidermal metaplasia without accompanying stromal fibrosis and vascularization. It depends on the nature of the irritation. The most common causes for such adaptation include chronic desiccation and mechanical irritation from eyelid diseases such as entropion or anomalous placement or direction of eyelashes. Desiccation may result from defective production of tears as in keratoconjunctivitis sicca, from improper distribution of tears because of improper eyelid structure or function, or because of ocular enlargement that prevents the lids from closing. Because the cornea is permitted to exist in its privileged state only because it is constantly bathed in a protective and nourishing tear film, the

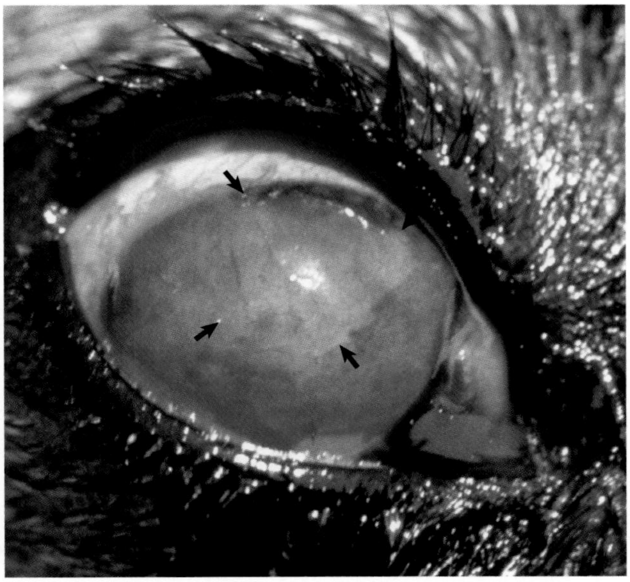

Fig. 20-59 Corneal cutaneous metaplasia, keratoconjunctivitis sicca, cornea, dog.
The diffuse corneal opacity *(outlined by arrows)* is caused by a combination of epithelial hyperplasia and keratinization, as well as stromal scarring and vascularization. (Courtesy Dr. B. Wilcock, Ontario Veterinary College.)

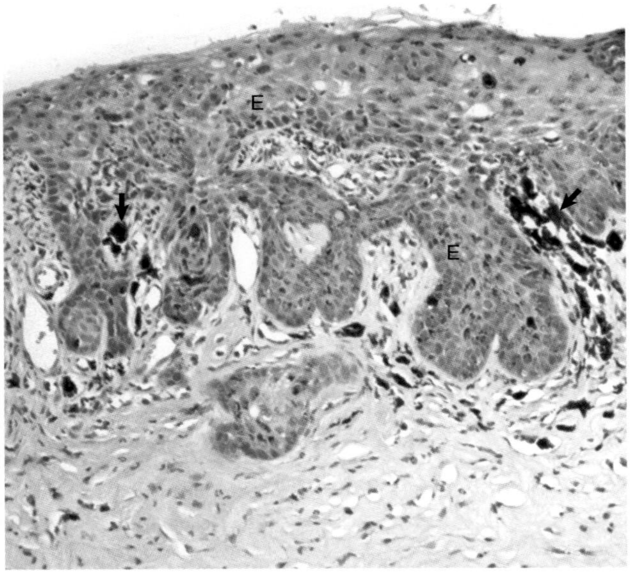

Fig. 20-60 Corneal cutaneous metaplasia, keratoconjunctivitis sicca, cornea, dog.
Chronic desiccation has caused adaptive epithelial hyperplasia *(E)*, epithelial and stromal pigmentation *(arrows)*, and stromal scarring. H&E stain. (Courtesy Dr. B. Wilcock, Ontario Veterinary College.)

partial or complete removal of that tear film represents a significant challenge to corneal homeostasis. If the change occurs slowly, the cornea successfully adapts by undergoing cutaneous metaplasia. If the desiccation occurs very rapidly, then the cornea will likely ulcerate.

Cutaneous metaplasia is a complex event that probably reflects the failure of conjunctival epithelial cells and stroma to acquire corneal phenotypes as they grow toward the center of the cornea to replace injured corneal tissue. The corneal epithelium has a finite number of replicative cycles. Persistent injury that exceeds the replicative ability of the corneal epithelium itself will require ingrowth of germinal cells that reside in the bulbar conjunctiva at the limbus. Similarly, injured corneal stroma often needs to recruit fibroblasts from the adjacent conjunctival lamina propria or sclera. Those chemical signals required to induce conjunctival or scleral tissue to undergo maturation into more appropriate "corneal" structure remain unknown.

Some of the lesions of cutaneous metaplasia are reversible, albeit only very slowly. Stromal fibrosis, however, is a permanent change, and the corneal stroma never again recovers complete transparency (see discussion on corneal wound healing). It is easy to think of corneal cutaneous metaplasia as an undesirable pathologic event, but in fact it is an eye-saving response to a pathologic change in the corneal environment. Failure to undergo cutaneous metaplasia would lead to corneal disintegration and subsequent destruction of all of the intraocular tissues.

Clinical entities characterized by corneal cutaneous metaplasia include pigmentary keratitis (corneal desiccation in brachycephalic dogs), keratoconjunctivitis sicca, band keratopathy secondary to eyelid closure defects, chronic keratitis secondary to irritation from eyelids or eyelashes, and chronic corneal desiccation as a consequence of chronic glaucoma.

Epithelial and/or Stromal Necrosis

Injuries to the cornea that occur too quickly or with too much severity to permit cutaneous metaplasia result in corneal necrosis. Because most of the injuries are from external insults, it is the corneal epithelium that is most commonly affected. The usual result is corneal ulceration. The causes are numerous, including rapidly progressing desiccation, severe mechanical injury, injury from exogenous chemicals, and a few niche-adapted infectious diseases such as herpesvirus infection in cats and *Moraxella bovis* infection in cattle.

After full-thickness epithelial loss, there is immediate osmotic absorption of water from the tear film into the anterior stroma, resulting in focal superficial stromal edema that is the clinical hallmark of corneal ulceration. The absorption of water increases the spacing between the stromal collagen fibers and results in increased scattering of light, which clinically appears as corneal opacity. Coloring the tear film with water-soluble dyes like fluorescein is a very common clinical diagnostic technique to accentuate the edema within the stroma. Within hours after injury, the early healing process begins and neutrophils from the tear film are also absorbed into the cornea (Fig. 20-61). In small "physiologic" numbers, they aid in defending the denuded cornea against opportunistic infection, provide growth factors for subsequent wound healing, and help with a small amount of corneal stromal débridement necessary for wound healing. If the wound becomes infected and the neutrophils migrate from the tear film and limbus in large numbers, their lytic enzymes create enough bystander injury to result in stromal destruction, known as suppurative keratomalacia (Fig. 20-62).

Corneal injuries of greater magnitude result in deep ulcers with substantial stromal loss, even to the point of disappearance of the entire stroma exterior to Descemet's membrane. This is most commonly seen in rapidly progressing ulcers contaminated with bacteria, resulting in neutrophil-induced keratomalacia. These ulcers, known as *melting ulcers,* may progress over just a day or two to full-thickness stromal dissolution. Descemet's membrane is the last barrier. It will bulge anteriorly into the defect created by the loss of the overlying stroma and epithelium to create a descemetocele (Fig. 20-63). In most instances, this fragile membrane (Descemet's membrane) ruptures, resulting in a perforating ulcer, which leads

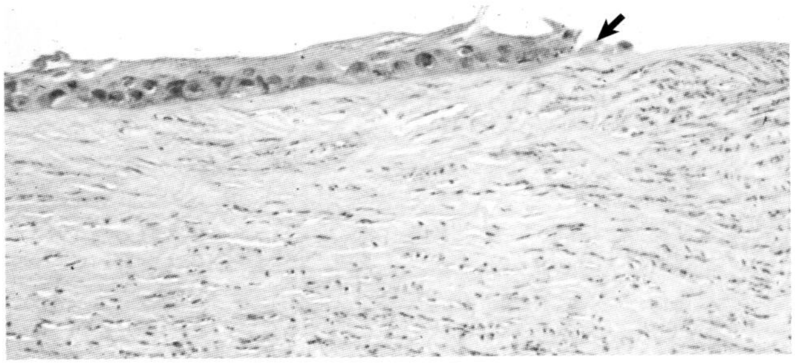

Fig. 20-61 Early healing, shallow ulcer, cornea, dog.
The corneal epithelium *(arrow)* is sliding along the surface of the denuded intact stroma that now has substantial staining pallor and separation of collagen fibers typical of edema. Numerous neutrophils have migrated into the stroma from the tear film. The neutrophils, although necessary in moderation, have the potential to cause enzymatic digestion of the stroma (keratomalacia) and are sources of fibroblastic and angioblastic growth factors. H&E stain. (Courtesy Dr. B. Wilcock, Ontario Veterinary College.)

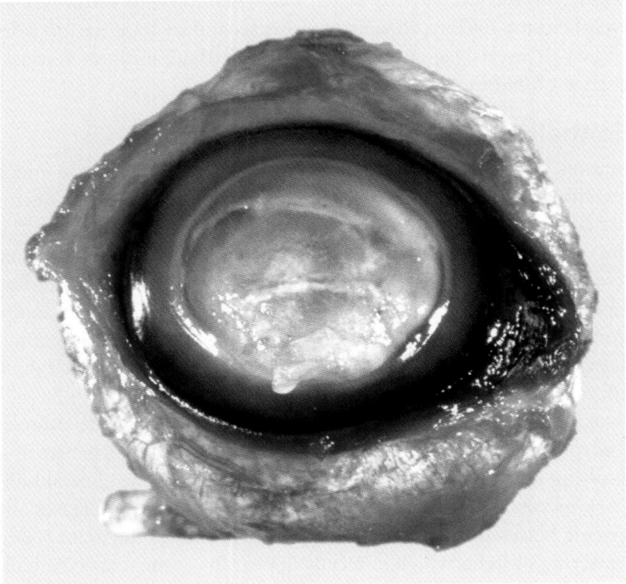

Fig. 20-62 Suppurative keratomalacia, enucleated globe, horse.
An initial corneal laceration became infected with *Pseudomonas* spp. The infection has resulted in proteolytic destruction of the stroma caused mostly by the release of digestive enzymes from neutrophils in the inflammatory exudate *(center to lower half of pupil)*. Healing will result in a large amount of stromal scarring. (Courtesy Dr. B. Wilcock, Ontario Veterinary College.)

to the loss of anterior chamber fluid and the strong probability of iris prolapse. Iris prolapse may also result from corneal perforation from trauma.

Keratitis is a common clinical term indicating inflammation of the cornea. Because the normal cornea is avascular, true inflammation cannot occur until later in the disease process, after the injured cornea has been vascularized as part of wound healing (see later discussion). Nonetheless, corneal ulcers are very susceptible to opportunistic infection from normal conjunctival flora or organisms from the environment. This is probably particularly true of mycotic keratitis in horses, particularly when the fungal infection is given an unfair advantage because of inappropriate use of antibiotics and/or corticosteroids in the management of minor corneal lacerations. The presence of such organisms within the cornea results in a marked acceleration of leukocyte immigration from the tear

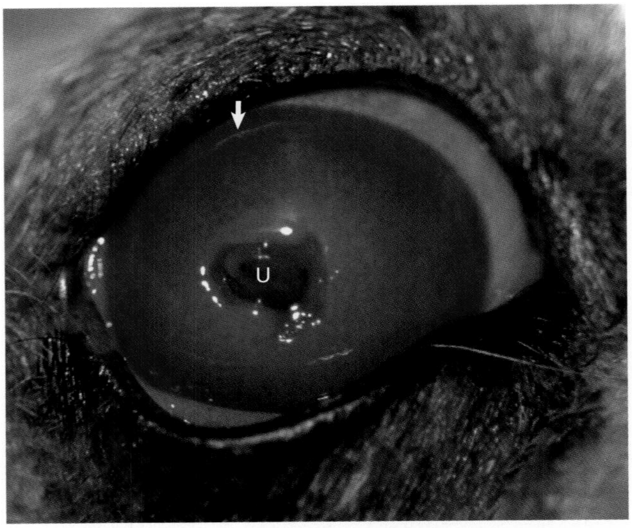

Fig. 20-63 Deep central corneal ulcer *(U)* (with descemetocele and early iris prolapse), dog.
Note the diffuse corneal edema (diffuse gray appearance) caused mostly by imbibition of tear fluid, with some contribution from the blood vessels which are growing (angiogenesis) into the injured cornea as part of wound healing (the circumferential red "brush border" from the limbus *[arrow]*). (Courtesy Dr. J. Wolfer, Islington Animal Clinic.)

film and blood vessels of the limbus. Although these leukocytes may be effective in neutralizing the infectious agent, they usually create substantial bystander injury to the stroma or the epithelium, resulting in a delay in wound healing and an increase in scarring.

Repair (Wound Healing)

Those injuries limited to just a portion of the epithelial thickness are rapidly repaired by epithelial sliding and eventual mitotic regeneration. Such injuries are unlikely to ever receive veterinary attention. Deeper defects that involve the full thickness of the epithelium and varying depths of stroma initiate a stereotypic series of events that are clinically significant, easily observed in clinical practice, and amenable to both medical and surgical intervention. Because the cornea is optically clear and readily accessible for continuous observation after injury, it is a favorite model for the in vivo study of the basic events of wound healing in mammalian tissue. From a pragmatic clinical perspective, the vast majority of corneal lesions encountered in clinical practice are already past the stage of initial injury and are at the stage of corneal wound healing. If healing is less than optimal, an array of antimicrobial agents, surgical procedures, and chemical agents to modify the wound healing response is commonly used.

Most models of corneal wound healing use a mild, controlled nonseptic epithelial injury. The sequence of events and the biochemical signaling involved in such injury are not necessarily the same as those in naturally occurring massive corneal injuries and subsequent infections seen in veterinary practice, but nonetheless these carefully controlled models provide the only information available.

After full-thickness destruction of a portion of the corneal epithelium, the sequence of events is depicted in Fig. 20-64. Briefly, the injured epithelial cells release cytokines, such as interleukin-1 and platelet-derived growth factor (PDGF). Within minutes of lethal epithelial injury, these chemical mediators cause necrosis and/or apoptosis of stromal cells within the very superficial corneal stroma. At the same time, injured epithelial cells at the margin of

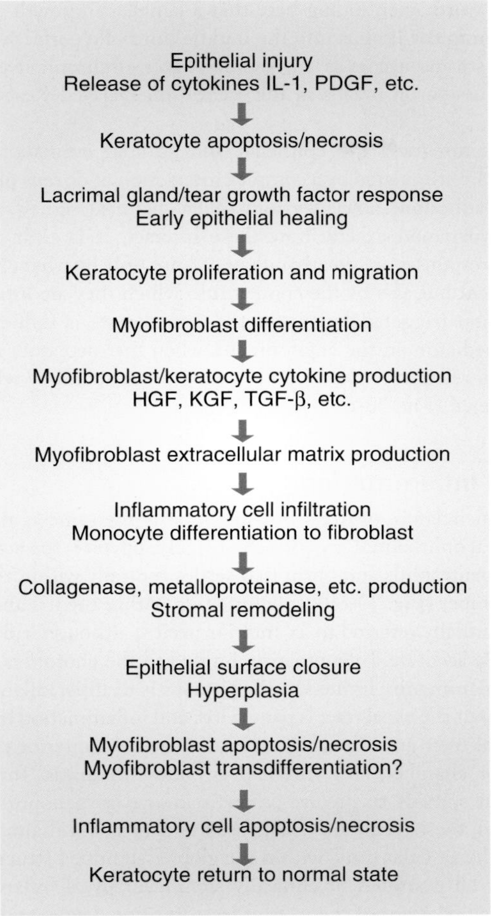

Fig. 20-64 Schematic diagram of the corneal wound healing cascade. *HGF,* Hepatocyte growth factor; *IL-1,* interleukin-1; *KGF,* keratocyte growth factor; *PDGF,* platelet-derived growth factor; *TGF-β,* transforming growth factor-β. (Redrawn from Klenkler B, Sheardown H: *Exp Eye Res* 79:677-688, 2004.)

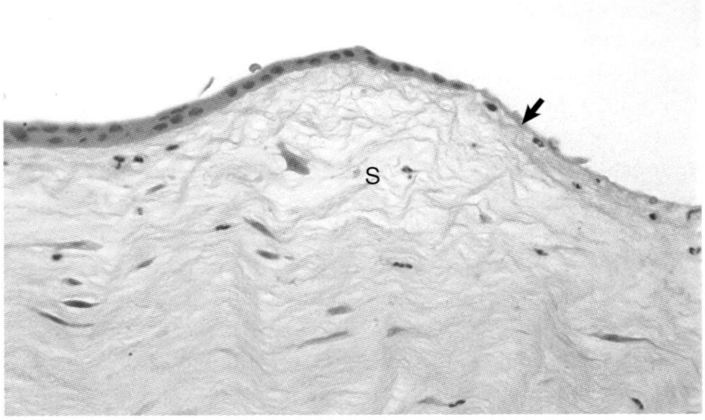

Fig. 20-65 Corneal epithelial cell migration (epithelial sliding), early wound healing, cornea, dog.
Corneal epithelial cells are migrating (sliding) to cover the corneal ulcer *(arrow)*. The stroma is edematous *(S)* and contains a few neutrophils derived from the tear film. H&E stain. (Courtesy Dr. B. Wilcock, Ontario Veterinary College.)

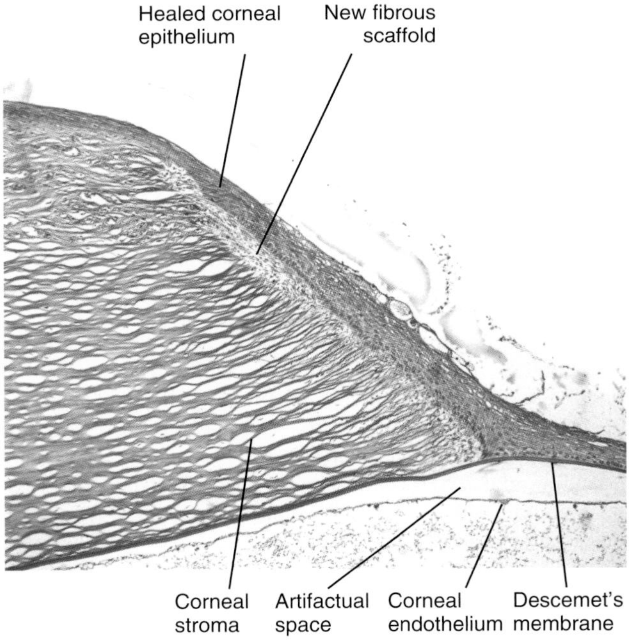

Fig. 20-66 Chronic descemetocele, cornea, dog.
On the right, at the site of a former deep corneal ulcer, the epithelium has healed by corneal epithelial cell migration (sliding) into the ulcer, with subsequent epithelial hyperplasia and return of the corneal epithelium to normal or even increased thickness. However, because there has been no replacement or remodeling of the stroma *(right),* the epithelium is positioned directly on the surface of Descemet's membrane instead of on a reconstituted fibrous stroma. This process is "unsuccessful" wound healing, because the "healed" cornea, lacking stroma, is too fragile to survive. Masson trichrome stain. (Courtesy Dr. B. Wilcock, Ontario Veterinary College.)

the ulcer release epidermal growth factor (EGF), keratocyte growth factor (KGF), and hepatocyte growth factor (HGF) to stimulate epithelial migration and proliferation. Additionally, the production of these growth factors is upregulated in the tear film. The increase in EGF and other growth factors results in flattening and sliding of viable suprabasilar epithelial cells from the adjacent intact epithelium. These cells dissolve their intercellular junctions and migrate across the exposed stromal surface, adhering to a temporary scaffold of fibronectin and other adhesion molecules (Fig. 20-65). As long as the underlying stroma is healthy enough to support epithelial migration, excessive numbers of neutrophils are not present, and if the event that caused the original corneal injury is no longer active, those epithelial cells slide with remarkable speed (as much as 1 mm per day) across the denuded surface in an attempt to close the defect. There are many other cytokines and adhesion molecules involved in corneal epithelial sliding and regeneration, suggesting that rapid sealing of the defect must be exceedingly important. Closure of the defect by even a thin layer of epithelium halts the continued recruitment of neutrophils, which are responsible for the keratomalacia, vision-impairing stromal fibroplasia, and vascularization from the limbus. Closure of the corneal defect also prevents further edema and limits access by potentially injurious infectious agents.

Lagging behind the epithelial activation and sliding, which occur within minutes to hours of injury, is rebuilding of the injured stroma, which starts within a few days. It is not clear how the cornea recognizes the need for stromal rebuilding. There are some cases in which even a deep stromal defect does not initiate ingrowth of fibroblasts and blood vessels to rebuild the stroma. Instead, the epithelium simply slides across whatever small amount of normal stroma remains. This results in an optically clear but precariously thin healed cornea (Fig. 20-66). Migration of neutrophils from the tear film and from the limbus into the corneal wound is a powerful stimulus for the recruitment of both blood vessels and fibroblasts from the limbus. Neutrophil immigration begins about 12 hours after mild injury in response to chemotactic factors released by injured epithelium and stroma. This delay in neutrophil recruitment presumably allows the epithelium to slide and seal small defects and thus prevents excessive immigration of neutrophils (and its negative consequences as outlined later). Additional stimulation of stromal fibroplasia and angiogenesis comes from release of growth factors, such as PDGF, vascular endothelial growth factor (VEGF), and transforming growth factor-β (TGF-β) from the injured epithelium, migrating neutrophils, and the injured stromal keratocytes. Not only does injury stimulate activation and migration of fibroblasts and angioblasts from the limbus, but it also changes the morphology and activity of the resident stromal fibroblasts (keratocytes). These cells undergo myofibroblastic metaplasia, become mobile and contractile, and produce increased amounts of various matrix proteins, growth factors, and metalloproteinases essential for stromal remodeling.

The histologic events of stromal rebuilding after significant injury are less complicated than the innumerable biochemical signaling interactions involved. Mild stromal injuries are repaired by in situ enlargement and sluggish proliferation of resident keratocytes, which undergo fibroblastic metaplasia. After significant stromal injury, however, repair using just local keratocytes/monocytes is not adequate. Such repair must await the arrival of reinforcements in the form of fibroblasts and blood vessels from the limbus. Histologically, enlargement and hyperchromasia of limbal fibroblasts and angioblasts is visible within a day or two of injury, but detectable migration is not evident until about 4 days. Fibroblasts and blood vessels, preceded by a halo of edema and stromal proteolysis, migrate with a maximum speed of 1 mm per day until they reach the site of injury (Fig. 20-67). Here, they rebuild the injured stroma to provide a scaffold suitable for the migration, adhesion, and eventual normalization of the epithelium. Over time, this fibroblastic-angioblastic matrix of granulation tissue matures to histologically resemble normal stroma. However, it is never able to replicate the very specific lamellar structure of normal stroma and even with optimal stromal wound healing, corneal clarity is permanently impaired.

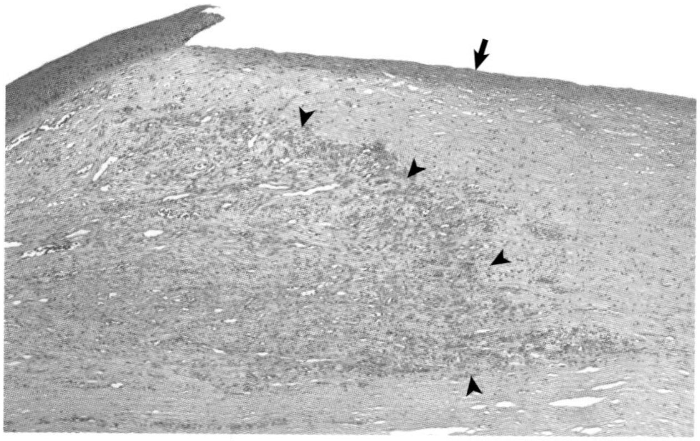

Fig. 20-67 Normal wound healing, cornea, dog.
Following shallow ulceration *(arrow)* that had damaged both the epithelium and the superficial stroma, the stroma is repaired and returned to near normal function by ingrowth of blood vessels and fibroblasts (wound healing) from the limbus *(leading edge of healing is shown by arrowheads)*. Such repair of the stroma is usually a prerequisite for epithelial regeneration following any large corneal ulceration. H&E stain. (Courtesy Dr. B. Wilcock, Ontario Veterinary College.)

It is worth mentioning here that a lamellar ingrowth of blood vessels from the limbus into the middle third of a perfectly normal corneal stroma occurs as a bystander effect of chronic uveitis (see the discussion on uveitis in the section on Delayed Responses to Injury).

To summarize, the epithelial and stromal events of wound healing are stimulated by a complex interaction of dozens of growth factors, adhesion molecules, and other chemical signals. It is far from understood exactly how these interact. It is clear that the cellular responses are greatly influenced not only by what chemicals are present but also by the context into which they are introduced. The action triggered by any of these mediators is influenced by other mediators in the environment, when the mediators are generated in relation to the wound healing process, and by what cells are targeted (Fig. 20-68).

UVEA

Uveal Inflammation

The nomenclature of uveal inflammation is the same as that used in clinical ophthalmology (Box 20-12). Hypopyon is the accumulation of neutrophils and fibrin that settles ventrally within the anterior chamber (Fig. 20-69). Inflammation within the iris and ciliary body is usually referred to as anterior uveitis, although iridocyclitis is equally accurate. Inflammation limited to the choroid is choroiditis; inflammation limited to the vitreous is hyalitis; inflammation throughout the uveal tract is panuveitis; and inflammation involving the uveal tract and the adjacent ocular cavities (anterior chamber, posterior chamber, and vitreous) is endophthalmitis. Inflammation that spreads to involve sclera is known as panophthalmitis. Although these terms are widely used in clinical ophthalmology, in reality, the vascular tunic within the globe is a unified structure and virtually all examples of clinically significant uveal inflammation involve all portions of the uvea at least to some degree and have at least a little bit of effusion into the ocular chambers. Furthermore,

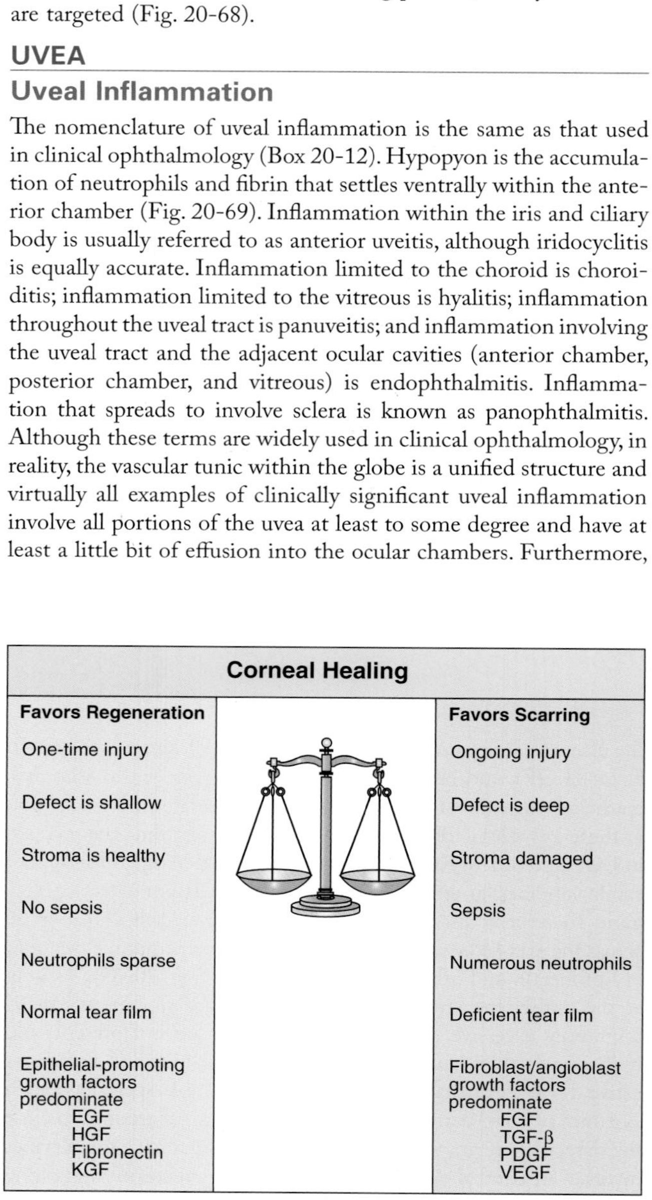

Fig. 20-68 Schematic diagram of corneal wound healing.
The outcome of corneal wound healing depends in part on the balance among growth factors coming from the tear film, injured epithelium and stroma, and immigrating leukocytes. *EGF,* Epidermal growth factor; *FGF,* fibroblast growth factor; *HGF,* hepatocyte growth factor; *KGF,* keratocyte growth factor; *PDGF,* platelet-derived growth factor; *TGF-β,* transforming growth factor-β; *VEGF,* vascular endothelial growth factor.

BOX 20-12 Histologic-Clinical Correlation in Uveitis

The uveal tract responds to inflammatory stimuli as do other tissues. The macroscopic manifestations detectable by clinical examination are as follows:

- Aqueous flare: an increase in protein content within the aqueous humor increases light scattering
- Iris swelling and color change: iris stromal hyperemia, edema, and leukocyte accumulation
- Conjunctival reddening: hyperemia of the superficial and deep conjunctival blood vessels in response to vasoactive chemicals generated by the nearby uveitis
- Hypopyon: the accumulation of neutrophils and fibrin that settles ventrally within the anterior chamber
- Keratic precipitates: small clusters of macrophages and/or neutrophils adherent to the corneal endothelium
- Peripheral corneal midstromal vascularization: persistent inflammation results in the generation of enough angiogenic growth factors to stimulate "accidental" migration of limbal blood vessels into the peripheral cornea

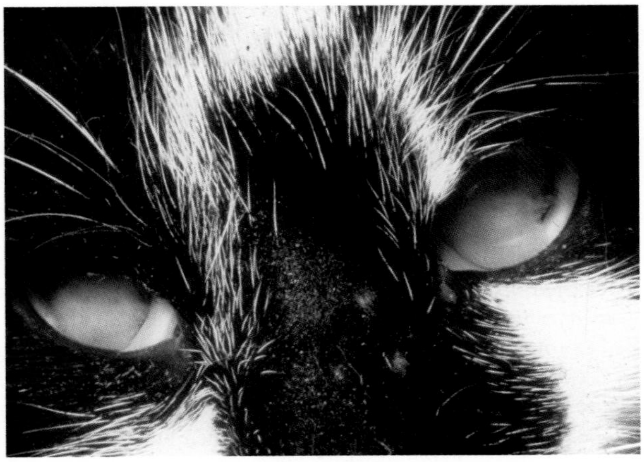

Fig. 20-69 **Hypopyon (bilateral), feline infectious peritonitis, cat.** A mixture of fibrin and neutrophils (white-gray opacity) is present within the anterior chamber of the eyes. (Courtesy Dr. B. Wilcock, Ontario Veterinary College.)

the globe is a sealed sphere filled with fluid, so that inflammatory mediators or toxic products of infectious agents are likely to be widely disseminated within the globe. Thus from a purely histologic perspective, virtually all cases of uveitis can be correctly classified as endophthalmitis.

A further source of confusion between histopathologic and clinical terminology is a consequence of identification of the predominant leukocyte in the exudate. As is true of lesions in many other tissues, histopathologic examination underestimates the number of rapidly migrating granulocytes and is misled by the gradual accumulation of nonemigrating mononuclear leukocytes. Neutrophils rapidly accumulate within the aqueous or vitreous humors where they can be detected by clinical or cytologic examination. Unless bound up in fibrin, those leukocytes are washed away during histologic processing, leaving only the predominantly mononuclear population within the uveal stroma. This is not unique to the globe: An identical opportunity for confusion exists in correlating cytologic and histologic lesions in immune-mediated joint disease, chronic rhinitis, and pyometra (among others).

Causes of Uveitis

Uveitis can be initiated by a wide array of infections, immune responses, and trauma. Tissues of the globe usually act as an integrated unit, so injury to one part almost always has at least some influence on the health of other parts of the globe. The globe is filled with fluid, thereby allowing chemical messengers generated in one part of the globe to be absorbed by distant intraocular tissue. The iris stroma, in particular, is highly reactive because there is free communication between it and the aqueous humor. Any toxins, chemical mediators of inflammation, or growth factors secreted into the aqueous are absorbed by the iris, causing that portion of the uveal tract to react. (See later discussion on preiridal fibrovascular membrane in the section on Delayed Responses to Injury).

Most of the infectious causes of uveitis are ocular responses to systemic viral, bacterial, or parasitic diseases in which the uveal tract is only one of many tissues affected. Endophthalmitis as the sole manifestation of infectious disease is usually seen only as a sequela to penetrating injuries or perforating ulcers that allow the entry of environmental organisms into the globe. There are no viral causes of endophthalmitis, although there are a few systemic viral infections that cause vasculitis or retinitis that result in a uveal inflammatory response. Aberrant migration of nematode or trematode larvae occasionally causes endophthalmitis, as does ocular colonization by a variety of protozoal parasites that cause systemic disease (toxoplasmosis and encephalitozoon in particular). Uveal involvement in systemic mycoses and protothecosis is particularly common in animals in certain geographic regions.

Immune-mediated uveitis is a particularly frequent finding. In only a few types is there a reasonable understanding of the pathogenesis, as in uveodermatologic syndrome and phacoclastic uveitis (see later discussion). In the great majority, there is a chronic lymphocytic-plasmacytic endophthalmitis with no demonstrable infectious agent and a moderately successful clinical response to immunosuppressive therapy (see the later discussion on idiopathic lymphonodular uveitis in the section on Diseases of the Uvea). The lesion is clearly the result of an immunologic response, but it is not known whether such a lesion reflects primary immune-mediated disease or simply a response to an elusive infectious agent that has long since disappeared.

Ocular trauma is a frequent cause of transient endophthalmitis. The uvea also responds to afferent neural signals and chemical factors released from an injured cornea, so that with any significant corneal ulceration or keratitis, one can expect to have at least a mild anterior uveitis.

Immediate Response to Injury: Uveitis

Because the uveal tract has a fibrovascular stroma similar to the lamina propria of intestine or the dermis of skin, it undergoes all of the usual inflammatory reactions. There is nothing at all unique about these reactions. What is unique, however, is the importance of the consequences of that inflammation for other parts of the globe.

Delayed Responses to Injury

What is most distinctive about uveitis is not the macroscopic or microscopic character of the inflammatory reaction itself, but the consequences of that inflammation for adjacent portions of the globe. These bystander effects, which include anterior and posterior synechiae, retinal detachment, cataract, corneal vascularization, preiridal fibrovascular membrane, and glaucoma, are clinically significant and are frequently the targets of therapeutic intervention.

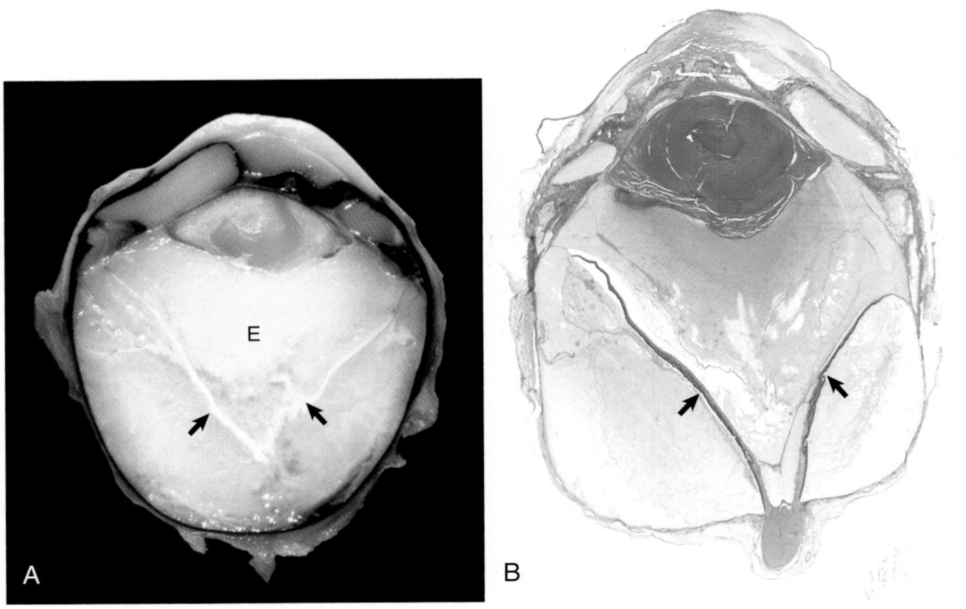

Fig. 20-70 Posterior synechia, pupillary block and iris bombé, eye, sagittal section, dog.
A, The iris has adhered to the lens, creating a pupillary block and subsequent iris bombé. Cloudy exudate *(E)* fills the vitreous, and its accumulation in the subretinal space has caused complete retinal detachment *(arrows)*. These changes occurred as a consequence of corneal perforation and secondary septic endophthalmitis. **B,** Same globe as **A.** The serous effusion from the choroid has caused retinal detachment *(arrows)*, which has serious implications for retinal survival. Additional lesions include posterior synechia, iris bombé, ciliary-lenticular adhesions, and circumferential cortical cataract. The combination of posterior synechia, pupillary block, iris bombé, and secondary peripheral anterior synechia is an exceedingly common sequence in the pathogenesis of glaucoma secondary to uveitis. H&E stain. (Courtesy Dr. B. Wilcock, Ontario Veterinary College.)

Synechiae are adhesions between the inflamed sticky iris and either the lens or cornea. Adhesion to the anterior capsular surface of the lens (in the normal globe, the iris lies against the lens capsule) is known as *posterior synechia.* The adhesion is initially fibrinous but will become a firm fibrous adhesion if allowed to persist. If that adhesion is sufficiently extensive around the pupillary margin (i.e., approaching the full circumference of the pupil), there is significant impairment of aqueous outflow from the posterior chamber to the anterior chamber (pupillary block) and inevitable secondary glaucoma. Increased pressure within the posterior chamber in the presence of a circumferential posterior synechia results in anterior bowing of the iris known as *iris bombé* (Fig. 20-70, *A*).

Anterior synechia is a focal-to-diffuse iridocorneal adhesion. Because the iris is not normally in proximity to the cornea, anterior synechia is much less prevalent than posterior synechia. It is most commonly seen as a sequela to iris prolapse, in which the flexible iris is literally "sucked up" into the corneal defect, where it then becomes anchored by fibrin and later by fibrosis. Peripheral anterior synechia commonly accompanies iris bombé and preiridal fibrovascular membranes (see later discussion).

Retinal detachment is a common sequela to uveitis and/or endophthalmitis by one of two mechanisms. Increased vascular permeability within the choroid results in effusion of fluid and cells into the subretinal space, resulting in so-called exudative detachment (Fig. 20-70, *B*). The normal retina is not actually adhered to the RPE. Fluid leaving the choroid during inflammation preferentially accumulates in the potential space between the retina and RPE because its only alternative would be to try to escape through the dense fibrous shell of the sclera. Alternatively, replacement of fibrinous exudates by fibrous tissue within the vitreous may result in tractional detachment. The immediate and delayed visual consequences of retinal detachment are discussed later (see section on Diseases of the Retina). If there is a lot of fibrovascular ingrowth as a consequence of organization of vitreal exudate, the maturing fibrovascular tissue routinely creates a dense membrane across the anterior surface of the vitreous (just posterior to the lens). This cyclitic membrane is anchored into the ciliary epithelium and often incorporates remnants of the detached retina.

Cataracts are frequent sequelae to uveitis, but the exact mechanisms are poorly understood. We do know that the avascular lens entirely depends on the aqueous humor for the delivery of nutrients and the removal of metabolic waste products. In eyes with uveitis, there is a notable drop in the production of aqueous humor (ocular hypotension is one of the clinical features of uveitis), resulting in lens "malnutrition." It is assumed that the lens is also susceptible to injury by mediators of inflammation and other toxic products in the aqueous humor of inflamed globes.

Corneal endothelialitis is characterized by an infiltration of neutrophils and/or lymphocytes into the corneal endothelium (Fig. 20-71). It usually is seen in globes with other lesions of chronic uveitis, but sometimes it is the most obvious histologic lesion of a uveitis that has almost disappeared (at least histologically) from other parts of the globe. It is much more prevalent in feline globes with feline infectious peritonitis (FIP) and idiopathic lymphonodular uveitis than in any others. Its pathogenesis is unknown. It was once a common lesion as a delayed sequela to vaccination with modified live vaccines containing canine adenovirus 1 and occasionally to canine adenoviral hepatitis. Complement-fixing antibodies against the virus were present within the endothelium as a result of a previous viral infection, resulting in attraction of neutrophils and subsequent bystander injury to the endothelium.

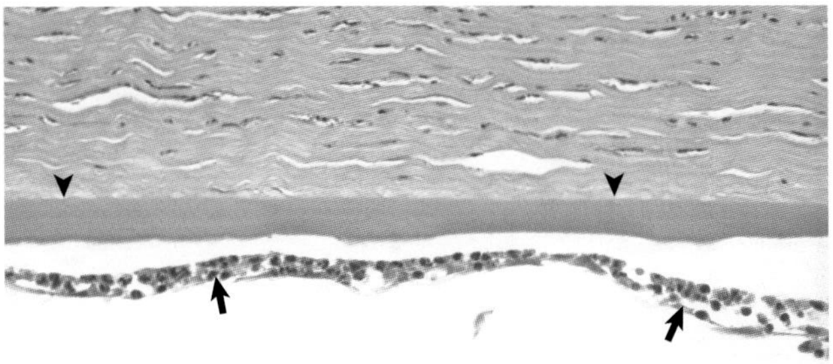

Fig. 20-71 Corneal endothelialitis, cornea, cat.
Neutrophils *(arrows)* adhere to and have accumulated on and in the corneal endothelium. When numerous, they separate the corneal endothelial cells from the adjacent Descemet's membrane *(arrowheads)*. This is a relatively frequent complication of anterior uveitis in cats and especially cats with feline infectious peritonitis. The leukocytes may be predominantly neutrophils or lymphocytes, depending on the pathogenesis and the duration of the uveitis. H&E stain. (Courtesy Dr. B. Wilcock, Ontario Veterinary College.)

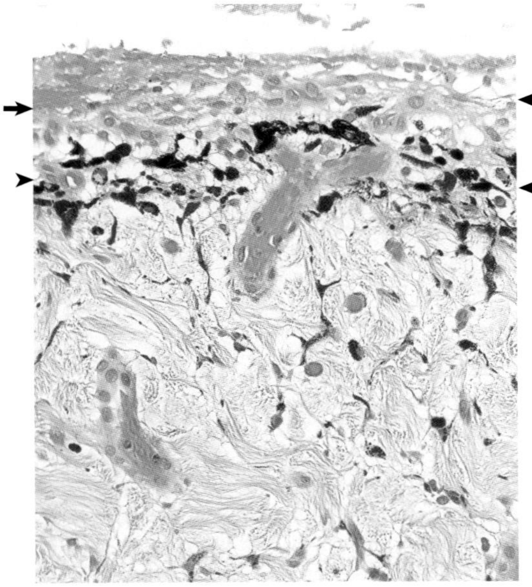

Fig. 20-72 Preiridal fibrovascular membrane, iris, dog.
A preiridal fibrovascular membrane *(between arrows)* formed by proliferating fibroblasts and capillaries has grown out from the iris stroma and has adhered to the anterior surface of the iris (represented here by the thin layer of pigmented melanocytes *[between arrowheads]*). These membranes form in response to growth factors within the aqueous humor, originating from such varied sources as intraocular neoplasms, or follow retinal detachment or chronic uveitis. H&E stain. (Courtesy Dr. B. Wilcock, Ontario Veterinary College.)

If the endothelial damage was of sufficient magnitude, the result was the development of severe and sometimes permanent corneal edema, commonly referred to as *blue eye*.

Preiridal fibrovascular membrane refers to a layer of granulation tissue on the anterior surface of the iris. It is created by budding and migration of capillaries from the iris stroma and recruitment of fibroblasts as a routine response to cytokine mediators of wound healing (Fig. 20-72). It is no different from granulation tissue anywhere else in the body, but in typical ocular fashion, it achieves special significance within the globe. If the granulation tissue migrates across the anterior face of the lens, it creates a pupillary block resulting in secondary glaucoma. Alternatively, this granulation tissue can also migrate across the anterior face of the filtration

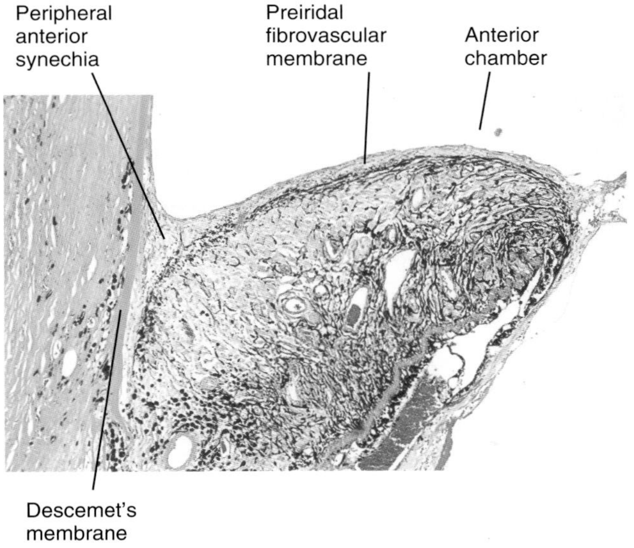

Fig. 20-73 Mature preiridal fibrovascular membrane, iris, dog.
A layer of mature granulation tissue (preiridal fibrovascular membrane) has adhered to the anterior surface of the iris. Contraction of the maturing membrane has distorted the shape of the iris and has caused it to adhere to the posterior surface of the cornea (peripheral anterior synechia). If extensive, the anterior synechia will result in secondary glaucoma. H&E stain. (Courtesy Dr. B. Wilcock, Ontario Veterinary College.)

angle to create a peripheral anterior synechia and once again cause secondary glaucoma (Fig. 20-73). Like any immature granulation tissue, it is also susceptible to hemorrhage and is a frequent cause of anterior chamber hemorrhage, known as *hyphema*. Wound healing after uveitis is only one of several mechanisms for the development of preiridal fibrovascular membranes, which are described in greater detail in the section on Glaucoma.

Midstromal corneal vascularization is an extremely common and clinically useful clue pointing to the presence of chronic uveitis. The vessels grow inwardly from the limbus. It has no known functional significance and appears to be a purely accidental lesion because the blood vessels of the limbus respond to angiogenic growth factors being produced within the globe as part of the ongoing inflammation and repair.

Phthisis bulbi refers to a shrunken, disorganized endstage globe. It is a sequela not only to uveitis, but also severe uveitis is the most common cause.

LENS

The stereotypic histologic response of the lens to injury is hydropic swelling of the injured lens fibers, fiber disintegration resulting in cortical liquefaction, and abortive efforts at regeneration. This combination of changes is essentially identical, regardless of pathogenesis. They all result in opacification of the lens, referred to by the generic term *cataract*.

In clinical ophthalmology, cataracts are extensively subclassified by location within the lens, by age of onset, by the macroscopic appearance, or by the state of progression. This gives rise to an exceedingly complicated list of purely descriptive adjectives that are not at all reflective of the pathogenesis. Such classification is used mostly when dealing with inherited cataracts in dogs to ensure that the data being collected about the frequency or behavior of a cataract in a specific breed are indeed referring to the same disease.

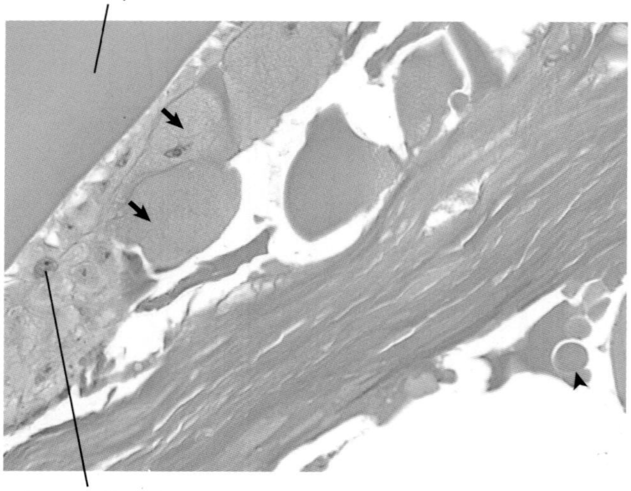

Fig. 20-74 Cataract, lens, dog.
There is epithelial hyperplasia of the lens with fibroblastic metaplasia, formation of bladder cells *(arrows),* and a Morgagnian globule *(arrowhead).* H&E stain. (Courtesy Dr. B. Wilcock, Ontario Veterinary College.)

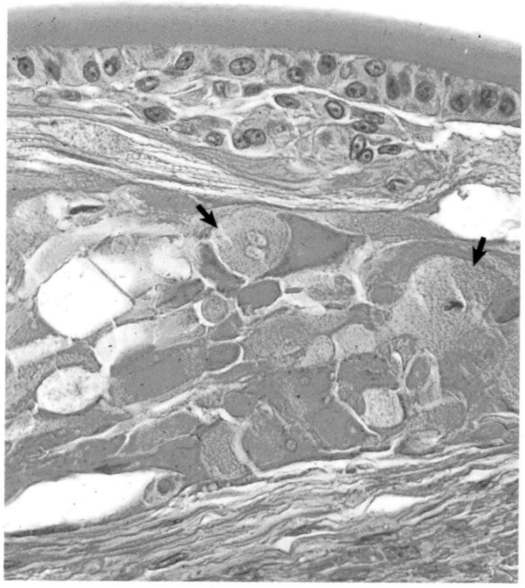

Fig. 20-75 Anterior cortical cataract, lens, fish.
Note the lens epithelial proliferation, fibroblastic metaplasia, and prominent bladder cells *(arrows).* (Courtesy Dr. B. Wilcock, Ontario Veterinary College.)

The stereotypic microscopic changes of cataracts (Figs. 20-74 and 20-75) are various combinations of the following, listed in order of overall frequency:

1. Fragmentation and liquefaction of cortical fibers, creating spherical globules of denatured lens protein known as Morgagnian globules.
2. Hydropic swelling of cells, known as *bladder cells,* attempting but failing to regenerate.

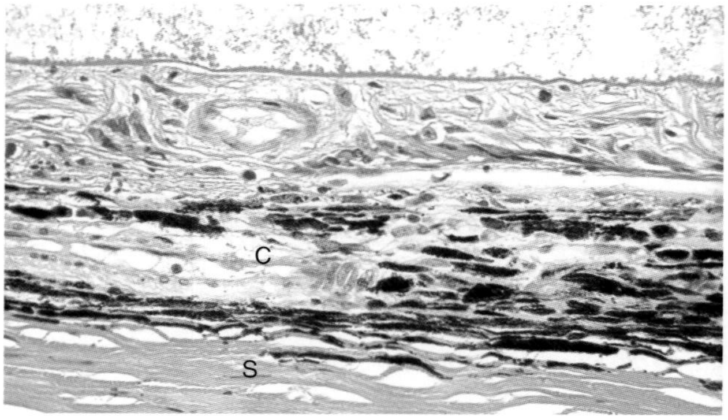

Fig. 20-76 Retinal atrophy (advanced), retina, dog.
There is virtually complete loss of all retinal layers, including photoreceptors, leaving only a few surviving blood vessels and glial cells. The impression of retinal fibrosis is mostly the result of fibrous astrocytosis originating within the inner nuclear layer. This lesion could be the end stage of almost any severe retinitis or retinal necrosis (including retinal detachment, retinal hypertension, glaucoma, or trauma). *C,* Choroid; *S,* sclera. H&E stain. (Courtesy Dr. B. Wilcock, Ontario Veterinary College.)

3. Hyperplasia and fibrous metaplasia of lens epithelium; the epithelial hyperplasia may create plaque-like thickening with or without fibroblastic metaplasia.
4. Posterior lens epithelial migration; the lens epithelium migrates from the equator to lie under the posterior lens capsule; the normal adult lens has no epithelium posterior to the equator.
5. More variable changes include lens swelling in acute cataracts, lens shrinking with wrinkling of the lens capsule in advanced ("hypermature") cataracts, and intralenticular mineralization.

The lens is capable of additional responses to injury other than those associated with cataracts, but these are much less frequent. As discussed in the section on phacoclastic uveitis, rupture of the lens capsule allows regenerative lens epithelium to escape from the lens, undergo fibroblastic metaplasia, and migrate within the anterior and posterior chambers, sometimes with devastating consequences. The same type of proliferation complicates cataract surgery, producing thick plaques of fibroblast-like epithelial cells that are aesthetically displeasing and reduce visual acuity.

RETINA AND VITREOUS

The general pathology of the retina resembles that of the brain. The neuronal elements of the adult retina of higher mammals do not regenerate; the outer segments of the photoreceptors, however, have a rapid turnover and have among the highest metabolic activity in the body. As long as the cell body within the outer nuclear layer remains viable, photoreceptors can be quickly regenerated.

The RPE remains mitotically active throughout life. Like other epithelia, it repairs itself, first by sliding viable cells into the area where cells have been lost and then by mitosis. Fibroblastic metaplasia is common (see later discussion).

The glial elements of the retina, particularly the astrocytes that reside within the inner nuclear layer (Müller cells), are exceedingly hardy and capable of proliferation. Repair of most cases of retinal necrosis occurs primarily by proliferation of Müller cells, which eventually form a dense glial scar, sometimes with a contribution from migrating RPE cells that can also undergo fibroblastic metaplasia (Fig. 20-76). Occasionally, the astrocytes proliferate along the vitreal face of the retina, forming a preretinal fibroglial membrane.

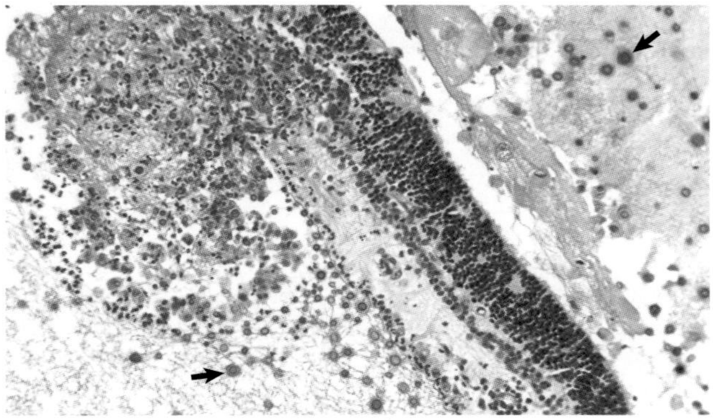

Fig. 20-77 Retinitis, retinal necrosis (with exudative retinal detachment), cryptococcosis, retina, dog.
Cryptococcus neoformans organisms *(arrows)* are numerous within the subretinal exudate. A mixture of fibrin, leukocytes, and organisms has replaced a portion of retina and created a focal preretinal exudate. Periodic acid–Schiff reaction. (Courtesy Dr. B. Wilcock, Ontario Veterinary College.)

Subretinal membranes (between the photoreceptors and the RPE) of a similar microscopic appearance are seen with chronic detachments and originate from migrating Müller cells or from retinal pigment epithelium that has undergone fibroblastic metaplasia.

The vast majority of retinal lesions fall into the following three categories:

1. Inflammation as a result of extension from endophthalmitis or encephalitis. Inflammation targeting the retina specifically is exceedingly uncommon. The character of the inflammation within the retina is exactly the same as it is within the brain: neuronal necrosis, perivascular cuffing, and gliosis. What is different about the retina, however, is its susceptibility to exudative retinal detachment. Fluid and cells escaping from inflamed retinal vessels are most likely to accumulate in the subretinal space and result in the separation of the photoreceptors from the RPE and the choroidal vasculature (Fig. 20-77). The photoreceptors are therefore likely to become necrotic, not only from the by-products of inflammation but also from ischemia and other forms of malnutrition resulting from their anatomic dislocation from the RPE (remember that the photoreceptors are entirely dependent on their intimate contact with the RPE and their proximity to the choroid for their nutrition). Serious photoreceptor damage occurs within days.
2. Noninflammatory photoreceptor degeneration from inherited metabolic disease, retinal detachment, or toxicity. Histologically, almost all of these photoreceptor diseases are indistinguishable from one another. The changes are the same regardless of whether the damage is from inborn metabolic errors (especially the innumerable inherited photoreceptor dysplasias of purebred dogs), excessive exposure to light or other radiation, or toxic chemicals.
3. Destruction of the neural elements of the inner retina (nerve fiber layer, ganglion cells, and inner nuclear layer) as a result of glaucoma. The pathogenesis of the inner retinal destruction and destruction of the optic nerve remain a source of great controversy and probably varies among species and with the type of glaucoma. Some of the damage is probably from pressure-induced collapse of retinal and even choroidal blood vessels, and some is probably the result of pressure-induced interference with the axoplasmic flow of nutrients within the optic nerve and nerve fiber layer (see the section on Glaucoma).

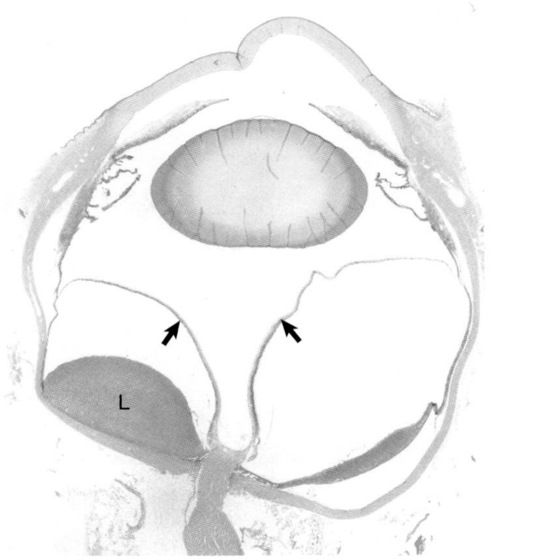

Fig. 20-78 Retinal detachment (complete), globe, sagittal section, dog.
Serous effusion from the growth of metastatic lymphoma *(L)* within the choroid and subretinal space has caused a complete retinal detachment *(arrows)*. H&E stain. (Courtesy Dr. B. Wilcock, Ontario Veterinary College.)

Retinal Detachment

The neurosensory retina (not including the RPE) is physically anchored only at the ora ciliaris and at the optic disc. It is held in apposition to the RPE partly by the physical presence of the gel-like vitreous and partially by the membrane forces related to the intricate interdigitations between photoreceptors and surface crevices in the RPE. The potential space between the photoreceptors and the RPE is the remnant of the lumen of the primary optic vesicle, and it persists throughout life. Retinal detachment (sometimes referred to as *retinal separation* by those who correctly point out that the retina is never really attached at all) is a frequent and serious complication of many different ocular diseases. It may be focal or more diffuse. The distance of separation between the photoreceptors and the RPE may only be slight (so-called flat detachments) or the entire retina may be separated and suspended in the vitreous (Fig. 20-78), supported only by its durable attachments to the ciliary body and optic nerve (so-called morning glory detachment because of its resemblance to a tubular flower when viewed by clinical examination through the pupil).

The most frequent types of retinal detachment are as follows:

1. Exudative retinal detachment: accumulation of serous, fibrinous, or cellular exudates (or hemorrhage) within the subretinal space as a consequence of choroiditis, retinitis, or retinal vascular hypertension (see Fig. 20-78).
2. Hematogenous retinal detachment: leakage of liquefied vitreous into the subretinal space through traumatic or degenerative breaks in the peripheral retina. This may occur secondary to trauma or to a very frequent aging lesion known as microcystoid peripheral retinal degeneration (Fig. 20-79).
3. Tractional retinal detachment: maturation of hemorrhage or fibrin within the vitreous, which pulls the retina away from the choroid. As it matures, the combination of fibrous tissue,

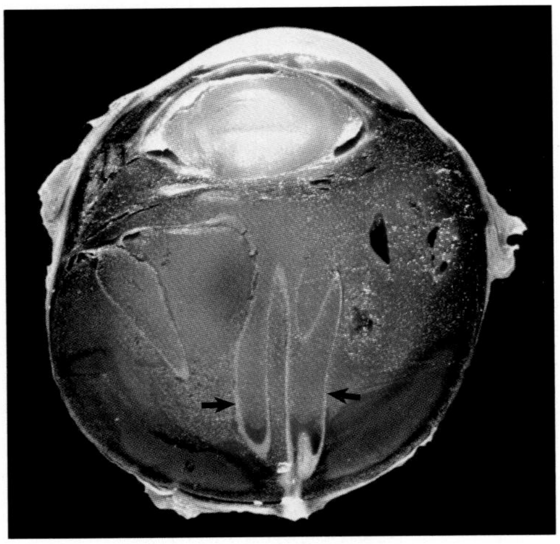

Fig. 20-79 Retinal detachment (traumatic), globe, sagittal section, dog. The detachment has been caused by accumulation in the posterior chamber of subretinal hemorrhage. The retina *(arrows)* remains attached only at the sites of true anatomic attachment: the optic disc and its junction with the pars plana of the ciliary body. (Courtesy Dr. B. Wilcock, Ontario Veterinary College.)

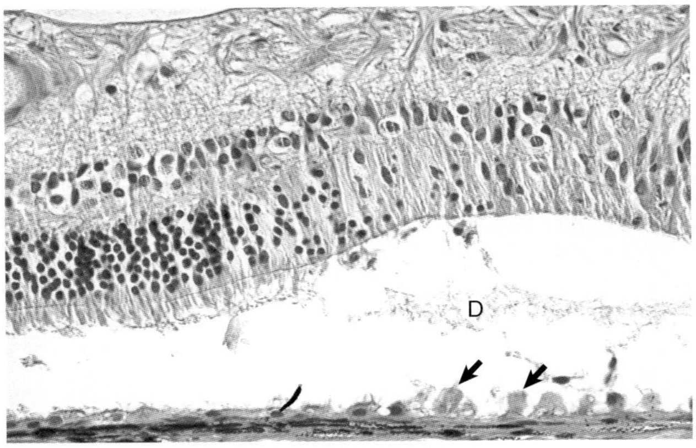

Fig. 20-80 Retinal detachment (serous), retina, dog. Floccular eosinophilic debris *(D),* the histologic counterpart of a serous exudate, has pushed the retina away from the retinal pigment epithelium (RPE). There is hypertrophy *(arrows)* of the RPE, degeneration of the photoreceptors, and focal loss of neurons from the outer nuclear layer. RPE hypertrophy occurs after just a few hours of detachment. The rapidity of progression of the photoreceptor degeneration depends on the magnitude of the detachment and the toxicity of the fluid within the subretinal space. H&E stain. (Courtesy Dr. B. Wilcock, Ontario Veterinary College.)

fibrin, and detached retina lies as a membrane stretching from ciliary body to ciliary body across the posterior surface of the lens, a lesion known as a *cyclitic membrane.*

Retinal detachment is immediately significant because the image on the retina is out of focus, but more serious is the rapidity with which the photoreceptors are damaged. The outer segments of the photoreceptors, responsible for light absorption and electrical signal generation, are lost within 2 weeks after experimental saline-induced flat detachment (Fig. 20-80). Histologic and clinical evidence in natural disease suggests that this degeneration occurs much more rapidly (a few days at most) in the presence of toxic by-products of inflammation, or when the distance between the retina and the RPE is great. The inner segments of the photoreceptors and the cell bodies within the outer nuclear layer are

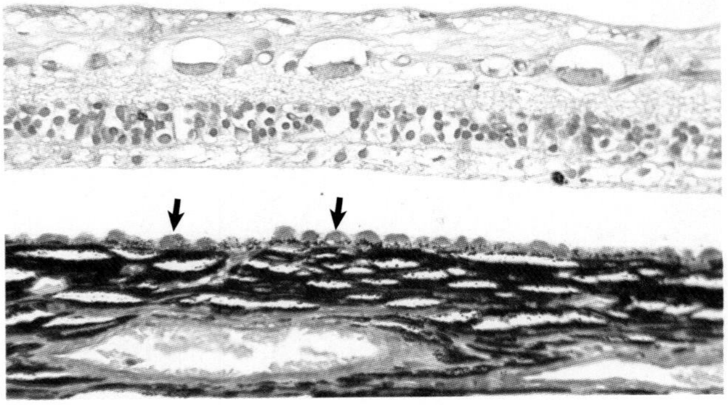

Fig. 20-81 Retinal detachment (chronic), retina, dog. There is hypertrophy of the retinal pigment epithelium *(arrows),* with loss of nuclei from the outer nuclear layer as well as disintegration of the photoreceptors. At this stage, the loss of vision from this portion of retina is irreversible. H&E stain. (Courtesy Dr. B. Wilcock, Ontario Veterinary College.)

much more resistant to injury and may remain viable for months (Fig. 20-81).

The retinal consequences of detachment probably vary by species, depending on how much intrinsic retinal vasculature is present. There is virtually no published information, but the almost avascular retina of horses should be much more susceptible to full-thickness ischemic injury than the well-vascularized retinas of dogs or cats (in which the inner half of the retina remains unaffected by detachment).

The detached retina in every species produces a variety of angiogenic growth factors presumably intended to increase its own blood supply. In species other than primates, however, there is little evidence of stimulation of retinal angiogenesis. Instead, these growth factors percolate through the vitreous and are absorbed into the iris stroma where they stimulate the production of a preiridal fibrovascular membrane. The result is a substantial risk of secondary glaucoma from either pupillary block or occlusion of the filtration angle (see the section on Glaucoma).

EYELIDS, CONJUNCTIVA, AND ORBIT

Eyelids

The responses of the eyelids to injury, the spectrum of potentially injurious agents, and the susceptibility to neoplasia are exactly the same as for skin and are not discussed further.

Although the responses of the eyelid itself to injury may be identical to those of skin elsewhere, there may be unique consequences for other parts of the globe, particularly the nearby conjunctiva and cornea. There may be direct spread of inflammation or neoplasia from the eyelid to the nearby conjunctiva or even to the cornea. Physical distortion of the eyelid from inflammation, scarring, or neoplasia may interfere with the ability of the eyelid to distribute the tear film, or to properly protect the cornea from injury. The abnormal eyelid may even cause mechanical injury by scraping the cornea that it was designed to protect.

There are only a few inflammatory diseases and neoplasms with a predilection for the eyelids, and these are discussed later under specific diseases. It is appropriate to be skeptical when attempting to prove an infectious cause for blepharitis in any species. There is a tendency to assume that whatever infectious agents are isolated from swabs of the eyelid margin or from expressed Meibomian secretion must be the cause of the blepharitis. This is flawed logic because ordinarily those same organisms are readily isolated from the conjunctival sac, or the eyelid margin, of perfectly healthy animals.

Conjunctiva

The reaction of conjunctiva to injury is the same as that of any other mucous membrane. It has a narrow spectrum of responses to injury and only seldom can an etiologic diagnosis be made by histologic examination of a conjunctival biopsy. The epithelium responds to acute injury with ulceration. With chronic mild injury, there is squamous metaplasia. In animals with pigmented conjunctivae, chronic irritation also stimulates hyperpigmentation, just as it often does in skin. If there is desiccation, the areas of squamous metaplasia are often keratinized.

The underlying lamina propria usually responds with a stereotypic lymphocytic-plasmacytic accumulation, with the development of hyperplastic lymphoid nodules if the stimulation is persistent. Neutrophils are seldom numerous within the tissue; if present at all, they are usually found migrating through the epithelium en route to the conjunctival sac where they will do battle with the infectious agents that might be present as opportunistic pathogens. Eosinophils are occasionally present in poorly defined allergic conjunctivitis in dogs, cats, and horses. They are present in greater numbers in the more discrete collagenolytic granulomas in horses with habronemiasis.

Looking for specific infectious agents in sections of conjunctiva is usually a waste of time. It is true that some of the viral diseases and chlamydial infections can leave specific footprints in the form of inclusion bodies, but these are usually present only very early in the course of these diseases, at a time before the lesion is assessed by conjunctival scraping or biopsy examination.

Orbit

There is nothing specific about the reaction of orbital tissues to injury. Each constituent (bone, fat, and muscle) reacts to injury in an identical fashion to that in the same type of tissue elsewhere. As has been a recurring theme in discussions of diseases in other parts of the globe and ocular adnexa, an event at one site almost always causes significant consequences for other parts of the globe, such as the following:

1. Accumulation of fluid, cellular exudates, or tumor cells in the orbit, resulting in protrusion of the globe (exophthalmus) with the resulting risk of corneal ulceration secondary to desiccation.
2. Destruction of orbital tissue and loss of fat from emaciation having the opposite effect; the globe sinks into the orbit, creating the risk of secondary entropion and resultant corneal irritation.
3. Injury to extraocular muscles, resulting in abnormal positioning of the globe, thus predisposing the cornea to ulceration from eyelid trauma or desiccation.
4. Significant damage to the function of the lacrimal gland, resulting in injury to the cornea via desiccation.
5. Space-occupying orbital lesions, particularly neoplasms, which may cause injury to the optic nerve and result in blindness.

DISORDERS OF DOMESTIC ANIMALS

ANOMALIES OF THE GLOBE AS A WHOLE

The globe has a complex embryogenesis involving carefully orchestrated interactions of neuroectoderm, surface ectoderm, and periocular mesenchyme throughout embryogenesis and in carnivores into the fifth or sixth week after birth. The opportunity for developmental error is thus substantial. This also means that all developmental errors, especially in carnivores, are not necessarily congenital. Because the globe is not essential for postnatal survival, even severe anomalies are encountered with considerable frequency. Selective breeding practices have increased the frequency of ocular anomalies. Those that are important or prevalent are discussed in sections dealing with diseases of the specific ocular segment affected.

As a general framework for understanding ocular anomalies, they are most conveniently divided into failures of initial induction, failures in remodeling, and late failures in atrophy. Included in this section are only those anomalies in very early induction that affect the eye as a whole. Those lesser anomalies that result from later defects in remodeling or atrophy are discussed in the sections devoted to diseases of the most severely affected components of the eye.

The eye begins very early in gestation as an outgrowth from the primitive forebrain. This primary optic vesicle grows outwardly from the brain toward the overlying surface ectoderm, remaining connected to the brain by the optic stalk. As the primary optic vesicle approaches the overlying ectoderm, it induces a focal thickening in that ectoderm, known as the *lens placode.* The placode thickens, separates from the surface ectoderm, and migrates inwardly to indent the spherical optic vesicle. As the lens pushes into that optic vesicle, the vesicle collapses on itself to form a bilayer optic cup (Fig. 20-82). When the lens vesicle separates from the surface ectoderm, that ectoderm re-forms over the lens and forms the presumptive corneal epithelium. The presence of the epithelium seems to act as a magnet to attract one or more waves of periocular mesenchyme that forms the primitive corneal stroma and endothelium. This periocular mesenchyme is derived from the neural crest and eventually also forms the sclera, the uveal stroma, and a well-developed but transient intraocular network of blood vessels (hyaloid artery and tunica vasculosa lentis) that nourish the developing retina and lens (Fig. 20-83). The eyelids, extraocular muscles, lacrimal gland, and orbit are formed more or less independent of the globe and are generally not affected by those diseases that impair development of the eye itself.

Anophthalmia is a very rare condition in which there is no detectable development even of the primary optic vesicle. It is usually bilateral. The vast majority of the cases clinically diagnosed as "anophthalmia" are in fact severe microphthalmia, and some vestige of a globe is found somewhere within the orbit.

Microphthalmia is the presence of a miniature, disorganized globe in an orbit of relatively normal size. In the great majority of cases, the anomaly does not reflect a primary maldevelopment but rather involution after some type of exogenous injury to a globe that up to that stage was normal in its development. This includes in utero trauma, ischemic injury, and infection. Such globes can be remarkably small; usually it is a tiny pigmented nodule somewhere within the abundant fat and muscle still present within the orbit (Fig. 20-84). Microscopically the most durable and therefore the most recognizable remnants of the previously normal globe are the pigmented ciliary processes. If they are present, then one can be sure that the globe had reached a reasonably advanced state of embryologic development before undergoing regression.

Congenital cystic eye results from the failure of the primary optic vesicle to invaginate under the influence of the developing lens.

Cyclopia and synophthalmia are perceived clinically as a single midline globe and virtually always occur in animals with other major developmental anomalies. They reflect failure of division of the very primitive optic primordium into paired symmetric optic

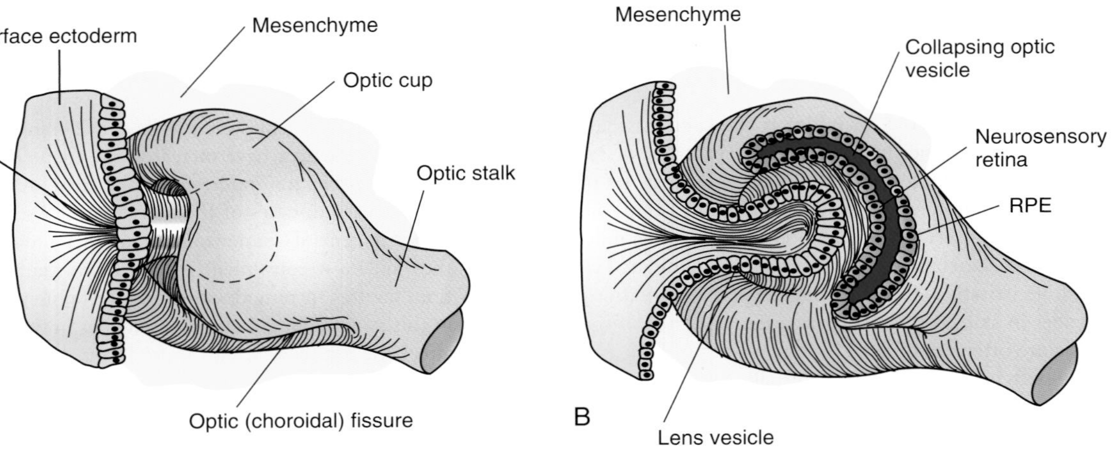

Fig. 20-82 Schematic diagram of the formation of the primary optic vesicle and optic cup.
Note that the optic fissure is present because the optic cup is not yet fused inferiorly. **A,** Formation of lens vesicle and optic cup with inferior choroidal or optic fissure. Mesenchyme surrounds the invaginating lens vesicle. **B,** Surface ectoderm forms the lens vesicle with a hollow interior. Note that the optic cup and optic stalk are of surface ectoderm origin. *RPE,* Retinal pigment epithelium. (From Cook CS, Sulik K, Wright K: Embryology. In Wright KW, ed: *Pediatric ophthalmology and strabismus*, St Louis, 1995, Mosby.)

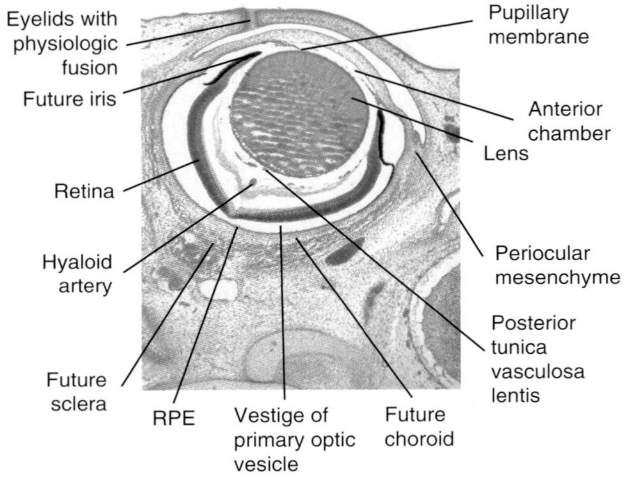

Fig. 20-83 Fetal globe, gestational age day 34, dog.
The periocular mesenchyme is organizing to form the choroid and sclera. The anterior chamber has been formed, but the anterior lip of the optic cup has not yet folded inwardly to induce the formation of the iris and ciliary body. The relatively large lens is surrounded by a rich vascular tunic derived from the hyaloid artery and pupillary membrane. *RPE,* Retinal pigment epithelium. H&E stain. (Courtesy Dr. B. Wilcock, Ontario Veterinary College.)

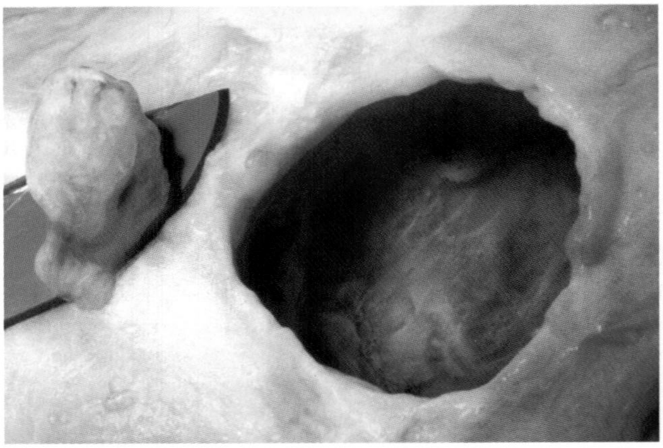

Fig. 20-84 Microphthalmia, globe and orbit, calf.
Note that the orbit *(right)* remains relatively normal, probably indicating that the initial development of the globe was normal and that its current small size *(on the scalpel blade, left)* is a result of in utero injury and subsequent atrophy (indicating so-called secondary microphthalmia rather than a primary failure of ocular development). (Courtesy Dr. B. Wilcock, Ontario Veterinary College.)

stalks and vesicles (or perhaps subsequent fusion), which therefore results in a single midline globe. Most examples have some degree of duplication of intraocular structures, such as the retina or lens, and are properly termed *synophthalmia* (Fig. 20-85). As naturally occurring developmental anomalies, cyclopia and/or synophthalmia are exceedingly rare. However, ewes grazing pastures of the alpine legume *Veratrum californicum* on day 15 of gestation give birth to lambs with this malformation. Ingestion of the plant before day 15 results in fetal death but no anomalies. Ingestion after day 15 results in various skeletal anomalies and cleft palate, but the globes are apparently normal. Similar ocular lesions have been experimentally induced in goats and cattle.

Coloboma is the least severe of the developmental abnormalities affecting the globe as a whole. When used in this context, the term refers to a defect in the closure of the optic fissure, which is a normal channel in the floor of the optic cup that remains open long enough to allow the entry of the blood vessels that form the hyaloid artery and the perilenticular vascular tunic. This fissure normally closes in the last third of gestation, persisting longest near the posterior pole of the globe just ventral to the optic disc. If it persists for too long, there is the possibility that the developing retina will accidentally grow outwardly through this defect (i.e., coloboma) to cause a retrobulbar cyst lined by retinal neuroectoderm (Fig. 20-86). This is a lesion made famous by its occurrence as one of the hallmarks of collie eye anomaly. The same defect occurs sporadically in other breeds of dogs and in horses, cattle, and cats. In Charolais cattle, colobomas at or near the optic disc are inherited as an autosomal dominant trait with incomplete penetrance.

The stepwise closure of the optic fissure appears to be orchestrated by soluble factors released from the retinal pigmented

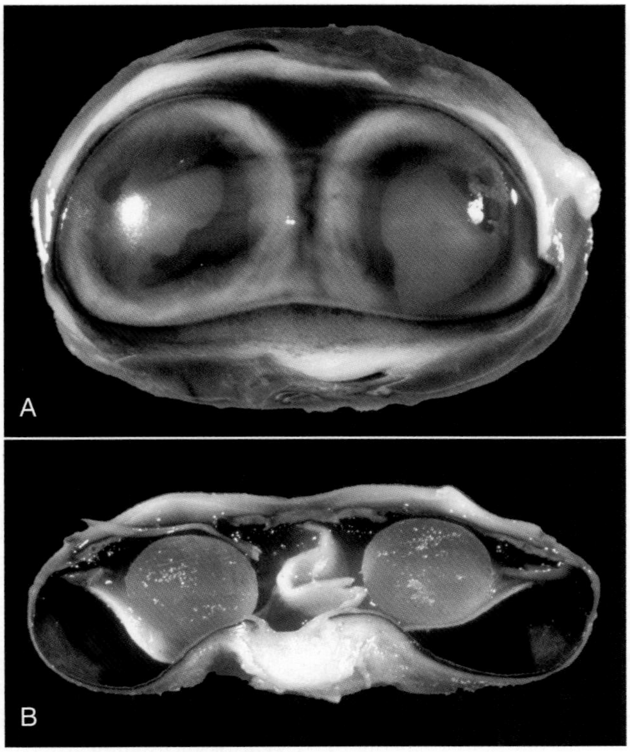

Fig. 20-85 Synophthalmia, globe, calf.
A, This fused globe has two lenses, two corneas, and partial duplication of the retina. **B,** Horizontal section of the fused globe revealing two lenses but a shared fused midline retina. (Courtesy Dr. B. Wilcock, Ontario Veterinary College.)

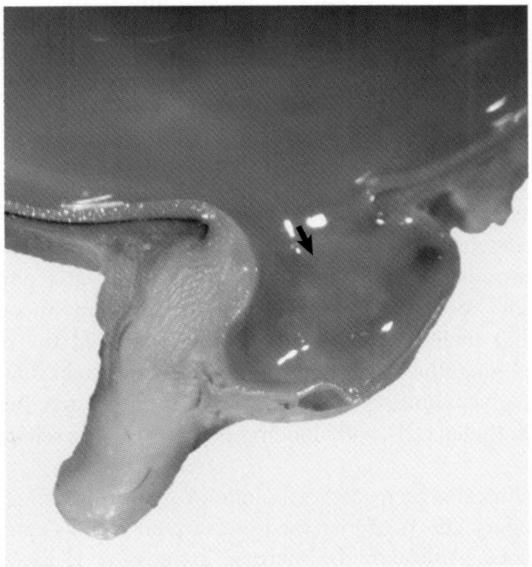

Fig. 20-86 Posterior polar coloboma, collie eye anomaly, globe, sagittal section, dog.
Failure of closure of the most posterior portion of the optic fissure has allowed outpouching *(arrow)* of the developing retina, adjacent to the optic nerve. The protruding retina is covered by sclera. This result has prevented proper local formation of choroid and sclera, resulting in so-called scleral ectasia. Such globes always have choroidal hypoplasia. (Courtesy Dr. B. Wilcock, Ontario Veterinary College.)

epithelium, which is developing from the neuroectoderm of the posterior layer of the primitive optic cup. Because such colobomas are most commonly found in color-dilute animals, we assume that the proper chemical signaling is somehow related to the proper acquisition of pigment (or pigment-producing capability) by this neuroectoderm (see later section on Choroidal Hypoplasia).

DISEASES OF THE GLOBE AS A WHOLE

Glaucoma

Glaucoma is not a single disease but a group of diseases sharing specific physiologic and structural characteristics. It is a clinical syndrome characterized by a sustained increase in intraocular fluid pressure that is detrimental to the health of the optic nerve and the retina, resulting in loss of vision and eventual blindness. Glaucoma causes changes in virtually every tissue within the globe, but changes in the retina and optic nerve are the most important. The syndrome is most prevalent in dogs, followed by cats and horses. It is rarely documented in other species but undoubtedly exists in all. Glaucoma is extremely prevalent as a cause for ocular pain and blindness in dogs, and it is by far the leading reason for surgical removal of the globe (enucleation). It is relatively less common in cats, yet it is still the leading cause for enucleation in that species. Its frequency in horses may be greatly underestimated because of its variable clinical presentation in that species and because ocular pressure is not routinely measured in horses.

Theoretically, glaucoma may result from an increase in the production of aqueous humor or a decrease in its removal. In practical terms, however, all examples of glaucoma in domestic animals result from impairment of aqueous outflow. Glaucoma is usually divided into primary and secondary glaucoma. Primary glaucoma refers to those examples occurring without any known acquired intraocular disease to explain the increase in pressure. The great majority of these result from developmental errors in the structure and function of the aqueous drainage pathways. Secondary glaucoma refers to those examples in which there are changes, such as lens luxation, pupillary block, or intraocular neoplasia, to explain the impairment of aqueous humor outflow.

The aqueous humor that fills the anterior and posterior chambers is a low-protein transparent fluid just slightly denser than water. It is formed continuously by a combination of plasma filtration and active secretion by ciliary epithelium. Its chemical composition varies somewhat among species, but it always has a very low total protein concentration (about 5% of total plasma protein) but an amino acid concentration 50% higher than that of plasma. It contains glucose and electrolytes in concentrations roughly equivalent to those in plasma. The aqueous humor produced within the ciliary body circulates past the lens to provide nutrients to it and remove waste products, enters the anterior chamber through the pupil, circulates within the anterior chamber to nourish corneal endothelium and stroma, and then exits through slitlike spaces at the junction between peripheral cornea and iris. This iridocorneal angle extends circumferentially around the globe and normally has tremendous reserve capacity to accommodate fluctuations in aqueous production and to provide a substantial margin of safety against the development of glaucoma secondary to partial blockage of the aqueous outflow by accumulations of blood or inflammatory debris.

The maintenance of intraocular fluid pressure is a balance between aqueous production and outflow and in domestic animals is influenced primarily by resistance to outflow. The rate of production varies from 2.5 μl per minute in dogs to 15 μl per minute in cats. The outflow pathway is through the iridocorneal angle and more specifically through a series of perforations in the connective tissue

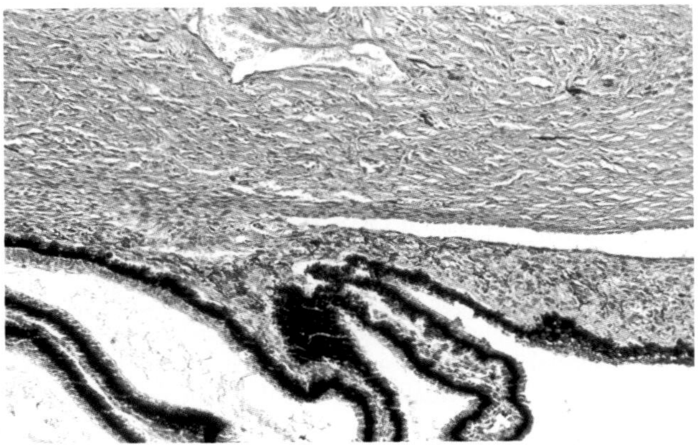

Fig. 20-87 Normal neonatal globe, immature ciliary cleft, trabecular meshwork and iris stroma, dog.
The trabecular meshwork will develop by rarefaction and remodeling of this ciliary cleft over a period of a few weeks during normal maturation. H&E stain. (Courtesy Dr. B. Wilcock, Ontario Veterinary College.)

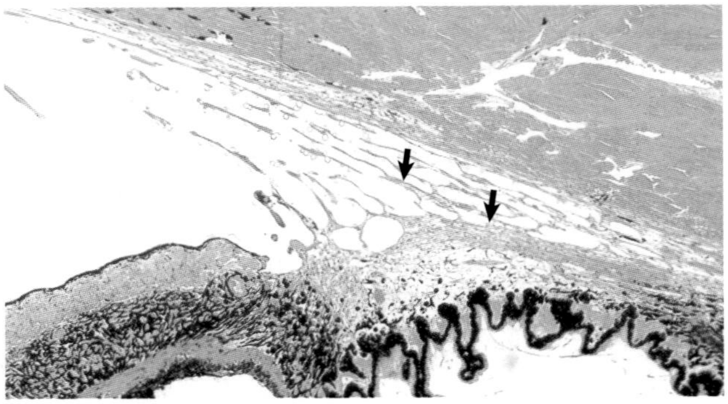

Fig. 20-88 Normal adult ciliary cleft, trabecular meshwork and other portions of the drainage pathway, cat.
The *arrows* indicate the predominant pathway for aqueous outflow in carnivores. H&E stain. (Courtesy Dr. B. Wilcock, Ontario Veterinary College.)

of the peripheral cornea, sclera, and iris stroma that makes up the trabecular meshwork. The microscopic anatomy of this outflow pathway varies by species, but all examples are quite similar in general design.

The trabecular meshwork is a series of mesenchymal sieves that occupies the iridocorneal angle and extends circumferentially around the globe. Embryologically, the trabecular meshwork is formed by rarefaction of the same mesenchyme that forms iris stroma. In carnivores this remodeling continues for several weeks after birth (Fig. 20-87). This area of perforated mesenchyme is referred to as the *ciliary cleft.* It is bordered externally by sclera, posteriorly by the muscles of the ciliary body, and internally by the iris stroma. Its anterior border, separating it from the anterior chamber, is formed by the pectinate ligament. With proper instrumentation (gonioscopy), the pectinate ligament is visible through the cornea as a series of cobweb-like branching cords (carnivores) or a fenestrated sheet (ungulates), stretching from the termination of Descemet's membrane to the anterior portion of the iris root (Fig. 20-88).

Ultrastructurally, the trabecular meshwork is a series of connective tissue beams covered (completely or incompletely, depending on the species) by a single layer of trabecular endothelial cells connected to each other by delicate cytoplasmic tendrils. The cells are phagocytic and are probably important in regulating the outflow of aqueous humor. Most of that flow is probably by transcellular movement of pinocytotic vesicles across the cytoplasm of the trabecular endothelium.

In most species, the most functionally significant portion of the trabecular meshwork exists in the deep peripheral corneal stroma and inner sclera, and is known as the corneoscleral meshwork. Aqueous humor passing through this portion of the meshwork then enters a network of large veins, known as the *scleral venous plexus,* which is embedded in the peripheral sclera. The aqueous humor entering these veins is then returned to the systemic circulation. A small percentage of the aqueous humor entering the filtration angle will exit via a more posterior route known as the uveoscleral meshwork, percolating into the veins of the ciliary body and choroid rather than into the scleral venous plexus (see Fig. 20-88). The proportion of aqueous humor leaving the globe by this more posterior route varies by species: 3% in cats, 15% in dogs, and a larger (but undetermined) percentage in horses. Differences in the proportion of fluid leaving the globe by different routes might explain differing susceptibilities to different types of glaucoma among the domestic animals, and it also creates at least the potential for different types of therapeutic interventions.

These outflow pathways are not just passive conduits through which the aqueous humor can flow. There is an important physiologic resistance to outflow responsible for the maintenance of normal intraocular pressure. The exact anatomic and physiologic constituents of this outflow resistance remain incompletely defined but include important contributions from the endothelial cells lining the collagen beams within the trabecular meshwork, the glycosaminoglycans embedded in the matrix supporting those endothelial cells, and blood pressure within the scleral venous plexus.

The clinical (macroscopic) lesions of glaucoma are related to the secondary effects of increased pressure on various components of the globe. Although the increase in pressure is the result of obstruction of outflow in the anterior chamber, the pressure elevation is distributed throughout the fluid medium of the globe, and the effects are thus felt by all parts of the globe. These effects are the same, regardless of the pathogenesis of the glaucoma, and they vary with the rapidity of onset, the magnitude of the pressure elevation, and the duration of the elevation. They are also influenced by the age of the patient and by the species. The most obvious of the macroscopic changes include ocular enlargement, corneal cloudiness because of edema, pupillary dilation, and excavation of the optic disc. The most frequent microscopic changes in glaucoma are listed in Box 20-13.

BOX 20-13 The Most Frequent Histologic Lesions in Glaucoma

Atrophy of the nerve fiber layer and ganglion cell layer of the retina
Loss of neurons from the inner nuclear layer
Collapse of the trabecular meshwork
Corneal edema
Cataracts
Optic nerve atrophy
Optic disc cupping
Atrophy of ciliary processes
Corneal striae

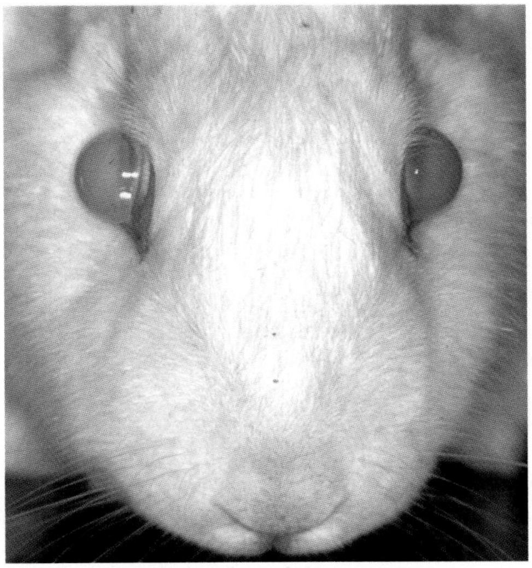

Fig. 20-89 **Bilateral primary glaucoma (inherited), eye, rabbit.** The eyes are protruding and have diffuse gray corneal opacity typical of edema. Distinguishing ocular enlargement caused by glaucoma from exophthalmos caused by a retrobulbar mass is based on clinical assessment of intraocular pressure, the ability to push the globe more deeply into the orbit (retropulsion), and the presence or absence of an orbital mass as detected by radiography or other imaging techniques. (Courtesy Dr. B. Wilcock, Ontario Veterinary College.)

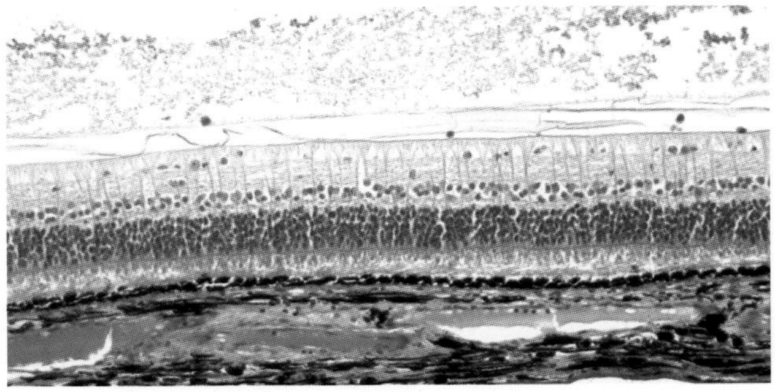

Fig. 20-90 **Retinal atrophy, glaucoma, retina, horse.** There is loss of density in the nerve fiber layer and loss of virtually all the ganglion cells *(top),* but excellent preservation of the outer nuclear layer and photoreceptors. Retinal microscopic changes in glaucoma vary with its severity and duration and with the species affected. H&E stain. (Courtesy Dr. B. Wilcock, Ontario Veterinary College.)

Morphologic Changes Secondary to Glaucoma

Buphthalmos (megaloglobus) is stretching of the globe secondary to increased intraocular pressure. It is most obvious in dogs and least obvious in horses (Fig. 20-89). Histologically the sclera becomes thin, and the anterior chamber increases in its anterior-posterior dimension. The enlargement is significant because it probably causes pain, and it prevents the eyelids from closing over the cornea, thus resulting in corneal desiccation, which can lead to either corneal cutaneous metaplasia or ulceration (depending on the speed of onset and the severity of the desiccation).

Corneal edema develops when the aqueous pressure exceeds the ability of the sodium pump within the corneal endothelium (in dogs, at about 40 mm Hg). More severe corneal edema then develops as a result of pressure-induced injury to that endothelium and that injury may become permanent if the endothelial injury is so extensive that it exceeds the capacity of the corneal endothelium to repair itself by sliding, usually when there is a loss of more than 50% of corneal endothelial cells. Corneal edema secondary to glaucoma is much more frequent in dogs than in cats for reasons that remain unclear.

Corneal striae are breaks in Descemet's membrane occurring secondary to corneal stretching. They are visible on clinical examination as serpentine tracts of deep corneal stromal opacity.

Atrophy of the iris and ciliary processes occurs late in the course of glaucoma, probably as a consequence of chronic pressure-induced ischemia. Atrophy of the iris causes the initial physiologic pupillary dilation typical of glaucoma to become permanent. Atrophy of the ciliary processes eventually leads to normalization of intraocular pressure and even eventual hypotony, seen as part of very endstage glaucoma.

Cataracts are common in glaucoma, presumably as a result of the stagnation of aqueous flow that results in inadequate delivery of nutrients to and impaired removal of metabolic waste products from the lens.

Lens luxation probably results from stretching of the zonules secondary to ocular enlargement. Pressure-induced degenerative change in the zonules is another possibility. The luxation may be into the anterior chamber or into the posterior chamber. Luxation into the posterior chamber requires that the vitreous has already liquefied. Such vitreal liquefaction is a common sequela to inflammation that may have preceded the glaucoma, and it also occurs as a sequela to the glaucoma itself. In globes with vitreal liquefaction, whether the dislocated lens moves anteriorly or posteriorly seems to be just a matter of chance.

Retinal degeneration is the most important secondary change in glaucoma and is the one against which most therapeutic efforts are directed. It is very important because it causes blindness as a result of damage to the ganglion cells, which cannot regenerate, even if the glaucoma is eventually brought under control. The exact pathogenesis for the characteristic retinal and optic nerve changes probably varies among species and among different types of glaucoma. At least some of the contributing factors include the following:

1. Pressure-induced ischemic damage after collapse of blood vessels in the retina, optic nerve, or choroid in response to increased pressure in the vitreous.
2. Interference with ganglion cell nutrition by impairment of axoplasmic flow caused by pressure-induced compression of the axons passing through the lamina cribrosa.
3. Direct damage to ganglion cells by elevated local production of excitatory amino acids, notably glutamate, from injured optic nerve and retina.

The degeneration characteristically causes atrophy of the nerve fiber layer and ganglion cells, and later loss of neurons from the inner nuclear layer. The hardy astrocytes within the inner nuclear layer (Müller cells) remain intact. In classic glaucomatous retinal atrophy, the outer nuclear layer and photoreceptors remain unaffected for years (Fig. 20-90). This pattern of "inner retinal atrophy" with sparing of the outer nuclear layer and photoreceptors is virtually unique to glaucoma (remembering that inherited, nutritional, and toxic retinopathies all target photoreceptors). In dogs with high-pressure glaucoma, however, it is common to also see destruction even of outer portions of the retina. Such destruction sometimes occurs quite quickly, presumably in response to pressure-induced collapse of the superficial choroidal blood vessels (choriocapillaris) responsible for the nutrition of the photoreceptors and outer nuclear layer. In such cases, there is also necrosis of RPE.

Optic nerve changes are among the most controversial lesions seen in glaucoma. Much of the controversy centers on whether the

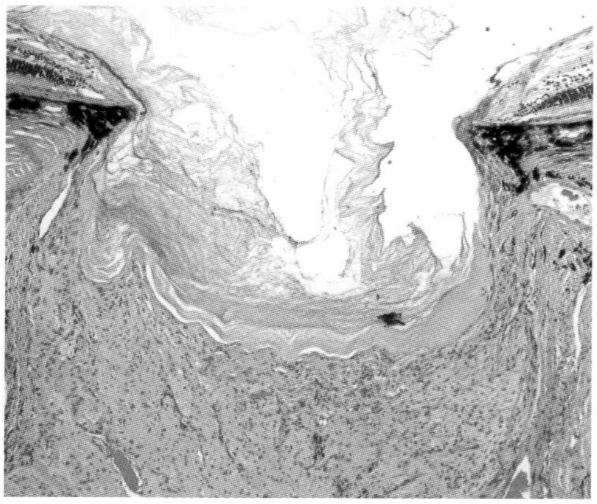

Fig. 20-91 Cupping of the optic disc, glaucoma, eye, dog. The exact pathogenesis for the cupping in response to increased intraocular pressure probably involves many mechanisms and varies from species to species and among the different types of glaucoma. H&E stain. (Courtesy Dr. B. Wilcock, Ontario Veterinary College.)

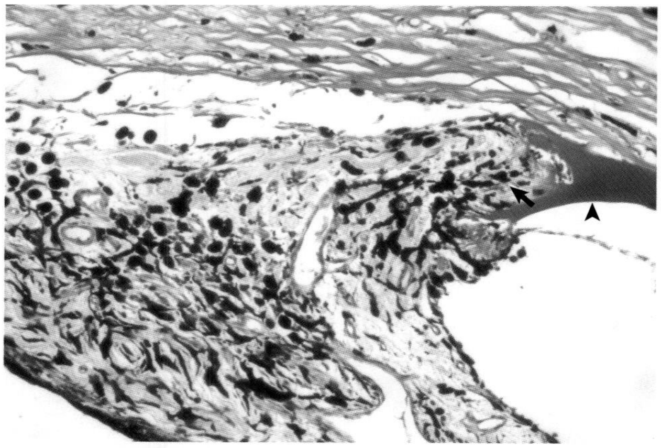

Fig. 20-92 Goniodysgenesis, primary glaucoma, dog. Note the absence of a normal pectinate ligament. Descemet's membrane *(arrowhead)* inserts directly into a broad band of stroma *(arrow)* continuous with the iris stroma. The rest of the trabecular meshwork is microscopically normal. Periodic acid–Schiff reaction. (Courtesy Dr. B. Wilcock, Ontario Veterinary College.)

optic nerve changes are just a consequence of glaucoma or whether they can occur independently of the pressure changes. The answer probably varies with the species and with the type of glaucoma under consideration. The situation is greatly confused by incautious extrapolation of the results from human glaucoma research. Glaucoma in humans is substantially different from that seen in most of our domestic animals. Microscopic changes in the optic nerve include degeneration of axons (Wallerian degeneration) and astrogliosis secondary to the loss of the ganglion cells and pressure-induced posterior displacement of the lamina cribrosa. Optic disc cupping is almost pathognomonic for glaucoma. It may occur very quickly as a result of pressure-induced posterior displacement of the lamina cribrosa or more slowly as a result of atrophy of the optic nerve itself from the loss of axons (Fig. 20-91).

The Classification of Glaucoma

Primary Glaucoma

Primary glaucomas are those glaucomas occurring without any significant contribution from disease elsewhere within the globe. Primary glaucomas are subdivided into those cases in which there is detectable maldevelopment of the trabecular meshwork (goniodysgenesis) and those cases in which there are no primary histologic lesions (open-angle glaucoma). A very small proportion of these are truly congenital glaucomas in which clinical signs of glaucoma are evident in the first few weeks of life. The vast majority, however, have no clinically detectable increase in pressure or clinical signs related to glaucoma until middle-age or even older. The reasons for this delay in clinical onset are unknown.

Goniodysgenesis

Goniodysgenesis is a general term denoting imperfect development of the trabecular meshwork. It reflects incomplete remodeling of the solid mass of anterior chamber mesenchyme that gives rise to the stroma of the cornea and anterior uvea. In carnivores, most of this remodeling occurs in the first few weeks of life and involves rarefaction of what was previously a solid mesenchymal mass. In truly congenital glaucoma, there may be virtually no rarefaction (so-called trabecular hypoplasia), but in the great majority of cases there is reasonably complete development of the trabecular meshwork and other portions of the drainage system. The most common histologic anomaly is failure of the most anterior portion

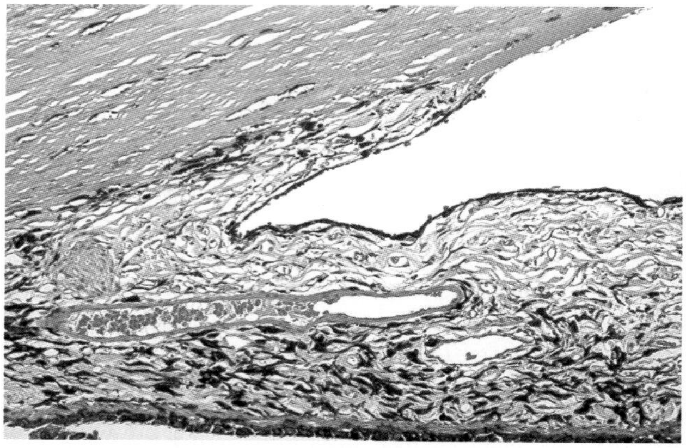

Fig. 20-93 Goniodysgenesis, primary glaucoma, dog. Note the almost complete hypoplasia of the trabecular meshwork, the result of a profound arrest in remodeling of the mesenchyme within the ciliary cleft. H&E stain. (Courtesy Dr. B. Wilcock, Ontario Veterinary College.)

of the trabecular meshwork to be adequately remodeled, resulting in what looks like an abnormal solid or imperforate pectinate ligament (Figs. 20-92 and 20-93). The majority occurs as inherited disease in purebred dogs, with at least 20 different breeds known to be affected. The correlation between the severity of the goniodysgenesis and the frequency of glaucoma varies among breeds. It is sometimes quite poor, suggesting that there are other factors, perhaps functional rather than morphologic, involved in the pathogenesis of glaucoma.

The reasons for the delay in the onset of clinical signs of glaucoma, often for 5 years or more, are poorly understood. There may be age-related changes in the composition of trabecular meshwork matrix components or in lens position that result in a small decrease in aqueous outflow. Such minor decreases would normally be insignificant, but they may be critical to a dog that already has impaired aqueous drainage. Alternatively, acquired changes, such as preiridal fibrovascular membrane or minor cellular infiltrates associated with a normally insignificant uveitis, might provide the "final straw" that triggers glaucoma in these predisposed individuals. There is no reason to presume that the triggering events are the same in each individual.

Primary open-angle glaucoma

Some examples of primary glaucoma in dogs, cats, and horses occur in globes in which there is no visible abnormality in the structure of the trabecular meshwork or other portions of the aqueous outflow pathways. The best known is open-angle glaucoma in beagles. It has been widely used as a laboratory model, but its frequency outside of the laboratory appears to be very low. These dogs develop increased intraocular pressure by about a year of age but usually do not have clinical signs of glaucoma (such as conjunctival congestion, corneal edema, and pupillary dilation) until they are between 2 and 4 years of age. In the early stages of glaucoma, all portions of the aqueous outflow pathways are histologically and ultrastructurally normal.

Secondary Glaucoma

Anything capable of obstructing the flow of aqueous through the pupil or its exit through the trabecular meshwork can cause secondary glaucoma. The most common are listed next more or less in the order of frequency in dogs, the species in which glaucoma is by far the most prevalent. These mechanisms are not mutually exclusive, and frequently several different mechanisms act together to produce glaucoma. It is also undoubtedly true that dogs with goniodysgenesis are particularly prone to the development of secondary glaucoma, even when the degree of pupillary or trabecular occlusion is less than would be required to produce glaucoma in normal dogs.

Pupillary block

The passage of aqueous through the pupil may be blocked by the anterior movement of the vitreous after primary anterior lens luxation by posterior synechiae as a sequela to fibrinous iridocorneal adhesions or by extension of a preiridal fibrovascular membrane (Fig. 20-94). Blockage may also occur from migration and fibroblastic metaplasia of lens epithelium that has been freed by rupture of the lens capsule or by massive swelling of the lens in what is known as intumescent cataract (Fig. 20-95). Displacement of the lens into the posterior chamber (posterior lens luxation) does not result in prolapse of the vitreous or in glaucoma.

Trabecular occlusion

The trabecular meshwork extends the full circumference around the iridocorneal angle, and no one is sure how much occlusion is required to produce glaucoma. The general consensus among ophthalmologists is that it must be at least 80%. The most common causes for this type of diffuse occlusion are infiltration by neoplastic cells (Fig. 20-96 and Box 20-14), peripheral iridocorneal adhesions by preiridal fibrovascular membranes (Fig. 20-97), or mechanical compression of the base of the iris by intumescent cataract or by large posterior chamber neoplasms. The tumors that most frequently cause glaucoma by infiltration of the trabecular meshwork are anterior uveal melanocytoma and metastatic lymphoma in dogs and diffuse iris melanoma and metastatic lymphoma in cats. Glaucoma caused by compression of the base of the iris is less frequent because it requires a very large tumor to cause the nearly circumferential occlusion. Only anterior uveal melanocytomas in dogs are likely to fulfill this requirement.

Very occasionally, glaucoma is caused by the occlusion of the trabecular meshwork by particulate material such as erythrocytes or leukocytes. It might seem that such occlusion would be prevalent,

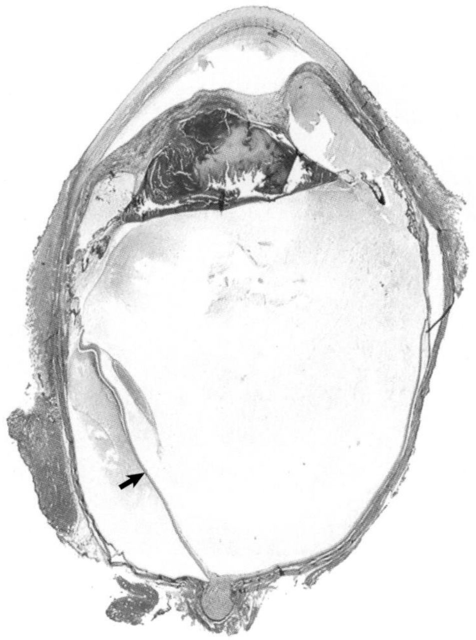

Fig. 20-94 Secondary glaucoma (from posterior synechia), iris bombé and peripheral anterior synechia, globe, sagittal section, dog.
The original injury was a penetrating wound of the cornea that caused phacoclastic uveitis. The inflamed iris adhered to the ruptured lens, causing a pupillary block and then iris bombé. The anterior displacement of the iris resulted in narrowing of the iridocorneal angle, in this case with adhesion of the base of the iris to the peripheral cornea (peripheral anterior synechia). Note the retinal detachment *(arrow)* and the abnormal shape of the lens (the latter resulting from loss of lens material at the time of perforation). Masson trichrome stain. (Courtesy Dr. B. Wilcock, Ontario Veterinary College.)

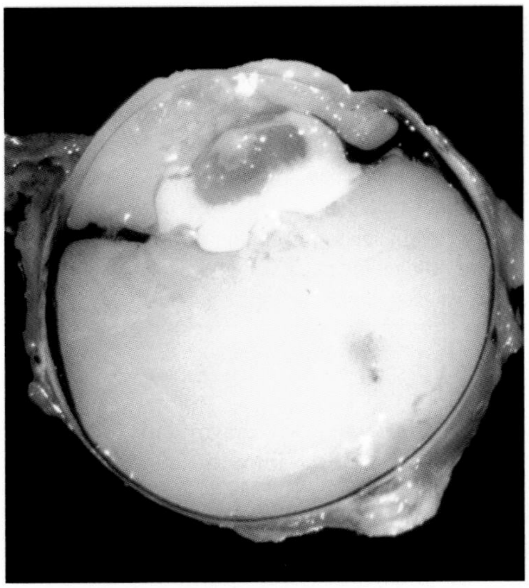

Fig. 20-95 Secondary glaucoma (from intumescent cataract), globe, sagittal section, dog.
Hydropic swelling of the lens (intumescent cataract) secondary to diabetes mellitus has caused the iris to be compressed against the peripheral cornea, resulting in a functional peripheral anterior synechia and a secondary glaucoma. The lens has subsequently ruptured, triggering a phacoclastic uveitis that explains the coagulated protein visible within the lens and ocular chambers. (Courtesy Dr. B. Wilcock, Ontario Veterinary College.)

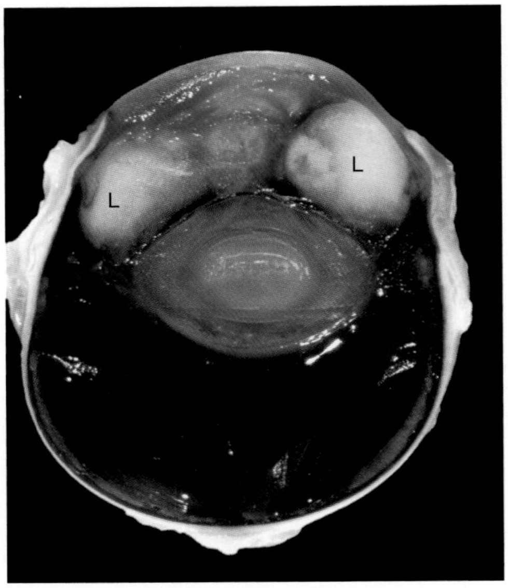

Fig. 20-96 Secondary glaucoma (from metastatic lymphoma), globe, sagittal section, dog.
The trabecular meshwork has been occluded by metastatic lymphoma *(L)* within the anterior uvea and anterior chamber. (Courtesy Dr. B. Wilcock, Ontario Veterinary College.)

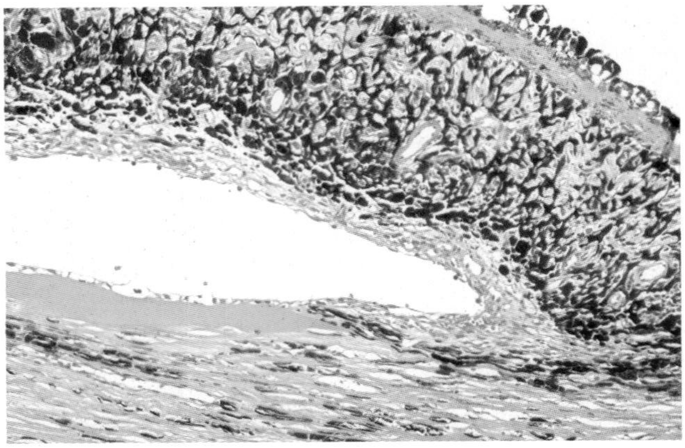

Fig. 20-97 Secondary glaucoma (from preiridal fibrovascular membrane), globe, sagittal section, dog.
The mature membrane has grown across the anterior surface of the pectinate ligament, creating peripheral anterior synechia. The trigger for the formation of the preiridal fibrovascular membrane was a small, otherwise insignificant iridociliary adenoma (not visible here). H&E stain. (Courtesy Dr. B. Wilcock, Ontario Veterinary College.)

BOX 20-14 How Intraocular Neoplasms Cause Glaucoma

Direct infiltration of the trabecular meshwork
- Feline diffuse iris melanoma
- Canine anterior uveal melanocytoma

Production of angiogenic growth factors that cause a preiridal fibrovascular membrane leading to pupillary block and/or trabecular occlusion
- Iridociliary adenoma/adenocarcinoma

Triggering of intraocular inflammation with posterior synechia and pupillary block or serous choroidal effusion with retinal detachment and preiridal fibrovascular membrane
- Metastatic carcinomas
- Malignant lymphoma

Primary intraocular neoplasms, with the exception of feline ocular sarcoma, have little metastatic risk and usually become medically significant by causing glaucoma.

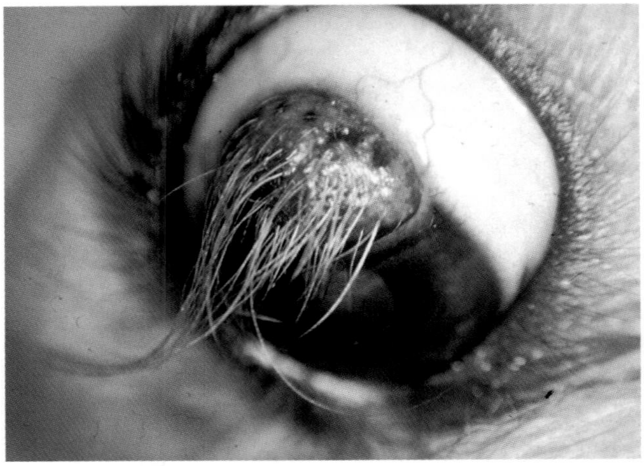

Fig. 20-98 Dermoid, cornea, dog.
A plaque of haired skin exists in place of the normal peripheral cornea. What triggers the failure of normal corneal maturation from pluripotential fetal ectoderm is unknown. Its clinical significance depends on how much corneal irritation is caused by the hair. Such dermoids may arise in cornea or, more commonly, bulbar conjunctiva. (Courtesy Dr. B. Wilcock, Ontario Veterinary College.)

but such material usually settles by gravity and temporarily occludes only the ventral portion of the filtration angle.

DISEASES OF THE CORNEA

Corneal Anomalies

Dermoid

Dermoid is the only corneal anomaly that is reasonably prevalent. It reflects the failure of the fetal ectoderm to undergo complete corneal "metaplasia," with the result that a portion of the cornea remains as skin. Clinically, it is visible as a focus of corneal opacity in which there is hair and histologically as a segment of cornea that is more or less identical to normal skin (Fig. 20-98). The degree of skinlike change varies from complete development of skin and hair follicles to a less extreme version in which only vestigial hair follicles are present.

Acquired Corneal Diseases

Superficial Stromal Sequestration/Canine Persistent Ulcer

In dogs, cats, and horses (and probably in other species), there is a syndrome in which injury to the corneal epithelium is followed by an increased amount of superficial stromal apoptosis above the small amount that normally follows any corneal epithelial injury. In dogs and horses, this results in an inability of the sliding corneal epithelium to properly adhere to the underlying stroma, which is a prerequisite for full epithelial regeneration. Initially, adhesion of the sliding epithelium is to fibronectin and other transient adhesion molecules, but permanent adhesion requires the reformation of basement membrane, hemidesmosomes, and hemidesmosomal anchoring filaments, which extend through the basement membrane to anchor into the superficial stroma. If that stroma is

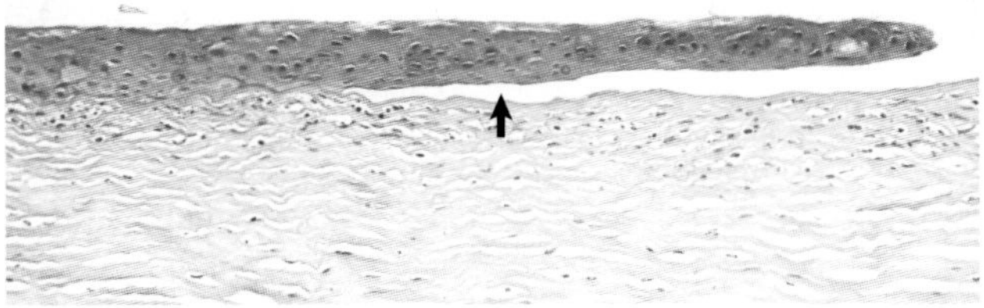

Fig. 20-99 Persistent ulcer, cornea, dog.
The epithelium is thickened and disorganized and has failed to adhere *(arrow)* to the adjacent corneal stroma. This failure of adhesion results in ineffective wound healing, seen clinically as either persistent or repeated ulceration. The failure of epithelial adhesion probably occurs because the hemidesmosomal anchoring filaments are unable to "anchor" in the injured stroma. H&E stain. (Courtesy Dr. B. Wilcock, Ontario Veterinary College.)

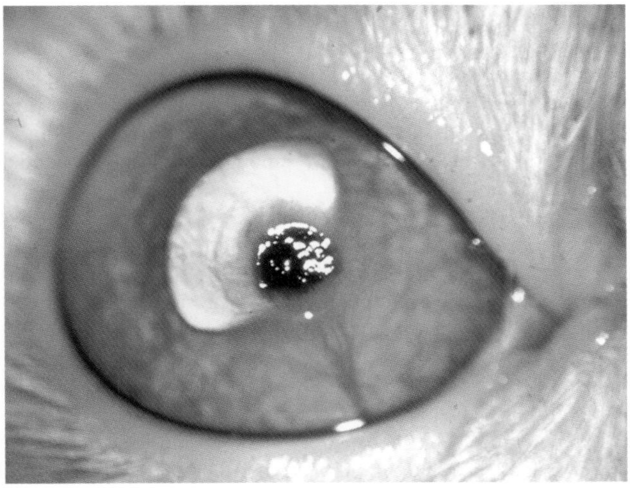

Fig. 20-100 Corneal sequestrum, cornea, cat.
The axial corneal ulcer has been accentuated by the absorption of a brown pigment, probably derived from porphyrins in the tear film. The gray halo of corneal edema and the prominent vascular ingrowth from the limbus to the edge of the ulcer are frequent but inconsistent features. (Courtesy Dr. M. Zigler, Mississauga-Oakville Veterinary Emergency Clinic.)

abnormal, these filaments cannot grip and the regenerating epithelium is easily swept away with even the mildest trauma (Fig. 20-99). The cause for the excessive amount and/or persistence of the superficial stromal degeneration is not known. The most effective therapy is to surgically remove the superficial stroma (i.e., superficial keratectomy) to permit the epithelium to anchor into the normal deeper stroma.

In cats, the magnitude of the stromal devitalization is much greater, and there is imbibition of brown-colored pigment (thought to be derived from porphyrins in the tear film) into the dead stroma. This results in a very characteristic central corneal dark brown pigmentation that is the predominant and essentially pathognomonic feature of this disease (Figs. 20-100 and 20-101). The overlying epithelium may be ulcerated as it is in dogs or horses, but in many cases, it re-forms over the surface of the dead stroma. The frequency of this disease is much higher in those breeds with flat faces and prominent eyes, such as Persians and Himalayans, presumably because these eyes are predisposed to desiccation and other types of mechanical corneal injury. In non-Persian breeds with normal facial configuration, there is some evidence that ulceration caused by the herpesvirus is the most common predisposing cause.

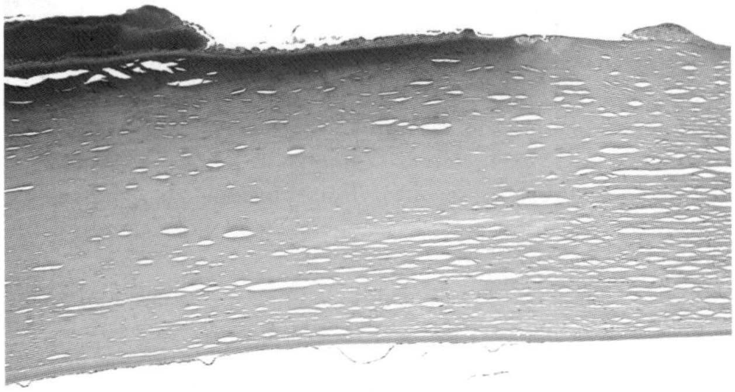

Fig. 20-101 Corneal sequestrum, cornea, cat.
Note the complete loss of epithelium on the right two thirds of the cornea (ulcer) and the necrosis of the remaining epithelium *(left third)*. The stroma under the ulcer is necrotic (deeper eosinophilic) to a depth of approximately half the thickness of the cornea. The necrotic epithelium, the thickened basement membrane, and some of the necrotic stroma are accentuated by brown porphyrin pigment from the tears. Corneal sequestra also occur in the dog and horse, but they do not become pigmented. H&E stain. (Courtesy Dr. B. Wilcock, Ontario Veterinary College.)

Suppurative Keratomalacia ("Melting Ulcer")

Ulcers that become contaminated with bacteria or fungi are prone to suppurative destructive keratomalacia. Most of the stromal dissolution is probably the result of bystander injury from neutrophils recruited because of infection, but part of the damage may be associated with proteases of bacterial or fungal origin. Pseudomonas and streptococcus are the bacteria most likely to cause suppurative keratomalacia, which sometimes rapidly progresses to descemetocele and corneal perforation (see Fig. 20-62). Contamination by opportunistic hyphal fungi (especially *Aspergillus* spp.) is a particularly frequent cause of keratomalacia in horses (see Equine Keratomycosis).

Infectious Bovine Keratoconjunctivitis

See the discussion on infectious bovine keratoconjunctivitis in the section on Disorders of Ruminants.

Feline Herpetic Keratitis

See the discussion on feline herpetic keratitis in the section on Disorders of Cats.

Eosinophilic Keratitis

See the discussion on eosinophilic keratitis in the section on Disorders of Cats.

Canine Pannus Keratitis (Chronic Superficial Keratitis, Uberreiter's Syndrome)

See the discussion on canine pannus keratitis in the section on Disorders of Dogs.

Equine Keratomycosis

See the discussion on equine keratomycosis in the section on Disorders of Horses.

Corneal Dystrophies and Depositions

Macroscopic examination of the cornea often reveals various types of colored or refractile stromal deposits. Some of these have already been discussed (superficial stromal pigmentation as part of cutaneous metaplasia or accumulation of leukocytes as part of stromal inflammation). Most other corneal deposits are composed of lipid and/or mineral. Among the domestic animals, they are most often seen in dogs. These deposits generally have characteristic clinical features (breed, age, exact anatomic location, and macroscopic appearance) that allow a diagnosis to be made without the need for histopathologic examination. They fall into two broad categories: inborn errors of metabolism known as *corneal dystrophies* and *acquired corneal deposits,* resulting from previous corneal disease or as incidental manifestations of systemic metabolic abnormalities that have "overflowed" into the cornea.

Genetically conditioned canine corneal stromal dystrophies include a seemingly endless array of lipid or mineral deposits somewhere within the corneal stroma. By definition, the defect is bilateral and congenital, even though the clinical or histologic manifestation of the abnormality may not be visible until later in life. The list of affected breeds grows daily. In each breed, the location, clinical character, and progression of the lesion are characteristic. In many, the exact nature of the deposit has not been characterized, but cholesterol, phospholipid, or lipid-calcium complexes, either alone or in combination, have been identified in some.

Corneal endothelial dystrophy is seen in several breeds of dogs as bilateral, diffuse corneal edema secondary to the progressive destruction of corneal endothelial cells. The edema is not accompanied by any evidence of inflammation or stromal fibrosis (Fig. 20-102) and usually begins at the lateral peripheral cornea and progresses over months-to-years to create diffuse edema. The microscopic lesion is extremely difficult to see because the corneal endothelial cells are generally not well preserved in histologic sections. Scanning electron microscopy and other specialized techniques demonstrate a progressive decrease in the number of corneal endothelial cells over time. The exact pathogenesis remains unknown.

Acquired corneal lipidosis (lipid keratopathy) results in milky or crystallin stromal deposits of serum lipids within the corneal stroma. The location depends on the pathogenesis. Any animal with an excessively high serum lipid concentration is predisposed to the deposition of neutral fat and cholesterol within the peripheral corneal stroma, reflecting an overflow from the limbal blood vessels. The lipid deposits become greatly accentuated if there is corneal inflammation because vascularization is increased and immature blood vessels are notoriously leaky.

The microscopic changes associated with corneal lipid deposition include the presence of the lipid material and variable degrees of reaction to those deposits. Stromal keratocytes may accumulate small lipid vacuoles, and clefts of cholesterol are usually found among the stromal fibers. In some cases there is virtually no inflammatory reaction, whereas in other dogs there is a well-developed granulomatous inflammatory reaction.

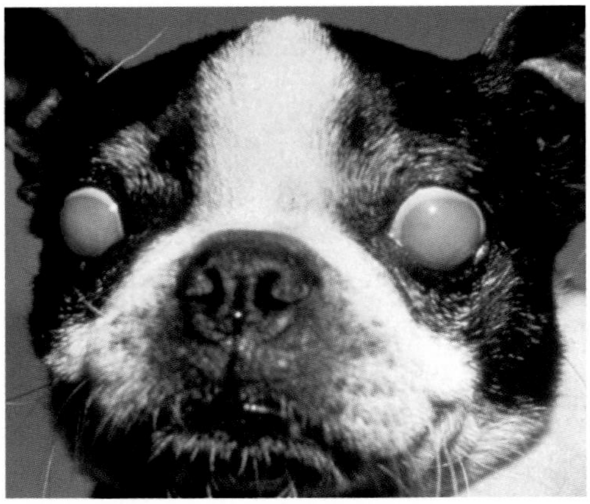

Fig. 20-102 Corneal endothelial dystrophy (inherited), cornea, Boston terrier, dog.

The blue-gray appearance of the corneas is due to severe diffuse corneal edema. The edema is secondary to progressive loss of corneal endothelial cells. The pathogenesis of this loss is unknown, but because these cells are critical in regulating the movement of water and electrolytes from the aqueous humor into the corneal stroma, their loss results in passive absorption of water into the cornea from the aqueous humor. (Courtesy Dr. M. Nasisse, Carolina Veterinary Specialists.)

DISEASES OF THE UVEA

Uveal Anomalies

The epithelium on the posterior surface of the iris, the inner surface of the ciliary body, and the retinal pigment epithelium on the inner surface of the choroid are all derived from portions of the original optic vesicle. The bulk of the uvea is fibrovascular stroma derived from the periocular mesenchyme that originates from the neural crest (see Fig. 20-83). After outgrowth and later invagination of the primary optic vesicle to form the optic cup, the intraocular migration of this mesenchyme and its subsequent remodeling seem to be guided by soluble factors released from the neuroectoderm; failures of proper induction, remodeling, and eventual atrophy of portions of this mesenchyme are among the most prevalent of ocular anomalies.

The anomalies of the uveal tract can be divided into those resulting from a failure of initial induction or migration, a failure of later remodeling, or a failure of eventual atrophy (Table 20-3). During early embryogenesis, there is a persistent gap between the anterior lip of the optic cup and the overlying corneal epithelium. Several waves of periocular mesenchyme migrate through this gap to form the corneal stroma and endothelium, the stroma of the anterior uvea, and the anterior portion of the perilenticular vascular tunic. The ingrowth of mesenchyme to form the iris stroma is guided by the infolding of the most anterior margin of the optic cup, which will form the two layers of the future iris epithelium. Later, papillary proliferation of that iris epithelium gives rise to the epithelium of the ciliary processes. Proper inward migration of the neuroectoderm at the anterior lip of the optic cup seems to be a prerequisite for the subsequent migration of the mesenchyme to form the stroma of the iris and ciliary body (Fig. 20-103). Similarly, proper maturation of the future retinal pigment epithelium from the posterior neuroectoderm of the optic cup is required for the proper maturation of the retina, choroid, and overlying sclera.

Iris Hypoplasia

Failure of ingrowth of the future iris epithelium results in the relatively rare anomaly of extreme iris hypoplasia, clinically referred to as *aniridia* (Fig. 20-104). This is relatively more frequent in horses than in other species. At least in some cases (and probably in most), it is inherited.

TABLE 20-3 Uveal Anomalies

Failure of Formation	Failure of Remodeling
Iris hypoplasia	Goniodysgenesis
Choroidal hypoplasia and sequelae	Persistent pupillary membrane
	Persistent hyaloid/primary vitreous
	Anterior segment dysgenesis

Lists are arranged from most prevalent to least prevalent.

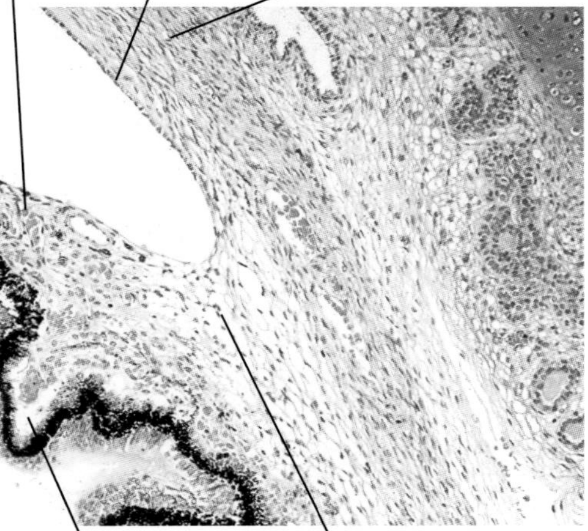

Fig. 20-103 Normal anterior uvea, 1-day-old puppy.
The iris is just beginning to be formed by ingrowth of neuroectoderm and associated mesenchyme from the anterior lip of the optic cup. Formation of the ciliary processes and trabecular meshwork will follow. H&E stain. (Courtesy Dr. B. Wilcock, Ontario Veterinary College.)

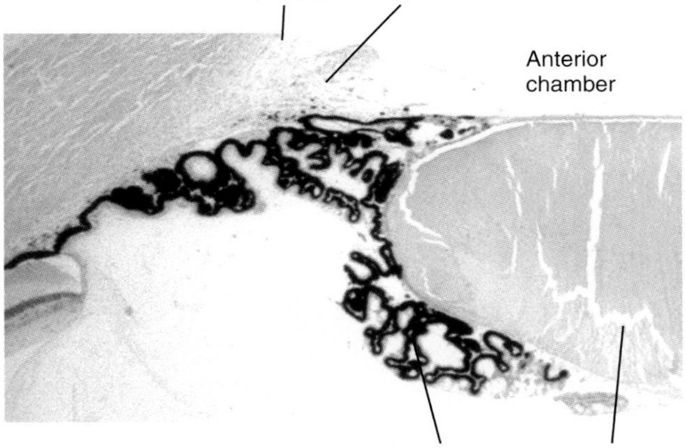

Fig. 20-104 Iris hypoplasia, piglet.
There is no ingrowth of iris epithelium, and the periocular mesenchyme has therefore not migrated inward to form the iris stroma. Unexpectedly, the ciliary processes have formed normally but have arrested maturation in that they have not retracted from the lens capsule. H&E stain. (Courtesy Dr. B. Wilcock, Ontario Veterinary College.)

Choroidal Hypoplasia

Choroidal hypoplasia is a common anomaly in the eyes of dogs and cats and is often associated with inadequate pigmentation of the retinal pigment epithelium and choroid. There are many examples in which lack of pigmentation and thinning of the choroid seems to have no effect on vision or any other aspect of ocular health (the so-called subalbinotic fundus). There is often an association between choroidal hypopigmentation, choroidal hyperplasia, and color dilution within the hair coat. Some are accepted as "normal for the breed" by genetic screening registries, although perhaps unwisely.

There are other instances in which choroidal hypoplasia is part of a significant developmental anomaly involving the choroids, retina, optic nerve, and sclera. By far, the most important example is collie eye anomaly. There are very similar anomalies in phenotypically related breeds, such as the Shetland sheepdog and Australian shepherd dog.

Collie eye anomaly was first described in 1953 as a widespread disease in smooth and rough collies in North America, Europe, and England. During the 1970s, it was found in more than 70% of collies within the United States, often with devastating consequences for vision. The multitude of anomalies can be explained by a single fundamental defect in the proper induction of the retinal pigment epithelium. The most basic and most prevalent of those inductive failures is hypoplasia and hypopigmentation of the choroid, which is why the disease is included here.

The fundamental defect in this anomaly appears to be improper inductive chemical signaling from the developing RPE. Choroidal development (in dogs and many other species) is in some way linked to the acquisition of melanin pigmentation. As a result of this defective signaling, the periocular mesenchyme destined to form the choroid and the sclera receives insufficient stimulation. In the choroid, this outcome is manifest as hypopigmentation and hypoplasia, including hypoplasia of the tapetum (Fig. 20-105). Within the fibrous tunic of the sclera, the most common manifestation is arrested growth, which results in delayed closure of the optic fissure along the ventral floor of the optic cup. This delay in closure allows the growing retina to bulge outwardly through the most posterior portion of this optic fissure. The outward protrusion of retina, usually just ventral to the optic disc, permanently prevents the proper closure of the embryonic fissure and sclera. The combined defect is referred to as posterior polar (or optic disc) coloboma, which produces a bulging of the sclera known as *scleral ectasia* (Fig. 20-106).

Other common defects in collie eye anomaly include mild microphthalmia, congenital retinal folding, tapetal hypoplasia, and retinal detachment. Detachment is usually delayed until the puppy is a few months of age and is not present at birth. Both the microphthalmia (which is usually just mild) and the retinal folding (see later discussion in the section on Retinal Dysplasia) probably represent improper coordination of the rates of retinal and scleral growth and may be another manifestation of improper signaling from the RPE. A retinal growth rate that exceeds that of the scleral shell inevitably results in folding of the redundant retina (interestingly, these retinal folds usually disappear as retinal and scleral growth eventually normalize). Conversely, normal growth of the scleral shell, accompanied by deficient retinal growth, stretches the retina and eventually results in complete retinal detachment (Fig. 20-107).

Other Uveal Abnormalities

Goniodysgenesis is maldevelopment of the filtration angle and is exceedingly common as a cause of primary glaucoma in dogs, but it is much less frequent in other species. It results from incomplete atrophy of the mesenchyme at the base of the iris. Most of this remodeling occurs in the first few weeks of life. For reasons that are poorly understood, clinical manifestations of glaucoma attributed to this developmental anomaly are not usually detected until middle-age or even later. Goniodysgenesis is described in more detail in the section on Glaucoma.

Persistent pupillary membranes and persistent primary vitreous refer to abnormal persistence of portions of the perilenticular vascular tunic or the vascular network within the developing vitreous. Such anomalies are common in dogs. The embryonic lens

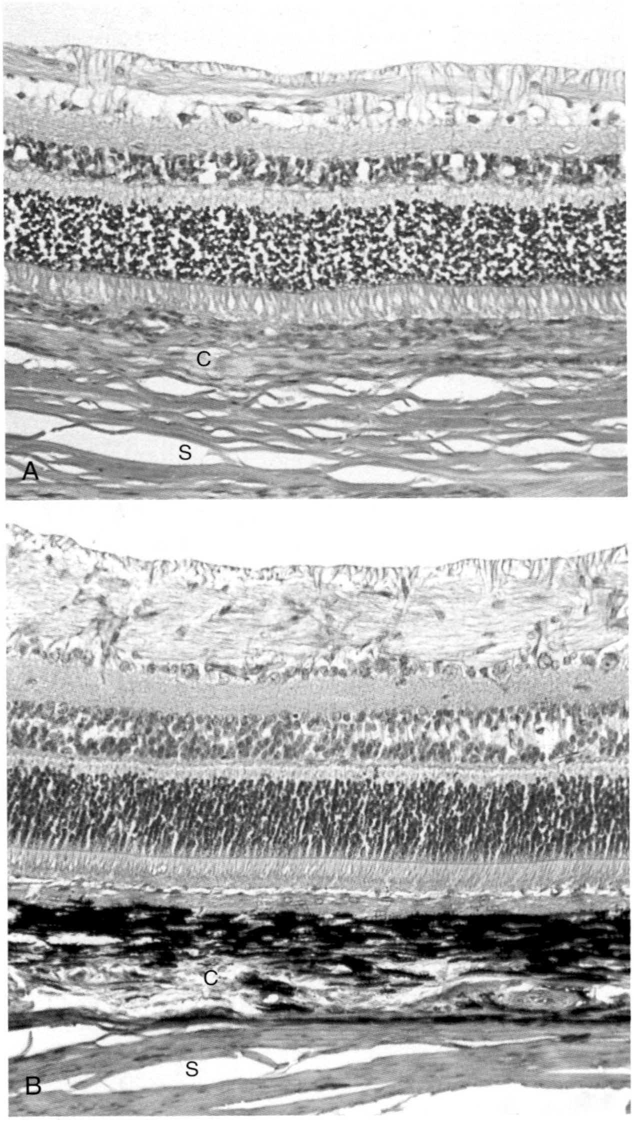

Fig. 20-105 Choroidal hypoplasia, collie eye anomaly, choroid, dog.
A, The choroid is only about half normal thickness and has no pigment. These lesions are the most consistent of those described for collie eye anomaly, but the molecular basis remains unknown. H&E stain. **B,** Normal canine retina and choroid, age-matched control. *C,* Choroid; *S,* sclera. H&E stain. (Courtesy Dr. B. Wilcock, Ontario Veterinary College.)

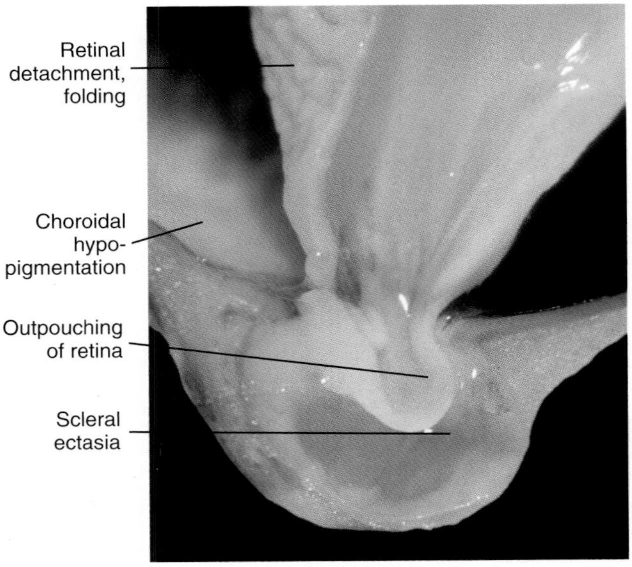

Fig. 20-106 Posterior polar scleral ectasia (at a site of coloboma), collie eye anomaly, eye, posterior pole, sagittal section, dog.
The retina protrudes through a defect in the posterior pole of the globe, a sequel to the delayed closure of the posterior margin of the embryonic fissure. The protruding retina is covered by sclera that also bulges posteriorly to accommodate the retinal protrusion. The lack of synchronization between the retinal and scleral growth rate that is part of collie eye anomaly causes retinal folding and, later, retinal detachment. (Courtesy Dr. B. Wilcock, Ontario Veterinary College.)

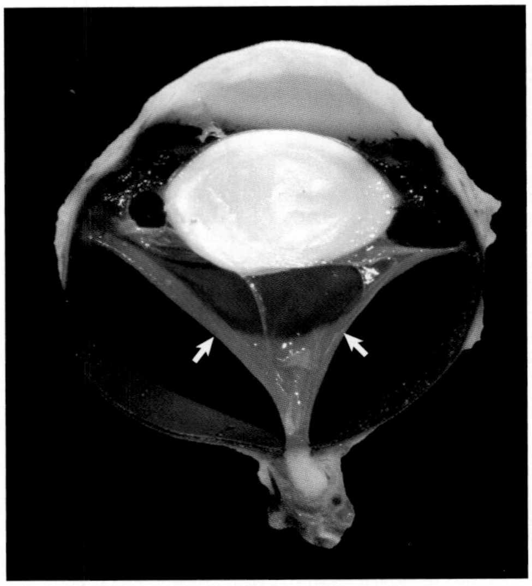

Fig. 20-107 Retinal detachment (complete), collie eye anomaly, globe, sagittal section, dog.
The retina *(arrows)* remains attached only at the sites of its true anatomic attachment: the optic disc and its junction with the pars plana of the ciliary body. (Courtesy Dr. B. Wilcock, Ontario Veterinary College.)

is encased in a network of blood vessels known as the *tunica vasculosa lentis* (Fig. 20-108). This network is created by contributions from the same mesenchyme that forms the iris stroma and from vasogenic mesenchyme growing into the developing vitreous through the posterior portion of the slowly closing optic fissure. The latter vessels, growing in from near the optic disc, are the hyaloid artery system (see Fig. 20-83). Together with other non-angiogenic mesenchymal elements, these vessels form the primary vitreous. This embryonic hyaloid artery system creates a temporary vascular network along the surface of the developing retina and also joins with the anterior chamber vessels to complete the tunica vasculosa lentis. All portions of this elaborate vascular system undergo atrophy before maturation of the globe. Persistence of one or more portions is common. The most common is persistence of the anterior portion of the tunica vasculosa lentis. This is usually referred to as persistent pupillary membrane. Macroscopically, these are seen as fine threads originating from the minor arterial circle of the iris. They are usually bloodless but are often pigmented. They may be inserted into the anterior stroma of the iris, or they may contact the surface of the lens (Fig. 20-109). Occasionally, in what is probably a more significant anomaly, they insert into the cornea. These membranes become clinically significant if they contact the

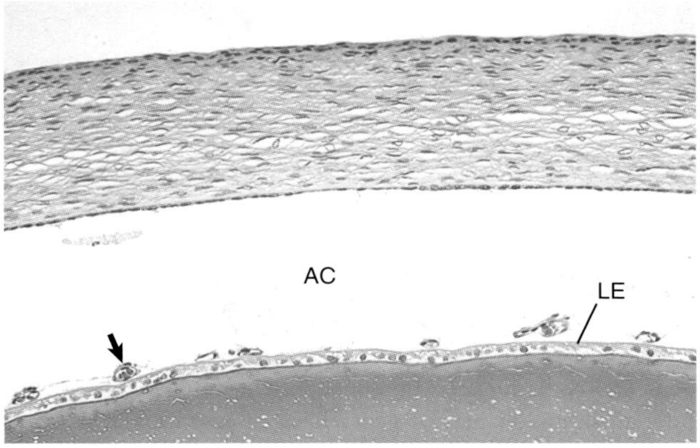

Fig. 20-108 Tunica vasculosa lentis (anterior portion [arrow]), 1-day-old kitten.
The vessels on the anterior surface of the lens will gradually disappear during the first few weeks of postnatal life. *AC,* Anterior chamber; *LE,* lens epithelium. H&E stain. (Courtesy Dr. B. Wilcock, Ontario Veterinary College.)

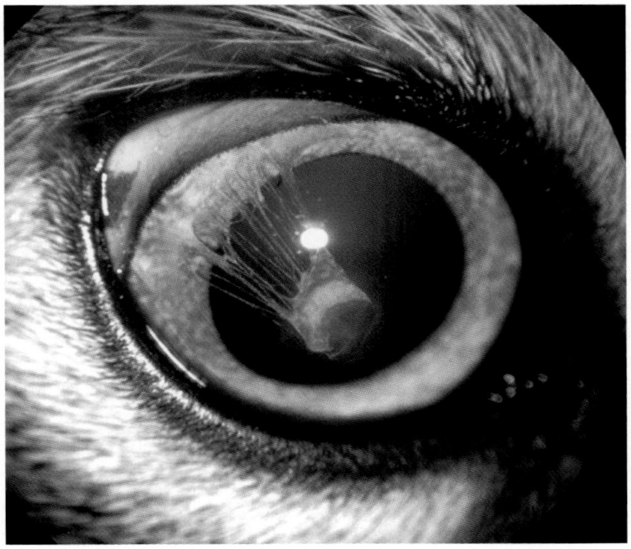

Fig. 20-109 Persistent pupillary membrane, 6-month-old dog.
These persisting portions of the tunica vasculosa lentis have adhered to the anterior surface of the lens, causing anterior polar lens opacity. (Courtesy pathology archives, Ontario Veterinary College.)

lens or cornea, where they interfere with proper development of corneal or lens epithelium, or their associated basement membranes (Descemet's membrane and lens capsule, respectively). Histologically, persistent pupillary membranes are thin endothelial tubes accompanied by varying amounts of mesenchymal stroma. At sites of corneal contact, they may cause fibrous metaplasia of the corneal endothelium. Where they contact the lens, there is usually epithelial proliferation and dysplasia of the lens capsule, resulting in a permanent focal cataract (Fig. 20-110). Those cases in which the pupillary membranes contact the cornea are probably more correctly classified as a minor expression of anterior segment dysgenesis (see later discussion).

Persistence of various portions of the hyaloid artery system, with or without other portions of the primary vitreous, include much less common anomalies known as persistent hyaloid artery, and persistent (hyperplastic) primary vitreous (Fig. 20-111). When persistent blood vessels are accompanied by hyperplastic

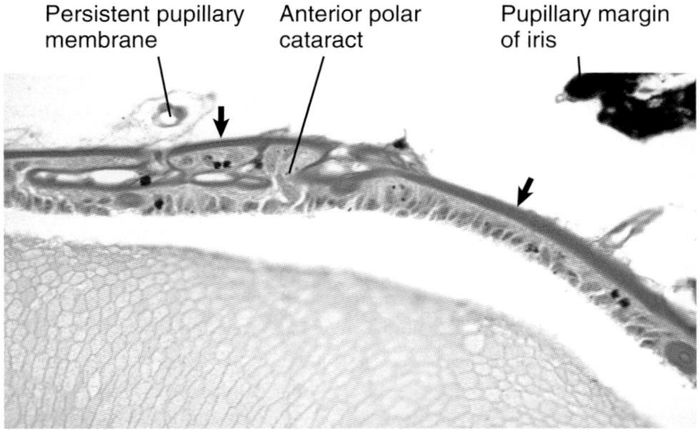

Fig. 20-110 Persistent pupillary membrane, dog.
These membranes *(arrows)* have adhered to the anterior lens capsule, resulting in disorganized proliferation of lens epithelium and lens capsule. The result is an anterior polar cataract. Periodic acid–Schiff reaction. (Courtesy Dr. B. Wilcock, Ontario Veterinary College.)

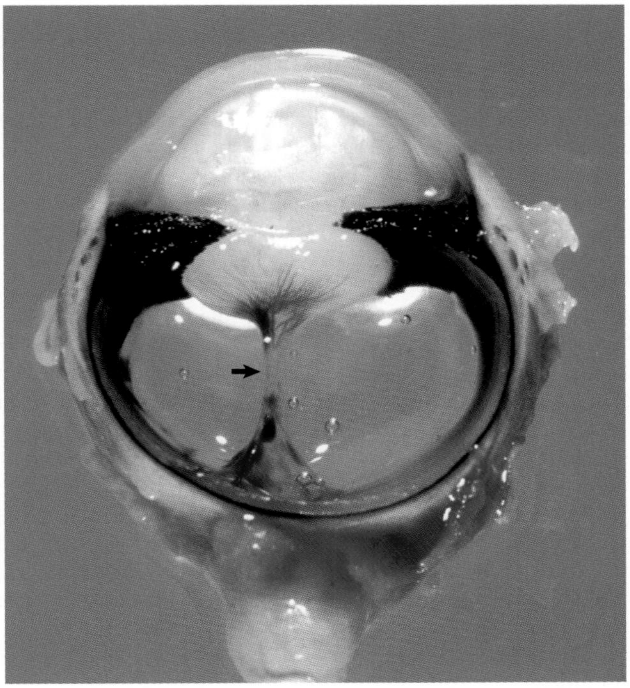

Fig. 20-111 Persistent hyaloid artery and posterior portions of the tunica vasculosa lentis, globe, sagittal section, dog.
A stalk *(arrow)* of fibrovascular tissue (the fetal hyaloid artery and associated mesenchyme) extends from the optic disc to ramify over the posterior surface of the lens. Opacity and deformity of the posterior pole of the lens are frequent complications. (Courtesy Dr. B. Wilcock, Ontario Veterinary College.)

nonangiogenic mesenchymal spindle cells, the resulting anomaly is known as persistent hyperplastic primary vitreous. It has been described as a prevalent familial lesion in several breeds of dogs, particularly Doberman pinschers. The nonangiogenic mesenchyme undergoes notable fibroblastic proliferation, sometimes with cartilaginous metaplasia. Most affected dogs have concurrent anomalies, such as persistent pupillary membrane, microphthalmia, congenital cataract, and abnormal lenticular shape. Many of the described cases do not have the full range of lesions required for the diagnosis of persistent hyperplastic primary vitreous. Most would be better classified as persistent posterior tunica vasculosa lentis because the "hyperplastic" lesions of vitreal mesenchymal proliferation are absent.

Anterior segment dysgenesis is a blanket term for a variety of rare anomalies in which there is a failure of remodeling of the periocular mesenchyme destined to create the corneal stroma, corneal endothelium, iris stroma, and the anterior portion of the tunica vasculosa lentis. The usual clinical observation is absence of anterior chamber and the apparent fusion of the iris stroma to the corneal stroma and no corneal endothelium or Descemet's membrane. The vast majority of these cases are not primary developmental anomalies but the result of perinatal corneal perforation. The loss of the anterior chamber is thus the result of a diffuse anterior synechia, usually secondary to traumatic corneal perforation or perforating ulcers that result in subsequent iris prolapse.

Acquired Uveal Diseases

There are in excess of 50 different etiologic types of uveitis in dogs alone, but in most of these the uveitis is only an incidental part of a systemic disease. The macroscopic or microscopic lesions within the globe are usually not distinctive, and diagnosis of the disease is rarely made on the basis of ocular lesions. Even when uveitis is the only clinical sign of disease, rarely is an etiologic diagnosis made. Many of the specific examples of uveitis listed in clinical textbooks are syndromes made distinctive by clinical features or by identification of a causal agent, rather than by distinctive histologic lesions. Listed next and in Table 20-4 are the most common and most important examples of uveitis that do have distinctive histologic features.

Idiopathic Lymphonodular Uveitis

Although not really a specific disease, idiopathic lymphonodular uveitis is by far the most common histologic pattern seen in uveitis. This may reflect in part a genuinely high frequency of immune-mediated uveitis. More likely, however, it is simply an indication of the chronicity of the uveitis because microscopic evaluation of globes with uveitis is usually done only in the chronic stages of disease, after all attempts at therapy have failed. Lymphonodular uveitis may therefore imply nothing more than a stereotypic endstage of uveitis that initially had a more distinctive and more variable histologic appearance. Lymphonodular uveitis was made famous by recurrent uveitis in horses. It is the only example of lymphonodular uveitis for which we have some insight into the actual cause, and for that reason it serves as the archetype for this group.

Equine Recurrent Uveitis

See the section on Disorders of Horses.

Feline Idiopathic Lymphonodular Uveitis

See the section on Disorders of Cats.

TABLE 20-4 Frequent Causes of Uveitis

Dog	Cat	Horse
Idiopathic causes	Idiopathic causes	Recurrent uveitis
Phacolytic uveitis	Cryptococcosis	
Trauma	Feline infectious peritonitis	
Foreign body		
Blastomycosis		
Phacoclastic uveitis		

Lists are arranged from most prevalent to least prevalent.

Canine Lymphocytic Uveitis

See the section on Disorders of Dogs.

Uveodermatologic Syndrome in Dogs (Vogt-Koyanagi-Harada Syndrome)

See the section on Disorders of Dogs.

Systemic Mycoses

Systemic mycoses, such as blastomycosis, cryptococcosis, histoplasmosis, and coccidioidomycosis, are frequent causes of severe uveitis in those geographic areas where the organisms are common environmental contaminants. Immunodeficient animals may develop endophthalmitis as part of generalized disease caused by saprophytic fungi such as *Aspergillus* spp. or *Candida* spp., but these cases are rare; these same agents occasionally cause endophthalmitis when introduced by penetrating plant foreign bodies.

The frequency with which endophthalmitis accompanies systemic mycosis is unknown. The majority of cases are found in dogs, except for the inexplicable predilection of cryptococcosis for cats. Ocular involvement is part of systemic disease, but fairly frequently, ocular disease is the only obvious clinical sign. Blastomycosis is by far the most prevalent example of an endophthalmitis caused by systemic mycosis, and it serves here as the prototype for this group.

Blastomycosis is the most frequently reported intraocular mycosis in dogs, but it is rare in cats. It is estimated that about 25% of dogs with the systemic disease have clinically obvious ocular disease: unilateral or bilateral endophthalmitis with a very high frequency of exudative retinal detachment. The microscopic lesion is severe diffuse pyogranulomatous endophthalmitis, which tends to be more severe in the choroid and subretinal space than in the anterior uvea. The greatest accumulation of both leukocytes and organisms is usually in the subretinal space. The disease is pyogranulomatous and very destructive. The organisms may be numerous or extremely sparse, probably depending on the duration of the disease and on therapy. They are either free or within the cytoplasm of macrophages and have the typical features of *Blastomyces* spp.: thick-walled yeast 4 to 20 μm in diameter, with occasional broad-based budding. The diagnosis can often be made by cytologic evaluation of subretinal exudates in eyes that are already blind because of retinal detachment (one would probably not dare to attempt aspiration of the subretinal space in a globe that still had vision). Other lesions in affected globes are those seen in any severe uveitis: intraocular hemorrhage, posterior synechia, preiridal fibrovascular membrane, or cataract. Spread into the optic nerve and even orbit is an infrequent complication.

Cryptococcosis is similar to blastomycosis in that the lesions are predominantly within the retina, choroid, and optic nerve. As mentioned earlier, ocular cryptococcosis is immeasurably more prevalent in cats than in dogs or any other domestic animal. As is typical of cryptococcosis in other feline tissue, the granulomatous inflammatory response is often minimal. Large collections of poorly stained pleomorphic yeasts, surrounded by wide capsular halos, impart a typical "soap-bubble" appearance in hematoxylin and eosin (H&E)-stained sections. The organisms are usually numerous and vary greatly in size and shape. In a few cases, the granulomatous reaction is much more severe and mimics that seen in blastomycosis. In such lesions, organisms are typically scarce.

The ocular disease caused by *Coccidioides immitis* resembles blastomycosis but is more suppurative, more destructive, and more prone to progress to outright panophthalmitis. Involvement of the anterior uvea is perhaps more common than in the other systemic mycoses. The disease is seen only in animals that live in (or have

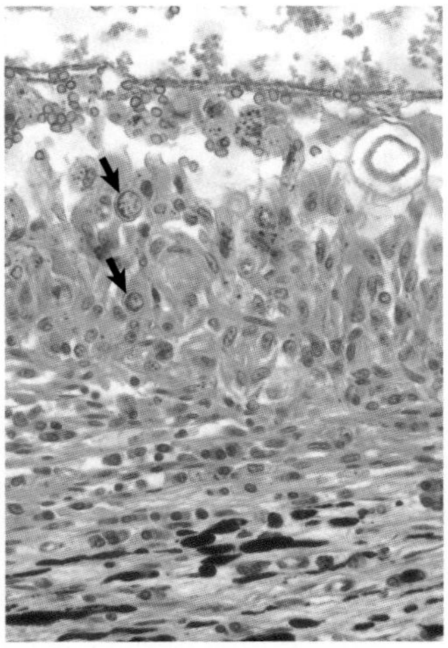

Fig. 20-112 Granulomatous choroiditis (destructive), coccidioidomycosis, choroid, dog.
The retina is absent because inflammatory exudate has caused retinal detachment. Organisms are usually difficult to find, but two spherules *(arrows)* are amid the macrophages. H&E stain. (Courtesy Dr. B. Wilcock, Ontario Veterinary College.)

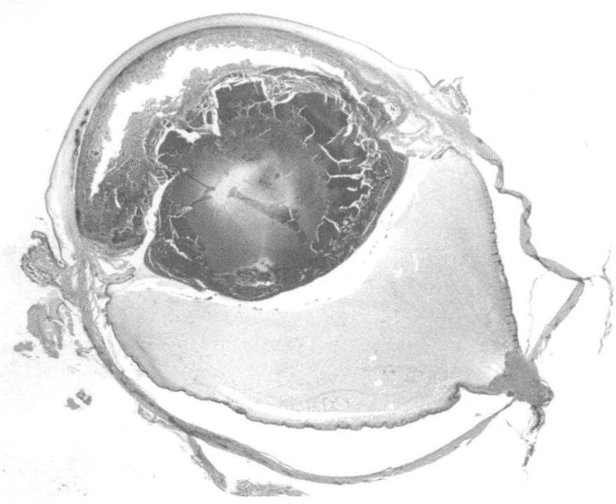

Fig. 20-113 Phacoclastic uveitis, encephalitozoonosis, eye, sagittal section, rabbit.
The anterior lens capsule has disintegrated, with substantial loss of lens material from the anterior cortex. The scalloped remnant of lens is now covered by a mixture of fibrin and leukocytes that fills the anterior chamber. In all species, the sudden release of intact lens protein triggers massive suppurative and granulomatous perilenticular inflammation that is typically delayed until 10 to 14 days after lens rupture. H&E stain. (Courtesy Dr. B. Wilcock, Ontario Veterinary College.)

visited) the very restricted geographic regions in which the organism is common. The great majority of cases are seen in dogs from the desert regions of the American Southwest (Fig. 20-112).

The lesions caused by ocular infection with *Histoplasma capsulatum* are distinctive and quite different from those of the other systemic mycoses. There is usually a diffuse granulomatous and lymphocytic choroiditis with little suppuration and without much of the destruction that characterizes blastomycosis and coccidioidomycosis. Organisms are usually very numerous and visible as small spherical bodies within the cytoplasm of macrophages.

Protothecosis is included here because the organisms can easily be mistaken for yeast and because the clinical and histologic features closely resemble those of the systemic mycoses described earlier. Prototheca are colorless saprophytic algae capable of causing enteric, cutaneous, or generalized granulomatous disease in a variety of mammalian species. Ocular lesions have been described only in dogs with the disseminated form of the disease. The lesions are essentially identical to those seen with blastomycosis and are distinguishable only by the detection of the pleomorphic algae (which usually are very numerous). In histologic section, the algae are free or within macrophages. The organisms are spherical to oval, from 2 to 20 μm in diameter, and have a refractile cell wall that stains with periodic acid–Schiff (PAS) reaction or Gomori's methenamine silver stain. Prototheca reproduces by asexual multiple fission, so that multiple daughter cells form enclosed within a single cell wall. There is no budding as with blastomyces and cryptococcus.

Feline Infectious Peritonitis–Associated Uveitis

See the section on Disorders of Cats.

Bovine Malignant Catarrhal Fever–Associated Uveitis

See the section on Disorders of Ruminants.

Lens-Induced Uveitis

Phacolytic uveitis is an extremely common, mild lymphocytic-plasmacytic anterior uveitis that occurs in a large proportion of animals with cataracts in which the lens protein is beginning to disintegrate and leak through the intact lens capsule. Although seldom significant as the cause of clinical signs, it significantly reduces the success of cataract surgery, unless the surgery is preceded by a course of antiinflammatory drugs.

Phacoclastic uveitis is predominantly an immune-mediated disease in response to the release of large amounts of intact lens protein through a traumatically ruptured lens capsule. The severity and character of the reaction seem to be influenced by the amount of lens material lost, the speed of the loss, the age of the animal, and the species. The disease is most commonly seen in dogs because of their habit of running into sharp objects or having unpleasant encounters with the neighborhood cat. Lens rupture may also occur after blunt trauma, in which case the rupture is usually of the thin posterior capsule. Phacoclastic uveitis also occurs after spontaneous lens rupture not associated with trauma. This occurs in rabbits as a result of penetration of the lens by *Encephalitozoon cuniculi* and in dogs with rapidly progressing diabetic cataracts.

The clinical syndrome is quite distinctive: the initial clinical signs are related to corneal perforation and uveitis as direct consequences of the penetrating injury and/or subsequent sepsis. Those are often managed successfully with antiinflammatory and antibiotic therapy, and everything seems to be healing very well until the development of a severe and therapeutically refractory anterior uveitis that most commonly occurs about 2 weeks after the initial injury. Once the phacoclastic uveitis is initiated, the prognosis for saving the globe becomes poor.

There are two different types of lesions of phacoclastic uveitis, and these usually occur concurrently. The typical lesions in acute disease include rupture of the lens capsule, accumulation of intralenticular neutrophils, and a perilenticular inflammatory reaction that is initially neutrophilic. With time, it becomes progressively more granulomatous but remains distinctly perilenticular (Fig. 20-113). After a few days, the inflammatory reaction is accompanied by proliferation, fibroblastic metaplasia, and perilenticular migration of lens epithelial cells that have escaped through the

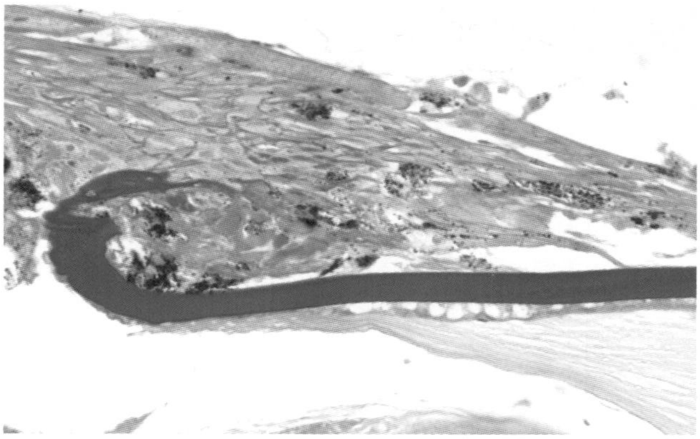

Fig. 20-114 Chronic phacoclastic uveitis, eye, horse.
The predominant lesion is now a plaque of fibroblast-like cells on the anterior surface of the lens adjacent to the site of capsular rupture *(lower left)*. This plaque is created by metaplasia of lens epithelium that has escaped through the capsular defect. These proliferating cells frequently cause pupillary blockage and secondary glaucoma. H&E stain. (Courtesy Dr. B. Wilcock, Ontario Veterinary College.)

site of perforation (Fig. 20-114). Because the perforating injuries causing phacoclastic uveitis may also implant bacteria or foreign material into the globe, it is not always possible to determine what part of the posttraumatic lesion is phacoclastic uveitis and what part is in response to a foreign body or infection. True phacoclastic uveitis is distinctly perilenticular, with minimal reaction in more distant portions of the uvea such as the choroid.

The pathogenesis of the inflammatory component of phacoclastic uveitis is probably an immunologic response to the release of large amounts of strongly antigenic lens protein into the aqueous humor. Although lens protein is not truly "foreign," the body has tolerance for only small amounts of lens protein. The sudden release of large amounts following capsular rupture overwhelms this immune tolerance, resulting in a suppurative-to-pyogranulomatous reaction centered on the lens. This immune pathogenesis explains the lag between lens rupture and development of the phacoclastic uveitis. It also explains why small perforations might not cause the disease and why removal of the injured lens shortly after perforating injury prevents the development of the disease.

The fibrous metaplasia and migration of lens epithelium are critical prognostic events. This epithelium, once out of the lens, recognizes no barriers to its proliferation and causes pupillary block, occlusion of the filtration angle, and secondary glaucoma. In cats, probably it is this same epithelium that undergoes malignant transformation to the clinically significant and uniquely feline entity of posttraumatic primary ocular sarcoma (see discussion on neoplasia).

Phacoclastic uveitis can be a serious complication of cataract surgery in which too much lens material is left behind within the lens capsular bag. In most instances, complications arise primarily from the migration and fibroblastic metaplasia of this residual lens epithelium. This can result in opacification of the pupil (and of any artificial lens implant) and possibly pupillary block, causing secondary glaucoma.

Neoplasms of the Uvea

Primary uveal neoplasms are common only in dogs and cats, but they are exceedingly important in both species and vie with glaucoma as the most common reason for enucleation (Table 20-5). Primary tumors (melanocytic tumors and iridociliary epithelial tumors) are considerably more prevalent than metastatic tumors

TABLE 20-5 Common Primary Intraocular Neoplasms

Dog	Cat	Horse
Anterior uveal	Diffuse iris melanoma	Medulloepithelioma
Iridociliary adenoma	Iridociliary adenoma	Melanocytoma
	Primary ocular sarcoma	

Lists are arranged from most prevalent to least prevalent.

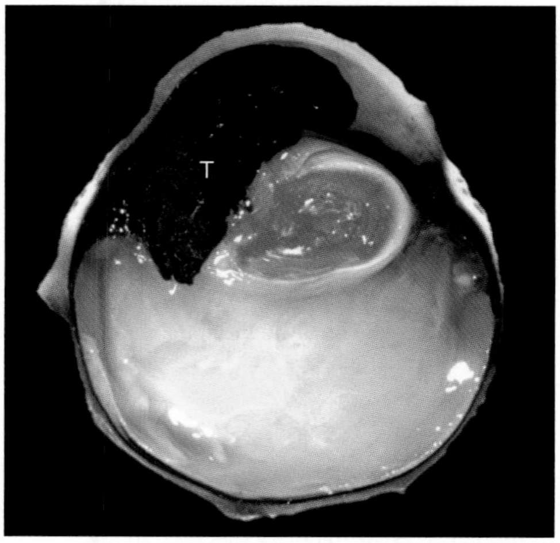

Fig. 20-115 Anterior uveal melanocytoma, eye, sagittal section, dog.
A large black tumor *(T)* has replaced the anterior half of the uvea and filled much of the anterior chamber. (Courtesy Dr. B. Wilcock, Ontario Veterinary College.)

in the globe, with the possible exception of metastatic uveal lymphoma in cats.

In all species, melanocytic tumors are by far the most common of all ocular tumors. Those tumors predicted to be behaviorally benign are referred to as melanocytomas; those predicted to be malignant are classified as melanomas. As with melanocytomas and melanomas elsewhere, there is substantial variation in biologic behavior, depending on species and location. These site and species variables are more important in establishing the prognosis than are many of the histologic and cytologic features.

Canine anterior uveal melanocytoma is by far the most common primary intraocular tumor of dogs, arising from the melanocytes within the stroma of the iris or ciliary body. They ordinarily form a solid, deeply pigmented mass that protrudes into the anterior or posterior chamber. Growth is expansive rather than invasive (Fig. 20-115). The typical tumor has an inconspicuous germinal population of cytologically bland and poorly pigmented spindle cells, and a much larger proportion of huge ballooned "plump cells" distended with pigment (Fig. 20-116), which are assumed to be postmitotic endstage neoplastic melanocytes. These tumors have very little metastatic potential, and the few that are likely to metastasize can be identified by a notable increase in the numbers of mitotic figures. Sooner or later, all of these tumors grow large enough to cause obstruction of aqueous outflow and secondary glaucoma.

Histologically identical melanocytoma occasionally arises within the choroid as a slowly expanding subretinal mass. They are significant because they cause retinal detachment.

Feline diffuse iris melanoma has a distinctive clinical presentation: unilateral coalescing hyperpigmentation of the iris that slowly (often over many years) progresses to diffuse iris thickening and

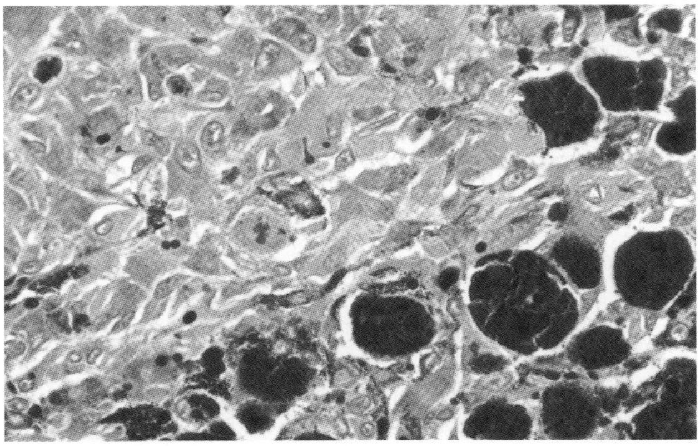

Fig. 20-116 Anterior uveal melanocytoma, iris, dog.
Large, heavily pigmented polygonal "plump cells" predominate *(lower right)*. The smaller number of lightly pigmented spindle cells are germinal cells. The paucity of mitotic figures is a predictor that the tumor is benign. H&E stain. (Courtesy Dr. B. Wilcock, Ontario Veterinary College.)

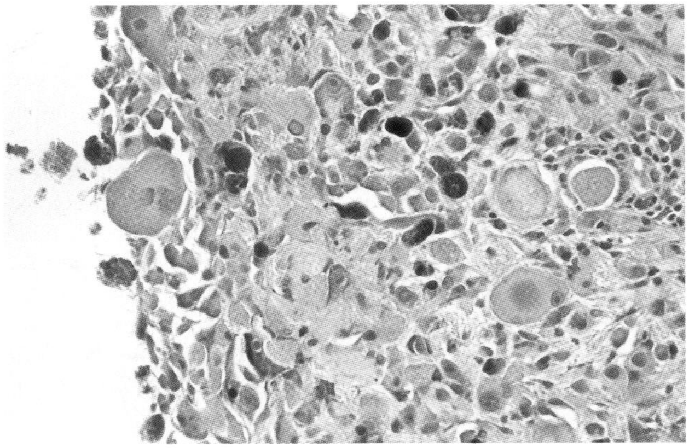

Fig. 20-118 Diffuse iris melanoma, iris, cat.
Note the extreme variation in cellular morphology: threefold variation in cellular size, nuclear gigantism, and variation in cell shape from round to spindle. The marked variation in the histologic and cytologic appearance of this tumor from case to case has no proven prognostic significance. H&E stain. (Courtesy Dr. B. Wilcock, Ontario Veterinary College.)

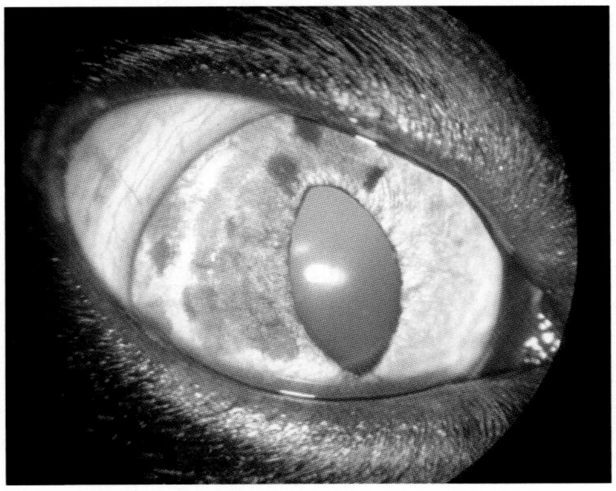

Fig. 20-117 Diffuse iris melanoma, eye, cat.
Coalescing areas of brown pigmentation have caused thickening of the iris. In many cats, the extent of the pigmentation and thickening progresses over many years, and eventually the tumor may cause glaucoma secondary to trabecular occlusion. Enucleation may then be necessary. (Courtesy pathology archives, Ontario Veterinary College.)

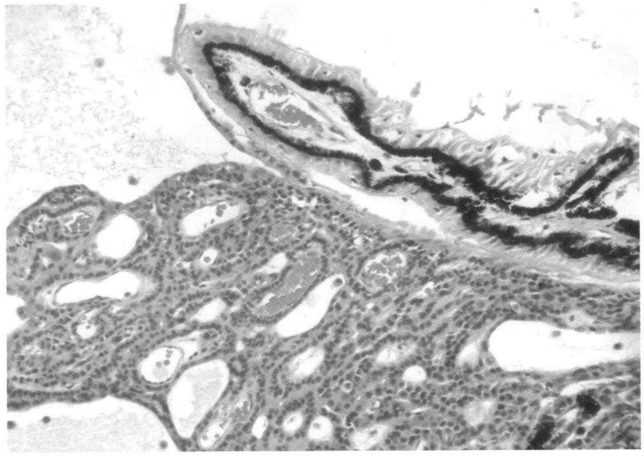

Fig. 20-119 Iridociliary adenoma *(lower half of image)*, well-differentiated, posterior chamber, dog.
Although almost always benign, even small tumors of this type may induce the formation of a preiridal fibrovascular membrane that leads to secondary glaucoma. H&E stain. (Courtesy Dr. B. Wilcock, Ontario Veterinary College.)

secondary glaucoma (Fig. 20-117). This is a uniquely feline disease. The tumor originates from the layer of melanocytes that forms the anterior border layer of the normal iris. The transformed cells have enlarged nuclei and hyperchromasia and proliferate slowly to replace the normal iris architecture. The fully developed tumor, as the name implies, results in a diffuse iridal infiltration by pleomorphic round-to-epithelioid melanocytes. Their appearance in cytologic preparations is extremely variable. Tumors vary from amelanotic to heavily pigmented, and from round cell to epithelioid to spindle cell (and mixtures of all of the above). Mononuclear gigantism is frequently seen (Fig. 20-118). None of these variables has any prognostic significance.

The prognosis has been the subject of great debate over the past 10 years. Retrospective studies that have attempted to establish histologic predictors of behavior have been thwarted by poor overall follow-up data (cats lost to follow-up, very few necropsies). Nonetheless, emerging from these studies is the general consensus that although these tumors are substantially more likely to eventually metastasize than are canine uveal melanomas, the overall risk of an affected cat developing clinical signs related to metastatic disease seems to be low. The probability that the affected eye will eventually develop glaucoma secondary to tumor infiltration of the trabecular meshwork is exceedingly high, although it may take years.

Rarely, cats develop canine-like nodular uveal melanocytomas (and dogs occasionally develop feline-like diffuse melanomas).

Iridociliary tumors vary from well-differentiated papillary adenomas to solid carcinomas. They all arise from the neuroectoderm of the posterior iris or ciliary body. The histologic distinctions have no apparent relevance to biologic behavior, because all of these tumors are benign. These are relatively common intraocular tumors in dogs (second in frequency only to melanocytoma), occasionally seen in cats, and infrequently seen in other species. They usually grow as discrete, expansile nodules that protrude into the posterior chamber and are thus visible through the pupil. They are populated by cuboidal and columnar epithelial cells resembling normal iridociliary epithelium and usually form cords and papillary structures reminiscent of disorganized ciliary processes (Fig. 20-119). Some have a more primitive cytologic and histologic appearance, but extraocular metastasis is so rare as to be nonexistent. Even small tumors may become clinically significant because they habitually produce fibroblastic and angiogenic growth factors that stimulate the development of preiridal fibrovascular membranes, causing secondary glaucoma or intractable hyphema.

Medulloepithelioma is a relatively rare congenital counterpart of iridociliary adenoma. It has the distinction of being the most common primary intraocular tumor of horses. The histologic appearance reflects its embryonic origin from primitive neuroectoderm still capable of both iridociliary and retinal differentiation. The tumor is populated by hyperchromatic cuboidal cells that make structures reminiscent of ciliary processes and sometimes tubular structures resembling the rosettes seen in retinal dysplasia. In horses, they often incorporate foci of cartilage, bone, and even brain tissue; these are known as *teratoid medulloepitheliomas.* Although they are by definition congenital tumors, their growth is slow and they may not be diagnosed until many years later.

Feline primary ocular sarcoma (posttraumatic sarcoma) is a high-grade spindle cell neoplasm that probably arises from lens epithelial cells that have escaped through ruptures in the lens capsule. These cells routinely undergo fibroblastic metaplasia as part of ineffective wound healing (see discussion on phacoclastic uveitis), but the metaplasia progresses to outright sarcoma only in cats. The tumor begins as a distinctly perilenticular mass and then grows to fill the globe (Fig. 20-120). As with histologically similar postvaccinal sarcomas, these tumors may have fibroblastic, osteoblastic, or cartilaginous areas in the same tumor (Fig. 20-121). The interval between trauma and detection of tumor can be many years, but the key word here is "detection." It is very common for cats with this tumor to be presented for veterinary attention only after the tumor has filled the globe. We do not know the rapidity of microscopic tumor development following injury. These tumors frequently invade the optic nerve and then extend into the brain. They are also capable of distant metastasis.

Neoplasms metastatic into the globe are much less frequent than tumors originating within the globe. Virtually any metastatic neoplasm can localize within the uveal tract and spread from there into other portions of the globe. Their histologic appearance is the same as that of the primary tumor. By far the most prevalent is lymphoma (lymphosarcoma), seen in many species but particularly prevalent in cats. It causes diffuse thickening and pallor of the iris and less frequently the choroid. It is clinically almost indistinguishable from severe idiopathic uveitis, and the distinction is usually made on the basis of additional clinical evidence.

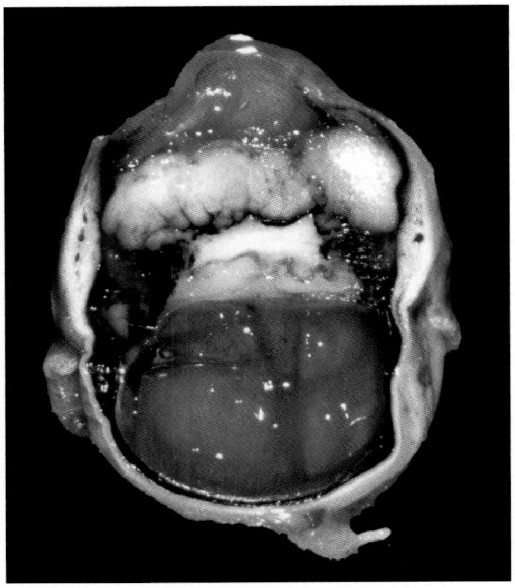

Fig. 20-120 Primary ocular sarcoma, eye, sagittal section, cat. A solid white stromal sarcoma surrounds remnants of a ruptured lens. Wrinkled remnants of the lens capsule are still visible near the posterior margin of the tumor. (Courtesy Dr. B. Wilcock, Ontario Veterinary College.)

DISEASES OF THE LENS

Anomalies of Lens

The lens is derived from the thickening of the ectoderm induced by contact with the primary optic vesicle. This lens placode then migrates inwardly to cause the optic vesicle to invaginate on itself to form the primary optic cup. As it does, the lens placode grows to become a lens vesicle and separates from the overlying ectoderm, which will become corneal epithelium (see Fig. 20-83). This vesicle initially is just a single layer of cuboidal epithelial cells surrounded by a very thin capsule. The epithelial cells along its posterior surface elongate to obliterate the lumen of this primitive vesicle, creating the primary lens fibers that persist throughout life as the lens nucleus. The subsequent development of the cortical fibers of the postnatal lens depends entirely on mitotic activity from the anterior lens epithelium. No epithelium remains along the posterior half of the lens any time after the stage of the primary lens vesicle.

Anomalies of the lens are of minor importance when contrasted with anomalies of other portions of the globe. The lens has a central inductive role in ocular development, so significant anomalies of the lens are almost always accompanied by multiple ocular anomalies such as microphthalmia. It is likely that many of the lens anomalies reflect acquired degenerative changes (even if occurring in utero), resulting in regression of what was a normally developing lens. Such changes include an abnormally small lens (microphakia), an abnormally shaped lens (lenticonus and lentiglobus), and a congenital lens luxation, which is presumably secondary to some congenital abnormality in the zonules.

Lens Luxation

Dislocation of the lens may be partial (subluxation) or complete (luxation). It may fall forward into the anterior chamber, or it may remain trapped in the posterior chamber. A completely dislocated lens is likely to develop a diffuse cataract, presumably because of its inadequate access to aqueous humor. Anterior lens luxation (Fig. 20-122) is much more significant because it predisposes to

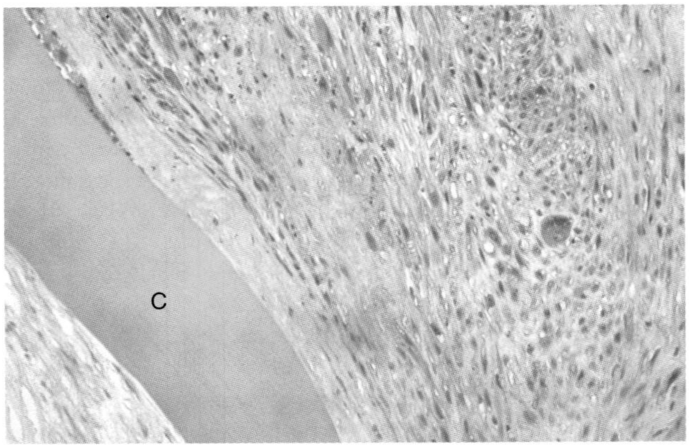

Fig. 20-121 Primary ocular sarcoma *(right half of image)*, eye, cat. Pleomorphic fibroblast-like cells, thought to be derived from lens epithelium, lie adjacent to remnants of lens capsule *(C)*. Virtually all cases are preceded by rupture of the lens capsule. H&E stain. (Courtesy Dr. B. Wilcock, Ontario Veterinary College.)

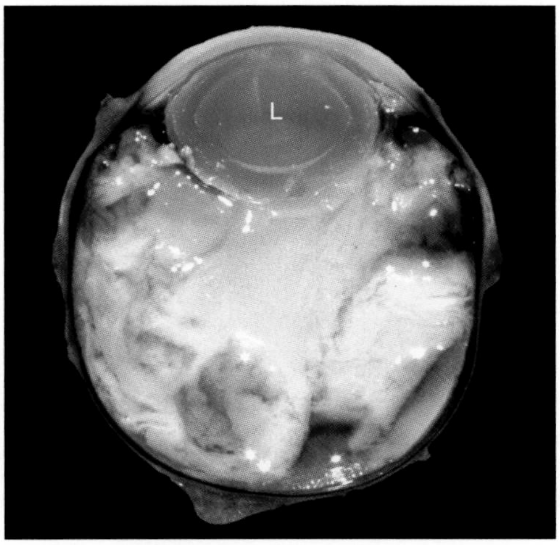

Fig. 20-122 Anterior lens luxation, eye, sagittal section, dog. The dislocated, swollen lens *(L)* has moved anteriorly to lie against the posterior surface of the cornea and has compressed the iris, creating pupillary blockage and secondary glaucoma. There is coagulation and opacification of the aqueous humor and the vitreous because of increased protein from inflammation. (Courtesy Dr. B. Wilcock, Ontario Veterinary College.)

glaucoma (see the section on Glaucoma). Lens luxation may be primary or secondary.

Primary lens luxation refers to that occurring without any known trauma or other ocular disease. It may be congenital or may be seen later in life. Congenital luxation is usually the result of a developmental error that causes abnormal or insufficient zonules. Much more prevalent are spontaneous luxations that occur in young adult dogs of specific breeds (notably terriers). The luxation is almost always bilateral, even if not simultaneous in onset. The ultrastructural and biochemical defect within the lens zonules have not been defined.

Secondary lens luxation is almost always a manifestation of blunt trauma that causes avulsion of the zonules, or excessive stretching of zonules within a globe that has become greatly enlarged secondary to glaucoma. It may also occur as a result of lysis of zonules by neutrophil enzymes or perhaps bacterial proteases in septic endophthalmitis.

The potential consequences of lens luxation are numerous, but the most significant is glaucoma. This is particularly frequent with anterior lens luxation. The pathogenesis may involve several factors including anterior dislocation of the vitreous causing pupillary block and accumulation of degenerate zonular material within the trabecular meshwork. It is sometimes impossible to decide whether the luxation caused the glaucoma, or the glaucoma caused the luxation.

Diabetic Cataract

Rapidly progressing bilateral cataracts develop in at least 70% of spontaneously diabetic dogs (but not in cats). Progression to complete cortical opacity usually occurs within a few weeks. The swelling may be so rapid that the lens actually ruptures. The pathogenesis of the cataract has traditionally been ascribed to the excessively high level of glucose within the aqueous. Glucose is normally the major energy source for lens fibers via anaerobic glycolysis. When the rate-limiting enzyme of this pathway, hexokinase, is overloaded with glucose, most of the excess glucose absorbed by the lens is shunted to the sorbitol pathway where it is transformed into the polyalcohol sorbitol, which is then slowly reduced to a ketose.

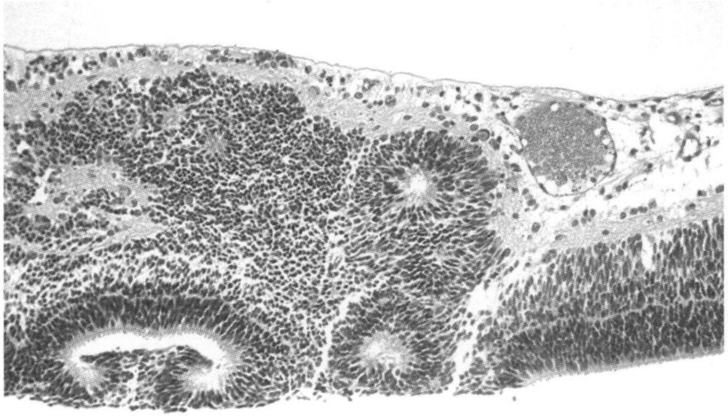

Fig. 20-123 Primary retinal dysplasia, retina, puppy. The cells of the retinal layers are poorly organized and arranged haphazardly, sometimes creating acinar-like structures known as retinal rosettes. H&E stain. (Courtesy Dr. B. Wilcock, Ontario Veterinary College.)

Sorbitol may accumulate to very high concentrations within the lens where it osmotically attracts water, resulting in rapid swelling of the lens and disruption of its critical architecture. Sorbitol-induced osmotic disruption alone is not sufficient to explain all of the structural and metabolic changes in sugar-induced cataracts. The efficacy of antioxidants in slowing the progression of such cataracts, the nature of intralenticular biochemical alterations, and detection of increased intralenticular oxidants all point to some kind of oxidative damage as an additional promoter of cataracts.

DISEASES OF THE RETINA

Retinal Anomalies

Retinal Dysplasia

Retinal dysplasia is a general term denoting an abnormal retinal differentiation characterized by jumbling of retinal layers. In the past, the term has been used rather loosely to include not only the rare genuine primary developmental anomalies but also postnecrotic and/or postinflammatory retinal scarring within the developing retina and retinal folding without any true disorganization. They should be considered as separate entities.

Primary retinal dysplasia is a rare anomaly that probably results from improper induction of retinal maturation by the RPE. Whether the failure relates to delayed and/or inadequate apposition between the two layers or a failure in the production of appropriate signaling molecules by the RPE is not known. The result is a retina with patchy-to-diffuse jumbling of the retinal layers (Fig. 20-123). Primary retinal dysplasia as the sole anomaly is seen as an inherited disease in a few breeds of dogs, but most examples are a part of multiple ocular anomalies. The significance of the lesion varies with the extent of dysplasia. Such retinas are prone to detachment (and in severe cases, the retina may never have been attached at all).

Postnecrotic retinal dysplasia is a much more frequent phenomenon, seen as a sequel to acquired retinal necrosis of the developing retina. In dogs and cats, the period of susceptibility extends for at least 6 weeks after birth, during which time the retina continues to develop. Most of the documented examples are sequelae to viral infection, but in theory virtually any kind of retinal injury during its development could result in postnecrotic retinal "dysplasia." In contrast to the adult retina, which retains no mitotic capability within the neurons of its various layers, the developing retina can still react with at least some neuronal regeneration. Such regeneration is usually mixed with glial scarring and does not restore perfect retinal architecture (Fig. 20-124).

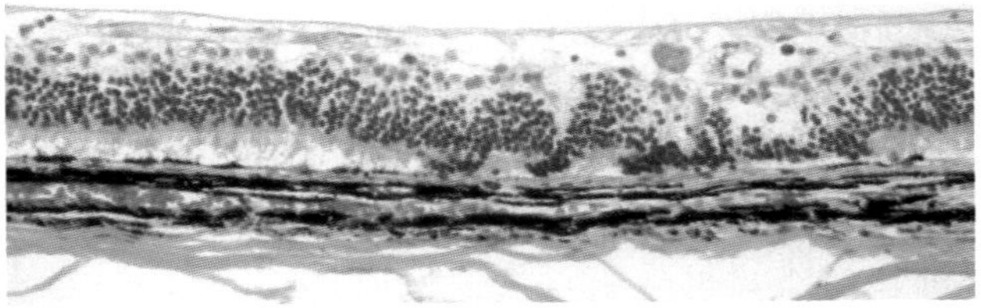

Fig. 20-124 Postnecrotic retinal dysplasia (so-called), in utero bovine viral diarrhea (BVD) virus infection, retina, calf.
There is loss of nuclei from all retinal layers as a sequela to the in utero destruction of retinal neurons by BVD virus. In some instances, this loss is followed by efforts at retinal regeneration, resulting in disorganization that may be considered as a retinal dysplasia. H&E stain. (Courtesy Dr. B. Wilcock, Ontario Veterinary College.)

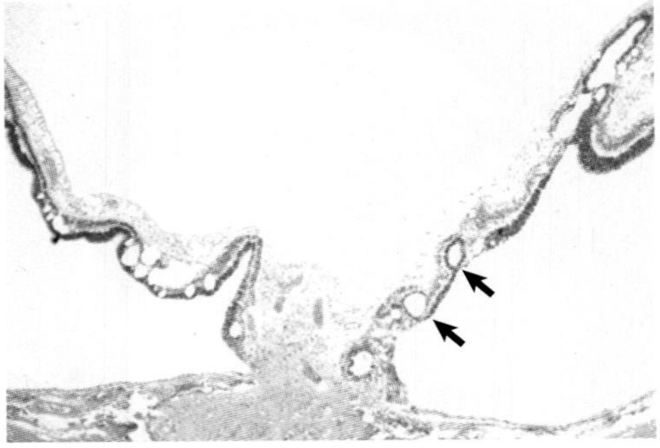

Fig. 20-125 Inherited retinal folds and retinal detachment, eye, posterior chamber, dog.
The acinar-like structures *(arrows)* within the detached retina are transverse sections through retinal folds. These folds probably arise because the growth rate of the retina temporarily exceeds that of the sclera, forcing the retina to fold on itself. H&E stain. (Courtesy Dr. B. Wilcock, Ontario Veterinary College.)

The viruses most often implicated in causing retinal dysplasia in domestic animals are bovine virus diarrhea (BVD) virus in cattle, bluetongue virus in sheep, herpesvirus in dogs, and both parvovirus and choroid virus in cats. The histologic lesions can be quite variable, but usually there is a combination of very subtle residual inflammation along with postnecrotic scarring in the retina, optic nerve, and perhaps the choroids. Only if these viral infections damage the retina while its neurons still have proliferative capacity, will there be additional findings of disorganized neuronal proliferations with blending of nuclear layers. Proliferation also occurs in the RPE, which may be stimulated to migrate into the overlying scarred retina or to proliferate in situ as plaques of fibroblast-like cells. The pathogenesis of the "dysplasia" is the same as for lesions caused by these agents in the brain: infection and subsequent destruction of neurons (and possibly other cell types). The dysplasia is not specific to the mechanism of the cellular injury; it reflects only the unsuccessful attempts at postnecrotic healing in a retina still capable of at least some neuronal replication.

The window of susceptibility for the development of retinal dysplasia depends on the species (simply because the timetable for retinal development varies with the species). Infection of calves with BVD virus between 79 and 150 days gestation regularly results in postnecrotic retinal dysplasia, which is the most frequent and certainly the most studied of the virally induced retinal dysplasias. The initial ocular lesion is necrotizing lymphocytic endophthalmitis with random retinal necrosis. The inflammation gradually subsides, so there is scant evidence of inflammation in fetuses aborted later or in dead neonatal calves. Those ocular structures (cornea, uvea, optic nerve) that are already well differentiated at the time of the endophthalmitis may remain normal or exhibit some postnecrotic scarring; only the retina will exhibit abortive efforts at regeneration. Because the peripheral retina remains mitotically active for several weeks after the central retina has matured, dysplastic lesions may be found only in the peripheral retina. It is said that all calves with BVD-associated retinal dysplasia also have cerebellar hypoplasia. The same is probably true of cats with retinal dysplasia caused by in utero or perinatal infection with panleukopenia virus.

Retinal folding is by far the most common type of so-called retinal dysplasia. The great majority of such lesions are seen in juvenile purebred dogs. Most examples are inherited as autosomal recessive traits (sadly, so common in some breeds that they are now accepted as "normal variants"). The ophthalmoscopic findings and effect on vision vary from breed to breed. The histologic lesion is different from true retinal dysplasia and postnecrotic retinal dysplasia in that there is no jumbling of retinal layers, and there is no scarring. The exact pathogenesis for these retinal folds has not been determined, and it may not be the same among all breeds. What seems logical, however, is that the retinal folds represent nothing more than buckling of excessive retina within a globe because growth of the retina has been greater than that of the surrounding choroidal/scleral shell (Fig. 20-125). Supporting this speculation is the observation that such retinal folds are often transient and disappear as the puppy ages (implying that the growth rate of the scleral shell finally "catches up" to that of the retina). The most severe examples occur in dogs with developmental retinal nonattachment. These have extensively folded retinas because the distance from optic disc to ora ciliaris in a straight line is shorter than the convex route taken by a normally attached retina.

Optic Nerve Hypoplasia

The true frequency of optic nerve hypoplasia is unknown. Most examples are seen in toy breeds of dogs, with the diagnosis being made by clinical examination. Because there is no apparent visual defect, these eyes are almost never available for histologic assessment and the exact nature of the defect (true hypoplasia versus atrophy) remains unknown. Genuine hypoplasia of the optic nerve is the expected result of prenatal or neonatal destruction of ganglion cells from any intraocular disease (including congenital glaucoma, viral infection, and neonatal septicemia with embolic endophthalmitis). The lesion should therefore be correctly classified as atrophy rather than hypoplasia, although the distinction becomes muddy when talking about injuries in the prenatal and perinatal periods.

A distinctly different pathogenesis explains optic nerve hypoplasia in calves born from cows with vitamin A deficiency or in young calves with persistent perinatal dietary deficiency. Atrophy of the nerve results from compression as it passes through an abnormally flattened foramen. The reason for the flattening is improper regulation of osteoblastic activity around the periphery of the developing foramen. Optic nerve damage is not seen if the deficiency in vitamin A occurs after 2 years of age.

Acquired Retinal Disease (Tables 20-6 and 20-7)

Canine Progressive Retinal Atrophy

See the section on Disorders of Dogs.

Photoreceptor Dysplasias

See the section on Disorders of Dogs.

TABLE 20-6 Acquired Retinal Diseases (Classified by Lesion)

Photoreceptor Atrophy	Ganglion Cell Atrophy	Full-Thickness Necrosis	Retinitis	Other
PRA	Glaucoma	High pressure glaucoma (dogs only)	Localization of systemic infections	Storage diseases
Retinal detachment	Optic nerve injury (dieback)	Ischemic injury	Bystander reaction to endophthalmitis	Anomalies
Light-induced retinopathy		Vascular hypertension		
Drug toxicity		Vascular occlusion (thromboemboli, tumor)		
Nutritional deficiency				
Choroidal ischemia				

PRA, Progressive retinal atrophy.

TABLE 20-7 Acquired Retinal Diseases (Classified by Pathogenesis)

Ischemia	Inflammation	Trauma	Toxic/Metabolic	Developmental Error
Glaucoma*	Hematogenous infection	Detachment	Inherited photoreceptor dysplasias/degenerations	Retinal dysplasia
Detachment	Infection via penetrating injury	Hemorrhage/infarction	Nutritional deficiency	
Hypertension	Bystander injury from endophthalmitis	Optic nerve trauma/dieback neuropathy	Light-induced retinopathy	
Thromboembolism/metastasis			Neuronal storage diseases	

*The role of ischemia in glaucomatous retinal atrophy is controversial and probably varies by type of glaucoma and by species.

Photoreceptor Degenerations

See the section on Disorders of Dogs.

Other Inherited Retinal Degenerations and Dysplasias

Inherited retinal dysplasias and degenerations have been reported as sporadic occurrences in a variety of cat breeds, but the syndrome has been adequately studied only in the Abyssinian breed. In this breed, there are two different diseases: early onset rod-cone dysplasia and late onset retinal degeneration affecting rods much sooner than cones. The early onset dysplasia is inherited as an autosomal dominant trait and is almost identical to the rod-cone dysplasia of Irish setter dogs. Retinal function deteriorates rapidly, with virtually all affected cats being blind before 1 year of age. In contrast, the late-onset retinal degeneration is inherited as an autosomal recessive, and affected cats usually show no clinical signs until about 2 years of age; they may retain at least some useful vision throughout life. The earliest structural changes are loss of neurons from the outer nuclear layer and disintegration of rod outer segments.

Congenital stationary night blindness in horses (nyctalopia) is a poorly documented disease affecting the Appaloosa breed (occasionally others). At least in Appaloosas, it seems to be inherited. The visual defects and associated behavioral abnormalities are seen in foals in dim light. In most cases, it does not progress sufficiently to cause obviously defective vision in daytime. Retinal histology is normal.

Other (Noninherited) Photoreceptor Diseases

Sudden acquired retinal degeneration (SARD) is an enigmatic, rapidly progressing, photoreceptor degeneration that is histologically identical to those of the inherited progressive retinal atrophies. Blindness occurs very rapidly (over a period of a few days to a few weeks). Affected dogs are adult or even elderly, and the disease can affect any breed or crossbreed. The funduscopic lesion is bilaterally symmetric and diffuse across the retina. Histologic studies of the early lesions are very few because there is no ethical justification for the surgical removal of these globes as the dogs are otherwise healthy. The disease has not been experimentally reproduced. The cause is unknown, but its occurrence is sometimes associated with polyuria, polydipsia, elevated serum cholesterol concentration, and increased serum alkaline phosphatase activity. Some but not even the majority of the affected dogs have adrenal cortical hyperfunction. How this malfunction causes the irreversible retinopathy, if indeed it does, is unknown. One small study demonstrated circulating, complement-fixing antibody to retinal S-antigen and interphotoreceptor retinoid-binding protein, raising the possibility that the disease is a cytotoxic autoimmune phenomenon.

Light-induced retinopathy is an important cause of blindness in animals maintained under inappropriate lighting conditions. The intensity and especially the duration of the light are important. Those species that are preferentially nocturnal in their natural habitat are particularly susceptible. The most susceptible group of all are deep-water fish maintained in aquariums with continuous artificial lighting or in shallow outdoor tanks without protection from sunlight. Outbreaks of blindness in different species of laboratory animals (especially albino rats) housed under continuous fluorescent lighting were the first to focus attention on this phenomenon.

The initial lesion is disruption of rod outer segment disks, followed by destruction of all photoreceptors and then their nuclei. At higher light intensities, but still within the range for "normal" room lighting, there may also be damage to neurons of the inner nuclear layer and to astrocytes and Müller cells. The histologic changes are the same as those for most other photoreceptor diseases, so this specific etiologic diagnosis is made based on the circumstantial evidence of abnormally bright light or an inappropriate balance between high-light and low-light intervals. The mechanism by which "ordinary" light damages the retina is still incompletely understood. Even normal vision is a "destructive" event, with light activation of photopigments generating a lot of free radicals and requiring physiologic replacement of photopigments and photoreceptor membrane discs during periods of sleep. The most popular theory is that of light-induced excessive oxidation of the very abundant polyunsaturated long-chain fatty acids of the rod discs, with the generation of free radicals. These cause cell membrane damage, and without adequate dark intervals there is reduced opportunity for regeneration.

Taurine deficiency as a cause for photoreceptor degeneration is seen only in cats. It is now largely a historical disease because all commercial feline diets are supplemented with taurine. Cats are unable to synthesize taurine from cysteine in amounts adequate for retinal function. Cats eating inappropriate diets (most often, stealing dog food) develop focal retinal atrophy in a horizontal streak dorsal to the optic disc. The disease, at least in some cases, progresses slowly to generalized retinal atrophy and blindness. The clinical features are identical to those of a historic disease known as *feline central retinal degeneration*. It is now assumed that the two diseases are the same but that may not be true in every single case. The histologic lesion is photoreceptor degeneration, initially involving cone outer segments, but eventually affecting rods as well. The rods of the peripheral retina are the last to degenerate.

Hypovitaminosis A as a cause for retinopathy is occasionally seen in groups of cattle or pigs receiving a ration deficient in vitamin A over a prolonged interval. Because most pastures have more than adequate vitamin A, deficiencies in cattle are likely to be seen only in animals raised in confinement and fed a poor quality ration (especially hay or grain that has been stored for a very long time). In adult animals, the effects of hypovitaminosis A first involve photoreceptor outer segments, slowly progressing to diffuse photoreceptor atrophy, loss of the outer nuclear layer, and eventually to complete retinal atrophy. These lesions have been reproduced in all domestic animals by feeding them specially formulated diets, but naturally occurring retinal lesions are seen almost exclusively in cattle. The deficiency of vitamin A results in a deficiency of rhodopsin within the photoreceptors. The initial ultrastructural lesion is swelling, followed by disintegration and fragmentation of the outer segments. Initially this can be reversed with vitamin A therapy until inner segments have also been affected.

Ischemic retinopathy may occur as a sequela to vascular occlusion within the retina itself or within the choroidal vasculature by tumor metastases or thromboemboli, as a sequela to retinal detachment, or as one of the mechanisms for retinal atrophy in glaucoma. Retinal ischemic injury may also occur subsequent to retinal or choroidal vasculitis associated with immune disease or a few infectious diseases such as thrombotic meningoencephalitis of cattle or Rocky Mountain spotted fever or ehrlichiosis in dogs (Fig. 20-126). The microvascular disease associated with diabetes mellitus is an exceedingly important cause of ischemic retinopathy in humans, but examples in domestic animals with spontaneous diabetes are rare.

Vascular hypertension is an additional and relatively common cause for devastating retinal ischemic damage in dogs and cats. It is usually secondary to chronic renal failure. At least 60% of dogs with chronic renal failure are hypertensive.

The clinical disease is characterized by hemorrhage within the retina or from the retina into the posterior vitreous and retinal detachment secondary to serous effusion from injured retinal and choroidal blood vessels. The histologic lesions are primarily in retinal and choroidal vessels, but they may be found throughout the uvea. Characteristic changes are most easily found in the small retinal muscular arteries and larger arterioles. The vessel lesions include mural edema that may progress to fibrinoid necrosis of the tunica media and perivascular fibrosis. Muscular hypertrophy may occur in larger vessels, particularly those of the choroid. Changes occurring as a consequence of the vascular damage include localized retinal necrosis, serous retinal separation with resultant atrophy of photoreceptors and hypertrophy of retinal pigmented epithelium, and intraretinal hemorrhage (Fig. 20-127). There may be necrosis and/or repair of cells of the RPE and sclerosis within the choroid. The severity of the retinal necrosis varies from focal infarcts in the inner retina to (more commonly) extensive full-thickness hemorrhagic infarcts in large segments of retina. The larger lesions probably reflect the effects of widespread choroidal and retinal vascular degeneration. At least some of the retinal lesions are not the direct result of vascular necrosis but are the result of exaggerated autoregulatory vasoconstriction of precapillary sphincters attempting to protect the retinal capillary bed from the systemic hypertension. Sustained vasoconstriction leads to ischemic necrosis of the deprived retina, RPE or choroid, and necrosis of vascular endothelium distal to the constricted precapillary sphincters. Any blood that does manage to pass through the constricted sphincters into the capillaries enters blood vessels already damaged by a drop in perfusion pressure, so there is inevitable transmural leakage of serum and even blood.

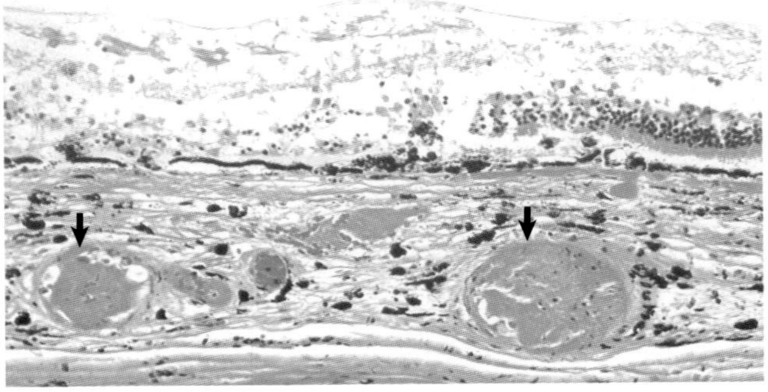

Fig. 20-126 Choroidal vasculitis with thrombosis, choroid and retina, horse.
Dilated choroidal blood vessels *(arrows)* contain fibrin thrombi and are surrounded by edema and some hemorrhage. There is ischemic necrosis of the overlying retina. The horse retina, with its very limited intrinsic vasculature, should theoretically be more susceptible to infarction secondary to choroidal vascular disease than the retina of any other domestic mammal. Such lesions are occasionally seen with disseminated intravascular coagulation regardless of the pathogenesis, as well as with idiopathic coagulopathies. H&E stain. (Courtesy Dr. B. Wilcock, Ontario Veterinary College.)

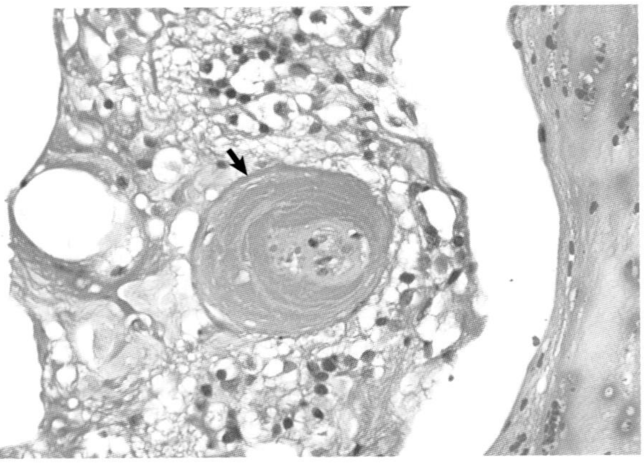

Fig. 20-127 Retinal hypertensive vasculopathy, retina, dog.
There is fibrinoid necrosis of the retinal arteriole *(arrow)* and nonselective ischemic necrosis of the surrounding retina. The dog had end-stage retinal disease. H&E stain. (Courtesy Dr. B. Wilcock, Ontario Veterinary College.)

Retinitis

Retinitis as the sole ocular lesion is rare. When it does occur, however, it is almost always in the course of neurotropic virus infections, such as canine distemper, rabies, and pseudorabies.

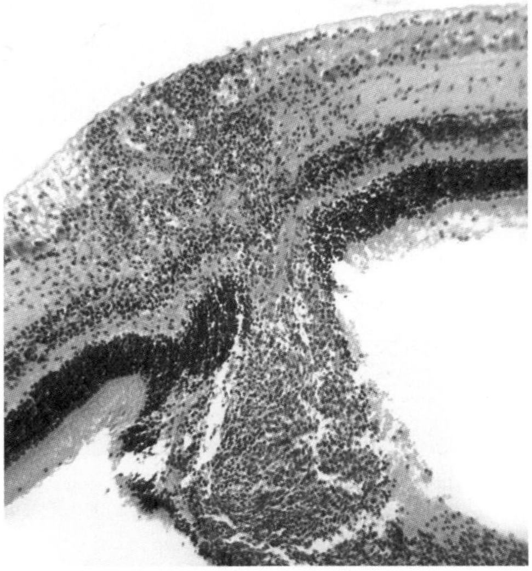

Fig. 20-128 Suppurative embolic retinitis, retina, steer. There is focal obliteration of the retina by a combination of necrosis and inflammation. The leukocytes extend through the outer nuclear layer into subretinal space. This lesion is common in bovine thrombotic meningoencephalitis but is occasionally seen in other bacteremic or septicemic diseases. H&E stain. (Courtesy Dr. B. Wilcock, Ontario Veterinary College.)

Additional diseases that frequently cause prominent retinal lesions (albeit virtually never retinal lesions alone) include toxoplasmosis, canine ehrlichiosis and Rocky Mountain spotted fever, and thrombotic meningoencephalitis of cattle (Fig. 20-128). The lesions in the retina are the same as those in any other tissue affected by these systemic diseases. Retinal lesions also occur in the course of visceral larval migrans caused by the migration of the larvae of *Toxocara canis* and *Baylisascaris procyonis*.

DISEASES OF THE EYELIDS

Developmental Anomalies

Anomalies in the formation of eyelids, including the shape of the palpebral fissure, are exceedingly common in dogs because "eye shape" has been so extensively manipulated during the evolution of the various breeds. In some instances, the "anomaly" is even a required feature for the breed (e.g., as with ectropion in bloodhounds and Saint Bernards). Most of these anomalies are not examined microscopically because they are macroscopically obvious. They are important in clinical ophthalmology and are considered in much greater detail in clinical textbooks than they are here.

Eyelid Agenesis and Coloboma

There may be partial or complete absence of an eyelid, particularly in cats. The most common by far is a partial defect (i.e., coloboma) involving only the upper eyelid. The notchlike defect results in localized corneal desiccation followed by cutaneous metaplasia.

Premature Eyelid Separation

The normal fusion of eyelids (known as *physiologic ankyloblepharon*) in carnivores is essential to protect the immature cornea from infection and desiccation. Premature eyelid separation (technically a "maldevelopment" because it occurs before the maturation of the globe) seriously predisposes the eye to infectious keratitis, desiccation, and even corneal rupture.

Entropion and Ectropion

Entropion is the inward rolling of the eyelid margin because of inadequate overall length. The usual result is irritation of the cornea by the eyelid skin, cilia, and/or hair. It is a very common anomaly in purebred dogs because they have been selected for breeding based partly on the shape of the palpebral fissure, which is a factor in determining facial "expression." The extent and magnitude of the defect varies greatly among individual animals but tends to be relatively uniform within an affected breed. Clinical textbooks have extensive accounts of the manifestations of entropion and ectropion in different breeds and the innumerable techniques for their repair. The outcome for the cornea varies from corneal cutaneous metaplasia to outright ulceration, depending on the severity of the irritation. Entropion may also be acquired as the result of inflammation and subsequent contracture of a scar in the eyelid.

Ectropion is created by undue laxity of an excessively long eyelid, resulting in an outward gaping of the eyelid margin. As with entropion, its extent and severity vary greatly among individual animals and among breeds. The lower eyelid is more frequently affected to a clinically significant degree than the upper, presumably because the effect of gravity on the upper eyelid makes ectropion there less obvious. The anomaly has less significance than entropion because there is no direct corneal irritation. The protruding conjunctiva may entrap debris and become chronically inflamed and because of the failure of the lids to close properly, there may be some chronic exposure keratitis.

Anomalies of Eyelashes: Trichiasis, Distichiasis, and Ectopic Cilia

Anomalies of eyelashes are prevalent in dogs and may or may not cause clinical signs, depending on whether they irritate the cornea or not. They are mentioned here only for the sake of completeness because these are almost never evaluated histologically. Distichiasis is the presence of an ectopic row of cilia originating from the ducts of the Meibomian glands. The defect is usually bilateral. It may be clinically silent or cause corneal irritation. Trichiasis is misdirection of the normal cilia so that they contact the cornea. Ectopic cilia are abnormally placed cilia within the lamina propria of the conjunctiva. Their emergence through the palpebral conjunctiva may result in profound corneal irritation.

Acquired Diseases

Chalazion is sterile granulomatous inflammation in response to the leakage of Meibomian secretion into the surrounding dermis. It is much more common in dogs than in any other species. Although it can theoretically occur in response to any type of injury to the Meibomian gland, in almost all cases, the inflammation is found adjacent to Meibomian adenomas. Histologically, the inflammation is an accumulation of large foamy macrophages and multinucleated cells around the abnormal Meibomian gland. Some of the lipid may occur in the form of extracellular lakes of unstained free lipid, especially in cats. The macrophages contain distinctive slender, birefringent, intracellular crystals, which are readily visible under polarized light.

Idiopathic granulomatous marginal blepharitis is seen only in dogs as a series of coalescing nodules that eventually create a diffuse thickening of one or both eyelid margins. The histologic lesion is a coalescence of suppurating granulomas in the subconjunctival tissue of the eyelid margin, without any proven association with any particular adnexal structure, such as a Meibomian gland or hair follicle. The lesion is very similar to those of cutaneous sterile pyogranuloma syndrome and other idiopathic granulomatous

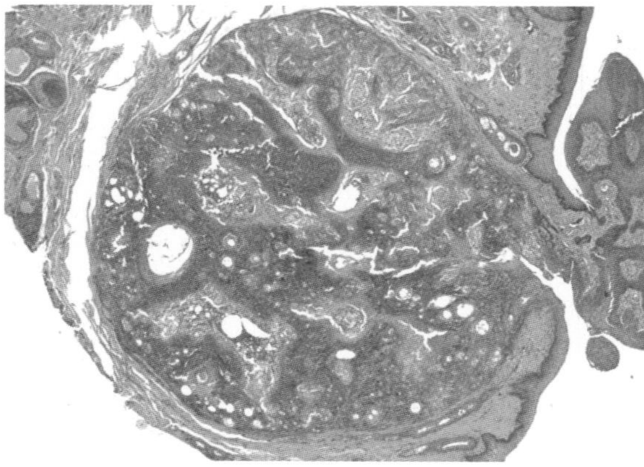

Fig. 20-129 Meibomian adenoma, eyelid, dog.
The tumor is a well-demarcated, encapsulated, expansile nodule consisting of intermingled basal and sebaceous cells. The accompanying papillary hyperplasia of the overlying epidermis is a common secondary reactive change. H&E stain. (Courtesy Dr. B. Wilcock, Ontario Veterinary College.)

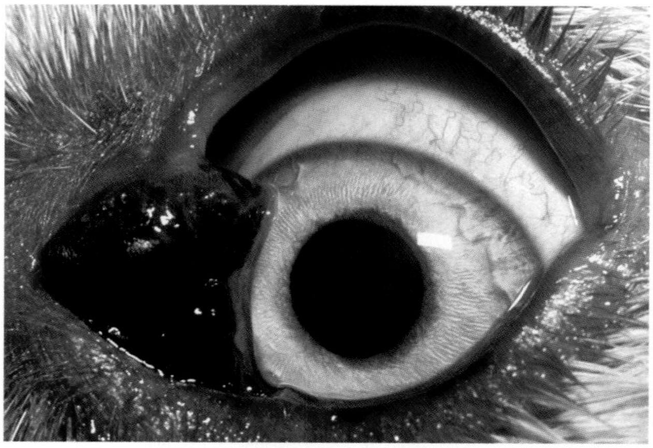

Fig. 20-130 Cutaneous melanocytoma, eyelid skin, dog.
A nodule of firm black tissue has replaced a wedge of the eyelid skin at its margin. Determining the exact location of the mass is clinically critical because a similar tumor arising even a few millimeters away on the palpebral conjunctiva would probably be behaviorally malignant. (Courtesy Dr. R. Peiffer, University of North Carolina.)

panniculitides, for all of which the pathogeneses are unknown. No infectious agent has ever been identified.

Neoplasms of the Eyelids

Meibomian adenoma is by far the most common tumor of the canine eyelid, accounting for in excess of 80% of all eyelid tumors in that species. Eyelid tumors in any other species are infrequent to rare. The tumor is an exact counterpart of sebaceous adenomas seen elsewhere in skin: a smooth expansile growth populated by intermingled basal cells and mature sebaceous cells. The tumor usually retains well-developed lobular architecture and in some cases differs from a normal gland only by its much greater overall size (Fig. 20-129). Many are populated almost exclusively by basal cells with just a few foci of sebaceous differentiation. Many contain substantial amounts of melanin pigment. Behaviorally, they are benign and are easily cured by excision.

Melanocytoma is the second most common tumor of the canine eyelid. It is identical in all respects to superficial dermal melanocytomas found elsewhere in the skin, and it is universally benign (Fig. 20-130).

Other neoplasms affecting the eyelid with greater-than-usual frequency include nerve sheath tumors in dogs and cats, squamous cell carcinoma and mast cell tumors in cats, and sarcoids in horses. They are identical in histologic appearance and behavior to those tumors occurring anywhere else in skin.

DISEASES OF THE CONJUNCTIVA

Developmental Anomalies

Conjunctival Dermoid

As with corneal dermoid, this is the presence of ectopic hair follicles and adnexal glands within the conjunctiva. Ordinarily, it is the bulbar conjunctiva that is affected. The ectopic tissue ranges from just a few scattered sebaceous glands to mature hair follicles with a full complement of adnexa.

Acquired Conjunctival Diseases

Infectious Diseases

Infectious bovine rhinotracheitis (bovine herpesvirus 1) is usually accompanied by serous to purulent conjunctivitis, which can be confused clinically with infectious bovine keratoconjunctivitis caused by *Moraxella bovis.* However, corneal involvement with rhinotracheitis is uncommon, and it is never the major presenting complaint and never reaches the severity seen in infectious bovine keratoconjunctivitis. After the acute serous conjunctivitis, hyperplasia of the resident conjunctival lymphoid nodules (follicular lymphoid hyperplasia) frequently occurs. Macroscopically, this is evident as a series of glistening gray-white protruding nodules a few millimeters in diameter, visible through the epithelium of the bulbar and palpebral conjunctiva.

Feline infectious conjunctivitis is caused by mycoplasma, chlamydia, or herpesvirus. The microscopic lesions are not specific except for the presence of inclusion bodies characteristic of the specific infectious agent. Unfortunately, inclusion bodies are present only during the first few days of disease and are almost never present by the time cytologic or histologic samples are obtained. Thus the presumptive diagnosis is usually based on the clinical characteristics of the conjunctival disease and especially on the presence of other clinical signs. Because these agents are all quite widely distributed in the healthy feline population, one must use great caution in interpreting a positive result of a serologic or polymerase chain reaction (PCR) test as indicating a causal role for that organism in the disease in that patient.

Feline herpesvirus 1 (FHV-1) causes a combination of conjunctivitis, keratitis, and upper respiratory disease when it first affects young cats, but it may cause conjunctivitis alone as a recurring infection in older cats that have recovered from the initial, more widespread disease. Herpesvirus is a more significant cause of keratitis in cats.

Mycoplasma felis and *Mycoplasma gatae* have been reported to cause suppurative, erosive conjunctivitis. However, a review of the available evidence suggests that it is more likely that these mycoplasmas, which are members of the normal feline conjunctival flora, act only as significant opportunists in disease initiated by herpesvirus or chlamydia.

Chlamydia psittaci usually causes unilateral conjunctivitis in cats of any age, without any other associated disease. The conjunctivitis is initially neutrophilic but rapidly becomes a subepithelial mixture of neutrophils, macrophages, lymphocytes, and plasma cells. Early in the disease (between days 7 and 14), typical intracytoplasmic inclusion bodies can be seen, and their detection is improved by immunofluorescent staining. Because the clinical signs are characteristic and disease is easily treated, histologic assessment is rarely required. By the time histologic assessment is required in the few cases not responding to therapy, it is too late because lesions have become completely nonspecific lymphonodular conjunctivitis with no visible inclusion bodies.

Thelazia are thin, rapidly motile nematodes 7 to 20 mm in length that inhabit the conjunctival sac and lacrimal duct of a variety of wild and domestic mammals. They are perhaps not exactly "normal" in the conjunctival sac, but only a small proportion of animals infected with the parasite have clinical disease. They are transmitted from animal to animal by face flies, which ingest larvae in lacrimal secretions. In North America, they are of minor significance as parasites of horses and cause only a mild lymphonodular conjunctivitis.

Habronemiasis is a far more significant disease in horses. It causes oozing eosinophilic granulomas, up to 1 cm in diameter, in the palpebral and bulbar conjunctivae. The macroscopic lesion is a firm nodule with yellow, caseous gritty debris in the center. The lesion is in response to nematode larvae deposited by a fly intermediate host, usually *Musca domestica* or *Stomoxys calcitrans*. They are attracted to this location by the moisture collecting in the medial canthus. Larvae of *Habronema muscae, Habronema microstoma,* or *Draschia (Habronema) megastoma* are also capable of causing the same histologic lesion that is identical to cutaneous habronemiasis, a chronic eosinophilic and granulomatous inflammation surrounding live or dead larvae that are difficult to find in histologic sections (Fig. 20-131).

Idiopathic and Immune Diseases

Idiopathic eosinophilic conjunctivitis is probably the conjunctival counterpart of the eosinophilic keratitis syndrome seen in cats and occasionally in horses. Rarely, the conjunctival lesion exists without any obvious corneal involvement. Lesions may be unilateral or bilateral. The microscopic lesions are greatly influenced by age and the previous antiinflammatory therapy, so it is hard to know what the "real" lesions are. In biopsy samples, the usual changes include ulceration, epithelial hyperplasia, squamous metaplasia, and a notable lymphocytic infiltration with a large number of eosinophils. The presence of eosinophils is a requirement for the diagnosis. They are not present as part of a granulomatous disease as in habronemiasis nor are they associated with collagenolysis as seen in insect bite reactions.

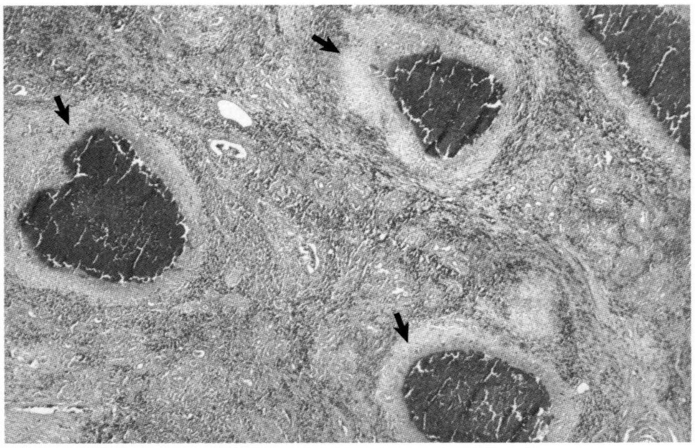

Fig. 20-131 Granulomatous conjunctivitis with eosinophils (focal), habronemiasis, conjunctiva, horse.

Note the multiple coalescing eosinophil-rich granulomas *(arrows)* within the conjunctival lamina propria. These granulomas are old larval migration tracts, but habronema larvae are rarely visible in them by the time such lesions are sampled for histological examination (usually to rule out neoplasia). H&E stain. (Courtesy Dr. B. Wilcock, Ontario Veterinary College.)

Protrusion and/or prolapse of the gland of the third eyelid is quite common in dogs and is thought to be the result of laxity in the connective tissue anchoring the gland to the cartilage of the third eyelid. Because the prolapsed mass is unsightly and resembles a neoplasm, it is sometimes excised and submitted for histologic examination, which reveals that the gland is usually completely normal or has mild nonspecific changes in response to desiccation or chronic edema.

Nodular granulomatous episcleritis (NGE) is a prevalent nodular lesion of the conjunctival lamina propria of dogs. It has been known by many names over the years, reflecting confusion about its exact status as an immune-mediated proliferative disease or a histiocytic neoplasm. Some of the synonyms include ocular nodular fasciitis, fibrous histiocytoma, or collie granuloma. It is not known whether this is one disease or several different diseases with the same histologic appearance. The disease is defined by its histopathologic changes: a discrete nodular accumulation of macrophages, fibroblasts, lymphocytes, and plasma cells anywhere in the conjunctival lamina propria. These cells are uniformly intermingled, without the formation of discrete granulomas. There is no collagenolysis, and usually there are not a significant number of granulocytes. The lateral limbus is the most frequent site, but the third eyelid is also frequently affected. In most instances, the lesion is unilateral and solitary, but bilateral involvement is not uncommon.

Necrotic scleritis is another canine idiopathic "immune-mediated" disease that may be mistaken for NGE. It often begins as a nodular thickening of the bulbar conjunctiva or underlying sclera just posterior to the limbus. Microscopically, however, it is a more destructive lesion with collagenolysis and (at least in the early disease) numerous eosinophils in addition to the macrophages, fibroblasts, and lymphocytes, which are also seen in NGE. It is a rapidly progressive and destructive lesion, capable of spreading rapidly to involve large areas of the sclera. Late in the disease it may spread into the globe, causing destructive coalescing granulomas throughout the uvea.

Neoplasms of the Conjunctiva

Squamous cell carcinoma is an exceedingly prevalent and economically significant neoplasm affecting the sunlight-exposed, nonpigmented epithelium of the eyelids, bulbar conjunctiva, usually at the lateral limbus and third eyelid of cattle living outdoors in sunny environments. The frequency is highest in areas in which livestock are likely to be exposed to ultraviolet radiation: areas with high altitude and lots of sunshine. Animals with poor pigmentation of eyelids and conjunctiva are particularly susceptible because this increases the risk of chronic cellular injury from solar radiation. Viruses, such as bovine papillomavirus and bovine herpesvirus 5, have been detected within bovine ocular squamous cell carcinomas, but their causal role has not been proven. An identical tumor occurs in horses living in the same environments.

As occurs with sunlight-induced squamous cell carcinoma in other cutaneous locations, the ocular tumor goes through a series of precancerous changes in response to actinic injury. The sequence of lesions is squamous plaque (acanthosis), keratoses (localized foci of hyperkeratosis), squamous papilloma, dysplasia, squamous carcinoma in situ, and eventually invasive squamous cell carcinoma (Fig. 20-132). Keratoses can sometimes develop into cutaneous horns. These are usually conical, can reach a length of a few centimeters, and consist of compacted laminated keratin (Fig. 20-133). Occasionally, they are on the surface of a papilloma. Like actinic

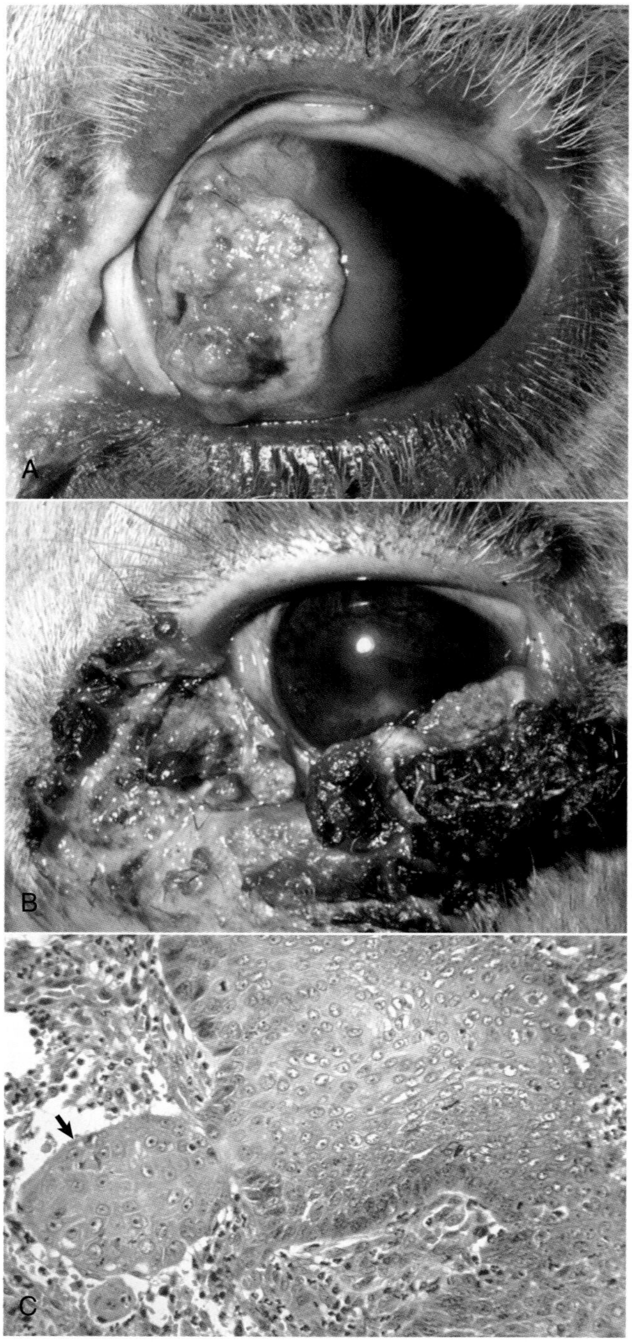

Fig. 20-132 **Squamous cell carcinoma, eye and eyelids, Hereford cow.** **A,** Medial limbus. The carcinoma has spread over the cornea as an exophytic growth from its original site on the medial limbus. Note the corneal edema *(gray area)* adjacent to the margin of the carcinoma. Pigmentation of the eyelids, as shown here, does not protect the conjunctiva or the limbus from developing an actinic (exposure to sunlight) squamous cell carcinoma. **B,** Third and lower eyelids. Note the early exophytic squamous cell carcinoma on the third eyelid, nodules of acanthosis on the lateral half of the lower lid conjunctiva and on the skin of the medial canthus, and keratoses on the lower lid. **C,** Early infiltrative squamous cell carcinoma, lower lid. A small group *(arrow)* of epithelial cells has infiltrated through the basement membrane of the mucosal squamous epithelium. Note that these cells are atypical. The basal cells have lost their polarity and now lie horizontal to the edge of the infiltrating mass instead of vertically, as do normal basal cells (perpendicular to the basement membrane). H&E stain. (Courtesy Dr. M.D. McGavin, College of Veterinary Medicine, University of Tennessee.)

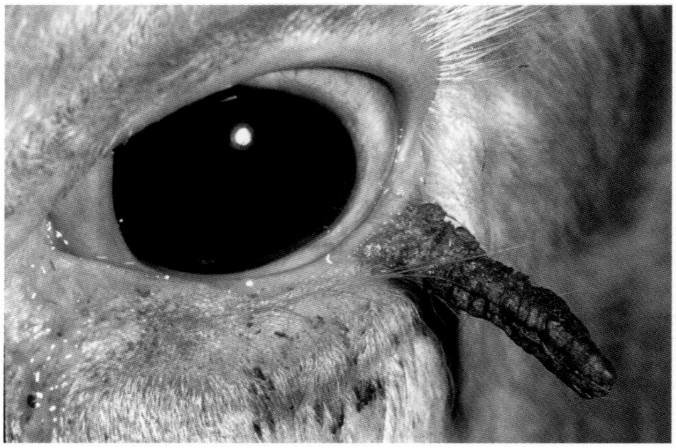

Fig. 20-133 **Cutaneous horn, lower eyelid, mucocutaneous junction.** The cutaneous horn on the lower lid is an exaggerated form of a keratosis. The unpigmented skin of the lower lid and medial canthus is erythematous, and the surface of the medial aspect of the lower lid is slightly roughed by white foci of acanthosis. (Courtesy Dr. M.D. McGavin, College of Veterinary Medicine, University of Tennessee.)

keratoses they are considered to be premalignant. The stepwise transition from acanthosis to eventual carcinoma in situ is characterized by increasing nuclear pleomorphism, hyperchromasia, and loss of polarity of the cells and maturational jumbling of cells within the stratum spinosum. The only absolutely unequivocal proof of malignant transformation is invasion by cords of malignant cells through the basement membrane into the underlying lamina propria (Fig. 20-132, *C*). The mass of invading cells is usually surrounded by an intense lymphocytic-plasmacytic inflammatory reaction, a reaction that is interpreted as an immune response to the developing tumor. Not all precursor lesions develop into carcinomas. The efficacy of the immune response in destroying precursor lesions and early carcinomas is unknown.

In cats, squamous cell carcinoma usually affects the skin of the eyelid itself rather than conjunctiva. Squamous cell carcinoma is inexplicably rare in either the eyelids or the conjunctiva of dogs.

Benign squamous papillomas with no inclination for malignant progression are frequent tumors of the bulbar conjunctiva of dogs. They are formed by multiple slender fronds consisting of conjunctival lamina propria covered by hyperplastic but otherwise orderly and mature stratified squamous nonkeratinized epithelium. There is often substantial melanin pigment within the basal cells and lamina propria, so these tumors can be mistaken on clinical examination for conjunctival melanomas. There is no evidence that these papillomas are caused by a viral infection.

Primary conjunctival melanomas arise within the epithelium of the bulbar conjunctiva of dogs and cats. In dramatic contrast to the benign melanotic tumors of the haired skin of the eyelid or those arising deeper within the stroma of the limbus (see later discussion), these are aggressively invasive with a high risk of metastasis. They resemble oral melanomas in histologic and cytologic appearance and in the frequency of being amelanotic. Microscopically, they form solid endocrine-like packets of 20 to 30 cells supported by a delicate fibrous stroma. Intraepithelial clusters (junctional activity) are often present. The cells generally are pleomorphic epithelioid cells with frequent nuclear gigantism and hyperchromasia. They are markedly invasive, a feature often visible in histologic sections. Postoperative recurrence is extremely frequent. Pigment, when present, is most frequently found in tumor cells within or near the epithelium.

Limbal melanocytomas are relatively common tumors in dogs. They are infrequent but not rare in cats. They arise from the pigmented cells within the limbus, which is the junction of the corneal stroma and sclera. They form a slowly expanding, heavily pigmented discrete nodule populated by heavily pigmented large plump cells identical to those seen in the more common anterior uveal melanocytoma. They have no metastatic potential, and surgical excision is curative. They may bulge outwardly to distend the overlying conjunctiva, but histologic examination reveals that they do not infiltrate the epithelium and are therefore easily distinguished from the more dangerous primary conjunctival malignant melanoma.

Hemangioma and hemangiosarcoma are vascular endothelial neoplasms arising within the conjunctival lamina propria at the lateral edge of the third eyelid, and in the lateral bulbar conjunctiva of dogs, cats, and (occasionally) horses. About 30% of canine cases are bilateral. The sites of predilection and the increased risk of disease in outdoor dogs in sunny climates and high altitudes suggest that this disease is probably triggered by chronic actinic radiation injury (as is true for at least some examples of cutaneous hemangioma and hemangiosarcoma in dogs). Those tumors that are well circumscribed and consist of bland endothelium are classified as hemangiomas, and those formed by hyperchromatic endothelium with at least moderate anisokaryosis and peripheral invasion are classified as hemangiosarcomas. However, there is a continuum in the histologic appearance from hemangioma to hemangiosarcoma. Many are intermediate, or even show a continuum of lesions from benign to malignant within the same tumor. Distinguishing benign from malignant is based primarily on the degree of peripheral invasion. At least in dogs (the species most often affected), this distinction appears to have no behavioral significance, as almost all are benign and surgically curable.

In horses, some (but not all) of the vascular tumors involving the third eyelid are solid primitive hemangiosarcomas. Some of these tumors are very invasive and have a high risk of metastasis to the regional lymph node.

Adenocarcinoma of the gland of the third eyelid is a tumor of very old dogs (rarely cats), which is usually seen as a well-differentiated, slowly expanding tubular adenocarcinoma at the dorsal margin of the third eyelid. It replaces the normal gland of the third eyelid but only slowly invades adjacent tissue. The risk of metastasis is very low.

Lymphoma (lymphosarcoma) occasionally arises within the lamina propria of the third eyelid in animals (most often in cats) that do not have any evidence of disseminated lymphosarcoma. The cells are similar in histologic appearance to those of lymphomas elsewhere, but it takes courage to make this diagnosis when the tumor appears to be present in only a single, unlikely location, such as the third eyelid.

DISEASES OF THE ORBIT

Orbital cellulitis is not a specific disease but inflammation of soft tissue in response to infectious agents introduced via a penetrating wound, a migrating foreign body, or an inflammatory focus from some adjacent tissue (often, a tooth root abscess). Only rarely does panophthalmitis extend into the orbit to cause orbital cellulitis because the sclera seems to be an effective barrier to the migration of leukocytes and infectious agents.

Lymphocytic interstitial dacryoadenitis is a progressive idiopathic lymphocytic inflammation of the lacrimal gland and/or gland of the third eyelid of dogs. It is present as a histologic lesion in most cases of spontaneous keratoconjunctivitis sicca. The initial lesion is an interstitial lymphocytic infiltration with epithelial necrosis, followed by glandular atrophy and extensive interstitial fibrosis with residual nests of lymphocytes. Because no infectious agent can be found and because the disease can be successfully managed with immunosuppressive therapy (particularly cyclosporin), it is assumed to represent a T lymphocyte–dependent autoimmune disease.

Orbital extraocular myositis affects all the extraocular muscles except the retractor bulbi. It is a rare disease of dogs. Histologically, there is a lymphocytic myositis that results in myonecrosis, followed by attempts at regeneration and eventually muscle atrophy and fibrosis. The acute disease causes enough swelling to result in pain and exophthalmos. In the chronic disease, there is a notable enophthalmos (retraction of the globe into the orbit). An immune-mediated attack directed specifically against the extraocular muscles is suspected to be the cause of this disorder. Because the extraocular muscles are a difficult site from which to obtain a biopsy, diagnosis is generally based on the typical clinical findings. Corticosteroid therapy is effective, but episodes can recur.

Orbital neoplasms are surprisingly frequent in dogs. They are rare in other domestic animals with the exception of cattle, in which malignant lymphoma occurs. Most orbital tumors are not discovered until they are large enough to cause exophthalmos or blindness, by which time the majority of cases are no longer amenable to surgical cure. Many different tumors in the orbit have been reported, but the only ones that are relatively frequent are optic nerve meningioma and multilobular osteochondroma in dogs, nasal carcinoma and gingival squamous cell carcinoma in dogs and cats, and malignant lymphoma in cattle. These tumors are all histologically identical to those in other locations.

DISORDERS OF HORSES

EQUINE KERATOMYCOSIS

Equine keratomycosis (mycotic keratitis) is probably always a manifestation of opportunistic contamination of corneal wounds by fungi that are common within the environment around horses. *Aspergillus* spp. is by far the most common agent isolated. Similar infection occurs much less frequently in dogs, cats, and other species. Alteration of the corneal defenses or the normal microbial environment by the prolonged use of antibiotics or corticosteroids in the management of corneal wounds is a strong predisposing factor in all species. In all species there are two different syndromes: (1) opportunistic infection of dead superficial stroma by huge numbers of fungal hyphae in the almost complete absence of inflammation or (2) deep stromal infection that evokes an intense suppurative keratomalacia that, if untreated, often progresses to corneal perforation and iris prolapse. The deep stromal keratitis in cases in which the stroma and epithelium have healed over the top of a deep stromal infection is referred to as a *stromal abscess.* The fungi exhibit strong tropism for Descemet's membrane (as they do for basement membranes in other tissues) and may be absent from the stroma of the superficial (anterior) half of the cornea (Fig. 20-134). This explains why confirmation of infection by means of corneal scrapings is often unsuccessful. It also explains why topical application of antifungal medication alone is rarely successful. In many cases, successful management of the disease requires surgical débridement of the cornea to remove most of the infected tissue and the damaging leukocytes. One peculiarity of this disease is that the infection virtually never spreads into the globe itself, even though the fungi can be seen dangling within the anterior chamber. There must be something unique to the corneal environment that is essential for fungal virulence or survival.

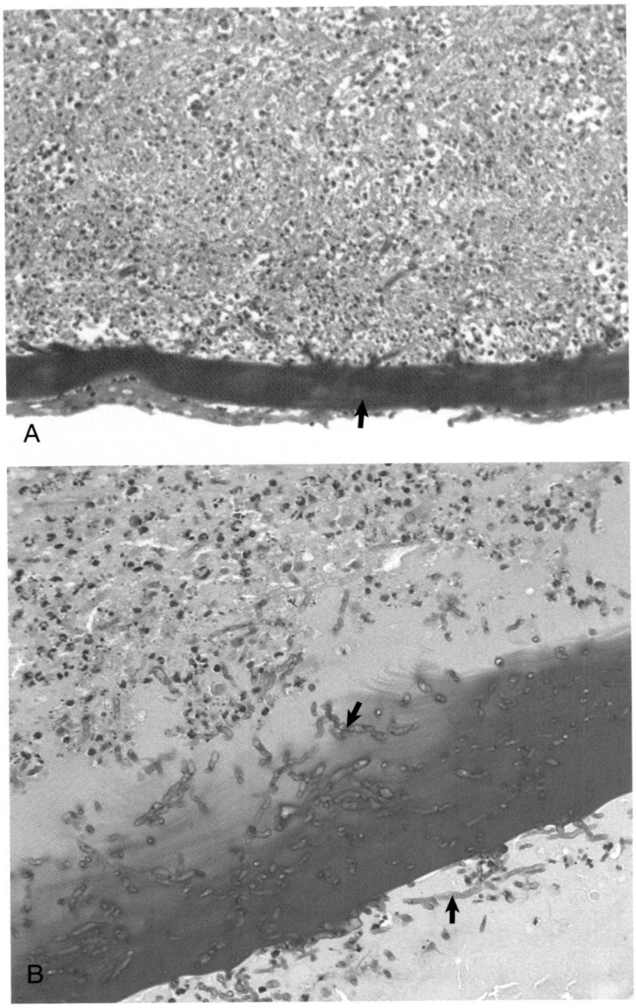

Fig. 20-134 Suppurative keratomalacia (deep stromal), posterior cornea, keratomycosis, horse.

A, The deep portion of the corneal stroma contains numerous neutrophils, resulting in stromal destruction (keratomalacia). Descemet's membrane *(arrow)* is thickened and irregular and contains fungal hyphae. This is the most common histologic form of the disease. H&E stain. **B,** Higher magnification to show fungal hyphae *(arrows)* within and adjacent to Descemet's membrane. Note the loss of the normal appearance of the stroma and the infiltration by neutrophils and edema fluid. H&E stain. (Courtesy Dr. B. Wilcock, Ontario Veterinary College.)

EOSINOPHILIC KERATITIS

Eosinophilic keratitis occurs predominately in cats and occasionally in horses (see the section on Disorders of Cats).

EQUINE RECURRENT UVEITIS

Equine recurrent uveitis (ERU), also referred to as periodic ophthalmia and moon blindness, is a frequent cause of blindness in horses. It is characterized by unpredictable episodes of severe uveitis with a tendency to become increasingly frequent and increasingly severe over time. It is likely that several different diseases are included under this diagnostic umbrella, but at least one of the causes is an immunologic reaction against intraocular leptospiral antigens. It is thought to be a delayed reaction to a systemic infection with *Leptospira interrogans* (most often serovar Pomona). The evidence supporting a role for leptospirosis in the pathogenesis of equine recurrent uveitis is substantial even if not absolutely conclusive:

1. Horses with high serum titers to *Leptospira interrogans* are 13 times more likely to have uveitis than horses with no such titers.
2. Antileptospiral antibodies rise during episodes of uveitis and decrease during quiescent phases.
3. The disease can be reproduced by infection of naive horses with *Leptospira interrogans* serovar Pomona. Not all infected horses developed uveitis, and the onset of ocular signs is usually delayed for a year or more after infection. In the original study, 22 of 36 of the eyes of Shetland ponies inoculated subcutaneously with small numbers of *Leptospira interrogans* serovar Pomona eventually developed classic recurrent uveitis. All ponies developed leptospiremia soon after inoculation, but none developed ocular disease until at least 50 weeks later.
4. There is cross-reaction between leptospiral antigens and various intraocular antigens, particularly those of the corneal endothelium and lens. This creates the possibility that the ongoing immune-mediated inflammation is not necessarily in response to persisting leptospiral antigens. Leptospirosis may cause the initial uveitis but may not be responsible for its perpetuation.

The most common alternative agent implicated in a syndrome clinically indistinguishable from leptospira-associated recurrent uveitis is *Onchocerca cervicalis.* Intraocular dead or dying microfilaria have been proposed as sources of antigen responsible for the disease.

The microscopic lesions depend on the stage of the disease and represent a continuum from anterior uveitis to endophthalmitis with retinal scarring or even phthisis bulbi. The earliest lesion is an anterior uveal inflammation that is transiently neutrophilic but rapidly becomes predominantly lymphocytic. Even during intervals in which the clinical disease is quiescent, the histologic lesions of perivascular lymphocytic anterior uveitis persist (Fig. 20-135). Peripheral corneal vascularization becomes increasingly prominent, eventually extending across the entire diameter of the corneal stroma. Choroidal inflammation is usually most obvious near the optic disc and may cause exudative retinal detachment. Even if the retina reattaches, there are residual lesions of photoreceptor loss or even full thickness retinal scarring as a result of ischemic injury during periods of detachment. This peripapillary retinal scarring is sometimes the only lesion seen in horses with a clinical history suggesting chronic, episodic ERU.

A characteristic lesion of chronic ERU is an eosinophilic hyaline membrane that seems to cover the ciliary epithelium. This material in fact lies within the apical cytoplasm of the nonpigmented ciliary epithelium and resembles amyloid. Its pathogenesis is unknown, but it serves as a useful marker for the disease.

DISORDERS OF RUMINANTS (CATTLE, SHEEP, AND GOATS)

INFECTIOUS BOVINE KERATOCONJUNCTIVITIS

Infectious bovine keratoconjunctivitis (commonly known as *pink eye*) is a worldwide contagious disease of considerable economic importance that has been recognized for more than 100 years. It is caused by specific strains of the Gram-negative bacillus *Moraxella bovis,* which is part of the normal conjunctival and nasal flora of cattle. Virulent strains have capsular pili, which facilitate corneal colonization, and most of the virulent strains are also hemolytic. In contrast, most of the strains recovered from the conjunctiva of healthy animals are nonhemolytic and nonpiliated. It is not

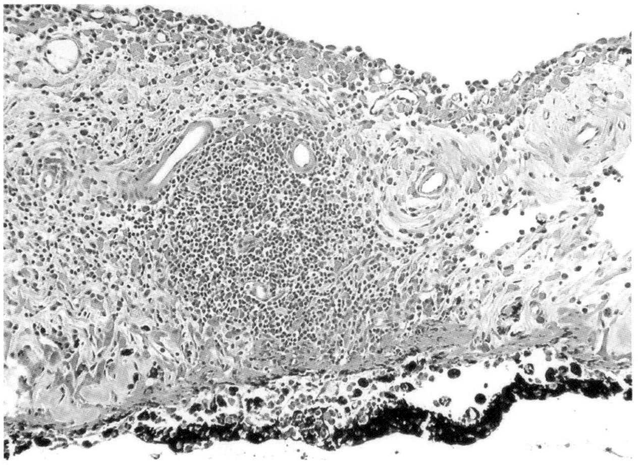

Fig. 20-135 Equine recurrent uveitis, iris, horse.
Perivascular lymphocytic-plasmacytic aggregates *(center of image)* within the iris stroma are typical of equine recurrent uveitis, but the same lesion is commonly seen in idiopathic uveitis in various species. H&E stain. (Courtesy Dr. B. Wilcock, Ontario Veterinary College.)

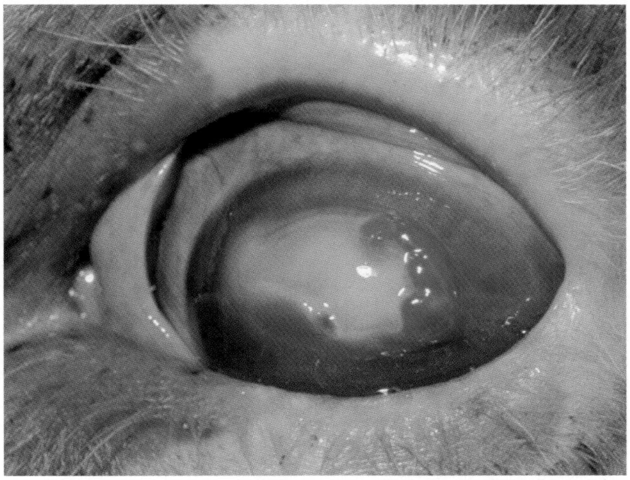

Fig. 20-136 Infectious bovine keratoconjunctivitis ("pink-eye"), cow.
The axial half of the ulcerated cornea is filled with neutrophils (suppurative keratomalacia) and surrounded by a border of red fleshy granulation tissue. The initial lesions are shallow corneal ulcers and foci of suppurative superficial stromal keratitis with conjunctival hyperemia, followed by circumferential superficial vascular ingrowth from bulbar conjunctiva toward the central ulcers. (Courtesy Dr. M.D. McGavin, College of Veterinary Medicine, University of Tennessee.)

clear exactly what is responsible for emergence of the virulent strains. *Moraxella bovis* is transmitted from animal to animal by mechanical vectors such as flies, by direct contact, and by fomites. In natural outbreaks, face flies *(Musca autumnalis)* appear to be the most important vectors. The concurrent presence of other infectious agents, such as *Mycoplasma* or infectious rhinotracheitis virus, often increases the severity of the disease.

The initial lesions are shallow corneal ulcers, which are probably the direct result of epithelial cytotoxin produced by adherent *Moraxella.* The organisms then gain access to the stroma, which results in attraction of large numbers of neutrophils from the limbus and from conjunctival blood vessels via the tear film. Inevitably, there is bystander injury from the degranulating neutrophils, but *Moraxella* also produces a potent cytotoxin, which accelerates neutrophil destruction. Lesions are initially unilateral but eventually become bilateral. Progression of a lesion is rapid during the initial 48 to 72 hours after infection and usually results in a shallow painful corneal ulcer and foci of suppurative superficial stromal keratitis that gradually heal over the next few weeks. There is usually severe conjunctival hyperemia, followed by circumferential superficial vascular ingrowth from bulbar conjunctiva toward the central ulcers (Fig. 20-136). Healing involves the usual events of fibrovascular ingrowth from the limbus, resulting in permanent central corneal scarring, which is usually not functionally significant. In severe cases, the ulcer may progress to descemetocele, iris prolapse, and destruction of the globe.

Similar clinical and histologic entities exist in sheep, goats, and pigs associated with corneal colonization by *Chlamydia* spp. and *Mycoplasma* spp.

BOVINE MALIGNANT CATARRHAL FEVER–ASSOCIATED UVEITIS

The majority of cattle with malignant catarrhal fever have prominent ocular lesions in the form of peripheral midstromal corneal vascularization and obvious anterior uveitis. These lesions help to clinically distinguish this disease from mucosal disease and acute severe BVD. The histologic lesions within the eye resemble those elsewhere in the body: arterial necrosis with perivascular and intramural accumulation of lymphoblasts, among which are a few with mitotic figures. The vasculitis is most often identified within the iris, but it can be found anywhere within the uveal tract or retina. The accompanying uveitis is predominantly lymphocytic right from the start. Of great diagnostic significance from a clinical perspective is a ring of peripheral corneal stromal vascularization extending into the cornea from the limbus. The vascular ingrowth is accompanied by notable corneal edema. Although this is a routine lesion seen in any chronic severe uveitis, it is not seen in keratoconjunctivitis associated with several other bovine infectious diseases. There may be a concurrent lymphocytic corneal endothelialitis contributing to the corneal edema.

The pathogenesis of the disease remains controversial. The appearance of the vasculitis suggests that it should be an immune-mediated vasculitis, yet intramural deposition of immunoglobulin or complement is not a significant feature of the vascular lesion. A T lymphocyte–dependent, type IV immune pathogenesis has been suggested.

SQUAMOUS CELL CARCINOMA

See the discussion on neoplasms of the conjunctiva in the section on Disorders of Domestic Animals.

DISORDERS OF DOGS

CANINE PANNUS KERATITIS (CHRONIC SUPERFICIAL KERATITIS, UBERREITER'S SYNDROME)

Pannus is a clinically and histologically distinctive superficial stromal keratitis seen primarily but not exclusively in German shepherd dogs. The disease usually begins at the lateral limbus as red conjunctival thickening. The lesion spreads toward the axial cornea as a superficial, fleshy, vascularized stromal infiltrate, involving both eyes (Fig. 20-137). Older lesions become intensely pigmented, and eventually the entire superficial stroma may be vascularized, scarred, and pigmented. The frequency and the severity of the disease increase proportionately as altitude increases, suggesting

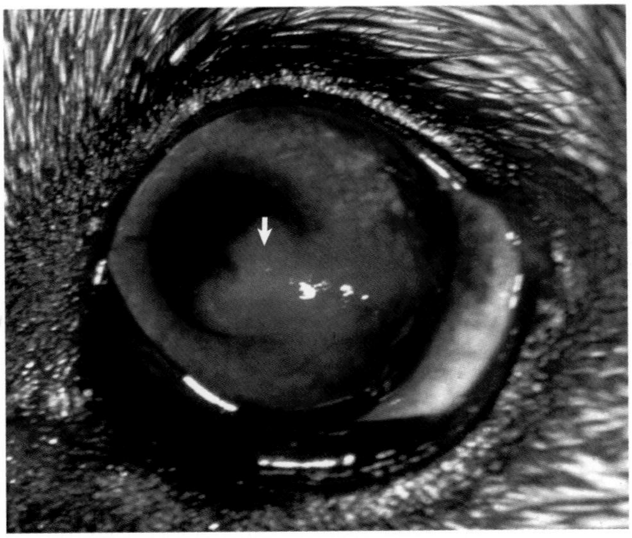

Fig. 20-137 Pannus keratitis, cornea, German shepherd dog. Note the fleshy gray-pink superficial stromal ingrowth *(arrow)* from the lateral limbus *(right)* into the anterior stroma of the cornea. This appearance is classic for pannus. (Courtesy Dr. B. Wilcock, Ontario Veterinary College.)

that sunlight exposure is important either in the initiation or the progression of the disease.

The histologic changes are almost identical to those seen in cutaneous discoid lupus, another disease with a predilection for German shepherds and related breeds. Discoid lupus is also exacerbated by sunlight. The early lesion is characterized by infiltration of plasma cells and smaller numbers of lymphocytes into the basilar half of the epithelium and the adjacent superficial corneal stroma near the limbus. There is vacuolation and then patchy loss of basal cells, followed by the dispersal of pigment from the injured epithelial cells. This is phagocytosed by macrophages, which accumulate within the superficial stroma. As the disease progresses, cellular infiltration is accompanied by corneal vascularization and fibrosis.

The disease is successfully treated (but never cured) by immunosuppressive therapy identical to that used to treat cutaneous discoid lupus. The inability to identify an infectious agent and the response to immunosuppressive therapy suggests that the disease has an immunologic pathogenesis, but the exact mechanism remains elusive.

COLLIE EYE ANOMALY

See the discussion on choroidal hypoplasia in the section on Disorders of Domestic Animals.

UVEODERMATOLOGIC SYNDROME IN DOGS (VOGT-KOYANAGI-HARADA SYNDROME)

Despite the exotic-sounding name, uveodermatologic syndrome is relatively frequent in the most susceptible breeds (Akitas, Siberian huskies, and Samoyeds). The clinical syndrome of facial dermal depigmentation and severe bilateral uveitis is distinctive, although many dogs with the uveitis do not have skin lesions. The canine syndrome closely parallels that of the human disease, except that the encephalitis, which is the least frequent part of the human syndrome, has not been confirmed in dogs. The histologic lesion is a destructive granulomatous endophthalmitis with abundant dispersal of melanin, a consequence of T lymphocyte–mediated destruction of melanin-producing cells of the RPE and urea. The disease is slowly progressive and is always eventually bilateral even though initially it may not affect both eyes.

CANINE PROGRESSIVE RETINAL ATROPHY

Progressive retinal atrophy is the traditional designation for a large group of inherited bilateral degenerative retinopathies of dogs. These have become widespread because of deliberate restrictions of genetic diversity imposed by current line-breeding practices in purebred dogs. Innumerable breeds are affected, and the list grows daily. They all have a similar clinical and microscopic appearance but that is where the uniformity ends. In reality, this group of diseases includes a genetically and biochemically diverse collection of photoreceptor dysplasias and degenerations that looked similar only when our methods of detection were limited to ophthalmoscopic evaluation and histopathologic examination. Its inclusion here as an acquired retinal disease rather than as a developmental disease is in deference to its clinical presentation and because at least some of this group are indeed true degenerations.

The stereotypic features seen by light microscopy are loss of photoreceptor outer segments followed by progressive loss of inner segments and eventually loss of neurons from the outer nuclear layer. The result is collapse and thinning of the retina. Other portions of the retina remain normal, and there is no inflammation.

Currently, these bilateral noninflammatory photoreceptor dysfunctions are divided into developmental photoreceptor dysplasias and later-onset, purely degenerative diseases. The classification of these various syndromes is under continuous review because in some cases what was once thought to be a degenerative disease affecting previously normal photoreceptors has been discovered to be an inborn biochemical error with a delayed phenotypic manifestation. The list of breeds in which photoreceptor dysplasia or degeneration has been described grows daily, so this brief discussion is not intended to be inclusive.

PHOTORECEPTOR DYSPLASIAS

The majority of the photoreceptor dysplasias cause clinical signs of bilateral, progressive blindness in juvenile dogs. The fundamental defect varies by breed; the defect may specifically target rods or cones or affect both. Most examples have a simple, autosomal recessive inheritance pattern. The most thoroughly studied is the combined rod-cone dysplasia of Irish setter dogs. It is beyond the scope of this text to discuss all of the various photoreceptor dysplasias, so this one example serves to illustrate the general model.

Rod-cone dysplasia of Irish setters is inherited as a simple autosomal recessive trait. Dogs homozygous for the defect have arrested differentiation and then deterioration of the rod external segments, with cones being much less affected. The defect is detected ultrastructurally as early as 16 days after birth, at which time the outer rod segments adjacent to the retinal pigment epithelium should be developing. There is essentially diffuse loss of all rod photoreceptors by 12 weeks of age. This is followed by loss of cones and cells of the outer nuclear layer. The central retina is affected earlier and more severely than is the peripheral retina. Biochemical abnormalities are detected as early as 1 week of age. There is a severe deficiency of the activity of the phosphodiesterase responsible for the continuous hydrolysis of cyclic guanine monophosphate (cGMP) within outer segments. This results in a tenfold excess of cGMP, which has been shown to be toxic to photoreceptors in vitro, and also inhibits photoreceptor development. The basic defect is defective messenger RNA in the gene encoding the outer segment-specific phosphodiesterase.

PHOTORECEPTOR DEGENERATIONS

Photoreceptor degeneration refers to an equally diverse group of diseases in which early development is (as far as we can currently detect) normal, and degeneration occurs later in life. Prototype for this group is a rod-cone degeneration in toy and miniature poodles (with virtually identical diseases seen in English and American cocker spaniels, Labrador retrievers, and Portuguese water dogs). This disease is classified as a true degeneration in that photoreceptor differentiation seems to be normal until 6 to 9 weeks of age. After this time and progressing at an unpredictable rate, photoreceptor outer segments degenerate. Rods are affected earlier and with greater severity than are cones. The disease progresses at an unpredictable rate; affected dogs may not have clinical or ophthalmoscopic evidence of disease until 3 to 5 years of age (which in breeding dogs means that they will already have passed on the genetic defect). The macroscopic and histologic lesions begin centrally, around the optic disc, but eventually (by 6 to 7 years of age), the entire retina is affected and the dog is blind. The biochemical basis for the degeneration remains unknown.

CANINE LYMPHOCYTIC UVEITIS

Canine lymphocytic uveitis has the most frequent histologic pattern of uveitis seen in dogs (as it is in cats and horses), a lymphocytic-plasmacytic panuveitis that tends to be more severe in the anterior uvea than in the choroid. It should not really be considered a specific disease but rather a histologic pattern that is probably shared by many different diseases. As in the other species, the disease may be unilateral or bilateral and tends to occur in multiple episodes interrupted by periods of quiescence. The cause remains unknown, and it is likely that there are multiple different agents capable of inducing this identical histologic change. In contrast to the situation in cats, it does not cause glaucoma. The main differential diagnosis is phacolytic uveitis, and indeed in some cases the histologic distinction is impossible.

CANINE ANTERIOR UVEAL MELANOCYTOMAS

See the discussion on neoplasms of the uvea in the section on Disorders of Domestic Animals.

MEIBOMIAN ADENOMAS

See the discussion on neoplasms of the eyelids in the section on Disorders of Domestic Animals.

MELANOCYTOMAS

See the discussion on neoplasms of the eyelids in the section on Disorders of Domestic Animals.

LIMBAL MELANOCYTOMAS

See the discussion on neoplasms of the conjunctiva in the section on Disorders of Domestic Animals.

DISORDERS OF CATS

FELINE HERPETIC KERATITIS

Feline herpesvirus 1 (FHV-1) is an exceedingly common cause of acute-to-chronic keratitis in cats. Viral infection of the corneal epithelial cells results in shallow intraepithelial branching tracts of necrosis, known as *dendritic ulcers.* FHV-1 can also cause a more severe delayed, deeper stromal accumulation of lymphocytes and plasma cells that appears to be a syndrome separate from the dendritic ulcers. In cats with deeper stromal keratitis, there is concurrent nondendritic regional epithelial ulceration, necrosis of superficial stroma, and an intense accumulation of lymphocytes and plasma cells that presumably have migrated from the limbus. The histologic pattern is nonspecific, and a more definitive etiologic diagnosis requires the demonstration of viral antigen within the injured epithelium or in the deep stromal lesion. Most cases of herpetic stromal keratitis probably result from activation of latent infections precipitated by concurrent disease or the topical application of corticosteroids. The specific etiologic diagnosis can be problematic because viral antigen can be difficult to demonstrate in chronic lesions laden with a lot of neutralizing antibody. In addition, many cats are asymptomatic carriers and so the mere demonstration of the FHV-1 (by immunohistochemistry or PCR done on diseased corneas) is not sufficient to establish causation.

EOSINOPHILIC KERATITIS

Eosinophilic keratitis is a unique disease that occurs predominantly in cats but has been seen occasionally in horses. The macroscopic appearance is characteristic: a granular white proliferative lesion extending inwardly along what seems to be the corneal surface from the medial or lateral limbus. Many cases have similar lesions in the adjacent conjunctiva, and in a few cases the lesions are exclusively conjunctival. Most begin as a unilateral disease, but soon both eyes are involved. The histologic lesion is a nonulcerative superficial stromal infiltration of a mixture of eosinophils, plasma cells, mast cells, and macrophages (Fig. 20-138). The percentage of each cell type within the lesion varies with the duration of the disease and is significantly influenced by therapy, but eosinophils are always present and are a requirement for the diagnosis. The granular appearance of the macroscopic lesion is created by the degranulation of eosinophils, which create a thick refractile eosinophilic coagulum along the surface of the lesion (see Fig. 20-138). The diagnosis is usually made on the basis of clinical appearance and the presence of eosinophils in a superficial corneal scraping. Even a few eosinophils in a superficial stromal keratitis with compatible clinical signs should be diagnosed as chronic eosinophilic keratitis, even though the majority of the leukocytes are plasma cells or other mononuclear leukocytes.

The cause and pathogenesis are unknown. Affected cats do not have concurrent skin lesions of eosinophilic granuloma complex or any other concurrent disease. Between 70% and 80% of lesions contain the DNA of FHV-1; the problem is that ocular

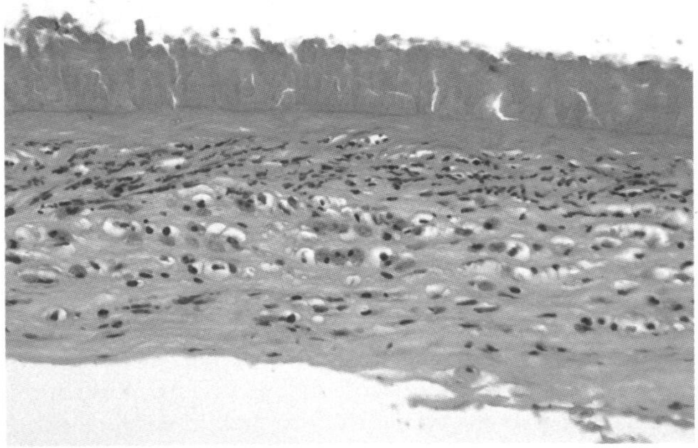

Fig. 20-138 Feline eosinophilic keratitis, cornea (keratectomy sample), cat.
The corneal epithelium and superficial stroma have been replaced by a coagulum of eosinophil granules. A mixture of leukocytes, predominantly eosinophils, has infiltrated the underlying stroma. The histologic changes are highly variable depending on the stage of the disease, but eosinophils are always present. H&E stain. (Courtesy Dr. B. Wilcock, Ontario Veterinary College.)

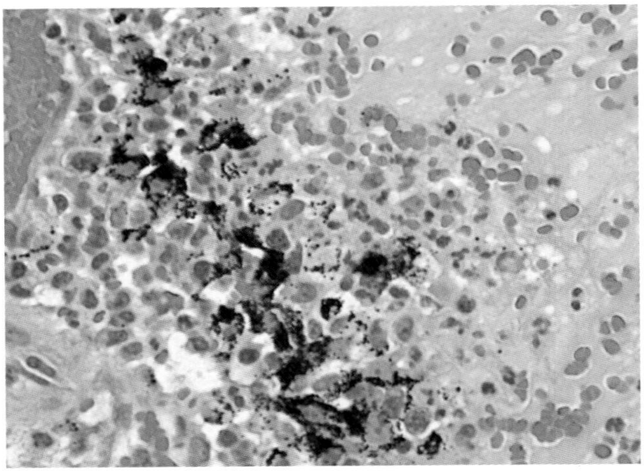

Fig. 20-139 Lymphocytic, granulomatous, and neutrophilic iridocyclitis (destructive), feline infectious peritonitis, ciliary body, cat. Lymphocytes and plasma cells tend to predominate within the uveal stroma *(left)*, whereas neutrophils, fibrin, and macrophages predominate within the adjacent aqueous humor of the posterior chamber *(right)*. These lesions are typical of feline infectious peritonitis. H&E stain. (Courtesy Dr. B. Wilcock, Ontario Veterinary College.)

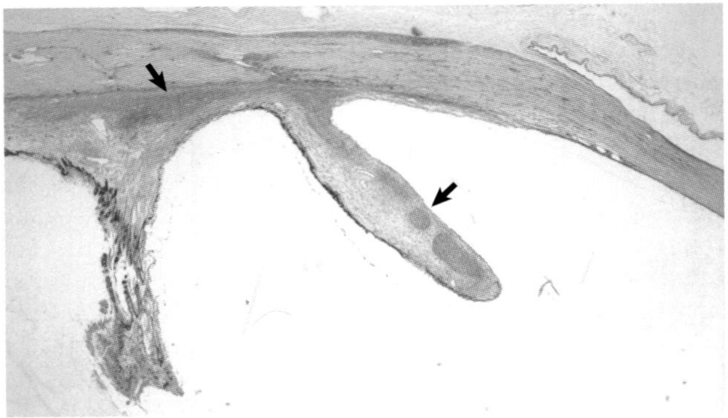

Fig. 20-140 Idiopathic lymphonodular uveitis, anterior uvea, cat. The iris and ciliary body contain numerous coalescing perivascular lymphocytic-plasmacytic nodules *(arrows)*. This lesion is the most common cause of glaucoma in cats (vying with diffuse iris melanoma for that distinction), but the mechanism by which it causes glaucoma is unknown. H&E stain. (Courtesy Dr. B. Wilcock, Ontario Veterinary College.)

herpesvirus infection is so common in cats that a definitive causal link is difficult to establish.

FELINE INFECTIOUS PERITONITIS–ASSOCIATED UVEITIS

The coronavirus of feline infectious peritonitis (FIP) causes a diffuse uveitis that is probably immune-mediated. The frequency of ocular lesions is unknown because the eyes are not regularly examined in cats with the disease. The histologic lesions in the globe are always bilateral and are similar to those seen in any other organ affected with the disease. As elsewhere, the lesions vary in the relative proportions of the different leukocyte types, the amount of fibrin, and the amount of necrosis. In most cases the disease is primarily an anterior uveitis with a mixture of lymphocytes, plasma cells, neutrophils, and macrophages. The often-repeated statement that FIP causes "pyogranulomatous" inflammation, especially within the globe, is greatly exaggerated. The exudate within the anterior chamber is usually predominantly neutrophilic, yet in the choroid the inflammation is usually lymphocytic-plasmacytic. Formation of keratic precipitates and a neutrophilic corneal endothelialitis are strong indicators of an FIP-associated uveitis (Fig. 20-139). In many cases, there are also typical histologic lesions in the orbital soft tissue adjacent to the sclera and in the meninges of the optic nerve. There is no other cause of uveitis in cats that is also routinely involved in orbital cellulitis. Classic necrotizing vasculitis is seen only rarely, and if present, it is likely to be in the retina. Sequelae such as pupillary block and secondary glaucoma are rarely seen, simply because cats with ocular lesions of FIP are usually in the advanced stages of the systemic disease and do not survive long enough for those potential sequelae to develop.

FELINE IDIOPATHIC LYMPHONODULAR UVEITIS

Feline idiopathic lymphonodular uveitis is by far the most frequent histologic pattern of the uveitis in cats. It is important as a cause of the clinical signs of uveitis itself, but it is even more important as a very common cause of glaucoma in cats. The mechanism by which the uveitis causes the glaucoma is unknown; it is not by the usual mechanisms of posterior synechia or preiridal membrane formation. At the initial clinical presentation, the lesion may be unilateral, but in most cases the uveitis eventually becomes bilateral.

The microscopic lesions are essentially identical to those seen in equine recurrent uveitis: perivascular accumulations of lymphocytes and plasma cells throughout the anterior uvea, and with less regularity, within the choroid and around small vessels in the retina. The iris tends to have the greatest accumulation, and here the lymphocytic-plasmacytic perivascular aggregates may become so large as to be clinically visible (Fig. 20-140). The degree of iris thickening and pallor may be sufficient to make this lesion macroscopically indistinguishable from that of lymphoma (lymphosarcoma).

The cause remains a complete mystery despite considerable investigation. The syndrome is presumed to be immune-mediated, but the identity of the antigen or antigens is unknown. Affected cats are no more likely to be seropositive or PCR-positive for the various feline systemic infectious agents (feline immunodeficiency virus [FIV], FIP, leukemia virus, etc.) than are healthy cats, but no credible cause has been demonstrated by immunohistochemical or PCR investigation of affected globes. Some believe strongly that a previous infection with *Toxoplasma* is somehow involved, but the evidence remains inconclusive.

FELINE DIFFUSE IRIS MELANOMA

See the discussion on neoplasms of the uvea in the section on Disorders of Domestic Animals.

FELINE PRIMARY OCULAR SARCOMA (POSTTRAUMATIC SARCOMA)

See the discussion on neoplasms of the uvea in the section on Disorders of Domestic Animals.

SUGGESTED READINGS

Information on this topic is available at evolve.elsevier.com/Zachary/McGavin/.

APPENDIX

Photographic Techniques in Veterinary Pathology

M. Donald McGavin

After the fourth edition of this book was published, the editors received numerous compliments on the quality of the photographs. The ability to take good gross photographs and photomicrographs should be part of the armamentarium of the pathologist. Although space is limited in this edition, we have included a brief overview of optimal techniques of specimen photography. Detailed descriptions on the techniques of gross specimen photography with a camera on a stand with photographic lamps, a hand-held camera with electronic flash, and photomicrography can be found at evolve.elsevier.com/Zachary/McGavin/.

GROSS SPECIMEN PHOTOGRAPHY

CAMERA STAND AND PHOTOGRAPHIC LAMPS

For many decades, obtaining the correct exposure was the overriding concern of those taking gross photographs of pathologic specimens. This problem has been solved in recent years by using cameras with automatic exposure devices and particularly by using digital cameras, which allow multiple exposures and automatic bracketing of exposures at half-stop intervals, virtually guaranteeing an optimal exposure. Thus the photographer now has a chance to be concerned with other factors of which the most important is lighting, particularly the angle of the main light and the position and intensity of the fill-in light. Correct lighting creates shadows on the surface of an organ to depict its modeling and texture (see Figs. 7-48 and 13-49). The worst possible lighting is axial, the type in which the light source is mounted close to the lens axis, for example, the flash unit on many "point-and-shoot" digital cameras. This type of illumination casts no shadows, and thus there is no rendition of the texture or modeling (see Figs. 1-40, *A,* and 7-46).

The better option for photographing gross specimens is to have a main light (the major source of illumination) and a fill-in light to illuminate the shadows cast by the main light (Figs. 1 and 2). The optimal lighting arrangement is based on that used for portrait photography. The axis of the main light is approximately 60° to the left and above the axis of the lens (see Fig. 1). Lights arranged in this manner cast a shadow downward and to the right that is similar to the position of the nose shadow in portrait photography. Also, it appears "natural" to us because the human brain has been programmed for millions of years to interpret visual images based on the assumption that there is only one light source and that light comes from above, as does the light from the sun. These requirements are met by positioning the lights as depicted in Fig. 1. The main light *(left)* is at the 10 to 11 o'clock position (as viewed along the lens' optical axis) and closer to the subject than the fill-in light to the right, so that the light from the main light is more intense (see Fig. 2). For increased rendition of surface texture, the angle between the axes of the light and camera lens can be increased from 60° to 70 to 80° (i.e. "to skim the surface"; Fig. 3).

The light from the fill-in light should not obliterate the shadows cast by the main light but should sufficiently illuminate details in the shadows. In lighting for portrait photography, the fill-in light is mounted close to the camera (axial illumination). However, this arrangement cannot be done with specimens mounted on glass because axial light is reflected directly back into the camera. Therefore the fill-in light should be placed at 45° to the right and approximately 1.5× to 3× times the distance of the main light from the subject. The 1.5× position is a good starting default position, but the optimal position of the fill-in light to illuminate shadows and still retain the texture of the surface is best determined by trial and error. The fill-in lamp-to-subject distance varies from subject to subject, depending on the color, height, and depth of the "hills and valleys" on the surface of the specimen. Different amounts of fill-in light should be tried by moving the fill-in lamp to the right, evaluating the images in the digital camera immediately, and adjusting the position of the fill-in light accordingly.

It should be noted that the arrangement with the lamps at the 3 o'clock and 9 o'clock positions and both lamps at a 45° angle to the lens axis used in many necropsy laboratories is a legacy of the "early days" when specimen photography was done on a copy stand designed for the photography of flat items, such as documents, and the major requirement was even illumination. Also, because early color films had little latitude and could record only a limited contrast range of less than 2:1, they required relatively even illumination. The new arrangement of the lamps, illustrated in

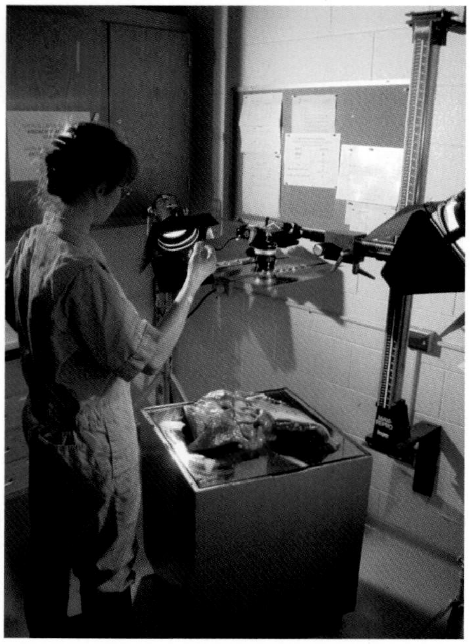

Fig. 1 Photographic unit-camera stand and photographic (studio) lamps.

Note the positions and angles of the lamps. The axis of the main light on the left is 60° from the lens axis and is at the 10 o'clock position, and the right lamp (fill-in lamp) is at 45° and further away from the specimen to reduce its intensity. The pathologist is using a cable release to avoid shaking the camera *(camera shake)*. (Courtesy Dr. L. Bowman, College of Veterinary Medicine, University of Tennessee.)

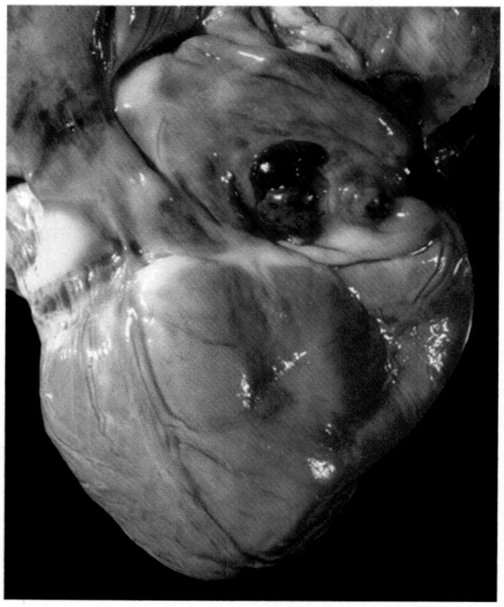

Fig. 2 Standard lighting method, right atrial hemangiosarcoma, heart, dog.

Note that the standardized lighting, as depicted in Fig. 1, has resulted in a three-dimensional (rounded) appearance of the heart and of the tumor projecting from the right auricle. (Courtesy Dr. M.D. McGavin, College of Veterinary Medicine, University of Tennessee.)

Fig. 1, requires little adjustment from the old copy stand position. The main light merely needs to be moved from the 9 o'clock position to the 10 o'clock position and be at an angle of 60° from the camera's lens axis instead of 45°, and the fill-in light needs to be moved to the right as described.

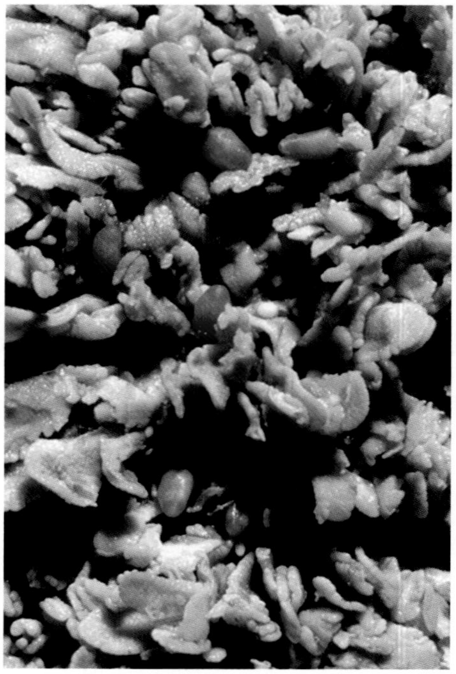

Fig. 3 Texture lighting, ruminal papillae and paramphistomes, cow.

The main light is positioned at the 11 o'clock position and the angle between the axis of the main light and the lens axis has been increased to 80° to emphasize the shadows between the papillae. The fill-in light is minimal and could have been a little more intense to give more detail in the depths of the shadows. (Courtesy Dr. M.D. McGavin, College of Veterinary Medicine, University of Tennessee.)

If the lighting is to appear correct in the photograph, the specimen must be placed in its correct anatomic position at the time of photography to ensure that the light comes from the anatomic "top" of the specimen. This means that a vertical (portrait) format must be used for a ventral or dorsal view of the body (see Fig. 11-62), and a horizontal (landscape) format is required for a lateral view (see Fig. 9-24). With high-resolution digital cameras, the standard horizontal (landscape) position can be used for both portrait- and landscape-oriented specimens, even though the frame may not be completely filled by a vertically oriented specimen.

Backgrounds

Colored backgrounds are a common problem; black or dark gray backgrounds cause the fewest problems. Colored backgrounds should be avoided because they distort the brain's perception of the colors in the specimen; for example, the complementary color of red (like flesh) is cyan (a blue-green). If a cyan background is adjacent to a specimen, it causes the brain to interpret the pinks and reds as being more saturated ("redder") than they are. Also, light reflected from the background can spill onto the specimen, causing a color cast. (The undesirability of blue and colored backgrounds is described in more detail on the Evolve website.)

Besides lighting and background, other important factors are exposure, focusing, depth of field (i.e., depth of the tissue in focus), and specular highlight control. These topics are discussed on the Evolve website. Even if photography is optimal, it is possible to end up with an excellent photograph of a poorly dissected and presented specimen.

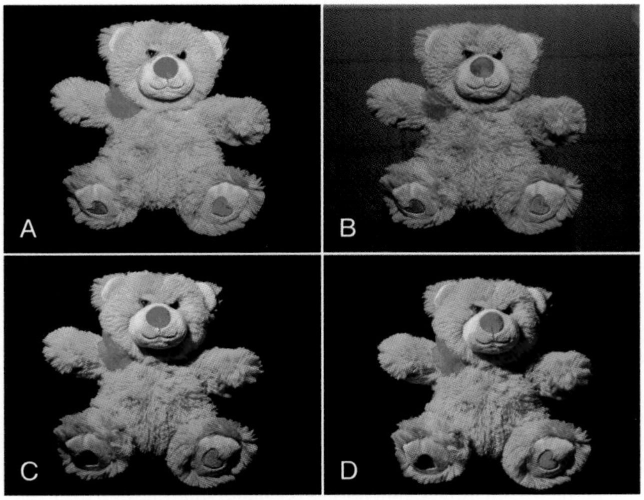

Fig. 4 Flash lighting.

Comparisons of the effects of locating the flash unit on the camera (**A** and **B**) and off the camera (**C** and **D**) and with direct (**A** and **C**) versus bounced diffused (**B** and **D**) flash lighting. **A,** Flash unit mounted directly on the top of the camera (axial lighting). Note the absence of shadows over most of the model and lack of texture in the hair. **B,** Flash unit mounted directly on top of the camera but with bounced-diffused lighting. A commercially available "bounce-flash diffuser" was attached to the flash unit, which was then tilted up vertically (90°). The result is that there is some shadow under the nose and better texture in the hair, the result of the diffused light from the flash unit and its higher position. **C,** Flash unit handheld approximately 2½ feet from the camera and to the upper left at the 10 o'clock position. Note the location of the shadows under and to the side of the chin and the good rendition of the texture of the hair. **D,** Flash unit held as in **C** but fitted with a bounce-flash diffuser as described in **B.** The shadows are better illuminated, and thus more detail is visible in them, and the rendition of the texture of the hair is excellent. (Courtesy Mr. P.D. Snow, College of Veterinary Medicine, University of Tennessee.)

FLASH PHOTOGRAPHY

Modern "point-and-shoot" digital cameras with automatic exposure determination, automatic color temperature selection, and built-in flash units can produce excellent gross photographs of pathologic specimens in situ in the necropsy room and are quick and simple to operate. However, their main defect is lack of rendition of surface texture and modeling, an inevitable consequence of the flash unit being in or on the camera body. Because of this arrangement, these cameras produce axial lighting (along with the lens axis) and thus result in a flat type of lighting without shadows (Fig. 4). Axial lighting is most successful in depicting lesions that have color differences between the lesions and normal tissues, for example, the red-purple diamond-shaped lesions of erysipelas on the skin of a white pig (see Fig. 17-51, *A*). The effects of on- and off-camera lighting and direct and bounced-diffused flash lighting are compared in Fig. 4. Also, automatic focusing results in photographs in which the point of interest is not always accurately in focus, particularly when depth of field is shallow (e.g., in close-up photographs). Thus the question is "Is there a way to have flash photography so that the lighting gives more modeling or texture in the surface of the specimen and not have the equipment become too cumbersome and difficult to use?" The answer is "yes," and this outcome can be accomplished by mounting the flash unit on a flash bracket on the left side of the camera and positioning the lighting axis of the flash unit built in the camera so it is above that of the lens axis (Fig. 5). Optimally, the main light's axis is 60° to the side and above the lens axis, but this position requires a fill-in light to illuminate the shadows. Most advanced, single-lens reflex cameras can use an external flash unit as the main light and the camera's built-in flash unit as a fill-in light to illuminate the shadows. Some of these cameras have the capability of regulating the amount of fill-in light needed to illuminate but not obliterate the shadows cast by the main flash unit, but this equipment can be cumbersome because of the length of the flash bracket required to position the main flash unit at 45 to 60°.

If only a single flash unit and no fill-in flash light is used (Fig. 6), the alternative is to move the flash unit to the side and above but not so far as to produce large shadows that are poorly illuminated (Figs. 7, 8, and 9). The light from a flash unit can be direct, bounced from a ceiling (which has to be white to avoid color casts), or diffused by a bounce-diffuser mounted on the flash

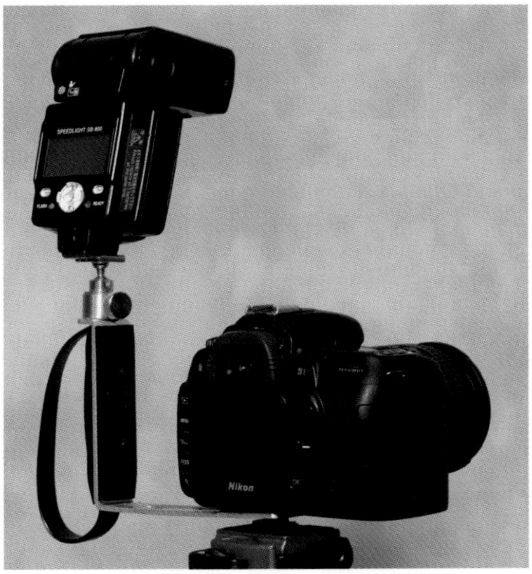

Fig. 5 Camera, flash bracket, and flash unit.

For simplicity, the synchronizer cable between the camera and the flash unit has been omitted. (Courtesy Mr. P.D. Snow, College of Veterinary Medicine, University of Tennessee.)

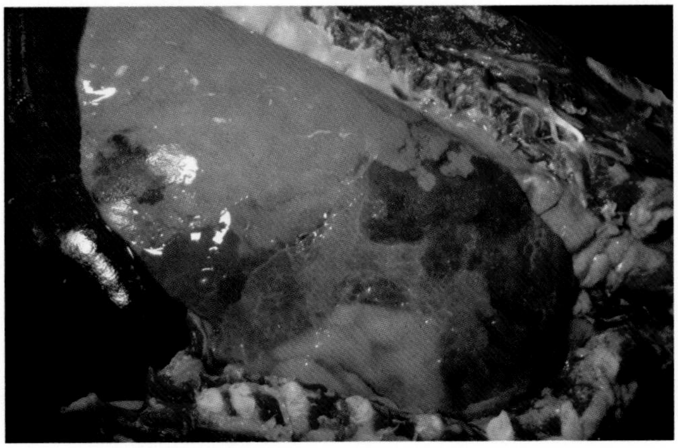

Fig. 6 Direct flash mounted on the camera, pneumonia, lung, sheep.

The different colors of the pneumonic areas have recorded well. However, because of the "flat" (axial) lighting, it is not possible to detect depressed areas in the surface and thus differentiate between atelectasis and red consolidation. (Courtesy Dr. M.D. McGavin, College of Veterinary Medicine, University of Tennessee.)

unit. Fig. 4, *B* and *D,* show the effects of using a bounce-diffuser mounted on the flash unit. Diffusing the light source often has the advantage of providing more illumination to the shadows and thus more shadow detail (see Fig. 4).

Selection of a flash unit is a balance between weight and light output (guide number = aperture × distance in either feet or meters). The light output must be adequate to allow the camera to be used at f-16, even with a dark subject at a distance of up to 6 to 8 feet, the distance required for photography of organs in situ in a large animal. This requirement calculates to a guide number of about 30 in metric units. Many flash units at an ISO setting of 100 to 200 meet this requirement, even if a bounce-diffuser is used, and are still relatively lightweight.

If the specimen is to show the texture and modeling from the flash when the lens subject distance is greater than several feet, then it is necessary to remove the flash unit from the bracket and hold it in the hand or have an assistant hold it above and to the side at an angle of 30° to 40° from the camera lens axis (see Fig. 4, *C* and *D,* and Figs. 7, 8, and 9). The effectiveness of this position and angle in revealing the surface topography and yet providing adequate shadow detail can be immediately evaluated in a digital camera's viewing screen, and additional exposures can be made with the flash unit in different positions.

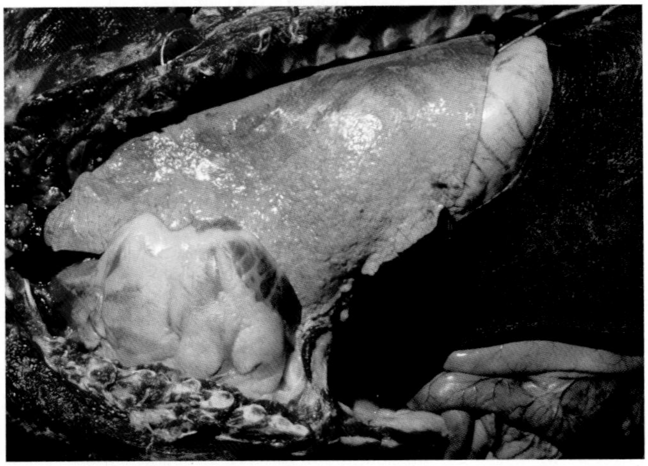

Fig. 7 Flash unit off the camera and handheld above and approximately 2½ feet to the left at 45° to lens axis, normal lung, horse.

The lung has partially collapsed, which occurred when the thorax was opened. Note the texture of the surface of the lung (lung lobules) and the fibrous tissue in the capsule of the spleen. (Courtesy Dr. M.D. McGavin, College of Veterinary Medicine, University of Tennessee.)

The more common and less complicated method is to use a single flash unit mounted on a bracket, with its lighting axis approximately 20° to 30° above and to the left of the optical axis of the camera (see Fig. 5). This approach also has the advantage of preventing so-called "red eye," which is the reflection of the light from the choroid plexus in humans, or "green eye" (or bluish green), which is the reflection of light from the tapetum lucidum in animals. Thus the advantages of the flash unit mounted on a bracket are (1) depiction of some modeling and texture to the surface, (2) reduction in direct reflections (specular highlights) from wet surfaces of the specimen and background and green eye, and (3) better illumination with darker subjects where some texture to the surface is essential. Once the camera settings are standardized (ISO setting, aperture [e.g., f-16 on the "aperture preferred" setting], and exposure bracketing), a single-lens reflex camera can be used as a point-and-shoot camera. Optimally, focusing should be manual because the automatic focusing mechanism can be misled because it will not know which portion of the specimen is of interest or whether the depth of field (the depth of the specimen in focus) is adequate.

The requirements of a necropsy photograph of gross specimens include the following:

1. Correct exposure
2. Correct focusing with adequate depth of field (see Fig. 5)
3. Appropriately dissected specimen (see Fig. 6)
4. Correct anatomically oriented specimen (see Figs. 2, 6, and 9)
5. Suitable framing so that anatomic landmarks are included and can be recognized and used for orientation by the viewer (see Figs. 6 and 9)
6. Lighting from above that renders surface modeling and texture (see Figs. 2, 3, 7, and 8)

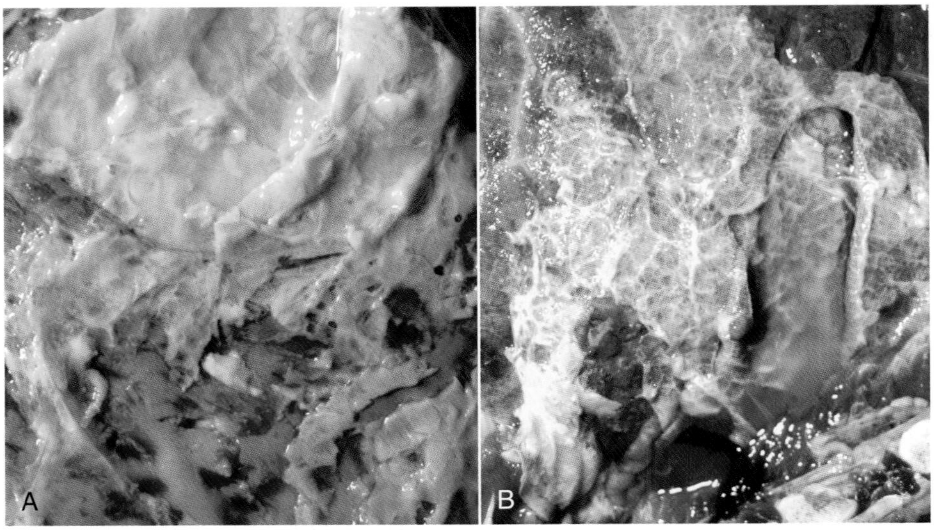

Fig. 8 Fibrinous exudate, texture lighting.

A, Camera stand and lights (i.e., main studio light) as used in Fig. 1. **B,** Electronic flash unit used. The axes of both the main studio light and the flash unit were approximately 75° to the lens axis (texture lighting). Even with the flash unit at this angle, it does not depict the gross appearance of fibrin as well as studio lighting (also see Fig. 3-4, *A1* and *A2*). (Courtesy Dr. M.D. McGavin, College of Veterinary Medicine, University of Tennessee.)

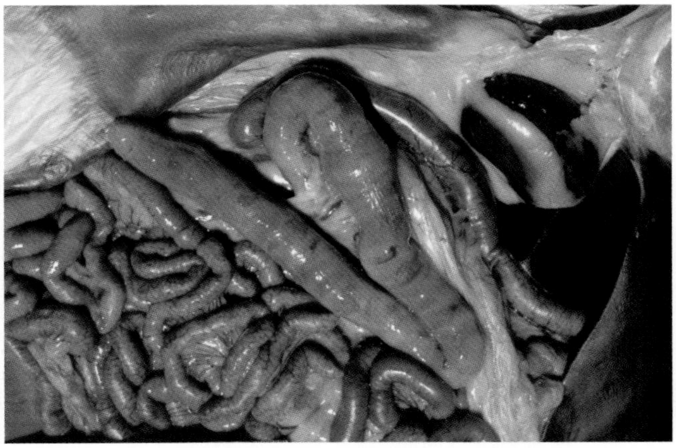

Fig. 9 Anatomic orientation and lighting, abdomen, colon, coccidiosis, sheep.

This specimen is in the correct anatomic position for photography, but the light comes from below. The shadows are cast craniodorsally and indicate that the flash unit was held too low and on the left. This type of lighting (called *spook lighting*) gives the picture a strange and in some cases, unnatural appearance. (Courtesy Dr. M.D. McGavin, College of Veterinary Medicine, University of Tennessee.)

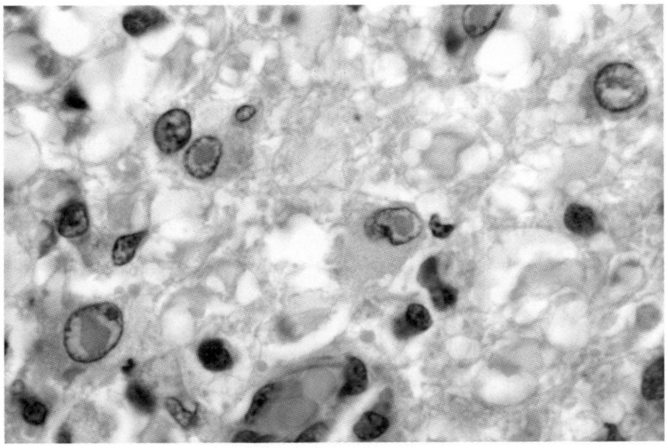

Fig. 10 Optimal resolution and contrast, photomicrography (H&E stain), brain, canine distemper, inclusion bodies.

Note the excellent resolution and contrast, the result of using a thin (4 μm thickness) section that was well stained with H&E, high-quality optical components (40× plan apochromatic objective and an achromatic-aplanatic condenser), Koehler illumination, and the aperture diaphragm set at 90% cone. H&E stain. (Courtesy Dr. M.D. McGavin, College of Veterinary Medicine, University of Tennessee.)

7. Interesting and aesthetically pleasing composition, if possible (see Figs. 3 and 6)
8. Unobtrusive backgrounds (no stainless steel table, grates, tiled floors, floor drains, or blue boards [see Fig. 2])

PHOTOMICROGRAPHY

Photomicrography has become a lot easier since the introduction of digital cameras and software that provide automatic exposure, focusing, and color balance. Additionally, biomedical journals now routinely accept color photomicrographs, which are far less demanding to produce than black and white photomicrographs. Focusing has also become easier because it is done on a computer monitor screen, which is far more successful than the previously used methods of focusing on an aerial image viewed in the microscope or in a side telescope.

However, there are still some features of microscopy that are essential for obtaining optimal function of the optical microscope and thus an optimal photomicrograph (Fig. 10; also see Fig. 14). One such feature is Koehler illumination, particularly the correct positioning of the aperture diaphragm (located on the condenser). Koehler illumination has two basic steps carried out after the microscope has been focused: (1) focusing the image of the field diaphragm in the microscope's field of view (easier to do than describe) and (2) setting the position of the aperture diaphragm whose control lever is usually on the condenser (Fig. 11). The aperture diaphragm controls three important features of the image: (1) resolution, the ability of the lens to separate adjacent points; (2) contrast, the differences between the light and dark tones (gray scale) of colors, and (3) depth of field, the thickness of the specimen in focus. Maximum resolution occurs when the aperture diaphragm is open so its circle of light in the rear focal plane (RFP) of the objective (visible only when the ocular has been removed [Fig. 12]) is the same diameter as the circle of light of the objective. This arrangement is called *100% cone* and is an expression of the relative diameters of the illuminated circles from the objective and condenser as viewed in the RFP. Closing the aperture diaphragm

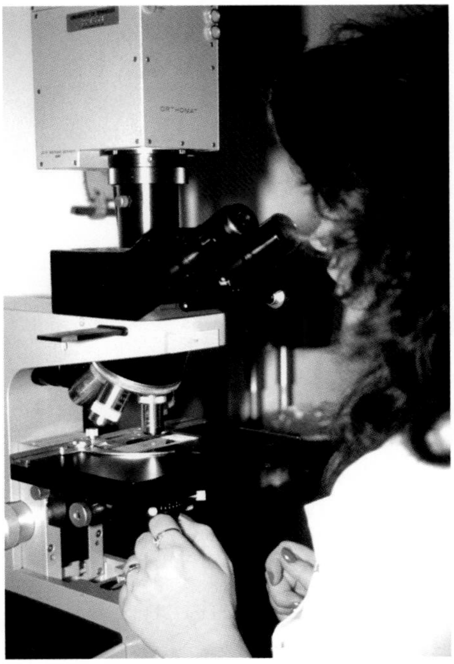

Fig. 11 Koehler illumination, aperture diaphragm.

The aperture diaphragm is opened and closed by moving the lever on the side of the condenser. (Courtesy Dr. M.D. McGavin, College of Veterinary Medicine, University of Tennessee.)

increases contrast (similar to "lowering" the condenser), but if the aperture diaphragm is closed too far, diffraction occurs and resolution is markedly reduced (Fig. 13). Thus the choice is a balance between resolution and contrast. There are some rules of thumb for obtaining maximum resolution. With thin specimens, such as blood smears and thin tissue sections (3 to 4 μm in thickness), open the aperture diaphragm to 90% to 100% of the RFP (i.e., the condenser's circle of illumination is just visible inside the circle of the RFP). For well-stained histologic sections, use 80% and

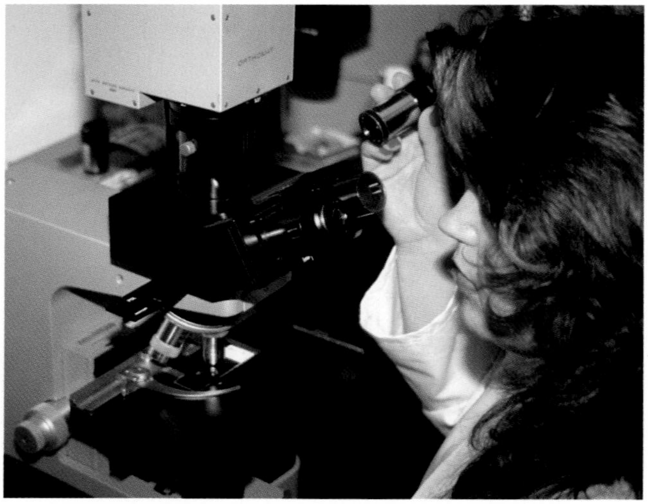

Fig. 12 Koehler illumination, circle of illumination, rear focal plane (RFP).

Removal of the eyepiece is necessary to allow observation of the circle of illumination of the condenser in the RFP of the objective and to select the diameter of the condenser's image (circle of light) relative to that of the objective. These steps can only be done after Koehler illumination has been set up correctly. For optimal results it is necessary that these adjustments be done each time an objective or slide is changed. (Courtesy Dr. M.D. McGavin, College of Veterinary Medicine, University of Tennessee.)

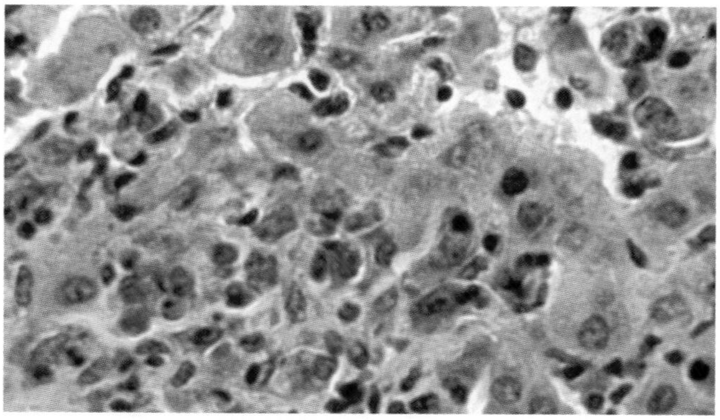

Fig. 13 Diffraction, 40× plan apochromatic objective.

The aperture diaphragm has been closed too far (in this case 50% cone) with a resultant loss of resolution. Note how the globules of hemosiderin are not clearly defined and separated. Also, the image has a smudgy or "oily" appearance. In extremely severe cases, diffraction can cause double outlines of thin fibrous strands and cell membranes. H&E stain. (Courtesy Dr. P.W. Ladds, James Cook University, Australia.)

try 70% to 90%, depending on the contrast of the stained section (Fig. 14, also see Fig. 10). For low-contrast specimens, it may be necessary to close the aperture diaphragm even more and risk diffraction if the specimen is to be visible. In pathology, the secret is to have well-stained sections with good color and tonal (gray scale) contrast (see Figs. 10 and 14). If the specimen is thick (7 to 9 μm in thickness) and to have the image in focus, it may be necessary to close the aperture diaphragm almost to the point of causing diffraction, particularly with high magnification objectives, which have the shallowest depth of field (i.e., depth of the tissue in focus).

EVALUATION OF PHOTOMICROGRAPHS

The pathologist should know how to evaluate the different features of a photomicrograph. These features include the following:

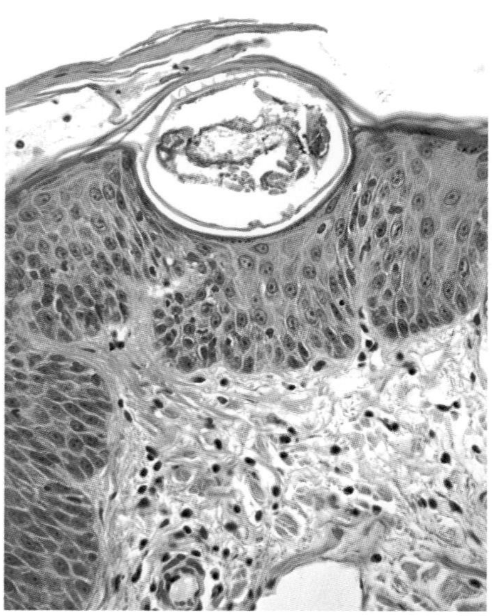

Fig. 14 Excellent photomicrograph, H&E staining, skin, sarcoptic mange, dog.

This section is correctly stained. The hematoxylin (Harris' hematoxylin) has stained the nuclei dark blue to black and has been correctly differentiated to remove excess hematoxylin and reveal internal nuclear chromatin. The eosin has also been differentiated; note the different reds and pinks in the erythrocytes, stratum corneum, dermis, and the cuticle of the *Sarcoptes* mite. Thus the section has both good color and gray-scale contrast. H&E stain. (Courtesy Dr. M.D. McGavin, College of Veterinary Medicine, University of Tennessee.)

1. **Focus.** The image should be in focus across the entire monitor. If it is out of focus at the edges ("fall off"), this appearance could be caused by poorly corrected flat field (or plan objectives) or by the incorrect positioning of the aperture diaphragm.
2. **Focusing.** Before the use of digital cameras and focusing on the screen of computer monitors, focusing was done on the aerial image, which was viewed either in the microscope or in a side telescope. This method meant that there had to be correction for the microscopist's vision and failure to do this would result in out-of-focus images. Another problem was that objectives with a large depth of field, such as the 4× and lower power objectives, were particularly difficult to focus on a plane, which would give the appearance of the whole field being in focus. The tendency was to focus on a single cell, which may or may not be in a plane that would render those cells above and below it, also in focus. However, focusing the image on the monitor's screen is relatively reliable and avoids these problems.
3. **Exposure.** Exposure is evaluated by looking at the microscope's clear background in the print or digital image. This background should be faint gray unless there is a color cast, which is undesirable. However, there should be a faint density, which when printed is slightly darker than the white of the blank page.
4. **Color cast.** The microscope's clear background should be white and have no color casts. The usual color casts, which were more frequent in the days of film cameras, were yellow, orange, or blue (from incorrect color temperature) because the color temperature of the light did not match that of the film. Occasionally, color casts were green, the result of a color cast either from a lens (usually in the lamp house) or in a specific brand of film. Some brands of older microscopes and films were notorious for

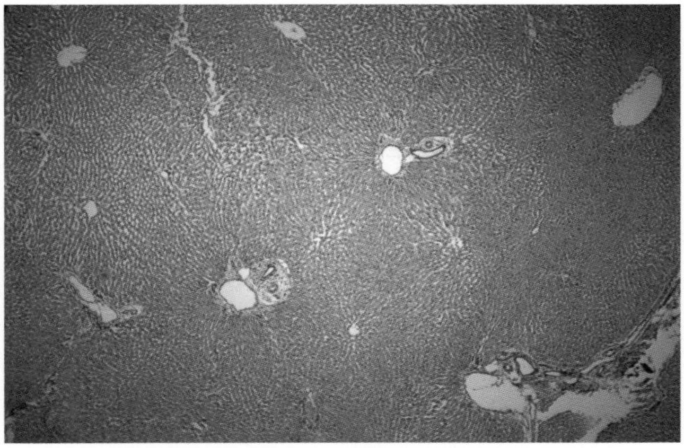

Fig. 15 Uneven illumination, 2.5× objective, liver, dog.
Uneven illumination is usually the result of failure to set up Koehler illumination correctly or because of inadequacy of components of the optical system, particularly of very low-power objectives and the condenser. Objectives of less than 4× magnification often require special condensers to obtain even illumination. H&E stain. (Courtesy Dr. M.D. McGavin, College of Veterinary Medicine, University of Tennessee.)

a green cast. Color casts can be easily prevented in the digital image by setting the white background before each exposure. This action is done differently in different microscopes and cameras, but one of the more convenient ways is to outline a box on the microscope's clear background and press the set white button.

5. **Uneven illumination.** Uneven illumination is more of a problem with low-power objectives. Frequently, to obtain even illumination with low-power objectives of less than 4× magnification, special condensers and highly corrected objectives have to be used (Fig. 15). Some digital photomicrographic cameras have a software program to neutralize uneven illumination, which is a useful addition.
6. **Contrast.** The factors involved in controlling contrast are as follows:
   - Quality and staining of the specimen and the specific stain chosen (e.g., trichrome [blue and red] vs. van Gieson [yellow and pink]).
   - Quality of the objectives (e.g., apochromatic objectives have far higher contrast than achromatic or planapochromatic objectives).
   - Koehler illumination and the positioning of the aperture diaphragm control the resolution, contrast, and depth of field (i.e., the depth of the specimen that is in focus). Its correct positioning is particularly important with high dry and 100× oil immersion objectives.
   - Cover glass and mountant thickness and mountant quality.
   - Digital camera quality.
   - Cleanliness of the surface of the cover slip.
   - Magnification of the objective: Lower magnification objectives and high-power objectives (i.e., high-dry and oil-immersion) have lower contrast than 10× and 25× objectives of the same optical correction (e.g., all apochromats or all achromats).

A description of the procedures to follow to obtain optimal results and to "troubleshoot" problems is involved and lengthy. Microscope instruction manuals sometimes apply to several related models and not to a specific model. Therefore the most convenient arrangement is for the operator to make a checklist that applies to the procedure for photomicrography with a specific microscope and digital camera. Checklists may be boring, but they are essential for ensuring the correct steps and sequence in Koehler illumination. Unfortunately, Koehler illumination is not an intuitive process. More information on these topics is available at evolve.elsevier.com/Zachary/McGavin/.

SUGGESTED READING

McGavin MD, Thompson SW: *Specimen dissection and photography*, Springfield, IL, 1987, Charles C Thomas.

This book was written before the era of digital photography, but the general principles of gross specimen photography, selection of backgrounds, preparation and color restoration in specimens, and the dissection methods to produce optimal specimens for photography still apply.

INDEX

Page numbers followed by *b* indicate boxes; *f*, figures; *t*, tables.
Page numbers preceded by *e* indicate material found on the Evolve web site.

E

F

H

I

J

K

M

N

P

T